Hunter's Tropical
Medicine
and Emerging
Infectious Diseases

Editors

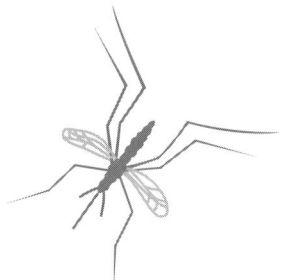

Hunter's Tropical Medicine
and Emerging
Infectious Diseases

Eighth Edition

G. Thomas Strickland
M.D., Ph.D., D.C.M.T., F.A.C.P.

Captain, Medical Corps, United States Navy (Retired)

Director, International Health Program; Professor of Epidemiology and
Preventive Medicine, Microbiology and Immunology, and Medicine,
University of Maryland School of Medicine, Baltimore, Maryland

Senior Associate, Department of Molecular Microbiology and Immunology,
The Johns Hopkins School of Hygiene and Public Health, Baltimore, Maryland

W.B. SAUNDERS COMPANY
A Division of Harcourt Brace & Company
Philadelphia   London   Toronto   Montreal   Sydney   Tokyo

W.B. SAUNDERS COMPANY
A Division of Harcourt Brace & Company

The Curtis Center
Independence Square West
Philadelphia, Pennsylvania 19106

Library of Congress Cataloging-in-Publication Data

Hunter's Tropical Medicine and Emerging Infectious Diseases—8th ed. / [edited by]
G. Thomas Strickland.

    p.   cm.

Includes bibliographical references and index.

ISBN 0–7216–6223–4

1. Tropical medicine.   I. Hunter, George W. (George William).
   II. Strickland, G. Thomas.
   [DNLM: 1. Tropical Medicine.   WC 680 T857 2000]

RC961.H84   2000

616.9′883—dc21

DNLM/DLC   98-13361

HUNTER'S TROPICAL MEDICINE AND EMERGING INFECTIOUS DISEASES   ISBN 0–7216–6223–4

Last digit is the print number: 9   8   7   6   5   4   3   2   1

Preface

Hunter's Tropical Medicine grew out of a World War II Army Medical School tropical and military medicine course taught at the Walter Reed Army Medical Center in Washington, D.C. The first edition, entitled a *Manual of Tropical Medicine,* was published in 1945 by three of the course instructors, Colonel Thomas T. Mackie, Major George W. Hunter III, and Captain C. Brooke Worth. A second edition was published by the same authors in 1954. Colonel Hunter was joined by co-authors from the Louisiana State University School of Medicine for the third, fourth, and fifth editions, published in 1960, 1966, and 1976, respectively. George Hunter's contribution was acknowledged by adding his name to the book title in the sixth edition, which I edited in 1984. I also edited the seventh edition, published in 1991.

The sixth edition of *Hunter's Tropical Medicine* was an entirely new book, and *Hunter's* purpose since that time has been to be the most detailed and comprehensive clinical tropical medicine textbook. It covers all the "tropical" infectious diseases and gives extensive information on other medical conditions, e.g., nutritional problems and deficiencies and snakebite, which occur commonly in the tropics and other developing countries.

There are four criteria for covering an infectious disease in *Hunter's Tropical Medicine:* (1) The disease occurs exclusively, or almost exclusively, in the tropics and nontropical developing countries, e.g., malaria, schistosomiasis, dengue fever; (2) it occurs much more commonly, or often has a different clinical presentation, in a developing country, e.g., tuberculosis, amebiasis, measles; (3) it is caused by parasites that may occur in temperate climates as well as the tropics, e.g., trichomoniasis, babesiosis, anisakidosis; and (4) it is transmitted by vectors or is a zoonotic disease, e.g., hantavirus infection, Lyme disease, leptospirosis, plague, dirofilariasis.

These criteria, particularly the fourth one, include all of the emerging and re-emerging infectious diseases with the exception of the increasing problem of the development of resistance to antibiotics by antimicrobial agents. In recognition of this extensive coverage of emerging and re-emerging infectious diseases, the title has been modified to *Hunter's Tropical Medicine and Emerging Infectious Diseases.* The chapters on human immunodeficiency virus and AIDS, viral hepatitis, the viral hemorrhagic fevers, cholera, tuberculosis, malaria, and leishmaniasis have been extensively rewritten and updated. Among the new chapters are those on human T-cell lymphotrophic virus infections, herpes virus infections, spongiform encephalopathies, diseases caused by hantaviruses, *Campylobacter* enteritis, *Heliobacter pylori* infections, ehrlichiosis, penicilliosis marneffei, and cyclosporidiosis.

The first part of the book, Clinical Practice in the Tropics, sets the stage for understanding medical practice in developing countries. It approaches illness by body systems and by clinical syndromes or problems, and the authors have attempted to describe medical practice in the tropics as it differs from practice in the more developed temperate climates. In this edition, we have added important chapters on maternal and child health, the integrated management of the sick child, traditional medicine, environmental health hazards in the tropics, and imaging in the tropics and the imaging of tropical diseases as well as updated chapters on pulmonary diseases, sexually transmitted diseases, surgery in the tropics, and heat-associated illness. We have found this part particularly useful to those from North America or Europe who become health care providers in developing countries.

The purpose of the tenth part of the book, Tropical Disease in a Temperate Climate, is the reverse of this. It is to assist the practitioner in a temperate climate who sees patients with illnesses that may have been contracted in the tropics. This is classic "traveler's medicine," and although there are textbooks and other materials available on this subject, we believe that a textbook of tropical medicine must have a section with this approach to patients with tropical diseases. Dr. Jay Keystone has again assisted in preparing this part; chapters on establishing a travel clinic and screening long-term travelers augment the chapters in the seventh edition on advice to travelers, fever in travelers, and diseases in immigrants. The chapter on global epidemiology of infectious diseases, prepared by Dr. Guénaël Rodier and his colleagues in the WHO's emerging and infectious diseases program, is particularly extensive and very useful, with up-to-date information on the global distribution of infectious diseases.

The parts on poisonous plants and animals, vector transmission and zoonoses, and laboratory diagnosis of parasitic diseases have been updated and presented in a format and detail suitable for the medical practitioner who is taking care of patients with tropical medical problems and emerging and re-emerging infectious diseases. *Hunter's Tropical Medicine and Emerging Infectious Diseases* focuses on clinical practice; it does not include extensive details covering the basic research of tropical infectious diseases. However, information on basic research is included if it adds to essential knowledge of the practicing physician, and additional readings on these topics are listed in the chapter's bibliography. *Hunter's Tropical Medicine and Emerging Infectious Diseases* is not referenced. The editors believe that a bibliography of publications that provide additional information for the clinician is more useful. Most chapter bibliographies are more extensive in the new edition. Extensive illustrations also make this book more useful to the practitioner. An additional two pages of color illustrations have been added. Despite increased text and illustrations, the eighth edition remains a single, and very useable, volume.

I wish to thank Raymond R. Kersey, David H. Kilmer, and Cass Stamato of W. B. Saunders Company for their editorial assistance. Constance Burton has smoothly and efficiently copy edited the book. The two associate editors, the five part editors, and the almost 200 contributors to *Hunter's Tropical Medicine and Emerging Infectious Diseases,* and I all hope that the readers will find the eighth edition as useful as they have found the earlier versions.

G. THOMAS STRICKLAND

Contributors

John Aaskov, Ph.D.
Lecturer, School of Life Sciences, Queensland University of Technology, Brisbane; Director, World Health Organization Collaborating Centre for Arbovirus Reference and Research, Brisbane, Queensland, Australia
Epidemic Polyarthritis

M. John Albert, M.D.
International Centre for Diarrhoeal Disease Research—Bangladesh, Dhaka, Bangladesh
Cholera and Other Vibrioses

Ray R. Arthur, Ph.D.
Medical Officer, Department of Communicable Diseases Surveillance and Response, World Health Organization, Geneva, Switzerland
Rift Valley Fever

David M. Asher, M.D.
Chief, Laboratory of Method Development, Division of Viral Products, Office of Vaccine Research and Review, Center for Biologics Evaluation and Research, U.S. Food and Drug Administration, Rockville, Maryland
Transmissible Spongiform Encephalopathies

Abdu F. Azad, Ph.D.
Professor of Microbiology and Immunology, University of Maryland Medical School, Baltimore, Maryland
Murine Flea-Borne Typhus; Injurious Arthropods; Ticks and Mites in Disease Transmission

Tariq Al-Azraqui, M.D.
Infectious Diseases Fellow, Centre for Tropical Diseases, Montreal General Hospital, McGill University, Montreal, Quebec, Canada
Tetanus

Robin Bailey, Ph.D., M.R.C.P., D.T.M.&H.
Senior Lecturer, Department of Infectious and Tropical Diseases, London School of Hygiene and Tropical Medicine; Honorary Consultant Physician, Hospital for Tropical Diseases, London, England
Trachoma and Inclusion Conjunctivitis

Ronald C. Ballard, M.I.Biol., Ph.D.
Associate Professor, Department of Clinical Microbiology and Infectious Diseases, University of The Witwatersrand, Johannesburg; Head, National Reference Centre for Sexually Transmitted Diseases, South African Institute for Medical Research, Johannesburg, South Africa
Gonococcal Infections

John G. Bartlett, M.D.
Professor and Chief, Division of Infectious Diseases, Johns Hopkins University School of Medicine, Baltimore, Maryland
Botulism; Gas Gangrene

James W. Bass, M.D.
Professor, Department of Pediatrics, Uniformed Services University of the Health Sciences, Bethesda, Maryland; Clinical Professor, Department of Pediatrics, John A. Burns School of Medicine, University of Hawaii, Honolulu; Senior Consultant in Pediatrics and Pediatric Infectious Disease, Tripler Army Medical Center, Honolulu, Hawaii
Pertussis

William R. Beisel, M.D., F.A.C.P.
Adjunct Professor, Department of Molecular Microbiology and Immunology, Johns Hopkins School of Hygiene and Public Health, Baltimore, Maryland
Interactions Between Nutrition and Infection

Thomas A. Bell, M.D., M.P.H.
Clinical Associate Professor of Epidemiology and Pediatrics, University of Washington, Seattle; Health Office, Conlitz, Lewis, and Wahkiakum Counties, Washington
Syphilis and the Endemic Treponematoses

Stephen Berman, M.D.
Professor of Pediatrics, University of Colorado School of Medicine, Denver; Attending Pediatrician, Children's Hospital, Denver, Colorado
Viral Respiratory Infections

Robert E. Black, M.D., M.P.H.
Professor and Chairman, Department of International Health, School of Hygiene and Public Health, The Johns Hopkins University, Baltimore, Maryland
Viral Diarrheas

William A. Blattner, M.D.
Professor, Department of Epidemiology and Preventive Medicine, University of Maryland at Baltimore School of Medicine; Associate Director, Institute of Human Virology, Medical Biotechnology Center, Baltimore, Maryland
Human T-Lymphotropic Virus Type I/II Infection

Gerard C. Bodeker, Ed.D.
Chair, Global Initiative for Traditional Systems of Health, Institute of Health Sciences, University of Oxford, Oxford, England
Traditional Medicine

C.L. Bolis
Consultant, Unit of Neurosciences, Division of Mental Health and Prevention of Substance Abuse, World Health Organization, Geneva, Switzerland
Neurologic Diseases

Robert C. Bollinger, Jr., M.D., M.P.H.
Associate Professor, Division of Infectious Diseases, Department of Medicine & International Health, Schools of Medicine and Hygiene and Public Health, The Johns Hopkins University, Baltimore, Maryland
Tetanus; Botulism; Gas Gangrene

Prasert Boongird, M.D.
Professor, Department of Medicine, Faculty of Medicine, Mahidol University, Bangkok, Thailand
Neurologic Diseases

Robert W. Bradsher, M.D.
Vice Chairman and Professor of Medicine; Director, Division of Infectious Diseases; University of Arkansas for Medical Sciences, Little Rock; John L. McClellen Veterans Administration Hospital, Little Rock, Arkansas
Blastomycosis

Joel G. Breman, M.D., D.T.P.H.
Deputy Director, Division of International Training and Research, Fogarty International Center, National Institutes of Health, Bethesda, Maryland
Measles; Poxviruses

Philippe Brouqui, M.D., Ph.D.
Professor of Medicine, Unité des Rickettsie, Faculté de Medicine, Université de la Medeterranée, Marseille; Tropical Medicine and Infectious Disease Department, CHU Houphouet Boijny, Marseille, France
Tick-Borne Rickettsioses of the Eastern Hemisphere

Joel D. Brown, M.D., F.A.C.P., D.T.M.&H.
Professor of Medicine, John A. Burns School of Medicine, University of Hawaii, Honolulu; Consultant in Tropical and Infectious Diseases, Tripler Army Medical Center; Associate Director, Medical Education, The Queen's Medical Center, Honolulu, Hawaii
Pyomyositis

Donald A. P. Bundy, Ph.D.
Professor of Parasite Epidemiology, Wellcome Trust Centre for the Epidemiology of Infectious Disease, Oxford University, Oxford, England
Nematodes Limited to the Intestinal Tract (Enterobius vermicularis, Trichuris trichiura, *and* Capillaria philippinensis); *Intestinal Nematodes That Migrate Through Lungs* (Ascariasis)

Danai Bunnag, M.D., D.T.M.&H.
Professor Emeritus, Department of Clinical Tropical Medicine, Mahidol University, Bangkok, Thailand
Intestinal Fluke Infections; Liver Fluke Infections; Lung Fluke Infections: Paragonimiasis

Thanongsak Bunnag, M.D., D.T.M.&H., M.P.H.&T.M., Dr.PH
Emeritus Professor of Tropical Medicine; Consultant, Faculty of Tropical Medicine, Mahidol University, Bangkok, Thailand
Gnathostomiasis; Angiostrongylus *Meningitis; Intestinal Fluke Infections; Liver Fluke Infections; Lung Fluke Infections: Paragonimiasis*

Brenton B. Burkholder, M.D., M.A.
Adjunct Associate Professor of Public Health, Rollins School of Public Health, Emory University, Atlanta; Chief, International Emergency and Refugee Health Branch, Centers for Disease Control and Prevention, Atlanta, Georgia
Health and Nutrition Among Refugees and Displaced Persons

Thomas Butler, M.D.
Professor of Internal Medicine and of Microbiology and Immunology, Texas Tech University Health Sciences Center, Lubbock; Chief of Infectious Diseases; Attending Physician, University Medical Center, Lubbock, Texas
Campylobacter *Enteritis; Relapsing Fever*

Benjamin Caballero, M.D., Ph.D.
Professor of Nutrition and International Health; Director, Center for Human Nutrition, The Johns Hopkins School of Hygiene and Public Health; Professor of Pediatrics, The Johns Hopkins School of Medicine, Baltimore, Maryland
Nutritional Problems and Deficiency Diseases: General Principles; Beriberi; Scurvy; Pellagra; Ariboflavinosis

Philippe Calain, M.D., Ph.D.
Visiting Scientist, Special Pathogens Branch, Centers for Disease Control and Prevention, Atlanta, Georgia
Ebola and Marburg Virus Infections

K. S. Chia, M.D.
Professor of Community, Occupational, and Family Medicine, National University of Singapore, Singapore
Environmental Health Hazards in the Tropics

James E. Childs, Sc.D.
Chief, Viral and Rickettsial Zoonoses Branch, National Center for Infectious Diseases, Centers for Disease Control and Prevention, Atlanta, Georgia
Zoonoses

Surgheel H. Choudhri, M.D.
Assistant Professor, Department of Medicine and Medical Microbiology, University of Manitoba School of Medicine, Winnipeg, Manitoba, Canada
Eosinophilia in Travelers and Immigrants

Stephen L. Cochi, M.D., M.P.H.
Director, Vaccine Preventable Disease Eradication Division, National Immunization Program, Centers for Disease Control and Prevention, Atlanta, Georgia
Poliomyelitis

Bradley A. Connor, M.D.
Clinical Assistant Professor of Medicine, Cornell University Medical College; Assistant Attending Physician, The New York Hospital–Cornell Medical Center, New York, New York
Cyclosporiasis; Diarrhea in Travelers

Edward Cooper, M.B.B.S., F.R.C.P.
Consultant Paediatrician, Homerton Hospital, London, England
Nematodes Limited to the Intestinal Tract (Enterobius vermicularis, Trichuris trichiura, *and* Capillaria philippinensis)

Philip J. Cooper, M.B.B.S., Ph.D., D.T.M.&H.
Fogarty Visiting Fellow, Laboratory of Parasitic Diseases, National Institutes of Health, Bethesda, Maryland
Onchocerciasis

John H. Cross, Ph.D.
Professor, Tropical Public Health, Department of Preventive Medicine and Biometrics, Uniformed Services University of the Health Sciences, Bethesda, Maryland
Trematode Infections: General Principles; Intestinal Fluke Infections; Liver Fluke Infections; Lung Fluke Infections: Paragonimiasis; Laboratory Diagnosis of Parasitic Diseases: General Principles; Examination of Stool and Urine Specimens; Examination of Blood, Other Body Fluids, Tissue, and Sputum

Rose D. Danella, Ph.D.
Research Assistant Professor, Division of Epidemiology and Prevention, Institute of Human Virology, University of Maryland at Baltimore, Baltimore, Maryland
Human T-Lymphotropic Virus Type I/II Infection

Kevin M. De Cock, M.D., F.R.C.P., D.T.M.&H.
Director, Division of HIV/AIDS Prevention—Surveillance and Epidemiology, National Center for HIV/STD/TB Prevention, Centers for Disease Control and Prevention, Atlanta, Georgia
Human Immunodeficiency Virus Infection and AIDS

James D. DeMaio, M.D.
Infectious Diseases Physician, Infections Limited, Tacoma, Washington
Glanders

David T. Dennis, M.D., M.P.H., D.C.M.T.
Chief, Bacterial Zoonoses Branch, Division of Vector-Borne Infectious Diseases, Centers for Disease Control and Prevention, Atlanta, Georgia
Plague; Tularemia; Lyme Disease

Nilanthi De Silva M.D., M.Sc.
Senior Lecturer in Parasitology, Faculty of Medicine, University of Kelaniya, Ragama, Sri Lanka
Intestinal Nematodes That Migrate Through Lungs (Ascariasis)

J. Fernando Diaz, M.D.
Research Assistant, Department of International Health, The Johns Hopkins School of Public Health and Hygiene, Baltimore, Maryland
Sparganosis; Coenuriasis

Joseph J. Drabick, M.D., F.A.C.P.
Department of Bacterial Diseases, Walter Reed Army Institutes of Research, Washington, D.C.; Associate Professor of Medicine, Uniformed Services University of the Health Sciences, Bethesda, Maryland
Free-Living Amebic Infections; Pentastomiasis

Françoise Dromer, M.D., Ph.D.
Chargé de Recherche, Unité de Mycologie, Institut Pasteur, Paris, France
Cryptococcosis

J. Stephen Dumler, M.D.
Associate Professor, Department of Pathology, Program in Cellular and Molecular Medicine, The Johns Hopkins University School of Medicine; Department of Molecular Microbiology and Immunology, The Johns Hopkins University School of Hygiene and Public Health; Director, Division of Medical Microbiology, Department of Pathology, The Johns Hopkins Hospital, Baltimore, Maryland
Rickettsialpox

John T. Dunn, M.D.
Professor of Medicine, University of Virginia School of Medicine, Charlottesville, Virginia; Secretary, International Council for the Control of Iodine Deficiency Disorders
Iodine Deficiency Disorders

Michael A. Dunn, M.D.
Assistant Chief, U.S. Army Medical Corps; Associate Professor of Medicine, Uniformed Services University School of Medicine, Bethesda, Maryland; Staff Gastroenterologist, Walter Reed Army Medical Center, Washington, D.C.
Hepatobiliary Diseases

Bertrand Dupont, M.D.
Professor and Director, Unité de Mycologie, Institut Pasteur, Paris, France
Cryptococcosis

Kathryn M. Edwards, M.D.
Professor of Pediatrics, Vanderbilt University Medical Center, Nashville, Tennessee
Cat-Scratch Disease

Carlton A. W. Evans, M.B.B.S., M.R.C.P.
Medical Research Council Clinical Training Fellow, University of Cambridge Clinical School and Trinity College, Cambridge; Infectious Diseases Specialist Registrar, Addenbrooke's Hospital, Cambridge, England
Cysticercosis

James L. Fishback, M.S., M.D.
Course Director, Pathology, University of Kansas School of Medicine; Attending Physician, University of Kansas Medical Center, Kansas City, Kansas
Toxoplasmosis

Susan P. Fisher-Hoch, M.D., M.R.C.Path.
Director, Laboratoire Jean Merieux, Fondation Marcel Merieux, Lyon, France
West Nile Fever; Lassa Fever; Crimea-Congo Hemorrhagic Fever

Alan D. Fix, M.D., M.S.
Assistant Professor, Department of Epidemiology and Preventive Medicine, University of Maryland School of Medicine, Baltimore, Maryland
Helicobacter pylori *Infections*

Alan F. Fleming, M.A., M.D., F.R.C.Path.
Formerly, Professor of Haematology, Almada Bello University, Zaria, Nigeria; University of the Witwatersrand, Johannesburg, South Africa; University Zambia, Lusaka, Zambia; Formerly, Director of Laboratory Services, University Teaching Hospital, Lusaka, Zambia
Hematologic Diseases

David O. Freedman, M.D.
Associate Professor, Division of Geographic Medicine, University of Alabama at Birmingham School of Medicine, Birmingham, Alabama
Filariasis

Jacob K. Frenkel, M.D., Ph.D.
Adjunct Professor of Pathology, University of New Mexico, Albuquerque, New Mexico
Toxoplasmosis; Sarcosporidiosis; Cystoisosporidiosis

Arthur M. Friedlander, M.D.
Clinical Associate Professor of Medicine, Uniformed Services University of the Health Sciences, Bethesda; Chief, Bacteriology Division, U.S. Army Medical Research Institute of Infectious Diseases, Frederick, Maryland
Anthrax

Hector H. Garcia, M.D.
Assistant Professor, Department of Pathology, Universidad Peruana Cayetano Heredia, Lima, Peru
Cysticercosis

John W. Gardner, M.D., Dr.P.H.
Professor, Department of Preventive Medicine and Biometrics, Uniformed Services University of the Health Sciences, Bethesda, Maryland
Heat-Associated Illness

Robert A. Gasser, Jr., M.D.
Infectious Disease Officer, Department of Immunology, Walter Reed Army Institute of Research, Washington, D.C.; Assistant Professor, Department of Medicine, Uniformed Services University of the Health Sciences, Bethesda, Maryland
Diphtheria

Vinodh Gathiram, M.B.Ch.B., M.D., F.C.P.
Professor, Department of Medicine, Head of Infectious Diseases, University of Natal Medical School, Durban; Senior Consultant, King Edward VIII Hospital, Congella-Durban, Kwazulu-Natal, South Africa
Amebiasis

Robert H. Gilman, M.D.
Professor, Department of International Health, The Johns Hopkins University School of Hygiene and Public Health, Baltimore, Maryland
Intestinal Nematodes That Migrate Through Skin and Lung; Cysticercosis; Cystic Hydatid Disease; Alveolar Hydatid Disease; Sparganosis; Coenuriasis

Armando E. Gonzalez, M.D.
Universidad Nacional Mayor de San Marcos, Lima, Peru
Cystic Hydatid Disease

Simin Goral, M.D.
Assistant Professor of Medicine, Vanderbilt University Medical Center, Nashville, Tennessee
Cat-Scratch Disease

Sandy Gove, M.D., M.P.H.
Research Associate, University of California, Berkeley, School of Public Health, Berkeley, California
Integrated Management of Childhood Illness

J. R. Graybill, M.D.
Professor, Division of Infectious Diseases, Department of Medicine, University of Texas Health Science Center, San Antonio, Texas
Coccidioidomycosis

Sharone Green, M.D.
Assistant Professor of Medicine, Center for Infectious Disease and Vaccine Research, University of Massachusetts Medical School, Worcester, Massachusetts
Dengue and Dengue Hemorrhagic Fever

Brian M. Greenwood, M.D., F.R.C.P.
Professor of Communicable Diseases, London School of Hygiene and Tropical Medicine, London, England
Acute Bacterial Meningitis; Meningococcal Disease

Duane J. Gubler, M.S., Sc.D.
Director, Division of Vector-Borne Infectious Diseases, Centers for Disease Control and Prevention, Fort Collins, Colorado
Insects in Disease Transmission

Roderick J. Hay D.M., F.R.C.P., F.R.C.Path.
Mary Dunhill Professor of Cutaneous Medicine, St. John's Institute of Dermatology, United Medical and Dental Schools, St. Thomas Hospital, London, England
Actinomycosis; Nocardiosis; The Mycoses: General Principles; Superficial Mycoses; Subcutaneous Mycoses: General Principles; Histoplasmosis; Other Opportunistic Mycoses

Neill C. Hepburn, M.D., F.R.C.P.
Consultant Dermatologist, Lincoln County Hospital, Lincoln, United Kingdom
Dermatologic Diseases

Barbara L. Herwaldt, M.D., M.P.H.
Medical Epidemiologist, Division of Parasitic Diseases, Centers for Disease Control and Prevention, Atlanta, Georgia
Babesiosis

David L. Heymann, M.D.
Executive Director, Communicable Diseases, World Health Organization, Geneva, Switzerland
Global Epidemiology of Infectious Diseases

James A. Higgins, Ph.D.
Microbiologist, U.S. Department of Agriculture— Agriculture Research Station, Beltsville, Maryland
Murine Flea-Borne Typhus

Eileen Hilton, M.D.
Associate Professor of Medicine, Albert Einstein College of Medicine, Bronx; Director, Travel and Immunization Center, Long Island Jewish Medical Center, New Hyde Park, New York
Establishing a Traveler's Clinic

Stephen L. Hoffman, M.D., D.T.M.&H.
Director, Malaria Program, Naval Medical Research Institute, Bethesda, Maryland; Adjunct Professor, Department of Preventive Medicine and Biometrics, Uniformed Services University of the Health Sciences; Visiting Professor of Tropical Medicine, Mahidol University, Bangkok, Thailand
Typhoid Fever

Alison Holmes, M.A., M.D., M.R.C.P., D.T.M.&H., M.P.H.
Senior Registrar in Infectious Disease, Imperial College School of Medicine, Hammersmith Hospital, London, England
Diseases of Immigrants

Dale J. Hu, M.D., M.P.H.
Medical Epidemiologist, International Activities Branch, Division of HIV/AIDS Prevention, Centers for Disease Control and Prevention, Atlanta, Georgia
Human Immunodeficiency Virus Infection and AIDS

Walter T. Hughes, M.D.
Arthur Ashe Chair for Pediatric AIDS Research, St. Jude Children's Research Hospital; Professor of Pediatrics and Preventive Medicine, University of Tennessee College of Medicine, Memphis, Tennessee
Pneumocystosis

Lisa A. Jackson, M.D., M.P.H.
Assistant Investigator, Immunization Studies Program, Center for Health Studies, Group Health Cooperative; Assistant Professor, Department of Epidemiology, School of Public Health and Community Medicine, University of Washington, Seattle, Washington
Trench Fever

Terry F. H. G. Jackson, Med.Tech.(SA); Ph.D.
Honorary Professor, Department of Medical Microbiology, University of Natal Medical School; Regional Executive, South African Medical Research Council, Durban, Kwazulu-Natal, South Africa
Amebiasis

Elaine C. Jong, M.D.
Clinical Professor, Department of Medicine; Co-Director, UW Travel and Tropical Medicine Service; Director, Hall Health Primary Care Center/UW Student Health Service, University of Washington, Seattle, Washington
Advice to Travelers

Benjamin Joseph, M.D., M.S., M.C.H.
Professor of Orthopedics, Kasturba Medical College, Karnataka State, India
Orthopedics

Dennis D. Juranek, D.V.M., M.Sc.
Associate Director, Division of Parasitic Diseases, Centers for Disease Control and Prevention, Atlanta, Georgia
Cryptosporidiosis

Kevin C. Kain, M.D., F.R.C.P.C.
Associate Professor, Department of Medicine, Division of Infectious Disease, University of Toronto; Director, Tropical Disease Unit, The Toronto Hospital, Toronto, Ontario, Canada
Skin Lesions in Travelers

John A. Kark, M.D.
Associate Professor, Department of Internal Medicine, Howard University Hospital, Washington, D.C.
Heat-Associated Illness

Jay S. Keystone, M.D., M.Sc.(CTM), F.R.C.P.C.
Professor of Medicine, University of Toronto; Staff Physician, Centre for Travel and Tropical Medicine, The Toronto General Hospital, Toronto, Ontario, Canada
Tropical Disease in a Temperate Climate: General Principles; Skin Lesions in Travelers; Eosinophilia in Travelers and Immigrants

Ali S. Khan, M.D.
Chief, Epidemiology Unit, Special Pathogens Branch, Centers for Disease Control and Prevention, Atlanta, Georgia
Diseases Caused by Hantaviruses

Christopher L. King, M.D., Ph.D.
Associate Professor, Department of Medicine, International
Health and Pathology, Case Western Reserve University;
Staff, Veterans Affairs Medical Center and University
Hospitals of Cleveland, Cleveland, Ohio
Filariasis

Amy Klion, M.D.
Staff Physician, Laboratory of Parasitic Disease, National
Institute of Allergy and Infectious Diseases, National
Institutes of Health, Bethesda, Maryland
Loiasis

Phyllis E. Kozarsky, M.D.
Associate Professor of Medicine, Emory University School
of Medicine; Adjunct Assistant Professor of International
Health, Emory University School of Public Health; Division
of Infectious Diseases, Emory Clinic, Atlanta, Georgia
Screening of the Long-Term Traveler

Thomas G. Ksiazek, Ph.D., D.V.M.
Chief, Disease Assessment Section, Special Pathogens
Branch, Centers for Disease Control and Prevention,
Atlanta, Georgia
*Ebola and Marburg Virus Infections; Diseases Caused by
Hantaviruses*

Eve Lackritz, M.D.
Medical Epidemiologist, International Activities Branch,
Division of HIV/AIDS Prevention, Centers for Disease
Control and Prevention, Atlanta, Georgia
Human Immunodeficiency Virus Infection and AIDS

Larry W. Laughlin, M.D., Ph.D.
Chairman, Department of Preventive Medicine and
Biometrics, Uniformed Services University of the Health
Sciences, Bethesda, Maryland
*Clinical Practice in the Tropics: General Principles; Urinary Tract
Diseases; Bartonellosis*

Thong P. Lee, M.D.
Formerly of the Malaria Program, Naval Medical Research
Institute, Bethesda, Maryland
Typhoid Fever

Ben M. Lee, M.D., M.P.H.
Research Assistant, Department of International Health, The
Johns Hopkins School of Public Health and Hygiene,
Baltimore, Maryland
Alveolar Hydatid Disease

Myron M. Levine, M.D., D.T.P.H.
Head, Divisions of Geographic Medicine, Infectious
Diseases and Tropical Pediatrics; Professor, Departments of
Medicine, Pediatrics, Epidemiology and Preventive
Medicine; and Microbiology and Immunology, University of
Maryland School of Medicine, Baltimore, Maryland
Shigellosis; Diarrhea Caused by Escherichia coli

Robert N. Longfield, M.D.
Clinical Associate Professor, Department of Medicine, The
University of Texas Health Science Center at San Antonio;
Clinical Director, Texas Center for Infectious Disease, San
Antonio, Texas
Anthrax; Nontyphoidal Salmonella *Infections*

Sebastian J. Lucas, M.D., F.R.C.P., F.R.C.Path.
Professor, Department of Histopathology, United Medical
and Dental Schools, St. Thomas Hospital, London, England
Human Immunodeficiency Virus Infection and AIDS

David C. W. Mabey, M.A., B.M., B.Ch., D.M.
Professor of Communicable Diseases, London School of
Hygiene and Tropical Medicine; Consultant Physician,
Hospital For Tropical Diseases, London, England
*Sexually Transmitted Diseases; Trachoma and Inclusion
Conjunctivitis; Chlamydial Infections*

Douglas W. MacPherson, M.D., M.Sc.(CTM), F.R.C.P.C.
Assistant Professor, Department of Pathology, McMaster
University; Director, Regional Parasitology Laboratory,
Hamilton Regional Laboratory Medicine Program; Director,
Infectious Diseases and Tropical Medicine Clinic, Hamilton
Health Sciences Corporation/St. Joseph's Hospital,
Hamilton, Ontario, Canada
Screening of the Long-Term Traveler

Alan J. Magill, M.D.
Head, Parasitology Division, U.S. Naval Medical Research
Institute, Walter Reed Army Institute of Research,
Washington, D.C.
American Trypanosomiasis; Leishmaniasis; Fever in Travelers

James H. Maguire, M.D., M.P.H.
Associate Professor of Medicine, Harvard Medical School;
Associate Professor of Immunology and Infectious Disease,
Harvard School of Public Health; Clinical Director, Division
of Infectious Diseases, Brigham and Women's Hospital,
Boston, Massachusetts
Diseases of Immigrants

Carl J. Mason, M.S., M.D., M.P.H.
Chief, Infectious Disease Research, Walter Reed Project,
Kenya Medical Research Institute, Nairobi, Kenya
Nontyphoidal Salmonella *Infections*

Joseph B. McCormick, M.D., M.S.
Director, Department of Epidemiology, Pasteur Mérieux
Connaught, Lyon, France
West Nile Fever; Lassa Fever; Crimean-Congo Hemorrhagic Fever

Kelly T. McKee, Jr., M.D., M.P.H.
Chief, Preventive Medicine Service, Womack Army Medical
Center, Fort Bragg, North Carolina
South American Hemorrhagic Fevers

Donald E. Meier, M.D.
Associate Professor, Department of Surgery, University of Texas Southwestern School of Medicine, Dallas, Texas
Surgery

Wayne M. Meyers, M.D., Ph.D., D.Sc. (Hon.)
Chief, Mycobacteriology Branch, Armed Forces Institute of Pathology, Washington, D.C.
Tropical Phagedenic Ulcer; Leprosy; Nontuberculous Mycobacterial Skin Infections; Miscellaneous Filarial Infections; Cutaneous Larva Migrans

Karen Midthun, M.D.
Adjunct Assistant Professor, Department of International Health, The Johns Hopkins University School of Hygiene and Public Health, Baltimore; Chief, Vaccines Clinical Trials Branch, Office of Vaccines Research and Review, Center for Biologics Evaluation and Research, Rockville, Maryland
Viral Diarrheas

James N. Mills, Ph.D.
Chief, Medical Ecology Unit, Division of Viral and Rickettsial Diseases, National Center for Infectious Diseases, Centers for Disease Control and Prevention, Atlanta, Georgia
South American Hemorrhagic Fevers

Patrick S. Moore, M.D., M.P.H., M.Phil.
Professor, Division of Epidemiology and Department of Pathology, Columbia University School of Medicine, New York, New York
Herpesvirus Infections

Pedro Morera, M.Q.C.
Full Professor of Medical Parasitology, School of Medicine and Institute of Health Research, University of Costa Rica, San José, Costa Rica
Abdominal Angiostrongyliasis

Pedro L. Moro, M.D.
Research Assistant, Department of Pathology, Universidad Peruana Cayatano Meredia, Lima, Peru
Cystic Hydatid Disease

J. Glenn Morris, Jr., M.D., M.P.H.&T.M.
Professor and Director of Hospital Epidemiology Division, Departments of Medicine and Epidemiology and Preventive Medicine, University of Maryland School of Medicine, Baltimore, Maryland
Cholera and Other Vibrioses; Helicobacter pylori *Infections*

K. Darwin Murrell, Ph.D.
Deputy Administrator, Agricultural Research Service, U.S. Department of Agriculture, Washington, D.C.
Trichinosis

James P. Nataro, M.D., Ph.D.
Associate Professor, Department of Pediatrics, Center for Vaccine Development, University of Maryland School of Medicine, Baltimore, Maryland
Diarrhea Caused by Escherichia coli

Eileen E. Navarro, M.D.
Fellow and Instructor, Division of Infectious Diseases, Department of Medicine, University of Maryland School of Medicine, Baltimore; Biotechnology Fellow, National Cancer Institute, Immunocompromised Host Laboratory, National Institutes of Health, Bethesda, Maryland
Histoplasmosis

Ronald C. Neafie, M.S.
Chief, Parasitic Diseases Pathology Branch, Department of Infectious and Parasitic Diseases, Armed Forces Institute of Pathology, Washington, D.C.
Tropical Phagademic Ulcer; Protothecosis; Miscellaneous Filarial Infections; Cutaneous Larva Migrans

Ricardo Negroni, M.D.
Professor of Microbiology, University of Salvador School of Medicine, Buenos Aires; Chief of Mycology Unit, Francisco Javier Muñiz Hospital, Buenos Aires, Argentina
Paracoccidioidomycosis

Ann M. Nelson, M.D.
Chief, Division of AIDS Pathology and Emerging Infectious Diseases, Armed Forces Institute of Pathology, Washington, D.C.
Protothecosis

Thomas B. Nutman, M.D.
Head, Helminth Immunology Section, Laboratory of Parasitic Diseases, National Institute of Allergy and Infectious Diseases, National Institutes of Health, Bethesda, Maryland
Onchocerciasis

M. Steven Oberste, Ph.D.
Microbiologist, Division of Viral and Rickettsial Diseases, Centers for Disease Control and Prevention, Atlanta, Georgia
Venezuelan Equine Encephalitis

Kimberly O. O'Brien, Ph.D.
Assistant Professor, Center for Human Nutrition, The Johns Hopkins University School of Hygiene and Public Health, Baltimore, Maryland
Rickets and Osteomalacia

Edward C. Oldfield III, M.D.
Professor of Medicine, Microbiology, and Immunology; Director, Division of Infectious Disease, Eastern Virginia Medical School, Norfolk, Virginia
Treatment of Systemic Mycoses

Sonja J. Olsen, Ph.D.
Division of Epidemiology, Columbia University School of Medicine, New York, New York
Herpesvirus Infections

James G. Olson, Ph.D.
Supervisory Research Biologist, Viral and Rickettsial Zoonoses Branch, Centers for Disease Control and Prevention, Atlanta, Georgia
Q Fever; Bartonella-Associated Diseases: General Principles; Rickettsial Infections: General Principles; Typhus: General Principles; Epidemic Louse-Borne Typhus; Scrub Typhus; Ehrlichiosis

Mark A. Pallansch, Ph.D.
Chief, Enterovirus Section, Centers for Disease Control and Prevention, Atlanta, Georgia
Acute Hemorrhagic Conjunctivitis

Philip E. S. Palmer, M.B., F.R.C.P., F.R.C.R.
Emeritus Professor of Radiology, University of California, Davis, California; Advisor in Radiology, World Health Organization, Geneva, Switzerland
Imaging in the Tropics and the Imaging of Tropical Diseases

D.M. Parkin, M.D.
Chief, Unit of Descriptive Epidemiology, International Agency for Research on Cancer, Lyon, France
Malignant Diseases

Jacques Pépin, M.D., F.R.C.P.C.
Associate Professor, Infectious Diseases Division; Director, Center for International Health, University of Sherbrooke, Sherbrooke, Quebec, Canada
African Trypanosomiasis

Peter L. Perine, M.D., M.P.H.
Professor of Epidemiology and Medicine, University of Washington; Attending Physician, Harborview Hospital, Seattle, Washington
Syphilis and the Endemic Treponematoses

Louis Polish, M.D., D.T.M.&H.
Associate Professor, Division of Infectious Diseases, Washington University School of Medicine, St. Louis, Missouri
Pasteurella

Bernadette L. Ramirez, Ph.D.
Associate Professor, Department of Biochemistry and Molecular Biology, College of Medicine, University of Philippines, Manila, Philippines
Schistosomiasis

Virginia F. Randall, M.D., M.P.H.
Clinical Associate Professor of Pediatrics, Uniformed Services University of the Health Sciences, Bethesda, Maryland
Maternal and Child Health in the Tropics

Stephen C. Redd, M.D.
Chief, Air Pollution and Respiratory Health Branch, National Center for Environmental Health, Centers for Disease Control and Prevention, Atlanta, Georgia
Measles

Steven G. Reed, Ph.D.
Associate Professor, Department of Pathobiology, University of Washington; Chief Scientific Officer, Corixa Corporation, Seattle; Senior Scientist, Infectious Disease Research Institute, Seattle, Washington
American Trypanosomiasis

Michael F. Rein, M.D.
Professor, Division of Infectious Diseases, Department of Medicine, School of Medicine, University of Virginia, Charlottesville, Virginia
Trichomoniasis

John Richens, M.A., M.B.B.S., M.Sc.
Lecturer, Department of Sexually Transmitted Diseases, University College, London Medical School, London, England
Granuloma Inguinale

Leon L. Robert, Ph.D., M.S., M.Ed.
Formerly, Assistant Professor, Department of Chemistry, United States Military Academy, West Point, New York
Control of Arthropods of Medical Importance

Guénaél R. Rodier, M.D., M.Sc., C.T.M.
Medical Officer, Department of Communicable Diseases Surveillance and Response, World Health Organization, Geneva, Switzerland
Global Epidemiology of Infectious Diseases

Pierre E. Rollin, M.D.
Chief, Pathogenesis Section, Special Pathogens Branch, Centers for Disease Control and Prevention, Atlanta, Georgia
Ebola and Marburg Virus Infections

Gustavo C. Román, M.D.

Nutritional Neuropathies

Allan R. Ronald, M.D., F.R.C.P.C.
Professor of Medical Microbiology and Internal Medicine, University of Manitoba, Winnipeg, Manitoba, Canada
Chancroid

Trenton K. Ruebush II, M.D.
Malaria Branch, Division of Parasitic Diseases, Centers for Disease Control and Prevention, Atlanta, Georgia
Vector Transmission of Diseases and Zoonoses: General Principles of Infectious Disease Transmission

Michael J. Ryan, M.D., M.P.H.
Medical Officer, Communicable Diseases, Department of Surveillance and Response, World Health Organization, Geneva, Switzerland
Global Epidemiology of Infectious Diseases

Arif R. Sarwari, M.D., M.S.
Assistant Professor and Consultant Physician, Infectious Diseases, Aga Khan University Hospital, Karachi, Pakistan
Dracunculiasis

Peter M. Schantz, V.M.D., Ph.D.
Epidemiology Branch, Division of Parasitic Diseases, Centers for Disease Control and Prevention, Atlanta, Georgia
Toxocariasis; Cestode Infections: General Principles; Tapeworm Infections; Polycystic Hydatid Disease; Parasitic Immunodiagnosis

Daniel A. Scott, M.D.
Enteric Diseases Program, Naval Medical Research Institute, Bethesda, Maryland
Miscellaneous Bacterial Enteritides

Uzi M. Selcer, M.D.
Division of Infectious Diseases, Departments of Internal Medicine and Pediatrics, Albert Einstein Medical Center, Philadelphia, Pennsylvania
Tuberculosis

Daniel J. Sexton, M.D.
Professor, Division of Infectious Diseases, Department of Medicine, Duke University School of Medicine, Durham, North Carolina
Rocky Mountain Spotted Fever

David R. Shlim, M.D.
Medical Director, The CIWEC Clinic Travel Medicine Center, Kathmandu, Nepal
Cyclosporiasis

Ellen K. Silbergeld, Ph.D.
Professor of Epidemiology and Preventive Medicine; Director, Program in Human Health and the Environment, University of Maryland Medical School; Adjunct Professor of Environmental Health, The Johns Hopkins School of Hygiene and Public Health, Baltimore, Maryland
Environmental Health Hazards in the Tropics

Thira Sirisanthana, M.D.
Associate Professor of Medicine and Chairman, Department of Medicine, Faculty of Medicine, Chiang Mai University, Chiang Mai, Thailand
Penicilliosis marneffei

Peter M. Small, M.D.
Assistant Professor, Division of Infectious Diseases and Geographic Medicine, School of Medicine, Stanford University, Stanford California
Tuberculosis

Raymond A. Smego, Jr., M.D., M.P.H., F.A.C.P., D.T.M.&H.
Professor and Chairman, Department of Infectious Diseases and Clinical Microbiology, Faculty of Health Sciences, University of the Witwatersrand; South African Institute for Medical Research, Johannesburg, South Africa
Cardiovascular Diseases; Actinomycosis; Nocardiosis

William A. Sodeman, Jr., M.D., J.D.
Professor of Medicine, Division of Gastroenterology, Medical College of Ohio, Toledo; Consultant Physician, Medical College Hospital, Toledo, Ohio
Poisonous Plants and Fish; Animals Hazardous to Humans: General Principles; Venomous Marine Animals; Leeches; Fish; Lizards; Bats; Mollusks Involved in Disease Transmission

Noel W. Solomons, M.D.
Scientific Director, Senior Scientist and Co-Founder, Center for Studies of Sensory Impairment, Aging, and Metabolism, Guatemala City, Guatemala
Zinc and Other Trace Mineral Deficiencies and Excesses

Alfred Sommer, M.D., M.H.Sc.
Professor of Ophthalmology, Epidemiology, and International Health; Dean, The Johns Hopkins School of Hygiene and Public Health, The Johns Hopkins University, Baltimore, Maryland
Ophthalmologic Diseases; Vitamin A Deficiency and Xerophthalmia

Daniel E. Sonenshine, Ph.D.
Professor (Eminent) of Biological Sciences, Department of Biological Sciences, Old Dominion University, Norfolk, Virginia
Ticks and Mites in Disease Transmission

Mark C. Steinhoff, M.D.
Professor, Departments of International Health, Epidemiology, and Pediatrics, The Johns Hopkins University School of Hygiene and Public Health, Baltimore, Maryland
Pulmonary Diseases

August H. R. Stich, M.D., M.Sc., D.T.M.&H.
Lecturer, Department of Tropical Medicine, Medical Mission Hospital, Würzburg, Germany
Lymphogranuloma Venereum

Rebecca J. Stoltzfus, M.S., Ph.D.
Associate Professor, Center for Human Nutrition, The Johns Hopkins University School of Public Health, Baltimore, Maryland
The Impact of Parasitic Infections on Nutrition

G. Thomas Strickland, M.D., Ph.D., D.C.M.T., F.A.C.P.
Director, International Health Program; Professor of Epidemiology and Preventive Medicine, Microbiology and Immunology, and Medicine, University of Maryland School of Medicine; Senior Associate, Department of Molecular Microbiology and Immunology, The Johns Hopkins School of Hygiene and Public Health, Baltimore, Maryland
Viral Hepatitis; Ehrlichiosis; Lyme Disease; Protozoal Infections: General Principles; Malaria; Helminthic Infections: General Principles; Intestinal Nematode Infections: General Principles; Schistosomiasis; Vector Transmission of Diseases and Zoonoses: General Principles of Infectious Disease Transmission; Zoonoses; Fever in Travelers

Robert H. Sudduth, M.D.
Gastroenterologist, The Doctors Clinic, Silverdale, Washington
Anisakidosis

Roland W. Sutter, M.D., M.P.H.&T.M.
Acting Chief, Technical Services Branch, Vaccine Preventable Disease Eradication Division, Centers for Disease Control and Prevention, Atlanta, Georgia
Poliomyelitis

Herbert B. Tanowitz, M.D., F.A.C.P.
Professor of Pathology and Medicine, Albert Einstein College of Medicine; Attending Physician, Associate Director of Parasitology Laboratory and Clinic, Jacobi Medical Center, Weiler Hospital of the Albert Einstein College of Medicine, Bronx, New York
Cestode Infections: General Principles; Tapeworm Infections

John L. Tarpley, M.D.
Professor of Surgery, Vanderbilt University School of Medicine; Chief, General Surgery, Veterans' Affairs Medical Center, Nashville, Tennessee
Surgery

David N. Taylor, M.D., M.Sc.
Infectious Disease Officer, Department of Enteric Infections, Division of Communicable Diseases and Immunology, Walter Reed Army Institute of Research, Washington, D.C.
Campylobacter *Enteritis*

Hugh R. Taylor, M.D., F.R.A.C.O.
Head, Department of Ophthalmology and Ringland Anderson Professor, University of Melbourne; Director of Eye Services, Royal Victorian Eye & Ear Hospital; Managing Director, Centre for Eye Research Australia, Melbourne, Victoria, Australia
Ophthalmologic Diseases; Trachoma and Inclusion Conjunctivitis

Terrie E. Taylor, M.D.
Associate Professor, Department of Medicine, School of Medicine, Michigan State University, East Lansing, Michigan
Malaria

Jean-Claude Theis, M.D., M.C.H. (Orth.), F.R.C.S. Ed. (Orth.), F.R.A.C.S.
Senior Lecturer, Orthopaedic Surgery, Dunedin School of Medicine, University of Otago, Dunedin; Orthopaedic Surgeon, Dunedin Hospital, Healthcare Otago, Dunedin, New Zealand
Orthopedics

David Thomas, M.D., M.P.H.
Associate Professor, Division of Infectious Diseases, Departments of Medicine and Epidemiology, The Johns Hopkins Medical Institutions, Baltimore, Maryland
Viral Hepatitis

Benjamin Torun, M.D., Ph.D.
Professor of Nutrition, INCAP/Universidad De San Carlos; Head, Human Nutrition Unit, Institute of Nutrition of Central America and Panama (INCAP), Guatemala City, Guatemala
Protein-Energy Malnutrition

Nadia M. F. Trugo, Ph.D.
Senior Lecturer, Departamento de Bioquimica, Instituto de Quimica, Universidade Federal do Rio de Janeiro, Rio de Janeiro, Brazil
Nutritional Macrocytic (Megaloblastic) Anemia

Theodore Tsai, M.D., M.P.H.
Wyeth-Lederle Vaccines and Pediatrics, Pearl River, New York
Viral Infections: General Principles; Chikungunya Fever; O'nyong Nyong Fever; Sindbis Fever; Sandfly Fever; Japanese Encephalitis; Rocio Encephalitis; Other Arboviral Encephalitides; Yellow Fever; Kyasanur Forest Disease

David W. Vaughn, M.D., M.P.H.
Chief, Department of Virus Diseases, Walter Reed Army Institute of Research, Washington, D.C.
Dengue and Dengue Hemorrhagic Fever

Athasit Vejjajiva, M.D.
Professor and President, Mahidol University, Bangkok, Thailand
Neurologic Diseases

Judy M. Vincent, M.D.
Associate Clinical Professor, John A. Burns School of Medicine, University of Hawaii, Honolulu; Chief, Pediatric Infectious Diseases, Department of Pediatrics, Tripler Army Medical Center, Honolulu, Hawaii; Clinical Assistant Professor of Pediatrics, Uniformed Services University, Bethesda, Maryland
Pertussis

Charles Vitek, M.D., M.P.H.
Medical Epidemiologist, Infant Immunization Activity, Child Vaccine Preventable Diseases Branch, National Immunization Program, Centers for Disease Control and Prevention, Atlanta, Georgia
Diphtheria

Thomas J. Walsh, M.D.
Chief, Immunocompromised Host Section, Pediatric Oncology Branch, National Cancer Institute, Bethesda, Maryland
Histoplasmosis

Brian J. Ward, M.Sc., M.D.C.M.
Associate Professor of Medicine, McGill University Medical School; Centre for Tropical Diseases, Montreal General Hospital, Montreal, Quebec, Canada
Psittacosis; Tetanus

David A. Warrell, M.A., D.M., D.Sc., F.R.C.P.
Professor, Division of Tropical Medicine and Infectious Diseases, Nuffield Department of Clinical Medicine, John Radcliffe Institute Hospital, Oxford University, Oxford, England
Rabies and Related Viruses; Animals Hazardous to Humans: Snakes

M. J. Warrell, M.B., M.R.C.P., F.R.C.Path.
Centre For Tropical Medicine, John Radcliffe Institute Hospital, Oxford University, Oxford, England
Rabies and Related Viruses

George Watt, M.D., D.T.M.&H.
Armed Forces Research Institute of Medical Sciences; Chief, Medicine Section, Retrovirology Department, Bangkok, Thailand
Scrub Typhus; Leptospirosis

Douglas M. Watts, Ph.D.
Scientific Director, U.S. Naval Medical Research Center Detachment, Lima, Peru
Mayaro Fever; Group C Virus Fevers; Oropouche Fever; Venezuelan Equine Encephalitis

Louis M. Weiss, M.D., M.P.H.
Associate Professor, Departments of Medicine and Pathology, Albert Einstein College of Medicine; Attending Physician, Infectious Diseases, Jack D. Weiler Hospital of Montefiore Medical Center, Bronx Municipal Hospital (Jacobi Medical Center), Bronx, New York
Microsporidiosis

Nicholas J. White, D.Sc., M.D., F.R.C.P.
Professor of Tropical Medicine, Faculty of Tropical Medicine, Mahidol University, and University of Oxford; Bangkok, Thailand; Consultant Physician, John Radcliffe Institute Hospital, Oxford, England
Melioidosis

Marianna Wilson, M.S.
Chief, Reference Immunodiagnostic Laboratory, Biology and Diagnostics Branch, Division of Parasitic Diseases, Centers for Disease Control and Prevention, Atlanta, Georgia
Parasitic Immunodiagnosis

Robert A. Wirtz, Ph.D.
Chief, Entomology Branch, Division of Parasitic Diseases, Centers for Disease Control and Prevention, Atlanta, Georgia
Injurious Arthropods

Murray Wittner, M.D., Ph.D.
Professor of Pathology and Parasitology (Tropical Medicine), Albert Einstein College of Medicine; Attending Physician; Director of Tropical Disease Clinic and Parasitology Laboratory, Jacobi Medical Center, Montefiore Medical Center, Bronx, New York
Cestode Infections: General Principles; Tapeworm Infections

Martin S. Wolfe, M.D., D.C.M.T., F.A.C.P.
Clinical Professor of Medicine, George Washington University Medical School and Georgetown University Medical School; Director, Traveler's Medical Service of Washington, D.C.
Miscellaneous Intestinal Protozoa

Michael T. Wong, M.D.
Department of Infectious Diseases, Wilford Hall Medical Center, Lackland Air Force Base, San Antonio, Texas
Vascular Angiomatosis

Bradley A. Woodruff, M.D., M.P.H.
Adjunct Assistant Professor, Rollins School of Public Health, Emory University; Medical Epidemiologist, International Emergency and Refugee Health Team, Centers for Disease Control and Prevention, Atlanta, Georgia
Health and Nutrition Among Refugees and Displaced Persons

Stephen G. Wright, M.B., F.R.C.P., D.C.M.T.
Honorary Senior Lecturer, Department of Infectious and Tropical Diseases, London School of Hygiene and Tropical Medicine; Consultant Physician, Hospital For Tropical Diseases, London, England
Gastrointestinal Diseases; Brucellosis; Giardiasis

Ray Yip, M.D., M.P.H.
Chief of Health and Nutrition, UNICEF China, Beijing, China
Iron Deficiency

Jonathan Zenilman, M.D.
Associate Professor, Division of Infectious Diseases, Department of Medicine, The Johns Hopkins University School of Medicine; Attending Physician, The Johns Hopkins Hospital, Baltimore, Maryland
Trichomoniasis

J. L. Ziegler
Mill Valley, California
Malignant Diseases

Contents

Color section follows page xxxii.

PART III
Bacterial Infections

 SECTION A **Infections of the Eye and Throat**

■ SECTION B **Respiratory Tract Infections**

■ SECTION C **Gastrointestinal Tract Infections**

■ SECTION D **Sexually Transmitted Diseases**

■ SECTION E **Infections Causing Neurologic Manifestations**

SECTION I **Mycobacterial Infections**

PART IV
The Mycoses

PART V
Protozoal Infections

■ SECTION A **Intestinal and Genital Infections**

■ SECTION B **Infections of the Blood and Reticuloendothelial System**

■ SECTION C **Tissue Infections**

PART VI
Helminthic Infections

PART VII
Poisonous and Toxic Plants and Animals

PART VIII
Nutritional Problems and Deficiency Diseases

PART IX
Vector Transmission of Diseases and Zoonoses

PART X
Tropical Disease in a Temperate Climate

PART XI
Laboratory Diagnosis of Parasitic Diseases

Hunter's Tropical
Medicine
and Emerging
Infectious Diseases

COLOR PLATES

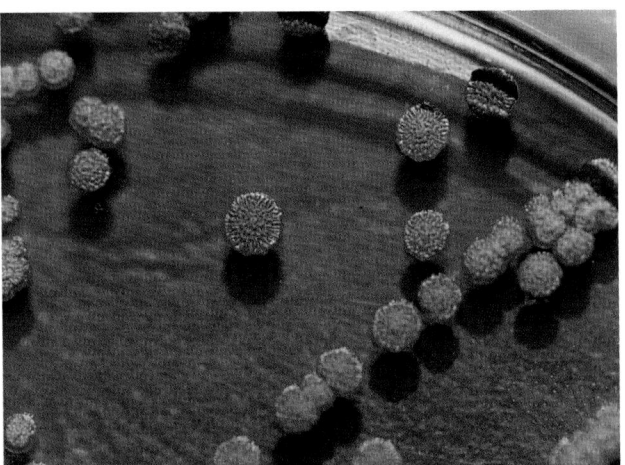

Figure 37–3. Cornflower head colonies of *B. pseudomallei* after several days' growth on Ashdown's selective agar.

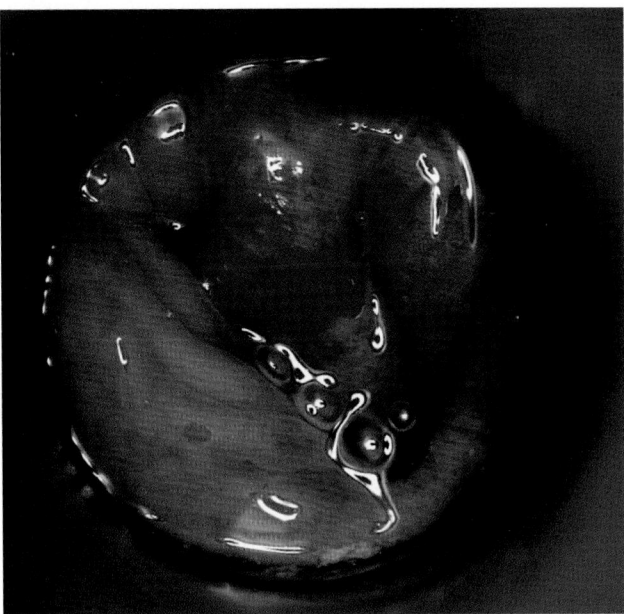

Figure 40–1. Proctoscopy of a patient with Shiga dysentery. Edema of the mucosa, copious mucus discharge, and focal hemorrhages are all evident.

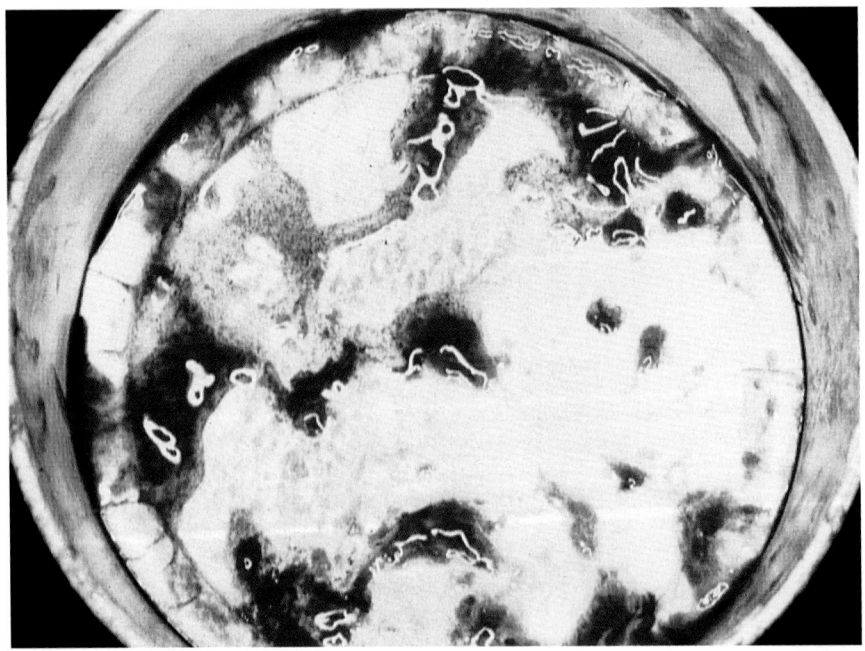

Figure 40–3. A typical dysenteric stool. Note the scanty discharge consisting almost entirely of blood and mucus. At the height of the dysenteric illness, patients can pass such stools at a frequency of every 1 to 2 hours, accompanied by severe tenesmus.

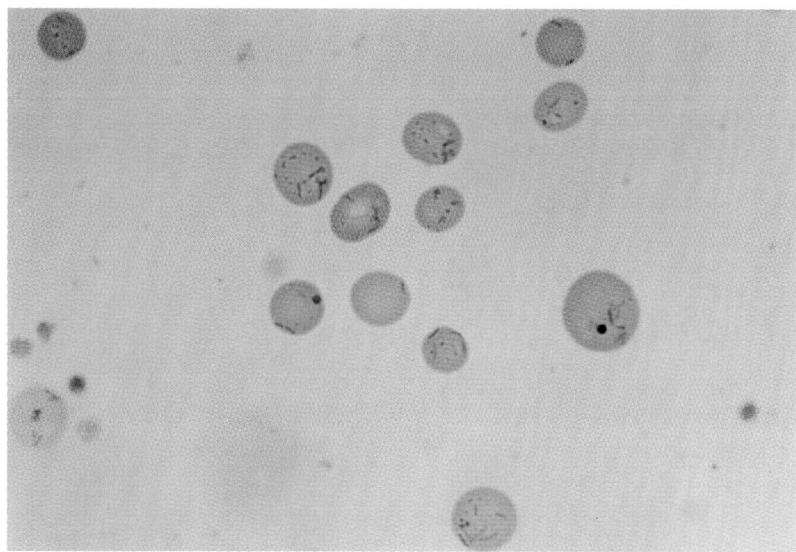

Figure 60–4. Bartonellosis. Thin Giemsa-stained blood film from a severely ill patient with 100% parasitemia. Note both bacillary and coccoid forms of *B. bacilliformis,* with multiple bacteria in each erythrocyte. The patient had severe anemia. (Courtesy of Evan R. Farmer, M.D.)

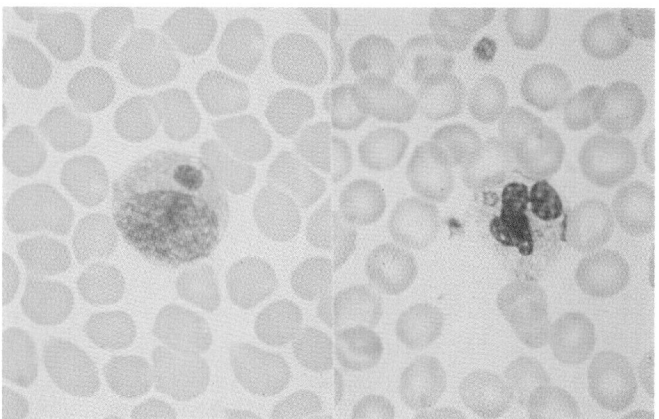

Figure 70–2. Morulae (*Ehrlichia* spp. microcolonies) in peripheral blood films stained with Giemsa. *Left, Ehrlichia chaffeensis* in a mononuclear leukocyte. (Courtesy of Christopher Paddock, M.D.) *Right*, HGE agent in a neutrophil. (Courtesy of Jesse L. Goodman, M.D.)

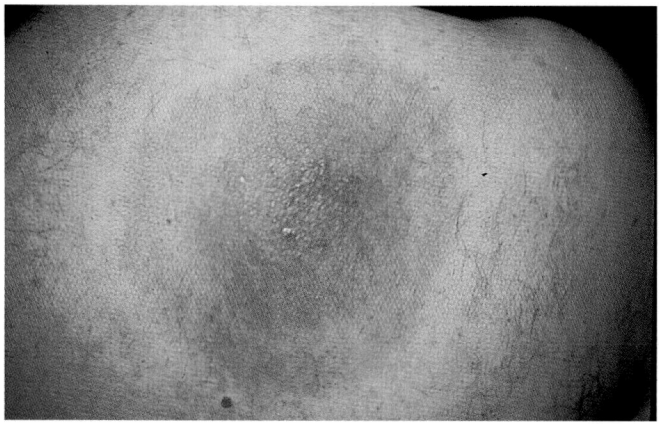

Figure 73–5. Erythema migrans lesion of early localized Lyme disease. Note the central punctum at the site of tick attachment and expanding concentric erythematous rings.

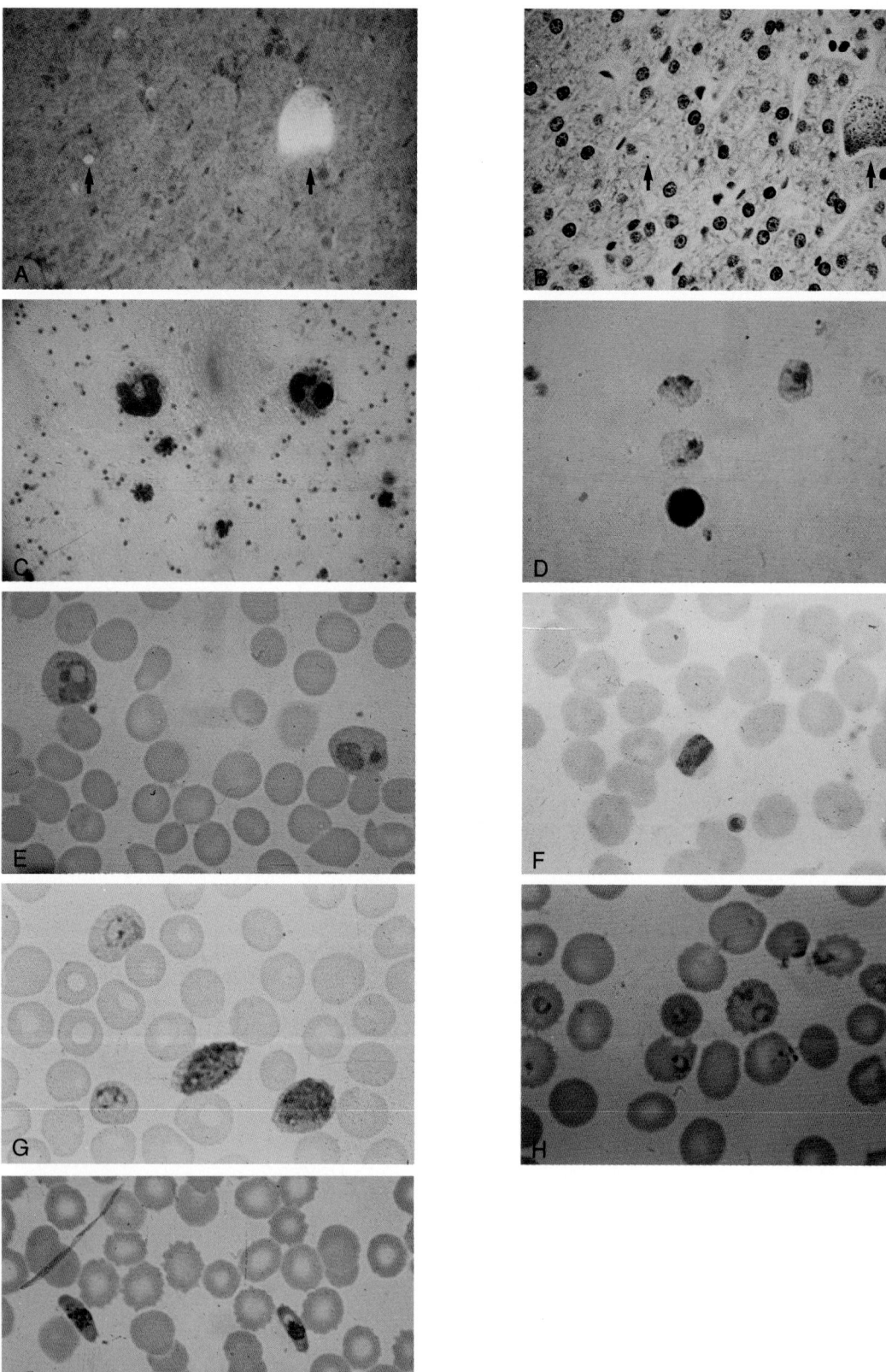

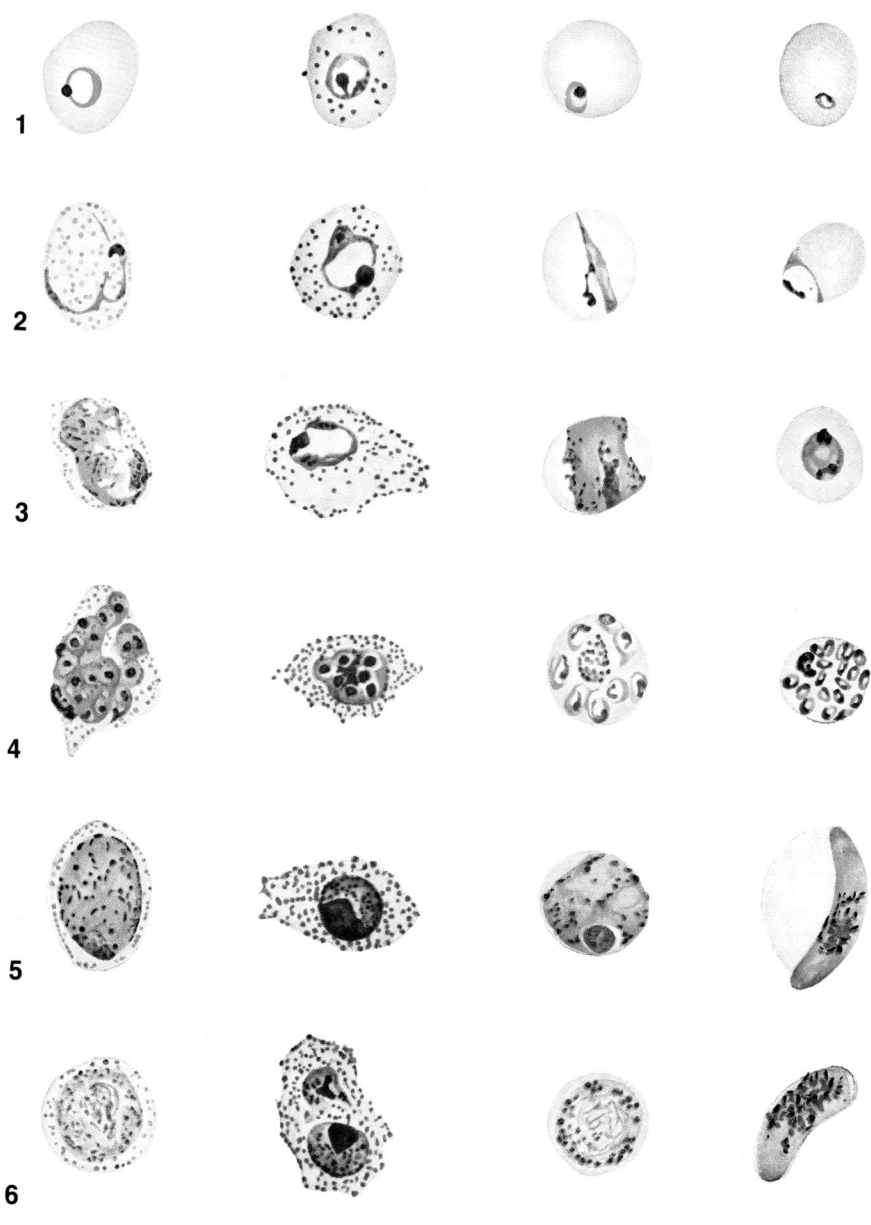

Figure 92–5. Rows *A, Plasmodium vivax; B, P. ovale; C, P. malariae; D, P. falciparum.* Rows *1,* Young trophozoites; *2,* growing trophozoites; *3,* mature trophozoites; *4,* mature schizonts; *5,* macrogametocytes; *6,* microgametocytes. (From Wilcox A: Manual for the Microscopical Diagnosis of Malaria in Man. Bulletin No. 180, National Institute of Health, 1942.)

1

2

3

4

5

6

A   **B**   **C**   **D**

Figure 92–4. All blood smears are stained with Giemsa stain. *A* and *B,* Schizont *(right arrow)* and hypnozoite *(left arrow)* of *Plasmodium cynomolgi bastianellii* in a liver biopsy specimen taken from a rhesus monkey that was inoculated intravenously with 12 million sporozoites 7 days before. *A,* Indirect immunofluorescence staining, using rhesus antibody to disrupted blood stages and a fluorescein-conjugated rabbit anti-rhesus IgG. *B,* After restaining with Giemsa-colophonium. The schizont is approximately 30 μm in diameter; the hypnozoite has a diameter of 5 μm (×500). (Courtesy of W. A. Krotoski.) *C,* Thick blood smear from a patient with heavy *Plasmodium falciparum* infection. Note the leukocytes, platelets, and numerous ring forms of the parasite. *D,* Thick blood smear from a patient with *Plasmodium vivax* infection. Note the three ameboid trophozoites and smaller ring form. Lymphocyte nucleus assists in estimating size of parasites. *E,* Thin blood smear from a patient with *P. vivax* infection. Note the ameboid trophozoites and Schüffner's dots in the enlarged erythrocytes. *F,* Thin blood smear from a patient with *Plasmodium malariae* infection. Note the band-shaped trophozoite in the normal-sized erythrocyte. *G,* Thin blood smear from a patient with *Plasmodium ovale* infection. Note the two ameboid trophozoites in the enlarged stippled erythrocytes and the two schizonts in oval (or elongated) erythrocytes. *H,* Thin blood smear from a patient with heavy *P. falciparum* infection. Note the normal-sized erythrocytes with multiple infections with small ring trophozoites and accolé forms (parasite present on the margin of the erythrocyte) (×290). *I,* Thin blood film showing *P. falciparum* microgametocyte *(left)* and macrogametocyte *(right).*

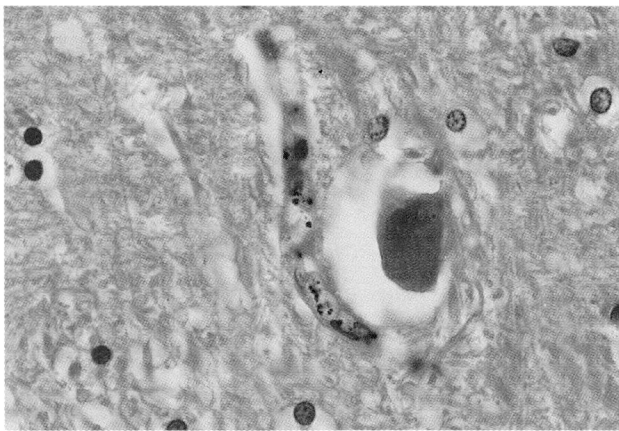

Figure 92–10. Late stages of asexual malaria parasites in erythrocytes adherent to wall of capillary in brain (H&E stain, ×250). (Courtesy of Ronald Neafie and the Armed Forces Institute of Pathology.)

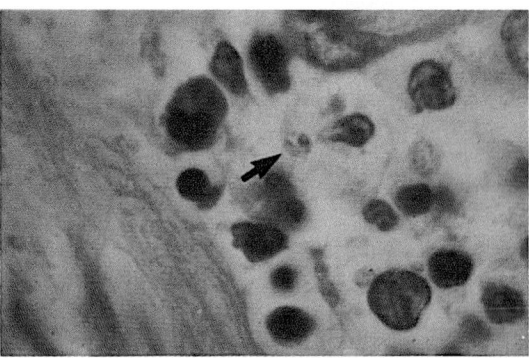

Figure 95–2. Skin biopsy specimen from a patient with cutaneous leishmaniasis. An amastigote is present in tissue macrophage *(arrow)*. Note the nucleus and kinetoplast (H & E stain, ×2600). (Courtesy of Ronald Neafie and the Armed Forces Institute of Pathology, Photograph Neg. No. 74-11632.)

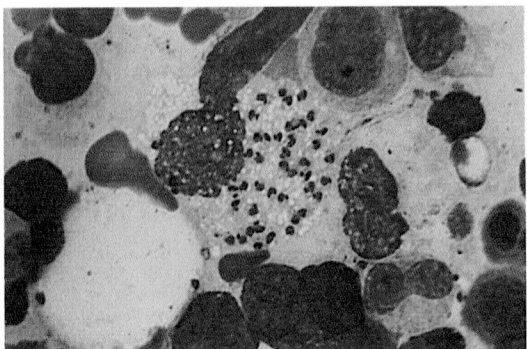

Figure 95–3. Bone marrow aspirate from a patient with visceral leishmaniasis. Note the numerous amastigotes in macrophage (Giemsa stain). (Courtesy of the Armed Forces Institute of Pathology.)

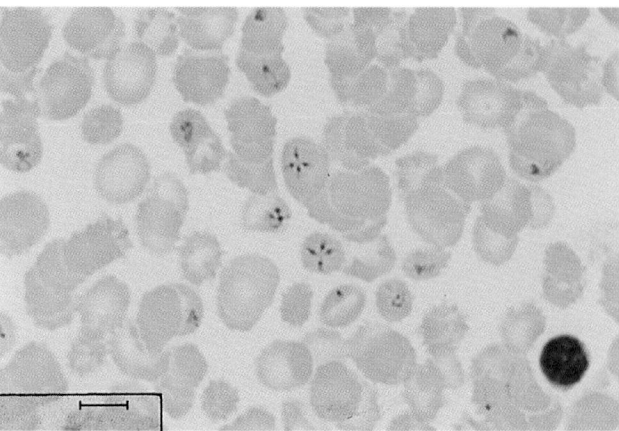

Figure 96–1. Babesiosis. Giemsa-stained blood smear from a patient infected with a WA1-type parasite in California. Note ring forms, which can be oval, round, or pear-shaped, and tetrad forms ("Maltese cross") within normal-sized erythrocytes.

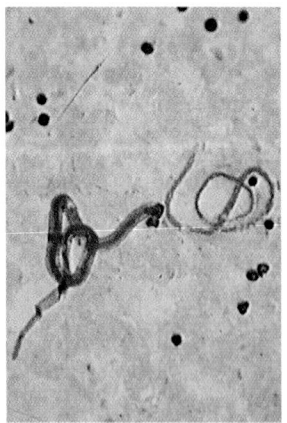

Figure 106–13. Filariasis. *W. bancrofti (left)* and *B. malayi (right)* microfilariae in Giemsa-stained blood film.

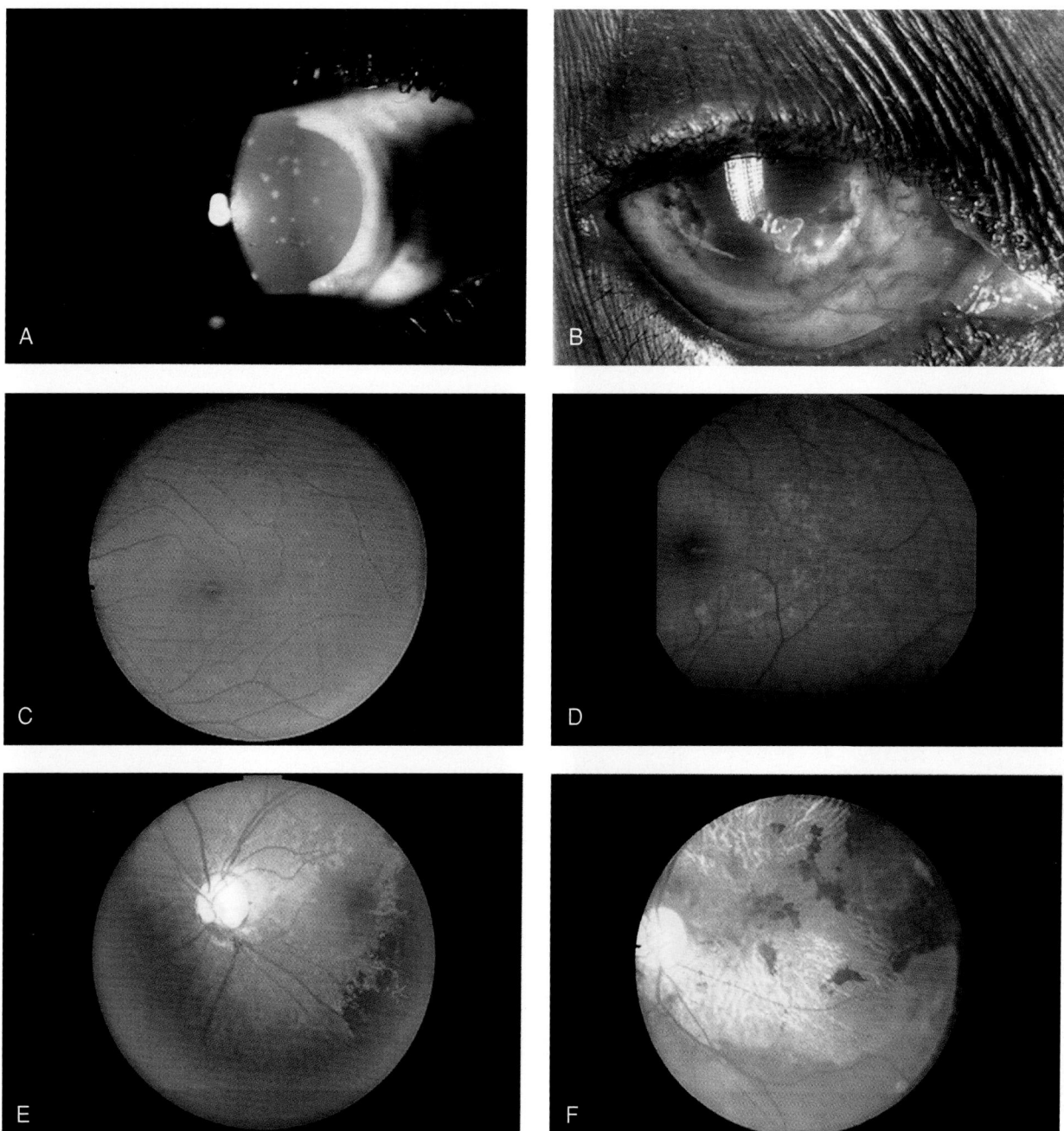

Figure 108–10. Ocular changes in onchocerciasis. *A*, Punctate opacities in the cornea. *B*, Sclerosing keratitis (Courtesy of Dr. I. Murdoch.) *C*, Early mottling of retina temporal to the macula. *D*, Mottling of retina temporal to macula (Courtesy of Dr. R. Proaño.) *E*, Postneuritic optic atrophy with peripapillary pigmentation and temporal chorioretinal scar. *F*, Postneuritic optic atrophy and geographic atrophy of the retinal pigment epithelium with choriocapillary atrophy. (Courtesy of Dr. I. Murdoch.)

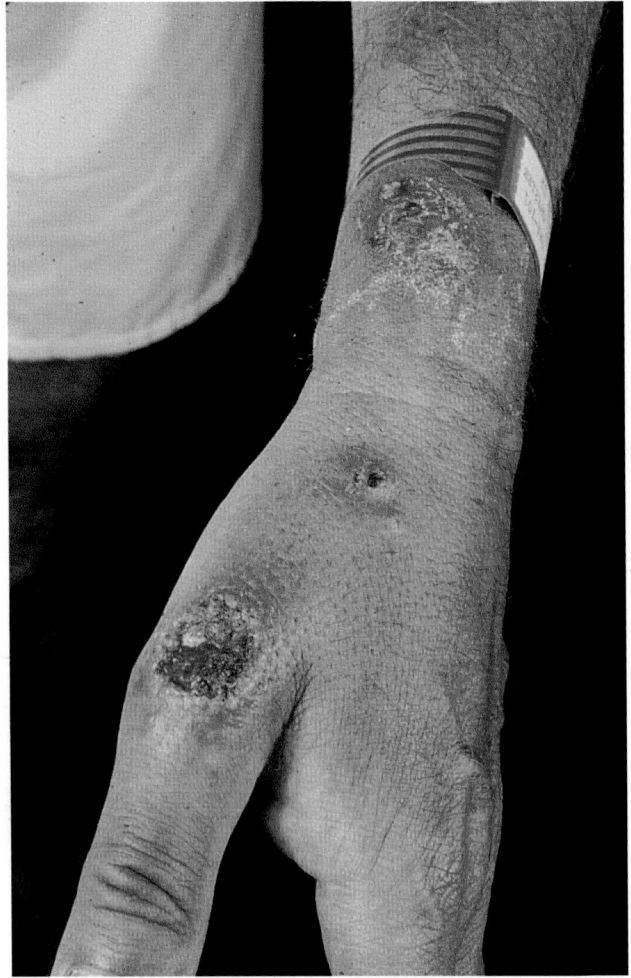

Figure 146–2. Cutaneous leishmaniasis presenting in a lympho-cutaneous fashion resembling sporotrichosis in a Guyanese male.

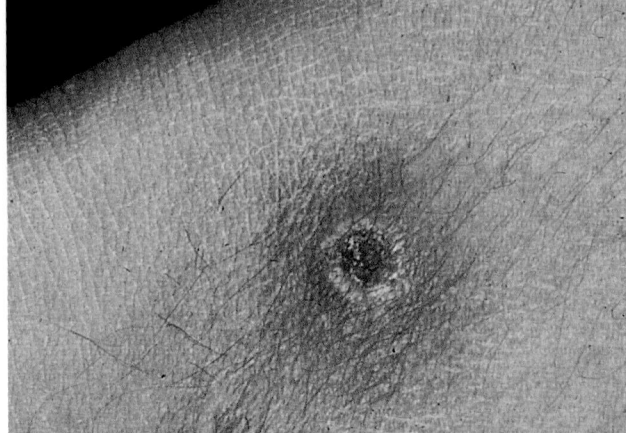

Figure 146–3. A tick eschar of African tick typhus on the leg of a young male recently returned from a safari in southern Africa

1 General Principles

Larry W. Laughlin

THE ART. Medicine in the tropics is exciting, fulfilling, and challenging, but complicated. Clinicians must understand the intricacies of managing the illness of a senior foreign government official or heir to the throne, referring patients or their bodily fluids to distant sophisticated medical centers. Clinicians must also be comfortable sitting on the ground on a torrid summer day drinking hot tea with a village headman while being "credentialed" to care for local patients. Clinicians must adjust to observing a young village child die of severe malaria because no quinine is available, and the next day be confident in interpreting an MRI film taken to detect minimal biliary tract enlargement in a healthy foreign diplomat with vague abdominal pain. Tropical clinicians practice medicine when the electricity is on, when the electricity goes off, and where there never has been any electricity. They must do the best they can with the resources they have. Patients must be cared for even if what is needed to deliver good care is not available. Clinicians must treat individual patients as well as tropical communities, including designing and implementing public health programs for populations of refugees and displaced persons. They must respect local health customs and local medical practice standards while maintaining the integrity of their own practice standards. They must coordinate their treatment program with the traditional healers' efforts and local cultural beliefs. In this edition, a new chapter on traditional medicine provides needed information and perspective in this area. Clinicians must comfort their patients and their families even when they do not speak their language and are unsure of their culture. The practice of medicine in the tropics is an art.

THE PRACTICE. The history of clinical tropical medicine practice is rich with heroes. As Europe colonized Asia, Africa, and South America the new cheap labor had to be kept on the job and the colonial supervisors shielded from the discomforts of local disease. Doctors with special knowledge and skills were needed. Schools and institutes of tropical medicine flourished in England, Germany, Holland, France, and Italy, staffed by returning colonial practitioners and scientists. Young physicians were frequently coerced by large trading companies or their governments and pressed into service "for the greater good." Military and religious organizations also contributed physicians to the practice of tropical medicine. It was also fashionable for the physician sons of aristocrats to practice in the tropics as a life-broadening adventure.

Although the United States had no colonies, the ecology and geography of the new country allowed tropical infectious diseases, e.g., malaria and yellow fever, to flourish. Prior to the maturation of public health, sanitation, and hygiene during the early 20th century, the United States was a developing country with tropical diseases, e.g., cholera, typhoid fever, and syphilis, running rampant. Tropical medicine, much as we know it today, was the normal practice of medicine in many parts of the United States before World War II.

Because of significant economic and social development, most of North America, Europe, and other temperate developed countries now practice a highly sophisticated and highly technical type of medicine. This type of medicine is not available to most tropical, less developed nations, the homeland for the majority of the world's population. There is still a need for the practice of "tropical medicine." As documented in a 1987 report published by the Institute of Medicine, the capacity to train physicians to practice tropical medicine has greatly diminished in the United States. One of the goals of this textbook is to facilitate the training of more physicians in the discipline of tropical medicine.

THE CLINICAL PRACTICE CHAPTERS. Most tropical medicine texts present information primarily by disease agent. While the knowledge of the etiologic agent is critical to diagnosis and specific therapy, patients do not present to you in clinic as *Trypanosoma cruzi* but rather as constipation or syncope. The clinician must be able to think in a matrix, with etiologic agents along one axis and body system complaints on the other axis. The clinical chapters attempt to assist tropical clinicians in initially approaching their patients and their systemic complaints. The clinician is also reminded that ordinary North American disease occurs in the tropics. New chapters on maternal and child health emphasize the importance of this high-risk family component. Nutrition and infectious diseases are prominent medical issues in populations of refugees and displaced persons—an increasing problem in tropical regions—and are given new emphasis. Environmental health threats have existed in the tropics for decades but have been suffocated by more obvious disease burdens. A new chapter deals with this neglected subject. The clinical practice chapters are intended to help practicing clinicians provide comfort and cure for their patients, support and improve their local communities, and improve their skills in tropical medicine.

2 Pulmonary Diseases

Mark C. Steinhoff

■ MAGNITUDE OF PROBLEM

In tropical regions, as elsewhere, respiratory infections are the most common illnesses encountered by health workers in clinics and hospital wards. The common mild upper respiratory infections of children are as frequent in tropical regions as in temperate zones. However, the incidence and mortality of severe lower respiratory tract infections are increased manyfold in the tropics (Fig. 2–1).

Table 2–1 displays a ranking of the important causes of morbidity and mortality for Ghana, showing that childhood pneumonia ranks third, after malaria and measles; and adult pneumonia ranks twelfth—higher than neonatal tetanus, typhoid, meningitis, and hepatitis. These data underscore the importance of pneumonia in all age groups in developing

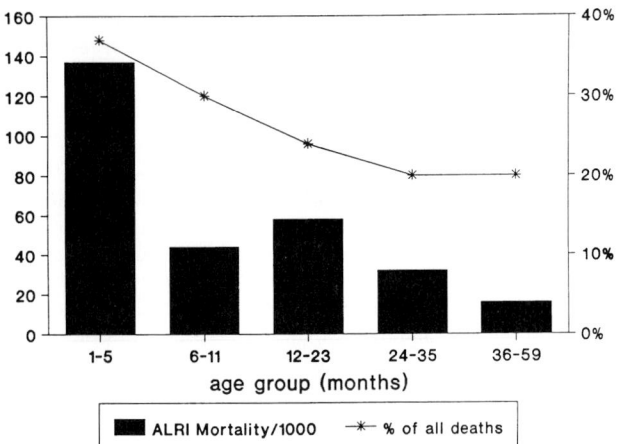

Figure 2–1. Acute lower respiratory infection (ALRI)–specific mortality rates, and proportionate mortality of ALRI in Bangladeshi children, by age. The left vertical axis denotes mortality per 1000 per year and the right axis denotes the proportion of all deaths. These data are from Teknaf, Bangladesh. (From Spika JS, et al: Ann Trop Pediatr 9:33, 1989.)

countries. Pneumonia is a major cause of mortality among infants and children who live in developing countries, as it was in North America and Europe 100 years ago.

The incidence of pneumonia in North America in children <5 years of age is estimated at 10 to 50/1000 per year; investigations of children in developing countries report pneumonia rates of 100 to 400/1000 per year, with the highest rates in the first and second years of life. One study from The Gambia noted an annual rate of 165 radiologically proved pneumonias per 1000 children <5 years of age. Admissions for respiratory diseases accounted for 17 to 24% of all hospital admissions in five African countries, with acute pneumonia exceeding tuberculosis in most of them. The higher incidence and increased severity of pneumonia in these regions may be due to the concentration of risk factors frequently present in developing countries: low birthweight and malnutrition, changes in weaning practices, zinc deficiency, industrial and domestic air pollution, incomplete immunizations, poor access to medical treatment, and crowding and other effects of poverty. It is estimated that the global toll of acute pulmonary infections is 3 to 4 million infant and child deaths per year, or approximately one-third of the total global infant and child mortality. The vast majority of these deaths occur in developing regions.

Virtually all microorganisms can cause lower respiratory tract disease, but only a few, e.g., *Bordetella pertussis* and respiratory syncytial virus, cause syndromes distinct enough to enable diagnosis on clinical grounds. Although the etiologic spectrum of pulmonary infections is wider in developing countries than in developed regions, the availability of diagnostic technology is more limited. If the microbial etiology is known, treatment is straightforward. In the usual clinical situation, however, a treatment decision must be made before the etiologic data are available.

■ PNEUMONIA

ETIOLOGY. Investigations using pulmonary needle aspiration of children hospitalized with pneumonia have shown that 50 to 60% had bacteria isolated and approximately 20% had viruses isolated. The common bacterial isolates were *Streptococcus pneumoniae*, *Haemophilus influenzae*, and *Staphylo-*

coccus aureus. The first two are important because they are now preventable by immunization. Among the viruses, respiratory syncytial virus (RSV) and influenza and parainfluenza viruses accounted for 60% of all viral isolates from lung aspirates, with adenoviruses, enteroviruses, and herpesviruses constituting the remainder. Numerous investigations of the virology of lower respiratory tract illness in children show that RSV is the single most important agent (Chapter 26). One study from Papua New Guinea suggests the possible importance of *Pneumocystis carinii* (Chapter 98), *Chlamydia trachomatis* (Chapter 46), cytomegalovirus (CMV), and *Mycoplasma pneumoniae* in infant pneumonia.

Though clinicians in the tropics recognize epidemics of the influenza syndrome, most hospital and clinic surveys of ill children show low isolation rates of influenza virus. However, seroepidemiologic surveys from Africa confirm the importance of this virus. Data from Kenya and The Gambia over a single epidemic season show primary infection rates of 30 to 50% in children <5 years of age, with similar rates in older children and adults.

MICROBIOLOGIC DIAGNOSIS. Determining a specific microbiologic etiology for lower respiratory disease is problematic. Sputum for Gram stain and culture is not available from infants and in adults may reveal oral flora that are unrelated to the pneumonia. Blood culture is positive in only 20% of lung aspirate–proved bacterial pneumonias. Needle aspiration of the affected pulmonary tissue is regarded as the diagnostic gold standard, yet it may be falsely negative in up to 20% of blood culture–positive cases.

There is an urgent need for better noninvasive tests for the diagnosis of bacterial pulmonary disease. Detection of bacterial antigen in blood or urine with commercial latex

TABLE 2–1. Disease Problems of Ghana—Ranked in Order of Days of Healthy Life Lost

Rank Order	Disease	Days of Healthy Life Lost*	Percentage of Total
1	Malaria	32,600	10.2
2	Measles	23,400	7.3
3	Childhood pneumonia	18,600	5.8
4	Sickle cell disease	17,500	5.5
5	Malnutrition (severe)	17,500	5.5
6	Prematurity	16,800	5.2
7	Birth injury	16,400	5.2
8	Accidents	14,900	4.7
9	Gastroenteritis	14,500	4.5
10	Tuberculosis	11,000	3.5
11	Cerebrovascular disease	10,400	3.3
12	Adult pneumonia	9,100	2.9
13	Neonatal tetanus	6,900	2.2
14	Cirrhosis	6,600	2.1
15	Congenital malformations	6,000	1.9
16	Complications of pregnancy	5,900	1.8
17	Hypertension	5,100	1.6
18	Intestinal obstruction	4,900	1.6
19	Typhoid	4,800	1.5
20	Meningitis	4,600	1.5
21	Hepatitis	4,600	1.5
22	Pertussis	4,600	1.5
23	Other birth diseases	4,600	1.5
24	Adult tetanus	4,500	1.4
25	Schistosomiasis	4,400	1.4
	TOTAL OF FIRST 25 DISEASES	270,200	94.9

*Per 1000 persons per year.
From Ghana Health Assessment Project Team, 1981.

TABLE 2–2. Suggested Initial Therapy for Acute Pneumonia, by Age Group

Age Group	Common Agents	Initial Empirical Therapy	
		Outpatient	*Inpatient*
0–2 mo	Enteric bacilli Group B streptococcus *Streptococcus pneumoniae* *Haemophilus influenzae* *Chlamydia trachomatis* *Staphylococcus aureus* Viruses	Not appropriate*	Ampicillin plus aminoglycoside PRSP† if *S. aureus* suspected Erythromycin if *C. trachomatis* suspected
3 mo–5 yr	*S. pneumoniae* *H. influenzae* *S. aureus* Viruses	TMP/SMX‡ or amoxicillin	Chloramphenicol PRSP plus aminoglycoside if *S. aureus* suspected
6 yr–adult	*S. pneumoniae* *H. influenzae* *S. aureus* Mycoplasma Viruses	Ampicillin, or amoxicillin, or erythromycin	Penicillin G PRSP if *S. aureus* suspected

*Most young infants with pneumonia should be admitted for parenteral therapy.
†PRSP, penicillinase-resistant synthetic penicillin (e.g., methicillin, cloxacillin, flucloxacillin).
‡TMP/SMX, trimethoprim-sulfamethoxazole.

agglutination kits appears to be sensitive and specific in invasive *H. influenzae* type b (Hib) infections, including pneumonia. The performance of similar commercial tests for *S. pneumoniae* antigens is not satisfactory.

For hospitalized patients, a blood culture and Gram stain of an adequate sputum sample (with ≥25 neutrophils, ≤10 epithelial cells/high-power field) or an antigen detection test is recommended to guide therapy.

RADIOLOGY. Although radiologic investigation may not be available or feasible for every patient, it should be used in the evaluation of hospitalized patients or those who do not improve on standard therapeutic regimens.

INITIAL CLINICAL MANAGEMENT. Since the microbial etiology of pneumonia is rarely ascertained, presumptive treatment must be decided on the basis of the clinical information available at initial presentation. An approach to pneumonia based on age is presented in Table 2–2 to aid initial management. Since it is not possible to distinguish viral from bacterial disease by clinical signs or simple laboratory tests, antibiotic therapy is advocated for all but mild cases, even though many cases of pneumonia may be caused by viruses (Chapter 26). If the bacterial etiology is determined from blood or sputum culture, therapy should be changed to the most appropriate agent.

Newborns and Young Infants. Newborns are most likely to have pneumonia due to enteric or genital tract gram-negative organisms, group B streptococci, or viruses acquired from the mother. Broad-spectrum antibiotic management is required to treat these organisms (Table 2–2). Pneumonia in infants beyond the second month is often caused by *S. pneumoniae*, *H. influenzae*, or viruses. Infection with *C. trachomatis* is associated with an afebrile pneumonia syndrome in young infants that will not respond to the foregoing treatment regimen. Erythromycin should be used to treat *C. trachomatis* infections.

Older Infants and Children. Pneumonia in infants and children aged 2 months to 5 years is associated with viruses, *S. pneumoniae*, and *H. influenzae*. In this age group, RSV is the most common cause of lower respiratory infections. The differentiation of pneumonia and bronchiolitis caused by RSV is often difficult. Infants and children who are not seriously ill can be adequately treated as outpatients with oral trimethoprim-sulfamethoxazole or amoxicillin. A simplified case management algorithm to diagnose childhood lower respiratory tract infections has been advocated by the World Health Organization (WHO) (Chapter 16). The accuracy of this algorithm in the prediction of physician-diagnosed pneumonia is quite high, with both sensitivity and specificity exceeding 80%. Use of simplified case-management algorithms by village health workers has reduced childhood respiratory mortality by 15 to 50% in community trials in Asia and Africa.

The child with more severe illness should be admitted to the hospital for therapy with chloramphenicol. Infants and children who do not improve with initial therapy may have staphylococci or other bacteria resistant to first-line antibiotic therapy; therefore, a combination of antibiotics (a penicillinase-resistant semisynthetic penicillin plus an aminoglycoside) is required for treatment. All severely malnourished children with pneumonia are at high risk of mortality and also should be treated with this combination of antibiotics. An important aspect of the supportive care of severe pneumonia is the provision of oxygen. Oxygen by nasal catheter or cannula is essential for infants and young children with pneumonia or bronchiolitis.

Older Children and Adults. The common causes of pneumonia in children >6 years of age and in adults are pneumococci, mycoplasmas, and viruses. Oral ampicillin, amoxicillin, or erythromycin is adequate therapy for outpatient management. Severely ill inpatients should receive parenteral therapy designed to treat pneumococci, *H. influenzae*, and staphylococci (Table 2–2).

Lobar Pneumonia

Community-acquired classic pneumococcal lobar pneumonia remains common in the tropics, a situation similar to the preantibiotic era in North America. The typical patient is a previously healthy young adult. In addition to the classic signs of fever, tachypnea, and a cough productive of purulent or rusty sputum, a tender and enlarged liver (in 60%), jaundice (in 20%), myalgia (in 68%), and diarrhea (in 25%) have been described as presenting symptoms in Nigerian patients with lobar pneumonia. Presumptive therapy with penicillin is necessary and adequate for pneumococcal lobar pneumonia. Single-dose, 3-dose, and other shortened penicillin regimens have been as effective as the traditional 5- to 7-day course of therapy in adults and older children. In Nigeria, 30% of patients with lobar pneumonia who eventually responded to penicillin therapy remained febrile for 3 or more days.

Pneumococcal strains resistant to penicillin are described from the Pacific, Asia, and Africa and have spread to other areas, including the United States. They are more common in patients who have been previously hospitalized or treated with penicillins. Treatment with erythromycin, vancomycin, or a third-generation cephalosporin is advised when penicillin-resistant pneumococci are suspected or when presumptive penicillin therapy is not successful. Otherwise, if no response is noted with the initial therapy, antibiotics for penicillin-resistant *S. aureus* and gram-negative organisms must be used; a penicillinase-resistant semisynthetic penicillin and chloramphenicol are suggested. Other organisms have been associated with lobar pneumonia, notably *Mycobacterium tuberculosis* (Chapter 77), *Klebsiella* species, and *S. aureus*. *M. pneumoniae* was present in 17% of lobar pneumonia cases in Nigeria.

Atypical Pneumonia

Atypical pneumonia describes a syndrome that is distinct from the acute lobar pneumonia syndrome. Usually, an older child or young adult presents with an illness of gradual onset and with constitutional symptoms of fever and malaise that are more marked than the respiratory symptoms; cough is often minimal with little sputum production. The causes of the atypical pneumonia syndrome include *M. tuberculosis* (Chapter 77), mycoplasmas, influenza viruses A and B, adenovirus, and RSV (Chapter 26). *Chlamydia pneumoniae* (Chapter 46) and *Legionella pneumophila* have been reported in this syndrome in developed societies and may also be important in developing regions. Erythromycin or trimethoprim-sulfamethoxazole is the recommended empirical therapy for adults with mild illness. Older children and adults who develop pneumonia after an influenza-like syndrome should be managed with penicillinase-resistant penicillin because of the possibility of staphylococcal disease.

DIFFERENTIAL DIAGNOSIS. The spectrum of differential diagnoses of pneumonia of the nonlobar type is very broad in tropical regions; the major causative organisms are discussed below (also see Chapter 26 for viral causes).

Bacteria. Airborne transmission of Q fever, in areas with sheep and goat animal husbandry and often following "lambing" in the spring, have caused sporadic cases and epidemics of atypical pneumonia (Chapter 34) *Salmonella typhi* not infrequently causes a bronchitis and also has been associated with a nonspecific bronchopneumonia (Chapter 75). The pneumonic form of plague should be considered when a severe, rapidly progressive bronchopneumonia is encountered in the regions endemic for *Yersinia pestis*. The bronchopneumonia may occur without buboes, is characterized by watery and bloody sputum, and has a high fatality rate unless antibiotic therapy is begun early in the course of disease with streptomycin or tetracycline (Chapter 61). A sputum Gram stain can be useful for diagnosis. About half of patients with leptospirosis have pulmonary disease with cough, hemoptysis, and patchy bronchopneumonia on radiograph (Chapter 72). Pulmonary disease caused by the soil saprophyte *Pseudomonas pseudomallei* is infrequently seen in residents or travelers in Southeast Asia. Melioidosis may present as an acute upper lobe pneumonitis or as chronic cavitary disease (Chapter 37).

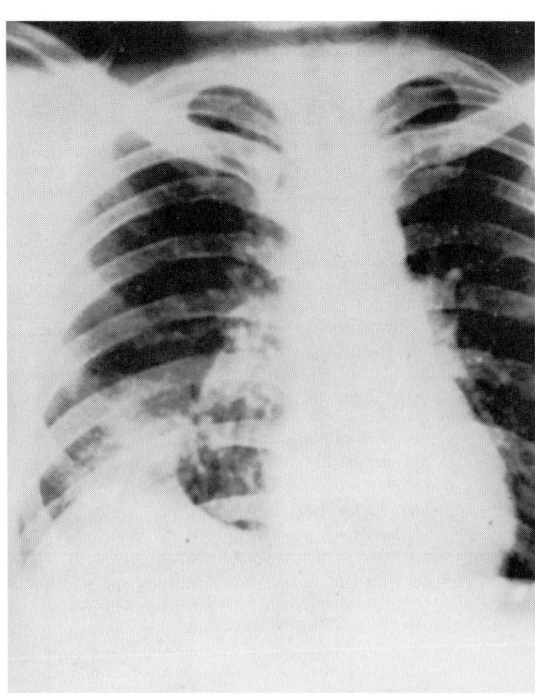

***Figure* 2–2.** Amebic liver abscess with pulmonary extension. (Courtesy of Dr. E. Barrett-Connor.)

Protozoa. Parasitic infections may be associated with pulmonary findings. Falciparum malaria infrequently causes a pneumonia-like syndrome of high fever and bloody sputum, with patchy infiltrates on radiography (Chapter 92). Hepatic abscess caused by *Entamoeba histolytica* may be associated with pneumonitis or pleural effusion due to sympathetic inflammation or to direct extension through the diaphragm. One should consider amebiasis when confronted with right-sided lower lobe disease or right-sided pleural fluid of obscure origin (Fig. 2–2; Chapter 86). Although reported more frequently from developed countries, *P. carinii* has been associated with illness in malnourished and immunosuppressed patients in tropical countries. It is characterized by nonspecific clinical findings and a diffuse alveolar or interstitial pneumonitis on radiograph (Chapter 98).

Helminths. Metazoan parasites may cause pulmonary disease by at least three mechanisms: (1) during the obligatory migration of larvae from the gut through the pulmonary capillaries to the alveoli and back to the gut, (e.g., ascariasis, strongyloidiasis, and hookworm infections); (2) by passage through the pulmonary vasculature as part of a blood-borne stage of the parasite's life cycle (e.g., schistosomiasis, filariasis, trichinosis); and (3) by residence of the adult or cyst form in pulmonary tissue (e.g., paragonimiasis, echinococcosis).

Pulmonary paragonimiasis is often asymptomatic but in the endemic regions of West Africa, Asia, and the Americas may present with chronic persistent cough with intermittent hemoptysis. Sputum or feces may reveal *Paragonimus westermani* eggs (Fig. 117–2C and Chapter 121), and radiographs may demonstrate peripheral or cystic nodular lesions (Figs. 2–3 and 121–5).

The lung is second only to the liver as the most common site for the hydatid cysts of *Echinococcus granulosus*. These may be associated with chronic cough, dyspnea, and hemoptysis. Chest radiograph classically reveals one or more round "cannonball" shadows (Figs. 2–4 and 124–8). Peripheral eosinophilia may or may not be present.

Measles-Associated Pneumonia. Up to 25% of all child-

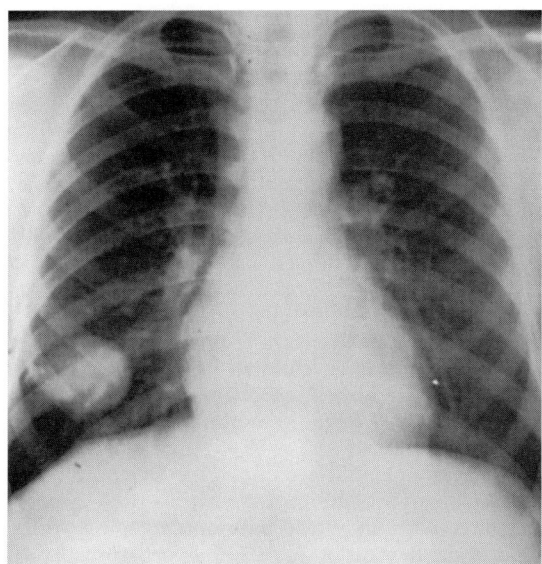

Figure 2–3. Pulmonary paragonimiasis. (Courtesy of Dr. E. Barrett-Connor.)

hood pneumonia in developing countries may be associated with measles, and pneumonia is the most frequent complication of measles infection (Chapter 25.1). Pneumonia occurring with the measles rash is likely to be primary measles giant-cell pneumonia. Pneumonia that has its onset after the rash has faded may be associated with bacteria (e.g., *S. pneumoniae, H. influenzae, S. aureus, Klebsiella, Pseudomonas,* and other gram-negative bacilli) or viruses (e.g., herpes simplex, adenovirus). Because of the high case-fatality rate of measles-associated pneumonia and the probability of bacterial etiology, these children should be admitted for inpatient therapy with broad-spectrum antibiotics (Chapter 16).

Eosinophilic Pneumonia Syndromes. Tropical pulmonary eosinophilia is associated with the host response to filarial infections (*Wuchereria bancrofti* and *Brugia malayi*); it is seen mostly in the Indian subcontinent, although it has also been reported from Africa and the Americas. The disease occurs more often in males and is characterized by a persistent cough and wheezing of insidious onset associated with a striking eosinophilia (Chapter 106.3). There is usually little systemic disturbance, but low-grade fever is common. The cough is often worse at night and is not productive of sputum. Physical examination reveals minimal pulmonary findings, hepatosplenomegaly, and generalized lymphadenopathy. Radiography shows diffuse coarse interstitial infiltrates and hilar lymphadenopathy. The absolute eosinophil count often exceeds 4000/mm³. This syndrome must be distinguished from other eosinophilic pulmonary syndromes; this is generally not difficult, given the geographic regions of occurrence and the rapid clinical and radiologic response to therapy with diethylcarbamazine.

The migration of parasite larvae from pulmonary capillaries to alveoli may be associated with a short-lived syndrome of pulmonary symptoms, transient radiologic infiltrates, and moderate peripheral eosinophilia, sometimes referred to as Löffler's syndrome. *Ascaris, Necator,* or *Ancylostoma* larvae may be present in sputum (Chapters 104 and 105). Immunocompromised hosts may have severe pulmonary disease and eosinophilia caused by *Strongyloides stercoralis* (Chapter 105.2). Acute infections with *Schistosoma mansoni* and *Schistosoma japonicum* may produce an acute eosinophilic syndrome caused by the passage of schistosomula through the pulmo-

nary vasculature, with diffuse nodules on radiography (Chapter 118). The migration of the ascarid larvae of *Toxocara canis* and *Toxocara cati* in pulmonary tissue as a manifestation of visceral larva migrans may be associated with hepatosplenomegaly, transient reticular radiographic infiltrates, and eosinophilia (Chapter 112).

Pneumonia in HIV-Infected Persons

Opportunistic pneumonia is a frequent occurrence in persons infected with the human immunodeficiency virus (HIV) (Chapter 22). In North America, these pulmonary infections constitute most of the AIDS-defining illnesses and cause a major proportion of mortality. *M. tuberculosis* reactivation or infection is frequently reported in AIDS patients in Africa. Unlike North America, where *P. carinii* pneumonia occurs in up to 50% of all AIDS patients, this organism has been described less frequently in people with AIDS in Africa and Asia. An increased incidence of pneumonia due to *S. pneumoniae* and *H. influenzae* has been reported in patients with AIDS in North America as well as increased rates of CMV infection, cryptococcosis, and pulmonary and systemic infection with the *Mycobacterium avium–intracellulare* complex. An aggressive diagnostic evaluation with sputum induction by inhalation of saline mist, bronchoscopic procedures, arterial blood gases, and lung biopsy may not be feasible in many developing country settings. Presumptive therapy for the bacterial causes should be instituted in AIDS patients who present with the sudden onset of pulmonary symptoms (Chapter 22). A more gradual onset of pulmonary symptoms should prompt diagnostic efforts and therapy for *M. tuberculosis* (Chapter 77), nontuberculosis mycobacteria (Chapter 79), or *P. carinii* infection (Chapter 98).

◼ BRONCHIECTASIS

Bronchiectasis remains common in developing regions, where the most frequent causes are infectious. Bronchiectasis may be a sequela of childhood measles or pertussis, may occur as a complication of bacterial pneumonia, or may be caused by compression of an airway by enlarged lymph

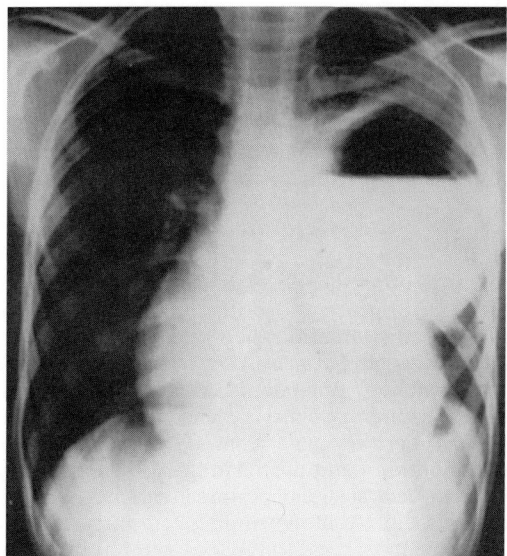

Figure 2–4. Ruptured pulmonary hydatid cyst. (Courtesy of Dr. E. Barrett-Connor.)

nodes. Although in North America cystic fibrosis is the most common cause of bronchiectasis, cystic fibrosis appears to be rare in most tropical countries.

Chronic cough productive of purulent sputum is the usual clinical presentation of this syndrome. Repeated episodes of acute pneumonia and evidence of chronic pulmonary disease (e.g., generalized wasting and clubbing of fingers) are often encountered. Plain chest radiographs may or may not be abnormal, and bronchographic studies are the definitive diagnostic test. Therapy consists of physiotherapy for drainage of sputum, antibiotic management of exacerbations, and surgery for localized disease.

■ ASTHMA

Although a common chronic illness in developing regions, asthma is often underdiagnosed and frequently undertreated. Nonproductive recurrent cough, especially in the evening, is an important symptom for the clinical diagnosis. The pathophysiology and clinical management of asthma in the tropics do not appear to be unique. Therapy with corticosteroids, symphthomimetics, methylxanthines, and the cromones must be tailored to the local availability and cost of these agents.

■ PLEURAL EFFUSION

Pleural effusions may be seen more frequently in developing regions than in developed regions, and the etiologic spectrum is more varied. A common etiology is *M. tuberculosis*, either as pleural disease without pulmonary parenchymal involvement or as part of more widespread pulmonary disease (Chapter 77). Pleural effusion or empyema is a common complication of pneumonia due to *S. pneumoniae, Streptococcus pyogenes, S. aureus,* and *Klebsiella pneumoniae.* A right-sided pleural effusion may be associated with amebic hepatic abscess (Fig. 2–2). Any syndrome associated with edema may also cause a pleural effusion: cardiac failure, cirrhosis of the liver, hypoproteinemia, endomyocardial fibrosis, and neoplastic disease should also be considered in tropical settings. Thoracentesis and pleural biopsy are the mainstays of diagnosis, and the results dictate treatment.

■ PREVENTION OF PNEUMONIA

Economic development with improved nutrition and better access to medical services, including immunizations, will be accompanied by a decreased incidence and mortality of pneumonia. In the interim, improved clinical management and immunization are the foundation of control programs.

Immunization

VIRUSES. Routine measles vaccination at 9 to 12 months of age is likely to prevent a sizable proportion of childhood pneumonia deaths. Immunization with newer measles vaccines at 6 to 9 months of age would probably prevent a still larger proportion of pneumonia. When safe and effective vaccines for respiratory syncytial and parainfluenza viruses become available, they will be useful in the prevention of childhood morbidity and deaths in the developing world.

BACTERIA. New acellular pertussis vaccines will be used to control this disease in developing countries. The bacteria pneumococcus and *H. influenzae* type b (Hib) cause at least 50% of all severe pneumonia cases. Annual incidence per 100,000 children <5 years of age for these bacteria are 240

and at least 60, respectively, in The Gambia, suggesting prevention will have a major impact on disease and mortality. A randomized double-blind trial of a 14-valent pneumococcal polysaccharide vaccine in adults in Papua New Guinea demonstrated an 85% reduction in pneumococcal pneumonia, proved by positive blood culture or lung aspirates, as well as a 44% reduction in all pneumonia mortality. A 13-valent pneumococcal vaccine was evaluated in novice miners in South Africa, whose incidence of pneumonia was 90/1000 per year. These studies showed a 50% reduction in radiologic pneumonia and an 80% decrease in bacteremia and pneumonia caused by serotypes included in the vaccine. The South African data led to the licensure of pneumococcal vaccine for high-risk adults and older children in the United States.

A randomized double-blind evaluation of pneumococcal vaccine in over 3000 6- to 36-month-old children in Papua New Guinea demonstrated a 59% reduction in deaths ascribed to pneumonia and a reduction in overall mortality of 19%. New pneumococcal polysaccharide–protein conjugate vaccines have been shown to be immunogenic in infants in many parts of the world. A recent report from the United States of the high efficacy of a conjugate vaccine against invasive disease in infants means that there will soon be an effective tool to prevent pneumococcal morbidity and mortality.

H. influenzae type b protein-conjugated polysaccharide vaccines have been proved safe and efficacious against meningitis and are licensed for universal use in children in North America and Europe. Studies of Hib vaccines in The Gambia and Chile have recently shown that they will reduce severe radiographic pneumonia by 20%, and WHO has recommended Hib vaccination for infants.

Specific Nutrients

Some authorities advocate vitamin A (200,000 IU by mouth ×2 doses in children >1 year of age) for all children with measles in regions where vitamin A deficiency is common (Chapter 131.1). This may reduce postmeasles pneumonia morbidity and mortality. Zinc supplementation in regions with zinc deficiency has been shown to be highly effective in reducing pneumonia morbidity (Chapter 132.3).

Bibliography

Barker J, Gratten M, Riley I, et al: Pneumonia in children in the Eastern Highlands of Papua New Guinea: A bacteriological study of patients selected by standard clinical criteria. J Infect Dis 159:348, 1989.

Campbell H, Lamont AC, O'Neill KP, et al: Assessment of clinical criteria for identification of severe acute lower respiratory tract infections in children. Lancet 1:297, 1989.

Cherian T, John TJ, Simoes E, et al: Evaluation of simple clinical signs for the diagnosis of acute lower respiratory tract infection. Lancet 2:125, 1988.

Cherian T, Simoes EAF, Steinhoff MC, et al: Bronchiolitis in tropical south India. Am J Dis Child 144:1026, 1990.

Ghana Health Assessment Project Team: A quantitative method of assessing the health impact of different diseases in less developed countries. Int J Epidemiol 10:73, 1981.

Gilks CF, Ojoo SA, Ojoo JC, et al: Invasive pneumococcal disease in a cohort of predominantly HIV-1 infected female sex-workers in Nairobi, Kenya. Lancet 347:718, 1996.

Jeena PM, Coovadia HM, Chrystal V: *Pneumocystis carinii* and cytomegalovirus infections in severely ill, HIV-infected African infants. Ann Trop Pediatr 16:361, 1996.

Kaplan JE, Hu DJ, Holmes KK, et al: Preventing opportunistic infections in human immunodeficiency virus–infected persons: Implications for the developing world. Am J Trop Med Hyg 55:1, 1996.

Kaschula ROC, Druker J, Kipps A: Late morphologic consequences of measles: A lethal and debilitating lung disease among the poor. Rev Infect Dis 5:395, 1983.

Lagos R, Horwitz I, Toro J, et al: Large scale post licensure, selective vaccination of Chilean infants with PRP-T conjugate vaccine: Practicality and effectiveness in preventing invasive *Haemophilus influenzae* type b infections. Pediatr Infect Dis J 15:216, 1996.

Lalitha MK, Pai R, John TJ, et al: Serotyping of *Streptococcus pneumoniae* by agglutination assays: A cost-effective technique for developing countries. Bull WHO 74:387, 1996.

Macfarlane JT, Adegboye DS, Warrell MJ: *Mycoplasma pneumoniae* and the aetiology of lobar pneumonia in northern Nigeria. Thorax 34:713, 1979.

McGregor IA: The epidemiology of influenza in a tropical (Gambian) environment. Br Med Bull 35:15, 1979.

Management of the Young Child with an Acute Respiratory Infection. Geneva, WHO, 1990.

Metselaar D: Machakos project studies; agents affecting health of mother and child in a rural area of Kenya. X. Haemagglutination inhibiting antibodies against influenza A (H2N2) and influenza B virus in sera from children living in the Machakos district of Kenya. Trop Geogr Med 30:523, 1978.

Mootsikapun P, Chetchotisakd P, Intarapoka B: Pulmonary infections in HIV infected patients. J Med Assoc Thai 79:477, 1996.

Mulholland K, Hilton S, Adegbola R, et al: *Haemophilus influenzae* type b–tetanus protein conjugate vaccine prevents pneumonia and meningitis due to *Haemophilus influenzae* type b in Gambian infants. Lancet 349:1191, 1997.

Pinkston P, Vijayan VK, Nutman TB, et al: Acute tropical pulmonary eosinophilia. Characterization of the lower respiratory tract inflammation and its response to therapy. J Clin Invest 80:216, 1987.

Respiratory Infections in Children: Management in Small Hospitals. Geneva, WHO, 1988.

Riley ID, Lehmann D, Alpers MP: Pneumococcal vaccine prevents death from acute lower respiratory tract infections in Papua New Guinean children. Lancet 2:877, 1986.

Shann F: Etiology of severe pneumonia in children in developing countries. Pediatr Infect Dis J 5:247, 1986.

Shann F, Walters S, Pifer LL, et al: Pneumonia associated with infection with pneumocystis, respiratory syncytial virus, chlamydia, mycoplasma, and cytomegalovirus in children in Papua New Guinea. Br Med J 292:314, 1986.

Spika JS, Munshi MH, Wojtyniak B, et al: Acute lower respiratory infections: A major cause of death in children in Bangladesh. Ann Trop Paediatr 9:33, 1989.

Steinhoff MC: *Haemophilus influenzae* type b infections are preventable everywhere. Lancet 349:1186, 1997.

Wall RA, Corrah PT, Mabey DCW, Greenwood BM: The etiology of lobar pneumonia in the Gambia. Bull WHO 64:553, 1986.

Warrell DA, Fawcet IW, Harrison BDW, et al: Bronchial asthma in the Nigerian Savanna region. Q J Med 174:325, 1975.

3 Cardiovascular Diseases

Raymond A. Smego, Jr.

The pattern of cardiovascular diseases varies between developed and developing countries (Fig. 3–1). Atherosclerotic or ischemic heart disease is the most common type of cardiovascular pathology in industrialized nations, whereas hypertension, rheumatic fever, and nutritional, toxic, and idiopathic conditions are major contributors to cardiovascular disease in developing regions. As for tropical medicine, cardiovascular diseases of infectious origin are much more common in developing countries. In higher socioeconomic populations within poorer countries, however, and in transition countries, ischemic heart disease is increasingly prevalent along with other "affluent" or "lifestyle" diseases. Furthermore, cardiovascular morbidity and mortality vary between adult and pediatric populations, with congenital heart disease being the most frequently encountered cardiovascular disease among children (Fig. 3–2).

For effective diagnosis and treatment, a physician must be familiar with the epidemiology of cardiovascular conditions within his or her region of practice. Chagas' disease needs to be considered in the rural environment of South and Central America. Pulmonary hypertension can be caused by restrictive cardiomyopathy in a Rwandan laborer, filariasis in a young Sri Lankan, schistosomiasis in an Egyptian farmer, and rheumatic mitral stenosis in a child from an urban slum. This chapter reviews the salient clinicoepidemiologic features

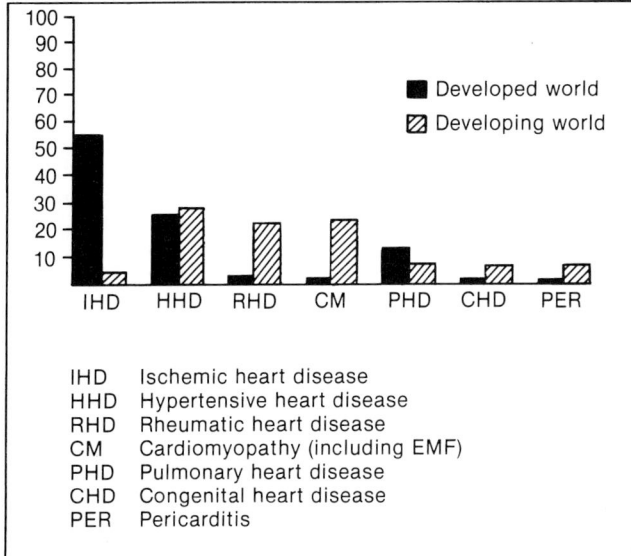

Figure 3–1. Profile of cardiovascular diseases in the context of developed and developing countries. Percentages indicate proportion of cardiac pathology for relevant environment.

of the most important diseases of the heart and aorta encountered in clinical practice in the tropics.

HYPERTENSIVE CARDIOVASCULAR DISEASE

Incidence and Etiology. Hypertension is the most serious cardiovascular problem worldwide. It affects both rich and poor and is present in almost every geographic region. Populations in which blood pressure does not rise with age are few, isolated, and small. Their members are often unacculturated and consume little or no salt. The highest incidence of hypertension is found in groups with the highest salt intake, e.g., Japanese fishermen. Even when racially similar groups are compared, e.g., New Guinea tribes, salt intake correlates with blood pressure, independent of body build or fatness. Careful multicenter "inter-salt" studies have shown that the salt-hypertension association is more complex; that large amounts of salt must be consumed over a considerable time to cause sustained hypertension; and that the diet must be practically devoid of salt to lower the blood pressure consistently in mild hypertension. Moreover, there is marked individual variation in the ability to handle salt. Many black hypertensive populations have delayed excretory capacity for salt.

Renal disease accounts for about 20% of hypertension in developing countries and is particularly likely to be the cause of severe hypertension in the younger age groups. Reno-

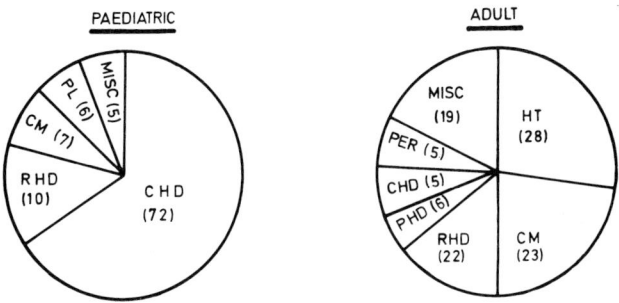

Figure 3–2. Cardiovascular morbidity in Nigeria. (See Figure 3–1 for key to abbreviations.)

vascular hypertension is usually due to fibromuscular dysplasia or atherosclerosis. There is no convincing evidence of an etiologic relationship between urinary schistosomiasis and hypertension.

Clinical Manifestations, Diagnosis, and Treatment. Of the three primary hypertension target organs, the heart is less susceptible than the brain or kidneys to the more devastating effects of severe and long-standing hypertension. Hypertension heart failure may be easily confused with chronic rheumatic heart disease or dilated cardiomyopathy, as the dysfunctional heart readily becomes fibrotic and dilated.

The goal of treatment is to prevent morbidity and mortality attributable to high blood pressure. This may involve the use of both nonpharmacologic and pharmacologic therapy. The success of the therapeutic alliance depends on individual motivation and effective communication between patient and health care provider. Projects for the community control of hypertension in developing countries have been started in pilot areas as part of integrated programs for the control of noncommunicable diseases. The emphasis is on primordial and primary prevention in these communities.

RHEUMATIC HEART DISEASE

Epidemiology. Streptococcal pharyngitis, rheumatic fever (RF), and rheumatic heart disease (RHD) can occur anywhere. RHD appears to be the leading form of acquired heart disease in the tropics in persons between 5 and 15 years of age. Fortunately, most children are not susceptible to the development of RF following an untreated episode of streptococcal throat infection. Perhaps 6 out of 100 children will develop RF if challenged repeatedly; about half of them will be left with heart murmurs that permit a retrospective diagnosis. Genetic factors may be important in determining susceptibility to RF. When a prevalence of chronic RHD of over 2% is encountered, an RF experience of over 4% is implied. Such percentages indicate that the population at risk has been saturated with streptococcal infection.

Bacteriologic and serologic surveys from many parts of the world confirm the ubiquity of streptococcal disease. Antistreptolysin O (ASO) surveys show that children living in crowded and poor conditions begin to experience streptococcal infections in infancy. Throat culture surveys in primary school children often show more than 3% with β-hemolytic streptococcus carriage. M-typing of these organisms has shown regional differences, but in some studies the majority of isolates could be typed (an indication of virulence), with more than one type detected in children from a single classroom. Infection with one M type does not confer immunity against others of the more than 60 identified. Consequently, repeated infection is almost inevitable. When such exposure and infection start in the first few years of life, RF and RHD often appear so early that valve calcification and stenosis are commonly seen in children and young adults.

Pathogenesis. That pharyngitis frequently precedes RF has been recognized for over a century; the importance of the streptococcus in the development of RF has been known for 50 years. However, only in recent years did it became apparent that group A β-hemolytic streptococcus is the sole etiologic agent of RF. Streptococcal pharyngitis is followed by RF, whereas streptococcal pyoderma is not. Some M types (5, 14, 24) appear to be especially likely to cause RF (i.e., rheumatogenic). It has been suggested that strains of group A streptococci are emerging that are both rheumatogenic and nephritogenic. The role of host (including genetic) factors is not clear, but no ethnic group seems either particularly prone or unusually resistant to RF. Good antibiotic prophylaxis programs work well everywhere—one reason for implicating the streptococcus as the sole agent of the disease.

Pathology. Although the rheumatic cardiac nodule, or Aschoff body, is considered the pathognomonic lesion of RHD, nonspecific changes, e.g., lymphocytic interstitial exudation and myocardial fibril fragmentation, predominate during the acute illness. The pericardial surface has a fibrinous exudate, and serosanguineous pericardial effusion is common. Adhesions subsequently form, but chronic constructive pericarditis does not occur even though pericardial calcification occasionally results. The endocardial involvement is most common in the mitral and aortic areas, with the tricuspid valve involved less often and the pulmonary valve rarely. Multivalvular involvement is seen in a substantial number of cases of RF. Fibrinous deposits are organized via granulation and fibrosis, which lead to regurgitation and/or stenosis of the affected valve(s). Persistence of the Aschoff body is more common in patients who subsequently develop mitral stenosis.

Clinical Manifestations. There is a belief that RF in the tropics is clinically different from that in temperate zones because severe carditis is more common and arthritis less frequent. A prospective study in Nigeria supports this, whereas a similar study in India does not. The earlier the onset of RF, the more likely the patient is to have carditis and the less likely to have arthritis. Sixty years ago in the United States, carditis and chorea were more common signs of RF than was arthritis. American medical students were taught that "rheumatic fever licks the joints but bites the heart"; this may be true in tropical Africa.

Symptomatology. In developing countries a child suffering from joint pain or swelling may be considered to have a hemoglobinopathy (sickle cell disease, Chapter 6), particularly if the symptoms are accompanied by fever. Although the child with carditis and congestive heart failure (CHF) is unlikely to be misdiagnosed, first presentation in hospital is usually delayed. In the tropics, many children have parasitic diseases that directly or indirectly place a burden on the heart. In such children, rheumatic carditis is an additional burden that can cause cardiac decompensation. In developing countries, many children with rheumatic carditis and CHF are likely to be experiencing their second or third episode of RF and are chronically, rather than acutely, ill.

There may be genuine racial differences in the response to streptococcal infection beyond the difference due to socioeconomic factors and age of onset. To the clinician the important point is that in the tropics the child presenting with RF is likely to have carditis with or without mitral insufficiency and is not likely to have migratory polyarthritis. Chorea is not common (with an incidence of less than 5%); subcutaneous nodules and erythema marginatum are also rare.

CARDIAC FAILURE. The incidence of cardiac failure reported in different series is extremely variable, ranging from below 5% to over 90%. When cardiac failure is present, there are obvious changes clinically and on the chest film. In addition to the murmur of mitral regurgitation, the child may have murmurs of aortic and tricuspid valve involvement, evidence of pulmonary hypertension, inappropriate tachycardia, and signs and symptoms of pericarditis. The electrocardiogram (ECG) and echocardiogram are useful in confirming the presence of complications, e.g., arrhythmias and pericardial effusion.

LEFT ATRIAL ENLARGEMENT. The involvement of the atrial wall in the rheumatic process in childhood is a reasonable explanation for the prominence of the left atrium and its appendage (LAA) in RHD. The LAA enlargement can be easily appreciated on the chest film (Fig. 3–3). The enlarging left atrium can protect the lungs against mitral regurgitation, so that some patients with mitral incompetence of rheumatic origin may not complain of significant dyspnea until they develop atrial fibrillation. This discrepancy between dramatic

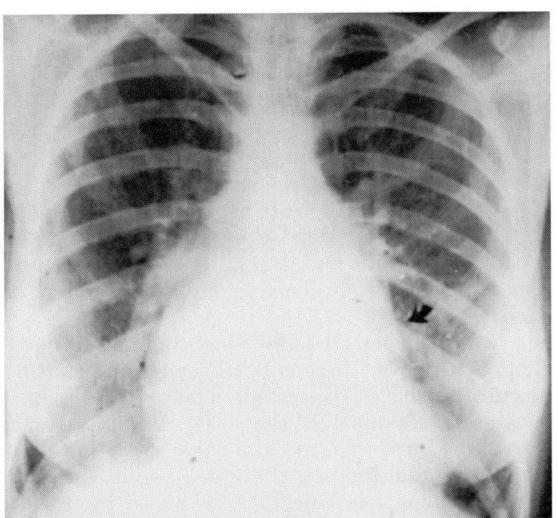

Figure 3–3. Posteroanterior chest film in patient with mitral insufficiency due to rheumatic heart disease. Arrow points to prominent left atrial appendage.

physical findings (i.e., very large hyperactive heart with a loud murmur and third heart sound) and minimal symptoms can exist for some years in a patient with moderate mitral insufficiency.

CHOREA. As mentioned previously, chorea is not a common manifestation of RF. It usually occurs, by itself or with carditis but not with arthritis, several months after the streptococcal infection. After puberty it occurs more frequently in girls. It may be associated with a normal temperature or normal erythrocyte sedimentation rate (ESR), and the ASO titer may be normal. This "pure" chorea does not respond to the usual treatment for RF and responds poorly to sedatives (diazepam, chlorpromazine).

Diagnosis. The diagnosis of RF is generally based on a constellation of major and minor clinical criteria, i.e., the Jones criteria (Table 3–1). The major criteria for the diagnosis of RF in the tropics are carditis, chorea, subcutaneous nodules, erythema marginatum, and migratory arthritis. However, children are sometimes presumed to have RF if fever, tachycardia, and severe migratory polyarthropathy are present, even without definite joint swelling.

Preceding Streptococcal Infection. Current criteria for the diagnosis of RF stress the importance of establishing whether there was an antecedent streptococcal infection. A history of

TABLE 3–1. The Modified Jones Criteria Used in the Diagnosis of Acute Rheumatic Fever*

Major Manifestations	Minor Manifestations
Carditis	Previous history of rheumatic fever or rheumatic heart disease
Polyarthritis	
Chorea	Fever
Subcutaneous nodules	Arthralgia
Erythema marginatum	Elevated ESR or C-reactive protein, or leukocytosis
	Prolonged P-R interval (first-degree AV block)

*A high probability of rheumatic fever is indicated by the presence of two major criteria or one major and two minor criteria, *plus* supporting evidence of preceding streptococcal infection (e.g., positive throat culture for group A streptococci, increased ASO titer or other streptococcal antibodies, or recent scarlet fever).

sore throat is of some help. A history of scarlet fever is specific, although unusual, but a negative culture does not exclude RF. A high and rising streptococcal antibody titer (e.g., ASO titer) is the most important laboratory confirmation of streptococcal infection (250 Todd units in adults, 300 Todd units in children). All but the most rudimentary laboratories have the ability to culture and identify β-hemolytic streptococcus and perform the ASO test. However, because these investigations are more often than not unavailable to doctors practicing in developing countries, increased reliance has to be placed on clinical skills and a high index of suspicion. The possibility of RF must always be considered in any child or young adult with fever, sore throat, and a heart murmur.

Differential Diagnosis. Deciding whether a patient with established valvular heart disease has RF is usually not too difficult, even in the absence of a typical history. Mitral stenosis, with or without regurgitation, is usually due to RF. Mitral valve disease in association with aortic valve disease is almost certainly rheumatic in origin. The presence of tricuspid valvular abnormalities with mitral disease suggests a rheumatic origin. Atrial fibrillation in a young patient with valvular heart disease favors a diagnosis of RHD or endomyocardial fibrosis (EMF). In patients with mitral incompetence, the larger the left atrium, the more likely a rheumatic etiology (Fig. 3–3). Patients with giant left atria (>40 mm diameter) are almost always in atrial fibrillation, have mitral incompetence, and frequently have RHD. The following conditions must be excluded in the differential diagnosis of rheumatic fever: typhoid fever (Chapter 75); bacterial septicemia, infective endocarditis, and tuberculosis (Chapter 77); sickle cell anemia (Chapter 6); nonspecific pancarditis with effusion and undulant fever (Chapter 64); and serum sickness, leukemia, rheumatoid arthritis, and systemic lupus erythematosus. A high index of suspicion, a careful history, and a critical assessment of the character of the fever, the arthritis, the murmur, and other cardiac abnormalities will distinguish RF from other conditions.

Treatment and Prophylaxis

Rest. Patients with active RF should be at rest. Those with CHF and severe carditis or arthritis will wish and need to stay in bed. Those with less serious symptoms should be at modified rest. The duration of disease activity, although masked by therapy, ranges from 2 to 4 months or as long as 6 to 12 months when chorea is a feature.

Anti-inflammatory Drugs. Aspirin has been used to treat RF since 1876 and is still the mainstay of therapy. For children, 100 mg/kg/day in five divided doses is standard. For adults, 6 to 8 g/day should be given, increasing this cautiously until side effects (salicylism) limit the dose. The fever, joint symptoms, and tachycardia should respond promptly. The C-reactive protein test should rapidly become negative, but the ESR is usually much slower to respond.

Corticosteroids should be used in patients with severe carditis, e.g., prednisone at a dose of 40 to 60 mg/day for adults and 2 mg/kg/day for children, even though controversy surrounds their presumed efficacy and the distinct possibility exists of rebound carditis on withdrawal. The rationale for steroids is the prevention of valvular damage in the early stages of disease. Steroids should be tapered off within a few weeks. Patients with mild carditis can be treated with either salicylates or steroids. A reasonable program is to start with steroids, reducing them during the third week while starting salicylates. CHF is treated with steroids plus diuretics and digitalis.

Antistreptococcal Therapy. A most important part of the original therapy is administration of the antistreptococcal dose of antibiotic. This should be given even if the throat cultures on admission are negative. Usually the most effective antistreptococcal therapy is 1.2 million U of benzathine penicillin G as a single IM injection for adults (600,000 to 900,000 U for children). Erythromycin, 250 mg four times daily for 10 days, is satisfactory therapy for individuals with penicillin sensitivity, but erythromycin plus aspirin frequently causes gastrointestinal symptoms. Sulfonamides are bacteriostatic, not bactericidal, and should not be used to treat streptococcal infection.

Prophylactic Therapy. Prophylaxis against further episodes of RF is mandatory in a patient with RF or RHD. The most effective prophylactic antibiotic is benzathine penicillin G, traditionally given once-monthly in a dose of 1.2 million U (600,000 U in children weighing <27 kg). Recent data from South Africa suggest that in highly endemic regions an every-3-week rather than once-monthly schedule may prevent recurrences of RF. Less reliable are sulfadiazine, 1.0 g once daily (0.5 g in children weighing <27 kg); penicillin V tablets, 250 mg twice daily; or erythromycin, 250 mg twice daily. If sulfadiazine is used, the white blood cell count should be checked every few weeks for the first several months. In children with carditis, prophylaxis should be continued indefinitely, certainly into adult life. In those without evidence of residual carditis, it should be continued into adult life.

Prognosis, Late Manifestations, and Control. Death from acute RF is unusual but can occur in severe CHF or with arrhythmias. Prognosis depends on the amount of residual cardiac damage and on recurrence of active disease. A child who has had RF experiencing another episode of untreated streptococcal infection is very likely to develop RF again. A child with badly damaged valves may do well for a short while but will eventually develop pulmonary hypertension and become symptomatic.

Surgery. Valve replacement is not available in many parts of the developing world. Even where it is available, the cost of the surgery is beyond the reach of most patients, and those patients with replaced valves often do poorly. The reasons for this poor outcome include the following: (1) Artificial valves may become infected and require replacement; (2) anticoagulation is often indicated in patients with artificial valves but is impossible in many areas; and (3) porcine replacement valves have generally not worked well in children. Whenever possible, cardiac surgeons favor valvuloplasty. In most developing countries, children with significant mitral or aortic insufficiency from RF are likely to have a normal life span; the majority having both lesions die young, principally from heart failure.

Children who develop mitral stenosis as the principal cardiac lesion after an attack of RF are likely to benefit from surgery (closed valvotomy). The problem is one of diagnosis, since mitral stenosis may escape detection unless it is specifically suspected. Dyspnea, hemoptysis, early age onset, a sudden cerebrovascular accident, or the appearance of atrial fibrillation is a more important clue. A loud first heart sound is the auscultatory hint to listen carefully for the opening snap and apical diastolic rumble. Embolic manifestations frequently precede atrial fibrillation. Echocardiography, when available, is diagnostic.

Prevention. Treatment of streptococcal pharyngitis is the key to prevention of RF. In an area where streptococcal infection and RF are common, it is better to overtreat nonstreptococcal causes of sore throat than to let RF develop.

In several areas of the developing world where there are good antistreptococcal treatment and RF prophylaxis programs, the incidence of RF has declined sharply over the past decade. This is despite lack of improvement in living conditions, indicating that when specific therapy is available, a disease can be controlled without social change. Such observations place a burden on physicians to prevent and control this major cause of cardiac disability and death.

CHAGAS' DISEASE. Chagas' cardiomyopathy has supplanted rheumatic fever as the most common form of heart disease and the leading cause of cardiac death in young adults in parts of South and Central America, particularly Chile, Argentina, and Mexico (Chapter 94). The pathophysiology of Chagas' heart disease is multifactorial, involving direct parasitic invasion and host fibrosis, autonomic neuropathy, and antiheart autoreactive and immunoregulatory mechanisms.

Acute Myocarditis. CHF is the most common form of presentation. Syncope is a frequent early symptom, and sudden death is not unusual. A pancarditis is present, but right-sided heart failure predominates. The heart is enlarged, and, in addition to the presence of regurgitant systolic murmurs, the second heart sound may be abnormally split. Patients may also have dysphagia or constipation caused by aperistalsis from autonomic neuropathic involvement of the esophagus or colon.

Chronic Cardiomyopathy. Conduction and rhythm abnormalities and CHF are the outstanding clinical features of chronic Chagas' disease. Atrioventricular blocks of all degrees, bundle branch block, intraventricular block, and premature ventricular contractions are often present in some combination on the ECG. Premature ventricular contractions (often multifocal) are the most common arrhythmia, and right bundle block with left anterior hemiblock is the most common conduction abnormality.

Cardiac Aneurysm. Another distinctive feature of Chagas' heart disease is the predilection for the formation of cardiac "aneurysms," usually located at the apex of the left ventricle, which predisposes these patients to atrial embolization. Postmortem findings show these aneurysms as herniations of endocardium at the cardiac apex.

Diagnosis. Chagas' disease often occurs where RHD, other forms of cardiomyopathy, and schistosomal cor pulmonale also exist. Typically, the patient with acute infection is young and from a rural area. Patients may have the symptoms of CHF or complain of dysphagia or abnormal bowel function. Most have an abnormal heart rhythm and an enlarged heart. There may be Stokes-Adams attacks and evidence of arterial embolization. In contrast, conduction disturbances other than atrial fibrillation are less common in chronic RHD. Laboratory diagnosis of Chagas' disease is made serologically, by visualization of trypanosomes in blood smears of patients with acute disease, or by xenodiagnosis (Chapter 151).

THE CARDIOMYOPATHIES. Two important varieties of heart disease have been identified in the tropics over the past four decades—idiopathic cardiomegaly and EMF. Both are now grouped as cardiomyopathies and on the basis of their effects on ventricular structure and function have been classified into dilated, restrictive, and hypertrophic forms. When the cause of heart muscle disease is known or there is some association with systemic disease, the disorder is classified under specific heart muscle disease and is designated by the etiology—viral, nutritional, alcoholic, toxic, and so forth.

Dilated Cardiomyopathy

Incidence and Etiology. This accounts for at least 10% (in children) and 30% (in adults) of acquired heart disease in many parts of tropical Africa. Subclinical viral myocarditis has been implicated in its pathogenesis in children. The majority of adults, however, have a background of undiagnosed or untreated hypertension with one or more superimposed factors: alcohol, malnutrition, thiamine deficiency, anemia, multiparity, and viral (e.g., coxsackie, echo) and protozoal (e.g., *Toxoplasma gondii*) infections.

Pathology. Macroscopically the heart is pale and flabby, with hypertrophy and dilatation of all chambers. Occasionally, only the left ventricle and atrium are involved. The atrioventricular rings are dilated and the trabeculae carneae flattened into a lacelike pattern, and there are focal areas of ventricular endocardial fibrosis. Mural thrombi may be present in the atrial appendage or ventricular apex in up to 50% of adults with this disease. Microscopically the cardiac muscle fibers are hypertrophied, and there are scattered areas of myocytolysis, replacement fibrosis, and lymphocytic collections. The coronary arteries are normal.

Clinical Manifestations. Only about 10% of children with this condition present with asymptomatic cardiomegaly. The rest exhibit fever, cough, tachypnea, signs of biventricular failure, an apical impulse, and a ventricular gallop with evidence of mitral regurgitation. In adults there is also evidence of CHF with signs of gross biventricular enlargement, functional atrioventricular incompetence, murmurs, and pulmonary hypertension in the absence of systemic hypertension. These patients are prone to systemic and pulmonary embolism and cardiogenic shock.

Laboratory Findings. Chest x-ray shows cardiomegaly, pulmonary arterial and venous hypertension, and edema. Various forms of arrhythmia may be evident on the ECG (atrial fibrillation, atrial or ventricular extrasystoles), or there may be both right and left ventricular hypertrophy. With time, heart failure supervenes with consequent clockwise rotation of the precordial leads and dominant S waves in V5 and V6.

Hemodynamic studies are useful in confirming primary heart muscle disease. There is reduction in the cardiac output and an increase in the end-diastolic pressures of both ventricles. Angiographic and echocardiographic studies show a large, dilated, poorly contractile left ventricle without septal hypertrophy or cavity obliteration. The coronary vessels are patent.

Association with Pregnancy. Dilated cardiomyopathy is occasionally seen in pregnancy, when it may present as heart failure toward term and up to 6 months post partum in women with no previous history of heart disease. The pathogenesis in some cases of peripartal heart disease is linked to volume overload from excessive salt consumption. It is also possible that previous myocardial damage is triggered into failure as a result of the metabolic demands of pregnancy and the puerperium.

Restrictive Cardiomyopathy

Etiology. This includes endomyocardial fibrosis (EMF) and Löffler's eosinophilic endomyocardial disease. EMF is typically found in the hot and humid areas of the tropics. Its etiology is obscure, but malnutrition, serotonin (from consumption of plantain or banana), vitamin E deficiency, filariasis and other helminthic infestations, lymphatic obstruction, and allergy are suspected causes.

Pathology. Structurally there is dense deposition of fibrous tissue in the walls of one or both ventricles, with involvement of the inflow tract and posterior cusp of the atrioventricular (AV) valves. This leads to restriction in ventricular filling with consequent decrease in cardiac output, simulating massive pericardial effusion or constrictive pericarditis.

Clinical Manifestations. The clinical features of right- and left-sided EMF are shown in Figure 3–4. The chest x-ray shows, with (R)EMF, a globular heart with oligemic lung fields. In (L)EMF there is either a normal cardiac silhouette or an enlarged left atrium with changes suggestive of pulmonary congestion, edema, and hypertension.

Laboratory Findings and Diagnosis. The ECG of (R)EMF shows low-voltage complexes in the event of a pericardial effusion. The rhythm is sinus, or there may be atrial fibrillation, and an rSr pattern may be seen in leads V1–V4. In

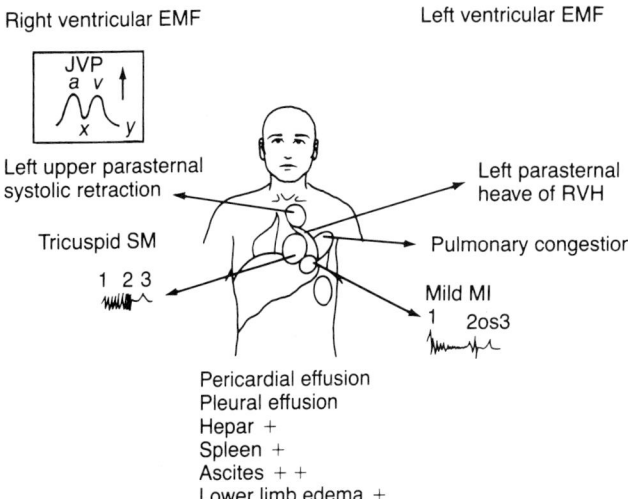

Figure 3–4. The clinical features of right and left restrictive cardiomyopathy (EMF). (From Akinkugbe OO, Falase AO: Cardiovascular Disease. Oxford, Blackwell Scientific Publications, 1987.)

(L)EMF there may be atrial fibrillation and evidence of left atrial or ventricular hypertrophy. Definitive diagnosis of EMF can be made by cardiac catheterization and angiocardiography. The pressure tracing in (R)EMF shows the "dip and plateau" configuration, indicating a restrictive filling defect. With angiocardiography there is a small right ventricle with irregular margins and dilated outflow tract. With (L)EMF, angiography shows a reduction in cavity size and obliteration of the apex.

Apart from the initial febrile illness with facial edema, progressive edema, and evidence of carditis as described, patients with EMF often have such extracardiac features as cyanosis, finger clubbing, oral gingival or periorbital pigmentation, parotid enlargement, and retarded growth.

Hypertrophic Cardiomyopathy (HCM). This is a much less common form of cardiomyopathy in the tropical setting. There is marked hypertrophy of the left and sometimes the right ventricular muscle, without obvious cause, predominantly involving the septum. This may occur with or without outflow obstruction. HCM is thought to be inherited as an autosomal dominant trait, with incomplete penetrance.

Treatment. Treatment of all these forms of cardiomyopathy is as for CHF: diuretics as necessary, digitalis in the presence of fast atrial fibrillation, and amiodarone in suppressing troublesome ventricular arrhythmias. Angiotensin converting enzyme (ACE) inhibitors and peripheral vasodilators may be indicated in severe heart failure to "unload" the left ventricle and its inotropic effects. Thromboembolic events may call for the use of anticoagulants. For EMF, a loop diuretic may need to be combined with thiazides to obtain effective results. Where the facilities exist for open heart surgery, resection of the fibrous tissue in one or both ventricles has been undertaken with prosthetic replacement of the AV valve. Beta-blocking agents are useful in angina associated with HCM.

INFECTIVE ENDOCARDITIS. The majority of cases of infective endocarditis occur in patients with congenital or acquired cardiac defects. The clinical course of bacterial endocarditis may be acute, subacute, or chronic depending on the pathogenicity of the organisms and the response of the host.

Etiology. The usual causative organisms are *Streptococcus viridans* and *Staphylococcus aureus*. Less common are *Enterococcus faecalis, Staphylococcus epidermidis, Escherichia coli, Klebsiella* and *Pseudomonas* spp., and rarely, fungal and atypical organisms, e.g., *Chlamydia, Coxiella,* and *Brucella.* Not infrequently the offending organism remains elusive despite repeated blood cultures. Persistently negative cultures may be due to previous indiscriminate use of antibiotics for unexplained fever. Primary sites of bacteremic infection leading to infective endocarditis include skin (cellulitis), bone (osteomyelitis), muscle (pyomyositis), and scalp. Some of the clinical lesions (e.g., cutaneous vasculitis, focal and diffuse glomerulonephritis) have an immunologic basis.

Clinical Manifestations. Generally, the mitral, aortic, and tricuspid valves are affected in that order of frequency. In acute infective endocarditis (usually due to *S. aureus*) there is extensive valvular damage with a rapidly progressive illness. The more common subacute form is characterized by low-grade fever, cardiac murmurs, and a raised ESR. There may also be arthralgia, anorexia, lassitude, weight loss, splenomegaly, subungual hemorrhages, finger clubbing, unexplained cardiac failure, or one of the consequences of peripheral embolization (e.g., strokes; cold, pulseless extremities; occult abscess formation). The telltale Osler nodes are not common in the tropics, nor are café-au-lait spots easily discernible on dark skin. Investigations often show a mild to moderate normochromic/normocytic anemia with a normal or increased white cell count. Hematuria may be present, and occasionally there is evidence of renal impairment. Chest films, ECGs, and echocardiograms are sometimes useful in monitoring progress.

Unexplained fever, heart failure that is out of proportion with the severity of the heart lesion or resistant to conventional therapy, persistent anemia, and hemoptysis should prompt a high index of suspicion for infective endocarditis.

Treatment and Prevention. Patients with valvular heart disease should be protected with prophylactic antibiotics at certain periods, e.g., during dental surgery, urogenital instrumentation, and abdominal operations. For definitive therapy, the antibiotic chosen should be bactericidal and parenteral; combination antibiotic therapy may be needed, depending on the bacterial pathogen. When the causative organism is difficult to determine, it may be necessary to initiate therapy with a combination of gentamicin with vancomycin, penicillin, amoxicillin, or an antistaphylococcal penicillin. The long-term prognosis is often determined by the late consequences of residual valve damage.

CONGENITAL HEART DISEASE

Incidence and Etiology. In the pediatric age group in practically all developing countries, congenital heart disease (CHD) accounts for over 70% of cardiac disease cases. Data from hospital records and community-based deliveries suggest an incidence of 6.6 per 1000 live births in the tropics, as opposed to 8.0 per 1000 in developed countries.

The most frequently diagnosed acyanotic malformations are ventricular septal defect (VSD), patent ductus arteriosus (PDA), pulmonary stenosis (PS), atrial septal defect (ASD), and coarctation of the aorta (CA), in that order. Of the cyanotic group, tetralogy of Fallot (TF) is the most common. With the exception of PDA and ASD (both of which show a female predilection) and VSD (which shows no gender bias), the defects are more prevalent in males. In areas of Latin America, Africa, and Asia that are above 1000 M in altitude, PDA and pulmonary hypertension are more common.

Clinical Manifestations and Prognosis. Many children are born at home. Neonatal surgery is seldom available, and thus infants with the more severe forms of CHD do not survive. The clinical features of these cardiac defects are similar to those reported elsewhere except that concomitant growth retardation is much more striking in tropical countries. Etiologic factors in CHD include intrauterine rubella and perina-

tal asphyxia. The low prevalence of CA and aortic stenosis in these communities has been linked with hypocalcemia.

PERICARDIAL DISEASE. Pericarditis of infectious origin develops secondary to either hematogenous seeding or direct extension from infection of structures contiguous with the heart.

Pericarditis in the tropics is typified by few reported cases of viral etiology and an increased prevalence of pyogenic and tuberculous involvement. The incidence of pericardial disease due to uremia, connective tissue disease (e.g., systemic lupus erythematosus), and malignancy is not as high as that reported for developed countries.

Pyogenic Pericarditis. Pyogenic pericarditis is more common in infants and children. In infants in particular, a pericardial rub may not be heard, and the ECG may not show ST-T changes (although the voltages will generally be low). The diagnosis should be considered in children with clinical deterioration following soft tissue infection, osteomyelitis, or post-measles or HIV-related pneumonia. The presence of a pericardial rub and ST-segment elevation on the ECG is helpful, but the appearance of a globular cardiac shadow on the chest film of an acutely ill–appearing child with evidence of cardiac tamponade is the traditional diagnostic confirmation of effusive pericarditis. Echocardiography, if available, is the best noninvasive method of determining the presence of pericardial fluid collection.

Pericardiocentesis will yield purulent fluid. Unless inhibited by prior antibiotic therapy, a causative organism can usually be cultured. Since the most common responsible bacteria are the pneumococcus and staphylococcus, therapy must include a bactericidal, penicillinase-resistant antibiotic. Appropriate antibiotic therapy plus surgical drainage usually results in cure of this otherwise universally fatal condition.

Tuberculous Pericarditis. Tuberculous pericarditis is an indolent disease, usually occurring in adults with or without HIV infection, that may present in an acute fibrinous form. Chronic constriction, with or without tamponade, is the rule for tuberculous pericarditis. Most patients have a pleural effusion, pulmonary infiltrate, and/or hilar adenopathy, but the pleurae, lungs, and mediastinum may all be radiologically normal. A positive tuberculin skin test is a helpful diagnostic aid, but a negative test does not exclude the diagnosis, especially in a patient with AIDS likely to be anergic. The pericardial fluid is usually serosanguineous, with a lymphocytic pleocytosis. Tubercle bacilli are usually not recovered from pericardiocentesis. In exceptional cases a pericardial biopsy will confirm the diagnosis, revealing tubercle bacilli or caseating granulomas. Where available, polymerase chain reaction (PCR) and adenosine deaminase determinations from pericardial fluid can be useful adjunctive diagnostic tests. As is often the case in extrapulmonary tuberculosis, a therapeutic trial may be required to establish the diagnosis (Chapter 77).

Amebic Pericarditis. Although sometimes confused with tuberculous pericarditis, amebic pericarditis is much less common and is rarely seen in nontropical areas. It deserves discussion, particularly since the well-known dictum that "amebic pericarditis has never been observed unassociated with amebic liver abscess" can be misleading.

Pathophysiology. Suppurative amebic pericarditis is probably always due to rupture of an amebic liver abscess into the pericardium (Chapter 86). However, such an abscess is likely to be in the left lobe of the liver (rather than the typical right lobe location) and may escape clinical detection. Therefore, the patient with amebic pericarditis may have cardiac tamponade without obvious clinical evidence of liver disease (Fig. 3–5).

Diagnosis and Treatment. Rapid diagnosis and treatment are

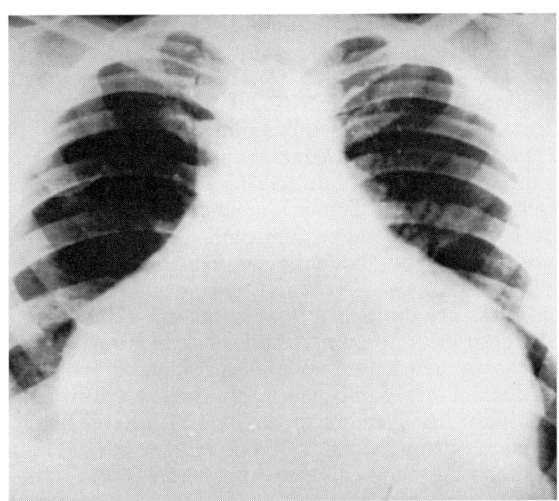

Figure 3–5. Posteroanterior chest film in patient with amebic pericarditis without evidence of liver abscess clinically or by scan. He received corticosteroids for "fever of unknown origin." Pulmonary oligemia is also evident.

lifesaving in a disease that is otherwise fatal. The diagnosis of amebic pericarditis is not likely to be made fortuitously, because these patients usually do not experience diarrhea or have amebas in the stool; nor is the organism likely to be seen in the pericardial aspirate. The pericardial fluid can be either purulent or a mixture of blood and pus. In amebic pericarditis, neutrophils predominate in the pericardial fluid, in contrast to tuberculous pericarditis, in which lymphocytes are predominant.

Diagnosis is established by performing a serologic test (e.g., IHA test) for amebiasis on either blood or pericardial/pleural aspirate. Treatment with metronidazole is the same as for liver abscess except that the pericardium should be surgically drained. Adequate pericardial drainage may obviate the need for laparotomy and subdiaphragmatic drainage.

ATHEROSCLEROTIC HEART DISEASE. In the early 1970s in Ibadan, Nigeria, only 10 cases of myocardial infarction were seen among 8000 necropsies over a 10-year period. Four of these were due to coronary embolism rather than atherosclerosis. In the past 2 decades, reports indicate a rising incidence in ischemic heart disease (IHD) in developing countries, particularly in the urban setting, with a rapidly changing social and dietary lifestyle. Attendant risk factors include the high consumption of saturated fats, cigarette smoking, sedentary habits, and lack of exercise. Hypertension and diabetes are also well-recognized predisposing factors. Cardiologic practice in many parts of the developing world would thus appear to be going through a transition phase of two populations of cardiac patients—one with CHF from diseases associated with infection and hypertension, and the other with complaints of chest pain from coronary heart disease.

Ischemic Heart Disease. This may lead to sudden death or, less commonly, to congestive heart failure (CHF). An antecedent history of angina is often lacking, and CHF patients often have the symptoms associated with fluid retention. Physical signs may be few and definitive diagnosis hampered by the paucity of investigative facilities (ECG, myocardial enzymes). Particular attention should be paid to controlling the blood pressure, as there is ample evidence to show that hypertension worsens the prognosis in blacks with end-organ damage.

It should be stressed that IHD is not an unavoidable concomitant of socioeconomic development. The decline in IHD mortality in many industrialized societies has been related to the reduction of risk factors through the adoption of healthier lifestyles.

SCHISTOMOSOMAL COR PULMONALE. Chronic cor pulmonale heart disease is secondary to disease of the respiratory system, e.g., fibrosis, emphysema, or pneumonia. Dyspnea is the cardinal presenting feature and is due to the increased work of breathing resulting from the mechanical effects of lung disease with right heart overload. In its chronic form, its differential diagnosis includes mitral stenosis and thromboembolic pulmonary hypertension.

Pathophysiology. Schistosomes seldom seriously injure the heart directly. An adult worm in a coronary artery at autopsy is rare. Ova in the myocardium can rarely elicit a granulomatous response and, when present in large numbers, can produce myocarditis. References to nonspecific "toxic" or "allergic" schistosomal myocarditis are suspect. Some of the antischistosomal drugs used in the past have been cardiotoxic (Chapter 118). Moreover, "toxic" schistosomal myocarditis has been reported principally in areas where Chagas' disease is also present. The principal way in which schistosomiasis causes cardiovascular disease is by leading to cor pulmonale.

Of patients dying with schistosomal hepatic fibrosis, 10 to 15% have right ventricular hypertrophy. Although ova are routinely found in the lungs of patients with *S. haematobium* infection, cor pulmonale is rare. It is also unusual in *S. mansoni* infection without hepatic involvement. Patients with schistosomal pulmonary hypertension usually have portal hypertension as well, suggesting that ova passing through collateral blood vessels may reach and obstruct pulmonary arterioles. The association between pulmonary hypertension and hepatic cirrhosis of other cause suggests that other factors may also cause pulmonary hypertension.

Clinical Manifestations. The usual patient is a farmer who complains of dyspnea on exertion. He may also experience exertional dizziness or syncope and oppressive chest or epigastric discomfort (right ventricular angina). Cough and wheezing are common. Hemoptysis is rare but ominous. Exertional palpitation is a frequent complaint. Premature atrial contractions may be present, but atrial fibrillation is unusual before the age of 40 years. The presence of syncope and the absence of hemoptysis and atrial fibrillation are important points in the diagnostic differentiation from RHD.

Physical examination of the patient with schistosomal cor pulmonale should be conclusive. The noncardiac findings are those of portal hypertension with hepatosplenomegaly and venous collaterals. Inspection shows visible neck vein activity, with a prominent *a* wave in early cases and a large *v* wave if tricuspid regurgitation is present. When the patient lies back, pulsations along the left upper sternal border indicate the presence of an enlarged pulmonary artery. On palpation, right ventricular heave and loud pulmonary valve closure may be felt. If tricuspid or pulmonary regurgitation has occurred, appropriate thrills may be felt. Auscultation confirms the presence of a loud pulmonary closure. If there are no murmurs, a right atrial S4 can be heard in the epigastrium (corresponding to the *a* wave in the neck) along with an ejection sound along the left sternal border. If present, the systolic murmur of tricuspid regurgitation should not be confused with that of a ventricular septal defect (which is usually rougher). The diastolic blow of pulmonary regurgitation secondary to the pulmonary hypertension with dilatation of the pulmonary artery (PA) sounds similar to the murmur of aortic regurgitation. The tricuspid valve flutters in the flow produced by the pulmonary regurgitation and produces a rumble that can be mistaken for tricuspid or mitral stenosis.

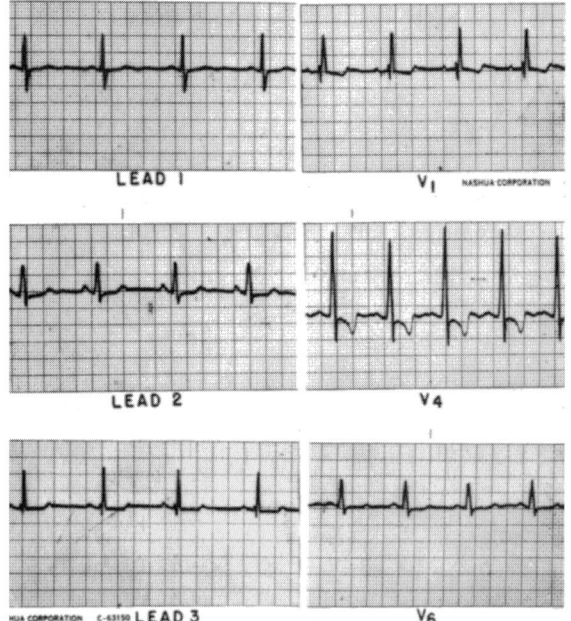

Figure 3–6. Electrocardiogram of patient with bilharzial cor pulmonale, showing a vertical axis and right ventricular hypertrophy and strain.

Laboratory Findings. The ECG shows normal sinus rhythm and right ventricular hypertrophy (Fig. 3–6). The chest film reveals the cardiac silhouette of right ventricular hypertrophy and a large PA. Sometimes, granulomas are visualized on the roentgenogram, being most noticeable in the lower fields. As the PA becomes aneurysmal, pulmonary regurgitation becomes inevitable. Huge PAs are commonly seen in farmers who continue to work in the fields during the progression of pulmonary hypertension (Fig. 3–7). At cardiac catheterization, these patients have lower PA pressures and higher right ventricular diastolic pressures than do patients with a lesser degree of PA enlargement.

Treatment and Progress. Since schistosomal cor pulmonale is a complication of hepatosplenic schistosomiasis and since patients with pulmonary hypertension of any cause do poorly, it is not surprising that those with schistosomal cor pulmonale have a poor prognosis. Cardiac catheterization can be hazardous. If angiographic demonstration of the pulmonary vasculature is desired, it is better done selectively. Treatment is also associated with some risks, since dead or dying worms can embolize to the lungs and complete the obstructive process. Thrombus in situ, particularly of the right PA, also occurs. Dissection of the aneurysm provokes sudden hemoptysis, chest pain, and death. Some patients die suddenly without obvious cause, possibly from arrhythmias. If a patient with schistosomal cor pulmonale can leave the fields and hard labor, he may live longer.

DISEASES OF THE AORTA

Primary Arteritis of the Aorta. This clinically distinctive arteritis of unknown etiology occurs in all continents but most often in Asia, Africa, and Latin America. It is most common in Asian women and has frequently been reported by Japanese investigators since its first description by Takayasu in 1908.

There is no definite association between this disease and infection, but there is some evidence implicating mycobacteria. Histologically, however, the disease does not resemble tuberculous infection but rather a nonspecific, nonatherosclerotic panarteritis. Current thinking favors an autoimmune etiology.

Clinical Manifestations and Diagnosis. Early symptoms of this arteritis include fever, weight loss, night sweats, and erythema nodosum. The tuberculin test may be positive. Such findings in a young Asian woman, coupled with tenderness and bruits over the carotid arteries and a very high ESR, clinically suggest the diagnosis of Takayasu's arteritis.

Later in the disease, when "pulselessness" is apparent, the diagnosis is obvious. Patients complain of visual or neurologic symptoms and sometimes note claudication in their arms. Pulses are difficult to feel in the arms and neck, and the retinal arteries are nonpulsatile. The femoral arteries are usually easily felt. Unless there is considerable involvement of the descending thoracic aorta, the pressure in the legs is usually high. Involvement of the carotid arteries below the carotid sinus also results in systemic hypertension. The renal arteries may be involved, producing stenosis and hypertension. Because of the high pressure in the ascending aorta and involvement of the aortic valve, patients with primary arteritis can develop aortic regurgitation. The combination of an aortic regurgitation murmur and weak, rather than bounding, pulses in the arms is a distinctive finding in this disease.

Treatment and Prognosis. Treatment consists of surgical correction of the lesion when feasible, but early involvement of the coronary or renal arteries carries a poor prognosis. Steroids have not been effective except in the early febrile phases of Takayasu's arteritis. Antituberculous drugs should be considered in patients with positive tuberculin skin tests, because of the possibility of an active tuberculous infection.

Aortic and Ventricular Aneurysms

Aorta. Aneurysms of the aorta may be saccular, fusiform, or dissecting. They may give rise to pressure symptoms depending on their size and location. Abnormal pulsation may be visible over the chest wall, but the diagnosis is best made on chest or abdominal x-ray confirmed by angiography.

A dissecting aneurysm usually results from a tear in the aorta such that blood leaks into the media, dissecting the aorta wall for a variable length. It becomes rapidly fatal if it eventually ruptures outside the aortic wall. The clinical picture of dissection is that of severe chest pain extending rapidly to the back, groin, and legs. Ischemia or infarction of organs may occur from blockage of arteries to the brain, kidneys and gastrointestinal tract, or limbs. Serial chest x-ray

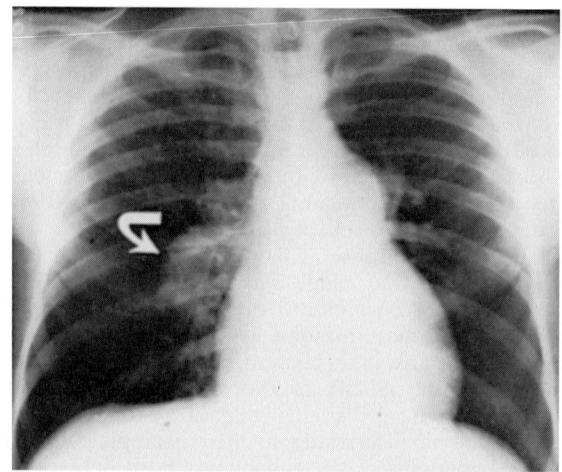

Figure 3–7. Chest film in patient with bilharzial cor pulmonale. Arrow points to dilated right pulmonary artery.

shows enlargement of the aorta, and an angiogram determines the site and extent of the dissection. Treatment, when possible, is by resection and graft replacement.

Ventricles. In many tropical areas, ventricular aneurysms are the subvalvular type, affecting more the mitral and aortic valve rings. Most of these patients are symptomless, but a few complain of palpitation or chest pain radiating to the neck and arm; some may have symptoms caused by pressure on neighboring structures. Emboli may arise from these aneurysms, giving rise to angina or pain over the spleen or kidneys. Physical signs may be confined to CHF, but there is sometimes a pansystolic mitral incompetence murmur with an audible third heart sound.

The chest x-ray shows an enlarged heart with an unusual bulge on the left cardiac border caused by the aneurysm. A left ventricular angiogram demonstrates its location and size. The only effective treatment is open heart surgery: resection of the aneurysm combined with valve replacement.

CARDIOVASCULAR SYPHILIS. Syphilitic involvement of the heart and arteries has become unusual in the industrialized world, but autopsy series from elsewhere (e.g., Khartoum) show syphilis accounting for over 10% of all cardiovascular deaths, just as it did in Europe a century ago. It has a male preponderance, and the common age spectrum is 20 to 40 years (Chapter 48.1). Aneurysms may occur in the ascending or thoracic aorta or, less commonly, in the abdominal aorta above the renal vessels. Pathologically there is endarteritis obliterans of the vasa vasorum of large vessels, leading to medial necrosis and disruption of the elastic tissue in the relevant part of the aorta.

Diagnostic clues include a history of chancre, angina in a young man with mild to moderate aortic insufficiency, and telltale neurologic stigmata (in about 40% of patients). Standard tests (e.g., the VDRL) may be negative in about a third of patients with cardiovascular syphilis, but the FTA-ABS test is almost always positive. Distinct clinical syndromes associated with cardiovascular syphilis include (1) asymptomatic uncomplicated aortitis, (2) aortic incompetence, (3) aneurysms (fusiform or saccular but not dissecting), and (4) coronary ostial stenosis. Although treatment with penicillin is routinely given, it is difficult to know what purpose it serves, since the disease is chronic and the changes are irreversible. Conversely, in very rare instances, treatment has been associated with the dramatic enlargement of a small aneurysm.

NUTRITIONAL HEART DISEASE

Protein-Calorie Malnutrition. PCM can lead to a heart with interstitial edema or with gradual disappearance of all pericardial fat and consequent atrophy. Clinically the cardiac output is reduced, and there is ECG evidence of S-T segment elevation and low voltage, and flat or inverted T waves. There may also be sudden cardiac arrest or fibrillation (Chapter 130).

Beriberi Heart Disease. With deficiency in dietary thiamine, the beriberi heart may develop, characterized by peripheral vasodilatation, high-output biventricular myocardial failure, and sodium retention. In its extreme form, cardiomegaly is associated with marked dyspnea, restlessness, and cyanosis. This condition improves rapidly when large doses of thiamine (50 mg) are given orally or parenterally. The skin temperature falls, and the cardiovascular decompensation improves to near-normal within a few days (Chapter 131.2).

Alcoholic Heart Disease. This is a form of cardiomyopathy that results from the direct toxic effect of alcohol on the heart in the relatively malnourished, thiamine-deficient individual. Certain additives in beer (e.g., cobalt) may complicate the picture. Patients have a long history of heavy alcohol intake and complain of palpitations followed by features of left- or right-sided heart failure. A chest x-ray shows a globular enlarged heart with evidence of pulmonary congestion. A wide variety of ECG abnormalities have been described, including arrhythmias (atrial and ventricular extrasystoles, atrial fibrillation, sinus tachycardia), abnormal P wave, low-voltage QRS complex, prolonged Q-T interval, and bizarre forms of T waves (dimpled, spinous, cloven flat, and negative). The blood pressure is normal, and there is no evidence of coronary or valvular heart disease.

Congestive heart failure is managed along conventional lines; complete abstinence from alcohol is mandatory. Some patients respond well to thiamine or vasodilator drugs.

Bibliography

Akinkugbe OO (ed): Cardiovascular Disease in Africa. Basel, Ciba Geigy, 1976.

Akinkugbe OO, Falase AO: *In* Clinical Medicine in the Tropics Series: I. Cardiovascular Disease. Oxford, Blackwell Scientific Publications, 1987.

Andrade ZA: Pathogenesis of Chagas' disease. Res Immunol 142:126, 1991.

Andy JJ, Ogunowo PO, Akpan NA, et al: Helminth-associated hypereosinophilia and tropical endomyocardial fibrosis (EMF) in Nigeria. Acta Trop 69:127, 1998.

Cheever AW, Kamel IA, Elwi AM, et al: *Schistosoma mansoni* and *S. haematobium* infections in Egypt. III. Extrahepatic pathology. Am J Trop Med Hyg 27:55, 1978.

Haffejee I: Rheumatic fever and rheumatic heart disease: the current status of its immunology, diagnostic criteria, and prophylaxis. Q J Med 84:641, 1992.

Lindsay J Jr: Diagnosis and treatment of diseases of the aorta. Curr Probl Cardiol 22:485, 1997.

Maher D, Harries AD: Tuberculous pericardial effusion: A prospective clinical study in low-resource setting—Blatyre, Malawi. Int J Tuberc Lung Dis 1:358, 1997.

Martin DR: Rheumatogenic and nephritogenic group A streptococci. Myth or reality? An opening lecture. Adv Exp Med Biol 418:21, 1997.

Mastroianni A, Coronado O, Chiodo F: Tuberculous pericarditis and AIDS: Case reports and review. Eur J Epidemiol 13:755, 1997.

Mota EA, Guimaraes AC, Santana OO, et al: A nine-year prospective study of Chagas' disease in a defined rural population in northeast Brazil. Am J Trop Med Hyg 42:429, 1990.

Pless M, Juranek D, Kozarsky P, et al: The epidemiology of Chagas' disease in a hyperendemic area of Cochabamba, Bolivia: A clinical study including electrocardiography, seroreactivity to *Trypanosoma cruzi*, xenodiagnosis, and domiciliary triatomine distribution. Am J Trop Med Hyg 47:539, 1992.

Shaper AG: Cardiovascular disease in the Tropics. II. Endomyocardial fibrosis. Br Med J 3:743, 1972.

Sieck JO, Awad M, Saour J, et al: Concurrent post-streptococcal carditis and glomerulonephritis: Serial echocardiographic diagnosis and follow-up. Eur Heart J 13:1720, 1992.

Strang JI: Tuberculous pericarditis. J Infect 35:215, 1997.

Suwan PK, Potjalongsilp S: Predictors of constrictive pericarditis after tuberculous pericarditis. Br Heart J 73:187, 1995.

Vaughan JP: A brief review of cardiovascular disease in Africa. Trans R Soc Trop Med Hyg 71:226, 1977.

Veasy LG, Hill HR: Immunologic and clinical correlations in rheumatic fever and rheumatic heart disease. Pediatr Infect Dis J 16:400, 1997.

4 Gastrointestinal Diseases

Stephen G. Wright

■ COMMON SYNDROMES OF GASTROINTESTINAL DISEASE IN THE TROPICS

Gastrointestinal problems are common in medical practice in the tropics and subtropics. The principal syndromes are acute diarrhea (less than 2 weeks' duration), chronic diarrhea (greater than 2 weeks' duration), abdominal pain, and abdominal distention.

Diarrhea

The majority of patients are children, but individuals of all ages can be affected. Increased frequency of bowel action and altered consistency of the stools are the usual symptoms. The duration of diarrhea is a guide to the range of conditions that must be considered. Most acute infections of the gut have resolved or are resolving within 2 weeks. Diarrhea that wakens the patient at night should always prompt thorough investigation, as it suggests an underlying organic cause.

ACUTE DIARRHEA. Intoxications, viral and bacterial pathogens, and *Cryptosporidium* cause diarrhea of shorter duration (Table 4–1). In a large study from Bangladesh, rotavirus was the most common cause of diarrhea in children under 2 years of age (Chapter 27.2).

Watery Diarrhea. Large-volume stools indicate a small bowel etiology, with cholera (Chapter 41) and enterotoxigenic *Escherichia coli* (Chapter 42) often implicated. Diarrhea induced by accumulation of malabsorbed solutes in the gut lumen also produces large-volume stools, and in children low stool pH may be an indicator of this. Toxin-induced secretory diarrhea will continue unaffected by food intake, whereas solute-induced diarrhea is reduced by reduced food intake. The passage of much rectal gas and frothy stools is an indication of malabsorption of carbohydrate in the small intestine and fermentation of unabsorbed substrates by colonic bacteria. *Cryptosporidium* causes short-lived and self-limiting diarrhea. Both small and large bowel can be involved, but the stools are nondysenteric. This infection in patients with impaired immune responses causes prolonged diarrhea (Chapter 88). *Cyclospora cayetanensis* is newly recognized as a cause of acute and more chronic diarrhea with abnormalities of intestinal absorption (Chapter 89).

Dysentery. Diarrhea with blood in the stools indicates inflammation and ulceration of the colonic wall. In acute illnesses, bacterial infection is usually the cause; the presence of pus cells in fecal smears supports this possibility. Colicky abdominal pain is more common with this group of infections, and tenderness over the colon, particularly the sigmoid

TABLE 4–1. Causes of Diarrhea Lasting Less Than 2 Weeks

Viruses
Rotavirus
Norwalk agent
Adenoviruses
Coronaviruses
(Probably more agents yet to be defined)

Bacteria
Intoxication
  Staphylococcal enterotoxin
  Clostridium perfringens enterotoxin
  Bacillus cereus enterotoxin
  Botulism (uncommon)
Infection
  Escherichia coli (enterotoxigenic, enteropathic, enteroinvasive)
  Vibrio cholerae
  Vibrio parahaemolyticus
  Campylobacter enteritis
  Salmonella species (nontyphoid)
  Shigella species
  Yersinia enterocolitica

Protozoa
Cryptosporidium species (immunocompetent host)
Cyclospora cayetanensis

TABLE 4–2. Causes of Diarrhea Lasting More Than 2 Weeks

Specific Infections
Cryptosporidiosis (immunodeficient)
Cyclosporiosis
Giardia lamblia
Amebic dysentery
Trichinella spiralis (rare)
Capillaria philippinensis (limited geographic distribution)
Strongyloides stercoralis (uncommon)

Malabsorption Syndromes
Giardiasis
Chronic calcific pancreatitis
Tropical sprue
Intestinal tuberculosis
Celiac disease (rare in indigenous populations)

Diarrhea in AIDS
Mild to moderate to severe

AIDS, acquired immunodeficiency disease.

colon, is often found. Amebic dysentery does not usually present acutely as a cause of dysenteric diarrhea.

CHRONIC DIARRHEA. Weight loss is the main clinical feature that separates disorders of intestinal motility and hypolactasia in the adult (in whom it is not solely responsible for significant weight loss) from disorders causing malabsorption (Table 4–2) or inflammatory and malignant disease of the gastrointestinal tract. When there is continuing diarrhea without systemic upset or weight loss, disorders of intestinal motility need to be considered.

Small Bowel Disorders. The passage of frequent, pale, offensive stools suggests malabsorption. Stool weight is a useful clinical indicator, greater than 200 g/24 hours being abnormal. Pancreatic disease in the tropics is not uncommon and often is unrelated to alcohol ingestion. Calcific pancreatitis can occur, even in young children. Tuberculosis is a cause of intestinal strictures that may cause malabsorption (Chapter 77). Immunoproliferative small intestinal disease (IPSID), also known as alpha chain disease, occurs widely throughout the tropics and should be considered as a cause of malabsorption. Hyperpigmentation, gross weight loss, finger clubbing, and edema are prominent clinical features in advanced cases (Chapter 12).

The acquired immunodeficiency syndrome (AIDS) commonly causes chronic diarrhea in patients in the tropics and the subtropics (Chapter 23). Clinicians in Uganda described "slim disease," manifested as continuing diarrhea with weight loss, as a recognized presentation of AIDS. Several intestinal parasites (e.g., *Cryptosporidium*, *Isospora belli*, Microsporidia) are commonly found in association with other infectious agents (e.g., cytomegalovirus, nontyphoidal salmonellae, *Shigella*, *Mycobacterium avium-intracellulare*, and *Mycobacterium tuberculosis*) in the gut of patients with AIDS.

LARGE BOWEL DISORDERS. Inflammatory bowel disease due to Crohn disease and ulcerative colitis is widely recognized throughout the temperate world; there are increasing numbers of case reports of these diseases in migrants from tropical areas and in indigenous tropical residents. Although this should be considered in patients with diarrheal disease, abdominal pain, weight loss, and mucosal abnormalities in the small or large intestine, specific infectious causes of inflammatory disease, e.g., amebiasis or tuberculosis, must first be rigorously excluded before nonspecific inflammatory diseases are diagnosed. Proctocolitis is a relatively common

TABLE 4–3. Causes of Abdominal Pain

Peptic ulceration (gastric or duodenal; benign or
  malignant, including gastric lymphoma)
Chronic pancreatic disease
Complications of heavy ascaris infection
Sickle cell disease with abdominal crisis
Intussusception
Intestinal volvulus
Incarcerated or strangulated hernia
Pelvic inflammatory disease
Ectopic pregnancy
Appendicitis

finding in homosexuals and patients with AIDS, although a specific infection is not always found. *Cryptosporidium* and cytomegalovirus are two well-recognized causes. Leishmaniasis may complicate recurrent perianal sepsis with circulating parasitized macrophages attracted to an area of chronic sepsis, and in AIDS severe infections occur.

Abdominal Pain

The range of causes is as wide as it is in temperate regions (Table 4–3). Duodenal ulcer is common in the tropics. Malignant lesions of the stomach, e.g., carcinoma and lymphoma, occur. Therefore, full investigation with endoscopic biopsy should be undertaken if indicated, where facilities exist. Chronic pancreatitis can be a cause of persisting epigastric pain. Pancreatic calcification may be seen on plain radiographs of the abdomen, and marked changes may be present on ultrasound scans. This disease occurs in children as well as adults.

Adult ascaris worms can migrate into the biliary and pancreatic ducts to cause upper abdominal pain as well as biliary tract obstruction, ascending infection of the biliary tree, liver abscess, or pancreatitis (see Fig. 104–3). A massive knotted bolus of worms can also cause intestinal obstruction and may be associated with volvulus of the intestine.

Sickle cell disease is common in many parts of the tropics and in migrants and their children moving from those areas to temperate regions (Chapter 6). Acute abdominal pain with physical signs as a manifestation of sickle cell crisis can be difficult to distinguish from acute appendicitis or other causes of acute abdominal pain. Intussusception is fairly common in the tropics. Pelvic inflammatory disease and ectopic pregnancy secondary to infection-induced damage to the fallopian tubes should also be considered in females with acute lower abdominal pain. Appendicitis is well recognized in the tropics. Actinomycosis can cause right iliac fossa inflammatory masses (Chapter 38).

Abdominal Distention

Abdominal distention can be caused by a wide range of diseases (Table 4–4). Ascites is frequently encountered, and examination of ascitic fluid is essential for diagnosis. Tuberculosis (Chapter 77) and chronic liver disease are among the most common causes. Spontaneous bacterial peritonitis may complicate ascites due to chronic liver disease (Chapter 5). Hepatosplenic schistosomiasis complicated by viral hepatitis–caused cirrhosis is a common cause of ascites in endemic areas (Chapter 118). Intra-abdominal malignancy may present with ascites, and cytologic examination of fluid may show cancer cells. Chylous ascites is uncommon. Heart disease due to endomyocardial fibrosis, rheumatic heart disease, and constrictive pericarditis can cause ascites as part of se-

vere heart failure (Chapter 3). Huge ovarian cysts can present with massive abdominal distention, but the central location of the swelling, presence of a fluid thrill, and absence of shifting dullness help to distinguish this from ascites. Occasionally, patients who have peritoneal dissemination of hydatid material from a ruptured hepatic cyst are seen with a massively distended abdomen in which numerous small lumps can be felt (Chapter 124.2). Eosinophilia is usual in these cases. Ultrasound scanning is especially useful in visualizing the numerous peritoneal cysts. Ultrasound is also particularly valuable in the investigation of intra-abdominal conditions.

Gaseous distention of the abdomen is a common complaint. It may relate to hypolactasia, which can be primary or secondary. It may be part of the irritable bowel syndrome. When abdominal distention develops acutely in a very ill patient with dysenteric diarrhea, toxic dilatation of the colon must be considered. This complication can occur in the course of any of the colitides related to infection and nonspecific ulcerative colitis or Crohn disease.

The Acquired Immunodeficiency Syndrome and the Gastrointestinal Tract

The acquired immunodeficiency syndrome (AIDS) due to infection with the human immunodeficiency virus (HIV) is commonly associated with gut disease, most often due to infections but also due to Kaposi sarcoma and intestinal lymphoma (Chapter 23). Gut involvement is summarized in Table 4–5.

ESOPHAGITIS. This is a common manifestation of AIDS, and *Candida albicans* is the most frequent cause (Chapter 81.3). It presents with dysphagia and is usually associated with florid oral candidiasis. Cytomegalovirus (CMV), herpes simplex, and, much less commonly, *Torulopsis glabrata* can also produce esophagitis.

ENTERITIS. Chronic diarrhea may be the presenting feature in AIDS, and "slim disease" described from Uganda is one manifestation of this. A wide range of viral bacterial and parasitic pathogens has been isolated from the intestines of infected patients with diarrhea, and often more than one pathogen, frequently among *Cryptosporidium*, *Isospora*, and *Microsporidia*, may be found. However, a recent study reported that 50% of patients with chronic diarrhea had no detectable gut pathogen.

Mycobacterial infections of the gut are fairly common; it should be noted that the clinical features and findings on investigation are similar to those seen in non–HIV infected

TABLE 4–4. Causes of Abdominal Distention

Fluid

Ascites due to
  Chronic liver disease (cirrhosis, hepatosplenic schistosomiasis)
  Intra-abdominal tuberculosis
  Intra-abdominal malignancy
  Disease of the heart or pericardium
  Lymphatic disease (chylous ascites)

Mass Effect

Huge ovarian cyst
Disseminated hydatid cysts into peritoneal cavity

Gaseous Distention

Hypolactasia
Bowel motility disorders
Toxic dilatation of the colon

TABLE 4–5. Gut Involvement in AIDS

Infection

  a. Esophagitis due to
    Candida albicans
    CMV
    Herpes simplex
    Torulopsis glabrata
  b. Enteritis due to
    Mild, nonspecific CMV
    Salmonellosis
    Campylobacter
    Tuberculosis (*Mycobacterium tuberculosis* and other organisms, esp. *Mycobacterium avium-intracellulare*)
    Cryptosporidium
    Isospora belli
    Microsporidia
    Leishmania (possible)
  c. Pancreatitis due to
    CMV
    Toxoplasma gondii

Malignancy

  Any location, due to
    Kaposi sarcoma
    Intestinal lymphoma

AIDS, acquired immunodeficiency disease; CMV, cytomegalovirus.

patients (Chapter 77). The disease responds to standard antituberculous therapy, but there are indications that reactions to these drugs may be more common. Atypical mycobacteria also cause intestinal tuberculosis in AIDS (Chapter 77). Colitis is recognized in AIDS, although it may be less common in Africa. Cytomegalovirus and *Cryptosporidium* are two causes.

PANCREATITIS. The pancreas may be infected with CMV. *Toxoplasma gondii* has also been identified in the pancreas. Abnormal endocrine and exocrine functions have been suggested, but studies from Uganda have failed to show defects in exocrine function.

MALIGNANCY. Kaposi sarcoma is the most common malignancy seen in AIDS and can occur anywhere in the gut (Chapter 12). Multicentric tumors are found. Lymphomas also occur.

■ DISEASES OF THE GASTROINTESTINAL TRACT COMMON TO THE TROPICS

Gastrointestinal diseases are among the most common encountered in the tropics. Table 4–6 lists some of those that are frequently found in tropical and temperate regions of the world.

Cancrum Oris

Gangrenous necrosis of the soft tissues of the lips and cheeks is the main feature of this condition. It is common in malnourished children. Measles and anemia are other predisposing conditions. The sequence of events is that an ulcer on the lip, perhaps due to herpes, becomes secondarily infected with the anaerobic bacteria *Fusiformis fusiformis* and *Borrelia vincentii*. An area of soft tissue necrosis spreads from the original ulcer, with these bacteria growing in the tissue at the extending margin. In most cases, there is an obvious line of demarcation between healthy and gangrenous tissues. Treatment with penicillin controls the infection, but necrotic tissues slough and surgical reconstruction is needed to correct the deformities.

Esophageal Disease

ESOPHAGITIS. Chemical burns of the esophagus are common in the tropics as a result of drinking corrosive substances, e.g., Lysol, sodium hydroxide, sulfuric acid, and nitric acid, either with suicidal intent or by accident. Two Nigerian proprietary medicines contain corrosive substances.

Severe pain, shock, esophagitis, and perforation of the esophagus are immediate effects of drinking such corrosive agents. There is a high mortality rate; those who survive often develop fibrous strictures, which cause dysphagia and necessitate periodic dilatation.

ESOPHAGEAL VARICES. Esophageal varices are relatively common in the tropics. The causes can be classified as prehepatic, hepatic, and posthepatic. Increased blood flow through the hepatic portal vein in the tropical splenomegaly syndrome and portal vein thrombosis are prehepatic causes. Cirrhosis, schistosomal periportal fibrosis, veno-occlusive disease of the liver, and Indian childhood cirrhosis are hepatic causes, whereas constrictive pericarditis and chronic congestive cardiac failure due to rheumatic heart disease and endomyocardial fibrosis are posthepatic causes. Bleeding from varices is a life-threatening complication, and management comprises restoration of circulating volume with blood transfusions and prevention of further bleeding by measures such as balloon tamponade, vasopressin (Pitressin) infusion, obliteration of bleeding varices by endoscopic sclerotherapy, and surgical decompression by shunting procedures.

MEGAESOPHAGUS. This is irreversible dilatation of the esophagus that may occur in chronic *Trypanosoma cruzi* infections owing to destruction of ganglion cells of the autonomic plexuses in the esophageal wall (Chapter 94). Contractile activity is lost, and patients complain of dysphagia. Aspiration pneumonia may also occur. There is no specific treatment for megaesophagus, but pneumonia requires antibiotic treatment.

Gastroduodenal Disease

PEPTIC ULCER. Gastric ulcer is relatively rare in Africa and Asia. An increased incidence of gastric ulcer has been reported from the highland regions of Papua New Guinea, but most of the ulcers found were prepyloric, conforming to

TABLE 4–6. Occurrence of Gastrointestinal Diseases in the Tropics

More Common in the Tropics	Less Common in the Tropics
Pyloric stenosis due to duodenal ulcer	Gastric ulcer
Gastrointestinal infections	Hemorrhage and perforation due to duodenal ulcer
Tuberculosis of the abdomen and intestine	Gluten-sensitive enteropathy
Malabsorption due to	Mesenteric vascular occlusion
Giardiasis	Diverticulosis
Tropical sprue	Nonspecific ulcerative colitis
Chronic calcific pancreatitis	Crohn disease
Malnutrition	Ischemic colitis
Alpha chain disease	
Hypolactasia	
Capillariasis	
Strongyloidiasis	
Specific inflammatory bowel disease	
Intestinal obstruction due to	
Ascariasis	
Intestinal volvulus	
Intussusception	

the pattern of duodenal ulcer. Duodenal ulcer is particularly common in West Africa, northern Tanzania, Ethiopia, southern and northeastern India, and Afghanistan. It is relatively common in the hilly areas of northwestern India. The ratio of duodenal ulcer to gastric ulcer in the tropics is higher than in developed countries.

HELICOBACTER PYLORI INFECTION. This is probably the most common infectious agent affecting the gastrointestinal tract (Chapter 45).

Etiology. *H. pylori* is an S-shaped, gram-negative, motile organism that grows slowly in culture. In vivo it is found adherent to the epithelium in the mucous layer. It secretes urease to help protect it against gastric acid and a protease. Infection can result in gastritis, increased gastric acid secretion, and gastric metaplasia in the duodenum. Infection by ingestion usually occurs early in life in the tropics and in later decades in the temperate regions.

Distribution and Incidence. Infection in childhood is common throughout the tropics with infection rates from 40 to 65% by the age of 5 years in a range of countries from north to tropical Africa and from 70 to 100% at age 25. In addition, migrants to temperate countries, e.g., Turks in Germany, have much higher infection rates than do the indigenous population. In the Gambia, infection in the first year of life has been documented.

DISEASES CAUSED BY *H. PYLORI* INFECTION. *H. pylori* is established as the cause of antral gastritis, gastric ulcer, duodenal ulcer, gastric cancer, and low-grade gastric lymphoma. Long-standing total gastritis leads to gastric atrophy and gastric ulcer with the possibility of later gastric cancer. Eradication of *H. pylori* is associated with (1) healing of peptic ulcer and relatively low rates of relapse when compared with treatment with H_2 receptor antagonists alone, which do not eradicate the organism; and (2) regression of low-grade gastric lymphoma. There is no such regression with gastric cancer.

Acute infection in adults causes hypochlorhydria which takes several months to resolve, and among Gambian children gastric acid secretion is reduced so that *H. pylori* may be relevant in reducing the effectiveness of the gastric acid barrier to gut infection. Those children acquiring infection early had poorer weight gain in the first year than those infected later. Maternal anti–*H. pylori* secretory IgA in breast milk had protective effects, delaying infection.

Clinical Manifestations, Complications, and Therapy. Epigastric pain after eating and waking the patient at night, relieved by food and antacids, are typical features. Symptoms wax and wane with time. Treatment should combine a drug to reduce gastric acid secretion, an H_2 receptor antagonist or proton pump inhibitor, and antibiotics (amoxicillin and metronidazole or tinidazole). The combination regimen should be taken for 2 weeks. Eradication of infection is associated with healing of ulceration or antral gastritis and a relatively low rate of relapse in contrast with high relapse rates when healing is produced by antacid drugs alone. Higher rates of nitroimidazole resistance to *H. pylori* are seen in the tropics, perhaps in relation to the more widespread use of these drugs in parasitic infections. There is some evidence to suggest that healing will occur with a nitroimidazole-containing regimen even though drug resistance occurs. With improved treatment leading to permanent cure, the complications of bleeding and pyloric stenosis should become less frequent.

Prevention and Control. As yet there are no specific methods to reduce infection rates since the source of infection is not defined, but the prospect of a vaccine against *H. pylori* that would prevent peptic ulcer disease, gastritis, gastric cancer, and lymphoma is exciting.

Intestinal Infection

Intestinal infection is a major cause of morbidity and mortality in the tropics and subtropics. Children are most often and most seriously affected. Dehydration is the main cause of death, whereas deterioration of nutritional state is the main cause of morbidity. The mortality rate among infants and young children from dehydrating diarrheal disease in the tropics is 55/1000 per year, compared with a rate of 0.4/1000 per year in Europe.

ETIOLOGY AND DISTRIBUTION. Rotavirus is the most common gut pathogen found worldwide in children under 2 years of age (Chapter 27.2). When all age groups are considered, enterotoxigenic strains of *Escherichia coli* are the most common pathogens (Chapter 42), responsible for almost one third of episodes of diarrhea in a large study from Bangladesh (Tables 4–1 and 4–2). A major study of the etiology of acute diarrhea in children under 3 years showed rotavirus and pathogenic *E. coli* in 16% each and *Shigella* in 11%. *Campylobacter* species have a worldwide distribution and are relatively common causes of infectious diarrheal disease wherever they are looked for (Chapter 43). Salmonellosis is the most common cause of food poisoning in developed countries. Varying incidences of salmonellosis have been reported from countries in the tropics (Chapter 76). Shigellae are common worldwide and cause diarrhea in all age groups (Chapter 40). *Escherichia coli* O:157 causes a dysenteric illness very similar to shigellosis. Recent decades have seen the spread of cholera due to the El Tor biotype; most African countries have now had epidemics (Chapter 41). *Vibrio cholerae* 0.139 caused acute watery diarrhea in the Indian subcontinent among both children and adults, indicating a lack of cross-protection between the newly recognized strain and the classic and El Tor strains. *Vibrio parahaemolyticus* is one of the few organisms limited in geographic distribution, with most cases in Japan and the countries of Southeast Asia. Sporadic cases occur in other areas (Chapter 41.3). *Aeromonas hydrophila* has been associated with both acute and more chronic diarrheal disease.

TRANSMISSION AND EPIDEMIOLOGY. Infection occurs by the ingestion of organisms in food and water contaminated by feces from a man or animal excreting the organism. This contamination is associated with inadequate public sanitation and low standards of personal hygiene. Defecation near pools and streams that are sources of water for domestic use is common, and simple sewage disposal systems often empty feces into the domestic water supply of the next house. Person-to-person spread of infection also occurs.

Seafoods such as shellfish, mussels, and crabs transmit viruses causing gastroenteritis, cholera, and *Vibrio parahaemolyticus*. Flies carry bacteria from feces to food on their mouth parts and legs. Low standards of kitchen hygiene in homes and public eating places also encourage transmission of intestinal infection. Precooked food kept warm for long periods, e.g., food bought from roadside food peddlers, may transmit a number of gut pathogens and contain enterotoxin formed by staphylococci growing in warmed food. Poultry and eggs are important sources of nontyphoid salmonellae. *Salmonella* and *Campylobacter* species are harbored in the gut of chickens.

An important and avoidable source of intestinal infection in infants results from misguided attempts at bottle-feeding with powdered milk solution instead of breast-feeding. Unsterilized bottles and nipples and contaminated water all contribute to the considerable risk of gut infection.

Most intestinal infections occur in children; 40% of all cases occur in those under 2 years old; 60% occur in children under 9 years of age. Lower socioeconomic groups are most often affected. Malnutrition is a predisposing factor, and diarrhea is prolonged in malnourished children. Reduced gastric acid secretion as a result of *Helicobacter pylori* infection, malnutrition, or surgery is also a predisposing factor. Further work is needed to determine a link between *H. pylori* infection and susceptibility to gut infection in the tropics.

PATHOGENESIS AND PATHOLOGY. Diarrhea can be defined as an increase in the water content of stools. Physiologically, the cause may be that (1) the small intestine secretes more fluid than it reabsorbs; (2) solute absorption in the small intestine is impaired so that the osmotic load retains fluid in the gut lumen; (3) the volume of fluid entering the colon exceeds its capacity for water absorption; (4) water- and electrolyte-reabsorbing capacity of the colon is reduced as a result of enterotoxigenic infection such as cholera; or (5) the water-reabsorbing capacity and motility of the colon are altered by localized or generalized colonic inflammation and ulceration. Protein-rich fluid is also lost through inflamed and ulcerated mucosa in any area of the gut. Infectious agents produce diarrhea by causing one or more of these effects.

Enterotoxin-Producing Bacteria. *V. cholerae* typifies those bacterial pathogens that cause diarrhea through the actions of enterotoxins. The cholera vibrio adheres to proximal small bowel epithelial cells but does not invade the mucosa. The cholera enterotoxin is secreted and binds to the GM$_1$ ganglioside component of the epithelial cell surface. The A subunit of the bound toxin is transported into the cell, where it activates the enzyme adenyl cyclase located in the basolateral regions of the cell. Increased amounts of cyclic adenosine monophosphate (cyclic AMP) are produced. This inhibits absorption of sodium, chloride, and water by villous epithelial cells and stimulates sodium-dependent secretion of chloride and possibly bicarbonate by crypt cells (Chapter 41). This is not the sole mechanism causing net fluid secretion in cholera. There is also evidence that local neurohumoral mechanisms are involved.

Enterotoxigenic *E. coli* produce two enterotoxins, designated heat-labile enterotoxin and heat-stable enterotoxin (Chapter 42). The former activates adenylate cyclase, and the heat-stable enterotoxin activates guanylate cyclase to produce cyclic guanosine monophosphate. There are some differences in the physiologic changes that ensue, but the result is net secretion of isotonic fluid. The enterotoxin of *Staphylococcus aureus* is thought to act through adenylate cyclase stimulation, and the *Shigella* enterotoxin may have a similar effect in the proximal small intestine. *Salmonella* enterotoxin causes intracellular accumulation of cyclic AMP with net secretion of isotonic fluid mediated by local synthesis of prostaglandins.

Colonic function in infectious diarrhea has not had the intense examination given to the small intestine. Research in cholera has shown defects in epithelial function, and new insights into the absorptive functions have shown the colonic epithelium to be actively involved in substrate absorption.

Invasive Bacteria. *Shigella*, *Salmonella*, and *Campylobacter* species are enteroinvasive organisms. *Campylobacter* can invade the mucosa at any site in the small or large intestine, whereas *Shigella* and *Salmonella* invade the colonic mucosa and terminal ileum. Histologically, the changes seen are epithelial ulceration, tissue edema, and acute inflammation.

Intestinal Protozoa. *Giardia lamblia*, *Cryptosporidium*, and *Entamoeba histolytica* frequently cause diarrhea; *Cyclospora cayetanensis* causes diarrhea in a proportion of those infected, whereas *Balantidium coli* infections are rare. Direct mucosal damage, malabsorption of nutrients, and secondary bacterial colonization contribute to diarrhea in giardiasis (Chapter 87). Histologic changes in the proximal small bowel are nonspecific, although trophozoites may be found in the intervillous

spaces. *Cryptosporidium* causes a short-lived, self-limiting diarrheal illness in immunocompetent persons. The mechanisms involved are poorly understood (Chapter 88).

Diarrhea in amebic dysentery results from ulceration in which amebas invade the colonic mucosa (Chapter 86). The cecum and rectum are favored sites of invasion. Amebas are found in the tissues at the edges of the ulcers. Necrosis of tissue around the amebas is usual, although there may be acute inflammatory responses in the mucosa due to secondary bacterial infection.

Balantidium coli is usually a parasite of pigs, but in communities where there is close contact with pigs, it invades the mucosa in humans to cause dysenteric diarrhea (Chapter 90.1).

CLINICAL MANIFESTATIONS AND COMPLICATIONS. Vomiting and diarrhea are the most common symptoms in gastrointestinal infection. The onset of symptoms can vary from a few hours after ingesting food containing *Staphylococcus aureus* enterotoxin, to several days after ingesting bacterial pathogens, to 2 or more weeks in giardiasis.

Profuse watery diarrhea suggests infection causing net secretion of fluid in the small intestine. *Vibrio cholerae*, enterotoxigenic *Escherichia coli*, rotavirus, and *Campylobacter* are common causes of watery diarrhea. Frequent bowel actions with small volumes of stool and the passage of blood suggest colonic infection. Continuous central abdominal pain often precedes the onset of diarrhea in *Campylobacter* infections. Colicky abdominal pain is common in many gut infections, but the patient with cholera usually has no pain. Fever, chills, and generalized myalgia are usually associated with infection by invasive organisms. Diarrhea that persists for weeks with offensive yellow stools may indicate giardiasis. Irregular bowel movements with stools that vary in consistency and contain blood and mucus are characteristic of amebic dysentery.

Dysentery. Patients infected with invasive organisms are often ill-looking and febrile. Most patients have generalized abdominal tenderness with increased bowel sounds. The findings on rectal examination may be abnormal in patients with dysenteric diarrheas, e.g., an edematous, roughened mucosa and blood on the examiner's glove. A smear from the material on the glove should be made for immediate microscopy. Diffuse inflammation, ulceration, and bleeding of the rectal mucosa are the usual appearance in invasive bacterial infections at proctosigmoidoscopy.

Dehydration. The most important physical signs to be elicited concern the assessment of hydration (Chapter 16); the patient should be weighed at first presentation, as weight gain or loss can be a valuable guide to the effectiveness of rehydration. Severe dehydration is most common in cholera and enterotoxigenic *Escherichia coli* infection.

Sequelae of Diarrhea. Dehydration is the most important cause of death in infants and children with gastrointestinal infection. The nutritional state of children often deteriorates because of anorexia, malabsorption of nutrients, and the practice of not feeding children with diarrhea. Hypolactasia is a sequela of many gut infections and may cause persisting diarrhea. Hemorrhage, perforation, and toxic dilatation of the colon may complicate diarrhea caused by invasive organisms. A hemolytic-uremic syndrome can complicate *Shigella dysenteriae* and *Escherichia coli* O:157 infections (Chapters 40 and 42). Reactive arthritis and Reiter syndrome can follow *Shigella*, *Salmonella*, *Campylobacter*, and *Yersinia* infections. Frequently, no specific pathogen can be related either to antecedent diarrheal disease or to continuing diarrhea. A child with persistent diarrhea is more likely to be malnourished. Cow's milk protein intolerance is one cause of persisting diarrhea in Europe, and it may also contribute to this relatively common entity in the tropics.

DIAGNOSIS. The range of laboratory tests and expertise needed to make a specific microbiologic diagnosis in most patients with intestinal infection requires facilities not often available in the tropics. Some simple tests can be useful in most circumstances. It is important to examine the stool sample for blood. Flecks of blood-stained mucus should be mounted in saline for direct microscopic examination for motile trophozoites of *Entamoeba histolytica* (Chapter 150). A smear of fluid stools should always be examined by direct microscopy for amebic trophozoites and trophozoites and cysts of *Giardia lamblia*. The presence of any cellular exudate in the smear should also be noted. The presence of polymorphonuclear leukocytes suggests infection with enteroinvasive bacteria, whereas a predominance of red cells is found in amebic dysentery. A proctosigmoidoscopy should be performed in patients with dysentery. Ulcerated or bleeding areas of mucosa should be scraped and the material examined immediately for amebic trophozoites.

TREATMENT AND PROGNOSIS. The mortality from dehydrating diarrheal diseases will decline if measures to correct and maintain hydration are started as early as possible.

Oral Rehydration. Oral rehydration with glucose electrolyte solution (ORS) has markedly reduced mortality from dehydrating diarrhea in communities in the tropics (Chapter 16). Community health providers can distribute ORS and teach others how to make up and give the solution. The standard formula recommended by the World Health Organization (WHO) is sucrose 40 g, sodium chloride 3.5 g, trisodium citrate dihydrate 2.9 g, and potassium chloride 1.5 g made up to 1 liter with clean water. The trisodium citrate has replaced sodium bicarbonate because the former gives better stability to the powdered mixture. An oral rehydration mixture made with rice flour as the carbohydrate source is also very effective and will reduce the volume of fecal effluent.

Antimicrobial Agents. Antimicrobial drugs have a limited role in the treatment of gut infections. Giardiasis (Chapter 87) and amebiasis (Chapter 86) will require specific treatment with metronidazole or tinidazole. Antibiotics should also be given to those patients who have fever, abdominal pain, toxicity, tenesmus, and frequent stools containing mucus and blood, the symptoms and signs of infection with enteroinvasive organisms. In the tropics children with bloody diarrhea should receive empirical antibiotic treatment according to standard WHO protocols (Chapter 16). Erythromycin is the drug of choice for *Campylobacter* infection, but the choice of agent for shigellosis and salmonellosis can be difficult because antibiotic resistance is common. Tetracycline treatment reduces the duration of diarrhea and fecal excretion of vibrios in cholera. The quinoline antibiotics are usually effective against enteroinvasive bacteria.

ADDITIONAL THERAPY. Intestinal sedatives reduce intestinal motility but do not affect the pathologic processes. The reduced frequency of bowel movements causes fluid stagnation in the gut lumen, encouraging proliferation of organisms and keeping organisms and their toxins in contact with the mucosa. The forward motion of fluid along the gut washing out organisms and toxins is lost.

The adverse effects of diarrhea on nutrition can be lessened by maintaining breast-feeding in infants and by the early reintroduction of feeding. Management of persistent diarrhea includes feeding as soon as patients, particularly children, want to eat. Energy-rich, low-osmolality foods should be given. Frequent small-volume meals may allow better absorption of nutrients than less frequent, large-volume meals. Trace element supplementation with zinc and vitamin A supplements are of value in prevention of diarrhea and in nutritional rehabilitation. If the possibility of cow's milk protein intolerance exists, withdrawal of cow's milk may be tried. There is no evidence that the routine use of antibiotics has any role in management.

PREVENTION AND CONTROL. Providing clean drinking water and proper sewage disposal reduces the incidence of gut infections. Tube wells are one means of providing clean water. The construction of acceptable latrines will help to break the cycle of fecal-oral transmission of gut pathogens. Health education regarding the importance of good sanitary practices and breast-feeding should be given by trained members of the community.

Vaccination has been of considerable value in controlling many communicable diseases in humans but hitherto has contributed little to the control of gut infections. Cholera vaccination has been used extensively, but the present parenteral preparation gives limited protection for a relatively short time. Oral immunization is the obvious route for vaccination against enteric pathogens. A variety of newer, more effective, and less toxic vaccines are now becoming available.

Control of epidemics of gastrointestinal infection includes finding the source(s) of infection, detection of cases, and treatment, as necessary, to prevent transmission of the disease. Handwashing prevents transmission of enteric infection, as does fly control. The latter may be difficult to maintain but is useful in epidemics, e.g., a shigellosis outbreak.

Malabsorption

Conditions that cause malabsorption in the tropics are listed in Table 4–7.

TROPICAL ENTEROPATHY. Minor degrees of malabsorption occur in patients following diarrhea owing to many causes and in residents of the tropics. Impaired absorption of D-xylose is the usual abnormality, and there are minor abnormalities of the jejunal mucosa. This is referred to as tropical enteropathy and is the usual state in most tropical residents. It is not a stage in the development of other conditions such as tropical sprue. An abnormal jejunal microflora has been found in some of these patients who remain symptomatic after leaving the tropics.

TROPICAL SPRUE

Definition. Tropical sprue (TS) has been defined as impaired absorption of two or more unrelated test substances with no recognized underlying cause. The diagnosis of TS is therefore made by the exclusion of other conditions. A disadvantage of this definition is that it includes no measure of the severity of intestinal dysfunction and so it includes patients with minor abnormalities of absorption who do not develop severe weight loss and the hematologic complications that are so common in TS. The variability of clinical presentations and the absence of a diagnostic test make the study of this condition difficult and raise the query that TS studied in different endemic areas may not be the same disease process.

TABLE 4–7. Causes of Malabsorption in the Tropics and Worldwide

Tropical sprue	Hypolactasia
Chronic calcific pancreatitis	Malnutrition
Parasitic infections	Alpha chain disease
Giardiasis	Intestinal tuberculosis
Cryptosporidiosis	
Strongyloidiasis	
Capillariasis	

Distribution and Incidence. Areas endemic for TS are Central and Southeast Asia, Puerto Rico, Cuba, Haiti, the Dominican Republic, Guatemala, Costa Rica, and Venezuela. Tropical sprue occurs in the Middle East but is rare in Africa. Epidemics of TS have occurred in India.

Both indigenous and expatriate populations are susceptible to TS in endemic areas. Upper and lower socioeconomic groups develop the condition. Black troops from West Africa serving in India were resistant to TS, whereas among Indian troops the incidence of TS was higher in vegetarians. Children are not commonly affected in endemic TS, although in epidemics they often develop it. Tropical sprue may follow a rapidly progressive course in women who are folate-deficient in late pregnancy or the puerperium.

Etiology and Pathogenesis. It is probable that several factors act together to cause TS. Patients often give a history of an acute gastrointestinal infection at the start of their illness, but no particular organism has been incriminated. Some persons affected in epidemic TS were found to be "resistant" to the condition in a second epidemic, suggesting that a single agent might have initiated both epidemics. If TS is simply a postinfective malabsorption syndrome, it is surprising that the condition is so uncommon in children, who have intestinal infections most often.

Gut Bacterial Flora. The jejunum is normally bacteriologically sterile. An abnormal jejunal microflora has been found in patients with TS studied in India and Puerto Rico and in Europeans with TS acquired in Asia and studied later in London. This microflora comprised enterobacteria, with higher yields of organisms from cultures of jejunal biopsy specimens than from aspirated jejunal fluid, suggesting that the organisms are adherent to the mucosa. Bacteria-free filtrates from cultures of these organisms produced net fluid secretion and mucosal changes in isolated loops of intestine in experimental animals. This abnormal microflora may therefore produce one or more toxins that damage the intestinal mucosa, impairing digestive and absorptive functions. Treatment with tetracycline usually eradicates the bacteria and is often associated with resolution of symptoms and intestinal abnormalities.

Reduced gastric acid secretion, which has been found in Indians with TS, and incoordinate to-and-fro movements of intestinal contents with prolonged intestinal transit may be factors that promote and maintain colonization. When fat is infused into the ileum, mouth to cecum transit is slowed. In individuals with TS this could help maintain bacterial colonization. Levels of gut hormones, i.e., enteroglucagon, motilin, and peptide YY, were markedly elevated in TS and these could also delay transit times. If steatorrhea is a major factor in promoting colonization through this ileal effect, it is a matter of speculation as to how this might occur in a patient who is usually anorexic owing to an acute gut infection.

Folic Acid Deficiency. British troops on tinned rations and pregnant and newly delivered women, two conditions causing reduction of folic acid levels, had enhanced susceptibility for TS. Folic acid alone will cure a proportion of patients with TS. Folic acid is a vital cofactor in deoxyribonucleic acid (DNA) synthesis and therefore in the processes of cell replication. Tissues with the highest folate requirements are the bone marrow and the intestinal epithelium. There is a similarity between erythropoiesis and the renewal of villous epithelial cells by crypt cell division. Both processes involve a stem cell compartment containing dividing cells that mature and enter the functional compartment. When folate deficiency is established in TS, disordered epithelial cell renewal may be analogous to disordered erythropoiesis. At this stage, the effects of folate deficiency on the gut may be the dominant abnormality. The cells of both the intestinal epithelium and the bone marrow are turning over rapidly, and so both tissues compete for available folate.

Malnutrition. Body wasting, hypoproteinemia, and depletion of vitamins and trace elements occur in severe TS, indicating malnutrition secondary to anorexia and malabsorption; however, malnutrition alone is not a primary cause of TS.

Immune Response. The prominent infiltrate of plasma cells and lymphocytes in the jejunal mucosa in TS suggests that immunologically mediated events may be occurring. These may be unrelated to the mucosal damage but may be evoked by antigens derived from the jejunal microflora and contribute to tissue damage.

Pathology. Impaired absorption of fat, D-xylose, and vitamin B_{12} is usual. Secondary hypolactasia is common in expatriates of European stock with TS. Red cell folate levels decline with increasing duration of symptoms, and serum vitamin B_{12} levels may be reduced. These changes are associated with macrocytosis in the peripheral blood and, later, megaloblastic anemia. Plasma albumin levels decline, and there is depletion of trace elements, e.g., magnesium and zinc. Protein-losing enteropathy contributes to the low plasma albumin levels.

Nonspecific changes comprising thickening of mucosal folds and dilatation of small bowel loops are seen in small bowel radiologic studies (Fig. 4–1).

Jejunal biopsies are abnormal. A ridged or convoluted mucosa is usually seen on dissecting microscopy (Fig. 4–2). Light microscopy shows reduced villous height with deeper crypts containing increased numbers of cells in mitosis (Fig. 4–3). There is a prominent infiltrate of plasma cells and lymphocytes in the lamina propria and of lymphocytes in the surface epithelium. A completely atrophic mucosa is

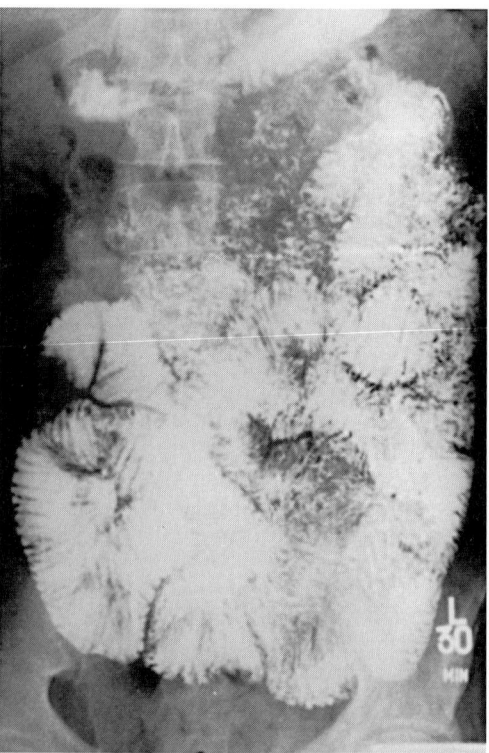

Figure 4–1. Widened loops of small bowel with thickened mucosal folds in a patient with tropical sprue. These are nonspecific signs and also occur in malabsorption due to giardiasis and celiac disease.

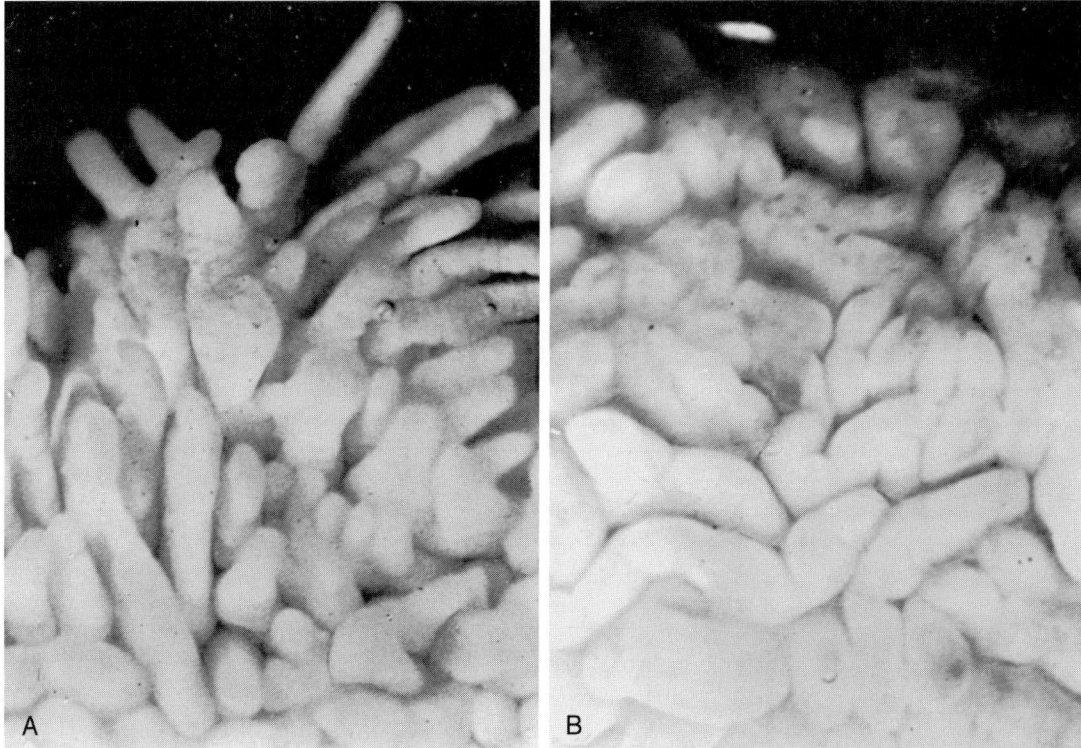

Figure 4–2. Dissecting microscopy of jejunal biopsies ($\times$ 60). *A*, Normal leaf- and finger-shaped villi. *B*, Thick, ridge-shaped, and convoluted villi from a patient with tropical sprue.

rarely seen in TS. The jejunal biopsy of an asymptomatic tropical resident is abnormal by North American standards but can be distinguished from TS by the greater degree of abnormality in TS.

Clinical Manifestations. The patient usually recalls an acute attack of diarrhea at the beginning of the illness, after which his or her bowel habit does not return to normal. Typically, the patient has several bowel actions in the early part of the day and the need may cause awakening from sleep in the early morning. The stools are soft, bulky, pale, and foul-smelling. Bowel actions are often accompanied by the passage of foul-smelling flatus. Abdominal distention and discomfort are commonly noticed. Appetite and energy decline, and the patient loses weight (Fig. 4–4). Patients with symptoms of several months' duration may have a sore tongue and mouth. Examination shows evidence of weight loss with mucosal pallor and glossitis in some patients. Abdominal distention and increased bowel sounds are often present. Rectal examination and sigmoidoscopy are normal.

Complications. The complications of TS are those of continuing diarrhea and malabsorption. Dehydration with electrolyte depletion is common among those patients with watery stools. Depletion of trace elements, e.g., zinc and magnesium, is common in patients having TS for several months. These deficiencies may contribute more to the clinical picture in severe TS than is appreciated at present. Low serum magnesium and calcium levels can cause tetany.

Severe megaloblastic anemia is most often caused by folic acid deficiency, with vitamin B_{12} deficiency being a less common cause. In a few of these patients, the hematologic features predominate, and gastrointestinal symptoms may be minimal or even absent. Subacute combined degeneration of the spinal cord has been seen in one patient with this form of tropical sprue.

Diagnosis. Diagnosis depends on the results of intestinal absorption tests together with abnormalities seen on jejunal biopsy (Figs. 4–2 and 4–3) and a history of residence in endemic areas. Table 4–7 lists other causes of malabsorption that occur worldwide, including the tropics.

Treatment

Diet. Provision of an adequate diet can cure TS. One third of a group of Indian patients were cured by diet alone. A low-lactose diet may control symptoms due to hypolactasia. Some patients are intolerant of fat, and thus a low-fat diet may be necessary. Avoidance of alcohol and foods seasoned with herbs and spices may also help alleviate symptoms.

Antibiotics and Folic Acid. Tetracycline, 250 mg 4 times daily, or doxycycline, 100 mg twice daily, for 1 to 3 months is often effective. Courses of up to 6 months' duration have been used in patients with prolonged TS. Physiologic doses of folic acid, 200 μg per day, will cure TS when there is folate deficiency, but it is usual to give 5 mg daily for a month or more. Tetracycline or doxycycline and folic acid are often given concurrently. A deficiency of vitamin B_{12}, if present, needs correction.

Prognosis. Within 3 months of starting treatment, most patients show considerable improvement (Fig. 4–4), and intestinal absorption and mucosal changes will have improved or returned to normal. Some patients notice an improvement in symptoms within 2 or 3 days of starting treatment. Symptoms and impaired absorption persist in a minority of patients despite all combinations of treatment, in which case the original diagnosis of TS must be reconsidered to ensure that no other cause has been overlooked.

The prognosis in tropical sprue is excellent, and most patients are completely cured. Deaths from TS were reported in the earlier part of this century and in epidemic TS before treatment could be given. The recurrence rate following cure is not known.

PARASITES AND MALABSORPTION. *Giardia lamblia, Cryp-*

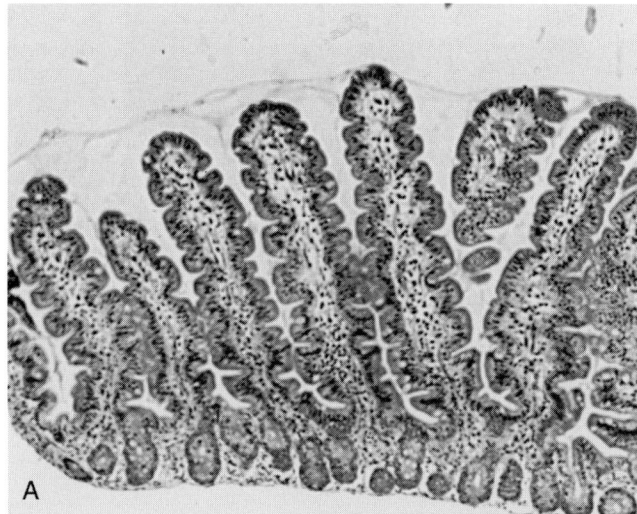

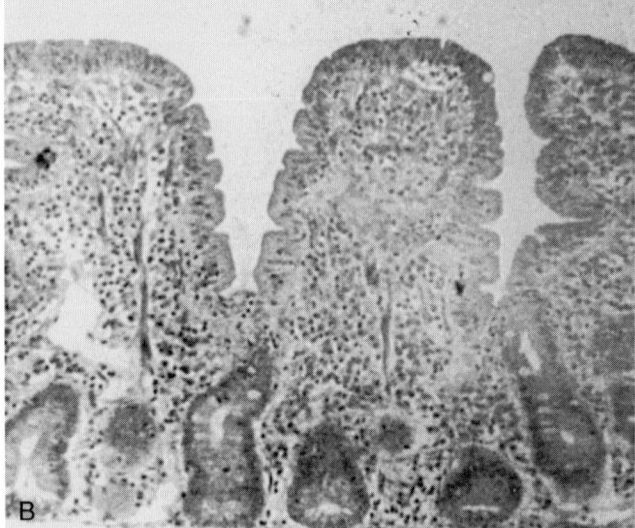

Figure 4–3. Histologic appearance of jejunal biopsies (H&E stain). *A,* Normal mucosa. *B,* Abnormal changes in a patient with tropical sprue of 4 months' duration.

worms in the gut, if sufficient numbers are present, impair food intake and result in declining weight gain. This seems likely to be caused by worm bulk in the gut causing more rapid satiation of appetite. Heavy trichuriasis causes stunting and even dysenteric diarrhea with evidence of increased levels of circulating tumor necrosis factor as a marker of the host inflammatory response in the gut mucosa. There is also concern that intestinal helminthiasis may have adverse effects on intellectual development. These various effects are reversible after effective anthelmintic therapy.

MALNUTRITION. Diarrhea in malnourished patients is caused by increased susceptibility to infections and abnormalities of digestion and absorption (Chapter 133.1). Mucosal changes found in jejunal biopsy specimens range from mucosal atrophy in kwashiorkor to a relatively normal appearance with reduced crypt cell replication in marasmus. An abnormal jejunal bacterial flora has been found in malnourished children with and without diarrhea, although net fluid secretion and reduced glucose absorption were found only in those with diarrhea. Brush border sucrase and lactase levels are reduced, but these increase after refeeding. Each of these functional abnormalities may contribute to diarrhea by the osmotic effects of a high solute load drawing water into the gut lumen. Steatorrhea can be caused by maldigestion of fat due to reduced secretion of pancreatic lipase and by defective fat absorption due to epithelial damage in the jejunum. Protein digestion and absorption are surprisingly well maintained owing to the considerable reserve capacity possessed by the gut. The practical importance of these changes concerns diets to be used in refeeding programs. Animal fats may be poorly tolerated, but vegetable fats can be used as a palatable source of calories in the diet.

CHRONIC CALCIFIC PANCREATITIS. Chronic calcific pancreatitis is a relatively common cause of malabsorption in

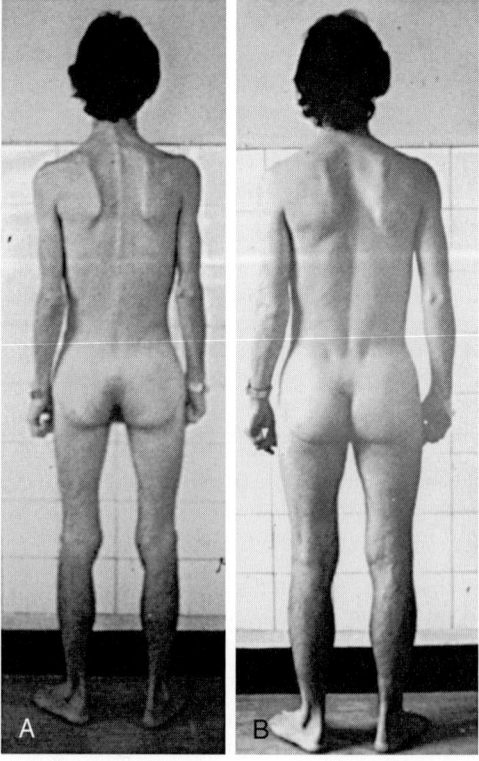

Figure 4–4. *A,* Patient with tropical sprue of 14 weeks' duration acquired during overland travels in Asia. *B,* The same patient 6 weeks after finishing a 6-week course of tetracycline and folic acid.

tosporidium, Cyclospora cayetanenis, Isospora belli, Strongyloides stercoralis, and *Capillaria philippinensis* have all been associated with malabsorption. There is reasonable evidence for this association with giardiasis, although only one fourth of infected patients have gastrointestinal symptoms and less than half of those have malabsorption. Capillariasis causes a severe diarrheal illness with malabsorption and dehydration in well-defined areas in the Philippines and Thailand (Chapter 103.3). Strongyloidiasis is an occasional cause of malabsorption (Chapter 105.2).

Helminths and the Gut. The availability of upper gastrointestinal endoscopy has led to the reporting of series of cases in which ascaris worms have been found in the bile or pancreatic ducts. Some of these patients had fibroscopic endoscopy for nonspecific colicky upper abdominal pain. A few had more severe upper abdominal pain, jaundice due to bile duct obstruction, and ascending biliary tract sepsis and septicemia. Worms can also be demonstrated in these ectopic sites by x-ray contrast studies and by ultrasound scanning (Fig. 104–3).

There is now good evidence to associate growth faltering and overt malnutrition with luminal helminthiasis. Ascaris

East and West Africa and on the Indian subcontinent. Calcific disease causing pain has been reported in children as young as 6 years. Presenting features include recurrent upper abdominal pain, diarrhea with steatorrheic stools, weight loss, and sometimes diabetes mellitus. There are no specific physical signs. Pancreatic calcification is seen on a radiograph of the abdomen in about 50% of cases. Steatorrhea, normal D-xylose absorption, and a normal jejunal biopsy are the usual findings.

Exocrine pancreatic function is abnormal, with reduced secretion of pancreatic enzymes and bicarbonate. There is extensive destruction of glandular acini with marked fibrosis. Diabetes mellitus results from the destruction of insulin-secreting cells. Stones may form in both small and large pancreatic ducts, and removing the stones may reduce symptoms. The cause is unknown, but viral infections, malnutrition, and the toxic effects of cyanide in cassava have all been suggested. Management consists of relief of pain, control of steatorrhea with pancreatic supplements, and insulin for diabetes mellitus.

HYPOLACTASIA. Lactose is a disaccharide and cannot be absorbed intact from the gut. The brush border enzyme lactase hydrolyzes it into glucose and galactose, monosaccharides that are absorbed separately. Lactose is an important source of calories in breast milk, and levels of the enzyme lactase are high at birth. Congenital absence of lactase is extremely rare. In the majority of the world's population, lactase synthesis declines under genetic control over the few years after breast-feeding ceases. Most of the indigenous populations of Africa, Asia, and South America conform to this pattern. Persistence of high lactase levels into adult life is usual among Europeans and North Americans of European ancestry and in Bedouins, Yemenis, the Tutsi of Uganda and Rwanda, and the Punjabis. Lactase is a noninducible enzyme, and therefore, enzyme levels cannot be increased by substrate feeding.

Clinical Manifestations. Nausea, abdominal pain, colic, abdominal distention, flatulence, and diarrhea after drinking milk or taking food containing dairy products are usual symptoms in persons with lactose intolerance from hypolactasia. Some who have hypolactasia as judged by an abnormal lactose tolerance test do not develop symptoms after drinking milk. Many persons are aware of their intolerance and avoid dairy products, whereas others who are intolerant learn this only when they follow a low-lactose diet. The osmotic effects of undigested lactose draw fluid into the gut lumen, causing diarrhea, and lactose is broken down by colonic bacteria, producing other osmotically active molecules, lactic acid, and gas. Children pass acid stools containing reducing sugars. The amount of lactose required to cause symptoms may in fact be relatively high, the equivalent of 240 mL of milk, and so more symptoms may be ascribed to hypolactasia than are actually caused by it.

Diagnosis. A lactose tolerance test can be performed. Capillary blood glucose levels are measured fasting and 15, 30, 60, 90, and 120 minutes after drinking 50 g of lactose dissolved in 400 mL of water. Children are given 2.0 g/kg of body weight. An increase in blood glucose level of less than 1.1 mmol/L (20 mg/dL) over the fasting value indicates hypolactasia. Brush border lactase levels can be measured in jejunal biopsy samples. Typical symptoms usually accompany the lactose tolerance test in patients with hypolactasia.

Treatment. Avoidance of lactose relieves symptoms arising from this condition. Gut infection may cause hypolactasia during the first year of life, when breast milk is essential for adequate nutrition. Enzyme levels will recover at this age, so that breast-feeding should be resumed as soon as the infant wishes.

ALPHA CHAIN DISEASES

Definition. Several names have been used for this disease entity, which is characterized by uncontrolled proliferation of a clone of B cells secreting an abnormal alpha heavy chain in the gut mucosa. A proportion of these cases progresses to develop lymphoma. Because of the geographic distribution of the early cases reported, the term "Mediterranean lymphoma" was used. Subsequently it became apparent that the condition was much more widespread and the term alpha chain disease (αCD) came into use. More recently, the term immunoproliferative small intestinal disease (IPSID) has been introduced, although in this section the older term, which is perhaps more widely known, is used.

Distribution and Epidemiology. The disease occurs most often in poor populations in the tropics and subtropics, with cases reported from the Middle East and the Mediterranean littoral; from West, Central and southern Africa; Asia; and Central and South America. Poverty, poor hygiene, and consequent exposure to gut infections seem to be predisposing factors. Children and young adults are most often affected with a slight predominance of males over females. Although αCD used to be seen in Jewish communities in the Middle East and Mediterranean region, the incidence has declined markedly in children of families that migrated to Israel from these areas, supporting the notion that environmental factors contribute to the etiology. αCD has, however, occurred in migrants who have lived in developed countries for many years. Evidence of genetic predisposition comes from studies that reveal associations with HLA-Aw19, B12, and A9. Chromosomal aberrations have also been documented.

Pathogenesis and Pathology. The disease is caused by uncontrolled proliferation of a clone of B cells derived from the IgA secreting cells of the gut. The cells secrete incomplete immunoglobulin comprising only heavy chains that are themselves deficient in the variable (V_H) and first constant (C_H1) regions. With the association between *Helicobacter pylori* and low-grade gastric lymphoma (Chapter 45), a similar role for organisms in the gut lumen in αCD is suggested in view of the good clinical responses following antibiotic therapy.

The second, third, and fourth parts of the duodenum and the proximal jejunum are areas of maximal involvement, although ileal or total small gut involvement has been reported. Stomach and colonic involvement is even rarer. The mucosa is grossly thickened with infiltrations producing a cobblestone appearance, localized nodules, or polypoid tumors.

The normal villous pattern of the gut is totally effaced by the massive infiltration of plasma cells. Villi are shortened but crypts remain small and are rather buried in the infiltrate. Dystrophic plasma cells are seen in the mucosa. Mature plasma cells occupy the superficial layers of the mucosa while dysplastic B cells are seen in the deeper layers. There may be involvement of mesenteric lymph nodes and liver and spleen but it is very rare for extension to occur outside the abdominal cavity. B-cell immunoblastic sarcoma is the most common transformation into an overtly malignant process, probably derived from the clone of cells exhibiting αCD as shown by the presence of messenger RNA common to both plasma cells and dysplastic cells.

Clinical Manifestations. The disease is characterized clinically by a severe malabsorption syndrome with diarrhea, pale offensive stools, weight loss, lethargy, abdominal distention, hyperpigmentation of the skin, and finger clubbing. Dependent edema and a palpable abdominal mass may also be present. Severe malabsorption is found on testing intestinal function. Anemia from folate deficiency and, less commonly, vitamin B$_{12}$ deficiency occurs. There is protein loss into the gut and serum albumin levels are low. Jejunal biopsy is grossly abnormal on both dissecting microscopy and histology showing the features previously described. Barium studies of the small intestine are abnormal with dilatation of small bowel loops, segmentation of barium and dilution of barium in the early stages, and polypoid tumors in the later stages after malignant transformation has occurred.

Diagnosis. The finding of heavy chains in biologic fluids is diagnostic and is present in up to 70% of cases. Plasma and urine are most readily examined for diagnostic purposes. Occasional cases of nonsecretory αCD are seen. The histologic features are, however, characteristic for this condition. Plasma immunoglobulin levels of all classes are generally reduced. It is common to find infection with several parasitic pathogens, particularly *Giardia lamblia*.

Treatment, Course, and Prognosis. In the early stages of this disease treatment with tetracycline, 2 g/day in divided doses, often has a dramatically beneficial effect. Steroids have often been given with the antibiotic. Abnormal tests of absorption return to normal, protein loss into the gut and symptoms regress markedly, sometimes for prolonged periods, but cure is not frequent and recurrence of disease, often with mass lesions indicating malignant transformation, is common. At this stage the abnormal heavy chains are no longer found, indicating the presence of a much less well differentiated cell type. Combination chemotherapy with potent cytotoxic agents can produce remission but cure is difficult to achieve. A case report of αCD occurring in a patient with *H. pylori,* colonization of the duodenum in whom the manifestations of αCD regressed when the *H. pylori* was treated, raises the possibility of a causative role for this organism in both low-grade gastric lymphoma and αCD.

GLUTEN-SENSITIVE ENTEROPATHY. This condition is uncommon in the tropics, although cases have been reported from Sudan, Saudi Arabia, Libya, and among Asians living in Britain. Diarrhea with pale, offensive stools, weight loss, and sometimes anemia due to folate deficiency are usual presentations. Absorption of D-xylose and fat is usually impaired, but vitamin B$_{12}$ absorption is normal. Severe mucosal atrophy is found in jejunal biopsy samples. Symptoms, functional abnormalities, and morphologic changes resolve when gluten is withdrawn from the diet. Definitive diagnosis is obtained by observing relapse of symptoms, functional impairment, and mucosal changes when gluten is reintroduced into the diet. Lifelong exclusion of gluten from the diet is required.

The usual infant feeding practices in the tropics, with prolonged breast-feeding and delayed introduction of mixed feeding, may protect against this condition.

Protein-Losing Enteropathy

A relatively small amount of protein is normally lost into the gut each day. Acute invasive infections of the gastrointestinal tract cause mucosal inflammation and ulceration, with increased protein loss into the gut. When there is extensive inflammation of the gut, the protein loss may be clinically significant. Protein-losing enteropathy occurs in (1) children with persistent diarrhea after measles; (2) intestinal tuberculosis; (3) obstruction of intestinal lymphatics as a result of tuberculous adenitis, malignancy, or filariasis; (4) granulomatous polyps (caused by *Schistosoma mansoni* infection); and (5) intestinal capillariasis.

Inflammatory Disease of the Large Bowel

The incidence of specific inflammatory disease of the large bowel in the tropics is far greater than that of nonspecific inflammatory bowel disease.

BACTERIAL INFECTIONS

Invasive Organisms. *Salmonella, Shigella, Escherichia coli, Campylobacter,* and *Yersinia* infections (Chapters 40, 42–44, and 76) can all involve the colon, causing diarrhea with blood and pus in the stools. Fever, diarrhea, colicky abdominal pain, dysentery, and tenesmus are presenting features that suggest colonic infection clinically. Generalized abdominal tenderness is a usual physical sign, and the colonic mucosa is abnormal, with inflammation and ulceration seen on proctosigmoidoscopy. An exudate of mucopus is present, and the mucosa bleeds where the instrument makes contact with it. Microscopy of fecal smears shows an exudate of pus cells with a few red cells. Culture of stool samples or rectal swabs gives the bacteriologic diagnosis. Specific antibiotic treatment is indicated in patients with marked symptoms and signs.

Antibiotic-Associated Pseudomembranous Colitis (AAPC). AAPC was first described in patients who had been given lincomycin (Chapter 44.3). During the course of treatment, these patients developed fever and diarrhea. Sigmoidoscopy showed an inflamed mucosa with pseudomembranous plaques adhering to the mucosa. Subsequently, AAPC has been reported in association with a range of antibiotics, including penicillin, ampicillin, co-trimoxazole, and metronidazole. The cause of AAPC is colonic overgrowth with *Clostridium difficile,* which secretes a cytotoxin that causes the pathologic changes. With the widespread use of antibiotics in the tropics, it would be surprising if cases did not occur. Management consists of replacement of lost fluids and oral vancomycin, which is not absorbed from the gut. Metronidazole is a cheaper alternative.

PARASITIC INFECTIONS. Amebic dysentery must always be considered in the differential diagnosis of patients with inflammatory bowel disease (Chapter 86). As with most infectious diseases, there is a range of severity of disease. This varies from mild cases, in which the patient reports a change in bowel habit, with stools that vary in consistency and often contain some blood-stained mucus, to severe cases, in which the patient is febrile and toxic and is passing uniformly blood-stained stools. Mucosal changes seen at sigmoidoscopy vary from the typical appearances of flask-shaped ulcers, with a sloughing base and a surrounding area of mucosal erythema scattered in an otherwise normal mucosa in those mildly affected, to a diffusely ulcerated bleeding mucosa in severe cases. More severe illness is usually associated with more extensive colonic involvement. Fecal smears and scrapes from the rectal mucosa should be examined for motile trophozoites of *Entamoeba histolytica*. Specific treatment with metronidazole or tinidazole produces rapid clinical improvement.

Postdysenteric ulcerative colitis has been described in patients who have been successfully treated for amebic dysentery. Diarrhea with blood and mucus in the stools is usual, and on sigmoidoscopy, an ulcerative colitis is found. Stool examinations for amebas and bacterial pathogens are negative. Histologic changes comprise ulceration of the epithelium, an infiltrate of lymphocytes and plasma cells in the mucosa, and, if full-thickness biopsies are obtained, destruction of the smooth muscle layer. Goblet cell depletion and glandular atrophy are not seen. Barium enemas show mucosal ulceration. Sulfasalazine may produce remission in these patients.

INTESTINAL TUBERCULOSIS. This can affect any part of the gastrointestinal tract, but the ileocecal region is an area of predilection (Chapter 77). Fever, night sweats, and loss of weight over a period of weeks or even months are symptoms that suggest tuberculosis, whereas abdominal pain, swelling of the abdomen due to ascites, diarrhea, malabsorption, and the presence of an abdominal mass raise the question of abdominal involvement. Abdominal tuberculosis is a common cause of ascites in the tropics. About half of patients with intestinal tuberculosis have open pulmonary disease, and therefore the patient's chest should be examined carefully. Tuberculin tests are usually strongly positive in those patients who are adequately nourished but are frequently negative in those whose nutritional state has deteriorated or who have an immunodeficiency. Sputum and gastric washings should be examined for tubercle bacilli. Ascitic fluid should be aspirated for examination, as tubercle bacilli can be found in the fluid; a high protein content with an exudate of lymphocytes suggests a tuberculous etiology. Peritoneal biopsies should be taken when diagnostic paracentesis is performed. Radiographic contrast studies of the gut show a range of changes, including mucosal ulceration, stricture formation, segmental narrowing, and fistula formation. Laparoscopy or laparotomy with microscopic examination and culture of biopsies may be the only means of establishing the diagnosis in some patients. If facilities for investigation are inadequate, it may be necessary to treat the patient on the basis of a clinical diagnosis.

NONSPECIFIC INFLAMMATORY BOWEL DISEASE. Cases of nonspecific inflammatory bowel disease, both ulcerative colitis and Crohn disease, continue to be reported from the tropics, with a progressive increase in the total number of countries from which these reports come. The specific causes of intestinal inflammation must always be considered first. In particular, Crohn disease should not be diagnosed in a patient who lives or has lived in the tropics without first excluding abdominal tuberculosis. In addition, amebiasis can be confused with ulcerative colitis.

Both the specific and the nonspecific causes of intestinal inflammation and ulceration can be complicated by hemorrhage, intestinal perforation, and toxic dilatation.

ENTERITIS NECROTICANS. This rare condition occurs worldwide in premature infants. It is a relatively common condition among children in the highland region of Papua New Guinea, where it seems to be associated with communal pig feasting. Infection with *Clostridium perfringens* type C occurs by ingestion of organisms. The β toxin (Chapter 44.3) is produced in the gut lumen, causing gross thickening, discoloration, or necrosis of the affected gut. The jejunum and ileum are usually affected, but colonic involvement also occurs. Fever, abdominal pain, and bloody diarrhea are usual presenting features; thickened loops of intestine may be palpable. Active immunization against *C. perfringens* type C β toxin has produced a dramatic decline in the incidence of this condition in New Guinea.

Stenosing Lesions of the Colon and Rectum

Stenosing lesions of the bowel can be caused by amebiasis, schistosomiasis, tuberculosis, and lymphogranuloma venereum. The last involves the rectum.

AMEBOMA. The cecum is the most common site for ameboma formation, but any part of the colon may be affected (Chapter 86). Occasionally, multiple amebomas occur in the same patient. Persisting diarrhea with blood in the stools and localized abdominal pain are the usual features, and one or more tender masses may be palpable in the abdomen. The lesion itself consists of granulation tissue with areas of necrosis and fibroblast proliferation. Amebas are often difficult to find, but serologic tests for amebiasis are positive in over 90% of cases. Rapid resolution follows specific treatment, and surgical excision is not required.

SCHISTOSOMIASIS. Granulomatous lesions of the colon due to schistosomiasis can cause narrowing of the bowel.

Early lesions are reversible with antischistosomal treatment. The rare fibrotic strictures that form require surgical removal.

Intestinal Obstruction

MEGACOLON. Colonic involvement with Chagas disease causes chronic constipation and fecal impaction and can predispose to volvulus of the sigmoid colon. These megalesions are irreversible.

ASCARIS OBSTRUCTION. Small bowel obstruction by a large mass of tangled *Ascaris lumbricoides* worms is a relatively common cause of obstruction in children in the tropics (Fig. 104–2).

OTHER CAUSES OF INTESTINAL OBSTRUCTION. Overall strangulated inguinal hernia is probably the most common cause of intestinal obstruction. Volvulus of the small intestine is common in some areas of India and East and South Africa, whereas volvulus of the sigmoid colon is relatively common in South and Central Africa, Brazil, western India, and Pakistan.

Intussusception

This is a relatively common cause of acute abdominal pain in adults in Africa. Cecocolic intussusception is usual in these cases. Amebomas, Burkitt lymphoma, and schistosomal granulomas may be at the apex of the intussusception. Colicky abdominal pain, vomiting, bloody diarrhea, and a palpable abdominal mass are usual clinical features. This condition is uncommon in adults in temperate regions. Among children in the tropics, intussusception is ileoileal or ileocecal, the types found in the temperate regions of the world. The incidence of this condition in childhood is similar worldwide.

Umbilical Hernia

This is a common condition in children of school age in tropical Africa and rarely causes symptoms. The majority of these hernias regress spontaneously.

Rectal Prolapse

This is a relatively common condition in the tropics. Contributing factors include recurrent diarrheal disease, malnutrition, and hyperinfection with *Trichuris trichiura*.

Bibliography

Banwell JG, Hutt MSR, Leonard PJ, et al: Exocrine pancreatic disease and the malabsorption syndrome in tropical Africa. Gut 8:388, 1967.
Cook GC: Tropical Gastroenterology. Oxford, England, Oxford University Press, 1980.
Ferguson A: Diagnosis and treatment of lactose intolerance. Br Med J 283:1423, 1981.
Gledhill T, Leicester RJ, Addis B, et al: Epidemic hypochlorhydria. Br Med J 290:1383, 1985.
Goodwin CS, Mendall MM, Northfield TC: Helicobacter pylori infection. Lancet 349:265, 1997.
Guerrant RL (ed): Diarrhoeal Disease. London, Ballière's Clinical Tropical Medicine and Communicable Diseases, 1989.
Holcombe C: Helicobacter pylori infection: The African enigma. Gut 33:429, 1992.
Reid NW: Diarrhoea, a failure of colonic salvage. Lancet 2:481, 1982.
Sanderson IR, Walker-Smith JA: Indigenous amoebiasis: An important differential diagnosis of chronic inflammatory bowel disease. Br Med J 289:823, 1984.
Speelman P, McGlaughlin R, Kabir I, Butler T: Differential clinical features and stool findings in shigellosis and amoebic dysentery. Trans R Soc Trop Med Hyg 81:549, 1987.
Stoll BJ, Glass RI, Huq MI, et al: Surveillance of patients attending a diarrhoeal disease hospital in Bangladesh. Br Med J 285:1185, 1982.
Suarez FJ, Saraiano DA, Levitt MD: A comparison of symptoms after the consumption of milk or lactose hydrolyzed milk by people with self-reported severe lactose intolerance. N Engl J Med 333:1, 1995.
Weaver LT: Helicobacter pylori infection, nutrition and growth in West African infants. Trans R Soc Trop Med Hyg 89:347, 1995.

5 Hepatobiliary Diseases

Michael A. Dunn

■ IMPORTANCE OF LIVER DISEASE

From ancient times, when the liver was regarded as the core of being by the Babylonians, to the present, when the profound influence of liver cell function on nearly all biochemical events is becoming clear, liver diseases have attracted great interest. This interest is intensified for students of tropical medicine for three reasons.

INCREASED MORBIDITY AND MORTALITY. In nearly all tropical regions, there is an impression that morbidity and death from liver disease are much greater than in other geographic areas. With few exceptions, verification of this impression is difficult, because rigorous population-based data for prevalence and attack rates of most liver diseases are lacking. The personal experience of clinicians and pathologists working in tropical areas supports the idea that most liver diseases are more prevalent in the tropics (Table 5–1). This predominance of liver disease in the tropics is easy to understand in the case of parasitic infections that require specific conditions for their transmission, e.g., schistosomiasis, hydatid disease, and clonorchiasis. It is also easy to account for the high prevalence of those diseases that are more easily transmitted under conditions of poor sanitation, crowding, and close personal contact, e.g., viral hepatitis and amebiasis. There remains a group of poorly understood liver diseases, e.g., as veno-occlusive disease, nonspecific portal fibrosis, and Indian childhood cirrhosis, whose prevalence is certainly greater in the tropics but whose causes and pathogenic mechanisms are poorly defined.

UNKNOWN ETIOLOGY. The second reason liver diseases attract interest in the tropics is that speculation on general causes and effects in liver disease is stimulated by the coexistence of attractive potential etiologic agents and unexplained end results. Perhaps the most intensely discussed topic in this regard has been the unproved concept of nutritional cirrhosis or chronic liver disease of any form resulting from dietary deficiency. One motivation that has fueled this discussion is the long debate on the mechanisms that cause cirrhosis in persons with chronic alcoholism in nontropical countries. The weight of evidence suggests that alcoholic liver disease is a direct result of the hepatotoxicity of alcohol and its metabolic products. However, the multiple effects of alcohol on nutrient absorption and metabolism make it difficult to prove or exclude a nutritional component in the evolution of alcoholic cirrhosis. In this context, the frequent occurrence of cirrhosis in nonalcoholic residents of tropical areas where nutrition is marginal has been used to support the idea of dietary deficiency as a cause of chronic liver disease. Although the concept of overall nutritional deficiency or lack of specific critical nutrients remains attractive to some workers as a possible cause of cirrhosis, the support for this proposal is as lacking in the tropics as it is elsewhere.

FOCAL DISTRIBUTION. The third factor that leads to interest in liver diseases in the tropics is the strikingly localized occurrence of some unique problems. This may be based on the limited geographic range of a parasite; e.g., the occurrence of cholestasis and hepatomegaly in a resident of northeastern Thailand can nearly always be explained by infection with the biliary fluke *Opisthorchis viverrini* (Chapter 120.1), which affects nearly half the population of Thailand's northernmost province. Geographic prevalence also applies strik-

ingly to some forms of nonparasitic disease, e.g., the hemosiderosis occurring in African Bantus, whose method of food preparation and brewing in cast-iron pots subjects them to an extraordinary load of absorbable iron.

■ GEOGRAPHIC DISTRIBUTION

Investigation of the causes of liver disease is more heavily influenced by geography than that of the causes of disease of any other major organ system. This results both from lack of specificity of the clinical manifestations of most liver diseases and from localized distribution of several important problems. The geographic ranges of the diseases covered in this chapter and a notation of other chapters dealing with liver diseases are shown in Table 5–1. Within broad geographic ranges, specific information can be very useful. For example, nearby pairs of villages and settlements in Egypt, the Caribbean, and Brazil have been shown to have very high prevalences or nonexistence of *Schistosoma mansoni* infection. Length of residence and habits of visitors to these regions are important as well: Anyone visiting the Nile delta who has had minimal water contact is unlikely to have hepatic schistosomiasis but may have viral hepatitis. A middle-aged lifelong resident of Haiti with acute hepatitis is unlikely to have hepatitis A, but this would be the most likely cause of acute hepatitis in a northern European visitor to the same country. In inhabitants of developing countries acute hepati-

TABLE 5–1. Liver Diseases Prevalent in the Tropics

Condition	Geographic Distribution
Noninfectious	
Bantu siderosis	Southern Africa
Veno-occlusive disease	Southern Africa, India, Middle East, Caribbean
Indian childhood cirrhosis	Indian subcontinent, Malaysia, Sri Lanka
Infectious	
Viral	
Hepatitis (A; B; C; D; E) (see Chapter 28)	
Yellow fever and other viral hemorrhagic fevers (see Chapter 31)	
Rickettsial, Bacterial, Spirochetal	
Q Fever, brucellosis (see Chapters 34 and 64)	
Syphilis, leptospirosis (see Chapters 48.1 and 72)	
Protozoal	
Amebiasis, malaria (see Chapters 86 and 92)	
Visceral leishmaniasis, toxoplasmosis (see Chapters 95 and 97)	
Helminthic	
Ascariasis, visceral larva migrans (see Chapters 104 and 112)	
Schistosomiasis (Chapter 118)	
Clonorchiasis, opisthorchiasis (see Chapter 120)	
Fascioliasis, dicroceliasis, hydatid disease (see Chapter 120)	

tis in children is frequently caused by hepatitis A or E infection; acute hepatitis in adolescents and adults is usually due to hepatitis B, C, or E virus (see Chapter 28). Although a specific cause of liver disease cannot often be assigned on geographic grounds, a knowledge of the liver diseases prevalent in any location weighs heavily in directing clinical evaluation of a given illness.

▪ CARDINAL MANIFESTATIONS OF LIVER DISEASES

The limited number of clinical responses to a wide variety of causes of liver injury is the same in both tropical and nontropical regions. Specific comments on some of these major findings are relevant.

SUBCLINICAL LIVER INJURY. The majority of the viral, bacterial, and parasitic infections discussed elsewhere in this text have the capacity to cause laboratory evidence of liver injury, not necessarily with direct invasion of the organ. In most cases, there are no clinical manifestations. In some infections, e.g., those with endotoxin-producing gram-negative bacteria, biochemical evidence of cholestasis can be followed by clinically recognizable jaundice that resolves as soon as the primary infection subsides. The main concern in dealing with multisystem infections that cause incidental minor liver injury is to maintain diagnostic and therapeutic focus on the primary problem and to follow the subclinical liver abnormalities to resolution. The orderly evaluation of persistently abnormal biochemical tests, including appropriate serologic tests, imaging procedures, and liver biopsy, is the same in tropical and nontropical areas. A heightened suspicion is in order in tropical residents for chronic active hepatitis, many of the causes of granulomatous hepatitis, secondary syphilis, and the inadvertent use of hepatotoxic drugs.

HEPATOMEGALY. Hepatomegaly in a person of average size is suggested on physical examination by a liver span in the right midclavicular line of more than 12 cm in a man or more than 10 cm in a woman. These limits are not absolute; their accuracy depends on individual skill and consistency in percussion and palpation, and imaging procedures sometimes fail to confirm the liver span measured on physical examination. In general, however, the same examiner will measure liver spans consistently. The character of a palpable liver edge on physical examination can be helpful when a definite finding exists, e.g., pulsations, tenderness, obvious coarse nodularity, or hardness. Findings such as fine nodularity often are not borne out under direct vision at surgery or autopsy. Point tenderness over an expanding amebic abscess is a very important finding that calls for ultrasound-guided therapeutic needle aspiration (see Chapter 86).

Ultrasound Evaluation. Reports from many tropical centers over the last 10 years emphasize the increasing importance of gray-scale ultrasound examination in the evaluation of hepatomegaly. This diagnostic method has become the most widely used supplement to physical examination in most tropical areas for several reasons. In initial investment and operating costs, ultrasound is within the economic reach of many centers in the developing world, whereas computed axial tomography is not. It has supplanted most isotopic imaging procedures in these same areas, where cost and timely delivery of isotopes are limiting factors (see Chapter 21). A major disadvantage of ultrasound over other imaging methods is its dependence on operator skill and experience for accuracy. With an experienced operator, however, accuracy of diagnosis is high for solid masses, e.g., as hepatocellular carcinomas, cystic masses, e.g., pyogenic and amebic abscesses, hydatid cysts that often have distinctive echogenic

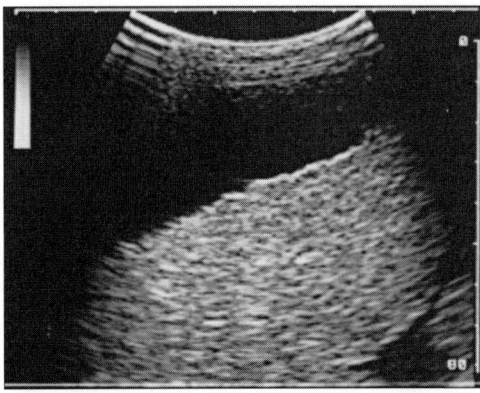

Figure 5–1. Abdominal ultrasonography showing severe cirrhosis with ascites (dark area at top), irregular surface of the liver, and a coarse bright echo pattern caused by the markedly increased fibrosis. (Courtesy of Professor Ahmed Medhat Nasr of Assiut University Faculty of Medicine, Egypt.)

walls and daughter cysts (Figs. 124–8 and 124–11), dilated intrahepatic bile ducts, and the distinctive echogenic patterns of cirrhosis (Fig. 5–1) and schistosomal liver fibrosis (Figs. 5–2 and 118–16). Ultrasonography has now provided the first accurate estimates of the prevalence and severity of Symmers periportal fibrosis in schistosome-infected populations. Serial examinations promise to be a noninvasive method of following the progression or stabilization of this key manifestation of the disease.

Blood Tests. Serum biochemical tests of aminotransferase and other enzyme activities are not often helpful in choosing the most likely cause of either diffuse hepatomegaly or a focal lesion. Plasma protein patterns are mainly useful in confirming that chronic liver disease exists. Positive serologic tests for antibody to hepatitis A, B, and C viruses are common in most tropical areas. The high prevalence of such viral markers limits the confidence with which one can implicate viral hepatitis as the cause of a given case of liver injury without tissue confirmation (Chapter 28). The most useful tests that help to confirm a specific diagnosis are an α-fetoprotein level of more than 400 ng/mL, which strongly

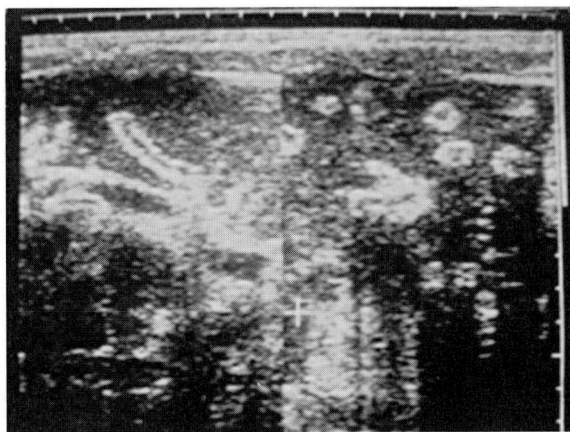

Figure 5–2. Abdominal ultrasonography showing grade III periportal fibrosis in an Egyptian patient with *Schistosoma mansoni* infection. Linear views of fibrosed portal tracts are seen on the left and in the right center; cross-sectional views are present on the right. (Courtesy of Professor Ahmed Medhat Nasr of Assiut University Faculty of Medicine, Egypt.)

suggests hepatocellular carcinoma, and a positive serologic test for invasive amebiasis. Serologic tests for schistosomiasis and echinococcosis are helpful in the diagnosis of individuals who have had only recent exposures to these infections, but their results are problematic in inhabitants from endemic areas. The presence of specific antibody represents only prior exposures to the agents; it does not mean that the patient is currently infected or that the current illness is caused by the parasite (see Chapter 152).

Diagnosis. History, physical examination, and an imaging procedure such as gray-scale ultrasonography help to determine whether hepatomegaly is focal or diffuse. In the case of focal lesions, imaging results and supplementary laboratory tests aid in selecting medical therapy, diagnostic or therapeutic needle aspiration, or surgical therapy for abscesses, tumors, or cysts. If diffuse hepatomegaly is not simply part of an obvious multisystem illness, e.g., malaria, visceral leishmaniasis, lymphoma, or right heart failure, strong consideration should be given to obtaining tissue by needle biopsy for accurate diagnosis and appropriate therapy.

JAUNDICE. The common mechanisms that govern the excretion and retention of bilirubin, bile salts, and other organic compounds have particular relevance to several tropical diseases. The normal daily production of unconjugated bilirubin is taken up in hepatocytes and conjugated to glucuronic acid before excretion into the bile ducts. In the event of failure of this excretion pathway, conjugated bilirubin that refluxes from hepatocytes into plasma can be filtered and excreted in the urine. The jaundice that occurs in a severe episode of malaria illustrates these principles. The hemolysis that results from heavy parasitemia or the severe hemolysis that sometimes results from administration of primaquine to persons with glucose-6-phosphate dehydrogenase deficiency (see Chapter 6) overwhelms the bilirubin uptake and conjugation capacity of even a normal liver. If liver blood flow falls below that required to maintain normal cellular perfusion, bilirubin conjugation and excretion are directly impaired. Any viral or bacterial illness that affects hepatic uptake and excretion of bilirubin may also cause jaundice, which can become especially prominent when renal impairment blocks the secondary pathway for bilirubin excretion, as in leptospirosis.

Diagnosis. Evaluation of the biliary tract for evidence of mechanical obstruction is appropriate in the event that jaundice is accompanied by hepatomegaly, chills, fever, or abdominal pain. Once again, gray-scale ultrasonography is the most convenient and reliable screening method to detect dilated bile ducts proximal to a mechanical obstruction. When required, direct contrast imaging by endoscopic retrograde cholangiography or fine-needle percutaneous cholangiography is performed, especially when surgical relief of mechanical duct obstruction is being planned. A stool examination may suggest that helminthic infection is responsible for bile duct obstruction. *Fasciola* (Fig. 5–3), *Dicrocoelium*, *Ascaris*, and *Clonorchis* can cause mechanical obstruction while alive; dead adult *Ascaris* and *Clonorchis* organisms in the ductal system can become a nidus for stone formation as well. Cholangiocarcinoma (Chapter 12) is a late complication of infection with *Clonorchis* and *Opisthorchis* biliary flukes.

ACUTE HEPATIC FAILURE. Fortunately, massive necrosis of a previously normal liver is a rare event. As in nontropical areas, a few persons with acute viral hepatitis, some immunologically deficient patients with opportunistic viral or fungal infection, and some victims of toxin ingestion, e.g., phosphorus or carbon tetrachloride, will die of acute hepatic insufficiency. Of specific interest is that acute hepatic failure occurs in some persons with Rocky Mountain spotted fever,

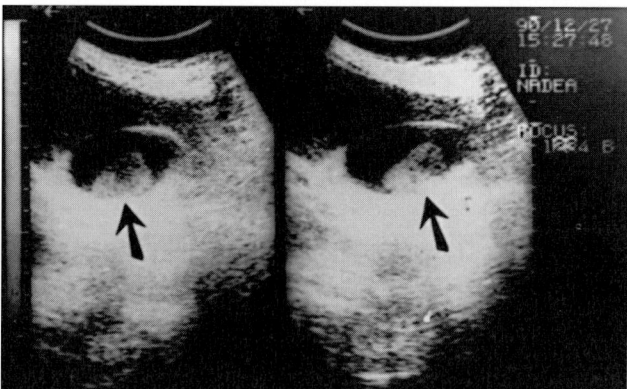

Figure 5–3. Abdominal ultrasound examination of Egyptian farmer demonstrating a *Fasciola hepatica* fluke in the gallbladder. (Courtesy of Gamal Esmet, M.D.)

yellow fever, and some of the other hemorrhagic fevers (see Chapter 31). In all these cases, intensive physiologic support with attention to correction of hypoxia, hypoglycemia, cerebral edema, and hemorrhagic tendencies is needed to promote recovery. When recovery occurs, liver structure and function return to normal.

CHRONIC LIVER INJURY. The bulk of morbidity and death from liver disease is associated with chronic liver injury, with permanent distortion of architecture and disturbance of normal circulation. The number of functioning hepatocytes in persons dying of chronic liver disease is usually more than sufficient to sustain life; failure of adequate circulation to these cells is of prime importance in the chronic liver failure of cirrhosis. Liver cirrhosis requires two components: (1) distortion of normal architecture and blood flow by an excessive deposition of fibrous tissue, and (2) the presence of regenerative nodules of liver cells. Because the cells within these regenerative nodules are not adequately perfused, their contribution to overall liver function is impaired.

The symptoms, findings, and supportive therapy of patients with cirrhosis in the tropics are the same as those for persons in other areas. A number of other chronic liver diseases occur in tropical areas; they sometimes cause changes such as portal hypertension without leading to the regenerative nodule formation of cirrhosis. Among these diseases are portal fibrosis and hepatic schistosomiasis (see Chapter 118).

Assignment of a specific etiology to explain the manifestations of chronic liver disease in a tropical population can be both difficult and critically important in planning control measures. Perhaps the most important current example of this problem is the occurrence of chronic liver failure in persons with *Schistosoma mansoni* infection. The normal liver architecture seen with schistosomal liver fibrosis (Fig. 5–2) should not be associated with any manifestations of chronic liver disease other than presinusoidal portal hypertension. When they occurred, hepatic encephalopathy, hemostatic defects, jaundice, and ascites were viewed as end stages of schistosomiasis in persons with this infection, without any clear explanation. We now know that the majority of schistosome-infected persons who present with these signs of chronic liver failure have coexisting hepatitis B or C infection, with chronic active hepatitis and cirrhosis on histologic examination. It is not yet clear whether this represents the additive effects of two common diseases or whether chronic schistosome infection and chronic hepatitis B or C infection, both immunosuppressive states, might predispose to mutual morbidity. The practical implications of answering this question are great; eradication of schistosomiasis has been a costly and largely unsuccessful venture in economically undeveloped regions. On the other hand, hepatitis B vaccination may afford lifelong protection against a substantial share of the morbidity once attributed to schistosomiasis alone. Clearer definition of the possible interactions between these two conditions will be critical in planning efforts directed at either one.

■ GEOGRAPHIC LIVER DISEASES

Portal fibrosis, idiopathic cirrhosis, Bantu siderosis, Indian childhood cirrhosis, and veno-occlusive disease are all tropical clinical problems that are addressed in detail elsewhere in this text.

PORTAL FIBROSIS. The normal portal tract contains a supporting framework of connective tissue, composed mainly of a family of structural proteins, the collagens. Portal tracts contain collagen types I and III, which are associated with nearly all interstitial supporting tissues, and additional collagens associated with basement membrane structures. Fibrosis can be defined as a net increase in the collagen content of an organ, which usually occurs in such a way as to distort normal architecture and circulation. In the case of hepatic schistosomiasis, the primary disturbance is disruption of normal portal inflow by extensive portal fibrosis. In cirrhosis, regenerative nodules of liver cells further disrupt normal architecture and circulation.

An incidental finding in many biopsy and autopsy liver specimens from tropical centers, especially in Africa, is an increase in portal tract connective tissue. As with all other examples of liver fibrosis, this increase includes all the collagen types normally present in the portal tract; there are no new or distinctive collagens associated with portal fibrosis. The degree of fibrosis present is usually not sufficient to interfere with normal circulation; clinically manifest portal hypertension is not usually a problem; and serum biochemical tests are normal. There is no evidence of inflammation or liver cell necrosis adjacent to the portal tract, as would be the case in chronic hepatitis. The finding is not present in nontropical residents of African descent, so that it appears to be acquired rather than inherited, in much the same way as the occurrence of the blunted-villus intestinal histology of asymptomatic tropical residents. Its cause is unknown; there is no evidence that it progresses to significant parenchymal liver disease; and no therapy other than reassurance is needed.

IDIOPATHIC CIRRHOSIS. The frequency of the finding of liver cirrhosis on autopsy in most tropical countries is considerably greater than it is in nontropical regions. In most cases, the architectural pattern is macronodular or mixed macronodular and micronodular. Before the development of serum and tissue markers for hepatitis B and C virus infection, no clear-cut cause could be assigned to the majority of these cases. As autopsy material is studied more intensively with the full range of viral tissue markers, the bulk of previously unexplained cirrhosis seems to be attributable to chronic hepatitis B and/or C infection in many tropical areas (Chapter 28). There remain a substantial number of cases of unexplained cirrhosis in the tropics. Their assessment awaits development of reliable tissue assays for other viral etiologic agents.

BANTU SIDEROSIS. Among the Bantu residents of southern Africa, there is a high prevalence of cirrhosis associated with iron overload. Use of cast-iron vessels for cooking and brewing beer leads to oral ingestion of huge quantities of absorbable iron that exceed the regulatory capability of the normal intestinal control mechanisms that limit iron absorption. Hepatic iron stores in Bantus with cirrhosis match those of persons with idiopathic hemochromatosis. The disease differs from inherited hemochromatosis in several important respects, however. There is extensive reticuloendothelial as well as parenchymal iron deposition in the liver in Bantu siderosis. Once cirrhosis develops, its rate of progression to liver failure and death is considerably more rapid than that of hemochromatosis, which tends to remain clinically stable over many years. The strong association of excessive alcohol consumption in concert with the iron loading makes primary assignment of alcohol or iron as the key injuring agent problematic. Although iron deposits in other tissues may sometimes occur in a similar pattern to that of idiopathic hemochromatosis, their extent and the occurrence of clinically significant organ damage such as diabetes and heart failure are much less common in Bantu siderosis than they are in idiopathic hemochromatosis.

INDIAN CHILDHOOD CIRRHOSIS. This important disease of children on the Indian subcontinent and in Malaysia, Burma, and Sri Lanka is a rapidly progressive illness of unknown cause that usually leads to death from hepatic failure within a year of the initial manifestations of liver injury. Its onset can resemble that of acute hepatitis, or it can present with failure to thrive and well-developed evidence of chronic liver failure and portal hypertension.

Indian childhood cirrhosis is generally believed to be a disease of dietary copper overload. There is a positive family history in one third of the cases. The histologic appearance of liver biopsy specimens is distinctive, with focal intralobular inflammation and necrosis; Mallory alcoholic hyaline, rapidly progressive fibrosis involving the whole lobular structure; and development of a micronodular cirrhosis with relatively little regenerative activity. There is striking cytoplasmic copper overload, with liver copper contents as high as those of Wilson's disease or biliary cirrhosis. Rhodamine stains for copper and orcein stains for copper-binding protein are positive. Unlike in Wilson's disease, however, there are no Kayser-Fleischer corneal rings or basal-ganglion abnormalities, and serum ceruloplasmin levels are normal. As with Wilson's disease, however, penicillamine therapy to remove the copper overload can stabilize and dramatically improve the status of affected patients. Therapy is more effective in precirrhotic disease, but is appropriate even in the presence of established cirrhosis.

VENO-OCCLUSIVE DISEASE. Postsinusoidal hepatic outflow tract obstruction can occur at any level from the hepatic venules to the right side of the heart. In a number of tropical regions, particularly the Middle East, Jamaica, India, and southern Africa, a common cause of hepatic outflow tract obstruction is occlusion of the small intrahepatic venules. In nearly all locations where veno-occlusive disease occurs, it has been associated with ingestion of pyrrolidizine alkaloids, plant-derived compounds found in herbal teas as well as in contaminated grain. Depending on the opportunity for toxin exposure, veno-occlusive disease is predominantly a pediatric problem. Clinical findings include rapidly progressive ascites (Fig. 5-4), tender hepatomegaly, clinically evident portosystemic collaterals, wasting, anorexia, and death from liver failure or variceal bleeding. There are a few reports of spontaneous resolution of the illness with restoration of normal liver function and development. A key finding on most adequate liver biopsy specimens is marked proliferation of the intima of the small hepatic venules. Presence of organized clots in larger hepatic veins can sometimes be seen in veno-occlusive disease, but they are more commonly found with more distal outflow tract obstructions such as the Budd-Chiari syndrome of hepatic vein thrombosis, membranous

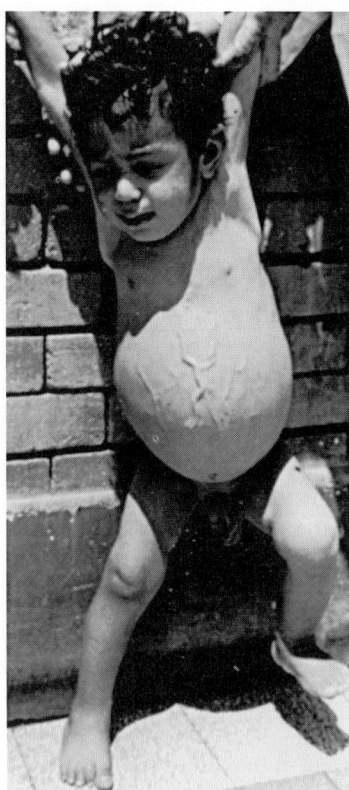

Figure 5–4. Egyptian child with acute onset of severe ascites and hepatomegaly due to veno-occlusive disease. In Egypt, the disease occurs more frequently in male children younger than 5 years of age from rural areas. They often have some evidence of malnutrition. Note distended collateral veins across the abdomen. (Courtesy of Professors I. M. Fayad and M. Safouh, Cairo University Faculty of Medicine.)

webs of the hepatic vein or vena cava, or constrictive pericarditis.

Evaluation should include an attempt to define the level of obstruction in order to exclude treatable alternative problems, such as vena cava webs and right-sided obstruction to cardiac inflow. When available, right heart and vena caval catheterization with pressure measurements and injection of contrast medium into the hepatic vein ostia is useful for this purpose. In theory, relief of the postsinusoidal portal hypertension by construction of a side-to-side portosystemic shunt might benefit patients who could tolerate extensive surgery, as has been proposed for therapy of the Budd-Chiari syndrome. However, at present, there is no basis of experience to recommend such a procedure in veno-occlusive disease.

HUMAN IMMUNODEFICIENCY VIRUS INFECTION. The acquired immunodeficiency syndrome (AIDS) pandemic caused by the human immunodeficiency virus (HIV) has had a devastating impact on health in many tropical areas (see Chapter 22). Liver involvement by Kaposi's sarcoma, lymphoma, and the usual opportunistic infections is evident in many patients, with hepatomegaly, abnormal hepatic blood tests, and liver biopsy abnormalities each present in at least two thirds of those with overt disease. The biopsy findings are generally either nonspecific or attributable to infectious or malignant processes that are clinically evident elsewhere. Death from liver failure is not a usual outcome of AIDS. Clinically severe visceral leishmaniasis (see Chapter 95) is being recognized with increasing frequency in HIV-infected

persons, in some cases many years after their last potential exposure to leishmanial infection. In such patients, it has been proposed that visceral leishmaniasis should be recognized as an AIDS-defining illness on the same basis as *Pneumocystis* pneumonia or Kaposi's sarcoma. An unusual syndrome of cholestasis in AIDS patients has been attributed to biliary tract infection with cytomegalovirus or cryptosporidia, leading to stenosis at the papilla of Vater and sclerosing cholangitis. Endoscopic sphincterotomy is often helpful in relieving itching and jaundice and minimizing recurrence of superimposed bacterial cholangitis.

Bibliography

Abdel-Wahab MF, Esmat G, Milad M, et al: Characteristic sonographic pattern of schistosomal hepatic fibrosis. Am J Trop Med Hyg 40:72, 1989.

Albrecht H, Sobottka I, Emminger C, et al: Visceral leishmaniasis emerging as an important opportunistic infection in HIV-infected persons living in areas nonendemic for *Leishmania donovani*. Arch Pathol Lab Med 120:189, 1996.

Bavdekar AR, Bhave SA, Pradham AM, et al: Long term survival in Indian childhood cirrhosis treated with d-penicillamine. Arch Dis Child 74:32, 1996.

Bras G, Brooks SEH, Walter DC: Cirrhosis of the liver in Jamaica. J Pathol Bacteriol 82:503, 1961.

Cook GC (ed): Imported Gastrointestinal Diseases. London, BMJ Publishing Group, 1995.

Higginson J, Gerritsen T, Walker ARP: Siderosis in the Bantu of South Africa. Am J Pathol 29:779, 1953.

Kamel MA, Miller FD, El Masry AG, et al: The epidemiology of *Schistosoma mansoni*, hepatitis B and hepatitis C infection in Egypt. Ann Trop Med Parasitol 88:501, 1994.

Lebovics E, Dworkin BM, Heier SK, Rosenthal WS: The hepatobiliary manifestations of human immunodeficiency virus infection. Am J Gastroenterol 83:1, 1988.

Lyra LG, Reboucas F, Andrade ZA: Hepatitis B surface antigen carrier state in hepatosplenic schistosomiasis. Gastroenterology 71:641, 1976.

Safouh M, Shehata AH: Hepatic vein occlusion disease of Egyptian children. J Pediatr 67:415, 1965.

Schneiderman DJ, Cello JP, Laing FC: Papillary stenosis and sclerosing cholangitis in the acquired immunodeficiency syndrome. Ann Intern Med 106:546, 1987.

Strickland GT: Gastrointestinal manifestations of schistosomiasis. Gut 35:1334, 1994.

Tandon BN, Tandon RK, Tandon HD, et al: An epidemic of veno-occlusive disease of the liver in central India. Lancet 2:271, 1976.

6 Hematologic Diseases

Alan F. Fleming

■ ANEMIA

Definition and Prevalence

The World Health Organization (WHO) has proposed levels of hemoglobin concentration considered normal for age, sex, and pregnancy status (Table 6–1). There is no evidence of racial differences in hemoglobin concentration in the absence of recognized genetic or environmental factors.

Anemia is possibly the most common manifestation of disease in the tropics, and is most prevalent during pregnancy and the first 5 years of life, periods during which it is estimated that over half the population is anemic (Table 6–2).

Anemias of Infection

MALARIA. About 40% of the world's population, or 2200 million people, are exposed to malaria, and there are 300 to 500 million clinical illnesses per year with about 2 million

TABLE 6–1. Hemoglobin Concentrations Below Which Anemia Is Likely in Populations Living at Sea Level

	Hemoglobin (g/L)
Newborn infants	140
6 months–6 years	110
6–14 years	120
Adult males	130
Adult females—nonpregnant	120
Adult females—pregnant	110

From World Health Organization: Nutritional anaemias. Technical Report Series No. 503. Geneva, WHO, 1972.

deaths, mostly due to *Plasmodium falciparum* infections of children in sub-Saharan Africa. Even these figures from the WHO are underestimates: In Garki, northern Nigeria, the average prevalence in five surveys was 90% for *P. falciparum* and about 40% for *Plasmodium malariae* among children aged 1 to 8 years; the infant mortality rate was 135/1000 per year and childhood mortality rate was 154/1000 per year. Antimalarial intervention (mass drug administration, insecticide spraying, and larvicide) reduced both infant and childhood mortality by 60%, demonstrating the large numbers of deaths due directly or indirectly to malaria. *P. falciparum* causes serious morbidity and mortality directly through cerebral malaria and anemia; the proportions of African children with life-threatening malaria who have severe anemia is between one fourth and one half.

Mechanisms. Anemia is an inevitable and serious complication of malaria, especially with *P. falciparum* infection (Chapter 92). The intracellular development of parasites results in the intravascular rupture of red cells, but anemia is always greater and persists longer than can be explained by the number of parasitized red cells. Other mechanisms of anemia are either hemolytic or through disturbed red cell production.

Following infection there is lymphoid and macrophage hyperplasia, with enhancement of phagocytic activity. The spleen becomes enlarged, and both nonparasitized and parasitized red cells are pooled in the spleen and phagocytosed. Up to 50% of patients with acute malaria show positive direct Coombs tests, due to the adsorption of immunoglobulin (Ig) G, immune complexes, and complement; in most patients,

this does not indicate an autoimmune hemolysis, but it could be contributory in patients whose hemolysis is prolonged for weeks after clearing parasitemia, especially during pregnancy.

During the stage of parasitemia, the release of reticulocytes from the bone marrow is suppressed. With recurrent malaria, there is severe dyserythropoietic disturbance: the red cell precursors, or normoblasts, show cytoplasmic vacuolation, basophilic stippling, intracytoplasmic bridges, nuclear fragmentation (karyorrhexis), incomplete and unequal nuclear division, and multinuclearity. Red cell production and release are suppressed. Possible mechanisms include the packing of marrow sinusoids with parasitized red cells or tumor necrosis factor (TNF) mediation.

Malaria is immunosuppressive and is often complicated by secondary bacterial or viral infection, especially of the respiratory and gastrointestinal tracts. Malarial anemia tends to be most severe in those with other infections. Coincidental infections with malaria and parvovirus B19 are probable causes of epidemics of profound anemia.

Clinical Manifestations. There are two major clinical patterns: (1) acute malaria in the nonimmune, and (2) recurrent malaria. With acute malaria, the hematocrit starts to fall 24 to 48 hours after onset of symptoms, and continues to decline during parasitemia and after the parasitemia is cleared. With recurrent malaria, there is splenomegaly and children present with anemia that may be severe but with only scanty asexual forms and some gametocytes in their peripheral blood films.

Hematologic Manifestations. The anemia of malaria in children and others who are nonimmune may be profound; hemoglobin (Hb) concentrations less than 20 g/L are not uncommon. The red cells show anisocytosis, with both microcytes and macrocytes; during recovery, in the second week, macrocytosis and polychromasia predominate. In the first 2 days, there is a neutrophilic leukocytosis, but later there is a moderate neutropenia. From the second week, there is often considerable neutrophilic leukocytosis, with the release into blood of young forms of neutrophils, with toxic granulation and vacuolation of the cytoplasm, especially if there are complicating bacterial infections; rarely, there is a myeloid leukemoid reaction. There is a monocytosis, frequently with vacuolated cytoplasm or cytoplasm containing malarial pigment. The lymphocyte count is raised, with numerous transformed cells with dark blue–staining cytoplasm (on Romanowsky stain), large nuclei with nucleoli, and occasional

TABLE 6–2. Estimated Prevalence of Anemia by Geographic Region, Age, and Sex (Circa 1980)*

	Children						Women						Men		
	0–4 Years			5–12 Years			(15–49 Years)						(15–49 Years)		
							Pregnant			All					
	Total	Anemic	%	Total	Anemic	%	Total	Anemic	%	Total	Anemic	%	Total	Anemic	%
Africa	85.7	48.0	56	96.6	47.3	49	17.9	11.3	63	106.4	46.8	44	116.8	23.4	20
South Asia	212.0	118.7	56	278.4	139.2	50	41.7	27.1	65	329.4	191.0	58	386.3	123.6	32
East Asia	16.1	3.2	20	25.4	5.6	22	2.7	0.5	20	46.9	8.4	18	55.8	6.1	11
Europe	33.4	4.7	14	55.0	2.7	5	5.7	0.8	14	117.5	14.1	12	147.2	3.0	2
North America	19.6	1.6	8	27.5	3.6	13	3.4	—	—	64.2	5.1	8	76.3	3.1	4
Developing regions	395.0	183.2	51	456.8	208.3	46	71.0	41.9	59	539.5	255.7	47	621.2	162.2	26
Developed regions	86.1	10.3	12	130.7	9.1	7	14.8	2.0	14	285.5	32.7	11	346.5	12.0	3
World	445.1	193.5	43	587.6	217.4	37	85.8	43.9	51	825.0	288.4	35	967.7	174.2	18

*Population data in millions. China excluded. Anemia is defined as hemoglobin concentration below World Health Organization reference values for age, sex, and pregnancy status. Modified from DeMaeyer E, Adiels-Tegman M: World Health Statistics Q 38:302, 1985.

plasma cells. There is invariably a moderate thrombocytopenia during the acute phase of malaria: severe thrombocytopenia is unusual. There is activation of the coagulation cascade and of natural anticoagulants (e.g., antithrombin III [AT III]), but progression to disseminated intravascular coagulation (DIC) is seen only rarely in disease with severe complications.

Examination of the bone marrow may show either erythroid hyperplasia or hypoplasia, and increasing degrees of dyserythropoiesis with recurrent malaria. A neutrophil precursor proliferation is seen whenever there is a secondary bacterial infection. Lymphocyte numbers are increased, with many showing activation or transformation to plasma cells. Monocytes and macrophages are increased, showing vacuolation and deposits of malarial pigment. Intracellular iron may be seen only in the macrophages with no sideroblasts, but is absent with coincidental iron deficiency.

In the acute phase response, serum iron is reduced, serum transferrin is normal or low, and serum ferritin is greatly increased. The red cell folate is raised, possibly because of synthesis by the plasmodia. The estimation of serum ferritin in assessment of iron stores and of red cell folate in the diagnosis of folate deficiency are almost valueless in children exposed to malaria. Serum nonconjugated bilirubin is high because of hemolysis, and serum haptoglobin is chronically low.

Malaria in the Partially Immune. In immune adults, recurrent malaria causes a constant moderate hemolysis with compensatory erythroid hyperplasia; the mean hemoglobin in such a population is around 20 g/L lower for both sexes at all ages than in populations not exposed. There is moderate anisocytosis, with some macrocytes and microcytes and occasional polychromatic red cells. This balance is disturbed in two conditions, namely, pregnancy and (less commonly) hyperreactive malarial splenomegaly (HMS).

Malaria in Pregnancy. Malaria is more severe in pregnant than in nonpregnant women (Chapter 92). Pregnant women with low or no immunity to *P. falciparum,* for example in southern Africa, present with severe acute malaria, often complicated by cerebral malaria, renal failure, blackwater fever, profound anemia, and DIC. There are high rates of abortion, premature delivery, and perinatal and maternal mortality.

In areas where malaria is hyper- or holoendemic and adults have high levels of immunity, the frequency of palpable splenomegaly approximately doubles in pregnant women of all gravidae classes, the peak frequency of palpable spleens being reached before 16 weeks of gestation (Fig. 6–1). In primigravidae, and in gravidae 2 where malaria is less stable, the frequency and density of malaria parasitemia increase also, to peak in the second trimester. However, parasite densities are not as great as those in childhood, and patients are either asymptomatic or have only minor complaints. The chief pathologic finding is extravascular hemolysis leading to anemia, most commonly in the second trimester (Fig. 6–1). Compensatory erythroid hyperplasia increases demands for folic acid so that the hemolytic anemia is complicated frequently by megaloblastic erythropoiesis. Anemia is often profound and life-threatening, but in the majority of patients there is a rapid response to antimalarials and folic acid. In about 25%, the hypersplenism of HMS makes a major contribution, and the hematocrit response to treatment is slow. In about 5%, there is an immune hemolysis, so that the hematocrit constantly falls, necessitating frequent transfusions of blood unless corticosteroids are given.

In general, there is no interaction between malaria and the human immunodeficiency virus (HIV); in pregnancy, however, *P. falciparum* parasitemia frequency and density and

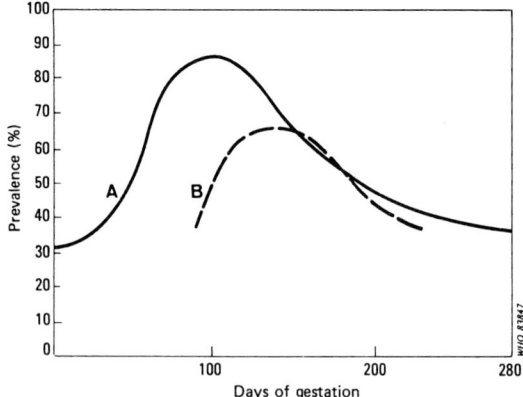

Figure 6–1. Prevalence of *P. falciparum* parasitemia *(A)* and hemolytic anemia associated with splenomegaly *(B)* in pregnancy. (From Brabin BJ: Bull WHO 61:1005, 1983. Reprinted by permission.)

infection of the placenta are all greater in HIV-infected than in noninfected women of all gravida classes.

Hyperreactive Malarial Splenomegaly (HMS). In the great majority of people exposed to endemic malaria, the spleen diminishes in size (although still remaining larger than the typical size in nonmalarial areas) once a degree of immunity has been acquired during childhood. A small proportion of adults living where malaria of any species is endemic have HMS. This is characterized by gross splenomegaly, hypersplenism, a polyclonal B-lymphocyte proliferation, excessively high IgM levels, and raised titers of antibodies against the predominant species of malaria. Other evidence associating the condition with malaria epidemiologically is an almost total protection afforded by sickle cell trait, and a slow but complete recovery with the administration of antimalarial prophylactics. The condition is more common in populations that have been exposed to endemic malaria for relatively few generations, and appears to be genetically determined. Subjects with HMS have a persistence of malaria-induced IgM lymphocytotoxic antibodies, which reduce the numbers of T-suppressor (CD8+) lymphocytes, allowing for an uncontrolled polyclonal proliferation of B lymphocytes (Chapter 92).

There is pooling in the spleen of granulocytes, platelets, and red cells up to one third of the total red cell volume, and an expansion of the plasma volume. There is a pancytopenia as a consequence of pooling, destruction in the spleen, and dilution of the circulating blood cells. The lymphocyte count is usually in the range of 1.0 to 4.0 × 10^9/L, but in about 15% of patients the peripheral blood lymphocyte count is from 40 to 100 × 10^9/L, and the condition may be mistaken for chronic lymphatic leukemia (CLL): the two conditions may be distinguished, inasmuch as IgM levels are low (unless there is a paraprotein) and the lymphocytes are unreactive to mitogens in CLL, with the opposite true in HMS.

It has been suspected for many years that HMS may be a premalignant condition liable to progress to a lymphoma. Recent evidence from Ghana suggests that some patients with HMS may develop splenic lymphoma with villous lymphocytes (SLVL).

VISCERAL LEISHMANIASIS. *Leishmania donovani* infects macrophages throughout the reticuloendothelial system. There is a progressive hyperplasia of macrophages and lymphocytes, massive production of IgG antibodies, and hepatosplenomegaly (Chapter 95). Spleen size, hypersplenism, and pancytopenia are all directly related to the duration of the infection. Pancytopenia is particularly severe in patients who are infected also with HIV. Other mechanisms of hemolysis have been postulated, but hypersplenism is certainly the main factor. The picture may be complicated by megaloblastic erythropoiesis secondary to high demands for folic acid. Neutropenia may be profound and lead to severe secondary infections, especially in children.

Thrombocytopenia can cause spontaneous epistaxis and bleeding from mucosal surfaces. Monocyte and lymphocyte counts are raised, occasionally to leukemoid levels. The bone marrow is generally hyperplastic; chronic kala-azar can be complicated by marrow hypoplasia, gelatinous transformation, dyserythropoiesis, or myelofibrosis with continued hypersplenism.

AFRICAN TRYPANOSOMIASIS. Infection by *Trypanosoma brucei rhodesiense* or *Trypanosoma brucei gambiense* is followed by proliferation of macrophages and lymphocytes, high production of IgM antibodies, splenomegaly, and hypersplenism (Chapter 93). Autoagglutination of red cells is common. Anemia and granulocytopenia are usually moderate but may be more severe with *T. brucei rhodesiense* infections. Lymphocyte and monocyte counts are elevated. Thrombocytopenia is sometimes severe in acute infections.

HELMINTH INFECTIONS

Mechanisms. Helminths cause several hematologic changes: (1) Invasion of tissues stimulates the production and release of eosinophils: prolonged eosinophilia has been implicated in the causation of endomyocardial fibrosis. Eosinophilia is pronounced only during the invasive migrating phase of those nematodes (hookworm, *Strongyloides*, and *Ascaris*) that establish themselves in the intestinal tract. (2) Chronic intestinal hemorrhage associated with hookworm infection may lead to iron deficiency. Other less common or less severe causes of chronic hemorrhage and iron deficiency are *Trichuris trichiura* in the gut, *Schistosoma mansoni* and *Schistosoma japonicum* in the colon, and *Schistosoma haematobium* in the bladder. (3) *S. mansoni* and *S. japonicum* can cause fibrosis of the liver, congestive splenomegaly, and hypersplenism. (4) Infections of the small intestine may deprive the host of nutrients; *Diphyllobothrium latum* occasionally causes megaloblastic anemia from vitamin B_{12} deficiency; *Strongyloides* and *Ascaris* lead to a more general and chronic malnutrition.

Hookworm. Approximately 1.2 billion individuals are infected by hookworm (Chapter 105.1). In the majority, infections are mild, but in 50 million to 100 million, the intensity is sufficient to cause anemia, making hookworm second only to malaria as an infectious cause of anemia, and an important health problem in farmers, women during reproductive life, and infants and children.

Ecology. In much of Africa west and north of the Niger River, generally only men and boys work in the fields, where they become heavily infected, with resultant iron deficiency anemia. In the remainder of Africa, women perform agricultural work and can be heavily infected. The women often are accompanied by small children, who play on the ground; the surface area exposed is large and the hookworm loads are heavy in proportion to body weight and stores of iron. Transplacental and transmammary transmission may explain neonatal *Ancylostoma duodenale* infections.

Pathophysiology. The daily loss of blood into the gut is 0.03 to 0.05 mL for each *Necator americanus* worm and 0.15 to 0.23 mL for each *A. duodenale* worm. In the iron-sufficient subject, iron loss is equivalent to approximately 0.5 mg/mL of blood; about 40% of the iron in the gut is reabsorbed. As iron deficiency develops, reabsorption increases to about 60% and the iron content of the blood is less. Because *N. americanus* produces fewer ova (9000/day per female) than does *A. duodenale* (30,000/day per female), a daily iron loss of 1 mg/

1000 ova/g of feces is a reasonable estimate of the burden of a hookworm infection, regardless of species.

Progress to iron deficiency depends on three factors: (1) the dietary intake of bioavailable iron, (2) the size of the iron stores in the body, and (3) the hookworm load (Chapter 105.1). When the diet is a poor source of bioavailable iron and the population has a high frequency of nutritional deficiency (e.g., in India, Mauritius, Mexico), almost any degree of hookworm infection will contribute to negative iron balance or deficiency. In populations with moderately good intake of iron (e.g., in Central America, southern United States, Fiji), a threshold of about 5000 ova/g of feces, equivalent to a loss of about 5 mg of iron per day, has to be reached before iron deficiency develops. In populations with a high intake of bioavailable iron (e.g., in western Nigeria), hookworm loads of more than 20,000 ova/g of feces with hemorrhage of 100 to 200 mL/day are needed before the men go into negative balance. Iron depletion and anemia always develop more rapidly in infected women (especially if pregnant or multiparous) and children than in men, because of their smaller reserves.

Infants infected with *A. duodenale* show melena, anorexia, listlessness, vomiting, and edema; intestinal hemorrhage and profound anemia lead to cardiac failure and a mortality rate of 4% to 12%. Young children can present with Löffler syndrome, abdominal pain, diarrhea, eosinophilia, and florid anemia from acute or subacute intestinal hemorrhage.

The iron deficiency anemia of hookworm infection can be profound (e.g., Hb of 20 g/L) and life-threatening; it can be distinguished clinically or hematologically from nutritional iron deficiency anemia only in a few details. Many patients show a loss of skin pigmentation (melanin) in addition to the pallor of anemia. In communities where heavy hookworm loads are required to induce iron deficiency, the loss of protein and zinc can lead to hypoalbuminemia and diminished serum zinc concentrations. The combination of eosinophilia and hypochromic anemia should alert the clinician to the probability of hookworm infection.

Trichuriasis. Infection by *Trichuris trichiura* (whipworm) is extremely common, about 1 billion persons globally, wherever young children come into contact with warm, moist, and polluted soil (Chapter 103.2). Blood loss is about 5 μL per worm, or 0.25 mL/1000 ova/g of feces. The majority of infections are harmless, but if there are more than 500 worms (16,000 ova/g of feces), the daily loss of blood may be 4 mL and of iron about 2 mg. This is sufficient to cause iron deficiency anemia in about 130 million young children, most commonly in Southeast Asia and Central America.

Schistosomiasis. About 300 million people are infected globally with *Schistosoma*, and numbers are increasing due to both large and small irrigation projects.

Urinary Schistosomiasis. Established infections with *Schistosoma haematobium* in the bladder cause hematuria, with a blood loss of up to 125 mL/day, and a mean loss of iron up to nearly 40 mg/day (Chapter 118). This loss of iron is usually short-lived, and the associated anemia is generally normocytic. However, high prevalences of iron deficiency anemia as a consequence of *S. haematobium* infection are found on the coastal plain of eastern Africa from Somalia to South Africa, affecting adolescent boys especially. Ureteral obstruction can lead to pyelonephritis, erythroid hypoplasia, and neutrophilic leukocytosis.

Intestinal Schistosomiasis. *Schistosomiasis mansoni* is a frequent cause of anemia in many countries, including Egypt (Chapter 118). The anemia has several mechanisms. (1) Ova lodged in the colon may lead to formation of polyps, from which there is chronic loss of blood and of iron up to 8 mg/day. (2) Ova carried to the liver result in hepatic fibrosis, leading to portal hypertension and to progressive splenomegaly with hypersplenism. This causes anemia, granulocytopenia, and thrombocytopenia; pancytopenia may be profound. (3) Acute hemorrhage from esophageal varices can cause acute anemia, with a diminution of the size of the spleen. The pathogenesis of disease due to *Schistosoma japonicum* is similar. (4) Adult schistosomes consume red cells for their nutrition.

Anemia of Chronic Disorders

Patients with chronic disease are often anemic. Infectious conditions that are associated with anemia include tuberculosis, pulmonary abscess, pelvic inflammatory disease, osteomyelitis, and bacterial endocarditis; noninfectious conditions include rheumatoid arthritis, systemic lupus erythematosus, sarcoidosis, and Crohn disease; patients with malignant disease (e.g., carcinomas, sarcomas, and lymphomas) are anemic even when there is no infiltration of the bone marrow. Mechanisms are complex: there is a reduction of and insensitivity to erythropoietin; iron is immobilized within the reticuloendothelial system, probably through the release from neutrophil granules of lactoferrin, which has a higher affinity for iron than transferrin and for which there are receptors in macrophages; and red cell survival is moderately reduced.

The anemia is usually moderate but may become severe with progression of chronic disease: It is normocytic and normochromic at first, but it may become microcytic and hypochromic when iron is immobilized. Serum iron declines, but the serum transferrin level remains normal or falls (in contrast to the raised transferrin levels of iron deficiency), so that the percentage saturation is reduced moderately to 15% to 25%. Serum ferritin is increased, sometimes to extremely high levels, as a reactive protein; except when there is coincidental iron deficiency, stainable iron is seen within the bone marrow macrophages, but not the normoblasts: there is often granulocytic proliferation and an excess of plasma cells in response to the underlying disease.

During the past decade, there has been a fundamental change in the pattern of severe anemias seen in sick patients attending hospitals and clinics in sub-Saharan Africa. Related to the rising incidence of tuberculosis and the pandemic of HIV, anemia of chronic disorders, often profound, is now the most common type of anemia seen in nonpregnant women and men seeking medical advice, and contributes significantly to the high prevalence of anemia in childhood and pregnancy.

TUBERCULOSIS. One third of the world's population is infected by *Mycobacterium tuberculosis*, and there are about 8 million cases of active tuberculosis per year, of which 4.5 million are in Asia (Chapter 77). About 7 million persons are infected with both HIV and *M. tuberculosis*: subjects with HIV infection are liable to reactivation of latent tuberculosis and have a greater than normal susceptibility to new infections by mycobacteria. Up to 60% of Africans with newly diagnosed tuberculosis are HIV infected and the incidence of tuberculosis has risen steeply to above 265/100,000 population per year, as a result not only of the pandemic of HIV, but also of such factors as urbanization, overcrowding, migrant labor, malnutrition, and substance abuse.

Patients with tuberculosis have the anemia of chronic disorders, which is more profound with extrapulmonary tuberculosis, granulomas of the bone marrow, and malnutrition. Patients with poor vegetarian diets enter a vicious cycle of malnutrition, depression of cell-mediated immunity, exacerbation of tuberculosis, anorexia and malabsorption, and further malnutrition. Pancytopenia results from splenomegaly with hypersplenism and from HIV infection. Disseminated or miliary tuberculosis results in severe anemia, often with leukocytosis that may be so high as to be a leukemoid reaction. Reactive thrombocytosis of around $1000 \times 10^9/L$ is common.

Therapeutic agents used in treatment can contribute to the anemia, through disturbed metabolism of pyridoxine, folate, or vitamin B_{12}; immune hemolysis; marrow hypoplasia; or hemolysis in subjects who are glucose-6-phosphate dehydrogenase (G6PD) deficient.

AIDS

Epidemiology. The full impact of the pandemic of HIV and the acquired immunodeficiency syndrome (AIDS) is still to come in the tropical world (Chapter 23). Among adults (aged 20–49 years) in sub-Saharan Africa, the annual number of new infections with HIV probably peaked in the early 1990s at about 1 million: the peak occurrence of AIDS will reach 750,000 per year in about the year 2005, and then decline slowly. Among adults in Asia, it is predicted that the annual number of new infections will peak at 1.3 million around the year 2000, with the occurrence of AIDS reaching 850,000 per year 10 years later.

The hematologic implications of the epidemic of HIV and AIDS are twofold. First, there is the impact on blood transfusion practices. Second, AIDS must now be considered in the differential diagnosis of any cytopenia.

Blood Transfusion. Transmission by blood transfusion had contributed about 10% to the prevalence of HIV infections in sub-Saharan Africa by the mid-1980s, when serologic testing first became available. Factors contributing to this high rate of HIV transmission included high prevalence among blood donors (most of whom were relatives of patients or paid donors) and the frequent need for blood transfusions in the management of profound anemia and exsanguination: groups at greatest risk were children with malaria and anemia, women with pregnancy-related hemorrhage or anemia, patients with sickle cell disease, and the victims of trauma. Blood transfusion services in Africa had been given low priority, but standards have improved enormously during the past decade, at least in larger centers, in response to the pandemic.

Strategies to reduce HIV transmission have included (1) donor selection, through policies to build up panels of volunteer nonremunerated donors recruited from sectors of the population with low seroprevalence; (2) HIV screening of units of blood, by the application of inexpensive but sensitive test-algorithms; (3) the appropriate use of blood; and (4) public health measures aimed at reducing the need for transfusions, such as the prevention of anemia in childhood and pregnancy, strengthening prenatal services, and maintaining the health of patients with sickle cell disease. (A fifth strategy, the inactivation of virus in plasma fractions, is not practiced in sub-Saharan Africa, where plasma fractions are imported if available at all, but methods of pasteurizing fresh-frozen plasma and cryoprecipitate would be most beneficial.) The transfusion of HIV-seronegative blood carries, however, a residual risk of being infectious, primarily because of donors being in the "window" between infection and seroconversion; this risk is probably between 2 and 5 units/1000 units of blood in sub-Saharan Africa, compared with about 2/100,000 units in North America and Europe, the risk being greater by a factor of over 10 from first-time compared with repeat donors.

The transmission of HIV by blood transfusion is potentially an even greater disaster in Asia than it has been in Africa. Remunerated blood donation is an organized profession in many Asian cities; selection is virtually nonexistent and many professional donors are intravenous drug users and/or commercial sex workers; screening for HIV and syphilis is often inaccurate, falsified, or not performed. Requirements for blood are high because of high incidences of acquired and inherited anemias, and of exsanguination. Already, 70% of multitranfused children with thalassemia major in Mumbai (Bombay) are reported to be HIV infected.

Hematologic Complications. Patients who develop the infectious mononucleosis-like illness at the time of early viremia and seroconversion show transient mild leukopenia with increased numbers of early neutrophils and thrombocytopenia. A fundamental feature of later HIV-related disease is lymphopenia and a specific loss of CD4 + T lymphocytes (Chapter 23). As well, anemia, granulocytopenia, and thrombocytopenia, singly or in combination, frequently complicate the course of HIV-related disease.

Thrombocytopenia may occur early and is sometimes the first manifestation of disease: about 30% of patients with AIDS have thrombocytopenia, and about 45% develop a lupus anticoagulant at some stage. The combination of these two is of clinical importance, because it leads to excessive hemorrhage during accidental trauma or following surgery.

Anemia and granulocytopenia develop later, and with the progression of disease, up to 80% of patients with AIDS have significant cytopenias. Because of the late attendance of patients in Africa, severe anemia may be the first presentation of AIDS, especially during pregnancy.

The red cells are normocytic and normochromic but commonly show anisocytosis and poikilocytosis. The reticulocyte count is usually normal or low. Hypergammaglobulinemia causes rouleau formation in red cells. Granulocytopenia is usually associated with a shift to the left of the neutrophils. Atypical lymphocytes with dark blue–staining cytoplasm and large nuclei with nucleoli occur with lymphopenia. Monocytes are frequently vacuolated.

Bone marrow examinations generally show nonspecific changes. Erythropoiesis is usually normoblastic but may be megaloblastic and dyserythropoiesis is common; activity is most variable, from hypoplastic to normal to hyperplastic. Myeloid hyperplasia is usual. There is often a striking plasmacytosis and aggregates of lymphocytes, secondary to dysregulation of B-cell proliferation and constant antigenic exposure; the appearance may lead to a misdiagnosis of myeloma. Patients with thrombocytopenia have normal or increased megakaryocytes. The iron in macrophages may be increased, a consequence either of inflammation following secondary infections or of alcoholism associated with a way of life that also carries a high risk of exposure to HIV.

MECHANISMS. The mechanisms of hematologic abnormalities are multiple and complex, involving both peripheral destruction of cells and disturbance of production. The synthesis of antiplatelet antibodies and the adsorption of nonspecific immune complexes onto platelets are important mechanisms in the early development of thrombocytopenia; anti–red cell antibodies and adsorbed immune complexes result frequently in a positive direct Coombs test with various antibody specificities, but hemolysis is not significant in most patients; similarly, neutropenia is associated with antigranulocyte antibodies. HIV has direct actions on (1) stem cells, (2) more mature marrow cells (e.g., megakaryocytes), and (3) marrow accessory cells (e.g., macrophages, fibroblasts, and T lymphocytes) leading to disturbance in the balances between hematopoietic regulatory or growth factors. Opportunistic or reactivated latent infections, especially *Mycobacterium tuberculosis*, result in the changes typical of anemias of chronic disorders. Parvovirus B19 infection may be uncontrolled because of immunodeficiency, causing chronic viral infection of proerythroblasts and pure red cell aplasia. Various nutritional deficiencies, e.g., vitamin B₁₂, folate, vitamin A, and pyridoxine, can contribute to the anemia and

other cytopenias; so can therapy, including overdosage of the antimicrobiologic folate antagonists trimethoprim and pyrimethamine, as well as treatment with antiviral or antineoplastic agents. Lymphomas as manifestations of AIDS are discussed in Chapter 23.

Treatment. Therapeutic options are limited in developing countries. Anemia may require transfusion with concentrated red blood cells. The effects of leukopenia can be countered by antibiotics, with varying success. Steroids are not recommended for the long-term treatment of thrombocytopenia associated with AIDS. Intravenous IgG is often effective in the control of hemorrhage or in preparation for invasive procedures, but is prohibited by cost and unavailability. The platelet count rises following splenectomy in many patients, but the operation could be foolhardy without adequate surgical facilities, antipneumococcal vaccine, long-term penicillin prophylaxis, and antimalarial prophylactics. Erythropoietin and granulocyte-monocyte colony-stimulating factor (GM-CSF) are reported to be effective in the treatment of anemia and neutropenia respectively, but are not generally available in developing countries.

PARVOVIRUS B19. The human parvovirus B19 is a nonenveloped virus containing a single-stranded DNA molecule. It is transmitted by droplets, transplacentally, and by blood transfusion. The virus has a tropism for erythroid progenitor cells, in which it replicates and is cytotoxic. Suppression of erythropoiesis correlates with viremia, when giant pronormoblasts are seen in the bone marrow. Most children are infected in the first 2 years of life in tropical countries; the infections are usually asymptomatic and the transient reduction of red blood cell production passes unnoticed; some develop erythema infectiosum or arthropathy at the time of the immune response. Infection by parvovirus B19 assumes hematologic importance in four situations. (1) Patients with chronic hemolytic anemia, such as sickle cell disease, thalassemia major or intermedia, and congenital spherocytosis, are dependent on a rapid rate of erythropoiesis, and will have aplastic crises precipitated by acute parvovirus B19 infections. (2) If acute malaria coincides with infection by parvovirus B19, severe life-threatening anemia is likely to follow. (3) Viremia is not controlled in immunocompromised subjects, so that both children and adults with AIDS will have a persistent infection of early erythroid precursors and chronic red cell hypoplasia. (4) Infection of nonimmune pregnant women can be followed by transplacental infection of the fetus, in whom severe anemia, cardiac failure, and edema (i.e., hydrops fetalis) develop, followed by abortion or stillbirth.

Nutritional Anemias

IRON DEFICIENCY. The iron found in food occurs in three main forms: (1) heme iron, (2) nonheme iron, and (3) extraneous iron (Chapter 132.1).

Heme in animal food (meat, poultry, and fish) is absorbed most readily as an intact metalloporphyrin by cells of the duodenal mucosa, and the iron is utilized. The nonheme iron of animal foods (with the exception of eggs, which contain phospholipids that block absorption) also has a high bioavailability, as absorption is enhanced by amino acids derived from the digestion of protein. Diets rich in animal protein generally meet the daily physiologic requirements for iron (see Table 132–2). Iron deficiency was infrequent in communities whose members had survived as hunter-gatherers into the twentieth century, e.g., the Hadza in Tanzania and the !Kung San in the Kalahari desert; encroachments of modern life, however, have marginalized such communities and driven them into states of severe malnutrition. Pastoralists such as the Masai in Kenya, who eat meat and drink blood, remain iron-sufficient communities. Nearly 50% of the iron in breast milk is absorbed, and deficiency is uncommon in mature breast-fed infants.

In contrast, nonheme iron of vegetable foods has low bioavailability. Absorption is inhibited by bulk, fiber, phytates, phosphates, polyphenols, and tannin. Ascorbic acid and amino acids are the main enhancers of absorption of nonheme iron, but sources of these are expensive or may not be eaten because of religious beliefs, e.g., the vegetarian diet of Hinduism. Much of the world's population subsists on diets based on the cereal staples—rice, wheat, maize, sorghum, and millet—from which sufficient iron cannot be absorbed to meet physiologic requirements, especially during early childhood, adolescence, menstruation, and pregnancy (see Table 132–4). Chronic hemorrhage and loss of iron from hookworm, schistosomal, and whipworm infection coincide frequently with low intake of bioavailable iron and contribute to the worldwide high prevalence of iron deficiency. Vitamin A appears essential for the utilization of iron, both newly absorbed or in storage form, and in deficient populations, vitamin A supplements enhance the effectiveness of iron supplements and therapy.

Iron deficiency is the most common nutritional disorder in all populations, and is the most common cause of anemia; probably 1 billion of the world's 5 to 6 billion inhabitants have iron deficiency anemia and an even greater number have depleted iron stores but have not reached the stage of anemia. Prevalences of iron deficiency anemia of over 50% are observed in preschool children and pregnant women in developing countries; other groups at risk include premature infants, the infants of iron-deficient mothers, and adolescent girls. Africa and south Asia have the highest regional prevalence rates (Table 6–2).

Clinical manifestations, laboratory diagnosis, treatment, and prevention of iron deficiency are discussed fully in Chapter 132.1. The principles of prevention are (1) supplements to groups at risk (premature infants, adolescent girls, pregnant women); (2) the prevention of transmission of hookworm and other helminths; (3) the fortification of commonly eaten staples with iron, most effectively in the form of sodium iron ethylenediaminetetraacetic acid (NaFeEDTA); and (4) changes in food preparation and the diet so as to increase the amount of bioavailable iron.

FOLIC ACID DEFICIENCY

Folate Metabolism. The core molecule of folic acid, pteroylglutamic acid, does not exist free in nature. In its active forms (folates) it is conjugated, reduced, and condensed (Chapter 131.7). Folates may be monoglutamates, such as $N5$-methyltetrahydrofolate in serum, or may be conjugated to form the polyglutamates found intracellularly. Folates are reduced to dihydro- or tetrahydrofolates by dihydrofolate reductase, which in mammals is a liver enzyme. Finally, the molecule is condensed with one-carbon radicals, e.g., methyl, methenyl, methylene, or formyl. Folates are essential cofactors in the transfer of one-carbon radicals in the synthesis of purines, pyrimidines, and nucleic acids. They are involved in amino acid intraconversions, e.g., histidine to glutamic acid, homocysteine to methionine, and glycine to serine. Folates are required in the conversion of uridine to thymidine in the synthesis of DNA. Folates are necessary, therefore, for all dividing cells, and the highest turnover is in tissues of rapid cell division, e.g., the bone marrow and the gastrointestinal tract.

Folate Sources and Requirements. Folates are widespread, and dietary sources are varied. Liver, kidney, and other meats, yeast products, eggs, yams, sweet potatoes, other tubers, plantain, bananas, mangoes, fresh green and red pep-

TABLE 6–3. Daily Dietary Requirements for Folates and Vitamin B$_{12}$

Nutrient	Group	Daily Dietary Requirement (µg)
Folate	0–6 mo	40–50
	7–12 mo	120
	1–12 yr	200
	≥13 yr	400
	Pregnant women	800
	Lactating women	600
Vitamin B$_{12}$	0–12 mo	0.3
	1–3 yr	0.9
	4–9 yr	1.5
	≥10 yr	2.0
	Pregnant women	3.0
	Lactating women	2.5

From World Health Organization: Nutritional anaemias. Technical Report Series No. 503. Geneva, WHO, 1972.

pers, locust beans, and green leafy vegetables are all rich sources of folates. Cereal grains, including rice, maize, sorghum, and millet, and roots, e.g., cassava, are poor sources. Folates are deconjugated and absorbed actively as monoglutamates in the jejunum. The liver is the main storage organ, but body stores normally are sufficient for only about 3 weeks. Folates are secreted in bile, urine, and breast milk. Physiologic requirements for folate are highest during periods of rapid growth, pregnancy, and lactation (Table 6–3).

Causes of Folate Deficiency. Deficiency of folate can follow (1) inadequate intake, (2) malabsorption, (3) high physiologic requirements, (4) high demands following hemolysis or other pathologic processes, and (5) disturbances of metabolism (Table 6–4).

Reduced Dietary Intake. Reduced dietary intake of folate may reflect a shortage of food but is frequently a result of inappropriate selection or preparation of food. Folates are water-soluble and heat-labile and so are leached out by boiling and destroyed by prolonged cooking. Soups or relishes added to bulky staple foods, e.g., maize-porridge, often contain foods that were originally folate-rich, e.g., spinach, peppers, meat, or fish. Prolonged boiling and reheating for each day's meal reduces active folate. For example, the frequency of folate deficiency is high in Indians, intermediate in Malays, and low in Chinese in Singapore, reflecting precisely their cooking practices. There are seasonal variations in the availability of folate and in the frequency of megaloblastic anemias in many countries. For example, folate deficiency is increasingly common in the late dry season and into the early rainy season in Nigeria, but the lifting of the new yam crop in August is followed almost immediately by a dramatic decline of megaloblastic anemia in pregnancy.

Folates and Infectious Disease. Infectious diseases disturb the folate balance through several mechanisms: (1) prolonged anorexia following intercurrent infections, e.g., malaria; (2) depressed absorption due to enteric infections and severe systemic diseases, including pneumonia, tuberculosis, and malaria; (3) erythroid hyperplasia following malaria, which is a major cause of severe folate deficiency in pregnancy; this mechanism, however, does not seem to be important in childhood; and (4) the enzyme dihydrofolate reductase is inactive at 39°C, a probable mechanism for acute megaloblastic arrest of erythropoiesis complicating infectious diseases of childhood and pregnancy.

Metabolic Inhibitors. The 2, 4-diaminopyrimidines, pyrimethamine and trimethoprim, are distant analogues of folic acid and are competitive inhibitors of dihydrofolate reductase. Their usefulness as antimalarials and antibiotics is due to their greater affinity for the enzymes of protozoa and bacteria than for those of humans. However, overdosage can occur and lead to megaloblastic anemias. This has been observed in infants receiving adult dosages of pyrimethamine and with self-medication with pyrimethamine plus cotrimoxazole.

Epidemiology. Folate deficiency in infancy and childhood commonly occurs in association with (1) prematurity; (2) inappropriate bottle-feeding with either boiled milk or goat's milk; (3) inappropriate weaning foods such as paps from maize or cassava; (4) diarrhea; (5) intercurrent infections; and (6) hemoglobinopathies. For example, folate deficiency contributed to one third of all anemias in children aged 3 months to 3 years in the north of Nigeria. One third of all Nigerian children with protein-energy malnutrition studied were also folate-deficient.

Folate deficiency frequently complicates the course of pregnancy because of (1) nutritional inadequacy; (2) the high demands of both the fetus and the mother; (3) enhanced catabolism of folate during pregnancy; and (4) hemolysis in primigravidae exposed to malaria. Megaloblastic erythropoiesis was observed in 55% of all primigravidae in northern Nigeria; it contributed to over 75% of severe anemias in Nigeria and to 66% in India. In southern Africa where maize is the common staple, severe deficiency of folate is seen often in lactating women around 6 months post partum, usually with a history of closely spaced pregnancies separated only by periods of breast-feeding.

In Africa, subjects with sickle cell disease are often folate-deficient when seen for the first time—the result of high demands due to constant erythroid hyperplasia and the effects of intercurrent infections.

Clinical Manifestations. Besides the symptoms and signs of anemia, folate-deficient subjects have increased susceptibility to infections owing to neutropenia and immune deficiency, and rarely may have hemorrhage from thrombocytopenia. With long-standing deficiency, there can be glossitis, angular cheilosis, mild malabsorption, hyperpigmentation most obvious on the palms and soles, mild peripheral neuropathy, depression or mood change, and retarded growth and development, especially in children with sickle cell disease. Deficiency at the time of conception or early pregnancy, or congenital disorders of folate metabolism (e.g., mutated methylenetetrahydrofolate reductase), lead to neural tube defects (e.g., spina bifida); deficiency in late pregnancy is a cause of anemia and intrauterine growth retardation.

Hematologic Manifestations. Folate deficiency is manifest as a macrocytic, megaloblastic anemia. The mean corpuscular hemoglobin concentration (MCHC) remains normal, but both the mean cell volume (MCV) and the mean cellular hemoglobin (MCH) are raised. The reticulocyte count is low or normal, unless raised when the primary lesion is hemolysis. The leukocyte count is most variable; the neutrophil count is often low with the characteristic hypersegmentation. However, with concurrent infections it may be raised, with release of early precursor cells from the bone marrow, to give a leukemoid reaction. The platelet count is reduced. The peripheral blood film shows considerable anisocytosis and macrocytosis with a few microcytes. In acutely developing anemias there is no poikilocytosis, but in more long-standing deficiencies there is ovalocytosis and poikilocytosis; polychromasia is more pronounced with hemolytic anemias, and there can be numerous nucleated red cells with megaloblastic features.

Smears of bone marrow aspirates show megaloblastic erythropoiesis and giant metamyelocytes. When there is un-

TABLE 6–4. Causes of Folate Deficiency

Inadequate intake	Excessive boiling of bottle feeds
	Goat's milk feeding of infants
	Inappropriate weaning food (PEM)
	Anorexia (recurrent infections)
	Prolonged cooking, reheating
	Seasonal food shortages
	Prolonged storage of food
	Famine
	Taboos
	Food fads
	Alcoholism
Malabsorption	Diarrhea in infancy
	Other enteric infections
	Systemic infections (pneumonia, tuberculosis)
	Acute tropical sprue
	Nontropical sprue
High physiologic demands	Premature infants
	Growth in infancy and adolescence
	Pregnancy
	Lactation
Pathologic high demands	Sickle cell disease
	Other chronic hemolytic diseases
	Recurrent malaria in pregnancy
	Burkitt lymphoma
	Choriocarcinoma
Disturbed metabolism	Pyrexia
	Overdosage of pyrimethamine, trimethoprim, methotrexate
	Congenital disorders

PEM, protein-energy malnutrition.

derlying hemolytic disease, changes are apparent earlier in the red cell than in the granulocyte series; in purely nutritional deficiencies, however, giant metamyelocytes may be the first feature. With the history and the presence of diseases known to deplete folate stores (Table 6–4), a diagnosis of folic acid deficiency can be made with a high degree of certainty. When there is doubt, folate deficiency and vitamin B_{12} deficiency must be distinguished by the assay of folate in serum and red blood cell, and vitamin B_{12} in serum. If these assays are not available, the hematologic response to physiologic doses (folic acid 50 μg/day or vitamin B_{12} 1 μg/day) can be followed with daily estimates of reticulocyte count and hemoglobin.

Treatment. Folic acid 5/mg day PO for 3 weeks is adequate for even the most severe deficiency; treatment needs to be prolonged if the cause of deficiency persists; intramuscular folate is rarely needed by patients with malabsorption; parenteral folinic acid is indicated when there is inhibition of dihydrofolate reductase.

Prevention. There are three strategies: supplementation, fortification, and change to the diet. Supplements are indicated for premature infants, infants with diarrhea (50 μg/day), pregnant women (500 μg/day combined with iron), and patients with chronic hemolysis (e.g., sickle cell disease; usually 5 mg/day). Fortification of a staple is advocated for the prevention of neural tube defects and for communities in southern Africa. Folate intake can be increased by eating more folate-rich foods, eaten raw or only lightly cooked.

VITAMIN B_{12} DEFICIENCY. The cobalamins, known collectively as vitamin B_{12}, are synthesized by microorganisms and found exclusively in animal food, not in vegetables (Chapter 131.7). Many of the functions of vitamin B_{12} remain obscure, but it is essential in conjunction with folate for the synthesis of purines, pyrimidines, and DNA. It is required by the cells of the central nervous system, such that deficiency leads not only to megaloblastic anemia but also to subacute combined degeneration of the spinal cord.

Dietary Sources. Dietary sources of vitamin B_{12} are liver and other animal tissues, eggs, and milk. Fecal contamination of well water is a major source of vitamin B_{12} in some impoverished vegetarian communities. Daily requirements are small (Table 6–3). Absorption depends on release of vitamin B_{12} in the stomach and binding to intrinsic factor (IF) secreted by parietal cells. The IF-B_{12} complex is absorbed by mucosal cells of the ileum, and the vitamin B_{12} is transported actively to the portal circulation. Transport is by transcobalamin II protein. The major storage site is in the liver; it is normally sufficient for about 2 years.

Causes of Vitamin B_{12} Deficiency. Deficiency of vitamin B_{12} can result from (1) inadequate intake; (2) gastric disease leading to a failure to secrete IF; (3) disease of the ileum; (4) competition by the fish tapeworm *Diphyllobothrium latum* (Chapter 123.1); and (5) metabolic blocks, which may arise acutely from nitrous oxide exposure or chronically from cyanide ingestion from eating poorly prepared cassava (Chapter 9).

Dietary Deficiency. A nutritional deficiency of vitamin B_{12} is difficult to achieve, as daily requirements are extremely low (Table 6–3) and are met by the smallest intake of animal food, including milk and milk products, or bacterially contaminated water. Women in southern India can be deficient as a consequence of low intake, malabsorption caused by chronic sprue, and the increased demands of pregnancy; the deficiency may be manifest in their infants, who are fed with vitamin B_{12}-free breast milk. Prisoners have developed severe vitamin B_{12} deficiency and megaloblastic anemia when fed for long periods on unrelieved vegan diets.

Malabsorption. Addisonian pernicious anemia is an autoimmune disease in which antibodies are formed against gastric parietal cells and IF; it is seen most commonly in those of northern European descent. It was thought to be rare in sub-Saharan Africa, but it is not uncommon in the black population of South Africa; there appears to be a change in epidemiology, as pernicious anemia is being diagnosed now in the more wealthy of Zimbabwe, Zambia, and Nigeria. Malabsorption can follow chronic infection with *Giardia lamblia* or severe enteritis. The fish tapeworm (*D. latum*) is transmitted by eating raw or undercooked freshwater fish, and infections have been reported on the shores of African lakes and elsewhere in the tropics. However, fewer than 1 in 1000 of those infected progress to deficiency.

Clinical Manifestations. The clinical presentation of vitamin B_{12} deficiency differs from that of folate deficiency in that there is a greater likelihood of neurologic complications and hyperpigmentation of the skin, best seen on the soles and the palms and across the knuckles.

Hematologic Manifestations. The hematologic findings of vitamin B_{12} deficiency are indistinguishable from those of folate deficiency; owing to the greater chronicity of vitamin B_{12} depletion, there is more likely to be poikilocytosis and thrombocytopenia. It is confirmed by a low serum vitamin B_{12} concentration. In many tropical communities the reference range of serum vitamin B_{12} is high (150 to 2500 pg/L) compared with Caucasian reference ranges, owing partly to genetically determined higher cobalamin-B_{12} binding. Malabsorption of vitamin B_{12} can be confirmed by measuring the absorption of radioactive cobalt-labeled vitamin, with and without the addition of IF; if radioactive vitamin B_{12} studies are not feasible, a diagnosis of pernicious anemia can be confirmed by the detection of parietal or IF antibodies.

Treatment. The preparation of choice is hydroxocobalamin,

administered intramuscularly 1000 μg six times over 2 weeks, followed by 1000 μg every 3 months to patients with malabsorption. Nutritional deficiencies can be treated orally. Some manufacturers still produce and some underdeveloped countries still import cyanocobalamin, which has the disadvantages of having to be given in larger initial doses and monthly for maintenance, and being totally ineffective in cyanide poisoning.

ANEMIA IN PROTEIN-ENERGY MALNUTRITION. Children with protein-energy malnutrition (PEM) usually have a moderate anemia (Hb of 75 to 100 g/L), which is normocytic and normochromic with low or normal reticulocyte counts (Chapter 130). The bone marrow is cellular and normoblastic. Erythropoietin levels are normal, and the cause of the anemia appears to be an impairment of erythropoiesis due to decreased reaction of erythroid progenitor cells to erythropoietin. In kwashiorkor, but not in marasmus, there is also a moderate shortening of red cell survival.

Anemia is more severe if there are complications, e.g., infections, which are common because of the impairment of immune mechanisms frequently associated with PEM. In some communities, e.g., West Africa, up to one third of children with PEM are folic acid–deficient; iron deficiency in early childhood is a common complication of PEM in almost any community.

Genetically Determined Anemias

BALANCED POLYMORPHISMS. There have been numerous mutations during human evolution causing inherited abnormalities in red blood cell hemoglobin, enzymes, and membranes. Some of these variations rendered the red blood cells a less perfect environment for the development of malarial parasites. Any gene conferring partial protection against malaria also would confer greater survival advantage; the genetic advantage of heterozygous inheritance would lead to increased gene frequency in each generation until a balance was reached between the genetic disadvantage of ill health and homozygous inheritance. This is illustrated most clearly by the HbS gene.

In its original global distribution before the transatlantic slave trade and modern travel, the HbS gene occurred at high frequency only in Africa and other parts of the world where *Plasmodium falciparum* malaria was endemic (Fig. 6–2). Subjects with sickle cell trait (HbAS) have a distinct survival advantage in regions where malaria is hyper- or holoendemic (Chapter 92); e.g., in Garki in the north of Nigeria the incidence of HbAS in newborns was 24%; this proportion rose to 29% by 5 years of age, at which prevalence it remained thereafter. The advantage of HbAS over the normal (HbAA) was the result of lower frequencies of *P. falciparum* parasitemia and, more importantly, lower densities of parasitemia between the ages of 6 months and 4 years. The partial protection against intense *P. falciparum* infection was shown clearly by the hospital observations that almost no one with sickle cell trait died from cerebral malaria.

Two mechanisms for limiting parasitemia have been demonstrated in vitro. (1) The consumption of oxygen by the early parasite forms in circulating red cells leads to sickling, and the preferential removal by the reticuloendothelial system of the parasitized sickled red cells. (2) In long-term cultures of *P. falciparum* at low oxygen tension, as experienced in the last 12 hours of the erythrocyte cycle in vivo, there is an inhibition of growth of mature parasites in red cells containing HbS compared with red cells containing HbA only. This inhibition could be accounted for by the jelling of deoxygenated HbS molecules. The protection of sickle cell trait extends to beyond early childhood: There are reduced para-

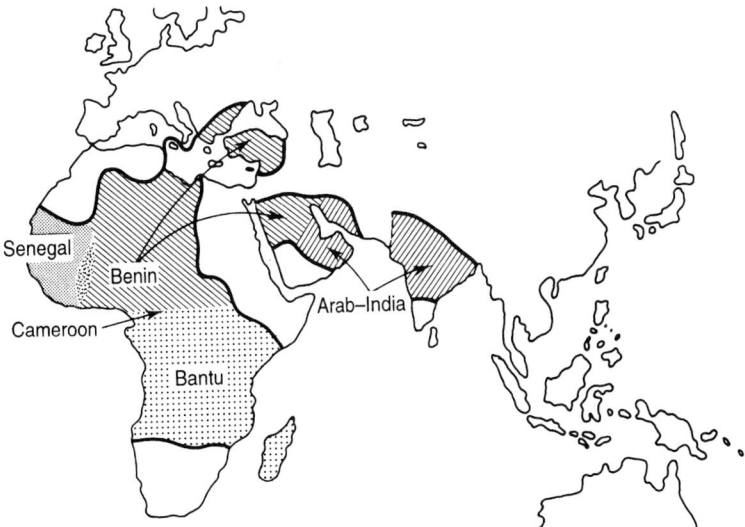

Figure 6–2. Areas of the Old World where HbS gene frequency is greater than 0.02, and the distribution of β^S haplotypes. (From Fleming AF: Haematological diseases in the tropics. *In* Cook GC [ed]: Manson's Tropical Diseases, 20th ed. London, WB Saunders, 1996, pp 101–173.)

sitemia during pregnancy, protection against hyperreactive malarial splenomegaly, and less inhibition by malaria on the antibody response to pneumococcal vaccine. Subjects with HbSS have the same limitation of *P. falciparum* parasitemia, but parasitemia is likely to precipitate hemolytic and infarctive crises, with high morbidity and mortality.

Genes that reach polymorphic frequency where malaria is, or was, endemic include hemoglobin S (Fig. 6–2); hemoglobins C, D, and E (Fig. 6–3); β-thalassemias (Fig. 6–7); α-thalassemias (Fig. 6–9); certain forms of G6PD deficiency (Fig. 6–10); Southeast Asian ovalocytosis and possibly elliptocytosis in West and North Africa (see Fig. 6–11).

SICKLE CELL DISEASE

Definition. Sickle cell disease results from the inheritance of two abnormal allelomorphic genes, at least one of which is the sickle cell gene, controlling the synthesis of the β-chains of hemoglobin. The most common form of sickle cell disease is sickle cell anemia or homozygous HbSS, but others include HbSC and HbS/β-thalassemia. HbSS is the most severe but is scarcely distinguished from HbS/β^0-thalassemia. HbSC is less severe, and HbS/β$^+$-thalassemia is relatively mild. The main description of sickle cell disease refers to HbSS as seen in Africa, unless stated otherwise.

Epidemiology. Between 1% and 2% of infants born in tropical Africa, or about 130,000 per year, have sickle cell disease, mostly HbSS, but HbSC and HbS/β$^+$-thalassemia are also common in West Africa (Figs. 6–2, 6–3, 6–7). Another 30,000 per year are born in other parts of the world, including India, the Mediterranean basin, the Americas, and Britain.

Pathophysiology. All pathology is derived from one mutation causing the substitution of the hydrophobic amino acid valine for the hydrophilic amino acid glutamic acid at position 6 on the β-chain of the adult hemoglobin (HbA) molecule. When deoxygenated, the sickle hemoglobin (HbS) has reduced solubility compared with HbA. Molecules of HbS jell, i.e., they adhere to each other to form long chains with 14 molecules in cross section. These polymers become aligned in parallel, thus distorting the red cell into the characteristic sickle form. At first, sickling is reversible with reoxygenation, but repeated sickling and unsickling leads to loss of cell membrane components, a decline in intracellular water and K$^+$, a rise in intracellular Ca^{2+}, and the formation of the irreversibly sickled cell. Sickled cells are rigid and have a tendency to adhere to each other and to endothelium, adherence being mediated by the von Willebrand factor, thrombospondin, fibrinogen, and fibronectin. Platelet counts tend to be high and the equilibrium of hemostatic mechanisms shifted toward thrombosis and coagulation. The pathology of sickle cell disease results from hemolysis and infarction from blocking of small blood vessels. Secondary effects include increased susceptibility to infections and retardation of growth and development.

Clinical Manifestations

Hemolysis and Anemia. In the steady state the Hb concentration usually ranges from 60 to 100 g/L in HbSS and HbS/β^0-thalassemia, and from 110 to 140 g/L in HbSC disease. There is constant moderate jaundice, with a serum bilirubin level of 35 to 140 μmol/L (2 to 8 mg/dL). About one fourth of patients over 15 years of age have pigment gallstones, but cholelithiasis is almost invariably asymptomatic.

There is a constant erythroid hyperplasia that leads to expansion of the bone marrow cavity and bossing of the bones of the skull (Fig. 6–4). The forehead is rounded, with an exaggeration of the line of the supraorbital sulcus. The bridge of the nose appears sunken because the bones around it are swollen. Expansion of the maxilla causes a forward

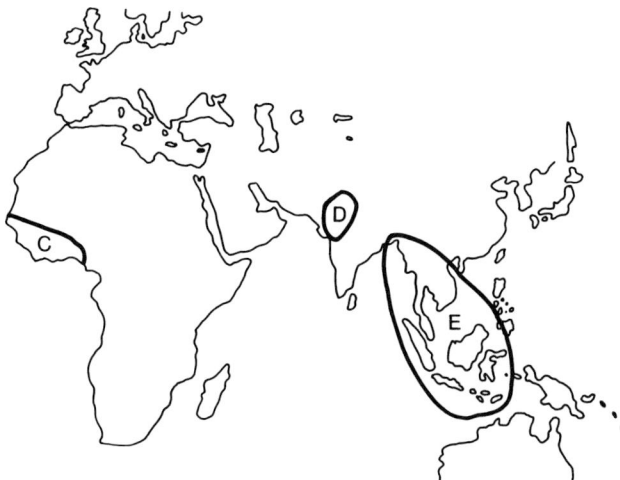

Figure 6–3. Areas of the Old World where HbC, HbD (Punjab or Los Angeles), and HbE reach polymorphic frequencies.

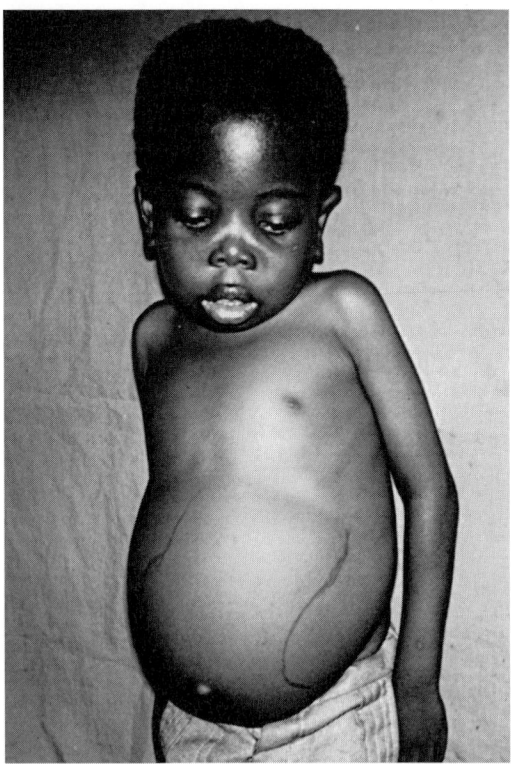

Figure 6–4. African child with HbSS having prominent frontal bossing and splenomegaly.

protrusion of the upper incisors (gnathopathy). Bossing of the vault of the skull is less common but can be dramatic, so that the head is grossly enlarged and the outer table is so thin as to be easily depressed on palpation. A radiograph of the skull can demonstrate the bossing and shows a "hair-on-end" picture of the bone marrow cavity of the vault (Fig. 6–5). As gross bossing is reversible with long-term antimalarial prophylaxis and as it is not observed in African Americans, it is probably due largely to the additional hemolysis of malaria.

The steady state can be interrupted by anemic crises, which may be caused by malaria, acute splenic sequestration, folate deficiency, or bone marrow aplasia.

Acute *P. falciparum* malaria can cause severe hemolytic crisis and profound anemia. Anemic cardiac failure with malaria is probably the most common cause of death in tropical Africa in children with HbSS not under medical supervision.

A splenic sequestration crisis is characterized by an acutely enlarging spleen with sequestration of a large proportion of the red cell mass and a catastrophic decline of the Hb by at least 20 g/L, but with an elevated reticulocyte count and erythroid hyperplasia in the bone marrow. This is believed to be precipitated by infection and a consequent alteration of the surface of the red cell membrane. It occurs most often in patients aged 6 months to 2 years but can be seen in older individuals who retain splenic function or who are pregnant. Its frequency in Africa is not defined, but in Jamaica, it is the single most common cause of death in early life.

Megaloblastic erythropoiesis with anemic crisis can interrupt the steady state as a consequence of any of the other causes of folate deficiency (Table 6–4) superimposed on the constant high demands due to erythroid hyperplasia. In West Africa, megaloblastic erythropoiesis is almost inevitable during pregnancy and occurs in over 10% of nonpregnant pa-

tients with HbSS disease who have not been receiving supportive therapy.

Any acute infection can depress erythropoiesis to some extent in an otherwise normal subject, usually without any significant clinical manifestations. However, such depression can be catastrophic in HbSS disease, in which the steady-state Hb level depends on a rate of erythropoiesis six to eight times normal. Many acute infections are followed by rapid declines in Hb and reticulocyte counts, but parvovirus B19 causes epidemics of severe aplastic crises among the populations with HbSS disease.

INFARCTIVE CRISES BONE PAIN. Infarction of sickled red cells in the small blood vessels of the small bones of the hands and feet is followed by tissue necrosis and an acute, painful, nonpitting swelling of the dorsa and digits, the so-called hand-foot syndrome (Fig. 6–6). This is the most common first clinical presentation, occurring in about 90% of children between the ages of 6 months and 2 years diagnosed as having HbSS disease in tropical Africa. In less than 10% of crises, there is a superimposed osteomyelitis, often with *Salmonella* as the infecting organism.

After about 2 years of age, the site of bone infarction shifts from the hands and feet to the long bones of the limbs. Pain is experienced most often around the large joints but can be present in any part of the limbs or bony skeleton. Pain has an acute onset and varies in severity from mild, lasting perhaps only a few minutes, to extremely severe, characteristically lasting 5 days. On physical examination, there is usually only mild pyrexia and no more than warmth and tenderness at the site of infarction. However, the paucity of signs should not lead to an underestimation of the severity of the patient's condition. Bone pain crisis is the first presentation in up to 40% of patients in tropical Africa; the most frequently recognized precipitating factors are malaria and various bacterial infections, but in many, no inciting factors are identi-

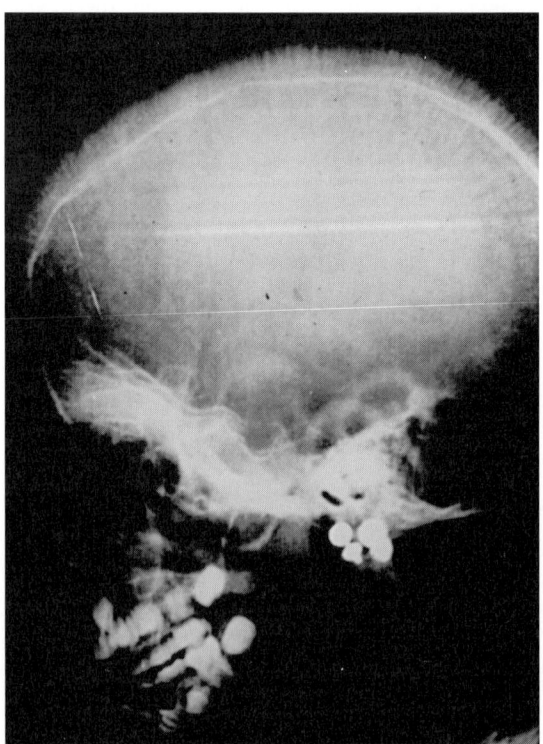

Figure 6–5. Skull radiograph of an African with HbSS, showing expansion of the vault with the "hair-on-end" appearance from erythroid hyperplasia.

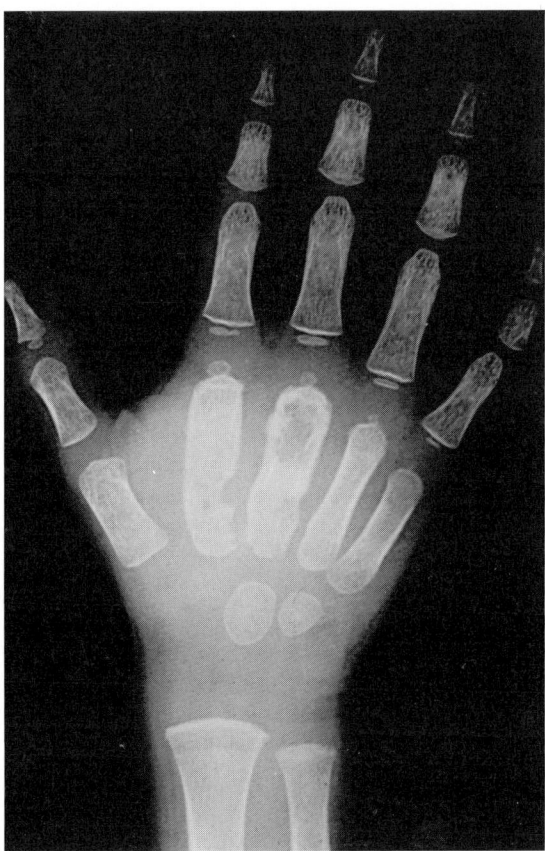

Figure 6–6. Multiple osteolytic lesions in the second and third carpal bones due to bone infarctions in an African child with HbSS disease.

fied. Bone pain crises usually resolve within 1 week, but their course may be complicated by fat or bone marrow embolism to lungs, brain, kidney, or other tissues or by osteomyelitis.

CHEST PAIN. Acute pain in the chest can result from pneumonia, pulmonary infarction, infarction into the thoracic cage, or, rarely, angina pectoris. The first two conditions are often impossible to distinguish, and as one may precede and precipitate the other, many clinicians refer to the complex as acute pulmonary episodes. The cumulative frequency of acute pulmonary disease in African patients is over 30%.

ABDOMINAL PAIN. Over two thirds of patients give a history of mild recurrent abdominal pain, and over 10% require admission to the hospital at some time because of severe abdominal pain. The pain of the acute abdominal crisis of sickle cell disease is usually central or epigastric. There may be vomiting and constipation: Bowel sounds are reduced or absent, and x-ray studies reveal gas and fluid levels. The etiology is obscure, but the probable cause is infarction in the mesenteric vessels. Usually, there is spontaneous recovery in about 5 days. Other causes of acute abdominal pain include splenic infarction, infarction in the lumbar spine, duodenal ulceration (usually in males over 25 years old), cholecystitis, and abdominal crises unrelated to sickle cell disease.

INFARCTIONS ELSEWHERE. Infarction can occur in any tissue and may be followed by a wide range of symptoms, signs, and pathology. For example, intracranial infarctions are fortunately uncommon but cause severe paralyses and alterations of cerebral function. Infarction into the skin around the ankles is followed by sickle cell ulcers; infarction into the corpora cavernosa results in priapism; and infarction in the kidneys causes hematuria and scarring.

Infections. Patients with sickle cell disease have a greater than normal susceptibility to bacterial infections as a result of (1) hyposplenism, which follows recurrent splenic infarction and fibrosis (autosplenectomy); (2) constant activation of the alternative pathway of complement by free hemoglobin in plasma, causing depletion of factor C3 and hence a deficit of opsonization; (3) colonization by bacteria of dead infarcted tissue; and (4) breaches in mucosal surfaces from infarction.

Patients with HbSS disease are particularly susceptible to *Streptococcus pneumoniae, Salmonella,* and other gram-negative organisms as well as *Haemophilus influenzae* type B. The major infectious cause of morbidity and mortality in temperate countries is the pneumococcus, whereas in tropical Africa it is *P. falciparum.* Pneumococcal septicemia, pneumonia, and meningitis occur most frequently below the age of 2 years and have a greater than 50% mortality in the absence of appropriate treatment. Other organisms commonly isolated from bacteremic children with HbSS disease include *Klebsiella, Salmonella, Pseudomonas aeruginosa, Escherichia coli, Staphylococcus* species, and *Streptococcus faecalis.*

At some stage, nearly 10% of patients develop an acute osteomyelitis at the site of bone infarction. In tropical Africa, organisms infecting bones are *Salmonella* (usually *S. typhi*) in 50%, other coliforms in about 45%, and *Staphylococcus pyogenes* in 20%; mixed infections are common.

Growth and Development. Before puberty, height and weight are well below average for age. The shortening is more evident in the trunk than in the legs. The limbs are characteristically long and thin, the abdomen protuberant, and the thorax barrel-shaped; the head and face show bossing (Fig. 6–4). After about age 11 years, skeletal maturation is slow and fusion of epiphyses may be delayed until after age 20 years. This allows subjects with HbSS disease to catch up on their growth during and after puberty, and some men may be excessively tall (over 190 cm [6 feet, 3 inches]).

Puberty is delayed. Menarche occurs in girls with HbSS disease later than normal. These females tend to be immature emotionally and to have prolonged dependence on parents. First pregnancies often are delayed until well after the age of 20 years. In contrast, in some cultures, the girls may be forced into marriage before they are physically or emotionally prepared for childbirth. Men are often impotent as a result of priapism leading to fibrosis.

Pregnancy. Women with the milder forms of sickle cell disease, e.g., HbSC disease, HbS/β+-thalassemia, or sickle cell anemia with favorable genetic or environmental factors, are likely to survive to adulthood and to be fertile. Women with sickle cell disease who are not under medical care are liable to develop extremely severe anemia during the second trimester of pregnancy, associated with malaria and folate deficiency. Other common complications include acute sequestration crises, bone pain crises near the time of delivery, preeclampsia during labor, operative deliveries necessitated by pelvic disproportion, bacterial infections, and wound sepsis. Perinatal mortality (up to 20%) and maternal mortality (up to 10%) remain high in Africa.

HIV and Sickle Cell Disease. There is a close geographic coincidence between regions where the HbS gene is frequent and those where HIV is epidemic (Chapter 23). HIV seropositivity may be as high as 20% among blood donors, and as a consequence, 5% to 20% of patients with sickle cell disease had become infected through blood transfusion in some cities by the mid-1980s, before HIV serology and donor screening became possible. The highest rates of infection had occurred where there had been no active maintenance of health but merely treatment of sickle cell crises, often with blood transfusions. Patients with sickle cell disease who are infected

TABLE 6–5. Maintenance of Health in Sickle Cell Disease

Early Diagnosis
a. Laboratory techniques
  HbS solubility
  Hb electrophoresis
b. Screening
  Pregnant women
  Newborn of mother with S gene
  Anemic children
  Siblings of patients
c. Clinical awareness

Education
a. Parents and patients
b. Health professionals
c. General public

Sickle Cell Clinics
a. Prevent infection
  Prophylactic antimalarials
  Immunization
  Prophylactic penicillin
b. Nutrition
  Folic acid supplements
  General nutritional advice
c. Advice
  Avoid cold, fatigue, dehydration, excessive alcohol
  No useless treatment
  Attend clinic regularly
  Report when ill
  Report when pregnant

Hospitals
  Prompt treatment of crises

Obstetrics
a. Supervision of pregnancy, delivery, puerperium
b. Family limitation to ≤3 viable children

with HIV present most commonly with generalized lymphadenopathy. Other common features are failure to gain (or loss of) weight, chronic lower respiratory tract infections, persistent watery diarrhea, oral candidiasis, and herpes zoster. Both onset of HIV-related disease following transfusion and progression to death appear rapid in the small series studied so far.

The advent of HIV and AIDS has made it more important than ever that (1) there be investment in maintenance of health of patients with sickle cell disease (Table 6–5), and (2) blood transfusions be given only when indicated. The relative size of this problem is clear when it is remembered that 1% to 2% of infants are born with sickle cell disease in tropical Africa each year, compared with only 1 in 10,000 born with hemophilia.

Prognosis. In rural Africa, where there is poor hygiene, no mosquito avoidance, and no modern medicine, less than 2% of children with sickle cell disease live beyond 4 years of age. In North America, in contrast, the median age of death is 42 years for men and 48 for women. There are both inherited and environmental factors that improve the prognosis.

Genetic Factors. The type of sickle cell disease is important. HbSS and HbS/β⁰-thalassemia carry the worst prognosis; HbSC is less severe, and HbS/β⁺-thalassemia is a relatively mild condition.

There are numerous polymorphisms of the β-globin gene cluster, referred to as the β-globin haplotypes. Four β-globin haplotypes are commonly associated with the βˢ mutation. The Senegal haplotype is found on the western seaboard of West Africa (Fig. 6–2). The Benin haplotype is prevalent in West Africa, from whence it has spread to the Mediterranean basin, Southwest Arabia, and Turkey. The Bantu haplotype is common in East and Central Africa and Madagascar. The Asian haplotype is prevalent around the Arabian Sea, including eastern Arabia and the Indian subcontinent. The Cameroon haplotype has a local frequency. These haplotypes are linked to determinants of levels of HbF persisting in HbSS anemia beyond infancy. The highest level of HbF (mean, 20%) is associated with the Asian haplotype. The Senegal haplotype has a higher HbF (mean, 12%) than do the other African haplotypes, Benin and Bantu (both average 8%). High levels of HbF lead to less jelling and sickling, longer red cell survival, and higher total Hb, hematocrit, MCV, and MCH. There is less infarction, less autosplenectomy, and generally milder disease.

Coincidental inheritance of homozygous α⁺-thalassemia (present in approximately 7% of the population of tropical Africa) with HbSS disease decreases the total Hb per red cell (low MCH); there are fewer sickled cells, longer red cell survival, increased red cell counts, lower reticulocyte counts, and lower serum bilirubin along with fewer complications, such as stroke and chronic organ damage in adults.

Environmental Factors. The genetic differences explain the wide variation in severity of sickle cell disease even within one family. In communities with high rates of intercurrent infection and malnutrition, however, the environmental factors are of far greater importance. Prognosis is improved greatly when families are able and willing to care for their children by protecting them from malaria, ensuring cleanliness and good hygiene, obtaining all immunizations, providing adequate nutrition, and seeking medical care. The role of health professionals is to support families in their attempts to maintain the health of their members born with this disorder. With proper care, patients with sickle cell disease lead full and active lives.

Maintenance of Health. Emphasis must be placed on maintaining the steady state in sickle cell disease through early diagnosis, education, and supportive care at sickle cell clinics, hospitals, and obstetric units (Table 6–5).

Diagnosis. Policies should be formulated and implemented for the widespread neonatal diagnosis of sickle cell disease. All pregnant women should be screened by the Serjeant HbS solubility test (not by commercial kits or the sickling test) followed by Hb electrophoresis if HbS is present. All infants born of women carrying at least one S gene should be tested at birth by electrophoresis on cellulose acetate at alkaline pH followed by electrophoresis on citrate agar at pH 6 to 6.5 if an abnormality is detected. Such a scheme would detect infants with HbSS, but would miss HbSC and HbS β-thal in infants who inherit the S gene from the father. In populations in which β-thalassemia is common, pregnant women should be screened with the one-tube osmotic fragility test. HbC can be detected only by electrophoresis, which is not cost-effective in prenatal screening.

Health Education. The condition should be explained to the parents and patients, verbally and by the use of pamphlets. Discussions at subsequent visits to the clinic reinforce the importance of disease prevention and health maintenance. Education should be extended to all medical and paramedical staff and to the general public.

Preventive Care. The most important intervention is the lifelong protection against malaria (Chapter 92). Patients should receive curative treatment at their initial clinic visit and at the first visit following any break in attendance, followed by prophylaxis for as long as they live where malaria is endemic. The choice of antimalarials is made difficult by the emergence of drug-resistant strains of *P. falciparum*. In much of sub-Saharan Africa sulfadoxine-pyrimethamine

(Fansidar), as first-line curative, and proguanil (Paludrine), as prophylactic, are effective. Compliance in taking white tablets (proguanil) and one yellow tablet (folic acid) has been excellent. A trial of atovaquone plus proguanil for prophylaxis in sickle cell disease is needed. Oral prophylactic penicillin is highly effective in preventing pneumococcal infection in the United States and the United Kingdom but has not received a trial in tropical Africa.

Another essential function of the sickle cell clinic is to provide a place where patients can report when sick, so that they can be assessed rapidly and be admitted to the hospital if necessary, and without becoming lost in the mass of patients attending the acute pediatric or medical outpatients' clinics.

Experimental Therapies. There are therapies under trial aimed at reducing the jelling of HbS in red cells; hydroxyurea and isobutyramide (an analogue of butyrate) raise the levels of HbF, and clotrimazole increases the water content of red cells. No results of trials in Africa have been published by 1998. Bone marrow transplant has, at present, no significant place in tropical Africa.

Management of Crisis

General Measures. Whenever a patient with sickle cell disease is seriously ill, a minimum of laboratory studies includes Hb (or hematocrit), reticulocyte count, total and differential white cell count, thick film for malaria, and urinalysis. If the patient has fever or if pneumonia, meningitis, or acute osteomyelitis is suspected, the blood should be cultured. A Gram stain and a sputum culture are required when there is an acute pulmonary disease. A lumbar puncture should be performed when there is even minimal meningism. Feces should be examined by microscopy and culture if there is diarrhea. Radiography of the chest is indicated when there is high fever or suspected pneumonia. After obtaining informed consent, serum should be tested for anti-HIV if there has been possible exposure, e.g., through blood transfusion, or if the clinical presentation suggests HIV-related disease.

It should be assumed that malaria is contributing to the crisis, and treatment should be started before results of microscopy of the blood are available (Chapter 92). Antimalarial prophylaxis and supplements of folic acid should be started or continued.

Treatment of Anemic Crises. The administration of antimalarials, folic acid, and antibiotics, if indicated, arrests the decline of hematocrit and is followed by recovery in most patients. Blood transfusion should be avoided whenever possible because of its dangers, including those of transmitting HIV, hepatitis B virus, and other infections. Transfusion is indicated (1) when there is incipient or established cardiac failure, which can develop when the Hb is less than 40 g/L; (2) when there is acute sequestration crisis, with Hb less than 60 g/L and falling rapidly; (3) when obstetric delivery is imminent and the Hb is less than 80 g/L; (4) following acute hemorrhage, when blood pressure and oxygenation cannot be restored by crystalloids or colloids; and (5) preceding or during emergency major surgery.

Donor blood should be subjected to the HbS solubility test, and HbAA blood donors should be selected: HbAS blood should be transfused only in emergencies and in the absence of suitable HbAA blood. Except for treating hemorrhage, concentrated red cells, *not* whole blood, should be transfused, 10 mL/kg body weight administered over 4 to 6 hours, preceded by intramuscular furosemide 1.0 mg/kg body weight when there is cardiac failure.

Other Indications for Blood Transfusions. Emergency exchange blood transfusions are administered by most clinicians in the treatment of acute cerebrovascular accident; they have been advocated also for severe priapism, acute chest syndrome, and acute abdominal crisis, but there is no convincing evidence that this treatment is advantageous. Elective exchange blood transfusions have been recommended to precede major surgery or contrast radiography, but patients do just as well with more conservative transfusion regimens and have less alloimmunization. In Africa, especially, transfusions should be limited as far as possible, so as to avoid infectious complications. The blood selected must be HbAA, HIV-, HBV-, and HCV-negative, and closely matched antigenically to the recipient. At least twice the patient's volume of blood is exchanged by an isovolumic procedure, with the aim of reducing the HbS to below 20% and giving a final Hb concentration of 140 to 150 g/L.

Hypertransfusion regimens have been proposed (1) in the management of pregnancy; (2) for 3 months following prosthetic joint surgery; (3) for 3 years following cerebrovascular accidents; (4) for recurrent life-threatening chest crises; and (5) when recurrent infarctive crisis prevents a normal life. There is no evidence that pregnant women or their fetuses do better on a hypertransfusion regimen, and this is not recommended in developing countries. Decisions to administer hypertransfusion treatment must be made on an individual basis and should not be embarked on unless (1) an adequate supply of suitable HbAA blood is ensured; (2) blood infected by HIV, HBV, or HCV can be excluded effectively; and (3) chances of alloimmunization can be kept to a minimum.

Treatment of Infarctive Crises. The principles of management are the control of pain, the maintenance of hydration and acid-base balance, and the treatment of infection. The physician must assess the severity of pain and prescribe analgesics at fixed dosages and regular intervals and not delegate decisions regarding pain control to nurses. Mild pain can be controlled by acetaminophen (paracetamol), moderate pain by dihydrocodeine tartrate, and severe pain by opiates. Patients should be encouraged to drink fluids if they are able to do so. More seriously ill patients may need nasogastric fluid or, if bowel sounds cannot be heard, intravenous fluid.

High-dose intravenous methylprednisolone is reported to decrease the duration of severe pain in children and adolescents, through its anti-inflammatory properties.

Treatment of Acute Infections. Antibiotics should be given only when they are needed, and then they must be administered quickly and in adequate dosage.

When a patient has fever higher than 39°C not accounted for by malaria, an acute pulmonary episode, or suspected meningitis, treatment should be started. Cefuroxime sodium, 150 mg/kg/day, or large doses of ampicillin or penicillin plus chloramphenicol are recommended. The initial treatment of acute osteomyelitis should be cloxacillin plus chloramphenicol.

Prenatal Diagnosis. Chorionic villous biopsy, DNA extraction, selective amplification of DNA fragments by polymerase chain reaction, and restriction endonuclease analysis allow for the prenatal diagnosis of sickle cell disease and β-thalassemia during the first trimester of pregnancy. There are several constraints preventing the large-scale application of prenatal diagnosis in developing countries. These include (1) the lack of trained staff and facilities for collection of chorionic villous biopsies; (2) the complexity and expense of gene analysis; (3) a lack of comprehension by most couples at risk; and (4) the illegality or ethical nonacceptance of therapeutic abortion. It is possible, however, that some centers in developing countries will be able to provide prenatal diagnosis of the hemoglobinopathies in the near future.

Sickle Cell Trait. This is essentially a benign condition. Microinfarcts in the renal medulla do have some consequences, however. There is a progressive loss of ability to concentrate urine, which increases the likelihood of dehydration: exertional heat illness, as experienced by military recruits in training, is a rare cause of death more common in carriers of HbAS. Significant bacteriuria during pregnancy is about twice as common as expected in women with sickle cell trait. Painless hematuria resulting from papillary necrosis has been reported. Early reports of splenic infarcts while flying in unpressurized aircraft were mostly in subjects with other conditions including HbSC, but splenic infarct can follow exertion at high altitude.

BETA-THALASSEMIAS. Depressions of synthesis of the β-chains of hemoglobin, conditions known collectively as the β-thalassemias, occur commonly throughout a broad belt from the Mediterranean to Oceania and on the Atlantic seaboard of West Africa (Fig. 6–7). Within this area, between 2% and 30% of the population are carriers of the abnormal genes, but β-thalassemia is seen sporadically in all racial groups. As much as 3% of the world's population, or over 150 million individuals, mostly in Asia, carry genes for β-thalassemia.

There are nearly 150 known mutations leading to β-thalassemia. Most are point mutations affecting rates of β-chain synthesis at any stage from initiation of transcription to translation, to messenger RNA (mRNA) function and mRNA processing, and only a few are deletions of the β-gene. About 20 alleles account for 90% of β-thalassemia genes. Different populations tend to have different groups of mutations, with a few common alleles and a variable number of rare ones.

The genes are expressed either as complete suppression of β-globin synthesis (β^0-thalassemia genes) or partial suppression (β$^+$-thalassemia genes).

Clinically, the thalassemias are classified according to their severity. *Thalassemia major* is a severe disorder in which the patient is dependent on blood transfusion for survival beyond early childhood. *Thalassemia intermedia* is characterized by anemia and splenomegaly, requiring blood transfusion only at irregular intervals. *Thalassemia minor* is the symptomless state, with moderate anemia only.

Beta-Thalassemia Major. Major disease arises from the homozygous or compound heterozygous inheritance of β^0- or most β$^+$-thalassemia genes. Over 50,000 infants are born each year with β-thalassemia major.

Etiology and Pathophysiology. As production of γ-globin declines in the first 6 months of postuterine life, it is not replaced with β-globin in infants with β-thalassemia. The

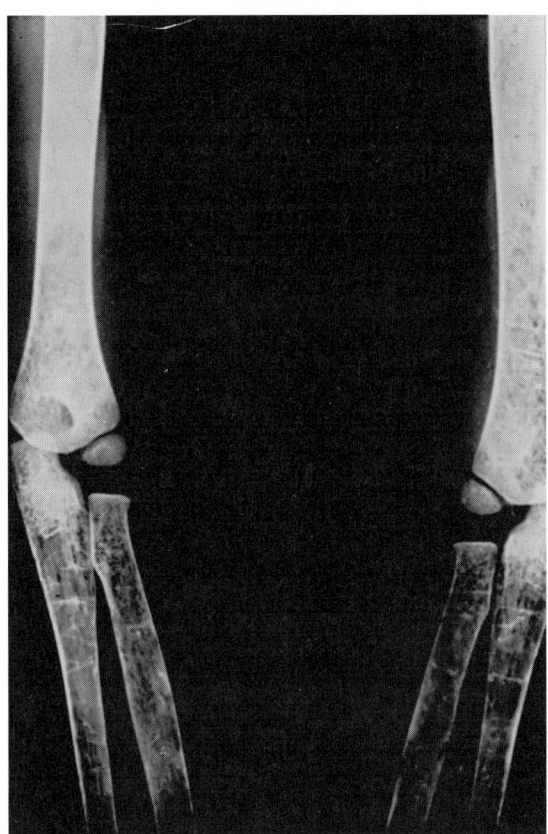

Figure 6–8. X-ray film of femur, tibia, and fibula of a patient with β-thalassemia major. Massive expansion of the bone marrow cavities due to erythroid hyperplasia has caused loss of calcification and cystic changes.

excess of α-globin chains form intracellular inclusions, which cause both ineffective erythropoiesis and hemolysis, especially from phagocytosis of erythrocytes in the spleen. There is gross erythroid hyperplasia with massive expansion of the bone marrow cavities (Fig. 6–8). Splenic hypertrophy leads to hypersplenism with further sequestration of red cells, granulocytes, and platelets and expansion of plasma volume. The absorption of iron is increased and it is poorly utilized in hemoglobin synthesis, so that iron accumulates in tissues. Some red cell precursors normally retain the ability to produce HbF ($\alpha_2\gamma_2$); the synthesis of these cells is increased in the hypertrophic bone marrow and they survive preferentially in the blood. As δ-chain synthesis is normal, there is a relative and absolute increase in HbA$_2$ ($\alpha_2\delta_2$).

Clinical Manifestations. Infants fail to thrive and have intermittent fevers, pallor, and splenomegaly. With no treatment, or only intermittent blood transfusions, there is severe retardation of growth and development throughout childhood. There is progressive enlargement of the spleen. Hypersplenism occurs and worsens the anemia and may cause hemorrhage as a complication of thrombocytopenia. There is gross bossing of all the bones of the skull, with poorly formed teeth and blockages of sinuses. Secondary infection of the middle ear may cause deafness. Skull radiographs show thinning of the outer table and spicules of bone in the expanded marrow cavity (i.e., "hair-on-end" appearance) (Fig. 6–5). Changes in the long bones are associated with pathologic fractures (Fig. 6–8). Severe drops in Hb concentration follow either infection or folic acid depletion.

The accumulation of iron leads to progressive hemosid-

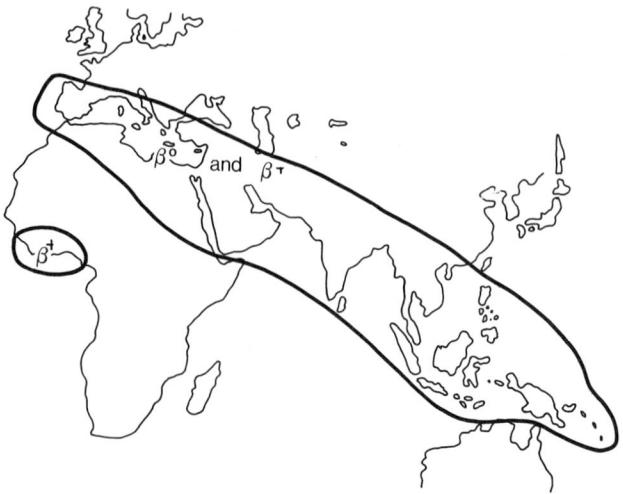

Figure 6–7. Areas of the Old World where various forms of β-thalassemia reach polymorphic frequencies.

erosis. This causes cardiac arrhythmias, pericarditis, and congestive heart failure; complex endocrine disorders include diabetes mellitus, hypoparathyroidism, hypothyroidism, adrenal insufficiency, and hypogonadism; hepatic cirrhosis develops with liver failure; in light-skinned people, there is bronze discoloration of the skin.

Other biochemical changes include hyperuricemia and secondary gout as well as depletion of ascorbate and vitamin E.

Without treatment, children die usually within the first 2 years from anemic heart failure. With intermittent treatment by blood transfusion, they are likely to succumb instead to overwhelming infection in childhood. If they survive beyond the age of puberty, the most common cause of death is cardiac failure from hemosiderosis.

Hematology. The hemoglobin is usually 20 to 80 g/L at the time of presentation. The MCH and MCV are reduced. The peripheral blood film is grossly abnormal, and characteristically there is considerable anisocytosis with macrocytes and microcytes, numerous target cells, poikilocytosis, fragmented red cells, marked hypochromia, nucleated red cells that may show megaloblastic change, and basophilic stippling. The reticulocyte count is usually only slightly elevated. The white cell counts may be high from infection or low from hypersplenism. Platelets may be decreased owing to hypersplenism. There is erythroid hyperplasia, often with megaloblastosis, and an excess of iron in the bone marrow.

Bilirubin levels, both conjugated and unconjugated, are high. There is an ahaptoglobulinemia. Serum iron and serum ferritin levels are raised. Patients with homozygous β^0-thalassemias have only HbF and HbA_2 and no HbA on Hb electrophoresis. Patients with β^+-thalassemias have 30% to 90% HbF, the rest being HbA except for less than 4% HbA_2.

Clinical observations, peripheral red cell appearance, and Hb electrophoretic patterns are diagnostic.

Treatment. The symptomatic treatment of β-thalassemia major depends on high blood-transfusion regimens, deferoxamine as an iron chelator, and splenectomy to counteract hypersplenism.

BLOOD TRANSFUSION. Shortly after the diagnosis is made, a hypertransfusion regimen should be implemented, with the aim of maintaining the hemoglobin at about 120 g/L. This may mean transfusion every 2 or 3 weeks. Red cells that are depleted of leukocytes by filtration, washing, or freezing are preferred because they cause fewer reactions from antileukocyte antibodies. This treatment effectively suppresses the patient's own abnormal erythropoiesis and allows for normal growth and development in childhood. However, as each milliliter of red cell contains 1 mg of iron, the progression of hemosiderosis is accelerated, and this will suppress the adolescent growth spurt and secondary sexual development. Death is usual in the second or third decade of life from progressive damage to the heart.

IRON CHELATION. Deferoxamine is an effective agent for enhancing the excretion of iron. A wide variety of routes of administration and dosages have been advocated for treating iron overload. One treatment regimen is to give deferoxamine, 6 and 12 g daily, by intravenous indwelling catheter. Iron overload can be prevented by the subcutaneous infusion of 2 g daily, starting at the same time as the high-transfusion regimen. All regimens are troublesome and expensive, and compliance is often poor. The oral chelator deferiprone (or L1) is efficacious, but carries a risk for agranulocytosis and other toxicities.

SPLENECTOMY. Increasing requirements for blood transfusions, along with leukopenia and thrombocytopenia, suggest hypersplenism and are, if severe, indications for splenectomy. The operation should be delayed until after the age of 5 years and should be followed by lifelong penicillin prophylaxis, and antimalarial prophylaxis in endemic areas.

These regimens have revolutionized the outlook for patients with β-thalassemia major; overall survival at 15 years is about 95%. Some women have had successful pregnancies. However, about 25 units of blood are needed for each patient per year, and the total cost of treating a patient in the United States can be over $30,000 per year. These are impossible burdens for the health resources of developing countries.

BONE MARROW TRANSPLANT. In selected patients who are in good health, bone marrow transplant is curative, but carries a 5% operative mortality.

EXPERIMENTAL THERAPIES. As with sickle cell disease, thalassemia may be ameliorated by agents that raise the levels of HbF, such as azacytidine, butyrate, hydroxyurea, and human recombinant erythropoietin.

PREVENTION. There are two approaches to prevention of β-thalassemia major.

HEALTH EDUCATION. In the first approach, carriers are identified and given genetic counseling about either the choice of marriage partner, or in the case of couples already married, the chances of infants being affected. This approach has not been conspicuously successful.

PRENATAL DIAGNOSIS AND ABORTION. The second approach is prenatal diagnosis by chorion biopsy at 10 to 12 weeks of pregnancy, fetal DNA analysis by the polymerase chain reaction (PCR) and reverse dot blotting, followed by therapeutic abortion of fetuses with major disease. Prenatal diagnostic services are well established in Greece, Cyprus, and Sardinia, and are being developed in Thailand. Widespread application of prenatal diagnosis in Asia would be most beneficial because of the severity of the disease and the limitations and cost of treatment.

Beta-Thalassemia Intermedia

Etiology. Intermediate disease arises from the inheritance of HbE β-thal, HbC β-thal, various $\delta\beta$-thalassemias, or Hb-Lepore disorders or from some homozygous β-thalassemias coinciding with α-thalassemia, homozygous β^+-thalassemia in West Africa, or the coinheritance of genes for enhanced HbF production.

Over 40,000 infants are born each year into the largest group, which is HbE β-thal in Southeast Asia (Figs. 6–3 and 6–7).

Clinical Manifestations. The spectrum of disease ranges from those who have only moderate anemia to those with Hb levels of 40 to 50 g/L, splenomegaly, folate deficiency, skeletal deformities, iron overload progressing with age, recurrent leg ulcers, gallstones, and increased susceptibility to infections.

Treatment. These patients need regular surveillance. For patients with more severe anemia, folic acid supplements are indicated, and antimalarial prophylaxis is required in endemic areas. Blood transfusions should be given to treat anemic crises, and regular transfusion regimens may have to be instigated for patients with growth retardation and serious bone deformities. Some develop hypersplenism and require splenectomy. Antibiotics are necessary to counteract infections.

Beta-Thalassemia Minor. The heterozygous inheritance of any of the β-thalassemia genes is usually symptom-free, but rarely there is mild splenomegaly. The Hb is generally 90 to 110 g/L, but in pregnancy it is often 20 g/L lower. The MCH and MCV are low. Red cells show anisocytosis, microcytosis, hypochromia, and occasional target cells. Sometimes basophilic stippling is seen in a few cells. The changes in the red cells are characteristically more than would have been expected from the Hb concentration. The bone marrow shows moderate erythroid hyperplasia. The frequency of iron deficiency reflects that of the general population. The HbA_2 is elevated to 4% to 6%, and this is the most valuable diagnostic observation. HbF is up to 3% in about half the subjects. Osmotic fragility is reduced; the one-tube osmotic fragility test is useful in population and antenatal screening.

Partial protection against *P. falciparum* parasitemia has been demonstrated in individuals from Liberia with β-thalassemia minor. The apparent protective effect may be related to greater expression of neoantigens on the surface of parasitized red cells, enhanced immune recognition, and hence clearance of parasitized erythrocytes.

Persistent anemia during pregnancy in women with β-thalassemia minor causes a degree of fetal hypoxia, compensatory placental hypertrophy, intrauterine growth retardation, low urinary estriol excretion, and an increased frequency of fetal distress during delivery. The resulting high frequency (about 12%) of 1-minute Apgar scores of 3 or less is not associated with any appreciable increase in infant mortality.

DELTA-BETA THALASSEMIAS. These are much less common than β-thalassemias. They arise from either gene deletion or crossing over between δ- and β-genes leading to the production of Hb-Lepore.

Homozygous $(\delta\beta)^0$ Thalassemia. This is characterized by an Hb of 80 to 100 g/L, moderate splenomegaly, and HbF of 100%. Anemia is more severe with infection and pregnancy. Heterozygotes are symptom-free; they have 5% to 20% HbF and normal HbA_2.

Homozygous δβ (Lepore). This presents generally as thalassemia intermedia. Electrophoresis shows only Hb-Lepore. Heterozygotes have characteristic thalassemic hematologic findings and 5% to 15% Hb-Lepore.

Hereditary Persistence of Hemoglobin F (HPHF). This is a group of conditions that are seen most commonly in Africa. Defective synthesis of β- and δ-chains is almost wholly compensated for by the continued synthesis of γ-chains. Homozygotes are not anemic but have a mild thalassemic red cell appearance and 100% HbF. Heterozygotes have no clinical or hematologic abnormality except HbF of 20% to 30%, distributed homogeneously in all red cells.

γδβ-Thalassemias. These conditions are rare, arising from deletions of γ- and δ- as well as β-genes. Homozygous inheritance is obviously incompatible with fetal survival. Heterozygotes have severe hemolytic disease of the newborn. Those who survive have a thalassemia minor with normal HbF and HbA_2.

ALPHA-THALASSEMIAS

Pathophysiology. The conditions that arise from genetically determined reductions in production of α-globin chains are known as the α-thalassemias. The α-globin genes are duplicated on chromosome 16, so that the normal individual has four active genes (αα/αα). Most α-thalassemias are the result of deletions of one ($-\alpha$ or α^+-thalassemia) or both genes ($-\alpha/-\alpha$ or α^0-thalassemia). Some α^+-thalassemias are nondeletional mutations effectively inactivating one α-gene through (1) abnormal splicing; (2) the synthesis of unstable α-chains; (3) interference with polyadenylation of mRNA; or (4) the slow synthesis of elongated chains (e.g., Hb-Constant Spring, which is present in 2% to 5% of the population of Thailand).

There are three genotypes that result in clinically asymptomatic states: (1) heterozygous α^+-thalassemia ($-\alpha/\alpha\alpha$); (2) homozygous α^+-thalassemia ($-\alpha/-\alpha$); and (3) heterozygous α^0-thalassemia ($--/\alpha\alpha$). There are two genotypes that cause symptomatic disease: (1) the double heterozygous α^+-thalassemia/α^0-thalassemia ($-\alpha/--$), in which three out of four genes are inactive, causing HbH disease; and (2) homozygous α^0-thalassemia ($--/--$), causing the Hb-

Barts hydrops syndrome. The pathophysiology of these conditions depends on the excess of γ-chains in fetal life combining to form tetrameres (γ_4) called Hb-Barts, and the excess of β-chains in postuterine life combining to form tetrameres (β_4) called HbH. The hemoglobins have excessively high oxygen affinity, causing tissue hypoxia. HbH is also unstable, being precipitated as inclusion bodies leading to hemolysis.

Clinical Manifestations

Asymptomatic States. The gene frequency (about 0.26) for α^+-thalassemia is remarkably uniform throughout tropical Africa, making this by far the most common variant of hemoglobin synthesis; 38% of the population is heterozygous and 7% homozygous. Frequencies are much more variable in Asia and Oceania and can be 80% in some populations (e.g., Nepal, Andra Pradesh, Papua New Guinea). These are wholly asymptomatic; hematologic changes are minimal and include slight anemia, reductions in MCV and MCH, and slight microcytosis on blood film appearance. Hb-Barts can be detected in trace amounts in only 10% of heterozygotes at birth and is about 2.5% of total Hb in all homozygotes. Only by DNA analysis or by measuring rates of globin-chain synthesis can α^+-thalassemia be diagnosed with certainty.

In Africa, α^+-thalassemia is significant because of (1) the high gene frequency accounting for an average reduction of Hb of 5 g/L in blacks in comparison with Caucasians; (2) causing a trimodal distribution of the proportion of HbS in subjects with sickle cell trait (i.e., mean HbS is 27% in α^+-thalassemia homozygotes, 35% in heterozygotes, and 41% in those with normal α-globin synthesis); (3) the amelioration of HbSS disease by homozygous α^+-thalassemia; and (4) the probability that α-thalassemia affords slight partial protection against malaria.

The strongest evidence that α-thalassemia provides partial protection against malaria is the geographic coincidence between high gene frequency and endemic malaria, implying selection for the gene. Survival, genetic, or parasitologic advantages have not been demonstrated convincingly: one possible mechanism is that malaria-induced neonatal antigens are more strongly expressed in α-thalassemia erythrocytes, similar to the clinical picture in β-thalassemias.

Heterozygous α^0-thalassemia is hematologically identical to homozygous α^+-thalassemia; each has two active globin genes. Thirty million subjects in Southeast Asia and southern China are carriers for α^0-thalassemia.

Hemoglobin-H Disease. The most common genotype leading to HbH disease is α^+-thal/α^0-thal, but the disorder arises also from α^+-thal/Hb-Constant Spring in Southeast Asia and homozygous inheritance of severe nondeletion α^+-thalassemias occurs in Saudi Arabia. About 60,000 affected infants are born each year in Thailand alone. The condition presents with a variable degree of anemia and splenomegaly. The course is usually mild, but rarely children have significant growth retardation and skeletal changes. Severe hemolytic anemic crises are associated with infection, pregnancy, and exposure to oxidant drugs. Patients survive into adult life, often with progressive pancytopenia due to hypersplenism.

At birth, there is up to 25% Hb-Barts; after the first year of life, there is 5% to 40% HbH, with HbA and low levels of HbA_2. The hemoglobin is 70 to 100 g/L in the steady state; the peripheral blood film shows a typical thalassemic picture. The reticulocyte count is usually slightly raised. There are numerous inclusion bodies of precipitated HbH in the preparation of red cells stained with cresyl blue. Following splenectomy, these inclusions are much more numerous.

Patients should be seen in medical clinics at regular intervals. They should be warned against the use of oxidant drugs

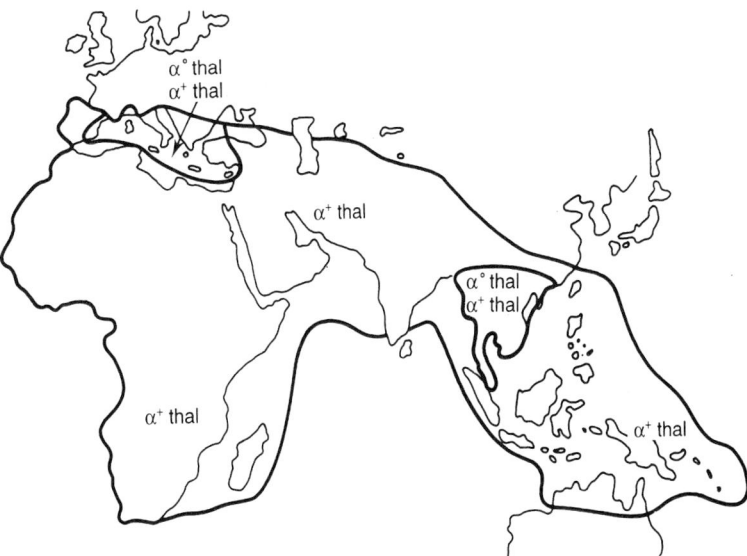

Figure 6–9. Areas of the Old World where the different forms of α-thalassemia reach polymorphic frequencies. (From Fleming AF: Haematological diseases in the tropics. *In* Cook GC [ed]: Manson's Tropical Diseases, 20th ed. London, WB Saunders, 1996, pp 101–173.)

and advised to report when unwell or pregnant. Splenectomy may become necessary with progressive hypersplenism.

Hemoglobin Barts Hydrops Syndrome. The homozygous inheritance of α^0-thalassemia occurs commonly in Southeast Asia, Greece, and Cyprus (Fig. 6–9). Over 20,000 affected infants are delivered each year. The infants are stillborn at 28 to 40 weeks of gestation or die shortly after delivery. They are pale and edematous and have massive hepatosplenomegaly. The placenta is enlarged and friable. The Hb is 60 to 80 g/L, and the blood picture is typically thalassemic. Electrophoresis reveals about 80% Hb-Barts and about 20% embryonic Hb-Portland ($\zeta_2\gamma_2$).

The mother frequently suffers from preeclampsia or even eclampsia. Both parents have the mildly abnormal hematologic findings of α^0-thalassemia trait.

There is a strong case to be made for the identification of couples at risk, the prenatal diagnosis by chorion biopsy and DNA analysis, followed by the termination of pregnancies with affected infants. This would avoid the obstetric complications and psychologic trauma of delivery of stillborn hydropic infants.

GLUCOSE-6-PHOSPHATE DEHYDROGENASE DEFICIENCY

Pathophysiology. About 90% of glucose in red cells is degraded by the Embden-Meyerhof pathway to produce adenosine triphosphate and release energy for cellular metabolic processes. The remaining 10% is degraded via the hexose monophosphate shunt (pentose shunt), with reduction of nicotinamide adenosine dinucleotide phosphate (NADP) to NADPH, which is the main H donor in other enzymatic reactions, including the maintenance by glutathione reductase of glutathione (GSSG) in its reduced form (GSH). GSH

protects components of the red cells from autooxidation. Failure of the system leads to oxidation of hemoglobin to methemoglobin or to the intracellular precipitation of globin as Heinz bodies, and oxidation of lipids and proteins in the membrane. A common cause of failure and consequent hemolysis is the congenital deficiency of activity of glucose-6-phosphate dehydrogenase (G6PD), the first enzyme of the hexose monophosphate shunt. The enzyme is found normally, and may be deficient, in a wide range of cells of the body, including the hepatocytes, as well as in red cells.

Over 440 variants of G6PD have been identified by thermostability, chromatography, and kinetic properties. They have been classified according to clinical manifestations and enzyme activity (Table 6–6). This discussion is confined to those enzymes that achieve polymorphic frequency in large populations. The most common, or normal, enzyme is GdB of class IV (normal activity). Variants with normal activity include GdA, common throughout Africa. Variants with moderately reduced activity (class III) include GdA$^-$, the common deficient enzyme of Africa (Fig. 6–10). The most common variant with severely deficient activity (class II) is Gd^{Mediterranean}.

The inheritance of G6PD synthesis is sex-linked. The hemizygous male, who inherits an abnormal gene ($\bar{X}Y$), will have all red cells containing the variant enzyme, as will the homozygous female ($\bar{X}\bar{X}$). Heterozygous females ($\bar{X}X$) will have, on average, half of all red cells with the variant and half with the normal enzyme.

Geographic Distribution and Malaria. The first evidence that G6PD deficiency confers some advantage against malaria is the worldwide coincidence between populations in which deficient enzymes are frequent and areas of the world where *P. falciparum* malaria is, or was until recently, endemic

TABLE 6–6. Variants of Glucose-6-Phosphate Dehydrogenase

Class	G6PD Activity	Clinical Presentation	Polymorphic Variants
I	Near-absent	Congenital nonspherocytic hemolytic disease	—
II	Severe <10%	Intermittent hemolysis	Mediterranean, Mali, Union
III	Moderate 10–60%	Less severe intermittent hemolysis	A$^-$, Canton, Mahidol
IV	Normal activity 60–150%	None	B (the normal enzyme), A, Gambia
V	Increased activity >150%	None	—

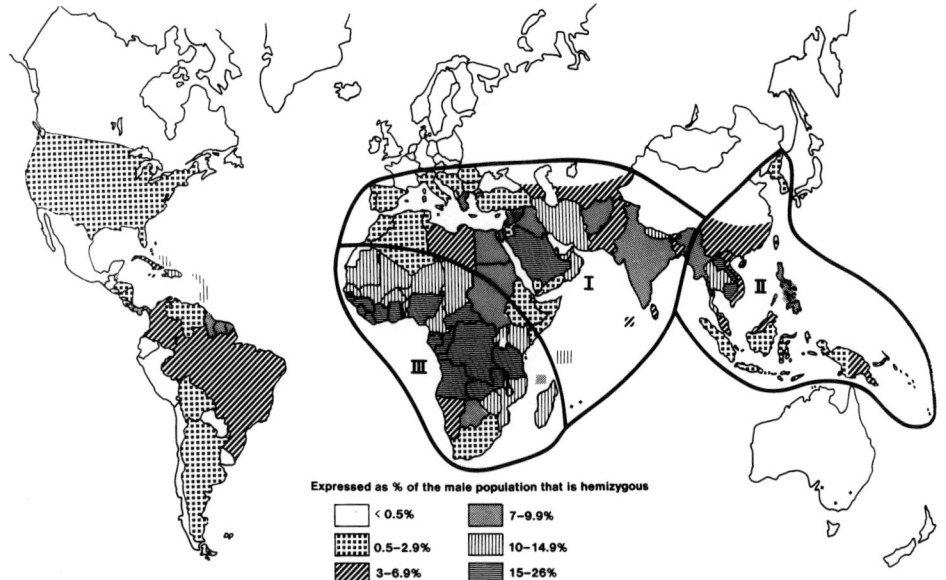

Expressed as % of the male population that is hemizygous

< 0.5%	7–9.9%
0.5–2.9%	10–14.9%
3–6.9%	15–26%

Figure **6–10.** World distribution of glucose-6-phosphate dehydrogenase (G6PD) deficiency. Superimposed are three zones where different G6PD variants reach polymorphic frequencies. Zone I, Gd^{Mediterranean}; zone II, Gd^{Canton}, Gd^{Union}, Gd^{Mahidol}, and eight or nine other variants; zone III, GdA$^-$. In the Americas, GdA$^-$, Gd^{Mediterranean}, and the different Asian variants reflect descent of the populations. (Reproduced by permission of WHO from: Glucose-6-phosphate dehydrogenase deficiency. Bulletin of the World Health Organization 67:601-611, 1989.)

(Fig. 6–10). The Old World can be divided broadly into three zones. In zone I, from the Mediterranean basin to the Indian subcontinent, Gd^{Mediterranean} with severely defective activity has high prevalence and Gd^{Aures} is also seen among Arabs and in Spain; frequencies are highest in Arabian countries (up to 50% of males in the Eastern Province of Saudi Arabia), Iran, south Asia, and Greece. In the zone II, covering Southeast Asia and southern China, there is great heterogeneity of enzyme variants, including variants of both severely deficient activity (Gd^{Union}) and moderately deficient activity (Gd^{Mahidol}, Gd^{Canton}); G6PD deficiency of all types is found in 12% to 15% of males in Indochina. The common deficient enzyme of zone III, sub-Saharan Africa, is GdA$^-$ with moderately deficient activity; frequency is highest at 32% of males among the Luo in the Lake Victoria region of Kenya, and declines as one moves west or south from Lake Victoria. The variant GdA with normal activity is found in the same populations at slightly greater frequency, e.g., 25% of males in Nigeria; Gd^{Mali} (severe deficiency) and Gd^{Gambia} (normal activity) reach polymorphic frequency locally.

Within these broad areas, micromapping has shown clear correlations between the frequencies of G6PD deficiencies and the intensity of transmission of malaria, e.g., in Sardinia, Greece, East Africa, and Papua New Guinea. Other evidence that G6PD deficiency confers partial protection against *P. falciparum* are (1) decreased parasite densities in deficient subjects compared with controls; (2) in Nigerian girls with malaria and heterozygous for Gd^B/GdA$^-$, there were fewer parasites in deficient than in normal red cells; (3) both hemizygous male and heterozygous female African children have about 50% protection against cerebral malaria or profound malarial anemia; and (4) parasites grow less well in vitro in G6PD-deficient than in normal red cells.

Clinical Manifestations. In the absence of factors triggering hemolysis, red cell survival is normal with class III (e.g., GdA$^-$) and only slightly reduced in class II enzyme deficiencies (e.g., Gd^{Mediterranean}) (Table 6–6). Severe or moderately severe G6PD deficiency is associated with the following clinical hemolytic conditions: (1) neonatal jaundice; (2) infection-induced hemolysis; (3) favism and other food-induced hemolysis; and (4) drug-induced hemolysis. Hemolysis is both more frequent and more severe with enzymes of class II than with class III, and in male hemizygotes and female

homozygotes than in female heterozygotes. Nearly 5 million infants born per year are at risk of the complications of G6PD deficiency.

Neonatal Jaundice. Severe jaundice with serum bilirubin levels above 250 µmol/L (15 mg/dL) on about the fourth day of life is seen commonly in hospitals throughout the Mediterranean basin, Asia, tropical Africa, and the Caribbean, although few accurate estimates of prevalence are available; in Hong Kong before the introduction of preventive measures, 12% of all newborn infants developed hyperbilirubinemia. Etiology is often multiple, the three most commonly identified factors being sepsis, prematurity, and G6PD deficiency. Other less common causes include fetomaternal ABO incompatibility, the resorption of hematomas, rhesus incompatibility, and intrauterine infections. GdA$^-$ is rarely the sole identified cause of neonatal jaundice in Africa but is almost always associated with sepsis, prematurity, or maternal ingestion of modern or traditional oxidative medications (Table 6–7). GdA$^-$ is not a major cause of neonatal jaundice in African Americans in the absence of prematurity or exposure to oxidant drugs. The contribution made to neonatal jaundice by G6PD deficiency varies widely in different populations; estimates have been 34% in Saudi Arabia, up to 5% among Chinese populations, over 10% in Thailand, 9% in Sardinia, 82% in Greece, 33% to 80% in West Africa, and 21% in Jamaica.

Jaundice is chiefly the result of impaired hepatic function, especially in premature infants. The infant's blood picture is most variable; changes include anisocytosis, spherocytosis, polychromasia, and numerous nucleated red cells. Anemia is either absent or mild (Hb <130 g/L). Serum bilirubin levels may rise rapidly to above 300 µmol/L, especially with Gd^{Mediterranean}, at which levels kernicterus can develop with permanent brain damage.

MANAGEMENT. Treatment while serum bilirubin levels are less than 300 µmol/L is by ultraviolet phototherapy; appropriate equipment can be extemporized with seven or more 20 watt fluorescent tubes placed 40 cm above the naked infant, or if necessary, by exposure to sunlight as long as the infant is cooled and the eyes are protected. When the serum bilirubin is above 300 µmol/L, the treatment is by double-volume exchange transfusion using blood compatible with both mother and infant, and which is G6PD normal. In in-

TABLE 6–7. Drugs and Chemicals Associated with Hemolysis in G6PD-Deficient Subjects

	Strong Association	Weak Association*
Antimalarials	Primaquine, pamaquine, pentaquine	Chloroquine
Sulfonamides	Sulfanilamide, sulfacetamide, sulfapyridine, sulfamethoxazole	Sulfamethoxypyridazine, sulfadimidine
Sulfones	Thiazolesulfone, diaminodiphenylsulfone (DDS, dapsone)	
Nitrofurans	Nitrofurantoin	
Antipyretic/analgesic	Acetanilid	
Others	Nalidixic acid, naphthalone, niridazole, phenylhydrazine, toluidine blue, trinitrotoluene, methylene blue, phenazopyridine	Chloramphenicol Vitamin K analogues

*Significant hemolysis occurs only in subjects with variants with severely deficient activity, or in neonates, or with greater than therapeutic dosage. (Adapted from Luzzatto L, Mehta A: In Scriver CR, et al (eds): The Metabolic Basis of Inherited Disease. Vol 2, ed 6, New York, McGraw-Hill, 1989. Reprinted by permission.)

fants of low birthweight or who are ill, treatment should be more vigorous, with phototherapy started earlier and exchange transfusion administered at lower bilirubin levels.

PREVENTION. Neonatal jaundice is largely preventable by good prenatal care, nontraumatic obstetric delivery, and hygienic precautions in the puerperium, thereby reducing the frequency of prematurity, sepsis, and hematomas. Oxidant drugs should not be prescribed during pregnancy unless absolutely essential and unless there are no alternatives. A national campaign in Singapore has dramatically reduced the impact of G6PD deficiency; all newborns have been screened for enzyme activity; deficient infants have been observed and jaundice treated early and vigorously; deficient individuals have been issued with cards identifying them and advising on drugs to be avoided; the general public and the health professionals have been educated.

Infection-Induced Hemolysis. Jaundice due to both hemolysis and hepatocellular failure may complicate the course of pneumonia, infectious hepatitis, typhoid, paratyphoid, and other septicemias or viremias in G6PD-deficient subjects. A possible mechanism is the release of active oxygen species from activated phagocytes. The clinical severity of this complication will be greater if there is pre-existing anemia, impaired hepatic or renal function, and the simultaneous administration of oxidant drugs. A patient may enter into a vicious circle of impaired renal function, superimposed urinary tract infection, hemolysis, administration of an oxidant drug, more intravascular hemolysis, hemoglobinuria, tubular obstruction, and renal failure.

Favism and Other Food-Induced Hemolysis. Acute hemolysis may be precipitated by the ingestion of the fava bean (*Vicia faba*), commonly in the Mediterranean basin, North Africa, and western and eastern Asia. Fresh beans in the spring are more potent than dried or frozen beans, but the chemical trigger to hemolysis has not been identified. Hemizygous males and homozygous females for Gd^Mediterranean and other severely deficient enzymes are affected most, but mild hemolysis is seen in heterozygous females and in Africans with GdA⁻. Children aged 2 to 6 years are affected most commonly, and hemolysis has been observed in breast-fed infants of mothers who have eaten fava beans. Some individuals with severe G6PD deficiency never show favism although exposed to the beans, and an additional necessary genetic factor is postulated.

Acute hemolysis starts 24 to 48 hours after the ingestion of the beans. There is pallor, jaundice, and hemoglobinuria. The anemia may be severe, and patients may progress to acute renal failure. There is no specific treatment; blood transfusion is indicated in the most profound anemias. Further

episodes are prevented by avoiding eating beans or inhaling the pollen.

Outbreaks of hemolysis have been described following eating red suya, peppered kebab-like meat, in Nigeria; coloring the meat with Orange RN (monosodium 1-phenylazo-2-naphthol-6-sulfonic acid) was responsible.

Drug-Induced Hemolysis. The ingestion of certain oxidant drugs (Table 6–7) by G6PD-deficient subjects is followed by intravascular hemolysis after 2 to 3 days. There is pallor, jaundice, and hemoglobinuria. Peripheral red cells show Heinz bodies. Once the oldest red cells, with the lowest G6PD activity, are destroyed, the hemolysis is generally self-limiting. Anemia is worst at about 7 to 8 days, after which there is a reticulocyte response and the Hb rises. Hemolysis and anemia can be prolonged with the more severely deficient enzyme activity or with higher dosage of the drug.

Often with GdA⁻, it is not necessary to withdraw the drug, and it is possible to continue with treatment when this is essential; for example, in the treatment of leprosy with dapsone, the patient has a clinically unimportant compensated hemolysis. In some patients, hemolysis and anemia may be more severe or complicated by hemolysis triggered by infection or renal failure; the only specific treatment is withdrawal of the drug. Prevention is by avoiding prescribing oxidant drugs (Table 6–7), especially during pregnancy.

Diagnosis. G6PD activity of red cells can be measured by several methods depending on the production of NADPH. The level of activity in young red cells is higher than in old cells, so that immediately after an acute hemolysis episode, total activity may be in the normal range. The problem can be overcome by centrifuging the red cells and measuring separately the activity in the red cells from the top (young cells) and from the bottom (older cells) of the column. Alternatively, measurement of activity can be delayed until about 6 weeks after any episode of acute hemolysis.

OVALOCYTOSIS AND ELLIPTOCYTOSIS. Several inherited abnormalities of spectrin or other proteins of the cytoskeleton of the red cells cause the cells to have an oval or elliptical shape and a membrane more rigid than normal.

Congenital ovalocytosis achieves high polymorphic frequency in Malaysia, Indonesia, the Philippines, Papua New Guinea, the Solomon Islands, and other Melanesian, Polynesian, and Micronesian islands (Fig. 6–11). The highest prevalences are up to 50% in Sulawesi and 27% on coastal Papua New Guinea. The molecular lesion is a deletion of nine amino acids from transmembrane protein 3, which results in the oval-shaped red cells with rigid membranes. Southeast Asian ovalocytosis does not cause hemolysis or anemia, but the red cells are characteristically oval (with a long axis less than

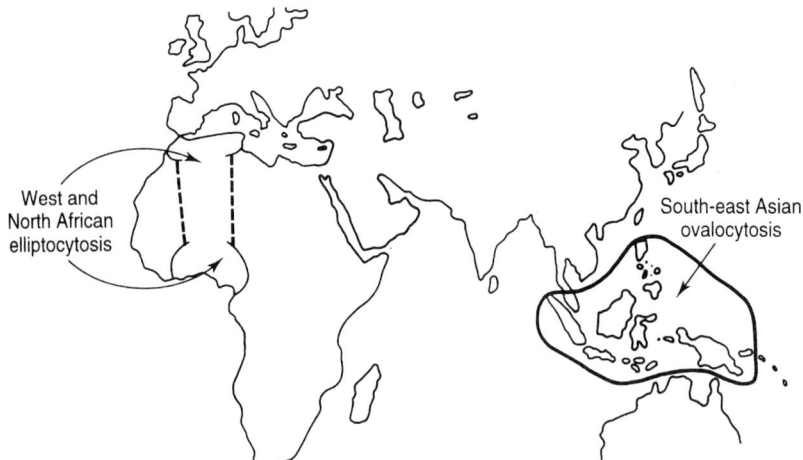

Figure 6–11. Areas of the Old World where congenital ovalocytosis and elliptocytosis are common. (From Fleming AF: Haematological diseases in the tropics. *In* Cook GC [ed]: Manson's Tropical Diseases, 20th ed. London, WB Saunders, 1996, pp 101–173.)

twice the transverse axis) and have decreased osmotic fragility. The rigid membrane seems to prevent penetration by the merozoites of both *P. falciparum* and *P. vivax*, and hence provides a partial protection against malarial parasitemia.

Congenital elliptocytosis (with a long axis more than twice the transverse axis) is seen in up to 3% of West African populations, in Tuaregs in the Sahara, and in inhabitants of the Magreb of North Africa (Fig. 6–11). Several variants of spectrin have been described in this area and it is not at all clear why there should be so many mutations in neighboring populations. Some elliptical red cells have been shown to be resistant to invasion by *P. falciparum*. Elliptocytosis may be symptomless but there may be mild hemolysis: occasional patients show severe anemia, but this could be from coincidental causes.

Pathophysiology of Anemia

Anemia has three grades of severity: (1) compensated anemia, in which the Hb is generally above 70 g/L; (2) uncompensated anemia, with the Hb usually below 70 g/L; and (3) anemic heart failure, which may develop when the Hb falls below 40 g/L. The Hb level is not the only determinant of the severity of anemia. Compensation is less effective and the pathology of anemia more advanced with (1) increasing age, children being better able to withstand anemia than adults; (2) rapidly developing anemia, more chronic disease allowing time for the compensating mechanisms to become effective; (3) hypervolemia of splenomegaly or pregnancy; and (4) intense muscular activity, e.g., obstetric delivery.

COMPENSATED ANEMIA. Individuals with moderate anemia are breathless only on exertion. Their maximal work capacity and ability to sustain work are directly related to their hemoglobin concentration. Productivity, earnings, and ability to look after home and children are all reduced. The family, the community, and the national economy all suffer.

The major compensatory mechanism at this stage in a rise in the intraerythrocyte concentration of 2,3-diphosphoglycerate, which has the function of fixing hemoglobin in the deoxygenated state and hence making oxygen more readily available for uptake by the tissue. Cardiac output is increased on exertion by a more rapid heart rate.

UNCOMPENSATED ANEMIA. Individuals with more severe anemia are breathless even at rest and are wholly unable to perform their usual work. It is at this stage that many patients in developing countries seek medical advice. Cardiac output is increased by both a large stroke volume and a rapid heart rate. Anemia of this severity is not by itself a

cause of death but is commonly contributory, as patients are less able to withstand other conditions, e.g., hemorrhage or infection. Uncompensated anemia in pregnancy contributes to approximately half of maternal deaths in the developing countries.

ANEMIC HEART FAILURE. The myocardium is no longer able to increase its work when its oxygenation becomes further impaired. The jugular venous pressure is raised. Pulmonary edema, peripheral edema, or ascites may develop. Without appropriate treatment, anemic heart failure is commonly fatal. Twenty percent of maternal deaths were due directly to anemia in Nigeria and India before the introduction of blood transfusions, and severe anemia must continue to contribute largely to maternal mortality in remote areas.

ASSOCIATED CAUSES OF MORBIDITY. The morbidity of anemia is often made worse by the morbidity of the primary cause of the anemia, e.g., malaria and hemoglobinopathies. Iron deficiency further reduces work capacity through diminished activity of iron-dependent oxidative enzymes. Both iron and folate deficiencies may be associated with impaired cell-mediated immunity and increased susceptibility to some infections.

ANEMIA IN PREGNANCY. Maternal anemia has adverse effects on the infant besides being a cause of maternal morbidity. With even moderate anemia, there is a degree of fetal hypoxia and a compensatory placental hypertrophy. This compensation is often inadequate, and there is intrauterine growth retardation. Maternal malaria causes additional growth retardation through parasitization of the placenta (Chapter 92). Anemia, folate deficiency, and malaria all cause premature delivery and hence further lowering of the birthweight. In pregnancies complicated by severe anemia due mainly to malaria and folate deficiency, perinatal mortality can be over 35%, and about half of all surviving infants can have very low birthweight (<2000 g). These small infants have immature immune systems and poor reserves of iron and folate and show high frequencies of neonatal jaundice, infections, malnutrition, anemia, and infant mortality.

ANEMIA IN INFANCY AND CHILDHOOD. Children in the tropical environment enter a vicious circle. Infections, e.g., malaria and measles, depress immunity and thus lead in particular to secondary infections of the respiratory and intestinal tracts (Chapters 133.1 and 133.2). Infections can cause malnutrition through the mechanisms of repeated periods of anorexia, malabsorption, and disturbances of metabolism. PEM and deficiencies of iron and folate further reduce immune responses. Nutritional anemias and anemias of infection are outcomes of this vicious circle (Chapter 131.7). Children with hemoglobinopathies enter the circle readily, as they have impaired immunity and folate deficiency.

Iron deficiency anemia in infancy and childhood has consequences of (1) impaired motor development and coordination; (2) impaired cognitive abilities and language development; (3) psychologic and behavioral disturbances; and (4) decreased physical activity (Chapter 132.1). It is probable that if iron deficiency develops in early infancy, these consequences are largely irreversible by iron therapy.

Treatment of Anemia

The first principle of treatment of the anemic patient is to diagnose the causes of the anemia. If diagnostic facilities are inadequate and treatment should not be delayed, it is often necessary to direct initial therapy against the causes that are known to be most probable from previous experience or research. The initial management of anemia in pregnancy or childhood in the tropics is likely to include the treatment of malaria (Chapter 92), antibiotics as indicated from clinical findings, oral iron (Chapter 132.1), and folic acid (Chapter 131.7).

When anemia has a treatable cause, blood transfusion is necessary only when the patient is in danger of dying of anemic heart failure during the approximately 5 days it takes for the Hb to rise following appropriate medication. Since the advent of HIV, it is even more important that strict criteria for blood transfusion be applied. Blood transfusion is indicated when (1) there is incipient or established heart failure due to anemia; (2) obstetric delivery is imminent and the Hb is below 70 g/L; or (3) emergency major surgery is essential, the Hb is below 80 g/L, and a blood loss of more than 500 mL is anticipated. Cardiac overload is avoided by giving concentrated red cells (not whole blood) 10 mL/kg body weight, transfusing slowly over 4 to 6 hours, and by administering a rapidly acting diuretic, e.g., intramuscular furosemide 1.0 mg/kg body weight, before the transfusion.

The role of blood transfusion in congenital anemias has been discussed earlier. Other absolute indications include (1) exchange blood transfusions for neonatal jaundice with serum bilirubin above 300 µmol/L; and (2) whole blood transfusion for acute hemorrhage of more than 30% of the total blood volume, when blood pressure and oxygenation cannot be maintained by crystalloids or colloids.

Prevention of Anemia

The prevention of anemia in pregnancy and childhood ought to be followed by significant reductions in maternal, infancy, and childhood morbidity and mortality rates. Prevention of anemia has an essential role in AIDS control programs through reducing the need to transfuse blood.

ANEMIA IN PREGNANCY. Measures to be taken at prenatal clinics include (1) therapeutic antimalarials at first attendance followed by prophylactics throughout pregnancy; and (2) supplements of iron and folic acid. At family planning clinics, first pregnancies can be delayed until growth is completed and subsequent pregnancies spaced in time.

JAUNDICE AND ANEMIA IN INFANCY. During pregnancy, maternal anemia and malaria should be prevented, and oxidant drugs avoided when the frequency of G6PD deficiency is high. At delivery, small women should be supervised carefully and birth trauma and infant hemorrhages avoided by assisted deliveries. Placenta-infant transfusion should be allowed before cutting the umbilical cord so that the infant retains the hemoglobin-iron. Perinatal sepsis must be prevented by cleanliness. Infants should be screened for G6PD deficiency in populations where this is common. Breast-

feeding is to be encouraged for all infants. Iron and folic acid supplements should be given to the premature infant after 2 weeks. When infants have diarrhea, breast-feeding should be continued with oral dehydration therapy and folic acid supplements. Hemoglobinopathies should be diagnosed shortly after birth.

ANEMIA IN CHILDHOOD. Prevention of anemia in childhood starts with the prevention of anemia and malaria in pregnancy. Breast-feeding should be encouraged for up to 2 years. Solid foods should be introduced early and should be rich in energy, protein, bioavailable iron, and folate. At the maternal-child health clinics, children should be weighed and measured and malnutrition, malaria, and hemoglobinopathies identified. Schedules of immunizations should be followed strictly.

ANEMIA IN THE COMMUNITY. Preventive measures should not be confined to the prenatal, family planning, pediatric, and hemoglobinopathy clinics but introduced as well in the community and at primary health care posts. Strategies to be encouraged include (1) mosquito control and avoidance (e.g., insecticide-impregnated bed nets) to reduce malaria; (2) the construction and use of latrines (e.g., the Zimbabwe VIP) to interrupt transmission of hookworm; (3) supplying clean water; and (4) making immunizations accessible. Nutrition can be improved through encouraging (1) breast-feeding; (2) gardening; (3) poultry-keeping; (4) fish-farming; and (5) inexpensive changes in food preparation and eating habits that would improve the availability of iron, folate, and other nutrients. Primary health care workers and traditional birth attendants can be trained to administer regimens of antimalarials and hematinic supplements to pregnant women, premature infants, infants with severe diarrhea, and children with hemoglobinopathies.

FOOD FORTIFICATION. It is feasible to add fortificants to a commonly eaten staple only if there is a developed centralized food processing and marketing system, e.g., the milling of corn (maize)-meal in southern and central Africa; fortification is not a strategy that can be applied among subsistence farmers selling their small surpluses in village markets. Iron fortification with NaFeEDTA of wheat flour, corn (maize)-meal, soybean, legume products, sugar, salt, fish sauce, soy sauce, or spices is expected to be most efficacious (Chapter 132.1). Fortification with folic acid should reduce the incidence of megaloblastic anemias and neural tube defects in many populations (Chapter 131.7).

◼ LEUKOCYTES

The reference ranges for total and differential leukocyte counts in peripheral blood vary with age, sex, pregnancy state, and race. These differences need to be appreciated, especially by physicians working in the tropics, where half the population may be aged less than 15 years, women are seen frequently with complications of pregnancy, and Caucasian reference ranges are inappropriate for the community.

Variations and Distributions

NEUTROPHILS

Age. At birth, there is a transient high neutrophilic leukocytosis (Table 6–8) and a high count of nonsegmented cells (up to 1.8×10^9/L); this declines, however, and lymphocytes are more numerous than neutrophils in the blood after 24 hours. The percentage and absolute number of neutrophils increase with age until adult life, when they are normally 40% to 75% of the total count in Caucasians (Table 6–8).

Sex. Women aged 18 to 47 years have counts on average

TABLE 6–8. Leukocyte Counts (× 10⁹/L): Means and 95% Confidence Limits

	Total Counts		Neutrophils		Eosinophils		Monocytes		Lymphocytes	
	Mean	*Range*	*Mean*	*Range*	*Mean*	*Range*	*Mean*	*Range*	*Mean*	*Range*
Caucasians										
Age 12 hr	22.8	13.0–38.0	15.5	6.0–28.0	0.5		1.2		5.5	2.0–11.0
Age 1 yr	11.4	6.0–17.5	3.5	1.5–8.5	0.3		0.6		7.0	4.0–10.5
Age 6 yr	8.5	5.0–14.5	4.3	1.5–8.0	0.3		0.5		3.5	1.5–7.0
Adults	7.4	4.5–11.0	4.4	1.8–7.7	0.2	0–0.4	0.3		2.5	1.0–4.8
Pregnancy	9.0	5.2–16.1	6.8	2.3–13.7						
Black Africans										
Adults	5.1	2.6–10.2	2.8	1.1–7.1	0.5	0–2.0	0.2	0–1.3	1.7	0.7–4.5

$0.66 \times 10^9/L$ higher than men. They show cyclical changes with two peaks coinciding with peaks of estrogen secretion and a fall following menstruation.

Pregnancy. The total leukocyte and neutrophil counts rise during pregnancy to plateau in the second trimester (Table 6–8). There is a shift to the left, and up to 3% are metamyelocytes or myelocytes. There is a high neutrophilic leukocytosis during labor, when the total count may reach $40.0 \times 10^9/L$ even in the uninfected individual. Counts return to nonpregnant levels by the sixth day following delivery.

Race. Black Africans and individuals of black African descent, Arabs, and Yemeni Jews normally have a relative neutropenia during adult life according to Caucasian standards (Table 6–8).

Total body neutrophils are the same in all races, but Caucasians have a greater number in circulation and black Africans have larger bone marrow storage pools. The neutrophil count rises to the same level in both races following provocation either artificially by hydrocortisone or naturally by infection. This racial difference is not present at birth but is apparent by 6 months of age. It is probably genetically determined, but hypersplenism may contribute where malaria is endemic.

Response to Infections. The usual response to infections is an increase in neutrophil release and production by the bone marrow, especially in older children and adults (Table 6–9). Total counts may be as high as $40.0 \times 10^9/L$ with 95% neutrophils. There can be numerous immature nonsegmented cells released into the blood. The cytoplasm of these cells often contains numerous azurophilic primary granules (toxic granulation). Degenerative changes can occur as well. The nuclei may show irregular staining and pyknosis, while the cytoplasm is ragged and contains vacuoles and Döhle bodies (condensed RNA). Overwhelming infections, including typhoid and other gram-negative septicemias, lead to leukopenia, especially in elderly and debilitated individuals; HIV is now a common cause of neutropenia (see previous text).

EOSINOPHILS

Age. Eosinophil counts are relatively high at birth and decline steadily with age during childhood. The eosinophil count in the normal adult uninfected by helminths is less than $0.4 \times 10^9/L$ (Table 6–8).

Pregnancy. The eosinophil count declines during pregnancy, and these cells vanish almost entirely from the blood during delivery, even when there is an initially high eosinophilia.

Eosinophilia. Eosinophilia is associated with three groups of conditions that raise serum IgE concentrations: (1) helminth infections; (2) type I allergic conditions; and (3) miscellaneous conditions (Table 6–9). Symptom-free individuals in tropical countries frequently exhibit eosinophilia due to subclinical infections with helminths (Table 6–8). Counts are higher in rural populations and in poorer socioeconomic groups (Chapter 147).

BASOPHILS. The basophil count in the peripheral blood is normally low, and small changes cannot be detected except by automated differential cell counters. A raised count is highly suggestive of myeloproliferative disease, but slight increases may occur with allergic responses. Counts are diminished by stress, corticosteroids, and some acute infections as well as during pregnancy.

MONOCYTES. The monocyte count is normally highest in the first 2 weeks of life (Table 6–8). Counts do not alter during pregnancy but fall at the time of delivery. Counts are lower in symptom-free black Africans and Arabs than in Caucasians.

Monocyte counts are high during viral, protozoal, rickettsial, and subacute or chronic bacterial infections (Table 6–9). Erythrophagocytosis, vacuolation, or malarial pigment may be seen following malaria and may be of diagnostic importance if parasitemia has been cleared naturally or by self-

TABLE 6–9. Reactive Causes of Leukocytosis

Neutrophilia	Viral infections: poliomyelitis
	Bacterial infections: staphylococci, streptococci, gram-negative sepsis
	Tissue damage: trauma, burns, cardiac infarction
	Hemorrhage
	Hemolysis
	Malignancy
	Miscellaneous: drug reactions, chemicals, renal failure
	Pregnancy and delivery
Eosinophilia	Helminth infections: during larval migration of *Ascaris*, and tissue invasion by *Schistosoma*, *Toxocara*
	Type I allergic disease: rhinitis, bronchial asthma, dermatitis, food and drug reactions
	Viral and other infections during convalescence
	Miscellaneous: postsplenectomy, familial, lead ingestion, pulmonary aspergillosis, rheumatoid arthritis
	Malignancy: Hodgkin disease, cytotoxic therapy
Monocytosis	Protozoal infections: malaria
	Rickettsial infections
	Subacute/chronic bacterial infections: tuberculosis, brucellosis
Lymphocytosis	Infection in childhood generally
	Protozoal infections: malaria, toxoplasmosis
	Viral infections: measles, influenza, rubella, hepatitis, chickenpox, infectious mononucleosis

medication. Exceptionally high counts are seen occasionally with tuberculosis.

LYMPHOCYTES

Age. The lymphocyte count in the peripheral blood is highest in the first year of life and declines slowly during childhood (Table 6–8).

Pregnancy. The total lymphocyte count is slightly lower during pregnancy. Of much greater importance is the alteration of function and depression of cell-mediated immunity, which is a physiologic response during pregnancy.

Racial or Environmental Differences. Symptom-free Africans and inhabitants of the Arabian peninsula have a relative lymphocytosis that is due to their neutropenia (Table 6–8). T cells, B cells, and null cells are intermingled in the blood in approximate proportions of 80%, 10% to 15%, and 5% to 10%, respectively, and CD4 and CD8 T cells are in a ratio of 2:1 in adults in industrialized countries. Inhabitants of the tropics have lower T-cell and higher B-cell counts, B-cell counts being highest in rural inhabitants, probably the result of recurrent malaria and other infections.

Response to Infections. Peripheral blood lymphocytosis is seen more commonly as a response to infection in childhood than in adult life (Table 6–9). Absolute lymphocyte counts are high during protozoal disease, especially malaria; activated lymphocytes with basophilic cytoplasm, large nuclei containing nucleoli, and plasma cells (Türk's cells) are seen commonly. Atypical lymphocytes, often with large nuclei and slate gray cytoplasm, are more characteristic of viral infections. Infection by HIV is followed by a progressive decline of the total lymphocytes and CD4 T cells, and a rise in CD8 cells (Chapter 23).

Leukemias

Leukemias are not uncommon in tropical countries. Because of the large patient populations being served, individual doctors are likely to see far more patients with leukemia than they would in practice in a developed country. There are epidemiologic differences in the distribution by age and sex, problems of clinical presentation and diagnosis, and limitations to the management of patients unique for developing countries (Chapter 12).

ACUTE LYMPHOBLASTIC LEUKEMIAS. The identification of cell-surface markers has led to the classification of acute lymphoblastic leukemias (ALL) according to their probable cell of origin. Immunophenotyping distinguishes ALL into (1) pre–B-ALLs, which include null-ALL, common or c-ALL, and pre–B-ALL; (2) B-ALL; and (3) T-ALL, which is further subclassified according to the maturity of the cell of origin.

Epidemiology. ALL is seen most often in childhood, although it may occur at any age. There are three epidemiologic patterns in the world (Table 6–10). First, where both clinical and laboratory facilities are inadequate, the rate of diagnosis of leukemias is extremely low. Second, where facilities have been established, there emerges a peak of frequency of ALL between 5 and 14 years, with T-ALL being the most common subtype. Third, c-ALL has a peak incidence between 2 and 5 years of age in white children in Europe, the Americas, Australasia, and South Africa. A similar peak has emerged in Asia, including Japan, Taiwan, Malaysia, and Arabia, associated with improvements in socioeconomic status; recent reports are of c-ALL being seen in young African children in South Africa, Zimbabwe, Zambia, and Nigeria in a significant incidence for the first time. It is probable that much of the difference between pattern I and pattern II can be accounted for by improved diagnosis following development of specialized centers but without any significant changes in the lifestyle of the general population (Table 6–10). On the other hand, it is accepted that the rarity of c-ALL, e.g., in tropical Africa, is actual. It is hypothesized that there is a "childhood leukemia virus," which is transmitted widely among young children where hygiene is poor; infection causes few or no symptoms; when standards of living rise, the age of first exposure tends to be later until a significant number of women are infected for the first time during pregnancy; transplacental transmission could be one step in the causation of c-ALL in early childhood. There has been no association between leukemia and HIV infection.

Males are affected about twice as often as females.

Clinical Presentation. The symptoms and signs of ALL are the consequences of anemia, hemorrhage and thrombosis, loss of immunity and infection, and malignant infiltration (lymphadenopathy, hepatosplenomegaly, and bone pain or tenderness). Presentation is essentially the same as in temperate countries. The diagnosis may be overlooked in a tropical pediatric clinic, in which a large proportion of acutely ill patients have anemia, infection, lymphadenopathy, and hepatosplenomegaly.

Diagnosis. The total leukocyte count is 20 to 50 $\times$ 10^9/L in about 70% of patients but is normal or low in the remainder. Lymphoblasts are present in the peripheral blood, and 70% to 95% of nucleated cells in the bone marrow are blasts. Anemia is always present, and thrombocytopenia is usual.

The peripheral blood picture may resemble ALL during lymphocytic responses to acute infections, especially malaria in early childhood. Other conditions that may mimic ALL include miliary tuberculosis, measles, pertusses, chickenpox, syphilis, and infectious mononucleosis (Table 6–9). These leukemoid reactions are differentiated from ALL by positive diagnosis of the infection, by recovery with appropriate antimicrobial treatment or spontaneously, and by the absence of blastic infiltration of the bone marrow.

ALL is classified on Romanowsky staining and light microscopy into three types:

L1—The blast is small and uniform; the nucleus is regular in shape and staining; nucleoli are absent or inconspicuous; and the cytoplasm is scanty and pale-blue staining.

L2—Cell size, nuclear shape and staining, and nucleoli are more variable, and the cytoplasm is more abundant. The distinction between L1 and L2 has no bearing on the immunophenotypic classification of ALL. L2 is the most common type in Africans.

TABLE 6–10. Epidemiologic Patterns of Childhood Acute Lymphoblastic Leukemia (ALL)

Pattern	Socioeconomic Status	Incidence of ALL	Examples
I	Low	Low: <0.1/10^5/yr	Tropical Africa generally
II	Intermediate	Uncommon: <1/10^5/yr T-ALL peak: 5–14 yr	North Africa, Arabs in Gaza Strip Blacks and colored in South Africa; Nigeria, Kenya
III	High	High: 2–3/10^5/yr c-ALL peak: 2–5 yr	Whites in the Americas, Europe, Australasia, South Africa; Japanese

L3—The cell is large; the nucleus has uniformly granular chromatin; nucleoli are conspicuous; the cytoplasm is deep-blue staining, and there are prominent vacuoles in the cytoplasm and the nucleus. L3 cells are blasts of B-ALL and indistinguishable from Burkitt lymphoma cells (see Fig. 12–9).

L2 ALL can be distinguished from M1 acute myeloid leukemia (AML) by the Sudan black or myeloperoxidase stains, which are negative with ALL and positive with AML. T-ALL cells stain positive with acid phosphatase.

Treatment and Prognosis. Supportive treatment should be given in the absence of specific treatment or while awaiting transfer to a specialized center. Anemia and thrombocytopenia can be countered with appropriate transfusions of concentrated red cells and platelets. All patients should receive curative followed by prophylactic antimalarials where malaria is endemic. Antibiotics should be given as indicated. Survival averages about 20 weeks without specific therapy.

Long-term remissions, which are probably cures, are achieved now in over 50% of children in centers specializing in the treatment of ALL in childhood. Regrettably, the benefits of these advances are not available to most children in developing countries. First, cytotoxic agents are expensive, and supplies are likely to be intermittent and insufficient; radiotherapy is available in only a few centers and liable to failure from unreliable electricity supplies and lack of maintenance. Second, many features carrying poor prognosis have high prevalence; these include late presentation, poor subsequent attendance, high leukocyte and low platelet counts, mediastinal masses, and T-cell rather than c-ALL markers. Thirdly, Africans and African Americans may have an independently determined poor prognosis. Low density expression of CD10, a surface cell marker of c-ALL, could be associated with this bad prognosis.

ACUTE MYELOBLASTIC LEUKEMIAS. The FAB classification of AML on Romanowsky stain is as follows: type M1, AML with predominantly myeloblasts that have few or no granules in the cytoplasm; M2, AML with blasts that have granules and Auer rods, and some promyelocytes; M3, promyelocytic leukemia of hyper- and hypogranular variants; M4, myelomonocytic leukemia; M5, monocytic leukemia; M6, erythroleukemia; and M7, megakaryocytic leukemia; M0 refers to leukemia that shows myeloid surface markers but is myeloperoxidase negative.

Epidemiology. In the Western world, there is a gradually rising age-specific incidence of AML from childhood to old age; ALL is about four times more common in childhood than AML. In tropical Africa, AML and ALL have equal frequency in children below the age of 15 years, owing in part to the low incidence of ALL but also probably to a true high incidence of AML. It has been postulated that there are two forms of AML in tropical Africa. One is associated with low socioeconomic status, childhood, presentation with chloromas, and a male-female ratio of 2:1. The second type conforms to the pattern in developed countries being seen most often in adults, affecting males and females equally, and showing no association with low social class.

Exposure to benzene is known to increase the probability of developing AML. Unofficial vendors siphoning gasoline into motor vehicles in Nigeria have high frequencies of anemia, neutropenia, and thrombocytopenia. It may be predicted that they will show a greater than normal frequency of AML.

Alkylating agents have a leukemogenic effect. In tropical countries, Burkitt lymphoma, other non-Hodgkin lymphomas, Hodgkin disease, multiple myeloma, and chronic lymphatic leukemia (CLL) all occur in the young or relatively young and are treated almost exclusively by cytotoxic drugs, especially alkylating agents, e.g., cyclophosphamide. It can be expected that some patients will develop AML.

Clinical Presentation. AML in Africa cannot be distinguished clinically from ALL, or from acute leukemias in general, except for the one feature of chloroma. About 25% of East African and 10% of West African patients present with a solid tumor, usually around the face and most commonly in the orbit. Chloromas are most frequent in male children. The tumors are histologically myeloblastic tissue. The name chloroma is derived from a characteristic green color of the freshly cut surface, which fades on exposure to air but may be renewed by adding a reducing agent such as ascorbic acid.

Diagnosis. The only infection that can cause a blood picture resembling any of the types of AML is severe pulmonary or extrapulmonary tuberculosis, when a monocytic or myelomonocytic leukemoid reaction may be present (Table 6–9).

Sudan black and myeloperoxidase stains give positive reactions in blast cells of AML. The nonspecific esterase reaction is positive with myelomonocytic (M4) and strongly positive with monocytic (M5) leukemias.

Treatment and Prognosis. Supportive treatment should be given as for ALL. Without specific treatment, survival is on average about 2 months.

Modern treatment involves marrow ablation followed by bone marrow transplant, the financial and technical resources for which are simply not available in developing countries. Useful and enjoyable life can be prolonged, however, by regimens of cytotoxic drugs given in rotation so as not to cause intolerable depression of normal bone marrow activity. Average survival in one center in Nigeria was about 9 months.

CHRONIC GRANULOCYTIC LEUKEMIA. Over 90% of chronic granulocytic leukemias (CGL) show the Philadelphia (Ph[1]) chromosome, an anomaly that consists of a translocation of the long arm from chromosome 22 with chromosome 9. The Abelson proto-oncogene (Abl) of chromosome 9 is juxtaposed with a breakpoint cluster (bcr) of chromosome 22; the chimeric RNA produced translates for a tyrosine kinase enzyme that confers independence from cytokine control of proliferation. Ph[1]-negative CGLs often show Abl/bcr. Juvenile CGL is an embryonic malignancy.

Epidemiology. The epidemiology of CGL appears to be uniform throughout the world, with a gradually increasing age-specific incidence from late childhood. Peak frequency is in the fifth decade in Europe and North America. In developing countries with younger populations, more patients are seen under the age of 40 years than above that age, and nearly 10% of CGL occurs in childhood. CGL is the third leukemia of childhood, contributing 15% of the total in Nigeria.

Clinical Presentation. Onset is insidious, and presentation is usually with gross hepatosplenomegaly, some lymphadenopathy, emaciation, and anemia.

Diagnosis. The leukocyte count is up to $500 \times 10^9/L$ with predominantly mature neutrophils (sometimes eosinophils and, rarely, basophils) and metamyelocytes, myelocytes, promyelocytes, and a few blast cells. The distribution of cells in the bone marrow is similar, and usually this investigation contributes little to the diagnosis.

Chronic granulocytic leukemoid reactions can occur with tuberculosis, meningococcal meningitis, septicemia, severe megaloblastic anemia in pregnancy, eclampsia, acute hepatic necrosis, amebic liver abscess, burns, mercury poisoning from skin-lightening ointments, and severe hemorrhage; infants infected with *Ancylostoma duodenale* can have eosinophilic leukemoid reactions (Table 6–9). CGL is differentiated by there being (1) often a gap in the progressive leukocyte count, i.e., numerous myelocytes and neutrophils but few metamyelocytes; and (2) low leukocyte alkaline phosphatase reaction. Leukemoid reactions do not show the hiatus in progression from blasts to mature neutrophil, have strongly positive leukocyte phosphatase reactions, and are associated with features of the primary disease.

Treatment and Prognosis. Supportive treatment should include curative followed by prophylactic antimalarials in malaria-endemic areas. Modern treatment has tended to be increasingly aggressive or to involve bone marrow transplant, with the aim of achieving long-term remission, but for most centers in tropical countries, this approach is not advisable.

Interferon-α is probably the drug of choice for CGL in the chronic phase, but it is prohibitively expensive for most patients in developing countries. CGL can be effectively controlled and active life prolonged by treatment with hydroxyurea, which is preferable to busulphan, with allopurinol during the remission-induction period. Treatment with busulphan, however, is easier to control and should be prescribed to patients who are believed to be attending for treatment at frequent intervals. Response is monitored easily by the total and differential leukocyte count, with the aim of keeping the total below $20 \times 10^9/L$. Patients survive on average 3 years, but active life of over 10 years can be achieved. Blastic transformation to AML or ALL is the usual terminal event.

CHRONIC LYMPHATIC LEUKEMIA. The majority of CLLs arise from mature B cells, but T-CLL occurs as well, especially in Asia. Other variants include prolymphocytic leukemia and hairy-cell leukemia.

Epidemiology. In Europe and North America, CLL is seen rarely under the age of 40 years; above that age there is a rapidly rising age-specific incidence and a male-female ratio of 2:1.

In tropical Africa, there is similar epidemiology of CLL after the age of 40 years, but there is also another condition closely resembling CLL clinically and hematologically, and seen as commonly. It is observed as early as the second and up to the fifth or sixth decades of life. The male-female ratio is 1:2 and it occurs predominantly in middle-aged women, exclusively in rural populations or in those of low socioeconomic status. Patients present with massive splenomegaly, but no or minimal lymphadenopathy. The lymphocytes, in Ghanaian patients, have the immunophenotypic markers of splenic lymphoma with villous lymphocytes (SLVL) (a condition that in the Western world is seen predominantly in elderly men), and not the markers typical of B-cell CLL.

It is hypothesized that recurrent malaria and other infections greatly enlarge the B-cell pool and so increase the probability of mutation. The greatest enhancement of the B-cell pool occurs (1) in those living in poor hygienic conditions; (2) in grande multiparae, whose cell-mediated immunity has been depressed repeatedly during pregnancy; and (3) in subjects with HMS. A second mutagenic event could follow infection by an unidentified virus, whose transmission is greater with overcrowding, and whose proliferation is more rapid with depression of immunity by malaria and pregnancy. The human T-cell lymphotropic virus type I (HTLV-I) shows a higher than expected prevalence in patients with B-CLL in Jamaica and Nigeria, but the mechanism of this association is not understood and it does not contribute to the frequency of a CLL-like condition in younger African adults (Chapter 24).

Clinical Presentation. The onset is gradual. The condition may be discovered incidentally, or patients may present with hepatosplenomegaly, lymphadenopathy, and emaciation. The clinical picture is the same in the developed countries as in the tropics, except that splenomegaly is often much more pronounced where malaria is endemic.

Diagnosis. The lymphocyte count is raised usually above $40 \times 10^9/L$. The predominant cell is a mature lymphocyte. In malarial regions, two populations of lymphocytes can be identified in the peripheral blood, one identical with cells infiltrating the bone marrow and presumably the malignant clone, and the other looking like reactive lymphocytes and presumably the result of a response to malaria. The raised nonmalignant lymphocyte count of HMS may be confused with that of CLL.

Treatment and Prognosis. All patients living where malaria is endemic should receive curative antimalarials at the time of diagnosis, followed by lifelong prophylaxis. It has been shown that proguanil alone reduces spleen size and leukocyte count, supporting the view that CLL and malaria interact. Specific therapy is not always required. Chlorambucil 0.1 mg/kg/day should be given for about 4 to 6 weeks and then in maintenance doses to keep the total leukocyte count below $20 \times 10^9/L$. This regimen can be monitored safely with limited facilities. Average survival after diagnosis is about 4 years.

Lymphomas

Non-Hodgkin lymphomas, including Burkitt lymphoma, Hodgkin disease and myeloma (Chapter 12), HIV-related lymphomas (Chapter 23), and HTLV-I and adult T-cell leukemia/lymphoma (Chapter 24) all have epidemiologies distinct from those seen in the industrialized countries.

■ HEMOSTASIS

REFERENCE VALUES

Age. Vitamin K is not detectable in umbilical cord blood, and in infants the vitamin K–dependent coagulation factors (factors II [prothrombin], VII, IX, and X) are only 25% to 70% of adult values. The prothrombin times (PT) and partial thromboplastin times (PTT) of cord-blood plasma are moderately prolonged compared with values for adult plasma. In preterm infants the PT can be up to 4 seconds longer than the adult range (11 to 14 seconds) and the PTT up to 15 seconds longer than the adult range (23 to 35 seconds). These factors decline further to reach a nadir of 5% to 20% of adult activity at 48 to 60 hours of life. Early feeding and colonization of the intestines by vitamin K–producing microorganisms normally supply sufficient vitamin for the infant liver to synthesize the coagulation factors and correct the defect by 72 to 120 hours of life. However, a few infants, especially those who are preterm, may progress to hemorrhagic disease of the newborn.

Other hemostatic functions at birth do not differ from adult values to any clinically significant degree.

Pregnancy. There are profound changes in the hemostatic mechanisms during pregnancy, which are probably beneficial at the time of parturition and separation of the placenta.

Platelets. There is a progressive decline of platelet count with period of gestation to around 80% of nonpregnant adult values (150 to $400 \times 10^9/L$), reflecting the expansion of plasma volume. Platelet function is unchanged, except for a greater availability of phospholipid platelet factor 3.

Coagulation. The coagulability of the blood increases throughout pregnancy. The factors of the rapidly acting extrinsic pathway (thromboplastin of the uterus itself, factors VII and X), plasma phospholipid, and fibrinogen show rises greater than the factors of the slowly but massively acting intrinsic pathway (factors XII, XI, IX, and VIII). Hypercoagulability is enhanced by a fall in antithrombin III, protein S, and protein C activities. The PT, PTT, and clotting times are accelerated. Fibrin monomers are detected in plasma in about half of normal pregnancies. Any tendency toward DIC is counteracted to some degree by a decline to about one half of factor XIII activity.

Fibrinolysis. Plasminogen levels double during pregnancy in parallel with fibrinogen. However, spontaneous fibrinolytic activity of plasma is progressively reduced during the second and third trimester to reach zero at term, owing to the action of the placenta in suppressing plasminogen-activator release from maternal endothelial cells. Only small quantities of fibrinogen/fibrin degradation products (FDPs) are present during the third trimester.

Parturition and the Puerperium. The potentials for coagulation and fibrinolysis, which are latent during normal pregnancy, are released at parturition. Vascular constriction and uterine contraction are major factors in the control of hemorrhage once the placenta has separated. There is deposition of fibrin over the whole inner surface of the uterus, followed by decreases in plasma fibrinogen, platelets, and factors II, V, and VIII. Plasminogen activators are released from the inhibitory effect of the placenta, and FDPs reach a maximum 1 to 4 hours post partum.

Platelet numbers and their activity rise in the first week of the puerperium. Platelet, coagulation, and fibrinolytic values return to nonpregnant levels by 2 weeks.

ENVIRONMENTAL AND GENETIC VARIATIONS

Platelets. Platelet counts at birth have not been found to differ between ethnic groups or geographic location. Symptom-free adults living in malaria-endemic areas have a mild thrombocytopenia, e.g., 73 to 370 $\times$ 10^9/L in male blood donors in northern Nigeria, in comparison with the internationally accepted reference range of 150 to 400 $\times$ 10^9/L. The most likely explanation is increased pooling of platelets in subclinically enlarged spleens.

Adhesion. Ristocetin-induced platelet agglutination (RIPA) in vitro depends on the receptor sites for the von Willebrand factor involved in platelet adhesion to collagen. RIPA is greatly reduced or even absent in rural nonelite Nigerians, whereas elite Nigerians show agglutination intermediate between that of nonelite Nigerians and that of Europeans. This inhibition of RIPA is due to plasma factors—probably high concentrations of macroglobulins, including IgM and fibrinogen. Platelet adhesion measurement has been reported to be less in black than in white South Africans.

Aggregation and Release. The platelets of inhabitants of tropical countries can show a relative resistance to aggregation induced by adenosine diphosphate, thrombin, collagen, and arachidonic acid in vitro. This is due also to inhibition by plasma factors, probably macroglobulins. In contrast, platelet factor 3 is reported to be more readily available, possibly owing to a younger population of circulating platelets when there is enhanced splenic pooling.

Coagulation. In general, PTT, PT, and thrombin times (TT) do not show racial or geographic differences. However, subpopulations of adults can be identified, e.g., in Africa and Papua New Guinea, who have prolonged PT and TT, probably as the result of subclinical hepatic disease.

Fibrinogen levels are high in nonelite populations in the tropics (e.g., 2.0 to 8.4 g/L in rural northern Nigerians) compared with elite groups and Caucasians. The higher levels are probably the result of more intense and more frequent muscular exercise.

In Africans, factor VIII coagulant activity is greater than 150% and factor VIII–related antigen is up to 460% of the values of pooled European plasma; in contrast, factor VII coagulant activity is about 25% less in Africans than Europeans. These are likely to be genetically determined differences.

Fibrinolysis. High plasminogen-activator levels and high spontaneous fibrinolytic activity are reported in nonelite groups in sub-Saharan Africa and Papua New Guinea. These are likely to be the normal response to active life and prolonged muscular exercise, as urbanization in Africans and rising social class in African Americans are associated with declining fibrinolytic activity.

Hemorrhage, Atheroma, and Thrombosis. Intercurrent malaria and other infections leading to hypersplenism and high plasma concentrations of IgM and other macroglobulins, diets low in saturated fatty acids and high in fiber, and frequent muscular exercise are associated with low platelet counts, diminished platelet adhesion, early disaggregation of platelets, and active spontaneous fibrinolysis. There is no apparent impairment of hemostasis in response to trauma, but these qualities of the blood of nonelite groups in rural areas of the tropics are likely to contribute importantly to the low incidence of atheroma and thrombotic disease. Factor V Leiden is a genetically determined risk factor for thrombosis which is common in Europe, Arabia, and north India, but its absence in Africa, East and Southeast Asia, and the original inhabitants of the Americas and Australasia may contribute to the rarity of thromboembolic disease in these populations.

ACQUIRED DISORDERS OF HEMOSTASIS.

The congenital disorders of hemostasis are better known by members of the medical profession, but the acquired disorders are much more common and of greater clinical importance in communities in the tropics.

Purpuras. There are three groups of disorders leading to disturbances of the initiation of hemostasis and to purpura: vascular disorders, diminished platelet function, and thrombocytopenia. The bleeding time is a simple, highly sensitive, and specific test for deficiencies in the initiation of hemostasis.

Vascular Purpuras. The endothelium may be damaged as a result of infections, through (1) direct toxicity, e.g., viremias and septicemias; (2) early immune reactions following the common childhood infections, e.g., rubella; and (3) late immune reactions leading to Henoch-Schönlein purpura or purpura fulminans. Dengue hemorrhagic fever is the most common and widespread of the viral hemorrhagic fevers (Chapters 29.1, 29.10, and 31). The common pathogenesis in all is damage to endothelial cells; this can lead secondarily to consumption of platelets (unusual in Lassa fever) and DIC; the hepatic damage of Ebola and Marburg virus infections results in failure of production and depletion of clotting factors. Idiosyncratic reactions to drugs, e.g., any antibiotics, are relatively common causes of vascular purpura.

Defective Platelet Function. Purpura due to disordered platelet aggregation can complicate the course of uremia and the acute leukemias or can result from large doses of salicylates.

Thrombocytopenia. The platelet count may be decreased either by diminished production or by increased destruction or consumption. Causes of diminished production include (1) exposure to drugs, e.g., co-trimoxazole and pyrimethamine, or chemicals, e.g., benzene in gasoline siphoned by illicit vendors of fuel; (2) acute infections, e.g., typhoid or other septicemias; (3) chronic inflammatory disease, e.g., tuberculosis; (4) primary and secondary aplastic anemias; and (5) bone marrow infiltration, e.g., by leukemia. Platelet destruction can be due to nonimmune mechanisms, e.g., acute malaria, trypanosomiasis, hypersplenism, chronic hepatic disease, or due to immune mechanisms primarily, e.g., idiopathic thrombocytopenic purpura, exposure to drugs (including quinine, mefloquine, and penicillin), AIDS, lymphomas, and CLL. Platelets are consumed in DIC, including some viral hemorrhagic fevers.

A form of immune thrombocytopenia called *onyalai* is endemic to northern Namibia and neighboring southern Angola, where it accounts for about 1% of all hospital admissions. It occurs at all ages and in both sexes. It is characterized by hemorrhagic bullae of the mucous membranes of the mouth and by other manifestations of purpura. Hemorrhagic shock accounts for mortality of about 10%. There is gross thrombocytopenia associated with IgG and IgM autoantibodies specific to glycoproteins IIb/IIIa on platelets. The condition is usually self-limiting but can become chronic. Treatment of acute disease is with the transfusion of whole blood and platelets, and supportive measures such as oral hygiene; mortality has been reduced to about 3%. Prednisolone or splenectomy has not been effective. Vincristine or intravenous immunoglobulin has been beneficial, but is expensive.

Increased pooling and destruction of platelets is a feature of hypersplenism from any cause, e.g., acute malaria, HMS, and portal hypertension following hepatic fibrosis as a result of *Schistosoma mansoni* infection or hepatic cirrhosis. A moderate thrombocytopenia is an invariable feature of acute malaria, but purpura is unusual; recovery follows resolution of the parasitemia.

Thrombocytopenia can be recognized by the absence or near-absence of platelets on a well-spread and stained film of the peripheral blood, as a confirmation of, or instead of, the platelet count.

Hypoprothrombinemia. Deficiencies of factors II, VII, X, and IX occur together as a result of vitamin K deficiency, hepatic disease, and anticoagulant therapy. The PT is prolonged.

Vitamin K Deficiency. Vitamin K is not available in hemorrhagic disease of the newborn or if the bowel has been sterilized by antibiotics. The fat-soluble vitamin is not absorbed in conditions of malabsorption. Parenteral vitamin K reverses the defect within 1 hour.

Hepatic Disease. The PT is prolonged frequently in patients with hepatic cirrhosis or fibrosis or in acute hepatic failure. Hemorrhage may follow trauma or surgery. Vitamin K should be administered but is usually ineffective, and replacement therapy with cryosupernate or fresh-frozen plasma may be necessary. (Cryosupernate is the plasma fraction removed from cryoprecipitate.)

Disseminated Intravascular Coagulation. Three groups of conditions can lead to the uncontrolled activation of coagulation mechanisms: (1) endothelial damage triggering the intrinsic coagulation cascade; (2) release of thromboplastins into the blood, triggering the extrinsic coagulation pathway; and (3) procoagulant venoms.

Etiology. Endothelial damage and DIC are features of the viral hemorrhagic fevers, septicemias (especially meningococcal and gram-negative bacterial) and *Trypanosoma brucei rhodesiense*. Severe *Plasmodium falciparum* parasitemia is only rarely further complicated by DIC. Other causes of extensive endothelial damage include heat stroke, hypotensive shock, diabetic ketosis, eclampsia, and the hemolytic uremic syndrome.

Excessive thromboplastins are released into the circulation following abruption of the placenta, amniotic fluid embolus, retention of a dead fetus, trauma, acute hemolysis (e.g., ABO incompatibility, hemolytic disease of the newborn), acute hepatic necrosis, burns, and certain malignancies (e.g., adenocarcinoma of the prostate, promyelocytic leukemia). The likelihood and severity of DIC are greater during pregnancy, owing both to obstetric accidents and to the hypercoagulability of the blood.

Snakebite. The venoms of various snakes contain powerful procoagulants (Chapter 126.5). The most important in Asia include the vipers *Echis carinatus* and *Daboia russelli* (Russell's viper) and the pit viper *Calloselasma rhodostoma*. In Africa, incoagulable blood results from the bite of *E. carinatus*. The venom of the puff adder *(Bitis arientans)* damages endothelium and may be complicated by thrombocytopenia, DIC, and spontaneous hemorrhage. Bites of *Naja nigricollis* (the spitting cobra) cause necrosis of tissue, which, when extensive, may be complicated by DIC. The venom of the boomslang *(Dispholidus typus)* contains procoagulants and spontaneous hemorrhage starts around 2 days after envenomation, but the snake is not aggressive and bites are rare except in snake handlers.

The rattlesnakes of tropical America with procoagulant venoms include *Bothrops atrox* and *Bothrops jararaca*. Australian species are *Notechis scutatus* (tiger snake), *Oxyuransu scutellatus* (taipan), and *Pseudonaja textilis* (eastern brown snake).

Pathology. The activation of the coagulation cascade causes (1) consumption of platelets and coagulation factors, including fibrinogen; (2) widespread deposition of fibrin with microvascular obstruction; and (3) activation of plasmin, with fibrinolysis and digestion of coagulant factors. As a result of consumption of clotting factors, hypofibrinogenemia, fibrinolysis, and circulating FDPs, the blood is partially or wholly incoagulable. There are spontaneous hemorrhages, which may be massive.

In subacute DIC, vascular obstruction causes death of tissue, which may lead to circulatory collapse and renal failure. Chronic DIC is characterized by microangiopathic hemolytic anemia resulting from the rupture of red cells when forced across fibrin strands.

Diagnosis. In acute disease, the patient shows the features of the primary condition, complicated by purpura or hemorrhage. In some, it is so serious that the blood fails to clot at all following collection. The TT, PT, and PTT or kaolin-cephalin clotting time are all prolonged, and FDPs are present at high concentrations in plasma. Subacute or chronic DIC is diagnosed when there are thrombocytopenia, FDPs in plasma, and schistocytes in the peripheral blood.

Treatment. The primary condition should be diagnosed and treated. Appropriate therapy of bacterial and protozoal infections and snakebite leads to a rapid cessation of DIC.

Transfusion of whole blood or red cells may be required to maintain blood volume and oxygenation. Cryoprecipitate, fresh-frozen plasma, or platelets may be necessary to replace the missing factors.

In subacute or chronic conditions for which there is no effective treatment, e.g., virus infections, it may be necessary to control the coagulation process with intravenous heparin 100 U/kg body weight/4 hr; treatment is monitored by repeated estimates of the clotting time, which should be kept at about 15 minutes.

CONGENITAL DEFECTS OF COAGULATION. The inherited abnormalities of clotting are not more rare in tropical countries than they are in the temperate zone. Globally, the incidence per 10^6 population for hemophilia A (factor VIII deficiency) is 100 (or 1 per 5000 male births); for von Willebrand disease the incidence is greater than 100; and for hemophilia B (factor IX disease) it is 20 (or 1 per 25,000 male births).

The clinical manifestations show no geographic differences, except that practices of circumcision are obviously important. In the tropics, cerebral hemorrhages are common possibly due to raised pressure from coughing, and pyoarthritis is not infrequent. Milder forms of the diseases are seen more often, probably because those with severe disease die undiagnosed.

The best specific treatments for bleeding episodes and surgical procedures are factor VIII concentrates for hemophilia A and factor IX concentrates for hemophilia B. These are now treated so as to inactivate viruses, removing the risk of transmission of HIV, hepatitis, and most other viral diseases. They have a long shelf life but are expensive and not often available in developing countries. Factors VIII and IX produced by recombinant DNA technology are expected to replace human plasma concentrates in the near future.

Cryoprecipitate can be prepared cheaply and simply even in small hospitals, by separating donor plasma and freezing at -20^0C overnight. The cryoprecipitate can be stored at -20^0C for up to 6 months and is effective in the treatment of hemophilia A, von Willebrand disease, DIC, and the bleeding of uremia.

The cryosupernate can also be stored at -20^0C for up to 6 months. Cryosupernate or fresh-frozen plasma is effective in controlling bleeding in patients with hemophilia B and hypoprothrombinemia unresponsive to vitamin K. Desmopressin is a preferred treatment of patients with mild von Willebrand disease.

Bibliography

Bates I, Bedu-Addo G, Rutherford T, Bevan DH: Splenic lymphoma with villous lymphocytes in tropical West Africa. Lancet 340:575–577, 1992.

Beutler E: G6PD deficiency. Blood 84:3613–3636, 1994.

Carper E, Kurtzman GJ: Human parvovirus B19 infection. Curr Opin Hematol 3:111–117, 1996.

Charache S: Treatment of sickling disorders. Curr Opin Hematol 3:139–144, 1996.

Chin J: Scenarios for the AIDS epidemic in Asia. Asia Pac Popul Res Rep 2:1–4, 1995.

Davis BR, Zauli G: Effect of human immunodeficiency virus infection on haematopoiesis. Baillieres Clin Haematol 8:113–130, 1995.

DeMayer EM, Dallman P, Gurney JM, et al: Preventing and Controlling Iron Deficiency Anaemia through Primary Health Care. Geneva, World Health Organization, 1989.

Dupuy E, Fleming AF, Caen JP: Platelet function, factor VIII, fibrinogen, and fibrinolysis in Nigerians and Europeans in relation to atheroma and thrombosis. J Clin Pathol 311:1094–1101, 1978.

Embury SH, Heppel RP, Mohandas N, Steinberg MH (eds): Sickle Cell Disease: Basic Principles and Clinical Practice. New York, Raven Press, 1994.

Fleming AF: Haematological manifestations of malaria and other parasitic diseases. Clin Haematol 10:983–1011, 1981.

Fleming AF: Possible aetiological factors in leukaemias in Africa. Leuk Res 12:33–43, 1988.

Fleming AF: The presentation, management and prevention of crisis in sickle cell disease in Africa. Blood Rev 3:18–28, 1989.

Fleming AF: Tropical obstetrics and gynaecology. 1. Anaemia in pregnancy in tropical Africa. Trans R Soc Trop Med Hyg 83:441–448, 1989.

Fleming AF: Chronic lymphocytic leukaemia in tropical Africa: A review. Leuk Lymphoma 1:169–173, 1990.

Fleming AF: Agriculture-related anaemias. Br J Biomed Sci 51:345–357, 1994.

Fleming AF: HIV and blood transfusion in sub-Saharan Africa. Transfus Sci 18:167–179, 1997.

Griffin TC, McIntire D, Buchanan GR: High-dose intravenous methylprednisolone therapy for pain in children and adolescents with sickle cell disease. N Engl J Med 330:733–737, 1994.

Hesseling PB: Onyalai. Baillieres Clin Haematol 5:457–473, 1992.

Hill AVS: Molecular epidemiology of the thalassaemias (including haemoglobin E). Baillieres Clin Haematol 5:209–238, 1992.

Ho NK: Neonatal jaundice in Asia. Baillieres Clin Haematol 5:131–142, 1992.

Hoffbrand AV, Pettit JE: Essential Haematology, 3rd ed. Oxford, England, Blackwell Scientific, 1992.

International Committee for Standardization in Haematology: Recommendations for neonatal screening for haemoglobinopathies. Clin Lab Haematol 10:335–345, 1988.

International Nutritional Anemia Consultative Group (INACG): Iron EDTA for food fortification. Washington, DC, The Nutrition Foundation Inc., 1993.

Knox-Macaulay HHM: Tuberculosis and the haemopoietic system. Baillieres Clin Haematol 5:101–129, 1992.

Nagel RL, Fleming AF: Genetic epidemiology of the β^s-gene. Baillieres Clin Haematol 5:331–365, 1992.

Nathwani AC, Tuddenham EGD: Epidemiology of coagulation disorders. Baillieres Clin Haematol 5:383–439, 1992.

Nurse GT, Coetzer TL, Palek J: The elliptocytoses, ovalocytosis and related disorders. Baillieres Clin Haematol 5:187–207, 1992.

Phillips RE, Pasvol G: Anaemia of *Plasmodium falciparum* malaria. Baillieres Clin Haematol 5:315–330, 1992.

Piomellli S: Recent advances in the management of thalassemia. Curr Opin Hematol 2:159–163, 1995.

Rush D: Preconceptional folate and neural tube defect. Am J Clin Nutr (Suppl) 59:511S–516S, 1994.

Savage D, Gangaidzo I, Lindenbaum J, et al: Vitamin B$_{12}$ deficiency is the primary cause of megaloblastic anaemia in Zimbabwe. Br J Haematol 86:844–850, 1994.

Sutcharitchan P, Embury SH: Advances in molecular diagnosis of inherited hemoglobin disorders. Curr Opin Hematol 3:131–138, 1996.

Thurnham DI: Vitamin A, iron and haemopoiesis. Lancet 342:1312–1313, 1993.

Weatherall DJ, Ledingham JGG, Warrell DA (eds): Oxford Textbook of Medicine, 3rd ed. (Disorders of the Blood, Vol 3, Section 22.) Oxford, England, Oxford University Press, 1996, pp 3373–3702.

7 Urinary Tract Diseases

Larry W. Laughlin

Urinary tract disease is frequently occult and underreported in developing countries. Therefore, clinical reports are sparse, focus on clinically obvious disease, and usually cannot be extrapolated to the general population.

Common urinary tract problems of the temperate, developed world also occur in the tropics. Disease frequency, individual impact, and outcome will vary in the tropics based on environmental factors, sociocultural practices, and economic status (Tables 7–1 and 7–2). Differences among ethnic and racial groups are nearly always due to one of these determinants, although genetically determined susceptibility may influence outcome following exposure to environmental insults, e.g., poststreptococcal glomerulonephritis. In addition, a few genetic disorders that occur more frequently in the tropics, e.g., sickle cell disease, may be associated with renal disorders.

Clinical features of the renal syndromes encountered in the tropics are, for the most part, similar to those seen in temperate zones; unusual features relate mainly to those environmental or etiologic factors that are peculiar to tropical countries (see Tables 7–1 and 7–2). However, many patients seek medical care at advanced stages of disease.

■ ACUTE NEPHRITIS SYNDROMES

DEFINITION. Acute nephritis is the sudden onset of glomerular inflammation, and to a much lesser extent tubular inflammation, most often caused by immune injury. Although this process is frequently transient, it is usually severe enough to allow red blood cells and plasma proteins to pass into the urinary tract. Gross or microscopic hematuria, red blood cell casts, and proteinuria are hallmarks of this syndrome. Clinical manifestations center around the acute reduction in glomerular filtration rate (GFR), oliguria, salt and water retention, and progressive azotemia. Patients present with abrupt-onset hypertension and its attendant complications, facial and peripheral edema, hematuria, and proteinuria.

ACUTE POSTSTREPTOCOCCAL GLOMERULONEPHRITIS. This prototypical acute nephritis is the delayed sequela of pharyngeal or cutaneous infection with particular "nephritogenic" strains of group A betahemolytic streptococci (types 1–4, 12, 25, 49, 57, 59–61).

Epidemiology. Of all cases of acute glomerulonephritis,

TABLE 7–1. Differences Between Common Renal Diseases in North America and the Tropics

Disease	North America	Tropics
Acute glomerulonephritis	Decreasing frequency	Frequency stable
	Detection high	Detection low
	Throat infections	Skin infections
Nephrotic syndrome	Minimal change	Proliferative
	Steroid-sensitive	Steroid-resistant
	Uncommon in adults	Common in adults and children (*P. malariae, S. mansoni,* amyloidosis)
Acute renal failure	Uncommon	Common (trauma, severe infection, dehydration, snake venom, agrichemicals)
	Prognosis good	Prognosis poor (paucity of emergency medical care)
Chronic renal failure	Uncommon	Common (poor detection, more infectious etiologies)
	Prognosis good (dialysis)	Prognosis poor (dialysis/transplant and other support not widely available)
Urinary tract infection	Common	Probably common (poor detection)
	Few complications	Frequent complications

streptococcal infection can be associated with approximately 25% of adult cases and more than 75% of childhood cases. During circumscribed epidemics, e.g., in Africa, the Caribbean, aboriginal Australia, and the Middle East, virtually 100% of cases are streptococcus-related. Because of the hot, humid climate of the tropics and prevalent poor hygiene, skin infections, particularly impetigo and secondarily infected scabies, cause poststreptococcal glomerulonephritis more commonly than in temperate developed regions.

Histopathology. Poststreptococcal glomerulonephritis is characterized histopathologically by diffuse exudative and proliferative lesions of the glomerular tufts, resulting from the deposition of specific streptococcal antigen-antibody complexes and activation of the complement cascade. Low levels of C3 occur; deposits of C3 and IgG are demonstrated by specific immunofluorescence as electron-dense "humps" on the epithelial side of the glomerular basement membrane, consistent with complement-mediated immune complex injury.

NONSTREPTOCOCCAL GLOMERULONEPHRITIS. Some patients with a clinically identical illness show no evidence of an antecedent streptococcal infection. The natural history of nonstreptococcal glomerulonephritis presumably involves infections that are currently prevalent in the tropics. Pneumococcal pneumonia, typhoid fever, diphtheria, Q fever, leptospirosis, syphilis, toxoplasmosis, varicella, hepatitis B, mononucleosis, measles, mumps, falciparum malaria, and enteroviral, adenoviral, and togaviral infections have been incriminated.

TABLE 7–2. Uniquely Tropical Renal Disease Seen in Endemic Populations

Urinary schistosomiasis (*S. haematobium*):
  Gross hematuria, hydronephrosis, bladder polyps, and calcification
Schistosomal nephrotic syndrome (*S. mansoni*):
  Proteinuria, edema, hypoproteinemia, and hyperlipidemia
Salmonella bacteriuria (*Salmonella* spp.):
  Chronic fever, with urinary schistosomiasis only
Malarial nephrotic syndrome (*P. malariae*):
  Proteinuria, edema, hypoproteinemia, and hyperlipidemia
Bladder stones: Bladder infection and obstruction, hematuria, nutritional association, low-protein diets, young boys
Chyluria: Lymphatic obstruction:
  Chronic bancroftian filariasis, tuberculosis, malignancy
Renal tuberculosis (*Mycobacterium tuberculosis* and *M. bovis*):
  Painless hematuria, culture-negative pyuria, fever

DIFFERENTIAL DIAGNOSIS. Unless the patient has received specific antibiotic therapy, *Streptococcus pyogenes* can often be isolated from the pharynx or from skin lesions. Streptococcal exoenzyme titers may be discriminating when positive, but titers are not always elevated and the assays not always available. Infective endocarditis must also be considered, although the presence of a low-grade fever is usually distinguishing. Systemic lupus erythematosus and other autoimmune connective tissue disorders (Henoch-Schönlein anaphylactoid purpura, polyarteritis nodosa, Goodpasture's syndrome) can be differentiated only with specific immunologic tests during the course of disease. Mesangiocapillary glomerulonephritis and focal glomerulonephritis with recurrent hematuria must also be excluded.

LABORATORY TESTS. Blood agar cultures for *Streptococcus* must be taken from the pharynx and all suspicious skin lesions immediately. For the throat, rough brushing with two untreated cotton-tipped wooden swabs for a minimum of 10 seconds each will yield the best results. Skin lesions should be washed and lightly debrided, then cultured near the edge of the scabbed area, elevating the crusted edge where possible. Streptococcal skin lesions may appear uninflamed, without purulence, or nearly healed. Streptococcal exoenzyme titers, including antistreptolysin O (ASO), antistreptokinase (ASK), antideoxyribonuclease B (ADNase B), antinicotinyl adenine denucleotidase (ANADase), and antihyaluronidase (AH), are often helpful in diagnosis. ASO titers are usually highest in pharyngeal infections and absent in cutaneous infections, whereas AH, ADNase, and ANADase responses are most evident in cutaneous infections. Urinary sediment, erythrocyte sedimentation rate, and serum complement levels will be abnormal but diagnostically nonspecific; however, they can be used to follow the progression and resolution of acute disease. By far the most clinically profound diagnostic test is the renal biopsy, which provides the best evidence to distinguish between transient self-resolving nephritis and disease associated with progressive renal failure.

TREATMENT AND PROGNOSIS. Treatment is supportive. Salt and fluid restriction and diuretics will frequently suffice for mild hypertension and edema. Circulatory overload manifest as severe hypertension, hypertensive encephalopathy, and congestive heart failure must be treated immediately with antihypertensive drugs and digitalis. Profound oliguria may require dialysis and/or treatment with ion exchange resin, especially if significant hyperkalemia exists. Immunosuppressive therapy, e.g., steroids and cytotoxic agents, is not useful. Penicillin or erythromycin antibiotic therapy is customary; it will eradicate persisting streptococcal infection but will have no impact on the renal disease. Prognosis in those from developed countries is variable, relating to whether the patient is a child or an adult and whether the case was sporadic or epidemic, epidemic disease in children having the most favorable outcome and sporadic disease in adults having the worst prognosis. However, mortality rates are less than 1%, and only 2% show residual renal abnormalities. Comparable data from the tropics are unavailable; collective wisdom suggests similar trends but higher acute mortality rates in patients with cardiocirculatory and electrolyte complications because of the unavailability of intensive medical care.

▪ NEPHROTIC SYNDROME

DEFINITION AND ETIOLOGY. Nephrotic syndrome is characterized by generalized edema (most clinically evident in the face), proteinuria of greater than 3.5 gm/day, hypoproteinemia, and hyperlipidemia (Fig. 7–1). The primary renal lesion results from glomerular basement membrane injury due to immunologic, toxic, or vascular pathologic processes, all producing increased capillary permeability with striking losses of protein into the glomerular filtrate. Etiology usually cannot be determined clinically. Exact diagnosis depends on immunopathologic evaluation of renal biopsy findings in the context of the patient's medical and environmental background.

QUARTAN MALARIA NEPHROSIS. *Plasmodium malariae* infection has long been associated with nephrotic syndrome in Africa. Renal biopsy reveals specific malaria antigen in complex with IgG, IgM, and C3. Studies from Nigeria suggest that certain glomerular lesions are morphologically specific for "quartan malarial nephrotic syndrome" (Figs. 7–2 and 7–3). Reports from the Ivory Coast and Senegal confirm the frequency of the lesion on biopsy but fail to support the contention that the findings are pathognomonic for quartan

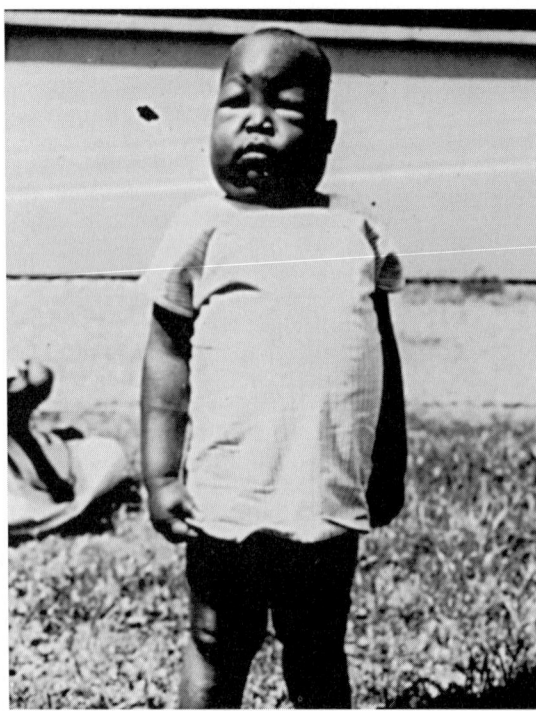

Figure 7–1. African child with the nephrotic syndrome with edema. (Courtesy of Dr. Philip Marsden.)

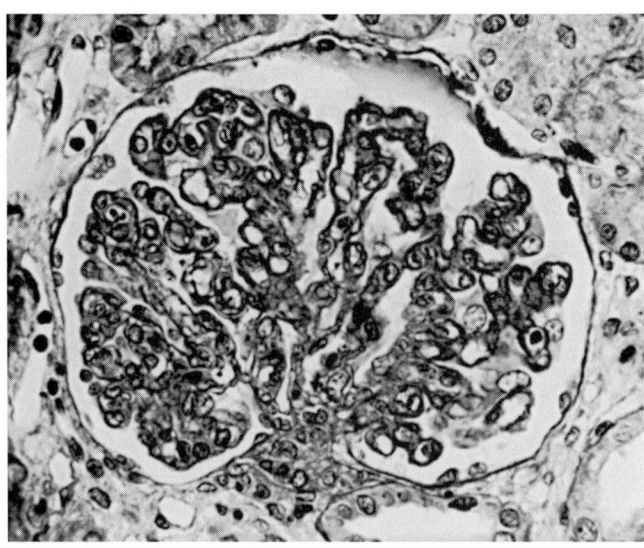

Figure 7–2. Renal biopsy from West African child with the nephrotic syndrome. Glomerulus showing the changes of "tropical nephropathy." There is irregular thickening of the capillary wall, which has a twisted, plexiform appearance. (Courtesy of Dr. Renee Habib.)

malaria, suggesting instead nonspecific trapping of IgM in the glomerulus. There is, however, acceptance by most investigators that quartan malaria may be followed by the nephrotic syndrome and that this occurs through the deposition of immune complexes rather than other immunologic mechanisms, e.g., antigenic resemblance between basement membrane and malarial products.

A recent report from Turkey attributes two cases of nephrotic syndrome to *P. vivax*. This new disease association needs confirmation from other areas endemic for vivax malaria.

SCHISTOSOMA MANSONI NEPHROSIS. Typical nephrotic syndrome may also occur with *Schistosoma mansoni* infection. Renal biopsy specimens show specific deposits of schistosomal polysaccharide, IgG, IgM, and C3. Immune complex glomerulonephritis has been induced in animals experimentally infected with *S. mansoni.* Pathologic changes are more likely to occur in the presence of large worm burdens and may parallel the development of portal obstruction with collateral circulation.

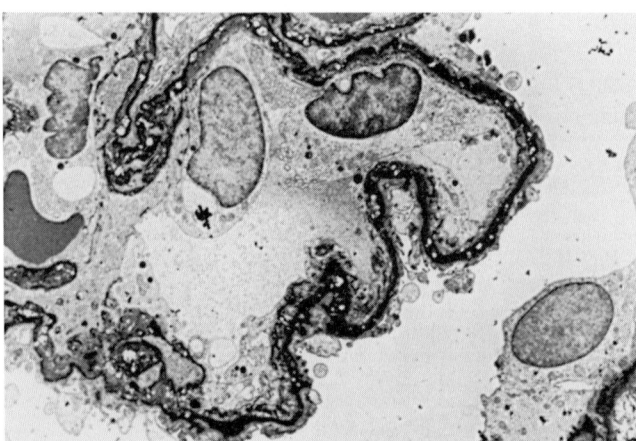

Figure 7–3. Electron micrograph of glomerulus from African child with the nephrotic syndrome. The basement membrane is irregular and contains many lacunae. (Courtesy of Dr. Renee Habib.)

MISCELLANEOUS INFECTIONS. Immune complexes are present in low concentrations in the serum of many apparently healthy inhabitants of the tropics, reflecting the frequency and variety of chronic infections. Intravascular deposition of specific complexes in many infectious diseases, e.g., kala-azar, lepromatous leprosy, toxoplasmosis, and hepatitis B, can be readily demonstrated. Skin-lightening creams may produce membranous nephropathy. There is little evidence, however, that these individual cases are important in the overall prevalence of the nephrotic syndrome in the tropics.

PATHOLOGY AND PATHOGENESIS. Histologic examination of a satisfactory biopsy specimen show changes consistent with minimal-change glomerular disease (lipoid nephrosis), focal glomerulosclerosis, membranous glomerulopathy, or proliferative glomerulonephritis; the last condition may be further characterized as acute exudative, mesangial, extracapillary (crescentic), or mesangiocapillary (membranoproliferative).

Biopsies of African children with the nephrotic syndrome have revealed a rather distinct lesion that may be diffuse or focal; it is distinguished by an irregular thickening of the glomerular capillary wall, which displays a twisted plexiform or double-outline appearance (Fig. 7–2). On electron microscopy, lacunae may be noted in the basement membrane (Fig. 7–3).

After the glomerular injury and protein leak are established, the remainder of clinical disease follows expected physiologic changes. Sustained heavy proteinuria, the hallmark of nephrosis, is eventually followed by hypoproteinemia via processes of excessive urinary losses, increased renal catabolism, and inadequate hepatic synthesis of albumin. The resulting decreased plasma oncotic pressure leads to fluid migration into tissue spaces, i.e., edema. Hepatic lipoprotein synthesis increases, probably stimulated by low plasma oncotic pressure, resulting in hyperlipidemia. This lipid aberration probably contributes to the accelerated atherosclerosis seen in nephrotic syndrome patients. Urinary losses of functionally important plasma proteins besides albumin have medical impact ranging from misleading thyroid function tests to anemia, vitamin D deficiency, trace mineral deficiency, hypercoagulable states, and increased susceptibility to infections because of the loss of specific protective immunoglobulins.

LABORATORY FEATURES. Gross proteinuria, frequently above 5 g/day, is the hallmark of nephrotic syndrome. Plasma albumin may fall below 1.0 g/dL; hyperlipidemia involves cholesterol, triglycerides, and phospholipids but with variability in each component. Renal biopsy with immunopathologic staining provides the most precise functional diagnosis and is rarely contraindicated.

Differential permeability of the glomerular membrane, with selective loss of smaller protein and lipid molecules, is thought to reflect a better prognosis than does a pattern of generalized protein excretion. This distinction can be made, when laboratory facilities permit, by correlation of plasma and urinary protein electrophoretic patterns. The ratio of urinary IgG to transferrin is a useful index, with values less than 0.15 denoting high selectivity of protein loss and a generally favorable prognosis.

CLINICAL MANAGEMENT. Generalized "soft" edema, particularly evident in the face, is the clinical sine qua non of nephrotic syndrome. As this extravascular fluid accumulation intensifies, ascites and pleuropericardial effusions accumulate, to become difficult management problems in late-stage disease. Pharmacologic diuresis is tempting to the clinician but can be dangerous and is rarely of long-term benefit. Albumin infusion is similarly deceptive; most administered proteins will be excreted within 48 hours. Generally, treatment of edema should be reserved for severe refractory anasarca or profound postural symptoms.

Hyperlipidemia is nearly constant, but not absolutely associated with increased morbidity or mortality. Most lipid-reducing agents are either too toxic or so poorly tolerated that treatment is rarely indicated.

Thromboembolic complications are common. Renal vein thrombosis is most often noted, with a striking clinical syndrome of flank/loin pain, gross hematuria, reduced GFR, asymmetry of renal size, scalloping of the ureters (due to collateral circulation), and evidence of pulmonary embolic disease. Oral anticoagulation is required.

The precise role of immunosuppressive therapy in nephrotic syndrome is unknown. Relating most directly to classification by renal biopsy, nephrosis either progresses to chronic renal failure or spontaneously remits. Immunosuppressive agents speed the process of spontaneous recovery but probably do not increase the absolute number of resolved cases. However, steroids probably reduce the amount of protein lost in the urine in unremitting disease. Therefore, most patients with nephrotic syndrome are given at least a trial of immunosuppressive drugs; the positive impact on outcome may not outweigh the negative complications of long-term steroid treatment.

DIFFERENTIAL DIAGNOSIS. Systemic conditions associated with the nephrotic syndrome are primary or secondary amyloidosis, diabetes mellitus, myelomatosis, and renal vein thrombosis. Quartan malaria (*Plasmodium malariae* infection) (Chapter 92) has been associated with the nephrotic syndrome in Nigeria, Uganda, other regions of West and Central Africa, and Guyana. *S. mansoni* infection (Chapter 118) in Brazil has been causally linked to the nephrotic syndrome through demonstration of specific antigens in the glomerular immune complex deposits. Secondary amyloidosis associated with chronic tuberculosis (often extrapulmonary) (Chapter 77) or lepromatous leprosy (Chapter 78) accounts for a variable proportion of cases in tropical countries.

TREATMENT AND PROGNOSIS IN CHILDREN. In temperate climates, most children (90% or more) show minimal glomerular lesions on biopsy, have a selective pattern of protein loss, and respond well to steroid therapy. This is not true of some tropical situations. Studies in the Sahel region of Africa have revealed structural glomerular lesions in most children with the nephrotic syndrome, even the very young, who might be expected to have minimal-lesion disease. A typical example may be seen in the biopsy of a West African child with the nephrotic syndrome; changes characteristic of "tropical nephropathy" include irregular capillary wall thickening (Fig. 7–2). Even so, corticosteroid therapy is usually recommended along with appropriate dietary and symptomatic management. Cyclophosphamide therapy has not been successful in West African cases, and azathioprine may adversely affect survival. Despite therapeutically induced remission, more of these children develop renal failure than do those from temperate climates. The natural history of the disease in Africa and elsewhere in the tropics requires much more investigation.

TREATMENT AND PROGNOSIS IN ADULTS. Many studies from tropical countries attest to the surprisingly high prevalence of the nephrotic syndrome in young adults. Proliferative glomerulonephritis predominates in reported renal biopsies, although minimal-lesion and membranous glomerulopathies may be more common in some areas, as in the Ryukyu Islands. In Singapore, more than 30% of glomerulonephritis cases, some associated with the nephrotic syndrome, are related to specific deposition of IgA complexes. Corticosteroid or other immunosuppressive therapy is not likely to be effective in other than minimal-lesion glomerulopathy; membranous or proliferative glomerular disease is usually not altered and requires symptomatic management as the disease runs its course.

ACUTE RENAL FAILURE

DEFINITION AND ETIOLOGY. Acute renal failure occurs when there is a sudden loss of the kidneys' contribution to body metabolism, associated with ineffective salt and water homeostasis, deficient hydrogen ion excretion, and accumulation of nitrogenous waste products in the plasma. The syndrome, manifested usually by acute oliguria and occasionally anuria, has many causes and always represents a medical emergency.

PREVALENCE IN THE TROPICS. Acute renal failure is a common clinical emergency in most tropical countries. Common to all areas are the frequency of trauma and infections and the delay in initiating effective antibiotic therapy or fluid replacement. Trauma, often with crush injuries, is becoming increasingly common with industrialization. In underdeveloped countries, a major cause of acute renal failure is untreated septic abortion; it may also complicate typhoid fever, leptospirosis (Weil's disease), pyomyositis, coliform septicemia, cholera, yellow fever, viral hemorrhagic fevers, and falciparum malaria (Chapter 92). Blackwater fever, characteristically seen in partially immune expatriates in areas of endemic malaria and thought to be precipitated by quinine administration, remains a highly fatal, if uncommon renal complication of malaria. Reports from South India emphasize the frequency of the hemolytic-uremic syndrome in children with bacillary dysentery (Chapter 40); in Vellore, such cases accounted for nearly 40% of acute renal failure in patients under the age of 15 years.

PATHOLOGY AND PATHOGENESIS. The causes of acute renal failure are usually classified as prerenal, renal, and postrenal. Hypovolemia with poor renal perfusion due to prerenal pathologic events (e.g., severe hemolysis or hemorrhage, extensive trauma or burns, various forms of septicemia, including black water fever, and severe dehydration from gastrointestinal disease or environmental conditions) may result in acute tubular necrosis, usually reversible with proper acute care. Examination by light microscopy of renal biopsies from such cases shows interstitial edema and dilated tubules containing casts, with varying degrees of tubular epithelial necrosis. Acute renal failure may be caused by direct injury to the kidneys (e.g., from poisoning by nephrotoxic chemicals carelessly introduced into the environment, certain drugs and local plant products, or snake venom), with acute tubular necrosis of greater severity. Postrenal causes include obstruction of urinary flow by bilateral renal calculi, bilateral ureteral schistosome granulomas, bladder stones, and malignant growths or other causes as well as neurogenic mechanisms.

CLINICAL MANAGEMENT. Patients seen during the early oligemic phase have care focused on the treatable underlying disease, hypovolemia, and shock or infection. The ensuing oliguric phase, generally associated with tubular necrosis, may last from a few days to more than a month. During this time, progressive uremia with hyperkalemia, acidosis, and overhydration becomes life-threatening and requires meticulous monitoring of fluid balance and nutrient intake. Peritoneal dialysis or hemodialysis may be lifesaving, and as tropical tertiary care centers gain experience mortality rates have declined. Gastrointestinal hemorrhage and intercurrent infection are the most important complications. The diuretic phase usually begins 10 to 14 days after onset but may be delayed. Beginning with functional nephrons, healing may continue until improved tubular function leads to an outpouring of urine rich in sodium and chloride, which usually lasts about 10 days. Obligatory loss of water may produce severe deficits of electrolytes during this period, in sharp contrast to accumulations during the oliguric phase. Prognosis is influenced by careful monitoring, competent management, and the underlying disease process.

CHRONIC RENAL FAILURE

DEFINITION. Chronic renal failure is the result of slow but progressive destruction of renal tissue by a variety of pathologic processes. The end-stage kidney is characterized by an inadequate number of functional nephrons with failure of glomerular and tubular function, loss of homeostasis, and progressive uremia.

ETIOLOGY AND PREVALENCE IN THE TROPICS. Owing to the relatively quiet onset, the infrequent availability of autopsy and biopsy material, and poor population health statistics in the tropics, the relative importance of different diseases as causes of chronic renal failure is difficult to estimate. Chronic glomerulonephritis, representing the end stage of the various histologic types, appears to predominate. In Kampala, Uganda, about 5% of necropsies (excluding infants) showed some form of progressive glomerulonephritis. Similar findings have been reported from Nigeria and New Guinea. These figures reflect the frequency of acute glomerulonephritis and the nephrotic syndrome in these populations. Chronic pyelonephritis appears to be an unimportant cause of chronic renal failure in Africa. Renal vascular disease and diabetes mellitus are uncommon causes except in certain groups, e.g., the Indian immigrant population in South Africa. Amyloidosis is the most common cause of death in lepromatous leprosy in some areas, but it is relatively rare in the general population.

Hydronephrotic atrophy and chronic pyelonephritis are well-known complications of *Schistosoma haematobium* infection, caused by inflammation and scarring (Fig. 7–4; Figs. 118–18 and 118–19) from deposition of eggs in the tissues of the lower urinary tract. The frequency of obstructive uropathy that proceeds to endstage renal disease in these cases increases with worm burden and with age. Although long-term studies on infected patients are generally inadequate, *S. haematobium* infection must account for many cases of chronic renal failure in areas of endemicity.

Chronic obstructive uropathy due to urethral stricture or neglected prostatic hyperplasia in men or advanced pelvic carcinoma in women is as common in the tropics as in temperate climates.

CLINICAL MANAGEMENT. Tropical patients with end-stage renal disease do not display unusual or unique clinical features but do present formidable problems in management. Long-term dialysis and transplantation programs are inadequate in most developing countries. Even when developed countries make dialysis available to tropical populations, cultural factors can neutralize expected benefit. In Kenya renal replacement therapy is provided, but the cost burden has impacted upon the more basic public health programs for malnutrition and infection.

Therapy usually consists of symptomatic management of hypertension, azotemia, and anemia, with correction of obstruction and treatment of infection as feasible. Specific measures in the management of the azotemic patient include: (1) judicious protein restriction and perhaps alkalinizing therapy for correction of acidosis, and (2) restriction of sodium intake to 25 to 35 mEq/day, with water intake between 1800 and 3500 mL/day. Therapeutic goals are necessarily limited, but

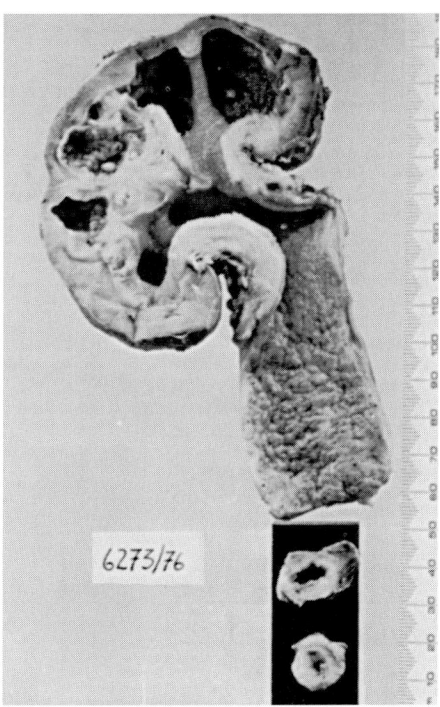

Figure **7–4.** Hydronephrotic atrophy of kidney associated with thickening of the ureteric wall due to *Schistosoma haematobium* infection.

proper therapy will improve the quality of life and often add months of useful activity. However, renal failure is nearly always progressive, even when there are no serious complications. The terminal stage is often defined as the point at which the plasma creatinine level exceeds 10 ml/dL. Experience in a modern hospital setting suggests that about 20% of patients with terminal renal failure stabilize and exhibit improvement with careful management, but 80% will not survive beyond 5 months without dialysis, with half of these succumbing within 2 months.

■ HEMATURIA

ETIOLOGY. Symptomatic recurrent hematuria in the tropics is usually associated with grossly visible pathologic lesions (e.g., tumors, stones) or is the result of schistosomiasis haematobia (Chapter 118). Gross hematuria rarely results from microscopic abnormalities of the kidney or lower urinary tract.

PATHOGENESIS AND PREVALENCE. Hematuria that results from diffuse renal disease, sometimes grossly visible but usually microscopic, is almost always accompanied by proteinuria. Hematuria resulting from local diseases of the genitourinary tract is rarely associated with protein excretion in excess of a few hundred milligrams daily, whereas in diffuse disorders of the kidney, the proteinuria may approach 10 gm/day. One of the diffuse renal diseases that produce episodic painless hematuria is IgA nephropathy of Berger, characterized by deposits of IgA in the mesangium, with resultant mesangial proliferation. An unusually high prevalence of this entity, said to be provoked by upper respiratory infections or undue physical exertion, has been reported from Singapore. Painless hematuria is seen in sickle cell disease, probably resulting from small renal infarctions (Chapter 6). Gross bleeding associated with trauma, hemorrhagic cystitis,

stones, genitourinary tumors, and hemorrhagic disorders such as thrombocytopenic purpura is common. Gross painless hematuria, a classic sign of urinary schistosomiasis, is regional in distribution (see Chapter 118). Diagnosis rests upon standard urologic procedures, usually including cystoscopy.

■ CHYLURIA

Frequently found in conjunction with hematuria, chyluria is the draining of lymphatic material directly into the urinary tract, resulting in a characteristic milky-tan urine. Chyluria is usually intermittent, asymptomatic, and caused by chronic bancroftian filariasis; it requires no specific therapy (Chapter 106.1). Its pathogenesis is obstructed lymphatic ducts and retrograde duct engorgement and dilation, with rupture or fistula formation into the urinary tract, frequently the renal pelvis. Rarely, chyluria may be severe, with massive urinary lipid excretion resulting in uncontrollable weight loss and renal colic from ureteral fibrin clots. In such cases surgical repair of the fistula, if it can be located, is curative; otherwise, a fat-restricted diet can be instituted to ameliorate symptoms. Diagnosis is established by Sudan III staining of the urine to identify fat globules or by allowing the urine to stand for 72 hours to separate into a top creamy layer, a red bottom deposit, and a cloudy intermediate layer that may clot. Other uncommon causes of chyluria are echinococcosis, urinary schistosomiasis, tuberculosis, and neoplastic infiltration of the retroperitoneal spaces.

■ URINARY CALCULI

Urinary tract stones may be asymptomatic, associated with infection, or manifested by episodes of excruciatingly severe colic and gross hematuria. They consist of crystalline aggregates of urinary salts or acids, precipitated within the urinary tract as a result of excessive excretion or changes in the physiochemical milieu of the urine. The primary distinction must be made on the basis of chemical composition, which often provides a clue to the underlying metabolic or endocrine disturbance; however, useful separation can be made clinically between stones of renal origin and primary bladder stones.

BLADDER STONES. These occur endemically among children in some less developed agricultural countries such as Thailand, Indonesia, Yemen, and the Sudan. Malnutrition, vitamin A deficiency, and low-protein diets are common in these areas but cannot be specifically incriminated. It is clear, however, that improved socioeconomic conditions result in amelioration of the problem.

The radiologic curiosity "fetal head" calcification of the bladder is sometimes seen in patients with chronic urinary schistosomiasis (see Fig. 118–21). Submucosal deposition of schistosome eggs with calcification leads to a thin layer of calcification involving the entire bladder.

KIDNEY STONES. North Americans and Europeans living in the tropics have increased rates of ureteral stone formation, attributed to unaccustomed dehydration and consequent urinary concentration. A curious situation exists in Fiji, where renal calculi are uncommon except among immigrant Indians, who suffer from "curry kidney," attributed locally to excessive ingestion of curries, pickles, and spices. Epidemiologic or physiologic studies to substantiate these impressions have yet to be reported. A tertiary care center in Accra, Ghana, reports a urinary tract stone incidence of 2 per 100,000, with men being at twice the risk of women.

■ URINARY TRACT INFECTION

DEFINITION AND EPIDEMIOLOGY. Urinary tract infections in the tropics, as elsewhere, are common, more frequent in women than in men, and strongly associated with structural abnormalities, e.g., congenital malformations, stasis, stones, foreign bodies, or diseases that disrupt bladder mucosal integrity (bladder carcinoma, urinary schistosomiasis). While there is a paucity of pertinent epidemiologic and postmortem pathologic studies, it is believed that urinary tract infections seldom lead to chronic pyelonephritis and renal failure, although they undoubtedly contribute heavily to morbidity. Asymptomatic bacteriuria, defined as quantitative counts of more than 10^5 organisms/mL in freshly voided specimens, is a largely unacknowledged entity in the tropics, as the required bacteriologic culture methods are available only in the most modern medical centers.

ETIOLOGY AND PATHOGENESIS. Urinary tract infections are much more common in women than in men, probably owing to anatomic differences (i.e., urethral length and vulnerability to coital trauma) and childbearing. Acute and chronic pyelonephritis may follow infection of the lower urinary tract, depending on the presence of vesicoureteral reflux, obstruction, stones, congenital abnormalities, and other acquired or hereditary factors. As elsewhere, gram-negative bacterial organisms are most commonly isolated, usually introduced from intestinal flora but sometimes from the environment.

Salmonella Bacteriuria. Chronic *Schistosoma haematobium* infection usually results in disruption of bladder mucosa and/or some degree of urinary obstruction with stasis. Under these circumstances, salmonella bacteriuria (with or without bacteremia) is seen in unexpectedly high rates. The pathogenesis of this entity is complex (Chapter 118). Curative therapy requires both antischistosomal and antibacterial agents.

Renal Tuberculosis. Tuberculosis is extraordinarily prevalent in most underdeveloped countries. Genitourinary tuberculosis is one of the common extrapulmonary manifestations of the disease. It results from hematogenous spread, usually with a delayed reactivation of lesions in the renal parenchyma (see Chapter 77). Involvement of the prostate, seminal vesicles, and epididymides may occur secondarily in the male, whereas involvement of the female pelvic organs is usually the result of direct spread to the fallopian tubes. Sterile pyuria in a patient with chronic fever, frequency, dysuria, or hematuria should suggest the possibility of renal tuberculosis. Cultures obtained from early-morning urine specimens will confirm the diagnosis.

Bibliography

Barton EN, Williams W, Morgan AG, Burden RP: A prospective study of ward referrals for renal disease at a Jamaican and a United Kingdom hospital. West Indian Med J 45:110, 1996.

Bennett E, Manderson L, Kelly B, Hardie I: Cultural factors in dialysis and renal transplantation among aborigines and Torres Strait Islanders in north Queensland. Aust J Public Health 19:610, 1995.

Coovadia HM, Adhikari M, Morel-Maroger L: Clinico-pathological features of the nephrotic syndrome in South African children. Q J Med 189:77, 1979.

Edwards BD, Eastwood JB, Shearer RJ: Chyluria as a cause of haematuria in patients from endemic areas. Br J Urol 62:609, 1988.

Hendrickse RG: Epidemiology and prevention of kidney disease in Africa. Trans R Soc Trop Med Hyg 74:8, 1980.

Hendrickse RG, Adeniyi A: Quartan malarial nephrotic syndrome in children. Kidney Int 16:64, 1979.

Hutt MSR: Renal disease in a tropical environment. Trans R Soc Trop Med Hyg 74:17, 1980.

Johansen MV, Simonsen PE, Butterworth AE, et al.: A survey of *Schistosoma mansoni* induced kidney disease in children in an endemic area of Machakos District, Kenya. Acta Trop 58:21, 1994.

Klufio GO, Bentsi IK, Yeboah ED, Quartey JK: Upper urinary tract stones in Accra, Ghana. West Afr J Med 15:173, 1996.

Lyrdal F, Hofvander Y: Urinary bladder stones. Their occurrence in children in South-East Asia. Trop Doct 18:102, 1988.

Martinelli R, Pereira LJ, Brito E, Rocha H: Clinical course of focal segmental glomerulosclerosis associated with hepatosplenic schistosomiasis mansoni. Nephron 69:134, 1995.

Mate-Kole MO, Yeboah ED, Affram RK, et al.: Hemodialysis in the treatment of acute renal failure in tropical Africa: A 20-year review at the Korle Bu Teaching Hospital, Accra. Ren Fail 18:517, 1996.

Mate-Kole MO, Yeboah ED, Affram RK, Adu D: Blackwater fever and acute renal failure in expatriates in Africa. Ren Fail 18:525, 1996.

Mathai E, John TJ, Rani M, et al.: Significance of Salmonella typhi bacteriuria. J Clin Microbiol 33:1791, 1995.

Naqvi R, Ahmad E, Akhtar F, et al.: Predictors of outcome in malarial renal failure. Ren Fail 18:685, 1996.

Oner A, Demircin G, Bulbul M: Post-streptococcal acute glomerulonephritis in Turkey. Acta Paediatr 84:817, 1995.

Vijeth SR, Dutta TK, Shahapurkar J: Correlation of renal status with hematologic profile in viperine bite. Am J Trop Med Hyg 56:168, 1997.

Were W, McLigeyo SO: Cost consideration in renal replacement therapy in Kenya. East Afr Med J 72:69, 1995.

Whittle HC, Abdullahi MT, Fakunle F, et al.: Scabies pyoderma and nephritis in Azria, Nigeria. Trans R Soc Trop Med Hyg 67:349, 1973.

8 Dermatologic Diseases

Neill C. Hepburn

Three groups of skin diseases are common in the tropics: (1) common dermatoses, which are similar throughout the world, e.g., psoriasis, viral warts, and alopecia areata; (2) dermatoses that occur throughout the world but that may be more common or differ clinically in the tropics because of heat, humidity, malnutrition, lack of appropriate therapy and concomitant diseases e.g., lupus vulgaris and acne; and (3) dermatoses that occur as a consequence of residence in the tropics, e.g., cutaneous leishmaniasis and myiasis. Scabies, insect bites, pyoderma, and dermatitis constitute a large part of dermatologic practice in the tropics. Because the skin is directly exposed to the environment, it is considerably affected by climatic conditions, local living conditions and customs, microorganisms, and exposure to noxious chemicals both at home and work, and local "cures."

■ APPROACH TO THE PATIENT

HISTORY. A good history provides a foundation for an accurate diagnosis. Practice in the tropics often involves large numbers of patients per clinician, leading to short patient interviews, and frequently compounded by language differences. Thus, detailed historical data are frequently inadequate. The following information should be recorded:

1. *Duration of the disease.* How long has it been since the earliest symptom? Is it days, weeks, months, or years?
2. *Initial body site(s) involved.*
3. *Description of the earliest lesion.* What did it look like before it evolved, was scratched, or treated?
4. *Distribution of the lesions.*
5. *Cutaneous symptoms.* Have itches, rashes, or pain been noted?
6. *Recurrences.* Are the lesions part of a cyclic phenomenon, possibly with disease-free intervals?
7. *Associated symptoms.* Are there any associated systemic symptoms, e.g., fever, arthritis, diarrhea?
8. *Prior therapy.* What has the patient tried and what was

the result? This may modify the appearance and natural history of the lesion.

PHYSICAL EXAMINATION. The patient should be undressed so that the entire skin surface can be easily examined. Clues to the diagnosis may be found at sites remote from the area of concern to the patient. The mucous membranes, hair, and nails should also be examined. Good, preferably natural, lighting is essential and a magnifying glass may help appreciate fine detail.

Definitions. The differential diagnosis of skin disease is based on the morphology of the lesions and their distribution over the body. The terms used are as follows:

1. A *macule* is an area of altered skin color without change in texture, elevation, or depression.
2. A *papule* is a raised solid area of skin less than 10 mm in diameter.
3. A *plaque* is a solid elevation of skin with a flat surface resembling a plateau.
4. A *nodule* is a solid lesion measuring greater than 10 mm in diameter and may vary in location from subcutaneous tissue to the skin surface.
5. A *vesicle* is a fluid-filled cavity raised above the skin surface measuring less than 10 mm in diameter. The terms *bulla* or *blister* may be used when the lesion is greater than 10 mm in diameter. If it contains pus (white blood cells) it is known as a *pustule.*
6. A *wheal* is a transient, localized area of edema that may or may not have an alteration in color.
7. An *ulcer* is a localized area of loss of epidermis leaving raw, denuded skin.
8. *Scale* is thickened stratum corneum, whereas a *crust* is composed of dried serum and pus.

Distribution. The pattern of the individual lesions should then be noted: Are they randomly distributed, grouped in clusters, or do they take on a geometric arrangement, such as linear or annular (ring-shaped)? Finally, the distribution over the body surface should be noted: Are they generalized, localized to various body sites, or do they follow the distribution of the dermatomes?

LABORATORY AIDS. The following simple tests, which require a minimum of equipment, are useful in confirming or refuting a diagnosis:

1. A *potassium hydroxide (KOH) preparation* is used to detect fungal infections. It is made by gently scraping scales from the lesion with the edge of a scalpel blade onto a glass slide, adding a drop or two of 10% KOH in water and covering with a cover slip. The slide is gently warmed with a match or candle until the preparation just begins to boil. After cooling it is examined with a microscope with the condenser in the down position or the diaphragm partially closed, when hyphae or spores of fungi may be seen.
2. A *smear* is useful in the diagnosis of viral or bacterial diseases and can be made by scraping the base of a lesion with a scalpel blade and transferring the serum and cellular debris to a glass slide. After fixation by either heat or alcohol, the specimen can be stained and examined locally or sent to a reference laboratory.
3. A *skin biopsy* is useful in the diagnosis of most skin diseases and can be processed at a later time if facilities are not readily available. A representative lesion is selected, cleaned thoroughly with an antiseptic solution, then infiltrated with a local anesthetic such as 1 or 2% lidocaine. If the lesion has an annular configuration and appears to be enlarging, the advancing border is the best place to biopsy; otherwise the center of the lesion, provided it is not necrotic, usually yields the best results. The specimen may be obtained with either a punch or an ellipse cut with a scalpel. It is important to take the specimen down to and including the subcutaneous tissue. Sutures may be used to close the wound if it is over 4 mm in diameter. The specimen may be divided into several pieces if cultures are desired. The specimen for histologic examination should be placed into 10% buffered formalin. Once in the fixative it may be stored indefinitely and processed at any time.

■ DIFFERENTIAL DIAGNOSIS OF DERMATOLOGIC DISEASES

The most frequently encountered dermatologic diseases discussed in this chapter can be grouped according to their appearance (Table 8–1), as this is often helpful in establishing a differential diagnosis.

Macules

POSTINFLAMMATORY PIGMENTATION. The development of hyperpigmentation, hypopigmentation, or various combinations of altered skin color is a common sequela to any cutaneous inflammatory process. Thermal burns, lichen planus, lupus erythematosus, insect bites, and dermatitis are frequently followed by pigmentary change. The diagnosis of these diseases may be suspected by the pattern of pigmentation. It is not possible to predict whether a given patient will develop hyper- or hypopigmentation following a given inflammatory process although, as a general rule, the darker a patient's skin the more likely it is that hyperpigmentation

TABLE 8–1. Dermatologic Diseases in the Tropics

Macules	Nodules	Vesicles	Papules	Ulcers	Pustules
Hypopigmented	Leprosy	Dermatitis	Scabies	Tropical ulcer	Pyoderma
Postinflammatory	Kaposi sarcoma	Pemphigus foliaceus	Tungiasis	Leishmaniasis	Paracoccidioidomycosis
Vitiligo	Myiasis		Flea bites	Leprosy	Acne
Tinea versicolor	Chromomycosis		Onchocerciasis	Buruli ulcer	
Leprosy	Sporotrichosis		Cutaneous larva migrans	Cancrum oris	
Onchocerciasis	Maduromycosis		2° syphilis	1° and 3° syphilis	
Pinta	Paracoccidioidomycosis		Leprosy	Sporotrichosis	
Hyperpigmented	Keloids		Myiasis	Tuberculosis	
Postinflammatory	Acne		Kaposi sarcoma	Diphtheria	
Mongolian spots	Tuberculosis		Acne	Pyoderma	
Malnutrition			Dermatitis	Tuberculosis	
Pellagra			Tuberculosis		

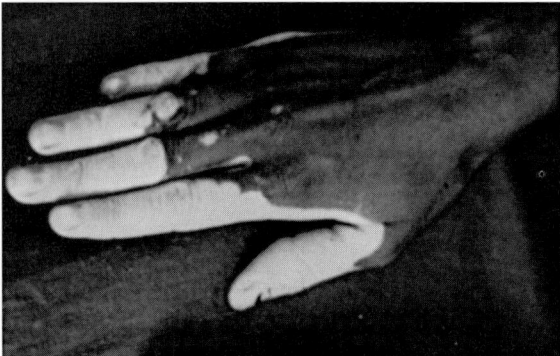

Figure 8–1. Vitiligo. Acral hypopigmentation is well developed in this Ethiopian woman.

will develop. The diagnosis of postinflammatory pigmentation is based on the history of a prior inflammatory process at that site. Postinflammatory pigmentary change tends to improve over months or years but resolution is rarely complete. Hyperpigmentation may be treated with daily application of 1 to 2% hydroquinone but the results are generally poor and if used for longer than 6 months it may cause a paradoxical increase in pigmentation. Cosmetic camouflage of hypopigmented areas can be achieved with the frequent application of aniline dyes.

VITILIGO. Vitiligo is a common idiopathic disorder characterized by well-demarcated, depigmented, white macules that gradually enlarge and coalesce (Fig. 8–1). It is not preceded by an inflammatory process, nor is there any scaling or scarring. Approximately 30% of patients have at least one affected family member. Hairs within the lesion may become white or retain their normal pigmentation. Lesions tend to develop around the orifices; over the extensor bony surfaces, particularly the digits, elbows and knees; and along the lower back. The natural history is unpredictable, although lesions tend to enlarge progressively. Spontaneous resolution can occur. The diagnosis is established by the characteristic skin lesions and the absence of a prior inflammatory process. Since vitiligo in the tropics carries a social stigma, because of similarities to leprosy and other diseases, most patients wish to be treated. Cosmetic camouflage may be achieved with repeated applications of aniline dyes. Repigmentation may be achieved in some cases by oral or topical psoralens, which sensitize the skin to ultraviolet A (UVA) light. A common therapy is oral trimethylpsoralen, 0.6 to 0.8 mg/kg, followed 2 hours later by exposure of the affected areas to 15 minutes of midday sunlight on 3 days each week, but not on consecutive days. The time of exposure should be increased by 5 minutes each day until faint erythema remains at 24 hours. Repigmentation usually requires 30 to 50 treatments to appear, and up to 300 treatments are needed for complete repigmentation. The treatment duration for repigmentation is unpredictable. Alternatively, psoralen plus ultraviolet A (PUVA; 8-methoxypsoralen) 0.6 mg/kg orally followed by artificial UVA irradiation is more predictable and easier to control but involves expensive equipment. Eye protection from UVA exposure must be used for 24 hours after taking psoralens to prevent damage to the lens.

TINEA VERSICOLOR. Tinea versicolor is a common chronic superficial mycosis caused by the overgrowth of *Pityrosporum orbiculare,* which is part of the normal skin flora. It is characterized by asymptomatic, well-defined, scaly macules of variable color, most of which tend to be hypopigmented (Fig. 81–8). They tend to coalesce, forming large patches, particularly on the upper trunk. It affects up to 40% of the popula-

tion in the tropics, particularly young adults and those taking corticosteroids. The diagnosis is established by the characteristic lesions and by the demonstration of spores and hyphae using the KOH test. The lesions are difficult to treat because of the high recurrence rate. Localized disease may be treated topically with 2.5% selenium sulfide shampoo, applied neatly and left overnight, or 1% clotrimazole cream, both for 2 weeks. Treatment failures and those with extensive disease, or follicular infections, may be given a 5- to 7-day course of systemic itraconazole or ketoconazole. Hypopigmented lesions take several months to resolve after successful treatment.

LEPROSY. Leprosy is a chronic disease caused by *Mycobacterium leprae* that predominantly affects the skin and peripheral nerves. The clinical characteristics reflect the state of the patient's immune response to the organism. In general, greater resistance is associated with more localized disease and vice versa. Early lesions commonly consist of one, or a few, slightly hypopigmented or erythematous macules, a few centimeters in diameter, with a poorly defined margin. Sensation and hair growth are usually normal. The lesions most often occur on the face, buttocks, or trunk (Fig. 78–6). This is known as indeterminate leprosy and may persist unchanged for many years, spontaneously resolve, or evolve. In tuberculoid leprosy a small number of lesions are present, either anesthetic macules or well-defined erythematous plaques that are hairless and dry (Fig. 78–7). It is important to look for enlarged nerves (Fig. 78–8), as this clinical finding predates a sensory peripheral neuropathy. In lepromatous leprosy there are numerous lesions; small erythematous macules, papules, or nodules—or all of these may be seen (Figs. 78–9 to 78–13). Initially, hair growth and sensation are normal. Later, the skin becomes very dry and ulcers may form. Ulcers more commonly occur as a result of repeated minor trauma in anesthetic areas, especially on the hands and feet. They may become very large through secondary infection and neglect.

MONGOLIAN SPOTS. A Mongolian spot is a blue-black macule or patch that usually occurs on the lumbrosacral area. It is present at birth in most mongoloid babies and many dark-skinned people. It generally fades before the age of 5 years. The diagnosis is established by the characteristic appearance. No treatment is necessary.

PINTA. Pinta is a contagious, nonvenereal treponematosis caused by *Treponema carateum,* which is endemic in Central and South America. It is spread by direct contact with skin and mucous membranes, and predominantly affects infants and children. The initial lesions are slightly scaly, erythematous papules on exposed sites. These enlarge by peripheral extension, or by the development of satellite lesions, to form scaly plaques that may be as large as 20 cm in diameter (Figs. 48–9 to 48–11). They may persist for months or years and often overlap with the secondary lesions, known as "pintides." These can be hypochromic, pigmented, or erythrosquamous macules that frequently merge together to produce the tertiary stage, which is characterized by patchy pigmentary change, hyperkeratosis, and then atrophy. Untreated, the eruptions persist unchanged or progressively enlarge. Generalized lymphadenopathy occurs during the later stages. The diagnosis is made on the basis of the characteristic mottled pigmentation in a patient from an endemic areas together with positive serologic test results or demonstration of the organism from lymph nodes by dark-field microscopy.

MALNUTRITION. In severe protein-calorie malnutrition (marasmus) the skin becomes dry, loose, and wrinkled. There is substantial loss of subcutaneous tissue and the skin appears too large for the patient. In contrast, in protein-calorie malnutrition with relative carbohydrate excess (kwashiorkor), the principal features are hypopigmentation, scaling, and edema (Fig. 130–3). Individual lesions start as erythematous macules that become reddish-brown with marked exfoliation. In mild cases the skin may be flaky or have a "crazy-paving" appearance and in severe cases it may progress to erosions. The changes are more pronounced in skin flexural areas. In both marasmus and kwashiorkor the hair becomes sparse.

PELLAGRA. Pellagra is a clinical syndrome caused by a deficiency of niacin that produces the triad of dermatitis, diarrhea, and dementia. Lesions start as redness with superficial scaling, which may then progress to vesiculation and crusting. A brownish-red pigmentation then develops. The lesions occur on sun-exposed sites; e.g., as the neck ("Casal's necklace"), and resemble sunburn (Figs. 131–10 and 131–11). The oral and genital mucous membranes are often affected but this may be due to associated deficiencies of zinc and other group B vitamins. The diagnosis is established on the basis of the clinical features: a diet consisting predominantly of maize and the rapid clinical response to niacin.

Papules

SCABIES. Scabies is a very common, itchy skin disease occurring worldwide in both sexes and in all age groups. It is caused by infection with, and sensitization to, the mite *Sarcoptes scabiei hominis.* The mites burrow into the keratin and epidermis at a rate of 3 to 4 mm/day. The infection is asymptomatic for the first 3 to 4 weeks, but reinfection is followed by immediate symptoms. Once sensitization to the mite and its products occurs severe itching develops, the burrows become erythematous, and inflammatory papules and nodules develop. Lesions are most commonly seen on the wrists, borders of the hands, sides of the fingers and in the finger web spaces, on the instep of the feet, on the genitalia in men, and the breasts in women (Figs. 8–2 and 128–9). Babies and small infants, but not adults, get scabietic lesions on the head. The diagnosis is suggested by the characteristic history of an itchy eruption, worse at night, together with the appearance of the lesions. Confirmation is by extraction of a mite. The mite can be identified as a gray dot at the nonscaly end of a burrow and it may be extracted either with a needle or by scraping the burrow with a blunt scalpel blade, placing it on a slide, adding a drop of KOH, and then examining it under a microscope. Many patients develop a widespread dermatitis, which is frequently secondarily infected.

Treatment consists of killing the mites and ova, and treating the dermatitis and secondary infection. Treatment of choice is either an aqueous emulsion of lindane 1% or permethrin 0.5%, which should be applied all over the body, except the head in adults, after a thorough shower or bath. It should be left on for 12 to 24 hours. A second application may increase the cure rate. Alternatives include sulfur 10% in yellow soft paraffin, malathion 0.5%, and benzyl benzoate 25%. They are best applied with a 2-inch paint brush. All clothing should also be washed. Itching may persist for 2 to 6 weeks after a successful cure and can be controlled by crotamiton cream. Secondary infection should be treated with a systemic antibiotic such as erythromycin.

A rare variant of scabies is crusted, or Norwegian, scabies, which is characterized by infection with millions of mites covering the whole body surface. It causes intense scaling and crust formation. The patients do not itch and therefore do not scratch. It occurs in patients with mental deficiency, dementia, severe physical disability, or immunosuppression.

TUNGIASIS. Tungiasis is a skin disease caused by the tiny burrowing flea *Tunga penetrans*, or jigger. The female flea burrows into the skin to lay eggs beneath the toenails and along the sides of the sole of the feet. The genitalia, buttocks, and hands may occasionally be affected. The lesion is a small papule with a central black dot that gradually enlarges becoming inflamed and painful (Fig. 128–5). The diagnosis may be confirmed by teasing out the flea with a sterile needle. Lesions should be treated by excision or by removal of the insect with a needle or application of turpentine. Secondary bacterial infection should be treated with systemic antibiotics.

FLEA BITES. Flea bites are a common problem throughout the tropics and are caused by infestation with *Pulex irritans*. Fleas that are generally host-specific to other animals, e.g., dog, cat or rat, may also infest man in the absence of their natural host. Flea bites tend to involve the exposed surfaces of the skin but may become widespread. Individual lesions are small, discrete papules with central puncta. There may be an erythematous ring or wheal surrounding each lesion. The lesions tend to cluster, probably caused by bites from a single flea. Excoriations and secondary bacterial infections are common. Bites from other insects cause similar lesions, and the identification of the specific offending insect can only be made by finding it, although it may be suspected from the history and distribution of the lesions. Therapy consists of killing the fleas with an insecticide, such as permethrin, and treatment of the secondary bacterial infection. The source

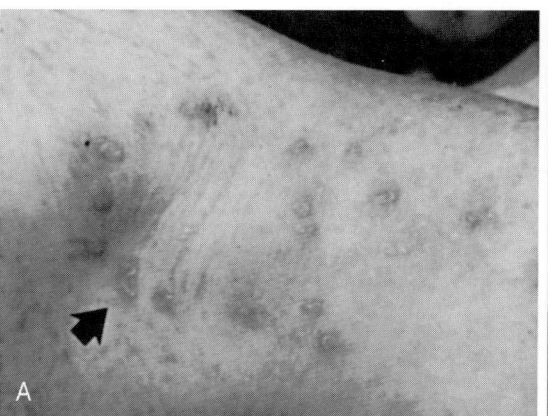
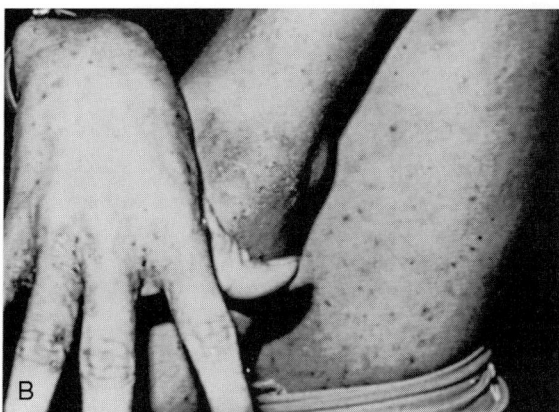

Figure 8–2. Scabies. *A,* The arrow points to a typical burrow in the axilla of a child. Nodules and papules are also present. *B,* The typical distribution of papules and excoriations in scabies: web spaces, elbows, and flanks. (*A,* Courtesy of Dr. Antoinette Hood; *B,* courtesy of Dr. Stanford Lamberg.)

of the fleas in the environment should also be eradicated. Itching may be alleviated by the use of a topical corticosteroid or calamine lotion.

CUTANEOUS LARVA MIGRANS. Cutaneous larva migrans, or creeping eruption, is a clinical term for a distinctive cutaneous eruption that has numerous causes. The prime features are lesions that creep or migrate due to the presence of moving parasites in the skin. Causes include *Ancylostoma braziliense, Uncinaria stenocephala, Ancylostoma caninum* and *Bunostomum phlebotomum,* which are all nonhuman parasitic hookworms. *Strongyloides stercoralis* also causes a distinctive form of cutaneous larva migrans in which a pruritic maculopapular rash, or a rapidly migrating linear urticaria, occurs at the site of penetration (Fig. 115–1). *Loa loa* causes migratory swellings. Hookworm larvae, present in animal feces, penetrate skin, usually on the feet, hand, or buttocks where they migrate at 3 to 50 mm/day leaving an elevated serpiginous, threadlike line about 3 mm wide. The lesion is exceedingly itchy and secondary bacterial infection and dermatitis from scratching are common. Large numbers of larvae may be active at the same time forming a disorganized series of loops. The diagnosis is established by the typical clinical appearance. The disease is self-limiting but it may persist for some months. Treatment is topical thiabendazole, two 0.5-g tablets homogenized into 10 g of petrolatum and applied twice daily. Alternatively, oral thiabendazole twice daily for 2 days can be given but it is less effective and more toxic. Albendazole 400 g twice daily by mouth for 3 days is safer and often effective. Alternatively, physical treatment with liquid nitrogen or ethyl chloride applied in front of the advancing burrow may be effective.

MYIASIS. Myiasis is the infestation by larvae of several types of diptera (two-winged flies). The site of infestation is usually the skin but it can also affect mucous membranes, the gastrointestinal tract, and the urinary tract. The larvae are deposited on the skin by the adult fly directly or indirectly via clothing, soil, or even by other insects. Depending on the species, the larvae may penetrate normal skin or may invade through an open wound. The initial lesion is an edematous, pruritic papule, which may enlarge into a nodule or may develop into a migratory lesion. The patient characteristically reports movement or "something alive" within the lesion. The larvae may also protrude through the top of the lesion and be observed by the clinician (Figs. 8–3 and

128–6). The diagnosis is established by the characteristic skin lesion. The larvae may be extracted through the dilated opening by pressing on the sides of the lesion and grasping the insect with fine forceps. Excision biopsy is rarely necessary.

ONCHOCERCIASIS. Onchocerciasis is a chronic filarial disease caused by *Onchocerca volvulus*, which is transmitted by the *Simulium* black fly. It characteristically affects the skin and the eyes. In the early stages patients present with severe pruritus, mainly around the pelvic and shoulder girdles. This is followed by a nonspecific edematous papular rash, often associated with fever and arthralgia. The pruritus leads to scratching producing excoriations and secondary bacterial infection, and later to lichenification. Lymphadenopathy is common. After several years the initial lesions resolve to leave characteristic spotty depigmentation, atrophy, and fine wrinkling ("leopard skin") (Fig. 108–6). The skin is dry but not itchy, and resembles tissue paper. The differential diagnosis lies between other pruritic conditions, such as scabies and dermatitis. It can be confirmed by identifying microfilariae in the early stages by skin snip and in the late stages, when the organisms lie deep in the dermis, by skin biopsy. Treatment is ivermectin 100 to 200 µg/kg given orally in a single dose.

SYPHILIS. Syphilis is a common, generally sexually acquired, infection with *Treponema pallidum*. Infection is characterized by 3 stages: (1) the primary lesion, or chancre, is usually single and occurs 3 weeks after infection at the site of inoculation, most commonly on the genitalia, anus, or mouth. It is a round, well-demarcated, indurated but painless, ulcer with a clean base. There is associated lymphadenopathy. (2) The second stage occurs about 8 weeks after infection and involves the skin and mucous membranes. There is a symmetrical pleomorphic, coppery-red rash that may be widespread, but commonly involves the palms and soles (Figs. 8–4 and 48–2). The basic lesion is a firm 0.5-cm papule but macular lesions also occur. Hypertrophic coalesced papules occur on the genitalia and anus, known as condylomata acuminata (Fig. 48–1). Eroded erythematous or gray patches occur in the mouth and on the genitalia. Hair loss may occur. These eruptions may remit and relapse for several years and are associated with nonspecific tiredness, fever, and generalized lymphadenopathy. (3) The tertiary stage follows after a latent period of around 20 years and may also involve the skin. The two common lesions are a painless but destructive ulcer known as a gumma, or groups of firm coppery-red nodules that tend to form incomplete rings. The diagnosis is by demonstration of the organism on dark-field microscopy in early lesions or by serologic testing. Treatment is with long-acting penicillin.

KAPOSI SARCOMA. Kaposi sarcoma is a multifocal neoplasm that presents as multiple macules, vascular papules, nodules, or plaques in the skin and internal organs. It is endemic in Zaire, Uganda, and Rwanda but occurs sporadically worldwide. There is a 9:1 male predominance. In Africa it has a peak incidence in the first decade of life, few cases in the second decade, then a gradually rising incidence throughout adult life; elsewhere it is usually seen in elderly men. In 1979 an epidemic of Kaposi sarcoma was identified in the homosexual community in New York and it has become firmly associated with the later stages of infection with the human immunodeficiency virus (HIV), but occurring much more commonly in homosexuals than drug abusers or hemophiliacs. The lesions start as dark blue macules, resembling bruises, which then enlarge to become papular or nodular. They usually start on the extremities, most often the feet, and are frequently accompanied by edema of the limb. Lesions may involute to leave pigmented scars, or become eroded, ulcerated, or fungating (Fig. 12–4). In HIV-associated

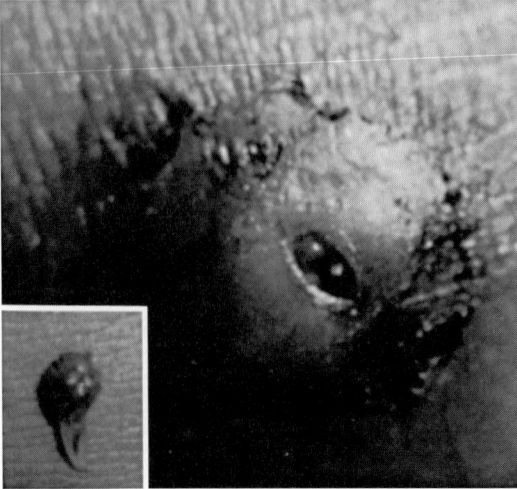

***Figure* 8–3.** Myiasis. Nodular lesion of myiasis demonstrates a central pore with the larva protruding. *Inset,* Intact larva has been extracted from the lesion. (Courtesy of Dr. E. Farmer.)

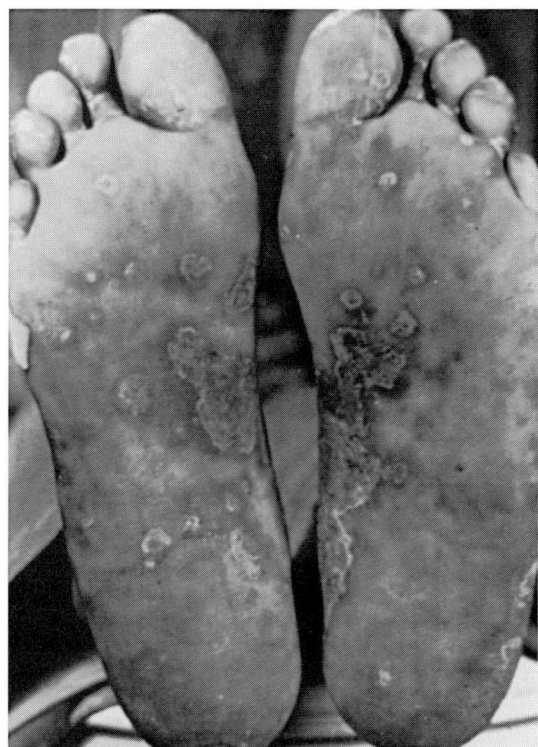

Figure 8–4. Secondary syphilis. Brown keratotic papules and plaques on the soles are characteristic of secondary syphilis. (Courtesy of Dr. E. Farmer.)

Kaposi sarcoma the signs are much less florid than in the classic disease. The diagnosis is established by biopsy. Treatment is by excision or localized radiotherapy.

Nodules

KELOIDS. A *keloid* is an overgrowth of dense fibrous tissue that develops in the skin as a result of trauma, e.g., surgery. A hypertrophic scar is similar but it will gradually involute. The etiology is unknown, although predisposing factors have been identified and it is more common in blacks (Table 8–2). Exuberant scar tissue may appear as early as 3 to 4 weeks after the injury. The scar becomes raised and thickened; it spreads out beyond the original injury to form a well-defined, firm, pink plaque. After 2 to 3 months it becomes tender. Growth usually continues for a few months but occasionally continues for years. Diagnosis is based on the history and appearance. There is no effective treatment; surgical excision will lead to recurrence. Lesions may be softened, and occasionally reduced in size, by injections of a steroid, e.g., triamcinolone acetate.

TABLE 8–2. Factors Predisposing to Keloid Formation

Type of trauma	More common after burns and scalds; also following surgery.
Wound infection	
Foreign material	Hair or suture material at site.
Site	Common sites are earlobes, chin, neck, shoulders, upper trunk, and legs.
Family history	
Racial background	More common in blacks.
Age	More common between puberty and age 30 years.

CHROMOMYCOSIS. Chromomycosis is a chronic granulomatous disease of the skin and mucous membranes caused by infection with various pigmented fungi. It predominantly affects agricultural workers, and the legs are the usual site. Following inoculation of the spores, usually from vegetation or through open wounds, a warty papule develops that slowly enlarges to form a brown warty plaque, which frequently ulcerates (Figs. 82–4 and 82–5). The lesion, which is painless, then becomes covered with a hyperkeratotic crust that may be 1 to 3 cm thick. Satellite lesions are produced by scratching. Treatment is with antifungal chemotherapy such as itraconazole given for 6 to 9 months. Alternatives include flucytosine either alone or in combination with amphotericin B. Very small lesions may be surgically excised but this should be combined with chemotherapy. Local warming has led to cure.

SPOROTRICHOSIS. Sporotrichosis is a chronic granulomatous disease of the skin and lymphatics caused by infection with *Sporothrix schenckii* (Chapter 82–2). It occurs throughout the world, predominantly affecting agricultural workers and gardeners, usually on the extremities. The infection may remain localized to the point of inoculation producing a nodule, a warty plaque, or an ulcer. More commonly, a nodule or pustule develops which ulcerates; this is followed by spread along the draining lymphatics resulting in a chain of nodules linked by a hard lymphatic cord (Fig. 8–5). These nodules subsequently soften and ulcerate. New nodules appear every few days and the regional lymph nodes may enlarge and ulcerate. The diagnosis is established by fungal culture of infected tissue; it is not usually possible to identify spores by direct microscopy. Treatment is with potassium iodide, which is continued for 3 to 4 weeks after clinical cure. A saturated solution is used and administered by mouth three times per day starting at a dose of 5 drops but progressively increased to 50 drops until lesions have healed. An alternative is itraconazole, 100 to 200 mg daily for 3 to 4 weeks.

PARACOCCIDIOIDOMYCOSIS. Paracoccidioidomycosis (South American blastomycosis) is a chronic granulomatous fungal infection caused by *Paracoccidioides brasiliensis* which affects the skin, mucous membranes, lymph nodes, and internal organs (Chapter 83–4). It occurs in South America, most commonly Brazil, and usually affects adult men. It probably enters the body through the lungs. It affects the mouth producing severe ulcerating stomatitis with loss of teeth. Skin lesions usually occur on the face at the mucocutaneous junctions by direct extension. They have a variable appearance consisting of papules, nodules, ulcers, and crusts. Subcutaneous abscesses result from hematogenous or lymphatic spread. The cervical lymph nodes enlarge, become painful and adherent to the overlying skin, and may suppurate with chronic sinus formation. Diagnosis is established by the clinical appearance and identification of the organism by microscopy and fungal culture. Treatment is with either itraconazole or ketoconazole for 3 to 6 months.

MADUROMYCOSIS. Maduromycosis (mycetoma, madura foot) is a very destructive chronic granulomatous disease of skin and underlying bone caused by infection with various fungi or actinomycetes. Infection follows inoculation, usually on the feet or lower legs of laborers who work barefoot (Fig. 82–1). A firm painless nodule appears followed by others which ulcerate and discharge pus containing grains. The lesions grow slowly over years and are relatively painless, but the infection progressively extends to the underlying bone and joints causing periostitis, osteomyelitis, and arthritis (Fig. 82–2). Cavities are formed associated with multiple sinus tracts draining pus. Diagnosis is based on the radiographic findings and direct demonstration of the organism

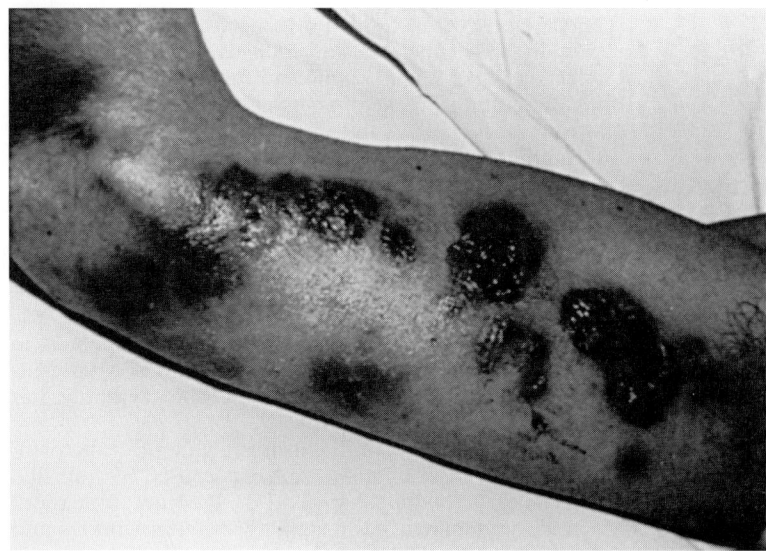

Figure 8–5. Sporotrichosis. Ulcerative nodular lesions are arranged in a linear fashion on the arm extending to the axilla in this South African man. (Courtesy of Dr. Michael Radowsky.)

in the exudate or confirmed by skin biopsy or fungal culture. Treatment, except for secondary bacterial infection, has not been particularly successful. Localized lesions should be surgically excised and amputation may be required for larger lesions. Although results are often poor, chemotherapy should be considered before amputation. For cases caused by actinomyctes use co-trimoxazole or dapsone and streptomycin. Itraconazole, griseofulvin, or ketoconazole should be used for cases caused by fungi.

Vesicles and Bullae

DERMATITIS. Dermatitis (eczema) means inflammation of the skin and does not imply a specific cause. It is common throughout the world and most cases can be categorized as endogenous (atopic, seborrhoeic, pompholyx, or stasis) or exogenous (irritant, allergic, or photodermatitis). The lesions are pleomorphic; in acute cases a poorly demarcated erythema and swelling associated with vesicles, papules, exudation, and crusting are seen. It is extremely itchy, thus excoriations and lichenification are common. Secondary bacterial infection is particularly common in tropical climates and if unrecognized or untreated is a common reason for therapeutic failure. The diagnosis is made clinically. Treatment consists of removing allergens and irritants, treatment of any secondary bacterial infection with systemic or topical antibiotics, topical (or for short periods, systemic) steroids and emollients, e.g., white soft paraffin or aqueous cream, applied liberally at least twice daily. The frequency of relapses can be reduced by the regular use of emollients and adopting protective measures.

PEMPHIGUS FOLIACEOUS. Pemphigus foliaceous is an immune-mediated disorder of unknown cause. It is a very rare disease occurring in the elderly except in Brazil where it is a disease of adolescents living in rural areas. It is characterized by flaccid blisters that rupture easily forming eroded areas with peripheral erythema and that heal with crusting and scaling (Fig. 8–6). Many patients progress to generalized erythroderma with an associated pyrexia that is often worse in the evenings. In chronic cases hyperpigmentation and hyperkeratosis may be prominent features. The diagnosis is made by skin biopsy. Treatment is with high-dose systemic steroids (e.g., prednisolone 60 mg daily initially). If untreated it has a 40% mortality in 2 years.

Pustules

ACNE. Acne is a common inflammatory disorder of the pilosebaceous glands occurring primarily in adolescents and young adults. It is characterized by the formation of comedones (blackheads and whiteheads), erythematous papules and pustules, nodules and cysts and, sometimes, scarring. Those prone to acne frequently deteriorate if they go to hot, humid climates and their acne becomes more inflammatory with pustules and papules. Treatment is with topical antibiotics, keratolytics, systemic antibiotics (e.g., tetracycline), and isotretinoin.

PYODERMA. Pyoderma is a general term that refers to any purulent skin disease. Although these conditions occur in temperate climates, their very high prevalence in the tropics accounts for many of the differences between tropical and temperate dermatologic practice. Furthermore, the presence of secondary bacterial infection modifies the presentation and management of many other conditions. Pyoderma is generally caused by infection of the skin with group A β-hemolytic streptococci, *Staphylococcus aureus,* or a mixed flora of both organisms with additional pathogens. The infection

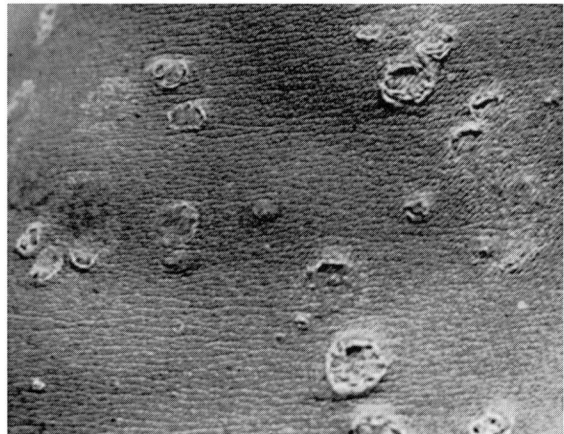

Figure 8–6. Pemphigus foliaceous. Ruptured flaccid bullae with peripheral rolls of epidermis are scattered on the trunk of an Ethiopian boy. (Courtesy of Dr. E. Farmer.)

may develop on normal skin but more commonly appears as a complication of wounds, insect bites, dermatitis, or other skin disease. Malnutrition and poor hygiene are predisposing factors in its development.

Specific names are given for the various clinical presentations of pyoderma. *Impetigo* presents as small pustules or vesicles which evolve into yellow crusts that heal without scarring. *Bullous impetigo*, more common in young children, is characterized by large bullae (blisters) that, when ruptured, develop brown crusts instead of the yellow crusts of impetigo. *Ecthyma* is a deep infection of the skin presenting as ulcers covered by an adherent, brown hemorrhagic crust. It usually occurs on the legs and may begin as pustules or arise in an open wound. Ecthyma heals with scarring. *Folliculitis* is characterized by pustules developing within the openings of the hair follicles. If superficial the pustules develop yellow crusts similar to those of impetigo. If the infection is in the deep portion of a hair follicle, forming an abscess, the term *furuncle* is used. A *carbuncle* refers to a localized aggregation of furuncles. *Erysipelas* is an infection within the skin in which a well-demarcated, warm, tender erythematous plaque appears suddenly. It enlarges peripherally and small vesicles may appear at the advancing edge. *Cellulitis* is similar but the infection lies in the subcutaneous tissues, so that the lesions are less well demarcated. In contrast to other forms of pyoderma, patients with erysipelas and cellulitis are systemically sick with fever, chills, and malaise. Lymphadenitis and lymphadenopathy are common associated findings and recurrent attacks of erysipelas and cellulitis, particularly on the extremities, lead to lymphatic obstruction and the development of lymphedema.

The diagnosis of the various forms of pyoderma is established by the clinical appearance and may be confirmed by bacterial culture of pus or blister fluid. Swabs taken from intact skin are rarely of value. However, swabs taken from the nose or perineal areas are often helpful. Systemic antibiotics are the treatment of choice. Penicillin, flucloxacillin or erythromycin, depending on the sensitivities, should be given in full dosage for at least 10 to 14 days. Attention to hygiene with regular bathing and possibly the use of an antiseptic should be considered. In recurrent cases the patient and the household should be examined and nasal and perineal swabs taken to identify a carrier.

Ulcers

LEISHMANIASIS. Cutaneous leishmaniasis is a chronic granulomatous disease of the skin and mucous membranes. It is caused by the protozoa *Leishmania*, which are transmitted by sandflies. Cutaneous leishmaniasis can generally be divided into 2 types, i.e., Old World (Oriental sore) or New World (American leishmaniasis) reflecting differences in their geographic occurrence and natural history. Lesions usually occur on exposed sites, especially the face. They begin as small papules which enlarge and develop a crust that subsequently separates to reveal an ulcer. Lesions vary in size from 0.5 to 5 cm in diameter, the ulcer base may be dry or moist, and there is an indurated margin (Fig. 92–10). Oriental sores often heal spontaneously within a year, whereas American leishmaniasis tends to be more persistent (Figs. 92–12 and 92–13). Mucous membrane involvement is much more common in American leishmaniasis and often presents months or years after the primary lesion (Fig. 92–14). It is characterized by ulceration which may lead to destruction of the nose and mouth. Dermal leishmaniasis following kala-azar is a pleomorphic eruption, characterized by macules, papules, nodules, or plaques that usually occur in patients who have been treated for visceral leishmaniasis (Fig. 92–7).

It may be persistent. Cutaneous leishmaniasis is diagnosed by demonstrating the organism from a skin biopsy, from a smear taken from the indurated margin of a lesion, or by culture (Fig. 92–12). Treatment is with pentavalent antimonials.

BURULI ULCER. A Buruli ulcer is a skin ulcer, caused by *Mycobacterium ulcerans*, which is common in Uganda and Zaire. It affects children predominantly. The lesion, which usually occurs on the legs, begins as a small nodule that rapidly breaks down to form a large, shallow necrotic ulcer surrounded by induration (Fig. 79–1). Characteristically the lesions are painless and there is no regional lymphadenopathy. The diagnosis can be established by a skin biopsy demonstrating the organisms directly or by culture. Healing may occur in 6 to 9 months but it is often prolonged. Scarring and deformity are common (Fig. 79–2).

TROPICAL ULCER. Tropical ulcer is a rapidly growing painful ulcer that is usually found on the legs of malnourished children. It is probably caused by a synergistic infection with at least two organisms, one of which is a fusobacterium, usually *Fusobacterium ulcerans*. It occurs in poor social circumstances, with filth and malnutrition thought to be important contributory factors. Lesions start as papules or bullae at sites of potential trauma; these rapidly enlarge and break down over 2 to 3 weeks to form sharply defined ulcers. They measure 2 to 4 cm in diameter, have an indurated raised margin, and the base contains gray slough (Fig. 59–1). There is no lymphadenopathy. Untreated, the ulcers persist for many years and squamous cell carcinoma has been reported to develop after 10 years. Healing occurs with fibrosis but the scar is very delicate (Fig. 59–2). Diagnosis is made by the clinical appearance together with the rapid onset and clustering of cases. Spiral organisms may be identified from the ulcer base (Fig. 59–3). Tropical ulcer must be distinguished from venous ulceration, Buruli ulcer, and mycoses. Treatment is rest, elevation of the affected limb, and local cleaning of the ulcer with silver nitrate solution to remove necrotic debris followed by bland applications. Penicillin and metronidazole should be given, and an adequate diet is important. Lesions that have been present for only a few months heal rapidly. Chronic lesions respond much less well and skin grafting may be necessary.

CANCRUM ORIS. Cancrum oris is a disorder characterized by rapidly developing necrotic ulceration of the face, occurring in malnourished children. It is thought to be due to infection by *Borrelia vincentii* and *Bacillus fusiformis*. Many of these children also have malaria, measles, kala-azar, or other systemic diseases. The ulceration is usually unilateral and tends to involve the mouth. Large defects may quickly develop and death may occur in untreated patients (Fig. 13–5). The lesions are quite painful, with variable systemic symptoms. The diagnosis is made by the characteristic clinical appearance and the exclusion of other diseases such as bacterial abscesses, actinomycosis, and maduromycosis. Treatment is systemic penicillin combined with cleaning the lesion and a balanced diet high in calories and protein. Reconstructive surgery may be required for extensive defects.

CUTANEOUS DIPHTHERIA. Cutaneous diphtheria is caused by infection with *Corynebacterium diphtheriae* (Chapter 33). It frequently colonizes other lesions and can be identified in up to 60% of skin lesions, such as impetigo, yaws and abrasions, in some tropical rural areas. Its pathogenic role in these cases is unclear. The primary lesion is a superficial ulcer with a clearly defined overhanging edge; the ulcer base contains an adherent gray membrane. As the lesion develops it becomes deeper, the edge becomes rolled and avascular, and regional lymphadenopathy appears. In contrast to faucal diphtheriae, little toxin is produced in the cutaneous forms.

Untreated, it may persist for 6 to 12 weeks healing with scar formation. Diagnosis is made by bacteriologic culture. Treatment is with specific antitoxin and penicillin.

CUTANEOUS TUBERCULOSIS. Cutaneous tuberculosis occurs in 10% of all cases of extrapulmonary tuberculosis and it can take many forms (Chapter 79). Inoculation of *Mycobacterium tuberculosis* into the skin may produce a *chancre*, a brown papule that ulcerates with undermined edges and a granular hemorrhagic base, associated with regional lymphadenopathy. It heals over several months. Alternatively, an indolent warty plaque may form, known as tuberculosis verrucosa cutis. The skin may be involved secondary to tuberculosis elsewhere. Scrofuloderma refers to the involvement and breakdown of the skin overlying a tuberculous focus, usually a lymph gland (Fig. 79–6). It starts as a brown nodule which ulcerates, often forming numerous interconnecting fistulas. Orifacial tuberculosis refers to the infection of mucosa or skin adjacent to orifices in patients with advanced tuberculosis; small edematous red nodules occur which rapidly break down to form shallow painful ulcers. In miliary tuberculosis profuse crops of bluish papules, vesicles, pustules, or hemorrhagic lesions may appear in a patient who is obviously sick; they may progress to ulcers. A tuberculous gumma presents as a firm subcutaneous nodule that slowly softens and ulcerates to form an undermined ulcer, often with sinuses. Lupus vulgaris occurs in patients with a moderate or high degree of immunity. It is a plaque composed of several nodules that have an "apple-jelly" (reddish-brown) appearance interspersed with scarring. The lesion has a soft, almost gelatinous consistency. It may occur at the site of inoculation but most commonly occurs in normal skin (Fig. 79–5). In Europe it is most common on the face but in India it is more common on the trunk and buttocks. The tuberculitides form in response to internal forms of tuberculosis and clear with antituberculous therapy. They may be papules, ulcers, or indurated red plaques, e.g., erythema nodosum and erythema induratum. The diagnosis of cutaneous tuberculosis is made by histologic examination of tissue. Treatment should be with standard regimens of antituberculous therapy; the vogue in the past for using isoniazid alone is no longer recommended.

Bibliography

Burns DA: The treatment of human ectoparasite infection. Br J Dermatol 125:89, 1991.
Champion RH, Burton JL, Ebling FKG (eds): Textbook of Dermatology, 5th ed. London, Blackwell Scientific, 1992.
Fahal AH, Hassan MA: Mycetoma. Br J Surg 79:1138, 1992.
Ramesh V, Misra RS, Saxena U, Mukherjee A: Comparative efficacy of drug regimens in skin tuberculosis. Clin Exp Dermatol 16:106, 1991.
Restrepo A: Treatment of tropical mycoses. J Am Acad Dermatol 31 (3 pt 2):S91, 1994.

9 Neurologic Diseases

C. L. Bolis, Athasit Vejjajiva, and Prasert Boongird

Neurologic problems are common in tropical areas and contribute substantially to mortality and morbidity. Diseases of the nervous system that are often seen in developed countries are also encountered in the tropics, albeit less frequently. Bacterial meningitis, cerebral malaria, cerebral parasitosis, tetanus, and cerebrovascular disease are leading causes of death and disability. Tropical countries are not homogeneous with regard to disease patterns, but certain features of neurologic illness are common to many areas. Important factors determining the pattern of neurologic illness include a high prevalence of infectious disease, poverty, ignorance, malnutrition, and local habits and beliefs. There is also a larger proportion of children in the population, and a relative paucity of the degenerative diseases of old age. Many of the common neurologic disorders in the tropics are diseases of the socially and economically disadvantaged.

Certain diseases, e.g., trypanosomiasis, rabies, poliomyelitis, and leprosy, are confined to or are much more common in the tropics; other neurologic diseases are rarer in the tropics than in temperate climates (Table 9–1).

The reactions of the nervous system to disease are relatively limited; many different pathogenic agents produce well-defined clinical syndromes, e.g., acute meningoencephalitis, hemiplegia, and paraplegia. In medical practice in the tropics, the differential diagnosis of the neurologic clinical syndromes is wider because it includes disorders of the nervous system that may be encountered anywhere as well as those that are almost always confined to the tropics. Generally, diagnostic facilities are less available than in temperate areas. The physician's objectives of prevention and early diagnosis and treatment are often unattainable because of inadequate primary care, late presentation, and poor public health services. High mortality rates and permanent neurologic damage are commonplace in the tropics.

▪ ACUTE CONFUSIONAL STATES

The common causes of acute confusional state (acute organic brain syndrome) in adults are shown in Table 9–2.

ACUTE INFECTIONS. Confusion, disorientation in time and space, clouding of consciousness, agitation, and hallucinations are seen as a result of severe febrile illness, e.g., malaria (Chapter 92), pneumonia (Chapter 2), or typhoid fever (Chapter 75). In these states, there is no macroscopic evidence of brain inflammation. Similar findings may mark the onset of meningitis (Chapter 52), encephalitis, or a metabolic encephalopathy. Lumbar puncture may be necessary to distinguish these conditions from meningitis.

ACUTE METABOLIC AND TOXIC ENCEPHALOPATHIES. Certain metabolic disorders and toxins cause confusion,

TABLE 9–1. Differences in the Incidence of Neurologic Illness in the Tropics and in Europe and North America

More Common in Tropics	Less Common in Tropics
Pyogenic meningitis	Subacute combined degeneration
Tuberculous meningitis	Multiple sclerosis
Arbovirus encephalitis	Prolapsed disk syndromes
Tetanus	Neurologic syndromes associated with malignancy, Meniere disease, and trigeminal neuralgia
Poliomyelitis	
Rabies	
Nutritional and toxic neuropathies	
Neurologic complications of malaria, trypanosomiasis, relapsing fever, amebiasis, hemoglobinopathies, hepatic failure, hydatid disease, cysticercosis, schistosomiasis, and Burkitt lymphoma	Degenerative disorders of old age, e.g., Parkinson disease, Alzheimer disease
Pyomyositis	

TABLE 9–2. Common Causes of Acute Confusional State (Acute Organic Brain Syndrome) in Adults

Systemic Disorders	Intracranial Disorders
Alcohol ingestion	Purulent meningitis
Hypoglycemia (often associated with alcohol ingestion or malaria)	Head injury (post-traumatic states)
	Cerebral malaria
Lobar pneumonia	Encephalitis
Hemorrhage or shock with peripheral circulatory failure	Subdural hematoma
	Cerebrovascular accident
Typhoid fever	Epilepsy (postictal state)
Renal failure	
Hepatic failure	
Hypovitaminosis	

coma, and, sometimes, recurrent convulsions. However, in contrast to acute infectious encephalitis, fever is usually absent and the cerebrospinal fluid (CSF) is normal. The delay in seeking or obtaining medical care contributes to the increased frequency of these problems in developing countries.

DEHYDRATION. Severe dehydration from diarrhea is common in children; usually, there is a balanced loss of water and electrolytes. In perhaps 5 to 10% of those with severe dehydration, excessive loss of electrolytes or replacement with water results in hyponatremic dehydration with circulatory failure, shock, and osmotic swelling of the brain, causing headaches, seizures, and coma. The intravenous administration of full-strength normal saline solution or even 3% NaCl is needed in severe cases, but correction of hyponatremia should be done cautiously to avoid precipitating the syndrome of acute central pontine myelinosis. Less commonly in the tropics, severe hypernatremia with plasma sodium levels above 150 mEq/L results from diarrhea, causing coma and seizures. These patients need to be treated with intravenous hypotonic solutions.

HEPATIC FAILURE. In countries with poor sanitation, viral hepatitis has a high incidence. In a few, it assumes a fulminant form, causing liver failure, particularly in pregnant women (Chapter 28). Some herbal toxins also cause acute liver failure. The outlook is grave, but full recovery without permanent liver damage is possible if the patient is treated with intravenous glucose solutions, neomycin (1 g orally every 6 hours to sterilize the gut), and laxatives or lactulose and is protected from secondary infection. Intravenous cimetidine may diminish gastrointestinal bleeding, a frequent complication in these patients.

Chronic liver damage by cirrhosis is a common cause of hepatic coma, which may be initiated by hemorrhage, alcohol consumption, infection, hypovolemia and electrolyte imbalance due to diarrhea, too-aggressive use of diuretics, or excessive removal of ascitic fluid. Mental changes, flapping tremor, and fetor hepaticus are danger signals in these patients. Precipitating causes need to be corrected and treatment for hepatic coma started.

HYPOGLYCEMIA. Patients in the tropics may be particularly liable to hypoglycemia owing to malnutrition and liver damage, which cause low hepatic glycogen stores. They also have difficulty obtaining emergency treatment. Common causes of hypoglycemia include (1) alcoholic intoxication; (2) viral hepatitis and hepatoma; (3) excessive insulin therapy for diabetics, who may have irregular food intake and energy output; (4) the vomiting sickness of Jamaica caused by the unripe akee fruit that contains hypoglycin A and B; (5) acute falciparum malaria; and (6) protein-energy malnutrition. A high index of suspicion is necessary in patients with these problems, and intravenous glucose should be given promptly if hypoglycemia is likely.

REYE SYNDROME. An encephalopathy with fatty degeneration of the liver causes death in children in association with aflatoxin and administration of acetylsalicylic acid. There is an acute onset, with vomiting, convulsions, coma, and decerebrate posturing. Pallor, hypoxia, hepatomegaly, hypoglycemia, elevated blood ammonia, and abnormal results on liver function tests also occur. Progressive coma and death ensue in many; survivors may have mental retardation, paralyses, and seizures. Intensive care with correction of hypoglycemia, acidosis, hypoxia, and electrolyte imbalance improves the outcome.

■ CENTRAL NERVOUS SYSTEM INFECTIONS

Syndromes associated with infections of the central nervous system (CNS) include acute encephalitis, acute meningitis (Chapter 52), chronic meningoencephalitis, and brain abscess. Important points in differentiating these syndromes are changes in mental status, the presence or absence of nuchal rigidity, and pleocytosis of the CSF. Fever with the relevant symptoms and signs suggests an infectious etiology. The country of origin of the patient may also provide important clues.

ACUTE ENCEPHALITIS. Acute encephalitis implies inflammation of the brain, which can be accompanied by meningeal inflammation. Viruses are often responsible, and pathologically they produce chromatolysis of neurons followed by necrosis and neuronophagia, microglial proliferation (Fig. 30–10), perivascular inflammation (Figs. 30–2 and 30–9), and inclusion bodies in nerve (Fig. 30–3) or glial cells.

Acute encephalitis usually begins as a nonspecific, febrile illness followed by involvement of the CNS, with increasing headache, mental disturbance, and sometimes delirium. Drowsiness, coma, and seizures may ensue. Focal pyramidal and brain stem disturbances and hyperpyrexia sometimes occur. If the meninges are involved, nuchal rigidity will be present. Permanent disabilities, e.g., mental retardation and spasticity, are not infrequent. Differentiation from bacterial meningitis by lumbar puncture is essential. In viral encephalitis, there may be very few, and sometimes no, cells in the CSF. In viral meningitis, there is usually an increase in CSF protein concentration and lymphocytes (10 to 1000 cells/mm³), but the glucose content is normal (50 to 75 mg/dL).

Important causes of encephalitis in the tropics include arboviruses (Chapter 30), poliomyelitis (Chapter 27.1), cerebral malaria (Chapter 92), rabies (Chapter 30.1) and African and American trypanosomiasis (Chapters 93 and 94). An acute encephalitic state with seizures is often due to cerebral malaria and, less frequently, to relapsing fever (Chapter 71). Sometimes, infections with helminths may involve the brain and cause acute encephalitis. This may occur in trichinosis (Chapter 11), cysticercosis (Chapter 124.1), and toxocariasis (Chapter 112), and rarely, after treatment of onchocerciasis (Chapter 108) or loiasis (Chapter 107) with diethylcarbamazine. *Angiostrongylus cantonensis* causes eosinophilic meningitis (Chapter 114.1).

All the postinfectious or postvaccination types are also found in the tropics. Measles is widespread and virulent, and encephalitis sometimes ensues (Chapter 25.1); vaccination at 9 months of age is now part of the worldwide program of expanded immunization against the major childhood infections (poliomyelitis, tetanus, whooping cough, diphtheria, tuberculosis), but there are major problems of cost and cold storage. Encephalomyelitis and peripheral neuropathy following vaccination against rabies using the Semple type vaccine may be as frequent as 1 in 500. Neurologic complications would disappear if human diploid cell vaccine were in universal use.

CHRONIC MENINGOENCEPHALITIS. Chronic meningoencephalitis is characterized by a gradual evolution and relentless progression over weeks, months, or years. The earliest symptoms are usually intellectual deterioration progressing to organic dementia, affective changes (particularly depression), and headache. Motor and sensory changes, tremors, convulsions, and urinary and fecal incontinence appear in the course of the disease; disturbances of consciousness and, finally, coma are terminal signs. The CSF usually shows increased protein and lymphocytic cells. In areas where African trypanosomiasis (Chapter 93) exists, it must be considered the most common cause of chronic meningoencephalitis, and lumbar puncture must be performed. General paresis, a form of neurosyphilis, is a chronic meningoencephalitis resulting in gradual but progressive loss of cortical function, leading to organic dementia (Chapter 48.1). Fortunately, it is a rare complication of syphilis, meningovascular neurosyphilis being more common in the tropics. Dementia is a chronic complication of Lyme disease (Chapter 73). However, infection with *Borrelia burgdorferi* has been rarely reported outside of the United States and Europe. Subacute sclerosing panencephalitis (SSPE), a sequela to measles infection characterized by psychomotor and developmental deterioration, myoclonus, and periodic electroencephalographic (EEG) changes, is rare in tropical Africa despite the high prevalence of measles. On the other hand, well-documented studies in Peru have shown that SSPE frequently occurs in that country as a cause of neurologic sequelae in children.

■ INTRACRANIAL TUMORS AND SPACE-OCCUPYING LESIONS

Signs and symptoms of raised intracranial pressure, e.g., headache, vomiting, and diminished vision; progressive focal neurologic signs; mental changes, including dementia; epilepsy; and endocrine changes due to pituitary or hypothalamic involvement are characteristic of CNS space-occupying lesions. Intracranial neoplasms have not been extensively investigated in many areas of the tropics because of a lack of

neurosurgical facilities and postmortem examinations but are probably as common as in temperate regions. Meningiomas may be relatively more common and gliomas less common in Africa than in Europe and North America. Tuberculomas may account for up to 10% of cerebral tumors diagnosed in the tropics, detection being aided by their intracranial calcification (Chapter 77). Pituitary tumors are relatively easily diagnosed when simple radiology is available. The possibility of a brain abscess, a hydatid cyst, cerebral cysticercosis, toxoplasmosis, or a hematoma should always be seriously considered as a nonmalignant cause of intracranial masses.

BRAIN ABSCESS. This may be more common than in temperate climates because of the frequency of neglected otitis media and chronic suppurative lung disease in the tropics. The symptoms and signs of cerebral tumor are present, but these evolve rapidly over days rather than weeks. Drowsiness is seen at an early stage, and signs of infection, e.g., fever and leukocytosis are found but may not be prominent. A primary source of sepsis in ears, lungs, paranasal sinuses, or heart valves is found in over 70% of patients. A brain abscess may present as meningitis secondary to rupture into the subarachnoid space. The role of anaerobic bacteria has been emphasized, and metronidazole has been employed in treatment in conjunction with antibiotics and surgery. In Europe and the United States, neurosurgical drainage and abscess removal after accurate localization by computed tomography (CT) has improved the gloomy prognosis. Prolonged chemotherapy and drainage may be required when this advanced technology is not available.

PARASITIC LESIONS OF THE CNS. Parasitic infections may present as intracranial masses (sometimes progressing rapidly), as focal or generalized epilepsy, as acute encephalopathies, or as organic dementia (Table 9–3). In the spinal cord, paraplegia due to cord compression or a transverse myelitis is the usual presentation. Diagnosis may be difficult, because although a space-occupying lesion is suspected from radiographic studies, the parasitic nature may not be revealed until exploratory operation. Parasitic infection elsewhere in the body, e.g., subcutaneous nodules, positive serologic tests, and eosinophilia may be helpful diagnostic clues. Surgery is usually the treatment, but sometimes, e.g., in cysticercosis, the cysts are multiple and inoperable. The availability of newer and safer drugs has increased the possibili-

TABLE 9–3. Parasitic Diseases Causing Lesions in the Nervous System

Disease	Parasite	Remarks
Amebic brain abscess	*Entamoeba histolytica*	Cerebral abscess—rare, usually fatal.
Primary amebic meningoencephalitis	*Naegleria* or *Acanthamoeba* species	Meningitis due to free-living ameba. Probable infection via nose while bathing—usually fatal.
Toxoplasmosis	*Toxoplasma gondii*	Frequent cause of encephalitis in the immunosuppressed, e.g., with AIDS.
Trypanosomiasis	*Trypanosoma gambiense/rhodesiense*	Encephalitis
Trichinosis	*Trichinella spiralis*	Epilepsy (usually) and encephalitis (sometimes) with focal features.
Angiostrongyliasis	*Angiostrongylus cantonensis*	Eosinophilic meningitis, granulomatous lesions in brain.
Gnathostomiasis	*Gnathostoma spinigerum*	Cerebral and cord lesions, and eosinophilic meningitis.
Schistosomiasis	*Schistosoma japonicum*	Epilepsy: CNS granulomas.
	Schistosoma mansoni *Schistosoma haematobium*	Transverse myelitis, spinal cord granulomas, and anterior spinal arteritis.
Paragonimiasis	*Paragonimus westermani*	Epilepsy: CNS granulomas (3%).
Cysticercosis	*Taenia solium*	Multiple cerebral cysts. Epilepsy is most common manifestation: may cause organic dementia, hydrocephalus, or focal signs.
Hydatid disease	*Echinococcus granulosus*	Space-occupying lesions in brain or spinal cord (2%).
Dracontiasis	*Dracunculus medinensis*	Cord compression due to extradural location—rare.
Coenuriasis	*Coenurus cerebralis*	Cerebral tumor—rare, usually fatal. Cord compression, paraplegia—rare.

TABLE 9–4. Causes of Coma in the Tropics, with Incidence in the Tropics Compared with That in Temperature Regions

More Common	As Common	Less Common
Cerebral malaria	Diabetic ketoacidosis	Sedative intoxication
Bacterial meningitis	Hypoglycemia	
Arbovirus encephalitis	Uremia	
Hepatic failure	Alcohol poisoning	
Hyperpyrexia	Head injury	
Poisoning with insecticides	Cerebrovascular accident	
Trypanosomiasis		

ties of medical treatment for CNS manifestations in parasitic diseases. In suspected schistosomiasis of the brain or spinal cord (Chapter 118) or amebic brain abscess (Chapter 86), schistosomicidal or amebicidal drugs should be given as soon as the diagnosis is made. Most immunosuppressed patients with toxoplasma encephalitis will respond to treatment if the diagnosis is made and therapy is initiated in a timely fashion (Chapter 97). Albendazole has been used in treating hydatid disease (Chapter 124.2), and praziquantel is efficacious in treating cerebral schistosomiasis, cysticercosis (Chapter 124.1), and paragonimiasis (Chapter 121).

HEAD INJURY AND INTRACRANIAL HEMATOMA. Head injury is frequent in the tropics. In many places, automobile and motorcycle accidents are the main cause, but assault and falls, e.g., from coconut trees, are also common. Subdural hematoma must be considered in coma and stroke, for a history of injury may not be obtained. Head injury is a significant cause of epilepsy in the tropics.

■ COMA

The diagnosis and management of coma are basically the same worldwide. However, the usual causes of coma are rather different in many parts of the tropics (Table 9–4).

It is important to diagnose inflammatory conditions of the nervous system by examination of the CSF and to consider cerebral malaria, cysticercosis, or toxoplasmosis, as specific therapy can be crucial.

■ EPILEPSY

Epilepsy is a significant medicosocial problem in developing countries. It is more common than in developed countries; estimates of the prevalence of chronic epilepsy vary from 5 to 40 per 1000 population. Birth injuries due to primitive midwifery, residua of repeated febrile convulsions, meningitis, encephalitis, and parasitic infections partially explain the increased prevalence of chronic epilepsy. Febrile convulsions are frequent because of the great number of febrile illnesses, including malaria, suffered by children in the tropics. Prolonged febrile convulsions may lead to permanent neurologic damage and chronic epilepsy. Severe and prolonged convulsions should be treated with anticonvulsants (i.e., diazepam, phenobarbital, or paraldehyde) and by cold sponging and antipyretics. Children under 18 months of age with recurrent febrile convulsions in whom antipyretic measures fail to prevent seizures should be given at least a year's treatment with phenobarbital or valproic acid, although it has been established that the adverse effects of phenobarbital on cognition may outlast by several months the period of adminis-

tration of the drug. Cerebral malaria and meningitis must be considered as possible causes of febrile convulsions.

Sufferers from epilepsy in tropical countries have serious social difficulties. Ignorance, prejudice, and erroneous beliefs about the nature of the illness lead to exclusion from school, loss of marriage prospects, and even divorce. Epilepsy is sometimes believed to be due to bewitchment or diabolic possession and is considered infectious by breath, saliva, or flatus. Thus, there is concealment of the illness, recourse to traditional healers, social isolation, and depression. Treatment is often sporadic, increasing the danger of status epilepticus. Burns from falling on open fires are a particular hazard. Management is often difficult because of the lack of drugs and the patient's inability to appreciate the need for prolonged treatment. Repeated explanations to the patient and the relatives are necessary to obtain cooperation.

■ CEREBROVASCULAR DISEASE

Cerebrovascular disease (CVD) is becoming as prevalent as in developed countries and is now a leading cause of mortality and morbidity in developing countries. Indeed, it is said to be the most common certified cause of death in Jamaican adults, accounting for 12% of all deaths in those over 15 years of age, and in China and Ecuador CVD has been documented to be a frequent cause of death. There are fewer older people (with increased risk of CVD) in the tropics, but in many areas, e.g., West Africa, the West Indies, and Southeast Asia, hypertension is prevalent and predisposes to CVD. Although hypertension is the most important factor, diabetes mellitus is also a contributor.

Rheumatic heart disease is extremely common in the tropics; severe cardiac valvular involvement occurs at an early stage and causes cerebral emboli (Chapter 3), as do tropical cardiomyopathies and Chagas disease (Chapter 94). Nonembolic ischemic cerebrovascular disease is the most common variety of CVD. The following are frequently observed in CVD in the tropics: (1) Hemorrhage strokes occur in young people with hypertension. (2) Cerebrovascular occlusions and subarachnoid hemorrhage are complications of sickle cell disease. (3) Arteriovenous congenital malformations are more common than berry aneurysms as the cause of subarachnoid hemorrhage in Malaysia and Thailand. (4) In Japan and areas of Southeast Asia, an aortic arch syndrome known as Takayasu arteritis, or pulseless disease, is a cause of cerebral infarction (Chapter 3). (5) Meningovascular syphilis is a significant cause of ischemic CVD in some parts of the tropics (Chapter 48.1). (6) Malignant trophoblastic disease in women of childbearing age (Chapter 12) is a great imitator of stroke and may, in fact, present as cerebral hemorrhage.

The best way to prevent CVD is to detect and treat hypertension. The relatively high incidence of CVD in tropical Africa exists in parallel with a relatively low incidence of coronary heart disease.

NEUROLOGIC COMPLICATIONS OF HEMOGLOBINOPATHIES. In those diseases in which the erythrocytes sickle under hypoxic conditions, the CNS may be affected by microcirculatory obstruction and profound anemia (Chapter 6). Neurologic disturbances may be precipitated by crisis, childbirth, blood transfusion, or general anesthesia. Lesions found at autopsy include diffuse microcirculatory stasis, large vessel obstruction, dural sinus thrombosis, pericapillary hemorrhages, subarachnoid hemorrhage, and subdural hematoma.

Patients in crisis may be mentally disturbed, and the EEG often shows generalized abnormalities even when there are no overt neuropsychiatric symptoms. There may be drowsiness proceeding to coma, meningismus, and convulsions.

Less commonly, hemiparesis due to vascular occlusion, subarachnoid hemorrhage, paraparesis, and cranial nerve palsies occur. Patients with hemoglobin SS disease are susceptible to pneumococcal meningitis because of depressed immune responses; polyvalent pneumococcal vaccine should be given prophylactically. Sudden blindness due to occlusion of the central artery of the retina is rare; chronic retinopathy is more common.

Patients with major thalassemia syndromes have an increased prevalence of strokes, convulsions, recurrent focal cerebral ischemia, and proximal myopathy.

■ CRANIAL NERVE DISORDERS

OPTIC ATROPHY. The etiology of optic atrophy is often obscure, with the disorder being referred to as tropical nutritional amblyopia. Occasionally, there is some improvement in the early stages after treatment with B complex vitamins. It may be associated with tropical ataxic neuropathy, beriberi, and pellagra. Bilateral retrobulbar neuritis is seen in Nigeria and may be associated with transverse myelitis (the syndrome of neuromyelitis optica), although multiple sclerosis is rare except in South America, where it is increasingly being reported. Other causes of optic atrophy are meningitis, trypanosomiasis, onchocerciasis, syphilis, Lyme disease, epidemic dropsy due to argemone oil, and methanol poisoning resulting from illicit alcohol production. Drugs used in the tropics that occasionally cause optic atrophy include quinine, chloramphenicol, isoniazid, para-aminosalicylic acid, and tryparsamide.

OPHTHALMOPLEGIA. A self-limiting, painful ophthalmoplegic syndrome of unknown etiology with an acute onset, spontaneous remission, and a tendency to recur has been described from parts of the tropics, including India, Zimbabwe, and West Africa. It responds to steroid therapy and must be differentiated from ophthalmoplegia due to berry aneurysms. The syndrome has been reported from temperate climates but appears to be more common in tropical areas. Elapid snakebites can cause ptosis and ophthalmoplegia, the former being an early sign of envenomation, requiring treatment with antivenin (Chapter 126.5).

FACIAL NERVE PARALYSIS. Lower motor neuron paralysis is usually due to Bell palsy; middle ear disease and diabetes should be considered as well. This is a frequent manifestation of Lyme disease (Chapter 73).

EIGHTH NERVE DISTURBANCES. Nerve deafness may follow pyogenic (Chapter 52) and tuberculous (Chapter 77) meningitis and may accompany tropical ataxic neuropathy. Meniere disease is rarely seen in tropical countries, but vestibular neuronitis is not uncommon. Hearing loss may follow the use of quinine, chloroquine (in large doses), aminoglycoside antibiotics, and furosemide.

MISCELLANEOUS. Acute bulbar palsy may be due to poliomyelitis (Chapter 27.1), diphtheria (Chapter 33), or elapid snakebite (Chapter 126.5). Nasopharyngeal carcinoma is common in Malaysia, Hong Kong, and parts of Kenya and sometimes causes multiple lower cranial nerve paralyses (Chapter 12). Trigeminal neuralgia is rare in most tropical countries. Burkitt lymphomas can cause polyneuritis cranialis.

■ SPINAL CORD DISEASE

Paraparesis and tetraparesis are the most common manifestations of spinal cord disease. They may be of gradual or sudden onset and may be associated with sphincter disturbances, sensory changes, and radicular, motor, and sensory signs. The prognosis is often poor because of late presentation, pressure sores, urinary infections, and lack of specialized medical facilities. The common causes of spinal cord syndrome are tuberculous osteitis, intraspinal canal neoplasms, tropical "nutritional" myelopathy, myelopathy associated with retroviral infections (human T-cell lymphotrophic virus-I, human immunodeficiency virus) (Chapters 22 and 23), parasitic infections, trauma, and spondylitic myelopathy. As a cause of lower motor neurone paralysis, poliomyelitis is on the decrease and has disappeared from the American continent (Chapter 27.1): cases of acute lower motor neurone paralysis have been reported from India and Thailand following outbreaks of acute hemorrhagic conjunctivitis due to EV70 virus (Chapter 27.3).

TUBERCULOSIS OF THE SPINE. This is a leading cause of paraplegia of subacute or insidious onset. A spinal deformity is usually obvious, but occasionally *Mycobacterium tuberculosis* involves the spinal cord meninges without bone involvement and causes an arachnoiditis (Chapter 77).

TRAUMA TO THE SPINE. This often occurs in automobile and motorcycle accidents. Falling out of trees while gathering coconuts is a tropical hazard. Falls while carrying heavy loads on the head sometimes cause paraplegia with injury at the C4–5 level.

OTHER CAUSES. Burkitt lymphoma is the most common childhood malignancy in tropical Africa and often causes either paraplegia due to involvement of the spinal cord or a meningoencephalitis (Chapter 12). Other tumors causing paraplegia are neurofibroma, meningioma, schwannoma, ependymoma, astrocytoma, and ganglioneuroma. Neuroplastic involvement of the cord may be secondary to primary lesions in the prostate, breast, thyroid, or liver or to Hodgkin's lymphoma or multiple myeloma. Neuromyelitis optica with paraplegia is sometimes found, although, as stated, multiple sclerosis is a rarity. Transverse myelitis has been associated with *Schistosoma mansoni* and *Schistosoma haematobium* infections (Chapter 118), and *Gnathostoma spinigerum* can cause an eosinophilic myeloencephalitis with pain and paralysis (Chapter 113). Fluorosis may cause spinal cord compression in parts of India (Chapter 132.3), and congenital atlantoaxial dislocation with quadriplegia is mysteriously frequent in India, Sri Lanka, and Thailand. Less common causes of spinal cord disease include epidural abscess, cysticercosis, dermoid cyst, and *Histoplasma duboisii* infection in Africa (Chapter 83.1). The migration of larvae of *Traenia solium* to the spinal cord may produce a clinical picture that mimics amyotrophic lateral sclerosis.

TROPICAL ATAXIC NEUROPATHY/MYELOPATHY. A myeloneuropathy resembling the syndrome first described among Jamaicans at the end of the nineteenth century has been reported from most parts of Africa including Nigeria, Senegal, Kenya, Uganda, and Natal. The syndrome includes myelopathy with or without visual and hearing impairment. Because ataxia is prominent, the disorder is often referred to as tropical ataxic neuropathy (Fig. 9–1). In Nigeria, Tanzania, and Mozambique, strong circumstantial evidence has accrued in the last four decades suggesting that the syndrome of tropical ataxic neuropathy is causally related to chronic cyanide intoxication of dietary origin, riboflavin deficiency, and possible low plasma ceruloplasmin levels. Epidemics of spastic paraparesis linked to cassava cyanide poison have been described in Tanzania, Mozambique, and Zaire.

The syndrome of tropical ataxic neuropathy (TAN) comprises myelopathy with predominant involvement of the posterior columns, bilateral optic atrophy, perceptive deafness, and symmetrical peripheral polyneuropathy, with evidence of more diffuse degenerative lesions in the neuraxis consisting of cerebellar degeneration, parkinsonism, motor neu-

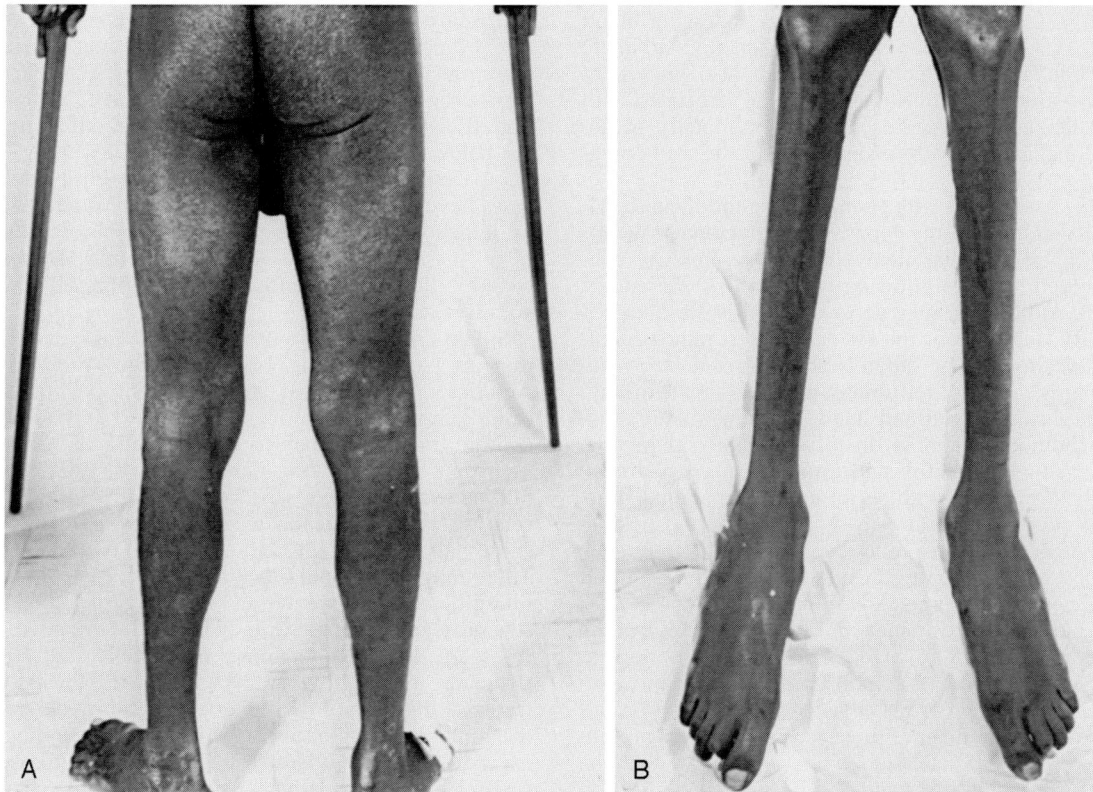

Figure 9–1. *A* and *B,* Patients with ataxic neuropathy.

ron disease, dementia, and schizophreniform psychosis in various combinations. CSF is normal. The disease affects all age groups and the sexes equally but is rare in the first decade of life. Familial cases accounted for 40% of patients in one series, but there was no evidence of genetically determined predisposition. Patients subsisted mainly on a cassava diet, and the cyanide content of food items of cassava derivatives was high. Plasma levels of thiocyanate (a detoxification product of cyanide) and cyanide and urinary thiocyanate excretion were high. The levels fell when the patients were fed on a hospital diet low in cassava and rose again when they reverted to cassava meals. Levels of free cyanide in blood were raised. Sulfur-containing amino acids were absent in the plasma of 60% of the patients and were greatly reduced in others. The levels of serum and tissue (hepatic) cyanocobalamin (another product of cyanide detoxification) were high. Total serum and hepatic vitamin B_{12} levels were normal, however.

Neuroepidemiologic studies in Nigeria showed correlation of the prevalence of the disease with the intensity of cassava cultivation, frequency of cassava meals, and plasma thiocyanate levels. Those who handled cassava roots, e.g., cassava farmers and processors, had the highest risk of developing the disease.

Cassava diet has been incriminated as a cause of some form of diabetes mellitus in young people in the tropics. The evidence is tenuous. No increase in frequency of glucose intolerance or diabetes mellitus has been seen in cassava-associated TAN.

Some tropical staple foods contain cyanogenetic glycosides, particularly cassava (manioc) but also sorghum, maize, and millet. These neuropathic syndromes occur particularly, but not exclusively, in individuals whose main diet consists of cassava. The actual intake of cyanogens depends on methods of cooking and preparation. Soaking the root and discarding the water markedly lowers cyanogen content, as does pressing it into a farina.

Tropical ataxic neuropathy is not explained by cyanide poisoning in all areas; vitamin deficiencies may play a part. The prognosis for complete recovery is poor. Treatment with vitamin B_{12} and other B vitamins has not been beneficial. If possible, the patient should stop eating cassava or at least should receive instructions on the safest way of preparing it. Smoking and alcohol may increase cyanide sensitivity and should be prohibited in these patients. Prevention involves replacement of cassava as a staple, ensuring proper preparation of the root drop, and cultivating strains with a low cyanide content. Early detection of minimal neuropathy may enable dietetic correction and prevention of serious disease.

Tropical Spastic Paraparesis. Throughout the tropics, geographic isolates of another type of spinal cord syndrome have been described and referred to as tropical spastic paraparesis (TSP). Clusters of the disease have been reported in many countries, including islands in the Caribbean, Colombia, the Seychelles, Ivory Coast, Senegal, and Ethiopia. The disorder is characterized by chronic spastic myelopathy of slow onset and progression accompanied initially by lumbalgias, foot dysesthesias, increased urinary frequency, and constipation. The predominant pyramidal tract involvement leads to spastic gait with hyperreflexia and Babinski sign. The syndrome is now established as causally related to human T-cell lymphocytic virus-I (HTLV-I), an association first reported from Martinique and subsequently well documented among the Japanese (Chapter 23). CSF pleocytosis and elevated protein are present in 15 to 40% of patients. HTLV-I virus has been isolated from the CSF. It is distinguished from cassava-induced TAN, in which spasticity is less obvious and perceptive deafness and optic atrophy are more frequently present.

Acute-onset HTLV-I–associated myelopathy following blood transfusion, HTLV-I infection, HTLV-I–associated subacute meningoencephalitis, and polymyositis are also known to occur. HTLV-I–associated myelopathy may be associated with adult T-cell leukemia, vasculitis, uveitis, pulmonary alveolitis, monoclonal gammopathy, Sjögren syndrome, and cryoglobulinemia.

Myelopathy Associated with Human Immunodeficiency Virus (HIV). HIV-associated myelopathy is characterized neuropathologically by vacuolar demyelination resembling subacute combined degeneration of vitamin B_{12} deficiency (Chapter 22). Although it may occur alone, it is often associated with HIV dementia or the HIV-associated minor cognitive motor syndrome. The latter is characterized by symptoms and signs, e.g., forgetfulness, slowness of thinking, reduced concentration, gait and hand clumsiness, and slowness of psychomotor response. In HIV-associated dementia, psychomotor slowing, apathy, and impaired memory are severe enough to interfere with social and occupational functioning and positive frontal release signs (snout, sucking, grasp, palmomental reflexes) may be present. The frequency of HIV-associated myelopathy in patients with the acquired immunodeficiency syndrome (AIDS) may be as high as 20%. Symptoms and signs predominate in the lower limbs, but the upper limbs may also be involved. There is usually no sensory level. Myelography (a spinal magnetic resonance imaging and CT scan where available) is normal. CSF abnormalities include mononuclear pleocytosis, raised protein concentration, and HIV isolation. Table 9–5 shows that the range of neuropsychiatric manifestations in HIV infection is protean.

TABLE 9–5. Neuropsychiatric Associations with Human Immunodeficiency Virus Infection

HIV-Associated Cognitive Motor Complex
  HIV-1–associated dementia
  HIV-1–associated myelopathy
  HIV-1–associated minor cognitive motor syndrome

HIV-Associated Mental and Behavioral Disorders
  Delirium
  Acute psychotic disorders
  Affective disorders
  Adjustment disorders
  Acute stress reactions
  Suicide

Other HIV-Associated CNS Disorders
  Progressive encephalopathy of childhood
  Meningitis (aseptic)

HIV-Associated Peripheral Nervous System Disorders
  Inflammatory polyneuropathy
  Predominantly sensory neuropathy
  Myopathy

Neuropsychiatric Disorders due to Opportunistic Processes in HIV-Infected Subjects
  Progressive multifocal leukoencephalopathy
  Cerebral toxoplasmosis
  Cryptococcal meningitis
  Cytomegalovirus encephalopathy
  Cytomegalovirus neuropathy
  CNS tuberculosis
  Herpes zoster/simplex encephalitis
  Varicella zoster radiculitis
  Other syndromes due to opportunistic infections
  Primary CNS lymphoma

CNS, central nervous system.

Obscure Tropical Paraplegias. The cause of as much as 20% of paraplegias in the tropics remains obscure. These cases are labeled tropical spastic paraplegia. Many of these cases progress, and many become arrested, but few improve. The disease is usually of insidious onset, afflicting individuals below the age of 40 years and presenting as spastic paraparesis with or without "posterior column" deficit. Many cases have normal myelography and are unrelated to retroviral infections, probably representing an autoimmune mechanism. In some patients, adhesions around the cord are detected radiologically or found at operation. This is known as adhesive arachnoiditis.

Spinal Cord Adhesive Arachnoiditis. This condition is common in parts of India, Sri Lanka, the West Indies, South America, and Africa. It is seen in Europe but is rare and diminishing in incidence. The patient has a subacute or chronic transverse myelitis or ascending radiculomyopathy. There may be paralysis, paresthesias, bladder disturbances, muscle wasting, and sensory root pain. In rare cases, ascending paralysis leads to respiratory paralysis. The CSF shows an elevated protein level and minimal pleocytosis. There may be a spinal block syndrome. Myelography shows filling defects, fragmentation of the dye, or a total block over several segments. The etiology is usually unknown, but some cases are due to tuberculosis or syphilis, and some follow pyogenic meningitis, trauma, spinal anesthesia, or the intrathecal injection of radiopaque dyes for myelography. Laminectomy is often necessary to confirm the diagnosis and exclude tumor. Division of adhesions or decompression rarely benefits the patient. Any suspicion of schistosomiasis as a cause of paraplegia should lead to prompt chemotherapy.

Lathyrism. Lathyrism is a spastic paraplegia associated with the consumption of large amounts (e.g., 200 to 300 g) of the chickpea, *Lathyrus sativus*. The toxic factor in the pea is an unusual amino acid, β-oxalyaminoalanine. This substance can be destroyed by boiling in a large volume of water or by parboiling before cooking. Heavy consumption of the chickpea takes place during severe food shortages, and lathyrism has occurred in India, Algeria, and Ethiopia. In lathyrism, there is fairly sudden onset of an upper motor neuron type of paralysis of the legs, which is usually permanent. At autopsy, demyelination of the lateral spinal cord is found. No specific therapy is known.

■ DISEASES OF PERIPHERAL NERVES

In a large proportion of cases of peripheral neuropathy (30 to 60%), no specific etiology is found. However, the common causes include leprosy, Lyme disease, nutritional deficiencies, Guillain-Barré syndrome, metabolic and toxic conditions (especially diabetes mellitus), drugs, and trauma. As a nosologic entity, leprosy is the most common cause of neuropathy in the world, affecting 15 million people, most of them resident in the tropics (Chapter 78). In certain areas, neuropathy is widespread and associated with malnutrition and exposure to toxic factors. There are many classifications of peripheral neuropathy. Asbury described 5 main patterns according to the clinical features. Some diseases, e.g., diabetes, appear in more than one pattern.

SYNDROME OF ACUTE ASCENDING MOTOR PARALYSIS WITH VARIABLE DISTURBANCE OF SENSORY FUNCTION. Acute idiopathic polyneuritis (Landry syndrome, Guillain-Barré syndrome) may follow viral or bacterial infection. Death results in 10 to 15% of patients owing to respiratory paralysis. Vital capacity should be monitored and respiratory assistance given if it falls below 1 L in an adult. Rarely, the syndrome follows viral hepatitis or diphtheria. Plasma exchange, where the facilities are available, is now accepted as efficacious in treatment of the Guillain-Barré syndrome if the patient is seen early and the disease is severe enough to warrant respiratory assistance. Acute motor paralysis has also occurred following exposure to triorthocresyl phosphate (TOCP), sometimes a contaminant of cooking oil and pesticides in the tropics, e.g., in Morocco and the Philippines.

SYNDROME OF SUBACUTE SENSORIMOTOR PARALYSIS. When symmetrical, this is often associated with calf tenderness and absent deep tendon reflexes. In the tropics, this may be due to alcoholism or beriberi (Chapter 131.2), may be associated with pellagra, or may occur following shigellosis or typhoid fever. Certain drugs, e.g., isoniazid, dapsone, nitrofurantoin, and nitrofurazone, can also be responsible. The incidence of diabetes is increasing in the tropics and is often undiagnosed or poorly controlled. It is a leading cause of this syndrome, and neuropathy is sometimes asymmetrical.

SYNDROME OF CHRONIC SENSORIMOTOR POLYNEUROPATHY. Tropical ataxic neuropathy, leprosy, uremia, beriberi, and diabetes are acquired causes of this syndrome. Carcinomatous neuropathic syndromes are reported less often in the tropics than in temperate zones, partly because of the low incidence of carcinoma of the bronchus. Genetic causes are rare but include peroneal muscular atrophy.

SYNDROME OF CHRONIC RELAPSING POLYNEUROPATHY. This is rare but may respond to corticosteroids; acute intermittent porphyria is rare, but porphyria cutanea tarda is not uncommon in South Africa and may be associated with a neuropathy.

SYNDROME OF MONONEUROPATHY OR MULTIPLE NEUROPATHIES. Pressure neuropathies include a radial palsy following drunken slumber. Cervical and lumbar disk root pressure due to prolapsed intervertebral disks is diagnosed less often than in developed countries. Leprosy causes inflammatory destruction of individual nerves, e.g., the ulnar and median nerves (Chapter 78).

Adverse reactions to drugs include polyneuropathies. Among the drugs commonly used in the tropics that can cause nerve damage are quinine, chloroquine, isoniazid, metronidazole, clioquinol, phenytoin, arsenicals, streptomycin, para-aminosalicylic acid, ethambutol, and pentamidine. Intramuscular quinine injections have caused sciatic palsies by local damage.

THE BURNING FEET SYNDROME. The burning feet syndrome is a distressing affliction that occurs in the nutritional, alcoholic, drug-induced (isoniazid) and diabetic neuropathies; in the sensory neuropathies associated with HIV infection; and often in patients without any objective signs of peripheral nerve dysfunction. The pathogenesis of pain in the peripheral neuropathies is not well understood. Pain may occur when the degeneration affects predominantly the large fibers in the peripheral nerves subserving modalities of proprioception (vibration, joint position sense), which should predispose to pain or dysesthesia, as well as the small fibers subserving perception of pain. Pain in diabetic neuropathies may diminish with normalization and stabilization of blood glucose levels, as hyperglycemia is a major factor in the pathogenesis of pain. The use of sorbinil (an aldose reductase inhibitor that theoretically should lower tissue sorbitol concentration by inhibiting conversion of glucose to sorbitol) may, or may not, relieve pain. Drugs beneficial in the symptomatic treatment of painful neuropathies include imipramine, carbamazepine, phenytoin, and intravenous lidocaine (5 mg/kg body weight), which may bring relief of pain for 3 to 21 days after a single injection. Recently, mexiletine, an analogue of lidocaine (which can be given by mouth 150 mg daily for 3 days, then 300 mg daily for 3 days, then 10 mg/kg body weight daily), was found to be efficacious in treatment of chronic painful diabetic neuropathy.

Anecdotal reports regarding the beneficial effects in herpetic neuralgia and the painful neuropathy of HIV infection of a cream containing 0.075% capsaicin (trans-8-methyl-N-vanillyl-6-nonenamide) have been made. Capsaicin is a naturally occurring substance derived from plants of the family Solanaceae, which apparently selectively affects unmyelinated C sensory fibers. It has no effect on discriminatory senses, e.g., touch, pressure, or vibration at the site of application. It causes a release and subsequent depletion of substance P, thereby impeding the conduction and transmission of peripheral pain impulses.

■ DISORDERS OF NEUROMUSCULAR TRANSMISSION

Myasthenia gravis and the myasthenic syndrome of Lambert and Eaton appear to be equally frequent in Southeast Asian countries, e.g., Thailand as in the West. The former is encountered in association with hyperthyroidism more frequently (15% vs. 5%) than reported in the United States or Europe. It is also noteworthy that thyrotoxic hypokalemic periodic paralysis, often prevalent in males, is similarly more encountered among Chinese and Thai people. In the northeastern part of Thailand and neighboring countries, namely Laos and Cambodia, hypokalemic periodic paralysis is not uncommonly seen in association with renal tubular acidosis.

■ PRIMARY MUSCLE DISEASES

PYOMYOSITIS. Muscle diseases are not uncommon (Table 9–6). The most common type is pyomyositis, widely reported in tropical Africa (Chapter 58). It affects young adults; the abscesses are either intra- or intermuscular and may be multiple. Staphylococci and coliforms are the organisms most frequently isolated. The muscle groups usually involved are the quadriceps femoris, hamstrings, gastrocnemii, erector spinae, latissimus dorsi, and trapezius. Treatment with drainage and antibiotics achieves cure in about 95% of cases.

OTHER CAUSES. Of the genetic myopathies, Duchenne, limb-girdle, facioscapulohumeral, and dystrophia myotonica are the types commonly seen. Autoimmune disease is rarely reported in Africans; however, polymyositis is occasionally encountered, and, similar to migraine, it shows a female preponderance. It may be associated with lymphoma, rheumatoid arthritis, multiple myeloma, and retroviral infections.

TABLE 9–6. Etiology of Primary Muscle Diseases as Seen in Ibadan, Nigeria

Disease	No. of Cases	Percentages
Pyomyositis	372	67.5
Genetic	76	13.8
Duchenne type	31	
Limb-girdle	28	
Facioscapulohumeral	12	
Dystrophia myotonica	5	
Polymyositis/dermatomyositis	60	10.9
Myasthenia gravis	32	5.8
Other*	11	2.0
Total	551	100.0

*Includes thyrotoxic, hypocalcemic and McArdle's myopathy in 6, 4, and 1 cases, respectively.

From Osuntokun BO: J Neurol Sci 12:417, 1971. Reprinted by permission.

■ PSYCHIATRIC DISEASE IN THE TROPICS

There are relatively few psychiatrists and mental hospitals in the tropics, and the general physician has to cope with many psychiatric problems. It is probable that psychiatric disease is as big a problem in the tropics as in temperate zones. Mental oddity is well tolerated in most simple farming communities, and there is often good family support for the mentally ill. Mental illness is often attributed to supernatural influences or witchcraft, and therefore, traditional healers are consulted rather than "Western medicine men."

Schizophrenia is probably as common as in Europe but may have a better prognosis because of better family support. Depressive illness often presents with somatic symptoms. Failure to have children often causes depression in women, who complain of abdominal pains. Acute, agitated, transient hallucinatory states are sometimes precipitated by fear of bewitchment. Recovery frequently occurs after sedation for a few days. Organic causes are frequently responsible for acute psychotic states and must always be excluded. Neurosis is perhaps more common in urban dwellers and students than in farmers, and societies in a state of rapid social change with increasing urbanization are subject to considerable mental stress. On migration to the town, there may be unemployment, loss of family support, and unfulfilled aspirations. New ideas and concepts are thrust on the individual, and the conflicts with ingrained beliefs can be traumatic. Students are under great pressure to succeed and thus often develop tension headache, inability to concentrate, poor memory, and reduced visual acuity—the West African brain fag syndrome. There is considerable fear of heart disease; the palpitations or chest pain of an anxiety state may be attributed to heart disease. Classic hysterical syndromes, sometimes epidemic in schools, are probably more common than in Europe or the United States.

KORO, LATAH, AND RUNNING AMOK. Three mental states peculiar to the tropics are koro, latah, and running amok. These are mainly seen in the Far East. In koro, the patient believes that his penis is withdrawing into his abdomen and that if this should happen, death will result. Latah is a fright neurosis with hysterical elaborations, including coprolalia, echolalia, and compulsive movements. In running amok, which usually occurs in Malaya, the victim runs wild and attacks those around him with murderous intent. It is suggested that this is a Malay form of suicide.

EXPATRIATE PSYCHONEUROSIS. Expatriate workers in the tropics and their wives may be under stress and are prone to neurotic illness, depression, and alcoholism. Frequently, there are frustrations, dissatisfaction with living and working conditions, worries about children and parents at home, heat intolerance, and boredom. Proper selection of personnel, enlightened management, reasonable leave arrangements, and organized recreation can help prevent these problems.

■ PREVENTION OF NEUROLOGIC DISEASE

Treatment of neurologic disease is often unsatisfactory, and recovery is sometimes slow and incomplete. Children are often victims and may be disabled for life. There is need and scope for preventive measures in tropical neurology. Improved primary care facilities would permit earlier diagnosis and treatment of meningitis, malaria, and metabolic derangements. Early oral rehydration in gastroenteritis prevents hyponatremia and hypernatremia. Improved midwifery could diminish birth injuries and neonatal and postpartum tetanus. There are many problems associated with vaccination in the tropics, including cost, the cold chain, lack of trained personnel, and depression of the immune response by concurrent infection or malnutrition. However, tetanus, poliomyelitis, measles, and selective meningococcal vaccination would considerably lessen neurologic illness. Detection and treatment of hypertension would diminish cerebrovascular disease. Health education is important in preventing and understanding epilepsy, tetanus, rabies, and other diseases that may affect the nervous system.

Bibliography

Alvarez G, Castillo JL, Ruiz F, et al: Multiple sclerosis in Chile. Acta Neurol Scand 85:1, 1992.

Bharucha NE, Bharucha EP, Dastur HD, Schoenberg BS: Pilot survey of the prevalence of neurologic disorders in the Parsi Community of Bombay. Am J Prev Med 3:293, 1983.

Dalal PM: Strokes in the young in West Central India. Adv Neurol 25:339, 1979.

Gout O, Cressain A, Bolgert F, et al: Chronic myelopathies associated with human T-lymphocytic virus type I. Arch Neurol 46:255, 1989.

Gray F, Gherardi R, Scaravilli F: The neuropathology of the acquired immune deficiency syndrome. Brain 111:245, 1988.

Howlett WP, Nrya WM, Mmuni KA, Missalek WR: Neurological disorders in AIDS and HIV disease in the northern zone of Tanzania. AIDS 3:289, 1989.

Kurtzke JF: MS epidemiology worldwide: One view of current status. Acta Neurol Scand 91 (S161):23, 1995.

Lambo TA: Stroke—a world-wide health problem. Adv Neurol 25:1, 1979.

Li SC, Schoenberg BS, Wang CC, et al: Cerebrovascular disease (CVD) in the People's Republic of China: Epidemiologic and clinical features. Neurology 35:1708, 1985.

Mesulam MM: Schizophrenia and the brain. N Engl J Med 322:842, 1990.

Ndekei DM: Psychiatric phenomenology across countries. Psychol Med 16:33, 1986.

Osuntokun BO, Adeuja AOG, Schoenberg BS, et al: Neurological disorders in Nigerian Africans: a community-based study. Acta Neurol Scand 75:13, 1987.

Pavlakis SG, Prohovnik I, Piomelli S, DeVivo DC: Neurologic complications of sickle cell disease. Adv Pediatr 36:247, 1989.

Roman GC, Spencer PS, Schoenberg BS: Tropical myeloneuropathies: The hidden endemias. Neurology 35:1158, 1985.

Sartorius N, Jablensky A, Korten A, et al: Early manifestation and first contact incidence of schizophrenia in different cultures. Psychol Med 16:909, 1986.

Schmutzhard E, Boongird P, Vejjajiva A: Eosinophilic meningitis and radiculomyelitis in Thailand caused by CNS invasion of *Gnathostoma spinigerum* and *Angiostrongylus cantonensis*. J Neurol Neurosurg Psychiatry 51:80, 1988.

Shorvon SD, Palmer PJ: Epilepsy in developing countries. Epilepsia 29(Suppl):536, 1988.

Spillane J: Tropical Neurology. London, Oxford Medical Publications, 1973.

Swift CR, Asuni T: Mental Health and Disease in Africa. Edinburgh, Churchill Livingstone, 1975.

Vejjajiva A: Parasitic diseases of the nervous system in Thailand. Clin Exp Neurol 15:92, 1978.

Vejjajiva A: Acute hemorrhagic conjunctivitis with nervous system complications. *In* Vinken PJ, Bruyn GW, Klawans HL (eds): Handbook of Clinical Neurology, revised series. Vol 12, Viral Disease. Amsterdam, Elsevier Science Publishers, 1989, pp 349–354.

Wadia NH: Myelopathy complicating atlanto-axial dislocation. Brain 90:449, 1967.

White NJ, Looareesuwan S, Phillips RE: Single dose phenobarbitone prevents convulsion in cerebral malaria. Lancet 2:64, 1988.

WHO Collaborative Study: Assessment of depressive disorders. Psychol Med 10:743, 1980.

WHO Study Group: Peripheral Neuropathies. Technical Report Series 654. Geneva, World Health Organization, 1980.

10 Ophthalmologic Diseases

Hugh R. Taylor and Alfred Sommer

THE MAGNITUDE OF BLINDNESS. Blindness remains one of the major disabilities affecting humans. The vast majority of blind people live in developing areas (Table 10–1). In the developed countries, blindness most commonly occurs in the

TABLE 10–1. Distribution and Characteristics of Blindness on a World Scale

	Developing World	Developed World
Number of blind (in millions)*	38.9–51.6	3.4–5.5
Blindness rate*	11–14/1000	3–5/1000
Major causes	Trachoma	Senile degeneration
	Cataract	Glaucoma
	Xerophthalmia	Cataract
	Onchocerciasis	Diabetes
	Corneal scarring	Congenital diseases
Primary anatomic area	Anterior segment	Posterior segment
Age at onset	All ages	Predominantly elderly
Percentage preventable	80%	20%
Etiology	Usually well known	Poorly understood

*World Health Organization: Available Data on Blindness. WHO/PBL/94, 38, 1994.

elderly and is usually caused by conditions that are, by and large, poorly understood and for which preventive treatment is not entirely satisfactory. In many ways, the rate of blindness in developed countries represents a baseline of unavoidable blindness about which relatively little can be done with the available technology and forms of treatment.

Blindness in the developing areas presents a totally different picture. Superimposed on the baseline of "unavoidable blindness" is a tremendous overburden of "unnecessary blindness." Millions of people in the developing areas are blinded by diseases that are either preventable or treatable. What is needed is a proper awareness of the problem and a rejection of the myth that only ophthalmologists are competent to deal with ocular disease. Trained field workers are crucial for the control of blinding infections, malnutrition, and filariasis; for primary care of simple trauma and acute glaucoma; and for the recognition and referral of cases of chronic glaucoma, cataracts, and the more complicated of the diseases requiring surgery.

The eye is made up of tissues that have similarities to tissues elsewhere in the body, and the eye responds to inflammation and injury in much the same way as other organs do. Inflammation of the eye produces pain, redness, swelling (and often discharge), and heat and is frequently attended by at least a partial loss of function. Whether from trauma or infection, ocular inflammation often leads to scarring. Since the eye depends on transparency of the ocular media (cornea, aqueous, lens, and vitreous) for normal function, it can be rendered useless by a relatively small, axially located scar or other opacity. Infection in the eye needs to be treated like infection elsewhere, with appropriate hygienic and antibiotic therapy. Foreign bodies usually must be removed from the eye, as is the case in other parts of the body.

There are, however, a number of specific conditions that involve only the eye. These conditions include cataract, glaucoma, and macular degeneration, which will be discussed later in this chapter.

THE OPHTHALMIC EXAMINATION. In ophthalmology, as in other fields of medicine, the most important steps in assessing a patient's problem involve taking a careful and appropriate history and performing a proper examination. It is important to elicit a history of the onset, duration, and characteristics of the presenting complaint, together with a review of the patient's general health and individual and family history. Specific information concerning vision—such as blurring, flashes or floaters, double vision, visual field loss, and night blindness—should be sought, and questions about ocular discharge, pain, and discomfort should be asked.

A basic part of the ophthalmic examination is the assessment of visual acuity, which is traditionally measured with a letter test chart, placed 6 M away from the patient. The acuity of small children can be assessed by determining their ability to fixate upon and follow a target, such as a light, with one eye at a time while the other eye is covered.

Simple observation of the eye will often give much information, especially in terms of the presence and site of infection or trauma, the alignment and movement of the eyes, or their possible displacement (Figs. 10–1 and 10–2). Careful examination of the front of the eye with a hand light will reveal gross corneal or conjunctival disease, including xerophthalmia, trachoma, foreign bodies, and corneal ulcers. It also reveals much about the anterior chamber and lens, the presence of blood or pus in the eye, acute glaucoma, and significant lens opacities (cataract). Whenever possible, the front of the eye should be examined with some magnification, such as a ×2 or ×3 loupe, or a direct ophthalmoscope using the +10 diopter lens. The diagnosis of mild trachoma requires examination of the conjunctiva on the undersurface of the upper lid, which is accomplished by everting the eyelid (Fig. 10–3). The pupils can also be examined with a hand light, taking note of their size, shape, and response to light. It is usually easier to examine the pupils in a somewhat darkened room. A direct ophthalmoscope is essential for examining the back of the interior eye, to search for abnormalities of the optic disc, macular region, blood vessels, and other areas.

■ DIFFERENTIAL DIAGNOSIS OF THE PAINFUL, RED EYE

The painful, red eye is one of the most common ocular problems. Many such patients have conjunctivitis, but all should be examined carefully, because a number of serious eye conditions can present with a similar picture. In almost every case, the correct diagnosis can be made from the history and a simple ocular examination.

The most important conditions that present as a painful, red eye are conjunctivitis, keratitis (including keratoconjunctivitis), corneal trauma and foreign bodies, anterior uveitis, and acute angle–closure glaucoma (Table 10–2).

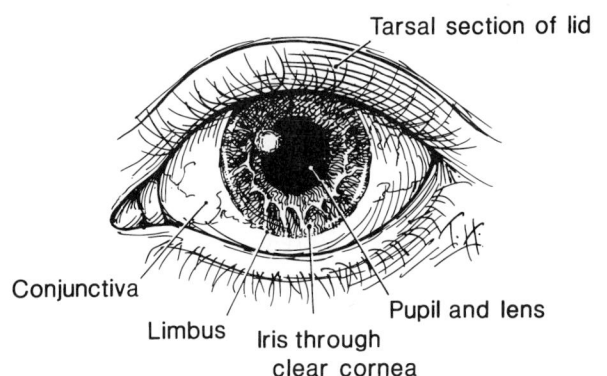

Figure 10–1. The front of the eye, showing the important landmarks.

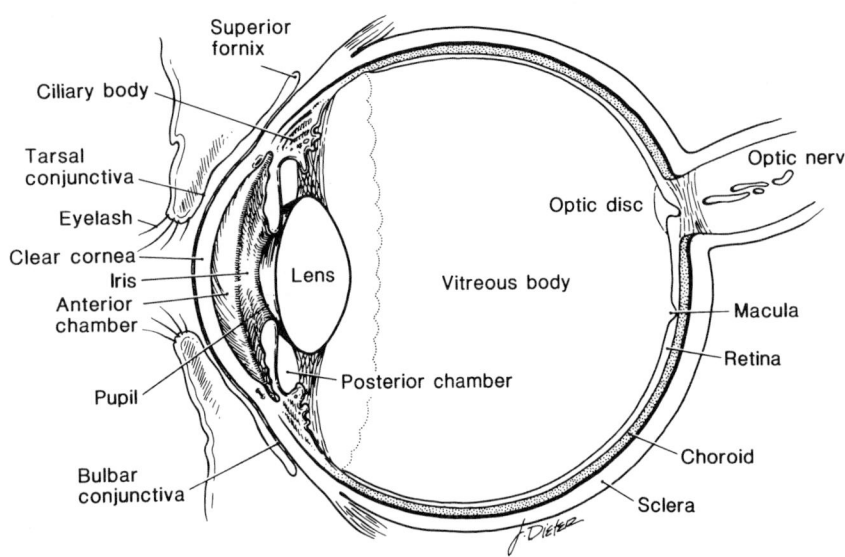

Figure **10–2.** Cross-sectional diagram of the eye.

CONJUNCTIVITIS. Conjunctivitis is the most common cause of red eyes bilaterally. It is usually infective, although conjunctivitis may be allergic or traumatic. It is commonly bilateral; a unilateral red eye increases the likelihood of other diagnoses. Infectious conjunctivitis usually has an acute onset, which is accompanied by ocular discharge. In viral and chlamydial conjunctivitis, the discharge is usually thin and watery. With bacterial conjunctivitis or secondary bacterial infection, the discharge is mucopurulent or purulent. A frankly purulent discharge is especially common in gonococcal infections. Mucopurulent and purulent discharges frequently accumulate on the eyelashes and lid margins, causing the lids to stick together.

The most consistent sign of conjunctivitis is conjunctival injection. The superficial and tortuous vessels of the conjunctiva appear dilated and bright red or pink, giving rise to the common term "pink eye." The conjunctival injection of the globe (bulbar conjunctiva) is most prominent in the fornices and is less marked at the limbus (the junction of the cornea and the sclera). The conjunctiva underneath the eyelids (tarsal conjunctiva) is frequently brick red. With severe inflammation, red blotches of subconjunctival hemorrhage may occur. These are seen more frequently in pneumococcal conjunctivitis and in some viral conjunctivides, such as epidemic hemorrhagic conjunctivitis (Chapter 27.3). In severe inflammation, pseudomembranes, or even true membranes, may be present. These are seen as dirty gray sloughs on the tarsal conjunctiva. In viral and chlamydial conjunctivitis, follicles are frequently present (Fig. 32–3). Giant, fleshy papillae may occur in allergic conjunctivitis. A detailed description of trachoma and inclusion conjunctivitis is provided in Chapter 32.

Visual acuity is usually not affected in conjunctivitis. The cornea is clear and bright; the pupil is circular and reacts normally; and the anterior chamber is clear and of normal depth.

Bacterial conjunctivitis usually requires specific antibiotic treatment. Antibiotics, such as chloramphenicol, may be given topically as 0.5% drops every 1 or 2 hours during the day and as 1.0% ointment at night. Alternatively, and especially in children, antibiotic ointment, such as 1.0% tetracycline, may be used four times a day and continued for 1

TABLE 10–2. Differential Diagnosis of the Painful, Red Eye

	Acute Conjunctivitis	**Keratitis**	**Anterior Uveitis**	**Acute Angle–Closure Glaucoma**
Occurrence	Very common	Common	Uncommon	Uncommon
Age	All ages, especially the young	All ages	Adolescents and adults	Elderly
Onset	Gradual	Sudden (trauma) or gradual	Gradual	Sudden
Pain	Itching, irritation	Moderate to severe	Moderate	Severe, with nausea
Vision	Normal	Blurred	Blurred	Marked reduction, with halos
Injection	Conjunctiva, bright red	Ciliary* or diffuse	Ciliary	Ciliary, purple
Discharge	Moderate to marked, watery to purulent	Variable, mild to marked	None	None
Cornea	Clear and bright	Abrasion, opacity, foreign body	Clear; keratic precipitates	Steamy
Pupil	Normal	Variable	Small, irregular, sluggish	Large, oval, unresponsive
Intraocular pressure	Normal	Normal	Usually normal	Markedly elevated

*Ciliary injection, A ring of redness at the limbus because of inflammation of the ciliary body and iris.

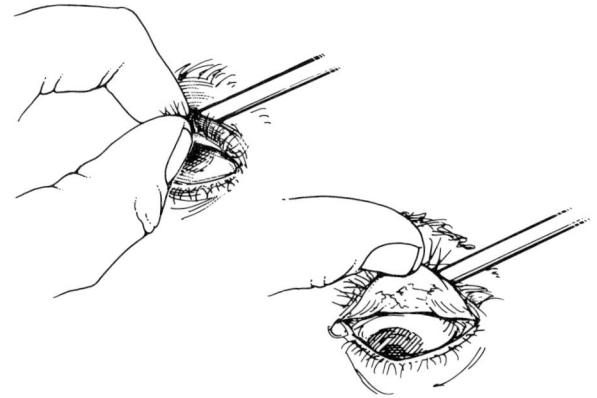

Figure 10–3. Eversion of the upper eyelid. With the patient looking down to relax the upper eyelid, gently grasp the eyelashes and lift the lid margin forward and upward over a probe placed above the tarsal plate. The tarsal plate is about 0.5 inch high, and its upper edge corresponds to the superior lid fold. The lid can be kept everted by holding the lashes against the brow. When the patient blinks, the lid will return to its normal position.

week. Patients should be cautioned to keep their eyes clean by washing away accumulated discharge. They should wash their hands carefully and not share towels or clothes with others, to avoid spreading the infection.

Neonatal gonococcal conjunctivitis is a medical emergency. The infant should be hospitalized and intravenous crystalline penicillin administered in a dose of 50,000 U/kg/day in two doses for 7 days. Saline irrigation of the eyes should be performed immediately and then at hourly intervals for as long as necessary to eliminate the purulent discharge.

Chlamydial conjunctivitis should be treated with systemic erythromycin. For neonates, a dose of 50 mg/kg/day in four divided doses should be used for 2 weeks. In adults, doxycycline (100 mg/day for 2 weeks) is preferred, although erythromycin should be used in pregnant women. A new, long-acting agent, azithromycin, is probably the drug of choice. Administer 1 g, in single or divided doses, once in 24 hours.

Viral conjunctivitis does not respond to antibiotics: Therefore, this form of treatment is usually contraindicated. Significant symptomatic relief can be obtained with the use of cold compresses and local vasoconstrictors, which also can be used for patients with allergic conjunctivitis. Topical steroids should never be used without the direct supervision of an ophthalmologist.

KERATITIS AND CORNEAL ULCERATION. These are common causes of painful, red eyes and are usually uniocular. Severe photophobia is often the main symptom, and the vision is usually blurred. Secondary uveitis may develop and cause ciliary injection. Ciliary injection shows a ring of redness, which is most intense around the limbus, and is a sign of inflammation of the ciliary body and iris. A history of trauma can often be elicited. At other times, a corneal ulcer and, more especially, keratitis may occur as a result of viral or severe bacterial conjunctivitis, in which case the signs of conjunctivitis may coexist. Sometimes, corneal ulcers develop spontaneously, especially with herpetic keratitis and in young children with vitamin A deficiency; in Africa it is particularly common following measles.

The most important diagnostic sign is the appearance of a corneal defect—either an opacity, which will obscure underlying iris details, or a surface defect, which will distort the surface reflex. If an ulcer penetrates the cornea, the globe may collapse and the intraocular contents may be expelled, or the hole in the cornea may be plugged with a knuckle of iris, which then shows as dark tissue in the base of the ulcer. A small ulcer, such as a dendritic ulcer caused by herpes simplex, is best seen if fluorescein is instilled and the eye is observed with a blue light. Large infective ulcers frequently are filled with white sloughed material and other debris. At times, pus may accumulate in the anterior chamber as a hypopyon.

Most corneal ulcers are medical emergencies. Proper management frequently requires a microbiologic diagnosis of the infectious agent, using isolation cultures. Intensive systemic and local antibiotics are used. For bacterial keratitis, commercially available antibiotic drops, e.g., chloramphenicol, tobramycin, or ofloxacin, can be used every hour. Fungal keratitis is usually treated with either topical natamycin or amphotericin drops. Doses of some commonly used subconjunctival antibiotics are penicillin, 1 megaunit; ampicillin, 100 mg; methicillin, 100 mg; carbenicillin, 100 mg; and gentamicin, 20 mg. The volume injected is usually 0.5 ml. These patients should be under the care of an ophthalmologist.

If a characteristic dendritic figure can be seen on the cornea and if the cornea has decreased sensation, a presumptive diagnosis of herpetic keratitis can be made. Dendritic ulcers are most appropriately treated with topical antiviral agents, e.g., trifluthimadine drops or acyclovir ointment applied every 4 hours for 1 week. A mydriatic, such as 5% homatropine three times a day, should be used until the ulcer has healed.

Again, as with conjunctivitis, steroids should not be used in patients with corneal ulcers and keratitis.

CORNEAL NECROSIS. A number of systemic conditions are associated with corneal ulceration and necrosis, including collagen vascular diseases, leukemia, and granulomatoses. In developing countries, nutritional keratopathy (xerophthalmia, keratomalacia) is the most common cause of childhood blindness (Chapter 131.1). In many Asian countries, measles is an important precipitating event for xerophthalmia (Chapter 25.1). Even in well-nourished Western children, measles causes a mild, superficial, self-limiting keratitis that does not require therapy. In much of Africa, however, measles itself is considered an important blinding condition. The mechanism is not entirely clear. In many instances it represents precipitation of acute xerophthalmia, as in Asia. In others it appears to represent secondary herpetic infection, which also accounts for accompanying stomatitis and skin ulcers. In still others, corneal damage is a chemical keratitis or bacterial infection secondary to the common practice of placing herbal and other traditional medicines in the eyes of measles patients.

CORNEAL TRAUMA. With trauma, ocular signs and symptoms are usually unilateral and the onset is sudden. A history of trauma or foreign bodies is usually present. Conjunctival foreign bodies cause pain and a feeling of having "something in the eye." Conjunctival vascular injection and some watering of the eye are usually present. A foreign body may be seen with a simple external examination. At other times, however, conjunctival foreign bodies lodge behind the upper eyelid and are not seen until the lid is everted, at which time they can be easily removed.

A corneal foreign body usually produces more severe pain and photophobia. After some time, it will often cause a secondary inflammation with ciliary-limbal injection. Most corneal foreign bodies can be removed fairly easily with a cotton-tipped swab, but if this is not possible, the case should be referred to an ophthalmologist. Frequently, patching the eye for 24 hours after the removal of a foreign body will give symptomatic relief and hasten healing of the corneal epithelium. A single application of antibiotic ointment should be used prophylactically.

In tropical environments in particular, corneal abrasions from plant matter, whether or not they leave a foreign body behind, carry a high risk of subsequent fungal infection. These can be notoriously difficult to treat and should be watched for closely.

Chemical burns to the eyes are best treated with immediate, thorough, and copious irrigation. Ideally, sterile saline solution should be used, but rather than delay irrigation, tap water should be used if saline is not available. The damage caused by an acid burn can usually be determined immediately. Because alkali continues to penetrate the eye, alkaline burns are frequently much more severe than initially realized. All chemical burns should be assessed by an ophthalmologist.

Conjunctival hemorrhages, which may be traumatic or spontaneous, require no treatment and will resolve in 1 to 2 weeks. Minor conjunctival lacerations do not require suturing and will heal in a few days. Topical antibiotics are usually given until the eye has healed.

All cases of penetrating trauma to the eye and lacerations to the globe, including corneal lacerations and intraocular foreign bodies, are medical emergencies that require prompt referral to and careful assessment by an ophthalmologist.

ANTERIOR UVEITIS. Anterior uveitis is a relatively uncommon cause of a sore, red eye. The term is used to describe inflammation of the anterior uveal structures—the iris and the ciliary body. "Anterior uveitis" is usually preferable to the terms describing inflammation in each of these structures individually, i.e., iritis, cyclitis, and iridocyclitis, because at least some inflammation is almost always present in both these tissues. Uveitis may occur as a primary event, either in isolation or in association with some underlying systemic disease. It also may occur as a result of other ocular pathology. Secondary uveitis is commonly seen with corneal trauma and ulceration.

Primary anterior uveitis has a gradual onset, with moderate to severe pain and some blurring of vision. It may be unilateral or bilateral, and the patient may have a history of similar episodes. Ciliary injection is the most important feature. This injection decreases with distance from the limbus, and the conjunctiva of the fornices and lids is not inflamed. There is usually no discharge.

The other important sign in anterior uveitis is a pupillary change. The pupil is usually small and reacts poorly to light. Frequently, the pupil is irregular because of adhesions, called posterior synechiae, between the pupillary margin and the lens. On examination with a slit lamp, keratic precipitates or inflammatory cells may be seen on the back of the cornea and also inflammatory cells and an aqueous "flare" in the anterior chamber. In severe cases, these changes may be recognized during the examination of the front of the eye with an ophthalmoscope, using the +10 diopter lens.

Uveitis may occur as an isolated ocular condition, but it also is often associated with underlying systemic disorders such as arthropathy, collagen diseases, and other systemic illnesses. For this reason, patients with anterior uveitis, especially those with recurrent episodes, should be examined in detail to exclude the possibility of such an underlying condition.

Treatment involves cycloplegia and mydriasis obtained with topical drops, such as atropine. One percent atropine drops may be given three times a day. A systemic analgesic, such as aspirin, will often give symptomatic relief. Topical steroids are frequently indicated, but they should be given only at the direction of an ophthalmologist. In severe uveitis and in chronic uveitis, secondary cataracts and secondary glaucoma may develop. These conditions require specific treatment.

ACUTE ANGLE–CLOSURE GLAUCOMA. Acute angle–closure glaucoma is a relatively uncommon cause of a painful, red eye, although its diagnosis is of great importance because (without prompt treatment) irreversible blindness can result. Acute angle–closure glaucoma is characterized by a sudden increase in intraocular pressure when the drainage channels for the intraocular fluid (aqueous humor) are obstructed. The persistence of elevated intraocular pressure can cause permanent and total loss of vision within 1 to 2 days. The condition is most frequent in Asian populations.

Acute angle–closure glaucoma usually starts with sudden and severe ocular pain, often severe enough to cause nausea and vomiting. Vision is markedly reduced, and the patient often complains of seeing halos, or colored rings, around lights. On examination, there may be ciliary injection, but the most striking features are the "steamy" or hazy cornea and the greatly increased intraocular pressure. The corneal changes are due to corneal edema. Intraocular pressure can be assessed by gently palpating the globe through the closed upper lid and comparing the degree of resilience of the affected eye with that of the other eye or with that of the eye of a person with normal vision. Increased intraocular pressure causes the eye to feel firmer, or hard.

The anterior chamber is usually very shallow in angle-closure glaucoma, and the iris appears to be almost touching the cornea. The pupil is frequently found to be semidilated and unreactive, and it may have an irregular or vertically oval shape.

Medical attempts to reduce intraocular pressure in such patients should be started without delay. Hyperosmotic agents, such as oral glycerin, 3 mL/kg, should be given, followed by frequent use of 2 to 4% topical pilocarpine drops, 1 drop every 15 minutes for four doses, then every half hour for 1 hour, and then every 1 to 2 hours, and oral carbonic-anhydrase inhibitors, such as acetazolamide, 500 mg orally or intravenously. These patients require referral to an ophthalmologist. An iridectomy or iridotomy is generally indicated to prevent further episodes. Pilocarpine 1 to 2% should be initiated twice daily in the fellow eye to reduce the risk of an acute attack until definitive surgical prophylaxis.

■ CHRONIC DISEASES

Cataracts, glaucoma, and macular degeneration are major causes of blindness in aged populations of both developed and developing countries.

CATARACT. Opacification of the lens interferes with transmission of clear images to the retina by both decreasing and scattering the light rays as they pass through. To the examiner, the pupillary area may look opaque and whitish or dark greenish brown on hand-light illumination, and fundus details will be obscured when viewed with the direct ophthalmoscope. Aside from cataracts of rare congenital origin and those that result from chronic inflammation, most cataracts are lumped together under the heading "senile." These are undoubtedly of multifactorial origin. Because the precise causes of such cataracts are as yet unknown, preventive measures do not now exist. Cataracts can be surgically removed, however, with a high degree of technical success and likelihood of return of useful vision.

In general, cataracts are the leading cause of blindness in developing countries. Visually disabling cataracts appear to occur earlier in life in some cultures than in others. More importantly, surgical therapy is commonly unavailable to large segments of the population. Some countries are overcoming the paucity and maldistribution of ophthalmologists by conducting intensive rural "cataract camps"; others are doing so by training properly supervised paramedical personnel to remove cataracts. Because the potential for intraoperative complications and postoperative infections is high under these circumstances, these approaches require careful consideration and detailed organization. However, as no other recourse exists, these methods require further development and extension.

Merely removing an advanced cataract can improve vision, but removal alone will not restore reading acuity. Some form of aphakic correction, most commonly spectacles or intraocular lenses, is also required.

GLAUCOMA. There are two major forms of glaucoma—acute and chronic. As already discussed, the acute form, with its red, injected, painful eyes, is the more dramatic. Chronic open-angle glaucoma, however, is much more common and is the more important cause of blindness.

Chronic elevation of intraocular pressure, at levels below those reached in acute angle–closure glaucoma, results in progressive destruction of the optic nerve. After many years (usually 10 to 20), this painless, asymptomatic destruction of the optic nerve results in loss of visual field, detectable by careful visual-field examination. Antiglaucoma therapy may delay or prevent further damage, but it cannot replace the vision that has already been lost. Unfortunately, patients are usually unaware of the problem until late in the course of the disease, when central acuity is finally involved and little vision or optic nerve remains to be saved.

Glaucoma is the classic disease in which screening methods have played an important role. Unfortunately, the simplest technique, that of demonstrating by tonometry that the intraocular pressure is greater than 21 mmHg, is far from infallible. Half of those with established glaucomatous field loss will have a normal pressure on a single casual screening test, and only 1 in 20 or 30 persons with an elevated pressure will already have field loss. The higher the pressure, however, the greater the likelihood of having, or soon developing, field loss. Screening is improved by combining tonometry with examination of the optic disc (by direct ophthalmoscopy or, preferably, with a slit lamp and contact lens). Deep, large, asymmetric optic-disc cupping, equal to or greater than 0.6 disc diameter, or loss of nerve fiber layer striations, suggests glaucomatous damage.

Ultimately, diagnosis requires demonstration of classic changes in the visual fields.

Treatment consists of lowering the intraocular pressure below 21 mmHg or to whatever level prevents further damage. A number of topical medications may accomplish this: Beta blockers such as betaxolol and timolol have the fewest side effects and are often the first agents of choice, though they are also the most expensive. An alternative initial agent is dipivylepinephrine (Propine), an epinephrine-like agent with fewer local side effects than epinephrine itself. Like β-blockers, epinephrine works primarily by decreasing aqueous formations. Pilocarpine, a parasympathomimetic agent, increases aqueous drainage and has had the most extensive use. It is usually the least expensive agent but requires application four times a day and results in severe miosis, which may degrade vision, particularly at night. As one agent proves inadequate, even at maximum dosage, others may be added to the regimen. Oral carbonic anhydrase inhibitors, such as acetazolamide, are often effective and have an additive effect to that of the topical agents.

Glaucoma management requires careful monitoring of pressure and visual field and frequent adjustment of dosage and regimen, while compliance of patients with the treatment plan is generally poor.

When visual-field loss continues, even on "maximum" medical therapy, the patient requires filtering surgery. A small channel is produced through the tough outer coats of the eye, so that some of the aqueous may percolate out of the eye into the subconjunctival space, where it is absorbed. Such artificial channels are at least temporarily successful, after one or more operations, in 85% of Caucasian patients. Because of their greater tendency for scarring, which closes the new channel, black patients do not fare so well, although concomitant local use of antimetabolites increases success.

Despite the potential for preventive measures, glaucoma is an especially difficult clinical problem in tropical countries; screening and diagnostic procedures are time-consuming and complex, and medical therapy is expensive, requires careful monitoring, and usually is attended by poor compliance. Although results of surgery are less than ideal, when available, surgery is probably the only practical treatment for patients who live in depressed rural communities of developing countries.

MACULAR DEGENERATION. In temperate climates, macular degeneration is the first or second leading cause of blindness. Because it is difficult to diagnose without a dilated-pupil fundus examination and is virtually impossible to treat, macular degeneration has received little attention in the tropics.

Of the many disease processes that can cause macular destruction, two are paramount—diabetes and age-related macular degeneration (AMD).

As its name implies, AMD comes on with aging, and at least some cases appear to be familial. Whether one or more causes are involved is unknown. Early in the disease, scattered, white, deep-retinal dots, known as drusen, can be seen concentrated in the macular area. Some, but not all, persons with these signs eventually develop progressive degeneration of their retinal pigment epithelium and the underlying choroid. Loss of vision is gradual, unpredictable, and almost always confined to loss of fine reading acuity. Such patients rarely develop "black blindness" (total loss of vision) and can usually care for themselves. In some, a net of new blood vessels pushes its way up from the choroid, and these vessels lie above or below the pigment epithelium. Such nets occasionally can be treated with a laser, perhaps delaying the sudden and dramatic loss of vision that can accompany leakage of fluid or blood. In any event, the benefits of therapy are far from dramatic, even when available.

Diabetic retinopathy includes a wide, complex spectrum of changes. Because few long-time diabetics survive in the rural, depressed communities of developing countries, diabetic retinopathy is of most concern in the developed countries and in increasingly affluent urban communities elsewhere. Again, the major treatable component of the disease is the growth of neovascular membranes, in this instance out into the vitreous from the surface of the optic nerve or retina. Photocoagulation, by either white light or laser therapy, provides substantial benefit to some groups of patients with this condition. It also benefits patients with fluid accumulation in the macula (macular edema) if they are treated early.

Bibliography

Buck AA (ed.): Onchocerciasis. Symptomatology, Pathology, Diagnosis. Geneva, World Health Organization, 1974.

Dawson CR, Jones BR, Tarizzo ML: Guide to Trachoma Control. Geneva, World Health Organization, 1981.

Diabetic Retinopathy Study Research Group: Photocoagulation treatment of proliferative diabetic retinopathy: The second report of diabetic retinopathy study findings. Ophthalmology 85:82, 1978.

Early Treatment Diabetic Retinopathy Study Research Group: Photocoagulation for diabetic macular edema. Early Treatment Diabetic Retinopathy Study Report Number 1. Arch Ophthalmol 103:1796–1806, 1985.

Fraunfelder F, Roy FH: Current Ocular Therapy. Philadelphia, WB Saunders, 1980.

Gass JDM: Stereoscopic Atlas of Macular Diseases. Diagnosis and Treatment. St. Louis, CV Mosby, 1977.

Guidelines for Programmes for the Prevention of Blindness. Geneva, World Health Organization, 1979.

Kolker AE, Hetherington J: Becker-Shaffer's Diagnosis and Therapy of the Glaucomas. St. Louis, CV Mosby, 1976.

Methods of Assessment of Avoidable Blindness. Geneva, World Health Organization, WHO Offset Publication No. 54, 1980.

Newell FW: Ophthalmology, Principles and Concepts. St. Louis, CV Mosby, 1978.

Sommer A: Field Guide to the Detection and Control of Xerophthalmia. Geneva, World Health Organization, 1982.

Sommer A: Nutritional Blindness. New York, Oxford University Press, 1982.

Vaughan D, Asbury T: General Ophthalmology. Los Altos, California, Lange Medical Publications, 1980.

World Health Organization: Conjunctivitis of the Newborn. Geneva, World Health Organization, 1986.

11 Sexually Transmitted Diseases

David Mabey

DEFINITION AND ETIOLOGY. In the golden era of microbiology in the late 19th and early 20th centuries, the microbial causes of five diseases clinically recognized as being transmitted predominantly by sexual intercourse—syphilis (hard chancre), gonorrhea, chancroid (soft chancre), lymphogranuloma venereum, and granuloma inguinale—were identified. Only syphilis and gonorrhea were recognized as major public health problems and became known as the major venereal diseases; the others were of "minor" public health concern. After World War II, new diagnostic techniques and clinical and epidemiologic studies in North America and Europe established that more than a dozen other microbial species could be sexually transmitted and were potentially pathogenic. Most have probably affected human beings since antiquity, but others may be newly evolved species. Among the latter are human immunodeficiency viruses (HIV) 1 and 2, agents of the current pandemic of the acquired immunodeficiency syndrome (AIDS).

Recognizing that multiple microorganisms cause symptomatic infections at the same anatomic site, most venereologists prefer a syndromic approach to the diagnosis of sexually transmitted diseases (STDs) (Table 11–1). Treatment regimens should be chosen with the recognition that several pathogens may be simultaneously infecting the same genital site and that several drugs may be required.

EPIDEMIOLOGY. In some developing countries, 10 to 20% of adult patients attending government health facilities do so because of an STD (Table 11–2). Based on hospital cases, the incidence of gonorrhea is estimated to be 3000/100,000 total population/year in some countries of sub-Saharan Africa, compared with less than 50/100,000 population in England and Wales. Yet this figure is almost certainly a considerable underestimate, since many, perhaps most, STDs in developing countries are not treated in the official health sector, patients preferring to visit traditional healers, quacks, pharmacists, or private practitioners, who are often more accessible and less judgmental in their attitudes.

Antenatal clinic attenders in several African cities have a high prevalence of laboratory-confirmed STDs, with over 10% of women having active syphilis, 5 to 10% gonorrhea, 5 to 10% chlamydial infection, and over 20% trichomoniasis. These diseases are of major public health importance in pregnant women, since they frequently result in perinatal morbidity and mortality as well as post-partum endometritis and salpingitis, often leading to infertility or subsequent ectopic pregnancy. Yet they are often asymptomatic and therefore, in the absence of screening programs, unsuspected and untreated.

In addition to the morbidity that they cause directly, the treatable bacterial STDs facilitate the transmission of HIV through heterosexual contact. This has been particularly well documented in the case of genital ulcer disease. HIV-infected men with urethritis also secrete higher levels of HIV RNA in their seminal fluid. The World Bank has estimated that the bacterial STDs are responsible for an extremely heavy burden of disease in developing countries, especially in sub-Saharan Africa. The treatment of these diseases is one of the most cost-effective health interventions in these regions.

The epidemiology of STDs is tied to human sexual behavior (Table 11–2). STDs are most prevalent in adolescents and young adults, in those with many sexual partners, in commercial sex workers and their clients, and in mobile population groups who are often separated from their families, e.g., sailors, truck drivers, and soldiers. Historically, STD control in Europe and North America has focused on these groups, with STD clinics being established in ports and by the military authorities. The explosive growth in the tourist industry in the past 30 years means that holiday makers are now by far the largest group of international travelers, making STD control a truly global issue.

The prevalence of the treatable bacterial STDs is also greatly influenced by access to medical services, since early and effective treatment will prevent further transmission in addition to preventing sequelae. Consequently, STDs are much more prevalent in developing countries and in impoverished and marginalized groups in the inner cities of developed countries. Poverty and population pressure in developing countries have led to vast human migrations, with young men from rural villages moving to cities in search of work, often leaving their families behind. This creates a demand for commercial sex, which is met by women (often themselves migrants from rural areas) who have no other way to support themselves and their children. Because effective treatment is expensive and often unavailable to these high-risk groups, the transmission of STDs continues.

The treatment of gonorrhea and chancroid has become increasingly difficult in many developing countries, owing to widespread resistance of *Neisseria gonorrhoeae* and *Haemophilus ducreyi* to commonly available and cheap antimicrobial agents. In many countries in Asia and Africa, more than 50% of gonococcal isolates are resistant to penicillin and tetracycline. Quinolone resistance is also widespread in some parts of Asia and has been reported in central Africa.

The incidence and prevalence of an infectious disease depends on its basic reproductive rate, R_0, which is the average number of subjects infected by an index case. For an STD, this in turn depends on the number of sexual partners, the duration of infectivity, and the probability of transmission per sexual contact. The first parameter is susceptible to behavioral interventions; the second can be reduced by early and effective treatment; and the third is an intrinsic biologic attribute of the particular infection, which can be reduced by the use of condoms. In many developed countries, a combination of behavior change and easy access to treatment has reduced R_0 to <1. In these circumstances, the disease would be expected to disappear. For example, chancroid and lymphogranuloma venereum (LGV), which are usually symptomatic and are not easily transmissible, are now very rare in many countries.

Even when R_0 <1 in the general population, an STD can

TABLE 11–1. Selected Syndromes and Complications With Corresponding Sexually Transmitted Etiologic Agents*

Syndrome or Complication	Sexually Transmitted Etiologic Agent
Acquired immunodeficiency syndrome (AIDS)	Human immunodeficiency viruses (HIV) 1 and 2
Adult T-cell lymphoma/leukemia; tropical spastic paraparesis, chronic progressive myelopathy	Human T-cell lymphotropic viruses (HTLV) 1 and 2
Pelvic inflammatory disease	*N. gonorrhoeae, C. trachomatis, M. hominis*
Infertility	
Post salpingitis, post partum, post abortion	*N. gonorrhoeae, C. trachomatis, M. hominis*
Spontaneous abortion, fetal wastage	Herpes simplex virus, *T. pallidum, N. gonorrhoeae, U. urealyticum, C. trachomatis*
Post epididymitis	*N. gonorrhoeae, C. trachomatis*
Congenital and perinatal infections	
TORCHES complex†	Cytomegalovirus (CMV), herpes simplex virus, *T. pallidum*
Other infant and childhood morbidity	
Sepsis, death	Group B streptococcus, herpes simplex virus
Eye infection	*C. trachomatis, N. gonorrhoeae*
Pneumonia	*C. trachomatis, T. pallidum,* CMV, *U. urealyticum*
Otitis media	*C. trachomatis*
Neurologic impairment	CMV, herpes simplex virus, *T. pallidum*
Male urethritis	*N. gonorrhoeae, C. trachomatis, U. urealyticum*
Epididymitis	*N. gonorrhoeae, C. trachomatis*
Lower urogenital tract infection in women	
Female urethritis	*N. gonorrhoeae, C. trachomatis*
Vulvitis	*C. albicans,* herpes simplex virus
Vaginitis	*T. vaginalis, C. albicans, G. vaginalis*
Cervicitis	*N. gonorrhoeae, C. trachomatis,* herpes simplex virus
Venereal warts, genital carcinomas	Human papillomaviruses
Genital ulceration	Herpes simplex virus, *T. pallidum, H. ducreyi, C. granulomatis, C. trachomatis* (LGV)
Proctitis	*N. gonorrhoeae,* herpes simplex virus, *C. trachomatis, E. histolytica*
Acute arthritis with genital infection	*N. gonorrhoeae, C. trachomatis*
Hepatitis	Hepatitis A, B, C, D, and E viruses, CMV
Kaposi's sarcoma	Human herpesvirus 8

*For each of the syndromes and complications, a variable proportion are not sexually transmitted, and some cannot yet be ascribed to pathogenic etiologic agents.
†TORCHES complex refers to congenital infection caused by toxoplasmosis, rubella, cytomegalovirus, herpes simplex virus, and syphilis.

be maintained in that population by the existence of a core group who change their sexual partners more frequently than the general population. The core group concept was originally put forward by Hethcote and Yorke, who used it to model the transmission dynamics of gonorrhea. It has been used to predict the theoretical impact and cost-effectiveness of control strategies in high-risk groups compared with the general population.

CONTROL. Since no vaccines are yet available for the bacterial STDs and no durable natural immunity is acquired after infection, prevention strategies depend on health education to modify risky sexual behavior. This means provision of condoms for primary prevention. Early and effective treatment, including the treatment of sexual partners of index cases, is needed to prevent further transmission (secondary prevention). In women, STDs are often asymptomatic, and passive case detection is often supplemented by active screening and case finding. The most common example is syphilis screening in pregnant women. In some countries mandatory screening programs have been implemented for certain high-risk groups, e.g., sex workers. Sometimes the targeting of high-risk groups leads to stigmatization, which

drives the target group (e.g., sex workers or men who have sex with men) underground, and the impact of public health programs is lost.

CLINICAL MANAGEMENT OF STDs. Prompt and effective treatment prevents further transmission and should be the cornerstone of an STD control program. Yet STD treatment services have until recently been accorded very low priority by health planners and ministries of health in most developing countries. If treatment for STDs is to be widely accessible in developing countries, it must be provided at the point of first contact with health services. It should be available at health centers and dispensaries in rural as well as urban areas. STD specialists and referral centers are best utilized to treat intractable cases, to train rural health workers, and to serve as a laboratory reference center to monitor antibiotic resistance.

History Taking and Examination. If clinical STD services are to be acceptable to populations at risk, certain criteria must be met: (1) privacy; an adequate sexual history and clinical examination can be taken only in private, (2) sympathy; patients rarely attend clinics where staff treat them in a hostile or judgmental manner.

Time is often short in health facilities in developing countries, but there are certain minimum requirements for the management of STD patients. The history should include details of the present complaint, including treatment already received; details of sexual partners since the onset of symptoms and in the preceding month; and past history of STDs. Examination should include inspection of the mucous membranes, palms, and anogenital region; palpation of the inguinal glands, penis, and scrotum in men, with retraction of the

TABLE 11–2. Reasons for High Prevalence of STDs in the Tropics

Demographic factors	Polygamy
Urban drift	Lack of medical facilities
Migrant labor	Misuse of drugs
Prostitution	Antibiotic resistance

Urethral discharge (with microscope)

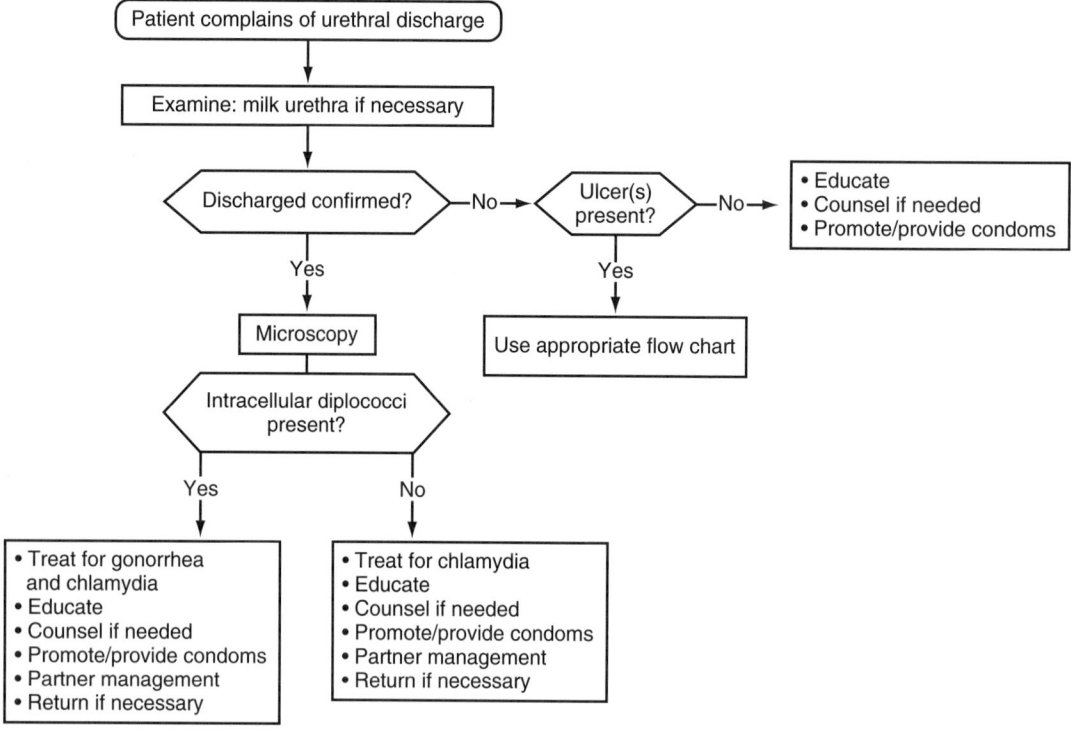

Figure 11–1. Management of urethral discharge. (From Recommendations for the Management of Sexually Transmitted Diseases. GPA/TEM/94.1. Geneva, World Health Organization, 1994.)

foreskin, if present. In women, a speculum examination to visualize the cervix and a bimanual examination are required. The examination should be performed in private in a good light, and gloves should be worn.

Counseling. This is an essential component of clinical management. STD patients should be advised that they are placing themselves at risk of HIV infection and encouraged to reduce their number of sexual partners. They should be encouraged to avoid sex while symptomatic or to use condoms. Condoms should also be recommended for high-risk future contacts; use should be demonstrated and free samples provided. The importance of complying fully with treatment

and of referring sexual contacts for treatment should be emphasized. Patients should be advised to return to the clinic promptly for treatment if they should develop symptoms of STD in the future.

The Syndromic Approach. Most health centers and dispensaries in developing countries lack adequate laboratory facilities for the diagnosis of STDs. The World Health Organization (WHO) has recommended that STDs be treated syndromically, according to suggested treatment algorithms for the common STD syndromes (urethral discharge, genital ulcer, vaginal discharge, pelvic inflammatory disease, inguinal bubo, and painful, swollen scrotum) (Figs. 11–1 to 11–5).

Genital ulcers

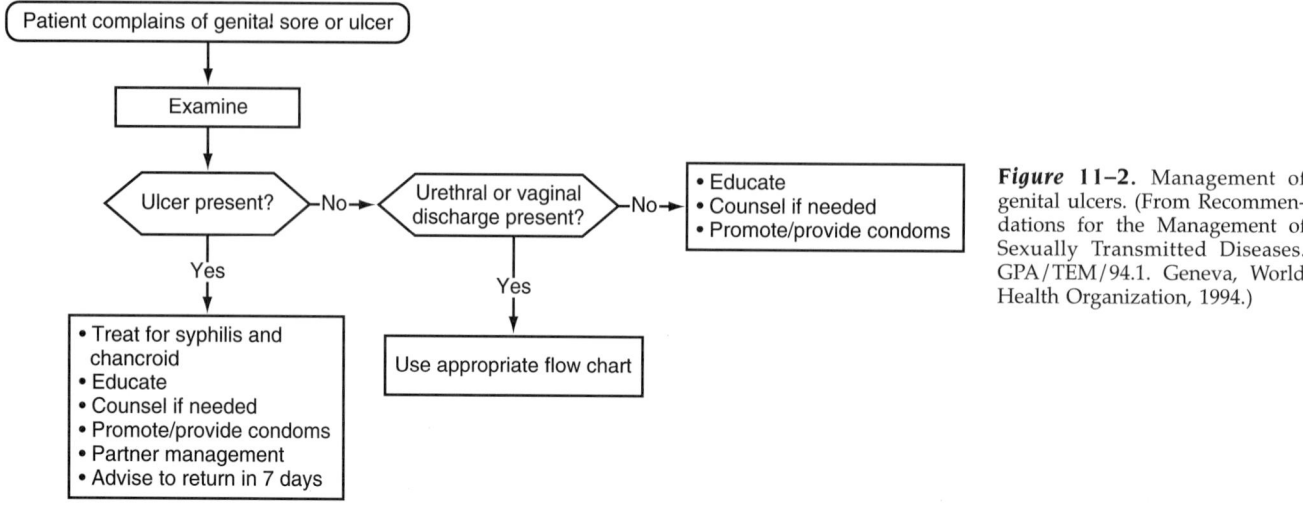

Figure 11–2. Management of genital ulcers. (From Recommendations for the Management of Sexually Transmitted Diseases. GPA/TEM/94.1. Geneva, World Health Organization, 1994.)

Vaginal discharge (with speculum)

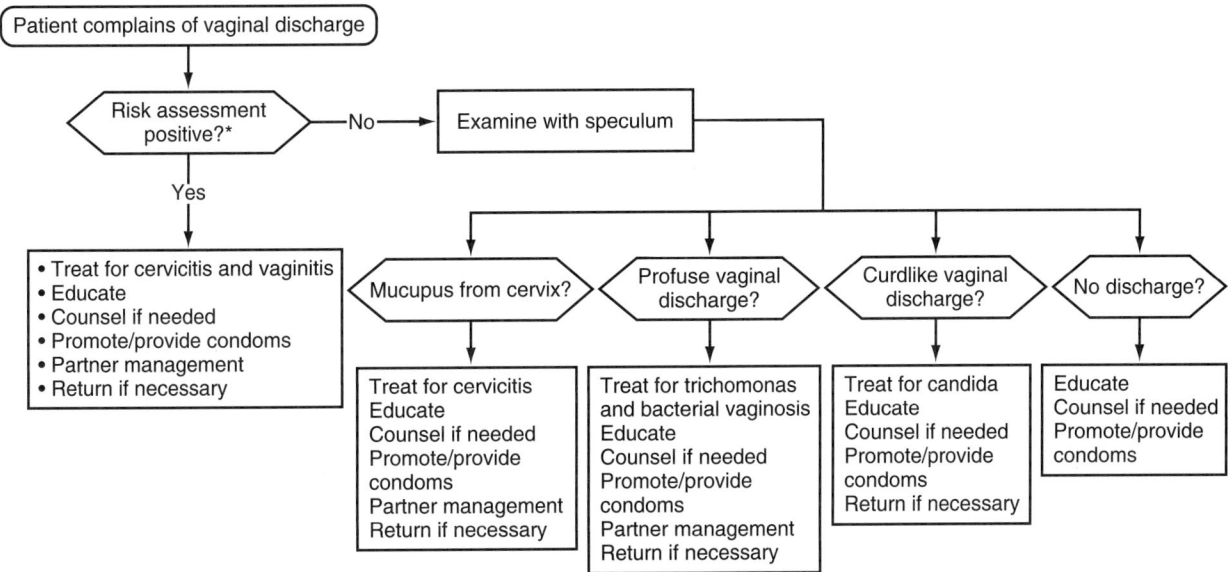

* Positive = partner symptomatic or any two of: age <21 years; single; >1 partner;
new partner in past 3 months

Vaginal discharge (with speculum and microscope)

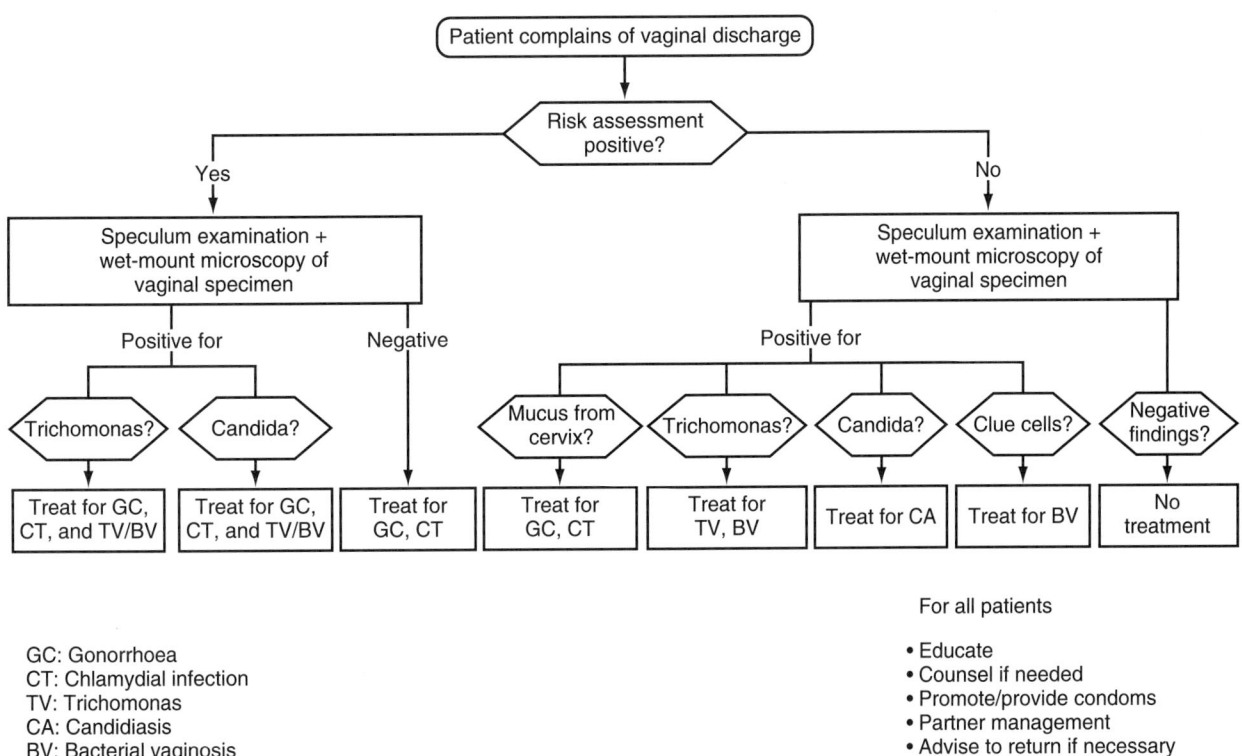

GC: Gonorrhoea
CT: Chlamydial infection
TV: Trichomonas
CA: Candidiasis
BV: Bacterial vaginosis

For all patients

• Educate
• Counsel if needed
• Promote/provide condoms
• Partner management
• Advise to return if necessary

Figure 11–3. Management of vaginal discharge. (From Recommendations for the Management of Sexually Transmitted Diseases. GPA/TEM/94.1. Geneva, World Health Organization, 1994.)

The principle underlying syndromic management is that treatment for all likely causes of a syndrome at the first visit will prevent further transmission and prevent sequelae in the patient.

The syndromic approach has been successfully used by nurses in rural health centers and dispensaries in Zimbabwe for over 10 years. Less than 5% of cases are referred to a doctor. A community-randomized trial in the Mwanza region of Tanzania showed that syndromic STD treatment, using medical assistants and nurses in rural health centers using

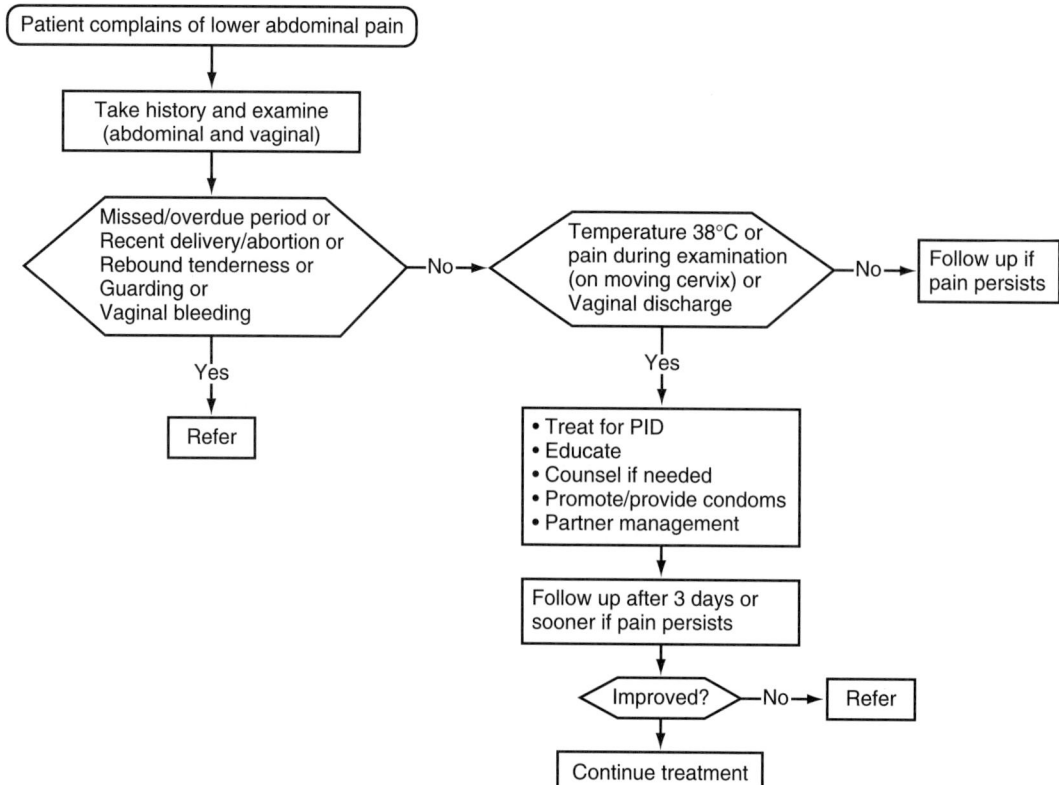

Figure 11–4. Management of lower abdominal pain. (From Recommendations for the Management of Sexually Transmitted Diseases. GPA/TEM/94.1. Geneva, World Health Organization, 1994.)

drugs of proven efficacy, was associated with a reduction in the incidence of HIV infection by 42%.

Urethral Discharge. Most male patients presenting with urethral discharge will have urethritis, defined as the presence of ≥5 polymorphonuclear leukocytes per high-power field on a Gram stain of a urethral swab, caused by one of four pathogens (Table 11–3). Although, in general, gonococcal urethritis has a shorter incubation period (3 to 7 days) than

nongonococcal urethritis (5 to 21 days) and gives rise to more acute symptoms and a more profuse purulent discharge, the two cannot be reliably differentiated clinically (Fig. 11–1). In developing countries, most cases of urethritis seen at health facilities are gonorrhea (Chapter 49).

If a microscope is available, the diagnosis of gonorrhea can be confirmed by the presence of intracellular gram-negative diplococci on Gram stain (Fig. 49–1). The recommended treat-

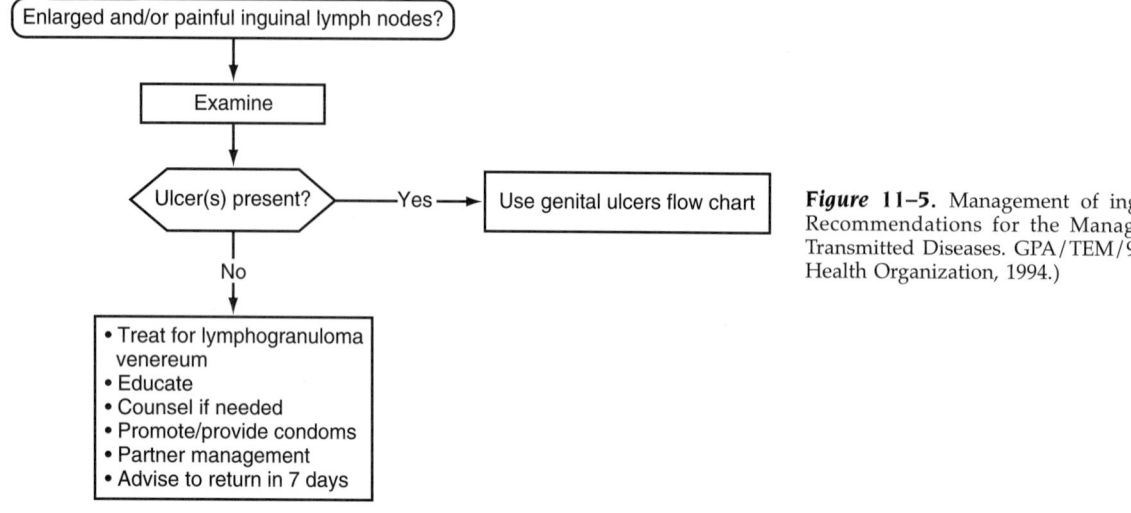

Figure 11–5. Management of inguinal bubo. (From Recommendations for the Management of Sexually Transmitted Diseases. GPA/TEM/94.1. Geneva, World Health Organization, 1994.)

TABLE 11–3. Causes of Urethritis

Neisseria gonorrhoeae	*Ureaplasma urealyticum*
Chlamydia trachomatis	*Trichomonas vaginalis*

TABLE 11–5. Common Causes of Vaginal Discharge

Vaginitis	**Cervicitis**
Trichomonas vaginalis	*Chlamydia trachomatis*
Candida albicans	*Neisseria gonorrhoeae*
Bacterial vaginosis	

ment of gonorrhea depends on the antimicrobial susceptibility of local isolates and on the local availability of drugs. Since mixed infections are common, patients with gonorrhea should also be treated for chlamydial urethritis (Chapter 46). If no microscope is available, men with urethral discharge should be treated for both gonorrhea and chlamydial infection. Treatment for chlamydial infection is also effective against most cases of nonspecific urethritis. In case of treatment failure, therapy for *Trichomonas vaginalis* should be considered (Chapter 91).

Genital Ulcer. There are five common causes of genital ulceration (Table 11–4). In most parts of Africa, the majority of genital ulcers are due to either syphilis (Chapter 48.1) or chancroid (Figs. 50–1 and 50–2), which cannot be reliably differentiated on clinical examination. Patients with ulcers should be treated for both infections (Fig. 11–2). Local epidemiologic data are important in the syndromic strategy of STD treatment; for example, in Papua New Guinea, chancroid is rare, but granuloma inguinale (donovanosis) (Figs. 51–1 and 51–2) is common.

Vaginal Discharge. A valid criticism of the syndromic approach to STD treatment is that it inevitably leads to overtreatment, since, although mixed infections may be common among high-risk groups, there will be many patients who have a single infection. This is especially true of women with vaginal discharge (Table 11–5), most of whom are suffering from vaginal infections (trichomoniasis [Chapter 91], candidosis [Chapter 81.3], or bacterial vaginosis); in some studies less than 10% of women presenting with vaginal discharge are infected with *N. gonorrhoeae* (Chapter 49) or *Chlamydia trachomatis* (Chapter 46). Yet because of the serious public health implications of these two infections, WHO recommends that syndromic treatment for vaginal discharge include treatment for these as well (Fig. 11–3). This greatly increases the cost of treatment.

A possible alternative, currently being explored in a number of studies in different countries, is to quantitate risk for gonorrhea and chlamydial infections. Risk assessment questionnaires are administered to women presenting with vaginal discharge, and results are correlated with laboratory-confirmed cases. Unfortunately, preliminary results suggest that this "risk score" approach is unlikely to be more than 70% sensitive or specific.

Pelvic Inflammatory Disease (PID). Infection of the upper female genital tract is commonly due to *N. gonorrhoeae* or *C. trachomatis*, in combination with normal vaginal flora, e.g., *Streptococcus* spp., anaerobes. PID often follows trauma to the cervix caused by termination of pregnancy, insertion of an intrauterine contraceptive device, or vaginal delivery. Gonococcal PID usually has a more acute onset and more severe symptoms than chlamydial PID, but either may cause irreversible damage to the fallopian tubes, leading to infertility or ectopic pregnancy. In developing countries, the diagnosis

of PID is usually clinical and associated with lower abdominal and cervical motion tenderness (Fig. 11–4). Laparoscopy is helpful when it is available. Important differential diagnoses include ectopic pregnancy, appendicitis, and endometriosis. Treatment should cover *N. gonorrhoeae* (Chapter 49), *C. trachomatis* (Chapter 46), and anaerobic bacteria.

Inguinal Bubo. Inguinal lymphadenopathy is a common feature of chancroid (Fig. 50–1), lymphogranuloma venereum (LGV) (Fig. 47–1), and syphilis (Chapter 48.1). Syphilitic adenopathy is usually painless and does not suppurate, in contrast to the buboes of chancroid and LGV. In males, a genital ulcer is usually visible when a bubo results from one of these conditions, although the primary lesion of LGV is often small, painless, and transient (Fig. 11–5). In women, the ulcer may be overlooked unless a careful speculum examination is performed. The differential diagnosis includes inguinal hernia, septic lesions of the lower limb, HIV infection with generalized lymphadenopathy, filariasis, tuberculosis, and plague.

Epididymitis. This is an important complication of gonococcal (Chapter 49) and chlamydial (Chapter 46) urethritis. It presents as a painful swelling of the scrotum, usually unilateral; the onset is usually more acute in gonococcal than in chlamydial disease. Torsion of the testis is an important differential diagnosis, requiring urgent surgical repair. In men over 50 years of age, epididymitis is more likely to be secondary to a bacterial urinary tract infection than to urethritis, at least in developed countries.

Partner Notification. Even in the case of easily treatable STDs, control is difficult because of the high prevalence of asymptomatic infection in both men and women. Partner identification and treatment is an important approach to a frequently asymptomatic, high-risk population. In developing countries resources are not usually available for the notification of partners by the health care provider. Patients must be relied on to refer their contact(s). It is important that the clinician spend time explaining the importance of treating partners, both to avoid re-infection and to prevent sequelae in the partner and any future children. Many clinics give contact notes to index cases to pass on to their sexual partners. Unfortunately, partner notification rarely results in the treatment of more than a small number of individuals.

Screening. In view of the serious consequences of syphilis in pregnancy, serologic screening for active syphilis is recommended for all antenatal clinics. Fiscal constraints limit implementation of this program in many developing countries. Risk factor questionnaires to identify gonorrhea and chlamydial infections have been tested in several antenatal clinics, with disappointing results. There is an urgent need for simple, cheap diagnostic tests (e.g., dipsticks) for these infections that could be used as screening tests in health facilities without laboratory support.

Ocular Prophylaxis. The prevention of ophthalmia neonatorum (ON) should be a simple matter. More than 100 years ago, Credé prevented the disease by the instillation of 1% silver nitrate drops into the eyes of infants at delivery. More recently, 1% tetracycline ointment, which is cheap, widely available, and easy to store, was shown to be equally effective. Given the high incidence of ON and its devastating consequences (Fig. 49–2), this simple measure is one of the

TABLE 11–4. Sexually Transmitted Diseases Causing Genital Ulceration

Chancroid	Granuloma inguinale
Syphilis	Lymphogranuloma venereum
Herpes simplex	

most cost-effective health interventions available. Yet there are very few developing countries in which ON prophylaxis is systematically carried out.

CONCLUSION. The great differences in the incidence and prevalence of the treatable bacterial STDs between developed and developing countries demonstrate that many STDs can be controlled and in some cases eradicated. Now that treatment of the bacterial STDs has been shown to reduce the incidence of HIV infection and to be highly cost-effective in terms of cost per healthy life-year saved, it is hoped that STD control will be given higher priority in developing countries.

Bibliography

Arya OP, Lawson JB: Sexually transmitted diseases in the tropics. Epidemiological, diagnostic, therapeutic and control aspects. Trop Doct 7:51, 1977.

Cates W, Farley TM, Rowe PJ: Worldwide patterns of infertility: Is Africa different? Lancet 2:596, 1985.

De Schryver A, Meheus A: Epidemiology of sexually transmitted diseases: The global picture. Bull WHO 68:639, 1990.

Grosskurth H, Mayaud P, Mosha F, et al: Asymptomatic gonorrhoea and chlamydial infection in rural Tanzanian men. Br Med J 312:277, 1996.

Grosskurth H, Mosha F, Todd J, et al: Impact of improved treatment of sexually transmitted diseases on HIV infection in rural Tanzania: Randomised controlled trial. Lancet 346:530, 1995.

Laga M, Plummer FA, Piot P: Prophylaxis of gonococcal and chlamydial ophthalmia neonatorum. A comparison of silver nitrate and tetracycline. N Engl J Med 318:653, 1988.

Latif AS, Mbengeranwa OL, Marowa E, et al: The decentralisation of the sexually transmitted disease service and its integration into primary health care. Afr J Sex Trans Dis 2:85, 1986.

Mabey DCW: Sexually transmitted diseases in developing countries. Trans R Soc Trop Med Hyg 90:97, 1996.

Mayaud P, Grosskurth H, Changalucha J, et al: Risk assessment and other screening options for the identification of gonorrhoea and chlamydial infection in rural Tanzanian antenatal clinic attenders. Bull WHO 73:621, 1995.

Moses S, Manji F, Bradley JE, et al: Impact of user fees on attendance at a referral centre for sexually transmitted diseases in Kenya. Lancet 340:463, 1992.

Muir DG, Belsey MA: Pelvic inflammatory disease and its consequences in the developing world. Am J Obstet Gynecol 138:913, 1980.

Over M, Piot P: Health sector priorities review: HIV infection and sexually transmitted diseases. In Jamison D, Mosley WH (eds): Disease Control Priorities in Developing Countries. New York, Oxford University Press, 1991.

Pepin J, Plummer FA, Brunham RD, et al: The interaction of HIV and other sexually transmitted diseases: An opportunity for intervention. AIDS 3:3, 1989.

Recommendations for the management of sexually transmitted diseases. WHO advisory group meeting on sexually transmitted diseases treatments. WHO/GPA/STD/93.1. Geneva, World Health Organization, 1993.

Schulz KF, Cates W, O'Masra PR: Pregnancy loss, infant death, and suffering: Legacy of syphilis and gonorrhoea in Africa. Genitourin Med 62:320, 1987.

Temmerman M, Mohamed Ali F, Fransen L: Syphilis prevention in pregnancy: An opportunity to improve reproductive and child health in Kenya. Health Policy Plan 8:122, 1993.

Vuylsteke B, Laga M, Alary M, et al: Clinical algorithms for the screening of women for gonococcal and chlamydial infection: Evaluation of pregnant women and prostitutes in Zaire. Clin Infect Dis 17:82, 1993.

World Development Report 1993: Investing in Health. New York, Oxford University Press for the World Bank, 1993.

12 Malignant Diseases

D.M. Parkin and J.L. Ziegler

Cancer is estimated to account for about 22% of deaths in developed countries in 1993, compared with 9% in the developing countries. Much of this disparity is the result of differences in the age profile of developed and developing countries and the burden of infectious disease and perinatal mortality in young children in the developing world. Cancer

appears to occur at younger ages in tropical countries, with one fifth of cancers occurring before age 45 years (Table 12–1). However, this is a reflection of the young age structure of the population, with over 80% aged under 45 years in tropical countries, compared with only two thirds in developed countries. The actual mortality rates between developed and developing countries from cancer are similar when stratified by age.

It is difficult to obtain accurate statistics on cancer in developing countries. Systems of civil registration of deaths, including medical certification of the cause of death, are present in parts of Latin America and a few of the smaller countries of Asia so that, overall, some 4 to 5% of the population of developing countries is covered by mortality statistics. Another important source of information is the cancer registry. Although cancer registries generally cover limited geographic areas (about 3% of the population of developing countries), they are present in many countries and provide vital clues to the current cancer profile and its evolution over time. Based on these sources of information, it is possible to estimate the worldwide cancer burden in terms of incidence (new cases) and deaths (Table 12–2).

Cancer will become an even more important problem for tropical health services in the coming decades. This is not so much because of the increases in the actual risk to individuals but rather because of the aging of the population. In the 25 years after 1990, the world population over 65 years of age (at highest risk of cancer) will more than double, so that, with no change in the rates of incidence, the number of new cancer cases will also double. However, exposures to the major environmental and lifestyle determinants of cancer, particularly infections, tobacco use, and diet, will undoubtedly contribute to increases in cancer rates. Thus, the relative immunity of many populations to certain major cancers (e.g., lung, large bowel, and breast) is likely to change with increasing urbanization (43% of the world population in 1990, 56% projected in 2015) and the related westernization of lifestyles.

The molecular understanding of oncogenesis has advanced rapidly in recent years. Thus, cancer has been associated with mutated, deleted, translocated, or otherwise altered genes whose normal function is regulation of cell growth, differentiation, or death. Two types of such oncogenes are recognized—one associated with excessive cell growth (e.g., overproduction of growth factors, their receptors, their intracellular second messengers, or genes that control the cell cycle); the other is linked to the checkpoints that ensure DNA integrity before cell division (e.g., p53, a protein that temporarily stops cell division in G1 to permit DNA repair or directly induces apoptosis). Either unrestrained cell growth (e.g., translocated *c-myc* in Burkitt's lymphoma), or removal of growth inhibitors (e.g., mutated p53 in many types of tumor) may result in neoplasia. Most cancers result from a concatenation of genetic accidents that occur over time. One of the best examples is colon cancer, in which an accumulation of gene changes (i.e., deletions, mutations) leads first to adenoma and ultimately to carcinoma. Genetic changes can be inherited (e.g., a defective version of the tumor suppressor gene RB in retinoblastoma) or acquired (e.g., a point mutation of p53 by aflatoxin in hepatocellular carcinoma).

Only a small proportion of cancers are the result of inheritance of major susceptibility genes, e.g., the genes responsible for familial breast cancer (BRCA 1 and 2). These account for a relatively small proportion of breast cancers, but their discovery has permitted genetic testing and counseling of high-risk family members. Quantitatively more important are the genetic polymorphisms, inherited differences in a variety of genes controlling metabolic pathways (e.g., the cytochrome

TABLE 12–1. Population Structure and Cancer Mortality, By Age, 1985 in Developed[1] and Tropical Areas[2]

Age Group	Population (%)		Cancer Deaths (%)		Mortality Rate ($\times 10^5$)	
	Developed	*Tropical*	*Developed*	*Tropical*	*Developed*	*Tropical*
0–14	22.0	37.3	0.7	3.1	5.9	6.7
15–44	44.6	45.6	5.2	17.2	22.2	29.1
45–64	21.8	12.9	33.5	43.3	291.7	258.9
65+	11.4	4.2	60.5	36.4	999.8	674.6
All ages	100% (1174×10^6)	100% (3564×10^6)	100% (2.22×10^6)	100% (2.75×10^6)	189.5	77.3

[1]Europe, North America, Japan, Australia/New Zealand.
[2]Africa, Central America and Caribbean, tropical South America, China, Southeast Asia, South Asia, Western Asia, Pacific islands.
Modified from Pisani P, et al: Int J Cancer 55:891, 1993.

p450 family). These explain some of the interindividual differences in susceptibility to carcinogens, which result from differential rates of activation or metabolism. The potential uses of tests to identify such individual determinants of cancer risk remain to be seen. Tests that identify altered oncogenes (or, more importantly, their products, e.g., abnormal p53 protein) may be useful in diagnosis and estimating prognosis (e.g., *n-myc* levels and disease severity of neuroblastoma). Finally, cancer treatment can be refined to attack specific proteins that are defective (e.g., management of promyelocytic leukemia with retinoic acid that bypasses the defective retinoid receptor and leads to complete remissions).

While these discoveries hold great promise for developed countries, cancer management in many tropical areas is less advanced. Here, the essential questions for proper clinical management remain: "What is the tumor diagnosis?" "Where has the tumor spread?" "What is the tumor doing to the patient?" Modern imaging technology may not be available, but standard x-ray, contrast x-ray, and ultrasound can be very helpful (Chapter 21). Endoscopy and cytology can speed the diagnosis. In addition to the surgeon, the availability of a medical oncologist and radiotherapist will often determine the treatment options. The arrival of hospices in many tropical areas, with its emphasis on palliation and pain control, has greatly assisted care of the dying. In management of cancer patients, there is always something that can be done to relieve suffering and improve quality of life.

The major cancers occurring in developing countries are described below, omitting those for which epidemiology, clinical features, and treatment show no features peculiar to such regions, and including a few that are relatively frequent in the tropics but not elsewhere.

■ CARCINOMA OF THE ORAL CAVITY AND PHARYNX

DEFINITION. This consists of squamous cell carcinomas arising in the mucosa of the mouth (including cheek, lips, and palate), in the gums, in the tongue, and in the oropharynx and hypopharynx.

EPIDEMIOLOGY AND ETIOLOGY. Cancers of the mouth and pharynx are the eighth most common cancer in the developing world, with about 360,000 new cases each year. Although a diverse group, tumors of the oral cavity and pharynx have risk factors in common and tend to have similar geographic patterns. Tumors of the tongue and mouth are most frequent in the Indian subcontinent and in some areas represent a third of all cancers in men. The explanation lies in the widespread and diverse use of oral tobacco in the region. The most common exposure is the chewing of betel

quid (a mixture of betel leaf, areca nut, lime, and tobacco in varying proportions), as well as use of powdered tobacco (snuff) taken orally in varying formats. The chewing habit is common in other populations (e.g., Papua New Guinea, parts of Southeast Asia) as well as in many migrant groups originally from the Indian subcontinent; elevated cancer rates are also observed in such groups. The other major risk factors for oral and pharyngeal cancers are tobacco smoking and alcohol (especially spirits); together they have a multiplicative effect on risk. These probably account for the relatively high rates observed in Caribbean countries, parts of South America (especially Brazil), and East and Southeast Africa. Reverse smoking (lighted end inside the mouth) is not common but results in cancers of the palate.

Cancer of the lip, involving the vermilion border, is more frequent in white-skinned populations, in whom it is associated with sunlight exposure and outdoor occupations.

DIAGNOSIS AND TREATMENT. Patients generally present with slightly elevated red mucosal lesions with irregular borders, a visible and palpable mass, or a malignant ulcer, often at advanced stages, with involvement of regional lymph nodes, bone, and skin.

Carcinomas of the oral cavity coexist with, or are preceded by, a variety of premalignant lesions that share the etiologic factors of oral cancer—particularly tobacco use. Leukoplakias are white patches that occur frequently in persons who chew and/or smoke; they have a similar intraoral location to invasive cancers. The risk of malignancy, overall about 1 to 5%, varies with the clinical subtype (nodular, ulcerated, and homogenous, in descending order). Erythroplakia is a much rarer condition, in which probability of malignant transformation is much higher (tenfold in some series). Submucous fibrosis appears to be specifically linked to areca nut use; it manifests as mucosal rigidity and fibrous bands, with restricted mouth opening and tongue mobility. Malignant transformation is common.

Treatment of premalignant lesions is difficult, as their presence indicates carcinogenesis, and there is a high probability of recurrence following excision or diathermy. Natural or synthetic analogues of retinoids given in high doses can induce remissions but are associated with toxic side effects and high relapse rates after therapy ceases.

For early-stage cancers of the oral cavity, both surgery and radiotherapy produce comparable results in controlling the primary disease. The choice of treatment depends upon factors, e.g., the site and clinical extent of disease, general health of the patient, functional and cosmetic results anticipated, preference of the patient, and availability of facilities. Although a limited local excision may prove curative for small lesions of the lip or buccal mucosa, more extensive resection

TABLE 12–2. Estimated Age Standardized Rates of Cancer Incidence by Site, Sex, and Area, 1990

	Mouth/Pharynx (140–149) M	F	Esophagus (150) M	F	Stomach (151) M	F	Colon/Rectum (153–154) M	F	Liver (155) M	F	Pancreas (157) M	F	Larynx (161) M	F	Lung (162) M	F	Melanoma (172) M	F
Eastern Africa	16.9	10.4	17.4	4.8	14.1	13.3	6.5	3.9	21.8	9.5	2.8	2.1	3.3	0.4	5.5	1.3	5.3	8.3
Central Africa	18.7	10.9	4.7	0.7	20.8	13.3	6.1	6.5	20.7	10.6	1.3	2.1	2.5	1.2	9.4	1.7	9.6	9.4
Northern Africa	12.4	7.2	5.3	1.7	5.8	3.4	7.9	7.9	5.9	2.7	3.2	1.7	15.4	2.0	20.7	5.5	1.3	0.9
Southern Africa	13.4	3.4	40.7	12.1	12.9	6.0	11.9	9.3	14.7	4.8	4.7	3.2	7.4	0.9	35.5	7.6	2.1	2.0
Western Africa	3.5	2.6	1.2	1.6	7.5	4.2	2.5	2.5	22.6	7.7	1.0	1.2	1.5	0.2	2.5	1.1	1.1	1.3
Caribbean	13.3	4.0	6.6	2.0	14.6	7.3	14.9	14.5	3.6	2.8	5.2	3.7	7.9	1.5	34.1	11.1	1.2	1.0
Central America	5.7	2.4	3.3	1.4	18.4	11.6	9.6	8.7	2.3	1.4	4.6	2.8	5.0	0.8	18.3	6.5	1.4	1.5
South America (tropical)	13.6	2.8	8.1	1.8	32.6	18.1	13.1	8.9	3.1	3.3	4.0	3.7	8.3	1.2	26.9	5.4	2.4	1.8
Eastern Asia: China	11.6	6.4	33.5	16.1	50.6	25.7	16.1	13.3	37.0	15.2	3.6	2.8	3.3	1.3	48.8	20.0	0.5	0.6
Southeastern Asia	16.2	11.0	3.5	1.5	8.9	5.3	10.4	10.0	18.7	6.7	1.9	1.2	4.0	1.0	27.2	8.5	0.6	1.0
Southern Asia	31.8	17.0	10.1	7.9	7.9	4.0	4.9	3.8	3.1	1.7	1.1	0.7	9.4	1.6	16.7	2.6	0.3	0.3
Western Asia	10.0	7.5	4.0	3.0	12.2	8.7	10.2	11.2	5.3	2.9	3.6	3.2	16.5	2.3	50.2	8.3	1.7	1.9
Melanesia	47.0	25.6	3.0	2.8	8.6	3.9	9.6	4.1	21.3	9.3	1.5	0.1	3.7	1.3	4.8	2.7	6.1	3.9
Micronesia/Polynesia	10.0	4.6	3.4	0.8	9.4	5.2	11.0	7.7	8.5	2.6	4.1	1.8	3.8	0.4	34.8	10.8	2.3	1.7
United States	4.5	2.6	5.3	1.4	7.9	3.9	46.6	33.5	3.5	1.5	8.7	6.4	7.5	1.3	75.8	34.7	10.5	8.6
Europe	5.3	6.1	6.1	1.2	16.7	7.5	33.8	23.7	5.8	2.0	6.1	3.9	8.8	0.5	55.6	10.3	4.6	6.5

	Breast (174) F	Cervix (180) F	Corpus Uteri (182) F	Ovary (183) F	Prostate (185) M	Bladder (188) M	F	Kidney (189) M	F	Lymphoma (200–203) M	F	Leukemia (204–208) M	F	All Sites Excluding Skin (140–208) M	F
Eastern Africa	19.4	49.2	4.8	7.8	27.4	8.0	4.5	1.6	1.3	7.5	4.5	2.5	1.5	186.5	180.7
Central Africa	26.3	38.0	9.3	7.1	31.5	9.6	2.3	1.4	0.8	12.7	7.9	2.2	0.7	212.1	199.0
Northern Africa	57.1	11.4	1.6	3.3	5.0	25.6	6.9	1.7	1.5	11.1	7.1	3.6	1.9	157.0	156.4
Southern Africa	28.8	46.8	4.1	5.5	20.7	8.4	2.1	2.0	1.1	3.7	2.1	5.0	3.4	215.7	166.9
Western Africa	11.1	22.0	1.9	6.0	11.5	4.6	1.0	1.4	1.7	5.1	2.9	1.3	2.6	82.2	89.9
Caribbean	36.6	21.6	6.4	5.4	31.4	8.9	2.6	2.5	1.4	4.1	4.0	5.2	5.3	186.6	163.5
Central America	29.3	39.5	6.8	6.1	26.0	7.3	1.9	3.5	2.2	6.0	3.9	5.9	4.3	161.9	172.4
South America (tropical)	25.8	36.2	6.2	6.8	27.9	9.9	1.8	3.6	1.9	6.4	4.2	6.2	4.1	213.4	181.1
Eastern Asia: China	20.5	14.7	5.5	5.0	2.3	7.7	2.4	2.5	2.1	4.7	3.2	7.3	6.6	251.2	205.3
Southeastern Asia	25.3	29.1	3.3	7.1	4.9	4.1	1.6	1.3	1.0	4.9	4.2	4.0	4.4	134.7	146.8
Southern Asia	21.9	27.8	1.6	5.2	4.1	3.5	0.8	1.4	0.8	3.5	1.9	2.9	2.1	127.9	122.3
Western Asia	37.8	7.4	9.4	8.2	8.8	16.3	3.8	3.0	2.1	6.2	4.8	5.4	3.9	194.1	169.2
Melanesia	20.3	39.9	7.7	7.1	2.8	1.9	0.5	0.9	0.8	8.4	4.1	4.0	2.1	159.7	162.6
Micronesia/Polynesia	28.8	16.5	6.8	4.8	10.4	3.5	0.8	1.5	1.3	4.1	2.5	8.0	5.3	135.9	120.3
United States	87.5	10.3	16.4	12.1	72.0	23.3	6.3	11.2	5.2	21.2	13.9	10.0	6.5	354.6	286.0
Europe	60.9	10.2	10.7	9.6	28.5	18.8	3.4	8.6	3.9	16.8	9.5	8.3	5.5	268.4	196.4

may be required for similar lesions in the tongue, floor of the mouth, or gingivae, resulting in disfigurement and functional loss. Small accessible lesions of the lip, cheek mucosa, tongue, and floor of the mouth may be effectively treated with interstitial irradiation. External irradiation may result in troublesome dryness of the mouth caused by salivary gland damage. Five-year survival in early oral cancer, treated with surgery or radiotherapy, ranges from 60 to 70%.

Patients with moderately advanced cancers of the oral cavity benefit from combined therapy involving both surgery and radiotherapy, with 5-year survival ranging from 20 to 40%. Radiotherapy with external irradiation from a telecobalt or 4-b MeV linear accelerator is the mainstay of treatment for cancers of the oro- and hypopharynx because surgery would entail extensive tissue loss and functional deficit. Radical neck dissection is the choice of treatment for metastatic neck nodes and may be supplemented by pre- or postoperative radiotherapy. Chemotherapy has only a limited role in the management of head and neck cancers. Although responses have been observed with single-drug or combination chemotherapy involving agents, e.g., cisplatin, bleomycin, mitomycin, methotrexate, fluorouracil, and doxorubicin, long-term survival has not improved.

Control of pain, bleeding, and other symptoms of advanced cancers may be achieved by palliative radiotherapy or chemotherapy. Oral morphine is effective in relieving pain not amenable to these procedures and to conventional analgesics.

PREVENTION. Success in convincing Indian populations to reduce their tobacco habits by vigorous, locally targeted health education programs has been demonstrated in several field projects. The value of chemoprevention with vitamin A or its analogues in individuals with precancerous lesions is under investigation.

Screening for early oral cancers, or precursor lesions, by visual inspection of the mouth, using trained paramedical workers, has been feasible in India and Sri Lanka. Whether this type of screening can actually reduce mortality rates from oral cancer is being studied.

■ NASOPHARYNGEAL CARCINOMA

Nasopharyngeal carcinoma (NPC) is an epithelial neoplasm, arising in the squamous epithelium overlying nasopharyngeal lymphoid tissue. Most of the tumors are undifferentiated, comprising small cells with heavy lymphoid infiltration.

EPIDEMIOLOGY AND ETIOLOGY. About 58,000 NPCs occurred worldwide in 1990, the majority (40%) in China, and specifically the provinces of southern China. Here, incidence rates may be around 20 to 30 per 100,000. Moderate incidence rates are seen in Southeast Asia, in northern Africa (Algeria and Tunisia), and in American Indian populations (from Alaska to Bolivia). The high rates of NPC in migrant populations from southern China as well as in their offspring strongly suggest that genetic factors are important in causation. An association with certain HLA types was noted some years ago, and more recently family studies have indicated the presence of a not yet identified susceptibility gene. Some dietary factors are important promoters of NPC; salted fish in Chinese populations (especially if consumed very early in life) and certain spices (harissa) in North Africa.

Epstein-Barr virus (EBV) has long been believed to play a part in the etiology of NPC. Antibodies to various viral components are found in higher titers in the sera of NPC patients than in control subjects, and viral nucleic acid has been found in nuclei of the tumor cells. However, EBV infec-

tion is virtually universal, so it is difficult to prove this "cause" of NPC, and the elevated antibody titers found in patients (suggesting viral activation or replication) have not been demonstrated before tumor development. NPC occurs at a relatively younger age than most epithelial tumors, with incidence increasing from age 15 to 24 years in high-risk populations. In North Africa, there is an early peak in incidence (age 15–19 years), followed by a fall and a later rise (≥50 years), so that it is a relatively common tumor of childhood (10–20% of cancers), although it is rare in children elsewhere.

DIAGNOSIS AND TREATMENT. Patients with NPC often present with symptoms and signs of regional lymph node metastasis—the so-called bull neck (Fig. 12–1). Because of tumor proximity to the exit foramina of cranial nerves IX to XII, cranial neuropathy may be present. Local symptoms, e.g., pain, regurgitation, blocked eustachian tubes, and nasal stuffiness, may occur. Diagnosis can be established by nasopharyngoscopy or lymph node biopsy. Care must be taken to distinguish the epithelial malignancy amid the infiltrating lymphocytes.

Treatment consists of radiotherapy, and 5-year survival ranges from 30 to 60%. Transverse myelitis and xerostomia are complications of radiotherapy. Up to 75% of patients with advanced disease will respond to chemotherapy, notably cisplatin, methotrexate, bleomycin, and fluorouracil in various combinations as well as to interferon-α, although survival is not improved. Owing to the advanced stage of disease on presentation, the prognosis in endemic countries with limited therapeutic options is generally poor.

PREVENTION. Early detection of NPC by screening for elevated antibody titers to EBV has been performed in the high-risk populations of southern China, but the effectiveness of screening in preventing death from the disease has not been evaluated.

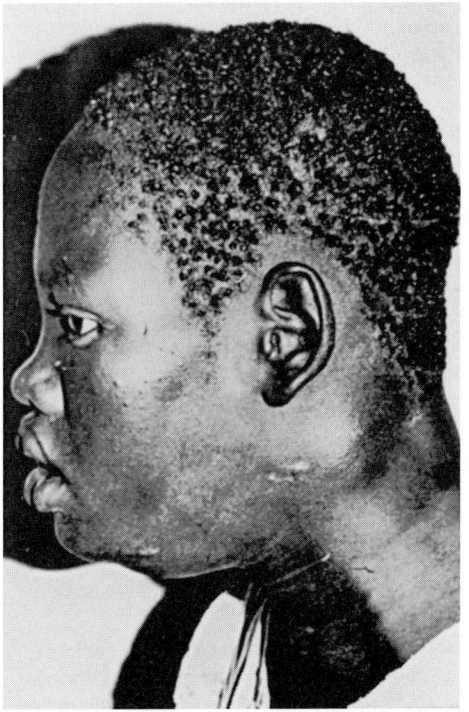

Figure 12–1. Enlarged cervical lymph nodes in a patient with nasopharyngeal carcinoma. (Courtesy of M. A. O. Malik, Khartoum.)

ESOPHAGEAL CARCINOMA

DEFINITION. Most of these are squamous cell carcinomas, arising in the lower third of the esophagus. Recently, there has been an increase in relative and absolute numbers of adenocarcinomas in Western countries, associated with Barrett's esophagus. The profile of genetic mutations is different in these two histologic subtypes, suggesting different etiologies.

EPIDEMIOLOGY AND ETIOLOGY. Esophageal cancer shows enormous geographic variability. The highest risk areas of the world are in the Asian "esophageal cancer belt" stretching from northern Iran through the central Asian republics to north-central China, with incidence rates as high as 200 per 100,000 and, in some areas, a female predominance. High rates are also present in parts of East and South East Africa (Uganda, Zimbabwe, Natal, Transkei) and eastern South America (southern Brazil, Uruguay, Paraguay, northern Argentina). Migrant studies suggest that when these populations move to areas of low risk they lose their high rates, confirming the importance of environmental factors in causation.

Studies in Western countries have consistently shown the etiologic importance of tobacco and alcohol—particularly in combination. Although they have been important in some studies, (e.g., South American and African), other factors must determine the striking geographic patterns. Nutritional deficiency (especially of micronutrients) has long been suspected to be the major factor in the Asian high-risk areas, although the results of recent vitamin supplementation trials have shown little benefit. In Africa a role for fumonisins (mycotoxins) and contaminants of home-brewed alcohol has been suggested as a risk factor, while in South America, the drinking of maté, the herb tea, is a well-established hazard.

DIAGNOSIS AND TREATMENT. Virtually all patients with this disorder complain of dysphagia, first to liquids and later to all foods, with accompanying weight loss. The next most common symptoms are vomiting and retrosternal chest pain. Cough and aspiration pneumonia may occur following regurgitation of foods. Early diagnosis using esophagoscopy or barium swallow may disclose resectable lesions, but the recurrence rates are high.

Surgery or radical radiotherapy may occasionally be effective in localized disease, with no involved nodes or metastases, but these patients constitute less than 10% of those presenting with disease. Overall survival with either treatment is around 5%, but some selected surgical series report 5-year survival rates of 20 to 30%. Radiotherapy, endoscopic laser therapy, endoscopic dilatation, endoscopic intubation, or a bypass operation provides temporary relief from dysphagia in subjects with widespread local tumor.

PREVENTION. Better nutrition will probably prevent many of the Central Asian cases (incidence rates in high-risk Linxian province in China are falling). Tobacco and alcohol control is clearly important. Screening by balloon cytology is purely experimental.

STOMACH CANCER

DEFINITION. The great majority of stomach cancers are adenocarcinomas.

EPIDEMIOLOGY AND ETIOLOGY. Stomach cancer is the most common malignancy in developing countries. Overall, the sex ratio is 1.7:1, with the highest incidence areas in eastern Asia (Korea, China) and South and Central America (particularly the Andean areas and southern Brazil). In Af-

rica, rates are generally higher in the west and in certain highland areas (Kilimanjaro, Rwanda/Burundi).

Chronic gastritis is an important precursor of stomach cancer; in this context, the role of long-term infection with *Helicobacter pylori* has attracted much attention (Chapter 45). However, *H. pylori* infection occurs at high prevalence in many developing countries, so the relatively low incidence in many areas (e.g., India, North Africa) appears paradoxical. Dietary factors may play an important role in the development of stomach cancer. Green and yellow vegetables and fruits have consistently been protective, whereas pickled, preserved, or salty foods pose a hazard.

The almost universal decline in stomach cancer risk is probably related to better nutrition (e.g., more fruits and vegetables in diets) and food preservation methods (refrigeration) and to the declining prevalence of *H. pylori* infection.

DIAGNOSIS AND TREATMENT. Gastric pain, vague abdominal discomfort, and anorexia and weight loss are the presenting features of stomach cancer, accompanied by vomiting (distal lesions) or regurgitation (proximal lesions). Hematemesis occurs in 20%. Definitive diagnosis rests on endoscopy and biopsy.

Surgery is the mainstay of treatment, although the cure rate is low owing to frequent lymph node metastasis by the time of presentation. Partial gastrectomy is recommended for distal tumors (antrum and pylorus), whereas total gastrectomy is usually necessary for proximal tumors (cardia, fundus). Regional lymph node dissection is done in both procedures.

Adjuvant postsurgical chemotherapy has been advocated by some groups, but this approach is not advisable outside an oncology center. Chemotherapy of advanced stomach cancer using mitomycin C, cisplatin, methotrexate, etoposide, and fluorouracil in combination yields partial remission in about 20%. Overall survival is poor—about 18% at 5 years in Europe and 7% in India. Five-year survival by stage in the U.S. SEER registries was 60% (localized tumors), 22% (regional spread), and 2% (distant spread).

PREVENTION. Fortunately, existing dietary trends will continue to reduce the risk. Studies are under way to investigate the effect of dietary supplements (vitamins) as well as treatment of *H. pylori* (with antibiotics and acid secretion blockers). These seem unlikely to become useful community interventions. There is very active research in progress to develop a vaccine for *H. pylori*.

Mass screening by contrast radiology has proved successful in Japan, but the benefits are probably small in relation to the huge costs involved, and it is not a practical policy option elsewhere (Chapter 21).

CARCINOMAS OF COLON AND RECTUM

DEFINITION. Almost all of these are adenocarcinomas, the great majority developing in the colon on the basis of a preexisting polyp.

EPIDEMIOLOGY AND ETIOLOGY. Incidence rates of these cancers in tropical countries are much lower than in the United States or in Europe, especially in Africa and India (Table 12–2). Migrant studies have shown that moving to a high-risk country can rapidly increase the probability of developing large bowel cancers. This is almost certainly the result of dietary change because many studies have pointed to the association between diets low in fiber and high in animal protein and fat and elevated risk. Incidence in developing countries is likely to increase, as traditional diets are replaced by more highly refined and packaged foods. Several cancer registries—even in Africa—suggest that incidence rates are rising.

DIAGNOSIS AND TREATMENT. Narrowing of stool caliber, constipation, anemia, and rectal bleeding are the cardinal signs of lower bowel cancer. Vague abdominal pain and an abdominal mass may be presenting features. Endoscopy, biopsy, and surgical resection constitute the diagnosis and therapy. Overall, the postsurgical 5-year survival is 50%. Patients with Duke's stage B or more advanced tumors may benefit from adjuvant chemotherapy with levamisole and fluorouracil. These tumors most frequently metastasize to the liver, where resection can be successfully performed on solitary secondary tumors, and palliation can be achieved with fluorouracil.

PREVENTION. A healthy diet is the best protection, but commercial dietary pressures will increasingly work against this. Studies are investigating the possible role of dietary supplements (vitamins, fiber, calcium) in offsetting this trend. The observation that consumption of nonsteroidal anti-inflammatory drugs (e.g., aspirin) can apparently lower the risk of colon cancer has awakened interest in their use as chemopreventive agents.

Screening is a feasible option but not a reasonable policy where rates are low. The method used for detecting early cancers is regular testing for fecal occult blood. Screening by sigmoidoscopy to detect and remove precursor adenomatous polyps is more promising, but the cost and acceptability of this procedure, even in high-risk populations, are questionable.

■ CANCER OF THE LIVER

DEFINITION. Most primary liver tumors involve the hepatocytes (hepatocellular carcinoma) or the epithelial lining of the intrahepatic bile ducts (cholangiocarcinomas).

EPIDEMIOLOGY AND ETIOLOGY. Over 80% of the 440,000 annual cases of liver cancer worldwide occur in developing countries. It is particularly common in East and Southeast Asia and sub-Saharan Africa, with moderate rates in the Middle East (Table 12–2). The male:female ratio in these high-risk areas is around 3:1. For hepatocellular carcinoma, the most important etiologic agents are the hepatitis viruses (Chapter 28). Over 80% of cancers are associated with underlying cirrhosis. About 60% of the cases in developing countries occur in persons who are chronic carriers of the hepatitis B virus (HBV), so that the risk of liver cancer closely follows the prevalence of HBV infection (Fig. 28–5). Infection with the virus of hepatitis C is less common, and the resulting chronic hepatitis and cirrhosis are estimated to cause about one quarter of cases. Consumption of aflatoxins in contaminated foods (especially maize and peanuts) is also an important etiologic determinant in tropical countries. The role of alcohol consumption is probably quantitatively small in developing countries.

Cholangiocarcinoma is not related to any of these factors. It is, however, a common tumor where chronic infection with liver flukes (*Opisthorchis* and *Clonorchis*) occurs, particularly in parts of Thailand, Korea, and China (Chapters 118.1 and 118.2).

DIAGNOSIS AND TREATMENT. Similar to other visceral tumors, in developing countries hepatocellular carcinoma usually presents in advanced stages (Fig. 12–2). Tumors as small as 1 cm can be detected by ultrasound. Although a clinical diagnosis has a sensitivity of about 95%, liver biopsy is recommended when there are no contraindications. Diagnosis can also be reinforced by an elevated (≥40 ng/dL) serum α-fetoprotein level.

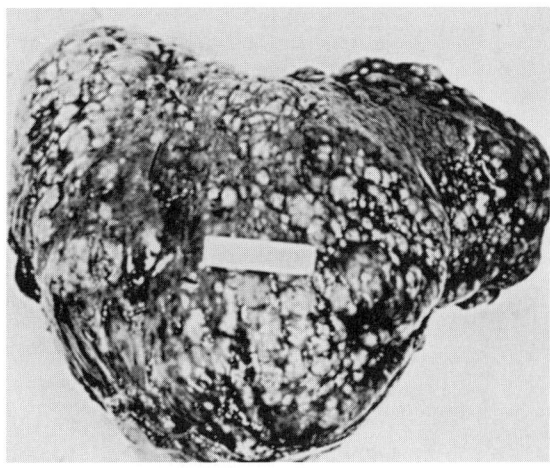

Figure 12–2. Multiple nodules of liver cell carcinoma, involving both lobes, in a cirrhotic liver.

When the tumor is localized to a single lobe, partial hepatectomy can be attempted, but even in experienced centers, the operative mortality is high. Ethanol injection into the tumor can be undertaken in centers where interventional radiography is available (Chapter 21). In Japan, the use of retinoid "chemoprevention" has reduced recurrences after successful extirpation of small tumors. Chemotherapy with doxorubicin (60–75 mg/m²) in a slow intravenous infusion once every 3 weeks can yield partial remissions in up to 25%. In specialized centers, hepatic artery embolization or infusions with fluorouracil can retard disease progression. Prognosis is poor, however, with 90% dying in the first year of diagnosis.

PREVENTION. Most liver cancer could be prevented by vaccination against hepatitis B virus. Trials of the effectiveness of hepatitis B vaccine in preventing liver cancer are underway in The Gambia and China (Qidong), and the vaccine is being introduced into immunization programs whenever resources permit. Avoiding aflatoxin contamination of foodstuffs requires changes in agricultural practices and food storage, which may be expensive and difficult. Drugs aimed to prevent metabolism of aflatoxin to its carcinogenic metabolites probably have no practical role. Screening for liver cancer by detection of raised serum titers of α-fetoprotein is not effective in reducing mortality.

■ LUNG CANCER

DEFINITION. Almost all lung cancers are of epithelial origin (mesotheliomas are tumors of the pleura). In men, squamous cell carcinomas are usually more common than adenocarcinomas, with the reverse being the case in women. Small cell carcinomas constitute around 10 to 20% of tumors.

EPIDEMIOLOGY AND ETIOLOGY. Patterns of lung cancer occurrence are determined almost entirely by past exposure to tobacco smoking. Of the 440,000 annual cases reported in developing countries, 76% of those in men and 24% of those in women are due to smoking. This pattern reflects the earlier adoption of smoking by men with highest rates where the habit has been longest established, i.e., in the Middle East, China, the Caribbean, South Africa and Zimbabwe, and the Pacific (Table 12–2). In most developing countries, women rarely smoke. Since the risk of smoking is greater for squamous cell tumors than for adenocarcinomas, high smoking prevalence and high incidence rates are generally accompa-

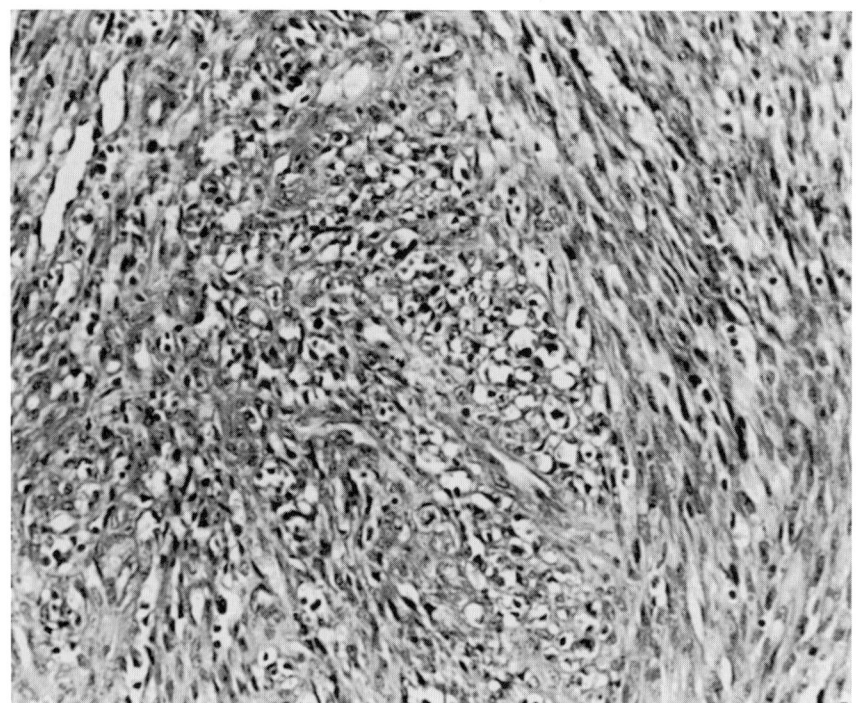

Figure **12–3.** Typical "sievelike" pattern of interlacing bundles of angioformative spindle cells from a patient with Kaposi's sarcoma. (H & E stain, × 250.)

nied by a higher proportion of squamous cell tumors. Tobacco consumption has been rising, at least in men, in most developing countries so that it is easy to predict a continuing evolution of the epidemic.

Chinese women, although few of them smoke, have a modestly raised incidence of lung cancer, possibly because of exposure to environmental smoke, particularly cooking fumes. But they may be at genuinely higher risk, too. Genetic mechanisms define susceptibility to tobacco smoke, possibly through controlling metabolism of carcinogens, and it could be that the genes responsible for susceptibility are differentially distributed by ethnic group. Other factors known to increase risk of lung cancer are occupational exposures to asbestos, some metals (e.g., nickel), mixtures of polycyclic aromatic hydrocarbons, and ionizing radiation.

DIAGNOSIS AND TREATMENT. Bronchogenic carcinoma is readily diagnosed by chest x-ray (Chapter 21) and bronchoscopy or by sputum cytology. Treatment of small cell carcinoma (about 20% of lung cancers) is with chemotherapy; a variety of regimens can induce complete remissions of varying duration. Management of non–small cell carcinoma is restricted to surgical resection and/or radiotherapy. Chemotherapy of this form of lung cancer is confined to specialized centers. Prognosis is poor.

PREVENTION. Although individuals can be convinced to give up smoking, and adolescents persuaded not to start, this is very difficult in the absence of reinforcing social pressures, to make smoking unattractive, and legislative framework, to make smoking expensive and difficult. The opposing pressures (agricultural and finance ministries, tobacco companies) are enormous. Although x-ray screening for lung cancer continues to attract enthusiasts, it is a useless procedure for reducing mortality.

■ KAPOSI'S SARCOMA

DEFINITION. The precise cell of origin for this tumor has been debated for many years. It is currently believed to be an endothelial cell, probably lymphatic. Despite its wide geographic distribution and varied clinical features, the histology of Kaposi's sarcoma (KS) is remarkably uniform (Fig. 12–3).

EPIDEMIOLOGY AND ETIOLOGY. KS has long been recognized as slowly progressive skin lesions arising generally on the lower limbs and affecting mainly middle-aged and elderly men (sex ratio about 5:1) in central Africa. The highest rates of this "endemic" form were found in eastern Zaire, Rwanda, Burundi, and western Uganda, and local variations in incidence were quite marked.

With the advent of the AIDS epidemic, the situation has entirely changed (Chapter 23). KS now occurs in an "epidemic" form related to infection with the human immunodeficiency virus (HIV); affecting primarily young adults (peak age around 35 years in men, and 30 years in women); and occurring as generalized skin lesions, often involving mucous membranes, lymph nodes, lung, and gastrointestinal (GI) tract.

By the early 1990s, KS was responsible for about 50% of tumors in men in Kampala, Uganda, and 25% in Harare, Zimbabwe, and it accounted for 20% and 10% of cancers in women, respectively. Epidemiologic studies among patients with AIDS in the United States suggested that KS was caused by an infectious agent, possibly sexually transmitted, with development of the tumor being facilitated by HIV-induced immunosuppression. The discovery of DNA from a type of herpes virus (KSHV or HHV8) in KS tissue, and its apparently higher prevalence in subjects from areas where KS was known to be endemic, suggests that the candidate agent has been identified (Chapter 24.2).

CLINICAL MANIFESTATIONS. Endemic KS is a pleomorphic tumor of the skin of the distal extremities, exhibiting a nodular, infiltrative, or sarcomatous ("florid") morphology (Fig. 12–4).

AIDS-associated epidemic KS appears most commonly on the skin, often in symmetric patches, macules, or nodules. Lesions are frequently multiple and asymptomatic, appearing on the face, truck, arms, and legs. Enlarged regional lymph

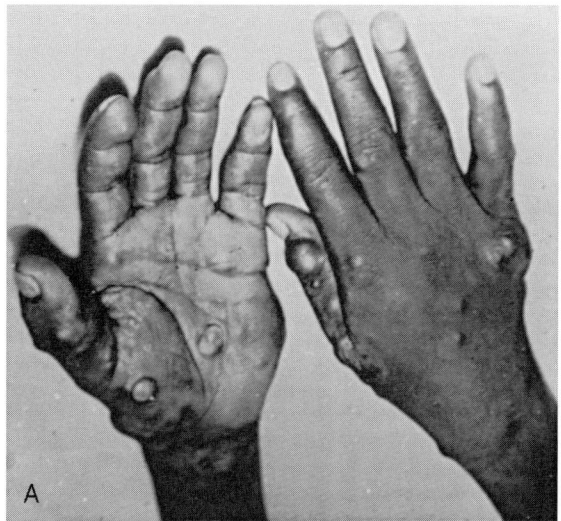

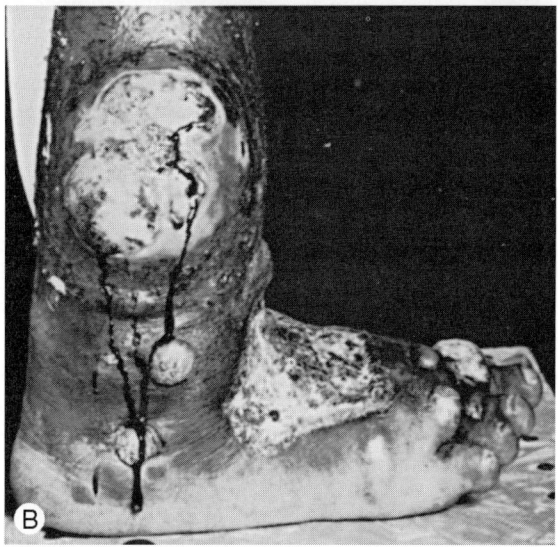

Figure 12–4. *A,* Nodular form of Kaposi's sarcoma on the hands of an African male. *B,* Florid form of Kaposi's sarcoma on the lower leg. Nodular lesions are also present, and there is some lymphedema. (*A,* Courtesy of Dr. E. H. Williams.)

nodes usually contain tumor when biopsied. Lesions are often edematous, with occasionally dramatic lymphedema (Fig. 12–5*A*). In addition to cutaneous involvement, KS appears in the mouth (tongue, palate, tonsil), lung, GI tract, penis, rectum, and liver (Fig. 12–5*B*).

Children develop lymphadenopathic oral and visceral lesions with a predilection for the head and neck or for the groin and anogenital region. Children respond to chemotherapy and may achieve durable remissions.

TREATMENT AND PROGNOSIS. Treatment of KS can be local (surgery, intralesional chemotherapy), regional (radiotherapy), or systemic (chemo- or biotherapy). The choice of treatment must be individualized and depends on the location of lesions, the degree of immunosuppression, the presence of concomitant opportunistic infection, and the local treatment facilities. Where available, radiotherapy affords the best palliative response in cutaneous lesions, and a single dose of 800 cGy is effective. Chemotherapy usually consists of single agents, e.g., doxorubicin, 50 mg/m² IV every 3 weeks, etoposide (oral or intravenous), vincristine or vinblastine (often alternating weekly), or a combination of these

drugs (etoposide, doxorubicin, and bleomycin is favored). Interferon-α, an expensive biotherapy often associated with unpleasant side effects, also produces remissions in about 50% of patients.

Because KS is responsive to a variety of therapies, remission can be achieved in 80% of patients, and some remissions are prolonged. The outcome often depends on the degree of immunosuppression and the presence of other infections, but remissions of 6 to 12 months' duration are possible.

PREVENTION. Currently, prevention of KS is through protection from HIV infection.

■ MALIGNANT MELANOMA

DEFINITION. The tumor arises from the melanocytes of the skin, retina, and, very rarely, other sites.

EPIDEMIOLOGY AND ETIOLOGY. Malignant melanoma of skin is a tumor of the white-skinned races. Where they are exposed to the strong ultraviolet irradiation of tropical areas, incidence rates can be very high—as observed in whites in Zimbabwe, for example. Benign nevi, induced by ultraviolet (UV) irradiation, particularly in childhood, are important precursor lesions.

Dark-skinned races have a low risk of melanoma. In both Africa and South America, the frequency with which melanomas appear on the sole of the foot (Fig. 12–6) has attracted much attention, but the incidence at this site is not high; rather the incidence elsewhere on the skin is very low. Asians have a low risk of melanoma despite their paler skins; nevi in Asian peoples, though common, are predominantly of the acral-lentiginous type, with low malignant potential.

TREATMENT AND PROGNOSIS. Because malignant melanoma in dark-skinned people in the tropics occurs most often on the foot, excisional surgery is the treatment of choice. Most evidence is against regional lymph node excision. Malignant melanoma is generally radioresistant. Chemotherapy for metastatic melanoma has not been successful; dacarbazine remains the drug of choice, but only 25% of patients are likely to experience tumor responses.

PREVENTION. White-skinned populations should take precautions to limit the exposure of their skin to UV radiation by using hats, appropriate clothing, and sunscreens.

■ NONMELANOMA SKIN CANCER

DEFINITION. Most of these arise in the epithelium, from squamous cells or basal cells. Other rarer tumors include sweat gland tumors and dermatofibrosarcomas.

EPIDEMIOLOGY AND ETIOLOGY. There are few good statistics on nonmelanoma skin cancer, since cases are not recorded in conventional cancer registries. White-skinned populations exposed to UV radiation are particularly at risk, and incidence rates in such groups (e.g., in Australia or Zimbabwe) are extremely high. Most tumors are basal cell carcinomas of the head and neck (e.g., face, ear); squamous cell carcinomas are one quarter to one third as common and usually also involve the head, neck, and upper limbs.

In Asian populations, squamous cell tumors are relatively more common. Whereas basal cell tumors occur mainly on the head and neck, squamous cell carcinomas are more common on the limbs, especially on the legs in Asians. This pattern is even more marked in Africans, in whom basal cell tumors are very rare, and squamous cell tumors occur predominantly on the legs. Squamous cell carcinomas often arise in chronic ulcers, sinuses, or old burns. Epitheliomas

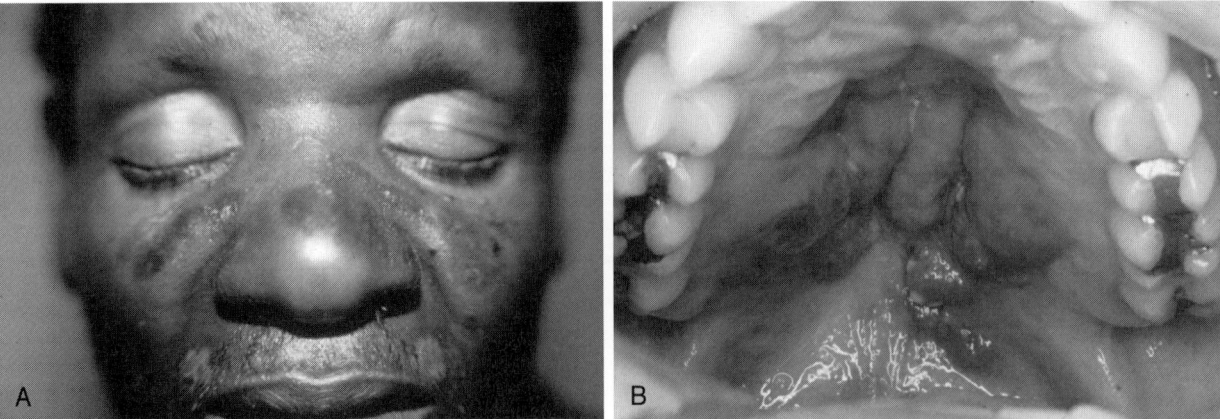

Figure 12–5. *A*, Epidemic Kaposi's sarcoma of the face. Note symmetry and edema. *B*, Epidemic Kaposi's sarcoma of the palate.

developing at the site of chronic tropical ulcers (Fig. 12–7) are becoming less common in Africa than in the past.

Treatment is by local surgery or by radiotherapy.

PREVENTION. White-skinned subjects and albinos living in the tropics should wear protective clothing and sunscreens during the midday, when UV light is most intense. Solar keratoses should be treated and the skin observed regularly for early carcinoma.

■ BREAST CANCER

DEFINITION. Most breast cancers are classified as adenocarcinomas or intraductal carcinomas.

EPIDEMIOLOGY AND ETIOLOGY. Although breast cancer is thought of as a mainly Western disease, it is also the most common cancer of women in developing countries. Within the tropical areas, the highest rates are seen in North Africa, the Middle East, and the Caribbean (Table 12–2).

The risk of breast cancer is related to reproductive factors. Thus, incidence increases fastest during the reproductive years, so that young age at menarche and older age at menopause, by lengthening the reproductive period, lead to higher overall risk. Each pregnancy leads to a temporary increase in the risk, followed by a permanent decrease, so that after reproductive life is over, highly fertile populations have lower incidence rates. Reproductive factors cannot explain the international differences or the change in disease risk following migration; dietary factors may be important, although their role is controversial. A small proportion of breast cancers ($\cong$3% in developed countries) are the result of inheritance of one of the breast cancer susceptibility genes (BRCA1 and 2), the carriers of which have a very high risk of developing breast cancer (70% by age 70 years for BRCA1). The prevalence of carriers of these genes has not been studied in developing countries, so corresponding estimates are not available.

DIAGNOSIS. The hallmark of successful breast cancer man-

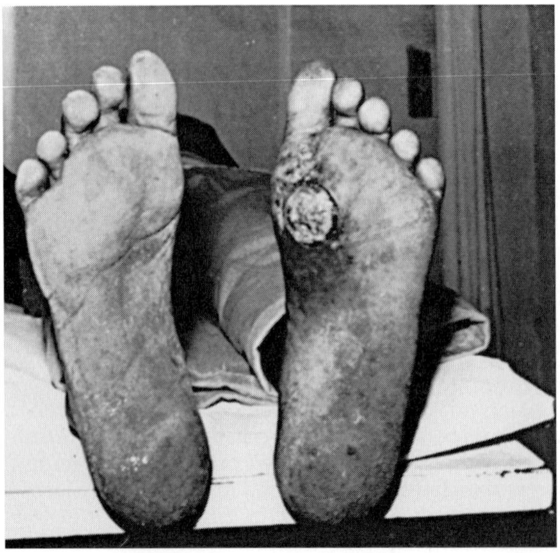

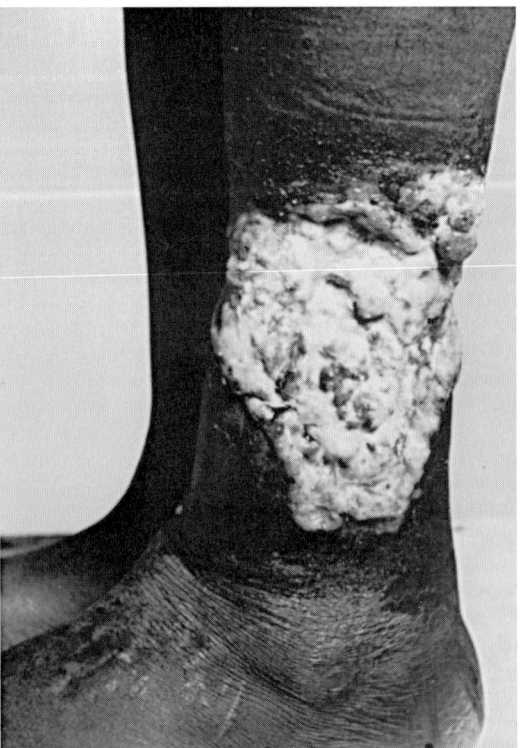

Figure 12–6. Malignant melanoma on the sole of the foot in an adult African. (Courtesy of Dr. E. H. Williams.)

Figure 12–7. Malignant change (squamous cell carcinoma) arising in the scar of an unhealed tropical ulcer.

agement is early detection. When a new breast cancer mass is detected, mammography, followed by needle aspiration or excisional biopsy, is recommended; a portion of the tumor should be set aside for estrogen receptor assay, if available. A suspicious breast mass should always be diagnosed, because 30% of breast tumors thought clinically to be malignant are benign, and 10% of benign tumors turn out to be malignant.

TREATMENT AND PROGNOSIS. Primary therapy depends upon the availability of radiotherapy. Breast-conserving management (partial mastectomy or lumpectomy) accompanied by axillary lymph node dissection and postoperative radiotherapy yields results equivalent to those of older, more radical procedures. Where radiotherapy is not available, partial mastectomy and axillary dissection should be done.

Breast cancer staging depends on the results of surgery and estrogen receptor presence, and subsequent management is dictated by stage. Patients with stage II cancer (any nodal involvement or large tumors without node involvement) should receive adjuvant chemotherapy. A standard regimen is cyclophosphamide 600 mg/m², methotrexate 40 mg/m², and fluorouracil 600 mg/m² IV on days 1 and 8. This CMF regimen should be repeated monthly for 6 months at full dose. Postmenopausal patients should receive tamoxifen, 10 mg orally, twice a day. Palliative therapy for patients with stage IV (metastatic) disease may employ radiotherapy (e.g., for specific bone or brain lesions), tamoxifen or bilateral ovariectomy (for premenopausal women), or chemotherapy. The most effective agents are CMF, doxorubicin, and a new agent, Taxol.

The prognosis for women with early breast cancer is excellent, with cure achievable in over half of stage II and one quarter of stage III patients, given proper management. Stage IV cancer can be palliated with hormonal therapy or chemotherapy, but survival is not affected. Five-year survival is about 50 to 60% in India and 70% in Shanghai, China.

PREVENTION. It has been difficult to find measures to prevent breast cancer. The antiestrogen tamoxifen, which has long been used in treatment of women whose tumors have estrogen receptors, has been shown in a clinical trial to reduce the incidence of breast cancer in women at high risk (e.g., with a strongly positive family history or prior breast lesions). Natural antiestrogens, e.g., in soy products, may prove useful.

Screening for breast cancer by mammography is effective in reducing death rates in women over 50 years. There is controversy, however, over the size of the benefit in routine service, and the expense of implementing such programs limits their potential to high-incidence, affluent populations. Less costly alternatives are screening through self-examination and by physical examination by trained nurses. Both are unproved at present but are undergoing evaluative trials.

■ CANCER OF THE CERVIX

DEFINITION. The majority of these tumors are squamous cell carcinomas, arising in the epithelium of the transition zone, close to the external os. These tumors are signaled by a sequence of precursor lesions, which demonstrate progressively increasing atypia of cells and gradual involvement of the whole thickness of the epithelium from the basal layer outward (cervical intraepithelial neoplasia [CIN] grades I–III). About 10% of tumors are adenocarcinomas, arising in the glands of the cervical canal.

EPIDEMIOLOGY AND ETIOLOGY. Cervix cancer is the second most frequent cancer of women in developing countries. High incidence rates are found in east, Southeast, and southern Asia; sub-Saharan Africa; Latin America and the Caribbean; and the Pacific islands. Only in Middle Eastern countries are relatively low incidence rates observed. Epidemiologic studies have long indicated that the disease could involve a sexually transmitted factor. Thus, it is associated with the age at first intercourse, number of sexual partners, and sexual activity of husband/partners. Barrier contraceptives reduce the risk.

Human papillomaviruses (HPVs) of certain oncogenic subtypes (16, 18, 31, 33, 35) are the causative agents. Infection by these subtypes predicts a very high probability of developing CIN. HPV proteins E6 and E7 bind to two tumor suppressor proteins (p53 and RB, respectively) and permit unimpeded cell proliferation. HPV infection is very common in young women and, at least in the United States, prevalence relates to sexual experience. Prevalence declines with age, and it is presumably long-term, persistent infections that are most relevant to cancer development. There is some suggestion that prevalence of HPV infection varies geographically in the same way as cervix cancer, but this has never been systematically investigated. Although HIV infection is associated with an increased risk of CIN, no increase in cervix cancer has been observed in areas where HIV is pandemic.

DIAGNOSIS AND TREATMENT. In developing countries many patients present in advanced stages, with uterine bleeding, anemia, pelvic obstructive symptoms, and pain. The usual gynecologic procedure is an examination under anesthesia to determine clinical stage (Table 12–3) and operability. Preoperative procedures also include a chest x-ray and contrast urography.

For stage IA, cervical conization is adequate, followed by simple hysterectomy. For stages IB and IIA, radical hysterectomy with pelvic lymph node dissection is recommended. Intracavitary irradiation with a radioactive isotope such as cesium or radium results in cure rates comparable to surgery in stages I and IIA. For stages IIB, III, and IV, radiotherapy is administered. In patients with advanced or recurrent cervical cancer, response rates of up to 90% are reported using cisplatin-based regimens, but overall survival has not improved. Five-year survival ranges reported in the West are: stage IA, 90%; stage IB/IIA 80–90%; stage IIB, 65%; stage III, 40%; and stage IV, 20%.

PREVENTION. Prevention of cervix cancer is a high priority in many developing countries, as it affects women in their forties and fifties with heavy social and economic responsibilities. Although the immunology of HPV is complex, prophylactic vaccines are being prepared for testing and hold the best long-term promise for control of the disease.

Screening by cervical cytology is effective in reducing the incidence of invasive cancer and hence mortality. However, the logistics of taking, preparing, and reading smears; of maintaining quality control in cytology laboratories; and of providing the necessary follow-up are complex and expensive. As a result, almost no well-organized programs exist in

TABLE 12–3. Clinical Staging of Cervical Cancer

Stage	Tumor Extent
Stage IA	Confined to uterus, microinvasive disease
Stage IB	Larger than IA, grossly visible
Stage IIA	Involves upper 2/3 of vagina but not pelvic sidewall
Stage IIB	Lateral extension to parametria
Stage IIIA	Lower 1/3 of vagina
Stage IIIB	Pelvic sidewall or ureter (hydronephrosis)
Stage IVA	Involvement of bladder or rectum
Stage IVB	Distant metastasis

developing countries. Alternative strategies, such as screening by visual inspection of the cervix alone (without cytology), may be cheaper but are much less accurate and are probably ineffective in practice.

CHORIOCARCINOMA

DEFINITION. This is a malignant tumor of the chorionic trophoblastic epithelium and hence of embryonal origin.

EPIDEMIOLOGY AND ETIOLOGY. Choriocarcinoma is a rare tumor. Most cases follow molar pregnancies. High rates are found in Southeast Asia and some populations of sub-Saharan Africa. This may relate in part to high fertility rates, but there is probably also a genetic component to the higher risk.

TREATMENT AND PREVENTION. About 1 in 125 pregnancies will result in hydatidiform mole, usually associated with excessive vomiting and uterine bleeding at 6 to 8 weeks. Occasional vaginal passage of grapelike vesicles is diagnostic of molar pregnancy. About 5% of hydatidiform moles become malignant.

When fully developed, choriocarcinoma is diagnosed by clinical examination (pelvic mass or the presence of large pulmonary metastases), by ultrasound (with a characteristic echogenic pattern), and by the presence of high choriogonadotropin levels (>100,000 IU/24 hr) in the urine. Metastatic choriocarcinoma is responsive to 2-week courses of chemotherapy with methotrexate (15 mg/m^2 daily for 4 days) and dactinomycin (0.04 mg/kg weekly) followed by a 2-week rest period. Eighty-five percent of cases can be cured with chemotherapy. Choriocarcinoma can be prevented by the routine administration of methotrexate, 15 mg daily for 1 week, following the extraction of a molar pregnancy.

PROSTATE CANCER

DEFINITION. Prostate cancer is an adenocarcinoma of glandular origin. Many tumors remain intraductal or localized and are discovered only on incidental histologic examination of surgical tissue or at autopsy.

EPIDEMIOLOGY AND ETIOLOGY. Prostate cancer is a common cancer of men (fourth in frequency worldwide), although rather more rare in some developing countries. Rates are especially low in Asian populations and in North Africa and the Middle East. In the United States and Brazil, incidence is highest in black populations, although recorded rates in sub-Saharan Africa are lower than those observed in North America. In developed countries this is probably because of the large excess of small, latent cancers detected following prostatectomy for benign hypertrophy or as a result of screening. In fact, clinical invasive cancer of the prostate is the most common cancer in African men over the age of 60 years. Etiologic factors remain obscure. A diet of fat and meat confers risk, whereas physical exercise is protective. The reason for the higher risk in men of African descent may relate to their genetically determined pathways of testosterone metabolism within the prostate gland.

DIAGNOSIS. The earliest urinary obstructive symptoms of prostate cancer (i.e., urgency, frequency, nocturia and hesitancy) are difficult to distinguish from those of benign prostatic hypertrophy in older men. Thus, cancer is often diagnosed incidentally following transurethral prostate resection to relieve urinary obstruction (stage A). Alternatively, a prostatic mass may be palpated on rectal examination, or back pain may develop because of spinal metastases. The discovery of elevated levels of prostate-specific antigen (PSA) (>4 ng/mL) also permits a diagnosis, but the test is not widely available in the tropics.

TREATMENT AND PROGNOSIS. There is controversy over optimal management of early (stage B) cancer confined to the prostate gland. Radical prostatectomy and pelvic lymph node dissection and radiotherapy yield similar survival but are associated with different side effects. Radiation therapy is reserved for stage C (periprostatic tissue involved), and hormone therapy (orchiectomy or diethylstilbestrol) for stage D (metastatic) cancer. Chemotherapy (weekly doxorubicin is best) or alternative antiandrogenic hormones (leuprolide, flutamide) also can be used in advanced disease. The approach to management depends on the facilities available (radiation therapy, PSA assay) and any co-morbidity present in the patient.

Prognosis is unusually good; 5- to 10-year survival rates for early prostate cancer are close to those of the general population, whereas survival for more advanced cases depends on the development and site of metastases.

PREVENTION. Asymptomatic cancers can be detected by screening, with measurement of PSA as the primary test, followed by ultrasonically directed biopsy. Enthusiasm for this procedure is high in North America and resulted in an enormous rise in apparent incidence of prostate cancer in the late 1980s and early 1990s. It is far from certain whether there is any ultimate benefit, in the form of reduced death rates; this information must await the outcome of ongoing trials.

PENILE CANCER

EPIDEMIOLOGY AND ETIOLOGY. Penile cancer is rare in developed countries but is not uncommon in some parts of Africa (Uganda, Kenya), Latin America (northeast Brazil), India, and Southeast Asia. The similar geographic distribution to cervix cancer as well as the higher than expected occurrence of penile cancer and cervix cancer in husband and wife suggests a common etiology, and indeed HPV has been identified in up to 50% of penile cancers. The disease is also related to penile hygiene (it is rare in circumcised individuals) in East Africa and India, and the declines in incidence in recent years may relate to improved washing facilities.

TREATMENT AND PROGNOSIS. Carcinoma of the penis is treated by surgical amputation, with delayed removal of inguinal nodes. Recurrent lesions may respond to radiotherapy, but chemotherapy has not been systematically evaluated. Five-year survival following surgery approximates 50%.

CANCER OF THE BLADDER

DEFINITION. Most bladder tumors arise in the transitional cell epithelium. Many, if not most, cases arise in papillomas, and microscopic examination of some apparently benign papillomas shows areas of hyperplasia or frankly malignant cells and even areas of microinvasive disease. This makes enumeration of "bladder cancer" incidence by cancer registries difficult. In areas of endemic urinary schistosomiasis, squamous metaplasia of the bladder epithelium caused by *Schistosoma haematobium* is followed by squamous cell carcinomas (Chapter 118).

EPIDEMIOLOGY AND ETIOLOGY. Bladder cancer is predominantly a tumor of males (sex ratio 3.5:1). The well-known risk factors for bladder cancer are tobacco smoking (responsible for about a quarter of the cases in men in developing countries) and occupational exposures such as to dyestuffs and industrial rubber and coal products. An additional

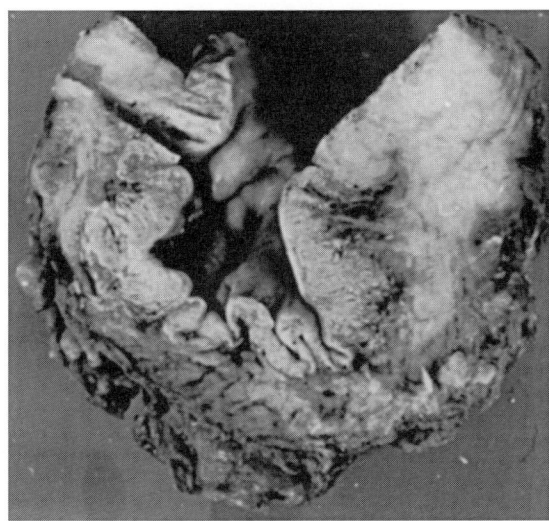

Figure 12–8. Invasive squamous cell carcinoma in a bladder with heavy *Schistosoma haematobium* infection.

factor in developing countries is chronic infection with *S. haematobium*, which accounts for the relatively high incidence rates in North Africa (Egypt) and the Middle East (Iraq, Iran) as well as in parts of sub-Saharan Africa (Malawi, Zambia, Zimbabwe, West Africa). In these three areas, schistosomiasis causes about one third of bladder cancers (Fig. 12–8).

DIAGNOSIS AND TREATMENT. For squamous cell tumors, the common presentation is hematuria, pyuria, or even necroturia (elimination of tumor fragments in the urine). At the National Cancer Institute in Cairo, first-line therapy is surgical, combined with a variety of ureteral diversion procedures tailored to the individual situation. Radiotherapy is palliative as is systemic chemotherapy, including cisplatin, etoposide, and cyclophosphamide. For patients with stages I to III bladder cancer, 5-year survival is about 65%.

Transitional carcinomas, if small, may be treated with transurethral resection, and recurrences can be controlled using intravesical chemotherapy, with or without immunotherapy with bacillus Calmette-Guérin (BCG). In developing countries, where such procedures may not be available, bladder resection with urinary diversion is often performed. Radiotherapy is palliative for advanced cases.

PREVENTION. Preventive measures include avoidance of smoking, appropriate industrial hygiene measures, and control of schistosomiasis. Screening (with urinary cytology) is not a practical proposition.

■ CANCERS OF THE EYE

DEFINITION. There are three principal eye cancers. Retinoblastomas affect young children (mainly those ≤ 7 years of age). Melanomas occur through the adult age range, arising in melanocytes of the uveal tract. Squamous cell tumors are largely derived from the conjunctival epithelium.

EPIDEMIOLOGY AND ETIOLOGY. About 40% of retinoblastomas are hereditary, the infant inheriting one chromosome with a defective retinoblastoma gene and a spontaneous mutation in its partner resulting in the tumor. Many of these cases are bilateral. The incidence of retinoblastoma is about 50 to 100% higher in African and some Asian populations than in Europe and North America, with most of this excess due to unilateral, and hence probably noninherited, tumors.

Ocular melanoma does not show any marked geographic variation, and studies do not suggest a strong link with sunlight, as in the case of melanoma of the skin. In contrast, squamous cell tumors of the conjunctiva are more common where solar UV radiation is high, and especially in African populations. The latter tumor is also strongly associated with HIV infection.

TREATMENT. In developing countries, ophthalmologic surgery is the treatment of choice for retinoblastoma and ocular melanoma. The rising incidence of squamous cell carcinoma of the conjunctiva associated with HIV infection requires special vigilance, as these tumors are easily cured if treated early.

■ LYMPHOMA

DEFINITION. Hodgkin's disease (HD) is relatively easily distinguished from other lymphomas by its characteristic histologic features, presence of Reed-Sternberg cells, and certain clinical features. Among the non-Hodgkin lymphomas (NHLs), Burkitt's lymphoma (BL) constitutes a distinct clinicopathologic entity, distinguished by its morphology (small round noncleaved cells of B-cell lineage) and specific cytogenetic features involving breakages or translocations of chromosome 8. These translocations appear to result in activation of the cellular oncogene *c-myc*, probably an important step in the malignant process. The other NHLs are classified by their appearance on light microscopy (cell size and appearance, lymph node architecture) and by immunologic features (T or B cells involved). It is not clear whether these distinctions have much etiologic relevance. About 85% of NHLs are of B-cell origin, probably reflecting the high proliferation and turnover of these cells.

EPIDEMIOLOGY AND ETIOLOGY

Hodgkin's Disease. In tropical countries, there is generally a first peak in incidence around age 5 to 9 years and a further rise in incidence after age 40 to 45 years. In developed countries, the childhood peak is replaced by an increase in incidence in young adults about 25 to 30 years of age. There are histologic differences, too, with childhood disease being mainly lymphocyte-depleted or mixed cellularity type, and young adults having a nodular sclerosing pattern. These patterns have been ascribed to differences in exposure to the Epstein-Barr virus (EBV) (Chapter 24.1). Such exposure occurs early in life in the more crowded, less hygienic conditions of tropical countries but may be delayed to adolescence in developed societies; it is manifested clinically as infectious mononucleosis. The genetic material of the EBV can be identified in quite a high proportion of tumors—around 70% in childhood (80% in developing countries), 20% in young adults, and 70% after age 45 years, correlating with the histologic features noted earlier. Studies have shown that abnormally high titers of certain anti-EBV antibodies (notably anti-VCA) precede the diagnosis of HD. All these features suggest that the virus has a causative role in perhaps half of the cases in developing countries, although the precise mechanism causing the tumor is unclear. However, HD is very rare in Asian populations (China, Japan, Southeast Asia), where it is confined to the older age groups, and is uncommon in children and in young adults.

Burkitt's Lymphoma. BL was first described in tropical Africa; the zone of high incidence coincided with that of holoendemic malaria and, hence, was absent in high-altitude regions. It occurs at similarly high incidence in Papua New Guinea, especially in the coastal areas, where malaria is most intense. The link with malaria is also shown by the somewhat lower risks of urban populations, in the altered risks of migrants moving to areas of differing malaria endemicity,

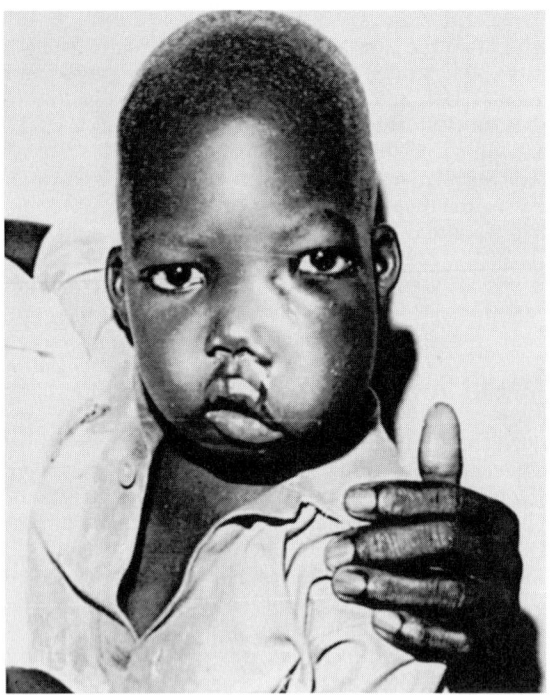

Figure 12–9. Left maxillary tumor in a child with Burkitt's lymphoma. (Courtesy of Dr. E. H. Williams.)

and in the reduced risk in malarious areas during chemoprophylaxis. In these areas, BL occurs mainly in boys (ratio 2:1) with peak occurrence at age 5 to 8 years and with up to half the tumors involving the face or jaw (Fig. 12–9). Over 95% of these cases demonstrate DNA of the EBV in the tumor, and raised antibody titers to EBV were observed in Ugandan children who subsequently developed the disease (Chapter 24.1). Malaria is thought to stimulate the immune system, causing proliferation of B cells and suppression of T cells. This results in dysregulation of EBV control, leading to further B-cell proliferation, from which clonal lymphoma may develop (Chapter 92).

Awareness of the characteristics of BL has allowed its identification throughout the world, and it is now clear that it constitutes a significant proportion of childhood NHL elsewhere—about 20 to 25% in the United States, for example.

Outside of Africa and Papua New Guinea, BL is rare after age 15 years and virtually never occurs after age 40 years. The proportion of cases associated with EBV also varies. In North Africa, it is rather high ($\cong$80%); in tropical South America, intermediate (50%); and in temperate countries, only about 15 to 25% of BL cases. The "sporadic" form of temperate countries is more evenly distributed by age, and the precise breakpoints on chromosome 8 are in different places than in the endemic or African form.

Other Non-Hodgkin's Lymphomas. In general, incidence rates of NHL are not very high in tropical areas. The relatively low rates of other cancers (lung, GI, cervix) in some areas of the Middle East and North Africa and consequently high prevalence in clinical series (e.g., 7 to 12%) make the lymphomas appear to be relatively more important than they actually are. However, there is a genuine excess of extranodal lymphomas in children. Although the existence of immunoproliferative small intestinal disease (IPSID), or "Mediterranean lymphoma," is well known, this condition has recently become rare, accounting for few of the apparent excess cases

of childhood lymphomas in the southern and eastern Mediterranean regions.

In North America and Europe, NHLs—particularly immunoblastic lymphoma, primary lymphoma of the central nervous system (CNS), and BL—are a presenting feature of about 3% of AIDS cases and develop at some time during the illness in up to 10% of cases (Chapter 22). This has resulted in a marked increase in the incidence of these malignancies in some areas of the United States. However, in tropical Africa, despite the high incidence of AIDS, no notable increase of NHL has been observed. This may be because lymphoma occurs relatively late in the course of AIDS, and other fatal complications (especially tuberculosis) have supervened before a lymphoma is recognized.

DIAGNOSIS AND TREATMENT

Hodgkin's Disease. This tumor requires a biopsy, because proper diagnosis depends on the identification of the characteristic Reed-Sternberg cells in the histologic specimen. HD may not be easily distinguished from NHL on clinical grounds, except that the tumors are almost always nodal, more frequently involve the mediastinal and hilar lymph nodes, and tend to spread in a contiguous pattern. Clinical staging divides nodal tumors into local (stage I), regional (stage II), above and below the diaphragm (stage III), and extranodal (stage IV).

Treatment consists of radiation therapy for early stages and alternating courses of combination chemotherapy for more advanced disease. The recommended regimen in 1996 was MOPP (nitrogen mustard or cyclophosphamide, vincristine, procarbazine, and prednisone) alternating every 3 to 4 weeks with ABVD (Adriamycin, bleomycin, vinblastine, and dacarbazine). The treatment is given for two courses beyond complete response. The prognosis is excellent, with greater than 90% complete response and 75% long-term survival.

Non-Hodgkin's Lymphoma. These tumors may be nodal or extranodal. BL in Central Africa develops in the jaw or face (Fig. 12–9), in the abdominal organs, or in the bone marrow and along the spinal cord and grows rapidly to large size within a few weeks. Adult lymphomas are more heterogeneous but commonly present as cervical lymphadenopathy that is sometimes massive. The differential diagnosis must include tuberculosis, although lymphomatous nodes are firm and rubbery whereas tuberculous nodes are soft and mobile.

Because of delays in histologic reporting in the tropics, the best method of diagnosing NHL is by aspiration cytology, by making imprints of freshly excised tumor ("touch preps"), or by cytologic examination of pleural fluid or ascites. An experienced hematologist, examining Giemsa-stained preparations, should be able to detect a lymphoma, although the histologic type (based on nodal architecture) would not be evident. BL, histiocytic lymphoma, and lymphocytic lymphoma can be distinguished cytologically, and treatment can begin without delay.

The best therapy for BL is cyclophosphamide, in a single intravenous dose of 1000 mg/m^2, repeated for two doses beyond complete remission. If available, methotrexate (15 mg orally daily for 3 days) and vincristine (2 mg IV) should be given along with cyclophosphamide (COM therapy). In patients with suspected renal tumors or kidney impairment, fluid intake should be encouraged to avoid the tumor lysis syndrome (impaired renal excretion of necrotic tumor components such as potassium, urates, and phosphates). Allopurinol, 100 mg twice daily, can be given to avert urate nephropathy in patients with large tumors.

The best therapy for all other NHLs is a combination of cyclophosphamide (750 mg/m^2 IV, day 1), doxorubicin (50 mg/m^2, day 1), vincristine (2 mg IV, day 1), and prednisone

(100 mg/m² daily) for 5 days. This so-called CHOP regimen is repeated every 3 weeks, for two courses beyond complete remission. Again, adequate hydration should be maintained throughout therapy.

The prognosis for chemotherapy of the NHLs is excellent, and oncologic assistance should be sought whenever this diagnosis is suspected. The rates of complete remission are 80 to 90%, and the cure rate is over 50%. Therefore, every effort should be made to achieve an early diagnosis and to institute appropriate therapy, even in the tropical setting.

■ LEUKEMIA

DEFINITION. The leukemias are distinguished by cell type of origin (lymphoid, myeloid, monocytic) and by their clinicopathologic features (acute, subacute, chronic).

EPIDEMIOLOGY AND ETIOLOGY. In general, the incidence rates of leukemias are lower in tropical countries than in the United States and Europe (Table 12–2), although the differences are not large. In part, this may relate to underdiagnosis in tropical countries; there are, however, some distinct differences in epidemiology of specific leukemias.

Acute Leukemia. Acute lymphocytic leukemia (ALL) is the most common childhood cancer of developed countries, with a marked peak in incidence at age 2 to 3 years. Immunologically, the cell type in ALL among this age group is "common" lymphocytes, derived from B-cell precursors. This peak is absent or much reduced in many developing countries, and its amplitude depends on the level of socioeconomic development, both between populations and over time. These observations suggest that some environmental exposure is responsible for childhood ALL; one current hypothesis is that ALL represents a rare response to delayed exposure to a common infectious agent. The incidence of myeloid leukemia increases gradually with age, as does the sex ratio. Incidence rates seem to be similar in different areas, although high rates have been reported in Pacific island populations. In Africa, about 10 to 25% of children with acute myeloid leukemia (AML) present with chloroma.

AML and ML are caused by exposure to ionizing radiation as well as to some drugs (e.g., chloramphenicol) and chemicals (e.g., benzene), although the fraction of cases attributable to such agents is very small.

Chronic Leukemia. Chronic lymphocytic leukemia (CLL) is a disease of the elderly, in whom it is frequently discovered as an incidental finding during investigations for other complaints. Thus, it may be less frequently diagnosed in developing countries than in those where white blood counts in the elderly are routinely performed. In addition, CLL is genuinely rare in populations in East and Southeast Asia.

DIAGNOSIS AND TREATMENT

Acute Leukemia. The acute leukemias are rare in the tropics but can be cured with chemotherapy. Unfortunately, the clinical signs and symptoms (anemia, abnormal bleeding, fever) can mimic many other disorders. The determination must be made on blood films and bone marrow examination, a diagnostic capability that is often not available. For ALL, complete remissions can be readily obtained with vincristine and prednisone. Postremission consolidation and maintenance require polychemotherapy (methotrexate, mercaptopurine, arabinosyl cytosine, asparaginase, and others) along with chemoradioprophylaxis of the CNS. AML is treated with daunorubicin and arabinosyl cytosine to eradicate marrow myeloblasts, and the resulting marrow hypoplasia requires extensive hematologic and antibiotic support. Successful in the West, bone marrow transplantation is not feasible in most tropical countries.

Chronic Leukemia. Patients with chronic leukemias present with splenomegaly, fever, and anemia—also common manifestations of other tropical disorders—and require a bone marrow examination for diagnosis. CLL is treated with prednisone and chlorambucil, whereas CML is managed with hydroxyurea and busulfan. Although neither condition is curable, such therapy can palliate symptoms for many years.

Bibliography

Berrino F, Sant M, Verdecchia A, et al (eds): Survival of Cancer Patients in Europe: The EUROCARE Study. IARC Sci Publ 132; 1995.

Bracken MB, Brinton LA, Hayashi K: Epidemiology of hydatidiform mole and choriocarcinoma. Epidemiol Rev 6:52, 1984.

de Thé G, Geser A, Day NE, et al: Epidemiological evidence for causal relationship between Epstein-Barr virus and Burkitt's lymphoma from Ugandan prospective study. Nature 274:56, 1978.

Fleming AG: The epidemiology of leukaemias and lymphomas in Africa—an overview. Leuk Res 9:35, 1985.

Garnick MB: Prostate cancer: Screening, diagnosis and management. Ann Intern Med 118:804, 1993.

Greaves MF: Speculations on the cause of childhood acute lymphoblastic leukaemia. Leukemia 2:120, 1988.

Kelsey JL, Gammon MD: Epidemiology of breast cancer. Epidemiol Rev 12:228,1990.

Kosary CL, Gloeckler Ries LA, Miller BA, et al: SEER Cancer Statistics Review, 1973–1992.

Miller AB (ed): Cervical Cancer Screening Programmes: Managerial Guidelines. Geneva, World Health Organization, 1992.

Newton R, Ferlay J, Reeves G, et al: Effect of ambient solar ultraviolet radiation on incidence of squamous-cell carcinoma of the eye. Lancet 347:1450, 1996.

Niloff JM: Cancer of the uterine cervix. N Engl J Med 334:1230, 1996.

Parkin DM, Stiller CA: Childhood cancer in developing countries: Environmental factors. Int J Pediatr Hematol Oncol 2:411, 1995.

Parkin DM, Pisani P, Ferlay J: Estimates of the worldwide incidence of eighteen major cancers in 1985. Int J Cancer 54:594, 1993.

Pisani P, Parkin DM, Ferlay J: Estimates of the worldwide mortality from eighteen major cancers in 1985. Implications for prevention, and projections of future burden. Int J Cancer 55:891, 1993.

Pontén J, Adami HO, Bergström R, et al: Strategies for global control of cervical cancer. Int J Cancer 60:1, 1995.

Sankaranarayanan R, Black R, Parkin DM (eds): Cancer Survival in Asia, Africa and Latin America. IARC Sci Publ 145, 1998.

13 *Surgery*

John L. Tarpley and Donald E. Meier

■ GENERAL PRINCIPLES

The authors' 1996 survey of physicians practicing surgery in hospitals in Africa, the Middle East, and Asia concluded that the major challenges to adequate surgical care were poverty, shortage of supplies, maintenance of equipment, and the lack of trained surgeons and anesthetists. The ubiquity of the human immunodeficiency virus (HIV) was assumed and hardly mentioned. These physicians reported an operative case frequency very different from their colleagues in the developed world. The elective procedures most frequently performed were herniorrhaphy, hysterectomy, cesarean section, prostatectomy, and skin grafting. The most often performed emergency procedures were cesarean section, laparotomy for acute abdomen, laparotomy for ectopic gestation, operations for incarcerated or strangulated hernia, and trauma or fracture wound care. Because of unreliable epidemiologic studies and deficient diagnostic capabilities, comparisons among disease occurrence frequencies between the developing and developed worlds are of limited value; however, definite differences do exist. Other related observations were the collapse of national health care systems, the emigration of trained national surgeons, and the late presentation of patients seeking care. The estimated number of surgeons per 100,000 population is only 7 for Colombia, 1.5 for the Philippines, and 0.5 for West Africa, as compared with the United States with 51 surgeons per 100,000 persons; therefore, in developing countries physicians with minimal or no surgical training as well as nonphysicians perform operations.

In the past decade the poverty gap between the developed and developing worlds has increased by 30%. An estimated 30,000 university-trained medical personnel left Africa during the 1980s as a consequence of failing economies and vanishing support for education and research. Compounding the depletion of human resources and the economic downturn are increasing HIV disease, civil wars, burgeoning refugee populations, and the prevalence of land mines planted for warfare purposes. On the other hand, some Pacific nations (e.g., Malaysia) have demonstrated economic and social development over the past decade with a more Western pattern of disease (e.g., intestinal obstruction) emerging. Thus the tropics is a heterogeneous geographic region, with some countries expanding their economies and others, largely sub-Saharan Africa, being stagnant or deteriorating. Heterogeneity also exists within an individual country. High-level government officials, the national elite, and members of the international community have access to health care resources, which are not readily available to the average citizen. Many developing countries spend less than $10 per capita each year for health needs.

▪ PRACTICAL ASPECTS OF SURGERY IN DEVELOPING COUNTRIES

The essentials for a tropical surgical service are basic equipment, sterile supplies, and anesthesia. Infrastructural necessities include water, electricity, anesthesia equipment and supplies, sterilization capability, a dynamic supply system, and adequate personnel. Laboratory, transfusion, radiology, and histopathology services are desirable but not essential to the tropical surgeon, whose most reliable diagnostic tools are clinical experience and judgment predicated on history, physical examination and, at times, operative exploration. Alternating rainy and dry seasons with relatively high average temperatures year-round are the norm; therefore, attention must be paid to providing acceptable working conditions and to protecting supplies and equipment from extremes of humidity, dust, heat, dryness, and insect infestation. Air conditioning, refrigeration, dehumidifiers, equipment covers, and other strategies for dealing with these adverse conditions must be considered and instituted as finances allow.

WATER. Public utilities, even if available, might not supply water reliably. Entrapment and holding systems (cisterns), wells, bore holes, and pumps for rivers or ponds can serve as primary or supplementary water sources.

ELECTRICITY. Hospitals in developed countries maintain back-up generators to ensure uninterrupted electrical supply during power failures. These generators may also serve as the sole source of electricity or as a supplement to public power. On-line stabilizers and circuit-breaking systems are strongly recommended to protect electrical equipment from destructive current fluctuations.

STERILIZATION TECHNIQUES. Four sterilization techniques can be used to meet differing needs: soaking in an antiseptic solution, boiling, steam autoclaving, and gassing with ethylene oxide. A steam autoclave powered by electric-

ity, gas, wood, coal, or kerosene is preferred for sterilizing instrument sets. Because disposable gowns, drapes, and linens are prohibitively expensive, surgical linens are sterilized using a steam autoclave. Soaking solutions will sterilize scissors, blades, and needles without the attendant dulling or rusting caused by steam autoclaving. Boiling, which does not kill spores, is not routinely employed but can serve as a "flash" technique for a dropped instrument. Commercially available small ethylene oxide ampule systems (e.g., Anpro) allow repeated sterilization of rubber and plastic tubes, catheters, drains, electrical cords, and instruments such as diathermy pencils and power drills.

ANESTHESIA. Anesthetic options range from vocal and hypnotic techniques to acupuncture, to local or regional conduction and dissociative and general anesthetic techniques. The choice of a particular method depends on the patient, the procedure, the availability of drugs and trained personnel, and the preference of the patient and surgeon. Of prime importance in all anesthetic techniques is airway management. The 11 golden rules of anesthesia must be followed regardless of the level of medical sophistication (Table 13–1). Pulse oximeters, durable and relatively affordable, greatly increase the safety of anesthesia delivery by allowing continuous monitoring of oxygenation and early detection of problems, which often can be corrected by simple airway repositioning. A pulse oximeter should become standard equipment in all tropical operating rooms and not be viewed as a high-tech luxury. Most elective operations below the diaphragm can be performed using spinal anesthesia. Operations on the upper extremity can be performed with an axillary block or intravenous regional technique. Local anesthetics with or without supplemental sedation can be used in many cases, including herniorrhaphy, in selected patients. General anesthesia capability necessitates additional equipment and personnel. Inhalational anesthetic systems that are technologically appropriate for the tropics have been developed. Drawover units, exemplified by the ubiquitous EMO (Epstein Macintosh Oxford) ether vaporizer, do not require compressed gases or electricity and have been modified for use with halothane. Because halothane has a cardiodepressant action, it should be given with oxygen enrichment. Portable oxygen concentrators can supply up to 6 L oxygen/minute to supplement these drawover systems (Fig. 13–1). Air compressors employed in combination with Boyle-type units can provide freshly compressed air as the carrier gas,

TABLE 13–1. The Eleven Golden Rules of Anesthesia

1. Perform an adequate history and physical examination.
2. Perform operations on fasting patients. For abdominal emergencies, empty the stomach with a nasogastric tube and use a crash induction.
3. Place the patient on a tilt-top table.
4. Check the anesthetic equipment BEFORE you begin.
5. Always have suction capability available.
6. Keep the airway clear and open.
7. Be prepared to control the patient's ventilation. (Have an ambu-type bag available.)
8. Have a good IV line (optional in some instances of local anesthesia or IM ketamine).
9. Monitor the patient frequently.
10. Have someone around to help.
11. Be ready with equipment and agents to manage resuscitation from a cardiopulmonary arrest.

IM, intramuscular; IV, intravenous.
Concepts covered in King M (ed): Primary Anaesthesia. Oxford, England, Oxford University Press, 1986.

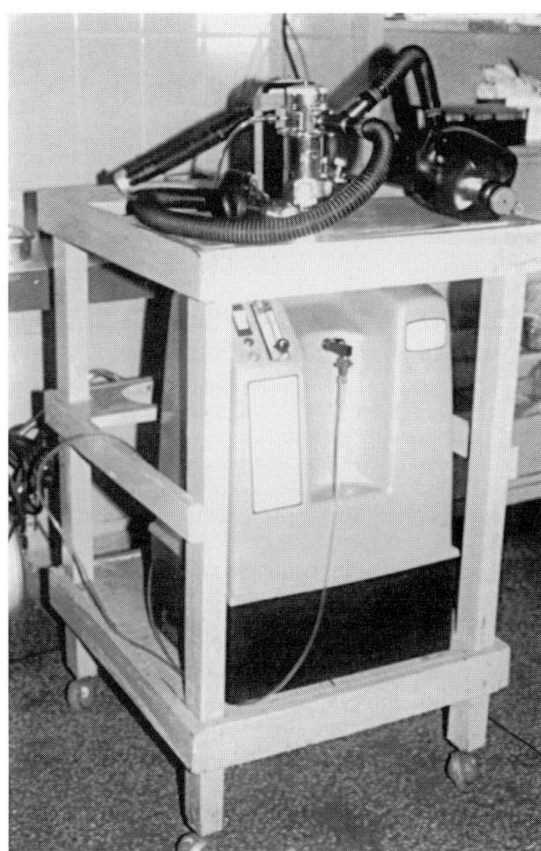

Figure 13–1. Drawover vaporizer and oxygen concentrator: inhalational general anesthesia without commercial gas cylinders.

thus eliminating the need for expensive and hard-to-find nitrous oxide.

Ketamine, a neuroleptic agent, provides dissociative anesthesia. It is used extensively in the developing world because of its effectiveness, availability, relatively low cost, and presumed safety. Airway monitoring is mandatory. In a prospective study using pulse oximetry the arterial oxygenation saturation of hemoglobin (SpO_2) dropped below 90% in one fifth of children and below 85% in one eighth. These drops occurred more often after intramuscular than after intravenous injections and were abrupt without premonitory signs. Eighty-three percent of children with lowered SpO_2 responded to airway manipulation with a jaw thrust, and only 3% of the total series required supplemental face mask oxygen. None required intubation or positive pressure ventilation. Ketamine does not provide muscle relaxation. It may serve as the sole anesthetic agent, as an induction agent, or as one part of a balanced technique when combined with a muscle relaxant, control of the airway, and controlled ventilation. Intramuscular ketamine safely anesthetizes children for dressing or cast changes, burn wound care, herniorrhaphy or, with repeated injections, for even longer procedures such as clubfoot operations. For adults, intravenous ketamine is especially useful as a short-duration anesthetic for dressing changes or incision and drainage procedures. Benzodiazepine co-medication decreases emergence phenomena in adults. Because ketamine does not lower the blood pressure, it is useful for induction of general anesthesia in emergency situations.

Emergency intra-abdominal procedures present an anesthetic problem. Gastric decompression to minimize the risk of aspiration is obligatory before delivery of any anesthetic in such situations. Intrathecal (spinal) anesthesia can be used for emergency procedures below the diaphragm; however, hypovolemia must be corrected before anesthesia delivery because the spinal technique abolishes the sympathetic tone of the lower extremities, increases the capacitance, and produces hypotension. A general anesthetic with a controlled airway is safer in emergency situations if appropriate equipment, agents, and personnel are available.

EQUIPMENT AND SUPPLIES. Equipment decisions are based on the surgeon's needs in relation to the hospital's capability to acquire and maintain technologically appropriate materials. Operating room essentials, in addition to a pulse oximeter, include an adjustable table, a lighting system, suction, and instruments. Nonessential but useful are an electrocautery, a fiberoptic headlight, and a table-mounted self-retaining retractor for upper abdominal procedures.

Laparoscopy as a minimally invasive technique for diagnosis and treatment is being introduced throughout the tropics, in part to compensate for the nonavailability of computed tomography (CT) and magnetic resonance imaging. Diagnostic laparoscopic procedures using nondisposable equipment and locally crafted dissectors can permit a reduction in nontherapeutic laparotomy, especially in the sexually active female when pelvic pathology is difficult to distinguish from appendicitis. Creative surgeons in India have decreased the instrument cost to $1.20 per patient. Laparoscopy is especially appealing for decision making in obstetrics and gynecology. Three obstacles to broader introduction of laparoscopy include equipment cost, subsequent maintenance, and the training of the surgical team.

Conditions in the tropics vary from hospital to hospital, but expense, erratic availability, pilferage, deterioration, and lack of domestic production complicate the maintenance of an adequate central store for supplies and drugs. The tropical surgeon must decide which supplies and drugs are essential and then obtain them locally when possible, import them, or improvise from local materials. Nylon fishing line can substitute for monofilament suture and carpet or sewing thread can substitute for multifilament suture. Plastic food storage bags serve as inexpensive barrier-protection gloves when handling dressings, examining wounds, and performing digital rectal examinations. For centuries, worn sheets and cloth have been converted into rolled bandages. Towels can be cut to serve as lap pads. Organization, frugality, improvisation, repeated use of "disposable" equipment, and the encouragement of local manufacture can improve the supply system.

PERSONNEL. The tropical surgeon must recruit, train, and motivate physicians, nurses, and technicians to perform at the highest level possible. Anesthesia personnel constitute a striking example; some countries, e.g., Malawi, may have only one or two physician-anesthesiologists for the whole nation. The general surgeon or general medical practitioner along with a personally trained nurse or technician is the anesthesia department in most tropical hospitals. Small group identity emphasizing each member's sense of responsibility, worth, and importance is key in developing a viable surgical service.

TRANSFUSION SERVICE. The transfusion service is largely a blood typing and collecting station and not a blood storage facility because transfusions often involve on-the-spot donor recruitment and immediate transfusion. The blood bank is heavily used by the obstetric unit owing to multiparity, short intervals between parturition, poor nutrition, and peripartum hemorrhage. Vehicular trauma victims are another major user. Children may have chronic or acute anemia of nutritional, hemolytic, hemoglobinopathic, or unknown origin and often require transfusion. Local customs and beliefs can inhibit blood donation; therefore, establishing and maintaining a blood bank in such areas is always difficult and often impossible. "Walking" blood banks, whereby volunteers in an institution, organization, or community are typed, can provide a measure of emergency supply. Potential transmission of hepatitis and HIV is a major consideration in determining blood banking policies worldwide. Unfortunately, even in highly endemic areas, some centers do not screen for either hepatitis or HIV. Increasingly, but not uniformly, HIV screening has been implemented throughout the tropics. Expense and the unreliable availability of testing kits interfere with compliance, thus substantially increasing the risk to the recipient. In parts of central, eastern, and southern Africa, one third of women attending antenatal clinics are seropositive for HIV. Hepatitis screening remains more problematic because of the complexity, expense, and requirement for trained technicians. Currently in the United States, the risk of HIV transmission via transfusion is placed at 1 per 493,000 persons; hepatitis B virus (HBV) risk is 1 per 63,000 persons; hepatitis C virus (HBC) risk is 1 per 103,000 persons; and the risk of bacterial infection is 1 in 25,000 persons. This risk in Third World hospitals is much greater. Malaria parasite transmission is quite common and Chagas' disease can also be transmitted in blood products. Alternatives to transfusion are few, because hemoglobin substitutes and volume expanders other than crystalloid solutions are not usually available. Autotransfusion has been much touted but infrequently practiced in most tropical medical centers. For some elective procedures with an anticipated transfusion requirement, patients can donate a unit of blood at weekly intervals for 2 or 3 weeks before the operation, take hematinics, follow a good diet in the interim, and then receive their own banked blood at the time of operation. This delayed autotransfusion has only limited application, however, because most transfusion requirements occur in emergencies or in debilitated patients.

LABORATORY. Physician interest and involvement are important determinants of laboratory function and quality control. In the authors' 1996 survey of tropical hospitals the laboratories had the following capabilities: one half, blood urea nitrogen or creatinine tests; two fifths, liver function tests; one fourth, blood cultures and electrolyte determinations; and one eighth, coagulation studies (e.g., prothrombin time, partial thromboplastin time, and INR); and almost none, arterial blood gases. Encouragingly, almost all could screen for HIV, but reagents and test kit availability were problematic. Hepatitis screening was not uniformly available.

IMAGING AND ENDOSCOPY. Outside of teaching hospitals and certain urban medical centers, the tropical surgeon rarely encounters radiologists, functioning fluoroscopic units, or interventional technique capability (Chapter 21). Ultrasound offers a diagnostic modality that is relatively inexpensive, noninvasive, portable, easy to maintain but, unfortunately, quite operator dependent. The accuracy, dependability, and reproducibility are proportional to the interest and competence of the operator, whether it is the physician or a locally trained technician. Ultrasound is especially useful in assessing the pelvis for obstetrics, but it also can provide the surgeon with important anatomic information about the biliary tree, liver, pancreas, and kidneys. Ultrasonography can detect ascites, distinguish solid from cystic masses, and localize intra-abdominal abscesses; and it is having an increasing role in the diagnosis and follow-up of parasitic diseases, e.g., schistosomiasis, hydatid cysts, amebic liver abscess, and lymphatic filariasis.

Endoscopic capability has become more widespread, and flexible fiberoptic esophagogastroduodenoscopy is sometimes found even in peripheral areas. Initial cost and equipment maintenance, however, limit the availability of this valuable diagnostic tool.

HISTOPATHOLOGY. Frozen-section capability is usually unavailable. Unless specimens are processed locally, the turnaround time for histopathologic reports can take months. Decisions relating to diagnosis, adequacy of margins, or institution of chemotherapy (e.g., antitubercular or antineoplastic) must therefore be made on clinical grounds alone or deferred for unacceptably long periods.

■ DIFFERENCES IN SURGICAL PRACTICE BETWEEN TROPICAL AND TEMPERATE SETTINGS

Patients in the developing world tend to be younger than patients in the developed world, but they present with more advanced disease. They tend to be undernourished instead of overnourished and have less comorbid disease, especially atherosclerotic vascular disease and smoking-related pulmonary disease. Few operative candidates are immunocompromised by steroids, concomitant cancer chemotherapy, or cyclosporine; however, the rising prevalence of HIV disease is a constant consideration. Distance, inconvenience, expense, and lack of a perceived need limit follow-up for subsequent evaluation, treatment, and physiotherapy. The physician's knowledge of treatment outcomes is therefore severely limited, and information sharing by surgeons is often anecdotal.

PROCEDURE PROFILES. Trauma, infection, and obstetric emergencies crowd elective cases and consume most of the surgeon's time. Operating rooms in developing countries often have poor illumination and climate control, with dust and flying insects a normal part of the operating room environment. Operative cases tend to be of short duration and are made as simple as possible.

■ AN OVERVIEW OF SURGICAL PRACTICE IN THE TROPICS

GENERAL SURGERY. Trauma, infections, neoplasms, and abdominal problems including groin hernias constitute the four major areas of general surgery. Endocrine procedures are generally limited to the thyroid. Vascular procedures are for trauma only; and transplants, until recently, have been exceptional.

Trauma. In many tropical wards half of the surgery beds are filled by trauma victims: vehicular, penetrating, thermal, falls, farming-industrial related, and warfare (including land mine) injuries. Although mortality is high, morbidity and disability in the survivors also pose great economic and social costs for families and society. The proximity of a medical facility to major highways will determine the volume of accident victims treated. Some of the world's highest traffic fatality rates are reported from tropical countries. Accident scene and transport care is generally rendered by untrained "good Samaritans" without regard for spinal injuries. Emergency rooms and trauma centers, if available, are seldom equipped or staffed adequately. Human factors account for at least 85% of vehicular accidents with overloading and overcrowding in cars, vans, open trucks, and matutus. Vehicle and roadway maintenance is grossly deficient. South African physicians report a disturbing change in the pattern of penetrating torso trauma in KwaZulu/Natal over the past decade with a 30% decline in stab wounds and a greater than 800% increase in gunshot wounds. Wound care and coverage comprise much of a tropical surgeon's daily work. Muscle, myocutaneous, and fasciocutaneous flap techniques

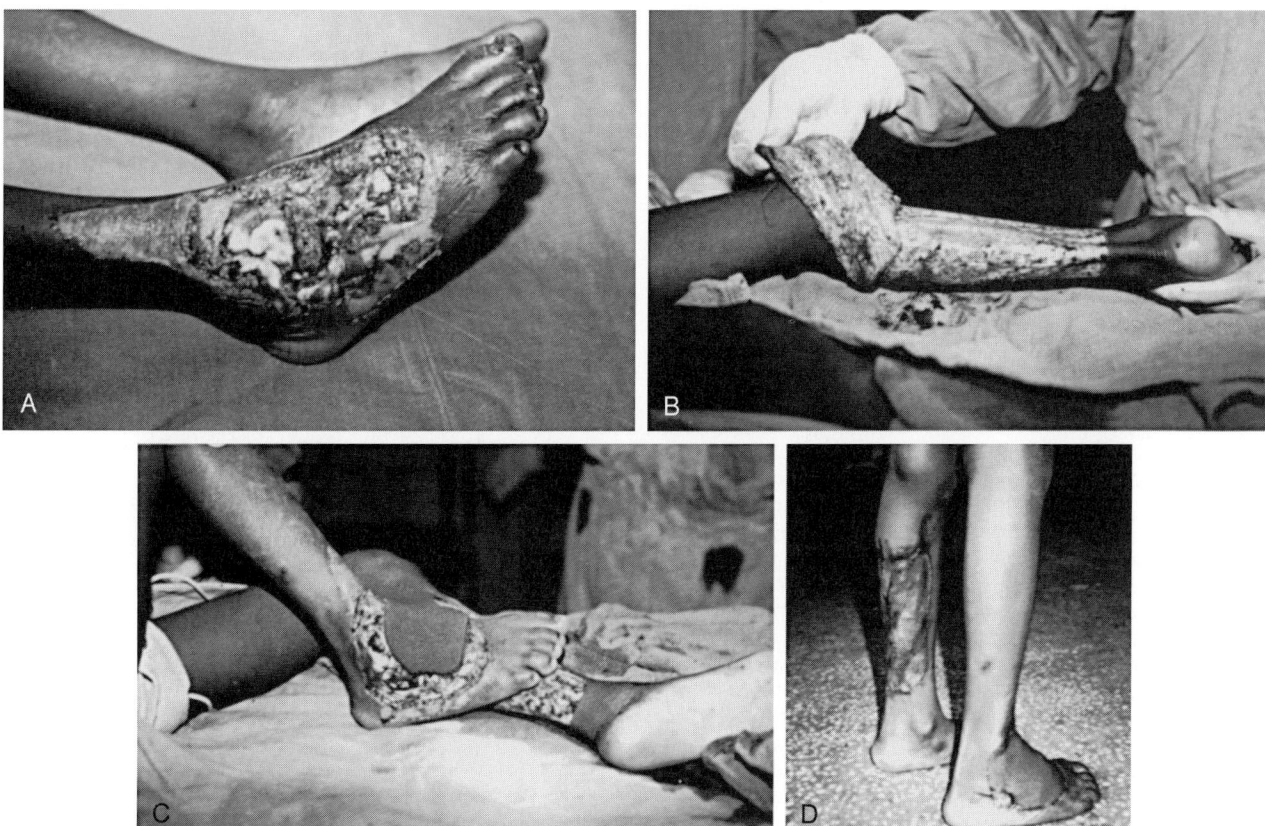

Figure 13–2. A 5-year-old boy's right foot traumatized by a taxi. *A,* Preoperative view with exposed ankle joint, tarsal joints, and soft tissue defect. *B,* Fasciocutaneous flap elevated from the left calf. *C,* Cross-leg flap placed to cover right foot defect. *D,* Postoperative result: full coverage and function.

not requiring a microscope appreciably expand the surgeon's options in dealing with wound coverage problems (Fig. 13–2).

It is estimated that 100 million land mines are currently deployed in the world in over 60 countries. Land areas needed for agriculture are potential "killing fields" for farmers in Southeast Asia, Mozambique, Angola, and much of the Third World. In Cambodia, one of every 235 civilians in a recent survey had a loss secondary to a land mine injury. There are an estimated 200,000 amputees in Vietnam. Eighty percent of the world's amputees live in the developing world. After initial treatment, rehabilitation and acquisition of a prosthesis offer the only hope for future self-sufficiency for the victim. Prosthesis production is not a one-time job, but an ongoing process since prostheses will in time require repair and replacement. Artificial limbs produced for dysvascular amputees are expensive even for Americans and Europeans and are out of financial reach for developing world amputees. Prostheses like the Jaipur limb and foot can be improvised locally to meet basic ambulation needs for amputees in the developing world.

Bites. Human bites as well as dog, cat, wild animal, snake, spider, and insect bites and scorpion stings cause local and systemic problems. Human bites are often underrated and mismanaged. Many bites are near hand joints with possible joint violation. Infections frequently occur. A common offender is *Eikenella corrodens,* a gram-negative rod that is sensitive to penicillin. The hand joints must be examined closely, opened if there is any suspicion of violation, irrigated, and left unsutured. The patient should be admitted for antibiotic administration and extremity elevation. Dog and cat bites

often inoculate *Pasteurella multocida,* which is sensitive to ampicillin or penicillin (Chapter 63). Rabies is a major concern with dog and wild animal bites (Chapter 30). Poisonous snakebites vary in incidence and type by topography and locale (Chapter 125.5). Considerations are for local and systemic (antivenom) treatment. Wound excision and fasciotomy may be required to treat local and vascular compartment problems. Procaine infiltration, ice, and analgesics can relieve the pain of scorpion envenomation. Hypersensitivity reactions are a threat to individuals stung by bees and wasps, and resuscitative measures should include epinephrine administration in cases of anaphylaxis. Black widow spider bites produce generalized muscle spasms, whereas brown recluse spider bites produce a local ulcer with ischemic necrosis (Chapter 127.3).

Abscesses. Abscesses of the skin, subcutaneous tissue, muscles (pyomyositis; Chapter 58), bones (osteomyelitis), joints (pyarthritis), thorax (empyema), and pericardial sac occur frequently and require drainage. *Staphylococcus aureus* is the most frequent etiologic agent. Multiple abscesses are common and may occur synchronously or metachronously. Early and wide drainage, preferably with antibiotic coverage, minimizes the hematogenous spread of infection. Hand infections pose a special difficulty because most patients delay seeking medical care. Even after drainage, antibiotics, elevation, and physiotherapy, residual hand deformity is the rule. Recent reports from Uganda associate tropical pyomyositis with HIV infection and suggest it as a sign of stage III to IV HIV disease.

Mycoses. Subcutaneous and deep mycotic infections occur throughout the tropics. The clinically important mycoses include mycetoma, aspergillus granuloma, phycomycosis, histoplasmosis, and chromoblastomycosis. Mycetoma (Madura foot) is a clinically defined lesion with three cardinal signs: swelling (chronic inflammation), multiple sinuses, and discharge of granules (Figs. 82–1 and 82–2). The disease is common in the thorny semidesert zones lying on either side of the fifteenth parallel north of the equator. Surgical treatment options include observation, local excision through healthy tissue, and amputation.

Cancer. More people die of cancer in the developing world than in the developed world (Chapter 12). Accurate statistics on the occurrence of cancer are not widely available for developing countries. Cancers of the cervix, stomach, breast, and prostate predominate. Increases in tobacco production and use in the developing world have been accompanied by corresponding increases in tobacco-related illnesses including lung cancer.

ABDOMINAL SURGERY. Changing disease patterns have been noted by gastrointestinal surgeons in the tropics. Appendicitis is more prevalent than 20 years ago, and intestinal obstruction is assuming a more Western pattern with adhesions and neoplasms joining hernias as common causes. Abdominal problems can be infectious, congenital, mechanical, obstructive, vascular, inflammatory, neoplastic, or a combination of these. Appendiceal perforation, strangulated bowel (intestinal obstruction, hernia, volvulus), typhoid perforations of the ileum, and perforation of duodenal ulcers are leading causes of secondary bacterial peritonitis and carry a high mortality rate because of advanced sepsis due to delays in seeking medical care. Primary hepatocellular carcinoma is more frequent in the high HBV-HCV areas of the world where aflatoxin might be another cofactor of oncogenesis. Spontaneous rupture of liver tumors can be a leading cause of hemoperitoneum. Amebic liver abscesses sometime rupture into the peritoneal cavity or into the pleural space, and necrotizing amebic colitis can mimic ischemic colitis or a toxic megacolon. Groin hernias frequently cause intestinal obstruction (Fig. 13–3). Because many persons seek care only for complications of a hernia, strangulation and peritonitis are not uncommon, sometimes causing fatalities. Appendicitis often progresses to perforation with abscesses or peritonitis by the time the patient seeks treatment.

Volvulus. Sigmoid volvulus is a frequent abdominal problem and in areas of East Africa constitutes a leading cause of intestinal obstruction. Previously healthy patients present with marked abdominal distention and tympany to percussion but without peritonitis unless strangulation or perforation has occurred. Although colonoscopic or sigmoidoscopic deflation can be attempted, operation is the usual treatment because the colon is often strangulated. If at laparotomy the bowel is viable, a rectal tube can be guided safely, the loop deflated, and the volvulus manually reduced. After a bowel preparation, an interval sigmoid resection should be performed to avoid the recurrence that is likely after simple reduction. Alternatively, with viable bowel, an on-table lavage can be performed, the sigmoid resected, and alimentary continuity can be re-established by a colorectostomy. When the sigmoid is strangulated, resection of the dead bowel with the creation of an end colostomy and mucus fistula or Hartmann pouch is recommended. Not infrequently, a loop of small bowel is caught up in a twist of the sigmoid colon mesentery, producing a concomitant closed-loop obstruction and strangulation of the small bowel, the so-called compound volvulus or ileosigmoid knotting. A small bowel resection and reanastomosis must be performed in addition to correction of the colonic volvulus.

Intestinal Obstruction and Inflammation. Although perforation and bleeding may complicate peptic ulcer disease, the

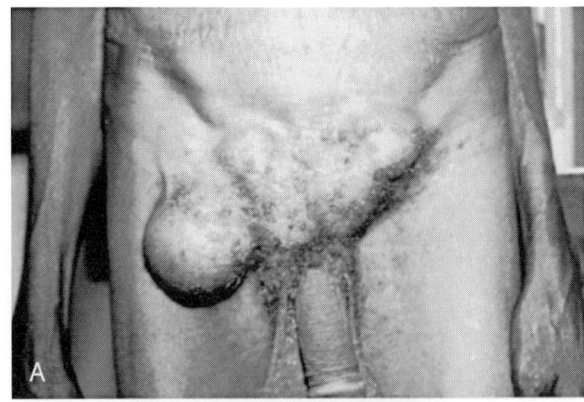

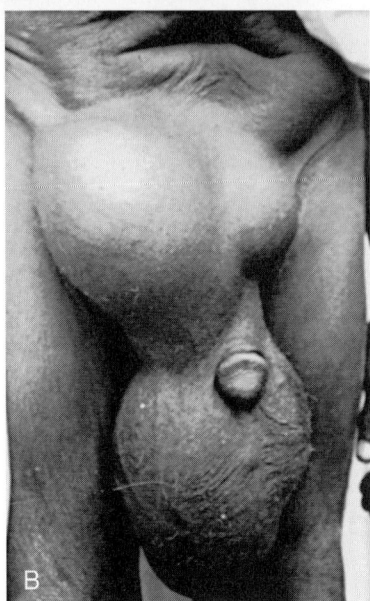

Figure 13–3. *A*, Femoral and inguinal hernias. *B*, Inguinoscrotal hernias.

leading operative indication in the developing world is gastric outlet obstruction. *Helicobacter pylori* has been called the most common bacterial infection in Africa (Chapter 45). *H. pylori* seropositivity of 57% to 80% was noted in Nigerian children, and it was 85% for adults in a random survey in northeast Nigeria. Mesenteric vascular diseases are not common. Although not diagnosed frequently in blacks, inflammatory-type bowel diseases mimicking regional enteritis or ulcerative colitis now occur in patients with HIV infections but usually prove to be infectious, not idiopathic. Enteritis necroticans (pig-bel), a particular problem in the highlands of New Guinea, is a necrotizing enteritis produced by *Clostridium perfringens* toxin (Chapter 44.3); operation and resection may be required to remove necrotic bowel.

Biliary Disease. Operative hepatobiliary and pancreatic diseases are not so often encountered in sub-Saharan Africa, although they are frequent in Asia, often secondary to ascarids and liver flukes obstructing the biliary or pancreatic ducts (Chapter 104). Cholecystitis appears to be increasing in the tropics; a 10-fold increase in the frequency of cholecystectomy over a 10-year period was reported in Saudi Arabia. Acalculous cholecystitis is a problem in the tropics. Gallbladder stones develop in patients with hemoglobinopathies.

Bezoars. Bezoars are concretions formed in the stomach. They are trichobezoars if they consist of hair and phytobezoars if composed of vegetable fibers. Bezoars are seen in edentulous patients with deficient mastication, in some young females, in patients after partial gastrectomy, and in psychiatric patients. Bezoars may occlude the stomach, produce a mass, and limit nutrition. They may also cause intestinal obstruction, ulceration, bleeding, or perforation. Although enzymatic dissolution of phytobezoars can be tried, the treatment for most patients is operative removal with subsequent counseling.

OBSTETRICS-GYNECOLOGY. Lack of antenatal care, obstructed labor, eclampsia, peripartum hemorrhage, ruptured ectopic gestations, and infertility are problems commonly seen by the tropical obstetrician. Most deliveries are performed in the patient's home with traditional birth attendants (TBAs) or older women supervising the delivery. Young age at first pregnancy, dietary deficiencies, and small stature increase the incidence of cephalopelvic disproportion. Not only does prolonged labor lead to an increased chance of infection and fetal and maternal loss, but it can also produce ischemia of the genital canal and adjacent tissues with eventual pressure necrosis and creation of a fistula. The incidence of vesicovaginal fistula in a community is an inverse indicator of the local level of obstetric care. Most obstetric fistulas are vesicovaginal and produce a continuous urine leak through the vagina, which results in an offensive odor and skin excoriation leading to exclusion and desertion by the husband, other family members, and friends. The majority of vesicovaginal and rectovaginal fistulas can be repaired through a vaginal approach using local tissues. Some larger fistulas and those with urethral loss may require labial flaps or a gracilis muscle flap to provide adequate support and to promote continence.

Close spacing between successive children, multiparity, and inadequate nutrition compromise the obstetric patient's health, resilience, and hemoglobin level. In areas where society demands many children and places a high priority on the production of a son and heir, the infertile woman or couple presents an obstetric challenge. Sexually transmitted diseases, conflicts between traditional and Western mores and practices, and the increasing incidence of criminal abortions affect obstetric practice. The tropical gynecologist routinely sees patients with fistulas, prolapse, and myomata. Neoplasms must be treated without sophistocated chemotherapeutic agents and without access to radiotherapy. Widespread public attention focuses on female circumcision and unsafe abortions. Female circumcision raises cultural, religious, and ethical issues; one in seven maternal deaths worldwide are related to unsafe abortion.

The United Nations Children's Fund recently reported that the difference between developed and developing countries is greater for maternal mortality rates than for any other commonly used index of health—a 15-fold difference of 30 versus 450 maternal deaths per 100,000 live births. They estimated that 585,000 women die each year in pregnancy and childbirth, with 18 million women suffering debilitating illness or obstetric injuries. One in 13 women in sub-Saharan Africa and 1 in 35 in South Asia die of causes related to pregnancy and childbirth, compared to 1 in 3200 in Europe, 1 in 3300 in the United States, and 1 in 7300 in Canada.

ORTHOPEDICS. Musculoskeletal problems in the tropics are ubiquitous and are covered in Chapter 14.

UROLOGY. Urologic problems may be congenital, infectious, obstructive, or neoplastic.

Congenital Lesions. Undescended testes, hypospadias, posterior urethral valves, and torsion of the testis (cord) are congenital anatomic problems. Histologic changes are noted in undescended testes by 18 months; orchiopexy by 18 months maximizes the chances for spermatogenesis. Children with hypospadias should not be circumcised because the foreskin can be utilized later for a flap when a surgeon with expertise in hypospadias repair can be consulted. Posterior urethral valves are diagnosed during the early months of life in males from the history of difficulty in initiating urination and a very weak urinary stream. A voiding cystourethrogram is the definitive test. Treatment consists of valve destruction, either endoscopically or through a perineal approach. A vesicostomy provides temporary treatment until a more definitive procedure can be performed. Torsion of the testis in a male with a tender scrotum-testis can be excluded only by direct observation. In societies in which procreation is nearly mandatory, all males without progeny who present with a swollen, tender scrotum-testis should undergo scrotal exploration for diagnosis. Although the ipsilateral testis with torsion often is unsalvageable, the contralateral testis can be protected by suturing the tunica albuginea testis to the tunica dartos at three sites.

Urinary Obstruction. Renal and ureteric stones are not prevalent among blacks, but Arabs in the Sudan and Yemen have frequent stone problems. Lithotomy is indicated for obstruction complicated by pain, progressive renal damage, or persistent infection. Because endoscopic and ultrasound techniques are generally not available, open operation is the usual procedure. Lower urinary tract obstructions in older men generally result from benign prostatic hypertrophy, prostatic carcinoma, or urethral stricture secondary to prior gonococcal urethritis. Benign prostatic hypertrophy is treated by prostatectomy, usually open rather than transurethral. Urethral stricture can be managed by repeated bougienage, suprapubic tube cystostomy, direct vision internal urethrotomy, or urethroplasty.

Urinary Tract Malignancies and Infections. Cancers of the kidneys, bladder, prostate, and penis (squamous cell carcinoma) are generally seen at an advanced, nonoperative stage (Chapter 12). Urinary tuberculosis should be considered in patients with acid pyuria or sterile pyuria (Chapter 77). Infection by *Schistosoma haematobium* may produce granulomas of the ureters and bladder and result in bleeding, obstructive uropathy, pyelonephritis, or carcinoma of the bladder (Chapter 118). Fournier's gangrene is a spontaneous gangrene of the skin of the scrotum and penis. The pathogenesis remains speculative. Multiple organisms have been cultured, including *C. perfringens*. The onset is sudden and painful, often in the dependent scrotum, and is accompanied by fever and toxemia. A partial- or full-thickness slough of the scrotum occurs after a few days, frequently exposing the testes. Penicillin, local wound care, and, at times, split skin grafts constitute treatment.

EAR-NOSE-THROAT AND DENTAL SURGERY. Foreign bodies, neoplasms, infections, allergic conditions, maxillofacial trauma, and congenital anomalies are all seen in a tropical surgical practice. Tuberculous cervical adenitis (Fig. 13–4), Ludwig's angina, dental abscesses, and otitis media with or without mastoiditis are common infections of the head and neck. Croup and laryngotracheobronchitis, especially as a complication of measles, may so compromise a child's airway that tracheostomy is mandatory. If nursing care, suctioning, and humidification are deficient, serious complications may accompany tracheostomy. Cancrum oris, or noma, usually seen in malnourished children, is a destructive, necrotic process (Fig. 13–5) that can produce oronasocutaneous fistulas and ankylosis of the temporomandibular joint. Once infarction, infection, and inflammation respond to debridement, penicillin, and diet, the resultant fibrosis and tissue defects present a formidable reconstructive challenge. Myocutaneous flaps such as the pectoralis major island flap can be used to repair these complex problems.

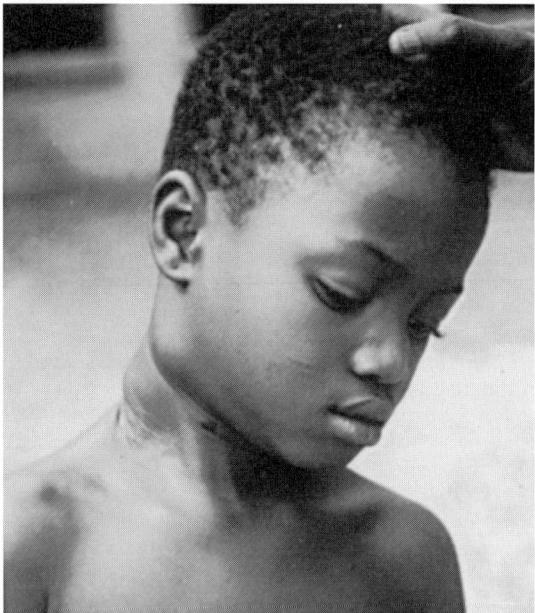

Figure 13–4. Tuberculous cervical lymphadenitis (scrofula) in an 8-year-old Yoruba boy.

Dental care is often extractive rather than preservative and preventive in nature and is not available in many rural areas. In a national survey in Nigeria, the percentages of decayed teeth were 30% in 12-year-olds, 43% in 15-year-olds, and 44% in adults 35 to 44 years old. It is estimated that 7 million Nigerians (estimated population 100 million) need extractions, and that about 23 million need conservative dental care.

PLASTIC SURGERY. Wound care occupies a significant percentage of the tropical surgeon's time as he or she attempts to deal with large, infected, neglected wounds using a minimum of equipment and supplies.

Burn Care. Thermal burns occur daily and often receive inadequate initial treatment with resultant high mortality from renal failure and burn wound sepsis. In acute burn survivors, residual contractures and hypertrophic scarring are often crippling. Skin-grafting capability for burn wound care is essential. Grafts may be taken freehand or with a drum or electric dermatome. The meshing technique of Tanner is recommended to allow expansion of the graft and to improve graft "take." Early tangential excision and skin grafting should be considered except for very extensive burns.

Hand Surgery. Burns of the hands are especially debilitating, but improved functional results can be obtained with early tangential excision and grafting, proper splinting, and conscientious physiotherapy. Infections and nonthermal hand injuries are very common and require prompt treatment to avoid fibrosis and contractures. The technique of groin-flap coverage is particularly helpful in dealing with hand injuries.

Cleft Lip and Palate. A common congenital abnormality is cleft lip with or without a palatal defect. The incidence of cleft lips is high in the Philippines and low in sub-Saharan Africa. Access to corrective procedures and rehabilitation is often poor. Parents, disturbed by the neonate's deformity, want immediate repair. Counseling is indicated because lip repairs traditionally are not undertaken until "10 weeks of age, 10 pounds of weight, and a hemoglobin level of at least 10 g/dL." Palatal repair is delayed until about 1 year of age

but should be performed before speech develops in order to prevent a nasalized speech pattern.

NEUROSURGERY. The imaging techniques, equipment, and personnel to detect and treat tumors, arteriovenous malformations, and various congenital abnormalities are rarely available (see Chapter 21). CT scanners are becoming available at a very few teaching hospitals and private clinics in the tropics, but scanner maintenance is a task.

Head Trauma. Tropical neurosurgery focuses on trauma. Without benefit of sophisticated diagnostic equipment, head injury victims who have deterioration in their level of consciousness or who develop lateralizing neurologic signs should undergo exploration through burr holes with drainage if an epidural or subdural hematoma is found. Patients with open, depressed skull fractures require operation for debridement, hemostasis, elevation, and closure and coverage of the dura. Pond fractures can be simply observed or elevated using an obstetric vacuum extractor.

Spinal Injuries. Spinal injuries, which often ensue from vehicular accidents or falls from trees, are a major cause of morbidity and mortality. Spinal cord injury rehabilitation programs are almost nonexistent in developing countries; and if the para- or quadriplegic patient survives the in-hospital period of stabilization by traction, he or she often will succumb to urinary or decubitus ulcer–related sepsis after discharge to home. Tuberculosis is also a common cause of paralysis. If deterioration of neurologic function in a patient with Pott's disease is recent or if it continues while the patient is receiving adequate antituberculous chemotherapy, drainage of the paraspinal abscess with spine stabilization should be considered (Chapters 14 and 77).

Pediatric Surgery. Special concerns in tropical pediatric surgery include the congenital anomalies of imperforate anus, bowel atresia, esophageal atresia, abdominal wall defects, and neural tube defects. Recent surveys in urban Pretoria and rural Transvaal reveal that the incidence of congenital anomalies in black South African neonates is as high as in other First World and Third World countries and in the rural areas may constitute a "silent epidemic" yet to be meaningfully addressed. These anomalies are apparent at birth, and parents may seek no treatment for such neonates and refuse operative intervention if it is offered. Hirschsprung's disease, urinary tract abnormalities, and pediatric tumors, on the other hand, are usually detected after the

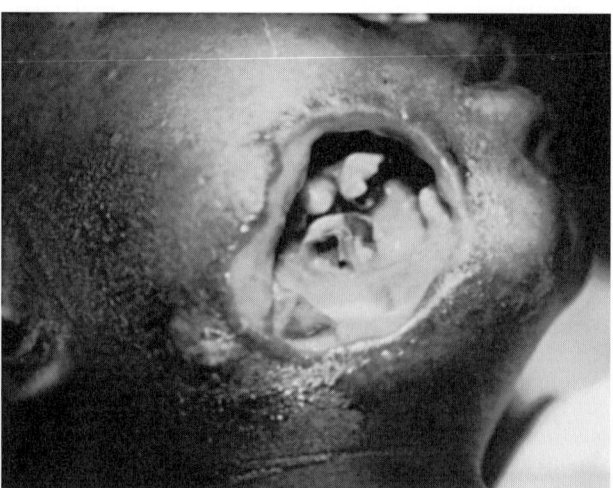

Figure 13–5. Cancrum oris (noma). Gangrenous stomatitis with soft tissue and bone defect producing an orocutaneous fistula in a 5-year-old malnourished boy.

child has been named and officially recognized as a family or clan member; thus surgical help is sought although stomas are often refused. Intussusception is the leading cause of intestinal obstruction in children 3 months to 2 years of age. Hydrostatic reduction is not routinely employed because of the uncertainty of adequate reduction as well as the scarcity of barium, film, and fluoroscopy units. Operative reduction is the usual management for intussusception, and a nonviable intussusceptum is common. The mortality rate is soberingly high.

CARDIOTHORACIC SURGERY. Pump oxygenators and the technological and financial support they require might be found at one or two medical centers in a developing country. Rheumatic fever with resultant valvular problems, congestive failure, congenital heart diseases, endomyocardial fibrosis and other cardiomyopathies, e.g., Chagas' heart disease, and the pericardial problems of constriction (tuberculosis) and effusion (pyopericardium) are the major problems facing the cardiologist and cardiac surgeon (Chapter 3). The noncardiac thoracic surgeon deals primarily with tuberculosis (Chapter 77), thoracic empyema (especially after measles), hemoptysis from destroyed lung, bronchiectasis, and lung abscess. Lung cancer has not been as widespread as in developed countries but is increasing as tobacco use increases. Hydatid cyst of the lung is focally prevalent in some areas with animal husbandry using dogs (Chapter 123.2).

OPHTHALMOLOGY. Eighty percent of the world's preventable blindness occurs in patients living in the developing world. Blindness results from trauma, trachoma (Chapter 32), onchocerciasis (Chapter 108), corneal scarring, xeropathia (dryness and vitamin A deficiency) (Chapter 130.1), and cataracts. The primary anatomic area is the anterior segment and the etiology is usually well-known. Cataracts blind 18 million persons in the Third World and this number is doubling every 20 to 25 years. A nation may have one or more major eye treatment centers, but only a select population has access to such care. Most people with treatable eye diseases never see an ophthalmic surgeon.

▪ SPECIFIC TOPICS OF SHARED INTEREST TO PHYSICIANS AND SURGEONS

TETANUS (Chapter 53). Even with expanded immunization programs, many in the tropics remain unprotected from tetanus. Neonatal tetanus remains a lethal, frequent problem in many areas. Certain injuries are more tetanus-prone than others, but without prior immunization and appropriate wound care, even trivial injuries are potentially lethal. Initial treatment for all patients with tetanus includes thorough wound debridement. A large neglected wound of the extremity may require amputation, and tetanus secondary to a septic abortion may necessitate a hysterectomy. Active and passive immunization should accompany debridement in the initial treatment of the unimmunized patient. Most deaths from tetanus result from asphyxia, aspiration, or pneumonia. A tube gastrostomy can be used to meet the accelerated nutritional needs of these patients without rendering the gastroesophageal sphincter incompetent as a nasogastric tube does.

TYPHOID (Chapter 75). Hemorrhage from and perforation of ileal ulcers are potentially fatal complications of typhoid fever. After prolonged periods of fever, catabolism, undernutrition, and immunosuppression, the patient often develops secondary bacterial peritonitis (Fig. 13–6). A properly randomized, prospective study to evaluate the comparability of operative versus nonoperative treatment for these exceedingly ill patients has not been reported. Published data sup-

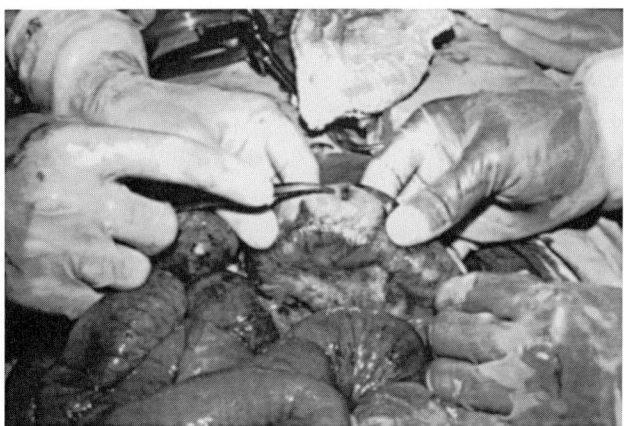

Figure 13–6. Perforation of the ileum in typhoid fever with secondary bacterial suppurative peritonitis.

port resuscitation followed by operative intervention to limit further contamination and to cleanse the peritoneal cavity. Simple two-layer closure in a transverse axis with chromic catgut and silk is adequate for one or two perforations. Multiple perforations require segmental resection with retention of the ileocecal valve if possible. Copious irrigation of the entire peritoneal cavity with saline is recommended. Operative mortality, although as low as 3% to 5% in some centers, is often in the 30% range. The perforation-to-operation interval and adequacy of resuscitation are important determinants of outcome. The aphorism "recognize, resuscitate, repair, recover, recuperate, rehabilitate" is applicable.

LEPROSY (Chapter 78). Patients with Hansen's disease may require surgical intervention to prevent or treat complications of the feet, hands, and eyes. Ulcers of the feet with or without accompanying osteomyelitis of the underlying bones demand bed rest, debridement, antibiotics, adequate footwear, and a change of lifestyle. Occasionally, ulcers necessitate a transtibial amputation. Tendon transfers can improve the pinch or intrinsic muscle function of a hand or counter a dropfoot gait, thus enhancing limb function and rehabilitation (Chapter 14).

TUBERCULOSIS (Chapter 77). Sub-Saharan Africa and Southeast Asia are the areas with the highest incidence of tuberculosis, which is compounded by drug resistance, the HIV epidemic, outmoded methods of treatment, and noncompliance with therapy. Pulmonary tuberculosis with cavities, empyema, and destroyed lung remains the primary presentation for *Mycobacterium tuberculosis*. Tuberculous adenitis (Fig. 13–4), abdominal and hepatic tuberculosis, Pott's disease with or without neurologic deficit (Chapter 14), urinary tuberculosis, and tuberculous arthritis are important differential diagnoses for the surgeon to consider in patients with failure to thrive, masses, or fever. Gastrointestinal tuberculosis and tuberculous peritonitis must be considered along with neoplasms in patients with weight loss, ascites, and an abdominal mass. Tuberculosis of the skin and breast may masquerade as carcinoma.

The diagnosis of pulmonary tuberculosis depends on symptoms, radiologic signs, and positive organism identification. The surgeon obtains material for diagnosis (bronchoscopy, lymph node biopsy) and treats complications. Tube thoracostomy is employed to treat pneumothorax, empyema, and pyopneumothorax. Elective resections are employed for bronchostenosis, bronchiectasis, destroyed lung, giant emphysematous bullas, resistant organisms, and recalcitrant patients with sputum-positive, localized open cavities. Elective pericardiectomy may be required in patients with constrictive pericarditis. Emergency thoracotomy with lobectomy or pneumonectomy is required in cases of life-threatening hemoptysis, a not unusual sequela of smoldering inflammation. Thoracoplasty procedures are not routine for residual pleural space conditions, but the Eloesser flap permits patients with space problems to go without a tube.

SCHISTOSOMIASIS (Chapter 118). Granuloma formation with bleeding, fibrosis, and stricture occurs in the lower gastrointestinal tract and the genitourinary tract.

Gastrointestinal Lesions. Intestinal polyps sometimes develop and require removal during colonoscopy because of bleeding. Schistosomiasis is the world's leading cause of portal hypertension. Periportal fibrosis following deposition of schistosomal ova in small portal venules increases presinusoidal resistance to portal blood flow. Treatment options for life-threatening variceal bleeding include medical management (vasopressin), balloon tamponade, injection sclerotherapy, variceal ligation, esophageal transection, and portal decompression. Because of better liver function, patients with schistosomiasis do better following shunt procedures than do those who bleed from alcoholic cirrhosis. Repeated hemorrhage, however, remains a frequent complication. A long-term follow-up of a Brazilian randomized trial comparing three operative options for treating portal hypertension from schistosomiasis found esophagogastric devascularization with splenectomy to be superior to either proximal or distal splenorenal shunting by virtue of the absence of encephalopathy and the lower mortality rate.

Urinary Tract Lesions. Urinary schistosomiasis can cause an obstructive uropathy with progressive renal failure. Intraluminal obstruction of the distal ureter and damage to the ureteric muscle with loss of peristalsis produce hydronephrosis. Preoperative assessment entails detection and treatment of active infection, assessment of renal function, and definition of anatomic lesions by radiologic methods. Operative options for an abnormal distal ureter include ureteroneocystostomy and a ureteric reconstruction (Boari flap or ileal ureter). Cystoplasty using sigmoid, cecal, or ileal bowel segments may be indicated in patients with a contracted bladder and can be combined with a ureteric replacement. Urinary schistosomiasis is a cause of carcinoma of the bladder (Chapter 12). Because such patients are often first seen with advanced disease, obstruction, and renal failure, few are candidates for total cystectomy. Urinary diversion, most frequently with a ureterocolostomy to avoid a stoma and appliance, may provide palliation.

HYDATID CYST (Chapter 123.2). Open surgical resection remains the treatment of choice for some patients with cystic hydatid disease (*Echinococcus granulosus* infection), although some excellent results following ultrasound-guided percutaneous aspiration (and injection of scolicides) of hydatid cysts in the liver have been recently reported. Hypertonic saline solution or 0.1% cetrimide is recommended as the operative scolicide in preference to formalin. The operative goal is removal of the cyst without (1) fluid leakage, which may cause toxic or anaphylactic reaction; (2) spillage of scolices or germinal epithelium, which may produce new cysts; or (3) bleeding and secondary infection. Alveolar hydatid disease of the liver (*E. multilocularis* infection) requires a partial hepatectomy for treatment (Chapter 123.3). Surgical resection, when possible, is recommended for polycystic hydatid disease (*E. vogeli* infection; Chapter 123.4).

AMERICAN TRYPANOSOMIASIS (Chapter 94). The "megasyndromes" cause either dysphagia from megaesophagus or constipation from megacolon. Surgical treatments for megaesophagus include partial or total resection of the esophagus, cardioplasty, and myotomy. However, a recent report from Brazil noted a 62% incidence of complications in patients operated on for chagasic megaesophagus, with one third requiring reoperation, and 88% having either a complication or postoperative dysphagia. Sigmoid resection is the operative treatment for megasigmoid. Toxic megacolon from Chagas' disease warrants total colectomy.

FILARIAL ELEPHANTIASIS (Chapter 106). Bancroftian, Malayan, and Timorian filariasis can produce secondary lymphedema and the chronic obstructive signs of elephantiasis involving the subcutaneous tissues of the scrotum and the lower extremities. Scrotal elephantiasis can be treated with excision of redundant tissue and placement of the testes in upper thigh adductor pockets or in a newly constructed scrotum. More than 20 operative procedures for the relief of chronic lower extremity lymphedema are extant, in itself an indication that none is superior. Operations for edematous extremities should be recommended only with hesitancy. The procedure employed most often at present is that of Charles (1912), in which the involved skin and lymphedematous subcutaneous tissue are excised down to deep fascia, and the fascia then skin-grafted.

ASCARIASIS

Intestinal Obstruction. In former decades small bowel obstruction was frequently attributed to a heavy ascaris worm burden (Fig. 104–2). Recent reviews attest that, although intestinal obstruction can occur, its incidence is low. In the patient exhibiting signs of partial bowel obstruction with a putty-like mass palpable on abdominal examination, a nonoperative trial of intravenous fluids and nasogastric suction is warranted to allow the obstruction to decompress; after the acute episode, vermicides are given to relieve the patient of the worm load. In the unusual instance of total intestinal obstruction, a history of recent anthelmintic use implies that the dead or dying worms have converted a partial obstruction into a complete obstruction requiring operative intervention. Options during laparotomy include milking the worm mass bolus into the cecum and right colon, enterotomy with manual worm removal and decompression, and, in rare instances, resection of compromised bowel.

Biliary Obstruction. Whereas intestinal obstruction requires a sizable nematode biomass, a single ascaris in the common bile duct can precipitate biliary tract obstruction with secondary jaundice or cholangitis. Biliary ascariasis is difficult to diagnose preoperatively without radiology and endoscopic retrograde cholangiopancreatography (Fig. 104–3). When infection is suspected, nonoperative management (intravenous fluids, nasogastric suction, antibiotics, and antispasmodics, with anthelmintic administration after the acute attack has subsided) can be successful. If a trial of nonoperative management is unsuccessful (deepening jaundice, increasing fever, peritonitis, increasing colic), common bile duct exploration is required for operative removal of the worm(s) and any associated calculi.

Ascaris has also been incriminated as a cause of volvulus, intussusception, appendicitis (Fig. 104–4), intestinal perforation, granulomatous peritonitis, pancreatitis, pyogenic cholangitis, acute cholecystitis, and perforation of the bile ducts. Considering the prevalence of this ubiquitous nematode, the actual number of patients who suffer surgical complications from ascariasis is extremely small.

ESOPHAGOSTOMIASIS (HELMINTHOMA). Reported from northern Ghana and Uganda, the nematode *Oesophagostomum*, a hookworm relative, can provoke an inflammatory reaction of the bowel in humans when larvae are ingested and penetrate the bowel mucosa. Tumor-like masses, granulomas, and abscesses may ensue, usually in the cecum and right colon, although the stomach, ileum, and even the abdominal wall may be involved. The disease may mimic appendicitis by the right lower quadrant presentation or may be confused with carcinoma or inflammatory lesions such as ameboma, ileocecal tuberculosis, or pyomyositis of the abdominal wall. Most helminthomas subside with nonoperative treatment, although complications (abscesses, intestinal obstruction, peritonitis) or uncertainty of diagnosis may require exploration.

HIV DISEASE AND NOSOCOMIAL VIRAL TRANSMISSION. Seropositivity for HIV in hospitalized adults may approach or exceed 50% in some tropical countries. In many tropical hospitals supplies are short and reuse of equipment is the rule. Open wards are crowded, water is often in short supply, and disposable gloves are not available. Serotyping kits are often reserved for the screening of blood for transfusion, not for diagnostic or confirmatory patient testing. Tropical wards and operating rooms float in a sea of secretions. Endoscopy equipment must be carefully and effectively cleaned to prohibit viral transmission while not damaging the fiberoptic units. Postoperative infections are increased several fold in HIV-positive patients compared with infection rates prior to the HIV era, especially in orthopedic procedures. Observing Universal Precautions is the ideal, because all blood and body secretions of all patients are considered potentially infectious for HIV as well as HBV, HCV, and other blood-borne pathogens. As was recently reported from Nigeria when three physicians and 19 others died from Lassa fever, there is a high price for poor medical practice. Likewise, Ebola outbreaks in Zaire point out the necessity of high standards of practice. Additional patients and health care providers will suffer without attention to rules for safe practice, surveillance, and continued medical education. Polypharmacy techniques using parenteral treatment for trivial conditions accompanied by a prime concern for profit are inimical to sane practice in this era of viral transmission. With Lassa and Ebola fevers, the outcome is acute and dramatic; with HIV transmission the time line, though measured in years, will result in an outcome as lethal.

Bibliography

Adegbembo AO, el-Nadeef MA, Adeyinka A: National survey of dental caries status and treatment needs in Nigeria. Int Dent J 45:35, 1995.

Adeloye A: Surgical services and training in the context of national health care policy: the Malawi experience. J Trop Med Hyg 96:215, 1993.

Ansaloni L: Tropical pyomyositis. World J Surg 20:613, 1996.

Arreola-Risa C, Mock CN, Padilla D, et al: Trauma care systems in urban South America: the priorities should be prehospital and emergency room management. J Trauma 39:457, 1995.

Arrowsmith SD: Genitourinary reconstruction in obstetric fistulas. J Urol 152:403, 1994.

Bagarani M, Conde AS, Longo R, et al: Sigmoid volvulus in West Africa: a prospective study on surgical treatments. Dis Colon Rectum 36:186, 1995.

Bassett MT, Chokunonga E, Mauchaza B, et al: Cancer in the African population of Harare, Zimbabwe, 1990–1992. Int J Cancer 63:29, 1995.

Boffetta P, Parkin DM: Cancer in developing countries. CA Cancer J Clin 44:81–90, 1994.

Cobey JC: Medical complications of antipersonnel land mines. Bull Am Coll Surg 81:7, 1996.

Delport SD, Christianson AL, van den Berg HJS, et al: Congenital anomalies in black South African liveborn neonates at an urban academic hospital. S Afr Med J 85:11, 1995.

Fisher-Hoch SP, Tomori O, Nasidi A, et al: Review of cases of nosocomial Lassa fever in Nigeria: the high price of poor medical practice. Br Med J 311:857, 1995.

Golding J, Jones L: Factors to be considered in devising an effective programme for the reduction of road traffic accidents. West Indian Med J 43:69, 1994.

Heim S: Advances in prosthetic and orthotic education and training in developing countries: a personal view. Prosthet Orthot Int 19:20, 1995.

Holcombe C: Surgical emergencies in tropical gastroenterology. Gut 36:9, 1995.

King M (ed): Primary Anaesthesia. Oxford, England, Oxford University Press, 1986.

Lee SH, Ong ETL: Changing pattern of intestinal obstruction in Malaysia: a review of 100 consecutive cases. Br J Surg 78:181, 1991.

MacGowan WAL: Surgical manpower worldwide. Bull Am Coll Surg 72:5, 1987.

Maine D, Karkazis K, Bolan N: The bad old days are still here: abortion mortality in developing countries. J Am Med Wom Assoc 49:137, 1994.

Martins P, Morais BB, Cunha-Melo JR: Postoperative complications in the treatment of Chagasic megaesophagus. Int Surg 78:99, 1993.

Meier DE, Coln CD, Rescorla FJ, et al: Intussusception in children: international perspective. World J Surg 20:1035, 1996.

Meier DE, OlaOlorun DA, Nkor SK, et al: Ketamine: a safe and effective anesthetic agent for children in the developing world. Pediatr Surg Int 11:370, 1996.

Meier DE, Tarpley JL, Imediegwu OO, et al: The outcome of suprapubic prostatectomy: a contemporary series in the developing world. Urology 46:40, 1995.

Meier DE, Tarpley JL, OlaOlorun DA, et al: Hematogenous osteomyelitis in the developing world: a practical approach to classification and treatment with limited resources. Contemp Orthop 26:495, 1993.

Muckart DJJ, Meumann C, Botha JBC: The changing pattern of penetrating torso trauma in KwaZulu-Natal—a clinical and pathological review. S Afr Med J 85:1172, 1995.

Narita A, Taylor HR: Blindness in the tropics. Med J Aust 159:416, 1993.

Nmadu PT: Trends in staffing an academic department of surgery in a tropical hospital: past, present, any future? Br Med J 312:1345, 1996.

Odero W: Road traffic accidents in Kenya: an epidememiological appraisal. East Afr Med J 72:229, 1995.

Ogbonna BC, Obekpa PO, Momoh JT, et al: Laparoscopy in developing countries in the management of patients with an acute abdomen. Br J Surg 79:964, 1992.

Persanna M, Singh K, Kumar P: Early tangential excision and skin grafting as a routine method of burn wound management: an experience from a developing country. Burns 20:446, 1994.

Raia S, da Silva LC, Gayotto LCC, et al: Portal hypertension in schistosomiasis: a long-term follow-up of a randomized trial comparing three types of surgery. Hepatology 20:398, 1994.

Raiga J, Kasia JM, Canis M, et al: Introduction of gynecologic endoscopic surgery in an African setting. Int J Gynaecol Obstet 46:261, 1994.

Schreiber GB, Busch MP, Kleinman SH, Korelitz JJ: The risk of transfusion-transmitted viral infections. N Engl J Med 334:1685, 1996.

Udwadia TE, Udwadia RT, Menon K, et al: Laparoscopic surgery in the developing world: an overview of the Indian scene. Int Surg 90:371, 1995.

Venter PA, Christianson AL, Hutamo CM, et al: Congenital anomalies in rural black South African neonates—a silent epidemic? S Afr Med J 85:15, 1995.

14 Orthopedics

Jean-Claude Theis and Benjamin Joseph

Most employment in developing countries requires manual labor. Thus, injury or chronic disease of the musculoskeletal system leading to disability will compromise the lives and livelihoods of those concerned, because orthopedic and rehabilitative facilities are sparse and medical insurance nonexistent.

■ SPECTRUM OF ORTHOPEDIC DISEASES IN THE TROPICS

Diseases of the musculoskeletal system are a common cause of morbidity in developing countries. As the spectrum of diseases is different from that in developed countries, orthopedic surgeons must be familiar with the epidemiology of orthopedic disorders in the tropics (Table 14–1). Certain diseases related to poverty, poor hygiene, and malnutrition, e.g., bone and joint infections, poliomyelitis and leprosy, are confined to or are much more common in developing countries. Other orthopedic conditions related to advanced age and sedentary lifestyle, e.g., osteoporosis and degenerative arthritis, are rarer in the tropics than in temperate climates.

Congenital dislocation of the hip is rare in the tropics

TABLE 14-1. Prevalence of Musculoskeletal Diseases and Injuries in the Tropics

More Common	Less Common
Osteomyelitis	Degenerative arthritis
Tuberculosis	Rheumatoid arthritis
Poliomyelitis	Osteoporosis
Leprosy	Back pain
Pyomyositis	Secondary bone tumors
Fungal infections	Congenital hip dislocations
Sickle cell disease	Spina bifida cystica
Congenital talipes equinovarus	Sports injuries
Neglected trauma	

due to genetic and environmental factors. Owing to natural selection, spina bifida cystica and cerebral palsy are rare conditions in tropical countries. Children born with myelodysplasia die in the neonatal period from meningitis and tetanus. Cerebral palsy is relatively uncommon because neonates with a low Apgar score do not survive, as resuscitation facilities are usually not available. On the other hand, the prevalence of congenital talipes equinovarus is much higher in developing countries. There appear to be racial and geographic variations in the incidence of Perthes disease. It is rare among Africans but common in rural parts of southwest India.

Infection of the musculoskeletal system is the most common cause of orthopedic disability in developing countries. *Salmonella* osteomyelitis, rarely seen in developed countries or in individuals with normal hemoglobin levels, is common in children with sickle cell disease (Chapters 75 and 76). Chronic osteomyelitis following compound fractures or hematogenous osteomyelitis is prevalent as a result of inadequate and delayed treatment. Bone and joint tuberculosis is a major health problem in Africa, Asia, and South America (Chapter 77). In these continents the incidence has been estimated at 25 to 35 per 100,000 per year. For comparison, in developed countries the incidence is much less and varies between 0.3 and 3 per 100,000 per year. Poliomyelitis has become an exclusively tropical disease, as it has been virtually eradicated from developed societies by immunization. In India alone, up until recently 150,000 new cases were reported yearly, and the incidence has been estimated at 20 to 30 per 100,000 per year (Chapter 27.1). The incidence of leprosy is highest in Africa and India, where the disease affects 1% to 4% of the population in certain areas.

Sickle cell disease (HbSS, SC) is endemic in many African and Caribbean countries and may lead to orthopedic complications (Chapter 6).

Primary osteoarthritis of the hip is rarely seen among Chinese and Indians, whereas the same condition is common in the knee and probably associated with squatting. Rheumatoid arthritis is seldom seen among the black population of rural South Africa but is not uncommon in those living in urban areas. Osteoporosis is rare in the tropics, most likely because of continuous physical activity until late in life.

The rarity of hallux valgus in Indians and Africans is probably due to the fact that closed footwear is not common. Nevertheless, hallux varus, a very rare condition in developed countries, is occasionally encountered in unshod persons.

A clear idea of epidemiologic aspects of trauma in the tropics is also important. There is a higher incidence of road traffic and industrial accidents because of a total lack of, or neglect of, safety regulations. Trauma due to gunshot and knife wounds as well as explosions is more common because of frequent political unrest. Many spinal injuries are secondary to falls from trees. Nonunion, malunion, and osteomyelitis following compound fractures are frequent problems.

Practical Considerations

The principles of orthopedic surgery in developing countries are the same as in developed countries: prevention, treatment, and rehabilitation. However, orthopedic practice depends largely on the patient and the available facilities. Patients with bone and joint problems are slow to seek medical assistance and often present with major deformities of the limbs. Surgery should aim at improvement of function, as cosmesis is less important than in developed societies. Established treatment methods are not necessarily appropriate on account of social and cultural factors. For example, total hip and knee replacements are of little use in many rural areas, as they are not designed to flex beyond 90 degrees, which is insufficient for squatting. Available facilities vary, and orthopedic practice must be adapted to the local conditions.

RADIOLOGY. If radiodiagnostic facilities are not available, the surgeon must rely on clinical signs in the assessment of orthopedic patients. It is possible to determine clinically if a fracture is reduced by checking the bony landmarks and comparing the length of the fractured limb with the opposite one.

ANESTHESIA. Local and regional (epidural or spinal) anesthesia is appropriate for most of the common orthopedic procedures because it is cheap, safe, and reliable. When a fully trained anesthetist is not available, the anesthesia can be administered by the surgeon or a trained nurse.

ASEPSIS AND ORTHOPEDIC IMPLANTS. Asepsis in the operating room must be the main concern if orthopedic implants are used. Sterilization facilities and operating room ventilation are often poor and subject to regular breakdowns. Treatment of orthopedic disorders is further complicated by the fact that the vast majority of implants and instrumentation used in reconstructive procedures are expensive and often in short supply. Therefore, closed treatment of fractures may be preferred to internal fixation. The importance of preparing the patient for the operation should be emphasized.

REHABILITATION. Physiotherapy services very often are nonexistent, and it depends on the surgeon to organize them. Orthoses and prostheses can be made locally at a reasonable cost.

Congenital Malformations

Congenital talipes equinovarus, or clubfoot, is the most common congenital foot deformity in the tropics. The deformity (varus or equinus of the hindfoot and adduction inversion of the forefoot) is rigid in the intrinsic and mobile in the extrinsic type. The rigid type, associated with calf wasting, is probably due to neuromuscular imbalance. In the mobile type, owing to a postural malposition in utero, the calf muscles are normal. Before treatment the spine should be examined to exclude myelodysplasia.

Although in some parts of the tropics children with clubfeet do not receive medical attention until they are several months old, in areas where health care is more advanced infants are seen soon after birth.

The treatment of the deformity in infancy consists of serial manipulation and maintenance of the correction by strapping, splints, or casts. In planning the treatment it is necessary to adopt a schedule that entails the fewest possible appointments at the clinic; these visits also have to be spaced appropriately, as patients often must travel great distances.

It has been the authors' practice to use plaster casts after each manipulation, changing them only at fortnightly intervals. If the feet do not respond to these measures by 3 to 6 months of age, soft tissue release operations are done without undue delay so that treatment can be completed by the time the child is ready to walk. The use of corrective footwear after surgery may be appropriate only in urban areas.

Treatment of children presenting later includes initial soft tissue release operations and possibly bony procedures such as calcaneal osteotomy or calcaneocuboid fusion. In children older than 12 to 14 years, triple fusion is done to obtain a plantigrade foot. Occasionally young adults present with a clubfoot deformity. In this case it is debatable whether surgery should be performed, as the foot may become painful following the operation. Weight bearing in adulthood is generally good, allowing an acceptable and pain-free gait.

Tumors of the Musculoskeletal System

Unless there is pain, tumors of the soft tissue and bone often attain a large size before the patient seeks treatment (Fig. 14–1). All types of benign bone tumors occur in the tropics and seldom pose problems in treatment.

GIANT CELL TUMORS. Giant cell tumors of bone are seen frequently in some areas. They affect adults between the ages of 20 and 40. The tumor arises from supporting connective tissue of the marrow and is characterized by multinuclear giant cells. The majority develop in the lower end of the femur, the upper end of the tibia, and the lower end of the radius. Patients present late with a painful large swelling around the joint; x-ray study shows an osteolytic lesion involving the epiphyseal end of the bone, with thinning and expansion of the overlying cortex. Giant cell tumors are classified as benign but 30% recur after surgery. Occasionally they metastasize and become malignant. After the diagnosis has been established by biopsy, the tumor is treated by curet-

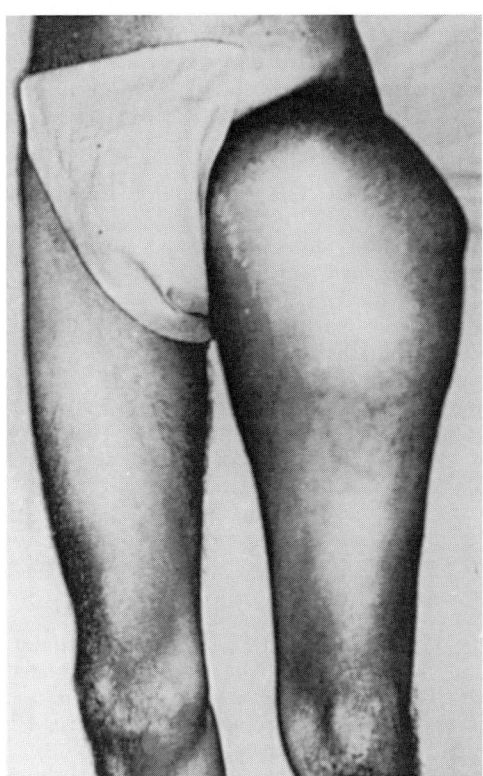

Figure 14–1. Patient with a large synovial sarcoma of the hip.

tage of the lesion and bone grafting if it has not breached the cortex. If the tumor recurs or if it has already breached the cortex at the time of presentation, excision of the involved segment of bone with massive bone grafting is performed, sacrificing the involved joint. In lesions involving expendable bones such as the metatarsals or fibula, primary excision is indicated.

MALIGNANT BONE TUMORS. Treatment of malignant bone tumors such as osteosarcoma and Ewing tumor is extremely frustrating. The patients often present late in the course of illness and even those who are seen early can seldom afford the prohibitively expensive multidrug chemotherapy used in developed countries. There is also little role for limb saving surgery in these conditions, as custom-made prostheses for resected bones are not available. The mainstay of treatment is ablative surgery, although amputation may often be refused by the patient.

Poliomyelitis

Although the orthopedic surgeon is usually called on to treat the residual permanent paralysis and sequelae of poliomyelitis (Chapter 27.1), it is imperative that he or she be aware of both preventive measures and treatment in the acute stage of the disease.

EARLY TREATMENT. An important aspect of treatment in the acute stage is correct posturing. This minimizes fixed deformities and contractures. The joints should be put through a full range of passive movement daily. This should be maintained for 6 weeks. Progressive recovery of muscle power occurs over the next 12 months. During this period appropriate calipers are provided to support the paralyzed limb and prevent deformities.

TREATMENT OF RESIDUAL PERMANENT PARALYSIS. The basic principles of treatment include correction of deformities, restoration of muscle power, stabilization of joints, and orthotic management.

Correction of Deformities. The two main causes of deformities in poliomyelitis are faulty posture and muscle imbalance. As a consequence of either factor, various deformities can develop with contractures of tendons and fascia. In long-standing cases, adaptive bony changes also occur. In the early stages, correction of the deformities may be achieved by release of the contracted fascia and tenotomy or lengthening of tendons. In the older child, bone surgery is often necessary in addition to these procedures.

Hip Deformity. The most common hip deformities are flexion, abduction, and external rotation. If these deformities are severe and bilateral, bipedal gait is impossible until the contractures are released. The main offending structure is the iliotibial band, which can be released quite easily at its proximal attachment. In a patient with long-standing and severe deformity it may be necessary to release the glutei and rectus femoris from the ilium. In severe cases, any residual deformity after a radical release can be treated by a corrective osteotomy of the femur at the subtrochanteric level.

Knee Deformity. The common deformities of the knee include genu valgum and flexion deformity. Minor degrees are due to a contracted iliotibial band. This is released just proximal to the knee along with the lateral intermuscular septum. If the flexion deformity at the knee is more marked, the hamstring tendons need to be lengthened surgically or by serial wedging of plaster casts.

Ankle and Foot Deformities. Various deformities around the ankle and foot are seen following poliomyelitis. Balancing of muscle power and stabilization of joints are required to correct most of these deformities. The equinus deformity of the ankle can be corrected by lengthening the Achilles tendon combined with capsulotomy of the ankle joint in severe case.

Restoration of Muscle Power. If a neighboring tendon can be spared without jeopardizing function, it can be transferred to replace the paralyzed muscle. Such tendon transfers additionally remove the deforming force at the joint. For example, in patients with paralyzed peronei and tibialis anterior muscles, an equinovarus deformity develops owing to unopposed action of tibialis posterior and triceps surae. Transfer of the tibialis posterior to the dorsum of the foot not only restores the power of dorsiflexion but also removes the deforming varus force.

Prior to planning tendon transfers, careful assessment of muscle power of every muscle is carried out. Because postoperative muscle re-education is necessary, tendon transfers are usually deferred until the child is over 7 years of age.

Stabilization of Unstable Joints. The majority of stabilization operations are done for instability around the foot and ankle and (less commonly) for shoulder paralysis. Most of these procedures are applicable only when the child is approaching skeletal maturity. The advantages of stability of joints, particularly the more proximal joints, should be weighed against the disadvantage of loss of mobility. A fused shoulder may be an asset for a manual laborer, whereas it may be a hindrance to a housewife who cannot comb her hair.

Orthotic Management. Orthotic appliances for poliomyelitis can be fabricated from inexpensive, locally available cheap materials with minimal equipment. Below-knee calipers (ankle-foot orthosis [AFO]) are used for instability of the foot and ankle. Above-knee calipers (knee-ankle-foot orthosis [KAFO]) are used when the quadriceps muscle is weak. A pelvic band is added (hip-knee-ankle-foot orthosis [HKAFO]) when the hip is also very weak.

All children with weak limbs in whom a deformity might develop should be encouraged to wear calipers until their growth is complete even if they can walk without support. Once skeletal maturity has been attained, unstable joints of the foot should be stabilized so that below-knee calipers can be discarded. In patients who need bilateral calipers, a walking aid is also required. Bilateral calipers are of little use to those with weakness of the upper limbs, as they will be unable to use crutches. These patients require a wheelchair (Fig. 14–2).

Tuberculosis

BONE AND JOINT TUBERCULOSIS. The majority of the 15 to 20 million individuals with active tuberculosis live in

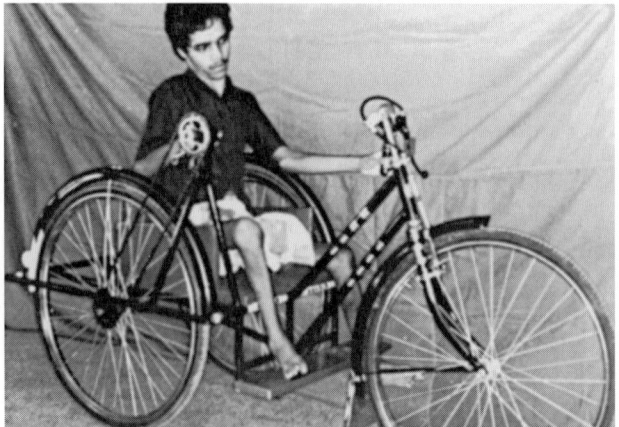

Figure 14–2. Hand-propelled tricycle used in the rehabilitation of patients with severe poliomyelitis.

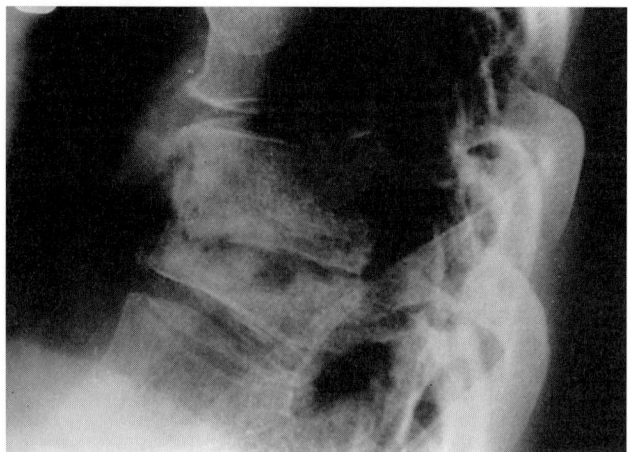

Figure 14–3. X-ray showing vertebral body destruction in the thoracic spine due to tuberculosis. (Courtesy of Professor A.K. Jeffery, Otago University, Dunedin, New Zealand.)

developing countries. Estimates of the proportion of those with illness due to tuberculosis who have bone and joint tuberculosis vary from 5% to 10%, indicating at least 750,000 active cases of bone and joint tuberculosis. Approximately 50% are spinal, 15% in the hip, 15% in the knee, 10% in other joints, and 10% in bone without joint involvement. Most cases occur in adolescents and young adults. The incidence is unknown for most tropical countries but is probably similar to the Asian immigrant population of Great Britain: 35 per 100,000 per year.

Musculoskeletal tuberculosis arises following hematogenous spread from a primary focus. Pathology of the bone lesions is similar to that of other tissues. Osteoclastic activity is not a particular feature of bone tuberculosis, although monocytes have the ability to resorb bone.

In the absence of diagnostic facilities, management is often based on clinical suspicion. An elevated erythrocyte sedimentation rate and bone destruction characterized by severe regional osteoporosis with little surrounding sclerosis and swelling of soft tissue on x-ray study is characteristic of tuberculosis. Antituberculous chemotherapy should be started (Chapter 77).

TUBERCULOSIS OF THE SPINE. Spinal tuberculosis is common in developing countries and may lead to severe disabilities. Most of those infected are young adults and children. The thoracic and lumbar vertebrae are most frequently involved, and paraplegia or other neurologic involvement is present in 30 to 40% of patients when they first seek medical assistance.

The characteristic lesion involves the vertebral bodies with destruction of the intervening disk (Fig. 14–3). As destruction proceeds, kyphosis develops. Soft tissue abscesses, composed of debris and lined by tuberculous granulation tissue, form. These may remain paravertebral, spread to the extradural space, or track to form a distinct abscess in paraspinal, psoas, buttock, or thigh muscles. Paraplegia with active disease is caused by extradural tuberculous abscess and formation of a kyphosis (Fig. 14–4).

Back pain, stiffness, kyphosis, and occasionally paraparesis or paraplegia in a young child or adult is usually due to tuberculous disease. Radiologic evidence of vertebral body destruction or paravertebral abscess formation makes the diagnosis virtually certain. In the absence of other diagnostic possibilities, antituberculous treatment should be started.

The results of clinical trials conducted by the Medical Research Council Working Party on Tuberculosis of the Spine

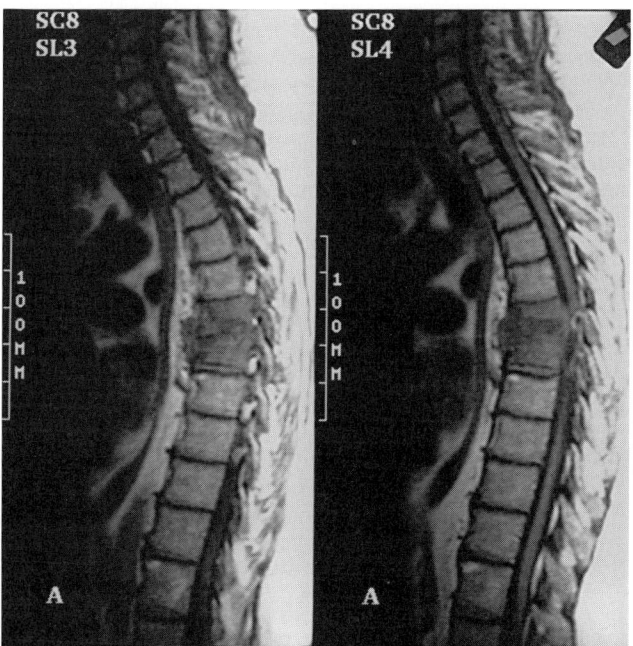

Figure 14–4. MRI scans showing tuberculosis of the thoracic spine causing spinal cord compression.

in different parts of the world clearly indicate that the mainstay of treatment of spinal tuberculosis is adequate chemotherapy (Chapter 77). The role of the surgeon is largely for diagnostic purposes. These studies have shown that there is no additional benefit from bed rest, wearing a plaster-of-Paris jacket, or simple surgical debridement of the diseased area. Although radical anterior surgery has the advantage of minimizing the kyphosis, such elaborate surgery is often not possible. The recent reports of clinical trials with short-term chemotherapy has shown that excellent results can be obtained with a 6- or 9-month course of isoniazid and rifampin. These results are comparable with that obtained previously with an 18-month triple-drug regimen.

Ten percent of spinal tuberculosis is complicated by paraplegia. The distinction between paraplegia of early and late onset is less important than formerly. The real distinction is between paraplegia arising in the presence of active infection in the vertebral bodies and that arising from healed disease, which is always of late onset. Many lesions associated with active disease respond to conservative treatment. However, pressure on the front of the dura mater by caseous material is the most common cause of paraplegia, and surgical relief of that pressure usually leads to a rapid resolution of the paralysis. Surgery is indicated in rapidly progressive paresis, slowly progressive paresis despite adequate chemotherapy, total paralysis not responding to 3 weeks of adequate chemotherapy, and "cord tumor–like" syndrome. The spine can be decompressed by a radical anterior resection or anterolateral decompression when adequate facilities are lacking. Laminectomy, although still performed by some surgeons, is no longer recommended. Paraplegia in patients with healed disease is more difficult to treat. The paralysis is attributed to stretching of the spinal cord over the angle at the back of the affected bodies, the so-called internal gibbus, leading to chronic ischemia. Surgery, if indicated, should be performed only in specialized centers.

TUBERCULOUS ARTHRITIS. Although any synovial joint can be affected by tuberculosis, the hip and knee are the most common sites. Diagnosis often relies on clinical judgment. A painful, swollen, and stiff joint with radiologic evidence of localized osteoporosis or joint destruction is most likely due to tuberculosis (Fig. 14–5). A good clinical response to antituberculous chemotherapy is a valuable diagnostic test.

Standard chemotherapy in all active cases is the keystone of treatment. Orthopedic management depends on the stage of disease. Early disease presents with regional osteoporosis and minimal joint space loss or bone destruction. Advanced disease is characterized by total joint space loss, severe bone destruction, and instability or subluxation. Early in the disease a good range of movement is normally preserved. Treatment consists of early mobilization and protected weight bearing. Later, when there is marked muscle wasting and joint stiffness, immobilization in a position of function is the accepted treatment. Either the joint will ankylose spontaneously or a painful, unstable, and deformed joint will result. In that case, two options are available: surgical arthrodesis or joint excision arthroplasty. The latter procedure should be performed only in adults. Arthrodesis is unacceptable in many countries, and excision arthroplasty (hip and elbow) may relieve pain with preservation of an acceptable range of movement. Unstable knees and ankles are best treated by arthrodesis.

Orthopedic Aspects of Leprosy

Leprosy is often a chronic disease of the peripheral nerves due to infection by *Mycobacterium leprae* (Chapter 78). The bacilli multiply in the Schwann cells, leading to a chronic granuloma that slowly infiltrates the nerve. This causes edema and ischemia, gradually resulting in fibrosis of the nerve. Pain is present in the early stages; later a sensory

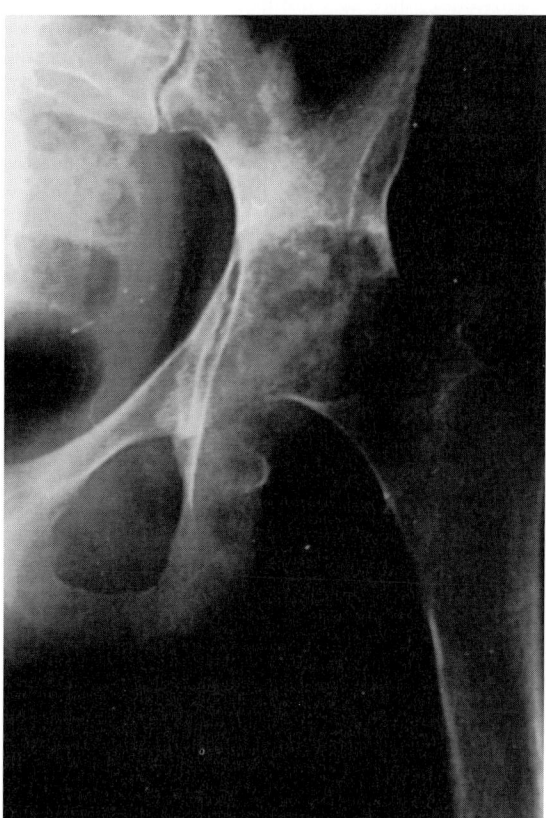

Figure 14–5. X-ray showing destruction of the hip due to tuberculosis. (Courtesy of Professor A.K. Jeffery, Otago University, Dunedin, New Zealand.)

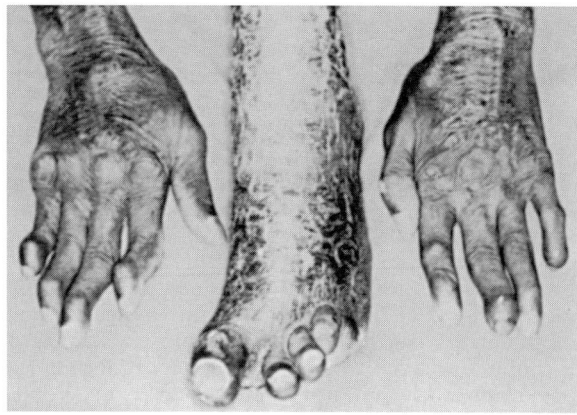

Figure 14–6. Finger and toe deformities in a patient with leprosy.

neuropathy is followed by paralysis. The small nerve fibers of the skin, bone, and vessels are also involved, explaining the chain of events leading to neurotrophic complications, e.g., skin ulceration and bone and joint destruction. Hands and feet are commonly involved, and secondary bone infection leads to further damage (Fig. 14–6).

The orthopedic management of leprosy includes prevention of deformities secondary to nerve damage, correction of established deformities, prevention and treatment of neuropathic ulceration, and management of neuropathic joints.

PREVENTION OF IRREVERSIBLE NERVE DAMAGE. It is now generally accepted that it is possible to minimize the extent of permanent nerve damage if appropriate treatment is instituted in the early stage of neuritis. Systemic steroids if administered early can minimize the nerve damage. If a nerve abscess develops it is surgically drained by incising the nerve sheath. In the case of the ulnar nerve, anterior transposition may help in reducing trauma to the inflamed nerve.

PREVENTION OF DEFORMITIES. Adequate treatment of the neuritis itself may help in preventing deformities. In addition, the limb needs to be splinted during the acute stage of neuritis. When the common peroneal nerve is affected, a footdrop splint is provided.

TREATMENT OF ESTABLISHED DEFORMITIES. Deformities in leprosy are primarily caused by muscle imbalance. These deformities are supple to begin with but gradually become rigid if appropriate passive stretching is not performed. For example, a footdrop secondary to paralysis of the dorsiflexors of the ankle may progress to become a rigid equinus deformity.

The nerves involved in the upper limb are the ulnar, median, and radial nerves in that order of frequency. Occasionally two nerves are affected, whereas all three are rarely affected. Ulnar nerve involvement causes clawing of the medial two fingers, median nerve involvement causes clawing of the lateral two fingers and an ape-thumb deformity, and radial nerve paralysis causes a wristdrop. Fortunately the sites of involvement of the nerves are never at the same level, and hence almost invariably there are unaffected muscles available for performing tendon transfers for correction of the deformities. Tendon transfers will only work if the joints are supple. Hence, if the deformity is a fixed one owing to joint contractures, initial physiotherapy before surgery is essential. Many of the tendon transfers devised for leprosy can be performed under local anesthesia with very few instruments.

The nerves affected in the lower limb are the common peroneal nerve and the tibial nerve. The common deformities encountered are footdrop, fixed equinus, and equinovarus deformities. The choice of treatment for a footdrop is an ankle foot orthosis or a tibialis posterior tendon transfer.

PREVENTION OF NEUROPATHIC ULCERATION. The patient must understand the significance of lost "protective feeling." He or she should be taught to inspect the soles of the feet daily so that trivial injuries can be recognized and treated early. Insensitive feet must be protected with footwear with a soft insole that evenly distributes pressure and a hard undersole that prevents penetration by sharp objects. Often protective footwear is not well accepted by the patient. The risk of plantar ulceration is high if the foot is rigidly deformed. Hence all deformities of the foot must be corrected. Over 90% of plantar ulcers in leprosy occur in the forepart of the foot and only 10% occur over the heel. Ulcers under the heads of the first and fifth metatarsals are common in patients with footdrop, and ulcers under the base of the fifth metatarsal are common in those with an equinovarus deformity.

TREATMENT OF PLANTAR ULCERATION. Plantar ulcers may be classified as incipient ulcers, simple ulcers, and complicated ulcers. Incipient ulcers are treated by rest until all the signs of inflammation subside. Simple ulcers are treated by cleaning and dressing after a foot soak daily until the floor of the ulcer is clean. If the edge of the ulcer is hyperkeratotic the ulcer is saucerized. The foot is then immobilized in a plaster-of-Paris molded double rocker shoe or a below-knee cast for a period of 3 to 6 weeks, during which time weight bearing is permitted. In a complicated ulcer there is often underlying osteomyelitis. Debridement and excision of infected tissues including the bone is needed. Once the wound granulates the treatment is the same as that for a simple ulcer.

TREATMENT OF NEUROPATHIC JOINTS. Tarsal disintegration with disorganization of the joints of the foot may occur in leprosy. Amputation may be justified in these patients especially if plantar ulceration is also present. A Syme amputation is indicated if the heel pad is healthy; otherwise a below-knee amputation is needed.

Salmonella Osteomyelitis

Bone and joint complications after *Salmonella* infections are relatively rare. However, there is an association between these infections and sickle cell disease. In these patients, multiple sites of infection are common involving hands, feet, and long bones. Many species have been identified, but *Salmonella choleraesuis* is particularly prone to cause bone infections. Children under 5 years of age have the highest incidence of salmonella osteomyelitis and clinically present with painful and swollen limbs associated with pyrexia and toxemia. An aseptic bone infarct in a patient with sickle cell disease may have a similar presentation. Most patients seek medical assistance late in the illness, with a soft tissue abscess, discharging sinuses, or pathologic fractures. Radiographs (Fig. 14–7) show extensive bone destruction and sequestration of the diaphysis surrounded by periosteal new bone formation.

Acute infections respond well to appropriate antibiotics (Chapters 75 and 76) and immobilization. The presence of an abscess, causing poor clinical response, requires surgical exploration. Chronic osteomyelitis, characterized by multiple recurrences despite adequate surgical debridement, is best treated by extensive "guttering." In this technique the entire medullary canal is deroofed, followed by a split skin graft once adequate granulation tissue has formed. However, amputation is often the final outcome.

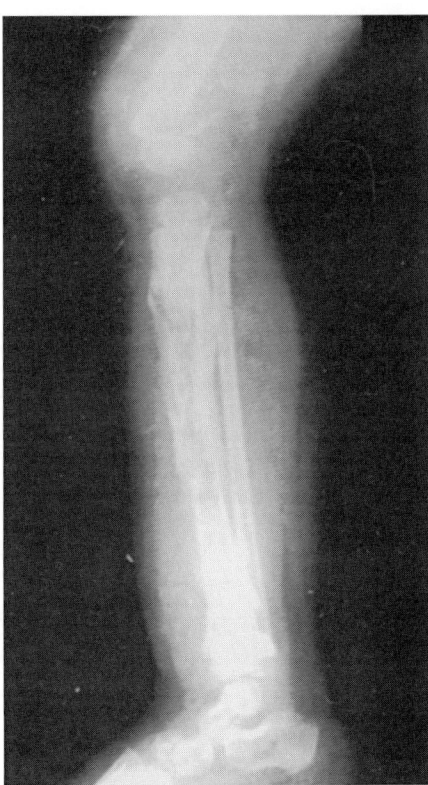

Figure 14–7. X-ray showing destruction of the midshaft of the tibia due to salmonella osteomyelitis in a child.

Miscellaneous Infections

PYOMYOSITIS. No accurate figures are available for the incidence of pyomyositis. It is common in tropical countries but rare elsewhere (Chapter 58). Many patients present with a fully developed intramuscular abscess. The route of bacterial spread is presumed to be hematogenous from skin and other lesions. Over 90% of cases are caused by *Staphylococcus aureus,* the remainder being caused by *Streptococcus* species. Trauma has been suggested as a potential predisposing factor. The majority of abscesses occur in the lower limbs and trunk. Many patients have multiple abscesses. Pyomyositis is occasionally associated with guinea worm (*Dracunculus medinensis*) infection. Local signs usually predominate, but occasionally patients have systemic symptoms. The management is based on surgical drainage and antibiotic therapy. Abscesses draining up to 5 L of pus have been described.

FUNGAL INFECTION OF BONES AND JOINTS. Mycetoma is endemic in the Sudan and some parts of India (Chapter 82.1). It usually involves the foot and less commonly the hand (Fig. 14–8). The lesions extend deep into subcutaneous tissues and eventually invade bone. They suppurate, and pus drains through multiple sinuses. The pus contains granules of various colors depending on the etiologic agent. The causative agent may be among at least six actinomycetes (false fungi) or 16 species of true fungi. The lesion spreads slowly, but treatment is difficult. Often the infected foot requires amputation.

ORTHOPEDIC COMPLICATIONS OF SICKLE CELL DISEASE. With the exception of salmonella osteomyelitis, avascular necrosis of the hip is the main orthopedic problem in sickle cell disease (Chapter 6). Avascular necrosis of the femoral head is a disabling complication predominantly affecting children and adolescents. The disease varies in incidence from 1 to 3% and seems to be more common in sickle cell

SC disease. The severity of hip symptoms varies with the amount of femoral head necrosis and collapse. The prognosis in children is better than in adults, as the epiphysis is remodeled following revascularization. Treatment is symptomatic, but in an adult resection arthroplasty (excision of the femoral head and neck) may be performed if the hip is stiff and painful.

Trauma Management in Developing Countries

TRAFFIC ACCIDENTS. The incidence of major traffic accidents is increasing in developing countries because of construction of paved roads, the increasing number of motor vehicles, and absence of safety precautions. Mortality and morbidity of multiply injured patients is high owing to isolation and lack of organized ambulance services, which results in delayed treatment. If the patient has severe head, chest, or abdominal injuries, the chances of survival are poor unless he or she is evacuated to a major medical center.

INDUSTRIAL ACCIDENTS. Lack of safety regulations leads to frequent industrial accidents, resulting in crush injuries and traumatic amputations of fingers and hands. The incidence of flexor tendon injuries due to knife and machete wounds is high. These injuries, especially the machete type, often are associated with damage to neurovascular structures and bone. Treatment is difficult, and the results are disappointing.

WOUNDS. Gunshot and explosion injuries frequently occur during civil unrest. Half the wounds result in fractures, which are often followed by wound infections and osteomyelitis. Damage to neurovascular structures is common, occurring in one third of cases. Low-velocity gunshot wounds, not producing damage to vital structures, should be left open to heal. High-velocity wounds or those with possible damage to vital structures should be explored, debrided, and left open. Additionally, tetanus and antibiotic prophylaxis must be given. Fractures are best stabilized with external fixation followed by secondary wound closure. Skin grafting or reconstructive plastic surgery procedures may be indicated.

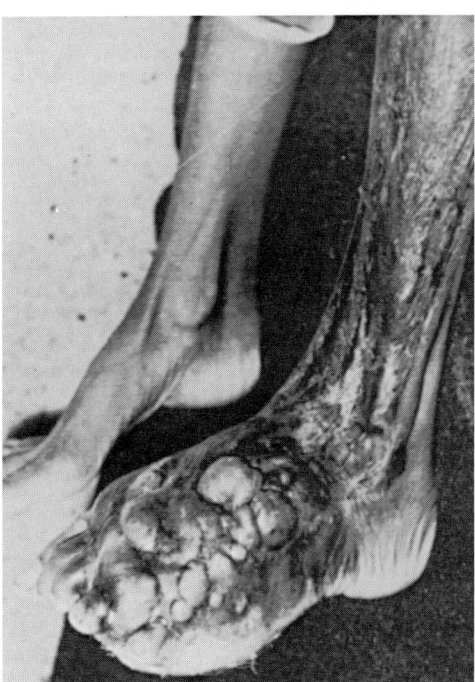

Figure 14–8. Granulomatous tumor of the foot due to mycetoma infection.

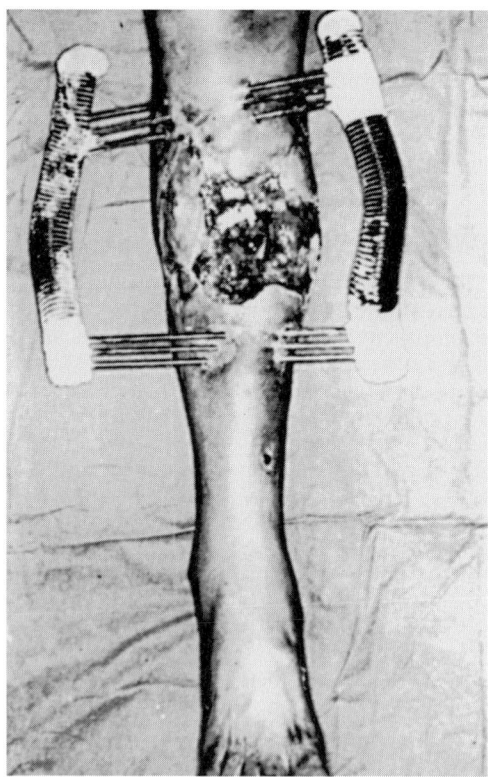

Figure 14–9. A locally fabricated external fixator made of PVC (polyvinyl chloride) tubing and dental acrylic used to treat an open fracture of the tibia.

FALLS. Falls from trees (e.g., coconut during harvesting) are a frequent cause of spinal injuries. Fractures are managed with bed rest followed by plaster immobilization. Management of spinal injuries with paraplegia or quadriplegia is very difficult in developing countries because of insufficient nursing and rehabilitation facilities. The morbidity and mortality are very high in these patients. Fractures of the neck of the femur and distal radius in the elderly is very rare in developing countries because the incidence of osteoporosis is low.

Therapy. The treatment of fractures in developing countries should be conservative. Internal fixation devices are often not available or are in short supply and should not be used unless expertise and clean surgical facilities are available. Closed stable fractures are treated in plaster. If the fracture is unstable, traction or external fixation is used. Locally made external fixators are cheap and usually satisfactory (Fig. 14–9). Open fractures with minor skin and soft tissue damage are debrided and treated in the same way as a closed fracture. In patients with major soft tissue and neurovascular damage, amputation is often the only alternative. Infection and nonunion after compound fractures are common complications and lead to secondary amputation in many cases. Malunion interfering with function should be treated by osteotomy if facilities are available.

Bibliography

Adeyokunnu AA, Hendrickse RG: Salmonella osteomyelitis in childhood. Arch Dis Child 55:175, 1980.
Brand PW: Paralytic claw hand with special reference to paralysis in leprosy and treatment by the sublimis transfer of Stiles and Bunnell. J Bone Joint Surg 40B:618, 1948.
Chacko V, Joseph B, Mohanty SP, Jacob T: Management of spinal cord injury in a general hospital in rural India. Paraplegia 24:330, 1986.
Griffiths DL, Seddon HJ, Roaf R: Pott's Paraplegia. Oxford, England, Oxford University Press, 1956.
Hodgson AR, Stock FE, Fang HSY, Ong GB: Anterior spinal fusion. Br J Surg 48:172, 1960.
Huckstep RL: Poliomyelitis: A guide for Developing Countries, Including Appliances and Rehabilitation for the Disabled. Edinburgh, Churchill Livingstone, 1975.
Iwegbu CG, Fleming AF: Avascular necrosis of the femoral head in sickle cell disease. J Bone Joint Surg 67B:28, 1985.
Kazen RO: Management of plantar ulcers—Theory or practice? Lepr Rev 64:188, 1993.
Kelsey JL: Epidemiology of Musculoskeletal Disorders. Monographs in Epidemiology and Biostatistics, Vol 3. New York, Oxford University Press, 1982.
MRC Working Party on Tuberculosis of the Spine: Controlled trial of short-course regimens of chemotherapy in the ambulatory treatment of spinal tuberculosis. Results at three years of a study in Korea. J Bone Joint Surg 75B:240, 1993.
Reddy CRRM, Rao PS, Rajakumari K: Giant-cell tumors of bone in South India. J Bone Joint Surg 56A:617, 1974.
Sim-Fook L, Hodgson AR: A comparison of foot forms among non-shoe and shoe-wearing Chinese population. J Bone Joint Surg 40A:1058, 1958.
Tuli SM, Mukherjee SK: Excision arthroplasty for tuberculous and pyogenic arthritis of the hip. J Bone Joint Surg 63B:29, 1981.

15 Maternal and Child Health in the Tropics

Virginia F. Randall

MATERNAL AND CHILD HEALTH PROGRAMS

Health Needs. Maternal and child health programs are those that identify, prioritize, address, and monitor the unique health care needs of women of childbearing age and children in that society. Specific health care needs of the mother-child unit include (1) family planning and well woman care; (2) prenatal care of the mother; (3) a healthy pregnancy and a safe delivery for mother and child; (4) adequate nutrition for the child; (5) prevention of communicable diseases through immunizations, sanitation, and hygiene; (6) identification and care of children with chronic illnesses and disabilities; (7) identification and care of abused children; (8) promotion of developmentally appropriate child-rearing practices; and (9) delivery of adolescent health programs including education about high-risk behaviors.

Public health programs in developing countries rarely focus on chronically ill and disabled children, and, if they do, provide services only in the most urbanized settings. The thrust of the maternal and child health programs reflects the level of economic development of the country; the status of education and health of the general population; the adverse effects of war, drought, famine, or epidemic; and the resulting public policies to prioritize and finance health programs for women and children.

Public Health Surveillance. Accurate population demographics and surveillance of the population's health are important cornerstones of an effective maternal and child health program. Statistics, e.g., birth rate, infant mortality rate (IMR), maternal mortality rate, prevalence of endemic and chronic diseases, and immunization rates, are data that reflect the health of the mother-child unit. A system that gathers, forwards, compiles, and interprets health statistics is crucial.

Infant Mortality Rate. Lesser developed countries almost always have a very high IMR. In the case of Zaire, it is 15-fold that of the United States (Table 15–1). IMR is the most often used maternal and child health indicator; however, it requires an accurate recording of all births and deaths in the

TABLE 15–1. Infant Mortality Rates in 1994 (Deaths During the First Month of Life/1000 Live Births)

Calculated		Estimated	
Singapore	4.3	Thailand	27
Israel	7.8	Vietnam	35
United States	8.0	Kenya	61
Cuba	9.4	India	79
Malaysia	11.6	Uganda	111
Costa Rica	13.0	Nigeria	114
Guatemala	41.3	Zaire	120

From Wegman ME: Infant mortality: Some international comparisons. Pediatrics 98:1020, 1996.

first year of life. In many developing and least developed countries, recording of births and deaths of children does not take place and population trends are difficult to follow. Economic and political disruptions add to this dilemma.

The IMR is sensitive to the economic conditions, distribution of resources, and political decisions of the country. The highest IMRs are found in countries with the highest fertility rates and the poorest economic conditions. Birth rates fall when the IMR and childhood mortality rates fall. Deaths in childhood fall when political and economic conditions improve and when primary health care is provided. Thus, the World Health Organization (WHO) has emphasized the importance of immunization, nutrition, family planning, care of children and mothers, proper use of drugs, and safe water as priority programs whose impact will decrease IMR.

Social and Economic Factors. These are primary determinants of the health of mothers and children (Fig. 15–1). Maternal literacy is associated with a decline in birth rate, a decline in IMR, an increase in immunization rates, and a decrease in prevalence of malnutrition. The mother-child unit is most vulnerable to the health-related effects of poverty, pollution, famine, and endemic disease. Providing clean water and encouraging literacy may improve health more than monies directed specifically to medical care.

UNDERSTANDING PUBLIC HEALTH REALITIES. Physicians from developed countries must understand the public health realities of the developing countries where tropical diseases are leading causes of morbidity and mortality in childhood. In many areas a large proportion of child deaths are due to malaria and/or the interaction between poor nutrition, a lack of basic resources, e.g., safe water, and infectious disease. Laboratory diagnosis, extensive cold-chains for providing immunizations and medications, tertiary medical care, and antibiotics are not available to the majority of the population. Successful prevention of illness depends on the availability of primary health care and low-cost, low-tech innovations, e.g., insecticide-impregnated mosquito netting to reduce malaria morbidity, community workers to directly observe tuberculosis treatment, and encouragement of infant breast-feeding.

Bibliography

Gessler MC, Msuya DE, Nkunya MHH, et al: Traditional healers in Tanzania: the perception of malaria and its causes. J Ethnopharmacol 48:119, 1995.

Hart RH, Belsey MA, Tarimo E: Integrating Maternal and Child Health Services with Primary Care. Geneva, World Health Organization, 1990.

Holland WW, Detels R, Knox G (eds): Oxford Textbook of Public Health, 2nd ed. Vol 2: Methods of Public Health; Vol 3: Applications in Public Health. Oxford, England, Oxford University Press, 1991.

Kasonde JM, Martin JD (eds): Experience with Primary Health Care in Zambia. Geneva, World Health Organization, 1994.

Magnani RJ, Rice JC, Mock NB, et al: The impact of primary health care services on under-five mortality in rural Niger. Int J Epidemiol 25:568, 1996.

Tarimo E, Webster EG: Primary Health Care Concepts and Challenges in a Changing World. WHO Division of Strengthening of Health Services. Geneva, World Health Organization, 1995.

Wegman, ME: Infant mortality: Some international comparisons. Pediatrics 98:1020, 1996.

Wilkinson D, Davies GR: Coping with Africa's increasing tuberculosis burden: Are community supervisors an essential component of the DOT strategy? Trop Med Int Health 2:700, 1997.

Winch PJ, Makemba AM, Makame VR, et al: Social and cultural factors affecting rates of regular retreatment of mosquito nets with insecticide in Bagamoyo District, Tanzania. Trop Med Int Health 2:760, 1997.

World Health Organization: Alma-Ata 1978, Primary Health Care. Geneva, World Health Organization, 1978.

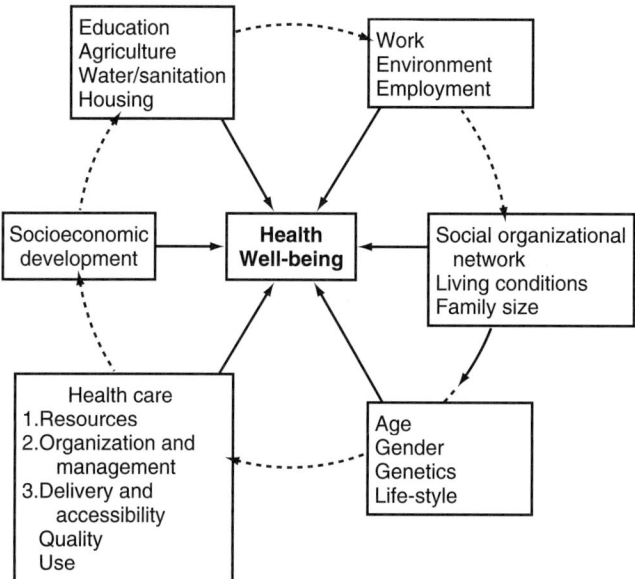

Figure 15–1. Determinants of health. (From Tarimo E, Webster EG [eds]: Primary Health Care Concepts and Challenges in a Changing World: Alma-Ata Revisited. Geneva, World Health Organization, 1995.)

16 Integrated Management of Childhood Illness*

Sandy Gove

Infant and young child mortality remains unacceptably high in developing countries, with >12 million deaths occurring annually in children <5 years of age. Seven in every 10 of these child deaths are due to diarrhea, pneumonia, measles, malaria, or malnutrition—and often to a combination of these conditions (Fig. 16–1). In addition to this substantial mortality, these conditions are the reason for seeking care at a health facility in at least 3 out of 4 sick children. Health facility staff are already treating these conditions and adequate clinical skills are essential to improving care.

The World Health Organization (WHO) guidelines for integrated management of childhood illness (IMCI) have been

---

*This chapter summarizes the technical basis of ICMI based on many contributions from the WHO Department of Child and Adolescent Health and Development and the WHO Working Group on Guidelines for Integrated Management of the Sick Child.

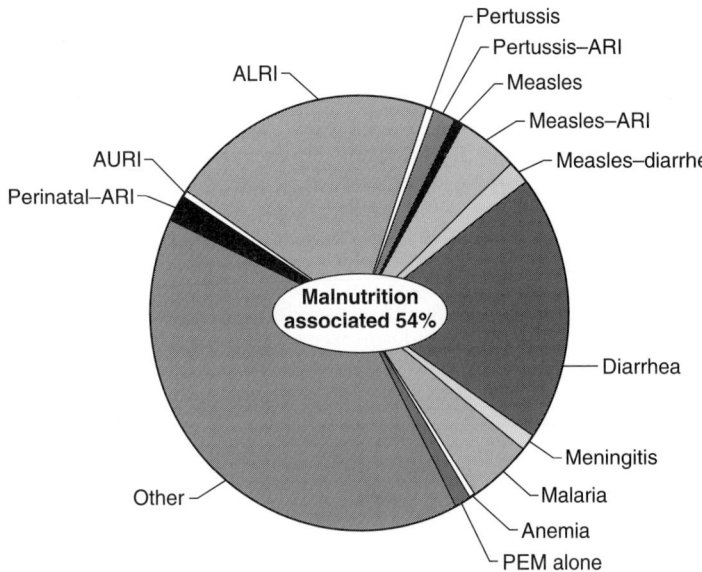

***Figure* 16–1.** Causes of 12.4 million deaths in children <5 years of age in developing countries. ALRI, acute lower respiratory infection; ARI, acute respiratory infection; AURI, acute upper respiratory infection; PEM, protein-energy malnutrition. (From GBD study, Bull WHO 73:735, 1995.)

chosen because they are expected to be applicable in the majority of developing countries where infant mortality is >40 per 1000 live births and where there is transmission of *Plasmodium falciparum* malaria. The WHO case management guideline charts contain a basic assessment and classification algorithm that has greatly simplified the management of the most common pediatric illnesses and has deliberately concentrated on the diseases that make the greatest contribution to mortality in children <5 years of age (Table 16–1).

Because there is considerable overlap in the signs and symptoms of several of the major childhood diseases, a single diagnosis for a sick child is often inappropriate. Focusing on the most apparent problem may lead to an associated, and potentially life-threatening, condition being overlooked. Treating the child also may be complicated by the need to combine therapy for several conditions.

This situation argues for child health programs that address not single diseases but the sick child as a whole. Much has been learned from disease-specific control programs in the past 15 years and these lessons have been used to develop a single, more efficient and effective approach to managing childhood illness. A number of programs in WHO and the United Nations Children's Fund (UNICEF) have collaborated in developing this approach, now referred to as Integrated Management of Childhood Illness (IMCI). These efforts are

coordinated by the WHO Division for Child Health and Development (CHD).

As potentially fatal illnesses in children are often brought to the attention of health workers at first-level health facilities, the initiative to improve care for the sick child is focusing first on improving the clinical performance of workers through training and support. The guidelines and training materials are appropriate for any health worker providing care in an outpatient facility—doctors, medical assistants, nurses, and literate paramedical workers. At the same time, work is ongoing on approaches to changing family behavior in relation to sick children and the development of guidelines and training materials for hospital care at the referral level.

In the WHO/UNICEF course *Management of Childhood Illness*, these integrated guidelines are presented on four wall charts, the contents of which are also reproduced as a booklet that can serve as a work aid. The case management process as laid out in the charts involves the following steps:

1. The health worker first *assesses* the child, by assessing danger signs, asking about four main symptoms in all children (cough or difficult breathing, diarrhea, fever, and ear problem), and carrying out further assessment if a main symptom is reported, then assessing the nutritional and immunization status in all children. The guidelines rely on detection of cases based on simple clinical signs and empirical treatment, without laboratory tests, as described for cough or difficult breathing (Fig. 16–2). A careful balance has been struck between sensitivity and specificity using as few clinical signs as possible and signs that health workers of varying backgrounds can be trained to recognize accurately.

2. Then the health worker *classifies* the child's illnesses. The classification of illness is based on a color-coded triage system with which many health workers are already familiar through use of the WHO case management guidelines for diarrheal disease (DD) and acute respiratory infection (ARI). This classifies each illness according to whether it requires:
   • Urgent referral
   • Specific medical treatment and advice, or
   • Simple advice on home management
   Action-oriented classification, rather than exact diagnoses, are used.

TABLE 16–1. Child Health Interventions Included in Integrated Management of Childhood Illness Guidelines

Case Management Interventions	Preventive Interventions
Pneumonia	Immunization during sick child visits
Diarrhea	Nutrition counseling
Dehydration	Breastfeeding support (including the
Persistent diarrhea	assessment and correction of
Dysentery	breastfeeding technique)
Meningitis, sepsis	
Malaria	
Measles	
Malnutrition	
Anemia	
Ear infection	

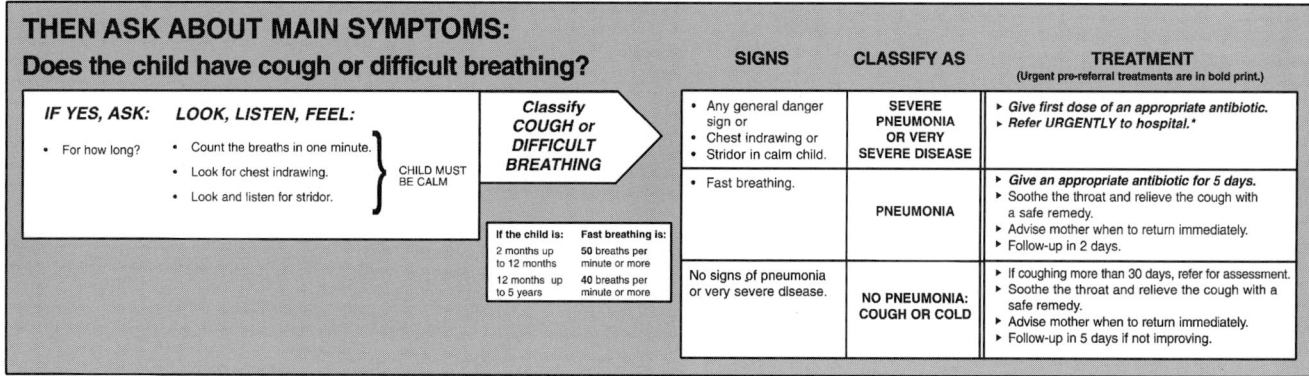

Figure 16–2. Assessment and classification of the sick child age 2 months to 5 years of age for the symptom of cough or difficult breathing. (From World Health Organization, Division of Diarrheal and Acute Respiratory Disease Control: Management of Childhood Illness. Chart booklet. Geneva, WHO, 1995, p 2.)

3. After classifying, *specific treatments are identified.* If the child is being referred urgently, health workers give only the urgent treatments before departure. Because most children have more than one illness classification, an integrated treatment plan is developed.

4. Practical *treatment instructions* are followed, including teaching the mother how to administer oral drugs (Fig. 16–3), to increase fluids during diarrhea, Plans A and B (Fig. 16–4), and to treat local infections at home. The mother is advised on which signs indicate the child should immediately be brought back to the clinic and when to return for scheduled follow-up.

5. Feeding is assessed (Fig. 16–5) and *counseling on feeding* problems (Figs. 16–6 and 16–7) is provided. The course emphasizes training the health worker to communicate well with mothers, based on asking questions using language that the mother understands, praising, giving appropriate and prioritized advice, then checking the mother's understanding using checking questions.

6. *Follow-up instructions* for various conditions are laid out in detail for return visits to the clinic.

■ SUMMARY OF THE INTEGRATED MANAGEMENT OF CHILDHOOD ILLNESS CASE MANAGEMENT AND PREVENTION GUIDELINES AND THEIR TECHNICAL BASIS

Pneumonia

COUGH OR DIFFICULT BREATHING (Fig. 16–2). Case detection of pneumonia is based on the WHO guidelines for ARI case management, which have been developed over the past decade. These guidelines divide children presenting with cough or difficult breathing into three groups: (1) those who require admission for severe pneumonia; (2) those who require antibiotics as outpatients because they are likely to have pneumonia; and (3) those who simply have a cough or cold and do not require antibiotics. This division is based on two key clinical signs: (a) respiratory rate, which distinguishes children who have pneumonia from those who do not and (b) lower chest wall indrawing, which indicates those with severe pneumonia who require hospital admission. Children with cough or difficult breathing and a danger sign (e.g., not able to drink or lethargic) should also be referred. No distinction is made between children with bronchiolitis and those with pneumonia.

Multiple studies using different definitions of "pneumonia" have shown that the sensitivity of fast breathing defined with age-specific respiratory rate thresholds is from 60 to 85%. It is probable that a higher proportion of children with potentially fatal pneumonia are successfully treated with this approach. No clinical sign has a better combination of sensitivity and specificity to detect this group than fast breathing. Even expert auscultation is less sensitive as a single sign, although when combined with fast breathing (requiring fast breathing *or* crepitations), the two signs together are more sensitive than either one alone but less specific. If both are required (fast breathing *and* crepitations), the two signs together are more specific but lose sensitivity. Thus, for primary care workers, fast breathing is clearly the best sign to teach pneumonia case detection, whereas for physicians skilled in the use of the stethoscope, their clinical assessments could be greatly improved by the addition of respiratory rate to the signs they already use.

A problem with the use of this simplified approach to the use of antibiotics for pneumonia is its modest specificity. Although some overtreatment results, it is small compared with current use of antibiotics for all children with an ARI, as occurs in many clinics.

Lower chest wall indrawing defined as inward movement of the bony structure of the chest wall with inspiration is a

TEACH THE MOTHER TO GIVE ORAL DRUGS AT HOME

Follow the instructions below for every oral drug to be given at home. Also follow the instructions listed with each drug's dosage table.

- ▶ Determine the appropriate drugs and dosage for the child's age or weight.
- ▶ Tell the mother the reason for giving the drug to the child.
- ▶ Demonstrate how to measure a dose.
- ▶ Watch the mother practice measuring a dose by herself.
- ▶ Ask the mother to give the first dose to her child.
- ▶ Explain carefully how to give the drug, then label and package the drug.
- ▶ If more than one drug will be given, collect, count and package each drug separately.
- ▶ Explain that all the oral drug tablets or syrups must be used to finish the course of treatment, even if the child gets better.
- ▶ Check the mother's understanding before she leaves the clinic.

▶ Give an Appropriate Oral Antibiotic

▶ FOR PNEUMONIA, ACUTE EAR INFECTION OR VERY SEVERE DISEASE:

FIRST-LINE ANTIBIOTIC: _____

SECOND-LINE ANTIBIOTIC: _____

AGE or WEIGHT	COTRIMOXAZOLE (trimethoprim + sulphamethoxazole) ▶ Give two times daily for 5 days			AMOXYCILLIN ▶ Give three times daily for 5 days.	
	ADULT TABLET 80 mg trimethoprim + 400 mg sulphamethoxazole	PEDIATRIC TABLET 20 mg trimethoprim + 100 mg sulphamethoxazole	SYRUP 40 mg trimethoprim + 200 mg sulphamethoxazole per 5 ml	TABLET 250 mg	SYRUP 125 mg per 5 ml
2 months up to 12 months (4 - < 10 kg)	1/2	2	5.0 ml	1/2	5 ml
12 months up to 5 years (10 -19 kg)	1	3	7.5 ml	1	10 ml

▶ FOR DYSENTERY:

Give antibiotic recommended for Shigella in your area for 5 days.

FIRST-LINE ANTIBIOTIC FOR SHIGELLA: _____

SECOND-LINE ANTIBIOTIC FOR SHIGELLA: _____

AGE or WEIGHT	COTRIMOXAZOLE (trimethoprim + sulphamethoxazole) ▶ Give two times daily for 5 days	NALIDIXIC ACID ▶ Give four times daily for 5 days
		TABLET 250 mg
2 months up to 4 months (4 - < 6 kg)	See doses above	1/4
4 months up to 12 months (6 - < 10 kg)		1/2
12 months up to 5 years (10 - 19 kg)		1

▶ FOR CHOLERA:

Give antibiotic recommended for Cholera in your area for 3 days.

FIRST-LINE ANTIBIOTIC FOR CHOLERA: _____

SECOND-LINE ANTIBIOTIC FOR CHOLERA: _____

AGE or WEIGHT	TETRACYCLINE ▶ Give four times daily for 3 days	COTRIMOXAZOLE (trimethoprim + sulphamethoxazole) ▶ Give two times daily for 3 days	ERYTHROMYCIN ▶ Give four times daily for 3 days	FURAZOLIDONE ▶ Give four times daily for 3 days
	TABLET 250 mg		TABLET 250 mg	TABLET 100 mg
2 months up to 4 months (4 - < 6 kg)		See doses above	1/4	
4 months up to 12 months (6 - < 10 kg)	1/2		1/2	
12 months up to 5 years (10 - 19 kg)	1		1	1/4

Figure 16–3. Oral antibiotic treatment administered at home. (From World Health Organization, Division of Diarrheal and Acute Respiratory Disease Control: Management of Childhood Illness. Chart booklet. Geneva, WHO, 1995, p 7, with modification.)

GIVE EXTRA FLUID FOR DIARRHEA AND CONTINUE FEEDING
(See FOOD advice on COUNSEL THE MOTHER chart)

▶ Plan A: Treat Diarrhea at Home

Counsel the mother on the 3 Rules of Home Treatment:
Give Extra Fluid, Continue Feeding, When to Return

1. **GIVE EXTRA FLUID** (as much as the child will take)

    ▶ TELL THE MOTHER:
      - Breastfeed frequently and for longer at each feed.
      - If the child is exclusively breastfed, give ORS or clean water in addition to breastmilk.
      - If the child is not exclusively breastfed, give one or more of the following: ORS solution, food-based fluids (such as soup, rice water, and yoghurt drinks), or clean water.

    It is especially important to give ORS at home when:
      - *the child has been treated with Plan B or Plan C (see Fig. 16–9) during this visit.*
      - *the child cannot return to a clinic if the diarrhea gets worse.*

    ▶ TEACH THE MOTHER HOW TO MIX AND GIVE ORS. GIVE THE MOTHER 2 PACKETS OF ORS TO USE AT HOME.

    ▶ SHOW THE MOTHER HOW MUCH FLUID TO GIVE IN ADDITION TO THE USUAL FLUID INTAKE:
      Up to 2 years   50 to 100 ml after each loose stool
      2 years or more   100 to 200 ml after each loose stool

    Tell the mother to:
      - Give frequent small sips from a cup.
      - If the child vomits, wait 10 minutes. Then continue, but more slowly.
      - Continue giving extra fluid until the diarrhea stops.

2. **CONTINUE FEEDING** ⎫
                              ⎬ See COUNSEL THE MOTHER chart
3. **WHEN TO RETURN** ⎭

▶ Plan B: Treat Some Dehydration with ORS

Give in clinic recommended amount of ORS over 4-hour period

▶ DETERMINE AMOUNT OF ORS TO GIVE DURING FIRST 4 HOURS.

AGE*	Up to 4 months	4 months up to 12 months	12 months up to 2 years	2 years up to 5 years
WEIGHT	< 6 kg	6 - < 10 kg	10 - < 12 kg	12 - 19 kg
In ml	200 - 400	400 - 700	700 - 900	900 - 1400

* Use the child's age only when you do not know the weight. The approximate amount of ORS required (in ml) can also be calculated by multiplying the child's weight (in kg) times 75.

- If the child wants more ORS than shown, give more.
- For infants under 6 months who are not breastfed, also give 100-200 ml clean water during this period.

▶ SHOW THE MOTHER HOW TO GIVE ORS SOLUTION.
  - Give frequent small sips from a cup.
  - If the child vomits, wait 10 minutes. Then continue, but more slowly.
  - Continue breastfeeding whenever the child wants.

▶ AFTER 4 HOURS:
  - Reassess the child and classify the child for dehydration.
  - Select the appropriate plan to continue treatment.
  - Begin feeding the child in clinic.

▶ IF THE MOTHER MUST LEAVE BEFORE COMPLETING TREATMENT:
  - Show her how to prepare ORS solution at home.
  - Show her how much ORS to give to finish the 4-hour treatment at home.
  - Give her enough ORS packets to complete rehydration. Also give her 2 packets as recommended in Plan A.
  - Explain the 3 Rules of Home Treatment:

1. **GIVE EXTRA FLUID** ⎫
                              ⎬ See Plan A for recommended fluids and
2. **CONTINUE FEEDING** ⎬ See COUNSEL THE MOTHER chart
                              ⎬ (Figs. 16–5 to 16–7)
3. **WHEN TO RETURN** ⎭

Figure 16–4. Increased fluids for diarrhea. ORS, oral rehydration salts. (From World Health Organization, Division of Diarrheal and Acute Respiratory Disease Control: Management of Childhood Illness. Chart booklet. Geneva, WHO, 1995, p 12, Plans A and B, with modifications.)

FOOD

Counsel the Mother to Assess the Child's Feeding

Ask questions about the child's usual feeding and feeding during this illness. Compare the mother's answers to the *Feeding Recommendations* for the child's age in the box (see Fig. 16–6).

ASK -

► Do you breastfeed your child?
 - How many times during the day?
 - Do you also breastfeed during the night?

► Does the child take any other food or fluids?
 - What food or fluids?
 - How many times per day?
 - What do you use to feed the child?
 - If very low weight for age: How large are servings? Does the child receive his own serving? Who feeds the child and how?

► During this illness, has the child's feeding changed? If yes, how?

Figure 16–5. Feeding assessment. (From World Health Organization, Division of Diarrheal and Acute Respiratory Disease Control: Management of Childhood Illness. Chart booklet. Geneva, WHO, 1995, p 17, with modifications.)

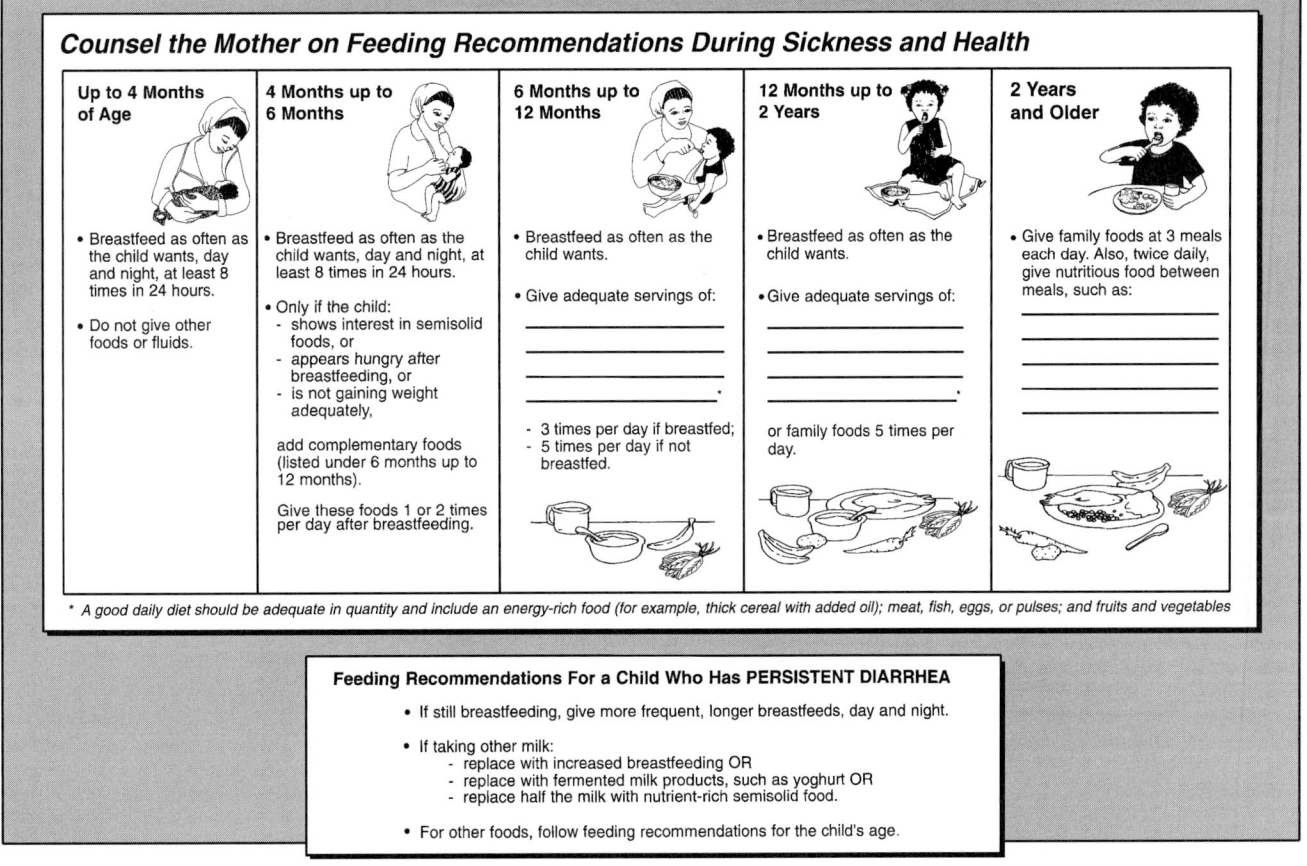

Counsel the Mother on Feeding Recommendations During Sickness and Health

Up to 4 Months of Age	4 Months up to 6 Months	6 Months up to 12 Months	12 Months up to 2 Years	2 Years and Older
• Breastfeed as often as the child wants, day and night, at least 8 times in 24 hours. • Do not give other foods or fluids.	• Breastfeed as often as the child wants, day and night, at least 8 times in 24 hours. • Only if the child: - shows interest in semisolid foods, or - appears hungry after breastfeeding, or - is not gaining weight adequately, add complementary foods (listed under 6 months up to 12 months). Give these foods 1 or 2 times per day after breastfeeding.	• Breastfeed as often as the child wants. • Give adequate servings of: ——————— ——————— ——————— ——————— * - 3 times per day if breastfed; - 5 times per day if not breastfed.	• Breastfeed as often as the child wants. • Give adequate servings of: ——————— ——————— ——————— ——————— * or family foods 5 times per day.	• Give family foods at 3 meals each day. Also, twice daily, give nutritious food between meals, such as: ——————— ——————— ——————— ———————

* *A good daily diet should be adequate in quantity and include an energy-rich food (for example, thick cereal with added oil); meat, fish, eggs, or pulses; and fruits and vegetables*

Feeding Recommendations For a Child Who Has PERSISTENT DIARRHEA

• If still breastfeeding, give more frequent, longer breastfeeds, day and night.

• If taking other milk:
 - replace with increased breastfeeding OR
 - replace with fermented milk products, such as yoghurt OR
 - replace half the milk with nutrient-rich semisolid food.

• For other foods, follow feeding recommendations for the child's age.

Figure 16–6. Feeding recommendations. (From World Health Organization, Division of Diarrheal and Acute Respiratory Disease Control: Management of Childhood Illness. Chart booklet. Geneva, WHO, 1995, p 18.)

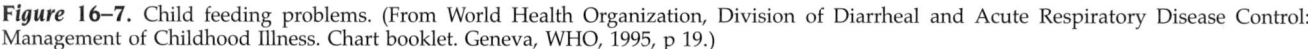

Counsel the Mother About Feeding Problems

If the child is not being fed as described in the above recommendations, counsel the mother accordingly. In addition:

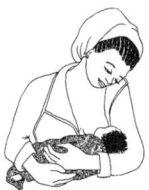

▸ **If the mother reports difficulty with breastfeeding, assess breastfeeding.**
(See *YOUNG INFANT* chart, Figs. 16–11 and 16–12)
As needed, show the mother correct positioning and attachment for breastfeeding.

▸ **If the child is less than 4 months old and is taking other milk or foods:**

- Build mother's confidence that she can produce all the breastmilk that the child needs.
- Suggest giving more frequent, longer breastfeeds, day and night, and gradually reducing other milk or foods.

If other milk needs to be continued, counsel the mother to:

- Breastfeed as much as possible, including at night.
- Make sure that other milk is a locally appropriate breastmilk substitute.
- Make sure other milk is correctly and hygienically prepared and given in adequate amounts.
- Finish prepared milk within an hour.

▸ **If the mother is using a bottle to feed the child:**

- Recommend substituting a cup for bottle.
- Show the mother how to feed the child with a cup.

▸ **If the child is not being fed actively, counsel the mother to:**

- Sit with the child and encourage eating.
- Give the child an adequate serving in a separate plate or bowl.

▸ **If the child is not feeding well during illness, counsel the mother to:**

- Breastfeed more frequently and for longer if possible.
- Use soft, varied, appetizing, favourite foods to encourage the child to eat as much as possible, and offer frequent small feedings.
- Clear a blocked nose if it interferes with feeding.
- Expect that appetite will improve as child gets better.

▸ **Follow-up any feeding problem in 5 days.**

Figure 16–7. Child feeding problems. (From World Health Organization, Division of Diarrheal and Acute Respiratory Disease Control: Management of Childhood Illness. Chart booklet. Geneva, WHO, 1995, p 19.)

useful indicator of severe pneumonia. It is more specific than "intercostal indrawing," and thus results in the classification of a smaller number of sicker children as having indrawing (and thus needing referral to the hospital).

Children who have stridor when calm have a substantial risk of obstruction and should be referred. Some children with mild croup have stridor only when crying or agitated. This should not be the basis for referral.

CHOICE OF ANTIBIOTICS FOR PNEUMONIA (Fig. 16–3). Co-trimoxazole and amoxicillin are the two most common oral antibiotics used for the outpatient treatment of pneumonia (and ear infection). Amoxicillin is much preferred to ampicillin, which has erratic absorption and is now more expensive than amoxicillin. If the child is not able to drink, intramuscular chloramphenicol is recommended prior to referral. The choice of antibiotic is based on the well-established finding that most childhood pneumonia of bacterial origin is due to *Streptococcus pneumoniae* or *Haemophilus influenzae.* Amoxicillin, ampicillin, trimethroprim-sulfamethoxazole, injectable penicillin G (but not penicillin V, which is poor against *H. influenzae*), and chloramphenicol are usually effective treatment for these two bacteria. A single injection of benzathine penicillin, although long-lasting, does not provide adequate levels of penicillin to treat *H. influenzae.* Tetracycline is *not* adequate treatment.

Diarrhea (Fig. 16–8)

All outpatient health workers should be prepared to manage the three leading contributors to diarrheal disease mortality: (1) acute watery diarrhea (including cholera): (2) dysentery (bloody diarrhea) and (3) persistent diarrhea (diarrhea that lasts ≥14 days). Rehydration therapy is provided to treat clinically apparent dehydration or to prevent its developing. Dysentery is treated with an oral antibiotic effective for *Shigella.* Careful nutritional management is provided for persistent diarrhea, as well as treatment of extraintestinal infections that may be contributing to the persistent diarrhea. The WHO control of diarrheal disease (CDD) guidelines for these conditions are both practical and effective in the global effort to reduce mortality and serious morbidity caused by diarrhea in young children, and are incorporated within the IMCI guidelines.

MANAGEMENT OF DEHYDRATION. The assessment and classification of dehydration has been simplified, drawing on years of clinical experience with the CDD case management chart. It now relies on the child's general condition, how fast the skin pinch returns, the presence or absence of sunken eyes, and how the child drinks (Fig. 16–8).

Patients with *severe dehydration* have a fluid deficit equaling >10% of their body weight, and patients with *some dehydration* have a fluid deficit equaling 5 to 10% of their body weight. The latter category includes both "mild" and "moderate" dehydration, which are descriptive terms used in many textbooks. Patients with diarrhea but no signs of dehydration usually have a fluid deficit, but equal to <5% of their body weight. Although these patients lack distinct signs of dehydration, they should be given more fluid than usual to prevent signs of dehydration from developing.

Dehydration Not Present. Plan A (Fig. 16–4) summarizes treatment for a child who has no signs of dehydration, centered on the three rules of home treatment: give extra fluids, continue feeding, and advise the mother when to return (bring the child back to the health worker if the child devel-

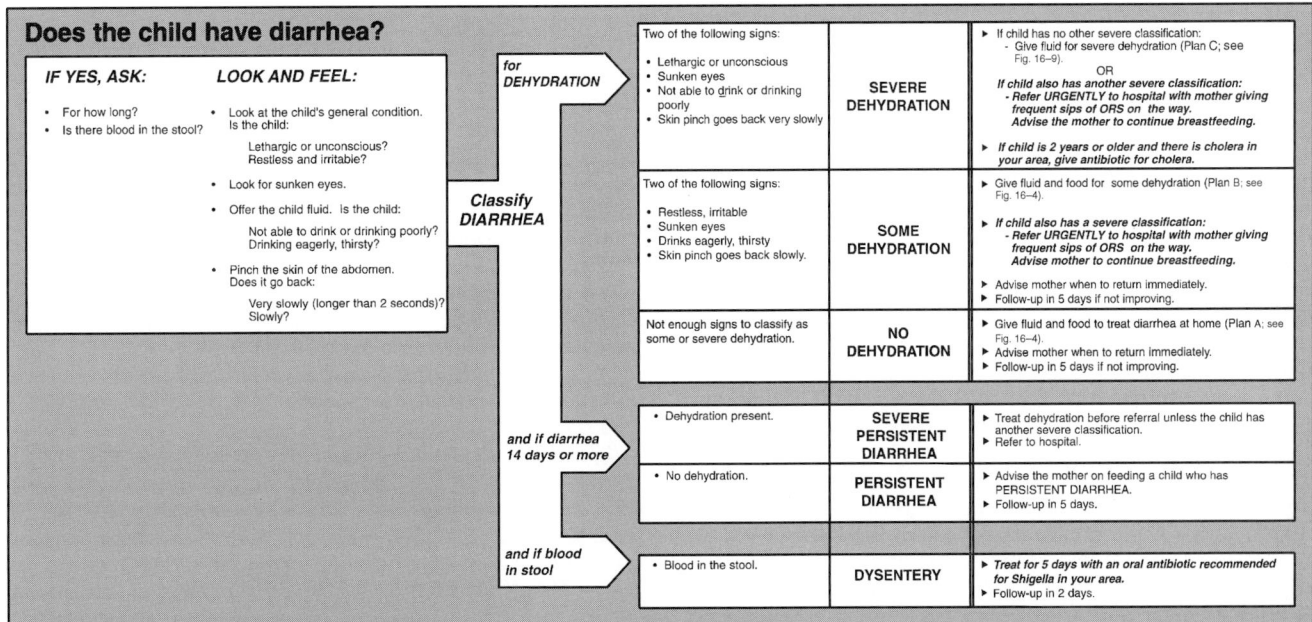

Figure 16–8. Management of diarrhea. (From World Health Organization, Division of Diarrheal and Acute Respiratory Disease Control: Management of Childhood Illness. Chart booklet. Geneva, WHO, 1995, p 3.)

ops blood in the stool, drinks poorly, becomes sicker, or is not better in 3 days). Fluids should be given as soon as diarrhea starts and the child should take as much as he or she wants. Correct home therapy can prevent dehydration in many cases. Adequate counseling of the mother is essential for effective use of Plan A. In addition to the specific advice in the chart summary, it is important that mothers of exclusively breast-fed children know they should resume limiting intake to breast milk alone after the diarrhea resolves.

Oral rehydration salts [or solution] (ORS) in water is recommended by WHO for the treatment of dehydration caused by diarrhea. The standard WHO recommended formulation contains (in grams per liter) sodium chloride, 3.5; trisodium citrate dihydrate, 2.9 or sodium bicarbonate, 2.5; potassium chloride, 1.5; and glucose, 20.0. Recent data suggest shifting the composition of ORS to a lower osmolarity solution (245 mOsm/L). Using the lower osmolarity formulation requires no change in the instructions for using ORS.

In nearly all developing countries, a major effort is being made to provide the whole population with access to treatment with ORS solution by trained health workers. ORS may also be used at home to prevent dehydration. However, other fluids that are commonly available in the home may be less costly, more convenient and nearly as effective, especially when given with food.

Some fluids and foods are especially effective, and thus should be promoted; a few should be avoided. Home fluid should be:

Safe when given in large volumes. Very sweet tea, soft drinks, and sweetened fruit drinks should be avoided. These are often hyperosmolar owing to their high sugar content (>300 mOsm/L). They can cause osmotic diarrhea, worsening dehydration and hypernatremia. Also to be avoided are fluids with purgative action and stimulants (e.g., coffee, some medicinal teas or infusions).

Easy to prepare. The recipe should be familiar and its preparation should not require much work or time. The required ingredients and measuring utensils should be readily available and inexpensive.

Acceptable. The fluid should be one that the mother is willing to give freely to a child with diarrhea and that the child will readily accept.

Effective. Fluids that are safe are also effective. However, some are more effective than others, depending on their composition. Most effective are fluids that contain carbohydrate and protein and some salt. However, nearly the same benefit may be obtained when water and other salt-free fluids are given freely along with weaning foods that contain salt.

Most fluids that a child normally takes can also be used for home therapy. They must, however, be considered acceptable by the mother for use during diarrhea. Some fluids are especially useful because they contain salt. Whenever possible, a fluid should be promoted that contains salt and sugar, starch or protein. The possibilities include ORS solution, a salted soup, or a salted drink. ORS solution should be promoted if ORS packets are readily available and affordable, and mothers know, or will be taught, how to mix and give ORS solution.

Teaching mothers to add salt (about 3 g/L) to an unsalted soup or drink during diarrhea is also possible, but requires a substantial and sustained educational effort. The cost and feasibility of this effort should be carefully considered before adopting this strategy. Sugar-salt solution (SSS) has been promoted previously for home therapy, but has not proved satisfactory in most countries. This is because mothers often forget the recipe, or are unable to obtain sugar or salt. Moreover, mistakes in mixing SSS can cause the concentrations of sugar and salt to be dangerously high. In most countries, SSS should not be promoted.

One or more fluids that are prepared without salt should also be promoted. These are often the most widely used home drinks and are the fluids most likely to be given in greater amounts than usual to a thirsty child. Some common examples are plain clean water, water in which a cereal has been cooked, e.g., (unsalted) rice water, soup, or yogurt-based drinks, green coconut water, weak (unsweetened) tea, or fresh fruit juice.

Plain clean water is the most widely given home fluid. Most mothers give water to children with diarrhea. Water should always be one of the promoted home fluids. Specific home fluid recommendations can be added to Plan A during the adaptation of course materials.

Moderate Dehydration. Plan B is summarized in Figure 16–4. Plan B includes an initial treatment period of 4 hours in the clinic. During these 4 hours, the mother slowly gives the recommended amount of ORS, by spoonfuls or sips. Breast-feeding should continue. It is helpful to set up an oral rehydration therapy (ORT) corner to facilitate this. After 4 hours, the child should be reassessed and reclassified for dehydration and feeding should begin. If the signs of dehydration are gone, the child is put on Plan A. If there is still some dehydration, Plan B should be repeated. If the child now has severe dehydration, the child should be put on Plan C.

Severe Dehydration. Plan C is summarized in Figure 16–9. Treatment depends on whether IV fluids can be given immediately in the clinic; if not, urgent referral to the hospital for IV treatment should be recommended. If referral takes more than 30 minutes, fluids should be given by nasogastric tube. If none of these are possible and the child can drink, ORS should be given by mouth. Ringer's lactate solution is the preferred commercially available solution. Early provision of ORS and early resumption of feeding are important to provide required amounts of potassium and glucose. Normal saline does not correct acidosis or replace potassium losses but can be used. Plain glucose or dextrose solutions are *not* acceptable for the treatment of dehydration.

MANAGEMENT OF DYSENTERY

Definitions. A child should be classified as having dysentery based on maternal report of blood in the stool. It is not necessary to examine the stool or perform laboratory tests to diagnose dysentery. Stool culture, to detect pathogenic bacteria, is rarely possible. Moreover, at least 2 days are required before results of a culture are available, whereas a decision on antimicrobial therapy must be made immediately. Although clinical texts often use the term *dysentery* to describe the syndrome of bloody diarrhea with fever, abdominal cramps, rectal pain and mucoid stools, these features do not always accompany bloody diarrhea, nor do they necessarily define its etiology or determine appropriate treatment. Bloody diarrhea in young children is usually a sign of invasive enteric infection that carries a substantial risk of serious morbidity and death.

Epidemiology. About 10% of all diarrheal episodes in children <5 years of age are dysenteric, but these cause up to 15% of all diarrheal deaths. Dysentery is especially severe in infants and in children who are undernourished, develop clinically evident dehydration during their illness, or are not breast-fed. It also has a more harmful effect on nutritional status than acute watery diarrhea. Dysentery occurs with increased frequency and severity in children who have measles or have had measles in the preceding month, and diarrheal episodes that begin with dysentery are more likely to become persistent than those that start with watery stools.

Etiology. The most important and most frequent cause of acute dysentery is *Shigella*, especially *Shigella flexneri* and *Shigella dysenteriae* type 1 (Chapter 40). *Shigella* is estimated

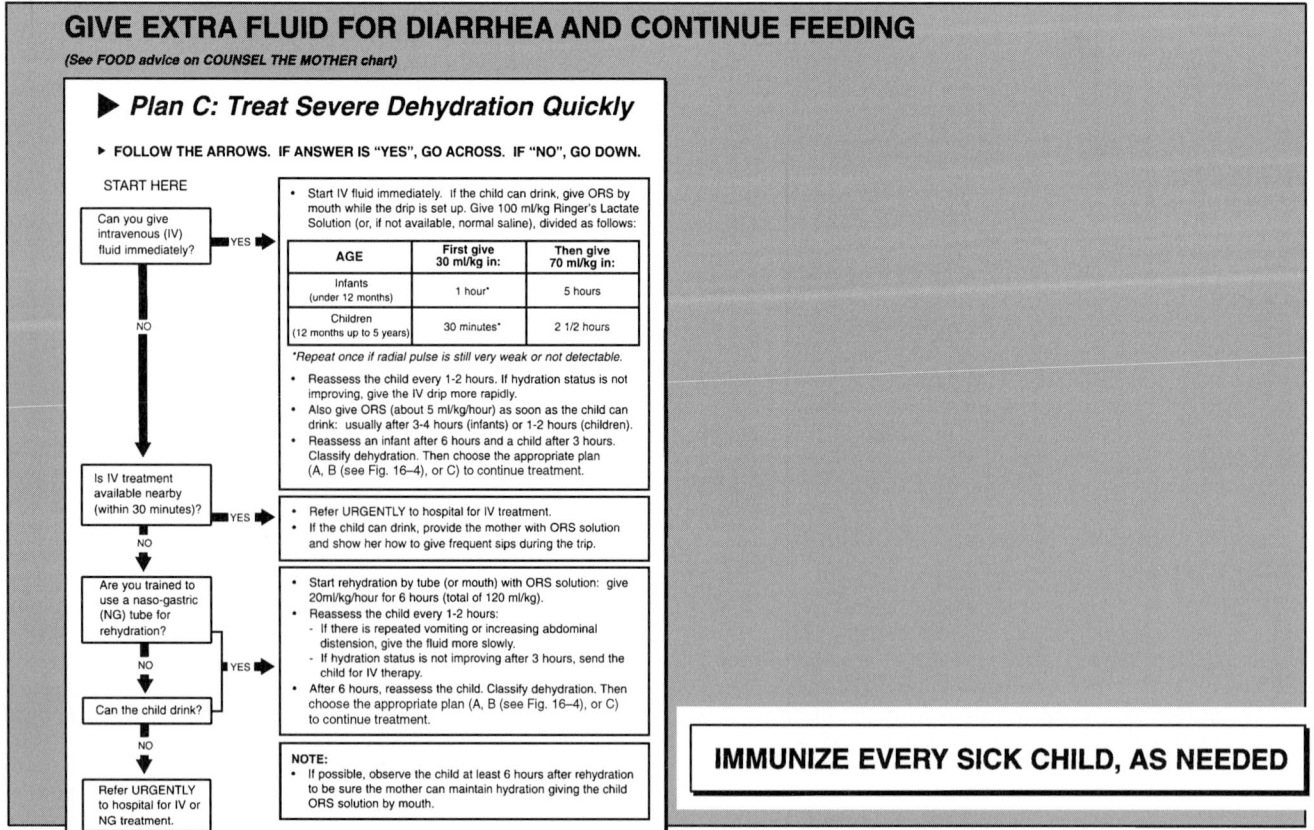

Figure 16–9. Treatment of severe dehydration. ORS, oral rehydration salts [solution]. (From World Health Organization, Division of Diarrheal and Acute Respiratory Disease Control: Management of Childhood Illness. Chart booklet. Geneva, WHO, 1995, p 13.)

to cause approximately 50% of all episodes of bloody diarrhea in young children, and a much higher proportion of episodes that are clinically severe. Other causes include *Campylobacter jejuni*, especially in infants (Chapter 43), and, less frequently, *Salmonella* (Chapter 76); dysentery caused by the latter agents is usually not severe. Enteroinvasive *Escherichia coli* are closely related to *Shigella* and may cause dysentery (Chapter 42). However, infection with this agent is uncommon. *Entamoeba histolytica* causes dysentery in older children and adults, but rarely in children <5 years of age (Chapter 86).

Therapy. All children with bloody diarrhea should be treated promptly with an antimicrobial effective against *Shigella* because:

1. Bloody diarrhea in this age group is caused much more frequently by *Shigella* than by any other pathogen.
2. Shigellosis is more likely than other causes of diarrhea to result in complications and death if effective antimicrobial therapy is not begun promptly.
3. Early treatment of shigellosis with an *effective* antibiotic substantially reduces the risk of severe morbidity or death.

Young infants (aged <2 months) with dysentery should be referred for hospital assessment and treatment, because (1) dysentery is uncommon in young infants and blood in the stool is more likely to be the sign of a surgical problem, and (2) in this age group treatment of shigellosis may require daily injection of ceftriaxone. Nalidixic acid and ciprofloxacin should not be used in infants <2 months of age.

The four key components of the treatment of dysentery are antibiotics, fluids, feeding, and follow-up. Early treatment of shigellosis with an appropriate antibiotic shortens the duration of the illness and reduces the risk of serious complications and death. However, such treatment is effective only when the *Shigella* are sensitive to the antibiotic that is given. If treatment is delayed or an antibiotic is given to which the *Shigella* are not sensitive, the bacteria may cause extensive damage to the bowel and enter the general circulation causing septicemia, prostration, and sometimes septic shock. These complications occur more frequently in children who are undernourished or in infants, and may be fatal.

As the antibiotic sensitivity of the infecting strain of *Shigella* is not known for each case, it is important to use an oral antibiotic to which most *Shigella* in the area are known to be sensitive. Resistance to ampicillin and co-trimoxazole, formerly the drugs of choice, is now widespread, particularly among *S. dysenteriae* type 1, but also in many areas among *S. flexneri*. Nalidixic acid, formerly used as a backup drug to treat resistant shigellosis, is now the drug of choice in many areas, but resistance to that drug is also appearing. Although treatment is recommended for 5 days, there should be a substantial improvement, i.e., less fever, pain, and fecal blood, and fewer loose bowel movements, after 2 days of treatment with the first-line antibiotic. If this does not occur, the antibiotic should be stopped and a different one used (second-line antibiotic). Selection of an antibiotic should be based on sensitivity patterns of strains of *Shigella* isolated in the area. Antibiotics should be selected to which most strains are susceptible, that are effective when given by mouth, that are affordable, and that are readily available, or can be rapidly obtained.

Antimicrobials that are not effective for shigellosis include metronidazole, streptomycin, tetracyclines, chloramphenicol and sulfonamides, to which *Shigella* are usually resistant in vitro. Agents that are effective in vitro but ineffective clinically because they penetrate poorly the intestinal mucosa where invasive *Shigella* must be killed include nitrofurans

(nitrofurantoin, furazolidone), aminoglycosides (gentamicin, kanamycin), first- and second-generation cephalosporins (cephalexin), and amoxicillin.

The IMCI guidelines recommend that all sick children with dysentery should return in 2 days for follow-up. This was done to simplify the guidelines and avoid requiring the health worker to consider whether the child is high risk in recommending referral. If there are many cases of dysentery and/or if follow-up is difficult, that follow-up should be focused on those at highest risk: infants <12 months, those dehydrated at the initial visit, and those with measles within the last 3 months.

If there is no improvement after 2 days of treatment with the second-line antibiotic, the patient should either be referred to the hospital for further evaluation or, if this is not possible, treated for possible amebiasis, which can only be diagnosed with certainty when trophozoites of *E. histolytica* containing red blood cells are seen in a fresh stool sample. Young children with dysentery should *not* be treated routinely for amebiasis. Treatment should only be given when *E. histolytica* trophozoites containing red blood cells are identified in feces or when bloody stools persist after consecutive treatment with two antibiotics that are usually effective for *Shigella*. The preferred treatment for amebic dysentery is metronidazole. If dysentery is caused by *E. histolytica* an improvement will occur within 2 to 3 days of starting treatment.

DETECTION AND TREATMENT OF CHOLERA. Antibiotics are recommended for patients >2 years with severe dehydration due to suspected cholera (Chapter 41). An effective antibiotic can reduce the volume of diarrhea in patients with severe cholera and shorten the period during which *Vibrio cholerae* is excreted. In addition, it usually stops the diarrhea within 48 hours, thus reducing the period of hospitalization. Selection of first- and second-line antibiotics for cholera should be based on the sensitivity pattern of strains of *V. cholerae* serogroup 01 isolated in the area.

PERSISTENT DIARRHEA. Persistent diarrhea is an episode of diarrhea, with or without blood, that begins acutely and lasts at least 14 days. It usually accounts for up to 15% of all episodes of diarrhea but is associated with 30 to 50% of deaths. It is usually associated with weight loss and, often, with serious nonintestinal infections. Many children who develop persistent diarrhea are malnourished and this greatly increases the risk of death. Persistent diarrhea almost never occurs in infants who are exclusively breast-fed.

Persistent diarrhea is associated with extensive changes in the bowel mucosa, especially flattening of the villi and reduced production of disaccharidase enzymes; these cause reduced absorption of nutrients and weight loss and may perpetuate the illness after the original infectious cause has been eliminated. Other contributing factors include poor food intake owing to anorexia or withholding of food, or substituting dilute, low-energy foods. Patients are also likely to become deficient in various vitamins and minerals: those of special importance because of their role in the renewal and repair of the intestinal mucosa and/or their role in normal immunologic responses include folate, vitamin B_{12}, vitamin A, and zinc.

Nutritional Therapy. Proper feeding is the most important aspect of treatment for most children with persistent diarrhea. Many can be treated on an ambulatory basis with food available in the home; however, some require specialized care in the hospital. The goals of nutritional therapy are to:

- Temporarily reduce the amount of animal milk (or lactose) in the diet.
- Provide a sufficient intake of energy, protein, vitamins, and minerals to facilitate the repair process in the damaged gut mucosa and improve nutritional status.

- Avoid giving foods or drinks that may aggravate the diarrhea.
- Ensure that the child's food intake during convalescence is adequate to correct any undernutrition and prevent its recurrence.

The general guidelines for feeding during and after diarrhea given in treatment Plan A (Fig. 16–4) should be followed. Young infants <2 months of age or any sick child with persistent diarrhea plus evidence of dehydration should be rehydrated (unless the child is severely malnourished) and referred to the hospital for further management. These children may require special efforts to maintain hydration, and replacement of animal milk with lactose-free or artificial milk formula. For other children, the mother should be instructed to continue breastfeeding (Fig. 16–6). If yogurt is available, give it in place of any animal milk usually taken by the child; yogurt contains less lactose and is better tolerated. If animal milk must be given, limit it to 50 mL/kg/day; greater amounts may aggravate the diarrhea. Mix the milk with the child's cereal. Do not dilute the milk. In many cases, these steps cause the diarrhea to subside rapidly.

Ensure a full energy intake for the child (i.e., about 110 kcal/kg/day) by giving thick cereal with added vegetable oil; mix this with other foods, e.g., well-cooked and mashed pulse, vegetables, and if possible, meat or fish. Avoid low energy foods that are dilute or bulky. At least half of the child's energy intake should come from foods other than milk or milk products. Avoid foods that are hyperosmolar (these are usually foods or drinks made very sweet by the addition of sucrose, such as soft drinks or commercial fruit drinks); these can make the diarrhea worse. Give food in frequent, small meals, at least six times a day.

Identify and Treat Specific Infections. Routine treatment of persistent diarrhea with antimicrobials is not effective. Some children, however, have nonintestinal (or intestinal) infections that require specific antimicrobial therapy. The persistent diarrhea of such children will not improve until these infections are diagnosed and treated correctly.

Every child with persistent diarrhea should be examined for nonintestinal infections, e.g., pneumonia, sepsis, urinary tract infection, and otitis media. Treatment of these infections should follow standard guidelines.

Persistent diarrhea with blood in the stool should be treated with an oral antimicrobial effective against *Shigella*. Treatment for amebiasis should only be given if the diagnostic criteria are met. Treatment for giardiasis should be given only if cysts or trophozoites are seen in the feces.

Supplementary Multivitamins and Minerals. Micronutrient deficiencies are common in malnourished children and are exacerbated by losses from diarrhea. This is why micronutrient supplementation plays an important role in the therapy of persistent diarrhea. All children with persistent diarrhea should receive supplementary multivitamins and minerals each day for 2 weeks. Locally available commercial preparations are often suitable; tablets that can be crushed and given with food are least costly. These should provide as broad a range of vitamins and minerals as possible, including at least twice the recommended daily allowances (RDAs) of folate, vitamin A, iron, zinc, magnesium, and copper.

USE OF ANTIDIARRHEAL DRUGS. A wide variety of drugs or combinations of drugs is sold for the treatment of acute diarrhea and vomiting. Antidiarrheal drugs including antimotility agents (e.g., loperamide, diphenoxylate, codeine, tincture of opium), adsorbents (e.g., kaolin, attapulgite, smectite), live bacterial cultures (e.g., *Lactobacillus, Streptococcus faecium*), and charcoal are not useful in the treatment of childhood diarrhea and some are associated with adverse reactions. Antiemetics include phenergan and chlorpromazine. *None* of these has provided practical benefits for children with acute diarrhea, and some may have dangerous side effects. These drugs should *never* be given to children <5 years of age.

Antibiotics also should not be used routinely. Antibiotics or other antimicrobials given "blindly" are *not effective* treatment for diarrhea in young children. This is because most diarrheal episodes are caused by agents for which antimicrobials are not effective, e.g., viruses, or by bacteria that must first be cultured to determine their sensitivity to antimicrobials. Culture, however, is costly and requires several days. Moreover, most laboratories are unable to detect many of the important bacterial causes of diarrhea. In practice, antimicrobials should only be given for bloody diarrhea (suspected shigellosis) and suspected cholera. Antiparasitic drugs are rarely indicated.

The overuse of antidiarrheal and antiemetic drugs, antibiotics, and antiparasitic agents often delays the initiation of ORT or a visit to the health facility to seek help; it also consumes precious financial resources of the family unnecessarily.

Fever

MANAGEMENT OF FEVER IN MALARIOUS AREAS. Children are considered to have fever if they have either a history of fever or a body temperature above 37.5°C axillary (38°C rectal) or, in the absence of a thermometer, if they feel hot. The malarial case management guidelines summarized in Figure 16–10 present a simplified system for outpatient settings in which microscopic results are either not promptly available or are reserved for children who fail the first-line oral antimalarial.

Children with fever with a stiff neck or a general danger sign may have severe malaria, meningitis, or another very severe febrile disease. They should be referred urgently to the hospital, after prereferral treatment with an effective antibiotic and intramuscular quinine (Chapter 92).

Management of febrile children without these severe signs depends on whether the risk of malaria is high or low. The decisions on whether a site is high or low risk must be made in order to adapt the IMCI guidelines to national conditions, based on knowledge of the seasonality of malaria locally and an estimate of the proportion of children presenting to the clinic with fever who have parasitemia. To guide antimalarial therapy in the absence of routine microscopy, a *high malaria risk setting* has been defined as a situation in which >5% of cases of febrile disease in children aged 2 to 59 months are malarial disease. A *low malarial risk setting* is a situation in which ≤5% of cases of febrile disease in children aged 2 to 59 months are malarial disease, but in which the risk is not negligible. If malaria transmission does not normally occur in the area, and imported malaria is uncommon, the setting is considered to have *no malaria risk*.

It is the responsibility of national malaria control programs to define high and low malaria risk settings (these may be geographic areas and/or seasons) and to inform health services of the malaria risk. If these investigations are not possible, and malaria is known to exist in the catchment area of the health facility, then it is better to assume high malaria risk.

In a high malaria risk area or season, presumptive treatment for malaria should be provided to all children with a fever in the clinic or a history of fever during this illness. Although a substantial number of children who are treated for malaria in fact have another febrile illness, presumptive treatment for malaria is justified given the high rate of ma-

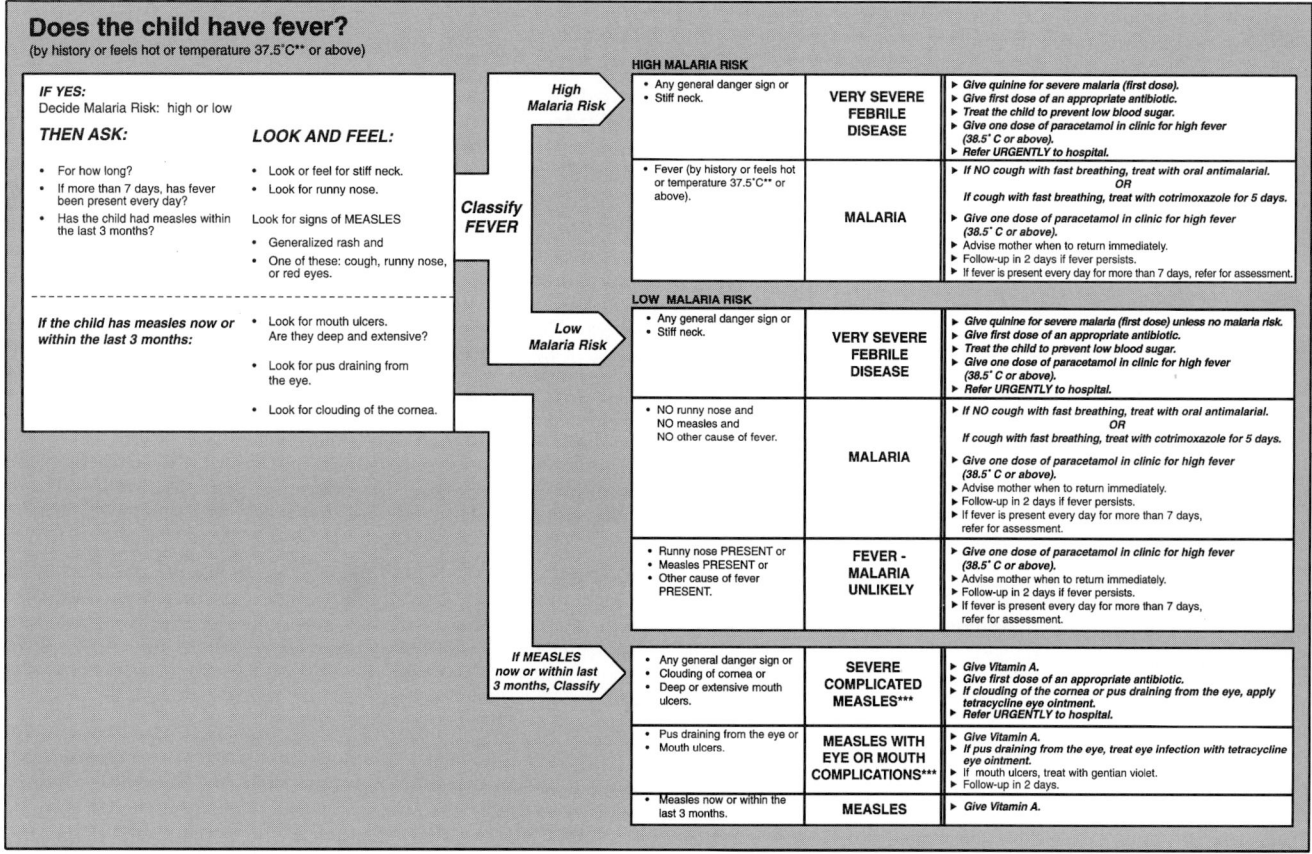

** These temperatures are based on axillary temperature. Rectal temperature readings are approximately 0.5° C higher.

*** Other important complications of measles - pneumonia, stridor, diarrhea, ear infection, and malnutrition - are classified in other tables.

Figure 16–10. Management of fever in malarious areas. (From World Health Organization, Division of Diarrheal and Acute Respiratory Disease Control: Management of Childhood Illness. Chart booklet. Geneva, WHO, 1995, p 4.)

laria parasitemia and the possibility that another illness might cause the malaria infection to progress.

In a low malarial risk area or season, children with fever or a history of fever are given an antimalarial only if they have no runny nose (a sign of ARIs), measles, or other apparent cause of fever. Evidence of another infection lowers the probability that the child's illness is due to malaria.

Any child with a fever every day for >7 days should be referred for assessment for typhoid and other causes of prolonged pyrexia.

Adaptations are required if malaria species besides falciparum are common; if falciparum malaria is not transmitted; if good quality microscopic results are available during the clinic session; and/or if there are other important causes of fever, e.g., relapsing fever or dengue hemorrhagic fever. Co-trimoxazole twice daily for 5 days has been shown to be an efficacious antimalarial for young children in some areas. Given the overlap in clinical presentation and the treatment of pneumonia and malaria, co-trimoxazole alone for the treatment of children presenting with cough, fast breathing, and fever. However, co-trimoxazole is only effective for the treatment of falciparum malaria when the parasites are sensitive to sulfadoxine-pyrimethamine and when compliance with a 5-day course of co-trimoxazole is likely. When this is not the case, cases presenting with fever, cough, and fast breathing need the conventional antimalarial treatment combined with the recommended antibiotic for pneumonia.

In a high malaria risk setting, all children with *anemia*, whether or not there has been fever during the current ill-ness, should be given an antimalarial. If there is significant resistance to the first-line oral antimalarial, the second-line oral antimalarial should be used.

USE OF ANTIPYRETICS. A child with a fever in the clinic (either an axillary temperature of 37.5°C or above, or if the child feels hot) or a history of fever by the mother should receive a further assessment for malaria and measles. Acetaminophen is recommended for the treatment of high fever only, defined as an axillary temperature >39.5°C or a rectal temperature >39°C. In the generic IMCI guidelines, children are given a single dose of acetaminophen only in the clinic, rather than dispensing several doses for continued use at home.

MEASLES CASE MANAGEMENT. Fever is also the starting point for the classification of measles (Chapter 25.1). Acute (current) measles is detected based on fever with a generalized rash *plus* red eyes, runny nose, or cough. The mother is also asked about the occurrence of measles within the last 3 months. Despite substantial success in improving immunization coverage in many developing countries, many measles cases and deaths continue to occur. Although the current vaccine is recommended to be given at 9 months of age, immunization is often delayed. In addition, many measles cases are seen at 6, 7 and 8 months of age, especially in urban and refugee populations.

The case-fatality rate of measles can be reduced by using vitamin A and by good case management of the common complications. Measles deaths occur from pneumonia and laryngotracheitis (67%), diarrhea (25%), measles alone, and a few from encephalitis. Other, usually nonfatal, complications include conjuctivitis, otitis media, and mouth ulcers. Significant disability can result from measles including blindness, severe malnutrition, chronic lung disease (bronchiectasis and recurrent infection), and neurologic dysfunction. Other than vitamin A administration, the management of pneumonia, diarrhea, and ear infection complicating measles is basically the same as in children without measles. If a child with pneumonia fails to improve by the follow-up visit on day 2, that child is referred to the hospital. In some countries, it may be possible to refer *all* children with measles and pneumonia to the hospital.

Measles increases the risk of pneumonia, persistent diarrhea, failure to thrive, and malnutrition for months after the acute infection. Studies in West Africa and Kenya suggest that the increased risk of death may extend for a full year; this has not been documented elsewhere. Studies in India have shown slower weight gain, a higher rate of infection, and a higher rate of hospitalization in the 6 months after a measles infection. Early complications from measles are usually due to the measles virus itself or to decreased vitamin A levels. Later complications are often caused by secondary viral and bacterial infections. Measles damages the epithelial surfaces and the immune system, and lowers vitamin A levels. This results in increased susceptibility to infections caused by pneumococcus, gram-negative bacteria, and adenovirus. Recrudescences of herpesvirus, *Candida*, and malaria can occur during measles infection. In high malaria risk settings, malaria treatment is given to children with measles with fever.

Stomatitis is a common problem in measles. In most children, this is limited to the early onset of a sore mouth without ulcers. This does not require specific treatment. Stomatitis with mouth ulcers that are not deep or extensive can be treated by cleaning with saline then applying gentian violet. This is usually a half-strength formulation with a concentration of 0.25%, compared with the full-strength concentration of 0.5%, which can be applied to the skin. This was recommended because of concern that full-strength gentian violet actually causes mouth ulcers. Severe stomatitis with deep or extensive mouth ulcers requires referral to the hospital, where nasogastric feeding may be required. Stomatitis can be due to the measles virus itself, herpesvirus, or *Candida*. Some of the variation in the rate of severe stomatitis complicating measles may be due to variations in the rate of herpes infection in children.

Ear Infection

The IMCI guidelines are designed for settings in which otoscopy is not available. Some cases of acute otitis media can be detected based on the mother's report that her child has ear pain or pus draining from the ear for <14 days. Acute ear infection is treated for 5 days with the same first-line antibiotic as for pneumonia; the child is then seen in follow-up on day 5.

An ear infection is classified as chronic if drainage has been present for ≥14 days. Chronic ear infections are treated by wicking them dry; some countries may adapt these guidelines to include at least a single course of antibiotics and referral care if wicking is not successful. Children with tenderness *and* swelling of the mastoid bone are referred to the hospital for treatment of suspected mastoiditis.

Managing Malnutrition

After looking for the presence of danger signs and assessing the four main symptoms (cough or difficult breathing, diarrhea, fever and ear problem), the nutritional status of *all* sick children should be assessed (Chapter 130). In an outpatient setting dealing with sick children, a key reason for assessing nutritional status is to identify children with severe acute malnutrition who have an elevated risk of *acute* mortality and who may respond to acute treatment. Visible severe wasting (marasmus) and/or edema of both feet (kwashiorkor) identify children with severe malnutrition who are at increased risk of acute mortality and need urgent referral to the hospital where they can be observed, treated, and fed day and night. Visible severe wasting (defined as severe wasting of the shoulders, arms, buttocks, and legs with ribs easily seen) is as effective as very low weight-for-height in identifying children with a significantly increased acute risk of mortality and is much easier to assess, not requiring use of a height board.

Most malnourished children presenting to the clinic are chronically malnourished, with suboptimal growth resulting from ongoing deficits in dietary intake plus repeated episodes of infection (Chapters 133.1 and 133.2). The usual outcome of this process during the first 2 years of life is stunting; in many developing countries, 30 to 60% of children have some degree of stunting and most children who are low weight for age will be so based on stunting rather than wasting. In an attempt to improve growth and reduce stunting, the IMCI course teaches health workers to focus nutritional counseling on children <2 years of age and to focus follow-up (with monitoring of weight gain and further help in resolving feeding problems) on those children with feeding problems and those who are very low weight-for-age (Z score less than −3).

NUTRITIONAL COUNSELING. The assessment of feeding (Fig. 16–5) is based on identifying common, important problems with feeding that are amenable to change. Health workers need to be trained to provide effective counseling on the most common feeding problems (Fig. 16–7) and to provide effective and acceptable feeding recommendations based on the child's age (Fig. 16–6), if the mother is not already adequately feeding the child.

To try to achieve an impact on child nutrition, nutrition counseling focuses on helping to solve the most common and important remediable feeding problems, rather than providing general nutritional advice. Local adaptation of these feeding recommendations and identification of common, modifiable feeding problems is recommended for each country.

Sick child encounters provide an opportunity for the delivery of sound consistent advice on the nutrition of the young child both during and after illness which may have a significant impact in reducing the adverse effect of infections on nutritional status. This includes the promotion of breast-feeding and improved weaning practices with locally appropriate energy- and nutrient-rich foods. Specific appropriate complementary foods are recommended and the frequency of feeding by age is clearly laid out. The type of complementary foods or fluids should be checked to assess their potential adequacy in terms of nutrient and energy density, by comparing them with the locally adapted age-specific feeding recommendations (Fig. 16–6). The frequency of feeding should be checked to determine its adequacy in terms of ability to fulfill the child's energy requirements.

Exclusive breast-feeding is encouraged for the first 4 to 6 months, use of bottles is discouraged at any age, and guidance is provided to solve important problems with breast-feeding. This includes assessing the adequacy of attachment and suckling, if difficulties with breast-feeding are reported or if a young infant (age <2 months) is low weight for age or is taking other foods (Fig. 16–11). If problems are found,

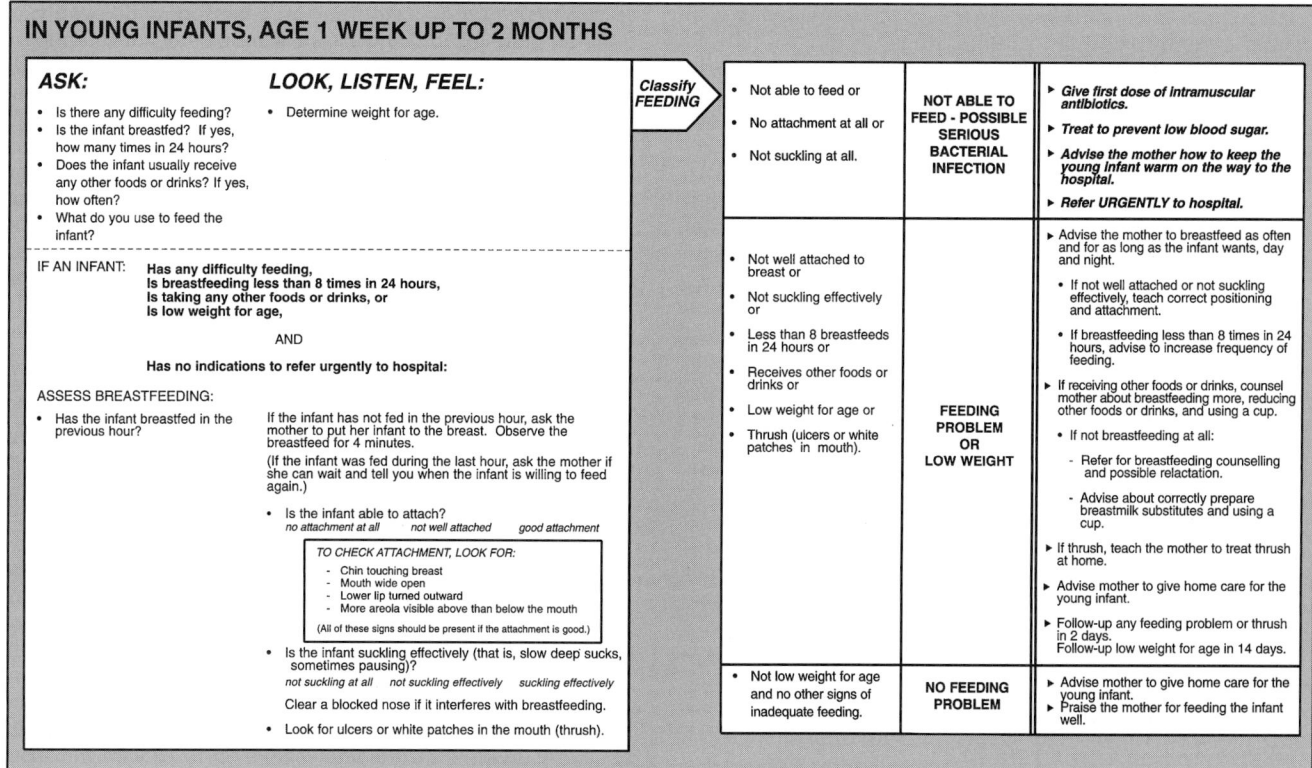

Figure **16–11.** Breast-feeding assessment. (From World Health Organization, Division of Diarrheal and Acute Respiratory Disease Control: Management of Childhood Illness. Chart booklet. Geneva, WHO, 1995, p 24.)

health workers should assist the mother to improve the positioning and attachment (Fig. 16–12).

The frequency of breast-feeding is checked, as it has been found to be a good predictor of the duration of breast-feeding. Low frequencies (<6 to 8 feedings/day) may be associated with insufficient intakes by the infant and may lead to early termination of breast-feeding. The presence of night feeding may have additional benefits to frequency in terms of milk production. The most frequent cause reported for premature introduction of complementary feeding is the mother's perception of her milk's inadequacy in terms of quality or quantity. In the majority of the cases the perception of inadequate quantity does not reflect reality if an adequate frequency of feeding is maintained. There is little variation in the quality of mother's milk outside of the extremes of nutritional deprivation. The experience of lactation clinics is that with adequate positioning and attachment and frequent breast-feeding, in addition to building up the confidence of the mother, adequate exclusive breast-feeding can be reestablished. If not, complementary foods are required. Mothers should be advised on their correct preparation, safety, and quantity.

Determining how the child is being fed is important. Feeding bottles have been shown in various studies in developing countries to be highly contaminated and difficult to clean; their use is associated with a higher incidence of diarrheal disease. Cup feeding is safer and experience in several countries indicates that even very young infants can be successfully fed with cups, if a complementary food is required. Health workers should be prepared to teach mothers how to use a cup.

If the weight is low for the child's age, additional information should be sought on causes of low food intake: the size of the servings, the child sharing the food serving with others and who feeds the child and how, trying to determine whether passive feeding by the caretaker may be the cause of low intake. Active feeding is important. A passive attitude of the caretaker in relation to the child's feeding, often based on the perception that the child will know how much he or she should eat, can lead to low intakes and malnutrition.

Figure **16–12.** Correct positioning for breast-feeding. (From World Health Organization, Division of Diarrheal and Acute Respiratory Disease Control: Management of Childhood Illness. Chart booklet. Geneva, WHO, 1995, adapted from p 28.)

Teach Correct Positioning and Attachment for Breastfeeding

▶ Show the mother how to hold her infant
  - with the infant's head and body straight
  - facing her breast, with infant's nose opposite her nipple
  - with infant's body close to her body
  - supporting infant's whole body, not just neck and shoulders.

▶ Show her how to help the infant to attach. She should:
  - touch her infant's lips with her nipple
  - wait until her infant's mouth is opening wide
  - move her infant quickly onto her breast, aiming the infant's lower lip well below the nipple.

▶ Look for signs of good attachment and effective suckling. If the attachment or suckling is not good, try again.

The chart recommends some active feeding behaviors, which should be complemented with local examples.

Changes in diet during illness should be assessed, to identify problems that appeared as part of the caretaker's management of illness and that might require specific counselling. Anorexia accompanies many illnesses, particularly diarrhea, and those associated with fever. Breast milk intake is usually well maintained during the illness and should therefore be offered in increased frequency. The child's refusal to eat and low intake at each meal can be partially compensated by increasing meal frequency and offering foods that besides being nutritious are likely to be better accepted by the ill child. Reassuring the mother that appetite will approve with the end of illness is important in helping her to sustain her efforts. A blocked nose can interfere with adequate feeding, particularly among infants.

SPECIFIC FEEDING RECOMMENDATIONS. Recommendations were prepared for five age groups for which specific feeding behaviors could be identified as practical and likely to lead to good nutrition (Fig. 16–6). For effective nutritional counseling, it is important to use locally adapted age-specific feeding recommendations. The *Adaptation Guide* provides guidance on how to adapt the feeding recommendations, including a short protocol.

Up to 4 Months of Age. The recommended feeding for these infants is exclusive breast-feeding. This is based on several epidemiologic studies indicating the adequacy of growth and the lower rate of morbidity in infants who are exclusively breast-fed in this age group. Except when they have diarrhea, no other foods or fluids are required by these infants if exclusively breast-fed, even in hot and dry climates.

4 Months Up to 6 Months. Most infants in this age group will have adequate growth and less morbidity if they are exclusively breast-fed. Some infants, however, will already need supplements in order to maintain adequate growth. These infants can be identified based on insufficient weight gain, hunger after breast-feeding, or reaching for food. These infants should be offered the same complementary foods as the child aged 6 months up to 12 months, after breast-feeding.

6 Months Up to 12 Months. Breast-feeding is still a major source of nutrients in this age group and should be promoted, particularly for the sick child who tends to reject other types of food. Locally available and affordable nutrient and energy-rich complementary foods are recommended for these children, at least 3 times per day if they are breast-fed and 5 times per day if they are not. Complementary foods are considered to be energy-rich when their energy density is equal or greater than 100 kcal/100 g. This is greater than the energy density of breast milk (just <70 kcal/100 g) and most soups and liquids offered to young children. Thick porridges, particularly if they contain oils or fats, are energy-dense. If foods from animal sources, e.g., chicken liver, fish, meat, milk or eggs, are added to the porridge, its nutrient density will be improved.

The recommended frequencies reflect results from work in Peru that indicate that if size of the portion offered is not limited, 5 meals per day of food with at least 70 kcal/100 g would satisfy the energy needs of children in this age range. It was assumed that breast-fed children would have at least two breastfeedings per day.

12 Months Up to 2 Years. Breast milk can still make a significant contribution to the diet of these children, particularly during illness, and also reduces the risk of morbidity (evidence is available for *Shigella* infection and cholera). In addition to the previously recommended complementary feeds, these infants should be introduced to the family foods, which are usually energy-dense and often adequate in nutrients.

2 Years and Older. Recommendations for these children are aimed at providing them with adequate energy and nutrient intakes while recognizing that time and other resources may be a limiting factor in their active feeding by the caretaker or the preparation of special foods. Snacks, e.g., biscuits and bread, are commonly used and tend to be energy and nutrient-rich foods in many settings. They are well accepted by children and caretakers and a useful solution to the constraint represented by caretakers' time. Snacks should be offered twice per day to complement three recommended meals.

Anemia

Children need referral to the hospital for possible transfusion if they have severe anemia with cardiopulmonary decompensation or if they are at high risk from any further decrease in hemoglobin (Chapter 6). A significant proportion of malaria deaths in young children are associated with severe anemia. Severe palmar pallor is present in a high proportion of children with severe anemia requiring referral to the hospital for possible transfusion. In the IMCI algorithm, children with severe anemia are referred urgently to the hospital on the basis of several clinical criteria: severe palmar pallor; cough or difficult breathing with chest indrawing; or general danger signs.

Children with less severe anemia usually need iron treatment (Chapter 132.1). Detecting anemia based on some palmar pallor will identify children with moderate or severe anemia but not those with mild anemia. It is acceptable for the clinical detection to be less specific because iron treatment is usually not harmful and many children have underlying iron deficiency without clinical signs of anemia. It is also acceptable for the clinical signs to detect anemia to have lower sensitivity because a child with malarial anemia will recover even without iron replacement. Children with some palmar pallor should be treated with oral iron for 2 months. The child should be seen every 2 weeks, at which time an additional 14 days of iron treatment is given. The mother should be cautioned to keep the iron tablets out of the reach of children and to expect black stools. If there is no response in pallor after 2 months, the child should be referred to the hospital for further assessment. Iron should not be given to children with severe malnutrition.

MEBENDAZOLE FOR TREATMENT OF ANEMIA AND PREVENTION OF MALNUTRITION. A 500-mg dose of mebendazole is recommended for all children, 2 years of age or older, who are anemic, if they live in areas where hookworm and/or whipworm are significant public health problems and if they have not been treated with mebendazole in the last 6 months (Chapters 103.2 and 105.1). Mebendazole can be given without microscopic examination of the stool. Hookworm (*Ancylostoma*) and whipworm (*Trichuris*) are significant contributors to anemia, mainly due to gut leakage of blood, especially in heavily infected children.

In addition to anemia, there is evidence that hookworm, whipworm, and ascaris are contributors to malnutrition and treatment with anthelmintics can improve nutrient intake and anthropometric indicators in some settings (Chapter 133.2). In these countries, the guidelines can be adapted to recommend regular deworming with mebendazole every 4 to 6 months. Mebendazole is inexpensive and safe in young children.

Sick Young Infant (Age 1 Week Up to 2 Months)

Separate guidelines are provided for the case management of sick young infants because the signs of illness differ and illness can progress rapidly to death. Every sick young infant is assessed for signs that may indicate a possible serious bacterial infection: fast breathing, severe chest indrawing, grunting, nasal flaring, bulging fontanelle, convulsions, fever, hypothermia, many or severe skin pustules, umbilical redness extending to the skin, pus draining from the ear, lethargy, unconsciousness, or less than normal movement. Young infants with any of these signs should be referred urgently to the hospital after giving intramuscular benzylpenicillin (or ampicillin) plus gentamicin, treatment to prevent hypoglycemia, and advice to the mother on keeping the young infant warm. If the young infant has only a few skin pustules or an umbilicus which is red or draining pus, but without redness extending to the skin, that young infant can be treated at home with oral antibiotics but should be seen in follow-up in 2 days.

Management of diarrhea differs somewhat from the older child. It is not reliable to assess thirst by offering a drink, so drinking poorly is not used as a sign for the classification of dehydration. All young infants with persistent diarrhea or blood in the stool should be referred to the hospital, rather than managed as outpatients.

Special guidelines are presented for assessing the adequacy of feeding and the technique of breast-feeding (Figs. 16–11 and 16–12).

Immunizing the Sick Child

Each sick child's immunization status should be checked and vaccinations given as needed. Illness is not a contraindication to immunization. Indeed sick children may be even more in need of protection provided by immunization than well children. The ability of vaccines to protect is not diminished in sick children. The importance and safety of immunizing sick children who are not being referred to the hospital needs to be consistently taught and reinforced, resulting in fewer missed opportunities for immunization.

Only very limited contraindications to immunization of sick children are needed. Immunizations should be deferred in children who are being referred urgently to the hospital. Live vaccines (bacille Calmette-Guérin [BCG], measles, polio, yellow fever) should not be given to children with immune deficiency diseases, or to children who are immunosuppressed due to malignant disease, therapy with immunosuppressive agents, or irradiation. However both measles and oral poliomyelitis vaccines as well as other nonlive vaccines (diphtheria-tetanus-pertussis [DTP], hepatitis B) *should* be given to children with human immunodeficiency virus (HIV) or AIDS. Children with symptomatic HIV infection should not be immunized with BCG and yellow fever vaccines because of the risk of a severe reaction. All the vaccines, including BCG and yellow fever, should be given to children who have or are suspected of having HIV infection but are not yet symptomatic.

Vitamin A Supplementation

In countries where vitamin A deficiency is a problem, sick child encounters can be used as an opportunity to update vitamin A supplementation (Chapter 131.1).

Referral of Severely Ill Children

Successful referral of severely ill children to the hospital depends on effective counseling of the mother. If she does not accept referral, consider options available to treat the child by repeated clinic or home visits. If she accepts referral, she should travel with a short, clear referral note. She needs

---

Treat the Child to Prevent Low Blood Sugar

▶ **If the child is able to breastfeed:**

Ask the mother to breastfeed the child.

▶ **If the child is not able to breastfeed but is able to swallow:**

Give expressed breastmilk or a breastmilk substitute.
If neither of these is available, give sugar water.
Give 30-50 ml of milk or sugar water before departure.

To make sugar water: Dissolve 4 level teaspoons of sugar (20 grams) in a 200-ml cup of clean water.

▶ **If the child is not able to swallow:**

Give 50 ml of milk or sugar water by nasogastric tube.

Figure 16–13. Treatment for hypoglycemia. (From World Health Organization, Division of Diarrheal and Acute Respiratory Disease Control: Management of Childhood Illness. Chart booklet. Geneva, WHO, 1995, p 11.)

---

clear counseling on what to do during referral transport, particularly if the hospital is distant.

Urgent prereferral treatments include providing the first dose of an appropriate antibiotic, and intramuscular quinine when severe malaria is a possibility. Certain prereferral treatments are especially important for high-risk children. Special attention should be paid to making sure that severely malnourished children and young infants are kept warm. Children who may have meningitis, severe malaria, severe malnutrition, or young infants with a possible serious bacterial infection are susceptible to hypoglycemia and should be given breast milk or sugar water (Fig. 16–13). Nonurgent treatments, e.g., wicking a draining ear or providing oral iron treatment, should be deferred, so as to not delay referral or confuse the mother.

■ EXPECTED IMPACT

According to the World Bank calculations of the total global burden of disease, WHO improved IMCI guidelines, implemented both at the outpatient and referral care level, is likely to have the greatest impact in reducing the global burden of disease. IMCI ranks high among the most cost-effective health interventions in both low- and middle-income countries (Fig. 16–14). In estimating the potential benefit of integrated management of the sick child in this analysis, both outpatient treatment and the benefit of inpatient management possible at a small hospital were considered but not the contributions to preventive interventions, e.g., raising immunization coverage levels by avoiding missed opportunities, increasing the coverage of vitamin A supplementation by using sick child encounters to give supplements in areas with vitamin A deficiency, or improving infant and child feeding and growth by nutritional counseling.

Integrated management of the sick child incorporates several child health interventions. For some of the interventions, there is substantial evidence for potential mortality reduction. Community-based intervention studies have demonstrated the potential impact of ARI case management in neonates, infants, and young children; vitamin A administration; and measles immunization. Clinical trials have demonstrated mortality reduction in young children with measles treated with vitamin A. For diarrheal disease, severe malaria, severe

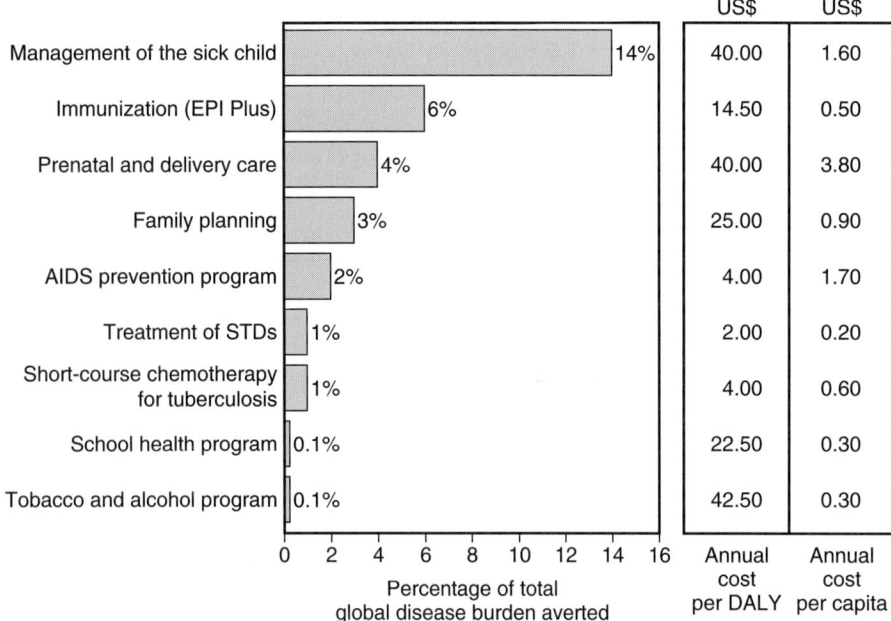

	US$	US$
Management of the sick child 14%	40.00	1.60
Immunization (EPI Plus) 6%	14.50	0.50
Prenatal and delivery care 4%	40.00	3.80
Family planning 3%	25.00	0.90
AIDS prevention program 2%	4.00	1.70
Treatment of STDs 1%	2.00	0.20
Short-course chemotherapy for tuberculosis 1%	4.00	0.60
School health program 0.1%	22.50	0.30
Tobacco and alcohol program 0.1%	42.50	0.30
Percentage of total global disease burden averted	Annual cost per DALY	Annual cost per capita

Figure 16-14. Cost-effective packages of public health interventions and essential clinical services in low-income and middle-income countries. DALY (Disability Adjusted Life Year), EPI, Expanded Programme of Immunization; STDs, sexually transmitted diseases. (From Bull WHO 73:735, 1995; data derived from World Bank: World Development Report 1993: Investing in Health. New York: Oxford University Press, 1993, p 1.)

pneumonia and severe malnutrition, case-fatality rates have been observed to decrease following the institution of effective standardized case management guidelines. Extensive clinical experience and several analyses of national diarrheal mortality rates have suggested an impact of ORT on diarrheal mortality related to dehydration. For other interventions, clinical experience indicates a relationship to mortality reduction (e.g., oxygen treatment in severe hypoxemia or glucose in the treatment of hypoglycemia) or an estimation that their implementation will result in the reduction of a known, important risk factor for mortality (e.g., lack of breastfeeding).

References

Brown KH et al: Optimal complementary feeding practices to prevent childhood malnutrition in developing countries. Food Nutr Bull 16:320, 1995.

International Working Group on Persistent Diarrhoea: Evaluation of an algorithm for the treatment of persistent diarrhoea: A multicentre study. Bull WHO 74:479, 1996.

World Health Organization Programme for the Control of Acute Respiratory Infections: Acute Respiratory Infections in Children: Case Management in Small Hospitals in Developing Countries—A Manual for Doctors and Other Senior Health Workers. Document WHO/ARI/90.5. Geneva: WHO, 1990.

World Health Organization: The Rational Use of Drugs in the Management of Acute Diarrhoea in Children. Geneva, WHO, 1990.

World Health Organization Programme for the Control of Diarrhoeal Disease: Management of the Patient with Cholera. Document WHO/CDD/SER/92.16. Geneva, WHO, 1992.

World Health Organization, Programme for the Control of Acute Respiratory Infections (Programme for the Control of Acute Respiratory Infections), Malaria Control Programme and Special Programme for Research and Training in Tropical Diseases: The overlap in clinical presentation and treatment of malaria and pneumonia in children: report of a meeting. Documents WHO/ARI/92/3; WHO/MAL/92.1065. Geneva, WHO, 1992.

World Health Organization Programme for the Control of Acute Respiratory Infections: The Management of Fever in Young Children with Acute Respiratory Infections in Developing Countries. Document WHO/ARI/93.30. Geneva, WHO, 1993.

World Health Organization Programme for the Control of Diarrhoeal Disease: The Selection of Fluids and Food for Home Therapy to Prevent Dehydration from Diarrhea: Guidelines for Developing a National Policy. Document WHO/CDD/93.44. Geneva, WHO, 1993.

World Health Organization Programme for the Control of Diarrhoeal Disease: The Management of Bloody Diarrhoea in Young Children. Document WHO/CDD/94.49. Geneva, WHO, 1994.

World Health Organization, Malaria Control Programme: A Standard Protocol for Assessing the Proportion of Children Presenting with Febrile Disease Who Suffer From Malarial Disease. WHO/MAL/94.1069. Geneva, WHO, 1994.

World Health Organization CDR: Integrated management of the sick child. Bull WHO 73:735, 1995.

World Health Organization, Division of Diarrheal and Acute Respiratory Disease Control: Management of Childhood Illness. Chart booklet. Geneva, WHO, 1995.

World Health Organization: Integrated Management of Childhood Illness. A WHO/UNICEF Initiative. Bull WHO 75(suppl 1):1, 1997.

World Bank: World Development Report 1993: Investing in Health. New York, Oxford University Press, 1993.

World Health Organization Department of Child and Adolescent Health and Development: Adaptation guide: A guide to identifying necessary adaptions of clinical policies and guidelines and to adapting the charts and modules for the WHO/UNICEF course Integrated Management of Childhood Illness. WHO/CHD/98.1, Geneva, WHO, 1998.

17 Heat-Associated Illness*

John W. Gardner and John A. Kark

DEFINITION. Heat illness encompasses a spectrum of metabolic disorders deriving from the combined stresses of heat exposure, exertion, and thermoregulation. These include classic (environmental) and exertional heat stroke, heat exhaustion, heat injury, dehydration, heat cramps, acute renal failure, hyponatremia, and rhabdomyolysis. In addition, there are some minor heat-associated illnesses, such as heat rash, heat edema, parade syncope, and sunburn. Heat illness represents primarily a continuum of multisystem illness related to elevation of core body temperature and the metabolic and circulatory processes (including changes in fluid and electrolyte balance) that are brought about by heat exposure, exercise, and the body's thermoregulatory response.

PATHOPHYSIOLOGY. The physiologic responses to heat stress in humans are controlled by a sensitive and efficient thermoregulatory system. Optimal body temperature is maintained through a balance of environmental temperature, endogenous production of heat, and effective loss of body heat. In hot environments thermoregulation is accomplished primarily by redistribution of blood flow to carry internal

---

*All the material in this chapter is in the public domain, with the exception of any borrowed figures or tables.

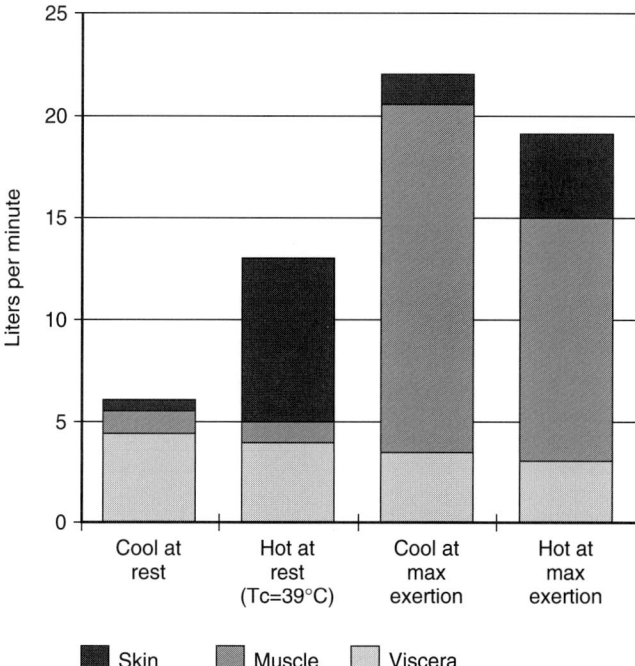

Figure 17–1. Estimated distribution of blood flow to the muscle, skin, and viscera as fraction of cardiac output at rest and with maximum exertion under cool and hot conditions. (Adapted from Rowell LB: Human cardiovascular adjustments to exercise and thermal stress. Physiol Rev 54:75, 1974.)

thermal energy to the skin, where heat dissipation occurs through conduction, convection, radiation, and evaporation. Figure 17–1 shows the estimated distribution of blood flow to the muscle, skin, and viscera as a fraction of cardiac output at rest and with maximum exertion under cool and hot conditions. A large temperature differential between the skin and its surroundings provides efficient heat dissipation under cool conditions, requiring only about 5% of resting cardiac output going to the skin. However, under hot conditions there is inefficient heat dissipation and blood flow to the skin increases dramatically even at rest, requiring a large increase in cardiac output (shown when rectal temperature has increased to 102°F [39°C], implying maximum thermoregulatory effort). This contributes to the fatigue one may feel even at rest in the heat.

Environmental Effects. Optimal thermal balance can work effectively within certain limits. Wind, solar radiation, and humidity play important roles in the efficiency of heat dissipation through convection, radiation, and evaporation. Even at rest in cool environments the body loses about 2 L of fluid per day through respiration and perspiration; this may be imperceptible in dry or windy weather conditions. As more body heat must be dissipated, these fluid losses increase due to heavier sweating, which may exceed 2 L/hour (up to a maximum of 12 to 15 L/day). Heat losses from the body to the environment through radiation, conduction, and convection are markedly reduced when the ambient temperatures rise above 86°F [30°C]. Under such circumstances, sweating becomes the most important means of heat loss. Evaporation is severely hampered by high ambient humidity. Thus, the combination of high ambient temperatures and high relative humidity sets the stage for the development of heat illness.

Impact of Exercise. With strenuous exercise there is a three- to six-fold increase in cardiac output due to increased blood flow to exercising muscle (Fig. 17–1). Exercise gener-

ates large amounts of heat and elevates body temperature, since about three fourths of the metabolic energy used by muscle during exercise is converted into heat within the body. As body temperature elevates, more blood flows to the skin for heat dissipation. Under cool conditions there is efficient heat dissipation, and the amount of blood flow to the skin increases only marginally. However, under hot conditions there is less efficient heat dissipation and a larger amount of blood flow goes to the skin. This produces peripheral pooling of blood, which decreases total cardiac output and further limits blood flow to muscle, thus reducing peak exercise performance in hot environments. These circulatory demands of sustained exercise and heat stress may also encroach on visceral blood flow to the extent of producing organ dysfunction or cellular injury, e.g., watery or bloody diarrhea often seen in marathon runners, and perhaps acute renal failure and encephalopathy often seen in heat stroke.

Acclimatization. Heat exposure and/or regular strenuous exercise, which raises core temperature and provokes heat-loss responses, produces heat acclimatization that improves the body's response to heat stress within a few days. The acclimatization achieved is a process of changes in circulation, sweating, and sodium and water balance, as well as a gradual increase in metabolic efficiency of energy utilization. Most of the physiologic improvement in heat tolerance occurs within 10 days of combined heat exposure and regular exercise. In acclimatized individuals blood volume increases, the heart rate is lower due to increased stroke volume, sweating begins earlier with a higher sweat rate and low sodium content, and the threshold for cutaneous vasodilatation is reduced. These changes improve transfer of body heat from the core to the skin and enhance heat dissipation at the skin. Although sodium is conserved with heat acclimatization, the need for water replacement is not reduced because sweat volume increases.

Water losses in exercising individuals are universal, but salt loss is excessive primarily in unacclimatized individuals. Thus, hypertonic fluid losses occur primarily during the first 2 weeks of training in a hot environment. Acclimatized individuals excrete large volumes of sweat with minimal salt content, and hypotonic fluid losses predominate. Dehydration may thus be due to isotonic, hypotonic, or hypertonic fluid loss.

EPIDEMIOLOGY AND PREVENTION. Numerous risk factors have been identified for heat illness, which relate primarily to weather and training circumstances; clothing and shade; acclimatization; physical fitness and body type; illness, medications, and alcohol; water and salt; and personal education. These factors are directly related to the occurrence and severity of heat illness, and attention to them can greatly reduce its morbidity and mortality and minimize the impact of heat stress exposure.

Weather and Training Circumstances. Temperature, humidity, and solar and wind conditions greatly influence the body's ability to maintain thermal balance. The wet bulb globe temperature index (WBGT = 0.7 × wet bulb temperature + 0.2 × black globe temperature + 0.1 × dry bulb temperature) was developed as a weather index that is linearly related to sweat rates during moderate exercise. It has therefore been adopted as a practical index of risk for heat illness during exercise in hot weather conditions. Exertional heat illness rates can be minimized by progressively limiting the level of exercise, increasing rest periods, increasing hydration, and reducing heat-retaining clothing as the WBGT rises above 70°F [21°C]. These modifications are implemented in a standard manner in U.S. military training for four categories of high WBGT (green flag, 80° to 85°F [26.7° to 29.4°C]; yellow flag, 85° to 88°F [29.4° to 31.1°C]; red flag, 88° to 90°F

[31.1° to 32.2°C]; black flag, 90°F [32.2°C] or higher). As a rough guide, regulations allow exercise to continue with caution during green flag, strenuous exercise (e.g., "marching at standard cadence") is suspended for unacclimatized individuals during yellow flag, strenuous exercise is curtailed for all individuals during red flag, and all outdoor physical training is suspended during black flag conditions. These guidelines were designed to minimize the risk during marching (at a metabolic rate about six times basal). An adjustment is necessary to protect individuals who are running (at 12 to 14 times the basal metabolic rate); under these circumstances risk for exertional heat illness increases dramatically as the WBGT rises above 65°F [18.3°C]. Restrictions are generally recommended at lower WBGT levels in athletic programs, and detailed recommendations have also been made for categories of industrial work, including criteria at which work should stop (see Bell and Watts in Bibliography).

Clothing and Shade. In mild to moderately severe weather, minimizing heat retention by clothing is an important benefit. Light, loose-fitting clothing with head cover or umbrella protects from sunburn, the radiant heat of the sun, and allows air circulation to enhance evaporation of sweat. During extreme heat with sun exposure, cover by loose-fitting clothing also reduces heat uptake and permits tolerance of a longer work period. Provision of shade and air movement is important. One large tree may cool as much as five 10,000 BTU air conditioners. An example is the provision of shade by planting trees in the mountainous area of Arafat in Saudi Arabia, where about a million pilgrims gather annually in a 10 km² area. Individuals required to perform heavy exertion in the heat will have much lower risk for heat illness if they spend most of their time in a cool environment, ideally with shade, ventilation, and low humidity, as may be provided by reflective shielding, heat insulation, or air conditioning. Other methods of providing a cool individual environment include cooling vests and suits used in special industrial operations.

Acclimatization. The physiologic changes of acclimatization increase the capacity for and efficiency of heat dissipation. Due to increased sweating, water intake requirements go up. There is no hot weather training that decreases water requirements. A sensible program for rapid acclimatization to heavy work in a hot climate is to perform at about half-maximal effort for 2 hours per day while resting in a cool place otherwise. This should be accompanied by generous hydration and a temporary increase of salt in the diet (as salty food, not salt tablets). Although the benefits of acclimatization can be seen within 2 to 4 days, full acclimatization requires 2 to 4 weeks.

Physical Fitness and Body Type. Poor physical fitness and obesity are interacting risk factors for exertional heat illness. In male U.S. military recruits beginning basic training, those in the slowest quartile of run-time had a 5.6-fold higher risk for heat illness than those in the fastest quartile. Those who were in the highest quartile of body mass index (BMI) had 3.6-fold higher risk for heat illness than those in the lowest quartile. Morbid obesity provides even higher risk for heat illness, and individuals with marginal cardiac reserve are particularly susceptible.

Illness, Medications, and Alcohol. Chronic illness is a primary predisposing factor, and the epidemics of heat-related deaths (often several hundred) seen during heat waves are due primarily to classic heat stroke in individuals with marginal cardiac reserve who are unable to maintain cool surroundings and/or adequate hydration. The largest group at high risk is elderly persons of low socioeconomic status.

Certain medical conditions and medications can put an individual at high risk for developing heat illness. These can make adjustment to hot environments more difficult, and include acute illness, especially infections and febrile conditions, chronic illness, prior history of heat stroke, pregnancy, obesity, skin disorders, sunburn, and uncleanliness. Medications, alcohol, caffeine, nicotine, loss of sleep, large meals, and missed meals can also predispose to heat illness and may nullify the effects of acclimatization. Drugs that interfere with thermoregulatory mechanisms are listed in Table 17–1. Individuals with diffuse skin disease and anhidrosis (Fig. 17–2) are particularly susceptible to severe heat illness. They

TABLE 17–1. Drugs That Interfere With Thermoregulatory Mechanisms

Drug Class—Examples	Physiologic Effect
Diuretics—furosemide, thiazides, caffeine	Water and electrolyte loss
Antihistamines—chlorpheniramine	Suppress sweating
Anticholinergics—atropine	Suppress sweating
Antiparkinsonian—procyclidine	Suppress sweating
Phenothiazines—chlorpromazine	Suppress sweating, anhydrosis
Tricyclics—tranylcypromine	Suppress sweating, hyperpyrexia
Butyrophenones—haloperidol	Suppress sweating, thirst suppression
Monoamine oxidase inhibitors	Suppress sweating
Sympathomimetics—amphetamine	Suppress sweating, hyperpyrexia
Nicotine	Inhibit vasomotor control
Antihypertensives—propranolol, methyldopa, guanethidine	Inhibit vasomotor control
Thyroid hormones—thyroxine	Hyperpyrexia
Hallucinogens—LSD	Hyperpyrexia
Salicylates, barbiturates	Hyperpyrexia
General anesthetics—halothane	Hyperpyrexia
Alcohol	Unknown

LSD, lysergic acid diethylamide.

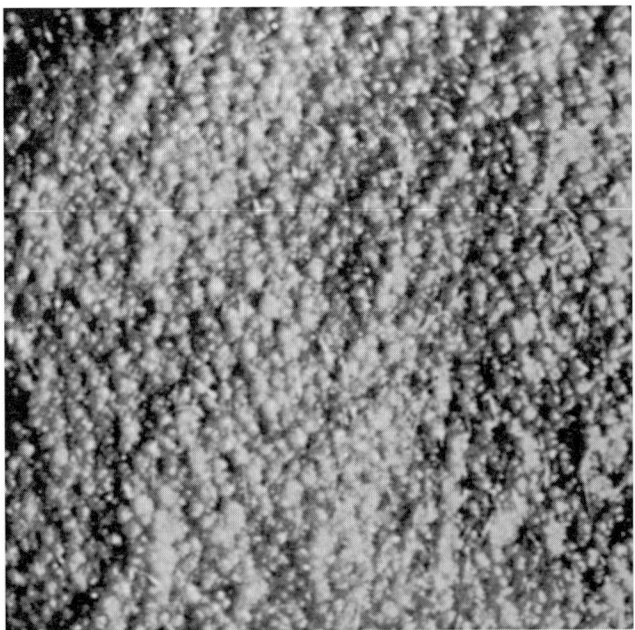

***Figure* 17–2.** An enlarged picture of human skin showing miliaria profunda. Notice the goose flesh–like appearance. (From Horne GO, Mole RH: Trans R Soc Trop Med Hyg 44:465, 1951. Reprinted by permission.)

may not be able to perform even a small amount of work in the heat without inducing heat stroke.

Water and Salt. Prevention of heat illness requires proper provision for water and salt requirements. Water must be available and palatable, and water intake must be monitored. Water requirements are not reduced by any form of training or acclimatization. Tolerance to dehydration cannot be developed, and water supplies are as important for survival as are food and shelter. For full-time outdoor activity in a hot environment, water intake should be about 1 L/hour. For planning purposes, 16 to 24 L of potable water per person per day are needed for drinking and cooking, and at least another 16 to 24 L for washing and bathing. Thirst is not an adequate guide to water needs because it starts only after losses of about 1 L occur. Urine volume and color, body weight changes, and orthostatic blood pressure changes can all be used as guides to adequate hydration. The advantages of carbohydrate/electrolyte beverages beyond their palatability are controversial. High sugar solutions may impede water absorption. Salt losses should be made up (during the first 2 weeks in a hot environment) with a high salt diet, not with salt tablets. *Replace water losses hour by hour, and salt losses day by day.* Sustained water replacement much beyond 1 L/hour may result in symptomatic hyponatremia, particularly if heat illness has already affected renal function.

Personal Education. Each individual must be fully aware of heat illness, its signs, and its prevention. Personal awareness and use of common sense will avoid most problems. Individuals should understand the early symptoms and signs of heat illness, and increased susceptibility with use of certain medications (including alcohol) and during and after recovery from acute (even minor) illness. It is important to avoid excessive fatigue, get adequate sleep, maintain calories and adequate salt in the diet, and avoid alcohol, nicotine, and caffeine. Each individual must maintain adequate water intake, which requires drinking when not thirsty and monitoring urine volume and color, weight changes, and so on. The individual must be aware of the need to hydrate ahead of thirst and before and during exercise. Individuals should wear appropriate clothing, seek shade and cool environments, utilize rest periods, and adjust the intensity and duration of exercise according to environmental conditions and their own sense of well-being. Buddies can recognize the symptoms and signs in each other, assisting in early recognition and management.

Heat Illness Syndromes

The spectrum of major heat illness represents a continuum of multisystem illness which may be divided into three main levels. The most severe are heat stroke (characterized by encephalopathy), rhabdomyolysis (characterized by muscle necrosis, with liver necrosis as a variant), and acute renal failure. The milder syndromes are categorized as heat exhaustion, and those with intermediate severity are called heat injury. Authors differ on the criteria used to describe each syndrome. Differentiation of heat illness syndromes by rectal temperature is popular in medical texts and emergency rooms, but this is unreliable for assessing severity of heat illness.

Classic (environmental) heat stroke is generally associated with extensive exposure to a hot environment in the absence of strenuous exercise, and is a different illness from exertional heat stroke. It has been associated with anhidrosis (absence of sweating), but anhidrosis is not a consistent finding in exertional heat stroke and consequently is not a useful criterion for categorizing heat illness.

Classification of the continuum of heat illness must be made on the basis of neurologic symptoms and evidence of organ damage or dysfunction. The neurologic symptoms in heat illness are those of a generalized encephalopathy, which range from lethargy, confusion, and disorientation to delirium, obtundation, and coma. The organ damage or dysfunction in heat illness is usually manifest as dehydration, electrolyte disturbances, metabolic acidosis, acute renal failure, and/or muscle or liver necrosis. It is valuable to provide an accurate assessment of each patient for encephalopathy, dehydration, metabolic acidosis, electrolyte disturbance, renal failure, tissue necrosis, and in severe disease, disseminated intravascular coagulation (DIC).

HEAT STROKE. Heat stroke is a life-threatening, progressive multisystem disorder reflecting collapse of the thermoregulatory system accompanied by severe neurologic symptoms with or without organ damage. The severe neurologic symptoms of heat stroke include delirium, obtundation, or coma and are usually apparent early in the course of illness (within the first hour); consequently, there is little difficulty in recognizing this end of the continuum of heat illness. Signs of organ damage may be more subtle and develop more slowly, requiring close monitoring of vital signs and laboratory studies. Progressive heat stroke often involves rhabdomyolysis and acute renal failure, occasionally involves liver necrosis and, in advanced stages, DIC. Severe hypotension or sudden cardiovascular collapse occur in about 5% of cases.

Individuals with heat stroke often have rectal temperatures exceeding 106°F [41°C]. Extreme hyperthermia per se may cause tissue damage at temperatures above 108°F [42°C]. High temperatures also change the kinetics of enzyme and other chemical reactions in the body. However, short-term rectal temperatures of 110°F [43°C] are seen in exertional heat stroke patients with no long-term sequelae if cooling and rehydration occur rapidly, and survival without permanent residua has been reported in at least one patient with a maximum rectal temperature exceeding 115°F [46°C]. In addition, cases of exertional heat stroke also occur at lower rectal temperatures, and many patients with high rectal temperature do not manifest the severe neurologic symptoms or organ damage that define heat stroke.

The temperature elevation in heat stroke is referred to as hyperthermia, not fever. In fever the primary event is an elevation of the thermoregulatory set point. In hyperthermia the regulatory set point remains normal but the thermoregulatory system is overwhelmed and unable to maintain the set-point temperature. When the fundamental cause of hyperthermia is sustained exposure to heat stress with little contribution from exercise, the case is considered *classic heat stroke.* It usually develops gradually, often over a period of days, with slow progression of dehydration and obtundation. Patients often present with marked hyperthermia, hot dry skin, and coma. Classic heat stroke occurs primarily in older people who have diminished cardiovascular reserve, and it has a high mortality. When the fundamental cause of hyperthermia is heavy exercise in hot weather, the resulting illness is considered *exertional heat stroke.* Typically, onset is abrupt, occurring during or shortly after exertion, with orthostatic manifestations (faintness, staggering, and/or visual disturbance) leading to collapse (with or without syncope), followed by confusion, combativeness, delirium, obtundation, and/or coma. This syndrome frequently evolves in minutes. If it is treated immediately by aggressive cooling and rehydration, severe organ damage and mortality are almost always prevented.

Water and electrolyte depletion, acute renal failure, and rhabdomyolysis are common components of heat stroke, and patients must be closely monitored and aggressively treated to minimize morbidity and mortality. Uncommon complications include hepatic necrosis, gastrointestinal bleeding, hypoxemia, pulmonary edema, shock, and DIC. Life-threatening cardiovascular collapse may occur early during the hyperthermic phase, emphasizing the need for immediate cardiac resuscitation capability.

EXERTIONAL RHABDOMYOLYSIS. Exertional rhabdomyolysis is caused by skeletal muscle damage with release of cellular contents into the circulation, including myoglobin, potassium, phosphate, creatine kinase (CK), lactic acid, and uric acid. These usually peak 24 to 48 hours after onset of illness. The severity of rhabdomyolysis can vary from asymptomatic elevation of serum skeletal muscle enzymes to muscle weakness, pain, tenderness, and stiffness with associated myoglobinuria, which can culminate in life-threatening metabolic acidosis, acute renal failure, DIC, and cardiovascular collapse. Although exertional rhabdomyolysis most often occurs as part of exertional heat stroke or heat injury, severe episodes without hyperthermia or encephalopathy are not uncommon.

Severe rhabdomyolysis may present without early muscle pain or tenderness, and muscle numbness may be the only symptom in the first few hours. Most patients develop remarkable muscle tenderness and pain on use, but there is great variability in muscle symptoms despite CK levels as high as 10,000 to 60,000 IU/L. Exercising military trainees frequently develop CK values ranging from 300 to 700 IU/L, but seldom above 1000 IU/L in the absence of heat illness. Other serum tests or enzymes that may be elevated include uric acid, lactate dehydrogenase (LDH), and aspartate transaminase (AST).

If skeletal muscle necrosis is extensive it produces a tissue lysis syndrome with lactic acidosis, hyperkalemia, hyperuricemia, hyperphosphatemia, hypocalcemia, dehydration, acute renal failure, and hypotension. These complications can become life-threatening, especially if DIC produces further organ damage. Fatal complications include acute hyperkalemia, hyperuricemia, hyperphosphatemia, disturbances of calcium metabolism, metabolic acidosis, advanced renal failure, shock, bleeding, myocardial ischemia, and secondary infections. It is extremely important to closely monitor fluid and electrolyte and acid-base status, because early aggressive parenteral correction of dehydration and electrolyte disturbance is the only effective treatment. The clinical picture may be deceptive, since the patient may manifest minimal clinical symptoms in the presence of profound metabolic abnormalities.

EXERTIONAL ACUTE RENAL FAILURE. The syndrome of isolated acute renal failure with hyperosmolar hypernatremia was often seen when salt tablets were in common use. By restricting oral salt replacement to mealtime consumption of salty foods this syndrome has become quite rare.

EXERTIONAL HYPONATREMIA. In recent years several clusters of cases of hyponatremia (Na < 130 mEq/L) have been noted in association with exertional heat illness. These can be severe or fatal, often presenting with nausea and vomiting, followed by seizures and associated brain swelling. This is a form of water intoxication due to excessive water drinking and inappropriate renal retention of water, perhaps due to dehydration and the simultaneous triggering of thirst and vasopressin secretion. This illness occurs primarily in the setting of forced water drinking (>15 L/day) for prevention of heat illness or to treat early symptoms of heat illness. If rehydration in exertional heat illness requires more than a liter or two of fluid, it should be accompanied by assessment of serum electrolyte levels.

EXERTIONAL HEAT INJURY. Exertional heat injury is a progressive multisystem disorder reflecting collapse of the thermoregulatory system accompanied by organ dysfunction, usually metabolic acidosis, acute renal failure, and/or muscle or liver necrosis. Patients with exertional heat injury often have milder neurologic symptoms. The absence of delirium, obtundation, or coma distinguishes exertional heat injury from exertional heat stroke. As in heat stroke, organ damage frequently is not manifest at the time of presentation of the patient. During the first hours of illness it may not be possible to distinguish exertional heat injury from heat exhaustion. Therefore, it is essential that all patients with heat illness be thoroughly evaluated for organ dysfunction before release from medical care, with re-evaluation often necessary on the following day.

HEAT EXHAUSTION. Heat exhaustion is a functional multisystem disorder reflecting inability of the circulatory system to meet the demands of thermoregulatory, muscular, and visceral blood flow. It represents primarily a syndrome of dehydration without serious metabolic complications. Heat exhaustion is typically thought of as producing minor elevations of rectal temperature (<104°F [40°C]), but it can be associated with subnormal or very high rectal temperatures. Increased circulatory demand (the result of increased muscle and thermoregulatory needs) and reduced effective blood volume (the result of thermoregulatory expansion of peripheral intravascular volume and depletion of water and electrolytes through respiration and sweating) result in metabolic acidosis and loss of orthostatic blood pressure control, which often produce exertional (heat) syncope.

Heat exhaustion most often includes both water and salt depletion, and most patients have nearly normal serum sodium levels. Patients need free water replacement, as well as isotonic solutions. In predominant water depletion there are characteristically intense thirst, fatigue, weakness, impaired judgment, hyperventilation with paresthesias, tetany, and hypernatremia. In predominant salt depletion there are characteristically headache, nausea, vomiting, giddiness, generalized muscle cramps, and hyponatremia. However, symptom patterns do not reliably reflect relative deficits of water or salt, and most patients benefit from hydration with normal or half-normal saline.

The symptoms of heat exhaustion can be quite varied (Table 17–2) and are rapidly improved by water and salt replacement, a cool environment, and rest. Rapid cooling to a body temperature below 102°F [39°C] is essential. Since heat exhaustion is a functional illness, with no organ or tissue damage, rapid improvement is the rule. Heat exhaustion may progress to heat injury or heat stroke if appropriate measures of rest, rehydration, and cooling are not instituted.

HEAT CRAMPS. Heat cramps are painful migratory skeletal muscle spasms occurring mainly in conditioned persons, at the end of the working day, or in the shower as muscles cool. They are attributed to salt depletion and resultant hyponatremia, and are rapidly reversed with water and salt replacement, usually by oral solutions containing electrolytes or infusion of normal saline. Prevention is through adequate water replacement and a high salt diet.

Minor Heat-Associated Syndromes

HEAT RASH, PRICKLY HEAT, MILIARIA RUBRA. Heat rash (also known as prickly heat or miliaria rubra) is a pruritic red papular rash, located particularly in areas of restrictive clothing and heavy sweating. It is one of the most common skin problems in hot climates, causing considerable irritation and discomfort. It is caused by inflammation of the sweat glands and blockage of the sweat ducts, perhaps as a result of maceration of the stratum corneum from continuous wetting of the skin by persistent sweating. The rash is an ery-

TABLE 17–2. Clinical Manifestations of Heat Illness

Nonspecific Symptoms

Thirst	Hyperventilation	Headache
Weakness	Lack of concentration	Nausea
Fatigue	Impaired judgment	Vomiting
Myalgia	Anxiety	Diarrhea
Cramps	Hysteria	

Progressive Orthostatic Symptoms

Faintness	Wobby legs
Dizziness (not vertigo)	Stumbling gait
Visual—blurred vision, tunnel vision, scotomata, blackness	
Collapse (without loss of consciousness)	

Exertional (Heat) Syncope:

Collapse with brief loss of consciousness

Severe Symptoms

Orthostatic or sustained hypotension, shock, cardiovascular collapse, pulmonary edema, acute respiratory distress syndrome

Metabolic Complications

Lactic acidosis	Rhabdomyolysis/ myoglobinuria
Electrolyte imbalances	
Acute renal failure	DIC/bleeding diatheses
	Hepatic necrosis

Neurologic Symptoms

Slow or altered mentation	Agitation, combativeness,
Poor concentration	lethargy, obtundation,
Drowsiness, dazed affect	delirium, coma, amnesia,
Confusion, disorientation	vertigo, seizures, ataxia

DIC, disseminated intravascular coagulation.

thematous epidermal vesicular eruption that is pruritic and accompanied by a prickling sensation ("prickly heat") when sweating is provoked. It may interfere with sweating and can therefore be a risk factor for more serious heat illness. Sleeplessness (due to itching) and secondary infection may further aggravate thermoregulation. Treatment is by cooling and drying the affected skin, controlling infection, and managing pruritus, with resolution of the rash over 7 to 10 days. Rare severe cases with generalized and prolonged rash, *miliaria profunda,* which has the appearance of goose flesh (Fig. 17–2), may require evacuation to a cooler environment to restore normal sweat gland function.

HEAT EDEMA. Travelers to the tropics may have temporary swelling of the feet and ankles, which is usually mild and disappears within a few days. Edema is due to expansion of blood volume during acclimatization and does not indicate excessive water intake or cardiac, renal, or hepatic disease. Management is to loosen clothing and elevate the legs.

PARADE SYNCOPE. Parade syncope is fainting during prolonged standing, due to inadequate venous blood return to the heart and brain. It can occur in the absence of heat illness, although it may be more common in a hot environment. Syncope occurring during or after work in the heat should be considered evidence of heat exhaustion or heat injury, warranting evaluation of fluid and electrolyte status. Parade syncope is managed by restoring normal blood circulation and minimizing peripheral pooling through a brief period of recumbence in a cool place. Allowing individuals to move about will help prevent parade syncope, and provision of chairs and/or railings will decrease the risk of injury from falling.

SUNBURN. Sunburn reduces the thermoregulatory capacity of the skin and should be prevented through adequate sun exposure protection. It should be managed as any other burn, and heat stress should be avoided until the burn has healed.

Clinical Presentation and Management

SYMPTOMS AND SIGNS. Table 17–2 lists, in order of progressive severity, the wide variety of symptoms associated with heat illness. Early in the course of illness weakness, fatigue, headache, thirst, hyperventilation, impaired judgment, or abdominal or muscle symptoms may predominate. As the illness worsens orthostatic symptoms develop (e.g., faintness, stumbling gait, blurred vision, narrowed or tunnel vision, or scotomata). Collapse may occur with or without loss of consciousness. Collapse with a brief period of loss of consciousness during or immediately after strenuous exercise is a fainting episode referred to as exertional (or heat) syncope. Syncope must be distinguished from a seizure or coma.

Neurologic symptoms are characteristic in heat illness, particularly in exertional heat stroke. These symptoms are not neurologic deficits relating to specific cranial or peripheral nerves, but represent a generalized encephalopathy affecting mental status. The symptoms range from lethargy and drowsiness through confusion and disorientation to delirium, obtundation, or coma. Amnesia is frequent and there are occasionally seizures and/or persistent ataxia.

CLINICAL MANAGEMENT. Heat stroke is a medical emergency. Early recognition and prompt treatment of heat stroke dramatically reduce the mortality rate. Rectal temperature should be obtained immediately and rapid cooling initiated if above 102°F [39°C]. In addition, there must be close monitoring of vital signs and mental status, aggressive replacement of fluid and electrolytes, and appropriate laboratory workup. Even in milder forms of heat illness immediate measurement of rectal temperature is necessary to help assess severity, the need for rapid cooling, and prognosis.

In controlled settings emergency medical care for heat illness should be arranged in advance through immediate access to medical support, including capability for measurement of rectal temperature, clinical assessment, and ice water cooling. In settings where heat illness is common, strenuous exercise or work should not be conducted without medical capability present on-site. Delay in treatment may result in much more severe illness, with resultant complications, organ damage, and increased morbidity and mortality.

Cooling. Body cooling should be accomplished as quickly as possible, using whatever means are available under the circumstances. The clothing should be loosened or removed, and evaporative cooling maximized. Methods for cooling include immersion in cold water, showering, and soaking the clothing, as well as using ice bags or a cooling blanket. The cooler the water the more rapidly the cooling process progresses, and ice bags placed over major arteries may enhance cooling. Briskly massaging the body helps prevent cutaneous vasoconstriction, which may impede core heat dissipation. Fanning can be accomplished manually, using electric fans, or by placing the patient under rotating helicopter blades (a military field expedient that appears to be very effective). There has been controversy concerning whether use of tepid water with fans or use of ice water is clinically appropriate. Clinical experience suggests that ice water may cause coronary spasm in people with coronary atherosclerosis but is not harmful in those without such disease. Ice water has been demonstrated to lower rectal temperature about twice as rapidly as use of tepid water with fans. We therefore recommend that ice water be used first on patients under 35 years of age and that tepid water be used first on older patients, especially those with a history of angina or coronary heart disease.

TABLE 17–3. Recommended Laboratory Workup for Heat Illness

Blood Count (CBC)	Hemoglobin, hematocrit, white blood cell count, platelet count
Urinalysis	Specific gravity, pH, evidence of myoglobin
Serum Chemistries (Heat Panel)	Sodium, potassium, chloride, bicarbonate, glucose, blood urea nitrogen, creatinine, uric acid, creatine kinase, aspartate transaminase, lactate dehydrogenase, alanine aminotransferase
If Severe	Arterial blood gases; calcium, phosphate; prothrombin time, partial thromboplastin time, fibrin split products, fibrinogen

Rapid cooling should continue until the rectal temperature remains below 102°F [39°C]. After reaching this temperature, cooling can proceed more slowly until the rectal temperature remains below 100°F [38°C]. Regardless of the method of cooling, the degree of organ damage and metabolic and neurologic complications is directly related to the magnitude and duration of elevated body temperature—patients who cool slowly tend to have more serious illness.

Rehydration. Rapid parenteral administration of 1 to 2 L of normal saline has been shown to enhance cooling. Rehydration should include restoration of water and electrolytes and re-establishment of normal acid-base balance. Generally 1 L of isotonic fluid is given immediately, with an additional 2 or 3 L as required. Some free water replacement is necessary, as well as normal saline solutions. A clinical decision to give more than 2 L of IV fluids constitutes an indication for laboratory determination of serum electrolytes. Management plans should include prompt laboratory evaluation, setting a desired level of fluid intake, maintaining records of fluid intake and output, and frequently monitoring vital signs to confirm that postural blood pressure control is returning to normal.

LABORATORY EVALUATION. In the circumstance of exercise-induced mental dysfunction, prompt laboratory evaluation is necessary to identify significant metabolic problems that may initially be asymptomatic: (1) exertional rhabdomyolysis, (2) acute renal failure, (3) depletion of electrolytes and water, (4) exertional hypoglycemia, and (5) metabolic acidosis. Close monitoring of vital signs and serum chemistries is essential, since clinical symptoms may not reflect profound metabolic abnormalities. The recommended labora-

tory workup includes a complete blood count, urinalysis, and serum chemistries (Table 17–3). These assess dehydration, electrolytes, acid-base balance, renal function, and muscle and liver cell lysis. Maximum laboratory abnormalities often do not appear until 24 to 48 hours after the onset of illness, necessitating follow-up laboratory assessment the next day, except in mild cases.

The standard measures for handling an unconscious or confused patient should be taken. Severely ill patients will require invasive monitoring and management in an intensive care unit. Classification in terms of severity in each major organ system is more useful than classification by specific syndrome and helps to guide clinical management (Table 17–4). This scheme applies to otherwise healthy young adults, and may require adjustment for elderly or very young patients.

Many patients appear to have mental and perhaps physical impairment for several days following even a moderate episode of heat illness. This requires activity restriction and continued follow-up. Patients having only moderately severe heat illness have been reported to have poor judgment and difficulty concentrating lasting at least 3 days following the episode, despite appearing completely well.

Bibliography

American College of Sports Medicine: Heat and cold illnesses during distance running: American College of Sports Medicine Position Stand. Med Sci Sports Exerc 28:i, 1996.

Armstrong LE, Crago AE, Adams R, et al: Whole-body cooling of hyperthermic runners: comparison of two field therapies. Am J Emerg Med 14:355, 1996.

Austin MG, Berry JW: Observations on one hundred cases of heatstroke. JAMA 161:1525, 1956.

Bell CR, Watts AJ: Thermal limits for industrial workers. Br J Ind Med 28:259, 1971.

Cantu RC, Micheli LJ: ACSM's Guidelines for the Team Physician. Philadelphia, Lea & Febiger, 1991.

Costrini A: Emergency treatment of exertional heatstroke and comparison of whole body cooling techniques. Med Sci Sports Exerc 22:15, 1990.

Costrini AM, Pitt HA, Gustafson AB, Uddin DE: Cardiovascular and metabolic manifestations of heat stroke and severe heat exhaustion. Am J Med 66:296, 1979.

Gardner JW, Kark JA: Fatal rhabdomyolysis presenting as mild heat illness in military training. Mil Med 159:160, 1994.

Gardner JW, Kark JA, Karnei K, et al: Risk factors predicting exertional heat illness in male Marine corps recruits. Med Sci Sports Exerc 28:939, 1996.

Grossman RA, Hamilton RW, Morse BM, et al: Nontraumatic rhabdomyolysis and acute renal failure. N Engl J Med 291:807, 1974.

Kark JA, Burr PQ, Wenger CB, et al: Exertional heat illness in Marine Corps recruit training. Aviat Space Environ Med 67:354, 1996.

Knochel JP: Environmental heat illness: an eclectic review. Arch Intern Med 133: 841, 1974.

Knochel JP: Heat stroke and related heat stress disorders. Dis Mon 35:301, 1989.

TABLE 17–4. Classification and Stratification of Heat Illness

Category	Dehydration	CNS	Renal	Lysis
1	Nonspecific symptoms	Normal	Cr: ≤1.4 mg/dL	CK: <700 IU/L
2	Orthostatic symptoms	Lethargic, slow mentation	Cr: 1.5–1.7 mg/dL	CK: 700–1200 IU/L
3	Exertional syncope	Amnesia, confusion	Cr: 1.8–1.9 mg/dL	CK: 1200–4,000 IU/L
4	Orthostatic hypotension	Delirious, ataxia/vertigo	Cr: ≥2.0 mg/dL	CK: 4–10,000 IU/L Progressive muscle symptoms
5	Shock	Seizure, obtunded, coma	Acute renal failure	CK: ≥10,000 IU/L Metabolic changes

Clinical Management

Category 1: Follow-up is not usually needed.
Category 2: Clinic and/or laboratory follow-up may be indicated.
Category 3: Clinic and laboratory follow-up is probably indicated.
Category 4: Hospitalization may be indicated.
Category 5: Hospitalization is indicated.

CNS, central nervous system; CK, serum creatine kinase; Cr, serum creatinine.

Malamud N, Haymaker W, Custer RP: Heat stroke: a clinico-pathologic study of 125 fatal cases. Mil Surg 99:397, 1946.
Rowell LB: Human cardiovascular adjustments to exercise and thermal stress. Physiol Rev 54:75, 1974.
Schrier RW, Hano J, Keller HI, et al: Renal, metabolic, and circulatory responses to heat and exercise: studies in military recruits during summer training, with implications for acute renal failure. Ann Intern Med 73:213, 1970.
Shibolet S, Lancaster MC, Danon Y: Heat stroke: a review. Aviat Space Environ Med 47:280, 1976.

18 *Traditional Medicine*

Gerard C. Bodeker

DEFINITION. The local health traditions of developing countries and of indigenous communities are commonly referred to as *traditional medicine*. Since most have a theoretical basis, a materia medica, a range of therapeutic modalities, an empirical approach to treatment, and a tradition of training, a more appropriate term is *traditional health systems*. These systems have been described by the World Health Organization (WHO) as "*holistic*—i.e., that of viewing man in his totality within a wide ecological spectrum, and of emphasizing the view that ill health or disease is brought about by an imbalance, or disequilibrium, of man in his total ecological system and not only by the causative agent and pathogenic evolution." Traditional health systems are "one of the surest means to achieve total health care coverage of the world population, using acceptable, safe, and economically feasible methods."

GENERAL PRINCIPLES. The paradigms of traditional health systems emphasize the integration of the individual and the environment, the integration of mind and body, the value of complex mixtures of medicinal plants, physical therapies such as massage, and the use of meditation, diet, and exercise programs as means of preventing and treating disease. The essence of traditional health care approaches is that a healthy, integrated lifestyle is the basis of effective treatment and prevention.

This chapter presents an overview of the major health traditions of regions in which tropical and traditional health systems interface. Survey chapters typically provide breadth of coverage at the expense of depth. However, the bibliography lists publications that provide deeper coverage of the traditions, their treatment modalities, and their efficacy.

THE SYSTEMS. Two broad categories for classifying traditional medicine are used in ethnomedical literature, i.e., the personalistic and the naturalistic.

Personalistic. Medical knowledge in a community is concentrated in an individual or individuals who have acquired their skills and knowledge through the training of a previous traditional practitioner, personal revelation, and experience. Treatments can include spiritual, mental, emotional, herbal, and physical modalities. Recognized "power of the hand" or individual healing ability is the basis for confidence in a practitioner. The indigenous traditions of Africa and Latin America are generally considered as personalistic traditions.

Naturalistic. This approach originates in a comprehensive, documented, theoretical framework based on empirical investigation of anatomy, nutrition, medicinal plants, and mind-body-spirit interaction and includes a systematic tradition of training and a documented materia medica. The traditional medical systems of Asia—the Ayurvedic system of India, Oriental medicine, Vietnamese medicine, and the Islamic Unani system—are considered naturalistic traditions.

UTILIZATION. The treatment strategies utilized in traditional health systems include the use of herbal medicines; mind-body approaches, e.g., meditation, physical therapies including massage, acupuncture and exercise programs; and approaches that address both physical and spiritual well-being. Although traditional health systems have long been accorded marginal status by health planners and personnel, the majority of the population of most developing countries rely on these systems for their everyday health care. The WHO estimates that approximately 80% of these populations, particularly poorer, rural sectors of society, rely on traditional health care as their first resort for preventing and treating illness.

Reasons for utilization vary. For many people in rural areas, traditional medicine is the only form of health care available. Economic factors are a significant consideration as well. The nearest clinic may be 1 or 2 days away and the cost of not working while traveling to and from a clinic, combined with the cost of the medicines prescribed, can serve as a significant incentive to seek treatment locally. Others may adopt a pluralistic approach, selecting traditional health care for what may be perceived as the underlying cause of a condition and modern medicine for symptomatic relief. Modern medicine is often utilized for acute conditions and traditional medicine for chronic conditions. People will often resort to either modern or traditional health care when they believe the other system has failed them.

Urban areas in Africa are witnessing an increased demand for traditional medicines and large urban herbal medicine markets flourish in the major cities of many African countries. A survey of 800 households conducted by the African Development Bank and the United Nations Children's Fund in Abidjan, Ivory Coast, found that 14% of households had turned to traditional medicine for their health care following devaluation of the local currency. Reasons given included the higher prices of modern medicines and a substantial overall increase in the cost of living. In households headed by women, the rate of increase in traditional medicine utilization was 17%. As part of health sector policy reform in many countries, international lenders, e.g., the World Bank, have insisted that countries introduce user fees for health services. In Tanzania, less than 1 year after user fees were introduced, there was a drop in attendance at some hospital outpatient clinics of up to 90%. Poorer members of society were using traditional medicine for obvious economic as well as cultural reasons.

Traditional Herbal Remedies. Approximately one fourth of the active components of medicines currently prescribed in North America and Britain were initially identified in higher plants. An increasing proportion of the populations of industrial countries regularly use herbal medicines for both preventing and treating disease. In developing countries, herbal medicines form an important mainstay of traditional medical practice. The plants in an environment are well known to local communities and most rural people treat themselves first before seeking help from either modern or traditional medical practitioners. Herbal medicines offer inexpensive, early intervention in the emerging stages of disease. Investigations in Thailand showed that the most effective use of traditional herbal medicines in primary health care is in their role in self-medication.

Traditional pharmacologies emphasize a principle of synergistic activity among the components of herbal mixtures. This assumes that, just as the body extracts multiple components from food, the body is also designed to do the same from medicinal plant materials. Traditional medicines typically use more than a single plant, favoring complex mixtures of plant materials, including leaves, roots, bark, and sap of plants, according to the condition being treated.

A study on the market value of medicinal resources from tropical forests estimates that "the value of traditional medical products, which are used by billions of people around the world, comprises billions of dollars each year." In the past decade, the search for molecules from traditional remedies or medicinal plants—known as "bioprospecting"—has become a feature of the traditional medicine landscape. In the face of bioprospectors' quests for a single, patentable molecule, traditional resource rights have emerged as a contentious issue, where debate centers on ownership and use of traditional knowledge.

The use of plants for medicines in both developed and industrial countries is placing pressure on wild stocks of plants. International agencies and scholars have drawn attention to the need for planning and conservation of the rain forests to ensure a future supply of important plants and their habitats.

RELATIONSHIPS BETWEEN MODERN AND TRADITIONAL HEALTH SYSTEMS. Under colonial influence, traditional health systems were frequently outlawed. In the postcolonial era the attitudes of Western-trained medical practitioners and health officials have largely maintained the marginal status of traditional health care providers in many countries, despite the role that traditional practitioners play in providing basic health care to the rural majority.

Traditional medicine and modern medicine have interfaced with each other in four broad ways:

1. *Monopolistic.* Modern medical doctors have the sole right to practice medicine.
2. *Tolerant.* Traditional medical practitioners are not officially recognized but are free to practice on condition that they do not claim to be registered medical doctors.
3. *Parallel.* Practitioners of both modern and traditional systems are officially recognized and they serve their patients through equal but separate systems (e.g., India).
4. *Integrated.* Modern and traditional medicine are merged in medical education and are jointly practiced within a unique health service (e.g., China, Vietnam).

A number of projects and policies have promoted a collaborative relationship between the traditions. In the Integrated Health Care System in Mangarivo, Madagascar, traditional healers and modern medical doctors work together in diagnosing and treating diseases with traditional and/or modern medicines according to the disease. The Foundation for Revitalization of Local Health Traditions in India educates villagers in the value of local medical formulas and in the cultivation and conservation of medicinal plants. Through a system of electronic databases, training courses, and research activities, modern medical practitioners are educated in the scientific basis of local traditions. A growing number of countries are using their local health traditions as a potential source of cost-containment in health care.

REGIONAL TRADITIONS AND TRENDS

Africa. African traditional medicine has been defined as a system that uses acquired and/or inherited indigenous knowledge and skills with the aim of improving the health and welfare of the individual and/or the community. In African health traditions, the distinction between personal misfortune and illness is essentially absent in most groups. This is characteristic of many traditional health systems and is reflected in cosmologies that take into account mind, body spirit, and environment. Accordingly, treatments emphasize both spiritual approaches as well as natural approaches, e.g., the use of medicinal plants and herbal preparations. Al-

though there are very few systematic data on the ratio of traditional health practitioners to population, one national survey in Uganda found a distribution of practitioners to population of between 1:200 and 1:400. In terms of available local health resources this contrasts with the availability of trained medical personnel in which the ratio is typically 1:20,000 and upward. In Lesotho in 1986, there were reportedly about 7800 traditional practitioners for a population of 1.4 million. In Swaziland, there were between 5000 and 7000 for a population of 700,000.

A 1986 Commonwealth meeting of experts on the evaluation of traditional medical practices in Africa identified the following categories of traditional practitioners: (1) diagnosticians/diviners; (2) herbalists; (3) midwives; and (4) other practitioners, including bone setters and traditional massage specialists.

The great majority of traditional practitioners are herbalists, with only 5% being estimated to be diviners or spiritualists. Accounts at the African Regional Meeting of the Global Initiative for Traditional Systems of Health indicated that the majority of the herbalists are women, although men are typically the organizers of the associations of traditional medicine. Women also serve as traditional birth attendants (TBAs), who are responsible for approximately 70% of deliveries in Africa. Through their role as mothers and caregivers, women also serve as the preservers and purveyors of cultural knowledge of health practices. Mothers are the first line of health intervention, often administering plants for childhood ailments and family health problems, passing on treatment that they learned from their own mothers. As the keepers of domestic gardens, women also have a significant role in medicinal plant conservation and cultivation.

The importance of women as TBAs in Africa has been addressed by a number of agencies, including the African Development Bank in its "Gender" paper and WHO, which has developed guidelines for the training of TBAs. TBAs often constitute the only available midwife service. In the context of safe motherhood initiatives, it is important that training be provided to TBAs. Training should emphasize issues of sanitary and safe delivery practices but should not attempt to change customary traditional delivery procedures if they are safe. The use of herbal medicines to induce labor can be effective, but with lack of dosage control, this can cause complications. Education regarding dosage of herbal medicines is another important step toward strengthening the role of TBAs in safe and effective midwifery.

The Americas. The health traditions of the Americas are highly variable. Common to most is the belief that spiritual factors contribute to the state of imbalance (dis-ease) that has produced vulnerability to sickness. Spiritual, herbal, and physical therapies are all utilized in treatment. A number of South American nations have established departments or divisions of traditional medicine within their health ministries.

In Mexico, whose population includes 9 million indigenous people, there has been a comprehensive program to revitalize the indigenous health traditions. The *curanderismo* traditions of Mexico have commonalities with other traditions of Latin America. *Curanderismo* embodies elements of Greek humoral theory, medieval Spanish medicine, Aztec medical traditions, the herbal practices and medicinal plants of Europe, and spiritual beliefs and practices from indigenous traditions of the region.

Ethnomedical and pharmacognostic research has identified over a thousand traditional medicines. The government and indigenous organizations have established training centers to communicate traditional medical knowledge to new generations of health care workers. Hospitals of traditional medicine have been established in a number of rural areas.

During the war in Nicaragua, the international economic blockade resulted in a severe shortage of medical and pharmaceutical supplies. In 1985, Nicaragua reappraised its herbal traditions as a potential means of addressing national medical needs. The government established a new department of indigenous medicine which undertook a program of ethnobotanical research. In the context of developing training and services in traditional health care, more than 20,000 people were interviewed concerning their use of traditional herbal remedies, methods for preparing these, and the locations and plants from which medicines were derived.

In Brazil, practitioners of the Afro-Brazilian traditions use herbal and traditional psychotherapeutic interventions in treating disease. Health organizations are collaborating with these healers in developing an effective and culturally appropriate AIDS prevention message.

The Canadian Midwifery Act (Bill 56) of 1994 formally exempted aboriginal midwives from its jurisdiction and regulatory process, resulting in the revitalization of traditional midwifery in Canada.

In the United States, many Native American communities incorporate traditional forms of treatment into Indian Health Service (IHS) alcohol rehabilitation programs. An analysis of 190 IHS contract programs found that 50% offered a traditional sweat lodge at their site or encouraged its use. Treatment outcomes were better for alcoholic patients when a sweat lodge was available and the presence of medicine men or healers greatly improved the outcome when used in combination with the sweat lodge.

Asia. Throughout Asia, the traditional health sector serves as the principal provider of health care to the poor and to rural communities and has been incorporated into most national health systems for two or three decades. The Indian and Chinese traditional systems, which account for the traditional medical sector of more than half of the world's population, contain a range of specific preventive methodologies that have direct application to lifestyle and preventive health issues. In cardiovascular prevention and treatment there are integrative exercise programs such as Tai Chi and yoga, vegetarian diets, and stress reduction through meditation. Not only has research found many of these to be safe and effective preventive methodologies, they are culturally familiar, hence increasing compliance prospects and contributing to a strengthening rather than a westernization of traditional cultures and their health knowledge.

Ayurveda. This is the ancient natural health care system of India. In Sanskrit, *ayur* means *life* and *veda* means *knowledge*, the science of life. It is a system designed to promote optimal human development throughout the life span. The Ayurvedic practitioner uses a range of different diagnostic procedures to determine the state of balance in the individual's mind and body. All are noninvasive, and the principal means is a system of pulse diagnosis, which uses a greatly expanded range of information than that typically gathered in taking a radial pulse.

Individual constitutions are classified according to three basic organizing principles, or *doshas*: (1) *vata*, which governs flow and motion and is said to be at the basis of the locomotor system's activity; (2) *pitta*, which is related to bodily functions associated with heat and metabolism; and (3) *kapha*, which is responsible for the structure and coordination of the physiology. Therapeutic modalities include mental (meditation), physical (yoga, therapeutic massage), herbal, and dietary approaches to both preventing and treating disease.

The Indian Medicine Central Council Act of 1970 gave an official place in national health programs to the Ayurvedic and Unani medical systems of India. India now has over 200,000 registered traditional medical practitioners. Most of these practitioners are graduates of degree-granting government colleges of Ayurvedic or Unani medicine. In Sri Lanka, where there is widespread use of the Ayurvedic system of medicine, the Health Ministry has a Department of Ayurveda. Nepal has a college of Ayurvedic education in Katmandu and a Department of Ayurveda within the Health Ministry.

The Unani Medical System. This is the Islamic medical tradition that was introduced into India in Mughal times. Unani, which derives from Greek medicine, uses humoral theory as the basis of diagnosis and treatment. Herbal medicines and mineral preparations are common in Unani. Pakistan and Bangladesh both have departments of traditional medicine within their health ministries, and universities and colleges offer degrees in Unani medicine.

Traditional Chinese Medicine. China established its policy of integrating traditional medicine into national health care in the 1960s. Under this system, modern and traditional medicine are combined as formal components of national health care provision. China has modernized traditional medicine, and extensive research on the safety, efficacy, and standardization of traditional medical treatments is being conducted at traditional medicine institutes throughout the country.

Fundamental concepts of traditional Chinese medicine reflect a broad framework for classifying matter and energy. They include a characterization of two underlying principles, *yin* and *yang*, which are considered as paired opposites that can be used to express concepts of normal physiology as well as pathology. *Five phases* are described to express the movement or dynamism within the components of physiologic and mental functioning. The concept of *qi* refers to subtle energy or life force and is further described in categories that govern nourishment, defense systems, flow of energy, physiologic functioning of organs, respiration, and circulation. Therapeutic procedures include acupuncture and moxibustion (a heat treatment)—both designed to affect movement of *qi*—massage, herbal medicine, diet, and *qigong*, a set of integrative exercise, breathing, and meditative practices.

Traditional Chinese medicine provides the underlying theoretical and clinical framework for the medical traditions of Japan, Korea and Vietnam, which have also developed regional variations and adaptations of concepts, practice, and materia medica. Official policy in these countries supports standardized training in traditional medicine, laboratory and clinical research, and a formal system of licensure.

Western Traditional Medicine. Current trends in Western health care are increasingly emphasizing the prevention of illness through health-promoting exercise, diet and nutrition, and stress reduction programs. Cardiovascular research has shown that a combination of vegetarian diet, mild exercise (yoga), and stress reduction (a meditation program) produced a significant reduction in the size of coronary artery lesions. Reductions in stress-related disorders and health care utilization result from a meditation program—the transcendental meditation program, including an 87.3% lower rate of hospital admissions for heart disorders and a 63.2% lower rate of hospital admissions for tumors than for the general public.

TRAINING. Several models of training are used in traditional medicine.

Recording the Traditional Heritage. In some countries, written, audio, and video records are gathered from the remaining custodians of traditional medical knowledge. The material is used to develop training programs for large groups of new traditional practitioners. Vietnam has an extensive "heritage" program sponsored by the government. The Inuit Women's Association of Canada had developed a program to revitalize traditional birth practices. Video recordings of women who were midwives for many years in their own communities are used to train young Inuit women in the use of traditional delivery methods in combination with modern training in hygiene and safety.

Training Primary Health Care Workers. WHO has promoted training traditional practitioners to become providers of primary health care. This training has been associated with improvements in health education, family planning, oral rehydration therapy use, personal hygiene, and environmental sanitation.

Although this is an obvious approach to provide primary health care and can clearly have benefits, it is important to note its risks. Insensitive training can weaken the traditional role of practitioners when they provide services in which they are not familiar. A hybridization of traditional and modern medical knowledge can result, undermining the original theory and clinical practice. By contrast, when trained to give a health education message in the context of their traditional role, traditional healers have welcomed training and have been successful in Brazil, Zambia, and Mozambique in giving effective AIDS prevention messages.

Formal Training for Traditional Health Practitioners. In many countries in Asia (e.g., India, China, Bangladesh, Korea, Sri Lanka, Nepal) the government regulates curriculum standards and certification for traditional medical practitioners to ensure professional standards of practice and training in traditional medicine. In addition to the training of traditional health practitioners, courses have been developed to orient modern medical health care providers to the health care practices that the majority of their patients are utilizing.

Training for Biomedical Health Professionals. A 1993 UNDP Workshop on Medicinal Plants, held in Eskisehir, Turkey in 1993, recommended that an introductory course on traditional medicine should be included in the curricula of faculties of medicine. Training in traditional medicine prepares medical students to understand the health care practices that the majority of their patients will be using. In Vietnam, for instance, every medical student takes 16 courses in traditional medicine whether he or she specializes in this field or not. In planning and evaluating training in traditional health care, assumptions about traditional health care and the goals of training must be made explicit. Fundamental questions include training in what, by whom, and for what purpose? Appropriate training should preserve and apply traditional health knowledge safely and effectively. Traditional systems can become viable and affordable components of national health care and can foster collaboration between modern and traditional health care providers in the interests of patient welfare.

TROPICAL DISEASE AND TRADITIONAL MEDICINE. Traditional health care practitioners in tropical regions are consulted by people seeking relief from a wide range of medical illness, including diarrheal diseases, malaria, tropical ulcer, and acute and chronic wounds. Results of investigations indicate the need for a comprehensive program to evaluate the clinical effects of traditional treatments in tropical diseases.

Malaria. In Africa, where 70% to 80% of the world's cases of malaria occur and it is the principal cause of death, conventional drugs have produced mutated forms of the malaria parasite and drug resistance has created a new crisis in malaria control (Chapter 92). In the Americas, almost 700 million people live in areas conducive to the transmission of malaria. Indigenous communities in remote rural areas have suffered the worst, with malaria afflicting 358/1000 popula-

tion in the Brazilian Amazon. Traditionally, societies afflicted by malaria have used local plants—either alone or in the form of complex mixtures—to prevent and treat malaria. Anecdotal and research data support the potential of locally growing plants as treatments for new, drug-resistant strains of malaria. Research in the Northern Amazon, conducted by the Royal Botanical Gardens, Kew, found that 80 species of plants are used by the Yanomami people to treat malaria.

In Uganda, where malaria remains the most important cause of morbidity and mortality, traditional and modern health practitioners have established collaborative clinical and research programs in treating malaria and other diseases. A study of the clinical effectiveness of southwest Ugandan antimalarials found that complex mixtures of antimalarial plants were effective in treating malaria, even in cases that were resistant to conventional drug treatment.

Both China and Vietnam have developed independent programs to produce a plant-based antimalarial, artemisinin. Artemisinin is derived from *Artemisia annua*, which has been used traditionally in Asia to control fever. Artemisinin has been effective in controlling drug-resistant *Plasmodium falciparum* on the Burma/Thai border.

Research in Africa points to the potential of the plant *Phytolacca dodecandra* as a means of controlling breeding patterns of mosquitoes. Warrell has emphasized the importance of expanding the search for new antimalarials to include clinical evaluation of single plants and complex mixtures used by communities to treat malaria. Such an approach would not necessarily aim to develop a single new antimalarial drug. Rather, it would serve to identify and promote existing local solutions that may provide sustainable, affordable, and locally available treatments.

Wound Healing and Skin Infections. In rural areas of developing countries, wounds and dermatologic conditions are very common reasons for people to seek medical care. People living in rural areas sustain injuries working in the fields, burns from cooking and from sleeping near fires, leg ulcers resulting from untreated wounds, injuries incurred in conflicts, and, increasingly, injuries resulting from traffic accidents (Chapter 13). Some countries have formal systems of traditional health care which provide traditional herbal remedies in the care of wounds. The Le Huu Trac Institute of Burns in Hanoi, Vietnam, emphasizes a combination of modern and traditional medicine for the treatment of burns. The Institute has an active program of research to develop medicines from traditional sources.

These medications have been found to be effective in generating membrane formation, inhibiting bacterial growth, and stimulating the formation of scar tissue on burn lesions. The treatment time with traditional medicine is markedly shorter than with conventional burn medication. In many cases, medical staff use traditional medical treatments by preference because they are found to be more effective than conventional burn treatments with respect to sepsis, healing time, scarring, pain, and patient comfort. Research conducted by our group at Oxford has found that honey, which is used historically in Africa, the Middle East, and Asia as a wound healing agent, is an effective means of treating cutaneous leishmaniasis. Antiviral effects of honey have also been observed. In tropical Africa, *Aristolochia bracteata* is used widely in treating chronic ulcers and eczema. In India, the same plant is used to treat scabies. Extracts from the root of the plant have antimicrobial properties against *Staphylococcus aureus* and other bacteria.

In Ghana, skin diseases have been identified as conditions for which traditional medicines are superior to, or are suitable substitutes for, modern medicine. Conditions identified include coccal and fungal infections, allergy, and herpes zoster. In Uganda, the AIDS Commission and the Joint Clinical Research Centre have worked with traditional healers in evaluating traditional treatments used for opportunistic infections associated with the human immunodeficiency virus and AIDS. Traditional medicines have been reported to be better suited for treatment of herpes zoster, chronic diarrhea, and weight loss. In Nigeria, the root of the woody perennial shrub *Borreria verticillata* (L.) G.F.W. Mey (Rubiaceae)—also known as the African borreria—is used to treat a range of skin diseases. In Senegal, the leaves are used topically and orally in the treatment of leprosy.

INTERACTION BETWEEN TRADITIONAL AND WESTERN HEALTH SYSTEMS. Traditional health systems are used by the majority of people in developing countries. Patients seeking care from a health professional will often have already used traditional medicine for their illness. In the United States more than 70% of Americans who use alternative forms of medicine do not inform their physician of its use. This failure to communicate about seeking out traditional health care may be even more prevalent in tropical regions because of bias against traditional forms of health care.

The tropical health professional will need to know what traditional medicines are being used, the effectiveness of local treatments—herbal and otherwise—and how best to use the strengths of traditional treatments and practitioners when health resources are scarce. Most national universities have anthropology or chemistry departments with some research expertise in the study of local health traditions and their medicines. The University of Illinois' database, NAPRALERT, is accessible through Medline and contains thousands of references on the chemistry and pharmacological properties of traditional medicines and medicinal plants.

Where training is undertaken, it is important that this be two-way, as each tradition—traditional and Western—can learn from the other. Training in health education is effective and is an important method for delivering a health message to traditional and rural communities. This should reinforce the value of local traditions in health care. Recognition should be given to the preventive strategies provided by traditional health systems, e.g., cultural and household dietary practices, exercise, and the regular use of medicinal herbs as food, as these may offer culturally acceptable and effective means of preventing disease.

Bibliography

Balick MJ, Elisabetsky E, Laird SE (eds): Medicinal Resources of the Tropical Forest: Biodiversity and Its Importance to Human Health. New York, Columbia University Press, 1996.

Bitahwa N, Tumwesigye O, Kabariime P, et al: Herbal treatment of malaria—four case reports from the Rukararwe Partnership Workshop for Rural Development, Uganda. Trop Doct 27(Suppl 1):17, 1997.

Boedeker G, Bhatt KKS, Burley J, Vantomme P (eds): Medicinal Plants for Forest Conservation and Health Care. FAO Non-Wood Forest Product Series No. 11, Food and Agriculture Organization, Rome, 1997.

Editorial: Pharmaceuticals from plants: Great potential, few funds. Lancet 343:1513, 1994.

Hall RL: Alcohol treatment in American Indian populations: An indigenous treatment modality compared with traditional approaches. Ann NY Acad Sci 472:168, 1986.

Hoff W: Traditional Practitioners as Primary Health Care Workers: An Evaluation of the Effectiveness of Four Training Projects in Ghana, Mexico, and Bangladesh. Geneva, World Health Organization, 1995.

Micozzi M (ed): Fundamentals of Alternative and Complementary Medicine. New York, Churchill Livingstone, 1995.

Orme-Johnson DW: Medical care utilization and the transcendental meditation program. Psychosom Med 49:493, 1988.

Ornish D, Brown SE, Scherwitz LW, et al: Can lifestyle changes reverse coronary heart disease? World Rev Nutr Diet 72:38, 1993.

Price RN, Nosten F, Luxemburger C, et al: Effects of artemisinin derivatives on malaria transmissibility. Lancet 347:1654, 1996.

Shankar D: Conserving the medicinal plants of India: The need for a biocultural perspective. J Alternat Complement Med 2:3, 1996.

Sofowora A: Medicinal Plants and Traditional Medicine in Africa. Ibadan, Nigeria, Spectrum Books Limited, 1993.

Trung LT: Vietnamese Experience in the Treatment of Burns. Hanoi, The Goi Publishers, 1992.

Warrell D: Herbal remedies for malaria. Trop Doct 27(Suppl 1):5, 1997.

World Health Organization: Traditional Medicine. Geneva, WHO, 1978.

World Health Organization: Guidelines for the Evaluation of Herbal Medicines. Manila, WHO Regional Office, 1993.

Zeina B: Effect of honey on leishmaniasis: An in vitro study. Trop Doct 27(Suppl 1):36, 1997.

Zeina B, Al-Assad S, Othman O: Effect of honey on rubella virus versus thyme survival in vitro. J Alternat Complement Med 2:3, 1996.

19 Health and Nutrition Among Refugees and Displaced Persons

Bradley A. Woodruff and Brenton B. Burkholder

■ GENERAL PRINCIPLES

The term *complex emergency* has been coined to describe situations that usually involve a combination of war or civil strife, food shortages, and population displacement, and that result in significant excess mortality. Persons who are displaced from their normal residence can be either refugees (those fleeing to another country because of persecution) or internally displaced persons (those fleeing for similar reasons but remaining within their country of origin). In 1995, there were more than 15 million refugees in need of international protection and assistance. In addition, more than 20 million people were displaced within their country of citizenship.

A common feature of the acute phase of almost all humanitarian crises, whether caused by war, famine, or natural disaster, is an elevated mortality rate. The average crude mortality rate in settled populations in developing countries is usually less than 0.5 deaths/10,000 population per day and for children <5 years of age is 1.0/10,000 per day. Rates more than double these are considered emergencies, and in many past situations, crude mortality rates have been 5 to 15 times normal. In emergency situations, curative and preventive care are often quite different from care delivered in developed countries. Medical care must be decentralized to reach everyone in the displaced population. Diagnoses are often made quickly without laboratory or radiologic support. For common medical conditions, detailed protocols are often used to simplify and standardize medical care. Case definitions for epidemiologic surveillance and clinical diagnosis should be simple and easily applied (Table 19–1).

With the exception of the trauma that occurs during conflicts, the causes of death are often similar to the causes of death during normal times in the same population (Fig. 19–1). Diarrheal disease, lower respiratory infection (LRI), measles, malaria, and undernutrition may account for 60 to 95% of all mortality. Additional mortality can be due to specific diseases, e.g., bacillary dysentery, cholera, meningococcal disease, and hepatitis E, which occur in rapidly spreading outbreaks. Although each emergency situation is somewhat different, these health problems have been responsible for substantial excess mortality in many past humanitarian emergencies in developing countries and must be anticipated in future emergencies. Moreover, the excess mortality after population displacement almost always disproportionately affects children <5 years of age.

TABLE 19–1. Typical Case Definitions Used for Epidemiologic Surveillance*

Medical Condition	Case Definition
Diarrhea	Three or more loose stools in a 24-hr period
Cholera	Watery diarrhea in an area with known cholera, *or*
	Dehydrating diarrhea in an older child or adult
Dysentery	Diarrhea with visible blood in the stool
Lower respiratory infection	Fever and cough
Measles	Rash and fever plus cough, coryza, or conjunctivitis
Malaria	Fever without cough
Meningitis	Sudden onset of fever and stiff neck
Hepatitis	Jaundice

*Clinical or diagnostic case definitions may be different.

■ DISEASES OF HIGH PRIORITY DURING THE ACUTE PHASE OF EMERGENCIES

DIARRHEAL DISEASE. Diarrheal disease is one of the most frequent causes of morbidity and mortality in the developing world (Chapter 4). The most common causative agents are viruses and bacteria; however, determining a specific diagnosis is usually impossible in emergency situations because of the lack of laboratory facilities. Nonetheless, in the midst of an outbreak in which a large proportion of cases are due to the same agent, the diagnosis in individual cases can often be inferred from epidemiologic evidence. The case-fatality rate from diarrheal disease can vary from <1 to 50%, depending on the etiologic agent, the preexisting condition of the patient, and the medical treatment received. Figure 19–2 shows the number of cases of diarrhea and the case-fatality rate for diarrheal disease during the first few weeks after 750,000 Rwandan refugees arrived in Goma, Zaire. In Goma and in other past emergencies involving displaced populations, cholera (Chapter 41) and dysentery (Chapter 40) caused a large proportion of morbidity and mortality (Fig. 19–3).

A major component of therapy for diarrheal disease is oral administration of fluids because, with the exception of dysentery, the predominant cause of mortality is dehydration. Antibiotic therapy is not warranted for most uncomplicated cases of diarrhea, and intravenous fluid administration, even if available, requires a high degree of supervision by trained health workers and may pose a risk of nosocomial infection. Oral rehydration therapy (ORT) is very effective in preventing dehydration and treating moderate dehydration (Chapter 16). Only patients who cannot take oral fluids as a result of severe vomiting or obtundation need to have fluids administered intravenously. A simple protocol for assessing dehydration and the appropriate administration of fluids has been published by the World Health Organization (WHO) and should be used in humanitarian emergencies. Health workers not familiar with ORT should receive specific training before attempting to treat diarrheal disease in emergencies. Diarrhea may exacerbate poor nutritional status, which in turn increases the severity of the next bout of diarrhea. To stop this cycle, feeding, especially breast-feeding for infants, should be continued during diarrheal illness. Small frequent meals may be better tolerated; after illness, young children should be given an extra meal each day for at least 2 weeks to recover lost weight. In addition, malnourished children with diarrhea can be referred to special feeding programs. Antisecretory, antiperistaltic, or bulk-forming agents should not be used and should *never* be sent as relief supplies.

Because most infections causing diarrheal disease are acquired from contaminated food or water, providing adequate clean water, soap, and facilities for feces disposal should be of the highest priority early in the emergency. In addition, because measles can cause diarrhea, vaccination against measles can prevent some diarrheal disease (Chapter 25.1).

CHOLERA. Cholera outbreaks are common in much of the developing world (Chapter 41.1). Explosive outbreaks of cholera have occurred in many displaced populations and have killed tens of thousands of people. The case-fatality rate among patients with untreated severe illness can exceed 50%, but can be decreased to <1% with fluid replacement therapy. In most outbreaks, more than 90% of hospitalized patients can be managed using only ORT (Chapter 16). The WHO protocol for assessing and treating dehydration should be

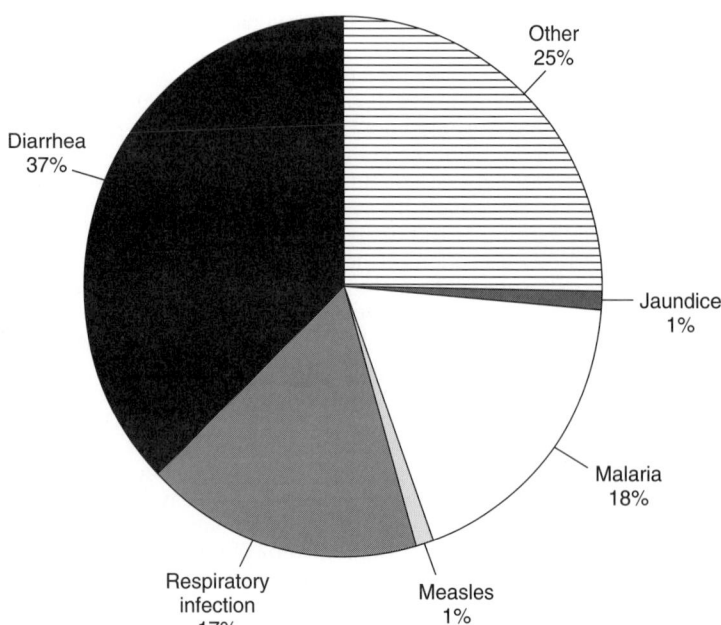

Figure **19–1.** Percentage of displaced persons <5 years of age presenting to health facilities with various health conditions, Khartoum, Sudan, 1988.

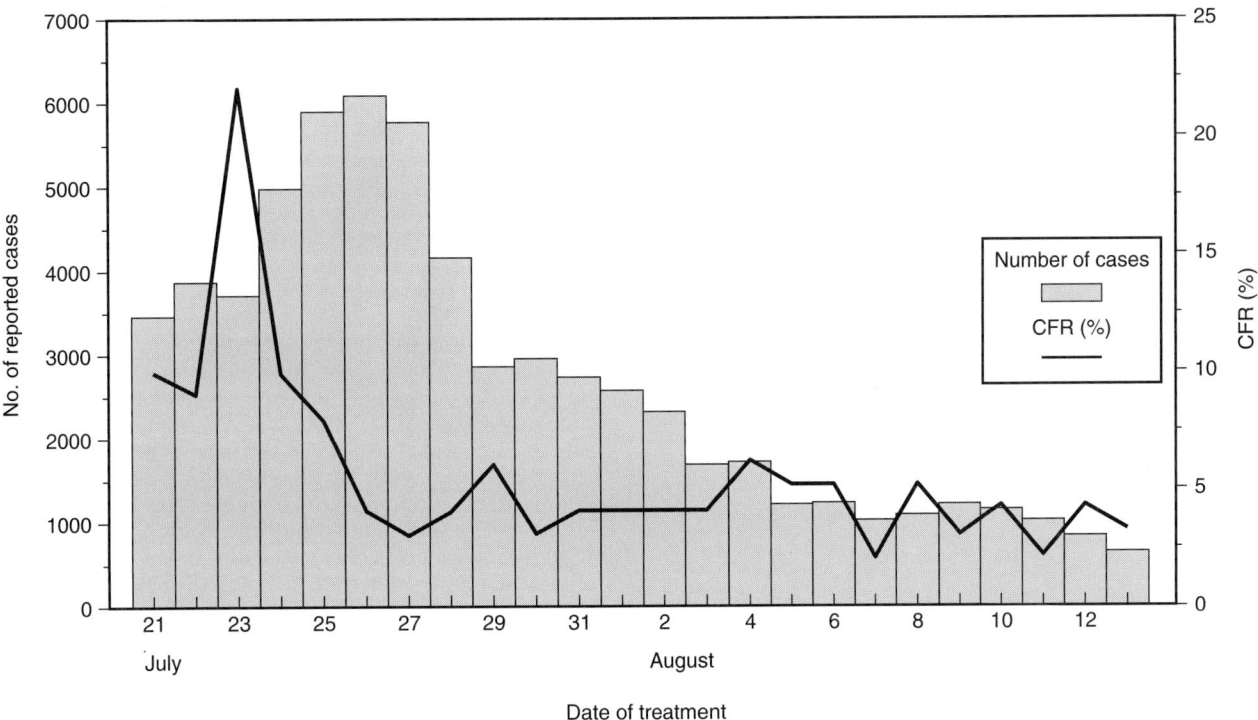

Figure 19–2. Number of reported cases of diarrhea and diarrhea case-fatality ratio (CFR), Goma, Democratic Republic of the Congo, 1994. (From The World Health Organization.)

used to treat cholera in emergency settings. Antibiotic treatment may shorten the course of illness but should be of only secondary importance and used primarily in patients with severe dehydration. The WHO-recommended treatment for adults is 300 mg of doxycycline given orally as a single dose. However, *Vibrio cholerae* serogroup 01, which caused recent outbreaks in displaced populations in Central Africa, has been relatively resistant to doxycycline.

Most infections are asymptomatic or result in mild illness; therefore, cholera may already be well established in a displaced population by the time the first clinical cases are detected. Early detection of epidemics and rapid mobilization of resources require good epidemiologic surveillance. An increase in the incidence of watery diarrhea or one case of dehydration from watery diarrhea in an older child or adult

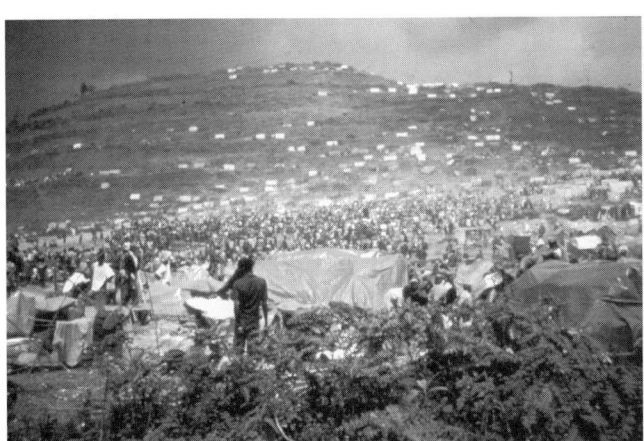

Figure 19–3. Overview of Rwandan refugee camp in Goma, Democratic Republic of the Congo, August 1994.

should alert health authorities to the possibility of cholera (younger children can have dehydrating watery diarrhea from other causes). Laboratory testing of the first few specimens in the beginning of an outbreak can confirm the presence of *V. cholerae* 01 and determine the antibiotic sensitivity pattern, but determining the diagnosis in individual patients thereafter should depend only on the presence of large-volume watery stools.

Rapid mobilization of resources and implementation of control measures are easiest if epidemic preparedness plans have been formulated in advance by all organizations working in the health, water, and sanitation fields. The plan should (1) identify potential resources, e.g., supplies of oral rehydration solution (ORS), intravenous fluids, and antibiotics; (2) outline the responsibilities of each type of health worker and each relief organization; (3) describe specific diagnostic and treatment protocols; and (4) organize health services, e.g., establish rehydration tents and cholera hospitals.

Because the infectious dose is relatively high, person-to-person transmission is not usually important, and control programs need not concentrate on this mode of transmission. Nonetheless, stringent precautions for handling stool and stool-contaminated material should be followed in any facility where cholera patients are treated. In the acute phase of an emergency, when the supply of clean water may be inadequate, chlorine can be added to household containers when water is obtained. Because fatal dehydration can occur within hours, rapid access to rehydration services is a major factor in reducing cholera-specific mortality. In recent outbreaks in refugee populations, as many as one half of the deaths from cholera occurred in patients who were never seen by a health worker. In large outbreaks, well-organized centers devoted exclusively to treating cholera can efficiently deliver rehydration (Fig. 19–4).

In emergency situations, antibiotic prophylaxis of house-

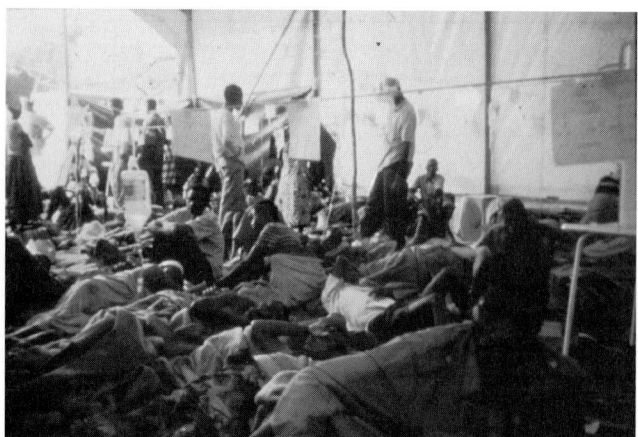

Figure 19–4. Patients with cholera and other diarrheal illnesses receiving rehydration and other therapy in a cholera tent, Goma, Zaire, August 1994.

hold contacts is not generally recommended because such contacts probably share exposures with the index patient, and prophylaxis programs may divert scarce resources away from more effective activities. Currently available vaccines against *V. cholerae* are not practical in emergency situations because outbreaks often spread too rapidly. Even if a timely vaccination campaign could be mounted, protective antibodies would not develop quickly enough to prevent the majority of infections. For example, among Rwandan refugees in Goma in July and August 1994, it was estimated that the entire displaced population was infected within 3 weeks.

DYSENTERY. In most developing countries, epidemic dysentery, or bloody diarrhea, is usually caused by *Shigella* species, especially *Shigella dysenteriae* type 1 (Chapter 40). The parasite *Entamoeba histolytica* also causes sporadic cases of bloody diarrhea, but it does not cause outbreaks of dysentery. Although other species of bacteria, e.g., certain serotypes of *Escherichia coli*, can also cause bloody diarrhea, outbreaks of dysentery in displaced populations in developing countries should be assumed to be due to *S. dysenteriae*, unless proved otherwise. The case-fatality rate for dysentery due to *S. dysenteriae* can be as high as 10%, especially among the very young, the elderly, and malnourished people.

Appropriate antibiotics, which can shorten the course of illness and prevent complications, are usually recommended for all patients with dysentery due to *S. dysenteriae*. Nalidixic acid, 1 g four times a day for 5 days for adults, is the WHO-recommended empiric therapy until the results of antibiotic sensitivity testing are known. However, in Central Africa, many strains, including the strain that caused the large outbreak of dysentery among Rwandan refugees in Goma, have high-level resistance to trimethoprim-sulfamethoxazole ampicillin, tetracycline, metronidazole, chloramphenicol, and nalidixic acid. Only antibiotics that belong to the quinolone family, which are expensive and in short supply in developing countries, remain effective in these areas. When the supply of effective antibiotics is insufficient to treat all cases of dysentery, treatment should be reserved for those at highest risk for death: children <5 years of age, adults ≥50 years of age, malnourished people, and patients with complications, including dehydration and convulsions. Because immediate treatment may be needed for life-threatening complications, including shock and convulsions, referral systems should be in place to provide more sophisticated treatment for those who need it.

Outbreaks of dysentery in displaced populations can be explosive due to poor sanitary conditions and a limited water supply. Epidemiologic surveillance is essential to identify outbreaks in order to implement control measures. A stool specimen for culture should be obtained from the first patients in whom cases of dysentery are suspected in order to confirm the etiology and determine the antibiotic sensitivity spectrum. Unlike cholera, *S. dysenteriae* is easily transmitted from person to person because the infectious dose is very small. Because the lack of water and soap restricts handwashing, supplying soap and an adequate quantity of water are important interventions to prevent dysentery, as is access to clean latrines.

ACUTE LOWER RESPIRATORY INFECTION. Lower respiratory infection is one of the most common causes of illness and death in young children in both displaced and settled populations in the developing world (Chapter 2). Such infections, if untreated, can lead to sepsis and death within 3 to 5 days after the onset of illness. The case-fatality rate for pneumococcal pneumonia in children in the preantibiotic era was 12 to 41% and may be higher among children compromised by undernutrition or other diseases.

Respiratory infections are diagnosed using simple methods. A well-tested algorithm that uses only clinical observation has been formulated by WHO to distinguish between children with LRI and those with less dangerous upper respiratory infections (Chapter 16). This algorithm can also be used to distinguish between children with severe pneumonia and those with less severe pneumonia. Identifying the causative agent, even in a small sample of cases, is usually not possible because specific bacteriologic diagnosis requires lung aspirate or blood culture, techniques that are not generally available. Because of the predominance of bacterial causes and the rapidity of disease progression, the key to the treatment of LRI is the prompt administration of appropriate antibiotics solely on the basis of symptoms and signs. Among children >2 months of age, the antibiotic chosen should be effective against *Streptococcus pneumoniae* and *Haemophilus influenzae*. WHO recommends a 5-day course of oral cotrimoxazole, amoxicillin, or ampicillin or intramuscular procaine penicillin. Virtually every emergency drug-supply kit contains at least one of these antibiotics. Among infants <2 months of age, the diagnostic criteria are somewhat more complex. These children should be treated with parenteral antibiotics covering a broader spectrum of gram-negative and gram-positive bacteria. WHO recommends a combination of injectable penicillin and gentamicin.

As with children with diarrheal disease, children with LRI should continue to receive feedings during the acute illness and to receive increased feedings during convalescence. In areas where falciparum malaria is endemic, children with suspected LRI should also receive therapy for malaria. If the assessment of respiratory difficulty shows wheezing, bronchodilators should be given. Serious upper respiratory infections, e.g., bacterial otitis media or mastoiditis, should be treated with appropriate antibiotics.

LRI is probably due to aspiration of nasopharyneal bacteria, especially *S. pneumoniae* and *H. influenzae* and carriage of these organisms may be more common among displaced populations than among settled populations because of crowding, poor heating, mucous membrane irritation from smoke, impeded immunologic resistance, and other factors. Moreover, the case-fatality rate may be higher in displaced populations due to compromised immunity and lack of access to prompt medical treatment.

Although preventing LRI may be more difficult than preventing other communicable diseases in children, one quarter or more of the cases of LRI can be eliminated by vaccination against measles, diphtheria, and pertussis. Enhancing overall immunologic status by reducing the prevalence of undernutrition and administering vitamin A may decrease the incidence of LRI and lower its case-fatality rate. Although not proved in displaced populations, reducing indoor smoke pollution by minimizing wood fires or by increasing ventilation may also help prevent infection. Safe and effective vaccines against *S. pneumoniae* and *H. influenzae* are available; however, their applicability in developing countries has yet to be determined. Conjugate vaccines against *S. pneumoniae* that are currently under development may protect younger children better than the currently available vaccine.

MEASLES. Measles, a leading cause of illness and death among children in developing countries (Chapter 25.1), is spread rapidly in crowded populations. In addition, the breakdown of vaccination programs that occurs during emergencies can leave a large cohort of young children unvaccinated. The case-fatality rate, as high as 5% in stable populations in developing countries, has been as high as 33% in displaced populations as a result of protein-calorie undernutrition, vitamin A deficiency, and lack of access to medical care. Acute protein-calorie undernutrition (Chapter 130) often occurs in children with measles who have marginal nutritional status and may result from the metabolic stress of acute infection and stomatitis, which interferes with a child's ability to eat. In addition, vitamin A deficiency resulting from measles may progress to xerophthalmia and may leave children more susceptible to other infections as a result of compromised immunity (Chapter 131.1).

The clinical diagnosis of measles relies on the signs of fever, cough, conjunctivitis, coryza, and the characteristic rash. In addition, knowledge of the patient's measles vaccination status and the distribution of measles in the general population may aid in diagnosis. WHO recommends that children with clinical measles receive two doses of oral vitamin A given on subsequent days. Children with measles should also have their nutritional status carefully monitored, be given extra food, be enrolled in a feeding program if necessary, and continue to receive prophylactic vitamin A. If possible, children with measles should be isolated from other children and checked daily for complications, which should be treated according to standardized protocols (e.g., ORT for diarrhea and dehydration, antibiotics for pneumonia, and vitamin A for signs of vitamin A deficiency).

Epidemiologic surveillance is a critical part of measles control. Early detection of cases of measles allows rapid implementation or expansion of emergency vaccination programs. In addition, cases of measles can indicate vaccine failure, poor local vaccine coverage, or other program deficiencies. As with other diseases of epidemic potential, an epidemic control plan can facilitate rapid mobilization of resources once an outbreak is suspected. Although a simple surveillance case definition should be formulated (Table 19–1), in many cultures measles is so endemic that it can be readily recognized by both health workers and mothers. Measles vaccination should be assigned the highest priority early in an emergency situation. Vaccination should *not* be delayed until a health infrastructure has been created, other childhood vaccines are available, or cases of measles appear. Because of overcrowding and increased susceptibility, measles vaccination is required even if most children are already vaccinated; outbreaks have occurred in displaced populations in which measles vaccine coverage exceeded 80%. Vaccination has also been recommended after the beginning of measles outbreaks. All necessary materials and equipment for emergency measles vaccination, including measles vaccine, sterile injection equipment, cold storage and transport boxes, refrigerators, vehicles, and fuel, should be immediately acquired locally or delivered in the very first relief shipments.

Vaccination programs generally should be organized and implemented by experienced personnel who are familiar with vaccine and equipment shipping and handling, cold chain maintenance, and personnel training and supervision.

All children 6 months to 5 years of age should be vaccinated, regardless of evidence of prior vaccination. Children vaccinated before 9 months of age should be revaccinated on reaching this age. The target age range should be extended to 12 years for undernourished or ill children. Because it is rarely sufficient to offer vaccine only at stationary facilities, measles vaccine is often delivered initially by mobile teams that distribute prophylactic vitamin A and other services at the same time. However, these additional duties must not delay the vaccination process.

MALARIA. Malaria (Chapter 92) is a major health problem in most displaced populations. People lacking immunity because they have lived in a less endemic area may be newly exposed during travel through or into areas of higher endemicity. Malaria control programs may be disrupted by civil unrest. In addition, the movement of large numbers of infected people may result in reestablishing malaria in formerly nonendemic areas. Displaced populations often settle near water or are forced to relocate on less desirable land, which may pose a higher risk for malaria infection. Poor housing provides less protection from mosquitoes, and crowding facilitates mosquito-borne transmission. Moreover, the case-fatality rate may be higher in displaced populations because of anemia from poor diets, the lack of prompt medical treatment, and relative immunosuppression due to undernutrition. Malaria is often especially severe in children, and death from *Plasmodium falciparum* infection can occur as a result of cerebral malaria or severe anemia within a few days of the onset of symptoms. Nonetheless, the prognosis with early and appropriate treatment is excellent.

The clinical diagnosis of malaria may be difficult to determine because of the nonspecific nature of the clinical manifestation. Ideally, thick and thin blood smears should be taken from all patients for whom malaria is considered; however, in emergency situations in which health personnel and equipment are limited and there are a large number of patients to care for, use of blood smears to determine the diagnosis for all patients may be impossible. An initial survey of 50 to 100 patients presenting with fever can estimate the relative importance of malaria and determine the predominant species of parasite. If malaria is seasonal, blood film surveys should be repeated at different times of the year. Later in the emergency, if blood film diagnosis is still unavailable for all patients, blood smears should be done on a proportion of patients to monitor the accuracy of clinical diagnosis. Treatment for *Plasmodium malariae, P. vivax,* and *P. ovale* infections is simpler because of the relative lack of drug resistance in these species. In contrast, *P. falciparum* infections are usually more severe and may be resistant to antimalarials. Recent information regarding drug sensitivity in the affected area is extremely valuable. National treatment policies in the country of origin and the country of asylum may not accurately reflect actual drug resistance patterns and should not be automatically followed in displaced populations. For example, in spite of widespread high-level resistance to chloroquine, it continues to be frequently used in many African countries. Although outpatient treatment delivered by community health workers is sufficient for treating most cases of malaria, referral mechanisms should allow emergency hospitalization of patients with severe or complicated illness. Treatment effectiveness can be evaluated by following the clinical course of the patient and by repeating a blood film 7 days after commencing treatment.

Data from epidemiologic surveillance for malaria can be

used to monitor trends in disease incidence, indicate the start of outbreaks, and evaluate the effectiveness of control activities. The typical surveillance case-definition of "unexplained fever" overestimates the incidence of malaria, especially if malaria is not a common cause of morbidity or mortality. Information about the local vector mosquito is necessary to plan malaria prevention programs and may be available from the local or national health authorities or representatives of WHO, other United Nations agencies, or relief organizations. In displaced populations in which malaria is a serious health problem, chemoprophylaxis can prevent placental infection and should be a routine part of prenatal care for pregnant women. Widespread chemoprophylaxis is not recommended. If feasible, mass presumptive treatment of displaced, repatriated, or relocated persons moving to an area free of malaria from an area with malaria transmission may be useful in preventing the reintroduction of malaria.

MENINGOCOCCAL DISEASE. Infection with *Neisseria meningitidis* causes acute bacterial meningitis and septicemia (Chapters 52 and 74). Case-fatality rates for meningococcal meningitis, even in patients receiving prompt and appropriate treatment, may be as high as 5 to 15%. Meningococcal sepsis, which can make up 20% of severe illness during outbreaks of meningococcal infection, can be fatal within hours of the onset of symptoms. The definitive diagnosis of meningococcal meningitis requires performing a lumbar puncture and culture of cerebrospinal fluid (CSF) to identify the species, serogroup, and antibiotic sensitivity pattern of the causative organism. Testing CSF or serum with latex agglutination kits can also identify the meningococcus and its serogroup. In acute humanitarian emergencies in which sufficient laboratory facilities may not be available, the clinical diagnosis of individual cases in the midst of an outbreak of meningococcal disease may depend solely on signs and symptoms or on noting turbidity in CSF.

Because of the severity and rapidity of disease progression, a case of meningococcal meningitis or sepsis should be considered a medical emergency. Although many antibiotics, including penicillin, ampicillin, amoxicillin, and some cephalosporins, can provide effective treatment when given intravenously, maintaining venous access and administering multiple doses may be difficult when resources are scarce. A single 6-mL (3-g) intramuscular dose of chloramphenicol in oil (Tifomycin) is as effective as intravenous antibiotic therapy; however, chloramphenicol in oil is not effective against the other major causes of bacterial meningitis (i.e., *Streptococcus pneumoniae* and *Haemophilus influenzae* type b). Chloramphenicol treatment may need to be repeated if no improvement is seen after 24 hours. Long-acting penicillin and ceftriaxone are also effective when given as single doses. Supportive therapy, including intravenous or nasogastric rehydration, treatment of shock, administration of anticonvulsants and antipyretics, and reduction of intracranial pressure, is often necessary.

Respiratory transmission of meningococcus occurs among crowded displaced populations living in inadequate housing. As a result, such populations are at increased risk for outbreaks of meningococcal disease, and these outbreaks may have higher attack rates. Outbreaks have occured in several recent humanitarian emergencies in displaced populations within or near the "meningitis belt" in sub-Saharan Africa, as well as in other developing countries in Africa and Asia. In this meningitis belt, outbreaks occur in the dry season, and the onset of rains may rapidly halt transmission. An outbreak preparedness plan should be prepared early in the emergency if meningococcal disease is a potential risk. This plan should identify laboratories capable of performing CSF

culture and serogroup identification, specify the possible sources of antibiotics and medical equipment, and describe specific diagnostic and treatment protocols. In addition, knowledge of the area-specific seasonality of meningococcal disease can help predict when outbreaks are most likely.

Safe and effective vaccines against meningococcus serogroups A and C are available. Although routine vaccination in nonepidemic periods is not generally recommended because of the limited duration of protection, particularly in children, mass vaccination can halt meningococcal epidemics within weeks. Epidemiologic surveillance for meningitis is critical to detect outbreaks in order to determine whether vaccination is required. A purely clinical surveillance case definition (Table 19–1) is sensitive but cannot distinguish among various causes of meningitis. Surveillance for meningitis in people 10 to 45 years of age is more specific for meningococcal disease because other causes of meningitis are less common among people in this age group. In situations in which the population size is known and incidence rates of meningitis can be calculated, an incidence rate greater than 15/100,000 population per week for 2 consecutive weeks may predict an epidemic. If the population is not known, as is the case in many emergencies involving displaced persons, a doubling of the number of cases each week for 3 consecutive weeks may indicate an outbreak. When the chosen threshold has been exceeded, an investigation should be done to (1) confirm the diagnosis of meningitis; (2) collect specimens to determine the causative organism, its serogroup, and its antibiotic sensitivity pattern; (3) quantify existing cases by time, person, and place to target subsequent vaccination; and (4) assess local resources for treatment and prevention. Because vaccination programs cannot be implemented until the serogroup has been determined, specimen collection and testing should be a very high priority during this investigation. Initially, the vaccination program should target geographic areas and, if resources are limited, those age groups with the highest attack rates. Often all people <30 years of age, including infants, are vaccinated. Throughout the outbreak, periodic testing of CSF specimens from a small sample of patients can detect rare midepidemic shifts in serogroup. Mass vaccination can be terminated when the incidence rate of meningitis falls to the preepidemic level for at least 2 consecutive weeks. In general, chemoprophylaxis of contacts of persons with meningococcal disease or of population subgroups should be discouraged because such programs divert health resources from more important activities.

Nutrition and Food Supply

Although nutritional deficiencies are common in many developing countries, acute protein-energy undernutrition (Chapter 130) is especially prevalent in emergency situations due to displacement of people from their normal food sources, breakdown in food distribution systems and markets, and use of food as a weapon in civil conflict. Children <5 years of age are often at greatest risk of undernutrition. In these children, undernutrition is often exacerbated by acute communicable diseases, and, in turn, undernutrition increases the susceptibility and severity of many communicable diseases (Chapter 133.1). Enhancing nutritional status can break this cycle of illness. Undernutrition has occurred in other high-risk groups, especially among the elderly and disabled, in recent humanitarian emergencies in Europe and Central Asia. In addition to protein and calories, micronutrients are also essential in the diet (Chapters 131 and 132). Unfortunately, donated relief food is often deficient in micronutrients. Outbreaks of vitamin A deficiency, scurvy, pellagra, and beriberi have occurred in displaced populations dependent on relief rations. Moreover, iron deficiency anemia is highly endemic among women and children in many populations.

The nutritional status of individuals in displaced populations is usually assessed by anthropometric measurement and clinical examination. For children <5 years of age, the ratio of weight-for-height is relatively independent of age and is the best measure of acute undernutrition. For a specific child, that child's weight is compared with the distribution of weights in the NCHS/WHO/CDC reference population for children of the same height. Each child's deviation from the reference population can be described either as the number of standard deviations (SD) from the reference median or as the percentage of the reference median. Use of SD, expressed as Z-scores, has become the preferred method. Moderate undernutrition is defined as being 2 to 3 SD less than the median for the reference population or 70 to 80% of the reference median. Severe undernutrition is defined as being more than 3 SD below the reference median or <90% of the reference median. If age is available, height-for-age can be used as an indicator of chronic undernutrition. Weight-for-age is less useful because it is a composite measure of acute and chronic undernutrition. If weight or height cannot be measured, mid–upper arm circumference (MUAC) can be used as a rough screening procedure to identify children who may be undernourished. Because MUAC changes with age, the cutoff points used to define undernutrition should be adjusted for age or height. Clinical examination should always be a component of nutritional status assessment. Children with pretibial edema from kwashiorkor may have normal weight-for-height but should be classified as severely undernourished. In addition, examination for clinical signs (e.g., night blindness or Bitot's spots for vitamin A deficiency and swollen bleeding gums and swollen painful large joints for scurvy) is often the only way to estimate the prevalence of micronutrient deficiencies in emergency situations.

Adult nutritional status is assessed using the body mass index (BMI), the ratio of a person's weight in kilograms to the square of their height in meters. A normal BMI is 18.5 or greater; a BMI 17.0 to 18.4 indicates mild undernutrition; 16.0 to 16.9 indicates moderate undernutrition; and <16.0 indicates severe undernutrition. Cutoffs for pregnant women are 1 to 2 units higher. As with children, persons with edema not attributable to other causes should be considered extremely undernourished.

Feeding programs for displaced populations generally fall into three categories: (1) general ration distribution to the entire population; (2) supplementary feeding targeted to nutritionally vulnerable groups; and (3) therapeutic feeding for intensive nutritional rehabilitation of severely undernourished individuals. On the basis of a typical age and sex distribution of a population, WHO and the United Nations High Commissioner for Refugees (UNHCR) recommend that the general ration distribution be sufficient to provide at least 2100 kcal/day per person. At least 20% of this energy requirement should be given in the form of edible fats or oils, and the diet should contain at least 46 g of protein. Additional food may be needed if the population has a larger proportion of adults, is in poor nutritional condition, or has extra energy needs due to physical activity or a cold climate. Fresh fruit, vegetables, and other dietary sources of micronutrients can be supplied by encouraging food exchange or purchase in local markets, and some relief foods can be fortified with niacin, iron, and iodine. Targeted micronutrient supplementation can include young children, who should receive vitamin A when they are vaccinated against measles, and pregnant and lactating women, who can be given iron and folate. Treatment with antihelmintics may decrease the rate of iron loss. Because food distribution is often inequita-

ble in displaced populations, measures should be taken to ensure that vulnerable population groups, e.g., children <5 years of age, persons in female-headed households, pregnant or lactating women, the elderly, and the disabled, receive an appropriate share.

Supplementary feeding is meant to treat moderate undernutrition and can consist of "dry" take-home rations or "wet" on-site feeding. In addition to providing extra calories and protein, feeding programs can provide oral micronutrient supplements, antihelmintic treatment, and measles immunization. Target groups for supplemental feeding programs include moderately undernourished children, pregnant and lactating women, the elderly, and people with chronic illness. Supplemental feeding programs targeting undernourished children should be set up when any of the following criteria are met:

1. More than 10% of children 6 to 59 months of age have acute undernutrition.
2. Among children 6 to 59 months of age, 5 to 10% have acute undernutrition and any of the following are present: (a) the general ration is insufficient; or (b) the crude mortality rate is greater than 1/10,000 per day; or (c) there are epidemics of measles or pertussis; or (d) the incidence of respiratory infection or diarrheal disease is high.

Universal supplementary feeding for all children <5 years of age and pregnant or lactating women should be implemented when the prevalence of acute undernutrition exceeds 20%, or if the prevalence of undernutrition is 10 to 19% and any factors listed in 2 a–d are present. Therapeutic feeding should target children with severe undernutrition, including those with edema from kwashiorkor and children referred by health workers for nutritional rehabilitation. Therapeutic feeding is a highly specialized medical treatment and should be implemented by people with appropriate knowledge and experience.

Monitoring the nutritional status and food supply of displaced populations can be done by routine epidemiologic surveillance or periodic surveys. Surveillance can include measuring all children 6 to 59 months of age on admission to the camp, recording the number of children admitted to feeding programs, and monitoring growth in child clinics. Especially early in the emergency, nutritional status is often assessed by weighing and measuring children 6 to 59 months of age or adults in randomly chosen households. Such surveys can also include examination for micronutrient deficiency, assessment of household food supply, questioning about access to food distribution and markets, and other measures of nutritional status and food security. One of the most useful methods for choosing such a sample is by using the cluster sampling methodology initially developed to measure vaccine coverage in rural Africa.

■ AFTER THE ACUTE PHASE OF EMERGENCIES

After the death rate drops to the preemergency level and health services have adequately addressed infectious and nutritional diseases, additional health interventions are required to achieve the goal of delivering comprehensive primary care and adequate preventive services. Interventions in this post–acute phase may include (1) vaccination against the other vaccine-preventable diseases, including diphtheria, pertussis, tetanus, polio, and tuberculosis; (2) prevention of human immunodeficiency virus infection; (3) prevention and treatment of other sexually transmitted diseases; (4) prevention and treatment of tuberculosis; and (5) provision of complete maternal and women's services, including family planning, prenatal care, and obstetric care.

Bibliography

Bloland P, Sexton J, Beach R, et al: Malaria control during mass population movements and natural disasters: Review and recommendations. Atlanta: Centers for Disease Control and Prevention, 1996.

Centers for Disease Control: Famine-affected, refugee, and displaced populations: Recommendations for public health issues. MMWR 41(RR-13), 1992.

Centers for Disease Control: Annex A: Guidelines for collecting, processing, storing, and shipping diagnostic specimens in refugee health-care environments, September 1992. Atlanta: Centers for Disease Control and Prevention, 1992.

World Health Organization: Guidelines for cholera control. Geneva: WHO, 1993.

World Health Organization: The management and prevention of diarrhoea: Practical guidelines, 3rd ed. Geneva: WHO, 1993.

World Health Organization: Control of epidemic meningococcal disease: WHO practical guidelines. Lyon, France: Fondation Marcel Merieux, 1995.

World Health Organization: Guidelines for the control of epidemics due to *Shigella dysenteriae* type 1. WHO/CDR/95.4. Geneva: WHO, 1995.

World Health Organization: The management of acute respiratory infections in children: Practical guidelines for outpatient care. Geneva: WHO, 1995.

World Health Organization: Manual on the management of nutrition in major emergencies. Geneva: WHO, 1996.

20 Environmental Health Hazards in the Tropics

Ellen K. Silbergeld and K.S. Chia

■ GENERAL PRINCIPLES

Understanding environmental and occupational health risks offers to clinicians and public health officials opportunities to reduce the incidence and prevalence of preventable diseases through the identification and management of controllable risks.

Occupational and environmental health are distinguished primarily by the setting in which exposures and intoxication occur and secondarily by the populations at risk. Although in most countries separate regulatory systems and clinical disciplines are involved in the diagnosis, treatment, and prevention of occupational and environmental health risks, in many cases these exposures cross over the physical line between the workplace and the nonoccupational setting, particularly in countries with weak health protection policies. Not only are the same chemical and physical risks often found in both the workplace and the nonoccupational environment, in some cases environmental pollutants arise from industrial releases. Despite this overlap, the outcomes of occupational and environmental exposures in populations may differ for two reasons: First, in many instances, although not always, exposures are more intense in occupational settings, so that the risks of disease are often greater; and second, in the nonoccupational setting the groups exposed can include pregnant women, the elderly, and the infirm, who are not usually employed. These distinctions are not always clear: For example, unregulated cottage industries (such as battery recycling in Jamaica) expose workers and their families equally to chemical risks. In many tropical countries, children are employed in industries such as mining, textiles, and agriculture, where they can be exposed to toxic chemicals (e.g., pesticides, metals, and solvents) that may be particularly hazardous to the developing nervous, reproductive, and immune systems.

Recently, the International Labor Organization (ILO), a bureau of the United Nations, published an encyclopedic reference on toxicology, work practices, clinical medicine, worker protection, policy, and other aspects of occupational and environmental safety and health. This document, which is available on CD-ROM, is a fundamental reference for knowledge and practice related to the identification and prevention of occupational and environmental disease.

Environmental and occupational risks in the tropics may be modified by other conditions affecting human health and the physical chemical context. It has been suggested that health risks in the developing world can be distinguished from those of the developed world (the health transition model) (Table 20–1). In the former, exposures are likely to be acute and excessive, resulting in acute intoxication, including death, whereas in the latter, exposures are likely to be chronic and low-level, resulting in subclinical physiologic changes or increased risks of chronic diseases, e.g., cancer. However, populations are often exposed to both types of risks. More importantly, in many developing countries, conditions in and outside the workplace are significantly different from those in temperate countries, as discussed below. The epidemiologic contexts in which humans encounter these conditions are also important: Undernutrition, chronic infectious disease, high fecundity rates, and heat and dehydration can affect response to chemical and physical stressors. And, in turn, environmental risks may modulate human response to these factors, resulting in complex interactions among health risks. Heat and humidity may reduce workers' willingness to use protective clothing and respirators. Social structures also influence the outcomes of similar exposures in different countries. In many tropical countries, rapid industrialization occurs in small-scale establishments, where health and safety facilities are limited or nonexistent. Workers and employers may be untrained in safe work practices and uninformed as to chemical and physical hazards. Hazardous technologies and banned substances are sometimes transferred from developed countries to tropical countries in development because these industries have difficulty operating in countries with more stringent and effectively enforced occupational and environmental standards (e.g., manufacture of naphthylamine and benzidine dyes, which are known to cause cancer, now takes place largely in Africa and India after bans were instituted in the United States and Western Europe). Hazardous wastes are often exported to developing countries, blatantly for hard currency payments. The economic need for hard currency has also affected agriculture in many tropical countries, which have shifted to producing specialized non-native crops for export that require use of chemical fertilizers, herbicides, and pesticides. Floriculture, the intensive growing of flowers in greenhouses, exposes workers to a range of pesticides; a study in Colombia indicated increased risk of spontaneous abortions, prematurity, and fetal malformations in women greenhouse workers.

■ ENVIRONMENTAL MODIFICATIONS AND HUMAN HEALTH

Environmental risks range from physical alterations of the environment that can affect the distribution of parasite vectors, to the discharge of toxic chemicals and pesticides that can pollute air, water, and foods. Recent concerns have arisen about the impact of human activity on a global scale. According to international panels of scientific experts, there is now good evidence that human activity is causing two types

TABLE 20–1. Distribution of Loss of Useful Years of Life (Disability-Adjusted Life Years)* in Several Regions of the World, by Percentage†

Cause	World	Sub-Sahara	India	Latin America and Caribbean	Developed Countries‡
Communicable disease	45.8	71.3	50.5	42.2	9.7
Cancer	5.8	1.5	40.4	42.8	19.1
Neuropsychiatric disease	6.8	2.8	6.2	4.6	15.0
Cerebrovascular disease	3.2	3.3	6.1	8.0	5.3
Ischemic HD	3.1	0.4	2.8	2.7	10.0
COPD	1.3	0.2	0.6	6.7	1.7
Injuries	11.9	9.3	9.1	15.0	11.9

*DALY, An economic measure of the value of useful years of life lost owing to disability or death adjusted for life expectancy and severity.
†Each number is expressed as percentage of total DALY losses for the region.
‡OECD countries.
Abbreviation: COPD, chronic obstructive pulmonary disease; HD, heart disease.
Source: World Bank: Investing in Health: World Development Report. Oxford, England, Oxford University Press, 1992.

of damage to climate: destruction of the tropospheric ozone layer and warming of the earth's surface. These effects are, respectively, associated with the release of reactive chemicals that break down ozone (chlorofluorocarbons and other agents) and excess release of carbon dioxide from a range of sources, mostly biomass burning, accompanied by depletion of natural carbon sinks such as the world's forest ecosystems. Both these global modifications are likely to affect health in tropical areas before temperate areas. Depletion of the ozone layer increases the amount of UV radiation incident on the earth's surface, and higher levels of UVB have been measured in several areas in Latin America. Although no health consequences have yet been demonstrated to result, increased exposure to UVB is associated with increased risks of blindness and melanoma and decreased immune function. Increases in surface temperature and changes in the patterns of rainfall and drought have been indicated as factors in the change in distribution of vectors of disease and in seasonality of algal growth cycles that are associated with cholera virulence. Increased temperature may also increase desertification in arid areas and result in salt intrusion into groundwater in coastal regions as freshwater is evaporated. Global warming is predicted to cause sea levels to rise, which will inundate low-lying areas, e.g., Bangladesh, and submerge island nations, e.g., the Seychelles and Fiji. All these effects are likely to occur more rapidly and with greater consequences in tropical areas.

Other physical changes of the environment occurring in many tropical areas are resource extraction, deforestation, urbanization, and diversion of water resources for energy generation and agricultural irrigation. Many of these changes are consequent to rapid population growth and shifts of population from rural to urban centers. The rapid growth of what are called megacities (populations in excess of 10 mil-

lion) places great stress on infrastructure to provide a healthful environment: The provision of safe drinking water, fuels for cooking and heat, and the safe management of household wastes and sewage is often difficult to ensure under conditions of explosive population growth and physical expansion. These conditions result in increased burdens of both infectious and chronic disease (Table 20–2). In a study of Brazzaville, Republic of the Congo, increased malaria transmission occurred in those areas where population density increased most rapidly. Not all physical changes that affect human health are due to anthropogenic disturbance of the environment. The sudden releases of carbon monoxide from lakes in Cameroon and the unanticipated volcanic eruption of Mt. Pinatubo in the Philippines caused many deaths.

Environmental exposures occur through contamination of air, water, soils, and food. Knowledge of the fate and pathways of environmental contaminants is important in identifying populations at risk and assessing health implications. The physical chemical nature of the toxic chemical is a major determinant of fate and transport, but pollutants released into one medium may eventually contaminate other media. Volatile chemicals (solvents) and chemicals with high vapor pressure (mercury) are easily transported by air and may travel long distances from points of release to deposition in soils and surface waters. Highly persistent chemicals (DDT, polychlorinated biphenyls) tend to accumulate in environmental compartments, e.g., sediments, and in biota. If these persistent chemicals are also lipophilic (i.e., they are not water soluble and partition into fat), they may be accumulated by organisms and concentrated within a food chain, whereby organisms that are "top predators" (e.g., large piscivorous fish, birds of prey, or humans) end up with the most intensive exposures and highest body burdens. Within organisms, physical chemical parameters determine toxicoki-

TABLE 20–2. Impact of Poor Environments on Health in Tropical Countries

Disease	Environmental Factors	Burden, in Terms of Loss of Useful Life
Tuberculosis	Crowding	46
Diarrhea (cholera, dysentery, typhoid)	Inadequate sanitation, unsafe water	99
Schistosomiasis, typanosomiasis, filariasis, malaria	Sanitation, garbage, vectors breeding near home	8
Respiratory problems	Indoor air pollution, poor ambient air quality	119
Chronic respiratory diseases	Indoor air pollution	41
Cancer of respiratory tract	Air pollution	4

From World Bank: World Development Report, 1993. Oxford, England, Oxford University Press, 1993.

netics, or the uptake and distribution of toxic chemicals. Lipophiles, e.g., the organochlorine insecticides DDT, methoxychlor, and dieldrin, are stored in fat and unless they are metabolized, they are slowly excreted. Lipophilic chemicals also tend to be secreted in breast milk. Bone-seeking elements, e.g., lead and cadmium, are stored in the skeleton over decades.

CHARACTERISTICS OF ENVIRONMENTAL AND OCCUPATIONAL HEALTH PROBLEMS IN THE TROPICS

In tropical countries, traditional industries, small-scale industries, and new industrialization involving highly sophisticated technologies often coexist, as in Thailand, India, Brazil, and Mexico. These activities present different types of risks. Traditional industries, including artisanal activity, can involve the use of materials that are quite hazardous. The traditional ceramicists of West Africa and Latin America use lead-based glazes, which present high hazards to workers and their families. Small-scale or cottage industries can create particular problems when hazardous activities are conducted in a household setting. Battery recycling (involving the breaking of storage batteries and crude smelting to recover lead) can be done in simple backyard hearths; in Jamaica there have been episodes of serious lead intoxication of whole families. In Brazil, crude refining of gold/mercury amalgams is sometimes done in kitchens, using propane heat sources, resulting in high immediate mercury exposures and local area contamination (Fig. 20–1).

Rapid industrialization and the global migration of industry from the developed to the developing world have also changed the context of occupational and environmental health. Some of these developments have had tragic consequences, as in the explosion of the Union Carbide facility at Bhopal, India, where the immediate and delayed rates of death and disease were substantially increased because housing was built close to the factory. Chemical exposures arise from the production, use, and disposal of products, including releases of wastes during production. Waste disposal itself can cause environmental pollution, especially when management practices are poorly suited to the toxic constituents of the waste stream.

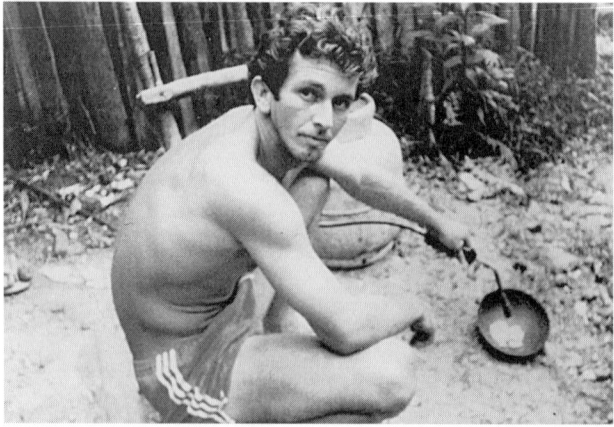

Figure 20–1. Crude refining of gold-mercury amalgams in Amazonian Brazil. This process results in acute exposures to inorganic mercury and releases of mercury to the environment. (Courtesy of Dr. D. Cleary.)

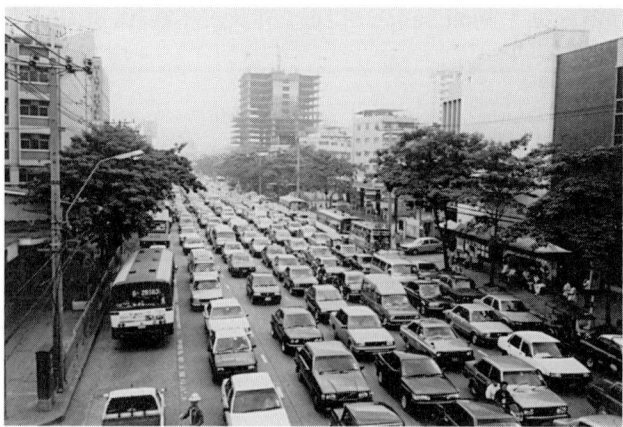

Figure 20–2. Traffic in Bangkok, Thailand. Rapid social change and urban growth have brought too many cars for available roadways, and air pollution (particulates, sulfur oxides, nitric oxides, ozone, lead, and polycyclic aromatic hydrocarbons) is dangerously high.

MAJOR PROBLEMS IN ENVIRONMENTAL AND OCCUPATIONAL HEALTH

Air Pollution

Air pollution is a major environmental health problem in most countries. Air quality is affected by particles and by chemicals released in the air by stationary facilities, including factories and incinerators; mobile sources, e.g., cars and trucks; and more generalized activities, e.g., forest burning, methane emissions from agriculture, and dusts from aridified areas. In many tropical countries, rapid urbanization has resulted in substantial increases in toxic air pollution in cities, including carbon monoxide, small particulates, ozone, oxides of nitrogen and sulfur, and incompletely combusted products of gasoline fuels (polycyclic aromatic hydrocarbons, benzene, and solvents). Traffic in Bangkok is among the most intense in the world, causing major problems from airborne lead from gasoline, particulates, sulfur oxides, and polycyclic aromatic hydrocarbons (Fig. 20–2). Levels of some of these pollutants in the megacities of the tropics and subtropics can be very high, and exposed populations are adversely affected in terms of both morbidity and mortality.

The health effects of these pollutants include exacerbation of asthma, increased morbidity and mortality from cardiovascular disease, and lung cancer. Tropical climate can also exacerbate urban air pollution by increasing the rate of formation of photochemical oxidant smog because of higher solar energy inputs. In addition, the continued use of certain energy sources, e.g., leaded gasoline for transportation and biomass fuels for cooking, add to the exposures of urban residents in many tropical countries. It has been estimated that exposure to small particulates in homes with poorly ventilated biomass stoves can be 60 to 100 times higher than ambient air levels in industrialized cities.

Waste Disposal

Much of the burden of disease and premature death in tropical countries is associated with unsafe drinking water and poor sanitation. A common element in many tropical countries is the lack of a functional infrastructure to manage waste disposal in order to prevent contamination of water and residential areas by biologic and industrial wastes. Sometimes these risks coincide. The mismanagement of occupational chemicals and processes in tanneries in Kanpur, India, results in releases of tannery wastes, containing acids, dyes, and biologic wastes, throughout the neighboring community. In peninsular Malaysia, the Juru River has been polluted by both untreated domestic sewage and industrial discharges. The main industrial sources for the Juru River are complex: electroplating and microelectronics fabrication (metals, solvents); tanneries (acids and dyes, including carcinogens, e.g., formamides and chromates, acids); textile mills (carcinogenic dyes); food processing (biologic wastes and pesticides); and chloralkali production (mercury). Specialized waste treatment facilities are needed to handle these materials, but these are rarely available in developing countries. Some of these wastes can poison the biologic treatment processes of sanitary wastewater treatment plants.

Hazardous wastes also come into tropical countries from developed nations, as the costs of disposal in the latter have increased as the result of stringent regulation. For example, 3800 metric tons of chemical wastes were dumped by Italian ships in the port of Koko on the Niger River in 1990. Economic pressures often drive this trade: Guinea-Bissau and Benin are two African countries that have sought contracts to receive toxic wastes from Europe and the United States in return for hard currency.

Lead Poisoning

Lead is a common environmental and occupational hazard in many countries as well as a leading cause of disease in children and workers throughout the world. Lead exposure causes infertility in men, miscarriage, renal failure, hypertension, anemia, and toxicity to the central and peripheral nervous systems. In tropical countries, both new industrial and traditional cultural practices may result in lead exposures that cross over from the workplace to the nonoccupational environment. The use of lead in gasoline results in substantial increases in lead in ambient air, which results in intoxication of populations in heavily trafficked areas. Lead also enters the environment from uncontrolled industrial sources, from battery recycling operations, and from the use of lead arsenicals as pesticides. Cottage industries, e.g., brass making in India and battery recycling in the Caribbean, expose workers and their families to high levels of lead. Home-based secondary lead smelting is a common sight in many developing countries. Children and women are often seen collecting scrap lead, especially from discarded car batteries. The lead plates are removed and smelted in open pots and pans, often in a kitchen with poor ventilation. In rapidly industrializing countries, migrant workers engage in secondary lead smelting at the end of the working day to supplement their income. Fortunately, most smelting takes place in open spaces but there are occasions when this is done indoors, especially during bad weather. In addition, many countries still permit the use of lead for plumbing, which can result in contamination of drinking water. Some cultures use lead-based glazes for ceramics (Mexico and West Africa) and lead-based products as traditional cosmetics and medicines (azarcon in Mexico, bint al zahab in Yemen, kohl in India). Cooking and storing food in lead-glazed ceramic vessels is a major risk for lead exposure.

Lack of adequate controls on primary and secondary lead smelters and industries, e.g., battery manufacturing, also results in environmental contamination. The exposure of children, who are especially sensitive to lead toxicity, may result in impaired intelligence and behavioral disorders. Rates of lead poisoning in tropical countries are not known, but available data indicate high rates of excess exposure, particularly in children (Table 20–3).

A case of lead poisoning in Singapore illustrates the problems in identifying and preventing exposures. A young Malay worker complained of lethargy and was found to be clinically anemic. He had been working as a production operator in a factory manufacturing polyvinyl chloride (PCV) stabilizers for the past 3 years. There are several types of PVC stabilizers, the most common being inorganic lead. The work process begins with the smelting of lead ingots and oxidation of the metal into lead oxide (litharge). The litharge is then combined with sulphuric acid into lead sulphate or with stearic acid into lead stearate. These salts are then packed or mixed before packing. Workers are exposed to lead fumes at the smelting process and lead dust at the packing and mixing area. A visit to the workplace found that the workers often failed to use respiratory protectors and gloves. Although smoking was not permitted in the production area, there was a canteen where workers could smoke and have their meals. The Malays often prefer to eat food with their bare hands rather than using forks, spoons, or chopsticks. Although they wash their hands before consuming food, it is difficult to remove fine lead oxide particles from the hands by cursory washing. Furthermore, significant amounts of lead dust are trapped under fingernails. Lead overexposure was primarily due to poor work practices. The worker was removed from further exposure and advised to stop work in the factory. Two years later, his hemoglobin increased to 12 g/100 mL, and his blood level of lead was down to 15 μg/dL.

Mercury

Mercury is another toxic metal that enters the environment from a range of sources, both local and long distance. Mercury affects intrauterine development of the nervous system, causing profound mental retardation and motor disorders at

TABLE 20–3. Blood Lead Levels in Different Populations in the Americas

Country	Population	n	Age (yr)	Average Blood Lead	Percent >10 μg/dL*
Brazil	Adults, urban	156	15–49	11.8	45
	Children, urban/industrial	199	4–5	9.6	30
Ecuador	Children, urban	64	7	29.8	100
	Pregnant women, urban	83	—	18.4	60
Mexico	Children, urban	200	<5	9.0	28
	Adults, urban	3,309	15–45	10.6	42
Nicaragua	Children, near industry	50	1–6	11.5	45
Trinidad	Mothers, urban	94	—	4.8	2
Tobago	Children near battery recycling facility	20	<2	72	100

*10 μg/dL is the advisory level set by US CDC and WHO for intervention to prevent toxicity.
Data from IOM-NIPH (1996).

high doses. In adults, mercury causes damage to liver, kidney, skin, and the nervous system. Mercury also impairs immune response and may reduce host resistance to pathogens. Mercury can enter the environment from industrial activities, particularly chloralkali production, in which mercury is used as a catalyst, and in agriculture, in which phenylmercurials are used as fumigants. Deforestation of some tropical ecosystems, as in Amazonia and Papua New Guinea, during mining and clearing for development, can result in release of mercury from soils. A particularly intensive local source of mercury comes from its use in extracting gold from sediments (artisanal mining). Amalgamation in artisanal mining occurs in many tropical countries, and tons of mercury are released each year to rivers and streams from gold mining. In Zimbabwe, for example, it was recently estimated by the United Nations that over 100,000 people are engaged in these mining activities; in Brazil, another country with a high level of artisanal mining, it was estimated in 1990 that about 100 metric tons of mercury were released each year in Amazonia. Workers are exposed directly by handling mercury (which vaporizes at ambient temperature), by forming the amalgam, and during crude refining. But the hazards of mercury from this source are not limited to settings where gold mining is taking place. In Alta Floresta, Brazil, refining of gold amalgams is so intensive that increased levels of mercury in ambient air have been detected.

The tropical environment may enhance the risks of mercury in two ways: First, elevated ambient temperatures increase the rate at which mercury is vaporized and then transported; second, tropical aquatic ecosystems may convert metallic or inorganic mercury into the more toxic methylated form more rapidly than occurs in temperate zones. In aquatic ecosystems, methylated mercury is absorbed and retained by fish, and as larger fish consumer smaller fish, levels of mercury increase exponentially. In some tropical ecosystems, the population structure of fish is complex, and high levels of mercury may be achieved, comparable to those found in large pelagic piscivorous fish of the oceans (e.g., swordfish) but rarely found in landlocked ecosystems in temperate zones. Nonmining communities may be exposed to highly toxic methyl mercury residues in fish, sometimes at considerable distance and long after releases from industry or mining.

Pesticides

Pesticide poisonings are a leading cause of intoxication and death in many tropical countries, resulting from both occupational and environmental exposures. Pesticides are substances utilized to control unwanted organisms that may interfere with agriculture or act as reservoirs or vectors of infectious disease, including fungi, plants, insects, rodents, and other animals. Pesticides range from natural compounds and extracts, e.g., the pyrethroids and arsenicals, to highly complex synthetic organic compounds, e.g., the organophosphates and halogenated hydrocarbon insecticides. Pesticides present risks of both acute and chronic toxicity. Some pesticides have a high acute toxicity (usually to reproductive organs or the nervous system) but are relatively nonpersistent; others have low acute toxicity but are carcinogenic in animals and are poorly metabolized or broken down and thus accumulate within organisms, including humans, and the environment. While newer pesticides have been developed with selective toxicity and newer methods of application that can reduce unintended exposures, it is generally the case that pesticides are toxic to a broad range of organisms, including humans. Many of the halogenated hydrocarbon insecticides cause cancer and hepatotoxicity in laboratory animals. Occupational exposures to pesticides occur in the

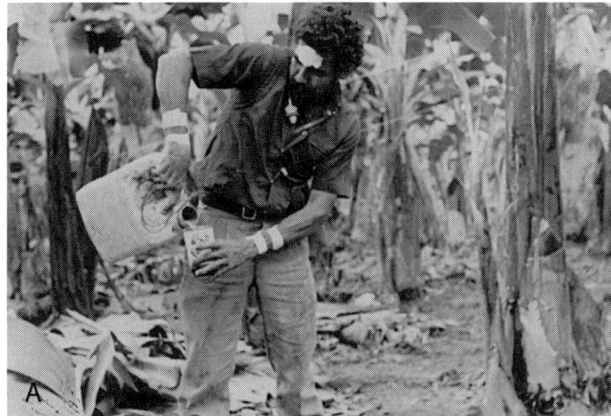
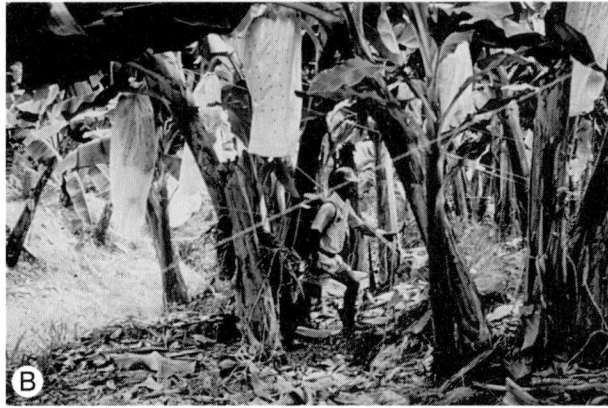

***Figure* 20–3.** Pesticide application in Costa Rica. Inadequate protection for workers during *(A)* mixing and *(B)* spraying results in frequent poisonings (Courtesy of Dr. H. Kromhout.)

manufacture, formulation, mixing, and application; nonoccupational exposures result from uncontrolled application, runoff into surface- and groundwater, improper reuse of pesticide containers, and contamination of food. Conditions of pesticide use in the tropics are often unsafe for both workers and others nearby (Fig. 20–3). Heat and humidity reduce the acceptability of protective gear, such as respirators and impermeable suits.

Contamination of food results from improper application and harvest of crops before chemicals dissipate. This has been responsible for thousands of cases of poisoning in Africa, South America, and Asia. The incidence of acute pesticide poisonings from occupational and nonoccupational exposures (including suicides) is unknown but is estimated in the millions of cases per year (Table 20–4). These figures suggest that preventable intoxications are a significant portion of the health problems experienced by tropical populations.

Although 80% of pesticide use is in the developed countries, over 90% of pesticide-caused deaths occur in developing countries. There are many reasons for this situation: First, conditions of pesticide use are often different in tropical regions, where, because of the types of crops grown for export and the complex ecology of pests, pesticides may be applied two to four times each month; second, there is a lack of information, infrastructure, and legal authority to control conditions of pesticide manufacture, use, and disposal; third, young children are often involved in agricultural production; fourth, pesticides are a frequently used method of suicide; and fifth, many pesticides banned or restricted in the developed nations are still used extensively (many of these pesti-

TABLE 20–4. Acute Pesticide Poisoning in Some African Countries, 1989

Country	Population (millions), 1989	% Labor Force in Agriculture	Annual Incidence of Poisoning
Sudan	24	80	384,000
Tanzania	23	85	368,000
Kenya	22	80	350,000
Uganda	17	80	272,000
Mozambique	15	70	240,000
Zimbabwe	10	80	160,000
Ivory Coast	10	80	160,000
Malawi	8	85	128,000

From Jeyaratnam J (ed): Occupational Health in Developing Countries. New York, Oxford University Press, 1992.

cides originate in the United States; in 1994, over 9 million pounds of unregistered, banned, suspended, or discontinued pesticides were exported from the United States).

Asbestos

Asbestos is a class of mineral fibers that differ slightly in chemical form and physical structure. Inhaled asbestos causes mesothelioma, a cancer of the pleural cavity, and debilitating and often fatal respiratory disease (asbestosis). For years, asbestos has been used because of its properties as an insulator, flame retardant, and easily workable material. In the United States, Canada, and the European Union, both occupational and environmental health authorities have concluded that no exposure to asbestos is safe, and the use of asbestos has been banned or severely restricted. Extensive precautions are required for use and removal of asbestos. However, in developing countries its use continues, often promoted by producing countries where asbestos use is restricted. Occupational exposures are gross, without adequate worker protection. At the same time, even more disturbing uses of asbestos involve housing and cooking, where discards of asbestos are used by communities to construct housing and there is little if any management of friable wastes (Fig. 20–4). Attempts to impose recommendations on use of asbestos in developing countries have been highly controversial. Based on experience in the United States and England, these failures to contain asbestos use and disposal can be expected to result in a significant burden of disease and premature death in countries such as India and Mexico.

▪ METHODS IN OCCUPATIONAL AND ENVIRONMENTAL MEDICINE

The identification, treatment, and prevention of disease from environmental and occupational exposures depend upon careful case histories and knowledge of specific situations in which exposures can occur. Very few chemicals cause "signature" diseases such that etiology can be deduced without ascertaining exposure. Information on exposure must be obtained by case history, combined with knowledge of industrial processes or the environmental context of an individual or group. In some instances, biologic monitoring can confirm reports or other information indicating an exposure. In the occupational context, such monitoring is often useful when exposures are likely to be recent or continuing. In the environmental context, where exposures may be highly variable, monitoring may be less informative and descriptive

information on residence, diet, and other factors is necessary. Sampling of environmental media—air, water, or soils—may be required to determine levels and likelihood of exposures.

Workplace factors can be a direct cause of disease, or they may combine with other risk factors in multifactorial causation of diseases. The term *work-related diseases* was recommended by a WHO Expert Committee to describe diseases in which workplace factors play a contributory role in causation. Occupational diseases are at one end of the spectrum when the relationship to specific workplace causative factors is well established. At the other end of the spectrum are general diseases, in which the relationship with workplace factors is weak, inconsistent, and unclear. Work-related diseases are those in which workplace factors are possibly causal, but the strength and magnitude of their associations vary. It may be difficult to quantify the role of workplace factors in work-related diseases, since the strength of the workplace factors can vary in time and place and the importance of these factors may be modified by other risk factors such as smoking, diet, and genetic differences. Epidemiologic studies in work-related diseases may not clearly identify a role for occupational factors. In the clinical situation, the decision must often be based on subjective judgment derived from knowledge of the degree of exposure and the known health effects of the hazard. Confirmation can be made when the patient improves upon removal from the hazard. However, in the case of chronic diseases, e.g., cancer, this may not be observable.

Another issue concerning the identification of work-related diseases involves patients with coexisting nonoccupational risk factors. For example, a patient with poorly controlled

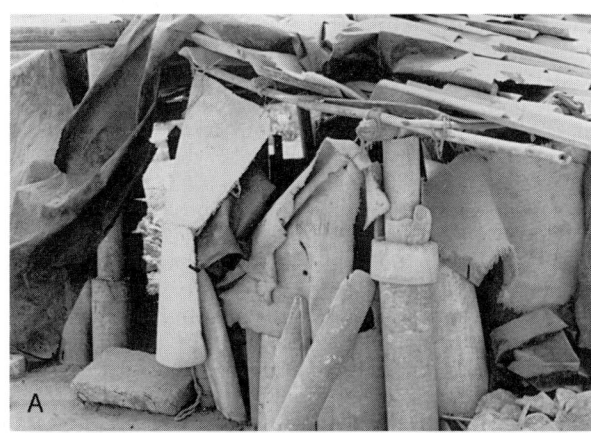

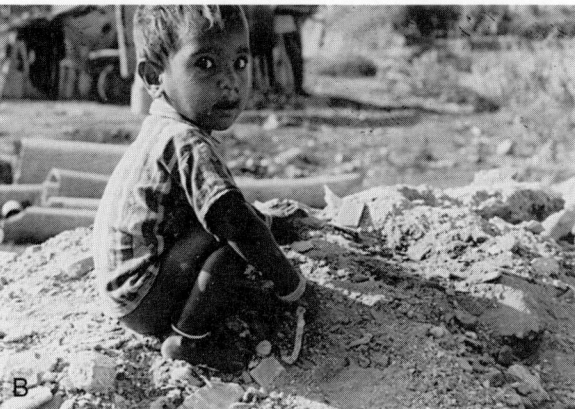

Figure 20–4. Asbestos problems in the developing world. Asbestos discards used for (A) housing and (B) children's play in India (Courtesy of Dr. B. Castleman.)

diabetes mellitus may be employed in a job with exposure to a nephrotoxic chemical, e.g., lead or cadmium. The functional reserve capacity of the kidneys may have already been compromised by diabetes. Exposure to the nephrotoxin may further impair the kidney, contributing to earlier onset of disease.

Work History

Bernardino Ramazzini, the Father of Occupational Medicine, stated ". . . to the questions recommended by Hippocrates, (the doctor) should add one more—What is your occupation?" He recognized that diagnosis may be incorrect and treatment inadequate if the occupation is ignored. In today's context, Ramazzini's exhortation is incomplete. Most patients, when asked for their occupation, will give a job title that is uninformative as to the type and degree of exposure to workplace hazards. For example, a common title is "production operator." A production operator in a car battery plant has very different exposure from a similar worker in an electronics factory. A full occupational history includes a careful description of the nature of work in all previous occupations. Most occupational diseases have long patent periods, so that information on the present occupation is often insufficient.

It can be difficult for the doctor to understand the working conditions described by the patient without visiting the workplace. It is not possible to manage ill health among workers without some firsthand experience of the workplace. Undercounting of occupational disease is an international problem. For example, a worker was diagnosed with adult-onset asthma without consideration of his occupational history. Only 9 years after diagnosis was an attempt made to evaluate the contribution of the work environment. He was subsequently transferred to another section of the factory; within 1 year his asthma improved dramatically, and after 2 years he had no further asthmatic attacks.

In clinical practice, it is therefore important to identify occupational or environmental factors when disease of this type is suspected. Attempts have been made to compile lists of so-called sentinel diseases, or conditions that suggest that exposure to an occupational or environmental risk has occurred (Table 20–5). Some diseases are so rare that a single case can provoke suspicion; e.g., if a worker is diagnosed with mesothelioma, the occupational history is then taken retrospectively to determine past exposure to asbestos. Patterns of disease can suggest an environmental cause; e.g., grain releases from storage silos in Barcelona were found to be the cause of episodic asthma, based on timing and location. It is also crucial to evaluate the role of occupational factors in a suspected work-related disease, in that a worker who is an asthmatic may have several different triggering factors. Some of these are in the home environment and others in the workplace. For effective management of these asthmatic attacks, all related factors have to be identified and controlled.

Registries and Surveillance

The systematic collection of information on individuals or cohorts into registries can provide health authorities with valuable information to follow the consequences of exposure and evaluate the likelihood of exposures in similar settings. In many countries, registries of workers are used to follow cohorts exposed to well-characterized toxic chemicals, e.g., asbestos, benzidine dyes, and heavy metals. Special episodes of exposure, e.g., the contamination of cooking oil by PCBs in Taiwan, have been followed up by surveillance programs to determine long-term consequences of exposure. Medical surveillance programs can also detect sentinel events or diseases that indicate excessive exposure to chemicals (Table 20–5). The sentinel approach is useful because it can alert health authorities to the need to identify and control risk factors even without comprehensive health surveillance data on a population. A classic example is the detection of an unusual incidence of small cell carcinoma of the lung, which alerted public health officials to the hazards of bischloromethyl ether in a chemical factory in the United States. However, in the absence of sentinel signs or detection systems, it can be difficult to determine the cause of such outbreaks, as has been the case in "toxic oil syndrome" in Spain.

Surveillance of workers' health in developing countries should not be limited to occupational diseases but should also be used for work-related as well as general diseases of the working population. This is because the main health problems among workers in some countries in Africa and Asia may involve the interaction of occupational problems with other diseases, e.g., infectious diseases. Collecting all relevant information is useful for the planning and allocation of health care resources.

In addition, a registry of factories and work processes, as opposed to a disease registry, can be useful. This registry obtains information from all factories, including work processes and materials used, that is updated periodically when new work processes or materials are introduced. Such registration is sometimes required by national legislation, but it is important to enforce the legislation in a comprehensive manner. For small-scale industries, such registration is often bypassed. Simple field surveys and assessments of the types of industry and the state of working conditions can provide basic information.

■ MANAGEMENT AND PREVENTION OF DISEASES ASSOCIATED WITH ENVIRONMENTAL OR OCCUPATIONAL RISKS

The management of environmental and occupational disease depends upon careful history taking and information on the likely risks present in specific occupations and environments. In occupational disease, information must often be available on the details of work practices and processes in order to discern exposures associated with specific jobs and in specific locations within industries. Management of the affected person almost always first requires reduction of exposure through removal from the occupational or environmental setting, or effective controls upon the source in the workplace or general environment. Treatment of specific disabilities or systemic dysfunction may also be needed, even in the absence of etiologic diagnosis. For some chemical toxicants, specific therapies are available, e.g., chelation treatment for heavy metal poisoning. However, in many instances, it is essential to administer these agents only after ongoing exposures are controlled, since these drugs can increase absorption of metals from the GI tract. Prophylaxis for chemical toxicants is not generally available; prevention of excess exposure is the most appropriate method.

Prevention of environmental and occupational disease requires control of exposures to levels that do not adversely affect health. Prevention demands knowledge of the hazards of toxic agents and other stressors, information on sources and pathways of exposure, and the sociolegal infrastructure that enables public health officials and others to ensure that exposures do not exceed acceptable levels. In principle, all environmental and occupational diseases can be prevented, but in most instances failure to accurately evaluate the risks

TABLE 20–5. Abbreviated List of Sentinel Health Events (Occupational)—Occupationally Related Preventable Diseases, Disability, and Untimely Death

Condition	Industry/Occupation	Agent
Pulmonary tuberculosis	Physicians, medical personnel	*Mycobacterium tuberculosis*
Plague, tularemia, anthrax, rabies, and other infections	Farmers, ranchers, hunters, veterinarians, laboratory workers	Various infectious agents
Rubella	Medical personnel, intensive care personnel	Rubella virus
Hepatitis	Daycare center staff, orphanage staff, medical personnel	Hepatitis A virus, hepatitis B virus
Ornithosis	Bird breeders, pet shop staff, poultry producers, veterinarians, zoo employees	*Chlamydia psittaci*
Malignant neoplasm of nasal cavities	Woodworkers, cabinet, furniture makers	Hardwood dust
	Radium chemists and processors	Radium
	Nickel smelting and refining	Nickel
Malignant neoplasm of larynx	Asbestos industries and users	Asbestos
Malignant neoplasm of trachea, bronchus, and lung	Asbestos industries and users	Asbestos
	Topside coke oven workers	Coke oven emissions
	Uranium and fluorspar miners	Radon daughters
	Smelters, processors, users	Chromates, nickel, arsenic
	Mustard gas formulators	Mustard gas
	Ion exchange resin makers, chemists	Bis(chloromethyl)ether
Mesothelioma	Asbestos industries and users	Asbestos
Malignant neoplasm of bone	Radium chemists and processors	Radium
Malignant neoplasm of scrotum	Automatic lathe operators, metal workers	Mineral/cutting oils
	Coke oven workers, petroleum refiners	Soots and tars
Malignant neoplasm of bladder	Rubber and dye workers	Benzidine, naphthylamine, auramine, 4-nitrophenyl
Malignant neoplasm of kidney	Coke oven workers	Coke oven emissions
Acute lymphoid leukemia	Radiologists, rubber industry	Ionizing radiation
Acute myeloid leukemia	Occupations with exposure to benzene	Benzene
	Radiologists	Ionizing radiation
Erythroleukemia	Occupations with exposure to benzene	Benzene
Nonautoimmune hemolytic anemia	Whitewashing and leather industry	Copper sulfate
	Electrolytic processes, smelting	Arsine
	Plastics industry	Trimellitic anhydride
Aplastic anemia	Explosives manufacture	TNT*
	Radiologists, radium, chemists	Ionizing radiation
Agranulocytosis or neutropenia	Explosives and pesticide industries	Phosphorus
	Pesticides, pigments, pharmaceuticals	Inorganic arsenic
Toxic encephalitis	Battery, smelter, and foundry workers	Lead
Parkinson's disease (secondary)	Manganese processing, battery makers, welders	Manganese
Inflammatory and toxic neuropathy	Pesticides, pigments, pharmaceuticals	Arsenic and arsenic compounds
	Furniture refinishers, degreasing operations	Hexane
	Plastics, rayon industries	Methyl butyl ketone, copper disulfide, other solvents
	Explosives industry	TNT*
	Battery, smelter, and foundry workers	Lead
	Dentists, chloralkali plants, battery makers	Mercury
	Plastics industry, paper manufacturing	Acrylamide
	Microwave and radar technicians	Microwaves
	Radiologists	Ionizing radiation
	Blacksmiths, glass blowers, bakers	Infrared radiation
	Moth repellent formulators, fumigators	Naphthalene
Noise effects on inner ear	Many industries	Excessive noise
Raynaud's phenomenon	Lumberjacks, chain sawyers, grinders	Whole body, segmental vibration
	Vinyl chloride polymerization industry	Vinyl chloride monomer
Extrinsic asthma	Jewelry, alloy, and catalyst makers	Platinum
	Polyurethane, adhesive, paint workers	Isocyanates
	Plastic, dye, insecticide makers	Phthalic anhydride
	Foam workers, latex makers, biologists	Formaldehyde
	Bakers	Flour
	Woodworkers, furniture makers	Red cedar and other wood dust
Pneumoconiosis of coal workers	Coal miners	Coal dust
Asbestosis	Asbestos industries and utilizers	Asbestos
Silicosis	Quarrymen, sandblasters, silica processors, mining, ceramic industries, and foundries	Silica
Talcosis	Talc processors	Talc
Chronic beryllium disease of the lung	Beryllium alloy workers, ceramic and cathode ray tube makers, nuclear reactor workers	Beryllium
Byssinosis	Cotton industry workers	Cotton, flax, hemp, and cotton-synthetic dusts
Acute bronchitis, pneumonitis, and pulmonary edema due to fumes and vapors	Alkali and bleach industries	Chlorine
	Silo fillers, arc welders	Nitrogen oxides
	Paper, refrigeration, oil industries	Sulfur dioxide
	Plastics industry	Trimellitic anhydride
Toxic hepatitis	Solvent users, dry cleaners, plastics industry	Carbon tetrachloride, chloroform, trichloroethylene
	Explosives and dye industries	Phosphorus, TNT*
	Fumigators, fire extinguisher formulators	Ethylene dibromide
Acute or chronic renal failure	Battery makers, plumbers, solderers	Inorganic lead
	Electrolytic processes, smelting	Arsine
	Battery makers, jewelers, dentists	Inorganic mercury
	Fire extinguisher makers	Carbon tetrachloride
	Antifreeze manufacturers	Ethylene glycol
Male infertility	Formulators and applicators	Dibromochloropropane
Contact and allergic dermatitis	Leather tanning, poultry dressing plants, packing, adhesives and sealant industry, boat building and repair	Irritants (e.g., cutting fish oils, solvents, acids, alkalis, allergens)

*TNT indicates 2,4,6-trinitrotoluene.

of chemicals and other exposures has interfered with our ability to accomplish these goals. Since many exposures are associated with industrial, agricultural, and other activities that have significant social and economic value, the costs of reducing risks is usually balanced by considerations of these benefits within the sociopolitical calculus of each society.

Infrastructure for Environmental and Occupational Health

The management of environmental and occupational health risks requires a specific set of policies directed at protecting specific resources, e.g., air or drinking water, and at regulating specific activities, e.g., the use of pesticides or waste discharges. In addition, implementation of these policies and mandates requires a high degree of technical expertise and resources to monitor compliance with laws and regulations, in addition to the availability of technology to support pollution control or source reduction. Population monitoring and health surveillance are also important parts of environmental health programs. There is a troubling discrepancy between the availability of resources for the study and management of environmental risks to health and the intensity of those risks. In the developing world, few resources are available for either research or prevention. In addition, the legal and political infrastructure to identify and manage these risks is often nonexistent. Thus, even programs such as the PIC (prior informed consent) convention proposed by the United Nations Commission on Environment and Development (UNCED) cannot contribute much to national programs unless an informed and empowered authority exists to receive and utilize information on toxic chemicals being imported into or used in developing countries. Conventions have been promulgated to prevent transfer of risks from the developed to the developing world (e.g., the Basel Convention, which prohibits shipments of hazardous wastes without adequate assurance as to knowledge and capacity in the receiving country). Some international resources are available to provide limited support, usually in the form of information sharing and limited technical assistance: the agencies of the World Health Organization (International Labor Organization, International Programme on Chemical Safety, International Registry of Potentially Toxic Substances), United Nations Environment Programme, Food and Agriculture Organization, the international development banks and donor organizations (World Bank, International Bank for Reconstruction and Development, UNIDO, UNICEF), and some nongovernment organizations (World Wildlife Fund, Pesticide Action Network). Recently, some national aid agencies in the United States, Canada, and the European Community have focused on environmental health as an area for assistance—sometimes on specific environmental risks, such as reducing lead exposures due to the use of lead in gasoline, and sometimes in terms of capacity building. New developments in international trade (the World Trade Organization) are generating pressures for greater harmonization among national risk assessment procedures and practices.

Bibliography

Castleman B: Asbestos: Medical and Legal Aspects. New Jersey, Aspen Law and Business, 1996.
Chia KS, Jeyaratnam J, Lee J, et al: Lead induced nephropathy: Relationship between various biological exposure indices and early markers of tubular dysfunction. Am J Ind Med 27:883, 1995.
Chia SE, Chia KS, Jeyaratnam J: Baker's asthma: A case report. Ann Acad Med Singapore 19:407, 1990.
Chia SE, Chia KS, Jeyaratnam J: Ethnic differences in blood lead concentration among workers in a battery manufacturing factory. Ann Acad Med Singapore 20:758, 1991.
Chivian E, McCally M, Hu H, Haines A: Critical Condition: Human Health and the Environment. Boston, MIT Press, 1993.
Cleary D: Anatomy of the Amazon Gold Rush. London, Macmillan, 1990.
Commission on Health Research for Development (CHRD): Health Research: Essential Link to Equity in Development. Oxford, Oxford University Press, 1990.
Foundation for Advancements in Science and Education (FASE): Exporting Risk: Pesticide Exports from US Ports, 1992–1994. Los Angeles, FASE.
Giannasi BEF, Thebaud-Mony A: Occupational exposures to asbestos in Brazil. Int J Occup Med Environ Health 3:150, 1997.
Goettsch W, Garasen J, Deijns A, et al: UV-B exposure impairs resistance to infection by *Trichinella spiralis*. Environ Health Perspect 102:298, 1994.
Howson CP, Hernandez Avila M, Rall DP: Lead in the Americas. Washington, DC, Institute of Medicine, 1996.
International Labour Organization Encyclopedia of Occupational Health and Safety (4 volumes), 2nd ed. Geneva, ILO (BT), 1997.
Jeyaratnam J (ed): Occupational Health in Developing Countries. New York, Oxford University Press, 1992.
Landrigan PJ, Baker D: The recognition and control of occupational disease. JAMA 266:676, 1991.
Miguel AH, et al: Characterization of indoor air quality in the cities of Sao Paulo and Rio de Janeiro, Brazil. Environ Sci Technol 29:338, 1995.
Ory FG, Rahman FV, Shukla A, et al: Industrial counseling: Linking occupational and environmental health in tanneries of Kanpur, India. Int J Occup Med Environ Health 2:311, 1996.
Patz JA, Epstein PR, Burke TA, Balbus JM: Global climate change and emerging infectious disease. JAMA 275:217, 1996.
Restrepo M, Munoz N, Day NE, et al: Prevalence of adverse reproductive outcomes in a population occupationally exposed to pesticides in Colombia. Scand J Work Environ Health 16:232, 1990.
Rutstein DD, Mullan RJ, Fazier TM, et al: Sentinel health effects (occupational): A basis for physician recognition and public health surveillance. Am J Public Health 73:1054, 1983.
Trape JF, Zoulani A: Malaria and urbanization in Central Africa: The example of Brazzaville. Trans R Soc Trop Med Hyg 81(Suppl 2):19, 1987.
van Wendel de Joode BN, de Graaf IAM, Wesseling C, Kromhout H: Paraquat exposure of knapsack spray operators on banana plantations in Costa Rica. Int J Occup Med Environ Health 2:294, 1996.
White JC (ed): Global Atmospheric Change and Public Health. New York, Elsevier, 1990.
World Bank: World Development Report 1993. Oxford, Oxford University Press, 1993.
World Health Organization: Identification and Control of Work-Related Diseases. WHO Technical Report Series No. 714. Geneva, WHO, 1985.
World Health Organization: Epidemiology of Work-Related Diseases and Accidents. WHO Technical Report Series No. 777. Geneva, WHO, 1989.

21 Imaging in the Tropics and the Imaging of Tropical Diseases

Philip E. S. Palmer

Although in some places in the tropics and lesser developed countries there are trained radiologists and radiographers using excellent equipment, the facilities for any sort of imaging are unsatisfactory in many small tropical hospitals. The World Health Organization (WHO) estimates that clinical imaging is unavailable to about two thirds of the world's population. Imaging equipment is expensive to purchase and maintain; films and chemicals as well as contrast drugs and darkroom equipment are costly; and the supplies of these necessities are often inadequate, intermittent, and sometimes incorrectly chosen. Specialist radiologists, if there are any in the country, are in the major cities, and experienced radiographers and sonographers are in equally short supply.

CHOICE OF IMAGING EQUIPMENT. Because it is one of the most expensive items for any hospital or clinic, the choice of imaging equipment must depend on the volume of patients, their imaging needs, and the clinical facilities available. Imaging may be helpful not only to decide on treatment but also to determine whether the patient can be treated locally or should be referred to a larger hospital.

In developing countries, the majority of patients will have suffered trauma or have pulmonary disease, particularly pneumonia or tuberculosis. There is a strong probability, especially in the tropics, that they are also infected by one or more parasites. Many of the women are pregnant, and others have pelvic inflammatory disease. AIDS complicates the clinical spectrum of many diseases, makes infections worse, and increases the risk of malignancies, especially lymphoma and Kaposi sarcoma. In women, the other common malignancy in the tropics (with or without AIDS) is carcinoma of the uterine cervix, and the complications from often advanced tumors are another reason why imaging is needed.

Three different levels of diagnostic imaging are recommended in the tropics. Primary (first-referral) hospitals or clinics, district (second-referral) hospitals, and tertiary care hospitals. Most district and tertiary care hospitals also provide primary and acute care.

FIRST-REFERRAL HOSPITALS OR CLINICS. WHO recommends that all first-referral hospitals or clinics (the first health care facility to which the patient may be sent for imaging or to see a physician) have imaging facilities that meet or exceed the specifications of the World Health Imaging System (WHIS) and the WHO General Purpose Ultrasound Unit (WH-GPUS).*

Radiographic Units. The radiographic equipment (the WHIS-RAD) must provide very high quality chest radiographs and a comprehensive range of high-quality skeletal examinations (Fig. 21–1). Abdominal radiology should include plain, supine, and erect radiographs; contrast urography; cystography; and cholecystography. Equipment for fluoroscopy is *not* recommended unless it will be used by a radiologist or physician who has received adequate training. Adding facilities for image-intensified fluoroscopy increases the initial costs as well as the expense for maintenance and spare parts: There are very few indications for fluoroscopy at the first-referral level, and it is a totally unreliable way to examine the lungs.

Electrical Supply. The WHO is aware that many hospitals and clinics in the tropics have a variable and unreliable electrical supply. Extensive field trials in Africa and elsewhere have shown that the WHIS-RAD specifications, which include a very reliable battery-powered x-ray generator, will produce high-quality radiographs, e.g., high kV, small focus, grid chest radiographs. A WHIS-RAD will continue to function for several weeks in a small hospital, even if no electrical power is available; it is quickly recharged whenever the electrical service is on, regardless of voltage or other fluctuations. The WHIS-RAD is not designed only for the developing world. It has been installed in several university towns in Sweden and elsewhere, where it has been used extensively.

Ultrasound. Similarly, the WHO-GPUS specifications provide a wide range of high-quality sonography, recording more information than is usually required by other than expert sonologists. The WHO has repeatedly and strongly emphasized that however good the ultrasound equipment, the users must have proper training. The WHO Manual of Ultrasound is user-friendly and comprehensive, but it is not meant to be a substitute for proper training and supervised experience. Without adequate training, sonography can be very misleading and potentially dangerous because of misinterpretation.

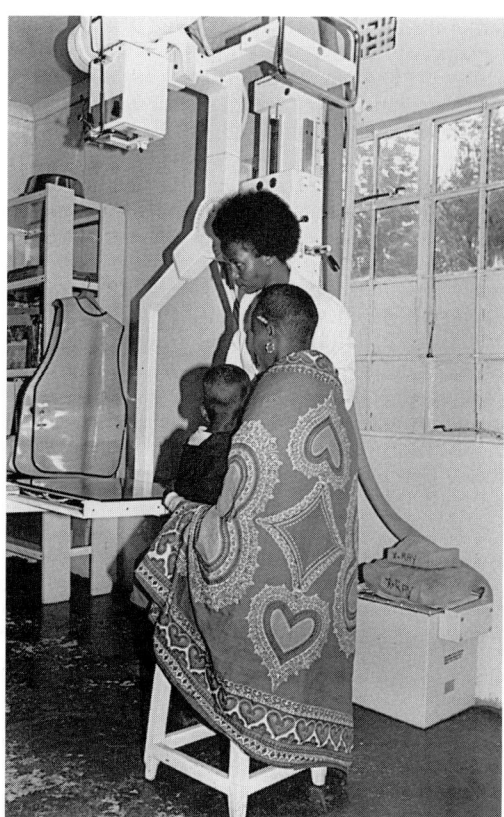

Figure 21–1. A WHO-designed x-ray unit in an African mission hospital. (Courtesy of WHO and D. Gibson.)

Darkroom and Other Accessories. WHO imaging system specifications are also available for all darkroom and accessory supplies, and there is a WHO Manual of Radiographic Technique and another for Darkroom Technique. There is also the Manual of Radiographic Interpretation for General Practitioners (as well as the Manual for Diagnostic Ultrasound).

Radiography/Ultrasound—Which Comes First? Radiography has more general uses than ultrasound and must be the first choice except in hospitals dedicated to obstetrics. The majority of patients in all hospitals in the tropics and lesser developed countries will need skeletal x-rays for trauma and chest x-rays for pulmonary infections. Neither can be provided by ultrasound. But, wherever possible, there should be both radiography and ultrasound, because many tropical diseases require imaging of the soft tissues, e.g., the liver, spleen, uterus, kidneys, pelvis, and gallbladder. In addition, ultrasound is useful for guiding drainage of an abscess, locating ascites or a pleural effusion for aspiration, and for directing tissue biopsy. Properly designed needles and training are necessary for all ultrasound-guided interventional procedures.

SECOND-REFERRAL (DISTRICT) HOSPITAL. The next level of imaging assumes that there will be a specialist radiologist, qualified radiographers, and, usually, ultrasonographers. The equipment recommended by the WHO at this level includes the WHIS-RAD and GPUS for the majority of imaging but adds fluoroscopy, linear tomography, and the capability for minimal peripheral angiography. Sonography includes endoscopic and Doppler scanning. The choice of equipment depends on the specialists and staff available in the imaging department and the clinical facilities of the hos-

---

*Full specifications for the World Health Imaging System can be obtained from Radiation Medicine, World Health Organization, 1211 Geneva 27, Switzerland, or through a regional or local WHO office or any of the United Nations bookstores.

pital. Radionuclide studies may be added if radioisotopes are readily available.

TERTIARY REFERRAL HOSPITALS. The tertiary level of imaging includes all the above but adds CT (preferably spiral CT) as well as angiography for invasive procedures, with advanced sonography and, if possible, magnetic resonance imaging (MRI). But, as at other levels, the choice of equipment must depend on the needs of the patients, the imaging specialists, and the clinical specialists available to provide the proper treatment. The more complex the equipment, the more essential it is to have an adequate power supply and readily available maintenance service.

CHOICE OF EQUIPMENT. The make and specifications of the equipment to be purchased at any level of hospital must be guided by prime requirements for high-quality images. Many mistakes in interpretation occur when images are of poor quality. No portable or ward x-ray unit is suitable for general radiography (and should not be used except in the ward or operating room), especially when there is not a trained radiographer available. Mobile x-ray units seem relatively inexpensive and easy to use. They are advertised as being "capable of every radiographic procedure," but the quality of the images is poor and the radiation exposure to the patient (and sometimes the staff) is much higher than from fixed equipment (e.g., the WHIS-RAD). Equally important, the purchasing contract should include 5 years of regular maintenance and the guarantee that spare parts will be readily available. The most expensive unit that anyone can buy is one that does not work.

THE FUTURE. Technical advances now permit high-quality "filmless" direct radiography, the conversion of x-ray energy into electrical signals without any intermediate steps. The images are then displayed on high-resolution, high-quality viewing screens; they can be transmitted or stored; and the densities can be manipulated while the images are viewed. At least one company has produced an x-ray unit with a rotating arm and mobile patient support very similar to the WHIS-RAD format. Technical results and ease of operation are excellent: What is not yet known is the reliability of the system in small hospitals and under tropical or other stressful climatic conditions. The standard WHIS-RAD is reliable and well tested; it will give good service until this new technology becomes more firmly established and less expensive.

CHOICE OF IMAGING TECHNIQUE. At the first-referral level, 90% of all imaging will be radiographs for the chest and skeleton (particularly for trauma) and obstetric ultrasonography.

Chest Imaging. Radiography of the chest is most commonly needed for tuberculosis (Figs. 77–3 and 5–8) and bacterial or mycotic (Figs. 83–5, 83–11, and 83–13) pneumonia in Southeast Asia, paragonimiasis (Figs. 2–4; 121–4 and 121–5) and melioidosis (Fig. 37–1), and in immunosuppressed persons, pneumocytosis (Fig. 98–4). However, it is often overused, particularly in the follow-up of chest infections, especially tuberculosis. No chest x-ray should be routine: There should be good clinical indication, even for repeat chest radiographs. Provided that a high kV, grid technique is used for radiography, only a frontal film will be required; an additional routine lateral projection at the first examination is seldom helpful in any tropical disease. After the frontal film is reviewed, occasionally a lateral projection may be added. Radiography in small children is very difficult, and when tuberculosis is suspected, an additional lateral view to demonstrate lymphadenopathy may be useful. Unfortunately, the accurate differentiation of many infections, e.g., tuberculosis vs. paragonimiasis or melioidosis, or pyogenic abscess vs. amebic lung abscess (Figs. 2–4 and 86–10), is not possible on chest radiographs alone. In some instances, a

knowledge of the geographic distribution of infectious diseases is very useful (Chapter 149).

For cardiac disease, echocardiography should be the first imaging used, provided that the user has special training. Plain chest radiographs often provide less information about the heart than is expected. Although the radiographic appearance of some of the cardiac myopathies is almost diagnostic, the differential diagnosis of an enlarged heart can seldom be made from a radiograph (Chapter 3). A good clinical examination, including the history, may be more useful. Ultrasound is the best way to image pericardial or subphrenic fluid and to see diaphragmatic movement. Pleural thickening may be mistaken for pleural fluid unless proper techniques are used, but ultrasound is useful to guide aspiration or biopsy of the pleura or of some peripheral pulmonary lesions. Apart from these very peripheral lesions, ultrasound has a negligible role in pulmonary disease.

The real problem in both pulmonary and cardiac imaging in the tropics is that there are many conditions with very similar appearances, making the differential diagnosis on a chest radiograph extremely difficult. It can usually be shown that something is wrong with the lungs, but it is not always possible to identify the etiology.

Many parasites, e.g., guinea worms, filariae, and cysticerci as well as calcified hydatid cysts may live in the muscles overlying the lungs and be mistaken for pulmonary lesions, as can exotic earrings or other social jewelry. The outline of the calcification or density is usually characteristic, but if there is doubt, a lateral or oblique projection will be very useful, after removing the adornments.

Skeleton. Skeletal radiographs, other than for trauma, are required for osteomyelitis, whether caused by tuberculous (Fig. 77–4), mycotic, hydatid, or more common pyogenic or enteric infection. Skeletal radiographs are also helpful in the hemoglobinopathies (Figs. 5–6, and 6–8); nutritional diseases, e.g., rickets (Fig. 131–9), scurvy, fluorosis; and to show soft tissue calcification resulting from parasites (Figs. 124–1 and 124–3).

Perhaps surprisingly, ultrasound is extremely useful in the diagnosis and management of early osteomyelitis; by enabling early and accurate antibiotic therapy it can prevent the disastrous bone disruption that can result (Chapter 14). It can also be used to assess the progress of callus formation after limb fractures but does not replace radiography.

Abdomen. In any small hospital there are 3 ways to image the abdomen, and each has specific indications. Plain abdominal radiographs are important to confirm the diagnosis of intestinal obstruction, to locate calculi or foreign bodies, to show calcification in the bladder (Fig. 118–21) and ureters in schistosomiasis, and to locate calcified hydatid cysts (Fig. 124–9).

Intravenous contrast urography will give more information about urinary schistosomiasis (Figs. 118–18 and 118–19) and renal tuberculosis and their complications. Oral or intravenous cholecystography will demonstrate biliary calculi or a nonfunctioning gallbladder.

Abdominal ultrasonography is of major importance in tropical diseases because it is the easiest way to demonstrate hepatic abscesses (amebic, pyogenic, ascaris; Fig. 68–7), liver flukes (Fig. 5–3), noncalcified hydatid cysts (Figs. 124–8 and 124–11), and all varieties and stages of hepatic schistosomiasis (Figs. 5–2 and 118–16). Sonography is the best way to demonstrate biliary calculi and ascaris and should be the first choice for imaging the kidney. It is an excellent way to recognize the bladder changes in schistosomiasis (Fig. 118–20) but is less reliable in the early stages of ureteric infections. Sonography is an accurate way to recognize splenomegaly but does not always indicate the cause. It is important in the diagnosis of pelvic inflammatory disease and the recognition of localized amebic or tuberculous abscesses in the pelvis. With experience, direct bowel involvement by amebiasis, tuberculosis, or schistosomiasis can be demonstrated by ultrasound, and it is the most reliable method for demonstrating ascites. Some bowel tumors may be seen.

Ultrasound has been used effectively in epidemiologic surveys of echinococcosis and schistosomiasis.

Soft Tissues. Sonography is an accurate way to locate soft tissue abscesses, particularly those in the paraspinal regions (tuberculosis, brucellosis, and pyomyositis) and early soft tissue abscesses elsewhere due to guinea worm or pyomyositis. The movement of filaria can be seen. It is a reliable way to recognize abdominal and cervical lymphadenopathy, but does not demonstrate the etiology. It does not provide useful information for patients with elephantiasis, guinea worm infestation, or ulcers of any sort.

Obstetric and Neonatal Scanning. Sonography should entirely replace radiography for all obstetric and neonatal imaging, but this does require extra skill and training. If ultrasound is not available, radiography should not be used until the last trimester, and then only for the diagnosis of a difficult fetal presentation or when there is hydramnios or other evidence of fetal abnormality. A single erect lateral film of the abdomen in the last 2 weeks of pregnancy can be helpful if disproportion is suspected.

Ultrasound is very useful in the first months of life in assessing and following the progress of neonatal and early childhood meningitis, cerebral tuberculosis, and abscesses. When the fontanelles have closed, only CT scanning or MRI can be used to investigate cerebral lesions.

ADVANCED (SPECIALIST) IMAGING. At the second or tertiary level of care, plain radiography and sonography are still essential for the majority of imaging, and the same WHIS and GPUS can be used.

Fluoroscopy. Where there is a radiologist or specially trained physician, fluoroscopy can be added, but it is of importance only in the examination of the GI tract. How much fluoroscopy is used depends on the endoscopic skills available. Rectal biopsy can be more accurate than a barium enema, for example. Fluoroscopy is totally unreliable in the diagnosis of any chest infection at any stage, even with image intensification. If chest disease is suspected, clinical examination and a chest radiograph should be used to make the diagnosis and assess progress, if necessary. Because ultrasound is useful to confirm and aspirate pleural effusions and to observe diaphragmatic movement, it should be used instead of fluoroscopy.

In most hospitals, skilled fluoroscopy using barium contrast (because the hygroscopic effect of some liquid contrast media makes them dangerous in the GI tract, especially in dehydrated patients and young children) is the reliable way of demonstrating strictures in the esophagus, whether due to neoplasm, caustic ingestion, or other cause. If there is a fistula and there is leakage of barium from the esophagus into the mediastinum, this does not alter the patient's prognosis. Fluoroscopy with contrast can demonstrate advanced esophageal varices but is unreliable in the recognition of early varices.

Gastrointestinal Imaging. All gastrointestinal examinations must be conducted with fluoroscopy, because without it, the alimentary tract can appear normal and yet have a major lesion. Equally important, a kink in the bowel or stomach appearing on a single radiograph may suggest an abnormality that is not present. With proper fluoroscopy, barium studies can demonstrate ascaris (Fig. 104–3), and in the large bowel, amebiasis, tuberculosis, and schistosomiasis (Fig. 118–17). In the small bowel the inflammatory and edematous changes of enteritis can be demonstrated (Fig. 4–1), but without considerable experience it is not usually possible to make a definite differential diagnosis. However, it is possible to demonstrate the extent of the disease and to monitor therapy and complications, e.g., the fistulae of lymphogranuloma venereum, the double volvulus of maize eaters, and the varying levels of intussusception that are so common in some populations (Chapter 13). With experience, a fluoroscopically controlled barium or air enema can be used safely to reduce ileocolic or colocolic intussusception.

Abdominal masses, whether imaged by radiography or ultrasound, are difficult to diagnose. Inflammatory masses due to parasites, e.g., ameboma, bilharzioma, or tuberculoma, appear very similar to neoplasm. Knowledge of the geographic epidemiology of these infectious diseases may be more significant in some patients than the imaging findings. Bowel neoplasia, idiopathic ulcerative colitis, and regional ileitis are very uncommon in some parts of the world (Chapter 4). The accuracy of all contrast and sonographic abdominal examinations depends very much on the experience and skill of the examiner.

Central Nervous System (CNS) Imaging. There is very little indication for plain skull radiography in any tropical disease, except in the third stage of treponematosis or when there is a localized tuberculous or mycotic bone infection. Ultrasound is very useful for imaging meningitis or cerebral abscess in neonates, but for little else. At any age, it can show a psoas abscess but cannot demonstrate the spinal lesions. Calcified intracerebral parasites can be better detected by CT scanning than by plain radiography of the skull (Figs. 124–3 and 124–4). Both CT and MRI will accurately show cerebral and spinal infections (including parasites) and other masses (Fig. 77–4). Scans may often reliably suggest the diagnosis, e.g., hydatid disease, cysticercosis, toxoplasmosis (Figs. 97–4 and 97–6), sparganosis, and paragonimiasis. Tuberculosis must be included in the differential diagnosis of almost all intracerebral masses.

There are no special indications for cerebral angiography in tropical diseases.

Spinal cord lesions are best imaged by MRI or CT. If scanning is not available, myelography will demonstrate almost all spinal masses but may not be able to differentiate infection from tumor. Myelography requires fluoroscopy and should not be used without it. There is no contraindication to myelography in active spinal tuberculosis: On the contrary, accurate localization of the lesion is important because, in spite of the level of vertebral infections shown on the plain radiograph, it may not be matched exactly by the extent of the abscess or other cause of the CNS symptoms.

Choice of Imaging When CT and MRI Are Available. Except for pulmonary, skeletal, or CNS lesions, ultrasound should precede CT or MRI in the investigation of tropical diseases. There are very few hepatic, splenic, or other soft tissue diseases that are not well demonstrated by ultrasound. Sometimes, follow-up CT or MRI may provide a little more information, because the early stages of some liver or other soft tissue infections do not always show any echogenic change. If the initial ultrasound study is inconclusive and there is strong clinical suspicion, sonography should be repeated after a few hours (even up to 24 hours), but if it is necessary to make a diagnosis quickly and the equipment is available, CT or MRI should be used.

Both CT and MRI are of particular importance for investigating the brain and spine. CT is a sensitive way to detect tissue calcification; MRI is not, but it is the most reliable way to scan soft tissue and joint lesions. Even when a soft tissue abscess (including the liver and spleen) has been first diagnosed using CT or MRI, it is usually best to monitor progress with ultrasound.

DIFFERENTIAL DIAGNOSIS OF TROPICAL DISEASES. Because the images of many tropical infections are very similar, the clinical history becomes extremely important for correct interpretation. It is equally important to know whether the patient has lived in an endemic area for some time or only paid a brief visit. Many infections, e.g., schistosomiasis, amebiasis, tuberculosis, and malaria, have a different natural history in those who have lived for an extended period in an endemic area, and this is reflected in the images. For example, bladder changes that have been described in schistosomiasis in Egypt may not occur in West Africa, and vice versa (Chapter 118). Local variations must be known. For example, the metacarpal index for sickle cell disease used in the United States and West Africa would suggest that almost all the Luo people of Kenya have sickle cell disease (Chapter 6). Nearly every baseline standard, from serum proteins to cell counts, shows regional differences. These base levels will not change immediately on moving to another country. Without understanding these variations, neither a clinician nor a radiologist will be able to interpret the images correctly. One example is the very wide differential diagnosis of an enlarged liver. To the relatively few common possibilities, e.g., fatty alcoholic livers, primary tumors, metastatic tumors, pyogenic abscess, and heart failure, must now be added the tropical differential of hydatid cysts, amebic liver abscess, and a whole range of tumors, e.g., Burkitt's lymphoma, as well as ascaris, mycosis, liver flukes, schistosomiasis, leishmaniasis, cirrhosis due to hepatitis viruses, malaria, and a host of other infectious and cardiac diseases.

An additional challenge in developing countries is that many patients have more than one disease concurrently and often complain of something different to what is actually detected by imaging or by laboratory tests. Where schistosomiasis is endemic, for example, few patients complain of the earliest symptoms of infection, e.g., hematuria or mucus and blood in the stool, since they are not disabling and occur in such a large proportion of the population that they are not considered abnormal (Chapter 118). *Ascaris* and other worms are also regarded as normal in many countries, and hydatid cysts are often asymptomatic. For the physician, finding evidence of a parasitic infection by imaging may distract from the undetected disease that is the real clinical problem.

Geographic variations and, therefore, differences in imaging are not reflected only in infectious and malignant diseases. For example, the patterns of intussusception, volvulus, and hernias vary all over Africa and certainly cannot be used as guidelines anywhere else in the tropics (Chapter 13). The surgeon who finds femoral hernias common in his or her practice in one locality may, on moving, wonder if he or she

is missing them, because they seldom turn up in the new practice. Particularly important examples are the common causes of intestinal obstruction in each area. These causes differ between West and East Africa, and neither would apply in southern Africa or North Africa, let alone in South America. Anatomic and genetic differences are not the sole explanation: Differences in clinical presentations are due to multiple variations in diet, parasites, and that mysterious but all important entity, "the way of life." There are even inexplicable variations between men and women, who apparently share everything else in their lives.

CONCLUSION. The most important imaging equipment is a high-quality general purpose radiography unit for examining the skeleton, chest, and abdomen, together with a general purpose ultrasound unit. This will provide for almost all the imaging needs in small clinics in first-referral hospitals where there is a physician or someone trained to interpret and act on the results of the imaging. Fluoroscopy is not necessary and not recommended.

In tropical countries, images will not be interpreted correctly unless the local pattern of disease, the patient's background, clinical information, and laboratory tests are available. With few exceptions, diagnostic imaging will clearly show the abnormality but will not establish the exact diagnosis. Experience is exceedingly important for the correct interpretation of the radiographs and scans; for ultrasound in particular, practical training is essential.

Bibliography

Agenant DMA: The basic radiological system. Trop Geogr Med 40:85, 1988.
Agenant DMA: The Simavi-BRS Project. A Successful WHO Project. Haarlem, Simavi, 1991.
Cockshott WP, Palmer PES: Exotic diseases in travelers. Curt Imag 2:142, 1990.
de Lacey G: Plain film radiography: The BRS solution. Clin Radiol 44:786, 1989.
Holm T, Palmer PES, Lehtinen E: Manual of Radiographic Technique. Geneva, World Health Organization, 1986.
Palmer PES: Imaging equipment for small hospitals. Trop Geogr Med 45:100, 1993.
Palmer PES, Holm T, Hanson GP: Radiology worldwide. *In* Pettersson M (ed): Global Textbook of Radiology. Oslo, The Nicer Institute, 1995, pp 85–100.
Palmer PES, et al: Manual of Radiological Interpretation for General Practitioners. Geneva, World Health Organization, 1985.
Palmer PES, Reeder MM: The Imaging of Tropical Diseases with Epidemiological, Pathological and Clinical Correlation. Heidelberg, Springer. In press.
World Health Organization: The hospital in rural and urban districts. Tech Rep Series 819, Geneva, WHO, 1992.
World Health Organization: Manual of Diagnostic Ultrasound. Geneva, WHO, 1995.
World Health Organization: A rational approach to radiodiagnostic investigation. Tech Rep Series 689. Geneva, WHO, 1983.
World Health Organization: The rational use of diagnostic imaging in paediatrics. Tech Rep Series 757. Geneva, WHO, 1987.
World Health Organization: Effective choices for diagnostic imaging in clinical practice. Tech Rep Series 795. Geneva, WHO, 1990.

General Principles

Theodore Tsai

Although many tropical viral infections are transmitted uniquely in that geographic zone, others exhibit specific clinical manifestations or particular epidemiologic patterns that differ from their characteristics in temperate regions. Yet others are as recognizable in the tropics as elsewhere. Numerous arthropod-borne viral (arboviral) infections transmitted in ecological niches limited to the tropical region, e.g., some of those listed in Table II–1, are examples of the first category. Although these principally zoonotic diseases may have been viewed as exotic in the past, the increasing prevalence of vector-borne infections in North America (e.g., Lyme disease), and the growing numbers of travelers who as part of an adventure experience knowingly place themselves at risk for these infections, have forced astute clinicians everywhere to include zoonotic diseases in their diagnostic repertoire. Two herpesviruses, Epstein-Barr and varicella viruses, provide examples of the second category: the particular association of Epstein-Barr virus infection (Chapter 24.1) with Burkitt lymphoma in Africa may be linked to local accessory factors, although the reportedly lower incidence of childhood varicella infections in tropical locations is unexplained. In better-defined examples, transmission patterns in tropical populations leading to early infection and acquired immunity are well known to underlie the lower frequencies of symptomatic adult polio (Chapter 27.1) and icteric hepatitis A (Chapter 28.1) cases in developing countries.

It is worth noting that the tropical region has been the source of several novel viruses with global public health significance. Worldwide transmission of human immunodeficiency virus (HIV) (Chapter 22), the specter of an influenza H5N1 pandemic (Chapter 26), and the celerity of African viral hemorrhagic fever viruses (Chapters 31.2 and 31.4) have highlighted the vulnerability of people everywhere to the rapid spread of infections from distant sources. From an evolutionary perspective, Africa was the source of HIV and also, putatively, the ancestral progenitor of yellow fever (Chapter 31.1), dengue (Chapter 29.1), and other flaviviruses.

In choosing the viral diseases addressed in the following chapters, we have described those that are particularly prominent in the tropics, emphasizing features that distinguish their occurrence there—in transmission pattern, incidence, or clinical manifestations—from those in other locations. Certain cosmopolitan infections, e.g., genital herpesvirus infection, are described elsewhere in their appropriate clinical contexts (Chapter 11).

■ ARBOVIRAL AND ZOONOTIC INFECTIONS

More than 150 arboviruses or related zoonotic viruses are known to be pathogenic in humans (Table II–1). Although an etiologic diagnosis ultimately requires laboratory confirmation, the choice of appropriate diagnostic tests and a systematic approach to clinical diagnosis are simplified by evaluating the clinical syndrome in the context of the patient's itinerary and activities within a typical incubation period of 3 to 21 days. Other relevant factors include the season of exposure and illness—since many zoonotic infections are transmitted only in specific months—often in conjunction with the rainy season, and the exceptionally short or long incubation periods associated with certain infections (e.g., the initial symptoms of Venezuelan equine encephalitis (Chapter 30.2) can appear within a day of exposure and Rift Valley fever retinitis (Chapter 29.10) may be delayed for >3 weeks after the initial infection). In addition, vaccination with commercially available vaccines for yellow fever, Japanese encephalitis (Chapter 30.3) and tick-borne encephalitis (Chapter 30.5) may militate against these diagnoses, or interfere with the interpretation of serologic tests. Often a patient will volunteer a history of tick exposure or tick bite, exposure to rodents, or other clue to a specific category of vector exposure. Table II–1 should be used by first evaluating the clinical syndrome within the possibilities in the geographic region of exposure, then by assessing the relative frequencies of the individual disease possibilities, and, if known, the mode of vector-borne transmission.

TABLE II–1. Arboviral and Zoonotic Viral Infections by Geographic Area, Mode of Transmission, and Clinical Syndrome

Location and Virus	Febrile Illness			Meningoencephalitis	Hemorrhagic Fever	Other
	Nondescript	With Rash	With Arthritis			
North America						
Mosquito-borne						
Cache Valley				○		
California encephalitis				○		
Dengue 1–4		●			●	Hepatitis
EEE				○		
Everglades (VEE type II)				○		
Jamestown Canyon				○		Respiratory symptoms
Keystone				○		
LaCrosse				●		
StLE				●		
Snowshoe hare				○		
Tensaw				○		
Trivittatus				○		Respiratory symptoms
VEE (sylvatic subtypes 1D and 1E)	○			○		Pneumonitis
Western equine encephalitis				●		Perinatal illness after congenital third-trimester infection
Sandfly-borne						
Vesicular stomatitis (New Jersey and Indiana)	○			○		Respiratory illness
Tick-borne						
Colorado tick fever	●			○	○	
Powassan				○		
Salmon River	○					
Zoonoses						
Lymphocytic choriomeningitis	○			○	○	Pneumonia, parotitis, orchitis, arthritis; congenital infection leads to CNS malformation
Bayou, Black Creek Canal						Noncardiogenic pulmonary edema, nephrosis, myositis
Modoc				○		
New York, Sin Nombre						Noncardiogenic pulmonary edema
Rabies				○		
Rio Bravo	○			○		Pneumonia, orchitis
Seoul						Interstitial nephritis
Central and South America						
Mosquito-borne						
Bussuquara	○					
Cache Valley	○					
Catu	○					
Cotia	○					
Dengue 1–4		●		○	●	Hepatitis, perinatal illness after congenital third-trimester infection
EEE				○		
Fort Sherman	○					
Group C viruses (Apeu, Caraparu, Itaqui, Madrid, Marituba, Murutucu, Nepuyo, Oriboca, Ossa, Restan)	○					
Guama	○					
Guaroa	○			?		Hepatitis
Ilheus	○			○		
Mayaro		●	●			
Mucambo (VEE type IIIA)	○			○		
Piry	○					
Rocio				●		
StLE	○			○		
Tacaiuma	○					Two cases with concurrent malaria were fatal
Tonate (VEE type IIIB)	○					
Tucunduba				○		
VEE (epizootic subtypes IA, IB, IC)	●			●		Abortion, CNS malformation after first-trimester infection

TABLE II–1. Arboviral and Zoonotic Viral Infections by Geographic Area, Mode of Transmission, and Clinical Syndrome
Continued

Location and Virus	Febrile Illness			Meningoencephalitis	Hemorrhagic Fever	Other
	Nondescript	*With Rash*	*With Arthritis*			
VEE (sylvatic subtypes 1D, 1E, and 1F)	○			○		Pneumonitis
Western equine encephalitis				●		
Wyeomyia	○					
Xingu	○					Hepatitis?
YF	●				●	Hepatitis
Sandfly- and/or midge-borne						
Alenquer	○					
Candiru	○					
Chagres	○					
Changuinola	○					
Morumbi	○					
Oropouche	●	○		○		
Punta Toro	○					
Serra Norte	○					
Vesicular stomatitis (New Jersey and Indiana)	○			○		
Vesicular stomatitis (Alagoas)				○		
Zoonoses						
Andes, Laguna Negra						Noncardiogenic pulmonary edema, nephrosis
Guanarito				○	●	
Junin				○	●	Fatal congenital infection
Machupo				○	●	Fatal congenital infection
Rabies				○		
Rio Bravo	○			○		Pneumonia, orchitis
Sabia					○*	
Europe						
Mosquito-borne						
Batai	○			○		
Inkoo	○			○		Respiratory illness
Sindbis (Ockelbo)	●	●	●			
Snowshoe hare				○		
Tahyna	●			○		Respiratory illness
West Nile	○	○	○	●		Hepatitis, pancreatitis
Sandfly-borne						
Sandfly fever (Naples)	●					
Sandfly fever (Sicilian)	●					
Toscana	●			●		
Tick-borne						
Bhanja	○			○		
Central European encephalitis†	●			●		Hepatitis, thrombocytopenia
Congo-Crimean hemorrhagic fever					●	
Dhori	○			○*		
Kemerovo				○		
Lipovnik				○		
Louping ill				○		
Thogoto	○			○		Hepatitis, optic neuritis
Tribec				○		
Zoonoses						
Erve				○		Thunderclap headache
Lymphocytic choriomeningitis	●			●	○	Pneumonia, arthritis, orchitis, parotitis; congenital infection leads to CNS malformation
Dobrava	○				○	Interstitial nephritis, pantropic
Puumula	●			○	○	Interstitial nephritis, myocarditis
Rabies				○		
Seoul	○				○	Interstitial nephritis, pantropic
Asia						
Mosquito-borne						
Batai	○			○		
Beijing				●		
Chandipura	○			○		
Chikungunya	●	●	●	○	○	
Dengue 1–4	●	●		○	●	Hepatitis common; perinatal illness after third-trimester infection
Gansu				●		

Table continued on following page

TABLE II–1. Arboviral and Zoonotic Viral Infections by Geographic Area, Mode of Transmission, and Clinical Syndrome
Continued

Location and Virus	Febrile Illness			Meningoencephalitis	Hemorrhagic Fever	Other
	Nondescript	*With Rash*	*With Arthritis*			
JE				●		Abortion after congenital first- and second-trimester infection
Kunjin	○		○	○		
Semliki Forest (MeTri)				○		
Sindbis	●	●	●	○	○	
Snowshoe hare				○		
Tahyna	●			○		Respiratory illness
West Nile	●	●	●	○		Hepatitis, pancreatitis
Yunnan	○					
Zika		●				
Sandfly-borne						
Chandipura	○			○		
Sandfly fever (Naples)	●					
Sandfly fever (Sicilian)	●					
Tick-borne						
Alma-Arasan	○					
Banna				●		
Congo-Crimean hemorrhagic fever					●	
Dhori	○			○*		
Ganjam	○					
Issyk-kul	○					
Karshi	○					
Kemerovo				○		
Kyasanur Forest				●	●	Pneumonia, retinitis
Negishi				○		
Omsk hemorrhagic fever				●	●	Pneumonia
Powassan				○		
Russian spring-summer encephalitis				●		
Syr-Darya Valley		○				
Tamdy	○					
Wanowrie				○	○	
Zoonoses						
Hantaan					●	Pantropic, interstitial nephritis
Lymphocytic choriomeningitis	○			○		Pneumonia, arthritis, orchitis, parotitis; congenital infection leads to CNS malformation
Rabies				●		
Seoul					●	Pantropic, interstitial nephritis
Africa						
Mosquito-borne						
Babanki	●	●	●			
Bangui		○				
Banzi	○					
Bhanja	○			○		
Bunyamwera		●		○		
Bwamba		●		○		
Chikungunya		●	●	○	○	
Dengue 1–4	●	●		○	●	Hepatitis; perinatal illness after congenital third-trimester infection
Germiston		○		○		
IgboOra			○			
Ilesha		●		○	○	
Koutango		○				
Lebombo	○					
Ngari				○		
Nyando	○					
O'nyong-nyong		●	●			
Orungo	●					
Pongola			○			
Rift Valley fever	●			●	●	Hepatitis, retinitis
Semliki Forest	○			○		
Shokwe	○					
Shuni	○					
Sindbis		●	●		○	

TABLE II–1. Arboviral and Zoonotic Viral Infections by Geographic Area, Mode of Transmission, and Clinical Syndrome
Continued

Location and Virus	Febrile Illness			Meningoencephalitis	Hemorrhagic Fever	Other
	Nondescript	With Rash	With Arthritis			
Spondweni		○				
Tahyna	●			○		Respiratory illness
Tataguine		●				
Usutu		○				
Wesselsbron	○					Hepatitis
West Nile	●	●	●	●		Hepatitis, pancreatitis
YF	●				●	Hepatitis
Zika		○				
Sandfly-borne						
Chandipura	○			○		
Sandfly fever (Naples)	●					
Sandfly fever (Sicilian)	●					
Tick-borne						
Abadina	○					
Bhanja	○			○		
Congo-Crimean hemorrhagic fever					●	
Dhori				○*		
Dugbe	○			○		
Nairobi sheep disease	○					
Quaranfil	○			○		
Thogoto	○			○		Hepatitis, optic neuritis
Zoonoses						
Dakar bat	○					
Duvenhage				○		
Lassa				○	●	Pantropic; abortion, hearing loss; fatal congenital infection
Lymphocytic choriomeningitis	○			○	●	Pneumonia, arthritis, orchitis, parotitis; congenital infection leads to CNS malformation
Mokola				○		
Monkeypox		●				
Rabies				●		
Tanapox		○				
Unknown mode of transmission						
Ebola (Democratic Republic of Congo, Sudan, Ivory Coast)		●			●	Pantropic; abortion
Kasokero	○					
LeDantec				○		
Marburg		●				Pantropic
Australia and Oceania						
Mosquito-borne						
Barmah Forest			●	○		Glomerulonephritis
Dengue 1–4	●	●				Hepatitis; perinatal illness after congenital third-trimester infection
Edge Hill			○			
GanGan			○			
JE				○		
Kokobera			○			
Kunjin			○	○		
Murray Valley				●		
Ross River		●	●	○		Glomerulonephritis
Sepik	○					
Sindbis	○	○	○			
Trubanaman	○					
Zoonoses						
Ballina (rabies)				○		
Hendra				○		Fatal pneumonia

Key: ○, rare, sporadic; ●, frequent, epidemic. Only arboviruses causing illness after natural infection are listed; viruses causing illness after laboratory exposure only are indicated by footnote.
*Illness reported only after laboratory-acquired infection.
†Also transmitted by ingestion of infected milk products.
CNS, central nervous system; EEE, eastern equine encephalomyelitis; JE, Japanese encephalitis; StLE, St. Louis encephalitis; VEE, Venezuelan equine encephalitis; YF, yellow fever.
Adapted from Tsai T, Niklasson B, Goujon C: Arboviruses and zoonotic viruses. *In* DuPont HL, Steffen R (eds): Textbook of Travel Medicine and Health. Philadelphia, BC Decker Inc, 1997, pp 200–214.

22 Human Immunodeficiency Virus Infection and AIDS

Kevin M. De Cock, Eve Lackritz, Dale J. Hu, and Sebastian J. Lucas

DEFINITION. Human immunodeficiency virus (HIV) infection causes progressive impairment of cellular immunity and is associated with a wide spectrum of disease manifestations. The acquired immunodeficiency syndrome (AIDS) is the most advanced stage of this infection and is characterized by severe immunodeficiency and increased incidence of tuberculosis, bacterial infections, other opportunistic infections, and certain malignancies. In the industrialized world, most countries have adopted the Centers for Disease Control and Prevention (CDC) surveillance case definition for AIDS or a minor modification of it (Table 22–1). Many of the criteria in the CDC case definition are impractical in the developing world because of lack of diagnostic facilities, and the World Health Organization (WHO) has therefore proposed clinical case definitions for the purposes of epidemiologic surveillance in developing countries (Table 22–2).

HISTORY. Since its recognition in the United States in 1981 among men who had sex with men, AIDS has rapidly emerged as a problem of global public health importance. The causative virus was isolated by workers at the Institut Pasteur in Paris in 1983, and blood tests detecting antibodies to HIV-1 were licensed in 1985. In 1986, French workers discovered another AIDS-associated human retrovirus, HIV-2, in persons from Guinea Bissau and Cape Verde Islands.

Although the origins of the AIDS epidemic remain uncertain, molecular and serologic tests on stored sera suggest that HIV was present in the Democratic Republic of the Congo (formerly Zaire) as early as 1959. Testing of stored serum specimens for HIV antibody from rural areas of the same country revealed that HIV was present at a low prevalence in 1976. The HIV epidemic escalated rapidly in the developing world, particularly in Africa, in the late 1970s and early 1980s, driven primarily by heterosexual transmission. Epidemic spread in Asia began later and has resulted from injection drug use as well as heterosexual transmission. In the mid- to late 1990s, the most rapid spread of HIV has occurred in southern Africa, South and Southeast Asia, and Eastern Europe, fueled in the latter regions by injection drug use.

Research in developing countries demonstrated that other sexually transmitted diseases (STDs) enhance the transmission and acquisition of HIV infection, and that their control may reduce HIV transmission at a population level. Epidemic tuberculosis has accompanied the emergence of HIV, and has been one of the most severe consequences of the spread of HIV. The social, economic, and demographic impact of HIV and AIDS has been most apparent in sub-Saharan Africa, which has seen greatly increased mortality, disruption of family structures, large numbers of orphans, and jeopardy to development and economic stability.

Research has clarified the spectrum of disease associated with HIV infection in different regions so that more logical approaches to treatment and prophylaxis for opportunistic infections have become apparent. Major advances in the 1990s include the introduction of effective antiretroviral drugs that have increased the survival of persons with HIV and AIDS in industrialized countries, reduced the progression to AIDS in persons with HIV infection, and lowered the

TABLE 22–1. Conditions Included in the CDC Surveillance Case Definition for Acquired Immunodeficiency Syndrome*

Bacterial infections, multiple or recurrent (any combination of at least two within a 2-year period of the following types affecting a child ≤13 years of age: septicemia, pneumonia, meningitis, bone or joint infection, or superficial skin or mucosal abscesses, caused by *Haemophilus*, *Streptococcus* including pneumococcus), or other pyogenic bacteria (2)
Candidiasis of bronchi, trachea, or lungs (1)
Candidiasis, esophageal (1, 3)
CD4+ T-lymphocyte count $<200/\mu L$ or $<14\%$ of total lymphocyte count (2)
Cervical cancer, invasive (2)
Coccidioidomycosis, disseminated or extrapulmonary (2)
Cryptococcosis, extrapulmonary (1)
Cryptosporidiosis, chronic intestinal (>1 mo duration) (1)
Cytomegalovirus disease (other than liver, spleen, or nodes) (1)
Cytomegalovirus retinitis (with loss of vision) (3)
Encephalopathy, HIV-related (2)
Herpes simplex: chronic ulcer(s) (>1 mo duration); or bronchitis, pneumonitis, or esophagitis (1)
Histoplasmosis, disseminated or extrapulmonary (2)
Isosporiasis, chronic intestinal (>1 mo duration) (2)
Kaposi sarcoma (4)
Lymphoid interstitial pneumonia and/or pulmonary lymphoid hyperplasia (LIP/PLH complex) affecting a child <13 yr of age (1, 3)
Lymphoma, Burkitt (or equivalent term) (2)
Lymphoma, immunoblastic (or equivalent term) (2)
Lymphoma, primary, of brain (5)
Mycobacterium avium complex or *M. kansasii*, disseminated or extrapulmonary (1)
M. tuberculosis, any site (pulmonary or extrapulmonary) (2)
Mycobacterium, other species or unidentified species, disseminated or extrapulmonary (2, 3)
Pneumocystis carinii pneumonia (1, 3)
Pneumonia, recurrent (2)
Progressive multifocal leukoencephalopathy (1)
Salmonella septicemia, recurrent (2)
Toxoplasmosis of brain (1, 3)
Wasting syndrome due to HIV (2)

[1]Considered AIDS-defining without laboratory evidence regarding HIV infection if diagnosed definitively.
[2]Considered AIDS-defining with laboratory evidence of HIV infection if diagnosed definitively.
[3]Considered AIDS-defining with laboratory evidence of HIV infection if diagnosed presumptively.
[4]For patients <60 years of age, as (2); for persons with laboratory evidence of HIV infection of any age, as (3) and (4).
[5]For patients <60 years of age, as (2); for persons with laboratory evidence of HIV infection of any age, as (3).
*Adapted from Centers for Disease Control and Prevention: Revision of the CDC surveillance case definition for acquired immunodeficiency syndrome. MMWR 36:1S, 1987; and CDC: 1993 revised classification system for HIV infection and expanded surveillance case definition for AIDS among adolescents and adults. MMWR 41(RR-17):1, 1992.

rate of transmission of HIV from mother to child; these advances thus far have had little influence on the situation in developing countries. Although trials of candidate HIV vaccines have started in certain developing countries, no vaccine is currently available for public health use.

By the end of 1998, the Joint United Nations Programme on HIV/AIDS (UNAIDS) estimated that more than 33 million persons worldwide were infected with HIV, of whom 95% were living in developing countries. Over the past decade, the AIDS epidemic has threatened gains made in improved life expectancy and child survival in many developing countries, especially in Africa. In 1998 alone, an estimated 2.5 million people died of AIDS. Without an effective, affordable vaccine, the contrast between the harsh realities of HIV-

TABLE 22–2. World Health Organization (WHO) Case Definitions for AIDS

WHO Case Definition of AIDS in Adults and Adolescents

For the purposes of AIDS surveillance an adult or adolescent (>12 yr of age) is considered to have AIDS if at least 2 of the following major signs are present in combination with at least 1 of the minor signs listed below, and if these signs are not known to be due to a condition unrelated to HIV infection. This WHO case definition does not require HIV serologic testing, making it simple and inexpensive, but having low sensitivity and specificity, particularly with respect to tuberculosis.

Major signs
- Weight loss ≥10% of body weight
- Chronic diarrhea for more than 1 mo
- Prolonged fever for >1 mo (intermittent or constant)

Minor signs
- Persistent cough for >1 mo*
- Generalized pruritic dermatitis
- History of herpes zoster
- Oropharyngeal candidiasis
- Chronic progressive or disseminated herpes simplex infection
- Generalized lymphadenopathy

The presence of either generalized Kaposi sarcoma or cryptococcal meningitis is sufficient for the diagnosis of AIDS for surveillance purposes.

For patients with tuberculosis, persistent cough for >1 mo should not be considered a minor sign.

Expanded WHO Case Definition for AIDS Surveillance

For the purpose of AIDS surveillance an adult or adolescent (≥12 yr of age) is considered to have AIDS if a test for HIV antibody gives a positive result and one or more of the conditions listed below. This WHO AIDS case definition *requires an HIV serologic test,* and includes a broader spectrum of clinical manifestations of HIV.
- ≥10% body weight loss or cachexia, with diarrhea or fever, or both, intermittent or constant, for at least 1 mo, not known to be due to a condition unrelated to HIV infection
- Cryptococcal meningitis
- Pulmonary or extrapulmonary tuberculosis
- Kaposi sarcoma
- Neurologic impairment that is sufficient to prevent independent daily activities, not known to be due to a condition unrelated to HIV infection (e.g., trauma or cerebrovascular accident)
- Candidiasis of the esophagus (which may be presumptively diagnosed based on the presence of oral candidiasis accompanied by dysphagia)
- Clinically diagnosed life-threatening or recurrent episodes of pneumonia, with or without etiologic confirmation
- Invasive cervical cancer

WHO Clinical Case Definition of AIDS in Children

Major signs
- Weight loss or failure to thrive
- Chronic diarrhea (>1 mo)
- Prolonged fever (>1 mo)

Minor signs
- Generalized lymphadenopathy*
- Oropharyngeal candidiasis
- Repeated common infections (otitis, pharyngitis, etc.)
- Persistent cough (>1 mo)
- Generalized dermatitis
- Confirmed maternal HIV infection

Pediatric AIDS is suspected in an infant or child presenting with at least 2 major signs associated with at least 2 minor signs in the absence of known causes of immunosuppression.

*Generalized lymphadenopathy = known lymph nodes measuring at least 0.5 cm and present in 2 or more sites, with bilateral lymph nodes counting as 1 site.
From World Health Organization: Wkly Epidemiol Rec 61:69, 1986; and World Health Organization: Wkly Epidemiol Rec 69:273, 1994.

AIDS in developing countries and the cautious optimism in industrialized countries can only become more stark.

ETIOLOGY

HIV-1 and HIV-2. Two distinct retroviruses, HIV-1 and HIV-2, cause HIV infection in humans. Both, as well as the related simian immunodeficiency viruses (SIV) of monkeys, are enveloped positive-strand RNA viruses belonging to the lentivirus subfamily. These RNA viruses integrate their genetic material into host cells causing a long course of chronic infection and disease (Fig. 22–1).

HIV-1 is the predominant type of HIV throughout the world. HIV-2 was first identified in persons originating from West Africa in the mid-1980s and is still found primarily among persons from that part of the world, although infection has spread to a limited degree in southwestern India, Angola, Mozambique, and Portugal. HIV-2 is closely related genetically to SIV$_{SM}$, even more closely than to HIV-1, and represents a zoonotic infection with a virus originating in sooty mangabeys and then established in humans. Recently published evidence suggests HIV-1 may be most closely related to a naturally occurring form of SIV in chimpanzees. HIV-1 and HIV-2 are structurally similar, are transmitted by the same routes, and are diagnosed with comparable serologic or virologic assays. Cross reactivity between HIV-1 and HIV-2 on serologic assays is common and virus-specific assays are required to distinguish the two infections.

HIV-2 has proved to be a less aggressive virus than HIV-1 both in terms of transmission and pathogenesis. Both sexual and perinatal transmission rates of HIV-2 are lower than those of HIV-1. Although the HIV-1 epidemic has increased dramatically over the past decade, the prevalence of HIV-2 has remained relatively stable and localized in West Africa. Although HIV-2 is associated with similar disease as HIV-1, progression of immune deficiency is slower than in HIV-1 infection.

HIV Subtypes. Based on viral genetic sequences, HIV-1 and HIV-2 isolates have been classified into a number of subtypes (also termed clades or genotypes). HIV-1 subtypes, designated by uppercase letters of the alphabet, constitute the major group (group M) and are the predominant viruses responsible for the global HIV pandemic. Some divergent, or "outlying" strains of HIV-1 have been identified, primarily among persons from different countries in central Africa, and have been provisionally categorized as groups O and N. Many commercially produced serologic assays were modified following the discovery that some HIV-1 group O infections were not detected by standard serologic screening tests. HIV-2 has been classified into five subtypes, although to date only a limited number of specimens have been evaluated. Distinguishing between HIV variants is complicated by the potential for co-infection and genetic recombination between distinct viral strains.

HIV-1 subtype B is the predominant subtype in the United States and Europe and has been the most widely studied. In Thailand, HIV-1 subtype E is most common among persons who have a history of prostitute or other heterosexual contact. Thai subtype B used to be the most prevalent among persons who inject drugs, although subtype E is now responsible for an increasing proportion of new infections in this population. Studies of non-B subtypes, particularly in Africa, have often been based on convenience sampling without the benefit of a systematic evaluation. Most of the 10 HIV-1 subtypes have been reported in sub-Saharan Africa. Subtype A appears to be the most common subtype in Central, West, and East Africa, with a large proportion of subtype D in East Africa. In Central Africa, a wide diversity of group M subtypes has been described. The prevalence of group O is also highest in Central Africa, particularly in Cameroon, Nigeria,

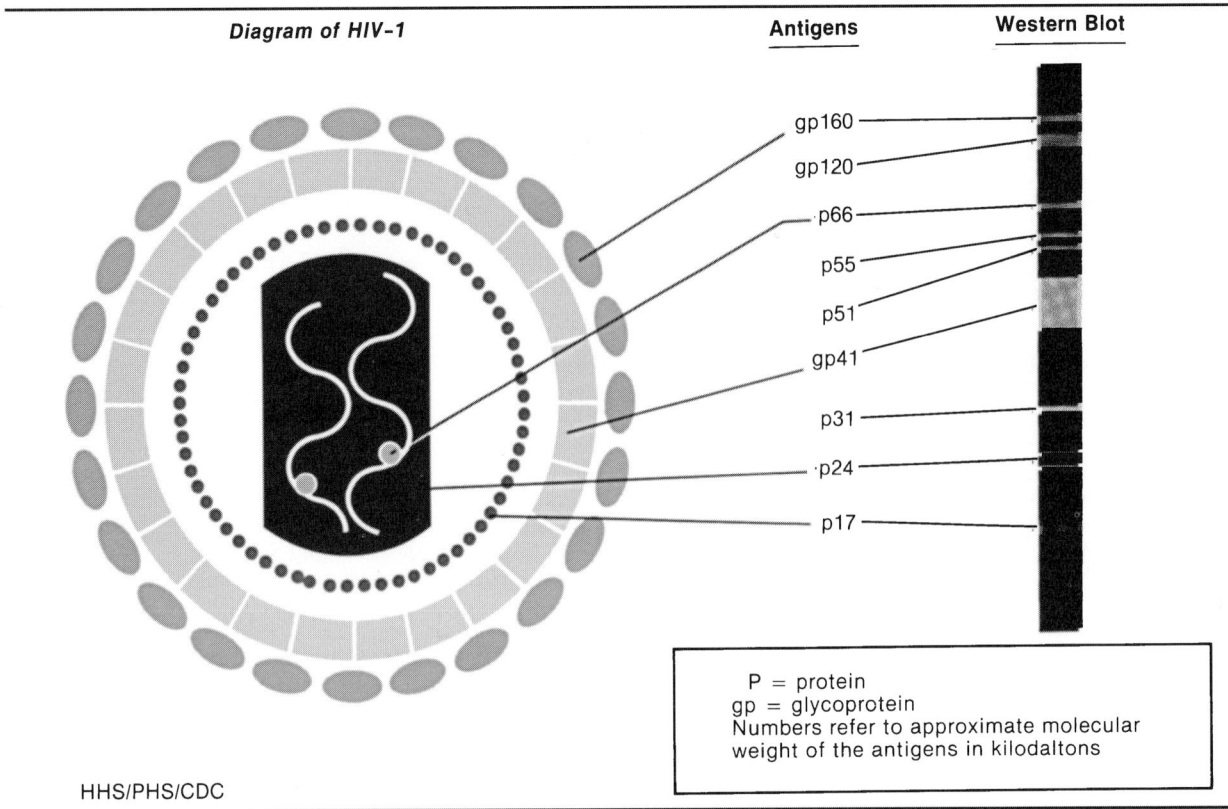

Diagram of HIV-1   <u>Antigens</u>   **Western Blot**

gp160
gp120
p66
p55
p51
gp41
p31
p24
p17

P = protein
gp = glycoprotein
Numbers refer to approximate molecular
weight of the antigens in kilodaltons

HHS/PHS/CDC

Figure **22–1.** Schematic representation of HIV-1. The virus consists of an outer envelope and an inner core containing the genetic material. Viral protein products coded for by individual genes elicit specific antibody responses in the infected host, which can be demonstrated on Western blot (see text). Envelope proteins are gp160, gp120, and gp41, coded for by the *env* gene; *gag* gene products are the core proteins p55, p24, and p17. The reverse transcriptase and endonuclease proteins, coded for by the *pol* gene, are p66 and p31.

and Gabon, although even in these countries group O viruses account for only 1 to 2% of all HIV isolates.

Research is ongoing to elucidate the significance, if any, of HIV genetic variation for transmission and pathogenesis. The extremely wide genetic variation among HIV isolates, as exemplified by the highly divergent HIV-1 groups O and N, poses a continuing challenge for the development of diagnostics, and perhaps for HIV vaccine development. Many commercial genomic assays for HIV DNA or RNA do not have equal sensitivity for non–subtype B as for subtype B infec-

tions. These assays must be evaluated and modified as they are introduced into the developing world for the purpose of patient management and diagnostics.

EPIDEMIOLOGY. The global epidemiology of HIV is dynamic and the prevalence of HIV infection, populations at risk, and predominant modes of transmission vary considerably by country and by region (Fig. 22–2; Table 22–3). It is estimated that in 1998 alone, 5.8 million new infections occurred, of which approximately 50% were among young adults 15 to 24 years of age, and 40% were in women.

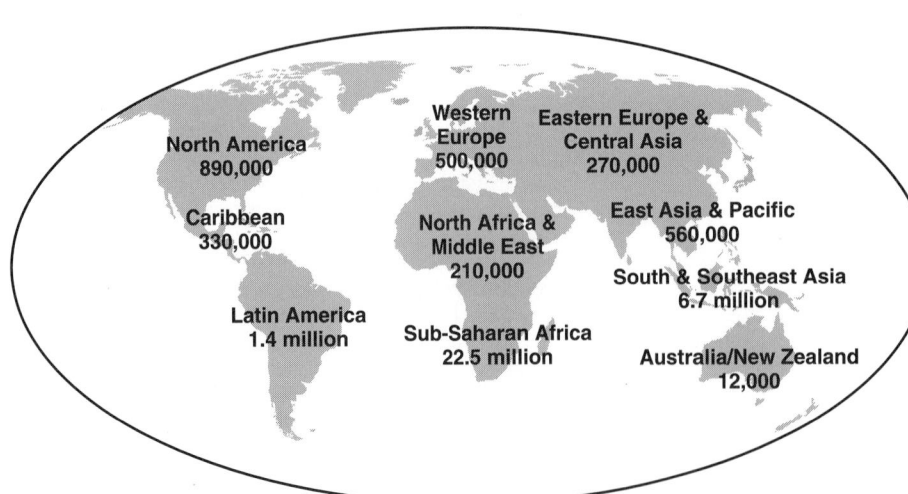

North America
890,000

Western Europe
500,000

Eastern Europe &
Central Asia
270,000

Caribbean
330,000

North Africa &
Middle East
210,000

East Asia & Pacific
560,000

Latin America
1.4 million

Sub-Saharan Africa
22.5 million

South & Southeast Asia
6.7 million

Australia/New Zealand
12,000

Figure **22–2.** Adults and children estimated to be living with HIV/AIDS at the end of 1998. Total: 33.4 million. (Source: UNAIDS.)

TABLE 22–3. Regional HIV/AIDS Statistics and Features (December 1998)

Region	Epidemic Started	Adults and Children Living With HIV/AIDS	Adults and Children Newly Infected With HIV	Adult Prevalence (%)*	Percent of HIV-Positive Adults Who Are Women	Main Mode(s) of Transmission† for Adults Living With HIV/AIDS
Sub-Saharan Africa	Late '70s–early '80s	22.5 million	4.0 million	8.0	50	Hetero
North Africa and Middle East	Late '80s	210,000	19,000	0.13	20	IDU, Hetero
South and Southeast Asia	Late '80s	6.7 million	1.2 million	0.69	25	Hetero
East Asia and Pacific	Late '80s	560,000	200,000	0.07	15	IDU, Hetero, MSM
Latin America	Late '70s–early '80s	1.4 million	160,000	0.57	20	MSM, IDU, Hetero
Caribbean	Late '70s–early '80s	330,000	45,000	1.96	35	Hetero, MSM
Eastern Europe and Central Asia	Early '90s	270,000	80,000	0.14	20	IDU, MSM
Western Europe	Late '70s–early '80s	500,000	30,000	0.25	20	MSM, IDU
North America	Late '70s–early '80s	890,000	44,000	0.56	20	MSM, IDU, Hetero
Australia and New Zealand	Late '70s–early '80s	12,000	600	0.1	5	MSM, IDU
TOTAL		33.4 million	5.8 million	1.1	43	

*The proportion of adults (15 to 49 years of age) living with HIV/AIDS in 1998, using 1997 population numbers.
†MSM (sexual transmission among men who have sex with men); IDU (transmission through injection drug use); Hetero (heterosexual transmission).

HIV infection is transmitted by sexual contact; from mother to child during pregnancy, delivery, and breast-feeding; and by injection drug use or other percutaneous needle exposure, transfusion of blood or blood products, or transplantation of infected organs or tissues. Heterosexual transmission is the predominant mode of transmission in the developing world, and accounts for over 70% of HIV infections worldwide. The heterosexual epidemic has been fueled by urbanization and other forms of population movement, which promote commercial sex and other STDs, with subsequent HIV epidemics in high-risk groups, e.g., sex workers and their clients. Secondary epidemics then develop in women of childbearing age and children, and in recipients of unscreened blood products. Injection drug use has also played an important role in the HIV epidemic in South and Southeast Asia. In Latin America and the Caribbean, HIV was initially transmitted primarily among homosexual and bisexual men, but later by heterosexual contact and by injection drug use. Among children, at least 90% of all HIV infections are transmitted from mother to child, with most of the remainder accounted for by transfusion of infected blood or blood products.

Global Surveillance of HIV and AIDS. Because the surveillance case definition for AIDS was introduced by CDC before serologic tests for HIV infection were available, it allows for some specific conditions to be considered indicative of AIDS in the absence of laboratory evidence of HIV infection. The greatly increased use of HIV testing has made the diagnosis of AIDS without concomitant diagnosis of HIV infection rare. Table 22–1 lists the major conditions considered AIDS-defining. Overall, surveillance for AIDS in industrialized countries has yielded higher-quality epidemiologic information than is available for any other condition.

In contrast, surveillance for AIDS in developing countries has been problematic. Lack of health care infrastructure, limited training of health care professionals, and difficulties in diagnosing AIDS-defining illnesses because of inadequate laboratory capacity for clinical diagnosis and HIV serologic testing have resulted in underdiagnosis of AIDS cases. Weak public health infrastructure, underreporting, and concerns about confidentiality and stigmatization have further hampered AIDS surveillance efforts. Although WHO developed clinical AIDS case definitions (Table 22–2) for adults and children, the sensitivity and specificity of these definitions are limited, particularly in areas that lack the capacity for HIV testing. Much of what we know about the severity of HIV-AIDS epidemics in the developing world is based on unlinked, anonymous HIV serosurveys of sentinel populations, e.g., blood donors and persons attending STD clinics, drug treatment centers, and antenatal clinics, where residual blood samples collected for other purposes are tested for HIV in an anonymous fashion. Although sentinel populations are not representative of the general population, serosurveys have been key in aiding our understanding of the trends in the HIV epidemic in many developing countries.

Regional Epidemiology of HIV-AIDS

Africa. Sub-Saharan Africa is the most heavily affected area of the world. Although accounting for <10% of the world's population, sub-Saharan Africa accounts for two thirds of all HIV-infected persons. Young adults are the most affected; over 8% of all Africans aged 15 to 49 years are infected with HIV. Because of high rates of HIV infection in young women, high fertility rates, and poor access to perinatal prevention methods, an estimated 90% of the world's perinatal HIV infections occur in Africa. The HIV epidemic in Africa has been fueled by male urban migration and by mobile populations (e.g., truck drivers and migrant workers having frequent contact with commercial sex workers) with subsequent spread to the general population. Male-to-male sex is not unknown but is considered uncommon. Although several African cities and ports are being recognized as important transit points for the international distribution of illegal drugs, HIV infection associated with injection drug use in Africa is also considered infrequent.

Rates of HIV infection vary widely across Africa, and the epidemic is at different stages of maturity in different countries. Urban areas of East and southern Africa are among the most severely affected, with 20 to 43% of women of childbearing age infected (Fig. 22–3). Recently, many areas of southern Africa have continued to experience increasing rates

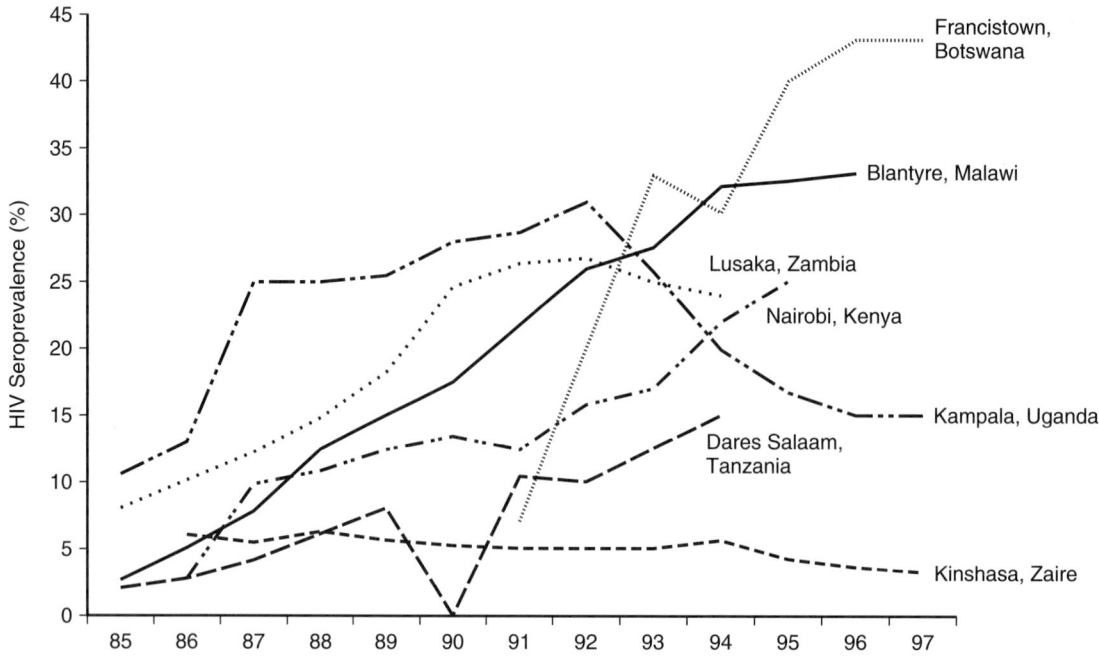

Figure 22–3. HIV seroprevalence among pregnant women in selected urban areas of Africa: 1985–1997. (Source: Health Studies Branch, U.S. Bureau of the Census.)

of HIV infection, whereas in eastern and central Africa a plateau in seroprevalence may have been reached. Uganda has shown a decline in seroprevalence over recent years, accompanying changes in reported sexual behaviors, and a strong national commitment to HIV education and prevention.

South and Southeast Asia. The HIV epidemic in Asia varies enormously by region, in terms of incidence, prevalence, and modes of transmission. In general, the epidemic is more recent in Asia than in Africa; many countries, e.g., Vietnam, China, and Myanmar, face emerging epidemics, primarily among injection drug users and commercial sex workers, with some early evidence of spread to the general population. In other countries, e.g., India and Cambodia, HIV may have been present longer but epidemics continue to escalate, fueled by commercial sex and injection drug use. Thailand suffered an explosive HIV epidemic in the late 1980s and early 1990s, introduced through two distinct outbreaks among commercial sex workers and persons using injection drugs. With a strong national "100% condom campaign," the nation is now seeing declines in HIV prevalence among several sentinel populations. Some areas of Southeast Asia, e.g., Indonesia, Malaysia, the Philippines, and Singapore, continue to have low seroprevalence rates. The reasons for such wide disparities between countries are incompletely understood.

Latin America and the Caribbean. In Latin America and the Caribbean, the HIV epidemic is also not uniform. Socially marginalized and economically challenged populations are often the most affected, including men who have sex with men and injection drug users. Spread to the heterosexual population has become more prominent in the Caribbean and in certain areas of Latin America, e.g., Honduras and Brazil.

Other Regions. Areas of Eastern Europe and the former Soviet Union have very recently been affected by a rapid rise in HIV infections, primarily among commercial sex workers and injection drug users. Epidemic increases of STDs have also been documented recently. In the midst of rapid political, social, and economic change, public health infrastructure is often not adequate to address such newly emerging epidemics.

Modes of HIV Transmission

Sexual Transmission. The estimated probability of HIV being transmitted by a single heterosexual contact is 0.03 to 0.09% for insertive and 0.05 to 0.15% for receptive vaginal intercourse. The risk of transmission, however, is modified by a number of virologic, host, and environmental factors. STDs facilitate HIV transmission. Genital ulcer disease (largely attributable to chancroid, syphilis, and herpes simplex) are highly prevalent in the tropics and significantly increase HIV infection risk. In addition, nonulcerative STDs, e.g., gonorrhea, chlamydial infection, and trichomoniasis, have been identified as risk factors for infection with HIV. STDs are believed to facilitate HIV transmission through disruption of normal barriers of the skin and genital mucosa, as well as by recruitment of CD4+ target cells to the affected genital area. In addition, more recent studies have demonstrated increased genital shedding of HIV by both men and women in the presence of ulcerative and nonulcerative STDs.

High plasma viral load, found to correlate with increased genital shedding of HIV, is also associated with increased risk of HIV transmission. Plasma viral load tends to be high soon after HIV infection and late in infection with loss of immune function. Male circumcision appears associated with a decreased risk of acquiring HIV infection, even when controlling for differences in sexual practices and other risk behaviors between circumcised and uncircumcised populations. Geographically, the highest seroprevalence areas of central and southern Africa are those areas where circumcision tends not to be practiced, although the public health implications of this observation remain unclear, and other factors may confound this ecologic association.

Mother-to-Child Transmission. Mother-to-child HIV transmission occurs during pregnancy (in utero), during labor and delivery (intrapartum), and postpartum via breast-feeding. Rates of perinatal transmission vary, generally ranging from 14 to 25% in industrialized countries and 25 to 40% in developing countries. The majority of infections occur around the time of labor and delivery. Although HIV has been found in fetal tissue as early as 8 weeks' gestation, in utero transmission of HIV is not a frequent event. Detection of HIV by polymerase chain reaction (PCR) at birth, believed to represent in utero transmission, is found in approximately one third of HIV-positive formula-fed infants. Studies among breast-feeding women in the Democratic Republic of the Congo and Rwanda found that an estimated 23% of HIV-infected children were infected in utero, 65% during the intrapartum and early postpartum period, and 12% in the late postpartum period. Breast-feeding, however, may make a considerably greater contribution to the risk of mother-to-child HIV transmission than previously believed. Studies in Kenya and the Ivory Coast suggest that as many as 12 to 40% of HIV-positive infants are infected by breast-feeding. Some middle-income countries have invested in the provision of formula for infants born to HIV-positive women. In Africa, however, where exclusive breast-feeding is often the norm and clean water is often not available, more work is needed to define if replacement feeding would be safe and acceptable. In many settings, considerable stigma is associated with HIV infection and avoidance of breast-feeding.

Factors associated with an increased risk of HIV transmission from mother to child include high maternal plasma viral load, low CD4+ count, presence of STDs and, in some studies, vitamin A deficiency. Prolonged rupture of membranes and increased exposure to blood and vaginal secretions during delivery, associated with invasive obstetric procedures, episiotomy, and scalp electrode placement, increase an infant's risk of HIV infection. Use of antiretroviral drugs is associated with decreased maternal plasma viral load and decreased risk of perinatal HIV transmission. Results of studies on the effects of cesarean section have been variable but generally have found an associated reduction in transmission. Neither vitamin A therapy nor vaginal disinfectants at the time of delivery affect perinatal transmission rates.

Transmission by Blood and Blood Products. In industrialized countries, recruitment and retention of low-risk blood donors, questioning of blood donors about risk behaviors ("donor deferral"), blood banking, and screening of blood donations with increasingly sensitive serologic tests have resulted in a very safe blood supply. In the developing world, however, this most preventable mode of HIV transmission may account for as much as 10% of all HIV infections. Multiple obstacles exist for the development and sustainability of effective blood safety programs, particularly in more economically disadvantaged areas. Adequate resources are often not available for blood collection, banking, and screening. Shortages of equipment, reagents, consumables (e.g., blood bags and needles) are common. It is often difficult to maintain a regular power supply and clean water. A study conducted in East Africa, for example, reported a national shortage of HIV test kits for a 4-week period. When test kits were available, 30% of HIV-positive donations were not removed from the blood supply due to poor laboratory techniques and record keeping, lack of adequate training and supervision, test kits stored and transported in ambient temperatures, and lack of adherence to universal screening.

Although transfusion use varies according to region and type of health care facility, young children often receive over half of all transfusions in malaria-endemic areas of Africa. Women of childbearing age are also frequent recipients of blood for treatment of severe anemia due to nutritional deficiencies and complications of pregnancy. A smaller proportion of transfusions are for trauma and other surgical conditions.

Patients with severe anemia in the tropics, particularly young children in malaria-endemic areas, are at high risk of death. Reliance on family donors, often used when adequate supplies of stored blood are not maintained, promotes collection from high-risk donors and does not provide blood to patients in a timely manner. Studies of transfused children in Kenya and the Ivory Coast found that transfusion was associated with decreased mortality only when used early in the course of hospitalization for severe anemia (hemoglobin < 5.0 g/dL) and when clinical signs of cardiac or respiratory distress were present. Adherence to these transfusion criteria would have reduced the rate of pediatric transfusions by half.

Transmission by Injections. Despite the frequent use of injections in developing countries, often with unsterile needles, little information is available about the contribution of percutaneous needle exposure to HIV transmission. Health care workers, who often receive little training in safe clinical practices, as well as laboratory staff are at risk for needlestick injury or other nosocomial exposures. In industrialized countries, the risk of acquiring HIV infection from a contaminated needlestick is approximately 3 per 1000. It is likely that in developing countries with high rates of HIV infection, some health care workers are acquiring HIV infection nosocomially.

NATURAL HISTORY AND CLINICAL FEATURES IN ADULTS

Pathophysiology and Immune Response. HIV antigen may appear transiently in the serum following acute infection, to reappear in some cases years later when immunosuppression is advanced. Seroconversion for antibody to HIV usually occurs within 3 to 6 weeks after infection, but in isolated instances has been delayed for many months. In advanced disease, HIV antibody levels may again fall and false negative serologic tests have been documented on rare occasions. A recent advance has been the development of assays to measure HIV RNA in plasma ("viral load"), which is a strong predictor of disease progression. It is likely that the amount of HIV RNA in plasma is also closely related to the degree of infectivity. At present, commercial assays have been produced only for HIV-1.

The immunologic hallmark of progressive HIV disease is decline in the CD4+ T-lymphocyte count. A sharp reduction in the CD4+ lymphocyte count can occur at the time of seroconversion, sometimes accompanied by clinical manifestations of immune deficiency, e.g., oral candidiasis. An infectious mononucleosis–like illness ("seroconversion illness") may also occur around this time, which is rarely diagnosed in resource-poor settings. High levels of viral load are found during this initial phase and the level at which HIV-RNA stabilizes ("set point") after acute infection influences the rate of subsequent progression of immune deficiency.

Clinical manifestations are closely related to the CD4+ T-lymphocyte count, which in industrialized countries declines in HIV-infected persons not on antiretroviral treatment at the rate of approximately 75/μL/yr. Symptoms of immune deficiency are absent at CD4+ lymphocyte counts of 500/μL and rare above 350/μL. As the level falls below this, general symptoms, e.g., weight loss and mucocutaneous manifestations, e.g., candidiasis, gradually develop and the risk for other opportunistic infections increases. The median CD4+ lymphocyte count in persons with HIV-associated tuberculosis in different studies has been of the order of 200 to 300/μL, and this common condition is one of the more aggressive diseases in terms of its incidence at relatively preserved immune function. Other bacterial infections, e.g., pneumococcal disease, also tend to occur relatively early (as well as later in the course of the illness), and there is a predictable and increasing susceptibility to different conditions as immune deficiency progresses. Although a substantial proportion of persons may have no symptoms until later, the risk of major disease and death is high when the CD4+ lymphocyte count falls below 100 to 150/μL. In Africa, patients dying of HIV/AIDS have CD4+ T-lymphocyte counts of 50 to 100/μL, whereas in industrialized countries patients with access to therapy for opportunistic infections die with counts close to zero.

From HIV Infection to AIDS. Although it is often stated that progression from asymptomatic HIV infection to AIDS is more rapid in Africa than in the industrialized world, there are few data to support this statement. Few long-term cohort studies have been conducted in developing countries, and even fewer with persons whose dates of infection were known accurately. Assessment of natural history is further complicated by the varying frequency in different regions of AIDS-defining illnesses, the different levels of immune deficiency at which these occur, and the variable standards of prophylaxis available to HIV-infected persons in different regions. Progression of immune deficiency is usually fastest in infants and older persons and slowest in adolescents and young adults.

The median period to AIDS in seroincident cohorts in the industrialized world has been about 10 years. The reported median times to AIDS in the few seroincident studies that have been performed in Africa among HIV-1–infected persons range from 2 to 7.5 years, but the possible reasons for this shorter interval are diverse. A study comparing the progression of immune deficiency and disease progression in African and non-African patients in London showed no significant differences in the natural history of disease in the two populations. There is currently no evidence that differences exist in the natural histories of infection with any of the different HIV subtypes. The progression of immune deficiency and disease in persons infected with HIV-2 is significantly slower than that in persons with HIV-1 infections.

Despite uncertainty about differences in incubation periods for AIDS in industrialized compared with developing countries, it is clear that once persons have AIDS, survival is significantly worse in resource-poor settings. Median survival in the industrialized world before the advent of highly active antiretroviral therapy has been of the order of 12 to 18 months, but this is variable according to the country of study and the nature of the AIDS-defining condition, and is now longer in patients receiving modern antiretroviral therapy. In developing countries, survival after an AIDS diagnosis is usually less than 6 months. The possible reasons for these international differences are many but late presentation and lack of access to diagnostic and treatment facilities are undoubtedly relevant.

Geographic Pathology and Spectrum of Disease in Adults. It was evident from early in the epidemic that the clinical and pathologic manifestations of HIV disease differ considerably in different countries; relevant factors influencing the local spectrum of disease are shown in Table 22–4.

General Features and Opportunistic Infections. Diarrhea is common in immunosuppressed HIV-infected persons everywhere. The causes, apart from direct HIV infection of intestinal mucosa, include many opportunistic infections and the systemic effects of tuberculosis. Relevant infections include *Cryptosporidium parvum*, *Isospora belli*, microsporidial infections, *Leishmania*, and cytomegalovirus (CMV) infection. All are documented in all continents, although *I. belli* is mainly restricted to South and Central America and parts of Africa. Cryptosporidiosis is common everywhere, and microsporidiosis—although difficult to diagnose—has been present in >20% of advanced HIV-infected patients with diarrhea in the United States, Europe, and Africa.

The major "standard" AIDS-defining diseases (Table 22–1,

TABLE 22–4. Determinants of the Local Spectrum of HIV Disease

Age and sex
Route of HIV transmission
Race/ethnicity
Diet
Type of HIV
Acquired community infections
Acquired latent infections
Medical factors, e.g., prophylaxis of opportunistic infections, access to treatment of opportunistic diseases, access to antiretroviral chemotherapy

CDC criteria) characterizing HIV disease occur globally, but in very different proportions. This variation is not only between countries and continents but within nations, according to socioeconomic criteria. Table 22–5 shows the similarities and contrasts between opportunistic diseases in a population well-served by medical care and with high living standards (the United States) and a population without such benefits (Abidjan, the Ivory Coast, in West Africa).

Certain diseases occur with similar frequency: cryptococcosis, bacterial pneumonia, and CMV infection (although the severity is greater outside of Africa, particularly in rates of CMV encephalitis). In industrialized countries, substantial variations occur in disease frequency by gender, race/ethnicity, and drug use. Certain diseases are notably more frequent in resource-poor settings: tuberculosis, both systemic and with meningitis; bacteremia with nontyphoid *Salmonella* and pneumococcal infections; and the HIV wasting syndrome ("slim disease," characterized by wasting, chronic diarrhea, and fever; Fig. 22–4), some of which may be associated with occult tuberculosis. The overwhelming importance of tuberculosis in HIV disease is best documented in Africa but extends to other resource-poor settings. Published autopsy studies from India show systemic tuberculosis in up to two thirds of HIV-infected patients, with gastrointestinal tuberculosis in 14% and central nervous system (CNS) involvement in 12%. In the later stages of HIV disease, the form of tuberculosis is disseminated and multibacillary.

TABLE 22–5. Prevalence of Specific Diseases in HIV-Positive Persons at Autopsy, West Africa and North America

	West Africa (%)	United States (%)
Systemic tuberculosis	37	8
Pyogenic pneumonia	29	24
CMV infection	19	23
Toxoplasmosis	18	7
Bacteremia	16	—
Kaposi sarcoma	8	22
TB meningitis	7	—
Bacterial meningitis	5	—
HIV encephalitis/dementia	4	10
Nocardiosis	4	—
Lymphoma	3	7
Cryptococcus	3	5
Pneumocystis	3	45
Mycobacterium avium	2	25
Wasting syndrome	40	24

CMV, cytomegalovirus; TB, tuberculosis.
From Lucas SB, Hounnou A, Peacock C, et al: The mortality and pathology of HIV infection in a West African city. AIDS 7:1569, 1993; and Chan ISF, Neaton JD, Saravolatz LD, et al: Frequencies of opportunistic diseases prior to death among HIV-infected persons. AIDS 9:1145, 1995.

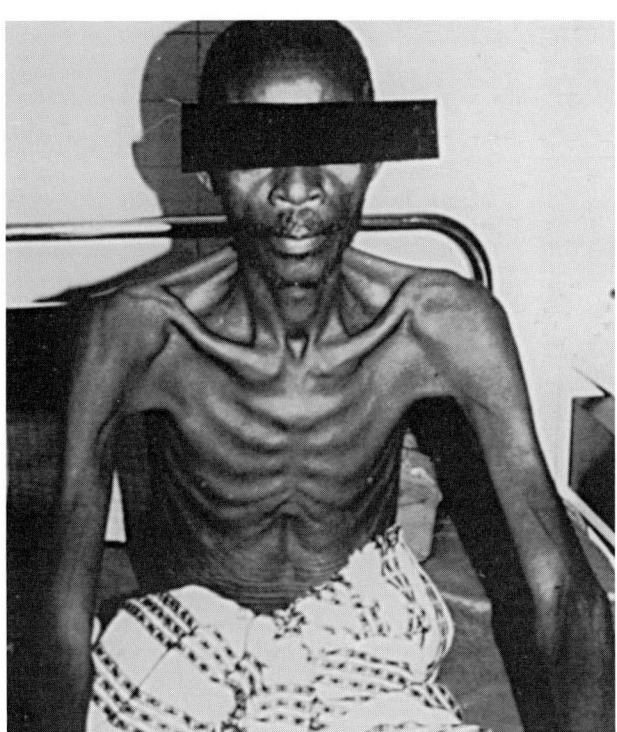

Figure 22–4. African AIDS: a patient with AIDS from the Ivory Coast. Profound weight loss, chronic diarrhea, fever, and oral candidiasis are the most common manifestations of AIDS in Africa. In Uganda, the term "slim" has been widely used to describe the disease. Weight loss exceeds that seen in almost all other diseases.

Disseminated infection with *Mycobacterium avium* complex and pneumonia due to *Pneumocystis carinii* are unquestionably less frequent in HIV-infected patients in Africa and other resource-poor settings despite the fact that both infections are prevalent in the environment. The reason may relate to survival; to develop pneumocystosis and disseminated *M. avium* infection requires a persistent low cell-mediated immunity, typically with a CD4+ lymphocyte count <50/µL. This explanation is not completely satisfactory, however, because toxoplasmosis occurs with high incidence in some settings and is also associated with advanced immune deficiency. The prevalence of latent infection with *Toxoplasma gondii* varies geographically according to dietary habits (eating raw or undercooked meat) and is highest in France and West Africa. Toxoplasmosis manifests as cerebral lesions, usually with focal neurologic signs or epilepsy, sometimes leading to coma. In parts of Africa with high rates of latent infection, cerebral toxoplasmosis is over 10 times more frequent than the other main cause of cerebral focal lesions, lymphoma. Lymphoma (high-grade B cell, mostly related to Epstein-Barr virus infection) is more frequent in industrialized countries, again perhaps related to survival duration.

The prevalence of Kaposi sarcoma is highly variable globally, depending both on sexual behavior (high rates occur among men who have sex with men, low rates among injection drug users) and geography. Classic, endemic Kaposi sarcoma in HIV-negative persons is most common in central African countries (Zambia, Democratic Republic of the Congo, Zimbabwe, Uganda, Rwanda, Burundi). HIV-associated Kaposi sarcoma, which is much more aggressive and disseminated (Figs. 22–5 and 22–6), is most frequent in these same areas and is less common in western and southern African countries. It is uncertain how this heterogeneity re-

lates to levels of infection with the putative causative virus of Kaposi sarcoma, human herpesvirus 8 (HHV8). Kaposi sarcoma is uncommon in Asia. Other frequent skin lesions and mucosal lesions include varicella zoster (sometimes multidermatomal, sometimes threatening vision by involvement of the ophthalmic branch of the trigeminal nerve); candidiasis (oral, esophageal, and vaginal); and pruriginous dermatitis, an initially papular rash that leaves pigmented, macular lesions (Fig. 22–7).

Certain opportunistic diseases are geographically restricted. Visceral leishmaniasis occurs in parts of sub-Saharan Africa, around the Mediterranean Sea, on the Indian subcontinent, and in South America. Where it coincides with HIV infection, an aggressive form of visceral leishmaniasis develops in co-infected people. In Southeast Asia, infection with the fungus *Penicillium marneffei* occurs. It is an intramacrophage infection and is frequently encountered as a systemic infection in HIV-infected people, notably in Thailand. HIV co-infection with other microbial agents that infect macrophages throughout the body (such as *Leishmania*, *Histoplasma capsulatum*, and *P. marneffei*), cause multiorgan disease, including skin lesions. *H. capsulatum* is widely distributed in the southern United States, the tropics, and subtropics, but is absent from Europe. Where prevalent, the latent infection recrudesces in late HIV disease, causing multiorgan damage. All these infections may be imported by HIV-infected travelers into nonendemic countries.

HIV encephalitis is much more commonly diagnosed in industrialized countries than in Africa, with South American surveys indicating intermediate levels of prevalence. The reasons for these differences may also relate to differences in late-stage survival. The relationship of the pathologic encephalitis to the HIV-associated dementia complex is much debated, and other subtle neuropathologic phenomena may underlie the dementia.

Route of HIV Transmission, Gender, and Age. The route of HIV infection and demographic factors, e.g., age and gender, influence subsequent clinical disease. Pediatric disease differs from that in adults because of the innate immaturity of the immune system in young children as well as the limited opportunity for exposure to many pathogens. HIV-infected

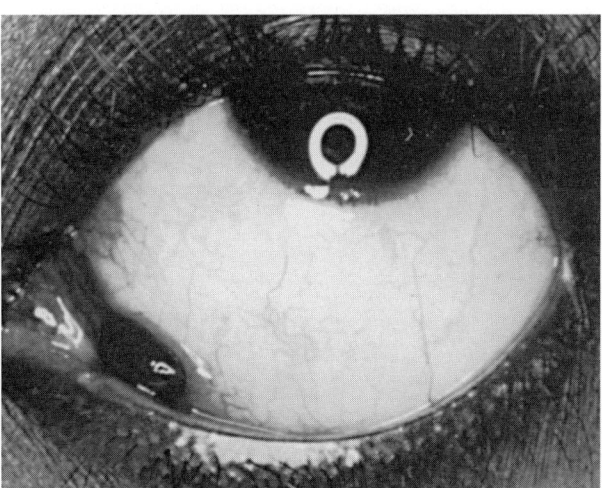

Figure 22–5. Kaposi sarcoma affecting the lower eyelid. Kaposi sarcoma may appear anywhere on the body. Careful examination of the whole skin and all mucous membranes is required for detection of the typical lesions. These are red-violet when involving the mucosa, and brown-violet on black skin. Occasionally, external lesions are absent despite extensive visceral involvement.

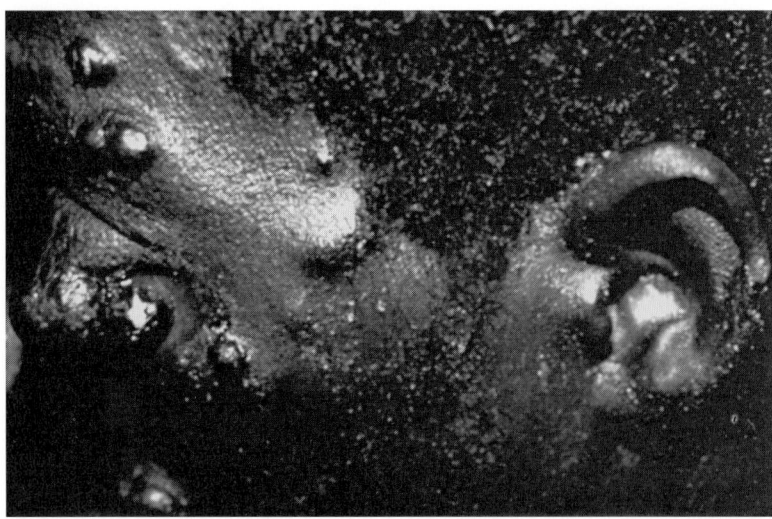

Figure 22–6. Kaposi sarcoma nodules on the face. Extensive nodular involvement of the face is seen in this patient with disseminated Kaposi sarcoma secondary to HIV infection. AIDS-related Kaposi sarcoma in Africa does not always produce these aggressive appearances; it sometimes resembles the classic variety of the tumor.

persons with hemophilia rarely develop Kaposi sarcoma, which is also uncommon in injection drug users. Conversely, drug users frequently develop systemic bacterial infections, in part from the use of infected needles. Men who have sex with men are more likely to acquire human papillomavirus (HPV) infection and to develop anal neoplasia; they are also more likely to acquire other gastrointestinal infections transmitted by feco-oral contact.

The systemic disease patterns in women with advanced HIV differ slightly from those in men, with Kaposi sarcoma being less frequent. Gynecologic disease, e.g., pelvic inflammatory disease, is more severe and frequent in women with HIV infection. Cervical intraepithelial neoplasia is more frequent in women with HIV, reflecting the increased frequency of HPV infections that predispose to malignancy. However, there is little or no evidence that invasive carcinoma of the cervix is more frequent among women with HIV. Particularly striking is the lack of an epidemic of HIV-associated cervical carcinoma in Africa, where the tumor was already a major

cause of cancer mortality before the HIV pandemic. It may be that women with HIV are dying before the invasive disease develops.

Viral Type. HIV-1 is the dominant global infection and most clinicopathologic descriptions pertain to it. HIV-2 infection progresses more slowly from infection to disease and death than HIV-1, although there is substantial variation. Once severe immune deficiency has developed, the pattern of HIV-2 disease is similar to that observed in HIV-1 infection. However, one study in West Africa showed a marked excess of HIV encephalitis among HIV-2–infected cadavers. This is compatible with longer survival in an advanced immune deficiency state for persons infected with HIV-2, although an alternate explanation is that the two viruses are not equally neurotropic.

Host Genetic Factors. Although environmental factors are probably more important overall, there are a few examples of host genetic factors influencing disease progression or presentation. For example, different host co-receptors may

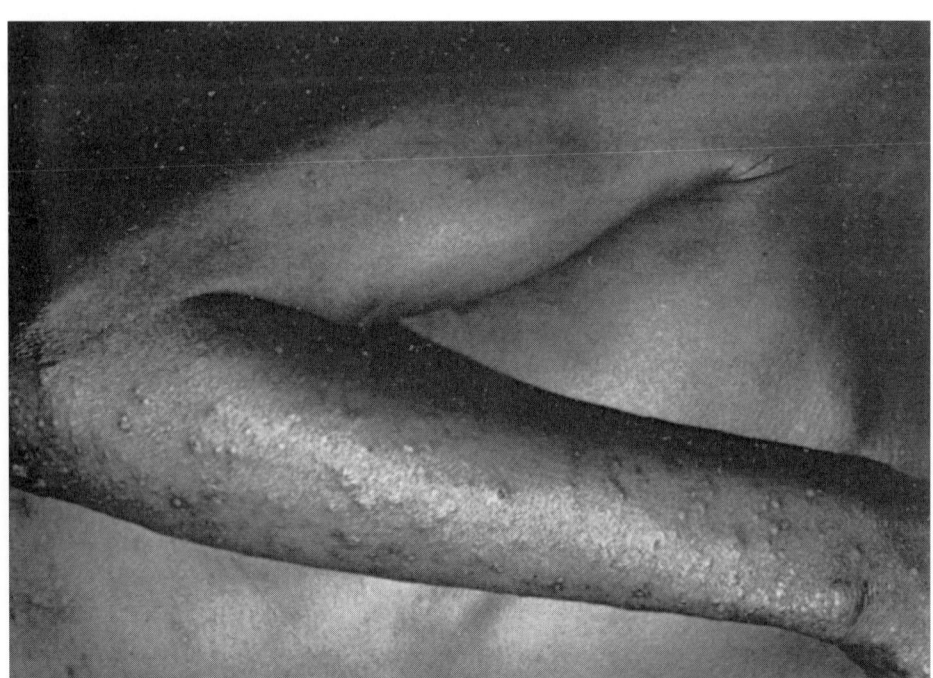

Figure 22–7. Pruriginous dermatitis. A condition of unknown cause, it is seen in many African AIDS patients and is highly predictive of HIV infections. Initially, itchy papules, which eventually leave a hyperpigmented, macular rash, appear. Scratching probably affects the appearance of the lesions. Histologic features are nonspecific.

be associated with variability in initial transmissibility and subsequent disease progression. A deletion in the chemokine receptor CCR-5 has been associated with lower susceptibility to infection and slower progression. This deletion mutation has to date only been found in low frequency among Caucasians.

Although opportunistic infections and tumors may affect the kidney in all populations, HIV-associated nephropathy (HIVAN) is essentially restricted to persons of black African race or ethnicity. This lesion comprises a progressive glomerulosclerosis, interstitial inflammation, and tubular dilatation. Clinically, it presents as nephrotic syndrome and renal failure. The etiology is unclear, but HIV is detectable in glomeruli and tubules; presumably, racial genetic determinants are required for this lesion to progress. It occurs in industrialized as well as tropical countries and is not related to malaria.

Prophylaxis and Antiretroviral Therapy. In view of the importance of tuberculosis and bacterial infections in HIV-infected adults in resource-poor countries, the opportunities for simple prophylaxis are being evaluated using treatments, e.g., isoniazid and co-trimoxazole. If effective use becomes widespread, there might be a shift toward the patterns of disease observed in industrialized countries. In countries of southern Europe, where tuberculosis is prevalent but there is access to care, the spectrum of disease associated with HIV is intermediate between that in developing and other industrialized countries.

In industrialized countries, highly active antiretroviral therapy (HAART) has reduced the incidence of AIDS in HIV-infected persons and increased their survival. Substantial side effects can occur and include pancreatitis, neuropathy, bone marrow suppression, hepatotoxicity, myopathy, lipodystrophy, hyperlipidemia, and atherosclerosis. By increasing immune function, HAART has been effective in preventing and treating many opportunistic infections, e.g., CMV disease, microsporidiosis, cryptosporidiosis, and JC virus infection; it may reverse lesions of Kaposi sarcoma, and it is expected to have an impact on the incidence of tuberculosis. Another manifestation of HAART is immune restoration disease, in which HAART-induced immunologic reactivity can precipitate clinical lesions from previously inapparent infections; the most frequent manifestation of this is *M. avium* lymphadenitis.

Relation to Endemic Tropical Diseases. Study of the relationship between HIV infection and the classic tropical diseases has been limited but some further insights have been gained recently.

Malaria. Malaria does not act as an opportunistic disease and there is no evidence that the clinical course in HIV-positive patients with malaria is different from that in HIV-negative persons. An important indirect association has been the transmission of HIV through blood transfusions for malarial anemia, especially in childhood. HIV infection may be associated with increased frequency and severity of *Plasmodium falciparum* parasitemia in pregnancy, and with increased frequency of malarial infection of the placenta and the newborn. It has also been suggested that placental malaria may facilitate the transmission of HIV from mother to child but this remains unproved.

Leishmaniasis. Visceral leishmaniasis (due to infection with *Leishmania donovani, L. infantum,* or *L. chagasi*) is increased in frequency in patients infected with HIV. Clinical features are mostly typical but case reports exist of disease affecting unusual sites, with prominence of intestinal disease. Relapse after treatment is frequent and maintenance therapy (e.g., with monthly pentavalent antimony) is usually required. Individual cases of cutaneous leishmaniasis (due to *L. aethiopica*) in HIV-infected persons have been reported but this has received little study. The majority of cases of leishmanial infections in HIV-infected persons have been reported from the Mediterranean littoral (France, Spain, Portugal). As with all latent infections, disease may present long after initial exposure.

Leprosy. Clinical leprosy is no more frequent in HIV-positive than in HIV-negative persons. The clinical and histologic expression of disease at presentation, particularly the frequency of paucibacillary and multibacillary disease, is similar in both groups. One interaction between HIV and *Mycobacterium leprae* that is yet to be confirmed is an increased frequency or severity of upgrading reversal reactions. There are several case reports of this paradoxical phenomenon.

Trypanosomiasis. Several studies in Africa have examined whether an association exists between African human trypanosomiasis and HIV infection, all with negative results. Several cases have been reported of Chagas' disease in HIV-infected persons but it is uncertain whether the incidence of this disease or its clinical manifestations are altered by HIV infection.

Filariasis and Schistosomiasis. Abundant epidemiologic opportunity exists for filariasis and schistosomiasis to occur in persons with HIV infection. No evidence exists of an increased incidence or altered clinical course for these diseases.

NATURAL HISTORY AND CLINICAL FEATURES IN CHILDREN

UNAIDS has estimated that 590,000 children <15 years old acquired HIV infection in 1998, that by the end of that year 1.2 million children were living with HIV-AIDS, and that since the beginning of the epidemic some 3.2 million children have died from AIDS. A major problem in assessing the magnitude of the epidemic of pediatric AIDS globally is the lack of a sensitive and specific, simple case definition for use in resource-poor countries. The symptoms and signs of HIV disease in children resemble those of many common pediatric problems in developing countries, and many children die before HIV infection can be reliably diagnosed serologically, because maternal antibody passively transferred transplacentally can persist for 12 to 15 months. Although data are limited, spontaneous abortion and stillbirth appear to be more frequent among HIV-infected women; HIV-infected women tend to have infants of lower birth weight; and women with advanced HIV disease have reduced fertility.

Studies in the United States and Europe have defined two extremes of pediatric disease, possibly relating to the time of infection and severity of HIV infection in the mother during pregnancy. Infants with a rapid course, accounting for about one quarter of HIV-infected infants, show fast progression of immune deficiency, with high rates of encephalopathy and severe opportunistic infections, e.g., *P. carinii* pneumonia early in life; approximately half die before the age of 3 years. Children with the slower course of infection survive considerably longer, and suffer milder complications, e.g., lymphocytic interstitial pneumonitis (LIP) and bacterial infections. The course of pediatric HIV disease in industrialized countries is being altered by antiretroviral therapy.

A surprising finding from autopsy studies in West and southern Africa has been the finding of *P. carinii* pneumonia as a cause of as many as 20% of HIV-infected infant deaths. The spectrum of disease in African children with HIV infection is relatively similar to that in HIV-negative children. In Abidjan, the Ivory Coast, six syndromic presentations accounted for more than 80% of HIV-positive as well as HIV-negative pediatric admissions to the city's university hospitals. These were (1) acute respiratory infection, (2) malnutrition, (3) diarrheal disease, (4) anemia, (5) malaria, and (6) meningitis. Malnutrition and respiratory infections were significantly more frequent in HIV-infected children, and ma-

TABLE 22–6. Major Clinical Features of Pediatric HIV Disease in Developing Countries

Pneumonia
Encephalopathy
Failure to thrive, growth failure, delayed puberty
Persistent fever
Parotitis
Recurrent gastroenteritis
Lymphadenopathy
Tuberculosis
Chronic lung disease
Kaposi sarcoma

laria was proportionately less frequent as a cause of hospitalization. Common clinical features (Table 22–6) are included in the pediatric AIDS case definition proposed by the WHO (Table 22–2), but the predictive value of this definition is limited.

HIV-infected children frequently show low weight for age, marasmus being more common than kwashiorkor. Growth retardation and delayed psychomotor development are frequent. Common childhood infections, e.g., measles, varicella, and other viral illnesses, are more frequent and more severe. Tuberculosis is undoubtedly more frequent in HIV-infected children than in HIV negatives but does not have the same importance in children as in HIV-infected adults, possibly because many children die before ever having been infected with *M. tuberculosis*. A syndrome common in African children frequently mistaken for tuberculosis is LIP, which typically occurs in the second year of life and is characterized by parotid enlargement, lymphadenopathy, and abnormal chest radiographs with diffuse pulmonary infiltrates.

Malignancies associated with HIV are not as common in children as in adults. Lymphoma associated with HIV is rare in children, and Burkitt lymphoma is not increased in frequency in the HIV infected. Kaposi sarcoma has increased in the pediatric age group since the onset of the HIV-AIDS epidemic, and there are case reports of mother-child couples having Kaposi sarcoma.

Infant mortality in children born to HIV-infected women in Africa is increased approximately three- to fivefold, and overall infant mortality is therefore strongly influenced by the local prevalence of maternal HIV infection. In children shown to be HIV-infected themselves, infant mortality is increased as much as 10-fold. One estimate from West Africa is that about 50% of HIV-1–infected children are dead by the age of 2 years, and probably three fourths of HIV-infected children in Africa die before their fifth birthday. Early death in uninfected children born to HIV-positive women was slightly increased in some African studies.

Data on the pathology of pediatric HIV disease are relatively scarce. Table 22–7 compares autopsy findings concerning the frequency of different respiratory diseases in HIV-infected children in Africa and Asia. Pneumocystosis is an important HIV-associated lung disease in children and is strikingly absent in children who are not immunosuppressed. Bacterial and CMV infections are also frequent. The rarity of tuberculosis at autopsy in children dying of AIDS correlating with the 1 to 2% annual incidence of *M. tuberculosis* infection in such resource-poor countries suggests that much of the clinically and radiologically diagnosed tuberculosis in HIV-infected children may be due to other pathologies.

Comparative information on the cerebral pathology of HIV disease in children is more scarce. Studies from the United States emphasize the frequency of HIV encephalitis, with a prevalence of up to 38% in combined series of children (median age of 30 months); toxoplasmosis is rare; and cerebral lymphoma may be present in up to 5%. Conversely, in West Africa (children with median age of 18 months), HIV-encephalitis and toxoplasmosis were uncommon (6% and 4%, respectively), lymphoma was absent, and bacterial meningitis was more common (14%).

DIAGNOSIS. Case definitions for AIDS were introduced for surveillance purposes; for clinical work the essential questions concern the diagnosis of HIV infection and the staging of HIV disease. Although symptoms and signs may be highly suggestive of HIV disease, it is desirable whenever possible that HIV infection be serologically diagnosed.

Serologic Testing. HIV testing has become far more widely available in developing countries than had been predicted when tests were first introduced. The most common test system used is an enzyme immunoassay (EIA). Although specific EIAs exist for HIV-1 and HIV-2, for most purposes mixed tests capable of recognizing both infections are appropriate. Although modern tests are highly sensitive and specific, the predictive value of a positive test is nevertheless related to the prevalence of the infection in the population, and it is conventional to submit positive specimens to a supplemental ("confirmatory") assay. The most widely used supplemental test has been the Western blot (WB). It has been recognized in recent years that supplemental testing can be satisfactorily performed using simple tests including other EIAs or synthetic peptide–based tests, instead of the more expensive WB test (Table 22–8). The optimal testing strategy depends to a large extent on the specific purposes for which testing is being performed. Other advances in testing technology include the development of rapid tests that can be used in combination and can provide results as reliable as traditional strategies, that take a few minutes to perform, and that can usually be done without access to running water or electricity. In addition, assays have been developed that can be performed on saliva and urine. Sero-

TABLE 22–7. Respiratory Disease at Autopsy in HIV-Infected Children in Africa (Three Cities) and Thailand (One City)

Location	Bulawayo (1)	Durban (2)	Chiang Mai (3)	Abidjan (4)
Mean age	10 mo	4.3 mo	NA	18 mo
PCP	16%	52%	55%	14%
CMV	7%	52%	48%	31%
TB	5%	3%	3%	1%
LIP	9%	NA	NA	1%
Bacterial infection	87%	26%	NA	42%

CMV, cytomegalovirus; LIP, lymphoid interstitial pneumonitis; NA, not available; PCP, *Pneumocystis carinii* pneumonia; TB, tuberculosis.
Sources: (1) Ikeogu MO, Wolf B, Mathe S: Pulmonary manifestations of HIV serpositivity and malnutrition in Zimbabwe. Arch Dis Child 76:124, 1997. (2) Jeena P, Coovadia HM, Chrystal V: Pneumocystis carinii pneumonia and CMV infections in severely ill, HIV-infected African infants. Ann Trop Paediatr 16:361, 1996. (3) Bhoopat L, Thamprasert K, Chaiwun B, et al: Histopathologic spectrum of AIDS-associated lesions in Maharaj Nakorn Chiang Mai Hospital. Asian Pac J Allergy Immunol 12:95, 1994. (4) Lucas SB, Peacock CS, Hounnou A, et al: Disease in children infected with HIV in Abidjan. Br Med J 312:335, 1996.

TABLE 22–8. Algorithms for Serologic Diagnosis of HIV Infection in Resource-Poor Settings

Strategy	Application
(I) Single EIA or rapid test	Transfusion Surveillance if HIV prevalence > 10% Surveillance if HIV prevalence ≤ 10%
(II) Screening EIA or rapid test. If negative, specimen is considered negative. If positive, a supplemental EIA or rapid test is performed using a different antigen preparation or test principle. If supplemental assay is negative, specimen is considered negative; if supplemental assay is positive, specimen is considered positive.	HIV diagnosis in patients with clinical symptoms and signs HIV diagnosis in asymptomatic persons if HIV prevalence > 10%
(III) As algorithm II, but requires a third test based on different antigen or test principle if second assay is positive. If all 3 tests are positive, the specimen is considered positive. A specimen positive on the first 2 tests but negative on the third is considered equivocal.	HIV diagnosis in asymptomatic persons if HIV prevalence ≤ 10%

EIA, enzyme immunoassay.
From World Health Organization: Global Programme on AIDS: Recommendations for the selection and use of HIV antibody tests. Wkly Epidemiol Rec 67:142, 1992.

logic tests also exist for HIV antigen but these are of limited use clinically.

Virus Culture and Molecular Diagnosis. Virus culture remains the gold standard for proof of infection with any virus, but is generally restricted to research and plays no role in routine clinical work. Gene amplification using the PCR has become widely used for research, e.g., for diagnosis of infection before the development of specific antibody and for the diagnosis of HIV infection in infancy. PCR assays exist for integrated proviral DNA as well as for HIV RNA. Commercially available assays exist for the quantification of HIV-1 RNA in plasma using PCR or other techniques, although these may not perform equally well for all non-B subtypes; such techniques are not currently available commercially for HIV-2.

Immunologic Staging. The most important laboratory marker of the degree of immune deficiency is the CD4+ T-lymphocyte count, which is usually measured indirectly using flow cytometry to determine the proportion of total lymphocytes that bear the CD4+ receptor. The equipment and reagents are expensive and relatively complex, and in many resource-poor settings are available only in privileged research settings. Simpler, low-technology assays for CD4+ T-lymphocyte counts have been introduced but not widely assessed or used. The total lymphocyte count is lowered in severe immune deficiency, as is the hemoglobin level. Other markers associated with immune deficiency are increased serum levels of β_2-microglobulin and neopterin, but these are rarely used clinically.

Diagnosis of HIV Infection in Infancy. Diagnosis of HIV infection in the newborn is complicated by the fact that maternal antibodies to HIV cross the placenta. HIV antibody tests in children are only indicative of HIV infection with certainty after 15 to 18 months of age, following loss of maternal antibody. HIV-1 p24 antigen testing of newborns is sometimes insensitive because of antigen-antibody complex formation. PCR testing at 6 months of age, or 3 months after cessation of breast-feeding, is the gold standard for diagnosis of HIV infection in children <15 months of age. Early diagnosis is important in areas where prophylaxis of pediatric opportunistic infections is recommended.

The clinical case definition for AIDS in children, analogous to the clinical case definition for adults, was introduced by WHO for surveillance purposes (Table 22–2). Unfortunately, because of the low sensitivity and positive predictive value of this clinical case definition, its utility is very limited. The difficulty of early diagnosis in developing countries, com-

bined with high mortality of HIV-infected infants, means many children die of HIV disease, especially in Africa, without HIV infection being diagnosed.

MANAGEMENT. The complexity of HIV-AIDS care in industrialized countries cannot be replicated in most developing nations, and care for HIV disease in resource-poor settings has been one of the most neglected aspects of the HIV-AIDS epidemic. In situations in which voluntary testing for HIV infection is scarce, patients mostly present with advanced disease. Studies have shown that most patients hospitalized with HIV-AIDS for the first time generally have severe immune deficiency (median CD4+ lymphocyte counts <200/μL) and suffer high mortality rates at first hospitalization. Expectations of what can be offered to such patients must be realistic, because whatever their presenting opportunistic illness, their degree of immunodeficiency determines to a major degree what the outcome will be.

Care Across the Continuum. This concept emphasizes four essential aspects of care—nursing, counseling, medical treatment and prophylaxis, and social support—but few countries have addressed the needs for HIV-AIDS care in an organized manner. Despite this, however, there have been outstanding examples of commitment and innovation by some nongovernmental, religious, and voluntary organizations, and approaches to care will continue to evolve.

Syndromic HIV-AIDS Care. Because of the difficulties in making specific diagnoses, guidelines for syndromic management of HIV disease have been developed covering issues, e.g., indications for hospitalization of HIV-infected persons (Table 22–9), essential drugs for HIV-AIDS care in resource-poor settings (Table 22–10), and providing algorithmic flow charts for diagnosis and treatment for specific conditions depending on the level of care available. These guidelines

TABLE 22–9. Indications for Hospitalization of Patients With HIV-AIDS in Resource-Poor Settings

1. Investigations not feasible as outpatient (e.g., lumbar puncture, surgical biopsy)
2. Severe illness
3. Special treatment not feasible as outpatient (e.g., regular intravenous fluids)
4. Special nursing or rehabilitation requirements (e.g., altered level of consciousness, physiotherapy)
5. Special social reasons (e.g., to give respite to regular caregivers, intensive palliative care)

TABLE 22–10. Example of Essential Drugs List for HIV-AIDS in Resource-Poor Settings (Excluding Antiretroviral Drugs)

Antituberculosis drugs
Antibiotics (specific, e.g., penicillin and metronidazole; broad spectrum, e.g., ampicillin)
Co-trimoxazole (antibiotic and prophylactic against PCP, toxoplasmosis, and bacterial infections)
Antifungal agents (topical, e.g., nystatin; oral, e.g., ketoconazole, fluconazole)
Corticosteroids (e.g., prednisolone)
Antihistamines (e.g., chlorpheniramine)
Analgesics (e.g., codeine, aspirin, acetaminophen, morphine)
Antidiarrheal agents (e.g., codeine phosphate)
Sedatives (e.g., chlorpromazine, diazepam)
Gentian violet
Hydrocortisone cream
Calamine lotion
Intravenous fluids (normal saline, 5% dextrose)

PCP, *Pneumocystis carinii* pneumonia.

have not been widely implemented or evaluated, however. Organized HIV-AIDS services are rare in developing countries and patients tend to be cared for by generalists or internists. In some settings, clinical subspecialists follow patients; pulmonary medicine specialists, for example, tend to see patients with pneumonia, gastroenterologists care for patients with chronic diarrhea.

Home Care. Overcrowding of hospital wards and shortage of facilities led many groups to propose that persons with HIV-AIDS remain in their own homes, involving the family and community in nursing and terminal care. An advantage of this approach is that it can focus on the overall social, spiritual, and material needs of persons ill with HIV-AIDS, rather than just on their medical conditions. Potential disadvantages of home care include its expense, especially when home care support teams must travel large distances, and the increased demands imposed on the usual caregivers, who invariably are women.

Prophylaxis for Opportunistic Infections. Because a substantial proportion of deaths in persons with HIV-AIDS in developing countries is attributable to conditions for which prophylaxis might be effective, it is surprising that more attention has not been paid to this topic (Table 22–11).

Tuberculosis. The results of several placebo-controlled trials indicate that prophylaxis with isoniazid (INH) significantly reduces tuberculosis incidence in HIV-infected persons with a positive tuberculin skin test. Because tuberculin testing is unlikely to be feasible on a wide scale in most developing country settings, INH prophylaxis may be offered to all HIV-infected persons after exclusion of active tuberculosis. The duration of protection is uncertain but likely depends on the

risk of reinfection with *M. tuberculosis;* although in the future lifelong prophylaxis may be recommended, based on current knowledge and recommendations, it seems reasonable to advise a 6-month course of therapy.

Pneumocystosis, Toxoplasmosis, and Bacterial Infections. Although pneumocystosis is uncommon in HIV-infected persons in Asia and sub-Saharan Africa, toxoplasmosis is frequent in some settings, and bacterial infections are especially common, including those with gram-negative organisms (particularly nontyphoid *Salmonella* species), pneumococcus, and, more rarely, nocardiosis. Depending on local antibiotic sensitivity patterns, co-trimoxazole may be useful for preventing many of these infections. Clinical trials in the Ivory Coast showed a significant lowering of morbidity in HIV-infected persons with moderately advanced disease and a 44% reduced mortality in tuberculosis patients receiving co-trimoxazole prophylaxis in addition to standard antituberculous chemotherapy. Table 22–12 shows regimens commonly used for the prophylaxis of opportunistic infections in industrialized countries.

The Essential Minimum in Resource-Poor Settings. A minimum level of care, which even the poorest health service should aim to provide, includes access to reliable HIV testing, counseling, information about HIV-AIDS, psychologic and social support, and basic symptomatic care. At more developed facilities, specific diagnosis and treatment should be provided for the common opportunistic infections, especially bacterial diseases and tuberculosis. Symptomatic treatment and terminal care should be seen as essential components of such treatment services. Prophylaxis for opportunistic infectious diseases should be considered once these other essentials are in place.

Specialist HIV-AIDS Care. Specialist HIV-AIDS services are available in very few countries, although in some countries they are available through the private sector. Antiretroviral drugs are not widely used but are purchasable in most capital cities. The specifics of modern HIV-AIDS care are beyond the scope of this text. Tables 22–12 and 22–13 summarize prophylactic and treatment regimens, respectively, for the major specific HIV-associated conditions.

The major change in the approach to HIV-AIDS in the industrialized world over the last few years has been the introduction of highly active antiretroviral therapy, now given in combinations that usually include a protease inhibitor and that typically are started in all patients with symptomatic disease, in persons with CD4+ lymphocyte counts below 500/μL, and in those with high viral load (Table 22–14). Regimens not including three drugs are increasingly considered suboptimal and likely to lead to treatment failure and drug resistance. Antiretroviral therapy is likely to be used more often in developing countries for prevention of mother-to-child transmission of HIV, and it is inevitable that

TABLE 22–11. Approaches to Prophylaxis Against Opportunistic Infections in HIV-Infected Persons in Resource-Poor Settings

Disease	Prophylaxis	Status
Tuberculosis	Isoniazid (6 mo)	Recommended for persons with positive tuberculin skin test after exclusion of active tuberculosis
Bacterial infections Toxoplasmosis *Pneumocystis carinii* pneumonia	Co-trimoxazole (lifelong)	Reduced mortality demonstrated in tuberculous patients with advanced immune deficiency
Pneumococcal infection	23-Valent polysaccharide vaccine	Recommended in industrialized countries for persons with CD4+ T-lymphocyte counts ≥200/μL; offered to more immunosuppressed persons; under further study

TABLE 22–12. Drug Regimens for Primary and Secondary Prophylaxis for Opportunistic Diseases in HIV-Infected Adults

Pathogen	Indication	First Choice	Alternatives
Primary Prophylaxis			
Pneumocystis carinii	CD4+ count <200/μL; oropharyngeal candidiasis; unexplained fever >2 wk	TMP 160 mg, SMZ 800 mg PO daily	Dapsone, 100 mg PO daily, *or* aerosolized pentamidine, 300 mg q 4 wk
Mycobacterium tuberculosis	Tuberculin skin test ≥5 mm; or contact with case of active tuberculosis	Isoniazid 300 mg PO daily for 6–9 mo	Isoniazid, 300 mg 2×/wk by DOT for 6 mo, *or* rifampin, 600 mg plus pyrazinamide, 2 g PO daily for 2 mo
Toxoplasma gondii	IgG antibody to *T. gondii* and CD4+ count <100/μL	TMP 160 mg, SMZ 800 g PO daily	Dapsone, 50 mg PO daily plus pyrimethamine, 50 mg PO every week plus leucovorin, 25 mg PO every week
Mycobacterium avium complex	CD4+ count <50/μL	Clarithromycin, 500 mg PO bid, *or* azithromycin, 1200 mg PO weekly	Rifabutin, 300 mg PO daily, *or* rifabutin, 300 mg PO daily plus azithromycin, 1200 mg PO every week
Streptococcus pneumoniae	All patients	Pneumococcal vaccine, 0.5 mL IM ×1	None
*Secondary Prophylaxis**			
P. carinii	Prior PCP	As for primary prophylaxis	
T. gondii	Prior toxoplasmic encephalitis	Sulfadiazine, 500–1000 mg PO qid plus pyrimethamine, 25–75 mg PO daily plus leucovorin, 10 mg PO daily	Clindamycin, 300–450 mg PO q 6–8 hr plus pyrimethamine, 25–75 mg PO daily plus leucovorin, 10–25 mg PO daily
M. avium complex	Documented disseminated disease	Clarithromycin, 500 mg PO bid plus ethambutol, 15 mg/kg PO daily, +/– rifabutin, 300 mg PO daily	Azithromycin, 500 mg PO daily plus ethambutol, 15 mg/kg PO daily, +/– rifabutin, 300 mg PO daily
Cytomegalovirus	Prior end organ disease	Ganciclovir, 1000 mg PO tid	Ganciclovir, 5–6 mg/kg IV 5–7 days/wk, *or* foscarnet, 90–120 mg/kg IV daily
Cryptococcus neoformans	Documented disease	Fluconazole, 200 mg PO daily	Amphotericin B, 0.6–1.0 mg/kg IV 1–3 times weekly, *or* itraconazole, 200 mg PO daily
Histoplasma capsulatum	Documented disease	Itraconazole, 200 mg PO bid	Amphotericin B, 1.0 mg/kg IV weekly, *or* fluconazole, 400 mg PO daily
Salmonella species	Bacteremia	Ciprofloxacin, 500 mg PO bid for several months	None
Herpes simplex	Frequent or severe recurrences	Acyclovir, 200 mg PO tid, *or* 400 mg PO bid	
Candida albicans	Frequent or severe recurrences	Fluconazole, 100–200 mg PO daily	Ketoconazole, 200 mg PO daily, *or* itraconazole, 200 mg PO daily
Cryptosporidium parvum	If benefit from acute treatment	Paromomycin, 500 mg PO bid	Azithromycin, 600 mg PO daily
Isospora belli	If benefit from early treatment	TMP-SMZ, 160/800 mg PO bid 3 days/wk	Pyrimethamine, 25 mg PO daily plus leucovorin, 5–10 mg PO daily

*To prevent recurrence after acute disease.
DOT, directly observed therapy; TMP-SMZ, trimethoprim-sulfamethoxazole; +/–, with or without.

if the benefits of treatment are sustained in industrialized countries, access to these drugs in developing countries will increasingly dominate discussion. Table 22–15 lists drugs currently licensed in the United States, some regimens for initiating treatment, and drug dosages and side effects. Before antiretroviral drugs are initiated, patients should ideally have a complete blood count, chemistry profile, CD4+ T-lymphocyte count, and plasma HIV RNA measurement performed.

A particularly complex subject is that of drug interactions, especially frequent with protease inhibitors. The most important example of drug interactions is that with antituberculous rifamycins (rifampin, rifabutin, rifapentine). Rifamycins induce liver enzymes that may lower bioavailability of certain antiretrovirals; conversely, ritonavir inhibits cytochrome P450 activity, which can lead to increased blood concentration of rifabutin and increased toxicity, e.g., uveitis. Patients with tuberculosis receiving treatment with protease inhibitors or non-nucleoside reverse transcriptase inhibitors should either have rifampin replaced with rifabutin (contraindicated in persons on ritonavir), or be treated with a 9- to 12-month regimen containing streptomycin.

PREVENTION OF HIV INFECTION

Prevention of Sexual Transmission. A number of successful strategies have been identified to prevent HIV infection

TABLE 22–13. Treatment of Opportunistic Infections in HIV-Infected Adults

Pathogen	First Choice	Duration	Alternatives
Mycobacterium tuberculosis	Isoniazid, 300 mg PO daily; *and* rifampin, 600 mg PO daily; *and* pyrazinamide, 2.0 g PO daily; *and* ethambutol, 1600 mg PO daily; all for 2 mo; then rifampin *and* isoniazid for 4–7 mo	Total 6–9 mo	If protease inhibitors used, substitute rifabutin, for rifampin* *or* Streptomycin, 1 g IV or IM daily; *and* isoniazid, 300 mg PO daily, *and* pyrazinamide, 2.0 g PO daily *and* ethambutol, 1600 mg PO daily, all for 2 mo; then isoniazid, 900 mg PO, *and* pyrazinamide, 2.5 g PO, *and* streptomycin, 1.5 g IV or IM, all 3×/wk for 7 mo
Pneumocystis carinii	TMP-SMZ, 5/25 mg/kg IV or PO q 8 hr; *or* clindamycin, 600 mg IV or PO tid; *and* primaquine, 30 mg po daily	14–21 days	Pentamidine isethionate, 3–4 mg/kg IV daily
Toxoplasma gondii	Pyrimethamine, 200 mg PO in divided doses first day, *then* 50–75 mg PO daily; *and* leucovorin, 10–20 mg PO or IV or IM daily; *and* sulfadiazine, 1 g PO q 6 hr;	4–6 wk	Pyrimethamine and folinic acid (as first choice); *and* clindamycin, 600 mg PO or IV qid
Cryptococcus neoformans	Amphotericin B, 0.7–0.8 mg/kg IV daily for 2 wk; *then* fluconazole, 400 mg PO daily for 6–8 wk	Total 8–10 wk	Amphotericin B (as first choice) *plus* flucytosine, 25 mg/kg PO or IV qid; then as first choice *or* For mild disease fluconazole alone, 400 mg PO daily
Histoplasma capsulatum	Amphotericin B, 0.7–0.8 mg/kg IV for 2 wk; *then* itraconazole, 400 mg PO daily for 10 wk	Total 12 wk	Itraconazole, 400 mg PO daily
Cryptosporidium parvum	None proved effective; paromomycin, 500 mg PO qid, *or* azithromycin, 1200 mg PO daily	4 wk	
Isospora belli	TMP-SMZ, 160/800 mg PO qid	10 days	Pyrimethamine, 50–75 mg PO daily for 2–4 wk plus folinic acid, 5–10 mg PO daily
Candida albicans	Fluconazole, 50–400 mg PO daily; *or* ketoconazole 200–400 mg PO daily	2 wk	Clotrimazole, 50 mg PO daily; *or* itraconazole, 200 mg PO daily
Herpes simplex	Acyclovir, 200 mg PO 5× daily, or 5–10 mg/kg IV tid	10 days	Foscarnet, 40 mg/kg IV tid
Cytomegalovirus	Ganciclovir, 5 mg/kg IV q 12 hr	14–21 days	Foscarnet, 60–90 mg/kg IV bid
Mycobacterium avium complex	Clarithromycin, 500 mg PO bid; *or* azithromycin, 500 mg PO daily; *and* ethambutol, 15–25 mg/kg PO daily; *and* one or more of the following: rifampin 600 mg PO daily; *or* rifabutin, 450–600 mg PO daily; *or* ciprofloxacin, 500 mg PO bid; *or* clofazimine, 100–200 mg PO daily; or amikacin, 7.5 mg/kg IV daily (for 2 wk)	Total 12 wk	See *Mycobacterium tuberculosis* for caution regarding concurrent use of protease inhibitors and rifamycins

*However, usual dose should be reduced from 300 mg to 150 mg PO daily with indinavir and nelfinavir and upward to 450 mg PO daily with efavirenz. Rifabutin dosage is less certain with soft-gel saquinavir and nevirapine. It should not be given with ritonavir or delavirdine.
TMP-SMZ, trimethoprim-sulfamethoxazole.

in developing countries. In countries, e.g., Thailand and Uganda, having a strong national commitment to prevention of HIV, widespread HIV education to reduce the numbers of sexual contacts, and condom promotion have contributed to reducing the population burden of HIV. Counseling and testing programs have played an important role in some countries, e.g., Uganda, Rwanda, and the Democratic Republic of

TABLE 22–14. Indications for Initiation of Antiretroviral Therapy in Persons With Established HIV Infection

Clinical	CD4+ T-Lymphocyte Count and HIV-1 RNA Level	Comment
Symptomatic	Any	Treat
Asymptomatic	CD4+ T cells <500/μL and/or HIV-1 RNA ≥10,000 copies/mL	Treat
Asymptomatic	CD4+ T cells ≥500/μL and HIV-1 RNA <10,000 copies/mL	Uncertain

Potential Benefits of Early Treatment	*Potential Reasons for Delayed Treatment*
Reduced viral replication and burden	Development of drug resistance may be reduced
Prevention of immune deficiency	Inconvenience and reduced life quality avoided
Greater possibility of immune reconstitution	Drug toxicity avoided
Increased AIDS-free and overall survival	Long-term toxicity uncertain Long-term effectiveness unknown

the Congo, to reduce the numbers of casual sexual contacts and increase condom use. A randomized community trial in Tanzania showed that enhanced treatment services for STDs resulted in a reduction in HIV infection incidence. Although a more recent study in Uganda showed that mass treatment failed to show any effect, control of STDs is still perceived as an HIV control strategy.

Comprehensive programs that include treatment of STDs have reduced HIV infection rates among commercial sex workers and the general community in a cost-effective manner. However, there is a need for increased education of health care providers to improve detection and appropriate syndromic management of STDs, as well as for increased availability of STD treatments. Because the heterosexual epidemic in many developing countries has been fueled by high HIV prevalence among commercial sex workers, targeting condom promotion and distribution, along with aggressive STD management, toward this core population, especially in the early phase of an epidemic, can have an important impact on the further spread of HIV.

Prevention of Perinatal Transmission. Prevention of HIV in newborns would best be accomplished by effective primary prevention of HIV infection among women of childbearing age. Increased access to counseling and testing services, linked to family planning services, will improve women's knowledge of their HIV status and enhance prevention of unplanned pregnancies. The regimen of zidovudine use in

TABLE 22–15. Licensed Antiretroviral Drugs, Daily Dosages, and Commonly Used Regimens for Initiating Treatment

Protease Inhibitors (PI)
Indinavir
Ritonavir
Saquinavir
Nelfinavir

Nucleoside Analogue Reverse Transcriptase Inhibitors (NRTI)
Zidovudine (ZDV)   Lamivudine (3TC)
Didanosine (ddI)   Stavudine (d4T)
Zalcitabine (ddC)   Abacavir (ABC)

Non-Nucleoside Reverse Transcriptase Inhibitors (NNRTI)
Nevirapine
Delavirdine
Efavirenz

Commonly Used Regimens for Initiating Treatment
1 PI + 2 NRTI (e.g., indinavir + ZDV + 3TC)
1 NNRTI + 2 NRTI (e.g., nevirapine + d4T + ddI)*

Drug	Adult Dosage	Major Toxicity
Zidovudine	300 mg bid or 200 mg tid	Bone marrow suppression, especially anemia and neutropenia; GI upset; headache; muscle wasting; asthenia
Didanosine	≥60 kg, 200 mg bid <60 kg, 125 mg bid	Pancreatitis; peripheral neuropathy; nausea; diarrhea
Zalcitabine	0.75 mg tid	Peripheral neuropathy; stomatitis
Stavudine	≥60 kg, 40 mg bid ≤60 kg, 30 mg bid	Peripheral neuropathy
Lamivudine	150 mg bid	Minimal
Abacavir	300 mg bid	Hypersensitivity reactions
Nevirapine	200 mg qd for 14 days, then 200 mg bid	Rash; hepatitis; raised liver enzymes
Delavirdine	400 mg tid	Rash; headache
Efavirenz	600 mg qd (evening)	Rash, CNS symptoms (e.g., bad dreams)
Indinavir	800 mg q 8 hr, 1 hr before or 2 hr after meals	Nephrolithiasis; GI upset; headache; asthenia; rash; metallic taste; blurred vision; dizziness; hyperlgycemia; lipodystrophy; thrombocytopenia
Ritonavir	600 mg q 12 hr	GI upset (nausea, vomiting, diarrhea); paresthesia (e.g., circumoral); hepatitis; asthenia; altered taste; hyperglycemia; hypertriglyceridemia; lipodystrophy
Saquinavir, hard gel caps	600 mg tid, with meal	GI upset; headache; abdominal pain; raised liver enzymes; lipodystrophy; hyperglycemia
Saquinavir, soft gel caps	1200 mg tid, with meal	
Nelfinavir	750 mg tid, with snack or meal	Diarrhea; hyperglycemia

*Non-PI containing regimens are less likely to achieve sustained viral suppression. This may not be true for regimens containing efavirenz.
GI, gastrointestinal.

pregnancy, as developed in the AIDS Clinical Trial Group (ACTG) 076 study, has been widely implemented in industrialized countries and has reduced the rate of perinatal transmission dramatically. This regimen entails daily zidovudine from the second trimester of pregnancy, intravenous therapy during labor and delivery, and 6 weeks of zidovudine therapy for the newborn. The complexity and cost of this regimen ($600 per patient) has placed it out of reach of many economically restricted countries. A recent study conducted in Thailand of a shorter, simpler regimen of oral zidovudine, given from 36 weeks' gestation with frequent oral doses during labor and delivery (Table 22–16), resulted in a 50% reduction in perinatal transmission in this non–breast-feeding population. HIV-infected women who can safely provide alternatives to breast-feeding must be advised to use such replacement feeding methods.

Implementation of short-course zidovudine will require substantial investment to improve women's access to prenatal care, to develop counseling and testing in the antenatal clinic setting, and to provide family planning following delivery. Extensive work is still needed to evaluate the safety, acceptability, and risk of stigmatization associated with use of replacement feeding in areas where breast-feeding is viewed as the only acceptable method of infant feeding. Research is needed to identify if use of antiretrovirals among lactating women or early weaning can reduce the high rate of postpartum perinatal HIV transmission.

Prevention of Parenteral Transmission. Comprehensive blood safety programs are needed to improve collection and banking of blood from low-risk donors, reliable infectious disease screening, and the appropriate use of blood. Increasing reliance on volunteer donors is an important step in improving the safety of the donor pool. Even in countries

TABLE 22–16. Zidovudine (ZDV) Regimens for the Prevention of Mother-to-Child Transmission of HIV

Regimen	Details
ACTG 076	*Antepartum:* ZDV, 100 mg 5 times daily, initiated at 14–34 weeks' gestation, continued throughout pregnancy until onset of labor *Intrapartum:* ZDV, 2 mg/kg body weight IV over 1 hr, followed by continuous infusion, 1 mg/kg body weight/hr until delivery *Postpartum:* Oral ZDV syrup, 2 mg/kg body weight every 6 hr for first 6 wk of life, beginning 8–12 hr after birth (for infant)
CDC/Thai "short course" regimen	*Antepartum:* ZDV, 300 mg twice daily, initiated at 36 weeks' gestation continued throughout pregnancy until onset of labor *Intrapartum:* Oral ZDV, 300 mg at onset of labor and then every 3 hr until delivery

with high rates of HIV infection not all persons are at equal risk, and recruitment of donors with low-risk characteristics is feasible even in resource-poor settings. Development and implementation of transfusion guidelines are required to promote the appropriate use of blood, and especially to eliminate unnecessary transfusions. Because severe anemia is generally preventable and treatable, strengthening of efforts in the primary health care system to detect and treat the causes of anemia, particularly among young children and pregnant women, is needed. Use of effective antimalarials, e.g., pyrimethamine-sulfa combinations, among young children in areas where chloroquine-resistant *P. falciparum* is prevalent, is an important strategy to decrease anemia-associated mortality and the frequent need for blood.

Finally, little attention has been given to decreasing the frequent use of injections in areas with high HIV prevalence. In addition to eliminating unnecessary injections, increased attention to sterilization techniques and improved clinical practices would serve to decrease risks to both patients and health care providers.

Bibliography

Buve A, Carael M, Hayes R, Robinson NJ: Variations in HIV prevalence between urban areas in sub-Saharan Africa: Do we understand them? AIDS 9(suppl A):S103, 1995.

Carpenter CCJ, Fischl MA, Hammer SM, et al: Antiretroviral therapy for HIV infection in 1998: Updated recommendations of the International AIDS Society—USA panel. JAMA 280:78, 1998.

Centers for Disease Control and Prevention: 1997 USPHS/IDSA guidelines for the prevention of opportunistic infections in persons infected with human immunodeficiency virus. MMWR 46(RR-12):1, 1997.

Centers for Disease Control and Prevention: Public Health Service Task Force recommendations for the use of antiretroviral drugs in pregnant women infected with HIV-1 for maternal health and for reducing perinatal HIV-1 transmission in the United States. MMWR 47(RR-2):1, 1998.

Centers for Disease Control and Prevention: Report of the NIH Panel to define principles of therapy of HIV infection and guidelines for the use of antiretroviral agents in HIV-infected adults and adolescents. MMWR 47(RR-5):1, 1998.

Centers for Disease Control and Prevention: Management of possible sexual, injecting-drug-use, or other nonoccupational exposure to HIV, including considerations related to antiretroviral therapy: Public Health Service statement. MMWR 47(RR-17):1, 1998.

Centers for Disease Control and Prevention: Prevention and treatment of tuberculosis among patients infected with human immunodeficiency virus: Principles of therapy and recommendations. MMWR 47(RR-20):1, 1998.

De Cock KM: The emergence of HIV/AIDS in Africa. Rev Epidemiol Sante Publique 44:511, 1996.

Grant AD, Djomand G, De Cock KM: Natural history and spectrum of disease in adults with HIV/AIDS in Africa. AIDS 11(suppl B):S43, 1997.

Kaplan JE, Hu DJ, Holmes KK, et al: Preventing opportunistic infections in human immunodeficiency virus–infected persons: Implications for the developing world. Am J Trop Med Hyg 55:1, 1996.

Laga M, De Cock KM, Kaleeba N, Mboup S, Tarantola D (eds): AIDS in Africa, 2nd ed. (Reprinted from AIDS, Vol. 11, Supplement B, 1997.) London, Rapid Science Publishers, 1997.

Lucas SB, Hounnou A, Peacock C, et al: The mortality and pathology of HIV infection in a West African city. AIDS 7:1569, 1993.

Mann JM, Tarantola D (eds): AIDS in the World, II. New York, Oxford University Press, 1986.

Sande MA, Volberding PA (eds): The Medical Management of AIDS, 6th ed. Philadelphia, WB Saunders. In press.

World Health Organization, Global Programme on AIDS: Recommendations for the selection and use of HIV antibody tests. Wkly Epidemiol Rec 67:145, 1992.

23 Human T-Lymphotropic Virus Type I/II Infection

Rose D. Danella and William A. Blattner

DEFINITION. Human T-lymphotropic virus type I (HTLV-I), an oncovirus (cancer-forming), is a member of a family of mammalian retroviruses with a tropism for CD4+ T lymphocytes. HTLV-I has been associated with several clinical syndromes and causes two well-defined diseases (Table 23–1). The first is adult T-cell leukemia/lymphoma (ATL), a malignant and often aggressive and fatal tumor of CD4+ T lymphocytes (Chapter 6; ATL was the first human cancer shown to be caused by a retrovirus). The second is HTLV-I-associated myelopathy/tropical spastic paraparesis (HAM/TSP), a chronic, progressive degenerative neurologic disorder (Chapter 9).

HISTORY. Retroviruses, discovered almost 100 years ago through research done on animals, were early identified as the etiologic agents of certain malignancies (leukemias, lymphomas, sarcomas, brain tumors, breast tumors) and immunologic diseases in various animal species. HTLV-I was identified and successfully isolated in 1980 in the United States from a T-lymphoblastoid cell line established from a patient diagnosed with cutaneous T-cell lymphoma.

ATL was first described as a distinct disease in Japan in 1977 and was thought to be confined to sections in the southern part of that country. The etiologic link between HTLV-I and ATL was established in 1982. HAM/TSP, initially described in 1956 as a subgroup of Jamaican neuropathy with primarily spastic but also ataxic symptoms, was associated with HTLV-I antibodies in patients from the West Indies in 1985 and in Japan in 1986.

EPIDEMIOLOGY

Distribution. The distribution of HTLV-I varies by geographic region, race, ethnicity, and risk factors. Three major types have been identified: the Cosmopolitan (worldwide), Melanesian (Papua New Guinea, Melanesia, and among Australian aborigines), and the Congo strains (Africa). The major subtypes of the Cosmopolitan strain are A (occurring in Japan, the Caribbean, Colombia, Chile, and India); B (Japan

TABLE 23–1. HTLV-Associated Diseases

Disease	HTLV-I	HTLV-II
Childhood		
Infective dermatitis	+ + + +	No
Persistent lymphadenopathy	+ +	No
Adult T-cell leukemia/lymphoma	+	No
HTLV-associated myelopathy	+ +	+
Adult		
Adult T-cell leukemia/lymphoma	+ + +	No
HTLV-associated myelopathy	+ + + +	+ +
Large cell granulocytic leukemia	No	Possible
Infective dermatitis	+ + +	Eczema?
Polymyositis	+ +	Unknown
Uveitis	+ + +	Unknown
HTLV-associated arthritis	+ + +	Possible
Sjögren syndrome	+ + +	Unknown
Strongyloides	+ +	Unknown
Pulmonary infiltrative pneumonitis	+ +	Asthma
Invasive cervical cancer	+ + +	Unknown

and India); C (Caribbean and West Africa); D (central Africa); and E (Papua New Guinea).

Prevalence. The number of people infected with HTLV-I worldwide has been estimated at between 10 million and 20 million. The virus is remarkable by virtue of its propensity to cluster tightly in endemic pockets of infection: HTLV-I is endemic in southern Japan, the South Pacific, and West Africa as well as in African populations of the Western Hemisphere. Prevalence rates vary even within endemic areas; e.g., in Japan the prevalence rate in nonendemic areas is from 0 to 1.2%, but in Okinawa, an endemic area, it is as high as 35%. The concordance of virus prevalence and ATL for these areas was one of the major factors in establishing an etiologic relationship between ATL and HTLV-I.

Transmission. HTLV-I transmission occurs in three ways: from mother to child, through sexual contact, and parenterally from infected blood and blood products (see Table 23–1).

Mother-to-infant transmission may account for up to 15% of all infections. Infected mothers can transmit the virus to the fetus or newborn most often through infected lymphocytes in breast milk and in rare cases through transplacental passage. In Japan, where mother-to-infant transmission has been most widely studied, seroconversion rates are 20% among breast-fed babies and 1 to 2% for bottle-fed babies. The subsequent recommendation that Japanese carrier mothers refrain from breast-feeding led to an extremely effective policy that resulted in a reduction of HTLV transmission.

HTLV-I is more efficiently transmitted from male to female during sexual intercourse through HTLV-I-infected cells in semen. However, there are documented instances of female-to-male sexual transmission, often augmented by coincident sexually transmitted diseases (STDs).

HTLV-I infection is most efficiently transmitted through contaminated blood (15–35% for 1 U of whole blood) or cellular blood products. Plasma and plasma derivatives, e.g., coagulation factors, do not transmit the virus. In recent years, HTLV transmission has been increasing among intravenous drug users (IDUs) sharing needles and syringes contaminated with infected blood lymphocytes, but this transmission is mostly of HTLV-II, not HTLV-I.

BIOLOGY

HTLV-I. This is classified in an as yet unnamed genus of the family Retroviridae. Based on morphology and disease association it is most closely related to the animal oncoviruses.

HTLV-I is approximately 100 nM in diameter with a thin electron-dense outer envelope and an electron-dense, roughly spherical outer core. The total RNA provirus genome contains 9032 nucleotides with two identical sequences in the long terminal repeats (LTRs) at the 5' and 3' ends of the genome. The encoding genes of the virus are *gag* (group-specific antigen) *pol* (protease/polymerase/integrase), *env* (envelope), and a series of accessory genes that regulate virus expression. The *gag* proteins function as structural proteins of the matrix, capsid, and nucleocapsid. The *pol* gene encodes for several enzymes: (1) Protease cleaves *gag* and *gag-pol* peptides into proteins of the mature virion; (2) reverse transcriptase generates a double-stranded DNA from the RNA genome; and (3) integrase integrates viral DNA into the host cell chromosomes. The *env* gene encodes the major components of the viral coat. There are two regulatory genes, *tax* and rex: tax enhances transcription of viral and cellular products; rex modulates the splicing and transport from the nucleus of viral RNA.

The virus replication cycle begins with its attachment to a cell surface receptor followed by uncoating. The target cell surface receptor is unknown, but it preferentially infects CD4 + T-helper cells, although cells with other functional phenotypes may be infected. Viral RNA is then transcribed by reverse transcriptase into a double-stranded DNA; this is integrated into the genome of the host cell, resulting in cell infection that may be lifelong. HTLV-I infection does not result in reduced numbers of CD4 + cells, although infected cells may show reduced helper and suppressor cell function in vitro. When the DNA provirus is expressed, viral proteins are made by the cell. Detection of antibodies to these structural viral proteins is the basis of serologic diagnosis of infection.

HTLV-II. Serologically related to HTLV-I, HTLV-II has not yet been associated with any disease (Table 23–1). HTLV-II infection has a high prevalence among IDUs. Archived sera collected from many IDU populations in the United States have HTLV-II infection rates ranging from 10 to 15% and higher. HTLV-II infection has been documented among American Indians in North, Central (Guaymi in northeastern Panama), and South America and from natives in equatorial Africa. Infected persons were not IDUs, and there was no clustering of seropositivity in family units, which would be against sexual and perinatal transmission. HTLV-II has also been isolated from two patients with hairy cell leukemia; however, most patients with the disease are seronegative for HTLV-II.

Immune Responses. ATL and HAM/TSP rarely occur in the same person. This may be related to host immune response in infection or to the involvement of different pathogenic pathways. Disruption of the host immune function by HTLV-I infection may affect the development and course of diseases other than ATL and HAM/TSP. Concurrent infection with HTLV-I/II and HIV is particularly common among IDUs and may alter the expression of HIV disease: Some studies show an acceleration of progression to AIDS; other studies show protection against progression.

SEROLOGY. The most sensitive screening assay for HTLV-I antibody is an enzyme-linked immunosorbent assay (ELISA) that uses whole disrupted virus, sometimes augmented with recombinant antigen; also available is a particle agglutination assay. These assays have high sensitivity but have poor type specificity owing to cross reactivity between HTLV-I and HTLV-II. The problem has been resolved by a Western blot (WB) test that uses a combination of whole virus and recombinantly produced peptides. This technique can confirm positive ELISAs and distinguishes between the two virus types. WB confirmation requires the presence of antibody to the *gag* protein product p19 and p24 and one of the HTLV-I *env* protein products, gp46 or gp61. Sera with no reactivity to viral protein bands are considered negative; sera with partial reactivity are called indeterminate. The vast majority of indeterminate sera are negative by polymerase chain reaction (PCR) and continue to be negative in the follow-up.

Because the virus is highly cell associated, additional tests are sometimes needed to demonstrate antibody to the *env* encoded components of the virus. *Env* antibodies are selectively picked up by radioimmunoprecipitation assay (RIPA) based on virus-infected whole cells. Confirmation by immunofluorescence assay is also useful for distinguishing type I from type II. Quantificative titration of antibody requires modifications to the ELISA and particle agglutination tests.

Another technique used for detection of HTLV-I/II is nucleic acid detection using PCR, which can both identify and quantitate specific virus types. It is especially useful in enigmatic situations. Antigen capture assays are currently being developed to detect circulating viral antigens.

PREVENTION AND CONTROL. Guidelines for prevention and counseling have been developed for HTLV-I/II by a Centers for Disease Control and Prevention (CDC) Working

Group. Standard prevention approaches are similar for both viruses: screening blood; proscribing recreational use of intravenous drugs; eliminating breast-feeding for known infected mothers and, where not feasible, restricting breast-feeding to the first 6 months of life; and using condoms for discordant couples. When counseling HTLV-I/II seropositive patients, a clear distinction must be made between HTLV and HIV infection and attendant disease associations.

The development of an effective vaccine is possible; whether the disease burden associated with the virus warrants a vaccine is the subject of an ongoing debate. In Japan, *spontaneous* declines in the prevalence rate of infections in different birth cohorts and declining rates among children have been ascribed to changing breast-feeding patterns, low STD rates, frequent condom use, and (perhaps) socioeconomic factors.

■ ADULT T-CELL LEUKEMIA/LYMPHOMA

EPIDEMIOLOGY. In Kyoto, Japan in 1977, 4 years before the discovery and isolation of HTLV-I, ATL was characterized as an aggressive leukemia/lymphoma of mature T lymphocytes. Although the cases were diagnosed in Kyoto, most of the patients were born in the southern Japanese islands of Kyushu, Shikoku, and the Ryukyu Archipelago, including Okinawa. Systematic organization of case findings by the Japanese T- and B-Cell Leukemia/Lymphoma Group demonstrated a pattern of disease clustering, particularly in southern Japan. This finding was confirmed by descriptive epidemiologic surveys, which advanced the idea that a transmissible agent (later identified as HTLV-I) would explain the disease clustering. Subsequent clusters were identified among patients of West Indian ancestry in Great Britain and blacks in the United States and in the West Indies.

Cases of HTLV-I–associated leukemia/lymphomas have been identified in North and South America, Africa, Europe (among migrants from endemic areas), the Middle East, Australia (among aboriginal people who harbor the HTLV-I Melanesian variant), the Caribbean Basin, and Japan. In endemic areas, e.g., southern Japan and the Caribbean Islands, the annual incidence of virus-associated leukemia is approximately 3 per 100,000 per year and may account for more than 50% of the adult lymphoid malignancies.

The possibility of an infected person developing adult T-cell leukemia/lymphoma over a lifetime is 1 to 5%; early life exposure is the single greatest risk for subsequent disease. The male:female ratio is approximately 1. The risk of HTLV-I as a cause of leukemia/lymphoma peaks from age 40 to 50 years and thereafter declines, with peak incidence in Japan occurring approximately a decade later than that observed in the Caribbean. Cases have been observed in children as young as 5 and 6 years, but this is extremely rare.

PATHOGENESIS. Molecular and virologic studies have provided much information about the pathogenesis of HTLV-I-associated ATL. In the initial stages, HTLV-I binds to an undefined receptor with subsequent uncoating, reverse transcription, and production of a DNA provirus. Although HTLV-I may exist for years as a latent virus, its genes promote cell proliferation and in the process promote the expression of viral antibodies and cytotoxic T cells targeted at viral antigens. After a long latent period (years to several decades), polyclonal and monoclonal HTLV expansion leads to proliferation, immune dysregulation, and the development of ATL or HAM/TSP (Fig. 23–1).

PATHOLOGY. In persons with ATL, CD4+/CD25+ malignant cells frequently are observed in the peripheral blood as circulating lymphocytes with irregular multilobulated nuclei (flower cells). These circulating cells have scant, agranular cytoplasm, occasionally with vacuoles. The chromatin of the nucleus is condensed with a vesicular to coarse pattern, and the nucleus may contain up to three (usually inconspicuous) nucleoli. Lymph node morphology shows lymphoma that is diffuse rather than nodular, and the underlying structure of the node is usually preserved. From patient to patient, however, there is considerable cytomorphologic pleomorphism. In the histologic classification system proposed by the Japanese Lymphoma Study Group, tumors are subclassified as small cell, medium-sized cell, mixed cell, pleomorphic, or other.

Malignant lymphocytes may infiltrate multiple sites, including the spleen, liver, meninges, and, occasionally, mediastinum. No recognized histologic pattern correlates with a given clinical outcome. Infiltrative skin lesions contain malignant cells in dense dermal nodules that resemble Pautrier's microabscesses, seen in classic mycosis fungoides. Lytic bone lesions usually contain areas of fibrosis and increased osteoclastic activity rather than malignant cells. When malignant

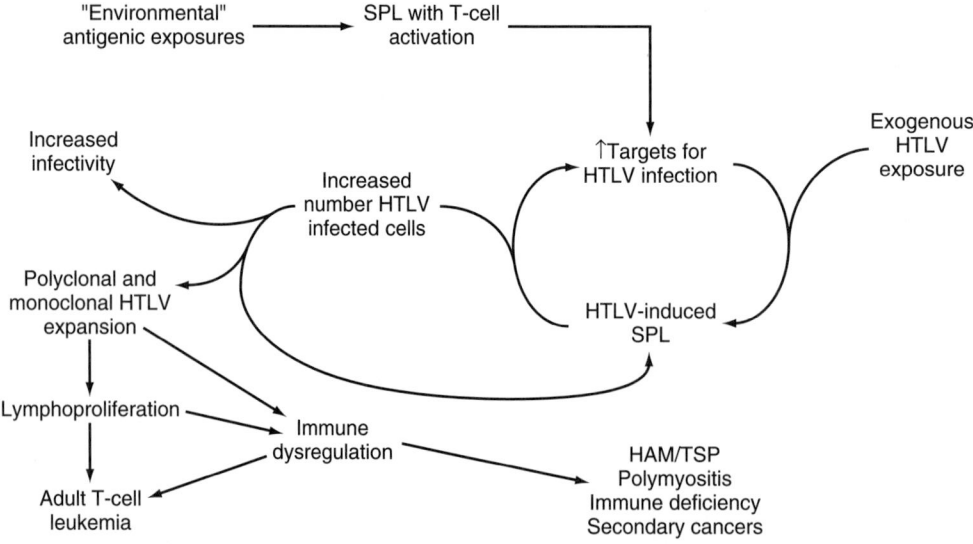

Figure 23–1. Interaction of HTLV and spontaneous proliferation of lymphocytes (SPL).

infiltration of the bone marrow occurs, it is always diffuse rather than paratrabecular. In the primary pulmonary disease of ATL, both leukemic infiltrates and diffuse fibrosis have been observed.

CLINICAL MANIFESTATIONS. In 1977, Takatsuki characterized ATL as an aggressive leukemia/lymphoma of mature T lymphocytes with varied clinical manifestations: generalized lymphadenopathy, visceral and cutaneous skin involvement, lytic bone lesions, hypercalcemia, and, in a large number of cases, pleiotropic features in peripheral blood cells. The Lymphoma Study Group in Japan classified ATL into four clinical subtypes based on clinical features and cell morphology: acute, chronic, smoldering, and lymphoma/leukemia types.

Acute ATL. The acute type (50–60% of ATL patients) is referred to as prototypic ATL. Patients exhibit increased numbers of ATL cells, skin lesions, systemic lymphadenopathy, and hepatosplenomegaly. Initial symptoms often include fever, rash, cough, malaise, weakness, and abdominal distention and pain. These patients often have tachypnea and dyspnea, which may progress to pulmonary failure. Opportunistic pathogens, e.g., *Pneumocystis carinii*, cytomegalovirus, *Cryptococcus*, *Candida*, and various bacterial and mycobacterial agents, also have been associated with pulmonary disease, especially in patients receiving combination chemotherapy. Central nervous system (CNS) abnormalities, due to leptomeningeal involvement, manifest as meningeal signs or as an altered level of consciousness. The skin lesions may appear as papules, nodules, tumors, generalized maculopapular rashes, parapsoriatic rashes, or generalized or localized erythroderma. Generally, the cutaneous lesions are not pruritic.

Hypercalcemia, occasionally in association with lytic bone lesions, occurs in up to 75% of patients with the acute pattern. Although some patients initially may have a lymphoma-like syndrome, most eventually become leukemic, often with marked leukocytosis and lymphocytosis; 10% or more of the lymphocytes may contain multilobulated nuclei. Eosinophilia may develop, but usually anemia and thrombocytopenia are either absent or mild. Glucose and protein in cerebrospinal fluid (CSF) are usually normal, but there may be a minimal increase in the number of cells, mostly lymphocytes.

Chronic ATL. Chronic type ATL, 20% of ATL cases, resembles chronic T-lymphocytic leukemia: Cells have a characteristic cleaved morphology called buttock cells, the white blood count is increased, and skin lesions are evident. Some patients manifest mild lymphadenopathy and hepatosplenomegaly, and serum lactate dehydrogenase is sometimes elevated. Serum calcium levels are normal.

Smoldering ATL. Smoldering ATL, 5% of the total cases, may clinically resemble mycosis fungoides/Sézary syndrome, with cutaneous involvement presenting as erythema or as infiltrative plaques or tumors, and with Pautrier's microabscesses.

Lymphoma Type ATL. Twenty percent of ATL cases, and the majority of cases in the Caribbean, present as a T-cell non-Hodgkin's lymphoma without leukemia. They have often other clinical features of ATL, e.g., hypercalcemia and monoclonal integration of HTLV-I in the proviral DNA of the tumor cells. These cases are called lymphoma type and are indistinguishable from peripheral T-cell lymphomas.

Prognosis. Patients usually present at an advanced stage of the clinical disease and die within 6 months of diagnosis, particularly if coincident hypercalcemia or opportunistic infections exist. The cause of death is usually an explosive growth of tumor cells, hypercalcemia, bacterial sepsis, or opportunistic infections.

In general, the smoldering type of ATL is the least aggressive. The chronic type has a relatively poor prognosis, with death occurring within a few years of diagnosis. The acute and lymphoma types are more virulent, with death occurring within 6 months of diagnosis.

DIAGNOSIS. A diagnosis of ATL and other HTLV-I related diseases (see Table 23–1) is established by testing serum for HTLV-I antibodies and finding leukemic T cells with the provirus in the blood or biopsy specimens. Acute ATL can be diagnosed with confidence in persons with a diffuse T-cell non-Hodgkin's lymphoma, skin lesions, hypercalcemia, leukemic cells, and reactive HTLV-I serologic test results. Patients with less acute illness, however, may be difficult to differentiate from persons with a cutaneous T-cell lymphoma e.g., mycosis fungoides or Sézary syndrome. Typical cutaneous T-cell lymphoma lesions spread less rapidly and less extensively than those of ATL, and they are typically band-like and sparsely infiltrated compared with the dense nodules of ATL. Also, patients with cutaneous T-cell lymphoma rarely have metabolic bone disease, lymphocytic invasion of the leptomeninges, and opportunistic infections. T-cell chronic lymphocytic leukemia and peripheral T-cell lymphoma also may be difficult to differentiate from chronic ATL. The differential diagnosis of ATL, therefore, must rely on the combination of clinical, pathologic, serologic, and epidemiologic features.

TREATMENT. ATL and other diseases caused by HTLV-I are difficult to treat and consequently have a poor prognosis. All forms of ATL are refractory to most conventional and experimental chemotherapeutic regimens, often having an initial brief response followed by rapid relapse.

Patients with chronic or smoldering type ATL are usually not treated or are treated with prednisone with or without cyclophosphamide. When treated aggressively, patients with these more indolent forms of ATL have high rates of complicating infections due to therapy-related bone marrow damage. The acute and lymphoma types progress rapidly; some cases respond to multidrug regimens with prolonged remission. In Japan, some short-term success has been achieved with trials of vincristine, cyclophosphamide, prednisolone, and doxorubicin. Phase I trials with topoisomerase inhibitors and dioxopiperazine have shown some promise. Other trials using a combination of antiretrovirals and interferon have reported remissions in some cases. If corroborated, these data would indicate that the oncogenic events are controllable or reversible and can provide opportunities for gaining an understanding of the mechanisms of oncogenic transformation.

■ HTLV-I ASSOCIATED MYELOPATHY/TROPICAL SPASTIC PARAPARESIS (HAM/TSP)

EPIDEMIOLOGY. HTLV-I is associated with HAM/TSP, a progressive immune-mediated disorder of the CNS characterized by demyelination of the long motor neurons of the spinal cord (Chapter 9). Evidence for this association includes (1) a 60 to 100% prevalence of HTLV-I antibodies in HAM/TSP patients; (2) intrathecal synthesis of HTLV-I antibody; (3) the finding in some patients of multilobulated cells in the peripheral blood and CSF; and (4) isolation of HTLV-I from peripheral blood lymphocytes and CSF mononuclear cells.

HAM/TSP is sporadic, occurring in adults (median age 40 to 50 years) and predominantly in females. Onset is usually after age 30 years and rarely after age 60 years. It is sometimes familial and is rarely found in children. It is the most common form of paraplegia in some areas of the tropics and Japan. The incidence of TSP/HAM is estimated to be approximately half the rate of ATL, but prevalence is greater because of longer survival of patients with TSP/HAM. The lifetime risk of HAM/TSP among HTLV-I infected persons is 1% or less, and the latency period may be shorter than for ATL. Genetic susceptibility may also be a risk factor.

PATHOGENESIS. The natural history of the disease begins with perturbation of the immune function by activated T lymphocytes, the indirect effect of cytokines, molecular mimicry, or cell-mediated immune responses directed against neural tissue caused by HTLV-I infection. The high virus loads suggest the inability of the host to control viral proliferation.

PATHOLOGY. Patients with HAM/TSP have axonal degeneration and myelin loss in the pyramidal tracts of the spinal cord. Changes are most prevalent at the thoracic and lumbar levels. A chronic meningomyelitis, predominantly at the spinal cord level but also involving the midbrain, the cerebellum, and the cerebrum, is typical. Although the degree of inflammation varies from patient to patient, perivascular lymphocytic infiltration, fibrosis, and hyaline arteriolar thickening are usually observed in the affected parts of the nervous system.

CLINICAL MANIFESTATIONS. Early diagnosis is difficult, since initial manifestations are often nonspecific (e.g., leg pain, back pain). A single symptom or physical sign may be the only clue of early HAM/TSP. The disease follows a slow course: Symptoms often begin with a stiff gait, progressing slowly to increased spasticity and weakness in the lower extremities. Patients may complain of sensory symptoms, e.g., tingling, a pins-and-needles sensation, and burning. Vibration sense may be impaired.

Physical examination reveals hyperreflexia of the lower limbs, and sometimes of the upper limbs, as well as an exaggerated jaw jerk; ataxia develops occasionally. Nuclear magnetic resonance scans can sometimes detect isolated lesions of the CNS. The syndrome is significantly different from classic multiple sclerosis (MS). HAM/TSP follows a slowly progressive course without the waxing and waning of symptoms characteristic of MS and without the changes in affect. HAM/TSP usually progresses over a decade or so, but it can be rapid, especially in older persons and in those infected by transfusion of HTLV-I-positive blood. Eventually patients are unable to walk even with crutches.

DIAGNOSIS. The diagnosis is suspected in unexplained CNS disease with loss of pyramidal tract functions and is confirmed by testing sera for HTLV-I antibodies. A diagnosis of HAM/TSP should always be considered for patients with these findings and a history of blood transfusion.

TREATMENT. Treatment with corticosteroids benefits some patients, particularly those with rapidly progressive disease. Treatment with danazol, an androgenic steroid, has resulted in improvement in urinary and fecal incontinence but not the underlying neurologic deficit.

Bibliography

Blattner WA: Human lymphotropic viruses: HTLV-I and HTV-II. *In* Richman DD, Whitley RJ, Hayden FG (eds): Clinical Virology. New York, Churchill Livingstone, 1997, pp 683–705.
Cann AJ, Chen SY: Human T-cell leukemia virus types I and II. *In* Fields BN, Knipe DM, Howley PM (eds): Field's Virology, 3rd ed. Philadelphia, Lippincott-Raven, 1996, pp 1849–1880.
Mueller NE, Blattner WA: Retroviruses—human T-cell lymphotropic virus. *In* Evans AS, Kaslow R (eds): Viral Infections in Humans: Epidemiology and Control, 4th ed. New York, Plenum Publishing, 1997, pp 785–813.
Osame M, Arimura K, Nakagawa M, et al: HTLV-I associated myelopathy (HAM). Review and recent studies. Leukemia (Suppl) 3:63, 1997.
Poiesz BJ, Ruscetti FW, Gazdar AF, et al: Detection and isolation of type C retrovirus particles from fresh and cultured lymphocytes of a patient with cutaneous T-cell lymphoma. Proc Natl Acad Sci USA 77:7415, 1980.
Tajima K: The fourth nation-wide study of adult T-cell leukemia/lymphoma

(ATL) in Japan: Estimates of risk of ATL and its geographical and clinical features. Int J Cancer 45:237, 1990.
Takatsuki K (ed): Adult T-Cell Leukaemia. New York, Oxford University Press, 1994.
Tsukasaki K, Ikeda S, Murata K, et al: Characteristics of chemotherapy-induced clinical remission in long survivors with aggressive adult T-cell leukemia/lymphoma. Leuk Res 17:157, 1993.
Waldmann TA, White JD, Carrasquillo JA, et al: Radioimmunotherapy of interleukin-2R alpha-expressing adult T-cell leukemia with yttrium-90-labeled anti-Tac. Blood 86:4063, 1995.
Yoshida, M: Molecular biology of HTLV-I: Deregulation of host cell gene expression and cell cycle. Leukemia 11(Suppl 3):1, 1997.

24 Herpesvirus Infections

Sonja J. Olsen and Patrick S. Moore

Eight herpesviruses currently are known to naturally infect humans (Table 24–1). Their clinical presentations in tropical and temperate areas do not differ; however, an important epidemiologic distinction is that herpesvirus infections frequently occur at an earlier age and infect a higher proportion of the population in developing, compared with developed, countries. This trend may be due to lower socioeconomic standards and crowded living conditions, which enhance transmission for most herpesviruses. Only those herpesviruses having distinct presentations in developing countries will be discussed in this chapter.

HERPES SIMPLEX TYPE II. This is a sexually transmitted virus that reaches high seroprevalence only in select risk groups in North America (e.g., prostitutes). In some African countries, however, as many as 75% of the adult population may be HSV-II infected. An exception is varicella-zoster virus infection, which generally occurs at an older age in tropical countries.

HERPES B VIRUS. This is the only nonhuman herpesvirus known to be highly pathogenic to humans. Infection is not known to occur routinely in any human population; the rare reported cases usually have occurred in laboratory workers or others after direct contact with nonhuman primates. The virus is transmitted from the saliva of Old World monkeys to humans, usually through bites; however, several episodes of person-to-person transmission have been documented. Untreated human infection causes encephalomyelitis and death in over 75% of cases, but antiherpesviral drugs, specifically acyclovir, may be effective if treatment is implemented early in the course of disease.

Two human herpesviruses, Epstein-Barr virus (EBV) and Kaposi's sarcoma–associated herpesvirus (KSHV), with unique links to human cancers with high incidence rates in the tropics, are the focus of this chapter.

24.1 Epstein-Barr Virus (EBV/HHV4)

DEFINITION. Epstein-Barr virus (EBV or human herpesvirus 4 [HHV4]) was first isolated from tumor tissue excised from an African patient with Burkitt's lymphoma (BL) in the 1960s (Chapter 12). EBV is a double-stranded DNA virus 172 kb in length, consisting of a long and a short unique segment divided by internal repeat sequences and flanked by terminal repeat sequences. The gammaherpesvirus is associated with

TABLE 24–1. Human Herpesviruses and Disease Associations

Formal Name	Descriptive Name	Subfamily	Disease Associations*
Human herpesvirus 1 (HHV1)	Herpes simplex virus I (HSV1)	Alpha	Oral fever blisters Encephalitis
Human herpesvirus 2 (HHV2)	Herpes simplex virus II (HSV2)	Alpha	Genital lesions Encephalitis
Human herpesvirus 3 (HHV3)	Varicella-zoster virus (VZV)	Alpha	Chickenpox (varicella) Shingles (herpes zoster)
Human herpesvirus 4 (HHV4)	Epstein-Barr virus (EBV)	Gamma	Burkitt's lymphoma Nasopharyngeal carcinoma Infectious mononucleosis Post-transplant lymphoproliferative disease Leiomyosarcoma Hodgkin's disease
Human herpesvirus 5 (HHV5)	Cytomegalovirus (CMV)	Beta	Mononucleosis Hepatitis
Human herpesvirus 6 (HHV6)		Beta	Exanthem subitum Febrile seizures
Human herpesvirus 7 (HHV7)		Beta	?
Human herpesvirus 8 (HHV8)	Kaposi's sarcoma–associated herpesvirus (KSHV)	Gamma	Kaposi's sarcoma Primary effusion lymphoma Multicentric Castleman disease

*Limited to prominent or well-documented disease associations.

infectious mononucleosis as well as several malignancies (BL, nasopharyngeal carcinoma [NPC], some forms of Hodgkin's disease, and post-transplant lymphoproliferative disorders and leiomyosarcoma in immunosuppressed persons).

Serology. IgG antibody titers to the EBV viral capsid antigen (VCA) are markedly higher in African BL cases than in either African controls or American BL cases, whereas titers in American cases are similar to those of matched controls. A large prospective study in Uganda detected higher titers months to years prior to BL development and an association with a 30-fold greater tumor risk. IgG antibodies to early antigen (EA) and VCA are elevated in NPC patients, and high IgA EA or VCA antibody titers may be predictive of NPC development or recurrence.

Transmission. EBV is primarily transmitted through infected oral secretions and is shed into saliva for years after infection. In developed countries, transmission can be delayed until adolescence, primarily because of improved living standards. Primary infection at an older age frequently results in clinically apparent mononucleosis, whereas in Africa most people are asymptomatically infected with EBV before the age of 3 years. EBV also can be transmitted perinatally, either in utero or during delivery; however, this is rare in developed countries. Immune tolerance due to perinatal infection has been suggested as a possible contributing factor to development of African BL.

BURKITT'S LYMPHOMA. Because of the ubiquitous nature of EBV infection, it has been difficult to determine whether the virus plays a causal role in BL, a B-cell lymphoma. Based on descriptive epidemiologic and clinical characteristics, BL is subdivided into endemic and sporadic types. BL is endemic in equatorial Africa and Papua New Guinea, with an annual incidence of approximately 6 to 7 cases per 100,000 per year. African BL never appears before the age of 1 year and has a peak incidence at 6 or 7 years, with a threefold higher rate in boys until the teenage years. The majority of childhood BL cases in Africa present with facial and jaw tumors (Fig. 12-9), although abdominal masses can also occur. EBV is detectable in virtually all tumors from endemic BL patients.

Sporadic BL is a rare tumor occurring in developed countries and is associated with EBV infection in less than a third of the cases. It occurs at a later age (often in AIDS patients) and generally presents with abdominal rather than jaw tumors. BL incidence is intermediate in Pakistan and South America, where these tumors also show evidence of EBV infection at a rate intermediate between endemic (high) and sporadic (low) BL.

Endemic BL is less frequent in tropical highland areas, and some studies have found a seasonal pattern, with more cases occurring in the wet season, suggesting that a vector-borne disease, specifically malaria, is a cofactor. However, epidemiologic studies have failed to demonstrate a clear link between malaria and BL, and further studies are needed to clarify the role of malaria, if any, in BL pathogenesis.

Virtually all examples of BL have a translocation involving the *c-myc* oncogene, which frequently places *c-myc* under a highly active promoter, leading to its overexpression in tumor cells. This translocation may represent an example of oncogene collaboration, in which *c-myc* overexpression acts in concert with EBV-encoded oncogenes to induce transformation of the B cell. Molecular biologic studies based on viral terminal repeat analysis demonstrate that among BL tumors infected with EBV, the virus is monoclonal (as are the tumor cells), thereby providing evidence that the virus serves an initiating function in generating the tumor.

NASOPHARYNGEAL CARCINOMA. NPC is a second EBV-associated cancer with a high incidence in some tropical areas (Chapter 12). Histologically, NPC is characterized by neoplastic epithelial cells infiltrated with a variable reactive lymphocytosis. NPC frequently escapes early detection because of its hidden location in the nasopharynx, and as a result patients often present at an advanced stage with lymph node and cranial nerve involvement (Fig. 12–1). EBV is present in all tumor cells of infected NPC lesions, and terminal repeat analysis and EBV antigens in premalignant lesions demonstrate that EBV is likely to be an initiating factor in NPC as it is in endemic BL. The highest NPC incidence rates are found in southern China (>20 cases/100,000/year); followed by moderate rates among North African Arabs and Alaskan, Canadian, and Greenland Inuit; and extremely low rates in North American and European Caucasians (<1/

100,000 persons/year). NPC incidence peaks at age 50 years with two- to threefold higher rates in men than in women. Environmental and dietary risk factors appear to play a large role in the genesis of NPC. Immigration studies show that Chinese and Inuits retain an elevated risk after moving to the continental United States, suggesting either a genetic or an environmental risk factor incurred early in life. Risk factor analyses in Chinese and Malaysian populations disclose an increased risk associated with eating salted fish, especially during early childhood. Cellular mutagenesis due to carcinogenic nitrosamines in salted fish has been suggested to act in concert with EBV to initiate this cancer.

OTHER EBV-ASSOCIATED MALIGNANCIES. Other neoplastic diseases associated with EBV include some forms of Hodgkin's disease, post-transplant lymphoproliferative disorders, and leiomyosarcomas occurring in immunosuppressed persons. It is unknown whether these disorders occur at higher rates in tropical countries.

24.2 *Kaposi's Sarcoma–Associated Herpesvirus (KSHV/HHV8)*

DEFINITION. Kaposi's sarcoma–associated herpesvirus (KSHV or human herpesvirus 8 [HHV8]), the most recently identified human herpesvirus, was found by DNA isolation without direct culture. KSHV is a 165 kb double-stranded DNA virus consisting of a single unique coding region approximately 140 kb in length flanked by terminal repeat sequences high in G+C content. KSHV is a gammaherpesvirus similar to EBV and infects endothelial cells and CD19+B lymphocytes. KSHV infection has been linked to three clinical disorders: Kaposi's sarcoma (KS; Chapter 12), B-cell body cavity–based lymphomas, and a subset of Castleman's disease (angiofollicular hyperplasia).

VIROLOGY. Unlike most human herpesviruses, the KSHV genome contains a number of genes with high sequence similarity to cellular genes, including known human proto-oncogenes. Viral genes with potential for promoting cell proliferation and oncogenesis include those similar to cellular genes encoding cyclin D, bcl-2, interleukin 6, interferon regulatory factors (IRF), and an IL-8-like receptor. Although this virus lacks the oncogenes associated with EBV-induced cell transformation, there is a close functional correspondence between many of the cellular genes induced by EBV infection and similar viral genes in the KSHV genome. The KSHV cytokine viL-6 induces B-cell proliferation in vitro and may contribute to the B-cell hyperplasia characterizing the plasma cell variant of Castleman's disease. KSHV can be cultured in vitro in body cavity–based lymphoma cells, but thus far, attempts to propagate the virus from KS cells have been unsuccessful. Despite this, KSHV is consistently linked to KS and is likely to be a necessary cofactor for this tumor.

SEROLOGY. Serologic assays have been developed to detect antibodies to both latent and lytic phase antigens based on both whole-cell and recombinant technologies. These assays are still experimental and achieve only approximately 80% sensitivity in detecting virus infection. Unlike EBV, KSHV is an uncommon infection in developed countries. High seroprevalence rates have been found in HIV-infected homosexual and bisexual men (30–35%) with low rates in HIV-infected patients from other risk groups. Seroprevalence rates in Mediterranean countries, where KS is endemic, are higher than in Northern Europe and North America. In Saudi Arabia, KS is the most frequent post-transplantation neo-

plasm, which may reflect high rates of endemic KSHV infection in this population. In this setting, the tumor presumably arises during immunosuppression among persons infected with KSHV prior to transplantation. Seroprevalence studies from Uganda and Zambia suggest that KSHV infection is common in both men and women. Infants and children can be infected, and the seroprevalence in adulthood may be as high as 60 to 70% (Fig. 24–1).

TRANSMISSION. The precise mechanism of KSHV transmission is currently unknown. Risk factor studies of men with KS from developed countries suggest that the main mode of transmission is sexual, through either infected semen or feces. Oral viral secretion frequently occurs among KS patients and also may contribute to transmission. Transmission through organ transplantation has been documented, although this does not account for most cases of post-transplantation KS. The high HSHV seroprevalence in Africa may be due to post-partum horizontal transmission in young children and adolescents.

KAPOSI'S SARCOMA. KS typically manifests with cutaneous lesions (Fig. 12–4), although mucosal and lymph node involvement may occur (Fig. 12–5). KS can be classified into four subtypes based on epidemiologic and clinical differences: classic (sporadic) KS, African (endemic) KS, post-transplant or immunosuppression-related KS, and AIDS (epidemic) KS. The classic form of the disease usually occurs in elderly men of Mediterranean descent and generally follows an indolent course. In eastern and central Africa, KS has very high incidence rates. It is a slow-growing tumor in adults but is rapidly fatal in children, in whom a lymphadenopathic form predominates. KS can also occur among KSHV-infected patients receiving immunosuppressive therapy, particularly after transplantation, but complete regression may follow cessation of immunosuppression. The most recently described subtype, AIDS-KS, is aggressive and often dissemi-

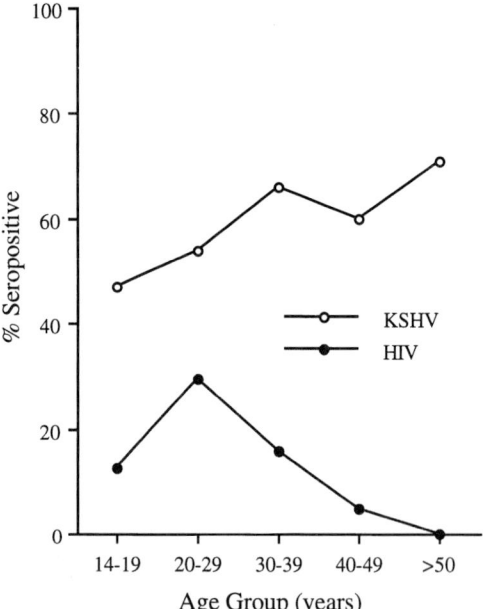

Figure 24–1. Age-specific KSHV and HIV seroprevalence rates in a hospital-based population from Lusaka, Zambia, 1985. KSHV seroprevalence increased linearly with age, consistent with the well-established infection in the population, possibly transmitted through nonsexual routes. In contrast, HIV seroprevalence was highest in 20- to 29-year group, consistent with the introduction of a sexually transmitted agent. (From Olsen S, et al: AIDS. In press.)

nates to oral, genital, and intestinal mucosa as well as lymph nodes and skin. Anecdotal reports indicate that tumors in AIDS-KS patients whose immune status is stabilized by highly effective antiretroviral therapy may regress.

The AIDS epidemic has dramatically increased the incidence of KS in some African countries. Equatorial Africa has the highest incidence rates of KS in the world, and in Uganda KS now accounts for almost 50% of all tumors in men reported to central cancer registries. This KS epidemic may be directly attributable to the high rate of AIDS-related diseases in these countries, although there are some indications that KS rates are increasing among HIV-negative portions of affected populations as well. In the adult form of endemic KS without HIV co-infection, radiation therapy and some combined drug therapies can provide excellent palliation and frequent tumor remission. Palliation and remission are far less successful among AIDS-KS patients without adequate antiretroviral therapy. Studies are ongoing to determine whether antiherpesviral drugs affect the course of KSHV-related tumors. In vitro studies indicate that the virus is relatively resistant to acyclovir but is sensitive to foscarnet and cidofovir.

Studies of AIDS and immunosuppressed transplant patients make clear that KSHV and related tumors are under strict immunologic control and that the majority of KSHV-infected individuals with intact immune systems do not develop tumors. KSHV DNA is present in 95% of all forms of KS lesions and is generally absent from control tissues of persons without KS. Serologic and DNA detection–based studies show that KSHV infection precedes onset of disease and is predictive of KS development. No immunologic defects have been found in classic and African endemic KS patients, although the disease may be associated with nonspecific age-related declines in immune function. The high rates of KS in central African countries is likely to be due to widespread KSHV infection in the general population. In contrast, KS and presumably KSHV infection are rare in Southeast and East Asia.

Little is known about the occurrence of other KSHV-related lymphoproliferative disorders in developing countries. Body cavity–based lymphomas and Castleman's disease can occur among North American AIDS patients as a consequence of KSHV infection, but these lymphoproliferative disorders also rarely occur in the absence of HIV infection. Hospital studies suggest that both lymphomas and Castleman's disease can occur in African KS patients, and it is likely that these disorders are more common in highly KSHV-endemic areas than in the United States.

Bibliography

Chang Y, Cesarman E, Pessin MS, et al: Identification of herpesvirus-like DNA sequences in AIDS-associated Kaposi's sarcoma. Science 265:1865, 1994.
de-Thé G: The epidemiology of Burkitt's lymphoma: Evidence for a causal association with Epstein-Barr virus. Epidemiol Rev 1:32, 1979.
Schulz T, Chang Y, Moore PS: Kaposi's sarcoma–associated herpesvirus (human herpesvirus 8). In McCance DJ (ed): Human Tumor Viruses. Washington, DC, ASM Press, 1998, pp 87–132.

25 Viral Infections With Cutaneous Lesions

25.1 Measles*

Stephen C. Redd and Joel G. Breman

DEFINITION. Measles (rubeola) is an acute, highly contagious viral disease, which usually affects children and is characterized by fever, a generalized maculopapular rash, cough, coryza, and conjunctivitis. The disease is a major cause of death in children, especially in developing countries, where most are afflicted before 5 years of age, and case-fatality rates may be 5% or greater. Measles vaccination is highly efficacious and may be the single most cost-effective preventive health intervention.

ETIOLOGY. Measles is a paramyxovirus in the morbillivirus genus. The virion is pleomorphic with a diameter of 120 nm to 250 nm. The virus has an outer lipid envelope that encloses glycoproteins and an inner nucleocapsid of protein and negative-sense, nonsegmented, single-stranded RNA. The RNA codes for six proteins from the 3' to 5' end, nucleoprotein (NP), phosphoprotein (P), matrix protein (M), fusion protein (F), hemagglutinin protein (H), and large polymerase protein (L). The genome has a molecular weight of about 4.5 × 10⁶ D and contains about 16,000 nucleotides. The measles virus is most closely related to the viruses causing canine distemper, rinderpest, and *peste des petits ruminants.* Like other members of the morbillivirus genus, none of the measles virus proteins contains neuraminidase activity. The measles virus genome differs from other morbilliviruses by 10 to 20%.

Measles virus is fragile under certain environmental conditions. The virus loses titer rapidly when exposed to light, while drying on fomites, and at pH 5. Lyophilization renders the virus more stable at higher temperatures and is the common method of preservation in vaccine production and shipping. Because infective virions survive in droplet nuclei, the infection can be spread as an aerosol.

HISTORY. Measles probably became an endemic human disease no earlier than about 3000 to 5000 B.C. Since measles produces lifelong immunity and the infectious period lasts only about a week, the disease requires a substantial birth cohort of susceptible persons in order to remain endemic. A fixed population of around 200,000 to 1 million, which would produce an annual birth cohort of between 10,000 and 40,000 persons, is required to sustain measles virus transmission. Human populations of this size did not exist before the urban civilizations of Mesopotamia. From its likely origins in the Middle East, measles probably spread throughout the eastern Mediterranean and the Roman Empire through about 500 A.D. At the same time the disease probably had also spread to Africa and to India and China. The disease spread to the New World through contact with Europe following Columbus's voyages to America.

The earliest surviving account of the clinical features of measles was written by Rhazes, a Persian physician, in 910 A.D. In Japan, the disease was described as distinct from smallpox in a treatise published in 998 A.D. Similar accounts are also found in China from the 11th century A.D. onward.

The significance of measles infection was gradually elucidated over the ensuing centuries. Peter Panum, a Danish physician, made a series of important observations during

*All the material in this chapter is in the public domain, with the exception of any borrowed figures or tables.

an epidemic of measles on the Faroe Islands in 1846. He described the primary mode of transmission and the incubation period, gave a complete clinical description of the illness, demonstrated higher mortality among the very young and very old, and discovered that measles disease confers lifelong immunity.

The virus was first grown in primary human kidney and rhesus monkey kidney cells by Enders and Peebles in the early 1950s. These investigators described characteristic cytopathic effects that occur in tissue culture, including the formation of multinucleate giant cells, vacuolization in the syncytial cytoplasm, and the presence of eosinophilic intracytoplasmic and intranuclear inclusion bodies.

The importance of measles in developing countries was widely publicized by Morley and colleagues in the 1960s. They studied childhood diseases in Imesi, Nigeria, a community of about 1000 persons. In this population, the mean age of measles patients was 15 months; the case-fatality rate was 7%, and biennial epidemics occurred during the dry season. Morley showed that the clinical and epidemiologic characteristics of measles were similar to those observed in Scotland in the late 1800s, thus providing epidemiologic evidence against the theory that the measles virus had mutated into a more virulent form in the tropics.

Vaccine trials in Burkina Faso, formerly Upper Volta in the early 1960s laid the foundation for mass vaccination campaigns against measles and smallpox in West and Central Africa. While the success of smallpox control in this program led to the eventual global eradication of that disease, measles proved a more difficult challenge. Only in The Gambia, a small country in West Africa, was the transmission of measles clearly interrupted. Unfortunately, when external funding for measles control ceased in the early 1970s, the epidemiology of measles reverted to its pre-interruption pattern. Nevertheless, the demonstration that mass vaccination efforts could interrupt the transmission of the virus set a benchmark for future efforts to control measles.

With the successful eradication of smallpox in 1977, worldwide control of measles, along with diphtheria, pertussis, tetanus, tuberculosis, and polio, became a major effort of the World Health Organization's (WHO) Expanded Program on Immunizations (EPI). In 1990, the attainment of full vaccination of 80% of the world's children, an achievement known as universal childhood immunization, represented a major triumph for public health. In that same year, at the World Summit for Children held in New York, the goals of reducing measles cases to 90% and deaths due to measles to 95% below prevaccination levels were set.

EPIDEMIOLOGY

Distribution and Incidence. Until the 1990s, measles was present in every country throughout the world. In 1995, an estimated 44 million cases, representing one third of the entire global birth cohort, occurred, and 1.1 million deaths in children under 5 years of age were attributed to measles. The incidence of measles is directly related to population immunity. Children not vaccinated against measles become susceptible at 3 to 15 months of age, when the maternal antibody against measles decays to nonprotective levels. Before the development of an effective vaccine, measles was a universal disease.

The age-specific incidence of measles depends on contact patterns within the population, the age distribution of susceptibility in the population, and immigration patterns. Measles is a reportable disease in most, but not all, countries, although only 1 million to 2 million cases are reported each year, significantly underestimating the health burden of this disease.

Transmission. Humans, the only reservoir of measles, are infectious for only a 7- to 10-day period beginning with the onset of symptoms. Infected persons develop lifelong immunity following the disease. Measles affects both sexes equally. Infectious patients transmit the disease to susceptible contacts by coughing droplet nuclei or disseminating aerosols. The CD46 molecule, a membrane surface protein found exclusively on primate and human cell membranes, is the receptor for measles virus, explaining the limited host specificity of measles. Other primates may be infected with measles virus and on rare occasions have transmitted the disease to humans.

It is one of the most contagious of infections. Approximately 90% of susceptible persons in close contact, e.g., siblings in a household, will develop measles. Contact with an infectious person at school, in a doctor's office or dispensary, on a bus, or even with an aerosol of virus is sufficient for transmission to occur. There have been documented instances of transmission in a doctor's office when the susceptible contact was exposed to virus in an examining room occupied 2 hours earlier by an infectious individual. The most infectious period is during the 2- to 4-day prodrome before the onset of the characteristic rash. This observation means that chains of transmission can be difficult to trace, since an individual may acquire measles through exposure to a person in the prodromal phase of disease but before the illness is recognized as measles.

Measles is a seasonal disease, with most cases occurring in the late winter or spring or, in tropical countries, during the dry, cool season. The reasons for this seasonality are not fully understood but probably involve social factors, e.g., increased exposure to other persons in enclosed settings in winter, and biologic factors, e.g., increased susceptibility because of pharyngeal mucosal changes or increased survival of measles virus in aerosols in dry, cool environments.

Prevaccine Measles. In the absence of vaccination, measles is typically an epidemic disease that recurs in patterns ranging from every year to every 3 years. The interepidemic period is determined chiefly by the size of the population and the rate of contact between susceptible children. The more frequent the epidemics, the lower the median age of measles cases. In settings of annual epidemics, the median age of onset can be as low as 15 months, as in Nigeria during the 1960s. Typically, urban areas in developing countries have had more frequent epidemics and a lower median age of onset compared with rural areas or developed countries.

Persons in areas with limited exposure to the outside world, e.g., in remote traditional populations or on isolated islands, can go for decades without a measles epidemic. When measles virus is imported into these communities, the result can be devastating, with a very high proportion of persons acquiring the disease in a short time.

Postvaccine Measles. With the widespread implementation of vaccination programs throughout the world during the 1980s, the epidemiology of measles changed. In populations with single dose vaccination coverage of 80 to 95%, the interval between epidemics lengthened from 1 to 3 years before vaccination to 5 or even 10 years, and the median age of disease onset increased. Measles occurred in persons who failed to develop protective immunity after vaccination; when vaccination coverage rates were very high, sometimes the majority of cases occurred among vaccinated persons. This often caused unfounded concern about reduced vaccine efficacy. In partially vaccinated populations, outbreaks of measles occur in schools, daycare settings, other institutions (e.g., prisons), in persons or groups opposed to vaccination for religious or other reasons, and in groups of children who have not been vaccinated. The critical epidemiologic factor that allows an outbreak to occur is the accumulation of susceptible persons. Susceptible persons accumulate for two reasons: failure to receive vaccination and failure to develop protective immunity in response to vaccination. The reduced chance of exposure to measles virus resulting from partial population immunity explains the older age at disease onset in partially vaccinated populations.

In the last decade, several countries, including virtually all countries in the Western hemisphere and several European countries, have implemented vaccination strategies that have effectively interrupted transmission of the virus. All have required giving more than a single dose of vaccine, and all have required extraordinary efforts to achieve coverage levels high enough to prevent ongoing transmission.

PATHOGENESIS. Measles is a systemic infection. In susceptible persons, measles virus enters the lymphoid tissue of the pharynx and reproduces locally. After 2 to 3 days, a brief viremia occurs, seeding the rest of the lymphoid tissue and infecting mononuclear and macrophage cells. After another 5 to 7 days, a second viremia occurs, disseminating the virus throughout the body and leading to the characteristic prodromal fever and cough. After an additional 2 to 4 days, the characteristic rash occurs, marking the development of an effective immune response.

At the molecular level, the fusion and hemagglutinin proteins bind to the CD46 molecule on the host cell membrane and promote entry of the virus into the cell. Initially, measles virus causes remarkably little disruption to normal cellular processes.

Pathology. The major pathologic findings of measles are in the skin and mucous membranes, the lymphoid tissue, and the respiratory system. The skin lesions typically include dyskeratosis and spongiosis with a lymphocytic infiltrate. The most characteristic finding, seen primarily in the lymphoid tissues and the respiratory epithelium, is multinucleate giant cells (Fig. 25–1). Such cells, which may measure up to 100 μM in diameter and contain 50 to 100 nuclei, are known as Warthin-Finkeldey cells. Characteristic eosinophilic intracytoplasmic inclusions are also seen, and intranuclear inclusions may occur. Intranuclear inclusions consist primarily of self-assembled nucleoprotein structures. The intracy-

toplasmic inclusions are generally known as fuzzy nucleocapsids and are composed of RNA, nucleoprotein, phosphoprotein, and matrix protein; the matrix protein is believed to impart the fuzzy appearance. More phosphoprotein is present in the intracytoplasmic inclusions than in the free virus.

Koplik spots, whitish raised papules on the buccal mucosa and conjunctiva, contain small necrotic foci with perivascular infiltrates of mononuclear cells, similar to the pathologic features of the rash.

Humoral Immune Response. The humoral immune response to measles becomes detectable around the time of rash onset with the production of IgM and, later, IgG antibodies. These antibodies are capable of preventing measles virus from infecting susceptible cells in cell culture. Using an IgM capture enzyme immunoassay, IgM antibodies are detectable in about 80% of persons with measles in the first 72 hours after rash onset and in nearly all persons from 3 through 28 days. IgM antibodies peak between 7 and 14 days after rash onset. IgG antibodies peak at about 30 days and then gradually decline, most rapidly over the next 6 months. The humoral immune response does not appear to be essential to prevent complications from measles, as children with agammaglobulinemia recover from measles uneventfully.

Cell-Mediated Immunity (CMI) and Measles Infection. The immune response to measles begins as a CMI response and shifts to a humoral response, with suppression of CMI about a week after rash onset. The initial CMI response is characterized by increases in β-interferon, soluble CD8 indicating effector–target cell interaction, and soluble interleukin-2 receptor. These findings suggest that the CMI response is the primary means by which measles virus is cleared. As the rash clears, approximately a week after onset, CMI is suppressed: Interleukin-4 levels increase; interleukin-12 levels are downregulated; and soluble CD8 levels decline to normal. The result of these changes is to shift the immune response from a Th-1 type to a Th-2 type response.

The suppression of CMI by measles produces a variety of abnormalities in laboratory tests, e.g., suppressing delayed type hypersensitivity skin tests. This immune suppression

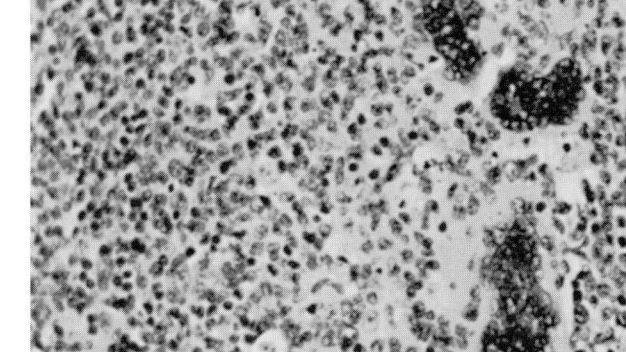

Figure 25–1. Lymph node from patient with measles showing Warthin-Finkeldey giant cells in reactive center (× 260). (Courtesy of Armed Forces Institute of Pathology, Photograph Neg. No. 57-1921.)

can cause reactivation of latent tuberculosis and can make tuberculin skin tests negative for several weeks, even in the presence of tuberculosis.

CLINICAL MANIFESTATIONS

Acute Illness. The incubation period is 10 to 12 days, with a range of 8 to 16 days, corresponding to the period between the local infection of the pharyngeal lymphoid tissues and the second viremia. Following the incubation period, the classic signs of cough, conjunctivitis, and coryza begin almost simultaneously, with a concurrent temperature rise to 38°C to 40°C. Diarrhea is a frequent sign of acute measles in young children and is a particularly serious complication in children who are already malnourished.

Measles-induced diarrhea can become chronic and exacerbate malnutrition. Excretion of measles virus may be prolonged among children with diarrhea who are malnourished. Vaccination against measles may prevent as many as 25% of deaths due to diarrhea, including some that would not be prevented with oral rehydration therapy.

The relatively nonproductive cough increases in severity as the rash develops to its fullest, 2 to 4 days after onset of symptoms. Cough generally lasts the entire duration of the illness, 7 to 10 days. Disease may be more prolonged and severe in younger and debilitated children. Coryza and nonpurulent conjunctivitis, often accompanied by photophobia, continue through day 6 to 8. Koplik spots begin on day 1 to 3 of illness, before rash onset. They are found on the buccal mucosa adjacent to the molar teeth and in the conjunctiva. Inexperienced clinicians may miss or misinterpret Koplik spots.

The maculopapular rash of measles first appears as an erythematous papular eruption behind the ears or at the hairline on the forehead and then spreads inferiorly during the next 2 to 3 days. The papules frequently coalesce, forming splotchy macules. The individual is sickest during the second through fourth days after rash onset, until the fever subsides. In black children, the sandpaper-like texture of the rash can be helpful in diagnosis, since the erythematous changes may be difficult to appreciate.

When the rash is totally coalescent, desquamation frequently occurs (Fig. 25–2). This can begin at the end of the first week of illness and can continue through the following

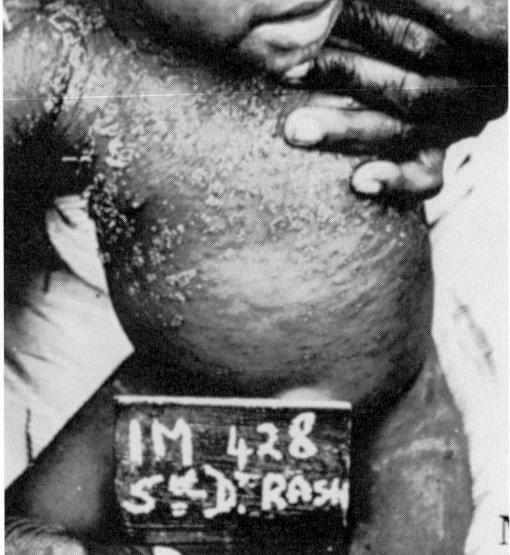

***Figure* 25–2.** Desquamation on fifth day of rash due to measles in black child. (Courtesy of Institute of Child Health, D. Morley.)

week. Anorexia and malaise are common throughout the illness, and generalized lymphadenopathy and hepatosplenomegaly can occur. For most patients, the signs and symptoms begin to abate rapidly when the temperature falls on day 6 or 7. Recovery from the acute illness is usually complete within 10 to 14 days.

Acute measles is associated with a drop in serum vitamin A levels. Although the mechanism is not fully understood, vitamin A depletion may result from the effects of measles infection on epithelial cells. Subclinical vitamin A deficiency resulting from measles may explain, in part, late complications.

Complications. Measles may cause several infectious complications, which result either from measles infection itself or from secondary infection.

Direct Effects of Measles. Among complications that are the direct effect of measles, abnormalities of the mucosal surfaces are the underlying cause in most instances. Stomatitis is frequent and may interfere with eating. Cancrum oris, a painful oral lesion developing concurrently with measles, is not infrequent and makes eating and drinking difficult. Laryngitis or laryngotracheitis may cause severe airway obstruction, requiring prompt tracheostomy if respiration is severely impaired. Xerophthalmia and keratomalacia leading to blindness may occur; blindness is a particularly common complication in regions where vitamin A deficiency is widespread. Measles pneumonia is characterized by interstitial infiltrations on chest radiograph. This complication is much more frequent in persons with an underlying immunodeficiency, e.g., leukemia. Diarrhea is the most common complication of measles in some developing countries. Abnormalities on electrocardiogram (ECG) may occur, e.g., inverted T-waves or prolongation of the P-R interval. Clinically apparent myocarditis is rare. Elevation of liver enzymes may occur with acute measles and is more common in adults. Renal dysfunction is unusual. Measles acquired during pregnancy is associated with fetal loss, but congenital abnormalities have not been reported.

Acute Postinfectious Encephalitis. Postmeasles encephalitis, or measles encephalitis, occurs with a reported frequency of 1 to 4 in 1000 measles cases and typically begins 2 to 6 days after rash onset. The course varies between mild and rapidly fulminant and can result in death within 24 hours. About 15% of patients with measles encephalitis die, and sequelae, e.g., mental retardation, seizures, and behavioral and learning disorders, may occur in as many as 25%. Neurologic involvement is probably more prevalent than is indicated by the incidence of overt acute encephalitis; changes in the electroencephalogram (EEG) and pleocytosis of the cerebral spinal fluid (CSF) are not uncommon in acute measles. Measles virus is not found in the central nervous system (CNS) of persons who die of acute measles encephalitis. The demyelination characteristic of measles encephalitis is caused by the host's immune response to infection. Postinfectious encephalitis is distinct from measles inclusion body encephalitis; the latter is a direct infection of the CNS, usually occurring within months of acute infection in immunocompromised persons.

Secondary Infections. These are a significant cause of morbidity attributed to measles. Otitis media is one of the most common complications of measles and should be suspected when fever lasts more than 5 to 7 days after rash onset. Mastoiditis resulting from untreated otitis media may occur. Secondary bacterial pneumonia associated with measles is a frequent cause of death; secondary viral pneumonia may also complicate recovery from measles. Among causes of bacterial pneumonia, *Haemophilus influenzae, Streptococcus pneumoniae,* and *Staphylococcus aureus* are the pathogens most commonly isolated. Diarrhea occurring 1 to 2 weeks after acute measles is frequently bloody and may indicate infection with *Shigella* spp.

Subacute Sclerosing Panencephalitis (SSPE). This is a late neurologic complication of measles, occurring 2 to 15 years after measles infection. Progressive behavioral changes and intellectual deterioration are usually associated with motor incoordination; fever is not present. SSPE is more common when the preceding measles infection is acquired within the first 2 years of life. Among the typical laboratory findings are an extremely high serum measles antibody titer with detectable antibody in the CSF. Measles virus can be isolated from brain tissue or CSF, although patients with SSPE are not infectious. A characteristic spike-and-wave pattern is seen on EEG. Death generally occurs with 6 months of symptom onset. The pathologic findings include patchy demyelination and intranuclear and intracytoplasmic inclusions in both neuronal and glial cells. Widespread vaccination has decreased the incidence of this complication dramatically, although cases of SSPE have occurred in vaccinated individuals, probably because of wild-type measles infection before vaccination. Genetic studies of measles viruses isolated from the brain tissue of persons with SSPE have shown that the virus is genetically distinct from usual wild-type virus, with an alteration in one of the membrane proteins responsible for budding of the virus (usually the matrix protein). Until recently, treatment of SSPE was supportive. Reports of therapy with intrathecal α-interferon have suggested that the progressive downhill course can be altered. Some investigators have combined intrathecal interferon with ribavirin, an antiviral drug, or Isoprinosine, an antimetabolite. Treatment with these drugs would be costly and impractical to use in developing countries.

PROGNOSIS. Case-fatality rates from measles vary, depending on the age and nutritional status of the patient and the type and severity of complications. Studies in Africa have shown that secondary household cases, which presumably have more intense exposure to the virus, tend to have more severe disease and a greater likelihood of dying than primary cases, suggesting that the size of the inoculum contributes to the severity of disease. Household exposure has not been associated with more severe disease in developed countries. In most developed countries, the case-fatality rate is about 1 per 1000 cases. Between 1989 and 1991 during a nationwide measles epidemic in the United States, the case-fatality rate was 3 per 1000 reported cases. In West Africa and Asia, case-fatality rates as high as 25% have been reported, although rates of 1 to 5% are more common. The highest case-fatality rates are reported from hospitals where the most severe cases are treated. Death is usually due to bacterial pneumonia, malnutrition, or diarrhea.

Immunocompromised persons, e.g., those with acute leukemia or congenital immunodeficiency or patients being treated with immunosuppressive drugs, are at greater risk for complications and death than persons with normal immune function. Persons with HIV infection are also at increased risk of death from measles, with case-fatality rates in small series reported to be 25 to 60%. Measles in children younger than 12 months of age is associated with a higher risk of complications and death than in older children. The lowest risk of death is in children between 5 and 16 years of age. Adults are at increased risk of death (and encephalitis) compared with 5- to 16-year-old children but at lower risk of death than children in the first year of life. Vitamin A deficiency is a risk factor for death due to measles, and many of the complications of measles appear to be mediated through depletion of vitamin A occurring as a result of measles.

Several investigators have reported a persistent increased risk of mortality in the months after acquiring measles among children in developing countries compared with children of similar age who did not contract measles. This effect is known as delayed excess mortality and has been corroborated by studies showing that measles vaccination improves child survival between 25 and 30%, larger than could be accounted for by the mortality attributed to acute measles infection alone. However, investigation and follow-up of several more recent measles epidemics have not found delayed excess mortality.

DIAGNOSIS. Measles is easily diagnosed when several children in a community who have not had measles or been vaccinated against measles have fever, cough, conjunctivitis, coryza, and a morbilliform rash. The clinical diagnosis is more difficult in populations with high vaccination coverage because the clustering of cases that is characteristic when large numbers of susceptible persons are exposed may not be evident. In countries with highly successful vaccination programs, younger physicians may not have seen cases of measles and may not recognize the characteristic clinical syndrome.

Differential Diagnosis. Measles may be confused with many other illnesses that cause rash and fever. Such common illnesses include scarlet fever, rubella, parvovirus B19 infection (fifth disease, or erythema infectiosum), human herpes virus 6 infection (roseola infantum), enterovirus infection (especially echovirus 16 and coxsackieviruses 4, 6, and 9), mucocutaneous lymph node syndrome (Kawasaki disease), meningococcemia, typhus and tick fever, secondary syphilis, and infectious mononucleosis. Scarlet fever is accompanied by a sore throat and pharyngeal exudate, and the rash has a sandpaper texture that blanches on diascopy. Rubella is a milder illness with a shorter course than measles. The rash associated with rubella fades as it spreads and is accompanied by prominent posterior cervical lymphadenopathy. Infection with parvovirus B19 results in a rash that begins with a "slapped cheek" appearance, which may not be present in adults, followed by a symmetric reticular rash on the extensor surfaces and, finally, an evanescent rash. The clinical course of roseola infantum includes 2 to 3 days of high fever followed by the appearance of a rash after defervescence. The rash begins on the trunk, neck, or behind the ears and may spread but rarely involves the arms or legs.

Skin reactions to antimicrobial drugs may be erroneously diagnosed as measles. Reactions to amoxycillin, other penicillins, co-trimoxazole, and sulfonamide drugs are most commonly confused with measles. This causes particular problems, since patients with the nonspecific prodromal symptoms of measles may be treated with one of these antimicrobial drugs.

Laboratory Diagnosis. *Serology.* Testing serum specimens for antibody to measles virus is the foundation of the laboratory diagnosis. Detection of measles IgM antibody after rash onset is becoming the standard method to diagnose measles. One of the major advantages of IgM testing is the need for only a single specimen, in contrast to testing for total or IgG antibody, in which acute and convalescent serum specimens are required. Recent work has led to the development of a radioimmunoassay test for detecting measles IgM antibody in oral secretions. This test was developed in the United Kingdom and is used routinely there. A fourfold rise in antibody titer against measles may be demonstrated with an enzyme immunoassay (EIA), hemagglutination inhibition (HIA), or plaque reduction neutralization testing. None of the diagnostic methods that are based on detection of antibody can distinguish an immune response following measles disease from an immune response following vaccination. If measles vaccine has been given within 6 to 45 days of the collection of the specimen, measles IgM antibody may indicate a response to vaccination rather than a response to infection.

Virus Isolation. Techniques in virus isolation have been improved, and methods to automate the genetic sequencing of measles viruses have been developed. These advances have made it possible to isolate and sequence the genomes of isolated measles viruses and to compare these genetic sequences. In many cases, the results can determine the probable origin of the virus. Chains of transmission can be traced using these techniques, even when the source of exposure is unknown. Virus isolation and genotyping can also be used to distinguish adverse reactions, e.g., fever and rash, caused by measles vaccination from infection with wild-type measles.

TREATMENT AND PROGNOSIS

Vitamin A. Treatment for measles is largely supportive, although evidence suggests that vitamin A therapy for children hospitalized with measles may prevent a significant proportion of deaths in developing countries. A double-blinded, placebo-controlled trial in hospitalized South African children convincingly demonstrated a benefit of vitamin A therapy, with a reduction in mortality of 40% in those randomized to receive vitamin A. Clinical vitamin A deficiency was not common in the area where the study was carried out. Currently, the WHO recommends that children with measles be treated with vitamin A, with the dose based on the age of the child. Children 0 to 5 months of age should receive 50,000 IU on each of the first 2 days after diagnosis (100,000 IU total) and an additional 50,000 IU no sooner than 2 weeks after the first dose. Children 6 to 11 months of age should receive 100,000 IU on each of the first 2 days after diagnosis (200,000 IU total) and an additional 100,000 IU no sooner than 2 weeks after the first dose. Children over 12 months of age should receive 200,000 IU on each of the first 2 days after diagnosis (400,000 IU total) and an additional 200,000 IU no sooner than 2 weeks after the first dose. These recommendations are for children who require hospitalization as well as for those less severely ill. In many developing countries, vitamin A supplementation programs that call for supplementary vitamin A to be administered at 3- to 4-month intervals have been established. One of the clearest benefits of these supplementary programs is a reduced case-fatality rate from measles.

Antiviral Drugs. Ribavirin, a nucleoside analogue effectively prevents replication of measles virus in cell culture, and limited clinical experience with ribavirin therapy for measles suggests that it may be beneficial. This experience has largely been in immunosuppressed patients with severe measles infection, although two clinical trials have shown a benefit. The high cost of ribavirin will limit its use in developing countries.

Supportive Care. Alert supportive care is needed, as complications, e.g., pneumonia or diarrhea, may occur suddenly, especially in young children. Rest, hydration, adequate nutrition, antitussives, and meticulous attention to therapy of bacterial complications are needed. The eyes should be carefully rinsed daily with sterile saline solution or, lacking this, with clean water. There should be daily examination for otitis media, pneumonia, and secondary bacterial skin infections, for which antimicrobial drug therapy is indicated. Routine prophylaxis with antimicrobial drugs has not prevented bacterial complications. For postinfectious encephalitis, general supportive care is needed, including anticonvulsant drugs to manage seizures. Gamma globulin and steroids have been assessed but offer no benefit in the management of measles or its complications.

PREVENTION AND CONTROL OF MEASLES

Passive Immunization. Passive immunization with gamma globulin (0.25 mg/kg, up to a total dose of 15 mL) is effective in preventing measles if given within 6 days of exposure. This is recommended to protect those at high risk of complications after exposure, e.g., pregnant women, immunosuppressed persons, children under the recommended age for vaccination, and those with tuberculosis, leukemia, or known HIV infection. Postexposure prophylaxis with gamma globulin is rarely possible in developing countries because of the cost and the difficulties of administering gamma globulin to persons for whom it is indicated within 6 days of exposure.

Immunization Using Standard Vaccines. Measles vaccine is one of the safest and most effective of all vaccines. The vaccine was originally developed in the late 1950s and early 1960s. Several strains of live attenuated measles virus vaccine, Schwarz, Moraten, Edmonston-Zagreb, and AIK-C, are currently in use. Seroconversion rates and rates of adverse events are roughly similar for all strains. These vaccine strains are genetically quite similar and differ from wild-type strains.

Vaccine Administration. Measles vaccines are frequently given in a combined product with other live attenuated vaccines—with rubella vaccine (as MR vaccine) or with rubella and mumps vaccine (as MMR vaccine). The addition of rubella and mumps vaccines to measles does not alter the rate of seroconversion or frequency of side effects to any of the three vaccines compared with giving each vaccine individually.

Routine measles vaccination must be integrated into the routine primary health care system of every country. Adequate record keeping, provision of sterile injections, and confidence in the health care system are critical components in achieving reductions in measles incidence and mortality. Achieving a high level of coverage with measles vaccine is one of the most effective public health interventions to prevent death in children.

Vaccine Effectiveness. The rate of seroconversion to measles vaccine is highly dependent on the age at which vaccination is administered. For children immunized at 15 months or older, seroconversion rates of over 95% are expected. The seroconversion rate in children given measles vaccine at 9 months of age is usually 80 to 85%, although some studies have reported higher percentages. Maternal antibody protects children from measles in the first 3 to 12 months of life but also interferes with immunization with measles vaccine. The age at which maternal antibody decreases to negligible levels varies in different populations. In some developing countries, significant loss of maternal antibody occurs in the first 3 to 6 months of life. Children born to mothers who experienced measles disease receive higher titers of transplacentally transferred measles antibody than do children whose mothers were vaccinated; therefore, children born to mothers who had measles become susceptible to measles at an older age than do children whose mothers were vaccinated. Determining the proper age for measles vaccination requires balancing the known risk of contracting measles, which increases with age, with the risk of not responding to vaccination, which decreases with age. The WHO's EPI program recommends vaccination at 9 months of age to prevent measles in the great majority of children in developing countries.

Vaccine failure can be divided into two types. Primary vaccine failure is the absence of any response to measles vaccination. The best understood cause is persistent maternal antibody to measles although use of impotent vaccine must be considered. Children reimmunized after primary vaccine failure generally respond with a normal primary immune response, including the production of IgM antibodies and protective levels of IgG antibody. Revaccination of children with primary vaccine failure results in seroconversion in 80 to 95% of children and appears to be equally successful when given at any age from 18 months through adulthood. Secondary vaccine failure occurs when vaccination initially produces an immune response but, over time, antibody levels decline until insufficient to provide protection. Most cases of vaccine failure are the result of primary vaccine failure.

Contraindications to Immunization. Children who have a mild illness, e.g., upper respiratory tract infection or diarrhea, may be safely and effectively immunized with measles vaccine. Data are inadequate to determine whether children with high fever or more severe illnesses would respond equally well to vaccination.

Measles vaccination is contraindicated for persons with severe immunosuppression, e.g., persons with leukemia or lymphoma or those undergoing immunosuppressive therapy. Persons with HIV infection should receive measles vaccine unless there is evidence of severe immunosuppression; some authorities recommend measles vaccine to all HIV-infected persons because of the high case-fatality ratio for measles among persons with HIV infection. Measles vaccination should not be given to pregnant women because of the theoretical risk of fetal infection. Persons who are known to have had an anaphylactic response to neomycin or gelatin should not be given measles vaccine because the vaccine contains these substances.

Adverse Events. Adverse events seen after measles vaccination are generally mild; fever up to 39°C and transient rash may occur between the seventh and twelfth days after vaccination and are observed in 5 to 15% of vaccine recipients. Fever following vaccination has been associated with febrile seizures, which are self-limited and do not increase the risk of a subsequent seizure disorder. Clinically evident thrombocytopenia occurs in between 1 in 25,000 and 1 in 40,000 vaccine recipients. There has been concern about the possibility of measles vaccination causing acute encephalopathy. Studies from the 1960s estimated the risk of encephalopathy or encephalitis at 1 per 1 million doses of vaccine administered. This is lower than the risk of encephalopathy or encephalitis of unknown etiology in unvaccinated children and suggests that there is not a causal relationship between vaccination against measles and either of these disorders. Measles vaccination has reduced the rate of SSPE to nearly undetectable levels. Although vaccinated persons have acquired SSPE, the very low rate of occurrence suggests that these cases resulted from undetected or inapparent prior wild-type measles virus infection rather than vaccine virus.

Atypical Measles. Persons vaccinated with killed measles vaccine, produced during the 1960s, are at risk for an unusual clinical presentation following exposure to wild-type measles. This syndrome, known as atypical measles, is characterized by high fever, headache, abdominal pain, cough, rash, elevated liver enzymes, and nodular pneumonitis. The rash begins on the extremities and spreads centrally; it may be maculopapular but more frequently is petechial and vesicular with edema. The syndrome is caused by a severe delayed hypersensitivity reaction resulting from an abnormal immune response caused by lack of antibody response to the fusion protein. Killed measles vaccines were withdrawn from production in the late 1960s. Persons who were vaccinated with a killed measles vaccine should be revaccinated with a live vaccine to prevent atypical measles.

Immunization With New Vaccines. In the mid-1980s, research was carried out into a vaccine that would be effective in children who still had maternal antibodies. This effort was believed to be essential to control measles, especially in densely populated urban areas, where measles virus continued to circulate among preschool age children despite vaccine coverage levels as high as 80%. The Edmonston-Zagreb measles vaccine, given in titers 10 to 100 times higher than standard-titer measles vaccine produced seroconversion in up to 95% of children immunized as young as 4 months of age. This finding led to a recommendation by the WHO in 1980 that high-titer Edmonston-Zagreb vaccine be used in areas where a substantial proportion of measles cases occurred among children under 9 months of age.

Later, in follow-up studies in Senegal, investigators found an increased risk of death in girls who had received high-titer vaccines compared with those who had received standard-titer vaccines. Although initially doubted, the same finding was observed in studies conducted in Guinea-Bissau and Haiti. The finding was never fully explained; no consistent clinical picture emerged; no immunologic abnormalities were demonstrated; and no risk factor other than female sex was determined. The effect was seen most frequently with high-titer Edmonston-Zagreb vaccine, although it was observed in one study in which high-titer Schwarz vaccine was used. These results led the WHO to rescind the recommendation for use of high-titer vaccines.

New Immunization Strategies. New strategies to control measles have been developed and widely implemented over the past decade and are based on the recognized need to prevent the accumulation of children susceptible to measles. Success following implementation of the strategies has rekindled enthusiasm for efforts to achieve global eradication of measles.

A mass vaccination approach to control measles was developed in Cuba in the late 1980s, building on work done in the late 1960s in West Africa. Despite high vaccination coverage levels with a single dose of measles, cases of measles continued to occur in Cuba. With the goal of eliminating measles, in 1987 the Cuban Ministry of Health conducted a mass vaccination campaign with measles vaccine. Every child from 12 months to 15 years of age was targeted for vaccination regardless of history of vaccination or disease. This strategy would render susceptible children immune to measles, whether that susceptibility was the result of failure to receive measles vaccine or failure to respond to measles vaccination. Following a campaign in which coverage was estimated to be 98%, the incidence of measles dropped abruptly. In 1992 a follow-up campaign was conducted vaccinating children 2 to 5 years of age, who would not have been immunized in the first campaign. The last confirmed measles case in Cuba occurred in 1993. Following the success of measles control efforts in Cuba, countries of the English-speaking Caribbean, with technical assistance of the Pan American Health Organization (PAHO), conducted a mass vaccination campaign in 1991, known in the Caribbean as the Big Bang. Again, the incidence of measles fell dramatically.

The PAHO strategy is composed of three major elements: (1) initiating a catch-up campaign, in which all children 9 or 12 months of age through 14 years of age are vaccinated; (2) changing the age for routine immunization to 12 months and achieving and maintaining routine vaccination coverage levels at 90% or higher; and (3) conducting periodic follow-up campaigns to keep the accumulation of susceptible persons below the level that would be required for a measles epidemic to occur. The current recommendation for conducting follow-up campaigns is that they take place whenever the number of susceptible children 12 months of age and older is equal to or greater than the number of children born in a year. In practice, depending on routine vaccine coverage levels, campaigns are recommended every 3 to 5 years. Based on the success in controlling measles, the Pan American Sanitary Conference in 1994 declared a goal to eliminate

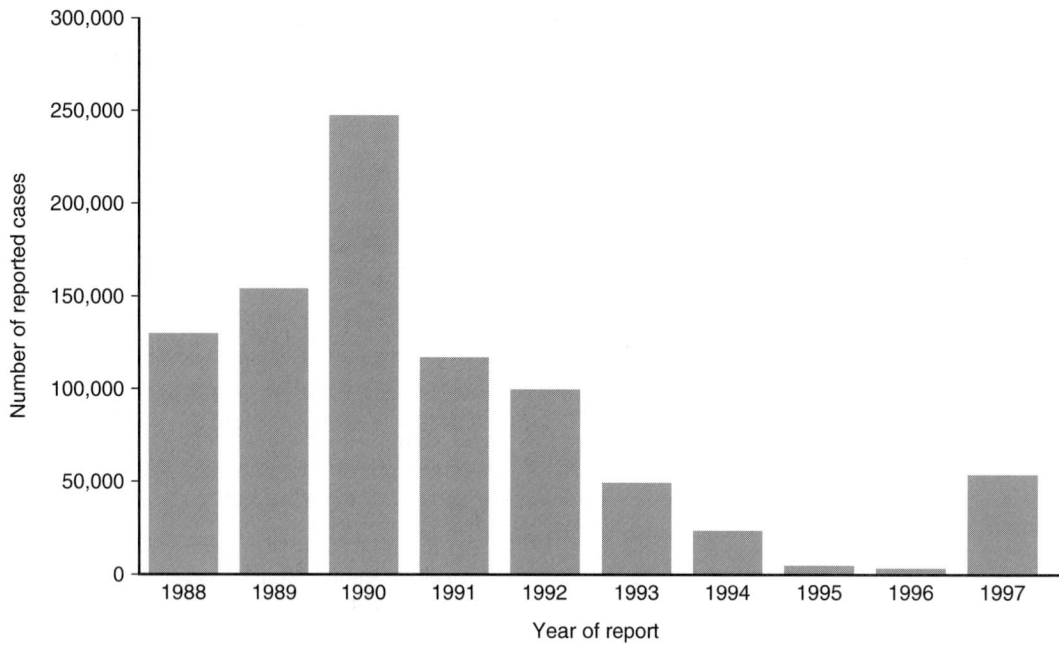

Figure 25–3. The reduction in reported cases of measles in the Western Hemisphere since the institution of the mass vaccination campaign by PAHO in 1991.

measles from the Western Hemisphere by the year 2000. PAHO member countries reported 2109 cases of measles in 1996, compared with 246,607 in 1990 (Fig. 25–3). The number of measles cases identified in the United States reported to have a source in another PAHO member country fell dramatically as a result of the drop in measles cases. No imported measles cases from countries of South or Central America were reported in the United States between 1994 and 1996. In 1997, a number of countries in the Americas reported measles outbreaks and the number of reported cases during 1997 was 52,618. In Brazil, migration of susceptible persons, older than the age recommended for inclusion in the mass vaccination campaigns and from rural areas with historically low rates of measles, were, in part, responsible for the urban measles outbreaks. In some settings, targeted vaccination of high-risk adults may be appropriate.

An alternative strategy uses an initial catch-up campaign followed by a standing recommendation for each child to receive a second dose of measles-containing vaccine by the time of school entry. Implementation of this strategy provides a second dose of measles vaccine to school-age children in a brief mass vaccination campaign and then sets in place a requirement for children who were too young to participate in the campaign, or not yet born, to receive a second measles vaccination by the time of school entry. Canada and the United Kingdom have been able to achieve routine coverage in excess of 90% with a single dose of measles vaccine.

Surveillance and Outbreak Control. Surveillance of measles cases is a critical tool to improve measles control programs and will be an essential element of a complete strategy to achieve sustained elimination of measles virus transmission. For countries that have vaccination coverage levels below 80%, surveillance should be used to improve routine vaccination activities by demonstrating the burden of disease and identifying geographic and population groups at greatest risk for measles and measles-related mortality. For countries that are implementing strategies designed to interrupt transmission of measles, laboratory confirmation of cases becomes essential. In such countries, all isolated measles cases and at least one case in each chain of transmission must be laboratory confirmed. Developing the capacity to provide laboratory confirmation of cases will be a major challenge for measles elimination efforts. In countries attempting to interrupt transmission, tracking chains of transmission will be a major focus of effort. The goal of such tracing is to document the absence of endemic measles transmission despite recurrent importations of measles from countries with less developed measles control programs.

Unlike smallpox eradication, which was largely achieved with a surveillance containment approach, measles eradication cannot be achieved only by isolating infectious patients through quarantine or by providing vaccination in response to outbreaks. Measles is too contagious and spreads too quickly for case-containment measures to be very effective in the absence of a high background level of population immunity. In situations in which a high level of population immunity to measles exists, measles vaccination should be provided to susceptible contacts of confirmed measles cases but must be given within 3 days of exposure to prevent measles disease. In institutional exposures, e.g., schools and prisons, rapid implementation of vaccination programs probably reduces transmission.

Bibliography

Bellini WJ, Rota JS, Rota PA: Virology of measles virus. J Infect Dis 170(Suppl 1):S15, 1994.

Brody JA, Bridenbraugh E: Prophylactic α-globuln and live measles vaccine in an island epidemic of measles. Lancet 2:811, 1964.

Clemens JD, Stanton BF, Chakraborty J, et al: Measles vaccination and childhood mortality in rural Bangladesh. Am J Epidemiol 128:1330, 1988.

Cliff A, Haggett P, Smallman-Raynor M: Measles: An Historical Geography of a Major Human Viral Disease. Cambridge, MA, Blackwell Publishers, 1993.

de Quadros CA, Olivé JM, Hersh BA, et al: Measles elimination in the Americas: Evolving strategies. JAMA 275:224, 1996.

Dörig RE, Marcil A, Chopra A, et al: The human CD46 molecule is a receptor for measles virus (Edmonston strain). Cell 75:295, 1993.

Enders JF, Peebles TC: Propagation in tissue cultures of cytopathogenic agents from patients with measles. Proc Soc Exp Biol Med 86:277, 1954.

Feacham RG, Koblinsky MA: Interventions for the control of diarrhoeal disease among young children: Measles immunization. Bull WHO 61:641, 1983.

Garenne M, Beau FP, Sene I: Child mortality after high-titre measles vaccines: prospective study in Senegal. Lancet 338:903, 1991.

Griffin DE, Ward BJ, Esolen LM: Pathogenesis of measles virus infection: An hypothesis for altered immune responses. J Infect Dis 170(Suppl 1):S24, 1994.

Halsey NA: The optimal age for administering measles vaccine in developing countries. In Halsey NA, de Quadros CA (eds): Recent Advances in Immunization. A Bibliographic Review. Washington, DC, Pan American Health Organization (publication 451), 1983, pp 4–17.

Hummel KB, Erdman DD, Heath J, Bellini WJ: Baculovirus expression of the nucleoprotein gene of measles virus and utility of the recombinant protein in diagnostic enzyme immunoassays. J Clin Microbiol 30:2874, 1992.

Hussey GD, Klein M: A randomized controlled trial of vitamin A in children with severe measles. N Engl J Med 323:160, 1990.

Mathias RG, Meekison WG, Arcand TA, Schechter MT: The role of secondary vaccine failures in measles outbreaks. Am J Public Health 79:475, 1989.

Nokes DJ, Williams Butler AR: Towards eradication of measles virus: Global progress and strategy evaluation. Vet Microbiol 44:333, 1995.

Panum PL: Observations Made During the Epidemic of Measles on the Faroe Islands in the Year 1846. New York; American Public Health Association, 1940, pp 1–110.

Robbins FS: Measles: Clinical features. Am J Dis Child 103:266, 1962.

Rota JS, Heath JL, Rota PA, et al: Molecular epidemiology of measles virus: Identification of pathways of transmission and implications for measles elimination. J Infect Dis 173:32, 1996.

25.2 *Poxviruses**

Joel G. Breman

DEFINITION. The family Poxviridae comprises the subfamilies Chordopoxvirinae and Entomopoxvirinae, containing

---

*All the material in this chapter is in the public domain, with the exception of any borrowed figures or tables.

the vertebrate poxviruses and insect poxviruses, respectively. The genome of Poxviridae has a single linear double-stranded DNA molecule of 130 to 375 kb pairs, with replication occurring in the cytoplasm of cells. Genera are related genetically and antigenically. Poxviruses have similar morphology, often brick-shaped by electron microscopy, about 220 to 450 nm in length and 140 to 260 nm in width and depth. Of the eight genera within the Chordopoxvirinae, the orthopoxviruses are the most important for humans (Table 25–1); Parapoxvirus, yatapoxvirus, and molluscipoxvirus also cause human disease but are of less clinical and public health importance.

Smallpox, caused by variola virus, was the most treacherous of the poxvirus diseases until its eradication in 1977. Currently, the major biologic, clinical, and public health poxvirus issues are the use of vaccinia and other poxviruses as expression vectors for other vaccines, the resemblance of human monkeypox, discovered in the early 1970s, to smallpox; and the destruction of variola virus, scheduled for June 1999.

Variola (Smallpox)

HISTORY. Smallpox was an acute exanthematous viral infection with a characteristic papulovesicular eruption. Variola major caused the most severe disease, with death occurring in about 10 to 30% of patients, whereas the genetic variant variola minor (alastrim) had a case-fatality rate of less than 2%. Smallpox was known in Egypt since at least 1157 B.C., when it probably caused the death of Ramses V; it may have

TABLE 25–1. Chordopoxvirinae: Host and Geographic Range of Orthopoxviruses and Others Affecting Humans*

Poxvirus Genus and Species	Reservoir Host	Animals Infected Naturally	Range in Laboratory Animals	Geographic Range of Natural Infections
Orthopoxvirus				
Camelpox	Camels (?)	Camels (?)	Narrow	Africa and Asia
Cowpox	Rodents	Carnivores, cows, elephants, gerbils, humans, okapi, rats	Broad	Europe, including Russia
Ectromelia	Rodents	Mice, voles	Narrow	Europe; infection of laboratory rodents
Monkeypox	Squirrels	Anteaters, great apes, humans, monkeys, squirrels	Broad	Western and central Africa
Raccoonpox	Raccoons (?)	Raccoons (?)	Broad	USA
Skunkpox	Skunks (?)	Skunks (?)	Unknown	Unknown
Taterapox	Gerbils	Gerbils (*Tatera kempi*)	Narrow	Western Africa
Uasin gishu	Unknown	Horses	Medium	Kenya, Zambia
Vaccinia	Unknown	Buffalo, cows, humans, pigs, rabbits	Broad	Formerly worldwide
Variola	Humans	Humans (eradicated)	Narrow	Formerly worldwide
Volepox	Voles	California voles	Broad	USA
Parapoxvirus				
Bovine papular stomatitis	Cattle	Cattle, humans	Unknown	Worldwide
Orf	Sheep	Other ruminants	Unknown	Worldwide
Pseudocowpox	Cattle	Cattle, humans	Unknown	Worldwide
Yatapoxvirus				
Tanapox	Rodents	Humans, rodents	Unknown	Eastern and central Africa
Yabapox	Monkeys	Humans, monkeys	Unknown	Western Africa
Molluscipoxvirus				
Molluscum contagiosum	Humans	Humans	None	Worldwide

*Modified from Fenner F: Poxviruses. *In* Fields BN, Knipe DN, Howley PM (eds): Fields Virology, 3rd ed. Philadelphia, Lippincott-Raven, 1996; and Jezek Z, Fenner F: Human Monkeypox. New York, Karger, 1988.

caused a "plague" in India in about 1346 B.C. Following the occurrence of the last endemic case in Merka, Somalia, on October 26, 1977, the disease was declared eradicated by the WHO in May 1980. This was the result of an intensified, WHO-coordinated eradication program that began in 1967.

Eradication. Smallpox vaccination with vaccinia virus was one of the most effective of all public health preventive measures. By 1972, the WHO program had advanced from essentially a mass vaccination strategy, whereby the goal was to cover 80% of the entire population in a country, irrespective of the location of smallpox cases, to that of vigorous and prompt case detection and containment. Selective epidemiologic surveillance and containment were used throughout all endemic areas in Africa and Asia by the mid-1970s. Tens of thousands of surveillance workers searched actively for cases in high-risk areas until every last focus was identified and eliminated. The last cases of endemic smallpox occurred in South America (Brazil) in 1971, in Asia (Bangladesh) in 1975, and in Africa (Somalia) in 1977.

After eradication, the WHO recommended discontinuation of vaccination. The risk of complications from the vaccine, although small, completely outweighed the nonexistent risk from endemic smallpox. The cost to the United States for the successful 10-year campaign to eradicate smallpox was about $30 million. Since smallpox was eradicated in 1977, the total investment has been returned to the United States every 26 days, mainly by elimination of routine smallpox vaccination, costs for treatment of complications from vaccination, and health surveillance at the borders.

There has been a scientific debate on whether variola virus should be destroyed. Proponents of destruction argue that cloning and sequencing of reference strains of variola virus will give adequate information for comparisons with other poxviruses. All possibility for reappearance of smallpox would be eliminated, including that caused by biologic warfare or terrorist actions. Opponents of destruction contend that research questions remain that can be answered only with variola virus, including why variola virus is uniquely a human pathogen. Opponents also maintain that destruction of variola virus could set a bad precedent; eradication of dracunculiasis and poliomyelitis are expected in the near future.

Vaccinia

Vaccinia virus is smallpox vaccine; it is an orthopoxvirus that is genetically distinct from variola virus and other orthopoxviruses (Fig. 25–4). Edward Jenner's original vaccine administered in 1796 is thought to have been cowpox, but the origin of many other smallpox vaccines used worldwide is obscure. There have been at least 35 strains of vaccinia virus studied during the 20th century, and several have been used as vaccines against smallpox. These vaccine strains have differences in genetic composition, pathogenicity in biologic systems, and adverse effects following vaccination in humans.

Vaccinia virus is used widely in biomedical research to study the mode of action of viral genes and cytokine expression and as a vector for recombinant gene expression. With the increased use of vaccinia virus as a vector of foreign genes, it is important to develop guidelines for using standard vaccinia viral strains, a biosafety level 2 infectious agent, in modern research. In addition to development of an effective oral recombinant vaccinia virus wildlife rabies vaccine, there are several veterinary and human vaccine trials in progress or planned using recombinant poxviruses. Immunogenicity and pathogenicity considerations have led to use of avian poxviruses and genetically altered strains of vaccinia in vectored-vaccine research.

Monkeypox

Monkeypox virus is genetically distinct from other orthopoxviruses (Fig. 25–4). Outbreaks of monkeypox in nonhuman primate colonies in laboratories had been reported between 1958 and 1968; however, human monkeypox was first discovered in Zaire in 1970. This caused alarm because the disease resembled smallpox clinically and was discovered in an area where smallpox had been eliminated over a year previously. From 1970 to 1986, the year when active surveillance stopped, 404 cases of human monkeypox were recorded from forested areas of western and central Africa, and over 95% of them occurred in the Democratic Republic of the Congo (formerly Zaire).

CLINICAL MANIFESTATIONS. The cutaneous eruption caused by monkeypox includes macules, papules, vesicles, pustules and crusts; lesions evolve in the same stage, similar to smallpox (Fig. 25–5). The major differences between smallpox and monkeypox are (1) pronounced postauricular, submandibular, cervical, and inguinal lymphadenopathy in a large majority of patients with monkeypox, not noted with smallpox; (2) occurrence of monkeypox cases in small, forest villages in western and central Africa, whereas smallpox was cosmopolitan; (3) through the 1980s, predominance of

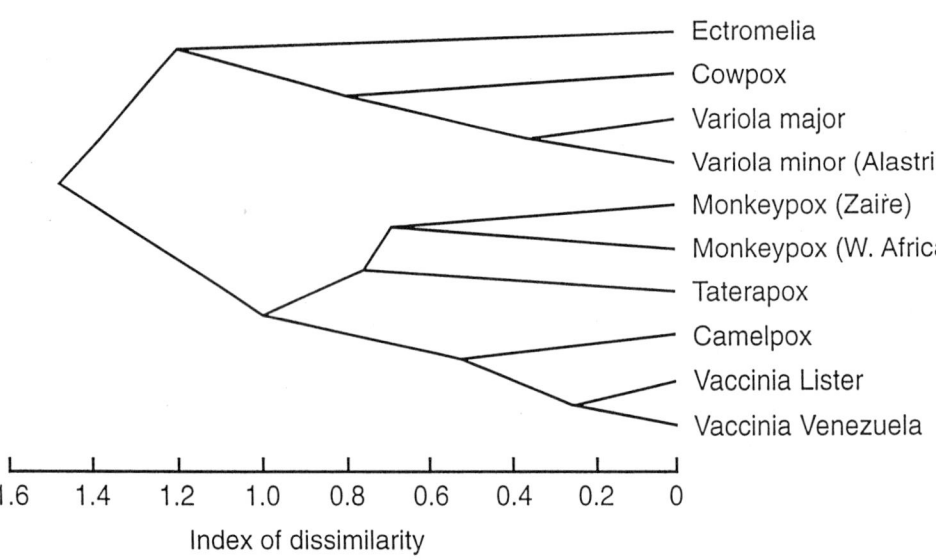

Figure 25–4. Dendrogram illustrating the similarities and differences between the DNAs of orthopoxviruses for which restriction sites are shown.

Ectromelia
Cowpox
Variola major
Variola minor (Alastrim)
Monkeypox (Zaire)
Monkeypox (W. Africa)
Taterapox
Camelpox
Vaccinia Lister
Vaccinia Venezuela

1.6   1.4   1.2   1.0   0.8   0.6   0.4   0.2   0

Index of dissimilarity

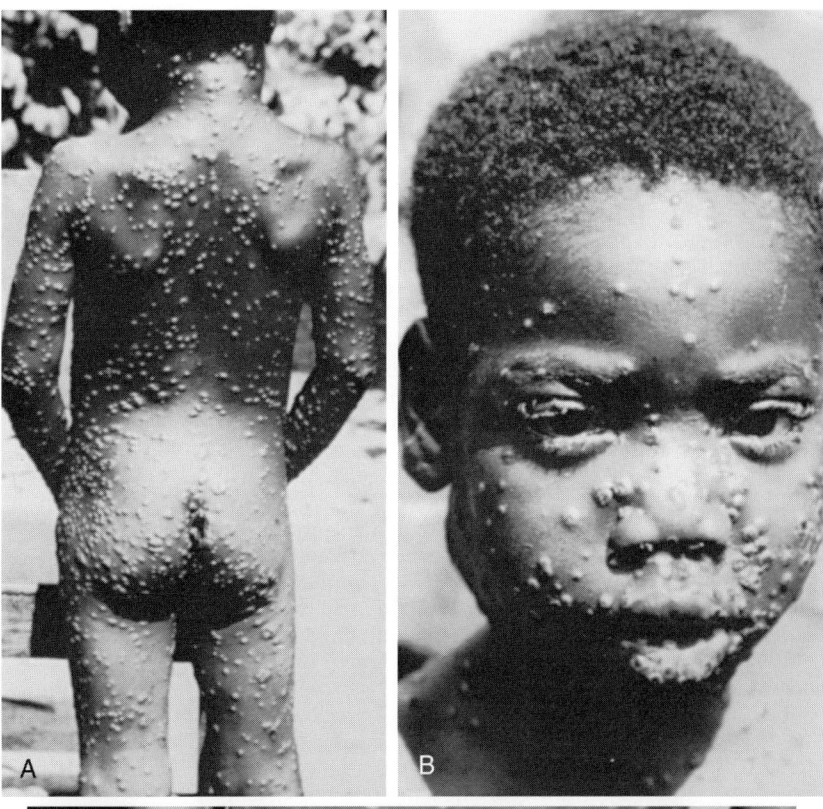

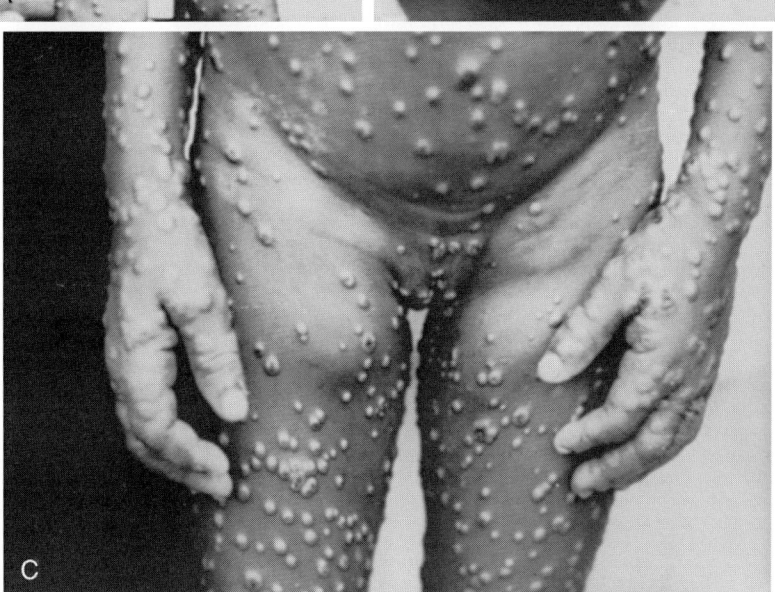

Figure 25–5. Monkeypox on eighth day of rash. *A*, The eruption resembles smallpox. *B*, Lesions on eyelid, nares, and lips. *C*, Note inguinal lymphadenopathy and dense concentration of lesions on hands. (Courtesy of World Health Organization, M. Szczeniowski.)

children with monkeypox (median age of 4 years), whereas smallpox would affect unvaccinated persons of all age groups; this is changing as the entire at-risk population becomes susceptible to orthopoxviruses following the cessation of smallpox vaccination; (4) relatively poor interhuman transmission of monkeypox; the secondary attack rate in susceptible family contacts is about 10% as compared with 25 to 40% for smallpox; and (5) interhuman spread to a fourth generation is rare with monkeypox; smallpox spread was by continuous person-to-person transmission. The case-fatality rate for monkeypox has been about 10 to 15%, the same rate as seen previously with smallpox in western and central Africa. Vaccination with vaccinia protects against monkeypox. A recent prolonged outbreak in the central Demo-

cratic Republic of the Congo indicates that more intense transmission may be occurring. Varicella and monkeypox have been confirmed in the same communities, causing difficulties in defining the situation.

Other Poxvirus Infections

Excepting *molluscum contagiosum*, the other Chordopoxvirinae infections of humans are zoonoses (Table 25–1).

PARAPOXVIRUS. Orf virus (contagious pustular dermatitis, contagious ecthyma, scabby mouth) causes disease in sheep. Pseudocowpox virus (milker's nodule, paravaccinia) and bovine pustular dermatitis virus (BPDV) cause disease of dairy cattle and beef cattle, respectively. Rarely, humans are infected by parapoxviruses of camels and seals. Orf and pseudocowpox are occupational dangers to sheep handlers and cattle handlers, respectively.

YATAPOXVIRUS INFECTIONS. Tanapox causes an acute febrile illness with one or two papulovesicular lesions, usually on the extremities. Persons with this disease have been found only in Kenya (the Tana River Valley) and Zaire. The virus is difficult to culture; clinical, epidemiologic, and serologic information is needed to confirm the diagnosis. The natural reservoir and vector are unknown, although it is speculated that mosquitoes may be involved, because more cases seem to occur during the rainy season in populations living along the banks of flooding rivers. A variant of tanapox, called Yaba-like disease virus, Yaba-related disease virus, and Oregon "1211" poxvirus, has caused outbreaks in macaque monkeys in U.S. primate centers, causing lesions on the hands of animal handlers. Yaba monkey tumor virus has been recovered from skin tumors in a colony of rhesus monkeys in Nigeria. Infections have not been found in the wild.

MOLLUSCIPOXVIRUS. Molluscum contagiosum virus is characterized by multiple (0.2 to 0.4 cm) thick-walled, noninflamed, "pearly white," unbilicated pustules in the skin. The lesions are predominant in the genital or anal regions in adults but may be scattered over the body in children. There is little inflammatory and immunologic response to infection and disease. Spread is by sexual and other person-to-person contact, and patients may have lesions for weeks or years. The disease has been important as a complication in patients with AIDS. Although the DNA of this virus has been characterized and shows the three genomic subtypes, the virus has only recently been cultured in foreskin explants and mouse renal capsule tissue.

Bibliography

Breman JG, Arita I: The confirmation and maintenance of smallpox eradication. N Engl J Med 303:1263, 1980.

Breman JG, Henderson DA: Poxvirus dilemmas—monkeypox, smallpox and biologic terrorism. N Engl J Med 339:556, 1998.

Centers for Disease Control and Prevention: Human monkeypox-Kasai Orientale, Zaire, 1996–1997. MMWR 46:304, 1997.

Esposito JJ, Massung RF: Poxvirus infections in humans. In Murray PR, Baron EJ, Pfaller MA, et al (eds): Manual of Clinical Microbiology, 6th ed. Washington, DC, American Society for Microbiology, 1995.

Fenner F: Poxviruses. In Fields BN, Knipe DN, Howley PM (eds): Fields Virology, 3rd ed. Philadelphia, Lippincott-Raven, 1996, p 2673.

Fenner F, Henderson DA, Arita I, et al: Smallpox and Its Eradication. Geneva, World Health Organization, 1988.

Hopkins DH: Princes and Peasants: Smallpox in History. Chicago, University of Chicago Press, 1983.

Jezek Z, Arita I, Szczeniowski M, et al.: Human tanapox in Zaire: Clinical and epidemiological observations on cases by laboratory studies. Bull WHO 65:1027, 1985.

Jezek Z, Fenner F: Human Monkeypox. New York, Karger, 1988.

Massung RF, Esposito JJ, Liu L, et al: Potential virulence determinants in terminal regions of variola smallpox virus genome. Nature 366:748, 1993.

Moss B: Poxviridae: The viruses and their replication. In Fields BN, Knipe DN, Howley PM (eds): Fields Virology, 3rd ed. Philadelphia, Lippincott-Raven, 1996, p 2637.

Moss B: Genetically engineered poxviruses for recombinant gene expression, vaccination and safety. Proc Natl Acad Sci USA 93:11341, 1996.

Porter CD, Blake NW, Cream JJ, Archard LC: Molluscum contagiosum virus. In Wright D, Archard LC (eds): Molecular and Cell Biology of Sexually Transmitted Diseases. London; Chapman and Hail, 1992 p 233.

26 Viral Respiratory Infections

Stephen Berman

Acute viral respiratory infections are the most frequent type of self-limited childhood illness throughout the world. A small percentage of these infections progress to severe and even fatal disease (Chapter 2). In children less than 5 years of age living in the developing world, approximately 1 in 400 cases of respiratory syncytial virus (RSV) infection and 1 in 600 cases of parainfluenza virus infection result in death (Table 26–1). An estimated 4 million deaths occur in children under 5 years of age from acute lower respiratory infections, most often pneumonia. Approximately 50% have a bacterial etiology and 35% are caused by viruses. Although the risk of death with untreated bacterial pneumonia is greater than 50 times the case fatality rate for viral pneumonia, the estimated number of pneumonia deaths due to bacterial infections alone is only 2.7 times higher than the number due to viral infections because of the much higher frequency of viral infection. The site of the viral infection determines the clinical manifestations. The clinical manifestations are used to classify respiratory infections into clinical syndromes.

■ CLINICAL SYNDROMES

Acute viral infections are classified into clinical syndromes that reflect lower, middle, or upper respiratory tract involvement (Table 26–2). When multiple areas of the respiratory tract are involved, there is considerable overlap. Acute viral respiratory infections initially present with upper respiratory tract findings because the portal of entry is the nose, mouth, or eyes. The three syndromes can be manifested initially by nonspecific symptoms of cough, fever, malaise, and anorexia. Progression of the infection to the middle and lower tract usually occurs within 2 to 4 days. A number of viral respiratory agents can produce any of the clinical syndromes.

UPPER RESPIRATORY TRACT SYNDROMES. Rhinoviruses, a type of picornavirus, cause approximately 50% of upper respiratory infections or colds but rarely if ever are

TABLE 26–1. Frequency With Which Viral Pathogens Result in Severe Disease and Death

Clinical Severity of ARI*	Relative Frequencies of Viral Infections by Clinical Severity	
	RSV	Parainfluenza Viruses
Upper respiratory infection (common cold)	300	500
Lower respiratory infection not needing hospitalization	100	100
Lower respiratory infection needing hospitalization	10	10
Death	1 (0.24%)	1 (0.16%)

From Institute of Medicine: New Vaccine Development: Establishing Priorities. Vol 2: Diseases of Importance in Developing Countries. Washington, DC, National Academy of Science Press, 1986.
*Acute respiratory infection.
RSV, respiratory syncytial virus.

TABLE 26–2. Clinical and Epidemiologic Characteristics of Viral Agents

Characteristic	RSV	Parainfluenza Type 2	Parainfluenza Types 1 and 3	Influenza	Adenovirus
Highest age-specific infection rate	<1 yr	<1 yr	1–5 yr	>5 yr	1–5 yr
Most common lower respiratory clinical syndrome	Bronchiolitis Pneumonia (tachypnea, wheezing, rales)	Bronchiolitis Pneumonia (tachypnea, wheezing, rales)	Croup LTB (stridor, sore throat)	Tracheobronchitis Pneumonia (high fever, headache, sore throat, myalgias, tachypnea, rales)	Pneumonia (fever, tachypnea, rales)
Activity pattern	Epidemic peak	Variable	Variable	Epidemic peak	Endemic

RSV, respiratory syncytial virus; LTB, laryngotracheobronchitis.

directly involved in the lower respiratory syndromes. However, these infections can trigger acute episodes of respiratory distress in individuals with reactive airway disease or asthma. Infection initially involves the ciliated and nonciliated epithelial cells of the upper respiratory tract. Viral replication, which peaks at about 24 hours, may persist for up to 3 weeks. The inflammatory response producing interleukins, bradykinins, and prostaglandins results in vasodilatation of the nasal blood vessels, nasal secretions, and stimulation of sneeze and cough reflexes. The signs and symptoms include fever, nasal congestion, coryza, cough, and sore throat. In most cases the clinical illness, in the absence of secondary bacterial infection, e.g., sinusitis or otitis, resolves within 7 to 10 days.

Sinusitis and otitis media usually indicate secondary bacterial infection. Sinusitis presents with cough, fever, purulent nasal discharge, and bad breath. Headache and pain over the face are more common in older patients than in children with sinusitis. In the absence of ear discharge, otitis media, or inflammation of the middle ear space, is diagnosed best with pneumatic otoscopy. Findings of otitis media include inflammation of the tympanic membrane (red and/or yellow color), bulging contour with absent bony landmarks, and diminished or absent tympanic membrane mobility.

MIDDLE RESPIRATORY TRACT SYNDROMES. The viral middle respiratory syndromes are acute laryngitis, laryngotracheobronchitis, croup, and tracheobronchitis. Laryngitis presents with hoarseness. Laryngotracheobronchitis presents with hoarseness, barking cough, and stridor. Tracheobronchitis is difficult to diagnose and is associated with the auscultatory finding of rhonchi, a harsh respiratory sound. Rhonchi are often difficult to clinically distinguish from sounds related to nasal congestion or discharge transmitted from the upper airway. Older children and adults with tracheobronchitis may cough up purulent sputum, but this finding is not present in young children.

LOWER RESPIRATORY TRACT SYNDROMES. The viral lower respiratory tract syndromes are pneumonia and bronchiolitis, which usually present with rapid breathing and retractions. Pneumonia (inflammation of the pulmonary interstitial space or alveoli) is often associated with auscultatory findings of rales, crackles, or crepitations. Bronchiolitis (inflammation of the small airways or bronchioles) presents as wheezing due to airway obstruction. Rales, crackles, or crepitations may also be heard in cases with bronchiolitis because of atelectasis distal to bronchiolar mucous plugging.

ETIOLOGY

Although many viral agents produce acute respiratory infections, the most important viral respiratory pathogens are RSV; parainfluenza viruses 1, 2, and 3; influenza viruses A and B; and adenovirus (Table 26–2). RSV is the most frequent cause of lower respiratory infection during infancy and early childhood, whereas influenza is the most important pathogen in older groups.

These four respiratory viruses produce the majority of cases of lower respiratory disease in developing countries (Table 26–3). The incidence rates for acute lower respiratory infections vary from 0.4 to 8.1 new episodes per 100 child-weeks. Borrero and associates followed 340 children from birth to 18 months in Cali, Colombia, with home visits. Overall incidence of viral middle and lower respiratory infection was 0.32 episode per child per year, with RSV accounting for 0.2, parainfluenza viruses 0.07, influenza viruses 0.033, and adenovirus 0.02 episodes per child per year.

RSV. RSV, a paramyxovirus, is the most frequent cause of pediatric lower respiratory infections in developing countries (Tables 26–2 to 26–4). RSV is a negative-stranded RNA virus with two antigenic subgroups based on the composition of surface glycoproteins. In children under 5 years, RSV infections are two to four times more frequent than other viral respiratory agents. Although RSV infections occur throughout childhood, the incidence is highest in the first 2 years of life. Seventy-five percent of RSV-related childhood deaths in developing countries occur in infants under 1 year of age. Primary RSV infection in the first 6 months of life often results in severe lower respiratory illness with bronchiolitis or pneumonia, or both. Subsequent reinfection usually produces less severe illness because infection provides partial immunity. Transmission of RSV is by contact or droplet spread, the nose, eyes, and mouth being the portals of entry. RSV can survive on hard surfaces and be transmitted by fomites.

In most developing countries, RSV appears to have characteristic epidemic peaks of activity that recur at yearly intervals. However, the seasonal pattern of these peaks varies in different areas of the world. In temperate climates the peaks occur during the winter months. In tropical areas the peaks follow no common pattern and can occur during wet or dry seasons. An epidemic of bronchiolitis and pneumonia that primarily affects infants is a strong indication of RSV activity in the community.

PARAINFLUENZA VIRUSES. These are paramyxoviruses with three serotypes: 1, 2, and 3. Following RSV, these viruses are the most frequently identified viral respiratory pathogens (Tables 26–3 and 26–4). Parainfluenza 1 and 3 are the most frequent cause of croup. Parainfluenza 2 is the second most common cause (after RSV) of pediatric bronchiolitis and pneumonia. Transmission of parainfluenza viruses is by contact or large droplets as well as by fomites. There is considerable variation in the pattern of activity for parainfluenza in developing countries. Whereas epidemic peaks of activity are noted in some countries, in others the virus appears to be endemic. Infection with one serotype provides no protection

TABLE 26–3. Viral Etiology of Acute Lower Respiratory Infection in Children Under 5 Years of Age

Country*	Setting†	No. of Cases	Percent of Acute Lower Respiratory Infection Cases According to Viral Agent					
			RSV	Parainfluenza	Influenza	Adenovirus	Other‡	Total
Argentina	H	1002	18.2	2.0	1.3	2.7	5.8	30.0
Bangladesh	I	401	14.4	1.2	3.7	NA	3.4	22.7
Bangladesh	I	601	17.1	0.8	3.2	0.8	NA	21.9
Chile	I	614	38.9	NA	NA	NA	NA	NA
Colombia	C	340	19.7	7.0	2.9	1.4	NA	31.0
India	H	809	13.1	4.4	0.6	1.4	NA	19.5
Pakistan	O	816	30.5	1.2	1.3	2.5	NA	35.5
Pakistan	I	676	35.7	0.4	1.3	1.1	NA	38.5
Philippines	I	537	12.2	6.3	3.9	5.0	1.8	29.2
Philippines	C	311	12.8	5.1	2.2	3.5	4.1	27.7
Thailand	H	596	20.3	13.0	4.1	6.7	4.3	48.4
Thailand	I	738	19.1	11.4	6.4	6.4	4.7	48.0

*All studies were carried out from 1984–1988.
†H, hospital inpatient and outpatient clinic; I, inpatient only; O, outpatient clinic; and C, community.
‡Other agents include enterovirus, herpes simplex, and cytomegalovirus.
NA, data not available; RSV, respiratory syncytial virus.

against infection with another serotype; and protection against re-infection with the same strain is incomplete.

INFLUENZA VIRUSES. These orthomyxoviruses circulate as three types: A, B, and C; type C however rarely causes clinical disease. Influenza viruses have a spherical shape and contain eight negative-sense RNA molecules in the genome. The viruses have two types of glycoprotein, i.e., hemagglutinin and neuraminidase, which play important roles in pathogenesis. Hemagglutinin is needed for attachment of the virus to the host cell membrane and neuraminidase is needed to release the virus from infected cells. In addition influenza viruses change their antigenic character at irregular intervals by altering their hemagglutinin and/or neuraminidase amino acid sequences.

Influenza viral infections have a worldwide distribution (Tables 26–3 and 26–4) and tend to produce illness in older children and adults (Table 26–2). The incubation period for influenza is 18 to 72 hours. Person-to-person transmission is principally by small-particle aerosols generated by coughing and sneezing. Onset is abrupt, with fever, chills, generalized malaise, myalgias, and headache. Fever and systemic symptoms subside within several days, at which time respiratory symptoms, including cough, nasal obstruction and discharge, and pharyngitis, increase. Symptoms subside over 4 to 5 days, but cough may persist for weeks. Although this is the most common presentation, the clinical spectrum of infection is quite broad, as influenza viruses can cause middle and lower respiratory syndromes indistinguishable from other viral respiratory pathogens. Patients with underlying cardiac and pulmonary disease are at high risk for fatal infection.

TABLE 26–4. Viral Etiology of Acute Middle and Lower Respiratory Syndromes in Children Under 5 Years of Age

Country*	Setting†	No. of Cases	Percent of Middle/Lower Respiratory Syndrome Cases According to Viral Agent					
			RSV	Parainfluenza	Influenza	Adenovirus	Other‡	Total
Pneumonia								
Thailand	H	267	22.0	8.6	1.8	6.3	NA	38.7
Bangladesh	I	520	16.5	0.7	2.8	0.9	NA	20.9
India	H	178	19.1	8.4	1.6	34.2	6.1	69.4
Uruguay	I	204	29.9	2.5	0.5	1.5	2.0	36.4
Bronchiolitis								
Thailand	H	25	36.0	NA	4.0	NA	NA	40.0
Bangladesh	I	61	24.5	1.6	6.5	NA	NA	32.6
India	H	116	57.7	11.2	0.8	3.4	2.5	75.6
Bronchitis								
Thailand	H	241	19.5	10.3	4.5	8.7	NA	43.0
Bangladesh	I	13	7.6	NA	NA	NA	NA	7.6
India	H	14	14.2	14.2	7.1	14.2	NA	49.7
Croup								
Thailand	O	63	9.5	46.0	6.3	3.1	NA	64.9
Bangladesh	I	5	20.0	NA	NA	NA	NA	20.0
India	H	8	NA	62.5	NA	NA	12.5	75.0

*All studies were carried out from 1984–1988.
†H, hospital inpatient and outpatient clinic; I, inpatient only; O, outpatient clinic.
‡Other agents include enterovirus, herpes simplex, and cytomegalovirus.
NA, data not available; RSV, respiratory syncytial virus.

Influenza is known to predispose to the development of secondary bacterial pneumonia.

Influenza occurs in an epidemic form, usually at intervals of 2 to 3 years. Pandemics, resulting from the appearance of new antigen subtypes, occur at longer intervals (10 to 15 years). In the 1969 influenza A (Hong Kong H3N2) epidemic in Belém, Brazil, absenteeism in all establishments rose from 10.7% during the first 6 weeks of the year to 40.8% during the next 6 weeks. During this period there was an excess mortality of 45%.

ADENOVIRUS. These are double-stranded DNA viruses with 42 antigenic types. Adenoviral infections occur throughout the developing world (Tables 26–3 and 26–4). This virus causes respiratory infections throughout all age groups. Adenoviral infections can produce a wide range of clinical illness including upper respiratory colds, exudative pharyngotonsillitis, pharyngeal-conjunctival fever, bronchiolitis, a pertussis-like syndrome, pneumonia, and necrotizing bronchiolitis or bronchiolitis obliterans (Table 26–4). Although adenovirus usually causes a self-limited lower respiratory infection, the infection can progress to necrotizing bronchiolitis. If this severe infection does not result in death, survivors have severe chronic lung disease. Transmission is similar to that of RSV. Usually adenoviral infections have an endemic activity pattern, occurring throughout the year.

ENTEROVIRUSES. Enteroviruses, e.g., coxsackievirus and echovirus, have been identified in cases of acute viral respiratory infection less frequently than the other three agents. Coxsackievirus infection can cause herpangina, a syndrome of sore throat and fever associated with punched out ulcers and/or vesicles in the posterior pharynx. This virus is also associated with hand, foot, and mouth disease; it is characterized by a vesiculopapular rash on the hands and feet as well as ulcerative or vesicular lesions in the mouth. The role of echovirus and coxsackievirus infections in cases with croup, bronchiolitis, and pneumonia is not clear.

■ DIAGNOSIS

Viral respiratory agents can be diagnosed by tissue culture isolation or rapid diagnostic techniques. Tissue culture isolation is expensive to maintain and technically difficult. Specimens should be collected by nasal pharyngeal aspirate and transported in viral transport media. Specimens should be inoculated as soon as possible, as RSV is quite labile. The best isolation results are obtained when multiple cell lines, such as HEP2, MDCK, MRC, and LLCMK2, are used. Clinical usefulness is limited because tissue culture isolation takes 2 to 14 days.

Rapid viral diagnostic techniques have greater clinical usefulness because results can be available in hours. However, the identification of a viral agent does not rule out a mixed viral-bacterial infection. The three methods currently available are immunofluorescence, enzyme immunoassay (EIA), and monoclonal antibody tests. Although rapid diagnostic techniques are very effective in identifying RSV infections, they are less sensitive in diagnosing the other respiratory viruses.

■ PATHOGENESIS

Complex interactions between the host, viral and bacterial pathogens, and environmental factors produce respiratory disease. Knowledge of the pathogenesis of acute respiratory infections in developing countries has been complicated by the number of potential pathogens, by the need for sophisticated laboratories for diagnosis, by a potentially large number of host risk characteristics, and by diverse social, cultural, and environmental factors. The incidence and severity of acute lower respiratory infections relate to four pathogenic interactions: (1) the effectiveness of the host defenses against the respiratory viral pathogens; (2) the degree of selectivity with which the inflammatory response destroys the pathogen while minimizing lower airway obstruction and damage to lung tissue; (3) the integrity of repair mechanisms that determine the rate of tissue recovery; and (4) the ability of the host to maintain adequate respiratory function.

The effectiveness of the host defenses against the viral pathogen is impaired by factors that promote pathogen transmission and increase the size of infecting dose, promote replication and spread, and inhibit host defenses. Neutrophil dysfunction resulting from the infection predisposes to secondary bacterial infections, especially when other risk factors are present in populations living in developing countries. Large family and household size, crowding, inadequate sanitation, and poor personal hygiene facilitate transmission and increase the size of the infecting dose. Increasing birth order is also an important risk factor for severe viral lower respiratory infection. Indoor smoke pollution from biomass fuels alters the integrity of the respiratory mucosal lining, disrupts mucociliary function, and promotes viral penetration and spread.

The pathogenic mechanisms of viral respiratory infection have been clarified by the description of viral regulation of apoptosis. Apoptosis or "programmed cell death" is a physiologic mechanism of cell death that includes the clearance of cellular debris by phagocytes. When viral infection inappropriately stimulates apoptosis, the immune response against infection may be impaired. When it blocks apoptosis, the life of the host cell is prolonged and viral replication may be enhanced. Thus, the viral regulation of apoptosis may affect the balance between viral replication and antiviral immunity.

The inflammatory response produced by the child's immune system on the lung tissue can be more significant than the direct toxic effects of the pathogen. Viral respiratory pathogens infect and disrupt the epithelial lining of the respiratory tract. The inflammatory response produces increased airway secretions, vascular engorgement, and smooth muscle contraction. This results in airway obstruction. The immune defense mechanisms that fight infection are the same mechanisms of inflammation that damage functioning lung tissue. Factors that exaggerate the inflammatory response beyond what is needed to control the pathogen are counterproductive. The most obvious example of this occurs in a child with asthma or other allergies. Coexisting parasitic infections that have a migratory phase through the lung may also increase the inflammatory response and cause more severe disease. Smoke pollution may increase the inflammatory response and/or make the lung tissue more susceptible to damage.

The severity of a respiratory infection will be affected by the underlying state of the lung. If the lung is exposed to another infection before it has fully recovered from an earlier insult, the damage is likely to be considerably more extensive. Therefore, it is important to understand factors that limit tissue repair and the subsequent recovery of respiratory functions. These include protein-calorie malnutrition; deficiencies in vitamin A and elemental minerals such as iron, copper, and zinc; and underlying disease of the lungs or heart. Conditions that predispose to frequent recurrent infections (e.g., as crowding and smoke pollution) will also affect recovery rates.

Several factors affect the ability of the host to maintain adequate respiratory function in the presence of acute respiratory infection. Age is a significant factor. Prematurity is associated with muscle weakness and fatigue that predispose the host to respiratory failure. Malnutrition impairs respiratory function by causing muscular weakness, blunting of the hypoxic response, and decreasing respiratory drive. Infants have a compliant chest wall that leads to inefficient respiratory function; in addition, the upper airway of infants is more susceptible to obstruction than that of adults. The respiratory drive center of young infants is more sensitive than that of older infants and children. RSV infection is often associated with apnea in young infants, especially premature infants.

■ PREVENTION AND CONTROL

IMMUNIZATION. Advances in the prevention of viral respiratory infection in childhood await the successful development of effective vaccines against RSV and parainfluenza. Early attempts at formaldehyde inactivation and more recently developed attenuated vaccines have not been effective. Successful prophylaxis for these agents requires a better understanding of the immunology of mucosal infections and the chemistry of glycoprotein antigens. RSV vaccines selectively activate different types of CD4+ T-helper lymphocytes. This may explain why some vaccine formulations have not been effective or have been associated with vaccine-enhanced illness. Work is currently underway to develop an effective vaccine that can be safely administered to very young infants. Oral adenovirus types 4 and 7 vaccines have been developed and tested on military recruits, but their benefit in children has not been assessed. Influenza vaccine, usually containing both type A and type B virus, is widely used in developed countries for persons with chronic illness and advanced age. The use of influenza vaccine in developing countries is limited by the high cost, the need for frequent revaccination because of antigenic shift, and the fact that the target population is the elderly rather than the young.

MEDICAL THERAPY/MANAGEMENT. Specific antiviral therapies are currently available—amantadine or rimantidine, ribavirin, and RSV immune globulin intravenous. Oral amantadine (adult dose: 200 mg total, 100 mg twice daily for 5 days) or rimantidine is effective treatment for influenza if given early in the disease course. It also may be used prophylactically. Ribavirin is an aerosolized drug used to treat severe RSV infections. Its effectiveness is unclear because of methodologic problems with clinical trials that used inappropriate controls. The drug must be delivered with a special small-particle aerosol generator unit. Its use in developing countries is limited because of the very high cost of the drug, technical difficulties in drug delivery, and lack of data from developing countries on preventing death. Intravenous RSV gamma globulin has been approved for prophylaxis in infants and children with high-risk conditions. However, its extremely high cost almost always precludes its use in developing countries.

Signs of respiratory distress that require hospitalization for oxygen and supportive care include respiratory rate greater than 70, severe retractions with decreased air exchange unresponsive to bronchodilators, or cyanosis. Correction of hypoxia with oxygen can be lifesaving in severe viral lower respiratory infection.

Bibliography

Abramson JS, Wheeler JG: Virus-induced neutrophil dysfunction: Role in the pathogenesis of bacterial infections. Pediatr Infect Dis J 13:643, 1994.

Avendano LF, Larranaga C, Palomino MA, et al: Community- and hospital-acquired respiratory syncytial virus infections in Chile. Pediatr Infect Dis J 10:564, 1991.

Berman S: Epidemiology of acute respiratory infections in children of developing countries. Rev Infect Dis 13(Suppl 6):S454, 1991.

Borrero IH, Fajardo LP, Bedoya AM, et al: Acute respiratory tract infections among a birth cohort of children from Cali, Colombia, who were studied through 17 months of age. Rev Infect Dis 12(Suppl 8):S950, 1990.

Campbell H: Acute respiratory infection: A global challenge. Arch Dis Child 73:281, 1995.

Collins M: Potential roles of apoptosis in viral pathogenesis. Am J Respir Crit Care Med 152:S20, 1995.

Ghafoor A, Nomani NK, Ishaq Z, et al: Diagnoses of acute lower respiratory tract infections in children in Rawalpindi and Islamabad, Pakistan. Rev Infect Dis 12(Suppl 8):S907, 1990.

Hortal M, Mogdasy C, Russi JC, et al: Microbial agents associated with pneumonia in children from Uruguay. Rev Infect Dis 12(Suppl 8):S915, 1990.

Huq F, Rahman M, Nahar N, et al: Acute lower respiratory tract infection due to virus among hospitalized children in Dhaka, Bangladesh. Rev Infect Dis 12(Suppl 8):S982, 1990.

Institute of Medicine: New Vaccine Development: Establishing Priorities. Vol 2: Diseases of Importance in Developing Countries. Washington, DC, National Academy of Science Press, 1986.

John TJ, Cherian T, Steinhoff MC, et al: Etiology of acute respiratory infections in children in tropical southern India. Rev Infect Dis 13(Suppl 6):S463, 1991.

Puthavathana P, Wasi C, Kositanont U, et al: A hospital-based study of acute viral infections of the respiratory tract in Thai children, with emphasis on laboratory diagnosis. Rev Infect Dis 12(Suppl 8):S988, 1990.

Rahman M, Huq F, Sack D, et al: Acute lower respiratory tract infections in hospitalized patients with diarrhea in Dhaka, Bangladesh. Rev Infect Dis 12(Suppl 8):S899, 1990.

Suwanjutha S, Chantarojanasiri T, Watthana-Kasetr S, et al: A study of nonbacterial agents of acute lower respiratory tract infection in Thai children. Rev Infect Dis 12(Suppl 8):S923, 1990.

Tupasi TE, deLeon LE, Lupisan S, et al: Community-based studies of acute respiratory tract infections in young children: Patterns of acute respiratory tract infection in children—a longitudinal study in a depressed community in Metro Manila. Rev Infect Dis 12(Suppl 8):S940, 1990.

Tupasi TE, Lucero MG, Magdangal DM, et al: Etiology of acute lower respiratory tract infection in children from Alabang, Metro Manila. Rev Infect Dis 12(Suppl 8):S929, 1990.

Weissenbacher M, Carballal G, Avila M, et al: Hospital-based studies on acute respiratory tract infections in young children: Etiologic and clinical evaluation of acute lower respiratory tract infections in young Argentinian children—an overview. Rev Infect Dis 12(Suppl 8):S889, 1990.

27 Enteric Viral Infections

27.1 Poliomyelitis

Roland W. Sutter and Stephen L. Cochi

DEFINITION. Poliomyelitis is an acute infectious and communicable disease caused by poliovirus. Three serotypes of poliovirus are transmitted primarily by person-to-person contact, which usually results in inapparent infection or mild nonspecific illness. Rarely, the virus invades the central nervous system (CNS), where viral replication in motor neurons causes cell destruction and permanent paralysis or weakness in the affected muscles. Widespread use of poliovirus vaccines has effectively controlled poliomyelitis in industrialized countries since the 1960s and has brought about considerable progress toward global poliomyelitis eradication.

ETIOLOGY. Polioviruses are classified in the enterovirus genus of the Family Picornaviridae (pico, implying small; RNA, the nucleic acid component). Polioviruses are small, nonenveloped, icosahedral viruses (27 to 30 nm in diameter), containing an RNA genome of 2.5×10^6 daltons. The poliovirus genome is a single-stranded messenger molecule containing about 7500 nucleotides that is covalently linked to a small protein. Single-stranded RNA constitutes approximately 30% of the virion, and the remainder consists of four major (VP1-4) and one minor (VPg) proteins (present in copies of 60 each of VP1 and VP3 and 58 or 59 copies of VP2 and VP4). There are three antigenic types (serotypes 1, 2, and 3) whose physical properties are nearly identical. Neutralizing antibody is directed toward VP1, VP2, and VP3, of which VP1 is the immunodominant antigen. There are at least four epitopes located on the surface of the virion.

HISTORY. The written history of poliomyelitis can be traced to the first description of the disease by Michael Underwood in 1789, although an Egyptian stele from the 18th Dynasty (1580–1350 B.C.) depicts a "crippled young man, apparently a priest, with a withered and shortened left leg, and with his foot held in a typical equinus position characteristic of the flaccid paralysis" typical of poliomyelitis. The term "poliomyelitis anterior acuta" is based on the characteristic anatomic location of lesions within the spinal cord (Fig. 27–1) and is constructed from the Greek *polios* (gray), and *myelos* (marrow, the gray matter of the spinal cord) with the ending *itis* to imply inflammation.

In the late 19th and early 20th centuries, a change in the epidemiology of poliomyelitis from a predominantly endemic to an epidemic form was observed in Sweden and Norway, heralding similar changes in other industrialized countries. Our understanding of these epidemiologic changes was greatly aided by groundbreaking investigations of the three largest poliomyelitis outbreaks of the time that occurred in Rutland County, Vermont, in 1894; in Sweden in 1905; and in New York in 1916.

Landsteiner and Popper determined in 1908 that a "filtrable agent" (i.e., virus) was the cause of poliomyelitis. The construction of the Drinker respirator ("iron lung") beginning in 1928 and its widespread use in the 1930s and 1940s increased the likelihood of survival for those with bulbar forms of poliomyelitis. Burnet and MacNamara demonstrated in 1931 that more than one strain of virus could cause poliomyelitis and that immunity to one strain did not confer immunity to another. Enders, Weller, and Robbins in 1949 grew poliovirus in non-nervous, human embryonic tissue,

work that was later honored with the Nobel Prize. Two years later, three distinct poliovirus strains, designated as types I, II, and III, were identified as causing poliomyelitis. Thus, the determination of the number of poliovirus strains, the ability for large-scale growth of the virus, and the finding that circulating antibody has a protective effect against poliomyelitis were essential pre-conditions for the development of effective poliovirus vaccines. Two approaches for vaccine development pursued at the time were successful: inactivation of poliovirus by formalin, pioneered by Dr. Jonas Salk and licensed as inactivated poliovirus vaccine (IPV) in 1955; and the attenuation of the three serotypes of poliovirus by Dr. Albert Sabin, licensed in 1961 as monovalent oral poliovirus vaccine and, in 1963, as trivalent oral poliovirus vaccine (OPV).

DISTRIBUTION AND INCIDENCE. Poliomyelitis is a ubiquitous, highly contagious, seasonal viral disease (with more pronounced seasonality in temperate zones than in the tropics) that, in the absence of vaccination, infects nearly every person in a given population, usually by 5 to 10 years of age. Poliovirus type 1 appears to be the most neurovirulent of the three serotypes. Most epidemic and endemic cases of poliomyelitis are caused by poliovirus type 1, followed by type 3, then type 2. Peak transmission occurs among infants and young children in tropical areas and, in school-age children in temperate zones. The distribution and incidence of poliomyelitis changed substantially over the last century as the epidemiology changed gradually from an endemic to an epidemic (pre–vaccine era), and finally to a vaccine-era pattern.

Epidemic Transmission. The delay in median age of poliovirus exposure permitted the accumulation of sufficient children susceptible to poliomyelitis that periodic outbreaks occurred. The generally accepted explanation is that economic development and correspondingly improved resources for community sanitation and household hygiene in temperate-zone climates postponed exposure to polioviruses. Epidemic transmission became the primary epidemiologic pattern in temperate climate countries until poliomyelitis was brought under control with the introduction of effective vaccines.

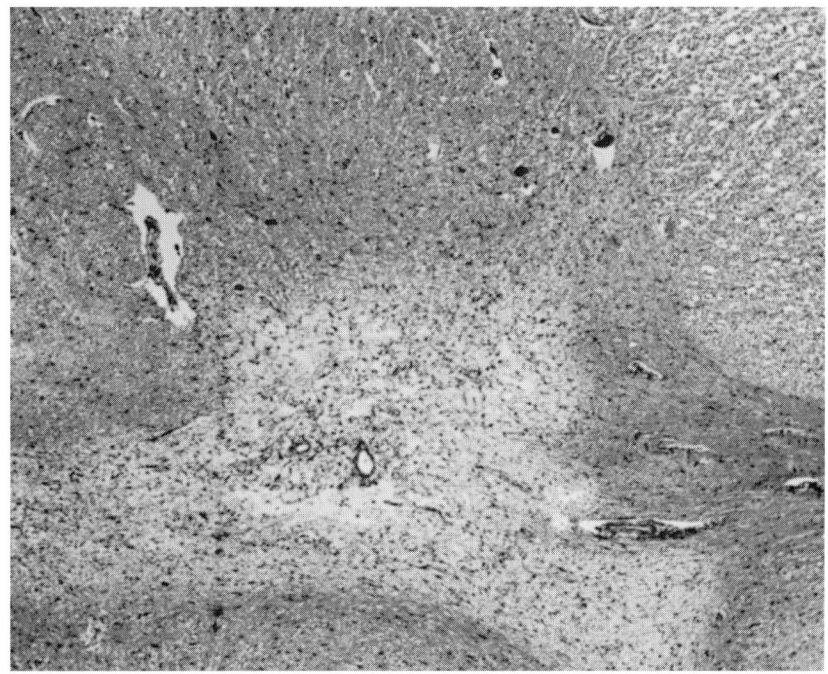

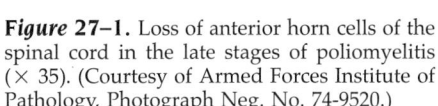

Figure **27–1.** Loss of anterior horn cells of the spinal cord in the late stages of poliomyelitis (× 35). (Courtesy of Armed Forces Institute of Pathology, Photograph Neg. No. 74-9520.)

Endemic Transmission. In developing countries and particularly in tropical areas, an endemic epidemiologic pattern predominated until recently with poliovirus exposure occurring early in life. In the last three decades, a series of lameness surveys were conducted in many developing countries that reported between 5 and 10 lameness cases per 1000 children in the age group studied, suggesting that approximately 1:100 to 1:200 children will acquire paralytic disease attributable to poliovirus in the absence of a vaccination program.

Postvaccine Transmission

Inactivated Poliovirus Vaccine. The incidence of paralytic poliomyelitis in the United States decreased by 86% from 18,308 reported cases in 1954 to 2499, only 3 years after the availability of IPV in 1957. Widespread use of IPV in other countries was followed by substantial decreases in the incidence of poliomyelitis and, in some European countries, including Finland, the Netherlands, and Sweden, resulted in the apparent elimination of indigenous wild poliovirus transmission.

Oral Poliovirus Vaccine. Although live-attenuated oral poliovirus vaccine was developed in the United States, the first large-scale production as well as large field trials that proved the safety and efficacy of the vaccine took place in the Soviet Union. A mass immunization program that was initiated in the Soviet Union in 1959 and completed in 1960 covered 77.5 million people, or 36.7% of the entire population. This was followed by a sharp decrease in the incidence of poliomyelitis. Similar declines in the incidence of poliomyelitis were observed in other European countries, Australia, New Zealand, Canada, and the United States following the introduction of OPV. In the United States, the effect of administering OPV to a population that already had high immunity levels generated by previous natural infection or vaccination with IPV was impressive and rapid. Epidemic poliomyelitis also was brought under control, with the last outbreak in the general population occurring in Texas along the United States–Mexico border in 1970, followed by small outbreaks occurring in 1972 and 1979 among religious groups whose members object to vaccination. The last indigenously acquired case of poliomyelitis due to the wild poliovirus was detected in 1979. Since 1980, aside from less than one imported case of poliomyelitis per year, all cases have been vaccine-associated.

Use of Poliovaccines in Developing Countries. Cuba interrupted wild poliovirus transmission following two rounds of mass vaccination campaigns in 1962. In many other developing countries, however, national vaccination programs were not operational until the late 1970s and early 1980s, and not until 1990 did global OPV coverage with three doses among children aged 1 year reach 80%. Wherever moderately high levels of OPV coverage were achieved, the incidence of poliomyelitis decreased, but endemic transmission of polioviruses and cases of poliomyelitis continued.

While poliomyelitis outbreaks in industrialized countries can be prevented with overall population immunity levels of approximately 80%, outbreaks in developing countries with poor sanitation and hygiene could still occur with immunity levels as high as 97%. These findings may be helpful in explaining why there was no spread to the general population following the outbreaks in the Netherlands, Canada, and the United States and why there was widespread transmission among fully vaccinated children in many outbreaks in developing countries.

TRANSMISSION. Poliomyelitis is transmitted by person-to-person spread via fecal-oral (developing countries) and oral-oral routes (industrialized countries) or rarely by a common vehicle (e.g., milk, water). Persons remain most infectious immediately before and 1 to 2 weeks after onset of paralytic disease, although poliovirus replicates for substantially longer periods and is excreted for 3 to 6 weeks in feces and approximately 2 weeks in saliva. Secondary infection rates of susceptible household or institutional contacts are >90%, probably mediated by fecal-oral spread.

Events Following Exposure. The incubation period between infection and the minor first symptoms is 3 to 6 days; the interval from infection to onset of paralytic disease is usually 7 to 21 days, with a range of 3 to 35 days. Most exposures to polioviruses result in inapparent infections. Based on serologic surveys in the prevaccine era and lameness surveys in developing countries, approximately 1 out of 200 (0.5%) unprotected children will develop paralytic disease following exposure to polioviruses.

PATHOGENESIS AND PATHOLOGY

Determinants of Severity. Besides older age and being unvaccinated or inadequately vaccinated, intramuscular injections with diphtheria-tetanus toxoids and pertussis vaccine (DTP) or antibiotics, strenuous exercise, injury (e.g., fractures), and pregnancy have been shown to increase the risk of acquiring paralytic manifestations. Removal of tonsils and adenoids predisposes to bulbar poliomyelitis. Lower socioeconomic status is a risk factor for paralytic poliomyelitis in developing countries, probably because the children experience more intense exposure to poliovirus with a resulting higher virus inoculum; these children are also at higher risk for primary vaccine failure after OPV because of more frequent concurrent enterovirus infections.

Viral Replication and Dissemination. The pathogenesis of poliovirus infection indicates that prevention through immunization can be accomplished by inhibiting replication at and dissemination from the gastrointestinal tract, inhibiting the viremia that follows, or both. Following oral exposure to poliovirus, the virus attaches and enters specific cells that express the poliovirus receptor (PVR). The virus replicates locally at the sites of virus implantation (e.g., tonsils, intestinal M cells, and Peyer's patches of the ileum) or at the lymph nodes that drain these tissues. The first approach requires the presence of local secretory IgA antibody. The second approach—because spread occurs primarily by way of the blood stream to other susceptible tissues, namely, other lymph nodes, brown fat, and the CNS, or by way of retrograde axonal transport to the CNS—requires the presence of neutralizing antibody.

The host range of poliovirus and tissue tropism is determined by expression of the PVR. Tissue tropism refers to the ability of poliovirus to replicate in specific cells. In situ hybridization with nucleic acid probes of PVR in transgenic mice suggested a limited expression of the PVR to the CNS (Fig. 27–1), thymus, lung, kidney, and adrenal glands and in mononuclear phagocytes. Even within the CNS, PVR expression is restricted to neurons.

CLINICAL MANIFESTATIONS AND COMPLICATIONS. Poliovirus exposure in a susceptible person results in one of the following consequences: (1) inapparent infection without symptoms, (2) minor illness, (3) nonparalytic poliomyelitis (aseptic meningitis); or (4) paralytic poliomyelitis.

Inapparent Infection. Infection without symptoms is the outcome in >95% of individuals.

Minor Illness. This is the most frequent form of the disease, characterized by transient illness associated with a few days of fever, malaise, drowsiness, headache, nausea, vomiting, constipation, or sore throat, in various combinations.

Nonparalytic Poliomyelitis. Aseptic meningitis is a relatively rare outcome of poliovirus infection. It usually begins as a minor illness characterized by fever, sore throat, vomiting, and malaise. One to two days later, signs of meningeal irritation become apparent, including stiffness of the neck or back, vomiting, severe headache, and pain in limbs, back, and neck. This form of the disease lasts from 2 to 10 days, and recovery is usually rapid and complete. In a small proportion of these cases, the disease advances to transient mild muscle weakness or paralysis.

Paralytic Poliomyelitis. This occurs in <1% of poliovirus infections among susceptible persons. Its clinical course is characterized by a minor illness of several days' duration and a symptom-free period of 1 to 3 days; these are followed by rapid onset of flaccid paralysis with fever and progression to the maximum extent of paralysis within a few days. After temperature returns to normal, there is usually no further progression of paralysis. If paralysis of an extremity is not complete, it is more pronounced proximally. Paralysis is usually asymmetric, associated with diminished or complete loss of deep tendon reflexes and an intact sensory system. Paralytic manifestations in extremities begin proximally and progress to involve distal muscle groups (i.e., descending paralysis). Depending on the anatomic location of motor neuron damage in the spinal cord or brain stem, spinal, mixed spinal-bulbar, or bulbar paralysis involving primarily respiratory muscles, respectively, may be observed. The anterior horn cells (and brain stem cells), just like other nerve cells of the CNS, cannot be regenerated or replaced, and paralysis is permanent. The case-fatality rate is variable and depends primarily on the age groups affected, but it is commonly between 5 and 10%. The highest case-fatality rates were reported among older persons during epidemics in the early 20th century.

Postpolio Syndrome. The PPS, a term crafted in the early 1980s, refers to late manifestations of acute paralytic poliomyelitis. After an interval of 15 to 40 years, 25 to 40% of individuals who contracted paralytic poliomyelitis in childhood may experience muscle pain and exacerbation of existing weakness or may develop new weakness or paralysis. Factors that enhance the risk of PPS include (1) prolonged interval since acute poliovirus infection, (2) presence of permanent residual impairment after recovery from the acute illness, and (3) female gender. The pathogenesis of PPS is thought to involve late attrition of oversized motor units that developed during the recovery process of paralytic poliomyelitis.

DIAGNOSIS. Paralytic poliomyelitis has become rare in the United States and many other countries. Therefore, physicians may not be familiar with the disease or may fail to consider the diagnosis of poliomyelitis until other more frequent causes of acute flaccid paralysis have been ruled out (Table 27–1). The diagnosis of paralytic poliomyelitis is dependent on (1) clinical course; (2) virologic testing; (3) special studies; and (4) residual neurologic deficit at least 60 days after onset of symptoms.

Clinical Characteristics. The clinical course is helpful in ruling in or ruling out paralytic poliomyelitis. Several studies in developing countries have assessed the sensitivity and specificity of different clinical case definitions for paralytic poliomyelitis and compared these with virologically confirmed patients based on poliovirus isolation from stool specimens. The largest study reported a sensitivity of 64% and a specificity of 82% for a case definition that included age <6 years, fever at onset, and rapid progression to maximum extent of paralysis within 4 days. The addition of a specific pattern of paralysis (proximal, unilateral, or absence of paralysis in all four extremities) increased the specificity with varying degrees of loss in sensitivity.

The clinical case definition for paralytic poliomyelitis requires a residual neurologic deficit at 60 days or more after onset of paralysis. Such a neurologic deficit may manifest as complete flaccid paralysis of one or more extremities or partial paralysis or weakness of muscles or muscle groups.

Culture. Because other enteroviruses and other diseases may cause acute flaccid paralysis, laboratory confirmation is critical to establishing the diagnosis of poliomyelitis. The most important is the recovery of poliovirus and the characterization of virus isolates as wild-type or vaccine-related. Poliovirus may be recovered from stool, throat swabs, or less commonly, cerebrospinal fluid (CSF) taken soon after the onset of illness and from stool specimens collected for up to 3 to 6 weeks following paralysis onset. Isolation of poliovirus from CSF suggests a causal relationship between a poliovirus serotype and paralytic disease. WHO recommends that two stool samples be collected at least 24 hours apart to confirm the diagnosis, because excretion of virus can be intermittent and the sensitivity of isolation is <100%. It is recommended that stool specimens be collected as soon as the diagnosis of poliomyelitis is suspected and ideally within 14 days of paralysis onset to maximize the likelihood of isolating poliovirus. After the serotype is determined, intratypic differentiation of poliovirus isolates as vaccine-related or wild-type should be considered.

Serology. Serologic testing may be helpful in establishing the diagnosis but often does not contribute and sometimes may cause confusion, because (1) antibody rises have already occurred by the time the first specimen has been collected; (2) antibody to one or more serotypes may be present owing to previous or recent vaccination; (3) heterotypic responses may be observed to one serotype after exposure to another serotype; and (4) lower motor neuron paralysis of another etiology could occur coincidentally in a child with asymptomatic recent poliovirus infection. There are no reliable means of distinguishing antibody induced by vaccine-related virus and that induced by wild-type poliovirus. Paired serum specimens are required to demonstrate a fourfold or greater rise in antibody titer between acute and convalescent sera. The first serum specimen should be collected as soon as possible after onset of paralytic manifestations, and the second specimen should be collected 2 to 3 weeks later. Neutralizing antibodies appear early and are usually already detectable at the time of onset of paralysis. However, if the first specimen is taken early enough, a rise in titer may be demonstrated during the course of the disease.

Laboratory Testing. Nerve conduction and electromyography studies can point to the anatomic location of the paralysis—destruction of anterior horn cells in the spinal cord vs. a demyelinating process in the peripheral nerves—helping to exclude Guillain-Barré syndrome (GBS), the most frequent cause of acute flaccid paralysis. Magnetic resonance imaging (MRI) has been used infrequently, but in at least one patient with poliomyelitis, MRI has highlighted the anterior column of the spinal cord. Analysis of spinal fluid may be helpful in ruling out other causes. In paralytic poliomyelitis, the CSF contains an increased number of leukocytes—usually 10 to 200/mL and seldom more than 500/mL. At the onset of CNS signs, the ratio of polymorphonuclear cells to lymphocytes is high, but within a few days the ratio is reversed. The total white blood cell count slowly subsides to normal levels. The protein content of the CSF initially is elevated only slightly. Glucose levels are usually within the normal range.

TREATMENT. There is no specific treatment for poliomyelitis. By the time the paralytic consequences of CNS viral replication are apparent, administration of immunoglobulin or use of antiviral compounds is not helpful. The specific objectives of therapy during the acute phase of the illness are (1) to prevent further progress of paralysis with mandatory bed rest; (2) to ensure respiratory sufficiency in cases of

TABLE 27–1. Distinguishing Features of Four Common Diagnoses of Acute Flaccid Paralysis

Feature	Poliomyelitis	Guillain-Barré Syndrome	Traumatic Neuritis (Following Injection)	Transverse Myelitis
Development of paralysis	24-48 hours' onset to full paralysis	From hours to 10 days	From hours to 4 days	From hours to 4 days
Fever at onset	High, always present at onset of flaccid paralysis; gone next day	Not common	Commonly present before, during, and after flaccid paralysis	Rarely present
Flaccid paralysis	Acute, usually asymmetric, principally proximal	Generally acute, symmetric, and distal	Asymmetric, acute and affecting only one limb	Acute, lower limbs, symmetric
Progression of paralysis	"Descending"	"Ascending"		
Muscle tone	Reduced or absent in affected limb	Global hypotonia	Reduced or absent in affected limb	Hypotonia in affected limbs
Deep tendon reflexes	Decreased or absent	Globally absent	Decreased or absent	Absent in lower limbs early hyperreflexia late
Sensation	Severe myalgia, backache, no sensory changes	Cramps, tingling, hypoanesthesia of palms and soles	Pain in gluteus; hypothermia	Anesthesia of lower limbs with sensory level
Cranial nerve involvement	Only when bulbar involvement is present	Often present, affecting nerves VII, IX, X, XI, XII	Absent	Absent
Respiratory insufficiency	Only when bulbar involvement is present	In severe cases, enhanced by bacterial pneumonia present	Absent	Sometimes
Autonomic signs and symptoms	Rare	Frequent blood pressure alterations, sweating, blushing, and body temperature fluctuations	Hypothermia in affected limb	Present
Cerebrospinal fluid	Inflammatory	Albumin-cytologic dissociation	Normal	Normal or mild in cells
Bladder dysfunction	Rare	Transient	Never	Present
Nerve conduction velocity: third week	Abnormal: anterior horn cell disease (normal during first 2 weeks)	Abnormal: slowed conduction, decreased motor amplitudes	Abnormal: axonal damage	Normal or abnormal; no diagnostic value
EMG at 3 weeks	Abnormal	Normal	Normal	Normal
Sequelae at 3 months and up to a year	Severe, asymmetric atrophy; skeletal deformities developing later	Symmetric atrophy of distal muscles	Moderate atrophy, only in affected limbs	Flaccid diplegia atrophy after years

Adapted from Global Program for Vaccines and Immunization. Field Guide for Supplementary Activities Aimed at Achieving Polio Eradication. Geneva, World Health Organization, 1996.

bulbar paralysis, if necessary with ventilatory assistance; and (3) to relieve pain and discomfort, particularly with the application of wet heat to the affected muscles. The specific objectives during the subacute (after body temperature has returned to normal) and chronic phases (after hospital discharge) are: (1) to strengthen the remaining functional muscles with physiotherapy to compensate for paralyzed or weak muscles; (2) to prevent deformities following paralysis of muscles and limbs with proper positioning of trunk and limbs, regular movements of limbs, and use of splints to ensure proper position of joints; (3) to assist with ambulation by proper use of splints, leg braces, crutches, and wheelchairs, when appropriate; and (4) to correct contracted muscles or shortened tendons with surgical procedures (Chapter 14). Antiviral compounds, particularly pleconaril, may be used to eliminate chronic enterovirus infections in immunodeficient patients (e.g., patients with agammaglobulinemia), including persistent infections caused by poliovirus.

PROGNOSIS. The prognosis depends upon the extent of weakness or paralysis at initial presentation, the degree of recovery achieved during the first 6 months after onset of paralysis, and the underlying medical condition. For example, the prognosis is more guarded in patients with underlying immunodeficiency disorders. However, most patients, except those with complete paralysis of a limb, will be able to compensate for loss of some muscle function by strengthening the remaining functional muscles.

PREVENTION AND CONTROL. Prevention of poliomyelitis depends on immunization with poliovirus vaccines. Two effective vaccines are available: IPV (Salk vaccine) and OPV (Sabin vaccine). Each of these vaccines has advantages and disadvantages.

Oral Poliovirus Vaccine. OPV, a live-attenuated viral vaccine, closely mimics natural infection; it replicates in the gastrointestinal tract and induces a broad immune response that includes both mucosal immunity and humoral immunity. Mucosal immunity is important in decreasing the circulation of poliovirus in the community. In addition, OPV-derived virus is excreted and can infect contacts of vaccinees, indirectly "vaccinating" those persons not directly reached by vaccination programs. However, as a rare consequence of OPV administration, the virus contained in the vaccine can revert to neurovirulence and cause vaccine-associated paralytic poliomyelitis (VAPP). Since OPV-derived virus is approximately 10,000-fold less neurovirulent than wild poliovirus, approximately 1 VAPP case/3 million doses of OPV administered would be expected. The specific qualities of OPV—superior mucosal immunity and the potential for secondary infection and indirect immunization, in addition to ease of administration by oral drops—make it the vaccine of choice for the global polio eradication initiative.

Inactivated Poliovirus Vaccine. IPV is very effective in inducing humoral immunity, but less efficient in inducing mucosal immunity. There are no known serious adverse effects of IPV administration.

Vaccination Schedules. These depend on the epidemio-

TABLE 27–3. Poliovirus Vaccine Schedule Recommended by the Expanded Program on Immunization (EPI), World Health Organization

Age	Vaccine
Birth*	OPV
6 weeks	OPV
10 weeks	OPV
14 weeks	OPV

*The dose is reserved for polio-endemic countries.

logic situation and specific objectives of the immunization program (Tables 27–2 and 27–3). In polio-endemic countries, the specific objectives are (1) to prevent further morbidity, disability, and mortality; and (2) to eliminate the circulation of poliovirus as part of the global polio eradication initiative. In industrialized countries, the objectives are (1) to ensure high-population immunity levels to prevent re-introduction of poliovirus; and (2) to minimize the potential for serious adverse events associated with the vaccines and the vaccination schedule used. For industrialized countries, use of IPV and OPV in a sequential schedule may offer the best balance by reaping the benefits of both vaccines and minimizing the potential for adverse reactions that rarely follow OPV use.

POLIO ERADICATION INITIATIVE. The global polio eradication objective, a goal established by the World Health Assembly in 1988 to be accomplished by the year 2000, recommends that the following four strategies be implemented in all polio-endemic countries to achieve the eradication target: (1) achieve and maintain high levels of routine coverage with vaccine in infants <1 year of age (Table 27–3) to prevent accumulation of susceptible infants; (2) conduct biannual national immunization days (NIDs), targeting all children <5 years of age regardless of previous immunization history to eliminate widespread circulation of poliovirus; (3) establish sensitive systems for poliomyelitis surveillance using acute flaccid paralysis as a screening case definition to target supplemental immunization activities and monitor the disappearance of poliovirus; and (4) initiate "mopping-up" activi-

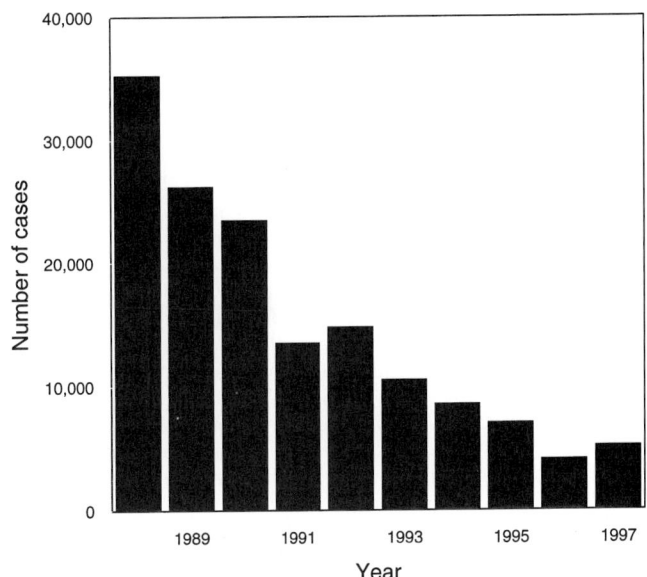

Figure 27–2. Number of reported poliomyelitis cases globally, 1988–1997.

TABLE 27–2. Current Poliovirus Vaccine Schedules in the United States, 1998

| Schedule | Month/Year of Age | | | | |
	2 Months	4 Months	6–18 Months	12–18 Months	4–6 Years
Sequential IPV/OPV	IPV	IPV		OPV	OPV
OPV only	OPV	OPV	OPV		OPV
IPV only	IPV	IPV	IPV		IPV

ties, mass campaigns that administer OPV by house-to-house visits to reach children who have been missed by the routine immunization program and NIDs.

Implementation of these strategies has resulted in ~90% reduction in reported poliomyelitis worldwide since 1988 (Fig. 27–2); the certification of the Western Hemisphere as free of indigenous wild poliovirus in 1994; the elimination of wild poliovirus from the Western Pacific Region (that includes China) of WHO in 1997; and rapid progress toward polio eradication in virtually all polio-endemic countries, with a few exceptions due to internal strife, civil war, or the absence of organized governmental structure.

Bibliography

Centers for Disease Control and Prevention: Poliomyelitis prevention in the United States: Introduction of a sequential vaccination schedule of inactivated poliovirus vaccine followed by oral poliovirus vaccine. Recommendations of the Advisory Committee on Immunization Practices. MMWR 46(RR3):1, 1997.

Centers for Disease Control and Prevention: Progress toward global eradication of poliomyelitis, 1997. MMWR 47:414, 1998.

Cochi SL, Hull HF, Sutter RW, et al: Status report on the Global Poliomyelitis Eradication Initiative. J Infect Dis (Suppl)S1, 1997.

Dalakas MC, Bartfeld H, Kurland LT: The post-polio syndrome: Advances in the pathogenesis and treatment. Ann NY Acad Sci 753:1, 1995.

Global Program for Vaccines and Immunization: Field Guide for Supplementary Activities Aimed at Achieving Polio Eradication. Geneva, World Health Organization, 1996.

Paul JR: A History of Poliomyelitis. New Haven, Yale University Press, 1971.

Sutter RW, Cochi SL, Melnick JL: Live attenuated poliovirus vaccines. In Plotkin SA, Mortimer EA, Orenstein WA (eds): Vaccines, 3rd ed. Philadelphia, WB Saunders, 1999.

27.2 Viral Diarrheas

Karen Midthun and Robert E. Black

The term viral diarrheas has been used to describe acute, self-limited illnesses characterized by diarrhea and often by vomiting for which bacterial enteropathogens could not be identified. Rotaviruses are a leading cause of severe diarrheal illness in infants and young children worldwide, whereas Norwalk-like viruses are an important cause of outbreaks of vomiting and diarrheal illness in older children and adults. Adenoviruses, astroviruses, and caliciviruses also have been identified as etiologic agents of diarrhea.

◾ ROTAVIRUS DIARRHEA

DEFINITION. Rotavirus diarrhea is an acute infectious disease characterized by watery diarrhea and vomiting; it occurs primarily in children less than 2 years of age.

ETIOLOGY AND HISTORY. Rotavirus was identified in 1973 by Australian workers using thin-section electron microscopy to examine duodenal mucosa biopsy specimens from children with diarrhea. Subsequently, researchers in several countries detected viral particles by direct electron microscopic examination of feces from children with diarrhea. The term rotavirus, derived from the Latin *rota* (wheel), was suggested by the appearance of the virus as a wheel with spokes radiating from a hub.

Rotaviruses are classified as a genus in the family *Reoviridae* and are etiologic agents of diarrhea in many animal species as well as in humans. They are spherical, are 70 nm in diameter, and have an inner and outer capsid (Fig. 27–3). The genome consists of 11 segments of double-stranded RNA

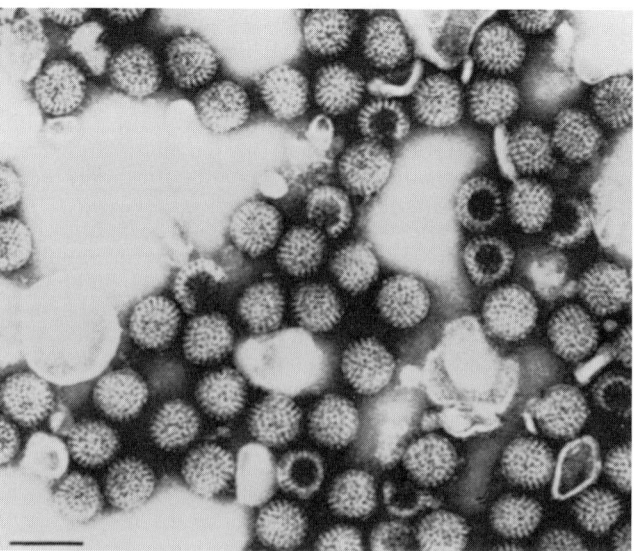

Figure 27–3. Rotavirus particles in a stool filtrate from an 11-month-old child with diarrhea. The particles appear to have a double-shelled capsid, and occasional "empty" particles are seen. (Electron micrograph by Dr. A. Z. Kapikian.) (Bar represents 100 nm.)

that encode six structural and five nonstructural proteins. Rotaviruses possess three important antigenic specificities: group, subgroup, and serotype. Most rotaviruses are classified as group A because they share a common antigen on VP6, the major inner capsid protein. Several rotaviruses that do not share the group A common antigen have been detected and classified into groups B through G. Both group B and group C rotavirus infections have occurred in humans, but they are not considered important causes of diarrhea.

Most group A rotaviruses belong to subgroup I or II, based on subgroup-specific antigens that are also located on VP6. The VP4 and VP7 outer capsid proteins of group A rotaviruses induce neutralizing antibodies and determine P and G serotype specificity, respectively. Although ten G and six P serotypes have been recovered from humans, it appears that the majority of epidemiologically important strains bear G1, 2, 3, or 4 specificity and P1A or 1B specificity. The G1 serotype is most prevalent worldwide, constituting approximately 60% of human isolates.

Rotavirus particles remain structurally stable after exposure to heat (37°C for 1 hour) or ambient temperature for 24 hours, ether, and mild acids but are disrupted by acid treatment at a pH of less than 3. Proteolytic enzymes, e.g., trypsin, pancreatin, and elastin, enhance viral infectivity and are essential for growth of human rotaviruses in cell cultures.

DISTRIBUTION AND INCIDENCE. Rotaviruses have a worldwide distribution and are important causes of diarrhea in every area of the world. In developed countries, they are the leading cause of severe childhood diarrhea and have been detected in approximately 40% of infants and young children hospitalized with acute diarrheal illness. In North American family surveillance studies, 10 to 23% of diarrheal episodes in infants and young children were related to rotavirus. In 57 studies conducted in health facilities in developing countries in the last two decades, rotavirus was detected in a median of 20% (range 5 to 49%) of children under 5 years of age with diarrhea. Studies of hospitalized children usually found a higher percentage with rotavirus infection than did studies done in outpatient clinics. Rotavirus either was the most frequent enteropathogen identified or was second to bacterial agents, particularly enterotoxigenic and enteropathogenic *E. coli*. In 22 community-based studies in developing countries, rotavirus was detected in 6% (range 2 to 29%) of diarrheal episodes in children.

Among children under 5 years of age in the developing world, it has been estimated that rotaviruses cause over 125 million cases of diarrhea annually, of which 18 million are moderately severe or severe and 873,000 lead to death. In the United States, rotavirus infections cause an estimated 3 million cases of diarrhea, 65,000 hospitalizations, and 125 deaths per year in infants and young children. The preeminence of rotavirus among children hospitalized with diarrhea in developing and developed countries undoubtedly is related to the greater degree of dehydration associated with rotavirus diarrhea than with most other types of childhood diarrhea.

In community-based studies in rural Bangladesh, the incidence of rotavirus diarrhea was highest between 3 and 23 months of age and reached a peak in the second 6 months of life; no rotavirus case was noted in children older than 24 months (Fig. 27–4). In the same area, treatment center visits for rotavirus diarrhea also reached a peak for children 6 to 11 months of age, whereas those for older children and adults were low. This and other studies of rotavirus incidence from communities in rural Bangladesh and Guatemala suggest that rotavirus diarrhea occurs once or twice in children during the first 2 years of life.

EPIDEMIOLOGY. In temperate climates, rotavirus diarrhea is seasonal, with the greatest prevalence in cold weather. During winter, rotavirus has been found in up to 70% of children hospitalized for diarrhea, whereas in summer it is detected infrequently. In tropical climates, rotavirus infections occur throughout the year, although the incidence may be higher during the cooler and drier months.

Community-wide epidemics primarily involve young children, although all age groups have been affected. Outbreaks of rotavirus diarrhea have been reported in a variety of settings, e.g., primary schools, daycare nurseries, hospitals, and nursing homes. Several large outbreaks of non–group A rotavirus diarrhea affecting adults have been described in China.

Hospitalized Patients and Neonates. Nosocomial infections occur frequently in pediatric wards. In one study in the United States, 17% of 60 pediatric patients hospitalized for nondiarrheal disorders developed rotavirus diarrhea more than 72 hours after admission. In another hospital study in Canada, approximately 20% of rotavirus infections appeared to be hospital-acquired. Nosocomial infections have been described in many neonatal nurseries around the world, and in some nurseries the same strain has circulated for extended periods. For unknown reasons, neonatal infections are usually subclinical. It has been suggested that maternally acquired antibody, breast-feeding, host factors, and characteristics peculiar to neonatal strains may contribute to this phenomenon.

Adult Infections. Adults are also susceptible to rotavirus diarrhea. Illnesses, which are usually mild, are often associated with exposure to infected children either in the hospital or at home. Studies of the adult household contacts of children with rotavirus diarrhea revealed a high rate of infection, but fewer than one third of infected adults developed diarrhea. Also, adults may experience rotavirus diarrhea when traveling in developing countries. In 14 studies of traveler's diarrhea, a median of 2.5% (range 0 to 36%) of diarrheal illnesses was associated with rotavirus. In these cases, the etiologic significance is unclear, since patients with rotavirus were frequently infected with other pathogens, and a high proportion of asymptomatic control subjects were also infected with rotavirus.

Serology. Seroepidemiologic studies in both developing and developed countries show an initial high prevalence and titer of serum antibody in infants, which falls by 6 months of age. By age 2 years, nearly all children have serum rotavirus antibody; titers remain elevated until late adulthood. The initial titers represent maternal antibodies, and the rise in early childhood is due to one or more rotaviral infections. Furthermore, evidence from a Bangladeshi longitudinal study indicates that many transient infections not associated with diarrhea stimulate an increase in serum antibodies.

Transmission. Rotavirus infection spreads by the fecal-oral route. When given orally, infectious particles from diarrheal feces have reproduced the disease in volunteers. The usual mode of transmission is probably by direct person-to-person contact or contact with contaminated objects. The virus is relatively resistant to adverse environmental conditions and can remain on surfaces for prolonged periods. It also maintains structural integrity in water, and water-borne transmission is a possibility. The respiratory symptoms associated with rotaviral diarrheal illnesses, the rapid acquisition of serum antibody during the first few years of life regardless of hygienic conditions, and the failure to document fecal-oral spread in a few large outbreaks have led to speculation that rotavirus can be transmitted by the respiratory route. However, rotaviruses have been detected infrequently in respiratory secretions. Animal-to-human transmission has not been documented. Although a high degree of homology between certain human and animal strains suggests that this may occur, it does not appear to be of clinical or epidemiologic importance.

IMMUNITY. Children over age 2 years and adults have substantial resistance to rotavirus diarrhea. Natural immunity probably follows one or more illnesses in early childhood and repeated asymptomatic exposures to the virus. Although reinfection within the first few years of life is a common event, most infants who have had a severe case of rotavirus diarrhea usually experience milder illness upon reinfection. Likewise, adults who experience re-infections are usually asymptomatic. The protective effect of natural infection was also demonstrated in children who had been infected as neonates. These children had significantly fewer episodes of severe rotavirus diarrhea than did their uninfected counterparts, although the incidence of rotavirus infection was similar in the two groups during 3 years of surveillance.

The immunologic correlates of protection against disease are not well understood. Serum or fecal antibody to rotavirus may be associated with, but does not consistently confer, protection from infection or disease. Antibody passively ad-

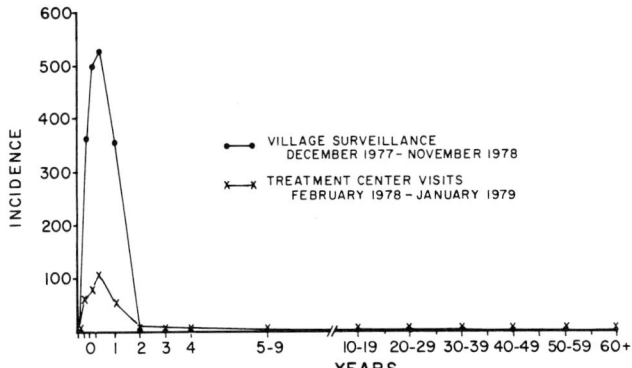

Figure 27–4. Annual age-specific incidence of rotavirus diarrhea per 1000 persons assessed by village surveillance and by treatment center visits. (From Black RE, et al.: Lancet 1:141, 1981.)

ministered via the alimentary tract has been shown to alter the susceptibility to disease.

PATHOGENESIS. Rotaviruses replicate in the mature villous epithelial cells of the small intestine. Small bowel biopsies from children with rotavirus diarrhea have revealed shortening and blunting of villi, flattening of epithelial cells, and infiltration of the lamina propria with mononuclear cells. Abnormalities have ranged from mild to severe and have tended to be patchy.

The mechanism whereby rotaviruses induce diarrhea is not completely understood. There is a net secretion of water, sodium, and chloride that has been attributed in part to the transient replacement of the absorptive villous tip cells with immature crypt cells, which retain some of their secretory characteristics. Studies in a murine model suggest that rotavirus may cause diarrhea through a toxin-like effect upon virus-cell contact. Rotaviral diarrheal stools contain 30 to 40 mEq/L of sodium, and the sodium concentration does not increase with higher rates of stool loss. Stool potassium losses also range from 30 to 40 mEq/L.

Rotavirus infection also results in decreased brush border disaccharidase activity. Children with rotavirus diarrhea may have increased fecal reducing substances, indicating some sugar malabsorption during illness. On the basis of the lactose–breath hydrogen test, 15 (29%) of 51 children studied on the fifth to nineteenth day after onset of rotavirus diarrhea were classified as malabsorbers of lactose. There was significantly more lactose malabsorption in children who continued to excrete rotavirus until the day of study compared with children whose stools had become rotavirus-negative. Follow-up studies of subjects originally diagnosed as malabsorbers showed marked improvement.

CLINICAL MANIFESTATIONS

Symptoms. Rotavirus infection may be asymptomatic or may cause diarrheal disease that ranges from mild to severe. The incubation period for rotavirus diarrhea ranges from 1 to 5 days but is usually less than 48 hours. The illness is characterized by the abrupt onset of watery diarrhea and vomiting. Vomiting is present in up to 90% of patients, may precede the onset of diarrhea, and usually stops within the first 2 days of the disease. Low-grade fevers have been found in 50 to 100% of cases.

The majority of children with rotavirus diarrhea have a mild self-limited illness lasting 3 to 8 days. However, dehydration develops in a substantial proportion of cases. Children with rotavirus diarrhea have more frequent and severe dehydration than do children with other types of diarrhea. The rate of dehydration in association with rotavirus diarrhea is second only to that of cholera.

Laboratory Findings. Clinical laboratory findings in children with rotavirus diarrhea may include elevations in blood urea nitrogen, urine and plasma specific gravity, and hematocrit. A metabolic acidosis, usually partially compensated, is a common finding. Serum electrolytes are usually normal, but low sodium and potassium levels are common; hypernatremia also occurs. Peripheral white blood cell counts are usually normal. Fecal leukocytes (9 to 31%) are less common than in diarrhea associated with invasive bacterial pathogens.

COMPLICATIONS. Severe, life-threatening dehydration occurs in only a small percentage of children with rotavirus diarrhea, but it is nonetheless an important cause of mortality among children under 2 years of age in developing countries. In Bangladesh it was estimated that 42% of deaths from watery diarrhea in this age group were due to rotavirus and that another 35% were caused by enterotoxigenic *E. coli*. These two illnesses alone were thought to result in an annual mortality rate of 6.5/1000 children. Occasional deaths from rotavirus diarrhea have also been documented in developed countries. In a 5-year study in Canada, 21 deaths in children 4 to 30 months of age were attributed to rotavirus.

Although most rotaviral illnesses resolve within 7 days, a small percentage have a longer duration. Viral shedding in the stool frequently continues for 10 days after onset of illness and may be associated with lactose malabsorption. Children with primary immunodeficiency syndromes can develop chronic symptomatic diarrhea with prolonged shedding of rotavirus. Likewise, rotavirus can cause especially severe gastroenteritis in individuals who are immunosuppressed for bone marrow transplantation. Rotavirus infection was not more common or severe in HIV-infected infants than in non–HIV infected infants hospitalized with diarrhea in Zambia. Rotaviruses do not appear to play an important role in HIV-infected adults with diarrhea.

Single cases of Reye syndrome, encephalitis, and aseptic meningitis following rotavirus diarrhea have been reported, but a causal relationship is unclear. Other central nervous system disorders, e.g., altered mental status and seizures, are probably due to hypoglycemia or electrolyte abnormalities. A temporal association of rotavirus infection with intussusception, Henoch-Schönlein purpura, hemolytic-uremic syndrome, sudden infant death syndrome, Kawasaki syndrome, and exanthema subitum has been noted, but a causal link remains to be determined.

DIAGNOSIS

Differential Diagnosis. The watery diarrheal illness due to rotavirus can be partially distinguished from diarrhea due to bacteria (e.g., enterotoxigenic or enteropathogenic *E. coli, Vibrio cholerae*) by its characteristic early vomiting and fever. Epidemiologic clues are its relative restriction to children under 2 years of age and its greater prevalence during the cool season in some settings. There are no features of this illness that would distinguish it from other viral diarrheas, e.g., those due to Norwalk-like agents or adenovirus.

Laboratory Diagnosis. Diagnosis requires the demonstration of rotavirus in the feces or an increase in serum antibody to rotavirus; routine diagnosis is usually based on the detection of virus in feces. Stools from the first to fourth day of illness are optimal for rotavirus detection, although shedding may continue for 3 weeks or longer. Methods to detect rotavirus in feces include electron microscopy (EM), enzyme-linked immunosorbent assay (ELISA), reverse passive hemagglutination assay (RPHA), latex agglutination (LA), counterimmunoelectrophoresis, RNA gel electrophoresis, dot hybridization, and polymerase chain reaction (PCR). The ELISA is the most commonly used because it is both sensitive and easy to perform. Commercially available tests for the detection of group A rotavirus include ELISA, RPHA, LA, and RNA electrophoresis. EM and RNA gel electrophoresis have the added advantage that they can detect both group A and non–group A rotaviruses. ELISAs have been developed for the detection of human group B or group C rotaviruses, but reagents for these assays are limited to research settings. Human rotavirus can be isolated in cell culture from approximately 75% of stool specimens shown to contain virus by other test procedures. However, this is impractical and has poor sensitivity when compared with other methods.

The determination of serotype is not usually clinically important but is of interest in epidemiologic studies and the evaluation of rotavirus vaccines. Methods to determine the G and P serotypes of group A isolates include a neutralization assay in cell culture, solid-phase immune EM, ELISA, and, most recently, PCR.

Rotavirus infection can also be diagnosed by serologic assays, e.g., complement fixation, immune EM, and ELISA. Rotavirus-specific IgG, IgM, and IgA levels in serum, intestinal fluid, feces, and saliva can be measured by ELISA. Neutralization assays in cell culture and epitope-blocking ELISA are important techniques in defining serotype-specific responses.

TREATMENT AND PROGNOSIS

Oral Rehydration. The most important principle of therapy of watery diarrhea, including that caused by rotavirus, is replacement of water and electrolytes that are lost in the diarrheal stool. This is necessary to prevent (or correct) dehydration and electrolyte imbalance. Most patients, even those with dehydration and vomiting, can be managed with an oral sugar-electrolyte solution (Chapter 16). The oral rehydration solution (ORS) recommended by the WHO can be prepared by adding the following to 1 L of water: sodium chloride 3.5 g, trisodium citrate dihydrate 2.9 g (or sodium bicarbonate 2.5 g), potassium chloride 1.5 g, and glucose 20 g. The resulting solution contains sodium 90 mmol/L, potassium 20 mmol/L, citrate 10 mmol/L (or bicarbonate 30 mmol/L), and glucose 111 mmol/L. After correction of the estimated fluid loss with ORS, fluids, e.g., water, breast milk, or some other form of low-solute feeding should be given in addition to ORS to replace losses from ongoing diarrhea and to provide normal daily fluid requirements. Sucrose (40 g/L) can be substituted for glucose in the ORS with only minimal loss of efficacy; rice-based solutions have been effective also.

Diarrhea is an important cause of malnutrition, and withdrawal of breast milk and other food during illness may be one reason for this adverse consequence. Thus, during diarrhea, children should continue to receive breast milk and other staple foods, e.g., rice. There is no need for routine dilution of milk or formula, but exceptional cases of lactose intolerance should be identified and managed by reducing the concentration of milk feeds for a short period. Antidiarrheal agents that alter the motility of the gut are not indicated.

Intravenous Fluids. Patients with severe dehydration, excessive vomiting, or other infrequent complications should be treated with intravenous fluid replacement. With prompt and appropriate treatment, mortality is negligible (Chapter 16).

Immunotherapy. Chronic rotavirus infection in immunodeficient children has been treated successfully with human milk containing rotavirus antibodies; also, persistent rotavirus diarrhea in two infants was cleared by the oral administration of human immunoglobulin. Colostrum or milk concentrate from cows immunized with human rotavirus was not effective in the treatment of children with acute rotavirus diarrhea, but one study reported that oral immunoglobulin shortened the duration of diarrhea, viral excretion, and hospital stay in children hospitalized for acute rotavirus gastroenteritis.

PREVENTION AND CONTROL. Preventive measures include immunization with rotavirus vaccine, sanitary waste disposal, avoidance of feces-contaminated water and objects, and hygienic practices, e.g., handwashing. The significant morbidity associated with rotavirus diarrhea during the first 2 years of life, regardless of hygienic conditions, underscores the need for vaccination in early infancy.

All rotavirus vaccine candidates tested in efficacy studies to date have been live, attenuated rotavirus strains administered by the oral route. In earlier trials, bovine (RIT4237, WC3) or rhesus (RRV) rotavirus vaccine candidates were shown to be safe and immunogenic, but they induced highly variable rates of protection against rotavirus diarrhea. These studies led to the concept that a multivalent vaccine that represented each of the four epidemiologically important G serotypes might be necessary to induce protection in young infants.

Human-animal rotavirus reassortants that derived the gene encoding VP7 from the human rotavirus parent but the remaining genes from the animal rotavirus parent were developed as vaccine candidates. The greatest experience with a multivalent vaccine to date has been with a tetravalent preparation containing RRV (G serotype 3) and human-RRV reassortants of G serotype 1, 2, and 4 specificity. A three-dose regimen administered to young infants in the United States showed an efficacy of 57% against any rotavirus disease and 82% against very severe disease over a 2-year observation period. Trials using a 10-fold higher dose (4×10^5 pFu/dose) of this vaccine were conducted in the United States, Finland, and Venezuela and yielded similar efficacy results. In 1998, the US FDA licensed this vaccine (Rotashield) for the prevention of rotavirus gastroenteritis and recommended oral administration at 2, 4 and 6 months of age.

■ DIARRHEA DUE TO NORWALK VIRUS GROUP AND OTHER CALICIVIRUSES

DEFINITION. The Norwalk group of viruses and other human caliciviruses cause diarrhea and vomiting of abrupt onset and short duration.

ETIOLOGY AND HISTORY. Norwalk virus was first visualized in 1972 by immune electron microscopy (IEM) of fecal material derived from an outbreak of gastroenteritis that had occurred in Norwalk, Ohio, in 1968 (Fig. 27–5). In that outbreak, half the students and teachers in an elementary school developed vomiting and diarrhea. Since no enteropathogens could be detected by direct methods, a bacteria-free filtrate of one patient's feces was administered orally to adult volunteers. The illness produced was identical to the disease seen in the school epidemic. In further studies in adult volunteers, it was found that the same agent can cause a spectrum of symptoms. In some, diarrhea occurred without vomiting, whereas others had vomiting without diarrhea. Most had

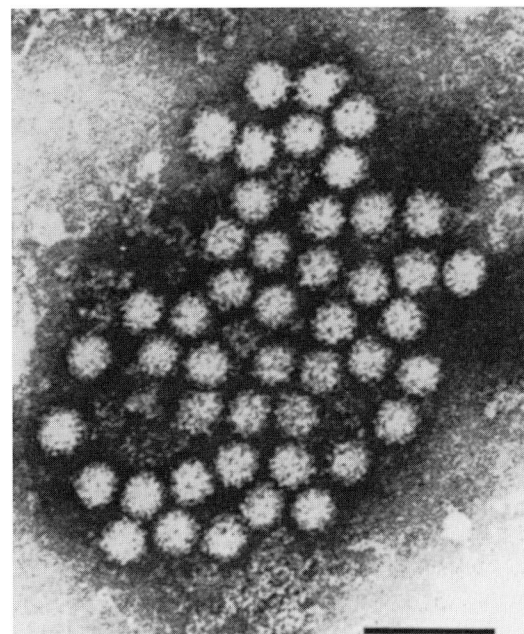

Figure 27–5. Immune aggregate of Norwalk virus in stool from an adult volunteer who developed diarrhea after ingesting a filtrate of a rectal swab specimen from an adult who was affected by a diarrhea outbreak in Norwalk, Ohio. (Electron micrograph by Dr. A. Z. Kapikian.) (Bar represents 100 nm.)

both manifestations. Most naturally and experimentally infected individuals developed a serologic response to the virus by IEM, providing evidence that the viral isolate was the etiologic agent of Norwalk gastroenteritis.

The Norwalk virus is the prototype strain of a group of small round structured viruses (SRSV) that have been associated with outbreaks of acute gastroenteritis. There are at least four distinct serotypes within this group, represented by the Norwalk, Hawaii, Snow Mountain, and Taunton viruses. The Norwalk and Norwalk-like viruses are members of the *Caliciviridae* family and have been classified into four genogroups on the basis of their RNA polymerase gene. They range in size from 26 to 35 nm and have a single-stranded RNA genome and a single structural protein of 59–62 kDa. They are unable to grow in cell culture.

Another group of human caliciviruses that have the more classic calicivirus morphology (cup-shaped indentations that form a six-pointed star with a central hollow) have usually been associated with mild cases of pediatric gastroenteritis; they have, however, also been implicated in outbreaks of gastroenteritis in adults, especially among elderly individuals. Five distinct serotypes, UK 1 to UK 4 and human calicivirus Japan, have been identified in this group by IEM.

DISTRIBUTION AND PREVALENCE. Norwalk virus has a worldwide distribution. In the United States, it has been associated serologically with approximately one third of acute gastroenteritis outbreaks in which no bacterial pathogen could be identified. In 558 unselected outbreaks approximately 10% were thought to be associated with Norwalk-like virus. Norwalk-associated outbreaks have occurred at all times of year and in all age groups but primarily have affected older children and adults. They have occurred in recreational camps, community or family settings, cruise ships, and nursing homes and frequently could be attributed to a common contaminating source, e.g., water or food. Some adults who have had diarrhea after traveling to developing countries have had serologic responses to Norwalk virus.

In developed countries serum antibody prevalence increases gradually during childhood, and the majority of adults have antibody. However, acquisition of antibody to Norwalk virus in Bangladesh, Ecuador, and the Philippines occurs early in life, suggesting that these infections may cause diarrheal illnesses in young children. A prospective study in rural Bangladesh found a high prevalence of elevated Norwalk antibody titers among children in their second and third years and demonstrated that children who seroconverted had a higher incidence of diarrhea than those who did not. It was estimated that Norwalk virus may cause 1 to 2% of episodes of diarrhea during a child's first 5 years. Serologic studies also have shown rapid acquisition of antibody to caliciviruses belonging to the UK and Japan serotypes; in daycare centers in the United States caliciviruses cause approximately 3% of diarrheal episodes. However, Norwalk virus and other human caliciviruses do not appear to be important etiologic agents of severe diarrheal disease in infants and young children, as they are rarely detected in the stools of children hospitalized with gastroenteritis.

TRANSMISSION. Norwalk-like viruses are transmitted by the fecal-oral route. Virus has been identified in vomitus, suggesting the possibility that aerosolization of virus during vomiting results in airborne spread. Transmission via a common source, e.g., feces-contaminated water and food (primarily shellfish) has been reported frequently, and secondary transmission by person-to-person contact is relatively common.

PATHOGENESIS AND PATHOLOGY. Volunteers ingesting Norwalk or Hawaii viruses develop histologic abnormalities in the proximal small bowel, including broadening and blunting of the villi, mononuclear cell infiltrate, and cytoplasmic vacuolization of epithelial cells. The virus has not been detected within mucosal cells, presumably because of its small size and the patchy distribution of the lesions. The mucosal changes in the small bowel return to normal within 2 weeks. The gastric and rectal mucosa remains normal during infection.

During experimentally induced Norwalk virus illness, small intestinal brush border enzymes are decreased; malabsorption of fat and xylose has been demonstrated. These alterations may persist for several days after diarrhea has stopped and may occur during asymptomatic infections.

CLINICAL MANIFESTATIONS AND COMPLICATIONS. The incubation period for Norwalk disease averages between 24 and 48 hours. Illness is usually mild and lasts between 24 and 60 hours. The majority of patients and experimentally infected volunteers have nausea, vomiting, or diarrhea or a combination of these. Additional symptoms may include anorexia, fever, headache, myalgias, and abdominal cramps. In outbreaks, vomiting is more common than diarrhea in children, whereas the opposite is true of adults. Stools are usually loose and watery and without blood, mucus, or leukocytes.

DIAGNOSIS. It cannot be distinguished from other viral diarrheal illnesses, e.g., that due to rotavirus. However, Norwalk-like viruses should be considered a possible etiologic agent in vomiting or diarrhea in an older child or adult, especially when other individuals with the same exposure history develop gastrointestinal illness.

Laboratory diagnosis is by identification of viral particles in stool obtained early in the illness or by a serologic response to viral antigen. Diagnostic tests, which include IEM, RIA, ELISA, and PCR, are still research procedures, since reagents are not available commercially.

TREATMENT AND PROGNOSIS. Treatment consists of replacement of fluids and electrolytes, as indicated for rotavirus diarrhea. Since most illnesses are mild and self-limited, the prognosis is excellent.

PREVENTION AND CONTROL. Interruption of fecal-oral transmission is the primary means of prevention. Volunteer studies have demonstrated that short-term homologous resistance to disease develops after Norwalk agent infection. The occurrence of long-term immunity is less clear, and the protective mechanisms are unknown. These uncertainties and the inability to grow the viruses in tissue culture have prevented development of a vaccine, although recently an abundant source of viral antigen has been generated using a baculovirus recombinant.

■ OTHER VIRAL AGENTS ASSOCIATED WITH DIARRHEA

ADENOVIRUSES. Enteric adenoviruses are the second most common cause, after rotavirus, of viral diarrhea requiring hospitalization in infants and young children. Adenoviruses are 70 to 80 nm in diameter and have a double-stranded DNA genome. They are classified into six groups (A–F) and comprise 47 distinct serotypes. Enteric adenoviruses belong to group F and include two serotypes, types 40 and 41.

Epidemiology. Enteric adenoviruses have a worldwide distribution; acquisition of serum antibody occurs early in life and has been detected in approximately 50% of children by 4 to 5 years of age. In 20 health facility–based studies in developing countries, a median of 3% (range 0 to 6%) of diarrheal episodes in infants and young children was associated with enteric adenoviruses. Most cases of diarrhea caused by adenovirus occur in children under 2 years of age. In contrast to rotavirus, enteric adenovirus infections show no seasonal variation. The mode of transmission has not been clearly documented but is presumably by the fecal-oral route.

Clinical Manifestations. Disease develops after an incubation period of 8 to 10 days and is characterized by watery diarrhea that lasts for an average of 10 days. Vomiting, fever, and dehydration may occur but are usually mild. Secondary lactose malabsorption has been reported. Respiratory symptoms were common in one study but rare in others. Enteric adenoviruses have not been detected in the respiratory secretions of children with adenovirus diarrhea.

Diagnosis. The diagnosis of diarrhea secondary to enteric adenovirus requires the identification of the virus in the stool specimen. Adenoviruses in stool can be detected by IEM (Fig. 27–6) or ELISA. An ELISA that specifically identifies types 40 and 41 using monoclonal antibodies is commercially available. The group F enteric adenoviruses differ from groups A–E adenoviruses in that the former will not grow in the conventional cell cultures used to propagate the latter.

ASTROVIRUSES. Astroviruses have been detected characteristically in stools of pediatric patients with mild gastroenteritis. They are 28 nm in diameter; up to 10% of particles have a distinctive stellate appearance on EM. They have a single-stranded RNA genome; seven serotypes have been identified in humans to date.

Epidemiology. Human astroviruses have a worldwide distribution. They appear to be more prevalent in the winter months, and serotype 1 strains are detected most often. Serum antibody to astrovirus is acquired in early childhood and is present in over 70% of children by 5 years of age. The development of an ELISA using astrovirus-specific monoclonal antibodies has allowed epidemiologic investigations of astroviruses. In a study of outpatient pediatric gastroenteritis in Thailand, astrovirus was detected in 9% of cases, whereas rotavirus was detected in 19% and enteric adenovirus in 3% of cases. In a 2-year longitudinal study of ambulatory children in Guatemala, astrovirus was detected in 7% of diarrheal episodes. In both studies, astrovirus infections occurred most often in children less than 1 year of age. A study conducted in daycare settings in the United States detected astrovirus in 4% of children with diarrhea. Thus, astroviruses are a relatively common cause of mild pediatric gastroenteritis but not an important cause of severe gastroenteritis, as they have been detected rarely in the stools of infants and children hospitalized with gastroenteritis.

Astroviruses have also been implicated in occasional outbreaks of diarrhea in newborn nurseries; pediatric wards; community settings, affecting children and adults; and nursing homes, affecting both patients and staff. Astroviruses are transmitted by the fecal-oral route. Two volunteer studies have suggested that astrovirus is readily transmissible but of low pathogenicity in healthy adults. Astrovirus infection early in life provides long-lasting immunity, since astrovirus gastroenteritis mainly affects infants and young children.

Clinical Manifestations. In two volunteer studies the incubation period was 3 to 5 days, but it was only 24 to 36 hours in secondary cases during an outbreak of astrovirus gastroenteritis in Japan. Illness is usually mild, characterized by diarrhea or vomiting, or both; fever, abdominal pain, and dehydration may occur. Illness has usually lasted for 2 to 3 days in several outbreaks affecting 5- to 6-year-old children, adults, and the elderly. In infants and younger children, illness usually lasts 4 to 5 days. The diagnosis of astrovirus infection has been limited to the research setting, where EM, ELISA, immunofluorescence assay, and PCR have been used to detect and type astrovirus in stool specimens.

■ OTHER VIRAL AGENTS

A variety of other virus-like particles have been observed by EM in diarrheal stool. Further research is needed to determine the significance of these other virus-like agents. Although the majority of diarrheal episodes can now be associated with a bacterial or viral enteropathogen, there remains an important minority of episodes for which no etiologic agent can be found.

Bibliography

Ando T, Jin Q, Gentsch JR, et al: Epidemiologic applications of novel molecular methods to detect and differentiate small round structured viruses (Norwalk-like viruses). J Med Virol 47:145, 1995.

Avery ME, Snyder JD: Oral therapy for acute diarrhea. The underused simple solution. N Engl J Med 323:891, 1990.

Bern C, Martines J, de Zoysa I, et al: The magnitude of the global problem of diarrhoeal disease: A ten-year update. Bull WHO 70:705, 1992.

Black RE, Lanata CF: Epidemiology of diarrheal diseases in developing countries. *In* Blaser MJ, Smith PD, Ravdin I, et al (eds): Infections of the Gastrointestinal Tract. New York, Raven Press, 1995, p 13.

Black RE, Merson MH, Huq I, et al: Incidence and severity of rotavirus and *Escherichia coli* diarrhoea in rural Bangladesh: Implications for vaccine development. Lancet 1:141, 1981.

Brandt CD, Kim HW, Rodriguez WJ, et al: Pediatric viral gastroenteritis during eight years of study. J Clin Microbiol 18:71, 1983.

Brandt CD, Kim HW, Rodriguez WJ, et al: Adenoviruses and pediatric gastroenteritis. J Infect Dis 151:437, 1985.

Cruz JR, Bartlett AV, Herrmann JE, et al: Astrovirus-associated diarrhea among Guatemalan ambulatory rural children. J Clin Microbiol 30:1140, 1992.

Cruz JR, Caceres P, Cano F, et al: Adenovirus types 40 and 41 and rotaviruses associated with diarrhea in children from Guatemala. J Clin Microbiol 28:1780, 1990.

Greenberg HB, Valdesuso J, Kapikian AZ, et al: Prevalence of antibody to the Norwalk virus in various countries. Infect Immun 26:270, 1979.

Grimwood K, Carzino R, Barnes GL, et al: Patients with enteric adenovirus gastroenteritis admitted to an Australian pediatric teaching hospital from 1981 to 1992. J Clin Microbiol 33:131, 1995.

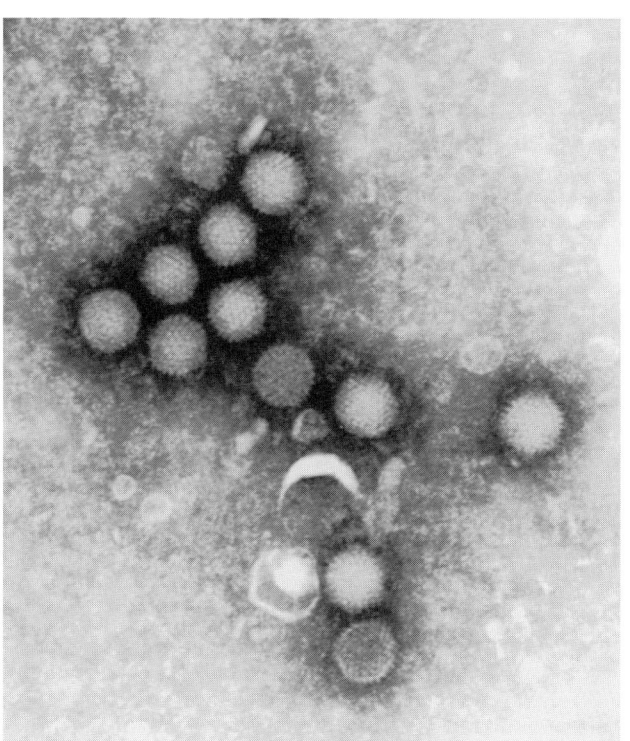

Figure 27–6. Adenovirus particles in a stool filtrate from a patient with diarrhea (× 142,500). (Electron micrograph by Dr. A. Z. Kapikian.)

Grohman GS, Glass RI, Pereira HG, et al: Enteric viruses and diarrhea in HIV-infected patients. N Engl J Med 329:14, 1993.

Haffejee IE: The epidemiology of rotavirus infections: A global perspective. J Pediatr Gastroenterol Nutr 20:275, 1995.

Herrmann JE, Taylor DN, Echeverria P, et al: Astroviruses as a cause of gastroenteritis in children. N Engl J Med 324:1757, 1991.

Huilan S, Zhen LG, Mathan MM, et al: Etiology of acute diarrhoea among children in developing countries: A multicentre study in five countries. Bull WHO 69:549, 1991.

Hung T, Chen G, Wang C, et al: Waterborne outbreak of rotavirus diarrhoea in adults in China caused by a novel rotavirus. Lancet 1:1139, 1984.

Kapikian AZ: Viral gastroenteritis. JAMA 1993;269:627.

Kapikian AZ, Chanock RM: Rotaviruses. In Fields BN, Knipe DM, Howley PM, et al (eds): Fields Virology, 3rd ed. Philadelphia, Lippincott-Raven, 1996, p 1657.

Kapikian AZ, Estes MK, Chanock RM: Norwalk group of viruses. In Fields BN, Knipe DM, Howley PM, et al (eds): Fields Virology, 3rd ed. Philadelphia, Lippincott-Raven, 1996, p 783.

Kaplan JE, Gary GW, Baron RC, et al: Epidemiology of Norwalk gastroenteritis and the role of Norwalk virus in outbreaks of acute nonbacterial gastroenteritis. Ann Intern Med 96:756, 1982.

Matsui MM, Greenberg HB: Astroviruses. In Fields BN, Knipe DM, Howley PM, et al (eds): Fields Virology, 3rd ed. Philadelphia, Lippincott-Raven, 1996, p 811.

Midthun K, Kapikian AZ: Rotavirus vaccines: An overview. Clin Microbiol Rev 9:423, 1996.

Parker SP, Cubitt WD, Jiang XJ, et al: Seroprevalence studies using a recombinant Norwalk virus protein enzyme immunoassay. J Med Virol 42:146, 1994.

Rennels MB, Glass RI, Dennehy PH, et al: Safety and efficacy of high-dose rhesus-human reassortant rotavirus vaccines—report of the national multicenter trial. Pediatrics 97:7, 1996.

Rodriguez WJ, Kim HW, Arrobio JO, et al: Clinical features of acute gastroenteritis associated with human reovirus–like agent in infants and young children. J Pediatr 91:188, 1977.

Smith JC, Haddix AC, Teutsch SM, et al: Cost-effectiveness analysis of a rotavirus immunization program for the United States. Pediatrics 96:609, 1995.

Treanor JJ, Clark HF, Pichichero M, et al: Evaluation of the protective efficacy of a serotype 1 bovine-human rotavirus reassortant vaccine in infants. Pediatr Infect Dis J 14:301, 1995.

Uhnoo I, Olding-Stenkvist E, Kreuger A: Clinical features of acute gastroenteritis associated with rotavirus, enteric adenoviruses, and bacteria. Arch Dis Child 61:732, 1986.

Ward RL, Bernstein DI: Protection against rotavirus disease after natural rotavirus infection. J Infect Dis 169:900, 1994.

Woods PA, Gentsch J, Gouvea V, et al: Distribution of serotypes of human rotavirus in different populations. J Clin Microbiol 30:781, 1992.

27.3 Acute Hemorrhagic Conjunctivitis

Mark A. Pallansch

DEFINITION. Acute hemorrhagic conjunctivitis (AHC) is a highly contagious epidemic disease characterized by painful conjunctivitis, subconjunctival hemorrhages, and, in rare cases, neurologic symptoms.

ETIOLOGY AND HISTORY. AHC first appeared almost simultaneously in 1969 in Ghana and Indonesia, and within 3 years epidemics swept through North and East Africa, India, and Asia, with scattered outbreaks extending into Europe. From this first pandemic, two novel enteroviral agents were isolated. Enterovirus 70 (EV70) was isolated in 1971 in Japan and shown to be a new enterovirus, unrelated serologically to other picornaviruses. The second virus was an antigenic variant of coxsackievirus A24 (CA24v) and was first isolated from Southeast Asia during epidemics in 1970. Although EV70 has been responsible for most cases, AHC caused by CA24v and adenovirus 11 are clinically nearly indistinguishable. In 1980 a new pandemic due to EV70 began in Asia, and by 1981 epidemics appeared for the first time in South and Central America, the Caribbean, and the southern United States. CA24v was introduced into the Western Hemisphere for the first time in 1986 during renewed worldwide activity of this virus. Both viruses have continued to cause periodic

epidemics in many parts of the world; most recently, EV70 outbreaks occurred in 1996 in parts of Asia and the Middle East.

DISTRIBUTION AND INCIDENCE. The distribution is worldwide, covering most tropical and semitropical areas. Hot, humid, crowded conditions with a low level of sanitation favor transmission, and outbreaks have occurred primarily in coastal towns and cities. Cases of enterovirus AHC in temperate regions can almost always be traced to travelers to epidemic areas. Morbidity estimates are imprecise, although it is estimated that tens of millions of cases occurred in Africa and Asia between 1969 and 1972. In a study conducted in Ghana, a low prevalence of neutralizing antibodies was found in sera collected before the 1969 epidemic, and prevalence rates of 50 to 60% were detected after the epidemic. Similar high infection rates were detected serologically in outbreaks in American Samoa, Singapore, and Taiwan. The disease remains endemic in many tropical areas and is distinctly characterized by focal outbreaks in parts of a community, rather than by sporadic cases. The incidence of neurologic manifestations has been estimated at 1 case per 10,000 to 15,000 persons with AHC.

TRANSMISSION. AHC is highly contagious and most likely is spread by contaminated fingers, towels, cosmetics, and clothing as well as possibly by respiratory droplets. Transmission by flies is possible but conjectural. As with many enterovirus infections, secondary spread within households occurs readily and seems facilitated by the presence of young household members and crowding. Iatrogenic transmission (in eye clinics) is also of importance. There has been no recognizable pattern to the temporal, geographic, or etiologic findings in AHC epidemics, and previous infection offers only partial protection against disease from later infections.

The origin of these enteroviral agents is problematic. Studies on the viral genome of EV70 isolates have confirmed that all isolates are related, and extrapolation of differences over time predict a common ancestor that arose in the mid-1960s. It is possible that EV70 is a human virus that escaped from some segregated population, whence it was spread to other parts of the world. The origin of CA24v is also conjectural. The possibility that these agents have an animal reservoir has received some attention, and neutralizing antibodies have been found in cattle and sheep in West Africa.

CLINICAL MANIFESTATIONS AND COMPLICATIONS. The incubation period is 12 to 48 hours, followed by acute onset of lacrimation, severe pain, chemosis and periorbital edema, photophobia, conjunctival hyperemia, and, in 10 to 100% of patients in various series, mild to severe subconjunctival hemorrhages (Fig. 27–7). The disease is primarily bilateral, beginning in one eye and rapidly spreading to the other. Preauricular lymphadenopathy, a scant purulent discharge, punctate epithelial keratitis, and conjunctival follicular hypertrophy are variably present. Secondary bacterial infection may complicate recovery. Studies done during outbreaks of AHC due to CA24v have indicated that nonspecific upper respiratory symptoms may be more common with this virus than during infection with EV70.

Anecdotal reports indicate that AHC may be followed by a neurologic syndrome or generalized malaise, occasional fever, and bilateral lumbosacral radiculomyelitis characterized by severe bilateral root pain and signs of asymmetric lower motor neuron dysfunction, including weakness, hypotonia, and diminished reflexes, especially involving the proximal muscles of the lower extremities. Sensory function is preserved. The syndrome is more common in adults than in children, and full recovery is the rule. Isolated unilateral facial palsy has also been described.

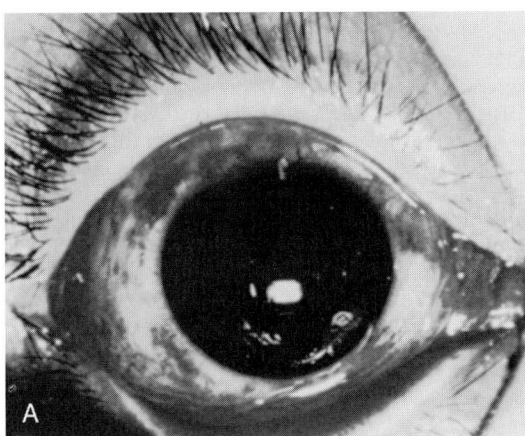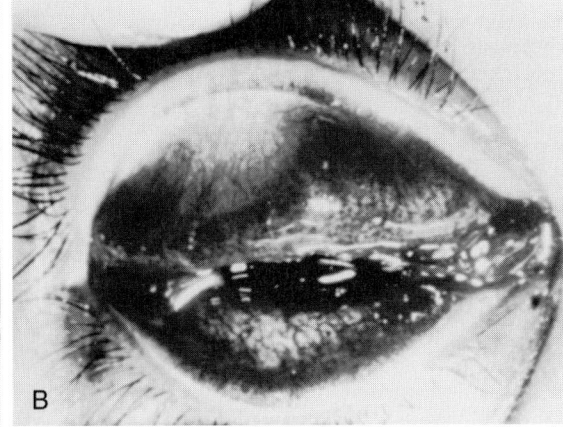

Figure 27–7. Subconjunctival hemorrhage *(A)* and inflammation and eyelid edema *(B)* 2 days after onset of acute hemorrhagic conjunctivitis due to enterovirus 70. (From Hung T-P, Kono R: Handbook of Clinical Neurology, Vol. 38. Amsterdam, North-Holland Publishing Co, 1979. Reprinted by permission.)

TREATMENT AND PROGNOSIS. AHC is a self-limited disease, and full recovery occurs within 10 to 14 days. Treatment is symptomatic and includes astringent eyedrops and cold soaks. Interferon may provide effective prophylaxis, but its therapeutic value is questionable. The clinical efficacy of specific antivirals is under investigation but has not been demonstrated. Steroid and antibiotic preparations should be avoided unless bacterial superinfection is suspected, in which case specimens for bacterial cultures should be obtained and antibiotic therapy instituted.

DIAGNOSIS. The clinical diagnosis is relatively straightforward in the setting of an epidemic with prominent subconjunctival hemorrhage. EV70, CA24v, and adenovirus 11 may produce an identical clinical illness, and outbreaks may be of mixed etiology. Specific diagnosis depends upon virus isolation or detection from conjunctival swabs or serologic testing. Eye swab specimens may be collected in transport medium (tryptose phosphate broth containing 0.5% gelatin) and should be shipped on ice as rapidly as possible to a competent virus laboratory. Virus isolation of CA24v is readily accomplished in human embryonic lung fibroblast cell cultures or other cell lines of human origin. Since 1982, isolation of EV70 has been rare regardless of the cell types employed for isolation. Prior to that time, isolation of EV70 was often obtained in a variety of human and primate cell lines, but the virus has undergone a poorly understood change that has rendered it cultivatable in only 5% of attempts. Evidence of a specific virus in conjunctival specimens also can be demonstrated by detecting antigen, using indirect immunofluorescence, or detecting the virus genome using the polymerase chain reaction (PCR). EV70 and CA24v infections also can be diagnosed serologically by demonstrating a rise in neutralizing antibody titers between paired acute and convalescent sera. In addition, tests are available that measure specific IgG, IgA, and IgM antibodies to EV70 and CA24v using a capture enzyme-linked immunosorbent assay, although the serotype specificity of these tests is not high. Specific diagnosis of the neurologic syndrome is often complicated by the difficulty of virus isolation. The presence of antibodies to one of these viruses in cerebrospinal fluid and a recent history of AHC is presumptive evidence for an etiologic association.

PREVENTION AND CONTROL. Spread of AHC with familial groups and eye clinics may be limited by scrupulous handwashing and disinfection of fomites.

Bibliography

Bern C, Pallansch MA, Gary HE Jr, et al: Acute hemorrhagic conjunctivitis due to enterovirus 70 in American Samoa: Serum-neutralizing antibodies and sex-specific protection. Am J Epidemiol 136:1502, 1992.

Hierholzer JC, Hatch MH: Acute hemorrhagic conjunctivitis. *In* Darrell RW (ed): Viral Diseases of the Eye. Philadelphia, Lea & Febiger, 1985, pp 165–196.

Ishiko H, Takeda N, Miyamura K, et al: Phylogenetic analysis of a coxsackievirus A24 variant: The most recent worldwide pandemic was caused by progenies of a virus prevalent around 1981. Virology 187:748, 1992.

Uchio E, Yamazaki K, Aoki K, et al: Detection of enterovirus 70 by polymerase chain reaction in acute hemorrhagic conjunctivitis. Am J Ophthalmol 122:273, 1996.

Wadia NH, Wadia PN, Katrak SM, et al: Neurologic manifestations of acute haemorrhagic conjunctivitis. Lancet 2:528, 1981.

Wright PW, Strauss GH, Langford MP: Acute hemorrhagic conjunctivitis. Am Fam Physician 45:173, 1992.

28 *Viral Hepatitis*

David Thomas and G. Thomas Strickland

DEFINITION. At least five viruses belonging to five different families cause hepatitis in humans. Each has a unique epidemiology. Two, hepatitis A virus (HAV) and hepatitis E virus (HEV), are acquired chiefly through ingestion of fecally contaminated food or beverage and cause a self-limited illness. Others, hepatitis B virus (HBV), hepatitis C virus (HCV), and hepatitis delta virus (HDV), are transmitted in varying degrees by blood and by percutaneous, perinatal, and sexual exposures, which may lead to either self-limited or chronic hepatitis. Additional hepatotropic viruses are suspected, and recently a candidate, GB virus C (GBV-C) or hepatitis G virus (HGV), has been proposed. Other viruses, e.g., Epstein-Barr virus (EBV) and cytomegalovirus (CMV), also may cause human hepatitis, but it is not their principal clinical characteristic. The impact of the hepatitis viruses has been strongly influenced by changes in human ecology and by socioeconomic status. In some cases this has resulted in diminished disease, whereas marked increases in disease due to viral hepatitis have occurred in other circumstances. Worldwide, viral hepatitis is a major public health problem because of the morbidity and occasional fatalities from acute infection and, even more importantly, the long-term consequences of chronic infection with HBV and HCV, e.g., cirrhosis and hepatocellular carcinoma (HCC).

PATHOLOGY. Common to all types of acute viral hepatitis are focal hepatocyte necrosis and histiocytic periportal inflammation. The reticulin framework of the liver is well preserved, except in cases of massive and submassive necrosis. Hepatocyte necrosis varies in form and intensity and is usually multifocal, with the most severe changes occurring in the centrilobular areas. Individual hepatocytes may be swollen (balloon) but can also constrict, giving rise to acidophilic bodies. For HBV, eosinophilic "ground-glass" cytoplasm is seen, as are orcein-staining cells. However, fatty changes are uncommon.

A mononuclear cellular infiltration, which is particularly marked in the portal zones, is accompanied by some proliferation of bile ducts. Kupffer cells and endothelial cells proliferate, and the Kupffer cells often contain lipofuscin pigment. Cholestasis may occur in the early stages of viral hepatitis, and plugs of bile thrombi may be found in the bile canaliculi. Lesions in patients with anicteric hepatitis are generally less severe, consisting of focal inflammation and necrosis.

Repair occurs by regeneration of hepatocytes: Frequent mitoses, polyploidy, atypical cells, and binucleated cells are seen in biopsy material. There is a gradual disappearance of the mononuclear cell infiltrate from the portal tracts, but elongated histiocytes and fibroblasts may persist. The short-term outcome of acute viral hepatitis may be complete resolution or fatal massive hepatic necrosis. Chronic hepatitis may follow HBV infection and is the rule after acute hepatitis C (Fig. 28–1). Cirrhosis and HCC may occur in 10 to 30 years in those who have persistent HBV or HCV infections.

CLINICAL MANIFESTATIONS. The particular virus causing hepatitis can rarely be clinically ascertained. However, hepatitis viruses have a tendency to manifest differently.

Clinical Symptoms and Signs. Characteristically, there are four phases to an episode of viral hepatitis. After exposure, the virus *incubates* for from 2 to 6 weeks for HAV and HEV and from 4 to 10 weeks for HBV and HCV. Then, there may be flulike symptoms or a *prodromal illness,* characterized by fever, chills, headache, fatigue, malaise, rash, arthritis, right upper quadrant pain, or a tender liver. Several days later and often coincident with an improvement in systemic symptoms, the patient will have more pronounced anorexia, nausea, vomiting, weight loss, and right upper quadrant abdominal pain. *Jaundice,* occurring more frequently with acute

hepatitis A and hepatitis E and least often with hepatitis C, is detected by icteric sclera. Jaundice usually persists for several weeks and is associated with dark urine, light (clay-colored) stools, and severe pruritus. Often the patient begins to feel better following the onset of jaundice. Most symptoms of viral hepatitis abate within 1 to 3 weeks. However, during the *convalescent phase,* significant malaise, fatigue, anorexia, and other symptoms may persist for months, especially in adults. This characteristic clinical presentation occurs in the minority of viral hepatitis cases, especially among infants and children who generally have mild or no symptoms.

Laboratory Studies. Laboratory abnormalities are common, occurring even in asymptomatic cases. The classic laboratory findings for viral hepatitis are elevated serum aminotransferases, which often are 10 to 20 times the normal range. The alanine aminotransferase (ALT, SGPT) elevation is generally greater than the aspartate aminotransferase (AST, SGOT), a finding that distinguishes viral hepatitis from alcohol-induced liver disease. The serum bilirubin is usually elevated, often peaking at 10 to 15 times normal and with levels >3.0 mg/dL correlating with clinical jaundice. Bilirubin may also be detected in the urine. There may be mild elevations in the alkaline phosphatase, and atypical lymphocytes are usually present in the peripheral blood film. The leukocyte count is usually normal.

Complications. Viral hepatitis may be fulminant and associated with altered mental status, coagulopathy, and severe jaundice. This occurs in <0.5% of HAV infections, and it is even rarer with acute hepatitis C. Acute HBV infection may cause fulminant hepatitis, especially when there is concurrent HDV infection. HEV is unique among viral hepatitis agents in causing fatal fulminant hepatitis in pregnant women. Acute fulminant HEV hepatitis has been reported in 10 to 25% of pregnant women during the third trimester, but this estimate is elevated owing to a patient selection bias in hospital-based published reports.

With hepatitis A and E, acute cases resolve; with HBV, HCV, and HDV, infections may persist, causing chronic hepatitis leading to cirrhosis and HCC. The frequency of persistence varies with the virus and the host and inversely correlates with the severity of acute infection. As a rule, infants and young children and immunocompromised adults who have less severe episodes of acute hepatitis have high rates of persistence when infected with these viruses. HBV infection persists in <5% of those infected as adults but in >80% of those infected as infants. HCV infection is symptomatic less frequently than hepatitis B but persists in 85% of infections.

DIAGNOSIS. The cause of viral hepatitis is ascertained through serologic testing. Each virus elicits a characteristic antibody response. Detection of virus-specific IgM class immunoglobulins generally represents acute infection, while IgG antibodies may be found years after resolution of disease. Recognition of viral antigens or nucleic acid represents ongoing infection and usually correlates with transmissibility.

TREATMENT AND PREVENTION. There is no pharmacologic treatment for acute viral hepatitis. Supportive care, including rest, is considered important. Secondary transmission should be prevented through active and passive immunization and behavior modification. Counseling regarding prognosis and follow-up is also necessary, especially for HBV, HCV, and HDV infections, which can persist. Interferon-α has been used to treat patients with chronic hepatitis due to HBV and HCV infections, with varying, but usually low, success rates. The addition of ribavirin to 12 months of interferon-α has increased sustained response rates to ~35%. Daily oral administration of lamivudine has recently been shown beneficial in treating chronic hepatitis B. Pharmaceutical companies are developing other antiviral drugs for treat-

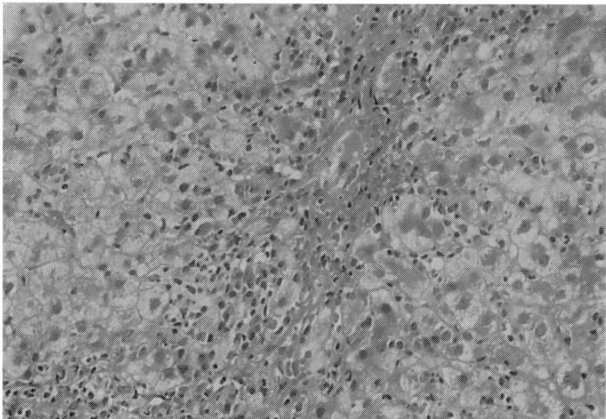

***Figure* 28–1.** Histologic illustration of chronic hepatitis from a patient with chronic hepatitis C virus infection. Note bridging fibrosis and piecemeal necrosis.

ing chronic hepatitis, which may further improve the success of treating HBV and HCV infections.

Highly effective vaccines are available for preventing HAV and HBV infections. Phase I vaccine trials should be started before the year 2000 to evaluate vaccines to prevent HCV, and a vaccine for HEV should be ready for phase III trials before then. HDV infections, requiring HBV replication, can be prevented by immunization for HBV.

Bibliography

Alter MJ, Mast EE: The epidemiology of viral hepatitis in the United States. Gastroenterol Clin North Am 23:437, 1994.

Darwish MA, Faris R, Clemens JD, et al: High seroprevalence of hepatitis A, B, C, and E viruses in residents in an Egyptian village in the Nile delta: A pilot study. Am J Trop Med Hyg 54:554, 1996.

Ghabrah TM, Strickland GT, Tsarev S, et al: Acute viral hepatitis in Saudi Arabia: Seroepidemiological analysis, risk factors, clinical manifestations, and evidence for a sixth hepatitis agent. Clin Infect Dis 21:621, 1995.

Lemon SM, Thomas DL: Vaccines to prevent viral hepatitis. N Engl J Med 336:196, 1997.

Purcell RH: Hepatitis viruses: Changing patterns of human disease. Proc Natl Acad Sci USA 91:2401, 1994.

28.1 Hepatitis A Virus Infection

DEFINITION AND HISTORY. Hepatitis A virus (HAV) causes *short-incubation infectious hepatitis* that is transmitted by the fecal-oral route and has the potential of causing epidemics, particularly when it contaminates the water supply. Most infections in developing countries occur early in life and cause few or no symptoms, whereas infections in transitional or developed countries often lead to acute viral hepatitis in adolescents and adults. Unlike hepatitis B and C viruses, HAV never causes chronic infection.

Although *epidemic jaundice* has been recognized from epidemics of "campaign jaundice" that affected armies during the Middle Ages up until the Korean and Vietnam conflicts, HAV was not identified until 20 or 25 years ago. Diagnostic serologic tests were subsequently developed and are now commercially available, and an effective vaccine is now licensed.

VIROLOGY. HAV is a small, unenveloped, RNA-containing virus recently classified as a hepatovirus in the family Picornaviridae.

Physical Properties. The complete virion (Fig. 28–2) is 27 to 32 nm in diameter, has icosahedral symmetry, a sedimentation coefficient of 156S, and a buoyant density of 1.32 g/cc³ in CsCl. The HAV genome, which is approximately 7.5 kb in length, encodes four capsid proteins (VP1, VP2, VP3, and VP4) whose conformation determines seroreactivity, and nonstructural peptides including an RNA-dependent RNA polymerase and a protease. Although there are four HAV genotypes recognized in humans, there is only one HAV serotype such that neutralizing antibody to any HAV strain will protect against infection worldwide.

As an unenveloped virus, HAV is resistant to solvents, e.g., 20% ether, chloroform, dichlorodifluoromethane (Freon), and trichlorotrifluoroethane (Arklone). HAV is also relatively resistant to acidity and heat, being stable at pH 3.0 for 3 hr at 25°C; in perchloracetic acid (300 mg/L) for 15 min and at 60°C for 60 min. Inactivation of HAV is successfully achieved by incubation at temperatures above 85°C, iodine, chlorine, sodium hypochlorite, ultraviolet radiation, formalin, and potassium permanganate.

Culture Characteristics. HAV can be propagated in primate epithelial and fibroblast cells. Growth of HAV in cell culture

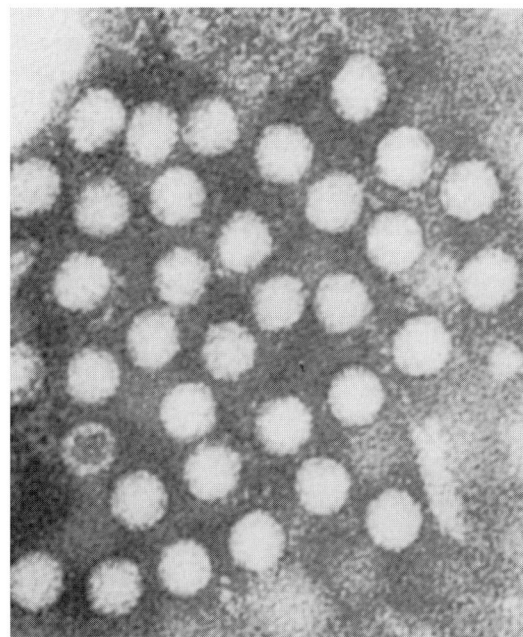

Figure 28–2. Hepatitis A virus particles in a fecal extract obtained from a patient during the late incubation period of the infection. The particles measure 25 to 27 nm in diameter and possess cubic symmetry (× 300,000).

is slow compared with other picornaviruses and does not produce a cytopathic effect. Adaptation occurs after passage with more rapid production of intracellular antigen and with higher final yields. Virus isolation is not a practical diagnostic technique in most laboratories.

EPIDEMIOLOGY

Age and Pattern of Infection. Although HAV infection occurs worldwide, the epidemiology differs according to conditions, e.g., water purification, sewage disposal, and crowding. Nearly all inhabitants of some economically developing countries are infected with HAV during their first 2 or 3 years, when infection occurs with no or few symptoms. In contrast, in economically developed nations HAV infection occurs sporadically throughout life, leaving a substantial segment of the adolescent and adult population susceptible. Consequently, large outbreaks of hepatitis A may occur in these economically developed nations, generally because of exposure to a common source of contaminated food or water. In addition, HAV infection is a threat to persons traveling from nonendemic to endemic areas. An intermediate pattern of HAV infection is also recognized. As countries undergo economic transformation, HAV infection may be delayed to the second and third decades, paradoxically becoming a larger public health problem, since infection in older individuals is more severe.

Routes of Transmission. HAV is principally transmitted person-to-person by a fecal-oral route. Transmission requires more than casual contact, e.g., exposures that might occur within a family or between playmates. Asymptomatic transmission between children and then to a parent is especially characteristic, illustrating why daycare centers may be implicated in the spread of infection. Food- and water-borne HAV infection also occurs, often involving a food handler with hepatitis A who failed to observe handwashing protocol after defecation. Contamination of inadequately chlorinated water sources has led to both epidemic and sporadic HAV infections. Shellfish are particularly associated with HAV transmission, since they concentrate the virus by filtering large volumes of contaminated water. A massive epidemic of HAV occurred in Shanghai in 1988 following ingestion of undercooked shellfish. The short period of viremia before the onset of symptoms makes parenteral transmission possible. Transmission from contaminated blood products has been demonstrated but contributes little to the total number of hepatitis A cases.

Specific risk factors for HAV infection in developed countries include contact with another person with hepatitis or jaundice, homosexuality, travel to a less developed country, contact with children attending daycare centers, and intravenous drug abuse. HAV infection remains endemic among Native Americans in the western states and Alaska.

CLINICAL MANIFESTATIONS. After a susceptible person ingests HAV, viral replication occurs principally in the liver. Virions can be detected in stool and blood before the onset of symptoms (Fig. 28–3). Serum transaminases increase several days after viral replication begins, indicating that hepatocellular damage may be immunologically mediated.

Symptomatology. Up to 2 weeks after viral excretion and 15 to 50 days after exposure (average incubation period, 25 to 30 days), prodromal symptoms may occur. The prodrome, which has an abrupt onset and consists of fever, fatigue, malaise, anorexia, and nausea and vomiting, occurs in >60% of adults but is uncommon among young children. After several days, flulike symptoms give way to jaundice, which occurs in >60% of adults and <25% of children. About 60% of symptomatic children have diarrhea, which occurs in 20% of adults with hepatitis A. Within 2 weeks of the onset of jaundice, HAV is generally not detected in stool. The serum bilirubin peaks after 7 to 10 days at a level usually <10 mg/dL, although concentrations up to 20 mg/dL may occur. Within 2 to 4 weeks of the onset of prodromal symptoms, jaundice resolves and transaminases return to normal. Posthepatitis A convalescence (generally malaise, fatigue, and anorexia) may be prolonged for months. Hepatic failure occurs in 1 in 300 to 350 hepatitis A cases and generally does not result in death or the need for liver transplantation.

Atypical Manifestations. These include relapsing hepatitis, induction of autoimmune hepatitis, and a prolonged cholestatic syndrome. Relapsing hepatitis occurs in up to one fifth of adult patients. Within 6 months of the resolution of the acute illness, a similar syndrome may recur, along with viral excretion and elevated transaminases. Variations include asymptomatic resurgence in liver enzymes, which may persist for as long as a year, and more than one relapse. Prolonged cholestasis with fever, pruritus, and diarrhea can last for months. Although the acute illness may be prolonged, there is no chronic liver disease after HAV infection.

DIAGNOSIS. HAV infection is generally diagnosed by detecting IgM antibodies to the virus (IgM anti-HAV) in the blood. IgM anti-HAV can be detected at the onset of symptoms, peaks 4 to 6 weeks after exposure, and persists for 3 to 12 months. IgG HAV antibodies, which can be detected 1 week after the IgM response, have neutralizing activity and may persist for life (Fig. 28–3). Thus, IgG anti-HAV, when present without IgM anti-HAV, represents past HAV infection and means that an individual is protected against recurrent infection. IgG anti-HAV may also be detected after immunoglobulin (IG) administration or HAV vaccination. The duration of detectable IgG anti-HAV after IG administration is 2 to 6 months, depending upon the volume injected. The length of protection afforded by HAV immunization remains to be determined but is probably >10 years. HAV infection can also be recognized by detection of the virus in stool by electron microscopy. Liver biopsy is rarely useful in the diagnosis of acute hepatitis A.

PREVENTION AND CONTROL

Sanitation. Worldwide, the most important measures to reduce HAV infection involve improvements in sewage disposal, crowding, and general hygiene. Food handlers who are ill and certainly those with hepatitis A or unexplained jaundice should be restricted from work, and handwashing should be strictly enforced. Persons recognized with HAV infection should be thoroughly instructed regarding means of preventing transmission. If hospitalization is necessary, enteric isolation is recommended for 1 week after the onset of jaundice, coinciding with the highest quantities of viral excretion in stool. Additional precautions need be applied only in special cases, e.g., with an incontinent or demented patient.

Immunization. When exposure has occurred or is anticipated, HAV infection can also be prevented through immunization: (1) passive immunoprophylaxis using IG that contains at least 100 IU/mL of anti-HAV and (2) vaccination with inactivated HAV.

Passive Immunoprophylaxis. Since it may take weeks to achieve reliable protection after HAV vaccination, IG administration (0.02 mL/kg) is recommended when prompt protection is required, e.g., with persons who had intense exposure to someone with HAV infection. Since the risk of HAV infection is not increased unless the exposure is heavy, casual contact with cases, including those by health care workers, does not require IG.

Active Immunization. The two vaccines licensed in the United States are formalin-inactivated viral particles produced in infected human diploid fibroblasts. These and others available worldwide are safe and effective means of preventing HAV infection. Protection from vaccination is sustained for 10 or more years, an important feature for susceptible persons living in, or traveling frequently to, developing countries.

Adverse events, e.g., mild soreness at the injection site and, fever, are rare. Neither vaccine is approved for use in children under 2 years of age. Over 95% of healthy adults develop anti-HAV antibodies within a month after receiving a single dose of the vaccine. A booster dose, recommended 6 months after the first dose, raises the anti-HAV titer to levels easily detected by commercial ELISAs. In clinical trials, a single 25 U dose of vaccine completely prevented symptomatic HAV hepatitis in heavily exposed children 18 days or more after immunization. Because immunization restricts hepatic viral replication, it should reduce fecal viral shedding and interrupt viral transmission. Travelers to regions where HAV is endemic should receive a first dose of vaccine at least 1 month before departure. The major limitation to more extensive use of the current HAV vaccines is their high cost. When

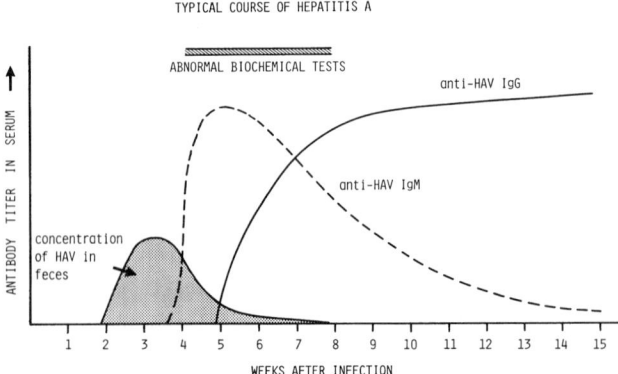

Figure 28–3. Typical course of hepatitis A. (From McCollum RW, Zuckerman AJ: Med Virol 8:1, 1981.)

they become less expensive, the criteria for their use can be broadened; universal immunization has the potential to markedly reduce HAV transmission and national rates of infection.

Bibliography

Clemens R, Safary A, Hepburn A, et al: Clinical experience with an inactivated hepatitis A vaccine. J Infect Dis 171 (Suppl 1):S44, 1995.

Hoke CH Jr, Egan JE, Sjogren MH, et al: Administration of hepatitis A vaccine to a military population by needle and jet injector and with hepatitis B vaccine. J Infect Dis 171 (Suppl 1):S53, 1995.

Innis BL, Snitbhan R, Kunasol P, et al: Protection against hepatitis A by an inactivated vaccine. JAMA 271:1328, 1994.

Krugman S, Giles JP, Hammond J: Infectious hepatitis: Evidence for two distinctive clinical, epidemiological and immunological types of infection. JAMA 200:365, 1967.

Lemon SM, Robertson BH: Current perspective in the virology and molecular biology of hepatitis A virus. Semin Virol 4:285, 1993.

Poovorawan Y, Tieamboonlers A, Chumdermpadetsuk S, et al: Control of a hepatitis A outbreak by active immunization of high risk susceptible subjects. J Infect Dis 169:228, 1994.

28.2 Hepatitis B Virus and Hepatitis D Virus Infections

DEFINITION AND HISTORY. Up until the late 1960s the diagnosis of *long-incubation serum hepatitis* was made on the basis of jaundice and other symptoms and signs of hepatitis occurring 60 to 120 days following the injection of human blood or plasma fractions or the use of inadequately sterilized syringes and needles. Serum hepatitis followed vaccination for smallpox in the 19th century and became more prevalent with the increasing use of syringes and needles to treat syphilis in the first half of the 20th century. During the 1940s, epidemics of hepatitis followed the administration of yellow fever vaccines stabilized by adding human serum.

In 1965, the Australia antigen was discovered by Blumberg and colleagues, who subsequently associated its presence in the sera of patients with hepatitis B virus (HBV) infection. The discovery of Australia antigen, which became hepatitis B surface antigen (HBsAg), and other antigens and antibodies associated with HBV infection has led to considerable knowledge about the transmission and natural history of HBV in the past 30 years and has permitted the development of a very effective vaccine for its prevention.

VIROLOGY. HBV is a small, enveloped, incompletely double-stranded DNA virus of the family Hepadnaviridae. In a HBV-infected person, there are three distinct viral particles, including the complete 42 nm virion, smaller 22 nm diameter spheres, and rodlike particles 22 nm by 200 nm (Fig. 28–4). The HBV genome, which has only 3200 bases, has four open reading frames (ORFs). The products of one ORF, the S gene and prior regions (pre-S1 and pre-S2), compose the HBsAg that is contained in the surface envelope of the intact virion and subviral particles. Large, middle, and small polypeptides are encoded by, respectively, the S alone; S and pre-S1; and S, pre-S1, and pre-S2 sequences.

A second gene, the core, encodes the major core or nucleocapsid polypeptide and a smaller protein, the hepatitis e antigen (HBeAg). If core gene translation begins at the first (pre-C) initiation codon, the truncated HBeAg is made. When translation begins at the second (core) codon, the full core protein is expressed. A third gene, which spans approximately 75% of the genome, encodes a protein with DNA polymerase (and reverse transcriptase) activity. The fourth

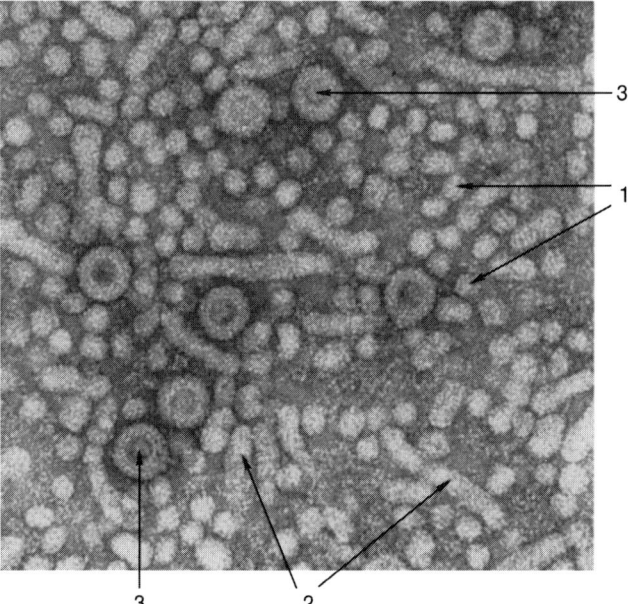

Figure 28–4. Electron micrograph showing the complex morphology of hepatitis B virus in serum: (1) Small spherical particles of hepatitis B surface antigen about 22 nm in diameter, (2) tubular structures of the surface antigen, and (3) large spheroidal particles about 42 nm in diameter. This is the complete virus particle, which may be solid or double-shelled ($\times$ 252,000).

gene, the X gene, product is a small protein that has transactivation potential.

HBV replication occurs by reverse transcription, an unusual process for a DNA virus and one that predisposes to mutations. Mutation in the pre-core region of the genome interrupts translation of mRNA into HBeAg. Viral replication and synthesis of core polypeptide still occur, as indicated by the presence of HBV DNA in plasma, but HBeAg is not detected. HBV envelope mutants have also been described. A single amino acid substitution inhibits expression of the "a" subtype protein, which may affect the immunogenicity of HBV vaccines consisting of this antigen.

Surface Antigen. The HBsAg consists of a group-specific determinant (a) shared by all HBsAg preparations, and two pairs of subtype determinants (d,y and w,r). Eight recognized strains of HBV are denoted by the universal determinant "a" as well as various combinations of subtype determinants, e.g., adw and adr. Further complexity is reflected in additional permutations of subtypes. Antibodies to HBsAg are neutralizing. Recognition of a particular HBV subtype may be useful for tracking viral transmission. The major subtypes have differing geographic distribution. For example, in northern Europe, the Americas, and Australia, subtype adw predominates. Subtype ayw occurs in a broad zone that includes northern and western Africa, the eastern Mediterranean, Eastern Europe, northern and central Asia, and the Indian subcontinent. Both adw and adr are found in Malaysia, Thailand, Indonesia, and Papua New Guinea, whereas subtype adr predominates in other parts of Southeast Asia, including China, Japan, and the Pacific Islands.

Physical Properties. Studies of the chemical stability of HBV have been limited by difficulties in propagating the virus in vitro. However, using direct chimpanzee inoculation methods, the following were shown to effectively eliminate transmission of HBV: 0.1 aqueous glutaraldehyde at 24°C for 5 min; 80% ethyl alcohol at 11°C for 2 min; heat at 98°C for

2 min; aqueous sodium hypochlorite (500 mg free available chlorine/L); mixture of 2% glutaraldehyde and 7% phenol (Sporidin); 70% aqueous isopropyl alcohol; and an iodophor detergent disinfectant (Wescodyne; 80 mg available iodine/ L). Procedures that have been unsuccessful in reducing HBV transmission from contaminated sera include heat treatment at 60°C for 10 hours and drying and storage at 25°C for 1 week. HBV also withstands exposure to ultraviolet radiation and extraction with ether, benzalkonium chloride, and alcohol.

EPIDEMIOLOGY. The WHO estimates that there are 350 million carriers of HBV (the majority in China, sub-Saharan Africa, and other developing countries) and that >1 million deaths annually are due to HBV-associated cirrhosis and HCC.

Geographic Distribution. There are marked geographic differences in the prevalence of HBV infection (Fig. 28–5) and principal routes of transmission. The prevalence of HBV infection remains higher in developing than in developed countries. In most areas it has been reduced by the use of serologic tests to screen blood transfusions and blood products and by the availability and use of disposable syringes and needles. Despite this reduction in transmission in developed countries during the past 20 to 25 years, HBV remains a major cause of chronic liver disease. This is partially because of the delay (15 to 30 years on average) between infection and severe medical complications. However, in many developing countries, blood and blood products are not always screened, and disposable syringes and needles are reused. Hepatitis B is endemic (antibody to hepatitis B core antigen [anti-HBc] prevalence of 30 to 60% and/or HBsAg rates of 5 to 15%) in sub-Saharan Africa and in much of Asia. HBV infection also occurs with greater frequency in Central and South America and the Caribbean and in North Africa and the Middle East than it does in the United States and Western Europe. HBV exposures are more common in southern Europe than in northern Europe, and in eastern Europe and the former USSR than in western Europe. Major outbreaks of hepatitis B due to the reuse of unsterilized syringes and needles have occurred in Eastern Europe and the former Soviet Union. In the United States, the HBV carrier state is higher in refugees, particularly those from Southeast and East Asia, and their children are at a greater risk of infection than the general population. In most areas, higher HBV rates are found in persons of low socioeconomic status.

Modes of Transmission. HBV transmission is facilitated by the large human reservoir (those who are HBsAg seropositive), estimated at 350 million HBV carriers. The virus can be transmitted by transfusions and injections of blood products; by needlestick either by medical or dental accidents or by illicit intravenous drug abusers sharing needles; by heterosexual or homosexual activities; and from mothers to their unborn or newborn infants. It is the most infectious of the blood borne viruses. In Asia about half of HBV transmission is from mother to infant, whereas in sub-Saharan Africa and other developing countries hepatitis B is generally acquired in the first decade of life through horizontal transmission within families and among playmates or, later, by heterosexual sex. In the United States, Europe, and other developed nations, homosexual and heterosexual exposures and use of illicit drugs are the most important risk factors for HBV infection. The marked increase in these activities during the past 30 to 40 years has accounted for the increased prevalence of HBV (and HCV) infections in developed countries among high-risk groups.

Blood transfusions were once important vehicles for HBV transmission. However, owing to careful screening of blood donations, the incidence has dropped to <1 in 100,000 units in the United States. However, this is still an important mode of transmission where screening of blood prior to transfusion is inadequate or is not done. HBV also may be transmitted to patients or health care workers through hemodialysis (via contaminated equipment or the environment), by tattoos,

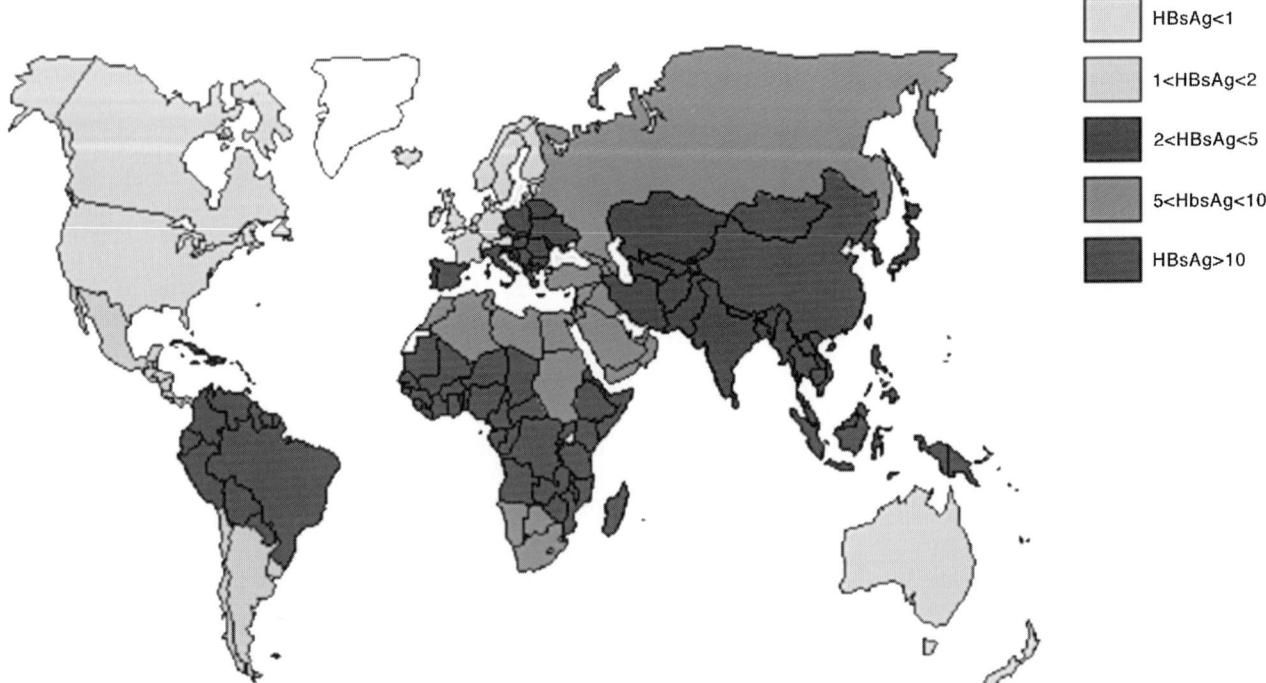

Figure 28–5. Geographic distribution of chronic hepatitis B virus infection as manifested by prevalence of hepatitis B surface antigen (HBsAg) rates in the general population. (Courtesy of the Centers for Disease Control and Prevention.)

TABLE 28–1. Interpretation of Results of Serologic Tests for Hepatitis B

HBsAg	HBeAg	Anti-HBe	Anti-HBc IgM	Anti-HBc IgG	Anti-HBs	Interpretation
+	+	–	–	–	–	Incubation period
+	+	–	+	+	–	Acute hepatitis B
+	+	–	–	+	–	Persistent carrier state
+	–	+	+ / –	+	–	Persistent carrier state
–	–	+	+ / –	+	+	Convalescence
–	–	–	–	+	+	Recovery
–	–	–	+	–	–	Infection with hepatitis B virus without detectable HBsAg
–	–	–	–	+	–	Recovery with loss of detectable anti-HBs
–	–	–	–	–	+	Immunization without infection. Repeated exposure to antigen without infection, or recovery from infection with loss of detectable anti-HBc

From Zuckerman AJ: Priorities for immunisation against hepatitis B. Br Med J 284:686, 1979.

acupuncture, surgery, barbers during shaving, male and female circumcisions, or human bite. Multiple investigations have failed to establish a role for vector-borne transmission.

The patterns of HBV transmission relate to the relative presence of infectious virions in body fluids, exposure to those fluids, and the environmental stability of the fluids. The highest concentration of HBV (up to 10 billion/mL) is found in the blood of HBeAg-positive patients. HBsAg and presumably infectious virions have also been detected in saliva, semen, menstrual fluid, pleural fluid, ascitic fluid, cerebrospinal fluid, tears, urine, feces, and breast milk. HBV-containing blood remains infectious when stored for over 1 week at room temperature. In experimental settings, HBV transmission has been demonstrated with percutaneous but not oral inoculation of semen and saliva. Oral inoculation of high concentrations of virus from serum may cause mild infection. Thus, nonparenteral transmission requires high concentrations of virus or a break in mucosal barriers, e.g., as might occur with anal receptive intercourse, in someone with a genital ulcer, and between children with ulcerative skin lesions. Exposures to other body fluids, e.g., urine, do not cause HBV infections.

CLINICAL MANIFESTATIONS

Acute Infections. From 1 to 4 months after exposure, prodromal symptoms may be experienced, although this occurs in <50% of HBV infections. Approximately 15% of adult patients have a serum sickness–like illness characterized by fever, malaise, symmetric distal joint pain, and urticaria; jaundice occurs in 25 to 35%. There may be right upper quadrant tenderness with an enlarged liver. Uncommonly, acute hepatitis B becomes fulminant, associated with a shrinking liver as noted by palpation or ultrasound, increased abdominal pain, fever, vomiting, and encephalopathy. Although <1% of HBV infections are fulminant, this occurs more frequently in the elderly and in those with hepatitis delta (HDV) co-infection.

Chronic Infections and Complications. Acute HBV infection is self-limited in 95% of adults but persists in up to 80 to 95% of infants. The chronic carrier state also ensues with a greater frequency in immunosuppressed children and adults who are infected with HBV. Since clinical illness is directly related to the immune response to the HBV virus, those having no or minimal symptoms are more likely to become chronic carriers of HBV than are those who have acute viral hepatitis. This reverse relationship between symptoms and persistent infection is highly influenced by age at onset of infection during childhood. Some of those with persistent HBV infection have waxing and waning of symptoms and serum levels of liver transaminases with eventual

progression to cirrhosis and liver failure. The disease may also progress without apparent symptoms or remain indolent for 10 to 20 years. Approximately 5% of patients with hepatitis B–related cirrhosis will develop HCC, which is characterized by right upper quadrant tenderness, weight loss, hepatomegaly, and elevated serum α-fetoprotein (Chapter 12). HBV infections are also associated with a variety of extrahepatic syndromes including polyarteritis nodosa, membranous glomerulonephritis, and papular acrodermatitis.

Chronic Hepatitis. Most patients with persistent HBV infection are asymptomatic and have little histologic evidence of liver damage by biopsy. These "healthy" carriers are HBsAg-positive but generally lose HBeAg, developing anti-HBe in association with a transient exacerbation of liver disease. The 5-year survival of carriers with chronic persistent hepatitis is 97%. Other patients progressively develop liver disease, sometimes in association with systemic symptoms, e.g., fatigue and malaise. Long-term complications of this progression include liver failure and HCC. Evidence of persistence can generally be detected histologically. In one study, the 5-year survival was 86% in patients with chronic active hepatitis and 55% once cirrhosis was evident.

Hepatocellular Carcinoma. Patients with chronic HBV infection develop HCC at a rate of 0.5 to 1.0% per year. The risk of HCC is higher in males and in patients with cirrhosis. These tumors present with weight loss, right upper quadrant pain, and occasionally fever or gastrointestinal bleeding. Hepatomegaly and ascites are common, but a discrete mass is often not palpable. Tumors are slow-growing and uncommonly metastasize.

HCC has a multifactorial etiology (Chapter 12). HBV infection increases its risk by 100 to 200 fold, implying that it has a primary role. Possible mechanisms include increasing malignant transformation of cells indirectly by increasing cell turnover and fibrogenesis and the induction of oncogenes or proto-oncogenes.

DIAGNOSIS. A simplified guide to the interpretation of the test results is shown in Table 28–1.

Detection of HBV Antigens and Antibodies. During the incubation period (4 to 8 weeks before biochemical evidence of liver dysfunction or the onset of jaundice), HBV DNA, HBsAg, and HBeAg can be detected in the plasma (Fig. 28–6). Detection of HBeAg correlates closely with the number of virus particles and relative infectivity. Anti-HBc is found in the serum 2 to 4 weeks after the appearance of HBsAg. Core antibody of the IgM class becomes undetectable within 6 months of the onset of uncomplicated acute infection, but IgG core antibody persists for many years, possibly for life. Antibodies to the surface (anti-HBs) and e (anti-HBe) anti-

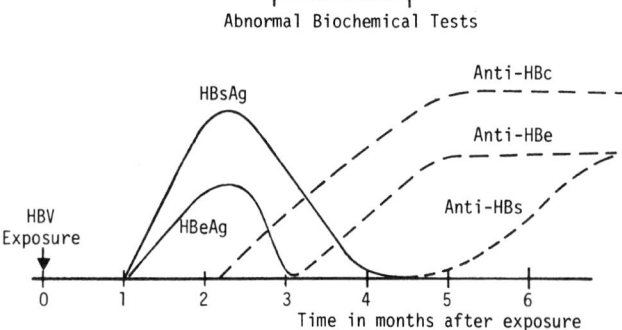

Figure 28–6. Diagram showing serologic course of uncomplicated acute hepatitis B with recovery. (From McCollum RW, Zuckerman AJ: J Med Virol 8:1, 1981.)

gens then appear, with anti-HBe indicating low infectivity and resolving infection. The presence of pre-S proteins in serum has been associated with high HBV replication, while antibodies to pre-S2 have been reported as markers of viral clearance and recovery.

Detection of HBV DNA. This may be detected in serum using direct hybridization techniques or the polymerase chain reaction (PCR); DNA fingerprinting has been used to investigate HBV transmission in endemic areas. As with HBV-related antigens, the presence of HBV DNA represents viral replication and infectivity and is present early in acute cases of HBV and persistently in chronic cases. In addition, the loss of HBV DNA has been used as a marker of successful therapy.

ANTIVIRAL THERAPY. Treatment of HBeAg-positive patients with α-interferon increases the sustained suppression of viral replication. A meta-analysis of 15 studies reported that 33% and 37% of interferon-treated patients had undetectable levels of HBeAg and HBV DNA compared with 12% and 17% among those given placebo. The nucleoside analogue lamivudine, which has been used to treat HIV infection, reduces HBV replication and appears to increase the rate of HBeAg clearance and decrease hepatic inflammation. However, in many patients the effect is not sustained when the drug is discontinued. Multiple additional reverse transcriptase inhibitors are being developed. Clearance of HBeAg following treatment has been associated with improved clinical outcomes.

PREVENTION AND CONTROL. HBV infection can be prevented by reducing exposures, by passive immunoprophylaxis, and by immunization. Dramatic reductions in posttransfusion HBV infection have been achieved by screening donated blood and blood products for HBsAg and surrogate markers. Infection control policies to prevent transmission in hemodialysis units and health care centers also have reduced nosocomial transmission. Reductions in high-risk sexual and drug-related practices (usually due to fear of contracting AIDS) is presumed responsible for declining rates of HBV infection in some homosexual and drug-using populations.

HBV Vaccination. Vaccination is also an important means of reducing HBV transmission. Two types of HBV vaccine are widely used: heat-inactivated or chemically inactivated subviral particles derived from chronic HBsAg carriers (plasma-derived vaccine) and HBsAg particles expressed from recombinant DNA in the yeast *Saccharomyces cerevisiae* (recombinant vaccine). Combination vaccines that contain recombinant HBsAg coupled with *Haemophilus influenzae* and other childhood vaccines are being developed, as are recombinant vaccines that include pre-S and S antigens.

Hepatitis B vaccines are among the safest and most immunogenetic products available. Mild injection-site reactions occur in about 20%, but fever and other systemic symptoms are uncommon. Protection titers (>10 mIU/mL) develop in more than 95% of healthy infants, children, and adults. Vaccine immunogenicity is reduced in patients who are >40 years of age, on hemodialysis, HIV-infected, obese, or cigarette smokers. Decreased immunogenicity also is associated with low-dose subcutaneous injection (vs standard dose intramuscular) and freezing of vaccine. Although the recommended schedule includes 3 doses at 0, 1, and 6 months, minor alterations in the timing of vaccine administration do not substantially reduce the immunogenicity. Generally, immunization schedules include a booster dose 4 to 6 months after primary immunization in order to obtain higher antibody titers and more durable protection.

Vaccine Efficacy. The efficacy of both plasma-derived and recombinant HBV vaccine has been demonstrated. In homosexual male cohorts, HBV incidence was reduced 90% by vaccination. Protection is evident within weeks of the second dose of vaccine and correlates with anti-HBs titers above 10 mIU/mL. It is important to realize that up to 50% of persons who initially developed anti-HBs titers >10 mIU/mL after vaccination no longer have protective antibody titers 5 to 10 years later. Nevertheless, symptomatic HBV infection is rare in initial responders, who mount a protective amnestic antibody response on re-exposure to the virus. A nationwide HBV vaccination program in Taiwan has markedly reduced the prevalence of HBsAg carriage in that nation. This program, which was started in 1984, had already markedly reduced the incidence of HCC in Taiwanese children by 1994.

Vaccine Administration. Strategies vary depending on the national or regional HBV prevalence. Especially in areas of endemicity, the WHO advocates inclusion of HBV vaccination in routine immunization programs for infants. Even in North America, Europe, and other areas with low HBV incidence, the high risk of chronic disease resulting from HBV infection occurring in childhood, the difficulty reaching persons at risk later in life, and other factors make universal vaccination of infants a rational strategy.

Mutant HBV strains that do not express the S protein present in many recombinant formulations have been found in infants not protected by HBV vaccination and immunoglobulin administration. The public health importance of those strains and the protection conferred by recombinant vaccines containing additional pre-S antigens remain to be demonstrated.

Global Immunization Strategy. More than 80 countries will have introduced HBV immunization into their national immunization programs by 1998. The WHO's goal is to reduce the incidence of new carriers by 80% by 2001 and eventually eliminate the >1.0 million deaths that occur annually from HBV-associated cirrhosis and HCC. Owing to the 350 million carriers of HBV, the infection cannot be eradicated in the near future. However, in countries where HBV immunization has been incorporated into national immunization programs, horizontal transmission can be almost eliminated, since 85 to 95% of vaccine recipients will become immune.

Postexposure Prophylaxis. HBV infection can also be prevented after exposure has occurred. Common examples include perinatal exposure, sexual contact, and needlestick accidents. Once exposure to HBV is established or judged possible, the person's HBV susceptibility must be ascertained. Anti-HBsAg should be assessed in individuals who have been vaccinated or who are at high risk of infection. Those with anti-HBs titers >10 mIU/mL can be reassured. Previously vaccinated persons with anti-HBs titers <10 mIU/mL should receive HBV-enriched immunoglobulin (HBIG) and a dose of vaccine. Individuals without prior HBV vaccination or infection should receive HBIG and three doses of vaccine.

The effectiveness of postexposure prophylaxis has been demonstrated in many settings. The incidence of HBV infection in infants born to HBeAg-positive mothers can be reduced from 90% to <10% by HBIG and HBV vaccine. Similarly, HBV infection after occupational and sexual exposures can be substantially reduced. Postexposure prophylaxis is beneficial even when delayed by more than a week but is most effective within 48 hours of exposure. In most countries, pooled IG is less effective than HBIG, but it may be substituted when HBIG is not available.

Hepatitis Delta Virus

HISTORY AND ETIOLOGY. In 1981 an outbreak of severe hepatitis was investigated among Amerindians inhabiting villages southwest of Maracaibo, Venezuela. The disease, characterized by severe hepatitis and a high mortality, especially among young children and adolescents, was shown to be due to delta agent. The clinical and epidemiologic features of the outbreak were similar to those in previous reports of Labrea hepatitis (black fever) in the upper Amazon river basin along the Purus and Juruá Rivers in Brazil.

Hepatitis delta virus (HDV) is an unclassified RNA virus that is dependent on HBV envelope proteins for replication. HDV is distinct from known antigenic determinants of HBV and is localized in the nuclei of liver cells of patients with HBV infection. HDV RNA encodes for two forms of the nucleocapsid protein, the delta antigen (HDAg). The two HDAg products function differently, the short form being necessary for viral replication while the longer is required for packaging the genome and suppressing replication. A method of efficiently propagating HDV in vitro has not been developed. Animal models of HDV include hepadnavirus-infected chimpanzees (HBV) and woodchucks (woodchuck hepatitis virus).

EPIDEMIOLOGY. The distribution and transmission of HDV infection has three patterns: (1) endemic and associated with nonparenteral spread in Italy, other Mediterranean countries, and the Middle East; (2) endemic-epidemic in the Amazon area and other remote areas of South America; and (3) sporadic and associated with parenteral transmission in almost all other geographic areas examined. Like HBV, HDV is parenterally transmitted. HDV in developed countries is most prevalent in certain high-risk groups, e.g., illicit intravenous drug users. There is good evidence that it can be transmitted both sexually and through nonsexual household contacts; the latter is believed to be the most common route of transmission in indigenous populations in South America, Africa, and parts of Central and Southeast Asia.

CLINICAL MANIFESTATIONS AND NATURAL HISTORY. HDV infection can occur with acute HBV infection (co-infection) or in a patient chronically infected with HBV (superinfection). After an incubation of 4 to 8 weeks, there is a viral hepatitis syndrome that is generally more severe than with other hepatitis viruses and may be fulminant. When HDV and HBV co-infection occurs, recovery is the rule. In contrast, HDV superinfection of chronic hepatitis B persists in more than 60% of patients and is associated with a threefold increased rate of progression to cirrhosis.

DIAGNOSIS. Acute HDV and HBV co-infection is recognized by transient detection of HDAg or, more often, antibody (IgG or IgM) to HDAg (anti-HD) with the typical serologic profile for acute HBV infection. Within months of infection, there may be no serologic evidence of HDV co-infection. HDV superinfection occurs in a HBsAg-positive patient and is recognized by anti-HD (IgG or IgM) and/or

HDV RNA or HDAg. Persistent detection of these HDV markers generally signifies chronic infection.

PREVENTION. HDV infection is deterred by prevention of HBV infection. There is no HDV vaccine to prevent infection of the estimated 350 million patients infected with HBV worldwide. Natural infection appears to prevent reinfection.

Bibliography

Alter MJ, Hadler SC, Margolis HS, et al: The changing epidemiology of hepatitis B in the United States: Need for alternate vaccination strategies. JAMA 264:2231, 1990.

Beasley RP, Hwang LY, Lin CC, Chien CS: Hepatocellular carcinoma and hepatitis B virus: A prospective study of 22,707 men in Taiwan. Lancet 2:1129, 1981.

Beasley RP, Hwang L-Y, Lin C-C, et al: Incidence of hepatitis B virus infection in preschool children in Taiwan. J Infect Dis 146:198, 1982.

Chang M-H, Chen C-J, Lai M-S, et al: Universal hepatitis B vaccination in Taiwan and the incidence of hepatocellular carcinoma in children. N Engl J Med 336:1855, 1997.

Chen HL, Chang MH, Hsu HY, et al: Seroepidemiology of hepatitis B virus infection in children: Ten years of mass vaccination in Taiwan. JAMA 276:906, 1996.

Chisari FV, Ferrai C: Hepatitis B immunopathogenesis. Annu Rev Microbiol 13:29, 1995.

Frank AL, Berg CJ, Kane MA, et al: Hepatitis B infection among children born in the United States to Southeast Asian refugees. N Engl J Med 321:1301, 1989.

Hadler SC, de Monzon M, Ponzetto A, et al: Delta virus infection and severe hepatitis: An epidemic in the Yucpa Indians of Venezuela. Ann Intern Med 100:339, 1984.

Kane M: Global programme for control of hepatitis B infection. Vaccine 13 (Suppl 1):S47, 1995.

Larouze B, Saimot G, Lustbader ED, et al: Host response to hepatitis-B infection in patients with primary hepatocellular carcinoma and their families: A case/control study in Senegal, West Africa. Lancet 2:534, 1976.

Lau JY, Wright TL: Molecular virology and pathogenesis of hepatitis B. Lancet 342:1336, 1993.

Liaw Y-F, Chiu K-W, Chu C-M, et al: Heterosexual transmission of hepatitis delta virus in the general population of an area endemic for hepatitis B virus infection: A prospective study. J Infect Dis 162:1170, 1990.

Ljunggren KE, Patarroyo ME, Engle R, et al: Viral hepatitis in Colombia: A study of the "hepatitis of the Sierra Nevada de Santa Marta." Hepatology 5:299, 1985.

McMahon BJ, Alward WLM, Hall DB, et al: Acute hepatitis B virus infection: Relation of age to the clinical expression of disease and subsequent development of the carrier state. J Infect Dis 151:599, 1985.

Rizzetto M, Ponzetto A, Forzani I: Epidemiology of hepatitis delta virus: Overview. Prog Clin Biol Res 364:1, 1991.

Seeff LB, Beebe GW, Hoofnagle JH, et al: A serologic follow-up of the 1942 epidemic of post-vaccination hepatitis in the United States Army. N Engl J Med 316:965, 1987.

Stevens CE, Beasley RP, Tsui J, Lee W-C: Vertical transmission of hepatitis B surface antigen in Taiwan. N Engl J Med 292:771, 1975.

Stevens CE, Taylor PE, Tong MJ, et al: Yeast-recombinant hepatitis vaccine: Efficacy with hepatitis B immune globulin in prevention of perinatal hepatitis B virus transmission. JAMA 257:2612, 1987.

Taylor JM: The structure and replication of hepatitis delta virus. Annu Rev Microbiol 46:253, 1992.

Whittle HC, Maine N, Pilkington J, et al: Long-term efficacy of continuing hepatitis B vaccination in infancy in two Gambian villages. Lancet 345:1089, 1995.

28.3 Hepatitis C Virus Infection

DEFINITION AND HISTORY. Hepatitis C virus (HCV) is the principal cause of parenterally transmitted non-A, non-B hepatitis. Since its discovery in 1989, there has been an explosion of information regarding the epidemiology and, more recently, the biology of this virus. HCV has been cloned and sequenced, and assays have been developed to detect HCV RNA and antibodies. The epidemiology of HCV has largely been characterized. It is now apparent that parenteral exposures, e.g., sharing of needles by injecting drug users or transfusion of blood products prior to screening procedures, account for most hepatitis C cases in developed countries. Risk factors for infections in developing countries are less clear, but parenteral exposures from injections, shaving, dental work, male and female circumcisions, and tattoos are suspected offenders. Approximately 85% of acute HCV infections persist and may progress over 10 to 30 years to cirrhosis and HCC. HCV is the leading cause of chronic liver disease in many countries, including the United States, Egypt, and Japan.

VIROLOGY

Properties of the Virion. HCV is classified along with pestiviruses and flaviviruses as genera of the Flaviviridae family. It is a spherical enveloped virus approximately 50 nm in diameter. Its buoyant density in sucrose is only 1.06 g/cm^3, but much of the virus in chronically infected individuals is bound to antibody, with a higher density of 1.17 g/cm^3. HCV clones have been developed that are infectious in chimpanzees, the only animal model for HCV infection. Efforts to obtain long-term cell cultures of HCV have been unsuccessful.

Properties of the Genome. The HCV genome, a single-stranded linear RNA of positive sense, is approximately 9.5 kb in length and is composed of 5′ and 3′ noncoding regions and genes for core (C), envelope 1 (E1), envelope 2 (E2), and nonstructural 2-5 (NS2-NS5) glycoproteins (Fig. 28–7). The noncoding regions may affect translation, while the heavily glycosylated E1-2 proteins are present in the lipid envelope. Nonstructural regions encode protease, a helicase, and an RNA polymerase.

Genetic Heterogeneity. Within an individual there are innumerable HCV variants that constitute a quasispecies, whose presence often confounds the immune response and complicates vaccine development. In addition, HCV isolates from different people may have as little as 50 to 60% nucleic acid identity. Based upon this genetic heterogeneity, HCV strains can be divided into major groups, called genotypes. Some genotypes of HCV appear to be geographically restricted; others have worldwide distribution. Types 1 and 2 predominate in the United States and Europe; type 4 is found almost exclusively in Egypt and other parts of Africa.

EPIDEMIOLOGY

Distribution. Although the prevalence of HCV in the adult population of most countries is 1 to 2%, infection rates increase with age and are much higher in high-risk groups in developed countries. The WHO estimates that 3% of the world's population has been infected with HCV and that >170 million persons are chronic carriers. There may be 10 million carriers in Egypt alone. Nearly 4 million Americans are infected with HCV, with about 30,000 new infections each year. HCV is estimated to be responsible for the deaths of 10,000 Americans annually. In some villages in Egypt and Japan, HCV rates of 20 to 40% have been reported.

Transmission. HCV is principally transmitted by exposure to blood. Accordingly, the highest prevalence (40 to 90%) is found among persons injecting illicit drugs, hemodialysis patients, hemophiliacs, and others who received multiple transfusions of blood or plasma products in the past. HCV infection may occur after blood transfusion. In countries such as the United States, where donors are screened for HCV antibody, this has become rare. However, in some developing countries with high rates of HCV infections, transfusions remain risky because there is inadequate or no screening of blood or blood products for HCV. From 2 to 8% of infants born to HCV-infected mothers develop hepatitis C. Perinatal transmission is more likely when the mother is dually infected with HIV-1 and, as with HBV, when there are high quantities of maternal virus. There are no data to suggest that breast-feeding is an important transmission route. Assessment of infant HCV infection should include HCV RNA detection, since antibody-negative infection has been documented and maternal HCV antibodies are passively transferred to infants. Sexual transmission of HCV also occurs but with low frequency. In over one third of HCV infections that occur in the United States, no specific exposure is identified. However, factors that suggest unacknowledged drug use can often be detected.

The high prevalence in Egypt is believed to be due to various percutaneous exposures. For example, from the 1950s through the 1970s the government sponsored a national schistosomiasis control program that used intravenous tartar emetic in a mass treatment campaign. Parenteral exposure to blood by injections from conventional and traditional village health workers, dental procedures, cuts from barbers, male and female circumcisions, and other activities are believed to continue HCV transmission in these communities with a large HCV reservoir.

PATHOLOGY. Individuals with chronic hepatitis C generally have lymphocytic inflammation with lymphoid aggregation in portal tracts (Fig. 28–1). There may also be microvesicular fatty changes and damage to bile ducts and acidophilic changes in hepatocytes—histologic findings that may also occur with HBV infection but are more characteristic of hepatitis C. Cirrhosis may also be present, being found more often in persons with a long duration of infection and possibly more frequently in those with genotype 1b.

Immunity and Resistance to Infection. HCV infections usually persist, owing at least in part to the rapid replication of the virus and its tendency to mutate, hence forming variants not contained by the immune response. The resulting population of viral strains are referred to as the HCV quasispecies. Although antibodies in pooled Ig may neutralize (prevent transmission of) some variants, other members of the quasispecies may still transmit HCV infection. Chimpanzees can be experimentally re-infected with inoculates of HCV and

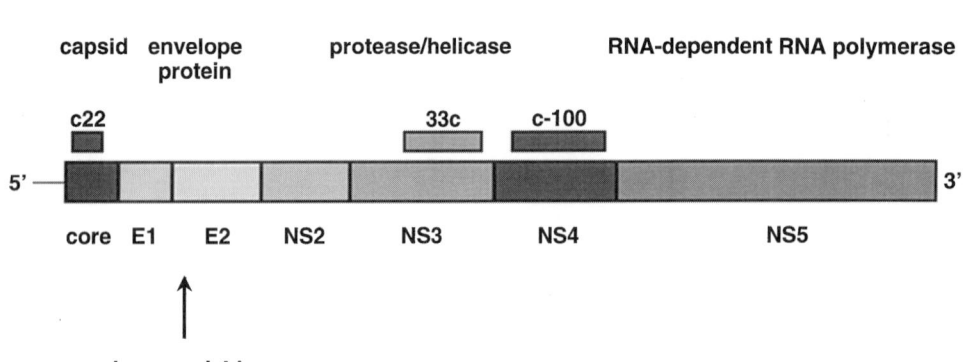

Figure **28–7.** The hepatitis C virus genome. (From the Centers for Disease Control and Prevention.)

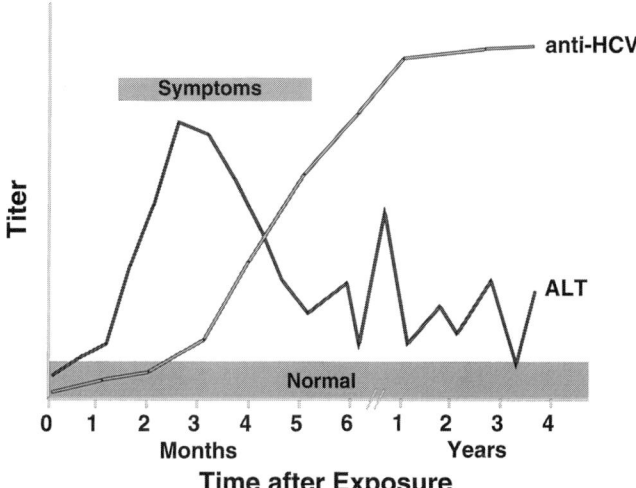

Figure 28–8. Typical course of symptomatic infection with hepatitis C virus. (From the Centers for Disease Control and Prevention.)

natural re-infections have been reported in children with thalassemia who receive multiple blood transfusions.

CLINICAL MANIFESTATIONS AND COURSE. The onset of HCV infection is often unrecognized, and the early course is most frequently indolent and protracted.

Acute Infections. Within 1 to 3 weeks of exposure, HCV RNA can be detected in blood. Transaminases become elevated 3 to 9 weeks later (average 50 days after exposure), but only 25 to 35% of those infected are jaundiced or are symptomatic (Fig. 28–8). When symptoms are experienced, there is a prodrome indistinguishable from that caused by other hepatitis viruses but that tends to have a gradual onset and to be mild. The mean incubation period until the onset of symptoms is 7 weeks. HCV is the cause of 20 to 25% of the cases of acute viral hepatitis in the United States and the Middle East. Clinical illness usually lasts from 2 to 12 weeks. Fulminating hepatitis from HCV infection is exceedingly rare. In patients having acute self-limiting disease, aminotransferases return to normal and HCV RNA becomes undetectable within that time.

Chronic Infections. HCV RNA can be persistently detected in 85% of patients with acute hepatitis C, most of whom will also have intermittent elevations in transaminases (Fig. 28–8). Not all viremic patients have elevated ALT levels. Liver biopsies in HCV-positive patients with persistently normal ALT levels usually reveal evidence of inflammation. Nevertheless, the prognosis in these patients is considered better than if ALTs were elevated. Clinical symptoms or signs of liver disease tend to initially be nonspecific, mild, and intermittent: fatigue described as lethargy, malaise, lack of energy. Other less frequent symptoms include anorexia, nausea, arthralgia, myalgia, weakness, and weight loss.

Some individuals have no symptoms from HCV infection and die of other conditions. The duration of infection and the occurrence of putative cofactors, e.g., use of alcohol, concurrent HIV-1 infection, or the HCV genotype causing the infection, may affect hepatitis C prognosis. However, although persistence and progression appear to be the rule, it remains difficult to predict the outcome for an individual patient.

Cirrhosis. From 10 to 20% of HCV-infected patients develop cirrhosis over a period of 20 years. Once cirrhosis develops, marked fatigue, muscle weakness and wasting, fluid retention with edema and ascites, easy bruising, dark urine, jaun-

dice, itching, and upper gastrointestinal hemorrhage can occur. Hepatic failure is more likely to occur in those having additional causes of liver disease, e.g., schistosomiasis and alcoholic liver disease. Chronic alcoholism promotes HCV disease progression.

Hepatocellular Carcinoma. The annual incidence of HCC is 2 to 3% in those who have been HCV carriers for 30 years, particularly in the elderly, who can develop liver cancer sooner. There are geographic differences in the incidence of HCC in those having HCV infections; perhaps this is due to the length of time that HCV has been transmitted in the local area or to differences in the prevalence of other HCC-causing cofactors. HCV-related HCC usually occurs in the context of cirrhosis. In some areas of the world, e.g., Egypt, chronic HCV with cirrhosis is the most important risk factor for HCC.

Extrahepatic Complications. HCV infection has been associated with several extrahepatitic syndromes, including essential mixed cryoglobulinemia (EMC, with or without vasculitis) and membranoproliferative glomerulonephritis. There are also reported correlations of HCV infection with arthritis, keratoconjunctivitis sicca, lymphoma, Hashimoto's thyroiditis, lichen planus, and porphyria cutanea tarda (PCT). PCT occurs in several types of chronic liver disease, often in association with iron overload. Chronic hepatitis C is a major cause of PCT in some areas.

Hepatitis C appears to be the most common cause of EMC, a syndrome marked by varying combinations of fatigue, myalgia, arthralgia and arthritis, hives, purpura or vasculitis, neuropathy, and glomerulonephritis. Cryoglobulins, composed of immune complexes of HCV and anti-HCV, immunoglobulins, rheumatoid factor, and complement, are present in the serum. Cryoglobulins are detectable in up to one third of patients with chronic hepatitis C, but the clinical syndrome of EMC occurs in <2% of patients. EMC sometimes improves with treatment of the HCV infection.

Non-Hodgkin Lymphoma (NHL). HCV has been shown to be lymphotropic as well as hepatotropic. Case series have had a higher than expected prevalence of NHL in patients with EMC and chronic HCV infection and of HCV infections in case series of NHL. It is probable that chronic HCV infection is a risk factor for both NHL and HCC.

DIAGNOSIS

Enzyme Immunoassay (EIA). Hepatitis C infections are principally diagnosed by detection of anti-HCV in plasma or serum. About 70 to 80% of those who are positive by the second- or third-generation EIA tests are also positive by RIBA and RT-PCR and are considered to have HCV infections. The remaining 20 to 30% of anti-HCV positive subjects who are RIBA and/or RT-PCR negative usually represent false positive antibody tests. However, if there is a high clinical suspicion, or if acute infection is suspected, testing should be repeated. Anti-HCV assays, which combine various structural and nonstructural HCV recombinant or synthetic peptides, detect HCV antibody 4 to 12 weeks after the onset of symptoms (Fig. 28–8). False positive antibody assays have been reported, especially when the first-generation assays were applied in low-prevalence populations, e.g., with blood donors or among persons with autoimmune diseases. Additional specificity has been achieved with subsequent generations of assays, which combine recombinant proteins from nonstructural (c100-3, NS-5, and c33) domains and structural (c22-3) core regions of the HCV genome. Anti-HCV correlates with infectivity and ongoing infection. Generally, anti-HCV persists. However, seroreversion has been documented and may correlate with resolution of infection. Differentiation of the IgM and IgG response to HCV has not been diagnostically useful.

Recombinant Immunoblot Assay. RIBA, or MATRIX, now

in a third generation, may be used to enhance the specificity of HCV screening by revealing antibody binding to each of the HCV-encoded antigens or superoxide dismutase immobilized on nitrocellulose strips. Depending on which generation of EIA is used, the prevalence of HCV in the population being tested, and the optical density cutoff used, immunoblot assays usually confirm 40 to 95% of specimens repeatedly positive by ELISA.

Reverse Transcriptase Polymerase Chain Reaction. The only readily available method to directly assess HCV infection is through detection of HCV RNA. Several methods have been developed to detect HCV RNA. Many rely on reverse transcription of the RNA to cDNA, then amplification by polymerase chain reaction (PCR). Some HCV RNA assays are difficult to perform, and marked lab-to-lab variability has been reported. Nonetheless, these assays are widely used to (1) confirm HCV infection following positive serologic results; (2) resolve samples that are indeterminate by RIBA; (3) provide early diagnosis of infection prior to seroconversion; (4) monitor viremia following antiviral treatment; (5) detect HCV in immunosuppressed patients who do not produce HCV antibodies; and (6) determine HCV genotypes.

Detection of HCV RNA indicates ongoing infection and transmissibility. Studies of perinatal hepatitis C have demonstrated that anti-HCV positive, HCV RNA negative mothers do not transmit infection to their infants, whereas HCV RNA positive mothers can. Quantitation of the level of viremia can be performed using branched DNA (bDNA) signal amplification. The quantity of HCV RNA correlates with perinatal and sexual transmission. HCV RNA may rarely be detected in anti-HCV negative individuals. Patients who have sustained responses to interferon-α therapy generally have lower pretreatment levels of HCV than do nonresponders. Thus, HCV RNA assays can help select HCV patients likely to benefit from treatment.

TREATMENT, PREVENTION, AND CONTROL. In the United States α-interferon injected subcutaneously three times weekly for 6 to 12 months is licensed to treat HCV infection. This regimen clears HCV infection in about 50% of cases, possibly leading to improved liver histology and a lower incidence of cirrhosis. However, HCV infection recurs in 50 to 60% of initial responders, and α-interferon is expensive and inconvenient to use. Clinical trials employing treatment earlier in the course of infection, longer durations of therapy, daily dosing, and combinations with ribavirin are under way and indicate that 30 to 50% sustained response rates can be achieved. The combination of ribavirin and interferon is increasingly being used to treat HCV infection, and for genotypes 2 and 3 may be used for 6, rather than 12, months. Novel antivirals being prepared specifically for HCV, with or without immunologic stimulation with therapeutic vaccines, may prove useful for treating patients with persistent HCV infections.

Dramatic reductions in post-transfusion hepatitis C occurred in the United States after the institution of screening of blood donors for HCV antibodies. Similar reductions would be expected in Egypt and other highly endemic areas as modes of transmission are delineated. Activities in the communities, e.g., cuts from barbers, dental procedures, and injections from traditional healers as well as health care providers, all may transmit HCV and can be influenced by appropriate health education. The relatively high percentage of cases that occur without identifiable exposures complicates preventive efforts.

It is essential for those who have chronic HCV infections to drink little or no alcohol. The combination of HCV and alcoholic liver disease is detrimental. Use of IG to prevent HCV infection appears to be ineffective. There is no available vaccine to prevent HCV infection, and, owing to the extent of viral heterogeneity, a universally effective HCV vaccine will be difficult to develop. However, some HCV epitopes produce neutralizing antibodies in experimental animals, and primates have been protected from challenge from homologous strains when immunized with recombinant antigens. A vaccine that does not prevent HCV infection but hinders the development of chronic infections would also be valuable.

Bibliography

Alter HJ, Purcell RH, Shih JW, et al: Detection of antibody to hepatitis C virus in prospectively followed transfusion recipients with acute and chronic non-A, non-B hepatitis. N Engl J Med 321:1494, 1989.

Alter HJ: New kit on the block: Evaluation of second-generation assays for detection of antibody to the hepatitis C virus. Hepatology 15:350, 1992.

American Academy of Pediatrics Committee on Infectious Diseases: Hepatitis C virus infection. Pediatrics 101:481, 1998.

Bukh J, Miller RH, Purcell RH: Genetic heterogeneity of hepatitis C virus: Quasispecies and genotypes. Semin Liver Dis 15:41, 1995.

Choo QL, Kuo G, Weiner AJ, et al: Isolation of cDNA clone derived from a blood-borne non-A, non-B hepatitis genome. Science 244:359, 1989.

DiBisceglie AM, Goodman ZD, Itoki HG, et al: Long-term clinical and histo-pathological follow-up of chronic posttransfusion hepatitis. Hepatology 14:969, 1991.

Estaban JL, Estaban R, Viladomiu L, et al: Hepatitis C virus antibodies among risk groups in Spain. Lancet 2:294, 1989.

Farci P, Alter HJ, Wong D, et al: A long-term study of hepatitis C virus replication in non-A, non-B hepatitis. N Engl J Med 325:98, 1991.

Farci P, Alter HJ, Govindarajan S, et al: Lack of protective immunity against reinfection with hepatitis C virus. Science 258:135, 1992.

Gretch D, Corey I, Wilson J, et al: Assessment of hepatitis C virus RNA levels by quantitative competitive RNA polymerase chain reaction: High titer viremia correlates with advanced stage liver disease. J Infect Dis 169:1219, 1994.

Hayashi J, Kishihara Y, Yamaji K, et al: Transmission of hepatitis C virus by health care workers in a rural area of Japan. Am J Gastroenterol 90:794, 1995.

Houghton M, Weiner A, Han J, et al: Molecular biology of the C viruses: Implications for diagnosis, development and control of viral disease. Hepatology 14:381, 1991.

Honda M, Kanedo S, Sakai A, et al: Degree of diversity of hepatitis C virus quasispecies and progression of liver disease. Hepatology 20:1144, 1994.

Kiyosawa K, Tanaka E, Sodeyama T, et al: Transmission of hepatitis C in an isolated area in Japan: Community acquired infection. The South Kiso Hepatitis Study Group. Gastroenterology 106:1596, 1994.

Kobayashi M, Tanaka E, Sodeyama E, et al: The natural course of chronic hepatitis C: A comparison between patients with genotypes 1 and 2 hepatitis viruses. Hepatology 23:695, 1996.

Kuo G, Choo QL, Alter HJ, et al: An assay for circulating antibodies to a major etiologic virus of human non-A, non-B hepatitis. Science 244:362, 1989.

Lai ME, Mazzzoleni AP, Argiolu F, et al: Hepatitis C virus in multiple episodes of acute hepatitis in polytransfused thalassemic children. Lancet 343:388, 1994.

Lau JYN, Davis GL, Kniffen J, et al: Significance of serum hepatitis C virus RNA levels in chronic hepatitis C. Lancet 341:1501, 1993.

Management of hepatitis C. NIH Consensus Statement 15 (3):1, 1997.

Shara AI, Hunt CM, Hamilton JD: Hepatitis C. Ann Intern Med 125:658, 1996.

Tassopoulos NC, Hatzakis A, Delladetsima I, et al: Role of hepatitis C virus in acute non-A, non-B hepatitis in Greece: A 5-year prospective study. Gastroenterology 102:969, 1992.

Tong MJ, El-Farra NS, Reikes AR, Co RL: Clinical outcomes after transfusion-associated hepatitis C. N Engl J Med 332:1463, 1995.

28.4 Hepatitis E Virus Infection

DEFINITION AND HISTORY. In 1983 HEV was visualized by immune electron microscopy (IEM) in stool from infected patients. It was then transmitted to a human volunteer and cynomolgus monkeys, thereby establishing its role in enterically transmitted non-A, non-B (NANB) hepatitis. Since it could not be cultured and the amount of virus recoverable from stool from a naturally infected human and experimentally infected monkeys was small, progress was slow. This changed in 1990, when the genome of HEV was cloned and viral antigens encoded by this RNA genome were expressed by recombinant DNA technology. This led to the rapid development of specific diagnostic tests, and a protective vaccine is expected to be commercially available early in the 21st century. HEV was retrospectively recognized as a cause of fecal-oral transmitted NANB hepatitis when the newly developed serologic testing was used to investigate clinical samples collected during epidemics of water-borne hepatitis in India in the 1950s and 1960s.

VIROLOGY. HEV is a single-stranded positive-sense RNA virus that remains unclassified but has characteristics of caliciviruses and alphaviruses. It is an icosahedral, unenveloped virus 32 to 34 nm in diameter that was first identified in 1983 by IEM in feces of patients with enterically transmitted NANB hepatitis. The 7.2 kb genome consists of three ORFs. ORF-1 encodes proteins for viral replication, while an approximately 70 kb polypeptide from ORF-2 forms the capsid and is included in assays to detect HEV antibody. ORF-3 may also be a structural protein. Although genomic variability has been noted among geographically distinct isolates, HEV has a least one major cross-reactive epitope. The virus is relatively sensitive, being inactivated by CsCl, freeze-thawing, and pelleting. HEV has a sedimentation coefficient of 183S and buoyant density of 1.29 g/cc³ in CsCl. Conventional cell culture systems are not permissive for HEV.

EPIDEMIOLOGY. HEV is transmitted by a fecal-oral route and is the principal cause of enteric NANB hepatitis. HEV infections are very rarely contracted in the United States and other developed countries. However, sporadic cases of HEV have been recognized in most developing countries, and major water-borne epidemics have been reported in India, Pakistan, and Nepal. HEV is endemic to the remainder of Central and Southeast Asia, the Middle East, Africa, and Central America. In these areas HEV is the etiologic cause of 20 to 30% of cases of acute viral hepatitis and even more in the Indian subcontinent and during outbreaks. Children often have asymptomatic or anicteric infections, while the clinical attack rate is higher in the 15 to 40 year age group. HEV is a risk to travelers to endemic areas, albeit less so than HAV. Without travel to an endemic country, HEV infection is rare.

Although sharing the same basic route of transmission as HAV, HEV infection occurs more often in the second and third decades of life, while HAV infection is almost universal in the first decade. Also, the secondary attack rate is lower for HEV than for HAV. Although not completely explaining the differences in transmission, lower quantities of HEV are excreted in the stool for shorter periods of time.

HEV infection also occurs in large outbreaks. Links to a common source of contaminated water are not uncommon, and these epidemics often follow heavy rains. As with HAV, HEV infection can occur after exposure to contaminated blood products, owing to the viremia that occurs during acute infection. There has been considerable recent interest in HEV infections occurring in animals, and investigations are ongoing to determine whether HEV is a zoonosis. HEV has been isolated from pigs, rats, and other animals.

CLINICAL FEATURES AND COURSE OF INFECTION. The course of HEV infection is similar to that of hepatitis A (Fig. 28–9). The incubation period averages 40 days (range 15 to 60 days). After oral inoculation the virus principally replicates in the liver and produces cytopathic changes. HEV can be detected in stool and blood 3 to 4 weeks after ingestion, prior to the onset of symptoms and for 1 to 2 weeks after. Like hepatitis A, there are more asymptomatic and anicteric infections with HEV than diagnosed cases of acute viral hepatitis. Children are more likely to have anicteric infections, whereas young adults have the most clinical illness, and severity of illness increases with age.

Symptoms and signs are similar to those caused by other

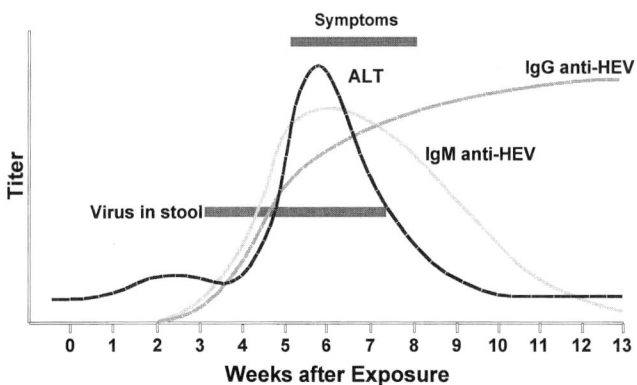

Figure 28–9. Typical course of symptomatic infection with hepatitis E virus. (From the Centers for Disease Control and Prevention.)

types of viral hepatitis: malaise, fatigue, anorexia, nausea and vomiting, jaundice and dark urine, abdominal pain, fever, and hepatomegaly. The most common laboratory findings include elevated bilirubin, ALT, AST, and alkaline phosphatase. Histopathologic findings in biopsies from patients with HEV hepatitis have included both cholestatic hepatitis and classic acute viral hepatitis.

Symptoms, hyperbilirubinemia, and elevated aminotransferase levels generally resolve within 1 to 6 weeks after onset of illness. Jaundice may be prolonged with HEV infection, which may also cause fulminant hepatitis. For unknown reasons, 10 to 20% of pregnant women in the third trimester who are hospitalized with acute HEV infection during outbreaks develop fatal fulminant hepatitis. As with HAV, HEV infection does not persist as chronic hepatitis.

DIAGNOSIS. Acute HEV infection can be diagnosed by detecting IgM HEV antibody, high titers of IgG anti-HEV, or increasing titers of total HEV antibody in the plasma of a patient with concurrent or recent hepatitis. The titer of IgM anti-HEV declines rapidly but can be detected in some patients for 5 to 6 months. IgG HEV antibodies persist and have been detected in persons from regions without recognized infection. Thus, their presence must be coupled with the appropriate clinical and epidemiologic presentation. Previously used diagnostic tests (e.g., fluorescent antibody blocking assay, Western blot assay) have been superseded by commercial EIAs (which in 1998 are not yet FDA approved in the United States) using recombinant-expressed proteins or synthetic peptides depicting immunodominant epitopes of the structural regions of the virus.

Acute HEV infection can also be diagnosed by detection of HEV particles in stool using IEM, by detection of HEV RNA in the stool or blood amplified with PCR, or by detecting HEV antigen in the liver using an immunofluorescent probe. HEV RNA has been detected in the stool and blood of 14 of 67 Nepalese patients with acute viral hepatitis who did not have either IgM or IgG antibodies to HEV.

PREVENTION AND CONTROL. HEV infection rarely occurs in developed countries. The primary means of control is through improvements in hygiene, especially by providing noncontaminated food and potable water. Immunoglobulin prepared from donors in nonendemic regions would not protect against infection. However, studies in primates show that infection can be ameliorated and prevented through preinoculation of immunoglobulin containing HEV antibodies, and immunization with recombinant HEV proteins can prevent HEV infection. Immunization with a vaccine based on the ORF-2 protein protected rhesus monkeys from intravenous challenge with both homologous and heterologous

HEV. Thus, a candidate HEV vaccine will probably proceed to clinical trials before the year 2000.

Bibliography

Bryan JP, Tsarev SA, Iqbal M, et al: Epidemic hepatitis E in Pakistan: Pattern of serologic response and evidence that antibody to hepatitis E virus protects against disease. J Infect Dis 170:517, 1994.

Clayson ET, Myint KSA, Snitbhan R, et al: Viremia, fecal shedding, and IgM and IgG responses in patients with hepatitis E. J Infect Dis 172:927, 1995.

Clayson ET, Shrestha MP, Vaughn DW, et al: Rates of hepatitis E virus infection and disease among adolescents and adults in Katmandu, Nepal. J Infect Dis 176:763, 1997.

Kane MA, Bradley DW, Shrestha SM, et al: Epidemic non-A, non-B hepatitis in Nepal. Recovery of a possible etiologic agent and transmission studies in marmosets. JAMA 252:3140, 1984.

Khuroo MS: Study of an epidemic of non-A, non-B hepatitis. Possibility of another human hepatitis virus distinct from post-transfusion non-A, non-B. Am J Med 68:818, 1980.

Khuroo MS, Teli MR, Skidmore S, et al: Incidence and severity of viral hepatitis in pregnancy. Am J Med 70:252, 1981.

Khuroo MS, Rustgi VK, Dawson GJ, et al: Spectrum of hepatitis E virus infection in India. J Med Virol 43:281, 1994.

Mast EE, Krawcznski K: Hepatitis E: An overview. Annu Rev Med 47:257, 1996.

Mast EE, Kuramoto K, Favorov MO, et al: Prevalence of and risk factors for antibody to hepatitis E virus seroreactivity among blood donors in northern California. J Infect Dis 176:34, 1997.

Tsarev SA, Tsareva TS, Emerson SU, et al: Successful passive and active immunization of cynomolgus monkeys against hepatitis E. Proc Natl Acad Sci USA 91:10198, 1994.

Tsarev SA, Tsareva TS, Emerson SU, et al: Recombinant vaccine against hepatitis E: Dose response and protection against heterologous challenge. Vaccine 15 (17–18):1834, 1997.

28.5 Non-A-to-E Hepatitis

From 2 to 20% of acute hepatitis cases do not appear to be due to any of the well-described hepatitis viruses. Induction of hepatitis in primates with plasma from some non-A-to-E patients suggests that at least some are caused by an infectious disease. A novel RNA virus has been recognized in the plasma of humans with acute non-A-to-E hepatitis, persons injecting illicit drugs, dialysis patients, and blood donors; it has been provisionally named hepatitis G virus (HGV) or GB virus C. This agent is a single-stranded, positive-sense RNA virus with approximately 25% nucleic acid identity with HCV. Its occurrence in humans can be demonstrated by detection of RNA and antibody to the viral envelope. HGV/GBV-C infection appears to persist with a frequency intermediate between those of HBV and HCV. The association of HGV/GBV-C with liver disease has not been shown, and the virus is probably not hepatropic. The virus has been detected in cases of fulminant hepatitis not due to other recognized viruses. However, there are no data suggesting that it causes either acute or chronic liver disease.

Bibliography

Linnen J, Wages J Jr, Zhang-Keck Z-Y, et al: Molecular cloning and disease association of hepatitis G virus: A transfusion-transmissible agent. Science 271:505, 1996.

29 Viral Febrile Illnesses

29.1 Dengue and Dengue Hemorrhagic Fever

David W. Vaughn and Sharone Green

DEFINITION. Classic *dengue fever* ("breakbone fever") is an acute self-limited illness with fever, headache, arthralgia, myalgia, rash, lymphadenopathy, and leukopenia caused by four distinct serotypes of dengue virus, a mosquito-borne flavivirus. Thrombocytopenia and hemorrhage may be seen in dengue fever but are not prominent features. *Dengue hemorrhagic fever* (DHF) is distinguished from classic dengue by plasma leakage and simultaneous thrombocytopenia. The plasma leakage is manifested by hemoconcentration and, in severe cases, circulatory failure, shock (*dengue shock syndrome* [DSS]), and death in a proportion of cases. DHF and DSS result from infection with any of the four serotypes of dengue virus; immunopathologic mechanisms are postulated to play a role in the genesis of the disease.

HISTORY. The clinical syndrome was first described in 1780 as "breakbone fever" by Benjamin Rush in Philadelphia. The term "dengue" was first applied in 1828 during an epidemic in Cuba. Until the 20th century, the similar diseases dengue and Chikungunya often were confused. Since the 18th century, dengue has caused recurrent epidemics worldwide. *Aedes aegypti* was first implicated as the vector in 1903 by H. Graham. In 1907, P. M. Ashburn and Charles Craig demonstrated that the virus was in human plasma by transmitting the infection to human volunteers. Prototype dengue types 1 and 2 viruses were isolated, characterized, and adapted to mice by Albert Sabin and his colleagues in 1944–1945; similarly dengue types 3 and 4 viruses were recovered by William Hammon in 1956. Although hemorrhagic phenomena were described in earlier epidemics, DHF gained nosologic status (as Philippine hemorrhagic fever) in 1954 and subsequently became endemic and epidemic in many areas of tropical Asia (Thai and Singapore hemorrhagic fever). In 1981 DHF occurred in epidemic form in the Caribbean for the first time.

ETIOLOGY. The four dengue viruses (types 1 to 4) constitute a distinct antigenic complex within the *Flavivirus* genus of the family *Flaviviridae*. Dengue serotypes are distinguishable by complement fixation and neutralization tests using hyperimmune antisera or by immunofluorescence tests using monoclonal antibodies. Despite the close antigenic relationship of these viruses, cross-protection in humans is incomplete and short-lived.

Dengue virions are small (40 nm) spherical particles composed of a lipoprotein envelope and nucleocapsid of single-strand RNA genome with positive polarity. The three viral structural proteins are C, the nucleocapsid or core protein; M, a membrane-associated protein; and E, the major envelope glycoprotein, which is exposed on the virion surface and contains type-specific and group-reactive antigens. At least seven nonstructural proteins also are formed during infection, of which at least one (NS1) is present on the surface of infected cells and may play a significant role in immunologic responses of the host. Many strains of dengue are nonpathogenic or only minimally pathogenic for suckling mice unless adapted by repeated passage. A variety of mammalian cell lines may be used for isolation and assay, but mosquito cells or intrathoracic inoculation of living mosquitoes are more sensitive.

DISTRIBUTION AND INCIDENCE. The distribution of dengue corresponds roughly to that of the principal vector, *Ae. aegypti,* and includes tropical and subtropical regions of Asia, the Americas, Africa, and Australia. During and after World War II, *Ae. aegypti* became more widely distributed and more prevalent in Asia. All four serotypes of dengue virus have long been endemic in Asia; *Ae. aegypti*–infested areas of the southern United States experienced large epidemics of dengue until 1945. Sporadic outbreaks have occurred again recently in Texas. In the 1980s, *Ae. aegypti* reinvaded Brazil, Ecuador, Paraguay, and Bolivia, with resulting large epidemics. Dengue type 2 virus was first isolated in the Americas in 1953, and dengue type 3 virus in 1963. Dengue type 1 virus first appeared in the Caribbean in 1988, and dengue type 4 virus in 1981. All four dengue virus serotypes have been isolated in Africa. Sporadic cases compatible with DHF have been reported, although epidemic DHF has not been recognized in Africa to date.

Dengue fever epidemics attack many thousands of person (e.g., over 1 million were infected in Rio de Janeiro in 1986) and are characterized by infection rates as high as 75 to 80%. Immunity is serotype-specific and long-lasting (probably for life). Repeated outbreaks of dengue in a geographic area result from introductions of new serotypes or recurrence of infection with the same serotype in susceptible segments of the population, e.g., those born after the last epidemic.

Dengue fever and DHF incidence have increased dramatically in the past 40 years, owing to expanding urbanization and *Ae. aegypti* populations and to increased movements of viremic travelers by airplane. Although 250,000 cases of DHF are officially reported, it is estimated that 100 million cases of dengue fever occur annually. Dengue hemorrhagic fever is a perennial problem in parts of Southeast Asia, where it is a leading cause of hospitalization of children. In the 5-year period from 1986 to 1990, 1.1. million cases of DHF and over 10,000 deaths were officially reported from Thailand, Indonesia, Vietnam, and Burma alone; these incidence data are widely accepted as a gross underestimate.

TRANSMISSION AND EPIDEMIOLOGY. The transmission cycle is simple, involving humans as the viremic host and the *Ae. aegypti* mosquito as the vector. In certain areas, other vectors (e.g., *Aedes albopictus* and *Aedes polynesiensis*) play a role in transmission. The extrinsic incubation period in mosquitoes (time between ingestion of infectious blood and ability to transmit) is 8 to 11 days; mosquitoes remain infective for life. *Ae. aegypti* breeds in peridomestic containers, e.g., water storage jars, flower pots, tin cans, and discarded tires. Its flight range is generally limited, although the mosquito is capable of flying long distances if breeding sites are not readily available. Interrupted probing and feeding are common and one mosquito may infect a number of household members.

Most dengue virus infections of nonimmune adults result in clinically apparent disease (dengue fever). However, most infections of young children are inapparent or mild enough to escape medical attention. At the same time, although most adults are immune to multiple dengue virus serotypes, DHF is predominantly a disease of children. In tropical areas, dengue outbreaks coincide with the monsoon or rainy season. Dengue virus has been experimentally passed vertically in *Aedes* mosquitoes but the epidemiologic significance of transovarial transmission is uncertain. A jungle cycle of dengue (analogous to yellow fever), involving forest mosquitoes and wild monkeys, has been documented in Malaysia and in West Africa. The role of enzootic dengue as a source of human infections is presently unknown.

PATHOGENESIS. After the bite of an infected mosquito, the virus replicates in regional lymph nodes and is dissemi-
nated via the lymph and blood to other tissues. Replication in the reticuloendothelial system and skin produces a viremia that is detectable in most patients early in the illness. In the majority of dengue virus infections, the disease is self-limited; however, a small proportion of infections lead to a more severe illness, dengue hemorrhagic fever–dengue shock syndrome (DHF-DSS). The hallmarks of DHF-DSS are abnormalities in capillary permeability and in coagulation and hemostasis. Ninety percent of cases of DHF-DSS occur during secondary infections. In primary DHF-DSS, a subpopulation of cases occurs in infants under the age of 1 year who are born to dengue-immune mothers. Based on these epidemiologic data, the immune status of the host is believed to play an important role in determining the course of dengue infections and the subsequent development of DHF-DSS. The presence of non-neutralizing antibodies to a heterologous dengue virus may form virus-antibody complexes that enhance dengue virus entry into Fc receptor–bearing lymphoid cells. This mechanism is known as antibody-dependent enhancement. The increased number of infected cells, e.g., monocytes, stimulate cross-reactive memory CD4+ and CD8+ lymphocytes as evidenced by elevated serum levels of tumor necrosis factor alpha (TNF-α), soluble interleukin-2 (IL-2) receptors, and soluble CD8 seen in children with DHF. In addition, the complement system is activated with elevated levels of C3a and C5a fragments. It is possible that certain dengue virus serotypes or genotypes may have differing propensities to induce DHF either by a direct mechanism or via HLA-regulated pathways. Studies in Thailand have shown that the class I HLA-A2 haplotype is associated with DHF.

PATHOLOGY. Microscopic changes in skin lesions of patients with dengue fever include perivascular edema, endothelial cell swelling, and mononuclear cell infiltration. The pathologic changes in fatal cases of DHF are not extensive or impressive and do not reflect the profound physiologic disturbances or cause of death. Pathologic findings include megakaryocytic arrest in the bone marrow; active proliferation and lymphocytolysis of germinal centers in lymph nodes and spleen; focal midzonal necrosis, fatty changes, swelling, hyaline necrosis of hepatocytes and occasional Councilman bodies; and glomerulonephritis (possibly due to immune complex deposition). Hemorrhages are generally minor and not life-threatening; occasionally, major gastrointestinal bleeding, which is more frequent in adolescents and adults, may be clinically significant.

CLINICAL MANIFESTATIONS AND COMPLICATIONS

Classic Dengue. The incubation period is usually 3 to 8 days, followed by abrupt onset of fever, chills, headache, eye pain, and lumbosacral aching. A transient, generalized erythematous flush–like rash may be present during the first 24 to 48 hours (Fig. 29–1). Generalized myalgia and arthralgia increase in severity and other symptoms, e.g., anorexia, nausea, vomiting, respiratory symptoms, marked lassitude, cutaneous hyperesthesia and altered taste, appear on the second to the fourth day. The physical examination may reveal relative bradycardia and generalized lymphadenopathy. Marked leukopenia (as few as 1500 cells/mm^3) and neutropenia are typical, and thrombocytopenia may occur on the third to eighth day. On the third to fifth day, fever abates and a morbilliform rash appears on the trunk, spreading centripetally to the face and extremities, sometimes accompanied by a brief (12 to 24 hour) recrudescence of fever (Fig. 29–2). Hemorrhagic phenomena, particularly petechial hemorrhages and epistaxis, may occur during the course of the illness; in the absence of signs of plasma leakage these patients do not meet the criteria for having DHF.

Dengue Hemorrhagic Fever. This syndrome, characterized

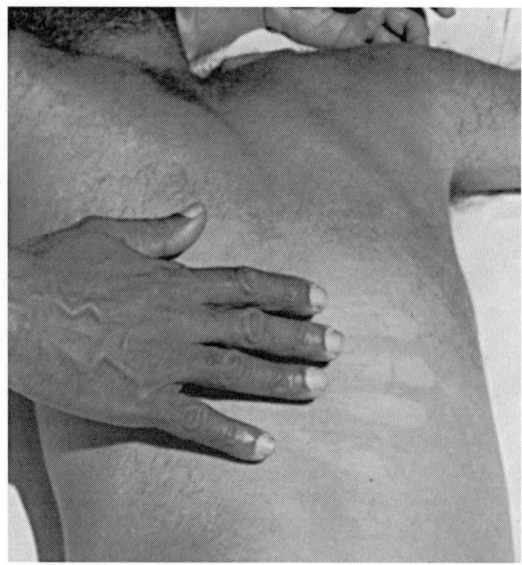

Figure 29–1. Pressure blanching of erythematous, macular rash of dengue. (Courtesy of Dr. Telford H. Work.)

the right lung field), and petechiae, ecchymoses, and other spontaneous hemorrhages including gastrointestinal hemorrhage, metromenorrhagia, and epistaxis. Enlargement and tenderness of the liver may be noted. Some patients manifest signs of restlessness, abdominal pain, and shock (cold and clammy extremities, diaphoresis, circumoral cyanosis, irritability, or change in mental status). These cases, known as DSS, are characterized by hypotension or narrowing of the pulse pressure to <20 mmHg (often with a normal systolic blood pressure), or in the most severe cases, undetectable blood pressure. This rapid deterioration typically occurs on the second to fifth day of illness, usually around the time of defervescence. Laboratory findings seen in DHF include hypoproteinemia and mildly elevated serum aspartate aminotransferase and urea nitrogen levels. Evidence for disseminated intravascular coagulation (DIC), prolonged prothrombin and partial thromboplastin times, and reduced fibrinogen and clotting factors II, V, VII, X, and XII are found in up to 25% of patients with shock. Metabolic acidosis may be present. Without treatment, up to 50% of such patients die. Patients with less severe illness or those successfully treated recover rapidly after a 1- to 2-day period of acute illness.

Other Manifestations. There are rare reports of encephalopathy, impairment of renal function, and fulminant hepatitis associated with dengue infection.

PROGNOSIS AND THERAPY. After recovery from classic dengue, convalescence may be prolonged for several weeks by weakness, depression, and occasional cardiac symptoms (palpitations, ventricular extrasystole, and bradycardia). The case-fatality rate in severe DHF-DSS is high in patients who are not hospitalized and treated promptly, but with good medical management <1% of these patients die.

Treatment of classic dengue is symptomatic, e.g., acetaminophen, bed rest, and oral (rarely parenteral) fluid replacement (Fig. 29–4). In cases of DHF without shock, dehydration and hemoconcentration may be managed by oral rehydration on an outpatient basis. In patients with signs of moderately decreased intravascular volume or vomiting, intravenous fluid replacement consisting of 5% dextrose in half normal

by increased capillary permeability and hemostatic derangements, occurs more frequently in children. Cases of DHF can be characterized into four grades of disease severity as defined by World Health Organization (WHO) guidelines (Fig. 29–3). The minimum diagnostic criteria for DHF are a positive tourniquet test or spontaneous hemorrhages, thrombocytopenia (<100,000 cells/mm³), and evidence of plasma leakage (increase in hematocrit by 20% or more from baseline, ascites, or pleural effusion).

Early in the illness, these children are clinically identical to those with classic dengue but around the time of defervescence, DHF patients enter a second phase of illness with variable ascites or pleural effusion (more commonly seen in

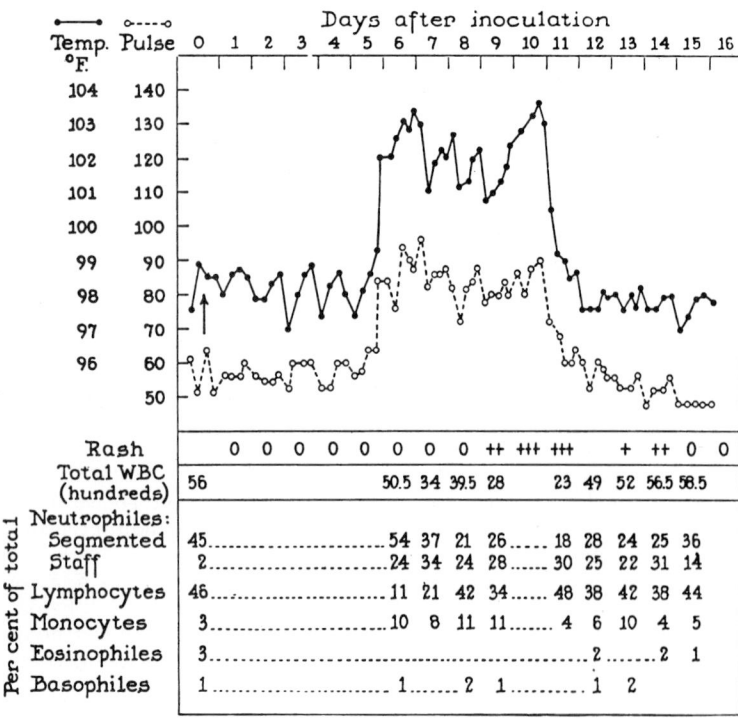

Figure 29–2. Graphic representation of temperature and pulse rate of a human volunteer inoculated experimentally with the Hawaiian strain of dengue virus by means of the bites of eight infected *Aedes aegypti* mosquitoes; arrow indicates day on which the patient was bitten. Time of appearance of rash is also indicated as well as total and differential blood counts. (From Sabin AB: *In* Rivers TM, Horsfall FL Jr: Viral and Rickettsial Infections of Man, 3rd ed. Philadelphia, JB Lippincott, 1959. Used by permission of the National Foundation.)

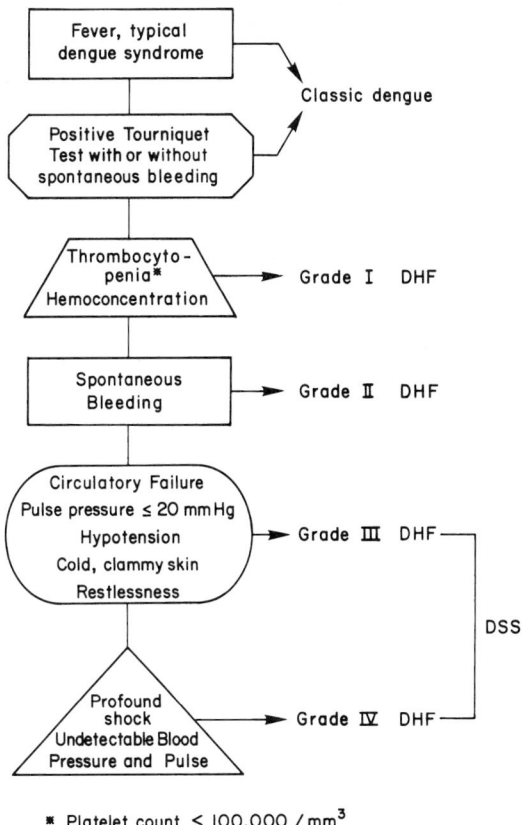

Figure 29–3. Algorithm for the diagnosis and grading of dengue, dengue hemorrhagic fever (DHF), and dengue shock syndrome (DSS).

saline or Ringer's lactate may be given in the hospital. Acetaminophen should be used to control fever, as salicylates are contraindicated because of the bleeding diathesis. Vital signs, hematocrit, and platelet counts should be monitored. The early recognition of DHF with shock, followed by intensive care in the hospital and proper management, is essential. Immediate replacement of fluids with normal saline or lactated Ringer's solution is necessary. In continued or prolonged shock, plasma or other colloid may be added (10 to 20 mL/kg/hr). Careful and repeated estimation of volume status is essential and is obtained by measuring vital signs, urine output, and hematocrit or serum protein concentration. Oxygen should be given to patients in shock. Blood gases and serum electrolytes should be monitored and acidosis should be treated. Because the acid-base disturbance in DHF-DSS is usually a mixed respiratory alkalosis and metabolic acidosis (both of which lower the plasma HCO_3 concentration), $NaHCO_3$ should be administered only after determination of blood pH. To avoid fluid overload and pulmonary edema, parenteral fluid therapy should be stopped when the hematocrit drops to approximately 40% and clinical signs and urine output improve (generally after 24 to 72 hours). If the hematocrit falls without corresponding clinical improvement, one should suspect gastrointestinal hemorrhage. If there is laboratory evidence of DIC and/or intractable bleeding it should be managed by the administration of fresh blood or fresh-frozen plasma.

Corticosteroids have been used to treat DHF-DSS; however, comparative therapeutic trials have yielded conflicting results. Corticosteroids have not been shown to be beneficial once plasma leakage has become overt. At present, there is no specific drug therapy for DHF beyond supportive care, as outlined previously.

DIAGNOSIS

Virus Isolation. The virus should be sought from serum obtained during the febrile phase of illness. Serum should be aseptically collected and kept at refrigerator temperatures (wet ice) for delivery to a virus laboratory within 24 to 48 hours or should be frozen on dry ice if a longer delivery time is anticipated. Virus isolation in cell cultures, e.g., *Ae. albopictus, Aedes pseudoscutellaris,* or LLC-MK2 cells, is confirmed by development of cytopathic effect, plaques, or immunofluorescence (IF) antigen detection. Alternatively, live mosquitoes, e.g., *Toxorhynchites* or *Ae. aegypti,* may be intrathoracically inoculated and examined for virus by IF testing after incubation for 7 to 14 days. Dengue virus serotypes are identified by neutralization test, using hyperimmune antisera or by IF with type-specific monoclonal antibodies. Reverse-transcriptase polymerase chain reaction (RT-PCR) may extend the interval during which a virologic diagnosis may be made, as it relies on the detection of viral RNA rather than viable virus.

Serology. Serologic diagnosis is achieved by demonstrating a rise in hemagglutination-inhibition, complement fixation, or neutralizing antibody titers in appropriately timed paired sera drawn 7 to 14 days apart. In patients with primary dengue infection and no previous exposure to related flaviviruses, e.g., yellow fever, St. Louis encephalitis, Japanese encephalitis, and West Nile fever, the serologic responses are relatively type-specific, whereas persons with prior dengue or nondengue flaviviral exposure have a more rapid, high-titered, and broadly cross-reactive antibody response. The IgM antibody-capture enzyme-linked immunosorbent assay (ELISA) has improved dengue serodiagnosis. By 2 days following defervescence, patients with primary or secondary infections have detectable IgM antibodies. These antibodies wane relatively rapidly, so that by 2 to 3 months the majority of patients are seronegative; thus, tests on a single serum sample may indicate recent infection. IgM antibodies are relatively specific for dengue (minimal cross reactions with heterologous flaviviruses) but do not readily distinguish infections with the individual dengue serotypes.

PREVENTION AND CONTROL. Several live attenuated dengue vaccines, prepared in Thailand and the United States, have undergone successful preliminary testing in human volunteers. Because of the potential for severe disease in individuals sequentially exposed to wild dengue viruses, it will be necessary to simultaneously immunize against all or multiple serotypes. Considerable progress has been made on the molecular structure of flaviviruses in general, and dengue viruses in particular. Dengue viral genes for protective antigens of the envelope and NS1 proteins have been cloned and expressed in several recombinant systems, including vaccinia, baculovirus, and bacteria, and these approaches offer promise for the development of diagnostic reagents and vaccines.

Prevention of dengue fever outbreaks can be achieved by reducing vector mosquito populations (principally *Ae. aegypti*) through elimination of breeding sites and use of larvicides. Emergency control of dengue or DHF epidemics uses ground or aerial ultra-low-volume sprays of an effective mosquito adulticide. Such emergency measures have generally been undertaken without studies to determine efficacy, and recent research indicates that ultra-low-volume adulticides have little impact on *Ae. aegypti* adults resting indoors.

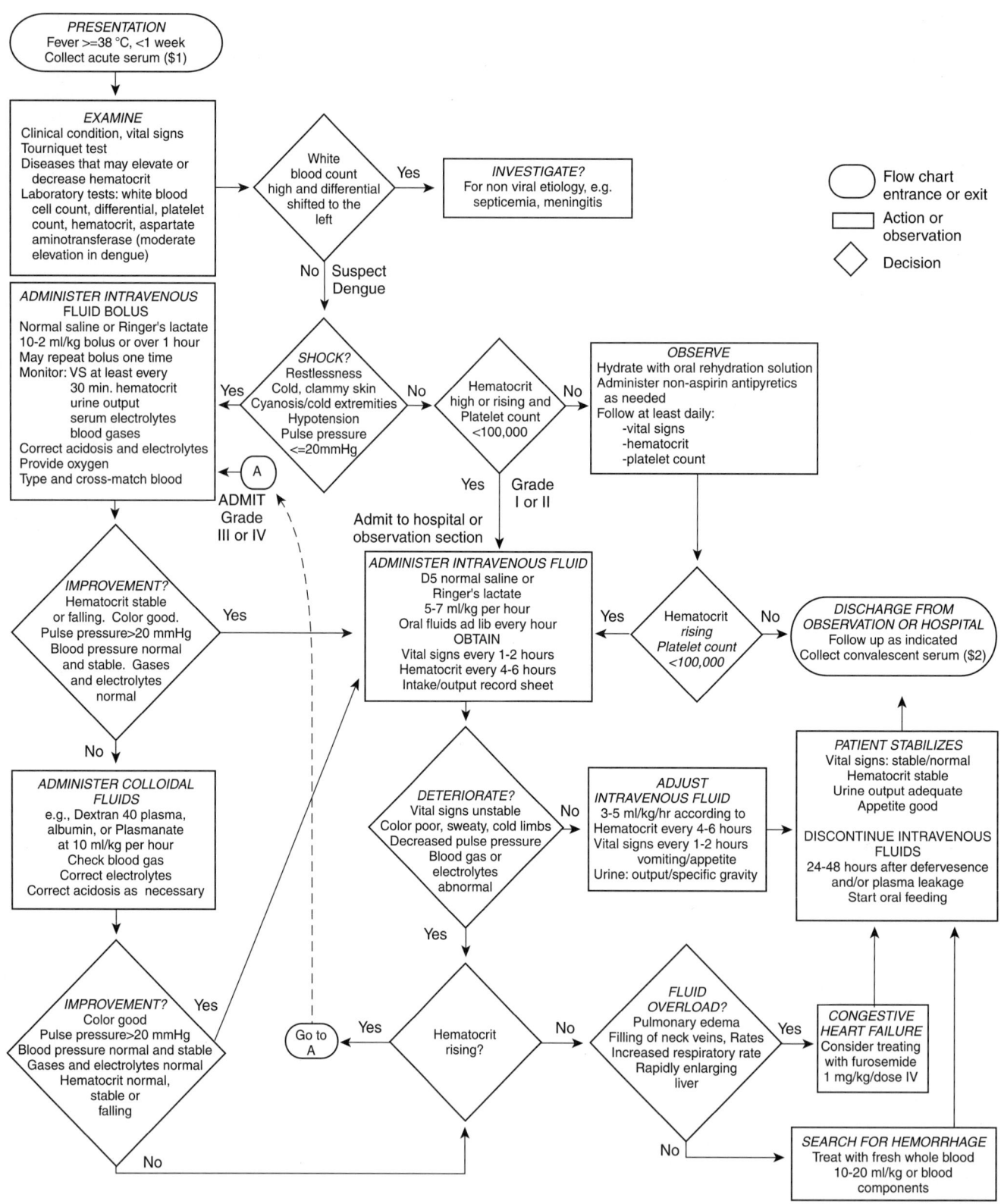

Figure 29–4. Algorithm for the treatment of dengue hemorrhagic fever. (Modified from Dengue Hemorrhagic Fever: Diagnosis, Treatment, and Control. Geneva, WHO, 1988.)

Bibliography

Gubler DJ: Dengue. *In* Monath TP (ed): The Arboviruses: Epidemiology and Ecology, Vol II. Boca Raton, FL, CRC Press, 1988, pp 223–260.

Halstead SB: Pathogenesis of dengue: Challenges to molecular biology. Science 239:476, 1987.

Halstead SB, Nimmannitya S, Margiotta MR: Dengue and chikungunya virus infection in man in Thailand, 1962–1964. II. Observations on disease in outpatients. Am J Trop Med Hyg 18:972, 1969.

Innis BL: Dengue and dengue hemorrhagic fever. *In* Porterfield JS (ed): Kass Handbook of Infectious Diseases: Exotic Viral Infections. London, Chapman and Hall Medical, 1995.

Kurane I, Ennis FA: Cytokines in dengue virus infections: Role of cytokines in the pathogenesis of dengue hemorrhagic fever. Semin Virol 5:443, 1994.

Monath TP: Dengue: The risk to developed and developing countries. Proc Natl Acad Sci USA 91:2395, 1994.

Sabin A: Research on dengue during World War II. Am J Trop Med Hyg 1:30, 1952.

Vaughn DW, Green S, Kalayanarooj S, et al: Dengue in the early febrile phase: Viremia and antibody responses. J Infect Dis 176:322, 1997.

World Health Organization: Dengue Haemorrhagic Fever: Diagnosis, Treatment and Control. Geneva, WHO, 1986.

29.2 West Nile Fever

Susan P. Fisher-Hoch and Joseph B. McCormick

DEFINITION. West Nile (WN) virus is a mosquito-borne flavivirus. Although it is widely distributed and causes many human infections, most are asymptomatic or mild. Disease, when it occurs, consists of acute fever, sometimes with a rash and occasionally encephalitis, especially in the elderly. Hemorrhagic disease with hepatitis has been reported.

VIROLOGY. The virus was first isolated from a febrile woman in 1937, and is named after the West Nile province of Uganda where the patient lived. It is antigenically related most closely to Murray Valley encephalitis, St. Louis encephalitis, and Japanese encephalitis viruses. Like other flaviviruses, WN RNA is enveloped and measures about 45 nm. It has a positive-sense RNA genome of about 4×10^6 kb, composed of 10,960 nucleotides, complexed with a single species of capsid protein. A viral polyprotein is translated from a single, long open-reading frame. Structural and nonstructural proteins, which are synthesized from this polyprotein by cleavage processes involving viral and cellular enzymes, accumulate in large amounts in infected cells. There are three structural proteins, C, M, and E. The E protein, a large membrane-associated, variably glycosylated protein, with a molecular mass of about 50 kDa, is responsible for hemagglutination. There are also seven nonstructural proteins.

ECOLOGY. WN virus has been isolated from a wide range of birds and mammals in the Old World. It has been found throughout Europe as far west as Portugal, the Middle East, the former Soviet Union, and South Asia. Birds have been demonstrated experimentally to sustain viremia sufficient to infect mosquitoes and are therefore considered the primary reservoir. Infection in wild birds is common. In a study conducted in the Punjab, Pakistan, 27% of 317 wild birds captured had neutralizing (strain-specific) antibody to WN virus. Virus has also been isolated from wild birds in the Caucasus and central Asian republics. A wide range of bird species have evidence of natural infection. In experimental studies, 13 species of birds from South Africa and 5 from Egypt sustained viremia for at least 3 days. Many wild and domestic mammals may be infected with WN virus both naturally and experimentally. However, prevalence of antibody in mammals in the wild is lower than in birds, and mammals do not sustain viremia at levels thought to make them as ecologically important as birds.

WN virus has been isolated from a wide variety of mosquitoes; however, bird-feeding hemipteran bugs, mites, and ticks may also be infected. Various *Culex* species are the mosquitoes most frequently implicated in epidemics, the most prominent being *Culex univittatus*, *Culex pipiens*, and *Culex neavei*. In India and Pakistan, *Culex vishnui*, *Culex tritaeniorhynchus*, and *Culex quinquefasciatus* are vectors. In a novel urban epidemic in Bucharest, Romania, in 1996, *C. pipiens* was the suspected vector. WN virus has been isolated from wild ixodid and argasid ticks in central Asia. WN virus is most active in temperate and subtropical areas but is also found in the tropics. Peak activity usually occurs during the hottest time of year, and is probably related to high mosquito vector density and capacity. Although infection in most animals and birds is silent, WN virus occasionally has been recovered from horses with encephalitis in Egypt and France, and disease, and even death, has resulted from experimental infections in some birds. Although humans, like equines, can develop encephalitis, neither are part of the natural transmission cycle of the virus and are therefore dead-end hosts.

EPIDEMIOLOGY. The endemicity of WN virus and its ability to cause human epidemic disease was first described in Egypt in the 1950s. Endemic disease has now been reported in many other countries including Uganda, Nigeria, South Africa, France, Portugal, Pakistan, India, and countries of the former Soviet Union. Interpretation of prevalence based on surveys using serologic assays is confounded by extensive cross reactions with other flaviviruses. Reported seroprevalence rates range from 15% to over 80%. Seropositivity increases with age but varies with time and place. Adjacent geographic areas often have markedly different human seroprevalences, probably resulting from differing local ecological conditions. Furthermore, in a given area, population antibody prevalence has been observed to wane over a period of 10 to 15 years, presumably setting the stage for new epidemics.

The lack of specificity of serologic assays also makes uncertain the final interpretation of all outbreaks in which virus was not isolated. Nevertheless there are data that support the ability of the virus to cause major epidemics. Between 1951 and 1957, epidemics in Israel involved hundreds of cases. An attack rate of 64% was documented in an outbreak in a military camp. An epidemic was reported as far west as southern France (the Camargue) in 1962. The largest outbreaks on record have occurred in South Africa: in 1974 in the high veldt of the Transvaal and Orange Free State, and in 1983 and 1984 in the Pretoria area. In the 1974 outbreak, it was estimated that 18,000 persons were infected with the virus among a population of 30,000. However because inapparent infections are common, these estimates may not be accurate. Endemic and epidemic disease has been recorded in Romania for many years, and in 1996 an outbreak starting in Bucharest at the end of July resulted in about 450 cases of reported neurologic illness, over 300 of which were confirmed serologically. Further confirmation of the etiology of this outbreak by viral isolation would facilitate tracing the virus's genealogy, possibly an African source.

PATHOLOGY AND PATHOGENESIS. There is generalized involvement of the brain and spinal cord with diffuse inflammation, perivascular cuffing with small hemorrhages, and neuronal degeneration. The virus is widely disseminated to most organs. There may be variation in pathogenicity between strains; antigenic differences have been demonstrated between strains from India and those from Africa and the Middle East, and variation occurs even within these regions.

The immune response to WN virus is complex and the phenomenon of immune enhancement described in dengue hemorrhagic fever may occur. There is experimental evidence that IgG1 and IgG3 antibodies at subneutralizing concentrations may enhance infection by inducing virus attachment to the macrophage cell surface via Fc receptors. In the presence of complement, IgM may enhance replication of the virus. On the other hand, the role of the macrophage in defense against central nervous system (CNS) invasion has been demonstrated in mice, and neutralizing antibody is protective and probably acts extracellularly by inhibiting the uncoating of virus. The CNS pathology may be immunopathologic. WN virus induces the expression of major histocompatibility complex (MHC) molecules on the surface of astrocytes, suggesting possible T-cell–mediated damage to neural tissue.

CLINICAL MANIFESTATIONS AND COMPLICATIONS. Most WN infections in humans are asymptomatic. In those who do develop symptoms, the incubation period is between 2 and 6 days, and the patient is viremic during the first 24 to 48 hours of illness. Detailed observations made in 21 terminal cancer patients therapeutically injected with WN virus as immunotherapy showed that only 7 developed detectable viremia. Symptoms were only observed during viremia, and virus was only recovered from blood, never from throat washings, urine, or stool. The disease resembles other arbovirus infections with sudden onset; fever is accompanied by anorexia, nausea, vomiting, malaise, eye pain, myalgia, rash, diffuse lymphadenopathy, and occasionally conjunctivitis and pharyngitis. One third of patients have sore throat. Rash occurs in about half of patients. The rash consists of discrete roseolar spots, diffuse small spotted exanthem, or mottling of the skin, described as typhoid-like and more frequently is seen in young children. Spleen and liver may be enlarged in WN fever, but this observation in malaria-endemic areas is of questionable specificity. Lymphopenia is common. WN fever is therefore similar in many respects to other flavivirus infections, especially dengue fever, and is difficult if not impossible to distinguish on clinical grounds alone.

WN virus invades the CNS in a small proportion of patients. In a study conducted in Cairo, it was responsible for illness in 5% of patients admitted to the hospital with aseptic meningitis or encephalitis. Symptoms variously reported include nuchal rigidity, somnolence, papillitis, confusion, dysarthria, convulsions, and leg weakness. Absent or abnormal reflexes and paraparesis have been described. The cerebrospinal fluid (CSF) may be clear and pressure normal, but the white blood cell (WBC) counts may reach 400 cells/mm³, with increased protein. CSF glucose is within normal limits.

A single case of pancreatitis has been reported. Hepatitis with hemorrhagic manifestations has been described in three patients in the Central African Republic infected by WN viral strains identical by DNA and serologic analysis. These strains were also closely related to tick and mosquito isolates.

PROGNOSIS AND THERAPY. As with many viral diseases, convalescence may be prolonged and associated with lassitude and depression. The typical disease is self-limited, with full recovery expected. Neurologic sequelae are not described. There is no specific therapy. The potential severity of encephalitis in the elderly is reflected in a 10-fold higher incidence in persons >60 years of age, and the preponderance of fatal cases in the elderly.

DIAGNOSIS. WN virus is pathogenic for suckling and weanling mice inoculated intracerebrally and intraperitoneally, chick embryos, hamsters, and a wide variety of cell cultures. Virus may be isolated from serum during the acute febrile phase or during the incubation period (1 or 2 days before onset) by intracerebral inoculation of suckling mice or tissue culture. Serologic methods include complement fixation (CF), hemagglutination-inhibition and neutralization tests. CF tests are useful in distinguishing between infections

with closely related flaviviruses that cause extensive cross reactions. ELISA methods are sensitive and specific, but a rise in titer is required for diagnosis. Antibody-capture ELISA performed on serum and/or CSF is sensitive and is somewhat specific. It is likely that molecular techniques such as RT-PCR for detection of viral RNA, already in use for dengue and other flaviviruses, may offer the most accurate and rapid approach to diagnosing WN virus infections.

PREVENTION AND CONTROL. No vaccine is available. Mosquito control is effective, and in some areas, surveillance may be warranted to implement mosquito control efforts. Emergency mosquito adulticide spraying should be considered in the event of an epidemic.

Bibliography

Ben Nathan D, Huitinga I, Lustig S, et al: West Nile virus neuroinvasion and encephalitis induced by macrophage depletion in mice. Arch Virol 141:459, 1996.

Castle E, Leidner U, Nowak T, Wengler G: Primary structure of the West Nile flavivirus genome region coding for all nonstructural proteins. Virology 149:10, 1986.

Coldblum N, Sterk VV, Paderski B: West Nile fever: The clinical features of the disease and the isolation of West Nile virus from the blood of nine human cases. Am J Hyg 59:89, 1954.

Draganescu N, Duca M, Girjabu E, et al: Epidemic outbreak caused by West Nile virus in the crew of a Romanian cargo ship passing the Suez Canal and the Red Sea on route to Yokohama. Virologie 28:259, 1977.

Gollins SW, Porterfield JS: A new mechanism for the neutralization of enveloped viruses by antiviral antibody. Nature 321:244, 1986.

Hayes CG, Baqar S, Ahmed T, et al: West Nile virus in Pakistan: I. Seroepidemiological studies in Punjab Province. Trans R Soc Trop Med Hyg 76:431, 1982.

King NJ, Maxwell LE, Kesson AM: Induction of class I major histocompatibility complex antigen expression by West Nile virus on gamma interferon–refractory early murine trophoblast cells. Proc Natl Acad Sci USA 86:911, 1989.

Luby JP: St. Louis encephalitis, Rocio encephalitis and West Nile fever. *In* Porterfield JS (ed): Exotic Viral Infections. London, Chapman and Hall Medical, 1995, pp 183–202.

Marberg K, Goldblum N, Sterk VV, et al: The natural history of West Nile fever: I. Clinical observations during an epidemic in Israel. Am J Hyg 64:259, 1956.

Mathiot CC, Georges AJ, Deubel V: Comparative analysis of West Nile virus strains isolated from human and animal hosts using monoclonal antibodies and cDNA restriction digest profiles. Res Virol 141:533, 1990.

McIntosh BM, Jopp PG, Dos Santos I, Meenehan GM: Epidemics of West Nile and Sindbis viruses in South Africa with *Culex* (Culex) *univittatus* Theobald as vector. S Afr J Sci 76:295, 1976.

Peiris JS: West Nile fever. *In* Beran GW (ed): Handbook of Zoonoses, 2nd ed. Boca Raton, FL, CRC Press, 1996, pp 139–398.

Peiris JS, Gordon S, Unkeless JC, Porterfield JS: Monoclonal anti-Fc receptor IgG blocks antibody enhancement of viral replication in macrophages. Nature 289:189, 1981.

Smithburn KC, Hughes TP, Burke AW, Paul JH: A neurotropic virus isolated from the blood of a native of Uganda. Am J Trop Med 20:471, 1940.

Taylor RM, Work TH, Hurlbut HS, Rizk F: A study of the ecology of West Nile virus in Egypt. Am J Trop Med Hyg 5:579, 1956.

Work TH: On the Japanese B–West Nile virus complex or an arbovirus problem of six continents. Am J Trop Med Hyg 20:169, 1971.

Work TH, Hurlbut HS, Taylor RM: Indigenous wild birds of the Nile Delta as potential West Nile virus circulating reservoirs. Am J Trop Med Hyg 4:872, 1955.

29.3 Chikungunya Fever

Theodore Tsai

DEFINITION AND ETIOLOGY. Chikungunya (CHIK) fever is an acute symmetric polyarthropathy with fever, rash, and rarely, generalized hemorrhages and CNS symptoms. The *Alphavirus* causing CHIK is placed in the Semliki Forest antigenic complex and is only differentiated from o'nyong nyong (ONN) virus by cross neutralization tests. Oligonucleotide maps of viral strains from Asia and Africa have differentiated the geographic origin of strains and may be of value in tracing viral and epidemic movements.

HISTORY. Chikungunya takes its name from a Kimakonde root verb meaning "to dry up" or "to become contorted," which appropriately describes the bent position of patients attempting to guard their painful joints against movement. The local use of the term chikungunya before the first outbreak known to Western medicine was described in Tanganyika in 1952 indicates that the disease had occurred previously. Oral history and results of serosurveys confirm the likelihood of earlier outbreaks.

DISTRIBUTION AND INCIDENCE. CHIK virus is widely distributed in Africa, the Middle East, and Asia. Historical accounts of epidemic denguelike illnesses suggest that CHIK may have been carried to the New World with the slave trade; however, the virus has never been isolated in the Western Hemisphere. CHIK is transmitted in an endemic pattern in Africa resulting in high seroprevalence rates that vary locally from 30 to 100%. Regional outbreaks in East and South Africa occurred between 1952 and 1977 and spread with high (50%) attack rates from village to village but were not reported.

In Asia, transmission occurs in long cycles of emergence followed by the virus's disappearance for variable intervals. When the virus is introduced into a susceptible urban population, epidemic infection attacking 30 to 80% of the residents may follow. During the Madras outbreak in 1964, 400,000 cases were estimated and postepidemic serosurveys indicated 38% of the population had been infected. Similar seroconversion rates were observed in Bangkok in 1962. No cases were reported from Thailand between 1988 and 1995 when a series of outbreaks re-emerged. An age cohort effect has been seen in serosurveys of areas with prior outbreaks, e.g., antibodies were present only in adults >50 years of age among Calcutta residents tested in 1994.

TRANSMISSION AND EPIDEMIOLOGY. In Africa, the CHIK virus is transmitted by forest mosquitoes to monkeys, humans, and possibly other mammals, analogous to the respective sylvan cycles of yellow fever in East, West, and South Africa. When introduced into villages, *Aedes aegypti*–borne human-to-human transmission had led to rapidly spreading epidemics. Whether because of poor surveillance or other factors, such outbreaks have not been reported recently, although seroprevalence studies indicate the continued occurrence of cases. In Asia, sylvatic viral reservoirs have not been defined; however, antibodies have been demonstrated in nonhuman primates and the virus has been isolated from bats in southern China. Highly visible epidemics have recurred in southern Asia but the virus's fate during interepidemic intervals is unknown. Continued low-level interhuman transmission may occur. *Ae. aegypti* is the principal epidemic vector, but *Ae. albopictus* and *Ae. vittatus* also may have roles in transmission.

PATHOGENESIS AND PATHOLOGY. After an infectious mosquito bite, CHIK virus appears in the blood between the second and fifth days of illness. Virus has not been recovered from other body fluids or sites and descriptive pathology is available only from examination of skin and lymph node biopsies. Perivascular infiltrate and red cell extravasation from capillaries are seen in the upper dermis; lymph node capsules are thickened by a mild inflammatory infiltrate and their internal architecture is disorganized by reticuloendothelial cell proliferation. Pathologic changes in acutely inflamed joints have not been described, but joint fluid of patients with chronic arthritis has exhibited reduced viscosity, poor mucin clot formation, and WBC counts from 2000 to 5000/mm³, and biopsies have disclosed pannus formation with acute and chronic synovial inflammation. The pathogenesis of the hemorrhagic diathesis is unstudied; however, in vitro experiments showed viral binding to platelets.

CLINICAL MANIFESTATIONS. After an incubation period of 2 to 10 days, there is a precipitous onset of fever and severe pain affecting both muscles and joints. There may be chills, headache, mild conjunctivitis, and pharyngitis as well. The joints may be so inflamed that normal activities, posture, and walking become impossible. Arthropathy is symmetric, affecting the extremities and less often the shoulders and hips. Previously injured joints are often the most sensitive. Periarticular swelling, pain, redness, and limitation of movement are pronounced and definite effusions are present in about 10% of cases. Examination reveals conjunctival and pharyngeal injection, diffuse (sometimes prominent) lymphadenopathy, and a faint macular or irritating fine papular rash, which spreads centrifugally, often to the palms and soles. The rash may appear concurrently with the defervescence of fever. The illness may be biphasic interrupted by a remission of several days. Joint pains typically are milder and may be entirely absent in children.

Complications include mild hemorrhages from mucosal surfaces and rarely, severe gastrointestinal bleeding leading to shock, myocarditis, and neurologic involvement. In a few cases, meningismus or convulsions in infants suggested the possibility of CNS infection; however, CSF examination in several cases showed no pleocytosis and in only one case, elevated protein. Acute polyneuropathy also has been reported. Acute illness in children and infants rarely has been fatal.

DIAGNOSIS. Differentiation of CHIK from dengue fever may be difficult, especially in children in whom joint symptoms may be mild or absent. More prominent lymphadenopathy and acute evolution of illness have been cited as helpful signs in children; in adults, conspicuous joint involvement differentiates the disease from dengue, in which musculoskeletal pain is more diffuse. Clinical differentiation from ONN is even more difficult, although lymphadenopathy may be more pronounced in ONN. Other viruses producing acute symmetric polyarthropathy, e.g., Sindbis, West Nile, rubella, parvovirus, hepatitis A and B, mumps, Epstein-Barr virus (EBV), and enteroviruses, should be considered as well as serum sickness, Henoch-Schönlein purpura, enteroarthritis, disseminated gonococcal infection, and acute rheumatoid arthritis.

Routine laboratory examinations are not specific. The erythrocyte sedimentation rate (ESR) may be prolonged to 20 to 50 mm/hr with an elevated C protein. Low titers of rheumatoid factor (1:5) may appear. The infection can be confirmed by isolating the virus or identifying genomic products in acute-phase blood specimens or, serologically, by demonstrating specific IgM or fourfold changes in other antibodies. Cross reactions with ONN virus are a limitation of serologic testing.

TREATMENT AND PROGNOSIS. Symptomatic treatment with nonsteroidal anti-inflammatory drugs and rest should provide relief from the acute symptoms. Arthropathy, usually limited to pain and limitation of movement, may persist for months or, in one third of cases, for 1 year or more. Residual symptoms are more common in adults and especially in elderly patients. Destructive arthritis has not been reported, but patients with persistent joint pain may need long-term analgesic and anti-inflammatory therapy.

PREVENTION AND CONTROL. An experimental live-attenuated vaccine has been shown to produce high levels of neutralizing antibody in human volunteers but efficacy has not been tested. Mosquito repellents are recommended for persons traveling to endemic or epidemic areas. Community programs of *Ae. aegypti* control for dengue and yellow fever also will reduce risk of CHIK transmission.

Bibliography

Kennedy AC, Fleming J, Solomon L: Chikungunya viral arthropathy: A clinical description. J Rheumatol 7:231, 1980.

Moore DL, Reddy S, Akinkugbe FM, et al: An epidemic of chikungunya fever at Ibadan, Nigeria, 1969. Ann Trop Med Parasitol 68:59, 1974.

Nimmannitya S, Halstead SB, Cohen SN, Margiotta MR: Dengue and chikungunya virus infection in man in Thailand, 1962–64: I. Observations on hospitalized patients with hemorrhagic fever. Am J Trop Med Hyg 18:954, 1969.

Thiruvengadam KV, Kalyanasundaram V, Rajgopal J: Clinical and pathological studies on chikungunya fever in Madras city. Indian J Med Res 53:729, 1965.

29.4 O'nyong Nyong Fever

Theodore Tsai

DEFINITION AND ETIOLOGY. O'nyong nyong (ONN) fever is an acute symmetric polyarthropathy resembling chikungunya (CHIK) in its clinical features and human-to-human transmission but limited in its distribution to Africa. The virus is closely related to CHIK virus, from which it can be differentiated antigenically and by genomic sequencing. Viral strains from the first recognized outbreak in 1959 and from the most recent emergence in 1995 share a 90% homology with Igbo-Ora virus, a related alphavirus isolated from West Africa.

HISTORY. The disease name, derived from an Acholi term meaning "very painful and weak," characterizes the illness's principal symptom of acute debilitating joint pain. The illness came to light with an explosive outbreak that began in Uganda in 1959 and subsequently spread over a 3-year interval to the remainder of sub-Saharan Africa. An estimated 2 million persons were infected before disease activity disappeared from recognition. Although epidemic studies proved a mosquito-borne person-to-person mode of transmission, the viral reservoir never was determined. Serosurveys in Kenya indicated the virtual cessation of viral transmission and only rare viral isolations from mosquitoes were recovered in subsequent field studies. The disease re-emerged in 1995 in an epidemic in Uganda not far from the virus's first recognized source. Retrospective serologic studies indicate that the virus had been circulating in Kenya in 1994 to 1995 suggesting that surveillance may have missed focal ongoing transmission during the previous apparently silent interval. The close relationship of ONN and Igbo-Ora viruses also suggests that continued transmission may have escaped notice, since, at least in Nigeria, there was evidence of ongoing transmission of the latter virus to animals.

DISTRIBUTION AND INCIDENCE. Evidence of viral transmission has been reported in the triangle defined roughly by Kenya, Senegal, and Mozambique. During the initial recognized outbreak, epidemics spread explosively, attacking 30 to 90% of exposed populations from village to village at a rate of 1.7 miles/day. Oral accounts suggesting an earlier outbreak in 1905 were confirmed by an age cohort effect of reduced attack rates in adults >50 years of age.

TRANSMISSION AND EPIDEMIOLOGY. *Anopheles gambiae* and *Anopheles funestus*, the principal epidemic vectors, rapidly transmit the virus from viremic humans to susceptible humans until their numbers are "exhausted" by immunity. Saltatory spread by viremic individuals traveling long distances by train or vehicles has occurred. ONN vectors also are the principal malaria vectors in areas experiencing outbreaks. Where surface waters are available, they breed throughout the year with expansions of vector populations during the rainy season. Risk factors for acquiring infection are similar to those for malaria. Similar to CHIK, clinical illness may be milder in children than in adults.

The fate of the virus during interepidemic intervals still is unknown, but viral transmission in a silent cycle among animal hosts, possibly involving other arthropod vectors, with only an occasional involvement of epidemic vectors, explain the apparent rarity of human infections.

CLINICAL MANIFESTATION. After a brief incubation period of less than a week, fever, chills, headache, backache, and muscle and joint pains begin abruptly, in the most severe cases, leading to excruciating joint pain and incapacity to work, walk, or even sit. Arthropathy typically is symmetric involving most or all joints, especially those in the extremities. Severe conjunctivitis and suffusion are common and in two thirds of cases, a morbilliform rash, similar to measles, appears on the fourth day of illness or with remission of other symptoms. Pharyngitis was a feature of Igbo-Ora infection. Pronounced lymphadenopathy is a principal clinical feature; nodes, especially in the cervical chains, may be massively enlarged. Epistaxis occurs in some patients but other hemorrhagic manifestations have not been prominent. Other complications have not been reported. Recovery may be prolonged by weakness for several weeks; little is known about the chronicity of joint symptoms.

DIAGNOSIS. Individual cases cannot be differentiated easily from acute arthropathy due to CHIK and other causes; to date, cases have been detected only during epidemics (Chapter 29.3). Virus can be recovered from blood obtained during the first 6 days of illness by inoculating Vero or mosquito cell lines; the virus kills suckling mice only after several blind passages. Rapid diagnosis also is possible by polymerase chain reaction (PCR) detection of genomic sequences or ELISA detection of viral-specific IgM in acute-phase blood samples.

TREATMENT, PREVENTION, AND CONTROL. The illness is self-limited, but therapy with nonsteroidal anti-inflammatory drugs benefits joint symptoms. Preventive measures against exposure to malaria vectors, e.g., bednets and residual indoor insecticides, also should be effective in controlling epidemic ONN.

Bibliography

Johnson BK: O'nyong nyong virus disease. *In* Monath TP (ed): The Arboviruses: Epidemiology and Ecology, Vol III. Boca Raton, FL, CRC Press, 1988, p 217.

Rwaguma EB, Lutwanma JJ, Sempala SDK: Emergence of epidemic O'nyong nyong fever in southwestern Uganda after an absence of 35 years. Emerg Infect Dis 3:77, 1997.

Shore H: O'nyong nyong fever: An epidemic virus disease in East Africa: III. Some clinical and epidemiological observations in the northern province of Uganda. Trans R Soc Trop Med Hyg 55:361, 1961.

Williams MC, Woodall JP, Gillett JD: O'nyong nyong fever: An epidemic virus disease in East Africa: VII. Virus isolations from man and serological studies up to July 1961. Trans R Soc Trop Med Hyg 59:186, 1965.

29.5 Sindbis Fever

Theodore Tsai

DEFINITION. Mosquito-borne Sindbis fever produces a self-limited febrile illness with rash and polyarthropathy.

ETIOLOGY AND HISTORY. Sindbis, Western equine encephalitis, and other chiefly mosquito-borne viruses form a serocomplex within the *Alphavirus* genus. Antigenic varieties have been described from Australia, Europe (Ockelbo), and West Africa (Babanki) but no associated clinical or epidemiologic differences have been elucidated. The virus was first isolated in 1952 from *Culex univittatus* mosquitoes in Egypt and was shown to be a human pathogen when it was recovered from ill patients in Uganda.

DISTRIBUTION AND INCIDENCE. Illness is recognized principally in Africa, the Middle East, and northern Europe but sporadic cases and viral isolates have been reported from Australia and Asia. Outbreaks in South Africa have been associated with simultaneous epidemics of West Nile fever, a flaviviral infection transmitted in a similar *Cx. univittatus*–avian cycle. Enzootic viral transmission varies regionally, leading to a wide range of human seroprevalence from 1 to 50%. Outbreaks in South Africa have led to thousands of cases and in 1982, the disease was recognized for the first time in Europe when a series of small outbreaks was reported from Fenno-Scandinavia. The disease, called Ockelbo fever in Sweden, now is known to be an endemic infection affecting principally berry pickers, mushroom gatherers, and naturalists entering the virus's sylvatic habitat in the spring and early summer. Scores of cases are reported annually and seroprevalence rates range from 10 to 50% in the narrow range of latitudes where the virus is transmitted. Genetic sequences of Scandinavian strains indicate dissimilarities from Egyptian and Australian strains and a closer relationship with South African isolates, indicating their possible introduction by migratory birds. Little is known about viral transmission patterns in Australia and the Far East. Isolated cases, but no outbreaks, have been reported from Australia, Malaysia, the Middle East, and India but the mild nondescript nature of the illness easily could have escaped notice.

TRANSMISSION AND EPIDEMIOLOGY. The virus is transmitted in an avian-mosquito cycle with the participation of various *Culex* species as the principal enzootic vector in different locations. *Cx. univittatus* transmits the virus in inland locations of Africa but *Cx. neavei* is a more important vector along coastal South Africa. Although the virus is the most widely distributed mosquito-borne virus collected in Australia and New Guinea, human cases are recognized rarely; *Cx. annulirostris* is the principal vector. The virus has been isolated from *Cx. tritaeniorhynchus*, *Cx. bitaeniorhynchus*, and anopheline species in Asia. In northern Europe, Sindbis virus is transmitted in the enzootic cycle by *Culiseta morsitans* and *Cx. torrentium* with *Aedes cinereus* and *Ae. communis* functioning as bridging vectors. Numerous avian species have been shown by experimental studies and from field studies to be effective viral amplifiers. The virus also has been isolated from ticks collected from migratory birds and from mites.

Cases in Scandinavia occur mainly from July to September, whereas outbreaks in South Africa have occurred during the austral summer from December to April.

PATHOLOGY AND PATHOGENESIS. The difficulty in isolating virus from acute blood samples indicates a brief low-level viremia. In a patient from whom virus was isolated from a skin vesicle, endothelial damage, lymphocytic infiltration edema, hemorrhage, and occasional cellular necrosis were seen histopathologically. The immunohistochemical distribution of viral antigen has not been reported. Levels of circulating immune complexes during the acute phase of illness have not correlated with clinical severity and C3 and C4 levels were normal, suggesting no direct role of immune complexes in the pathogenesis of arthritis. Destructive changes in the muscles, tendons, and connective tissue of experimentally infected mice suggest that viral infection of these structures in humans may underlie the musculoskeletal symptoms.

CLINICAL MANIFESTATIONS. The incubation period has not been reported. Although fever, rash, and polyarthropathy constitute the full disease syndrome, in more than one third of cases no fever is reported and in other cases, no rash is present. Associated symptoms include malaise, headache, myalgias, and occasionally, conjunctivitis and pharyngitis. The severity of joint pain and the number of involved joints vary widely, but any and all joints, including the spine, may be involved. The fingers, ankles, wrists, elbows, and knees are most frequently affected, usually in a symmetric distribution. Joint effusions may be present, but more often arthropathy is manifested by periarticular swelling, pain, and limitation of movement. Nerve entrapment may produce paresthesias. The rash evolves from a macular eruption of the trunk and limbs to a papular and sometimes vesicular rash that often becomes pruritic. Lesions are smaller than those in chickenpox and in contradistinction to chickenpox, evolve and fade over several days in synchrony. In one case, cutaneous hemorrhagic bullae developed.

In 58% of cases joint symptoms resolve over a period of weeks, but symptoms persist for up to 2 years or longer in one third of cases. Infection has not been associated with permanent destructive arthritis.

CNS infection has been reported in sporadic cases from China.

THERAPY. Symptomatic therapy with nonsteroidal anti-inflammatory drugs and rest provide relief of joint symptoms, but response may vary with individual drugs.

DIAGNOSIS. Virus and genomic products are recovered from blood and skin vesicular fluid in rare instances only. The diagnosis is confirmed serologically, by demonstrating fourfold or greater antibody titer changes or by detection of viral-specific IgM. IgM-capture ELISA is highly sensitive; cross reactions occur with other western equine encephalomyelitis complex viruses but their geographic distributions differ.

The differential diagnosis includes serum sickness, rubella, and infections with other agents that produce a symmetric polyarthritis, including human parvovirus, *Mycoplasma pneumoniae*, hepatitis A and B, EBV, and enteroviruses; and post- and parainfectious enteroarthritis, disseminating gonococcal infection, rheumatic fever, Henöch-Schonlein purpura, and Reiter syndrome. The illness also could mimic the early presentation of rheumatoid arthritis.

PREVENTION AND CONTROL. No vaccine is available. Individual protection against mosquito exposure and mosquito bites is recommended.

Bibliography

Horling J, Vene S, Franzen C, Niklasson B: Detection of Ockelbo virus RNA in skin biopsies by polymerase chain reaction. J Clin Microbiol 31:2004, 1993.

Lundstrom JO, Vene S, Espmark A, et al: Geographical and temporal distribution of Ockelbo disease in Sweden. Epidemiol Infect 106:567, 1991.

McIntosh BM, McBillivray GM, Dickinson DB, et al: Illness caused by Sindbis and West Nile viruses in South Africa. S Afr Med J 39:291, 1964.

Nikalsson B, Espmark A, Lundstrom J: Occurrence of arthralgia and specific IgM antibodies three to four years after Ockelbo disease. J Infect Dis 157:832, 1988.

29.6 *Epidemic Polyarthritis*

John Aaskov

DEFINITION AND HISTORY. Epidemic polyarthritis is caused by a mosquito-borne *Alphavirus*, Ross River virus. The first recorded outbreak of what is believed to have been epidemic polyarthritis occurred in 1926 in New South Wales.

TABLE 29–1. Average Annual Notifications of Epidemic Polyarthritis From Australian States (1992–1995)

State	No. of Cases	Incidence (per 100,000 Residents)
Queensland	2852	89.2
New South Wales	354	5.8
Australian Capital Territory	2	0.7
Victoria	357	8.0
Tasmania	0	0
South Australia	221	15.0
Western Australia	311	18.3
Northern Territory	285	166.5

Data provided by the Communicable Diseases Branch, Commonwealth Department of Health, Canberra, Australia.

Serologic confirmation of Ross River virus infection only became possible after the virus was isolated from *Aedes vigilax* mosquitoes in 1963. The steady increase in the number of reported cases up to 1989–1990 reflects the increase in the number of laboratories performing diagnostic serology for Ross River virus infection. The clinical illness is characterized by arthritis, fever, and rash.

EPIDEMIOLOGY

Distribution. Epidemic polyarthritis is endemic in Australia and New Guinea and possibly New Caledonia. Most of Australia's 5000 annual cases occur in the northern and coastal regions with frequent outbreaks along the major river networks (Table 29–1).

Epidemics of Ross River virus infection occurred in Fiji, Samoa, Tonga, and the Cook Islands in 1979–1980, but no disease has been reported from these islands since then—presumably due, in part, to a high "herd immunity." Cases of epidemic polyarthritis have also occurred in Europe and the United States in tourists returning from Australasia.

Incidence. The ratio of subclinical to clinical infections varies from 15:1 in endemic areas to 2:1 during epidemics. Earlier estimates of 80:1 for the ratio of subclinical to clinical infection in endemic areas were inaccurate due to the absence of comprehensive serodiagnostic facilities.

In those parts of northern Australia where disease is endemic, approximately 1.5% of the population are infected with Ross River virus each year, whereas in southern areas where disease is more epidemic, the average infection rate is 0.5% or less per annum. This constant rate of infection, most of which is subclinical, may explain the steady decrease in clinical infections in those >40 years of age.

Transmission. Ross River virus has been isolated from five genera of mosquitoes (*Aedes, Culex, Anopheles, Mansonia, Coquillettidia*), and although this does not prove they are vectors, 19 species have been shown, in laboratory experiments, to be able to transmit this virus.

As might be expected from the wide range of habitats occupied by this group of mosquitoes, human disease occurs throughout Australia. Serologic surveys indicate that a wide range of native and domestic animals are infected with Ross River virus, and epidemiologic data suggest that this virus can exist in zoonotic cycles. However, most clinical disease occurs in people living in urban areas suggesting that, as was the case in the epidemic in Fiji in 1979, the virus also moves very efficiently in human-mosquito-human cycles.

PATHOPHYSIOLOGY

Pathology. The pathogenesis of the arthritis following Ross River virus infection is unknown. Those with the HLA-DR7 haplotype are 3.3 times as likely to develop clinical disease

following infection as those without. There is no correlation between anti–Ross River virus antibody titers and the presence or duration of disease. Virus has never been recovered from the joint of a patient, although viral antigen has been demonstrated in mononuclear cells in joint exudate. The inflammatory response in both synovium and joint fluid consists of predominantly mononuclear leukocytes at all stages of disease, and neither immune complexes nor complement split products have been detected in joint fluid.

Immunity. A virus-specific T-lymphoproliferative response has been detected in the peripheral blood of epidemic polyarthritis patients, but neither its magnitude nor its duration correlated with disease symptoms. $CD8^+$ virus-specific cytotoxic T cells have not been detected in blood from patients, but a strong correlation was observed between changes in peripheral natural killer (NK) cell activity and symptoms. Functional NK cells were also recovered from the knee of an epidemic polyarthritis patient.

CLINICAL MANIFESTATIONS. Epidemic polyarthritis is characterized by arthritis, particularly in the joints of the hands and feet and in the knees. Approximately 50% of patients experience fever and/or chills lasting 2 to 4 days, and a similar proportion develop a maculopapular rubella-like rash that may cover the whole body. This triad of symptoms may occur in any sequence. Patients may also develop a range of other nonspecific signs and symptoms (e.g., myalgia, lethargy, headache) (Table 29–2). Clinical symptoms occur less commonly in children and adolescents than in adults and are usually less severe and of shorter duration. Epidemic polyarthritis is seldom diagnosed in febrile patients without arthritis.

The interval from infection to onset of symptoms varies from 2 to 21 days, with a range of 7 to 9 days being most common. Virus can be isolated from the peripheral blood from some patients for up to 7 days after onset of symptoms.

The arthritis commonly lasts 30 to 40 weeks in adults, and 25% of patients have symptoms a year after onset. The arthritis is usually intense during the first 1 or 2 weeks after onset, after which it steadily decreases in severity with asymptomatic periods varying in duration from a few days to a week or two. Patients may also experience relapses of severe arthritis for a week or more during the recovery period. Once recovery is complete, there are no long-term sequelae and there are no confirmed reports of a second clinical infection.

There are very rare reports of glomerulonephritis and signs of CNS pathology following Ross River virus infection. The virus also has the ability to cross the placenta during pregnancy (approximately 3% of infected mothers) but without any detectable effect on the fetus.

DIAGNOSIS. Most patients are diagnosed by detecting anti–Ross River virus IgM antibody in serum collected within a month of onset of symptoms compatible with a Ross River virus infection. ELISA kits to perform these assays are now available commercially. Although isolation of virus or the detection of fourfold rises in antibody titer in paired sera

TABLE 29–2. Common Symptoms of Epidemic Polyarthritis

Symptom	Approximate Frequency (%)
Arthritis	100
Rash	50
Myalgia	50
Fever/chills	36
Headache	33
Paresthesia	25
Nausea	20

may be more accurate diagnostic procedures, they are rarely performed outside reference laboratories attempting to resolve some unusual diagnostic issues. Patients with EBV, cytomegalovirus, malaria, or *Coxiella* infections sometimes display extensive polyclonal B-lymphocyte activation that can result in production of IgM antibody to Ross River virus, so care should be taken when interpreting serologic data in the absence of clinical information because the patients may have a current or recent infection with any of these four organisms. There are also well-documented cases of Ross River virus IgM production continuing for years after the initial infection.

There are a number of other alphaviruses (Barmah Forest, Sindbis) and flaviviruses (Kunjin, Kokobera, and Edge Hill) in the region that cause symptoms that may be indistinguishable clinically from those of a Ross River virus infection. Rubella and human parvovirus infection should also be considered when making a differential diagnosis.

TREATMENT. There is no specific therapy for epidemic polyarthritis. Rest, but not to the point of losing significant muscle tone, is beneficial to most patients. Aspirin or indomethacin provides significant relief from arthritic symptoms. The dose and duration of medication require regular monitoring by a medical practitioner.

PREVENTION. Although a killed Ross River virus vaccine will go to clinical trial in 2000, the only effective protection against Ross River virus infection is mosquito avoidance—screening of houses, use of personal repellents, and covering of exposed parts of the body—in conjunction with well-planned vector control programs by local authorities.

Bibliography

Doherty RL, Whitehead RH, Gorman BM, et al: The isolation of a third group A arbovirus in Australia with preliminary observations on its relationship to epidemic polyarthritis. Aust J Sci 26:183, 1963.

Fraser JRE: Epidemic polyarthritis and Ross virus disease. Clin Rheum Dis 12:369, 1986.

Kay BH, Aaskov JG: Ross River virus (epidemic polyarthritis). In Monath TP (ed): The Arboviruses: Epidemiology and Ecology, Vol IV. Boca Raton, FL, CRC Press, 1986, p 93.

Mudge PR, Aaskov JG: Epidemic polyarthritis in Australia, 1980–81. Med J Aust 2:269, 1983.

29.7 Mayaro Fever

Douglas M. Watts

DEFINITION. Mayaro fever is an acute, self-limited, mild to moderately severe, febrile, mosquito-borne viral disease, usually manifested by fever, chills, headache, myalgia, and arthralgia.

ETIOLOGY AND HISTORY. Mayaro virus, of the family *Togaviridae* and the genus *Alphavirus*, is a member of the Semliki Forest antigenic complex. Mayaro virus was first isolated in 1954 from five sporadically occurring human cases. Epidemics were described in 1955 among quarry and forest workers in Para, Brazil and among Okinawan forest workers in eastern Bolivia, and during 1977 and 1978 among residents of a rural town in Belterra, Para, Brazil. More recently, five outbreaks between 1991 and 1993 were recognized in Brazil. In 1994, Mayaro virus was isolated for the first time in Peru from eight patients with febrile illness in the Northwestern Pacific coastal plains and Amazon basin region. Confusion of Mayaro fever with other febrile illnesses, e.g., dengue fever, is likely to have underestimated the public health importance of this disease.

Cases of Mayaro fever based on virus isolations have been reported from Trinidad, Suriname, Brazil, Bolivia, and Peru. The virus also has been isolated from mosquitoes, lizards, and marmosets in Brazil; mosquitoes in Panama and Trinidad; and from a migrating bird in Louisiana. More recently, Mayaro virus was isolated from a febrile female patient in Ohio, apparently infected while visiting Iquitos, Peru. A survey conducted during the 1954 and 1955 Bolivian epidemic suggested that 10 to 15% of febrile illness in 200 people was caused by Mayaro virus. In the 1978 outbreak in Belterra, Brazil, 20% of 4000 residents were infected, with about 80% developing clinical illness. Sero conversions to Mayaro virus were demonstrated among 2 to 5.3% of 874 Dutch soldiers who were deployed for 1 year in Suriname.

TRANSMISSION AND EPIDEMIOLOGY. Mayaro fever epidemics in Brazil occurred during the rainy season, which corresponded with an apparent increase in the abundance of the mosquito vector(s). Working and/or residing in or near forested areas appeared to be the greatest risk for contracting this disease. Antibody rates vary, but generally increase with age to high levels among older adults, especially men. The sylvan transmission cycle involves nonhuman primates and *Haemagogus* mosquitoes in the tropical forest of South America. Although the transmission cycle appears to be analogous to that of yellow fever, an urban cycle has not been documented for Mayaro virus.

PATHOLOGY AND PATHOGENESIS. The pathogenesis of Mayaro fever among humans is unknown. Infection of mice produced necrosis of skeletal muscle, periosteum, and perichondrial tissues, which may account for myalgia and arthralgia observed during human disease.

CLINICAL MANIFESTATIONS AND COMPLICATIONS. After an incubation period of about 7 to 12 days, illness begins with an abrupt onset, usually accompanied by a fever of 2 to 4 days' duration, chills, headache, myalgia, and arthralgia. Other clinical manifestations include epigastric pain, backache, nausea, vomiting, photophobia, vertigo, dizziness, eye pain, rash, and diarrhea. Clinical manifestations appear during the viremic phase, and usually last from 2 to 5 days. However, arthralgia, the most prominent and severe clinical feature, may persist for up to 2 months in some cases. Joint pain involves the wrists, ankles and toes, and occasionally the elbows and knees. Swelling of affected joints is noted in about 20% of cases and lasts from 4 to 5 days, up to 2 months in some cases. A maculopapular or micropapular rash occurs in up to two thirds of patients, usually appearing on about the fifth day after onset and persisting for 3 to 4 days. Rash is more common in children and more prominent on the trunk and limbs than on the face. Other features include inguinal lymphadenopathy and leukopenia with mild lymphocytosis during the first week of illness.

All observed cases of Mayaro fever have recovered without long-term sequelae. Illness ranges from mild to severe and in some cases may be briefly incapacitating. Treatment is symptomatic.

DIAGNOSIS. The diagnosis can be made by isolating the virus from blood or serum during the acute phase of illness or by demonstrating a rise in viral-specific antibodies 1 to 3 weeks after onset. Virus can be isolated from serum taken during the first 3 to 4 days after onset by inoculating infant mice or hamsters, chicken eggs and cell cultures, including C6/36, VERO, HeLa, BHK-21, and primary baby chicken and duck embryo cells. Viral isolates can be identified by IF and neutralization tests. Available serologic tests include hemagglutination-inhibition, complement fixation, neutralization, and ELISA assays.

PREVENTION AND CONTROL. Although there are no specific measures to prevent the disease, persons at risk should avoid mosquito bites by use of repellents and protective clothing, and by sleeping under bednets. During outbreaks, application of ultra-low-volume insecticides to communities adjacent to forested areas may be considered.

Bibliography

Hoch AL, Peterson NE, LeDuc JW, et al: An outbreak of Mayaro virus disease in Belterra, Brazil: III. Entomological and ecological studies. Am J Trop Med Hyg 30:689, 1981.

LeDuc JW, Pinherio FP, Travassos da Rosa APA: An outbreak of Mayaro virus disease in Belterra, Brazil: II. Epidemiology. Am J Trop Med Hyg 30:682, 1981.

Pinherio FP, Freitas RB, Travassos da Rosa APA, et al: An outbreak of Mayaro virus disease in Belterra, Brazil: I. Clinical and virological findings. Am J Trop Med Hyg 30:674, 1981.

Pinherio FP, LeDuc JW: Mayaro virus disease. *In* Monath TP (ed): The Arboviruses: Epidemiology and Ecology, Vol. III, pp 137–150. Boca Raton, FL, CRC Press, 1988.

Pinherio FP, Travassos da Rosa APA: Mayaro fever. *In* Beran GW (ed): Handbook of Zoonoses. Section B: Viral. Boca Raton, FL, CRC Press, 1994, pp 201–203.

29.8 Group C Virus Fevers

Douglas M. Watts

DEFINITION. The group C viral fevers are caused by at least 13 antigenically related viruses. All cause undifferentiated self-limited febrile illnesses characterized by headache, vertigo, backache, muscle and joint pain, nausea, and photophobia.

ETIOLOGY AND HISTORY. The 13 group C viruses comprise four antigenic complexes, including (1) Caraparu, types Caraparu, Apeu, Vinces and Bruconha, and subtype Ossa; (2) Madrid virus, type Madrid; (3) Marituba, types Marituba, Nepuyo, and Gumbo Limbo, and subtypes Murutucu and Restan; and (4) Oriboca, type Oriboca and subtype Itaqui. As members of the genus *Bunyavirus* and family *Bunyaviridae*, the virions are spherical, 90 to 100 nm in diameter, and contain a single-strand, three-segmented, negative-sense RNA genome. The segmented genomes may allow for genetic reassortment among these viruses, which may explain their genetic diversity.

The first five group C viruses were isolated during 1954 from sentinel *Cebus* monkeys in forested areas near Belem, Brazil. Subsequently, eight other viruses of this group were obtained from mosquitoes, humans, sentinel hamsters, rodents, marsupials, and bats in forested or forest fringe areas in Brazil, Trinidad, Panama, French Guiana, Suriname, Peru, Honduras, Mexico, Guatemala, and Venezuela. Also, one strain, Gumbo Limbo, was isolated from a migrating bird in Florida. More recently, an unidentified group C virus was isolated during 1994 from a human case of febrile illness near Iquitos, Peru. Persons whose occupation involves activities in the forest are at greatest risk for infection. Although the viruses have not been associated with epidemics or fatal disease, they are a common cause of sporadic, mild to severe, self-limiting febrile illness.

EPIDEMIOLOGY

Distribution. The geographic distribution of the group C viruses includes Florida, Central America, northern South America, and Brazil. Most foci are within or on the fringe of forested areas in swampy habitat in association with their specific mosquito vector(s) and vertebrate hosts. Among the 13 recognized group C viruses, 10 have been associated with human illness, including Oriboca, Caraparu, Murutucu, Restan, Nepuyo, Ossa, Apeu, Marituba, Itaqui, and Madrid viruses.

Incidence. The incidence of disease is not known. On the basis of virus isolations, >50 cases have been diagnosed among adult patients. Although epidemics have not been reported, antibody prevalence rates as high as 38% have been reported. Also, the incidence of infection among Dutch military personnel stationed for 1 year in Suriname was as high as 22% among some units, suggesting that disease may be more prevalent than viral isolations suggest.

Transmission. The roles of season, age, sex, and race on risk for acquiring group C viral infections are unknown. Cases have been documented primarily among young adult males, which likely reflects increased risk associated with occupational activities in forested areas. Most patients had a history of exposure in or adjacent to forested areas during the evening. The group C viruses are transmitted by forest mosquitoes, principally *Culex melanoconium* spp. Forest rodents, marsupials, and possibly bats are the primary vertebrate hosts.

PATHOLOGY, PATHOGENESIS, AND CLINICAL MANIFESTATIONS. The pathology and pathogenesis are not understood. Fatal human cases have not been reported. Infection of laboratory mice produces encephalitis and hepatitis.

After an incubation period of approximately 10 days or less, fever begins abruptly, occasionally is biphasic, and lasts from 2 to 5 days. Illness is accompanied by severe headache, vertigo, backache, generalized malaise, myalgia, joint pain, nausea, and photophobia. Rash has not been reported, but conjunctival injection has been noted occasionally. Severely ill patients may be prostrate. Leukopenia has been recorded in some patients. Recovery may be prolonged with weakness and anorexia lasting 1 to 2 weeks, but without sequelae. All cases of illness associated with group C viral infection have recovered without sequelae. Treatment is symptomatic.

DIAGNOSIS. Group C viruses can be isolated from blood or serum obtained during the acute phase of illness in a variety of cell cultures and by intraperitoneal and intracerebral inoculation of suckling mice. Virus can be identified by neutralization and indirect fluorescence (IF) tests. A serologic diagnosis can be made by demonstrating a rise in antibody titer by hemagglutination-inhibition, complement fixation, or neutralization tests.

PREVENTION AND CONTROL. Personal protection measures include the avoidance of mosquito bites by the use of mosquito repellents and bednets, especially from dusk to dawn in forested areas.

Bibliography

Gibbs CJ Jr, Bruckner EA, Schenker S: A case of Apeu virus infection. Am J Trop Med Hyg 13:108, 1964.

Pinheiro FP, Bensabath G, Andrade AHP, et al: Infectious diseases along Brazil's Trans-Amazon Highway: Surveillance and research. Bull PAHO 8:111, 1974.

Pinheiro FP, Travassos da Rosa APA: Group C bunyaviral fevers. *In* Beran GW (ed): Handbook of Zoonoses, Section B. Boca Raton, FL, CRC Press, 1994, pp 212–214.

Shope RE, Woodall JP, Travassos da Rosa A: The epidemiology of disease caused by viruses in group C and Guama (*Bunyaviridae*). *In* Monath TP (ed): The Arboviruses: Epidemiology and Ecology, Vol III. Boca Raton, FL, CRC Press, 1988, pp 37–42.

29.9 Oropouche Fever

Douglas M. Watts

DEFINITION. Oropouche (ORO) fever is an acute undifferentiated febrile illness characterized by an abrupt onset of fever, chills, severe headache, myalgia, arthralgia, dizziness, anorexia, weakness, and photophobia.

ETIOLOGY AND HISTORY. ORO virus is a member of the Simbu serogroup of the genus *Bunyavirus*, family *Bunyaviridae*. The serogroup is comprised of 25 antigenically related viruses from North and South America, Europe, Africa, Asia, and Australia. ORO virus is the only important human pathogen among Simbu serogroup viruses. The virion is enveloped, 90 to 100 nm in diameter, with helical capsid symmetry and three segments of single-strand negative-sense RNA. These viruses are genetically distinct from all other bunyaviruses sequenced to date, and only slight genetic differences were noted among six different ORO strains isolated during the past 4 decades.

ORO virus was originally isolated in 1955 from a febrile forest worker in Trinidad. The virus was later isolated from sylvan mosquitoes and from a sloth (*Bradypus tridactylous*) in Trinidad and Brazil. The first recognized epidemic affected about 11,000 persons in Belem, Brazil in 1961. Subsequent epidemics from 1967 to 1996 occurred in urban communities of the Amazon region of Brazil and Peru, and in the Isthmus of Panama, producing as many as 100,000 cases. The transmission of ORO, as well as all other viruses of the Simbu serogroup, has been linked to biting midges and/or mosquitoes.

EPIDEMIOLOGY

Distribution. ORO virus has been isolated from cases of human disease in Trinidad, Brazil, Panama, and Peru, and seropositive monkeys have been found in Colombia. ORO fever has been mistaken for dengue during several outbreaks, indicating that its distribution may be much wider than previously recognized. Attack rates have ranged from 18 to 42% during selected epidemics in Brazil, and from 0 to 28% in various communities in the Amazon basin of Peru, suggesting that transmission is highly focal.

Incidence and Transmission. Estimates of the size of epidemics in Brazil have ranged from several hundreds to more than 100,000 cases. Epidemics occurred primarily during the rainy season. All ages and both sexes appeared to be equally susceptible; however, in other outbreaks, infection rates were higher among females, and most cases occurred among children and young adults. The apparent to inapparent infection ratio is believed to be as high as 63%. A biting midge, *Culicoides paraensis*, is the primary vector, and viremic humans were considered to be the primary vertebrate host during epidemics in Brazil. *Culex quinquefasciatus* mosquitoes also were suspected as epidemic vectors in urban areas. A forest cycle involving primates, sloths, and birds as vertebrate hosts, and an unidentified arthropod vector has been proposed as a mechanism for vital maintenance during interepidemic periods.

PATHOLOGY AND PATHOGENESIS. ORO fever has not caused any human fatalities. Infection of monkeys and sloths produces a viremia, but no signs of illness, and laboratory mice and hamsters infected by the intracranial and intraperitoneal routes develop fatal encephalitis. Hamsters develop hepatic necrosis with cellular changes occurring as early as 6 hours after infection.

CLINICAL MANIFESTATIONS. Clinical features include an abrupt onset of fever, accompanied by chills, headache, arthralgia, myalgia, anorexia, nausea, vomiting, photophobia, dizziness, and generalized malaise. Meningitic symptoms have been reported in some cases. Rash is seldom present, but leukopenia is common. The acute phase of illness usually ranges from 2 to 5 days; however, asthenia and occasionally dizziness may persist for 3 to 4 weeks. The severity of illness varies, and a prolonged convalescence may follow the acute phase, with weakness, fatigue, and other nonspecific clinical features. During some outbreaks, up to 60% of patients relapsed with original signs and symptoms 2 to 10 days after

they became afebrile. Recurrent illness tended to occur more frequently among persons who resumed strenuous activities.

Treatment is symptomatic. Although abortions have occurred among pregnant women during ORO outbreaks, controlled studies were not conducted to verify the association.

DIAGNOSIS. A diagnosis can be made by isolating virus from blood or serum obtained during the acute phase of illness. Inoculation of infant mice, adult hamsters, and a variety of cell cultures have been used successfully. A serologic diagnosis can be made by demonstrating rising antibody titers by hemagglutination-inhibition, IF, neutralization, or ELISA assays. Virus can be identified by complement fixation, IF, and/or neutralization tests.

PREVENTION AND CONTROL. Currently, there is no vaccine for ORO fever. Vector control, including the destruction of *Culicoides paraensis* larval habitat and the reduction of adult midge populations with insecticides may be effective during epidemics.

Bibliography

LeDuc JW, Pinheiro FP: Oropouche fever. *In* Monath TP (ed): The Arboviruses: Epidemiology and Ecology, Vol IV. Boca Raton, FL, CRC Press, 1988, pp 1–14.

Pinheiro FP, Travassos da Rosa APA: Oropouche fever. *In* Beran GW (Ed): Handbook of Zoonoses. Section B: Viral. Boca Raton, FL, CRC Press, 1994, pp 214–217.

Tesh RB: The emerging epidemiology of Venezuelan hemorrhagic fever and Oropouche fever in tropical South America. Ann NY Acad Sci 740:129, 1994.

29.10 Rift Valley Fever

Ray R. Arthur

DEFINITION. Rift Valley fever is a viral zoonotic disease in Africa that primarily affects sheep and cattle. Infections in humans are usually restricted to periods of intense epizootic activity. The human disease may be characterized by a nonspecific influenza-like syndrome or, in severe cases, by retinitis, encephalitis, or hemorrhagic fever.

ETIOLOGY AND HISTORY. Rift Valley fever virus is classified in the *Phlebovirus* genus, one of the five genera of the family *Bunyaviridae*, an enveloped group of viruses with single-strand RNA genomes consisting of three segments. Phylogenetic analysis of Rift Valley fever virus strains from different parts of Africa has shown two major lineages, Egyptian and sub-Saharan. The virus has a wide host range; it grows to high titer in a variety of cell lines and is pathogenic for infant and adult mice, hamsters, and rats by the intracerebral and intraperitoneal inoculation routes. Inbred rat strains show differing susceptibility to visceral and encephalitic infection with the virus and can be used to study variation in virulence among virus strains.

The disease in sheep, cattle, and humans was first described and a virus etiology proved in 1930 in Kenya when the virus was isolated from sheep on a farm on the shores of Lake Naivahsa in the Great Rift Valley of Kenya. Disease outbreaks in the early 1900s in Kenya are retrospectively attributed to Rift Valley fever virus. In 1944, the virus was isolated from wild-caught mosquitoes in Uganda. Epizootics in southern and East Africa in the 1950s, 1960s, and early 1970s were associated with human cases, which were characterized as self-limited undifferentiated febrile illnesses. The first recognition of severe and fatal infections (hemorrhagic fever) occurred in South Africa in 1975. In 1977 to 1978, the first large human epidemic was recorded in the Nile Delta of Egypt; many cases were complicated by hemorrhagic fever, encephalitis, or retinitis. A second less severe epidemic occurred in Egypt during 1993 and 1994. In 1987 and again in 1998 epizootic epidemics occurred in southern Mauritania. The largest reported epidemic in East Africa began in late 1997 and continued into early 1998. Although epizootics occur regularly in Kenya, many cases of hemorrhagic fever were reported for the first time in Kenya and Somalia.

DISTRIBUTION AND INCIDENCE. Rift Valley fever virus is widely distributed throughout sub-Saharan Africa. The virus has been isolated in Burkina Faso, the Central African Republic (where it was first called Zinga virus), Guinea, Kenya, Mozambique, Namibia, Nigeria, Senegal, Mauritania, Somalia, South Africa, Sudan, Tanzania, Uganda, Democratic Republic of the Congo, Zambia, and Zimbabwe. Serologic evidence suggests virus activity in many other countries. Epizootics affecting livestock have been most frequent in South Africa, Zambia, Zimbabwe, Kenya, Tanzania, and Uganda, but have been associated with a relatively low incidence of human disease. In contrast, the recent outbreaks in Egypt, Mauritania, and East Africa were characterized by high attack rates in livestock and humans and by severe human disease. In the 1977 to 1978 Egyptian epidemic, more than 18,000 human cases and 598 deaths were officially reported, but other estimates indicate an incidence of at least 200,000 cases. The second epidemic in Egypt (1993 to 1994) was less severe; retinitis was the most frequent complication, although a small number of encephalitis and hemorrhagic fever cases were reported. In the 1987 to 1988 Mauritanian epidemic, 224 deaths were reported; considerably fewer deaths were reported in 1998. Initial estimates for the 1997 to 1998 epidemic in East Africa are 89,000 cases with approximately 200 deaths.

TRANSMISSION AND EPIDEMIOLOGY. Infection of domestic livestock is the result of transmission by mosquitoes. Many mosquito species belonging to five genera have yielded virus isolations. Cattle and sheep develop high-titer viremias and serve as the source of infection for mosquitoes. Epizootics coincide with periods of heavy rainfall and high vector density. Direct contact, mechanical transmission by biting and nonbiting insects, or milk-borne spread may also play a role in animal infection.

Transmission to humans may occur by the bite of infected vectors or by direct contact with body fluids (particularly blood or amniotic fluid from aborting animals), carcasses, tissues, and organs of infected animals; butchers, ranchers, veterinarians, and others with frequent exposure to animals are at highest risk of infection. Aerosol infection can occur under both natural and laboratory conditions.

In the Egyptian epidemics, where many persons acquired Rift Valley fever without direct exposure to animals, arthropod-borne infection was considered a probable means of transmission. Virus isolations were made from *Culex pipiens* mosquitoes during the 1977 to 1978 outbreak. Humans develop high-titer viremias, raising the possibility of human-mosquito-human transmission. Virus can also be recovered from the throat, and interhuman spread by contact or aerosol transmission and mechanical spread by flies and fomites must be considered, but definitive evidence for this mode of transmission is absent.

The reservoirs that maintain the enzootic cycle of Rift Valley fever virus in sub-Saharan Africa are mosquito species of two subgenera of *Aedes*. In the primary cycle, eggs infected by transovarial transmission persist over the long dry season and hatch during periods of inundation of larval habitats. These mosquitoes infect domestic livestock, which serve as amplifying hosts. An important geologic feature of the enzootic East African focus is the "dambo," a shallow depression that collects ground water and serves as a breeding site for

Aedes. In years of prolonged and excessive rainfall, the initial emergence of *Aedes* vectors is followed by successive waves of secondary vectors, species of *Anopheles* and *Culex*, which further amplify the rate of virus transmission and cause recognized epizootics. It is under these conditions that infections spill over into the human population. Identification of dambos and monitoring changes in groundwater and vegetation by means of satellite remote sensing have provided new approaches to predictive surveillance.

The 1977 to 1978 Egyptian epidemic was the result of introduction of the virus into naive livestock and human populations from an enzootic focus. The extensive irrigation system provides conditions suitable for high densities of mosquitoes. The known reservoir species of floodwater *Aedes* mosquitoes are not present in Egypt and during the interval between the 1977 and 1993 outbreaks, surveillance failed to detect any viral activity. Before the discovery of transovarial transmission, studies searched for other vectors and hosts involved in transmission during intraepidemic periods. This is still a fertile area of investigation, especially in areas, e.g., Egypt where epidemics occur sporadically and known reservoir species of *Aedes* are not found.

PATHOGENESIS AND PATHOLOGY. Rift Valley fever virus is highly hepatotropic. The most extensive lesions are seen in newborn lambs and are characterized by massive hepatic necrosis. Councilman-like bodies and intranuclear eosinophilic inclusions are also described. Lymphocyte necrosis in lymph nodes, widespread serosal and visceral hemorrhages, and renal glomerular and tubular changes are present. These pathologic features are also seen to a lesser degree in adult sheep and in cattle. Laboratory rodents provide useful models of the hepatitis and encephalitis associated with human Rift Valley fever. Only limited pathologic studies of human cases have been reported. Changes include severe hepatic necrosis and hemorrhages, myocardial fiber degeneration, and interstitial pneumonitis.

CLINICAL MANIFESTATIONS AND COMPLICATIONS

In Animals. The disease in sheep and cows is characterized by fever, listlessness, leukopenia, vomiting, melena, and blood-stained nasal discharge. Mortality is 70 to 90% in newborn lambs and kids, 10 to 70% in adult sheep and calves, and usually less than 10% in adult cattle, goats, and buffaloes. Abortions are common. Equines and pigs are refractory to disease, and infection in camels is usually inapparent except for abortions in pregnant animals. It should be noted that for different outbreaks, reports of disease in some species of domestic livestock, e.g., goats and camels, attributed to Rift Valley fever vary and often lack laboratory confirmation.

In Humans. Disease onset is sudden and occurs 3 to 6 days after exposure. Uncomplicated illness (observed in 98 to 99% of symptomatic cases) is characterized by fever, malaise, chills, headache, lumbosacral pain, generalized myalgia, anorexia, nausea with epigastric discomfort, vomiting, retro-orbital pain and photophobia. Upper respiratory tract symptoms are absent. Physical findings include relative bradycardia and conjunctival injection. Clinical laboratory tests may show an initial leukocytosis followed by leukopenia; results of liver function tests are normal. The disease runs its course in 4 to 7 days and recovery is complete.

The disease in <1% of infected individuals progresses to a hemorrhagic syndrome, with hematemesis, melena, petechiae, and occasionally jaundice. In <1% of cases, signs of meningoencephalitis and elevated CSF lymphocyte counts develop 1 to 3 weeks after onset of fever and may result in permanent neurologic deficits. Fatalities are recorded in patients with both the hemorrhagic and, more rarely, the encephalitic forms.

Ocular complications develop 1 to 3 weeks after fever

onset. They occur more frequently (1 to 2% of cases) than either the hemorrhagic syndrome or encephalitis and take the form of macular, paramacular, and extramacular retinal lesions; hemorrhages; and vasculitis. The characteristic appearance of these lesions is easily recognized by ophthalmologists familiar with Rift Valley fever retinopathy and has led to the recognition of disease outbreaks that may have gone otherwise unnoticed. Central visual loss may be permanent. Presently there is no evidence for or against an increased risk of abortion in humans.

DIAGNOSIS. During the acute phase of illness, Rift Valley fever virus may be isolated from blood by inoculation of cell cultures or mice. Viral nucleic acid sequences can be detected in acute sera or tissues by the polymerase chain reaction (PCR) test. The utility of PCR as a rapid diagnostic test was demonstrated in the 1997 to 1998 East African epidemic. Viral antigens can be detected in postmortem liver tissues by immunohistochemical staining techniques. A serologic diagnosis is made by testing acute sera by IgM antibody-capture ELISA or paired acute and convalescent phase sera by IgG ELISA, hemagglutination-inhibition, complement fixation, or IF antibody tests. IgM antibodies are locally produced in the CNS in patients with encephalitis and may be measured in cerebrospinal fluid.

TREATMENT AND PROGNOSIS. Treatment of Rift Valley fever is symptomatic. Drugs that are potentially hepatotoxic or may exaggerate the bleeding diathesis should be avoided. In patients with jaundice and hemorrhage, measures to counteract shock may be required. Estimates of the case-fatality rate in hemorrhagic fever cases vary widely and may be as high as 50%. An antiviral drug, ribavirin, as well as interferon, interferon inducers, and passive antibody have demonstrated efficacy in experimental systems but remain to be tested in humans.

PREVENTION AND CONTROL. Rift Valley fever can be prevented by a sustained program of animal vaccination. Both live-attenuated and killed vaccines have been developed for veterinary use. The live vaccine offers the advantage that only one dose is required to produce long-lived immunity, but the presently available vaccine may cause abortion if given to pregnant animals. Formalin-inactivated cell culture–propagated vaccine has been used to protect laboratory and field workers and military troops; there have been several thousand recipients of this vaccine. Adequate serologic responses occur in over 95% of vaccinated persons, with only a few minor local reactions. However, the vaccine has not been licensed and is not available commercially. A live mutagen-attenuated vaccine has been shown to be safe and effective in experimental studies in pregnant animals but has not been carefully evaluated in large field trials. Human trials of this vaccine are being conducted.

Mosquito control measures are indicated in the setting of epizootic epidemics. Insecticides are effective if conditions allow access to mosquito breeding sites. Public health measures also include advice to the general public and to high-risk groups to avoid contact with sick or dead livestock. This is particularly important in cultures that practice ritual methods of slaughter, which involve only a single act of slaughtering and bleeding. For personal protection against mosquitoes, individuals should wear protective clothing, e.g., long shirts and trousers, use insect repellent, and avoid outdoor activity at peak biting times of the vector species. Surveillance, animal quarantine, and animal vaccinations are important in preventing spread of the disease.

Bibliography

Abdel-Wahab KSE-D, El Baz LM, El Tayeb EM, et al: Rift Valley fever infections in Egypt: Pathological and virological findings in man. Trans R Soc Trop Med Hyg 72:392, 1978.

Daubney R, Hudson JR, Garnham PC: Enzootic hepatitis or Rift valley fever: An undescribed disease of sheep, cattle and man from East Africa. J Pathol Bacteriol 34:545, 1931.

Meegan JM, Bailey CL: Rift Valley fever. *In* Monath TP (ed): The Arboviruses: Epidemiology and Ecology, Vol VI. Boca Raton, FL, CRC Press, 1988, pp 51–76.

An outbreak of Rift Valley fever—Eastern Africa. Wkly Epidemiol Report 73:105, 1998.

Swanepoel R, Coetzer JAW: Rift Valley fever. *In* Coetzer JAW, Thomsom GR, Tustin RC (eds): Infectious Diseases of Livestock. Cape Town, South Africa, Oxford University Press, 1994, pp 688–717.

Wilson ML: Rift Valley fever virus ecology and the epidemiology of disease emergence. Ann NY Acad Sci 740:169, 1994.

29.11 Sandfly Fever

Theodore Tsai

DEFINITION. Sandfly fevers (papataci fever, phlebotomus fever, three-day fever) are brief, self-limited, undifferentiated febrile illnesses caused by sandfly-borne viruses belonging to the phlebotomus fever serogroup. Toscana viral infection is exceptional in producing chiefly CNS infection.

ETIOLOGY AND HISTORY. At least 38 registered viruses belong to the phlebotomus fever serogroup and constitute the *Phlebovirus* genus of the family *Bunyaviridae*. Of these, eight viruses have been recovered from infected persons (sandfly fever Naples, sandfly fever Sicilian, Chagres, Candiru, Punta Toro, Toscana, Alenquer, and Rift Valley fever) (Chapter 29.10). Sandfly fever Naples, sandfly fever Sicilian, and Toscana virus are the most medically important members of the group.

Sandfly fever was delineated and transmission of the causative agent by *Phlebotomus papatasi* was described by the Austrian Military Commission in Dalmatia in 1909, but the viruses (Naples and Sicilian serotypes) were not isolated until 1943 to 1944. During the 1960s and 1970s, a large number of other phlebotomus fever serogroup viruses were isolated, mainly in the neotropics. The history of sandfly fever is closely tied to military campaigns. Toscana virus initially was isolated from sandflies in the Tuscan region of Italy and in 1983 from CSF of an aseptic meningitis patient.

DISTRIBUTION AND INCIDENCE. The distribution of Naples and Sicilian viruses overlaps that of the *P. papatasi* (Fig. 29–5), and Toscana virus, the distribution of *P. perniciosus*. Although these areas overlap geographically, antibody prevalence rates for Toscana and for sandfly fever Naples and sandfly fever Sicilian viruses often diverge, reflecting local differences in their transmission cycles. Sporadic cases, mainly in children, occur in these endemic areas. Serologic studies show acquisition of high titers of antibody early in life, and most infections escape medical attention. Sandfly fever has assumed great importance when large numbers of nonimmune persons (military troops, refugees) enter endemic areas. Nearly 20,000 cases were reported in U.S. soldiers during World War II (1.8 cases/1000 troops stationed overseas); British Middle East forces suffered an incidence of 21.5 cases/1000 troops in 1942. More recently, outbreaks occurred among United Nations soldiers on Cyprus and Russian troops in Afghanistan.

Chagres and Punta Toro viruses have been isolated in Panama and Candiru and Alenquer viruses in Brazil. The maximum prevalence of antibodies to Chagres and Punta Toro viruses in residents of Panama is 17 and 35%, respectively. Only sporadic cases of illness have been recognized.

Toscana virus occurs in the Mediterranean region where it is a frequent cause of meningoencephalitis in adults and children. Many patients give a history of outdoor exposure

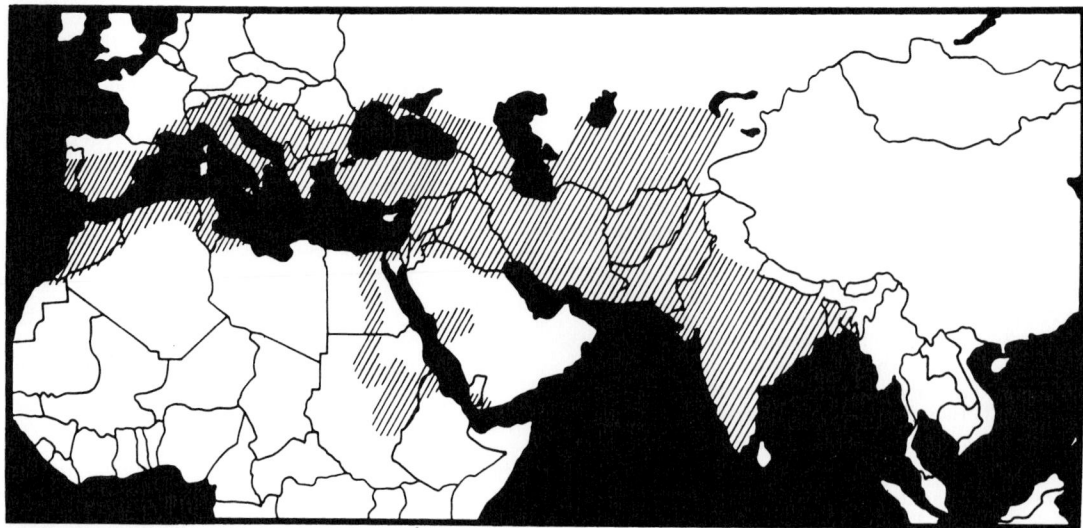

Figure 29–5. Distribution of *Phlebotomus papatasi*, which closely parallels areas affected by sandfly fever. (From Tesh RB, Saidi S, Gajdamovic SJ, et al: Bull WHO 54:663, 1976. Reprinted by permission.)

while gardening, fishing, or in other avocational or occupational activities. In central Italy, Toscana virus is the leading cause of acute childhood CNS infection. Antibody prevalence rates of 20 to 50% indicate high levels of viral transmission and frequent asymptomatic infections. Sporadic cases and outbreaks have been recognized among foreign travelers to popular tourist destinations in the Mediterranean (Fig. 29–6).

EPIDEMIOLOGY AND TRANSMISSION. *P. papatasi* is the principal vector of Naples and Sicilian viruses, and *P. perniciosus* is the chief vector of Toscana virus. These nocturnal biting midges avidly feed on humans and are closely associated with human habitation. They breed in organic debris and loose soil near houses; adults rest during the day in dark areas and crevices in and around dwellings. Only the adult females bite; they are small (2 to 3 mm) and readily pass

through bednets and screens. Sandfly fever viruses are transovarially transmitted in their vector species. This mechanism probably accounts for virus maintenance, although horizontal transmission involving viremic humans or wild and domestic vertebrates may play a secondary role. Anthroponotic transmission (sandfly-borne transmission between humans) may contribute to high epidemic attack rates. Sandfly abundance and activity may be quite focal and strongly influenced by rainfall. In some endemic areas high rates of viral infection (1:150 infected female sandflies) are found, with a high relative risk of human infection.

Punta Toro and Chagres viruses have been isolated from the Panamanian sandflies, *Lutzomyia trapidoi* and *Lutzomyia ylephilator*. Both male and female sandflies have yielded virus, indicating transovarial transmission of these viruses. *L. trapi-*

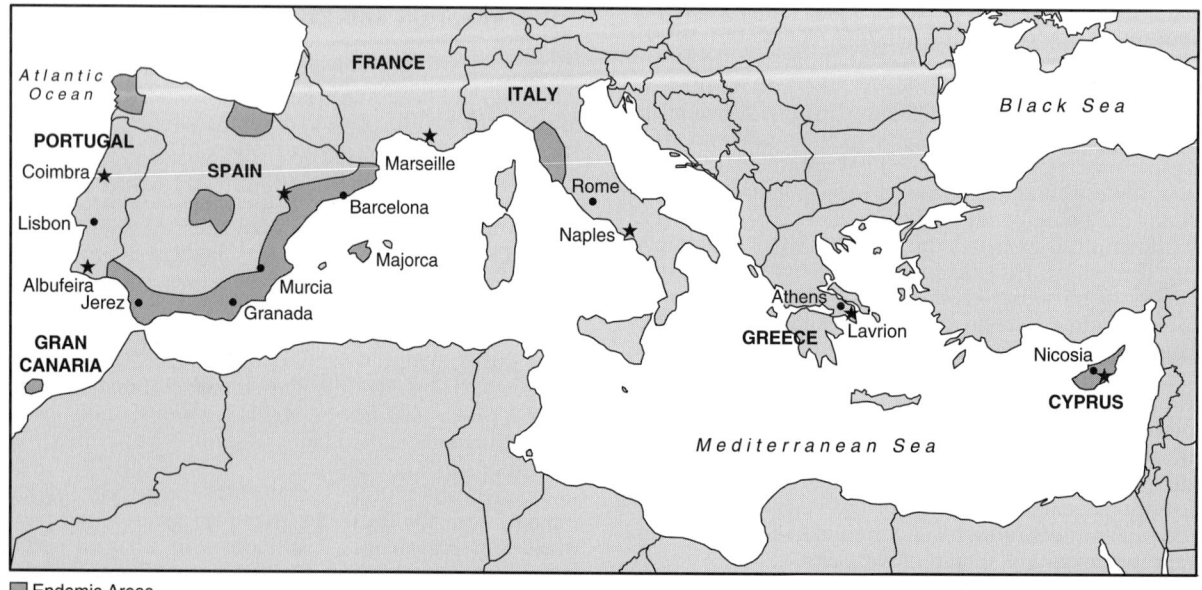

Endemic Areas
★ Cases

Figure 29–6. Areas of endemic Toscana virus transmission established by serosurveys and locations of serologically confirmed cases in travelers.

doi is a highly anthropophilic species. Toscana virus has been recovered from both male and female *P. perniciosus* in Italy and Portugal.

PATHOLOGY AND PATHOGENESIS. No fatal human cases are reported. Mice inoculated intracerebrally develop encephalitic lesions.

CLINICAL MANIFESTATIONS AND COMPLICATIONS. Illness begins abruptly after an incubation period of 3 to 6 days. Symptoms include fever, generalized malaise, headache, retro-orbital pain, photophobia, gastrointestinal symptoms (nausea, vomiting), and myalgia. The absence of rash, lymphadenopathy, and respiratory symptoms may help in differentiating the illness from other viral syndromes. The total WBC count is typically depressed, principally because of a neutropenia.

The acute febrile illness lasts approximately 3 days but may be followed by a period of weakness, fatigue, and depression lasting 1 to 2 weeks.

Homologous immunity is probably lifelong; however, neutralizing antibody titers wane significantly after 20 years. Infection with Naples virus does not confer protection against the Sicilian serotype or vice versa. Because both viruses occur together in endemic areas, clinical reinfections are reported. The clinical disease associated with the neotropical sandfly fever viruses is probably similar, but descriptions are incomplete.

Neurologic infection with Toscana virus usually results in an aseptic meningitis syndrome of acute fever, stiff neck, headache, vomiting, and photophobia, and changes in mental status and seizures, including status epilepticus, characterizing encephalitis also occur. The CSF cell count is moderately elevated with 30 to 1200 predominantly mononuclear cells/mm³. CSF protein may be slightly elevated. Electroencephalographic tracings show slowing in some cases, but both electrical and clinical abnormalities resolve without sequelae.

DIAGNOSIS. Specific diagnosis depends on serologic tests (hemagglutination-inhibition, ELISA, neutralization) on paired sera or isolation of the virus from blood, although it may be suspected on clinical and epidemiologic grounds. Detection of Toscana viral genomic sequences in CSF by PCR is positive in two thirds of cases, and virus can be recovered from CSF in 15% of cases.

PROGNOSIS AND THERAPY. Sandfly fever is self-limited. Treatment is symptomatic. Patients with Toscana CNS infection may require intensive supportive care.

PREVENTION AND CONTROL. No vaccines have been developed. Use of residual insecticides has resulted in effective control of *P. papatasi*–transmitted sandfly fever. Visitors to forested areas of the New World tropics may be advised to use repellents to protect against the bites of sandflies. Although ordinary screens are too coarse to exclude sandflies, they are highly effective when impregnated with permethrin. Oral ribavirin is an effective prophylactic agent in experimental sandfly fever.

Bibliography

Braito A, Corbisiero R, Corradini S, et al: Toscana virus infections of the central nervous system in children: A report of 14 cases. J Pediatr 132:144, 1998.

Hertig M, Sabin AB: Sandfly fever. *In* Preventive Medicine in World War II, Vol VII. Washington, DC, Office of the Surgeon General, Department of the Army, 1964, pp 109–174.

Srihongse S, Johnson C: Human infections with Chagres virus in Panama. Am J Trop Med Hyg 23:690, 1974.

Tesh RB, Saidi S, Gajdamovic SJ, et al: Serological studies on the epidemiology of sandfly fever in the Old World. Bull WHO 54:663, 1976.

30 *Viral Encephalitis*

30.1 *Rabies and Related Viruses*

M.J. Warrell and D.A. Warrell

DEFINITION. Rabies is a zoonosis of wild and domestic mammals that may be transmitted to humans, usually by the bite of a rabid dog. In humans, rabies encephalitis is almost invariably fatal. The disease is enzootic in mammals throughout most parts of the world, involving different species of carnivores and bats in different regions. The problem of human rabies is most severe in tropical developing countries where the disease is uncontrolled in domestic dogs. Rabies virus and five other morphologically and immunologically related viruses are members of the genus *Lyssavirus* of the Rhabdoviridae.

ETIOLOGY. Rabies virus is a rhabdoid or rod-shaped virus approximately 180 by 75 nm (Fig. 30–1). The nucleocapsid contains a single negative strand of RNA, nucleoprotein, phosphoprotein, and an RNA polymerase required for production of positive messenger RNA. The envelope contains lipid, matrix protein, and a glycoprotein, which forms the spiky surface projections. Repeated intracerebral passage in animals of "street virus" from naturally infected species results in a "fixed virus" of uniformly shortened incubation period and reduced pathogenicity, which is used in vaccine production. Strains of rabies virus from different vector species have been identified using panels of monoclonal antibodies or nucleotide sequence analysis. In the laboratory, rabies can be isolated and cultivated by intracerebral inoculation of suckling mice, in mouse neuroblastoma cell cultures, and in other tissue culture cell lines. The virus is inactivated by heat (56°C for 1 hour), ultraviolet light, detergents and soap solution, ethanol, iodine, quaternary ammonium compounds, chloroform, and acetone.

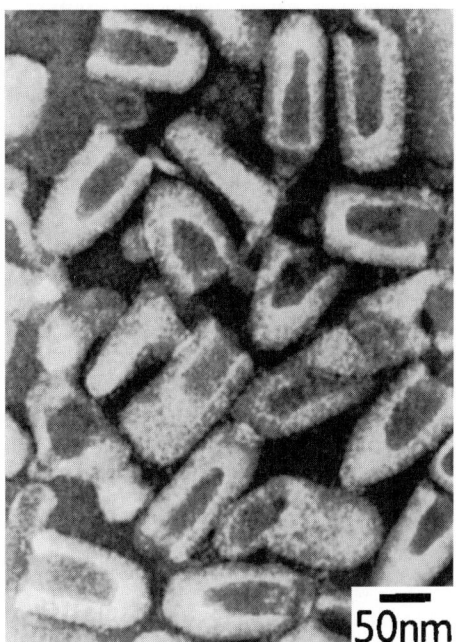

Figure 30–1. Rabies virus visualized by electron microscopy. (Courtesy of G. J. Smale.)

Nine rabies-related viruses have been isolated from shrews, bats, rodents, other mammals, and insects in Africa, Europe, and Australia (Table 30–1).

DISTRIBUTION AND INCIDENCE. Rabies is enzootic worldwide, except for Australia, Antarctica, most of Scandinavia, and a number of islands including the British Isles, Iceland, New Guinea, New Zealand, Japan, Taiwan, Singapore, Mediterranean islands, some Caribbean islands, and the Iberian peninsula. Human rabies is generally underreported. An annual mortality of 50,000 in India now seems probable. Annual mortalities in Bangladesh, Nepal, and Sri Lanka are 1.8, 1.1, and 0.6 per 100,000, respectively. Other countries reporting a high incidence of human rabies are Pakistan, Vietnam, the Philippines, Indonesia, Mexico and Ethiopia. In the United States, there have been 32 cases in the last 16 years; 53% were due to bat rabies viruses, and 38% were imported dog rabies strains.

TRANSMISSION AND EPIDEMIOLOGY. Human rabies usually results from inoculation of virus-bearing saliva through the skin by the bite of a rabid dog. Scratches, abrasions and other wounds, and intact mucosal membranes can be contaminated with infected saliva. Rare modes of infection are inhalation of virus aerosols, created in caves inhabited by bats or as a result of laboratory accidents; accidental injection of vaccines containing live rabies virus (rage de laboratoire); and transplantation of infected corneal grafts. In the ten cases of transplant rabies, the donors had died of unsuspected rabies.

The major reservoir and vector of urban rabies is the domestic dog. Sylvatic rabies occurs predominantly in skunks, foxes, raccoons, and insectivorous bats in North America; foxes in the Arctic; mongooses in some Caribbean islands; vampire bats in Latin America and Trinidad; wolves, jackals, and small carnivores in Africa and Asia; and foxes, wolves, and raccoon dogs in Europe. Each species forms its own ecologic compartment with a distinct strain of rabies virus. Transmission between sylvatic and urban populations and between different species occurs when, for example, wild Canidae come into towns, scavenging for food, or when a carnivore eats or is bitten by a sick bat. In countries, e.g., the United States, where control of rabies in domestic animals has been successful, wild animals, e.g., insectivorous bats, skunks and raccoons now constitute the main threat for spread to humans. Vampire bats (*Desmodontinae*) are confined to Southern Texas, Mexico, Central and South America, and some Caribbean islands, e.g., Trinidad and Margarita. While taking their blood meals from cattle they transmit a form of paralytic rabies responsible for the loss of 1 to 2 million cattle per year. In Trinidad, 89 human cases of vampire bat–transmitted paralytic rabies were identified between 1925 and 1935; others have been described from Mexico, Guyana, Brazil, Bolivia, and Argentina. The vectors and distribution of rabies-related viruses are listed in Table 30–1. It has been suggested that infection by rabies-related viruses, such as Mokola virus in cats and dogs in Zimbabwe, may have conferred some protection against rabies.

PATHOGENESIS AND PATHOLOGY. After entering a susceptible host the rabies surface glycoprotein attaches to a cell which it enters by endocytosis. The virus envelope fuses with the vesicle membrane and the ribonucleoprotein enters the cytoplasm. Local replication may occur in striated muscle near the site of the bite, but there may also be direct invasion of nerve cells. Postsynaptic nicotinic acetylcholine receptors at neuromuscular junctions are important binding sites but the receptors on other cell types are unknown. Once inside peripheral nerves, the virus is carried in the flow of axoplasm at the rate of about 3 mm/hr to the dorsal root ganglia where replication may be responsible for prodromal paresthesia at the site of the bite. On reaching the central nervous system (CNS), there is massive replication with viral budding from intracellular membranes of neurons and transsynaptic transmission of virus from cell to cell. Passive centrifugal spread of virus from the CNS in the axoplasm of many efferent nerves, including those of the autonomic nervous system, spreads the virus to the salivary glands (whence it is shed and in the case of infected animals spread by the bite) and to lacrimal glands and a variety of other tissues. In animals, centrifugal spread to the skin is detectable before development of symptoms. In human victims of rabies, histopathologic changes may be surprisingly mild. In furious rabies, the midbrain and medulla are mainly involved and in paralytic rabies, the spinal cord. The brain, spinal cord, and peripheral nerves may show ganglion cell degeneration, perineural and perivascular mononuclear cell infiltration (Fig. 30–2), neuronophagia, and formation of glial nodules. Negri bodies, the characteristic intracytoplasmic inclusion bodies (Fig. 30–3) contain viral components, mainly ribonucleoprotein and fragments of cellular organelles such as ribosomes. They are most numerous in pyramidal cells of the hippocampus, in Purkinje cells of the cerebellum, and in the medulla and ganglia. Extraneural changes include focal degeneration of salivary and lacrimal glands, pancreas, adrenal medulla, and lymph nodes and an interstitial myocarditis with round cell infiltration, which may explain the cardiac arrhythmias and other cardiovascular abnormalities sometimes observed in patients.

IMMUNOLOGY. Immunity to infection was thought to depend largely on neutralizing antibody induced by viral glycoprotein. Nucleoprotein antigens can stimulate protective immunity in the absence of neutralizing antibody. In unvaccinated patients with rabies encephalomyelitis, no antibody response is detectable in serum or cerebrospinal fluid (CSF) for about 7 days after the first symptom, suggesting immune evasion or immune suppression by rabies virus. Intrathecal

TABLE 30–1. Rabies-Related Viruses Causing Human Disease

Lyssavirus Genotype	Virus	Source	Geographic Range	Human Disease
3	Mokola	Shrew, mouse, cat, dog	Nigeria, Cameroon, Central African Republic, Zimbabwe	
		Human	Nigeria	Pharyngitis, fatal encephalitis
4	Duvenhage	Insectivorous bat, human	South Africa	Fatal furious rabies
5	European bat lyssavirus 1	Insectivorous bat	Germany, Denmark, Netherlands, Russia, Poland, France, Spain	
		Human	Russia	Fatal furious rabies
6	European bat lyssavirus 2	Insectivorous bat	Netherlands, Denmark, Switzerland	
		Human	Finland	Fatal furious rabies
7	Australian bat lyssavirus	Flying fox	Australia	Fatal encephalitis

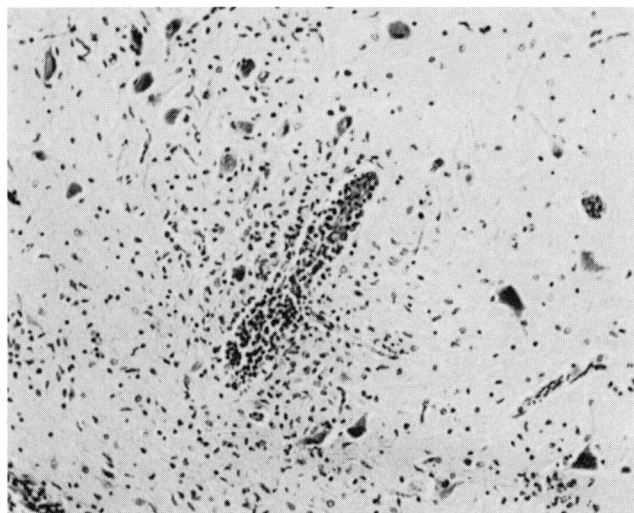

Figure 30–2. Perivascular cuffing by lymphocytes, histiocytes, and plasma cells in the brain stem of a patient dying of rabies (× 165). (Courtesy of Armed Forces Institute of Pathology, Photograph Neg. No. 73–12328.)

production of rabies IgG is detectable in some patients whose survival is prolonged by intensive care. After symptoms of encephalitis have developed, the role of antibody is uncertain. In experimental animal models, low levels of antibody may produce "early death," perhaps by enhancing viral replication. Low levels of interferon are sometimes detectable in human victims, but large amounts have been found in animal brains.

CLINICAL MANIFESTATIONS AND COMPLICATIONS

In Animals. In dogs, the incubation period is usually between 2 weeks and 4 months (extreme range, 5 days to 14 months). The illness may start with 2 to 3 days of prodromal symptoms, e.g., a change in behavior, fever, and intense irritation at the site of the bite. Dogs with the less common but more familiar furious form of the disease become aggressive, wander away from home, and may develop convulsions, dysphagia, pharyngeal paralysis causing an altered

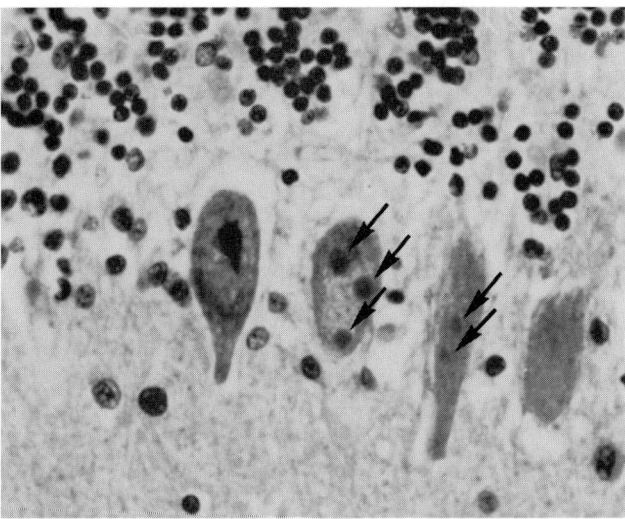

Figure 30–3. Negri bodies *(arrows)* in Purkinje cells of the cerebellum of a patient dying of rabies (× 615). (Courtesy of Armed Forces Institute of Pathology, Photograph Neg. No. 73–12332.)

bark, and hypersalivation. Those with paralytic or "dumb" rabies hide themselves away and develop paralysis of the jaw, neck, and hind limbs. Dysphagia and drooling of saliva may raise the suspicion of a foreign body stuck in the throat. Virus may be excreted in the saliva for 2 or 3 days before there are signs of rabies and the animal usually dies within the next 7 days. A small proportion of infected animals recover and may continue to excrete virus for long periods. Horses, cats, Mustelidae, and Viverridae usually exhibit furious symptoms, whereas paralytic disease is the rule in foxes and bovines. Hydrophobia is not seen in animals but inability to drink is a common symptom of rabies.

In Humans. The incubation period is usually between 20 and 90 days (extreme range, 4 days to >19 years). Relatively short incubation periods are observed after facial and severe multiple bites, transmission by corneal grafts, and accidental inoculation of live virus (rage de laboratoire). The prodromal symptom most suggestive of rabies encephalitis is paresthesia, especially itching, at the site of the healed bite wound. Other early symptoms include fever, mood changes, and nonspecific upper respiratory tract or gastrointestinal symptoms. The two distinct clinical forms of rabies, furious (agitated) and paralytic (dumb), may be determined by the strain of rabies virus or the immune response.

Furious Rabies. This is the more commonly recognized presentation. After a few days of prodromal symptoms, the pathognomonic symptom and sign of hydrophobia or aerophobia develops (Fig. 30–4). A forceful jerky inspiratory spasm is provoked either by attempts to drink water or by a draft of air on the face. Both reflexes are associated with a compelling but inexplicable terror. The spasms involve the diaphragm and accessory muscles of inspiration, particularly the sternomastoids; the head is thrown back; the arms are raised; and a generalized extension response may ensue, resulting in opisthotonus and generalized convulsions with cardiac or respiratory arrest. Splashing water on the skin, irritation of the respiratory tract, or, by conditioning, the sight, sound, or even the mention of water may provoke a hydrophobic spasm. Patients also experience episodic generalized arousal during which they become wild, hallucinated, and sometimes aggressive. During lucid intervals, they cerebrate normally and are aware of their terrible predicament. Neurologic abnormalities include meningism, cranial nerve lesions, upper motor neuron lesions, fasciculation, and involuntary movements. Generalized hyperesthesia or hyperacusis is described. Hypersalivation (Fig. 30–5), lacrimation, sweating, fluctuating blood pressure and body temperature, and inappropriate secretion of antidiuretic hormone (ADH) or diabetes insipidus suggest disturbances of the hypothalamus or autonomic nervous system. Lesions of the amygdaloid nuclei result in increased libido, priapism, and spontaneous orgasms. Without intensive care, most patients die within a few days of developing hydrophobia. About one third of patients die during a hydrophobic spasm, whereas the others lapse into coma with abnormalities of respiratory rhythm, e.g., periodic or cluster breathing with prolonged apneic periods.

Paralytic Rabies. This is less distinctive than furious rabies and is undoubtedly underdiagnosed. Almost all the cases of rabies transmitted by vampire bats in Latin America and the Caribbean were of this type, as were the cases of rabies caused by vaccination with live virus and inhalation of fixed virus. Paralytic rabies may develop in patients and experimental animals who have a low but unprotective level of immunity. After the usual prodromal symptoms, especially fever, headache, and local paresthesia, flaccid paralysis develops (usually in the bitten limb) and ascends symmetrically or asymmetrically, with pain and fasciculation in the affected

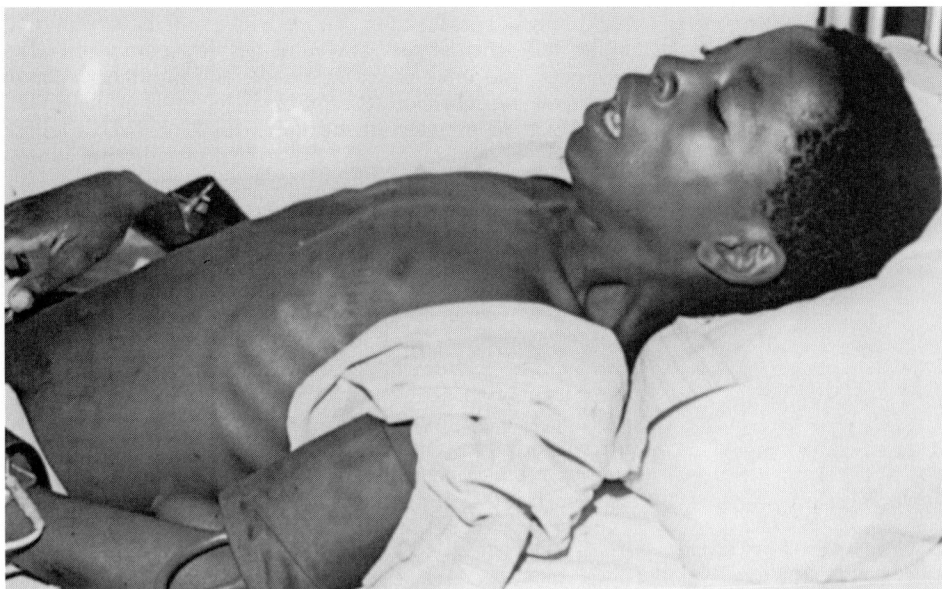

Figure **30–4.** Hydrophobic spasm in a Nigerian boy with furious rabies. Note forceful contraction of the diaphragm (depressing the xiphisternum) and sternocleidomastoid muscles. (Copyright D. A. Warrell.)

muscles and mild sensory disturbance. Paraplegia and sphincter involvement then develop and finally fatal paralysis of deglutitive and respiratory muscles. Hydrophobia is rare. Patients may survive for a month even without intensive care.

Complications of Prolonged Survival. Patients with rabies whose lives are prolonged by intensive care may develop a wide range of complications, including aspiration pneumonia, pneumothorax, respiratory failure, cardiac arrhythmias, hypotension, pulmonary edema, myocarditis with congestive cardiac failure, generalized convulsions, cerebral edema, polyneuropathy, and hematemesis associated with ulceration or tears in the mucosa of the upper gastrointestinal tract.

Infections by Rabies-Related Viruses. Two cases of Mokola virus infection were reported in children in Nigeria. A

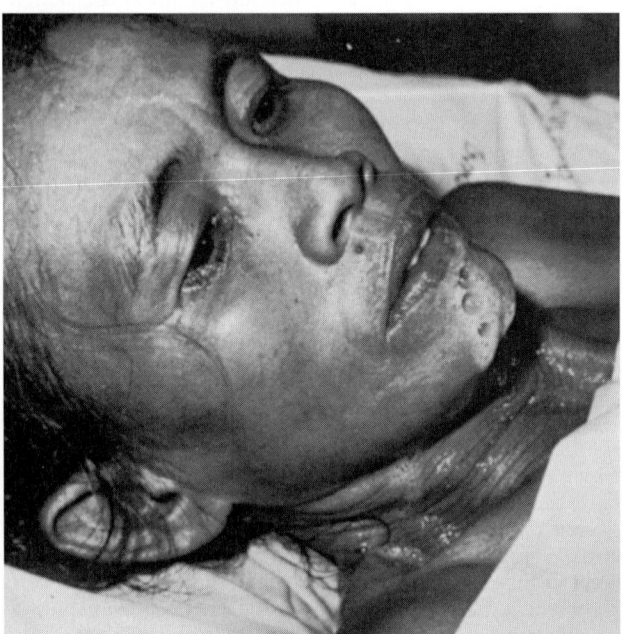

Figure **30–5.** Sweating and hypersalivation in a Thai woman with furious rabies. (Copyright D. A. Warrell.)

3½-year-old girl presented with febrile convulsions and mild congestion of the pharynx. The CSF was entirely normal and so the original description of "aseptic meningitis" was incorrect. She recovered in 48 hours. The other patient, a 6-year-old girl, was admitted to the hospital drowsy and with generalized flaccid paralysis and died 3 days later. The South African case of Duvenhage virus infection was clinically indistinguishable from furious rabies. The Swiss zoologist who died in Finland of European bat lyssavirus infection had ascending paralysis followed by hyperexcitability and spasms. Two Russian girls died of bat-transmitted furious rabies; European bat lyssavirus was isolated from one of them. An Australian bat handler died of encephalitis due to Australian bat lyssavirus infection. These infections may not be detected by routine diagnostic rabies immunofluorescent antigen detection tests.

PROGNOSIS AND TREATMENT. In patients who develop signs of rabies encephalomyelitis, the prognosis remains virtually hopeless. One patient who inhaled fixed virus developed paralytic rabies despite pre-exposure immunization, but no postexposure treatment. He survived with severe neurologic sequelae. This case is the only fully documented human survival from the infection, but the diagnosis was serologic. One patient in the United States and one in Argentina who had been given postexposure duck embryo and suckling mouse brain rabies vaccine, respectively, developed severe neurologic symptoms from which they recovered after intensive care. In neither case could rabies virus be demonstrated, but a diagnosis of rabies encephalitis rather than postvaccinal encephalitis was based on very high titers of rabies antibody in the CSF. In Mexico, two boys aged 9 and 12 years developed rabies encephalitis after multiple severe bites, despite starting cell culture vaccine 1 and 5 days after exposure, but with no hyperimmune globulin. Both survived for long periods (34 months in one case) but with severe neurologic sequelae.

Intensive care is the only known method for prolonging the lives of patients with rabies encephalomyelitis. Life-threatening complications, e.g., cardiac arrhythmias, cardiac and respiratory failure, raised intracranial pressure, convulsions, fluid and electrolyte disturbances, and hyperpyrexia can be prevented or treated. Immunosuppressive agents, including corticosteroids, rabies hyperimmune serum, antiviral agents, and interferon, have not proved effective. If intensive care is not possible or is considered inappropriate, heavy sedation and analgesia should be given to relieve the agonizing symptoms.

DIAGNOSIS

Differential Diagnosis. Rabies should be suspected in any patient who develops neurologic symptoms a week or more after being bitten by an animal. However, in up to 16% of cases no history of exposure can be elicited. Rabies is often misdiagnosed. In patients with furious rabies, the alteration in mood, hallucinations, and bizarre behavior may raise suspicions of psychiatric disease, hysteria, or malingering. Other patients are sent to otolaryngologists because of their upper respiratory tract symptoms. Rabies phobia or pseudohydrophobia is usually manifest as a caricature of popular conceptions of rabies with an emphasis on aggression and spitting. The interval between the mammal bite and the appearance of symptoms is usually short.

The spasms of tetanus may resemble hydrophobia, especially if they involve the pharyngeal muscles (hydrophobic tetanus), and this disease can also complicate an animal bite (Chapter 53). Severe tetanus is distinguished by its shorter incubation period (usually less than a week), by the presence of trismus, and the persistence of muscular rigidity between spasms. Tetanus does not cause an encephalitis and the CSF is usually normal. The combination of severe brain stem encephalitis with full consciousness in rabies is rare in other encephalitides, but has been described in serum sickness. In a case of an anaphylactic reaction to an insect sting, paroxysms of muscle spasms, tachycardia, sweating, and rage were attributed to brain stem dysfunction analogous to the "rage reaction" produced experimentally in animals by diencephalic damage or stimulation.

Various poisons, drugs, and plant toxins can produce syndromes of muscle spasm, agitation, hallucinations, psychiatric disturbances, signs of autonomic nervous system stimulation, and convulsions. These include strychnine, phenothiazines, atropine-like compounds, and cannabis. Delirium tremens may also be included in a differential diagnosis of furious rabies. Paralytic rabies should be considered in patients with rapidly ascending (Landry type) flaccid paralysis, suspected Guillain-Barré syndrome, and transverse myelitis. In the many tropical developing countries where Semple-type and suckling mouse brain rabies vaccines are still used, the most important differential diagnosis is postvaccinal encephalomyelitis. This usually develops within 2 weeks of the first dose of vaccine, but a delayed-onset cerebral type with psychiatric symptoms has been described in Japan. Poliomyelitis is distinguished by the lack of sensory abnormalities. Herpes simiae (B virus) encephalomyelitis, transmitted by monkey bites, has an incubation period of only a few days. Vesicles may be found in the monkey's mouth and at the site of the bite. The diagnosis can be confirmed virologically and the patient treated with acyclovir.

Laboratory Diagnosis. In humans, rabies encephalitis can be confirmed during life by immunofluorescence of skin and brain biopsies, but the corneal impression smear technique is too often falsely negative to be useful. Early in the illness, rabies virus can be isolated from saliva, brain, CSF, and even spun urine, but not from blood. Virus can be isolated in neuroblastoma cell cultures in 2 to 4 days and in 2 to 3 weeks using intracerebral inoculation of suckling mice. Viral RNA detection in CSF and other samples by PCR is possible in a few laboratories. The presence of rabies antibody in CSF or serum is diagnostic of rabies encephalitis unless the patient has been vaccinated or given rabies immune globulin. In postvaccinal encephalomyelitis, rabies neutralizing antibody leaks across the blood-CSF barrier but a very high titer (as in

three of the patients thought to have survived rabies) suggests rabies encephalitis. The most reliable method for distinguishing rabies from postvaccinal encephalomyelitis while the patient is alive is by demonstrating rabies antigen by immunofluorescence in skin or brain biopsies. In rabies encephalitis, pleocytosis was absent in 40% of patients in the first week, and 13% in the second week of illness. The average pleocytosis is about 75 lymphocytes/µL, but rarely exceeds a few hundred cells. A neutrophil leukocytosis of 20,000 to 30,000/µL is commonly found in the blood.

In the mammal responsible for the bite, rabies can be confirmed within a few hours by immunofluorescence of acetone-fixed brain or spinal cord impression smears, a technique that has replaced the classic Seller's stain for Negri bodies, which is less specific. A simple enzyme-linked immunosorbent assay (ELISA) test can be used if fluorescent microscopy is not available, and a sensitive avidin-biotin peroxidase method can detect antigen in formalin-fixed histologic sections. Rapid examination of CNS tissue in animals suspected of being rabid is now preferred to observing them in isolation for 10 days.

PREVENTION AND CONTROL

Local Measures. Bite wounds (Fig. 30–6), scratches, or abrasions that may have been contaminated by infected saliva should be scrubbed with soap or detergent and generously rinsed under running water for at least 5 minutes. Foreign material and dead tissue should be removed under anesthesia. Wounds should be irrigated with a virucidal agent, e.g., 20% soap solution, povidone-iodine, 0.1% aqueous iodine, or 40 to 70% alcohol. Quaternary ammonium compounds, hydrogen peroxide, and mercurochrome are not recommended. Suturing should be avoided or delayed wherever possible as it may inoculate virus deeper into the tissues. The risk of other viral, bacterial, fungal, and protozoal infections associated with mammal bites should be considered and in particular tetanus prophylaxis may be required. Amoxicillin–clavulanic acid, cefoxitin, or tetracycline are recommended antimicrobials for mammal bite wounds.

PROPHYLAXIS

Postexposure (Table 30–2). Specific prophylaxis includes the use of both active immunization with vaccine and passive immunization with hyperimmune serum. Cell culture and purified avian embryo vaccines are now the vaccines of

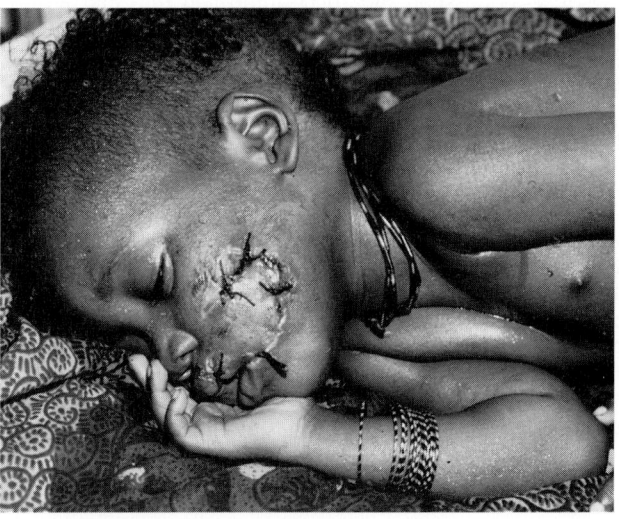

***Figure* 30–6.** Severe facial bite inflicted by a rabid dog on a 3-year-old Fulani girl. Early suturing of bite wounds should be avoided when possible. (Copyright D. A. Warrell.)

TABLE 30–2. Specific Postexposure Prophylaxis for Use in a Rabies-Endemic Area*

Exposure	Treatment
Minor Exposure Licks of broken skin Minor scratches or abrasions without bleeding	*Start vaccine:* Stop treatment if animal remains healthy for 10 days or if laboratory test on animal's brain proves negative
Major Exposure Licks of mucosa Transdermal bites or scratches	*Serum and vaccine:* Stop if domestic cat or dog remains healthy for 10 days, or if laboratory test on animal's brain proves negative

*Following an unprovoked attack by cat or dog or an attack by wild animal. From World Health Organization: Expert Committee on Rabies. Eighth Report. Technical Report Series 824. Geneva, WHO, 1992.

choice, but nervous tissue vaccines (e.g., Semple and suckling mouse brain) are still the most widely used throughout the tropical rabies endemic area. These vaccines are of variable potency and carry a risk of neuroparalytic reactions.

Currently available cell culture and avian embryo vaccines include human diploid cell strain vaccine (introduced in 1973), purified vero cell rabies vaccine, and purified chicken and duck embryo cell vaccines. These vaccines are given by IM injection (deltoid muscle or anterolateral aspect of the thigh but not the gluteal region) on days 0, 3, 7, 14, and 28. The initial dose should be doubled or given at eight sites intradermally, if there has been a delay of more than 48 hours in starting postexposure prophylaxis; if passive immunization was given 12 hours or more before active immunization; if patients are elderly, have chronic diseases, e.g., hepatic cirrhosis, or are likely to be immunodeficient, immunosuppressed, or severely malnourished; and if hyperimmune serum is not available. An economical regimen inducing a rapid immune response, recommended by the World Health Organization, consists of intradermal injections of 0.1 mL (one tenth of the usual IM dose) given at eight sites (deltoids, suprascapular, abdominal, and thighs) on day 0; 4 sites on day 7; and single sites on days 28 and 90.

Passive immunization consists of equine antirabies serum (40 IU/kg body weight) or, preferably, human rabies immune globulin (20 IU/kg). This should be given at the same time as the first dose of vaccine but at a different site. As much of the dose as possible should be infiltrated into and around the bite wound, and any remainder is given intramuscularly. Care is needed when injecting into tight tissue compartments (e.g., in a digit).

Those who have received pre-exposure vaccination do not require passive immunization if they are then exposed to rabies. A booster course of two doses of cell culture vaccine is required by IM or intradermal injection on days 0 and 3.

Pre-exposure. Immunization with safe tissue culture vaccines is recommended for high-risk groups, e.g., veterinarians, health care personnel, laboratory workers, dog catchers, zoologists, other field workers, foresters, cave explorers, and those whose work involves walking and cycling in urban and rural areas of India, Southeast Asia, and Latin America. In the areas with a high prevalence of canine rabies there may be a case for including rabies vaccine in the expanded program on immunization for children. Three doses are given on days 0, 7, and 28, either 1.0 mL IM or 0.1 mL intradermally. A single booster given 1 year later may produce sustained immunity for 5 to 8 years. Alternatively, a booster dose can be given every 2 years if the neutralizing antibody levels fall and continued protection is needed. People working with rabies virus in laboratories should have their anti-

body titer checked every 6 months and further booster injections given when indicated. A failure of pre-exposure vaccination by the intradermal route was found in American Peace Corps workers who were immunized in the tropics while taking chloroquine for antimalarial prophylaxis. The intradermal course should therefore be completed before starting chloroquine administration or the vaccine should be given in the full dose intramuscularly.

Efficacy of Postexposure Prophylaxis. Combined active and passive immunization given on the day of the bite, with optimum wound care, can reduce the risk of rabies from about 15 to 60% in untreated cases to practically zero with tissue culture vaccines. The risk varies with the biting species and the site and severity of the bites and is highest following head bites by rabid wolves. Prophylaxis may fail if nervous tissue vaccine of uncertain potency is used, if vaccination is delayed, if wound cleaning and passive immunization are neglected, and if the vaccine is not normally immunoresponsive. Conventional rabies vaccines may be less effective against the rabies-related viruses, Duvenhage and European bat lyssavirus, and ineffective against Mokola virus because of antigenic differences from rabies.

Complications of Rabies Vaccines. Tissue culture vaccines cause only mild local or transient influenza-like symptoms in a small minority of vaccinees. However, in the United States, 6% of pre-exposure booster injections were associated with mild immune complex disease 3 to 13 days later. Neuroparalytic accidents complicate 1 in 220 courses of Semple vaccine and 1 in 27,000 courses of suckling mouse brain vaccine. Clinical forms include Gullain-Barré syndrome (especially after suckling mouse brain vaccine), mononeuritis multiplex, dorsolumbar transverse myelitis, and encephalitis. The overall mortality is 10 to 20%. If symptoms of a neuroparalytic reaction develop, vaccination with nervous tissue vaccines should be stopped immediately, corticosteroids should be given in high dosage, and the postexposure course should be continued with a cell culture vaccine.

Control of Animal Rabies. Domestic dogs, including strays, are responsible for urban rabies. The size of stray dog populations is determined by the amount of food, water, and shelter available. Muzzling, restricting movement of owned dogs, and killing strays were effective in eradicating rabies from some islands and peninsulas (e.g., Britain, Japan, and West Malaysia). However, in many tropical endemic zones, attempts to eliminate stray dogs are difficult, unpopular, and inefficient. In several large cities in South America, intense mass vaccination programs, aimed at immunizing 60 to 80% of the entire dog population, including strays, were dramatically effective in reducing the incidence of canine rabies and eliminating human disease. Control of wildlife rabies by reducing populations of important species such as foxes in Europe and skunks in Canada were of limited benefit, costly, and at odds with current principles of ecology and conservation. However, the use of oral live attenuated or vaccinia recombinant rabies vaccines in baits has reduced the prevalence of fox rabies in several European countries and Canada, and recombinant vaccines have produced promising results in raccoons and coyotes in the United States. Oral vaccines for a variety of other species in America (e.g., skunks) and Africa (e.g., black-backed jackals) are being developed. A recombinant oral vaccine for stray dogs might have a major impact on rabies epidemiology in the future.

Bibliography

Baer GM (ed): The Natural History of Rabies, 2nd ed. Boca Raton, FL, CRC Press, 1991.
Bernard KW, Fishbein DB, Miller KD, et al: Pre-exposure rabies immunization

with human diploid cell vaccines: Decreased antibody responses in persons immunized in developing countries. Am J Trop Med Hyg 34:633, 1985.

Callaham M: Controversies in antibiotic choices for bite wounds. Ann Emerg Med 17:1321, 1988.

Campbell JB, Charlton KM (eds): Rabies. Boston, Kluwer, 1988.

Centers for Disease Control: Rabies prevention—United States, 1991. Recommendations of the Immunization Practice Advisory Committee (ACIP). MMWR 40: RR-3, 1991.

Helmick CG, Tauxe RV, Vernon AA: Is there a risk to contacts of patients with rabies? Rev Infect Dis 9:511, 1987.

Hurst EW, Pawan JL: An outbreak of rabies in Trinidad: Without history of bites, and with the symptoms of acute ascending myelitis. Lancet 2:622, 1931.

Koprowski H, Dietzschold B: Rabies: Lessons from the past and a glimpse into the future. In Peterson PK, Remington JS (eds): In Defense of the Brain: Current Concepts in the Immunopathogenesis and Clinical Aspects of CNS Infection. Malden, MA. Blackwell, 1997.

Meslin F-X, Kaplan MM, Koprowski H (eds): Laboratory Techniques in Rabies, 4th ed. Geneva, WHO, 1996.

Rupprecht CE, Dietzschold B, Koprowski H (eds): Lyssaviruses. Berlin, Springer-Verlag, 1994, pp 145–160.

Smith JS: New aspects of rabies with emphasis on epidemiology, diagnosis and prevention of the disease in the United States. Clin Microbiol Rev 9:166, 1996.

Thomson G, King A (eds): Rabies in Southern and Eastern Africa. Onderstepoort J Vet Res 60:263, 1993.

Tsiang H: Pathophysiology of rabies virus infection of the nervous system. Adv Virus Res 42:375, 1993.

Warrell DA: The clinical picture of rabies in man. Trans R Soc Trop Med Hyg 70:188, 1976.

Warrell DA, Davidson NMcD, Pope HM, et al: Pathophysiologic studies in human rabies. Am J Med 60:180, 1976.

Warrell MJ, Nicholson KG, Warrell DA, et al: Economical multiple-site intradermal immunisation with human diploid-cell-strain vaccine is effective for post-exposure rabies prophylaxis. Lancet 1:1059, 1985.

World Health Organization: Expert Committee on Rabies. Eighth Report. Technical Report Series 824. Geneva, WHO, 1992.

World Health Organization recommendations on rabies post-exposure treatment and the correct technique of intradermal immunization against rabies. WHO 1997. WHO/EMC/ZOO. 96.6.

30.2 Venezuelan Equine Encephalitis

Douglas M. Watts and M. Steven Oberste

DEFINITION. Venezuelan equine encephalitis (VEE; "peste loca") is an acute viral disease characterized by fever, chills, headache, myalgia, lumbosacral pain, prostration, nausea, and vomiting, which may progress to encephalitis, especially in children.

ETIOLOGY AND HISTORY. VEE viruses are alphaviruses in the family Togaviridae. The serogroup is comprised of six VEE virus subtypes (I to VI); subtype I is further divided into five varieties, and subtype III into three varieties. Subtype I viruses AB and C have been associated with epidemics and equine epizootics. The others have reduced equine pathogenicity and are considered sylvatic viruses causing sporadic human cases and rare equine outbreaks.

Periodic epidemics and epizootics involving tens of thousands of humans and hundreds of thousands of equines have been reported since 1936 primarily in northern South America. IAB/C viruses are transmitted among equines by a variety of mosquito species. Sylvatic subtype ID viruses in Colombia, Panama, and Peru; subtype II (Everglades virus) in southern Florida; subtype IIIA (Mucambo virus) in Brazil, Venezuela, and Surinam; and subtype IIIB (Tonate virus) in French Guiana are transmitted in a cycle among Culex (Melanoconion) mosquitoes and small rodents. Human infections occur in an endemic pattern.

EPIDEMIOLOGY

Distribution. VEE IAB and/or IC viruses have been isolated in Venezuela, Colombia, Ecuador, Guyana, Peru, Trinidad, Costa Rica, Nicaragua, El Salvador, Honduras, Guatemala, Belize, Mexico, and Texas. IAB virus also was isolated in Argentina following the use of an inadequately inactivated VEE vaccine. Enzootic virus subtypes are distributed throughout tropical and subtropical regions of the Americas from Florida to Argentina.

Incidence. The size of epidemics caused by IAB and IC viruses between 1936 to 1973 can be appreciated by considering the IC virus outbreaks from 1962 to 1964 in Venezuela as examples. There were 23,283 human cases, including 960 with neurologic symptoms and 156 deaths. Attack rates among humans ranged from 183 to 291 per 1000 persons per month among children under 15 years of age to 73 per 1000 persons per month in older persons. Neurologic manifestations typically occur in 4 to 14% of cases, with overall fatality rates of <1%. Mortality rates have varied from 19 to 83% among equines.

In 1995, the first major VEE outbreak since 1973 led to >100,000 human cases in Venezuela and Colombia, with more than 20 VEE-associated deaths. VEE type IC was isolated from human and equine cases. The attack rates exceeded 50% in some towns, affecting all ages equally.

Transmission. Equines are the principal amplifier hosts in outbreaks due to type IAB/C viruses. Humans and horses are infected by a wide variety of mosquito vectors, including *Psorophora, Aedes,* and *Mansonia* species and mechanically by other hematophagous insects (Fig. 30–7). Although VEE virus has been isolated from serum and throat washings of patients, and viremia exceeds the threshold level required to infect mosquitoes, neither human-mosquito-human transmission nor person-to-person transmission has been documented.

The transmission cycle of enzootic VEE virus subtypes involves small wild rodents and *Culex* (Melanoconion) mosquitoes in tropical rain forest and swamp habitats. Transmission appears continuous and highly focal; humans are infected on entering the sylvatic foci.

PATHOLOGY AND PATHOGENESIS. Pathologic changes in the brain consist of congestion, perivascular cuffing and hemorrhage, glial nodule formation, and focal necrosis. Changes are most prominent in the substantia nigra and basal ganglia, but also affect the deep cerebral white matter and cerebral cortex. In congenitally infected fetuses, there is massive and widespread necrosis, hemorrhage, and resorption of brain tissue, resulting in cystic changes and hydranencephaly.

After replicating in extraneural tissues, circulating virus invades the CNS from the blood or possibly through the olfactory apparatus. Sites of extraneural viral replication in humans are uncertain, but in equines and laboratory rodents, skeletal muscle and hematopoietic and lymphoid tissues have been implicated. Acute VEE deaths in hamsters have been related to virus-induced depression of the reticuloendothelial system, necrosis of Peyer's patches, and endotoxic shock. Impaired glucose tolerance and insulin release have been described in experimental animals as long as 1 year after VEE infection, but there are no reports of a diabetogenic effect in humans.

CLINICAL MANIFESTATIONS AND COMPLICATIONS

Febrile Illness. Inapparent infections are rare. Typically, VEE appears as a grippe-like disease with sudden onset 2 to 5 days after infection. Fever, chills, malaise, severe headache, myalgia, lumbosacral pain, nausea, vomiting, and prostration occur initially and may be followed by diarrhea and sore throat. There are few physical findings other than fever, pharyngitis, conjunctival congestion, facial hyperemia, and, rarely, lymphadenopathy. Some patients exhibit somnolence, photophobia, and mild confusion, but no progression or localization of neurologic signs occurs. Abortions and fetal deaths may result when infection occurs during pregnancy. Congenital infection with CNS malformations has been reported in

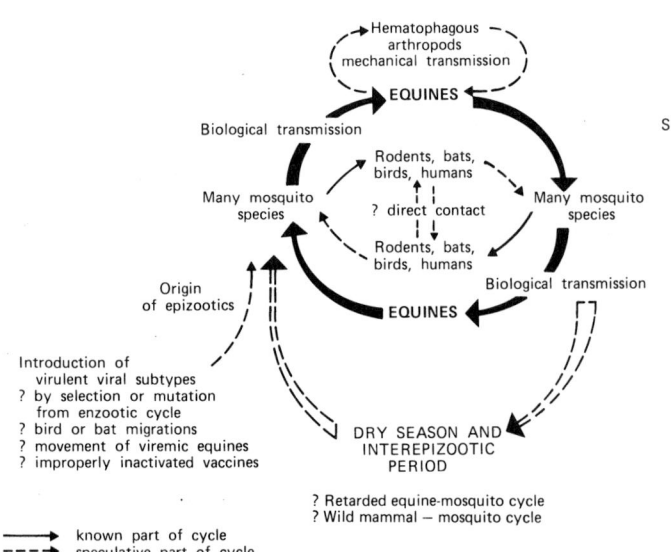

Figure **30–7.** Transmission cycle of epizootic subtypes of Venezuelan equine encephalitis virus.

some cases. The duration of illness is generally 2 or 3 days with a prolonged convalescent phase of lethargy and weakness lasting 1 to 2 weeks. Illness may be biphasic in some cases.

Neurologic Illness. Neurologic symptoms occur in approximately 4% of infected children <15 years of age, but rarely in adults. CNS manifestations include nuchal rigidity, stupor, coma, delirium, seizures, cranial nerve palsies, nystagmus, pathologic reflexes, and spastic paralysis. Involuntary movement disorders, tremors, and visual field defects are unusual or absent. A decrease in lymphocytes or both granulocytes and lymphocytes is a frequent finding 1 to 3 days after onset. Eosinopenia and abnormal vacuolated monocytes have been described. CSF mononuclear pleocytosis with a normal glucose concentration is usual. Elevated levels of serum aspartate aminotransferase and lactate dehydrogenase have been reported.

PROGNOSIS AND TREATMENT. Non-neurologic infections are self-limited, with complete recovery within several weeks after onset. The overall fatality rate in encephalitic cases is approximately 20%, ranging from 6 to 9% in older children and young adults to 35% in 0- to 5-year-old children. A prolonged convalescence is common, with recurrent headaches, forgetfulness, and asthenia lasting up to 1 month after recovery. Long-term sequelae, e.g., dysarthria, motor disorders, pathologic reflexes, abnormal electroencephalograms, and affective disorders may occur among recovered children.

Specific therapy is unavailable. In encephalitic patients, supportive care will reduce mortality. Prompt administration of anticonvulsants may be needed to treat protracted seizures. Dehydration and electrolyte imbalance caused by fever, vomiting, insufficient oral intake, and inappropriate ADH secretion should be corrected by fluid management. Airway management and respiratory support in semicomatose and comatose patients are essential. The contribution of cerebral edema to the pathogenesis is uncertain; where intensive supportive modalities are available, intracranial pressure should be monitored and controlled. Prevention and treatment of secondary bacterial infections are considered critical to prognosis.

DIAGNOSIS The geographic and epidemiologic setting of an ongoing equine epizootic should suggest the diagnosis. Examination and culture of the CSF are essential elements of the diagnostic procedure. A specific diagnosis of VEE may be made by isolating virus from blood or serum or a throat swab taken within 1 to 3 days after onset. A variety of laboratory animals, e.g., mice, hamsters, and avian or mammalian cell cultures are susceptible. Virus can be identified by ELISA, immunofluorescence, and neutralization tests. A diagnosis also can be made by demonstrating fourfold changes in serum antibody titer.

PREVENTION AND CONTROL. VEE outbreaks in equines and humans can be prevented by mass vaccination of equines. During epizootics, equines should be vaccinated in unaffected areas threatened by the epizootic. Large-scale (usually aerial), ultra-low-volume applications of insecticides may reduce the population of adult mosquitoes.

Attenuated live (TC-83) and formalin-inactivated (C-84) vaccines are used to protect laboratory workers, but are not licensed for use in the general public. Safety of these vaccines has not been assessed in children.

Bibliography

Dietz WH, Peralta PH, Johnson KM: Ten clinical cases of human infection with Venezuelan equine encephalomyelitis virus, subtype 1D. Am J Trop Med Hyg 28:329, 1979.

Johnson KM, Martin DH: Venezuelan equine encephalitis. Adv Vet Sci Comp Med 18:79, 1974.

Leon CA, Jaramillo R, Martinez S, et al: Sequelae of Venezuelan equine encephalitis in humans: A four year follow-up. Int J Epidemiol 4:131, 1975.

Walton TE, Grayson MA: Venezuelan equine encephalomyelitis. *In* Monath TP (ed): The Arboviruses: Epidemiology and Ecology, Vol IV. Boca Raton, FL, CRC Press, 1988, pp 203–231.

Weaver SC, Bellew LA, Rico-Hesse R: Phylogenetic analysis of alphaviruses in the Venezuelan equine encephalitis complex and identification of the source of epizootic viruses. Virology 191:282, 1992.

Weaver SC, Salas R, Rico-Hesse R, et al: Re-emergence of epidemic Venezuelan equine encephalomyelitis in South America. Lancet 348:436–440, 1996.

30.3 *Japanese Encephalitis*

Theodore Tsai

DEFINITION. Japanese encephalitis (JE), a severe mosquito-borne infection of the CNS, is a leading cause of childhood encephalitis in Asia and also is an important veterinary infection, producing abortions in swine and epizootic encephalitis in horses.

ETIOLOGY AND HISTORY. The flavivirus is related antigenically to St. Louis encephalitis virus, Murray Valley encephalitis, and West Nile virus. Four genotypes have been delineated by genomic sequencing but no associated clinical or epidemiologic differences have been documented and immunity extends to viruses throughout the region. Molecular determinants of neurovirulence have been defined partially by sequence comparisons of wild-type and derived attenuated viruses and by the introduction of mutations in infectious viral cDNA clones and chimeric viruses. Several important mutations have been identified in envelope and nonstructural proteins and noncoding regions. The virus was isolated from human brain of an epidemic case in Japan in 1934 in a period when summer outbreaks numbering several thousand cases recurred annually in Japan and Korea. The disease and virus were classified as Japanese B encephalitis in deference to von Economo's A encephalitis. The virus' mosquito-borne mode of transmission was proved in 1938. Recurrent epidemics in Japan, Korea, and Taiwan were brought under control with the licensure and distribution of an inactivated vaccine in 1956.

DISTRIBUTION AND INCIDENCE. JE occurs across the entire Asian landmass from areas of Pakistan in the west to maritime Siberia (Fig. 30–8). The virus is transmitted in the southeast Asian archipelagoes and twice has appeared on islands in the western Pacific. In 1995, JE invaded and has since persisted on the Torres Strait islands of Australia. In 1998, further spread to Cape York peninsula, including a human case, has led to concern that the virus may become established on the mainland. Within temperate areas of China, Korea and Japan, JE is transmitted seasonally in the late summer and fall (July to September); epidemics occur sporadically and annual incidence is low. In subtropical Asia, enzootic viral transmission begins several months earlier and ends later (March to October) and incidence rates are severalfold higher (approximately 3 to 10 per 100,000). Local hy-perendemic transmission can produce incidence rates exceeding 100 per 100,000. Viral transmission occurs year round in tropical Asia (e.g., Indonesia) where viral activity and disease incidence fluctuate more with irrigation schedules than with natural rainfall patterns. Although reported disease incidence rates are lowest in tropical locations, surveillance has not been rigorous; alternatively, the circulation of naturally attenuated JE viral strains has been proposed as a contributing factor to the paucity of recognized disease.

TRANSMISSION AND EPIDEMIOLOGY. The virus is transmitted by *Culex vishnui* complex mosquitoes to aquatic birds and pigs, which are the principal viral amplifying hosts. Adult pigs remain asymptomatic while circulating high levels of virus for several days; infected pregnant sows abort or deliver stillbirths, however. Horses, like humans, develop encephalitis after infection but they are dead-end hosts. The principal JE vectors use ground pools for their larval stages. Rice paddies are highly productive of vector mosquitoes, especially *Culex tritaeniorhynchus*, the principal vector species in most areas. Risk for infection is highest in rural locations where rice paddies and pigs both are prevalent; however, zoning restrictions may not apply in some Asian cities and urban cases and outbreaks occur. The principal vector species are exophilic and crepuscular (feed outdoors in the evenings) and prefer animal to human hosts.

Only one in several hundred infections results in clinical disease, so in areas where viral transmission is enzootic, infections occurring at an early age result in immunity in over 80% by the end of the second decade. The peak incidence of infection is in children from 2 to 10 years of age with a slightly greater proportion of cases among boys, presumably reflecting an increased risk of exposure. In Asian populations protected by childhood immunization, cases occur principally in the elderly which may be a result of waning immunity and biologic factors associated with increased susceptibility to neuroinvasion.

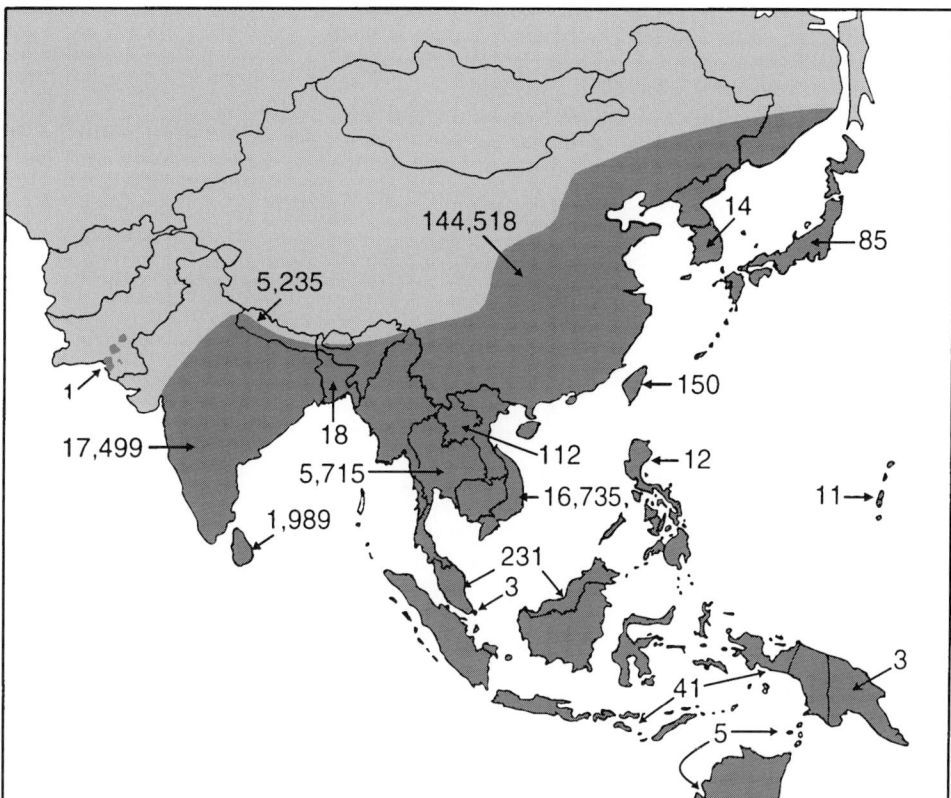

***Figure* 30–8.** Reported Japanese encephalitis cases by country, 1990–1996, and regions where viral transmission is proved or suspected. 1997–1998 provisional cases from Australia and Papua New Guinea are included.

Travelers from developing countries generally lack naturally acquired protective antibodies and risk is equal among young adults and children. The absence of reported cases from developed countries with high childhood vaccination coverage is potentially disarming since enzootic viral transmission can persist in the absence of human disease. Overall, risk of illness in travelers is estimated to be as low as 1 per 150,000 person-months of exposure, reflecting the low proportion of vector mosquitoes that are infected (0.5%) and the small proportion of all infections that are symptomatic (0.3%).

PATHOLOGY AND PATHOGENESIS. After an infectious mosquito bite, the virus propagates locally and in regional lymph nodes. Viremia leads to widespread infection including the brain unless the infection is cleared or modulated by a timely immune response. Neuroinvasion probably occurs as the virus grows through vascular endothelial cells to the parenchymal side. The meninges and cut surface of the brain appear congested and may exhibit focal hemorrhages. Microscopic changes of neuronal degeneration and necrosis, perivascular inflammation, and microglial reaction are seen in widespread distribution (Fig. 30–9). Viral antigen is seen in neurons and later in phagocytic cells as they clear the infection. Lesions are distributed in the thalamus, basal ganglia, brain stem, cerebellum, hippocampus, and cerebral cortex. Delayed CNS vital clearance has been suggested by the isolation of virus, demonstration of antigen, or persistence of CSF IgM antibodies several weeks after the onset of illness. Viral antigen also has been found in peripheral blood mononuclear cells months after clinical recovery, but the significance of these findings still is unclear.

CLINICAL MANIFESTATIONS AND COMPLICATIONS. The incubation period is estimated to be 4 to 14 days. A prodrome of malaise, headache, fever, myalgias, nausea, and vomiting usually precedes the onset of CNS signs. A change in consciousness or behavior is the most consistent neurologic abnormality but ataxia, motor weakness, and acute seizures also can herald CNS involvement. Involuntary movements, changes in tone, slurred speech and bulbar paralysis, and extrapyramidal signs often are present. Most patients develop coma, and respiratory failure is common.

The most frequent complications are hyponatremia due to inappropriate ADH secretion and secondary infections, chiefly pneumonia during the acute phase of illness and infected decubitus ulcers, urinary tract and other nosocomial infections during the often prolonged interval of convalescence.

A peripheral leukocytosis may be present and liver enzymes may be mildly elevated. CSF pleocytosis with a median of several hundred leukocytes is usual. Imaging studies frequently disclose only cerebral edema, but specific lesions in the thalamus, basal ganglia, pons, and cerebellum may be seen. Hemorrhages into the thalamus frequently can be detected. Electroencephalograms disclose a pattern of diffuse delta wave activity consistent with thalamic damage. A neurogenic pattern of electromyographic activity suggests anterior horn cell involvement.

TREATMENT AND PROGNOSIS. No specific therapy has been proved. The efficacy of α-interferon or interferon inducers has not been evaluated systematically. Fatality rates have varied widely with the availability of supportive care. Mannitol is generally used to control intracranial pressure; in a controlled trial, however, dexamethasone therapy did not improve outcome. Anticonvulsant therapy may be needed and trihexphenidyl has been used to treat extrapyramidal symptoms. Neurologic and respiratory intensive care has reduced mortality to 5 to 10% in some locations. In areas where sophisticated modalities are unavailable, fatality rates may exceed 35%. The reported frequency of neurologic and psychologic sequelae has varied from 10 to 75% in long-term follow-up. Psychologic disturbances, e.g., behavior disorders and mental retardation predominate; however, motor disturbances and convulsions are not uncommon.

DIAGNOSIS. Virus can be isolated from blood only during the first few days of illness, usually preceding the onset of neurologic symptoms. Virus usually is isolated from CSF only in patients with a poor prognosis who have low intrathecal antibody levels. Preliminary reports of polymerase chain reaction (PCR) analysis of CSF show poor sensitivity. Detection of viral-specific IgM in CSF or serum is a well-standardized and sensitive procedure. Cross reactions with dengue are controlled by comparing absorbance values. Other serologic procedures may be substituted with the same caution to rule out cross reactive flaviviral antibodies.

PREVENTION AND CONTROL. Inactivated mouse brain–derived vaccine is widely used in Asia where childhood vaccination has controlled the disease in Japan, Korea, and Taiwan. The vaccine is licensed for travelers in Europe and the United States; however, it is associated with a high rate of allergic side effects and only expatriates and travelers at high risk for acquiring infection should be immunized (three doses on days 0, 7, and 30). A live attenuated cell culture–derived vaccine (SA$_{14}$ 14-2 strain) has been used safely and with high effectiveness in China but it is not approved internationally. Unvaccinated travelers should protect themselves against mosquito bites with bed netting and repellents. Larvicides and agricultural pesticides can reduce vector mosquito populations but control programs have been limited by the scale of application.

Bibliography

Hoke CH, Vaughn DW, Nisalak A, et al: Effect of high-dose dexamethasone on the outcome of acute encephalitis due to Japanese encephalitis. J Infect Dis 165:631, 1992.

Innis BL, Nisalak A, Nimmannitya S, et al: An enzyme-linked immunosorbent assay to characterize dengue infections where dengue and Japanese encephalitis cocirculate. Am J Trop Med Hyg 40:418, 1989.

Rojanosuphot S, Tsai TF (eds): Regional workshop on control strategies for Japanese encephalitis. Southeast Asian J Trop Med Public Health 26:1, 1995.

Tsai TF, Chang GJ, Yu YX: Japanese encephalitis vaccines. In Plotkin S, Orenstein WA (eds): Vaccines, 3rd ed. Philadelphia: WB Saunders, 1998, pp 672–710.

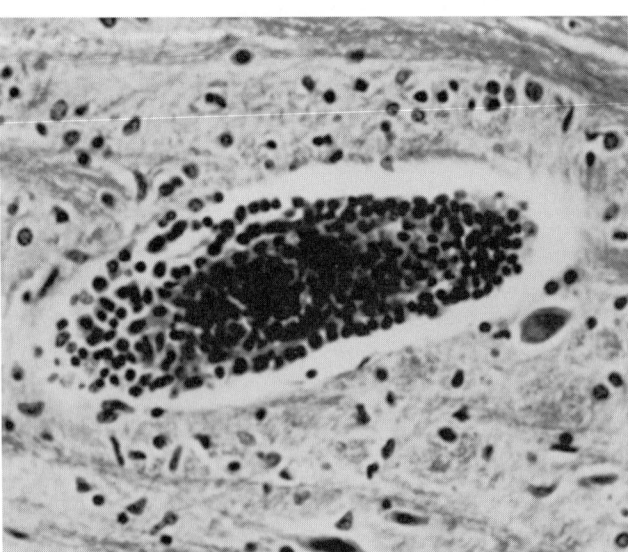

Figure 30–9. Perivascular cuffing by lymphocytes in brain of patient dying of Japanese encephalitis (× 305). (Courtesy of Armed Forces Institute of Pathology, Photograph Neg. No. 73–12327.)

30.4 Rocio Encephalitis

Theodore Tsai

DEFINITION. Rocio encephalitis is an acute mosquito-borne CNS infection transmitted in southern coastal Brazil.

ETIOLOGY AND HISTORY. The disease first came to light in 1975 when a severe outbreak of encephalitis was reported in coastal areas of São Paulo state, Brazil. Epidemic transmission continued in 1976 and 1977, after which only sporadic cases were recognized, the last confirmed case in 1980. Asymptomatic infections were recognized in serosurveys as recently as 1987, however. The flavivirus, isolated from brain of a fatal case, was shown to be related antigenically and genetically to St. Louis encephalitis virus. The sudden emergence of the outbreak and the subsequent disappearance of the disease has suggested the possibility that a viral mutation resulted in a novel agent poorly adapted to available ecological niches.

DISTRIBUTION AND INCIDENCE. Until 1996, the disease has been recognized only in coastal areas of São Paulo state, in the Ribeira Valley and Santista lowlands and, an adjacent area of Paraná state. More than 1000 cases were reported between 1975 and 1977 with incidence rates ranging between 47 to 200 per 100,000 inhabitants. In 1996, eight cases in Bahia state, 1500 km to the north occurred under unexplained circumstances.

TRANSMISSION AND EPIDEMIOLOGY. Only one viral isolate from a field-collected mosquito (*Psorophora ferox*) has been made and the enzootic transmission cycle is still undetermined. The involvement of *Aedes scapularis* is suspected because of its abundance in the area and its capacity to transmit the virus in experimental studies. The virus has been isolated from sentinel mice and a captive wild bird. Experimental infections suggest that wild birds and possibly chickens may contribute to viral amplification. Humans appear to be dead-end hosts. Epidemic attack rates were highest among adult men of working age, particularly fishermen, and others with outdoor occupations.

PATHOLOGY AND PATHOGENESIS. No viral isolates from human blood have been recovered despite numerous attempts. Neuropathologic findings in fatal cases consist of diffuse meningeal inflammation and congestion, focal brain hemorrhages, and neuronal degeneration with parenchymal and perivascular inflammatory infiltrates and microgliosis. The distribution of lesions is widespread involving the thalamus, dentate nucleus of the cerebellum, basal ganglia, brain stem, and anterior horn of the spinal cord.

CLINICAL MANIFESTATIONS AND COMPLICATIONS. The incubation period is estimated to be 7 to 14 days. The onset usually is abrupt with fever, headache, malaise, and neck stiffness, frequently accompanied by nausea, vomiting, and abdominal distention. Mental confusion and signs of meningeal irritation are the most frequently reported neurologic signs but they often are accompanied by tremor, slurred speech, motor weakness and incoordination, abnormal reflexes, and convulsions. Occasional patients have presented with urinary retention or arterial hypertension. The clinical course may be fulminant resulting in respiratory failure and coma. The CSF shows a pleocytosis of several hundred leukocytes, with a lymphocytic predominance and elevated protein. A moderate peripheral leukocytosis is present in half of cases but leukopenia also is observed.

PROGNOSIS AND TREATMENT. Overall, 5% of cases are fatal but mortality rates are higher in children (30%) and in the elderly. Significant neurologic sequelae consisting of motor impairment, loss of sphincter control, bulbar palsy, and visual and auditory impairment are reported in 20% of recovered cases. The value of intensive supportive care was shown in the reduction of case-fatality rates from 15 to 20% to 4% with the early recognition of cases and admission to hospital care.

DIAGNOSIS. The virus has been recovered from at least nine fatal cases; however, the virus has not been isolated from blood of acutely ill patients. Application of PCR or other direct detection techniques in the acute phase of illness has not been reported. The diagnosis usually is confirmed serologically by demonstrating viral-specific IgM in CSF or serum, typically using an IgM capture technique. Fourfold changes in hemagglutination inhibition (HI), complement fixation, or neutralizing antibody titers also are diagnostic. Serologic results may be difficult to interpret because of cross reactions with dengue and other co-circulating flaviviruses.

Clinical features of Rocio encephalitis are similar to those produced by other CNS infections, which include agents with a special distribution in the tropics as well as common infections, e.g., enteroviruses, herpes simplex virus, and respiratory viruses.

PREVENTION AND CONTROL. A formalin-inactivated mouse brain–derived vaccine was administered to 1800 subjects; however, only 22% of vaccinees developed low titered antibodies after three doses. Vector control measures, e.g., larviciding ground pools and campaigns to apply insecticides around houses via truck and air were implemented during previous outbreaks.

Bibliography

Iversson LB: Rocio encephalitis. *In* Monath TP (ed): The Arboviruses: Epidemiology and Ecology, Vol IV. Boca Raton, FL, CRC Press, 1988, pp 78–92.

Iversson LB, Travassos da Rosa APA, Rosa MDB: Ocorrencia recente de infeccao humana por arbovirus Rocio na regiao do Vale do Ribeira. Rev Inst Med Trop (São Paulo) 31:28, 1989. Lopes OS, Pinheiro F, Iversson LB: Arboviral zoonoses of Central and South America. *In* Beran GW (ed): Handbook of Zoonoses, 2nd ed. Section B: Viral. Boca Raton, FL, CRC Press, 1994, pp 201–226.

Lopes OS, Sacchetta LA, Coimbra TLM: Emegence of a new arborvirus disease in Brazil. I. Isolation and characterization of the etiological agent, Rocio virus. Am J Epidemiol 107:444, 1978.

30.5 Other Arboviral Encephalitides

Theodore Tsai

CENTRAL AND SOUTH AMERICA. CNS symptoms may complicate arboviral infections principally associated with milder illnesses (e.g., Oropouche and dengue fevers) and for others, the potential for CNS infection has been shown only in special circumstances of experimental human infection (Ilheus virus). Arboviral infections that are familiar causes of encephalitis in North America exhibit different transmission cycles in the Southern Hemisphere and human cases typically are sporadic and associated with forest exposure. The North American subtype of eastern equine encephalitis (EEE) virus is the cause of occasional epizootics in Central America and rarely has been associated with small epidemics (Jamaica, Dominican Republic, Cuba, and Trinidad). The South American EEE viral subtype is transmitted in an enzootic pattern, leading to occasional equine cases and epizootics; although antibody surveys have documented variable rates of human infection, clinical cases have not been reported. Western equine encephalitis (WEE) virus epizootics with small numbers of concurrent human cases have been reported from Rio Negro province, Argentina and viral activity has been recognized in Mexico, Guyana, Brazil, and Uruguay. A sylvatic subtype of WEE virus also is transmitted in Chaco province, Argentina. In contrast to its epidemic potential in North America, St. Louis encephalitis has been recognized in only 12 sporadic cases in South America. The virus is transmitted in a forest mammal-mosquito cycle. Meningoencephalitis has been reported to complicate infection with Rio Bravo virus, a bat-associated zoonosis.

AFRICA. Among the large array of arboviruses causing specific syndromes of hemorrhagic fever or nonspecific febrile illnesses, many also are associated with CNS manifestations (Table II–1). A few deserve specific mention: Semliki Forest virus produced fatal encephalitis in one laboratory-associated case, and in naturally acquired infection it causes severe persistent headache in humans and encephalitis in horses. A greater role in undiagnosed CNS infection may be unrecognized. Rift Valley fever rarely can be complicated by meningoencephalitis and optic neuritis, usually presenting as late events. CNS symptoms and optic neuritis also have been reported with tick-borne Thogoto viral infection; and West Nile virus is a cause of epidemic meningoencephalitis, with an age-related increase in severity similar to St. Louis encephalitis.

ASIA. In the Mediterranean basin, Toscana virus, a sandfly-borne phlebovirus, appears to be a common cause of mild CNS infection in local children and also in travelers. In Asia proper, several viruses have been associated serologically with CNS infection, including Me Tri virus, a subtype of Semliki forest virus; snowshoe hare virus, a member of the California serogroup of bunyaviruses; and Sindbis virus. Single cases of Reye syndrome due to Chandipura virus, which can be both sandfly- or mosquito-borne, and hemorrhagic fever with encephalitis due to Wanowrie virus, which can be tick- or mosquito-borne, have been reported. After JE, perhaps the most prevalent arboviral CNS pathogen in China is a mosquito-borne coltivirus, also transmitted by the principal JE virus vector, *Culex tritaeniorhynchus*. There may be several such related agents with a wide geographic distribution in China, among which Banna virus also has been isolated from ticks. Tick-borne Russian spring-summer encephalitis virus has been known to be transmitted in temperate areas of Asia, including Manchuria, but recently two human cases were reported from Hokkaido Island, Japan. Langat virus, an antigenically related flavivirus isolated in Southeast Asia, produced primary encephalitis in experimentally infected cancer patients, but illness due to naturally acquired infection has not been reported. Tick-borne Bhanja virus, which has been associated with meningoencephalitis in Europe, has been isolated in India although human illnesses have not been reported there. The roles of chikungunya and dengue viruses as direct agents of CNS infection or indirect causes of CNS symptoms arising from petechial hemorrhages, shock, or high fever still are unclear.

AUSTRALIA. Mosquito-borne flaviviruses in the JE antigenic complex, Murray Valley encephalitis (MVE), and Kunjin viruses cause sporadic cases and occasionally small epidemics of encephalitis in Australia and New Guinea, sometimes called simply Australian encephalitis, because of similarities in their clinical features and transmission cycles. Outbreaks in 1917, 1918, 1922, and 1925 were reported as "Australian X" disease until, during an epidemic in 1951, the etiologic agent was isolated and named after the epicenter in the Murray Valley. During the last major outbreak in 1974, 58 cases were reported over a wide geographic area of Australia and New Guinea but 39 cases were from the Murray Valley region. All subsequent reported cases however, have occurred sporadically in northern Australia, 29 of 47 cases in northern areas of Western Australia. Enzootic MVE viral transmission evidently is maintained among wading birds

and *Culex annulirostris* mosquitoes in northern Australia, and sporadically when introduced to the inland river basins, infections are transmitted in epidemic proportions. *Aedes tremulus* mosquitoes may have a role in maintaining virus during the dry season in the north. Clinically, illness severity varies from mild confusion with variable neurologic impairment to a severe encephalitis with seizures, early onset of coma, muscle and respiratory paralysis, and death in 30% of cases. Residual neurologic deficits complicate recovery in one third of patients. Serologic determinations may be obscured by cross reactions from numerous sympatric flaviviruses including Alfuy, Kokobera, and JE viruses, the latter recently having been recognized to occur in the Torres Strait islands above Queensland. An extensive chicken surveillance system is maintained to monitor risk of epidemics; MVE immune globulin is under investigation for immune prophylaxis of at-risk populations.

Bibliography

Beran GW (ed): Handbook of Zoonoses, 2nd ed. Section B: Viral. Boca Raton, FL, CRC Press, 1994.

Richman DD, Whitley RJ, Hayden FG (eds): Clinical Virology. New York, Churchill Livingstone, 1997.

30.6 Transmissible Spongiform Encephalopathies*

David M. Asher

DEFINITION. The transmissible spongiform encephalopathies (TSEs) are a group of slowly progressive and invariably fatal diseases of the CNS in humans and animals (Table 30–3) associated with vacuolation of gray matter (Fig. 30–10) and accumulation of host-encoded amyloid protein in the brain and caused by infection with incompletely characterized agents now called TSE agents, or prions.

ETIOLOGY AND PATHOGENESIS. The nature of the TSE

---

*All the material in this chapter is in the public domain, with the exception of any borrowed figures or tables.

TABLE 30–3. Transmissible Spongiform Encephalopathies (TSEs) of Humans and Animals

Disease	Naturally Infected Hosts
Creutzfeldt-Jakob disease (CJD)	Humans
Familial CJD (fCJD)	
Iatrogenic CJD (iCJD)	
Sporadic CJD (sCJD)	
New-variant CJD (vCJD)	
Gerstmann-Sträussler-Scheinker syndrome (GSS)*	Humans
Fatal familial insomnia syndrome (FFI)†	Humans
Kuru	Humans
Bovine spongiform encephalopathy ("mad cow" disease/BSE)	Cattle, zoo ungulates; zoo felines, domestic cats‡
Chronic wasting disease	Deer, elk
Scrapie	Sheep, goats
Transmissible milk encephalopathy (TME)	Mink

*Might be considered equivalent to fCJD with prominent amyloid plaques.
†Transmission to mice claimed; not successfully transmitted to primates.
‡Some authorities classify the new TSE of house cats and felines in zoos as a separate feline spongiform encephalopathy (FSE).

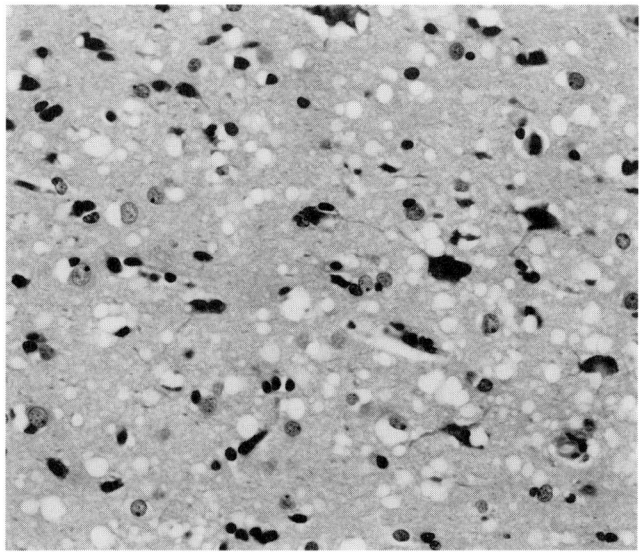

Figure 30–10. Vacuolation (spongiform change) in the cerebral cortex of a patient with the Gerstmann-Sträussler-Scheinker syndrome.

agents is still disputed. Although several studies suggested that their minimal size may fall within the range of very small viruses, no virus-like particles associated with TSE infectivity have been consistently recognized. TSE agents are extremely resistant to inactivation by a variety of chemical and physical treatments. This characteristic, as well as their partial sensitivity to protein-disrupting treatments and their consistent association with an abnormal amyloid protein, stimulated the hypothesis that the TSE agents are probably subviral in size, composed of protein and devoid of nucleic acid. Prusiner suggested the term "prion" for such agents and concluded that the amyloid protein found in brain tissues of humans and animals with TSEs was the prion or a component of it. The prion hypothesis proposes that the etiologic agent propagates itself by some self-replicating change in folding of a host-encoded amyloid protein (prion protein, or PrP) associated with a transition from an alpha-helix-rich structure in the native protease-sensitive conformation (designated PrP^C or PrP-sen) to a mainly beta-sheet structure in the protease-resistant conformation (PrP^{Sc} or PrP-res) associated with infectivity. The existence of a second host-encoded protein—a "protein X" that participates in the transformation—was postulated to explain certain otherwise puzzling findings. The prion hypothesis has been widely accepted and was recognized by the awarding of the Nobel Prize for Physiology and Medicine to Prusiner in 1997. However, the hypothesis has not been universally accepted; its postulated genome-like coding mechanism based on differences in folding of a degraded host protein is not understood at a molecular level and does not yet account for the many biologic strains of the TSE agent.

Studies by Prusiner and colleagues convincingly demonstrated that PrP must be expressed for an individual to be susceptible to infection with a TSE agent and that overexpression of an abnormal form of PrP causes a disease resembling a TSE. It remains unclear if the abnormal PrP overexpressed by genetically engineered animals actually replicates like an infectious TSE agent.

The pathogenesis of scrapie and other TSEs of animals resembles that seen in some infections with conventional viral agents: the agent first replicates in lymphoid tissues, not causing apparent injury, before spreading to the CNS.

Some studies suggested that TSE agents also spread to the CNS through peripheral nerves.

HISTORY

TSEs of Animals. Scrapie has been known for more than 200 years to affect European sheep; it was transmitted to normal sheep and goats in the 1930s. Scrapie accidentally entered the United States and other countries in the 1940s. Sheep in Australia and New Zealand are now free of scrapie, but the disease remains in the United States and Europe. Transmissible mink encephalopathy (TME) is a similar disease of mink; no outbreaks of TME have been seen in the United States since 1985. A scrapie-like chronic wasting disease (CWD) affects deer and elk in the United States, mainly in captive animals in Colorado and Wyoming; CWD was recently recognized in hunter-killed animals in the same area. A large outbreak of a bovine spongiform encephalopathy (BSE, or mad cow disease) that probably began in 1985 and peaked in 1992 has already affected more than 170,000 cattle in Great Britain and smaller numbers of native-born cattle in several continental European countries. BSE has a wider natural host range than do other TSEs and has infected nonbovine ungulates and felines as well as people. In spite of active surveillance by public health and agricultural authorities, BSE has never been detected in the United States.

TSEs of Humans. Kuru ("trembling") was first described by Gajdusek and Zigas in 1957 among the Fore people living in what is now the Eastern Highlands province of Papua New Guinea (Fig. 30–11). Two years later, similarities in epidemiology, clinical illness, and histopathology suggested that kuru might be an unusual slow infection similar to scrapie. Kuru was successfully transmitted to chimpanzees in 1966 and later to other nonhuman primates. Creutzfeldt-Jakob disease (CJD) was first described in 1921, and its histopathologic similarity to kuru was noted in 1959. Sporadic CJD was first transmitted to animals in 1968; subsequently all other variants of CJD, including iatrogenic CJD (iCJD), new-variant CJD (vCJD), familial CJD (fCJD), and the Gerstmann-Sträussler-Scheinker syndrome (GSS) as well as the fatal familial insomnia syndrome (FFI) were also found to be associated with similar transmissible agents.

DISTRIBUTION, PREVALENCE, TRANSMISSION, AND EPIDEMIOLOGY

Kuru. This once affected Fore boys and girls aged ≥4 years as well as many women and a few adult men. The disease gradually disappeared among the Fore and now occurs only very rarely among older adults exposed as children to infected tissues by cannibalism, which ended in the late 1950s. There has been no evidence of transplacental spread of kuru or by nursing mothers to their offspring, or of any other mechanism of natural transmission except cannibalism.

Sporadic CJD. This occurs in all populations studied throughout the world with a recognized annual incidence of about 1 case per million; geographic foci of CJD with much higher incidence are attributed to fCJD, which usually accounts for no more than 10% of cases in other populations. GSS and FFI are extremely rare and always familial. In families with fCJD, GSS, and FFI, the disease is expressed in an autosomal dominant pattern of inheritance, segregating with 1 of more than 10 mutations in or increased numbers of duplications in an octapeptide region of the gene encoding PrP, discussed earlier.

Iatrogenic CJD. This has been accidentally transmitted by preparations of human-cadaveric pituitary hormones (most often growth hormone), by transplants of human corneas and of dura mater, and by contaminated cortical electrodes and other instruments used in neurosurgery. A few medical personnel may have gotten CJD from exposure to infected

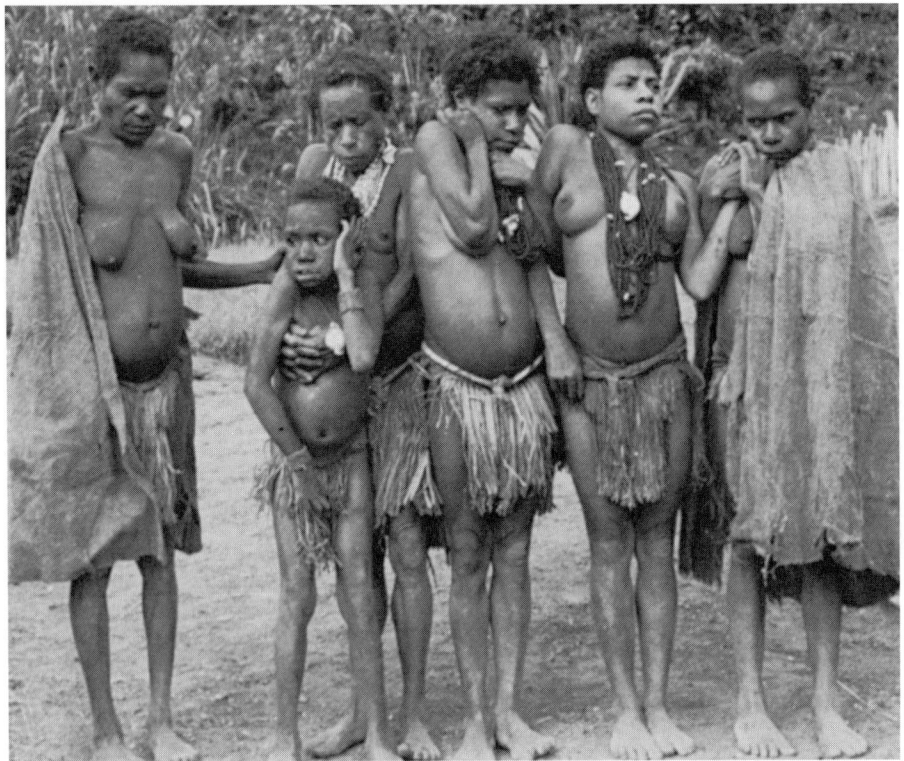

Figure **30–11.** Six kuru patients from one village in the South Fore. Their postural instability may be seen from the activity of muscle groups in their legs and feet. To maintain their posture and also damp down involuntary movements, their arms are held closely and firmly against each other. The girl shows a left convergent strabismus. (Courtesy of Dr. D. Carleton Gajdusek, National Institutes of Health, and Am J Med 26:447, 1959.)

human tissues. CJD has not been recognized in children born to mothers with iCJD.

New-Variant CJD. This was most likely transmitted to humans by exposure to some beef product contaminated with the BSE agent, perhaps carried into meat with bovine CNS tissue; the cattle themselves were apparently infected by ingesting BSE agent–contaminated meat and bone meal added to their feed. It has been postulated that the BSE agent arose when a strain of sheep scrapie with an unusually broad host range accidentally entered the rendered animal protein that comprises meat and bone meal. None of the TSEs—with the possible exception of scrapie—seems to be contagious by ordinary contact among individuals. The agents of scrapie and other animal TSEs, excepting BSE, have not been recognized to cause disease in humans.

PATHOLOGY. With the exception of FFI, in which pathology is largely restricted to thalamic nuclei and neuronal vacuolation is minimal, all the TSEs are characterized by a marked spongiform change in the cerebral cortex (Fig. 30–10), variable loss of neurons in the cerebral cortex and cerebellum, and hypertrophy and proliferation of astrocytes. Amyloid plaques (Fig. 30–12) are found in the cerebellum, and sometimes in the cerebral cortex, of about 70% of patients dying with kuru; perhaps 10% of those with sCJD; many with fCJD; and all subjects diagnosed with GSS. The plaques contain PrP-res, as evidenced by staining with labeled antibodies; PrP-res also accumulates in areas of the brain parenchyma not containing visible plaques; small amounts are sometimes in lymphoid tissues as well. Unique findings in vCJD are consistent presence of "florid" (flower-like) amyloid plaques surrounded by halos of vacuoles in the cerebral cortex and exceptionally dense accumulation of PrP-res in brain and lymphoid tissues. (The finding of PrP-res in lymphoid tissues may be useful for premortem diagnosis of vCJD without recourse to brain biopsy.)

CLINICAL MANIFESTATIONS

Onset. The TSEs all have a relatively long asymptomatic incubation period that varies from about 18 months in sub-

jects accidentally infected with CJD agent during surgery and 4 years for some Fore children exposed to cannibalism during early infancy to more than 30 years. Onset of illness is insidious. Most patients with kuru first noticed changes in coordination that were not apparent on physical examination. Cerebellar ataxia may be the presenting complaint of patients with iCJD. Sporadic CJD typically begins with confusion that may progress over a few weeks to frank dementia. Patients with vCJD, who are much younger than those with sCJD

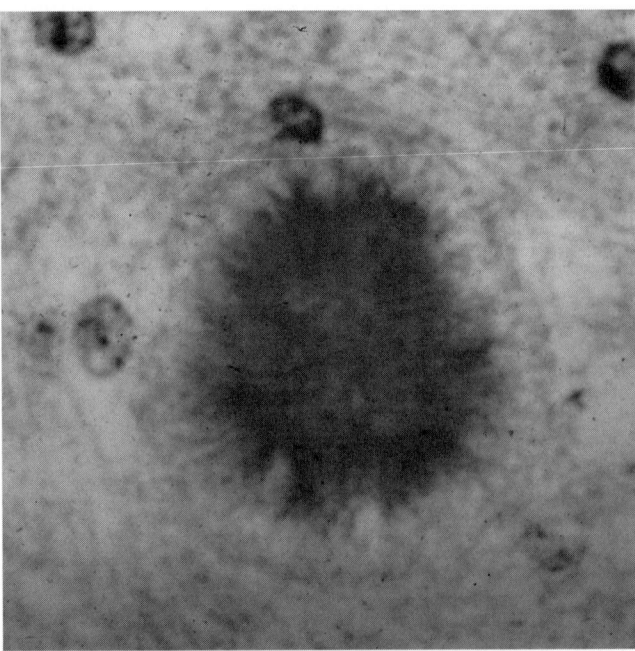

Figure **30–12.** An amyloid plaque in the cerebellum of a patient with kuru.

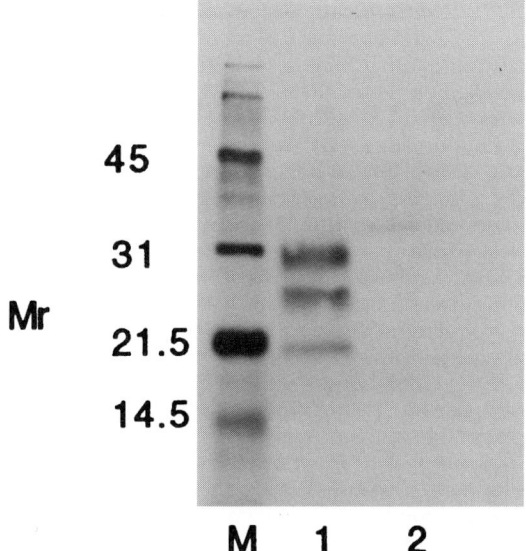

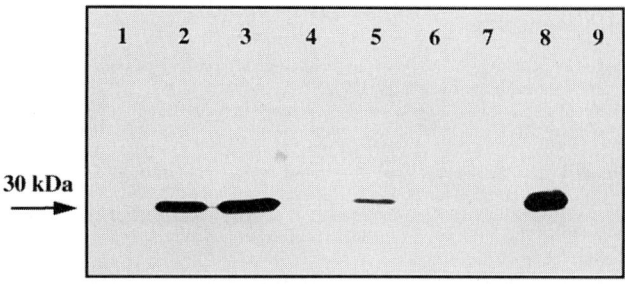

Figure 30–14. Specimens of CSF from patients with CJD *(lanes 2, 3, 5, and 8)* Western blotted with antibody to the 14-3-3 protein. CSF from other patients do not contain detectable protein. (From Hsich G, et al: N Engl J Med 335:924, 1996.)

Figure 30–13. Protease-resistant prion protein *(lane 1)* separated by electrophoresis and Western immunoblot with labeled antibody to show its three glycoforms. Prion protein extracted from a normal brain *(lane 2)* is not detected.

(Table 30–4), have subtle changes in behavior—originally thought to be psychiatric—and complaints of dysesthesias at onset.

Course. Kuru progressed over the course of several months with the appearance of ataxia and apraxia, shivering truncal and limb tremors, and a variety of cranial nerve signs including strabismus and dysarthria, without frank dementia or myoclonic jerks. Death in kuru resulted from inanition, pneumonia, infected skin ulcers or accidental burns, usually in less than a year after onset. In all variants of CJD, dementia progresses to akinetic mutism and coma. Myoclonic jerks are common. Most patients with CJD live for less than a year after onset, although a few have survived for several years; patients with vCJD tend to live longer than those with other forms of CJD.

PROGNOSIS AND TREATMENT. The TSEs are fatal. Only supportive treatment is available. Postexposure treatment regimens based on experimental studies of the pathogenesis of TSE in animals were recently recommended for humans, but these have yet to be validated in clinical practice.

DIAGNOSIS AND PREVENTION. The diagnosis of TSEs is mainly based on clinical features during life and examination of CNS tissues obtained from cerebral cortical biopsy (when indicated for differential diagnosis or other compelling reason) or from brain tissue at autopsy. Both conventional histopathologic examination (Figs. 30–10 and 30–12) and testing for the presence of PrP-res by immunohistochemistry, Western immunoblotting (Fig. 30–13), or by immunogold-labeling negative-stain electron microscopy of extracted PrP have been helpful in different laboratories. Testing for PrP-res in more accessible tissues, e.g., tonsils or nictitating membrane, may eventually prove useful for improved premortem diagnosis of TSEs of animals but nothing comparable has been attempted with humans. A nonspecific surrogate test for TSE based on the appearance of detectable amounts of a normal neuronal protein (the 14-3-3 protein, Fig. 30–14) in the CSF of patients with CJD has been useful to rule out a diagnosis of Alzheimer disease and to help confirm the diagnosis of vCJD. At some time during the course of CJD, most patients have a typical electroencephalographic pattern of periodic high-voltage complexes on a generalized slow background that aids in diagnosis; this finding has been absent during the course of vCJD.

TABLE 30–4. Clinical and Histopathologic Features of Patients With New-Variant Creutzfeldt-Jakob Disease (vCJD) and Typical Sporadic CJD

Clinical Feature	New-Variant CJD (N = 10)	Sporadic CJD (N = 185)
Age* at death (yr): average (range)	29 (19–41)	65
Duration* of illness (mo): average (range)	12 (8–23)	4
Presenting clinical signs	Abnormal behavior, dysesthesia	Dementia
Later clinical signs	Dementia, ataxia, myoclonus	Ataxia, myoclonus
Electroencephalogram: periodic high-voltage complexes	None	Most
PRNP† Codon 129 Met/Met	100%	83%
Histopathologic changes	Vacuolation, neuronal loss, astrocytosis, amyloid plaques (100%)	Vacuolation, neuronal loss, astrocytosis, amyloid plaques (~15%)
"Florid" amyloid plaques‡	100%	None
PrP-res§ glycosylation pattern	BSE-like¶	Not BSE-like

*Median age and duration for vCJD; averages for sporadic CJD.
†Gene encoding prion protein.
‡Dense plaques, pale periphery, surrounded by halo of vacuoles.
§Protease-resistant prior protein.
¶Predominantly diglycosylated PrP-res (Collinge et al: Nature 383:685, 1996).
Modified from Will RG, Ironside JW, Zeidler M, et al: A new variant of Creutzfeldt-Jakob disease in the UK. Lancet 347:921, 1996.

Bibliography

Aguzzi A, Collinge J, Hill AF, et al: Post-exposure prophylaxis after accidental prion inoculation. Lancet 350:1519, 1997.

Asher DM: Slow viral infections of the human nervous system. *In* Scheld WM, Whitley RJ, Durack DT (eds): Infections of the Nervous System, 2nd ed. New York, Raven Press, 1997, pp 199–221.

Brown P: The "brave new world" of transmissible spongiform encephalopathy (infectious cerebral amyloidosis). Molec Neurobiol 8:79, 1994.

Brown P, Gibbs CJ Jr, Rodgers-Johnson P, et al: Human spongiform encephalopathy: The NIH series of 300 cases of experimentally transmitted disease. Ann Neurol 35:513, 1994.

Bruce ME, Will RG, Ironside JW, et al: Transmissions to mice indicate that 'new variant' CJD is caused by the BSE agent. Nature 389:498, 1997.

Chesebro B: BSE and prions: Uncertainties about the agent. Science 279:42, 1998.

Collee JG, Bradley R: BSE: A decade on. Lancet 349:636, 715, 1997.

Collinge J, Sidle KC, Meads J, et al: Molecular analysis of prion strain variation and the aetiology of 'new variant' CJD. Nature 383:685, 1996.

Gajdusek DC, Zigas V: Kuru: Clinical, pathological and epidemiological study of an acute progressive degenerative disease of the central nervous system among natives of the Eastern Highlands in New Guinea. Am J Med 26:442, 1957.

Hsich G, Kenney K, Gibbs CJ, et al: The 14-3-3 brain protein in cerebrospinal fluid as a marker for transmissible spongiform encephalopathies. N Engl J Med 335:924, 1996.

Prusiner SB: Prion diseases and the BSE crisis. Science 278:245, 1997.

Schonberger LB: New variant Creutzfeldt-Jakob disease and bovine spongiform encephalopathy. Infect Dis Clin North Am 12:111, 1998.

Will RG, Ironside JW, Zeidler M, et al: A new variant of Creutzfeldt-Jakob disease in the UK. Lancet 347:921, 1996.

31 Viral Hemorrhagic Fevers

31.1 Yellow Fever

Theodore Tsai

DEFINITION. Yellow fever (YF) is an acute mosquito-borne infection of variable severity complicated by the triad of hepatitis, hemorrhagic diathesis, and proteinuria. The flavivirus is transmitted only in South America and Africa.

ETIOLOGY. The virus is the type species of arboviruses in the *Flavivirus* genus, family *Flaviviridae*. Hepatitis C virus exhibits a similar genomic and physical structure and is classified in the same family; however, it shares no antigenic relationships with viruses in the *Flavivirus* genus. Virions are spherical, approximately 40 nm in diameter, and enveloped by a lipid bilayer containing a matrix protein and an envelope (E) glycoprotein. The single 11-kb positive-strand RNA is complexed with a capsid protein. The three structural and eight nonstructural proteins are encoded in a single open-reading frame that is cotranslationally processed. The E protein (53 kDa) is variably glycosylated and mediates important biologic functions, e.g., attachment to cellular membranes, hemagglutination, and viral neutralization. The E protein is a homodimer with head-to-tail configuration, lying horizontally on the virion surface with conformationally dependent epitopes at various sites along the external face of the rodlike structure. Viral assembly takes place in the cytoplasm, but RNA is replicated in the perinuclear reticular network with the mediation of NS1, a glycosylated dimer that also is secreted and elicits protective antibodies. Other nonstructural proteins exhibit enzymatic activities required for viral replication. NS5 appears to be an RNA-dependent polymerase.

Taxonomic analyses of E protein–associated sequences have defined two major genotypes representing strains from West and central Africa and from East Africa. Similarity among the 20 strains from a 67-year interval was above 89%. Strains from South America were closely related to those of West African origin, confirming previous conjectures that YF virus was introduced to the Western Hemisphere from Africa. A second South American subtype was defined from differences in viral 3' noncoding region sequences. Genomic sequences of strains within each geographic area were highly conserved, indicating little mixing between strains from East and West Africa.

HISTORY. In the previous two centuries, YF was a major epidemic disease in the Western Hemisphere and Europe, spread from city to city by infected humans and mosquitoes aboard trading ships. Outbreaks occurred on the eastern seaboard of the United States and inland along the Mississippi, the last major outbreak occurring in New Orleans in 1905. In Europe, notable outbreaks were reported in Lisbon, Gibraltar, and Swansea, Wales. The mosquito-borne mode of transmission proposed by Carlos Finlay in 1881 was proved by the U.S. Army commission led by Walter Reed in 1900. Acting on this information, Gorgas rapidly eliminated YF from Havana by a systematic mosquito eradication program. Epidemic transmission largely had been interrupted in Central America before the virus was isolated in 1927 in rhesus monkeys from a viremic Ghanese man named Asibi.

DISTRIBUTION AND INCIDENCE. YF occurs only in South America and Africa (Fig. 31–1). In the Western Hemisphere, the virus is transmitted in tropical forests, maintained in a jungle cycle among monkeys and sylvatic mosquito vectors. A relatively constant number of sporadic cases and occasional outbreaks in occupationally exposed adults are reported each year (Fig. 31–2). As a result of the successful *Aedes aegypti* eradication campaign in the Western Hemisphere, the last major urban epidemic occurred in 1942 in Acre State, Brazil; however, the threat of epidemic transmission has resurfaced in newly reinfested locations. Sylvatic infections occur under similar circumstances in forested areas of West, Central, and East Africa, but in areas where human habitations are clustered near the forest, or in the moist savanna, where monkeys are numerous, a high level of endemic infection occurs (Fig. 135–2). The number of such cases is poorly quantified, and usually only outbreaks come to attention. Both rural and urban outbreaks occur at intervals, with recognized cases sometimes numbering in tens of thousands of cases (Fig. 31–3). However, when epidemics have been investigated systematically, actual incidence estimates have exceeded official reports by up to 40-fold. For example, during the interval from 1984 to 1993, Nigeria reported more than 20,000 cases and 4000 deaths, but extrapolating from field studies, at least 1 million cases are estimated to have occurred. The resurgence of cases in West Africa since 1983 is the latest wave in a succession of periodic epidemic activity observed since the colonial era.

The absence of YF from Asia, despite the presence of competent *Ae. aegypti* vectors, is not fully understood but may be explained in part by cross-protective immunity from endemic dengue infections.

TRANSMISSION AND EPIDEMIOLOGY. Epidemic (urban) YF is transmitted from human to human by *Ae. aegypti* mosquitoes. The jungle cycle transmitted among sylvatic mosquito vectors and forest primates serves as a viral reservoir and is a source of infection for humans only when they intrude on active foci (Fig. 135–2).

After an infectious bite, humans become viremic for a period of several days during which they can serve as a source of infection for other mosquitoes. Unlike other viral hemorrhagic fevers, direct person-to-person spread does not occur in YF. After taking an infectious blood meal, viral

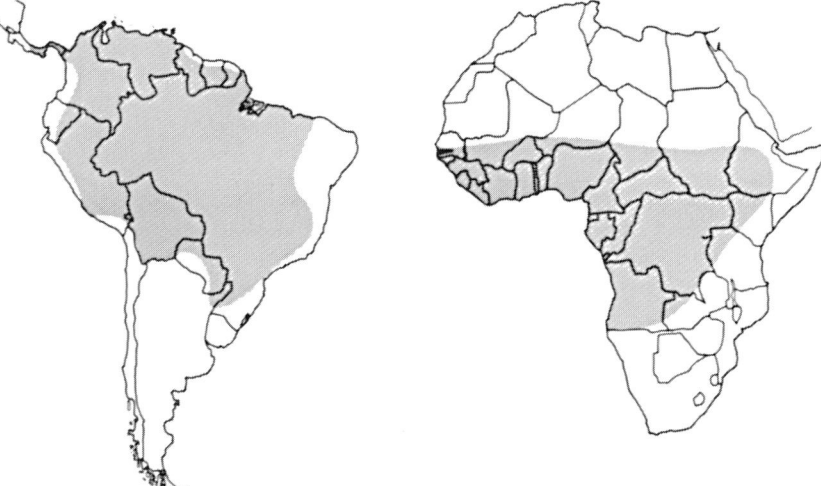

Figure 31–1. Regions of tropical America and Africa endemic for yellow fever or experiencing intermittent epidemics. Travelers to these areas should receive yellow fever immunization. Yellow fever does not occur in Asia, Australia, or the Pacific.

infection must disseminate in the mosquito over a period of 9 to 12 days (extrinsic incubation period) before the mosquito can transmit the virus in future feedings. Epidemic interhuman transmission occurs in villages and urban locations where human population density is high and *Ae. aegypti*, adapted to the human environment, breed in peridomestic containers holding rainwater, e.g., discarded cans, flower dishes, tires, and in uncovered storage containers where drinking water is stored. Highly infested villages (e.g., Breteau indices >50 larval-positive containers per 100 houses) are at high risk for epidemic transmission should a viremic person introduce the virus.

South America. The sylvatic cycle of YF in South America is maintained by diurnal *Haemagogus* sp. mosquitoes and forest monkeys in moving epizootics along riverine gallery forests. A sufficiently large population of vertebrate amplifying hosts must be available to support continued viral transmission, because acquired immunity and, in the case of *Alouatta* sp. (howler) monkeys, deaths from the infection, would otherwise exhaust the susceptible reservoir. Maintenance of viral transmission most likely is supplemented by other mechanisms, e.g., vertical infections in mosquitoes. Cases occur mainly in the rainy season from January to March among unvaccinated persons entering forests to fell trees and construct roads, and among settlers in the tropical frontier. Thus, most cases are in adults and more cases are seen in males than in females. These are dead-end infections

acquired from sylvatic vectors, although small outbreaks may be seen in groups exposed to a common sylvatic source or during periods of hyperenzootic transmission.

Africa. In Africa, humans are tangentially infected when exposed to a similar sylvatic cycle maintained among monkeys and *Aedes africanus* (Fig. 135–2). In the open vegetation zones characterized by forest-savanna mosaic and moist savanna, however, an active cycle of endemic and enzootic infections is maintained during the rainy season by *Aedes furcifer*, *Ae. luteocephalus*, and other tree-hole mosquitoes to both humans and monkeys. A high level of endemic infection results from exposures occurring in childhood. Perennial viral transmission in this cycle is a potential source for viral introduction to an *Ae. aegypti*–borne epidemic cycle and thus its significance as the "zone of emergence." There is evidence that virus is maintained over the dry season by vertical transmission in mosquitoes or infected ticks.

PATHOLOGY AND PATHOGENESIS. The incubation period after an infectious mosquito bite is 3 to 6 days. Viral replication occurs initially in regional lymph nodes and after viremic spread to other organs, principally in liver, spleen, and bone marrow. Viral antigen has been found in degenerating hepatocytes and Councilman bodies, kidney, and myocardium. Intranuclear inclusions, or Torres bodies, occasionally may be seen. Hepatocellular degeneration is concentrated in the midzone, sparing hepatocytes surrounding the central vein and portal triad and with preservation of the reticulum

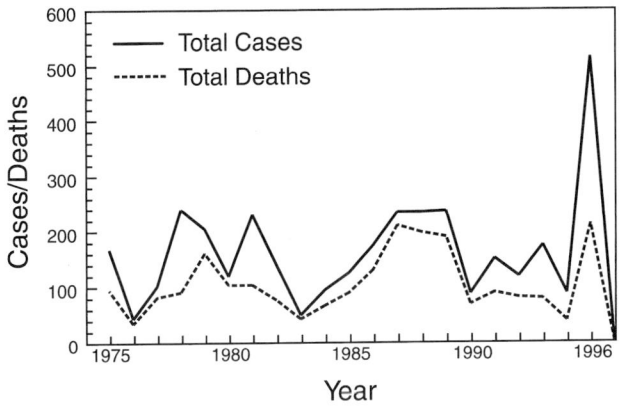

Figure 31–2. Reported yellow fever cases, South America, 1975–1996.

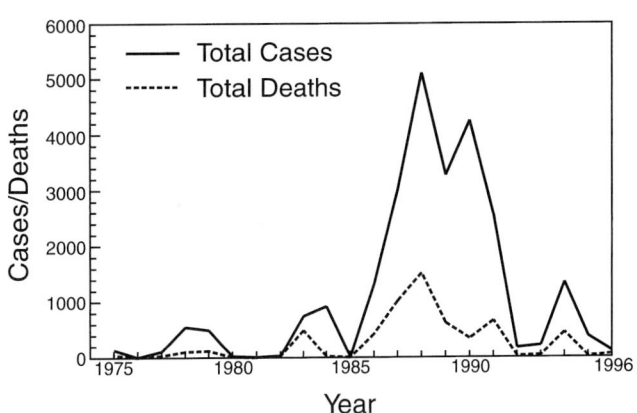

Figure 31–3. Reported yellow fever cases, Africa, 1975–1996.

(Fig. 31–4). Microvesicular fatty changes and deposition of ceroid pigment are prominent, but there is a scant mononuclear inflammatory response. Hepatic histopathologic findings overlap those of other African hemorrhagic fevers. The kidneys are edematous with tubular epithelial and glomerular endothelial cell swelling and mesangial proliferation. The brain also appears swollen and may exhibit petechial bleeding. Hemorrhages are found on mucosal surfaces of the gastrointestinal tract and abdominal and pleural serosae with bleeding into the gastrointestinal tract and the abdominal and pleural cavities. Degenerative myocardial changes with fatty infiltration also are a consistent finding. The pathogenesis of the bleeding diathesis reflects depletion of hepatic clotting factors, intravascular coagulation, and platelet dysfunction. Shock and fatal illness result from a combination of direct parenchymal damage to the myocardium, kidneys, and other organs, and to the effects of vasoactive cytokines.

CLINICAL MANIFESTATIONS. Illness in the majority of cases is a self-limited grippe with fever and myalgias but is fatal in 25 to 50% of cases with the full syndrome of hemorrhages, jaundice, and renal disease. After the abrupt onset of fever, headache, and myalgias (period of infection), the illness may resolve or remit briefly for a few hours or several days (period of remission), followed by the resumption of high fever, lumbosacral back pain, nausea, vomiting, abdominal pain, and changes in consciousness (period of intoxication). The patient is prostrated and lethargic and usually is dehydrated due to protracted vomiting and poor intake. The pulse may be slow in proportion to the temperature (Faget sign), the conjunctivae injected, and the facies flushed. Jaundice may be evident and epistaxis, oral mucosal bleeding, hematemesis, and petechial or purpuric hemorrhages may be prominent. Clinical deterioration progresses to combined hepatitis and renal failure and hypotension from fluid loss, capillary dysfunction, and bleeding. Signs of encephalopathy or coma are not uncommon, resulting from metabolic disturbances and cerebral edema; death usually occurs within 7 to 10 days after onset.

Early in the illness, the blood count discloses neutropenia and later, thrombocytopenia. Prolonged prothrombin, partial thromboplastin, and clotting times are seen in cases with severe illness, and in some patients fibrin degradation products have been detected. Proteinuria is a signature of the illness, and renal failure may lead to an exacerbation of electrolyte disturbances due to emesis. Hepatic transaminases and bilirubin are elevated; azotemia may be of prerenal origin in dehydrated patients or may reflect renal failure. Cerebrospinal fluid (CSF) examination discloses an elevated protein count without pleocytosis. ST-T wave changes and arrhythmias may be seen on electrocardiogram (ECG).

The critical phase of the illness usually resolves within a week or, rarely, after 2 weeks, during which secondary bacterial infections resulting in pneumonia or sepsis are frequent complications. Recovery of icteric patients has not been reported to be complicated by chronic hepatitis.

TREATMENT. No specific therapy is available but attentive monitoring and correction of potentially life-threatening physiologic disturbances resulting from the infection are critical. Evaluation and treatment of dehydration and electrolyte disturbances are important in the early phase of illness, and differentiation of prerenal and renal failure may be difficult at the stage of intoxication when acute renal tubular dysfunction may occur. Data and experience are insufficient to evaluate the role of disseminated intravascular coagulation in the illness and the value of heparin therapy. Secondary bacterial complications should be anticipated and attention should be

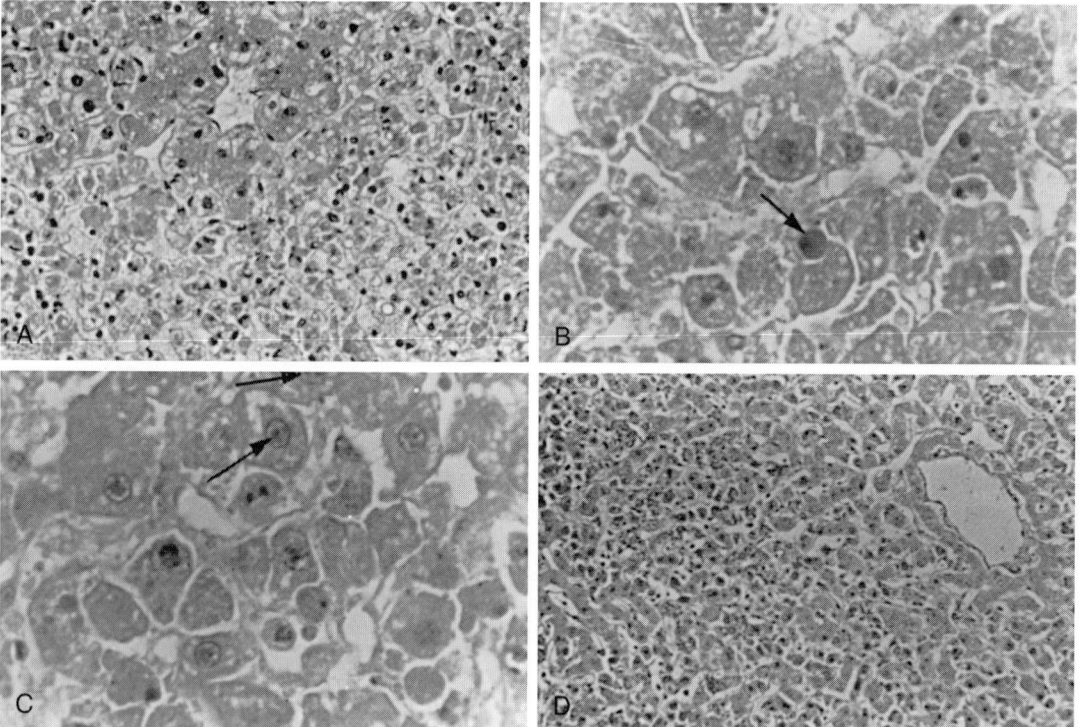

Figure 31–4. Fatal yellow fever: histopathologic changes in the liver. *A,* Central zone of a liver lobule, showing cytoplasmic degeneration, sinusoidal Councilman bodies, and sparing of hepatocytes around central vein. *B,* Acidophilic cytoplasmic degeneration of hepatocytes with Councilman body formation *(arrow). C,* Amorphous amphophilic mass in nucleus (Torres body, *arrows):* these are not viral inclusions, but are derived from host cell nuclear proteins. *D,* Midzonal necrosis of liver lobule. (*A* and *D,* courtesy of Armed Forces Institute of Pathology.)

given to prompt recognition and therapy and to the prevention of nosocomial infection.

DIAGNOSIS

Differential Diagnosis. The diagnosis should be considered in unvaccinated persons with onset of illness within a week of exposure to an enzootic location. Severe YF is similar clinically to other viral hemorrhagic fevers occurring in Africa and South America, and laboratory confirmation is required to make the diagnosis. Confirmation of the specific diagnosis is important because precautions against nosocomial and secondary person-to-person spread should be instituted for several of the other viral hemorrhagic fevers and because the diagnosis of a YF case may signal the need for a vaccination campaign and vector control. Important clues can be gathered from a description of the patient's activities and itinerary; from the occurrence of cases suggesting secondary transmission (as might occur in Congo-Crimean, arenavirus, or filovirus hemorrhagic fevers); a concurrent febrile illness outbreak suggesting dengue; and from certain clinical features, e.g., rash, suggesting Ebola or Marburg viruses or dengue infection. Other conditions that should be considered in the differential diagnosis include leptospirosis, viral hepatitis, malaria, typhoid, typhus, relapsing fever, acute fatty liver in pregnancy, and toxin-related hepatitis.

Diagnostic Tests. Laboratory methods to detect viral genomic sequences or viral antigen in acute-phase blood samples have been described, but their application to clinical samples has not been reported. Virus in blood samples taken within the first 12 days of illness can be isolated in susceptible cell cultures (e.g., C636, AP61, Vero) or by intrathoracic inoculation of mosquitoes or intracerebral inoculation of suckling mice. Viral recovery from individual patients, or in the event of an outbreak, from at least several patients, is highly desirable to prove the etiology because cross reactions often obfuscate the interpretation of serologic tests. IgM-capture enzyme-linked immunosorbent assay (ELISA) is the preferred serologic test because of its sensitivity and relative specificity (comparable to complement fixation). However, in persons with previous flavivirus infections, heterologous reactions frequently interfere with interpretation. The neutralization test provides the highest specificity, but usually it is available only in reference laboratories and results are unavailable for a week or more.

Organ samples from fatal cases (especially liver) should be examined immunohistochemically to provide a specific diagnosis because pathologic changes in YF are not specific and cannot be differentiated reliably from those due to other causes of hepatitis and hemorrhagic fever. Liver biopsy during the period of intoxication is dangerous and is contraindicated because of the possibility of hemorrhage. Viral isolation and direct detection of viral antigen or genomic sequences also should be attempted from pathologic specimens.

PREVENTION AND CONTROL

Travelers. Live-attenuated vaccine made from the 17D strain is safe and provides protective immunity in 95% of vaccinees within 10 days after vaccination. One subcutaneous dose provides decades-long immunity, but reimmunization at 10-year intervals is required for travel. Side effects are mild and rare except in infants, in whom encephalitis is a potential complication. Eighteen cases of vaccine-related encephalitis have been reported, all in infants and children and the majority in infants <4 months of age. The vaccine is contraindicated in infants <4 months old and should be given to 4- to 9-month-old infants only if they are traveling to areas with high risk. The vaccine is grown in chick embryos, and persons with egg allergy should be tested for sensitivity before vaccination (see package insert). Congenital infection without malformation or disease was reported in

one case when vaccine was given in the first trimester of pregnancy. The vaccine has been given safely to human immunodeficiency virus–infected persons with CD4 cell counts >200/mm³ and to individuals on mild immunosuppressive regimens (e.g., alternate-day steroids for arthritis), but in general the vaccine is contraindicated in immunosuppressed patients. For pregnant women and immunosuppressed persons, vaccine recommendations should be individualized based on the risk for exposure during travel and the theoretical risks of vaccination. Exacerbations of multiple sclerosis and ketoacidosis in a diabetes mellitus patient after vaccination have been reported anecdotally.

Travelers to and from YF enzootic zones (Fig. 31–1) should be immunized according to international health regulations, keeping in mind that disease risk exists in enzootic areas even when none is reported. Two cases in travelers to an unpublicized epidemic focus in Brazil, one in an unvaccinated U.S. citizen, underscore this point. YF vaccine can be given together with chloroquine, immune globulin, measles, diphtheria-tetanus-pertussis (DTP), polio, hepatitis A or B, or intramuscular typhoid vaccines without interference (the last has an adjuvant effect). Other preventive measures, e.g., use of insect repellents and mosquito netting, are recommended if there is a high risk of exposure.

Endemic Areas. In areas of Africa where the disease is endemic, universal childhood vaccination through the World Health Organization's Expanded Programme of Immunization (EPI) (coadministered with measles vaccine) has been recommended since 1988, but coverage rates are low (9% overall). Neutralizing antibodies are detected in only 15% of vaccinated asymptomatic HIV-infected children, and it is unknown whether they are protected.

The emergency response to an epidemic should focus on mass vaccination in the epidemic area and surrounding susceptible population. Control of *Ae. aegypti* should be initiated by eliminating breeding sites in discarded containers and potable water reservoirs and by applying insecticides.

Bibliography

deBrito T, Sigueira SAC, Santos RTM, et al: Human fatal yellow fever—immunohistochemical detection of viral antigens in the liver, kidney and heart. Path Res Pract 188:177, 1992.
Freestone DS: Yellow fever vaccine. In Plotkin SA, Mortimer EA (eds): Vaccines, 2nd ed. Philadelphia, WB Saunders, 1994, pp 741–779.
Monath TP: Yellow fever: A medically neglected disease. Report on a seminar. Rev Infect Dis 9:165, 1987.
Monath TP: Yellow fever and dengue—the interactions of virus, vector, and host in the re-emergence of epidemic disease. Semin Virol 5:133, 1994.

31.2 Lassa Fever

Susan P. Fisher-Hoch and Joseph B. McCormick

DEFINITION. Lassa virus, the cause of the hemorrhagic disease Lassa fever, is an arenavirus. Members of this family of viruses are natural parasites of rodents, in whom they establish a chronic but silent, lifelong infection. High titers of the virus are present in rodent urine, and exposed humans may become infected as accidental hosts. Although Lassa fever was first described in West Africa in the 1950s, the virus was not isolated from a patient until 1969. Lassa fever occurs from Nigeria to Guinea, resulting in as many as 5000 deaths annually.

VIROLOGY. Lassa virus belongs to the *Arenaviridae* family of viruses consisting of a single genus, *Arena virus*. They are enveloped viruses with a mean diameter of 110 to 130 nm.

The virion density in sucrose is 1.17 g/cm³. The arenaviruses contain two segments of RNA (large, L and small, S) encoding at least four gene products in ambisense arrangements in both segments. L-strand RNA encodes the negative-sense viral polymerase; this is a 2210 amino acid protein with a calculated molecular weight of 254,529 in the case of the closely related lymphocytic choriomeningitis virus (LCMV). Mutations in this gene affect LCMV plaque morphology, lethality in guinea pigs, and ability of the variant strain to suppress the cytotoxic T-cell response and initiate persistent infection. A newly described positive-sense Z gene codes for a 10-kDa zinc finger protein. It appears that for LCMV at least, the genes on the L strand are critical elements controlling virus replication, virulence, and persistence. Furthermore, the arenavirus polymerase is unique, bearing little resemblance to other RNA virus polymerases. The 3' half of the S-strand RNA encodes a positive-sense, nucleoprotein, and the 5' half encodes a negative-sense glycoprotein precursor. The viral envelope is composed of two glycosylated proteins (GP1 and GP2), which are created by enzyme cleavage after translation. GP1 (molecular weight, 35 to 38) makes up the amino end and GP2 (molecular weight, 44 to 64), the carboxyl end of the precursor. The single nucleocapsid protein of the *Arenaviridae* range in molecular weight from 54 to 68 kDa and the viral polymerase is usually about 200 kDa in size.

EPIDEMIOLOGY AND ECOLOGY. The modes of transmission from rodent to human are not precisely known. Arenaviruses are stable, especially with low humidity. Virus transmission is a function of the interaction of humans with rodents or their excretions, e.g., urine. Transmission is also a result of close human to human interaction involving contact with infected human secretions. Direct contact of cuts and scratches on hands and feet with articles and surfaces contaminated by virus may be an important and consistent mode of transmission.

Transmission

Rodent to Human. The only known reservoir of Lassa virus is *Mastomys natalensis*, one of the most common rodents in Africa. At least two species of *Mastomys* (diploid types with 32 and 38 chromosomes) inhabit West Africa, and both harbor Lassa virus. A third diploid type (with 36 chromosomes) in southern Africa, carries the closely related, Mopeia virus, which is not virulent for humans. These rodents, especially the species with 32 chromosomes, are highly commensal with humans, and are a common domestic rodent in West Africa. Rodent movement within a village is limited usually to the area near the house the rodents occupy. Infection rates are higher in household members when the house is occupied by infected rodents, particularly if numbers are large. As all age groups and both sexes are affected, and antibody prevalence increases with age, it is assumed that most virus transmission to humans takes place in and around the homes. Rodent-to-human infection is highly associated with indiscriminate food storage and catching, cooking, and eating rodents.

Person to Person. Spread of Lassa virus in households is common, although it is less frequent than rodent to human spread. Risk of infection is associated with direct contact with, nursing care of, or possibly sexual contact with someone during the incubation or convalescent phases of illness.

Nosocomial Spread in Hospitals. This is a prominent mode of transmission in medical facilities with poor safety practices. Furthermore, increasing use of injections and intravenous therapy in West African hospitals with inadequate needle and syringe supplies has led to deadly epidemics among patients. Staff become infected when they practice inadequate barrier nursing techniques. Infection is usually due to injuries with needles and other sharp instruments, ill-advised surgery on infected patients, and exposure to blood. Nevertheless, it has been demonstrated that nosocomial transmission is effectively prevented by attention to clean needles and syringes and simple isolation and barrier nursing techniques.

Prevalence. Estimates of prevalence of antibody to Lassa virus range from 4 to 6% in Guinea to 15 to 20% in Nigeria, although in some villages in Sierra Leone, as many as 60% of the population have evidence of past infection. In prospective studies, seroconversion to Lassa virus ranged from 5 to 20% of susceptible (seronegative) Sierra Leone villagers. Most of those infected were asymptomatic. However, antibody prevalence was only 1.4% in villagers in the community surrounding a Nigerian hospital with a recent nosocomial outbreak with very high fatality (76%). These data suggest some strains may vary in virulence.

In Sierra Leone, illness to infection ratios range from 1:4 to 1:5, and the proportion of all febrile illnesses associated with seroconversion was found to range from 5 to 14% in prospective, village-based studies. Five to 8% of infected people were hospitalized, and, although overall fatality was as low as 2 or 3%, it rose to 15 to 20% in hospitalized case, and to 30% or more in women in the third trimester of pregnancy. Case-fatality rates in hospitalized children <15 years of age were 12 to 15%. In two hospitals in Sierra Leone, Lassa fever accounted for 10 to 15% of all adult admissions and 30% of adult deaths, peaking during the dryer months. Lassa fever is therefore common and probably results in more than 100,000 infections per year in West Africa. With so many living in poor-quality, rodent-infested housing and, with the increasing indiscriminate use of needles in hospital practice, community and hospital epidemics continue to occur. Because the Eastern Province of Sierra Leone, where the major studies were carried out, has been devastated by civil war with major disruption of populations and deteriorating living conditions, it is likely that Lassa fever will continue to be rampant.

PATHOPHYSIOLOGY

Pathology. Although the outcome in Lassa fever is directly associated with levels of virus replication, tissue destruction is not a major component. The most frequent and consistent microscopic lesions in fatal human Lassa fever are variable hepatocyte necrosis with regeneration and focal necrosis of adrenal glands and spleen, with little, if any, lymphocytic inflammatory response. Although high virus titers occur in brain, ovary, pancreas, uterus, and placenta, no significant pathologic lesions have been observed in these organs.

Pathogenesis. The critical events in fatal disease are intractable hypovolemic shock, severe central nervous system (CNS) involvement, bleeding, and gross edema of the head and neck with pulmonary edema and respiratory distress. Some of these manifestations are due to disturbances in the intravascular compartment, particularly increased endothelial cell permeability. Although circulating platelet numbers are moderately well conserved (usually about 100,000 × 10⁹/L), platelet dysfunction correlates with severity of illness, and a marked decrease in prostacyclin production by endothelium has been measured in primates infected by Lassa virus. An inhibitor of platelet function has been identified in the serum of patients and nonhuman primates with severe Lassa fever. Disseminated intravascular coagulation is not a significant component of fatal Lassa fever; circulating platelet numbers are maintained, and, in primates with severe Lassa infection, platelet and fibrinogen turnover have been normal, and there is no increase in fibrinogen breakdown products in humans. No clear evidence of virus replication and damage to endothelium has been demonstrated, so it must be concluded that shock and bleeding are due to disturbances in the functional homeostatic mechanisms of the intravascular compartment rather than simple activation of the coagulation cascade.

Immunity. The rapid development of antibodies to Lassa virus is accompanied by lymphopenia and absence of tissue infiltration by lymphocytes, suggesting that some impairment may occur in the T-cell arm of the immune response. In primates, the response to nonspecific antigens is markedly reduced during the acute phase of fatal infection. Lassa virus does not induce neutralizing antibodies in humans or primates during the acute or early convalescent phases of illness. In a minority of patients, neutralizing activity may occasionally be detected several weeks or months into the illness. These antibodies do not appear to be associated with virus clearance nor with immunity to reinfection. The cell-mediated immune response to Lassa virus may be assumed to be critical to virus clearance and presumably protects against reinfection. An experimental vaccine of the glycoprotein of Lassa virus expressed in vaccinia virus protects nonhuman primates, despite no production of neutralizing antibodies, although killed vaccine, which produces high titered antibodies to all proteins, is not protective.

CLINICAL MANIFESTATION

Symptoms and Signs. Following an incubation period of 7 to 18 days, Lassa fever begins insidiously with fever, weakness, and malaise. More than 50% of patients then experience joint and lumbar pain and 60% or more have a nonproductive cough. Most patients also have severe headache, usually frontal, and a painful sore throat. Many also develop severe retrosternal chest pain, and about half have vomiting or diarrhea and abdominal pain. On physical examination, respiratory rate, temperature, and pulse rate are elevated and blood pressure may be low. About a third have conjunctivitis and more than two thirds have pharyngitis, half of whom have exudates with diffusely inflamed and swollen posterior pharynx and tonsils but with few if any petechiae.

Hospital Course. Up to a third of hospitalized patients progress to a prostrating illness 6 to 8 days after onset of fever. They are often dehydrated and the hematocrit is elevated on admission. Bleeding occurs in only 15 to 20% of patients, limited primarily to the mucosal surfaces or occasionally conjunctival hemorrhages or gastrointestinal or vaginal bleeding. In severe disease, edema of the face and neck carries a poor prognosis. In the absence of peripheral edema, this may indicate capillary leakage rather than cardiac dysfunction or impaired venous return. About half of all patients have diffuse abdominal tenderness but there are no localizing signs, and bowel sounds are usually active. Proteinuria occurs in two thirds of patients, and blood urea nitrogen level may be moderately elevated.

Pulmonary and Cardiac. Crepitations in the lungs and pleural and pericardial rubs develop usually in early convalescence in about 20% of patients, occasionally in association with congestive heart failure. Severe retrosternal or epigastric pain seen in many patients may be due to pleural or pericardial involvement. More than 70% of 32 patients had abnormal ECGs. The changes included nonspecific ST-segment and T-wave abnormalities, ST-segment elevation, generalized low-voltage complexes, and changes reflecting electrolyte disturbance. None of the abnormalities correlated with clinical severity of disease, serum aminotransferase levels, or eventual outcome.

Neurologic. CNS signs are infrequent but also carry a poor prognosis, progressing from fine tremors and confusion to severe encephalopathy with or without generalized seizures, but without focal signs. CSF is usually normal, but there may be a few lymphocytes. Virus titers are lower in the CSF than in the serum.

Hematologic. The most significant hematologic changes are in platelet function. Thrombocytopenia is moderate even in severely ill patients, and function is markedly depressed or even absent. This abnormality is usually maximal on admission to the hospital, and is characteristically present even when circulating platelet numbers remain normal. A circulating inhibitor of platelet function has been associated with severe disease; it specifically inhibits platelet-dense granule and adenosine triphosphate release, relatively sparing the thromboxane pathways.

The mean white blood cell (WBC) count in Lassa fever on admission to hospital is $6000/mm^3$ and there is characteristically early lymphopenia, relative thrombocytopenia, and sometimes a relative or absolute neutrophilia. Neutrophil counts as high as $30,000/mm^3$ have been recorded in severe disease. The inhibitor activity of platelet function is also associated with poor generation of the chemotactic peptide N-formyl-methionyl-leucyl-phenylalanine (FMLP)–induced superoxide generation in neutrophils.

Prognosis. Serum aminotransferase levels >150 IU/L on admission are associated with a case-fatality rate of 50%. The level of viremia, i.e., a blood virus level $>1 \times 10^3$ mL, median tissue culture infective dose ($TCID_{50}$) per milliliter, is also associated with an increasing case fatality. Both factors together carry a mortality risk of 80%.

COMPLICATIONS

Maternal and Fetal Morbidity. Lassa fever is a common cause of maternal mortality in many areas of West Africa. Two studies have shown that the case-fatality rate in pregnant women is about 20%. In the case of women infected during the third trimester of pregnancy, the case fatality approaches 30%, even with good obstetric care, and virus titers in the placenta are as high as 10^9 $TCID_{50}/mL$. A fourfold reduction in mortality was noted among women who spontaneously or were therapeutically aborted. Fetal loss is over 87% and does not vary by trimester.

Deafness. Another important complication of Lassa fever is acute eighth nerve deafness. Nearly 30% of patients with Lassa fever infection have an acute loss of hearing in one or both ears. About half of the patients have a near or complete recovery, but in many the deafness is permanent. Other less frequent complications are uveitis, pericarditis, orchitis, pleural effusion, and ascites. Renal and hepatic failure are not seen.

DIAGNOSIS

Clinical Diagnosis. All ages including children can be infected, and Lassa fever is difficult to diagnose because its manifestations are so general and easily confused with early manifestations of many common infections, e.g., malaria, arbovirus infections, and typhoid fever. In young babies, marked edema has been reported. In older children, the disease may manifest as diarrhea or as pneumonia or simply as an unexplained prolonged fever. Among adults in an endemic area, fever with pharyngitis, proteinuria, and retrosternal chest pain had a positive predictive value for Lassa fever of 81% and a specificity of 89%. However, this triad's diagnostic sensitivity was only 50%. Bleeding and sore throat have a sensitivity and specificity for fatal outcome of about 90%.

Laboratory Diagnosis

Specimen Collections. All procedures must be carried out wearing gloves, mask, and gown, with provision of freshly made disinfectant (e.g., 10% hypochlorite) for immediate discard of contaminated materials. Particular care must be taken with all sharp instruments, e.g., needles. Specimens should be drawn into a vacuum tube system if available to minimize risk of spill, and blood should be allowed to clot at room temperature. Laboratory manipulations should be carried out within an exhaust vented cabinet if this is available. If not, all procedures must be in the hands of an experienced person who is aware of the risks of parenteral exposure and equipped with gloves and disinfectant. Glass must be avoided. The serum is separated and placed in a screw cap plastic vial for storage and/or transfer. Urine should be mixed with an equal amount of bovine serum albumin at pH 7.4 before freezing. Other fluids should be frozen undiluted. All of these specimens keep best if they are frozen at −70°C or lower as soon as possible. More hazardous in the laboratory are routine hematologic and biochemical assays, particularly if they fall into the hands of technicians unaware of the suspected diagnosis and the potential risks of virus-infected blood. Overall, if specimens are handled with the same precautions afforded HIV-infected samples, the risk to staff is minimal.

Antigen or Genome Detection. Reverse transcriptase polymerase chain reaction techniques (RT-PCR) detecting fragments of the S gene of the virus coding for the glycoprotein have been used successfully. The technique is rapid and accurate and the RNA extraction techniques effectively inactivate the virus, so that the procedure has minimal laboratory hazards. Antigen detection techniques include ELISA, immunofluorescent antibody assay of direct smears of liver biopsy, or viral strains isolated in cell cultures.

Antibodies. The most tried and safe method for the laboratory is detection of virus-specific antibody by indirect fluorescent antibody (IFA). Slides of inactivated Lassa virus–infected tissue culture cells may be stored at −20°C for 6 months or at −70°C for several years. Generally, an IgG titer of at least 16 and an IgM titer of 4 are considered specific for Lassa infection. At least 50% of Lassa fever patients have measurable IgG or IgM IFA antibodies by day 5 of illness, and virtually all have antibodies by days 12 to 14. The IgG antibodies are directed against the glycoprotein and nucleocapsid of Lassa virus; they are often present simultaneously with high levels of viremia and during the most severe stage of illness.

Virus Isolation. Virus may be isolated from serum specimens taken from acutely ill patients. Lassa virus isolation requires laboratory biosafety level 4 (BSL4) facilities, and any manipulation of high titer virus in tissue cell cultures should be performed in very specialized facilities. Lassa virus may easily be isolated in cell culture (the E6 clone of Vero cells) or suckling mice. Tissue cell cultures should be harvested after 7 days, and tested by IFA for presence of virus. Mice are killed after 7 to 9 days and the brain harvested. Infected animals present by far the highest laboratory risk to personnel, particularly since arenaviruses persistently and silently infect rodents, and are excreted in high titers in their urine. All animal experiments must be performed in BSL4 facilities.

Viremia in Lassa fever may be as high as 10^{6-8} TCID$_{50}$/mL and sustained up to 3 or 4 weeks in severe disease. Serum virus titers in clinically milder cases are lower and of short duration. Lassa virus has been isolated from throat swabs during acute illness, but the titer is low and recovery variable. Virus has also been isolated from breast milk, spinal fluid, pleural and pericardial transudate, and autopsy material. Virus may be recovered for 1 to 2 months in urine during convalescence albeit at low titer, and its presence in urine during acute disease is sporadic.

Virus may be inactivated for safe laboratory manipulation for antibody studies by using heat (56°C for 30 minutes), β-propiolactone, formalin, and ultraviolet radiation. Antigenic properties are best conserved by inactivation with gamma irradiation. Disinfection can be accomplished by washing with 0.5% phenol in detergent (e.g., Lysol), 10% hypochlorite solution, formaldehyde, or peracetic acid.

TREATMENT AND MANAGEMENT

Antiviral Therapy. Ribavirin, a guanosine analogue, is effective in treating acute Lassa fever. When therapy was given within the first 6 days of illness, a 5- to 10-fold decrease in the case-fatality rate was demonstrated in patients treated with ribavirin compared with untreated patients. A smaller but still significant decrease in fatality also was demonstrated in patients treated later in illness. Hospitalized patients in whom elevated aspartate transaminase and viremia levels were risk factors for fatal outcome experienced a 5 to 9% case-fatality rate when treated within the first 6 days of illness. Those with the same risk factors receiving treatment >6 days after the onset of illness had a 26 to 47% fatality compared with mortality rates of 52 to 78% in untreated patients. Furthermore, patients treated with ribavirin had a significant reduction in viremia regardless of outcome. The drug was given intravenously as a 2-g loading dose, followed by 1 g every 6 hours for 4 days, and then 0.5 g every 8 hours for 6 more days. There is some evidence that oral ribavirin may also be effective, particularly when given early in milder cases.

Supportive Therapy. Fluid, electrolyte, respiratory, and osmotic imbalances should be corrected to prevent clinical shock. However, even vigorous support of this kind may be insufficient to prevent fatal progression of advanced disease when antiviral treatment is started late in infection. Furthermore, the tendency of these patients to develop pulmonary edema may be gravely exacerbated by injudicious fluid replacement.

Vaccines. A candidate Lassa fever vaccine, made by cloning and expressing the Lassa virus glycoprotein gene in vaccinia virus, has proved highly successful in preventing severe disease and death in monkeys challenged with a lethal dose of Lassa virus. It is hoped that such a vaccine may eventually be tested in humans. A vaccine may be the most realistic and practical approach to control of this disease.

Hospital Control. Although nosocomial transmission of Lassa virus occurred during the first recognized outbreaks, basic barrier nursing methods (gloves, gowns, and masks) are highly effective in preventing secondary spread of the infection. Strict isolation with rigorous barrier nursing should be combined with full medical care, including surgery if indicated, to ensure the safety of the staff and survival of the patient. Extensive nosocomial epidemics may result from reuse of inadequately sterilized equipment (e.g., needles, syringes, gloves) during surgery or midwifery. In this context, the importance of awareness by medical teams of the possibility of Lassa fever in patients cannot be overemphasized. Early recognition is the key to early treatment and prevention of nosocomial transmission, and to community based-public health action.

Bibliography

Auperin DD, McCormick JB: Nucleotide sequence of the Lassa virus (Josiah strain) S genome RNA and amino acid sequence comparison of the N and GPC proteins to other arenaviruses. Virology 168:421, 1989.

Centers for Disease Control: Management of patients with suspected viral hemorrhagic fever. MMWR 37(Suppl 3):1, 1988.

Cummins D, Bennett D, Fisher-Hoch SP, et al: Electrocardiographic abnormalities in patients with Lassa fever. J Trop Med Hyg 92:350, 1989.

Cummins D, Bennett D, Fisher-Hoch SP, et al: Lassa fever encephalopathy: Clinical and laboratory findings. J Trop Med Hyg 95:197, 1992.

Cummins D, McCormick JB, Bennett D, et al: Acute sensorineural deafness in Lassa fever. JAMA 264:2093, 1990.

Fisher-Hoch SP: Stringent precautions are not advisable when caring for patients with viral haemorrhagic fevers. Rev Med Virol 3:7, 1993.

Fisher-Hoch SP, McCormick JB: Pathophysiology and treatment of Lassa fever. Curr Top Microbiol Immunol 134:231, 1987.

Fisher-Hoch SP, McCormick JB, Auperin D, et al: Protection of rhesus monkeys from fatal Lassa fever by vaccination with a recombinant vaccinia virus containing the Lassa virus glycoprotein gene. Proc Natl Acad Sci USA 86:317, 1989.

Fisher-Hoch S, McCormick JB, Sasso D, Craven RB: Hematologic dysfunction in Lassa fever. J Med Virol 26:127, 1988.

Fisher-Hoch SP, Mitchell SW, Sasso DR, et al: Physiologic and immunologic disturbances associated with shock in a primate model of Lassa fever. J Infect Dis 155:465, 1987.

Fisher-Hoch SP, Price ME, Craven RB, et al: Safe intensive-care management of a severe case of Lassa fever with simple barrier nursing techniques. Lancet 2:1227, 1985.

Fisher-Hoch SP, Tomori O, Nasidi A, et al: Review of cases of nosocomial Lassa fever in Nigeria: The high price of poor medical practice. Br Med J 311:857, 1995.

Jahrling PB, Peters CJ: Passive antibody therapy of Lassa fever in cynomolgus monkeys: Importance of neutralizing antibody and Lassa virus strain. Infect Immun 44:528, 1984.

Johnson KM, McCormick JB, Webb PA, et al: Clinical virology of Lassa fever in hospitalized patients. J Infect Dis 155:456, 1987.

McCormick JB: Epidemiology and control of Lassa fever. Curr Top Microbiol Immunol 134:69, 1987.

McCormick JB, King IJ, Webb PA, et al: Lassa fever: Effective therapy with ribavirin. N Engl J Med 314:20, 1986.

McCormick JB, King IJ, Webb PA, et al: A case-control study of the clinical diagnosis and course of Lassa fever. J Infect Dis 155:445, 1987.

McCormick JB, Webb PA, Krebs JW, et al: A prospective study of the epidemiology and ecology of Lassa fever. J Infect Dis 155:437, 1987.

Monath TP, Newhouse VF, Kemp GE, et al: Lassa virus isolation from *Mastomys natalensis* rodents during an epidemic in Sierra Leone. Science 185:263, 1974.

Price ME, Fisher-Hoch SP, Craven RB, McCormick JB: A prospective study of maternal and fetal outcome in acute Lassa fever infection during pregnancy. Br Med J 297:584, 1988.

Walker DH, McCormick JB, Johnson KM, et al: Pathologic and virologic study of fatal Lassa fever in man. Am J Pathol 107:349, 1982.

31.3 South American Hemorrhagic Fevers*

James N. Mills and Kelly T. McKee, Jr.

DEFINITION AND HISTORY. Argentine, Bolivian, and Venezuelan hemorrhagic fevers are clinically similar, rodent-borne diseases caused by closely related viruses of the family *Arenaviridae*. The respective etiologic agents are among 14 currently recognized New World arenaviruses (the Tacaribe complex). Most New World arenaviruses are associated with rodents of family *Muridae*, subfamily *Sigmodontinae*. Sabiá virus, a recently identified member of the group, has been recognized as a cause of only one naturally acquired case of hemorrhagic fever and two laboratory infections; its reservoir is unknown. Although the South American hemorrhagic fevers represent geographically and virologically distinct entities, their clinical, pathophysiologic, and (to the extent known) epidemiologic features are strikingly similar.

Argentine hemorrhagic fever (AHF) was first recognized in 1953, and the etiologic agent, Junín virus, was isolated in 1958. Bolivian hemorrhagic fever (BHF) was described after clusters of cases were observed in northern Bolivia in 1959; its etiologic agent, Machupo virus, was isolated in 1965. An outbreak of hemorrhagic fever among rural inhabitants of the Venezuelan llanos led to the isolation of Guanarito virus, causative agent of Venezuelan hemorrhagic fever (VHF), in 1989. Sabiá virus was isolated from a human case that occurred near São Paulo, Brazil, in 1990.

EPIDEMIOLOGY AND EPIZOOTIOLOGY. A hallmark of the arenaviruses is their maintainance in nature by a single rodent species in which chronic infection leads to long-term shedding of infectious virus in secretions and excreta. The specificity of this virus-host relationship restricts the geographic distribution of each arenavirus to the range of its particular rodent reservoir. For unknown reasons, the endemic areas for South American hemorrhagic fevers are more limited than the recognized ranges of the host species. Unlike the Old World arenaviruses, Lassa virus and lymphocytic choriomeningitis virus (LCMV), which are reported to be transmitted vertically within their respective reservoir populations, New World arenaviruses may be spread principally by horizontal transmission. Human infections with South American hemorrhagic fever viruses are acquired primarily via the inhalation of infectious aerosols of rodent excreta or via percutaneous or mucous membrane inoculation after direct contact with virus-contaminated surfaces. Person-to-person transmission can occur through contact with infected body fluids (e.g., sexual transmission), and nosocomial infections, although infrequent, have occurred. Overall mortality in untreated cases may exceed 30%.

Argentine Hemorrhagic Fever. In the 1950s, the AHF-endemic area encompassed approximately 16,000 square kilometers around the town of Junín, in Buenos Aires Province on the central Argentine pampa. Subsequently, the disease-endemic area has expanded progressively toward the north and west and now includes approximately 150,000 square kilometers of farmland covering parts of four provinces. In general, disease incidence is much higher along the periphery of the expanding endemic area (epidemic zone) than in areas where AHF has been endemic for many years (historic zone).

The principal viral reservoir, the corn mouse (*Calomys musculinus*), prefers relatively stable border habitats (fencelines, roadsides, railroad rights-of-way), but enters crop fields to feed. It is rarely captured in or around human dwellings. The prevalence of infection in reservoir populations is highly variable in space and time. Although the species is widespread throughout northern and central Argentina and Paraguay, infected *C. musculinus* have not been found outside of the AHF-endemic area. Field studies indicate that AHF incidence is correlated with local reservoir population levels; disease incidence increases with climatic conditions that allow rodent populations to reach unusually high densities.

Although AHF occurs year-round, a prominent autumn disease peak coincides with harvest of the summer corn and soybean crop and with the period of maximum reservoir population density. Male farm workers 20 to 60 years of age, the group at greatest risk of infection, are infected by contaminated aerosols generated by mechanical grain harvesters and exposure to crop borders frequented by *C. musculinus*. Prior to the introduction of a live-attenuated Junín vaccine in 1991, 200 to 1000 AHF cases were reported each year; annual incidence has declined considerably since then.

Bolivian Hemorrhagic Fever. Naturally acquired BHF has been documented only from the department of Beni, in northern Bolivia; 2000 to 3000 cases have been recognized, mostly prior to 1975. Like AHF, BHF is a seasonal disease occurring in the dry season, at the peak of agricultural activity. The preponderance of sporadic cases are in adult men in rural areas; however, family and community clusters have affected both sexes and all age groups. Larger epidemics have been associated with high densities of the rodent host, *Calomys callosus*. This species generally frequents grassland and forest ecotones; however, it also has peridomestic affinities. In 1963–1964, a BHF epidemic in the village of San Joaquín resulted in 637 cases and 113 deaths among the town's 3000 residents. The outbreak ended abruptly after 2 weeks of continuous trapping in homes, during which 3000 *C. callosus* were captured.

Organized rodent surveillance and control programs have effectively eliminated epidemic BHF in the Beni region. Between 1975 and 1992, no BHF cases were reported; 1 case was identified in 1993 and 9 cases occurred in 1994, 7 of which involved a family outbreak. Several clusters of BHF appear to have resulted from person-to-person transmission

---

*All the material in this chapter is in the public domain, with the exception of any borrowed figures or tables.

following primary cases. Five health care workers who had exposure to the index case or a secondary case contracted BHF in a hospital in Cochabamba in 1971. In the 1994 family outbreak, a farm worker transmitted the disease to six of eight family members. Although the index case patient survived, all 6 family members died.

C. callosus is distributed across northern Argentina and Paraguay, through eastern Bolivia to east-central Brazil. However, the BHF-endemic area is restricted to a small part of northern Bolivia. The extent of infection in the reservoir population and whether infection is present outside of the known-endemic area are unknown. The prevalence of infection in reservoir populations has ranged as high as 77% among a sample of animals trapped during the San Joaquín outbreak to 5% in subsequent rodent serosurveys in areas where no disease had occurred for at least 2 years. During a recent investigation of a sporadically acquired human case, the population density of *C. callosus* was very low (19 captures during 2250 trap nights) and no seropositive rodents were found.

Venezuelan Hemorrhagic Fever. VHF was recognized after an outbreak of severe hemorrhagic illness in the municipality of Guanarito, Portuguesa State, Venezuela, in 1989. About half of the approximately 165 VHF cases reported to date occurred during the initial outbreak years of 1989 to 1991. Although few cases occurred between 1992 and 1996, a trend toward increasing disease incidence was observed in late 1996 and 1997. As noted for AHF and BHF, children and adults of both sexes are susceptible to infection; however, risk is highest among adult male farm workers. Although cases of VHF have been observed throughout the year, epidemics appear to have a seasonal peak in November to January.

To date, human cases of VHF have been largely restricted to southwestern Portuguesa State. The primary host for Guanarito virus is the cane mouse (*Zygodontomys brevicauda*). Although the species is found from southeastern Costa Rica through northern Brazil, Guanarito virus has not been detected in cane mice outside of the VHF-endemic area.

Sabiá Virus. Nothing is known of the natural reservoir and disease-endemic area for Sabiá virus. Two infections with Sabiá virus have been acquired following laboratory mishaps, emphasizing the importance of limiting work with this and related viruses with human pathogenic potential to laboratories with maximum (biosafety level 4) containment facilities.

PATHOGENESIS. Common to all arenavirus hemorrhagic fevers is disruption of vascular endothelial integrity, most likely resulting from the release of endogenous mediators after infection of macrophages and perhaps endothelial cells. The resulting extravasation of fluid into extravascular spaces and activation of hematologic and immunologic cascades produce the characteristic clinical and laboratory features. High levels and prolonged circulation of interferon and other mediators (e.g., tumor necrosis factor alpha) probably contribute to the observed clinical and pathologic changes. In AHF, exceptional elevations of serum α-interferon (1,000 to 16,000 IU/mL) have been documented, and patients with higher levels tend to have poorer prognoses. In fatal cases of AHF, BHF, and VHF, organ histopathology tends to be relatively unimpressive. Consistent findings include congestion, petechiae, and relatively minor foci of necrosis in lymphoreticular, hematologic, renal, and hepatic tissues. Observations in experimental animals and humans suggest that viral invasion of the brain may be responsible for the sometimes prominent CNS symptoms in some cases.

A fatal guinea pig model using Pichindé virus (an arenavirus that is not pathogenic for humans) has disclosed an initial viral tropism for macrophages and epithelial cells. Minor histopathologic damage includes focal necrosis of the liver, adrenals, and spleen; interstitial pneumonitis; and an intestinal lesion associated with infection of mucosal macrophages. Death results from a dramatic decrease in cardiac output brought about by soluble mediators, including leukotrienes, platelet-activating factor, and endorphins, which decrease heart function.

CLINICAL MANIFESTATIONS. Human infection with Junín, Machupo, or Guanarito viruses generally results in symptomatic illness, the clinical features of which are remarkably similar. After an incubation period of 1 to 2 weeks, there is a gradual onset of fever, malaise, myalgia, and anorexia, followed within 3 to 4 days by severe prostration, headache, dizziness, back pain, and gastrointestinal disturbances. Conjunctival injection, edema, and flushing of the face; orthostatic hypotension; petechiae on the palate and axillae; and congestion and bleeding of the gums reflect damage to the vascular bed. Hemorrhage along the gingival margin is a characteristic finding. Neurologic manifestations are common and most frequently include tremor of the tongue and hands, diminished deep tendon reflexes, lethargy, and hyperesthesia.

After 1 to 2 weeks, most patients begin to improve. About a third progress to a more serious phase, however, with illness evolving along 1 of 3 lines: (1) a pronounced hemorrhagic diathesis with diffuse echymoses, bleeding from puncture wounds, and oozing from mucous membranes; (2) severe neurologic deterioration characterized by delirium, coma, and convulsions; or (3) a mixed hemorrhagic-neurologic syndrome with shock. Case-fatality rates among untreated patients can be ≥30%. Among survivors, convalescence typically takes 1 to 3 months, with weight loss, fatigue, autonomic instability, and occasionally hair loss.

Laboratory findings early in the course of disease nearly always include leukopenia (white blood cell count <4000/mm^3) and thrombocytopenia (platelet count <100,000/mm^3). Proteinuria is also common and may be accompanied by microscopic hematuria. Serum enzyme values (aspartate aminotransferase and alanine aminotransferase) are usually normal or slightly elevated, and routine clotting studies are normal except in severe cases.

DIAGNOSIS. Laboratory samples from suspected cases should be handled under biosafety level 4 containment until treated chemically or with ionizing radiation to inactivate virus. Antigens prepared for diagnostic tests and suspect sera can be inactivated by gamma irradiation so that serologic tests can be performed on the benchtop. Laboratory diagnosis of South American arenaviral infections is made by serologic methods, including IFA, ELISA, or plaque-reduction neutralization test (PRNT); antigen-capture ELISA; or viral isolation. Antibody generally appears during the third week of illness (1 to 2 weeks later than with Lassa virus and LCMV). IFA and ELISA are broadly cross reactive among Tacaribe complex arenaviruses but PRNT readily distinguishes most arenaviruses. Virus can be isolated from blood or serum samples obtained 2 to 14 days after onset, or from postmortem tissue samples. Virus can be isolated in Vero cells or by intracranial inoculation of suckling mice or hamsters. Cocultivation of peripheral blood mononuclear cells with Vero cells improves sensitivity. Antigen-capture ELISA of blood, serum, or tissue homogenates may provide the earliest diagnostic results for acute-phase patients.

TREATMENT. Aggressive supportive treatment with careful attention to fluid and electrolyte balance is critical to the successful management of patients with arenaviral hemorrhagic fevers. The administration of high-titer, convalescent-phase plasma to patients has been successful in the treatment of AHF, resulting in mortality reduction from 15 to 20% to less than 1%. Plasma must be given within 8 days of disease onset to be effective; its administration is associated with a curious late neurologic syndrome of uncertain etiology in about 10% of survivors. The syndrome begins 4 to 6 weeks after treatment and is characterized by fever, headache, ataxia, and tremors but is usually benign. Convalescent-phase plasma has been used in BHF patients as well, but its efficacy is unproved.

Preliminary studies suggest that intravenous ribavirin therapy may be beneficial in AHF. Two BHF patients treated with intravenous ribavirin recovered uneventfully, but additional studies are needed to demonstrate its efficacy. Recent experience with early ribavirin treatment following a laboratory exposure to Sabiá virus was also encouraging.

PREVENTION AND CONTROL. The peridomestic affinities of *C. callosus*, and the favorable resolution of the San Joaquín outbreak of BHF, suggest that rodent control is a viable approach to reduce disease transmission. The absence of epidemic disease in the Beni region since 1974 may be due, at least in part, to active public health surveillance and rodent control. The reservoirs for Junín and Guanarito viruses are rarely found in association with towns or in human dwellings, making their control much less tractable. *C. musculinus* depends on the relatively stable linear habitats of roadsides, fencelines, and railroad rights-of-way that crisscross the pampa. This feature suggests that the practice of burning or cutting these habitats could reduce the reservoir populations and lower the incidence of AHF.

A live-attenuated Junín virus vaccine (Candid #1) has been shown to be safe and highly efficacious against AHF. Since its introduction in the AHF-endemic area in 1991, there has been a marked decrease in AHF incidence. Candid #1 was shown to prevent BHF in rhesus macaques, but its effectiveness has not been tested in humans. The same vaccine did not protect guinea pigs or macaques challenged with Guanarito virus.

Bibliography

Barrera Ora JG, Maiztegui JI, McKee KT Jr, et al: Protective efficacy of a live-attenuated vaccine against Argentine hemorrhagic fever. J Infect Dis 177:277, 1998.

Barry ML, Russi M, Armstrong L, et al: Brief report: Treatment of a laboratory-acquired Sabiá virus infection. N Engl J Med 333:294, 1995.

Childs JE, Peters CJ: Ecology and epidemiology of arenaviruses and their hosts. In Salvato MS (ed): The Arenaviridae. New York, Plenum Press, 1993, pp 331–384.

De Manzione N, Salas RA, Paredes H, et al: Venezuelan hemorrhagic fever: Clinical and epidemiological studies of 165 cases. Clin Infect Dis 26:308, 1998.

Mills JN, Ellis BA, McKee KT, et al: A longitudinal study of Junín virus activity in the rodent reservoir of Argentine hemorrhagic fever. Am J Trop Med Hyg 47:749, 1992.

Peters CJ, Buchmeier M, Rollin PE, et al: 1996. Arenaviruses. In Fields BN, Knipe DM, Howley PM (eds): Virology. Philadelphia, Lippincott-Raven, 1996, pp 1521–1551.

Peters CJ, Johnson ED, McKee KT Jr: Filoviruses and management of viral hemorrhagic fevers. In Belshe RB (ed): Textbook of Human Virology. St. Louis, Mosby Year Book, 1991, pp 699–712.

Tesh RB, Jahrling PB, Salas R, et al: Description of Guanarito virus (Arenaviridae: Arenavirus), the etiologic agent of Venezuelan hemorrhagic fever. Am J Trop Med Hyg 50:452, 1994.

Vainrub B, Salas R: Latin American hemorrhagic fever. Infect Dis Clin North Am 8:47, 1994.

Weissenbacher MC, Laguens RP, Coto CE: Argentine hemorrhagic fever. Curr Top Microbiol Immunol 134:79, 1987.

31.4 Ebola and Marburg Virus Infections*

Pierre E. Rollin, Philippe Calain, and Thomas G. Ksiazek

DEFINITION AND HISTORY. The filoviruses Marburg and Ebola, which have been recognized only in the last 30 years, cause similar diseases characterized by high mortality and frequent nosocomial transmission in hospital and laboratory settings.

Marburg Virus. The first described member of the family *Filoviridae* was isolated in 1967 in Marburg and Frankfurt, Germany, and in Belgrade, former Yugoslavia, during a severe outbreak of a syndrome that included fever and hemorrhage. Thirty-three cases and seven deaths occurred among vaccine-production laboratory workers, medical personnel, and some family members attending the patients. Isolated cases of Marburg hemorrhagic fever occurred in 1975 in Zimbabwe (index and two secondary cases), 1980 in Kenya (index and one secondary case), and in 1987 in Kenya (a single fatal case).

Ebola Virus. In 1976, two concomitant massive hemorrhagic fever epidemics occurred in the northern Democratic Republic of the Congo (estimated 318 cases) and southern Sudan (estimated 284 cases) with estimated case-fatality rates of 88% and 53%, respectively. Two serologically distinct viruses were isolated from patients in these outbreaks and were named Ebola virus (after a small river in the northwest Democratic Republic of the Congo). A severe case associated with laboratory contamination was reported the same year in England; a fatal case occurred in 1977 in the Democratic Republic of the Congo not far from the location of the original outbreak; and in 1979, at the site of the 1976 outbreak in Sudan, 34 cases (with 22 deaths) of Ebola hemorrhagic fever were confirmed. No further evidence of Ebola virus circulation in Africa occurred for the next 15 years. In November 1994, a primate ethologist was infected with a new serotype of Ebola virus while performing a necropsy on a chimpanzee that died in a national park in the western Ivory Coast. Then, in May 1995, a massive epidemic affected the residents in and around Kikwit, in the central Democratic Republic of the Congo. The epidemic started in the town in January but remained unnoticed until late April when it rapidly amplified as a result of pervasive nosocomial spread in the local general hospital. The epidemic resulted in approximately 300 cases, with an 80% mortality. In nearby Gabon, three separate outbreaks occurred in late 1994 and in February and July 1996, each caused by slightly different strains of the subtype of Ebola virus from the Democratic Republic of the Congo.

Primate Outbreak. In a U.S. primate quarantine facility, in 1989, several cynomolgus macaques (*Macaca fascicularis*) recently imported from the Philippines started to die; a clinical picture of viral hemorrhagic fever and simian hemorrhagic fever (SHF) virus was suspected as the cause. Unexpectedly, in addition to SHF virus, a new serotype of Ebola virus called Reston Ebola virus was isolated. Epidemiologic investigations traced the origin of this outbreak to a facility in the Philippines owned by an exporter of nonhuman primates. The same source was again responsible for subsequent exportation of Ebola virus–infected monkeys to the United States in 1990, to Siena, Italy in 1992, and again to the United States in 1996. The origin of the contamination of this exporter's facility remains unknown.

ETIOLOGY. Marburg and Ebola viruses, the only members of the family *Filoviridae*, are composed of a helical nucleocapsid covered by an envelope with glycoprotein spikes protruding from the virion surface. As seen in electron microscopy preparations, both Ebola and Marburg viruses appear as

---

*All the material in this chapter is in the public domain, with the exception of any borrowed figures or tables.

long, filamentous, and sometimes branched forms (Fig. 31–5). The length of virions varies greatly, but the diameter is uniform (80 nm). The virion contains one molecule of noninfectious, linear, negative-sense, single-stranded RNA coding for seven structural proteins. Four of them (the nucleoprotein [NP], VP30, VP35, and the polymerase [L]) are associated with the RNA to form a ribonucleocapsid complex. The three remaining structural proteins are membrane associated: the glycoprotein (GP), VP24, and VP40. No subtypes are known among the Marburg viruses, but there are four subtypes (Republic of Congo, Sudan, Reston, Ivory Coast) of Ebola viruses. The infectivity of a virus suspension is stable at room temperature, especially if the solution contains proteins, as found in serum or blood, but virus is inactivated by heat, lipid solvents, gamma irradiation, β-propiolactone, hypochlorite, and phenolic disinfectants.

EPIDEMIOLOGY. All the Marburg and Ebola virus episodes were followed by ecological investigations. None succeeded in finding the source of virus infection for the index human case. Nevertheless, in several instances, nonhuman primates were identified as the source of human infection, acting as a bridge that linked humans to the hypothetical reservoir. Early serologic studies, using an IFA, showed a high prevalence of filovirus antibodies among wild-caught and laboratory-bred monkeys. However, it was subsequently demonstrated that the antibodies actually were directed against phylogenetically related viruses, most likely paramyxoviruses. The spread of virus from nonhuman primates to humans as with episodes of human-to-human transmissions has occurred during unprotected contact with blood, secretions, and excretions of an acutely infected individual, or with tissues during surgery or necropsy procedures (Table 31–1). Virus could be found at very high concentration in blood and all organs examined, including the lungs, the gastrointestinal tract, and the skin. The presence of Ebola virus in the pneumocytes and even free in the alveoli are the best arguments in favor of aerosol transmission of the virus. In addition, this mode of transmission remains a hypothesis to explain consecutive infections among animals during nonhuman primate outbreaks. However, no epidemiologic evidence exists to support aerosol transmission during human epidemics, suggesting that direct contact with patients or their biologic fluids in the later stages of illness or after death is the principal means of transmission. These facts support the use of strict barrier nursing measures and recommended personnel protection devices with high-efficiency particulate air (HEPA)–filtered respirators when caring for suspected or proved filovirus-infected patients or in handling nonhuman primates in quarantine facilities. The unexpected presence of high concentrations of Ebola antigen in the dermis and the sweat glands could explain some cases of transmission by contact. Skin biopsy provides a safe and easy procedure for retrospective diagnosis in suspected filovirus-associated deaths. The persistence of virus for at least several weeks in the semen was suspected when a secondary infection occurred in the spouse of a Marburg virus–infected convalescent patient. Virus was later successfully isolated from patients during the early convalescent phase of Marburg and Ebola hemorrhagic fevers.

During human outbreaks, which are predominantly nosocomial, human-to-human filoviral transmission occurs by direct contact with blood and excretions of a known patient during the clinical phase of the disease. Needlestick injuries are certainly the most efficient way to transmit the virus. Unprotected necropsy or processing of meat from infected nonhuman primates is also a source of exposure that can lead to disease. Experimental aerosol transmission has been demonstrated, but has not been implicated in human outbreaks to date.

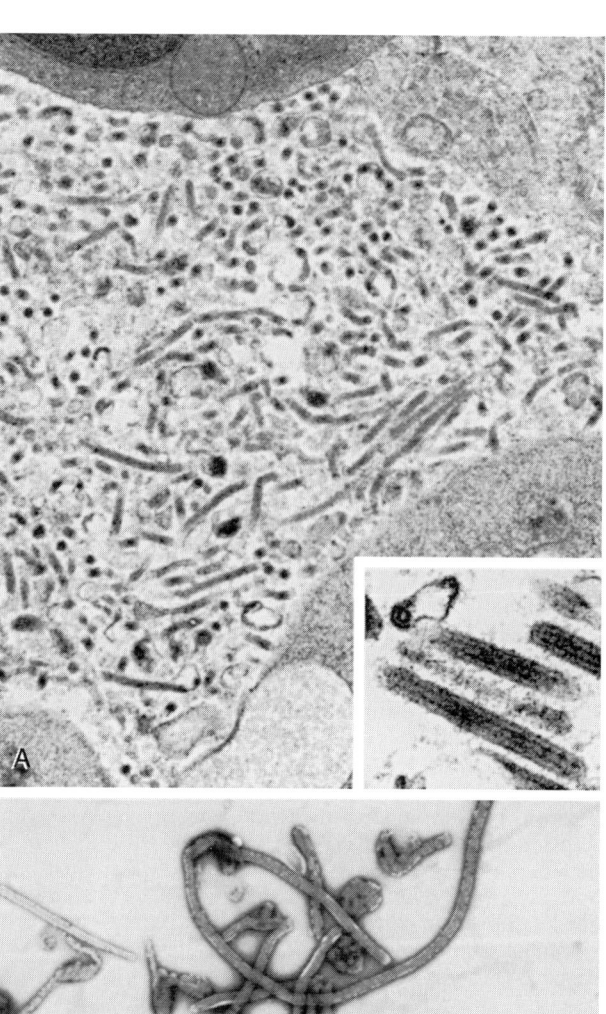

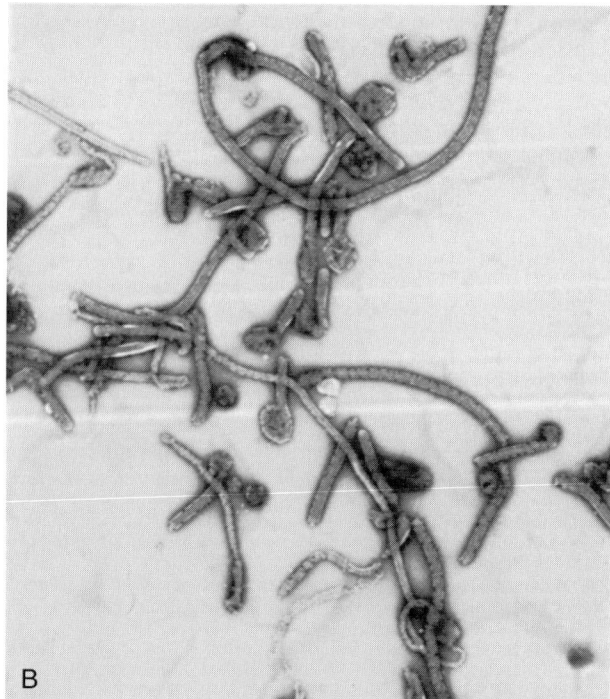

Figure 31–5. *A,* Thin-section electron micrograph of lymph node tissue (× 14,000). Ebola virions can be 10 μm in length and pleomorphic. *Inset,* Viral envelope around cylindric nucleocapsid at higher magnification (× 40,000). *B,* Ebola virus. Negative-stain electron micrograph (× 15,340) showing highly pleomorphic quality of extracellular viral particles, including elongated and branched forms. (*A,* courtesy of Dr. John D. White; *B,* courtesy of B. Geisbert.)

PATHOGENESIS. The virus spreads via infection of circulating monocytes and shortly afterward intensively replicates in endothelial and Kupffer cells. Vascular leakage through lysis of the endothelial cells is only one of the pathophysiologic parameters. Production and secretion of a number of

TABLE 31–1. Risk of Transmission of Ebola Virus by Degree of Person-to-Person Contact (Sudan, 1976 and 1979)

	1976			1979		
	Contacts	**Cases**	**%**	**Contacts**	**Cases**	**%**
Nursing care	48	39	81	60	24	40
Physical contact only	28	5	23	26	3	12
Entered room (no contact)	Not available			23	0	0

cytokines by infected monocytes and macrophages, among them tumor necrosis factor alpha (TNF-α), may also play a role in the increased vascular permeability, coagulopathies, and the development of a shock syndrome in the late phase of the disease. Sequential studies of the cascade of pathologic events in nonhuman primate models remain to be done to understand the different components of shock seen in filovirus-infected patients. Only the consequences of this devastating infection are seen in the extensive visceral effusions, pulmonary interstitial edema, and liver involvement; and enormous disseminated deposits of viral antigen are observed post mortem. Viral persistence in the anterior chamber of the eye and in the semen was demonstrated in some survivors, several weeks after the end of the clinical phase.

CLINICAL MANIFESTATIONS

Symptoms and Signs. After an incubation of usually 4 to 10 days, the onset of Marburg and Ebola virus disease is sudden, with fever, headache, myalgia, sore throat, and extreme fatigue (Table 31–2; Fig. 31–6). Gastrointestinal signs are usual with nausea, vomiting, and profuse diarrhea. A maculopapular rash is frequent, and is obvious on white skin, but more difficult to see on dark skin. Hemorrhagic manifestations occur during the peak of the illness (days 5 to 7) in fewer than half of patients and include epistaxis, gum-bleeding, hematemesis, melena, petechiae, and hemorrhages from needle sticks and other puncture wounds. Dehydration and prostration are frequent. A poor prognosis is

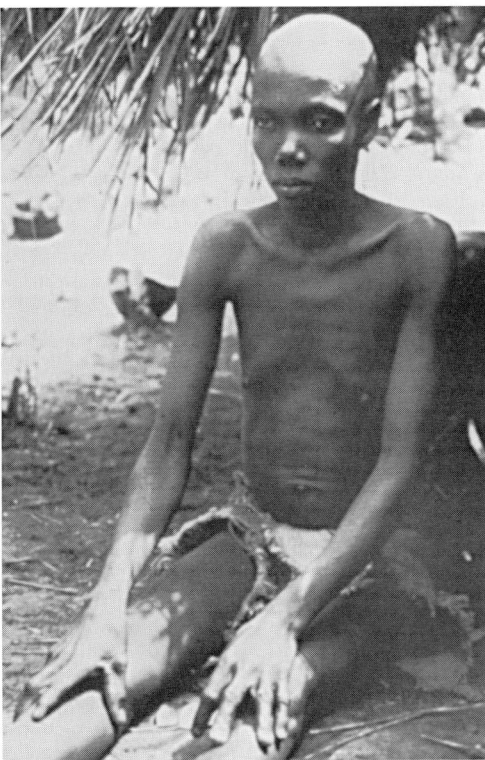

Figure 31–6. A case of Ebola virus disease in the Republic of the Congo, 1976, showing the ghostlike facies typical of this highly lethal disease. The patient died 24 hours later.

marked by hemorrhagic signs, as well as oliguria or anuria, chest pain, shock, tachypnea (possibly caused by a metabolic acidosis), and neurologic symptoms, e.g., sudden hearing loss, blindness, and painful paresthesia. Clinical laboratory findings, when available, show an early lymphopenia and a thrombocytopenia. Liver function enzyme levels (AST and ALT) are elevated. Recovery takes several weeks and is sometimes associated with arthritis, conjunctivitis, hearing loss, or orchitis.

Differential Diagnosis. Outside of the course of a known epidemic, in which clinical suspicion can be sustained by epidemiologic context, other possible diagnoses of nonspecific febrile illness are difficult to eliminate clinically. Treatable infectious diseases should be excluded or covered by specific therapy; among the wide range of bacterial, rickettsial, and viral diseases to be considered, malaria, typhoid fever, meningococcemia, and shigellosis head the list. The occurrence of clusters of cases with evidence of person-to-person transmission among close contacts and hospital staff should be sufficient to make a presumptive diagnosis of Ebola or Marburg hemorrhagic fever and for instituting strict barrier nursing procedures.

LABORATORY DIAGNOSIS

Specimen Collection and Handling. Acute-phase sera, blood, or tissue specimens from patients contain a high concentration of virulent filoviruses and should be processed with a maximum of safety precautions. Gowns, gloves, goggles, and HEPA-filtered respiratory protection should be used to collect and process specimens. Specimens for diagnosis should be sent to a high-containment (BSL4) laboratory. International Airlines Transportation Association (IATA)–approved shipping containers and preapproved import permits are required by most of the airline carriers and countries of destination. Heating (56°C for 30 minutes) or addition of

TABLE 31–2. Frequency of Symptoms and Signs in Fatal and Nonfatal Ebola Infections (Democratic Republic of the Congo, 1976)

	Fatal Infections			Nonfatal Infections		
	N	**Frequency**	**%**	**N**	**Frequency**	**%**
Symptoms						
Fever	231	226	98	34	20	59
Headache	210	202	96	34	20	59
Abdominal pain	201	163	81	34	17	50
Sore throat	207	164	79	34	11	32
Myalgia	206	163	79	34	16	47
Nausea	178	117	66	30	10	33
Arthritis	193	102	53	34	13	38
Signs						
Diarrhea	228	180	79	34	15	44
Bleeding	223	174	78	34	6	18
Oral/throat lesions	208	154	74	34	9	27
Vomiting	225	146	65	34	12	35
Conjunctivitis	208	121	58	34	12	35
Cough	208	75	36	34	6	18
Abortion	73	18	25	9	1	11
Jaundice	191	10	5	34	0	0

detergents only partially reduce the infectivity of blood and, therefore, gamma irradiation or formalin should be used to inactivate blood and tissues.

Virus Isolation and Antigen Detection. Filoviruses are found at very high titer and are well preserved in the serum, plasma, and blood of patients during acute illness. Vero E-6 cell lines are used for isolation by most laboratories, although other diploid cell lines have been used with success. Cytopathic effects are not obvious in all cell types and specific immunofluorescence is used to confirm the infection. ELISAs have been used with success for early detection of Ebola antigens in blood or suspensions of tissues obtained during necropsies. Reverse transcriptase polymerase chain reaction (RT-PCR) has been validated and shown to be highly sensitive for detecting viral RNA in acute-phase sera or postmortem tissues of laboratory-infected nonhuman primates. RT-PCR was also used in investigations of the recent human epidemics in the Republic of the Congo and Gabon and is potentially useful in the search for the viral reservoir. In addition to being an excellent diagnostic tool for specialized laboratories, this new technique provides genetic epidemiologic markers of the species and strain of virus. During the 1995 outbreak of Ebola hemorrhagic fever in the Republic of the Congo, an immunohistochemical assay was developed that made a retrospective, specific diagnosis possible. Ebola antigens are present in high quantities in all the organs tested, including the skin, leading to the development of a skin-biopsy surveillance kit, now under field evaluation during the postepidemic period in the Republic of the Congo.

Serology. As for other viral hemorrhagic fevers, IFA previously was used for the diagnosis of suspected filovirus infections. However, during acute infection, the rise of antibodies detected by IFA is delayed and during animal and/or human serosurveys, specificity problems have been noted. IgG and IgM capture ELISAs, validated in animal models and in human infection, were superior in sensitivity and specificity. Capture IgM and antigen ELISA for early diagnosis in suspected human infections and ELISA IgG for serosurveys are now recommended. Current assays for antibodies use native viral antigens that are inactivated for safe use and assays using recombinant antigen are under development.

TREATMENT. No effective antiviral drug is available. Transfusion of human convalescent-phase plasma or blood has been tried but to date no clinical or experimental data support its efficacy. Supportive therapy is the only alternative presently available. Symptomatic treatment should be administered whenever possible by the oral route to maintain cutaneous integrity and to limit the risk of needlestick injury among the medical staff. Unfortunately, vomiting and diarrhea make the ingestion of food, liquids, or drugs difficult; therefore, the use of the intravenous route is sometimes unavoidable. All invasive procedures should be performed carefully by experienced personnel.

PREVENTION AND CONTROL. No vaccine is available to protect against Marburg or Ebola virus infection. Laboratory personnel working with suspected specimens and viruses in central Africa or in various maximum containment laboratories would benefit from such a vaccine, but its efficacy will be difficult to assess. Recommendations for reducing person-to-person transmission during epidemics are more important and already are available. These include strict-barrier nursing protocols, disinfection and/or destruction of contaminated medical devices (e.g., needles), early laboratory confirmation of suspected cases, and tracking and surveillance of suspected contacts.

Bibliography

Centers for Disease Control: Management of patients with suspected viral hemorrhagic fever. MMWR 37(S-3):1, 1988.

Centers for Disease Control: Update: Ebola-related filovirus infection in nonhuman primates and interim guidelines for handling nonhuman primates during transit and quarantine. MMWR 39:22, 1990.

Dalgard DW, Hardy RJ, Pearson SL, et al: Combined simian hemorrhagic fever and Ebola virus infection in cynomolgus monkeys. Lab Anim Sci 42:152, 1992.

Feldmann H, Klenk H-D, Sanchez A: Molecular biology and evolution of filoviruses. Arch Virol (Suppl) 7:81, 1993.

Hayes CG, Burans JP, Ksiazek TG, et al: Outbreak of fatal illness among captive macaques in the Philippines caused by an Ebola-related filovirus. Am J Trop Med Hyg 46:664, 1992.

Martini GA, Siegert R (eds): Marburg Virus Disease. Berlin, Springer-Verlag, 1971.

Muyembe T, Kipasa M, the International Scientific and Technical Committee, World Health Organization Collaborating Centre for Haemorrhagic Fevers: Ebola haemorrhagic fever in Kikwit, Zaire. Lancet 345:1448, 1995.

Peters CJ, Sanchez A, Rollin PE, et al: Filoviridae: Marburg and Ebola viruses. In Fields BN, Knipe DM, Hawley PM (eds): Virology, 3rd ed. Philadelphia, Lippincott-Raven, 1996, p 1161.

World Health Organization/International Commission to Sudan: Ebola hemorrhagic fever in Sudan, 1976. Bull WHO 56:247, 1978.

World Health Organization/International Commission to Zaire: Ebola hemorrhagic fever in Zaire, 1976. Bull WHO 56:271, 1978.

World Health Organization: Ebola hemorrhagic fever—A summary of the outbreak in Gabon. Wkly Epidem Rec 72:7, 1997.

31.5 Crimean-Congo Hemorrhagic Fever

Joseph B. McCormick and Susan P. Fisher-Hoch

DEFINITION AND HISTORY. Crimean hemorrhagic fever is a tick-borne viral disease first described in the Soviet Union in the 1930s. A virus isolated in 1967 from an ill child in what is now Kisingani, Republic of the Congo (formerly Stanleyville in the Belgian Congo) was found to be identical to a virus isolated later in the Crimea and eventually was named Crimean-Congo hemorrhagic fever (CCHF) virus. The disease is now known to occur from Eastern Europe through Asia, the Middle East, the steppes and dry subtropics of middle Asia, and all of Africa. In China, the Xinjiang strain of CCHF virus causes a disease known locally as Xinjiang fever. Humans may be infected directly from the bite of a tick, by contact with blood or tissues from infected domestic animals, or by person-to-person spread via direct contact with blood or secretions from an infected person.

ETIOLOGY. CCHF virus is a member of the *Nairovirus* genus of the *Bunyaviridae*, a large family of viruses, most of which are transmitted between animals by insect or tick vectors. The spherical virions are 85 to 100 nm in diameter, with a unit membrane and regular surface projections. Like all bunyaviridae the nairoviruses possess a tripartite negative-sense (i.e., noninfectious) RNA genome. The nairoviruses differ from other bunyaviridae genera in the molecular weights of the respective genomic segments, which are approximately 4.3, 1.5, and 0.6×10^6, and in their antigenic profile. The nucleocapsid core protein is about 50 kDa, and the two glycosylated surface and membrane proteins 75 kDa and 30 kDa, respectively. The CCHF agent is the prototype of the nairovirus taxon. It is assumed that the small (S) RNA species encodes the nucleocapsid protein; that the middle (M) RNA segment encodes the glycoprotein precursor, which is post-translationally cleaved to make the two virion glycoproteins; and that the large (L) RNA segment encodes the virus-directed RNA polymerase.

ECOLOGY

Vectors and Reservoirs. CCHF virus is a parasite of ixodid (hard) ticks. It is likely that ixodid ticks serve as both reservoir and vector of this agent. CCHF viruses have been isolated from at least 24 species and subspecies of ixodid ticks, belonging to seven distinct genera. Among these are one-, two-, or three-host ticks, with a wide mammalian host range. In South Africa, native ixodid ticks belonging to *Hyalomma*, *Rhipicephalus*, and *Amblyomma* species were shown to be capable of transmitting CCHF virus, but argasid species failed to do so. *Hyalomma* species appear to be the most efficient transmitters of CCHF virus and transovarial, trans-stadial, and horizontal transmission have been recorded.

The best-studied tick hosts and most important vectors to humans are *Hyalomma* spp., including *H. marginatum marginatum* of southeastern Europe and Caspian region and *H. anatolicum anatolicum*, found in drier areas in south central Asia (Chapter 135). These are two-host species whose larva molt to a nymph on the same animal. The nymph feeds, then falls away to molt to an adult, which must find a new host. Adult *H. m. marginatum* prefer large domestic animals and avidly attack humans, whereas immature stages usually parasitize small ground-living or ground-feeding vertebrates, including birds. In contrast, all stages of *H. a. anatolicum* feed mostly on large domestic animals.

Tick bites are the source of CCHF virus for many domestic and wild animals, all of which are apparently asymptomatic and probably only briefly viremic. Some birds, e.g., rooks, are not susceptible to tick-borne infection. Other data suggest, however, that birds, e.g., ostriches, may become viremic and function as amplifying hosts; human infection has been associated with ostrich farming. Transport of infectious ticks by birds may contribute to the wide geographic distribution of CCHF virus. Mammals, e.g., hares, cattle, sheep, and goats, develop low levels of viremia. The role, if any, of such viremia in amplifying the virus in tick populations is unclear. The most important reservoirs as well as vectors of CCHF are infected ticks, which can also survive winter cold and transmit the virus to subsequent generations through transovarial passage.

EPIDEMIOLOGY

Transmission. Transmission of CCHF virus to humans occurs from bites of infected ticks or through contamination by blood or infected material from animals or other humans. In endemic areas, the high prevalence of anti-CCHF antibodies in domestic animals and the relatively lower prevalence in humans show transmission from animals to humans to be infrequent. Animals have brief and low viremia and, therefore, would only occasionally transmit infection to humans, depending on the type of human-animal interaction. It is clear that tick bites are frequent in those living among domestic animals in CCHF endemic areas. The relatively low frequency of primary human CCHF infection suggests that a minority of these bites result in infection, either because of low infection in ticks or inefficiency of virus transmission.

Seasonality. The seasonality of CCHF depends on climate and local tick hosts. In the lower Volga and Don river basins of Russia where *H. m. marginatum* is the main vector, the disease occurs almost exclusively in the spring months of April to June when adult ticks become active. Similar patterns are seen in South Africa, where cases are most frequently observed in spring and fall. In the rest of Africa, sporadic mostly nonhemorrhagic human illness has been observed without a clear seasonal pattern. Although more cases are generally registered in the warmer months, seasonality is much less pronounced in the Balkans, central Asia, and the Middle East, where the vectors, *H. a. anatolicum* and other ticks, feed exclusively on domestic animals. Sheep shearing may be a risk factor. Throughout the Eastern Hemisphere CCHF has emerged in arid farming areas that have high tick populations, with peaks of disease in the spring and fall coinciding with maximal tick infestation.

Prevalence of Disease. Most primary CCHF infections are sporadic. In some areas, cases occur with regularity; for example, in Bulgaria, about 25 cases are hospitalized each year. In South Africa, also, cases occur perennially following clear seasonal patterns. Little is known about the illness to infection ratio of CCHF, although this appears to be high in some areas. In southern Russia, about one fifth of infections resulted in a clinical illness sufficient for individuals to seek medical attention. In South Africa, 70% of those with evidence of past infection are hospitalized with CCHF disease. These varying observations may be explained by poor identification of illness or infections in some areas, or possibly, differences in pathogenicity of viruses in different geographic areas. Antibody prevalence in seminomadic tribes in Senegal ranges from 1 to 21%, and 2 to 70% in sheep in the same area, emphasizing the focality of transmission. In the Kimberley region of South Africa, antibody prevalence in domestic animals was high: 15% of sheep, 39% of cattle, and 53% of goats. In the same study, evidence of human infection was only 2.7%, and all positive individuals had daily animal exposure. In Baluchistan, Pakistan, human antibody prevalence of 5% has been detected.

Occupational Exposure. CCHF in Russia is a disease of adults who handle or milk cattle, and any sex difference is a function of gender differences in agricultural practice. Milkmaids in some areas and sheep handlers in others appear to be at greatest risk. Epidemics are usually focal and numbers small, but as recently as 1989, as many as 90 cases were reported in an outbreak in Kazakhstan. Two thirds of the cases were infected shearing sheep, but there were also secondary cases and infections resulting from transfusion of infected blood. CCHF equally infects males and females and persons of all age groups in central Asia and Iraq. This is explained by the "peridomestic" nature of the disease, which occurs even in urban areas, where people live in close daily proximity to sheep, goats, and camels and their associated infected ticks. A case-control study of risk factors in human infections in South Africa did not show a positive association with tick infestation or animal slaughter, but handling young sheep and goats for vaccination, castration, ear notching, or tail docking was associated with disease transmission. However, CCHF disease in Saudi Arabia has been described in slaughterhouse workers and butchers.

Although they constitute only a minority of cases, the most noticeable infections result from nosocomial transmission. CCHF has repeatedly infected unwary surgeons, nursing staff, and other medical attendants. In all reported outbreaks, direct contact with blood, needlestick or other injury, or failure to observe simple barrier techniques were recorded. Airborne spread in a hospital setting is not a risk.

Human Disease. Most primary infections are from tick bites or animal blood exposure. Humans are accidental, dead-end hosts for CCHF virus, and surprisingly, appear to be the only species in whom CCHF virus produces severe disease. Even nonhuman primates have asymptomatic infections. Following infection from ticks or viremic animal blood, the incubation period of CCHF is relatively brief, generally 2 to 5 days (Fig. 31–7). This brevity is probably a consequence of direct hematogenous infection. The infectious dose of virus delivered by ticks is not known. Nosocomial infections generally have an incubation period of 4 to 9 days, but there is at least one report of as few as 48 hours elapsing between medical personnel administering mouth-to-mouth resuscitation to a bleeding patient and onset of fever.

The case-fatality rate also appears to vary in different locations, reflecting, in part, a variable availability of medical and diagnostic services. There may be important strain differences in virulence, but there is no objective evidence for this or even for the presence of more than one CCHF virus strain able to infect humans. In southern Russia, where disease

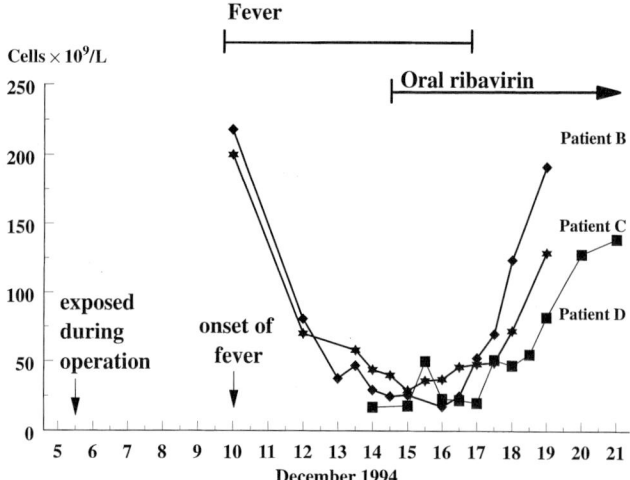

Figure 31–7. Incubation period of Crimean-Congo hemorrhagic fever. (From Fisher-Hoch SP, Khan JA, Rehman S, et al: Crimean-Congo haemorrhagic fever treated with oral ribavirin. Lancet 346:472, 1995.)

surveillance is more complete, milder disease forms are often noted and case-fatality rates rarely exceed 5 to 10%. In South Africa from 1981 to 1986, the reported case-fatality rate was 35% in an area with both good surveillance and medical facilities. In central Asia and the Middle East, case-fatality rates of 35 to 50% or more are recorded, with highest rates in nosocomial outbreaks. Virus variation, route of inoculation, and dose may all be important in determining severity of disease.

PATHOPHYSIOLOGY AND PATHOLOGY. Viremia, thrombocytopenia, and lymphopenia are features of the acute disease process. As with other viral hemorrhagic fevers, raised AST may be seen. Features predictive of fatal outcome are a platelet count of $\leq 20 \times 10^9$/L, partial thromboplastin time of ≥ 60 seconds, AST of ≥ 200 IU/L, and ALT of ≥ 150 IU/L. Prothrombin times and ALT are relatively normal, underscoring that the disease process although it involves the liver, is not primarily hepatic. In the terminal stages, however, generalized hepatorenal and cardiac failure may be observed. At autopsy, eosinophilic necrosis of the liver (Councilman bodies) is present, but without inflammatory infiltrate. Indeed, there is generalized lymphoid depletion with significant necrosis of red and white pulp in the spleen. Hemorrhages are widely distributed in many organs, and death may be partially attributable to blood loss. The pathology most resembles Marburg and Ebola disease. Although it is possible that disseminated intravascular coagulation (DIC) is important in the final stages of illness, definitive hematologic studies and pathologic evidence at autopsy for this are lacking. As with other viral hemorrhagic fevers, marked weight loss with generalized muscle wasting occurs over a period of just a few days.

CLINICAL MANIFESTATIONS

Symptoms and Signs. Onset is abrupt with severe headache, high fever, chills, and myalgia strongly localized to the lower back, joint pains, and epigastric pain. Patients have described the body pains as insupportable. Conjunctivitis and a mild flushing of the face and chest, pharyngeal hyperemia, and petechiae on the palate are frequent. Bradycardia is typical. Some patients may have watery diarrhea. Hemorrhage may begin as early as 3 to 5 days after onset, usually manifest in the first instance as hematuria, nosebleeds, and bleeding from the gut. Epistaxis and gum-bleeding are common, with small ecchymotic lesions on the skin. Hematuria, proteinuria, and azotemia are associated with severe disease and a poor prognosis. Bleeding may occur at any mucosal surface as well as from venipuncture sites, often with development of ecchymoses (Fig. 31–8). Some patients develop uncontrolled bleeding, and some may have severe hepatic impairment. Pulmonary edema and hypovolemic shock, due to capillary leakage and blood loss, portend a fatal outcome. A variety of neurologic signs suggest encephalopathy rather than viral encephalitis, meningitis, or myelitis. Patients are anorectic, irritable, or obtunded. Changes in affect and mood, including aggressive behavior and depression, are frequently described, particularly in the convalescent phase. Recovery may be slow and convalescence prolonged.

Laboratory Findings. The WBC count is low (<2000/mm³) early in illness, with proteinuria and hematuria. Lymphopenia persists throughout the illness, while later a rise in neutrophils may be observed. Severe thrombocytopenia with counts <20,000/mm³ is frequently encountered. AST is raised. Prior to death, there may be biochemical evidence of hepatic or renal impairment.

DIAGNOSIS

Specimen Collection. The serum is separated and placed in a screw-cap plastic vial for storage and/or transfer. Other fluids should be frozen undiluted.

Laboratory Hazards. Precautions similar to those used for Lassa fever should be followed (Chapter 31.2). The virus is labile and not spread by aerosol.

Virus Detection. CCHF is a disease that develops rapidly following infection, and patients frequently die before the development of an antibody response. Rapid diagnosis of the acute disease rests on detection of the agent in blood or biopsy material. Recently, the development of reverse transcriptase polymerase chain reaction techniques (RT-PCR) detecting relatively well conserved sequences in the S gene of

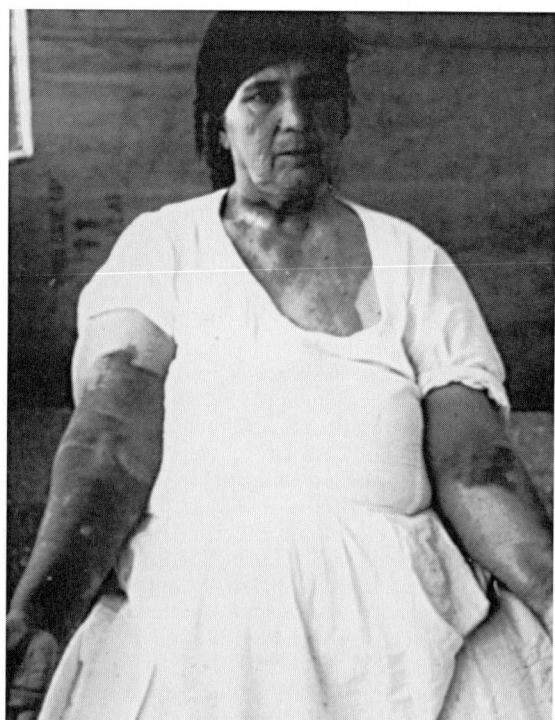

Figure 31–8. A patient with Crimean-Congo hemorrhagic fever, former Soviet Union. Of all the viral hemorrhagic fevers, CCHF is characterized by the most severe ecchymoses.

the virus has been used successfully. The reliable application of this technique has enormous advantages. It is rapid, accurate, and the RNA extraction techniques effectively inactivate the virus, so that the procedure has minimal laboratory hazards.

Other antigen detection techniques employ ELISA, IFA of direct liver biopsy smears, or virus isolation. Intracerebral inoculation of suckling mice is the most reliable method for primary virus isolation. CCHF virus can be recovered from brain of these animals 3 to 6 days following inoculation and identified by a number of methods including hemagglutination-inhibition (HI), ELISA, neutralization, or IFA.

Several types of cultured cells may be used to isolate virus strains, but in most cases infection is not cytolytic, and the virus is present in low titer and may be difficult to detect, particularly on first passage. The virus is fairly stable, but only in blood, for up to 10 days at 4°C. However, transport at −170°C or lower is important for preservation of live virus, or for RNA for RT-PCR assays.

Antibody Detection. Acute and convalescent serum pairs are used to demonstrate an increase in virus-specific IgM or IgG antibodies by ELISA or IFA tests. These antibodies may be present 7 to 10 days after infection with CCHF virus, reaching high titers months later, but decreasing over ensuing years to undetectable levels by some methods. On the other hand, neutralizing antibodies appear by days 14 to 16, and persist for many years.

MANAGEMENT

Specific Measures. Immune plasma therapy had little efficacy when used by Russian workers to treat CCHF. They observed no difference in duration of viremia, fever, or clinical outcome of 61 persons given plasma containing CCHF antibodies compared with 88 subjects who received normal plasma. More recently, CCHF specific purified immunoglobulin has been successful in a small number of patients in Bulgaria. Ribavirin, a drug that is effective against several RNA viruses, is active against CCHF virus in vitro and in vivo, and the drug has been used to treat acute CCHF. Data from South Africa suggest efficacy with intravenously administered ribavirin. Three CCHF patients with poor prognostic indicators were treated with oral ribavirin and survived, but numbers are too small to evaluate efficacy. Ribavirin is well absorbed from the gastrointestinal tract and would be expected to attain therapeutic blood levels. Treatment regimens should deliver a 2-g loading dose, then 4 g/day divided into four 6-hourly doses for 4 days, dropping to 2 g/day for 6 days. This dose can be tolerated over a short period, given the life-threatening nature of the disease. The regimen is in line with experience gained during treatment studies of Lassa fever in West Africa, and should produce virucidal serum levels in CCHF patients. Oral ribavirin treatment provides a simple, inexpensive alternative in areas where medical facilities may be limited.

As with all viral diseases, efficacy of the antiviral depends on rapid institution of therapy. This requires that physicians diagnose the disease rapidly, and institute immediate therapy on reasonable suspicion of CCHF disease.

Supportive. In addition to the careful management of fluid and electrolyte dynamics during the acute stages of disease, whole blood, platelets, and fresh plasma may be indicated. Care must be taken to avoid overhydrating the patient because the disease may be associated with a leaky capillary syndrome, and pulmonary edema may result from fluid overload despite clinical hypovolemia and dehydration.

Patient Isolation. Together with Lassa, Marburg, and Ebola viruses, CCHF is the hemorrhagic fever virus best known for nosocomial and intrafamilial secondary infection. Infectious blood and vomitus are the most likely vehicles of such transmission. Surgery and needlestick injuries must be avoided. The combination of abdominal pain and hematemesis have led to laparotomy in several instances. The patient has always died, and in some instances so have the surgeon and other theater personnel. Strict isolation, restriction and education of attendant personnel and visitors, and observance of simple precautions using gloves, gowns, masks, care with sharp instruments, and thorough disinfection are the essentials. Procedures, e.g., mouth-to-mouth resuscitation, which have been featured in published reports of CCHF outbreaks, must be avoided. In poor communities where families culturally and of necessity are involved in direct patient care, time must be given to educating and equipping people to protect themselves from the fate of their relatives.

Prophylaxis. Postexposure prophylaxis with oral ribavirin should be offered to anyone with a high-risk history of exposure to CCHF virus. High risk constitutes direct exposure to blood either on cuts or abrasions, mucous membranes, or by needlestick or other penetrating injury.

PREVENTION AND CONTROL. Avoidance of tick bite or contact with blood from infected engorged ticks is the most effective strategy to prevent infection. Repellents applied to skin, or better, soaked into clothing prior to its use, are the methods of choice. Slaughter of potentially viremic animals is also a hazard, and care should be taken to avoid contamination of cuts or mucous membranes by blood from viremic animals or from infected ticks during such procedures as shearing, dehorning, or castration.

Reports from Russia have described the use of 2% hypochlorite to control virus-transmitting ticks. When used to dip dairy cattle, it reduced tick infestation and CCHF infection rates among milkmaids. Reasonable control of adult ticks was achieved for about 6 weeks when it was applied at the rate of 50 to 100 L/hectare to pastures. Longer-lasting results were achieved with immature stages, which are the virus transmitters in subsequent years. In the Rostov region of Russia, an exceptionally cold winter in 1968 to 1969 was followed by a fourfold reduction in disease in 1969 and the complete absence of human infection in 4 of the succeeding 5 years. *H. m. marginatum* virtually disappeared, but the cold-resistant *Rhipicephalus rossicus*, which rarely attacks humans, showed no such decline and continued to maintain CCHF. Since 1975, both *H. m. marginatum* and human disease have again increased.

A formalin-inactivated CCHF vaccine produced from brains of suckling mice has been used in Bulgaria in high-risk groups, e.g., farmers and border guards, but no efficacy data are available.

Bibliography

Bishop DH: Infection and coding strategies of arenaviruses, phleboviruses, and nairoviruses. Rev Infect Dis 11(Suppl 4):S722, 1989.

Centers for Disease Control: Management of patients with suspected viral hemorrhagic fever. MMWR 37:S1, 1988.

Chapman LE, Wilson ML, Hall DB, et al: Risk factors for Crimean-Congo hemorrhagic fever in rural northern Senegal. J Infect Dis 164:686, 1991.

Chumakov MP, Smirnova SE, Tkachenko EA: Relationships between strains of Crimean haemorrhagic fever virus and Congo viruses. Acta Virol 14:82, 1969.

Fisher-Hoch SP, Khan JA, Rehman S, et al: Crimean-Congo haemorrhagic fever treated with oral ribavirin. Lancet 346:472, 1995.

Fisher-Hoch SP, McCormick JB, Swanepoel R, et al: Risk of human infections with Crimean-Congo hemorrhagic fever in southern Africa. Am J Trop Med Hyg 36:120, 1987.

Hoogstraal H: The epidemiology of tick-borne Crimean-Congo hemorrhagic fever in Asia, Europe, and Africa. J Med Entomol 15:304, 1979.

Joubert JR, King JB, Rossouw DJ, Cooper R: A nosocomial outbreak of Crimean-Congo haemorrhagic fever at Tygerberg Hospital. Part III: Clinical pathology and pathogenesis. S Afr Med J 68:722, 1985.

Shepherd AJ, Swanepoel R, Leman PA: Antibody response in Crimean-Congo hemorrhagic fever. Rev Infect Dis 11(Suppl 4):S801, 1989.

Shepherd AJ, Swanepoel R, Leman PA, Shepherd SP: Comparison of methods for isolation and titration of Crimean-Congo hemorrhagic fever virus. J Clin Microbiol 24:654, 1986.

Shepherd AJ, Swanepoel R, Leman PA, Shepherd SP: Field and laboratory investigation of Crimean-Congo haemorrhagic fever virus (Nairovirus, family Bunyaviridae) infection in birds. Trans R Soc Trop Med Hyg 81:1004, 1987.

Swanepoel R: Nairovirus infections. *In* Porterfield JS (ed): Exotic Viral Infections. London, Chapman and Hall Medical, 1995, pp 285–293.

Swanepoel R, Gill DE, Shepherd AJ, et al: The clinical pathology of Crimean-Congo hemorrhagic fever. Rev Infect Dis 11(Suppl 4):S794, 1989.

Swanepoel R, Shepherd AJ, Leman PA, et al: A common-source outbreak of Crimean-Congo haemorrhagic fever on a dairy farm. S Afr Med J 68:635, 1985.

Swanepoel R, Shepherd AJ, Leman PA, et al: Epidemiologic and clinical features of Crimean-Congo hemorrhagic fever in southern Africa. Am J Trop Med Hyg 36:120, 1987.

van de Wal BW, Joubert JR, van Eeden PJ, King JB: A nosocomial outbreak of Crimean-Congo haemorrhagic fever at Tygerberg Hospital. Part IV: Preventive and prophylactic measures. S Afr Med J 68:729, 1985.

Wilson ML, Leguenno B, Guillaud M, et al: Distribution of Crimean-Congo hemorrhagic fever viral antibody in Senegal: Environmental and vectorial correlates. Am J Trop Med Hyg 43:557, 1990.

Yu CY, Ling KX, Ling L: Characteristics of Crimean-Congo hemorrhagic fever virus (Xinjiang strain) in China. Am J Trop Med Hyg 34:1179, 1985.

31.6 Diseases Caused by Hantaviruses*

Ali S. Khan and Thomas G. Ksiazek

DEFINITION AND HISTORY. Hantavirus diseases are undoubtedly ancient disorders, readily recognizable from reports of epidemic hemorrhagic fever, especially during military campaigns from the turn of the century. Western attention to these diseases was directed during the Korean conflict when over 3000 United Nations troops were afflicted with a disease characterized by hemorrhagic fever associated with renal failure and shock. A concerted effort to delineate the etiology, epidemiology, pathogenesis, and ecology of these diseases led to the recognition of a spectrum of clinical illnesses caused by newly identified and distinct hantaviruses, each with specific rodent reservoirs. This effort culminated in the unification of a number of diseases with regional distributions under the rubric of hemorrhagic fever with renal syndrome (HFRS). These diseases are caused by the Old World hantaviruses (Hantaan, Seoul, Dobrava, Puumala) and associated Old World rodent hosts. A distinct clinical entity, hantavirus pulmonary syndrome (HPS), is caused by the New World hantaviruses (Sin Nombre, Bayou, Black Creek Canal, Andes, Juquitiba, and others) and their associated rodent hosts. Diseases caused by these viruses can occur worldwide and are best conceptualized in term of the geographic niche and phylogenetics of the associated rodent hosts (Table 31–3; Fig. 31–9). Thus, these diseases should be included in the differential diagnosis of most patients with unexplained febrile nephropathies or noncardiogenic pulmonary edema.

ETIOLOGY. Like other members of the family *Bunyaviridae*, hantaviruses are enveloped viruses with a negative (complementary) sense RNA genome that consists of tripartite, single-stranded segments designated S (small), which encodes the nucleocapsid protein; M (medium), which encodes a polyprotein that is cotranslationally cleaved to yield the envelope glycoproteins G1 and G2; and L (large), which encodes the L protein, the functional viral transcriptase/replicase. Hantaviruses replicate exclusively in the host cell cytoplasm. Entry into host cells is thought to occur by attachment of virions to cellular receptors and subsequent endocytosis.

These viruses have highly specific rodent hosts although

spillover infection has been detected in sympatric species. There appears to be a long-term virus-host relationship with evidence of chronic infection. The patterns of viral excretion by the natural hosts are not fully known, but, with the exception of a recent study, the infection is not thought to be deleterious to survival or reproduction of the rodent reservoir. Transmission from rodent to rodent is believed to occur primarily after weaning and through direct contact, perhaps after aggressive contact with accompanying combat wounds.

DISTRIBUTION

Eastern Hemisphere. Four genetically distinct Old World hantaviruses are recognized and well-characterized causes of HFRS. Hantaan virus, the prototype member of the genus, causes the most severe clinical form. Hantaan virus is endemic in Asia and is associated with the Manchurian striped field mouse (*Apodemus agrarius*). Dobrava virus is endemic in the Balkans, causes a severe form of HFRS, and is associated with the yellow-necked field mouse (*Apodemus flavicollis*). Seoul virus is associated with a less severe form of HFRS and is found worldwide, reflecting the distribution of its rodent hosts, the black rat (*Rattus rattus*) and the Norway rat (*Rattus norvegicus*). Puumala virus is endemic in western Europe, Scandinavia, and Russia, to the west of the Ural Mountains. This virus is the etiologic agent of a mild form of HFRS known as nephropathia epidemica and is carried by the European bank vole (*Clethrionomys glareolus*). The most severe forms of HFRS are associated with murine rodents, whereas Puumala virus is maintained in an arvicoline rodent. Numerous other hantaviruses have been identified from arvicoline rodents, including Prospect Hill virus, which is associated with meadow voles (*Microtus pennsylvanicus*) in the United States but which has never been implicated in human disease.

Western Hemisphere. HPS, first recognized following the investigation of a cluster of unexplained respiratory deaths in the southwestern United States during the spring of 1993, is characterized by a febrile prodrome and acute noncardiogenic pulmonary edema presenting as acute respiratory distress syndrome. In the United States, HPS is caused by at least three newly identified hantaviruses: Sin Nombre, Black Creek Canal, and Bayou viruses. The identified sigmodontine rodent reservoirs for these viruses—*Peromyscus maniculatus* and *Peromyscus leucopus* (deer and white-footed mouse) for Sin Nombre virus and its variants, *Sigmodon hispidus* (cotton rat) for Black Creek Canal virus, and *Oryzomys palustris* (rice rat) for Bayou virus—collectively extend across most of North America. Cases caused by Sin Nombre virus have been identified in Canada within the ecological range of deer mice and also are assumed to occur in Mexico. HPS has also been recently identified in Argentina, Brazil, Paraguay, Chile, and Uruguay (Fig. 31–9). Although Juquitiba virus and related viruses have been identified as the cause of Brazilian clusters of illness and as a cause of HPS, the specific sigmodontine rodent hosts for these viruses have not been defined. Thus, the complete geographic extension of HPS in South America remains in flux. Conversely, by using sophisticated molecular techniques, numerous new hantaviruses have been identified in additional sigmodontine rodents; these viruses are of unknown human pathogenicity.

TRANSMISSION. The exact mechanisms of human infection are unknown, although infective aerosols are known to be dangerous and are likely the major route of transmission. Thus, it is believed that hantaviral infection is spread to humans, who are dead-end hosts, through aerosolization or direct contact of the virus from urine or other excreta of chronically infected rodents and rarely through bites. Outbreaks from contact with infected laboratory rodents are well described and support aerosols as the major route of human transmission. Nosocomial or person-to-person transmission

---

*All the material in this chapter is in the public domain, with the exception of any borrowed figures or tables.

TABLE 31–3. Taxonomic Relationship Between Rodent Species and Their Related Hantavirus Species Plus Associated Human Diseases (If Any)

Order Rodentia	
Suborder Sciurognathi	Genus *Hantavirus* / Family *Bunyaviridae*
Family *Muridae*	
Subfamily *Arvicolinae*	
Genus *Clethrionomys*	
Species *glareolus* (European bank vole)	Puumala (Nephropathia epidemica / HFRS)
Microtus	
arvalis (common vole)	Tula
pennsylvanicus (meadow vole)	Prospect Hill
californicus (California vole)	Isla Vista
rossiaemeridionalis (eastern European vole)	Tula
Sigmodontinae	
Peromyscus	
maniculatus (deer mouse)	Sin Nombre (HPS)
leucopus (white-footed mouse)	New York-1 (HPS)
Oryzomys	
palustris (rice rat)	Bayou (HPS)
Reithrodontomys	
megalotis (western harvest mouse)	El Moro Canyon
mexicanus (Mexican harvest mouse)	Rio Segundo
Sigmodon	
alstoni	Caño Delgadito
hispidus (hispid cotton rat)	Black Creek Canal (HPS)
Oligoryzomys	
flavescens	Lechiquanes (HPS)
longicaudatus	Andes Joran (HPS)
microtis (pigmy rice rat)	Rio Mamore
Calomys	
laucha (vesper field mouse)	Laguna Negra (HPS)
?	Juquitaba (HPS)
Murinae	
Apodemus	
agrarius (striped field mouse)	Hantaan (HFRS)
flavicollis (yellow-necked field mouse)	Dobrava / Belgrade (HFRS)
Rattus	
norvegicus (Norway rat)	Seoul (HFRS)

HFRS, hemorrhagic fever with renal syndrome; HPS, hantavirus pulmonary syndrome.

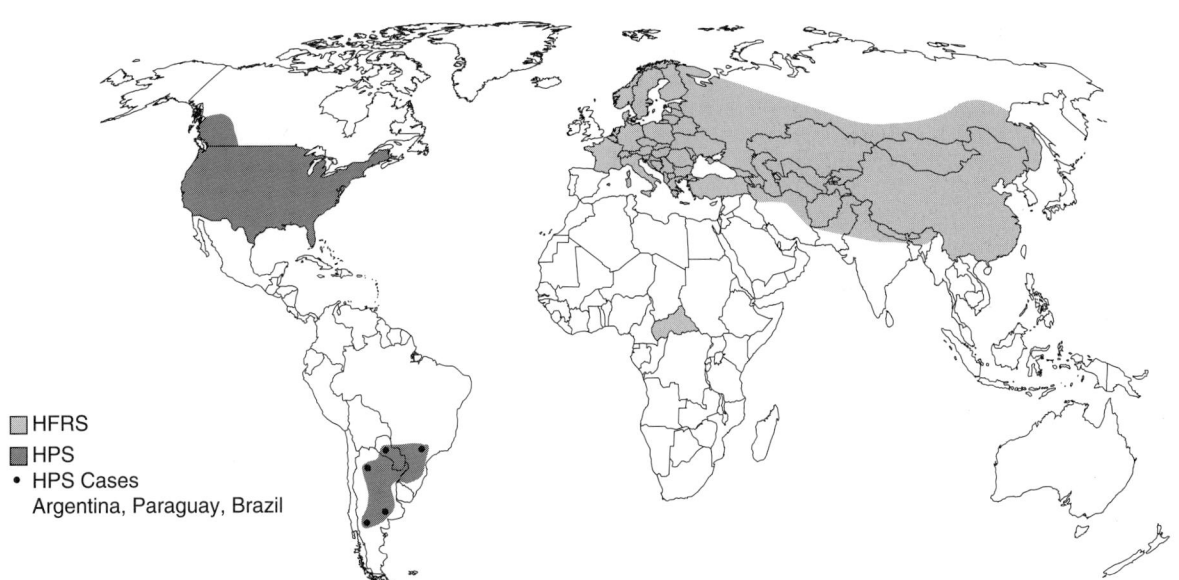

■ HFRS
■ HPS
• HPS Cases
Argentina, Paraguay, Brazil

Figure 31–9. Geographic distribution of hemorrhagic fever with renal syndrome (HFRS) and hantavirus pulmonary syndrome (HPS).

of HFRS has never been reported, which is consistent with the difficulty of culturing virus from infected persons. However, nosocomial and person-to-person transmission of HPS has been reported with Andes virus infection in southern Argentina.

DIAGNOSIS. Antibody detection using traditional IFA and neutralization assays for the Old World hantaviruses is being supplanted by ELISA assays that use native or newer recombinant antigens with a marked improvement in sensitivity and retained specificity. These assays are the standard for detection of the New World or HPS-causing hantaviruses. IgM antibodies are invariantly detectable on presentation by using specific antigens. A Western blot assay, using Sin Nombre recombinant antigens and isotype-specific conjugates to differentiate IgM from IgG, also has been developed. Its results are generally in agreement with those of the IgM-capture format.

Immunohistochemical testing of formalin-fixed tissues with specific monoclonal and polyclonal antibodies can be used to detect hantavirus antigens and has proved to be a sensitive method for retrospective and postmortem laboratory confirmation of hantaviral infections. Detection of hantaviral RNA has been useful for diagnosis when fresh-frozen lung tissue, blood clots, or the buffy coat are tested by RT-PCR. However, serum does not appear to be as useful for amplification of viral RNA as clots or nucleated cells from the blood. Isolation of hantaviruses from human sources is difficult, and therefore virus isolation is not a consideration for diagnostic purposes. In suspected cases, specimens should be forwarded after consultation to the regional World Health Organization collaborating center for viral hemorrhagic fevers.

PREVENTION AND CONTROL

Rodent Exclusion. Prevention of hantaviral diseases centers on reducing the frequency of rodent-human interactions. This emphasis applies to all rodents because visual inspection of the rodents rarely allows speciation of competent hantaviral rodent hosts and never allows determination of infectiousness. The analogy to standard precautions would be to consider every rodent as potentially infected with a hantavirus. Rodent control efforts in rural environments are futile because it is impossible to eliminate the rodent reservoir. The same can be said for occupational exposures that are predominantly rural, e.g., farming, in which rodent exclusion is impossible. The thrusts of prevention efforts for peridomestic rodents are to eliminate their access and to make domestic settings uninhabitable by proper storage, which effectively removes all sources of food and water. Additionally, hantaviruses are sensitive to heat, acid pH, detergents, formalin, and lipid solvents, and can therefore be inactivated with the use of commercially available cleaning products.

Immunization. Humoral response alone appears sufficient for protection from hantavirus infection. However, a cell-mediated response also appears protective and may be cross protective. Therefore, an efficacious vaccine targeted to the at-risk population provides the best prospects for control of HFRS in Eurasia. A formalin-inactivated Hantaan virus vaccine from infected suckling mouse brain and other inactivated tissue cultures are commercially available, but no effectiveness data are available. Phase II human trials using a recombinant vaccinia virus that expresses both the M and S segments for Hantaan virus are underway to assess effectiveness, complications, the permanence of the immune response, and the cross protection against viral subtypes and related strains.

Hantavirus Pulmonary Syndrome

EPIDEMIOLOGY. Although the high-profile investigation of this syndrome emphasized public health authorities' warn-

ings about new and emerging infectious diseases, HPS has turned out to be a newly identified, not a "new" disease. It is best characterized as a sporadic zoonosis with episodic regional increases tied to rodent abundance, which in turn is linked to meteorologic and resulting ecological conditions. The earliest case-patient confirmed by serology developed an HPS-compatible illness in July 1959. As of March 1999, the Centers for Disease Control and Prevention confirmed 211 cases of HPS in the United States; 131 cases had occurred since January 1, 1994, with a case-fatality of 34% and an overall fatality of 43%. Although most of the initial cases were recognized among Native Americans, HPS also occurs in Caucasians and African Americans. The mean age of cases is 37 years (range 11–69 years), and approximately half are male. The temporal distribution of cases shows a major peak that corresponds to the initial 1993 outbreak in June and July, minor peaks in 1994 and 1998, and a spring-summer seasonality, although cases occur throughout the year. Cases have now been identified in 30 U.S. states, most of which are west of the Mississippi River. About 75% of patients with HPS have been residents of rural areas. HPS has also been identified in Canada, Argentina, Brazil, Chile, Paraguay, and Uruguay, making this syndrome a Pan-American viral zoonosis (Fig. 31–9). In South America, HPS is characterized by variant clinical and epidemiologic features, e.g., more infection and disease among children.

Although little is known about activities that lead to a greater risk of infection, an early case-control study suggests that (1) entering rarely opened or seasonally closed buildings may contribute to infection and (2) increased numbers of rodents in the household are the strongest risk factor for infection. Among cases of HPS for which exposure information is available, 70% had exposures closely associated with peridomestic activities in currently inhabited homes that showed signs of rodent infestation. Manufactured housing features prominently in these infestations. Four clusters of HPS with two to four persons each have been documented for which exposure probably occurred within an enclosed structure. Only 4% of HPS cases have had solely occupational exposure, and 17% have had combined occupational and peridomestic exposure to rodents. Additionally, very few professionals who work with rodents have serum antibodies reactive to Sin Nombre virus, but risk of infection increases with increasing rodent contact.

PATHOLOGY AND PATHOGENESIS. The pathologic lesions are primarily vascular with variable degrees of generalized capillary dilatation and edema. Morphologic changes of the endothelium are uncommon and, when present, consist of prominent and swollen endothelial cells. Histopathologic lesions are mainly seen in the lung and spleen. The lungs, in most cases, reveal a mild to moderate interstitial pneumonitis with variable degrees of congestion, edema, and mononuclear cell infiltration. The cellular infiltrate is composed of a mixture of small and enlarged mononuclear cells with the appearance of immunoblasts. Focal hyaline membranes, as well as extensive intra-alveolar edema, fibrin, and variable numbers of inflammatory cells, are observed. Neutrophils are scanty, and the respiratory epithelium is intact in typical cases, with no evidence of cellular debris, nuclear fragmentation, or type II pneumocyte hyperplasia. Other typical histopathologic findings are seen in lymphoid tissues of HPS patients and include the presence of immunoblasts within the red pulp and periarteriolar sheaths of the spleen and paracortex, and within sinuses of lymph nodes.

Functional impairment of vascular endothelium is central to the pathogenesis of HPS. However, the pathogenesis is complex, and it is unclear how the shock syndrome relates to factors, e.g., viral distribution and immunologic and pharmacologic mediators of capillary permeability. There appears to be compartmentalization of a selective immune response in the lungs of HPS patients in combination with extremely high levels of viral antigens in the pulmonary vasculature. This feature suggests that the mechanism of inflammatory cell recruitment in the lungs of HPS patients may result from specific attraction and adherence of a selective population of inflammatory cells to an activated pulmonary microvascular endothelium. Immunohistochemical examination has shown that viral antigens are distributed primarily within the endothelium of capillaries throughout various tissues from patients with HPS. Marked accumulations of hantaviral antigens are seen in the pulmonary microvasculature and in follicular dendritic cells within the lymphoid follicles of spleen and lymph nodes. Hantaviral nucleic acids can also be localized to endothelial and inflammatory cells in tissues from HPS cases by using in situ hybridization. Electron micrographic studies confirm the infection of endothelial cells and macrophages in the lungs of patients. Typical hantaviral inclusions are seen frequently in pulmonary endothelial cells and their identity can be confirmed by immunolabeling.

CLINICAL MANIFESTATIONS

Symptoms and Course. Patients usually present after a brief 3- to 5-day febrile prodrome associated with myalgia, headache, cough, nausea or vomiting, and chills. Malaise, diarrhea, shortness of breath, and dizziness or light-headedness are also reported by approximately half of the patients with less frequent reports of arthralgias, back pain, and abdominal pain. Within 24 hours of initial evaluation, most patients develop some degree of hypotension and progressive evidence of pulmonary edema and hypoxia, usually requiring mechanical ventilation. The rapidity of this decompensation is a hallmark of HPS. Patients who do not survive had severe hypotension, frequently terminating with sinus bradycardia, electromechanical dissociation, or ventricular tachycardia or fibrillation. This terminal hemodynamic compromise can be independent of oxygenation status and occurs a median of 5 days after onset. Multiorgan dysfunction syndrome is rarely seen. Survivors usually undergo diuresis prior to convalescence, if they were in positive fluid balance, and improve almost as rapidly as they decompensate. Chronic sequelae are not reported.

Asymptomatic and mild infections have been reported both in the United States and Chile. Virus-specific variants are being recognized, e.g., renal disease and myositis appear more prominent with Bayou and Black Creek Canal virus infections.

Signs. The physical examination is usually normal on presentation except for fever, tachypnea, and tachycardia. Rashes, conjunctival or other hemorrhages, throat or conjunctival erythema, and peripheral or periorbital edema are absent. The rapidly progressive respiratory and hemodynamic compromise reflects the serial clinical findings of increasing tachypnea, hypotension, and chest findings of pulmonary edema and pleural effusions. Profuse exudate from the endotracheal tube is common. Petechiae and overt hemorrhage are being reported in patients from South America.

Laboratory Findings. Notable hematologic findings on presentation or shortly thereafter include neutrophilic leukocytosis with increased myeloid precursors, circulating immunoblasts, thrombocytopenia, and hemoconcentration, which is most pronounced in patients with florid pulmonary edema. The presence of the complete tetrad may help in early diagnosis. Hypoalbuminemia, proteinuria, and mild to moderate elevations of transaminases, creatine phosphokinase, amylase, and creatinine have also been reported. Other abnormalities mirror the hemodynamic and pulmonary involvement, including the development of metabolic acidosis, rising serum lactate levels, and prolongation of prothrombin and partial thromboplastin times. Marked renal insufficiency has mainly been noted among cases from the southeastern United States, although mild serum creatinine elevations are now recognized in up to 15% of cases. Although prolongation of prothrombin and activated partial thromboplastin times does occur, suggesting a consumptive coagulopathy, elevated fibrin split products and decreased fibrinogen levels, commonly seen in DIC, are uncommon.

Initial chest radiographs in almost all patients are abnormal, with findings indicative of interstitial edema, specifically, Kerley B lines, hilar indistinctness, or peribronchial cuffing with normal cardiothoracic ratios. A third of patients also have evidence of air space disease on the initial radiograph. By 48 hours, all patients have evidence of interstitial edema and two thirds have developed extensive air space disease that is initially bibasilar or perihilar with some degree of pleural effusions (Fig. 31–10). The initial absence of peripherally distributed air space disease, the prominence of interstitial edema, and the presence of pleural effusions early in the disease process are in contrast to the typical radiographic findings in acute respiratory distress syndrome of other etiologies.

DIFFERENTIAL DIAGNOSIS. Diagnostic confusion can occur with sepsis and severe pneumonia, caused by *Streptococcus pneumoniae*, *Chlamydia pneumoniae*, *Mycoplasma pneumoniae*, or *Legionella pneumophila*; influenza; adenovirus; and other viral pneumonias. Also to be excluded, depending on history, are plague, tularemia, leptospirosis, Q fever, ehrlichiosis, coccidioidomycosis, histoplasmosis, and diffuse pulmonary hemorrhage, as in Goodpasture syndrome.

TREATMENT. Treatment of patients with HPS remains supportive in nature. Early intensive care management is imperative, with prompt correction of electrolyte, pulmonary, and hemodynamic abnormalities. Flow-directed catheterization of the pulmonary artery is helpful not only in intensively monitoring and clinically managing the patient but also in verifying the normal-to-low pulmonary wedge pressure, decreased cardiac index, and increased systemic vascular resistance in patients who progress to shock. This pattern of shock is in contrast to the typical hemodynamic profile for septic shock of increased cardiac index and low systemic vascular resistance. Fluid administration should be limited to correct hypovolemia so as to prevent worsening pulmonary edema. The early use of inotropic agents, e.g., dobutamine, can be used to treat hypotension. Given that patients who recover from this syndrome do so rapidly, salvage therapy with extracorporeal membrane oxygenation, if available, should be considered for patients with poor prognostic indicators.

An open-label trial of treatment with intravenous ribavirin—which is effective in treating HFRS—failed to document a dramatic improvement in mortality but a placebo-controlled trial is in progress.

Hemorrhagic Fever With Renal Syndrome

EPIDEMIOLOGY

Distribution. Clinical disease caused by hantaviruses has been described in many parts of the world and they are major pathogens in such countries as China, where 60,000 to 150,000 cases are reported each year (Fig. 31–9). Most cases are described in Korea, China, Japan (Hantaan, Seoul-associated), Scandinavia, Holland, Great Britain, France, Belgium, Russia (Puumala-associated), and the Balkans (Puumala-, Hantaan-, and Dobrava-associated). However, serologic evidence of infection has also been reported from Nigeria, Central African Republic, India, Iran, Gabon, Argentina, and

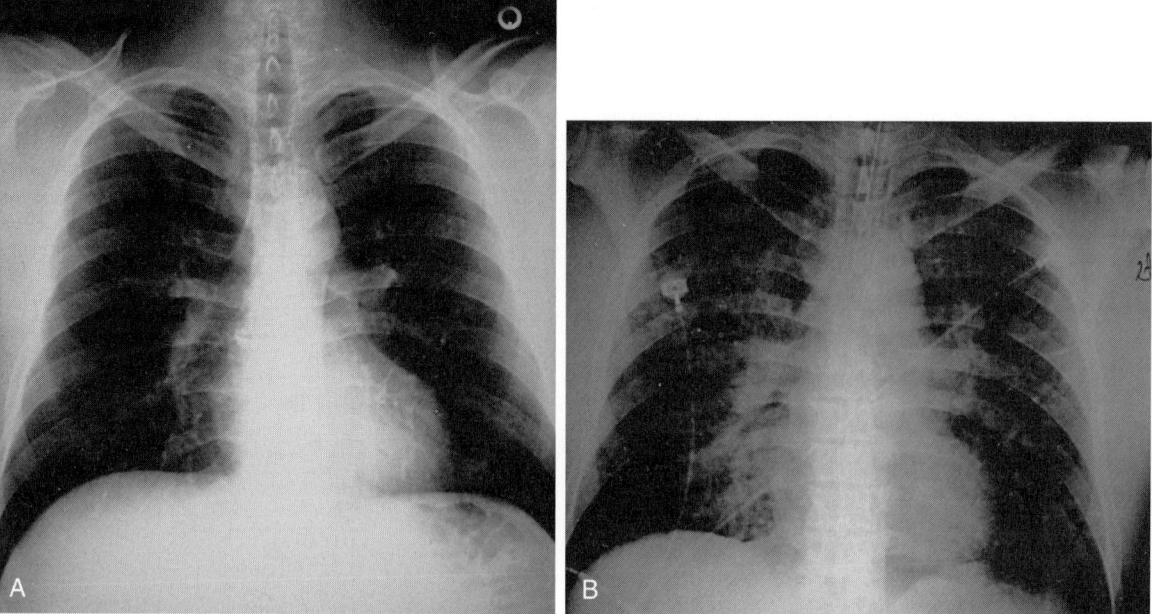

Figure 31–10. Serial chest radiographs from a patient with hantavirus pulmonary syndrome. *A,* On presentation; *B,* 24 hours later.

Bolivia. In addition, three cases associated with Seoul virus infection have been reported from Baltimore, Maryland.

Patterns of Transmission. Three epidemic patterns of HFRS are recognized: (1) *Rural type*: Patients are primarily farmers, soldiers, and construction workers, who work or reside in the field. Two seasonal peaks are usually superimposed on endemic transmission. (2) *Urban type*: This type is usually connected with *Rattus* species. A hundred cases are reported annually in Seoul and other major Korean cities. Disease is endemic with an increase in the fall and winter. (3) *Animal-room type*: Patients have become infected from colonized experimental rats or captured field rodents. Numerous outbreaks have been reported in Korea, Japan, and Russia among personnel in animal rooms where no experiments were being conducted on Hantaan or Seoul virus. Screening of introduced animals, whether or not they are feral, can prevent infection within a colony. Appropriate infection control practices, including cesarean section and foster rearing with hantavirus-negative mothers, can be used to clear the virus from an infected colony.

PATHOLOGY AND PATHOGENESIS. Generalized capillary damage is the hallmark of these diseases: vascular tone is impaired and vascular permeability is increased. A spectrum of host response reflects a unified underlying disease mechanism for the different viruses. Widespread vascular dilatation and engorgement with hemorrhage involving the kidney, heart, and anterior pituitary are characteristic. The most striking abnormalities are in the kidneys, which show a pale swollen cortex with a sharp demarcation from a variably hemorrhagic medulla. The most common histopathologic abnormality is acute tubulointerstitial nephritis with interstitial edema, extravasation of red blood cells, and inflammatory infiltrates.

As discussed for HPS, pathogenesis of HFRS is also complex, and it is unclear how the syndrome relates to factors, e.g., viral distribution and immunologic and pharmacologic mediators of capillary permeability. The presence of an active immune response at the time of disease onset has suggested an immunopathologic basis for this disease, although viral antigen is detectable in capillaries and virus isolations can be made with difficulty from acutely ill patients. This has focused previous attention on the deposition of immune complexes in glomerular capillary basement membranes, mesangium, tubular membranes, platelet surfaces, and elevation of IgE. Specific T-cell activation occurs close to disease onset, and there is persistent immune activation throughout convalescence. Activation of the classical and alternative complement pathways also appears to be an early event in HFRS pathogenesis that can lead to subsequent activation of the kinin, coagulation, and fibrinolytic pathways. Full clarification of the pathogenic mechanisms for HFRS and HPS will have to await refinement of animal models or detailed study of patients with modern methods.

CLINICAL MANIFESTATIONS

Classic Phases of Illness. The severest form of HFRS is caused by Hantaan and Dobrava viruses and is classically associated with five consecutive phases with a characteristic physiologic derangement: (1) *Febrile phase*: Onset is usually abrupt with fever, chills, lethargy, and weakness. Other associated symptoms include frontal or retro-orbital headache, which is occasionally associated with pain on eye movement; myalgia; lumbar aching; diffuse abdominal pain; blurred vision; and nausea and vomiting, which tend to occur a few days later. Within a few hours the patients are more or less prostrated and begin to have marked thirst and anorexia. (2) *Hypotensive phase*: Shock or hypotension occurs to varying degree during the last 24 to 48 hours of the febrile phase on or about day 5 of illness. (3) *Oliguric phase*: Blood pressure tends to normalize with occasional episodes of brief hypertension. Oliguria is the prominent feature in the majority of patients. Most symptoms start to abate during this phase, although nausea and vomiting can be troublesome and approximately 15% of patients develop overt hemorrhagic manifestations, e.g., epistaxis, ecchymoses, and subconjunctival hemorrhage and less commonly, gross hematuria, hemoptysis, and CNS and gastrointestinal bleeding. This phase reflects the overall severity of the illness and is associated with major electrolyte, fluid, and CNS abnormalities in addition to pulmonary complications. (4) *Diuretic phase*: Progressive improvement is heralded by the onset of diuresis, usually within 2 weeks of onset. (5) *Convalescent phase*: Convalescence is usually asymptomatic but associated with polyuria and loss of urine-concentrating ability. Increasing reports suggest long-term sequelae, e.g., renal tubular acidosis, renal hypertension, proteinuria, end-stage renal disease, and empty sella syndrome.

Variation in Clinical Illness. There is considerable variation in both the incidence of various manifestations and the severity of the individual phases, which may overlap. This is most apparent in Puumala virus infection, the mildest form of the syndrome, in which shock does not occur, skipping of phases is common, and overt hemorrhagic manifestations may be completely absent or consist of only scattered petechiae. However, severe hemorrhagic and fatal illnesses as well as a recently described association with Guillain-Barré syndrome can occur with Puumala infection. Disease caused by Seoul infection is intermediate in severity to these two presentations and more commonly associated with increased abdominal symptoms and hepatic involvement. Dividing these illnesses into a shock syndrome, acute renal failure syndrome, and an undifferentiated febrile illness is another analogous descriptive approach. Although the diseases are difficult to mistake in their classic polyphasic form, they may be confused with leptospirosis, scrub typhus, dengue fever, renal vein thrombosis, and other mild febrile illnesses. This is especially true for Puumala virus–associated infections.

Symptoms and Signs. Patients with severe HFRS appear acutely ill on presentation with an erythematous flush of the face and upper torso with blanching on pressure and dermatographia. Petechiae are present in axillary and waist folds and occasionally on the face and upper torso. Conjunctival injection is common. Conjunctival petechiae and hemorrhage occur on days 3 to 5 in some patients. The soft palate is also intensely and diffusely reddened. A mild generalized lymphadenopathy is noted on day 2. Tachycardia and hypotension are prominent during the hypotensive phase with development of bulbar conjunctival edema. Blood pressure normalizes during the oliguric phase with CNS and pulmonary abnormalities noted depending on the severity of oliguria and its associated hypertension, fluid overload, and uremia. Mortality ranges from 5 to 15% for Hantaan virus–associated disease to <1% for Puumala virus–associated illness.

Laboratory Findings. On presentation of acute severe HFRS, these are usually unremarkable but patients develop progressive thrombocytopenia and leukocytosis during the course of the febrile phase and into the hypotensive phase. An abrupt onset of proteinuria is usually noted on about day 5 of illness with isosthenuria (urine specific gravity of 1.010) and evidence of hemoconcentration. Evidence of renal insufficiency and electrolyte abnormalities are prominent during the oliguric phase.

TREATMENT. The cornerstone of therapy remains supportive in nature, with strict management of fluid and electrolyte abnormalities to prevent fluid overload during the early stages of the disease, and to keep up with fluid losses during the polyuric phase. Early hospitalization is recommended. Transportation and other trauma should be limited to prevent exacerbation of the underlying vascular injury. Hypotension is preferably treated with colloids, when volume expansion is indicated, and vasopressors if intravascular volume is judged to be normal. Dialysis can be life-saving. Attempts to modify the course with immunosuppressive agents have yielded contradictory results and steroids have not proved efficacious.

Intravenous ribavirin therapy in a double-blind, concurrent, placebo-controlled trial resulted in a sevenfold reduction in Hantaan virus–associated HFRS mortality when administered within 6 days of fever onset. The effect on mortality appears to be mediated through a reduction in the risk of experiencing oliguria; a reduction in hemorrhage also occurs. The need for early administration of ribavirin may explain the lack of apparent efficacy in HPS, in which onset of severe cardiopulmonary disease occurs after a very brief prodrome.

Bibliography

Bruno P, Hassell LH, Brown J, et al: The protean manifestations of hemorrhagic fever with renal syndrome: A retrospective review of 26 cases from Korea. Ann Intern Med 113:385, 1990.

Cosgriff TM: Mechanisms of disease in hantavirus infection: Pathophysiology of hemorrhagic fever with renal syndrome. Rev Infect Dis 13:97, 1991.

Duchin JS, Koster FT, Peters CJ, et al: Hantavirus pulmonary syndrome: A clinical description of 17 patients with a newly recognized disease. N Engl J Med 330:949, 1994.

Hallin GW, Simpson SQ, Cromwell RE, et al: Cardiopulmonary manifestations of hantavirus pulmonary syndrome. Crit Care Med 24:252, 1996.

Huggins JW, Hsiang CM, Cosgriff TM, et al: Prospective, double-blind, concurrent, placebo-controlled clinical trial of intravenous ribavirin therapy of hemorrhagic fever with renal syndrome. J Infect Dis 164:1119, 1991.

Khan AS, Khabbaz RF, Armstrong LR, et al: Hantavirus pulmonary syndrome: The first 100 US cases. J Infect Dis 173:1297, 1996.

Kim YS, Ahn C, Han JS, et al: Hemorrhagic fever with renal syndrome caused by Seoul virus. Nephron 71:419, 1995.

LeDuc JW, Childs JE, Glass GE: The hantaviruses, etiologic agents of hemorrhagic fever with renal syndrome: A possible cause of hypertension and chronic renal disease in the United States. Annu Rev Public Health 13:79, 1992.

Lee HW: Epidemiology and pathogenesis of hemorrhagic fever with renal syndrome. *In* Elliott RM (ed): The Bunyaviridae. New York, Plenum Press, 1996, pp 253–267.

McKee K, LeDuc JW, Peters CJ: Hantaviruses. *In* Belshe RB (ed): Textbook of Human Virology, 2nd ed. St. Louis, Mosby Year Book, 1991, pp 615–632.

Mustonen J, Brummer-Korvenkontio M, Hedman K, et al: Nephropathia epidemica in Finland: A retrospective study of 126 cases. Scand J Infect Dis 26:7, 1994.

Nichol ST, Spiropoulou CF, Morzunov S, et al: Genetic identification of a hantavirus associated with an outbreak of acute respiratory illness. Science 262:615, 1993.

Schmaljohn CS: Molecular biology of hantaviruses. *In* Elliott RM (ed): The Bunyaviridae. New York, Plenum Press, 1996, pp 63–90.

Zaki SR, Greer PW, Coffield LM, et al: Hantavirus pulmonary syndrome: Pathogenesis of an emerging infectious disease. Am J Pathol 146:552, 1995.

31.7 Kyasanur Forest Disease

Theodore Tsai

DEFINITION. Kyasanur Forest disease (KFD) is a severe, sometimes biphasic, febrile illness frequently complicated by gastrointestinal and other hemorrhages and a delayed neurologic syndrome.

ETIOLOGY AND HISTORY. Antigenically, the virus is a member of the tick-borne complex of flaviviruses that includes Powassan, tick-borne encephalitis, and Omsk hemorrhagic fever (OHF) viruses. The disease first came to light in 1957, when a cluster of deaths was reported in forest monkeys and humans living in nearby villages in the Shimoga District of Mysore (now Karnataka) state, India (Fig. 31–11). The clinical features of the illness and epizootic disease in monkeys initially suggested the first recognition of jungle yellow fever in Asia, but among field-collected arthropods, the virus was isolated only from ticks. The virus was shown to be a novel member of the tick-borne flavivirus complex and named after the location of the outbreak.

DISTRIBUTION AND INCIDENCE. The virus and disease have been recognized only in Karnataka state, India. The disease spread slowly from the initial epidemic focus in the Shimoga district and subsequently has appeared in several noncontiguous areas within the state, most recently in the

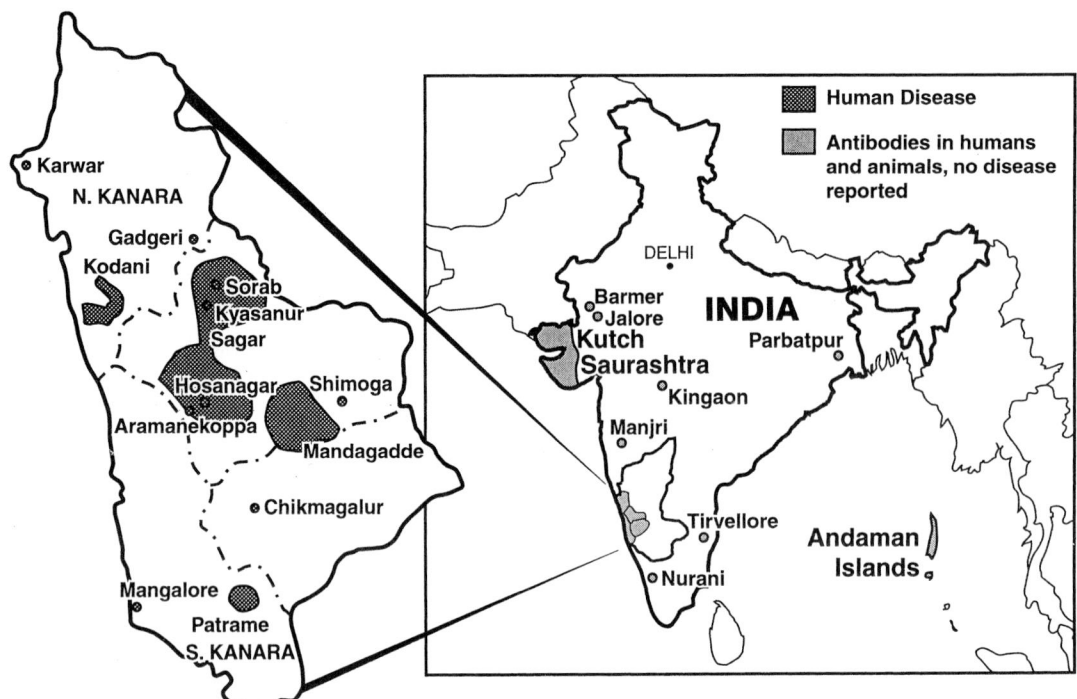

Figure 31–11. Kyasanur Forest disease: distribution in India.

South Kanara district. Within each epidemic focus, the disease has spread centripetally during several years to become locally hyperendemic. Several hundred cases are reported annually and more than 1000 cases were reported in 1976, 1977, and 1983. Approximately 5% of the population in the initial epidemic area in 1957 and 1958 were seropositive, but in some villages up to one third of residents had been infected. The epidemic foci have been situated on moist mountainous slopes and plains with high rainfall (>80 inches), mixed deciduous and evergreen forests, and thick vegetation supporting small wild mammals, pigs, porcupines, monkeys, and birds.

Serologic surveys that demonstrated KFD viral antibodies in animals and humans in Kutch and Sourashtra, semiarid to arid locations in northwestern India, far removed from the recognized enzootic area and with considerably different ecological conditions suggest the circulation of a related virus.

TRANSMISSION AND EPIDEMIOLOGY. The virus has been isolated from numerous species of forest tick; however, >90% of viral isolates have come from *Haemaphysalis spinigera*, which also are the predominant species on the forest floor. Infection is transmitted trans-stadially but not transovarially. Infected nymphs are principally responsible for human infection. Larval ticks feed on small rodents and birds; adult ticks rely on larger mammals, including livestock cattle. Because they develop low levels of viremia, cattle are not considered to have a role in viral amplification. Porcupines and flying squirrels, however, develop elevated viremias, are prevalent and mobile, and could have important roles in disseminating the virus. The virus is isolated easily from *Haemaphysalis* ticks during the dry months from December to May, but viral maintenance during the monsoon relies on unknown mechanisms, possibly involving *Ixodes* ticks, which are prevalent during this period.

Outbreaks have developed as a result of human activities within forests, mainly deforestation for the purpose of planting crops, commercial lumbering, and rearing cattle. The epidemic period from December to June corresponds to the period when nymphal ticks are most abundant. Year to year variations in tick abundance correlate with the number of human and monkey cases. Cases occur principally in young adults who are exposed occupationally in the forest; early cases were principally in males; however, recent cases in Belthangadi, south Kanara district, have occurred mainly in females (3:1 ratio). The emergence of outbreaks in noncontiguous areas may reflect the unmasking of previously silent viral enzootic foci or, possibly, novel introductions by infected ticks or animals during human movements.

PATHOGENESIS AND PATHOLOGY. The virus circulates in the blood between the second and twelfth days of illness with peak viral titers occurring between the fourth and seventh days. Infection disseminates widely, and in fatal cases, virus has been recovered from lung, liver, spleen, heart, kidneys, and skeletal muscle. In several cases, virus has been isolated from the CSF. Erythro-, leuko-, and thrombophagocytosis appear in the peripheral blood after the first week of illness, and similar findings are prominent in the liver and spleen, and in experimentally infected monkeys, in lymph nodes. Gross hemorrhagic consolidation of the lungs and evidence of massive gastrointestinal bleeding are present while other organs are grossly normal or exhibit mild congestion. Parenchymal and inflammatory changes are seen in areas of focal hepatitis, with rare coagulative necrosis and extrusion of Councilman bodies; congestion and tubular degenerative changes in the kidney; pleuritis, septal prominence, peribronchiolar inflammatory infiltrate and alveolar hemorrhage in the lungs; interstitial inflammatory changes consistent with myocarditis; and prominence of the splenic sinusoids with erythrophagocytosis. Although only cerebral edema has been demonstrated in patients dying early in the course of illness, in experimentally and naturally infected monkeys a pattern of disseminated focal encephalitis is present.

The biphasic course of illness and often late onset of neurologic symptoms, similar to that of louping ill, tick-borne encephalitis, Omsk hemorrhagic fever, and Rift Valley fever, reflect delayed infection of the CNS rather than a postinfectious etiology.

CLINICAL FEATURES. After an incubation period of 3 to 8 days, illness begins abruptly with fever, shaking chills, headache, and striking myalgias, leading to severe prostration. Eye pain, vomiting, diarrhea, abdominal pain, and hyperesthesia of the skin add to the intensity of illness. The initial examination discloses extreme prostration, a dulled sensorium, facial flushing, prominent conjunctivitis or suffusion, gingival hyperplasia, and cervical and occasionally generalized adenopathy. In more than half of cases, the illness evolves with more critical features of pneumonia, leading to death in 10 to 33% of cases. Hemorrhagic manifestations, usually epistaxis, bleeding from the gums, and passage of melanotic stools or hematemesis, develop within several days of the onset of illness. Pulmonary signs are present in half of cases and tender hepatomegaly is common, accompanied by jaundice in rare cases. A slowed pulse has indicated heart block in some cases. Diffuse neurologic involvement is suggested by an altered sensorium, meningismus, tremors, rigidity, and occasionally, pyramidal signs. Generalized convulsions signal a poor prognosis. Hemorrhagic pulmonary edema or pneumonia frequently leads to respiratory failure. Subarachnoid hemorrhage is a rare complication.

The peripheral blood count typically shows leukopenia, moderate thrombocytopenia and anemia. The pathogenesis of the hemorrhagic diathesis has not been defined, but prolonged prothrombin, bleeding, and clotting times have been demonstrated in some patients. Elevated hepatic transaminases and bilirubin are seen in some patients. Despite the prominence of neurologic symptoms, CSF is normal in the majority of cases, although lymphocytic pleocytosis and elevated protein are seen occasionally.

In about 15% of cases, recovery from the acute phase of illness is followed by an afebrile interval of 7 to 21 days, after which illness recurs with fever, headache, generalized myalgias, and variable dyspnea, bleeding, hepatosplenomegaly and neurologic signs, principally tremor, vertigo, meningismus, abnormal reflexes, and mental status changes. Deaths have occurred during the second phase of illness, which usually lasts 2 to 12 days. In patients exhibiting neurologic signs, CSF examination discloses a mild mononuclear pleocytosis.

DIAGNOSIS. A history of forest exposure in the endemic area within the known incubation period is the most important clue to diagnosis. The infection can be confirmed by isolating virus from acute-phase blood specimens or serologically, by demonstrating fourfold antibody changes between acute and convalescent phase specimens by hemagglutination-inhibition, complement fixation, or neutralization tests. Cross reactions due to previous flavivirus infections can complicate interpretation.

TREATMENT AND PROGNOSIS. No specific antiviral therapy is available. Intensive supportive care with specific attention to monitoring blood pressure, fluid and electrolyte balance, and respiratory exchange may be life-saving.

PREVENTION AND CONTROL. A formalin-inactivated chick embryo–derived vaccine is safe, immunogenic and in limited field studies, protective. The vaccine is used in high-risk groups and in response to epidemics in the recognized affected areas. Although tick-borne encephalitis vaccine elicits cross reactive antibodies, laboratory acquired cases in immunized workers have demonstrated the absence of efficacy. Area application of acaricides during the season when nymphs are most abundant could reduce risk of human infection. Personal protective measures, including the application of repellents and dressing in protective clothing, are recommended.

Bibliography

Bannerjee K: Kyasanur Forest disease. *In* Monath TP (ed): The Arboviruses: Epidemiology and Ecology, Vol III. Boca Raton, FL, CRC Press, 1988, pp 93–116.

Morse LJ, Russ SB, Needy CF, Buescher EL: Studies of viruses of the tick borne encephalitis complex. II: Disease and immune responses in man following accidental infection with Kyasanur Forest disease virus. J Immunol 88:240, 1962.

Prabha A, Prabhu MG, Raghuveer CV, et al: Clinical study of 100 cases of Kyasanur Forest disease with clinicopathological correlation. Ind J Med Sci 47:124, 1993.

Webb HE, Kakshmana Rao R: Kyasanur Forest disease: A general clinical study in which some cases with neurological complications were observed. Trans R Soc Trop Med Hyg 55:284, 1961.

PART III
Bacterial Infections

SECTION A Infections of the Eye and Throat

32 *Trachoma and Inclusion Conjunctivitis*

Robin Bailey, David C.W. Mabey, and Hugh R. Taylor

TRACHOMA

DEFINITION. Trachoma is a chronic follicular conjunctivitis prevalent in many resource-poor environments worldwide. The infection is usually acquired early in childhood. Progressive scarring and distortion of the upper eyelid may lead to corneal scarring and blindness, usually in late middle age.

ETIOLOGY. Trachoma is caused by infection with *Chlamydia trachomatis*, almost exclusively by serotypes A, B, Ba, and C. "Genital" serotypes D through K may cause disease indistinguishable from trachoma, but they do so rarely. A single infection with *C. trachomatis* usually produces a self-limiting follicular conjunctivitis (i.e., inclusion conjunctivitis). Repeated episodes of infection appear to be necessary for the development of intense inflammation and the characteristic scarring sequelae. Immunologic mechanisms rather than direct tissue damage by *C. trachomatis* are considered to be responsible for the pathologic features of the disease.

DISTRIBUTION AND PREVALENCE. Trachoma, one of the most common infectious diseases, has been estimated to affect 500 million people. It is the leading preventable cause of blindness worldwide; in 1995 WHO estimated that almost 6 million were blind as a result of trachoma. The global burden of trachoma is likely to increase owing to demographic trends. In severely affected communities, signs of trachoma can be found in over 90% of 1- to 2-year-olds; as many as 25% of those over 60 years may be blind as a result of it.

Trachoma is a disease of poverty, occurring in areas of poor personal and environmental hygiene. It was common in much of Europe and North America during the 19th century, disappearing as socioeconomic and public health improvements took place. Trachoma is found in North and sub-Saharan Africa, the Middle East, and the Indian subcontinent. There are also foci in parts of Central and South America, Australia, and the Pacific. It tends to be more common in arid areas, where water availability is limited.

EPIDEMIOLOGY

Reservoir of Infection. In trachoma-endemic communities, active trachoma is frequently found in children but is unusual in adults, indicating that acquired immunity modulates the occurrence or duration of disease episodes. The main reservoir of infection is the eye and possibly the nasopharynx and GI tract of children with active trachoma. Repeated reinfection is necessary for the development of trachomatous scarring, and the higher prevalence of active trachoma and

scarring sequelae found among women in most endemic areas is probably due to their closer contact with children.

Transmission. Most transmission of trachoma occurs within the family, as a result of close contact between young children and their mothers or other caregivers. Transmission is favored by poor environmental and personal hygiene. Lack of water for washing leads to the persistence of infected secretions on the face, hands, and clothing. Inadequate sleeping space and poor ventilation may also permit spread by direct contact, by transmission through fomites on bedding, or from the nasopharynx by coughing or sneezing. Inadequate disposal of rubbish or sewage, or the proximity of domestic animals, supports flies that can transmit infected ocular or nasal secretions. The relative importance of flies, fomites, and fingers probably varies from one community to another.

In some areas, such as North Africa, seasonal epidemics of bacterial conjunctivitis occur superimposed on endemic trachoma and may exacerbate its effects by producing more severe inflammation, accelerated development of conjunctival and corneal scarring, and copious ocular discharge that may increase transmission of chlamydiae.

PATHOGENESIS

Pathology. Intracytoplasmic inclusions in epithelial cells, which stain blue with Giemsa stain (Halberstaedter-Prowazek bodies), are characteristic of chlamydial infection. Inclusions are most common in conjunctival scrapings taken from patients with acute infection. Early in the disease, the conjunctiva shows an acute inflammatory response, but soon mononuclear cells and plasma cells are also present. The most characteristic histologic finding in trachoma is the presence of follicles in the superior tarsal conjunctiva. These are germinal centers surrounded by small lymphocytes. Often, the conjunctival epithelium is invaded by polymorphonuclear leukocytes and mononuclear cells, and it may thin to a single layer over the surface of a follicle. Later, necrosis in the follicles leads to subconjunctival scarring. Contraction of this scar tissue leads to distortion of the tarsal plate, producing entropion and trichiasis, which in turn lead to corneal opacification and blindness. Pannus is initially an inflammatory infiltrate, which is replaced by fibrous tissue and new blood vessels.

Immune Mechanisms. The pathogenesis of trachoma is not well understood. It seems clear that repeated reinfection is necessary for it to develop; this observation led to the concept of trachoma as a disease mediated by immune hypersensitivity. The role of specific chlamydial antigens in this process is disputed, and the mechanism of induction of pathology is unknown, but there is evidence that T-cell and macrophage cytokine products such as interferon gamma (IFN-γ), tumor necrosis factor alpha (TNF-α), and transforming growth factor beta (TGF-β) may have a role.

CLINICAL MANIFESTATIONS. Trachoma usually produces few symptoms until its final stages, when trichiasis (turning

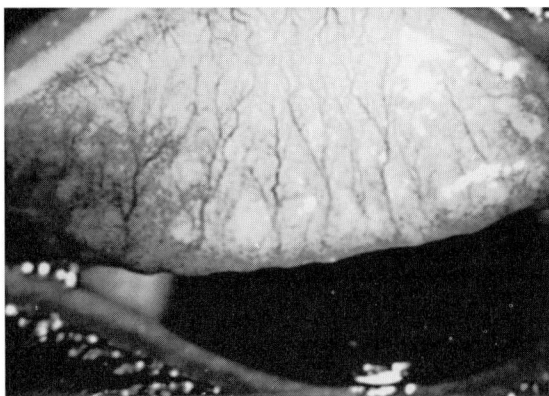

Figure 32–1. Superior tarsal conjunctiva of a child with trachoma. The upper lid has been everted, showing several large white follicles, especially along the upper border of the tarsal plate. The tiny dark dots are papillae.

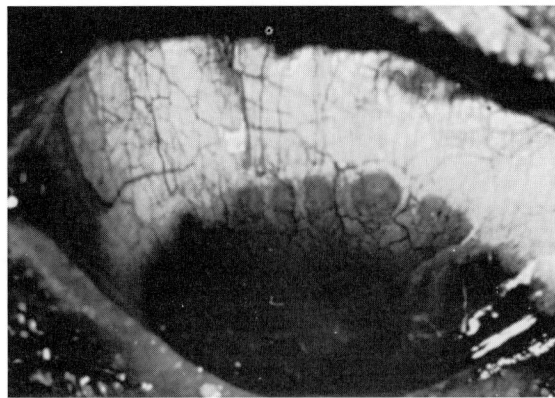

Figure 32–3. Superior cornea of a child with active trachoma showing large, gray, fleshy limbic follicles. Corneal pannus extends several millimeters into the cornea.

in of the eyelashes) develops. A superimposed bacterial conjunctivitis causes a mucopurulent discharge. In the absence of secondary conjunctivitis, the symptoms may be mild and are ignored (even if medical care is available) as are a purulent nasal discharge, chronic serous otitis media, and a productive cough, which also may be due to an initial chlamydial infection followed by secondary bacterial infection.

Active Inflammation Stage. The most obvious sign of trachoma during the stage of active inflammation is the follicle, either in the superior tarsal conjunctiva or at the corneal limbus (Figs. 32–1 and 32–2). Follicles are large pale yellow or white spots that may be slightly elevated and are 0.25 to 2 mm in diameter. Those on the limbus are often a dirty gray and may be semitranslucent (Fig. 32–3).

Active inflammation is also accompanied by marked thickening of the conjunctiva. This can be recognized when the tarsal blood vessels are obscured or conjunctival papillae are present. Papillae appear as small, pinpoint red dots (Fig. 32–1). They are not specific for trachoma. Papillae appear earlier than trachomatous follicles and may be the only sign of ongoing active inflammation in the eyes of young children or older persons, who usually have no follicular response. The papillary response increases dramatically with bacterial secondary infection. The intensity of the papillary response in the presence of follicles is a good index of the severity of the inflammation and infection.

Chronic Recurring Stage. Fine conjunctival scars gradually appear. Occurring first as small stellate figures, they gradually accumulate to form a basket-weave network (Fig. 32–5). With time, this consolidates to form strong bands of scar tissue (Fig. 32–6). Sometimes, an especially prominent band, Arlt's line, develops a few millimeters above and parallel to the lid margin. Follicles seem to blend into the scars and may be difficult to distinguish.

Trichiasis. Scarring of the conjunctiva impedes the normal protective role of this mucous membrane and leads to distortion and buckling of the tarsal plate. The scar tissue contracts like the string of an archer's bow, causing the lid margin to rotate inward, leading to entropion. The earliest sign of this is the irregular migration of the openings of the meibomian glands onto the inner surface of the lid (Fig. 32–6). This is followed by turning in of the lashes, which rub on the cornea, causing trichiasis (Fig. 32–7). The continual abrasion of the cornea rapidly produces corneal edema, ulceration, and scarring—the main route by which trachoma leads to blindness.

Superior Corneal Pannus. Inflammatory infiltrate and punctate keratitis may occur in the superior cornea during active inflammation; corneal stromal opacification and new vessels later develop to produce the superior corneal pannus characteristic of trachoma (Figs. 32–3 and 32–4). The pannus may extend several millimeters across the cornea and, in rare cases, may reach the central cornea and affect vision. More often, however, blood vessels will extend from the pannus to

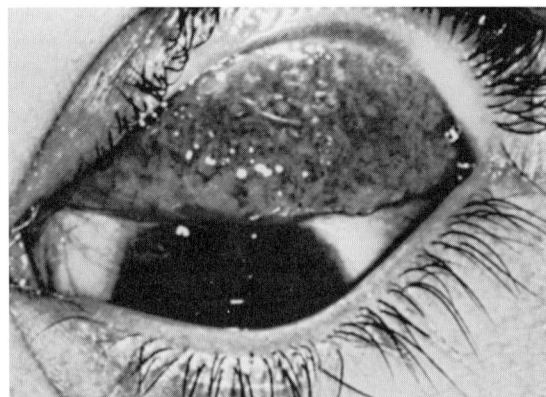

Figure 32–2. An intense inflammatory response to trachoma. Follicles extend over most of the superior tarsal conjunctiva; some are confluent. The inflammation and hyperemia have caused spontaneous hemorrhages.

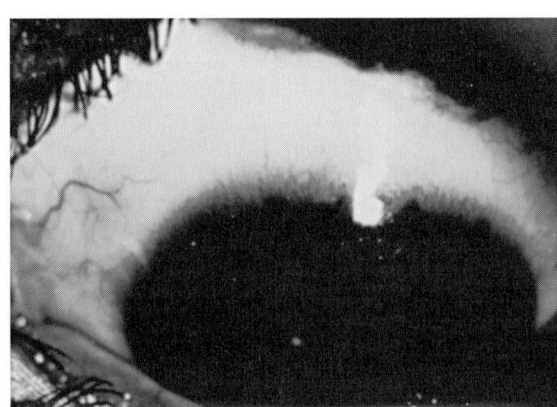

Figure 32–4. Superior limbus of a child with trachoma showing many Herbert's pits and about 1 mm of corneal pannus.

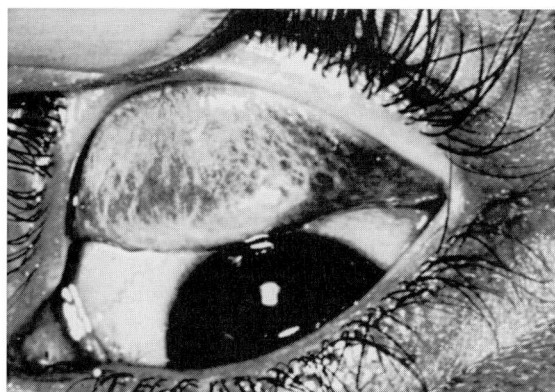

Figure 32–5. The superior tarsal conjunctiva of a child with trachoma, showing an extensive "basket-weave" network of conjunctival scarring. Although no follicles are obvious, active inflammation is indicated by the numerous papillae.

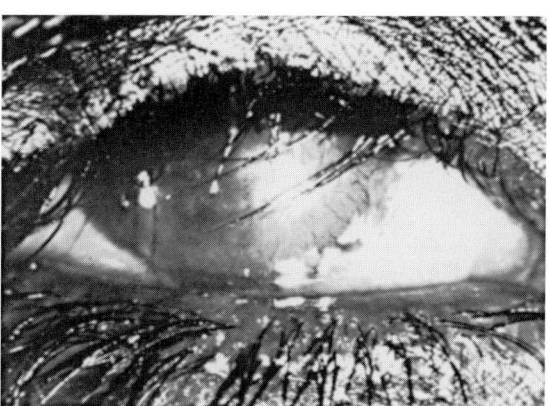

Figure 32–7. Early trichiasis in an adult with advanced cicatricial trachoma. The medial lashes of the upper lid rub on the cornea, which has become opaque and vascularized.

an area of corneal ulceration and lead to a vascularized leukoma. As the pannus advances across the cornea, it bypasses the sites of limbic follicles. After the follicles resolve, clear depressions are left, surrounded on three sides by pannus. These depressions are known as Herbert's pits (Fig. 32–4).

Reduced Tearing. A decrease in the tears in those with cicatrizing trachoma has been described, but no specific abnormality in tear function has been shown. The eyes are often more moist (watery) than usual, and there may even be maceration from chronic conjunctivitis. Signs of cicatrization (e.g., tarsal scarring, entropion and trichiasis, pannus, and Herbert's pits) indicates that the eye has had active inflammatory trachoma in the past. Follicles (either tarsal or limbic) and inflammatory thickening indicate an active inflammatory response at the time of examination. Trachoma and inclusion conjunctivitis present a spectrum of chronicity. Inclusion conjunctivitis develops following an isolated episode of infection, whereas repeated infection is needed to maintain trachoma. Putative relapses of trachoma are almost certainly due to reinfection.

DIAGNOSIS

Clinical Diagnosis. Trachoma is usually diagnosed on clinical grounds. A simplified grading scheme has been developed by WHO (Table 32–1) that is widely used for public health purposes. For more sophisticated studies, the detailed

system proposed by Dawson and colleagues in a 1981 WHO publication, which has a defined correspondence to the simplified scheme, may be useful.

Laboratory Diagnosis

Detection of Chlamydiae. Several tests can be used to make a laboratory diagnosis of trachoma. Previously, Giemsa staining of conjunctival scrapings was used to demonstrate characteristic chlamydial inclusions in epithelial cells. The organism can be cultured in embryonated hen's eggs or in one of several tissue culture systems, the best of which is McCoy cells treated with cycloheximide. Antigen detection methods using commercial kits have been applied in field studies for some years. In direct fluorescent antibody (DFA) cytology, chlamydial elementary bodies are detected in conjunctival smears using fluorescein-conjugated monoclonal antibodies (Fig 32–8), and enzyme immunoassay (EIA) methods use enzyme-linked antibodies to detect chlamydial antigens in conjunctival swabs. These tests are more sensitive than Giemsa cytology and cheaper than culture but are being superseded by DNA amplification methods, which are much more sensitive than either antigen detection or culture and can detect very low numbers of chlamydial genomes.

Detection of Chlamydial DNA. DNA amplification based on the polymerase chain reaction (PCR) or the ligase chain reaction (LCR) is the most sensitive method for demonstrating ocular chlamydial infection and is available commercially. Sensitivity has been improved by targeting sequences in the common plasmid pCT1 of *C. trachomatis*, multiple copies of which appear to be universally present in each bacterial cell. With these methods, sensitivities approaching the detection of a single chlamydial elementary body are feasible. Because

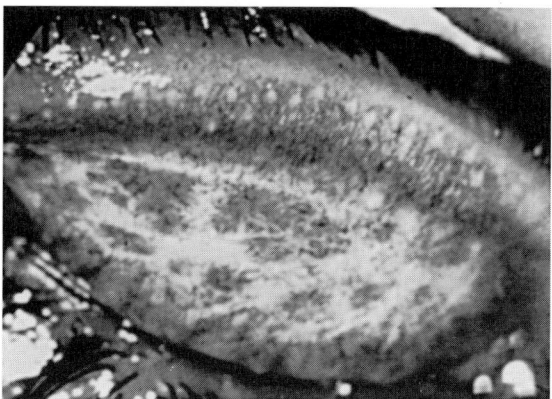

Figure 32–6. Strong, organized bands of scarring of the superior tarsal conjunctiva in an adult, with distortion of the line of openings of the meibomian glands as they are dragged onto the tarsal surface by scarring. (Courtesy of Professor F. C. Hollows.)

TABLE 32–1. World Health Organization Simplified Trachoma Grading Scheme

TF:	Trachomatous inflammation—follicular; 5 or more follicles ($\geq$0.5 mm) in the upper tarsal conjunctiva
TI:	Trachomatous inflammation—intense; inflammatory thickening of tarsal conjunctiva obscuring more than half of the normal deep tarsal vessels
TS:	Trachomatous conjunctival scarring; easily visible scarring in the tarsal conjunctiva
TT:	Trachomatous trichiasis; at least 1 eyelash rubbing on the eyeball
CO:	Corneal opacity; easily visible opacity over the pupil obscuring at least part of the pupil margin

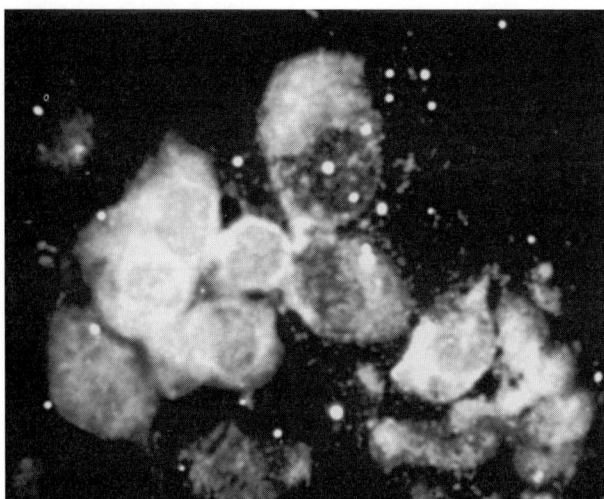

Figure 32–8. Direct fluorescent antibody (DFA) cytology preparation. The free chlamydial elementary bodies are stained brightly with a fluorescent-labeled monoclonal antibody.

the target sequences are unique to *C. trachomatis*, these tests are essentially completely specific as well as very sensitive. However, occasional discrepancies between amplified DNA methods and other tests can arise owing to the presence in the sample of inhibitors of the amplification reaction.

Detection of Chlamydial Antibodies. The presence of antichlamydial antibodies in serum or tears may reflect past infection and thus is not diagnostic for current infection. However, the presence of IgM antibodies in serum or the presence of sIgA antibodies in tears is suggestive of recent or current infection.

Differential Diagnosis. Trachoma may be confused with other conditions producing a follicular conjunctivitis or conjunctival scarring. Follicles may be found in the fornix conjunctivae in otherwise healthy eyes. This occurs most commonly in young children in whom the follicles are not associated with inflammation, especially in the inferior fornix, and do not involve the superior tarsus—a condition called folliculosis. Viral infection is the most common nonchlamydial cause of follicular conjunctivitis, but it is an acute and self-limiting infection that shows significant resolution within 2 weeks. A toxic follicular conjunctivitis may also occur in molluscum contagiosum, prolonged use of topical drugs, and allergy to eye cosmetics. The large papillae found in vernal conjunctivitis may be mistaken for trachomatous follicles. In Parinaud's oculoglandular syndrome, conjunctival follicles are involved with gross preauricular lymphadenopathy, fever, and malaise. It is associated with a number of infections, including syphilis, tuberculosis, tularemia, and lymphogranuloma venereum, and is the result of pathogenic invasion through the conjunctiva. The other differential diagnoses are inclusion conjunctivitis, which is due to chlamydial infection, and two conditions that are probably forms of mild trachoma and are presumed to be due to chlamydial infection: Axenfeld's chronic follicular conjunctivitis and Thygeson's chronic follicular keratoconjunctivitis.

Tarsal scarring likely to be confused with trachoma may be produced by trauma, a previous chalazion, and severe bacterial conjunctivitis.

TREATMENT AND PROGNOSIS

Antibiotic Therapy. Chlamydiae are sensitive to a number of antimicrobial agents including sulfonamides, tetracyclines, erythromycin and the newer macrolides, and rifampin. The mainstay of trachoma treatment has been topical 1% tetracycline ointment, which has been used in a number of regi-mens. For continuous treatment, twice-daily use for 6 weeks has been recommended by the WHO. Where the area to be treated is too large or populous to organize simultaneous continuous treatment, intermittent therapy for 5 to 7 consecutive days every month for 6 months has been found to be efficient and effective.

A number of systemic treatments have been efficacious when given for 2 to 3 weeks but have associated risks; e.g, tetracycline is inexpensive and safe but should not be given to pregnant women or children under 8 years of age (usually the prime group for treatment). Sulfonamides are effective systemically but have rare severe adverse effects, such as Stevens-Johnson syndrome. Rifampin is useful but should probably be reserved for treatment of mycobacterial diseases; moreover, in vitro resistance has been found to develop quickly in laboratory strains of *Chlamydia* exposed to rifampin. Erythromycin is safe and effective but must be given four times a day.

A number of macrolide antibiotics with altered pharmacokinetic properties resulting in greater tissue penetration and prolonged excretion relative to erythromycin are now available; they can be administered in regimens of one or a few doses. Azithromycin is foremost among these; in a randomized trial it was effective as a single oral dose of 20 mg/kg for trachoma treatment and gave similar results to 6 weeks of topical tetracycline. This has obvious advantages for compliance and convenience, but azithromycin is currently expensive and cannot be recommended for pregnant women, as there are no safety data in this context.

If significant bacterial conjunctivitis coexists, treatment should be with topical antibiotics. Although the therapies outlined above are effective for managing sporadic cases, treatment of patients in endemic areas is usually compromised by rapid reinfection, and mass treatment must be considered.

Treatment of Complications. Trichiasis should be treated. Single lashes can be epilated by the patient or a family member. However, relief is only temporary because the lashes promptly regrow. Lid surgery is needed to evert the lashes and prevent blindness; a number of procedures have been advocated, but the treatment of choice is probably tarsal rotation. In addition to relieving discomfort, it improves visual acuity.

PREVENTION AND CONTROL. The aim of prevention is to reduce transmission of infection and thereby reduce exposure to the extent that reinfection does not occur often enough to cause blinding trachoma. Measures to improve personal and community hygiene are likely to lessen trachoma. These include provision and proper use of adequate water supplies, housing, food storage, fly control, and rubbish and sewage disposal. Studies of community behavioral interventions to promote face washing in children have shown that with effort, reductions in trachoma transmission are possible, but the improvements are not sustained in the long term.

Antibiotic Treatment. This may be used to reduce transmission or to eliminate the infectious reservoir. Treatment of active cases with topical antibiotics, such as tetracycline, may reduce secondary bacterial infection and can temporarily clear the conjunctiva of chlamydiae. However, such a strategy usually results in rapid reinfection, presumed to be either endogenous from an extraocular reservoir or exogenous from members of the household or community who are subclinically infected, incubating infection, or harboring undetected disease. To reduce the infectious reservoir in a community, treatment must reach all infected or potentially infected members and must clear infection from all involved mucosal sites in an infected individual. The family, household, or whole community may need to be treated systemically. The extent to which endogenous reinfection contributes to re-emergent disease in a trachoma-endemic community is under investigation as is whether mass treatment with a systemic antibiotic such as azithromycin will reduce the rate of reinfection.

There is no vaccine available for trachoma prevention or control.

■ INCLUSION CONJUNCTIVITIS

DEFINITION. Inclusion conjunctivitis is an acute conjunctivitis caused by *C. trachomatis*. In neonates, it is typically purulent and severe and may be associated with extraocular infection, of which pneumonia is the most serious manifestation. In adults, it is often a more chronic follicular conjunctivitis and is usually associated with urogenital infection. The term *paratrachoma* has been used to refer to adult inclusion conjunctivitis.

DISTRIBUTION AND PREVALENCE. Inclusion conjunctivitis has a worldwide distribution. Its prevalence has been suggested to vary inversely with that of trachoma. In communities with low hygienic standards there is transmission of chlamydial infection from eye to eye (trachoma), but as hygienic standards improve this no longer occurs, and infection is transmitted mainly through sexual contact or from mother to infant (inclusion conjunctivitis). The relationship between the two has not been studied in depth, and there is little evidence as to whether significant cross-immunity underlies this observation.

ETIOLOGY. *C. trachomatis*, usually of the genital serotypes D through K, is the cause of of inclusion conjunctivitis. There is some overlap between "genital" and "ocular" serotypes: Trachoma serotypes A through C have been isolated from the eye and genital tract of subjects with presumed inclusion conjunctivitis, and the genital serotypes may be associated with clinical disease indistinguishable from trachoma. However, in trachoma-endemic areas, genital infection is usually caused by genital rather than ocular serotypes.

EPIDEMIOLOGY. Inclusion conjunctivitis usually results from inoculation of infected genital secretions into the eye. While transmission by eye-finger-eye contact can occur and classic outbreaks have been associated with communal bathing, most transmission is via the genital route. An infant born through a birth canal infected with *Chlamydia* has a 20% to 50% chance of developing chlamydial inclusion conjunctivitis, and in some studies up to 30% of pregnant women have been found to have chlamydial cervicitis. Neonatal inclusion conjunctivitis usually develops 5 to 21 days after birth. However, a few infants have signs of chlamydial infection at birth or develop them following cesarean section, indicating that intrauterine transmission can occur. Pneumonia may develop later, between 4 and 12 weeks after birth; it is not always associated with conjunctivitis and may lead to permanent lung damage (Chapter 46).

In adults, inclusion conjunctivitis is often associated with genital infection. The usual incubation period in adults is 7 to 14 days.

CLINICAL MANIFESTATIONS AND COMPLICATIONS

Neonates. In neonates, inclusion conjunctivitis is a mucopurulent conjunctivitis. It causes lid swelling and hyperemia and edema of the conjunctiva. Rarely, untreated cases develop some conjunctival scarring and corneal pannus.

Adults. In adults, inclusion conjunctivitis causes an acute follicular conjunctivitis, often with preauricular lymphadenopathy. Unilateral ocular involvement is a common presenting feature. There is usually a mild to moderate watery or mucopurulent discharge that is less severe than that of herpetic or adenoviral keratoconjunctivitis. Diffuse superficial punctate keratitis or, less often, subepithelial infiltrates may occur. Often, other evidence of chlamydial infection exists, such as genital infection or otitis media. Anterior uveitis is a rare manifestation.

DIAGNOSIS. Inclusion conjunctivitis is usually diagnosed clinically and confirmed by laboratory testing. Giemsa-stained conjunctival smears may show characteristic intracytoplasmic inclusions in epithelial cells. DFA cytology testing using a fluorescein-conjugated monoclonal antibody directed against the surface of the elementary body is more sensitive and specific than Giemsa staining (Fig. 32–8), but DNA methods based on amplification and detection of target sequences in the chlamydial plasmid by PCR or LCR are likely to become the method of choice.

The most important differentiation in neonates is gonococcal ophthalmia neonatorum, which is usually more severe, appearing within the first 8 days of life. The typical gram-negative intracellular diplococci are usually seen in smears and can be grown on chocolate agar in 5% carbon dioxide. Inclusion conjunctivitis should also be differentiated from adenovirus and herpes simplex keratoconjunctivitis.

TREATMENT AND PROGNOSIS

Neonates. Chlamydial infection in neonates is potentially serious and should be treated with a systemic antibiotic. Erythromycin 50 mg/kg/day in four divided doses for 3 weeks is the preferred treatment. The macrolide agents, e.g., azithromycin 20 mg/kg weekly for 3 doses, are also likely to be effective, although efficacy and safety data in neonates are limited. Topical treatment with tetracycline eye ointment can be used four times daily or more frequently (e.g., q2h) if there is marked discharge, to rapidly reduce the risk of contagious spread.

Adults. Adults should receive systemic treatment with a tetracycline or macrolide for 2 weeks. Tetracycline 500 mg 4 times daily, erythromycin 500 mg 4 times daily, or doxycycline 100 mg twice daily for 2 weeks are all effective therapies but require substantial compliance; azithromycin 1 g as a single dose, or weekly for 3 doses, is a useful alternative.

Topical antibiotics can be used if there is marked ocular discharge. Sexual partners should be examined and treated. Although persistent infection may ensue, recurrences are usually due to reinfection. Adults with inclusion conjunctivitis usually recover without sequelae, although in untreated patients scarring similar to that seen in trachoma has occurred.

PREVENTION AND CONTROL. Preventing inclusion conjunctivitis is difficult. The treatment of patients and their sexual partners and the identification and treatment of infected pregnant women are important. The application of silver nitrate drops to the eyes of infants as used for prophylaxis of gonococcal ophthalmia neonatorum does not prevent chlamydial infection. A single application of erythromycin ointment at birth has reduced the incidence of ocular but not of subsequent respiratory infection.

Bibliography

Bailey RL, Arullendran P, Whittle HC, et al: Randomised controlled trial of single-dose azithromycin in treatment of trachoma. Lancet 342:453, 1993.

Bailey RL, Hayes LJ, Hampton TJ, et al: Polymerase chain reaction for the detection of ocular chlamydial infection in trachoma-endemic communities. J Infect Dis 170:709, 1994.

Dawson CR, Jones BR, Tarizzo ML: Guide to Trachoma Control. Geneva, World Health Organization, 1981.

Francis V, Turner V: Achieving Community Support for Trachoma Control. Geneva, WHO Programme for the Prevention of Blindness, 1993.

Grayston JT, Wang S-P, Yeh L-J, et al: Importance of reinfection in the pathogenesis of trachoma. Rev Infect Dis 7:717, 1985.

Hollows FC: Community-based action for the control of trachoma. Rev Infect Dis 7:777, 1985.

Jones BR: The prevention of blindness from trachoma. Trans Am Ophthalmol Soc 95:16, 1975.

Reacher M, Foster A, Huber J: Trichiasis Surgery for Trachoma. The Bilamellar Tarsal Rotation Procedure. Geneva, WHO Programme for the Prevention of Blindness, 1993.

Reacher MH, Munoz B, Alghassany A, et al: A controlled trial of surgery for trachomatous trichiasis of the upper lid. Arch Ophthalmol 110:667, 1992.

Schachter J, Dawson CR: Human Chlamydial Infection. Littleton, MA, PSG Publishing, 1978.

Thylefors B, Dawson CR, Jones BR, et al: A simple system for the assessment of trachoma and its complications. Bull WHO 65:485, 1987.

West S, Munoz B, Lynch M, et al: Impact of face washing on trachoma in Kongwa, Tanzania. Lancet 345:155, 1995.

World Health Organization: Primary Health Care Level Management of Trachoma. Geneva, WHO Programme for the Prevention of Blindness, 1993.

33 Diphtheria*

Robert A. Gasser, Jr., and Charles Vitek

DEFINITION. Diphtheria is an acute infectious disease caused by toxin-producing strains of *Corynebacterium diphtheriae*. It is typically characterized by pharyngitis, by the development of a membrane in the throat, and by systemic illness, including myocarditis and neuritis, resulting from absorption of the toxin. Infection may be localized in the skin or in wounds.

ETIOLOGY. *C. diphtheriae* is a pleomorphic, gram-positive, non–acid fast, nonmotile, nonsporulating, slightly curved or club-shaped bacillus. The four subspecies of diphtheria bacillus—*mitis, gravis, intermedius,* and *belfanti*—as well as the related organism *Corynebacterium ulcerans* can each cause the disease. Bacteriophage-dependent production of a protein exotoxin is required to produce the classic systemic illness. Strains of *C. diphtheriae* that do not produce toxin may rarely produce invasive disease.

HISTORY. Diphtheria was known in the ancient Middle East, as indicated by references in Babylonian Talmud. Description of an illness, particularly severe in children, characterized by pharyngeal eschars, hoarseness, and suffocation if the lesions spread to the trachea, has been found in writings dating to the second century Roman Empire. Epidemics of similar illnesses were reported in 16th century Spain and 18th century New England. In 1826, Pierre Bretonneau, a French physician, adopted the term *diphtherite*, from a Greek root meaning hide or leather, to allude to the disease's characteristic pharyngeal membrane. In 1884, Friedrich Löffler proved that a bacillus was responsible for the illness and predicted that it must produce a toxin to cause lesions at sterile sites remote from the site of infection. He later showed that children could carry the bacterium in their throats without signs of illness, an observation essential for understanding the disease's transmission patterns. In 1888 Pierre Roux provided evidence of a toxin by inducing diphtheria-like illness in healthy animals injected with a bacteria-free filtrate of diphtheric membranes. Two years later, Emil von Behring demonstrated that serum from a rat that had survived diphtheria killed the bacillus. Between 1893 and 1894, Roux showed that immune serum, or antitoxin, cut mortality in pediatric diphtheria cases from 51 to 24%. In 1924, trials of a heat- and formalin-altered diphtheria toxin, or toxoid, effectively conferred immunity to diphtheria. This advance her-

alded a rapid, profound decline in the incidence of the disease. The near-eradication of diphtheria in developed countries brought confidence that this disease would pose little future threat. However, a massive diphtheria epidemic began in Russia and bordering countries in 1990. This outbreak demonstrated that diphtheria has great capacity for resurgence if constant measures to maintain high levels of immunity in a population are allowed to lapse.

EPIDEMIOLOGY. Human beings are the only known reservoir for *C. diphtheriae*. The organism remains widely endemic in economically less developed regions of the world, where immunization is not universal. Transmission of diphtheria occurs directly or indirectly by exposure to respiratory secretions or exudate from skin lesions. Respiratory tract carriers of *C. diphtheriae* transmit infection, but they do so less efficiently than individuals with disease. Transmission of infection from fomites has been demonstrated. Virulent organisms have been shown to persist for at least 13 weeks in floor dust, suggesting sustained potential for indirect transmission of infection. Occasionally, strains of *C. ulcerans*, a pathogen associated with livestock, acquire the bacteriophage carrying the toxin gene. Human infection with such toxigenic strains of *C. ulcerans* can cause clinical disease identical to that caused by *C. diphtheriae*. Infection with *C. ulcerans* may be acquired by drinking raw milk.

In tropical areas without established vaccination programs, cutaneous infections are often hyperendemic and are associated with high rates of naturally acquired immunity to diphtheria toxin within the first 3 years of life. When combined with transplacentally acquired antitoxin antibody, which protects infants under 6 months of age, this early acquisition of natural immunity results in low incidences of nasopharyngeal disease and severe clinical illness in local populations. Sporadic cases of diphtheria occur in young children, but epidemics are uncommon. After implementation of infant immunization programs, residual disease tends to shift to older age groups over time.

In temperate regions, in the prevaccine era, diphtheria was one of the leading childhood killers. High rates of severe clinical disease, with frequent epidemics, were seen in children. Childhood immunization programs have produced high rates of immunity to diphtheria toxin, and the prevalence of *C. diphtheriae* infection has diminished greatly. Furthermore, those organisms that do persist in these populations tend to lose the gene responsible for toxin production, thereby losing their potential to cause clinical diphtheria. Presumably this genetic loss occurs because of loss of the selective advantage that toxin production would naturally afford. Immunization alone, even when associated with high levels of circulating antitoxin antibody, does not confer absolute protection from diphtheria. Instead, disappearance of disease in populations with high rates of immunization results from several factors, including individual resistance to diphtheria toxin, the decreased efficiency with which immunized individuals transmit infection, and the diminished risk of exposure resulting from disappearance of toxigenic strains of *C. diphtheriae*.

Even populations with very high immunization rates remain vulnerable to limited diphtheria outbreaks if toxigenic strains of *C. diphtheriae* are introduced by travelers, immigrants, or refugees. This vulnerability is magnified if the protection achieved by immunizing children is not sustained by giving periodic booster immunizations to adults. The recent epidemic in Russia and its neighbors illustrates this point. At the onset of the epidemic, only 20% of Russian adults had received diphtheria toxoid immunization within 10 years, and childhood immunization rates had dropped below 70%. Between 1990 and 1995, 125,000 diphtheria cases

---

*All material in this chapter is in the public domain, with the exception of any borrowed figures or tables.

occurred, 70% of them in persons over 15 years of age. Adult populations in many other developed nations share this pattern of waning immunity.

PATHOGENESIS. *C. diphtheriae* infects the skin and/or the epithelium of the upper respiratory tract, most commonly the pharynx, but occasionally the nose, larynx, and tracheobronchial structures. Occasionally, wounds, conjunctiva, middle ear, umbilicus, vagina, or joints may be infected. The primary virulence factor is a protein exotoxin, an extremely potent inhibitor of cellular protein synthesis. Local damage from the exotoxin helps produce the characteristic thick, adherent pseudomembrane composed of bacteria, necrotic cells, phagocytes, and fibrin. Absorbed exotoxin causes tissue damage, which is most clinically evident in the heart and peripheral nerves. The gene *tox*, coding for this toxin, is carried by a bacteriophage. Strains of *C. diphtheriae* that have not been converted by the bacteriophage, i.e., nontoxigenic strains, may occasionally cause invasive disease, including pharyngitis, septic arthritis, and endocarditis. Nontoxigenic strains do not cause myocarditis, neuropathy, or other toxin-mediated manifestations of diphtheria.

CLINICAL MANIFESTATIONS. Disease of the upper respiratory tract, producing the classic clinical syndrome of diphtheria, and skin infection are the major clinical syndromes. Cutaneous diphtheria and respiratory tract diphtheria or carriage may occur simultaneously in the same patient.

Respiratory Tract Diphtheria. Asymptomatic nasal or pharyngeal carriage of *C. diphtheriae* occurs commonly after exposure to the organism and occurs in immune as well as nonimmune hosts. More than half of untreated carriers will spontaneously clear themselves of the organism by 10 days, but carriage can persist for over a month in up to 20%.

When respiratory tract disease does develop, the incubation is brief, generally 1 to 6 days. Onset of symptoms may be insidious or abrupt. Sore throat occurs in 85 to 100% of patients, and most have fever. Nausea and vomiting, pain on swallowing, neck edema, and headache are each seen in 10 to 40% of patients. Other symptoms can include hoarseness, nasal discharge or obstruction, cough, and a characteristic oral fetor. Pharyngeal redness, often accompanied by palatal, tonsillar or uvular edema, typically precedes development of a nonadherent exudate, which, in turn, evolves into the distinctive adherent membrane. The membrane may be absent in a substantial proportion of cases. When present, it can vary widely in appearance. Its color may range from creamy to grayish green. In location and extent, the membrane can vary from a small patch anywhere on the pharyngeal, palatal, nasal, or laryngeal mucosa to a large confluent structure covering the entire pharynx and extending into the larynx and tracheobronchial tree. Cervical adenopathy commonly develops; when combined with cervical edema it creates a "bull-neck" appearance. Nasal diphtheria usually causes a mucopurulent discharge, often unilateral, that may be blood-tinged.

In the absence of its membrane, diphtheritic pharyngitis is difficult to distinguish from streptococcal pharyngitis, although marked pharyngeal edema suggests diphtheria. Pharyngeal co-infection with group A streptococci is common in diphtheria; therefore, identification of streptococcal infection does not exclude diphtheria as a diagnostic consideration.

Cutaneous Diphtheria. Diphtheria of the skin is most readily recognized when it presents as an ecthymic lesion: a deep, punched-out ulcer with rolled margins, a gray or black membranous exudate on its base, and, occasionally, a distinctive foul odor. However, the vast majority of diphtheritic skin lesions are indistinguishable from skin lesions caused by other pyogenic bacteria. They are usually superficial and may resemble impetigo, eczema, burns, abrasions, or infected insect bites. Co-infection with streptococci and/or *Staphylococcus aureus* is typical. If untreated, cutaneous diphtheria may persist for many months. Such sustained infections are associated with the development of immunity to diphtheria toxin. Although cutaneous diphtheria has been commonly associated with the tropics, it occurs worldwide where there is poor hygiene.

Complications. The major complications of diphtheria are neuropathy, myocarditis, airway obstruction, and pneumonia. Neuropathy and myocarditis can occur in cutaneous diphtheria but are much more common and more likely to be severe in respiratory tract diphtheria. Extensive primary lesions, a low level of pre-existing immunity, and delay in initiating treatment increase the risk of developing complications. Both neuropathy and myocarditis may appear during improvement or after resolution of the primary diphtherial lesion.

Neuropathy. The reported incidence of neuropathy complicating diphtheria has varied widely in different outbreaks, from as low as 3% to as high as 43%. Neuropathy can develop even when diphtheria has been diagnosed and properly treated within 4 days of onset. Involvement of cranial nerves IX and X, causing palatal or posterior pharyngeal wall paralysis, manifests as dysphonia or regurgitation of liquids through the nose. This may begin as early as 10 days after the onset of illness. Dysfunction of other cranial nerves, including vagal palsies, may follow over the first 2 to 5 weeks. Peripheral neuropathy, predominantly motor in character, may emerge over weeks 3 to 8, even in the absence of preceding cranial nerve dysfunction. Weakness typically begins proximally, then spreads distally, accompanied by hyporeflexia or areflexia. Death due to respiratory failure can result when both the diaphragm and the intercostal muscles are paralyzed; fortunately, paralysis of this severity is rare. Sensory dysfunction, most commonly paresthesias, occasionally anesthesia, may occur.

Laboratory studies are of limited value. Cerebrospinal fluid (CSF) may show normal or elevated levels of protein. CSF pleocytosis, predominantly lymphocytic, may occur but is less common than elevated protein levels. Findings in CSF correlate poorly with the clinical course. Nerve conduction studies show a pattern consistent with acute demyelination.

Neuropathic symptoms may peak as late as 3 months into the illness. Duration of symptoms is proportional to their duration of onset and progression. Complete recovery of neurologic function occurs in most, if not all, survivors. Resolution usually occurs by 5 to 6 months but may take as long as 12 months.

Myocarditis. Clinically significant myocarditis occurs in 7 to 20% of respiratory tract diphtheria cases; pathologic or electrocardiographic (ECG) evidence of myocarditis has been identified in up to 65% of patients. In contrast, myocarditis occurs in only 0 to 5% of cutaneous diphtheria cases. Myocarditis can develop very rapidly. The first ECG abnormalities can appear within 3 days of the onset of illness. Cardiogenic death can follow within the first week. More typically, myocarditis appears within the first 2 weeks, occasionally taking as long as 7 weeks to emerge. Earlier onset is associated with higher likelihood of death. Diphtheritic cardiac disease can present as any of a wide variety of abnormalities. Angina, syncope, diminished heart sounds, new or altered murmurs, ectopic beats, cardiac enlargement, or hypotension may be noted. However, ECG abnormalities of major import may develop without obvious coincident symptoms or signs. At the benign end of the spectrum, ECG abnormalities that do not exceed ectopic supraventricular beats, sinus bradycardia, or first-degree AV block are associated with little, if any, increased risk of death. Of intermediate severity are blocks of a single bundle branch, QRS widening, ST-T segment shifts, T-wave inversions, prolonged QT intervals, and supraventricular tachycardias. These have been associated with mortality rates of 10 to 50%. Elevations of serum creatine kinase and aspartate aminotransferase (AST, SGOT) can accompany the onset of these ECG changes. Mortality rates may exceed 90% in patients with third-degree heart block, more than two ventricular premature contractions on ECG at time of first presentation, ventricular tachycardia, or congestive heart failure. Cardiac pacing appears to be of little value in diphtheria patients who develop third-degree heart block. These patients have suffered severe myocardial injury and die of heart failure or ventricular tachycardia. Death due to myocarditis tends to come early in disease, usually within the first 2 weeks. Abatement of ECG abnormalities reflects improving cardiac function and favors survival. Detectable cardiac injury may resolve entirely over months or years, but some survivors are left with persisting abnormalities.

Airway Obstruction. Extension of the diphtherial membrane into the larynx or tracheobronchial tree can cause airway obstruction, resulting in death from asphyxiation. Airway obstruction has been reported in 4 to 15% of respiratory diphtheria cases, with fatal outcomes in 40 to 100% of these. Laryngeal involvement should be suspected when croupy cough, stridor, hoarseness, dysphonia, or aphonia is observed. Dyspnea may signal the presence of laryngeal or tracheobronchial membrane. When either symptoms or the presence of a pharyngeal membrane suggest the possibility of a laryngeal membrane, laryngoscopy should be performed. Detection of a laryngeal or tracheal membrane should prompt consideration of early endotracheal intubation or tracheostomy. If the airway is not secured early, rapid progression of the membrane may preclude a later opportunity. Ongoing attention to the airway is essential, even if tracheostomy or intubation is not needed initially.

Pneumonia. Respiratory tract diphtheria is complicated by pneumonia in 2 to 7% of cases. Pneumonia occurs more frequently in patients with laryngeal or tracheal diphtheria, developing in perhaps a quarter of such cases. Although most diphtheria-associated pneumonias appear to be postobstructive, aspiration due to palatal or pharyngeal paralysis is also a frequent cause.

Prognosis. Overall mortality in respiratory tract diphtheria has ranged from 2 to 20% in various series, usually running about 10%. Cutaneous diphtheria is rarely lethal, but isolated deaths from myocarditis have been reported. In diphtheria patients with adequate prior toxoid immunization, the risk of mortality is cut by about 90% compared with the unimmunized. Immediate initiation of treatment with diphtheria antitoxin at the onset of illness may cut mortality 80% or more when compared with case fatality rates in those who first receive antitoxin after a week. More extensive diphtherial membranes, diphtherial membranes involving the larynx or lower airways, pneumonia, onset of abdominal pain with vomiting, leukocytosis, and early onset of myocarditis are associated with increased risk of death.

DIAGNOSIS

Culture. Diphtheria is confirmed by isolation of *C. diphtheriae* or *C. ulcerans*, and demonstration of the isolate's toxigenicity, from a patient with a compatible clinical syndrome. In respiratory tract disease, swabs of the membrane or of the mucosal surface beneath the membrane should be obtained. Culturing both nasal and pharyngeal sites improves rates of isolation. For skin lesions, surface swabs are of little value; deep samples, preferably from under any membrane present, should be obtained. Swabs should be immediately streaked onto proper media, including a tellurite-containing medium such as modified Tinsdale medium, blood agar, and a Löffler slant, then incubated at 35 to 37°C with or without added CO_2 for 48 hours. If delay in plating or shipment is unavoidable, the swab should be transported dry, then incubated overnight in broth containing plasma or blood before plating. A Gram stain of the original specimen should be prepared (Fig. 33–1). Characteristic morphology of the bacilli and the appearance of metachromatic granules, particularly with isolates on the Löffler medium, provide presumptive identification. Species identification is confirmed by biochemical testing or DNA hybridization. Antibiotic susceptibility testing should be considered; resistance to erythromycin has emerged in an epidemic setting.

Testing for Toxigenicity. Toxigenicity is demonstrated by immunodiffusion on solid culture media (Elek test), guinea pig inoculation with clinical isolates, cytotoxic effects of broth culture supernatants on tissue culture cells, monoclonal en-

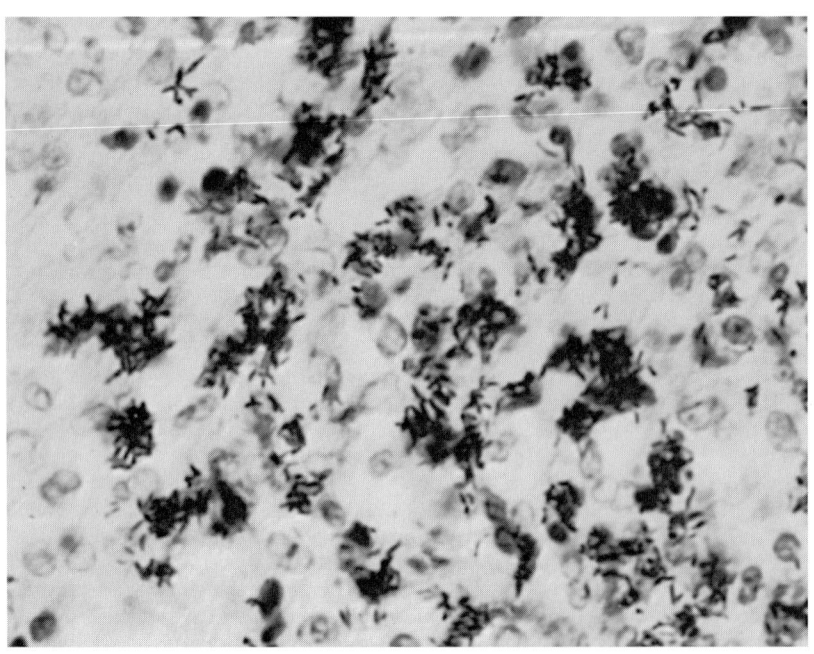

Figure 33–1. Cutaneous diphtheria of the scalp. Club-shaped *C. diphtheriae* gram-positive bacilli in the acute inflammatory reaction at the base of an ulcer (Brown and Brenn Gram stain, × 1200). (Courtesy of the Armed Forces Institute of Pathology. Photograph Neg. No. 76–7065.)

zyme immunoassay for toxin (EIA), or polymerase chain reaction (PCR) testing of the isolate's DNA, using primers for the *tox* gene. PCR testing might identify altered but inactive *tox* genes, implying toxin production when none is present. Such false positive findings are apparently rare. On balance, PCR testing for presence of *tox* seems the fastest, simplest, and most accurate test now available for toxigenicity. Because both toxigenic and nontoxigenic organisms may coexist in the same patient, at least ten colonies from a primary culture plate should be tested for toxigenicity.

Molecular Microbiologic Testing. A variety of additional techniques can be used to distinguish different strains of *C. diphtheriae.* Primarily useful for epidemiologic investigations, these methods include multilocus enzyme electrophoresis (MEE), ribotyping, use of cDNA probes to hybridize with restriction enzyme digests of a variety of bacterial or phage genes, and PCR single-strand conformation polymorphism analysis (PCR–SSCP).

TREATMENT. The fundamentals of treatment are protection of a threatened airway, immediate administration of diphtheria antitoxin, administration of antibiotics, and establishment of active immunity to diphtheria toxin.

Antitoxin. Diphtheria antitoxin works by neutralizing the toxin so that it does not bind to cell membrane surface receptors and cannot enter the cell. Because delays in administering antitoxin are associated with markedly increased risk of complications or death, antitoxin should be given to patients with suspected respiratory tract diphtheria immediately, without awaiting diagnostic confirmation. Respiratory tract carriers do not need antitoxin. The balance of antitoxin's risk and benefit in patients with uncomplicated cutaneous diphtheria is less clear. Antitoxin is a horse serum preparation, which may provoke severe hypersensitivity reactions. Therefore, a test dose of 50 to 100 U should be given subcutaneously 30 minutes prior to giving the therapeutic dose. If an immediate hypersensitivity reaction occurs, desensitization must be conducted before the full dose is given. The dose of antitoxin required varies from 20,000 to 100,000 U, in a single dose, depending on the severity of illness. Disease limited to the nose requires doses at the low end of this spectrum, given intramuscularly (IM). Uncomplicated disease limited to the pharynx or tonsils may be managed with intermediate doses, by IM, intravenous infusion (IV), or combined IM and IV routes. Extensive, late, or complicated disease should be treated with doses at the high end of this range, given either IV or by combined IM and IV routes. For patients with cutaneous diphtheria, if skin testing shows no immediate reaction, IM administration of 20,000 U is prudent. Following antitoxin treatment, serum sickness or febrile reactions occur in approximately 10% of patients.

Antibiotics. These are an adjunct, not a substitute, for antitoxin. Antibiotics are indicated because they quickly eradicate the pathogen, ending local invasive disease, further production of toxin, and transmission of infection. Penicillin and erythromycin are the agents of choice. Adult patients should receive 14 days of treatment with procaine penicillin G, 600,000 U, IM, twice daily, or penicillin V, 125 to 250 mg orally four times daily, or erythromycin 250 to 500 mg four times daily orally or IV. Children should get 14 days' treatment with procaine penicillin G, 25,000 to 50,000 U/kg/day in two divided doses, or erythromycin, 40 to 50 mg/kg/day, parenterally or orally, divided into four doses.

Adult carriers should receive a single dose of 1.2 million U benzathine penicillin G, IM, or erythromycin 250 mg four times daily for 7 to 10 days. Child carriers should receive a single IM dose of benzathine penicillin G, 600,000 U if younger than 6 years, 1.2 million U if older than 6 years. Alternatively, child carriers may be treated with oral erythro-

mycin, 40 to 50 mg/kg/day in divided doses for 7 to 10 days. Erythromycin, if taken as directed, is more effective in eradicating carriage, but this advantage must be weighed against ease of administration and certainty of compliance with injected penicillin.

Toxoid Immunization. Diphtheria may fail to induce effective immunity. The immunization history of patients should be determined. If indicated by the history, booster doses of toxoid or completion of a primary immunization series should be provided as the patient convalesces.

PREVENTION. Diphtheria is prevented by establishing population-wide immunity with a primary immunization series using toxoid, maintaining that immunity by periodic booster doses of toxoid, and promptly containing any outbreaks by isolating cases and treating patients and carriers.

Immunization. Diphtheria toxoid is formaldehyde-inactivated diphtheria toxin. In persons who have been fully immunized with toxoid, the risk of developing disease after exposure to *C. diphtheriae* is cut by 90%. In addition, in fully immunized persons who do develop diphtheria, the likelihood that the illness will be severe is greatly reduced. The only contraindication to toxoid is a history of immediate hypersensitivity or a neurologic reaction to a prior dose. Full-strength toxoid, in combination with tetanus and pertussis vaccines (DTP), or with tetanus toxoid alone (DT) if pertussis vaccine is contraindicated, is used for primary childhood immunization. The World Health Organization (WHO) recommends a three-dose primary immunization series given at 6, 10, and 14 weeks of age; in the United States, the first three doses are given at 2, 4, and 6 months. A booster dose should be given at 12 to 18 months of age, then another at 4 to 6 years of age. The adult toxoid dose (Td) is about one fifth to one third as potent as DT or DTP. This reduced dose is used in children older than 7 years and adults to avoid adverse reactions to the vaccine. Td should be given at about age 11 to 12 years if a child has not been reimmunized within the 5 preceding years and readministered every 10 years thereafter. Immunization history should be reviewed before international travel and, if needed, a booster dose administered. Adults who have never received a primary toxoid immunization series should be given a three-dose series of Td.

Isolation of Cases and Treatment of Carriers. Patients with respiratory tract diphtheria should be placed in strict isolation. If infection is limited to the skin, patients may be placed in contact isolation. Isolation should be maintained until therapy has been completed and until two cultures obtained at least 24 hours apart, starting 24 hours after completion of antibiotic therapy, are both negative. Close contacts, including health care workers, should be identified, observed for development of disease for 7 days, and tested with cultures of nose and pharynx. Carriers should be treated with antibiotics, and close contacts of carriers should be evaluated in the same manner as contacts of cases. Food handlers or those who work with children should be barred from work until carriage is excluded but need not be otherwise isolated. The immunization status of cases, carriers, and contacts should be assessed and toxoid booster doses or primary immunization series administered as needed.

Bibliography

Belsey MA, Sinclair M, Roder MR, LeBlanc DR: *Corynebacterium diphtheriae* skin infections in Alabama and Louisiana: A factor in the epidemiology of diphtheria. N Engl J Med 280:135, 1969.

Brainerd H, Bruyn HB: Diphtheria: The present day problem. Calif Med 75:290, 1951.

Clarridge JE, Spiegel CA: *Corynebacterium* and miscellaneous irregular Gram-positive rods, *Erysipelothrix,* and *Gardnerella. In* Murray PR, Baron EJ, Pfaller MA, et al (eds): Manual of Clinical Microbiology, 6th ed. Washington, DC, American Society for Microbiology, 1995, pp 357–378.

Dobie RA, Tobey DN: Clinical features in diphtheria of the respiratory tract. JAMA 242:2197, 1979.

Farizo KM, Strebel PM, Chen RT, et al: Fatal respiratory disease due to *Corynebacterium diphtheriae*: Case report and review of guidelines for management, investigation, and control. Clin Infect Dis 16:59, 1993.

Galazka AM, Robertson SE: Diphtheria: Changing patterns in the developing world and the industrialized world. Eur J Epidemiol 11:107, 1995.

Galazka AM, Robertson SE: Immunization against diphtheria with special emphasis on immunization of adults. Vaccine 14:845, 1996.

Harnisch JP, Tronca E, Nolan CM, et al: Diphtheria among alcoholic urban adults: A decade of experience in Seattle. Ann Intern Med 111:71, 1989.

Hoyne A, Welford NT: Diphtheritic myocarditis: A review of 496 cases. J Pediatr 5:642, 1934.

Liebow AA, MacLean PD, Bumstead JH, Welt LG: Tropical ulcers and cutaneous diphtheria. Arch Intern Med 78:255, 1946.

Mikhailovich VM, Melnikov VG, Mazurova IK: Application of PCR for detection of toxigenic *Corynebacterium diphtheriae* strains isolated during the Russian diphtheria epidemic, 1990 through 1994. J Clin Microbiol 33:3061, 1995.

Naiditch MJ, Bower AG: Diphtheria: A study of 1433 cases observed during a ten-year period at the Los Angeles County Hospital. Am J Med 17:229, 1954.

Popovic T, Kombarova SY, Reeves MW, et al: Molecular epidemiology of diphtheria in Russia, 1985–1994. J Infect Dis 174:1064, 1996.

Scheid W: Diphtherial paralysis: An analysis of 2292 cases of diphtheria in adults, which included 174 cases of polyneuritis. J Nerv Ment Dis 116:1095, 1952.

 SECTION B **Respiratory Tract Infections**

34 Q *Fever*

James G. Olson

DESCRIPTION. *Coxiella burnetii,* the etiologic agent of Q fever, is a small, coccoid bacterium belonging to the *Rickettsiaceae* family. *C. burnetii* replicates only within phagolysosomes of living cells, where it is uniquely adapted to the acidic conditions. However, the organism can survive extracellularly for long periods, during which it is resistant to desiccation and to many commonly used disinfectants.

TRANSMISSION. *C. burnetii* is unique among rickettsiae because, although arthropod-vector transmission occurs, most human infections are acquired by inhalation. The organism is highly infectious—a single inhaled bacterium can cause illness. An antigenic phase variation (phase I to phase II) occurs, and immune response to the two phases can differentiate acute from chronic infection.

EPIDEMIOLOGY. Q fever has a worldwide distribution, although <10 cases per year are reported in the United States. However, a serosurvey in Michigan found a 15 to 42% prevalence of antibody to *C. burnetii* among persons from urban and rural areas, suggesting frequent asymptomatic infection and/or undiagnosed illness.

NATURAL HISTORY. Q fever is classically associated with occupational exposure to livestock, especially sheep, although a variety of animal reservoirs exist. In maritime Canada and Maine, household outbreaks of Q fever have been associated with cats, and in one case, a dog. Most outbreaks are associated with a parturient animal, which is not surprising because *C. burnetii* is highly concentrated in placental and fetal tissues. Unpasteurized milk, including human milk, has also been implicated as a source of infection. Person-to-person transmission occurs rarely.

CLINICAL MANIFESTATIONS. The most common manifestation of Q fever is probably a self-limited acute febrile illness. After an incubation period of 1 to 6 weeks, patients have onset of fever as high as 41.1°C (106°F) lasting 5 to 10 days. Associated symptoms can include chills, headache, cough, and fatigue. Many patients have gastrointestinal symptoms including anorexia, abdominal pain, vomiting, and, less commonly, diarrhea. Acutely ill patients may develop pneumonia, hepatitis (Fig. 34–1), or less commonly, meningoencephalitis. The case-fatality rate is very low, approaching 0%; however, among hospitalized patients it may be 2%.

Chronic Q fever syndromes also occur. Patients with underlying structural heart disease can develop chronic Q fever endocarditis accompanied by systemic illness usually involving the liver, and in some reports, splenomegaly, aneurysm, osteomyelitis, or chronic hepatitis may occur. Chronic Q fever is rare, serious, and often fatal.

LABORATORY DIAGNOSIS. Abnormal laboratory findings

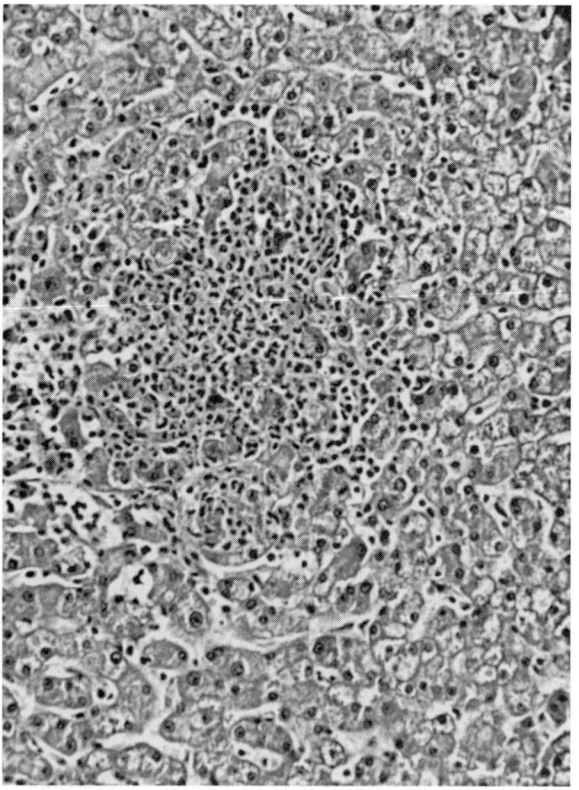

***Figure* 34–1.** Focal granulomatous lesions in the liver of a patient with Q fever. (From Dupont, HL, et al: Ann Intern Med 74:198, 1971.)

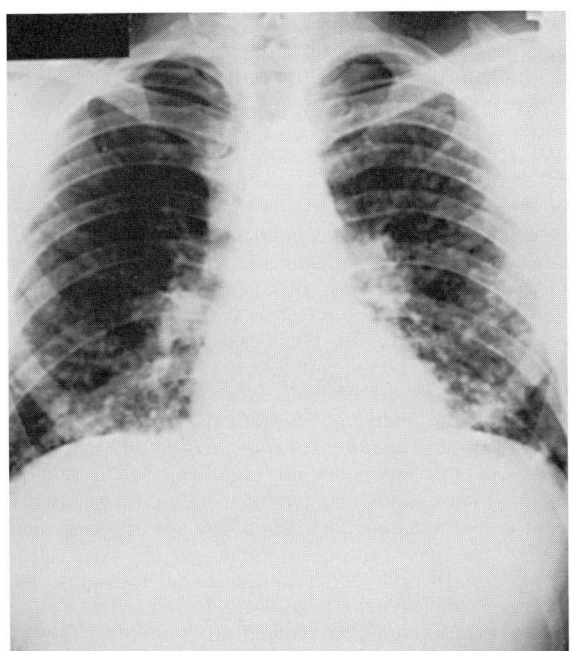

Figure 34–2. Chest radiograph of a patient with Q fever showing patchy densities predominantly in the lower lung fields 13 days after aerogenic exposure to *Coxiella burnetii*. (From Dupont HL, et al: Ann Intern Med 74:198, 1971.)

vary depending on the case series. Both leukopenia and leukocytosis are reported, and thrombocytopenia may occur. Liver function test abnormalities are usually limited to mild elevation of transaminases and lactate dehydrogenase. Typical radiographic findings show patchy infiltrates resembling *Mycoplasma pneumoniae* infection (Fig. 34–2).

Laboratory diagnosis of rickettsial diseases is routinely accomplished by serologic assay (indirect fluorescent antibody [IFA], enzyme immunoassay [EIA], or complement fixation [CF]) that detect antirickettsial antibodies. Early diagnosis of acute Q fever is problematic, as confirmation depends on detection of IgG antibody. Diagnosis generally depends on the demonstration of fourfold or greater increase in antibody titer between the acute-phase and convalescent-phase serum samples. With single serum specimens, CF titers of ≥16 in a clinically compatible case are also considered positive. With the IFA test, single titers of 256 are considered minimal for confirmation of Q fever. Antibodies to phase II antigen, which dominate the humoral immune response in acute infection, appear by the fourth week after onset of symptoms. With chronic Q fever infection, phase I antigen titers eventually equal or exceed phase II titers. Primary isolation of *C. burnetii* requires passage in animals, tissue culture, and/or embryonated eggs and is not recommended because of risk to laboratory personnel. Alternative procedures include isolation of rickettsiae from patient tissues and techniques aimed at detection of rickettsiae in tissue. However, the latter two methods are generally restricted to research laboratories.

Indirect Fluorescent Antibody Assays. The IFA procedure for the rickettsiae is similar to conventional IFA techniques, with inactivated yolk sac or tissue culture suspensions of *C. burnetii* being used as an antigen. IFA assays for diagnosis of Q fever have been used for many years with good results. IFA test are reasonably sensitive, although the subjectivity of endpoint determinations is an obvious disadvantage.

Complement Fixation. CF tests have been used for many years for the diagnosis of most rickettsial diseases. In general,

these tests are specific but less sensitive and more cumbersome than IFA or the agglutination assays and for these reasons are no longer used widely.

The CF assay for diagnosis of Q fever uses an ether extract of phase II *C. burnetii*. By the fourth week after the onset of symptoms from Q fever, >90% of patients have antibodies that fix complement in the presence of phase II antigen. Antigenic phase must be considered for the interpretation of serologic results for Q fever. In acute, self-limited Q fever infections, antibodies to the phase II antigen appear first and dominate the humoral immune response. With chronic Q fever infections, however, phase I titers eventually equal or exceed phase II titers. The detection of antibodies that fix complement in the presence of phase I antigen has been useful in recognition of subacute Q fever endocarditis.

Enzyme Immunoassays. Enzyme immunoassays for serologic diagnosis of Q fever have shown equal sensitivity and specificity as the IFA. Fourfold rises in titer are evidence of *C. burnetti* infections.

TREATMENT. Athough most acute Q fever infections resolve without treatment, antibiotics may prevent chronic infection. *C. burnetii* is sensitive in vitro to rifampin and fluoroquinolones, and usually to tetracyclines and trimethoprim. In cases of chronic endocarditis, prolonged treatment (several years) with a combination of drugs is recommended.

SPECIAL CONSIDERATIONS. Infection with *C. burnetii* during pregnancy, although not known to be teratogenic, can result in premature delivery or intrauterine death. The placenta, a fertile substrate for *C. burnetii* replication, becomes necrotic leading to placental insufficiency. Fetal infection has been demonstrated immunologically and may play a role in intrauterine death; however, healthy, uninfected infants have been delivered despite the recovery of *C. burnetii* from the placenta. Delivery room personnel are at risk for infection through aerosols.

PREVENTION. A vaccine to prevent Q fever has successfully protected high-risk abattoir workers, but its use is not indicated for children. Infection can be prevented by avoidance of contact with potentially infectious animal tissues, particularly products of conception and raw milk. Occupationally exposed persons may reduce their risk of infection with *C. burnetii* by wearing respirators that prevent aerosol infections.

Bibliography

Friedland JS, Jeffrey I, Griffin GE, et al: Q fever and intrauterine death. Lancet 343:288, 1994.
Mann JS, Douglas JG, Inglis JM, Leitch AG: Q fever: Person to person transmission within a family. Thorax 41:974, 1986.
Marmion BP, Ormsbee RA, Kyrkou M, et al: Vaccine prophylaxis of abbatoir-associated Q fever: Eight years' experience in Australian abbatoirs. Epidemiol Infect 104:275, 1990.
Newhouse VF, Shepard CC, Redus MD, et al: A comparison of the complement fixation, indirect flourescent antibody and microagglutination test for serological diagnosis of rickettsial diseases. Am J Trop Med Hyg 28:387, 1979.
Pinsky RL, Fishbein DB, Greene CR, Gensheimer KF: An outbreak of cat-associated Q fever in the United States. J Infect Dis 164:202, 1991.
Raoult D: Antibody susceptability of rickettsia and treatment of rickettsioses. Eur J Epidemiol 5:432, 1989.
Raoult D, Stein A: Q fever during pregnancy—A risk for women, fetuses, and obstetricians. N Engl J Med 330:371, 1994.
Richardus JH, Dumas AM, Huisman J, Schaap GJP: Q fever in infancy: A review of 18 cases. Pediatr Infect Dis 4:369, 1985.
Ruiz-Contreras J, Montero RG, Amador JTR, et al: Q fever in children. Am J Dis Child 147:300, 1993.
Sawyer LA, Fishbein DB, McDade JE: Q fever: Current concepts. Rev Infect Dis 9:935, 1987.
Sienko DG, Barlett PC, McGee HB, et al: An outbreak of Q fever probably due to contact with a parturient cat. Chest 93:98, 1988.
Uhaa IJ, Fishbein DB, Olson JG et al: Evaluation of the specificity of the indirect enzyme-linked immunosorbent assay for diagnosis of human Q fever. J Clin Microbiol 32:1560, 1994.

35 *Psittacosis*

Brian J. Ward

DEFINITION. Psittacosis is a systemic illness that most commonly manifests in humans as an atypical pneumonia. A rare but serious presentation of psittacosis is endocarditis, which can elude diagnosis for prolonged periods of time. The causative agent of psittacosis is *Chlamydia psittaci*, which can infect most bird species and a wide range of wild and domestic mammals (e.g., antelopes, cats, cows, goats, sheep, yaks) and even some marsupials (e.g., koala bears).

HISTORY. The first recorded description of psittacosis is that of Ritter who studied a Swiss outbreak of "pneumotyphus" in 1879. The name psittacosis was coined by Morange in 1892 when he recognized a link between the disease and exposure to sick parrots (*psittakos* in Greek). *C. psittaci* was isolated more or less simultaneously by several laboratories in 1930 and was initially thought to be a large virus. The organism was subsequently found to contain both DNA and RNA, leading to its recognition as a very small (0.3–1.0 μm), intracellular bacterium.

EPIDEMIOLOGY. *C. psittaci* is found throughout the world. Most human cases are sporadic but both large and small outbreaks occur frequently. In 1929–1930, a pandemic of psittacosis involving more than 700 cases in 12 countries was caused by the importation of infected birds from South America. Since *C. psittaci* infection is common in birds and several domestic animals, human populations at greatest risk include poultry farmers (particularly commercial turkey operations), bird importers and fanciers, pet shop employees, abattoir workers, and veterinarians. Exposure to birds is certainly the greatest risk and more than 70% of human cases can be linked directly to birds. Although some avian exposures are massive and relatively intimate (e.g., mouth-to-beak resuscitative attempts), even visiting a bird park or sharing a room with a sick bird for a few moments can result in transmission.

It is probable that all birds can be infected with *C. psittaci* and such infection has been documented in more than 130 species to date. These include domestic poultry, wild game birds, members of the parrot family, seabirds, finches, and pigeons. This lack of species specificity has led some to suggest that "ornithosis" would be a more appropriate name for the illness. Although studies of strain differences are just beginning, isolates associated with domestic poultry appear to be the most virulent for humans. Infected birds can be either asymptomatic or obviously ill. The latter are highly infectious and *C. psittaci* can be found in large numbers in their respiratory secretions and excreta as well as on their feathers and in cage-associated fomites. *C. psittaci* is vertically transmitted from parents to nestlings and about 10% of infected birds become chronic, asymptomatic carriers of the disease. Shedding of infective *C. psittaci* by carrier birds is intermittent, varying from a baseline of 5% to 10% to as high as 100% during extensive handling or transportation. Although the disease is most commonly transmitted by inhalation of bird-associated "dust" (i.e., dried excreta), transmission may also occur by biting or exposure to tissue aerosols generated in poultry processing plants.

Although most human cases can be linked to birds, 20% to 25% of psittacosis patients have no known avian exposures. Transmission of *C. psittaci* to humans has been documented from infected cats, cows, goats, and sheep. The organisms may be concentrated in the ovine placenta since human cases have been associated with both abortion and birthing in sheep. Although human-to-human transmission is rare, infectious elementary bodies are present in large numbers in the respiratory secretions of patients seriously ill or dying with psittacosis.

BIOLOGY OF THE ORGANISM AND PATHOLOGY. The infectious stage of the *C. psittaci* life cycle is the elementary body, which is found in virtually all secretions and tissues of diseased birds and the excrement of asymptomatic carriers. This life stage is metabolically inactive and highly resistant to desiccation. Elementary bodies can remain viable in dried excrement for at least 1 week at 20°C. On inhalation by a susceptible individual, the elementary body is phagocytosed by the host macrophage but resists phagolysosomal fusion. The organism then becomes metabolically active and grows as a cytoplasmic inclusion, the reticulate body. This stage is noninfectious and cannot survive outside of the host cell. Infected macrophages carry the organisms to the reticuloendothelial system where extensive replication takes place. Subsequent cell-associated bacteremia spreads the organism to the lungs, the heart, and other target organs. After 20 to 30 hours of growth and replication, cell wall formation begins and progeny elementary bodies are formed. The *C. psittaci* life cycle is completed when infectious elementary bodies are released by cell lysis.

Although *C. psittaci* pathology in birds is most prominent in the liver, spleen, and pericardium, the lungs are the predominant target organ in humans. Inflammation of the respiratory epithelium extends from the trachea to the alveoli with mononuclear cell infiltrates, epithelial cell hyperplasia, desquamation, and mucous plugging. Intracytoplasmic inclusions are readily detected by light microscopy. The hilar lymph nodes are enlarged and a lobar pattern of congestion, edema, and red-to-gray hepatization of the lung parenchyma is observed. Other affected tissues (e.g., brain, heart) also show prominent mononuclear cell infiltrates with edema and varying degrees of tissue destruction (e.g., fatty degeneration, subendocardial hemorrhage). The liver may show nonspecific hepatitis or granuloma formation. It is interesting that neither inclusion bodies nor chlamydial antigens can be demonstrated in the emboli that occasionally complicate *C. psittaci* endocarditis.

CLINICAL MANIFESTATIONS

General. The severity of psittacosis ranges from subclinical infection to life-threatening systemic disease. The incubation period usually ranges from 7 to 15 days but may be as long as 21 days. Clinical disease typically has a rapid onset with chills and high fever (up to 40°C), but psittacosis may also develop more insidiously with steadily increasing malaise and fever. As with other intracellular infections, there may be relative bradycardia for the degree of fever. Cough and fever are almost always present (70% to 100%) and headache, myalgias, and chills can be prominent symptoms (30% to 70%). Pharyngeal erythema, abnormal chest auscultation, and hepatomegaly are present in more than 50% of patients. A wide variety of other signs and symptoms including anorexia, abdominal pain with nausea, vomiting or diarrhea, arthralgias, ataxia, confusion and somnolence, dyspnea, chest pain, epistaxis and hemoptysis, rash, adenopathy, and splenomegaly occur in a minority of psittacosis patients. The initial clinical manifestations of psittacosis tend to be nonspecific and other diagnoses are frequently considered during the initial evaluation of a patient. For example, combinations of the common symptoms and signs outlined earlier may suggest a nonspecific viral infection, a mononucleosis-like syndrome, enteric fever, or an atypical pneumonia. More unusual combinations of symptoms and signs may lead to the consideration of endocarditis, hepatitis, gastroenteritis, meningitis, myocardial infarction, pulmonary embolism, and polymyositis, among others.

Pneumonia. Atypical pneumonia is the most frequently recognized manifestation of psittacosis. These patients usually present with several days of fever and malaise accompanied by a dry cough, occasionally with small amounts of mucopurulent or blood-tinged sputum, and fine crepitant rales. The physical findings often belie the pulmonary involvement demonstrated on the chest radiograph. Although no characteristic x-ray pattern can be used to make the diagnosis, consolidation of a single lower lobe is seen in 90% of the abnormal films. Radiologic resolution of abnormalities is slow and one third of psittacosis patients still have evidence of their disease on chest films at 12 weeks. Dyspnea and hypoxia are proportional to the degree of pulmonary involvement. A pleural rub can occasionally be heard but true pleurodynia is unusual in psittacosis. Similarly, pleural effusions can occur but are rare. Although it occurs less than half of the time, splenomegaly in a patient with an atypical pneumonia is strongly suggestive of psittacosis.

Nonpulmonary Manifestations. *C. psittaci* can infect both native and previously damaged heart valves and is one of the causative agents of "culture-negative" endocarditis. Organisms can be demonstrated histologically in infected heart valves and can be cultured from the blood of many patients with *C. psittaci* endocarditis. Other rare cardiac complications of psittacosis include myocarditis and pericarditis. Neurologic manifestations include meningitis, encephalitis, seizures, transverse myelitis, Guillain-Barré syndrome, and cranial nerve palsies. Although the cerebrospinal fluid (CSF) is typically normal in psittacosis, lymphocytes are sometimes present and CSF protein levels can occasionally be markedly elevated. Liver function tests are abnormal in half of psittacosis patients and may have a cholestatic pattern. Hepatitis is occasionally severe enough to produce jaundice. Joint involvement can manifest as arthralgias resembling rheumatic fever during the acute illness or as a reactive arthritis 2 to 4 weeks after resolution of the illness. The latter is typically polyarticular and may be associated with conjunctivitis and HLA-B27 (i.e., Reiter's syndrome). *C. psittaci* has been isolated occasionally from synovial fluid during the acute illness. Dermatologic manifestations include Horder spots (i.e., evanescent maculopapular eruptions similar to the rose spots of typhoid fever), erythema multiforme, erythema marginatum, erythema nodosum, and urticaria. Other very rare presentations of psittacosis include disseminated intravascular coagulation, thrombophlebitis, pancreatitis, panniculitis, acute renal failure, keratoconjunctivitis and a sarcoid-like illness (i.e., hilar adenopathy on chest x-ray film with noncaseating granuloma in the liver and skin).

LABORATORY FINDINGS. The laboratory findings in psittacosis are nonspecific. The total white blood cell count is typically normal or slightly increased. Most patients present with a left shift during the acute phase of the illness. Thrombocytopenia is seen only rarely. Approximately half of the patients have mild elevations of liver function tests, which can occassionally take a cholestatic pattern. An abnormal chest x-ray study is the most consistent (70% to 80%) finding in psittacosis and the degree of radiologic involvement is often disproportionate to the auscultatory findings. Consolidation of a single lower lobe is by far the most common (85% to 90%) presentation but reticular, homogeneous ground-glass, and patchy segmental patterns have been reported. Pleural effusions are present in almost half of the cases but are generally small and transient. Hilar adenopathy is evident in only a minority of cases and never occurs in isolation. The radiologic findings in psittacosis typically take 6 to 8 weeks to resolve, although abnormalities can persist in some individuals for more than 5 to 6 months.

DIAGNOSIS. In the classic pulmonary presentation, other causes of atypical pneumonia must be considered (e.g., legionellosis, *Chlamydia pneumoniae*, *Mycoplasma pneumoniae*, Q fever, viral pneumonitis). In patients presenting with a more systemic illness, the differential diagnosis is very broad and includes infectious mononucleosis, typhoid fever, brucellosis, acute human immunodeficiency virus (HIV) infection, tularemia, influenza, and subacute bacterial endocarditis. The most helpful clues to the diagnosis include a history of exposure and, when present, relative bradycardia, splenomegaly, epistaxis, hemoptysis, and Horder spots.

The laboratory diagnosis of psittacosis remains problematic. Although this organism can be grown easily in a modern microbiology facility, cultures of *C. psittaci* are highly infectious and this procedure should not be attempted except in specialized laboratories. Complement fixation (CF) is the most commonly used test for the confirmation of *C. psittaci* infection but no commercial kits are available. *C. psittaci* CF is typically performed in the virology laboratories of large centers using assays based on commercial antigen preparations. Either a fourfold rise in CF antibody titers or a single high titer ($\geq$ 1:32) in an individual with a compatible illness is thought to indicate infection. Although it is widely used, the CF test is neither very sensitive nor specific. In particular, CF testing cannot distinguish between the three *Chlamydia* species (i.e., *C. trachomatis*, *C. pneumoniae*, and *C. psittaci*), all of which can cause pulmonary disease. Recent data also suggest that CF antibodies wane quickly after infection such that almost 75% of patients have titers < 1:32 9 months after the diagnosis. Species-specific serology can be obtained using IgM microimmunofluorescence (micro-IF) but cross-reactions complicate the interpretation of these results as well. The micro-IF test is generally available only in reference and research laboratories (e.g., the Centers for Disease Control and Prevention Chlamydia Laboratory). Although polymerase chain reaction (PCR), direct fluorescence, and enzyme-linked immunosorbent assay have been reported for use in psittacosis, none has moved beyond the research laboratory as yet.

PROGNOSIS AND TREATMENT. Psittacosis is often a mild to moderate illness but mortality rates of 20% to 40% among those with severe infections in the preantibiotic era remind us that *C. psittaci* is an organism to be respected. Mortality rates have now declined to less than 1% with improved recognition of milder illness and modern antibiotic treatment. Patients with mild infections usually recover within a week but recovery from more severe infections may require 3 weeks or longer. The disease may be particularly virulent in pregnancy and in the elderly.

Tetracyclines (tetracycline hydrochloride 500 mg PO q.i.d. or doxycycline 100 mg PO b.i.d.) are the drugs of choice in nonpregnant adults. A clinical response to therapy is usually obvious within 24 hours but may take 2 to 3 days or longer. Therapy continuing for 10 to 14 days beyond defervescence may decrease the rate of relapse. Chloramphenicol has been used in the past but is less effective than tetracycline. Erythromycin is useful when tetracycline is contraindicated in pregnant women, young children, and those with drug allergy but may be less effective in severe cases. The newer macrolide antibiotics (clarithromycin, azithromycin) are active against *C. psittaci* in vitro but there are insufficient data to comment on their use in treating patients. Doxycycline (100 mg/day PO for 10 days) may be considered for prophylaxis following significant exposures in nonpregnant adults. Although successful nonsurgical treatment of *C. psittaci* endocarditis with a combination of erythromycin and rifampin has been reported, replacement of the diseased valve is usually necessary in addition to prolonged antibiotic therapy.

PREVENTION AND CONTROL. C. psittaci has both epizootic and epidemic potential. As a result, prevention and control measures must extend to both human and avian populations. Infected birds should be destroyed or treated for at least 45 days with a tetracycline. Shorter periods of treatment may only suppress C. psittaci shedding by infected birds. Human psittacosis is a reportable disease in many countries, allowing for epidemiologic investigations and bird quarantine and treatment during outbreaks. Respiratory isolation should be instituted for individuals hospitalized with serious C. psittaci pneumonia. Surfaces contaminated by infected birds or terminally infected humans should be thoroughly disinfected with phenolic compounds to destroy elementary bodies.

Bibliography

Centers for Disease Control and Prevention: Human psittacosis linked to a bird distributor in Mississippi, Massachusetts and Tennessee, 1992. MMWR 41:793, 1992.

Crosse B: Psittacosis: A clinical review. J Infect 21:251, 1990.

Esposito AL: Pulmonary infections acquired in the workplace. Clin Chest Med 12:245, 1992.

Essig A, Zucs P, Susa M, et al: Diagnosis of ornithosis by cell culture and polymerase chain reaction in a patient with chronic pneumonia. Clin Infect Dis 21:1495, 1995.

Harris RL, Williams TW: Contribution to the question of pneumotyphus: A discussion of the original article by J Ritter in 1880. Rev Infect Dis 7:119, 1985.

Hedberg K, White KE, Hedberg CW, et al: Persistence of Chlamydia complement fixation antibody after an outbreak of psittacosis. J Infect Dis 167:502, 1993.

Hughes P, Chidley K, Cowie J: Neurological complications of psittacosis: A case report and review of the literature. Respiratory Med 89:637, 1995.

Khatib R, Thirumoorthi MC, Kelly B, Grady KJ: Severe psittacosis during pregnancy and suppression of antibody response with early therapy. Scand J Infect Dis 27:519, 1995.

MacFarlane JT, Miller AC, Roderick Smith WH, et al: Comparative radiologic features of community acquired Legionnaires' disease, pneumococcal pneumonia, mycoplasma pneumonia and psittacosis. Thorax 39:28, 1984.

Reeve RVA, Carter LA, Taylor N, et al: Respiratory tract infections and importation of exotic birds. Lancet 1:829, 1988.

Wong KH, Skelton SK, Daugharty H: Utility of complement fixation and microimmunofluorescence assays for detecting serologic responses in patients with clinically diagnosed psittacosis. J Clin Microbiol 32:2417, 1994.

36 Pertussis

James W. Bass and Judy M. Vincent

DEFINITION. Pertussis (whooping cough) is a communicable infection of the respiratory tract characterized by repeated paroxysms of cough. In its most severe form, paroxysms may terminate in a gasping, musical, stridulous inspiratory effort with a "whooping"-like sound. This sound has given rise to the term *whooping cough*. The word *pertussis* means intensive cough. This designation is more appropriate than whooping cough, since not all patients with pertussis whoop.

ETIOLOGY AND HISTORY. The disease was first described by Baillou in 1578, and Sydenham reported epidemics in England in 1670 and 1680. The causative organism, *Bordetella pertussis*, was first isolated by Bordet and Gengou in 1900, but it was not until 1906 that *B. pertussis* was grown in the laboratory on artificial media and its morphology and cultural characteristics described. Including *B. pertussis*, six species of this genus have been described. *Bordetella parapertussis*

is a less common cause of a pertussis-like illness usually associated with a milder clinical course than that due to *B. pertussis*.

DISTRIBUTION AND INCIDENCE. Pertussis continues to be a disease of worldwide importance. An estimated 51 million cases with 600,000 deaths occur annually; it is the leading cause of death in infants unprotected by immunization. Even in the United States, where current pertussis vaccine acceptance has exceeded 90%, pertussis was reported from every state in 1995 and 1996. In 1994, the 4617 cases of pertussis reported in the United States totaled more than all other childhood vaccine-preventable diseases combined.

TRANSMISSION AND EPIDEMIOLOGY. Pertussis occurs year round in the tropics and subtropics, whereas in temperate climates it occurs more often in the late summer and fall. Significantly higher attack rates, morbidity, and mortality from pertussis are seen in females than in males, in contrast to other childhood infectious diseases.

The disease is spread by the airborne route, directly from droplet aerosols generated by the intense cough of affected persons. The highest attack rate occurs in individuals exposed to within several feet of coughing patients. Less often, infection may spread by handling objects freshly contaminated with nasopharyngeal secretions. Pertussis is one of the most communicable diseases of humans. Attack rates in susceptible contacts approach 100%.

Infections in Adults. Pertussis is a leading cause of sickness and death in countries where immunization with pertussis vaccine is not practiced, and it is also prevalent in industrialized countries where no vaccine or ineffective vaccines are used. Even in countries where effective whole-cell vaccines have been in use for the past five decades the epidemiology of the disease is changing. These vaccines were developed in the 1930s, field-tested in the 1940s, and accepted for general use since the 1950s. They were targeted at preschool children, in whom the disease was most often seen in the prevaccine era. Owing to concerns of possible vaccine reactions, primarily encephalopathy, booster immunization after 7 years of age has not been recommended. As a result, vaccine-induced immunity wanes, and little protection is present 7 to 12 years after the last booster is given. Accordingly, use of these vaccines led to a marked overall decrease in the incidence of pertussis in preschool children during the 1950s through the 1970s; however, the incidence in adolescents and young adults has increased since the 1980s. In these persons pertussis is atypical, usually manifested only as a chronic cough, often lasting several weeks or more.

Infections in Infants. Currently, in the United States, incompletely immunized young adults serve as the largest reservoir of *B. pertussis* infection and the major source of transmission. Spread is primarily to young infants less than 1 year of age who do not have passive immunity to pertussis from their mothers and who have not achieved active immunity from vaccine. These young infants, especially those under 6 months of age, also have atypical pertussis. The whoop is often absent, and cough may be overshadowed by episodes of apnea and cyanosis, often leading to hospitalization for intensive care. The diagnosis of pertussis may not be considered in these highly contagious infants; isolation precautions may not have been implemented; and epidemic spread to young susceptible adult health care providers frequently occurs.

PATHOGENESIS AND PATHOLOGY. Pertussis organisms are not invasive. In susceptible persons they adhere to the cilia of the epithelial cells lining the mucosal surface of the respiratory passages from the nasopharynx to the respiratory bronchioles in the lung, where they replicate. Their presence in large numbers on these surfaces is associated with elaboration of profuse, tenacious mucus. Ciliary function is impaired, resulting in the stagnation of mucus flow, inspissation of air passages, and secondary infection. Necrosis of the tracheal and bronchial epithelium is often present, producing perihilar atelectasis that is responsible for the "shaggy heart border" on the chest radiograph, a hallmark of the disease. Bronchitis is constant, and areas of bronchopneumonia are common. The bacterial pathogens implicated in these secondary infections (including acute otitis media and sinusitis) are the pneumococcus, *Haemophilus influenzae* type b, and, less often, *Staphylococcus aureus* and group A β-hemolytic streptococci.

B. pertussis organisms are not found beyond the cilia of the respiratory epithelium. Here, several biologically active surface components that play a role in the pathogenesis of the disease are elaborated and absorbed. The characteristic lymphocytosis associated with pertussis is stimulated by lymphocytosis-promoting factor (LPF), now called pertussis toxin (PT); filamentous hemagglutinin (FHA) is involved in the attachment of *B. pertussis* organisms to ciliated respiratory epithelial cells; agglutinogens are thought to be associated with type-specific immunity; and tracheal cytotoxins (TCTs) cause ciliostasis and epithelial cell death. PT and FHA are the primary antigens incorporated into effective acellular vaccines. TCT causes most of the destruction of the respiratory tract as well as the respiratory symptoms associated with the disease. As both secretory and humoral antibodies are produced in increasing quantity, the organism is gradually eliminated from the respiratory passages, ciliary movement is restored, tenacious mucus secretions are diminished, mucus inspissation is resolved, and the airway heals, usually without residua.

The exact cause of pertussis encephalopathy has not been determined. The fact that it is often seen in patients with hyperlymphocytosis suggests that PT may be causally related to this complication of pertussis. Whether the organism elaborates a neurotoxin or whether encephalopathy is due to intracranial hemorrhage or anoxia secondary to severe cough spasms is debatable. Edema, congestion, and scattered petechial hemorrhages, commonly found in brain tissue of patients who die from pertussis, are consistent with hypoxic brain damage.

CLINICAL MANIFESTATIONS. After an incubation period of 7 to 10 days (range 5–20 days), clinical illness evolves in three stages: (1) the catarrhal, prodromal, or preparoxysmal stage; (2) the acute paroxysmal or spasmodic cough stage; and (3) the convalescent stage.

The Catarrhal Stage. This is characterized by a period of one to several days of clear, serous, or mucoid rhinorrhea; nasal congestion; and sneezing followed by cough. During this time the disease is often indistinguishable from the common cold, and pertussis is seldom suspected unless classic clinical whooping cough has been observed in other members of the family or local community. Later in this period the cough grows more severe and persistent, particularly at night, and profuse nasopharyngeal secretions grow thick and tenacious. There is heavy shedding of pertussis organisms in these secretions; it is at this stage that the patient is most contagious and the organism is most easily cultured. The catarrhal stage may persist for up to 2 weeks, whereas in other cases it may be so mild that it goes unrecognized.

The Paroxysmal Stage. This rarely begins abruptly, without a preceding catarrhal stage. Violent, protracted bouts of coughing occur in distinct paroxysms lasting up to several minutes. There may be only 2 to 5 or up to 40 to 50 episodes a day. Toward the end of these paroxysms, patients often vomit previously swallowed thick, ropy secretions. Severe cough may produce a marked florid venous engorgement of

the head and neck. In younger, weaker infants, severe cough paroxysms may not be associated with the characteristic whoop but more often terminate in exhaustion, vomiting, aspiration, apnea, cyanosis, and loss of consciousness. Without resuscitation, these episodes may result in anoxic brain damage or death. In older children and adults with relatively larger upper airways, the characteristic whoop is also often absent. The paroxysmal stage of pertussis may last from only a few days to 3 to 4 weeks.

The Convalescent Stage. This begins when chronic cough replaces paroxysms. It usually lasts for 3 to 4 weeks with decrease in frequency and severity of cough. Rarely, the convalescent stage may persist for months.

COMPLICATIONS

Suppurative Complications. Secondary infections of the respiratory tract should be suspected in the patient who develops fever and toxicity, as uncomplicated pertussis is not associated with fever. Acute otitis media is common, as is sinusitis. Clinical and radiographic evidence of pneumonia develops in approximately 10% of infants with pertussis. This may be difficult to differentiate from atelectasis, which is usually present in varying degrees. Segmental or lobar atelectasis primarily affects the lower lobes, the right middle lobe, and the lingular segment of the left upper lobe. Serial radiographs may show frequent changes, as some segments re-aerate, whereas others collapse. If soft, fluffy infiltrates develop around these areas of atelectasis and the patient becomes toxic and febrile, secondary bronchopneumonia should be suspected. Treatment should be initiated against the bacterial pathogens most often causing these infections.

Nonsuppurative Complications. Increased intrathoracic pressure resulting from severe cough paroxysms, hypoxia, and persistent vomiting causes venous engorgement and hypoxemia with petechial hemorrhages, epistaxis, subconjunctival and scleral hemorrhages, and cerebral hemorrhages. Rarely, subarachnoid and subdural hemorrhages with convulsions, transient hemiplegia (Todd's paralysis), encephalopathy, and coma occur.

Marked prolonged increases in intrathoracic and intra-abdominal pressure with cough paroxysms have been associated with rupture of the diaphragm; interstitial, subcutaneous, or mediastinal emphysema; pneumothorax; umbilical and inguinal hernia; and rectal prolapse. Intractable vomiting may produce severe metabolic alkalosis with tetany, aspiration pneumonia, and inanition. Mortality is greater in the tropics than in developed countries. In the former, death is frequently due to secondary bacterial infections. Medical care, including the availability and proper use of antibiotics, is limited, and children who die frequently have concomitant medical problems, e.g., malnutrition or other infections.

DIAGNOSIS. The diagnosis of pertussis should be suspected in any child with severe cough, and it should be considered foremost if the cough occurs in severe paroxysms. It is helpful if there is a history of contact with a person known to have pertussis or if the disease is prevalent in the community. Lack of prior immunization or only partial immunization against pertussis should further increase the likelihood of the diagnosis.

Differential Diagnosis. The differential diagnosis includes respiratory infections caused by respiratory syncytial virus, influenza, parainfluenza, and adenoviruses. *Chlamydia trachomatis* pneumonia in infants is often confused with pertussis, as is perinatally acquired cytomegalovirus infection. Cystic fibrosis and laryngeal foreign body are often accompanied by persistent severe bouts of cough suggesting pertussis.

An absolute lymphocytosis involving small, mature lymphocytes with counts ranging from 20,000 to ≥100,000/mm³ is usually seen in the late catarrhal stage and throughout most of the paroxysmal stage. This characteristic lymphocytosis may not be present in infants less than 6 months of age, partially immunized individuals, and adults. The erythrocyte sedimentation rate in patients with uncomplicated pertussis is abnormally low.

Culture. Culture of *B. pertussis* organisms from respiratory tract secretions remains the gold standard for laboratory diagnosis of pertussis. Although this test is highly specific, it is not very sensitive. It is best accomplished with nasopharyngeal secretions obtained by aspiration during irrigation with phosphate buffered saline. Culture of calcium alginate swabs inserted through the nose deep enough to reach the posterior pharynx also yields excellent results. Dacron and cotton swabs are not as effective. Cough plate specimens and swabs taken from the oropharynx yield less reliable results, and these latter techniques are not recommended.

Nasopharyngeal secretions obtained by aspiration or from nasal calcium alginate swabs should be smeared directly onto Regan-Lowe (RL) medium with and without cephalexin, and/or fresh Bordet-Gengou (BG) medium with and without penicillin. RL medium is superior to BG medium when compared in the same study population, so RL medium should be selected if only one is used.

Culture plates should be streaked and sealed with masking tape to prevent desiccation during the prolonged incubation required for growth of *B. pertussis* organisms. Characteristic small pinpoint metallic-like colonies are first noted after incubation of 72 hours or more at 37°C. Most positive cultures are evident after 5 to 7 days; however, initial positive readings have been observed on plates held and read at 12 days. Positive cultures are obtained in only 35 to 80% of patients with obvious clinical pertussis, varying significantly with the skill and experience of laboratory personnel and with the timing of the culture. Organisms are most often cultured during the catarrhal stage of illness, when almost pure cultures are obtained. The incidence of positive cultures remains equally high throughout the first week of the paroxysmal stage. It decreases thereafter, and it is seldom possible to recover the organism more than 3 weeks after the onset of the paroxysmal stage of illness.

Direct Fluorescein-Labeled Antibody Test. Fluorescein antibody (FA) staining can quickly confirm the presence of *B. pertussis* organisms in nasal secretions. This method is compromised by interobserver variability. Both false positive and false negative results can occur; however, FA tests may be more sensitive than culture, and they often remain positive even after effective antibiotic treatment has cleared the patient of viable organisms. It is the best test currently used for immediate presumptive diagnosis of pertussis and permits early management decisions regarding isolation of the patient, pertussis vaccine administration, and antibiotic treatment and prophylaxis.

Serology. Enzyme linked immunosorbent assay (ELISA) tests for IgG antibodies to PT and FHA may reflect past infection or vaccine administration when a single serum speciman has levels of antibody above the reference range. An elevation of IgM antibody indicates concurrent or recent infection or vaccine adminstration. IgA antibodies are produced only with infection, not by vaccine administration. Since they are short-lived, the finding of IgA antibodies indicates recent infection; however, only about half of patients with *B. pertussis* infection develop IgA antibodies. A significant rise in any of these antibodies noted in paired acute and convalescent sera confirms recent infection with *B. pertussis.* An ELISA test for detection of secretory IgA antibody to PT in nasal secretions indicates current or recent infection. DNA hybridization and polymerase chain reaction (PCR) have been developed for identification of the organisms in naso-

pharyngeal secretions. Results of these tests are seldom available in time to guide patient management decisions; however, they are useful in epidemiologic studies. These tests are both highly sensitive and specific but they are not currently available for general use.

TREATMENT AND PROGNOSIS

Supportive Therapy. It is wise to hospitalize young infants with pertussis who have cough paroxysms terminating in episodes of cyanosis and apnea. Infants 1 to 4 months of age with these complications may die of asphyxia if immediate resuscitation is not available. When cough paroxysms occur, the infant should be positioned in a head-down or lateral decubitus position so that aspiration of secretions accumulating at the end of a paroxysm does not occur. Vomiting frequently ensues following severe paroxysms, and aspiration of vomitus by the weak, exhausted, hypoxemic infant must be prevented.

Suctioning and supplemental oxygen administration are indicated during and after severe bouts of paroxysmal cough. Experienced, efficient nursing care is probably the most important factor in survival. In situations in which nursing care is not optimal, the mother should be shown how to care for the child and allowed to stay at the bedside. Fluid depletion from suctioning of secretions, vomiting, and inadequate oral fluid intake may necessitate parenteral fluid and electrolyte administration. Although mist therapy is not helpful, supplemental administration of well-humidified oxygen is needed in some patients who have sustained hypoxemia. Blood gas determinations, if available, should be performed in patients with labored respirations, unstable vital signs, or alterations in mental status, who usually have complications, e.g., atelectasis or bronchopneumonia. Cough suppressants, expectorants, and sedatives have not helped in the treatment of pertussis.

Specific Therapy

Human Immune Pertussis Globulin. These preparations were commercially available from the late 1940s until 1981, when they were withdrawn from the market after controlled studies showed them to be of no benefit in preventing pertussis in exposed susceptible persons or in modifying severity of the disease in patients with pertussis. In a more recent controlled study a specific pertussis hyperimmunoglobulin was shown to be efficacious in reducing severity and duration of symptoms, but this preparation is not generally available.

Antimicrobial Agents. Treatment with antimicrobial agents that are active against *B. pertussis* results in eradication of the organisms from infected patients, provided that the drug diffuses in significant concentrations into respiratory tract secretions. No antimicrobial drug has been shown to alter the subsequent clinical course when given in the paroxysmal stage of disease. However, antibiotics can attenuate the disease when given in the catarrhal or preparoxysmal stage and abort or prevent disease in individuals during the incubation period. Their administration at any stage of pertussis regularly produces bacteriologic cure and may render the patient noncontagious. These are the rationale for the use of antimicrobials in pertussis. Erythromycin estolate is the most effective and least toxic of all drugs studied to date. Erythromycin may also be of value in prophylaxis in exposed susceptible individuals. The recommended dose is 40 to 50 mg/kg/day (maximum 2 g) orally in two divided doses for 14 days. Treatment for less than 14 days may be complicated by bacteriologic and clinical relapse. *B. pertussis* susceptibility to erythromycin has ranged from 0.2 to 0.5 mg/L over the past 30 years with no evidence of development of resistance.

The activity of clarithromycin against *B. pertussis* organisms and its concentration in serum and respiratory tract secretions are equal to—or greater than—those of erythromycin. Limited clinical trials indicate that this drug may be equivalent or superior to erythromycin for treatment of pertussis. It has a significantly longer half-life. The recommended dosage is 15 mg/kg/day in two divided doses, and it is better tolerated than erythromycin. With these advantages, clarithromycin may become the preferred drug for treatment of pertussis in situations in which it is affordable.

Trimethoprim-sulfamethoxazole may be an effective alternative to erythromycin for treatment of pertussis, but its efficacy has not been proved in controlled studies. Other antibiotics, such as the penicillins, including ampicillin, and first-generation cephalosporins, have some activity against *B. pertussis* in vitro but are clinically ineffective, probably owing to poor penetration into respiratory secretions.

Corticosteroids. Three controlled studies indicate that corticosteroids may reduce the number, severity, and duration of cough paroxysms in patients with pertussis, even when treatment is initiated after the paroxysmal stage has developed. Young infants with severe pertussis may benefit from treatment with hydrocortisone, 30 mg/kg/day; betamethasone, 0.075 mg/kg/day; or dexamethasone, 0.3 mg/kg/day; for 3 to 7 days.

Albuterol. Most controlled studies evaluating albuterol in the treatment of pertussis have shown a beneficial effect. Its use may be indicated in treatment of small infants with severe life-threatening paroxysms; 0.3 to 0.5 mg/kg/day in three divided doses is effective and well tolerated.

Prognosis. In developed countries where patients who develop pertussis are generally healthy, have an early diagnosis, appropriate treatment, and, in particular, skilled nursing care, the prognosis is good. In the United States the mortality has been ≤1% over the past several years; nearly all deaths have been in infants less than 1 year of age, most less than 6 months of age. Many deaths are from secondary bacterial infections, primarily pneumonia, and early diagnosis and proper antimicrobial treatment of this complication are major determinants for survival. Although convulsions occur in 1 to 3% of these infants, pertussis encephalopathy with stupor and coma develops in ≤1%. Among children with pertussis encephalopathy who become comatose, nearly half die; of those who survive, nearly half have permanent neurologic residua.

In developing countries the prognosis for patients with pertussis varies with the general health of the individual and the quality of health care in the community. In areas where there are no skilled health care providers and poor diagnostic and treatment facilities, the prognosis is guarded, especially in patients with poor nutrition, multiple parasitic infections, and a high prevalence of other acute and chronic diseases (Chapter 16). Mortality in the most primitive of these circumstances may be as high as 5 to 10% for young infants with severe pertussis.

PREVENTION AND CONTROL. The incidence and severity of pertussis have been markedly reduced in countries where effective vaccines have been utilized.

Immunization. In the United States, where whole-cell vaccines have been used since the 1950s, the incidence of the disease has decreased from 150,000 to 200,000 cases annually in the prevaccine era to a low of 1010 cases in 1976 (<99%). Since 1976 the incidence has increased.

Using present strategies, overall maximal benefit from use of whole-cell pertussis vaccine has already been achieved. Young adults with vaccine-induced waning immunity are a reservoir of pertussis, and newborn infants are a susceptible group who have life-threatening disease after exposure. Future strategies for control of pertussis will depend on development of acellular component vaccines that are highly immunogenic and minimally reactogenic, allowing booster

immunizations at appropriate intervals throughout life. This change in strategy would not only curb the development of epidemic pertussis that is occurring in populations using past strategies but could also lead to eradication of pertussis in these populations.

Isolation and Prophylactic Antibiotics. Protection against pertussis in exposed individuals as well as controlling its spread can be accomplished by isolation of individuals with the disease and administration of erythromycin. Since nearly all patients who receive this drug become culture negative after 5 days, isolation beyond this period does not seem indicated. Prophylactic administration of erythromycin to susceptible close contacts of these patients, including household/family members, health care providers, and attendees of daycare facilities, may minimize secondary spread of the disease.

Bibliography

Bass JW, Klenk EL, Kotheimer JB, et al: Antimicrobial treatment of pertussis. J Pediatr 75:768, 1969.

Bass JW, Wittler RR: Return of epidemic pertussis in the United States. Pediatr Infect Dis J 13:343, 1994.

Cattaneo LA, Reed GW, Haase DH, et al: The seroepidemiology of *Bordetella pertussus* infections: A study of persons aged 1–65 years. J Infect Dis 173:1256, 1996.

Deville JG, Cherry JD, Chistenson PD, et al: Frequency of unrecognized *Bordetella pertussis* infections in adults. Clin Infect Dis 21:639, 1995.

Farizo KM, Cochi SL, Zell ER, et al: Epidemiological features of pertussis in the United States, 1980–1989. Clin Infect Dis 14:708, 1992.

Gordon JE, Hood RI: Whooping cough and its epidemiological anomalies. Am J Med Sci 222:333, 1951.

He Q, Viljanen MK, Nikari S, et al: Outcomes of *Bordetella pertussis* infection in different age components of an immunized population. J Infect Dis 170:873, 1994.

Hoppe JE: Update on epidemiology, diagnosis, and treatment of pertussis. Eur J Clin Microbiol Infect Dis 15:189, 1996.

Jenkinson D: Natural course of 500 consecutive cases of whooping cough: A general practise population. Br Med J 310:299, 1995.

Marchant CD, Loughlin AM, Lett SM, et al: Pertussis in Massachusetts, 1981–1991: Serologic diagnosis, and vaccine effectiveness. J Infect Dis 169:1297, 1994.

Mink CM, Sirota NM, Nugent S: Outbreak of pertussis in a fully immunized adolescent and adult population. Arch Pediatr Adolesc Med 148:153, 1994.

MMWR 44:525, 1995. Pertussis—United States, January 1992–1995. JAMA 272:450, 1995.

Mulholland K: Measles and pertussis in developing countries with good vaccine coverage. Lancet 345:305, 1995.

Nennig ME, Shinefield HR, Edwards KM, et al: Prevalence and incidence of adult pertussis in an urban population. JAMA 275:1672, 1996.

Olson LC: Pertussis. Medicine 54:427, 1975.

Rosenthal S, Strebel P, Cassiday P, et al: Pertussis infection among adults during the 1993 outbreak in Chicago. J Infect Dis 171:1650, 1995.

Shefer A, Dales L, Nelson M, et al: Use and safety of acellular pertussis vaccine among adult hospital staff during an outbreak of pertussis. J Infect Dis 171:1053, 1995.

Wirsing von Konig CH, Postels-Mulrni A, Bloxk HL, Schmitt HJ: Pertussis in adults: Frequency of transmission after household exposure. Lancet 346:1326, 1995.

Wright SW, Edwards KM, Decker MD, Zeldin MH: Pertussis infection in adults with persistent cough. JAMA 273:1044, 1995.

37 *Melioidosis*

Nicholas J. White

DEFINITION. Melioidosis is an infection of humans, mammals, and birds caused by a motile aerobic gram-negative bacillus, *Burkholderia (Pseudomonas) pseudomallei.* Melioidosis means a resemblance to the distemper of asses, or glanders. Whitmore and Krishnaswami, who first recognized melioidosis in Rangoon in 1911, shrewdly noted the similarity between the two infections, but although *B. pseudomallei* and *B. mallei* (which causes glanders) are close genetically, there is no epidemiologic relationship between these two infections.

EPIDEMIOLOGY. Melioidosis is a tropical infection of mammals and birds occurring predominantly in countries between the latitudes 20 degrees north and 20 degrees south. *B. pseudomallei* is an environmental saprophyte that can be isolated from wet soils, streams, ponds, and, in particular, rice paddies in endemic areas. Although cases have been reported throughout the tropics, the majority of infections occur in east Asia and northern Australia. Sporadic cases in humans and animals have been reported from the United States (although nearly all these were imported from endemic areas), Mexico, Panama, El Salvador, Haiti, Puerto Rico, Ecuador, Brazil, Guyana, and Peru in the Americas; Iran and Turkey in central Asia; several countries from the east to the west of the African continent; and also Madagascar. In Europe a famous epizootic occurred in the animals of the Paris zoo in the mid-1970s. Melioidosis is being recognized increasingly in India, and has also been reported from Guam and Fiji. In northeastern Thailand, where the majority of cases in recent years have been reported, melioidosis accounts for approximately 20% of all community-acquired septicemias. The majority of these cases occur during the rainy season months in rice farmers (the major occupation), and most cases have an underlying condition (usually diabetes mellitus or renal disease) that predisposes to infection. Human immunodeficiency virus (HIV) infection does not appear to predispose to melioidosis. In endemic areas seroconversion starts as soon as children are exposed to wet soil, and occurs at approximately 25% per year between 6 months and 4 years of age. Most clinical infections therefore are not primary infections with *B. pseudomallei*. The average annual incidence of melioidosis in Ubon Ratchatani province in northeastern Thailand between 1987 and 1991 was estimated to be 4.4/100,000 population. Melioidosis is also a disease of veterinary importance affecting a variety of birds, sheep, goats, pigs, horses, camels, and also dolphins. Animals do not appear to represent a reservoir for the transmission of human disease. Melioidosis is acquired through soil or water contamination of skin abrasions, or by inhalation. There is no evidence that human disease may be acquired by ingestion. Although sexual transmission and nosocomial transmission of melioidosis are documented, these are very unusual.

CLINICAL MANIFESTATIONS. Melioidosis may occur at any age. The pattern of disease in children differs from that in adults, with parotid abscess accounting for 30% of pediatric cases, whereas this is a rare presentation in adults. In endemic areas the peak incidence of melioidosis is in the fifth and sixth decades, reflecting the age distribution of the conditions, e.g., diabetes mellitus and chronic renal diseases, that predispose to the infection. The incubation period of melioidosis has not been defined precisely, but may be very short (<3 days) after exposure to a large number of organisms (e.g., aspiration following near-drowning). Latent infection is also well recognized with a maximum interval between first exposure and disease of 26 years. In the majority of cases there is no obvious portal of entry such as an infected skin abrasion or penetrating wound.

Inapparent Infection. Most people exposed to *B. pseudomallei* in the environment do not become ill. In northeastern Thailand most of the rural population has serologic evidence of exposure to *B. pseudomallei* but no evidence of disease. Mild influenza-like illnesses associated with primary infections in adults have been reported in Australia.

Suppurative Parotitis. This is a unique clinical condition, possibly representing primary infection, which occurs almost exclusively in children. The child presents with unilateral or, less commonly, bilateral tense painful parotid swelling and fever. The skin overlying the abscess is often inflamed and edematous. Unless the parotid abscess is drained, suppuration breaks through either to the skin or to the external auditory meatus and may result in permanent lower motor neuron facial palsy. Unlike the other presentations of melioidosis, parotid abscess is not associated with underlying disease, and with incision, drainage, and appropriate antibiotics the long-term prognosis is good.

Acute Localized Suppurative Disease. Localized infections of subcutaneous tissue, lymph nodes, and occasionally other salivary glands may occur. There is pain, swelling, and localized lymphadenopathy, and often the spontaneous discharge of brown-yellow odorless pus.

Acute Septicemic Disease. Originally described by Whitmore and Krishnaswami in debilitated morphine addicts in Rangoon, septicemic melioidosis today is more usually seen against a background of pre-existing diabetes, renal failure, alcoholism, leukemia or lymphoma, or corticosteroid or other immunosuppressant use. This is a community-acquired septicemia and patients present with a high swinging fever, obtundation, and often shock. As in other causes of septicemia, absence of fever or leukocytosis carries a poor prognosis. In 2 to 5% of patients superficial skin or subcutaneous abscesses may be present. Gram-negative rods can be seen in the aspirated pus. Concomitant primary or metastatic pneumonia (Fig. 37–1) is common, as are hepatic and splenic abscesses and less commonly secondary lung abscesses. Metastatic abscess formation may also occur in skeletal muscle, joints, bones, kidneys, and, occasionally, the central nervous system (CNS). *B. pseudomallei* infection does not cause primary endocarditis or pyogenic meningitis although suppurative pericarditis is well recognized. A primary focus of infection is evident in 50% of cases, usually the lung or urinary tract or less commonly a skin or soft tissue wound. The chest radiograph

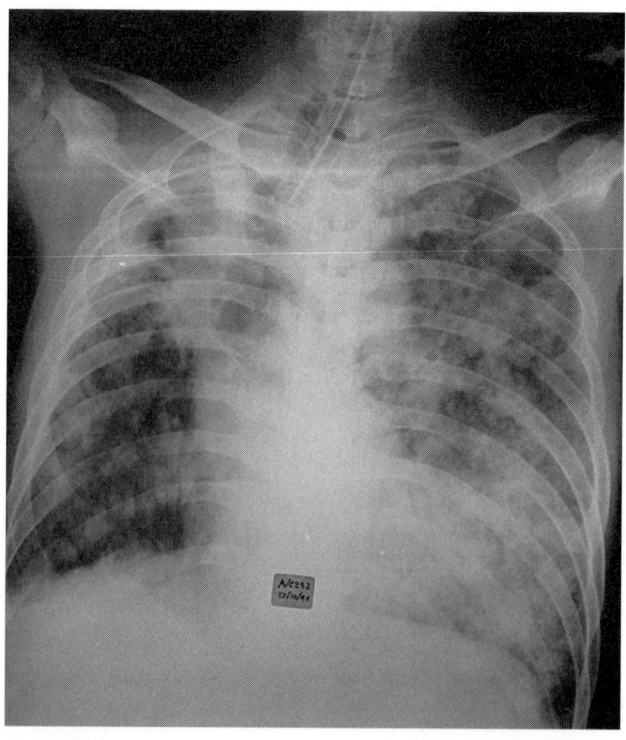

Figure 37–1. Extensive metastatic pneumonia in fulminant septicemic melioidosis.

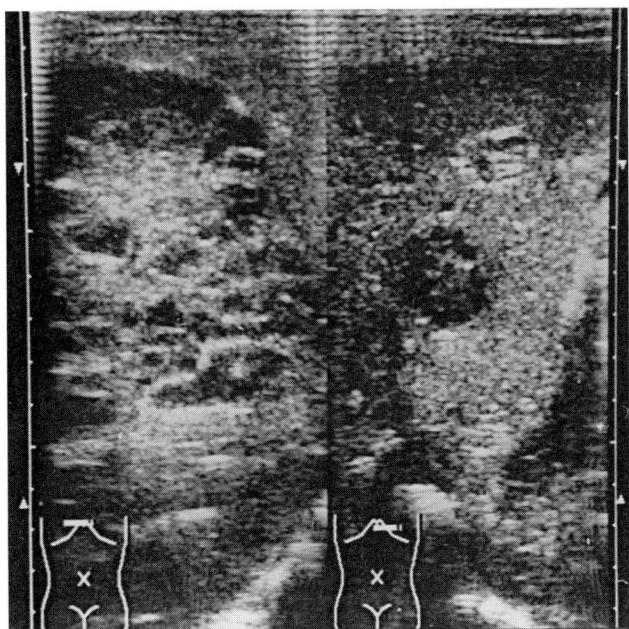

Figure 37–2. Multiple "Swiss cheese" liver abscesses in melioidosis.

often shows the features of "blood-borne pneumonia," and ultrasound examination of the abdomen commonly reveals single or multiple liver abscesses and often accompanying splenic abscesses.

Subacute Disease. Melioidosis may also present with sub-acute suppuration most commonly in the lung (abscess or empyema), liver (single or multiple abscesses giving a "Swiss cheese" appearance on ultrasound; Fig. 37–2), and spleen. Suppuration is associated with high swinging fever, marked constitutional features, and rapid weight loss. Pyomyositis may present subacutely and osteomyelitis, prostatitis, epidid-ymo-orchitis, septic arthritis, and lymphadenitis may also occur. Subacute subcutaneous abscesses, commonly on the scalp, presumably result from direct inoculation. Rapidly de-structive corneal ulceration also results from direct inocula-tion of the organism into the eye. Melioidosis may cause cerebral abscess with sometimes fatal secondary meningitis.

Latent Disease. Although most cases of melioidosis repre-sent primary infections, the organism may remain quiescent for many years following primary exposure, or resolution of a primary infection. Recrudescence is often provoked by intercurrent illness, surgery, trauma, development of diabetes or renal failure, or use of immunosuppressant drugs.

Nonmetastatic Encephalitis. Melioidosis may cause a neu-rologic syndrome manifest as brain stem encephalitis, aseptic meningitis, or peripheral motor neuropathy without demon-strable foci of infection in the CNS. The cerebrospinal fluid usually has increased protein and a mononuclear pleocytosis. Respiratory failure is a common complication and if the patient recovers from the acute phase there is often neuro-logic deficit. This syndrome has been ascribed to an as-yet unidentified neurotoxin. In the Northern Territory of Austra-lia this neurologic syndrome occurred in 13% of all cases of melioidosis, whereas in Thailand the incidence is less than 1%.

DIAGNOSIS. The syndrome of acute suppurative parotitis is distinctive, but otherwise melioidosis must be distin-guished from other causes of localized abscess or septicemia. The chest radiograph (Fig. 37–1) and ultrasound imaging of the abdomen (Fig. 37–2) are valuable investigations but ultimately the diagnosis rests on identification of the organ-

ism. Blood, sputum or throat swab, and pus cultures should be obtained. Direct immunofluorescence tests (using the same polyclonal antibody as in the latex test) on pus, sputum, or infected urine samples are 70% sensitive and 99% specific in comparison with culture and may provide the diagnosis within 1 hour. *B. pseudomallei* grows readily on most bacterio-logic media, although it may require 48 to 72 hours of incuba-tion and is therefore easily overgrown in mixed cultures on nonselective media. Preincubation in a selective broth is particularly valuable for cultures taken from sites with a normal flora such as sputum or open abscesses. *B. pseudomal-lei* is readily identified on the selective media described by Ashdown, which contains gentamicin, glycerol, and crystal violet. On Ashdown's agar the organism produces character-istic wrinkled, raised, or flat "cornflower head" purple colo-nies that have a silvery sheen and a pleasant musty or earthy odor (see Fig. 37–3 in color section). The organism is an oxidase-positive gram-negative rod that is characteristically resistant to gentamicin and colistin but sensitive to amoxicil-lin–clavulanic acid. Biochemical tests or a latex agglutination test using a rabbit polyclonal antibody may be used to con-firm identification. As background exposure is so common in endemic areas, serologic tests have not proved useful in diagnosis, although improved specificity has been claimed for more specific IgM antibody detection tests. The immuno-dominant antigen is the cell wall lipopolysaccharide, and this is remarkably conserved between strains. Four polymerase chain reaction methods have been described, all of which claim to be sensitive and specific although none of these are readily available.

TREATMENT. Severe melioidosis should be treated with intravenous ceftazidime (120 mg/kg/day). This has reduced the mortality of severe melioidosis to approximately 40%. Intravenous amoxicillin–clavulanic acid (160 mg/kg/day) is an effective alternative with a similar treated mortality, but a slightly higher rate of treatment failure. The imipenem-cilas-tatin combination is also effective clinically, but there is con-siderably less experience with its use. Intravenous treatment should be given for at least 10 days and continued until there is a clear symptomatic response. Melioidosis responds slowly to all treatments, with a median time to defervescence of 9 days. Many patients, particularly those with visceral or pulmonary abscesses, may have high swinging fevers for several weeks and respond very slowly to appropriate anti-microbial treatment. Oral maintenance treatment should be continued with either high dose amoxicillin–clavulanic acid or a combination of chloramphenicol (50 mg/kg/day for 2 months), trimethoprim-sulfamethoxazole (10 and 50 mg/kg/day), and doxycycline (4 mg/kg/day). The last two drugs should be continued for a total treatment duration of 20 weeks. Treatment courses of 8 weeks or less are associated with relapse rates of approximately 25%. Some authorities give doxycycline (the most active of the oral drugs) alone, as it is uncertain how much the other potentially toxic drugs contribute to efficacy. The fluoroquinolone antibiotics have intermediate activity against *B. pseudomallei* in vitro, but have been shown recently to be inferior to these other drugs for maintenance treatment.

Antimicrobial Resistance. All strains of *B. pseudomallei* are resistant to aminoglycosides and the majority of β-lactams. *B. pseudomallei* may develop simultaneous resistance to chlor-amphenicol, the tetracyclines, and trimethoprim-sulfameth-oxazole while on treatment. Extended-spectrum β-lactam re-sistance has also been described either through β-lactamase production, reduced penetration or binding, or in the case of amoxicillin–clavulanic acid through reduced β-lactamase inhibition by clavulanic acid. Resistance to ceftazidime occurs in less than 3% of strains.

PROGNOSIS. Melioidosis is difficult to treat. The overall mortality from hospitalized melioidosis is 50%. In endemic areas many patients present late and die rapidly, often before microbiologic confirmation of the diagnosis. Except for localized suppurative disease, which responds well to incision, drainage, and appropriate antibiotics, the therapeutic response is slow and metastatic abscess formation may develop despite appropriate antimicrobial therapy. The average time of hospitalization in survivors is 4 weeks. There is considerable weight loss during this period. Patients need lifelong follow-up. Recrudescence rates with 20 weeks of antimicrobial treatment should be less than 10%.

Bibliography

Chaowagul W, White NJ, Dance DA, et al: Melioidosis: A major cause of community-acquired septicemia in northeastern Thailand. J Infect Dis 159:890, 1989.

Dance DA: Melioidosis: The tip of the iceberg? Clin Microbiol Rev 4:52, 1991.

Leelarasamee A, Bovornkitti S: Melioidosis: Review and update. Rev Infect Dis 11:413, 1989.

Supputtamongkol Y, Hall AJ, Dance DAB, et al: The epidemiology of melioidosis in Ubon Ratchatani, North Eastern Thailand. Intl J Epidemiol 23:1082, 1995.

Whitmore A, Krishnaswami CS: An account of the discovery of a hitherto undescribed infective disease occurring among the population of Rangoon. Indian Medical Gazette 47:262, 1912.

38 Actinomycosis

Roderick J. Hay and Raymond A. Smego, Jr.

DEFINITION. Actinomycosis is a chronic, localized, suppurative, bacterial disease caused by species of *Actinomyces*. It is characterized by the formation of abscesses and multiple draining sinus tracts, through which colonies (sulfur granules) are discharged onto the surface.

ETIOLOGY. The most common cause of actinomycosis in humans is *Actinomyces israelii*, although other species are recognized pathogens (i.e., *Actinomyces naeslundii*, *Arachnia propionica*, and *Bifidobacterium eriksonii*). They are anaerobic members of the normal human flora, growing on the surfaces of teeth and in the tonsillar crypts, and as commensals of the gastrointestinal and female pelvic tracts. They have not been recovered from other natural habitats, and infections are consequently endogenous rather than exogenous in origin. In infected tissues, the agent appears as compact grains (sulfur granules) that are white or, more characteristically, yellow; rounded or lobulated; of a soft consistency; and up to 2 mm in diameter. Early stages of growth are by fine, branching filaments, 0.5 to 1 μm in diameter (Fig. 38–1), but the organisms may undergo extensive fragmentation in both tissues and cultures, so that their hyphal-like nature may not be readily recognized. Typically, they are closely associated with other anaerobic bacterial inhabitants of the colonized sites, including fusiform bacteria, anaerobic streptococci, and *Actinobacillus actinomycetemcomitans*. It is likely that these associated microorganisms act synergistically in establishing an infection.

EPIDEMIOLOGY. Actinomycosis occurs worldwide. Cases are sporadic and somewhat uncommon. Males are infected more frequently than females, but this sexual predilection has now become less evident with the recognition of a link between pelvic actinomycosis and intrauterine contraceptive

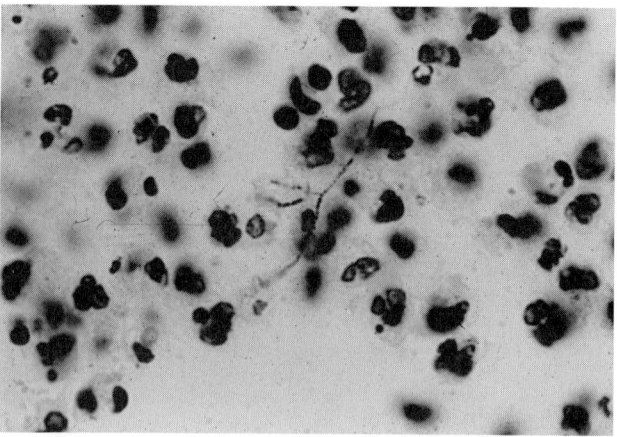

Figure 38–1. Fine, branching filaments of *Actinomyces israelii* in aspirate from a brain abscess; 500× magnification.

devices. Any age group may be affected, but the disease is rare in children under 10 years of age and generally occurs between the ages of 15 and 40. No racial or occupational susceptibilities are evident, although individuals with poor standards of oral hygiene may be more likely to acquire the disease.

PATHOGENESIS AND PATHOLOGY. Because the causal agents are normal members of the microflora of mouth and throat, the most common form of actinomycosis is cervicofacial. Infection becomes established when the agents invade mucous membranes of the mouth and pharynx, presumably through the gums, teeth, or tonsils. Initial signs of actinomycosis may originate in the pharynx, but the disease more commonly is first seen in the lower jaw. A history of dental disease or extraction is common.

If the bacteria are aspirated, infection becomes established in the lung, with extension to the pleura and chest wall. Abdominal actinomycosis probably originates from the intestinal flora. Once established, infection may extend through the diaphragm to the chest cavity. Metastatic spread may set up focal infections in a wide range of body sites. The causes of susceptibility are not understood, but as saprophytes, *Actinomyces* are generally of low pathogenicity and cause disease only in the setting of antecedent tissue injury.

The gross pathology may vary according to the rate of infection but usually is characterized by chronicity, fibrosis, suppuration, abscesses of varying size, scar formation, and sinus tracts that often interconnect. Sulfur granules consisting of interwoven and often fragmented hyphae, together with cellular debris and associated microorganisms, are surrounded by abundant neutrophils. Toward the periphery, hyphae are oriented radially and commonly have sheaths of eosinophilic material ("clubs"). Giant cells are uncommon. Macrophages containing fat may be present in sufficient numbers to impart a yellow color to the lesion, which is visible on gross examination.

Sulfur granules are distinctive and usually diagnostic, but are not unique to actinomycosis. They are also seen in soft tissue lesions of nocardiosis, chromomycosis, eumycetoma, and botryomycosis. Causative organisms are recognized by their particular morphologic features and cultural characteristics. Sulfur granules are clearly revealed in Gram-stained sections or in material stained by silver impregnation, but they may not be abundant and their detection may require a careful search of histopathologic sections (Fig. 38–1).

CLINICAL MANIFESTATIONS

Cervicofacial Lesions. Tissue swelling is not prominent in the early stages of cervicofacial actinomycosis. Skin overlying the lesion soon becomes inflamed and develops an uneven surface, and the tumor becomes indurated and woody. Localized lesions suppurate and drain through single and multiple sinus tracts, which may heal and reopen or be replaced by new ones. Extension to cranial bones, brain, meninges, and thorax may occur.

Thoracic Actinomycosis. Thoracic actinomycosis may involve the lungs, pleura, mediastinum, or chest wall; routes of infection include aspiration of oropharyngeal or gastric content, cervicofacial extension, or contiguous spread from the abdomen. Radiographs show large areas of perihilar or basilar consolidation (Fig. 38–2), often containing small abscess cavities. In contrast to tuberculosis, infection often is confined to the bases of the lungs. Common findings are cough, low-grade fever, weight loss, night sweats, and anemia; in addition, dysphagia may result from mediastinal invasion.

Abdominal Actinomycosis. Abdominal actinomycosis may initially mimic acute or subacute appendicitis, but primary lesions are usually palpable in the ileocecal region. As the infection progresses, there may be extension to the liver, ovaries, and urinary tract, with development of pyelonephritis or cystitis, or to the spine, resulting in compression of the cord and sometimes psoas abscess. Sinus tracts may develop in the abdominal wall. The most common single finding is a tender, palpable mass in the region of the appendix or in other parts of the abdomen. Chronic gastrointestinal actinomycosis may mimic other diseases with ileocecal predilection, including tuberculous enteritis, amebiasis, regional enteritis, and carcinoma of the cecum. Pelvic actinomycosis has been reported, particularly in women using intrauterine contraceptive devices for many years.

Central Nervous System (CNS) Actinomycosis. Infection of the CNS may take the form of brain abscess (accounts for 75% of all lesions), chronic meningitis or meningoencephalitis (resembling tuberculous meningitis), subdural empyema, actinomycoma, and spinal and cranial epidural abscess. CNS actinomycosis is usually secondary to hematogenous spread from primary infection in the lung, abdomen, or pelvis or less commonly from contiguous extension from infection of the head and neck.

DIAGNOSIS. The diagnosis of actinomycosis is supported by detection of sulfur granules in pus or tissue sections (Fig. 38–1) and by the isolation and identification of the agent. Image-guided aspiration of deep lesions may be useful. Cervicofacial actinomycosis or visceral forms of the disease with sinus tract formation usually present no difficulties with diagnosis. Abdominal or pelvic actinomycosis without abdominal wall involvement may be diagnosed only at laparoscopy or laparotomy.

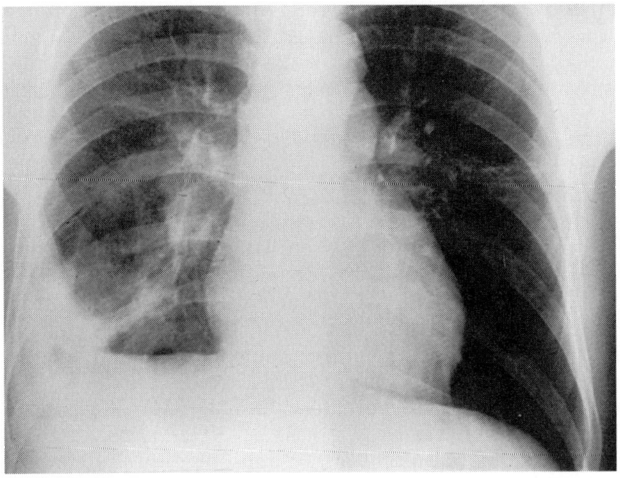

Differential Diagnosis. The condition may simulate several chronic diseases, including tuberculosis, osteomyelitis, carcinoma, and amebiasis.

TREATMENT. Penicillin is the drug of choice, the regimen depending on the extent and severity of the disease. High doses (5 to 10 million units daily) may be administered intramuscularly or intravenously for 6 weeks or until lesions have healed, followed by oral therapy with 2 to 5 million units of penicillin or 2 g of tetracycline daily for 2 to 12 months. Patients allergic to penicillin may be given tetracycline, erythromycin, or chloramphenicol. Surgical resection and incision and drainage of badly diseased tissues are valuable ancillary therapeutic procedures.

PROGNOSIS. Before the antibiotic era, the prognosis was very poor. Based on experience with penicillin, anticipated recovery rates are now about 90% for cervicofacial, 80% for abdominal, and 40% for thoracic forms of the disease. Prognosis is greatly improved when the condition is diagnosed early. Recovery with adequate penicillin therapy is common, but chronic abdominal infections and thoracic empyema may be difficult to eradicate.

PREVENTION. Prevention is not practicable; maintenance of good dental hygiene, however, may reduce the density or incidence of oropharyngeal colonization.

Bibliography

Brown JR: Human actinomycosis: A study of 181 subjects. Hum Pathol 4:319, 1973.

Cintron JR, Del Pino A, Duarte B, et al: Abdominal actinomycosis. Dis Colon Rect 39:105, 1996.

Fiorino AS: Intrauterine contraceptive device–associated actinomycotic abscess and *Actinomyces* detection on cervical smear. Obstet Gynecol 87:142, 1996.

Smego RA Jr: Actinomycosis of the central nervous system. Rev Infect Dis 9:855, 1987.

39 Nocardiosis

Roderick J. Hay and Raymond A. Smego, Jr.

Figure 38–2. Pulmonary actinomycosis with right lower lobe consolidation in a patient with *A. israelii* infection.

DEFINITION. Nocardiosis is an acute or chronic suppurative infection caused by aerobic, gram-positive filamentous bacteria of the order Actinomycetales and genus *Nocardia*. There are four species of *Nocardia* generally recognized as pathogenic in humans: *N. asteroides*, *N. brasiliensis*, *N. caviae*, and *N. madurae*. Of these, *N. asteroides* and *N. brasiliensis*, in that order, are the most frequent etiologic agents.

ETIOLOGY. *N. asteroides* most commonly produces pleuropulmonary infection, and has the tendency to hematogenously seed to many body sites, particularly the central nervous system (CNS). *N. brasiliensis*, however, is generally associated with infection of skin and soft tissue; pulmonary and other systemic diseases have been reported only infrequently. *N. asteroides* is geographically distributed widely in soil, while *N. brasiliensis* is found as a soil inhabitant predominantly in warmer subtropical or tropical regions of the world.

EPIDEMIOLOGY. Nocardiosis occurs in all age groups, but is more common in older subjects. Males are affected more commonly than females. There are no occupational or racial susceptibilities. Systemic nocardiosis occurs sporadically throughout the world in both temperate and tropical climates; skin and soft tissue nocardiosis is typically a tropical and subtropical disease. *N. asteroides* is increasingly recognized as an opportunistic pathogen in immunosuppressed patients, e.g., those with Hodgkin disease, malignant tumors, leukemia, and AIDS. In contrast, *N. brasiliensis* causes disease predominantly in immunocompetent individuals.

PATHOGENESIS AND PATHOLOGY. The primary route of infection for *N. asteroides* is via respiratory inhalation. In contrast, traumatic inoculation of the organism into skin is the most common mode of acquisition of *N. brasiliensis*. Once established, the agent appears in smears and histopathologic sections as spreading, delicate hyphae-like filaments 1 μm in diameter. Lesions are suppurative, characterized by abscesses of varying size. Generally, these are multiple and confluent, and their walls may be partially lined by fibrosing granulation tissue. The reaction is almost exclusively pyogenic, with little evidence of granuloma formation or giant cells. Systemic nocardiosis may be localized to the lungs or disseminated lesions may occur in brain, meninges, peritoneum, subcutaneous tissues, or muscle. Sections of lung show abundant abscesses with areas of chronic pneumonia lying adjacent to areas of suppuration. Caseation and tubercle formation are not present. The gram-positive filaments are found within macrophages or lying free in the pus. Although sulfur granules can exude from soft tissue lesions, they are not found in deep abscess or visceral specimens, as in actinomycosis.

CLINICAL MANIFESTATIONS. Nocardiosis can be an acute, subacute, or chronic suppurative infection that ranges from mild cutaneous or pulmonary disease to aggressive and often fatal dissemination. Pulmonary involvement and hematogenous spread of disease to other organs, particularly the CNS, are the major manifestations of *N. asteroides*.

Pulmonary Nocardiosis. Pulmonary nocardiosis is characterized by malaise, fever, weakness, night sweats, weight loss, dyspnea, and chest discomfort. Cough is unproductive initially, but mucopurulent sputum is eventually produced. Consolidation of one or more lobes is characteristic, and extension to the pleural space is common. The pleura may become markedly thickened, and the pleural space may be obliterated by suppuration. Cavitation may be prominent and associated with hemoptysis. Sinus tracts may be a prominent feature, occasionally penetrating the chest wall. The radiologic appearance may resemble upper lobe tuberculosis, bronchopneumonia, or unresolved pneumonia. Small scattered nodular opacities with cavitation may occur throughout both lung fields, suggesting other opportunistic infection or metastatic tumor.

Disseminated Lesions. Metastatic spread to the brain is common, the presenting symptoms being those of a space-occupying lesion (i.e., headache, nausea, vomiting, lethargy, mental confusion, convulsions, and paralysis, with or without fever). Computed tomography scans show intracranial abscesses and subependymal nodules (Fig. 39–1). Other sites include the meninges and peritoneum, and rarely heart and kidney. Bone infections are uncommon. Subcutaneous abscesses may result from early metastasis. If untreated, these eventually rupture, leaving chronically draining fistulas.

Cutaneous Nocardiosis. Primary cutaneous nocardiosis due to *N. brasiliensis* manifests as cellulitis, subcutaneous abscesses, pustules, pyoderma, and ulcerations typically resembling lesions caused by staphylococci and streptococci. Some persons may develop a lymphocutaneous syndrome that displays a sporotrichoid appearance. Worldwide, the most common cutaneous manifestation is actinomycetoma

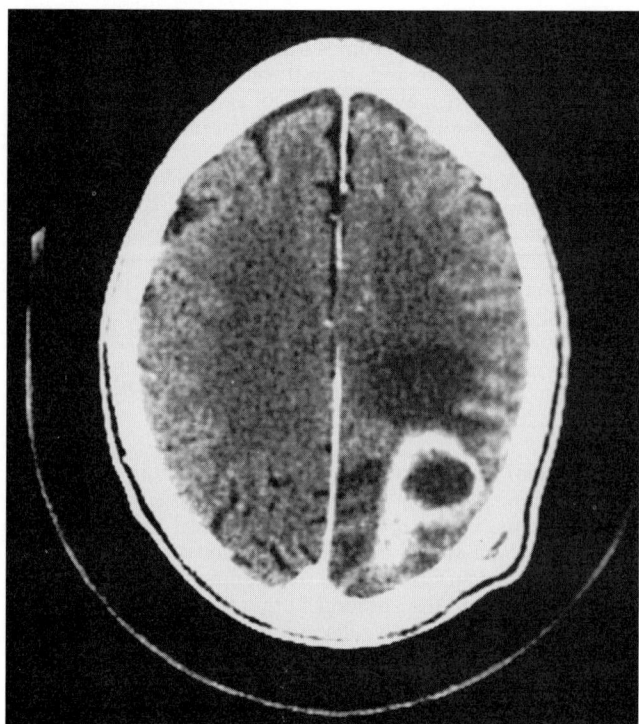

Figure 39–1. CT scan with contrast showing a left occipital brain abscess caused by *Nocardia asteroides*.

(see Chapter 82.1). Involvement of the skin with *N. asteroides* generally occurs as a result of blood-borne dissemination of the organism.

DIAGNOSIS. A positive diagnosis of nocardiosis depends on recognition of the slender, branching actinomycete filaments in exudates or tissue sections and on the isolation and identification of *Nocardia* species in culture. Partial acid-fastness using a cold-modified Kinyoun stain with sulfuric acid or hydrochloric acid decoloration distinguishes *Nocardia* from *Actinomyces*. Serologic testing is not commercially available.

Culture. The agent grows well on many types of media including sheep blood agar and chocolate agar, Sabouraud's medium, and most media used for isolation of tubercle bacilli. Speciation of *Nocardia* is difficult and requires the use of biochemical techniques.

Differential Diagnosis. Nocardiosis has many clinical forms and must be distinguished from a wide range of pulmonary, cerebral, cutaneous, and systemic diseases. Among these are tuberculosis, neoplasms, sarcoidosis, sarcoma, brain abscess, and actinomycosis.

TREATMENT. For almost 40 years, sulfonamides were the mainstay of therapy for nocardiosis. The fixed combination of trimethoprim-sulfamethoxazole (TMP-SMX), however, is the drug of choice for serious systemic infection, including CNS or disseminated disease. For patients with life-threatening *Nocardia* infection, it may be advisable to combine TMP-SMX with other antimicrobial agents. Older agents active against *Nocardia* include ampicillin, erythromycin, minocycline, and gentamicin. Various combinations of imipenem, amikacin, and ceftriaxone are more active and may be useful combined with or as alternatives to TMP-SMX. For patients with mycetoma due to *N. brasiliensis*, TMP or SMX alone, TMP-SMX plus streptomycin, or dapsone plus streptomycin may be the most effective drug regimens.

Given the tendency for *Nocardia* infections to recur, drug therapy is probably best continued for 3 to 12 months as judged by the clinical site and severity of disease, immune status of the patient, and potential time at risk for infection. Adequate drainage of abscesses, exploration and debridement of sinus tracts, and excision of necrotic tissues are all crucial surgical adjuncts to antimicrobial treatment.

PROGNOSIS. The prognosis is most favorable when the diagnosis is made early, before metastasis to the brain. In view of the ubiquity of the organisms, it is likely that humans have an innately high level of resistance.

Nocardiosis that is recognized early and treated promptly may be completely eradicated. However, the disease, particularly when disseminated, is often refractory to treat-

ment and has a poor prognosis, with a survival rate of about 50%.

PREVENTION. Prevention is not practicable.

Bibliography

Beaman RL, Burnside J, Edwards B, et al: Nocardial infection in the United States, 1972–1974. J Infect Dis 34:286, 1976.
Frazier AR, Rosenow EC, Roberts GD: Nocardiosis: A review of 25 cases occurring during 24 months. Mayo Clin Proc 50:657, 1975.
Poonwan N, Kusum M, Mikami Y, et al: Pathogenic *Nocardia* isolated from clinical specimens including those of AIDS patients in Thailand. Eur J Epidemiol 11:507, 1995.
Smego RA Jr, Gallis HA: The clinical spectrum of *Nocardia brasiliensis* infection in the United States. Rev Infect Dis 6:1184, 1984.
Smego RA Jr, Moeller MB, Gallis HA: Trimethoprim-sulfamethoxazole therapy for *Nocardia* infections. Arch Intern Med 143:711, 1983.

SECTION C Gastrointestinal Tract Infections

40 Shigellosis

Myron M. Levine

DEFINITION. Shigellosis is an acute bacterial infection of the intestinal tract, predominantly involving the terminal ileum, colon, and rectum, caused by organisms of the genus *Shigella*. The spectrum of illness is broad, extending from subclinical infections and mild watery diarrhea to fulminating dysentery manifested by high fever, chills, toxemia, tenesmus, and the passage of multiple scanty stools of blood and mucus. Strictly speaking, dysentery implies the presence of blood and mucus in stools, of which *Shigella* is the most common cause. However, bacillary dysentery has become synonymous with all clinical presentations of shigellosis.

ETIOLOGY. *Shigella* are nonmotile, gram-negative, rod-shaped bacteria within the family Enterobacteriaceae. Four species or groups of *Shigella* are recognized based on biochemical and serologic differentiation: *S. dysenteriae* (group A); *S. flexneri* (group B); *S. boydii* (group C); and *S. sonnei* (group D). Groups A, B, and C have multiple serotypes and subtypes, whereas only a single serotype of group D is recognized. *S. dysenteriae* type 1, so-called Shiga bacillus, is a unique serotype that causes the most severe clinical illness, manifests pandemic behavior, and is particularly difficult to isolate from clinical specimens. *S. flexneri* and *S. dysenteriae* serotypes predominate in the less developed world, while *S. sonnei* is the most frequent isolate in industrialized countries.

HISTORY. Bloody diarrhea accompanied by tenesmus and abdominal cramps was described by Hippocrates, who also recognized the seasonality of this disease, which peaked in summer. Throughout recorded history, bacillary dysentery has afflicted military units and played a decisive role in military campaigns. The outcome of many a battle has been influenced by a dysentery epidemic in one of the opposing armies, thereby altering the course of history. *Shigella* was first identified by Kiyoshi Shiga at the end of the nineteenth century, at a time when extensive epidemics were sweeping the islands of Japan accompanied by high case fatality.

DISTRIBUTION AND INCIDENCE. *Shigella* infections occur throughout the world, from the tropics to the Arctic, wherever personal hygiene is compromised. Thus, shigellosis is endemic among toddlers and preschool children in less developed countries, while in industrialized countries it occurs in custodial institutions for the mentally retarded and the mentally ill and in some daycare centers for preschool children.

Prospective household surveillance of cohorts of children for diarrheal disease in less developed countries has shown that the peak incidence of *Shigella* infections occurs in the second and third years of life. During this early age, approximately three to six episodes of diarrhea per child per year occur, and about 10% of the episodes are due to *Shigella*. Worldwide, shigellosis is a formidable public health problem. A study by the Institute of Medicine estimates that, annually, *Shigella* causes 250 million cases of diarrheal illness and 654,000 deaths throughout the world.

Pandemics of shigella (*S. dysenteriae* 1) dysentery have been observed in Central America in the late 1960s, Bangladesh in the early 1970s, Central Africa in the late 1970s, 1980s and 1990s, and south Asia in the mid-1980s (Table 40–1). The strains of *S. dysenteriae* type 1 responsible for these pandemics all harbored R-factor plasmids that confer resistance to multiple clinically important antibiotics and caused severe clinical illness and high case fatality in all age groups.

TRANSMISSION AND EPIDEMIOLOGY. Other than primates in captivity, humans serve as the only reservoir and natural host for *Shigella*. As few as 10 *Shigella* organisms can cause overt clinical illness in volunteers. This finding corroborates the epidemiologic observations that indicate the ready transmission of *Shigella* by direct fecal-hand-oral contact in propagated epidemics. The low inoculum required for transmission explains why spread of *Shigella* easily occurs wherever crowding, poor sanitation, and primitive personal hygiene coexist. Less commonly, *Shigella* is transmitted by contaminated food or water vehicles. Under certain conditions, as found seasonally in many less developed areas, *Shigella* may be transmitted by houseflies serving as mechanical vectors. Shigellosis has been recognized with increased frequency in male homosexuals, in whom the infection is transmitted by oral-anal contact.

TABLE 40–1. Epidemics of Shiga (*Shigella dysenteriae* Type 1) Dysentery Throughout the World Since the Late 1960s

Years	Countries Affected	Resistance to Clinically Relevant Antibiotics
1968–1970	Guatemala, El Salvador, Nicaragua, Honduras, Costa Rica, southern Mexico	Tetracycline, sulfas, chloramphenicol
1972	Mexico	Tetracycline, sulfas, chloramphenicol, ampicillin
1972–1977	Bangladesh	Tetracycline, sulfas, chloramphenicol, ampicillin (some strains)
1974–1978	Southern India	Tetracycline, sulfas, chloramphenicol, ampicillin
1979–present	Zaire, Rwanda, Burundi	Tetracycline, sulfas, chloramphenicol, ampicillin
1984–present	India, Burma, Nepal, Bangladesh, Thailand, southern China	Tetracycline, sulfas, ampicillin, trimethoprim-sulfamethoxazole

PATHOGENESIS AND PATHOLOGY. *Shigella* are notably more acid resistant than many other bacterial enteropathogens, which allows them to survive passage through the acid environment of the stomach; this explains why minute inocula can cause clinical illness and why direct contact transmission occurs. Two new enterotoxins have recently been discovered, *Shigella* enterotoxin 1 and 2 (ShET 1 and 2), which are responsible for small bowel secretion and the watery diarrhea that is prominent early in the course of clinical shigellosis. However, the predominant sites of pathology are in the terminal ileum and the colon, where one finds evidence of a cardinal feature of *Shigella*, i.e., its capacity to invade and multiply within mucosal epithelial cells (ultimately leading to cell death) and to elicit a striking polymorphonuclear leukocyte influx. The ability to invade epithelial cells involves both chromosomal genes and a large enteroinvasiveness plasmid that encodes the expression of several outer membrane proteins required for *Shigella* to gain entry into the colonocyte, to propel itself intracellularly, and to move to adjacent cells. The striking influx of polymorphonuclear leukocytes into the lamina propria accounts for many of the clinical and pathologic features of shigellosis. With progression of the mucosal infection, death of enterocytes leads to small ulcers, hemorrhage, microabscesses, and the presence of many leukocytes in the fecal material. *Shigella* that lose their invasive potential are no longer pathogenic.

S. dysenteriae type 1 expresses a highly potent exotoxin, the Shiga toxin. This toxin exhibits several biologic activities: it is cytotoxic for HeLa and Vero cells in nanogram quantities; following inoculation of guinea pigs, mice, or rabbits, hind limb paralysis becomes evident, thus Shiga toxin has been called a neurotoxin; inoculated into an ileal loop, it acts as an enterotoxin and induces intestinal secretion. Shiga toxin is a powerful inhibitor of protein synthesis. Only *S. dysenteriae* type 1 elaborates true Shiga toxin. Other *Shigella* serotypes elaborate small quantities of other cytotoxins. Whereas some of these other cytotoxins may be partially or even completely neutralized by Shiga antitoxin, demonstrating antigenic cross reactivity, these strains of other serotypes do not hybridize with DNA probes specific for the genes of true Shiga toxin. Thus, these other toxins, even if immunologically related, are genetically distinct from true Shiga toxin.

The exact role of Shiga toxin in the pathogenesis of shigella dysentery is not known. Animal experiments and volunteer studies show that mutants of *S. dysenteriae* type 1 that retain invasive potential while lacking the ability to elaborate Shiga

toxin cause diarrhea and dysentery which is virtually indistinguishable from that caused by Shiga toxin–producing strains. In neither humans nor monkeys was the amount of watery diarrhea diminished in infection with the strain lacking Shiga toxin, although in monkeys less blood in stools was seen. The most prominent effect of Shiga toxin in monkeys appeared to be the occurrence of vascular damage in the intestine. One report in humans suggests that among *Shigella* strains that elaborate cytotoxins other than Shiga toxin, those that show increased cytotoxin expression are associated with more severe clinical illness as measured by higher fever and more blood in stools.

A much-feared complication of shigellosis, the hemolytic-uremic syndrome, is attributed to the effects of Shiga toxin. This syndrome is an uncommon but often fatal complication seen with *S. dysenteriae* type 1 (Shiga bacillus) infection; it is rarely, if ever, observed with infection caused by any other serotype. Notably, in industrialized countries, enterohemorrhagic *Escherichia coli* (most commonly of serotypes O157:H7, O26:H11, and O111:H8) that elaborate Shiga toxins are important etiologic agents of the hemolytic-uremic syndrome.

Bacteremia is generally uncommon in shigellosis. Exceptions are *S. dysenteriae* type 1 infection in malnourished children and shigellosis caused by any serotype in AIDS patients.

When visualized by proctoscopy, the mucosa of the terminal ileum and the colon is edematous and covered with mucus and shows interspersed hemorrhages (see Fig. 40–1 in color section). Biopsy of a typical affected area reveals a striking polymorphonuclear leukocyte infiltration, congestion of blood vessels, edema, and ulceration of the overlying mucosa (Fig. 40–2).

CLINICAL MANIFESTATIONS. The spectrum of clinical illness due to *Shigella* includes asymptomatic infection; mild diarrheal illness indistinguishable from that caused by many other bacterial, viral, or protozoal agents; and severe dysentery. The incubation period is usually 1 to 4 days but may be as long as 6 to 8 days with *S. dysenteriae* type 1 infection. While any serotype can cause either mild diarrhea or fulminating dysentery, *S. sonnei* tends to be more frequently associated with mild ("catarrhal") enteritis, and *S. flexneri* and *S. dysenteriae* serotypes with more severe clinical illness. *S. dysenteriae* type 1 is particularly feared because of the severity of the clinical illness and the frequency of major complications. Shiga dysentery is often characterized by high fever,

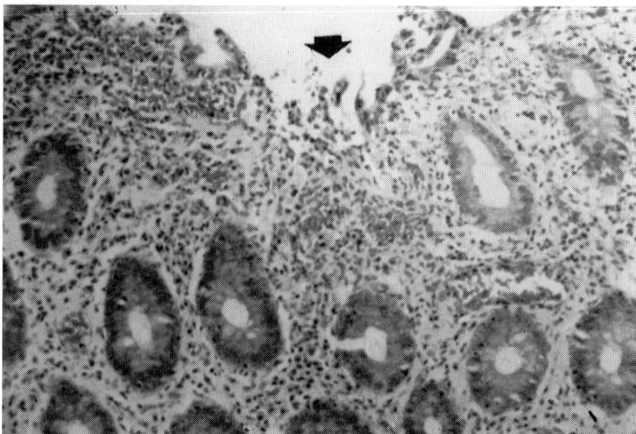

Figure 40–2. A rectal biopsy from the patient with Shiga dysentery whose proctoscopic examination results are shown in Figure 40–1. The biopsy reveals hemorrhage, vascular congestion, intense infiltration of the lamina propria with polymorphonuclear leukocytes, and a mucosal ulceration (*arrow*).

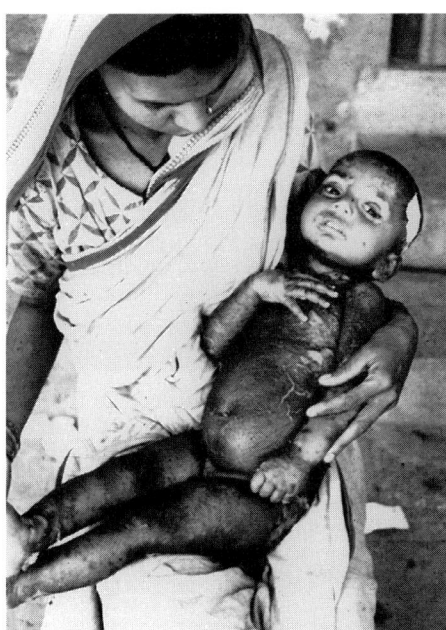

Figure 40–4. A Bangladeshi child with severe hypoproteinemia and acute onset of nutritional edema following Shiga dysentery. (Courtesy of Dr. M. Mujibur Rahaman.)

toxemia, disabling abdominal cramps, tenesmus, frequent bloody mucoid stools (see Fig. 40–3 in color section), vomiting, and convulsions (in pediatric patients).

In shigellosis there is typically a progression of disease through several fairly distinct phases. Toxemia, malaise, and high fever are often present at the onset of clinical illness, followed by some hours of watery diarrhea. When convulsions occur as part of shigellosis in children, they accompany the early phase of illness. Lastly, the dysenteric phase begins manifested by lower abdominal cramps, tenesmus, and the passage of scanty stools of blood and mucus (Fig. 40–3).

Complications. Diarrheal dehydration may accompany *Shigella* infection in infants and young children but is less common in older age groups. Convulsions may be considered an uncommon presentation of acute disease in children rather than as a complication per se.

The hemolytic-uremic syndrome, leukemoid reactions (with polymorphonuclear leukocyte counts exceeding 100,000/mm³), and severe hypoproteinemia are recognized complications of shigella dysentery. In hemolytic-uremic syndrome a disseminated intravascular coagulopathy occurs with massive hemolytic anemia, the presence of fragmented erythrocytes (schistocytes) in the peripheral blood smear, severe thrombocytopenia, and acute renal failure. Electron microscopic examination of the kidney in such patients reveals immune complexes, fibrin-platelet deposits, endocapillary cell lysis, and necrosis of glomerular and tubular epithelial cells. The exudation of proteins through the extensive mucosal damage in the intestine of young children with shigella dysentery can lead to a precipitous drop in plasma protein levels, resulting in an acute kwashiorkor syndrome characterized by edematous extremities (Fig. 40–4).

Rarely, Reiter syndrome follows shigellosis, particularly that due to *S. flexneri* serotypes. This hypersensitivity reaction, manifested by reactive arthritis (joint fluid cultures are sterile) and conjunctivitis or uveitis, is most frequent in patients having histocompatibility antigen HLA-B27. In infants or young children with severe shigellosis, rectal prolapse can

occur. *Shigella* also occasionally causes vaginitis in young girls.

DIAGNOSIS

Clinical and Laboratory. There are no characteristic features of shigellosis detectable on physical examination. Consequently, considerable emphasis is placed on the medical history. The white blood cell count is variable but often is elevated with a shift to the left.

Stool Culture. A specific diagnosis can usually be made within 48 hours by means of bacteriologic culture; however, special attention must be paid if *S. dysenteriae* type 1 is suspected, since this serotype is notoriously difficult to cultivate. Culture of a fresh stool is optimal. If this is not possible, buffered glycerol saline makes the best transport medium for rectal swabs, if *Shigella* is suspected. The combination of a selective medium such as xylose-lysine-deoxycholate (XLD) agar and a differential (noninhibitory) medium such as MacConkey agar should be used. Culture of two or more specimens from the patient increases the likelihood of isolating *Shigella*. If an outbreak of *S. dysenteriae* type 1 is suspected, Tergitol-7 agar is particularly useful in detecting this serotype, although XLD agar also functions quite well.

Serology. In investigation of outbreaks where the serotype is known but coprocultures may not be readily obtainable, the measurement of serum antibodies to the O antigen of the specific *Shigella* serotype by passive hemagglutination or by ELISA is very useful for serodiagnosis.

Stool Microscopy. Patients with a clinical syndrome suspicious for *Shigella* infection should have a drop of stool mucus mixed with a drop of saline, smeared and dried on a slide, lightly heat-fixed, stained with methylene blue or Gram stain, and examined by light microscopy for the presence of fecal leukocytes. Virtually all patients with shigellosis have polymorphonuclear leukocytes in abundance in such smears (Fig. 40–5). Although nonspecific, this test provides evidence that a bacterial pathogen has invaded the intestinal mucosa. Other

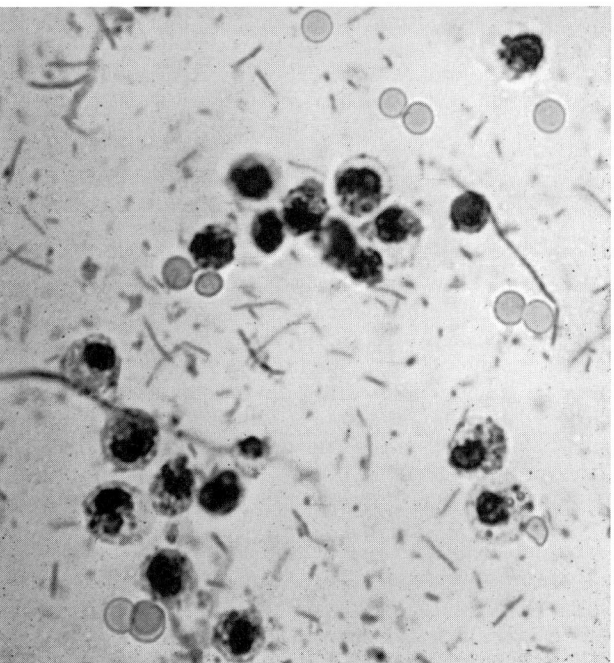

Figure 40–5. Demonstration of abundant fecal leukocytes and some red blood cells in stool mucus of a patient with dysentery due to *Shigella flexneri* 2a. Stained and examined under high dry lens (450 ×).

bacterial enteropathogens that cause a dysenteric syndrome and are associated with abundant fecal leukocytes are *Campylobacter jejuni* (Chapter 43), enteroinvasive *E. coli* (Chapter 42), *Yersinia enterocolitica* (Chapter 44.1), and *Salmonella* causing nontyphoidal infections (Chapter 76). The presence of fecal leukocytes in an acutely ill patient with clinical features of shigellosis provides sufficient indication to initiate therapy for shigellosis while awaiting the results of coprocultures. Stool microscopy in a patient with dysenteric stools will also differentiate amebic dysentery (Chapter 86) from enteroinvasive bacterial infection. The former does not exhibit abundant fecal leukocytes, but amebic trophozoites are visible.

Differential Diagnosis. Mild forms of shigellosis that are not accompanied by overt dysentery are indistinguishable from acute watery diarrhea due to any infectious etiology and should be treated, as any diarrhea, with oral rehydration (Chapter 16). Bacillary dysentery due to *Shigella* is clinically very similar to dysentery caused by *C. jejuni*, *Y. enterocolitica*, *Salmonella*, or enteroinvasive *E. coli*. Amebic dysentery does not manifest the high fever and constitutional symptoms of shigellosis. Furthermore, amebic infection can be differentiated by direct stool microscopy. Bacillary and amebic dysentery can also be distinguished by sigmoidoscopic examination. In shigellosis the observed mucosal ulcerations appear punched-out and are not undermined, as they often are in amebic infection (see Fig. 40–1 in color section).

TREATMENT AND PROGNOSIS. The therapy of shigellosis can be divided into four phases: emergency treatment of life-endangering complications, supportive measures, specific antimicrobial drugs, and health education.

Potentially Life-Endangering Emergencies. Shock accompanying severe diarrheal dehydration can occur in acute shigellosis, especially in infants. It must be vigorously combated with a rapid intravenous infusion of Ringer's lactate, isotonic saline, or a similar solution given as rapidly as possible. This bolus of fluid quickly expands the intravascular volume and begins to correct the signs of shock. Continuing rehydration in such patients must then proceed with either intravenous hypotonic electrolyte solutions or, preferably, oral glucose electrolyte solutions. Acidosis is corrected in the course of rehydration.

Convulsions are a well-recognized complication of shigellosis in infants and children. As with convulsions of any cause, aspiration, airway obstruction, and head trauma can occur during loss of consciousness and become more life-threatening than the underlying infection. Convulsions should be treated with intravenously administered diazepam (up to 10 mg) or phenobarbital (5 mg/kg body weight). The high fever usually associated with *Shigella* convulsions in children should be lowered with oral acetaminophen and by sponging the child in a tepid water bath.

Supportive Measures. Significant dehydration should be treated mainly with oral rehydration. Agents that suppress intestinal motility, such as diphenoxylate, loperamide, and tincture of opium, are generally to be avoided in known or suspected shigellosis. Such agents may prolong the duration of fever and excretion of *Shigella*. If antimotility agents are used to ameliorate the severe abdominal cramps of suspected shigellosis, only a single dose should be administered and always in conjunction with antibiotics active against *Shigella*.

There is no evidence that common antidiarrheal preparations such as kaolin-pectin formulas, lactobacilli, or bismuth subsalicylate have a significantly beneficial effect on the clinical or bacteriologic course of shigellosis. Nor is there evidence to suggest that these agents are deleterious and therefore contraindicated.

Specific Antimicrobial Therapy. Results of many controlled clinical trials have shown that appropriate antibiotics significantly decrease the duration of fever, diarrheal illness, and excretion of the pathogen in *Shigella* infections. This cumulative experience in conjunction with the fact that humans are the natural reservoir and host of this infection, which is transmitted by contact, provides a compelling rationale for treating all persons with shigellosis with antibiotics. This must be reconciled with the reality that only a few antibiotics have proven clinical efficacy in patients (even though many more show good activity in vitro against *Shigella*) and that widespread use of these effective antibiotics eventually leads to the emergence of resistant *Shigella* strains. Sulfonamides, the drugs of choice in the 1940s, were of little practical use by the mid-1950s because of resistance and were replaced by tetracycline. Widespread resistance to tetracycline resulted in ampicillin's becoming the drug of choice in the 1960s.

Trimethoprim-sulfamethoxazole replaced ampicillin as the most important antibiotic in the late 1970s and early 1980s because of widespread resistance to ampicillin. Treatment with trimethoprim-sulfamethoxazole is given for 5 days. The adult dosage is 160 mg of trimethoprim and 800 mg of sulfamethoxazole q 12 hr. Children should receive 10 mg/kg trimethoprim and 50 mg/kg sulfamethoxazole daily in two divided doses q 12 hr.

In the 1990s, members of the quinolone family of antimicrobials, e.g., nalidixic acid, ciprofloxacin, and norfloxacin, became mainstays in the treatment of *Shigella* infections that manifest resistance to other previously useful antibiotics. Particularly in dysentery due to *S. dysenteriae* type 1, the quinolones have proved invaluable. Nalidixic acid has been used in all age groups, including infants and young children. Whereas ciprofloxacin was initially used only in adults (500 mg q 12 hr for 5 days), it is increasingly being used in pediatrics to treat severely ill children with dysentery in areas where prevalent *Shigella* strains are known to be resistant to other antimicrobials. Parenteral ceftriaxone is a highly effective alternative for pediatric use when oral antibiotics cannot be tolerated; however, this regimen is costly for use in developing countries.

Health Education. Because *Shigella* is so readily transmitted from person to person by minute numbers of organisms, health workers must emphasize the importance of handwashing with soap after each defecation. Intervention studies have demonstrated the effectiveness of handwashing with soap and water in interrupting transmission of *Shigella*. Other studies have shown that the incidence of *Shigella* disease diminishes with increasing availability of water, even if the water is not potable.

PREVENTION AND CONTROL. Provision of adequate sanitation and proper hygiene practices minimize the chance of acquiring *Shigella*. In high-risk situations where local conditions favor transmission, attempts must be made to initiate a high standard of personal and food hygiene. This includes compulsive handwashing with soap and water after defecation and before food preparation. Food preparation and eating areas should be kept free of flies. The use of baited fly traps has proved effective in diminishing fly-borne transmission of shigellosis in areas where this mode of transmission is important.

Mass antibiotic therapy has been used with varying results in closed populations, such as in custodial institutions. While occasional successes have been reported, the general experience is that it usually fails.

For decades there have been attempts to prepare vaccines to prevent shigellosis. In the 1960s, streptomycin-dependent *Shigella* vaccines and the T_{32} colonial mutant (*S. flexneri* type 2a) strain were shown to be safe and protective when used as live oral vaccines. These vaccines suffered drawbacks, however, and never gained widespread usage. Research is continuing to develop improved *Shigella* vaccines that are well-tolerated and provide a high level of broad-spectrum, long-lived immunity following one or two doses. Encouraging results have been obtained with parenteral vaccines consisting of O polysaccharide of *S. sonnei* and *S. flexneri* type 2a conjugated to carrier proteins and with several new genetically engineered strains of *Shigella* used as live oral vaccines.

Bibliography

Bennish ML: Potentially lethal complications of shigellosis. Rev Infect Dis 4(Suppl 13):S319, 1991.

Cohen D, Green M, Block C, et al: Reduction of transmission of shigellosis by control of houseflies (*Musca domestica*). Lancet 337:993, 1991.

DiJohn D, Levine MM: Treatment of diarrhea. Infect Dis Clin North Am 2:719, 1988.

Gangarosa EJ, Perera DR, Mata LJ, et al: Epidemic Shiga bacillus dysentery in Central America. II: Epidemiologic studies in 1969. J Infect Dis 122:181, 1970.

Khan MU, Shahidullah M: Interruption of shigellosis by handwashing. Trans R Soc Trop Med Hyg 76:164, 1982.

Nataro JP, Seriwatana J, Fasano A, et al: Identification and cloning of a novel plasmid-encoded enterotoxin in enteroinvasive *Escherichia coli* and *Shigella*. Infect Immun 63:4721, 1995.

Raghupathy P, Date A, Shastry JCM, et al: Haemolytic uremic syndrome complicating *Shigella* dysentery in South Indian children. Br Med J 1:1518, 1978.

Rahaman MM, Khan MM, Aziz KMS, et al: An outbreak of dysentery caused by *Shigella dysenteriae* type 1 on a coral island in the Bay of Bengal. J Infect Dis 132:15, 1975.

41 *Cholera and Other Vibrioses*

M. John Albert and J. Glenn Morris, Jr.

DEFINITION. Cholera is a disease characterized by profuse, watery, typically "rice-water" diarrhea. Until recently, *Vibrio cholerae* strains belonging to serogroup O1 were regarded as the sole etiologic agents of cholera. However, since late 1992, *V. cholerae* serogroup O139 (synonym Bengal because of its first isolation from the coastal areas of the Bay of Bengal) has emerged as a second causative agent of cholera in the Indian subcontinent and neighboring countries. Both *V. cholerae* O1 and O139 strains can produce a protein enterotoxin known as cholera toxin (CT). Persons infected with toxin-producing strains of these organisms may become rapidly dehydrated; this dehydration, if untreated, may lead to death within 24 hours of onset of symptoms. *V. cholerae* of other O serogroups and other *Vibrio* species ("noncholera" vibrios) may cause diarrhea of mild to moderate severity. Some *Vibrio* species have also been implicated as a cause of wound infections and septicemia (Table 41–1).

41.1 *Cholera* (Vibrio cholerae O1 *and* O139 *Serogroups*)

ETIOLOGY. *V. cholerae* is a curved gram-negative rod with a characteristic rapid wobbly helical motility seen in dark-field or phase-contrast microscopy. While there have been multiple classification systems for the O antigen of *V. cholerae*, the system of Sakazaki and Shimada, which employs sera raised against killed organisms, is currently the one most

TABLE 41–1. *Vibrio* Species Implicated as a Cause of Human Disease

Species	Clinical Presentation		
	GI	**Wound/Ear**	**Septicemia**
V. cholerae			
V. cholerae O1	+ +	(+)	
V. cholerae O139	+ +		(+)
V. cholerae non-O1, non-O139	+ +	+	(+)
V. parahaemolyticus	+ +	+	(+)
V. fluvialis	+ +		?
V. mimicus	+ +	+	
V. hollisae	+ +		(+)
V. furnissii	+ +		
V. vulnificus	+	+ +	+ +
V. alginolyticus	?	+ +	?
V. damsela		+ +	?
V. cincinnatiensis			+
V. carchariae			+
V. metschnikovii	?		?

GI, gastrointestinal; + +, most common presentation; +, other clinical presentations; (+), rare presentation.

widely used; more than 150 different O groups have been identified with this system.

V. cholerae O1 has two biotypes, the classic and the El Tor. These differ in biochemical and epidemiologic parameters and by reason of El Tor's hemolytic characteristic (recent isolates from the seventh pandemic are nonhemolytic, with the exception of U.S. Gulf Coast isolates), agglutination of chicken erythrocytes, positive Voges-Proskauer reaction, polymyxin B resistance, milder spectrum of disease, resistance to Mukerjee's cholera phage IV but susceptibility to phage 5, and greater hardiness in the environment. Each biotype has two distinct and one intermediate serotype (Ogawa, Inaba, and Hikojima, respectively).

Recent molecular studies indicate that *V. cholerae* O139 is virtually identical genetically to seventh pandemic El Tor strains. However, O139 strains lack 22 kb of chromosomal DNA that encode the genes responsible for synthesis of the O1 antigen; in their place is a region of approximately 35 kb that encode expression of a polysaccharide capsule. Phenotypically, O139 strains are encapsulated, with a short O antigen side chain. The serotype distinctions seen in O1 strains (Ogawa vs. Inaba) do not occur in O139 strains. Biotype reactions of O139 strains are the same as those seen with El Tor strains, with the exception of resistance to cholera phages 4 and 5.

Survival of *V. cholerae* is facilitated by the ability of the organism to shift to a viable but nonculturable form, in which the bacterium "hibernates" until environmental or other signals trigger a return to a "normal" culturable state. The bacterium can also shift to a "rugose" morphology, producing an extracellular polysaccharide matrix that promotes adherence and biofilm formation and that protects the organism from adverse environmental conditions.

HISTORY. The classic work of John Snow during the London cholera epidemics of the 1830s elucidated many of the key characteristics of cholera epidemiology and illustrated the importance of providing hygienic water to prevent waterborne outbreaks. During the period, O'Shaughnessy pioneered chemical analyses of blood and stool in patients with cholera, and Thomas Latta of Leith was inspired by these analyses to conceive of replacing the water and salts lost in the copious cholera diarrhea by means of intravenous infu-

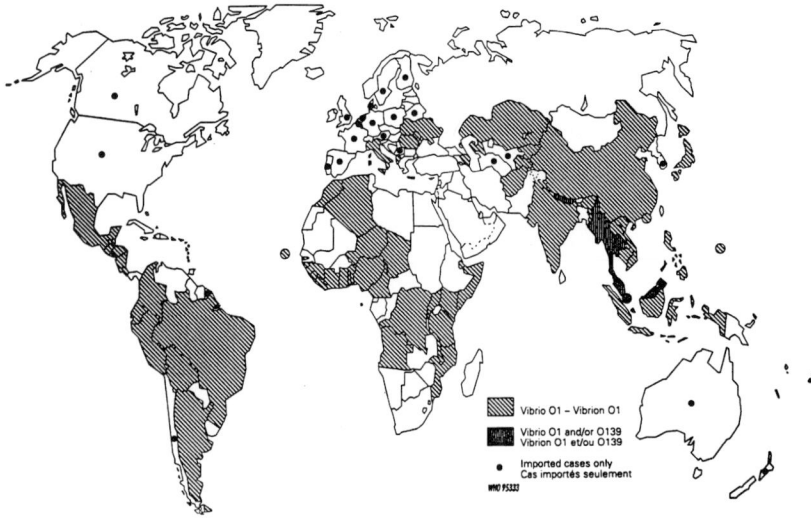

Figure **41–1.** Distribution of *Vibrio cholerae*, 1994. (From WHO, Wkly Epidemiol Rec 70:201, 1995.)

sions. These workers developed an infectious "principle," the nature of which awaited the later discovery of the vibrio by Pacini.

DISTRIBUTION AND INCIDENCE. Cholera has encompassed the globe in a series of pandemics. The seventh pandemic began in 1961 in the Celebes (Sulawesi) and has continued since, spreading through trade, tourism, and pilgrimage routes across Asia (the Philippines, Taiwan, Thailand, India, Pakistan, Bangladesh, Sri Lanka, countries of the former Soviet Union, and China) to Europe (Italy, Czechoslovakia, Spain), Africa (Tanzania, South Africa, Togo, Kenya, Congo, and other countries), and to the South Pacific. In January 1991, explosive cholera outbreaks occurred in cities along the Peruvian coast. Within a year, the majority of countries of South and Central America were affected. The Pan-American Health Organization estimates that by June 1993 there had been 830,000 cases of cholera in 20 Western Hemisphere countries accompanied by 7200 deaths, resulting in a striking increase in total reported global cholera cases and in the number of countries reporting cholera (Figs. 41–1 and 41–2).

V. cholerae O139 emerged as a cause of epidemic cholera in the Indian subcontinent in 1992. It caused an outbreak of

cholera in Madras in October of that year. In subsequent months, it spread to the rest of India (Fig. 41–3). It spread into Bangladesh to urban Dhaka in January 1993 following a large Muslim festival. Throughout 1993, *V. cholerae* O139 surpassed the El Tor strain as the predominant organism causing cholera in Bangladesh and other parts of the Indian subcontinent (Fig. 41–4). At the same time, *V. cholerae* O139 caused cholera in several neighboring countries, including Sri Lanka, Nepal, Burma, Thailand, Malaysia, China, Hong Kong, Pakistan, and Saudi Arabia, with imported cases re-

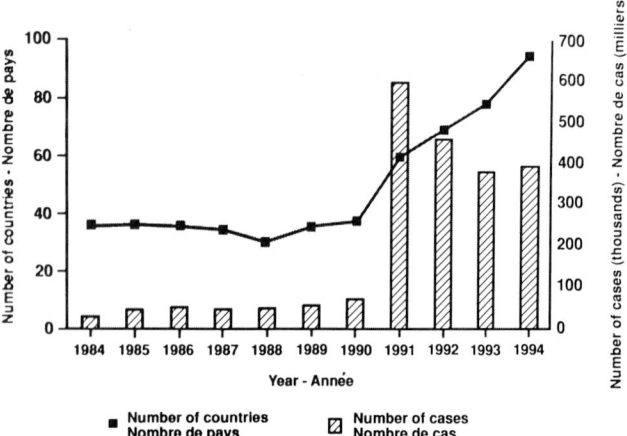

Figure **41–2.** Number of cases of cholera and number of countries reporting cholera, 1984–1994. (From WHO, Wkly Epidemiol Rec 70:201, 1995.)

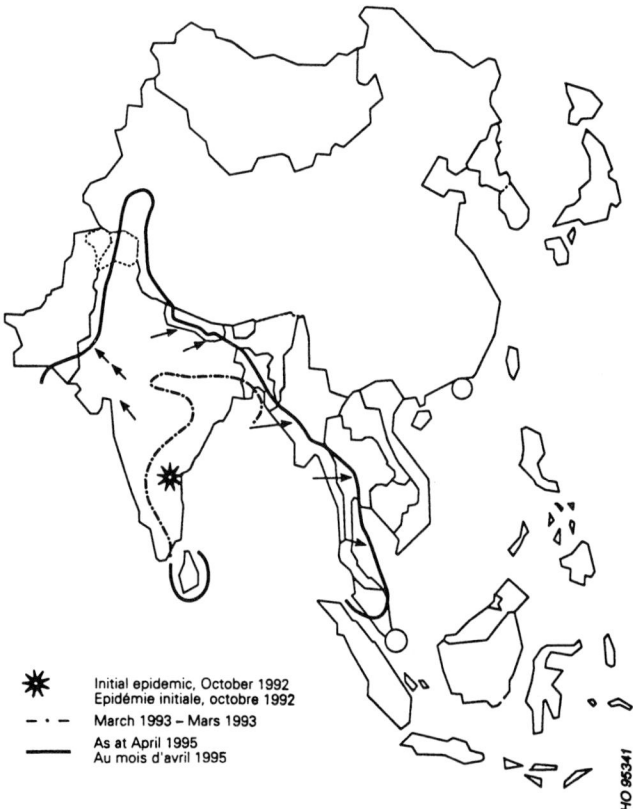

Figure **41–3.** Spread of *V. cholerae* O139 Bengal through the Indian subcontinent and Asia, 1992–1995.

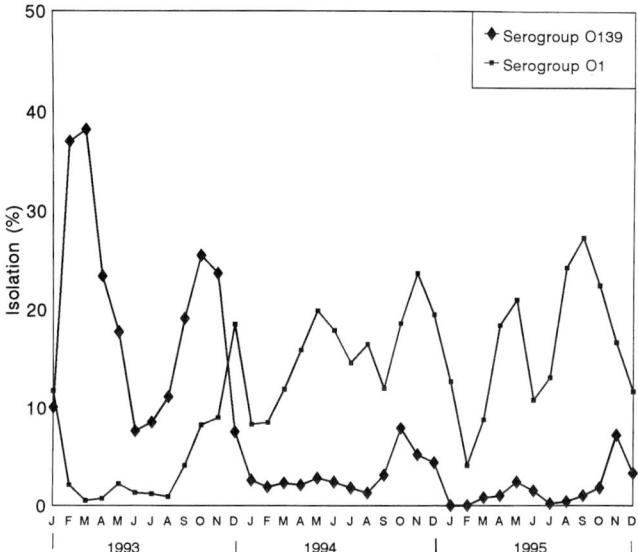

Figure 41–4. Percentage of total *V. cholerae* isolates within serogroups O1 and O139, respectively, in Dhaka, Bangladesh, 1993–1995.

ported from the United States, Japan, Germany, and the United Kingdom. El Tor strains have subsequently re-emerged as the predominant strain causing cholera in Bangladesh and India; the risk of pandemic cholera due to *V. cholerae* O139 remains to be determined,

Cholera has a worldwide distribution, with endemic foci of disease remaining in many, if not most, of the areas through which the epidemic wave of the seventh pandemic has passed (Fig. 41–1). In 1994, 94 countries reported a total of 384,403 cholera cases to the World Health Organization, including the dramatic cholera outbreak that devastated the Rwandan refugee camps in Goma, Congo in July. Major outbreaks also affected Afghanistan, Brazil, Guinea, Guinea-Bissau, and Somalia. A number of countries known to have endemic cholera did not report cases, however, and in some that did, the reported cases represent only a small fraction of the actual number of cases. In endemic areas, e.g., Bengal, clinical case-attack rates vary from 2 to 6 per 1000 population per year, but inapparent or asymptomatic infections are estimated to be 5 to 27 times more common.

EPIDEMIOLOGY. In endemic areas, cholera is rare under 1 year of age, because infants are protected by factors such as maternal antibodies acquired transplacentally or in breast milk. Weanling malnutrition (with associated hypochlorhydria) along with increasing contact with contaminated water leads to the peak incidence in the nonimmune 2- to 9-year age group. Up to 20% of cholera cases, however, occur in young adults in the child-rearing age group, and the nutritional and economic consequences of loss of a parent often prove fatal to surviving members of impoverished families. In nonendemic areas, or in areas into which a new strain is being introduced, cases tend to be distributed across all age groups. This latter pattern was seen in the initial spread of cholera across South and Central America and in the emergence of epidemic O139 disease in the Indian subcontinent and Asia.

For unknown reasons, persons with blood group O are significantly more likely to have severe disease. Factors that predispose to hypochlorhydria (malnutrition, gastrectomy, acid-reducing medications) also increase susceptibility to illness. The atrophic gastritis and hypochlorhydria of chronic *Helicobacter pylori* infection has also been associated with an increased risk of severe illness.

Marine and estuarine waters serve as the primary reservoir for *V. cholerae*, with the organism able to live and grow in the environment by adhering to chitinaceous fauna, certain algae, or higher aquatic plants, or as a free-living organism. In keeping with this concept, a single clone of *V. cholerae* has persisted for over 30 years in the U.S. Gulf Coast environment, in a setting in which there would be minimal opportunity for reintroduction of the bacterium from human sources.

TRANSMISSION. Water has traditionally been regarded as the primary vehicle of infection for cholera. However, *V. cholerae* concentrations in surface water of endemic areas ($\leq 10^2$ organisms/L) are usually far below doses (10^{11} organisms) needed to cause disease in most healthy normochlorhydric volunteers. Transmission may be facilitated by increased levels of susceptibility to infection in host populations, increased levels of contamination associated with sewage contamination of water and food supplies, or protection of the bacterium from the effect of stomach acid by ingestion with food. In volunteer studies, the infective inoculum of the El Tor biotype was lowered when given with milk or with rice and fried fish, similar to the diet in Bengal. Alkaline dietary residues, inhibition of acid secretion by dietary fats, or adsorption of vibrios to cells or to food particles (such as chitin) may all protect the bacterium from gastric acid.

Foods, usually those in contact with contaminated water, have been the source of outbreaks in many newly infected areas; these foods have included mussels (Italy), salted fish (Guam), raw cockles and water (Portugal), crab and coconut milk (United States), and possibly raw vegetables. Cooked rice appears to be a particularly effective vehicle, with rice implicated as the cause of a number of outbreaks in settings as diverse as meals served at African funerals, on a U.S. oil rig platform, and to a group of luxury cruise ship passengers in Thailand (the latter associated with an O139 strain). Cholera is not easily spread by person-to-person contact. Nosocomial transmission has been reported, and care should be taken to ensure that water and food served within a hospital are not contaminated with the organism.

Cholera displays a striking seasonality in endemic areas. In the Indian subcontinent, the seasonal peak in cases occurs earlier in the year as one moves westward, possibly linked to variations in monsoon onset and local ecologic factors. In East Bengal (Bangladesh), epidemics start at the end of the monsoon (August to September), when floodwaters are high, and peak during October to December as waters dry up. By January, cases have sharply diminished and few are seen until the smaller spring wave (April to June) begins. In West Bengal (Calcutta), in contrast, the spring wave is prominent and the winter wave is absent. In South America, cases are concentrated in the summer months of January and February.

It has been hypothesized that during interepidemic periods *V. cholerae* persists in surface waters as a viable but nonculturable form in association with plankton (copepods and blue-green algae). Just prior to the onset of cholera season in the postmonsoon period in Bangladesh, plankton blooms occur, which may trigger vibrios to transform into a culturable form and, in turn, initiate epidemics. In support of this hypothesis, nonculturable *V. cholerae* have been demonstrated in blue-green algae by a fluorescent antibody technique. However, further work is needed to define the environmental conditions that actually trigger the shift from nonculturable to culturable forms and to assess the role that this process plays in the epidemiology of the disease.

PATHOGENICITY AND PATHOPHYSIOLOGY. After ingestion and stomach transit, surviving vibrios must multiply and colonize the small bowel. The toxin-coregulated pilus (TCP) appears to be a key colonization factor: In volunteer studies, a strain containing a mutation in the gene encoding the TCP subunit (tcpA) failed to colonize and produce disease. Expression of tcpA is controlled by the *toxR* gene, which regulates expression of a variety of virulence-associated factors, including cholera toxin.

Cholera Toxin. A protein enterotoxin, cholera toxin (CT), is the primary factor responsible for the severe diarrhea seen in patients with clinical cholera. The cholera toxin gene (of which there may be multiple copies) is carried in the chromosome of toxigenic *V. cholerae* O1 and O139 strains. Cholera toxin consists of cyclase-activating (A) and five binding or light (B) subunits (choleragenoid) of 28,000 and 11,600 dalton molecular weight, respectively. The B subunit itself is nondiarrheagenic but binds the toxin molecule to GM_1 ganglioside in the cell membrane, permitting the active A moiety to enter the cell. Subsequently, adenyl cyclase activity inside the basolateral enterocyte border is enhanced by adenyl diphosphonucleotide (ADP) ribosylation of the enzyme. The resulting increase in cell cyclic adenosine monophosphate (cAMP) is associated with the net secretion of water and electrolytes into the gut lumen. The response to CT may also be mediated by prostaglandins, vasoactive intestinal peptide (VIP), and elements of the enteric nervous system. Other toxins that may contribute to diarrhea are zonula occludens toxin (Zot), accessory cholera enterotoxin (Ace), and hemolysin/cytolysin.

The genes encoding CT (*ctx*), Zot (*zot*), Ace (*ace*), an open reading frame of unknown function (*orfu*), and core-encoded pilus (*cep*) are located on a 4.5 kb region of the chromosome called the core region. The core region is flanked by one or more copies of a 2.7 kb sequence called RS1. Recombination between RS1 sequence can lead to tandem duplication and amplification of the core region as well as deletion of the core region. A similar arrangement of virulence genes in the core region of the chromosome has been shown for *V. cholerae* O139. Waldor and Mekalanos have demonstrated that the core region is part of a filamentous bacteriophage, related to coliphage M13, allowing for horizontal transfer of these genes among *V. cholerae* strains.

Although cholera toxin is the critical diarrheagenic factor in cholera, *V. cholerae* strains that do not carry the cholera toxin gene, or from which the cholera toxin gene has been deleted by genetic techniques, can cause diarrheal disease. Mechanisms remain unclear, although there are suggestions that diarrhea-associated CT-negative strains produce an increased inflammatory response in the gut.

LPS/Capsule. *V. cholerae* O1 has a typically smooth lipopolysaccharide (LPS) and upon SDS-PAGE, the LPS separates into a lipid A, core region, and a long side chain showing a ladder-like pattern.

Unlike *V. cholerae* O1, *V. cholerae* O139 has a polysaccharide capsule. Strains are able to undergo phase variation, shifting between an opaque colony morphology (encapsulated variant) and a translucent morphology (unencapsulated or minimally encapsulated). The capsule confers the property of serum resistance. Among non-O1 *V. cholerae* strains, the degree of encapsulation is positively associated with the risk of bacteremia; *V. cholerae* O139, which is "moderately" encapsulated, has been reported to cause bacteremia in some susceptible hosts (persons with underlying liver disease or who are immunocompromised). The capsule functions as an adherence factor of *V. cholerae* O139, as strains devoid of capsule are poor colonizers. The O139 strain arose from an O1 El Tor strain by deletion of the chromosomal region that encodes the O1 antigen specificity and acquisition of a novel chromosomal region that encodes the O139 antigen specificity.

IMMUNE RESPONSES. Infection-derived immunity exists in cholera. In volunteer studies, protection against disease conferred by an initial infection with a classic strain lasted

for at least 3 years, the longest interval being with the same biotype. Immunity is serotype specific, but cross-immunity occurs, chiefly when Inaba confers immunity against the Ogawa serotype. However, whereas an initial infection with a classic strain of *V. cholerae* is associated with complete protection, initial infection with an El Tor biotype is less protective.

Animal studies have shown that there is a synergistic effect of antibacterial and antitoxic immunity, with antibacterial immunity being the more important. Serum vibriocidal antibody titer correlates with protection in O1 strains, but no such correlation is seen with serum antitoxin titer. Most of the vibriocidal antibody is directed against LPS, and some against unidentified protein antigens. In addition, host antibody responses to a variety of antigens including pili, outer membrane proteins, and in vivo expressed antigens can be demonstrated. Even though TCP is the most important adhesion antigen, antibody response to it is rather poor.

Infection with *V. cholerae* O139 elicits antibodies to CT, LPS, and CPS. Studies in animals suggest that antibodies directed against the CPS are protective; rabbits immunized with a CPS tetanus toxoid conjugate showed protection against subsequent high-level challenge. Occurrence of O139 cholera, predominantly in adults, in O1 cholera–endemic areas of the Indian subcontinent, suggests that pre-existing immunity to *V. cholerae* O1 is not cross-protective against O139. This has been corroborated by animal studies.

PATHOLOGY

Histology. The small intestinal mucosa in patients with cholera seems histologically intact. Ultrastructural studies of small intestinal mucosal biopsies of O1 cholera patients in India have demonstrated several abnormalities; widening of the intercellular space and alteration of apical junctional complexes are prominent in the villus epithelium, whereas blebbing of the microvillus border and mitochondrial changes are more prominent in the crypt epithelium. There are no data on the histology of the small intestinal mucosa in cholera due to *V. cholerae* O139 in naturally infected subjects in cholera-endemic areas. In a volunteer model in North American volunteers, no histologic or ultrastructural abnormalities of the upper small intestine were evident.

Changes in Electrolyte Metabolism. The principal effect of cholera toxin in humans and in dogs is a 70% reduction in unidirectional influx of water and ions from gut lumen into gut mucosal cells. A slight increase in outflux from cell to lumen may also occur. The net sum of these two movements (influx and outflux) yields the net secretion observed. In canine jejunum, cholera toxin reduces unidirectional influxes of many molecules, including tritiated water and ^{14}C-labeled urea; the water becomes totally nonabsorbable. In short-circuited tissue preparations, chiefly chloride absorption is inhibited. Cholera toxin thus causes a diffuse decrease in gut mucosal permeability to a wide range of molecules, leading, in turn, to a shift from primarily absorptive to primarily secretory osmoregulating mechanisms. Net chloride and sodium absorption are absent, and net secretion is present during cholera; glucose, potassium, and bicarbonate absorption, however, remain intact in cholera and allied diarrheas, as does glucose-linked enhancement of sodium and water absorption. Thus, although plain salt water is nonabsorbable during cholera and aggravates the diarrhea, the addition of glucose renders the solution absorbable and thereby provides the physiologic basis of oral rehydration and maintenance therapy. Galactose and certain amino acids (glycine, alanine) have an effect similar to that of glucose. Fructose is ineffective.

CLINICAL MANIFESTATIONS. The clinical manifestations

of cholera due to *V. cholerae* O1 and O139 are virtually identical.

Symptoms. After an incubation period of about 45 hours, cholera diarrheal fluid accumulates, filling the small intestinal lumen to the point of causing gut distention, increased intestinal motility, decreased transit time, and diarrhea. All other clinical symptoms result entirely from the effects of loss of fluid and electrolytes in stool and vomitus. These changes lead to circulatory collapse, diminished total body water, and decreased plasma volume. The alterations, coupled with the acidosis that results from stool bicarbonate loss, lead to peripheral venospasm, pooling of remaining circulating blood volume in the heart and lungs, and ultimately circulatory failure and death. The cause and mechanism of vomiting in cholera and other intestinal infections are unknown; gut distention may be contributory. Toxin absorption plays no role in cholera pathogenesis.

Most cholera infections are, however, asymptomatic or cause only mild symptoms indistinguishable from those of other mild diarrheas; such patients rarely seek therapy. In most clinically apparent cases the first symptom is diarrhea, which, in severe cases, can proceed over several hours to assume a translucent, fishy-smelling, rice-water appearance. Typically, vomiting occurs early and abruptly; it occasionally begins before diarrhea and usually before dehydration or acidosis appears. Brief fever occurs in 25% of hospitalized cholera patients. Early symptoms that are more prominent in adults with cholera than in adults with *Escherichia coli* or rotavirus diarrhea include borborygmi and abdominal fullness, heralding emesis.

The diarrhea rate may quickly reach 500 to 1000 mL/hr, leading rapidly to tachycardia, hypotension, and vascular collapse due to dehydration. As dehydration progresses, the tongue becomes dry, urine production ceases, skin turgor and elasticity decrease, eyes become deeply sunken (Fig. 41–5), fingers become wrinkled, and the voice becomes raspy. Severe acidosis is associated with a Kussmaul breathing pattern. Although patients are prostrated and weak, they remain conscious, albeit sometimes obtunded. If coma occurs, further diagnostic workup is necessary to rule out complicating disorders.

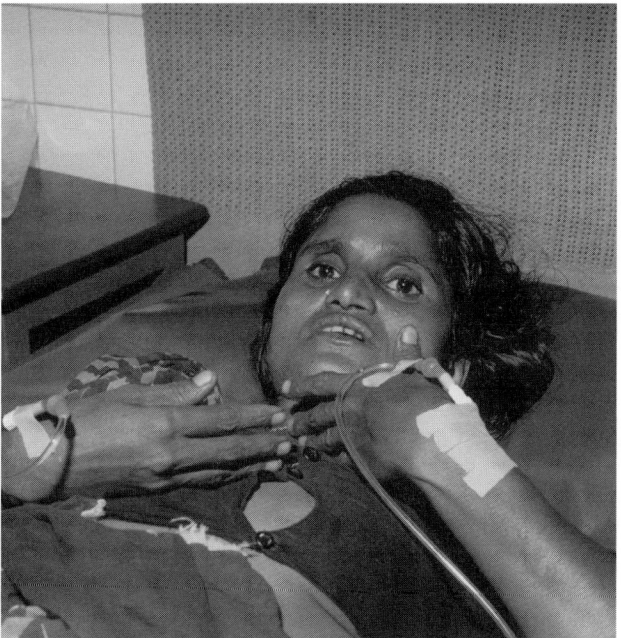

Figure 41–5. Cholera patient with severe dehydration.

Laboratory Abnormalities. Sodium and potassium loss from muscle accompanies electrolyte depletion and leads to cramps in the extremities and abdominal muscles. Water depletion is reflected by increased plasma protein concentrations and elevated hematocrit values; the plasma bicarbonate level falls, with progressive loss of plasma bicarbonate into stool. The resulting acidosis elevates plasma potassium levels despite overall body potassium depletion. Plasma sodium and chloride concentrations remain in the normal range. Cumulative potassium loss may result in severe potassium depletion with or without hypokalemia in convalescence; ventricular dysrhythmias, muscle weakness, paralytic ileus, and nephropathy may result. Hypoglycemia occurs in patients, mostly children, with cholera and may cause permanent brain damage. It appears to be primarily due to a failure of gluconeogenesis.

Complications. Complications consist chiefly of aspiration pneumonia after vomiting, especially in children, and the residual effects of improperly managed electrolyte deficits or hypoglycemia. Among properly treated patients, deaths are rare (<1%); death may, however, ensue in patients with coexisting pulmonary diseases and malnutrition.

DIAGNOSIS. The clinical diagnosis is based on the rapid onset of diarrhea and vomiting with dehydration and the profuse, rice-water stool. A presumptive bacteriologic diagnosis can be made by phase contrast or darkfield microscopy of a hanging-drop preparation of fresh liquid stool by detecting the characteristic helical vibrio motion. Stool spirochetes have a screwlike motion that experienced workers can easily distinguish from that of *V. cholerae*. The addition of a drop of group O1 and O139 antiserum to the slide stops the motility of the specific vibrios.

Culture. A fresh rectal swab or stool specimen should be plated directly on suitable selective media such as thiosulfate–citrate–bile salt–sucrose (TCBS) agar or taurocholate-tellurite-gelatin agar (TTGA; Monsur's medium). Suspected vibrio colonies are confirmed as *V. cholerae* O1 or O139 by slide agglutination with specific antisera to these serogroups. *V. cholerae* O1 serogroup can be further serotyped with Inaba or Ogawa by serotype-specific antisera. Enrichment broth is commonly used to recover vibrios from carriers, from patients late in the course of their disease, or from partially treated cases. Alkaline peptone water, the most commonly used enrichment broth, should be subcultured after 6 to 8 hours of incubation. When processing is delayed, specimens should be placed in Cary-Blair transport medium. Alternatively, filter paper should be soaked in liquid stool and sealed in airtight plastic bags. Vibrios preserved and transported in ambient temperature by these methods remain viable for 4 to 5 weeks.

DNA Probes and PCR Technique. Since *V. cholerae* O1 and O139 have identical *ctx* genes, these organisms can be rapidly identified by hybridization of colony blots or vibrios directly in the stool with DNA fragment probes and synthetic oligonucleotide probes for *ctx*. Radioactive labels have been superseded by nonradioactive labels, e.g., alkaline phosphatase. The PCR technique has been used to detect *ctx* sequence. Specific primers have been used that amplified a 302 bp region and could detect as little as 1 pg of DNA and three viable cells from broth culture after 40 cycles of amplification. The PCR technique was more sensitive than culture and a bead-ELISA (for CT) for diagnosis of *V. cholerae* O1; it was also superior for detection of the organism from contaminated foodstuffs.

Rapid Tests. Examination of cholera stools by darkfield or phase contrast microscopy for the characteristic darting motility and inhibition of motility by specific antisera is a less sensitive technique. Monoclonal antibody–based coagglutination tests for *V. cholerae* O1 and O139 (Cholera Screen for *V. cholerae* O1 and Bengal Screen for *V. cholerae* O139) (New Horizons Diagnostic Corp.), SMART (sensitive membrane antigen rapid test), a colloidal gold-based colorimetric test for *V. cholerae* O1 (cholera SMART) and O139 (Bengal SMART) (New Horizons Diagnostic Corp.), and a latex agglutination test for *V. cholerae* O1 (Denka Seiken, Tokyo) have been developed and are commercially available. These tests have comparable sensitivity and specificity to standard culture. Moreover, results are available in minutes and can be employed for field diagnosis.

Serology. After an acute episode of cholera due to *V. cholerae* O1 or O139, a sharp rise in antibody to cholera toxin occurs. Persons infected with *V. cholerae* O1 also show a vibriocidal antibody response to *V. cholerae* O1. In some volunteer studies, by using the standard vibriocidal assay patterned after *V. cholerae* O1, a vibriocidal response to *V. cholerae* O139 could not be demonstrated. However, by modifying the standard assay through the use of a lower inoculum of a lower protease-producing strain and by increasing the complement concentration, a vibriocidal assay for *V. cholerae* O139 has been developed that can demonstrate a vibriocidal antibody response in patients infected with the O139 serotype. Using this modified assay, it has been shown that O139 patients develop a vibriocidal antibody response. These patients do not mount a vibriocidal response to *V. cholerae* O1, and neither do O1 patients have a vibriocidal response to *V. cholerae* O139.

The identification of a sharp rise in the titer of vibriocidal and antitoxic antibodies between acute and convalescent sera is virtually diagnostic of cholera. In a single convalescent serum sample in a nonendemic area, the presence of an antitoxin by immunoglobulin G (IgG) ELISA at fourfold or greater titer than the negative control and a vibriocidal antibody titer >1280 are strong evidence for a recent infection. In endemic areas, high background levels of immunity render serologic testing of less utility, and caution should be expressed in interpretation based on a single serum sample. Serologic responses can also be influenced by cross reactivity with antigens from other species, including *Brucella*, *Citrobacter*, and *Yersinia*. Antibodies directed against *V. cholerae* O139 may also cross react with *V. cholerae* serogroups O22 and O155 or *Aeromonas trota*. Similarly, antitoxic antibodies directed against the heat-labile toxin (LT) of enterotoxigenic *E. coli* give positive responses in assays for anticholera toxin antibodies.

Subtyping of V. cholerae. Subtyping of *V. cholerae* is useful for epidemiologic studies. These include phage typing, *ctx* gene typing, multilocus enzyme electrophoresis (MEE), rRNA gene typing (ribotyping) and pulsed-field gel electro-phoresis (PAGE). The phage typing technique is limited to reference laboratories owing to the availability of only a small number of phage sets. There currently is not a consensus typing scheme and discrimination of strains is less than satisfactory. Restriction fragment length polymorphism (RFLP) analysis of *ctx* gene detects sequence divergence in genes flanking the *ctx* locus. This technique has yielded useful epidemiologic information on clonality of isolates from different geographic areas. Sequence divergence in the PCR-generated amplicons of *ctx*B has also been useful in discriminating among strains from the U.S. Gulf Coast, Australia, the seventh pandemic, and Latin America. MEE may not be useful in distinguishing strains within a single outbreak, but can assist in investigating the origin of new outbreaks of disease. Ribotyping yields greater diversity than MEE technique. In general, PFGE is as discriminating or sometimes more discriminating than ribotyping.

DIFFERENTIAL DIAGNOSIS. In epidemic settings, no other disease can consistently cause severe, life-threatening diarrhea and dehydration in adults. In individual cases, diarrhea that approaches the severity of cholera can be caused by other pathogens, including enterotoxigenic *E. coli* and strains of non-O1 *V. cholerae*. Among children, rotavirus also can be a cause of severe dehydrating diarrhea. These disorders respond to the same therapeutic fluid regimen as cholera.

Among noninfectious causes, acute arsenic poisoning is sometimes mistaken for cholera. Rare adenomas that produce vasoactive intestinal polypeptide (VIP) and related tumors may present with cholera-like diarrhea.

TREATMENT. The replacement, either intravenously or orally, of fluid and electrolytes lost through diarrhea and vomiting is the cornerstone of therapy for cholera. Most mild to moderately dehydrated cholera patients can usually be treated with oral rehydration solution (ORS) alone (Chapter 16). The composition of ORS approximates the water and salts contained in the diarrheal stool. Intravenous electrolyte solutions should be used only for the initial rehydration of severely dehydrated patients and in patients with constant vomiting.

Assessment. Patients are first assessed for dehydration according to the criteria given in Table 41–2. To guide rehydration therapy, each patient should be weighed on admission. This is helpful in calculating the individual's net fluid requirement. As a first step to therapy, the estimated volume needed for rehydration should be calculated. This is determined by the patient's body weight in kilograms and clinical estimate of dehydration. For example, a severely dehydrated adult weighing 50 kg will require 5 liters of rehydration fluid to correct rehydration (10% of 50 kg = 5 kg = 5 L).

Intravenous Therapy. Intravenous fluids should be given

TABLE 41–2. Assessment of Diarrhea Patients for Dehydration

Condition	No Dehydration	Some Dehydration	Severe Dehydration
General	Well, alert	Restless, irritable*	Lethargic or unconscious, floppy*
Eyes	Normal	Sunken	Very sunken and dry
Mouth and tongue	Moist	Dry	Very dry
Thirst	Drinks normally, not thirsty	Thirsty, drinks eagerly*	Drinks poorly or not able to drink*
Skin pinch	Goes back quickly	Goes back slowly*	Goes back very slowly*
Status	The patient has no signs of dehydration	If the patient has two or more signs, including at least one sign,* there is some dehydration	If the patient has two or more signs, including at least one sign,* there is severe dehydration

In adults and children older than 5 years, other signs for severe dehydration are absent radial pulse* and low blood pressure.* The skin pinch may be less useful in patients with marasmus or kwashiorkor or obese patients. Tears are a relevant sign only for infants and young children.

TABLE 41–3. Comparison of Cholera Stools in Adults and Children and of Intravenous and Oral Fluids Used in Cholera Treatment

				mmol/L	
Cholera Stools	Na$^+$	K$^+$	Cl$^-$	HCO$_3^-$	Glucose
Adults	130	15	100	45	—
Children	105	25	90	30	—
Intravenous fluids					
Ringer's lactate (Hartmann's fluid)	131	4	111	29	—
Diarrhea treatment solution (DTS)	118	13	83	48	50
Dhaka solution	113	13	98	48	—
2 saline:1 lactate	158	—	103	56	—
Normal saline	154	—	154	—	—
Half-Darrow's solution with 2.5% glucose*	61	17.5	52	26	150
Oral rehydration solution as recommended by WHO	90	20	80	30 (10 as citrate)	111

*Full-strength Darrow's solution contains too much potassium, while half-strength has too little sodium for correcting dehydration in cholera.

rapidly to cholera patients to quickly restore circulating volume. Half the estimated volume of fluid requirement in a severely dehydrated patient should be given in the first hour, initially as rapidly as possible until the radial pulse is palpable. The patient should be fully hydrated in 2 to 4 hours, at which time the IV line can be removed. Sometimes, it may be necessary to start an IV line at several sites simultaneously to restore circulation quickly. The compositions of ORS and IV fluids are given in Table 41–3. The composition by weight of the ORS solution is given in Table 41–4.

Oral Rehydration. ORS, rather than IV fluids, can be given for both initial rehydration and replacement of ongoing fecal losses for most patients with mild to moderate dehydration. Early in treatment, some patients may continue to vomit, and this may discourage ORS administration. However, with small, frequent drinks, most patients will retain enough fluid to become rehydrated (Fig. 41–6).

The adequacy of fluid replacement should be assessed by return of (1) radial pulse to normal, (2) normal skin turgor, (3) a feeling of comfort to the patient, (4) fullness to the neck veins, (5) urine output within 12 to 20 hours of initial rehydration, and (6) weight gain. A severely dehydrated patient should gain 8 to 10% of the body weight after adequate rehydration.

After the initial fluid and electrolyte deficit has been corrected, the ongoing losses should be replaced; this is known as maintenance therapy. For older children and adults, fluids

normally consumed (e.g., water) can be given as desired in addition to ORS. For infants and young children, breast-feeding should be continued, and to non–breast fed babies, other fluids should be offered at regular intervals.

Patients are easily treated while lying on a cholera cot (Fig. 41–7), since this allows convenient collection and measurement of stool and urine separately. While the volume of stool output is measured periodically (e.g., every 4 to 8 hours), it is important that an equivalent amount of ORS is taken by

TABLE 41–4. ORS Solution: Composition by Weight of Oral Rehydration Salts (ORS) (for Preparation of 1 L of ORS Solution)*

Ingredient	Weight (g)
Sodium chloride	3.5
Trisodium citrate, dihydrate	2.9
or	
Sodium hydrogen carbonate (sodium bicarbonate)	2.5
Potassium chloride	1.5
Glucose, anhydrous†‡	20.5

*The formula for oral rehydration salts (ORS) recommended by WHO.
†Or glucose, monohydrate, 22 g; or sucrose 4 g.
‡Fifty grams of rice powder can replace 20 g glucose. To prepare a rice powder solution, put 50 g rice powder (i.e., rice flour) in 1100 mL of water and bring it to boil. Continue boiling for approximately 7 minutes when the mixture becomes opalescent. Allow it to cool, then add and mix the three salts. Serve the solution warm. After 8 hours, discard and prepare a fresh batch.

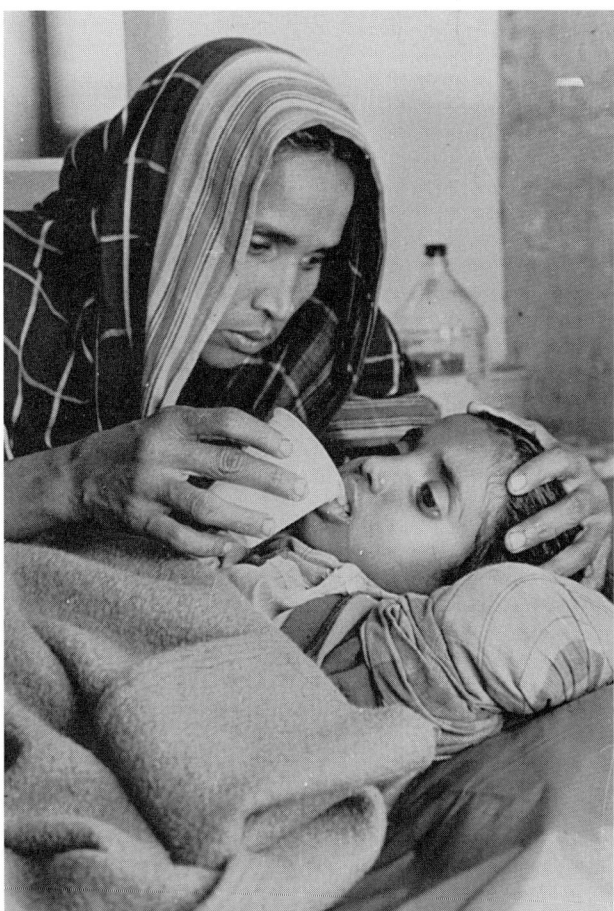

Figure **41–6.** Feeding of oral rehydration solution.

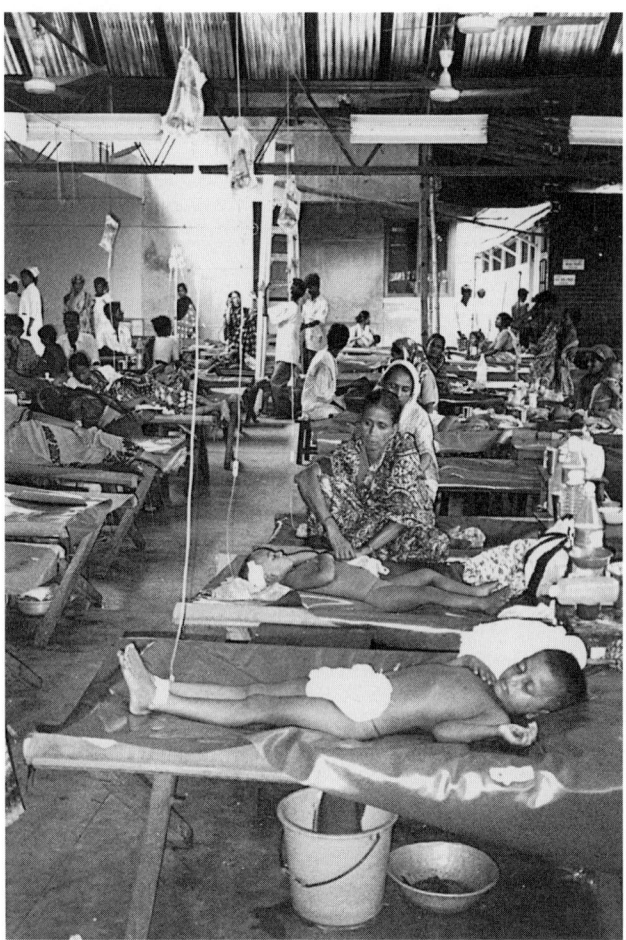

Figure 41–7. Dhaka treatment center, with cholera cots.

the patient. An input-output chart at the bedside should be maintained. In patients with heavy purging, signs of dehydration may recur while they are on oral maintenance therapy. In such cases, additional IV fluids are given, following which oral maintenance should be resumed.

Antibiotic Therapy. Antibiotics can reduce the volume and duration of diarrhea and shorten the period during which cholera organisms are excreted in stool. The choice of drug should take into account the local pattern of resistance of *V. cholerae* to different antibiotics (Table 41–5). Resistant organisms should be suspected if diarrhea continues after 48 hours of antibiotic treatment.

Complications of Therapy. Pulmonary edema is caused by

giving too much IV fluid, especially when metabolic acidosis has not been corrected. The latter is most likely to occur when normal saline is used for IV rehydration and ORS is not given at the same time. ORS is unlikely to cause pulmonary edema. Renal failure may result when there is inadequate rehydration or when shock is not rapidly corrected. Severe hypoglycemia rarely occurs; if it does, it is likely to be seen in children with malnutrition. If hypoglycemia is suspected, appropriate measures should be taken.

MANAGEMENT OF CHOLERA EPIDEMICS

Epidemiology and Prevention. A cholera outbreak should be suspected if there is a sudden increase in the number of patients with acute watery diarrhea, passing rice-water stools. The health authorities should be notified immediately. During cholera outbreaks in newly affected areas, people of all ages may contract the disease. However, the more mobile members of the community (usually adults) are more frequently affected because of their greater exposure to possible sources of contamination. In contrast, a preponderance of cases in children suggests that the disease is endemic in the area. When a suspected cholera epidemic occurs in an area where the disease has not been previously confirmed, bacteriologic and epidemiologic investigation should be promptly arranged to determine the cause of the outbreak. Case-control studies may help define the mode of transmission.

Since cholera is contracted from drinking water or eating food contaminated with cholera organisms, prevention is based on reducing the chances of ingesting vibrios. When cholera appears in a community, efforts must be intensified to promote the sanitary disposal of human waste, the provision of safe water, and safe practices in handling food. Mass chemoprophylaxis is ineffective and leads to antibiotic resistance. In an acute phase of an emergency, e.g., the cholera epidemic that occurred in Rwandan refugees in Goma, Congo, cholera vaccination is not likely to be useful and is not recommended. However, after the acute phase has passed, refugee camps may still have a substantial risk of cholera. In the stable phase, two uses of cholera vaccine may be considered: "pre-emptive" immunization, in which vaccine is given before an epidemic occurs, and "reactive" immunization, in which vaccine is given soon after an epidemic is recognized, in an attempt to shorten its course.

Management and Logistics. The principles of clinical management of individual patients during outbreaks of cholera are the same as previously described. If treatment centers are already established, efforts may have to be made to enlarge the inventory of rehydration supplies and to reorganize the medical staff to handle an increased number of patients. In the absence of treatment centers, temporary facilities can be established in huts, school buildings, or tents, and in favourable conditions, no buildings are needed at all. A team should be formed to organize the available resources and

TABLE 41–5. Antimicrobial Agents Used to Treat Cholera

Antimicrobial Agent	Dose	
	Children	*Adults*
Tetracycline	12.5 mg/kg, 4 times daily for 3 days	500 mg, 4 times daily for 3 days
Doxycycline	Not recommended for children	300 mg, single dose
Furazolidone	1.25 mg/kg, 4 times daily for 3 days	100 mg, 4 times daily for 3 days
Trimethoprim-sulfamethoxazole (TMP-SMX)	TMP 5 mg/kg and SMX 25 mg/kg, twice daily for 3 days	TMP 160 mg and SMX 800 mg thrice daily for 3 days
Erythromycin	10 mg/kg, 3 times daily for 3 days	500 mg, 4 times daily for 3 days
Norfloxacin	Not recommended for children	400 mg, 2 times daily for 3 days
Ciprofloxacin	Not recommended for children	500 mg, 2 times daily for 3 days

TABLE 41–6. Supplies Required for the Treatment of Cholera in Field Facilities

Intravenous solution (5–10 L/patient)
5–10 mL syringes
18-gauge needles for adults and 21- to 23-gauge needles for children
Tape, arm splints, poles to hang IV drips
Scalp vein sets*
Nasogastric tubes†
ORS packets (10–15 one liter packets/patient)
500 mL or 1 L bottles for ORS
Clean water for mixing ORS
Effective antimicrobial agents against the causative organism
Kidney dishes
Spirit lamps
Flashlights (or hurricane lantern)
Cotton
Alcohol
Soap
Disinfectant
Bleaching powder
If possible:
   Cholera cots
   Plastic drain sheets
   Plastic buckets
   Patient scales

*For use in small children for IV fluid therapy.
†For administration of ORS, if the patient is unable to drink and IV fluid therapy is not possible.

provide treatment to the people. A plan for this organization may already be part of a national diarrhea control program, or it may have to be formulated by the health or community health authorities. To estimate the number of cases that can be expected in a country or areas affected by a cholera epidemic, an attack rate of 0.2% can be used (i.e., 200 cases may be expected to occur in a population of 100,000). In a severe epidemic, the national attack rate may be higher. A list of supplies needed for establishing a treatment center is given in Table 41–6.

PROGNOSIS AND PREVENTION. Prompt therapy according to the listed guidelines yields a cholera case-fatality rate of less than 1%; the few deaths are in the aged or very young with major complicating (chiefly pulmonary) diseases. The diarrhea rate is higher in pregnant patients and in those who arrive in shock.

Vaccination. Since the parenteral vaccine consisting of phenol-killed *V. cholerae* O1 organisms generates only moderate short-lived protection, does not prevent asymptomatic infection, and is reactogenic, use of this vaccine has been abandoned. Three doses of two formulations of a killed oral vaccine (whole cell pilus B subunit [B-WC] or whole cell only [WC]) were tested in a field trial in Bangladesh in 1985. During the first 6 months of surveillance, the B-WC vaccine conferred 85% protection against cholera, and the WC vaccine 58%. However, over a 3-year follow-up, both vaccines gave approximately 50% protection and did not show any efficacy during the fourth and fifth years of follow-up. An attenuated strain of *V. cholerae* O1, CVD103-HgR, prepared from the classic Inaba strain 569B by recombinant DNA techniques with deletion of the gene encoding the A subunit of cholera toxin subunit offers great promise. This oral vaccine strain is safe and highly immunogenic. In volunteer challenge studies, it afforded 82 to 100% protection against challenge with strains of the classic biotype, and 62 to 67% protection against challenge with El Tor strains. Both CVD103-HgR and BS-WC vaccines have been licensed for

use in travelers. Live attenuated vaccines for *V. cholerae* O139 have been constructed and are being tested. A conjugate vaccine derived from purified O139 CPS has also been developed and shows promise in animal studies.

Bibliography

Albert MJ: *Vibrio cholerae* O139 Bengal. J Clin Microbiol 32:2345, 1994.
Albert MJ, Ansaruzzaman M, Bardhan PK, et al: Large epidemic of cholera-like disease in Bangladesh caused by *Vibrio cholerae* O139 synonym Bengal. Lancet 342:387, 1993.
Barua D, Greenough WB III (ed): Cholera. New York, Plenum Medical Book Co., 1992.
Carillo L, Gilman RH, Mantle RE, et al: Rapid detection of *Vibrio cholerae* O1 in stools of Peruvian cholera patients by using monoclonal immunodiagnostic kits. J Clin Microbiol 32:856, 1994.
Carpenter CCJ: The treatment of cholera: Clinical science at the bedside. J Infect Dis 166:2, 1992.
Centers for Disease Control and Prevention: Update: Cholera—Western Hemisphere. MMWR 42:89, 1992.
Clemens J, Albert MJ, Rao M, et al: Impact of infection by Helicobacter pylori on the risk and severity of endemic cholera. J Infect Dis 171:1653, 1995.
Comstock LE, Johnson JA, Michalski JM, et al: Cloning and sequence of a region encoding a surface polysaccharide of *Vibrio cholerae* O139 and characterization of the insertion site in the chromosome of *Vibrio cholerae* O1. Mol Microbiol 19:815, 1996.
Hasan JAK, Huq A, Nair GB, et al: Development and testing of monoclonal antibody–based rapid immunodiagnostic test kits for direct detection of *Vibrio cholerae* O139 synonym Bengal. J Clin Microbiol 33:2935, 1995.
Hasan JAK, Huq A, Tamplin ML, et al: A novel kit for rapid detection of *Vibrio cholerae* O1. J Clin Microbiol 32:249, 1994.
Islam MS, Miah MA, Hasan MK, et al: Detection of non-culturable *Vibrio cholerae* O1 associated with a cyanobacterium from an aquatic environment in Bangladesh. Trans R Soc Trop Med Hyg 88:298, 1994.
Kaper JB, Morris JG Jr, Levine MM: Cholera. Clin Microbiol Rev 8:48, 1995.
Khan WA, Begum M, Salam MA, et al: Comparative trial of five antimicrobial compounds in the treatment of cholera in adults. Trans R Soc Trop Med Hyg 82:103, 1995.
Mahalanabis D, Molla AM, Sack DA: Clinical management of cholera. *In* Barua D, Greenough WB III (eds): Cholera. New York, Plenum Medical Book Co., 1992, pp 253–283.
Mekalanos JJ, Sadoff JC: Cholera vaccines: Fighting an ancient scourge. Science 265:1387, 1994.
Qadri F, Hasan JAK, Hossain J, et al: Evaluation of the monoclonal antibody–based kit, Bengal SMART, for rapid detection of *Vibrio cholerae* O139 Bengal in stool samples. J Clin Microbiol 33:732, 1995.
Ries AA, Vugia DJ, Beingolea L, et al: Cholera in Piura, Peru: A modern urban epidemic. J Infect Dis 166:1429, 1992.
van Loon FPL, Clemens JD, Chakraborty J, et al: Field trial of inactivated oral cholera vaccine in Bangladesh: Results from 5 years of follow-up. Vaccine 14:162, 1996.
Wachsmuth IK, Blake PA, Olsvik O (eds): *Vibrio cholerae* and Cholera: Molecular to Global Perspectives. Washington, DC, ASM Press, 1994.
Waldor MK, Mekalanos JJ: Lysogenic conversion by a filamentous phage encoding cholera toxin. Science 272:1910, 1996.
World Health Organization: Cholera in 1994. Wkly Epidemiol Rec 70:201, 1995.
World Health Organization: Cholera outbreak among Rwandan refugees. Wkly Epidemiol Rec 69:221, 1994.
World Health Organization: Guidelines for Cholera Control. Geneva, WHO, 1993.
Yamamoto T, Nair GB, Albert MJ, et al: Survey of in vitro susceptibilities of *Vibrio cholerae* O1 and O139 to antimicrobial agents. Antimicrob Agents Chemother 39:241, 1995.

41.2 *"Noncholera"* or *"Nonepidemic"* Vibrio cholerae

During the past two decades there has been increasing recognition that *V. cholerae* strains outside the "epidemic" O1 and O139 serogroups can cause human disease. These strains can produce mild to severe diarrhea but, with rare exceptions, do not produce the life-threatening diarrheal purges seen in cholera.

DISTRIBUTION AND EPIDEMIOLOGY. Non-O1/non-O139 *V. cholerae* are part of the normal, free-living (autochthonous) bacterial flora in estuarine areas throughout the world; in areas such as the U.S. Gulf Coast, these strains are several orders of magnitude more common in the environment than O1 strains. Isolation has been reported from fresh water, and infections have occurred after exposure to freshwater inland lakes. Non-O1/non-O139 *V. cholerae* have also been isolated from a variety of wild and domestic animals, including 6% of seagulls sampled in England and 14% of dogs in Calcutta.

Non-O1/non-O139 strains are a common isolate from shellfish in the United States, particularly from filter-feeders such as oysters. In a study conducted by the U.S. Food and Drug Administration, these noncholera *V. cholerae* were isolated from 111 (14%) of 790 samples of freshly harvested oyster shellstock. While non-O1/non-O139 *V. cholerae* have been shown to be a frequent isolate in raw shellfish in other geographic areas, it is clear that the organism can be transmitted by a variety of routes. For example, in a study in the Ban Vinai refugee camp in Thailand, noncholera strains were isolated from 4% of vegetable samples, 39% of meat samples, and 16% of drinking water samples; in Cancun, Mexico, 86% of untreated well water samples were culture positive for non-O1/non-O139 strains.

Despite the frequency with which they have been identified in the environment, nonepidemic *V. cholerae* strains generally account for only a small proportion of cases of sporadic diarrheal disease in developing countries. In one study in Cancun, Mexico, non-O1/non-O139 *V. cholerae* were isolated from 16% of persons with diarrhea; in most other studies, isolation rates have ranged from <1.0 to 3.0% of persons with diarrhea.

PATHOGENICITY AND PATHOPHYSIOLOGY. The relatively low rate of isolation of non-O1/non-O139 *V. cholerae* from patients compared with the environment is a reflection of differences in virulence among strains; i.e., it is possible that only a minority of these strains carry the necessary virulence factors to cause human disease. Some nonepidemic strains produce cholera toxin, and studies of hospitalized patients in Bangladesh show that persons infected with cholera toxin–producing strains have more severe gastrointestinal symptoms than those infected with strains that do not produce cholera toxin. Other proposed virulence factors include the El Tor and Kanagawa hemolysins, a Shiga-like toxin, various cell-associated hemagglutinins, and a 17–amino acid, heat-stable enterotoxin (designated NAG-ST) that closely resembles the heat-stable toxin produced by enterotoxigenic strains of *E. coli*. Virulence is believed to depend on the ability of a non-O1/non-O139 *V. cholerae* strain to colonize the intestine, as demonstrated in rabbits using the removable intestinal tie–adult rabbit diarrhea (RITARD) model.

In contrast to *V. cholerae* O1, the majority of non-O1 *V. cholerae* (including *V. cholerae* O139) are able to produce a polysaccharide capsule. The degree of encapsulation is directly correlated with the ability of the strain to cause bacteremia. Heavily encapsulated strains have an opaque colony morphology, whereas unencapsulated or minimally encapsulated strains have a translucent morphology.

CLINICAL MANIFESTATIONS. Non-O1/non-O139 *V. cholerae* have been associated with gastroenteritis, wound and ear infections, and septicemia. Gastroenteritis can occur in normal healthy persons. When a nonepidemic *V. cholerae* strain that produced NAG-ST (but not cholera toxin) was administered to volunteers, six of ten developed diarrhea. Although illness was generally mild, one volunteer had over 5 L of diarrhea, with typical rice-water stools. The median incubation period in these studies was 10 hours (range 5.5–96 hours), with a median duration of illness of 21 hours (range 3.5–48 hours). These results are in agreement with reports from non-O1 *V. cholerae* foodborne disease outbreaks, in

which symptoms tended to be mild, with a short incubation period and a short duration of illness. Septicemia appears to occur primarily in persons who are immunocompromised or who have underlying liver disease; the mortality rate for persons with septicemia exceeds 50%.

DIAGNOSIS/THERAPY. Techniques for isolation of non-O1/non-O139 *V. cholerae* are identical to those used for *V. cholerae* O1, with non-O1/non-O139 strains differentiated by their failure to agglutinate in specific antisera. Persons with acute non-O1/non-O139 *V. cholerae* gastroenteritis do not have a rise in titer of vibriocidal antibodies.

Treatment of persons with severe diarrhea is the same as that used in management of cholera patients. No data on antibiotic efficacy are available, but use of tetracycline appears to be reasonable in severe cases.

Bibliography

Johnson JA, Panigrahi P, Morris JG Jr: Non-O1 *Vibrio cholerae* NRT36S produces a polysaccharide capsule that determines colony morphology, serum resistance, and virulence in mice. Infect Immun 60:684, 1992.

Morris JG Jr: Non-O group 1 *Vibrio cholerae*: A look at the epidemiology of an occasional pathogen. Epidemiol Rev 12:179, 1990.

Morris JG Jr, Takeda T, Tall BD, et al: Experimental non-O group 1 *Vibrio cholerae* gastroenteritis in humans. J Clin Invest 85:697, 1990.

41.3 Vibrio Parahaemolyticus

V. parahaemolyticus is a well-recognized cause of diarrheal disease throughout the world. In Japan, it is among the most common causes of food-borne illness. Illness tends to be mild, although cases of severe diarrhea and dysentery have been reported.

DISTRIBUTION/EPIDEMIOLOGY. As with *V. cholerae*, *V. parahaemolyticus* strains are part of the normal, free-living bacterial flora in estuarine areas throughout the world. They are halophilic (salt-loving) and a very common isolate from estuarine and marine water, sediment, suspended particulates, plankton, fish, and shellfish. In temperate climates isolation is seasonal, with *V. parahaemolyticus* apparently passing the winter in sediment and then proliferating as water temperatures rise.

In Japan, *V. parahaemolyticus* has been implicated as the etiologic agent in 24% of reported cases of food-borne disease. In the United States it has been associated with a number of major food-borne disease outbreaks, often involving mishandling of seafood after cooking. Reported isolation rates from patients with diarrhea vary widely, ranging from 11% in Calcutta and 10.7% in Thailand to 2.6 to 3.7% in Indonesia and 1.5% in Korea. Illness is frequently but not exclusively associated with eating seafood.

PATHOGENICITY AND PATHOPHYSIOLOGY. While the exact mechanisms by which *V. parahaemolyticus* causes human disease have yet to be determined, gastrointestinal pathogenicity has traditionally been correlated with hemolytic activity: In initial studies, over 95% of *V. parahaemolyticus* strains associated with gastroenteritis were hemolytic on Wagatsuma agar (the "Kanagawa phenomenon"), compared with 1% or less of environmental isolates. At least four hemolytic constituents have been described for *V. parahaemolyticus*, including a heat-stable and heat-labile direct hemolysin. The heat-stable direct hemolysin (Vp-TDH) has been most extensively studied. It is a protein with a molecular weight of 42,000 and an apparent subunit structure; it is lethal for mice; it is active in guinea pig skin bluing assays; it has enterotoxic activity in suckling mice; and deletion of the gene encoding Vp-TDH results in loss of enterotoxic activity in Ussing chambers and rabbit ileal loops.

Nonhemolytic strains are also able to cause gastrointestinal illness. One marker for pathogenicity in these strains is urease production, with hemolysin-negative, urease-positive strains implicated in several recent outbreaks, including those on the U.S. Pacific Coast.

CLINICAL MANIFESTATIONS. In a summary of eight culture-confirmed United States outbreaks, symptoms included diarrhea (98% of patients); abdominal cramps (82%); nausea (71%); vomiting (52%); headache (42%); fever, rarely above 38.9°C (27%); and chills (24%). Incubation periods ranged from 4 to 96 hours. Illness was usually self-limited, with a median duration of 3 days. A dysentery-like syndrome has been reported in association with *V. parahaemolyticus* cases in India and Bangladesh; the incubation period for the dysentery-like form of the disease may be as short as 2.5 hours (range 1–9 hours). While rare, cases of dysentery associated with *V. parahaemolyticus* have been reported in the United States. Septicemia due to *V. parahaemolyticus* occurs but is limited to persons with underlying host defense problems.

DIAGNOSIS AND THERAPY. *V. parahaemolyticus* grows well on blood agar and other nonselective media. Isolation from stool generally requires use of a selective medium such as TCBS; *V. parahaemolyticus* does not ferment glucose, and consequently colonies on TCBS are colored blue-green. Species identification is based on standard biochemical tests. The organism does not grow in 0% sodium chloride (as *V. cholerae* does) but will grow in salt concentrations as high as 6 and 8% NaCl. Strains having an increased potential for causing illness can be identified based on hemolytic activity on Wagatsuma agar; on hybridization with DNA probes for the gene encoding Vp-TDH; or on the basis of a positive assay for urease activity.

Patients with diarrhea should be managed as previously described for other diarrheal pathogens. No good data on antibiotic efficacy are available; use of tetracycline (or possibly one of the newer quinolones such as norfloxacin or ciprofloxacin) appears to be reasonable in severe cases.

Bibliography

Abbott SL, Powers C, Kaysner CA, et al: Emergence of a restricted bioserovar of *Vibrio parahaemolyticus* as the predominant cause of vibrio-associated gastroenteritis on the west coast of the United States and Mexico. J Clin Microbiol 27:2891, 1989.

Joseph SW, Colwell RR, Kaper JB: *Vibrio parahaemolyticus* and related halophilic vibrios. CRC Crit Rev Microbiol 10:77, 1983.

Shirai H, Ito H, Hirayama T, et al: Molecular epidemiologic evidence for association of thermostable direct hemolysin (TDH) and TDH-related hemolysin of *Vibrio parahaemolyticus* with gastroenteritis. Infect Immun 58:3568, 1990.

41.4 Vibrio Vulnificus

V. vulnificus is a halophilic *Vibrio* species that has been implicated as a cause of severe wound infections, septicemia, and possibly gastroenteritis. Biochemically it is very similar to *V. parahaemolyticus*, and some severe infections previously attributed to *V. parahaemolyticus* may have actually been due to *V. vulnificus*.

As with other *Vibrio* species, *V. vulnificus* is a free-living estuarine organism and is frequently isolated from water and shellfish, particularly oysters. In the United States it is the most common cause of serious vibrio infections. The incidence of *V. vulnificus* infections in coastal states approximates 0.5 cases/100,000 population/year, with primary septicemia accounting for two thirds of cases. *V. vulnificus* case series have been published from Taiwan and Korea, with anecdotal data suggesting that the incidence in Korea exceeds that in the United States.

Occurrence of primary septicemia due to *V. vulnificus* (i.e., septicemia without an obvious focus of infection) is associated with eating raw oysters. However, susceptibility appears limited to certain high-risk groups, particularly individuals with hemochromatosis, cirrhosis, hematologic, and other disorders associated with immunosuppression, renal failure, and diabetes. Wound infections are associated with contamination of wounds with seawater. While wound infections occur in otherwise healthy persons, deaths associated with wound infections have occurred almost exclusively among persons in these same high-risk groups.

One third of patients with primary septicemia present in shock or become hypotensive within 12 hours of hospital admission. Three fourths of patients have distinctive bullous skin lesions. Thrombocytopenia is common, and there is often evidence of disseminated intravascular coagulation. Complications such as gastrointestinal bleeding are not infrequent. Over 50% of patients with primary septicemia die; the mortality rate exceeds 90% for those who become hypotensive. Persons with septicemia often have symptoms of gastroenteritis, but the organism can cause gastroenteritis in the absence of septicemia.

V. vulnificus can be isolated on blood agar and other nonselective media, including that used in commercial blood culture systems. TCBS is the preferred medium for isolation from stool. Identification is based on standard biochemical tests; identity can be confirmed using DNA probes. Successful therapy depends on early administration of antibiotics. Tetracycline appears to be the drug of choice. Anticapsular antibodies are protective even after onset of symptoms in a mouse model; however, as antibodies are type-specific, any antisera used therapeutically must be multivalent.

Bibliography

Devi SJN, Hayat U, Powell J, Morris JG Jr: Immunoprophylactic and immunotherapeutic efficacy of antisera to capsular polysaccharide–tetanus toxoid conjugate vaccines of *Vibrio vulnificus*. Infect Immun 64:2220, 1996.

Klontz KC, Lieb S, Schreiber M, et al: Syndromes of *Vibrio vulnificus* infections: Clinical and epidemiological features in Florida cases, 1981–1987. Ann Intern Med 109:318, 1988.

Park SD, Shon HS, Joh NJ: *Vibrio vulnificus* septicemia in Korea: Clinical and epidemiologic findings in seventy patients. J Am Acad Dermatol 24:397, 1991.

Wright AC, Simpson LM, Oliver JD, Morris JG Jr: Phenotypic evaluation of acapsular transposon mutants of *Vibrio vulnificus*. Infect Immun 58:1769, 1990.

41.5 Other Vibrio Species

A number of other *Vibrio* species have also been associated with human disease (see Table 41–1). *V. fluvialis* is a species that includes strains previously designated at enteric group EF-6 or group F *Vibrios*. *V. fluvialis* was associated with a large outbreak of diarrheal disease in Bangladesh in 1976–1977. Reported clinical features included diarrhea (100% of cases), vomiting (97%), abdominal pain (75%), moderate to severe dehydration (67%), and fever (35%); 75% of patients had leukocytes and red blood cells in their stools. In the United States there has been at least one reported death associated with the organism.

V. mimicus, *V. hollisae*, and *V. furnissii* have also been associated with diarrheal disease. *V. mimicus* is a newly named species that includes isolates previously classified as sucrose-negative *V. cholerae*. Strains previously identified as enteric group EF-13 are now included in the species *V. hollisae*. *V. furnissii* includes aerogenic strains (strains that produce gas from glucose) that were classified as biovar II of *V. fluvialis*. *V. alginolyticus* and *V. damsela* have been implicated as the cause of infections in seawater-exposed wounds. There is a single report of isolation of *V. cincinnatiensis* from a patient with septicemia and meningitis. *V. carchariae* was isolated from a patient with an infected shark bite.

Diagnosis is based on isolation of the organism from stool, blood, or wound cultures. With the exception of *V. hollisae*, the medium of choice for isolation from stool is TCBS. Diarrheal disease is best managed with appropriate fluid therapy. Isolates are almost uniformly sensitive to tetracycline, with norfloxacin or ciprofloxacin providing a possible alternative therapy.

42 Diarrhea Caused by Escherichia coli

Myron M. Levine and James P. Nataro

DEFINITION. The bacterial species *Escherichia coli* plays an important role in maintaining normal gut physiology in humans. Nevertheless, there exist within this species primary pathogens that cause various syndromes of diarrheal disease, including watery diarrhea, dysentery, and hemorrhagic colitis, in different age groups under distinct epidemiologic settings. Collectively, these clinical gastrointestinal infections are referred to as *E. coli* diarrheal illness, even though the individual categories of diarrheagenic *E. coli* constitute discrete pathogens that can cause distinct clinical syndromes.

ETIOLOGY. *E. coli* are generally motile, gram-negative, rod-shaped bacteria within the family Enterobacteriaceae. Strains of *E. coli* that cause diarrhea are of six major categories: enterohemorrhagic, enterotoxigenic, enteroinvasive, enteropathogenic, enteroaggregative, and diffuse-adherent. In the 1940s, Kauffman proposed a scheme to differentiate *E. coli* on the basis of lipopolysaccharide O, flagellar H, and capsular polysaccharide K antigens. At present, more than 170 O serogroups and more than 60 H types are recognized. Together these designate the O:H serotype of isolates, which is important in studying the epidemiology and pathogenesis of *E. coli* infections. Each category of diarrheagenic *E. coli* has a different pathogenesis, possesses distinct virulence attributes, and comprises a separate set of O:H serotypes. The individual categories can cause distinctive clinical syndromes and exhibit characteristic epidemiologic patterns.

HISTORY. In the 1940s and 1950s, investigators in the United States and Europe found that *E. coli* strains of certain O:H serotypes were associated with sporadic cases of infant summer diarrhea and of epidemic gastroenteritis in hospital nurseries. The term enteropathogenic *E. coli* (EPEC) was coined to refer to these pathogens. Studies in adult volunteers in the 1950s in the United States and Japan confirmed the capacity of these strains to cause diarrheal illness, although the virulence mechanisms remained unknown.

In the late 1960s, largely based on investigations carried out in the Indian subcontinent, a new category of diarrheagenic *E. coli* was discovered that was associated with severe, cholera-like, watery diarrhea. These *E. coli* strains elaborated enterotoxins, including one that was found to share properties with cholera enterotoxin. These were referred to as enterotoxigenic *E. coli* (ETEC).

Also in the late 1960s, another category of *E. coli* pathogens was identified that in many ways resembled *Shigella*, particularly in its ability to invade epithelial cells and in its capacity to cause dysenteric illness. These were named enteroinvasive *E. coli* (EIEC). A multistate outbreak of hemorrhagic colitis in the United States in the early 1980s caused by organisms of serotype O157:H7 led to the discovery of another distinct category of diarrheagenic *E. coli*, enterohemorrhagic *E. coli* (EHEC).

In the 1980s it was found that *E. coli* strains that exhibit a unique pattern of adherence to HEp-2 cells in tissue culture, so-called aggregative adherence, were associated with diarrheal disease in infants in developing countries, particularly the syndrome of persistent diarrhea. These pathogens are referred to as enteroaggregative *E. coli* (EAggEC). In some epidemiologic studies, *E. coli* strains that manifest a diffuse pattern of adherence to HEp-2 cells in tissue culture have also been associated with nonbloody diarrheal illness in young children in developing countries. These putative pathogens have been called diffuse-adherent *E. coli* (DAEC).

DISTRIBUTION AND INCIDENCE. ETEC, EPEC, EIEC, and EAggEC are commonly isolated as agents of diarrheal disease among infants and young children in less developed countries. EPEC used to be a common cause of diarrheal illness in Europe and North America but largely disappeared in the 1970s. It remains an important cause of diarrhea in young infants (≤6 months of age) in many developing and newly industrializing countries, where it is particularly associated with bottle feeding as a risk factor. In many developing countries, ETEC is the second most common cause (after rotavirus) of diarrheal dehydration in infants of a severity that requires rehydration at treatment centers. ETEC is also the most common cause of traveler's diarrhea when adults from industrialized countries visit less developed countries. As a contrast in epidemiologic pattern, EHEC constitutes an emerging cause of diarrheal illness, hemorrhagic colitis, and hemolytic-uremic syndrome (the most severe complication of EHEC infection) in industrialized countries (North America, Europe, Japan, Australia), whereas EHEC disease is rather rare in developing countries. EAggEC has been identified as the single most important cause of persistent diarrhea among infants in Asia and South America. Reports from Germany and the United Kingdom suggest that EAggEC diarrhea may also be common in some industrialized countries. The geographic distribution of DAEC diarrhea is the least well mapped, with the most incriminating studies coming from Latin America (Mexico and Chile). In some epidemiologic studies in developing countries, DAEC was more common in the preschool age group (3–5 years of age), in contrast with EPEC, ETEC, and EAggEC, which manifest the highest incidence in the first year of life.

TRANSMISSION. EPEC is associated with bottle feeding of young infants in developing countries. ETEC is transmitted by contaminated food and water vehicles, and relatively large inocula (circa 10^6 viable organisms) appear to be required to cause clinical illness. EHEC can be transmitted by rather low inocula (10^1–10^2 organisms). Thus, although it is primarily transmitted by ingestion of contaminated beef and other food vehicles, EHEC can also be transmitted directly by contact spread. The modes of transmission of EAggEC and DAEC are not yet clearly defined.

PATHOGENESIS AND PATHOLOGY. The different categories of diarrheagenic *E. coli* have in common certain pathogenesis motifs that include attachment to and interaction with intestinal mucosa, the elaboration of enterotoxins (all except DAEC), carriage of plasmids that encode virulence attributes, and a set of O:H serotypes characteristic of each category. A brief summary of these properties for each category of diarrheagenic *E. coli* is shown in Table 42–1.

EPEC. These carry a circa 60 MDa plasmid that encodes bundle-forming pili (BFP) that foster the initial attachment of EPEC to intestinal epithelium. This plasmid also regulates expression of a chromosomal gene encoding intimin, a 94 kd protein that mediates intimate attachment to enterocytes. This is followed by actin condensation and other cytoskeletal changes in the enterocytes and by secretion. The consequence of this interaction between EPEC and intestinal mucosa is a pathognomonic "attaching and effacing" intestinal lesion observed by electron microscopy.

ETEC. These carry one or two plasmids circa 60 MDa in size that encode heat-labile (LT) or heat-stable (ST) enterotoxins (or both). These plasmids usually also encode one or more fimbrial colonization factor antigens (CFAs) or genes encoding regulatory proteins necessary for the high-level expression of CFAs encoded by chromosomal genes. LT closely resembles cholera enterotoxin in its primary sequence, tertiary structure, antigenicity, and mode of activity (ADP ribosylation). ST, which consists of peptides 18 or 19 amino acids in length, has a distinct mechanism of action (it activates guanylate cyclase, which results in an intracellular accumulation of GMP that leads to secretion) and is not immunogenic. Some ETEC strains capable of causing diarrhea express only LT or ST, whereas others elaborate both toxins.

EIEC. This closely resembles *Shigella* in its pathogenesis, which involves an early step of enterotoxin production leading to intestinal secretion and invasion of intestinal epithelium. EIEC possesses virtually the identical 140 MDa virulence plasmid as *S. flexneri*, which encodes an enterotoxin called *Shigella* enterotoxin 2 in *Shigella* and enteroinvasive *E. coli* toxin in EIEC. Invasion plasmid antigens (IPAs) mediate the uptake of EIEC into enterocytes; this is followed by a process of intracellular and intercellular spread of EIEC, ultimately leading to death of the enterocyte. EIEC infection, like *Shigella*, is characterized by an influx of polymorphonuclear leukocytes into the lamina propria of affected intestinal mucosa.

EHEC. This carries a ~ 60 MDa plasmid that appears to be involved in the expression of novel fimbriae. Phages carried by EHEC encode the powerful cytotoxins, Shiga toxin 1 or 2. Finally, many (albeit not all) EHEC express a 94 kd protein that resembles intimin of EPEC, with which it shares considerable homology in the N-terminal region. EHEC expressing this protein can cause attaching and effacing lesions of intestinal epithelial cells similar to those caused by EPEC.

EAggEC. This harbors a plasmid ~ 60 MDa in size that encodes fimbrial colonization factors that mediate the pathognomonic aggregative adherence to HEp-2 cells. EAggEC expresses at least two enterotoxins that appear to contribute to pathogenesis of clinical illness, including a cytotoxin circa 108 kd in size and the plasmid-encoded EAggEC heat-stable enterotoxin (EAST). Whereas EAST was initially identified in association with EAggEC, more recent studies have also found this toxin in a proportion of ETEC and EHEC strains.

DAEC. The pathogenesis of DAEC is the least understood of the different categories of diarrheagenic *E. coli*. The characteristic diffuse adherence to epithelial cells is mediated by fimbriae. Heretofore, no toxins specific for this category have been identified.

CLINICAL MANIFESTATIONS
EPEC. With rare exceptions, EPEC diarrheal illness is confined to the first 6 months of life. Full-blown EPEC disease is characterized by watery diarrhea with prominent mucus, toxemia, fever, and rapid onset of dehydration (Table 42–2).

ETEC. Clinical ETEC infection exhibits a wide range of severity in infants in developing countries as well as in adult travelers. Mild illness presents as mild diarrhea, low-grade fever in about 20%, nausea and mild abdominal cramps, and gurgling. In contrast, severe ETEC diarrhea closely resembles cholera because of the passage of voluminous rice-water stools that are rich in electrolytes; like cholera, severe ETEC diarrhea can rapidly lead to dehydration. Patients ill with ETEC often have nausea and vomiting for some hours, about 20% manifest moderate fever, and some exhibit muscle cramps. The main difference between severe ETEC diarrhea and cholera is the duration of copious purging, which is much more curtailed with ETEC diarrhea.

EIEC. EIEC has a predilection for colonic mucosa as the favored site of host-parasite interaction. Clinically, the illness is marked by fever, abdominal cramps, malaise, toxemia, and watery diarrhea. In approximately 10% of individuals who develop clinical illness during food-borne outbreaks of EIEC, overt dysentery occurs, manifested by scanty stools of blood and mucus (see Table 42–2).

EHEC. This also exhibits a wide spectrum of clinical illness. Mild cases manifest diarrhea indistinguishable from that caused by many other agents. One pathognomonic syndrome of EHEC is hemorrhagic colitis characterized by severe abdominal cramps and copious bloody diarrhea, with most patients not exhibiting fever (see Table 42–2). These features are points of differentiation from dysentery caused by EIEC, *Shigella*, and certain other pathogens in which the bloody stools tend to be quite scanty and fever is prominent. The second clinical syndrome that occurs with EHEC but not with infection by any other category of diarrheagenic *E. coli*

TABLE 42–1. Pathogenetic Mechanisms of Diarrheagenic *E. coli*

Category	Typical Size of Virulence Plasmid	Proteins Promoting Interaction with Mucosa	Characteristic Pattern of Attachment to HEp-2 Cells	Toxins
ETEC	60 MDa	CFA fimbriae	None	LT, ST
EPEC	60 MDa	BFP; intimin	Localized adherence	None
EIEC	140 MDa	IPAs	Invasion	ShET-2
EHEC	60 MDa	Novel fimbriae; intimin	None	Shiga toxin 1 and 2
EAggEC	65 MDa	AAF fimbriae	Aggregative adherence	EAST1, 108 kda toxin
DAEC	60 MDa	F1845 fimbriae; AIDA-I outer membrane protein	Diffuse adherence	None

CFA, Colonization factor antigen; LT, heat-labile enterotoxin; ST, heat-stable enterotoxin; BFP, bundle-forming pili; IPAs, invasion plasmid antigens; ShET-2, *Shigella* enterotoxin 2; AAF, aggregative adherence fimbriae; EAST1, enteroaggregative heat-stable enterotoxin 1.

TABLE 42–2. Clinical and Epidemiologic Characteristics of Diarrheagenic *E. coli*

Category	Characteristic Clinical Syndrome*	Predominant Geographic Distribution	Peak Age Incidence of Disease	Molecular Diagnostic Targets
ETEC	Watery diarrhea	Developing world	Infants, adult travelers	ST, LT genes
EPEC	Watery diarrhea	Developing world	Very young infants	EAF plasmid, BFP and intimin genes
EIEC	Dysentery†	Worldwide	Toddlers, preschool children	Inv plasmid
EHEC	Hemorrhagic colitis, HUS	Developed world, Latin America	Children 2–7 years of age	EHEC plasmid; intimin and Shiga toxin genes
EAggEC	Persistent diarrhea	Mainly developing countries	Mainly infants	AA plasmid
DAEC	Watery diarrhea	Unknown	Preschool children	F1845 fimbriae genes

*In mild cases, the clinical illness caused by any of the categories of diarrheagenic *E. coli* consists of watery diarrhea, low-grade fever, nausea, and mild abdominal cramps and is indistinguishable.

†Dysentery occurs in only 10% of patients; the other 90% exhibit watery diarrhea without blood.

is the hemolytic-uremic syndrome (HUS) or the variant seen in adults, thrombotic thrombocytopenic purpura. In HUS a disseminated intravascular coagulopathy occurs with massive hemolytic anemia, the presence of fragmented erythrocytes (schistocytes) in the peripheral blood smear, severe thrombocytopenia, and acute renal failure. This is an emerging health problem in industrialized countries but not in developing ones (although it is a problem in several rapidly industrializing nations such as Argentina and Chile). In less developed countries, HUS is more often seen as a complication of Shiga dysentery (Chapter 40).

EAggEC. In approximately 4% of infants in developing countries who present to treatment centers with acute diarrheal illness, the diarrhea continues unabated for more than 14 days, thereupon meeting the WHO definition of persistent diarrhea. The syndrome of persistent diarrhea carries a very poor prognosis for infants in developing countries, typically leading to malnutrition and often to death. An important breakthrough with public health implications was the recognition of EAggEC as the single most frequent agent associated with persistent diarrhea.

DAEC. This is associated with a fairly nonspecific clinical picture of watery diarrhea and low-grade fever. In developing countries this infection tends to occur more commonly in preschool children rather than in infants.

DIAGNOSIS

Indicative Clinical Features. EPEC—The presence of prominent mucus in the diarrheal discharges of a young, bottle-fed infant less than 6 months of age with toxemia should raise suspicion of EPEC in the differential diagnosis (rotavirus would be the other main suspect).

ETEC—Copious purging of rice-water stools should lead to a suspicion of severe ETEC infection as well as cholera. The main clinical feature that differentiates ETEC from cholera is the duration of purging of rice-water stools, which tends to be greater with cholera.

EIEC—In the absence of overt dysentery, clinical EIEC infection exhibits no characteristic clues. On the other hand, among patients with overt dysentery, EIEC must be one of the agents considered in the differential diagnosis. If mucus from a diarrheal stool with or without gross blood is stained and microscopic examination reveals large numbers of fecal leukocytes, EIEC should be considered in the differential diagnosis along with *Shigella, Salmonella,* and *Campylobacter jejuni; Yersinia enterocolitica,* which also results in many fecal leukocytes, is rare in the tropics.

EHEC—The occurrence of hemorrhagic colitis is indicative of EHEC infection. HUS in the tropics is more likely to be caused by Shiga dysentery; nevertheless, EHEC must be kept in mind in the differential diagnosis.

EAggEC—Persistent diarrhea in young infants in developing countries should lead the clinician to consider that EAggEC infection is responsible.

DAEC—There are no characteristic clinical features of DAEC diarrhea.

LABORATORY TESTS

Stool Culture. Some EIEC are late lactose fermenters (or even fail to ferment lactose) and some EHEC, particularly those of serotype O157:H7, do not ferment sorbitol. However, all other diarrheagenic *E. coli* are visually indistinguishable on the usual enteric media (e.g., MacConkey's and eosin methylene blue agar) from normal flora strains of *E. coli.* For this reason, diarrheagenic *E. coli* must be detected by examining typical coliform colonies for either phenotypic or genotypic properties that are characteristic of the different categories (e.g., LT and ST for ETEC).

Immunoassays. ELISAs have been described to identify ETEC, EPEC, EIEC, and EHEC using colony blots or culture supernatants. ELISAs that can be used directly on stool extracts are available to identify LT and Shiga toxins.

DNA Probes and PCR. Molecular diagnostic methods are widely used in the detection of diarrheagenic *E. coli,* since a single uniform molecular method can be adapted to detect genes for many different pathogen-specific genotypes. Polynucleotide and oligonucleotide assays are typically employed in epidemiologic studies. In such studies, colonies of *E. coli* are grown on or transferred to filter paper blots, their DNA is released, and the blots are reacted with the probes. Hybridization is then detected by radioisotopic or nonisotopic detection systems. Using this method, large numbers of *E. coli* can be tested at one time for several different gene targets. Polymerase chain reaction (PCR) for detection of pathogen-specific genes may be more difficult to perform in the setting of a very large epidemiologic study. In contrast, for the processing of a single clinical stool specimen, it is often more efficient to run a panel of PCR reactions using primers against diarrheagenic *E. coli* target genes. Specific DNA probes have been utilized with excellent success in epidemiologic field studies to test DNA extracted from colonies of *E. coli* for the presence of gene sequences specific for the different categories of diarrheagenic *E. coli.* PCR assays have also been described using primers specific for ETEC, EIEC, EHEC, EPEC, and EAggEC.

Adherence to HEp-2 Cells. The HEp-2 assay is one of the most useful phenotypic assays used in the detection of diarrheagenic *E. coli* (Figs. 42–1 to 42–3). The presence of the

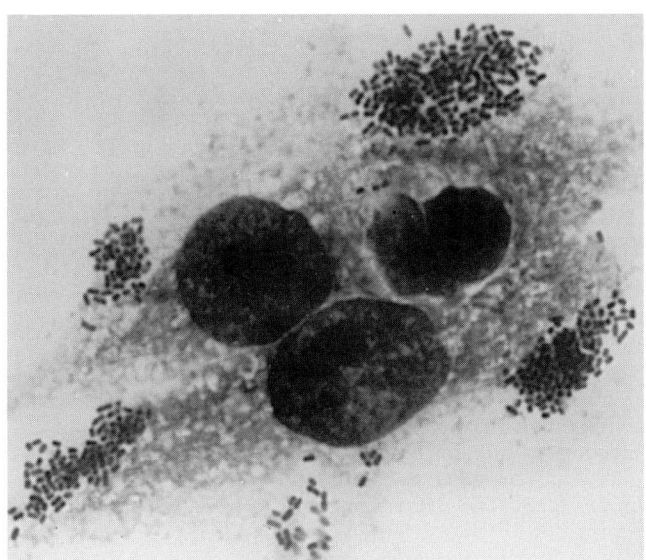

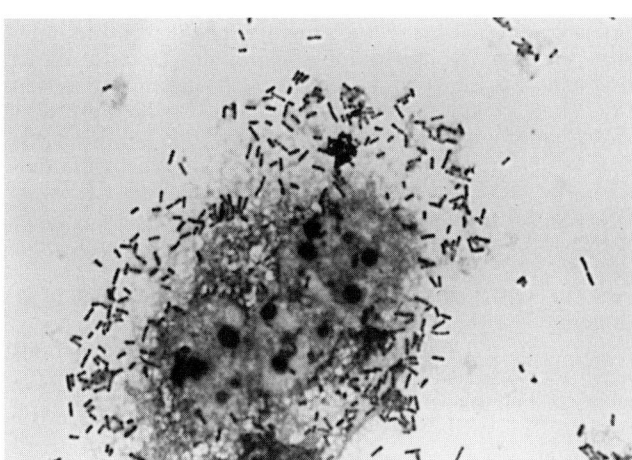

Figure 42–3. The diffuse pattern of adherence to HEp-2 cells that identifies diffuse adherence *E. coli* (DAEC). The bacteria are attached individually, interspersed over the surface of the entire HEp-2 cells.

Figure 42–1. The localized adherence pattern of enteropathogenic *E. coli* (EPEC) to HEp-2 cells in tissue culture. Focal clusters of bacteria are seen attached to one portion of the HEp-2 cells.

distinctive adherence pattern visualized by light microscopy after 3-hour co-incubation of bacteria with HEp-2 cells correlates well with the EPEC (localized), EAggEC (aggregative), and DAEC (diffuse) categories.

Serology. Following diarrheal infection with *E. coli*, rises in serum antibody against the O antigen of the infecting strain can be demonstrated. Many of the virulence attributes of the different categories are also immunogenic, although in almost all instances these remain research tools available only to reference laboratories. Thus, rises in serum or intestinal antibodies can be observed to BFP or intimin following EPEC infection, to LT and CFAs following ETEC infection, to IPAs following EIEC infection, and to AAFs following EAggEC infection. Only a small proportion of infected subjects manifest rises in serum antibody to Shiga toxins following EHEC infection.

Stool Microscopy. Patients with dysentery or suspected EIEC infection should have a drop of stool mucus mixed

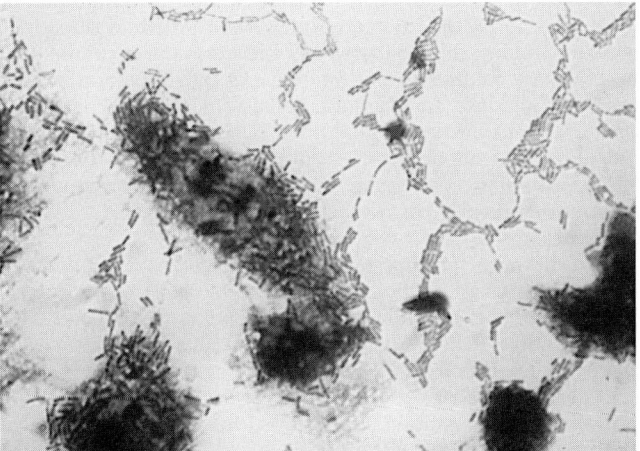

Figure 42–2. The aggregative pattern of adherence to HEp-2 cells diagnostic of enteroaggregative *E. coli* (EAggEC). Note the stacked brick appearance of bacteria attaching both to the tissue culture cells and to the glass slide in between the cells.

with a drop of saline, smeared and dried on a slide, lightly heat-fixed, stained with methylene blue or Gram stain, and examined by light microscopy for the presence of fecal leukocytes. Virtually all patients with EIEC have numerous polymorphonuclear leukocytes in such smears. Although nonspecific, this test provides evidence that a bacterial pathogen has invaded the intestinal mucosa. Other bacterial enteropathogens that cause a dysenteric syndrome and are associated with abundant fecal leukocytes are *Shigella* spp., *Campylobacter jejuni*, and *Salmonella* causing nontyphoidal infections. *Yersinia enterocolitica*, which also results in many fecal leukocytes, is rare in the tropics.

TREATMENT AND PROGNOSIS

Pediatric Patients. For infants with diarrheagenic *E. coli* infection, assessment of the state of hydration is the critical first step in evaluating the patient, and rehydration should be initiated if dehydration is evident. In patients with mild and moderate dehydration, oral rehydration usually suffices.

Specific Antimicrobial Therapy. In the few controlled trials reported, EPEC diarrhea in infants was significantly ameliorated by treatment with appropriate antibiotics. ETEC diarrhea in infants in developing countries responds adequately to rehydration therapy alone. Although there are no controlled trials of EIEC infection, because of its close resemblance clinically to shigellosis it is usually treated with the same antibiotics as used for *Shigella* infections in young children (oral trimethoprim/sulfamethoxazole, nalidixic acid, and ampicillin and parenteral ceftriaxone). There is disagreement on whether antibiotics are helpful in EHEC diarrheal illness or whether they actually increase the chance of developing HUS as a complication. Antibiotics are indicated in the treatment of persistent diarrhea caused by EAggEC. It is not known if antibiotics affect the course of DAEC diarrheal disease.

Adult Patients. Neither EPEC nor EAggEC is currently recognized as an important cause of diarrheal disease in adults, so there are few situations in which questions of treatment arise. Severe ETEC infections can lead to overt dehydration requiring aggressive rehydration. This is usually accomplished with oral rehydration, but occasionally several liters of intravenous fluids may be required to replace fluid and electrolyte deficits.

Specific Antimicrobial Therapy. ETEC diarrhea in adult travelers to developing countries should be treated with antibiotics (fluoroquinolones such as ciprofloxacin) early in the course of clinical illness. Such treatment significantly diminishes the severity and duration of illness. Because of its resemblance to shigellosis, clinical EIEC diarrhea or dysentery is treated with the same antibiotics as used in adults for *Shigella* infections (oral fluoroquinolones such as ciprofloxacin). As in children, there is disagreement on whether antibiotic therapy of EHEC diarrhea or colitis diminishes the severity or duration of illness or increases the propensity to develop HUS as a complication. It is not known if antibiotics affect the course of DAEC diarrheal disease.

PREVENTION AND CONTROL. The provision of adequate sanitation and proper hygiene practices minimize the chance of acquiring *E. coli* diarrheal infection. In high-risk situations in which local conditions favor transmission, attempts must be made to initiate a high standard of personal and food hygiene. This includes compulsive hand washing with soap and water after defecation and before food preparation. Food preparation and eating areas should be kept free of flies. To prevent ETEC diarrhea, travelers must be assiduous about what they eat and drink and must avoid drinks with ice, peeled fruits, salads with raw vegetables, sauces and dips kept at room temperatures, and cooked dishes that are not served piping hot (Chapter 144).

Considerable progress has been made to develop vaccines to prevent ETEC diarrhea. These vaccines aim to stimulate protective immune responses of both an antitoxic and an anticolonizing nature. The most advanced candidate vaccines under development include (1) inactivated ETEC expressing colonization factor antigens (CFAs) combined with B subunit of cholera toxin or LT; and (2) attenuated *Shigella* or *Salmonella typhi* live vectors expressing CFAs and LT B subunit or a mutant LT.

Bibliography

Bhan MK, Raj P, Levine MM, et al: Enteroaggregative *Escherichia coli* associated with persistent diarrhea in a cohort of rural children in India. J Infect Dis 159:1061, 1989.

Gicquelais KG, Baldini MM, Martinez J, et al: Practical and economical method for using biotinylated DNA probes with bacterial colony blots to identify diarrhea-causing *Escherichia coli*. J Clin Microbiol 28:2485, 1990.

Levine MM: *Escherichia coli* that cause diarrhea: Enterotoxigenic, enteropathogenic, enteroinvasive, enterohemorrhagic and enteroadherent. J Infect Dis 155:377, 1987.

Levine MM, Ferreccio C, Prado V, et al: Epidemiologic studies of *Escherichia coli* diarrheal infections in a low socioeconomic level periurban community in Santiago, Chile. Am J Epidemiol 138:849, 1993.

Nataro JP, Kaper JB: Diarrheagenic *Escherichia coli*. Clin Microbiol Rev. In press.

Nataro JP, Kaper JB, Robins-Browne R, et al: Patterns of adherence of diarrheagenic *Escherichia coli* to HEp-2 cells. Pediatr Infect Dis J 6:829, 1987.

Nataro JP, Seriwatana J, Fasano A, et al: Identification and cloning of a novel plasmid-encoded enterotoxin in enteroinvasive *Escherichia coli* and *Shigella*. Infect Immun 63:4721, 1995.

Nataro JP, Steiner T, Guerrant RL: Enteroaggregative *Escherichia coli*: An emerging cause of diarrhea and malnutrition. Emerging Infect Dis. In press.

Tacket CO, Losonsky G, Link H: Protection by milk immunoglobulin concentrate against oral challenge with enterotoxigenic *Escherichia coli*. N Engl J Med 318:1240, 1988.

Wolf MK, Taylor DN, Boedeker EC, et al: Characterization of enterotoxigenic *Escherichia coli* isolated from US troops deployed to the Middle East. J Clin Microbiol 31:851, 1993.

43 Campylobacter *Enteritis*

David N. Taylor and Thomas Butler

DEFINITION. *Campylobacter* enteritis is one of the most common causes of acute bacterial diarrhea throughout the world affecting mostly children in tropical countries, adult travelers to tropical countries, and adults and children in food-borne outbreaks in developed countries. It is caused by *Campylobacter jejuni* and less often by *Campylobacter coli*, thermophilic gram-negative bacilli that have their natural reservoirs in the intestinal tracts of wild and domestic (predominantly chickens and cattle) animals. Transmission of the infection to humans occurs through ingestion of contaminated chicken, other meats, milk, or by direct contact with animal feces. The disease is characterized by acute watery diarrhea or dysentery, fever, and abdominal pain that is usually self-limited over a few days.

ETIOLOGY. Previously classified as *Vibrio fetus* and "related vibrios," *Campylobacter* came to be recognized as a separate bacterial genus in the 1960s. The two species of human enteric pathogens are *C. jejuni* and *C. coli*, whereas *Campylobacter fetus* (previously *V. fetus*) is an opportunistic pathogen of immunocompromised patients and can be cultured from the blood. The importance of *Campylobacter* as a human pathogen was missed until the 1970s, because it does not grow on routine bacteriologic media for stool pathogens. The development of Butzler's and Skirrow's selective media took advantage of the natural antibiotic resistance and the microaerophilic and thermophilic (42°C) characteristics of *Campylobacter* to obtain its growth among the multitude of normal enteric flora.

Campylobacter species are gram-negative rods about 1.5 to 3.5 μm in length and 0.2 to 0.4 μm in width that have varied morphologies on Gram stain, including curved or comma-shaped rods, spirals, and "seagull" forms. One or more flagella impart a darting rapid motility easily observable when liquid stool is viewed by phase contrast or darkfield microscopy. The organisms grow well on blood or brucella agar supplemented with sheep blood and containing a combination of antibiotics. Skirrow's medium contains trimethoprim, polymyxin B, and vancomycin. A cephalosporin is also included in Butzler's medium and Campy-BAP. The plates are incubated at 42°C for 1 to 2 days under microaerophilic conditions (5 to 10% oxygen and 3 to 10% carbon dioxide), produced using microaerobic gas sachets or in a candle jar. Colonies are confirmed as *Campylobacter* by showing positive results in oxidase and catalase tests, sensitivity to nalidixic acid, and resistance to cephalothin. *C. jejuni* is distinguished from *C. coli* by its ability to hydrolyze hippurate. The more important enteric pathogen is *C. jejuni*, but many diagnostic laboratories do not distinguish between the species in routine work.

Two different serotyping schemes are used to distinguish among strains of *Campylobacter*. Over 100 Lior serotypes based on the heat-labile flagellar proteins have been described, and a scheme based on heat-stable or Penner serotypes has identified 60 different serotypes.

EPIDEMIOLOGY

In the Tropics. Among children less than 5 years old living in tropical and developing countries of Central and South America, Africa, and Asia, *Campylobacter* enteritis ranks with rotavirus, enterotoxigenic *Escherichia coli*, and shigellosis as a leading cause of acute diarrhea. Recent surveys of childhood diarrhea in the tropics showed that *Campylobacter* was isolated from the stool cultures of 4 to 35% of cases, with the highest rate of infection reported in infants with diarrhea. Older children and adults are infected less frequently because of immunity acquired in early childhood. Healthy children in tropical countries frequently have asymptomatic infection. Infections caused by *C. coli* are more likely to be asymptomatic than ones caused by *C. jejuni*. The ratio of cases of diarrhea to all persons infected with *Campylobacter* is highest in infancy and declines with increasing age. In rural Mexico there were over two episodes of *Campylobacter* infection per child per year and the case-to-infection ratio was 20% in children 1 to 6 months old and declined thereafter. Reinfections were due to different serotypes of *Campylobacter*. These high rates of infection in infancy in developing countries result in acquisition of anti-*Campylobacter* serum antibodies, which were shown in Thailand to reach a peak in children less than 2 years old. The acquisition of immunity may prevent symptoms or serve to decrease the severity of infection. Symptomatic infections in Mexican children were shown to be more protective than asymptomatic infections. The most prevalent Lior serotypes in Thai children are 4, 28, and 36. In all age groups, male cases outnumber females cases.

In Temperate Climates. In contrast to the hyperendemic situation in the tropics, *Campylobacter* infections in developed countries are less frequent, are rarely asymptomatic, and affect adults more often. Outbreaks are identified sometimes, affecting both children and adults, and may be traced to contaminated sources of drinking water, poultry, eggs, raw milk, and raw hamburger meat. *Campylobacter* is a common cause of diarrhea in travelers from developed countries who return from the tropics. Among American college students living in the United States this is the most frequent form of diarrheal illness. Among homosexual men in the United States, including some with AIDS, *Campylobacter* was recovered from 20% of diarrheal cases. The most prevalent Lior serotypes in American students were 1, 4, 9, and 33, and the most prevalent Penner serotypes were 1, 2, 3, and 5.

Seasonality. *Campylobacter* enteritis occurs during all seasons with little variation by season in tropical countries. In more temperate developing countries, e.g., North Africa, there is a higher prevalence during the wet winter months. In developed countries, there is an increased incidence of infection during summer months. In Singapore, the highest incidence of *Campylobacter* enteritis was in September.

Zoonotic Transmission. The distribution of *C. jejuni* in nature indicates it is a zoonotic infection; humans are an accidental host. These bacteria inhabit the intestinal tracts of a variety of birds, including chickens, turkeys, and water fowl; farm animals, including pigs, cows, sheep, goats, and horses; domestic dogs and cats; and wild rodents and monkeys. These animals are infected frequently and do not usually show signs of illness. For example, in Peru 61% of household chickens had infected feces.

Transmission of infection to humans occurs by ingestion of the organism. This occurs usually when food is contaminated, such as incompletely cooked chicken or other meats and unpasteurized milk. Direct contact with animal feces is probably important in tropical countries like Peru, where children are exposed to chicken droppings in and near their houses. Viable bacteria can survive in chicken droppings for about 4 days. Contact with cats and dogs is significant also, and waterborne outbreaks occur. Secondary spread of infection from person to person has not been documented, although household contacts of cases have higher rates of infection than persons living in houses without cases of infection. This increased rate of infection in household contacts is attributable to common sources of exposure to contaminated foods or animals. In developing countries, the highest rates of infection occur in homes of persons of low socioeconomic status living under unsanitary conditions, often with dirt floors and without running water. Food handlers who are asymptomatic excretors of *C. jejuni* are not a significant source of infection for the community.

PATHOGENESIS. To initiate infection, organisms must be ingested. The infective dose is estimated to vary from 800 to 10^6 bacteria. Volunteers who ingested inocula of these sizes became ill. *C. jejuni* is killed by acid at about pH 2.3, indicating that gastric acid is an effective barrier against infection and that ingestion of organisms with milk or other food that neutralizes acid may enhance infection by reducing the required inoculum. The incubation period varies from 1 to 7 days and is usually 2 to 4 days. During the incubation period, illness, and convalescence, *C. jejuni* multiplies in the intestine and is excreted in feces in quantities of 10^6 to 10^9 organisms/g of stool. The duration of fecal excretion varies from about 8 days in children 1 to 5 years old to 14 days in infants and up to 3 months in adults not treated with antibiotics.

After *C. jejuni* organisms have traversed the stomach, they adhere to the intestinal epithelial cells. Some of the bacteria invade epithelial cells, leading to ulcerated mucosa and bloody diarrhea. The regions of the intestine most affected are the jejunum, terminal ileum, and colon. Biopsies of infected intestines show inflammatory infiltrates in the lamina propria, crypt abscesses, and mucosal ulceration. Bacteria gain access to the blood stream, but bacteremia is uncommon because most strains of *C. jejuni* are susceptible to the bacteriolytic action of serum complement. Watery diarrhea during infection has been attributed to the action of cholera-like enterotoxin, but clinical and immunologic studies have cast doubt on the role of an enterotoxin in this disease. *C. jejuni* produces a cytotoxin also, which might play a role in epithelial cell destruction in the ulcerated mucosa. Bloody diarrhea is more likely to be caused by *C. jejuni* than *C. coli*.

C. jejuni infection has been identified as one of the triggers of Guillain-Barré syndrome (GBS), an acute demyelinating disease of peripheral nerves, and acute motor axonal neuropathy. Between 20 and 40% of GBS cases have serologic or microbiologic evidence of a *C. jejuni* infection usually within a month before the onset of neurologic symptoms. *C. jejuni* infection was significantly associated with a slower recovery and a poorer outcome than cases not associated with a *Campylobacter* infection.

CLINICAL MANIFESTATIONS. The three consistent clinical features of *Campylobacter* enteritis are fever, diarrhea, and abdominal pain. The diarrhea may be either watery or dysenteric with the presence of blood or mucus in liquid stool. In developing countries most children present with watery diarrhea rather than dysentery, whereas a larger portion of patients in developed countries report dysenteric disease. Fever, nausea, vomiting, and malaise may precede the onset of diarrhea by a day or more, and such nonspecific constitutional symptoms may be more severe than the diarrhea itself. The disease is usually self-limited and lasts 1 to 7 days. Severity of disease varies widely with stool frequency from once to more than eight times a day. Most cases are mild, but about 20% of cases have prolonged severe disease with high fever, grossly bloody stools, and relapses. The abdominal pain may be severe and because it is sometimes localized to the right lower quadrant, patients with this infection have been subjected to laparotomy for suspected appendicitis. Cases of toxic megacolon, pseudomembranous colitis, and massive rectal bleeding have been reported. In homosexual males, *Campylobacter* infection is associated with diarrhea more often than proctitis.

Although fatalities are rare from this illness, children in tropical countries with severe diarrheal syndromes commonly die. In Bangladesh, *Campylobacter* was the fourth most common cause of diarrhea in children who died, and most of these children showed severe colitis and the complicating conditions of pneumonia, septicemias with other organisms, and malnutrition. Less common complications reported in patients with *Campylobacter* enteritis include hypoglycemia, pancreatitis, peritonitis, and cholecystitis. A reactive arthritis may develop in patients who have the HLA-B27 haplotype.

DIAGNOSIS. The diagnosis of *Campylobacter* enteritis requires isolation of the bacterium from stool cultures. This requires selective media, such as Skirrow's or Campy-BAP, incubation at 42°C, and a microaerophilic environment, such as a gas sachet or a candle jar. Identification follows standard bacteriologic techniques. Fresh stool should be examined for the presence of leukocytes and to exclude the possible presence of trophozoites of *Entamoeba histolytica*. Often, a Gram stain of stool shows bacterial forms, including spiral or "seagull" shapes, suggestive of *Campylobacter* morphology.

Differential Diagnosis. As the differential diagnosis includes other enteric pathogens, stool should be cultured also for species of *Salmonella, Shigella, Vibrio,* and *Yersinia* and, when diagnostic facilities are available, for enterotoxigenic *E. coli* and rotavirus. Examination of diarrheal stools for other pathogens in the tropics is important, because it was shown in Bangladesh that most patients with *Campylobacter* infections were infected with other diarrheal pathogens.

Endoscopy is not advised routinely; however, when inflammatory bowel disease is considered in the differential diagnosis, colonoscopy with biopsy may be performed. The colonic mucosa shows erythema, superficial ulcerations, and friability, and biopsy reveals characteristically acute inflammation and crypt abscesses.

TREATMENT. As in other diarrheal diseases, rehydration with isotonic fluids or oral rehydration solutions (Chapter 16) is the most important therapeutic intervention. Severe dehydration is uncommon with *Campylobacter* enteritis and it is often a self-limited disease. Use of antibiotics is controversial. Clinical trials, in which treatment was delayed until *C. jejuni* was isolated, comparing erythromycin with a placebo, did not show significant differences in clinical responses. However, early treatment with erythromycin in children with dysentery showed a clear benefit. Therefore, presumptive clinical diagnosis or direct visualization of organisms in stool followed by specific therapy can be of clinical benefit. In patients with bloody diarrhea, fever, or worsening symptoms, treatment with a macrolide antibiotic such as erythromycin or azithromycin should be considered. Erythromycin is still considered the drug of choice because of its wide availability, efficacy, and safety, and it is much cheaper than azithromycin. However, erythromycin can cause significant gastrointestinal upset, so clinicians are often reluctant to prescribe it for a gastrointestinal illness. The recommended dosage of erythromycin for adults is 250 mg q.i.d. for 5 to 7 days; the recommended dosage for children is 30 to 50 mg/kg/day divided in four daily doses. Although ciprofloxacin, 500 mg b.i.d. for 5 to 7 days, is an attractive alternative therapy because of its activity against numerous enteric bacteria, strains of ciprofloxacin-resistant *Campylobacter* have emerged worldwide, especially in Southeast Asia. A presumptive diagnosis of ciprofloxacin resistance should be considered if the patient fails to improve after 24 to 48 hours of drug therapy and appropriate rehydration. Azithromycin has been evaluated as an alternative to ciprofloxacin for the treatment of *Campylobacter* enteritis acquired in Thailand by U.S. military personnel; 50% of the *Campylobacter* isolates in this study were resistant to ciprofloxacin. Azithromycin given at 250 mg b.i.d. for 3 days was as efficacious as ciprofloxacin in reducing the time of illness in ciprofloxacin-susceptible iso-

lates and better than ciprofloxacin for resistant isolates. Azithromycin was also superior to ciprofloxacin in decreasing the excretion of bacteria in the stool. Although the optimal dose and duration for azithromycin use in *Campylobacter* enteritis are yet to be determined, 500 mg/day for 3 days is likely to be effective.

PREVENTION AND CONTROL. Reducing the hyperendemic transmission of *Campylobacter* infection in developing countries requires improvements in basic hygiene and living conditions of the people. Because children acquire infection in infancy and early childhood by ingesting contaminated food and by direct contact with animals, household methods of food preparation must be improved, and animals, especially chickens, must be kept away from people's homes. Handwashing before meals is a good preventive measure against most enteric infections.

In developed countries, transmission of *Campylobacter* infection could be reduced by cooking meats thoroughly and avoiding contamination of other foods by the juices of uncooked meats. Travelers to tropical countries should take the usual precautions to avoid most uncooked foods and to ensure that their cooked food is served fresh and thoroughly cooked.

Bibliography

Allos BM, Blaser MJ: *Campylobacter jejuni* and the expanding spectrum of related infections. Clin Infect Dis 20:1092, 1995.

Butler T, Islam M, Azad AK, et al: Causes of death in diarrhoeal diseases after rehydration therapy: An autopsy study of 140 patients in Bangladesh. Bull WHO 65:317, 1987.

Chowdhury MNH, Al-Eissa YA: *Campylobacter* gastroenteritis in children in Riyadh, Saudi Arabia. J Trop Pediatr 38:158, 1992.

Coker AO, Adefeso AO: The changing patterns of *Campylobacter jejuni-coli* in Lagos, Nigeria after ten years. East Afr Med J 71:437, 1994.

Cruz JR, Cano F, Bartlett AV, et al: Infection, diarrhea, and dysentery caused by *Shigella* species and *Campylobacter jejuni* among Guatemalan rural children. Pediatr Infect Dis J 13:216, 1994.

Desheng L, Zhixin C, Bolun W: Age distribution of diarrhoeal and healthy children infected with *Campylobacter jejuni*. J Trop Med Hyg 95:218, 1992.

Kuschner R, Trofa AF, Thomas RJ, et al: Use of azithromycin for the treatment of *Campylobacter* enteritis in travelers to Thailand, an area where ciprofloxacin resistance is prevalent. Clin Infect Dis 21:536, 1995.

Lim YS, Tay L: A one-year study of enteric *Campylobacter* infections in Singapore. J Trop Med Hyg 95:119, 1992.

Marquis GS, Ventura G, Gilman RH, et al: Fecal contamination of shanty town toddlers in households with non-corralled poultry, Lima, Peru. Am J Publ Health 80:146, 1990.

Murga H, Guevara G, Huicho L, et al: Differential clinical and epidemiological features in children with *Campylobacter* diarrhoea, mixed-agent diarrhoea and *Campylobacter* diarrhoea plus parenteral infections. J Trop Pediatr 41:57, 1995.

Murga H, Huicho L, Guevara G: Acute diarrhoea and *Campylobacter* in Peruvian children: A clinical and epidemiologic approach. J Trop Pediatr 39:338, 1993.

Puthucheary SD, Parasakthi N, Liew ST, et al: *Campylobacter* enteritis in children: Clinical and laboratory findings in 137 cases. Singapore Med J 35:453, 1994.

Rees JH, Soudain SE, Gregson NA, Hughes RAC: *Campylobacter jejuni* infection and Guillain-Barré syndrome. N Engl J Med 333:1374, 1995.

Skirrow MB: *Campylobacter*. Lancet 336:921, 1990.

Taylor DN, Echevarria P, Pitarangsi C, et al: Influence of strain characteristics and immunity on the epidemiology of *Campylobacter* infections in Thailand. J Clin Microbiol 26:863, 1988.

Taylor DN: *Campylobacter* infections in developing countries. *In* Nachamkin I, Blaser MJ, Tompkins LS (eds): *Campylobacter jejuni*: Current Status and Future Trends. Washington, DC, American Society of Microbiology, 1992.

44 *Miscellaneous Bacterial Enteritides*

Daniel A. Scott

44.1 Yersinia enterocolitica *Infections**

DEFINITION. *Yersinia enterocolitica* is a facultatively anaerobic gram-negative rod bacterium. The most common clinical syndrome caused by this enteric pathogen is diarrhea, fever, and abdominal pain that at times may mimic acute appendicitis. Common pathologic lesions are acute enteritis and mesenteric lymphadenitis. *Y. enterocolitica* has its natural reservoir in the intestines of pigs, cows, and a wide range of other mammals. Humans become infected by ingesting contaminated food or water.

ETIOLOGY. *Y. enterocolitica* is a member of the bacterial order *Enterobacteriaceae*. Accordingly, it is a gram-negative rod, is oxidase negative, and grows on agars containing bile salts. On triple sugar iron agar and acid slant it produces acid but without hydrogen sulfide or gas. At 25°C it is motile with minimal nutritional requirements, whereas at 37°C it is nonmotile and has increased nutritional requirements. There are multiple O serotypes and the most common serotype isolated from humans varies geographically. In Europe and Japan serotypes O3 and O9 are most commonly associated with human disease, whereas serotype O8 has been the most common isolate in the United States. *Y. enterocolitica* causes disease by invading the gastrointestinal epithelium. The initial attachment and subsequent invasion is mediated by three chromosomally encoded proteins. Virulence also depends on the presence of a 70-kDa virulence plasmid (pYV) that is about 50% homologous with the very closely related plasmids of *Yersinia pseudotuberculosis* and *Yersinia pestis*. The plasmid codes for a group of highly conserved outer membrane proteins known as Yops, which are important in bacteria avoiding phagocytosis and destruction by macrophages and neutrophils. Other virulence factors include a heat-stable enterotoxin similar to that produced by *Escherichia coli*, and several proteins that bind iron or other iron-containing molecules.

EPIDEMIOLOGY. Infection caused by *Y. enterocolitica* is distributed worldwide but is more common in northern countries and appears to be an infrequent cause of tropical diarrhea. In the United States, infection with *Y. enterocolitica* is rare when compared with *Campylobacter*, *Salmonella*, and *Shigella* species and outbreaks are uncommon. However, in northern European countries, the incidence of infection is higher, approaching the rates for *Campylobacter* and *Salmonella*, and most of the disease is sporadic. Although adults and children are both susceptible to infection, illness occurs more commonly in children. The natural reservoirs of infection are farm animals, especially pigs, cows, goats, and other domestic animals, including dogs and cats. These animals harbor the bacteria in their intestines and excrete them in feces. Humans become infected by ingesting food or water contaminated by animal feces. Ingestion of improperly prepared pork or other swine products, e.g., chitterlings, are a major source of infection. Outbreaks have been associated with raw milk, and because of its ability to multiply at 4°C, even pasteurized milk was a source of infection, probably

from being contaminated at a dairy after pasteurization. *Y. enterocolitica* can also multiply in stored human blood collected from persons with bacteremia following a gastrointestinal infection. This very rare problem is generally seen when blood is stored for a long period resulting in the release of iron-containing heme. The bacteria can reach high levels in the blood and cause a rapid onset of sepsis after transfusion. Person-to-person transmission of infection seems to be rare. A seasonal increase in cases in the fall and winter has been described in Europe and the United States.

CLINICAL SYNDROMES

Diarrhea. This is the most common presentation of *Y. enterocolitica* and is particularly common in young children. Presenting symptoms frequently include fever and abdominal pain, and vomiting is common in children. Although the diarrhea is generally mild and nonbloody, it can present as a more invasive syndrome with blood and leukocytes in the stool. Most cases are self-limited with resolution of symptoms in 1 or 2 weeks. However, in adults there are reports of chronic diarrhea lasting months to years and presentations that resemble inflammatory bowel disease.

Pseudoappendicitis. In adults and older children a pseudoappendicitis syndrome is a frequent presentation of yersiniosis. The majority of these patients do not have diarrhea but present with severe abdominal pain that may localize to the right lower quadrant and be mistaken for appendicitis. On laparotomy surgeons find mesenteric lymphadenitis, terminal ileitis, and either a normal or only slightly inflamed appendix.

Other Manifestations. Other possible gastrointestinal complications include an ulcerative enteritis that can rarely lead to perforation, intussusception, actual appendicitis, and toxic megacolon but these are very rare. Some patients may develop extraintestinal complications, e.g., arthralgias, reactive arthritis, or Reiter syndrome, and erythema nodosum. As the synovial and cutaneous tissues in these syndromes are sterile, an immunologic reaction has been postulated to explain their pathogenesis. Individuals with HLA-B27 haplotype are more susceptible to reactive arthritis and Reiter syndrome. Most arthralgia and arthritis symptoms resolve quickly but some go on to have chronic symptoms. Septicemia is a rarer complication that occurs most commonly in patients with iron overload secondary to hemochromatosis, transfusion-dependent anemias, or therapy with an iron chelator, e.g., desferoxamine. Transfusion of *Y. enterocolitica*–infected blood may cause sudden onset of fever, hypotension, and diffuse pain.

DIAGNOSIS. The diagnosis requires the isolation of *Y. enterocolitica* from stool, blood, or surgical specimens. Isolation from the stool is typically on MacConkey agar with growth of nonlactose-fermenting colonies appearing after 48 hours' incubation at 25 to 28°C. Recovery may be enhanced by the use of cold-enrichment techniques or cefsulodin-irgasin-novobiocin (CIN) agar. A serologic diagnosis can be made by showing a rise in agglutinin titer in paired serum specimens but the assay is serotype-specific, thus limiting its usefulness. There is currently no stool polymerase chain reaction diagnostic test available but this would potentially be a very useful test for rapid diagnosis, particularly in patients presenting with a pseudoappendicitis syndrome. Diagnosis of *Yersinia* septicemia from transfusion may be made by Gram stain or culture of the infected unit of blood. It is important to suspect the diagnosis in patients with severe abdominal pain to avoid unnecessary surgery for appendicitis. Ultrasound may be helpful in the differential diagnosis.

TREATMENT. Infection with *Y. enterocolitica* is usually self-limited and so rarely diagnosed that there is little useful data to assess the benefits of antibiotic treatment. Most isolates are susceptible to aminoglycosides, tetracyclines, chloramphenicol, trimethoprim-sulfamethoxazole, fluoroquinolones,

---

*All the material in this chapter is in the public domain, with the exception of any borrowed figures or tables.

third-generation cephalosporins, imipenem, and aztreonam. They are resistant to ampicillin and the first-generation cephalosporin antibiotics. Empirical treatment at presentation is probably warranted for severe gastrointestinal disease and a fluoroquinolone would be the drug of choice. Treatment is also indicated for severe systemic infections, bacteremia, and localized suppurative complications. There are no clinical trials, but treatment options include fluoroquinolones, doxycycline, trimethoprim-sulfamethoxazole, and aminoglycosides probably in combination.

PREVENTION AND CONTROL. The major risk factor for *Y. enterocolitica* infection is the ingestion of contaminated pork and other foods. Initial prevention efforts should include procedures to decrease contamination of meat in the slaughterhouse. Public education efforts should stress proper handling and cooking of pork, chitterlings, and other meat or meat products. There is currently no human or animal vaccine to prevent disease or decrease colonization in farm animals.

Bibliography

Cover TL: *Yersinia enterocolitica* and *Yersinia pseudotuberculosis*. *In* Blaser MJ, Smith PD, Ravdin JL, Greenberg HB, Guerrant RL (eds): Infections of the Gastrointestinal Tract. New York, Raven Press, 1995, pp 811–823.

Doyle MP: Pathogenic *Escherichia coli, Yersinia enterocolitica,* and *Vibrio.* Lancet 336:1111, 1990.

Stolk-Engelaar VM, Hoogkamp-Korstanje JA: Clinical presentation and diagnosis of gastrointestinal infections by *Yersinia enterocolitica* in 261 Dutch patients. Scand J Infect Dis 28:571, 1996.

Van Noyen R, Selderslaghs R, Bekaert J, et al: Causative role of *Yersinia* and other enteric pathogens in the appendicular syndrome. Eur J Clin Microbiol 10:735, 1991.

Verhaegen J, Charlier J, Lemmens P, et al: Surveillance of human *Yersinia enterocolitica* infections in Belgium: 1967–1996. Clin Infect Dis 27:59, 1998.

44.2 Aeromonas *Infections**

DEFINITION. The aeromonads are a complex group of gram-negative, oxidase-positive bacteria that cause a variety of clinical syndromes in humans. Their role as gastrointestinal pathogens remains controversial but the evidence suggests some aeromonads cause gastrointestinal disease.

HISTORY. The first description of diarrhea attributed to an *Aeromonas* infection was published in 1964. In the late 1960s the role of *Aeromonas* in wound infections and septicemia was first recognized. Although numerous case-control studies have shown an association with diarrheal disease, some have not, and no outbreaks of *Aeromonas* gastroenteritis have been described. In the past it was believed that some of this confusion may have been due to the complex taxonomy and difficulty identifying pathogenic strains, but this does not appear to be the case. Although the taxonomy has undergone a fundamental change over the last 10 years, studies still find that the isolates from diarrhea cases and controls are from the three main species causing disease in humans. The best evidence that *Aeromonas* can cause diarrhea comes from a small number of well-described cases in which there was relatively severe disease, a pure culture of a single pathogen, and in some cases intestinal biopsy or serologic data that supported the diagnosis. At the present time some experts in the field believe that at least some strains of *Aeromonas*, perhaps when ingested at high inocula, can cause gastrointestinal disease.

MICROBIOLOGY. Aeromonads are gram-negative, facultatively anaerobic bacilli. Most are motile and have a single polar flagellum. There are many *Aeromonas* species, with only five main ones being associated with human disease, and three main species—*A. hydrophila, A. veronii,* and *A. caviae*—associated with diarrheal disease.

EPIDEMIOLOGY. The major reservoir for *Aeromonas* appears to be fresh water, and bacterial counts rise during the warmer months of the year. This is monitored by an increase in *Aeromonas*-associated diarrhea during those months. The highest attack rates of diarrhea are seen in children <3 years of age. The percentage of diarrhea cases attributed to *Aeromonas* varies widely from a low of <1% to a high of 50% in a study in Peru. The incidence of copathogens is quite high in a number of these studies. The only risk factors identified are ingestion of untreated water and prior antibiotic usage. Many recent case-control studies have showed a significant association between the presence of *Aeromonas* on the primary stool culture and gastrointestinal disease. However, unlike other food- and water-borne pathogens, there have been no clear outbreaks of diarrhea attributable to *Aeromonas*.

CLINICAL PRESENTATIONS. As with most enteric pathogens the gastrointestinal symptoms caused by *Aeromonas* are variable. Most common is a mild to moderate, acute, watery diarrhea. This can be associated with abdominal pain, fever, and vomiting. Symptoms are generally self-limited, lasting less than a week. In perhaps a quarter of the cases patients present with a dysentery-like illness with severe abdominal pain, fever, and bloody diarrhea. A third presentation is that of a more chronic, intermittent diarrhea that can last for months to years. Recently *Aeromonas* gastroenteritis has also been linked to the hemolytic-uremic syndrome. Other infections caused by *Aeromonas* include wound infections in normal hosts after trauma or burns, postoperative wound infections, spontaneous wound infection, and septicemia in compromised hosts. Wound infections can be related to exposure to fresh water. Respiratory and ocular infections have also been described.

DIAGNOSIS. During the acute phase of gastrointestinal illness *Aeromonas* is present in the stool in high concentration and is easily isolated. Most aeromonads grow well on most agars commonly used for stool cultures, e.g., MacConkey, xylose-lysine-deoxycholate, and Hektoen. However, some strains do not grow well and some are lactose-positive on MacConkey agar, so a nonselective media, e.g., blood agar, should also be used. In more chronic diarrhea cases the bacterial counts are lower and enrichment media, e.g., selenite broth or alkaline-peptone-water, should be used.

TREATMENT. Most *Aeromonas* species are susceptible to tetracyclines, aminoglycosides, trimethoprim-sulfamethoxazole, third-generation cephalosporins, and the fluoroquinolones. Results are variable with the first- and second-generation cephalosporins and they are generally resistant to ampicillin. There are no controlled clinical trials of antibiotic therapy for *Aeromonas* gastroenteritis; however, case reports suggest they may shorten the clinical course, particularly for patients with chronic diarrhea. Based on in vitro data and reported clinical responses, reasonable antibiotic choices include trimethoprim-sulfamethoxazole and the fluoroquinolones. Ciprofloxacin would be a particularly useful choice for empirical therapy because of its excellent activity and proved efficacy against a wide range of bacterial enteropathogens.

Bibliography

Janda JM, Abbott SL, Morris JG Jr: *Aeromonas, Plesiomonas,* and *Edwardsiella. In* Blaser MJ, Smith PD, Ravdin JL, Greenberg HB, Guerrant RL (eds): Infections of the Gastrointestinal Tract. New York, Raven Press, 1995, pp 905–917.

Janda JM, Abbott SL: Evolving concepts regarding the genus *Aeromonas:* An expanding panorama of species, disease presentations, and unanswered questions. Clin Infect Dis 27:332, 1998.

Kuhn I, Albert MJ, Ansaruzzaman M, et al: Characterization of *Aeromonas* spp.

---

*All the material in this chapter is in the public domain, with the exception of any borrowed figures or tables.

isolated from humans with diarrhea, from healthy controls, and from surface water in Bangladesh. J Clin Microbiol 35:369, 1997.

Pazzaglia G, Sack RB, Salazar E, et al: High frequency of coinfecting entero-pathogens in *Aeromonas*-associated diarrhea of hospitalized Peruvian infants. J Clin Microbiol 29:1151, 1991.

Yamada S, Matsushita S, Dejsirilert S, Kudoh Y: Incidence and clinical symptoms of *Aeromonas*-associated travellers' diarrhoea in Tokyo. Epidemiol Infect 119:121, 1997.

44.3 Clostridium difficile–*Induced Colitis**

DEFINITION. *Clostridium difficile* is a recently described enteric pathogen that is responsible for nearly all cases of antibiotic-associated colitis and approximately 20 to 25% of antibiotic-associated diarrhea.

HISTORY. Studies of antibiotic-associated colitis in the 1950s and early 1960s suggested that *Staphylococcus aureus* was the etiologic agent in most cases. Lack of histologic study, the presence of *S. aureus* in the fecal flora of healthy individuals, and the results of more recent studies cast doubt about the precise role of this microbe. In the early 1970s, the widespread use of endoscopy in patients with antibiotic-associated diarrhea permitted extensive studies of its incidence, pathology, and natural history. It was noted that *S. aureus* was rarely recovered from the stools of afflicted patients and that even if it was present, there was no clear cause and effect relationship. Studies in the later 1970s implicated *C. difficile* as the etiologic agent; a tissue culture assay was developed for detecting *C. difficile* toxin in stool, and vancomycin and cholestyramine became therapeutic modalities with established efficacy.

DISTRIBUTION. *C. difficile* is found in soil samples and in the stools of a number of animals. The carrier rate in stools is 30 to 60% for newborn infants, which decreases to approximately 3% in adults and in children >8 months of age. The high carrier rate in infants, originally thought to be due to maternal-child transmission, is now considered linked to nosocomial spread.

TRANSMISSION AND EPIDEMIOLOGY. Antibiotic-associated diarrhea due to *C. difficile* may occur sporadically or in epidemics. The latter occurs primarily in institutions, where there may be widespread contamination of the environment from stools of affected patients combined with extensive use of antibiotics. Environmental cultures near patients with *C. difficile*-induced diarrhea show that the organism is recovered in up to 30% of case-associated sites compared with only 1 to 3% of control sites. Recurrences of antibiotic-associated colitis due to *C. difficile* may in some instances be due to reinfection from environmental sources following successful elimination from the bowel. Outbreaks of disease have occurred in both acute and chronic care facilities.

Colitis most commonly follows parenteral or oral therapy with ampicillin, cephalosporins, and clindamycin, although most antibiotics, including antineoplastic antibiotics, have been implicated. Besides exposure to antibiotics, other risk factors include advanced age, female sex, antecedent bowel manipulations, and perhaps inflammatory bowel disease. Disease is rare in infants and in those with cystic fibrosis, even when they have large numbers of *C. difficile* and high titers of toxin in their stool. Lack of toxin receptors on the bowel mucosa or the presence of inhibitory substances, e.g., secretory antibody, may explain the low incidence in these groups.

C. difficile–induced colitis is recognized primarily in industrialized countries where toxin assays are available. It is assumed that this organism is also an important cause of enteric disease in developing countries where there is crowding of hospitalized patients and less stringent control of antibiotic use.

PATHOGENESIS AND PATHOLOGY. *C. difficile* is an enteric pathogen almost exclusively in the presence of antibiotic exposure. Endoscopy in patients with antibiotic-associated diarrhea shows a spectrum of pathologic changes ranging from an entirely normal colon to severe colitis, with the most characteristic lesion being pseudomembranous colitis (PMC). Typical findings in patients with PMC are multiple, elevated, yellowish-white plaques that vary in size from a few millimeters to 20 mm in diameter. Coalescence of these plaques, which consist of polymorphonuclear leukocytes, fibrin, epithelial cell debris, and mucin, produces the classic pseudomembrane. The intervening mucosa is normal or shows hyperemia and edema. In most instances, the entire colon is involved. Histologic studies show that the pseudomembrane arises from superficial ulceration on an intact mucosa and an acute or chronic inflammatory infiltrate in the lamina propria.

C. difficile toxin assays implicate this organism in nearly all cases of antibiotic-associated PMC and in 20 to 25% of "simple diarrhea" related to antibiotic usage. The carriage rate among healthy adults increases with antibiotic exposure, presumably reflecting ingestion from environmental sources. Both colonization and toxin production are enhanced by suppression of the competing colonic flora. Support for the importance of the normal flora comes from clinical studies indicating a close association with antibiotic usage as well as from experimental studies in rodents indicating that typical disease is readily induced only in neonates, gnotobiotes, and animals given a variety of antibiotics. The common denominator in these seemingly diverse settings is reduced or altered colonic flora.

C. difficile Toxins. *C. difficile*–induced enteric disease is toxin-mediated. The putative agent produces two toxins, designated toxin A and toxin B, which are large-molecular-weight proteins produced during logarithmic growth of the vegetative forms. Toxin A causes fluid accumulation and a profound hemorrhagic inflammation in the rabbit ileal loop assay. Toxin B is a potent cytopathic toxin that is detected in tissue cultures in concentrations as low as 100 pg/mL. Toxins A and B are both present in the stools of patients with colitis and may act synergistically to produce disease. Toxin A may play a permissive role, interacting with gut mucosa to facilitate the exit of toxin B from the intestinal lumen. Toxin A damages villous tips and the brush border membrane but has no demonstrable enzymatic activity. Toxin B activates guanylate cyclase and disrupts the mucosal cell's microfilament system. A motility-altering factor and adherence pili may be additional virulence factors.

CLINICAL MANIFESTATIONS. Nearly all antimicrobial agents that have an antibacterial spectrum of activity have been implicated in *C. difficile*–induced enteric disease. The diarrhea, which is generally large in volume and watery or mucoid, begins typically 5 to 7 days after the initiation of antibiotic therapy. It is first noted during antibiotic administration in two thirds of patients, and up to 4 weeks following discontinuation of the implicated agent in the remaining one third. Illness may be mild, but most patients with PMC experience abdominal cramps and tenderness, fever, and leukocytosis. Late and serious complications include severe dehydration, electrolyte imbalance, hypotension, and hypoalbuminemia and anasarca, toxic megacolon, and colonic perforation. Without therapy, the illness abates generally 1 to 3 weeks after removal of the offending antibiotic.

DIAGNOSIS

Endoscopy. The typical mucosal plaquelike lesions are visualized by endoscopy. Less specific changes include hemor-

---

*All the material in this chapter is in the public domain, with the exception of any borrowed figures or tables.

rhage, ulcerations, easy friability, erythema, and edema. These findings must be differentiated from those in other forms of colitis, e.g., idiopathic ulcerative colitis, shigellosis, and amebiasis.

Toxin Assays. The preferred method for confirming the diagnosis is to demonstrate *C. difficile* toxin or toxins in stool by observing in a tissue culture assay typical cytopathic changes that are neutralized by *Clostridium sordellii* or *C. difficile* antitoxins. Toxin neutralization with antisera to *C. sordellii* represents an antigenic cross-reaction. Over 90% of patients with *C. difficile*–associated colitis have cytotoxic activity in their stool. Toxin is found much less frequently in the stool of those with colitis without pseudomembranes and in those with diarrhea only. Alternative methods for antigen detection include counterimmunoelectrophoresis or an enzyme-linked immunosorbent assay procedure. Stool cultures may be done using a selective medium containing cycloserine and cefoxitin, but these are more laborious, may prove difficult in many clinical laboratories, and are less specific than the toxin assay.

TREATMENT AND PROGNOSIS. The natural course of the disease in patients with antibiotic-associated PMC is highly variable. Some patients have minimal symptoms that resolve rapidly when the implicated antibiotic is discontinued. Other patients have protracted or debilitating diarrhea with up to 30 stools per day. The overall mortality rate without specific therapy is approximately 20%. Therapeutic recommendations include antibiotics directed against the putative agent or anion exchange resins to bind *C. difficile* toxin. The most frequently used antibiotic is orally administered vancomycin, 125 to 500 mg, 4 times daily for 7 to 14 days. Nearly all patients respond, but approximately 20% relapse following discontinuation of this agent. Relapses may be due to the presence of *C. difficile* spores or to reinfection with *C. difficile*. Relapses may be treated with an additional course of vancomycin, or with alternative antibiotics, e.g., metronidazole (1500 mg/day orally or intravenously) or bacitracin (500 mg orally 4 times per day). The latter antibiotics are considerably less expensive than vancomycin and deserve consideration as primary therapies, at least for those with mild to moderate disease. Cholestyramine and colestipol, two anion exchange resins that bind or inactivate *C. difficile* cytotoxin, may be given in doses of 4 g, 3 times daily for 5 days. Compared with vancomycin, these resins have a less predictable response, but are also considerably less expensive, and patients who respond are less likely to have relapses.

PREVENTION AND CONTROL. The best control method is judicious use of antibiotics, especially those that are commonly associated with this complication. In view of evidence for spread within hospitals, it is recommended that hospitalized patients with *C. difficile*–induced disease be isolated and monitored with enteric precautions until diarrhea resolves or the toxin is eradicated in stools.

Bibliography

Bartlett JG: *Clostridium difficile:* History of its role as an enteric pathogen and the current state of knowledge about the organism. Clin Infect Dis 18(Suppl 4):S265, 1994.

Bartlett JG: *Clostridium difficile* infection: Pathophysiology and diagnosis. Semin Gastrointest Dis 8:12, 1997.

Kelly CP, LaMont JT: *Clostridium difficile* infection. Annu Rev Med 49:375, 1998.

Lyerly DM, Wilkins TD: *Clostridium difficile. In* Blaser MJ, Smith PD, Ravdin JL, Greenberg HB, Guerrant RL (eds): Infections of the Gastrointestinal Tract. New York, Raven Press, 1995, pp 867–891.

Manabe YC, Vinetz JM, Moore RD, et al: *Clostridium difficile* colitis: An efficient clinical approach to diagnosis (see Comments). Ann Intern Med 123:835, 1995.

44.4 *Enteritis Necroticans**

DEFINITION. Enteritis necroticans, also known as "pig-bel" and "Darmbrand," is a necrotizing enteritis caused by β toxin produced by *Clostridium perfringens* type C.

HISTORY. The first systematic study of enteritis necroticans was conducted during and shortly after World War II. At that time, there were hundreds of cases of "Darmbrand" (meaning "firebowels") in Germany and Norway; most of these were in malnourished individuals who often had a history of sudden dietary overindulgence. The disease was limited to the early years following World War II, peaking in incidence in 1948, and disappearing thereafter. The etiology was debated, but the likely mechanism centered on a toxin produced by *C. perfringens*. These organisms were classified originally as type F and then reclassified as type C by Oakley, who also detected antitoxin to the β toxin produced by this organism in convalescing patients. Antitoxin therapy was proposed but not used, because the epidemic resolved with improved nutritional status around 1949. Interest in this disease revived in the early 1960s when the same disease process, known locally as "pig-bel," was found to be endemic in the highlands of New Guinea. Extensive studies of enteritis necroticans at this location have provided most of the current information concerning the pathology, pathophysiology, detection, treatment, and prevention of this disease.

DISTRIBUTION. The organism appears to be widely distributed in soil, has been found in asymptomatic carriers, and may be found in the stools of animals, including pigs. Acquisition of the disease depends on a complex combination of circumstances, including contact with the organism, dietary habits, and undernutrition. Since World War II, enteritis necroticans has been found occasionally in Western countries, but most cases occur in developing countries along the equator, e.g., Uganda, Indonesia, Thailand, Malaysia, and New Guinea. Serologic studies in the highlands of New Guinea in 1963 and 1964 showed a prevalence of 50 cases per 10,000 with a mortality rate of 14 per 10,000. Enteritis necroticans was the most common cause of death in children >12 months of age in this location, whereas over 86% of adults in the high-incidence region had circulating antibody to the β toxin.

PATHOGENESIS. In the highlands of New Guinea, the disease is found commonly in children who have participated in the pig and sweet potato feast. The responsible toxin is a protein of approximately 48,000 D that is produced by *C. perfringens* type C. This exotoxin, which is produced in early logarithmic growth, is susceptible to destruction by proteases, including trypsin. The diet among inhabitants of the islands of Papua New Guinea is low in protein, with sweet potatoes accounting for up to 90% of calories. Contributory factors in the diet include a depression of proteolytic activity resulting from reduced protein consumption combined with trypsin inhibitors in the sweet potato staple. It is presumed that the organism is acquired by ingestion of contaminated pig or is present owing to prior colonization and that the toxin is not inactivated because of inadequate proteolysis. This theory is supported by the production of a similar disease in protein-deficient guinea pigs given sweet potato and a broth culture containing *C. perfringens* type C. Co-infection with intestinal parasites may be important also. *Ascaris lumbricoides*, present in 65% of cases of pig-bel, is a source of trypsin inhibitors, whereas another common intestinal helminth, *Strongyloides stercoralis*, may reduce intestinal motility and contribute to intestinal obstruction, or, by penetrating the intestinal mucosa, allow greater absorption of β toxin. Pig-bel is primarily a disease of children in New Guinea, with a peak incidence in children 4 years of age,

---

*All the material in this chapter is in the public domain, with the exception of any borrowed figures or tables.

apparently reflecting the fact that most adults have circulating antibody. The pathogenesis of enteritis necroticans may be different for disease occurring outside of New Guinea, especially when there is no history of pork or sweet potato ingestion or overeating.

PATHOLOGY. Enteritis necroticans is a segmental disease of the small bowel that might be restricted to a few centimeters or may involve the entire length of the small intestine. The external surface shows dilatation, with areas of erythema and fibropurulent exudate. The mucosa underlying segmental areas of peritonitis shows green, necrotic pseudomembranes that may be restricted to the mucosa but are more frequently of full thickness. With more advanced lesions, the bowel wall becomes thinned, friable, and subject to perforation. Microscopic sections taken from involved segments show mucosal infarction with edema, hemorrhage, and infiltration by polymorphonuclear leukocytes. The membrane consists of necrotic mucosal epithelium containing numerous gram-positive bacilli. This inflamed segment is sharply demarcated, with small-vessel thrombi at the junctional zone, suggesting thrombotic necrosis.

CLINICAL MANIFESTATIONS. The usual presenting symptoms are abdominal pain and distention, vomiting, and passage of a bloody or black, tarry stool. The usual incubation period is 48 hours following ingestion of the dietary source of the toxin, but this may vary from 24 hours to 1 week. There is considerable variation in the severity of the disease. Some patients have a fulminant course and die within 24 hours following the onset of symptoms, whereas mild cases may be difficult to distinguish from common forms of gastroenteritis. Occasionally, patients present with malabsorption or intestinal obstruction months or years after the acute episode.

DIAGNOSIS. The diagnosis of enteritis necroticans in the endemic area is based usually on clinical observations, sometimes accompanied by the demonstration of typical pathologic changes at surgery or autopsy. The responsible organism, *C. perfringens* type C, may be demonstrated in small bowel contents or stool using a fluorescein-stained antibody. Stool cultures are difficult to interpret, because the carrier rate of the putative agent in New Guinea is 50 to 100% for inhabitants of both the highland area, where the disease is endemic, and the coastal region, where the incidence is extremely low.

TREATMENT AND PROGNOSIS. Medical therapy includes intestinal decompression with nasogastric intubation; penicillin, or chloramphenicol given intravenously; and intravenous fluid support with appropriate monitoring of serum electrolytes and special attention to potassium depletion. The major indications for operative intervention are persistent toxicity, intestinal obstruction, suspected bowel perforation, and severe recurrent bleeding. Prolonged delays in therapy may result in a technically difficult operation, because the intestine becomes extremely friable with extensive adhesions. In New Guinea, approximately 50% of patients require surgery. The usual procedure is small bowel resection, usually 50 to 200 cm of jejunum. The mortality rate, excluding mild cases, is reported to be 15 to 40%.

PREVENTION. There is little prospect for reversing the dietary and social habits in the highlands of New Guinea to alter the unique combination of circumstances that promotes enteritis necroticans. However, immunization with toxoid prepared from culture filtrates of the putative agent confers protection. This is based on analogous experience with this disease in veterinary medicine, the low incidence of the disease in the endemic area among adults with circulating antibody, and, most importantly, a vaccine trial that demonstrated efficacy.

Immunization. The current recommendation is to administer β toxoid to children in the highlands of New Guinea at 2, 4, and 6 months of age, and to children in other populations outside of New Guinea in whom the disease is active. A tattoo is the suggested recording method, because conventional methods of record keeping have proved futile. The duration of protection is not known, and it is possible that booster injections may be needed.

Bibliography

Borriello SP: Clostridial disease of the gut. Clin Infect Dis 20(Suppl 2):S242, 1995.

Mpamugo O, Donovan T, Brett MM: Enterotoxigenic *Clostridium perfringens* as a cause of sporadic cases of diarrhoea. J Med Microbiol 43:442, 1995.

Murrell TG, Walker PD: The pigbel story of Papua New Guinea. Trans R Soc Trop Med Hyg 85:119, 1991.

Parkes G: Pig-bel in Nepal. Trop Doctor 21:180, 1991.

45 Helicobacter pylori *Infections*

Alan D. Fix and J. Glenn Morris, Jr.

DEFINITION. Since its isolation in 1982, *Helicobacter pylori* has been associated with several disease states. At the time of initial infection, *H. pylori* causes an acute, self-limited gastrointestinal illness that is usually undiagnosed. The almost invariable subsequent chronic infection has been associated with chronic gastritis, peptic ulcer disease (PUD), gastric carcinoma, gastric lymphoma, and Ménétrier's disease. Although controversial, evidence exists for the association of *H. pylori* with nonulcer dyspepsia in adults, as well as recurrent abdominal pain in children. These associated illnesses appear to be multifactorial, since the majority of persons infected by *H. pylori* do not develop them. Unless treated, *H. pylori* infection persists for decades, if not for life.

ETIOLOGY. *H. pylori* is a urease-producing, spiral, microaerophilic, gram-negative rod measuring 0.5×3.0 μm. It is motile, possessing two to six flagella. In addition to this culturable form, it can transform to a viable, nonculturable coccoid bacterium. *H. pylori* displays a particular trophism for normal gastric mucosa, especially in the antrum, and in areas of gastric metaplasia in the esophagus, intestine, rectum, and Meckel diverticulum. It is not found in areas of intestinal metaplasia in the stomach.

HISTORY. Although there were suggestions of the existence of such an organism in the gastric mucosa a century ago, the modern recognition of this pathogen dates only to the early 1980s. The key event was its successful isolation by Warren and Marshall in 1982, reports of which were met with initial skepticism from the medical community. Originally named *Campylobacter pyloridis*, with the elucidation of more of its characteristics it became evident that the organism did not belong in the genus *Campylobacter*, and it was renamed *Helicobacter pylori* in 1989. Shortly after its isolation, it was determined to be a cause of an acute gastrointestinal illness with accompanying hypochlorhydria, and the cause of previously reported instances of epidemic hypochlorhydria. Since that time, evolving knowledge about *H. pylori* has led to a radical change in the conceptualization of several chronic gastrointestinal illnesses, reassigning them to the realm of curable infectious diseases.

EPIDEMIOLOGY. *H. pylori* infection is postulated to be

one of the world's most common infections, if not the most common. Prevalence of infection is universally found to increase with age (Fig. 45–1). It is highly prevalent among populations in developing areas, with the vast majority becoming infected in childhood. In developed areas, it is less prevalent and infection occurs later, with an almost linear increase in seroprevalence, which peaks at about 60% by the seventh decade.

There is strong evidence of a cohort effect, with studies demonstrating decreasing seroprevalence for successive birth cohorts, presumably due to improvements in living conditions. A dramatic example is the sharp decline in seroprevalence in Japan for those born after 1950. However, there is also evidence for continuous exposure and infection throughout life, with incidence rates of up to 1% per year. In developed areas, reappearance of infection following treatment appears to be recrudescence of incompletely eradicated infection, whereas in developing areas ubiquitous infection favors reinfection as the cause for reappearance after treatment. Seroprevalence studies have indicated a drop in prevalence after the sixth or seventh decade, but this may represent loss of the organism's niche as the gastric mucosa undergoes atrophy.

Distribution. An inverse association with socioeconomic status has been a consistent finding across varying populations, and ethnic differences in prevalence may be attributable to differences in socioeconomic status. In developed nations, *H. pylori* is associated with low socioeconomic status and density of living conditions. In developing nations, the prevalence of infection is similarly associated with socioeconomic status only among children. Early childhood appears to be the critical period for acquisition (and possibly transmission).

Reservoir. Humans appear to be the major reservoir for infection. However, determination of reservoirs has been complicated by the difficulty involved in successful culturing of the organism. In vitro, the organism tends to transform to a viable, nonculturable form. There is some evidence that zoonotic reservoirs exist, with the organism having been found in some primates and domestic cats, as well as increased prevalence rates among those working with animals. Although reports of environmental reservoirs have been scant, there is evidence that it can remain viable and potentially infectious in water for some time, being culturable for more than 10 days and present in its coccoid form for more than a year.

Transmission. Transmission is primarily from person to person. Supporting this conclusion is the clustering of infection under conditions of crowding (e.g., intrafamilial, institutional, and among submarine crews). However, clustering is consistent with common source transmission as well.

Two routes of person-to-person transmission have been proposed: oral-oral and fecal-oral. The organism has been found in dental plaque and saliva, but the consistent lack of evidence for transmission between spouses is inconsistent with oral-oral transmission. The support for fecal-oral transmission has come from epidemiologic similarities with other pathogens transmitted in this manner (e.g., hepatitis A virus), as well as acquisition being predominantly in childhood, noting the frequency of fecal-oral transmission favored by hand-to-mouth habits of young children and recent reports of the isolation of *H. pylori* from stool. Shedding is probably greatest in the acute phase of infection (generally taking place in childhood), which explains why the major risk factor for acquisition of infection in adulthood is the presence of children in the household. A report linking infection to consumption of sewage-contaminated vegetables provides evidence for water-borne transmission, a route which may be significant in the developing world. No evidence for sexual transmission exists.

H. pylori Association With Clinical Illness. The similarities between both temporal and geographic epidemiologic patterns of *H. pylori* infection and those of gastritis, PUD, and gastric carcinoma have supported the association between these diseases and the organism. The decreasing prevalence among successive birth cohorts parallels the pattern of decreasing prevalence of gastritis, PUD, and gastric carcinoma in successive cohorts. Exceptions to the similarities of patterns exist, e.g., areas of Africa in which infection is highly prevalent but PUD and gastric carcinoma are not. These discrepancies have been partly explained on the basis of the multifactorial process in carcinogenesis, with cultural, host, and virulence variation influencing development of disease.

Chronic Gastritis. Despite humoral response to the infection, the organism is not cleared following the acute illness, and chronic infection results in superficial mucosal inflam-

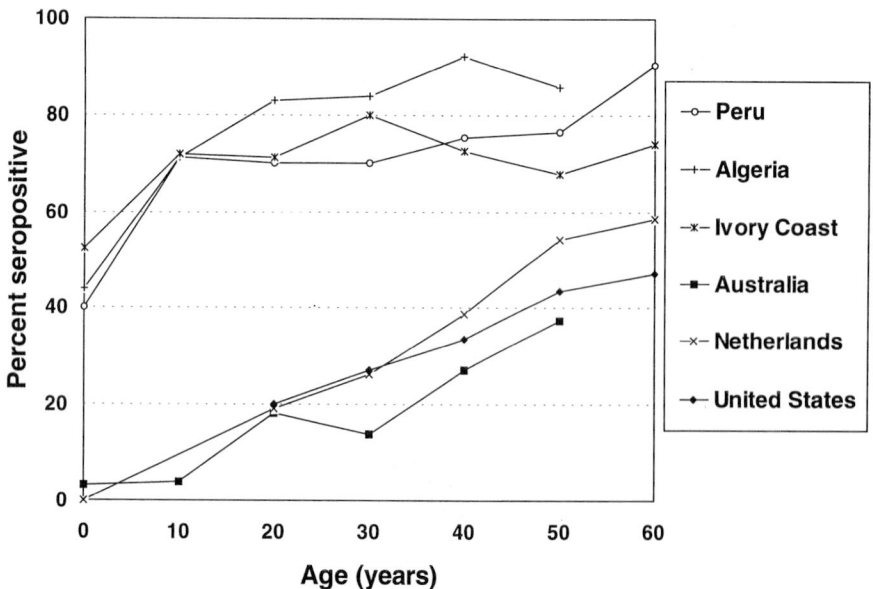

Figure 45–1. National variation in *H. pylori* seroprevalence. (From Hopkins RJ, Morris JG Jr: *Helicobacter pylori:* The missing link in perspective. Am J Med 97:265, 1994.)

mation. Antral gastritis has been noted in virtually all *H. pylori*–infected patients undergoing endoscopy, and most patients with gastritis have been found to be infected with *H. pylori*.

Peptic Ulcer Disease. The association of *H. pylori* infection and PUD is well established. Eradication of infection prevents recurrence of ulcer in most patients, and at least one of its complications, bleeding. This strong association exists for both duodenal ulcers and gastric ulcers, albeit somewhat less for gastric ulcers. It has been suggested that in the absence of other specific causes, *H. pylori* may be a sine qua non for duodenal ulcer. Nonetheless, the majority of infected individuals do not develop disease.

Because PUD is associated with both *H. pylori* and blood group O, there has been speculation regarding the association of *H. pylori* infection and blood group. There is evidence that the terminal fucose group of the H antigen of the ABO group and the Lewis[b] antigen acts as a receptor for *H. pylori*; however, epidemiologic studies have not found an association between *H. pylori* infection and either ABO group or secretor status.

Gastric Carcinoma. On the basis of accumulated evidence of the association between *H. pylori* and gastric carcinoma, *H. pylori* was declared a carcinogen by the International Agency for Research on Cancer of the World Health Organization in 1994. Several nested case-control studies within large cohorts have demonstrated an association between antecedent infection and subsequent development of gastric carcinoma. This association exists for carcinoma of both diffuse and intestinal types in the antrum and body of the stomach, but not the cardia. However, substantially less than 1% of those infected develop gastric carcinoma, one of the most common cancers in the world despite declining incidence in the past several decades.

Interestingly, those patients who develop duodenal ulcers generally do not develop gastric carcinoma, and there is an association with the age at acquisition: those with acquisition early in childhood having a greater risk of developing cancer, and those with acquisition later in childhood having an increased risk of developing PUD.

Gastric Lymphoma. Although healthy gastric mucosa normally does not contain lymphoid follicles, mucosa-associated lymphoid tissue (MALT), resembling Peyer's patches, has been described and ascribed to *H. pylori* infection. MALT is estimated to give rise to 20 to 30% of gastric lymphoma. *H. pylori* is, thus, associated with primary B-cell gastric MALT lymphoma, since over 90% of patients with these lesions have evidence of *H. pylori* infections. Several studies have indicated regression of low-grade MALT lymphomas following eradication of *H. pylori*.

Hypertrophic Gastropathy. *H. pylori* is also associated with Ménétrier's disease, or hypertrophic gastropathy. There is evidence of *H. pylori* infection in 90% of cases, as well as healing of the lesions following successful eradication of the infection.

Nonulcer Dyspepsia. The association of *H. pylori* with nonulcer dyspepsia remains controversial. A review of clinical trials investigating the association and resolution with anti–*H. pylori* therapy has found flaws with virtually all studies. Although methodologically sound evidence is lacking, it appears there is a subset of patients whose nonulcer dyspepsia is associated with *H. pylori* and who would benefit from eradication of the organism.

Childhood. Among children, *H. pylori* has been associated predominantly with nodular gastritis, and with PUD and recurrent abdominal pain in a subset of children, but these associations remain controversial.

PATHOGENESIS. *H. pylori*'s ability to infect and cause its particular spectrum of disease is dependent on its ability to colonize in the hostile environment of the stomach. Its unique ability to survive in the acid environment of the stomach allows it to avoid competition from other organisms. Its motility allows it to escape the contents of the gastric lumen quickly by penetrating the mucous layer that overlies the gastric mucosa.

Survival in the Stomach. The organism's urease activity results in a less acidic microenvironment in which it can survive. In fact, there is evidence that, in the presence of urea, an acid environment is necessary for the organism's survival. Most *H. pylori* remain free within the mucous layer, although some adhere to epithelial adherence pedestals.

Its colonization over the mucosa, without invasion, may be partly responsible for its evasion of host defenses, allowing it to become resident for the life of the host despite a host humoral response. Although circulating antibodies to *H. pylori* are not protective, observational evidence in breast-fed infants and experimental evidence in animals indicate that the presence of IgA in the stomach's lumen is protective.

Peptic Ulcer Disease. Local inflammation results from both products of the bacterium itself and the host response to the infection. In addition, *H. pylori* infection interferes with inhibition of gastrin secretion, with resultant inappropriately high acid levels. Increased duodenal acid loads may give rise to gastric metaplasia and subsequent *H. pylori* colonization, causing localized inflammation and ulcer in the duodenum.

Gastric Carcinoma. *H. pylori* is associated with the progressive stages in the pathogenesis of gastric carcinoma: chronic gastritis, atrophic gastritis, intestinal metaplasia, and dysplasia. The chronic inflammation due to *H. pylori* infection, and the products of that inflammation, are apparently key factors in the development of gastric carcinoma. *H. pylori* may initiate the process by causing chronic cellular proliferation, increasing the likelihood of mutagenic processes in the presence of carcinogenic substances (e.g., salt and nitrates in preserved foods) and in the absence of protective substances (e.g., ascorbic acid and β-carotene in fruits and vegetables). Gastric carcinoma appears to be a long-term complication of the chronic inflammation resulting from *H. pylori* infection. This has prompted Blaser and Parsonnet to dub *H. pylori* "the 'slow' bacterium."

Strain Heterogeneity. Differences in virulence between strains of *H. pylori* exist. Two genes have been identified, the products of which are associated with PUD; *cagA* is present in approximately 60% of *H. pylori*, and is invariably present in those strains associated with PUD. The other gene, *vacA*, is present in all *H. pylori*, but due to sequence divergence, only 50 to 60% of isolates produces the gene's product, which induces vacuolation in eukaryotic cells. Variations in distribution of these strains may be responsible for geographic variations in incidence of gastric carcinoma and PUD among varying populations with high prevalence of infection. Environmental and cultural factors may also play a part in these variations in disease. There are data to suggest that strains causing PUD cluster differently from those causing asymptomatic gastritis. Smoking may increase the progression from intestinal metaplasia to dysplasia.

CLINICAL MANIFESTATIONS. The disease states associated with *H. pylori* infection include an acute gastrointestinal illness, chronic gastritis, PUD, gastric carcinoma, gastric lymphoma, and Ménétrier's disease.

Acute Gastritis. The acute gastritis associated with *H. pylori* infection has been described from case reports of self-inoculation as well as outbreaks of hypochlorhydria among healthy volunteers undergoing secretion studies. This self-limited illness is marked by nausea, vomiting, and abdominal pain several days to a week following ingestion of the organism, with resolution generally within 1 week. Endoscopy demonstrates superficial gastritis. This acute illness is accompanied by hypochlorhydria, with acid production generally returning to normal over a period of months. During the period of hypochlorhydria, there is an increase in growth of other bacteria in stomach secretions. It has been suggested that acute infection with *H. pylori* in early childhood may make a significant contribution to chronic diarrhea and malnutrition in the developing world, initiating the cycle of gastrointestinal infection and malnutrition.

Other Symptom Complexes. The other clinical manifestations associated with, or purported to be associated with *H. pylori* are well described in standard textbooks. At present, no clinical features have been described that are peculiar to chronic gastritis, PUD, gastric carcinoma, MALT-type gastric lymphoma, hypertrophic gastropathy, nonulcer dyspepsia, and recurrent abdominal pain of childhood when associated with *H. pylori*.

DIAGNOSIS. Initially, diagnosis of *H. pylori* infection was dependent on endoscopy and biopsy, with culture and histology to establish the diagnosis. It is difficult to culture the organism, taking at least 4 days. The development of *Campylobacter*-like organism (CLO)-urease testing has provided a quick and reliable test, but still requires endoscopy. The test uses a gel pellet buffered to an acid pH and containing urea, phenol red, and a bacteriostatic agent. The action of preformed urease of *H. pylori* raises the pH within the gel, causing a color change. Serologic testing with enzyme-linked immunosorbent assays has proved both sensitive and specific, and is widely used for epidemiologic studies. As spontaneous resolution of the infection is apparently rare, a positive titer in an untreated patient is indicative of current infection. Titers decrease after eradication of the organism.

The urea-breath test is also sensitive and specific, and it has been proposed as a good tool for both assessing current infection and evaluating response to therapy. The breath test is based on the ingestion of ^{13}C-urea (nonradioactive isotope) or ^{14}C-urea (radioactive isotope) and subsequent breath sampling to detect labeled CO_2, the product of *H. pylori* urease. The combination of virulence markers, e.g., antibodies to cagA, may prove useful in defining a subset of seropositive individuals for eradication treatment.

TREATMENT. Effective treatment for the eradication of *H. pylori* exists, but indications for eradication are still evolving. The evidence that eradication of *H. pylori* prevents ulcer recurrence is convincing, and consensus exists for the treatment of patients with PUD who are infected. Eradication as a treatment for nonulcer dyspepsia remains controversial.

Eradication of infection in an attempt to prevent gastric carcinoma is not recommended. Screening and treatment of the asymptomatic population is not feasible, as the majority may be infected, and only a small fraction will develop gastric carcinoma. Identification and treatment of infected individuals who are at high risk for gastric carcinoma, e.g., those with family history of gastric carcinoma and those with endoscopic evidence of early mucosal changes, is probably justified, as is eradication of *H. pylori* in those with MALT and Ménétrier's disease.

Although treatment with bismuth subsalicylate (or subci-

trate) alone results in suppression of the organism, there is often recrudescence of the infection. Triple therapy with bismuth subsalicylate (two tablets four times a day), metronidazole (250 mg four times a day or 500 mg twice a day), and tetracycline (500 mg four times a day) has proved very effective, albeit the complicated regimen and side effects can affect compliance. Amoxicillin (500 mg four times a day or 1 g twice a day) can be substituted for tetracycline. Therapy for 2 weeks has been shown to be effective, but there is evidence that 1 week may suffice. A combination of omeprazole (20 mg twice a day), a proton-exchange inhibitor, and either clarithromycin (250–500 mg twice a day) or amoxicillin has also proved effective, but triple therapy with omeprazole and 2 antibiotics is more effective and may require only 1 week of therapy. The addition of an H_2 blocker is indicated when treating patients with active ulcers.

PREVENTION. Dramatic decreases in seroprevalence in different populations in developed countries are believed to be the result of improved living conditions and sanitation. A similar decrease is to be anticipated with improved conditions in the lesser developed countries. Recent advances in the development of oral vaccines for *H. pylori* show promise, and if inexpensive and effective vaccines can be developed, this may provide the best means of infection control and prevention on a population level. There is the possibility that such vaccines may also prove to be therapeutic in those already infected.

Bibliography

Blaser MJ, Parsonnet J: Parasitism by the "slow" bacterium *Helicobacter pylori* leads to altered gastric homeostasis and neoplasia. J Clin Invest 94:4, 1994.

Brown KE, Peura DA: Diagnosis of *Helicobacter pylori* infection. Gastroenterol Clin North Am 22:105, 1993.

Bujanover Y, Reif S, Yahav J: *Helicobacter pylori* and peptic disease in the pediatric patient. Pediatr Clin North Am 43:213, 1996.

Correa P: *Helicobacter pylori* and gastric carcinogenesis. Am J Surg Pathol 19:S37, 1995.

EUROGAST Study Group: Epidemiology of, and risk factors for, *Helicobacter pylori* infection among 3194 asymptomatic subjects in 17 populations. Gut 34:1672, 1993.

Feldman RA: Prevention of *Helicobacter pylori* infection. Baillieres Clin Gastroenterol 9:447, 1995.

Goodman KJ, Correa P: The transmission of *Helicobacter pylori*: A critical review of the evidence. Int J Epidemiol 24:875, 1995.

Hopkins RJ, Morris JG, Jr: *Helicobacter pylori*: the missing link in perspective. Am J Med 97:265, 1994.

Marshall BJ: The 1995 Albert Lasker Medical Research Awards. *Helicobacter pylori*: The etiologic agent for peptic ulcer. JAMA 274:1064, 1995.

NIH Consensus Development Panel on *Helicobacter pylori* in Peptic Ulcer Disease: NIH Consensus Conference. *Helicobacter pylori* in peptic ulcer disease. JAMA 272:65, 1994.

Salcedo JA, Al-Kawas F: Treatment of *Helicobacter pylori* infection. Arch Intern Med 158:842, 1998.

Sipponen P: *Helicobacter pylori*: a cohort phenomenon. Am J Surg Pathol 19:S30, 1995.

Soll AH: Consensus conference. Medical treatment of peptic ulcer disease. Practice guidelines. Practice Parameters Committee of the American College of Gastroenterology. JAMA 275:622, 1996.

Talley NJ: A critique of therapeutic trials in *Helicobacter pylori*–positive functional dyspepsia. Gastroenterology 106:1174, 1994.

Taylor DN, Blaser MJ: The epidemiology of *Helicobacter pylori* infection. Epidemiol Rev 13:42, 1991.

Thijs JC, Kuipers EJ, van Zwet AA, et al: Treatment of *Helicobacter pylori* infections. Q J Med 88:369, 1995.

Walsh JH, Peterson WL: The treatment of *Helicobacter pylori* infection in the management of peptic ulcer disease. N Engl J Med 333:984, 1995.

46 *Chlamydial Infections*

David C.W. Mabey

Chlamydiae are among the most successful bacterial pathogens. *Chlamydia trachomatis* is responsible for blindness (Chapter 32), pelvic inflammatory disease (PID), urethritis, epididymitis, infertility, and ectopic pregnancy in millions of people annually; it also causes lymphogranuloma venereum (Chapter 47), reactive arthritis, ophthalmia neonatorum, and infantile pneumonia. *C. pneumoniae* is among the most common causes of community-acquired pneumonia, and it may play a part in the pathogenesis of coronary heart disease. *C. psittaci* is a highly prevalent zoonotic infection with a wide host range (Chapter 35). It is of great economic importance and causes sporadic but sometimes devastating disease in humans.

HISTORY. The inclusion bodies characteristic of chlamydial infection were first described by Halberstaedter and von Prowazek in 1907, in conjunctival scrapings from patients with trachoma. Shortly after this, similar inclusions were observed in scrapings from the conjunctiva of a neonate with ophthalmia and in cervical scrapings from the infant's mother. *C. psittaci* was first isolated in 1930 by Bedson, in budgerigars, and *C. trachomatis* in 1957, in fertile hen's eggs by Tang and colleagues. The isolation of *C. trachomatis* in tissue culture in 1965 provided a less laborious and more sensitive diagnostic technique, which led to an appreciation that *C. trachomatis* is a genital tract pathogen of major importance. With the development of antigen and DNA detection methods since 1980, this impression has been confirmed in numerous studies in many populations. In 1986 an atypical strain of *Chlamydia*, first isolated in the 1960s from the eye of a child with trachoma, was found to be an important cause of community-acquired pneumonia in young adults in the United States. Unlike *C. psittaci*, it appeared to have no animal reservoir, and in 1989 it was designated the third chlamydial species, *C. pneumoniae*.

ETIOLOGY. The genus *Chlamydia* contains three species that cause human disease: *C. trachomatis*, *C. pneumoniae*, and *C. psittaci*. The chlamydiae have their own family (Chlamydiaceae), which is the only one in the order Chlamydiales, reflecting the uniqueness of these organisms. Chlamydiae are bacteria that are unable to synthesize adenosine triphosphate (ATP), since they lack enzymes of the cytochrome oxidase pathway; they are therefore "energy parasites," which can replicate only within a eukaryotic host cell. They have a unique life cycle when grown in tissue culture. The infectious elementary body (EB) is a metabolically inert, sporelike structure with a rigid cell wall 0.3 μm in diameter. The rigidity of the cell wall is conferred by extensive disulfide bonding within the cysteine-rich major outer membrane protein (MOMP), which makes up 60% of the cell wall.

After attachment to the host cell, EBs are actively ingested by host cells. *C. trachomatis* generally infects epithelial cells rather than specialized phagocytic cells, and it is not clear whether phagocytosis or receptor-mediated endocytosis plays the more important role in chlamydial uptake by infected cells. Some hours after ingestion the EB loses its structural rigidity and enlarges to form a metabolically active reticulate body (RB). RBs divide by binary fission before condensing to form new EBs. By 36 hours after infection, chlamydial inclusions, containing large numbers of RBs and EBs, can be observed in the cytoplasm of infected cells, and by 72 hours inclusion-containing cells are likely to have ruptured, releasing large numbers of infectious EBs. Inclusions of *C. psittaci* and *C. pneumoniae* differ from those of *C. trachomatis* in that they do not contain glycogen.

Fifteen serotypes of *C. trachomatis* were identified by the microimmunofluorescence test of Wang and Grayston. These 15 serotypes contain two biovars: trachoma and the more invasive lymphogranuloma venereum (LGV). Serotypes A through C cause trachoma, and serotypes D through K cause genital tract and neonatal infections (Table 46–1).

PATHOGENESIS. The clinical and pathologic hallmark of chlamydial infection is the lymphoid follicle. Follicles contain typical germinal centers, consisting predominantly of B lymphocytes, with T cells in the parafollicular region, which consists mostly of CD8+ cells. Fibrosis is the cause of the irreversible late sequelae of chlamydial infection seen, for example, in trachoma and PID. The histopathology of chlamydial infection suggests that much of its pathophysiology is of immunopathologic origin. Repeated reinfection and/or latent chronic infection are required to induce fibrosis. It is likely that fibrogenic cytokines are released locally by immune cells in response to continuing antigenic stimulation.

EPIDEMIOLOGY. *C. trachomatis* is the most prevalent sexually transmitted bacterial pathogen in developed countries

TABLE 46–1. Clinical Features of Chlamydial Infection

Chlamydial Species/Serotype	Clinical Association
Chlamydia trachomatis A–C	Trachoma (follicular conjunctivitis → cicatricial sequelae)
Chlamydia trachomatis D–K	Urethritis
	Cervicitis
	Acute salpingitis
	Chronic pelvic inflammatory disease
	Epididymo-orchitis
	Proctitis
	Infertility
	Ectopic pregnancy
	Reiter's syndrome
	Fitz-Hugh–Curtis syndrome
	Paratrachoma
	Neonatal ophthalmia
	Infantile pneumonia
Chlamydia trachomatis L_1–L_3	Lymphogranuloma venereum
Chlamydia pneumoniae	Community-acquired pneumonia
	Pharyngitis
	Sinusitis
	Myocarditis
	Association with atheroma/ischemic heart disease
Chlamydia psittaci	Pneumonia ± other organ
	Involvement ± avian contact

and is highly prevalent worldwide. Many studies have found between 3 and 10% of antenatal clinic attenders to have a chlamydial cervical infection, and up to 30% of patients in some urban clinics in developing countries have been found infected. It has been estimated that in the United States in the early 1980s there were approximately 2 million cases of chlamydial cervicitis per year and 300,000 cases of chlamydial PID, costing the country over $1 billion annually. The prevalence is invariably higher in younger women and is often lower than expected in high-risk groups, e.g., commercial sex workers, suggesting that protective immunity may eventually be induced by natural infection.

CLINICAL MANIFESTATIONS. The clinical syndromes caused by *Chlamydia* species are shown in Table 46–1. Trachoma and inclusion conjunctivitis are covered in Chapter 32, lymphogranuloma venereum in Chapter 47, and psittacosis caused by *C. psittaci* infections in Chapter 35.

Genital Tract Infections

In Males. *C. trachomatis* can be isolated from the urethra of 20 to 50% of men with nongonococcal urethritis; since it often coexists with *Neisseria gonorrhoeae* and does not generally respond to treatment for gonorrhea, it is also an important cause of postgonococcal urethritis. Chlamydial urethritis is generally milder than the gonococcal form, usually giving rise to a less profuse and more mucoid discharge, and the incubation period is typically longer (5–21 days). Epididymitis is the most important complication in men; in one study in the United States, *C. trachomatis* was shown to be the most frequent cause of this condition in men under 35 years of age. It is possible that *C. trachomatis* is a cause of chronic urethritis and urethral stricture. There is no evidence that it causes prostatitis.

In Females. In women the majority of chlamydial infections are asymptomatic, although they are often associated with mucopurulent cervicitis. Chlamydial cervicitis has been implicated as a possible cofactor for the heterosexual transmission of the human immunodeficiency virus (HIV). Infection of the urethra may give rise to dysuria and/or sterile pyuria.

Ascending infection is more common after cervical trauma, for example, that caused by termination of pregnancy or insertion of an intrauterine device. It may give rise to endometritis, salpingitis, or perihepatitis—the Fitz-Hugh–Curtis syndrome, which may mimic gallbladder disease clinically. Although the symptoms of chlamydial PID are usually less severe than those of gonococcal disease and may indeed be minimal or absent, sequelae are equally common and severe; infertility and ectopic pregnancy occur in a high proportion of cases.

Reactive Arthritis. Sexually acquired reactive arthritis or Reiter's syndrome may follow a chlamydial genital tract infection, usually in males. Despite the presence of chlamydial antigen and DNA in the joints of such patients, viable organisms have not been isolated, and the response to antibiotics is usually disappointing.

Adult Paratrachoma. This condition, caused by *C. trachomatis* serotypes D through K, usually coexists with genital tract infection and is presumed to result from accidental contamination of the eye with genital secretions. It usually presents as an acute follicular conjunctivitis, often unilateral and commonly accompanied by preauricular adenopathy. In long-standing cases punctate keratitis and even pannus, similar to that associated with trachoma, may be seen. Management of this condition includes investigation and treatment for genital tract infection, with partner notification.

Neonatal Infections. Up to 50% of women with cervical infections infect their infants at delivery. Neonatal infection may be asymptomatic or may give rise to ophthalmia neona-

torum (in approximately 30% of exposed infants) or pneumonitis (in approximately 10%).

Ophthalmia Neonatorum. Ophthalmia usually occurs within 3 weeks of birth and is characterized by mucopurulent conjunctivitis that is characteristically less severe than that caused by *N. gonorrhoeae* and is self-limiting. Chlamydial ophthalmia may be accompanied by otitis media, and *C. trachomatis* has been isolated from the middle ear.

Pneumonitis. This usually occurs between the ages of 4 and 12 weeks. Most, but not all, infants with chlamydial pneumonia will have previously suffered from ophthalmia. Typically there is a paroxysmal cough and tachypnea in the absence of fever, and there are few signs on auscultation. Chest x-ray reveals diffuse bilateral interstitial infiltrates and hyperinflation. An eosinophilia is sometimes present. Although neonatal chlamydial pneumonitis may be mild and often resolves without treatment, it may give rise to permanent pulmonary sequelae, since infants with this condition are at increased risk of obstructive airways disease in later life.

Chlamydia pneumoniae. *C. pneumoniae* was first detected as a novel ocular serovar in Taiwan in 1976. It has since become apparent that it is a distinct species on genetic, serologic, and morphologic criteria. Differing serovars of *C. pneumoniae* have yet to be described. It is primarily a respiratory pathogen, rarely if ever causing genital or ocular disease.

BRONCHITIS AND PNEUMONIA. *C. pneumoniae* is a common cause of bronchitis and community-acquired pneumonia. Seroepidemiologic surveys have shown that the majority of the population is exposed to *C. pneumoniae* infection, with the peak ages of seroconversion being 5 to 15 years. Most infection is subclinical or does not come to medical attention, but it can cause severe disease, especially in the elderly with pre-existing respiratory disease. Patients often report having a sore throat with onset a week or two prior to their respiratory illness, but there are no other distinguishing features in history, physical examination, or radiology that separate *C. pneumoniae* from other causes of community-acquired pneumonia.

ISCHEMIC HEART DISEASE. Seroepidemiologic surveys have shown an association between ischemic heart disease and elevated antibody titers to *C. pneumoniae*, with the findings confirmed in subsequent prospective studies. There have also been reports of the identification of *C. pneumoniae* EBs within diseased coronary arteries.

DIAGNOSIS. Since *C. trachomatis* is an intracellular pathogen, the diagnosis of genital tract chlamydial infection depends on the collection of a sample that contains an adequate number of epithelial cells from the site of infection: the cervix and/or urethra in women, and the urethra in men.

In the past, isolation in tissue culture has been regarded as the gold standard for the diagnosis of genital and ocular chlamydial infection. Since this is laborious and technically demanding, it is not widely available, and in many laboratories simpler antigen detection tests are used. The direct fluorescent antigen detection assay has the advantage that the adequacy of the specimen can be ascertained by performing a cell count, but it is laborious and subjective in its interpretation. Several enzyme immunoassays are commercially available.

Recently, diagnostic tests based on DNA amplification techniques—polymerase chain reaction (PCR) and ligase chain reaction (LCR)—have been licensed in the United States and Europe. Since their advent, it has become apparent that both isolation and antigen detection methods lack sensitivity, even in the best laboratories. DNA amplification assays have the added advantage that invasive sampling is not required: A first-void urine will suffice, in both men and women. These are now the diagnostic methods of choice, although they remain too expensive for use in most developing countries. They are also appropriate for the diagnosis of ocular infection.

The diagnosis of neonatal chlamydial pneumonia is made serologically, using the serotype-specific microimmunofluorescence test; the presence of IgM antibody to *C. trachomatis* is diagnostic. *C. pneumoniae* and *C. psittaci* infections are also generally diagnosed serologically, although seroconversion may not occur until several weeks after the onset of symptoms. Complement fixation tests do not distinguish between the chlamydial species; using this method, many cases diagnosed in the past as psittacosis are likely to have been due to *C. pneumoniae*. Recently, PCR-based diagnostic tests have been used to detect these organisms in throat swabs or sputum.

TREATMENT

Genital Infections. All chlamydial species remain, for practical purposes, universally sensitive to tetracyclines and macrolides. Recommended treatment regimens for uncomplicated genital infections include tetracycline hydrochloride 500 mg four times daily, doxycycline 100 mg twice daily, or erythromycin stearate 500 mg four times daily for 1 week. One study in pregnant women has shown that amoxicillin 500 mg three times daily for 1 week is equivalent to the standard course of erythromycin in the treatment of uncomplicated cervical infection and is better tolerated. A 2-week course of treatment is recommended for chlamydial PID.

Recently, a single 1 g dose of the azalide antibiotic azithromycin was shown to be as effective as the 7-day regimen in the treatment of uncomplicated lower genital tract infection; this is a major advance, since compliance can be ensured by giving treatment under supervision. As for the other sexually transmitted diseases, the treatment of sexual partners is essential both to prevent reinfection of the index case and to prevent sequelae in the partners.

Ocular Infection. *C. trachomatis* eye infections should be treated systemically. In the case of adults, this is because of the high likelihood of coexisting genital tract infection. In the case of infants, the purpose is to eradicate nasopharyngeal carriage and hence prevent pneumonia. *C. pneumoniae* and *C. psittaci* infection should be treated with a 2-week course of tetracycline hydrochloride or erythromycin stearate 500 mg four times daily for 2 weeks.

CONTROL. Chlamydial salpingitis and its sequelae of infertility and ectopic pregnancy have been described as a silent epidemic, because the symptoms are mild or absent in the early stages. A study in the United States has shown that a screening program for genital *C. trachomatis* infection at the primary health care level can reduce the incidence of upper genital tract infection and its complications in women. Now that noninvasive diagnostic tests and single-dose treatment are available, it is possible to prevent and treat individual infections and control the epidemic of genital chlamydial infection.

Bibliography

Alary M, Joly RR, Moutquin J-M, et al: Randomised comparison of amoxycillin and erythromycin in treatment of genital chlamydial infection in pregnancy. Lancet 344:1461, 1994.

Been MO, Saxon EM: Respiratory-tract colonization and a distinctive pneumonia syndrome in infants infected with Chlamydia trachomatis. N Engl J Med 296:306, 1977.

Berger RE, Alexander ER, Monda GD, et al: Chlamydia trachomatis as a cause of acute "idiopathic" epididymitis. N Engl J Med 298:301, 1978.

Brunham RC, Paavonen J, Stevens CE, et al: Mucopurulent cervicitis—the ignored counterpart in women of urethritis in men. N Engl J Med 311:1, 1984.

Chernesky MA, Lee H, Schachter J, et al: Diagnosis of Chlamydia trachomatis urethral infection in symptomatic and asymptomatic men by testing first-void urine in a ligase chain reaction assay. J Infect Dis 170:1308, 1994.

Grayston JT, Campbell LA, Kuo C-C, et al: A new respiratory tract pathogen: Chlamydia pneumoniae strain TWAR. J Infect Dis 161:618, 1990.

Kuo C-C, Shor A, Campbell LA, et al: Demonstration of Chlamydia pneumoniae in atherosclerotic lesions of coronary arteries. J Infect Dis 167:841, 1993.

Lee HH, Chernesky MA, Schachter J, et al: Diagnosis of Chlamydia trachomatis genitourinary infection in women by ligase chain reaction assay of urine. Lancet 345:213, 1995.

Martin DH, Mroczowski TF, Dalu ZA, et al: A controlled trial of a single dose of azithromycin for the treatment of chlamydial urethritis and cervicitis. N Engl J Med 327:921, 1992.

Martin DH, Pollock S, Kuo CC, et al: Chlamydia trachomatis infections in men with Reiter's syndrome. Ann Intern Med 73:569, 1984.

Schachter J: Chlamydial infections. N Engl J Med 298:428, 490, 540, 1978.

Scholes D, Stergachis A, Heidrich FE, et al: Prevention of pelvic inflammatory disease by screening for cervical chlamydial infection. N Engl J Med 334:1362, 1996.

Thom DH, Grayston JT, Siscovick DS, et al: Association of prior infection with Chlamydia pneumoniae and angiographically demonstrated coronary artery disease. JAMA 268:68, 1992.

Washington AE, Johnson RE, Sanders LLJ: Chlamydia trachomatis infections in the United States: What are they costing us? JAMA 257:2070, 1987.

Westrom L, Mardh P-A: Chlamydial salpingitis. Br Med Bull 39:145, 1983.

47 *Lymphogranuloma Venereum*

August H.R. Stich

DEFINITION. Lymphogranuloma venereum (LGV) is one of the five classic venereal diseases, together with gonorrhea, syphilis, chancroid, and donovanosis. Especially between the latter and LGV, there is considerable confusion about terminology. Various similar synonyms are used inconsistently in the literature; this is clarified in Table 47–1.

LGV is essentially a systemic disease with an aggressive nature. Its natural course has three distinct stages. The primary stage is normally an inconspicuous genital lesion. This stage is followed by a regional lymphadenopathy accompanied by systemic symptoms (secondary LGV). In special circumstances hemorrhagic proctocolitis, occasionally seen in women and mostly in homosexual men, can occur. Serious late complications may follow in the tertiary stage, e.g., genital elephantiasis, rectal or urethral strictures and lymphatic fistulas.

ETIOLOGY. LGV is a chlamydial infection. Chlamydiae are highly specialized, obligate intracellular gram-negative bacteria that cannot replicate outside a living host cell (Chapter 46). They are characterized by a unique reproductive cycle

TABLE 47–1. Terminology of Donovanosis and Lymphogranuloma Venereum

Accepted terminology	Donovanosis	Lymphogranuloma Venereum
Infectious agent	*Calymmatobacterium granulomatis*	*Chlamydia trachomatis* L$_{1-3}$
Synonyms	Granuloma inguinale Granuloma venereum	Lymphopathia venereum Lymphogranuloma inguinale Tropical bubo, climatic bubo Durand-Nicolas-Favré disease

with two distinct phases of development called "elementary body" and "reticulate body." The elementary body is the form adapted to extracellular survival. It acts as the infective agent and attaches to susceptible epithelial cells. In this process, heparan sulfate is used as a bridge to the epithelial surface of the host. After invasion of the target cell, usually by receptor-mediated endocytosis, the elementary body transforms into an intracellular reticulate body, which is capable of multiplication. The reticulate body divides to form a cytoplasmic inclusion, which ruptures after 48 to 72 hours releasing new infectious elementary bodies.

The genus *Chlamydia* (order Chlamydiales) contains three species sharing a common group antigen: *C. trachomatis*, an exclusively human pathogen, *C. pneumoniae* and *C. psittaci*. *Chlamydia trachomatis*, formerly called *Chlamydia*, is able to cause a wide range of different diseases. Only serovars L_1, L_2, and L_3 are able to cause LGV, with L_2 being the most prevalent. Whereas the other serovars of *C. trachomatis* all produce superficial epithelial infections of mucous membranes in the eyes, genitalia, or respiratory system, L_{1-3} serovars (LGV strains) have a distinct invasive behavior in lymphatic tissue. They grow rapidly in cell culture, show enhanced resistance to phagocytosis, and kill mice after intracerebral inoculation.

HISTORY. Following introduction of the first serologic tests for venereal diseases by Wassermann in 1906, it became possible to separate the distinct manifestations of LGV from those of syphilis. A first full description of the disease was given in 1913 by Durand, Nicolas, and Favré. Initially LGV was mainly observed in returnees from the tropics, e.g., in sailors, tradesmen, or soldiers. No pathologic agent could be isolated. By 1925, Frei introduced an intradermal skin test which gave positive responses in most LGV patients. The terms "climatic bubo" and "tropical bubo" were associated with the disease some years later when their common etiology was successfully demonstrated. Using the Frei skin test, the late complications of elephantiasis and rectal stricture could also be connected with LGV.

With the isolation and culture of chlamydiae in the 1930s and the introduction of specific serologic tests in the 1960s, the natural history of LGV was fully described. Advances in immunology and molecular biology in the 1980s and 1990s led to a new phase of understanding in the pathophysiology of the disease. DNA amplification tests began to replace the difficult-to-perform cell culture as the gold standard in diagnosis.

In spite of rapid progress in understanding this disease, the public health impact of LGV, especially in countries with limited health resources, is still unknown. Data of population-based surveys on its prevalence in areas where LGV is endemic are not available.

EPIDEMIOLOGY
Transmission. LGV is a sexually transmitted disease (STD). The major sources of infection are asymptomatic carriers, especially women with LGV endocervicitis. The percentage of asymptomatic carriers in endemic areas is shown to be very high as the diagnostic methods for their detection improve. The frequency of infection following exposure seems relatively low, although the actual risk of infection is unknown. Extragenital transmission, mostly laboratory infection, occasionally occurs. Autoinfection (conjunctivitis) is possible.

Geographic Distribution. LGV has a worldwide distribution but is more prevalent in tropical and subtropical regions. Apparently the global overall incidence is in a decline. LGV is sporadic in North America and Europe but is still highly endemic in parts of Africa, India, Southeast Asia, the Carib-

bean, and Brazil. In some places prevalence is reported to reach 20% of those attending health facilities.

Prevalence also varies according to the quality of the diagnostic facilities available. It had usually been overestimated when the data were based on the Frei skin test. On the other hand, in clinics with no adequate laboratory facilities LGV is only diagnosed in the late stages, thus giving again a false impression of its true prevalence in the population.

PATHOPHYSIOLOGY. The pathogenesis of chlamydial infections, leading to inflammation and tissue destruction, is only partly understood. Some of the pathology appears to be caused by the host immune response. The leading pathologic feature of LGV is a progressive thrombo- and perilymphangitis. Endothelial cells along the lymphatic vessel walls proliferate, finally causing stenosis and vessel obstruction. The lymph nodes are invaded by neutrophils and mononuclear macrophages leading to granuloma formation and to the characteristic stellate microabscesses. The architecture of the nodes is effaced until the infection finally resolves in progressive fibrosis and scarring.

CLINICAL MANIFESTATIONS. Like syphilis, LGV is a systemic disease that undergoes three distinct stages.
Primary LGV
Classical Lesion. Following a sexual contact, a small papule or ulcer develops at the site of infection (penis, labia, vagina, cervix) after a variable incubation period ranging from 3 to 30 days. Initially, the lesion might resemble genital herpes but is usually painless. This primary lesion ("haircut" lesion) is inconspicuous and frequently remains undetected by the patient. It is more often seen in men than in women, with a ratio of about 4:1. It heals spontaneously and without scarring after a few days.

Other Primary Manifestations. Receptive anal intercourse or contamination of the rectal mucosa with infected secretions may result in a primary anal or rectal infection. With the primary lesion in the urethra, symptomatic urethritis might result. Extragenital primary manifestations of LGV are rare. The best known is a conjunctivitis with preauricular lymphadenopathy and lymphedema of the eyelid ("Parinaud's oculoglandular syndrome").

Secondary LGV. From the site of the primary lesion, be it genital, urethral, anal, or rectal, the infection reaches the neighboring lymph nodes resulting in an extensive regional lymphadenitis. This feature is often the first presentation of the disease. In most patients, it might be noted at a time when the primary lesion has already healed. Thus, LGV is an important differential diagnosis of inguinal bubos without the presence of a genital ulcer.

Constitutional symptoms are common during the secondary stage of LGV indicating the dissemination of the infection. Fever, malaise, and myalgia are reported by most patients; meningism or arthralgia are less frequent complaints.

Extraregional manifestations, e.g., lymphocytic meningitis, sterile arthritis, hepatitis or erythema nodosum, are rare. In some cases the organism has been recovered from blood or cerebrospinal fluid.

Inguinal Syndrome. Most commonly, patients present with an "inguinal syndrome," a painful inguinal lymphadenopathy, which develops some 2 to 6 weeks, rarely later, after the initial infection. The inflammation usually starts unilaterally, but tends to spread in about one third of the cases to both sides. Progressive periadenitis involves the overlying skin, which becomes fixed and thinned over a matted mass of painfully enlarged lymph nodes. Small abscesses coalesce forming bubos that may rupture spontaneously. Multiple fistulas and sinuses break open and discharge purulent fluid. The enlargement of inguinal (above the inguinal ligament) and femoral (below the ligament) lymph nodes results in the characteristic "groove sign," which, however, is not specific for LGV (Fig. 47–1).

After several months spontaneous healing occurs leaving extensive scars and masses of fibrotic granulomatous tissue. A relapse occurs in about 20% of untreated cases.

Anorectal Syndrome. The anorectal syndrome is usually found in homosexual men and occasionally in women. On examination, patients present with a hemorrhagic proctitis or proctocolitis. The rectal mucosa has numerous small erosions and ulcerations. Macroscopically and histologically, LGV proctitis can resemble chronic inflammatory bowel disease. With a primary lesion in the rectum extensive lymphadenopathy might develop in the pelvic, obturator, or iliac area leading to complaints of lower abdominal and back pains. Retroperitoneal lymph node enlargement opens a wide range of possible differential diagnoses.

When untreated the anorectal syndrome may result in anorectal fistulas and perirectal abscess formation. A late complication is rectal stricture, which is most commonly located in the lower part of the rectum. Its differential diagnosis includes malignancies, but strictures following LGV proctitis usually have a long and more tubular appearance.

Tertiary LGV. The tertiary stage includes the late complications of untreated LGV, which develop months and years after the initial infection. Patients with these presentations are rare except in countries with limited health care facilities.

Chronic lymphangitis and lymphadenitis can lead to an excessive obstruction of lymphatic vessels resulting in lymphedema and elephantiasis of the external genitalia and sometimes even the lower limbs. Lymphatic filariasis is considered as a differential diagnosis. The overlying skin of the genital and inguinal region suffers severe damage. Fenestration of the labia may occur. Severe skin damage in combination with chronic hypertrophic enlargement or elephantiasis of the vulva or scrotum is called *esthiomène* (Greek, "eating away").

Other complications are chronic strictures of the urethra or rectum. Carcinoma of the rectum or vulva may be a complication as a result of a chronic LGV, but this is not proved, as yet.

DIAGNOSIS. Whenever LGV is clinically suspected, the definitive diagnosis requires confirmation by specialized laboratory examinations. A rational diagnostic approach is sophisticated and has to be evaluated locally. It depends on availability of laboratory facilities, personal expertise and resources, but also on the expected grade of endemicity of LGV and other chlamydial infections in the examined population.

Microscopy of Smears and Biopsies. Smears, scrapings, aspirated material or biopsies obtained from LGV suspected discharge or tissue can be Giemsa stained and examined under high resolution (oil immersion). This is the simplest but also the crudest diagnostic test. As *C. trachomatis* is an obligate intracellular pathogen, the detection of the blue-mauve–stained mass of inclusion bodies in the cytoplasm of macrophages indicates LGV. However, the cytologic diagnosis needs an experienced and skilled observer, and even then has a low sensitivity. Sensitivity and specificity can be improved when using a fluorescein-conjugated monoclonal antibody. On viewing the slide with a fluorescence microscope the inclusion bodies are more easily identified, thus enhancing their chance of detection.

In the pathohistologic examination, inclusion bodies (preferably stained with direct fluorescent antibodies) or the characteristic stellate microabscesses in biopsy material are highly indicative, but not unique for LGV.

Isolation in Culture. Isolation and strain differentiation of chlamydiae in cell culture, still the gold standard in diagnosis, is an expensive and technically demanding method, available only in specialized reference centers. Specific cell lines (HeLa or McCoy) and techniques are required. As *C. trachomatis* is an intracellular pathogen, material for detection of chlamydiae must contain epithelial tissue. Therefore pus and secretions of lymph nodes are less suitable for culture. When a specimen is obtained it should be placed in a special transport medium and refrigerated immediately. Under optimal conditions, the specificity of the method approaches 100%, the sensitivity 70 to 90%, according to quality and experience of the laboratory.

Amplification Tests. Amplification techniques for *C. trachomatis* DNA have been recently introduced. They are based on polymerase chain reaction (PCR) or ligate chain reaction and have a remarkably high sensitivity. Urine may be used, thus avoiding invasive diagnostic procedures. Their importance for the diagnosis of chlamydial infections could increase in the future as their cost becomes acceptable.

Antigen Detection Tests. An enzyme-linked immunosorbent assay for chlamydial antigen detection has been developed. As the method is easy to perform and can be used to test multiple samples, it can be used as a screening test. It is more reliable in patients with florid symptoms shedding high numbers of organisms than in those with asymptomatic

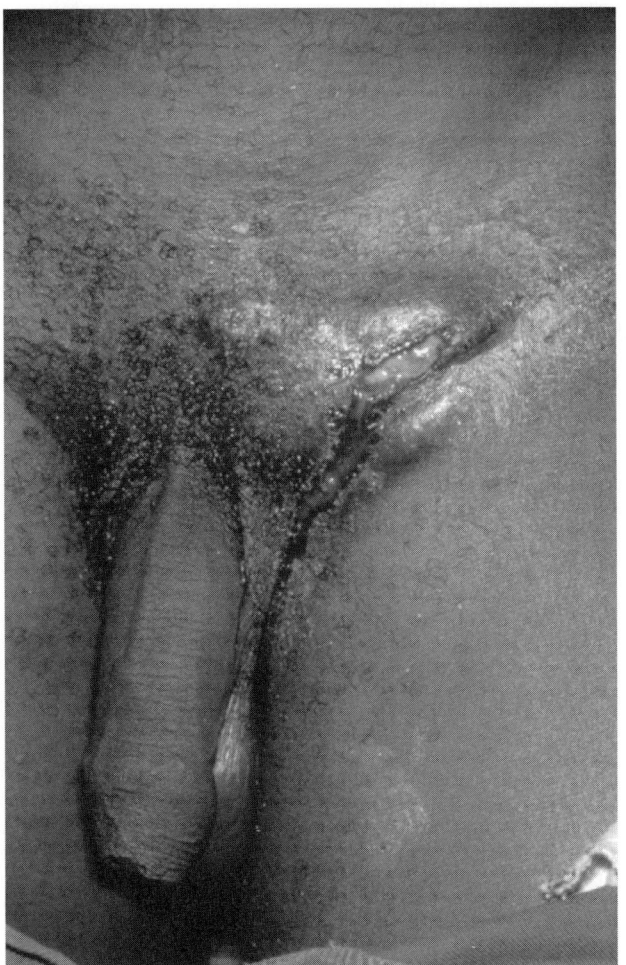

***Figure* 47–1.** Lymphogranuloma venereum. Bilateral inguinal buboes with separation of the matted left inguinal and femoral lymph nodes by the inguinal ligament, creating the pathognomonic sign of the "groove."

disease. In low-prevalence populations a significant proportion of those tested will be falsely positive. Therefore, the test has a much better positive predictive value in subjects at high risk for LGV, e.g., in STD clinics.

Antibody Detection Tests. Antibody detection tests are of limited value for diagnosing LGV. Normally a fourfold or greater increase in acute and convalescent serum sample is considered to be diagnostic. After successful treatment the titer falls rapidly. Several techniques are used and commercially available. Most lack acceptable specificity.

The complement fixation (CF) test uses a heat-stable antigen of *Chlamydia* which, being a common group antigen, is present in all species. Therefore the test is not indicative for *C. trachomatis*. The cutoff point for a positive titer is usually set at 1:64. The indirect fluorescent antibody technique (microimmunofluorescence, micro-IF) is a complex test with a much higher sensitivity and specificity for antibodies to *C. trachomatis*. The test is usually available only in specialized research laboratories. The cutoff point for the micro-IF titer is usually 1:512.

Skin Tests. Historically an intradermal skin test (Frei test) similar in principle and technique to tuberculin skin tests was used to detect previous LGV exposure. The original antigen was obtained from heat-inactivated pus aspirated from LGV bubos and later from cell cultures. The test is no longer produced commercially.

TREATMENT

Medical Treatment. The treatment of choice for LGV is tetracycline hydrochloride 500 mg q.i.d. for 21 days. Alternatively, doxycycline 100 mg b.i.d. can be given. Resistance to these antibiotics is unknown. Treatment failure is usually due to misdiagnosis, poor compliance, or reinfection.

If antibiotics of the tetracycline group are contraindicated, erythromycin 500 mg q.i.d. can be substituted, also given for 21 days. Chloramphenicol, rifampicin, or sulfisoxazole are other alternatives. Penicillins, cephalosporins, and aminoglycosides are not effective against chlamydiae. The effect of fluorinated quinolones is uncertain.

Surgical Treatment. Pus from bubos should be aspirated and drained. Fistulous openings should receive sterile dressing. The severe deformities of tertiary LGV can only be treated with plastic surgery, which occasionally provides remarkable results. Surgical interventions should only be performed after a prolonged course of antibiotics. Patients with extensive tissue scars should be monitored frequently. Regular biopsies of suspicious areas are recommended to detect any malignant change.

PREVENTION AND CONTROL. Prophylactic treatment of partners should be offered for all detected patients with LGV, as the duration of contagiousness can last for several months.

Bibliography

Centers for Disease Control and Prevention: Recommendations for the prevention and management of *Chlamydia trachomatis* infections, 1993. MMWR 42:1, 1993.

Grosskurth H, Mayaud P, Mosha F, et al: Asymptomatic gonorrhoea and chlamydial infection in rural Tanzanian men. Br Med J 312:277, 1996.

LeBar WD: Keeping up with new technology: new approaches to diagnosis of *Chlamydia* infection. Clin Chem 42:809, 1996.

Mabey D: Sexually transmitted diseases in developing countries. Trans R Soc Trop Med Hyg 90:97, 1996.

Perine PL, Osoba AO: Lymphogranuloma venereum. *In* Holmes KK, Mardh P-A, Sparling PE, et al (eds): Sexually Transmitted Diseases, 2nd ed. New York, McGraw-Hill, 1990, pp 195–204.

48 Syphilis and the Endemic Treponematoses

Peter L. Perine and Thomas A. Bell

DEFINITION. Syphilis and the endemic treponematoses—yaws, endemic syphilis, and pinta—are chronic diseases caused by three subspecies of *Treponema pallidum*. Venereal and nonvenereal syphilis are caused by *T. pallidum pallidum*, yaws by *T. pallidum pertenue*, and pinta by *T. pallidum carateum*. These closely related, morphologically identical treponemes elicit antitreponemal antibodies that cannot be differentiated by conventional tests. These species can be distinguished from each other only by their patterns of infection in human beings and in experimentally infected animals, by differences in geographic distribution (Fig. 48–1; Table 48–1), by nucleic acid sequencing, and perhaps by minor antigenic differences. All have three main disease stages.

ETIOLOGY. The pathogenic treponemes are corkscrew-shaped spirochetes that are 0.1 to 0.15 μm in diameter and usually about 12 μm long. They grow best in an environment with a low oxygen concentration and die rapidly when exposed to atmospheric oxygen, soaps, detergents, and mild antiseptic solutions. They cannot be routinely propagated in vitro, but male rabbits are susceptible to experimental infection. Injection of *T. pallidum pallidum* or *T. pallidum pertenue* into the rabbit testis causes acute orchitis.

These species die rapidly outside a host. They are transmitted by close personal contact, which is almost exclusively sexual in the case of venereal syphilis. Both *T. pallidum pallidum* and *T. pallidum pertenue* penetrate mucous membranes, but intact skin is a formidable barrier to infection. In yaws and perhaps in pinta, most infections occur by contamination of small cutaneous lacerations, abrasions, or insect bites with infectious exudate from primary or secondary lesions.

PATHOPHYSIOLOGY. The treponemes produce no known toxins and do not directly kill host cells. The immune response of the host to the treponeme causes much of their damage. Their favorite tissue location is in the perivascular lymph spaces, where immune lymphocytes cause an obliterative endarteritis and periarteritis.

The extent of damage varies by subspecies: *T. pallidum pallidum* damages any organ or tissue of the host, *T. pallidum pertenue* only skin and bone, and *T. pallidum carateum* only the superficial layers of the skin. This variation probably reflects an inherent property of the individual treponeme, because all three species can invade systemically.

48.1 Venereal Syphilis

HISTORY. Syphilis (*lues venerea*) was first described in Europe in the late 15th century, shortly after Columbus's return from America. Whether it was carried to Europe by the explorers or arose by mutation of indigenous treponemes remains controversial. Whatever its origin, in the 16th century, syphilis was thought to be a new disease—the "great pox"—and it spread rapidly. In early descriptions, the most prominent manifestations were skin lesions. Death in the early stages was common. Over the next five centuries, syphilis became less virulent and usually more of a chronic infection. Death and disability occurred in the tertiary stage after a quiescent or latent period of several years.

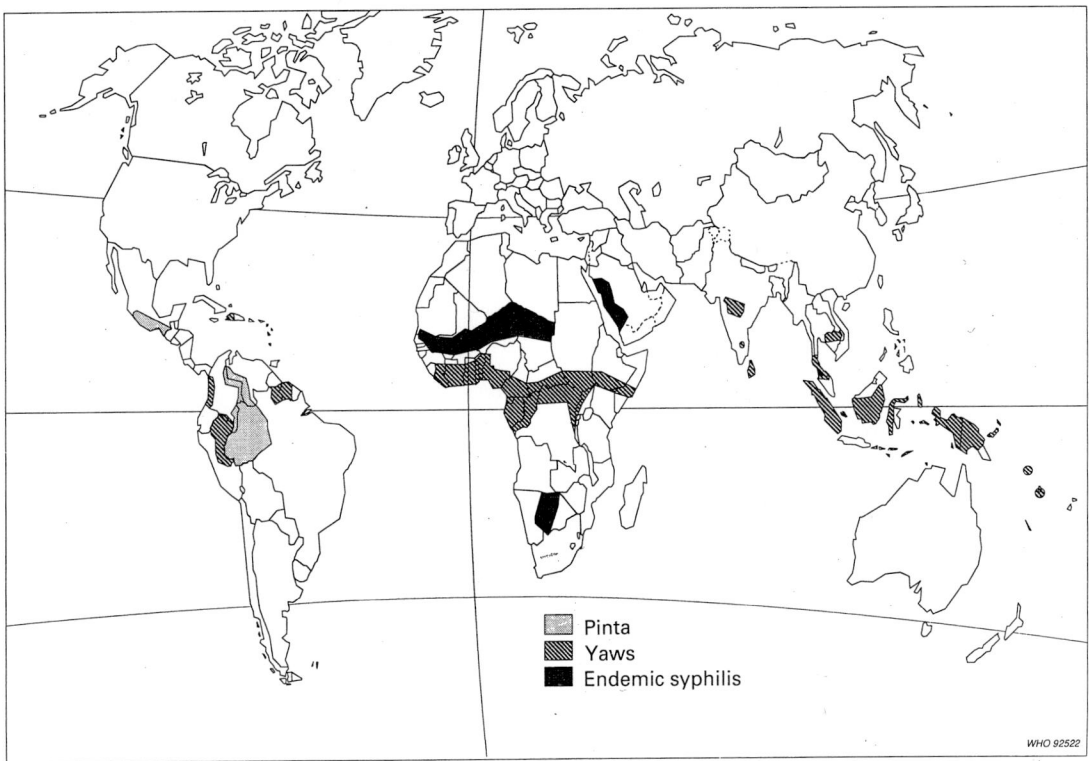

Figure 48–1. Global distribution of yaws, endemic syphilis, and pinta. Syphilis is global in distribution and more common in urban areas. (From Meheus A, Antal GM: World Health Stat Q 45:228, 1992.)

EPIDEMIOLOGY. Since 1860, the worldwide incidence of syphilis has declined steadily except for temporary increases during wars. In North America and Europe, venereal syphilis decreased more than 90% after the advent of penicillin therapy, and late stages became even rarer until the pandemics of human immunodeficiency viruses (HIVs). Incidence of venereal syphilis is increasing in many urban areas of Africa and Asia that were formerly relatively free of it. As with other sexually transmitted diseases, this increase is a result of urbanization and industrialization of many parts of the tropical world and, possibly, of increased sexual permissiveness and promiscuity. In Africa especially, the pandemics of HIVs and the epidemics of syphilis and other causes of genital ulcers are synergistic because they enhance each other's transmission.

Almost all cases of syphilis are contracted during coitus. The risk of infection after a single exposure is highly variable by geographic region. In North America, it is about 12%.

CLINICAL MANIFESTATIONS. The stages of syphilis are punctuated by variable periods of latency. Estimates of the proportions of persons in each stage of syphilis who progress to the next stage were made in the era before antibiotic therapy. Those estimates have little relevance to contemporary practice because the ubiquity of antibiotic treatment and the effect of concurrent HIV infection have changed the "natural" history of syphilis.

Primary Syphilis. T. *pallidum pallidum* penetrates intact mucous membranes or abraded skin. Systemic and central nervous system (CNS) invasion occur almost immediately. Treponemes enter the subcutaneous blood vessels and lymphatics at the site of primary invasion and disseminate to most organs and tissues within hours.

The characteristic primary lesion is the *chancre*, which develops at the site of invasion after an incubation period of 9 to 90 days (average, 3 weeks) (Fig. 48–2). A chancre begins as a small papule, but this is rarely the presenting complaint. It soon erodes to form a shallow, painless, crater-like ulcer with indurated margins and a diameter of between a few millimeters and 3 centimeters. A chancre usually is covered by a thin, easily removed crust. The serous exudate from its

TABLE 48–1. Epidemiologic Features of Syphilis and the Endemic Treponematoses

	Venereal Syphilis	Endemic Syphilis	Yaws	Pinta
Geographic area	Urban, worldwide	Rural, arid Africa, Asia	Rural, humid tropics	Rural, semiarid Central and South America
Seasonal variations	None	Increases rainy season	Increases rainy season	?
Peak incidence (age)	20–30	2–10	4–15	18–30
Transmission				
Congenital	Frequent	Rare, if ever	Never	Never
Venereal	Usual	Rare	Never	Never
Direct (skin)	Occasional	Common	Usual	Probable
Fomite (utensils)	Rare	Usual	?	Never

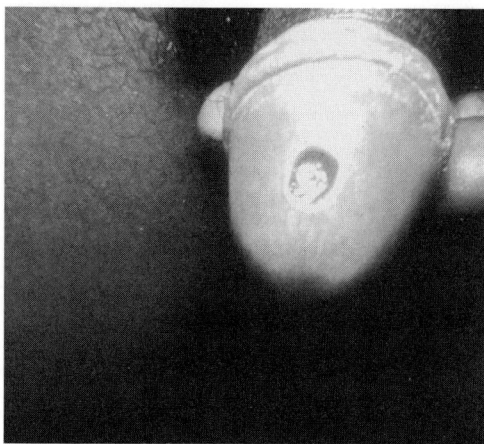

Figure 48–2. A chancre. Most are not so classic in appearance. (Courtesy of Centers for Disease Control and Prevention.)

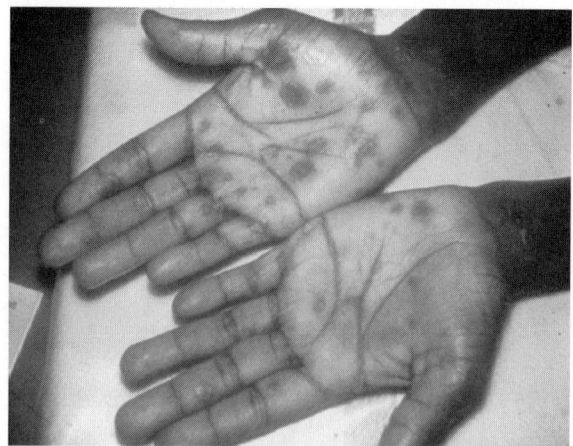

Figure 48–3. Rash of secondary syphilis. (Courtesy of Centers for Disease Control and Prevention.)

hard, granular base teems with spirochetes. The lymph nodes draining the lesion are often discrete, enlarged, firm, and painless. Among heterosexual men, most chancres are on the penis. Among women, chancres are usually on the cervix, vaginal wall, or posterior fourchette; they may also be on the labia or perineum. Multiple chancres occur infrequently and are usually clustered; these may result from multiple sites of infection or from autoinoculation. The "typical" chancre is atypical in appearance. Every genital ulcer should be evaluated for its possible syphilitic nature.

Extragenital chancres, usually caused by sexual contact, are rare and, unlike genital chancres, usually painful. They may occur anywhere on the body, the most common sites being the lips, nipples, fingers, and oral and rectal mucosa. They usually cause painless regional lymphadenopathy. Their appearance is more frequently atypical than is that of genital chancres.

Most chancres heal without scarring in 3 to 6 weeks in persons with competent immune systems, but healing sometimes takes longer in those with immunodeficiency. Afterward, the untreated infected person is immune to reinfection ("chancre immunity").

Secondary Syphilis. Secondary syphilis begins 3 weeks to 6 months (average, 6 weeks) after the chancre heals but sometimes is concurrent with the chancre. The clinical manifestations of secondary syphilis are protean, because any organ or tissue may be involved. The most common manifestations are rashes that are usually painless, nonpruritic, and almost never vesicular or bullous. The rash of secondary syphilis may be macular, papular, follicular, papulosquamous, or pustular and may involve both the skin and the mucous membranes. If generalized, it tends to be bilateral and symmetric and more prominent on the face and thorax. Involvement of the palms and soles is common, and any such rash should make the clinician suspect syphilis (Fig. 48–3).

Skin Lesions. Some types of cutaneous lesions are found typically in secondary syphilis. These include *condylomata lata*—broad, moist, grayish white, exudative lesions that appear in the intertriginous areas of the perineum, scrotum, vulva (Fig. 48–4), and axilla; *mucous patches*—oval, shallow ulcers often covered by a grayish white membrane that are found in the mouth and on the moist surfaces of the genitalia; *follicular syphilids*—small papular lesions involving hair follicles and causing temporary patchy hair loss (alopecia areata) of the eyebrows, beard, and scalp hair; *papulosquamous syphilids*—indurated papules with peripheral scales, usually found on the palms and soles; and *nummular syphilids*—

coinlike lesions with sharply defined borders that are usually on the face or perineum, especially in dark-skinned persons (Fig. 48–5).

Most rashes of secondary syphilis heal within a few weeks without scar formation, but some may persist for months. Up to 25% of untreated persons experience mucocutaneous relapses within 2 years of infection. Relapse lesions, such as condylomata lata or mucous patches, tend to be asymmetrically distributed and more exudative than the initial lesions.

General Symptoms. The constitutional symptoms of secondary syphilis include mild fever, malaise, headache, and anorexia, with or without cutaneous lesions. Generalized, discrete, nontender lymphadenopathy is common. The spleen is sometimes palpable. Acute meningitis, hepatitis, nephrosis, arthritis, periostitis, iridocyclitis, and anterior uveitis are rarer manifestations of secondary syphilis. Concurrent infection with HIV may promote CNS complications of secondary syphilis.

Latent Syphilis. The disappearance of the lesions of sec-

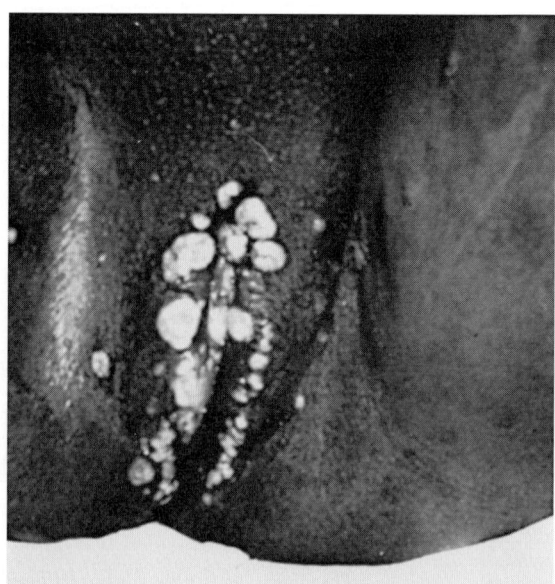

Figure 48–4. Venereal syphilis. Raised condylomata lata of secondary syphilis, which are usually found in the warm, moist areas of the body such as the perineum, anal cleft, and axilla.

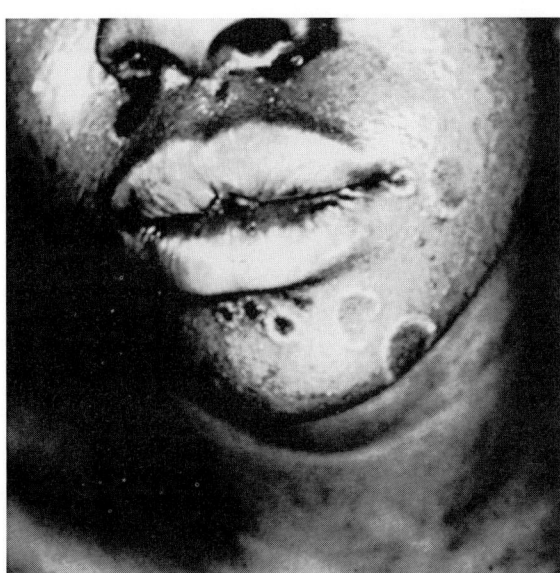

Figure 48–5. Coinlike, or nummular, secondary syphilis lesions on the face. These lesions characteristically occur in dark-skinned people.

ondary syphilis is followed by another period of quiescence, or latency, which may last for more than 20 years. The early latent period is the first year after infection, during which secondary lesions may recur. The late latent period is between 1 year and the appearance of tertiary manifestations. Persons with latent syphilis of unknown duration should be managed as though they have late latent syphilis. The only evidence of infection in latent syphilis is a reactive serologic test for syphilis.

Tertiary Syphilis. The three types of tertiary syphilis are cardiovascular syphilis, gummatous syphilis, and neurosyphilis, which in turn may be classified as meningovascular, parenchymatous, and gummatous (which is rare). All forms of tertiary syphilis were rarely diagnosed after the initial worldwide availability of antibiotic therapy for syphilis and many other infectious diseases, treatment for which serendipitously cured many cases of latent syphilis, even though many antibiotics may not attain treponemicidal concentrations in the CNS.

Cardiovascular Syphilis. Syphilis destroys the wall of the thoracic aorta by immune-mediated thrombosis (obliteration) of the vasa vasorum in its wall. Its elastic fibers are weakened, and an aortic aneurysm forms. If the dilatation occurs near the aortic valve, the valve cusps are separated, to cause aortic insufficiency. The left ventricle enlarges, and refractory congestive heart failure may ensue. The coronary ostia may be narrowed, and coronary circulation may be reduced.

Gummatous, or Late Benign, Syphilis. Gummas have become rare since the advent of penicillin therapy. Histologically, gummatous syphilitic lesions resemble tuberculomas. They are an area of coagulation necrosis surrounded by epithelioid cells and fibrous tissue. Gummas vary greatly in size and location. Although they may impair normal function as result of the fibrous tissue reaction, they are usually "benign," because they seldom cause physical disability unless they are in the CNS or bones. Gummas are most often found in the liver, where they form irregular lobules separated by fibrous bands. On the skin, they form round ulcers that resemble the lesion of yaws. Gummas of bone and cartilage may perforate the hard palate and nasal septum or cause other significant damage. In the heart, they may interrupt the conduction system and cause cardiac arrhythmias.

Meningovascular Neurosyphilis. Chronic meningitis occurs in most persons with CNS syphilis, but it is often asymptomatic. Overt disease is caused by an obliterative endarteritis in the CNS. Symptoms vary because lesions may involve any part of the nervous system and may be sharply focal or diffuse. Focal cerebral lesions commonly produce hemiplegia or a selective neuropathy, especially of the third cranial nerve. Diffuse cerebral lesions cause severe headache, mental changes, and convulsions. HIV infection may predispose to CNS infarcts, which may be the first manifestation of both syphilis and HIV infection.

Parenchymatous Neurosyphilis. This includes the tabetic and paretic forms and differs from meningovascular neurosyphilis by the absence of vascular lesions and by the lesions tending to be selectively distributed. Involvement of the spinal cord is common and usually affects the dorsal roots, causing pain, weakness of the lower limbs, flaccid paraplegia, and loss of sensation below the level of the lesion. Tabes dorsalis is characterized by attacks of "lightning" pains, paresthesias of the lower extremities, and ataxia. Pain sensation is lost, and painless arthropathies—Charcot joints—result from unrecognized trauma to the joint. Painless trophic ulcers of the feet that resemble those of diabetes mellitus are present more commonly. Tabetic crises are rare, paroxysmal, painful disorders of function of abdominal viscera that may resemble an acute surgical emergency. *General paresis* manifests as a progressive dementia accompanied by generalized or focal seizures with or without manifestations of tabes dorsalis. Before the advent of penicillin therapy, parenchymatous syphilis was a major cause of psychosis and dementia in North America and Europe.

The Argyll Robertson pupil, one of the most common abnormalities seen in neurosyphilis, is small, irregular, and fixed, with synechiae at the inner edge of the irides. It contracts with accommodation but not illumination. A fulminating degeneration of the optic nerve and blindness (*primary optic atrophy*) that produces arachnoiditis may occur in both meningovascular and parenchymatous neurosyphilis but is more commonly associated with tabes dorsalis.

Congenital Syphilis. Transplacental passage of *T. pallidum pallidum* may occur as early as the ninth week of gestation. The probability of congenital infection is highest during the secondary stage of syphilis and decreases with the duration of untreated infection in the mother. The combined fetal and perinatal death rate of untreated congenital syphilis is approximately 40%. In parts of Africa, syphilis is the most common cause of perinatal death, primarily because women receive inadequate prenatal care. Most often, the infected infant who survives is apparently normal.

Manifestations of congenital syphilis include a mucopurulent nasal discharge ("snuffles"); any of the rashes of secondary acquired syphilis, especially bullae and generalized desquamation; hepatosplenomegaly; ascites; pneumonia; osteoperiostitis of the long bones; anemia; hemorrhage; and failure to thrive. When it appears, early congenital syphilis usually does so between 3 weeks and 6 months of age. Latent congenital syphilis is usually manifested only by a reactive serologic test. The signs and symptoms of this stage may result from previous damage in utero or in early life. Late congenital syphilis may cause interstitial keratitis, dental abnormalities of permanent teeth, and auditory nerve deafness (Hutchinson triad) as well as any of the lesions of tertiary acquired syphilis. The secretions of infants with congenital syphilis can be highly contagious.

An infant should be evaluated for congenital syphilis if the mother has positive serologic tests plus inadequately treated syphilis, treatment during pregnancy with a drug other than penicillin, treatment with penicillin without an adequate serologic response, treatment less than 1 month before delivery, treatment before pregnancy without adequate documentation of serologic response, or undocumented treatment before pregnancy. If the mother was adequately treated during pregnancy, the infant should be examined periodically until nontreponemal antibody tests are normal.

DIAGNOSIS. Syphilis is known as the great imitator because it may mimic many diseases manifesting local or generalized symptoms and lesions. Syphilis often accompanies other sexually transmitted infections, which should be excluded by clinical and laboratory examination. Syphilis should be sought in any patient with a compatible genital lesion or skin, heart, aorta, or CNS disease. Pregnant women should be tested early in pregnancy or if they experience a fetal death after 20 weeks' gestation. In populations with a high prevalence of syphilis, such women should be tested again in the third trimester and at delivery.

Darkfield Microscopy. The most specific diagnostic test for infectious syphilis (primary, secondary, and early congenital) is a darkfield microscopic examination of exudate obtained from an appropriate lesion or aspirate from an enlarged lymph node. Its sensitivity can be low, especially if the patient has been partially treated with self-administered antimicrobials. *T. pallidum* is between 1 and 3 erythrocyte diameters long and appears as a thin, coiled silver thread on a dark background. It spins rapidly along its longitudinal axis. It often flexes in the middle, or "whiplashes," while keeping its corkscrew appearance. Lesions in the oropharynx, rectum, cervix, and vagina may contain saprophytic *Borrelia* or nonpathogenic treponemes that are difficult to distinguish morphologically from *T. pallidum*.

Serologic Tests. In all stages of acquired and congenital syphilis, the diagnosis is supported, but not established, by a reactive serologic test for syphilis, of which two general types are used.

***N**ontreponemal Antigen Tests.** The first and older is the nontreponemal antigen test, which uses cardiolipin, an alcoholic extract of beef heart and a normal constituent of mammalian cells, as antigen. Examples are the Venereal Disease Research Laboratory (VDRL), Kolmer, and rapid plasma reagin (RPR) tests, which detect antibodies by flocculation, complement fixation, and agglutination, respectively. The nontreponemal antigen tests do not vary significantly in their sensitivity or specificity for syphilis. They are excellent screening tests for most stages of syphilis, and when quantified, they provide good measurements of disease activity.

Many nontreponemal diseases induce antibodies to cardiolipin and cause false positive reactions (Table 48–2), but they, and anticardiolipin antibody, do not provide immunity to syphilis, which should be sought regardless of the presence of these other diseases. A positive test that uses a nontreponemal antigen result should always be confirmed by a more specific treponemal antigen test unless a darkfield examination is positive.

False negative tests may be caused by a delay in antibody production in primary syphilis; immunosuppression, especially by HIV; the prozone phenomenon of undiluted serum, especially in stages later than the primary and early latent; and immunologic "burnout," especially in tertiary syphilis. A quantitative nontreponemal test can be used to monitor the response to treatment.

***Treponemal Antigen Tests.** The second type of serologic test is the treponemal antigen test, which uses *T. pallidum pallidum* or closely related treponemes. These tests include the *T. pallidum* immobilization (TPI) test, in which treponemes are immobilized in vitro by antibody; the *T. pallidum* hemagglutinin assay (TPHA) test, which uses *T. pallidum* adsorbed to erythrocytes; and the fluorescent treponemal antibody (FTA)

TABLE 48–2. Causes of False Positive Nontreponemal Tests

Infectious
Viral
    Epstein-Barr virus
    Human immunodeficiency viruses
    Mumps
    Rubeola
    Varicella

Bacterial
    Endocarditis
    Borrelia infections
    Chlamydia psittaci
    Haemophilus ducreyi
    Leptospira
    Lymphogranuloma venereum
    Mycobacterium leprae
    Mycobacterium tuberculosis
    Scarlet fever
    Streptococcus pneumoniae pneumonia

Protozoan
    Malaria
    Trypanosoma cruzi

Noninfectious
    Blood transfusions
    Cancer
    Connective tissue diseases
    Injecting drug abuse
    Liver disease
    Pregnancy
    Tropical spastic paresis

test, which uses lyophilized *T. pallidum* in an indirect fluorescent antibody technique. To increase FTA specificity, a modification of the test, the FTA-ABS test, uses an extract of saprophytic treponemes to absorb antibody elicited by such organisms in the gut. Although these tests vary in their sensitivity, the FTA and TPHA tests rarely yield false positive results. The TPI is rarely used now because it is cumbersome. Treponemal tests generally remain positive for life and are not useful for monitoring the response to treatment.

***Other Detection Methods.** T. pallidum* can be detected by direct fluorescent antibody stains of appropriate specimens, or by detection of its nucleic acid sequences with a polymerase chain reaction (PCR) assay.

Laboratory Abnormalities. A mild polymorphonuclear leukocytosis, elevated sedimentation rate, hypergammaglobulinemia, rheumatoid factor activity, and cryoglobulinema may occur in late primary, secondary, congenital, and tertiary syphilis. Liver enzymes are elevated in syphilitic hepatitis. Anemia is common in early congenital syphilis.

Cerebrospinal fluid (CSF) abnormalities may occur during any stage of syphilis, and especially with congenital, meningovascular, or parenchymatous neurosyphilis. These include a mild mononuclear cell pleocytosis (<100 cells/µL), a reactive nontreponemal serologic test for syphilis, and increased protein concentration. The FTA test should not be used for diagnosing neurosyphilis, because it is nonspecific.

Histopathology. Syphilitic lesions may show pathognomonic changes. Spirochetes can be found with special stains. Concurrent HIV infection can either suppress the titers of nontreponemal tests or increase them.

Evaluation of the Infant for Congenital Syphilis. The infant who may have congenital syphilis may also require radiographic examination of the long bones and the lungs. Blood from the umbilical cord is both insensitive and nonspecific in comparison with blood from the infant. Passively acquired antibody detected in nontreponemal tests persists for approximately 6 months; that detected by treponemal tests lasts for as long as 12 months.

Examination of the CSF is indicated for infants born to women with gestational syphilis or with suspected or proven congenital syphilis. Protein and cell concentrations in the CSF of newborns are difficult to interpret. The VDRL is the preferred screening test. It may be negative in the presence of neurosyphilis and positive from passively acquired antibody if the mother has a high concentration of anticardiolipin in her serum.

TREATMENT. Whereas the treatment of other sexually transmitted diseases has evolved with counterbalancing development of drug resistance and new antimicrobials, the recommended treatment for syphilis has changed little over time. Parenteral penicillin G is still the drug of choice, so much so that desensitization of penicillin-allergic patients is indicated for treatment of some late stages of disease. Other antibiotics should be used for primary or later syphilis only if the patient has a definite penicillin allergy documented by history or skin testing. A treponemicidal blood level must be maintained for 7 to 10 days to cure an immunocompetent host. Thus, the longer acting penicillin preparations are preferred. Most antimicrobials used to treat *Neisseria gonorrhoeae*, *Chlamydia trachomatis*, and *Haemophilus ducreyi* eradicate incubating syphilis, but they should not be used as the only therapy for disease that has reached the primary stage unless penicillin in contraindicated. Aminoglycosides are not effective against syphilis.

Primary, Secondary, Early Latent Syphilis. Adults who are not pregnant and who are not infected with HIV should receive 2.4 million U of benzathine penicillin IM in a single dose. Children with acquired primary or secondary syphilis should be evaluated for sexual abuse and be treated with 50,000 U/kg of body mass, up to 2.4 million U.

Persons allergic to penicillin should be treated with one of the following oral regimens for 14 days: 500 mg of tetracycline or 500 mg of erythromycin four times daily; or 100 mg of doxycycline twice daily. Daily doses of 250 mg of cetriaxone in 1% lidocaine given IM for 14 days is probably effective also.

Late Latent and Tertiary Syphilis, Without CNS Involvement. Three doses of benzathine penicillin are required, at weekly intervals. Neurosyphilis must be excluded. Persons allergic to penicillin should be treated with doxycycline or tetracycline for 28 days.

Neurosyphilis. More intense therapy is required. A 10- to 14-day regimen of either aqueous crystalline penicillin G in a total daily dose of 12 to 24 million U, in equal IV doses every 4 hours; or procaine penicillin, 2.4 million U in a single IM dose daily, plus 500 mg probenecid given by mouth four times per day.

Penicillin Allergy and Desensitization. Persons allergic to penicillin present a special challenge. Whenever possible, they should be desensitized to penicillin and then given the standard regimen.

Only approximately 10% of persons with a history of severe allergy to penicillin remain allergic. Penicillin allergy should be confirmed by testing them with major and minor determinants of penicillin hypersensitivity. Penicilloyl poly-L-lysine is commercially available as the major determinant, and freshly prepared or fresh frozen benzylpenicillin G as the minor determinant. Use of these two agents may still fail to detect up to 10% of persons with allergy. Minor determinants (benzylpenicillin G, benzylpenicilloate, and benzylpenilloate) are present in aged penicillin.

The antigens should be diluted 100-fold for persons with a history of life-threatening reactions, and 10-fold for those with milder immediate, generalized reactions within the past year. The positive control is commercial histamine, 1 mg/mL, for epicutaneous testing; the negative is the diluent used to dissolve the other reagents. Drops of test materials and control reagents are placed in duplicate on the volar surface of the forearm. The underlying skin is pierced with a 26-gauge needle without inducing bleeding. The test is positive if the average wheal diameter is at least 4 mm greater than that of negative controls 15 minutes after injection. The positive control is affected by antihistaminic drugs.

If these epicutaneous tests are negative, a 26- or 27-gauge needle is used to inject 0.02 mL of each reagent intradermally and in duplicate in the volar surface of the forearm. A positive test is at least 2 mm larger than the initial wheal, and also the negative control, 15 minutes after injection.

Desensitization involves starting with an oral dose of 100 U of penicillin V and doubling the dose every 15 minutes until a dose of 640,000 U is administered (cumulative dose over 3.75 hours is 1,296,700 U). This must be done under strict medical supervision with resuscitation equipment and medications immediately available. Following desensitization, the appropriate penicillin regimen should be administered promptly.

Persons treated with doxycycline or tetracycline should be evaluated thoroughly after treatment. An equivalent regimen of ceftriaxone may be possible in persons without cross reactions from their penicillin allergies. Despite good penetration of the CSF, ceftriaxone may fail to eradicate neurosyphilis.

Pregnancy. Treatment with penicillin should be the standard dose for the stage of pregnancy. Additional treatment such as an additional 2.4 million U of benzathine penicillin is recommended by some experts, especially late in the last trimester and for those with secondary syphilis.

Women allergic to penicillin should be desensitized to, then treated with, penicillin. Doxycycline and tetracycline are contraindicated, and erythromycin does not provide reliable treatment of the fetus.

Congenital Syphilis. In the newborn period, congenital syphilis is treated as though it were neurosyphilis, either with a 10- to 14-day course of aqueous crystalline penicillin G (ACPG), 50,000 U/kg IV every 12 hours for the first 7 days of life and then 50,000 U every 8 hours for another 3 to 7 days; or with procaine penicillin G in a single daily dose of 50,000 U/kg IM for 10 to 14 days. ACPG produces higher concentrations in the CSF. A full course of treatment should be repeated if more than 1 day of therapy is missed. After the newborn period, the dose of ACPG is 200,000 to 300,000 U/kg/day, given IV or IM in doses of 50,000 U/kg every 4 to 6 hours for 10 to 14 days.

Children allergic to penicillin should be desensitized to, then treated with, penicillin. Doxycycline and tetracycline are contraindicated for children younger than 8 years.

Some experts treat congenital syphilis less aggressively. Some would treat an infant whose mother was treated inadequately but is otherwise normal with only a single dose of benzathine penicillin G, 50,000 U/kg IM. Some would treat an infant with documented congenital syphilis, mild or no physical abnormalities, and normal CSF with only benzathine penicillin G, 50,000 U/kg IM, at weekly intervals thrice. Such treatment regimens may be dictated by necessity in some situations.

Concurrent HIV Infection. Treatment of most stages should be the same as for persons without HIV, though some experts would treat primary and secondary stages as though such infections were tertiary syphilis. Early latent syphilis in persons with HIV should be treated as though it were late latent or tertiary. Examination of the CSF for evidence of neurosyphilis is warranted in the evaluation of latent and tertiary disease, probably of secondary disease, and possibly of primary syphilis. Persons allergic to penicillin should be desensitized to, then treated with, penicillin, regardless of the stage of infection.

Post-Treatment Observations. Pretreatment and post-treatment quantitative VDRL tests are the only means of detecting persisting infection or reinfection after cutaneous syphilitic lesions have healed. The patient should be warned that the initial dose of antibiotic may provoke a Jarisch-Herxheimer reaction: Chills, fever, headache, leukocytosis, and aggravation of local syphilitic lesions begin 6 to 12 hours after the injection of penicillin. No specific treatment is required.

Treponemes disappear from cutaneous syphilitic lesions within 48 hours of penicillin treatment, and the lesions heal rapidly. In rare cases of neurovascular and congenital syphilis, and more commonly in HIV-infected persons, viable treponemes persist in the CNS despite recommended doses of parenteral penicillin, prolonged or repeated courses of which may be required to cure such patients.

Most patients with seropositive primary and secondary syphilis become seronegative 6 to 12 months after treatment. For those who remain seropositive 18 to 24 months after treatment, spinal fluid examination should be repeated to detect possible CNS involvement. If clinical signs or symptoms of syphilis persist or recur, or if an initial high-titer nontreponemal antigen test fails to decrease fourfold within a year, or if the titer increases fourfold, the patient should be treated again with the same or a more intense regimen. An increase in the concentration of antibody measured by a nontreponemal test usually indicates reinfection rather than treatment failure. For patients with primary and secondary syphilis, the failure rates for penicillin treatment range from 0 to 4% after 1 year to as high as 11% after 2 years of observation. Failure rates are higher in HIV-infected persons.

Patients with latent and tertiary syphilis may remain seropositive ("serofast") with stable, low VDRL titers 2 years after treatment. This persistent seropositivity does not indicate treatment failure or reinfection, and these patients are likely to remain seropositive for life even if treated again. Much of the tissue damage in late congenital, CNS, and cardiovascular syphilis is irreversible.

The sera of infants with congenital syphilis should be tested at ages 3, 6, and 12 months after completion of treatment or until nontreponemal antibody disappears. CSF should be examined every 6 months until it is normal. Persistence of abnormalities at age 2 years indicates treatment failure and the need for another course.

PREVENTION AND CONTROL. Vigorous efforts should be made to find recent sexual contacts of patients with infectious (primary, secondary, early latent) syphilis and long-term sexual partners of persons with late latent or tertiary syphilis. Presumptive, or "epidemiologic," treatment should be given to persons who were sexual partners of the index case during the 3 months plus duration of symptoms if the index case is in the primary stage, 6 months plus duration of symptoms if in the secondary stage, and 1 year if in the early latent stage. For persons with secondary syphilis, contact tracing should include those of the previous 12 months. These individuals should be treated if serologic tests and continued observation are not feasible. An index case with a high titer of a nontreponemal test in the context of syphilis of unknown duration should be considered to have early syphilis.

In some situations, cluster treatment has been used to control the spread of syphilis because many infected persons have anonymous sexual contacts. This involves treated persons likely to have had sexual contact with the index case or a sexual contact of the index case, regardless of symptoms or

laboratory tests. In more developed countries, registries have been useful in monitoring persons infected with syphilis and in determining the significance of their serologic tests when they are repeated at another clinical facility.

Screening with a nontreponemal antigen test is important in the detection of gestational/congenital, latent, and tertiary syphilis. Appropriate strategies may include testing of all pregnant women, many hospitalized patients, persons with other sexually transmitted diseases, and those with vague or mysterious rashes or neurologic symptoms. Positive tests must be confirmed by a treponemal antigen test because the positive predictive value of a positive nontreponemal test may be low in such populations.

Bibliography

Aiken CG: The causes of perinatal mortality in Bulawayo, Zimbabwe. Centr Afr J Med 38:263, 1992.

American Academy of Pediatrics: Syphilis. *In* Peter G (ed): 1994 Red Book: Report of the Committee on Infectious Diseases, 23rd ed. Elk Grove Village, IL, American Academy of Pediatrics, 1994, pp 445–455.

Azimi PH, Janner D, Berne P, et al: Concentrations of procaine and aqueous penicillin in the cerebrospinal fluid of infants treated for congenital syphilis. J Pediatr 124:649, 1994.

Beall GN: Penicillins. Ann Intern Med 107:204, 1987.

Centers for Disease Control: Guidelines for the Prevention and Control of Congenital Syphilis. MMWR 37 (Suppl S-1):1, 1988.

Centers for Disease Control and Prevention: 1993 Sexually transmitted diseases treatment guidelines. MMWR 42 (RR-14):27, 1993.

Gadde J, Spence M, Wheeler B, Adkinson NF: Clinical experience with penicillin skin testing in a large inner-city STD clinic. JAMA 270:2456, 1993.

Delport SD: On-site screening for maternal syphilis in an antenatal clinic. S Afr Med J 83:723, 1993.

Goldmeier D, Hay P: A review and update on adult syphilis, with particular reference to its treatment. Int J STD AIDS 4:70, 1993.

Gordon SM, Eaton ME, George R, et al: The response of symptomatic neurosyphilis to high-dose intravenous penicillin G in patients with human immunodeficiency virus infection. N Engl J Med 331:1469, 1994.

Green EC: Sexually transmitted disease, ethnomedicine and health policy in Africa. Soc Sci Med 35:121, 1992.

Hook EW III, Marra CM: Acquired syphilis in adults. N Engl J Med 326:1060, 1992.

Ikeda MK, Jenson HB: Evaluation and treatment of congenital syphilis. J Pediatr 117:843, 1990.

Larsen SA, Steiner BM, Rudolph AH: Laboratory diagnosis and interpretation of tests for syphilis. Clin Microbiol Rev 8:1, 1995.

McDermott J, Steketee R, Larsen S, Wirima J: Syphilis-associated perinatal and infant mortality in rural Malawi. Bull WHO 71:773, 1993.

McFarlin BL, Bottoms SF, Dock BS, Isada NB: Epidemic syphilis: Maternal factors associated with congenital infection. Am J Obstet Gynecol 170:535, 1994.

Peterman TA, Zaidi AA, Lieb S, Wroten JE: Incubating syphilis in patients treated for gonorrhea: A comparison of treatment programs. J Infect Dis 170:689, 1994.

Rolfs RT: Treatment of syphilis, 1993. Clin Infect Dis 20 (Suppl 1): S23, 1995.

Wendel GD Jr, Stark BJ, Jamison RB, et al:: Penicillin allergy and desensitization in serious infections during pregnancy. N Engl J Med 312:1229, 1985.

48.2 Yaws

EPIDEMIOLOGY. Yaws (*framboesia tropica, pian, bomba*) occurs in warm, humid tropical regions of Africa, Asia, South America, and Oceania where little clothing is worn and hygiene is poor (Fig. 48–1). Areas of greatest prevalence currently are countries on the southern coast of West Africa, equatorial countries of Africa, parts of India and Sri Lanka, Kampuchea, southern Thailand, Indonesia, Papua New Guinea, islands of Oceania, Suriname, Guyana, Colombia, Peru, Ecuador, and some of the Antilles. Yaws is spread by direct contact with skin lesions or contaminated fingers and fomites. More than 90% of cases begin before the age of 15 years, and infection is common in endemic areas. Yaws was one of the world's most prevalent diseases before the World

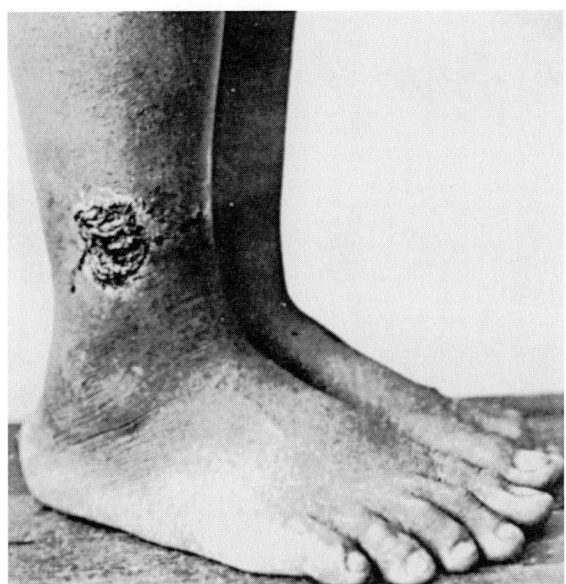

Figure 48–6. Yaws. The mother yaw, most frequent on the extremities, begins as a hyperkeratotic papilloma that later undergoes shallow ulceration. (Courtesy of the Armed Forces Institute of Pathology. Photograph Neg. No. 39207.)

Health Organization (WHO) began mass treatment campaigns with penicillin in 1949. After decades of successful control efforts, yaws has reappeared in some areas where it was believed to have been eradicated. Nomadic peoples in Africa may have contributed to its spread.

CLINICAL MANIFESTATIONS

Primary Lesions. Yaws is more contagious and invasive than pinta. It affects the skin and bones. Congenital transmission does not occur. T. *pallidum pertenue* cannot penetrate intact skin. After 2 to 8 weeks' incubation, the initial lesion—the "mother yaw"—appears as a papule at the site of a recent skin abrasion or laceration, usually on the legs or buttocks. The papule increases in diameter (3 to 5 cm) to become a papilloma, a raised lesion that resembles a raspberry. This lesion persists for 1 to 3 months and is often accompanied by regional lymphadenopathy (Fig. 48–6).

Secondary Lesions. Secondary papillomas erupt locally or elsewhere on the body before or several weeks after the mother yaw heals (Fig. 48–7). These lesions usually occur in crops, have a moist appearance around the nose and mouth (Fig. 48–8), and are hard, fissured, and painful on the palms and soles. Palmar and plantar yaws prevent normal gait and use of the hands; walking may be possible only by placing weight on the sides of the feet. The resulting gait resembles that of a crab ("crab" yaws) (Fig. 48–9). Bone involvement produces painful swelling of the fingers (dactylitis), nose, and tibia (osteoperiostitis). Secondary lesions may relapse repeatedly over a period of 5 years. They may leave "tissue paper" scars, especially if they are secondarily infected by other types of bacteria. In cooler regions, secondary lesions may appear only on warm parts of the body. Focally rarified areas of infected bone heal spontaneously over weeks to months. A "saber shin" deformity may ensue.

Tertiary Lesions. These develop 5 to 10 years after infection in about 10% of untreated persons, with or without an intervening latent period. The most common lesions are chronic ulcerations of the extremities (Fig. 48–10) and face that mutilate and disfigure. Another late lesion is "dry crab yaws," a hyperkeratosis with fissuring of the soles. Destructive bone lesions resemble syphilitic gummas. Destruction of the nasal bones produces gangosa (Fig. 48–11). The viscera, heart, and nervous system are spared.

DIAGNOSIS. Demonstration of T. *pallidum pertenue* by darkfield microscopic examination of exudate from a suspected lesion and seroreactivity in both nontreponemal and treponemal antigen tests serve to distinguish yaws from other conditions except those caused by other *Treponema* species.

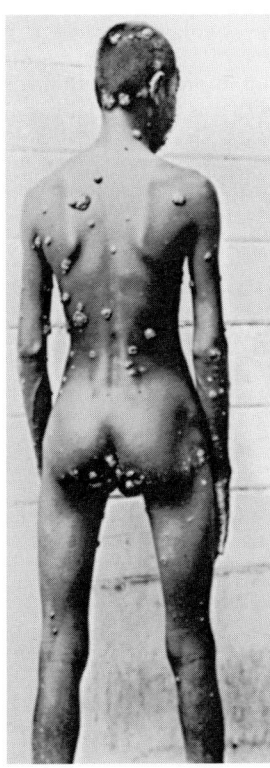

Figure 48–7. The elevated papillomatous nodules characteristic of early yaws are widely distributed and painless. (Courtesy of the Armed Forces Institute of Pathology. Photograph Neg. No. 39205.)

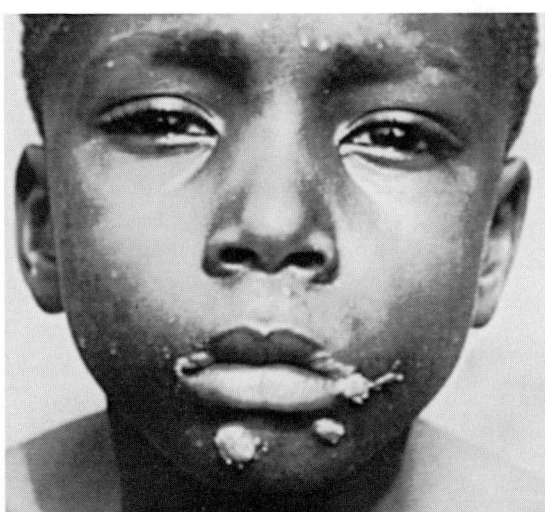

Figure 48–8. Early mucocutaneous yaws with papillomas on the chin and scattered papules elsewhere on the face. Identical mucocutaneous lesions are found in endemic syphilis. These lesions are highly infectious.

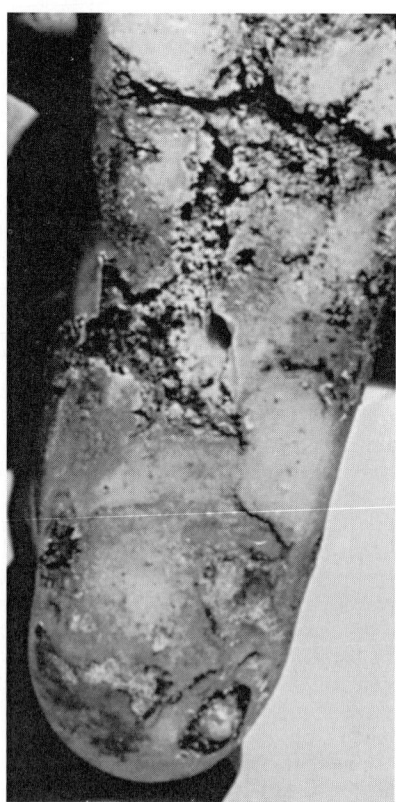

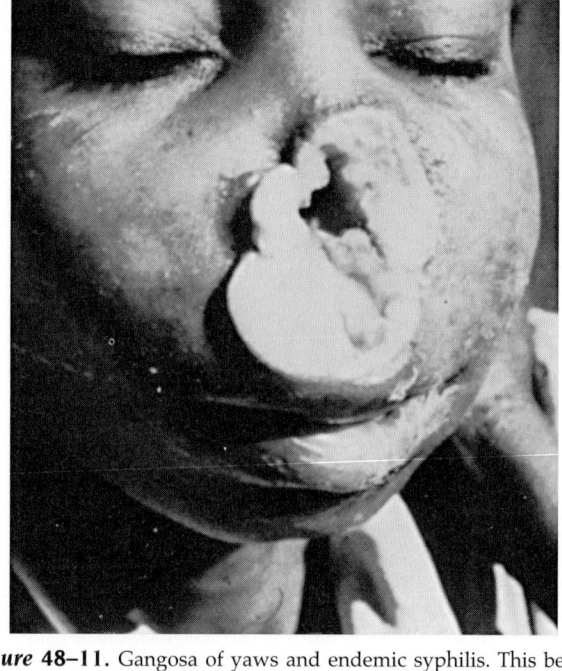

Figure 48–11. Gangosa of yaws and endemic syphilis. This begins as mucocutaneous lesions of the nares during the early stages of infection. Although a characteristic lesion of the late yaws and endemic syphilis, it may also occur in children who are infected for relatively short periods of time.

Figure 48–9. Early plantar or "crab" yaws. Yaws papillomas and hyperkeratoses are exquisitely painful and cause the patient to walk on the sides of the feet, which produces a gait resembling that of a crab.

TREATMENT AND CONTROL. Benzathine penicillin G, 2.4 million U IM in adults and half doses in children under 10 years of age, rapidly cures early lesions and prevents relapses. In populations with a prevalence rate of active yaws of at least 10% or higher, all members of a community should be treated. If the prevalence is less than 5%, only afflicted individuals and close contacts need treatment. Persons aller-

gic to penicillin can receive a tetracycline (erythromycin if less than 8 years old) in a dose similar to that used for venereal syphilis.

Control of yaws by conducting a mass penicillin treatment campaign requires careful coordination and planning; the aim is to create an ever-enlarging yaws-free area. Continuous surveillance for several years after the last clinical case is detected is important to prevent recrudescence of the disease. Recent resurgences of yaws, especially in West and Central Africa and islands in Oceania were caused by failure to maintain active surveillance and lack of integration of yaws control into rural health programs.

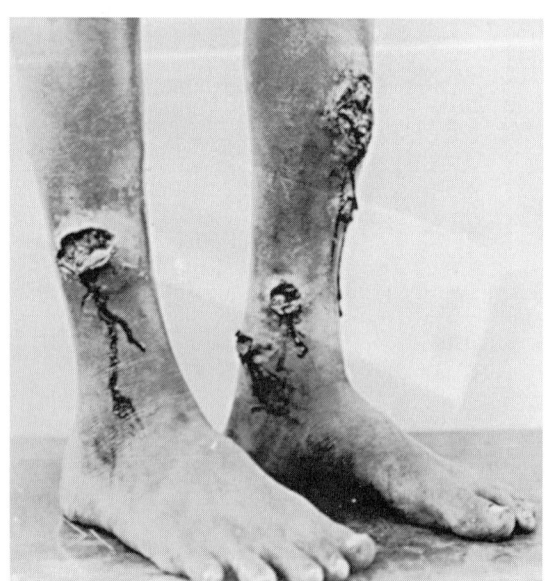

Figure 48–10. Two of the late complications of both yaws and nonvenereal syphilis are illustrated. The bowing deformity of the left leg is probably caused by hypertrophic periostitis. The deeply ulcerated draining lesions are gummas. (Courtesy of the Armed Forces Institute of Pathology. Photograph Neg. No. 40815.)

Bibliography

Meheus A, Antal GM: The endemic treponematoses: Not yet eradicated. World Health Stat Q 45:228, 1992.

Noordhoek GT, Engelkens HJ, Judanarso J, et al: Yaws in West Sumatra, Indonesia: Clinical manifestations, serological findings and characterisation of new *Treponema* isolates by DNA probes. Eur J Clin Microbiol Infect Dis 10:12, 1991.

Rothschild BM, Rothschild C: Treponemal disease revisited: Skeletal discriminators for yaws, bejel, and venereal syphilis. Clin Infect Dis 20:1402, 1995.

Vorst FA: Clinical diagnosis and changing manifestations of treponemal infection. Rev Infect Dis 7(Suppl): S327, 1985.

48.3 Endemic Syphilis

EPIDEMIOLOGY. Endemic nonvenereal syphilis (*bejel, njovera*) occurs in arid regions among nomadic and semi-nomadic peoples of the western Arabian Peninsula and sub-Saharan Africa, southern Africa, and some remote villages in Pakistan (Fig. 48–1). It is most common among children.

CLINICAL MANIFESTATIONS. The initial lesions are mucous patches of the secondary type localized to the oral mucosa and are similar to those of secondary syphilis. These are soon followed by moist papules in the axillae and skin folds. Other early lesions are macular or resemble those of secondary venereal syphilis. Palmar and planter hyperkeratoses occur commonly and are indistinguishable from those of yaws (Fig. 48–9). Late destructive lesions of the long bones (Fig. 48–10) and nasopharynx (gangosa) (Fig. 48–11) occur more frequently than in yaws. Isolated cases of cardiovascular syphilis and CNS system infection sometimes occur.

DIAGNOSIS, TREATMENT, AND CONTROL. These are similar in all respects to those of yaws.

Bibliography

Antal GM, Causse G: The control of endemic treponematoses. Rev Infect Dis 7(Suppl 2): S220, 1985.

Csonka G, Pace J: Endemic nonvenereal treponematosis (Bejel) in Saudi Arabia. Rev Infect Dis 7(Suppl 2): S260, 1985.

48.4 Pinta

EPIDEMIOLOGY. Pinta (*mal del pinto, carate, azul, boussarole, tine, lota, empeines*) is a nonveneral skin infection caused by *T. pallidum carateum*. It persists only in isolated aboriginal populations of southern Mexico and the Amazon River basin (Fig. 48–1). The exact mode of transmission is unknown, but prolonged close personal contact is required. Not very contagious, it is most common in early to middle adulthood.

CLINICAL MANIFESTATIONS. The primary lesion is a small, erythematous papule that appears within 10 days at the site of inoculation, which is usually on the legs or face. Over the next 2 to 3 months, the papule grows to become a flattened, scaly plaque up to 10 cm in diameter and with irregular margins. In 5 to 18 months, secondary lesions called pintids, develop. These are flat, bluish brown, hyperpigmented macules on the exposed surfaces (Fig. 48–12), including the face. The primary lesion merges with adjacent secondary pintids. As the lesions progress toward the tertiary stage they become hyperkeratotic and depigmented. The epidermis atrophies, and permanent cosmetic disfigurement results (Fig. 48–13). The disease is limited to the skin (Fig. 48–14). Except for occasional enlargement of regional lymph nodes,

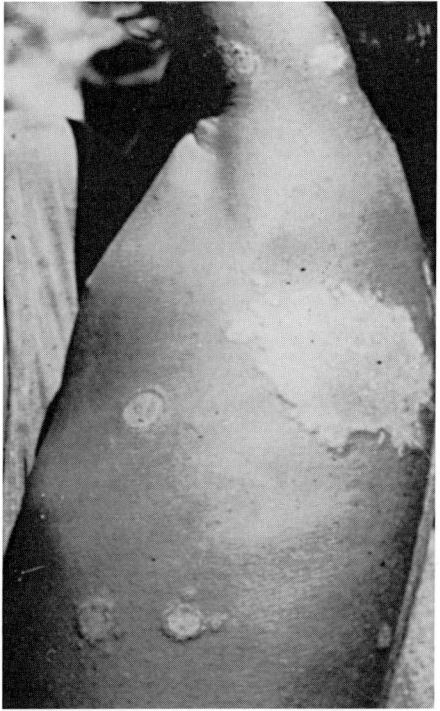

Figure 48–12. Pinta. Large primary and secondary lesions in a young child from Venezuela. (Courtesy of the Armed Forces Institute of Pathology. Photograph Neg. No. 75-5536-2.)

general clinical symptoms and signs are absent during all stages of infection.

DIAGNOSIS. Pintids may resemble psoriasis, lichen planus, leprosy, and other skin diseases. Symmetric vitiligo of the hands and feet is characteristic. Treponemes are easily seen

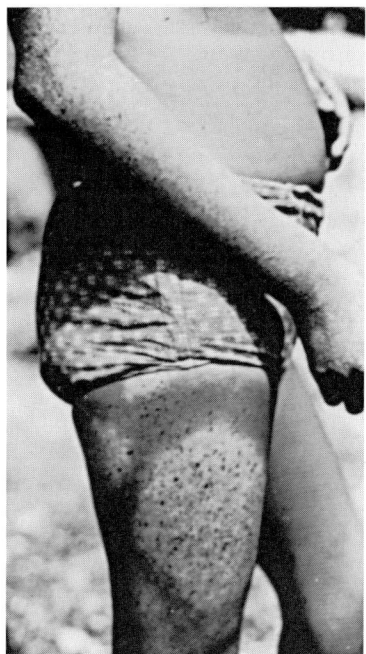

Figure 48–13. Late pinta. Hypopigmentation and hyperpigmentation of the right arm, forearm, and thigh. (Courtesy of the Armed Forces Institute of Pathology. Photograph Neg. No. 75-5536-3.)

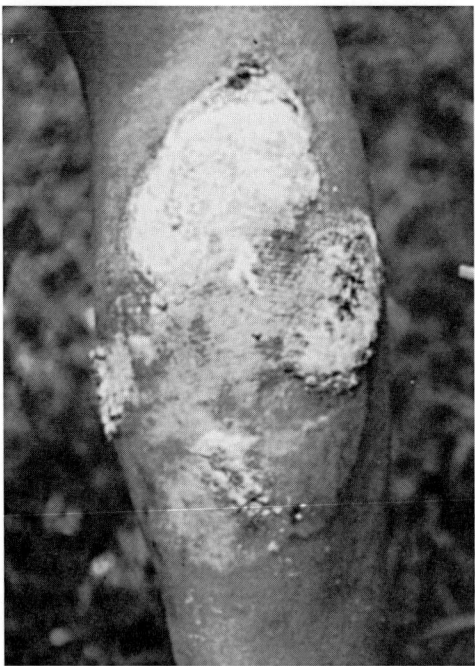

Figure 48–14. Pinta. Dyschromic lesion on the calf in various stages of healing. Only the dermis is involved, and the complications of pinta are cosmetic.

with darkfield microscopy of scrapings taken from the periphery of primary and early secondary lesions. The VDRL test is positive in approximately 60 to 75% of cases during the secondary stage and in most cases of tertiary pinta.

TREATMENT AND CONTROL. A single dose of benzathine penicillin G, 2.4 million U IM, is the treatment of choice. Children younger than 10 years of age receive 1.2 million U. Only family contacts require prophylactic penicillin treatment. Pigmented lesions heal rapidly. Vitiliginous areas of less than 5 years' duration often regain pigment.

Improved living conditions and better access to modern medicine have contributed to the eradication of pinta from much of its former range.

Bibliography

Dominguez-Soto L, Hojyo-Tomoka T, Vega-Memije E, Arenas R: Pigmentary problems in the tropics. Dermatol Clin 12:777, 1994.

49 Gonococcal Infections

Ronald C. Ballard

DEFINITION. Gonorrhea is caused by *Neisseria gonorrhoeae*, a gram-negative diplococcus that can infect a variety of mucosal surfaces lined by columnar epithelial cells. It remains the most frequently reported infectious disease in the United States—despite the fact that reported cases have more than halved in the past 20 years. Elsewhere in the industrialized world the decline in gonorrhea has been even more precipitous, with the disease nearing eradication in some Scandinavian countries. Unfortunately, this situation is not reflected in the majority of developing countries, where gonorrhea remains a significant public health problem.

Gonorrhea is transmitted almost exclusively by sexual contact, with adults under 30 years of age who have multiple sexual partners at the highest risk of infection. The sites most affected are the urethra in men and the uterine cervix and urethra in women. Rectal infection is common in both women and homosexual men, and gonococcal pharyngitis can occur in both sexes following orogenital contact. Although gonococcal vulvovaginitis in prepubertal girls can be the result of contact with fomites, sexual transmission is the most frequent cause of infection, even in young children. Complications include epididymo-orchitis and urethral stricture in men; bartholinitis, salpingitis, perihepatitis, chorioamnionitis, tubal infertility, and ectopic pregnancy in women; and bacteremia, arthritis-dermatitis syndrome, endocarditis, and meningitis in both sexes. Vertical transmission can result in conjunctivitis and infection of the pharynx, vagina, and rectum of babies born to infected mothers.

ETIOLOGY. *Neisseria gonorrhoeae* is a gram-negative diplococcus that forms small, mucoid, oxidase-positive colonies on chocolate agar. It is differentiated from other species of *Neisseria* by its ability to ferment glucose but not lactose, sucrose, or maltose. Confirmatory tests include coagglutination with monoclonal antibodies and DNA hybridization. The ultrastructure of the gonococcal cell envelope is similar to that of other gram-negative bacteria. Notably, the cell wall contains a number of antigenic proteins, lipopolysaccharide (in which resides endotoxic activity), and pili (which are filamentous structures that aid attachment to cell surfaces and enhance resistance to phagocytosis and killing by neutrophils).

Antigens and Immunity. The gonococcal pili, lipopolysaccharide, and the outer membrane proteins are antigenic; IgG and IgA antibodies to homologous isolates have been detected in mucosal secretions following uncomplicated infections. However, in practice, natural uncomplicated gonococcal infections do not confer any significant immunity, and reinfections are common. Patients with a congenital deficiency in one of the terminal components of complement (C7, C8, C9) may experience recurrent episodes of disseminated gonococcal infection. A variety of methods for gonococcal typing have been developed, including auxotyping (which is dependent upon determining amino acid and purine and pyrimidine requirements for growth), or protein I serotyping, or the two used in combination. By using both auxotyping and serovar analysis, gonococci have been divided into a large number of auxotype/serovar (A/S) classes that have been widely used as a discriminatory tool for the epidemiologic study of gonococcal infections. More recently, *opa*-typing has also been employed in gonococcal epidemiology.

Antibiotic-Resistant Strains. Plasmids encoding for the production of β-lactamases were first demonstrated in gonococci in 1976. These penicillinase-producing *N. gonorrhoeae* (PPNG) are now commonly isolated in Africa and Asia. In addition, gonococci may be resistant to penicillin/ampicillin/amoxicillin as a result of chromosomal mutations. These strains may also show decreased susceptibility to certain cephalosporins, tetracycline, and macrolide antibiotics. High-level resistance to tetracyclines associated with acquisition of a 25.2 Md tet-M plasmid has emerged in most regions of the world, and fluoroquinolone resistance has been detected in many Asian countriesas been documented sporadically in the United States, Europe, and Australia. Quinolone resistance is thought to result from mutations in genes encoding gonococcal DNA gyrase and changes in membrane permeability.

CLINICAL MANIFESTATIONS

Urethritis. The clinical features of gonococcal urethritis in men are a urethral discharge, which is often profuse and

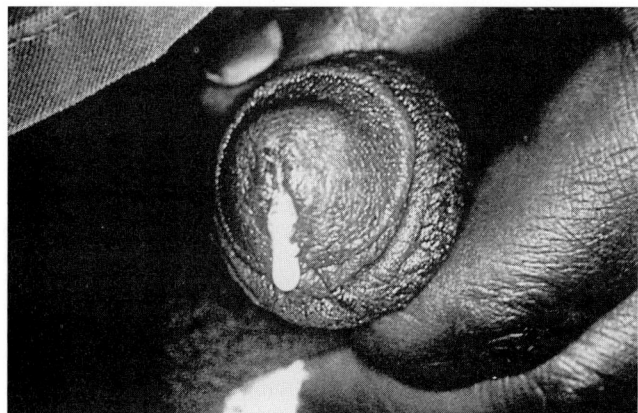

Figure 49–1. Purulent urethral discharge associated with gonococcal urethritis.

purulent (Fig. 49–1), dysuria, and frequency of micturition. The onset of symptoms is often sudden following an incubation period of 1 to 10 days, but in a minority of cases the disease may be asymptomatic. In rare cases, *N. gonorrhoeae* may spread to the epididymis and testis, the prostate, or Skene's and Littré's glands. These complications occur frequently as a sequel to asymptomatic or inapparent urethral infection.

Endocervical Infection. In contrast to men, most women with gonococcal infection are asymptomatic or minimally symptomatic. Those with symptoms may complain of a vaginal discharge or dysuria, which may be associated with an infection of the urethra. On examination, a purulent discharge may be seen arising from the endocervical canal, but in the majority of cases no visible endocervical mucopus can be detected on visual inspection. In many cases these infections may progress to salpingitis without any obvious symptoms.

Pelvic Inflammatory Disease (PID). *N. gonorrhoeae* may ascend from the endocervical canal to the endometrium, fallopian tubes, and eventually the peritoneal cavity, causing endometritis, salpingitis, and pelvic peritonitis. Symptomatic patients may report lower abdominal pain, which is usually bilateral. The severity of the condition may vary from being virtually asymptomatic to life-threatening. A characteristic PID gait has been described, namely, a patient walking slowly and grasping her lower abdomen. A profuse vaginal discharge, often with an offensive odor, is commonly noted and is often associated with dysuria. Abnormal uterine bleeding occurs in 35 to 40% of patients, probably as a result of endometritis.

Clinical findings include pyrexia, tachycardia, lower abdominal tenderness, and, depending on severity, pelvic or even generalized peritonitis. Vaginal examination reveals cervical excitation tenderness and, frequently, adnexal tenderness. Adnexal masses may be formed from tubo-ovarian abscesses or from omentum and bowel adherent to the inflamed tubes and ovaries. Occasionally a patient may present in extremis, with features of generalized peritonitis, septicemic shock, and disseminated intravascular coagulopathy. In some severe cases the liver capsule can become inflamed and attached to peritoneum by fine "violin-string" adhesions. This perihepatitis is also known as Fitz-Hugh–Curtis syndrome. Resolution of tubal infections may result in formation of fine scars that are associated with increased risk of ectopic pregnancy and tubal infertility.

Gonococcal Proctitis. The majority of cases of gonococcal proctitis are asymptomatic but may be associated with an anal discharge, blood and/or mucus in stools, and pain during defecation. Gonococcal proctitis is common in homosexual men who practice anal-receptive intercourse, and the disease is frequently associated with other sexually acquired enteric pathogens. Women may acquire gonococcal proctitis from heterosexual anal intercourse or as a result of spread from the adjacent vagina.

Gonococcal Pharyngitis. Pharyngeal gonococcal infection, in common with rectal infections, tends to be asymptomatic. However, a minority of patients may complain of a sore throat, and on examination a mucopurulent exudate may be present. Pharyngeal infections occur in those patients practicing fellatio or cunnilingus.

Ocular Infections. Ocular infections occur in neonates born to infected mothers during passage through an infected birth canal. It is characterized by edema of the lids, severe chemosis, and later a profuse purulent discharge (Fig. 49–2). The incubation period is usually very short (normally 1–4 days.) Occasionally, a severe, purulent keratoconjunctivitis is seen in adults following accidental exposure of the eye to genital discharges. Both neonatal and adult eye infections require prompt diagnosis and treatment in order to prevent sight-threatening sequelae that may ensue as a result of the formation of corneal opacities, scarring, or panophthalmitis and perforation.

Disseminated Gonococcal Infection. Disseminated gonococcal infection (DGI) occurs as a result of gonococcal bacteremia. The source of infection tends to be asymptomatic endocervical, pharyngeal, rectal, or urethral disease. The most common form of DGI is the dermatitis-arthritis syndrome, in which patients, usually women, develop arthralgias and macular, pustular, hemorrhagic, or necrotic skin lesions on the distal extremities. A minority of patients develop septic joints with a purulent effusion and associated fever. The disease normally affects isolated joints, which, without treatment, may be destroyed within a few days. Other manifestations of gonococcal bacteremia include endocarditis and meningitis. Fortunately, these complications are extremely rare.

LABORATORY DIAGNOSIS

The Gram Stain. The finding of intracellular gram-negative diplococci in Gram-stained smears of urethral or conjunctival material is generally regarded as sufficient evidence for a presumptive diagnosis of gonococcal infection in symptomatic men with acute urethritis and in patients with conjunctivitis (Fig. 49–3). However, whenever possible, the exudate should be cultured on a selective medium to confirm the diagnosis. Because of the large numbers of bacteria that can be mistaken for (or mask) *N. gonorrhoeae* or because of the presence of other *Neisseria* spp., especially in the oropharynx,

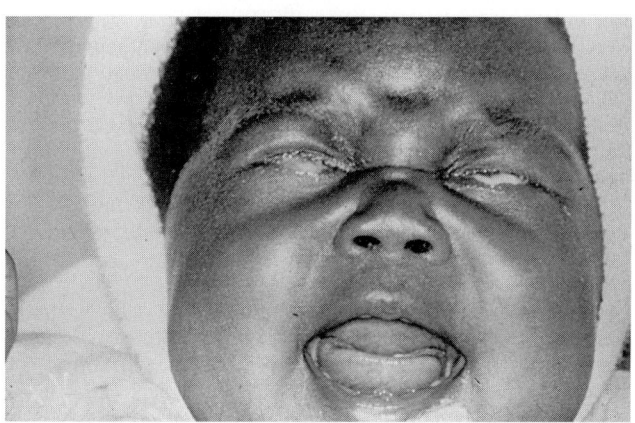

Figure 49–2. Gonococcal ophthalmia neonatorum.

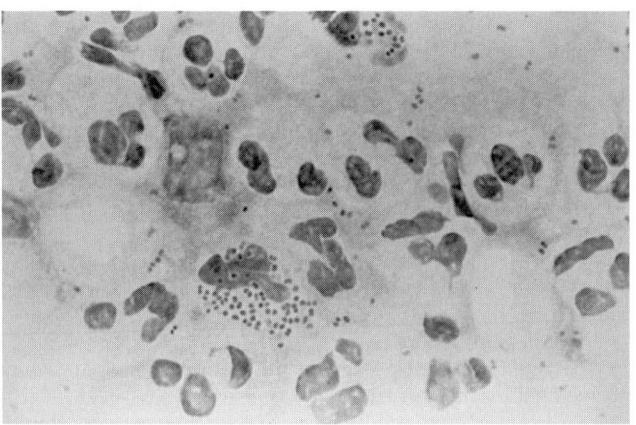

Figure 49–3. Gram-stained smear of urethral exudate showing gram-negative intracellular diplococci.

Gram-stained smears of genital secretions from women and from the rectum or pharynx of patients with suspected gonococcal infection are of questionable diagnostic value.

Culture. Specimens for culture of *N. gonorrhoeae* should be plated directly onto a medium such as Thayer-Martin or New York City medium, each of which is composed of a gonococcal (GC) or equivalent agar base, with additional growth supplements and antibacterial and antifungal agents to make it selective. If the specimen is obtained from a site that is usually sterile (e.g., blood or synovial fluid), it can be inoculated directly onto plates of nonselective chocolate agar. Inoculated plates can be stored at room temperature in a candle extinction jar for up to 6 hours without significant loss of viability. Alternatively, specimens may be sent to the laboratory in Stuart's or Amies' transport medium. After incubation for 24 to 48 hours at 35°C in an atmosphere of 10% CO_2 in air, isolated colonies can be identified on the basis of a Gram stain, oxidase test, and sugar fermentation reactions. *N. gonorrhoeae* produces oxidase and ferments glucose but not sucrose, lactose, or maltose. Alternatively, isolated organisms can be identified by using monoclonal antibodies in commercial co-agglutination tests.

Whereas endourethral swabs are the most suitable specimens for isolation of *N. gonorrhoeae* from men with urethral infection, endocervical, urethral, and rectal swabs should be taken from women to optimize detection rates. Likewise, oropharyngeal swabs should be taken from all patients with a history of recent orogenital contact.

Nonculture Tests. These are commercially available. They include antigen detection tests, e.g., ELISA assays, nonamplified nucleic acid probes, and amplified nucleic acid tests, e.g., the polymerase chain reaction (PCR) and ligase chain reaction (LCR). These amplified tests, although expensive, are more sensitive than culture and have the advantage that they can be applied to "noninvasive" specimens such as first-catch urine. Unfortunately, all nonculture tests share the disadvantage that they can detect nonviable *N. gonorrhoeae*. Therefore, they cannot be recommended for evaluation of tests of cure following treatment. At the present time there is no reliable serodiagnostic test available for acute, superficial gonococcal infections.

TREATMENT

Uncomplicated Gonococcal Infections. The choice of antimicrobial agents for the treatment of uncomplicated gonorrhea is influenced by a number of factors in addition to the antimicrobial susceptibilities of local gonococcal isolates. As a general rule, single-dose therapy is preferred in order to overcome problems associated with patient compliance.

However, in many countries where gonorrhea is common, the choice of treatment is limited by financial constraints and the availability of certain antibiotics. In addition, the likelihood of concurrent infection justifies the use of combination therapies active against all possible causes of the presenting disease "syndrome" (Chapter 11). This "syndromic approach" to the management of sexually transmitted infections has been actively advocated by the World Health Organization (WHO) for a number of years. As an example of this approach, since 1985 the treatment guidelines for gonorrhea published by the Centers for Disease Control (CDC) have recommended that single-dose treatments effective for eradication of *N. gonorrhoeae* be automatically followed by a 7-day course of a tetracycline or macrolide antibiotic, which would be expected to eradicate concomitant *C. trachomatis* infection and other causes of nongonococcal urethritis. In many countries with few laboratory facilities, routine treatment of acute urethritis in men is achieved with such double therapy, while routine therapy of sexually acquired vaginal discharge and PID is achieved by addition of multidose metronidazole to this regimen to eradicate trichomoniasis, bacterial vaginosis, and anaerobes associated with pelvic infection.

In the few regions of the world where antimicrobial resistance of *N. gonorrhoeae* is not a problem, single-dose treatment with either 4.8 million U of procaine penicillin G IM plus 1.0 g probenecid by mouth or 3.5 g ampicillin or 3.0 g amoxicillin plus 1.0 g probenecid, all by mouth, remains acceptable followed by a 7-day course of doxycycline 100 mg twice daily or tetracycline 500 mg four times daily, both by mouth. In areas where antimicrobial resistance is more common, ciprofloxacin 500 mg, ofloxacin 400 mg, or cefixime 400 mg as a single oral dose or ceftriaxone 125 mg or spectinomycin 2 g as a single IM injection may precede the 7-day treatment for other infections. Less expensive, and often less effective, alternatives used in some developing countries include combining antichlamydial therapy with either kanamycin 2 g as a single IM injection or with trimethoprim (80 mg)/sulfamethoxazole (400 mg), 10 tablets orally, once daily for 3 days. Sexual partners of patients with gonorrhoea should be treated simultaneously regardless of the results of laboratory investigations, in order to prevent reinfection and complications.

Epididymo-orchitis. Since the most important causes of sexually acquired epididymo-orchitis are identical to those of acute uncomplicated urethritis, namely, *N. gonorrhoeae* and *C. trachomatis*, the treatment for this complication is identical to that of uncomplicated disease. In most tropical regions this is achieved by providing appropriate single-dose therapy for gonorrhea plus a week-long course of doxycycline, tetracycline, or erythromycin.

PID and Other Genital Complications. In general, other complicated gonococcal infections require treatment for longer periods. Empirical therapy for PID is complicated by the diversity of organisms isolated from specimens obtained from the upper genital tract. The presence of *N. gonorrhoeae* in the endocervix does not automatically indicate that it is the main etiologic agent of the associated PID. Likewise, the presence of *N. gonorrhoeae* in the upper genital tract does not preclude a role for other pathogens in the etiology of the disease. Clinical experience determines which patients with PID should be treated on an outpatient basis and which ones require hospitalization and intravenous therapy. Hospital admission is warranted for a temperature >38°C, pelvic or abdominal peritonitis, or pelvic masses or when the diagnosis is in doubt. Outpatient therapies recommended by the WHO for treatment of PID in areas where gonococcal resistance is common include

1. Single-dose therapy normally recommended for uncom-

plicated gonorrhea plus doxycycline, 100 mg orally twice daily, or tetracycline, 500 mg orally four times daily for 14 days, plus metronidazole, 400 to 500 mg orally, twice daily for 14 days.

2. The alternative regimen, recommended for areas where single-dose therapy for gonorrhea is not available, is trimethoprim (80 mg)/sulfamethoxazole (400 mg), 10 tablets orally once daily for 3 days, and then 2 tablets orally twice daily for 10 days, plus doxycycline, 100 mg orally twice daily, or tetracycline, 500 mg orally, four times daily for 14 days, plus metronidazole, 400 to 500 mg orally twice daily for 14 days.

In cases of severe PID requiring hospitalization, the spectrum of causative organisms is even broader than that for milder disease that is treated on an outpatient basis. In order to provide adequate antimicrobial cover for *N. gonorrhoeae*, *C. trachomatis*, anaerobic bacteria (*Bacteroides* spp. and gram-positive cocci), facultative gram-negative rods, and *Mycoplasma hominis*, the WHO recommends the following treatment regimens:

1. Ceftriaxone, 500 mg by IM injection, once daily, plus doxycycline, 100 mg orally or by IV injection, twice daily, or tetracycline, 500 mg orally four times daily, plus metronidazole, 400 to 500 mg orally or by IV injection, twice daily, or chloramphenicol, 500 mg orally or by IV injection, four times daily.

2. Clindamycin, 900 mg by IV injection, every 8 hours, plus gentamicin, 1.5 mg/kg by IV injection every 8 hours.

3. Ciprofloxacin 500 mg orally, twice daily, or spectinomycin 1 g by IM injection, four times daily, plus doxycycline, 100 mg orally or by IV injection, twice daily, or tetracycline, 500 mg orally, four times daily, plus metronidazole 400 to 500 mg orally or by IV injection, twice daily, or chloramphenicol, 500 mg orally or by IV injection, four times daily.

Note: For all three regimens, therapy should be continued until at least 2 days after the patient has improved and should then be followed by either doxycycline 100 mg orally, twice daily for 14 days, or tetracycline, 500 mg orally, four times daily for 14 days.

Since intrauterine devices (IUDs) are recognized as a risk factor for PID, removal of the IUD is recommended soon after initiation of antimicrobial chemotherapy. When the IUD has been removed, appropriate contraceptive counseling should be provided.

Disseminated Gonococcal Infection. Prolonged therapy with ceftriaxone or spectinomycin has been recommended by the WHO: ceftriaxone, 1 g by IM or IV injection, once daily for 7 days, or spectinomycin, 2 g by IM injection, twice daily for 7 days.

Note: Repeated aspiration of fluid from any septic joint is recommended. For gonococcal meningitis and endocarditis, treatment with either of the above is recommended but for 14 days in the case of meningitis and 4 weeks in the case of endocarditis.

Gonococcal Eye Infections. Ocular infections in adults should be treated as for uncomplicated infections of the genital tract. In addition, the eyes should be irrigated frequently with sterile saline to prevent buildup of purulent discharge. Topical antibiotics alone are not considered sufficient therapy and should be avoided.

Neonates with gonococcal ophthalmia should, ideally, be hospitalized and isolated for 24 hours after initiation of therapy. Ceftriaxone 50 mg/kg (maximum 125 mg), spectinomycin 25 mg/kg (maximum 75 mg), or kanamycin 25 mg/

kg (maximum 75 mg) can all be given as a single IM injection. As with adults, the eyes of babies should be irrigated with sterile saline hourly to prevent buildup of discharge. Topical antibiotic preparations alone are not sufficient for therapy owing to pharyngeal gonococcal colonization and are unnecessary when appropriate systemic therapy is provided. Both parents of neonates with gonococcal ophthalmia must receive appropriate treatment. Gonococcal ophthalmia neonatorum may be prevented by the instillation of silver nitrate eyedrops at birth (Credé prophylaxis). However, since many cases of chemically induced conjunctivitis have been recorded following this procedure, many centers routinely use topical chloramphenicol or another suitable antibiotic eye ointment for ocular prophylaxis.

PREVENTION AND CONTROL. Prevention strategies for gonorrhea are identical to those used for other sexually transmitted diseases (STDs), namely, rapid diagnosis and provision of effective therapy together with early partner notification, condom promotion, and patient education programs about gonorrhea specifically and STDs in general. Since gonorrhea may act as a cofactor in the transmission of human immunodefiency virus (HIV), control strategies should form an integral part of AIDS-control activities (Chapter 22). In developing countries, targeted interventions aimed at high-risk populations, e.g., sex workers, military personnel, and migrant workers, may be productive. Broad-based case-finding programs using noninvasive techniques, e.g., testing of urine for specific gonococcal nucleic acid sequences by PCR or LCR, may be cost effective in more affluent settings, where there is a low prevalence of disease.

Bibliography

Sparling PF: Biology of Neisseria gonorrhoeae. *In* Holmes KK, Mardh P-A, Sparling PF, et al (eds): Sexually Transmitted Diseases. New York, McGraw-Hill, 1990, pp 131–147.

Whittington W, Ison C, Thompson S: Gonorrhoea. *In* Morse SA, Moreland AA, Holmes KK (eds): Atlas of Sexually Transmitted Diseases and AIDS. London, Mosby-Wolfe, 1996, pp 100–117.

World Health Organization: Management of Sexually Transmitted Diseases. WHO/GPA/TEM/94.1, Geneva, 1994.

50 Chancroid

Allan R. Ronald

DEFINITION. Chancroid is a genital ulcer caused by *Haemophilus ducreyi*. Ricord differentiated the primary hard chancre of syphilis from the soft chancre of chancroid in 1840 and Ducrey described the etiologic agent in 1889. Classic chancroid is an acutely painful, irregular ulcer occurring on the genitalia with associated inguinal lymphadenitis that may proceed to bubo formation.

ETIOLOGY. *H. ducreyi* is a small gram-negative bipolar staining organism which often has a "school of fish" arrangement on stain. The organism requires hemin and the amino acids glutamine and cystine. Its taxonomic placement is controversial but it is more closely related to the *Pasteurella* rather than the *Haemophilus* genus. *H. ducreyi* reduces nitrate and produces alkaline phosphatase. It possesses several characteristics that appear important for virulence including pili, a hemolysin, and a hemoglobin receptor.

PATHOGENESIS. As few as 30 *H. ducreyi* organisms can

produce ulceration following inoculation on the forearms of healthy human volunteers. Immunohistochemical analysis of the ulcerating lesions has shown that a cell-mediated Th 1 response consisting predominantly of T lymphocytes and macrophages, is present interstitially and perivascularly. Presumably, cytotoxins and hemolysins produced by *H. ducreyi* cause tissue destruction. The pathogenesis of the lymphadenitis and bubo formation is still not understood.

EPIDEMIOLOGY. Chancroid is endemic in most countries of the developing world with about 10 million cases occurring annually. In some tropical countries, as many as 1% of individuals attending for primary care and 20 to 50% attending a sexually transmitted disease (STD) clinic will have genital sores as their presenting complaints. Chancroid flourishes in societies in which many men are having sex with a few women who are often commercial sex workers, a substantial proportion of men are uncircumcised, and STD control programs are not well established. Male to female ratios average about 8:1 in most studies. Introductions occur in the industrialized world, particularly at seaports, leading to clusters of cases which usually can be readily controlled. Outbreaks in several cities, including New York City, have been ongoing among individuals who use cocaine or trade sex for drugs.

Reservoir. The reservoir for *H. ducreyi* is presumed to be women who have relatively asymptomatic genital ulcers and who continue to be sexually active. There does not appear to be an important reservoir of women or men who have positive cultures for *H. ducreyi* without clinically evident ulceration. The attack rate following unprotected intercourse is high with at least 50% of men acquiring genital ulcers. Secondary attack rates are also substantial with at least one half of subsequent partners infected. It appears that many men are sexually active despite genital ulcers.

Interaction with Human Immunodeficiency Virus (HIV). Numerous studies have demonstrated that *H. ducreyi* and HIV infection interact in several ways to increase heterosexual transmission of HIV while concomitantly altering chancroid. HIV seronegative men with chancroid have a fivefold greater risk of HIV seroconversion than men with urethritis following exposure to women who are known to be HIV-infected. Women with genital ulcers who sell sex are at much greater risk of acquiring HIV. The immune response to *H. ducreyi* recruits and activates macrophages and T-helper lymphocytes, which increases the susceptibility of individuals with ulcers to HIV infection. Excretion of HIV in genital discharge is markedly increased. As a result, genital ulcers become both the portal of HIV entry and exit. HIV-infected women are also more susceptible to *H. ducreyi* infection. Patients with chancroid who are HIV-infected more commonly fail treatment or relapse. As a result of these numerous interactions, a cycle of amplification between *H. ducreyi* and HIV can occur which markedly increases risks of transmission of HIV while enlarging the epidemic of chancroid.

CLINICAL FEATURES. After an incubation period of 3 to 7 days, a rapidly eroding ulcer develops. About one half of chancroid ulcers are classic and present as irregular, nonindurated, very painful lesions with an undermined edge and yellow-gray purulent exudative base which bleeds readily. The depth is variable but many of the ulcers are quite superficial. The skin surrounding the ulcer is usually not inflamed. Other presentations include giant ulcers formed when several smaller ones merge (Fig. 50–1); dwarf ulcers, which are tiny, shallow, round ulcers that mimic genital herpes; transient ulceration which resembles lymphogranuloma venereum; single painless ulcers which can be confused with syphilis; and beefy, raised, indurated lesions that clinically appear to be granuloma inguinale. The sensitivity and specificity of the

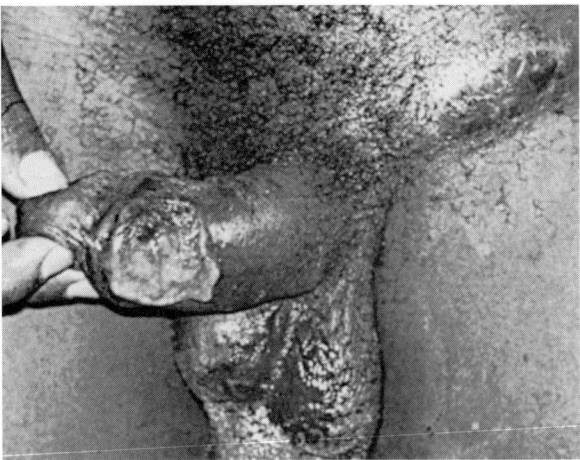

Figure 50–1. Chancroid. Large penile ulceration with a suppurative left inguinal bubo.

clinical diagnosis depends on the relative proportion of genital ulcers due to *H. ducreyi* in the population.

The site of ulceration on the genitalia varies, with about half the lesions occurring on the prepuce in uncircumcised men. Kissing lesions are common on adjacent cutaneous surfaces. In women, the majority of lesions are on the fourchette, labia, and perineal area (Fig. 50–2). About 40% of patients develop painful inguinal adenitis which can progress to bubo formation with overlying erythema. Buboes may rupture and produce an inguinal abscess.

Careful, definitive laboratory studies suggest that about 10 to 15% of patients with chancroid also have a second ulcerating pathogen, usually either herpes simplex or *Treponema pallidum*.

LABORATORY DIAGNOSIS. Cultures should be either plated directly or transported on a swab that is kept at 4°C for up to 6 hours. The culture should be plated on either gonococcal agar or Mueller-Hinton agar, each with added vancomycin, 3 mg/L to inhibit the growth of gram-positive bacteria with added 2% hemoglobin and 1% vitamin enrich-

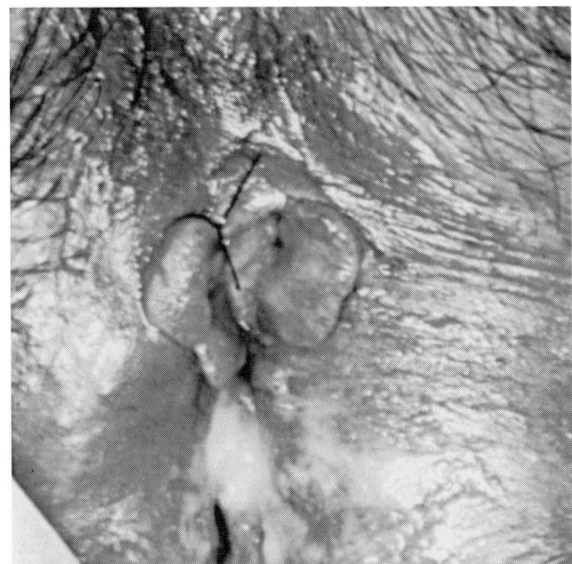

Figure 50–2. Chancroid. Labial lesion. (Courtesy of the Armed Forces Institute of Pathology, Photograph Neg. No. 82-9102.)

ment. Charcoal 0.25% is a satisfactory replacement for fetal calf serum. Incubation should be carried out at 32° to 33°C in a 100% humidity, CO_2-enriched environment. A candle extinction jar with a moist paper towel is adequate. After 2 to 5 days, small yellow-gray colonies of varying size appear on the culture plate. The colonies can be moved intact across the plate and when stained demonstrate gram-negative coccal bacilli in short chains.

Whenever possible, genital ulcers should be investigated with darkfield examination, serology for syphilis, and culture for herpes in addition to *H. ducreyi*. Numerous studies have confirmed the nonspecificity of the clinical diagnosis. The features of herpes, syphilis, lymphogranuloma venereum, and granuloma inguinale can all be mimicked by atypical chancroid presentations. As a result, syndromic diagnosis and treatment of genital ulcer disease is necessary for management and control interventions.

Polymerase chain reaction (PCR) has recently been evaluated for the diagnosis of *H. ducreyi* infection and it appears sensitive and specific. A commercial product will shortly be marketed which can be used to identify each of the three major pathogens—*H. ducreyi*, herpes simplex, and *T. pallidum*. Serologic studies have been used for the diagnosis of *H. ducreyi* but these are relatively insensitive and are best reserved for seroimmunologic investigation of populations.

TREATMENT. *H. ducreyi* is readily infected with plasmids and as a result antimicrobial resistance has developed and spread quickly in many societies. In most of the world, *H. ducreyi* is resistant to tetracycline, ampicillin, sulfonamides, and trimethoprim. Less commonly, plasmids that mediate resistance to kanamycin, streptomycin, and chloramphenicol may be present.

Erythromycin prescribed in a dose of 500 mg three times a day for 7 days has become the drug of first choice. No resistance is known to occur and treatment is almost uniformly effective. Azithromycin as a single 1-g dose regimen is more expensive but is an equally effective regimen. Ceftriaxone prescribed as a single dose of 250 mg IM is effective but with the spread of HIV in this population, treatment failures are more common. Ciprofloxacin and presumably other fluoroquinolones are also effective regimens for chancroid. Ciprofloxacin is usually prescribed in a dose of 250 mg twice daily for 3 days with very high rates of cure.

Fluctuant buboes should be incised or aspirated.

PREVENTION. With the increasing evidence that links chancroid to explosive heterosexual transmission of HIV, control and elimination of chancroid from populations is now a priority. Enhanced STD control strategies to include effective treatment regimens based on syndromic diagnosis at the point of first contact with the health care system, the increased use of condoms particularly with female sex workers, programs to provide care and treatment for prostitutes, and partner referral can all be markedly successful in controlling endemic infections. Sexual partners should be treated concurrently and empirically whether or not ulcers are present. Recently in Thailand a 10-fold reduction in chancroid has been reported. This was due to the availability of effective treatment regimens together with widespread use of condoms. Chancroid is one sexually transmitted disease that is susceptible to rapid control with appropriate targeted intervention.

Bibliography

Bogarts J, Vuylsteke B, Martinez-Tello W, et al: Simple algorithms for the management of genital ulcers: evaluation of a primary health care centre in Kigali, Rwanda. Bull WHO 73:767, 1995.
Cameron DW, Simonsen JEN, D'Costa LJ, et al: Female to male transmission of human immunodeficiency virus type 1: risk factors for seroconversion in men. Lancet 2:403, 1989.
DiCarlo RP, Armentor BS, Martin DH: Chancroid epidemiology in New Orleans men. J Infect Dis 172:446, 1995.
Hayes RJ, Schulz KF, Plummer FA: A cofactor effect of genital ulcers on the per-exposure risk of HIV transmission in sub-Saharan Africa. J Trop Med Hyg 98:1, 1995.
King R, Gough J, Ronald A, et al: An immunohistochemical analysis of naturally occurring chancroid. J Infect Dis 174:427, 1996.
Martin DH, Sargent SJ, Wendel GD, et al: Comparison of azithromycin and ceftriaxone for the treatment of chancroid. Clin Infect Dis 21:409, 1995.
Nasio JM, Nagelkerke NJD, Mwatha A, et al: Genital ulcer disease among STD clinic attenders in Nairobi: association with HIV-1 and circumcision status. Int J STD AIDS 7:410, 1996.
Ndinya-Achola JO, Kihara AN, Fisher LD, et al: Presumptive specific clinical diagnosis of genital ulcer disease (GUD) in a primary health care setting in Nairobi. Int J STD AIDS 7:201, 1996.
Orle KA, Gates CA, Martin DH, et al: Simultaneous PCR detection of *Haemophilus ducreyi*, *Treponema pallidum*, and herpes simplex virus types 1 and 2 from genital ulcers. J Clin Microbiol 34:49, 1996.
Plummer FA, D'Costa LJ, Nsanze H, et al: Epidemiology of chancroid and *Haemophilus ducreyi* in Nairobi. Lancet 2:1293, 1983.
Sivayathorn A: The use of fluoroquinolones in sexually transmitted diseases in Southeast Asia. Drugs 49:123, 1995.
Trees DL, Morse SA: Chancroid and *Haemophilus ducreyi*: an update. Clin Microbiol Rev 8:357, 1995.

51 *Granuloma Inguinale*

John Richens

DEFINITION, HISTORY, AND ETIOLOGY. Granuloma inguinale (donovanosis) is a chronic granulomatous infection, largely confined to the tropics, that produces anogenital and inguinal ulcers. Early descriptions of the disease refer to "serpiginous" or "lupoid" ulceration of the genitals and "lupoid" groin ulceration. Most recent publications use the term *donovanosis*, coined by Marmell in 1952 to avoid confusion with lymphogranuloma venereum which shares clinical and epidemiologic features. Unfortunately, Donovan's name is associated with two infections in which he discovered intracellular inclusions—leishmaniasis, in which the intracellular amastigotes are sometimes referred to as Leishman-Donovan bodies, and granuloma inguinale (which he believed to be caused by a protozoon), whose inclusions are now known as Donovan bodies.

Granuloma inguinale is transmitted primarily through sexual contact. The recognition of Donovan bodies in lesions was made independently by Flu, Siebert, and Donovan who examined material from Suriname, German New Guinea, and India, respectively. These countries continue to be important endemic foci of the disease, for which the main mode of diagnosis is still the identification of Donovan bodies, which are the intracellular forms of a pleomorphic gram-negative coccobacillus.

In 1942 Anderson isolated in the yolk sac of chick embryos an encapsulated gram-negative coccobacillus, using material from a patient with typical lesions of granuloma inguinale. This bacterium, originally named *Donovania granulomatis*, is now termed *Calymmatobacterium granulomatis*. Recent research has shown that this organism can be cultured in human peripheral blood mononuclear cells and HEp-2 cells. All reported isolates have been found nonpathogenic to animals and will not grow on solid media. The organism shares antigens with *Klebsiella*, and granuloma inguinale shows a close similarity to rhinoscleroma, the lesions of which contain intracellular organisms of *Klebsiella rhinoscleromatis* in a pattern reminiscent of granuloma inguinale. *C. granulomatis* shows a clear predilection for skin but is capable, in exceptional cases, of infecting deeper tissues, notably bone, liver, spleen, lung, upper genital tract of women, and epididymis.

EPIDEMIOLOGY

Distribution and Incidence. Granuloma inguinale is patchily distributed throughout the tropics. There are major endemic foci in Papua New Guinea, India, and Central and South America. It is notably absent in much of Africa with the exception of parts of South Africa (Natal, Swaziland, Eastern Transvaal). Small foci have been reported in Zambia, Zimbabwe, Vietnam, and among Australian aborigines. Large numbers of cases were formerly seen in the southeastern United States. The infection is much more frequently observed in black and dark-skinned peoples, but it is not known whether this can be attributed to genetic or environmental factors. Major epidemics of granuloma inguinale have occurred among tribes in New Guinea practicing ritual homosexual and heterosexual promiscuity. During these epidemics, the last of which occurred in the early 1950s, surveys indicated infection in up to 30% of adults in some villages.

Transmission. Granuloma inguinale has been observed most frequently among impoverished sectors of society in both urban and rural settings. An association with prostitution has often been noted, since transmission is primarily sexual. Most lesions occur in the anogenital area. A history of risky sexual exposure can usually be obtained from patients, and other sexually transmitted infections, especially syphilis, are often found concomitantly with granuloma inguinale. Small outbreaks have been traced back to a sexual exposure from a common source, and the major outbreaks in New Guinea were clearly associated with sexual promiscuity. Regular sexual partners of infected persons show evidence of infection in up to 50% of cases. Anal lesions have been linked specifically to receptive anal intercourse. Occasional instances of nonsexual transmission have been documented, and congenital transmission occurs in exceptional cases. Goldberg has proposed that *C. granulomatis* resides in the large bowel and is an opportunistic invader of the anogenital region, but evidence for this is based on a single reported isolation of the organism from stool. Infectivity of *C. granulomatis* is low, or individual susceptibility is highly variable. Individuals exposed over protracted periods by regular sexual contact have remained uninfected, and it is not known whether an asymptomatic carrier state exists.

CLINICAL MANIFESTATIONS. The incubation period reported by Clark in 1947 was between 3 and 40 days in 92% of 60 patients. The initial lesion was usually a soft, elevated nodule that soon ulcerated. The most common sites were the distal penis in men, and the vulva, especially the fourchette, in women. The clinical course of the ulcer was indolent both in causing little pain and in its progression. The advanced state of infection observed in so many patients is not due simply to the relatively painless nature of the lesions; it is also related to the stigmatization of patients with sexually transmitted diseases and the setting of poverty where the disease is most endemic. The ulcer may have a depressed base and flat edges, but usually the margins show some degree of hypertrophy; the base of the ulcer may be filled with hypertrophic granulomatous tissue that projects above the level of the surrounding skin. The color of the lesions is usually a striking, glistening, deep red (traditionally compared to raw beef). Occasionally pale, dry, warty lesions are observed. Ulcers have a tendency to extend in a linear fashion along skin folds, toward the anus and along the inguinal creases (Fig. 51–1).

Inguinal Lesions. Inguinal lesions (Fig. 51–2) are noted in about 10% of patients. Some believe that the infection does

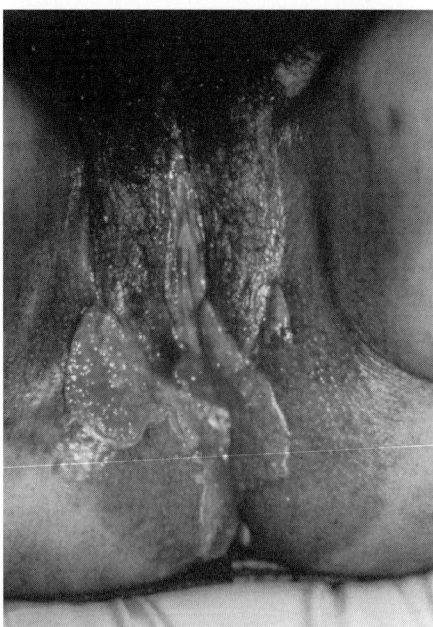

Figure 51–1. Granuloma inguinale: typical lesions in a female patient. (From Richens J: Donovanosis. *In* Oxford Textbook of Medicine, 3rd ed. Oxford, UK, Oxford University Press, 1996, p. 776. By permission of Oxford University Press.)

not involve the inguinal lymph nodes and that the inguinal lesions represent an ulcerating subcutaneous infection. However, spread of granuloma inguinale via the lymphatics to local nodes has been well documented. On reaching the nodes the infection has a strong tendency to move out into overlying subcutaneous tissue—hence the term *pseudobubo* to

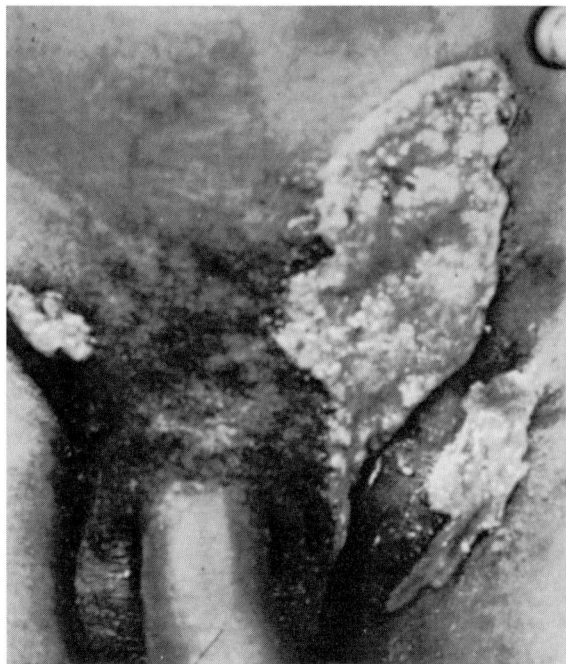

Figure 51–2. Granuloma inguinale. The subcutaneous granulomatous tissue has eroded through the skin in both inguinal areas. The surface of the granulation tissue glistens and is remarkably free of pus and necrotic debris.

describe a lesion centered on subcutaneous tissue rather than the node itself. This term has often been applied indiscriminately to any kind of inguinal lesion of granuloma inguinale. It was originally applied by Greenblatt and others specifically to a small number of patients who present with unruptured, fluctuant lesions in the groin and who, if left untreated, soon go on to develop the more familiar open, ulcerating lesions in the groin (see Fig. 51–2).

Vaginal Lesions. In women, lesions may occur in the vagina, where well-defined tufted lesions projecting from the vaginal wall may be observed. Cervical lesions may be indistinguishable clinically from carcinoma or tuberculous infection of the cervix. Involvement of the uterus, fallopian tubes, and ovaries can cause a firm pelvic mass, simulating pelvic malignancy, and in some cases cause obstruction of the ureters. Pregnancy is a strong stimulus to growth of genital lesions.

Extragenital Lesions. Donovanosis may occur extragenitally through primary inoculation or autoinoculation. Intraoral lesions are reasonably common, and infection may spread to the cervical nodes and ulcerate through the overlying skin, in a similar way to inguinal lesions. Lesions of the anus occur commonly in women through direct spread, whereas in men they are more likely to occur through primary inoculation. Infection of the rectum and colon is exceptionally unusual.

Disfiguring and mutilating complications occur in long standing cases. These include genital destruction (including autoamputation of the penis), secondary infection with fusospirochaetal organisms causing massive tissue destruction and fistula formation (especially in women), development of lymphedema of the genitalia, and the development of squamous carcinoma in chronic infections or in the scars of former lesions. Some patients develop a cicatrizing variant of the disease with extensive tracts of scar tissue. This is infrequent in Melanesians and more common in Indian patients. Hematogenous dissemination of infection is particularly associated with untreated lesions of the cervix in pregnant women. Tearing of the diseased cervix during vaginal delivery increases the likelihood of infection being disseminated through the blood to bone, liver, spleen, or lung. Death from granuloma inguinale is uncommon in comparison with the preantibiotic era. Congenital transmission has been well documented in an infected infant who presented some months following delivery with lesions of ears, umbilicus, and a long bone of one arm.

Natural History of Infection. Information about the natural history of granuloma inguinale is scanty. Spontaneous resolution of lesions has rarely been reported but may occur more frequently. Lesions healing spontaneously only to relapse during pregnancy have also been described. Extreme cases of infections persisting for 20 to 30 years or more have been recorded.

DIAGNOSIS

Microscopic Diagnosis. The diagnosis of granuloma inguinale is best made by demonstration of Donovan bodies in material taken from individuals with clinical features of granuloma inguinale (Fig. 51–3). This material can be prepared on a microscopic slide for rapid diagnosis or removed by biopsy for fixing and staining. Slides may be prepared by scraping the base or edge of an ulcer and smearing material onto the slide or, better still, by pinching off a small fragment of tissue and crushing this between two glass slides. Donovan bodies are easily seen with Giemsa, Wright's, or Leishman stains. For histologic specimens, Giemsa or silver stains are recommended, as Donovan bodies are difficult to recognize on hematoxylin and eosin–stained specimens. They are identified on the basis of their intracellular location within

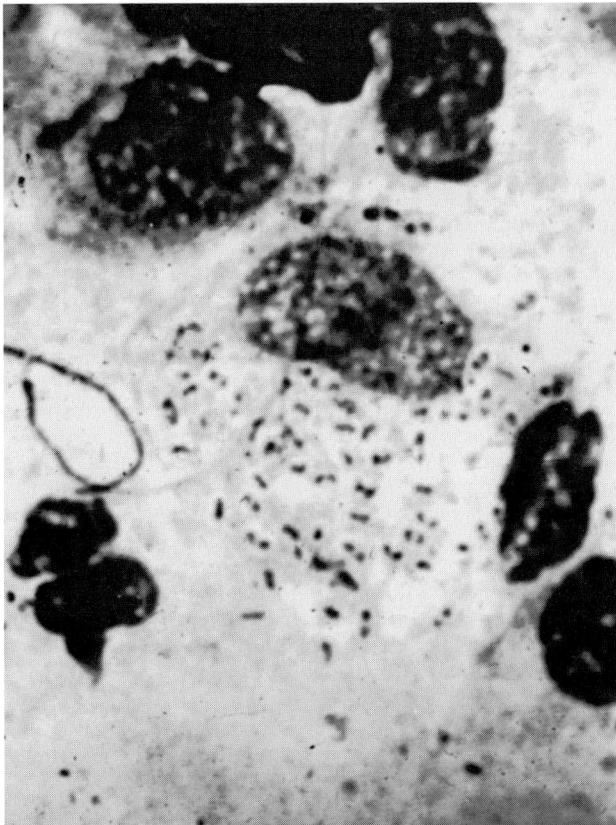

Figure 51–3. Granuloma inguinale. Donovan bodies in monocyte (Giemsa stain, × 2200). (Courtesy of the Armed Forces Institute of Pathology, Photograph Neg. No. TDS 106.)

monocytes and histiocytes; bipolar densities, giving a "closed safety pin" appearance; and the presence of a capsule (see Fig. 51–2). The number of organisms in lesions varies considerably. They are less prevalent in chronic lesions. In endemic areas, histologic or cytologic confirmation of the diagnosis is often achieved in only 60% of cases. Histologic features of the infection also include epithelial hyperplasia, sometimes pronounced enough to suggest squamous cell carcinoma, and a dense dermal infiltrate of plasma cells. The use of hematoxylin and eosin alone to stain biopsies of penile lesions has led on occasion to the misdiagnosis of granuloma inguinale as penile carcinoma, followed by inappropriate penile amputation.

Differential Diagnosis. In practice, the conditions most likely to be confused with granuloma inguinale are syphilis, chancroid, lymphogranuloma venereum, genital warts, cutaneous amebiasis, and carcinoma. The following would be appropriate for diagnosing a suspected case:(1) microscopy of unstained material for the presence of spirochetes and trophozoites of *Entamoeba histolytica;* (2) examination of Giemsa-stained smear or crush for Donovan bodies; (3) cultures for *H. ducreyi* and *C. trachomatis;* (4) serologic tests for syphilis, amebiasis, and lymphogranuloma venereum; and (5) biopsy for demonstration of carcinoma, warts, or Donovan bodies. It is important to notes that co-infection with syphilis occurs frequently in patients with granuloma inguinale and that nonpathogenic spirochetes are often found in the more extensive genital lesions of granuloma inguinale.

TREATMENT AND PREVENTION

Therapy. Many antibiotics have given good clinical results in the treatment of granuloma inguinale. No randomized comparisons of therapy have been reported, however. The choice of therapy should be guided by the safety and tolerability of available drugs and local experience of effectiveness. The most widely used antibiotics in recent years have been tetracycline, doxycycline, and co-trimoxazole (trimethoprim/sulfamethoxazole). Chloramphenicol, traditionally used for this infection in Papua New Guinea, gives excellent results. Aminoglycosides such as streptomycin and gentamicin are effective but seldom used. Ampicillin is of dubious value. Good results in the treatment of pregnant women have been reported with combined erythromycin and lincomycin; the use of combination therapies should probably be explored further for treatment of resistant or complicated cases. Good results have recently been reported with norfloxacin and, in South America, with thiamphenicol. All antibiotics are given in standard dosage and continued until lesions have healed and often a little longer. Relapse of chronic cases frequently occurs. Recent work from Australia suggests that azithromycin (500 mg daily or 1 g weekly) and ceftriaxone (1 g daily) are valuable in the management of patients who have failed on alternative treatments or who are poorly compliant.

Penicillin or soaking in potassium permanganate solution can help to relieve the discomfort and unpleasant smell in patients presenting with chronic extensive lesions. Plastic surgery may be required to deal with genital elephantiasis or strictures secondary to scarring disease.

Case Detection. Patients should be encouraged to refer sexual partners for examination. Treatment is usually reserved for partners with demonstrable lesions, but a 1-week course of doxycyline would be reasonable to offer to exposed contacts. The approach to epidemic donovanosis in Guinea was to use regular field surveys of affected populations to detect and treat cases until the epidemic was brought under control.

Bibliography

Bassa AG, Hoosen AA, Moodley J, Bramdev A: Granuloma inguinale (donovanosis) in women. An analysis of 61 cases from Durban, South Africa. Sex Transm Dis 20:164, 1993.
Bowden FJ, Mein J, Plunkett C, Bastian I: Pilot study of azithromycin in the treatment of genital donovanosis. Genitorurin Med 72:17, 1996.
Kharsany AB, Hoosen AA, Kiepiela P, et al: Culture of *Calymmatobacterium granulomatis*. Clin Infect Dis 22:391, 1996.
Latif AS, Mason PR, Paraiwa E: The treatment of donovanosis (granuloma inguinale). Sex Transm Dis 15:27, 1988.
Merianos A, Gilles M, Chuah J: Ceftriaxone in the treatment of chronic donovanosis in central Australia. Genitourin Med 70:84, 1994.
Parkash S, Radhakrishna K: Problematic ulcerative lesions in sexually transmitted diseases: Surgical management. Sex Transm Dis 13:127, 1986.
Ramanan C, Sarma PSA, Ghorpade A, Das M: Treatment of donovanosis with norfloxacin. Int J Dermatol 29:298, 1990.
Richens J: The diagnosis and treatment of donovanosis (granuloma inguinale). Genitourin Med 67:441, 1991.
Sehgal VN, Sharma HK: Donovanosis. J Dermatol 19:932, 1992.

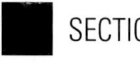

SECTION E Infections Causing Neurologic Manifestations

52 *Acute Bacterial Meningitis*

Brian M. Greenwood

DEFINITION. Acute bacterial meningitis is the condition that results from invasion of the meninges by bacteria that induce an acute inflammatory response. This acute inflammatory reaction, which involves the arachnoid and the pia mater, is characterized by a polymorphonuclear neutrophil leukocyte exudate.

ETIOLOGY. A large number of bacteria can cause acute bacterial meningitis (Table 52–1). However, studies carried out in many industrialized and developing countries have shown that three species of bacteria—*Haemophilus influenzae*, *Streptococcus pneumoniae*, and *Neisseria meningitidis*—nearly always head the list, although occupying different positions in the ranking in different epidemiologic situations. Figure 52–1 shows the typical pattern of meningitis in a tropical African hospital outside the African meningococcal meningitis belt. Nearly all cases of meningitis caused by *H. influenzae* are due to bacteria belonging to capsular serotype b (Hib). In contrast, many of the more than 80 different capsular serotypes of pneumococcus can cause meningitis. Meningococcal meningitis (Chapter 74) is usually caused by bacteria belonging to one of three capsular serogroups—A, B, or C. Bacteria other than these three are a cause of acute bacterial

meningitis most frequently in subjects with impaired immunity, e.g., the very young, or in those with malnutrition or other immunosuppressive diseases.

INCIDENCE AND DISTRIBUTION. Hospital surveys undertaken in several developing countries have shown that meningitis accounts for about 1% of all admissions. Few population data are available on the incidence of acute bacterial meningitis in tropical developing countries. Figures from Dakar, Senegal, suggest that the risk of a Senegalese child's being affected with acute bacterial meningitis before the age of 5 years is at least 1:500. This risk is probably higher in areas where outbreaks of meningococcal infection frequently

TABLE 52–1. Organisms Identified Most Frequently as a Cause of Bacterial Meningitis

Acute Meningitis	Chronic Meningitis
Streptococcus pneumoniae	*Mycobacterium tuberculosis*
Haemophilus influenzae	*Treponema pallidum*
Neisseria meningitidis	*Borrelia burgdorferi*
Escherichia coli	
Other gram-negative bacilli	
Listeria monocytogenes	
Salmonella species	
Leptospira species	
Staphylococcus aureus	
Group B streptococci	

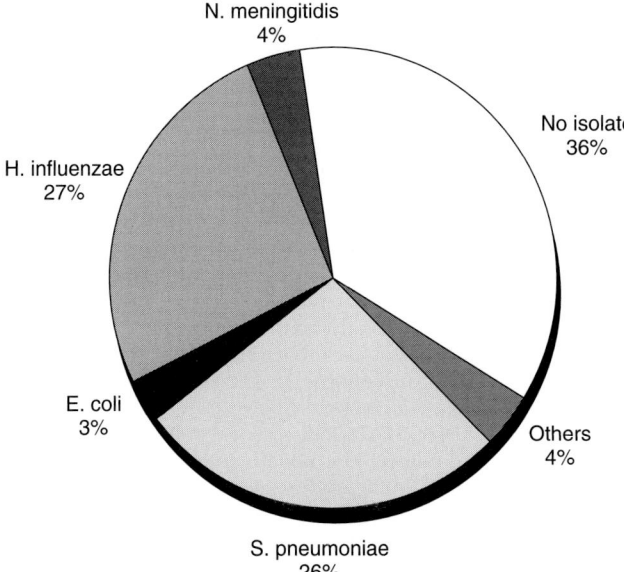

Figure 52-1. The causes of meningitis among children admitted to the pediatric wards of the Royal Victoria Hospital, Banjul, The Gambia, over a 4-year period. (Annual Reports of the Paediatric Department, the Royal Victoria Hospital.)

occur. Studies of deaths of children in a rural area of The Gambia suggest that as many as 1 in 200 die of acute bacterial meningitis before reaching age 5.

Infection with the pneumococcus or with *H. influenzae* occurs throughout both the wet and the dry tropics. Meningococcal infection is most prevalent in the northern savanna region of tropical Africa, where major outbreaks of this infection often occur (Chapter 74).

EPIDEMIOLOGY. The pneumococcus, the meningococcus, and *H. influenzae* are usually spread from person to person by respiratory droplets. Animal reservoirs of these infections are not known. Each of these three organisms can colonize the nasopharynx to produce an asymptomatic carrier. Asymptomatic carriers greatly outnumber cases of clinical disease and are the main source of infection. In many developing countries, most infants are colonized with the pneumococcus and with *H. influenzae* in the first few months of life.

Predisposing Factors. A number of factors predisposing to acute bacterial meningitis have been identified, but it is uncertain what determines whether an individual infected with a pneumococcus, a meningococcus, or *H. influenzae* becomes an asymptomatic carrier or a patient with clinical disease. The presence or absence of circulating antibody at the time of infection is one important factor. It is possible that damage to the local defenses of the nasopharynx by a virus (e.g., influenza virus) or by adverse climatic conditions predisposes to systemic infection. Patients with a primary or an acquired defect in humoral immunity show increased susceptibility to pneumococcal and meningococcal infection. An anatomic defect resulting from trauma or surgery that allows nasopharyngeal bacteria to gain access to the inside of the skull also predisposes to these infections. Sickle cell disease is an important factor predisposing to pneumococcal meningitis in areas of the tropics where this condition is prevalent. The incidence of pneumococcal infection is at least ten times higher in people with the hemoglobin genotype SS than in those with a normal genotype. HIV infection is another important predisposing cause of invasive pneumococcal disease, even during the early phase of infection before

the development of AIDS. Malnutrition predisposes to infection of the meninges with organisms of low virulence, such as nontyphoidal salmonellae, which rarely cause meningitis in healthy persons.

Age Distribution. Age has an important influence on susceptibility to different forms of acute bacterial meningitis (Fig. 52–2). Acute bacterial meningitis in neonates is most frequently caused by gram-negative bacilli such as *Escherichia coli* or, more rarely, by group B streptococci or pneumococci. The pneumococcus and *H. influenzae* are the main causes of meningitis in children younger than 1 year; meningitis due to *H. influenzae* is rare in subjects older than 5. In some tropical countries, meningitis attributable to *H. influenzae* occurs at an even earlier age than in Europe or the United States, with a peak incidence at about 6 months. The meningococcus is the most frequent cause of meningitis in older children, whereas the pneumococcus is the main cause of meningitis in the elderly.

Transmission. Pneumococcal, meningococcal, and *H. influenzae* infections are endemic in most communities. Small outbreaks of pneumococcal or *H. influenzae* infection may occur among subjects living in crowded conditions, but epidemics of these infections are rare. In contrast, large epidemics of meningococcal disease occasionally occur in communities in which the infection is usually endemic.

Person-to-person spread of infection often can be observed during the course of outbreaks of meningococcal disease. *H. influenzae* also can spread within households in a manner similar to that of the meningococcus. In contrast, secondary spread of pneumococcal disease within households is rare.

PATHOLOGY AND PATHOGENESIS

Pathology. The brain of a patient who has died of acute bacterial meningitis usually is covered with a thick exudate that extends inward along the perivascular spaces. An extradural effusion and medullary coning may be found. When the brain is cross sectioned, dilatation of the ventricles may be noted. On microscopy, the meninges show the characteristic features of an acute inflammatory response—a fibrinous exudate, hyperemia, and infiltration with polymorphonuclear neutrophilic leukocytes. Gram staining may show the causative organism within leukocytes or lying free in a fibrinous

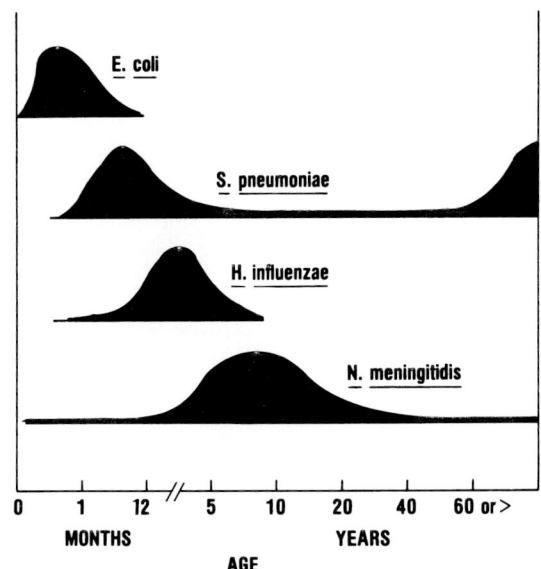

Figure 52–2. The age distribution of four important types of acute bacterial meningitis in a tropical African country where meningococcal meningitis is prevalent at a later age than in developed countries.

exudate. The lining of the ventricles may show acute inflammatory changes similar to those in the meninges. Inflammatory cells are sometimes seen in the brain substance of a patient who has died of meningococcal meningitis, indicating an associated encephalitis. Microscopy may show inflammatory changes in cerebral arteries and veins, especially if the patient has died of pneumococcal meningitis.

Post-mortem examination of the rest of the body may show foci of infection at other sites. Thus, otitis media or pneumonia may be found in a patient who has died of pneumococcal meningitis, and bone or joint lesions are sometimes found in a young child who has died of a systemic *H. influenzae* infection. Some of the pathologic features of acute meningococcemia (Chapter 74) may be present in cases of meningococcal meningitis.

Pathogenesis. The pathogenesis of many of the clinical features of acute bacterial meningitis is incompletely understood. It is probable that most cases of pneumococcal, meningococcal, and *H. influenzae* meningitis follow spread of infection from the nasopharynx into the systemic circulation, with subsequent seeding of bacteria to the meninges. Some pneumococcal meningeal infections, however, probably follow invasion of the blood stream by bacteria present in a consolidated area of lung.

Once bacteria reach the meninges, they initiate an acute inflammatory response. In the case of meningococcal and Hib infections, release of endotoxin may stimulate the production of mediators of inflammatory reactions such as tumor necrosis factor, interleukin-1, and interleukin-6. In the case of the pneumococcus, which does not possess an endotoxin, inflammatory changes are induced by cell wall components including peptidoglycans. Both endotoxin and some pneumococcal capsular polysaccharides can activate complement to produce chemotactic breakdown products such as C5a, which may attract more leukocytes to the inflamed meninges.

Acute bacterial meningitis may be accompanied by marked changes in cerebral metabolism. Transfer of glucose across the blood–brain barrier is defective, and a shift toward anaerobic carbohydrate metabolism occurs in the brain.

IMMUNITY. Epidemiologic and laboratory studies suggest that protection against pneumococcal, meningococcal, and *H. influenzae* infection is mediated mainly by antibody. The possible protective role of cell-mediated immunity in these infections has undergone little investigation. The formation of antibody to the capsular polysaccharide antigens of the meningococcus, the pneumococcus, and *H. influenzae* can be stimulated by asymptomatic nasopharyngeal carriage as well as by clinical infection. Antibody to the capsular polysaccharides of these three organisms can also be formed as a result of infection with harmless bacteria that share antigens with them. Thus, asymptomatic infection with *Neisseria lactamica*, a frequent commensal of the nasopharynx of young children, can induce the formation of antibodies that are bactericidal for virulent strains of meningococci.

As a result of one or another of these immunizing mechanisms, most adults possess bactericidal antibodies to meningococci, *H. influenzae,* and some serogroups of pneumococci. Prospective studies of American military recruits have clearly shown that adults who lack bactericidal antibodies to the meningococcus are susceptible to subsequent clinical infection with this organism.

CLINICAL MANIFESTATIONS

Symptoms and Signs. The usual presenting symptoms of acute bacterial meningitis are headache, backache, fever, and general malaise. Other common symptoms are photophobia and vomiting. Convulsions may occur, especially in young children. The onset of acute bacterial meningitis is usually sudden, and provided that transport is available, most patients reach the hospital within 2 or 3 days of the start of their illness. Several studies have shown that patients with a long history of this illness have a good prognosis, presumably because they have mild disease.

On initial examination, most patients with acute bacterial meningitis are febrile and have signs of acute meningeal inflammation. The neck is stiff, and Kernig's sign is positive (Fig. 52–3). Consciousness may be impaired to a degree that ranges from mild confusion to deep coma. Bradycardia and, in young infants, bulging of the anterior fontanelle may be present, indicating raised intracranial pressure, but papilledema is rare. A sixth cranial nerve palsy is the most frequently encountered localized neurologic sign. Third, seventh, and eighth cranial nerve palsies are encountered less frequently. Neurologic abnormalities may be detected in the limbs but are unusual.

General examination may show signs outside the central nervous system. Many patients with meningococcal meningitis have petechiae. In dark-skinned subjects, these are seen best in the conjunctiva (Fig. 74–3) or on the soft palate. A patient with meningococcal meningitis often has signs of myocardial damage, e.g., a third heart sound or an arrhythmia. Patients with pneumococcal meningitis may have signs

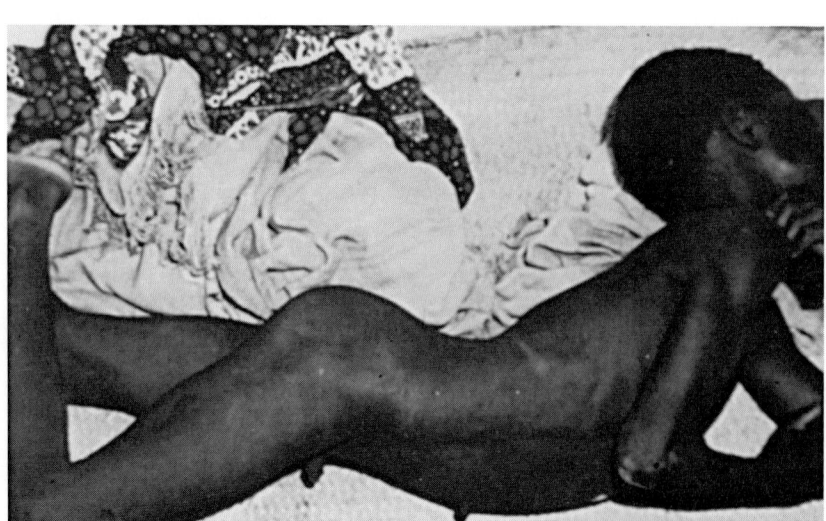

Figure 52–3. Acute bacterial meningitis in a 10-year-old Nigerian boy who had severe neck retraction.

of the sinusitis, otitis media, or pneumonia from which their infection derived. Focal neurologic signs are common in patients with meningitis caused by *Listeria*. Widespread dissemination of bacteria through the circulation may have produced pyogenic lesions at sites other than the meninges.

Blood Tests. A patient with acute bacterial meningitis usually has a polymorphonuclear neutrophilic leukocytosis. Thrombocytopenia may be noted, especially in patients with associated septicemia. Blood culture is positive in about two thirds of patients with *H. influenzae* meningitis, but a positive culture is obtained in a lower proportion of patients with pneumococcal or meningococcal meningitis.

Cerebrospinal Fluid. The cerebrospinal fluid (CSF) of patients with acute bacterial meningitis is usually turbid and under pressure. On laboratory examination, a high white blood cell count, mainly polymorphonuclear neutrophilic leukocytes, a high protein level, and a low glucose level are found. The CSF glucose content is usually lower than that of a blood sample collected at the time that lumbar puncture was performed. Examination of a spun deposit of CSF may show the causative organism directly, and culture is usually positive. Bacterial polysaccharide capsular antigens are frequently present.

Complications. Local complications of acute bacterial meningitis include the formation of an extradural effusion or empyema and thrombosis of cerebral vessels; both of these complications may result in deterioration of a patient's neurologic state. Raised intracranial pressure occasionally causes medullary coning. Widespread dissemination of the causative bacterium may produce pyogenic lesions at distant sites such as the joints and eyes.

About 10% of patients with meningococcal meningitis have arthritis, cutaneous vasculitis, episcleritis, or pericarditis. These late complications probably have an allergic cause.

Herpes simplex infection is a common complication of acute bacterial meningitis in adults or older children. Herpetic lesions usually appear around the mouth 2 or 3 days after a patient's admission to the hospital. The virus occasionally spreads extensively to involve the eyes or limbs. Activation of herpes infection in patients with acute pyogenic meningitis is probably a consequence of the generalized impairment of cellular immunity that is associated with this transient condition.

DIAGNOSIS

Clinical. A clinical diagnosis of acute bacterial meningitis can usually be made in adults and older children on the basis of their characteristic symptoms and signs. The characteristic clinical features of acute meningitis may be absent, however, in the very young and the old. Thus, meningitis must be considered as a possible diagnosis in any infant with febrile convulsions or who stops feeding and in any elderly patient who suddenly becomes confused. A malnourished child with meningitis may be afebrile. Meningism associated with an upper respiratory tract or other infection may suggest a clinical diagnosis of meningitis; if there is any doubt, lumbar puncture must be performed. A cerebral abscess usually causes more marked localized neurologic signs and less marked signs of meningeal irritation than acute meningitis. Differentiation of acute bacterial meningitis from cerebral malaria (Chapter 92) can be difficult, because consciousness may be impaired in both conditions and children with cerebral malaria may have neck retraction. The detection of malaria parasitemia does not confirm a diagnosis of cerebral malaria or rule out a diagnosis of meningitis. Lumbar puncture may be required to differentiate the two.

Acute bacterial meningitis usually can be differentiated clinically from tuberculous meningitis (Chapter 77) on the basis of a history of a sudden, short-lasting illness, but often it is not possible to differentiate acute bacterial meningitis from acute viral meningitis on clinical grounds alone. Cryptococcal infection (Chapter 83.5), common in patients with AIDS, may present as an acute meningitis but usually presents with a more chronic onset. Careful clinical examination may provide a clue to the cause of acute bacterial meningitis. The detection of petechiae suggests a diagnosis of meningococcal meningitis because petechiae are found only rarely in patients with other forms of bacterial meningitis, whereas the presence of otitis media or pneumonia favors a diagnosis of pneumococcal disease.

General examination may show features of a factor predisposing to acute bacterial meningitis such as sickle cell disease (Chapter 6). A firm diagnosis of acute bacterial meningitis can be established only by lumbar puncture, which should be performed whenever this diagnosis is seriously considered unless there is a firm contraindication such as papilledema or other signs of raised intracranial pressure. Opinion in developed countries is divided about whether it is necessary to perform lumbar puncture in all children with febrile convulsions. In developing countries, where meningitis is common, it is probably wise to do so unless an obvious alternative cause of their convulsions can be found.

Laboratory. A turbid CSF gives immediate confirmation of a clinical diagnosis of meningitis. A clear sample, however, does not preclude this diagnosis, because at least 200 cells/mm^3 must be present before CSF appears turbid to the naked eye. Thus, a CSF cell count must be made before a diagnosis of meningitis can be confidently excluded. Examination of a Gram-stained deposit allows the characteristics of the leukocytes present in the CSF to be determined. Polymorphonuclear neutrophilic leukocytes predominance occurs in patients with acute bacterial meningitis, whereas most white blood cells present in the CSF of patients with viral meningitis are lymphocytes. CSF obtained from patients with tuberculous meningitis usually contains cells of both types (Chapter 77). Caution is needed in interpreting CSF cell findings in patients who have acute meningitis and have received antibiotic treatment before lumbar puncture was performed, because CSF of partially treated patients with acute bacterial meningitis may contain both polymorphonuclear neutrophils and lymphocytes. A low ratio of CSF glucose to blood glucose is frequently found in patients with acute bacterial meningitis and tuberculous meningitis but not in patients with acute viral meningitis. Elevation of CSF levels of lactic acid and/or lactic acid dehydrogenase favors a diagnosis of acute bacterial meningitis as opposed to a diagnosis of acute viral meningitis. A raised serum level of C-reactive protein also favors a diagnosis of bacterial as opposed to viral meningitis, but this test has low specificity.

In laboratories with limited facilities, a dipstick developed for urinalysis can be used to detect changes in CSF cell count, protein, and glucose.

The cause of acute bacterial meningitis usually can be identified by Gram stain and by culture of a spun deposit of CSF, and the antibiotic sensitivities of the cultured organism can be determined. Staining with acridine orange rather than Gram stain increases the sensitivity of bacterial detection by microscopy. Difficulties may be experienced with both of these routine bacteriologic techniques. Gram stains may be misinterpreted, especially when performed by inexperienced staff in a clinical sideroom, and culture is frequently negative in patients who have already received an antibiotic. Diagnostic tests that depend on the detection of bacterial products in CSF rather than on the detection of live bacteria are especially useful in partially treated patients. Latex tests for the detection of polysaccharide antigens (Fig. 52–4), which require a minimum of equipment, are well suited for use in tropical

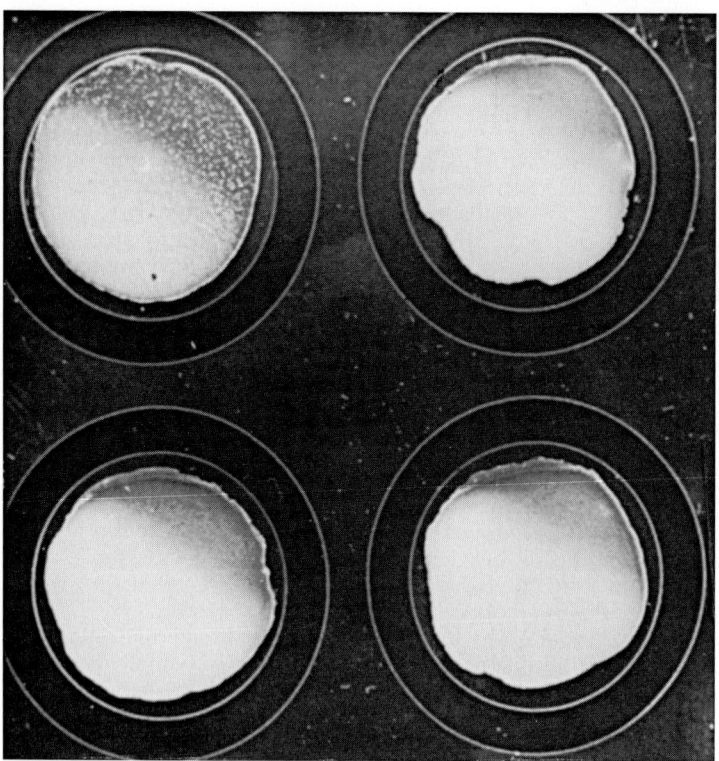

Figure 52–4. A latex test for the detection of bacterial antigens in CSF. A drop of CSF is mixed with latex particles coated with antibody to the meningococcus, pneumococcus, or *H. influenzae* type b. In this instance, agglutination *(top left corner)* has been produced by an antiserum to group A meningococcal capsular polysaccharide antigen.

developing countries and offer a means of establishing a bacterial cause of acute meningitis in small hospitals that lack a routine diagnostic bacteriology service. Their sensitivity is comparable to that of culture.

Bacterial DNA can be detected in the CSF of most patients with acute bacterial meningitis using polymerase chain reaction (PCR). This approach to diagnosis may prove to be especially useful in patients who have previously received antibiotics and have a sterile CSF, but appropriate assays for clinical use are still being developed.

TREATMENT

General Measures. Whenever possible, a patient with acute bacterial meningitis should be treated in a hospital. Unconscious patients should be nursed in a position that maintains their airway and should be turned regularly to prevent bedsores. In hot countries, patients with acute meningitis often are severely dehydrated by the time they reach the hospital because they are febrile and have stopped drinking. Thus, administration of intravenous or nasogastric fluids may be required. Headache may be severe, making a patient restless and difficult to nurse. Headache may be relieved by aspirin; some patients require stronger analgesics. Paraldehyde or diazepam may be needed to control convulsions.

Corticosteroids. Early trials suggested that corticosteroids were of no value in the management of acute bacterial meningitis, and until recently, they were little used for the treatment of this condition. However, experimental studies that have demonstrated the importance of cytokine and other inflammatory cascades in the pathogenesis of acute bacterial meningitis have led to a renewed interest in the potential role of this group of drugs in the management of this condition. Several studies have shown that the incidence of neurologic complications is reduced among children with Hib meningitis treated with dexamethasone, but most of these studies have involved only small numbers of patients and several have had flaws in study design. Thus, these findings are still not universally accepted. Studies undertaken in Egypt,

Mozambique, and Brazil have shown reductions in mortality among patients with acute bacterial meningitis treated with dexamethasone. Side effects associated with the use of dexamethasone for the treatment of meningitis have included an increased incidence of gastrointestinal bleeding. On balance, the evidence now available favors the administration of dexamethsone to patients with acute bacterial meningitis, if this can be afforded, but it is disputed whether it should be given to all patients or just to the most severely affected. Dexamethasone is given in a dose of 0.6 mg/kg for 2 to 4 days. It is not known for certain how dexamethasone exerts a protective effect. Reducing intracranial swelling may be one mechanism, and it has been suggested that glycerol given by mouth may be a cheaper and easier way of achieving this effect. However, a beneficial effect of treatment with glycerol has not been definitively established.

Antibiotics. Because the antibiotic treatment recommended for each of the main forms of acute bacterial meningitis is different, it is important that every effort be made to determine the cause of each case of bacterial meningitis and to prescribe treatment accordingly (Table 52–2). In developing countries, the choice of antibiotic used for the treatment of acute bacterial meningitis must frequently be influenced by cost and availability as well as by bacteriologic considerations.

Meningococcal Meningitis. Penicillin is still the preferred treatment for patients with meningococcal meningitis (Chapter 74). Chloramphenicol is an effective alternative for patients who cannot be given penicillin.

Hib Meningitis. Hib meningitis usually responds well to treatment with cephalosporins, and if available, a third-generation cephalosporin such as ceftriaxone is now the usual first choice of treatment for children with this condition. In many developing countries, however, only less expensive antibiotics such as chloramphenicol and ampicillin are available. Isolates of *H. influenzae* resistant to ampicillin and/or to chloramphenicol have been identified in many countries.

The prevalence of ampicillin resistance varies substantially from area to area, but few data are available on the prevalence of ampicillin resistance in the tropics. If it is known that the prevalence of ampicillin resistance in a community is low, this antibiotic can be chosen as the first line of treatment for Hib meningitis. If resistance is known to be prevalent and bacteriologic facilities are available, a reasonable approach is to start treatment with ampicillin and chloramphenicol until results of sensitivity tests become available and then to adjust treatment accordingly. No evidence shows that the drugs used together are any more effective than either used individually, provided that the bacterium is sensitive to the drug chosen, and some experimental evidence demonstrates that combination of these two drugs may actually reduce their efficacy.

Pneumococcal Meningitis. Until recently, penicillin could be recommended confidently as the first-line treatment for pneumococcal meningitis, with chloramphenicol as the second choice for patients unable to take penicillin. Unfortunately, this is no longer the case, because of a marked increase in the prevalence of penicillin resistance among pneumococci in the past few years. The distribution of penicillin resistance in industrialized countries is patchy, the level of resistance varying substantially from state to state within the United States and from country to country within Europe. Penicillin-resistant pneumococci are known to be prevalent in parts of South Africa and Pakistan, but there is no accurate information on their prevalence for many parts of the tropics. If the prevalence of penicillin resistance among pneumococci in a community is known to be low, then it is appropriate to start treatment of a patient with pneumococcal meningitis with high doses of penicillin given parenterally until the results of sensitivity testing become available or until it is apparent that the patient is not responding favorably. Most patients infected with a pneumococcus of intermediate resistance respond satisfactorily to high-dose penicillin treatment. If pneumococci with a high level of resistance are known to be prevalent in a community, a third-generation cephalosporin, such as ceftriaxone, is the recommended first line of treatment. However, treatment with ceftriaxone is at least five to ten times more expensive than treatment with parenteral penicillin. Unfortunately, some pneumococci are now resistant to cephalosporins as well as to many other antibiotics. Treatment of patients with meningitis caused by such bacteria that are resistant to many drugs is difficult, and treatment guidelines have not been clearly established. One recommendation is treatment with vancomycin and ceftriaxone. Unfortunately, vancomycin penetrates poorly into the CSF, espe-

cially if steroids are being given concurrently. Other regimens, such as treatment with imipenem, are being explored.

Culture-Negative Meningitis. In developing countries, physicians are frequently forced to make a choice of antibiotic treatment for a patient with acute bacterial meningitis without the benefit of an etiologic diagnosis because no bacteriologic facilities are available or because the patient has received prior antibiotics. In such circumstances, physicians have to make a guess about the likely cause based on the patient's age and clinical features and on their knowledge of the local epidemiology of acute bacterial meningitis. In such circumstances, it is important to choose an antibiotic with a wide spectrum of activity, and a third-generation cephalosporin is usually the first choice. If this is not available, chloramphenicol is probably the best alternative.

Assessment of the Response to Treatment. The temperature, level of consciousness, and neurologic state of a patient who is receiving treatment for acute bacterial meningitis should be carefully monitored. Failure of the patient to improve within 48 hours of the start of antibiotic therapy suggests that a localized collection of pus has formed or that an inappropriate antibiotic has been given. A patient who shows deterioration in neurologic state during the course of treatment should be investigated for the presence of a space-occupying lesion by any of the available appropriate diagnostic means. If it is impossible to perform such investigations and if there are strong clinical grounds for suspecting an extradural collection of fluid or pus, exploratory bur holes should be made. Unfortunately, fluid collections are not always found in such patients; a late deterioration in neurologic state may be caused by a vascular occlusion.

A secondary rise in temperature during the course of treatment should suggest the possibility of an extradural abscess, a collection of pus at another site to which the causative organism has seeded, a drug reaction, or, in a patient with meningococcal meningitis, the development of allergic complications.

Some physicians recommend that CSF changes be monitored regularly throughout the course of treatment. It is uncertain, however, whether repeated examinations of CSF add much to the information that can be obtained by regular and careful clinical examination. Nevertheless, a second lumbar puncture should be performed on any patient who fails to improve after 48 hours of antibiotic treatment, in case the initial bacteriologic diagnosis was incorrect or a resistant organism is present.

PROGNOSIS. The most important factor that determines

TABLE 52–2. Antibiotic Therapy Recommended for Initial Treatment of Patients With Acute Bacterial Meningitis*

Type of Meningitis	Antibiotic	Route	Dose		Duration (days)
			Adults	*Children*	
Meningococcal	Crystalline penicillin	IV or IM	2 megaunits q 6 hr	1 megaunit q 6 hr	5
Pneumococcal	Crystalline penicillin	IV or IM	4 megaunits q 6 hr	1–2 megaunits q 6 hr	10–14
	or				
	Ceftriaxone	IV	5 g daily	100 mg/kg daily	10–14
Haemophilus influenzae	Ceftriaxone	IV	—	100 mg/kg daily	7
	or				
	chloramphenicol	IV or IM then PO	—	25 mg/kg q 6 hr†	7
Undiagnosed	Ceftriaxone	IV	5 g daily	100 mg/kg daily	10–14
	or				
	chloramphenicol	IV or IM then PO	500 mg q 6 hr	25 mg/kg q 6 hr†	10–14

*Physicians should be prepared to change antibiotic treatment if a patient does not respond clinically or if a sensitivity test indicates that a change of treatment is needed.

†Neonates should not receive more than 50 mg/kg/day of chloramphenicol.

the course and prognosis of acute bacterial meningitis is the cause. Most patients with meningococcal meningitis treated promptly with an appropriate antibiotic make a rapid and uneventful recovery. Hospital-based surveys in developing countries have shown that the overall mortality rate of treated patients is usually in the range of 5 to 10%, a mortality rate little different from that in advanced centers. About 10% of patients with meningococcal meningitis develop allergic complications (Chapter 74). Some patients who recover from meningococcal meningitis are left with a degree of deafness, but other residual neurologic defects are unusual.

In contrast to the favorable prognosis for patients with meningococcal meningitis, the outlook for patients with pneumococcal meningitis is poor. Surveys performed in various parts of the tropics have shown that the overall mortality rate for this infection is about 50%, even when treated appropriately, and that about half of the survivors are left with a serious neurologic defect. Severe impairment of consciousness, a short history, and associated pneumonia all are poor prognostic signs. A few patients with pneumococcal meningitis have turbid CSF containing bacteria but few white blood cells; such patients rarely recover. Why the prognosis for patients with pneumococcal meningitis is so much worse than that for patients with meningococcal meningitis is not understood.

The outlook for patients with *H. influenzae* meningitis is worse in developing than in industrialized countries and lies between that of patients with pneumococcal or meningococcal meningitis; about 25% of patients die, and residual sequelae are common.

PREVENTION AND CONTROL. The use of chemoprophylaxis and vaccine to control meningococcal disease is covered in Chapter 74.

Chemoprophylaxis. Chemoprophylaxis has been used less widely in preventing pneumococcal and *H. influenzae* infections than in preventing meningococcal disease. Strong evidence, however, shows that penicillin gives some protection against pneumococcal infection in patients with sickle cell disease, and these patients should be given regular prophylaxis with penicillin until at least age 5 years.

Vaccination

Hib Meningitis. Dramatic progress in preventing Hib meningitis by vaccination has been recently made. Large-scale trials of Hib conjugate vaccines, made by linking the capsular polysaccharide of Hib to a protein carrier, have shown that Hib conjugate vaccines are remarkably effective at preventing Hib meningitis, even in the very young, and the vaccines have been rapidly introduced into the routine immunization programs of many industrialized countries. The results have been dramatic; Hib disease has virtually disappeared from several industrialized countries, even when only moderate levels of vaccine coverage have been achieved. This suggests that Hib conjugate vaccines can induce a herd effect, protecting those who have not been immunized, probably by reducing nasopharyngeal carriage. Until recently, it was not certain whether Hib conjugate vaccines would prove to be as effective in preventing Hib disease in developing countries as has been the case in the industrialized world, because the pressure of infection is likely to be higher in the more crowded conditions of much of the developing world. Fortunately, results of recent trials undertaken in The Gambia (Table 52–3) and Chile have shown that Hib conjugate vaccines are just as effective at preventing Hib meningitis in these communities as in industrialized societies and that they also prevent Hib pneumonia, a numerically more important condition than Hib meningitis in many developing communities. A strong case can now be made for including an Hib conjugate vaccine, preferably given as a combined vaccine

TABLE 52–3. The Effect of a *Haemophilus influenzae* Type b Conjugate Vaccine on the Incidence of *H. influenzae* Meningitis and Pneumonia in Young Gambian Children. Three Doses of a PRP/Tetanus Conjugate Vaccine Were Given at the Ages of 2, 3, and 4 Months as Part of a Routine EPI Schedule.

H. influenzae Type b Diseases	Vaccinated*	Controls
Meningitis	1	16
Pneumonia	0	10
Combined	1	26

From Mulholland K, et al: Randomised trial of *Haemophilus influenzae* type b tetanus protein conjugate for prevention of pneumonia and meningitis in Gambian infants. Lancet 349:1191, 1997.
*Received two or three doses.

with diphtheria-pertussis-tetanus, into the routine immunization programs of developing countries, but the cost is making this difficult to accomplish.

Pneumococcal Meningitis. Progress is also being made in the development of pneumococcal vaccines. For many years, the pneumococcal polysaccharide vaccines that have been available in industrialized countries have not been widely used among the target groups for which they have been recommended, which include the elderly and those with conditions predisposing to pneumococcal infection such as patients with heart failure, chronic lung disease, or liver disease. However, public health authorities in many industrialized countries are now making greater efforts to ensure that these risk groups are protected.

The demonstration that HIV-infected persons have a greatly increased risk of invasive pneumococcal disease, even early in the course of their infection, indicates another important at-risk group who need protection. Individuals with HIV infection should be immunized as soon as possible after diagnosis, because they respond best before their CD4 count declines. A controlled trial of pneumococcal polysaccharide vaccination in HIV-infected subjects is in progress in Uganda. In contrast to the situation in industrialized countries, the main impact of invasive pneumococcal disease in developing countries is in young children, who do not respond well to immunization with polysaccharide vaccines. Good progress is now being made in the development of pneumococcal polysaccharide/protein conjugate vaccines, however, and trials in both industrialized and developing countries have shown that these vaccines are immunogenic in young children. Experience with Hib conjugate vaccines suggests that these vaccines will be able to prevent pneumonia as well as meningitis. Large-scale efficacy trials in both industrialized countries and in Africa are now in progress. Unfortunately, the need to provide protection against several serotypes, probably about ten, means that pneumococcal conjugate vaccines will be costly and perhaps too expensive for many developing countries to afford, except for high-risk individuals, e.g., children with sickle cell disease. Some progress is being made with the development of pneumococcal protein vaccines that have a potential to provide protection against the many different capsular polysacharride serotypes that can cause invasive disease, and this approach to the prevention of pneumococcal disease might be less costly.

Bibliography

Fortnum HM: Hearing impairment after bacterial meningitis: A review. Arch Dis Child 67:1128, 1992.

Greenwood BM: The epidemiology of acute bacterial meningitis in tropical Africa. *In* Williams JD, Burnie J (eds): Bacterial Meningitis. London, Academic Press, 1987, p 61.

Moosa AA, Quortum HA, Ibrahim MD: Rapid diagnosis of bacterial meningitis with reagent strips. Lancet 345:1290, 1995.

Pecoul B, Varaine F, Keita M, et al: Long-acting chloramphenicol versus intravenous ampicillin for treatment of bacterial meningitis. Lancet 338:862, 1991.

Prasad K, Haines T: Dexamethasone treatment for acute bacterial meningitis: How strong is the evidence for routine use? J Neurol Neurosurg Psychiatry 59:31, 1995.

Quagliarello V, Scheld WM: Bacterial meningitis: Pathogenesis, pathophysiology, and progress. N Engl J Med 327:864, 1992.

Tunkel AR, Scheld WM: Acute bacterial meningitis. Lancet 346:1675, 1995.

53 *Tetanus*

Tarik Al Azraqùi, Robert C. Bollinger, Jr., and Brian J. Ward

DEFINITION. Tetanus is a potentially fatal disease caused by the action of tetanospasmin, a potent neurotoxin produced by the vegetative form of *Clostridium tetani*. This organism is an anaerobic, spore-forming, gram-positive bacillus. The spores have a characteristic drumstick appearance, are highly resistant to heat and disinfectants, and can survive for years in contaminated soil.

HISTORY. *C. tetani* has been a significant cause of human disease throughout recorded history. The classic symptoms of tonic muscle spasm disproportionately involving the head and neck (lockjaw) and trunk were recognized by Egyptian, Chinese, and Greek physicians. These ancient scholars also knew of the link between contaminated injuries and the subsequent development of fatal spasms. Many centuries passed before the toxin-producing anaerobic organisms were cultured from soil by Nicolaier in 1884. The first recorded attempt at active immunization with tetanus toxoid occurred as early as 1890, with material very similar to that in current use. It is sobering to acknowledge that tetanus is still a significant problem in many parts of the world more than a century later.

EPIDEMIOLOGY. The spores of *C. tetani* are ubiquitous and contaminate 2 to 23% of soil samples throughout the world. Soil contamination is greatest in areas with long histories of human activity, particularly agriculture.

Tetanus remains a major health problem in the economically deprived countries of the world, reflecting low immunization rates and poor hygiene. Mortality rates as high as 28:100,000 have been recorded in some regions of the developing world. The 1995 World Health Organization estimates for global incidence (1 million cases) and mortality (500,000 deaths) are therefore likely to be conservative. Neonatal tetanus is endemic in more than 90 countries in the developing world and accounts for more than 50% of tetanus-related deaths. The case-fatality rate approaches 90% in neonates, and as much as 25% of total neonatal mortality can be attributed to tetanus in many developing countries. Well-meaning but misguided perinatal interventions such as smearing dung or ghee (clarified butter) on the umbilical stump and circumcision wound without aseptic technique can be devastating for the children of unvaccinated mothers, in whom there is an inverse relationship between tetanus antibody titers and socioeconomic status.

The incidence of tetanus has declined precipitously in countries that have achieved a sustained antitetanus vaccination effort. For example, after more than 40 years of universal tetanus immunization in the United States, the incidence of tetanus has decreased to only 40 to 60 cases per year. Almost all of these cases occur in individuals who are either unvaccinated or incompletely vaccinated and/or who are inappropriately treated after a tetanus-prone injury. A health and nutritional survey demonstrated that 70 to 75% of elderly Americans have antitetanus antibodies less than 0.15 IU/mL. Therefore, it is not surprising that more than half of the cases in the United States occur in individuals older than 65 years.

PATHOGENESIS. Pathogenic strains of *C. tetani* produce toxins: tetanospasmin and tetanolysin. Tetanospasmin is a potent neurotoxin and appears wholly responsible for the pathogenic potential of this organism. The contribution of tetanolysin to the pathogenesis of tetanus is unknown.

Tetanospasmin is a 151-kD protein encoded on a plasmid present in all toxigenic strains of *C. tetani*. This heat-labile toxin is cleaved extracellularly by a bacterial protease into a 100-kD heavy chain that mediates binding to cell surfaces and transport proteins and a 50-kD light chain that mediates inhibition of neurotransmitter release. The two chains are connected by a disulfide bridge. Tetanospasmin is released when vegetative forms undergo autolysis. Under optimal conditions, the concentration of tetanospasmin can reach 10% of the total protoplasmic protein immediately before autolysis. Once released, tetanospasmin is taken up by peripheral terminals of lower motor neurons and is transported to the central nervous system (CNS) intra-axonally in membrane-bound vesicles at a rate of 75 to 250 mm/day. Once toxin enters the CNS, it acts presynaptically on afferent motor neurons to interfere with release of inhibitory neurotransmitters such as glycine and γ-aminobutyric acid. The absence of inhibition results in unrestrained neuronal firing with sustained muscle contraction. These effects stem from the selective cleavage of synatobrevin, a constitutively expressed small-vesicle protein with zinc-dependent metalloproteinase activity. Excitatory and autonomic systems can also be affected by tetanospasmin, but the toxin acts preferentially on inhibitory neurons.

CLINICAL MANIFESTATIONS. The clinical syndrome of tetanus requires the introduction of spores of toxigenic *C. tetani* at the site of injury, local tissue conditions that promote production of the toxin-producing vegetative form, and immunologic naïveté. Local factors that promote toxin elaboration at the site of injury include low oxygen tension (i.e., necrotic tissue), suppuration, and the presence of foreign bodies.

Approximately 30% of individuals with tetanus have either no obvious wound or have wounds that they consider to be trivial. The time between inoculation of spores and the first appearance of symptoms varies from 3 days to 3 weeks or longer. This incubation period depends on a number of factors including the site of the injury and its distance from the CNS and the nature of the wound (i.e., toxigenic conditions). As a general rule, the shorter the incubation period, the worse the prognosis. The clinical forms of tetanus are neonatal, generalized, cephalic, and localized.

NEONATAL TETANUS. This is largely restricted to economically deprived countries. Most cases (> 85%) arise as a result of unattended or "traditional" deliveries in unhygienic surroundings. The incubation period typically ranges from 2 to 10 days, and the initial symptoms are nonspecific. These include irritability, refusal to feed, and weak sucking, which progress quickly to more tetanus-specific symptoms such as spasticity, facial grimacing, and trismus. Most children (> 70%) rapidly develop complications such as sepsis or bronchopneumonia. Factors suggesting a poor prognosis include age younger than 10 days, rapid progression of symptoms, fever, and the presence of risus sardonicus (a bitter or sardonic smile). The consequences of neonatal tetanus are dire, with 80 to 90% mortality and significant developmental delay in most of the survivors.

GENERALIZED TETANUS. This is the most commonly recognized form of tetanus worldwide. Muscles served by nerves with the shortest neural pathways are usually the first to be affected, including facial, cervical, and masticatory muscles (trismus). As a result, the initial symptoms typically include localized or generalized weakness and difficulty swallowing or chewing. Patients are generally lucid throughout the illness and often suffer intense pain. The spasms may occur spontaneously but are frequently precipitated by aural, visual, or tactile stimuli. Involvement of the autonomic nervous system can lead to arrhythmias, extreme oscillations in blood pressure, diaphoresis, hyperthermia or hypothermia, and urinary retention. Only 60% of patients with uncomplicated generalized tetanus present with a temperature greater than 38°C. Rarely, generalized tetanus may be mistaken for an acute abdomen. Common complications include fractures from sustained muscle contractions, aspiration, pulmonary emboli, bacterial superinfections, dehydration, respiratory failure, and cardiac arrest. Long-term complications in survivors include irritability, sleep disturbances, myoclonus, seizures, decreased libido, orthostatsis, electroencephalographic abnormalities, and the consequences (e.g., osteoarthritis) of bone damage. Even with modern intensive care, mortality approaches 20% in these patients.

CEPHALIC TETANUS. This rare form of tetanus is most commonly associated with head injury or *C. tetani* infection of the middle ear. Trismus is a prominent feature, as is dysfunction of many cranial nerves, leading to difficulties with feeding, swallowing, and oral hygiene. The commonest initial presentation of cephalic tetanus is a seventh nerve palsy in a child with chronic otitis media or a recent head injury. More than two thirds of those with cephalic tetanus progress to the more generalized form. More than half of these patients have early, life-threatening bronchopneumonia, and the overall mortality rate is 20 to 30%.

LOCALIZED TETANUS. Most cases of localized tetanus progress to more generalized disease in a matter of days to weeks. Truly local disease is the rarest form of tetanus and may reflect partial immunity to tetanospasmin. These patients typically present with rigidity of muscles in the vicinity of a wound on an extremity. Weakness and loss of tone are frequently present in the most affected muscles (presumably as a result of local action of tetanospasmin at the neuromuscular junction). These symptoms usually resolve spontaneously but may occasionally persist for months.

DIAGNOSIS AND DIFFERENTIAL DIAGNOSIS. The diagnosis of tetanus is made by clinical observation. When the history includes an unattended delivery in the developing world or a grossly contaminated wound and the disease is advanced, the diagnosis is straightforward. However, in the absence of an obvious wound or earlier in the course of the illness, clinicians must maintain a high index of suspicion. Strychnine poisoning antagonizes the release of the neurotransmitter glycine and is the only condition that truly mimics tetanus. Other conditions that may be confused with tetanus include dystonic reactions to neuroleptic drugs, trismus caused by an oral abscess, mumps, meningitis, trichinosis, stiff-man syndrome, brain stem stroke, hypocalcemia, epilepsy, narcotic and alcohol withdrawal, and hysterical reactions. The spatula test (reflex spasm of the masseters when the posterior pharynx is touched) is thought to have high sensitivity (94%) and specificity (100%) in diagnosing tetanus. Absence of high fever and clear sensorium are other clinical clues that support a diagnosis of tetanus.

Antitetanus antibodies are not detectable in most patients with clinical disease, and tetanus can rarely occur in individuals with antibody titers greater than 0.01 IU/mL, the putative protective concentration. Cultures are usually not helpful because *C. tetani* can be isolated from wounds of only 30% of patients with clinical disease. Furthermore, few laboratories can test for the presence of the toxin-producing plasmid.

TREATMENT. Clinical management of tetanus usually requires intensive care if this is available. Treatment of tetanus has three major goals:

1. *Neutralization of circulating toxin and prevention of further elaboration.* Human tetanus immune globulin (HTIG: 500 units IM) can theoretically neutralize toxin that has not yet entered neurons. Prompt administration of HTIG can shorten the duration of symptoms and may also reduce the severity of the illness. Larger doses of HTIG do not appear to confer additional benefit. The use of intrathecal administration of HTIG is not effective in neonates but remains controversial in adults. Local infiltration of the wound has been recommended but is of unknown efficacy. Surgical debridement of devitalized tissues and removal of foreign bodies is critical to prevent the further elaboration and absorption of toxin. Metronidazole is the preferred antibiotic (2 g/day PO or parenterally), but alternative agents include erythromycin, tetracycline, and chloramphenicol.

2. *Symptomatic and supportive treatment of neurologic and autonomic disease.* Excellent nursing care and a wide range of supportive therapies may be necessary to save patients with established tetanus. Supportive therapies include avoidance of noxious stimuli, administration of benzodiazepines (diazepam or midazolam), neuromuscular blockade, tracheostomy and mechanical ventilation, administration of β blockers (labetalol), antiarrhythmics, and potent analgesics (morphine) to control the pain of spasms. Hypotension frequently requires intensive fluid therapy and inotropics. Other medications include anticoagulants, H_2 blockers or proton pump inhibitors to prevent stress ulceration, and antiseizure medications.

3. *Active immunization to provide long-term protection.* The development of effective immunity cannot be assumed even after a life-threatening episode of tetanus. Long-term protection against reinfection in these individuals is ensured by administration of a primary series of three monthly tetanus toxoid immunizations after recovery from the acute illness.

PROPHYLAXIS. Tetanus is a vaccine-preventable infection. Although the precise schedules and formulations vary from one country to another, a primary series of tetanus injections (minimum of three doses of absorbed toxoid at 1 to 2-month intervals) provides almost 100% protection for at least 5 years. Children younger than 7 years typically receive tetanus immunization in combination with other antigens (i.e., diphtheria, pertussis, *Haemophilus influenzae*, inactivated polio, hepatitis B) without compromise to immunogenicity. Individuals older than 7 years generally receive tetanus toxoid in combination with a lower dose of diphtheria toxoid. Data suggest that vitamin A deficiency may significantly impair tetanus antibody production and that calcium phosphate–containing preparations may be slightly more immunogenic than aluminum phosphate–based vaccines at a cost of slightly higher reactogenicity. There are no contraindications to tetanus immunization other than prior serious allergic response to the vaccine components. Extreme prematurity (< 29 weeks' gestation) is not an indication for delay in the tetanus immunization schedule; these infants respond well to routine vaccination at 2, 4, and 6 months of age.

The durability of vaccine-induced immunity against tetanus is not precisely known. Most children in developed countries receive four to five doses of a tetanus toxoid–containing vaccine before 10 years of age. This probably represents overvaccination for tetanus but is widely believed to be innocuous. In contrast, repeated (unnecessary) tetanus boosters in older individuals can result in marked reactogenicity. Boosting with a tetanus toxoid–containing vaccine is currently recommended every 10 years after completion of a primary series. However, data accumulating in the industrialized world suggest that a single midlife (55 to 65 years of age) booster may be adequate to provide lifelong immunity after a complete primary series in childhood. The relevance of these data to populations in economically deprived regions is uncertain.

Active immunization of tetanus-naïve women during pregnancy can significantly reduce the incidence of neonatal tetanus. If possible, at least two doses of tetanus toxoid should be delivered 4 to 6 weeks apart, such that the second dose is administered 4 weeks before delivery. Tetanus immunization during pregnancy is not associated with spontaneous abortion, stillbirth, or any known congenital malformation. Care should be taken to ensure that the primary series of tetanus immunization is completed in naïve mothers during pregnancy or after birth and that the child is not erroneously excluded from the routine infant vaccination schedule.

Immunocompromised patients may or may not respond to tetanus immunization with the production of protective levels of antitetanus antibodies ($\geq$ 0.01 IU/mL). HIV-positive patients typically retain good levels of antitetanus antibodies if a primary series is completed before the development of AIDS. A repeat primary series with tetanus toxoid should be considered for all long-term survivors of bone marrow transplantation.

Some injuries are particularly prone to contamination with *C. tetani* spores and the development of clinical tetanus. These include puncture wounds (e.g., from nonsterile injections), agricultural accidents, open fractures, burns, frostbite, crush injuries, and wounds contaminated with dirt, saliva, or feces. Inadequately immunized individuals who suffer these types of injuries should receive HTIG in addition to initiation of a primary series or administration of a booster. Although the simultaneous administration of HTIG and tetanus vaccine may reduce the final antibody titer achieved, the difference is not likely to be clinically significant.

Bibliography

Bennett J, Azhar N, Rahim F, et al: Further observations on ghee as a risk factor for neonatal tetanus. Int J Epidemiol 24:643, 1995.

Crone NE, Reder AT: Severe tetanus in immunized patients with high antitetanus titers. Neurology 42:761, 1992.

Dal-Ré R, Angel G, Gonzaloez A, Lasheras L: Does tetanus immune globulin interfere with the immune response to simultaneous administration of tetanus-diphtheria vaccine? A comparative clinical trial in adults. J Clin Pharmacol 35:420, 1995.

D'Angio CT, Maniscalco WM, Pichichero ME: Immunologic response of extremely premature infants to tetanus, *Haemophilus influenzae*, and polio immunizations. Pediatrics 96:18, 1995.

de Morales-Pinto MI, Oruamabo RS, Igbagiri FP, et al: Neonatal tetanus despite immunization and protective antitoxin antibody. J Infect Dis 171:1076, 1995.

Gergen PJ, McQuillan GM, Kiely M, et al: A population-based serologic survey of immunity to tetanus in the United States. N Engl J Med 332:761, 1995.

Montecucco C, Schiavo G: Structure and function of tetanus and botulinum neurotoxins. Q Rev Biophys 28:423, 1995.

Silveira CM, Caceres VM, Dultra MG, et al: Safety of tetanus toxoid in pregnant women: A hospital-based case-control study of congenital anomalies. Bull WHO 73:605, 1995.

Tetanus toxoid for adults—too much of a good thing. Lancet 318:1185, 1996.

54 Botulism

Robert C. Bollinger, Jr. and John G. Bartlett

DEFINITION. Botulism is a neuroparalytic illness of varying severity caused by neurotoxins produced by *Clostridium botulinum* and, rarely, other clostridia.

ETIOLOGY AND PATHOGENESIS

History. Outbreaks of botulism have been known in Europe since antiquity. In fact, the term *botulism* is derived from the early association with ingestion of spoiled sausages. In 1895, Van Ermengem isolated an anaerobic, spore-forming bacillus from raw ham and the post-mortem tissues of persons who died during an outbreak of botulism. He postulated the presence of an extracellular toxin, subsequently shown to be type B toxin, after he was able to reproduce the disease in animals following ingestion of the food vehicle or administration of culture filtrates. In parallel with the increase in commercial and home canning following World War I, numerous outbreaks of botulism were reported. Later, the ecology of *C. botulinum* was described, as well as the conditions favoring toxin production and those allowing destruction of toxin and spores during food processing. Application of these guidelines caused a dramatic decline in cases of botulism but did not eliminate those related to commercially prepared products. Today, food-borne botulism is associated most commonly with home-canned or home-processed food.

Organism and Toxins. *C. botulinum* is a diverse group of gram-positive, spore-forming obligate anaerobes that are widely distributed in nature. Although four biotypes have been described, *C. botulinum* is classified solely on the basis of the production of eight antigenically distinct toxins (A, B, C1, C2, D, E, F, and G), each with a molecular size of 150,000 daltons. Production of toxins by types C1 and D depends on infection of *C. botulinum* by specific bacteriophages. Most human disease is caused by types A, B, and E and rarely F and G. Types C1, C2, and D produce disease in mammals and birds. Each strain of *C. botulinum* usually produces but one toxin.

Spores of *C. botulinum* are regularly ingested by humans. During vegetative growth and lysis, the organism elaborates a neurotoxin that is among the most potent substances known. Some toxins (e.g., type E) may be elaborated in a precursor form that requires enzymatic activation. Spores, particularly types A and B, are heat stable and resist boiling for hours, especially at high altitudes. However, the neurotoxins are heat labile, providing the basis for the terminal heating of home-canned preparations. The neurotoxins are acid stable and resistant to digestive enzymes and thus are able to survive the mammalian gastric acid barrier, but germination and elaboration of toxin are inhibited at a pH less than 4.5. Alkali readily destroys the toxins. Food containing toxins of types A and B may appear and taste normal or spoiled.

Once absorbed, the neurotoxin disseminates hematogenously to peripheral presynaptic terminals, binding irreversibly to block the release of the neurotransmitter acetylcholine. Intoxication may result from ingestion of preformed toxin present in contaminated food or from absorption of toxin after vegetation growth of *C. botulinum* in the gastrointestinal tract or in an infected wound. Thus, at least four categories of botulism are now recognized: food-borne botulism, wound botulism, infant botulism, and botulism of undetermined classification.

DISTRIBUTION AND EPIDEMIOLOGY. Spores of *C. botuli-*

num are widely distributed in soil and aquatic environments throughout the world. Food-borne botulism occurs worldwide but is generally restricted to northern or temperate climates. The true incidence in developing countries is unknown because botulism may be misdiagnosed or underreported. In the United States, food-borne botulism has a distinctive distribution: more than 80% of type A outbreaks have occurred west of the Mississippi River, 63% of type B outbreaks have occurred east of the Mississippi River, and more than half of type E outbreaks have occurred in more northern areas, including the Great Lakes and Alaska. The distribution of clinical disease approximately parallels the distribution of *C. botulinum* spores in the soil.

From 1976 through 1984, 124 outbreaks of botulism were identified in the United States involving 308 persons (or 2.7 persons per outbreak). Sixty-eight percent involved only one person; 20% involved two persons; and 12% involved more than two persons. Outbreaks were reported in 30 states, but most occurred in Alaska, Oregon, Washington, and California. *C. botulinum* types A, B, and E were identified in 60%, 30%, and 10% of outbreaks, respectively. Vegetables, usually home canned, were implicated in 70% of cases and meat or fish in 30%. Home-processed fish or meat from marine mammals was responsible for all type E outbreaks, more than 90% of which occurred in Alaska, where dried or uncooked food is favored by the native populations. Meat and meat products are most frequently implicated in Europe, whereas dried fish is responsible most frequently in Japan, Scandinavia, and Russia. Fermented beans are most commonly implicated in China.

Commercially canned foods accounted for 3% of outbreaks from 1970 to 1984, whereas only 4% were related to food served in restaurants. However, restaurant outbreaks accounted for 42% of all cases of botulism during this period. Newly identified vehicles of food-borne transmission were observed, including sauteed onions, potato salad, chopped garlic, beef stew, and meat loaf, among others.

Wound botulism, infant botulism, and botulism of undetermined source are usually caused by *C. botulinum* types A or B and occasionally type F.

CLINICAL MANIFESTATIONS. Botulism is a neurologic disorder that is classically manifested as a bilaterally symmetric descending paralysis or weakness with prominent bulbar and respiratory involvement without sensory deficits. Patients are typically afebrile and bradycardiac, in the setting of hypotension.

Food-Borne Botulism. Symptoms of botulism begin usually 12 to 48 hours (range 6 hours to 8 days) after the ingestion of food containing preformed neurotoxins of *C. botulinum*. Symptoms of weakness, fatigue, and dizziness occur early. Sixty to 75% of those with disease due to type A or type B toxin have gastrointestinal symptoms, including nausea, vomiting, constipation, and abdominal cramps. Cholinergic blockade leads initially to bulbar dysfunction, with diplopia, dry mouth, dysphagia, dysphonia, and dysarthria. Although neurologic symptoms may be delayed for up to 3 days after the onset of illness, descending motor weakness and paralysis of the extremities develop with variable speed and severity. Respiratory muscles are involved, and breathing becomes difficult.

On physical examination, patients are mentally alert and afebrile but may exhibit orthostasis. Ocular findings are prominent, with bilateral ptosis, fixed, dilated pupils, and cranial nerve palsies, especially weakness of the sixth cranial nerves, leading to paralysis of lateral gaze (Fig. 54–1). The gag reflex is diminished, and nystagmus is occasionally seen. Mucous membranes and the tongue are dry and fissured. Motor dysfunction may be mild or severe. Deep tendon

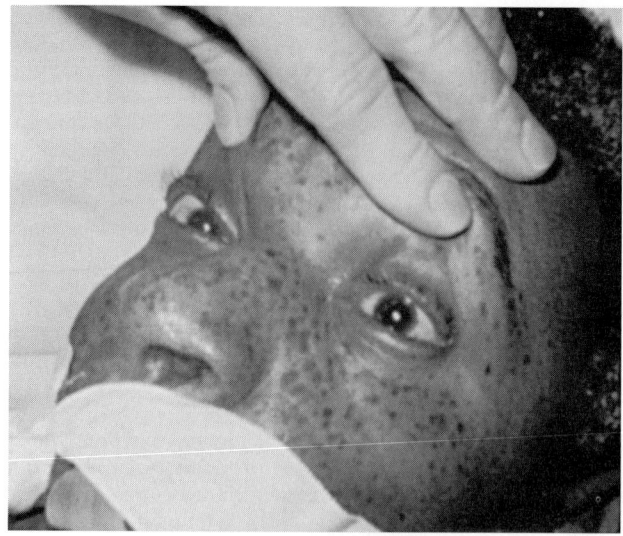

Figure 54–1. Bilateral palsies of the sixth cranial nerves and fixed, dilated pupils in an elderly woman on mechanical ventilation; the patient had lateral gaze paralysis bilaterally, although only left lateral gaze paralysis is shown.

reflexes are variably affected, but sensation usually remains intact. Pathologic reflexes are absent. Ileus and urinary retention may be present. Progression of respiratory muscle weakness may be mild and abortive or rapid and life threatening, requiring intubation and respiratory support. Recovery may be prolonged, and patients may be plagued with persistent fatigue, constipation, or a sicca syndrome.

Wound Botulism. This form of botulism is rare but probably underdiagnosed. Only 30 or 40 cases have been recorded since 1943, most occurring in the past 3 decades. Most patients have been young males who suffer a compound fracture or crush injury of an extremity with inoculation of *C. botulinum* spores. The incubation period ranges from 4 to 14 days (average, 10 days), gastrointestinal symptoms are infrequent, and single isolated cases are characteristic. Otherwise, the clinical syndrome is similar to that of food-borne botulism. A variant of wound botulism has been described in chronic intravenous drug abusers or is associated with sinusitis in intranasal cocaine use. Although the portal of entry is presumed to be sites of drug injection, 50% of these patients have no obvious wound infection.

Infant Botulism. This form of botulism was first recognized in 1976 as a cause of the floppy infant syndrome. Infants age 3 weeks to 11 months have been affected primarily. The disease has a unique pathogenesis: germination, in vivo multiplication, and elaboration of botulinal toxin in the gastrointestinal tracts of infants who have ingested spores of *C. botulinum* and rarely *C. butyricum* and *C. barati*. Approximately 50 to 200 cases are estimated to occur annually in the United States, making it now the most common form of botulism. Clinical disease varies considerably, from failure to thrive to sudden infant death syndrome. Constipation, a feeble cry, poor sucking, lethargy, and pooled oral secretions presage the onset of cranial nerve palsies, generalized flaccid paralysis, and apnea. The source of *C. botulinum* is unknown in most instances, but honey contaminated with *C. botulinum* spores has been incriminated as a vector in some cases. Rare cases associated with soil contamination have been reported.

Botulism, Classification Undetermined. Affected individuals are older than 12 months and develop botulism without an obvious source. It is likely that in some instances, in vivo elaboration of toxin by *C. botulinum* colonizing the gut occurs in a manner similar to that with infant botulism. A few of these individuals have received antibiotics before the onset of illness, suggesting that alterations in the normal gut flora may have allowed proliferation of *C. botulinum.*

DIAGNOSIS. The diagnosis of botulism should be suspected in any person who develops a neurologic illness characterized by a descending flaccid paralysis associated with gastrointestinal symptoms following ingestion of potentially contaminated food. Confirmation of the diagnosis depends on isolation of *C. botulinum* from stool, gastric contents, an antecedent wound, or incriminated food or on demonstration of botulinal toxin in the patient's serum, stool, gastric contents, or the incriminated food.

A sensitive enzyme-linked immunosorbent assay for type A toxin has been developed, but the most widely used method for assaying botulinal toxin is the mouse bioassay method. Identification of the toxin type and its quantitation may take up to 4 days and is usually performed in central or specialized laboratories. Stool cultures may be positive, and toxin can be excreted for 4 to 6 weeks after the disease onset. Presumptive clinical diagnosis is important for effective management but may be difficult. Lack of an obvious food vector, especially if not home prepared, the absence of other cases, and atypical features may make clinical diagnosis difficult. Paresthesias, asymmetric paralysis and ptosis, nystagmus, normal pupils, elevated cerebrospinal fluid protein levels, and a positive response to edrophonium chloride (Tensilon) testing have been reported in 8 to 25% of patients with botulism. However, the diagnosis should be strongly suspected in an alert, afebrile patient who develops bilateral sixth cranial nerve palsies, dilated and fixed pupils, a descending paralysis with respiratory weakness, orthostasis, and dry mucous membranes, supported by the findings of normal cerebrospinal fluid, typical changes on electromyography (an increase in the number of overall small-amplitude action potentials, facilitation of muscle-action potential after tetanic stimulation or following rapid-repetitive stimulation, and muscle fibrillation), and a negative response to edrophonium chloride testing. Differential diagnostic considerations include Guillain-Barré syndrome; myasthenia gravis; brain stem infarction; ingestion of anticholinergics (e.g., atropine or jimsonweed; tick paralysis; paralytic poliomyelitis; Eaton-Lambert syndrome; hypocalcemia; and paralytic shellfish poisoning.

TREATMENT AND PROGNOSIS

Supportive Therapy. Respiratory failure and superinfections are the principal causes of death in patients with botulism. Close monitoring of patients and early elective tracheal intubation or tracheostomy lowers the mortality rate for patients with diminishing vital capacities. Judicious use of antibiotics for nosocomial bacterial infections, nasogastric intubation and parenteral nutrition to relieve paralytic ileus, and bladder catheterization to relieve urinary retention are important to a successful outcome.

Toxin Neutralization. Efforts to remove neurotoxin from the gut and neutralize circulating toxin are indicated at any time during the course of illness, because toxin may persist in the gastrointestinal tract and serum for several weeks after onset. Cleansing enemas and cathartics given early may be beneficial in eliminating toxin from the body. The efficacy of equine trivalent botulinum antitoxin (containing antitoxins

A, B, and E) has been questioned in the past; however, retrospective studies show a lowered mortality rate and a shorter duration of illness for botulism due to types A and B when antitoxin is administered early in the disease. Two vials of antitoxin are administered immediately, one intravenously and one intramuscularly; if the disease is severe or if it progresses, two additional vials are given in 4 hours. Hypersensitivity to horse serum should be determined before administration of antitoxin, because 10 to 20% of patients have an adverse reaction. Although *C. botulinum* is susceptible to penicillin, the use of antibiotics to treat food-borne botulism is not recommended now. The efficacy of antibiotic therapy for patients with wound botulism is unclear. In an experimental animal model of wound botulism due to *C. botulinum* type A, antitoxin was superior to antibiotics in decreasing mortality rates; both improved survival over control animals. Aqueous penicillin G, 10 to 20 million units/day, is given intravenously. Infant botulism and food-borne disease in adults are usually not treated with antibiotics; in fact, there is some concern that such treatment would cause lysis of the organism with release of toxin.

Prognosis. In the United States, mortality rates for food-borne botulism, wound botulism, and infant botulism have been 7.5, 12.5, and 2.7%, respectively. In those with the diagnosis of botulism of undetermined classification, the mortality rate is 29%, perhaps reflecting a delay in diagnosis and the institution of appropriate therapy in the absence of an obvious source. Death is also more likely to occur in each of the following circumstances: age greater than 60 years, incubation period less than 36 hours, disease due to *C. botulinum* type A, delayed diagnosis, and single sporadic cases. Although mild cranial nerve dysfunction persists for a variable period during convalescence, the outlook for survivors is one of complete recovery.

PREVENTION. Although botulism is uncommon in the United States and mortality rates have declined in the past 30 years, the disease causes substantial mortality. Strict adherence to techniques of home canning can prevent food-borne botulism. Spores can be destroyed by heating food at 120°C for 30 minutes under pressure. Terminal heating at 80°C for 20 minutes or boiling for 1 minute inactivates the neurotoxin. Germination of *C. botulinum* can be prevented by refrigeration, freezing, drying, or the addition of salt or sodium nitrite. Wound botulism is best prevented by thorough surgical debridement of contaminated wounds and by avoiding chronic parenteral drug abuse. Some cases of infant botulism may be prevented by omitting honey from the diets of infants younger than 12 months.

Bibliography

Arnon SS: Infant botulism: Anticipating the second decade: J Infect Dis 154:201, 1986.

Dowell VR Jr: Botulism and tetanus: Selected epidemiologic and microbiologic aspects. Rev Infect Dis 6:S202, 1984.

Hughes JM, Blumenthal JR, Merson MH, et al: Clinical features of types A and B food-borne botulism. Ann Intern Med 95:442, 1981.

MacDonald KL, Cohen ML, Blake PA: The changing epidemiology of adult botulism in the United States. Am J Epidemiol 124:794, 1986.

MacDonald KL, Rutherford GW, Friedman SM, et al: Botulism and botulism-like illness in chronic drug abusers. Ann Intern Med 102:616, 1985.

Sakaguchi G: *Clostridium botulinum* toxins. Pharmacol Ther 19:165, 1983.

Tacket CO, Shandera WX, Mann JM, et al: Equine antitoxin use and other factors that predict outcome in type A foodborne botulism. Am J Med 76:794, 1984.

55 *Anthrax*

Arthur M. Friedlander, Jr. and Robert N. Longfield

DEFINITION. Anthrax is an acute bacterial zoonosis predominantly of herbivorous animals. It is caused by *Bacillus anthracis* and may be transmitted to humans by inoculation, inhalation, or ingestion.

In humans, the vast majority of cases involve the skin, and only very rarely are the respiratory and gastrointestinal (GI) tracts affected. Cutaneous anthrax is characterized by the development of a papule followed by a black eschar often surrounded by local edema. It may be complicated by septicemia and death in 5 to 20% of untreated cases. Inhalational anthrax is almost invariably fatal, and GI anthrax has a mortality of >50%. Cutaneous anthrax has been referred to as *malignant edema* or *pustule* and inhalational anthrax as *woolsorters'* or *ragpicker's disease*.

ETIOLOGY

Smear and Culture Characteristics. Anthrax bacilli are large (1.0 to 1.5 μm by 3 to 8 μm), nonmotile, gram-positive rods that possess a prominent capsule. Abundantly found in smears of blood and other tissues, bacilli occur singly or in short chains in host tissue. On sheep blood agar, 3- to 5-mm, gray-white, opaque, rough, nonhemolytic colonies become evident within 24 hours after infection and demonstrate the physical tenacity of beaten egg whites. The colonies have curled, irregular outgrowths giving a Medusa-head appearance. In the presence of carbon dioxide, the organism produces a capsule and the colony is round and mucoid. *B. anthracis* grows best aerobically but can grow under anaerobic conditions. It produces acid without gas from glucose and does not ferment lactose. Identification is confirmed by immunologic identification of the production of the protective antigen toxin component and the poly-D-glutamic acid capsule, susceptibility to specific bacteriophage, and virulence in mice and guinea pigs. Additional testing by polymerase chain reaction for the presence of the specific toxin and capsule genes is also available.

Spore Formation. *B. anthracis* develops central oval spores in culture or in soil. Spores do not develop in vivo unless the body or carcass has been opened to ambient air. Spores are somewhat resistant to heat and to many disinfectants. They are destroyed by boiling for 10 minutes, dry heat (140°C) for 3 hours, or autoclaving (121°C) for 15 minutes. Anthrax spores remain viable for years in dry soil. Cattle have become infected by grazing in fields where animals died of anthrax decades before. Sporulating cultures can represent a hazard to laboratory personnel.

EPIDEMIOLOGY

Incidence of Human Anthrax. Human infection with *B. anthracis* is infrequent and sporadic in the United States and most developed countries. Approximately 20,000 to 100,000 cases of human anthrax are estimated to occur annually throughout the world, although accurate figures are impossible to obtain. Careful descriptive studies of its occurrence in many developing countries are lacking; however, anthrax appears ubiquitous in rural agricultural nations that are economically dependent on animal husbandry. Epidemics of

human anthrax are rare. Large outbreaks of cutaneous anthrax occurred during wars in Zimbabwe in 1978 to 1980 and in Chad in 1988. The largest epidemic of inhalational anthrax occurred in 1979 in Sverdlovsk (Ekaterinburg), Russia, as a result of the accidental release of anthrax spores from a military research facility. The recent acknowledgment that Iraq produced anthrax spores for weapons use during the 1991 Gulf War raises the specter of the use of anthrax as a biologic weapon.

Zoonotic Anthrax. Anthrax is predominantly a disease of herbivores—cattle, sheep, horses, and goats. Animals are generally infected via the alimentary tract by grazing on contaminated pasture and rarely by direct contact with other infected animals. Before death, animals often contaminate the soil with infected saliva, blood, urine, or feces. Soil, forage, and to a lesser extent ground water are the major reservoirs of anthrax.

Geographic Occurrence. Neutral or alkaline soils in areas characterized by early spring rains and warm summers are particularly conducive to perpetuating anthrax spores. Historically, Louisiana, Arkansas, Mississippi, Texas, Oklahoma, Oregon, and California were regions of endemic anthrax; however, owing to intensive surveillance and control procedures, animal anthrax has been virtually eliminated in the United States, although outbreaks still occur. The disease remains endemic in some areas in Africa, India, Southeast Asia, the Middle East, Greece, Albania, southern Italy, Romania, France, countries of the former Soviet Union, and Central and South America. *B. anthracis* spores germinate in soil at 20°C to 44°C in areas with humidity of >85%. Germinated bacilli are thought to be destroyed then by other soil microbes. Therefore, in many tropical regions, animal anthrax occurs predominantly in the dry season, with some persistence into the early wet season. Although some replication may occur, it is likely that persistence in the soil results from amplification due to growth and sporulation in animal carcasses with subsequent contamination of the soil. Humans may be responsible for introducing anthrax into new areas by the importation of infected hides, hair, bristle, and bone, including bone meal fertilizer. In certain areas, vultures and nonbiting flies may be responsible for the geographic dissemination of anthrax.

Transmission. Generally, human anthrax is traced to agricultural, industrial, or, rarely, laboratory acquisition. There is no evidence of direct human-to-human transmission. Owing to occupational exposure, males are more often (3:1) infected than females, but anthrax has no predilection for age. In one outbreak of inhalational anthrax, children appeared to be at lower risk of infection.

Industrially Acquired Anthrax. In economically developed countries, e.g., the United States, it is estimated that industrial acquisition accounts for about 80% of cutaneous anthrax and almost all inhalational anthrax and occurs predominantly among tanners or leather workers and hair, wool, or bone meal fertilizer workers. Subclinical infection and seroconversion among workers in these industries may be more common than overt illness. Infections in developed countries are acquired often industrially from contaminated animal hides, hair, or bones imported from developing countries. Goat hair and wool from China, India, Pakistan, and Iran are more commonly contaminated with spores than are similar materials from Europe or Australia, reflecting the relative prevalence of zoonotic anthrax in these regions. Rough leather goods and bongo drums from Haiti and Morocco have been vehicles of anthrax transmission in the United States. In the past, facial lesions have been linked to natural-bristle shaving brushes and oral lesions to unsterilized toothbrushes.

Agriculturally Acquired Anthrax. In economically developed countries, direct contact with infected animals by farmers, butchers, and veterinarians is implicated in approximately 20% of cutaneous anthrax cases. Transmission by biting insects has been suspected but not conclusively demonstrated. Bone meal fertilizer has been implicated in sporadic cases of inhalational anthrax among home gardeners.

Anthrax Acquired in Developing Countries. In developing countries, human anthrax is usually acquired from sick animals or from fomites contaminated with their blood or body fluids. In the Gambia between 1970 and 1974, it was estimated that approximately 1.4% of the population of one area developed cutaneous anthrax, with most of the cases presenting in the dry season. Indirect human-to-human spread by the use of contaminated toilet articles or fomites was postulated also but not confirmed. GI anthrax was encountered rarely, perhaps because the people refrain from eating the meat of sick or dying animals. Serum antibodies were present in some people who denied prior cutaneous lesions, suggesting that asymptomatic infections may occur. During the 1978 to 1980 war in Zimbabwe, anthrax caused more than 10,000 human infections, essentially all cutaneous, with more than 100 deaths. Outbreaks of cutaneous and oropharyngeal anthrax have also been reported from Southeast Asia and of GI anthrax from Russia early in the 20th century.

PATHOLOGY

Cutaneous Anthrax. Lesions demonstrate acute inflammation with irregular epidermal ulceration and underlying coagulation necrosis. A fibrinopurulent covering or membrane that may be present, along with satellite bullous lesions, swarms with distinctive gram-positive bacilli; however, pus is not present unless superinfection occurs. The term *malignant pustule* is a misnomer. Beneath the epidermis, edema and exudate are prominent, especially for lesions of the head and neck. Massive hemorrhage into the dermis and subcutaneous fat may be evident, but voluntary muscle is involved rarely. Neural infiltration and degeneration may account for the characteristic hypalgesia of dermal anthrax. The blue-black eschar appears late and, rarely, may be inconspicuous.

Inhalational Anthrax. Woolsorters' disease is characterized by hemorrhagic edema and necrosis of mediastinal lymph nodes and connective tissue. No endobronchial ulcers or eschars are evident. Bronchi reveal hemorrhage, desquamation of cellular debris, and in rare instances bacilli. Focal hemorrhagic pneumonia has been reported in a minority of cases. Involved alveoli show a hemorrhagic exudate and only occasionally, in association with hemorrhage, bacilli. Polymorphonuclear leukocytes are usually absent. Alveolar capillaries contain widespread fibrin thrombi and bacilli. Hemorrhagic pleural effusions occur commonly. Hematogenous dissemination from the mediastinal nodes frequently ensues to the meninges, the spleen, the intestine, and other areas of the lungs. Anthrax bacilli may also rarely disseminate to the lungs from cutaneous lesions, producing focal hemorrhagic pneumonitis.

Gastrointestinal Anthrax. Hemorrhage, edema, and ulceration have been rarely reported in the stomach, cecum, and elsewhere in the intestinal tract. The intramural and regional lymphatics are extensively involved with hemorrhage and edema. Intestinal obstruction has been reported, and massive ascites, which can be hemorrhagic, may occur.

Central Nervous System Anthrax. Hemorrhagic meningitis is characteristic of central nervous system infection by *B. anthracis*. The leptomeninges reveal scant inflammatory cell reactions but widespread hemorrhages. The brain has hemorrhages and generalized cerebral edema. Subarachnoid hemorrhage may also occur.

PATHOGENESIS

Anthrax Virulence Factors. *B. anthracis* possesses three described virulence factors, a poly-D-glutamic acid capsule and two protein exotoxins. The polyanionic capsule, encoded on a 110-kb plasmid, is antiphagocytic and enables the vegetative bacillus to resist ingestion and killing by leukocytes. The anthrax toxins, encoded on a 60-kb plasmid, are composed of three proteins. These toxins are similar to other bacterial toxins in being composed of a eukaryotic cell receptor–binding protein and a second protein possessing the cytotoxic and usually enzymatic activity. In anthrax, the cell-binding protein, called *protective antigen*, is shared by both toxins. It combines with either edema factor, a calmodulin-dependent adenylate cyclase, to produce the edema toxin or, with lethal factor, to produce lethal toxin. The protective antigen is absolutely necessary for the binding and translocation of the cytotoxic proteins to their targets within the host cell cytosol. The edema toxin raises intracellular levels of cyclic adenosine monophosphate and has been shown to inhibit neutrophil function. It undoubtedly also contributes to the massive edema that may be seen clinically. In high concentrations, lethal toxin is lethal for experimental animals, and in some models macrophages appear to be the cellular target. Although the exact molecular mechanism of the lethal toxin is still unknown, in vitro it releases the cytokines interleukin-1 and tumor necrosis factor-α (TNF-α) from macrophages at low concentrations while being cytolytic specifically for these cells at higher concentrations. Thus, the toxins contribute to pathogenesis by interfering with host resistance mechanisms and possibly by causing uncontrolled release of toxic levels of cytokines.

Cutaneous Anthrax. Cutaneous anthrax follows the inoculation of spores, usually into a minor abrasion or scratch. Spores then germinate locally, multiply, and elaborate the antiphagocytic capsule and the two protein exotoxins that interfere with phagocytic cell functions, resulting in hemorrhagic necrosis. Hematogenous dissemination follows in 5 to 20% of untreated cases.

Inhalational Anthrax. Inhalational anthrax follows inhalation of spores 1 to 5 μm in diameter. Larger particles are cleared by the lungs' mucociliary mechanism and generally fail to cause infection. Spore aerosols may be encountered by workers handling contaminated batches of hair or wool and bone meal fertilizers. The aerosol infective dose required for human infection appears to be high. In certain animal hair mills, air sampling studies have estimated that nonimmune workers inhaled as many as 510 spores 5 μm or less in diameter, per 8-hour shift, without becoming ill. Studies of guinea pigs indicate that inhaled anthrax spores are ingested initially by alveolar macrophages and are then carried to tracheobronchial and mediastinal lymph nodes. The spores germinate to bacilli with production of capsule and toxins. This is followed by development of necrotic and hemorrhagic lymphadenitis with spread by efferent lymphatics to the systemic circulation. No primary mucosal lesions, analogous to cutaneous eschars, are found within the respiratory passages. Pneumonia is an uncommon finding in most reports but was noted in 25% of the cases in the Sverdlovsk outbreak.

Gastrointestinal Anthrax. Oropharyngeal and GI anthrax follow ingestion of spores, usually from poorly cooked, contaminated meat. There is no evidence that milk from infected animals transmits anthrax. An ulcer in the stomach or terminal ileum or cecum may be present with associated hemorrhagic abdominal lymphadenitis. Oropharyngeal forms are often marked by a local oral ulcer associated with cervical lymphadenopathy and edema of the neck.

Septicemic Anthrax. Generalized sepsis may follow cutaneous anthrax and almost invariably accompanies inhalational and GI anthrax. Vascular injury may be a result of the exuberant proliferation of the organism in the blood and the action of the exotoxins. The lethal and edema toxins may act directly on the vasculature or through the release of mediators such as TNF-α and interleukin-1 from macrophages. Widespread capillary thrombosis, circulatory failure, shock, and death ensue. Several human victims have demonstrated adrenocortical hemorrhage.

CLINICAL MANIFESTATIONS

Cutaneous Anthrax. Cutaneous anthrax accounts for >95% of human anthrax infections and commonly involves exposed areas of the face, neck, hands, and arms. The incubation period is from 12 hours to 7 days but averages 3 days. The initial lesion is a small erythematous macule or papule that resembles an insect bite or pimple. It turns brown and develops a surrounding ring of erythema and may form a pruritic vesicle or bulla. Vesicular satellite lesions may appear (Fig. 55–1A), and the initially clear vesicular fluid becomes blue-black from hemorrhage after a few days. Organisms are abundant on Gram stain and culture, but leukocytes are rarely seen unless there is superinfection. The papule ulcerates and develops a black eschar by the fifth to seventh day. Nonpitting, gelatinous edema may be prominent, extending occasionally to the iliac crest from lesions of the head and neck. This has been referred to as *malignant edema*, which in conjunction with a black eschar may be pathognomonic for anthrax. Mild tender regional lymphadenopathy may occur, but lymphangitis and cellulitis should suggest secondary bacterial infection. Generally, patients have few symptoms, e.g., malaise, headache, and low-grade fever. A few have a modest neutrophilic leukocytosis, and blood cultures are usually sterile.

Inhalational Anthrax. Inhalational anthrax (woolsorters' disease) accounts for <5% of reported cases and is often a

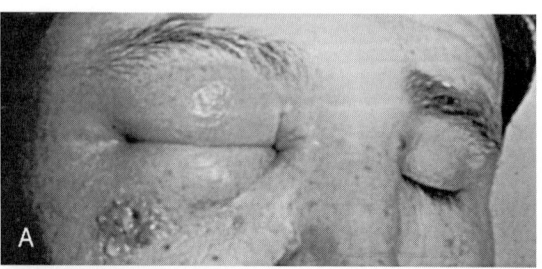

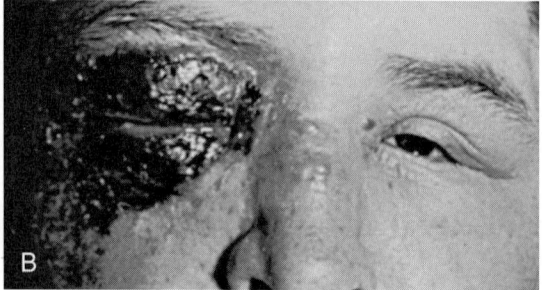

Figure 55–1. Cutaneous anthrax in a 45-year-old cattleman. *A,* Early facial lesion with prominent gelatinous edema and vesicular satellite lesions ("pearl wreath"), which revealed abundant anthrax bacilli on Gram stain and culture. *B,* Evolution of the cutaneous eschar despite antimicrobial therapy. (Courtesy of Dr. Alejandro Morales.)

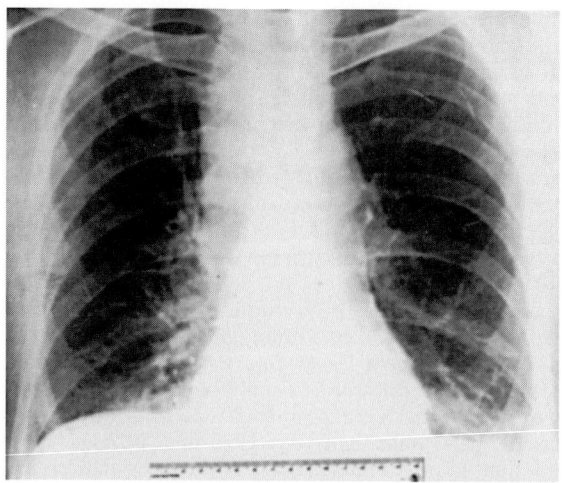

Figure 55–2. Chest radiograph on the second day of illness of a 51-year-old American laborer with occupational exposure to airborne anthrax. The combination of parenchymal infiltrate with striking mediastinal lymphadenopathy distinguishes inhalational anthrax. (Courtesy of the Armed Forces Institute of Pathology, Photograph Neg. No. 71–12790–2.)

biphasic illness. Initially nonspecific symptoms of mild fever, malaise, fatigue, and myalgia develop 1 to 5 days after exposure. Nonproductive cough and precordial oppression are often reported, and rhonchi may be heard. Patients may show brief improvement after several days or may directly develop the sudden onset of severe respiratory distress with dyspnea, cyanosis, diaphoresis, increased fever, and tachycardia. Stridor may be dramatic if enlarged mediastinal nodes impinge on the trachea. Diffuse rales and basilar dullness may be heard. Chest radiographs reveal symmetric mediastinal widening, pleural effusions, and in some cases patchy infiltrates (Fig. 55–2). Massive superficial edema of the head and neck may occur. Meningitis, often hemorrhagic, occurs in approximately 50% of cases. Pleural effusions may also be hemorrhagic. Cultures of blood, pleural fluid, and cerebrospinal fluid are usually positive.

Gastrointestinal Anthrax. Oropharyngeal and GI anthrax accounts for <5% of cases. Oropharyngeal anthrax presents with sore throat, an ulcer in the oral cavity, dysphagia, cervical and submandibular lymphadenopathy, and often dramatic neck edema. GI anthrax develops after an incubation period of 2 to 5 days. Patients have generalized abdominal pain, anorexia, nausea, vomiting, and in some cases hematemesis. Severe prostration accompanies the development of ascites, bloody diarrhea, toxemia, and shock. Subcutaneous edema may extensively involve the lower trunk. Survival has been reported but is rare.

Central Nervous System Anthrax. Anthrax meningitis follows bacteremia from a cutaneous, pulmonary, or intestinal source. These critically ill patients usually present with fever, meningismus, and rapidly deteriorating mental status. Lumbar puncture reveals hemorrhagic spinal fluid containing gram-positive rods. Bacteremia is documented in 70% of patients, and the usual survival is 2 to 4 days. In very rare cases, patients present with isolated meningitis without other evidence of disease.

DIAGNOSIS

Differential Diagnosis. The epidemiologic background of an industrial or agricultural exposure, the evolution of a pruritic then painless lesion unassociated with cellulitis or lymphangitis, and the dramatic appearance of the black eschar and extensive nonpitting edema help to distinguish anthrax from other bacterial skin infections. Small, early skin lesions may be difficult to recognize, however, and the edema often is not extensive. The initial symptoms of inhalational anthrax are nonspecific and may resemble influenza, bronchitis, or the common cold. The latter stage may mimic congestive cardiac failure or a cardiovascular catastrophe but should be suggested by mediastinal widening on chest radiographs in the setting of occupational exposure. Anthrax meningitis may be readily confused with other forms of bacterial meningitis or subarachnoid hemorrhage. GI anthrax with fever and severe abdominal pain may be confused with other causes of an acute abdomen.

Direct Smear and Culture Diagnosis. In cutaneous anthrax, the encapsulated bacilli can be identified on Gram- or Giemsa-stained smears and cultured on sheep blood or peptone agar. Nonpathogenic bacilli may be recovered from suspicious skin lesions; therefore, specific identification of isolates is necessary. Bacilli may also be abundant in Gram-stained smears of cerebrospinal or pleural fluid. Direct fluorescent antibody staining may enhance definitive, early identification of *B. anthracis* from vesicular fluid smears, tissue, or culture.

Serologic Diagnosis. Antibody to protective antigen or capsule, measured by enzyme-linked immunosorbent assay, develops in 67 to 94% of cases of cutaneous or oropharyngeal anthrax but is generally of value only retrospectively. More rapid diagnostic tests for detection of the protective antigen toxin component in body fluids have been developed and are currently being evaluated.

THERAPY AND MANAGEMENT

Antimicrobial Therapy. The key to successful therapy is prompt administration of an antimicrobial agent at the first suspicion of anthrax.

Cutaneous Anthrax. Untreated cutaneous anthrax can be associated with local malignant edema and can progress to septicemia, shock, renal failure, and death in 5 to 20% of cases. Virtually all cutaneous anthrax lesions are cured by antimicrobial therapy. An oral penicillin 1 to 2 g/day is the treatment of choice. Oral tetracycline 2 g/day is an alternative for penicillin-allergic patients and, although probably less effective than penicillin, regularly results in cure. Erythromycin, chloramphenicol, and streptomycin have also been used with success. In vitro sensitivities and testing in experimental animals suggest that fluoroquinolones should be highly effective, although no clinical experience has been reported. If severe systemic symptoms are present, intravenous penicillin in higher doses should be given.

Other Anthrax Syndromes. The treatment of choice for inhalational or GI anthrax is high-dose penicillin 18 to 24 million units/day. Some data in experimental animal models of anthrax suggest that the addition of streptomycin 2 g/day (or presumably other aminoglycosides) provides additional benefit. As noted earlier for cutaneous anthrax, fluoroquinolones are likely to be highly effective as well. Rare sporadic reports describe patients' surviving inhalational and GI anthrax or meningitis after receiving early, intensive antimicrobial therapy.

Supportive Therapy. The evolution of the anthrax skin lesion is not modified by antimicrobial treatment, although the lesion is rapidly sterilized; indeed, toxin-mediated edema may increase during the first 24 hours of therapy. Glucocorticoids have been used to reduce edema, but no controlled studies have been reported.

Isolation of Patients. Although direct human-to-human transmission has not been observed in any case of anthrax, standard and drainage/secretion precautions should be instituted for patients with cutaneous anthrax. Although pneumonia is very unusual in inhalational anthrax, respiratory isolation should be maintained in individuals producing bloody sputum until sputum cultures have been shown to be negative.

Antianthrax Serum Therapy. Before the development of antimicrobials, equine antianthrax serum therapy was believed to reduce mortality due to anthrax infections, but no carefully controlled studies have been reported. Anthrax antitoxin is no longer commercially available in the United States. Developments in our understanding of the pathogenic role of the anthrax toxins and the possible mediating role of cytokines may provide renewed interest in adjunctive antitoxin and cytokine-modulating therapies.

PROGNOSIS. Cutaneous anthrax is usually a self-limited disease. The 5 to 20% mortality rate of untreated patients is essentially eliminated by specific antimicrobial therapy. Inhalational and GI anthrax have almost always been fatal because of the difficulty of establishing the diagnosis and the rapidity of the course of disease despite antimicrobial therapy.

PREVENTION

Active Immunization. A human vaccine against anthrax licensed in the United States is made by adsorbing the sterile culture filtrate of an attenuated toxin-producing strain of *B. anthracis* to aluminum hydroxide. The major component of the vaccine is protective antigen, and it is available from the Michigan Biologic Products Institute (Lansing, Michigan). A vaccine similar to the currently licensed vaccine was shown in a controlled clinical trial to be effective in preventing cutaneous anthrax, but there were insufficient numbers of cases to determine its efficacy against inhalational anthrax. The currently licensed product has been shown to protect rodents and nonhuman primates against a lethal aerosol challenge. The recommended schedule for vaccination is 0.5 mL SC at 0, 2, and 4 weeks and again at 6, 12, and 18 months, followed by yearly boosters if the potential for exposure continues. The vaccine is recommended for workers exposed to potentially contaminated animal products such as wool, hair, hides, and bone. Individuals in direct contact with animals in parts of the world endemic for anthrax as well as laboratory workers should also be immunized.

A live attenuated, unencapsulated spore vaccine similar to the veterinary vaccine is available in countries of the former Soviet Union for human use. It is said to provide some efficacy against cutaneous anthrax and to be reasonably well tolerated.

Industrially Acquired Anthrax. Control of anthrax spores contaminating certain animal products would reduce human cases of anthrax. Sterilization of wool is not often economical or practical; however, bristles destined for shaving brushes may be readily sterilized before manufacture. Employee education, cleaning and disinfection of raw products, and routine vaccination of workers in the wool, hair, and bristle industries in Britain are thought to be responsible for the fourfold decline in anthrax between the periods of 1961 to 1965 and 1976 to 1980. Sporadic cases are still reported among transient factory workers and among hobbyists importing wool directly for their own use. Sterilization of bone meal fertilizer is difficult and uneconomical; however, many nations require that bags carry warning labels recommending that gloves be worn when using the product.

Zoonotic Anthrax. Disease should be diagnosed rapidly in animals; herds should be quarantined until 2 weeks after the last case. All animals in the herd should be vaccinated, and carcasses disposed of appropriately. A live attenuated, veterinary spore vaccine is available worldwide and has proved very effective in controlling the disease when it has been used.

Bibliography

Abramova FA, Grinberg LM, Yampolskaya OV, et al: Pathology of inhalational anthrax in 42 cases from the Sverdlovsk outbreak of 1979. Proc Natl Acad Sci U S A 90:2291, 1993.

Brachman PS: Inhalation anthrax. Ann N Y Acad Sci 353:83, 1980.

Brachman PS, Friedlander AM: Anthrax. *In* Plotkin SA, Mortimer EA Jr (eds): Vaccines. Philadelphia, WB Saunders, 1994.

Dutz W, Kohout E: Anthrax. Pathol Annu 6:209, 1971.

Gold H: Anthrax: A report of one hundred seventeen cases. AMA Arch Intern Med 96:387, 1955.

Kunmusont C, Limpakarnjanarat K, Foy HM: Outbreak of anthrax in Thailand. Ann Trop Med Parasitol 84:507, 1990.

Leppla SH: The anthrax toxin complex. *In* Alouf JE, Freer JH (eds): Sourcebook of Bacterial Protein Toxins. London, Academic Press, 1991.

Smego RA Jr, Gebrian B, Desmangels G, et al: Cutaneous manifestations of anthrax in rural Haiti. Clin Infect Dis 26:97, 1998.

Turnbull PCB: Anthrax vaccines: Past, present and future. Vaccine 9:533, 1991.

56 Glanders

James D. DeMaio

DEFINITION. Glanders is a rare zoonotic infection caused by *Burkholderia (Pseudomonas) mallei.*

EPIDEMIOLOGY. Horses, donkeys, and mules serve as the major animal reservoir. Infection in horses may present as either a suppurative pneumonia with systemic involvement (glanders) or a nodular lymphangitis with progressive subcutaneous ulceration (farcy). Spread to humans is presumed to occur via inhalation or contact with infected equine secretions. Sheep, goats, cats, and dogs may contract the disease but probably have a minor role as reservoirs.

During the early 1900s, protein extracts from *B. mallei* cultures (mallein) were used to skin test horse populations in North America and Western Europe. Destruction of infected animals led to eradication of disease in these areas. Glanders currently occurs sporadically in Asia, Africa, and South America.

ETIOLOGY. *B. mallei* is a nonmotile, oxidase-positive, gram-negative rod. The organism has been removed from the genus *Pseudomonas* and included within a new genus, *Burkholderia*, based on 16S rRNA homology.

CLINICAL MANIFESTATIONS AND DIAGNOSIS. The incubation period is thought to be brief (probably 1 to 5 days). Humans may present with sepsis and acute necrotizing pneumonia, acute focal abscesses, or chronic progressive subcutaneous abscesses. These clinical manifestations frequently overlap in individual patients.

B. mallei may be readily cultivated on MacConkey agar. Serologic tests are not commercially available.

TREATMENT. Sulfadiazine 100 mg/kg/day in divided doses has been considered the drug of choice. Patients should be treated for a minimum of 3 weeks. Animal experiments indicate that quinolones, ceftazidime, imipenem, and tetracyclines are reasonable alternatives in patients intolerant of sulfa drugs.

Bibliography

Antonov IV, Iliukhin VI, Popovtseva LD, et al: Sensitivity of *Pseudomonas* to currently used antibacterial drugs. Antibiot Khimioter 35:14, 1991.

Howe C, Miller WR: Human glanders: Report of six cases. Ann Intern Med 26:93, 1947.

Yabuuchi E, Kosako Y, Oyaizu H, et al: Proposal of *Burkholderia* gen. nov. and transfer of seven species of the genus *Pseudomonas* Homology Group II to the new genus, with the type species *Burkholderia cepacia* (Palleroni and Holmes 1981) comb. nov. Microbiol Immunol 36:1251, 1992.

57 Gas Gangrene

Robert C. Bollinger, Jr. and John G. Bartlett

DEFINITION. Gas gangrene is a rapidly progressive, often life-threatening infection associated with myonecrosis due to a toxin or toxins elaborated by species of clostridia, usually *Clostridium perfringens.* The term for gas gangrene is applied most accurately to a single entity, clostridial myonecrosis.

ETIOLOGY AND PATHOGENESIS. More than 150 species of clostridia have been recognized since the description of *C. butyricum* by Louis Pasteur in 1861. *C. welchii* was first recognized as a cause of gas gangrene in 1892 and later renamed *C. perfringens. C. perfringens* has been subsequently isolated from 80 to 90% of cases of gas gangrene, whereas two other histotoxic clostridia, *C. novyi* and *C. septicum*, have been implicated in 10 to 40% and 5 to 20% of cases, respectively. Patients may be infected with *C. histolyticum, C. bifermentans, C. fallax*, and *C. sporogenes*, but only rarely. These 7 species of clostridia produce more than 22 exotoxins, of which the most important is α toxin (α lecithinase; phospholipase).

Toxins. C. perfringens is the most important histotoxic species of clostridia and, in addition to α toxin, is known to produce at least 12 other tissue-active exotoxins. The species is divided into five types, designated A through E, on the basis of the production of four major toxins (α, β, ε, and θ). All five serotypes produce α toxin, but type A produces the greatest quantity. Only type A is present in both soil and intestine. Alpha toxin is oxygen stable and has a marked affinity for lipid membranes. As a result, severe hemolysis, platelet destruction, and widespread alterations in capillary permeability occur. Other toxins, in particular θ toxin, contribute also to local tissue necrosis and systemic toxicity, including shock.

Local Tissue Factors. Clostridia thrive in tissues with low oxygen tension. When tissue is damaged, its vascular supply is compromised and tissue tension is lowered. Settings favoring toxin elaboration are associated with clostridial myonecrosis, which usually results from the contamination of traumatic or surgical wounds by histotoxic clostridia under conditions of a decreased oxidation-reduction potential (Eh). Blood vessel trauma; intense edema; the use of tourniquets, pressure dressings, and vasoconstrictors; and the presence of foreign bodies, devitalized tissue, and other microorganisms contribute to vascular insufficiency and tissue hypoxia and the resultant toxin-mediated liquefactive necrosis of muscle and surrounding tissue.

INCIDENCE. Estimates of the frequency of occurrence of gas gangrene vary widely. In a large review of major open wounds, the incidence of gas gangrene ranged from 0.03 to 5.2%, depending on the type of wound and treatment. In the United States, 900 to 3000 cases per year are thought to occur. Trauma is associated with about half the cases of gas gangrene, and most other cases are associated with surgery. The incidence of gas gangrene in developing countries is likely higher.

DISTRIBUTION. Histotoxic clostridia are ubiquitous, exposure is universal, and infections occur worldwide. Soil samples universally harbor clostridia, including *C. perfringens*, at concentrations of 1000 organisms/g or greater. *C. perfringens* is commonly present also in water, meat, clothing, dust, air samples, and agricultural products. Most animals and humans harbor *C. perfringens* in the gastrointestinal tract at a mean concentration of 10^8 to 10^9 organisms/g of feces. As many as 80% of severe traumatic open wounds are contaminated with spores of *C. perfringens,* although gas gangrene occurs in fewer than 3%.

CLINICAL MANIFESTATIONS. Clinical settings associated with gas gangrene include the following: traumatic injuries and penetrating wounds; surgery, especially colonic resection or surgical wounds following a ruptured appendix, bowel perforation, or biliary tract surgery; uterine gas gangrene, most commonly following septic abortion, less commonly normal delivery, and least commonly necrosis of uterine fibroid tumors; soft tissue infections associated with vascular insufficiency and occasionally diabetes mellitus; and spontaneous (or nontraumatic) gas gangrene, a variant that arises without an apparent source.

Symptoms and Signs. Clinical manifestations of gas gangrene begin 3 to 5 days after a traumatic wound or a surgical procedure, with a range of 8 hours to 3 weeks. The sudden appearance of severe pain and tense edema and tenderness at the wound site is observed early. Initial skin pallor gives way to a blue, purple, or bronze discoloration, often accompanied by large, tense, hemorrhagic bullae filled with dark red or purplish fluid and cutaneous necrosis. As the lesion evolves, the scant, thin, watery discharge is replaced by a thick, profuse, sweet-smelling, serosanguineous discharge that contains abundant gram-positive bacilli and a paucity of inflammatory cells on microscopic examination. Spores are not seen with *C. perfringens.* Crepitance may be present, but its occurrence is irregular and noted often in the late stages of disease. Fever is usually low grade, but the pulse rate is usually increased far out of proportion to the temperature elevation. As the disease progresses, incisional or wound pain increases and circulatory collapse ensues, with the development of hemolytic anemia, hemoglobinuria with renal failure, and profound systemic toxicity. Remarkably, patients remain unusually alert and aware of their surroundings despite their severely toxic state. Indifference and apathy or extreme apprehension and a sense of doom may be noted. Coma and shock are terminal events.

Uterine Gas Gangrene. Postabortal and postpartum clostridial uterine infections and postoperative gas gangrene are more prevalent in developing countries than in the United States and Europe. Uterine gas gangrene begins 1 to 3 days after septic abortion, with the early onset of jaundice and renal failure caused by the massive intravascular hemolysis mediated by α toxin. Pigmenturia leads to acute renal cortical necrosis and anuria. Bacteremia is common, and hypotension and shock occur regularly. Pelvic findings may be minimal, although radiographs or computerized tomograms show gas in the myometrium.

Spontaneous Gas Gangrene. Nontraumatic gas gangrene occurs without apparent source and is distinctive for the absence of trauma, its clostridial etiology, and its rapidly progressive course. Extensive soft tissue gas that spreads far beyond the borders of necrotic muscle is characteristic. Hemolysis, renal failure, and shock develop early, and patients may die within 2 or 3 days of onset. Spontaneous gas gangrene is usually caused by *C. perfringens. C. septicum* commonly causes neutropenic enterocolitis as a complication of neutropenia or colon cancer.

DIAGNOSIS AND DIFFERENTIAL DIAGNOSES. The diagnosis of gas gangrene is usually based on a combination of characteristic clinical manifestations and supporting microbiologic studies. A history of trauma or surgery, the typical appearance of the wound in a severely toxic patient, the presence of acute hemolytic anemia, jaundice, and renal failure, and the observation of large gram-positive bacilli without spores on Gram stain ("boxcars") and *C. perfringens* on culture support the diagnosis of clostridial myonecrosis. The

great majority of patients with clostridia isolated from wound or blood cultures do not have gas gangrene, and thus the accompanying clinical features are important. A computed tomography scan may strongly support this diagnosis by demonstrating myonecrosis. Confirmation requires direct inspection of the involved muscle, which appears pale and edematous early in the disease. With progression, the muscle becomes beefy red, black, or friable and eventually gelatinous or even liquefied. Muscle contraction is absent on stimulation, and the cut surface fails to bleed. Radiographs of involved areas may show nonspecific gas collections. Blood cultures are positive in 15% of patients with gas gangrene, but the diagnosis can be established by the finding of myonecrosis at surgery or autopsy and typical organisms on Gram stain.

The differential diagnosis includes other soft tissue infections, particularly necrotizing fasciitis, streptococcal fasciitis, streptococcal myonecrosis, and synergistic necrotizing cellulitis. These distinctions can be made by the site of involvement (fascia versus muscle), Gram stain, and characteristic odor. *Vibrio vulnificans* and *Aeromonas* may cause serious soft tissue infections with hemorrhagic bullae in patients with typical exposures. Noninfectious causes of soft tissue gas include the effects of trauma, hydrogen peroxide irrigation, barotrauma, and prior extensive surgical procedures.

TREATMENT AND PROGNOSIS. Surgical exploration of the involved area with radical debridement of all necrotic tissue and delayed closure of open wounds are the most important therapeutic maneuvers. This usually involves excision of involved muscle, amputation of an extremity, or uterine curettage or hysterectomy. Although the efficacy of antibiotics in the treatment of established gas gangrene in humans is less well established, they are recommended as an adjunct to surgical debridement. Aqueous penicillin G should be given intravenously at a daily dose of 12 or 20 million units for 10 to 14 days; chloramphenicol, tetracycline, metronidazole, and clindamycin are effective alternatives and in murine models of gas gangrene have proved superior to penicillin G for prevention of disease. Cephalosporins are inadequate in preventing gas gangrene after severe open trauma.

Hyperbaric Oxygen. The value of hyperbaric oxygen in the treatment of gas gangrene remains unsettled after many years of scrutiny and discussion. Support for its efficacy is derived mainly from anecdotal experiences and uncontrolled or noncomparative studies. Proponents cite the dramatic improvement in some patients and the arrest and demarcation of the disease process, which help to facilitate surgical debridement. Most authorities would advocate the use of hyperbaric oxygen if facilities were available and this would not delay surgery. In experienced hands, oxygen toxicity has been minimal. Polyvalent gas gangrene antitoxin has proved worthless in the treatment of infected patients and is no longer available.

Prognosis. Supportive measures include fluid and electrolyte replacement, management of acidosis and hemolytic anemia, and measures to preserve renal function. Complications include superinfections, the adult respiratory distress syndrome, disseminated intravascular coagulopathy, acute tubular necrosis, myocardial irritability, thromboembolic disease, fat embolism, and tetanus. Overall mortality rates range from 20 to 60%, with an average of 25%. Mortality is highest in those patients with involvement of the abdominal wall, buttocks, and myometrium and in those with spontaneous (nontraumatic) gas gangrene. It is lowest in those with involvement of the distal extremity and the endometrium.

PREVENTION. If gas gangrene is suspected, early diagnosis and the avoidance of time-wasting and costly investigations are essential. Prompt and thorough debridement of traumatized tissue is a critical factor in the prevention of gas gangrene. Less delay in the institution of appropriate prophylactic antibiotics and prudent decisions about wound closure are important also. No effective means of active immunization exists.

Bibliography

Gorbach SL, Thadepalli H: Isolation of clostridium in human infections: Evaluation of 114 cases. J Infect Dis 131:S81, 1975.

Hart GB, Lamb RC, Strauss MB: Gas gangrene: I. A collective review. J Trauma 23:991, 1983.

Heimbach RD: Gas gangrene: Review and update. HBO Rev 1:41, 1980.

MacLennan JD: The histotoxic clostridial infections of man. Bacteriol Rev 26:177, 1962.

Smith LDS: The Pathogenic Anaerobic Bacteria, 2nd ed. Springfield, IL, Charles C Thomas, 1975, pp 109–176, 322–324.

Stevens DL, Maier KA, Laine BM, et al: Comparison of clindamycin, rifampin, tetracycline, metronidazole, and penicillin for efficacy in prevention of experimental gas gangrene due to *Clostridium perfringens*. J Infect Dis 155:220, 1987.

Stevens DL, Troyer BE, Merrick DT, et al: Lethal effects and cardiovascular effects of purified alpha- and theta-toxins from *Clostridium perfringens*. J Infect Dis 157:272, 1988.

58 Pyomyositis

Joel D. Brown

DEFINITION. Pyomyositis is a purulent infection of skeletal muscle that occurs without penetrating trauma or spread from a contiguous septic focus. This disease is common in the tropics and rare in the temperate zones, hence the synonym *tropical pyomyositis*. The infection often seems to appear spontaneously and can present a confusing diagnostic problem, particularly for physicians without experience in the tropics.

HISTORY. Pyomyositis was described in Japan by Scriba and Miyake at the turn of the century. *Staphylococcus aureus* was the usual pathogen, but streptococci and pneumococci were occasionally responsible. In the United States, William Osler wrote in 1892 of "septic cases in which diffuse purulent infiltration of the muscles of different regions occurs" and indicated that the muscle may be the primary source of infection. In 1947, Traquir reviewed the history of pyomyositis and emphasized that it was endemic throughout the tropics. Most patients were indigenous to the tropics, but colonial Europeans were not spared. In 1971, the disease was reported in patients immigrating from the tropics to North America. Occasional cases have been recognized in temperate regions among persons who have not been in the tropics; some of these patients had other associated, immunocompromising diseases.

ETIOLOGY. *S. aureus* causes 95% of the cases. *Streptococcus pyogenes* and various streptococcus species account for most of the remaining. Other pyogenic bacteria, such as *Streptococcus pneumoniae* and gram-negative organisms, are rarely responsible for pyomyositis.

Various bacteria can infect open, traumatized wounds. Clostridia species cause myonecrosis in wounds and occasionally infect a muscle during bacteremia from intestinal sources. A focus of infection (e.g., osteomyelitis, intra-abdominal abscess, or necrotizing fasciitis) can invade contiguous skeletal muscle. However, these well-known muscle infections are not considered in the usual definition of pyomyositis.

DISTRIBUTION AND INCIDENCE. Pyomyositis is common throughout the tropics, where it is familiar to local medical workers. Nearly 4% of all patients admitted to the surgical service of a major teaching hospital in Uganda, Africa, had pyomyositis. This infection is reported primarily from tropical Africa and Asia, but it is common also in Oceania and the Caribbean and occurs in Central and South America. Although initially described in Japan, pyomyositis has not been reported there recently. Most endemic regions are warm and humid, but pyomyositis occurs in warm, dry savanna regions as well. Most are young males, possibly because they encounter more trauma, but no age or gender is spared.

PATHOGENESIS. The mechanism by which bacteria establish infection in muscle and the reasons for the predominance of such infections in the tropics are unknown. Staphylococci, streptococci, and other pyogenic bacteria infect people throughout the world; however, these bacteria rarely infect normal skeletal muscle in patients outside the tropics, even during bacteremia.

Miyake designed an experimental rabbit model for staphylococcal pyomyositis. He injured a muscle by pinching, ligature venous stasis, or electrically induced tetanic spasm, then injected staphylococci intravenously. Animals that survived the initial septicemia developed abscesses only in the injured muscle. Clinical studies reveal a history of trauma to the involved muscle in as many as two thirds of cases. Pyoderma is common in the tropics and could be a source of bacteremia, which may seed skeletal muscle, particularly previously abnormal muscle. Patients often have pyoderma distal to the infected muscle, suggesting that bacteria from the skin may reach the muscle via the lymphatics. The muscle abscess may be a manifestation of bacteremia with multiple metastatic infections, or it may be the source of bacteremia.

Pyomyositis has been associated with other tropical diseases that may invade or damage the muscle, such as dracunculiasis, filariasis, aberrant nematode larvae, leptospirosis, sickle cell disease, scurvy, thiamine deficiency, and viral myositis. It is likely that pyoderma, plus some form of muscle damage, is important in the pathogenesis of pyomyositis. In developed countries, pyomyositis may occur in patients with diabetes, leukemia, aplastic anemia, asplenia, lupus erythematosus, the Felty syndrome, intravenous drug abuse, and AIDS. These case reports suggest that defects in host defenses may have a role in the pathogenesis.

PATHOLOGY. Pyomyositis usually involves one to several large skeletal muscles. The infection usually is subfascial but may be predominantly in the fascial space between the muscle groups. The muscle usually contains a solitary or multiloculated abscess with thick pus and necrotic muscle (Fig. 58–1). The muscle occasionally is diffusely infiltrated and hard, grossly mimicking a soft tissue tumor such as rhabdomyosarcoma. The abscess may spread to contiguous structures and spaces, leading to epidural abscess, meningitis, and peritonitis.

The histopathology consists of both acute and chronic inflammation, depending on the duration of the infection. Polymorphonuclear cells, lymphocytes, plasma cells, and eosinophils are present. The muscle may be diffusely infiltrated with inflammatory cells. It can have fibrosis or can contain microabscesses and macroabscesses.

CLINICAL MANIFESTATIONS. The disease can be mild and confined to one muscle or associated with sepsis. Pain, swelling, and tenderness develop rapidly over a few days or follow an indolent course over weeks. Fever is common but may be delayed for several days. A single large muscle of the lower extremity is usually involved, but abscesses may

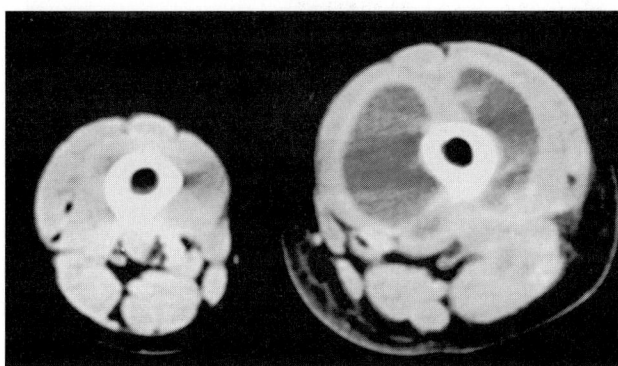

Figure 58–1. CT cross-sectional view of the thighs of a Micronesian boy who had fallen 1 month previously and developed staphylococcal abscesses in muscles of the thigh.

be found in many muscles of the arms or trunk. Skin redness and fluctuance of the muscle mass may not occur or may appear later, as the infection spreads from the muscle toward the surface. Diffuse inflammation and infiltration of the muscle without abscess formation are seen occasionally. A hard, woody, tumor-like quality of the affected muscle is typical of pyomyositis. Laboratory findings include leukocytosis and perhaps positive blood cultures. Muscle enzymes are usually normal. Eosinophilia may be present but is probably due to endemic parasites. The diagnosis can be easy in the tropics but confusing outside the endemic areas.

DIAGNOSIS. A history of recent muscle trauma and pyoderma, particularly when the latter is distal to the affected muscle, suggests pyomyositis. Aspiration of the area with a large needle and bacterial culture and Gram stain of the pus can be diagnostic. If needle aspiration is unrewarding, ultrasonography-guided aspiration or surgical exploration often confirms the diagnosis. Imaging with gallium and computed tomography (CT) scans (Fig. 58–1) may be useful in confirming the diagnosis or in detecting other sites of infection that need drainage. Pyomyositis without macroabscess may require muscle biopsy with cultures and tissue stains for microorganisms.

Pyomyositis may mimic muscle hematoma, septic arthritis, osteomyelitis, deep venous thrombosis, appendicitis, cellulitis, or muscle tumor (Fig. 58–2). When the skin becomes inflamed, a misdiagnosis of superficial cellulitis may be made, but the history of muscle pain preceding the skin changes suggests pyomyositis.

PROGNOSIS. Pyomyositis is usually confined to the muscle, but some cases may be septic. In a series of children reported from Nigeria, 25% had osteomyelitis and 14% had infections metastatic to other organs. The fatality rate in Africa is less than 1.5% but can be higher in the more serious cases with staphylococcal sepsis, endocarditis, pericarditis, pneumonia, or meningitis. These patients are referred to larger hospitals. Rhabdomyolysis with acute renal failure may occur in severe infections.

TREATMENT. Drainage of pus and debridement of necrotic muscle is required. Percutaneous catheter drainage may suffice, particularly if ultrasound or CT imaging is available for guidance and re-evaluation. Diffuse myositis without abscess may respond to antimicrobial agents alone, but abscesses may develop eventually and require drainage. Antimicrobial agents effective against penicillin-resistant staphylococci should be administered parenterally before drainage. The total dose of the antimicrobial agent and duration of therapy depend on the severity of disease and presence of complications.

Metastatic infections to bone or heart require 4 to 6 weeks of high-dose parenteral therapy. An uncomplicated case can be treated initially with parenteral antimicrobials and drainage of pus; oral antimicrobials may be substituted as the patient improves. Therapy should be continued until the wound is clean, the leukocyte count is normal, and the patient has been afebrile for several days. Penicillin, perhaps combined with clindamycin, should be used for proven streptococcal infections; therapy for the less common agents should be directed by laboratory studies. If laboratory support is unavailable and the patient fails to respond to initial antistaphylococcal management, broad-spectrum agents (e.g., cephalosporins) are justified. Methicillin-resistant *S. aureus* infections require treatment with intravenous vancomycin or perhaps trimethoprim-sulfamethoxazole. When resources are limited, oral chloramphenicol may be appropriate broad-spectrum therapy. Prognosis depends on the severity of the illness. Most patients have minimal sequelae.

PREVENTION. There are no proven preventive measures. Primary prevention or early treatment of pyoderma would probably reduce the incidence of pyomyositis. Early recognition and treatment of the disease may prevent complications.

Bibliography

Brown JD, Wheeler B: Pyomyositis: Report of 18 cases in Hawaii. Arch Intern Med 144:1749, 1984.

Chiedozi LC: Pyomyositis: Review of 205 cases in 112 patients. Am J Surg 137:255, 1979.

Echeverria P, Vaughn C: 'Tropical Pyomyositis': A diagnostic problem in temperate climates. Am J Dis Child 129:856, 1975.

Levin MJ, Gardner P, Waldvogel FA: 'Tropical Pyomyositis': An unusual infection due to *Staphylococcus aureus*. N Engl J Med 284:196, 1971.

Schlech WF III, Moulton P, Kaiser AB: Pyomyositis: Tropical disease in a temperate climate. Am J Med 71:900, 1981.

Schwartzman WA, Lambertus MW, Kennedy CA, Goetz MB: Staphylococcal pyomyositis in patients infected by the human immunodeficiency virus. Am J Med 90:595, 1991.

Traquir RN: Pyomyositis. J Trop Med Hyg 50:81, 1947.

Yousefzadeh DK, Schumann EM, Mulligan GM, et al: The role of imaging modalities in diagnosis and management of pyomyositis. Skeletal Radiol 8:285, 1982.

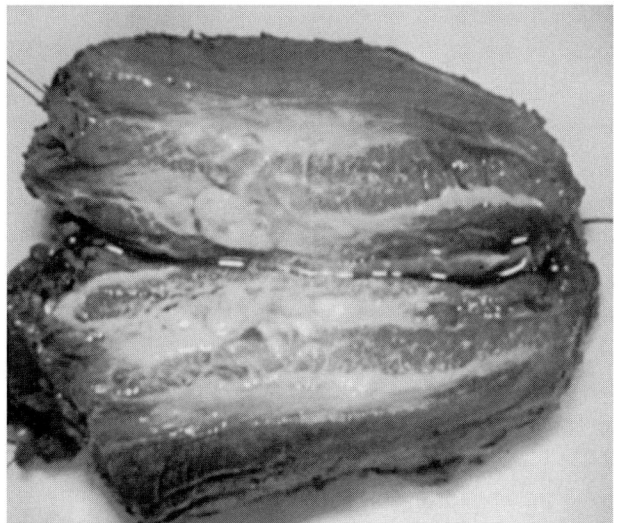

Figure 58–2. Infiltrating staphylococcal pyomyositis excised en bloc from a Samoan boy with a preoperative diagnosis of suspected rhabdomyosarcoma.

59 *Tropical Phagedenic Ulcer**

Wayne M. Meyers and Ronald C. Neafie

DEFINITION. Tropical phagedenic ulcer (TPU) is a painful, foul-smelling, necrotizing ulcer of the skin and subcutaneous tissue. Most ulcers are on the foot or leg.

ETIOLOGY AND HISTORY. Le Dante may have been the first to comment on the bacterial flora of lesions that were probably TPU. In 1884, he reported fusiform bacilli in ulcers in patients in Guiana but credited other observers with earlier clinical descriptions. The fusospirochetal etiology of TPU has long been suspected, and detailed microbiologic studies support this concept. Growing evidence, however, indicates that TPU is not caused by one or even two species of organisms but may be a remarkable example of the interaction of various microbes: fusobacteria (*? Fusobacterium nucleatum*), a spirochete (*? Treponema vincenti*), and other unidentified aerobic and anaerobic organisms, e.g., Tyzzer's bacillus (*Clostridium piliformis*).

EPIDEMIOLOGY AND DISTRIBUTION. TPU is virtually limited to the tropics and subtropics. The disease is more common in males, in rural environments, and in the rainy season. The major endemic areas are the tropical countries of Africa, Asia, and South America as well as New Guinea, the Pacific Islands, Central America, and the West Indies. Thus, most endemic areas are between 35° North and 10° South latitudes. Malnutrition and poor hygienic conditions are common in the endemic areas and may have a role in transmis-

---

*All the illustrations in this chapter are in the public domain.

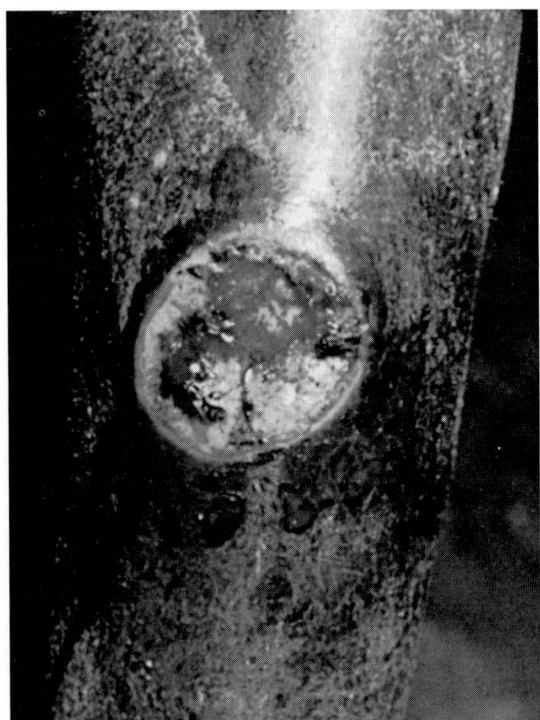

Figure 59–1. Typical early active tropical phagedenic ulcer over the lower one third of the pretibial area of an African patient. Note that the malodorous necrotic ulcer crater and the draining serous fluid have attracted flies. The ulcer margin is elevated by a hypertrophic epidermis. (Photograph by Dr. D. H. Connor. Courtesy of the Armed Forces Institute of Pathology. Photograph Neg. No. 68-658.)

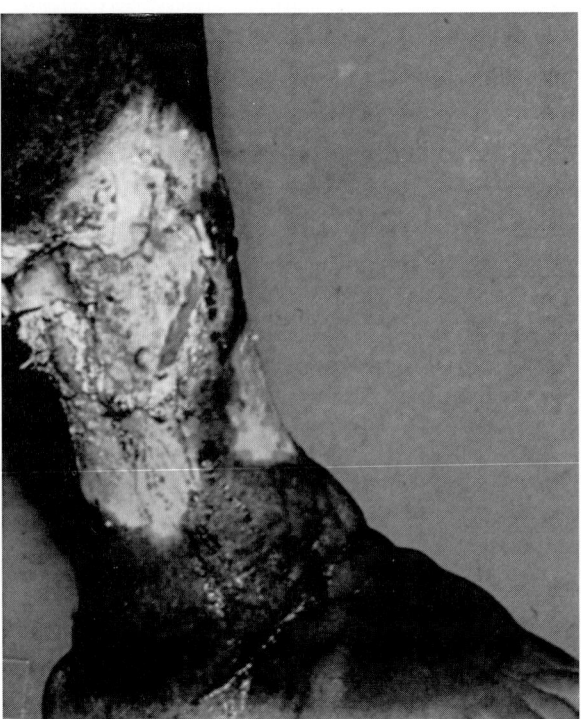

Figure 59–2. Old tropical phagedenic ulcer showing frayed scarring. The circumferential scar has caused lymphedema of the foot. (Photograph by Dr. D. H. Connor. Courtesy of the Armed Forces Institute of Pathology. Photograph Neg. No. 74-5309.)

sion and susceptibility; however, otherwise healthy individuals are often afflicted. The source of the infectious agent is unknown, but the fusospirochetal organisms found in the ulcers are similar to organisms that commonly inhabit the oral cavities of humans and some domesticated animals. Some authorities have speculated that there is a relationship between poor oral hygiene and TPU. Other investigators believe that the infectious agents are saprophytes in soil and mud. Patient-to-patient transmission is uncommon, but experimental inoculation of exudates from lesions of patients to healthy volunteers produces typical TPU.

PATHOGENESIS AND PATHOLOGY. A history of trauma or insect bite at the ulcer site can often be elicited. Perhaps contamination of this site by saliva or other materials introduces the infectious microorganism(s). The predominant, even nearly exclusive, location of advanced ulcers on the lower leg and foot may be related to exposure to contamination, dependency of the lower limb, and poor blood supply to the lower leg. Neglect of early lesions contributes to advanced ulceration and scarring. Once the microorganisms are sufficiently established in lesions, they may produce toxins that cause the typical excruciating pain and tissue necrosis of TPU. Butyrates elaborated by fusiform bacilli have been suggested as candidate toxins.

The histopathologic changes in early preulcerated lesions have not been reported, but sections through the margin and crater of the ulcerated area of a TPU reveal a necrotic coagulum of cellular debris and fibrin on the surface. This coagulum contains numerous fusiform and spirochetal organisms. Below this coagulum there is granulation tissue infiltrated by acute and chronic inflammatory cells. Many small blood vessels in the base of the ulcer are thrombosed, and others are narrowed by proliferating endothelial cells; however, the vasculitis does not appear to be primary. The margin of the ulcer is acanthotic or pseudoepitheliomatous, and dense fibrosis surrounds the lesion.

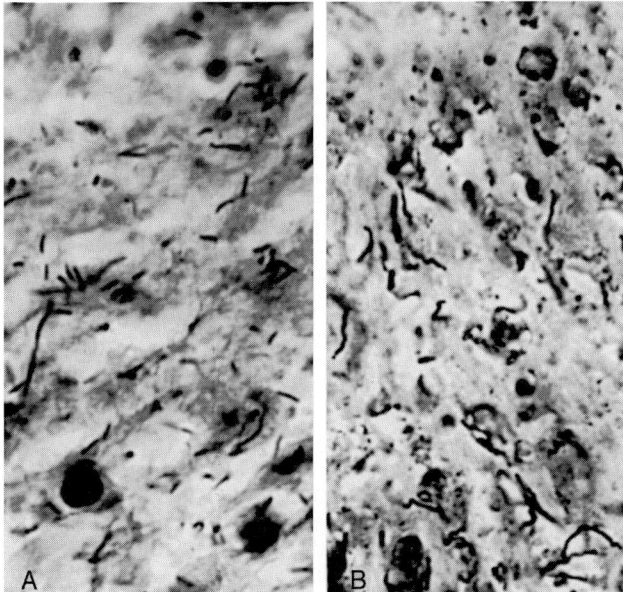

Figure 59–3. Exudates from the ulcer crater of active tropical phagedenic ulcers contain fusiform bacilli and spirochetes. *A*, Tissue Gram stain demonstrates the fusiform bacilli. Humberstone stain, × 1200. (Photograph Neg. No. 68-1876.) *B*, Warthin-Starry stain showing the spirochetal organisms. (Courtesy of the Armed Forces Institute of Pathology. Photograph Neg. No. 74-11309.)

CLINICAL MANIFESTATIONS. Lesions are nearly always single and begin as a small, painful, tender, erythematous, edematous area, which over 3 to 7 days becomes a 1- or 2-cm pustule that ulcerates and discharges sanguineous pus. The lesion is malodorous, and the base is covered by a necrotic slough. If untreated, tissue necrosis advances, forming an enlarging rounded ulcer, and may penetrate to underlying structures including fascia, muscle, tendons, and ultimately bone (Fig. 59–1). Regional lymphadenopathy and mild to moderate systemic symptoms may be present in the early stages. As the ulcer enters the chronic phase, the epithelium piles up at the margin and the base of the ulcer and surrounding tissues are scarred, frequently breaking down and becoming secondarily infected (Fig. 59–2). Without treatment, the average duration is several months, but ulcers may persist for as long as several decades. Most ulcers are 2 to 5 cm in diameter and rarely exceed 10 cm in diameter. A gradual nonpigmented re-epithelialization ordinarily occurs over the scarred base of the ulcer. If the ulcer is large, contractures may ensue. Squamous cell carcinoma sometimes develops at the ulcer site. This may be related to the chronic inflammation or to actinic stimulation of the nonpigmented epithelium at the healing or healed ulcer site.

DIAGNOSIS. "Once seen, once smelled, never forgotten" is a well-known maxim that physicians experienced in clinical tropical medicine have used in relation to TPU. The demonstration of fusiform bacilli and spirochetes in ulcer exudates or in histologic sections of an ulcer from the lower leg or foot is strong evidence for TPU (Fig. 59–3). The differential diagnosis is not usually a problem. TPUs are most frequently confused with Buruli ulcers, diphtheritic ulcers, and yaws; however, ulcers of *Mycobacterium ulcerans* are undermined and smears often reveal acid-fast bacilli; diphtheritic ulcers appear punched out, have a diphtheritic membrane, and contain diphtheroids; and ulcers caused by yaws have irregular contours and frequently demonstrable spirochetes. The histopathologic changes in all these lesions are often diagnostic.

TREATMENT AND PROGNOSIS. Early recognition followed by treatment is ideal but rarely possible. No published reports have outlined the therapy of early lesions, but one of the authors (WMM) treated several lesions in the preulcerative or very early ulcerative stage with penicillin intramuscularly. Rapid resolution of the lesion followed.

Unfortunately, most patients present with advanced, painful ulceration that has severely limited their activity and productivity. Much has been written about various topical treatments and dressings, but it is sufficient to clean the ulcer by routine methods (e.g., hydrogen peroxide), apply bland dry dressings, and give systemic antibiotics. Penicillin is usually administered, 500,000 to 1 million units IM daily for 7 to 20 days. Long-acting penicillin may be used as outpatient therapy. Metronidazole (800 mg b.i.d. for 1 or 2 weeks) is effective against fusobacteria and may accelerate healing.

Large ulcers should be skin grafted after successful systemic therapy and the development of healthy granulation tissue.

If carcinomatous changes are suspected, a biopsy specimen should be taken to establish the diagnosis. Squamous cell carcinomas developing in TPU lesions are locally invasive and eventually destroy soft tissue and bone, but metastases are rare. Local wide excision is the preferred treatment. Amputation is sometimes necessary with massive lesions or when bone is destroyed.

Bibliography

Adriaans RB: Tropical ulcer—a reappraisal based on recent work. Trans Soc Trop Med Hyg 82:185, 1988.

Conner DH, Neafie RC: Tropical phagedenic ulcer. *In* Binford CH, Connor DH (eds): Pathology of Tropical and Extraordinary Diseases. An Atlas. Washington, DC, Armed Forces Institute of Pathology, 1976, pp 199–201.

Falkler WA Jr, Montgomery J, Nauman RK, Alpers M: Isolation of *Fusobacterium nucleatum* and electron microscopic observations of spirochetes from tropical skin ulcers in Papua New Guinea. Am J Trop Med Hyg 40:390, 1989.

60 Bartonella-*Associated* Diseases

General Principles

James G. Olson

DESCRIPTION. The *Bartonella* genus consists of small, curved, pleomorphic, gram-negative rods with fastidious growth requirements. Hemin, 5% carbon dioxide, and prolonged incubation (1 to 8 weeks) are required for successful culture. Four pathogenic species have been identified: *B. bacilliformis*, *B. henselae*, *B. quintana*, and *B. elizabethae*.

B. henselae is, to date, the only species associated with cat-scratch disease, and has been identified by culture and polymerase chain reaction (PCR) from lymph nodes (Chapter 60.2). *B. henselae* bacteremia in otherwise well-appearing cats is common and can be prolonged. In a San Francisco study, 41% of pet and impounded cats were culture positive. The organism's mechanism of transmission is unknown, but probably involves fleas, at least from cat to cat.

B. quintana, the cause of louse-borne trench fever, and *B. henselae* have been recovered from the cutaneous lesions of bacillary angiomatosis (Chapter 60.3) and from the blood of febrile patients. A single isolate of *B. elizabethae* was identified in an immunocompetent adult with endocarditis. Animal reservoirs for *B. quintana* and *B. elizabethae* have not been identified; however, the agent has been recovered from an urban rat (*Rattus norvegicus*), and epidemiologic data suggest human infections in urban intravenous (IV) drug abusers. *B. bacilliformis* is transmitted by sandflies of the mountainous regions of South America and causes Oroya fever, a febrile hemolytic anemia, and verruga peruana, a red, wartlike rash not unlike bacillary angiomatosis (Chapter 60.1).

HISTORY. During the last decade, the etiology of cat-scratch disease was discovered, bacillary angiomatosis was recognized, and the relationship of these diseases to trench fever, an epidemic scourge of soldiers in the First World War (Chapter 68), was demonstrated. Because of recent microbiologic and genetic evidence, the etiologic agents of these diseases have been included in the genus *Bartonella*.

Recent progress in understanding of these diseases was stimulated by two observations in 1983. First, bacilli were seen in lymph nodes of patients with cat-scratch disease. Second, what is now known to be bacillary angiomatosis was described in a human immunodeficiency virus (HIV)–infected patient; cultures of affected tissues were negative but bacilli could be seen. The staining characteristics and morphologic appearance of the bacilli and the history of cat scratches given by patients with both diseases suggested that cat-scratch disease and bacillary angiomatosis might be caused by the same agent.

For more than 40 years following its first careful clinical description the etiologic agent of cat-scratch disease has eluded investigators. Researchers at Stanford University used eubacterial primers in a PCR to amplify bacterial 16S ribosomal gene fragments directly from tissue biopsies in bacillary angiomatosis. Specimens from several unrelated patients yielded a unique 16S gene sequence belonging to a pre-

viously uncharacterized microorganism most closely related to *Rochalimaea quintana*, the etiologic agent of trench fever, identified in 1969. Simultaneously, another group reported isolation, after lysis-centrifugation, of a gram-negative bacterium from the blood of febrile patients. The 16S ribosomal gene sequences identified in the tissue biopsies from patients with bacillary angiomatosis were identical or closely related to the 16S ribosomal gene sequence of this bacterium. The organism was classified as a new species of *Rochalimaea* and named *Rochalimaea henselae*. Recently, *R. henselae* and *R. quintana* have been placed in the genus *Bartonella* and classified as *Bartonella bacilliformis*.

CLINICAL AND EPIDEMIOLOGIC FEATURES. The bartonellae cause a wide spectrum of illness from self-limited fever and lymphadenopathy (e.g., cat-scratch disease) to prolonged or relapsing fever (e.g., trench fever). The case-fatality rate also varies from essentially zero (cat-scratch disease and trench fever) to as high as 88% (bartonellosis). Epidemiologic features for both immunocompetent subjects and for those whose immune status has been severely compromised are shown in Table 60–1.

Bibliography

Anderson B, Sims K, Regnery R, et al: Detection of *Rochalimaea henselae* DNA in specimens from cat scratch disease patients by PCR. J Clin Microbiol 32:942, 1994.

Brenner DJ, O'Connor SP, Winkler HH, et al: Proposals to unify the genera *Bartonella* and *Rochalimaea*, with descriptions of *Bartonella quintana* comb. nov., *Bartonella vinsonii* comb. nov., *Bartonella henselae* comb. nov., and *Bartonella elizabethae* comb. nov., and to remove the family *Bartonellaceae* from the order Rickettsiales. Int J Syst Bacteriol 43:777, 1993.

Koehler JE, Glaser CA, Tappero JW: *Rochalimaea henselae* infection: A new zoonosis with the domestic cat as reservoir. JAMA 271:531, 1994.

Relman DA, Loutit JS, Schmidt TM, et al: The agent of bacillary angiomatosis: An approach to the identification of uncultured pathogens. N Engl J Med 323:1573, 1993.

Spach DO, Candor AS, Dougherty MJ, et al: *Bartonella (Rochalimaea) quintana* bacteremia in inner-city patients with chronic alcoholism. N Engl J Med 18:708, 1995.

Zangwill KM, Hamilton DH, Perkins BA, et al: Cat-scratch disease in Connecticut: Epidemiology, risk factors, and evaluation of a new diagnostic test. N Engl J Med 329:8, 1993.

60.1 *Bartonellosis*

Larry W. Laughlin

DEFINITION. Bartonellosis is a three-stage clinical infectious disease caused by *Bartonella bacilliformis*, an aerobic, motile alpha-2 proteobacterium that infects erythrocytes and reticuloendothelial cells. Acute hematic bartonellosis frequently occurs in epidemics as a highly fatal acute febrile anemia. *Verruga peruana* manifests primarily as a characteristic chronic verrucous rash, whereas the most chronic and least well described form of bartonellosis is chronic asymptomatic bacteremia. Bartonellosis is most often reported from the Andean mountain valleys of South America and is thought to be vectored by the sandfly with humans who have chronic bacteremia serving as the reservoir host. Although the organism is sensitive to several antibiotics, treatment of the more chronic stages is difficult.

TABLE 60–1. Features of *Bartonella*-Associated Diseases

Etiologic Agent	Disease	Case-Fatality Rate Treated (Untreated)	Ecology of Exposure	Geographic Distribution
Immunocompetent Patients				
Bartonella bacilliformis	Verruga peruana, Oroya fever	<5% (40–90%)	Bite of infected sandfly, limited to western slopes of Andes Mountains	Bolivia, Chile, Colombia, Ecuador, Guatemala, and Peru (highlands of South and Central America)
B. quintana	Trench fever	Fatalities are rare	Infestations with the body louse (*Pediculus humanus*); crushed infected lice or louse feces introduced into cuts, abrasions, or through mucous membranes	Common in cold climates, particularly where laundering is infrequent and personal hygiene practices are poor
B. henselae	Cat-scratch disease	Fatalities are rare	Bite or scratch of cat allows infectious cat flea (*Ctenocephalides felis*) feces to penetrate skin	Well documented in the United States, South America, and Europe; probably worldwide
B. elizabethae	Endocarditis	Unknown	Unknown; may be associated with intravenous drug abuse and urban rats (*Rattus norvegicus*)	Urban United States; probably more widespread
Immunocompromised Patients				
B. quintana	Bacillary angiomatosis, visceral peliosis, bacteremia, endocarditis, lymphadenopathy	Fatalities are rare	Infestations with the body louse (*P. humanus*); crushed infected lice or louse feces introduced into cuts, abrasions, or through mucous membranes	Worldwide; more common in countries where HIV/AIDS is prevalent
B. henselae	Bacillary angiomatosis, visceral peliosis, bacteremia, endocarditis	Fatalities are rare	Bite or scratch of cat allows infectious cat flea (*C. felis*) feces to penetrate skin	Worldwide; more common in countries where HIV/AIDS is prevalent

HISTORY. Mummies from the pre-Colombian era have demonstrated verrucous lesions, and pre-Incan anthropomorphic pottery caricatures the disfiguring rash. Diaries of Spanish conquistadores carefully record the verrucous rash that befell 25% of the troops traversing the Peruvian Andes during the 16th century. The modern history of bartonellosis began in 1871 with a highly fatal epidemic that killed more than 7000 foreign laborers constructing a new railroad through the Rímac River valley connecting the cities of Lima and La Oroya. "Oroya fever" became synonymous with acute hematic bartonellosis.

In 1905, a Peruvian physician, Alberto Barton, described the presence of motile intraerythrocytic organisms in patients with Oroya fever. In 1913 Strong confirmed Barton's observations and named the agent *Bartonella bacilliformis*. The organism was first cultured in vitro by Noguchi in 1926, who also was able to produce septicemia experimentally in monkeys after IV inoculation and skin lesions after intradermal inoculation of cultured organisms. The phlebotomine sandfly was first suspected as the vector by Townsend in 1912, who named the species *Lutzomyia verrucarum*.

ETIOLOGY. *B. bacilliformis*, the only bacterium known to infect human erythrocytes and cause clinical disease, is a small (0.2 to 0.5 μm by 1 to 2 μm), motile, pleomorphic, gram-negative coccobacillus with multiple unipolar flagella. It is phylogenetically related to the causative agents of cat-scratch disease, bacillary angiomatosis, and trench fever. Based on unquantified visual observations of Giemsa-stained peripheral blood smears, bacillary forms appear to predominate in the early stages of the acute illness, and coccoid forms are more prevalent during convalescence. Organisms are found within the cytoplasm of erythrocytes and endothelial cells, sometimes appearing to lie inside vacuoles or attached to the inner surface of the cell membrane. They bind to human erythrocytes in vitro and produce substantial, long-lasting deformations in erythrocytic membranes. *B. bacilliformis* organisms appear as violet rods or cocci with Giemsa or Romanovsky stain and copper-brown with Warthin-Starry stain.

The *B. bacilliformis* genome has been physically mapped and consists of a 1600 kb, single circular DNA molecule. The molecular genetics of this organism is currently under extensive investigation, with early results providing insights into mechanisms of erythrocyte invasion and disease pathogenesis.

TRANSMISSION

Vector. Observations made earlier this century suggested that bartonellosis was a vector-borne disease transmitted by the sandfly, *L. verrucarum* (Fig. 139–7). However, biologic transmission was never demonstrated, and wild-caught sandflies from endemic regions have not yielded cultureable *B. bacilliformis*. With recent data suggesting transmission of other *Bartonella* species by other vectors, e.g., the flea (*B. henselae*), the body louse (*B. quintana*), and the tick (verruga peruana in Ecuador), and the documentation of clinical bartonellosis in Ecuador outside the usual mountain habitat of *L. verrucarum*, the previous certainty of sandfly transmission is being reconsidered.

The recent documentation of the close genetic relationship between *B. bacilliformis* and certain plant bacterial pathogens that cause verrucous-like plant lesions has given life to an Andean mountain "old wives' tale." Mountain clinicians have long suggested that the disease agent of bartonellosis is maintained in a local succulent plant, and that the sandfly while feeding on its juices becomes infected and later transmits the infection to a human while taking a blood meal.

There are no data to support this hypothesis, but studies in Peru are currently in progress.

Reservoir Hosts. An animal reservoir for bartonellosis has not been seriously entertained since early studies could not culture B. bacilliformis from the blood of several domestic and wild animals in the endemic area. However, a recent epidemic investigation in Ecuador documented sick or dying chickens and the presence of ticks within the house as risk factors for verrucous bartonellosis. These data plus the recent discovery of nonbacilliformis Bartonella species in wild rodents in the United States and Peru, some with verrucous-like lesions, reopen the issue of the role of an animal reservoir.

During the 1913 Harvard expedition to study bartonellosis in Peru, 53 asymptomatic humans from the endemic region had their blood cultured for B. bacilliformis; 5 were positive. Although rarely emphasized and never dealt with as a public health issue, the human was presumed to be the reservoir host. Over the next eight decades an occasional patient was reported to remain bacteremic for up to 15 months after acute bartonellosis, but the public health issue of a chronic asymptomatic carrier state was not studied until a population-based prospective study in an endemic region of Peru documented asymptomatic bacteremia in 0.7% of the inhabitants.

DISTRIBUTION. B. bacilliformis has been cultured only from patients living in elevated valleys of the Andes Mountains in Peru, Ecuador, and Colombia. Most disease is found at elevations from 800 to 3200 M above sea level where temperatures are moderate with little day-to-day variation throughout the year, and rainfall is sparse and occurs mostly from December to May. Bartonellosis is said to be seasonal (May to August); however, the minimal surveillance data that are available do not demonstrate seasonality. Collective community wisdom reports periodic epidemic years, when both the number of cases and disease severity increase. Bartonellosis may be increasing in frequency, and some attribute this to a decrease in use of the residual insecticide dichlorodiphenyltrichloroethane (DDT) in malaria and leishmania vector control programs. The geographic distribution and clinical manifestations of bartonellosis are reported to be changing. An aggressive verrucous bartonellosis has recently been reported from the western coastal desert region of Ecuador. Cases have been recorded in the jungle highlands of Peru.

Children <10 years of age are most often stricken by the acute and chronic forms of bartonellosis, with documented cases occurring in children 1 month old; adults who relocate from a nonendemic area to an endemic region are often infected. The age distribution of disease suggests that naturally acquired immunity may play a role in reduced acquisition. A noticeable number of pregnant women develop acute Bartonella infections in the third trimester of pregnancy and there have been reports of fetal wastage associated with maternal acute hematic disease. A clearly documented case in a traveler has been reported. ABO blood type, gender, and race do not appear to be risk factors.

CLINICAL MANIFESTATIONS AND COMPLICATIONS

Incubation Period. Because the mechanism of disease transmission is uncertain, the incubation period cannot be reliably calculated. Based on immigrant relocation to endemic regions, the incubation period for bartonellosis has been estimated to be from 7 to 100 days; typically it is 3 weeks in patients with Oroya fever. It is often longer in patients who manifest only skin lesions. There is no information to determine the incubation period of the asymptomatic bacteremic patient.

Pathogenesis. It is hypothesized that B. bacilliformis is inoc-

ulated into the subdermal vascular bed by a blood feeding vector. Presumably the organism has an affinity for vascular epithelium and erythrocytes and proliferation takes place until a sustainable infection is achieved. In acute hematic disease, virtually all of the peripheral erythrocytes of the severely ill patient may be infected, with individual cells showing as many as 20 bacilliform organisms. Entry of the organism into the erythrocyte has been associated with an extracellular protein, deformin, synthesized by B. bacilliformis, which causes specific deformation of erythrocyte membranes. Hemolysis follows invasion and may be abrupt and profound. A significant erythroid hyperplasia results in an outpouring of nucleated cells, a macrocytosis, and a profound reticulocytosis that may exceed 50%. Leukocyte counts are variable, but marked leukocytosis is rare. Thrombocytopenia may occur. In vitro studies suggest that bacteria multiply inside the erythrocyte, or multiple organisms may result from multiple invasions. The mechanism of hemolysis is not known, but presumably correlates with erythrocyte damage and subsequent removal by hepatosplenic erythrophagocytosis. Death is sometimes associated with central nervous system (CNS) symptoms; examination of the cerebrospinal fluid may show pleocytosis and B. bacilliformis.

After the acute disease stage B. bacilliformis organisms disappear from the blood and relocate in focal areas of subcutaneous tissues. Focal bacterial proliferation is obvious on pathologic examination of verruga peruana lesions. Lesions contain large numbers of organisms both inside vascular epithelial cells and in the extracellular spaces. Lesions are characterized by vascular proliferation, which in vitro has been associated with live B. bacilliformis and homogenates of live B. bacilliformis.

Acute Hematic Disease. The acute blood stage disease may begin insidiously with anorexia, malaise, headache, and intermittent low fever (37.5° to 38°C) or abruptly with chills, high fever, profuse sweating, prostration, and altered consciousness. Musculoskeletal discomfort is common and often severe. As the anemia and febrile state progress, weakness, dyspnea, vertigo, nausea, vomiting, and syncope are followed by complete prostration, often with delirium or CNS signs. Carditis has been documented, but pulmonary-specific disease is uncommon. Physical findings include apathy and profound pallor often mistaken for jaundice. Generalized nontender lymphadenopathy, tachycardia, and hemic murmurs, if anemia is prominent, are common. Severely ill patients display dehydration, peripheral circulatory collapse, delirium, and bleeding diathesis if thrombocytopenia develops.

Death may occur in ≤10 days but often is delayed for 3 or 4 weeks. If the patient survives without complication, the fever abates and the anemia stabilizes and slowly improves, but it sometimes takes months to regain normal blood counts. Convalescence is gradual, and the disease enters a latent stage that generally is followed by the development of cutaneous lesions or other late complications. Case-fatality rates vary greatly depending on availability of antibiotic therapy, co-infections, and epidemic state. Community epidemics which are complicated by salmonellosis and no access to antibiotics, report case-fatality rates of 90%, whereas patients with uncomplicated sporadic disease who present early and are quickly treated with antibiotics have a >95% chance of survival.

Complications. Salmonellosis is the most important and predictable complication of bartonellosis, commonly appearing during convalescence from acute hematic disease that has not been treated with antibiotics. Worsening of the patient's condition may be marked by renewed chills and prostration, high fever, gastrointestinal symptoms, and hepatosplenomegaly. Other terminal complicating infections include disseminated toxoplasmosis, staphylococcal sepsis, and reactivated histoplasmosis. The specific susceptibility of patients with acute hemolytic bartonellosis to intercurrent infection likely relates to nonspecific immunosuppression; hypotheses regarding mechanisms include reticuloendothelial blockade by erythrophagocytosis interfering with intracellular killing mechanisms, or the potentiation of free iron from hemolysis causing the pathogenesis of other organisms.

Epidemic cases of bartonellosis have an increased fatality rate, greater than that attributed to *Salmonella* co-infection and/or the absence of prompt antibiotic therapy. Local physicians believe that the organisms associated with epidemics are inherently more virulent. Recurrent episodes of acute bartonellosis may occur. A recent hospital case record review revealed that in 3 of 51 slide-proven cases, the patients had hospital-documented episodes of acute disease 4 to 6 years previously. No data are available pertaining to variations in the pathogenicity of individual strains of *B. bacilliformis* or the mechanisms of immune protection in humans.

Chronic Verrucous Disease. It is likely that chronic verrucous disease is the evolution of the relationship between the agent and the host, with a transition from an acute, highly fatal hemolytic disease to a teleologically sustainable chronic disease state. Little representative epidemiologic data exist to determine what percentage of acute disease patients evolve to this chronic stage. The clinical impression is that about 50% of acute patients develop chronic verrucous disease, whereas >50% of verrucous patients give no clear history of prior acute bartonellosis. In most cases of verrucous disease there is a prodrome, which is marked by various signs of subacute infection in a partially immune host, e.g., phlebitis, pleuritis, parotitis, meningoencephalitis, and erythemas. Transitory, but often severe, myalgias and arthralgia may occur, frequently with paresthesias and pruritus in this preeruptive stage.

In the verrucous phase skin lesions appear after 1 to several months of prodromal symptoms, arising as soft, round, movable nodules beginning subcutaneously and evolving to erythematous papules that rapidly enlarge to their final size. These are painful to palpation and warm to the touch. The rapid growth phase is analogous to the rapid vascular proliferation within a pyogenic granuloma, which they resemble. The lesions are most frequently present on extensor surfaces of the extremities or on the face, sometimes on the scalp or genitalia, and occasionally in a generalized distribution. Clinical designations are based on size and number: (1) miliary lesions are numerous, small (2 to 3 mm) papules resembling small pyogenic granulomas scattered over the body, mildly tender to palpation and movable (Fig. 60–1); (2) nodular lesions are fewer and larger, tend to occur over joints, and are painful (Fig. 60–2); and (3) large tumors, often measuring several centimeters in diameter, tend to ulcerate (often called "mular" after a large, similar-appearing growth in mules) (Fig. 60–3). The three forms may be seen together because the lesions appear in successive crops. Frequently one or more nodular lesions erupt into a markedly protuberant red raspberry–like lesion. The preponderance of lesions on exposed skin surfaces may be related to vector feeding sites. Mucosal lesions occur, and analogous lesions within the mesenchymal tissue of many organs have been reported at autopsy.

Verrucous lesions may bleed profusely after mild trauma or biopsy and become secondarily infected. All lesions regress over some months, and new lesions cease to arise. As healing occurs, they become less erythematous, flatten, and eventually leave a hypopigmented macule surrounded by a zone of hyperpigmentation. Verruga peruana has many clini-

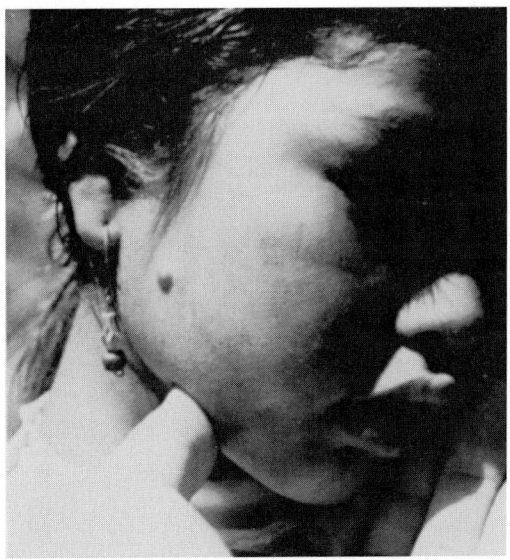

Figure 60–1. Bartonellosis. Characteristic papule on the face of a young Peruvian girl.

cal resemblances to bacillary angiomatosis, caused by *B. henselae* and most often seen in HIV patients in North America, and the clinical pathology of the two diseases is virtually identical.

DIAGNOSIS. The vast majority of cases of acute hematic bartonellosis are diagnosed in small regional hospitals or

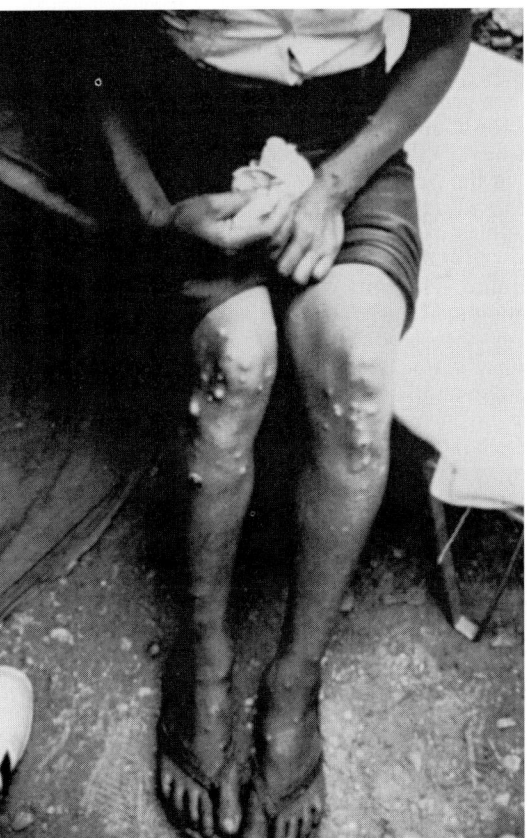

Figure 60–2. Bartonellosis. Numerous characteristic nodular lesions on the knees of a Peruvian woman.

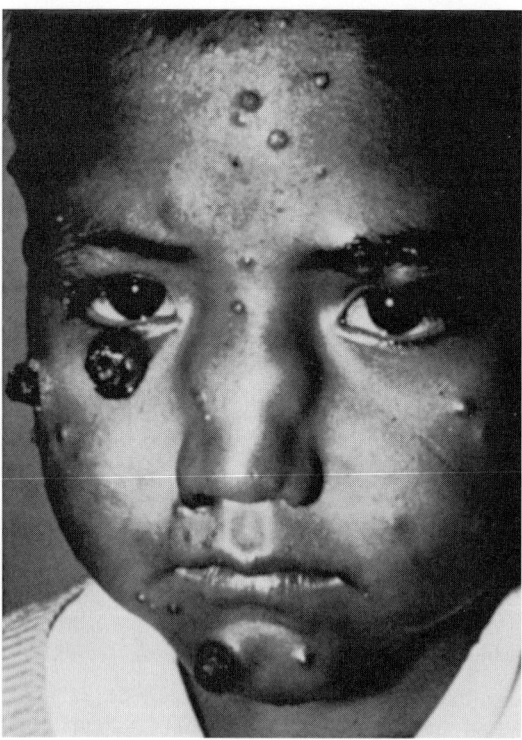

Figure 60–3. Bartonellosis. Large "mular" lesions with ulcerations on the face of Peruvian boy.

clinics in the Andes Mountains. Cases are identified by the clinical syndrome of fever, pallor, and residence in an endemic region, and by the demonstration of intraerythrocytic bacteria in a Giemsa- or Wright-stained thin blood film (see Fig. 60–4 in color section). Few regional laboratory technicians are provided the proper training for staining and reading blood films for *Bartonella*, and poorly stained smears are frequently incorrectly read as positive. Definitive diagnosis rests on the isolation of *B. bacilliformis* from blood culture, a procedure that is available only in sophisticated tertiary medical centers in the largest cities, away from the endemic regions.

Chronic verrucous disease is identified when multiple hemangioma-like cutaneous papules, nodules, or tumors (Figs. 60–1 to 60–3) appear on a person with or without a history of febrile anemia, who has been in the endemic area. The differential diagnosis of a solitary lesion includes hemangioma, pyogenic granuloma, molluscum contagiosum, and spindle cell and epithelioid nevus of Spitz. Skin biopsy and culture of a representative lesion with identification of characteristic organisms provides confirmation. Blood cultures are sterile and thin blood films are negative during this stage of disease.

Asymptomatic carriers of *B. bacilliformis* can only be identified by blood culture; thin blood films are negative. Colombia agar with 5% defibrinated human blood or semisolid nutrient agar with 10% fresh rabbit serum and 0.5% rabbit hemoglobin is an appropriate aerobic growth medium; growth occurs best at 28°C, small colonies becoming apparent in 7 to 10 days. Laboratory strains of *B. bacilliformis* grow well in Trager-Jensen in vitro malaria culture systems.

Some research laboratories offer serologic tests that use antigens prepared from cultured organisms for determination of antibodies by fluorescence antibody test, indirect hemagglutination, and enzyme immunoassay. It has been difficult to standardize these assays and correlate them to clinical

disease states. PCR assays to detect specific *B. bacilliformis* DNA are being tested on clinical specimens and may become a valuable diagnostic test.

TREATMENT AND PROGNOSIS. There have been no clinical trials to determine the efficacy of antibiotics in the treatment of any form of bartonellosis, and no standardized in vitro antibiotic sensitivity tests against *B. bacilliformis* are available. In clinical practice a variety of antibiotics, including penicillin, tetracycline, streptomycin, and chloramphenicol, have provided clinical remission of acute hematic symptoms. Chloramphenicol is the drug of choice for acute disease in endemic populations because it is readily available, inexpensive, and is effective against *Salmonella* infection, a feared complication. Blood transfusions and supportive measures are essential in severely anemic cases. With antibiotic therapy, defervescence occurs within 24 to 72 hours; organisms seen on blood films tend to become coccoid, and their numbers diminish. Blood cultures may continue to be positive in some patients after clinically adequate therapy. Opinions vary as to whether antibiotic therapy of acute disease protects against the later development of verrucous lesions.

Chronic verrucous disease responds poorly to most antibiotic therapy. Recent clinical experience suggests that rifampin reduces the size and pain of large lesions. Most patients with chronic verrucous disease do not seek medical attention because of the expense of antibiotics and the sublethal nature of the disease.

Bibliography

Alexander B: A review of bartonellosis in Ecuador and Colombia. Am J Trop Med Hyg 52:354, 1995.
Amano Y, Rumbea J, Knobloch J, et al: Bartonellosis in Ecuador: Serosurvey and current status of cutaneous verrucous disease. Am J Trop Med Hyg 57:174, 1997.
Birtles RJ: Differentiation of *Bartonella* species using restriction endonuclease analysis of PCR-amplified 16S rRNA genes. FEMS Microbiol Lett 129:261, 1995.
Caceres-Rios H, Rodriquez-Tafur J, Bravo-Puccio F, et al: Verruga peruana: An infectious endemic angiomatosis. Crit Rev Oncol 6:47, 1995.
Cooper P, Guderian R, Paredes W, et al: Bartonellosis in Zamor Chinchipe province in Ecuador. Trans R Soc Trop Med Hyg 90:241, 1996.
Garcia FR, Wojta J, Hoover RL: Interactions between live *Bartonella bacilliformis* and endothelial cells. J Infect Dis 165:1138, 1992.
Gray GC, Johnson AA, Thornton SA: An epidemic of Oroya fever in the Peruvian Andes. Am J Trop Med Hyg 42:215, 1990.
Ihler GM: *Bartonella bacilliformis*: Dangerous pathogen slowly emerging from deep background. FEMS Microbiol Lett 144:1, 1996.
Krueger CM, Marks KL, Ihler GM: Physical map of the *Bartonella bacilliformis* genome. J Bacteriol 177:7271, 1995.
Minnick MF, Mitchell SJ, McAllister SJ: Cell entry and the pathogenesis of *Bartonella* infections. Trends Microbiol 4:343, 1996.
Mitchell SJ, Minnick MF: Characterization of a two-gene locus from *Bartonella bacilliformis* associated with the ability to invade human erythrocytes. Infect Immun 63:1552, 1995.

60.2 *Cat-Scratch Disease*

Simin Goral and Kathryn M. Edwards

DEFINITION. Cat-scratch disease (CSD) in most patients is an acute, self-limited infection characterized by development of a papule at the site of inoculation by a cat, followed by regional adenopathy that may persist for 1 to 4 months. In a small percentage of patients serious systemic complications including involvement of the CNS, liver, spleen, lung, bone, eyes, and skin may arise.

HISTORY AND ETIOLOGY. Although CSD was recognized as a clinical entity in the 1930s, the first written report was not published until 1950 by Debre in France. The causative

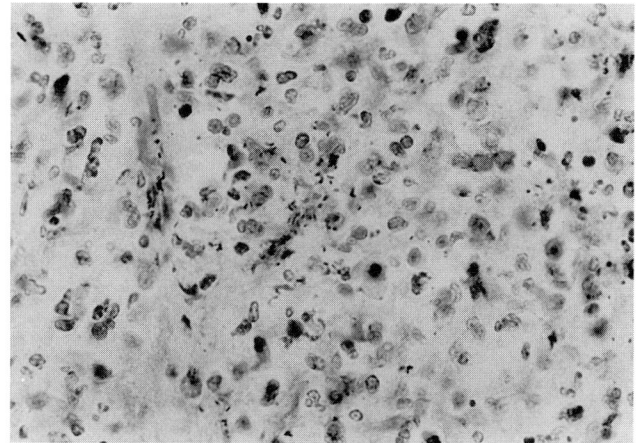

Figure 60–5. Warthin-Starry stain discloses cat-scratch bacilli.

agent of CSD has been sought for many years. In 1983, Wear and colleagues demonstrated small, pleomorphic, gram-negative bacilli in lymph nodes and skin papules from patients with CSD using a Warthin-Starry stain (Fig. 60–5). Initial attempts to culture the bacillus were unsuccessful. Subsequently, a bacterium was grown from CSD lymph nodes by English and colleagues and named *Afipia felis*. The discovery of bacillary angiomatosis (BA), the observation of similar organisms in tissue from BA and CSD patients, and the association of BA with *Bartonella* (formerly *Rochalimaea*) *henselae* stimulated further investigation of the role of this organism in CSD. In 1992, Regnery and colleagues showed elevated antibodies to *B. henselae* by indirect fluorescent antibody (IFA) test in serum samples from patients with suspected CSD. *B. henselae* has been cultured from lymph nodes obtained from patients with CSD. Purulent material aspirated from involved nodes was positive for *B. henselae* by PCR amplification and patients with CSD have IgM and IgG antibodies to *B. henselae*.

B. henselae, closely related to the trench fever agent *Bartonella quintana*, is a fastidious gram-negative rod. It is slow-growing and catalase- and oxidase-negative. Colony morphology is varied, ranging from small, dry, gray-white colonies to smooth, creamy yellow colonies.

EPIDEMIOLOGY AND TRANSMISSION. CSD occurs worldwide in all races, more often in males than in females. The Centers for Disease Control and Prevention (CDC) estimates that over 24,000 cases of CSD occur annually in the United States, of which approximately 2000 require hospitalization. The majority are reported in the fall and winter but patients can be infected during any season. About 90% of patients have a history of exposure to cats; CSD is strongly associated with owning a kitten, particularly a kitten with fleas, and a scratch or bite from a kitten. Although they remain asymptomatic, domestic cats serve as persistent reservoirs for *B. henselae*. Blood samples cultured from pet and impounded cats in the San Francisco Bay region grew *B. henselae* in 41% of these cats. *B. henselae* was detected in fleas from infected cats by both direct culture and PCR and cat fleas readily transmit *B. henselae* to cats.

PATHOLOGY

Inoculation Lesion. Examination of the primary inoculation lesion demonstrates dermal necrosis with variable numbers of histiocytes and occasional multinucleated giant cells accompanied by scattered microabscesses with neutrophils, eosinophils, lymphocytes, and plasma cells. The epidermal changes are nonspecific with parakeratosis, hyperkeratosis, edema, and exocytosis of inflammatory cells.

Adenopathy. Early in the course of infection lymph nodes show reactive lymphoid follicular hyperplasia with initial minute microabscesses adjacent to the subcapsular sinus. As the disease progresses, the histopathologic findings in involved lymph nodes characteristically reveal necrotizing granulomas with central microabscesses and palisading histiocytes. Most of the necrotic centers have a stellate configuration. Multinucleated giant cells in lymph nodes are either rare or absent. A perivascular neutrophilic infiltrate may be present. The Warthin-Starry or Steiner silver impregnation stains may reveal pleomorphic bacilli in clusters or short chains within the areas of central necrosis or around small vessels (Fig. 60–5). Although these histopathologic features are characteristic of CSD, they are not diagnostic and must be correlated to clinical findings and serologic studies. Other infections, e.g., tularemia, lymphogranuloma venereum, and fungal and mycobacterial infections may have a similar histology.

CLINICAL MANIFESTATIONS AND COURSE

Inoculation Lesion. The typical course of CSD begins with an erythematous papule or pustule at the inoculation site of a scratch or contact with a cat which usually persists for 1 to 3 weeks (Figs. 60–6 and 60–7A). An inoculation site may be detected in two thirds of patients. Within 2 weeks, lymph nodes draining the site of inoculation become enlarged and tender.

Regional Lymphadenitis. Lymphadenopathy occurs in >90% of patients with CSD; it usually resolves spontaneously within a period of several months. In about 50% of cases, regional lymphadenitis is the only manifestation of the

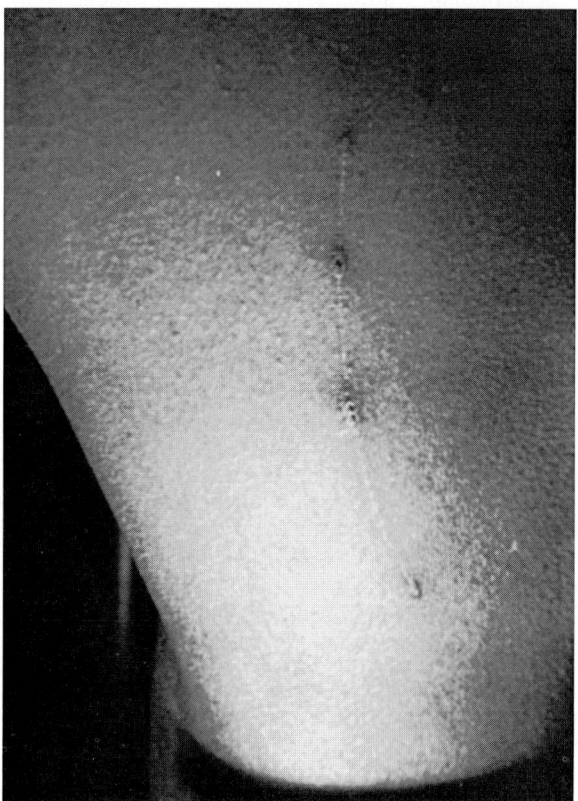

Figure 60–6. CSD in a 10-year-old boy with four crusted primary cat-scratch inoculation papules on left knee for 2 weeks. Inguinal lymphadenitis present for 10 days resolved spontaneously in 2.5 months. Cat-scratch skin test was positive. (Courtesy of A. M. Margileth.)

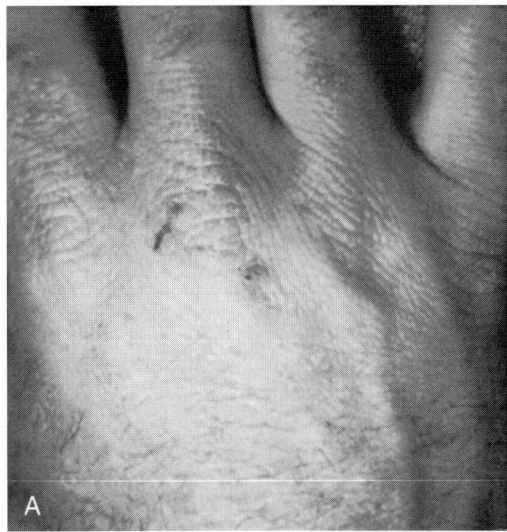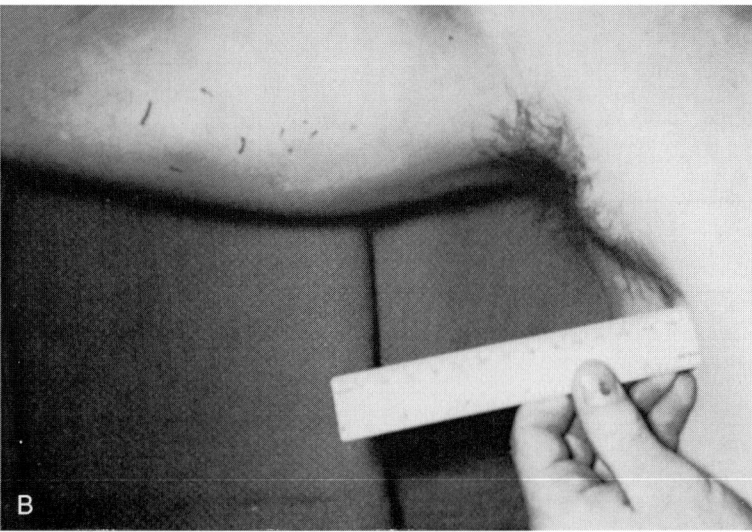

Figure 60–7. *A,* CSD in a 22-year-old male: three primary cat-scratch inoculation papules on hand for 4.5 weeks. *B,* Epitrochlear, brachial, and axillary lymphadenitis was present for 3 weeks along with fever, malaise, anorexia, and an 8-lb weight loss. Adenopathy resolved spontaneously in 6 to 7 months. (Courtesy of A. M. Margileth.)

disease. The adenopathy most commonly occurs in the head and neck area, followed by the upper and then the lower extremities (Fig. 60–7*B*). Suppuration of the involved lymph nodes occurs in about 10%. Constitutional symptoms of fever, anorexia, malaise, and headache accompany the lymphadenitis in 75% of patients, but in the majority these symptoms are mild.

Oculoglandular Syndrome. Atypical presentations occur in up to 15% of patients. Parinaud oculoglandular syndrome, the most common atypical feature, was first described by Henri Parinaud in 1889. It is characterized by ocular granuloma or conjunctivitis with preauricular lymphadenopathy and fever (Fig. 60–8). The affected eye is painless and nonpruritic and shows no evidence of discharge. Most patients recover spontaneously without any residua in 2 to 4 months.

Other Clinical Manifestations. These include encephalopathy, aseptic meningitis, seizures, neuroretinitis, transverse myelitis, osteolytic lesions, hepatic and splenic granulomas, thrombocytopenic purpura, hemolytic anemia, endocarditis, atypical pneumonia, pleural effusion, pulmonary nodules, breast mass, multiple granulomatous skin lesions, and recurrent adenopathy.

Neurologic Syndromes. In patients with CNS involvement, encephalopathy is the most common reported manifestation, occurring in 2 to 3%. Typically, 1 to 6 weeks after onset of lymphadenopathy, patients become abruptly confused and disoriented, rapidly progressing to coma. Cranial CT is generally normal, and cerebrospinal fluid shows minimal pleocytosis or elevation of protein. Electroencephalography is frequently abnormal. Neurologic recovery is almost always complete within 1 week, but persistent deficits have been reported.

Systemic CSD. There have also been reports of patients presenting with recurrent fever, malaise, fatigue, and weight loss without obvious site of focal infection. The symptoms may persist for weeks to months before the diagnosis is made.

DIAGNOSIS. Until recently, the clinical diagnosis of CSD required the presence of 3 of 4 criteria: (1) a history of contact with a cat and the presence of a scratch or primary dermal or eye lesion; (2) a positive CSD skin test; (3) negative serologic studies and cultures of aspirated pus or lymph nodes for other causes of lymphadenopathy; and (4) histopathologic

findings in a biopsy specimen consistent with CSD. The skin test antigen, first used in 1946, is prepared from lymph node aspirates from confirmed CSD patients and is 90 to 98% sensitive and specific for the diagnosis of CSD. However, use of the CSD skin test antigen is limited by both the absence of a standardized commercial source and by the potential risk of transmission of other infectious agents. New diagnostic techniques for detecting antibody and DNA, including IFA, enzyme immunoassay, and PCR, are safe, rapid, and reduce the need for skin testing and for biopsy. *B. henselae* can also be isolated from blood and from lymph nodes, liver, spleen, and skin lesions.

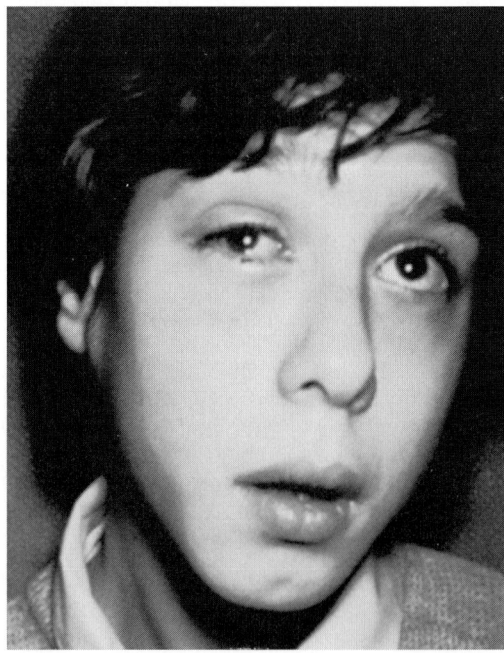

Figure 60–8. Oculoglandular syndrome of Parinaud in a 13-year-old; she had 2 weeks of fever, conjunctivitis, and a 5-mm ocular granuloma associated with preauricular adenitis. Adenopathy resolved after several months. (Courtesy of A. M. Margileth.)

The differential diagnosis of CSD includes lymphogranuloma venereum, syphilis, typical or atypical tuberculosis, other forms of bacterial adenitis, sporotrichosis, tularemia, brucellosis, histoplasmosis, sarcoidosis, toxoplasmosis, infectious mononucleosis, and benign or malignant tumors.

TREATMENT. In the majority of patients, CSD resolves spontaneously in 1 to 2 months.

Antibiotic Therapy. There are no controlled studies of antibiotic effectiveness. In Margileth's review of 202 patients with CSD, trimethoprim-sulfamethoxazole, ciprofloxacin, gentamicin, and rifampin appeared effective in 58 to 87% of cases, with rifampin having the highest response rate. Therapy with penicillins or cephalosporins does not appear effective. In vitro susceptibility data, particularly with beta lactam antibiotics, may not correlate with in vivo results. Treatment with erythromycin or doxycycline—either alone or in combination with rifampin—at standard doses but for longer duration (4 to 6 weeks) was also effective and safe in both immunocompetent and immunosuppressed patients. Currently, the role of systemic steroid therapy including for patients with neuroretinitis is not clear.

Local Treatment. Application of moist soaks, local heat, analgesics, limitation of activity, and aspiration of suppuration may help to relieve the pain and resolve the inflammation. Aspiration is preferred to surgical drainage which may lead to fistula formation or scarring.

PROGNOSIS AND PREVENTION. In typical CSD patients, complications are uncommon and the prognosis is excellent. Recurrent attacks are rare and systemic sequelae are unusual. Isolation is unnecessary. Currently, preventive measures with vaccines (either for humans or cats) are not available. Cat owners should be encouraged to take their pets to routine veterinary visits and prevent ectoparasite infections.

Bibliography

Bogue CW, Wise JD, Gray GF, et al: Antibiotic therapy for cat-scratch disease. JAMA 262:813, 1989.

Carithers HA: Cat-scratch disease: An overview based on a study of 1,200 patients. Am J Dis Child 139:1124, 1985.

Chomel BB, Wasten RW, Floyd-Hawkins K, et al: Experimental transmission of Bartonella henselae by the cat flea. J Clin Microbiol 34:1952, 1996.

Dolan MJ, Wong MT, Regnery RL, et al: Syndrome of Rochalimaea henselae adenitis suggesting cat scratch disease. Ann Intern Med 118:331, 1993.

Goral S, Anderson B, Hager C, et al: Detection of Rochalimaea henselae DNA by polymerase chain reaction from suppurative nodes of children with cat scratch disease. Pediatr Infect Dis J 13:994, 1994.

Koehler JE, Glaser CA, Tappero JW: Rochalimaea henselae infection: A new zoonosis with the domestic cat as reservoir. JAMA 271:531, 1994.

Margileth AM: Antibiotic therapy for cat-scratch disease: Clinical study of therapeutic outcome in 268 patients and a review of the literature. Pediatr Infect Dis J 11:474, 1992.

Regnery RL, Anderson BE, Clarridge JE, et al: Characterization of a novel Rochalimaea species, R. henselae sp. nov., isolated from blood of a febrile, human immunodeficiency virus–positive patient. J Clin Microbiol 30:265, 1992.

Regnery RL, Olson JG, Perkins BA, et al: Serological response to Rochalimaea henselae antigen in suspected cat-scratch disease. Lancet 339:1443, 1992.

Scott MA, McCurley TL, Vnencak-Jones CL, et al: Detection of Bartonella henselae DNA in archival biopsies from patients with clinically, serologically, and histologically defined disease. Am J Pathol 149:2, 1996.

Szelc-Kelly CM, Goral S, Perez-Perez GI, et al: Serologic responses to Bartonella and Afipia antigens in patients with cat scratch disease. Pediatrics 96:1137, 1995.

Zangwill KM, Hamilton DH, Perkins BA, et al: Cat scratch disease in Connecticut: Epidemiology, risk factors, and evaluation of a new diagnostic test. N Engl J Med 329:8, 1993.

60.3 *Vascular Angiomatosis*

Michael T. Wong

DESCRIPTION. Bacillary angiomatosis (BA) is a disease representing one aspect of the spectrum of infections due to the fastidious organisms *Bartonella (Rochalimaea) quintana* and *B. henselae*. More reliable diagnostic and identification methods are providing a better understanding of the ubiquitous distribution of both organisms and of the expanding spectrum and overlap of disease caused by these two organisms.

TRANSMISSION AND EPIDEMIOLOGY. BA usually occurs as sporadic infections and in most cases exposure to adult cats or kittens may be documented. However, clustered outbreaks and infection without any exposure to domestic pets have also been described, suggesting a potential arthropod vector.

B. quintana was first described as a cause of recurrent fevers in Ireland, and later found throughout Europe as the cause of trench fever in World War I. It had not been reported as a pathogen again until the mid-1980s. Since then, BA cases and *B. quintana* have been reported from every populated continent and the Pacific Rim. *B. henselae* has been similarly reported throughout North America, China, Sri Lanka, Australia, and Europe. In the United States, serologic and microbiologic culture data suggest a Pacific Coast predisposition for *B. quintana*, whereas *B. henselae* appears to be more widely distributed.

CLINICAL MANIFESTATIONS. BA most commonly presents as single or clustered, reddish papular lesions on the skin, but may also occur as brownish patches or subcutaneous nodules and may be confused with Kaposi sarcoma or disseminated fungal infections, e.g., *Cryptococcus neoformans* in the HIV-infected individual. Rarely, diffuse or isolated lymph node involvement can be seen without the characteristic rash. Systemic involvement may also occur, causing lytic bone lesions, peliosis hepatis, or dissemination to other visceral organs in more severe cases. Although descriptions of the disease were in patients with immune deregulation due to neoplastic processes, human immunodeficiency virus type I infection, or immunosuppressive therapy, BA has also been described in immunocompetent individuals. The severity of disease and presentation is related to the degree of immunologic competence of the host.

DIAGNOSIS

Histology. BA characteristically has vascular epithelioid hyperplasia, vascular lakes, and a mixed inflammatory response; interstitial bacillary elements are visualized by Warthin-Starry silver stain.

Serology. Serologic responses by IFA for antibodies to *B. quintana* and *B. henselae* may indicate recent infection. While the duration of antibody responses is not known, IFA reactivity has been documented to last for over 1 year in several longitudinally followed cases. PCR of the 16S ribosomal subunit or the citrate synthase gene with restriction fragment length polymorphisms has also been used for diagnosis.

Culture. Positive tissue and blood cultures are diagnostic but *B. quintana* and *B. henselae* are very slow growing and fastidious. The bacteria are pleomorphic, weakly gram-negative, and oxidase- and catalase-inert. Isolation may be achieved in a variety of liquid media, including HTM broth (BBL-Becton Dickinson). The highest yield of culture has been through Isolator (Wampole) lysis-centrifugation systems, although Bac-T-Alert and Bac-Tec blood culture systems may also support growth. In all cases, cultures must be held for up to 6 weeks, and isolation and subculture is performed with a high level of suspicion, as the growth-index readings do not register in the automated blood culture systems. The organisms are hemin-requiring with the highest success rates of subculture isolation on chocolate or CDC anaerobic blood agars, and occasionally on buffered-yeast charcoal-extract agar. Colony morphology may vary from dry, adherent whitish yellow colonies to somewhat moist, almost iridescent colonies. Identification may be made by measuring cellular fatty acid concentrations by gas-liquid chromatography demonstrating the characteristic C18:1, C18:0, and C16:0 fatty acids.

TREATMENT. BA requires systemic antimicrobial therapy, particularly when it occurs as an opportunistic infection in AIDS patients. Antimicrobial agents that develop high intracellular concentrations, e.g., doxycycline, rifampin, erythromycin, and the macrolides, and possibly trimethoprim-sulfamethoxazole, appear to have the best efficacy in treating and clearing infection. In severe cases, combination therapy with doxycycline or a macrolide and rifampin have been used with success. Minimal inhibitory concentrations for the fluoroquinolones are at the breakpoint and therefore may not be effective. The cell-wall active agents, including penicillins and cephalosporins, and aminoglycosides are ineffective. There is no clearly defined duration of therapy, although relapses have been seen with <4 weeks of treatment in both HIV patients and in others without evidence of immunosuppression.

Bibliography

Koehler JE, Quinn FD, Berger TG, et al: Isolation of *Rochalimaea* species from cutaneous and osseous lesions of bacillary angiomatosis. N Engl J Med 327:1625, 1992.

Tappero JW, Koehler JE, Berger TG, et al: Bacillary angiomatosis and bacillary splenitis in immunocompetent adults. Ann Intern Med 118:363, 1993.

Wong MT, Dolan MJ, Lattuada CP Jr, et al: Neuroretinitis, aseptic meningitis and lymphadenitis due to *Bartonella (Rochalimaea) henselae* in HIV infected and immunocompetent persons. Clin Infect Dis 21:352, 1995.

61 Plague*

David T. Dennis

DEFINITION. Plague is a zoonosis of rodents and their fleas caused by infection with *Yersinia pestis*. Natural cycles of plague occur in scattered, mostly rural foci in large areas of Asia, Africa, and the Americas. Infection results in an acute, often fatal disease that is notorious for its epidemic potential. Humans most often acquire infection by the bite of rodent fleas, less often by handling or ingesting infective animal tissues, and occasionally by airborne infection (Fig. 61–2). The principal clinical forms of plague are bubonic, septicemic, and pneumonic. Although the potential for rapid spread exists wherever plague occurs, epidemics can be prevented and controlled using standard public health measures.

HISTORY. The Justinian Pandemic (ca. 542–767 A.D.) began in Egypt and spread from there to Europe and Asia Minor, causing an estimated 40 million deaths. The Second Pandemic began in central Asia in the early 14th century, caused severe epidemics in China and India, moved along caravan routes to Constantinople, and spread through Persia and the Middle East to the Mediterranean region. Entering Sicily in

1347, it swept across Europe and the British Isles in successive waves over the next three centuries. Known as the "Black Death," medieval plague killed as many as a quarter or more of the affected populations at the height of its virulence. The latest pandemic, the Third (Modern) Pandemic, arose in southern China in the latter half of the 19th century, struck Hong Kong in 1894, and over the next several years spread by rat-infested steamships to major port cities throughout the world. Within 35 years of its appearance in Hong Kong, the Third Pandemic had resulted in an estimated 26 million plague cases and more than 12 million deaths, the vast majority occurring in India.

In 1894 Alexandre Yersin, in Hong Kong, isolated the plague bacillus from enlarged lymph nodes (buboes) of plague victims. In 1898, Paul-Louis Simond, a French scientist sent to investigate epidemic bubonic plague in Bombay, identified the plague bacillus in the tissues of dead rats and first proposed that the agent was transmitted from rat to rat, and from rats to humans, by rat fleas. Waldemar Haffkine, also working in Bombay, developed a crude vaccine of heat-killed bacilli to protect Indian populations against epidemic bubonic plague.

After 1900, the international spread of plague was largely halted by regulations that controlled rats in ports and required ships to be inspected and rat-proofed. However, by 1910 plague had become established in wild rodent populations in all inhabited continents other than Australia, resulting in many residual enzootic cycles of the plague bacillus that occur throughout the world today. For example, plague was imported into San Francisco in 1899, causing two major outbreaks in the city between 1900 and 1908. By 1908, plague was epizootic in ground squirrels in surrounding counties, and it has subsequently spread to various wild rodent populations throughout the western third of the United States.

Insecticides became widely available to control fleas in the 1940s, and antibiotics were first used to treat plague in the late 1940s. Since 1950, plague outbreaks have become mostly sporadic events that have been readily contained through surveillance, flea and rat control, and prompt diagnosis and treatment of plague patients. The major exception was the recurring rat-borne plague epidemics in war-torn Vietnam in 1962 to 1975.

Plague is 1 of 3 quarantinable diseases (plague, cholera, yellow fever) subject to the World Health Organization (WHO) *International Health Regulations*. In 1994, articles of these regulations were used to investigate reported outbreaks of plague in India, and to prevent spread of plague from India to other countries. Fear of plague in India evoked local panic and an exaggerated international response.

ETIOLOGY

General Microbiology. *Y. pestis* is a nonmotile, nonsporulating, gram-negative coccobacillus belonging to the family *Enterobacteriaceae*. It is microaerophilic, oxidase- and urease-negative, nonlactose fermenting, and biochemically unreactive. The organism is nonfastidious and is infective to laboratory rodents. It grows slowly, but well, on a wide variety of common liquid and solid microbiologic media (e.g., brain-heart infusion broth, sheep blood agar, chocolate agar, and MacConkey agar). It multiplies in a wide range of temperature (4° to 37°C) and pH (5.0 to 9.6), but grows optimally at 28°C and a pH of 7.4. Incubation of the plague bacillus at 37°C for 24 hours on agar plates results only in pinpoint, transparent, easily overlooked colonies; and, at 48 hours, the colonies are grayish, 1 to 2 mm in diameter, and have an irregular surface (hammered metal appearance) when viewed under magnification. In broth, *Y. pestis* grows in flocculent clumps, typically attached to the sides of tubes in a downwardly projecting stalactite fashion, and leaves a clear

---

*All the material in this chapter is in the public domain, with the exception of any borrowed figures or tables.

broth. Stained with a polychromatic stain, e.g., Wayson, Wright's, or Giemsa stain, plague bacilli obtained from clinical specimens demonstrate a characteristic bipolar appearance, often resembling "closed safety pins" (Fig. 61–1). *Y. pestis* is not truly encapsulated but produces an envelope that contains the unique fraction 1 (F1) glycoprotein surface antigen.

Although highly adapted to maintain its complex life cycle in rodent hosts and their fleas, the plague bacillus is not a saprophyte, and it is rapidly killed in nature by temperatures above 40°C and by desiccation.

Y. *pestis* Virulence Factors. *Y. pestis* possesses distinctive virulence factors important for survival in mammalian and flea hosts. The genes encoding these virulence factors are carried by three plasmids. The smallest (9.5 kb) of these is the pesticin or Pst plasmid, whose genes encode a plasminogen activator (Pla) and a bacteriocin (pesticin). Pesticin is thought to enhance iron uptake by *Y. pestis* in the mammalian host. The 70-kb low calcium response plasmid (Lcr) encodes gene products under low calcium environments. Plague organisms respond to low calcium environments by activating a group of virulence factors that include outer surface proteins (Yosp) and a soluble V antigen, which is essential for *Y. pestis* survival in macrophages. Lcr-positive strains are able to inhibit host production of gamma interferon and tumor necrosis factor alpha (TNF-α). Conversely, Lcr-negative strains are avirulent and do not inhibit cytokine activation in infected laboratory animals.

The pFra plasmid (110 kb) contains the genes encoding the F1 envelope antigen and the murine toxin. F1 antigen is produced only by organisms growing at ≥33°C. *Y. pestis* strains expressing the F1 antigen are resistant to phagocytosis in the absence of opsonizing antibodies. Murine exotoxin is highly toxic for mice and rats, but its effect in humans is not known.

Chromosomal genes encode several other virulence factors, including those associated with lipopolysaccharide endotoxin and with exogenous iron adsorption. The latter is manifest by pigment production when *Y. pestis* is grown on some media containing congo red, a heme analogue dye. Strains that do not produce pigment are usually avirulent to mammals and are unable to induce "blocking" of the flea gut. A chromosomally encoded product, the pH 6 antigen (Psa), is expressed under conditions of low pH and it may also inhibit phagocytosis of the plague bacillus.

Y. *pestis* Biotypes. Three biotypes of *Y. pestis,* classified on

TABLE 61–1. Reported Cases of Plague in Humans, by Country (1980–1994)

Continent	Country	No. of Cases	No. of Deaths
Africa	Angola	27	4
	Botswana	173	12
	Kenya	49	10
	Libya	8	0
	Madagascar	1390	302
	Malawi	9	0
	Mozambique	216	3
	South Africa	19	1
	Tanzania	4964	419
	Uganda	660	48
	Zaire	2242	513
	Zambia	1	1
	Zimbabwe	397	31
	Total	**10155**	**1344**
America	Bolivia	189	27
	Brazil	700	9
	Ecuador	83	3
	Peru	1722	112
	United States	229	33
	Total	**2923**	**184**
Asia	China	252	76
	India	876	54
	Kazakhstan	10	4
	Mongolia	59	19
	Myanmar	1160	14
	Vietnam	3304	158
	Total	**5661**	**325**
World Total		18739	1853

From World Health Organization: Human plague in 1994. Wkly Epidemiol Rec 22:165, 1996.

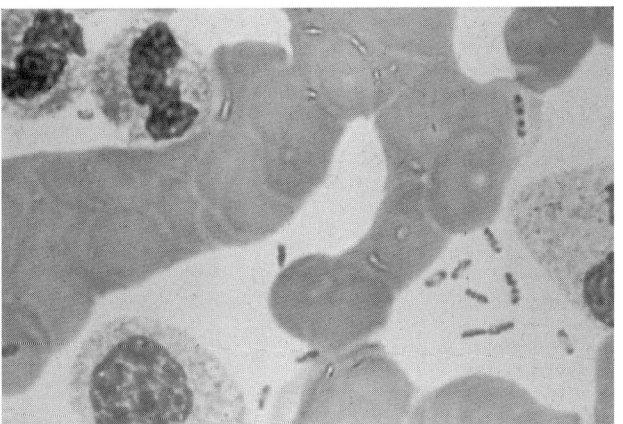

***Figure* 61–1.** Peripheral blood smear from a patient with fatal plague septicemia and shock, showing characteristic bipolar-staining *Yersinia pestis* (Wright's stain, oil immersion).

the ability to ferment glycerol and reduce nitrate, are correlated with the three major plague pandemics of history. These biotypes are named the antiqua, mediaevalis, and orientalis biotypes. The antiqua biotype occurs in parts of Africa, southeastern Russia, and central Asia; the mediaevalis biotype is found around the Caspian Sea; the orientalis biotype predominates in Asia, and it is the only biotype found in the Western Hemisphere. Ribotyping studies support these distinctions. In general, wild *Y. pestis* strains are stable and uniform in genetic complement and virulence throughout the world.

EPIDEMIOLOGY

Y. *pestis* Life Cycle. *Y. pestis* is maintained in rodents and their fleas in both wild rodent and domestic rodent cycles (Fig. 61–2). Humans become infected when they intrude into the natural wild cycle, or when domestic plague cycles become established. Person-to-person plague occurs as a result of close exposure to patients with respiratory plague, and very rarely as a result of direct skin or mucous membrane contact with infectious secretions or exudates. The transmission of infection from one person to another by fleas is controversial and, based on epidemiologic studies, its occurrence is considered to be rare.

Distribution of Human Plague. Plague foci are widely distributed throughout the world (Fig. 61–3), and human cases are reported in about 10 countries each year. The *International Health Regulations* require prompt reporting of plague cases to WHO. From 1980 through 1994, a total of 18,739 human plague cases (mean of 1249 per year) and 1853 (10%) deaths were reported by 24 countries to WHO (Table 61–1). More than half of the total number of cases were reported by countries in eastern and southern Africa, approximately a third in Asia, and the remaining sixth in the Americas. Recent outbreaks of plague have been reported by India, Vietnam, Myanmar, Tanzania, Democratic Republic of the Congo (DRC), Madagascar, Mozambique, and Peru. India, in 1994, reported its first cases of plague in nearly 30 years, when 876 bubonic and pneumonic plague cases and 54 deaths were reported from adjacent Maharashtra and Gujarat states, west-central India. Vietnam and Myanmar experienced both urban and rural plague and reported 1756 and 727 cases, respectively, in the period 1990 to 1994. Tanzania reported outbreaks involving 1293 cases in 1991 and 444 cases in 1994. DRC reported a total of 1397 cases in the period 1991 to 1994. Zimbabwe experienced outbreak activity involving 392 cases in 1994. Madagascar regularly reports cases, averaging 167 cases per year in the period 1990 to 1994; and, in 1995, 1996, and 1997, successive outbreaks of rat-borne bubonic plague occurred in the port city of Mahajanga.

In 1980 to 1994, the United States reported 229 plague cases (mean of 15 cases per year) and 33 (14%) deaths. Although enzootic and epizootic plague occurs in 17 of the contiguous western United States (Fig. 61–3), ≥80% of human cases occur in the southwestern states of New Mexico, Arizona, and Colorado, and approximately 10% in California. No plague cases have been reported by Canada or Mexico in recent decades.

Risk Factors for Human Plague. *Y. pestis* is universally infectious to humans.

Environmental Exposures. Differences in rates of infection and disease are determined by differences in environmental surroundings, human behaviors, and occupational and recreational activities that place persons at differing levels of exposure to infective fleas. Historically, persons with low socioeconomic status have been at greatest risk, especially for urban plague, since low standards of housing, environmental sanitation, and hygiene are associated with rat and flea infestations.

In the United States, more than half of all cases are thought to arise from plague cycles close to the patients' homes, especially in southwestern states where homes may be situated in natural surroundings that provide favorable habitat for plague-susceptible animals (e.g., rock squirrels and wood rats) or are situated near prairie dog colonies. In the Sierra Nevadas of California and Nevada, epizootic plague in chipmunks and ground squirrels poses a risk to visitors to public parks. Hikers, campers, and hunters in natural areas throughout the western states are at a small but definite risk of exposure, especially in the warmer months of the year.

Exposure to Infected Animals. Plague can be acquired as a result of skinning and handling carcasses of wild animals, e.g., rodents, rabbits and hares, prairie dogs, wildcats, and coyotes. Such direct inoculation is associated with an increased risk for primary septicemia and high fatality rates. In Mongolia and some areas of northeastern China, the hunting of marmots for fur and food is associated with an increased risk for plague. Furthermore, interperson pneumonic

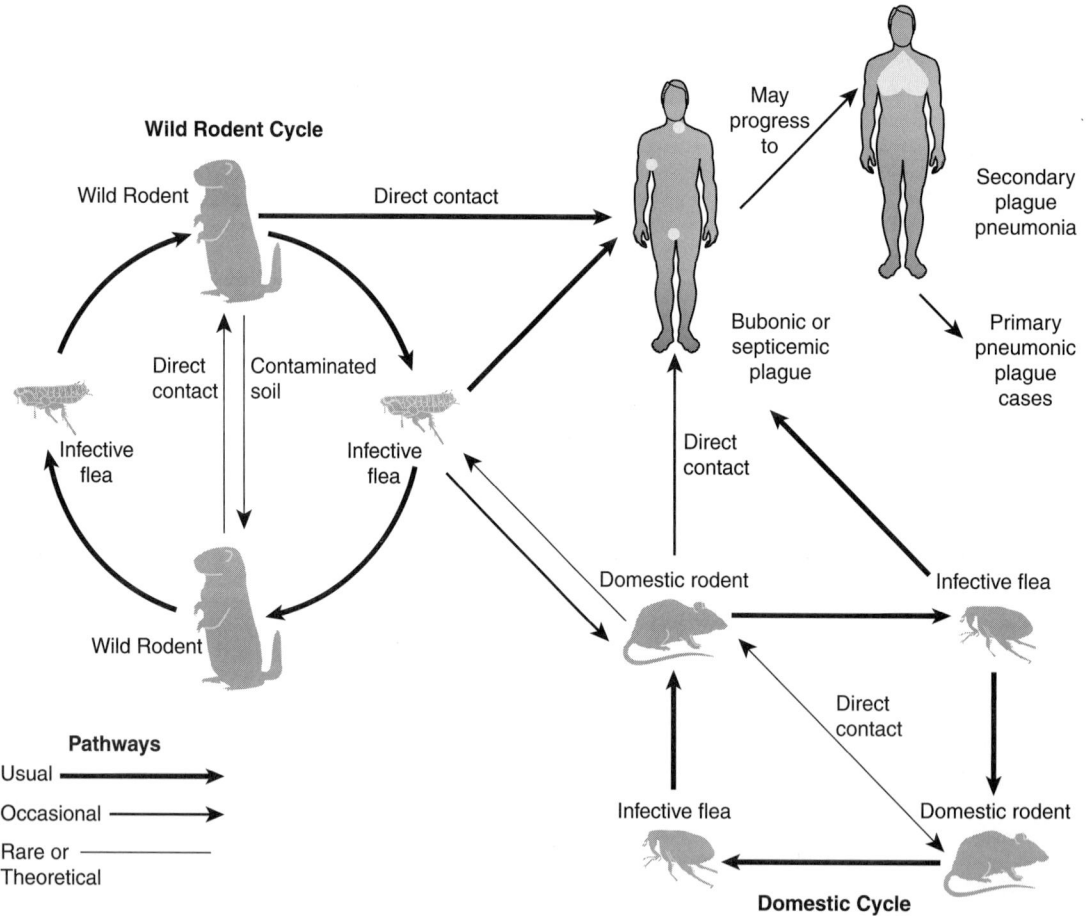

Figure 61–2. Animal and human plague transmission, demonstrating the interrelationship of the wild rodent and domestic rodent cycles and the routes of incidental infection of humans. (Adapted from Kartman L, Goldenberg MI, Hubbert WT: Recent observations on the epidemiology of plague in the United States. Am J Public Health 56:1554, 1966.)

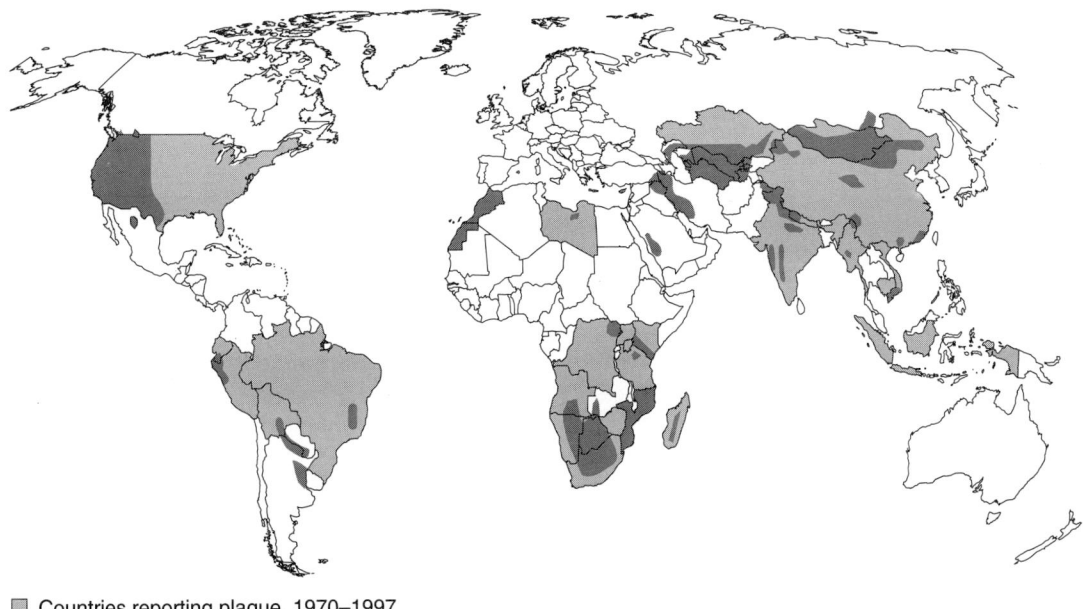

☐ Countries reporting plague, 1970–1997

■ Probable sylvatic foci

Compiled from WHO, CDC, and country sources.

Figure 61–3. Distribution of natural foci of plague. (Compiled from the World Health Organization, CDC, and other sources.)

spread is facilitated in the cramped living quarters of these nomadic hunters. Plague, including oropharyngeal plague, can result from the ingestion of undercooked contaminated meat and perhaps from the manual transfer of infected fluids to the mouth while handling infected animal tissues.

Exposures Influence Clinical Syndromes. In the United States, detailed information on clinical histories and infective exposures is available for plague cases. Among 364 evaluable patients reported in 1950 to 1994, 313 (84%) presented as primary lymphadenitic (bubonic) plague, almost all of which were thought to be associated with flea bites; 44 (12%) of these patients presented with primary septicemic plague, often following handling of infected animal tissues; and 7 (2%) patients presented with primary pneumonic plague with direct evidence that 5 cases had resulted from inhaling respiratory droplets expelled by infected domestic cats.

Respiratory Exposures. With the exception of outbreaks involving tens of thousands of cases of pneumonic plague in Manchuria in the early part of this century, respiratory spread of plague in the Third Pandemic and its aftermath occurred only sporadically and in limited clusters of close contacts of pneumonic plague patients, e.g., household members, patient visitors, and caregivers. A small outbreak of pneumonic plague occurred among household contacts and hospital staff caring for plague cases in Tanzania in 1991. *Y. pestis* does not disperse by aerosol but by respiratory droplet, and only those persons who have direct and close (2 m) respiratory exposure are at high risk of acquiring primary pneumonic plague. Primary plague pneumonia may, due to the watery nature of the sputum, be more contagious than secondary plague pneumonia.

Ecology. The natural history of *Y. pestis* is complex and habitat-specific, and a knowledge of the major ecologic factors supporting its life cycle is crucial in understanding the epidemiology of plague and its control and prevention. More than 200 species of mammals and 150 species of fleas have been found to be naturally infected with *Y. pestis*, although

relatively few are important in maintaining enzootic or epizootic cycles and fewer still pose a significant risk to humans.

Enzootic Plague. In its natural reservoir state, the plague bacillus is found in often silent or inapparent enzootic cycles involving relatively resistant rodents in mostly remote, sparsely populated areas of Asia, Africa, the Americas, and in limited rural foci in extreme southeastern Europe near the Caspian Sea (Fig. 61–3). These resistant rodents are able to circulate the organism in their blood and infect fleas that feed on them (Fig. 61–2). Although some of these rodents may sicken and die from plague, most tolerate the infection and population die-off does not occur. Other nonrodent mammals, although occasionally infected, do not contribute to the maintenance of these natural cycles. Cycles of enzootic transmission place humans at small direct risk, and cases that arise from enzootic exposures are typically infrequent and sporadic. Although these quiescent, enzootic cycles are often referred to as "sylvatic" plague, they most often occur throughout the world in campestral semiarid or arid grassland sites, e.g., the steppes of central Asia and the savannas of eastern Africa. Enzootic foci around the world have distinct ecological profiles, each with its own characteristic rodent and flea-host combinations.

Epizootic Plague. In epizootic plague, infection is spread rapidly in certain highly susceptible rodent populations by efficient and usually abundant flea vectors. Both rodents and fleas serve as amplifying hosts. Epizootics often result in local and sometimes widespread depopulation of affected rodents and a consequent dispersal of their fleas. Epizootic plague in rural foci may sometimes spread to rodent populations living in commensal association with humans (Fig. 61–2). Epizootics, therefore, pose a serious threat to humans. Historically, urban epidemics and pandemics of human plague have been associated with epizootics involving the commensal species, *Rattus rattus* and *Rattus norvegicus*. The smaller, domestic, roof or black rat (*R. rattus*) is considered the most dangerous host. This ubiquitous rodent has lived since ancient times in intimate domestic association with humans in many areas of Asia, the Middle East, and Africa. It first appeared in Europe in the Middle Ages, where it sustained the prolonged epidemics of plague, and spread to the New World during early periods of European colonization. The black rat lives in homes (from basements to attics), granaries, stables, warehouses, barns, and other places with ready harborage and food supplies. It travels easily with human cargo and baggage, and has, with its complement of fleas, been the principal agent of noncontiguous (per saltum) spread of plague.

R. norvegicus, the Norway rat, is larger and more aggressive than *R. rattus*. It is a burrowing rodent that mostly lives peridomestically around foundations of buildings, and frequents cellars, drains, sewers, alleyways, and refuse dumps. *R. rattus, R. norvegicus,* and the oriental rat flea, *Xenopsylla cheopis,* were instrumental in the global spread of plague during the Third Pandemic.

Although these domestic rats are the principal sources of infected fleas in human plague epidemics, they may not be capable of sustaining plague for long periods without reintroductions of *Y. pestis* from its natural sources. Enzootic wild rodent plague may spill directly into populations of rodents that live commensally with humans, or indirectly through intermediary rodent populations inhabiting agricultural sites adjacent to settlements. For example, recent investigations of plague in west-central India substantiated previously described "sylvatic" populations of gerbils *(Tatera indica)* as the probable reservoir source of plague. Where there is agriculture, they colonize cropland borders, and infection can spread by their fleas directly to *R. rattus* or indirectly through intermediary populations of bandicoot rats *(Bandicota bengalensis)* that are numerous in croplands surrounding rural villages.

The widely distributed oriental rat flea, *X. cheopis,* and the related species, *X. brasiliensis,* are efficient vectors of the plague bacillus between rats and are the most dangerous vectors to humans. At ambient temperatures of 28°C and below, *Y. pestis* can multiply exponentially in the gut of these fleas and result in a clotted bolus of organisms that blocks the passage of further blood meals at the level of the foregut. Regurgitation by a "blocked" flea while it feeds enhances transmission of the plague bacillus to a new host. The ability of *Y. pestis* to cause blockage has recently been shown to be plasmid mediated.

Incidental Animal Plague. In addition to rodent species that maintain enzootic and epizootic plague cycles, a diverse range of wild and domestic mammals become incidentally infected and can serve occasionally as sources of infection to humans, either through direct contact with infected tissues or exudates or by transport of infected rodent fleas into the peridomestic or domestic environment. Carnivores, especially felids, canids, and mustellids, are most notable in this regard. Infected felids, in contrast to canids, often become diseased, and domestic cats are an important source of human plague in the United States. Lagomorphs (rabbits, hares) can occasionally be a source of infection to hunters who handle contaminated carcasses. Ungulates, including antelope, deer, camels, and goats, can sicken and die from *Y. pestis* infection. Ingestion of undercooked infected goat and camel meat has been responsible for outbreaks of human plague in northern Africa, the Middle East, and in central Asia.

North American Plague Foci. Wild rodent plague has been reported west of the 100th meridian in 17 contiguous western states and in some areas of Canada and Mexico adjacent to U.S. plague foci. The major plague sites, however, are (a) the southwestern focus, comprising mainly semiarid grassland plateaus, foothills, and forested uplands of northeastern Arizona, most of New Mexico, southern Utah, and southern Colorado; (b) the Pacific coastal focus, comprising mostly valley grassland, foothill, and montane habitat of California and southern Oregon; (c) the Great Basin focus encompassing parts of Utah, Nevada, and southern Idaho; and (d) the Rocky Mountain and northern focus comprising mostly northern Colorado, Wyoming, and Montana.

Rodent Reservoirs. The principal rodent hosts in the southwestern focus are various burrowing ground squirrels *(Spermophilus* spp.), prairie dogs (primarily *Cynomys gunnisoni),* wood rats *(Neotoma* spp.), antelope ground squirrels *(Ammospermophilus* spp.), deer mice *(Peromyscus maniculatis),* and related species. The major rodent hosts in the various niches of the Pacific Coast focus include *Spermophilus* spp., especially the California ground squirrel *(Spermophilus beecheyi),* the golden manteled ground squirrel *(Spermophilus lateralis),* chipmunks (various *Tamias* spp.), deer mice and other *Peromyscus* spp., and voles *(Microtus* spp.). Other important hosts in the United States include various ground squirrels *(Spermophilus elegans, Spermophilus beldingi,* and *Spermophilus townsendi)* in the Rocky Mountain and Great Basin regions, and the black-tailed prairie dog *(Cynomys ludovicianus)* in the Great Plains region. Epizootics of plague have recently occurred in urban tree squirrel *(Sciurus niger)* populations in cities along the eastern foothills of the Colorado Rocky Mountains, but pose a small risk to humans because these squirrels are parasitized by fleas that rarely bite humans.

In the past several decades, *Y. pestis*–infected rodents have occasionally been found in large metropolitan sites (e.g., Tacoma, San Francisco, Los Angeles, Dallas). However, no widespread epizootics or human plague cases have resulted, possibly because rats collected in these cities have been infested with small numbers of fleas or with flea species that are inefficient vectors of *Y. pestis*.

Flea Vectors. The principal fleas transmitting plague among wild rodent epizootic hosts in the United States include various ground squirrel fleas *(Oropsylla montana* [*Diamanus montanus*], *Hoplopsyllus anomalus, Thrassis* spp., *Opisocrostis* spp., *Oropsylla idahoensis),* prairie dog fleas *(Opisocrostis* spp.), wood rat fleas *(Orchopeas* spp.), and chipmunk fleas *(Eumolpianus eumolpi). O. montana* is the most important vector of *Y. pestis* to persons in the United States because it is a competent host that readily feeds on a wide range of rodents and on other mammals, including humans.

South American Plague Foci. In South America, active enzootic plague foci exist in Brazil, Bolivia, Peru, and Ecuador, and have been described previously in Paraguay, Argentina, and Venezuela. *Y. pestis* infection in these foci has been variously found in commensal rats *(Rattus* spp.), cotton rats *(Sigmodon* spp.), rice rats *(Oryzomys* spp.), field mice *(Akodon* spp.) and cane mice *(Zygodontomys* spp.), wild cavies and domesticated guinea pigs *(Cavia* and *Galea* spp.). Domestic guinea pigs are reared in homes for food in the Andean region and have been considered a potential commensal risk of infection to humans; plague outbreaks in the Andean region, including a recent extensive bubonic plague epidemic in northern Peru, have been suspected to be associated with infected domestic guinea pigs as well as *R. rattus.* Fleas that serve as principal vectors in South American foci are *X. cheopis* on *Rattus* spp. and *Polygenis* and *Pleochaetis* spp. on wild rodents. *Pulex irritans,* the human flea (which also parasitizes domesticated guinea pigs), has been implicated as a potential transmitter of plague in some Andean outbreaks.

African Plague Foci. Widely scattered active plague foci exist in eastern and southern Africa, including DRC, Uganda, Kenya, Tanzania, Zambia, Zimbabwe, Mozambique, Botswana, South Africa, Namibia, and Angola, and on the island of Madagascar. Less active foci, most recently manifest as camel and goat associated human plague cases, exist in some northern Africa states (e.g., Libya) and on the Arabian Peninsula. The principal wild rodent hosts in Africa include gerbils (*Tatera* and *Desmodillus* spp.), swamp rats (*Otomys* spp.), various grass mice (*Arvicanthis* spp.), multimammate mice (*Mastomys* spp.), and commensal rats (*Rattus* spp.). One East African scenario describes plague in grassland gerbil populations spreading to multimammate mice in agricultural fields, and then to commensal rodents in villages, resulting in human plague outbreaks. The principal flea vectors of plague among wild rodent hosts are *Xenopsylla* and *Dinopsyllus* spp., while *X. cheopis* and *X. brasiliensis* are the principal flea species involved in transmission among commensal rats and to humans.

Asian Plague Foci. The most important Eurasian plague hosts are gerbils (*Meriones* spp.) in Iran, Kurdistan, Transcaucasia; ground squirrels (*Spermophilus* spp.) around the Caspian Sea and the plains of southeastern Russia; marmots (*Marmota* spp.) in central Asia, including northeastern China, Mongolia, Manchuria, and in Transbaikalia; ground squirrels (*Spermophilus* spp.) in Mongolia, north-central China, and some areas around the Caspian Sea; and gerbils (*Rombomis opimus*) in the deserts of central Asia. The primary flea vectors on gerbils are *Xenopsylla* and *Nosopsyllus* spp.; on marmots they are various *Oropsylla*, *Rhadinopsylla*, and *Citellopsylla* spp.; and on ground squirrels they are *Citellophilus* and *Neopsylla* spp.

In India, the gerbil, *T. indica*, has been described as the principal wild rodent maintenance host. Although it lives mostly in open grassland sites in its natural state, it does sometimes invade agricultural fields and village peripheries. Other maintenance hosts include *Mellardia meltada*, various field mice, and palm squirrels (*Funambulus* spp). The important commensal rat species are *Bandicota bengalensis*, *Bandicota indica*, *R. rattus*, and *R. norvegicus*. The primary vectors of plague in India are *X. cheopis* and *Xenopsylla astia*.

The principal rodent host in Indonesia is *R. rattus* (subspecies *diardii*); the Polynesian rat (*Rattus exulans*). *R. norvegicus* and the bandicoot, *B. indicus*, have been described as important hosts in Vietnam and Myanmar. The shrew, *Suncus murinus*, is possibly an important host of plague in Vietnam and Indonesia. *R. rattus* (subspecies *flavipectus*) is the principal host associated with human plague in southern China. *X. cheopis* is the major vector of plague in southern China, Myanmar, Vietnam, and Indonesia; *X. astia* (a less efficient vector) is also found on rats in Myanmar and Vietnam. *Stivalius cognatus* is considered to be an important secondary vector of plague in Indonesia.

PATHOGENESIS AND PATHOLOGY OF HUMAN PLAGUE

Molecular Basis of Disease. *Y. pestis* is among the most invasive bacteria known; both chromosomal- and plasmid-encoded gene products are associated with virulence. A lipopolysaccharide endotoxin is thought to be primarily responsible for the pathogenic effects of plague sepsis, systemic inflammatory response syndrome (SIRS), and associated adult respiratory distress syndrome (ARDS), cytokine activation, complement cascade and resultant disseminated intravascular coagulation (DIC) and bleeding, unresponsive shock, and organ failure. Before antibiotics became available, nearly all persons with septicemic or pneumonic plague died rapidly from toxemia and organ failure.

Tissue Invasion and Pathology

Cutaneous Exposure. *Y. pestis* organisms inoculated through the skin or mucous membranes are usually carried by lymphatics to regional lymph nodes, although direct blood stream dissemination may occur. In the early stages of infection, affected lymph nodes are edematous and congested and have minimal inflammatory infiltrates and vascular injury. Fully developed buboes, however, contain large numbers of infectious plague organisms, and show vascular damage and hemorrhage, necrosis, and a mild neutrophilic infiltration. The affected nodes are usually surrounded by serosanguineous effusion. When several adjacent lymph nodes are involved, a boggy, edematous mass can result. Abscess formation, spontaneous rupture, and suppuration may occur.

Primary septicemic plague results from direct entry of *Y. pestis* through broken skin or mucous membranes, or follows an infective flea bite in the apparent absence of a bubo; secondary septicemic plague occurs when lymphatic defenses are breached and the plague bacillus enters and multiplies within the blood stream. Newly inoculated plague bacilli, especially those producing the F1 antigen, survive phagocytosis and are disseminated by mononuclear cells to distant sites. *Y. pestis* can invade and cause disease in almost any organ, and untreated infection usually results in widespread and massive tissue destruction. A diffuse interstitial myocarditis with cardiac dilatation, multifocal necrosis of the liver, diffuse hemorrhagic splenic necrosis, and fibrin thrombi in renal glomeruli are common findings at autopsy. If DIC occurs, the result is thrombosis and vascular necrosis with widespread cutaneous, mucosal, and serosal petechiae and ecchymoses, and acral gangrene.

Respiratory Exposure. Pneumonic plague can result from inhalation of infective respiratory droplets from a person or animal with respiratory plague or secondary to hematogenous spread in a patient with bubonic or septicemic plague. It can result also from inhalation of *Y. pestis* in a laboratory accident. Primary plague pneumonia generally begins as a lobular process and then extends by confluence, becoming lobar and then multilobar (Fig. 61–6). Typically, plague bacilli are most numerous in the alveoli. Secondary plague pneumonia begins more diffusely as an interstitial process, with organisms most numerous in the interstitial spaces. In untreated cases of both primary and secondary plague pneumonia, the usual pathologic findings are diffuse pulmonary hemorrhage, necrosis, and scant neutrophilic infiltration.

CLINICAL MANIFESTATIONS

Bubonic Plague. Bubonic plague usually has an incubation period of 2 to 6 days, occasionally longer. Typically, the patient first experiences chills, fever that rises within hours to 38°C and higher, myalgias, arthralgias, headache, and a feeling of weakness. Soon, usually within 24 hours, tenderness and pain occur in one or more regional lymph nodes proximal to the site of inoculation of the plague bacillus. The femoral and inguinal groups of nodes are most commonly involved, followed in frequency of occurrence by axillary and cervical nodes, varying with circumstances of flea exposure. The enlarging bubo(es) becomes progressively swollen, painful, and tender, sometimes exquisitely so. Typically, the patient guards against palpation and limits movement, pressure, and stretching around the bubo. The surrounding tissue often becomes edematous, sometimes markedly, and the overlying skin may be erythematous, warm, and tense (Fig. 61–4). Inspection of the skin surrounding or distal to the bubo may reveal the site of a flea bite marked by a small papule, pustule, scab, or ulcer (phlyctenule). Larger ulcers or eschars indistinguishable from those caused by tularemia rarely occur. The bubo of plague is distinguishable from lymphadenitis of most other causes by its rapid onset, extreme tenderness, accompanying signs of toxemia, and absence of cellulitis or obvious ascending lymphangitis. Treated in the uncomplicated state with an appropriate antibiotic, bubonic plague usually responds quickly, with defervescence of fever and resolution of other systemic manifestations over

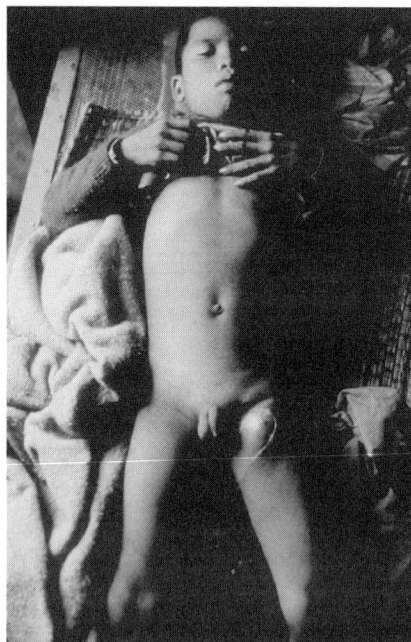

Figure 61–4. Patient with left inguinal and femoral buboes, demonstrating surrounding edema and overlying desquamation.

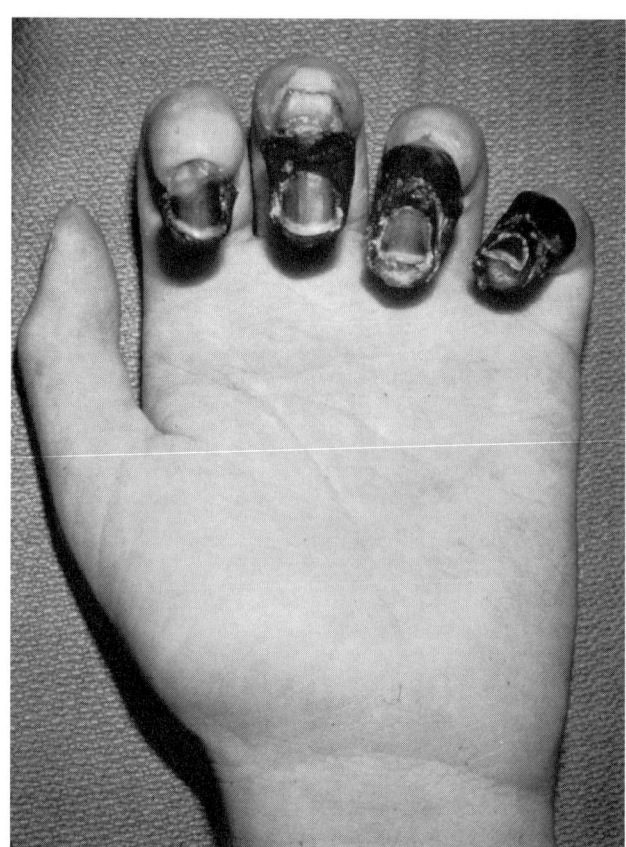

Figure 61–5. Septicemic plague, with acral gangrene of the terminal digits due to disseminated intravascular coagulation.

a 2- to 5-day period. Buboes often remain enlarged and tender for a week or more after treatment has begun and can become fluctuant. Without effective antimicrobial treatment, typical bubonic plague patients become increasingly toxic with fever, tachycardia, lethargy leading to prostration, agitation and confusion, and, occasionally, convulsions and delirium. Mild forms of bubonic plague, called pestis minor, have been described in South America and elsewhere; in these cases, the patients are ambulatory and only mildly febrile, and have subacute buboes.

Septicemic Plague. Septicemic plague is a rapidly progressive, overwhelming endotoxemia. Primary septicemia occurs in the absence of an apparent regional lymphadenitis, and the diagnosis of plague is often not suspected until preliminary blood culture results are reported by the laboratory. Further, patients with septicemic plague often present with gastrointestinal symptoms, e.g., nausea, vomiting, diarrhea, and abdominal pain, making misdiagnosis even more likely. If not treated early with appropriate antibiotics and aggressive supportive care, septicemic plague is usually fulminant and fatal. In the United States from 1950 to 1994, 64 septicemic plague cases and 18 deaths were reported, for a case-fatality rate of 28%. Progression of stages in the SIRS occurs. Petechiae, ecchymoses, bleeding from puncture wounds and orifices, and gangrene of acral parts are manifestations of DIC (Fig. 61–5); refractory hypotension, renal shutdown, obtundation, and other signs of shock are preterminal events. ARDS, which can occur at any stage of septicemic plague, may be confused with other conditions, e.g., hantavirus pulmonary syndrome.

Pneumonic Plague. Pneumonic plague is the most rapidly developing and fatal form of plague. The incubation period for primary pneumonic plague is usually 1 to 3 days, occasionally longer. The onset is most often sudden, with chills, fever, headache, body pains, weakness, dizziness, and chest discomfort. Cough, sputum production, increasing chest pain, tachypnea, and dyspnea typically predominate on the second day of illness and may be accompanied by hemoptysis, increasing respiratory distress, cardiopulmonary insuffi-

ciency, and circulatory collapse. In primary plague pneumonia, the sputum is usually watery or mucoid, frothy, and blood-tinged, but may become frankly bloody. Chest signs in primary plague pneumonia may indicate localized pulmonary involvement in the early stage; a rapidly developing segmental consolidation may be seen before bronchopneumonia occurs in other segments and lobes of the same and opposite lung (Fig. 61–6). Liquefaction necrosis and cavita-

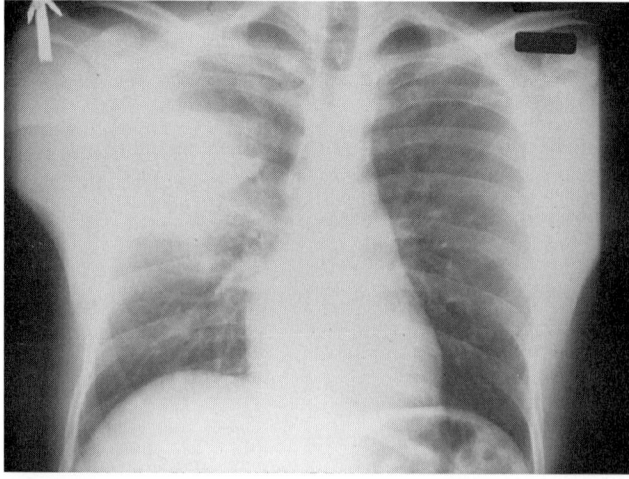

Figure 61–6. Chest radiograph of a patient with primary plague pneumonia, showing extensive infiltrates in right middle and right lower lobes.

tion may develop at sites of consolidation and leave residual scarring. Secondary plague pneumonia manifests first as a diffuse interstitial pneumonitis in which sputum production is scant. The sputum is more likely to be inspissated and tenacious in character than that in primary pneumonic plague. In the United States between 1950 and 1994, 39 cases of secondary pneumonic plague and 7 cases of primary pneumonic plague were reported, with no known secondary transmission to contacts and an overall case-fatality rate of 41%. Earlier observations of pneumonic plague remarked on minimal auscultatory findings, toxemia, and a high frequency of sudden death, as compared with patients with other bacterial pneumonias.

Meningeal Plague. Meningitis is an unusual manifestation of plague. In the United States, there were 12 (3%) meningitis cases among the total 373 plague cases reported in the 45-year period from 1950 through 1994. All cases were complications of treated bubonic plague and all survived. Although meningitis may be a part of the initial presentation of plague, its onset is often delayed and appears to be a consequence of insufficient antibiotic treatment of the primary illness. Chronic, relapsing meningeal plague over periods of weeks to months was described in the preantibiotic era. These patients typically presented with fever, headache, meningismus, and pleocytosis.

Pharyngeal Plague. Plague pharyngitis (an unusual condition) presents with fever, sore throat, cervical lymphadenitis and headache, and in its early stages may be clinically indistinguishable from more common infectious causes of pharyngitis. Characteristic cervical buboes may, however, precede the pharyngitis or develop secondary to the pharyngeal involvement. Health care providers working in plague-endemic areas must be alert to the possibility of plague pharyngitis to avoid misdiagnosis and delayed or inappropriate treatment.

DIAGNOSIS. Except in epidemic situations, a high index of clinical suspicion and a careful clinical and epidemiologic history and physical examination are required to make a timely diagnosis of plague. A delayed or missed diagnosis is associated with a high case-fatality rate, and infected travelers who seek medical care after they have left endemic areas (peripatetic plague cases) are especially at risk. When plague is suspected, close communication between clinicians and the diagnostic laboratory, and between the diagnostic laboratory and a qualified reference laboratory, is essential. Laboratory tests for plague are highly reliable when conducted by persons experienced in working with *Y. pestis*, but such expertise is usually limited to specialized reference laboratories.

Specimen Collection and Processing. When plague is suspected, specimens should be obtained promptly for microbiologic studies, chest roentgenograms taken, and specific antimicrobial therapy initiated. Appropriate diagnostic specimens for smears and culture include blood in all patients, lymph node aspirates in those with suspected buboes, sputum samples or tracheal aspirates in those with suspected pneumonic plague, and cerebrospinal fluid in those with suspected meningitis. A portion of each specimen should be inoculated onto suitable media (e.g., brain-heart infusion broth, sheep blood agar, chocolate agar, and MacConkey agar). Smears of each specimen should be stained with Wayson or Giemsa stain, and with Gram stain, and examined using light microscopy. If possible, the specimens should also be examined using direct fluorescent antibody (FA) testing using *Y. pestis* F1 antigen. An acute-phase serum specimen should be collected for *Y. pestis* antibody testing, followed by a convalescent-phase specimen collected 3 to 4 weeks later. For diagnosis in fatal cases, autopsy tissues should be collected for culture and FA testing, including buboes, samples

of solid organs (especially liver, spleen, and lung), and bone marrow. For culture, specimens should be sent to the laboratory either fresh or frozen on dry ice and not in preservatives or fixatives. Cary-Blair or a similar holding medium can be used to transport *Y. pestis*–infected tissues.

Plague patients typically have white cell counts of 15,000–25,000 per mm^3 with a predominance of polymorphonuclear leukocytes and a left shift. Leukemoid reactions with white cell counts as high as 100,000 per mm^3 can occur.

LABORATORY CONFIRMATION

Culture. Early laboratory confirmation of plague depends on isolation of *Y. pestis* from body fluids or tissues. When the patient's condition allows, several blood cultures taken over a 45-minute period prior to treatment usually results in successful isolation of the bacterium. *Y. pestis* strains are readily distinguished from other gram-negative bacteria by polychromatic and immunofluorescence staining properties, characteristics of growth on microbiologic media, biochemical profiles, and confirmatory lysis by the *Y. pestis*–specific bacteriophage. Laboratory mice and hamsters are susceptible to *Y. pestis* and are used in specialized laboratories to isolate organisms from contaminated materials and for virulence testing.

Serology. In the absence of cultural isolation of *Y. pestis*, plague cases can be confirmed by demonstrating a fourfold or greater change in serum antibodies to *Y. pestis* F1 antigen by passive hemagglutination (PHA) testing, or by detecting a serum antibody titer of ≥128 in a single serum sample from a patient with a compatible illness who has not received plague vaccine. The specificity of a positive PHA test is confirmed by F1 antigen hemagglutination inhibition testing. A few plague patients develop diagnostic levels of antibodies within as few as 5 days after the onset of illness, most seroconvert 1 to 2 weeks after onset, a few seroconvert ≥3 weeks after onset, whereas <5% fail to seroconvert. Early specific antibiotic treatment may delay seroconversion by several weeks. Following seroconversion, positive serologic titers diminish gradually over months to years. Enzyme-linked immunosorbent assays for detecting IgM and IgG antibodies to *Y. pestis* have been useful in identifying antibodies in early infection and in differentiating them from antibodies developed in response to previous vaccination. Various antigen-detection methods are currently being evaluated and standardized.

TREATMENT AND PROGNOSIS. Untreated, plague is fatal in >50% of patients with bubonic disease and in nearly all patients with septicemic or pneumonic plague. The overall mortality of plague cases in the United States in the past 25 years has been approximately 14%. Fatalities are almost always due to delays in seeking treatment, misdiagnosis, and delayed or incorrect treatment. Rapid diagnosis and appropriate antimicrobial therapy (Table 61–2) are essential.

Antibiotic Therapy. Streptomycin is the drug of choice for treating plague, although gentamicin is an acceptable substitute (Table 61–2). Tetracycline and chloramphenicol are effective alternatives to the aminoglycosides. Chloramphenicol is indicated for conditions in which high tissue penetration is important, e.g., plague meningitis, pleuritis, endopthalmitis, and myocarditis, and it may be used separately or in combination with an aminoglycoside. Penicillins, cephalosporins, and macrolides have a suboptimal effect and should not be used. Doxycycline may be as effective or more effective than other tetracyclines, but comparative evaluations have not been made. The fluoroquinolones have considerable in vitro activity against the plague bacillus, and appear to be promising candidates for clinical use. Trimethoprim-sulfamethoxazole has been used successfully to treat bubonic plague, but is not considered a first-line choice. In general, antimicrobial

TABLE 61–2. Plague Treatment Guidelines

Drug	Dosage	Interval (hours)	Route of Administration
Streptomycin			
Adults	2 g/day	12	IM
Children	30 mg/kg/day	12	IM
Gentamicin			
Adults	3 mg/kg/day	8	IM or IV
Children	6.0–7.5 mg/kg/day	8	IM or IV
Infants/neonates	7.5 mg/kg/day	8	IM or IV
Tetracycline			
Adult	2 g/day	6	PO
Children ≥9 yr	25–50 mg/kg/day	6	PO
Chloramphenicol			
Adults	50 mg/kg/day	6	PO or IV
Children ≥1 yr	50 mg/kg/day	6	PO or IV

From Dennis DT: Plague. *In* Rakel RE (ed): Conn's Current Therapy, 1996. Philadelphia, WB Saunders, 1996, p 124.

treatment should be continued for 10 days, or for at least 3 days after the patient has become afebrile and has made a clinical recovery. Patients begun on intravenous antibiotics may be switched to oral regimens as indicated by clinical response. Improvement is usually evident 2 to 3 days from the start of treatment, even though fever may continue for several more days.

Supportive Therapy and Treatment Response. Consequences of delayed treatment of plague include DIC, ARDS, and other complications of bacterial sepsis. Patients with these disorders require intensive monitoring and close physiologic support. Buboes may require surgical drainage if they threaten to spontaneously rupture. Abscessed nodes can be a cause of recurrent fever in patients who have otherwise had satisfactory recovery; the cause may be occult if intrathoracic or intra-abdominal nodes are involved. Viable *Y. pestis* organisms have been isolated from buboes 1 to 2 weeks after clinical recovery from acute disease. *Y. pestis* strains resistant to 1 or 2 drugs used to treat plague have rarely been identified, and have not been associated with treatment failures; however, a plasmid-mediated multidrug-resistant strain was recently isolated from a patient with bubonic plague in Madagascar. This finding underscores the need to maintain global surveillance for emerging antimicrobial-resistant strains.

PREVENTION AND CONTROL

Surveillance. Surveillance, education, and environmental management are the cornerstones of plague prevention and control. In the United States, a network of biologists and public health specialists coordinates these activities through local and state health departments and the Centers for Disease Control and Prevention. Surveys are conducted to determine sites of plague activity, using carnivore seropositivity as a sentinel of recent rodent plague epizootics, inspecting rodent habitat for signs of epizootics, collecting and testing fleas from abandoned burrows, trapping and testing of live rodents and their fleas for *Y. pestis* infection, and testing animals found sick or dead from suspected plague. Urban plague is monitored by trapping rats, determining species-specific flea indices on rats, and testing rats and fleas for *Y. pestis* infection.

Personal Protective Measures. These include avoidance of areas with known epizootic plague (these may be posted with warning signs); avoidance of sick or dead animals; use of repellents, insecticides, and protective clothing when there is a potential for exposure to rodent fleas; and use of gloves when handling animal carcasses.

Medical Care Precautions. Postexposure treatment for 7

days with a tetracycline or chloramphenicol is recommended for persons who have had a known close exposure to a suspected or known pneumonic plague patient in the prior 6 days. Short-term antibiotic prophylaxis may occasionally be recommended for persons who are unable to avoid visiting or residing in an area where a plague outbreak is in progress or who are caring for plague patients. To decrease the risk of pneumonic transmission, all suspected plague patients should be managed under respiratory precautions (appropriate to prevent droplet spread) during the first 48 hours of antibiotic treatment, following which standard precautions are adequate. Patients with suspected pneumonic plague should be managed under respiratory precautions until sputum cultures are shown to be negative. Persons caring for sick animals (especially cats) in plague-endemic areas should take precautions to avoid contamination with infectious exudates or expelled respiratory secretions. Plague in domestic cats often presents with oral ulceration and swollen, sometimes suppurative submandibular lymphadenopathy.

Environmental Management. Elimination of sources of rodent food (grains, garbage, animal feed, pet food) and harborage (brush piles, junk heaps, wood piles) in domestic, peridomestic, and working environments, and rat-proofing of buildings and food stores reduce plague risk. Controlling fleas with insecticides is a principal plague control health measure in situations in which epizootic plague activity places humans at high risk. This includes insecticidal dusting and spraying of rodent burrows, rodent runs, and other sites where rodents and their fleas are found. In known plague foci, persons should keep their dogs and cats free of fleas and restrained. The decision to control plague by killing rodents should be left to public health authorities and should only be carried out in conjunction with effective flea control. Killing rodents has no lasting benefit without environmental sanitation.

Control Measures During Epidemics. In the event of a plague epidemic, measures should rapidly be taken to control spread as described in international regulations and manuals of disease control. These measures include delineation of infected areas; enhanced surveillance, laboratory confirmation, and reporting of human and animal plague; rapid detection and treatment of cases and exposed contacts; isolation (quarantine) and surveillance of suspected human plague cases and case contacts; and control of fleas and rodents in plague-infected areas, in port facilities, and on ships and other conveyances as indicated. A surveillance system to identify and contain the possible introduction of pneumonic plague into the United States was rapidly established at major international airports at the time of the reported outbreaks of plague in India in 1994.

Plague Vaccine. A killed, whole-cell plague vaccine is available in the United States and some other countries. The efficacy of this vaccine in humans has not been evaluated in controlled studies, although reviews of vaccine use during the Vietnam War provide indirect evidence that it protects against bubonic plague. The vaccine does not fully protect against primary pneumonic plague. As recommended by the manufacturer, primary immunization consists of a series of three injections followed by booster doses (at 6-month or more prolonged intervals) as warranted. The degree and duration of the immune response vary, and persons with continuing risk may need to monitor their antibody levels. Adverse reactions after injection of the first dose are usually mild but may increase with repeated doses. With the exception of military personnel, plague vaccine is recommended only for persons at high risk of exposure, e.g., laboratory personnel who routinely work with *Y. pestis* and persons whose work brings them into regular contact with wild rodents and their fleas in plague foci. Vaccination is not routinely indicated for persons living in areas with enzootic plague, medical personnel, or travelers to countries having reported plague cases, or for controlling plague epidemics.

Bibliography

Bahmanyar M, Cavanaugh DC: Plague Manual. Geneva, World Health Organization, 1976.

Brubaker RR: Factors promoting acute and chronic diseases caused by yersiniae. Clin Microbiol Rev 4:309, 1991.

Butler T: A clinical study of bubonic plague: Observations of the 1970 Vietnam epidemic with emphasis on coagulation studies, skin histology, and electrocardiograms. Am J Med 53:268, 1972.

Butler T: Plague and Other Yersinia Infections. Plenum, New York, 1983.

Campbell GL, Hughes JM: Plague in India: A new warning from an old nemesis. Ann Intern Med 122:151, 1995.

Centers for Disease Control and Prevention: Fatal human plagues in Arizona and Colorado, 1996. MMWR 46:618, 1997.

Centers for Disease Control and Prevention: Prevention of plague. Recommendations of the Advisory Committee on Immunization Practices (ACIP). MMWR 45(RR-14):1, 1996.

Christie AB, Chen TH, Elberg SS: Plague in camels and goats: Their role in human epidemics. J Infect Dis 141:724, 1980.

Crook LD, Tempest B: Plague—a clinical review of 27 cases. Arch Intern Med 152:1253, 1992.

Dennis DT: Plague in India. Br Med J 309:893, 1994.

Gage KL, Lance SE, Dennis DT, et al: Human plague in the United States: A review of cases from 1988–1992 with comments on the likelihood of increased plague activity. Border Epidemiol Bull 19:1, 1992.

Hull HF, Montes JM, Mann JM: Septicemic plague in New Mexico. J Infect Dis 155:113, 1987.

Kartman L, Goldenberg MI, Hubbert WT: Recent observations on the epidemiology of plague in the United States. Am J Public Health 56:1554, 1966.

Mann JM, Martone WJ, Boyce JM, et al: Endemic human plague in New Mexico: Risk factors associated with infection. J Infect Dis 140:397, 1979.

Perry RD, Fetherston JD: Yersinia pestis—etiologic agent of plague. Clin Microbiol Rev 10:35, 1997.

Pollitzer R: Plague. WHO Monograph Series 22:1 Geneva, World Health Organization, 1954.

World Health Organization: International Health Regulations (1969). Geneva, WHO, 1983.

World Health Organization: Human plague in 1994. Wkly Epidemiol Rec 22:165, 1996.

62 Tularemia*

David T. Dennis

DEFINITION. Tularemia is an acute and potentially fatal bacterial zoonosis caused by *Francisella tularensis* (formerly *Pasteurella tularensis*). The natural cycle of the organism involves amplification in mammalian and tick reservoir hosts. Humans are incidentally infected by several modes, including bites by infective arthropods, direct handling or ingestion of infectious materials, and inhalation of contaminated aerosols or dusts. The disease occurs widely in temperate and subarctic regions of North America and Eurasia. Most commonly, the disease presents as fever, an indolent ulcer at the site of cutaneous inoculation, and regional lymphadenitis.

ETIOLOGY. *F. tularensis* is a small gram-negative coccobacillus. The organism has a lipidated capsule and is a hardy saprophyte that survives well in water, moist soil, and in decaying animal carcasses. It is extremely infectious and must be handled with care in the laboratory. *F. tularensis* strains may be divided into two main groups by virulence testing, biochemical reactions, and epidemiologic features.

Formerly, it was thought that strains of the more virulent type, termed Jellison type A (biovar *tularensis*), were found only in North America, but recent molecular studies have shown that some *F. tularensis* strains from central Asia and in Japan share significant genetic identity with *F. tularensis*. The less virulent Jellison type B strains (biovar *palearctica*) are the principal forms in Eurasia, and are also widely present in North America.

EPIDEMIOLOGY

Transmission. The principal zoonotic reservoirs of *F. tularensis* are numerous small and medium-sized mammals, especially lagomorphs (rabbits and hares), aquatic rodents (beaver, muskrats, water voles), field voles, ground squirrels, and other rodents, as well as various hard ticks. The organism is widespread in nature and has been found in more than 100 species of wild mammals, at least 9 species of domestic animals (including cattle, dogs, cats), numerous species of birds, in some amphibians and fish, and in more than 50 species of arthropods. However, in the zoonotic cycle, only mammals and blood-feeding arthropods are epidemiologically important. Species of hard ticks maintain the natural cycles of *F. tularensis* in wild hares and rabbits and certain terrestrial rodents (especially voles), whereas the cycle in aquatic rodents is maintained by direct animal-to-animal contact and by contaminated environmental sources (Fig. 62–1). Ticks serve as true reservoirs and amplifying hosts of *F. tularensis*; the bacillus multiplies within the tick, disseminates beyond the gut to various tissues (including the salivary glands), and is passed directly from one tick stage to the next. In contrast to ticks, biting flies and mosquitoes are not true hosts of *F. tularensis*; they act solely as mechanical vectors of organisms that contaminate their mouthparts after an interrupted feed on an infected animal. *F. tularensis* is readily isolated from water and soil contaminated by infected animals.

Palearctica. Cricetine rodents (especially field voles, lemmings, water voles, and muskrats), water and soil contaminated by these animals, hares (*Lepus* spp.) and bites by contaminated mosquitoes (especially *Aedes cinereus*, and *Aedes excruscians*) are important sources of human tularemia in Eurasia (Fig. 62–1). Mosquito-borne infection regularly occurs in forested and marshy Scandinavian and Baltic regions, and Sweden and Finland have reported large mosquito-borne outbreaks. Sporadic cases of tularemia also result there from bites by infected ticks and by blood-feeding flies, and by exposure to infected aerosols and dusts. The principal sources of infection in Russia have been reported to be voles (*Microtus* spp., *Arvicola* spp.) and muskrats (*Ondatra zibethica*). Outbreaks of tularemia have been described following respiratory exposures to dusts from contaminated stored and fresh-mown hay, to dusts from infected soils, and among workers in factories exposed to contaminated water sprays. In Japan, the disease has been historically associated with the trapping, handling, and eating of wild rabbits. Recent outbreaks of human tularemia in Italy and Spain have been associated with hunting of wild hares imported from Eastern Europe.

Neoarctica. The principal zoonotic sources of infection of humans in North America are the cottontail rabbit (*Sylvilagus* spp.) and wild hares, and to a lesser extent rodents (muskrats, beaver, voles, ground squirrels), and certain species of ticks that feed on them (Fig. 62–1). In the United States and Canada, the principal ticks that transmit *F. tularensis* to humans include the Lone Star tick (*Amblyomma americanum*), the American dog tick (*Dermacentor variabilis*), and the Rocky Mountain wood tick (*Dermacentor andersoni*). Lone Star tick bites account for most human tularemia in the South Central states. Outbreaks of tularemia due to bites by American dog ticks have repeatedly occurred in late spring and early

---

*All the material in this chapter is in the public domain, with the exception of any borrowed figures or tables.

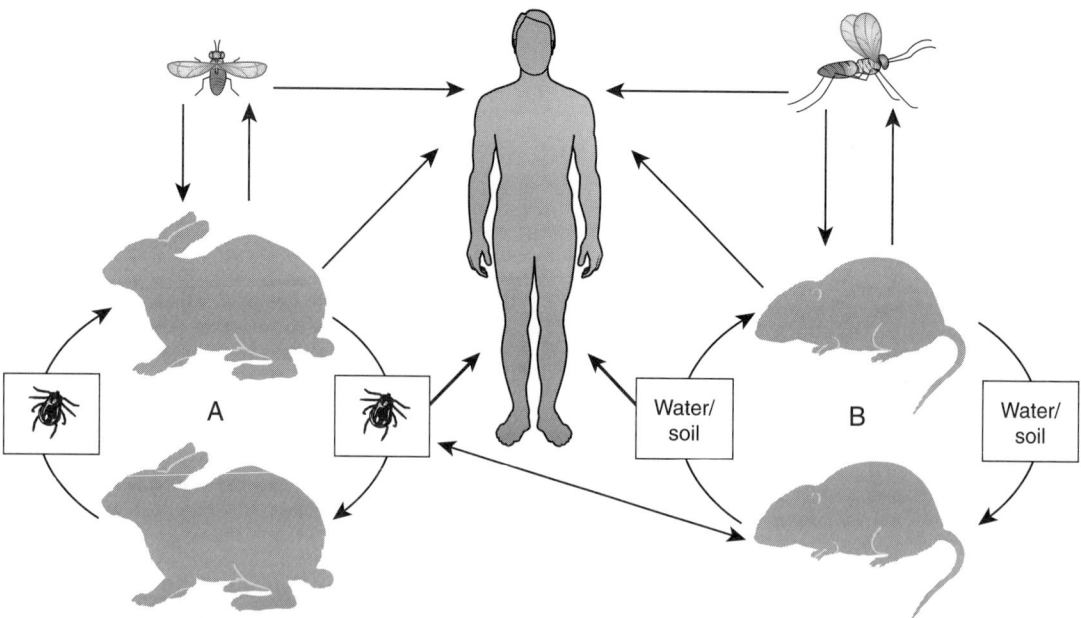

Figure 62–1. Two major life cycles of *Francisella tularensis* transmission. In cycle A, *F. tularensis* is maintained predominantly among lagomorphs and hard ticks; in cycle B, it is maintained among cricetine rodents, especially field voles, water voles, and other aquatic rodents, mostly through a contaminated environment. Humans are incidentally infected by tick vectors that "bridge" the natural cycle and incidental hosts, by the bites of flies or mosquitoes that have contaminated mouthparts, by direct contact with infected animal carcasses or contaminated soil or water, by ingestion of contaminated matter, or by inhalation of infectious aerosols or dusts. Cycle A is dominant in North America; cycle B is dominant in Eurasia.

summer among Native Americans in the Great Plains states, with cases most often presenting as mild glandular disease in children. The Rocky Mountain wood tick accounts for scattered human cases across the western United States.

Sporadic cases, small clusters, and occasional outbreaks of tularemia associated with bites by infected deer flies (*Chrysops discalis*) have been reported in some western states, especially in arid and semiarid areas of Utah, Nevada, and California.

Direct contact with infected cottontail rabbits was the principal cause of tularemia in the United States in the past, and still accounts for most cases in the southeastern region. Sporadic cases and outbreaks associated with direct exposures to muskrats, beaver, and water contaminated by them have been reported, including a large outbreak among muskrat trappers in the northeastern United States. Uncommon sources of tularemia in the United States include aerosols, especially among laboratory workers, and bites or scratches by cats.

The epidemiology of tularemia in North America has changed significantly since the 1930s, when the disease had a much higher incidence and when most cases were linked to hunting, dressing, and butchering of wild rabbits and hares rather than to arthropod bites. In many states, regulations were imposed to restrict rabbit hunting to winter months in order to reduce the risk of human exposure to infection; as well, the harvesting and marketing of wild rabbits for food is much less common now than in the past.

Seasonality. The seasonal distribution of tularemia cases is related to the activities of humans, susceptible animal hosts, and vector arthropods at sites where the disease is enzootic. As expected, mosquito-borne transmission in Eurasia peaks in the summer months. In the United States, a seasonal peak of tularemia cases in the spring and summer months is due to bites by contaminated ticks and blood-feeding flies, and a second peak in the late fall and winter is associated with

direct contact exposures to infected animals, especially among hunters and trappers of rabbits.

Populations at Risk. Humans become infected when they intrude into the natural cycle and are bitten by infectious ticks, biting flies, or mosquitoes; by handling or ingesting infectious animal tissues or fluids; by direct contact with, or ingestion of, contaminated water or soil; or by inhalation of infective aerosols or dusts. Person-to-person transmission has not been documented.

Tularemia is mostly a rural disease. It affects persons of all ages and both sexes. Persons at highest risk include hunters, trappers, wildlife specialists, animal skinners and dressers, butchers, and others who handle potentially infected animals; persons exposed to water, soils, and dusts contaminated by infected wild animals, especially meadow voles and aquatic mammals; and persons exposed to bites by certain hard ticks, tabanid flies, and mosquitoes. In the United States, the disease has been known as "rabbit fever" and "deer fly fever" because of its occurrence following direct contact with infected rabbits, and bites by contaminated deer flies, respectively; similarly, in Japan, the disease has been called "wild hare disease."

Geographic Distribution. Tularemia is endemic throughout much of the Northern Hemisphere between latitudes 30° North and 71° North. This includes all of North America from the Arctic Circle to northern Mexico, much of Eurasia, and some states of northern Africa along the Mediterranean littoral. In North America, cases have been reported from all continental United States, across Canada, and in Mexico as far south as Guadalajara. In Eurasia, tularemia occurs most frequently in Sweden, Finland, and Russia, where it often occurs in outbreaks. It also occurs sporadically throughout most of Europe, in some areas of the Near East, central Asia, and Mongolia. It has not been documented in Latin America, Australia, or Africa.

Disease Incidence. Worldwide incidence figures are not

available for tularemia. Cases are relatively common in Finland, Sweden, and Russia, where numbers vary greatly from year to year. Epidemics have been reported in Sweden involving more than 500 cases in a single year, and outbreaks involving thousands of persons have been reported from the former Soviet Union. Tularemia incidence is much more stable in the United States, where the disease has been in steady decline since 1945. A total of 1409 cases and 20 deaths were reported in the United States in the period 1985 to 1992, for a mean of 171 cases per year and a case-fatality rate of 1.4%. Of the 1298 cases in this period for which information was available, 942 (72.6%) occurred in males. Tularemia occurred among all age groups. Although cases have been reported from all states other than Hawaii, the south central states of Arkansas, Missouri, and Oklahoma now regularly report more than half of all cases in the United States.

PATHOLOGY. The principal pathologic changes in localized disease occur at the site of inoculation and in the involved regional lymph nodes; when disseminated, the lungs, spleen, lymph nodes, liver, and kidneys are most often involved. Secondary skin lesions have also been described, including papular and papulovesicular lesions, erythema nodosum, and erythema multiforme.

F. tularensis is a facultative intracellular organism, and the response to infection has a prominent cell-mediated immune component. Histologically, the disease is characterized by focal, suppurative necrosis, often very similar to the granulomatous reaction seen in tuberculosis. The central area of necrosis is comprised primarily of polymorphonuclear leukocytes and macrophages. In more advanced lesions, coagulative granular necrosis occurs, which is similar to caseation. A wall of fibroblasts may surround the acute inflammatory reaction; some may take the appearance of epithelioid cells and, occasionally, of giant Langhans cells. Smaller lesions may be indistinguishable from miliary tubercles. Almost half of pleuropneumonic cases have small (3 to 12 mm), yellowish, necrotic subpleural nodules. Bronchopneumonia occurs in about 30% of pleuropneumonic cases, and lobar pneumonia with consolidation of an entire lobe has been described in about 15%.

CLINICAL MANIFESTATIONS. Tularemia is a plaguelike disease. The major clinical forms of tularemia include the following: ulceroglandular (55 to 85% of cases); glandular (10 to 25%); oculoglandular (<5%); septic (<5%); oropharyngeal (<5%); and, pneumonic (<5%) (Table 62–1). All forms have similar onsets and underlying nonspecific constitutional manifestations. The incubation period is usually 3 to 5 days (range of 1 to 21 days). Onset is sudden: typically, the patient has a fever of 38° to 40°C and a constellation of manifestations including chills, headache, generalized body aches (often prominent in the lumbosacral region), cough, and chest pain. Without treatment, nonspecific symptoms usually persist for several weeks. Sweats, chills, progressive weakness, and weight loss characterize the illness. Any of the principal forms of tularemia may be complicated by bacteremic spread, leading variously to sepsis, tularemic pneumonia, and meningitis.

Ulceroglandular Tularemia. A local papule appears at the site of inoculation shortly after of the onset of generalized symptoms, becomes pustular, and then ulcerates within a few days of the papule's first appearance. The ulcer mostly has an indolent character and may be covered by an eschar (Fig. 62–2). By the time of ulceration, lymphadenitis is manifested as pain, tenderness, and swelling of one or a few adjacent nodes in the afferent pathway. In persons infected by handling contaminated materials, the epitrochlear (8%) and axillary (65%) nodes are most commonly affected. In persons infected by arthropod bites, femoral or inguinal

TABLE 62–1. Principal Clinical Presentations of Tularemia

Clinical Form	Characteristics
Ulceroglandular, oculoglandular	Local papule at inoculation site within days of exposure; ulcerates after several days; accompanied by fever, other constitutional symptoms, regional lymphadenitis
Glandular	As above, but without cutaneous ulcer
Septic (typhoidal)	Fever and systemic inflammatory response syndrome, including disseminated intravascular coagulation and bleeding, acute respiratory distress syndrome, organ failure, shock
Oropharyngeal	Exudative pharyngitis, tonsillitis, sometimes with ulceration of buccal or pharyngeal mucosa
Pneumonic	Fever; cough (sputum production minimal); pleuritic pain; dyspnea; occasionally hemoptysis. Infiltrates most often bilateral, often accompanied by enlarged hilar nodes, pleural effusions; lung abscess not uncommon

(64%), axillary (24%), and cervical (6%) nodes are most frequently affected. In unusual cases, abscessed nodes may suppurate and discharge purulent material. In *oculoglandular tularemia,* which follows contamination of the eye by infectious fluids, ulceration is localized to the conjunctiva. The conjunctiva may become severely inflamed, with marked chemosis and vasculitis.

Glandular Tularemia. This is more likely to follow an infectious arthropod bite than to occur by direct contamination of wounds of the hands and fingers of persons handling infected animal tissues and is not accompanied by a local cutaneous ulcer.

Tularemia Sepsis ("Typhoidal" Tularemia). This presents as an acute, sometimes fulminant illness without localizing signs, and the diagnosis is most often made by identifying *F. tularensis* in cultures of the blood. Abdominal pain, diarrhea, and vomiting may be prominent in the early illness. The systemic inflammatory response syndrome may ensue, accompanied by complications, e.g., disseminated intravascular coagulation and bleeding, adult respiratory distress syndrome, shock, and organ failure. Hematogenous spread to other organs may lead to pneumonia in more than half of septicemic patients, to involvement of the kidneys, and to meningitis. In some cases, the upper intestinal tract may be the principal target organ in typhoidal tularemia.

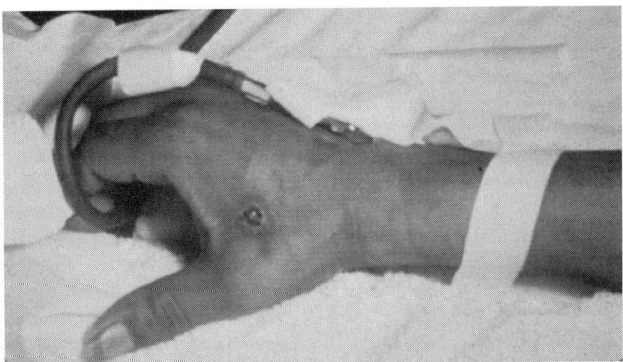

Figure 62–2. Tularemic ulcer with eschar formation, following percutaneous inoculation of *F. tularensis.*

Oropharyngeal Tularemia. This is acquired by ingesting contaminated food (almost always inadequately cooked meat) or water. Typically the patient develops exudative pharyngitis or tonsillitis, sometimes with ulceration, and cervical lymphadenopathy. Stomatitis occasionally occurs.

Pneumonic Tularemia. This is a common secondary complication of other forms of tularemia. Infrequently, primary pneumonia arises from exposure to an infective aerosol or dust. Pneumonic infiltrates of varying character may be seen in one or more lobes, and are often accompanied by pleural effusion, and by hilar lymphadenopathy. Lung abscesses are sometimes seen. Pulmonic manifestations include cough (usually with minimal sputum production), sometimes pleuritic pain, dyspnea, and, occasionally, hemoptysis.

DIAGNOSIS. The presumptive diagnosis of tularemia is made by clinical examination combined with information on potentially infective exposures.

Culture. The clinical diagnosis of tularemia is confirmed by cultural isolation of *F. tularensis*. Clinical suspicion of tularemia is critical in directing selection of the proper (cystine enriched) culture media. *F. tularensis* grows (slowly) on glucose cystine blood agar, thioglycolate broth, and buffered charcoal-yeast agar. Inoculated plates should be incubated at 37°C and held for up to 14 days. Colonies are pinpointed after 24 hours of incubation, and may be only 3 mm in diameter at 96 hours. Because of its slow growth, *F. tularensis* may be obscured in culture by more rapidly growing contaminants. In specialized laboratories, isolation of pure *F. tularensis* may be obtained from contaminated materials by passage through laboratory mice. In addition to culture, materials other than blood should be streaked on glass slides for presumptive diagnosis by direct fluorescent antibody testing.

Serologic Tests. The agglutination reaction for combined IgM and IgG immunoglobulins is the routine serologic procedure in use in most laboratories. Reference laboratories use microagglutination methods that are more sensitive than tube agglutination procedures. A fourfold rise in titer between acute and convalescent serum specimens, or a single titer of 1:160 or greater, is considered diagnostic for *F. tularensis* infection. Other potentially useful diagnostic procedures include enzyme-linked immunoassay and immunoblotting for IgM antibodies, polymerase chain reaction assays, and DNA probes, but these are still in the experimental stages of development. Many routine diagnostic laboratories have policies that exclude work on *F. tularensis*, because it readily aerosolizes and is notorious as a cause of laboratory-acquired infections. Biosafety level 2 precautions are essential for routine procedures, and biosafety level 3 precautions are needed for animal studies or for handling *F. tularensis* in large quantities, e.g., in reagent production. A skin test employing killed *F. tularensis* has been used to assist in the clinical diagnosis of tularemia in some countries.

Differential Diagnosis. Glandular and ulceroglandular tularemia must be distinguished from other forms of acute regional lymphadenopathy and fever, including plague, cat-scratch disease, rat bite fever, and lymphadenitis secondary to common skin infections, e.g., *Staphylococcus aureus* and *Streptococcus pyogenes*. Other diseases with or without cutaneous ulceration and regional lymphadenopathy include sporotrichosis, syphilis, anthrax, lymphogranuloma venereum, and chancroid. Oropharyngeal tularemia may resemble pharyngitis due to β-hemolytic streptococci, and other bacterial and viral causes of pharyngitis and cervical lymphadenopathy. Tularemia pneumonia may be difficult to distinguish from any of the atypical pneumonia syndromes, including those due to viruses, *Mycoplasma* and *Chlamydia* species, legionellosis, Q fever, and histoplasmosis. Typhoidal tularemia must be distinguished from typhoid fever, other salmonelloses, brucellosis, various rickettsial diseases, including ehrlichioses and Rocky Mountain spotted fever, and other causes of septicemia and febrile illness.

TREATMENT. Streptomycin, which is bactericidal, is the drug of choice. It is given to adults in a dosage of 7.5 to 10 mg/kg IM q 12 hr up to a total dose of 2 g a day for 7 to 10 days. Gentamicin, an acceptable alternative, is given in a dosage of 3 to 5 mg/kg/day IM in equal divided doses at 8-hour intervals for 10 days. Tetracycline or chloramphenicol may be used in place of an aminoglycoside, especially in less severely ill patients, but use of these bacteriostatic agents occasionally results in primary treatment failures, and dosage schedules longer than 10 days may be necessary to prevent relapses. Penicillins and cephalosporins are not effective and should not be used to treat tularemia. Universal precautions are required only for purposes of hospital infection control. Postexposure prophylactic antibiotic treatment of close contacts is not recommended because no human-to-human transmission has been reported.

PROGNOSIS. Prior to the availability of antibiotics, the overall mortality from infections with the more severe type A strains was in the range of 5 to 10%; however, a case-fatality rate as high as 40 to 60% has been reported for untreated typhoidal and pneumonic forms of disease. Untreated, type B strain infections were associated with a fatality of only 1 to 3%. In the United States, the case-fatality rate for all forms in recent years has been <2%.

PREVENTION. Tularemia is best prevented by avoiding recognized natural exposures to *F. tularensis*. Persons exposed in endemic areas to biting flies and ticks should when feasible wear protective clothing, tuck pants legs into socks, and apply repellents containing diethyltoluamide (DEET) to skin and clothing as directed by the manufacturer. Permethrin-based acaricides can be applied to clothing to kill ticks and biting flies on contact. Frequent examinations should be made for ticks on clothing and skin, and attached ticks promptly removed. Persons should always avoid handling sick or dead wild animals, and hunters, trappers, dressers, and butchers are advised to use impervious gloves when handling carcasses. Persons dressing and butchering animals also should wear gloves and notify authorities of any animals with suspicious nodular lesions in the liver and spleen. To reduce tick infestations in residential areas, pet dogs and cats should be restrained and kept tick-free using acaricides.

A live attenuated vaccine is available in the United States for limited use; it is recommended almost exclusively for laboratory personnel who routinely work with *F. tularensis*. Large-scale vaccination has, however, been an important component of prevention of disease in persons with high environmental risk in the former Soviet Union. Persons exposed to a laboratory accident possibly resulting in aerosolization of *F. tularensis* must be closely monitored for fever and other early signs of illness.

Bibliography

Boyce JM: Recent trends in the epidemiology of tularemia in the United States. J Infect Dis 131:197, 1975.

Capellan J, Fong IW: Tularemia from a cat bite: Case report and review of feline-associated tularemia. Clin Infect Dis 16:472, 1993.

Enderlin G, Morales L, Jacobs RF, Cross JT: Streptomycin and alternative agents for the treatment of tularemia: Review of the literature. Clin Infect Dis 19:42, 1994.

Evans ME, Gregory DW, Schaffner W, McGee ZA: Tularemia: A 30-year experience with 88 cases. Medicine 64:251, 1985.

Francis E: Tularemia. JAMA 84:1243, 1925.

Hopla CE: The ecology of tularemia. Adv Vet Sci Comp Med 18:25, 1974.

Hopla CE, Hopla AK: Tularemia. *In* Beran GW, Steele JH (eds): Handbook of Zoonoses, 2nd ed. Section A: Bacterial, Rickettsial, Chlamydial, and Mycotic. Boca Raton, FL, CRC Press, 1994, pp 113–126.

Jacobs RF, Narain JP: Tularemia in children. Pediatr Infect Dis J 2:487, 1983.

Klock LE, Olsen PF, Fukushima T: Tularemia epidemic associated with the deerfly. JAMA 226:149, 1973.

Markowitz LE, Hynes NA, de la Cruz P, et al: Tick-borne tularemia: An outbreak of lymphadenopathy in children. JAMA. 254:2922, 1985.

Rubin SA: Radiographic spectrum of pleuropulmonary tularemia. Am J Roentgenol 131:277, 1978.

Sunderrajan EV, Hutton J, Marienfield D: Adult respiratory disease syndrome secondary to tularemia. Arch Intern Med 145:1435, 1985.

Young LS, Bicknell DS, Archer BG, et al: Tularemia epidemic: Vermont, 1968. New Engl J Med 280:1253, 1969.

63 Pasteurella

Louis Polish

ETIOLOGY. Pasteurella organisms are non–spore-forming, nonmotile, bipolar staining, aerobic, facultatively anaerobic gram-negative coccobacilli. Pasteurella grows well at 37°C on blood, chocolate, and Mueller-Hinton agar but not MacConkey, and almost all species are both oxidase and catalase positive. DNA-DNA hybridization techniques have resulted in Pasteurella species' being segregated into a classification identified as Pasteurella sensu stricto (comprising 11 species) and those excluded from this grouping (6 species). Most human infections are caused by organisms identified as Pasteurella multocida subspecies multocida or by subspecies septica.

EPIDEMIOLOGY

Reservoirs of Infection. Pasteurella is relatively resistant and can remain viable in water or soil for approximately 3 weeks; however, exposure to direct sunlight for >10 minutes kills these organisms. P. multocida has been isolated from the nasopharynx or gastrointestinal tract of various domestic and wild mammals and birds including cats (50 to 90%), dogs (50 to 65%), swine (50%), Norway rats (14%), and buffalo (4%). Pasteurella infection in cats and dogs is generally asymptomatic; however, it is the cause of hemorrhagic septicemia in cattle, pneumonia in goats and sheep, cholera in waterfowl, and upper respiratory tract infections in rabbits.

Modes of Transmission. Infections in humans can be categorized as (1) those associated with animal bites or scratches, (2) those due to nonbite animal exposures, and (3) cases with no known animal exposure. Infections associated with bites or scratches most commonly follow exposures to cats or dogs, with 65% being caused by cats. Bites by other animals including opossums, rats, lions, rabbits, pigs, wolves, and Tasmanian devils have been rarely documented to cause Pasteurella infections.

Infections resulting from exposure to animal secretions are less common than those resulting from bites. Persons with frequent animal contact including pet owners, livestock handlers, and food processors may be at increased risk.

In 5 to 15% of patients with Pasteurella infections, no evidence of animal exposure can be elicited. Pasteurella has rarely been isolated from the upper respiratory tract of healthy veterinary students and animal handlers, indicating that Pasteurella may rarely be a normal inhabitant of the upper respiratory tract.

CLINICAL MANIFESTATIONS

Soft Tissue Infections. Localized soft tissue infections resulting from Pasteurella infection are most often characterized by the relatively rapid onset of erythema, increased warmth, pain, and swelling, generally within 48 hours after an animal bite. Although fever is not a prominent feature of these infections, low-grade fever occurs in approximately 20% of cases. Lymphangitis may be noted in as many as 20% of patients, and regional adenopathy in approximately 10%. In a large series reported by Weber, purulent drainage was reported in approximately 40% of patients. Fever resolved within 48 hours in the majority of patients receiving intravenous antibiotics.

Reported complications of Pasteurella soft tissue infections include septic arthritis, osteomyelitis, localized abscesses, tenosynovitis, and bacteremia. Rare manifestations of cutaneous Pasteurella infections reported in the literature have included penile ulceration, necrotizing fasciitis, and Ludwig's angina. Although physicians should be aware of the possibility that Pasteurella infection can follow animal bites, particularly bites by cats or dogs, open wounds that have been licked by these animals are also at risk of becoming infected with Pasteurella. Exposures to animals in the area surrounding the eye have resulted in conjunctivitis, corneal ulcers, and endophthalmitis.

Respiratory Tract Infections. The respiratory tract is the second most common site of Pasteurella infection. Otitis media, sinusitis, tonsillitis, bronchitis, pneumonia, empyema, and lung abscess are the most common manifestations. Epiglottitis has also been reported in several patients. In patients with chronic underlying pulmonary disease, Pasteurella has been isolated from the respiratory tract as a commensal organism.

Systemic Infections. Bacteremia has generally been attributable to localized sites of infection, most commonly secondary to intra-abdominal infections followed by meningitis, pneumonia, and wound infections. Approximately 30% of patients with Pasteurella sepsis have underlying liver disease, and the mortality in patients with cirrhosis and bacteremia may be 30 to 40%. Isolated cases of endocarditis, vascular graft infection, mycotic aneurysm, and purulent pericarditis have been reported. Waterhouse-Friderichsen syndrome was a documented complication of biliary sepsis in one patient with cirrhosis.

Central Nervous System Infections. These infections generally occur in patients at the extremes of age, and cerebrospinal fluid analysis usually shows >500 leukocytes/mm^3, low glucose levels, and increased protein concentration. In addition to meningitis, brain abscess and subdural empyema have been reported.

Intra-Abdominal Infections. P. multocida has also caused intra-abdominal infections including appendicitis with and without perforation, abdominal abscesses (retrocecal, omental, liver), postoperative surgical wound infections, and spontaneous bacterial peritonitis, which usually is present in patients with hepatic cirrhosis. Genitourinary infections have included a Bartholin's gland abscess, infected endometrial polyp, and both upper and lower urinary tract infections, including renal abscess. In addition, several reports have described infections during pregnancy, including in utero infection, with congenital pneumonia and acute chorioamnionitis leading to premature delivery and neonatal death.

DIAGNOSIS. Pasteurella infections should be considered in all patients who have had a bite or who have wounds that have been licked by an animal, particularly cats and dogs. Other possibilities in the differential diagnosis, especially if the incubation period is >24 hours, include staphylococcal, streptococcal, or anaerobic bacterial infection, tularemia, and plague. Because Pasteurella can be mistaken for other bipolar staining gram-negative rods such as Haemophilus, Neisseria, and Acinetobacter, the microbiology laboratory should be informed that Pasteurella is in the differential diagnosis.

TREATMENT. The treatment of choice for Pasteurella infections is penicillin. Other effective antibiotics are ampicillin, amoxicillin-clavulanic acid, trimethoprim-sulfamethoxazole, tetracycline, and ciprofloxacin. Parenteral agents with good activity include mezlocillin, piperacillin, cefuroxime, and cefotaxime. Antibiotics shown to have poor activity against *Pasteurella* include dicloxacillin, cephalexin, erythromycin, and clindamycin. For patients with a penicillin allergy, doxycycline is an effective alternative.

PREVENTION. Prevention of *Pasteurella* infections depends on reducing contact with animals. Bite wounds should be aggressively irrigated with normal saline, and all necrotic skin debrided. Wounds that are grossly infected or those that are treated later than 24 hours after the bite should not be closed. There is no clear consensus on the appropriate management of wounds that are not clearly infected on the initial visit or those that are treated 8 hours or less after the bite. Prophylactic antibiotic therapy is generally recommended for wounds that are seen within 8 hours in the following situations: crush injury or edema, bones or joints are involved, bites are on the hand, bite was inflicted by a cat, puncture wound (especially near a joint), wound near a prosthetic joint, or for patients with an underlying immunocompromising illnesses that would predispose them to serious infection.

Bibliography

Boyce JM: *Pasteurella* species. *In* Mandell GL, Bennet JE, Dolin R (eds): Principle and Practices of Infectious Diseases. New York, Churchill Livingstone, 1995, pp 2068–2070.
Goldstein EJC: Bite wounds and infection. Clin Infect Dis 14:633, 1992.
Kumar A, Devlin HR, Vellend H: *Pasteurella multocida* meningitis in an adult: Case report and review. Rev Infect Dis 12:440, 1990.
Weber DJ, Wolfson JS, Swartz MN, Hooper DC: *Pasteurella multocida* infections: Report of 34 cases and review of the literature. Medicine 63:133, 1984.

64 *Brucellosis*

Stephen G. Wright

DEFINITION. Brucellosis is a systemic infection with one of the species of *Brucella*, gram-negative coccobacilli: *B. abortus*, *B. melitensis*, and *B. suis*. This group of infections are zoonoses.

HISTORY. Brucellosis has been recognized in the Mediterranean littoral and the Red Sea basin for a long time. In his treatise "On Epidemics," Hippocrates (460 to 357 B.C.) described a prolonged febrile illness that had a tendency to spontaneous, periodic defervescence. The disease was known by many local geographic names. Because brucellosis could not be distinguished clinically from other causes of prolonged fever (e.g., typhoid), the diagnostic accuracy was poor. Marston in 1861 was able to distinguish between brucellosis and typhoid in autopsy studies by the consistent involvement of Peyer's patches in typhoid and their normal appearance in brucellosis.

The island of Malta had considerable strategic importance in the 19th and early 20th centuries. Brucellosis was common among both the military and civilian populations, including the large British garrison. In 1886, Bruce identified a "micrococcus" in fresh material from the spleen of a patient dying of the disease and in 1887 grew the organism from the spleen in another fatal case. In Copenhagen in 1895, Bang showed that contagious abortion in cattle was caused by a bacillus

that he referred to as the "bacillus of abortion" and subsequently *Bacillus abortus*. This organism was not then associated with human disease. The clinical features of brucellosis were clearly described by Hughes in his study "Mediterranean Fever" in 1897. The Mediterranean Fever Commission began its work as a result of the high incidence of brucellosis in Malta, and its findings, defining the clinical picture, the epidemiology, the etiologic agent, the reservoir of infection, the mode of transmission, and the means of control were published between 1904 and 1907. Themistocles Zammit found both antibodies to the organism in high titer and later the organism in the blood and milk of a goat. When troops were prohibited from drinking local milk, the incidence of the disease declined dramatically.

Alice Evans in 1918 created a major stir in the bacteriologic world when she reported the similarities between *B. abortus* and *Micrococcus melitensis*. She suggested that the former might be a human pathogen, and in 1924, Keefer proved her correct. Subsequently, the genus was named *Brucella*.

ETIOLOGY. The members of the genus are small, gram-negative, aerobic, nonmotile coccobacilli. It is this variation in shape and size that led to the organism isolated by Bruce to be named *M. melitensis*.

Species. *B. melitensis*, *B. abortus*, and *B. suis* are the species that cause disease in humans, and their virulence for humans decreases somewhat in the order given. Primarily a pathogen of dogs, *Brucella canis* occasionally causes human infections. *Brucella ovis*, a pathogen of sheep, and *B. neotomae*, which infects desert wood rats, are other members of the genus. These organisms are intracellular pathogens. The three principal species each have a number of biotypes; *B. melitensis* 3, *B. abortus* 9, and *B. suis* 5. This is the accepted classification, but DNA hybridization studies showed that the degree of homology among species and biotypes when compared with *B. melitensis* biotype 1 was great enough to raise questions about the validity of our views of *Brucella* taxonomy.

Culture, Biochemical Characteristics, and Antigens. Samples for culture are first inoculated into liquid medium, e.g., trypticase soy broth. The organisms grow slowly in culture, and blind subcultures should be made every 5 days onto solid medium, e.g., trypticase soy agar. Colonies are small, smooth, and circular. Growth is best at 37°C. An atmosphere containing 5% to 10% carbon dioxide is needed and is a distinguishing feature for most *B. abortus* isolates.

B. suis oxidizes L-arginine, DL-citrulline, L-lysine, and DL-ornithine, whereas *B. abortus* and *B. melitensis* do not. The latter two species can be distinguished by their oxidation reactions with ribose and galactose. These methods are used in reference laboratories. Phage typing is valuable in distinguishing species; the Tblisi phage lyses *B. abortus* but not *B. melitensis* or *B. suis*, whereas the Weybridge phage lyses *B. suis* and *B. abortus* but not *B. melitensis*. With AP12ONE test strips *B. abortus* has given reactions that led to incorrect identification as *Moraxella phenylpyruvica*.

Two antigens, *A* and *M*, have been defined in quantitative agglutination studies using smooth strains that are the forms isolated in initial culture. Rough strains cannot be used for these studies because they autoagglutinate. *A* antigen predominates in *B. abortus* and *B. suis*, whereas *M* predominates in *B. melitensis*. Serologic cross-reactivity exists between brucellae and *Escherichia coli* 0:116, *Francisella tularensis*, *Pseudomonas maltophila*, *Vibrio cholerae*, *Yersinia enterocolitica* serogroup 0:9, and *Salmonella urbana*.

EPIDEMIOLOGY

Reservoirs. Infected animals are the reservoirs from which humans are infected. The first pregnancy after infection of a cow ends in abortion, and the cow is likely to remain chronically infected thereafter. The animal's vaginal discharges, membranes, placenta, and fetus are all heavily contaminated with brucellae. Organisms survived for 20 weeks in fetal organs and placenta lying on the earth covered with leaves through winter and spring in the northeastern United States. Subsequent pregnancies can continue to term, but brucellosis recrudesces to infect the placenta, developing fetus, placental membranes, amniotic fluid, udders, and hence the milk. Contamination of pastures and fodder by any of these sources infects other animals. Abortion rates as great as 50% occur in newly infected herds. The cycle of transmission is similar in goats and sheep infected with *B. melitensis*. Among these animals, many recover spontaneously but those chronically infected may transmit the disease either congenitally or in the milk. Among pigs, infection localizes to the genitalia, and sows usually are infected by a common boar because brucellae are present in the semen. The economic effects of brucellosis in livestock are considerable, with reduced fecundity, fetal losses, and reduced milk production.

Transmission. Humans become infected by various routes. Ingestion of organisms in contaminated foods is common. Milk and milk products are common sources of infection. Survival of the bacteria is prolonged if milk and milk products are stored under optimal conditions to prevent souring. Brucellae are very acid sensitive, and so milk may neutralize gastric acid and thus protect the bacteria. Investigations in Malta clearly showed the relation between the amount of milk drunk and the risk of infection and the dramatic decline in incidence of the disease after prohibiting milk consumption.

Contact with infected animals or animal products also is important. Workers in the dairy industry, shepherds, farm workers, family members who have contact with animals around the home, abattoir workers, kitchen workers, and veterinarians all are at risk of infection. Cuts and abrasions on the hands and forearms are sites of entry of infected material. Aerosols of infected fluid also are sources of infection, and entry of organisms may take place across mucosal surfaces (e.g., the conjunctivae, oropharynx, or respiratory tract). Workers in microbiology laboratories who handle infected specimens are at particular risk. The attenuated S19 *B. abortus* or Rev-1 *B. melitensis* vaccine strains are attenuated only as far as the primary animal hosts are concerned and can cause disease when accidentally inoculated into humans.

The causes listed here account for most infections in humans. Brucellae are capable, however, of prolonged survival in the environment, so that viable organisms inhaled in dust may be infective. Blood transfusion, bone marrow transplantation, and possibly kidney transplantation are sources of infection. Sexual transmission in semen may occur. Because of the acid sensitivity of brucellae, anything that reduces gastric acidity may enhance susceptibility—for example, taking antacids, H$_2$ receptor antagonists, or proton pump inhibitors, as well as previous gastric surgery.

DISTRIBUTION AND INCIDENCE. Brucellosis has a worldwide distribution. The frequency of infection in animals is a guide to the likely occurrence in humans. Infection with the three species in animals is common in many parts of Africa, Asia (including the Middle East), and Central and South America. France and Spain have a moderate incidence of animal infections; in 1983, France had an incidence of 0.74 cases per 100,000 human population and Spain reported 1.04 cases per 100,000. Within France, the incidence is variable, ranging from 1.07 to 18.24 cases per 100,000 population in affected areas while many areas remain free of infection. The incidence in the United States declined from 0.15 to 0.06 cases per 100,000 population in the decade before 1984.

Brucellosis is common in the Middle East. The incidence reported from Kuwait rose from 1.15 to 42.78 cases per 100,000 population during a similar period. This probably represents an increased awareness of the disease by physicians, improved reporting of cases, and a true increase as well. These figures take no account of frequent subclinical infections occurring in perhaps as many as a quarter of the populations in endemic areas. Brucellosis is a major cause of morbidity in the endemic areas, but it has a low mortality. This infection is not commonly reported from Africa, although it certainly exists there. Control measures in animals and pasteurization have been major factors in reducing the incidence in temperate parts of the world, but infections still occur in these places as a result of importation by infected travelers or consuming infected imported foods, e.g., soft cheeses.

The disease is more common in males (male:female ratio, 1.6:1). Most cases occur in the second, third, and fourth decades of life, but no age is exempt. Cases in children younger than 10 years are not uncommon. About 6% of patients in a Kuwaiti series were age 50 years or older.

PATHOGENESIS AND PATHOLOGY

Invasion. How brucellae penetrate the mucosal surface is not understood. Having crossed the epithelial surface, brucellae are phagocytosed by neutrophils and macrophages, which then pass to local lymph nodes. Organisms are retained in this site but replicate intracellularly, and bacteria from lysed cells can infect other cells or disseminate throughout the body.

Immune Response. Naturally occurring opsonins in normal human serum are important in promoting phagocytosis. Complement possesses considerable opsonic activity. Heating normal human serum to 56°C abolishes opsonization and destroys complement, but the addition of guinea pig serum, a rich source of complement, increases opsonizing activity to only 50% of the normal value. About half of *B. abortus* and avirulent *B. melitensis* organisms are killed 4 hours after phagocytosis, but virulent *B. melitensis* organisms are not killed. Macrophages become infected early in the course of infection. Studies of murine infections with *B. abortus* have shown that at about 14 days after infection, the numbers of bacteria in the most heavily infected organs, the liver and spleen, decline markedly. This is thought to be due to T lymphocytes' activating macrophages. Cytokines are involved in controlling the infection at the molecular level, with the production of interferon turning on tumor necrosis factor (TNF) production as a likely final pathway. The specific subset of lymphocytes involved has a cytotoxic/suppressor phenotype. Those bacteria which persist may be responsible for the protracted course of the illness in untreated patients. Genetically controlled variation in expression of TNF may be a factor in determining the outcome of infection in brucellosis.

The role of antibodies in containing infection is difficult to assess. This is partly because of the intracellular localization of organisms sequestered from the actions of antibody. When organisms are released by rupture of infected cells, they are exposed to antibrucella antibody.

Pathology. The pathologic changes in brucellosis are characterized by granuloma formation in tissues (Fig. 64–1). All tissues and organs of the body can be involved, but liver and spleen are constantly affected. This applies to all three species that infect humans. The granulomas comprise epithelioid cells surrounded by lymphocytes and monocytes with fibroblasts. Giant cells are sometimes seen, but caseation does not occur. Necrosis with pus formation may be present, most often with *B. suis*, less commonly with *B. melitensis*, and rarely with *B. abortus*. Abscesses can occur in any tissue, but lymph glands and the spine are the more usual sites.

CLINICAL MANIFESTATIONS. The incubation period, most

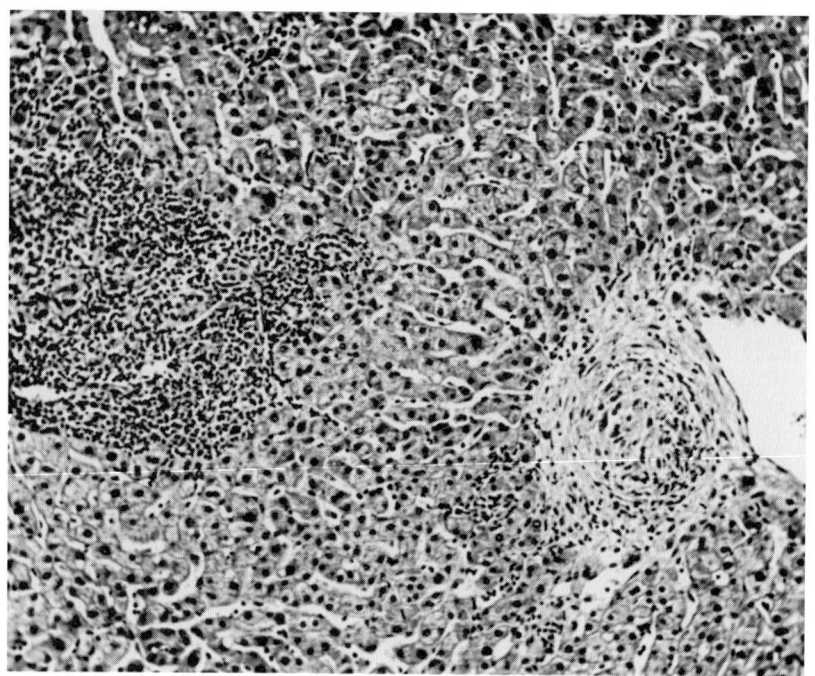

Figure **64–1.** Brucellosis. Liver biopsy showing small epithelioid cell granuloma and a large periportal lymphocyte infiltrate (H & E, × 130). (Courtesy of the Armed Forces Institute of Pathology, Photograph Neg. No. 73-918).

accurately gauged in accidental laboratory-acquired infections, is usually 3 to 4 weeks.

Acute Illness. The acute form is well recognized; fever, generalized aches and pains in the limbs, chills, night sweats, anorexia, and lethargy are typical features. A number of investigators have commented on the strong, moldy odor of the sweat, often noted by spouses and attendants rather than the patients themselves. Patients are unwell with these symptoms but may wait 3 weeks or more before seeking medical attention. Examination may show a febrile patient who is not very ill. Hepatosplenomegaly is common, being present in 27% of a large series with acute brucellosis. Relapse after treatment is a well-recognized occurrence in brucellosis, with similar though perhaps less marked clinical features.

Joint and Bone Involvement. Arthritis is common, often severe, and often disabling. Patients may be unable to walk because of back or hip pain. Inflammation and swelling of the intervertebral disk can compress spinal nerve roots, particularly in the lumbar region, and can cause sciatica. Large joints are commonly affected (i.e., lumbar spine, sacroiliac joints, hips, and knees). The cervical and thoracic vertebrae may be involved. Vertebral infection can produce an abscess that protrudes anteriorly, laterally, or posteriorly. Posteriorly sited abscesses can compress the spinal cord or cauda equina. Psoas abscess is seen, and bilateral psoas abscesses have occasionally been reported. Involvement of other joints (e.g., wrist, elbow, sternoclavicular joint) is well recognized. Inflammation at costochondral junctions can also occur. The nature of joint involvement is not always clear. Septic arthritis with organisms isolated from joint fluid occurs, and preexisting degenerative joint disease is a predisposing factor in older patients.

Other Localized Infections. Epididymo-orchitis is present in 5 to 9% of cases in different series. Pyelonephritis and glomerulonephritis have been documented, and brucellae can be excreted in the urine. Pulmonary involvement is not common. When it is present, it occurs early in the course of the illness, often in patients who have no history of drinking milk; this lends support to the notion of inhalation of contaminated dusts as the route of infection. Endocarditis that affects either a previously normal valve, usually the aortic, or a previously diseased valve, often the mitral, happens rarely. Pericarditis also is reported. Neurologic involvement has been reported in 2 to 7% of patients with diverse manifestations (Table 64–1) and, like many of the clinical manifestations of brucellosis, can occur in the course of acute disease, within days or weeks of the onset of symptoms, or much later after months of disease in chronically infected patients. The features of brucellar meningitis can resemble those of tuberculous meningitis. Lymphadenopathy is found in about 4% of cases, and abdominal lymphoid hyperplasia occasionally has led to surgery for appendicitis. Skin rashes are described, often papular lesions on the limbs and trunk. Ocular involvement, although uncommon, is recognized. Brucellosis in pregnancy can result in abortion, particularly in the first trimester of pregnancy. Whether this frequency (36%) is

TABLE 64–1. Neurologic Syndromes in Brucellosis

Cerebral

Papilledema
Cranial neuritis
Focal or diffuse cerebritis
Meningoencephalitis
Parkinsonian syndrome
Cerebellar disorders
Encephalopathy
Transient ischemic episodes/cerebral vasculitis
Ruptured mycotic aneurysm

Spinal

Acute poliomyelitis-like syndrome
Spinal cord compression due to abscess
Cauda equina syndrome
Myelitis
Myelopathy

Peripheral

Monoradiculopathy ⎫
Polyradiculopathy ⎬ Motor/sensory or mixed
Sciatica ⎭

greater than that caused by any septicemic illness in early pregnancy is not clear.

Chronic Infection. In addition to the wide range of clinical manifestations, chronicity of infection adds to the complexity of the disease. Alice Evans, the American microbiologist, suffered relapses of the infection for many years. In a large series reported from Kuwait, 77% had symptoms for 2 months or less, 13% had symptoms lasting 2 to 12 months, and 10% had symptoms for more than a year. The diagnosis in cases of protracted infection can be difficult. Fever may be present intermittently. Splenomegaly may be found. The history is particularly important; animal contact, occupational exposure, and raw milk drinking are valuable occurrences that prompt further investigation.

Laboratory. Routine blood counts usually show a normal or slightly reduced hemoglobin level. White blood cell counts are below $4.0 \times 10^9/L$ in a fifth of patients, and a lymphocytosis is present in almost half. Reduced platelet counts are found in 10%, and disseminated intravascular coagulation has been noted. Liver function tests show moderate abnormalities, with elevations of aminotransferases and alkaline phosphatase levels. The latter may relate to either granulomas in the liver or bone and joint involvement.

DIAGNOSIS

Culture. Blood culture is most commonly used to isolate the organism, yielding positive results in 14 to 30% of cases. The biphasic Castenada medium was developed specifically for *Brucella* isolation. The Bactec system has given good results with brucellosis, and the introduction of nonisotopic indications of growth is a further useful advance. Positive cultures are usually obtained at about 10 days and may be apparent within 1 week. If brucellosis is considered in the differential diagnosis, the laboratory must be informed so

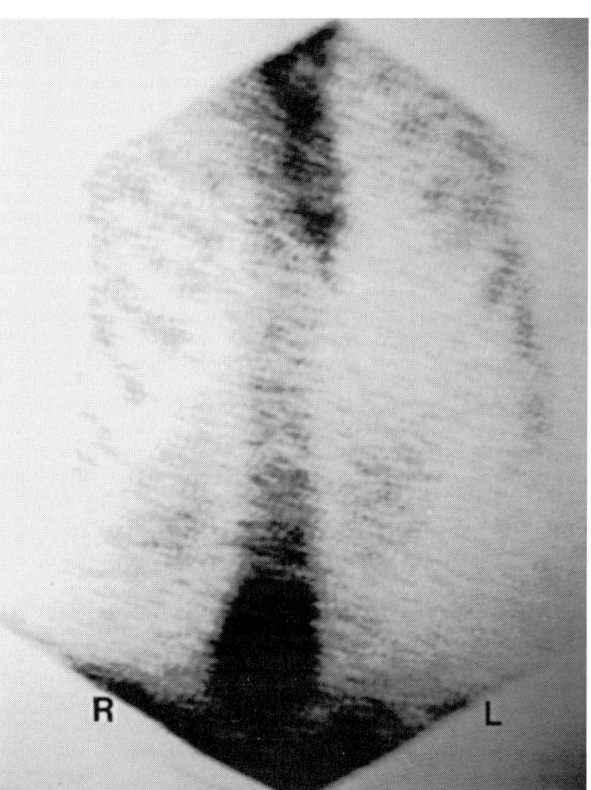

Figure 64–3. This is the technetium bone scan of the case illustrated in Figure 64–2. There is a marked increase in uptake of isotope in the lower lumbar spine. This nonspecific appearance is seen in any inflammatory spondylitis.

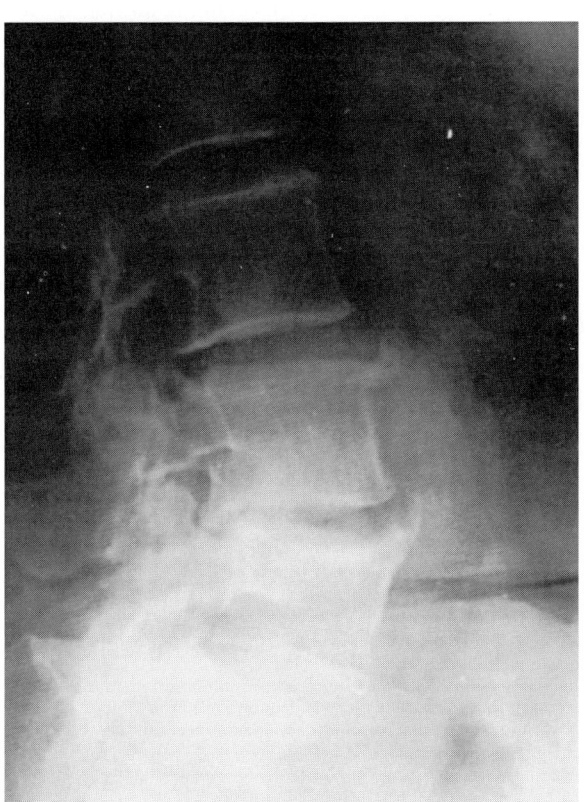

Figure 64–2. The fourth and fifth lumbar vertebrae are involved in this case of brucellar spondylitis. There is irregularity of affected vertebral bodies, loss of disk space, and osteophyte formation. There is also a soft tissue shadow in front of the spine.

that the cultures are retained for up to 6 weeks to give the maximum chance of finding this slow-growing organism. Clot culture also is frequently positive, but manipulating infected material presents risks of laboratory infection. Bone marrow culture has given yields as great as 90%. Any pus or tissue taken during biopsy should be cultured as well.

Polymerase Chain Reaction. PCR is very sensitive in detecting infectious agents and is particularly appropriate for this slow-growing organism that is highly infectious. Several sets of primers that have been devised are either genus or species specific. Studies of field applications are awaited, but preliminary results are promising. Need for isolation of the organism remains to monitor antibiotic sensitivities.

Serology. A serum agglutination test (SAT) titer of over 1:160 is suggestive of disease, but results can never be interpreted without relevant clinical data. Titers usually rise fairly early in the course of infection and are positive by 21 days of illness. Agglutinating antibody is initially IgM, but with increasing duration of infection IgG titers become higher and IgM declines. Use of enzyme-linked immunosorbent assay (ELISA) testing has shown a rise in IgA titers along with IgG with increasing duration of symptoms. After treatment, titers decline, only to rise in relapse. A persistently elevated titer in a treated patient who remains well is not usually significant.

The prozone phenomenon can cause a false-negative result because of the presence of blocking, nonagglutinating antibody. This effect occurs at low titer and is readily overcome by diluting out test samples. Laboratories performing these tests routinely set them up at low and high dilutions to prevent this source of false-negative results.

The agglutination test also can be performed after treating the sample with 2-mercaptoethanol (2-ME), which inactivates IgM so that early in the course of disease the SAT result is high but the 2-ME titer is much lower. The antiglobulin Coombs test result is positive in patients with chronic infections. Complement fixation tests also have been used. Among developments in serologic testing have been radioimmunoassay, which is not readily applicable in most endemic areas because of the need for isotopes, and ELISA using either whole organisms or subcellular fractions as antigen.

Radiology. Plain radiographs of affected bones and joints may show changes. The intervertebral disk space is narrowed, and bone destruction is seen at the epiphysis. This is accompanied by sclerosis and formation of osteophytes and syndesmophytes (Fig. 64–2), which may firmly ankylose adjacent vertebrae. Soft tissue swelling, which may include an abscess, can be seen anterior or lateral to the bony lesion on plain radiographs. Computed tomographic scans show bone destruction and associated inflammation. They also show psoas abscesses. Technetium isotope scans show increased activity at the sites of bone or joint lesions (Fig. 64–3). This may be present before radiographic changes are evident, although abnormalities persist for a considerable time after treatment. Therefore, changes in scan appearances cannot be used to monitor the response. Results of gallium scanning are also abnormal, and some evidence suggests that resolution of gallium scan abnormalities may correlate with a good response to treatment.

Differential Diagnosis. The differential diagnosis is wide and includes tuberculosis (Chapter 77) and typhoid (Chapter 75). Gastrointestinal symptoms usually are more prominent in typhoid, and the duration of fever is less except when it occurs in patients with schistosomiasis. Bone and joint involvement is not common in typhoid fever. The wide range of manifestations of tuberculosis makes it difficult to distinguish from brucellosis. Bone and joint involvement are features common to both infections. The dorsal spine is more commonly the site of spinal disease in tuberculosis. Lumbar spine involvement is more common in brucellosis, but any part of the spine can be affected in both diseases. Sacroiliitis is common in brucellosis. Both diseases affect the nervous system. Meningitis in the two infections can be similar, with similar changes in the cerebrospinal fluid (CSF). Protracted examination of CSF for tubercle bacilli may allow definitive diagnosis of tuberculous infection at the outset. Q fever (Chapter 34) is another condition capable of causing prolonged fever, hepatosplenomegaly with granulomatous liver disease, and epididymo-orchitis.

TREATMENT. Tetracycline and streptomycin were the mainstays of treatment for many years, and evidence shows greater efficacy for this combination, using doxycycline instead of tetracycline, than for the combination of doxycycline plus rifampicin, which has the advantage of oral administration (Table 64–2). The advantage may relate to synergistic activity between streptomycin and doxycycline. Patients' compliance is likely to be better if they need to take fewer drugs and if once- or twice-daily dosing regimens are used. Children younger than 8 years and pregnant women should not receive doxycycline; thus, rifampicin plus either streptomycin or co-trimoxazole should be given to younger children and rifampicin alone to pregnant women. Co-trimoxazole as monotherapy is associated with high relapse rates and should not be used. Cephalosporins, e.g., cefuroxime and ceftriaxone are effective against brucellae and are safe in pregnancy, although there is little experience with their use, but they may have a use in special situations. The fluorinated quinolones are active in vitro, but clinical experience has not yet produced compelling indications for their use. Chloramphenicol is effective and cheap and diffuses readily into the tissue of the central nervous system (CNS), but it is not used routinely.

TABLE 64–2. Antibiotic Treatment of Brucellosis*

Clinical Manifestations	Antibiotic Regimen
Systemic illness plus lymphadenopathy, enlargement of liver or spleen	Tetracycline, 500 mg q.i.d. for 6 wk *plus* Streptomycin, 1 g IM daily for 2 wk **or** Doxycycline, 100 mg b.i.d. for 6 wk *plus* Streptomycin, 1 g IM daily for 2 wk **or** Doxycycline, 100 mg b.i.d. for 6 wk *plus* Rifampicin, 900 mg daily for 6 wk
Localized disease, e.g., neurologic involvement and osteoarticular disease	Regimens as above, but the 6-wk dosage period is extended up to 12 wk

*This is not an exhaustive list of regimens but indicates generally accepted approaches to treatment. Some authors have used 6-wk regimens successfully for treatment of localized disease. These regimens are not used in children under age 8 or in pregnant women.

Six weeks of treatment is usually recommended for uncomplicated cases, but when there is specific organ localization, e.g., joint or CNS involvement, 12 weeks is needed. Treatment duration in children is similar. Endocarditis is difficult to manage but almost invariably requires valve replacement in addition to prolonged antibiotic treatment. Surgical drainage of pus is needed when abscesses have formed. This may be done at an open procedure, but percutaneous aspiration under imaging control may be possible.

PREVENTION. Prevention of brucellosis can be achieved by boiling milk before it is drunk or used to prepare milk products. This seems easy, but in many countries, it would require people to make a major change in their behavior. Pasteurization in commercial dairy practice achieves the same effect. Control of infection among the animal populations is of major importance and is achieved by testing animals to find which are infected, destroying infected animals with financial compensation to the farmer for loss of stock, vaccinating uninfected animals, and continuing surveillance thereafter to ensure the herd remains free of infection. The vaccines used are attenuated strains of *B. abortus* (S19), *B. melitensis* (Rev-1), and *B. suis*.

Bibliography

Acocella G, Bertrand A, Beytout J, et al: Comparison of three different regimens in the treatment of acute brucellosis. J Antimicrob Chemother 23:433, 1989.

Araj GF, Lulu AR, Mustafa MY, et al: Evaluation of ELISA in the diagnosis of acute and chronic brucellosis in human beings. J Hyg (Cambridge) 97:457, 1986.

Ariza J, Gudiol F, Valverde J, et al: Brucellar spondylitis: A detailed analysis based on current findings. Rev Infect Dis 7:656, 1985.

Baldwin CL, Winter AJ: Macrophages and brucella. Immunol Ser 60:363, 1994.

Bashir R, Al-Khawi MX, Harder EJ, et al: Nervous system brucellosis diagnosis and treatment. Neurology 35:1576, 1985.

Hall WH: Modern chemotherapy for brucellosis in humans. Rev Infect Dis 12:1060, 1990.

Jayakumar RV, Al-Aska AK, Subesinghe NA, et al: Unusual presentations of brucellosis. Postgrad Med J 64:118, 1988.

Lubani MM, Dudin KI, Sharda DC, et al: A multicentre therapeutic study of 1100 children with brucellosis. Pediatr Infect Dis J 8:75, 1989.

Lulu AR, Araj GF, Khateeb MI, et al: Human brucellosis in Kuwait: A prospective study of 400 cases. Q J Med 66:39, 1988.

Mousa ARM, Koshy TS, Araj GF, et al: Brucella meningitis: Presentation, diagnosis and treatment. Q J Med 60:873, 1986.

Solera J, Rodriguez ZM, Geijo P, et al: Doxycycline-rifampicin versus doxycycline-streptomycin in treatment of human brucellosis due to *Brucella melitensis*. Antimicrob Agents Chemother 39:2061, 1995.

Young EJ: An overview of human brucellosis. Clin Infect Dis 21:283, 1995.

65 *Rickettsial Infections: General Principles*

James G. Olson

DEFINITION. Rickettsiae, members of the order Rickettsiales, comprise a diverse group of organisms responsible for a large burden of morbidity that is largely unrecognized. A wide range of clinical entities are usually acute and self-limited and are distributed worldwide. Most are typhus-like diseases that are accompanied by nonspecific signs and symptoms; however, some produce a pathognomonic rash following systemic symptoms. More than 16 species in 4 genera (*Rickettsia, Ehrlichia, Coxiella,* and *Orientia*) of the family *Rickettsiaceae* are pathogenic for humans.

DESCRIPTION. Members of the order Rickettsiales are morphologically and biochemically similar to other gram-negative bacteria. They are short, rod-shaped or coccobacillary organisms, usually 0.4 to 2.0 μm long and 0.2 to 0.5 μm in diameter. They are typical of other gram-negative bacteria in that they have a cell wall, typical prokaryotic DNA arrangement with genome the size of *Neisseria,* frequently a slime layer or microcapsule (Fig. 65–1), and an independent metabolism. All are obligate intracellular parasites and may grow only within eukaryotic host cells. Multiplication is by transverse binary fission. *Coxiella burnetii* produce minute endospore-like structures that are resistant to heat and desiccation (Fig. 65–2). *Rickettsia* and *Coxiella* produce endotoxins similar to those produced by gram-negative bacilli.

INTERACTIONS WITH HOST CELLS. All have the ability to penetrate through host-cell plasma membrane into the cytoplasm, where they multiply (Fig. 65–3). Spotted fever group rickettsiae can penetrate the nucleus of the host cell. *Rickettsia typhi,* unlike *R. prowazekii,* can escape through the plasma membrane without requiring host cell destruction. *C. burnetii* is taken in by endocytosis and grows within a membrane-bound vacuole. These differences in host cell interaction may account for differences in disease patterns and immune response (Table 65–1).

NATURAL HISTORY
Transmission. With the exception of louse-borne typhus, all rickettsioses are zoonoses. They are maintained in nature in an enzootic cycle that includes vertebrate (usually mammalian) and invertebrate (usually arthropod) vectors (Fig. 65–4; Table 65–2). Humans are usually infected when they inadvertently come in contact with the vector. They are usually dead-end hosts and are not responsible for infecting other humans either directly or indirectly by infecting arthropods. Exceptions include louse-borne typhus, which can be transmitted both person-to-person and indirectly through infection of lice. Transfusion of blood and blood products may also be a rare source for the person-to-person transmission of rickettsiae. Vectors responsible for human infection may not be those involved in the enzootic maintenance cycle. Many species of ticks, fleas, mites, and lice may be capable of becoming infected and transmitting rickettsiae to the mammalian reservoir hosts, but only those with host feeding patterns that include humans are implicated as potential vectors of disease.

Mechanisms of transmission vary with the species of rickettsia and the vector. For the tick- and mite-transmitted rickettsioses, which include scrub typhus and the spotted fever group, the rickettsiae colonize the salivary glands of the vector and are transmitted to the host by bite. For louse- and flea-transmitted rickettsioses, which include the typhus group, rickettsiae multiply in the midgut epithelium of the vector and are excreted in the feces. Human infection depends on the contamination of the bite, breaks in the skin, or mucous membranes with infective feces or crushed lice. Rickettsiae remain infective in dried feces and lice for long periods. Abundant accumulation of feces on animal fur and of lice in clothing account for airborne spread of typhus group rickettsiae. Humans are highly susceptible to the airborne route of infection through the respiratory tract, mucous membranes, and conjunctiva.

Reservoirs. The vector is the primary reservoir for most rickettsiae transmitted by ticks and mites; the efficiency of transovarial transmission from generation to generation, and trans-stadial transmission from instar to instar, ensure survival of the rickettsiae. Ehrlichiae are an exception in that there is no evidence that transovarial transmission occurs. Those rickettsiae that either are incapable of transovarial

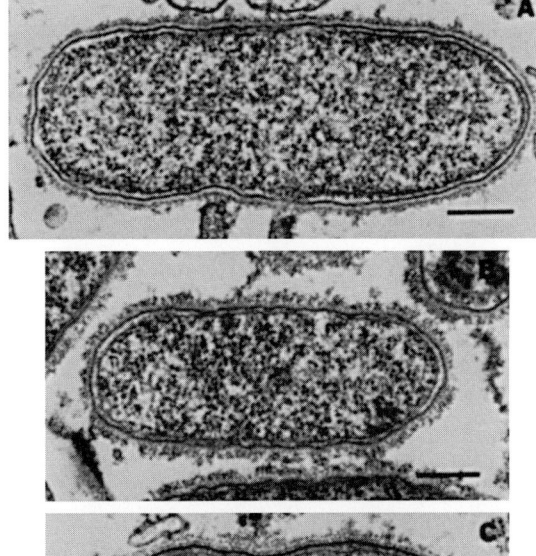

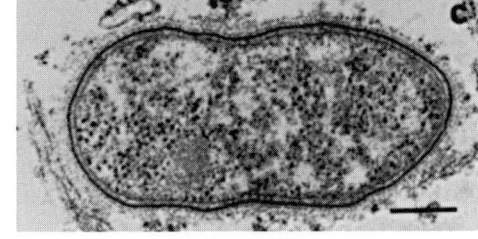

Figure 65–1. Comparison of ultrastructure as revealed by transmission electron microscopy of *R. prowazekii (A), R. rickettsii (B),* and *O. tsutsugamushi (C).* Note the small residual slime layer stabilized by antibody, the inner and outer membranes, and the internal ribosomal structures. This outer envelope of *O. tsutsugamushi* differs from the others in thickness of the outer leaflet of the outer membrane. (Bar = 0.25 μm.) (From Silverman DS, Wisseman CL Jr: Infect Immunol 21:1020, 1978. Reprinted by permission.)

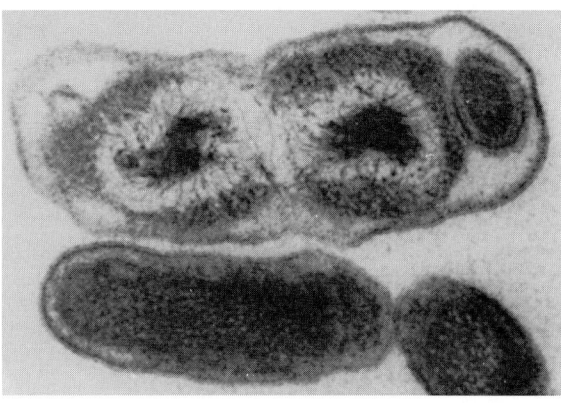

Figure 65–2. Transmission electron micrograph of *C. burnetii* showing small, dense, endospore-like structure. The small, dense forms are thought to account for the unusual stability of *C. burnetii*. (From McCaul TF, Williams JC: J Bacteriol 147:1063, 1981. Reprinted by permission.)

TABLE 65–1. Diversity in Human Rickettsioses Among Target-Cell Relationships, Basic Pathologic Lesions, and Type of Clinical Disease

Disease	Target Cell	Host-Cell Association	Basic Lesion	Clinical Manifestations
Typhus-like fevers				
Typhus group	Endothelial	Free intracytoplasmic	Vasculitis	Acute, self-limited fever
Scrub typhus	Endothelial	Free intracytoplasmic	Vasculitis	Acute, self-limited fever
Spotted fever group	Endothelial, smooth muscle	Free intracytoplasmic and intranuclear	Vasculitis	Acute, self-limited fever
Q fever	Reticuloendothelial	Intracytoplasmic vacuole	Granulomas	Acute, self-limited fever, atypical pneumonia, subacute hepatitis, endocarditis
Ehrlichiosis				
Human monocytic ehrlichiosis (HME)	Monocytes	Intracytoplasmic vacuole	Vasculitis	Acute, self-limited fever
Human granulocytic ehrlichiosis (HGE)	Granulocytes	Intracytoplasmic vacuole	Vasculitis	Acute, self-limited fever

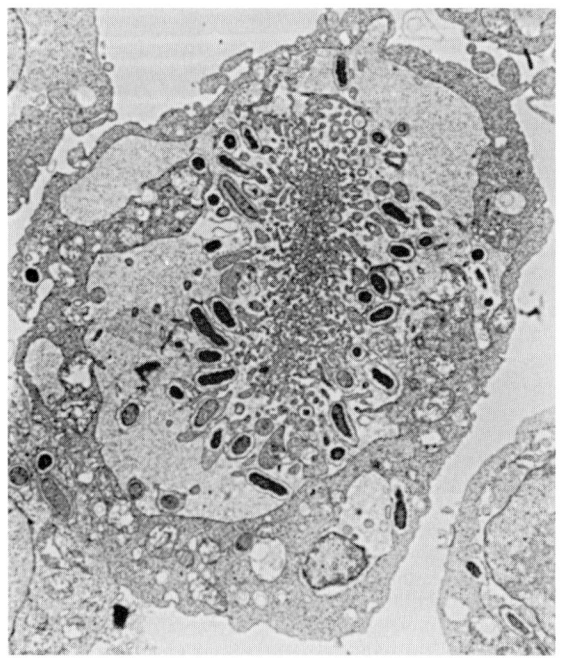

Figure 65–3. Transmission electron micrograph of chicken embryo fibroblast late in the infection cycle of *R. rickettsii*. Note the enormous swelling of the endoplasmic reticulum with entrapped organisms. Similar changes in the endoplasmic reticulum have been described in endothelial cells in a fatal case of RMSF. (From Silverman DS, Wisseman CL Jr: Infect Immunol 26:714, 1979. Reprinted by permission.)

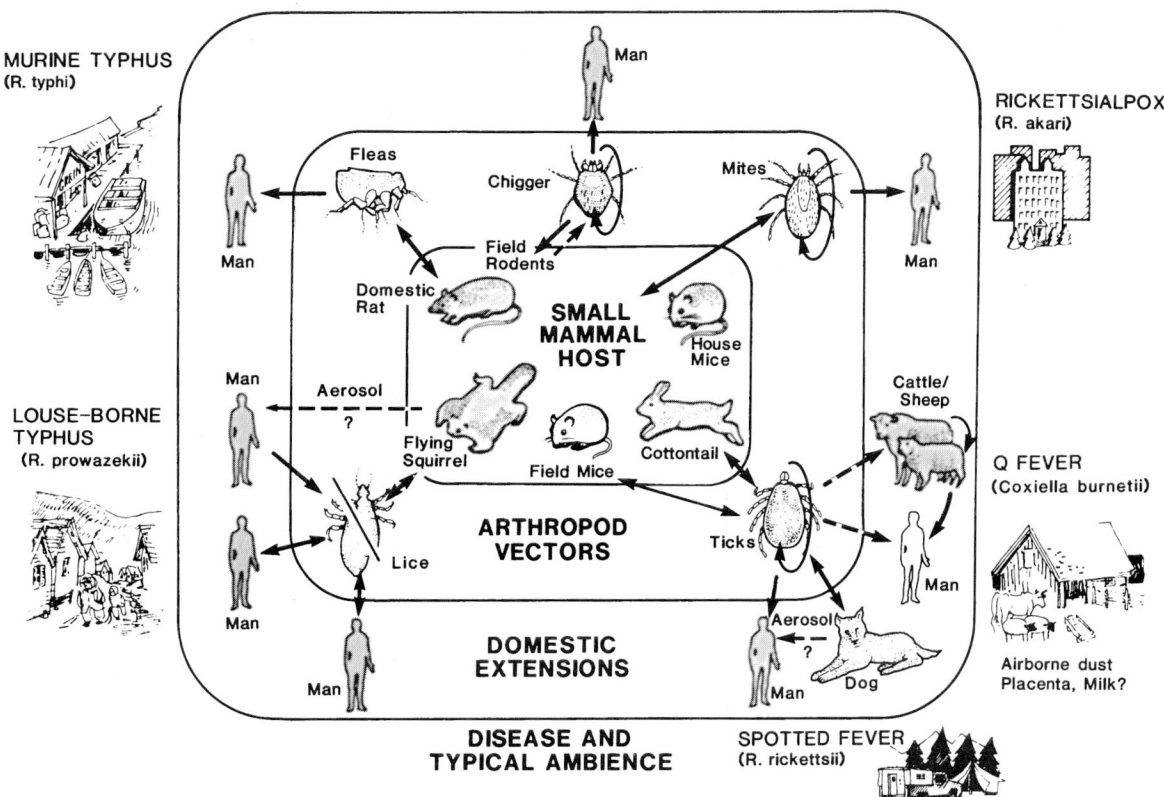

Figure 65–4. Schematic summary of some major interactions between rickettsial organisms, their small animal hosts and Arthropod Vectors, the participation of domestic animals, and examples of the typical ambience under which each rickettsial infection is contracted by man. Scrub typhus is transmitted in grassy, scrub, or transitional vegetation; by rickettsialpox in the incinerator areas of large apartment houses; by spotted fever through occupational or recreational activities in tick-infested terrain; by Q fever in the husbandry or use of sheep and cattle; by louse-borne typhus where human body lice are prevalent, now largely confined to poverty-stricken mountain villages in some developing countries; and by murine typhus in rat-infested grain/food storage structures and warehouses. (Courtesy of Dr. J.K. Frenkel, University of Kansas Medical Center, Kansas City, KS.)

transmission or for which it is an infrequent occurrence require a reservoir host to maintain the rickettsiae and infect the vector.

PATHOGENESIS. Similarities exist among the diseases caused by rickettsiae. In boutonneuse fever, African tick-bite fever, and scrub typhus, a visible lesion (eschar) (Fig. 69–1) develops at the inoculation site during the incubation period. Rickettsiae are introduced into the skin by the bite of the arthropod, through skin excoriation (crushed arthropod), or through the conjunctiva. Rickettsiae attach to vascular endothelial cells, are phagocytized, and then rapidly escape from the phagocytic vacuole to multiply freely in the cytoplasm. Infected endothelial cells are destroyed by direct injury, which often results in thrombosis of small vessels. Injury to endothelium results in an increase in vascular permeability, which is responsible for hypovolemia, edema, hypotension, and hypoalbuminemia.

Vasculitis. Disseminated focal infection occurs in the endothelium of small blood vessels of the skin, brain, lungs, heart, liver, kidneys, and other organs (Fig. 65–5). Multifocal, multiorgan vasculitis is the most important pathophysiologic feature of rickettsial diseases. Rickettsiae infect, multiply in, and damage endothelial cells, causing necrosis, hypertrophy, and proliferation. Loss of protein-rich fluid from the intravascular compartment into tissues across endothelium plays a

prominent role in the pathophysiology of these diseases. Infection is limited to endothelial cells in typhus and scrub typhus infections but may extend to all layers in Rocky Mountain spotted fever (RMSF), causing necrosis of the media. At the sites of endothelial damage, platelet-fibrin thrombi form, along with endothelial hypertrophy and proliferation that partially occlude the vascular lumen (Fig. 65–6). The typical perivascular inflammatory response develops at infection sites, with polymorphonuclear and monocytic cells early and macrophages, lymphocytes, and occasional plasma cells later, coinciding with the timing of the antibody response (Figs. 65–6 and 65–7). This sequence suggests that the infection may evolve through an early phase, with vascular damage as direct result of rickettsial infection, to a late phase, with additional vascular damage from immune mechanisms. An immunopathologic mechanism is consistent with patients with typhus and scrub typhus appearing more toxic and having greater vascular instability and mortality in the late phase of illness after antibodies are present. On the other hand, the more severe vascular lesions with little perivascular cellular response, no antibody response, and unresponsiveness to antirickettsial therapy in fulminant RMSF suggest that direct rickettsia-induced damage alone can cause irreversible pathophysiologic changes.

Pathology. The disseminated vascular lesions can account

TABLE 65–2. Summary Features of Selected Diseases Caused by Rickettsiae

Typhus Group Rickettsia

Disease	Etiologic Agent	Arthropod Vector	Ecology of Exposure	Geographic Distribution
Louse-borne (epidemic) typhus	Rickettsia prowazekii	Human body louse (Pediculus humanus)	Crowded, squalid conditions created by war and natural disasters that lead to body louse infestations; exacerbated by cold weather or following disruption of water supply for bathing	Endemic in highlands of Africa, Asia, and the Americas
Sylvatic (flying-squirrel) typhus*	R. prowazekii	Squirrel flea (Orchospea howardii)	Houses (e.g., attics) or other areas where flying squirrels nest	Eastern United States
Brill-Zinsser disease (recrudescent typhus)*	R. prowazekii	No vector; recrudescence from patients who have previously recovered from louse-borne typhus	Debilitation caused by stress, malnutrition, or illness in chronically infected person leads to recrudescence	Worldwide; most common in areas where louse-borne typhus occurs or has occurred in the past
Flea-borne (murine, endemic) typhus*	Rickettsia typhi	Fleas: Oriental rat flea (Xenopsylla cheopis) and cat flea (Ctenocephalides felis)	Urban and suburban areas where rats (Rattus spp.) and their fleas are common (in the U.S. most common during April–August)	Worldwide, particularly in coastal areas of tropics and subtropics
Cat flea typhus*	Rickettsia felis	Cat flea (Ctenocephalides felis)	Contact with cat fleas and opossums in suburban areas	California, Texas, and Oklahoma

Spotted Fever Group Rickettsia

Disease	Etiologic Agent	Arthropod Vector	Ecology of Exposure	Geographic Distribution
Rocky Mountain spotted fever*	Rickettsia rickettsii	Ixodid ticks: Dermacentor variabilis, D. andersoni, Amblyomma americanum, A. cajennense	Grassy areas, forest edge, roadsides, hiking trails, stream banks, unmowed areas around homes (in U.S., most common during May–September)	Throughout most of the U.S., Central America, and South America; most common in southeastern U.S.
Mediterranean spotted fever	Rickettsia conorii	Ixodid ticks: Brown dog tick (Rhipicephalus sanguineus)	Peridomestic; contact with buildings in which dogs have been kept	Southern Europe, Africa, and Asia
African tick-bite fever	Rickettsia africae	Ixodid ticks (Amblyomma spp.)	Camping, safaris, exposure in cattle farming areas	Eastern and sub-Saharan Africa, (South Africa, Zimbabwe, and Ethiopia)
Queensland tick typhus	Rickettsia australis	Ixodid tick (Ixodes holocyclus)	Outdoor activities that involve contact with vegetation harboring questing ticks	Australia
Flinders Island spotted fever	Rickettsia honei	Unknown vector	Outdoor activities that involve contact with vegetation harboring questing ticks	Eastern and sub-Saharan Africa, (South Africa, Zimbabwe, and Ethiopia)
Siberian tick typhus (North Asian tick typhus)	Rickettsia sibirica	Ixodid ticks (Dermacentor nuttallii, D. sylvarum, D. marginatus, Hamaphysalis concinna)	Outdoor activities that involve contact with vegetation harboring questing ticks	North Asia (including China and the former Soviet Union)
Japanese spotted fever (Oriental spotted fever)	Rickettsia japonica	Unknown tick vector	Outdoor activities that involve contact with vegetation harboring questing ticks	Japan
Rickettsialpox*	Rickettsia akari	Mouse mite (Liponyssoides sanguineus)	Contact with urban dwellings infested by house mice and their mites (occurs year round)	Worldwide; occasionally cases occur in large metropolitan centers in the U.S., especially New York City. Also reported from Croatia, Ukraine, South Africa, and Korea

Other Rickettsiae

Disease	Etiologic Agent	Arthropod Vector	Ecology of Exposure	Geographic Distribution
Human monocytic ehrlichiosis (HME)*	Ehrlichia chaffeensis	Lone Star tick (Amblyomma americanum)	Grassy areas, forest edge, roadsides, hiking trails, stream banks, unmowed areas around houses (most common during May–September)	Southeastern U.S. (most common in Oklahoma, Missouri, Tennessee, Arkansas, and Georgia); possibly Portugal, Mali, and Italy
Human granulocytic ehrlichiosis (HGE)*	Ehrlichia sp., the HGE agent (closely related or identical to E. equi or E. phagocytophila)	Ixodid ticks: black-legged tick (Ixodes scapularis), European sheep tick (I. ricinus)	Grassy areas, forest edge, roadsides, hiking trails, stream banks, unmowed areas around houses (most common during May–September)	Northeastern coastal areas and upper midwestern states of U.S. (most common in New York, Wisconsin, Minnesota, Connecticut, and Massachusetts); Europe (Slovenia and possibly Germany, Sweden, Switzerland, and UK)
Sennetsu ehrlichiosis	Ehrlichia sennetsu	No arthropod vector	Consumption of raw fish that may contain nematode intermediate host of ehrlichia	Japan
Scrub typhus	Orientia tsutsugamushi	Larval mites (chiggers): Leptotrombidium deliense	Walking in areas where regrowth of forest is occurring and contact with larval mites (chiggers) is common; plantations, clearing, building sites, river banks (most common during warmer temperatures in subtropics, and following onset of rains in tropics)	Asia (including southeastern Asia, Korea, China, far eastern Russia, Nepal, India, and Pakistan), Indonesia, northern Australia, and the Pacific islands (including Japan, Taiwan, Philippines and New Guinea)
Q fever	Coxiella burnetii	Arthropod vector not important	Inhalation of species or contact with infectious blood from infected animals	Worldwide

*Diseases endemic in the United States.

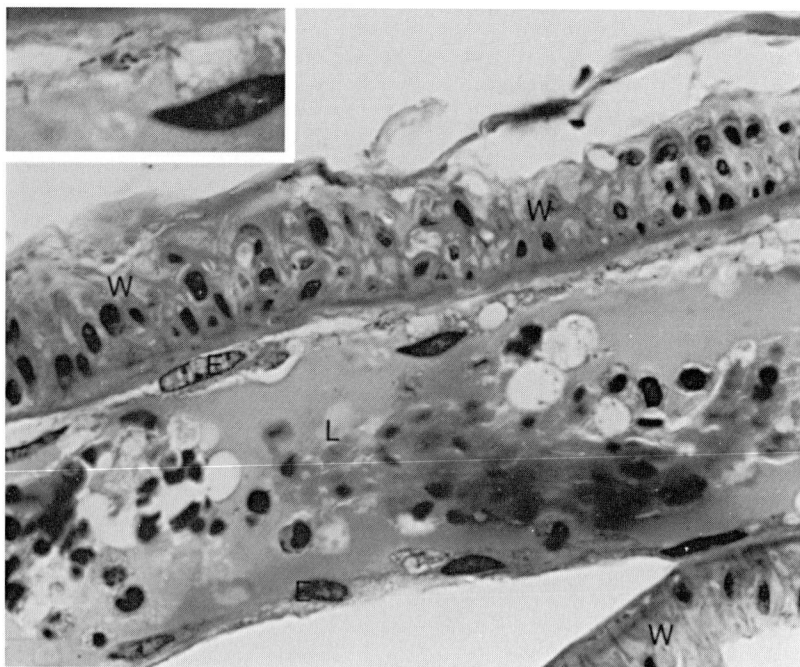

Figure 65–5. *R. rickettsii* within a vascular endothelial cell *(inset)* from a fatal case of human Rocky Mountain spotted fever (W = wall; E = endothelium; L = lumen). (Courtesy of Drs. Douglas Wear and Daniel Connor and the Armed Forces Institute of Pathology, Photograph Negative No. 79-15424.)

for multiorgan involvement and many clinical and pathophysiologic abnormalities, including rash, edema and increased extravascular fluid space, hypovolemia, hypotension, and gangrene in louse-borne typhus and RMSF. These lesions may also account for the clotting abnormalities in severe RMSF. The classic typhus nodules in the brain (Fig. 65–7) are of the same vascular origin and, along with edema, help explain mental changes and cranial nerve deficits. In RMSF, discrete microinfarcts may occur in the white matter of the brain (Fig. 65–8) with persisting electroencephalographic changes.

The heart often shows edema, a diffuse mononuclear infiltrate, and some muscle necrosis. Nonspecific electrocardiographic changes are common. Perivascular lesions occur in

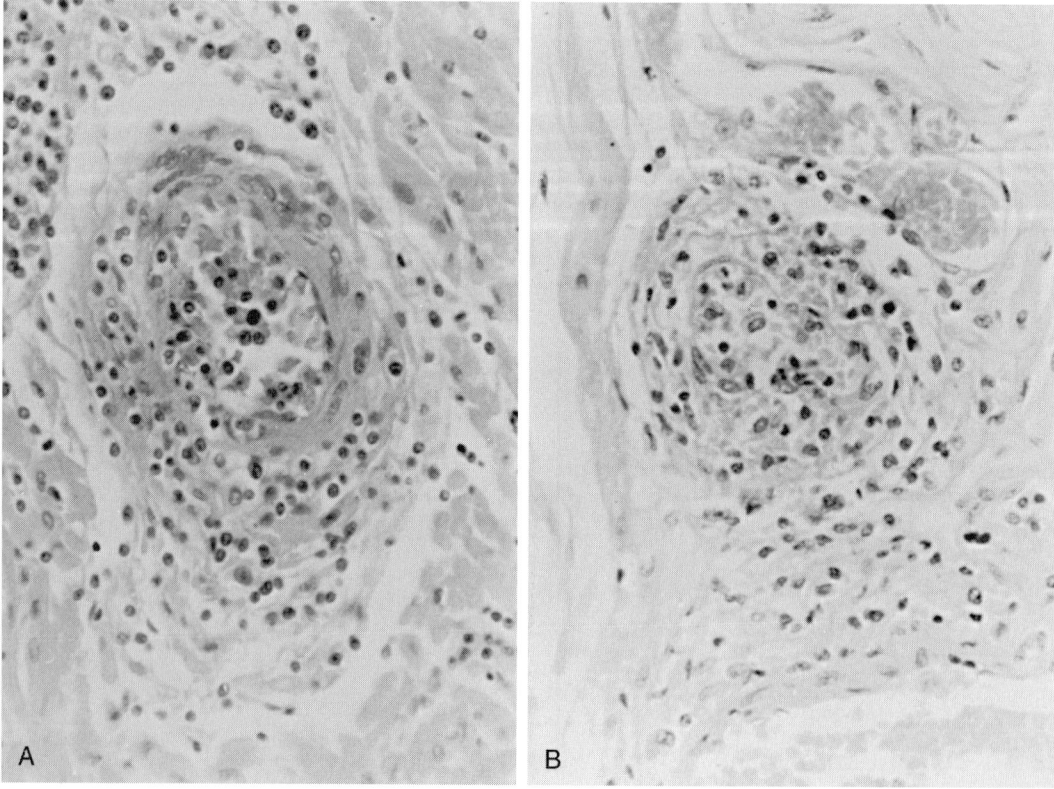

Figure 65–6. Comparison of vascular lesions in human louse-borne typhus fever *(A)* and Rocky Mountain spotted fever *(B).*

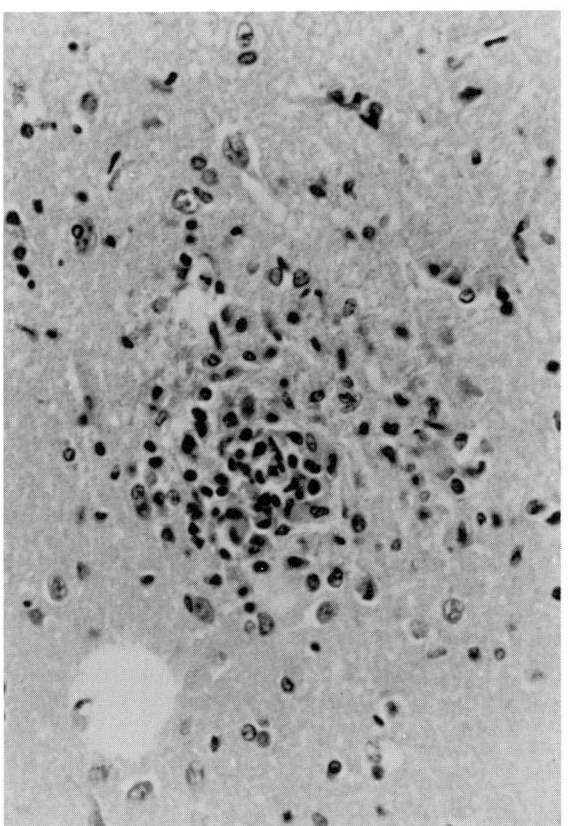

Figure 65–7. "Typhus nodule" in the brain of a patient with louse-borne typhus. Similar lesions are found in scrub typhus and, more rarely, in Rocky Mountain spotted fever.

the portal areas of the liver, along with nonspecific focal areas of fatty degeneration in hepatocytes. Blood levels of aminotransferases are elevated. Kidneys show focal interstitial vascular lesions involving only a few nephrons. The characteristic oliguria and azotemia of typhus are attributable to prerenal causes, including hypotension, hypovolemia, and tissue catabolism. Renal tubular necrosis is observed in severe RMSF. The lungs show interstitial pneumonitis on histologic examination and radiography.

Immune Response. Immunity to rickettsial infection is generally solid and lifelong, but viable rickettsiae may remain latent in tissues for months or years. Antibodies are detectable during the first week of illness but are not rickettsicidal and have little effect on rickettsial growth or control of disease. Instead antibodies probably opsonize extracellular rickettsiae and facilitate their destruction by macrophages. Cell-mediated immunity develops and is important in controlling intracellular parasitism.

GENERAL CLINICAL CONSIDERATIONS. Some clinical features of selected rickettsial diseases are presented in Table 65–3. Most typhus-like rickettsial diseases have common clinical features, including fever, headache (Fig. 66–1), cough, prostration, rash (Figs. 66–2 and 67–1), altered mental state (Figs. 66–3 and 66–4), hypotension, and a low white cell count.

DIAGNOSIS
Differential Diagnosis. The signs and symptoms at onset of illness are common to many infectious diseases; differential clinical diagnosis may be difficult. Early signs (e.g., eschar[s]) (Fig. 69–1), provide specific diagnostic information. Later signs indicative of rickettsial diseases include the appearance

of rash (Figs. 66–2 and 67–1), hypotension, and altered mental state (Figs. 66–3 and 66–4), but rickettsioses vary in severity and presentation. Practitioners must utilize epidemiologic and laboratory information to augment their clinical observations. Waiting for specific laboratory confirmation is impractical and dangerous. Many deaths from RMSF in the United States are directly attributable to delays in initiation of specific antimicrobial therapy.

Laboratory Diagnosis. Methods for confirmation of clinical diagnoses are well developed but not universally available. No satisfactory methods are available for etiologic confirmation during the acute phases of illness, when decisions on chemotherapy are necessary.

Direct Detection of Rickettsiae. Rickettsiae can be detected by immunofluorescence and immunohistochemistry in tissue biopsies obtained from the site of the arthropod bite (eschar) and from cutaneous lesions (rash). The assays are highly specific but less than 70% sensitive in patients with these lesions.

Rickettsiae can also be detected in circulating endothelial cells by direct immunofluorescence. This procedure has very high specificity and a sensitivity of 60%. The test can be completed in less than 3 hours and has great potential for use as a rapid diagnostic assay. Immunofluorescence and immunohistochemical tests are important for the retrospective etiologic confirmation on tissues collected post mortem. Polymerase chain reaction (PCR) is an important method for confirmation of ehrlichiosis and may have a use in other rickettsioses as well.

Serologic Tests. The standard for confirmation of rickettsioses is serologic testing for specific antibodies. Indirect immunofluorescence is the most frequently used and best standardized assay. Enzyme immunoassays have been developed

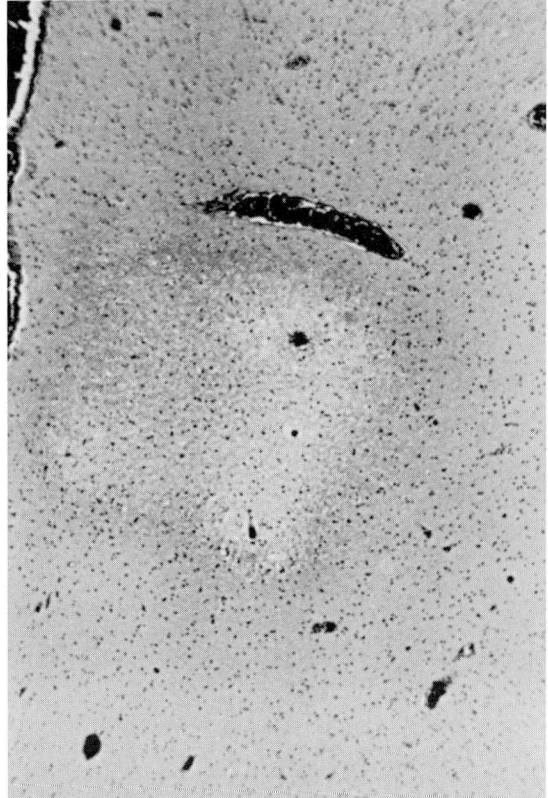

Figure 65–8. Microinfarct in white matter of the brain of a patient with Rocky Mountain spotted fever.

TABLE 65-3. Some Clinical Features of Selected Rickettsial Diseases

Disease	Usual Incubation Period (Days)	Eschar	Rash: Onset (Day of Disease)	Rash: Distribution	Rash: Type	Usual Duration of Disease* (Days)	Usual Severity†	Duration of Fever after Chemotherapy (Hours)
Typhus Group								
Murine typhus	12 (range: 8–16)	None	5–7	Trunk, extremities	Macular, maculopapular	12 (range: 8–16)	Moderate	48–72
Epidemic typhus	12 (range: 10–14)	None	5–7	Trunk, extremities	Macular, maculopapular, petechial	14 (range: 10–18)	Severe	48–72
Brill-Zinsser disease		None		Trunk, extremities	Macular	7–11	Relatively mild	48–72
Spotted Fever Group								
Rocky Mountain spotted fever	7 (range: 3–12)	None	3–5	Extremities, trunk, face	Macular, maculopapular, petechial	16 (range: 10–20)	Severe	<48–72
Boutonneuse fever	5–7	Often present	3–4	Trunk, extremities, face, palms, soles	Macular, maculopapular, petechial	10 (range: 7–14)	Moderate	—
Rickettsialpox	9–17	Often present	1–3	Trunk, face, buccal mucosa	Papulovesicular	7	Relatively mild	—
Scrub typhus (tsutsugamushi disease)	12 (range: 9–18)	Often present	4–6	Trunk, extremities	Macular, maculopapular	14 (range: 10–20)	Mild to severe	24–36
Q fever	19 (range: 10–26)	None		None		6‡ (range: 2–21)	Relatively mild	48 (occasionally slow)
Ehrlichiosis	10 (range: 0–34)	None	5 (range: 0–21)	Trunk, legs, arms, face	Petechial, erythematous	16 (range: 0–86)	Mild to severe	24–48

*Untreated disease.
†Severity can vary greatly.
‡Occasional chronic infections occur (e.g., hepatitis, endocarditis).

that show promise for laboratory confirmation early in disease. Weil-Felix testing is still frequently used because of its convenience, but it suffers from a lack of sensitivity and specificity.

TREATMENT
Antibiotics

Tetracyclines. In almost all clinical circumstances, tetracyclines are the drugs of choice. Tetracyclines are bacteriostatic against *Rickettsia* spp. and bactericidal against ehrlichia. Doxycycline is generally preferred over other tetracyclines because of its longer plasma half-life (18 hours). The most notorious side effect of the tetracyclines is their propensity to bind calcium, resulting in staining and hypoplasia of developing tooth enamel. For this reason, routine use of tetracyclines in children younger than 8 years has been discouraged. However, the benefit of tetracycline use in children with potentially life-threatening rickettsial and ehrlichial infections far exceeds the risks, and doxycycline remains the antimicrobial of choice in pediatric patients of any age. As the degree of dental staining is dose and duration dependent (the threshold for cosmetically perceptible staining appears to be 6 or more multiple-day courses of therapy), the risk of discoloration is minimal following a short course of doxycycline. Doxycycline is effectively administered orally in most cases. Intravenous therapy is given to hospitalized patients with vomiting, severe multisystem disease, or obtundation. Tetracyclines are contraindicated in pregnant women because of the risk of severe maternal hepatotoxicity and pancreatitis as well as interference with normal development of teeth and long bones in the fetus.

Chloramphenicol. This is an alternative therapy for the rickettsioses and has been used in pregnant patients with severe rickettsial disease. Oral chloramphenicol has been unavailable in the United States since 1995. The only systemic formulation of chloramphenicol currently available is parenteral sodium succinate. This drug provides broad-spectrum activity against other infectious agents that may mimic rickettsial infections (including *Neisseria meningitidis* and *Salmonella typhi*) and may be preferred in select critically ill patients when the diagnosis is uncertain and the differential diagnosis includes one or more of these pathogens. Chloramphenicol is neither bacteriostatic nor bactericidal against *Ehrlichia* spp. in vitro, and there are reports of treatment failures in some patients with ehrlichiosis. Idiosyncratic aplastic anemia, which occurs in 1 in 24,500 to 40,800 courses of treatment, is the most devastating adverse reaction caused by this antibiotic. There also appears to be a dose-response relationship between chloramphenicol use and some childhood leukemias (e.g., acute lymphocytic and nonlymphocytic leukemias). Chloramphenicol has a low therapeutic-to-toxic ratio, and a number of reversible, dose-related toxicities are associated with this drug, including bone marrow suppression (reticulocytopenia, granulocytopenia, and/or thrombocytopenia), cardiomyopathy, and gray baby syndrome in neonates. For this reason, serum concentrations should be routinely monitored, with the peak levels maintained between 10 and 20 µg/mL.

Other Drugs. Rifampin shows significant in vitro bactericidal activity against *E. chaffeensis* and the human granulocytic ehrlichiosis (HGE) agent, and anecdotal reports describe rapid clinical improvement in patients with HGE treated with rifampin in the second and third trimesters of pregnancy. These data should be interpreted cautiously, however, and should not be uniformly applied to other rickettsial infections. Indeed, treatment failures have been documented in clinical trials evaluating rifampin for the treatment of Mediterranean spotted fever (MSF).

The efficacy of currently available quinolones against the ehrlichioses and rickettsioses other than MSF have not been evaluated by clinical trials. There are anecdotal reports of rapid clinical response with ciprofloxacin in the treatment of flea-borne typhus and scrub typhus, and successful patient outcomes are well documented for MSF. Ciprofloxacin is not active against *Ehrlichia* spp. and should not be used to treat these infections. In vitro studies indicate that several newer quinolones possess bacteriostatic and/or bactericidal activities against spotted fever group rickettsiae (e.g., levofloxacin) and ehrlichia (e.g., trovafloxacin); however, these drugs have not been evaluated in patients with active disease.

Duration of Therapy. Although no consensus exists regarding optimal length of therapy for these infections, the best guide appears to be the clinical response: Most clinicians advocate continuing antibiotic coverage for at least 2 to 3 days following defervescence, for a minimum total course of 5 days. In general, patients become afebrile within 24 to 48 hours after initiation of effective therapy, and the total duration of treatment is 5 to 10 days. Shortened (i.e., single-dose) regimens have been successfully implemented during outbreaks of louse-borne typhus, and effective single-day therapy for MSF has been reported. However, disease relapses within 2 to 8 days following termination of therapy have been described for several rickettsioses, including RMSF, Israeli spotted fever, flea-borne typhus, and scrub typhus, particularly with abbreviated treatment regimens initiated very early in the course of infection. Relapses are more frequently associated with chloramphenicol use but have also been described with single-dose doxycycline. Longer courses of doxycycline (10 to 21 days) may be warranted in select patients with HGE if co-infection with *Borrelia burgdorferi* is suspected.

Precautions. Therapy with sulfa-containing antimicrobials is contraindicated; there is evidence that these drugs may increase the severity of several rickettsial infections, including RMSF, MSF, flea-borne typhus, and possibly ehrlichiosis.

Prophylactic therapy in individuals who are not ill but who have recent arthropod bites is not warranted. Administration of doxycycline prior to the onset of symptoms may only delay the onset of clinical disease with some rickettsial infections.

Antimicrobial Resistance. In vitro sensitivities are not routinely done on rickettsiae because isolation is attempted only in a few research laboratories and because intracellular rickettsiae require cell culture for antibiotic susceptibility testing.

Supportive Therapy

Corticosteroids. Use of high-dose corticosteroids late in the course of severe vasculotropic rickettsioses has been advocated by some, but there are no controlled trials to suggest the efficacy of this therapy.

Cardiovascular Complications. Severely ill patients may develop marked hypotension, oliguria, and shock from intravascular fluid losses. Close hemodynamic and electrolyte monitoring, coupled with careful fluid replacement and pharmacologic blood pressure support, is required in these patients. Marked anemia and thrombocytopenia can develop in some cases, requiring close attention to blood counts. Standard criteria for transfusion of red cells and platelets should be followed. The prominent features of typhus, scrub typhus, and spotted fevers are attributed to abnormalities of the cardiovascular system.

Other Complications. Bacterial pneumonia is common in epidemic typhus and should be treated according to the etiology and sensitivity patterns of the causative agent. Gangrene, decubitus ulcers, and thrombophlebitis are treated by appropriate surgical and medical methods. Personality changes, electroencephalographic changes, and deafness may persist in some patients.

Bibliography

Beltran RR, Herrero JIH: Evaluation of ciprofloxacin and doxycycline in the treatment of Mediterranean spotted fever. Eur J Clin Microbiol Infect Dis 11:427, 1992.

Clements ML, Dumler JS, Fiset P, et al: Serodiagnosis of Rocky Mountain spotted fever: Comparison of IgM and IgG enzyme-linked immunosorbent assays and indirect fluorescent antibody test. J Infect Dis 148:876, 1983.

Dasch GA, Halle S, Bourgeious AL: Sensitive microplate enzyme-linked immunosorbent assay for detection of antibodies against the scrub typhus rickettsia, *Rickettsia tsutsugamushi*. J Clin Microbiol 9:38, 1979.

Drancourt M, George F, Brouqui P, et al: Diagnosis of Mediterranean spotted fever by indirect immunofluorescence of *Rickettsia conorii* in circulating endothelial cells isolated with monoclonal antibody–coated immunomagnetic beads. J Infect Dis 166:660, 1992.

Halle S, Dasch GA, Weiss E: Sensitive enzyme-linked immunosorbent assay for detection of antibodies against typhus rickettsiae, *Rickettsia prowazekii* and *Rickettsia typhi*. J Clin Microbiol 6:101, 1977.

Levy PY, Drancourt M, Etienne J, et al: Comparison of different antibiotic regimes for therapy of 32 cases of Q fever endocarditis. Antimicrob Agents Chemother 35:533, 1991.

Newhouse VF, Shepard CC, Redus MD, et al: A comparison of the complement fixation, indirect fluorescent antibody, and micragglutination tests for the serological diagnosis of rickettsial diseases. Am J Trop Med Hyg 28:387, 1979.

Raoult D, Roux V: Rickettsioses as paradigms of new or emerging infectious diseases. Clin Microbiol Rev 10:694, 1997.

66 Typhus: General Principles

James G. Olson

Five clinical and epidemiologic entities constitute the established diseases of the typhus group: (1) primary epidemic louse-borne typhus (*Rickettsia prowazekii*); (2) its recrudescent form, Brill-Zinsser disease (*R. prowazekii*); (3) sporadic flying squirrel typhus (*R. prowazekii*); (4) flea-borne murine typhus (*R. typhi*); and (5) cat-flea typhus (*R. felis*). These diseases are similar clinically and pathologically but differ in intensity of certain symptoms and signs, severity, and case-fatality rates. Tables 65–1 through 65–3 summarize selected features of the rickettsiae and their associated diseases.

66.1 Epidemic Louse-Borne Typhus

James G. Olson

DEFINITION. Classic typhus fever is an acute infectious disease transmitted by the human body louse (*Pediculus humanus corporis*; Fig. 139–1) characterized clinically by the sudden onset of a sustained high fever of about 2 weeks' duration, a maculopapular rash, and altered mental state. Brill-Zinsser disease, a recrudescence of typhus that occurs months to years after primary infection, is caused by organisms persisting in tissues since the primary infection and clinically resembles a mild form of classic typhus.

ETIOLOGY AND EPIDEMIOLOGY. *R. prowazekii* is the etiologic agent of classic typhus fever, Brill-Zinsser disease, and sporadic flying squirrel typhus (Table 65–2; Fig. 65–1).

Epidemic Louse-Borne Typhus. The classic infection cycle is restricted to humans and the human body louse (*Pediculus humanus corporis*; Fig. 65–4 and Table 65–2). The louse acquires the rickettsiae by feeding on the blood of a typhus patient during the rickettsemic phase; large numbers of rickettsiae are excreted in louse feces. The organisms are not transmitted by bite. Instead, crushed infective lice or louse feces contaminate bite sites or other breaks in the skin, or airborne infective louse feces gain access through the respiratory tract.

Brill-Zinsser Disease (BZD). In most areas, humans, through the phenomenon of persisting infection and subsequent recrudescence, are the only known interepidemic reservoirs and the means by which lice are exposed to the rickettsiae (Table 65–4). Factors that precipitate recrudescence include poor nutritional status and debilitation caused by illness or stress. The frequency of recrudescence may be up to 15% in those having primary infections and may be higher among patients who receive incomplete antibiotic therapy. The efficiency of transmitting *R. prowazekii* to feeding lice is apparently less in BZD than in patients with primary typhus.

Distribution. Typhus can occur anywhere when political, socioeconomic, environmental, and cultural factors predispose to lousiness and the transfer of lice among people. These factors are currently present in some mountainous areas of both hemispheres as well as in equatorial regions, in deserts (Sahara and Arabian deserts) where heavy clothing is worn continuously, and in tropical regions among nearly naked populations whose waistbands or arm and leg ornaments provide harborage for lice. The present known distribution of louse-borne typhus fever includes the mountainous regions of Mexico and Guatemala, the Andean highlands of South America, the Himalayan regions (including Afghanistan and Pakistan), mountainous or highland regions of Africa (i.e., Ethiopia, Burundi, Rwanda, and Lesotho), and northern China. Reservoirs in the form of typhus convalescents occur on all continents, but reservoirs derived from typhus contracted during and after World War II are diminishing in number.

Depending on many factors, louse-borne typhus can occur as a truly epidemic disease, as a prolonged endemic-epidemic disease (e.g., in Ethiopia and Burundi), or as a high endemic infection with sporadic, often unrecognized infections, especially in young age groups, but sometimes with sharp, sporadic village outbreaks involving all age groups (e.g., in Andean countries).

IMMUNITY. Susceptibility to louse-borne typhus is universal. Convalescence from infection leads to long-lasting immunity against the disease, although second infections have been described. Both humoral and cellular immune responses to *R. prowazekii* are demonstrable for many years. The immunologic defect that permits recrudescence (BZD) to occur is unknown. Cross-immunity is strong against murine typhus, but not against Rocky Mountain spotted fever, with which there may be some serologic cross reactions.

PATHOLOGY. The general pathologic and pathophysiologic features are described in Chapter 65, Table 65–1, and Figures 65–6 and 65–7.

CLINICAL MANIFESTATIONS AND COURSE. The incubation period of primary louse-borne typhus usually is from 8 to 12 days but may be as short as 6 days or as long as 15 days. The disease may be divided into prodromal, early, and late phases.

Prodromal and Early Phases. Prodromes of vague malaise and headache are common. The early phase is usually ushered in by the abrupt onset of fever, severe headache (Fig. 66–1), myalgia of the back and legs, and chills or chilly sensations. The headache is intense and intractable and persists day and night. Over the first 2 or 3 days, the temperature attains a level of about 39° to 41°C, and continues until death or recovery. The skin is usually hot and dry. The face is flushed or dusky; the conjunctivae are suffused; photophobia is frequent. The mental state is dull. Weakness and prostration may be mild early after onset but may become profound after 2 or 3 days. Unproductive cough with sparse

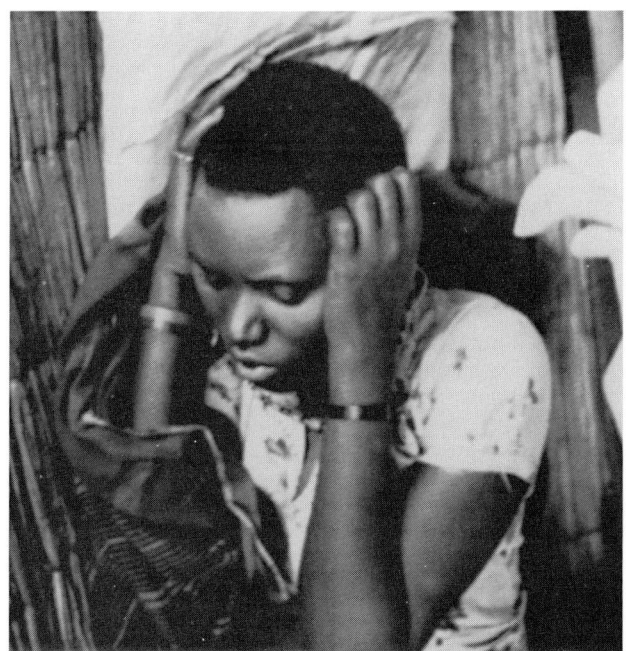

Figure 66–1. Louse-borne typhus fever. Headache, although not invariably a prominent feature, is commonly severe, constant, relentless, and incapacitating. Patients often describe it as the worst headache they ever experienced. Similar headache may be present in murine typhus, scrub typhus, spotted fever group infections, and Q fever. (Courtesy of Charles L. Wisseman, Jr.)

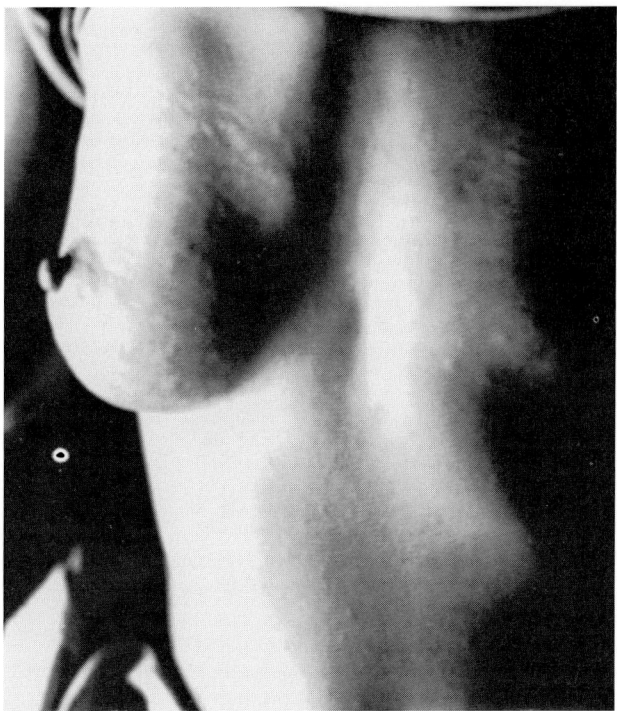

Figure 66–2. Louse-borne typhus fever. The rash in typhus is macular to maculopapular, pink and blanching under pressure early, and fixed and petechial late. The papular component may be seen under appropriate lighting conditions even when the erythema is masked in deeply pigmented skin. (Courtesy of Charles L. Wisseman, Jr.)

physical findings occurs in about two thirds of patients. Nausea, vomiting, and diarrhea occur but are uncommon. Constipation is usually present.

Late Phase

Rash. The characteristic rash appears between the fourth and seventh days and is the hallmark of the late phase of disease. In some instances, it is preceded by a diffuse, transient erythema. The lesions first appear on the trunk and axillary folds and spread to the extremities, sparing the face, palms, and soles, except in severely ill patients. At first, the lesions are pinkish-red macules that blanch on pressure. The evolution of the rash depends on the severity of the illness. In mild cases, it may fade completely in 1 or 2 days; in cases of moderate severity, it may become maculopapular, possibily hemorrhagic, changing to a reddish-brown color and lasting for 1 to 2 weeks before fading. In severe cases, the lesions may be numerous, almost confluent, quickly becoming hemorrhagic or purpuric. The rash may be absent in 5 to 10% of patients. With experience and proper lighting, the papular component may be seen without too much difficulty in dark-skinned persons (Fig. 66–2).

Cardiopulmonary Findings. At first, the pulse rate is slow in relation to the temperature, but by the end of the first week, it becomes rapid (110 to 140 beats/min), weak, and frequently undulating or irregular. The blood pressure is usually low, sometimes with a systolic pressure below 80 mm Hg, and there may be brief episodes of severe hypotension. Cyanosis may be present.

Neurologic Findings. The mental state progresses from dullness to stupor or, occasionally, coma (Fig. 66–3). The stupor may be interrupted by periods of delirium, excitement, or vigorous activity, during which time the patient may exhibit self-destructive action or wander off into the bush (Fig. 66–4). Cranial nerves are selectively and variably involved (e.g., causing tinnitus, deafness, dysphagia, and dysphonia).

Coarse tremors may appear. Urinary and fecal incontinence is encountered in moderately or severely ill patients.

Laboratory Findings. Oliguria, proteinuria, and azotemia are common. Jaundice is rare, but elevations in serum aminotransferases may appear early. The white blood cell count may show leukopenia early; in the second and third weeks of the disease, it is normal or only slightly elevated unless complications ensue. Eosinophils are absent or rare in the early stages of typhus. Anemia may develop in the second or third week.

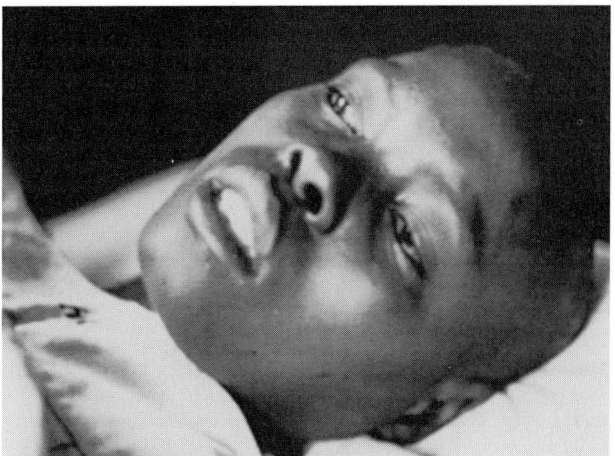

Figure 66–3. Louse-borne typhus fever. After a few days of untreated typhus fever, patients may sink into a semistuporous state with characteristic facies, lying immobile, staring unseeing, and responding only to strong external stimuli. (Courtesy of Charles L. Wisseman, Jr.)

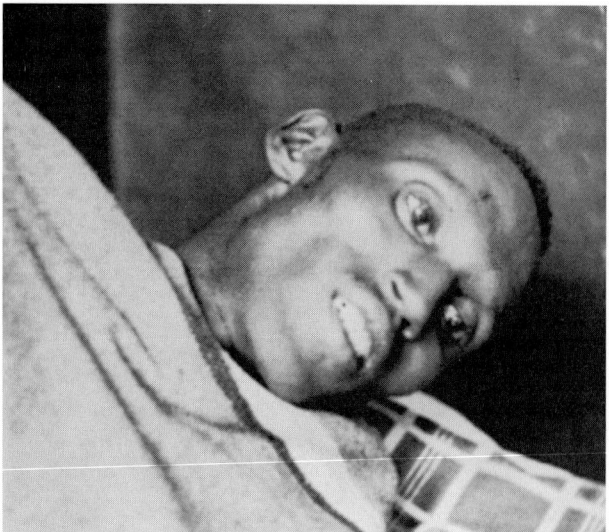

Figure 66–4. Louse-borne typhus fever. Delirium is a troublesome complication. (Courtesy of Charles L. Wisseman, Jr.)

Outcome. Death from untreated typhus usually occurs between the 9th and 18th days of illness. The terminal period is usually characterized by a profound stupor, peripheral vascular collapse, and severe renal failure. Among patients who recover, the temperature begins to decline after 14 to 18 days and reaches a normal level by rapid lysis in 2 to 4 days. The mental and physical states of the patient improve strikingly as the temperature falls, but strength returns more slowly, often taking 2 to 3 months (Fig. 66–5).

Complications. Secondary bacterial bronchopneumonia, otitis media, and parotitis are common in untreated patients. Thrombosis may affect the large arteries with major complications, e.g., hemiplegia. Thrombosis of small vessels in the skin may lead to gangrene, particularly of the toes, fingers, or earlobes (Fig. 66–6). Necrosis of the skin may occur over the bony prominences, especially over the sacrum or the greater trochanter.

Modified Disease. The severity of disease and the case-fatality rate increase with age, being less severe and often uncharacteristic in younger children, but increasing rapidly in those over the age of 40 years.

Brill-Zinsser Disease. Recrudescent typhus is similar to primary typhus except that it is milder. On the average, the fever is lower and of shorter duration, the rash is less intense and often absent, and the case-fatality rate is less than 1%.

LABORATORY DIAGNOSIS. *R. prowazekii* can be isolated from blood or tissues by inoculating guinea pigs or directly in tissue culture. Diagnosis is usually made by demonstrating a rise in antibody titer by a serologic test. The indirect immunofluorescence assay (IFA) test and the enzyme immunoassay (EIA) are most useful in distinguishing among current primary typhus (early IgM response), recrudescent typhus (BZD—accelerated dominant IgG response), and past typhus infection (unchanging dominantly IgG titers). Differentiation between louse-borne and murine typhus can be made with species-specific complement fixation (CF) tests, or absorption-type IFA tests. The microagglutination test is convenient for field use but does not reliably differentiate between louse-borne and murine typhus infections in humans. Antibodies persist for many years.

PROGNOSIS. Depending on host factors, e.g., age, stress, nutritional state, other concurrent diseases, and perhaps the past typhus history of the population, the case-fatality rate

in untreated typhus may range from 10% or less to 60%. Deep coma, severe hypotension, and tachycardia associated with falling body temperature are signs of a poor prognosis. However, even patients with these signs often respond dramatically to appropriate chemotherapy and supportive measures. Appropriate treatment reduces the frequency of mortality in ordinary severe typhus fever virtually to zero.

TREATMENT. Doxycycline is preferred over tetracyclines because of its reduced phototoxicity, safety in patients with renal insufficiency, reduced deposition in teeth and bone, and longer plasma half-life. Doxycycline is effectively administered orally in most cases. Intravenous therapy is given to hospitalized patients with severe multisystem disease or obtundation. Dosage is 200 mg in two divided doses per day. Clinical response is the best guide to duration of therapy. Most clinicians advocate continued antibiotic coverage for at least 2 days following defervescence, for a minimum total course of 5 days. The response of uncomplicated typhus to specific antirickettsial chemotherapy, whether begun early or late, is highly predictable. The temperature returns to normal within 48 to 72 hours, averaging about 60 hours, accompanied by progressive lessening of headache and improvement of mental status. Occasionally manifestations, e.g., deafness, may appear during response to early therapy but subsequently subside. The occasional recrudescence of fever is usually mild and self-limited, but more severe recrudescences respond to retreatment with the same drug and dose. Other

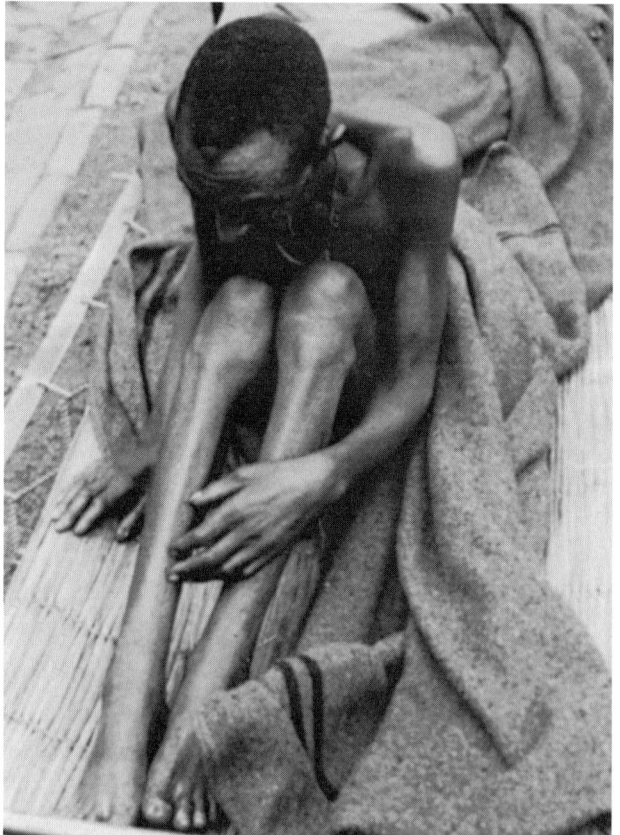

Figure 66–5. Louse-borne typhus fever. Three weeks after onset of disease, this formerly robust and well-developed young adult male shows the wasting, extensive loss of tissue mass, and debilitation typical of severe untreated typhus. Prompt early specific antirickettsial chemotherapy prevents this troublesome complication that needlessly prolongs convalescence. (Courtesy of Charles L. Wisseman, Jr.)

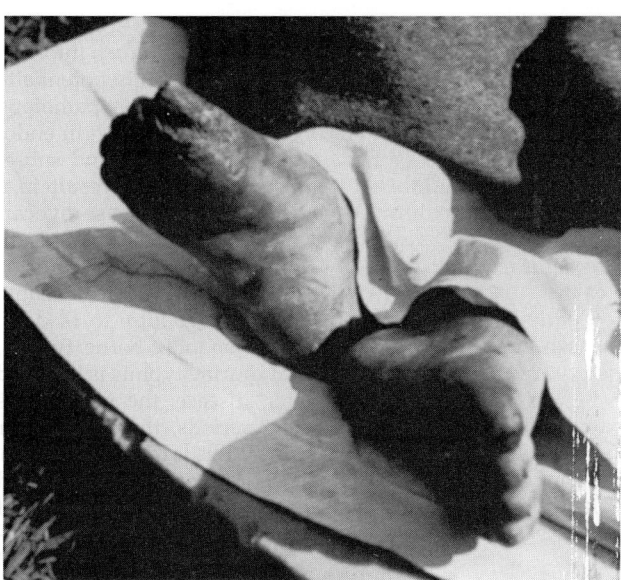

Figure 66–6. Louse-borne typhus fever. A small proportion of patients may develop some degree of dry gangrene, most commonly of the extremities. It may be limited to the tips of the fingers and toes but on occasion may involve all or part of the foot or even the entire lower leg. This patient shows gangrene of the distal part of the right foot and beginning necrosis of the left hallux. Partial debridement of the insensitive necrotic right hallux and foot was occurring during nightly visits of rats. (Courtesy of Charles L. Wisseman, Jr.)

concurrent or intercurrent infections are treated by appropriate methods; gangrene may require surgical intervention.

BZD is managed in an identical manner. Because louse-borne typhus, especially in epidemic form, tends to occur in circumstances under which even the most elemental components of conventional medical care may not be available, it is heartening to know that the simple expedient of administering a single 100- to 200-mg dose of doxycycline will cure almost all patients.

PREVENTION AND CONTROL

Decontamination. Infected lice and louse feces on a patient with typhus present a special hazard to all nonimmune contacts, including physicians and attendants, among whom infection is a common occupational hazard. Decontamination and delousing of the patient (including the head) and his or her clothing (including blankets and hats) are performed immediately on hospitalization. Clothing and bedding are best decontaminated by heat, because this kills the lice as well as the rickettsiae. After the patient is decontaminated and deloused, isolation and quarantine are not necessary. Depending on the circumstances, it may be necessary to apply insecticides at appropriate intervals to prevent reinfestation with lice.

Louse Control. Control of louse-borne typhus currently depends heavily on control of the louse vector. When simple hygienic measures, e.g., bathing and laundering of clothes in hot water with detergent, cannot be followed, the application of insecticide dusts (10% dichlorodiphenyltrichloroethane [DDT], 1% malathion, 1% lindane, or newer carbamates, depending on local louse resistance patterns) to fully clothed persons is effective in reducing louse populations and controlling disease in acute outbreaks (Chapter 139). Insecticide resistance among body lice is a widespread and growing problem. Kits for testing insecticide susceptibility are available from the World Health Organization. The older methods

of subjecting clothes and bedding to heat or fumigants, e.g., methyl bromide, are effective but cumbersome. It is possible but unproved that repellent-treated (e.g., with M-1960, permethrin, or diethyltoluamide) clothing reduces the chances of louse acquisition. Insecticides alone are less effective for long-term louse control in areas where conditions conducive to lousiness persist and where louse strains resistant to insecticides can be, and are, selected. Long-term louse control or eradication depends on correcting the complex environmental, economic, cultural, educational, and political factors that contribute to lousiness.

Vaccine. Conventional typhus vaccines composed of killed organisms are no longer available in the United States, pending development of improved vaccines of proved protective potency. The attenuated E strain of *R. prowazekii*, when used as a living vaccine, is protective but may produce a mildly symptomatic, self-limited infection in 10 to 15% of recipients.

Reduction of Exposure. Under current circumstances, the ordinary tourist is not likely to be exposed to louse-borne typhus, in contrast to murine typhus, even in endemic areas, nor are businesspersons, government representatives, archeologists, or engineering or construction workers likely to be exposed on assignment to most endemic zones if they maintain the usual separate households, pay attention to personal hygiene, and do not mix intimately with the affected local population. At high risk, however, are medical personnel and others who must treat or otherwise come into close contact with members of the affected populations. Depending on the circumstances, the wearing of insecticide- or repellent-treated clothing and the overnight exposure of clothing to a dichlorvos strip (No-Pest Strip) in an airtight bag may reduce exposure to lice.

Chemoprophylaxis. Under special short-term circumstances when it is necessary to keep personnel disease-free for a limited time, chemoprophylaxis with 100 mg of doxycycline once or twice a week might be effective. However, this has not been formally tested to determine the optimal spacing of doses and duration of administration to permit subclinical immunizing infection. Disease might develop after the drug is discontinued. Close medical surveillance and prompt chemotherapy on the first or second day of illness reduce typhus to a relatively minor inconvenience, with possible return after a few days to sedentary or light physical activity for the otherwise healthy young adult. The practice of administering a single dose of doxycycline to healthy contacts of patients with typhus to prevent typhus reveals an ignorance of the interplay between a rickettsiostatic antibiotic and the developing immunity that is essential to control the infection. Delay of disease onset is the likely outcome.

It is presumed that chemotherapy shortens the period of rickettsemia in louse-borne typhus as it does in scrub typhus. Under primitive or overwhelming conditions, when louse control may not be possible, chemotherapy is expected to limit the time a patient is infectious for lice. However, although the growth of rickettsiae in infected lice feeding on blood containing therapeutic levels of doxycycline is inhibited, the lice survive longer.

Bibliography

Gaon JA, Murray ES: The natural history of recrudescent typhus (Brill-Zinsser disease) in Bosnia. Bull WHO 35:133, 1966.

Raoult D, Ndihokubwayo JB, Tissot-Dupont H, et al: Outbreak of epidemic typhus associated with trench fever in Burundi. Lancet 352:353, 1998.

Wohlbach SB, Todd JL, Palfrey FW: The Etiology and Pathology of Typhus. Cambridge, MA, Harvard University Press, 1922.

66.2 *Murine Flea-Borne Typhus*

James A. Higgins and Abdu F. Azad

DEFINITION. Murine flea-borne, or endemic, typhus fever is an acute infectious disease caused by *R. typhi* and transmitted from rodents to humans principally by either the oriental rat flea (*Xenopsylla cheopis*; Fig. 139–11) or the cat flea (*Ctenocephalides felis*). This mode of transmission, and the lower case-fatality rate in infected individuals, distinguishes murine typhus from louse-borne typhus.

ETIOLOGY. *R. typhi* shares some common antigenic determinants (epitopes) with *R. prowazekii* and the spotted fever group of rickettsiae, but it differs in specific epitopes, host range, and other biologic properties. Significant cross-immunity between *R. typhi* and *R. prowazekii* is produced by infection. Both *R. typhi* and the recently discovered flea-borne *R. felis* exhibit substantial differences in DNA sequences for several genes from *R. prowazekii*. In the United States, *R. felis* occupies the same ecologic niche as *R. typhi* and has been linked to a human infection in Texas, with symptoms similar to murine typhus. Information on its prevalence and distribution is lacking. Differentiation between *R. typhi* and *R. felis* is currently only possible using molecular diagnostic procedures, e.g., polymerase chain reaction (PCR) and restriction fragment length polymorphism (RFLP). Experiments with laboratory rats have shown that infection with *R. typhi* can render them resistant to infection with *R. felis*, confirming that these species share antigenic properties.

EPIDEMIOLOGY

Transmission. Murine typhus is not communicable from person to person. It is a zoonosis maintained in nature in a cycle involving small mammals, primarily rats, and their fleas (Table 65–2; Fig. 65–4). It is thought that fleas become infected when feeding on a rickettsemic host and introduce the organisms to new hosts during subsequent feedings, probably by inoculation of infected feces (fleas tend to defecate during feeding) into the bite wound. Fleas are infected for life, and transovarial transmission of *R. typhi* has been documented in both rat and cat fleas. Typhus can be contracted through inhalation of infected flea or rat feces and in the laboratory by inhalation of concentrated rickettsial preparations; therefore, a history of flea bite may not be reported by all patients. The ecology governing the transmission of murine typhus is complex and may vary significantly from place to place with sporadic cases the rule, although well-delineated outbreaks have been reported.

Distribution and Exposure. Murine typhus is widely distributed over the world in areas populated by *Rattus rattus* and *Rattus norvegicus* and where the vector fleas exist. It is grossly underestimated as a cause of febrile human disease in many tropical and subtropical areas where, untreated, it may have substantial economic consequences. In some regions, the *Rattus* transmission cycle of *R. typhi* may be supplanted by one involving interactions with peridomestic animals. In the suburban United States, for example, infected cat fleas have been recovered from dogs, cats, opossums, and bobcats. Seasonal incidence of human infections correlates with the period of abundance of vector fleas, which is in the summer months in the United States. Rats are commensal animals closely associated with buildings or structures containing food (e.g., warehouses, markets, grain elevators, refuse dumps). Hence, in some areas, acquisition of murine typhus by humans is often associated with certain places and occupations; in others, as in some tropical areas where heavy rodent infestation of dwellings is universal, infection is acquired in dwellings.

PATHOLOGY. Although murine typhus is the second most frequently documented rickettsial disease, not much information is available regarding the pathology of this potentially fatal infection. As with other rickettsial infections, pathology is thought to be a consequence of rickettsial growth in endothelial cells (Fig. 65–5; Table 65–1). Colonization and subsequent lysis of endothelial cells by *R. typhi* can result in a characteristic vasculitis. Damage to lungs, kidneys, myocardium, brain, and liver has been observed at autopsy; death is thought to result primarily from interstitial myocarditis.

CLINICAL MANIFESTATIONS AND COURSE. The incubation period of murine typhus lasts from about 6 to 14 days. The symptoms are similar to those of louse-borne typhus, the principal differences being that murine typhus is believed to be a milder and shorter-lasting disease; the rash is less extensive and persists for shorter periods, there are fewer complications, and the case-fatality rate is lower (Table 65–3).

Although murine typhus is often referred to as mild, and truly mild cases do occur, on the average the degree of mildness is only relative to louse-borne typhus. On an absolute scale, it can be severe and debilitating, and untreated patients may require 2 to 3 months to regain strength and weight. High fever (40° to 41°C), excruciating headache, prostration, delirium, and stupor or coma may occur. Other patients may have a low-grade fever (38° to 39°C) and remain provisionally ambulatory.

DIAGNOSIS

Clinical Diagnosis. The diagnosis of murine typhus is problematic (nearly 90% of patients with murine typhus in south Texas were not identified at presentation) but may be suspected when a patient has sustained fever of several days' duration accompanied by headache, generalized aches and pains, and a macular or maculopapular rash appearing on the trunk on the fifth or sixth day after onset of fever. It is not unusual for patients to complain of gastrointestinal pain, diarrhea, and vomiting; pediatric patients may infrequently complain of headache. Diagnosis can be complicated by the fact that rash never develops in nearly one half of patients and may not be a presenting sign. Thrombocytopenia in children and adults is one consistent laboratory finding that can aid in diagnosis.

The patient may give a history of activities that brought him or her into contact with rats. However, there is often no definite recollection of a flea bite. Alternatively, the patient may receive flea bites continually due to flea infestation in a pet. Patients from suburban temperate areas should be asked if wild animals (e.g., opossums, feral cats, skunks) have been observed in proximity to their dwellings or pets.

Laboratory Diagnosis. Diagnosis can be confirmed by specific rickettsial serologic tests or by isolation of the agent. Confirmation may also be made by PCR amplification and RFLP analysis of rickettsial DNA from blood and tissue samples if facilities for molecular diagnostics are available.

IMMUNITY. Immunity to *R. typhi* is similar to that observed for other rickettsial infections; both cell-mediated and humoral responses are believed to play a role. Convalescent patient and animal sera recognize 120–135- and 17-kDa antigen bands on immunoblots, and occasionally a 68–70-kDa band. The former are surface proteins, whereas the 68–70-kDa polypeptide may be a heat shock–related protein. There is evidence from laboratory animals that immunity is not sterile and that viable rickettsiae may be sequestered in the host's tissues for extended periods of time following the initial infection, but documentation of this phenomenon in humans is lacking.

PROGNOSIS. The case-fatality rate is usually 6% in untreated patients and is virtually zero with rapid convalescence in patients with uncomplicated murine typhus treated with appropriate antirickettsial drugs.

TREATMENT. Treatment follows the guidelines presented in Chapter 65. A single dose of doxycycline may not effect a cure.

PREVENTION AND CONTROL. Individual preventive measures include avoiding endemic foci where rats and their fleas abound (e.g., warehouses, storage areas, grain elevators) and wearing repellent-treated clothing to prevent acquisition of fleas. Residents of suburban areas should reduce the contact between their pets and wild mammals by securing refuse in sealed containers, not putting food outdoors, and keeping pets indoors during the night. Flea control of pets is also encouraged.

A killed *R. typhi* vaccine was developed and tested but did not protect volunteers from challenge infections and therefore is of dubious efficacy. No vaccine for murine typhus is licensed for use in the United States.

Rodent and Flea Control. General control measures are directed at reducing rat and flea populations. These include, among others, ratproof construction and preventing rats access to food materials; reducing rat populations by poison baits (e.g., warfarin and α-naphthylthiourea), trapping, or infiltrating poison gases into burrows; and reducing the flea population through application of appropriate insecticides to rat runs or at bait stations. When contemplating a rodent control program, it is important to plan insecticide application for flea control prior to or simultaneously with the rodent control measures. This prevents the increased exposure of humans to fleas seeking alternative hosts. Resistance of fleas to insecticides is a growing problem.

Bibliography

Azad AF: Epidemiology of murine typhus. Annu Rev Entomol 35:553, 1990.

Baxter JD: The typhus group. Clin Dermatol 14:271, 1996.

Dumler SJ: Murine typhus. Semin Pediatr Infect Dis 5:137, 1994.

Dumler SJ, Taylor JP, Walker DH: Clinical and laboratory features of murine typhus in south Texas, 1980 through 1987. JAMA 2666:1365, 1991.

Higgins JA, Azad AF: The typhus fevers. *In* Rakel R (ed): Conn's Current Therapy. Philadelphia, WB Saunders, 1996, pp 168–170.

Raoult D, Drancourt M: Antimicrobial therapy of rickettsial diseases. Antimicrob Agents Chemother 35:2457, 1991.

Schriefer ME, Sacci JB Jr, Dumler SJ, et al: Identification of a novel rickettsial infection in a patient diagnosed with murine typhus. J Clin Microbiol 32:949, 1994.

Walker DH, Parks FM, Betz TB, et al: Histopathology and immunohistologic demonstration of the distribution of *Rickettsia typhi* in fatal murine typhus. Am J Clin Pathol 91:720, 1989.

67 *Spotted Fevers*

67.1 *Rocky Mountain Spotted Fever*

Daniel J. Sexton

DEFINITION AND ETIOLOGY. Rocky Mountain spotted fever (RMSF) is a potentially fatal tick-borne disease caused by *Rickettsia rickettsii*, a gram-negative coccobacillus that, is an obligate intracellular pathogen with a striking tropism for human endothelial cells (see Figs. 65–1*B* and 65–3). *R. rickettsii* exists in nature in close association with various species of ticks that are both reservoirs and vectors of the disease.

DISTRIBUTION AND INCIDENCE. The name Rocky Moun-

tain spotted fever can be misleading for those who are not aware of its widespread distribution throughout the Western Hemisphere.

Latin America. In Mexico the same disease is known as fiebre manchada; in Colombia it is called fiebre petequial; and in Brazil it has been São Paulo typhus, and fiebre maculosa brasiliensis (Brazilian spotted fever). In fact, human *R. rickettsii* infection occurs throughout the Americas from Canada to Brazil.

Serologic evidence of human spotted fever group rickettsial infection has been found in six Brazilian states ranging from Rio Grande do Sol in the south to Bahia in the north. *R. rickettsii* has been isolated from humans in Argentina, Brazil, Colombia, Costa Rica, Panama, and Mexico. The geographic distribution of RMSF in the tropics is still poorly understood, as only a few studies have been undertaken in the tropical region of the Americas during the last 25 to 30 years. Few of these studies utilized the sophisticated microbiologic and serologic methods that are necessary to distinguish infection by different members of the spotted fever group. It is possible that RMSF is substantially more common in the tropics and subtropical regions of the Americas than previously recognized. For example, a recent study of patients from southern Mexico who were clinically suspected of having dengue fever but who lacked convalescent phase antibodies against dengue virus revealed that 40% of 50 patients had serologic evidence of recent infection with spotted fever group rickettsiae.

United States. The incidence of RMSF in the United States varies in different regions and at different times of year. The geographic locations of highest incidence include the southeastern region, the west south central region (including Oklahoma and northern Texas), and selected areas of the northeast (e.g., Cape Cod and Long Island). The annual reported incidence of disease in the two states with the highest incidence (North Carolina and Oklahoma) ranges from 2 to 3 cases/100,000 population. It is likely that many cases of RMSF in the United States and the other endemic regions of the Western Hemisphere are not reported, not recognized, or treated empirically and never confirmed. A prospective study of *R. rickettsii* infection in residents of a known endemic area of North Carolina suggests that the annual incidence of RMSF may be as high as 42 cases/100,000 persons/year in the age group 5 to 9 years. Recent reports from Brazil suggest that *R. rickettsii* infection was unrecognized or unreported for decades in regions such as Espirito Santo. In temperate regions, RMSF is more prevalent in spring and summer, but in warmer regions of North America cases may occur in any month, including winter. In southern Brazil the disease is most common from October to February, but in the tropics, seasonal variation in incidence is less striking.

TRANSMISSION AND EPIDEMIOLOGY. *R. rickettsii* circulates in nature in a complex cycle consisting of ticks, rodents, and a few larger animals, e.g., dogs (Table 65–1; Fig. 65–5). The tick vectors and their host animals vary in different regions. For example, the two principal vectors of RMSF in North America are *Dermacentor variabilis* (in the eastern U.S. and Oklahoma) and *D. andersonii* (in the Rocky Mountain region and Canada). The principal vectors of RMSF in the tropics are *Rhipicephalus sanguineus* (in Mexico and Central America) and *Amblyomma cajennense* (in South and Central America). Other ticks including *A. cooperi, A. americanum, I. pacificus,* and *H. leporispalustris* have also been associated with *R. rickettsii* infection, but these arthropods are, at best, infrequent vectors for human infection. Serologic evidence of infection with spotted fever group rickettsiae has been detected in Brazil and Central and North America in a variety of small mammals and in wild and domestic animals, e.g., the capybara and the dog.

RMSF is primarily a disease of rural or suburban dwellers, although occasionally cases occur in highly urbanized regions, e.g., New York City. Disease is more common in males and in children, but any age group may be affected. Transmission is primarily via a tick bite, but rarely it occurs following contact of mucous membranes or skin with infectious tick tissues (e.g., during the process of crushing a tick) or via inhalation of similarly infectious aerosols. Many patients with RMSF do not recall a history of tick bite; thus the absence of a history of tick bite should not dissuade clinicians from considering a diagnosis of RMSF.

PATHOLOGY. Following inoculation of *R. rickettsii* into the skin, organisms attach to endothelial cells and then move intracellularly via induced phagocytosis (Table 65–1; Fig. 65–4). Soon thereafter rickettsiae escape from the cytosol, replicate by binary fission, and spread centripetally from endothelial cell to endothelial cell without producing cell lysis. By mechanisms that are still poorly understood, direct rickettsiae-induced vascular injury ensues, resulting in increased vascular permeability with movement of fluid to the interstitium and a secondary host cellular response (Fig. 65–6B). The culmination of this process is a generalized lymphohistiocytic vasculitis involving virtually every organ of the body (Figs. 65–7 and 65–8). Rickettsiae-induced vasculitis is responsible for the skin rash that is one of the classic signs of infection as well as highly variable degrees of cardiac, neurologic, hepatic, renal, and pulmonary dysfunction. RMSF tends to be more severe in adults, in males, and in individuals with glucose-6-phosphate dehydrogenase (G6PD) deficiency.

CLINICAL MANIFESTATIONS. The onset of RMSF is often abrupt (Table 65–3). Fever is present in virtually all patients with RMSF, and chills occur in many, but not all, patients. Headache is typically a prominent symptom in all except very young children. Myalgia is also a typical early symptom. These three nonspecific symptoms often lead to the mistaken conclusion that the cause of illness is a benign viral infection. In the early phases of illness, many patients do not have a skin rash. In a recent study only 39% of patients had a skin rash when they first sought medical attention, and only 18% had the classic triad of fever, rash, and a history of tick bite at the time they first consulted a physician. Gastrointestinal symptoms, e.g., nausea, vomiting, and abdominal pain, may be misleading and be predominant early, especially in children. A few patients have undergone appendectomy or cholecystectomy before the diagnosis of RMSF became obvious (usually after a typical skin rash appeared).

Skin Rash. Approximately 90% of patients manifest a skin rash at some point in their illness. In its classic form, skin rash begins as a maculopapular eruption on the ankles and wrists and then spreads centripetally to involve the trunk as well as the palms and soles and the rest of the extremties (Fig. 67–1). Later in the illness the rash often become petechial; rarely, frank purpura and, even more rarely, skin necrosis and gangrene of the extremities, scrotum, and ears may occur.

In approximately 10% of cases no rash occurs; some of these cases are not diagnosed until late in the course of infection or after death. Early antibiotic therapy can abort the illness before a rash appears, but in some untreated cases the rash does not occur until the ninth to twelfth day of illness, or it appears as a localized or extremely faint eruption. Unlike other spotted fever group infections, a localized eschar is rare in RMSF, although such lesions have been described.

Other Signs. In addition to fever and chills, many patients with RMSF develop neurologic signs that may include confusion, seizures, and focal neurologic deficits, e.g., cranial neuropathies, urinary or fecal incontinence, and paralysis. Rarely patients may develop hallucinations. Occasionally patients with RMSF develop a stiff neck, which if accompanied by headache, fever, or confusion, may mimic bacterial or viral meningitis. Diagnostic confusion in such cases may persist following lumbar puncture, as many patients with RMSF have a mild pleocytosis in their cerebrospinal fluid. Sinus tachycardia is common. Patients who develop vasculitis in the cardiac microcirculation may develop arrhythmias or signs of congestive heart failure. Jaundice may occur in severe cases. Children with RMSF may present with striking periorbital edema, and both children and adults may develop edema of their extremities.

LABORATORY ABNORMALITIES. The white blood cell count (WBC) is normal in most patients with RMSF. However, leukopenia or leukocytosis may occur in some patients; thus no WBC is characteristic of human *R. rickettsii* infection. Most patients with severe RMSF have thrombocytopenia, and a low platelet count is an important diagnostic clue to the diagnosis even in patients who do not appear acutely ill on initial evaluation. Anemia commonly develops in patients who are hospitalized with RMSF, and disorders of coagulation may manifest as elevated prothrombin and partial thromboplastin time. However, the classic laboratory markers of disseminated intravascular coagulation occur only rarely in patients with severe or fatal infections. Laboratory signs of hepatic and renal dysfunction are commonly present in

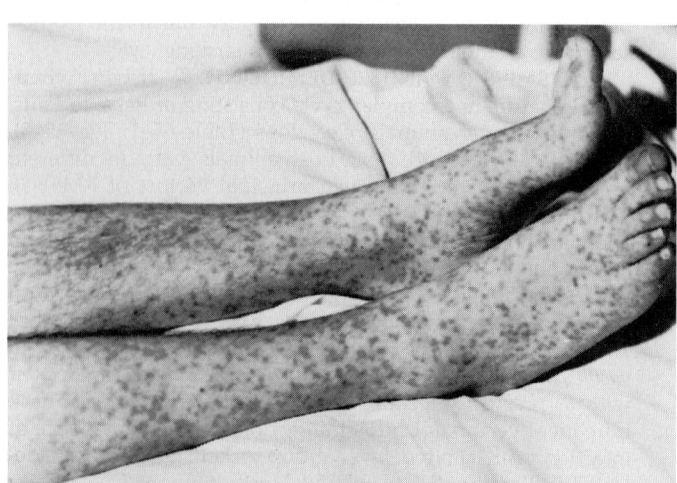

Figure **67–1.** Rash in Rocky Mountain spotted fever. Note also the discoloration of the right hallux suggestive of incipient gangrene. (Courtesy of the Armed Forces Institute of Pathology, Photograph Neg. No. 67987-3.)

severe cases. Hyperbilirubinemia and/or mild to severe elevations of serum asparatate aminotransferase enzyme and other hepatic enzyme levels may occur in severely ill patients and lead to diagnostic confusion. Elevations of serum creatinine and blood urea nitrogen are also common in patients with severe infection. These abnormalities may reflect both tubular and glomerular injury induced by rickettsial vasculitis. Hyponatremia is common in RMSF. In most patients this reflects salt and water depletion that will usually respond to judicious replacement of fluids and electrolytes.

DIAGNOSIS

Early Diagnosis and Treatment. Even experienced clinicians who practice in endemic areas often have difficulty recognizing RMSF when patients present in the early phases of their infection. Such patients often have nonspecific complaints that are compatible with a wide array of undifferentiated viral illnesses. In a study done in North Carolina (where RMSF is recognized as an important seasonal endemic disease by both physicians and patients), only 26% of patients with RMSF received effective antirickettsial therapy on the day of their first visit to a physician. It remains an important clinical axiom that the diagnosis of RMSF must be based on a combination of a suggestive epidemiologic history and a suggestive or characteristic clinical illness.

Therapy must be started empirically on the basis of these findings, because, at present, there is no completely reliable laboratory test on which to make or exclude the diagnosis of RMSF. A history of residence or travel in an endemic area during the season when ticks are active or a tick bite or exposure to potentially tick-infested environments is an important diagnostic clue in the evaluation of an individual with fever, headache, and myalgias. It is reasonable and often appropriate to initiate therapy for RMSF empirically on the basis of these types of exposures, even if a characteristic skin rash is absent.

Diagnostic Tests. Serologic testing is generally not useful early in the illness because antibodies against *R. rickettsii* antigens do not generally appear until the second or third week. Skin biopsy coupled with direct fluorescent antibody techniques can lead to a rapid diagnosis, but such techniques are useful only in patients with skin rash who are seen in specialized medical centers that stock diagnostic reagents and have facilities for fluorescent microscopy. Although the specificity of skin biopsy is nearly 100%, the sensitivity of this method is only about 70%; thus a negative skin biopsy should not deter a physician from initiating or continuing empirical treatment in patients with a high probability of having RMSF. *R. rickettsii* can be visualized in skin or other tissues using formalin-fixed tissues with immunoperoxidase stains, but such methods rarely have immediate clinical utility. Other methods of diagnosis, e.g., rickettsial cultures, polymerase chain reaction (PCR) technology and enzyme immunoassay techniques are available in a few research centers but either lack sensitivity or are too costly to be used for general care.

Serology. The indirect immunofluorescent antibody (IFA) test is the most widely used serologic technique to confirm the clinical diagnosis of RMSF. A fourfold antibody titer rise or a single convalescent antibody titer of 1:64 or greater (in patients with a recent illness suggestive of RMSF) is considered diagnostic. Other serologic techniques, e.g., the latex agglutination and hemagglutination inhibition antibody tests, and a defined epitope blocking enzyme immunoassay test (DEB-EIA) can be used to confirm that a recent illness was due to RMSF. The IFA test cannot distinguish between infection with *R. rickettsii*, *R. conorii*, and *R. sibirica*. Of available serologic tests, only the DEB-EIA test can distinguish

between infection with individual members of the spotted fever group of rickettsiae.

The Weil Felix test, which is based on a cross reaction between *Proteus* antigens and antirickettsial antibodies, is neither specific nor sensitive. This test is now primarily of historical interest, and its use has been supplanted by the IFA test.

Differential Diagnosis. In tropical or semitropical regions RMSF can mimic or be confused with a wide array of endemic diseases including dengue, measles, malaria, murine typhus, leptospirosis, and meningococcemia. In temperate regions RMSF may be confused with many of the same diseases as well a long list of common and rare diseases including nonspecific viral illnesses, other acute rickettsial infections, acute Lyme disease, staphylococcal sepsis, Kawasaki syndrome, thrombotic thrombocytopenic purpura, various forms of vasculitis, and drug reactions.

TREATMENT. Only two drugs have reliable activity against *R. rickettsii*: chloramphenicol and tetracycline. A tetracycline compound (usually doxycycline) is the drug of choice for most patients. Short courses of doxycycline can be safely given to children in whom the diagnosis of RMSF is considered possible or likely, even though repeated use of this drug or other forms of tetracycline can cause dental staining. Chloramphenicol is considered by many experts to be less effective than tetracyclines against *R. rickettsii*, but it has been successfully used as therapy for RMSF for decades; it remains the drug of choice for pregnant women and possibly for children less than 9 years of age with suspected RMSF in whom tetracyclines are contraindicated. Chloramphenicol is also useful as initial empirical therapy in patients in whom it is impossible to distinguish between meningococcemia and RMSF.

Seriously ill patients should receive parenteral therapy with either a tetracycline or chloramphenicol, but most patients can be treated with oral therapy. Duration of therapy for RMSF has not been critically studied. Although short courses of therapy (e.g., 3 days) have been shown to be effective in infection with *R. conorii*, most experts continue therapy for RMSF for at least 5 days or for 48 to 72 hours after defervescence has occurred. Patients with severe disease may be slower to respond to effective therapy, but most patients with uncomplicated RMSF become afebrile within 1 to 3 days after therapy is started. Relapse after successful therapy, which may occur in other rickettsial infections, is uncommon in RMSF.

Severely ill patients with RMSF may require intensive care and careful administration of intravenous fluids. Such patients may need therapy for hypotension; seizures or coma; renal, respiratory, or cardiac failure; and bleeding.

PROGNOSIS AND SEQUELAE. Prognosis is dependent on the time delay from onset to treatment, on host factors, and, perhaps, on poorly understood rickettsial virulence factors. Although fulminant illness with rapid progression to death occurs rarely, fatalities and complications in patients who are treated during the first 5 days of illness are unusual. Death usually occurs during the second week of illness if no therapy is given or if the onset of therapy is greatly delayed. However, the mortality rate of untreated RMSF may be as low as 10 to 25% in geographic areas such as the Snake River Valley in Idaho and the southeastern U.S. and as high as 80% in locales in Montana and Brazil. This geographic variation in mortality rates has been noted for nearly a century with no satisfactory explanation. Prognosis is also related to age and gender. Fatalities are more likely to occur in individuals older than 40 years and in males. Both children and adults with G6PD deficiency have a high mortality rate if they acquire RMSF.

Seriously ill patients who survive RMSF may have permanent neurologic sequelae including deafness, paralysis, incontinence, and mononeuropathies. Rarely, patients with severe disease may require amputation for gangrene of one or more extremities.

PREVENTION. At present there is no satisfactory strategy to prevent RMSF. Repeated attempts to develop an effective and practical vaccine have been unsuccessful, and as yet there is no vaccine commercially available. Strategies to control ticks are both economically and environmentally impractical, although tick control measures directed against household pets may have limited benefit. The best preventive measure against RMSF is prompt detection and removal of ticks, since infected ticks do not transmit their infection if removed within a few minutes to a few hours after attachment. Attached ticks should be removed using paper, cloth, or forceps, since tick tissues and fluids contains a large inoculum of *R. rickettsii*. It is possible that infected tick tissues could result in disease transmission if the arthropod is crushed during or after removal or if infective material is inoculated on mucous membranes or skin abrasions. The use of clothing treated with tick repellents has efficacy in temperate zones but is generally impractical for individuals living in the tropics and during the warm weather months in other geographic areas.

Bibliography

Archibald LK, Sexton DJ: Long-term sequelae of Rocky Mountain spotted fever. Clin Infect Dis 20:1122, 1995.

Calero MC, Nunez JM, Silva Gotyia R: Rocky Mountain spotted fever in Panama. Report of two cases. Am J Trop Med Hyg 1:631, 1952.

de Lemos ERS, Machado RD, Coura JR: Rocky Mountain spotted fever in an endemic area in Minas Gerais, Brazil. Mem Inst Oswaldo Cruz 89:497, 1994.

Dumler JS, Gage WR, Pettis GL, et al: Rapid immunoperoxidase demonstration of *Rickettsia rickettsii* in fixed cutaneous specimens from patients with Rocky Mountain spotted fever. Am J Clin Pathol 93:410, 1990.

Fuentes L: Ecological study of Rocky Mountain spotted fever in Costa Rica. Am J Trop Med Hyg 35:192, 1986.

Hattwick M, O'Brien RJ, Hanson BF: Rocky Mountain spotted fever: Epidemiology of an increasing problem. Ann Intern Med 84:732, 1976.

Kaplowitz LG, Robertson GL: Hyponatremia in Rocky Mountain spotted fever: Role of antidiuretic hormone. Ann Intern Med 98:334, 1983.

Kirk JL, Sexton DJ, Fine DP, Muchmore HG: Rocky Mountain spotted fever: A clinical review based on 48 confirmed cases, 1943–1986. Medicine 69:35, 1990.

Kirkland KB, Marcom PK, Sexton DJ, et al: Rocky Mountain spotted fever complicated by gangrene: Report of six cases and review. Clin Infect Dis 16:629, 1993.

Kirkland KB, Wilkerson WE, Sexton DJ: Therapeutic delay and mortality in cases of Rocky Mountain spotted fever. Clin Infect Dis 20:1118, 1995.

Massey EW, Thames T, Coffey CE, Gallis HA: Neurologic complications of Rocky Mountain spotted fever. South Med J 78:1288, 1985.

Newhouse VF, Shepard CC, Redus MD, et al: A comparison of the complement fixation, indirect fluorescent antibody, and microagglutination tests for the serological diagnosis of rickettsial diseases. Am J Trop Med Hyg 28:387, 1979.

Radulovic S, Speed R, Feng H, et al: EIA with species-specific monoclonal antibodies: A novel seroepidemiologic tool for determination of the etiologic agent of spotted fever group rickettsiosis. J Infect Dis 168:1292, 1993.

Sexton DJ, Corey GR: Rocky Mountain "spotless" and "almost spotless" fever: A wolf in sheep's clothing. Clin Infect Dis 15:439, 1992.

Sexton DJ, Corey GR, Dietze R, et al: Brazilian spotted fever in Espirito Santo, Brazil: Description of a focus of infection in a new endemic region. Am J Trop Med Hyg 49:222, 1993.

Sexton DJ, Kanj SS, Wilson K, et al: The use of polymerase chain reaction as a diagnostic test for Rocky Mountain spotted fever. Am J Trop Med Hyg 50:59, 1994.

Verne GN, Myers BM: Jaundice in Rocky Mountain spotted fever. Am J Gastroenterol 89:446, 1994.

Walker DH: Rocky Mountain spotted fever: A seasonal alert. Clin Infect Dis 20:1111, 1995.

Walker DH, Gay RM, Valdes-Dapena M: The occurrence of eschars in Rocky Mountain spotted fever. J Am Acad Dermatol 4:571, 1981.

Walker DH, Hawkins HK, Hudson P: Fulminant Rocky Mountain spotted fever. Arch Pathol Lab Med 107:121, 1983.

Walker DH, Henderson FW, Hutchins GM: Rocky Mountain spotted fever: Mimicry of appendicitis or acute surgical abdomen? Am J Dis Child 140:742, 1986.

Walker DH, Lesesne HR, Varma VA, Thacker WC: Rocky Mountain spotted fever mimicking acute cholecystitis. Arch Intern Med 145:2194, 1985.

Wilfert CM, MacCormack J, Kleeman K, et al: Epidemiology of Rocky Mountain spotted fever as determined by active surveillance. J Infect Dis 150:469, 1984.

Yagupsky P, Gross EM, Alkan M, Bearman JE: Comparison of two dosage schedules of doxycycline in children with rickettsial spotted fever. J Infect Dis 155:1215, 1987.

Zavala-Valazquez JD, Yu X-J, Walker DH: Unrecognized spotted fever group rickettsiosis masquerading as dengue fever in Mexico. Am J Trop Med Hyg 55:157, 1996.

67.2 *Tick-borne Rickettsioses of the Eastern Hemisphere*

Philippe Brouqui

ETIOLOGY. Rickettsiae are small gram-negative obligate intracellular bacteria that live in the cytoplasm of infected cells. Six new tick-transmitted rickettsiae have been isolated from humans in the Eastern Hemisphere during the last 12 years. The recognition of these agents and the diseases that they cause have resulted from a range of factors, including physicians' curiosity, and the introduction of new molecular tools, e.g., PCR gene amplication and subsequent DNA sequencing; 16s rRNA gene sequence analysis suggests that all tick-transmitted rickettsiae are closely related and are grouped together within the α_2 subdivision of Proteobacteria.

EPIDEMIOLOGY. These diseases are zoonoses, and therefore their spectrum, incidence, and distribution are consequences of the surrounding wild and domestic animal populations, e.g., dogs, deer, and cattle, that are reservoirs of infection. The tick vectors usually involved in the transmission of rickettsioses of the Eastern Hemisphere are *Rhipicephalus*, *Amblyomma*, *Dermacentor*, *Ixodes*, and *Haemaphysalis* species, and the distribution of the diseases is widespread (Tables 65–1 and 67–1).

PATHOPHYSIOLOGY. Rickettsiae are introduced into the skin by the bite of the tick, through skin excoriation (crushed tick), or through the conjunctiva. Rickettsiae attach to vascular endothelial cells, are phagocytized, and then rapidly escape from the phagocytic vacuole to multiply freely in the cytoplasm (Table 65–1). Infected endothelial cells are destroyed by direct injury, which often results in thrombosis of small vessels. Injury to endothelium results in an increase in vascular permeability, which is responsible for hypovolemia, edema, hypotension, and hypoalbuminemia.

DIAGNOSIS. The diagnosis of tick-borne rickettsioses is based upon clinical and epidemiologic findings. The diagnosis should be suspected in a febrile patient with a history of a tick bite, a rash and/or skin lesion consisting of a black necrotic area surrounded by erythema or a pseudofurunculus or a crust. Confirmation of the diagnosis may be assessed by specific serology or isolation or molecular identification of the causative organism. Microimmunofluorescence (IFA) is the reference technique for serology of rickettsial diseases. The presence of specific IgM antibodies or a fourfold increase in titer of IgG antibodies from acute-phase illness to the convalescent phase is considered diagnostic. Rapid detection by IFA of the rickettsiae in circulating endothelial cells is also very useful and may provide laboratory confirmation of the clinical diagnosis in 3 hours. Isolation with cultivation of the bacteria using the shell vial technique is limited by the availability of specialized laboratories.

Molecular tools have allowed identification of new pathogens and should be used in atypical cases, when available. PCR amplification of fragments of the genes encoding the

TABLE 67–1. Tick-Borne Rickettsioses of the Eastern Hemisphere: Rickettsia Species, Their Vectors, the Disease They Cause, and Its Geographic Location

Rickettsia	Vector	Human Disease	Country
R. conorti	*R. sanguineus*	Mediterranean spotted fever	Mediterranean and South Africa
R. sibirica	*D. nuttall, D. marginatus, D. silvarum, H. concinna*	North Asian tick typhus, Siberian tick typhus	Former USSR, Siberia, Mongolia, northern China
R. (unnamed)	*R. pumilio, R. sanguineus*	Astrakhan fever	Astrakhan (former USSR)
R. africae	*A. hebraeum, A. varlegatum*	African tick bite fever	South Africa and Zimbabwe
R. austalis	*I. holocyclus*	Queensland tick typhus	Northern Australia
R. honei	*I. tasmani*	Flinder's Island spotted fever	Flinder's Island (southern Australia)
R. japonica	*H. longicornis*	Japanese spotted fever	Japan
R. (unnamed)	*R. sanguineus*	Israeli tick typhus	Israel
R. mongolotimonae	Unknown	Marseilles tick bite fever	Southern France

190 kDa protein, 17kDA protein, rOMP A and rOMP B proteins, citrate synthase gene or 16 s rRNA has been used for laboratory confirmation and can be applied on preserved samples, e.g., skin biopsies, isolated circulating endothelial cells, or frozen leukocyte-rich plasma. Restriction fragment length polymorphisms analysis (RFLP-PCR) and base sequence determination of the PCR product have allowed the discovery of new pathogens.

TREATMENT. In adults, a single dose of 200 mg of doxycycline has been shown efficient in uncomplicated Mediterranean spotted fever (MSF). In the malignant form of the disease, 200 mg of intravenous doxycycline per day added to anticoagulant should be prescribed until complete recovery. In those allergic to tetracyclines, ciprofloxacin 1.5 g/day orally for 5 days or chloramphenicol 2 g/day for 7 to 10 days usually cures the infection. In infants, a single dose of doxycycline 5 mg/kg/day is efficient and has no consequences on tooth coloration. Alternatively, josamycin, 500 mg/day for 5 days, or chloramphenicol 50 mg/kg/day for 5 days, could be prescribed. In pregnant women, josamycin 3 g/day for 5 days is efficient and safe. Most *Rickettsia* species are also susceptible to rifampin in vitro, but failure of such therapy in vivo has been reported in Spain. A new *Rickettsia* species from Spain was rifampin-resistant in vitro, confirming clinical data and suggesting that some strains may be naturally resistant to this drug.

PREVENTION AND CONTROL. Prophylaxis is based on the prevention of tick bite. Removal of ticks, within 20 hours after attachment reduces the probability of infection. Antibiotic prophylaxis after tick bite is not recommended, as it only delays the onset of symptoms and may interfere with making a correct diagnosis.

Mediterranean Spotted Fever

EPIDEMIOLOGY. *R. conorii* is prevalent in southern Europe (below the 45th parallel), all Africa, and western and central Asia, including India. The tick vector and reservoir are mainly *Rhipicephalus sanguineus*, the dog brown tick (Tables 65–1 and 67–1). Regional names for boutonneuse fever depend on the region where it is diagnosed: MSF, Kenya tick typhus, or Indian tick typhus.

CLINICAL MANIFESTATIONS. The tick bite is usually painless and unnoticed by the patient. After an incubation period of 5 to 7 days, the disease begins with high fever (39°C), severe headache (56% of cases), and frequently malaise, myalgia, arthralgia, or back pain. Careful examination of the patient, including the scalp, the scrotum, and the armpit, should lead to the discovery of the "tache noire" in most cases. Patients who lack a tache noire often have unilateral or bilateral conjunctivitis that may represent the inoculation site of the rickettsia. Three to five days after the onset, the patient typically presents with fever (100% of cases), a maculopapular rash (97% of cases), and the tache noire (72% of cases) (Table 65–3). The disease can be mild or severe and is associated with a significant weight loss. Laboratory data frequently indicate elevated liver enzymes and lactate dehydrogenase (Table 67–2). In 5% of cases, a malignant form is observed, especially in the elderly or those with predisposing diseases, e.g., diabetes mellitus, alcoholism, G6PD deficiency, or cardiac insufficiency. Confusion, pneumonia, purpuric rash, thrombosis with pulmonary embolism, and oliguria associated with renal failure, hyponatremia, hypocalcemia, and thrombocytopenia with consumption coagulopathy are among the clinical manifestations (Tables 65–2 and 65–3). The specific IFA serologic test may confirm the diagnosis. Rickettsiae are susceptible to doxycycline, the first-line therapy. In most cases a single 200 mg dose is sufficient for cure, but prolonged therapy may be needed, especially in cases of the malignant form of MSF.

Other Tick-Borne Rickettsioses

MARSEILLES TICK-BITE FEVER. In March 1996, a new *Rickettsia* species was isolated from a Frenchwoman from Marseilles who presented with very mild boutonneuse fever and with a very discrete rash. This atypical MSF was due to *R. mongolotimonae*, a rickettsia previously isolated from a tick in Inner Mongolia.

AFRICAN TICK-BITE FEVER. During the 1930s, in South Africa, Pjiper described a very mild and frequently spotless disease transmitted by the bite of ticks of the *Amblyomma* complex in the bush. He isolated the causative agent and determined that is was different from *R. conorii* by cross-protection studies in guinea pigs. However, the isolate was lost and Pjiper's work forgotten. Shortly afterward, Gear isolated *R. conorii* from a patient with MSF in South Africa, and confusion arose between African tick-bite fever (ATBF) and MSF. In fact, two different tick-borne diseases have been reported in southern Africa: MSF, as described above, and ATBF, which is caused by *R. africae*, a rickettsia that infects *Amblyomma* ticks (Table 67–1). These ticks bite any animal, including humans, whereas *Rhipicephalus* ticks rarely bite humans. ATBF is milder than MSF, but multiple taches noire may be observed along with fever, a tender large lymph node, lymphadenopathy, lymphagiitis, and edema. The rash is often absent and, if present, is made up of few eruptive elements, some being vesicular (Fig. 67–2). *R. africae* can be

TABLE 67–2. Clinical, Laboratory, and Epidemiologic Characteristics of Patients With Mediterranean Spotted Fever, African Tick Bite Fever, Queensland Tick Typhus, or Flinder's Island Spotted Fever

	Mediterranean Spotted Fever	African Tick Bite Fever	Queensland Tick Typhus	Flinder's Island Spotted Fever
Fever	+ + +	+ + +	+ + +	+ + +
Presence of a tache noire	+ +	+ + +	+ + +	+ +
Multiple taches noire	−	+ + +	−	−
Lymphadenopathy	−	+ + +	+ + +	+ +
Lymphangitis	−	+ +		
Local edema	−	+ +		
Maculopapular rash	+ + +	Absent or mild and vesicular	Absent or vesicular	+ + +
Malignant forms	+	−		
Elevated ALT	+ +	−		
Thrombocytopenia	+ +	−		
Antirickettsia serum IgA	+	+ +		
Rural area	−	+ + +		
Urban area	+ + +	−		
Dogs	+ + +	−		
Cattle and wild mammals	−	+ + +		
Amblyomma ticks	−	+ + +		
Rhipicephalus spp. ticks	+ + +	−		

Legend : (−) rarely or not observed, (+) occasionally observed, (+ +) frequently observed, (+ + +) observed in most cases.

demonstrated using cross-absorption and immunoblotting of patient's sera and isolated from blood and skin biopsies. A recent study reported that the attack rate of ATBF among U.S. troops on exercise in Botswana was as high as 30%. ATBF is likely to be the most common imported rickettsiosis from southern Africa.

ASTRAKHAN FEVER. In Astrakhan on the Caspian Sea, an eruptive febrile disease, originally thought to be of viral origin, has been observed every summer since 1983. However, the presence of tache noire was reported in 20% of cases and alerted the rickettsiologists, who found this disease to be clinically indistinguishable from MSF. A new as yet unnamed species of *Rickettsia*, "Asktrakan fever agent," which is differ-

ent from *R. conorii* and is transmitted by the dog tick *Rhipicephalus pumilo*, has been identified as the etiologic agent.

JAPANESE SPOTTED FEVER. *R. japonica*, the causative organism is transmitted by the tick *Haemaphysalis longicornis*. The disease, clinically indistinguishable from MSF, is endemic in the southwestern part of Japan, where more than 100 cases have been described.

FLINDER'S ISLANDS SPOTTED FEVER AND QUEENSLAND TICK TYPHUS. In Australia, two spotted fevers are described: Queensland tick typhus, due to *R. australia* transmitted by *Ixodes holocyclus*, has been described in northeastern Australia. The skin eruptions associated with this disease are frequently vesicular, and there is an inoculation eschar (Table 67–2). Flinder's Islands spotted fever has been recognized on a very small island close to Tasmania in southern Australia and is due to the recently characterized rickettsia *R. honei*. It causes a summer febrile illness associated with a rash, being erythematous in the majority of cases, while being purpuric in two severe cases associated with thrombocytopenia. Patients have presented with a local lesion in half the cases and enlarged local lymph nodes in one half the cases. In fact, the main clinical difference between Queensland tick typhus and the Flinder's Islands spotted fever consists of the occurrence of a vesicular rash and of local lymph node enlargement in Queensland tick typhus (Table 67–2).

ISRAELI TICK TYPHUS. This is due to *R. conorii* variants that are transmitted by *Rhipicephus* spp. and cause a mild spotted fever without tache noire. It occurs in the northern part of the Caspian Sea in Russia and in Israel.

NORTH ASIAN TICK TYPHUS. Siberian or North Asian tick typhus is caused by *R. sibirica* and is prevalent in eastern Russia, Mongolia, and western China. It is a mild disease; patients present with fever, eruption, and tache noire. *R. sibirica* is transmitted by *Dermacentor* ticks.

Bibliography

Baird RW, Lloyd M, Stenos J, et al: Characterization and comparison of Australian human spotted fever group rickettsiae. J Clin Microbiol 30:2896, 1992.

Brouqui P, Harle JR, Delmont J, et al: African tick bite fever: An imported spotless rickettsiosis. Arch Intern Med 157:119, 1997.

Eremeeva ME, Beati L, Makarova VA, et al: Astrakhan fever rickettsiae: Antigenic and genotypic analysis of isolates obtained from human and *Rhipicephalus pumilio* ticks. Am J Trop Med Hyg 51:697, 1994.

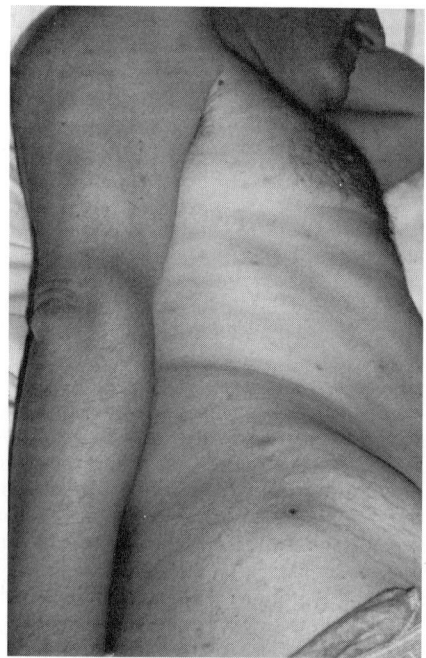

Figure 67–2. Mild papulovesicular rash and eschar in patient with African tick bite fever due to infection with *R. africae*.

Mahara F: Japanese spotted fever: A new disease named for spotted fever group rickettsiosis in Japan. Ann Rep Ohara Hosp 37:83, 1987.

Raoult D, Brouqui P, Roux V: A new spotted fever group rickettsiosis. Lancet 348:412, 1996.

Raoult D, Weiller PJ, Chagnon A, et al: Mediterranean spotted fever: Clinical, laboratory, and epidemiological features of 199 cases. Am J Trop Med Hyg 35:845, 1986.

67.3 *Rickettsialpox*

J. Stephen Dumler

DEFINITION. Rickettsialpox is a vasculotropic rickettsiosis that results in a mild to moderately severe but self-limited febrile illness associated with an eschar, a maculopapular to papulovesicular exanthem, and occasional systemic signs and symptoms. The rickettsial agent is transmitted to humans via the bite of an infected mite, and an eschar often is detected at the site of the arthropod bite.

ETIOLOGY. *Rickettsia akari* is a small obligate intracellular bacterium that contains LPS and protein antigens that cross react in serologic tests with other spotted fever group rickettsiae. However, significant differences in conformation-dependent species-specific epitopes on surface proteins and nucleotides that encode the immunodominant rickettsial outer surface proteins (rOsp) indicate that it is phylogenetically closer to *R. australis* than to other spotted fever group rickettsiae.

DISTRIBUTION AND INCIDENCE. Rickettsialpox has been reported from many of the cities in the northeast regions of the United States; in addition, cases have been described in various locations including the southwestern and midwestern United States, the Ukraine, Croatia, and South Africa. As of the last accumulated report in 1982, more than 800 cases had been identified, most reported within the 3 years after the discovery of the disease. It has been estimated that approximately one case is identified each year, but it is likely that many more cases go unrecognized or are diagnosed as other spotted fever group rickettsioses.

EPIDEMIOLOGY, ECOLOGY, AND TRANSMISSION. *R. akari* is transmitted via the bite of the mite *Lipnyssoides sanguineus*, in which the organism is maintained by transovarial transmission (Table 65–1). The role of horizontal transmission in a mite-mouse-mite enzootic cycle is not clear. The preferred host for the mite is *Mus musculus*, the house mouse (Fig. 65–5). The infectious agent is probably transmitted to humans only inadvertently when mice or other preferred hosts are unavailable. Control of mice and mites has presumably led to a significant reduction in incidence. Many cases are identified in urban environments in which the mouse hosts often reside.

PATHOGENESIS AND PATHOLOGY. The causative agent is transmitted via the saliva of infected mites. As local proliferation of *R. akari* occurs at the bite site, endothelial injury characterized by edema, erythrocyte extravasation, and fibrin deposition accumulates and leads to lymphoid and histiocytic inflammatory cell recruitment. The increasing inflammatory infiltrate and edema result in development of a papule. As the rickettsiae continue to grow, lymphatic and hematogenous dissemination occur and lead to early regional lymphadenopathy and a generalized maculopapular rash 4 to 7 days after onset of illness. Because of the local rickettsial proliferation and ongoing inflammatory reaction at the bite site, damage to the dermal vasculature results in lesions in the basal layer of the epidermis and the subsequent formation of a subepithelial vesicle. With time the dermis and overlying epidermis become necrotic and form an eschar. The disseminated maculopapular lesions may follow a similar course through extensive dermal lymphohistiocytic infiltrates and basal epidermal injury to form papulovesicles that heal by subvesicular epidermal regeneration. It is presumed that similar vascular injury occurs in other organs to a limited degree, accounting for the systemic signs and symptoms that accompany rickettsialpox.

CLINICAL MANIFESTATIONS. The incubation period for rickettsialpox is 9 to 14 days (Table 65–3). The eschar that develops is painless and often not recognized by the patient, although tender regional lymphadenopathy is often present. Within 1 week to 10 days, systemic manifestations are detected, including high fever (39 to 40°C), headache, myalgia, malaise, and—in less than half—rigors, sweats, photophobia, conjunctival injection, rhinorrhea, sore throat, cough, anorexia, nausea, and vomiting. Many patients have sparse (5 to 40) papulovesicles, red macules, and papules that develop approximately 3 to 7 days after the fever. An enanthem may be identified on the buccal mucosa. Laboratory findings are usually nonspecific but may include a slight leukopenia and a mild left shift in neutrophils.

DIAGNOSIS. The infection is usually identified on the basis of the characteristic clinical presentation; a distinctive eschar is followed by a papulovesicular eruption associated with systemic signs and symptoms. The proportion of individuals who do not develop the typical vesicular rash is not known. The vesicular lesions are confused most often with chickenpox (varicella-zoster virus) or herpes simplex virus. They can be distinguished by the concurrent presence of an eschar, the appearance of lesions simultaneously, and the relatively small number of lesions present.

A definitive diagnosis can be achieved by cultivation of *R. akari*, a procedure rarely attempted. This has been performed by animal inoculation, inoculation of embryonated chicken egg yolk sacs, and tissue culture. Generally, the diagnosis is confirmed by the demonstration of a serologic reaction with other spotted fever group rickettsial antigens, e.g., *R. rickettsii*. The exact identification by serologic means is difficult, but higher titers to *R. akari* than to other spotted fever group rickettsiae support the specific diagnosis. A skin biopsy method used to identify *R. rickettsii* in patients with Rocky Mountain spotted fever has also been used to identify *R. akari* within skin biopsies of papulovesicles by virtue of group-shared antigens. This method is the only tool currently available for diagnostic confirmation at the time of infection.

PROGNOSIS. Fatalities associated with rickettsialpox have not been reported. Many untreated patients experience spontaneous remittance after short periods of symptomatic disease. With specific treatment, symptoms usually abate within 12 to 48 hours. A degree of lassitude and headache may persist for a week or more after defervescence. Complications, sequelae, and recrudescence have not been reported.

THERAPY. The treatment of choice is a tetracycline antibiotic administered for 2 to 5 days. Either tetracycline given orally, 15 to 30 mg/kg/day in four doses, or doxycycline given orally, 100 mg/day for adults in two daily doses is adequate. Chloramphenicol is also effective and may be given in 4 divided daily doses at 50 mg/kg/day.

PREVENTION AND CONTROL. The continued, albeit infrequent, reports of rickettsialpox in urban environments attest to the continued potential for human disease. Simple control measures include ruling out *M. musculus* and the accompanying mites from human habitats. Such control is accomplished by antirodent measures and the application of acaricides to potentially mite-infested areas.

Bibliography

Brettman LR, Lewin S, Holzman RS, et al: Rickettsialpox: Report of an outbreak and a contemporary review. Medicine 60:363, 1981.

Kass EM, Szaniawski WK, Levy H, et al: Rickettsialpox in a New York City Hospital, 1980 to 1989. N Engl J Med 331:1612, 1994.

Radulovic S, Feng H-M, Morovic M, et al: Isolation of *Rickettsia akari* from a patient in a region where Mediterranean spotted fever is endemic. Clin Infect Dis 22:216, 1996.

68 *Trench Fever*

Lisa A. Jackson

DEFINITION. Trench fever (5-day fever, Wolhynia fever) is an acute febrile disease caused by infection with *Bartonella quintana*. The infection is classically characterized by fever, headache, muscle and bone pain, splenomegaly, and a maculopapular rash. It is usually self-limited, although relapses are not uncommon.

ETIOLOGY AND CLASSIFICATION. *B. quintana* is a fastidious, slow-growing, gram-negative bacillus. *B. quintana*, along with *B. henselae* (the agent of cat-scratch disease), *B. elizabethae* (which has been isolated from one patient with endocarditis), and *B. vinsonii* (the "Canadian vole agent," not known to be a human pathogen) was formerly classified under the genus *Rochalimaea*. Genotypic analysis indicated, however, that the members of the genus *Rochalimaea* are most closely related to *Bartonella bacilliformis*, the agent of Oroya fever and verruga peruana. The genus designation *Bartonella* now replaces the *Rochalimaea* designation.

EPIDEMIOLOGY, TRANSMISSION, AND DISTRIBUTION. *B. quintana* was first identified as a human pathogen during World War I, when epidemics of louse-borne trench fever affected an estimated 1 million troops in Europe. The disease also affected troops during World War II but to a lesser degree. Transmission via the human body louse *Pediculus humanus* has been experimentally documented and is believed to have been the primary route for epidemic trench fever (see Fig. 65–5). *B. quintana* is considered to have a global distribution, and cases of trench fever have also been reported from Mexico and North Africa (Table 65–1). Since the end of World War II, however, trench fever has been infrequently identified.

In the 1980s, *B. quintana* re-emerged as an opportunistic pathogen in HIV-infected persons. Among this population, *B. quintana* has been identified as a cause of bacillary angiomatosis, endocarditis, and bacteremia and has been isolated from AIDS patients in France and the United States (Chapter 60.3). *B. henselae* has also been identified as a cause of bacillary angiomatosis and bacteremia among HIV-infected persons and is probably a more common cause of these syndromes than *B. quintana*.

More recently, *B. quintana* has been identified as a cause of invasive infection among another population, HIV-negative, inner city, homeless, alcoholic persons. In 1993, ten cases of *B. quintana* bacteremia among homeless, alcoholic persons were identified in Seattle, Washington, within a 6-month period. These were the first confirmed cases of *B. quintana* infection among HIV-negative persons in the United States. Since that time three additional cases have been reported among HIV-negative, alcoholic, homeless persons in France.

The mode of transmission of *B. quintana* among homeless persons is not well defined. Lice were detected on one patient at the time of presentation, and five patients were reported to have been previously diagnosed with scabies. Lice, however, have not been associated with bacillary angiomatosis

among AIDS patients, although cat, and therefore possibly flea, exposure has been associated with bacillary angiomatosis and bacillary peliosis and with cat-scratch disease caused by *B. henselae*. Currently, the human body louse is the only known vector of *B. quintana*; the organism has no known nonhuman vertebrate reservoir.

PATHOLOGY. Little information is available on the pathology of classic trench fever, which was associated with a low case-fatality rate (Table 65–2). Many of the recent cases among urban homeless persons were associated with endocarditis. Examination of excised valves has revealed the presence of fibrinous vegetations and valve perforations.

CLINICAL MANIFESTATIONS AND COURSE

Classic Trench Fever. Classically, four clinical patterns of trench fever have been recognized: (1) asymptomatic or minimally symptomatic infection; (2) a single acute febrile attack lasting 3 to 4 days; (3) a periodic form, with multiple febrile paroxysms; and (4) a continuous form with weeks of fever. Studies involving inoculation of humans with *B. quintana* from infected louse feces show that the incubation period ranges from 5 to 20 days depending on the size of the inoculum. *B. quintana* may circulate in the blood for weeks after resolution of symptoms, and infection has been documented to last as long as a year. A typical episode is characterized by sudden onset of fever and chills; headache; ocular pain; pain in the bones, joints, and muscles; and malaise. A transient maculopapular rash may also occur.

Urban Trench Fever. The clinical spectrum of infection among HIV-negative, alcoholic, and homeless persons has varied. Of these 13 individuals with "urban trench fever," 5 developed endocarditis. All those patients had left-sided endocarditis, and four required valve replacement despite antibiotic therapy. One patient died 4 months after valve replacement surgery; one patient, who had a concurrent positive blood culture for *Streptococcus pneumoniae*, also died, presumably owing to pneumococcal sepsis. Many of the patients with *B. quintana* bacteremia presented with a subacute course of chronic fever, fatigue, and weight loss. Two patients had splenomegaly; however, other symptoms classically associated with trench fever, e.g., headache, rash, and bone pain, were not reported.

A seroprevalence study was conducted 1 year after the *B. quintana* outbreak among patients at a downtown Seattle clinic serving a primarily indigent and homeless population. It was reported that 20% of patients had microimmunofluorescence titers ≥ 64 to *B. quintana*. Interpretation of these results is limited by the high cross reactivity of the assay to *B. henselae*. The results suggest, however, that exposure to the organism was common among that population and that many infections may have been asymptomatic or minimally symptomatic.

DIAGNOSIS

Culture. *B. quintana* is a slow-growing bacterium that requires special culture methods for isolation. The use of Isolator (lysis-centrifugation) tubes improves the yield from blood cultures. Specimens should be plated on enriched media (blood or chocolate agar) incubated at 35 to 37°C in 5% CO_2 and high humidity and held for at least 4 weeks. The organism can also be isolated from blood using Bactec or resin-containing culture medium if the contents are stained with acridine orange after 1 week of incubation. All stain-positive bottles are then subcultured onto enriched media and processed as above. Co-cultivation of blood samples with endothelial cells has also been used for isolation of *Bartonella* species. With wider use of culture methods for the isolation of *Bartonella* species, the spectrum and extent of infections due to this organism may be expanded.

Serology. Enzyme-linked immunosorbent (ELISA) and immunofluorescence (IFA) assays are available for serologic diagnosis. Both these assays exhibit substantial cross reactivity between *Bartonella* species. The use of paired sera obtained 4 or more weeks apart is recommended for serologic diagnosis of infection. PCR amplification from infected tissues of DNA specific to *Bartonella* species has also been used to confirm the diagnosis.

TREATMENT. Minimal published data exist regarding antimicrobial therapy for *B. quintana* infections and in vitro susceptibility testing has proved unreliable. Erythromycin has been the drug of choice, although doxycycline, tetracycline, and azithromycin appear to be acceptable alternatives. At least 14 days of oral therapy is recommended for uncomplicated infection, and for bacteremia at least 4 weeks of therapy is indicated. Although the number of patients identified with *B. quintana* endocarditis are few, most have required cardiac valve replacement despite treatment. Therefore, initial parenteral therapy and a longer duration of treatment (2 to 3 months) should be considered for cases of suspected or confirmed *B. quintana* endocarditis.

Relapsing disease is well described, especially if therapy is terminated prematurely. In the Seattle outbreak, one patient who was noncompliant with therapy had bacteremia documented from blood cultures obtained over an 8-week period.

PROGNOSIS. In immunocompetent hosts, infection with *B. quintana* is usually self-limited. Many patients who develop endocarditis, however, have required valve replacement because of hemodynamic compromise. The course of disease is more severe in immunocompromised hosts and may progress to death.

Bibliography

Drancourt M, Mainardi JL, Brouqui P, et al: *Bartonella (Rochalimaea) quintana* endocarditis in three homeless men. N Engl J Med 332:419, 1995.

Jackson LA, Spach DH, Kippen DA, et al: Seroprevalence to *Bartonella quintana* among patients at a community clinic in downtown Seattle. J Infect Dis 173:1023, 1996.

Maurin M, Raoult D: *Bartonella (Rochalimaea) quintana* infections. Clin Microbiol Rev 9:273, 1996.

Spach DH, Kanter AS, Dougherty MJ, et al: *Bartonella (Rochalimaea) quintana* bacteremia in inner-city patients with chronic alcoholism. N Engl J Med 332:424, 1995.

Spach DH, Koehler JE: *Bartonella*-associated infections. Infect Dis Clin North Am 12:137, 1998.

Vinson JW, Varela G, Molina-Pasquel C: Trench fever. III. Induction of clinical disease in volunteers inoculated with *Rickettsia quintana* propagated on blood agar. Am J Trop Med Hyg 18:713, 1969.

69 *Scrub Typhus*

George Watt and James G. Olson

DEFINITION. Scrub typhus or tsutsugamushi fever is an acute, febrile zoonosis of rural Asia. The causative organism, *Orientia* (formerly *Rickettsia*) *tsutsugamushi* (Fig. 65–2C), is transmitted to humans by the bite of a larval mite (chigger) (Table 65–1). An eschar and regional lymphadenopathy often develop at the site of infection and may be followed by a systemic illness ranging in severity from inapparent to fatal. Most cases go undiagnosed, particularly those in which an eschar cannot be found, because symptoms and signs are often nonspecific and serologic confirmation is rarely available where most cases occur.

ETIOLOGY AND HISTORY. Scrub typhus gained prominence in World War II, when tens of thousands of soldiers in the Asiatic-Pacific theaters contracted the disease: Case-fatality ratios were as high as 35%. It was a serious problem in U.S. military personnel in Vietnam in the 1960s. Thousands of cases of scrub typhus still occur each year, and it is an important cause of febrile illness in endemic areas. The disease is transmitted in an extremely large geographic area, ranging from the coastal portions of North Australia to Asia and the Indian subcontinent and including Japan, Korea, southern China and Tibet, Vietnam, the Philippines, Indonesia, New Guinea, Sri Lanka, and the islands of the Chagos Archipelago. Habitats of *O. tsutsugamushi* range from sandy beaches and mountain deserts to equatorial rain forests. Thus, the term *scrub typhus* is a misnomer; chigger-borne rickettsiosis is a more accurate term.

EPIDEMIOLOGY. Despite their apparent diversity, scrub typhus habitats have one thing in common: All have experienced ecologic modifications by humans or nature that have resulted in transitional, nonclimactic vegetation (Fig. 65–5). Such areas bring together the classic scrub typhus triad, *Rattus* rats, *Leptotrombidium* mites, and *O. tsutsugamushi*. Chiggers (larval mites) of the *L. deliense* group are the principal vectors to humans, but other mite species are also vectors. *O. tsutsugamushi* is maintained in mites primarily by transovarial transmission. Although rats are hosts for the chiggers, they are not thought to contribute significantly to the maintenance of *O. tsutsugamushi*, except perhaps to occasionally infect a previously uninfected female mite that could pass the infection to its progeny.

Incidence figures for scrub typhus are generally unavailable because adequate surveillance systems are lacking. One study in Malaysia estimated the incidence there to be 3 to 4% per month. In a related study, 19.3% of all diagnosed febrile illnesses in a rural area of Malaysia were due to scrub typhus. Such a high incidence is not surprising, particularly when one realizes that infection with a given strain of *O. tsutsugamushi* does not confer immunity to many other strains. Multiple scrub typhus infections are common among occupationally exposed persons.

PATHOLOGY AND PATHOGENESIS. It has been appreciated for many years that severity and case-fatality rates vary markedly in different regions, but determinants of severity have not been clearly identified. Suspected virulence factors include variations in *O. tsutsugamushi* strain virulence, host factors, and regional differences in nutrition, access to medical care, and concomitant infections. Infection with the human immunodeficiency virus does not influence the clinical severity of scrub typhus. Like other rickettsial diseases, scrub typhus is a disseminated, multiorgan vasculitis (Table 65–2). This explains the great diversity of clinical manifestations that can be encountered.

CLINICAL MANIFESTATIONS

Symptoms and Signs. The chigger bite can occur on any part of the body and is usually unnoticed. An eschar forms at the bite site in about 60% of primary infections and less frequently in secondary infections. The eschar begins as a small, painless papule during the 6 to 18 (usually 9 to 12) day incubation period (Table 65–3). It enlarges, undergoes central necrosis, and acquires a blackened scab to form a lesion resembling a cigarette burn (Fig. 69–1). Regional lymph nodes are enlarged and tender. The eschar is generally well developed and healing at the onset of disease. Fever and headache begin abruptly and are frequently accompanied by myalgia, malaise, and weakness. More specific clues to the presence of scrub typhus are deafness and tinnitus, which occur in up to a third of cases, as well as conjunctival suffusion and lymphadenopathy, which are common. A macular rash is a helpful sign but is difficult to see on dark-skinned

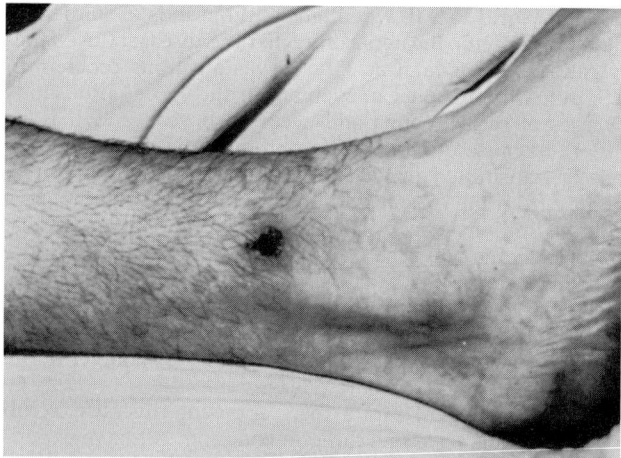

Figure 69–1. Eschar in scrub typhus. These may also be located on the trunk, neck, and arms and may be single or multiple. (Courtesy of the Armed Forces Institute of Pathology, Photograph Neg. No. D-4451.)

individuals. The rash appears on the trunk late in the first week of illness and then spreads peripherally and becomes maculopapular.

Complications. Pulmonary involvement frequently dominates the clinical picture in mild cases and is the principal cause of death in patients with severe disease. Cough, tachypnea, and infiltrates on chest x-ray are one of the most common presentations of scrub typhus. In severe cases, tachypnea progresses to dyspnea; the patient becomes cyanotic; and full-blown adult respiratory distress syndrome (ARDS) may ensue. Apathy, confusion, and personality changes in moderate cases of scrub typhus may give way to stupor, convulsions, and coma in severe cases. Severely ill patients can often have multiple organ failure.

Laboratory Findings. There is no constellation of laboratory test results that strongly suggests *O. tsutsugamushi* infection. Slight elevations of the total white blood cell count are typical, and mild rises in liver transaminases also occur. Laboratory findings are chiefly useful to rule out other infections.

DIAGNOSIS. Scrub typhus is usually confirmed by serologic tests, performed with the three prototype strains of *O. tsutsugamushi* (Karp, Gilliam, and Kato), as antigens. Currently, the indirect immunofluorescence assay is the method of choice, but the immunoperoxidase test, enzyme immunoassays, and passive hemagglutination assay have also been employed successfully. Minimum titers have not been established with certainty, and, therefore, tests of paired serum specimens showing a rise in antibody titer are recommended. Polymerase chain reaction (PCR) assays have confirmed *O. tsutsugamushi* infections in acute-phase blood of patients and may be of great potential use as a diagnostic tool.

Differential Diagnosis. This depends on the diseases prevalent in the area in which the illness originated. The importance of a careful search for an eschar cannot be overemphasized—its presence is pathognomonic for scrub typhus in much of Asia. Tularemia and anthrax can cause eschars but are rare. Eschars frequently occur in the genital region and can be confused with the ulcers of chancroid or lymphogranuloma venereum. A hemorrhagic rash, particularly if associated with leukopenia and thrombocytopenia, suggests infection with dengue rather than *O. tsutsugamushi*. Severe myalgia, jaundice, and raised serum creatinine levels suggest leptospirosis rather than scrub typhus, in which myalgia is generally mild. Typhoid fever and malaria also figure fre-

quently in the differential diagnosis, but parasites are generally detectable in blood films from Asian patients infected with *Plasmodium* sp. Febrile patients from urban areas are more likely to have murine than scrub typhus, although transmission of *O. tsutsugamushi* occurs in suburban Bangkok.

TREATMENT. Prompt antibiotic therapy is the single most important factor in shortening the disease, reducing mortality, and speeding convalescence. Treatment must often be presumptive, and the benefits of avoiding severe scrub typhus by early antibiotic administration generally far outweigh the risks of a 1-week course of tetracycline—the treatment of choice. Either tetracycline, 500 mg q.i.d., or doxycycline, 100 mg b.i.d., per day for 7 days can be used. Shorter treatment courses are curative but associated with recrudescences. Chloramphenicol (50 to 75 mg/kg/day) is also effective. Parenteral therapy should be used in patients who are vomiting or have severe disease. Scrub typhus is considered to be very susceptible to antibiotics, with patients generally becoming afebrile within 24 to 36 hours after beginning antibiotic therapy. However, a focus of antimicrobial-resistant scrub typhus has recently been identified in northern Thailand. Its geographic boundaries have not yet been defined, and the mechanism of resistance is unknown. Antibiotics effective against resistant strains in mice are currently undergoing human clinical trials. The treatment of pregnant women and children poses problems because tetracycline and chloramphenicol may be contraindicated. However, the benefits of short courses of tetracycline outweigh the risks of no treatment or inadequate treatment of scrub typhus.

Good supportive care and early detection of complications is important in severe cases if a good outcome is to be obtained. Severely ill patients are often hypotensive and have increased vascular permeability caused by vasculitis. They are at risk of pulmonary edema and present difficulties with fluid management. Careful monitoring of pulmonary wedge pressure is advisable to avoid fluid overload.

PROGNOSIS. Case-fatality ratios ranged from 0 to 50% in the preantibiotic era. Prompt antibiotic therapy markedly reduces mortality, but up to 15% of patients still die in northern Thailand. Death is attributable to a variety of factors, including late presentation, delayed diagnosis, and drug resistance. Some abnormalities, such as deafness and personality changes, may persist for months. Eventually, however, symptoms resolve completely in nonfatal cases.

PREVENTION. Weekly doses of 200 mg of doxycycline can prevent *O. tsutsugamushi* infection. Occupationally exposed nonimmune populations would benefit most from scrub typhus protection, but chemoprophylaxis should also be considered in high-risk travelers, such as those backpacking or trekking in endemic areas. Contact with chiggers can be reduced by not sitting or lying directly on the ground and by applying repellent to the tops of boots, on socks, and on the lower trousers. Unfortunately, these measures are rarely practical in those who are occupationally exposed. Safe, effective vaccines have not yet been developed to prevent scrub typhus.

Bibliography

Berman SJ, Kundin WD: Scrub typhus in South Vietnam: A study of 87 cases. Ann Intern Med 79:26, 1973.

Brown GW, Robinson DM, Huxsoll DL: Serological evidence for a high incidence of transmission of *Rickettsia tsutsugamushi* in two Orang Asli settlements in peninsular Malaysia. Am J Trop Med Hyg 27:121, 1978.

Brown GW, Shirai A, Jegathesan M, et al: Febrile illness in Malaysia—an analysis of 1,629 hospitalized patients. Am J Trop Med Hyg 33:311, 1984.

Chayakul P, Panich V, Silpapojakul K: Scrub typhus pneumonitis: An entity which is frequently missed. Q J Med 68:595, 1988.

Kantipong P, Watt G, Jongsakul K, Chuenchitra C: Infection with the human immunodeficiency virus does not influence the clinical severity of scrub typhus. Clin Infect Dis 23:1168, 1996.

Olson JG, Bourgeois AL, Fang RCY, et al: Prevention of scrub typhus. Prophylactic administration of doxycycline in a randomized double blind trial. Am J Trop Med Hyg 29:989, 1980.

Sugita Y, Yamankawa Y, Takahashi K, et al: A polymerase chain reaction system for rapid diagnosis of scrub typhus within six hours. Am J Trop Med Hyg 49:636, 1993.

Tamura A, Ohashi N, Urakami H, et al: Classification of *Rickettsia tsutsugamushi* in a new genus, *Orientia* gen. nov., as *Orientia tsutsugamushi* comb. nov. Int J Syst Bacteriol 45:589, 1995.

Traub R, Wisseman CL Jr: The ecology of chigger-borne rickettsiosis (scrub typhus). J Med Entomol 11:237, 1974.

Watt G, Chouriyagune C, Ruangweerayud R, et al: Scrub typhus infections poorly responsive to antibiotics in Northern Thailand. Lancet 348:86, 1996.

70 Ehrlichiosis

G. Thomas Strickland and James G. Olson

DEFINITION AND HISTORY. The human ehrlichioses are vector-borne zoonotic bacterial infections that cause nonspecific multisystem febrile illnesses. *Ehrlichia canis*, the type species of the genus, was first recognized in 1935 as a pathogen of dogs. It was assigned to the genus *Rickettsia*, and the disease was called canine rickettsiosis. Subsequently, members of the genus were found that cause diseases in a wide range of animal species. Canine ehrlichiosis was studied intensively in Vietnam in 1968–1970, when tropical canine pancytopenia, a severe hemorrhagic disease causing extensive morbidity and mortality in military working dogs, was found to be due to *E. canis*. It is now a well-recognized pathogen of dogs worldwide, especially in tropical and other warm climates where its vector, *Rhipicephalus sanguineus*, flourishes.

The first human pathogen of the genus, *E. sennetsu*, was isolated in Japan in 1954. Sennetsu fever, an infectious mononucleosis–like disease, remains restricted to localities in western Japan. Human monocytic ehrlichiosis (HME), caused by *E. chaffeensis* and detected because it serologically cross-reacted with *E. canis*, was identified in a patient who became ill following tick exposure in Arkansas in 1985. The agent was isolated in 1991 from a patient training at Fort Chaffee, Arkansas, and the agent was named for that geographic area. In 1994, human granulocytic ehrlichiosis (HGE), an illness similar to HME, was reported in the upper Midwest. Both *E. chaffeensis* and the HGE agent are limited by the geographic distribution of their principal hard tick vectors: *Amblyomma americanum* and *Ixodes scapularis*, respectively.

ETIOLOGY. *Ehrlichia* is a genus in the family Rickettsiaceae; the small, obligate intracellular bacteria in this genus multiply within the cytoplasm of white blood cells (WBCs) or platelets. The gram-negative pleomorphic bacteria appear as compact inclusions and proceed through elementary body, initial body, and morula stages. *Ehrlichia* are cultivatable on primary monocyte cultures and in continuous cell lines, e.g., canine histiocytoma (DH82), but do not grow in chick embryos or cell-free media. *E. sennetsu* has been isolated from blood, lymph nodes, and bone marrow.

By serology, genomic sequencing, and morphology (electron microscopy), the agent of HME is closely related but not identical to *E. canis*. The agent causing HGE is the same as, or closely related to, *E. phagocytophila* and *E. equi*, which are pathogenic for sheep, goats, dogs, horses, cattle, and deer. In addition to human diseases, *Ehrlichia* species cause a number of diseases of veterinary importance: Potomac horse fever (*E. risticii*), equine ehrlichiosis (*E. equi*), tick-borne fever in sheep (*E. phagocytophila*), and infectious cyclic thrombocytopenia of dogs (*E. platys*) and canine granulocytic ehrlichiosis of dogs (*E. ewingi*). Rarely, *E. ewingi* has caused human illness and *E. canis* has caused human infection.

EPIDEMIOLOGY

Distribution, Incidence, and Prevalence. Since the recognition of HME in the United States in 1986, more than 500 cases, including several fatalities, have been identified in 30 states, principally those where Rocky Mountain spotted fever (RMSF) is also found (Fig. 70–1). Most cases have been reported from the south central states (especially Oklahoma, Arkansas, Texas, Missouri, and Tennessee) and South Atlantic states from Georgia to New Jersey. HME incidence during active case detection in Oklahoma, Georgia, and Maryland was the same as or greater than RMSF; 5–10/100,000, depending upon whether the cases were detected in hospitals or in physicians' offices. Although most cases have been sporadic, outbreaks of HME occurred in a group of army reservists camping in a tick-infested field in New Jersey and in a golf-oriented retirement community in Tennessee.

At least 200 cases of HGE have been reported in the upper Midwest (Minnesota, Wisconsin), Northeast (Massachusetts, Connecticut, Rhode Island, and New York to Maryland), and California (where the vector is believed to be *I. pacificus*; see Fig. 70–1).

HME or HGE transmission occurs in Europe (e.g., Greece, Italy, Slovenia, Sweden, Switzerland, Russia) and Africa. Serologic evidence of possible exposures in Southeast Asia requires verification. Sennetsu fever is localized to focal areas in Japan and Malaysia.

Transmission. About two thirds to three fourths of patients report a tick bite or tick exposure 7 to 21 days before symptom onset; most cases have an onset between April and September. The geographic distribution of HME patients and experimental transmission studies indicate that *A. americanum* is the vector for HME; *E. chaffeensis* has been identified in ticks collected from endemic areas. Detection of the organism and experimental transmission in ticks and the geographic distribution of the infection all point to *I. scapularis* as the vector for HGE in the upper Midwest and eastern United States, *I. pacificus* in California, and *I. ricinus* in Europe. Sennetsu fever cases are detected in the summer and fall, suggesting that *E. sennetsu* is transmitted by an invertebrate vector, e.g., a tick. Latent infections occur in experimentally infected dogs, raising the possibility of their role as a reservoir host.

PATHOGENESIS. Although the clinical manifestations intimate a defect in microvascular integrity, the ehrlichioses differ from the vasculotropic rickettsial diseases in not including vasculitis. Both *E. chaffeensis* and the HGE agent are introduced into the dermis by the bite of an infected tick. They then are spread hematogenously throughout the body. Intracellular infection is established in phagosomes in macrophages (in the case of HME) and neutrophils or myeloid precursor cells (in the case of HGE). Morulae, cytoplasmic inclusions of *Ehrlichia*, are sometimes seen in monocytes (HME) and granulocytes (HGE) in stained peripheral blood films. Leukopenia and thrombocytopenia are characteristic; granulomas and lymphohistiocytic infiltrates have been detected in bone marrow examinations, which are usually hypercellular with a megakaryocytosis but are sometimes normocellular or hypocellular. The peripheral blood cytopenias are associated with sequestration with hemophagocytosis in the spleen, liver, lymph nodes, and bone marrow. Hepatic lesions range from focal hepatic necrosis to ring granulomas. Interstitial pneumonia, pulmonary hemorrhage,

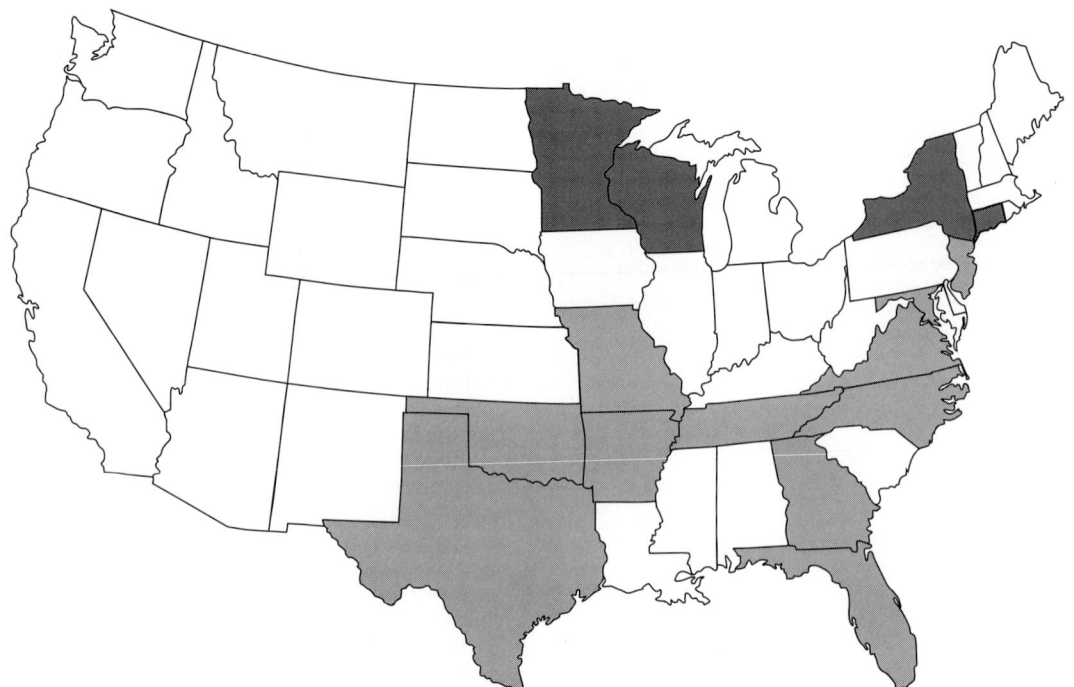

Figure 70–1. States reporting more than ten cases of ehrlichiosis, 1985–1996. Lighter shaded areas show human monocytic ehrlichiosis transmission, and darker shaded areas mark human granulocytic ehrlichiosis transmission.

and diffuse alveolar damage have been described in postmortem examinations.

The pathologic findings suggest that induction of nonspecific mononuclear phagocyte– or cytokine-mediated injury is a pathogenic mechanism. The presence of opportunistic infections suggest that suppression of host defense mechanisms plays a pathogenic role in severe infections.

CLINICAL MANIFESTATIONS

Spectrum of Disease. The clinical manifestations of HME and HGE are similar to those of RMSF and have been described as spotless RMSF. The disease-to-infection ratio is low. The majority of those infected probably have mild symptoms and do not seek medical attention. The next largest group have nonspecific influenza-like symptoms that are not diagnosed and are treated with analgesics and sometimes with antibiotics. The minority have severe enough clinical illnesses to require extensive diagnostic testing (which is essential for establishing the diagnosis) and/or hospitalization. Resistance to disease is inversely related to age, explaining why the mean age of HME and HGE case series is in the late 40s and 50s despite the fact that older people have no greater exposure than the young to tick bites.

Milder illness has best been described during investigation of an outbreak of ehrlichiosis in a group of army reservists; nine persons with serologic evidence of infection were identified. Only seven sought medical care; only three missed more than a day of work because of illness; and none was hospitalized. Arthralgia, myalgia, headaches, and anorexia were more common in persons with serologic evidence of ehrlichiosis; all three patients having WBC counts had fewer than 4000 leukocytes/μL.

Symptoms and Signs. Symptoms usually first occur 3 to 21 days following a tick bite or exposure (reported in 60 to 80% of diagnosed cases of ehrlichiosis). Onset is abrupt or subacute. Virtually all patients have a temperature greater than 38°C. Symptoms, nonspecific and resembling those of RMSF, include fever, chills, headache, stiff neck, sore throat, cough, dizziness, myalgia, arthralgia, anorexia, nausea, vom-

iting, diarrhea, and abdominal pain. Skin lesions are less common in ehrlichiosis than in RMSF. A rash, often small, erythematous, pruritic, and localized, was noted in about 20 to 30% of patients with HME but less often in HGE. The patient may be confused or drowsy, but the results of the physical examination are usually otherwise normal. A few patients with either HME or HGE have had peripheral neuropathies, including involvement of the brachial plexus or the ocular motor muscles.

Laboratory Evaluation. The complete blood count (CBC) reveals leukopenia and thrombocytopenia in 50 to 60% of clinically diagnosed patients, with one or the other being present in 80%; both neutropenia and lymphocytopenia are frequent findings. In one study, the median WBC count at admission to the hospital was 4450/μL and the median platelet count was 133,000/μL. Elevated hepatic transaminases (ALT, AST) are reported in more than 75% of hospitalized patients, but the degree of elevation is usually relatively mild at the time of admission (median ALT of 68 U/L and median AST of 62 U/L), becoming more elevated later in the clinical course. Mild anemia and jaundice with serum bilirubin in the 2 to 3 mg/μL range have been present in some patients. Hospitalized patients have had elevated serum creatinine. Half the patients having chest x-rays have pulmonary infiltrates. A few patients with clinical findings suggestive of aseptic meningitis have had cerebrospinal fluid (CSF) pleocytosis.

Complications. These include severe confusion, drowsiness, seizures and coma, peripheral neuropathies, gastrointestinal hemorrhage, fungal superinfection, and death. Mortality has been reported in as many as 7 to 10% of hospitalized patients with HGE. Severe human ehrlichiosis can become a multisystem disease like RMSF, with hepatitis, cholestasis, pancreatitis, renal failure, central and peripheral neurologic lesions, and pneumonia. The greatest risk is in the elderly, who may die from nosocomial infections including bacterial or fungal pneumonia and disseminated candidiasis.

Death may occur after pulmonary or gastrointestinal hemorrhage secondary to thrombocytopenia.

Co-morbidity with other tick-borne infections, particularly Lyme disease, has been a subject of recent interest. Clearly, dual infections occur more frequently than anticipated and patients may be sicker than they would be with a single infection. On the other hand, data from a population-based epidemiologic study suggest that HGE patients who have concurrent *Borrelia burgdorferi* infections are less ill than those patients with HGE alone. The same tick might transmit both infections (e.g., in the case of *I. scapularis* transmitting both HGE and Lyme disease); people bitten by one tick are more likely to be exposed to other ticks; and in the case of infections with variable penetrance of clinical illness, two infections would be more likely than one to make the individual sick enough to seek medical care and receive extensive medical evaluation. At least three patients with HME have been subjected to cholecystectomies because of mild jaundice, right upper quadrant abdominal pain, and elevated ALT (with incidental thickened gallbladder wall and/or gallstones demonstrated by abdominal ultrasound). One of these had severe bleeding during surgery and required multiple blood transfusions. She survived, but her convalescence was prolonged and complicated.

Sennetsu Ehrlichiosis. Sennetsu fever is characterized by fever, lymphadenopathy, and atypical lymphocytosis. The lymphadenopathy is generalized but is most prominent in the postcervical and postauricular regions, and some patients have hepatosplenomegaly. The incubation period is about 2 weeks following exposure. Onset is typically sudden and is manifested by fever and chills. Headache, myalgia, sore throat, and back and joint pain are common during the acute phase. The generalized lymphadenopathy is first noted 5 to 7 days following onset of symptoms. The involved lymph nodes are usually tender, but suppuration does not occur. Skin rash is rare; an eschar has been described. Tetracycline is effective therapy.

DIAGNOSIS

Diagnostic Suspicion. Diagnosing a patient with ehrlichiosis requires clinical suspicion. Laboratory confirmation often is available too late to be clinically useful. A patient of any age living in an endemic area who has a recent exposure to ticks and presents with nonspecific febrile symptoms from April through September should prompt the physician to consider ehrlichiosis. A CBC might show mild thrombocytopenia, leukopenia, and/or anemia. Characteristic morulae (*Ehrlichia* inclusion bodies; Fig. 70–2 [see color section]) can be best seen in the cytoplasm of granulocytes (HGE) or monocytes (HME) in stained buffy coat smears of a small proportion of patients. This usually requires careful microscopy; morulae are seen more frequently in HGE than in HME, and their absence does not rule out ehrlichiosis. The patient might have an ALT in the 50 to 100 U/L range, and the serum bilirubin might be slightly elevated as well. Other evidence of multisystem involvement supports the diagnosis. If the physician believes that the patient might have ehrlichiosis or RMSF and there are no contraindications to treatment with tetracyclines, doxycycline should be started based on the presumptive diagnosis. A rapid clinical response, i.e., within 36 to 48 hours, further favors the diagnosis of a rickettsial disease. A serum sample for a serologic confirmation test should be sent to the CDC or to one of the commercial laboratories providing this service. However, antibody response is often negative early in the illness, and the usual delay in obtaining test results from the reference laboratory directs that treatment be based upon clinical suspicion.

Serology. The most commonly used and most reliable test is an indirect immunofluorescence assay (IFA) using the HGE agent and *E. chaffeensis* antigens propagated in cell cultures. As noted above, these tests are often negative early in infection; there are some cross reactions between HME and HGE. Positive and negative predictive values of serologic tests in an outpatient setting with a low prevalence of infection remain unknown.

A fourfold increase or decrease in serum antibody titer from the acute to convalescent phase of illness in a patient whose disease is compatible with ehrlichiosis meets the CDC diagnostic criteria. A single serum antibody titer $\geq$1:64 in a patient with a compatible illness is strongly suggestive of ehrlichiosis.

Other Diagnostic Methods. Detection of ehrlichial DNA in a patient's blood or in ticks by polymerase chain reaction (PCR) has been successful in several research laboratories and is now becoming commercially available. The PCR may detect either HME or HGE DNA in blood early in the infection prior to the development of specific antibodies. The procedure is intricate since the organisms are in leukocytes and anticoagulated blood provides better specimens than serum collected after the blood clots.

Differential Diagnosis. Ehrlichiosis resembles a number of other tick-borne diseases, especially RMSF. When a tick-borne infection is suspected the differential diagnosis should include several other diseases (RMSF, tularemia, relapsing fever, acute Lyme disease, Colorado tick fever, and babesiosis) depending on the clinical presentation and geographic area of exposure. Some patients with ehrlichiosis are believed to have influenza, a mild viral hepatitis, or even infectious mononucleosis. Ehrlichiosis has been mistaken for pyelonephritis, gastroenteritis, and unexplained febrile illnesses with leukopenia or thrombocytopenia. Leptospirosis, typhus, dengue fever, and other vector-borne viral infections, e.g., Rift valley fever, have similar clinical presentations. At least three patients with HME had cholecystectomies for incidental cholelithiasis.

TREATMENT. Human ehrlichiosis responds to treatment with doses of tetracycline similar to those used for other rickettsial disease (Chapter 65). The recommended regimen for adults is doxycycline, 100 mg twice daily continued for a minimum of 5 to 7 days, or 3 days after defervescence. Children should receive 3 to 5 mg/kg body weight divided in two daily doses. Tetracycline can be given at 250 to 500 mg four times daily for the same period of time to adults and 25 mg/kg orally in divided doses to children. Parents of children under 8 years of age should be informed of the benefits of therapy as well as the complications associated with using tetracyclines in this age group. A 7-day treatment course is highly unlikely to cause dental staining. The response to doxycycline or tetracycline is rapid (usually within 48 hours). Untreated patients may die or have prolonged illness with complications (e.g., as occurs in inadequately treated RMSF); therefore, antibiotic therapy must be initiated based on a presumptive diagnosis. Chloramphenicol, although not as effective as tetracycline, has been shown to produce clinical improvement more rapidly than no treatment or treatment with other antibiotics. It should be given at a dose of 500 mg every 6 hours to adults or 75 mg/kg per day in divided doses every 6 hours to children. Very ill patients are often initially treated with intravenously administered doxycycline or chloramphenicol. Many antibiotics frequently used in clinical practice, e.g., penicillin, cephalosporins, aminoglycosides, macrolides, and sulfonamides, do not cure ehrlichiosis.

PREVENTION. Since ehrlichiosis is transmitted by ticks, recommendations for prevention are similar to those for RMSF (Chapters 65 and 137). Tucking the pants legs under the socks and treating clothing with permethrin before going into tick-infected areas and tick checks and removal of attached ticks after leaving these areas can reduce exposures.

Bibliography

Aguero-Rosenfeld ME, Horowitz HW, Wormser GP, et al: Human granulocytic ehrlichiosis: A case series from a medical center in New York State. Ann Intern Med 125:904, 1996.

Anderson BE, Dawson JE, Jones DC, Wilson KH: *Ehrlichia chaffeensis*, a new species associated with human ehrlichiosis. J Clin Microbiol 29:2838, 1991.

Anderson BE, Sumner JW, Dawson JE, et al: Detection of the etiologic agent of human ehrlichiosis by polymerase chain reaction. J Clin Microbiol 30:775, 1992.

Anderson BE, Sims KG, Olson JG, et al: *Ambylomma americanum*: A potential vector of human ehrlichiosis. Am J Trop Med Hyg 49:239, 1993.

Bakken JS, Dumler JS, Chen S-M, et al: Human granulocytic ehrlichiosis in the upper Midwest. A new species emerging? JAMA 272:212, 1994.

Bakken JS, Krueth J, Wilson-Nordskog C, et al: Human granulocytic ehrlichiosis (HGE): Clinical and laboratory characteristics of 41 patients from Minnesota and Wisconsin. JAMA 275:199, 1996.

Chen S, Dumler JS, Bakken JS, Walker DH: Identification of a granulocytotropic Ehrlichia species as the etiologic agent of human disease. J Clin Microbiol 32:589, 1994.

Dawson JE, Childs JE, Biggie KL, et al: White-tailed deer as a potential reservoir of Ehrlichia spp. J Wildlife Dis 30:162, 1994.

Dumler JS, Bakken JS: Ehrlichial diseases of humans: Emerging tick-borne infections. Clin Infect Dis 20:1102, 1995.

Fishbein DB, Kemp A, Dawson JE, et al: Human ehrlichiosis: Prospective active surveillance in febrile hospitalized patients. J Infect Dis 160:803, 1989.

Fishbein DB, Dawson JE, Robinson LE: Human ehrlichiosis in the United States, 1985–1990. Ann Intern Med 120:736, 1994.

Harkess JR: Ehrlichiosis. Infect Dis Clin North Am 5:37, 1991.

Harkess JR, Ewing SA, Crutcher JM, et al: Human ehrlichiosis in Oklahoma. J Infect Dis 159:576, 1989.

Petersen LR, Sawyer LA, Fishbein DB, et al: An outbreak of ehrlichiosis in members of an army reserve unit exposed to ticks. J Infect Dis 159:562, 1989.

Standaert SM, Dawson JE, Shaffner W, et al: A hyperendemic focus of human ehrlichiosis at a golf-oriented retirement community. N Engl J Med 333:420, 1995.

Walker DH, Dumler JS: Emergence of the ehrlichioses as human health problems. Emerg Infect Dis 2:18, 1996.

71 Relapsing Fever

Thomas Butler

DEFINITION. Relapsing fever is an acute febrile illness of humans caused by blood spirochetes belonging to *Borrelia* species. The two major kinds are louse-borne relapsing fever, for which humans are the reservoir and body lice are the vector, and tick-borne relapsing fever, for which rodents and other animals are the predominant reservoirs and ticks are the vectors. The relapsing fevers are distributed worldwide in both tropical and temperate climates. The natural course of relapsing fever consists of one or more phases of fever and spirochetemia, which last for several days and are separated by afebrile intervals of several days without spirochetemia. Relapsing fever is usually a self-limited disease, but high mortality rates have been recorded during epidemics of louse-borne relapsing fever.

ETIOLOGY. Relapsing fevers are caused by blood spirochetes of *Borrelia* species, which belong to the order of bacteria called Spirochaetales. *Borrelia* species differ from the other two genera of pathogenic spirochetes, *Leptospira* and *Treponema*, by structure, biochemical characteristics, and antigenic determinants.

Borrelia spirochetes are spiral organisms that measure 5 to 40 μm in length and about 0.5 μm in diameter. They are too thin to be seen reliably by light microscopy of wet prepara-

tions, but they are easily visible when viewed by darkfield or phase contrast microscopy. They are stainable with aniline dyes, such as Wright's and Giemsa stains, and can be visualized well in tissue by the application of silver stains, such as the Dieterle and Warthin-Starry stains. Like other bacteria, these spirochetes possess an outer cell wall (outer envelope) and an inner cytoplasmic membrane that contains muramic acid. Between the cell wall and cytoplasmic membrane are 15 to 20 flagella, the organelles of motility. They are anchored to the ends of the spirochete and wrap around its body until they meet at the middle region. In three dimensions, the spirochetes have a helical configuration consisting of about five to ten coils with amplitudes of about 1 to 4 μm. Under darkfield or phase contrast microscopy, *Borrelia* spirochetes display an active corkscrew-like motility, which consists of rotation and helical waves, giving translational movement to the organisms. Inside the cytoplasmic membrane are ribosomes, DNA, and RNA. These prokaryotic organisms divide by transverse binary fission.

Borrelia organisms are microaerophilic and fermentative in their growth characteristics. Like other pathogenic spirochetes, they require long-chain fatty acids for growth. They can be cultivated in Kelly's medium, which is a complex broth containing proteose peptone, tryptone, bovine serum albumin, rabbit serum, *N*-acetylglucosamine, citric acid, and pyruvate in addition to glucose and salts. *B. recurrentis*, the agent of louse-borne relapsing fever, is more fastidious than the tick-borne *Borrelia* species and requires the further addition of asparagine and choline to Kelly's medium or use of medium for culturing *B. burgdorferi*. The *Borrelia* organisms grow slowly, with doubling times of 18 to 26 hours.

The species names of the tick-borne *Borrelia* are derived from the species names of *Ornithodoros* tick vectors that carry them. The more common ones in North America are *B. turicatae*, *B. hermsii*, and *B. parkeri*; in Africa, *B. duttonii*. The classification of *Borrelia* is not based on biochemical or antigenic characteristics that could be standardized for laboratory diagnosis.

The relapsing feature of *Borrelia* infection has been attributed to antigenic variation in the infecting population of spirochetes. In experimental infections of rats with *B. hermsii*, separate serotypes emerged sequentially during relapses and specific antibody appeared in response to each of the antigenic variants. Each of 25 serotypes of *B. hermsii* expresses different variable major proteins that are encoded by genes located on linear plasmids of the spirochete.

HISTORY. The name *relapsing fever* was coined by Craigie in 1843 in Edinburgh. A year later in the same city, Henderson differentiated this disease from typhus fever. The etiologic agent of relapsing fever, however, was first established in Berlin in 1873 by Obermeier, who used a microscope to observe spirochetes in the blood of patients. The transmission of *Borrelia* spirochetes by arthropod vectors was suggested in 1891 by Flugge, who postulated the body louse as a vector, and in 1905 by Dutton and Todd, who demonstrated the infection in the *Ornithodoros* ticks of Africa. The genus name *Borrelia* was proposed in 1907 in honor of the French bacteriologist Amédée Borrel.

Relapsing fever is certainly a disease of antiquity, and its known epidemic potential—particularly in times of war, migrations, and other conditions that favor human crowding and poor hygiene—suggests that relapsing fever has had a major impact on human history. Before the advent of microscopic diagnosis, however, it was not possible to distinguish relapsing fever reliably from similar scourges of humanity such as malaria, typhoid fever, and typhus fever. Therefore, the history of relapsing fever before 1873 is only speculative. In the 20th century, Bryceson described evidence for seven major epidemics of louse-borne relapsing fever. These outbreaks occurred between 1910 and 1945 in Africa, Eastern Europe, and Russia. Cases were estimated to number 15 million, with >5 million deaths and case-fatality rates as high as 73%.

DISTRIBUTION AND INCIDENCE. The geographic distribution of the relapsing fevers is widespread, with occurrence in most continents of the world, including the Americas, Europe, Africa, and Asia. Epidemic relapsing fever is the louse-borne kind, and endemic or sporadic relapsing fever the tick-borne variety.

Epidemic Relapsing Fever. Louse-borne relapsing fever occurs in parts of South America, Europe, Africa, and Asia. From 1960 to 1993, louse-borne relapsing fever was documented in Ethiopia and Sudan. Although accurate statistics on the incidence of this disease are not available, Ethiopia appears to be the country with the highest prevalence, estimated to be 10,000 or more cases per year.

Endemic Relapsing Fever. Tick-borne relapsing fever occurs in endemic foci in southern British Columbia, in the western United States, in the plateau regions of Mexico, and in Central and South America. It is present in all areas of Africa except the Sahara Desert and the rain forest belt. It also occurs in Spain and Portugal. In Asia, infection has been reported in Cyprus, Israel, Syria, Turkey, Iraq, Iran, southern Russia, China, Afghanistan, and India. Accurate statistics are not available, but the sporadic nature of human contact with rodent ticks and the small numbers of established diagnoses suggest that this infection occurs less frequently in humans than louse-borne relapsing fever.

EPIDEMIOLOGY AND TRANSMISSION. The two types of relapsing fever, louse borne and tick borne, differ so much in their epidemiology that they must be considered separately.

Epidemic Relapsing Fever. The only species of *Borrelia* that causes louse-borne relapsing fever is *B. recurrentis*. Its vector is the human body louse, *Pediculus humanus humanus* (see Fig. 139–1), and the only known natural reservoir is humans. Thus, the cycle of infection is simply from person to person by means of the louse. Body lice acquire the infection by feeding on a spirochetemic person, and they remain infected for their entire life span, which is 10 to 61 days under laboratory conditions. The ingested spirochetes pass through the esophagus to the midgut, where they penetrate the gut epithelium to reach the hemolymph, in which they multiply. Spirochetes do not reach the salivary glands or ovaries of the lice. Therefore, infection is not transmitted to people by bites of lice, and infection cannot be transmitted transovarially to offspring of infected lice. Infection is believed transmitted after lice are crushed on the skin during scratching by patients. This allows liberated spirochetes to penetrate through a bite site or through intact skin. Body lice prefer the normal human body temperature of 37°C to higher temperatures; thus, lice are likely to leave the skin of a febrile patient to go to another person. This may explain, in part, the rapid transmission of infection during epidemics.

The persons at greatest risk for acquiring louse-borne relapsing fever are those living under crowded, unhygienic conditions that favor infestation with body lice. Migrant workers and soldiers in war are particularly prone to develop this infection. Males are at much greater risk than females. A strain-specific and short-lived acquired immunity develops after the infection. This immunity helps to explain why migrant workers coming into an endemic area are more susceptible to infection than are the permanent inhabitants. In some endemic areas, such as Addis Ababa, Ethiopia, the incidence increases during the cool winter season, when people wear heavier clothing that becomes louse infested. In lowland regions of tropical equatorial Africa, where people wear scantier clothing, this infection has been reported but seems to occur less frequently than at higher altitudes.

Endemic Relapsing Fever. The species of *Borrelia* that cause tick-borne relapsing fever are numerous and include *B. duttonii* in East Africa, *B. hispanica* in Spain, *B. persica* in Asia, and *B. hermsii* and *B. turicatae* in North America. The vectors of these organisms are soft-bodied argasid ticks of the genus *Ornithodoros* (Figs. 137–4 and 139–17). The major reservoirs of the tick-borne relapsing fevers are wild rodents, including squirrels, deer mice, rats, chipmunks, and rabbits and occasionally, lizards, toads, turtles, and owls. The infection is passed between the reservoir animals by tick bites, and humans become accidental hosts when they come into contact with infected animal ticks. The exception to the animal reservoirs may be *B. duttonii* in eastern Africa, which is carried by the domestic tick *Ornithodoros moubata* and for which humans appear to be the reservoir.

Ticks acquire the infection by biting and sucking blood from a spirochetemic animal. The spirochetes, after entering the hemocoelom, invade other tissues of the tick, including the salivary glands, the coxal glands on the legs, and the ovaries. Transmission of the infection to animals or humans follows either injection of infected saliva through the bite site or secretion of infected coxal fluid, which enters through the bite site or intact skin. Tick bites are painless and usually occur at night. Ticks are more durable vectors than body lice, being able to survive as long as 15 years between blood meals and to harbor viable spirochetes for years. In addition, female ticks can pass *Borrelia* spirochetes transovarially to their offspring, thus permitting ticks to be infective without having previously bitten an infected host.

Persons at greatest risk of infection are those who come into contact with infected ticks from wild rodents. In the United States, the largest outbreak of tick-borne relapsing fever occurred in 62 campers and employees in the National Park at the northern rim of the Grand Canyon, Arizona, in 1973. They had all slept in log cabins that were inhabited by wild rodents. Another outbreak in the state of Washington affected 42 Boy Scouts, who also camped out in a log cabin. In tropical countries, people who live in dwellings that are not rodent proof are prone to infection. In eastern Africa, where ticks have become domesticated and humans have become a reservoir of tick-borne relapsing fever, people living in the endemic areas develop immunity to the disease. Neonates have acquired infection from their mothers' blood. Transmission of spirochetes in these cases occurred presumably by the transplacental route before birth or by exchange of blood at the time of birth.

PATHOGENESIS AND PATHOLOGY

Pathogenesis. After exposure to an infected louse or tick, spirochetes enter the body through the skin and into the subcutaneous tissue, where they have access to the systemic and lymphatic circulations. No symptoms develop during the incubation period, estimated to last from 4 to 18 days, while the spirochetes are dividing in the blood plasma. No local lesions develop at the skin site of entry, and there is no evidence for an intracellular phase of multiplication. After the spirochetes have built up to a concentration of 10^6 to 10^8/ mL of blood, symptoms begin suddenly. At this early stage of illness, large numbers of spirochetes are regularly present in the plasma space. A small proportion of the spirochetes are within circulating polymorphonuclear phagocytes, and some spirochetes have been phagocytosed by fixed macrophages of the reticuloendothelial system of the spleen, liver, and bone marrow. Although occasionally found in other tissues (e.g., the brain, hepatic cells, kidneys, and subcutaneous tissues), spirochetes do not proliferate or elicit inflammatory reactions in these extravascular sites.

Although *Borrelia* spirochetes do not possess endotoxin or any identified exotoxins, the spirochetes themselves are pyrogenic. The pyrogenic principle resides in the body or outer envelope of the spirochete, is heat stable, and probably acts by stimulating mononuclear phagocytic cells to elaborate tumor necrosis factor and interleukins 1, 6, and 8. The thrombocytopenia of relapsing fever, which causes petechiae and sometimes other hemorrhagic phenomena, results from sequestration of platelets and disseminated intravascular coagulation. During acute relapsing fever, levels of serum complement, Hageman factor, and prekalikrein are decreased, suggesting that activation of certain plasma proteins contributes to the pathogenesis. Before and during the Jarisch-Herxheimer reaction (a rigor elicited by antibiotic treatment), blood levels of the inflammatory cytokines, tumor necrosis factor-α, and interleukins 6 and 8 rise.

Most patients with relapsing fever recover from their illness either with or without antibiotic treatment. Patients develop antiborrelial antibodies, which can agglutinate, kill, or opsonize spirochetes. In the presence of opsonizing antibody, spirochetes are rapidly phagocytosed and digested by polymorphonuclear leukocytes. These antibodies also participate in rendering patients immune to future infection with the same serotype of *Borrelia*.

Pathology. Autopsies performed in Ethiopia and Sudan in fatal cases of louse-borne relapsing fever showed characteristic lesions in the spleen, liver, heart, and brain. The spleen is enlarged to as much as 900 g, and the cut surface shows white microabscesses, which consist of necrosis and hemorrhage in the white pulp. Occasionally noted are splenic infarcts and splenic rupture. The liver is also enlarged, often to >2000 g. The midzonal regions show scattered necrosis and hemorrhage, and Kupffer cells are enlarged and numerous. The heart is normal in size but frequently shows myocarditis, with interstitial edema and a cellular infiltrate of lymphocytes and plasma cells. The brain usually shows cerebral edema, and in some cases, there is hemorrhage into the subarachnoid space or cerebrum. Thus, the immediate causes of death in relapsing fever are varied and, in any particular case, may be liver failure, cerebral hemorrhage, or acute cardiac arrhythmia due to myocarditis.

CLINICAL MANIFESTATIONS. The illness begins abruptly with shaking chills, fever, headache, and fatigue. Most patients have these symptoms almost continuously throughout the day, whereas some patients report the intermittent appearance of symptoms several times a day. Patients complain frequently of myalgias, arthralgias, anorexia, dry cough, and abdominal pains. Epistaxis occurs occasionally, and children may experience seizures. These symptoms are usually mild on the first day of illness and increase in intensity over a few days, leading to prostration and a visit to a physician. The nonspecific nature of these symptoms leads patients or their physicians to believe they have a flulike illness. In louse-borne cases, patients show poor personal hygiene and report pruritus, sometimes with excoriated skin due to scratching. In tick-borne cases, patients may have seen ticks on their bodies, but the tick bites are painless and rarely leave any mark.

In pregnant women, it is common for infection to induce labor, leading to abortion or preterm delivery with high mortality for the infants. Neonates may acquire congenital infection, with illness detected 4 to 12 days after delivery. The temperature is elevated, in the range of 38.5°C to 40°C, and the pulse rate is increased to about 115 beats/min. The blood pressure is lowered to about 105/70 mmHg. Patients appear lethargic. Physical signs that are common but not regularly present are conjunctival injection, petechial skin rash that is more apparent on the trunk than on the extremi-

ties, and palpable liver and spleen. Jaundice is present occasionally. Generalized muscle weakness is common. Some patients display mental confusion, delirium, or coma, and some have nuchal rigidity.

The laboratory results show a positive blood smear for spirochetes. The white blood cell count is usually normal, with increased band forms and decreased eosinophils. Platelet counts are often <50,000/mm³, and there may be prolongations of the prothrombin time and partial thromboplastin time and increased titers of fibrinogen-fibrin degradation products. Results of liver function tests are frequently abnormal, with serum alanine aminotransferase elevations and bilirubin elevations that are evenly divided between the conjugated and unconjugated fractions. Renal function tests often show mild abnormalities of the serum urea nitrogen and creatinine values, and patients may have proteinuria and microscopic hematuria.

DIAGNOSIS

Visualization in Peripheral Blood. Relapsing fever is readily diagnosed by obtaining peripheral blood by either fingerstick or venipuncture and preparing a thin film on a microscope slide. *Borrelia* spirochetes are stained blue by aniline dyes. Thus, a routine blood smear stained with Wright's or Giemsa stain is adequate. Blood smears, thin and thick, prepared for examination for malaria parasites are also satisfactory for spirochete examination. The spirochetes are 5 to 20 μm in length and lie in the plasma spaces between blood cells or may overlie the blood cells (Fig. 71–1). Febrile patients with relapsing fever typically have several spirochetes per high-power field. Patients who are afebrile in the interval between relapses have negative smears and should be re-examined when the fever reappears.

Spirochetemia may be detected alternatively by dark-field or phase contrast microscopy. A drop of fresh blood is diluted with another drop of 0.9% NaCl and covered with a coverslip. Spirochetes are readily identified by their characteristic rotational motility.

Culture or Animal Isolation. For purposes of special investigation or research, culture and animal inoculations can be used. Infected blood is inoculated into Kelly's broth and allowed to incubate for about a week. Likewise, infected blood can be inoculated intraperitoneally into laboratory mice or rats and the blood of these animals examined daily for 14 days for spirochetemia. Tick-borne *Borrelia* species are more readily cultivated in Kelly's medium and recoverable from laboratory animals than are the louse-borne *B. recurrentis*.

Epidemiology and Vector Examination. Louse-borne and tick-borne relapsing fever are distinguished by knowing the geographic distribution of the types of relapsing fever and obtaining information about contact with lice or ticks. If the vectors can be collected from the patient or the household, they can be dissected and the hemolymph or coxal fluid examined microscopically for the presence of spirochetes.

Serology. Serologic testing has been used in endemic areas for purposes of seroepidemiology. Serum of convalescent patients contains antibodies that produce agglutination and immobilization of living spirochetes and fix complement during reaction with spirochetal antigens. None of these tests, however, is standardized or commercially available for general use. Patients' sera produce false-positive reactions in serologic tests for Lyme disease (Chapter 73).

TREATMENT AND PROGNOSIS

Antibiotics. The relapsing fevers are effectively treated with tetracycline, erythromycin, or penicillin. Tetracycline is the treatment of choice except in children less than 7 years old and in pregnant women, in which cases tetracycline may stain developing teeth. Studies in Ethiopia indicate that a

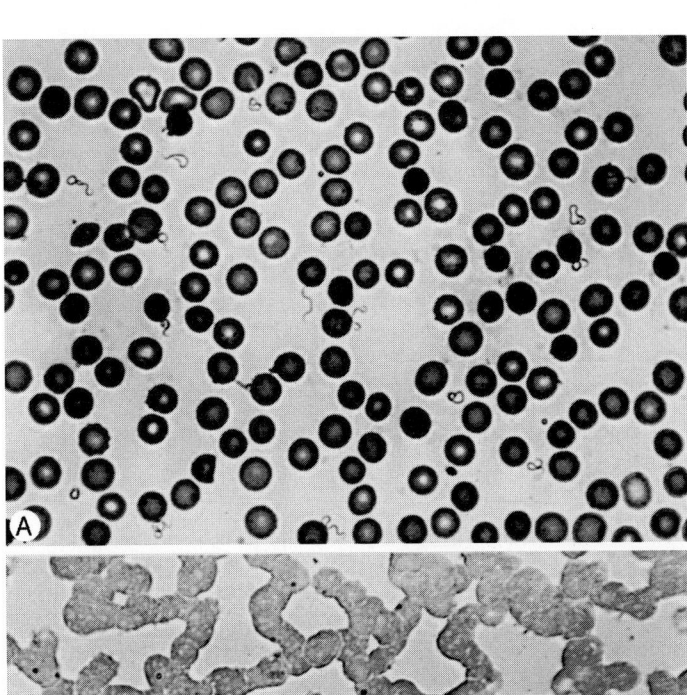

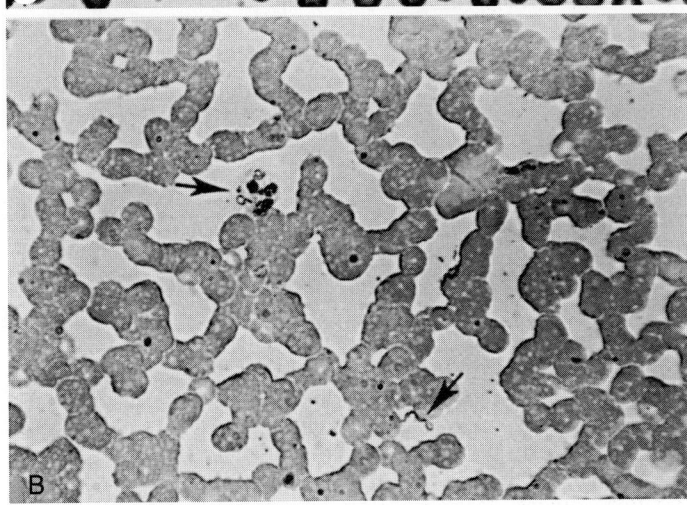

Figure 71–1. *A,* Blood smear from a patient with louse-borne relapsing fever stained with Wright's stain showing *Borrelia* spirochetes. *B,* Blood smear stained with Warthin-Starry stain after antibiotic treatment showing intracellular spirochetes in a polymorphonuclear leukocyte *(top arrow)* and a single extracellular spirochete *(bottom arrow).*

single 500-mg oral dose of tetracycline is as effective in clearing spirochetemia and preventing relapse as a longer course of treatment. Erythromycin, 500 mg PO as a single dose, is equally effective and is a satisfactory alternative to tetracycline. For patients unable to take oral medication, injections of 250 mg IV of tetracycline or erythromycin are curative. For children who weigh less than 30 kg, the dose of tetracycline or erythromycin should be reduced to approximately 10 mg/kg. Penicillin G has been used to treat relapsing fever, but its use has been associated with slow clearance of spirochetes and relapses after treatment. Good results have been reported from Africa with procaine penicillin G given as 400,000 or 600,000 units IM once or with the same dose repeated 12 hours later. Children should receive 30,000 units/kg. Some physicians use procaine penicillin fortified (3:1 ratio of procaine:benzyl) 800,000 units/day for adults and 30,000 units/kg/day for children for 5 days.

Jarisch-Herxheimer Reaction. In most patients with louse-borne relapsing fever and in some with tick-borne relapsing fever, antibiotic treatment provokes a distressing Jarisch-Herxheimer reaction. As depicted in Figure 71–2, which shows the mean values of 32 Ethiopian patients with louse-borne relapsing fever treated with erythromycin, a rigor occurred 2 or 3 hours after treatment in 28 patients. Temperature subsequently rose sharply, and blood pressure declined while spirochetes were cleared from the blood. Patients are extremely uncomfortable during the reaction, feeling very cold and having severe headache and myalgia. They often

express a sense of impending doom: "This is much worse than my illness was before treatment." During the Jarisch-Herxheimer reaction, blood leukocyte and platelet counts sharply decrease and spirochetes disappear from the plasma. Patients may require intravenous infusions of 0.9% NaCl to maintain adequate blood pressure. Deaths rarely occur during the reaction. For several hours, temperature declines and patients feel better. Attempts to ameliorate the severity of the reaction by giving antipyretic or anti-inflammatory drugs have not been useful. The best approach is to anticipate the reaction and to provide intensive nursing care and intravenous fluid support during the first day of treatment.

Prognosis and Relapses. The prognosis is favorable for complete recovery in 95% or more of treated cases of relapsing fever. Unfavorable prognostic signs are the presence of jaundice, coma, high spirochete counts in the blood, and hypotension. More than half of neonatal patients with relapsing fever die. The prognosis for untreated disease is grave in the case of louse-borne relapsing fever, for which mortality rates of 40% have been reported during epidemics. Untreated patients also experience relapses. In louse-borne relapsing fever, the first attack lasts about 6 days and is followed by an afebrile period of about 9 days. There usually is one relapse, which lasts only about 2 days. In tick-borne relapsing fever, the first attack lasts about 3 days and is followed by an interval of about 7 days, after which an average of three relapses occur, each lasting about 2 days. Relapses are usually milder in intensity than the first attacks.

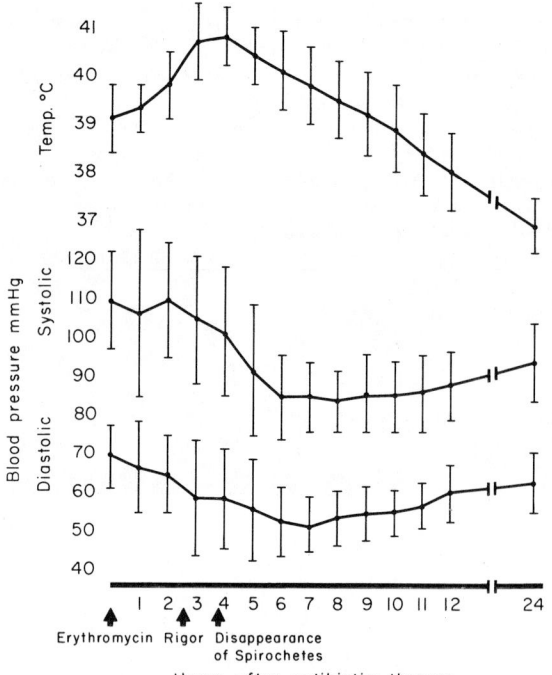

Figure 71–2. Changes in temperature and blood pressure during Jarisch-Herxheimer-like reaction. Thirty-two patients with louse-borne relapsing fever were treated with erythromycin, 500 mg orally.

PREVENTION AND CONTROL. Available approaches for the control of the relapsing fevers include the detection and treatment of human cases, vector control, rodent control, and public health education. Vaccines are not available.

Epidemic Relapsing Fever. For louse-borne relapsing fever, the detection and treatment of cases have the effect of reducing the reservoir of infection and, consequently, reducing transmission. More important is the control of louse infestation. Instructing people to bathe and wash their clothes is the rational approach, but compliance is likely to be low. Delousing of clothing should be done by insufflating powder containing 10% DDT or 1% malathion or 0.5% permethrin under the clothes (Chapter 139). Shaving and washing the body are useless. In known epidemic situations, prophylactic antibiotics are a temporary measure to contain spread of infection to persons at high risk.

Endemic Relapsing Fever. For tick-borne relapsing fever, the treatment of human cases has no impact on the animal reservoirs. It is not possible to control this infection in wild rodents. Campers and hikers going into endemic areas should be advised to avoid staying in cabins that are inhabited by rodents and their ticks and to apply topical tick repellents (35% diethyltoluamide [deet]) to their skin. In endemic areas of Africa, people need to be assisted in building rodent-proof houses.

Bibliography

Barbour AG, Hayes SF: Biology of *Borrelia* species. Microbiol Rev 50:381, 1986.
Barclay AJG, Coulter JBS: Tick-borne relapsing fever in central Tanzania. Trans R Soc Trop Med Hyg 84:852, 1990.
Borgnolo G, Denku B, Chiabrera F, et al: Louse-borne relapsing fever in Ethiopian children: A clinical study. Ann Trop Paediatr 13:165, 1993.
Borgnolo G, Hailu B, Ciancarelli A, et al: Louse-borne relapsing fever. A clinical and an epidemiological study of 389 patients in Asella Hospital, Ethiopia. Trop Geogr Med 45:66, 1993.
Bryceson ADM, Parry EHO, Perine PL, et al: Louse-borne relapsing fever. A clinical and laboratory study of 62 cases in Ethiopia and a reconsideration of the literature. Q J Med 39:129, 1970.
Butler T, Jones PK, Wallace CK: *Borrelia recurrentis* infection: Single dose antibiotic regimens and management of Jarisch-Herxheimer reaction. J Infect Dis 137:573, 1978.
Butler T, Hazen P, Wallace CK, et al: *Borrelia recurrentis* infection: Pathogenesis of fever and petechiae. J Infect Dis 140:665, 1979.
Colebunders R, DeSerrano P, Van Gompel A, et al: Imported relapsing fever in European tourists. Scand J Infect Dis 25:533, 1993.
Cutler SJ, Fekade D, Hussein K, et al: Successful in-vitro cultivation of *Borrelia recurrentis*. Lancet 343:242, 1994.
deJong J, Wilkinson RJ, Schaeffers P, et al: Louse-borne relapsing fever in Southern Sudan. Trans R Soc Trop Meg Hyg 89:621, 1995.
Fekade D, Knox K, Hussein K, et al: Prevention of Jarisch-Herxheimer reactions by treatment with antibodies against tumor necrosis factor α. N Engl J Med 335:311, 1996.
Gebrehiwot T, Fiseha A: Tetracycline versus penicillin in the treatment of louse-borne relapsing fever. Ethiop Med J 30:175, 1992.
Lovett MA, Goldstein EJC, Fleischmann J: Fever in a couple vacationing in the mountains of southern California. Clin Infect Dis 14:1254, 1992.
Mekasha A: Louse-borne relapsing fever in children. J Trop Med Hyg 95:206, 1992.
Negussie Y, Remick DG, DeForge LE, et al: Detection of plasma tumor necrosis factor, interleukins 6 and 8 during the Jarisch-Herxheimer reaction of relapsing fever. J Exp Med 175:1207, 1992.
Sundes KO, Haimanot AT: Epidemic of louse-borne relapsing fever in Ethiopia. Lancet 342:1213, 1993.
Warrell DA, Perine PL, Krause DW, et al: Pathophysiology and immunology of the Jarisch-Herxheimer–like reaction in louse-borne relapsing fever: Comparison of tetracycline and slow-release penicillin. J Infect Dis 147:898, 1983.
World MJ: Pestilence, war, and lice. Lancet 342:1192, 1993.

72 *Leptospirosis*

George Watt

DEFINITION. Leptospirosis is a zoonotic disease caused by the spirochete *Leptospira interrogans*. Infection can lead to asymptomatic infection, a nonspecific influenza-like febrile illness, a wide variety of severe clinical syndromes including severe icteric disease, hemorrhagic syndromes, renal failure, and death. Leptospirosis is of the greatest public health importance in the tropics, but most cases are not diagnosed because symptoms are nonspecific and confirmatory diagnostic testing is not available. Appropriate antibiotic therapy given early to patients with suspected leptospirosis may prevent severe complications from developing; it may also decrease the duration of illness in those with complications. Leptospirosis is known by a host of colorful descriptive terms, including peapicker's disease, swineherd's disease, canicola fever, and Fort Bragg fever. These names, which attempt to link specific serovars with distinct disease manifestations, are misleading and should be abandoned.

ETIOLOGY. Leptospires are tightly coiled motile spirochetes with an axial filament and hooked ends (Fig. 72–1). They are approximately 0.1 μm in diameter and from 6 to 20 μm in length and can pass through 0.2 μm pore-size filters. Leptospires are aerobic and utilize long-chain fatty alcohols as carbon and energy sources. Unstained organisms can be seen only by darkfield or phase contrast microscopy. Silver staining is the method of choice for demonstrating leptospires in tissue specimens.

The taxonomy of leptospires is evolving. At present, the genus has 2 species: *L. interrogans*, which is pathogenic to humans, and *L. biflexa*, which is saprophytic. Stable antigenic differences allow subclassification into serotypes, referred to in the literature as serovars (serovarieties). Antigens common to several serovars permit arrangement into broader sero-

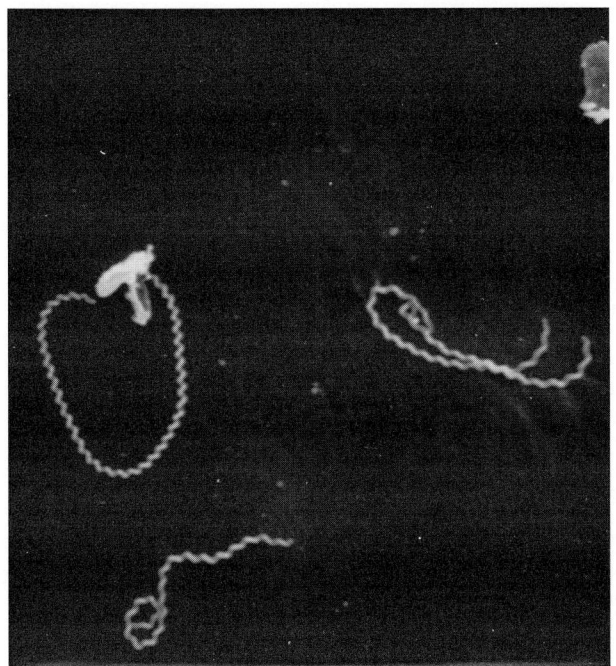

Figure 72–1. Typical leptospires viewed under electron microscopy at a magnification of 4000 ×. (Courtesy of J. Bruce McClain.)

groups. More than 200 serovars belonging to 23 serogroups have been identified for *L. interrogans*.

HISTORY. Leptospirosis is an ancient disease with wide geographic distribution. Weil is credited with the first description of severe cases of icteric disease (Weil's disease) that he recognized as a new clinical entity in 1886. The causative organism was first described in sections of kidney tissue taken from a patient dying during a yellow fever epidemic in 1907 by Stimson. Inada cultured the spirochete and proved its association with Weil's disease in 1915. Leptospires were recovered from a Norway rat in 1917, and the first human case connected with rat exposure was reported in 1922.

EPIDEMIOLOGY

Distribution and Prevalence. *L. interrogans* has a global distribution with greatest impact in the tropics, especially Latin America and Southeast Asia. An epidemic of severe hemorrhagic disease, initially thought to be dengue hemorrhagic fever, occurred in Nicaragua over a 2-month period in 1995; more than 2000 individuals were affected and there were at least 40 deaths. Although most cases are not specifically diagnosed, leptospirosis is a frequent cause of fever in the developing world with antibody positivity rates of 27% in Thailand, 23% in Vietnam, and 37% in rural Belize. It is primarily of veterinary importance in the United States, where 50 to 150 cases are reported annually, most from Hawaii. Sporadic urban transmission associated with exposure to rat urine has also been reported.

Animal Reservoirs. Pathogenic leptospires are found in the renal tubules of a wide variety of wild, peridomestic, and domestic animals, in which they are shed with the urine. They can survive for several months in the environment under moist conditions, particularly in the presence of ambient temperatures above 22°C and a relatively neutral (6.2 to 8.0) pH. These conditions are found year round in the tropics but only during the summer and autumn months in temperate climates. Survival is inhibited by contaminated water and by salinity. Among the 160 mammalian species harboring

organisms, rodents are the most important reservoir. Carrier rates of over 50% have been measured in Norway rats (*Rattus norvegicus*), which shed massive numbers of organisms for life without showing clinical illness. Some serovars appear to be preferentially adapted to select mammalian hosts. For example, *L. interrogans* serovar *icterohaemorrhagiae* is primarily associated with the Norway rat, *canicola* with dogs, and *pomona* with swine and cattle. However, a particular host species may serve as a reservoir for one or more serovar and a particular serovar may be hosted by many different animal species.

Transmission. Infection is usually transmitted from animals to humans through contact with contaminated water or moist soil. The streets of some crowded Asian cities that become submerged during the rainy season and have large rat populations provide ideal conditions for transmission, as do flooded rice fields. Jungle swamps and mud are rich sources of pathogenic organisms. Less frequently, leptospirosis is acquired by direct contact with the blood, urine, or tissues of infected animals. Transmission via laboratory accidents or breast milk has been reported but is rare. Organisms enter through abrasions of the skin or through the mucosal surface of the eye, mouth, nasopharynx, or esophagus.

Occupational Risk. People who work where rats or infected livestock contact water are especially prone to infection. Certain agricultural laborers are at high risk, and intense exposure to leptospires has been documented in rice, sugar cane, and rubber plantation workers. Others with hazardous occupations include abattoir workers, fish and poultry processors, butchers, ditch diggers, and sewer workers. Many residents of the tropics are infected by wading through streets flooded by leptospire-contaminated water. Epidemiologic patterns in the United States and United Kingdom have changed. Recreational exposure and animal contact at home have replaced occupational exposure as the chief source of disease.

PATHOGENESIS AND PATHOLOGY. There is a remarkable paucity of histopathologic lesions in the kidneys and livers of patients with marked functional impairment of these organs. This disparity suggests damage at the subcellular level. Icteric patients typically have marked leukocytosis but no leukocytic infiltrates in organs, suggesting the presence of a toxin. Patients who survive severe leptospirosis have complete recovery of hepatic and renal function—consistent with the lack of structural damage to these organs. Fatally infected animals and some human patients exhibit changes similar to those produced by the endotoxemia of gram-negative bacteremia. An endotoxin-like substance is present in the cell wall of leptospires but lacks the ketodeoxyoctonate of true endotoxin.

Kidneys. Renal failure due primarily to acute tubular necrosis is the most important cause of death in leptospirosis. Impaired renal perfusion constitutes the fundamental nephropathic change. Oliguria is rapidly reversed by intravenous fluid administration in many patients, suggesting that volume depletion is frequent. Hypovolemia is multifactorial: insensible water loss due to high fever, diminished intake of fluid, vomiting, diarrhea, and, infrequently, hemorrhage. A defect in the kidney's ability to concentrate urine is common and increases fluid loss. In some patients, widespread endothelial injury causes a shift of fluid from the intravascular to the extracellular space; hypotension of cardiac origin occurs rarely. Leptospires are frequently found in renal tissue (Fig. 72–2), but their role in mediating kidney damage is unknown. Interstitial nephritis occurs primarily in individuals who survive until inflammation has had an opportunity to

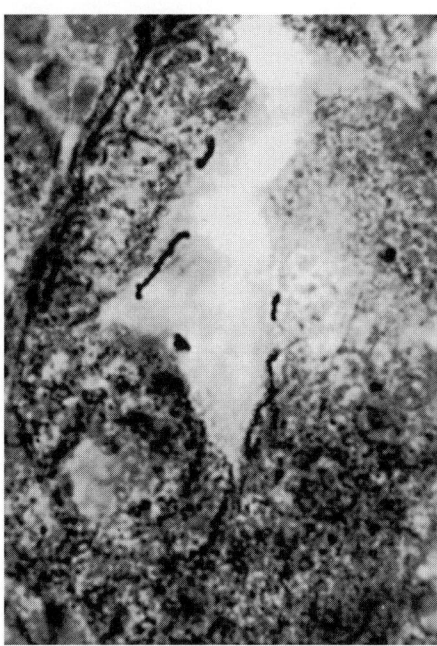

Figure 72–2. Leptospires in a renal tubule (Warthin-Starry stain, ×1320). (Courtesy of the Armed Forces Institute of Pathology, Photograph Neg. No. 60-1525.)

develop but is frequently absent in patients with fulminant disease.

Hemorrhage. A progressive severe hemorrhagic diathesis is a prominent feature of experimental leptospirosis. In humans, bleeding is generally restricted to the skin or mucosal surfaces; occasionally, however, massive gastrointestinal hemorrhage or bleeding into a vital organ occurs. Coagulopathy and thrombocytopenia occur together or separately in many patients with leptospirosis but do not adequately explain bleeding. By exclusion, capillary damage is the postulated mechanism, and toxins have been suggested as the mediators of endothelial injury.

Liver. Jaundice is the most noticeable clinical finding in cases of leptospirosis involving the liver, but its pathogenesis remains unexplained. Neither hemolytic anemia nor hepatocellular necrosis is a prominent feature of leptospirosis. The most severe hepatic pathologic changes are seen when organisms are difficult to demonstrate in tissue, suggesting subcellular toxic or metabolic effects.

Lungs. The importance of lung involvement was highlighted by frequent, severe pulmonary hemorrhages occurring during a 1995 outbreak of leptospirosis in Nicaragua. Early life-threatening pulmonary hemorrhage had previously been reported from China and Korea. Necropsy findings included massive intra-alveolar hemorrhage with or without diffuse alveolar damage. Leptospires were demonstrated in lung tissue. Localized or confluent hemorrhagic pneumonitis is the usual finding, with petechial and ecchymotic hemorrhages noted throughout the lungs, pleura, and tracheobronchial tree.

Meningitis. Organisms easily enter the cerebrospinal fluid (CSF) during leptospiremia, and this may explain the high incidence of meningitis. However, little meningeal reaction is elicited by these spirochetes, which are isolated frequently from CSF that is otherwise normal and from individuals without clinically detectable nervous system involvement. Symptoms of meningitis coincide with the development of antibodies and disappearance of leptospires from the blood

and CSF, suggesting an immunologic mechanism. Pathologic changes are minimal or absent, and the prognosis is excellent.

Heart. Focal hemorrhagic myocarditis has been reported, but hypovolemia, electrolyte imbalance, and uremia are more frequent causes of cardiac dysfunction. Minor electrocardiographic changes, particularly first-degree heart block, are common and resolve completely.

Skeletal Muscle. The myalgias typical of early disease appear to be due to invasion of skeletal muscle by leptospires. Muscle pain ends as antibody titers develop and organisms are cleared from the blood. Muscle biopsies in patients with early illness demonstrate vacuolation of the myofibrillar cytoplasm, loss of cellular detail, and fragmentation. Leptospiral antigen can be demonstrated by fluorescent antibody techniques. Pathologic changes are usually absent in the muscles of patients dying during the second week of disease.

Eye. The aqueous humor provides a protective environment for leptospires, which readily enter the anterior chamber of the eye during the leptospiremic phase of disease. There they can remain viable for months, despite the development of serum antibodies. Uveitis is frequent, appearing weeks or months after the onset of disease, and has been attributed to the persistence of organisms in the anterior chamber.

CLINICAL MANIFESTATIONS
General Features. Serologic surveys of workers at high risk confirm that subclinical infection is common. Among individuals unaware of illness due to leptospirosis, 16% of abattoir workers and 40% of rice farmers had antileptospiral antibodies. Less than 10% of symptomatic infections result in severe, icteric illness. Even relatively virulent serovars such as *L. icterohaemorrhagiae* lead more often to anicteric than to icteric disease.

After accidental laboratory exposure or immersion in contaminated water, the incubation period has varied from 2 to 26 days. The standard interval is 1 to 2 weeks, with a median of 10 days. The duration of the incubation has no prognostic significance. Once symptoms develop they follow a biphasic course: After an initial febrile illness, there is defervescence of fever and symptomatic improvement, followed by a second period of disease. However, a clear demarcation between the first and second stages is atypical of icteric leptospirosis; in mild cases the distinction can be unclear, or the second stage may never occur.

Anicteric Leptospirosis
Symptoms. The onset of symptoms is typically abrupt: Patients can time the beginning of their illness to within 1 or 2 hours. Headache, fever, chills, and myalgias are the most frequently reported initial symptoms. Headache is usually frontal, less often retro-orbital, and occasionally bitemporal or occipital. It is generally intense, persistent, and poorly controlled with nonprescription analgesics. Fever is high, with one or more daily peaks that often exceed 40°C (103°F) and are preceded by rigors. Muscle pain can be excruciating and occurs most commonly in the thighs, calves, lumbosacral region, and abdomen. Some patients with leptospirosis have intense abdominal wall pain, with tenderness and fever mimicking an acute surgical abdomen. There are numerous reports of inappropriate surgical interventions, particularly appendectomies. Myalgia adjacent to the cervical spine can cause nuchal rigidity and suggest meningitis in a patient with headache and fever. Lumbar puncture is often performed, but CSF obtained during the first week of illness is acellular with normal protein and glucose content. Leptospires can be isolated from the blood for 4 to 9 days after the onset of illness. During the "leptospiremic" phase of illness, many symptoms can occur (Table 72–1). Cough and chest

TABLE 72–1. The Most Common Clinical Manifestations of 208 Leptospirosis Patients in Puerto Rico*

	Anicteric (106 Cases)	Icteric (102 Cases)
Symptoms (% of cases)		
Fever	100	99
Myalgia	97	97
Headache	82	95
Chills	84	90
Sore throat	72	87
Nausea	71	81
Vomiting	65	75
Eye pain	54	38
Diarrhea	23	30
Decreased urine	20	30
Cough	15	32
Hemoptysis	5	14
Signs (% of cases)		
Conjunctival injection	100	98
Muscle tenderness	70	79
Hepatomegaly	60	60
Pulmonary findings	11	36
Lymphadenopathy	35	12
Petechiae and ecchymoses	4	29

*Adapted from Diaz-Rivera RS, et al: Zoonosis Res 2:159, 1963.

pain figure prominently in reports of patients from Korea and China. Up to a quarter of Korean patients present with pneumonia.

Signs. Conjunctival suffusion is the most characteristic and diagnostically helpful physical sign during the leptospiremic phase. It usually appears 2 or 3 days after the onset of fever and involves the bulbar conjunctiva. Redness decreases in intensity toward the cornea. It is not a conjunctivitis; pus and serous secretions are absent, and there is no matting of the eyelashes and eyelids. Suffusion gradually fades over a period of 3 days to 3 weeks. The marked variation in the reported incidence of this finding is due more to the diligence with which suffusion is sought than to true differences in the frequency with which it occurs. Unless specifically looked for, mild suffusion can easily be overlooked. Less common and less distinctive signs include pharyngeal injection, splenomegaly, hepatomegaly, lymphadenopathy, and skin lesions that may be macular, papular, erythematous, urticarial, or hemorrhagic.

Second Phase. Within a week most patients become asymptomatic, although occasionally disease persists for more than a month. After several days of apparent recovery, the illness resumes in some individuals. Manifestations of the second stage are more variable than those of the initial illness. Symptoms last from 2 to 4 days in most patients; fever is not so high; and myalgias and gastrointestinal disturbances are less severe. Leptospires disappear from the blood, CSF, and tissues but appear in the urine. Serum antibody titers rise—hence the term "immune phase."

Meningitis is the hallmark of this stage of leptospirosis. CSF pleocytosis can be demonstrated in 80 to 90% of all patients during the second week of illness, although only about 50% will have clinical signs and symptoms of meningitis. Pleocytosis usually lasts 1 to 3 weeks but occasionally may persist as long as 80 days. Meningeal signs can last several weeks but usually resolve within a day or two. Neurologic manifestations other than meningoencephalitis occur occasionally.

Uveitis is a late manifestation of leptospirosis. Although it is seen as early as the third week of illness, the average time of appearance is at 4 to 8 months, and intervals of up to 1 year have been reported. The anterior uveal tract is most frequently affected, and pain, photophobia, and blurring of vision are the usual symptoms. Iridocyclitis can be unilateral or bilateral; the prognosis is generally good.

Laboratory Findings. The white blood cell count may be low, normal, or elevated, but whatever the total count, neutrophilia is usually found. The erythrocyte sedimentation rate is consistently elevated. Urinalysis may show proteinuria, pyuria, and microscopic hematuria. Enzyme markers of skeletal muscle damage, e.g., creatinine phosphokinase and aldolase, are elevated in the sera of 50% of patients during the first week of illness.

Chest radiographs in patients with pulmonary manifestations show a variety of abnormalities, but none is pathognomonic of leptospirosis. The most common finding is small, patchy, snowflake-like lesions in the periphery of the lung fields, either restricted to a few intercostal spaces or widely disseminated. Other patterns include confluent infiltrates or massive consolidation, which represent hemorrhage, and solitary, patchy lesions with ill-defined margins.

Lumbar puncture during the second week of illness reveals changes characteristic of aseptic meningitis. CSF pressures and cell counts are generally less than 200 mm H_2O and 500 cells/mm³, respectively. There is an early, transient predominance of polymorphonuclear leukocytes, after which lymphocytes are the dominant cell type. Protein concentrations range from normal to 300 mg/dL, and glucose values are normal.

Icteric Leptospirosis (Weil's Disease). This dramatic, life-threatening illness is characterized by jaundice, renal dysfunction, hemorrhagic manifestations, and a high mortality rate; a clear-cut biphasic disease pattern is atypical. The key differences between icteric and anicteric leptospirosis are summarized in Table 72–2. The clinical picture is variable and may be dominated by symptoms of renal, hepatic, pulmonary, or vascular dysfunction. With adequate supportive care the case-fatality rate is less than 10%, but it is generally much higher in the tropics because facilities are lacking and patients present late in the course of illness.

Hepatic Findings. Although jaundice is the hallmark of severe leptospirosis, fatalities do not occur because of liver failure. The degree of jaundice has no prognostic significance, but its presence or absence does—virtually all leptospirosis deaths occur in icteric patients. Icterus first appears between the fifth and ninth days of illness, reaches maximum intensity 4 or 5 days later, and continues for an average of 1 month. Hyperbilirubinemia results from increases in both conjugated (direct) and unconjugated (indirect) bilirubin, but elevations of the direct fraction predominate. Other signs of hepatic dysfunction usually accompany jaundice. Prolongations of

TABLE 72–2. Salient Differences Between Icteric and Anicteric Leptospirosis*

	Icteric (Weil's Disease)	Anicteric
Jaundice	+ + +	+
Leukocytosis	+ + +	−
Hemorrhage	+	−
Renal failure	+	−
Death	+	−
Aseptic meningitis	−	+
Disturbances of consciousness†	+	+

*(−) = rare or absent; (+) = can occur; (+ + +) = characteristic.

†Due primarily to uremia in severe disease and to encephalitis in anicteric cases.

the prothrombin time occur commonly and are corrected by the administration of vitamin K; modest elevations of serum alkaline phosphatase are typical. Jaundice is not associated with marked hepatocellular necrosis; greater than fivefold increases of aminotransferase levels are exceptional. Hepatomegaly is found in the majority of patients (Table 72–1), and hepatic percussion tenderness is a reliable marker of continuing disease activity. There is no residual liver dysfunction in survivors of Weil's disease, consistent with the absence of structural damage seen on pathologic examination of this organ.

Bleeding Phenomena. Bleeding is occasionally seen in anicteric cases but is most prevalent in severe disease (Tables 72–1 and 72–2). Purpura, petechiae, epistaxis, bleeding of the gums, and minor hemoptysis are the most common hemorrhagic manifestations, and deaths due to subarachnoid hemorrhage and exsanguination from gastrointestinal bleeding occur. Adrenal hemorrhage is rare. Conjunctival hemorrhage is an extremely useful diagnostic finding and, when combined with scleral icterus and conjunctival suffusion, produces eye findings pathognomonic of leptospirosis.

Pulmonary hemorrhage is well recognized in the Far East. Forty patients died with acute pulmonary hemorrhage and respiratory insufficiency during an outbreak of leptospirosis in Nicaragua in 1995. Hemoptysis was common, and chest radiographs showed diffuse bilateral patchy small infiltrates; areas of consolidation progressed rapidly to a total whiteout in fatal cases.

Renal Abnormalities. Life-threatening renal failure is a complication of icteric disease, although all forms of leptospirosis may have mild kidney involvement. Prompt recognition with appropriate management of renal dysfunction in severe leptospirosis is the key to patient survival. Oliguria or anuria usually develops during the second week of illness but may appear as early as the third or fourth day. Despite extremely elevated serum creatinine levels, renal recovery can be achieved in most patients without dialysis provided that some urine output is present. Complete anuria is a grave prognostic sign, often seen in patients who present late in the course of illness with frank uremia and irreversible disease.

Most oliguric patients have decreased renal perfusion and respond to fluid challenge with increased urine output, but there is rapid progression to acute tubular necrosis and anuria if hypovolemia is not corrected. Signs of hypovolemia include flat neck veins, reduced ocular tension, poor skin turgor, and postural hypotension; urine specific gravity is high. Hypokalemia due to renal potassium wasting can occur. Occasional individuals have renal deterioration despite vigorous fluid therapy. Because renal failure develops very quickly in leptospirosis, symptoms and signs of uremia are frequently encountered. Anorexia, vomiting, drowsiness, disorientation, and confusion are seen early and progress to convulsions, stupor, and coma in severe cases.

Neurologic Changes. Disturbances of consciousness in a patient with severe leptospirosis are usually due to uremic encephalopathy, whereas in anicteric cases aseptic encephalitis is the most frequent cause (Table 72–2). Renal function eventually returns to normal in survivors of Weil's disease, although detectable abnormalities may persist for several months.

Laboratory Findings. In severe disease, laboratory abnormalites are nonspecific but helpful in the differential diagnosis. Jaundiced patients usually have leukocytosis in the range of 15,000 to 30,000/mm³. Extremely high counts have been reported, but whatever the absolute number of white cells, neutrophilia is constant. Anemia is common and multifactorial; blood loss and azotemia contribute frequently, intravascular hemolysis less often. Mild thrombocytopenia occurs often, but decreases in platelet count sufficient to be associated with bleeding are exceptional.

Childhood Disease. Pediatric leptospirosis shares many features with adult disease but has several distinct clinical features. Hypertension, acalculous cholecystitis, pancreatitis, abdominal causalgia, and skin lesions that may desquamate or become gangrenous have been reported. Cardiopulmonary arrest sometimes occurs. Deaths from pulmonary hemorrhage occur in children, and up to 80% of children hospitalized with leptospirosis have severe renal dysfunction. As in adults, antimicrobial therapy hastens recovery from renal failure.

Association With HIV Infection. Although the reported experience is limited, the risk of infection, severity of illness, response to therapy, or prognosis of leptospiral infection in HIV-infected persons or persons with AIDS does not appear to be appreciably different from those without HIV infection.

DIAGNOSIS

Differential Diagnosis

Anicteric Leptospirosis. The typical leptospirosis patient has a history of contact with animals or standing flood water, severe myalgias, and conjunctival suffusion. Atypical or mild cases are often confused with other entities, but because of a low index of suspicion and the disease's protean manifestations, the diagnosis is often missed even in typical cases. Infection with *L. interrogans* was included in the admitting differential diagnosis in less than 25% of over 1000 confirmed cases reported by the Centers for Disease Control since 1949. In another series of 483 proven cases, only 17% of patients were initially thought to have leptospirosis. Aseptic meningitis is the most common clinical impression in leptospirosis patients; fever of unknown origin, influenza, appendicitis, and gastroenteritis are other frequent diagnoses.

Weil's Disease. Viral hepatitis is a common misdiagnosis in patients with Weil's disease. Conjunctival suffusion, severe myalgias, and a history of water or animal contact are very helpful diagnostic clues in jaundiced patients, as they are in anicteric individuals. Leukocytosis, elevated serum bilirubin levels without marked transaminase elevations, and renal dysfunction are typical of leptospirosis but unusual in hepatitis. Malaria, typhoid fever, scrub typhus, and Hantaan virus infection (hemorrhagic fever with renal syndrome) are important differential diagnoses in the tropics. Marked leukocytosis and a negative malaria smear argue against *Plasmodium falciparum* infection; jaundice, severe renal dysfunction, and leukocytosis are atypical of typhoid fever. Differentiating leptospirosis from scrub typhus and Korean hemorrhagic fever in areas where these diseases coexist is more difficult. Both are associated with animals, and both can cause conjunctival suffusion. Splenomegaly and generalized lymphadenopathy are characteristic of scrub typhus but not leptospirosis; myalgia is typically mild and serum creatinine levels normal even in jaundiced patients infected with *Orientia tsutsugamushi*. Korean hemorrhagic fever is transmitted by infected rodent urine, and mixed infection with *L. interrogans* and Hantaan virus has been reported. Liver disease is not usually a prominent manifestation of Korean hemorrhagic fever. Leptospirosis with prominent hemorrhagic manifestations is easily misdiagnosed as dengue fever (this was the initial impression in the Nicaraguan outbreak).

Childhood Disease. Some features of pediatric leptospirosis, e.g., desquamation, myocardial involvement, and hydrops of the gallbladder, suggest Kawasaki's disease (mucocutaneous lymph node syndrome).

Laboratory Tests. The diagnosis of leptospirosis is usually based on serology. Culturing *L. interrogans* is not difficult, but growth is so slow that results may be delayed for up to 8 weeks—too late to benefit acutely ill patients. Animal inoculation offers no greater chance than culture for recovery of leptospires. Direct examination of blood or urine by dark-field microscopy is not only insensitive but often erroneous; it should not be performed except by highly skilled specialists.

Serology. The macroscopic slide agglutination test has long been commercially available, but both its sensitivity and its specificity have been questioned. Much progress has been made in the development of accurate, rapid diagnostic tests. ELISAs and dot-ELISA procedures have been field-tested and are becoming commercially available. There is a need for practical, affordable diagnostic kits in areas where leptospirosis is common.

The microscopic agglutination test is considered the serodiagnostic method of choice for leptospirosis, but its complexity limits its use to reference laboratories. Dilutions of patient sera are applied to live, pathogenic leptospires. The results are viewed under darkfield microscopy and expressed as the percentage of organisms cleared from the field by agglutination. To ensure detection of antibodies that may be provoked by any of the large number of different serovars, it is necessary to use a battery of antigens—usually 24. This test does not reliably identify the infecting serovar because of frequent cross reactivity.

The addition of antigen detection–based, rapid, "dipstick" diagnostic tests offers the first real opportunity for specific diagnosis in a clinically meaningful time frame. Although none of these assays has been approved by the United States Food and Drug Administration, they are commercially available in some regions.

Isolation Procedures. Isolation of leptospires from blood or CSF is possible during the first 10 days of clinical illness. Organisms usually appear in the urine during the second week and may persist for several months, thus permitting diagnosis by urine culture in untreated patients even after clinical illness is over. Leptospires are not difficult to isolate provided that specialized media are used. Organisms will not grow on standard media used for isolation of pathogens from blood or urine. If specialized media are not immediately available, leptospires will remain viable for up to 11 days in blood anticoagulated with sodium oxalate. Repeated attempts at isolation will increase the diagnostic yield. Isolations are usually made from urine, but too much urine inhibits its growth. Best results are obtained by diluting 0.1 mL of urine, obtained as sterilely as possible, with 0.9 mL of buffered saline and then making additional dilutions. These different concentrations are then inoculated into 5 mL of Fletcher's or EMJH semisolid medium and incubated at 28° to 30°C in the dark for at least 5 to 6 weeks. For either blood or CSF, the same procedures are followed beginning with from 1 to 4 drops of sample liquid. Isolates can be sent to reference centers for identification of the responsible serovar.

Molecular-Based Diagnostics. Reference laboratories have developed polymerase chain reaction (PCR) assays for the detection of leptospiral DNA in blood, serum, CSF, aqueous humor, and urine. Using PCR with arbitrary DNA primers also allows for rapid identification of serovars.

THERAPY

Supportive Therapy. Proper symptomatic treatment and supportive care are essential for a good outcome in cases of severe leptospirosis. Meticulous attention must be paid to fluid and electrolyte balance, and patients must be aggressively rehydrated when necessary. Ensuring adequate renal perfusion prevents renal failure in the vast majority of oliguric individuals. Rarely, patients present late in the course of disease with symptomatic uremia and anuria. Such individuals rarely respond to conservative measures and have a high mortality rate. Peritoneal dialysis is preferred to hemodialysis in patients who require it. Renal failure in leptospirosis is hypercatabolic, so frequent dialysis may be necessary.

Massive hemorrhage is uncommon in leptospirosis, but lesser amounts of bleeding occur frequently and decrease renal perfusion by worsening hypovolemia. A careful search should be made for sources of occult blood loss; blood should be transfused as necessary; and parenteral vitamin K should be administered in the event of a prolonged prothrombin time.

Meningoencephalitis is a nonfatal but extremely unpleasant complication of *L. interrogans* infection and is thought to be of immune origin. The possible role of corticosteroids as adjunctive therapy for meningitis needs evaluation by controlled trials. The management of pulmonary hemorrhage often requires prompt intubation and mechanical ventilation. Respiratory support to maintain adequate tissue oxygenation is essential, because in nonfatal cases complete recovery of pulmonary function can occur.

Antibiotic Treatment. A wide range of antibiotics, including penicillin, ampicillin, tetracyclines, some third-generation cephalosporins, and some quinolones, are active against *L. interrogans* both in vitro and in experimental infections in animals. In double-blind, placebo-controlled studies, doxycycline shortened the course of early leptospirosis, and intravenous penicillin decreased the duration of symptoms (Fig. 72–3) and renal dysfunction in severe, late disease. Antibiotics should therefore be given to all patients with leptospirosis, regardless of when in their disease course they are seen. Doxycycline is given at does of 100 mg orally twice a day for 1 week. Patients who are vomiting or are seriously ill require parenteral therapy: intravenous penicillin G, 1.5 million U every 6 hours, or ampicillin, 0.5 to 1.0 g every 6 hours, until the patient can tolerate oral therapy and is clearly improving. The Jarisch-Herxheimer reaction, if it occurs, is less prominent in leptospirosis than in other spirochetal illnesses, and antibiotics should not be withheld because of fear of a possible Jarisch-Herxheimer reaction.

PREVENTION. Doxycycline, 200 mg taken once a week, prevents infection by *L. interrogans*. Widespread use of doxy-

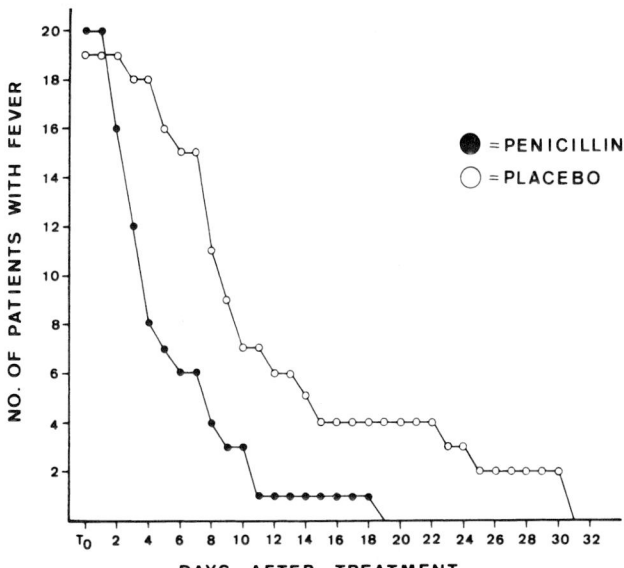

Figure 72–3. The effect of penicillin on the duration of fever in patients with Weil's disease. By day 4 more than half the penicillin-treated patients *(closed circles)* were afebrile, compared with only 1 of 19 patients in the placebo group *(open circles)*. (From Watt G, et al: Lancet 1:433, 1988.)

cycline prophylaxis is not indicated, but it can benefit those who are at high risk for a short time, e.g., military personnel and certain agricultural workers.

Infection by leptospires confers only serovar-specific immunity; second attacks due to different serovars can occur. Vaccines directed against regionally prevalent serovars are currently used in domestic animals and are a useful control measure. Immunization of groups of workers with high morbidity rates has successfully protected miners in Japan and Poland and rice field laborers in Italy and Spain. However, the efficacy and safety of human leptospiral vaccines have yet to be conclusively demonstrated. Surface decontamination, protective clothing, and rodent control are preventive methods applicable to some work environments.

Prevention of leptospirosis in the tropics is particularly difficult. The large animal reservoir of infection is impossible to eliminate; the occurrence of numerous serovars limits the usefulness of serovar-specific vaccine; and the wearing of protective clothing (e.g., rubber boots in rice fields) is both prohibitively expensive and impractical. Improved control will result only from a rise in the standard of living and betterment of general hygiene and sanitation.

Bibliography

Berman SJ, Tsai CC, Holmes KK, et al: Sporadic anicteric leptospirosis in South Vietnam. Ann Intern Med 79:167, 1973.

Brown PD, Gravekamp C, Carrington DG, et al: Evaluation of the polymerase chain reaction for early diagnosis of leptospirosis. J Med Microbiol 43:110, 1995.

Diaz-Rivera RS, Hall HE, Romos-Morales KY, et al: Leptospirosis in Puerto Rico. Clinical aspects of human infection. Zoonosis Res 2:159, 1963.

Edwards GA, Domm BM: Human leptospirosis. Medicine 39:117, 1960.

Faine S: Leptospira and Leptospirosis. Boca Raton, FL, CRC Press, 1994.

Farr RW: Leptospirosis. Clin Infect Dis 21:1, 1995.

Gussenhoven GC, van der Hoorn MA, Goris MG, et al: LEPTO dipstick, a dipstick assay for detection of Leptospira-specific immunoglobulin M antibodies in human sera. J Clin Microbiol 35:92, 1997.

Heath CW Jr, Alexander AD, Galton MM: Leptospirosis in the United States: Analysis of 483 cases in man, 1949–1961. N Engl J Med 273:915, 1965.

McClain JBL, Ballou WR, Harrison SH, et al: Doxycycline therapy of leptospirosis. Ann Intern Med 100:696, 1984.

Park SK, Lee SH, Rhee YK, et al: Leptospirosis in Chonbuk Province of Korea in 1987; A study of 93 patients. Am J Trop Med Hyg 41:345, 1987.

Watt G, Warrell DW: Leptospirosis and the Jarisch-Herxheimer reaction. Clin Infect Dis 20:1437, 1995.

Watt G, Padre LP, Tuazon L, et al: Placebo-controlled trial of intravenous penicillin for severe and late leptospirosis. Lancet 1:433, 1988.

Yasuda PH, Steigerwalt AG, Sulzer KR, et al: DNA relatedness between serogroups and serovars in the family Leptospiraceae with proposals for seven new Leptospira species. Int J Syst Bacteriol 37:407, 1987.

Zaki SR, Shieh WJ, and the Epidemic Working Group: Leptospirosis associated with outbreak of acute febrile illness and pulmonary haemorrhage, Nicaragua, 1995. Lancet 347:535, 1996.

73 Lyme Disease

David T. Dennis and G. Thomas Strickland

DEFINITION. Lyme disease (Lyme borreliosis) is a tickborne zoonosis caused by infection with the spirochete, *Borrelia burgdorferi*. Infection in humans results in an acute and chronic, multisystem inflammatory disease principally affecting the skin, joints, nervous system, and the heart. The disease complex, its epidemiology and ecology, were first described in the United States following investigations of an outbreak of "Lyme arthritis" in children in Lyme and sur-

rounding townships in coastal Connecticut in the mid-1970s. *B. burgdorferi* was isolated from ticks, white-footed mice, and humans in the early 1980s, and its zoonotic cycle was described. In its natural cycle, rodents and certain hard ticks belonging to the *Ixodes ricinus* complex are the principal reservoirs and amplifying hosts of *B. burgdorferi* infection; deer and some other large animals are the preferred maintenance hosts for adult vector ticks, and humans are incidentally infected when they intrude into the natural enzootic cycle. The disease occurs throughout much of the temperate Northern Hemisphere. In the United States, Lyme disease accounts for 95% of all reported cases of vector-borne disease. The incidence of Lyme disease in endemic areas of Europe is similar to that experienced in the United States, and it is the most common tick-borne disease in Europe and Russia.

ETIOLOGY. Lyme disease spirochetes were first identified in the midgut of the adult black-legged tick, *Ixodes scapularis* (deer tick, *Ixodes dammini*), and were cultured from ticks in a modified Kelly's medium, i.e., Barbour, Stoenner, Kelly (BSK) medium. They were shortly thereafter isolated from blood, skin, and cerebrospinal fluid (CSF) of patients with early Lyme disease, and were taxonomically described in 1984 as *B. burgdorferi* sp. nov.

Borreliae are flagellated helical bacteria comprised of a protoplasmic cylinder surrounded by an outer membrane that is loosely associated with the underlying structures. The outer surface membrane of *B. burgdorferi* and other borreliae is unique in that genes encoding its proteins are located on linear plasmids; these extrachromosomal genes determine molecular identity of the various strains and genomospecies of *B. burgdorferi* and are responsible for adaptive antigenic variability. *B. burgdorferi* is comprised of at least 30 different immunogenic proteins, including three major outer surface proteins, OspA (31 kDa), OspB (34 kDa), and OspC (23 kDa). A prominent 41-kDa antigen is located on the flagellum.

Genotypic Variations. A number of genetic differences have been described within and between *B. burgdorferi* genomospecies from Europe and the United States. The strain infecting humans in the United States is designated *B. burgdorferi*, sensu stricto, of which strain B31 is the prototype; the two dominant *B. burgdorferi* genomospecies in Europe and Asia are *B. garinii* and *B. afzelii* (Group V5461). These three genomospecies are associated with somewhat different disease expressions: arthritis occurs more frequently following infection with *B. burgdorferi*, sensu stricto; neurologic manifestations are more common in infections with *B. garinii;* and cutaneous manifestations occur more frequently in association with *B. afzelii* infection. A number of other genomospecies have been described from natural cycles in North America and in Eurasia, but none has so far been shown to cause infection and disease of humans.

ECOLOGY AND EPIDEMIOLOGY

Transmission. The basic elements in the life cycle of *B. burgdorferi* in North America (Fig. 73–1) are (1) small rodents, especially the white-footed mouse and the chipmunk in the northeastern and north central regions, and the dusky wood rat (pack rat) in the Pacific coastal region, are the principal reservoirs of *B. burgdorferi* infection for vector ticks; (2) three stages of tick (larva, nymph, adult) are involved in a life cycle that in most places takes 2 years to complete, and in each stage the tick usually takes a single blood meal; (3) trans-stadial transmission of *B. burgdorferi* from larva to nymph helps maintain the infective cycle, whereas transmission from an infected adult female to her eggs rarely occurs; (4) the efficiency of the cycle is enhanced in eastern regions of the United States by sequential feeding patterns in which nymphs, feeding in the spring, infect rodents that later in the year serve as sources of infection for larvae, which feed in

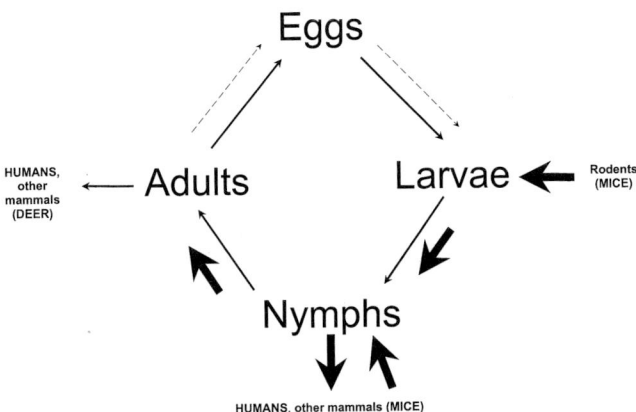

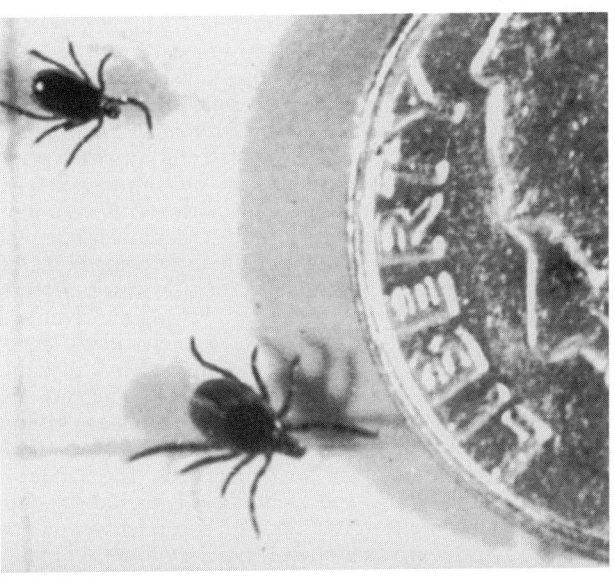

Figure 73–1. Schematic diagram of the enzootic cycle of *Borrelia burgdorferi*, showing the force of infection *(heavy arrows)* as ticks advance from one stage to another *(fine arrows)*. Infection moves from the rodent reservoir to larval and nymphal stages and trans-stadially from larva to nymph to adult tick. Trans-stadial transmission is important, whereas transovarial transmission is minimal and inconsequential.

Figure 73–3. Adult male *(upper)* and female *(lower) Ixodes scapularis.* (Courtesy of Dr. A. Main.)

the summer months; (5) deer, especially the white-tailed deer, and other large- and medium-sized animals, serve in the United States as the mating ground for adult ticks and provide adult female ticks the blood meal required for egg production. In Eurasia, the cycle is quite similar, although meadow voles and woodland mice serve as the principal rodent reservoirs of infection, and the roe deer, other wild cervids, cattle, and sheep typically serve as maintenance hosts for vector ticks.

Humans are incidental hosts of *B. burgdorferi*. Persons are most often infected by the bite of nymphal-stage ticks, usually in the late spring and early summer, and much less frequently by adult female ticks, which feed mostly in the late fall, but also in the winter and early spring.

Arthropod Vectors. Cycles of *B. burgdorferi* are found in the range of *I. ricinus* complex ticks (Fig. 139–18) throughout temperate North America and Eurasia (Fig. 73–2). *I. scapularis* is the principal vector in the eastern United States (Fig. 73–3); *I. pacificus* (the western black-legged tick) transmits *B. burgdorferi* in the western United States; *I. ricinus* (the castor bean, or sheep, tick) is the principal vector in western and central Europe; and *I. persulcatus* (the taiga tick) is the vector in

central and eastern Russia, China, and Japan. *I. ricinus* and *I. persulcatus* coexist in some areas of eastern Europe, and both tick species also transmit the tick-borne encephalitis (TBE) virus.

In the United States, spirochete rates in nymphal and adult ticks are often 20 to 50% in highly endemic areas of the northeastern and mid-Atlantic regions; infection rates are generally 10 to 20% in the less endemic north central region, 1 to 2% in the Pacific coastal region, and only 0 to 2% in southeastern and south central areas of the United States. Nymphal ticks are responsible for most Lyme disease transmission. Peak nymphal questing activity in late spring and early summer months strongly coincides with the peak incidence of disease onset in humans.

In the United States, the Lone Star tick, *Amblyomma americanum*, has been considered to be a potential vector of the Lyme disease spirochete. It is, however, an incompetent experimental vector of *B. burgdorferi*, and has never been found to maintain a cycle of the spirochete in nature. Although *B. burgdorferi* has been isolated from *A. americanum* and some blood-sucking insects, e.g., fleas, mosquitoes, and horseflies,

Figure 73–2. The global distribution of *Ixodes* spp. ticks able to transmit the agent of Lyme disease, *Borrelia burgdorferi*. (Modified from Filipova NA ed. Taiga Tick, *Ixodes persulcatus* Schulze [Acarina, Ixodidae]. Leningrad, Nauka Publishers, 1985.)

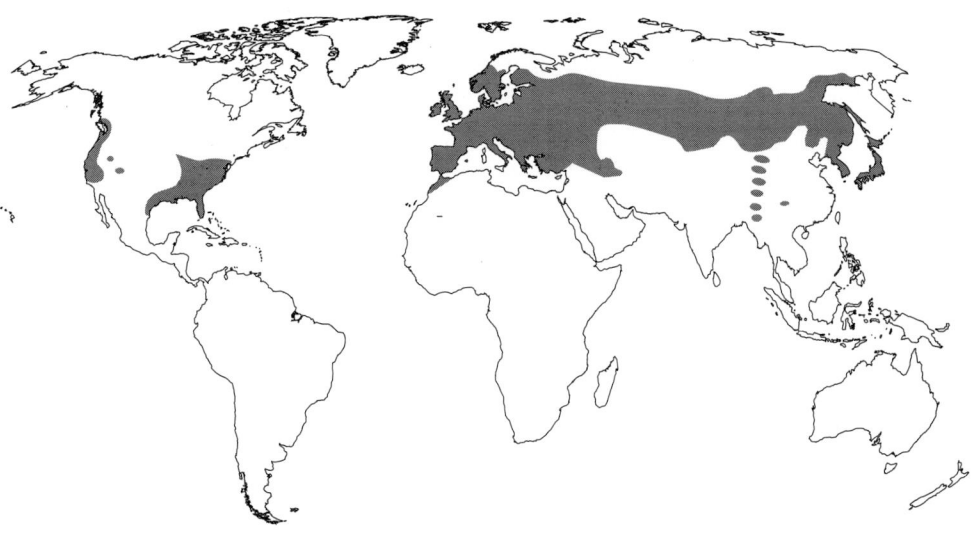

there is no evidence that the spirochete is adapted for survival in or transmission by these arthropods.

Environmental Factors. The ticks that transmit Lyme disease require shade, a high humidity in their microenvironment, and a ready access to preferred vertebrate hosts. *I. scapularis* is most often found in moist coastal and riparian areas. The landcover of northeastern coastal and island habitat is characterized by dense brush dominated by scrub oak, pine, bayberry bush and briar, and the inland northeastern and north central habitat by mixed deciduous succession forests with a sapling understory. A study of tick distribution on large suburban residential properties in a highly Lyme disease endemic area of New York found infective black-legged ticks on 60% of properties, with the greatest tick densities occurring in wooded areas, followed by fringe habitat, and much lesser densities among ornamental shrubbery and on lawns. Shaded leaf litter and humus provide a particularly favorable microenvironment for ixodid ticks. The habitat in southern Atlantic coastal and island areas is characterized by a landcover of complex mixed deciduous-conifer woodlands. *I. pacificus* in northern California is typically found in grassy, oak, and madrona woodland sites. In Europe, parks, woodlands, and nature preserves provide the most favorable habitat for the maintenance of enzootic cycles of *B. burgdorferi*.

Vertebrate Hosts. In the coastal northeastern United States, the white-footed mouse is the most competent vertebrate reservoir of *B. burgdorferi* and typically has infection rates of 80% or greater in highly endemic foci, maintains infection without apparent ill effects, and serves as the preferred vertebrate host for the immature stages of the tick vector. The chipmunk is also a competent reservoir host in the eastern United States and may be more important than the white-footed mouse in maintaining cycles of infection in the north central United States. Deer are a prerequisite for the establishment and maintenance of populations of black-legged tick populations in an area, and the explosive repopulation by white-tailed deer of the eastern United States in recent decades preceded the emergence of *I. scapularis* ticks and Lyme disease in this region. Alternate but less favorable tick maintenance hosts include raccoons, skunks, canids, and other medium- and large-sized mammals. The low infection rates of *Ixodes* vectors in the southern and western regions of the United States may be partly explained by the preferential feeding there of immature stages of vector ticks on lizards and skinks. These reptiles are incompetent reservoirs of *B. burgdorferi*, and thus act as diversionary, or zooprophylactic, hosts.

Several bird species serve as maintenance hosts for vector ticks and some may serve as lesser reservoir hosts of *B. burgdorferi*, and migrating birds may be responsible for establishing new enzootic foci. However, contiguous spread arising from movement of deer appear to be the principal factor in geographic spread in the United States. Seropositivity of dogs is a sensitive and reliable epidemiologic marker of the geographic distribution of *B. burgdorferi*, and dogs may be transient, secondary reservoirs of *B. burgdorferi* in the periresidential environment.

Tranmission of Infection to Humans. Lyme disease is transmitted in the saliva of feeding ticks, and possibly by regurgitation of tick midgut contents into the tick bite site. It is not transmitted from person to person. Transplacental infection of the fetus has been suggested by the finding of rare silver-stained spirochetal structures in fetal tissues; however, this has not been confirmed by cultural isolation. Although *B. burgdorferi* can be cultured from the blood in a small percentage of patients with early acute infection, and is able to survive in stored blood for prolonged periods, transfusion-acquired infection has not been documented.

Global Distribution. Lyme disease occurs in portions of the United States and Canada, the British Isles, Scandinavia, western, central, and eastern Europe, the Balkan states, and some states of the former Union of Soviet Socialist Republics, from the Baltic Sea east through northern forested areas of Russia to the Pacific coast, China, Korea, and Japan (Fig. 73–2). In Canada, Lyme disease is endemic only in southeastern Ontario Province, although *I. scapularis* is found in limited foci elsewhere in eastern Canada, and *I. pacificus* infected with *B. burgdorferi* has been found in British Columbia. In Japan, sporadic human cases occur mostly on Hokkaido Island and in central Japan (Nagano). In China, the disease is endemic in forested northeastern regions, and is found in a lesser frequency in scattered foci elsewhere. In the highly endemic areas of North America and Eurasia, Lyme disease incidence and epidemiologic patterns are similar. Suspect, unsubstantiated cases of Lyme disease have been reported from sub-Saharan Africa, South America, and Australia, but no transmission cycles of *B. burgdorferi* have been identified at these sites, and the Lyme disease spirochete has not been isolated there from patients or from nature.

Surveillance Statistics for the United States. Lyme disease accounts for more than 95% of all reports of vector-borne infectious disease in the United States. A total of 16,461 cases of Lyme disease were reported by 45 states in 1996, compared with 497 cases by 11 states in 1982 (Fig. 73–4). The national incidence of reported cases was 6.2 per 100,000 in 1996, ranging from 0 in several western states and in Hawaii to 94.8 per 100,000 in Connecticut. The distribution of cases by county shows geographic concentrations in the coastal northeastern and mid-Atlantic regions, in adjacent counties in western Wisconsin and eastern Minnesota, and in northern California. Incidences greater than the overall national rate were reported by eight states (Connecticut, Rhode Island, New York, New Jersey, Delaware, Pennsylvania, Maryland, Wisconsin, and Minnesota); these states accounted for 90% of the total number of reported cases, and New York alone accounted for one third of the total.

Lyme disease case reporting is limited by problems of misclassification, misdiagnosis, and under-reporting. Studies in some highly endemic areas of the United States suggest that Lyme disease is under-reported by 8- to 12-fold, and that many more patients are seen by physicians and treated for presumptive Lyme disease and for tick bite alone than patients meeting the Centers for Disease Control and Prevention (CDC) surveillance case criteria for reporting.

Lyme Disease Emergence. Lyme disease is one of the emerging diseases, including babesiosis and ehrlichiosis, transmitted by *Ixodes* ticks in the United States. Several localized outbreaks of Lyme disease have been described in the eastern United States since 1980. In the most highly endemic communities, annual Lyme disease incidence rates may reach 1 to 3%, and 5% or more of the population may have serologic evidence of prior infection with *B. burgdorferi*.

The buildup of Lyme disease to highly endemic levels in some states and regions since the mid-1970s is cause for concern, especially since there is no practical strategy to prevent expansion of the cycle of transmission in nature. The emergence has been most pronounced in suburban and rural areas in northeastern and mid-Atlantic states, and the disease is now endemic from coastal Maine to Maryland. Emergence has also been described in some north central states, e.g., Wisconsin and Minnesota. Lyme disease is more stable in the Pacific coastal region, where the majority of reported human cases occur in a few counties in northern California. Emergence of Lyme disease in Eurasia is less clear, and increasing numbers of reported cases may be due solely to a greater awareness and recognition of the disease.

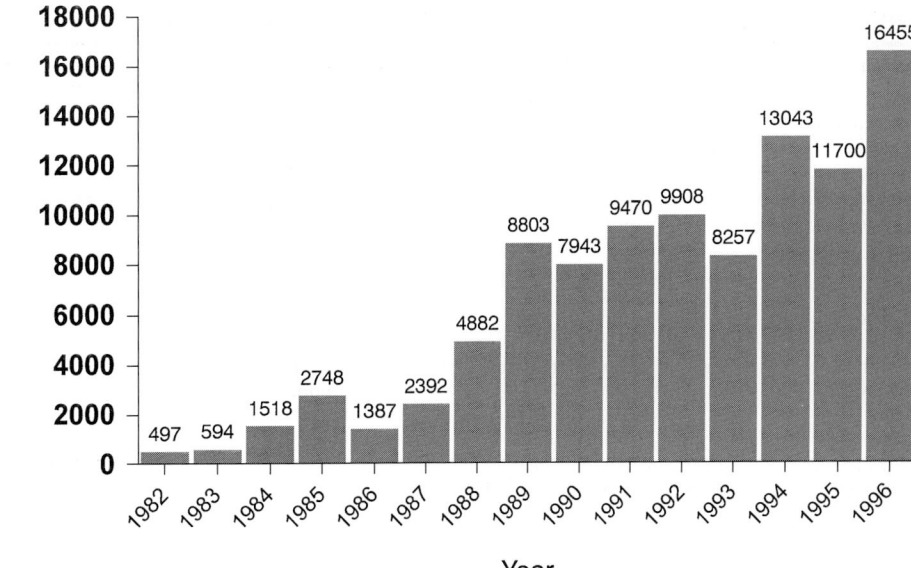

Figure 73–4. Number of reported Lyme disease cases by year in the United States, 1982–1996.

Areas with Unconfirmed Endemicity. The reporting of cases from areas where ticks are not known to transmit *B. burgdorferi* to humans, e.g., throughout many southern, midwestern, and mountain states, remains enigmatic. In the southern United States, *I. scapularis* has a low *B. burgdorferi* infection rate and rarely feeds on humans. Epidemiologic studies in Missouri and in North Carolina of persons with erythema migrans (EM)–like lesions suggest that the rash there is associated with the bites of ticks, but is not caused by *B. burgdorferi* or other known tick-borne infections. The EM-like lesions follow bites by the Lone Star tick, *A. americanum,* which is widely distributed throughout the southern and mid-Atlantic regions and is the most common human-biting tick in the South. Spirochetal structures have regularly been seen by darkfield microscopy in the midgut of 5% or less of adult, questing *A. americanum* ticks. However, *B. burgdorferi* has not been cultivated from questing *A. americanum* ticks or from biopsies of EM-like lesions from patients in the south central or southeastern United States. Recent studies using polymerase chain reaction (PCR) techniques did identify a new, uncultivable spirochete, *Borrelia lonestari,* sp. nov., in darkfield-positive *A. americanum,* but a causative link between this organism and disease in humans and animals has not been made. Cryptic cycles of *B. burgdorferi* involving *I. dentatus* ticks and rabbits in the eastern and southern United States and *I. spinipalpus* ticks and woodrats in the Rocky Mountain region, are not believed to pose a public health risk since these ticks rarely feed on humans.

There is no convincing evidence that enzootic cycles of *B. burgdorferi* occur in the Southern Hemisphere.

Risk Factors for Infection. Lyme disease is a disease of place. The principal risk factor for Lyme disease in the United States is permanent or seasonal residence in an area with high infestation with infected ticks, e.g., in some coastal lowland and island areas of New England and the mid-Atlantic states; selected wooded residential communities and natural areas further inland in these regions; in some rural, wooded areas of several states in the north central region; and in a few coastal counties of northern California. Exposures to infected ticks are most likely to occur in the parts of residential properties and their surroundings that are relatively undisturbed and provide forage and harborage for rodents and deer. Recreational activities in natural areas, e.g., gardening, hiking, camping, bird-watching, fishing, and hunting, may also expose persons to infective tick bites, especially during the late spring and summer months. As well, outdoor occupations, e.g., landscaping, brush clearing, forestry, and wildlife and parks management, may place persons at high risk in some areas. Ownership of cats has been found to be associated with an increased risk of acquiring Lyme disease in several small studies in the United States, and domestic cats have been observed to bring unattached nymphal ticks into homes. A study of dogs and persons living in the same households in highly endemic areas in Massachusetts showed that dogs were more likely to have serologic evidence of *B. burgdorferi* infection than their human co-residents, but dog ownership was not associated with an increased risk for their owners.

Lyme disease affects persons in all age groups, but highest rates are found in children <15 years of age and in adults ≥40 years of age. Males and females are nearly equally affected.

PATHOLOGY. Lyme disease is an inflammatory process that can be loosely categorized into early localized, early disseminated, and late disseminated stages of infection and disease (Table 73–1). The histopathologic findings in organs and tissues are generally not striking. The causative spirochetes are extremely sparse in tissues and difficult to identify, requiring tedious examination of silver-stained sections. The cellular reaction is characterized by infiltrates of lymphocytes and mononuclear phagocytes, as would be expected by an immunopathogenic disease mechanism. Biopsy specimens of the EM rash show intradermal perivascular round cell infiltrates with rare plasma cells and eosinophils (except at the point of tick attachment). There is no apparent endothelial damage, obliteration of vessel lumens, or fibrin deposits suggestive of a primary vasculitis. The most striking pathologic changes occur in affected joints. In chronic Lyme disease arthritis, the synovium is characterized by villous hypertrophy, fibrin deposition, and infiltrates of activated lymphocytes, plasma cells, macrophages, and mast cells. In early Lyme disease arthritis, radiographs may demonstrate intra-articular effusion, prepatellar bursal fluid collection, and infrapatellar fat edema. In late-stage chronic arthritis, a wide range of changes in the affected joints may be noted, including marked synovial hypertrophy; pannus formation; calcifications of periarticular ligaments, tendons, menisci, and patella; subchondral cysts; joint space narrowing; and osseous

TABLE 73-1. Common Manifestations of Lyme Disease by Stage of Infection

System	Early Localized Infection	Early Disseminated Infection	Late Infection
Constitutional symptoms	Fever, fatigue, anorexia	Severe malaise and fatigue	Fatigue
Skin	Erythema migrans	Secondary annular lesions, lymphocytoma	Acrodermatitis chronica atrophicans
Musculoskeletal system	Aches in muscles and joints	Migratory pain in joints, tendons, bursae, muscle, bone; brief arthritis attacks; myositis	Prolonged arthritis attacks, chronic arthritis, peripheral enthesopathy, periostitis or joint subluxations below lesions of acrodermatitis
Neurologic system	—	Meningitis, cranial neuritis, motor or sensory radiculoneuritis, subtle encephalopathy	Chronic encephalopathy, encephalomyelitis, subtle mental disorders, chronic axonal polyradiculopathy
Lymphatic system	Regional lymphadenopathy	Regional or generalized lymphadenopathy, splenomegaly	—
Heart	—	Atrioventricular nodal block, carditis	—
Eyes	—	Conjunctivitis	Keratitis

Adapted from Steere AC; Lyme disease. N Engl J Med 321:586, 1989.

changes of joint tissues. Erosion of joint surfaces infrequently occurs and is similar to that seen in many chronic inflammatory arthritides.

Almost no information is available on pathologic changes in the nervous system in persons with Lyme disease. The best available information comes from experimental infections in rhesus monkeys. These animals develop peripheral nervous system involvement characterized by electromyographic changes of a mononeuropathy multiplex with axonal loss. Histologic changes 3 months following infection include endoneural perivascular mononuclear cell infiltrates without necrosis; at 6 months, focal demyelination of the spinal cord and multifocal inflammation and fibrosis in peripheral nerve specimens have been noted. Evidence of central nervous system involvement includes CSF pleocytosis, chronic meningeal inflammatory cell infiltrate, and spinal cord lesions in some animals. Although *B. burgdorferi* has not been cultured from brain, spinal cord, or nerves of experimentally infected monkeys, specific bacterial DNA has been detected by PCR at each of these sites. These findings indicate that Lyme disease neuroborreliosis is associated with direct spirochetal invasion, and that the organism can persist for long periods in these tissues.

Inflammatory involvement of the heart in humans and in experimentally infected animals is characterized by perivascular and interstitial infiltrates of lymphocytes and plasma cells. These changes have been identified in the pericardium, myocardium, and the endocardium. Spirochetes were isolated from the myocardium of a patient with long-standing cardiomyopathy, and have been observed in the myocardium of fatal pancarditis in a patient with coexistent Lyme disease and babesiosis.

CLINICAL MANIFESTATIONS. The portal for infection with *B. burgdorferi* is the dermis, at the site of infective tick attachment. Following inoculation, infection may spread by cutaneous, lymphatic, and hematogenous routes. An incubation period of 3 to 30 days (typically 7 to 14 days) occurs between time of infection and onset of the characteristic EM rash that is the hallmark of early localized infection (see Fig. 73-5 in color section).

Early Localized Infection. This slowly expanding, annular, often large, erythematous rash (see Fig. 73-5 in color section), which is observed in 70 to 80% of symptomatic cases and in 90% of patients meeting objective clinical evidence of Lyme disease, is often accompanied by mild constitutional symptoms of fever, headache, fatigue, myalgia, arthralgia, and anorexia (Table 73-2). Not all Lyme disease patients remember a rash or other early manifestations. Flulike illness without localizing signs, subclinical, and asymptomatic infections (determined by serologic conversion) may occur in 20 to 30% of all infections with *B. burgdorferi*.

Early Disseminated Infection. This usually occurs days to weeks after onset of localized infection. The skin, nervous system, musculoskeletal system, and heart may be affected. Multiple, secondary EM lesions occur in about 15% of patients with early Lyme disease. Patients may show various neurologic signs and symptoms, most commonly associated with aseptic (lymphocytic) meningitis, cranial neuropathy (especially VIIth cranial nerve palsy), or radiculoneuritis. Many patients in the early disseminated stage of infection complain of migratory musculoskeletal pains without objective signs, although episodes of swelling and tenderness of one or a few joints sometimes occurs in this early stage. Rarely, persons with early Lyme disease develop cardiac conduction abnormalities, which are most often manifest as transient atrioventricular blocks of varying degree.

Late Disseminated Infection. Manifestations of late disseminated infection occur weeks to months after infection in untreated patients. The most common late-stage sequela is intermittent arthritis of one or a few joints, usually large, weight-bearing joints, especially the knee. Less frequently, a chronic encephalopathy with subtle memory deficit, sleep disturbance, fatigue, and personality disorders develop. Patients may also develop a chronic axonal polyneuropathy, which is most often manifest as distal paresthesia.

Untreated and inadequately treated infections result in mi-

TABLE 73-2. Most Frequently Reported Symptoms Accompanying Erythema Migrans, the Characteristic Rash of Early Lyme Disease (N = 314)

	No. of Patients (%)
Malaise, fatigue, and lethargy	251 (80)
Headache	200 (64)
Fever and chills	185 (59)
Stiff neck	151 (48)
Arthralgias	150 (48)
Myalgias	135 (43)
Backache	81 (26)
Anorexia	73 (23)

Adapted from Steere AC, et al: The early clinical manifestations of Lyme disease. Ann Intern Med 99:76, 1983.

crobial persistence, and *B. burgdorferi* has been isolated from skin lesions, myocardium, synovial fluid, or CSF months and even years, after the onset of symptoms in untreated persons. Genetic differences in susceptibility to infection have not been described, but chronic, antibiotic-refractory Lyme arthritis is associated with the major histocompatibility antigen, HLA-DR4, in some patients.

Morbidity can occasionally be severe, chronic, and disabling, especially if the disease is not treated adequately in its early stages. Maternal Lyme disease is not a proven cause of intrauterine death or congenital malformation, although this association has been suggested. Concurrent infections with *B. burgdorferi* and *Babesia microti* have been associated with a severity and duration of illness greater than that expected for either infection alone. A case of fatal Lyme disease pancarditis, in which spirochetes were seen in the myocardium, was reported in a patient who had concurrent babesiosis; however, there have been no deaths proven to be due to Lyme disease alone. Differentiating illness caused by *Borrelia*, *Babesia*, and *Ehrlichia* spp., and other as yet unidentified agents transmitted by the same tick vectors is important since treatments may differ, and babesiosis (Chapter 96) and ehrlichiosis (Chapter 70) may be fatal.

Persistent Symptoms After Therapy ("Chronic Lyme Disease," "Post–Lyme Syndrome"). Some patients have persistent symptoms following recommended courses of antibiotic therapy for Lyme disease. The first step in the evaluation of the patient is to determine whether there is evidence of persisting active infection. Although infection is almost always eliminated by a single course of appropriate antimicrobials in the treatment of early Lyme disease, some patients with late-stage neurologic or arthritic manifestations of Lyme disease may require more than one course of treatment to resolve active disease. A refractory response is most likely to occur in patients with Lyme disease arthritis who have HLA-DR4 specificity. Persons with late-stage encephalopathy may have subtle disturbances of memory, other cognitive functions, and personality changes that persist after treatment. There are, however, a number of reasons other than persisting infection that may account for post-treatment symptoms; these include the following: sterile inflammation due to dead organisms; permanent tissue damage not responsive to antibiotics; nonspecific factors related to chronic illness, especially chronic fatigue syndrome and fibromyalgia; molecular mimicry, or other tissue stimuli that may trigger postinfectious autoimmune responses; and, most commonly, misdiagnosis. Nonspecific or atypical symptoms, lack of objective signs of Lyme disease, lack of laboratory confirmation of infection, and lack of expected response to antibiotics suggest the misdiagnosis of Lyme disease.

DIAGNOSIS. The diagnosis of Lyme disease is easily made in persons who give a history of endemic exposure and who present with EM (Fig. 73–5 in color section) or other characteristic manifestations. History of recent tick bite significantly increases the pretest probability of a true diagnosis of early Lyme disease. Laboratory testing is generally unnecessary in persons with typical clinical presentations of early disease and known exposure to ticks in an area endemic for Lyme disease.

Serology. Serologic testing for antibodies directed against antigens of *B. burgdorferi* may be indicated when a clinical diagnosis and/or a history of tick exposure is not clear. The recommended test approach uses a sensitive first test, either enzyme immunoassay (EIA) or indirect fluorescent antibody (IFA) testing, followed by Western immunoblot (WB) testing of serum specimens equivocal or positive in the first test. Specific WB banding criteria have been recommended for both IgM and IgG antibodies. IgM antibodies to *B. burgdorferi*

can be detected within 2 weeks after EM onset, and usually peak between the third and sixth weeks of illness; IgG responses may arise early or be delayed for weeks, but are generally present at ≥6 weeks. Using the recommended two-test approach, sensitivity is generally 35 to 65% in early localized infection, 85 to 90% in early disseminated infection, and 95% in late disseminated infection. Specificity should be set at 98% or greater. Current serologic tests should not be used for clinical screening, since their use in persons with a low pretest probability yields a high rate of false positivity. Recent studies have identified inappropriate and costly overuse of serodiagnostic testing for suspected Lyme disease and tick bite exposures.

Patients with early disseminated disease (e.g., cranial neuritis or multiple EM) and with active later-stage disease (e.g., arthritis, radiculoneuritis, meningoencephalitis, and acrodermatitis chronicum atrophicans) almost always have strong serologic reactivity with expanded WB IgG banding patterns to diagnostic *B. burgdorferi* antigens. Antibiotic treatment in early localized disease may, however, blunt or abrogate the serologic response. Seronegative late-stage Lyme disease rarely occurs. Serum antibodies often persist for months and years following treated and untreated infection, and serologic reactivity cannot be used as a marker of disease activity. Also, the presence of antibodies does not indicate immune protection, and more than one occurrence of primary EM is not uncommon among persons at high environmental risk.

Culture. *B. burgdorferi* can be cultured from 80% of early EM lesions, but satisfactory isolation rates require skin biopsy, culture in BSK medium, and protracted observation of cultures; culture is, therefore, not a routine procedure.

DNA and Antigen Detection. PCR methods have been used to amplify genomic DNA of *B. burgdorferi* in blood, CSF, synovial fluid, and skin. The sensitivity of PCR is not as great as obtained by culture of organisms from blood and skin of untreated persons, but may be used to complement primary isolation procedures. As a research tool, PCR results have provided unique insights into the occurrence, sequestration, and persistence of borrelial DNA in various tissues and fluids. PCR is not standardized as a diagnostic tool for confirming infection with *B. burgdorferi*, and the procedure is fraught with the usual problems of amplicon contamination in the laboratory. Immunologic techniques for detecting antigens of *B. burgdorferi* in tissues and fluids are also unstandardized and experimental.

Differential Diagnosis. Although infection with *B. burgdorferi* most often results in objective signs and symptoms characteristic for the stage of infection and system involved, the range of manifestations is broad and may be nonspecific. The initial febrile illness in the absence of EM can be confused with influenza, viral gastroenteritis, infectious mononucleosis, ehrlichiosis, Rocky Mountain spotted fever, and other acute febrile infections. Even the characteristic EM rash may be confused with cellulitis, allergic reactions, and reaction to poisonous plants (e.g., poison oak and ivy). Cranial nerve palsies of Lyme disease must be distinguished from those caused by viral illness or idiopathic cause (e.g., Bell's palsy), and Lyme disease meningitis must be differentiated from the many causes of aseptic meningitis. Multiple sclerosis, amyotrophic lateral sclerosis, and other chronic CNS disorders may be confused with encephalomyelitis caused by *B. burgdorferi* infection. Chronic fatigue and the fibromyalgia syndrome are often confused with the diagnosis of Lyme disease; this is especially confusing since these syndromes may perhaps be triggered by Lyme disease. Autoimmune diseases (e.g., lupus erythematosus and rheumatoid arthritis) can mimic late-stage Lyme disease.

TREATMENT. Lyme disease can be treated successfully

with antibiotics in all of its stages. Early and uncomplicated disease may be satisfactorily treated with orally administered antibiotics; neurologic Lyme disease and late, complicated Lyme disease arthritis are best treated with parenteral cephalosporins or penicillin (Table 73–3).

Persons treated in the early stages of Lyme disease usually respond promptly and fully; inadequate or delayed treatment may result in microbial persistence and chronic, sometimes disabling sequelae. Late, complicated illness may respond slowly or incompletely, and more than one course of treatment may be required. Continuing or relapsing symptoms may be due to causes other than persisting infection. A small percentage of persons with Lyme disease arthritis, especially those with the HLA-DR4 allele, may respond poorly to antibiotics, and require anti-inflammatory medication and synovectomy. The majority of Lyme disease patients, however, have minimal or no residual illness following treatment.

PREVENTION

Avoidance and Personal Protection. Prevention of Lyme disease is based on avoidance of tick-infested areas, use of personal protective measures, environmental management, and early detection and treatment of disease manifestations. The public should be informed of tick-infested areas and avoid risky exposures, especially in spring and summer. Information on the distribution of ticks in an area can usually be obtained from health departments, park personnel, and agricultural extension services.

Protective Clothing and Tick Repellents. When in tick-infested areas, persons should wear light-colored clothing so that ticks can be spotted more easily and removed, and they should wear long-sleeved shirts and tuck trousers into socks or boot tops to prevent ready access of ticks to skin. Ticks, especially nymphs and larvae, quest close to the ground, and the wearing of high rubber boots may provide a simple means of protection for landscapers and persons clearing leaf litter and underbrush from wooded properties. Insect repellents containing diethyltoluamide (DEET) can be applied to clothes, and to exposed skin other than the face, and permethrin compounds (which kill ticks on contact) can be sprayed on clothing for longer-lasting protection.

Tick Checks and Removal. One of the most important preventive measures is the early detection and proper removal of attached ticks. Tweezers should be used to grasp the tick mouthparts, and the tick removed by steady, gentle backward traction. Transmission of *B. burgdorferi* from an infected tick is unlikely to occur before 36 hours of attachment. When in tick-infested areas, a daily check for ticks and their proper removal is an important measure to prevent infection. Antibiotic treatment to prevent Lyme disease after a known tick bite is not routinely warranted.

Prophylactic Antibiotics. The risk of asymptomatic infection or disease resulting from a recognized but untreated rick bite is less than 3%, even when the bite is by a known vector species in a highly endemic area. Risk of infection is, in most circumstances, below the cost-benefit threshold of prophylactic treatment. Considerable costs are incurred for inappropriate and unnecessary serologic testing and antibiotic treatment of persons with asymptomatic tick bite.

Landscape Management and Tick Control. In endemic residential areas of the northeastern United States, wood lots, stone fences, and unkempt edges of yards pose a greater risk of tick exposure than lawns and ornamental shrubbery areas. Removing leaf litter and woodpiles, and clearing trees and brush around houses and at the edges of yards to admit more sunlight and remove habitat suitable for deer, ticks, and rodent reservoirs of infection may reduce the numbers of ticks that transmit Lyme disease in the ensuing transmission seasons. Area application of pesticides to residential properties is highly effective in suppressing vector ticks, but raises environmental concerns. The distribution in yards of pesticide-impregnated cotton balls which mice then use for nest building has produced variable results. Fencing out deer, making properties less attractive to deer by removing gardens and ornamental plants favored as forage, and maintaining tick-free pets may reduce tick numbers in the periresidential environment.

There are no proven practical measures for controlling tick vectors or rodent reservoirs of infection over large areas, or for preventing their spread. Management of deer populations and control of ticks on deer would seem to be a logical strategy to reduce the intensity of transmission in already established foci and to limit spread to new areas. The killing

TABLE 73–3. Treatment of Lyme Disease

Manifestations	Antibiotic	Dose/Route		Duration
		Adult	**Child**	
Early Localized Lyme Disease				
Erythema migrans	Doxycycline	100 mg PO b.i.d.	(≥9 yr) 100 mg PO b.i.d.	14–21 days
	Amoxicillin	500 mg PO t.i.d.	25–50 mg/kg/d PO t.i.d. (max 2 g/day)	14–21 days
	Cefuroxime axetil	500 mg PO b.i.d.	15 mg/kg PO b.i.d.	14–21 days
	Erythromycin	500 mg PO q.i.d.	30–40 mg/kg PO q.i.d.	14–21 days
Early Disseminated and Late Disease				
Multiple erythema migrans	Early localized disease regimen but for 21 days' duration			
Facial palsy	Early localized disease regimen but for 21–28 days' duration			
Arthritis (uncomplicated)	Early localized disease regimen but for 21–28 days' duration			
Meningitis, encephalopathy or radiculoneuritis	Ceftriaxone	2 g/day IV	75–100 mg/kg/day IV (max 2 g/day)	21–28 days
	Penicillin G	20 million U/day IV	300,000 U/kg/day IV, in divided doses every 4 hr (max 20 million U/day)	21–28 days
Carditis with first-degree heart block	Early localized disease regimen for 21–28 days			
Carditis with advanced heart block or cardiomyopathy	Meningitis regimen for 21–28 days			
Arthritis, persistent or recurrent	Meningitis regimen for 21–28 days			

of ticks on deer using feeding stations at which deer rub against pesticide applicators is being evaluated in pilot trials in the eastern United States.

Vaccination. Vaccines against infection with *B. burgdorferi* have been developed for both dogs and humans. One commercial canine vaccine contains inactivated *B. burgdorferi*, which in laboratory experiments protects against challenge by inoculated live organisms as well as infected ticks. The vaccines under evaluation for human use, and a recently marketed canine vaccine, use a *B. burgdorferi* recombinant outer surface protein A (OspA) as immunogen. The recombinant OspA vaccines have been shown in phase I and phase II human trials to be safe and immunogenic. Phase III trials in the United States, involving approximately 20,000 adult participants by two manufacturers, indicate that, given in single doses at months 0, 1, and 12, the vaccines are safe and efficacious in adults. Studies are underway to evaluate the vaccine in children, and to determine the need for continuing boosters. A unique mechanism of action of the OspA vaccine is the killing of *B. burgdorferi* within the midgut of ticks feeding on immunized experimental animal hosts. Cost-benefit models of human Lyme disease vaccine use indicate that society benefits economically only when the vaccine is used to prevent disease in the highest at-risk populations. It is expected that recommendations for vaccine use will target persons living, working, or recreating in areas highly infested with vector ticks although many more will likely wish to receive the vaccine.

Bibliography

Baranton G, Postic D, Saint-Girons I, et al: Delineation of *Borrelia burgdorferi* sensu stricto, *Borrelia garinii* sp. nov., and Group V5461 associated with Lyme borreliosis. Int J Syst Bacteriol 42:378, 1991.

Barbour AG, Fish D: The biological and social phenomenon of Lyme disease. Science 260:1610, 1993.

Barbour AG, Maupin GO, Teltow GJ, et al: An uncultivable *Borrelia* sp in the hard tick, *Amblyomma americanum*: A possible agent of a Lyme disease–like disease. J Infect Dis 173:403, 1996.

Berglund J, Eitrem R, Ornsten K, et al: An epidemiologic study of Lyme disease in southern Sweden. N Engl J Med 333:1319, 1995.

Burgdorfer WA, Barbour AG, Hayes SF, et al: Lyme disease—a tick-borne spirochetosis? Science 216:1317, 1982.

Campbell GL, Paul WS, Schriefer ME, et al: Epidemiologic and diagnostic studies of patients with suspected early Lyme disease. Missouri J Infect Dis 172:470, 1995.

Centers for Disease Control and Prevention: Lyme disease—United States, 1996. MMWR 46:531, 1997.

Centers for Disease Control and Prevention: Recommendations for test performance and interpretation from the Second National Conference on Serologic Diagnosis of Lyme Disease. MMWR 44:590, 1995.

Coyle BS, Strickland GT, Liang YY, et al: The public health impact of Lyme disease in Maryland. J Infect Dis 173:1260, 1996.

Coyle PK (ed): Lyme Disease. Chicago, Mosby–Year Book, 1993.

Dressler F, Whalen JA, Reinhardt BN, et al: Western immunoblotting in the serodiagnosis of Lyme disease. J Infect Dis 167:392, 1993.

Eng TR, Wilson ML, Spielman A, et al: Greater risk of *Borrelia burgdorferi* infection in dogs than people. J Infect Dis 158:1410, 1988.

Fishbein DB, Dennis DT: Tick-borne diseases—a growing risk. N Engl J Med 333:452, 1995.

Fix AD, Strickland GT, Grant J: Tick bites and Lyme disease in an endemic setting: Problematic use of serologic testing and prophylactic antibiotic therapy. JAMA 279:206, 1998.

Frank DH, Fish D, Moy FH: Landscape features associated with Lyme disease risk in a suburban residential environment. Landscape Ecol 13:27, 1998.

Johnson BJB, Robbins KE, Bailey RE, et al: Serodiagnosis of Lyme disease: Accuracy of a two-step approach using a flagella-based ELISA and immunoblotting. J Infect Dis 174:346, 1996.

Johnson RC, Schmid GP, Hyde FW, et al: *Borrelia burgdorferi* sp. nov.: Etiologic agent of Lyme disease. Int J Syst Bacteriol 34:496, 1984.

Krause PJ, Telford SR, Spielman A, et al: Concurrent Lyme disease and babesiosis: Evidence for increased severity and duration of illness. JAMA 275:1657, 1996.

Lane RS, Piesman J, Burgdorfer W: Lyme borreliosis: Relation of its causative agent to its vectors and hosts in North America and Europe. Annu Rev Entomol 36:587, 1991.

Maupin GO, Fish D, Zultowsky J, et al: Landscape ecology of Lyme disease

in a residential area of Westchester County, New York. Am J Epidemiol 133:1105,1991.

Orloski KA, Campbell GL, Genese CA, et al: Emergence of Lyme disease in Hunterdon County, New Jersey, 1993: A case-control study of risk factors and evaluation of reporting patterns. Am J Epidemiol 147:391, 1998.

Piesman J, Maupin GO, Campos EG, et al: Duration of adult female *Ixodes dammini* attachment and transmission of *Borrelia burgdorferi*, with description of a needle aspiration isolation method. J Infect Dis 163:895, 1991.

Rahn DW, Evans J (eds): Lyme Disease. Philadelphia, American College of Physicians, 1998.

Spielman A: Prospects for suppressing transmission of Lyme disease. Ann NY Acad Sci 539:212, 1988.

Spielman A, Wilson ML, Levin JF, Piesman J: Ecology of *Ixodes dammini*-borne human babesiosis and Lyme disease. Annu Rev Entomol 30:439, 1985.

Steere AC: Lyme disease. N Engl J Med 321:586, 1989.

Steere AC, Dwyer E, Winchester R: Association of chronic Lyme arthritis with HLA-DR4 and HLA-DR2 alleles. N Engl J Med 323:219, 1990.

Steere AC, Malawista SE, Hardin JA, et al: Erythema chronicum migrans and Lyme arthritis: The enlarging clinical spectrum. Ann Intern Med 86:685, 1977.

Steere AC, Malawista SE, Syndman DR, et al: Lyme arthritis: An epidemic of oligoarticular arthritis in children and adults in three Connecticut communities. Arthritis Rheum 20:7, 1977.

Strickland GT, Karp AC, Mathews A, Pena CA: Utilization and cost of serologic tests for Lyme disease in Maryland. J Infect Dis 176:819, 1997.

Walker DH, Barbour AG, Oliver JH, et al: Emerging bacterial zoonotic and vector-borne diseases: Ecological and epidemiologic factors. JAMA 275:463, 1996.

Wormser GP: Prospects for a vaccine to prevent Lyme disease in humans. Clin Infect Dis 21:1267, 1995.

74 *Meningococcal Disease*

Brian M. Greenwood

DEFINITION. Meningococcal disease comprises various clinical syndromes that may follow infection with *Neisseria meningitidis*. These include septicemia, meningitis, arthritis, pericarditis, conjunctivitis, pharyngitis, pneumonia, urethritis, and proctitis.

ETIOLOGY. Meningococcal disease is caused by a gram-negative, bean-shaped diplococcus that grows on standard blood agar plates but grows best on enriched media such as Mueller-Hinton agar. Meningococci are delicate organisms that are sensitive to freezing or overheating. Thus, care is needed when samples for meningococcal isolation are collected in the field, because in the tropics, meningococci may be killed by exposure to ambient temperatures. Samples and plates should be kept cool but not frozen.

Meningococci are classified in various ways. The earliest classification characterized meningococci according to the structure of their capsular polysaccharide. Eight major serogroups are now recognized: A, B, C, X, Y, Z, W135, and 29E. Meningococci are also classified into serotypes and subgroups according to the structure of their outer membrane proteins. Thus, a meningococcus designated as B.15:P1.16 has a group B capsular polysaccharide and outer membrane proteins belonging to serotype 15 and subgroup 1.16. Other typing systems have been developed on the basis of allelic variations in bacterial enzymes, structural changes in lipopolysaccharide (LPS), and patterns produced on digestion with restriction endonucleases. Typing systems based on variations in a specific gene, detected using the polymerase chain reaction (PCR), have been developed also.

Typing of meningococci has two main uses. First, it allows identification of meningococci likely to be particularly pathogenic—for example, those belonging to serogroup A. Second, it allows the sequence of outbreaks to be monitored.

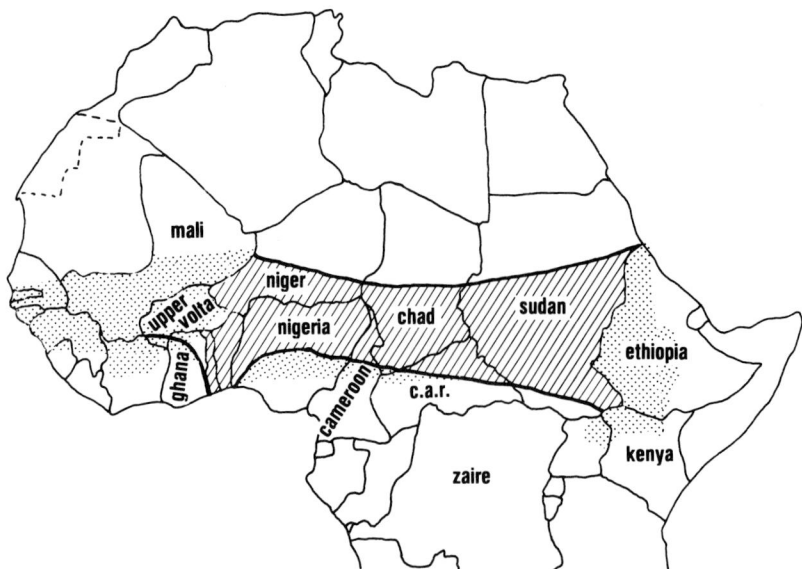

***Figure* 74–1.** The African meningitis belt. The shaded area indicates the area of the belt as originally defined by Lapeyssonnie. Dotted areas indicate regions where outbreaks of meningococcal disease with epidemiologic features characteristic of the African meningitis belt have sometimes been recorded. (Adapted from Lapeyssonnie L: Bull WHO 28(Suppl 3):3, 1963.)

Thus, typing may allow the spread of a strain of meningococcus within a household or community to be tracked. At a more global level, typing has allowed the spread of epidemic clones of meningococci from country to country to be observed. Thus, using electrophoretic typing, it was possible to document the spread of a clone of group A meningococcus (111–1) from Nepal in 1983 to Mecca in 1987 and then from Mecca to the African meningitis belt the following year.

DISTRIBUTION AND INCIDENCE. The meningococcus is a ubiquitous organism that causes meningitis throughout the world. In most tropical developing countries, the pneumococcus and *Haemophilus influenzae* type b (Hib) are more important causes of meningitis than the meningococcus (Chapter 52). However, this situation is reversed in an area of sub-Saharan Africa—the African meningitis belt—where major epidemics of meningococcal disease have been recorded every 5 to 10 years since the beginning of the century. The meningitis belt, first defined by Lapeyssonnie, extends from the Sudan and Ethiopia in the east to Senegal in the west (Fig. 74–1). To the north, the belt is bounded by the Sahara; to the south, by the rain forests of western and central Africa, where epidemics of meningococcal disease rarely occur. Major outbreaks of meningococcal infection have occasionally been recorded in many other parts of the tropics and subtropics, but in no other area of the world have epidemics occurred with the frequency or the severity recorded in the northern savanna region of Africa.

EPIDEMIOLOGY

Transmission. Meningococcal infection usually is transmitted from person to person by respiratory droplets, but occasional cases of sexual transmission have been recorded. Most infected persons become asymptomatic nasopharyngeal carriers rather than patients with clinical disease. The ratio of clinical to subclinical infections varies from situation to situation; it is highest during epidemics, but it is rarely <1:100. Spread of meningococci is favored by overcrowding, such as that in institutions or refugee camps, and the risk of infection is increased in close contacts of a patient with clinical disease, especially during epidemics.

Risk Factors. During outbreaks of meningococcal disease, attack rates are usually highest in the least privileged section of the community, implicating crowding and poverty as important risk factors. Smoking and prior exposure to a respiratory virus, particularly influenza virus, may predispose to

invasive meningococcal disease. Although the risk of invasive pneumococcal disease is increased many fold in HIV-positive individuals, this does not appear to be the case for meningococcal infection. Persons with complement deficiencies are at increased risk of meningococcal disease, and such individuals make a significant contribution to the overall burden of meningococcal disease in communities with a low level of endemic infection, but such patients are encountered rarely during outbreaks.

The majority of patients with meningococcal disease have no identifiable risk factor, although it is likely that genetic risk factors, e.g., those involving cytokine genes, will be found. During outbreaks, it is not infrequent for one community to be severely affected but another adjacent community to be spared, without any obvious explanation for this variability.

African Meningitis Belt. Within the African meningitis belt, the epidemiology of meningococcal infection differs from that observed elsewhere in a number of important respects (Table 74–1). Within this area, epidemics of meningococcal disease, usually caused by meningococci belonging to serogroup A or C, occur every 5 to 10 years. Such epidemics are often enormous. Approximately 50,000 cases of meningococcal disease with 5000 deaths were reported from countries in the center of the African meningitis belt in 1996; the true incidence is likely to have been several times higher. It is estimated that at least 1 million people have died of meningococcal infections in Africa during the past 50 years.

TABLE 74–1. Comparison of the Epidemiologic Features of Meningococcal Infection in the Northern Savanna of Africa and in Developed Countries

	Savanna of Africa	Developed Countries
Dominant serogroup	Group A > group C	Group B and group C
Pattern of infection	Epidemic	Endemic
Seasonal prevalence	Dry season	Winter
Maximal age incidence	5–14 yr	<5 yr
Pattern of spread	Child to child	Adult to infant

African epidemics show a marked seasonal association, nearly always starting during the middle of the dry season, when it is hot, dry, and dusty. They cease abruptly with the onset of the rains and flare up in adjacent areas during the following dry season (Fig. 74–2). Epidemics rarely spread into areas where the absolute humidity remains >10 g/m³ throughout the year. Studies in Upper Volta and in Nigeria have shown that the rate of nasopharyngeal acquisition of meningococci is not affected by seasonal changes. Thus, it is likely that environmental factors associated with the dry season alter the ratio of clinical to subclinical infection rather than causing an overall increase in the incidence of meningococcal infection. High temperature and low absolute humidity may damage the local defenses of the nasopharynx, favoring systemic infection.

During African epidemics, most cases of meningococcal disease occur in children age 5 to 14 years, in contrast to the much earlier onset of the infection in Europe and the United States. In Nigeria, the infection is uncommon in children younger than 2 years, and carriage as well as clinical infection is found most frequently in older children, suggesting that within the African meningitis belt spread of meningococcal infection is usually from child to child.

PATHOLOGY AND PATHOGENESIS

Pathology. Post-mortem examination of a patient who has died of acute meningococcemia may show only a few abnormalities. Petechiae are usually noted, and larger hemorrhages into organs such as the adrenals may be observed. Signs of encephalitis or pulmonary edema may be found. Microscopy may show extensive damage to small blood vessels. The pathologic features of meningococcal meningitis are characteristic of those of any form of acute bacterial meningitis (Chapter 52).

Pathogenesis. Meningococci produce large amounts of LPS endotoxin, which is probably responsible for the peripheral circulatory collapse characteristic of acute meningococcemia and which contributes to the pathogenesis of the acute meningeal inflammatory changes in patients with meningococcal meningitis. LPS binds to CD14 receptors on monocytes, macrophages, and other cells, stimulating them to release a number of cytokines, and elevated levels of tumor necrosis factor (TNF), interleukin-1 (IL-1), IL-6, IL-8, and IL-10 are found in patients with acute meningococcemia. TNF levels correlate with severity, and this cytokine, perhaps acting through the release of nitric oxide, probably has a major role in the pathogenesis of the clinical features of acute meningococcemia. Release of LPS also leads to activation of the kinin and coagulation pathways.

Extensive hemorrhage may be present in the adrenal glands of patients who have died of shock, but this lesion is sometimes found in patients who have died of acute meningococcemia but who have maintained normal blood pressure throughout their illness. Most patients with acute meningococcemia have elevated plasma cortisol levels and respond normally to stimulation with adrenocorticotropic hormone. Thus, it is likely that factors other than acute adrenocortical insufficiency are responsible for shock in most patients with this condition.

Patients with acute meningococcemia or meningococcal meningitis may have arthritis, cutaneous vasculitis, episcleritis, or pericarditis several days after the onset of illness, at a time when the early clinical features of the infection have resolved. Such lesions are usually sterile. Biopsy specimens of an affected area of skin or synovium show a vasculitis. This probably results from a local antibody-antigen reaction that has taken place at sites where meningococcal polysaccharide antigen was deposited during the acute phase of the illness. Serum levels of immune complexes are not markedly

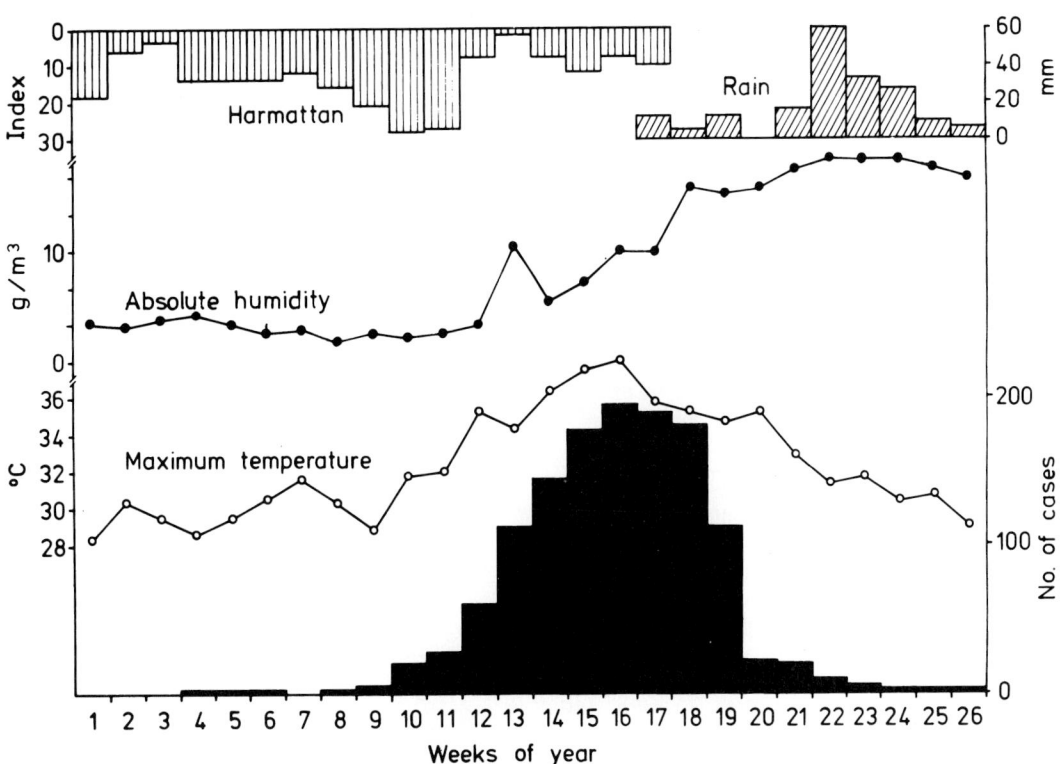

Figure 74–2. Relationship of an epidemic of meningococcal meningitis in northern Nigeria to seasonal climatic changes. The harmattan is a dry, dusty wind that blows from the Sahara. (From Greenwood BM, et al.: Trans R Soc Trop Med Hyg 73:557, 1979.)

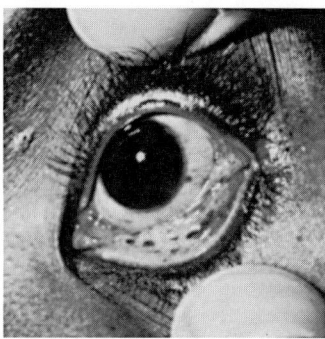

Figure 74–3. Conjunctival petechiae in a patient with meningococcal meningitis. (Photograph kindly provided by Professor D. A. Warrell.)

elevated in patients with meningococcal disease, and immune complex–mediated renal disease is seen rarely.

CLINICAL MANIFESTATIONS

Acute Meningococcemia

Symptoms. Acute meningococcemia can strike with frightening rapidity—a patient may be well at breakfast time but dead by the same afternoon. The early clinical features of the condition—fever, headache, and general malaise—are indistinguishable from those of many other less serious infectious diseases. Diarrhea is sometimes an early feature of acute meningococcemia, and it may be severe enough to suggest a diagnosis of acute gastroenteritis.

Signs. Initial clinical examination may show no abnormalities apart from fever and tachycardia. A nonspecific maculopapular rash may be noted. The appearance of petechiae often is the first indication of the potentially serious nature of a patient's illness. Petechiae may be present in the conjunctivae and on the palate, a useful diagnostic sign in patients with dark skin (Fig. 74–3). Later, more extensive ecchymoses may appear. Cardiovascular signs may be present when a patient is first seen, but they frequently do not appear until a few hours after a patient has been admitted to the hospital. A third heart sound may be heard, and the electrocardiogram often appears abnormal, showing features of myocarditis. The blood pressure may be low, and it may continue to fall despite treatment. Patients with acute meningococcemia frequently are confused, and their level of consciousness may deteriorate progressively.

Laboratory Findings. Examination of the blood usually shows a polymorphonuclear neutrophilic leukocytosis, but a severely ill patient may be leukopenic. Thrombocytopenia is usually present, and some patients have abnormalities, such as a raised level of fibrin degradation products, suggesting disseminated intravascular coagulation. Blood culture is frequently positive, and meningococcal capsular polysaccharide antigen sometimes can be detected in the serum. By definition, patients with acute meningococcemia have clear cerebrospinal fluid (CSF), but there may be a slight increase in the CSF white cell count.

Early Complications. Disseminated intravascular coagulation can occur as an early complication of acute meningococcemia, and it can lead to severe and sometimes fatal hemorrhage. Severe pulmonary edema may occur during the first few days of illness, and some patients remain unconscious for a prolonged period, perhaps because of an associated encephalitis. Acute renal failure may develop in a patient who has been severely hypotensive.

Late Complications. At least 10% of patients who survive the early phase of acute meningococcemia develop late allergic complications. These include a monoarthritis or a polyarthritis, cutaneous vasculitis and ulceration, episcleritis, and pericarditis. Vasculitis can occasionally be severe, leading to extensive ulceration (Fig. 74–4) and gangrene of distal extremities. Amputation of a digit or even a limb may become necessary. Accumulation of pericardial fluid can give rise to tamponade.

Meningitis. Patients with meningococcal meningitis show the characteristic clinical and laboratory features of patients with acute bacterial meningitis described in Chapter 52. Special characteristics of meningitis caused by the meningococcus are the presence of petecchiae, which are encountered only rarely in other forms of acute bacterial meningitis, the occurrence of late allergic complications, and a favorable prognosis, although about 5% of survivors are left with some sensorineural hearing loss.

A few patients present with clinical features of both meningitis and acute meningococcemia, but this is unusual.

Other Clinical Syndromes. Meningococcal infection of the nasopharynx is usually asymptomatic but can sometimes give rise to mild upper respiratory tract symptoms. A proportion of patients with meningococcal meningitis report a history of a preceding upper respiratory tract infection, perhaps due to meningococcal infection or perhaps to an antecedent viral infection. Meningococci are occasionally isolated from patients with pneumonia, urethritis, cervicitis, proctitis, or conjunctivitis; these syndromes have no characteristic clinical features. Chronic meningococcemia is a rare condition associated with persistent septicemia. It is characterized by intermittent fever, rash, arthritis, and splenomegaly.

DIAGNOSIS

Acute Meningococcemia. The early clinical features of acute meningococcemia are indistinguishable from those of

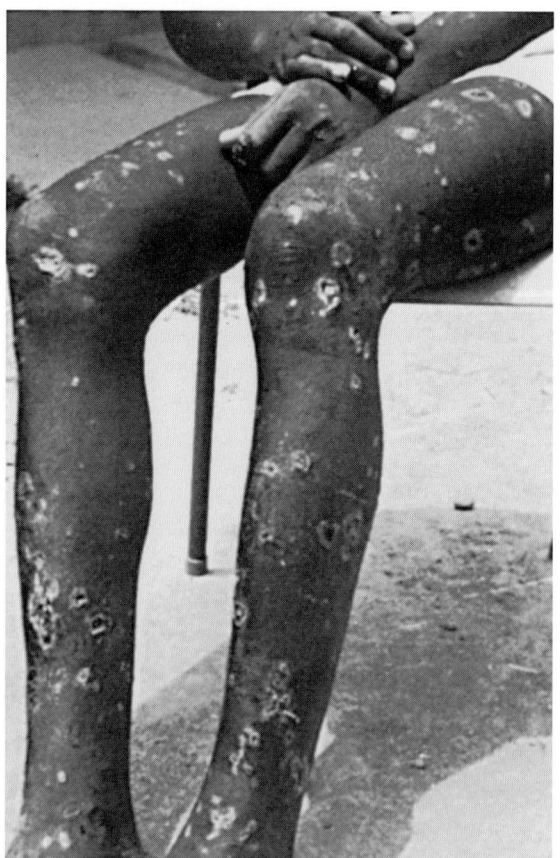

Figure 74–4. Cutaneous ulcerative skin lesions in a patient who had acute meningococcemia.

many other acute infections. Thus, clinical diagnosis is often impossible unless it is known that the patient has been in close contact with a case of meningococcal disease. The detection of petechiae in a febrile patient should suggest a possible diagnosis of acute meningococcemia, but many other organisms, for example rickettsial spotted fevers (Chapter 67), can cause a febrile illness associated with petechiae. A diagnosis of acute meningococcemia is confirmed by the detection of meningococcal antigen in the serum or by a positive blood culture. However, blood culture may be negative in patients who have received previous antibiotic therapy. Sensitive PCR techniques are being developed, and those may be especially useful in this group of patients. Meningococci can frequently be cultured from petecchiae. Meningococci in the nasopharynx are less sensitive to the action of systemically administered antibiotics than are bacteria in the blood. Thus, collection of a nasopharyngeal swab is a useful diagnostic test in a patient who has been started on treatment. If meningococcus is isolated from the nasopharynx of patients with clinical features of meningococcemia, it is likely that the strain of meningococcus obtained from the nasopharynx is the one responsible for their systemic illness.

Meningitis. The clinical and laboratory diagnosis of meningococcal meningitis is discussed in Chapter 52.

TREATMENT

Acute Meningococcemia

Supportive Therapy. A patient with acute meningococcemia should be treated in an intensive care unit whenever possible; assisted ventilation may be required. Fluid balance, acid-base status, and central venous pressure should be monitored whenever practicable. If a patient is hypotensive, infusion of plasma or dextran is required; 20 to 40 mg/kg should initially be given over 10 to 20 minutes. Further infusions may be required to maintain blood pressure, and because of the presence of a capillary leak, larger volumes of colloid may be required. Such large-volume infusions can precipitate pulmonary edema, and thus careful monitoring of the central venous pressure is required. To maintain peripheral perfusion, dopamine should be given in a dose of 2.5 to 5 µg/kg/min. If hypotension persists despite infusion of colloid and administration of dopamine, a further inotrope such as adrenaline 0.1 to 1.0 µg/kg/min can be given. Vasodilators, e.g., nitroglycerin, nitroprusside, and prostacyclin have been tried in resistant cases, but their role has not been established clearly.

The role of corticosteroids in the treatment of acute meningococcemia is uncertain. Because occasional patients with acute meningococcemia have low plasma cortisol levels, some physicians recommend that hydrocortisone or prednisone be given in conventional therapeutic doses to hypotensive patients with acute meningococcemia unless normal plasma cortisol levels can be demonstrated. Studies of animals have shown that corticosteroids have some prophylactic action against endotoxin shock but only when they are given in very large doses. Massive doses of methylprednisone (e.g., 1 or 2 g) have been given to patients with acute meningococcemia, but the value of this expensive form of therapy has not been clearly established.

Claims have been made that the lives of a number of patients with a poor prognosis have been saved by extracorporeal support, exchange transfusion, or by various forms of hemoperfusion. Because many of the clinical features of acute meningococcemia are probably due to endotoxin poisoning, this is a rational approach to therapy, but no controlled trials of this kind of treatment have been carried out. Such trials, which would probably need to be multicentered, are needed to allow the place of this expensive form of therapy to be established clearly. Administration of antiendotoxin antibod-

ies, anticytokine antibodies, or cytokine inhibitors offers an alternative approach to filtration techniques. Trials of antiendotoxin antibodies in patients with septic shock have not been successful, and the value of this overall approach to the treatment of endotoxin shock has not been validated.

Antibiotics. Although isolates of meningococci with a reduced sensitivity to penicillin have been described in a number of countries, penicillin resistance has not yet become a clinical problem and penicillin is still the antibiotic of choice for the treatment of acute meningococcemia. It should be given by intravenous infusion in high doses (4 megaunits every 6 hours for an adult) during the critical phase of the illness. In survivors, this can be changed subsequently to intramuscular injections. Penicillin is usually given for 7 days, but this is probably an unnecessarily long course of treatment. It is now recommended by some authorities that an intravenous or intramuscular injection of penicillin be given by the primary health care physician at the first suspicion of a diagnosis of acute meningococcemia, if necessary before any investigations are done, because some evidence suggests that this practice reduces mortality. However, this approach has not been validated in a large controlled trial. Chloramphenicol is an effective alternative for patients who cannot be given penicillin for any reason. Penicillin does not reliably eradicate meningococci from the nasopharynx, and thus a case can be made for treating all patients with rifampicin before they leave the hospital, to protect their close contacts.

Meningitis. The standard method of treatment of meningococcal meningitis is with crystalline penicillin (Chapter 52). During an epidemic, it may be necessary to establish temporary treatment centers in schools and similar buildings and to recruit untrained staff to help with patient care. In these circumstances, a treatment schedule that relies on a limited number of injections is required. An oily suspension of chloramphenicol (Tifomycine) given in a single injection (3 g for an adult) has been shown to be safe and effective. A single injection of ceftriaxone is a possible alternative, but this antibiotic is expensive.

PROGNOSIS. The outcome of acute meningococcemia is variable. Occasional patients have only a mild illness characterized by fever, petechiae, and a positive blood culture. In the savanna region of Africa, such cases are most frequently encountered toward the end of an epidemic. Unfortunately, the outlook for most patients with acute meningococcemia is grave. Various prognostic scores based on clinical and laboratory features have been established to allow patients at high risk to be identified early in the course of their illness. This may be helpful if transfer to special treatment facilities is possible or if an experimental therapy, such as hemoperfusion, is being considered. Mortality is especially high among patients who have neurologic signs or hypotension at the time of presentation. Death may result from shock or hemorrhage during the early phase of the infection, or it may occur later as a result of pulmonary edema, renal failure, or residual neurologic damage.

In contrast to the poor prognosis for patients with acute meningococcemia, the outlook for patients with meningococcal meningitis is good. Most series indicate a mortality rate from this infection of <10%, even in communities with limited health facilities. Residual neurologic damage is unusual, with the exception of deafness. Bacterial meningitis is a major cause of deafness in many developing countries, and deafness can prove to be a severe disability in a young child in a developing country where supportive facilities for the deaf are limited.

PREVENTION. Overcrowding and poor living conditions favor the spread of infections transmitted by respiratory

DETERMINE SEROGROUP AND MICROBIAL SENSITIVITIES OF THE ORGANISM RESPONSIBLE FOR THE

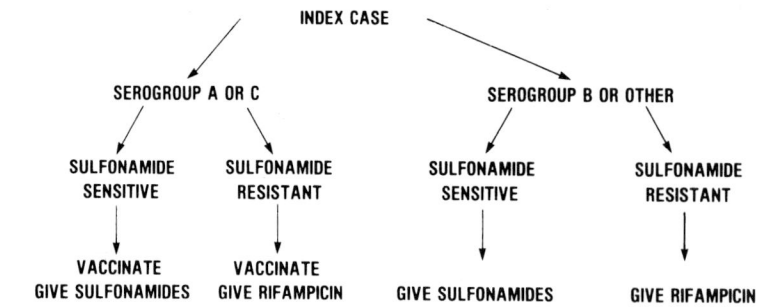

Figure **74–5.** Scheme for the management of close contacts of a patient with meningococcal disease.

Note: If the organism responsible for the outbreak cannot be identified, contacts should be vaccinated with A + C vaccine and given rifampicin.

droplets, and a general improvement in living standards has helped to reduce the incidence of meningococcal disease in industrialized countries during the past 50 years. During epidemics of meningococcal disease, a high attack rate may occur in residential institutions (e.g., boarding schools and military barracks), and it may be wise to close such institutions until the epidemic is over, although this carries the risk of disseminating the epidemic strain. It is doubtful whether other measures that have been adopted in the past, such as closure of markets and prevention of family gatherings, are of much value. Both chemoprophylaxis and vaccination have a role in the prevention of meningococcal disease. A scheme for the management of close contacts is shown in Figure 74–5.

Chemoprophylaxis. Chemoprophylaxis has been used widely in the past to control outbreaks of meningococcal infection in schools and barracks and to protect against infection of close household contacts of a patient. Sulfonamides, which are safe and inexpensive, eradicate sensitive strains of meningococci from the nasopharynx and thus interrupt transmission of the infection. Most strains of meningococci are now resistant to sulfonamides, however, and these drugs should no longer be used for prophylaxis unless it is known for certain that the outbreak strain is sensitive to this drug. Rifampicin is an alternative that is effective against sulfonamide-resistant meningococci, but the use of rifampicin for prophylaxis is usually followed by the rapid appearance of rifampicin-resistant strains of meningococci. Widespread use of rifampicin is not desirable in areas where tuberculosis is prevalent. Thus, rifampicin prophylaxis may have a place in the control of a local outbreak but not during a large epidemic. Both ceftriaxone given by injection and ciprofloxacin given by mouth are effective at eliminating carriage, but these drugs are expensive. Dosages of antimicrobials used in the prophylaxis of meningococcal disease are shown in Table 74–2.

Vaccination. Vaccines based on group A, C, Y, and W139 meningococcal polysaccharides have been available for a number of years, and groups A and C vaccines have been used extensively. These vaccines are very safe and relatively cheap. However, because they act as T-independent antigens, they induce little immunologic memory and are poorly immunogenic in the very young. Antibody levels decline rapidly after vaccination with polysaccharide vaccines in young children, and in children, clinical protection is probably lost 3 or 4 years after vaccination. For this reason, meningococcal polysaccharide/protein conjugate vaccines are being developed, and these should be much more immunogenic in young infants and should provide immunologic memory. Promising results have been obtained in pilot trials with the

first generation of groups A and C meningococcal conjugate vaccines (Fig. 74–6), but they have not yet been tested in efficacy trials.

It has not been possible to develop a vaccine based on the capsular polysaccharide of the group B meningococcus, because this antigen is poorly immunogenic in humans, perhaps because of a cross-reaction with human antigens. Thus, different strategies are being explored, and two group B vaccines, based on outer membrane proteins, have been developed in Norway and in Cuba, respectively. Both vaccines have given around 50% protection against group B meningococcal disease in clinical trials undertaken in Norway and in South America. Attempts are being made to develop more effective protein vaccines.

Because close contacts of a patient with meningococcal disease are at increased risk of infection, they should be vaccinated as soon as possible with a polysaccharide vaccine if the isolate that caused the initial case belonged to serogroup A or C or is unidentified. Because the risk to contacts is highest during the first few days after presentation of the index case, maximum protection is obtained if vaccination is combined with chemoprophylaxis.

Several studies have shown that groups A and C polysaccharide vaccines can be very effective at stopping epidemics. However, to achieve their maximum potential, they must be given as soon as possible after the outbreak has started; these vaccines frequently have been used too late, when the majority of susceptible persons had already been infected and the epidemic was already on the decline. Determining when an epidemic is imminent is not easy, but some guidelines have been developed for the countries of the African

TABLE 74–2. Recommended Dosages of Antimicrobials Used for the Chemoprophylaxis of Meningococcal Disease

	Sulfadiazine	Rifampicin	Ceftriaxone	Ciprofloxacin
Dose				
Adults	1 g	600 mg	250 mg	500 mg
Children 1–12 yr	500 mg	10 mg / kg	125 mg	250 mg
Infants <1 yr	125 mg	5 mg / kg	5 mg / kg	7.5 mg / kg
Route	PO	PO	IM	PO
Duration of Treatment	b.i.d. for 2 days	b.i.d. for 2 days	Single dose	Single dose

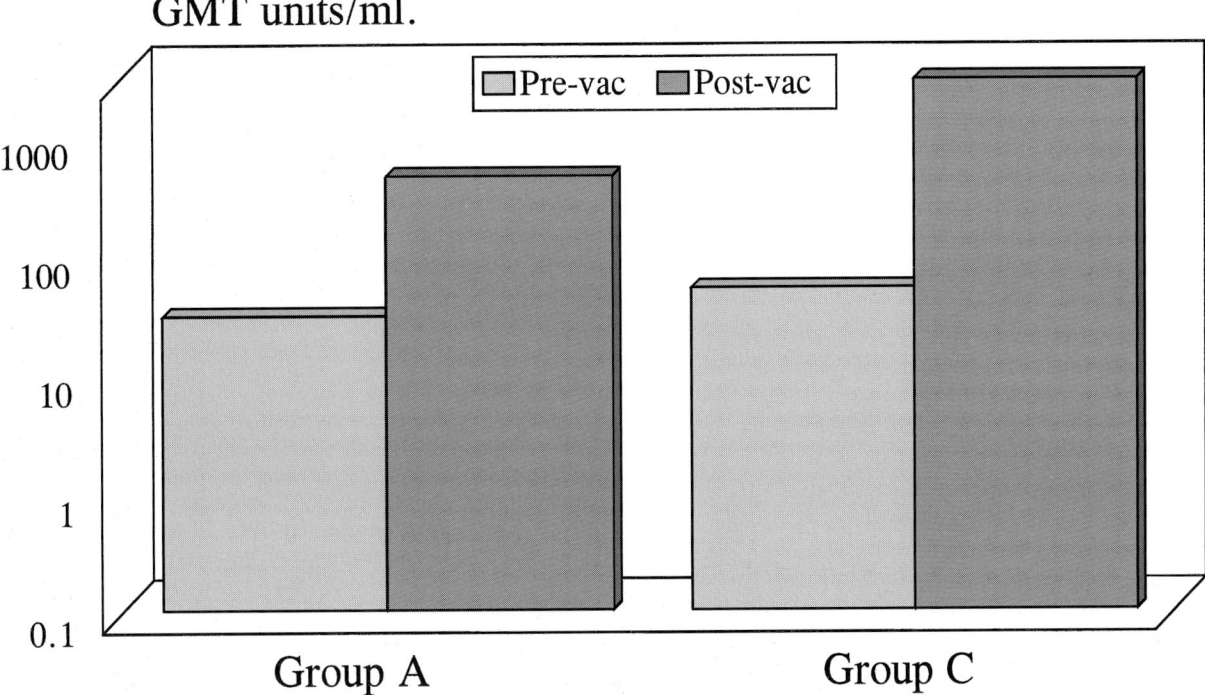

Figure 74–6. Geometric mean group A and group C meningococcal antibody titers, as measured by EIA, in African children immunized with a group A plus group C meningococcal polysaccharide CRM$_{197}$ protein conjugate vaccine at the ages of 2, 3, and 4 months. (From Twumasi PA Jr, et al: J Infect Dis 171:632, 1995.)

meningitis belt. Analysis of data collected in Burkina Faso has indicated that an outbreak is likely when the incidence rate exceeds 15 cases per 100,000 population per week averaged over a period of 2 weeks. Guidelines on the management of epidemics of meningococcal disease have recently been published by the World Health Organization.

Although meningococcal polysaccharide vaccines are effective at stopping epidemics of meningococcal infection, they do not provide a long-term solution to the problem of meningococcal diseases in areas where epidemics are frequent. It has been suggested that children living in the African meningitis belt should be given four doses of group A polysaccharide antibody during the first 5 years to maintain protective antibody levels. However, a more effective control strategy for such areas may prove to be the introduction of conjugate vaccines into routine infant immunization programs, supplemented with booster immunization at school age if this proves to be necessary.

Bibliography

Gardlund B, Sjolin J, Nilsson A, et al: Plasma levels of cytokines in primary septic shock in humans: Correlation with disease severity. J Infect Dis 172:296, 1995.

Gedde-Dahl TW, Bjark P, Høiby EA, et al: Severity of meningococcal disease: Assessment by factors and scores and implications for patient management. Rev Infect Dis 12:973, 1990.

Greenwood BM, Greenwood AM, Bradley AK, et al: Factors influencing susceptibility to meningococcal disease during an epidemic in the Gambia, West Africa. J Infect Dis 14:167, 1987.

Lapeyssonnie L: La meningite cérébrospinale en Afrique. Bull WHO 28(Suppl 3):3, 1963.

Moore PS, Plikaytis BD, Bolan GA, et al: Detection of meningitis epidemics in Africa: A population-based analysis. Int J Epidemiol 21:155, 1992.

Olyhoek T, Crowe BA, Achtman M: The clonal population structure of Neisseria meningitidis serogroup A isolated from epidemics and pandemics between 1915 and 1983. Rev Infect Dis 9:665, 1987.

Reingold AL, Broome CV, Hightower AW, et al: Age-specific differences in duration of clinical protection after vaccination with meningococcal polysaccharide A vaccine. Lancet 2:114, 1985.

Rey M: Treatment of purulent meningitis in developing countries. In Williams JD, Burnie J (eds): Bacterial Meningitis. London, Academic Press, 1987, p 211.

Robbins JB, Towne DW, Gotschlich EC, Schneerson R: "Love's labours lost": Failure to implement mass vaccination against group A meningococcal meningitis in sub-Saharan Africa. Lancet 350:880, 1997.

Twumasi PA, Kumah S, Leach A, et al: A trial of a group A plus group C meningococcal polysaccharide-protein conjugate vaccine in African infants. J Infect Dis 171:632, 1995.

Van Deuren M, van Dijke BJ, Koopman RJJ, et al: Rapid diagnosis of acute meningococcal infections by needle aspiration or biopsy of skin lesions. BMJ 306:1229, 1993.

Woods JP, Kersulyte D, Tolan RW Jr, et al: Use of arbitrarily primed polymerase chain reaction analysis to type disease and carrier strains of Neisseria meningitidis isolated during a university outbreak. J Infect Dis 169:1384, 1994.

World Health Organization: Control of Epidemic Meningococcal Disease: WHO Practical Guidelines. Geneva, World Health Organization, 1995.

75 Typhoid Fever*

Thong P. Lee and Stephen L. Hoffman

DEFINITION. Typhoid fever is an acute systemic illness caused by infection with *Salmonella typhi*. It is characterized by (1) prolonged fever, (2) sustained bacteremia without endothelial or endocardial involvement, and (3) bacterial invasion of and multiplication within the mononuclear phagocytic cells of the liver, spleen, lymph nodes, and Peyer's patches. Paratyphoid fever is a pathologically and clinically similar but generally milder illness that is caused by many serotypes of the species *Salmonella*, most commonly *Salmonella* serotype *paratyphi* A, serotype *schottmuelleri*, and sero-

---

*All the material in this chapter is in the public domain, with the exception of any borrowed figures or tables.

TABLE 75–1. Biochemical Differences Between *S. typhi*, *S. paratyphi A*, and *S. schottmuelleri*

	S. typhi	*S. paratyphi A*	*S. schottmuelleri*
Acid from glucose	+	+	+
Gas from glucose	−	+ (trace)	+
Hydrogen sulfide production	+ (trace −5%)	− (10% late +)	+
Citrate utilization	+	− (25% late +)	+
Lysine decarboxylase	+	−	+
Ornithine decarboxylase	−	+	+

type *hirschfeldii* (Chapter 76). *Enteric fever* refers to either typhoid or paratyphoid fever.

HISTORY. Although Hippocrates may have written about typhoid fever, it was not until the early 19th century that French workers described the clinical and pathologic features of the "dothoienenterite" (boil of the intestine) that was endemic in Paris. In 1829, Pierre Louis first called it typhoid, meaning "typhus-like," but he did not distinguish between the typhoid of Paris and typhus that was then common in Great Britain. Thus, both typhoid and typhus take their names from the Greek *typhos*, which means "smoke" and refers to the apathy and confusion associated with fever that are such prominent features of the fully developed clinical syndromes and also to the belief that the diseases had their origin in miasmic vapors. In 1837, William Wood Gerhard, a former student of Louis's working in Philadelphia, clearly differentiated typhoid from typhus fever, both clinically and pathologically. He wrote:

> The anatomical characters of these varieties of fevers are peculiar to themselves and it is (as) impossible to substitute the lesion of the follicles of the small intestine observed in typhoid fever from (for) the pathological phenomena of typhus as it is by other treatment or means to transform the eruption of measles into the pustules of smallpox.

In 1880, Eberth described *Bacillus typhosus* in histologic sections of mesenteric lymph nodes and the spleen. Four years later, Gaffky successfully cultured *S. typhi* and stressed that the infection was waterborne and not airborne. In 1896, Achard and Bensaude isolated *S. paratyphi* B and first used the term *paratyphoid fever*. In the same year, Widal described the Widal reaction and Wright from England and Pfeiffer from Germany introduced the first vaccination against typhoid.

Until 1948 there were no other major advances in typhoid research. Modifications of the first inactivated whole-cell vaccines were used for prevention, the Widal test and culture were used for diagnosis, and patient management was supportive, the outcome being highly dependent on the quality of nursing care. In 1948, Woodward and colleagues, who were working in Malaysia to determine whether chloramphenicol was effective for treating typhus, found that one of their patients suspected of having typhus had typhoid fever and that chloramphenicol rapidly cleared the bacteremia and markedly shortened the duration of the illness. Since then, chloramphenicol has been the antimicrobial agent of choice for treating both typhoid and paratyphoid fever. In the 1970s and 1980s, live oral attenuated and Vi capsular polysaccharide *S. typhi* vaccines were developed and shown to be effective in large field trials. By the mid-1990s, these vaccines replaced whole-cell vaccines in adults and children older than 2 years. In addition, in the 1990s, multidrug-resistant *S. typhi* has become endemic in many developing countries and is being increasingly reported from the developed world.

ETIOLOGY

Taxonomy and Classification. *Salmonella* is the most complex genus in the family Enterobacteriaceae, with more than 2200 serotypes previously described in the Kauffman-White schema. Salmonellae were previously classified as having three distinct species, *S. choleraesuis*, *S. typhi*, and *S. enteritidis*. Most of the described serotypes belonged to the species *S. enteritidis*. *Salmonella* was further grouped (A, B, C, and so on) on the basis of somatic O antigen and further divided into serotypes (1, 2, 3, and so on) on the basis of flagellar H antigens.

Based on DNA studies, in 1983, all *Salmonella* and *Arizona* isolates are now considered to be a single species, separated into seven distinct subgroups, I, II, IIIa, IIIb, and IV–VI. Subgroup I contains most of the *Salmonella* serotypes responsible for human diseases. Based on this new schema, all isolates should correctly be reported as, for example, *Salmonella* serotype *typhi*. However, because of wide clinical use and familiarity, it is still appropriate to address them as, for example, *Salmonella typhi*, as long as it is understood that these organisms are a serotype of the species *Salmonella* and not a distinct species.

All salmonellae grow on simple media; however, specimens are usually cultured on a selective medium, e.g., *Salmonella-Shigella* agar, to avoid the overgrowth of salmonellae by other enteric bacteria. The various salmonellae are differentiated on the basis of biochemical reactions and by serologic reaction—i.e., agglutination patterns with O, H, and Vi homologous antisera. The biochemical differences between *S. typhi*, *S. paratyphi* A, and *S. schottmuelleri* (paratyphi B) are summarized in Table 75–1. Serologic classification using the Kauffman-White agglutination schema of antigenic analysis is summarized in Table 75–2. Among the salmonellae, only *S. typhi* and *S. hirschfeldii* (paratyphi C) have the important K antigen called the *Vi antigen*. Vi stands for virulence, and *S. typhi* microorganisms with this antigen are thought to be more virulent than those without, possibly because the envelope protects the somatic O antigen from bactericidal antibody (Fig. 75–1).

Typhoid Fever. *S. typhi*, the etiologic organism, is similar to other salmonellae in that it is a gram-negative, flagellated, nonencapsulated, nonsporulating, facultative anaerobic bacillus. It ferments glucose; reduces nitrate to nitrite; synthesizes peritrichous flagellae when motile; has a somatic (O) antigen (oligosaccharide), a flagellar (H) antigen (protein), and an

TABLE 75–2. Antigenic Analysis by the Kauffman-White Schema of the Organisms Causing Typhoid and Paratyphoid Fever

	O Antigen Group	O Antigens	H Antigens Phase I	H Antigens Phase 2	K Antigens
S. paratyphi A	A	1, 2, 12	a		—
S. schottmuelleri	B	1, 4, 5, 12	b	1, 2	—
S. hirschfeldii	C	6, 7	c	1, 5	Vi
S. typhi	D	9, 12	d		Vi

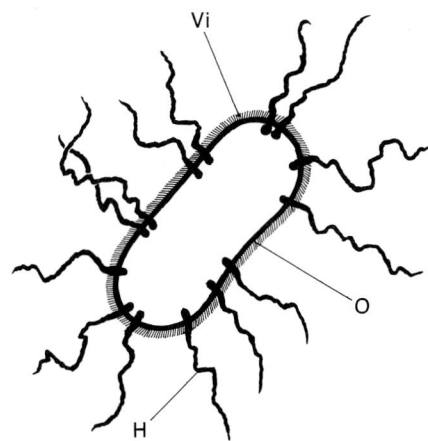

Figure 75–1. A schematic diagram of a single *Salmonella typhi* cell showing the locations of the H (flagellar), O (somatic), and Vi (K-envelope) antigens. (From Thomason BM, et al: J Bacteriol 74:525, 1957.)

envelope (K) antigen (polysaccharide); and has a lipopolysaccharide macromolecular complex called *endotoxin* that forms the outer portion of the cell wall (Fig. 75–1). The endotoxin is composed of three layers: outer (O-oligosaccharide), middle (R-core), and basal (lipid A). *S. typhi* is also capable of developing R-plasmid–transmitted antimicrobial resistance.

Paratyphoid Fever. Paratyphoid fever is caused by organisms of the formerly designated species *S. enteritidis*. The bacteria that most frequently cause paratyphoid fever are *Salmonella* serotype *paratyphi* A, *Salmonella* serotype *paratyphi* B, and *Salmonella* serotype *paratyphi* C, but they are commonly referred to as *S. paratyphi* A, *S. schottmuelleri*, and *S. hirschfeldii*, respectively (Chapter 76).

DISTRIBUTION AND INCIDENCE. Patients with typhoid fever are encountered in all parts of the world but are now primarily found in those countries where sanitary conditions are poor. In the Spanish-American War, one fifth of the United States troops had typhoid fever, with 1500 deaths. In the South African Boer Wars, the British Army lost more men to typhoid (8225 deaths) than it did to wounds (7582 deaths). When Sir William Osler published his first textbook of medicine in 1892, the first chapter was on typhoid, and in 1909 Osler estimated that there were 500,000 cases per year in the United States, with 35,000 to 40,000 deaths caused by typhoid. In 1988 there were 436 cases of typhoid fever in the United States, most commonly in travelers to Mexico and the Indian subcontinent. The yearly incidence of typhoid fever remained constant during the next 6 years, with 441 cases reported to the Centers for Disease Control (CDC) in 1994. There has been an equally dramatic decrease in the annual incidence of reported typhoid in most European countries.

Although not a major problem in the developed world, typhoid is considered by many to be one of the most important and underreported diseases in the developing world. The underreporting is due to the fact that a positive blood culture is often required for diagnosis, and many patients with typhoid are treated where there are no bacteriology facilities. However, studies in Chile, Nepal, South Africa, and Indonesia have documented annual blood culture–positive attack rates ranging from approximately 100/100,000 per year (Chile) to more than 1000/100,000 population per year (Indonesia). It has been estimated that the worldwide incidence (excluding China) of typhoid fever is approximately 12,500,000/year, with greater than 62% of cases occurring in Asia and 35% in Africa. In some areas, it has been estimated that typhoid fever is responsible for 2 to 5% of all deaths.

Hospital case-fatality rates for typhoid fever are still high (1 to 30%) in many parts of the developing world. Because typhoid frequently kills young adults, many of whom have recently finished school, entered the work force, and become parents, its economic and social impact on the family and society is often dramatic.

EPIDEMIOLOGY

Source of Infection. *S. typhi*, *S. paratyphi* A, and *S. schottmuelleri* infect only humans. Thus, all cases of typhoid fever and most cases of paratyphoid fever could theoretically be traced back to another infected human. The stool and, less commonly, the urine of carriers and those with or recovering from acute infections are the source of the organism. It is generally believed that 1 to 4% of patients with acute typhoid fever become carriers, but this rate is a function of the age and health of the patient. The carrier rate is higher in women and increases with increasing age and prevalence of gallbladder disease. Fecal carriers usually outnumber urinary carriers 10 to 1, but in areas endemic for *Schistosoma haematobium*, urinary carriers are often more common. The carrier rate within communities varies considerably.

Method of Transmission. The infection is most commonly acquired by ingestion of contaminated food or water but may rarely be transmitted by direct finger-to-mouth contact with the feces, urine, respiratory secretions, vomitus, or pus from an infected individual. The stools of chronic carriers usually contain from 10^6 to 10^9 organisms/g. *S. typhi* can survive for several weeks in water, ice, dust, or dried sewage and on clothing but survives in raw sewage for less than a week. It can also survive and multiply in milk or milk products without altering the appearance of the milk.

Food can be infected directly by water used to wash it or prepare it, by carriers, by fomites and dust, and probably by flies. In many cases, the initial concentration of organisms is too low to cause human disease, but under optimal environmental conditions the organisms can multiply in food. In the case of shellfish, e.g., oysters and mussels, the polluted water in which they live may not have a high enough concentration of organisms to cause disease in a swimmer who ingests small amounts of water. However, because shellfish filter up to 50 gallons of water per day and concentrate the microbial content, aficionados of raw shellfish from polluted water may be presented with an enormous dose of *S. typhi*.

Factors That Influence Infectivity. Studies of human volunteers using the Quailes strain of *S. typhi* showed that in healthy, previously unvaccinated male adults, ingestion of 10^5 organisms led to clinical disease in 25% of volunteers (ID_{25}); ingestion of 10^7 organisms caused disease in 50% (ID_{50}); and 10^9 organisms caused disease in 95% (ID_{95}). As the number of organisms increased, the incubation period decreased but the clinical syndrome was unchanged. Nothing is known about the relationship between differences in strains of *S. typhi* and infectivity except that strains that do not have Vi antigen are less infective and less virulent. A gastric pH less than 2 kills most of the organisms; those patients who chronically ingest antacids, have had a gastrectomy, or have achlorhydria due to aging or other reasons require lower numbers of organisms to produce clinical disease. Parenteral vaccination confers a fairly strong immunity, which may be overcome by increasing the infecting dose.

Patterns of Disease in the Community

Developed Countries. In industrialized nations with good sewage and water supply systems, most cases of typhoid fever are sporadic and either are imported or can be traced to contact with a chronic carrier. Intermittent epidemics are generally attributed to a common source exposure. In 1964, in Aberdeen, Scotland, 507 cases of typhoid fever were traced to ingestion of canned corned beef from Argentina. The leaky cans had been cooled in sewage-contaminated river water after canning. In 1973, there were 225 cases of typhoid fever in a migrant farm labor camp in Dade County, Florida. The laborers were infected by drinking from the camp water supply system, which had a defective chlorinator and probably had been contaminated by a mentally retarded girl who acquired the infection from a chronic carrier who lived next door to her. In 1981, 76 cases of typhoid fever occurred in San Antonio, Texas. They were traced to a tortilla shop where one employee had *S. typhi* in his stool. In 1986, 10 cases of typhoid fever were acquired in a fast-food restaurant in Silver Spring, Maryland. They were traced to a shrimp salad prepared by an 18-year-old asymptomatic carrier who worked in the restaurant.

Developing World. Epidemics also occur in the tropics and subtropics, but the majority of cases are reported in areas where typhoid fever is endemic. In these locations there are so many sick or recovering individuals that chronic carriers are less important in transmission than they are in the industrialized world. The incidence is frequently seasonal, with a peak in the hot, dry months of the year, when the concentration of organisms in water is increased—not diluted by rains. In some areas, the incidence is reported to peak during the rainy season, when flooding apparently breaks down the systems that separate sewage from drinking water.

In areas where typhoid fever is endemic, it is likely that more than 95% of patients are treated as outpatients by local physicians. Thus, hospital-based incidence figures may underestimate actual incidence by 15 to 25 times. In most areas of the developing world, the reported incidence of typhoid fever is at least two to three times that of paratyphoid fever, except during epidemics and in infants.

Age. The age-specific attack rates of typhoid fever must reflect exposure to the organism and the development of a protective immune response. In endemic areas, children between the ages of 1 and 5 years are at highest risk owing to waning passively acquired maternal antibody and lack of acquired immunity. Osler observed that typhoid fever was primarily a disease of late adolescence and early adulthood, and most current data derived from studies of hospitalized patients in the developing world support this observation. In more recent years, however, prospective studies of outpatients in endemic areas have shown that even where the incidence in inpatients is highest in adolescents and young adults, the overall incidence of blood culture–confirmed disease is generally highest in children age 3 to 9 years, declining significantly in late adolescence. The difference between hospital-based and outpatient studies may reflect the fact that older adolescents and young adults become more ill with *S. typhi* infection and require hospitalization more often than do children. Infants and children can certainly develop life-threatening typhoid fever, although the case-fatality rates for hospitalized children are generally lower than for adults.

Multidrug-Resistant Typhoid Fever (MDRTF) and S. typhi (MDRST). MDRST is epidemiologically defined as strains resistant to any two antibiotics in vitro, even if the antibiotics tested are known to be effective clinically (e.g., aminoglycosides, tetracycline, furazolidine). A more useful definition of MDRST should be reserved for strains resistant to all three first-line antibiotics, chloramphenicol, ampicillin, and trimethoprim-sulfamethoxazole.

S. typhi resistant to chloramphenicol was first reported in England in 1950, 2 years after this antibiotic was first successfully used in the treatment of typhoid fever. Outbreaks of chloramphenicol-resistant *S. typhi* occurred with increasing incidence in the developing world from the early 1970s to the mid-1980s. Since the late 1980s, outbreaks of MDRTF have been increasingly reported. MDRTF is now endemic in Southeast Asia, Africa, Latin America, China, and especially the Indian subcontinent. Incidence of MDRST strains reported in the Indian subcontinent and China currently ranges from 50 to 80% of all *S. typhi* isolates and approaches 100% during outbreaks.

Children with MDRTF are sicker and more toxic at admission, with a significantly higher incidence of life-threatening complications. Overall mortality for MDRTF is 7 to 16%, much higher than the 1 to 2% mortality common for susceptible typhoid fever. This finding is most likely due to delay in institution of effective antibiotics and not due to increased virulence in the MDRST strains.

PATHOGENESIS AND PATHOLOGY. The hallmark of the syndrome is bacterial invasion of and multiplication within the mononuclear phagocytic cells in the liver, spleen, lymph nodes, and Peyer's patches of the ileum. Our knowledge of the sequence of events following ingestion of an infective dose of *S. typhi* is derived from studies of human volunteers and chimpanzees experimentally infected with *S. typhi* and of mice infected with *S. enteritidis* and *S. typhimurium*. However, this information is incomplete, and the theories of pathogenesis are not well substantiated. For example, there is still no well-documented explanation for the pathogenesis of the mental confusion and other central nervous system (CNS) manifestations.

Proposed Sequence of Events

Mucosal Penetration. After ingestion, the organisms pass through the upper gastrointestinal tract to the small intestine, where they attach preferentially to the tips of the villi and either invade directly or multiply for several days before invading. Because fewer than 5% of the villi are involved, it is hypothesized that there are specific receptor sites on the villi, but these receptors have not been identified. Stool cultures are positive for several days after *S. typhi* ingestion and then become negative until after the onset of clinical illness. Studies of human volunteers have shown that invasion can take place in the jejunum, and animal studies suggest that it occurs in the ileum. The M cells, epithelial cells that overlie the Peyer's patches, are the potential sites where *S. typhi* are internalized and transported to the underlying lymphoid tissues. After penetration, the organisms pass to the intestinal lymphoid follicles and the draining mesenteric lymph nodes; some also pass into the systemic circulation, where they are filtered out by the reticuloendothelial cells of the liver and spleen. The salmonellae are able to prevent acidification of the phagosomes, survive, and multiply within the mononuclear phagocytic cells of the lymphoid follicles, lymph nodes, liver, and spleen. At this stage, subtle degenerative, proliferative, and granulomatous changes occur in the villi, crypt glands, and lamina propria of the small bowel and in the mesenteric lymph glands. These changes are reversible and unassociated with clinical symptoms.

Dissemination and Organ Invasion. At a critical point (which is probably a function of numbers of bacteria, bacterial virulence, and the host's immune response), a sufficient number of organisms and possibly other mediators that induce clinical symptoms are released from this sequestered intracellular habitat in the intestinal and mesenteric lymph system and pass through the thoracic duct and into the general circulation. This marks the end of the incubation period, which may last from 3 to 60 days but is usually 7 to 14 days.

During this bacteremic phase, the organisms may invade any organ but are most commonly found in the liver, spleen, bone marrow, gallbladder, and Peyer's patches in the terminal ileum. They invade the gallbladder either directly from the blood stream or from the bile and then reappear in the

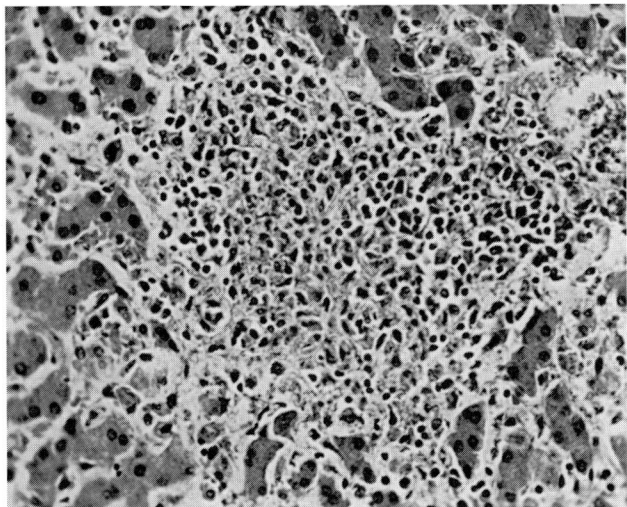

Figure 75–2. A typhoid nodule in the liver during the stage of active invasion. This lesion is principally composed of macrophages *(center)* with variable numbers of lymphocytes and plasma cells (periphery). (× 305.) (Courtesy of the Armed Forces Institute of Pathology. Photograph Neg. No. 72-4603.)

intestine, where they are excreted in the stool and reinvade through the intestinal wall. At most tissue sites, the organisms are again taken up by the mononuclear phagocytic cells, where they multiply.

Pathology. The basic histologic finding in typhoid fever is infiltration of tissues by macrophages (typhoid cells) containing bacteria, erythrocytes, and degenerated lymphocytes. Aggregates of these macrophages are called *typhoid nodules* (Fig. 75–2). They are most commonly found in the intestine, mesenteric lymph nodes, spleen, liver, and bone marrow but may be found in the kidneys, testes, and parotid glands.

Intestine. In the intestine there are four classic pathologic stages. *Hyperplastic* changes begin during the first week of illness and primarily involve Peyer's patches of the ileum and solitary lymphoid follicles of the cecum but may involve any lymphoid tissue in the intestine. Almost all infiltrative cells are mononuclear; typhoid nodules are common. If the hyperplasia does not resolve, *necrosis* of the intestinal mucosa develops, usually after 7 to 10 days of clinical illness (Fig. 75–3). Sloughing of the mucosa follows and results in the development of an *ulcer* that may bleed. The ulcers conform

in shape and distribution to the location of the lymphoid follicles, are largest in the ileum, and are almost always found on the antimesenteric border of the intestines. These ulcers may perforate into the peritoneal cavity. Perforations are single and measure less than 1 cm in 80% of cases; 90% are found within 60 cm of the ileocecal valve. When healing takes place, it is usually complete, without scarring.

Mesenteric Lymph Nodes, Spleen, and Liver. In the mesenteric lymph nodes, the sinusoids are enlarged and distended by large collections of macrophages and reticuloendothelial cells. The nodes become soft and swollen and often contain areas of focal necrosis. The spleen is enlarged, red, soft, and congested. Its serosal surface may have a fibrinous exudate. Microscopically, the red pulp is congested and contains typhoid nodules. The liver is usually enlarged. Hypertrophy and hyperplasia of the Kupffer cells produce the typhoid nodules. Frequently observed are focal hepatic necrosis and cloudy swelling of hepatocytes. The gallbladder usually is slightly hyperemic and may, in rare instances, show evidence of cholecystitis.

Other Organs. These are less frequently involved during typhoid fever and usually have lesions attributed to toxic factors. The heart may be flabby and have dilated ventricles, and often seen microscopically is a nonspecific pattern of necrosis with degeneration and fatty infiltration of the myocardial cells. The lungs show interstitial pneumonitis and bronchitis, and skeletal muscles may show Zenker's degeneration. The most common lesion found in the kidneys is swelling and albuminous degeneration of the proximal tubular epithelium, but interstitial nephritis, glomerulonephritis, and pyelonephritis have been noted. CNS changes have been poorly described, but ring hemorrhages, capillary thrombi, perivenous demyelinating leukoencephalitis, and meningitis have been reported. Focal lesions such as osteomyelitis, brain abscess, and spleen and liver abscesses have occasionally been reported. These lesions are almost always characterized by polymorphonuclear instead of mononuclear response. Salmonellae stimulate phagocytosis of neutrophils, red blood cells, and platelets by histiocytes within the bone marrow stroma. This may be the mechanism behind the pancytopenia commonly noted in typhoid fever.

Pathogenesis of Organ Dysfunction and Toxemia. A hypothesis for the pathogenesis of typhoid fever must explain (1) the inflammatory and necrotic changes at the sites of multiplication of the organism in the intestine, liver, spleen, and lymph nodes; (2) the prolonged pyrexia and toxemia; and (3) the pathologic changes and functional derangements

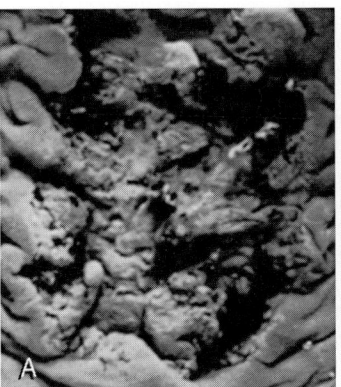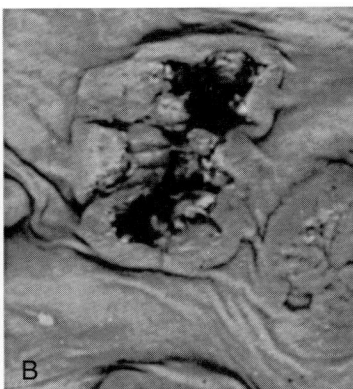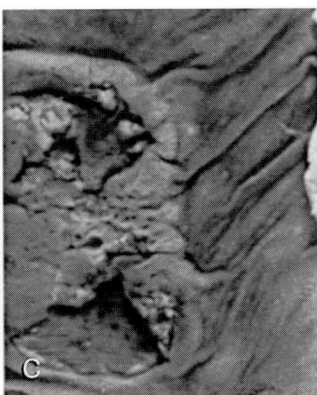

Figure 75–3. Peyer's patches in the ileum showing several stages in a single specimen. *A,* Active ulceration. *B,* Necrosis. *C,* The sloughing of necrotic tissue has left the muscularis bare. (Courtesy of the Armed Forces Institute of Pathology, Photograph Neg. No. 64-3208-2.)

in organs such as the heart, lungs, brain, and kidneys, where typhoid nodules and *S. typhi* are generally not found.

Until the 1970s, most authorities thought that the necrotic changes in the intestine, liver, spleen, and lymph nodes were the result of tissue hypoxia secondary to small vessel occlusion by typhoid nodules and that the systemic manifestations and dysfunction of other organs were caused by circulating endotoxin. Evidence now shows that neither small vessel occlusion nor circulating endoxin has a major role in the pathogenesis of typhoid fever.

Endotoxin. The role of endotoxin in the pathogenesis of typhoid fever is unclear. Investigators at the University of Maryland showed that when *S. typhi* endotoxin was initially injected into human volunteers, it produced chills, fever, headaches, myalgias, anorexia, nausea, thrombocytopenia, and leukopenia, as in typhoid fever. After these volunteers had received repeated injections of endotoxin, they became unresponsive (tolerant) to it, but when the tolerant individuals were challenged with *S. typhi,* they developed classic typhoid fever. Because typhoid fever is an unrelenting, sustained illness when not treated with antibiotics, the fact that the volunteers developed tolerance to endotoxin suggests that circulating endotoxin does not cause the symptoms and signs of naturally acquired typhoid fever. Furthermore, the facts that endotoxin-tolerant volunteers developed typhoid fever after rechallenge and that circulating endotoxin as detected by limulus assay is not present in many patients with typhoid make it even less likely that circulating endotoxin has a major role in the pathogenesis of the disease.

Immune Complexes and Other Immunologic Reactions. Several investigators have found circulating immune complexes in patients with typhoid fever, and others have noted immune complexes in renal biopsy specimens taken from typhoid-affected patients with glomerulonephritis and nephrotic syndrome. The significance of these complexes is unknown. Some investigators have hypothesized that some of the less common CNS manifestations of typhoid fever, e.g., Guillain-Barré syndrome, perivenous leukoencephalitis, and transverse myelitis, are due to an immune reaction.

Disseminated Intravascular Coagulation. Although several reports have described clinically classic disseminated intravascular coagulation (DIC) in patients with typhoid, this is a rare complication. On the other hand, research indicates that many patients with *S. typhi* infections have laboratory evidence of DIC without bleeding and may have localized DIC within organs.

Metabolic and Nutritional Factors. Various investigators have suggested that anemia, vitamin deficiencies, deficiencies of zinc and other trace metals, thyroid dysfunction, tryptophan metabolites, other amino acids, and the time of the day that infection occurs or treatment is initiated all are important in the pathogenesis of the disease and the host's ability to mobilize adequate defenses. Although it is likely that many of these may be important in determining the ultimate expression of the disease, it is unlikely that any of them is the major determinant of how the disease is expressed or how the host defends against the infection.

Proposed Pathogenesis. The unique feature of typhoid fever is the relationship between *S. typhi* and macrophages in the liver, spleen, intestinal lymphoid follicles, and mesenteric lymph nodes. Macrophages can produce an array of functionally active cytokines. These include tumor necrosis factor-α (TNF-α), interleukin-1 (IL-1), and interferon-α and β (IFN-α and -β). Macrophages are also an important source of arachidonate metabolites and reactive oxygen intermediates. These macrophage products can cause cellular necrosis, stimulation of the immune system, vascular instability, initiation of the clotting mechanism, bone marrow depression, fever,

and other abnormalities associated with typhoid fever. It is likely that *S. typhi* endotoxin stimulates the macrophages to release these substances, which locally mediate the intestinal and hepatocellular necrosis found in the disease and which, when released systemically, cause most of the other manifestations of the disease.

IMMUNOLOGIC RESPONSE. Typhoid fever induces both systemic and local humoral and cellular immune responses. Although many studies have described the immune responses associated with *S. typhi* infection and with immunization with typhoid vaccines, the roles of specific immune mechanisms in the development of resistance to reinfection with *S. typhi*, the pathogenesis of typhoid, and complete elimination of bacteria from infected individuals have not been clearly established. Some have suggested that infection with typhoid confers long-lasting immunity against reinfection, but the high incidence of typhoid fever in young adults in endemic areas and the results of volunteer studies indicate that this is not the case. Fifteen volunteers who had ingested 10^5 organisms and developed acute typhoid fever were rechallenged with 10^5 organisms (expected to cause infection in 25% of individuals) a mean of 20 months after the first infection. Five (33%) developed acute typhoid fever again. The fact that hospital-based studies indicate that the incidence of severe typhoid fever is higher in older adolescents and young adults than in young children suggests that an acquired immune response may have a role in the pathogenesis of severe disease. Relapse may reflect the inadequate development of an appropriate anti–*S. typhi* immune response.

Antibodies. *S. typhi*–specific secretory IgA in the small intestine may be important in determining whether mucosal penetration takes place. A study from India reported that patients with typhoid fever have lower levels of IgA in intestinal secretions than do control subjects. *S. typhi*–specific IgA has been demonstrated in the feces and intestinal fluid of volunteers immunized with the oral typhoid vaccine Ty21a.

Development of specific antibodies during typhoid fever has been well documented. Circulating IgG, IgM, and in some cases IgA, antibodies to *S. typhi* O, H, Vi, and porin antigens have been identified. Not all individuals with typhoid fever develop antibodies to these antigens. Fourfold titer rises to O, H, and Vi antigens were documented in 75%, 75%, and 40%, respectively, of volunteers experimentally infected with *S. typhi*. Immunization with the Vi antigen vaccine and the oral vaccine Ty21a induce IgG and IgA to Vi antigen and O antigen, respectively; immunization with the killed typhoid vaccines can induce antibodies to O, H, and Vi antigens. It has not been proved that these antibodies are responsible for the protective immunity found after administration of these vaccines. However, the developers of the Vi vaccine attribute the vaccine-induced protection to antibodies against Vi antigen. Interestingly, a study in Sweden showed that an O, H, and Vi antigen–free fraction of *S. typhi* induced serum antibodies in rabbits and that this serum protected chicken embryos against lethal doses of *S. typhi*. Research is beginning to determine the fine specificity of antigen-specific antibody responses.

Cellular Immune Responses. A major characteristic of typhoid fever is the activation of macrophages. Phagocytosis is a major host defense mechanism, and substances released from macrophages, including cytokines, reactive oxygen intermediates, and arachidonic acid metabolites, probably have a significant role in the pathogenesis of the disease. It has been proposed that the protective immunity induced by immunization with the oral typhoid vaccine Ty21a may be mediated by antibody-dependent cellular cytotoxicity involving IgA antibodies against *S. typhi* and CD4 + T cells, because volunteers immunized with Ty21a have been shown to develop this immune response.

CLINICAL MANIFESTATIONS. The clinical presentation of typhoid fever is variable, but nearly all patients have fever and most have a headache. The range of clinical manifestations and the severity of the illness vary, depending on the patient population. Clinicians who see outpatients in an endemic area of the developing world find that their patients with typhoid are moderately ill, that fewer than 10% require hospitalization, that complications are rare, and that the case-fatality rate is less than 1%. Hospital-based physicians in the same area see typhoid-affected patients who are much sicker and have a greater range of symptoms, signs, and complications; the case-fatality rate may approach 30%. If one sees patients with typhoid in the developed world, nearly all patients are hospitalized, but the clinical severity, complications, and case-fatality rates are comparable to those in outpatients in the developing world. In many cases, the most severely ill patients will have been sicker for longer periods than those who are moderately ill. The strain of *S. typhi*, the number of organisms ingested, the general and nutritional condition and immunologic status of the patient, and possibly the genetic makeup of the host may influence the clinical presentation.

Untreated Typhoid Fever. After ingestion of the organisms, 10 to 20% of patients have transient diarrhea. These patients, as well as all others, remain asymptomatic during the incubation period, which usually lasts 7 to 14 days but can be as short as 3 days and as long as 60 days, depending on the number of organisms ingested. As the stage of sustained bacteremia develops, the incubation period ends and the patient notices the onset of fever, which classically increases daily in a stepwise fashion but may be remittent or sustained. At this point, patients usually have a flulike syndrome with headache and malaise; frequently have a sore throat, anorexia, nausea, abdominal pain, and myalgias; but may have any of the symptoms listed in Table 75–3. By the end of the first week after the onset of symptoms, the fever is sustained and patients are often toxic and may have any of the symptoms and signs listed in Tables 75–3 and 75–4.

The fever remains sustained during the second week and by the third week begins to come down spontaneously by lysis. Intestinal perforation and/or hemorrhage can occur at any stage of the illness, but these findings classically occur during the third week. The illness can continue for several months, although by the end of the fourth week the temperature usually returns to normal, and except for individuals with metastatic foci in whom cholecystitis, osteomyelitis, and soft tissue abscesses may develop, most patients have recovered. It is at this stage that most relapses occur.

TABLE 75–3. Symptoms Expected on Admission in Hospitalized Typhoid Patients in Endemic Areas of the Developing World

Symptom	%	Symptom	%
Fever	99	Cough or chest discomfort	35
Weakness	99	Vomiting	35
Anorexia	85	Myalgia, arthralgia	35
Headache	85	Confusion	25
Dizziness	80	Sore throat	20
Abdominal pain	50	Decreased hearing	15
Nausea	50	Blood in stool or melena	12
Chills	50	Epistaxis	10
Diarrhea	45	Dysuria	2
Constipation	40	Seizures	2

TABLE 75–4. Physical Signs Expected on Admission in Hospitalized Typhoid Patients in Endemic Areas of the Developing World

Common		Less Common	
Sign	%	*Sign*	%
Fever	98	Disorientation	25
Coated tongue	95	Relative bradycardia	15
Apathy	70	Rales or rhonchi	15
Hepatomegaly	50	Delirium	15
Abdominal pain	45	Severely toxic	10
Rose spots	0–50	Decreased hearing	10
Moderately sick	45	Stiff neck	10
Toxic	45	Stupor	2
Splenomegaly	35	Focal neurologic findings	1

Clinical Course and Manifestations in Patients Who Receive Antimicrobials. Antimicrobials shorten the course, reduce the rate of complications if begun early, and reduce the case-fatality rate; though some antimicrobials may increase the relapse rate. During volunteer studies in Maryland, more than 400 patients with typhoid fever were treated within 3 days of the onset of fever, and the complication and case-fatality rates were 0.

Symptoms. The frequencies of symptoms expected in hospitalized patients in endemic areas are summarized in Table 75–3. Before hospitalization, most of these patients will have been ill for 6 to 12 days, most will have seen a health care provider at some point, and most will have received short courses of antibiotics, often with chloramphenicol. Fever is universal and, although present daily, is usually higher in the late afternoon and evening. Chills and dull frontal or diffuse headaches are common. The headaches often prevent patients from sleeping comfortably. Most patients are anorexic. They complain of abdominal pain but cannot localize it well. Both diarrhea and constipation are common; normal bowel function is unusual. Children frequently have diarrhea. Bloody dysentery is occasionally encountered. The incidence of cough and chest discomfort varies considerably. Sore throats are common during the first week of illness but less common later. Dysuria is more commonly encountered in parts of the world where *S. haematobium* is endemic. Epistaxis, which was a common finding in the preantibiotic era, occurs less frequently now. Seizures are occasionally reported, being more common in children younger than 5 years. If the family is interviewed, a history of intermittent confusion is frequently reported.

Signs. On physical examination, patients generally are moderately ill to toxic; however, 10 to 15% of patients are severely toxic and may be hyperpyrexic (Table 75–4). They lie apathetically immobile in bed, often staring blankly, but are arousable. About 10% of patients are severely agitated and 5% obtunded. Disorientation is common, as is frank delirium. Stupor and coma are infrequent. If patients are hypovolemic from blood loss or dehydration, hypotension or shock may be present. Characteristic gram-negative septic shock is uncommon on admission but does occur after intestinal perforation, in patients with severe typhoid fever without obvious perforation, and as a preterminal event. Relative bradycardia, once considered to be a classic finding in typhoid fever, is now encountered in fewer than 25% of patients. Rose spots, which are blanching, red maculopapular lesions measuring 2 to 4 mm, are most frequently found on the abdomen and chest but can be seen on the extremities and back. Rose spots are less frequently found in dark-skinned patients. The tongue is covered with a thick, furry, white-to-brown coating that spares the bright red tips and edges. The incidence of respiratory findings varies, but signs consistent with bronchitis (15%) are more common than those of lobar consolidation (1 to 8%).

The findings on abdominal examination are frequently difficult to interpret. In classic descriptions, the abdomen is said to be doughy, and the examiner easily palpates loops of bowel filled with air and fluid and finds diffuse lower quadrant tenderness. Diffuse abdominal pain with moderate guarding has often been described. It is frequently difficult for the examiner to be certain that perforation has not occurred. The spleen or liver is enlarged in 30 to 50% of patients, and although both organs can become quite large, they more commonly are moderately enlarged, with the liver palpable 2 or 3 cm below the right costal margin and the spleen palpable on deep inspiration or 1 or 2 cm below the left costal margin. Both organs are usually soft and moderately tender. Occult blood is found in the stool of 20 to 30% of patients.

Complications and Unusual Manifestations

Intestinal Perforation. Intestinal perforation occurs in about 3% of hospitalized patients. It usually occurs during the third week of illness but can happen during the first week. A patient with perforation has the usual symptoms of typhoid fever and complains of severe abdominal pain that often is localized to the right lower quandrant but may be diffuse. Bowel sounds are absent in 50% of cases. About 75% of patients have guarding, rebound tenderness, and rigidity, particularly in the right lower quadrant. Some patients have an absence of hepatic dullness because of free air in the abdomen, but a pneumoperitoneum is present on radiographs in only 50 to 70%. Perforation causes a marked sudden rise in pulse, fall in blood pressure, and onset of severe pain. In most patients, the diagnosis is not difficult. However, as noted earlier, approximately 25% do not have classic findings of peritonitis and perforation, and in these individuals it is difficult to decide whether they have perforation, impending perforation, or just severe typhoid abdominal pain. In the appropriate clinical setting, a rising white blood cell count with a shift to the left is suggestive of perforation but occurs in fewer than half of patients with perforation.

Intestinal Hemorrhage. Intestinal hemorrhage occurs in as many as 15% of cases. Patients may or may not be toxic. The bowel usually does not perforate, and bleeding is sometimes heavy enough to cause shock. If blood replacement can keep up with losses, the hemorrhaging is usually a self-limiting process, not requiring surgery. About 25% of patients with typhoid fever have minor bleeding that does not require transfusion.

Neuropsychiatric Manifestations. In the past 20 years, reports from India, Papua New Guinea, Indonesia, and Africa (particularly Nigeria) have documented a wide spectrum of neuropsychiatric manifestations of typhoid fever. In some series, half the patients have had disorders of mental status. The most common findings are disturbances of the level of consciousness that range from disorientation to delirium, obtundation, stupor, and coma. Delirium, stupor, and coma are grave prognostic signs associated with case-fatality rates that have exceeded 40%. Delirium often persists after the temperature and metabolic function have returned to normal, and there is no good explanation for its pathogenesis.

Other less commonly encountered CNS findings are seizures, typhoid meningitis, encephalomyelitis, transverse myelitis with spastic paraplegia, peripheral or cranial neuritis, and Guillain-Barré syndrome. Psychotic syndromes, including schizophrenia-like illnesses, mania, depression, and catatonia, have been described, especially in Africa.

Cardiovascular Manifestations. Myocarditis occurs in 1 to 5% of patients with typhoid, whereas nonspecific electrocardiographic changes occur in 10 to 15% of patients. Patients with myocarditis may have no cardiovascular symptoms or may have chest pains, congestive heart failure, arrhythmias, or cardiogenic shock. When myocarditis occurs in young children, it is frequently a serious complication. Electrocardiographic findings are the same as in any myocarditis. Pericarditis rarely occurs, but peripheral vascular collapse without other cardiac findings is being described increasingly. Deep venous and arterial thromboses are uncommon.

Hepatobiliary Manifestations. Asymptomatic typhoid hepatitis is a common finding; in fact, most patients have minor elevations of the serum enzymes (e.g., aspartate aminotransferase [AST] and alanine aminotransferase [ALT]). Jaundice with or without major elevations of hepatic enzymes occurs in 1 to 2% of patients, as does acute cholecystitis. Acute or chronic cholecystitis may occur months to years after an episode of typhoid fever. Culture of stones and/or bile yields *S. typhi* in these cases.

Genitourinary Manifestations. About 25% of patients excrete *S. typhi* in the urine at some point during their illness. Transient proteinuria is the most common urinary abnormality and in some cases is due to an immune complex–mediated glomerulonephritis. The glomerulonephritis may on occasion present as renal failure or nephrotic syndrome, and in these cases the prognosis is poor. Acute tubular necrosis may develop, and in patients with severe intravascular hemolysis, which may or may not be associated with glucose-6-phosphate dehydrogenase deficiency, renal failure can occur. Both pyelonephritis and cystitis occur in patients with typhoid.

Other Complications. DIC is rarely of clinical importance, but thrombocytopenia, hypofibrinogenemia, elevated prothrombin time (PT) and partial thromboplastin time (PTT), and elevated levels of fibrin degradation products can be found in most patients. The hemolytic-uremic syndrome and severe intravascular hemolysis have been reported. Because of the sustained bacteremia, focal infections can develop at any site of the body, but these are rare. The most common sites of infection are in the bones (extremities, spine, ribs), but infections have been reported in the brain, liver, spleen, muscles, breast, thyroid, salivary glands, and cervical lymph nodes. In the past, thrombophlebitis, parotitis, and decubitus ulcers were common complications, but they are now rare.

Relapse. Relapse occurred in 5 to 10% of patients in the preantibiotic era, and although initial reports in the 1950s and 1960s suggested that relapse increased to 10 to 20% in antibiotic-treated patients, most recent series have not reported increased relapse rates in appropriately treated patients. Fever generally returns about 2 weeks after the cessation of antibiotic therapy or in untreated patients about 2 weeks after defervescence. However, relapse can occur during convalescence when patients are afebrile but are still symptomatic and on antibiotics, and it has been reported several months after the initial illness. The relapse syndrome is usually but not always milder than the initial illness.

Typhoid in Children Younger Than 5 Years. *S. typhi* infections have been acquired congenitally, and many cases in neonates have been reported. The clinical presentation in children younger than 5 years, and especially younger than 1 year, is less predictable than in adults. It ranges from an extremely mild illness, often diagnosed as a viral infection but treated with antimicrobials, to severe typhoid fever with hospital mortality rates reaching 30%. Children with typhoid fever frequently have diarrhea and vomiting, and as many as 20% may have convulsions. Typhoid meningitis, although reported in adults and older children, is found almost exclusively in children younger than 5 years.

Geographic Variations. Reports from Papua New Guinea,

Indonesia, India, Nepal, and some areas of Africa have described patients with abnormal levels of consciousness or shock who have a much higher case-fatality rate than do those with normal mental status. These cases of severe typhoid fever with high mortality have rarely been reported from the Americas. It is not clear whether the difference in severity is a function of the host, bacteria, or epidemiologic factors. In areas of endemic schistosomiasis, a syndrome of prolonged, intermittent fever and *Salmonella* sp. bacteremia associated with chronic schistosomiasis has been documented (Chapter 118). The pathogenesis of this syndrome may be linked to the immune response in chronic schistosomiasis and/or the tegmental attachment of bacteria to the adult schistosome worm. Chronic *Salmonella* sp. urinary carriage is common in areas with endemic *S. haematobium* and is related to the obstructive uropathy of urinary schistosomiasis. These patients may experience intermittent fever and bacteremia secondary to the resultant pyelonephritis. Patients with opisthorchiasis (liver fluke infection) may have intrahepatic as opposed to gallbladder carriage, and these individuals may have asymptomatic carriage or recurrent cholangitis (Chapter 120.1).

Chronic Carriers. A person who excretes the organism in the stool 1 year after the initial illness is considered to be a carrier. Although 20% of typhoid patients excrete the organism for 2 months after the onset of illness, and 10% for 3 months, only 3% of patients go on to become carriers. The prevalence is higher in females and in the elderly and correlates with the prevalence of cholelithiasis. Most carriers are asymptomatic, and in some series as many as 25% could not give a history compatible with acute typhoid fever. Individuals with abnormalities of the genitourinary system have a much higher prevalence of urinary carriage than do those with a normal system.

Laboratory Findings. At the time of hospital admission, most patients are moderately anemic, have an elevated erythrocyte sedimentation rate, and have a platelet count reduced to about 150,000. The white blood cell count often is about 5000 to 6000/μm but may range from 1200 to more than 20,000/μm. The differential count is usually normal or shifted slightly to the left, but there may be a relative lymphocytosis, especially later in the disease. Most patients have slightly elevated PT and PTT, decreased fibrinogen levels, and circulating fibrin degradation products. Serum enzymes (e.g., AST and ALT) are usually elevated to values that are twice normal, as is the serum bilirubin. Hyponatremia and hypokalemia are commonly encountered but are usually not severe. Renal function is usually normal. The urine often has low levels of protein and a few white blood cells.

DIAGNOSIS. The diagnosis of typhoid fever is suspected by the clinician; is suggested by assays that identify *Salmonella* sp. antibodies, antigens, or DNA; and is confirmed by isolation of the organism. The Widal reaction is indicative of typhoid fever in only 40 to 60% of patients at the time of admission, and although the organism can be isolated from 95% of patients, identification takes at least 18 hours and often 4 days. Thus, investigations are under way to develop more sensitive laboratory methods for making the rapid, presumptive diagnosis of typhoid fever.

Isolation of the Organism
Bone Marrow Aspirates. Culturing bone marrow aspirates (BMA) is the single most sensitive method of isolating *S. typhi* from patients with typhoid fever. The diagnosis of typhoid cannot be excluded, and the sensitivity of other diagnostic techniques cannot be established without a BMA culture. These are positive in 80 to 95% of patients, even in those who have been taking antibiotics for several days, and regardless of how long they have been ill.

Blood Cultures. The blood culture is positive in 40 to 80% of patients. When experimentally infected human volunteers had daily cultures before antibiotic therapy (mean number of cultures was 5.8), only 75% had positive blood cultures. In the Dade County, Florida, epidemic, only 55% of hospitalized patients with typhoid fever had positive blood cultures. The sensitivity of blood cultures is greatest during the first week of illness, is reduced by prior ingestion of antibiotics, and is directly related to the quantity of blood cultured and the ratio of culture broth to blood. Repeating blood cultures may improve the yield. Reports from South Africa indicated that culturing blood clots in the presence of streptokinase was 50% more sensitive than culturing whole blood. This finding was not confirmed in studies in Indonesia. A major limitation of conventional culture techniques is that it takes a minimum of 48 hours, and often 72 hours, from specimen acquisition until identification of the organism in culture. Work carried out in Indonesia indicates that when the mononuclear cell fraction of blood is cultured, a procedure that concentrates organisms and presumably removes inhibitory serum factors, or when organisms are concentrated by lysis-centrifugation, 100% of cultured organisms can be identified within 18 hours of specimen acquisition.

Intestinal Fluid and Fecal Cultures. Culturing intestinal secretions collected on duodenal string capsule has a sensitivity of 60 to 80%. The sensitivity can be improved by culturing two specimens and leaving the string capsule in place overnight; sensitivity may increase during the third week of illness. A 1-g stool culture is reportedly more sensitive than a *rectal swab culture* but is much more difficult to obtain. A single admission rectal swab culture can be expected to detect *S. typhi* in 30 to 40% of patients; the sensitivity increases with length of illness. Because of irregular shedding, several stool cultures may be necessary to identify carriers.

Cultures of Other Biologic Samples. Urine cultures are positive in 5 to 10% of patients, except in areas endemic for *S. haematobium*, where the positivity rate increases markedly. *S. typhi* has been isolated from the cerebrospinal fluid, peritoneal fluid, mesenteric lymph nodes, resected intestine, pharynx, tonsils, abscesses, bone, and other sites. In a single study, culturing skin snips of rose spots had a sensitivity of 63%.

Culture Techniques. BMA and blood are cultured in a selective medium, e.g., 10% aqueous oxgall or a nutritious medium, e.g., tryptic soy broth, containing a complement and phagocytic inhibitor, e.g., sodium polyanetholesulfonate. One-half to 1 mL of BMA and 8 to 15 mL of blood are cultured at a 1:10 ratio in broth (e.g., 1.0 mL of BMA or 10 mL of blood in 9 mL or 90 mL of 10% oxgall, respectively). The cultures are incubated at 37°C for at least 7 days, and subcultures are made every day to one selective medium, e.g., MacConkey's and one inhibitory medium, e.g., Salmonella-Shigella agar. Suspected colonies are identified by standard biochemical reactions and by incubation with specific antisera. Rockhill and Lesmana have shown that a staphylococcal protein A coagglutination technique can be used to identify colonies as soon as they appear on culture plates.

After isolation, the organism should be tested for antimicrobial sensitivity. If it is resistant to chloramphenicol, it should be checked for the presence of R-plasmids.

Serologic and Other Tests
Widal Test. The standard serologic test in use for the diagnosis of typhoid fever is the Widal reaction, which measures agglutinating antibodies to the O and H antigens of *S. typhi*. Numerous studies have shown that the sensitivity, specificity, and predictive values of this test vary dramatically among laboratories. This wide variation is caused by differences in patient populations, antigens, and techniques. Thus, if

physicians do not know the sensitivity, specificity, and predictive values for the test in their laboratory and in their patient population, the results are almost uninterpretable. On the other hand, if these values are known, the Widal test can be useful.

The Widal test is inherently nonspecific because (1) all group D salmonellae have the same O antigens (9, 12) as *S. typhi* and all groups A and B salmonellae have the O antigen (12) (Table 75–2); (2) all group D salmonellae have the same d phase 1 H antigen as *S. typhi*; and (3) H antibody titers remain elevated for long periods after infection or immunization. The Widal test has a low sensitivity because (1) a significant number of culture-positive patients never develop detectable antibody as measured by this test and (2) in those who do develop an antibody titer, the titer frequently begins to rise before the onset of clinical disease, making it difficult to demonstrate a fourfold rise in titer.

Studies in endemic areas have shown the sensitivity of a single elevated O antibody titer (≥ 1:40 in Mexico and Indonesia, ≥ 1:480 in Rhodesia) to vary from 50 to 90% and the specificity of the same titer to vary from 70 to 99%. In Indonesia, an O antibody titer of 1:40 or greater measured by the rapid, Widal slide agglutination test (results available to the physician within 45 minutes of specimen acquisition) was shown to have a positive predictive value of 96%. Although not useful when negative, when the result was positive the health care provider could be 96% certain that the patient had typhoid fever. The sensitivity of a single H titer is similar, but the specificity is much lower. In endemic areas, a fourfold rise in O and/or H antibody titer is generally found in fewer than 40% of culture-positive patients. In nonendemic areas, the sensitivity is usually the same as in endemic areas, whereas the specificity is generally higher.

An agglutination reaction using O and/or H antigens from *S. paratyphi* A and *S. schottmuelleri* to diagnose paratyphoid fever has similar deficiencies. A Vi agglutination reaction has been used in screening for *S. typhi* carriers. The reported sensitivity and specificity are 70 to 80% and 80 to 95%, respectively.

Polymerase Chain Reaction. A nested polymerase chain reaction (PCR)–based test of blood specimens, using two pairs of oligonucleotide primers from a fragment of the *S. typhi* flagellin gene (*H1-d*), detected 11 of 12 culture-confirmed and 4 culture-negative, clinically suspected typhoid cases. This test only took 16 hours and could detect the presence of 10 organisms of *S. typhi*. The use of two sets of primers, one nonspecific and one specific for the *S. typhi* flagellin gene, allowed maximal amplification while minimizing inadvertent detection of a nontyphi *Salmonella, S. muenchen*. Extensive use of this PCR-based technique on culture-negative suspected typhoid cases at the Asan Medical Center in Korea has yielded a sensitivity of 93% and specificity of 100%. This assay has not been widely used worldwide and is not approved or available for use in the United States.

Another nested PCR based on the nucleotide sequences encoding the Vi antigen (ViaB region) was developed to detect *S. typhi* at single-cell level. This assay could potentially miss detection of *S. typhi* strains lacking the ViaB sequence and inadvertently detect other Vi antigen-containing organisms, *S. paratyphi* C, *S. dublin*, and *Citrobacter freundii* as *S. typhi*. There has not been as much experience with the Vi-antigen based PCR as with the flagellin-based PCR.

Differential Diagnosis

Endemic Areas. During the first week of illness, it is difficult to distinguish typhoid fever clinically from many other febrile illnesses. Thus, physicians must suspect typhoid fever, order appropriate cultures, and consider treatment before obtaining bacteriologic confirmation. During the second week of febrile illness, the range of possibilities is narrowed, particularly if the other locally prevalent diseases that can cause prolonged fever are known. These include other bacterial diseases, e.g., endocarditis, brucellosis, tularemia, tuberculosis, and abscesses; rickettsial infections, e.g., typhus; protozoan infections, e.g., malaria, visceral leishmaniasis, amebic liver abscess, and toxoplasmosis; and noninfectious diseases, e.g., connective tissue diseases and lymphoproliferative disorders.

Physicians practicing in the tropics frequently see patients who have fevers lasting for 7 to 10 days, who have nonspecific clinical findings compatible with typhoid and negative bacteriologic tests, and who recover either without antimicrobial treatment or after empirical treatment with a broad-spectrum antibiotic. It is likely that many of these patients have viral infections. It should be noted that the spleen in typhoid fever is generally smaller and softer than the spleen in malaria.

Developed Countries. In the absence of an epidemic, most cases are imported. Physicians must remember to take a travel history, suspect typhoid fever in febrile patients returning from endemic areas, and order appropriate cultures. The differential diagnosis includes those diseases prevalent in the areas visited as outlined earlier and all other causes of prolonged fever (Chapter 145). Typhoid should also be suspected in patients who have not traveled and who have prolonged fever.

If the diagnosis of typhoid fever is considered, and particularly if the patient is toxic and/or has had previous antibiotics, a BMA culture should be used as a primary diagnostic tool.

TREATMENT. In most cases of typhoid fever, successful treatment requires prompt diagnosis, use of an appropriate antibiotic, and bed rest at home. In many endemic areas, more than 90% of patients are treated in this way, and case-fatality rates for such patients are less than 1%. In some areas of Indonesia, India, Nepal, and a number of countries in Africa, 20 to 30% of patients who have typhoid and who are admitted to hospital are severely ill, and unless they receive intensive care, appropriate doses of corticosteroids, and surgery when indicated, may have case-fatality rates of 10 to 20%. Treatment of hospitalized patients requires (1) proper use of antibiotics; (2) attentive nursing care; (3) adequate nutrition; (4) careful attention to fluid and electrolyte balance; (5) prompt diagnosis and treatment of intestinal perforation, intestinal bleeding, and other complications; and (6) the use of high-dose corticosteroids in severely ill patients.

Antibiotics. Chloramphenicol is still the antibiotic most widely used for treating typhoid and is the standard for judging other antibiotics. It produces defervescence and relief of symptoms in most patients within 3 to 4 days, has reduced the preantibiotic era case-fatality rates of 10 to 15% to 1 to 4%, and cures approximately 90% of patients. Its major disadvantages are (1) it does not reduce the relapse rate; (2) it has no effect on the convalescent excretor or chronic carrier; (3) it causes aplastic anemia in 1 in every 10,000 to 50,000 patients; and (4) it is not useful for treating R-plasmid-mediated, chloramphenicol-resistant strains of *S. typhi*. Chloramphenicol's advantages are that it is inexpensive, widely available, and rarely associated with any short-term side effects noticeable to patients.

Although effective in vitro against *S. typhi*, sulfonamides, tetracyclines, and aminoglycosides are not useful therapy, probably because they are ineffective at the low pH of the phagolysosomes containing *S. typhi* within reticuloendothelial cells. Ampicillin, amoxicillin, and trimethoprim-sulfamethoxazole have been used successfully by a number of investigators in large series of patients. Trimethoprim alone has been effective in small groups of patients. In the past decade, third-generation cephalosporins, particularly ceftriaxone and cefoperazone, and fluoroquinolones including norfloxacin, ciprofloxacin, ofloxacin, and pefloxacin all have been shown in a number of studies to be at least as effective as chloramphenicol in treating typhoid fever. Studies of animals indicate that the third-generation cephalosporins are quite effective in the acid environment of reticuloendothelial cells and that cefoperazone in particular, but also ceftriaxone, is excreted in high concentration into the biliary tract. Fluoroquinolones also have intracellular antibacterial activity. The in vivo activity of these compounds against *S. typhi* has been attributed to these characteristics.

Most studies have shown that in acute chloramphenicol-sensitive *S. typhi* infections, chloramphenicol produces more rapid defervescence than do ampicillin, amoxicillin, and trimethoprim-sulfamethoxazole and a higher rate of clinical cure than does ampicillin. The use of amoxicillin or trimethoprim-sulfamethoxazole has generally been associated with clinical cure rates comparable to those of chloramphenicol as well as lower relapse and convalescent excretor rates. Reports thus far suggest that the rate of clinical cure is excellent, and relapse rates are quite low with fluorinated quinolones and cefoperazone.

Ampicillin, amoxicillin, and trimethoprim-sulfamethoxazole all are effective against *S. typhi* with R-factor–mediated resistance to chloramphenicol, but R-factor resistance to ampicillin has been reported. Presumably, these strains would also be resistant to amoxicillin, making a fluoroquinolone or trimethoprim-sulfamethoxazole the drug of choice for resistant infections. The dosage regimens listed in Table 75–5, if given for 7 to 10 days after defervescence, provide the best available cure rates and the lowest relapse rates. None of the available antibiotics can be considered ideal, because deaths and relapses still occur.

Antibiotics in the Treatment of MDRTF. The fluoroquinolones and the third-generation cephalosporins are the antibiotics of choice in treating MDRTF. Despite fears that fluoroquinolones might cause arthropathy in growing children, many studies have shown that a short course of these antibiotics in children is safe and efficacious in MDRTF. Duration of treatment of MDRTF with fluoroquinolones is recommended to be 10 to 14 days. This recommended treatment course has a cure rate of 100% and a negligible relapse rate. However, reports have described successful treatments of uncomplicated MDRTF with fluoroquinolones for a treatment course as short as 3 to 5 days. Two third-generation cephalosporins, ceftriaxone and cefoperazone, have been shown in trials to be equally effective for MDRTF, with cure rates of 92 to 95%. Cefotaxime is a less desirable alternative because of lower cure rates and higher relapse rates, despite prompt sterilization of blood cultures. Duration of treatment with the third-generation cephalosporins is recommended to be 7 to 10 days or at least 3 days after defervescence.

A ciprofloxacin-resistant *S. typhi* isolate was first reported from the United Kingdom in 1992 from a 1-year-old who acquired the infection in India and did not respond to therapy. Chromosomally mediated resistance to fluoroquinolones, associated with Vi phage type E1, was subsequently identified in other MDRTF isolates from patients returning from the Indian subcontinent.

Supportive, Nutritional, and Nursing Care. Toxic patients with typhoid fever are frequently immobile or agitated, anorexic or incapable of eating, and highly febrile. They must be turned and bathed frequently, fed intravenously or carefully by mouth, and cooled with a cooling blanket or by using tepid sponge baths supplemented by a fan to enhance evaporation. They must be protected against aspiration and observed for signs of intestinal perforation or hemorrhage and shock. Many authorities recommend avoidance of antipyretics, because they are reported to cause precipitous decline in temperature as well as hypotension; however, they may be used if the temperature remains greater than 39.5°C after other measures have been tried. Patients who do not have a paralytic ileus, suspected perforation, or severe abdominal pain should be encouraged to eat whatever they like, because maintenance of good nutritional status is more important than an unsubstantiated concern about some foods precipitating intestinal perforation or hemorrhage. Vitamin supplementation is recommended. Some patients may require total parenteral nutrition, but this is infrequent.

Fluid and Electrolyte Balance. Most cases can be managed without intravenous therapy. Patients with severe typhoid fever have poor oral intake, have high insensible water losses, and tend to become dehydrated with hyponatremia and hypokalemia. Vomiting or diarrhea exacerbates the situation. Initial fluid replacement therapy should provide for maintenance needs, insensible losses, and replacement for dehydration. A typical 50-kg patient who is not in shock requires 3 to 4 L of fluid the first day. Thereafter, records of input and output should be kept and used in treating the patient. If possible, electrolyte determinations should be performed frequently. If not possible, patients should receive liberal quantities of sodium, chloride, and potassium unless renal failure is suspected.

Corticosteroids. Since Woodward and Smadel's observa-

TABLE 75–5. Antimicrobial Treatment of Typhoid and Paratyphoid Fever

Antibiotic	Preferred Route of Administration	Daily Dose (mg/kg/day)	Doses per Day	Duration*
Chloramphenicol	PO/IV†	50	4	7–10 days after defervescence
Trimethoprim-sulfamethoxazole	PO/IV	6.5–10‡	2–3§	7–10 days after defervescence
Amoxicillin	PO	75–100	3	7–10 days after defervescence
Ampicillin	PO/IV/IM	100–150	4	7–10 days after defervescence
Ceftriaxone	IV/IM	50–80	2	7–10 days
Cefoperazone	IV	50–100	2	7–10 days
Cefotaxime	IV	100–150	3–4	10–14 days
Ciprofloxacin	PO/IV	20–30	2	14 days
Ofloxacin	PO/IV	10	2	14 days

*Many authorities recommended halving the daily dosage after the patient has been afebrile for 2 days.
†Absorption is poor and erratic if given intramuscularly.
‡The mg/kg dose refers to the trimethoprim component.
§Various recommendations are listed in the literature; most investigators have used the twice-daily lower dosage regimen.

tions in 1951, the use of corticosteroids in severe typhoid fever has been controversial. Corticosteroids dramatically shorten the toxic febrile stage in typhoid fever, but until 1982 there was no proof that they reduced mortality. Studies in Indonesia by Hoffman, Punjabi, and colleagues have shown that prompt administration of high-dose dexamethasone unequivocally reduces mortality in patients with severe typhoid fever without increasing the incidence of complications, carriers, or relapse among survivors. Patients with suspected typhoid fever who are delirious, obtunded, stuporous, comatose, or in shock (severe typhoid fever) should immediately receive dexamethasone or an equivalent corticosteroid. After antimicrobial therapy is started, an initial dose of 3 mg/kg of dexamethasone should be administered by slow intravenous infusion over 30 minutes. This is followed by 1 mg/kg of dexamethasone given at the same rate every 6 hours for eight additional doses, the total duration of corticosteroid therapy being 48 hours. Patients with normal mental and circulatory status do not require corticosteroids, but those with borderline mental and/or circulatory status should be monitored every 15 minutes in an intensive care unit. If their condition deteriorates, they should receive dexamethasone or an equivalent corticosteroid immediately, because a delay in institution of this therapy can significantly increase mortality.

Complications

Intestinal Perforation. Generalized peritonitis and large quantities of pus are often found in patients with intestinal perforation, but walling off of the perforation is infrequent. If a well-trained surgeon, anesthesiologist, and operating room staff and the necessary equipment are available, operative management of typhoid perforation is indicated (Chapter 13). If these are not available, the choice between operative and nonoperative management is controversial and must be individualized. No controlled trials have compared operative and medical management, but patients with clinical evidence of perforation have been successfully treated without surgery. Advocates of medical management point out that the intestinal lesions are friable, are sometimes larger than they appear, and tend to slough and that patients with perforation are usually very ill and withstand surgery poorly regardless of the sophistication of the surgeon and facilities.

In all cases, patients should be started on chloramphenicol or other appropriate antibiotics, depending on the local resistance pattern; placed on nasogastric suction; resuscitated with fluids, blood, and oxygen as needed; and given corticosteroids if severely toxic. In addition, further antibiotics need to be added to provide coverage for the gram-negative rods and anaerobes that make up the intestinal flora.

It is preferable to stabilize patients before surgery, but the operation should not be delayed for more than several hours after diagnosis. At operation, the ileum as well as the cecum and proximal large bowel should be examined for perforations, and one of several procedures should be performed, e.g., intestinal resection and primary anastomosis, or wedge excision or debridement of the ulcer with primary closure of the perforation (both single- and double-layer closures have been advocated). Most surgeons suture sites of impending perforation with serosa-to-serosa approximation. The peritoneal cavity is then lavaged, and the abdomen is closed, with or without drainage. Standard postoperative care is practiced. As the interval between perforation and surgery increases and the preoperative status of the patient worsens, the case-fatality rate increases. Mortality rates of 10 to 32% have been reported.

Intestinal Hemorrhage. In most cases, intestinal hemorrhage, even when massive, can be managed with general supportive care and vigorous replacement of blood. The use of platelets, fresh frozen plasma to replace clotting factors, or intestinal

resection is occasionally necessary, but this is uncommon. If a patient does not have an abnormal level of consciousness or shock, the case-fatality rate is 1%.

Other Complications. Renal failure, pneumonia, respiratory failure, myocarditis, arrhythmias, cardiac failure, shock, meningitis, localized abscesses, arthritis, osteomyelitis, hemolytic anemia, and cholecystitis all are occasionally encountered and should be managed with antimicrobials and standard medical and/or surgical practices. DIC may sometimes be clinically significant, in which case platelet, blood, and clotting factor transfusions may be necessary. There is no evidence that heparin therapy is useful in typhoid.

Relapse. Relapse should be treated in the same way as the first attack.

Carriers. In the absence of cholelithiasis, the majority of carriers can be cured by a course of oral ampicillin or amoxicillin, 100 mg/kg/day, plus probenecid, 30 mg/kg/day, or trimethoprim-sulfamethoxazole, two tablets twice daily, for 3 months. In the presence of cholelithiasis, the foregoing regimen should be tried before surgical intervention is considered; in most cases, however, antimicrobial treatment alone is not successful and cholecystectomy as well as the same antimicrobial regimen is required. A cure rate of 80 to 90% can be effected by combined surgical and antimicrobial treatment. Cure rates of approximately 80% have been reported with 28 days of ciprofloxacin 750 mg b.i.d. and with norfloxacin 400 mg b.i.d. Chronic urinary carriers of *S. typhi* infected with *S. haematobium* must have the schistosomiasis treated first before they respond to an antibiotic.

Prognosis. The prognosis depends on the patient population and the geographic area. In an epidemic in developed countries, patients are generally seen and treated promptly, have a case-fatality rate of less than 1%, and have a low incidence of complications. The majority of patients in endemic areas are treated as outpatients and have case-fatality and complication rates comparable to those expected in an epidemic in developed countries.

In Central and South America, hospitalized patients are reported to have mortality rates of less than 1%. In some endemic areas, including Indonesia, Nigeria, India, and Nepal, severe typhoid fever (abnormal level of consciousness or shock) is common among hospitalized patients. These patients with severe typhoid fever may have a mortality rate as high as 50% if they are not treated with high-dose dexamethasone therapy.

PREVENTION AND CONTROL

Nonendemic Areas. In developed countries, prevention is now the responsibility of sanitation, water supply, and public health officials. Individuals need not take any special precautions. Chronic carriers should be identified and treated. In the past, considerable time and money have been devoted to screening food handlers, but in many countries this is no longer considered necessary. In the event of an epidemic, the source of the infection must be identified and eliminated and any breakdown in the water delivery and sewage systems must be repaired. The general populace must be informed of the need to adhere to standard hygiene practices.

Endemic Areas. Individuals can minimize their chances of developing enteric fever by paying careful attention to the quality of the food and water they ingest and by receiving immunizations. *S. typhi* in water is killed by heating to 57°C, iodination or chlorination. *S. typhi* in food is killed at the same temperature, but the food must be heated uniformly for several minutes. Travelers to or residents of endemic areas should drink only boiled or bottled water; avoid eating fresh, uncooked vegetables or unpeeled fruits that have not been thoroughly washed in iodinated or chlorinated water; and use discretion when eating in restaurants or food stalls.

Reduction of endemicity depends on improvements in water supply and sewage systems and educating the populace about proper hygiene and food and water preparation practices. Mass immunization can be extremely useful.

Vaccines

S. typhi Vaccines. The first parenteral killed typhoid vaccine was introduced in 1896. By 1912, all United States military personnel were required to receive it, but it was not until the 1960s that the vaccine's efficacy was established in field trials. The World Health Organization (WHO) sponsored trials in typhoid-endemic areas of Poland, Yugoslavia, Guyana, and the Soviet Union and demonstrated that both phenol- and acetone-inactivated vaccines offered 51 to 88% protection to children and young adults. The acetone-inactivated vaccine, which preserves Vi antigen, was moderately more effective than the phenol-inactivated vaccine. In Poland and Guyana, one dose of the vaccine was as effective as two doses. This was probably because of vaccine stimulation of an immune system that had already experienced *S. typhi* infection.

Studies at the University of Maryland showed that the same vaccines used in the WHO studies gave 67% protection to volunteers who ingested an ID_{25} (10^5 organisms) of *S. typhi* but did not offer any protection to those who ingested an ID_{50} (10^7 organisms). At the ID_{25}, those who became infected had a longer incubation period, a milder illness, and a lower incidence of relapse than those who did not receive the vaccine. These volunteer studies also suggested that some efficacy may last as long as 12 years.

Thus, the standard typhoid vaccine is effective in individuals from endemic and nonendemic areas but offers only partial protection, is associated with local and systemic side effects in 25 to 50% of recipients, and must be given parenterally. Because of these drawbacks, other vaccines have been developed. A galactose epimerase (gal E) mutant of *S. typhi* (Ty21a) developed by Germanier is now being used as an oral vaccine. In volunteers in Maryland, five to eight doses conferred 87% protection against an ID_{50}. Field studies suggest an inverse relation between the level of transmission of typhoid in an area and protective efficacy. In 6- to 7-year-old Egyptians (incidence in controls, 46 cases/100,000 per year), the protective efficacy was 96% after 3 years. In 6- to 21-year-old Chileans (incidence in controls, 103 cases/100,000 per year) efficacy was 67% after 3 years; and in 3- to 19-year-old Indonesians (incidence in controls, 1206 cases/100,000 per year) efficacy was 53% after 2.5 years. In Chile, the protective efficacy has remained stable for 5 years. The vaccine does not contain Vi antigen and is thought to induce a protective cellular immune response.

A parenteral vaccine that includes the Vi antigen has been developed and studied by Robbins and coworkers. In 5- to 44-year-old Nepalese (incidence in controls, 654 cases/100,000 per year), a single injection of the vaccine was not associated with significant side effects and conferred a protective efficacy of 72% after 17 months. In South African schoolchildren (incidence in controls, 470 cases/100,000 per year), the Vi vaccine had a protective efficacy of 64% during 21 months of surveillance. It is thought that antibodies to Vi antigen are responsible for the protective immunity.

The TAB vaccine, which contains killed *S. typhi* (T), *S. paratyphi A* (A), and *S. paratyphi B* (B), is associated with more side effects than is the *S. typhi* vaccine and has never been shown to be of value in preventing paratyphoid fever. It is no longer recommended.

Vaccine Recommendations. Although no comparative studies have been carried out, current data indicate that both Ty21a and the Vi antigen vaccine are as effective, if not more effective, than the standard parenteral typhoid vaccine and are not associated with the side effects found after immunization with the latter. Both Ty21a (Vivotif Berna) and Vi antigen (Typhim Vi) are now available in the United States. Because the vaccines work through different mechanisms, some have advocated use of both in the same individual.

Routine typhoid vaccination should be given to laboratory workers likely to work with *S. typhi*, household contacts of known *S. typhi* carriers, and those traveling to or living in areas where typhoid is endemic. This includes most countries of the developing world. Routine vaccination is not recommended in those countries where incidence is low, as in the United States and Europe, not even during disasters or for family contacts. During disasters or in refugee camps in endemic areas, mass immunization should be considered, recognizing that provision of safe food and water is of primary importance.

TY21A. The only commercially available product is an enteric-coated formulation (Vivotif Berna). Four capsules should be given at 2-day intervals. The vaccine manufacturer recommends that Ty21a not be administered to children younger than 6 years. However, there are no data indicating that it is unsafe for such children. Because Ty21a is a live attenuated vaccine, it should not be given to immunocompromised persons, including those infected with HIV. Vaccination with Ty21a should be delayed for at least 24 hours after administration of mefloquine or any antibiotics that would inhibit growth of the live Ty21a strain. A booster dose is required every 5 years for continued protection against typhoid fever. Field studies suggest that a lyophilized preparation that is reconstituted in liquid just before ingestion and administered with sodium bicarbonate is more effective than the enteric-coated capsule. Current data indicate that vaccine efficacy lasts for at least 3 and perhaps 5 years.

VI ANTIGEN VACCINE. A single 0.5-mL (25-μg) dose is administered intramuscularly. This vaccine has not been studied in children younger than 1 year. The vaccine manufacturer does not recommend this vaccine for children younger than 2 years. Booster doses are recommended every 2 years.

Immunization

Standard Parenteral Vaccine. Adults and children 10 years and older are given 0.5 mL SC on two occasions 4 or more weeks apart. Children younger than 10 years receive half the dose on the same schedule. If there is insufficient time for two doses at the interval specified, one dose a week for 3 weeks may be given. A booster dose every 3 years is recommended. Repeat primary immunization is never necessary.

Bibliography

Acharya IL, Lowe CU, Thapa R, et al: Prevention of typhoid fever in Nepal with the Vi capsular polysaccharide of *Salmonella typhi*. N Engl J Med 317:1101, 1987.

Bitar R, Tarpley J. Intestinal perforation in typhoid fever: A historical and state-of-the-art review. Rev Infect Dis 7:257, 1985.

Butler T, Bell WR, Levin J, et al: Typhoid fever: Studies of blood coagulation, bacteremia, and endotoxemia. Arch Intern Med 138:407, 1978.

Butler T, Rumans L, Arnold K: Response of typhoid fever caused by chloramphenicol-susceptible and chloramphenicol-resistant strains of *Salmonella typhi* to treatment with trimethoprim-sulfamethoxazole. Rev Infect Dis 1 4:551, 1982.

Centers for Disease Control and Prevention: Typhoid immunization. Recommendations of the Advisory Committee on Immunization Practices (ACIP). MMWR 43(RR-14):1, 1994.

Fame TM, Englehard D, Riley HD Jr: Hemophagocytosis accompanying typhoid fever. Pediatr Infect Dis 5:367, 1986.

Gilman RH, Terminel M, Levine MM, et al: Relative efficacy of blood, urine, rectal swab, bone-marrow and rose-spot cultures for recovery of *Salmonella typhi* in typhoid fever. Lancet 1:1211, 1975.

Gulati PD, Saxena SN, Gupta PS, Chuttani HK: Changing pattern of typhoid fever. Am J Med 45:544, 1968.

Gulati S, Marwaha RK, Prakash D, et al: Multi-drug resistant *Salmonella typhi*: A need for therapeutic reappraisal. Ann Trop Paediatr 12:137, 1992.

Gupta A: Multidrug-resistant typhoid fever in children: Epidemiology and therapeutic approach. Pediatr Infect Dis J 13:134, 1994.

Hashimoto Y, Itho Y, Fujinaga Y, et al: Development of nested PCR based on the ViaB sequence to detect *Salmonella typhi*. J Clin Microbiol 33:775, 1995.

Hien TT, Bethell DB, Hoa NTT, et al: Short course of ofloxacin for treatment of multidrug-resistant typhoid. Clin Infect Dis 20:917, 1995.

Hoffman SL, Edman DC, Punjabi NH, et al: Bone marrow aspirate culture superior to streptokinase clot culture and 8 ml 1:10 blood-to-broth ratio blood culture for diagnosis of typhoid fever. Am J Trop Med Hyg 35:836, 1986.

Hoffman SL, Flanigan TP, Klaucke D, et al: The Widal slide agglutination test, a valuable rapid diagnostic test in typhoid fever patients at the Infectious Diseases Hospital of Jakarta. Am J Epidemiol 123:869, 1986.

Hoffman SL, Punjabi NH, Rockhill RC, et al: Duodenal string-capsule culture compared with bone-marrow, blood, and rectal-swab cultures for diagnosing typhoid and paratyphoid fever. J Infect Dis 149:157, 1984.

Hoffman SL, Punjabi NH, Kumala S: Reduction of mortality in chloramphenicol-treated severe typhoid fever by high-dose dexamethasone. N Engl J Med 310:82, 1984.

Hoffman TA, Ruiz CJ, Counts GW, et al: Waterborne typhoid fever in Dade County, Florida: Clinical and therapeutic evaluations of 105 bacteremic patients. Am J Med 59:481, 1975.

Hornick RB, Greisman S: On the pathogenesis of typhoid fever. Arch Intern Med 138:357, 1978.

Ivanoff B, Levine MM, Lambert PH: Vaccination against typhoid fever: Present status. Bull WHO 72:957, 1994.

Klotz SA, Jorgensen JH, Buckwold FJ, Craven PC: Typhoid fever. An epidemic with remarkably few clinical signs and symptoms. Arch Intern Med 144:533, 1984.

Klugman KP, Koornhof HJ, Schneerson R, et al: Protective activity of Vi capsular polysaccharide vaccine against typhoid fever. Lancet 2:1165, 1987.

Levine MM, Black RE, Ferreccio C, et al: Large-scale field trial of TY21A live oral typhoid vaccine in enteric-coated capsule formulation. Lancet 2:1049, 1987.

Meier DE, Imediegwu OO, Tarpley JL: Perforated typhoid enteritis: Operative experience with 108 cases. Am J Surg 157:423, 1989.

Murphy JR, Wasserman SS, Baqar S, et al: Immunity to *Salmonella typhi*: Considerations relevant to measurement of cellular immunity in typhoid-endemic regions. Clin Exp Immunol 75:228, 1989.

Osuntokun BO, Bademosi O, Ogunremi K, et al: Neuropsychiatric manifestations of typhoid fever in 959 patients. Arch Neurol 27:7, 1972.

Punjabi NH, Hoffman SL, Edman DC, et al: Treatment of severe typhoid fever in children with high dose dexamethasone. Pediatr Infect Dis J 7:598, 1988.

Rajagopalan P, Kumar R, Malaviya AN: Immunological studies in typhoid fever. I. Immunoglobulins, C3, antibodies, rheumatoid factor and circulation immune complexes in patients with typhoid fever. Clin Exp Immunol 44:68, 1981.

Rubin FA, McWhirter PD, Burr D, et al: Rapid diagnosis of typhoid fever through identification of *Salmonella typhi* within 18 hours of specimen acquisition by culture of the mononuclear cell/platelet fraction of blood. J Clin Microbiol 28:825, 1990.

Rubin FA, McWhirter PD, Punjabi NH, et al: Use of a DNA probe to detect *Salmonella typhi* in the blood of patients with typhoid fever. J Clin Microbiol 27:1112, 1989.

Soe GB, Overturf GD: Treatment of typhoid fever and other systemic salmonelloses with cefotaxime, ceftriaxone, cefoperazone, and other newer cephalosporins. Rev Infect Dis 9:719, 1987.

Song JH, Cho H, Park MY, et al: Detection of *Salmonella typhi* in the blood of patients with typhoid fever by polymerase chain reaction. J Clin Microbiol 31:1439, 1993.

Stanley PJ, Flegg PJ, Mandal BK, Geddes AM: Open study of ciprofloxacin in enteric fever. J Antimicrob Chemother 23:789, 1989.

Stuart BM, Pullen RL: Typhoid: Clinical analysis of three hundred and sixty cases. Arch Intern Med 1946; 78:629, 1946.

Tagliabue A, Villa L, De Magistris MT, et al: IgA-driven T cell–mediated anti-bacterial immunity in man after live oral Ty 21a vaccine. J Immunol 137:1504, 1986.

Wahdan MH, Serie C, Cerisier Y, et al: A controlled field trial of live *Salmonella typhi* strain Ty 21a oral vaccine against typhoid. Three-year results. J Infect Dis 145:292, 1982.

Woodward TE, Smadel JE: Management of typhoid fever and its complications. Ann Intern Med 60:144, 1964.

76 Nontyphoidal Salmonella Infections

Carl J. Mason and Robert N. Longfield

DEFINITION. Salmonellosis is a self-limited acute infection of the intestine and rarely other anatomic sites that occurs worldwide in many animal species and in humans. Infection is readily transmitted to humans by contaminated food or under conditions of poor personal hygiene. Clinical *Salmonella* syndromes include acute enterocolitis, enteric (paratyphoid) fever, and bacteremia with or without focal infection. These syndromes tend readily to overlap or to evolve. Transient asymptomatic intestinal infection is common; however, chronic intestinal, biliary, or urinary tract carriage occurs much less frequently than with *Salmonella typhi*.

ETIOLOGY. Salmonellae are nonsporulating, nonencapsulated, aerobic, gram-negative bacilli.

Classification. Formerly, *Salmonella* was considered to comprise three species: *S. typhi* (1 serotype) (Chapter 75), *S. choleraesuis* (1 serotype), and *S. enteritidis* (over 1700 serotypes or serovars), and the *Arizona* group was designated a separate genus. More recently, a single species, *Salmonella enterica*, with six subgroups or subspecies, has been proposed. Most common human pathogens fall within subgroup I, otherwise known as *S. enterica* ssp. *choleraesuis*.

Salmonellae, like other enteric gram-negative bacilli, possess lipopolysaccharide somatic (O) antigens, which have been grouped A to Z, with additional numbered categories; however, more than 90% of human isolates are included in groups A through E (Table 76–1). Rough strains lacking O antigens are often nonpathogenic. In most microbiology laboratories, clinical *Salmonella* isolates are identified as to species on the basis of fermentation reactions and group-specific O agglutinations.

Salmonellae also possess protein flagellar H antigens that exhibit phase variation under different culture conditions. A given phase 1 antigen is generally shared by only a few *Salmonella* serotypes, whereas a phase 2 antigen is more widely distributed and less serotype-specific. Using serologic methods developed by Kauffmann and White, large *Salmonella* typing centers can provide the identification of isolates necessary for an epidemiologic investigation. Bacteriophage typing may be feasible also for isolates of certain relatively common serotypes.

For convenience, *Salmonella* serotypes (also called serovars) are abbreviated as in the following example: the organism formerly known as *S. enteritidis* serotype *agona*, and now known as *S. enterica* ssp. *choleraesuis* serotype *agona*, is abbreviated as *S. agona*. In any given year, fewer than 200 *Salmonella* serotypes are responsible for human disease. In the United States in 1997, 10 serotypes represented over 70% of identified human isolates: *S. typhimurium, S. enteritidis, S. heidelberg, S. newport, S. thompson, S. hadar, S. infantis, S. montevideo, S. oranienburg,* and *S. agona. S. typhimurium* and *S. enteritidis* are the most common serotypes both in the United States and worldwide.

Cultural Characteristics. Most salmonellae ferment maltose, mannitol, and glucose, producing acid and gas, but do not ferment sucrose or lactose. However, in the 1970s, a strain of lactose-fermenting *S. typhimurium* was confused with *Escherichia coli* during an epidemic in Brazil. Most salmonellae also produce H_2S (except some strains of serotype *S. typhi*) and do not produce indole or urease. Except for *S. gallinarum*

TABLE 76–1. Kauffmann-White Classification of Common *Salmonella* Serotypes

Serotype	Group	O Antigens	H Antigens Phase 1	H Antigens Phase 2
S. paratyphi A	A	(1)*, 2†, 12	a	—
S. schottmuelleri	B	1, 4, (5), 12	b	1, 2
S. typhimurium	B	1, 4, (5), 12	(i)	1, 2
S. heidelberg	B	1, 4, 5, 12	r	1, 2
S. canada	B	4, 12	b	1, 6
S. saint-paul	B	1, 4, 5, 12	e, h	1, 2
S. hirschfeldii	C$_1$	6, 7	c	1, 5
S. bareilly	C$_1$	6, 7	y	1, 5
S. choleraesuis	C$_1$	6, 7	c	1, 5
S. montevideo	C$_1$	6, 7	g, m, s	—
S. oranienburg	C$_1$	6, 7	m, t	—
S. newport	C$_2$	6, 8	(e, h)	1, 2
S. typhi	D	9, 12	d	—
S. enteritidis	D	1, 9, 12	g, m	—
S. pullorum / gallinarum	D	(1), 9, 12	—	—
S. anatum	E	3, 10	e, h	1, 6
S. vancouver	I	16	c	1, 5

*Parentheses indicate that antigenic determinant may be absent or difficult to detect.
†*Italicized* number signifies major determinant of group.
  Modified from Rubin RR, Weinstein LT: Salmonellosis: Microbiologic, Pathologic, and Clinical Features. New York, Stratton Intercontinental Medical Book Corp., 1977.

and *S. pullorum*, all salmonellae exhibit motility by peritrichous flagella. Although salmonellae do not form spores, they readily remain dormant in a desiccated state, within living cells, or in necrotic tissue.

EPIDEMIOLOGY

Incidence and Distribution. Widespread among members of the animal kingdom, salmonellae are responsible for human disease on a global basis. Good data from systematic surveillance for the incidence and etiology of common diarrheal pathogens are lacking. Although the incidence of typhoid fever has declined in many developed nations, the incidence of nontyphoidal salmonellosis is rising. Despite identical mechanisms for reporting *Shigella* isolates to the

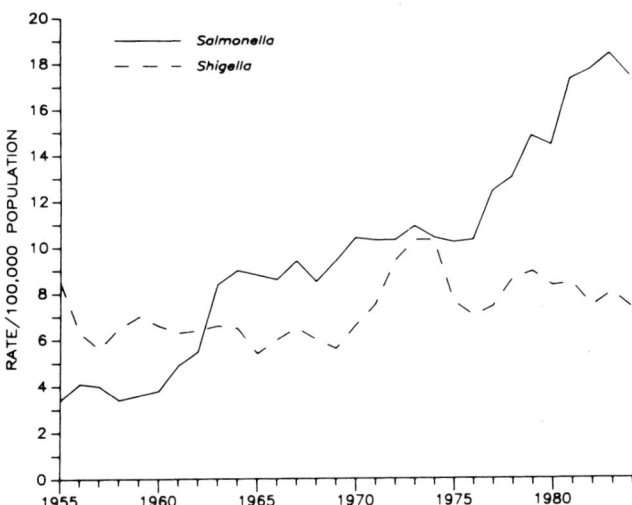

Figure 76–1. *Salmonella* (—) and *Shigella* (- -) infections reported to the Centers for Disease Control and Prevention, 1955 to 1984. Rates are per 100,000 population in the United States. *Salmonella* rate excludes infections due to *Salmonella typhi*. (From Chalker RB, Blaser MJ: Rev Infect Dis 10:111, 1988. Reprinted by permission.)

Centers for Disease Control (CDC), the number of human isolates of *Salmonella* has continued to rise disproportionately over the past 40 years (Fig. 76–1). In the United States, for example, over 40,000 human *Salmonella* isolations are now reported to the CDC annually. This figure may underestimate the actual incidence of salmonellosis by 100-fold or more. The World Health Organization (WHO) suggests that Salmonellosis is underreported by 350-fold or more.

Outbreaks. Coinciding with seasonal outbreaks of food poisoning, most human isolates in the temperate zones are obtained during the summer and fall. Although there is no preponderance by sex, children and the elderly are disproportionately represented among reported cases (Fig. 76–2). Most nontyphoidal *Salmonella* isolations occur in small sporadic epidemics, usually within households. Approximately one third of household contacts also become infected. Institutional outbreaks have occurred in acute care hospitals, pediatric wards, nurseries, and nursing homes. Communal banquet-, school-, restaurant-, and foodstore-related epidemics are not uncommon. In the past 20 years regional outbreaks caused by the commercial distribution of contaminated food have become increasingly important. A large outbreak from contaminated milk in the United States affected 285,000 people.

Although surveillance is lacking, *Salmonella* outbreaks have been reported in nearly all developing nations, and the occurrence of individual serotypes varies widely over time and from region to region. Contaminated water and fecal-oral transmission is important in these nations.

Reservoir Hosts. *S. typhi* and *S. paratyphi* infect humans exclusively. *S. schottmuelleri* (*S. paratyphi* B), *S. hirschfeldii* (*S. paratyphi* C), and *S. sendai* infect humans principally but may incidentally infect animals. Almost all other serotypes infect either humans or animals, and virtually any animal species may harbor these organisms. Past surveys in the United States have revealed *Salmonella* infection in chickens (50%), turkeys (41%), eggs (21%), swine (7 to 50%), and cattle (24%). Animals become infected from their environment or from contaminated feed. Infected animals may transmit salmonellosis among themselves during transport, holding, or

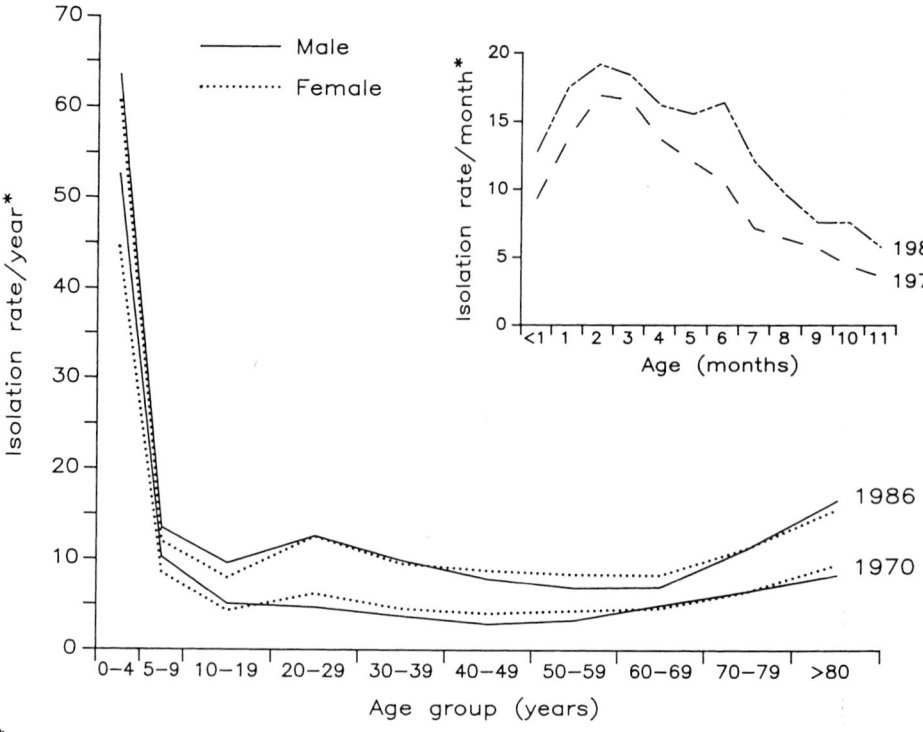

Figure 76–2. Rate of reported isolates of *Salmonella* by age in the United States, 1970 and 1986. (Courtesy of the Centers for Disease Control and Prevention, Atlanta, Georgia.)

*Per 100,000 population

butchering. Abattoir workers and food handlers may become infected readily and transmit *Salmonella.*

Conditions With Increased Incidence of Salmonella Infection

Hemolytic Disorders. Sickle cell anemia (SS) and other hemoglobinopathies (Chapter 6), acute bartonellosis (Chapter 60.1), and malaria enhance susceptibility to nontyphoidal *Salmonella* bacteremia. In patients with these disorders, increased hemolysis and the accompanying erythrophagocytosis by macrophages may impair their ability to clear blood-borne salmonellae. In one study in Africa, 44% of patients with *Salmonella* bacteremia or meningitis were found to have SS, whereas the incidence of SS in the general population was only 2%. *Salmonella* accounts for <1% of hematogenous osteomyelitis in normal hosts but is a frequent cause of such infections in patients with SS.

Schistosomiasis. Chronic or recurrent *Salmonella* bacteremia has been reported among patients with schistosomiasis in Egypt and Brazil (Chapter 118). In the urinary tract, fibrosis, scarring, and stone formation induced by *Schistosoma haematobium* promote chronic urinary carriage of salmonellae.

Other Chronic Conditions. *Salmonella* sepsis occurs more frequently in patients with serious underlying diseases, e.g., alcoholism, hepatic cirrhosis, inflammatory bowel disease, systemic lupus erythematosus, leukemia, lymphoma, other neoplasms, and chronic granulomatous disease. Patients with human immunodeficiency virus (HIV) infection (Chapter 22) and renal transplant recipients have an increased incidence of nontyphoidal *Salmonella* bacteremia and local suppuration. AIDS-associated salmonellosis has been reported from all groups at increased risk for AIDS. The presence of scarred, necrotic, or recently traumatized tissue, e.g., tumors, cysts, bone infarcts, hematomas, effusions, and arterial aneurysms, favors the localization of blood-borne salmonellae.

Transmission

Food. Contaminated food is the most frequent vehicle for transmission of salmonellosis (Table 76–2). Outbreaks are often traced to commercially processed meat and meat products, inadequately cooked poultry, eggs, and unpasteurized milk or dairy products. Food may become tainted during preparation on working surfaces or with utensils contaminated previously with salmonellae. Poultry products are responsible for over half of the common source epidemics. Salmonellae may be found on the shells of fecally contaminated eggs, between the shell and shell membrane, or in yolks of intact eggs from hens with ovarian infection. Pooling of eggs for freezing or drying increases the risk of contamination. Pork, beef, and lamb have also been implicated in salmonellosis epidemics.

Animals. Pets, e.g., dogs, cats, birds, turtles, and lizards, have been implicated in outbreaks of salmonellosis. Turtle-related salmonellosis has been virtually eliminated in the United States and Canada by legislation banning the distribution and sale of pet turtles <4 inches in carapace diameter.

Other Causes. Flies and other insects, gastrointestinal endoscopes, and even human breast milk have been reported to transmit *Salmonella.* Pharmacologic products implicated in

TABLE 76–2. Mode of Transmission in 500 Outbreaks of Human Salmonellosis in the United States (1966–1975)

Source	% Total
Poultry	17
Meat	13
Person to person	10
Eggs	6
Dairy products	4
Pets	3
Miscellaneous	19
Unknown	28
TOTAL	100

Data from the Centers for Disease Control, Atlanta, Georgia, 1977.

transmission include carmine dye, bile salts, pepsin, gelatin, vitamins, and extracts of liver, pancreas, thyroid, pituitary, and adrenal cortex. Even contaminated marijuana and the ingestion of capsules of dried, ground rattlesnake meat have been responsible for scattered cases of enterocolitis in the United States.

Fecal-Oral Route. Direct human-to-human transmission of salmonellosis via the fecal-oral route, although less common than with shigellosis, has been underestimated and may play a significant role in the amplification of infection under crowded, unhygienic conditions. Nursery and pediatric ward outbreaks have occurred in which direct cross-infection between neonates was the likely mode of spread. Neonates may become infected also by fecal-oral spread during labor or delivery, by direct contact with contaminated persons, by fomites, e.g., feeding tubes, by food, and, possibly, by aerosol transmission. Neonates convalescing from salmonellosis are a hazard to other family members: 50% are culture-positive at 3 months, and 10% may be positive for 1 to 2 years.

Nosocomial Salmonellosis. Often due to contaminated food or medicine with subsequent person-to-person spread, hospital-associated salmonellosis outbreaks carry a high mortality rate (7 to 9%).

International Spread. The mass production of food and animal feeds and their global distribution have contributed to the spread of *Salmonella* serotypes, some with disturbing antimicrobial resistance. *S. agona,* a rare isolate prior to 1970, was recovered from human cases in Peru in 1971 and subsequently produced epidemics of enterocolitis in Europe and the United States. In 1998, a subsequent outbreak in the United States of *S. agona* linked to a widely distributed breakfast cereal involved 209 reported cases in 11 states. Contaminated Peruvian fishmeal, used as poultry feed, proved to be the source. *S. eastbourne,* also an uncommon serotype, was introduced into the United States and Canada in 1974 in chocolate from contaminated African cocoa.

Infected travelers may spread *Salmonella* serotypes also. In an early epidemic in 1969, antibiotic-resistant *S. wien* was first encountered among patients in a large Algerian pediatric hospital. Extensive outbreaks of gastroenteritis occurred around the Mediterranean, and two small outbreaks in the United States were associated subsequently with persons arriving from Europe. Nontyphoidal *Salmonella* causes a small but significant proportion of diarrhea among travelers to developing nations.

Antibiotic-Resistant Strains. In the past 40 years, several serotypes of *Salmonella* causing clinical infection have acquired persistent, high-level resistance to ampicillin, chloramphenicol, trimethoprim-sulfamethoxazole (TMP-SMZ), and other commonly used antibiotics. Antibiotics added to animal feed as growth enhancers are believed to have contributed to the emergence of some antibiotic-resistant *Salmonella* strains.

In the United States, studies using restriction endonuclease "fingerprinting" of the DNA from antibiotic-resistant (R) plasmids from *Salmonella* isolates helped to clarify the relationship between resistant strains encountered in animals and those causing human disease. Identical or nearly identical R plasmids were found in salmonellae isolated from animals and persons in widely separated regions. Geographically dispersed human cases clustered in time, suggesting dissemination of a common source item by the food distribution system.

The presence of subsequent acquisition of antimicrobial resistance has characterized many reported outbreaks in both developed and developing nations. A particularly ominous multidrug-resistant *S. typhimurium* DT 104 was first reported in the United Kingdom in 1988. It is characterized by resistance to ampicillin, chloramphenicol, streptomycin, sulfamethoxazole, and tetracycline (ACSSuT) and often associated with resistance to other antibiotics. By 1995, 55% of human cases of *S. typhimurium* in Scotland and Wales were multidrug-resistant DT 104. The National Antimicrobial Resistance Monitoring System in the United States reported that during 1997, 63% of *S. typhimurim* isolates were resistant to one or more antibiotics and 35% had the ACSSuT resistance pattern associated with DT 104.

Chronic Carriers. The majority of *Salmonella* stool isolates from asymptomatic persons represent quiescent infection or transient convalescent carriage. *S. typhi, S. paratyphi,* and *S. schottmuelleri* induce chronic biliary or urinary tract carriage in 1 to 3% of infected patients. Women are three times as likely as men to become chronic carriers. Infection with other serotypes rarely results in true chronic carriage (excretion of the organism for 12 months or more). The prevalence of asymptomatic carriage of these serotypes is approximately 0.2%; however, 5.4% of children under 2 years of age continue to excrete nontyphoidal salmonellae 12 months after infection. Schistosomiasis and infection with the liver fluke *Opisthorchis sinensis* are also associated with chronic carriage of *Salmonella.*

PATHOLOGY. *Salmonella* enterocolitis contributes to mortality primarily in infants, the aged, and persons with underlying disease. At autopsy, the mucosa of the ileum and colon is red and swollen with petechial hemorrhages. Ulceration of Peyer's patches occurs less frequently than in typhoid fever. In neonates, the stomach and small bowel may be involved also, with extensive inflammation, ulceration, hemorrhage, and edema. Intestinal lesions are often absent in patients succumbing to primary *Salmonella* bacteremia. Localized metastatic infections manifest the characteristic histopathology of abscess, osteomyelitis, endarteritis, and meningitis.

In experimental primate infection, hyperemia of the colon with abundant mucus and microscopic acute colitis are present 24 hours after initial *Salmonella* infection. Blood, lymph node, liver, and other organ cultures may be positive at this time. With overwhelming infection, death results from septic shock, and acute colitis may be the only histologic lesion. Pancreatitis and renal tubular necrosis may develop with protracted shock.

PATHOGENESIS. *Salmonella* may proliferate rapidly in contaminated food that is either improperly heated or inadequately refrigerated. Exposure to such food appears quite common, and the presence or absence of clinical infection depends on the inoculum ingested, the virulence of the *Salmonella* strain, and the status of the human host. Infection may be asymptomatic or may present as acute enterocolitis, enteric fever, or bacteremia with or without local suppuration.

Inoculum. The dose of nontyphoidal *Salmonella* required to produce enterocolitis in normal adults has been estimated to be 10^5 to 10^8 bacilli. In general, the ingestion of 10^3 to 10^4 bacilli causes transient asymptomatic carriage; however, common source epidemics have occurred in which 10^2 to 10^3 bacilli produced symptomatic illness. The reported infective dose varies widely for different *Salmonella* serotypes, e.g., *S. newport:* 10^5; *S. anatum:* 5×10^6; *S. melagridis:* 5×10^7 and; *S. pullorum:* 5×10^9.

Virulence. Considerable differences in virulence exist among serotypes, e.g., *S. anatum* commonly causes inapparent infection or enterocolitis whereas *S. choleraesuis* more commonly causes bacteremia or local suppuration. Within a given *Salmonella* serotype dramatic differences in virulence by strain may be evident. In one outbreak of *S. typhimurium,* 60% of patients had dysentery and unusually prolonged symptoms (mean 10.8 days). A single *Salmonella* strain may produce either asymptomatic or rapidly fatal illness, depending on the host's status.

Protective Factors. Host gastric acidity is an important defense mechanism, as salmonellae are rapidly killed at a pH of 2.0. Because salmonellosis occurs in patients with normal gastric function, a large inoculum and the buffering of gastric acid or the physical protection of bacilli by food may nullify the gastric acid barrier. Oral antacids and gastrectomy or an increased rate of gastric emptying reduces the infective dose. Water-containing low inocula of salmonellae (10^2 to 10^3) may pass rapidly through the stomach and induce infection.

Mucosal Attachment and Invasion. Salmonellae that survive the transit through the stomach and upper intestine may localize and multiply in the ileum and colon. The normal bacterial flora are thought to exert anti-*Salmonella* activity by the elaboration of short-chain fatty acids and perhaps other substances. Antimicrobials that inhibit colonic flora substantially reduce the inoculum of *Salmonella* required to cause infection. The preferential attachment of bacilli to the villous tips of the ileal and colonic mucosa suggests a specific receptor. On attachment, salmonellae induce local degeneration of mucosal cell microvilli, advance into a vacuole that migrates through the cell to the basal membrane, and are discharged directly into the lamina propria. Polymorphonuclear leukocytes (PMN) attracted to the lamina propria may damage the colon secondarily by the release of lysosomal enzymes. Inflammation of the lamina propria and resultant smooth muscle spasm are responsible for the cramping abdominal pain and tenesmus. Mucosal damage is rarely sufficient to produce dysentery.

Immunity. The nature of the immune response elicited in the lamina propria determines whether *Salmonella* infection remains localized or becomes disseminated. Unlike *S. typhi*, which induces a mononuclear response with early invasion of lymphatics, regional lymph nodes, and the blood stream, nontyphoidal *Salmonella* elicits a PMN response and generally remains confined to the lamina propria in healthy adults. Infants experience bacteremia more frequently than adults, ostensibly because their bacteria-localizing immune defenses are immature.

In Infants. The inoculum of *Salmonella* required to infect neonates is lower than that for adults. During the newborn period, infection is promoted by a high average gastric pH, frequent milk feedings, which buffer gastric acid, and relatively rapid gastric emptying. The incidence of *Salmonella* enterocolitis is generally reduced in breast-fed infants, perhaps because they are not exposed to contaminated bottles. Mothers who have been naturally infected with or immunized against *Salmonella* secrete species-specific O and H agglutinins in colostrum and breast milk. Although agglutinins appear to retain their specific activity in the gut, they are neither bactericidal nor bacteriostatic in vitro. Maternal IgG antibodies transmitted to the fetus in late pregnancy may actually suppress the development of active humoral immunity in those neonates who subsequently develop *Salmonella* enterocolitis; however, no adverse consequences have been demonstrated.

Mechanism of Diarrhea. Invasion of the lamina propria appears to be a prerequisite for diarrhea in nontyphoidal *Salmonella* infections, because large inocula of killed salmonellae fail to evoke diarrhea. Using the infant mouse and rabbit ileal assays for the heat-stable enterotoxin of *E. coli*, a delayed-acting (18 to 24 hours), heat-labile enterotoxin has been isolated from nontyphoidal *Salmonella*. The toxin is active in vitro against Chinese hamster ovary cells and is neutralized by cholera antitoxin, indicating that its mechanism of action probably involves the adenyl cyclase system (Chapter 41). In experimental animals, pretreatment with the pros-

taglandin synthesis inhibitor indomethacin abolishes both fluid secretion and the adenyl cyclase activation induced by *Salmonella*. PMN in the lamina propria may synthesize and release prostaglandins, resulting in adenyl cyclase activation and secretory diarrhea. There is no evidence in salmonellosis that any portion of the intestine leaks fluid passively, nor is there any discernible defect in fluid absorption.

Local Suppuration. Localized *Salmonella* infection generally involves typical abscess formation with a PMN response, even in abscesses due to *S. typhi*. Any organ or tissue may be involved.

Sickle Cell Anemia. *Salmonella* is more common than *Staphylococcus aureus* as an etiologic agent of osteomyelitis in patients with SS who characteristically incur bony infarction. These individuals frequently acquire infarction-related autosplenectomy during childhood. In one study, heat-labile serum factors (principally components of the alternative pathway for complement activation) that are necessary for the opsonization of *S. typhimurium* were found to be deficient in 12 of 28 patients with SS.

Acquired Immunodeficiency Syndrome. Recurrent nontyphoidal *Salmonella* bacteremia may be the initial manifestation of AIDS or complicate the course of established AIDS. Patients may present with bacteremia and fever without the expected accompanying enterocolitis. Patients may also present with extraintestinal focal infections. Although both zidovudine and TMP-SMZ may prevent relapse, relapse follows standard antibiotic therapy with an increased frequency in AIDS.

Relapse and Chronic Carriage. Relapse in typhoid fever is thought to be due to the intracellular persistence of organisms in macrophages or in bone marrow. Except in the setting of AIDS, relapse tends to occur less commonly with nontyphoidal *Salmonella* that produces clinical enteric fever.

CLINICAL MANIFESTATIONS. Following the ingestion of contaminated food, an incubation period of 8 to 48 hours is required for *Salmonella* multiplication and mucosal invasion.

Enterocolitis. Transient nausea and vomiting are common early symptoms. An initial chill occurs in 30% of patients and a fever of 38° to 39°C is a common, if not invariable, finding. Most patients experience colicky periumbilical and lower quadrant abdominal pain, with a few to as many as 40 stools per day. Abdominal pain is severe occasionally and, when associated with hyperactive bowel sounds and local rebound tenderness, may suggest appendicitis. Surgery in this setting often yields a normal appendix; however, ileitis or appendicitis, with or without perforation, may be encountered. Frequently, stools test positive for occult blood but rarely demonstrate the gross blood or mucus of *Shigella* dysentery. Acute proctitis and colitis, heralded by tenesmus and small-volume blood stools, may be confirmed by sigmoidoscopy in a minority of patients. Intestinal perforation and toxic megacolon are rare. Patients exhibiting "cholera-like," watery diarrhea are exceptional; however, fluid and electrolyte depletion may be profound and may lead to hypovolemic shock. The symptoms of enterocolitis subside usually in 2 to 5 days; therefore, fever and diarrhea persisting beyond 7 days should suggest a suppurative complication of salmonellosis or an alternative diagnosis. Bacteremia follows enterocolitis in 1 to 4% of adults.

Routinely, children experience symptoms for a longer duration (mean of 8.7 days) and manifest dysentery and profound dehydration more frequently than adults. Enterocolitis develops in 25 to 50% of neonates exposed to *Salmonella* and may be chronic and indolent or acutely necrotizing with high mortality. Six of 91 infants studied prospectively with *Salmonella* enteritis had a positive blood culture. Other studies place the bacteremia rate among such patients at 14 to 45%.

Paratyphoid Fever. The incubation period of enteric (paratyphoid) fever, usually 6 to 18 days, may be as long as 30 to 60 days and is inversely proportional to the number of organisms ingested. Although any serotype may do so, *S. paratyphi, S. schottmuelleri, S. hirschfeldii, S. heidelberg, S. typhimurium,* and *S. choleraesuis* characteristically produce human enteric fever. Often preceded by symptoms of enterocolitis, fever becomes sustained and increases in a stepwise fashion. Associated symptoms include malaise (90%), cough (90%), anorexia (80%), myalgias and arthralgias (up to 60%), headache (34%), and pharyngitis (20 to 40%). Rose spots occur less frequently than with *S. typhi.* Rare complications include hepatitis, hepatomegaly, seizures, and an illness similar to Guillain-Barré syndrome. Paratyphoid fever is generally of shorter duration and milder and causes less mortality than typhoid fever (Chapter 75).

Primary Bacteremia. *Salmonella* bacteremia cannot be distinguished clinically from other causes of sepsis. Protracted, hectic fever, recurrent chills, anorexia, and weight loss are present; however, gastrointestinal symptoms, rose spots, and leukopenia are often absent, and stool cultures are negative.

Endovascular Infection. When more than 50% of the blood cultures of a given patient are positive (high-grade bacteremia) or when *Salmonella* bacteremia recurs after apparently adequate treatment, an endovascular focus, e.g., as endocarditis or mycotic aneurysm, should be suspected.

Mycotic Aneurysm. Persistent fever following enterocolitis and the presence of a known aortic aneurysm or the development of chest, back, or abdominal pain should suggest this diagnosis. Salmonellae occasionally seed atherosclerotic aneurysms of the thoracic or abdominal aorta or iliac vessels. Less commonly, infection may extend directly to the aorta from adjacent vertebral osteomyelitis or complicate prosthetic vascular grafts. *S. choleraesuis* is the most common isolate. Often fatal outcome is due to arterial rupture or a surgical complication. Iliac arteritis carries a better prognosis than aortic mycotic aneurysm. *Salmonella* infection has been reported with patent ductus arteriosus, coarctation of the aorta, arteriovenous fistula, idiopathic cystic medial necrosis, syphilitic aortitis, prosthetic valves, vascular grafts, and rarely with normal arteries.

Endocarditis. *Salmonella* endocarditis produces rapid and extensive valvular destruction and perforation. Myocardial abscesses, purulent pericarditis, and major emboli are common. Mural endocarditis occurs much more typically with *Salmonella* than with other organisms. *S. choleraesuis* and *S. typhimurium* are frequent isolates. Mortality is high despite combined surgical and antimicrobial therapy.

Pulmonary Infections. Pneumonia and empyema are most often present in the elderly and in patients with diabetes mellitus, malignancy, cardiac or pulmonary disease, or AIDS.

Central Nervous System Infections. In 95% of cases *Salmonella* meningitis occurs in neonates and children <2 years of age. In a recent study from Brazil, *Salmonella* accounted for 2.3% of all cases of bacterial meningitis but 52% of all cases due to gram-negative enteric bacilli. Fever and meningismus may be absent in patients at both extremes of age. Prematurity, the presence of an immune deficiency, and obstetric trauma increase the risk of neonatal *Salmonella* meningitis. Subdural or epidural empyema, brain abscess, ventriculitis, and obstructive hydrocephalus are common complications. *S. choleraesuis, S. typhimurium, S. enteritidis,* and *S. schottmuelleri* are frequent cerebrospinal fluid isolates.

Osteomyelitis. Conditions predisposing to bone infection include SS and other congenital hemoglobinopathies, diabetes mellitus, systemic lupus erythematosus, and corticoste-

roid therapy. Any bone may be infected; however, the long bones, spine, and costosternal junctions are involved most frequently. Often infection involves both the diaphysis and epiphysis with frequent erosion into an adjacent joint space. Vertebral osteomyelitis due to *Salmonella* is indistinguishable clinically and radiographically from that due to other agents. Disk spaces are involved early, bony lesions appear late, and mediastinal or paravertebral abscesses are common. *S. choleraesuis* and *S. typhimurium* are the prevalent organisms.

Arthritis. Pyogenic arthritis is a complication in 0.2 to 0.3% of patients hospitalized with salmonellosis. Many patients are <12 months of age, and 55% are <6 years of age. Antecedent diarrhea is reported in only half of the patients. Commonly involved joints include knees, shoulders, hips, and sacroiliac joints. Hematogenous seeding occurs more frequently than does direct extension of *Salmonella* infection from adjacent osteomyelitis. Prosthetic joint implants may become infected occasionally following *Salmonella* bacteremia. Male adults, predominantly with clinical enterocolitis due to *S. typhimurium,* may manifest Reiter's syndrome rarely. Urethritis has been inconspicuous in most reported cases, with many of these patients bearing histocompatibility antigen HLA-B27.

Genitourinary Tract Infections. Urinary tract infections with *Salmonella* are infrequent accompaniments of urolithiasis or underlying structural abnormalities. Testicular abscesses and epididymitis in males and ovarian abscesses and salpingitis in females constitute the most common genital sites of involvement.

Other Local Infections. Splenic abscesses are rare; however, *Salmonella* is implicated in 15% of reported cases. Soft tissue abscesses afflict <1% of patients hospitalized with salmonellosis in the United States. Surgical wound infection due to *Salmonella* has been reported to follow cholecystectomy in chronic carriers.

DIAGNOSIS
Differential Diagnosis
Enterocolitis. On initial clinical and laboratory examination, it is often difficult to distinguish acute diarrheal disease due to *Salmonella* from that due to other infectious or noninfectious causes. The presence of fecal PMNs favors the diagnosis of other invasive organisms. PMNs are observed also in patients with acute inflammatory bowel disease. Salmonellosis should be included in the differential diagnosis of the acute abdomen and of acute colitis.

Paratyphoid Fever and Local Suppuration. As with diarrheal disease, bacteremia and local suppuration due to *Salmonella* are best differentiated from those due to other etiologic agents by cultural isolation of the organism. Postdysenteric reactive arthritis has also been reported with *Shigella, Yersinia,* and *Campylobacter jejuni* infections. *Salmonella* osteomyelitis can clinically and radiographically mimic intraosseous sickling, and bone biopsy may be required for the diagnosis.

Culture. The diagnosis of *Salmonella* enterocolitis requires isolation of the organism from stool. Culture of 4 to 5 g of stool yields more consistent recovery than does a rectal swab. Contaminated specimens (stool, urine, sputum) require inoculation on an assortment of differential and selective media. MacConkey's agar (MC) and either Hektoen enteric (HE) or xylose-lysine deoxycholate (XLD) agar are appropriate solid media for initial isolation. Small numbers of salmonellae may be missed occasionally by direct plating of specimens. Prior to plating on selective media, inoculation of selenite or gram-negative enrichment broth enhances recovery. Enrichment broth should be employed routinely for serial stool specimens from suspected *Salmonella* carriers. On isolation, lactose-negative colonies (MC), which produce black pigment (H_2S with HE or XLD agar), are selected for confirmatory biochemical identification and O serogrouping. In one study, bismuth sulfite was the most sensitive selective medium for the detection of *S. arizonae* strains from subgroup IIIa and the lactose-positive *Salmonella* strains.

Salmonellae may be isolated readily from normally sterile body sites using simple, nonselective media, e.g., blood agar, chocolate agar, and nutrient broth. Selective media might inhibit growth and prevent recovery of organisms from usually sterile sites. In enteric fever, stool cultures are positive during the prodromal and convalescent phases; positive blood and urine cultures coincide with the febrile phase; and biopsy of rose spots may yield the causative organism on culture.

Blood Tests. Blood leukocyte counts are often normal in enterocolitis, reduced in enteric fever, and elevated in localized suppuration. Results of the O agglutination test are highly variable and are not helpful in the diagnosis of nontyphoidal salmonellosis. Critical studies are lacking to determine the specificity and clinical significance of positive or rising agglutinin serologic tests.

Treatment. Successful therapy of patients with nontyphoidal salmonellosis depends on diligent supportive care and antimicrobials for specific septic or suppurative complications. Antibiotic therapy for patients with entercolitis without underlying disease and without significant systemic manifestations is not warranted.

Supportive Therapy. Central to the successful management of *Salmonella* enterocolitis is the correction of fluid and electrolyte imbalance and the prevention of circulatory collapse. Oral rehydration with isotonic glucose-electrolyte solutions is an economical and practical alternative to intravenous rehydration for most patients. Inhibitors of bowel motility may delay excretion of the organism, prolong symptoms, and enhance the likelihood of *Salmonella* bacteremia and are not recommended except in limited amounts for control of severe abdominal cramps. Opiates and atropine-like antimotility agents may mask serious extracellular fluid losses by causing sequestration of large volumes of fluid in the intestinal lumen. Oral or parenteral nutritional supplementation can be critical in children and in patients who are malnourished at the onset or who have prolonged salmonellosis.

Antimicrobial Therapy

Enterocolitis. Many antimicrobials have been employed to treat enterocolitis; none has proved to hasten recovery, and all prolong convalescent carriage, presumably by suppressing normal fecal flora. Consequently, antimicrobials are contraindicated for the majority of patients, including neonates, with *Salmonella* enterocolitis. Patients with enterocolitis and hemoglobinopathies, AIDS, other serious underlying diseases, or suspected bacteremia should receive appropriate parenteral antimicrobials.

Paratyphoid Fever. Fluoroquinolones (ciprofloxacin, norfloxacin, orfloxacin) or third-generation cephalosporins (ceftriaxone, cefoperazone, or cefotaxime) are the antibiotics of choice for paratyphoid or enteric fever. For example, ciprofloxacin, 500 mg twice daily orally for 14 days, or ceftriaxone, 1 to 2 g once daily intravenously for 14 days, are recommended. For sensitive strains, a regimen of ampicillin, 100 mg/kg/day for 14 days in 3 or 4 divided doses, often will be effective; however, ampicillin resistance is encountered frequently. TMP-SMZ (10 mg/kg/day [TMP] and 50 mg/kg/day [SMZ]), given orally in divided doses every 12 hours for 14 days, is also an alternative regimen for susceptible strains.

Primary Bacteremia and Local Suppuration. Fluoroquinolones (ciprofloxacin) are the initial agent of choice for *Salmonella* bacteremia and local suppuration. The initial dose, 500 mg twice daily orally for adults, may be continued for 2 to 6

weeks, depending on clinical response and the adequacy of surgical drainage. If the strain is sensitive to them, amoxicillin or ampicillin may be satisfactory. Prosthetic replacement of the involved valve is often required. Mycotic aneurysms of the thoracic or abdominal aorta require surgical resection and intensive antimicrobial therapy. Four to 6 weeks of parenteral therapy have been recommended for the initial management of *Salmonella* osteomyelitis. Unfortunately, relapse of infection and chronic osteomyelitis occur in 40 to 50% of patients. Ciprofloxacin is well absorbed after oral administration, and the prolonged administration of this or a similar agent may treat or suppress localized *Salmonella* infections. Long-term suppression may become necessary in the setting of relapsing renal transplantation or AIDS-associated salmonellosis. Third-generation cephalosporins, including cefotaxime, ceftazidime, ceftriaxone, and moxalactam, have cured patients with *Salmonella* meningitis or osteomyelitis. These agents also represent acceptable alternative antimicrobials for the treatment of multiresistant salmonellosis. Aminoglycosides, tetracyclines, cephalosporins, polymyxins, and paromomycin demonstrate in vitro activity against *Salmonella* but generally have been ineffective in treating patients.

Chronic Carriers. Chronic biliary carriers of nontyphoidal *Salmonella* are managed as typhoid carriers. Cholecystectomy and therapy with a first-line antimicrobial has often resulted in the eradication of carriage. The benefits of eliminating asymptomatic carriage must be weighed against the risk and expense of surgery. Failure to eradicate carriage may be due occasionally to sequestration of the organism outside the gallbladder.

PROGNOSIS. *Salmonella* enterocolitis is rarely fatal in healthy adults. Infants, the elderly, and patients with serious underlying disease incur a greater risk of mortality. The case-fatality rate approaches 20% in patients with *S. choleraesuis* bacteremia. However, patients who have bacteremia due to other nontyphoidal *Salmonella* have a lower case-fatality rate in general than do patients with sepsis due to other *Enterobacteriaceae*. Salmonellosis causes unusually severe mortality in hospital-associated outbreaks, with the rates being 2.3% overall, 7.0% in newborn nurseries, and 8.7% in nursing homes. Neonatal meningitis results in an 85% mortality rate despite early specific therapy. Endocarditis and mycotic aneurysm due to *Salmonella* carry a poor prognosis also.

PREVENTION

Sanitation. The control of human-to-human spread of salmonellosis depends on good personal hygiene; a reliable, uncontaminated water supply; proper sewage disposal; the identification, treatment, and follow-up of chronic carriers; and the isolation of acute cases. Known chronic carriers should not be employed as food handlers or as health care or child care providers. Owing to the gravity of nosocomial outbreaks, particular attention should be paid to the application of enteric precautions for patients hospitalized with enterocolitis. Breast-feeding protects neonates and infants against *Salmonella* infection.

Vaccines. No immunization is available currently to prevent nontyphoidal salmonellosis. Parenteral or oral immunization with killed nontyphoidal *Salmonella* vaccines has not proved effective in preventing disease in humans.

Zoonotic Spread. Detection and control of salmonellosis among animals and reduction in the contamination of food products will not be easily accomplished. Heat treatment or pasteurization of animal feeds has curtailed the spread of *Salmonella* in some instances but may not be economical on a widespread basis. Improvement in the hygienic conditions encountered in the transport, holding, and slaughtering of animals and in food processing, distribution, and preparation remains a constant challenge. The continued use of antibiotics to control *Salmonella* infections in herds and flocks may promote the development of multidrug resistance.

Bibliography

Black PH, Kunz LH, Swartz MN: Salmonellosis: A review of some unusual aspects. N Engl J Med 262:811, 864, 921, 1960.

Chalker RB, Blaser MJ: A review of human salmonellosis. III. Magnitude of *Salmonella* infection in the United States. Rev Infect Dis 10:111, 1988.

Cohen JI, Bartlett IA, Corey CR: Extra-intestinal manifestations of *Salmonella* infections, Medicine 66:349, 1987.

Finlay BB: Molecular and cellular mechanisms of *Salmonella* pathogenesis. Curr Top Microbiol Immunol 192:163, 1994.

Gomez TM, Motarjemi Y, Miyagawa S, et al: Foodborne salmonellosis. Who Dir Health Stat Q 50:81, 1997.

LeMinor LL, Popoff MY: Designation of *Salmonella enterica* sp. nov., nom rev. as the type and only species of the genus *Salmonella*. Int J Syst Bacteriol 37:465, 1987.

O'Brien TF, Hopkins ID, Gillece ES, et al: Molecular epidemiology of antibiotic resistance in *Salmonella* from animals and human beings in the United States. N Engl J Med 307:1, 1982.

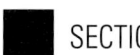 SECTION I **Mycobacterial Infections**

77 *Tuberculosis*

Peter M. Small and Uzi M. Selcer

■ DEFINITION

Tuberculosis (TB), a chronic infection usually affecting the lungs, claims more lives worldwide than any other infectious disease. Each year it causes an estimated 3 million deaths, the vast majority of which occur in developing countries. It is caused by bacilli of the *Mycobacterium tuberculosis* complex (*M. tuberculosis, M. bovis, M. africanum,* and *M. microti.*) The disease affects people in all parts of the world; its distribution, however, is very uneven. Developing nations have higher numbers of infected people and active cases than industrialized nations. Because of the growing global burden of TB, and the recognition that it is one of the most neglected health problems worldwide, in 1993 the World Health Organization (WHO) declared TB a global health emergency. Indeed, although the metaphor of TB as "the captain of all these men of death" was thought to be reaching obsolescence, we are currently in a period of resurgence of the disease. Even developed nations, in which the risk of infection had decreased steadily over the last 50 years, have seen increases in TB cases in the early 1990s. This has been attributed largely to the human immunodeficiency virus (HIV) epidemic, although neglect of control programs, immigration from poorer countries, and other social changes have been important factors.

The clinical manifestations of TB can be extremely varied, and may reflect involvement of any organ or system. In immune-competent hosts, a brisk granulomatous response attempts—and in most cases succeeds—to stop the progression of the infection. In 10 to 20% of infected individuals, depending on factors, e.g., age, immune status and, perhaps, genetic susceptibility, infection results in tuberculous disease, either as a result of primary progression or after reactivation later in life. The vast majority of cases primarily affect the lungs, and approximately half of these will be sputum smear positive and hence very infectious. If left untreated, chronic pulmonary cases pursue a destructive course, with the formation of a cavitary lesion in which large numbers of viable mycobacteria replicate. Approximately 60% of patients with the disease die unless adequate treatment can be instituted.

The enormous burden of TB in the developing world makes it one of the most important medical problems faced in poorer countries, in which 25% of all preventable deaths can be attributed to this disease.

■ HISTORY

Biologic and genetic data suggest that the human pathogen *M. tuberculosis* evolved from *M. bovis* some time after the domestication of cattle approximately 15,000 years ago. Neolithic development of urbanization and population concentration favored the airborne transmission of TB. Subsequently, as *M. tuberculosis* spread in epidemic waves around the globe, the pathogen was sequentially introduced to functionally discrete populations. The earliest recorded epidemic began in Europe at least 400 years ago, where the epidemic grew and spread. At its peak in the 1800s tuberculosis accounted for 25% of European deaths. Over time, these epidemics waned within a population, presumably as a consequence of progressive improvement in living conditions, segregation of infectious cases in sanatoria, attenuation in the genetic virulence, or natural selection of host resistance, availability of effective chemotherapy, and the intrinsic transmission dynamics of epidemics.

The 1990s have been notable for a global reawakening to the fact that a preventable and treatable disease accounts for 8 million illnesses and 3 million deaths each year. Furthermore, the misuse of antibiotics has led to epidemics of drug-resistant TB organisms that have the potential to become virtually untreatable. These realizations resulted in efforts, spearheaded by the WHO, to assist national TB control programs in administering directly observed therapy to tuberculous patients.

■ MICROBIOLOGY

Conventional

SPECIES. The term tubercle bacillus refers to organisms of the *Mycobacterium tuberculosis* complex, which includes *M. tuberculosis* (MTB); *M. bovis* and its attenuated form, bacille Calmette-Guérin (BCG); *M. africanum*; and *M. microti.* Most cases of tuberculosis are caused by MTB; however, in certain regions infection with *M. bovis* is also seen. There is such a degree of DNA homology between MTB and *M. bovis* that, although they differ in biochemical characteristics and host range, they are regarded by some as subspecies rather than as distinct species. This similarity, coupled with supporting paleopathologic and historical evidence, has led some authors to hypothesize that MTB evolved in humans from *M. bovis* as a result of the domestication of cattle.

ACID-FAST AND FLUORESCENT STAINING. The principal characteristic of the genus *Mycobacterium* is the staining feature of "acid fastness." This refers to the fact that once stained with carbolfuchsin in Ziehl-Neelsen or Kinyoun stains, these organisms resist decoloration by an acid-alcohol mixture. Hence, when counterstained with methylene blue, they appear as red rods on a blue background. Mycobacteria may also be visualized with fluorescent stains, e.g., auramine-rhodamine. The brilliant colors of organisms stained with this technique can be seen at lower magnification, thus allowing for a more rapid and sensitive examination of specimens. However, this method requires specialized, expensive fluorescent microscopes not available in most health care facilities. Also, because of the increased occurrence of staining artifacts, positive slides should be confirmed by traditional, nonfluorescent acid-fast stains.

CULTURE CHARACTERISTICS. *M. tuberculosis* is a slender, straight or somewhat curved, nonmotile rod. It is a non–spore-forming, obligate aerobe, measuring 1 to 4 μm in length and 0.2 to 0.5 μm in width. It grows extremely slowly, with a doubling time of 15 to 20 hours; thus it generally takes from 3 to 6 weeks to produce visible colonies on egg-based media, e.g., Löwenstein-Jensen. Because of this slow growth rate, faster growing bacteria and fungi present in sputum may overgrow the culture medium. To avoid this, and taking advantage of the fact that mycobacteria are heartier than most clinically relevant bacteria, decontamination and liquefaction of sputum samples with sodium hydroxide, *N*-acetylcysteine, or quaternary ammonium compounds is widely used. Growth may be evident up to a week earlier when translucent agar-based media, e.g., Middlebrook 7H10 is examined with a magnifying lens. Colonies are nonpigmented and niacin positive. MTB reduces nitrate and produces a small quantity of a heat-labile catalase. The combination of these cultural and biochemical characteristics serves to identify the majority of isolates of MTB. However, they require initial growth in solid media and subsequent subculture and hence they may take 3 to 6 weeks for definitive identification of the organism. To overcome these delays, culture systems using radiometrically labeled liquid media have been devised. The radiometric BACTEC system (Johnston Laboratories, Towson, MD) utilizes ^{14}C-labeled palmitate as the sole carbon source. The radioactive carbon dioxide (CO_2) liberated as a result of mycobacterial growth is measured by a detection device and thus positive cultures are identified. This method may decrease the time required for identification by 50%. Also, because the growth of MTB is inhibited by NAP (*p*-nitro-α-acetylamino-β-hydroxypropiophenone), growth in media containing NAP essentially rules out organisms of the MTB complex. As discussed later, these radiometric systems are well adapted for use in susceptibility testing.

DNA PROBES. The identification of unique genetic sequences in different mycobacterial species has allowed the development of DNA probes that hybridize to rRNA from MTB or other mycobacterial species and form highly specific complexes. These probes, labeled radioactively or nonisotopically, can be used for the rapid and specific identification at the species level. Although their current low sensitivity precludes their use on direct uncultured specimens, they are widely used for speciation once adequate growth has been obtained in either solid or liquid media. Results are obtained in a matter of hours.

Drug Susceptibility Testing

Drug susceptibility testing of MTB is currently recommended in the United States for all initial isolates and for subsequent isolates in persistently culture positive and relapsed cases, and in developing nations this should be a routine part of TB control program surveillance. Because these tests are complicated and require a great deal of expertise, they are best performed in reference laboratories that process a significant number of samples on a regular basis. Many methods exist, all of which can be performed directly from the original clinical specimen or indirectly from the primary culture isolated. Direct methods provide results sooner, and the inoculum is a true representation of the bacterial population in the clinical sample. Indirect methods allow for the easier preparation of a uniform inoculum and hence, their results are more reproducible. Care must be taken, however, to avoid selecting a predominant population of resistant or susceptible organisms.

Three different methods are commonly used. The *absolute concentration method* evaluates the growth of a standard inoculum in several concentrations of the drug to be tested as well as in a drug-free control. This technique most closely resembles a minimal inhibitory concentration (MIC) test. Results are expressed in terms of the minimal concentration of the drug that inhibits growth of the inoculum. The *resistance ratio method* compares the MIC of the test strain to that of a known susceptible control strain and expresses the result as a ratio of the test-strain MIC to that of the control. Ratios of 2 or less are usually considered susceptible and ratios of 8 or more indicate resistance. The *proportion method* is the most widely used technique in the United States. Mycobacteria are diluted to an inoculum that, when plated on drug-free media, yields approximately 100 individual colonies. This same inoculum is then plated on media containing a single concentration of each antibiotic. By comparing the amount of growth on media with and without antibiotic the proportion of the population that is resistant to the drug can be quantified. If more than 1% of the population is resistant, the isolate should be considered resistant to the drug being tested. The critical concentrations recommended by the U.S. Centers for Disease Control and Prevention for testing with the proportion method are as follows: for isoniazid (INH), 0.2 μg/mL; for streptomycin, 2.0 μg/mL; for ethambutol, 5.0 μg/mL; for rifampin, 1.0 μg/mL. Because pyrazinamide (PZA) is active at pH 5.5, and isolates of MTB may not grow at this low pH in solid media, it is recommended that susceptibility testing for PZA be performed by the radiometric BACTEC method. This newer method relies on the detection of radioactively labeled carbon as a reflection of bacterial growth. When growth occurs in the presence of critical concentrations of a test drug, it indicates resistance to that drug. The main advantage of the method is that results are frequently available in half the time required for conventional testing. Using radiometric methods, a well-equipped and functioning laboratory can now provide identification and susceptibility results in 4 weeks.

Molecular Diagnostics

To circumvent the time delays and biohazards inherent in conventional microbiology, several amplification techniques using target or signal amplification have been adapted for detecting mycobacteria in clinical specimens. These techniques (e.g., the polymerase chain reaction (PCR) or tran-

TABLE 77–1. Estimated Tuberculosis (TB) Incidence and HIV-Attributable TB Cases in 1990, 1995 and 2000, by Region

	1990			*1995*			*2000*		
Region	Total TB Cases	Rate*	HIV-Attributed TB Cases	Total TB Cases	Rate*	HIV-Attributed TB Cases	Total TB Cases	Rate*	HIV-Attributed TB Cases
Southeast Asia	3,106,000	237	66,000	3,499,000	241	251,000	3,952,000	247	571,000
Western Pacific†	1,839,000	136	19,000	2,045,000	140	31,000	2,255,000	144	68,000
Africa	992,000	191	194,000	1,467,000	242	380,000	2,079,000	293	604,000
Eastern Mediterranean	641,000	165	9,000	745,000	168	16,000	870,000	168	38,000
Americas‡	569,000	127	20,000	606,000	123	45,000	645,000	120	97,000
Eastern Europe§	194,000	47	1,000	202,000	47	2,000	210,000	48	6,000
Industrialized countries¶	196,000	23	6,000	204,000	23	13,000	211,000	24	26,000
TOTAL	7,537,000	143	315,000 (4.2%)	8,768,000	152	738,000 (8.4%)	10,222,000	163	1,410,000 (13.8%)
Increase since 1990				16.3%			35.6%		

*Crude incidence rate per 100,000 population.
†Includes all countries of the Western Pacific Region of WHO, except Japan, Australia, and New Zealand.
‡Includes all countries of the American Region of WHO, except USA and Canada.
§Eastern European countries, and independent states of the former USSR.
¶Western European countries, USA, Canada, Japan, Australia, and New Zealand.
From Dolin PJ, Raviglione MC, Kochi A: Global tuberculosis incidence and mortality during 1990–2000. Bull WHO 72:213, 1994.

scription mediated amplification) do not depend on growth of the organism but instead amplify minute quantities of mycobacterial nucleic acid to detectable levels. Although these techniques are potentially very sensitive and specific, currently available assays vary significantly in their positive and negative predictive values and presently have limited utility in clinical diagnosis. Moreover, the high cost of these techniques will probably limit their widespread application in resource-poor countries.

Molecular techniques for identifying specific strains of mycobacteria are also available for epidemiologic studies of TB outbreaks and to elucidate transmission dynamics in populations. These methods exploit polymorphism in the number and genomic location of repetitive DNA sequences in MTB to generate "fingerprints" specific for individual strains. The identification of individuals infected with bacteria that have the same fingerprints is used to infer epidemiologic links.

■ EPIDEMIOLOGY

INCIDENCE, PREVALENCE, AND DISTRIBUTION. TB is the most extensive infectious epidemic affecting the world today.

One third of the world population—1.7 billion people—is thought to harbor the infection. The number of incident cases was estimated at 7.5 million in 1990 and 8.8 million in 1995 and is projected to reach 10.2 and 11.9 million in the years 2000 and 2005 respectively, an increase of more than 57% in 15 years (Table 77–1). Even the most optimistic scenarios estimate that in the 10-year period from 1990 to 1999 more than 88 million people will develop tuberculosis and more than 30 million will die from it (Figs. 77–1 and 77–2). In fact, the annual death toll of 3 million people is the greatest of any single infectious agent and represents 25% of all preventable deaths in developing nations. Many reasons explain the failure to control this epidemic despite the fact that TB control is one of the most cost-effective public health interventions, on a par with measles vaccination. Much of this is attributable to a lack of political commitment to establishing and maintaining effective control strategies. In addition, control efforts are now hampered by co-infection with HIV which makes tuberculosis more common, more complicated to diagnose, and more difficult to treat. Indeed, approximately 10% of incident cases of tuberculosis between 1990 and 1999 and 14% of the annual deaths predicted for the year 2000 are

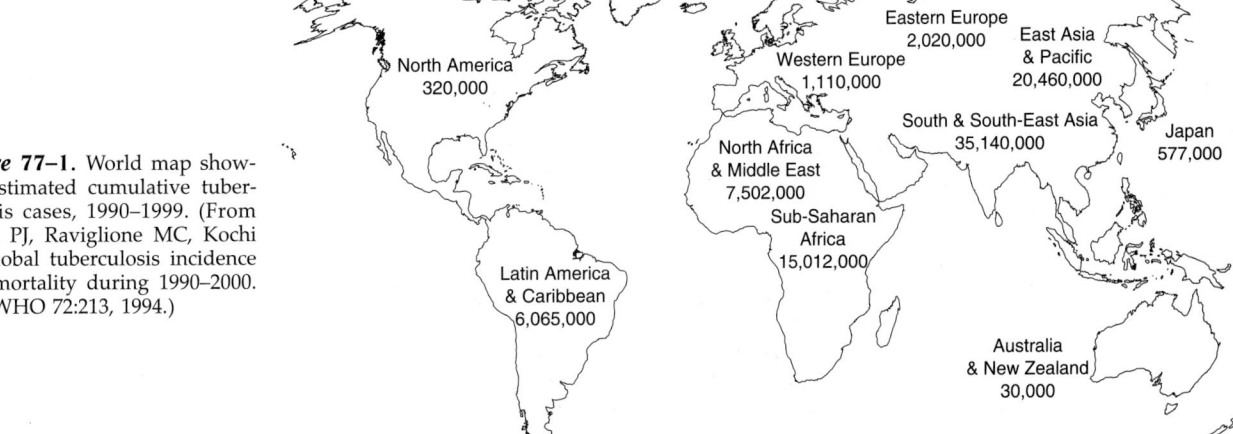

Figure 77–1. World map showing estimated cumulative tuberculosis cases, 1990–1999. (From Dolin PJ, Raviglione MC, Kochi A: Global tuberculosis incidence and mortality during 1990–2000. Bull WHO 72:213, 1994.)

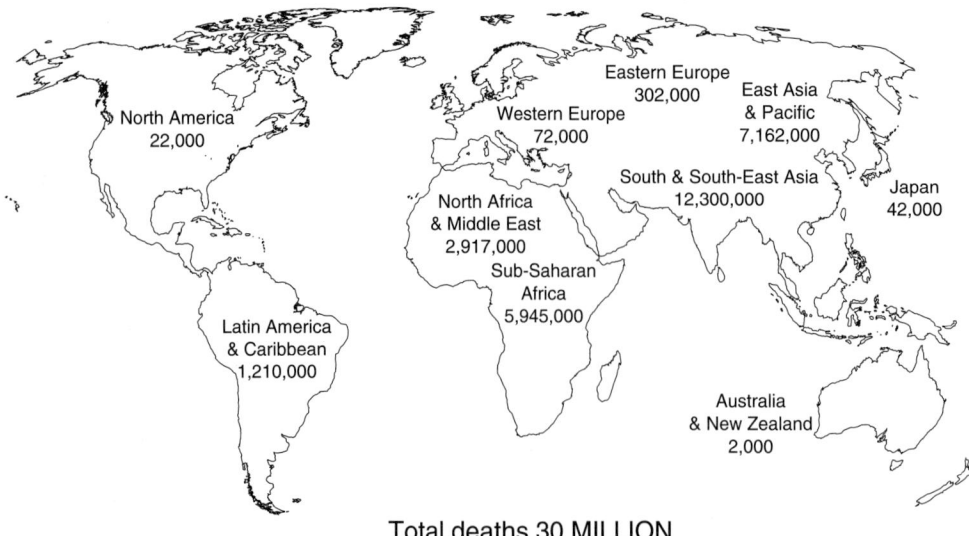

Figure 77–2. World map showing estimated cumulative tuberculosis deaths, 1990–1999. (From Dolin PJ, Raviglione MC, Kochi A: Global tuberculosis incidence and mortality during 1990–2000. Bull WHO 72:213, 1994.)

estimated by the WHO to be attributable to HIV infection (Table 77–2).

Although TB affects people all over the world, its distribution is very uneven, with the major burden of morbidity and mortality falling on the lesser developed nations. In 1990, the TB rates as estimated by WHO, ranged from 237 cases per 100,000 population for Southeast Asia to 23 cases per 100,000 in western European and other industrialized nations (Table 77–1).

TB has always been linked with poverty, particularly in the urban setting. Within developed nations, in an analogous fashion to the uneven world distribution, cases are also concentrated in certain at-risk populations. These include the homeless, injection drug users, HIV-infected people, prisoners, immigrants from high incidence regions, migrant farm workers, and residents of inner cities and other areas marginalized from health care and social services.

Transmission

The transmission cycle begins when an infectious particle is generated by a tuberculous patient (Fig. 77–3). In the vast majority of cases this occurs through the forced expiration that occurs when a sputum smear–positive person coughs, sneezes, sings or speaks, aerosolizing respiratory droplets of varying sizes. Infection by aerosolization is particularly efficient in patients with cavitary or laryngeal disease. Most of these particles are relatively large and not effectively transmitted because they rapidly settle to the ground or are eliminated by the recipient's mucociliary clearance mechanism. However, each cough also generates thousands of smaller particles on the order of 1 to 5 μm, known as "droplet nuclei," which contain from one to three viable mycobacteria. These particles remain suspended in the air, like smoke particles, for hours or even days. Sputum smear–negative persons can also serve as the source of droplet nuclei, although they are considerably less efficient and are consequently less likely to be the source for subsequent transmission. Other sources of infectious particles (e.g., power cutting tools during an autopsy, the use of high pressure irrigation of a tuberculous soft tissue abscess) have been described but occur much less commonly.

RESPIRATORY TRANSMISSION. Transmission occurs when as few as one infectious particle is subsequently in-

TABLE 77–2. Estimated Total Tuberculosis Deaths and HIV-Attributable Tuberculosis Deaths in 1990, 1995 and 2000, by Region, Assuming That Regional Treatment Coverage Rates Remain at Their 1990 Level

Region	Deaths in 1990		Deaths in 1995		Deaths in 2000	
	Total	Attributed to HIV	Total	Attributed to HIV	Total	Attributed to HIV
Southeast Asia	1,087,000	23,000	1,225,000	88,000	1,383,000	200,000
Western Pacific*	644,000	7,000	716,000	11,000	789,000	24,000
Africa	393,000	77,000	581,000	150,000	823,000	239,000
Eastern Mediterranean	249,000	4,000	290,000	6,000	338,000	15,000
Americas†	114,000	4,000	121,000	9,000	129,000	19,000
Eastern Europe‡	29,000	<200	30,000	<600	32,000	<900
Industrialized countries§	14,000	<500	14,000	1,000	15,000	2,000
All regions	2,530,000	116,000 (4.6%)	2,977,000	266,000 (8.9%)	3,509,000	500,000 (14.2%)
Increase since 1990			17.7%		38.7%	

*Excluding Japan, Australia, and New Zealand.
†Excluding USA and Canada.
‡Eastern Europe and independent states of former USSR.
§Western Europe, USA, Canada, Japan, Australia, and New Zealand.
From Dolin PJ, Raviglione MC, Kochi A: Global tuberculosis incidence and mortality during 1990–2000. Bull WHO 72:213, 1994.

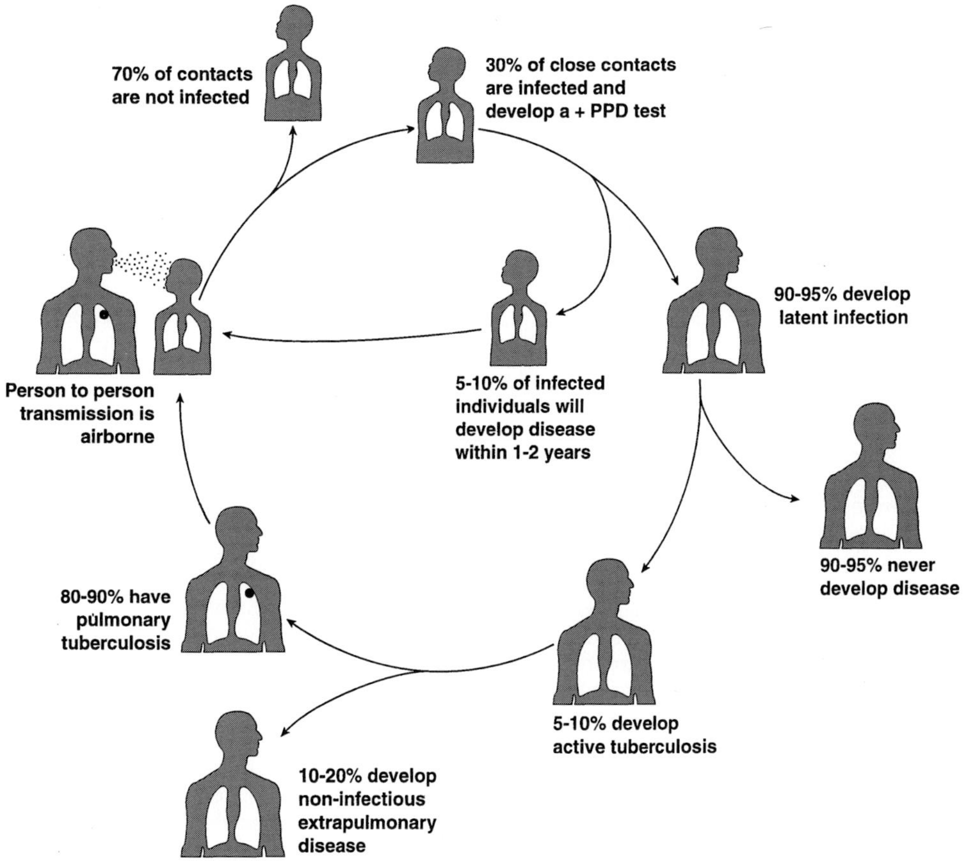

Figure 77–3. Tuberculosis transmission: 'life cycle' view. In high-prevalence areas, most infections are acquired early in life and result from the close contact of children or young adults with cases of active pulmonary TB. Only the minority of contacts are infected, and of these, the majority never develop active disease. Children under 5 years of age, HIV-infected individuals, and other immunosuppressed individuals are at much higher risk of developing active disease once infected.

70% of contacts are not infected

30% of close contacts are infected and develop a + PPD test

90–95% develop latent infection

5–10% of infected individuals will develop disease within 1-2 years

Person to person transmission is airborne

90–95% never develop disease

80–90% have pulmonary tuberculosis

5–10% develop active tuberculosis

10–20% develop non-infectious extrapulmonary disease

haled and deposited in the terminal alveoli of another person. The likelihood of this occurring is a function of the concentration of droplet nuclei containing viable bacilli and the quantity of infected air that is inhaled. Thus, transmission is most likely to occur with prolonged contact in poorly ventilated environments. Airborne bacilli are killed by sunlight and ultraviolet radiation or removed by high efficiency particle filtration. Conversely, expired air may remain infectious for prolonged periods of time in dark, poorly ventilated enclosures. Although transmission requires only the inhalation of a single bacterium, in general, transmission of TB is rather inefficient. It is estimated that overall approximately 30% of household contacts of a person with active pulmonary disease become infected. However, the actual amount of transmission from an individual case is highly variable. Transmission during some outbreaks has been extremely efficient. For example, a patient with laryngeal TB infected 50 people during a 6-hour visit to an emergency room; in another case, 17 health care workers whose purified protein derivative (PPD) was previously negative were exposed to an infectious patient for up to 10 hours. On follow-up evaluation 13 had been infected and 3 of them developed active disease.

BOVINE TUBERCULOSIS. Although aerosol generation from pulmonary cases accounts for the majority of MTB transmission, other mechanisms also occur. Transmission of *M. bovis* most commonly occurs through ingestion of unpasteurized milk from infected cattle. This was a significant cause of morbidity in Europe and the United States in the past, and sporadic cases are still identified in developed countries. However, the almost complete elimination of affected herds in the United States and Europe has resulted in the near disappearance of this phenomenon. The same is not

true for most developing nations where bovine TB in humans is a problem proportional to both the prevalence of affected cattle and the human consumption of unpasteurized milk products.

OTHER MODES OF TRANSMISSION. Direct inoculation has been described when infected cadaveric organs are transplanted, resulting in rapid and frequently fatal disease. Laboratory personnel who work with mycobacteria may contract TB through direct inoculation, generally resulting in a soft tissue abscess or cutaneous disease. Congenital TB, acquired either transplacentally or through the birth canal, may also occur.

■ IMMUNE RESPONSE: INFECTION OR DISEASE

PRIMARY INFECTION. Following transmission, infection occurs when MTB is phagocytozed by an alveolar macrophage. Mycobacteria have a variety of mechanisms that allow them to resist killing by the inactivated macrophage, and thus proliferate, essentially unchecked in this intracellular environment. Mycobacteria subsequently spread locally resulting in a pneumonic process, referred to as *primary tuberculosis*. The location is dictated by the site of implantation, and thus most commonly occurs in the well-ventilated lower lung fields. Over a period of weeks (a pace dictated by the slow growth rate of MTB), bacteria spread to local and regional lymph nodes and are carried by the blood stream to virtually all organs of the body. During this phase clinical manifestations of TB are mild and nonspecific and generally go undiagnosed.

LATENT INFECTION. In the majority of cases the infectious process is arrested by the host's generation of a cell-mediated immune (CMI) response. The sequence of events that ensues after phagocytosis of mycobacteria by macrophages involves the interaction of different T-cell subsets and their soluble products, as well as macrophages and other inflammatory cells. Once the mycobacteria are internalized by inactivated macrophages they continue to proliferate by evading intracellular killing mechanisms. At the same time, antigenic epitopes of the microorganism are processed for presentation to and recognition by T cells. This T-cell recognition and the subsequent release of cytokines leads to a state of macrophage activation and granuloma formation that, in the majority of cases, results in the suppression of mycobacterial proliferation. Two important populations of CD4+ T cells can be identified in the response to mycobacterial infection: Th1 cells produce interleukin 2 (IL-2) and γ-interferon (IFN-γ), which act as effector and regulatory elements in the cellular immune response; and Th2 cells produce IL-4, IL-5, IL-6, and IL-10, and provide help to B cells in the production of different immunoglobulins and the regulation of the humoral immune response. Other cytokines, such as IL-3, tumor necrosis factor alpha (TNF-α) and granulocyte-macrophage colony stimulating factor (GM-CSF), are secreted by both Th1 and Th2 subsets. The degree of the resulting T-cell activation and the local concentration of antigen determine the outcome of TB. In over 95% of cases this immune response achieves the containment of MTB but does not completely eradicate it (Fig. 77–3). This leaves the person infected with bacilli. During this period of "latent" infection individuals are asymptomatic and noninfectious. The only evidence that they harbor viable bacilli is the presence of CMI, detectable by tuberculin skin testing, in which the intradermal injection of a purified protein derivative of MTB elicits an immune response manifest by induration at the injection site. Efforts are underway to develop serologic assays to detect tuberculous infection.

ACTIVE DISEASE. Progression from latent infection to active disease is dictated by the balance between the virulent properties of the organism and the host defenses. Infection remains controlled in 90% of infected persons, who will live their whole lives oblivious to the fact that they harbor viable mycobacteria. However, other patients progress to active disease when the balance is tipped in favor of the bacilli (Fig. 77–3). Overall, 5% of patients progress to disease within 2 years of infection, and another 5% do so during the remainder of their lives. These numbers are dramatically different in patients who have compromised CMI systems. Direct progression to disease at the time of initial infection is particularly common in children <5 years of age. The likelihood of progressing to active disease over the patient's lifetime is increased by a factor of 2 to 3 in persons with moderately immunocompromising conditions, e.g., diabetes. The most profound increase in disease rates is seen in persons with advanced HIV infection. In such patients, progression to disease within 3 months of infection occurs in as many as one third of cases and the rate of subsequent progression is 7 to 10% per year. There is also some suggestion from epidemiologic studies that the genetic composition of certain ethnic groups, e.g., those of African descent, may confer an increased susceptibility to infection. Characteristics that may confer partial resistance to infection include previous infection with MTB, infection with atypical mycobacteria, and immunization with BCG.

■ CLINICAL MANIFESTATIONS
Pleuropulmonary Tuberculosis

In the vast majority of cases of TB, the lung is both the primary site of infection and of disease manifestation. Also, virtually all new infections are the result of transmission from a person with active pulmonary disease. Hence, pulmonary TB is the most important form of the disease both in terms of clinical manifestations and control issues.

PRIMARY INFECTIONS. Initial infection with MTB does not usually produce symptoms, although it may cause mild, self-limited fever and malaise. This phase of the infection is most often undetected and radiographic changes are minimal or not present. On occasion, and particularly in children, enlargement of hilar, mediastinal, or subcarinal lymph nodes may be apparent (Fig. 77–4). Partial or complete obstruction of the airway may lead to segmental hyperinflation or atelectasis (Fig. 77–5). Although hematogenous and lymphogenous spread is common during primary infection, the process is usually contained by the development of CMI. Cutaneous manifestations have been reported during primary infection and may include erythema nodosum and erythema induratum, but these are rare.

Pulmonary TB may occur soon after infection (*primary tuberculosis*) or well after the primary focus has been contained (*reactivation* or *postprimary disease*). In the former case, failure of the host's immune response to contain the initial focus of infection results in progressive disease at the site of initial implantation. Lower lobe infiltrates are common and ipsilateral hilar adenopathy is often a feature (Fig. 77–4); cavitation is infrequent early on but may be present as the disease progresses. Atelectasis, resulting from impingement of enlarging lymph nodes on the airway, is a common presenting picture in children. Associated pleural effusions are also frequent. Primary TB has been typically described as a disease of children, although in developed countries it has increasingly been identified in adults. This fact is partly a function of the changing epidemiology of the disease and the shift to a later age of acquisition of infection in low prevalence areas. Increasing rates of HIV infection, which causes

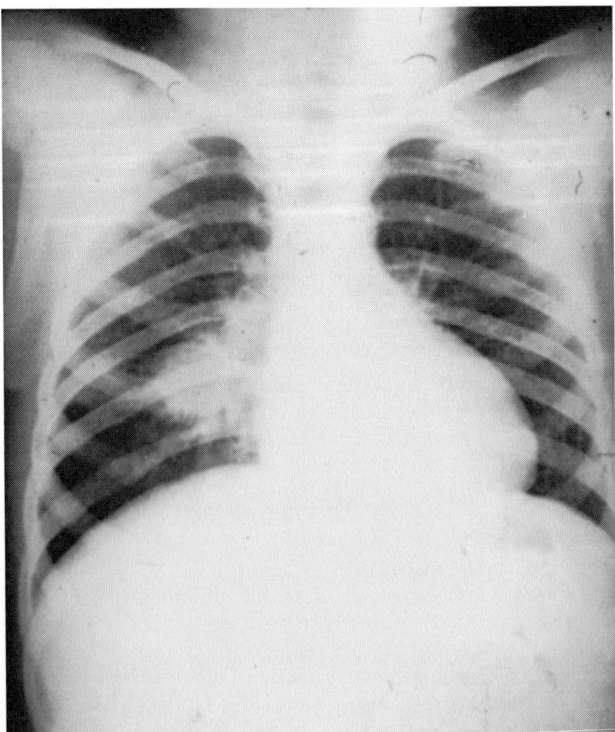

Figure 77–4. Primary infection. Posteroanterior chest roentgenogram shows an infiltrate in the periphery of the right middle zone of the lungs, with enlargement of lymph nodes in the right hilum.

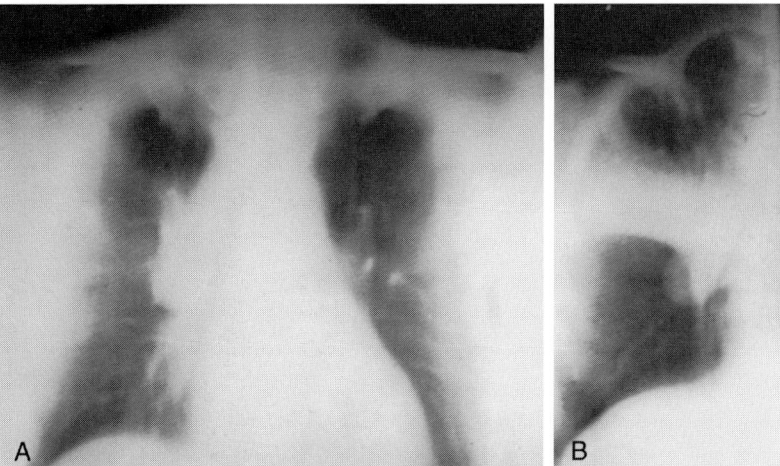

Figure 77–5. Adenopathy and bronchial obstruction. Chest tomograms show right hilar and paratracheal adenopathy *(A)* with right middle lobe collapse due to extreme pressure on the bronchi *(B)*.

profound CMI defect and predisposes to progression of primary infection, have also contributed to this trend.

REACTIVATION OR POSTPRIMARY TUBERCULOSIS. This is the result of the proliferation of organisms in a previously dormant focus of infection, usually implanted during the primary dissemination phase of the infection, often in the distant past. As opposed to primary disease, which may occur anywhere in the lung, *reactivation disease* most often affects the apical posterior segments of the upper lobes, followed by the superior segments of the lower lobes (Fig. 77–6). The characteristics of this form of the disease are chronicity and progressive worsening. Adenopathy is uncommon and nodular infiltrates and cavities (Fig. 77–7) are frequently seen; as the disease progresses fibrosis becomes a prominent feature. This is the most common form of TB, occurring in up to 90% of adult, non–HIV infected patients.

SYMPTOMS. The onset of constitutional and pulmonary symptoms is often insidious but they increase with disease progression. However, even patients who have extensive radiographic evidence of bilateral, cavitary, or multilobar disease may present with minimal symptoms. The most common symptom referable to the lung is cough, which in the early stages is often nonproductive. With increasing extension of the lesions, involvement of the airways also increases, and sputum production occurs. Cough may be mild and may occur only in the morning, when secretions accumulated during the night are more likely to be expectorated. Frank hemoptysis is unusual early in the course of the disease but may be a feature when extensive necrosis of the lung parenchyma has occurred. It may also result from erosion of cavitary lesions into adjacent blood vessels or from residual bronchiectasis. Uncommonly, hemoptysis may result from the rupture of an affected lymph node into the airway. Occasionally, an old cavity hosts an aspergillus fungus ball which may erode through the fibrotic walls, resulting in hemoptysis. Although TB is currently a rare cause of massive hemoptysis

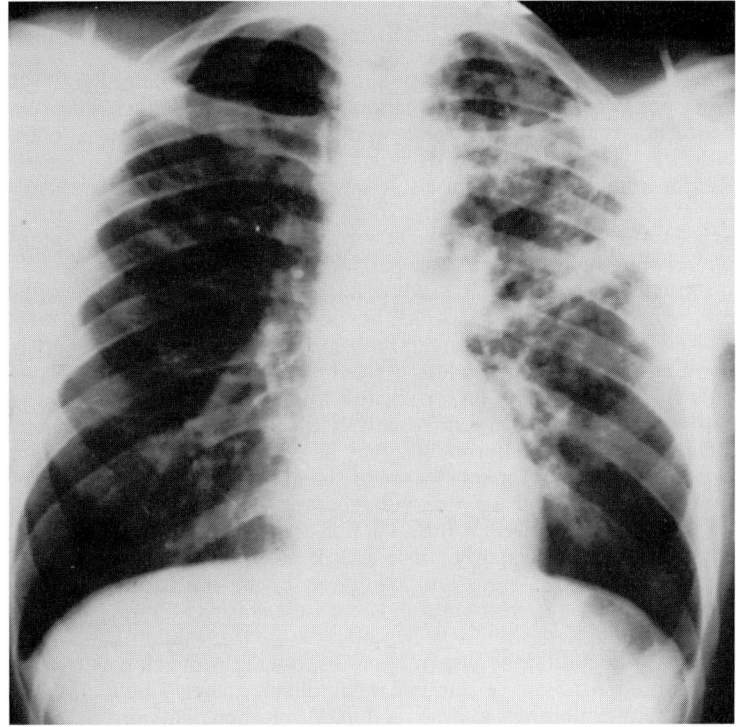

Figure 77–6. Adult recrudescent tuberculosis. Posteroanterior chest roentgenogram reveals nodular and linear infiltrates in the left and middle zones of the left lung.

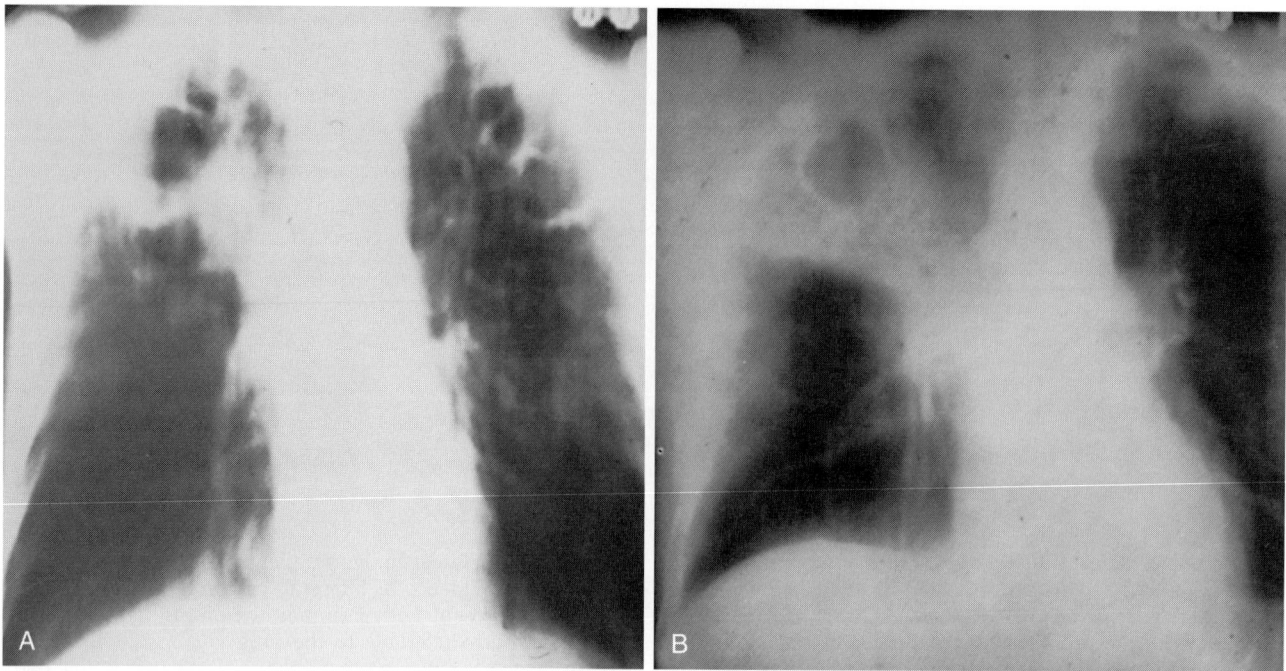

Figure **77–7.** Chronic cavitary tuberculosis. The chest tomograms show tuberculous disease in both lungs (*A* and *B*). It is more marked in both right lungs with cavitation at the apex.

in affluent countries, it was its most common cause before the advent of antituberculous chemotherapy and may still be an important cause in parts of the world where delayed diagnosis is common. Dyspnea is an unusual symptom unless extensive lung destruction has occurred or a large pleural effusion is present. Occasionally, the rupture of a caseous lesion into a bronchus results in rapid endobronchial spread of disease and respiratory failure. Chest pain is unusual and when present signifies localized pleural inflammation. The rare occurrence of spontaneous pneumothorax may result in acute pleuritic chest pain and dyspnea.

The most readily quantified systemic manifestation is fever, but this sign may be conspicuously absent early in the process; conversely, patients who are febrile on presentation are more likely to be symptomatic and have a higher incidence of cavitation and positive sputum smears. Fever has been variously reported to occur in 35 to 80% of patients. Weight loss and fatigue are also commonly reported, and a recent prospective study found them to occur in 74% and 68% of 188 patients, respectively. In the same study, night sweats were reported in 55% of patients.

LABORATORY FINDINGS. Hyponatremia, which in the prechemotherapy era was deemed a poor prognostic factor, is likely to be mediated through the action of an antidiuretic hormone–like substance released from affected lung tissue. This abnormality has been reported in up to 11% of patients and is probably more common with extensive lung involvement. Hematologic abnormalities may be varied and primarily consist of slight leukocytosis and anemia, although leukemoid reactions and leukopenia have also been reported.

PREDISPOSING DISEASES. TB frequently occurs with other diseases, particularly those associated with immunosuppression. Hence, signs and symptoms of the concurrent illness may mask or confound those of tuberculosis. A high index of suspicion should be maintained when evaluating patients with conditions known to predispose to the development of tuberculosis, e.g., chronic renal failure, diabetes mellitus, malnutrition, neoplasms, and HIV infection. Patients

with silicosis—a common condition in areas where mining is a prevalent activity—develop TB with a higher frequency than their normal counterparts, and their chest radiographs are often abnormal at baseline and difficult to evaluate.

PHYSICAL FINDINGS. The physical examination is not usually very helpful in establishing the diagnosis of pulmonary TB, since findings are neither sensitive nor specific. Crackles may be heard over areas of infiltration, and may be elicited early in disease by auscultation of the supraclavicular region. Amphoric or cavernous breath sounds are sometimes associated with areas of cavitation. Occasionally, an endobronchial lesion results in localized wheezing, which may be accentuated during forced expiration. Extrapulmonary physical findings are encountered in less than 5% of patients with pulmonary TB without HIV infection (and in 25% of patients with concomitant HIV). The most frequent sites of involvement are lymph nodes, bones and joints, and the urinary system.

Extrapulmonary Tuberculosis

Although TB most often affects the lungs, it is a systemic infection that may involve any organ. Extrapulmonary TB affected approximately 15% of all TB patients in the United States before the HIV era. In HIV-infected individuals, both the absolute and relative rates of extrapulmonary involvement are markedly increased. Several series show that extrapulmonary involvement, either alone or coexisting with lung involvement, affects up to two thirds of HIV patients with TB. Extrapulmonary involvement is also more frequent at the extremes of age, disproportionally affecting children <3 years of age and the elderly. Because of the relative inaccessibility of extrapulmonary sites, TB outside the lungs may present difficult diagnostic problems, and because clinicians may be less familiar with these forms of the disease, the diagnosis may be delayed. In developing areas of the world where TB is very prevalent, it may account for a significant proportion of cases of meningitis, osteomyelitis, arthritis, pericarditis, uveitis, and other diseases not often thought of as TB in the more developed regions of the world.

Tuberculous Adenitis

Lymph node TB is the most common form of extrapulmonary involvement, affecting up to 10% of all patients in some areas and occurring in more than 40% of those with extrapulmonary involvement. Although the nontuberculous mycobacteria cause a large proportion of mycobacterial lymph node infections in developed countries, organisms of the MTB complex account for the majority of cases in parts of the world where TB is more prevalent. Tuberculous lymphadenitis is primarily a disease of children in most developing countries where the incidence of TB in childhood is high. In the United States and other developed nations, childhood TB is uncommon, and most cases of lymphadenitis occur in the second and third decades of life. Both ethnic origin and sex seem to affect the risk of developing TB of the lymph nodes. Many studies report a 2:1 female:male ratio, and several surveys from the United States, Great Britain, and Australia point to a predisposition for the syndrome in patients from the Indian subcontinent, Southeast Asia and Africa, as well as in Native American and Hispanic patients. Also, HIV infection is a strong risk factor for extrapulmonary involvement in general and lymphatic tuberculosis in particular.

CLINICAL MANIFESTATIONS. More than 90% of palpable tuberculous lymph nodes are in the head and neck region (see Fig. 12–4). Commonly, several nodes within a group are affected, and bilateral involvement is not unusual, particularly in children. Generalized lymphadenopathy and hepatosplenomegaly are uncommon, occurring in 10 to 15% of cases of childhood miliary TB. Involvement of the axillary, epitrochlear, or inguinal nodes is rare and usually signifies the presence of a distal primary focus of infection on an extremity. Although most adults who present with tuberculous adenitis have no evidence of intrathoracic adenopathy, that is not the case in children with cervical lymphadenopathy, in whom intrathoracic involvement is present in up to 80%.

Cervical lymphadenopathy usually manifests as a painless, slowly growing neck mass that develops over weeks to months. If left untreated, most patients develop a chronically draining sinus tract, and this may be a common presenting complaint in tropical regions of the world. Systemic symptoms may or may not be present but are usually not very prominent, except when lymphadenitis presents in the context of miliary spread in children or immunocompromised patients, or when very enlarged hilar nodes cause bronchial obstruction leading to lobar atelectasis or lung collapse. This last scenario is more frequent in children, and the right middle lobe is most commonly affected.

DIAGNOSIS. Although the differential diagnosis of lymphadenitis is extensive and includes many infectious, neoplastic, and collagen vascular diseases, in most developing regions of the world TB is the most common cause of chronic, painless lymphadenopathy. Although the definitive diagnosis requires the isolation of MTB in culture, the histopathologic features of epithelioid cell granuloma with or without giant cells and caseation necrosis are very suggestive of the diagnosis (Fig. 77–8). Fine-needle aspiration is the diagnostic procedure of choice. Incisional biopsies should be avoided because of the high frequency of sinus tract formation.

THERAPY. The treatment of choice is short-course chemotherapy (see under Treatment of Pulmonary Tuberculosis), although in the past both surgical treatment and prolonged (18 months) courses of chemotherapy were advocated.

Genitourinary Tuberculosis

TB of the genitourinary tract is one of the most common forms of extrapulmonary involvement, representing up to 15% of all extrapulmonary cases and 2% of all TB cases in the United States.

PATHOPHYSIOLOGY. Renal TB is the result of hematogenous seeding, usually from a pulmonary focus. Initial infection occurs in the capillaries of the renal cortex because of the large proportion of the cardiac output that traverses them and the high oxygen tension at this site. After the initial infection is contained by the development of CMI, a fibrous scar can form and harbor viable bacilli for indefinite periods. These foci may then reactivate, giving rise to postprimary renal disease. During active disease, granuloma formation and tissue necrosis result in the shedding of bacilli into the tubular lumen and spread of infection deeper into the medulla. Progressive tissue destruction may lead to cavitation and involvement of the renal papillae. Bacilli appear in the urine and "sterile" pyuria and hematuria may result. On

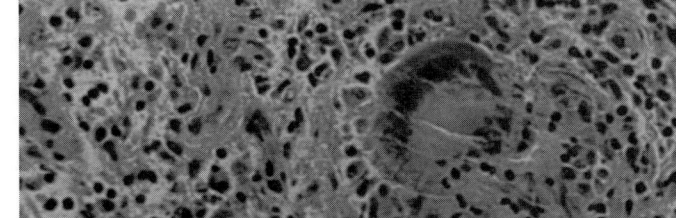

Figure 77–8. Caseating granuloma with multinucleated giant cells at the periphery.

occasion, debris may lead to caliceal and even ureteral obstruction. Deformity of the involved kidney results from a combination of necrosis, fibrotic scars, and mass lesions (tuberculomas). Calcifications are often seen, both in progressive disease and in healed lesions. When severe hydronephrosis results from ureteral obstruction, the renal parenchyma may be only a thin shell surrounding large calcified caseous lesions that fill the renal pelvis. Total loss of function of the involved kidney, so called autonephrectomy, may result. In the male, the disease may involve the seminal vesicle, epididymis, or prostate. Many patients with renal tuberculosis are asymptomatic, and early in the disease radiologic signs may be absent. It is not unusual for patients to come to medical attention because of incidental findings such as sterile pyuria or occult hematuria. At such times, the evaluation may disclose extensive necrosis, even before the development of any symptoms. When present, the most common symptoms are referable to the urinary tract rather than constitutional. A recent series of 81 patients from Spain reported local symptoms, e.g., dysuria, urgency, and flank pain in more than 90% of patients, whereas fever, the most common constitutional symptom, was present in only 35.

DIAGNOSIS. Urinary tract TB should be suspected whenever unexplained urinary symptoms are present or when persistent urinary sediment abnormalities, e.g., sterile pyuria are noted. In such instances, several early-morning urine specimens should be cultured for mycobacteria, since these are positive in more than 80% of patients. Acid-fast smears are much less frequently positive, and false positive smears may result from nonpathogenic mycobacteria in the external genitalia.

Radiographic abnormalities are usually present, except very early in the course of the disease. The intravenous pyelogram is the procedure of choice for evaluating renal TB; the retrograde pyelogram is sensitive for detecting abnormalities of the collecting system. CT scans may be very sensitive for early nodular lesions and for identifying nonfunctioning segments of the kidney, and an abdominal ultrasound examination of the kidneys, ureters, and prostate can usually detect abnormalities if present. The ultrasound may be the most readily available diagnostic procedure in smaller hospitals in developing countries.

FEMALE GENITAL TRACT TUBERCULOSIS. This is an unusual form of extrapulmonary involvement. It most often results from hematogenous spread but may rarely be due to intercourse with a partner with active disease. The fallopian tubes and endometrium are almost always affected, whereas the ovaries and cervix are involved in 20% and less than 1% of cases, respectively. Infertility and pelvic pain are common presenting complaints. The diagnosis requires endometrial curettage, ultrasound, laparoscopy or laparotomy.

Disseminated Tuberculosis

The terms miliary or disseminated TB are used interchangeably for the diffuse multiorgan involvement that occurs when inadequate host defenses cannot contain TB infection. This may occur either at the time of initial infection (primary dissemination) or later after containment of the initial infection. Although the term miliary was originally coined to describe the typical millet seed pattern seen in pathologic specimens, it has now come to be associated with the radiographic appearance of the lung involvement, which shows many small (2 mm) nodular interstitial infiltrates (Fig. 77–9). The same type of involvement, reflecting massive hematogenous seeding, can usually be found in most organs in the body.

PATHOLOGY. The gross appearance of involved organs is

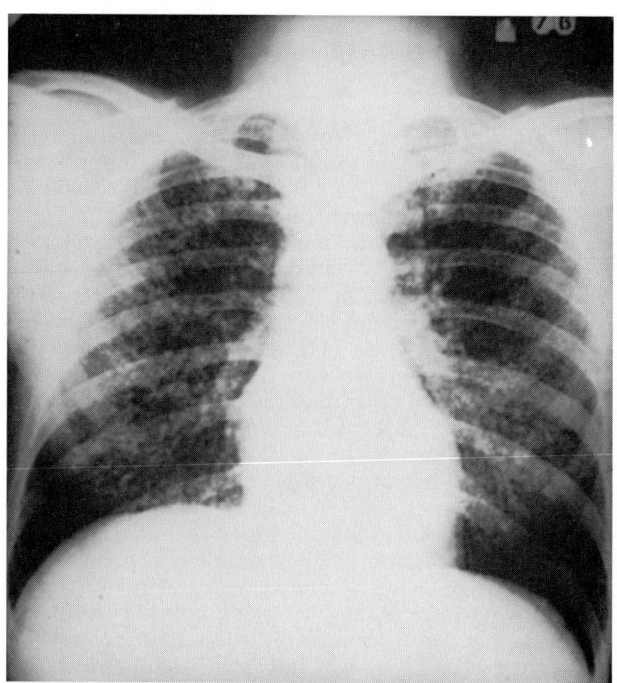

Figure 77–9. Miliary tuberculosis. Posteroanterior chest roentgenogram shows extensive bilateral miliary nodulations.

that of a tissue studded with small, punctate lesions, of uniform size and even distribution. Lesions can often be demonstrated in the spleen, liver, bone marrow, kidneys, adrenals, and eyes. Less frequent sites of involvement include the pancreas, thyroid, prostate, heart, testes, and pituitary.

EPIDEMIOLOGY. The incidence of miliary tuberculosis has decreased significantly in most developed nations since the advent of modern chemotherapy, both in absolute terms and as a proportion of all TB cases. In the United States miliary TB was reported in only 1.3% of all TB cases between 1969 and 1988. In sharp contrast is the observation from the prechemotherapy era, when at Boston City Hospital, 20% of all autopsied cases of TB had evidence of miliary spread. A recent increase in the relative incidence of miliary TB has been described in the United States and elsewhere and is largely due to the increased susceptibility of HIV-infected patients to dissemination of the infection. Although in affluent nations miliary TB has become a disease of the elderly, in high-incidence areas of the world where tuberculous infection is usually acquired early in life, most cases of miliary disease occur in children. Miliary spread is also more frequently seen in populations with poor access to treatment.

CLINICAL MANIFESTATIONS. The clinical manifestations of miliary TB are varied and range from the adult respiratory distress syndrome (ARDS) and multiorgan system failure to fever of unknown origin without obvious localizing findings. Fever and weight loss are the most commonly presenting symptoms. Other reported symptoms include cough, dyspnea, headache, hemoptysis, and weakness (Table 77–3). Establishing the diagnosis is very important, since the untreated disease is almost uniformly lethal. In the mid 1980s in the United States, almost 20% of cases of miliary TB were not diagnosed until after death. The typical patient presents with a febrile wasting syndrome of several months' duration and often has a coexisting debilitating illness. Severe malnutrition is often a common predisposing factor. Although the typical chest film pattern is that of many tiny nodular lesions, no abnormalities may be apparent on presentation, particu-

TABLE 77–3. Reported Presenting Symptoms in Miliary Tuberculosis

Symptom (%)	Gelb et al (N = 109)	Munt (N = 67)	Prout and Benatar (N = 59)	Kim et al (N = 38)
Fever	85	84	44	89
Weight loss	87	85	59	66
Cough	69	66	63	55
Weakness	NR	93	42	53
Headache	16	10	17	5
Hemoptysis	12	6	8	10
Dyspnea	29	<1	37	50

NR, not reported.

From Gelb AF, Leffler C, Brewin A, et al: Miliary tuberculosis. Am Rev Respir Dis 108:1327, 1973; Munt PW: Miliary tuberculosis in the chemotherapy era. Medicine 51:139, 1972; Prout S, Benatar R: Disseminated tuberculosis: A study of 62 cases. S Afr Med J 58:835, 1980; Kim JH, Langston AA, Gallis HA: Miliary tuberculosis: Epidemiology, clinical manifestations, diagnosis and outcome. Rev Infect Dis 12:583, 1990.

larly in patients with CMI defects. Miliary TB may present as ARDS. In a 1985 series from South Africa, miliary TB accounted for 2% of all ARDS cases during a 4-year period. Disseminated TB should be carefully ruled out in all HIV-infected patients presenting with diffuse alveolar infiltrates and hypoxemia, particularly if steroids are to be administered as part of the therapy for *Pneumocystis carinii* pneumonia.

Uveal choroidal tubercles are highly suggestive of disseminated TB but may also be present in localized pulmonary TB. Palpable organomegaly is variable and more commonly seen in children. Histologic involvement of the liver, however, is very frequent. In a large autopsy series, 50% of the eyes examined had choroidal involvement and 97% of examined livers exhibited granulomas, the majority of which were caseating (Fig. 77–8). Signs of hepatic involvement are often present, usually in the form of an alkaline phosphatase level elevation. A cholestatic picture is rarely seen. Urinary tract involvement may manifest as proteinuria, microscopic hematuria or pyuria, but frank renal failure is rarely seen. Clinical involvement of the central nervous system (CNS) has been reported in 16 to 30% of patients, and meningeal involvement and granulomatous involvement of the adrenals was present in almost half of postmortem examinations. Clinical adrenal insufficiency, however, occurs in about 1% of cases of disseminated TB.

DIAGNOSIS. A miliary pattern is seen on the initial chest film in more than half of presenting cases, and this pattern may develop up to several weeks later in some patients. Although there are many possible causes for a miliary radiographic pattern in a febrile patient, TB is its most common one in areas of the world where this disease is endemic (Table 77–4). Sputum cultures are only positive in up to 30% of cases and a similar yield can be expected for urine cultures. Histologic demonstration of typical granulomatous involvement is helpful and can be achieved by sampling the liver, bone marrow or the lung, as well as any involved serosal surface.

THERAPY. The treatment of miliary TB should be as for pulmonary disease and should, when possible, be guided by the result of drug susceptibility testing. A 6-month course appears adequate when organisms are fully susceptible and patients are immunocompetent. In HIV-co-infected patients therapy should be given for 9 months or, when documentation is possible, for 6 months after culture conversion. When meningeal or bone and joint dissemination is present, therapy may also need to be extended.

Osteoarticular Tuberculosis

Seeding of long bones, joints, and vertebral bodies usually occurs at the time of the initial bacillemia and is more common when primary infection occurs early in life. Bone and joint involvement may occasionally result from contiguous spread from affected adjacent tissues. Disease may occur soon after the *primary infection* or during *reactivation*. In the developing world osteoarticular disease most often occurs in children and young adults, whereas in more developed nations it has been primarily a disease of the elderly.

CLINICAL MANIFESTATIONS. Tuberculous arthritis can occur in any joint but most often involves the weight-bearing joints affecting, in descending order of frequency, the hip (see Fig. 13–6), knee, ankle, and foot. Non–weight-bearing joints commonly affected include those in the spine, the shoulder, elbow, and wrist. The spine is the most common site of bony involvement, accounting for more than 40 to 60% of all cases of skeletal tuberculosis. The thoracolumbar region is most commonly affected (see Fig. 13–4), with the cervical vertebrae affected in 2 to 3% of patients. Pott disease, as vertebral TB is called, usually begins as a diskitis, with one intervertebral disk and the adjacent vertebral end plates affected. It then progresses to cause disk space narrowing, vertebral end-plate destruction, and anterior vertebral body collapse (Fig. 77–10). The infection often extends to the paraspinal tissues, forming cold abscesses that may be paravertebral (see Fig. 13–5), in and around the psoas muscles or retropharyngeal, depending

TABLE 77–4. Miliary Infiltrates With Fever— Differential Diagnosis

  I. Infectious diseases
    A. Mycobacterial
      1. *M. tuberculosis**
      2. Atypical mycobacteria in immunocompromised hosts
    B. Fungal
      1. Histoplasmosis*
      2. Coccidiomycosis*
      3. Blastomycosis*
      4. Cryptococcosis
    C. Viral
      1. Varicella*
      2. Influenza*
      3. Measles*
      4. Cytomegalovirus infection
    D. Bacterial
      1. Mycoplasma infection
      2. Nocardiosis
      3. *Legionella micdadei* infection
      4. Brucellosis
      5. *Staphylococcus aureus*
      6. Melioidosis
      7. Psittacosis
      8. Tularemia
    E. Parasitic
      1. Schistosomiasis
      2. Toxoplasmosis
      3. Strongyloidiasis
  II. Neoplastic diseases
    A. Lymphoma
  III. Inflammatory diseases
    A. Hypersensitivity pneumonitis*
    B. Sarcoidosis
    C. Goodpasture syndrome
    D. Other alveolar hemorrhage syndromes

*More common causes.

From Baker SK, Glassroth J: Miliary tuberculosis. *In* Rom WN, Garay SM (eds): Tuberculosis. New York, Little, Brown, 1996.

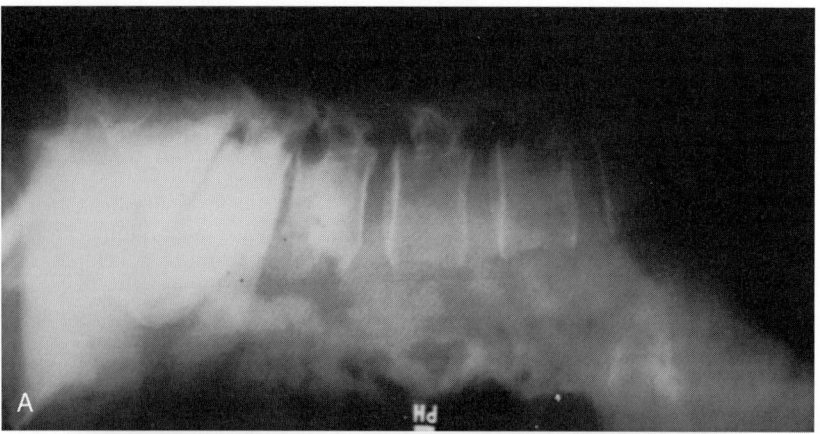

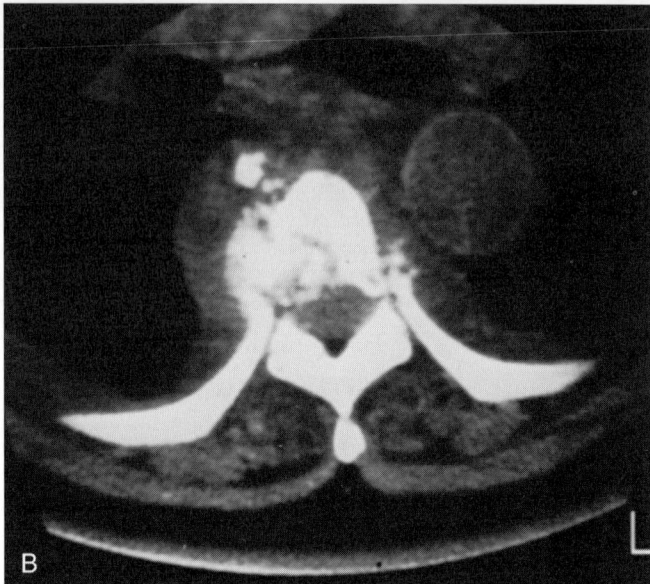

Figure **77-10.** Pott's disease. *A*, Lateral roentgenogram of the spine shows destruction of the body of the fourth lumbar vertebra; *B*, CT scan of the fourth lumbar vertebra reveals considerable destruction.

on the site of disease. Severe gibbus deformity and paraplegia are unfortunate complications that are still commonly seen in high-incidence regions of the world.

DIAGNOSIS. The diagnosis of osteoarticular TB should be suspected whenever monoarticular arthritis or a clinical picture suggestive of osteomyelitis is encountered in any patient with a likelihood of past tuberculous exposure. Joint effusions should be tapped and, when possible, synovial biopsy performed. Acid-fast smears are positive in only 20% of cases, but cultures yield the diagnosis in up to 80% of cases when synovial fluid is used and in more than 90% of cases when the synovium is cultured. Granulomatous involvement of the synovium is highly suggestive of tuberculosis. In vertebral disease, the best diagnostic yield is achieved through the use of CT-guided needle biopsy of the affected vertebra or an adjacent abscess.

THERAPY. Most cases of osteoarticular TB can be successfully treated with conventional short-course chemotherapy. For appendicular TB, surgery is indicated only as a diagnostic tool and to drain abscesses unresponsive to medical therapy. Surgery may be indicated for patients with vertebral TB complicated by neurologic deficits, spinal instability, or large paravertebral or psoas abscesses. Although no controlled trials have addressed the appropriate duration of antituberculous chemotherapy in vertebral disease, most authorities recommend extending the course for 9 to 12 months.

Central Nervous System Tuberculosis

TUBERCULOUS MENINGITIS. This is the most common form of CNS involvement in TB. Although CNS disease may occur at any age, the peak incidence is seen in infants and children <4 years of age. It also occurs with greater frequency in HIV-infected individuals, in whom brain tuberculomas are also noted with appreciable frequency. CNS disease represents approximately 5% of extrapulmonary cases and affects males and females with the same frequency.

Meningeal involvement results from seeding and proliferation of tubercle bacilli during hematogenous dissemination, either at the time of initial bacillemia or when there is breakdown of an old pulmonary or extrapulmonary focus. Breakdown of a previously inactive parameningeal or subependymal focus may also directly seed the subarachnoid space.

CLINICAL MANIFESTATIONS. Patients may have varying degrees of meningitis, myelitis, and encephalitis. The inflammation and bacillary invasion of the blood vessels may give rise to arteritis and thrombotic vascular occlusion, leading to localized ischemia and cerebral infarction. Formation of fibrous tissue, particularly at the base of the brain, may lead to complications, e.g., cranial nerve palsies, hydrocephalus, and spinal block. Symptoms at presentation usually include headache, decreased level of consciousness, and neck stiffness, with or without evidence of cranial nerve involvement. The duration of symptoms prior to presentation is quite variable and depends in part on involvement of other sites, but the disease can often pursue a subacute or indolent course. In most series the majority of patients have coexisting chest film abnormalities, either from old or active pulmonary TB. Miliary involvement is often present. Up to 50% of patients with tuberculous meningitis may have positive sputum cultures, suggesting that pulmonary or systemic complaints may be commonly found in addition to those referable to CNS involvement. Focal ischemic symptoms may be prominent in patients in whom arteritis is the predominant manifestation of meningitis.

DIAGNOSIS. The physical examination offers no specific findings for tuberculous meningitis, with the exception of the funduscopic examination, which may reveal the presence of choroidal tubercles. Although this last sign is very suggestive of TB, it is often not present or is missed. Hence the diagnosis is made on examination of the cerebrospinal fluid (CSF). The characteristic findings include increased opening pressure, pleocytosis and increased protein concentration, and low glucose concentration. The cell count is usually between 100 and 1000, and lymphocytes are the predominant cell type in more than 70% of patients. The protein concentration is almost always elevated, but when it is very high (> 300 mg/dL) it may indicate obstruction of CSF flow and portends a poor prognosis. Microscopic examination reveals acid-fast bacilli in only 10 to 20% of patients, and cultures are positive in 50 to 80%. Because tuberculous meningitis often coexists with other forms of TB, the organism may be isolated from other foci. The isolation of MTB from any site in the setting of compatible CSF findings should be sufficient to diagnose tuberculous meningitis.

THERAPY. The treatment of tuberculous meningitis should follow the same principles as that of lung disease, except that ethambutol at the usual doses does not achieve adequate CSF levels; hence streptomycin should be used. Prognosis is related in part to the duration of the disease, and hence any delay in initiation of treatment should be avoided. Although 6 to 9 months of treatment is adequate for most forms of extrapulmonary disease, 12 months of treatment are recommended for meningitis. The addition of corticosteroids has a beneficial effect on the outcome of tuberculous meningitis, especially when cerebral edema or severe inflammation are present.

The mortality of tuberculous meningitis is high even in the context of adequate chemotherapy; reported rates vary between 20 and 50%. Morbidity in survivors is also high, with neurologic sequelae seen in up to 30%.

TUBERCULOMA. This is the second most common form of CNS involvement in TB. It usually presents with a more indolent course than meningitis, and the predominant symptoms are those of a slowly enlarging brain mass. Increased intracranial pressure in the absence of focal findings may also occur. The CSF is usually normal and the diagnosis is suspected after the mass is revealed by imaging with CT scanning or magnetic resonance imaging (MRI). Subsequent resection or aspiration of the lesion confirms the diagnosis but is not necessary for adequate treatment since the response to antituberculous chemotherapy is good. Transient enlargement of the lesion after treatment has been instituted occurs with some frequency but usually reverts without any change in management. Corticosteroids should be used when intracranial pressure is increased, focal neurologic findings are present, or symptoms worsen during antitubercular chemotherapy.

Pericarditis

Tuberculous pericarditis is a rare but severe presentation of TB. Although this disease represents only 2 to 3% of all extrapulmonary cases and accounts for no more than 4% of acute pericarditis in the industrialized world, its impact is much greater in areas where TB is endemic. In recent reports from Transkei, South Africa, TB accounted for 80% of pericarditis cases.

CLINICAL MANIFESTATIONS. Pericardial TB may occur as a result of direct extension from adjacent infected lymph nodes or pleuropulmonary tissues, or it may result from hematogenous seeding. The initial granulomatous reaction gives rise to a serous or serosanguineous effusion, and the pericardial surfaces become thickened and gray. Fibrosis and constrictive pericarditis may ensue. At the beginning the pericardial fluid contains primarily polymorphonuclear cells, but after a few days lymphocytes predominate. Total cell counts range from 500 to 10,000 cells/mL. Low glucose and high protein are common findings. Massive effusions, of up to 4 L, have been described. The patient usually complains of substernal chest pain and shortness of breath. Cardiac tamponade may be present, manifested as neck vein distention, hepatomegaly, edema, and pulsus paradoxus. The most important physical finding of pericarditis is a pericardial friction rub, but this sign may be absent when effusions are large.

DIAGNOSIS. TB pericarditis should be suspected when cardiac symptoms coexist with night sweats, malaise, and the epidemiologic likelihood of TB in someone in or from a developing country. On chest films, the cardiac shadow may be enlarged in the acute stage but may be normal or small in the chronic phase. The electrocardiogram may show global ST-segment elevation and a characteristic PR-segment depression. Echocardiogram is crucial to the diagnosis of pericardial effusion, and pericardiocentesis with pericardial biopsy usually confirms the tuberculous etiology.

THERAPY. The risk of death from untreated pericardial TB may exceed 80%, and even when adequate treatment is instituted, mortality ranges between 14 and 40%. Chemotherapy for this condition should include corticosteroids, as they decrease mortality in acute cases. Doses of 60 to 80 mg/day of prednisone for 8 to 11 weeks have been used. Invasive surgical procedures should be considered for patients with acute cardiac tamponade, those with recurrent or progressive effusion or pericardial thickening, and those with constrictive pericarditis (Chapter 13).

Abdominal Tuberculosis

PREVALENCE. Although an uncommon disease in developed countries, abdominal TB remains a significant problem in most of the world. Tuberculosis can involve virtually any intra-abdominal site, but presents most commonly as diffuse peritonitis and focal intestinal disease. However, because there are no pathognomonic symptoms, signs, laboratory or radiographic findings, abdominal TB can be very difficult to diagnose.

The disease has become rare (less than 1 case per 100,000) in developed countries, where it is generally diagnosed in patients who are alcoholic, coinfected with HIV, or immigrants from high-prevalence countries. Accurate epidemiologic data are scarce from most low-income countries, but in some high-prevalence countries, e.g., India, abdominal TB may account for almost 1% of hospital admissions.

PATHOPHYSIOLOGY. Mycobacteria gain access to abdominal organs by ingestion and direct implantation in the gastrointestinal tract or by hematogenous seeding. In the prechemotherapy era abdominal TB was relatively common (occurring in about one quarter of patients with advanced pulmonary TB), presumably as a consequence of ingesting infected sputum. Consumption of infected dairy products is postulated to account for most cases of gastrointestinal *M. bovis.* In settings with good TB control programs and where milk products are pasteurized, abdominal TB is more likely due to reactivation of latent foci that were seeded at the time of initial infection.

CLINICAL MANIFESTATIONS. Tuberculous peritonitis commonly presents with the insidious onset of abdominal pain, swelling, fever, weight loss and anorexia, although any subset of these may be absent. The clinical presentation is particularly nonspecific in alcoholics, who have comparable symptoms as a result of underlying cirrhosis. The overlap between the clinical presentation of TB and other complications of HIV makes the diagnosis of tuberculosis particularly difficult in HIV-infected persons. The combination of abdominal pain and fever in patients with ascites should always prompt an evaluation for an infectious etiology.

DIAGNOSIS. Physical examination may reveal the characteristic "doughy abdomen" but most commonly is not helpful in establishing the diagnosis. Laboratory tests are consistent with chronic disease with anemia and an elevated erythrocyte sedimentation rate. Ascitic fluid is generally exudative, with a protein concentration exceeding 50% of the serum level and 50 to 10,000 leukocytes/μL (with a lymphocytic predominance). Acid-fast bacilli (AFB) are rarely seen on microscopic examination of fluid, and mycobacterial cultures yield *M. tuberculosis* in only 50% of cases. The yield of mycobacteriologic examination was improved to 83% in one study in which approximately 1 L of fluid was cultured. Radiographic evaluation with CT or ultrasound generally demonstrates ascites and may reveal adhesions suggestive of tuberculous peritonitis, but do not exclude other causes for these nonspecific findings. Laparoscopic examination (with histologic and mycobacteriologic examination of biopsy material) is currently the method of choice for diagnosing tuberculous peritonitis.

Tuberculosis may involve any region of the gastrointestinal tract from mouth to anus, but most commonly involves the ileum and cecum. Nonspecific complaints, e.g., abdominal pain, weight loss, fever, and diarrhea are common, and a significant number of patients present with bowel obstruction. Physical examination generally reveals tenderness and perhaps a mass. As in tuberculous peritonitis, laboratory evaluation is generally consistent with chronic disease, but there are no findings characteristic of intestinal TB. Barium studies of the gut and CT are useful steps in the evaluation of patients suspected of having gastrointestinal TB, but are rarely diagnostic. Endoscopic examination is the easiest and most direct method for diagnosing tuberculous colitis. When combined with histologic and mycobacterial examination of multiple biopsies of abnormal sites, the yield approaches 80%. Because the definitive diagnosis usually requires biopsy, the diagnosis is sometimes made only at the time of laparotomy.

THERAPY. Standard chemotherapy is adequate for the treatment of abdominal tuberculosis. Although most experience is with 9- and 12-month regimens, there is no reason that patients who are infected with organisms susceptible to first-line agents and who are compliant with therapy should not respond to the standard 6-month regimen. Patients with complete obstruction or perforation require surgical intervention, but the majority of patients with radiographically demonstrated strictures respond to medical therapy alone.

Tuberculosis and AIDS

Infection with HIV is the most potent risk factor for progression from tuberculous infection to active disease (Chapter 22).

PREVALENCE. Approximately 5 million people are esti-mated to harbor HIV and TB co-infection (Tables 77–1 and 77–2). It has been calculated that 14% of cases of TB occurring by the year 2000 will be attributable to HIV infection.

PATHOPHYSIOLOGY. CD4+ T lymphocytes and macrophages, which play a central role in the immune response against mycobacterial infection, are selectively and progressively depleted in the course of HIV infection. This results in a profound immunodeficiency state that sets the stage for the myriad opportunistic infections and neoplasms that have come to be associated with AIDS. In turn, infection with MTB can accelerate the course of HIV infection. The interaction of TB and HIV may increase the viral burden, accelerating the progression to advanced stages of HIV disease.

CLINICAL MANIFESTATIONS. Because MTB is a virulent organism in HIV infected people, it often causes disease early in the course of the infection, and TB is a common AIDS-defining condition in many developing nations. HIV infection predisposes patients to many conditions that may mimic the signs and symptoms of TB. Hence, although HIV may not alter the presentation of TB, it makes its symptoms (i.e., fatigue, weight loss, fever, cough, and anorexia) less specific. TB in HIV-infected people is often atypical when advanced immunosuppression is present. These patients have a high incidence of extrapulmonary disease, unusual radiographic images, and are frequently anergic. On the other hand, classic TB may be observed when the disease occurs before the development of severe immune deficit.

DIAGNOSIS. Because CMI is central to the response to intradermal PPD, anergy becomes increasingly common as the immune defect increases. Negative Mantoux skin tests should not be used to rule out the possibility of disease, and 5 mm of induration should be considered a positive test in this population. Whenever TB is suspected on clinical grounds, appropriate smears and cultures of all affected sites should be obtained. When sputum samples are negative or expectorated specimens cannot be obtained in patients clinically suspected of having pulmonary TB, bronchoscopy with bronchoalveolar lavage and transbronchial biopsy is indicated.

THERAPY. Therapy for TB in the HIV-infected patient yields very good results, contrary to the case with most other HIV-associated opportunistic infections. Standard short-course chemotherapy was effective in both retrospective reviews and prospective, controlled trials. In a recent study conducted in Haiti, a fully intermittent, directly observed antituberculous regimen was administered for 6 months to both HIV-infected and seronegative patients with pulmonary TB. In this study, the regimen was equally efficacious in both groups, resulting in cure rates of more than 80% and relapse rates of about 5%. Although short-course therapy may often be adequate, reported treatment failures have led to the recommendation that treatment be given for a minimum of 9 months and for at least 6 months after the patient has become culture negative. As in all cases of TB, directly observed therapy is strongly recommended because poor compliance is the strongest predictor of treatment failure.

Frequent symptom review and blood testing should be used to monitor patients receiving therapy, since adverse drug reactions are more frequently observed in HIV-infected patients. In addition, antituberculous chemotherapy may result in frequent adverse interactions with other medications commonly used in the course of HIV infection. Notably, rifampin may decrease ketoconazole, fluconazole, and clarithromycin serum levels. The complex interactions between protease inhibitors and other antiretroviral drugs and the rifamycins (rifampin, rifabutin, and rifapentene) require significant adjustments in patients receiving both classes of drugs.

CHEMOPROPHYLAXIS. Prevention of TB through the use of INH chemoprophylaxis can decrease the high rate of disease progression in HIV-infected people with positive PPD tests. Many issues regarding the appropriate length of chemoprophylaxis, as well as the role of secondary prophylaxis, remain unresolved.

■ DIAGNOSIS

Because of the protean nature of TB, its diagnosis depends on a high degree of suspicion on the part of clinicians. In areas of high prevalence of the disease, e.g., most tropical regions of the world, tuberculosis should be considered in the differential diagnosis of almost any chronic or acute pulmonary or systemic disease. Pulmonary TB should be carefully ruled out in any patient presenting with prolonged cough, whether or not any other signs or symptoms are present. Since physical findings are very nonspecific and have poor sensitivity, the definitive diagnosis rests on the results of the microbiologic examination of the sputum. In addition, evaluation of the chest radiographs plays a central role in both the diagnosis as well as in the determination of the extent and nature of pulmonary TB.

Chest Radiographs

Although no pathognomonic radiologic sign exists for TB, radiographic abnormalities are commonly present in pulmonary disease, and certain abnormalities can be highly suggestive of the disease. Patchy or nodular infiltrates in the apical and posterior segments of the upper lobes are most suggestive of reactivation disease (Fig. 77–6), particularly if the process is bilateral or cavitary (Fig. 77–7). Because plain radiographs may not fully delineate abnormalities, apical lordotic views may aid in the diagnosis of apical disease. Similarly, CT scans can be helpful in the evaluation of mediastinal structures and areas of the lung, e.g., the upper segment of the lower lobe, that may be obscured by the heart shadow. In addition, their higher resolution may reveal areas of nodular infiltration, sometimes with necrotic centers or early cavitation. Air-fluid levels are very rare in upper lobe cavitary TB but occur occasionally in cavities in the upper segments of the lower lobes. When cavities containing infectious caseous material erode into the bronchial tree, bronchogenic spread may result in the radiographic finding of multiple, discrete, fluffy infiltrates throughout both lungs. Lobar or segmental consolidations may also result from this process, but they seldom progress and usually resolve to smaller, more discrete lesions with regular edges. Although upper lobe cavitary changes are typical of TB (Fig. 77–7), other infectious and noninfectious processes, e.g., pyogenic bacterial pneumonias (particularly when caused by *Staphylococcus aureus, Klebsiella pneumoniae,* and anaerobes), fungal and nontuberculous mycobacteria infections, Wegener granulomatosis, and squamous cell carcinoma may also cause them.

Fibrotic scars, often exuberant, can be seen both in long-standing disease and in spontaneously healed TB. They frequently retract, producing a loss of pulmonary volume that is apparent in the chest film. In patients with spontaneously healed TB, changes in these abnormalities may indicate relapse, even after they have been stable for long periods of time.

The absence of these typical radiographic findings does not rule out the diagnosis. Even before the AIDS epidemic, atypical roentgenographic features were reported in up to one third of patients diagnosed with pulmonary TB. Findings, e.g., hilar and mediastinal adenopathy, pleural effusion, and lower lung zone infiltrates, are particularly common in primary disease. Other abnormalities include atelectasis (Fig. 77–5), single or multiple nodules (tuberculomas), miliary patterns (Fig. 77–9), and, rarely, pictures compatible with ARDS. The increase in the numbers of TB patients who are co-infected with HIV in many developing nations has led to an increase in the proportion of cases with an atypical radiographic presentation. In general, the degree of immunosuppression correlates with the radiographic appearance of TB; patients who develop TB early in the course of HIV infection tend to demonstrate roentgenographic findings typical of *reactivated disease*, whereas those who develop it in the later stages of HIV disease have abnormalities more suggestive of *primary tuberculosis* or even normal radiographs.

Microbiologic Evaluation

The definitive diagnosis of TB requires the isolation of MTB from the affected site. Isolation of the organism in culture is of paramount importance in settings in which drug resistance rates are high.

SPUTUM EXAMINATION. In the case of pulmonary TB, the obvious specimen of choice is sputum. Because of limited resources, the vast majority of persons in lesser developed nations are diagnosed solely on the basis of microscopic examination of sputum. However, this approach misses up to 50% of persons who are smear negative. Thus, whenever possible, and particularly in patients who are likely to harbor drug-resistant bacilli, culture and susceptibility testing is preferable. Sputum should be obtained as soon as TB is suspected, and if the initial smear is negative for acid-fast bacilli, additional specimens should be collected. Collection of sputum on arising results in the best yield, and single morning specimens have lower rates of contamination than pooled specimens. The optimal number of specimens is three, there being little improvement in the yield from two additional specimens, and no increase with more than five specimens.

When patients do not spontaneously produce sputum, several techniques can be used to procure a sample. The least invasive means is by inducing sputum production with the inhalation of aerosolized hypertonic (3 to 5%) saline solution. The resulting sputum is clear and thin and resembles saliva. Although this procedure is usually well tolerated, it may on occasion result in bronchospasm. Also, since sputum induction results in the production of high numbers of infectious particles, this should be carried out in well-ventilated, negative air pressure rooms to avoid the nosocomial spread of infection.

GASTRIC ASPIRATION. In patients for whom these measures are impractical, e.g., young children, aspiration of gastric contents through a nasogastric tube is another alternative. However, this procedure is uncomfortable and often requires an overnight stay in the hospital. Gastric aspiration should be performed in the early morning before arising and after an 8- to 10-hour fast. The stomach contents should be aspirated first and then 50 to 75 mL of sterile water should be used to irrigate and lavage the stomach. This second aspirate should be added to the first and the whole sample should undergo prompt acid neutralization with 10% sodium carbonate or 40% anhydrous sodium phosphate.

BRONCHOSCOPY. When the previous methods have failed to yield the diagnosis, and depending on the clinical situation and the available resources, bronchoscopy is another option, during which transbronchial biopsy should be considered to maximize the yield (particularly when miliary TB is suspected). In the evaluation of patients infected with HIV this approach has the added advantage of high yields for other pathogens, e.g., *Pneumocystis carinii*.

Pathologic Evaluation

When no readily available material exists for cultures and microscopic examination, particularly in the evaluation of extrapulmonary disease, a biopsy may be performed and tissue submitted for pathologic evaluation. The typical findings associated with TB are granuloma formation with palisading histiocytes and epithelioid, multinucleated giant cells, with or without caseation necrosis (Fig. 77–8). AFB may be observed within the granulomas but are usually few and may be completely absent. These features are not pathognomonic of TB, as they may be seen in other conditions, e.g., infection with nontuberculous mycobacteria or fungi as well as in noninfectious inflammatory diseases including sarcoidosis. Conversely, some immunocompromised patients present with very little tissue reaction and atypical pathologic findings even in the face of extensive TB.

Tuberculin Skin Testing

Dermal reactivity to PPD is the hallmark of CMI to tuberculosis and the single most important marker of prior infection with MTB. Although many preparations of tuberculin have been used historically, currently only the use of intermediate-strength PPD is recommended (5 tuberculin units of PPD-S, used in the United States, are equivalent to 2 tuberculin units of RT-23, used elsewhere). Other preparations of PPD having one fifth and 50 times the activity of intermediate-strength PPD, respectively are termed first-strength and second-strength PPD. Testing with these preparations is not standardized and should not be used.

METHOD. The standard technique for administration of PPD is the Mantoux method: injection of 0.1 mL of PPD into the most superficial layer of the dermis, on the volar surface of the arm, in such a way that a wheal is raised. A short-beveled 26- or 27-gauge needle should be used with a 1-mL graduated syringe. By convention, the reading is performed 48 to 72 hours after placement of the test, although induration persists for 7 days in 90% of tuberculin reactors, so the test can be read for up to 1 week. The reaction is read by inspecting and palpating the area where the test was administered and recording the area of induration in millimeters. The amount of erythema should be disregarded, as it does not constitute part of the CMI response.

INTERPRETATION. Although the tuberculin skin test is widely used as an aid in the diagnosis of TB, its limitations need to be understood. A positive tuberculin reaction merely indicates infection and not necessarily disease. Because in most developing nations the majority of adults are infected with MTB, but only a few of them have active disease, a positive skin test may not add significantly to diagnostic certainty. On the other hand, the false negative rate in patients with active disease is appreciable, reaching more than 20% when extensive disease is present. Moreover, false negative tuberculin skin tests are seen in the majority of patients with advanced HIV disease. Hence, a negative result may not be particularly helpful in excluding the diagnosis. Thus, in many clinical settings, the tuberculin skin test is better suited for epidemiologic purposes than for the diagnosis of individual cases.

Therapeutic Trial

When insufficient diagnostic data exist to confirm the presence of TB in a patient whose clinical presentation is sugges-

tive of this diagnosis, clinicians can use the clinical response to antituberculous therapy as evidence of TB. To ensure the accuracy of this approach, an objective assessment of the therapeutic response, e.g., elimination of symptoms, weight gain, radiographic improvement in the context of several months of therapy, should be used.

■ TREATMENT

Basic Principles

The introduction of effective antimicrobial agents in the 1940s and 1950s heralded dramatic changes in the management of TB.

NONPHARMACOLOGIC INTERVENTIONS. Diet modification, bed rest, and change of climate have been shown not to affect the outcome of treatment and are no longer recommended. Surgical interventions are indicated only in the most refractory cases. Appropriate chemotherapy rapidly renders patients noninfectious, obviating the need for prolonged isolation. Hospitalization, once an essential component of treatment, does not offer significant advantage over home treatment.

CHEMOTHERAPY—ANTIBIOTIC RESISTANCE. A great deal has also been learned about the limitations of chemotherapy, one of the earliest being the need to treat patients with multiple antituberculous agents. In 1945, initial enthusiasm about the curative effect of streptomycin was tempered by the realization that MTB can quickly become resistant to antituberculous agents. Following a marked initial improvement, patients were noted to worsen or relapse with organisms that had become resistant to streptomycin. This was particularly common in patients with extensive pulmonary involvement and cavitary disease. Similar results were found when isoniazid (INH) was first used as monotherapy for pulmonary TB. In 1952 the British Medical Research Council showed that although patients on INH monotherapy had impressive initial improvements, resistance to the drug developed in 11%, 52%, and 71% of cases at 1, 2, and 3 months, respectively. The addition of a second antibiotic to the regimen resulted in a marked decrease in relapses with resistant organisms. This phenomenon is attributable to the presence of small numbers of spontaneously resistant bacteria in any wild population of MTB. Indeed, the frequency of drug-resistant mutants in unselected populations of MTB has been calculated to be 3.5×10^{-6} for INH, 3.8×10^{-6} for streptomycin, 3.1×10^{-8} for rifampin, and 0.5×10^{-4} for ethambutol. Since it is estimated that the number of viable organisms within a cavitary lesion is likely to be in excess of 10^9, it is obvious that most such cases harbor organisms resistant to any single agent and that this population will proliferate unchecked when treated with only one antimicrobial agent. However, the likelihood of a wild population harboring organisms resistant to two agents is 10^{-10} to 10^{-14}. This principle underlies what has become the basic tenet of antituberculous therapy; patients should always be treated with at least two drugs to which the organism is susceptible, and a single drug should never be added to a failing regimen.

PROLONGED THERAPY. Another basic tenet is the need for prolonged therapy. Although great progress was made in shortening therapy with the addition of rifampin and pyrazinamide (PZA), the minimum acceptable duration of therapy remains 6 months. Shorter courses have unacceptable rates of failure, frequently associated with the emergence of drug resistance.

PATIENT COMPLIANCE. With current therapies, the major impediment to achieving cure rates in excess of 95% is ensur-

TABLE 77–5. Dosage Recommendation for the Initial Treatment of Tuberculosis in Children* and Adults

Drug (mg/kg)	Dosage					
	Daily Dose		**Twice-Weekly Dose**		**Thrice-Weekly Dose**	
	Children	Adults	Children	Adults	Children	Adults
Isoniazid	10–20; max 300 mg	5; max 300 mg	20–40; max 900 mg	15 max; max 900 mg	20–40; max 900 mg	15 max; max 900 mg
Rifampin	10–20; max 600 mg	10; max 600 mg	10–20; max 600 mg	10; max 600 mg	10–20; max 600 mg	10; max 600 mg
Pyrazinamide	15–30; max 2 g	15–30; max 2 g	50–70; max 4 g	50–70; max 4 g	50–70; max 3 g	50–70; max 3 g
Ethambutol†	15–25	15–25	50	50	25–30	25–30
Streptomycin	20–40; max 1.0 g	15; max 1.0 g	25–30; max 1.5 g	25–30; max 1.5 g	25–30; max 1.5 g	25–30; max 1.5 g

*Children ≤12 years of age.
†Ethambutol is generally not recommended for children whose visual acuity cannot be monitored (<8 yr of age). However, ethambutol should be considered for all children with organisms resistant to other drugs when susceptibility to ethambutol has been demonstrated or susceptibility is likely.
From American Thoracic Society: Treatment of tuberculosis and tuberculosis infection in adults and children. Am J Respir Crit Care Med 149:1359, 1994.

ing that patients adhere to treatment regimens. Prescription of inappropriate drugs and intermittent use of appropriate medications are associated with high rates of treatment failure and leads to the development of drug resistance. Thus, ensuring patient adherence with therapy is an important responsibility of anyone treating TB patients. This can be facilitated by combined pills and intermittent therapy administered under direct observation (DOT).

Antituberculous Drugs (Tables 77–5 and 77–6)

ISONIAZID (ISONICOTINIC ACID HYDRAZIDE). INH is the most widely used antituberculous medication. It is inexpensive and highly bactericidal against MTB. The mechanism of action is incompletely understood, but most likely involves the inhibition of mycolic acid formation. The drug requires intracellular activation by mycobacterial catalase and strains that lack this activity are resistant to it. Low level resistance has been associated with mutations in the *inhA* gene and high level resistance with mutations in the *katG* gene. INH inhibits both intracellular and extracellular organisms, partic-

ularly those that are rapidly replicating. It is well absorbed from the gastrointestinal tract and peak serum concentrations are achieved 1 and 2 hours after ingestion. INH diffuses readily into all body tissues and cells resulting in concentrations similar to those achieved in serum. The serum half-life of the drug varies between 2 to 4 hours in slow acetylators and 0.5 to 1.5 hours in rapid acetylators, but this difference has minimal clinical relevance.

Although INH is usually administered orally, a preparation for intramuscular administration is available for use when oral therapy is not an option. The same dosages apply as for the oral route.

INH is a very well tolerated and safe drug. Adverse reactions occur in only 5.4% of people receiving the drug. The most serious reported side effect is hepatotoxicity, including potentially fatal hepatitis. The rate of INH-associated hepatitis is directly associated with advancing age. In a large survey of patients receiving INH alone as preventive therapy, Kopanoff and coworkers found the incidence to be 0% for people younger than 20 years of age, 0.3% for those 20 to 34 years of age, 1.2% for people 35 to 49 years of age, and 2.3% for

TABLE 77–6. Second-Line Antituberculosis Drugs*

Drug	Dosage Forms	Daily Dose in Children and Adults†	Maximal Daily Dose in Children and Adults	Major Adverse Reactions	Recommended Regular Monitoring
Capreomycin	Vials: 1 g	15–30 mg/kg IM	1 g	Auditory, vestibular, and renal toxicity	Vestibular function, audiometry, BUN, and creatinine
Kanamycin	Vials: 75 mg, 500 mg, 1 g	15–30 mg/kg IM	1 g	Auditory and renal toxicity, rare vestibular toxicity	Vestibular function, audiometry, BUN, and creatinine
Ethionamide	Tablets: 250 mg	15–20 mg/kg PO	1 g	Gastrointestinal disturbance, hepatotoxicity, hypersensitivity	
Para-aminosalicylic acid	Tablets: 500 mg, 1 g Bulk powder Delayed-release granules	150 mg/kg PO	12 g	Gastrointestinal disturbance, hypersensitivity, hepatotoxicity, sodium load	Hepatic enzymes
Cycloserine	Capsules: 250 mg	15–20 mg/kg PO	1 g	Psychosis, convulsions, rash	Assessment of mental status

*These drugs are more difficult to use than first-line antituberculous drugs. They should be used only when necessary, and they should be given and monitored by health providers experienced in their use.
†Doses based on weight should be adjusted as weight changes.
BUN, blood urea nitrogen.
From American Thoracic Society, Am J Respir Crit Care Med 149:1359, 1994.

those 50 years of age or older. Other factors that may predispose to INH-associated hepatotoxicity are regular alcohol consumption, intravenous drug use, and a history of previous liver damage. Asymptomatic transaminase elevations may occur in up to 20% of patients early on in the course of treatment but most often return to baseline as treatment continues. Asymptomatic elevations of up to five times of normal values are tolerated and should not result in changes in therapy. On the other hand, any sign or symptom of liver toxicity, e.g., prolonged nausea, vomiting, anorexia, fatigue, abdominal discomfort, icterus, light-colored stools, or dark-colored urine, should raise the suspicion of hepatotoxicity and should prompt the immediate discontinuation of the medication.

The second most important side effect reported with INH is peripheral neuropathy, which especially affects patients already at risk for developing neuropathy from other illnesses, e.g., diabetes mellitus, alcoholism, uremia, and malnutrition. This adverse reaction can be prevented or reversed by the administration of pyridoxine.

The simultaneous administration of INH and phenytoin results in elevated serum levels of both drugs. Hence, when such therapy is necessary, the phenytoin serum concentration should be monitored and its dose adjusted accordingly.

RIFAMPIN. RIF is a broad-spectrum antibiotic whose addition to the antituberculous armamentarium has contributed to the reduction in the length of treatment from the formerly recommended 18 to 24 months to the currently accepted standard of 6 to 9 months. It is bactericidal for MTB, relatively nontoxic, and quickly absorbed from the gastrointestinal tract. It penetrates well into tissues and cells and achieves therapeutic levels in the CSF in the presence of meningeal inflammation.

RIF inhibits bacterial RNA synthesis by interacting with the beta subunit of RNA polymerase, and resistance to this drug is most often mediated by point mutations in the *rpoB* gene.

RIF is safe and well tolerated. The most common untoward reaction encountered with RIF is gastrointestinal upset. Other side effects include rash; hepatitis, found in 3.1% of patients in a U.S. Public Health Service study of 6 months of INH-RIF treatment; and rarely, thrombocytopenia. Administration of doses larger than 10 mg/kg in the course of twice-weekly treatments has been associated with immunologically mediated reactions, e.g., thrombocytopenia, hemolytic anemia, acute renal failure, and a flulike syndrome. Patients on intermittent therapy who develop mild allergic reactions can usually be switched to daily dosing with resolution of the symptoms. As with other drugs, HIV-infected patients may experience a higher rate of adverse reactions. RIF is a potent inducer of hepatic microsomal enzymes and hence it accelerates the metabolism of many drugs, e.g., digoxin, warfarin, and oral contraceptives. Of note is RIF interaction with azole antifungal agents, e.g., ketoconazole and itraconazole, as well as the recently described interaction with clarithromycin. Doses of these medications should be monitored and adjusted when concurrent therapy is required. RIF imparts an orange tinge to urine and other body fluids and may stain contact lenses; patients should be apprised of this fact.

PYRAZINAMIDE. PZA is bactericidal for MTB, particularly in the acid intracellular environment of the macrophage. Absorption from the gastrointestinal tract is almost complete. It is well distributed in all tissues and in patients with tuberculous meningitis, CSF levels equal those in serum. The most important adverse reaction of PZA administration is hepatotoxicity, which appears to be dose related. However, when used in the initial intensive phase at the recommended doses, it does not increase the overall rate of hepatotoxicity

of short-course combinations. PZA inhibits renal tubular secretion of urate and causes serum uric acid elevation in most patients. A related polyarthralgia occurs in up to 40% of patients but usually responds to analgesics or anti-inflammatory agents and does not require the discontinuation of the drug. Skin rashes and gastrointestinal upset may also occur.

The mechanism of action of PZA is not well understood but it requires the presence of the enzyme pyrazinamidase and an acidic environment. Hence, organisms that lack this enzyme, such as *M. bovis*, are not inhibited by PZA.

PZA is a crucial component of short-course therapy. Several studies have shown that the addition of PZA to the intensive phase of 6 month regimens significantly reduces the rate of relapse at 2 and 5 years.

STREPTOMYCIN. STM is not absorbed from the gut, and hence must be given parenterally, seriously limiting its usefulness. It is bactericidal for MTB in an alkaline environment. The drug has good tissue penetration but will only enter the CSF in the presence of meningeal inflammation. Dosages should be carefully adjusted in renal failure. The most common serious adverse effect of STM is ototoxicity, which usually results in vertigo but may also cause hearing loss. STM causes occasional nephrotoxicity, and this adverse effect may be more common in persons with pre-existing renal disease or with concurrent use of other nephrotoxic agents. Both these toxicities are more common in patients >60 years of age. Cumulative doses of more than 120 g should be avoided unless no other therapeutic option exists, as they are associated with increased side effects. A rare but potentially life-threatening adverse effect is neuromuscular blockade, thought to be mediated at the level of the motor end plate.

Like other aminoglycosides, STM exerts its effects by binding to the 30S subunit of bacterial ribosomes. Hence it reduces protein synthesis and induces misreading of mRNA. Resistance to STM in MTB is mediated through certain known mutations and through other, as yet uncharacterized mechanisms.

ETHAMBUTOL. EMB is considered bacteriostatic at the doses recommended for daily regimens, although it may be bactericidal at the higher doses used for intermittent therapy. CSF concentrations of EMB are usually low, even in the presence of inflamed meninges.

EMB has a low frequency of adverse reactions, the most common and serious one being optic neuritis. Symptoms include blurred vision, central scotomas, and red-green color blindness. The complication is dose dependent; it occurs in less than 1% of patients receiving a daily dose of 15 mg/kg, in up to 5% of patients when the dose is 25 mg/kg, and in 15% of patients receiving 50 mg/kg per day. Whenever possible, ethambutol should be avoided in children too young to evaluate for visual acuity and color discrimination. The mechanism of action of this drug is not known.

THIACETAZONE. This second-line agent is rarely used in the United States and other developed nations but, because of its low cost, has been widely used in resource-poor countries. It is a bacteriostatic agent for MTB and it is well absorbed from the gastrointestinal tract.

The most frequent side effects are nausea, vomiting, and diarrhea. Less frequent reactions include bone marrow depression, agranulocytosis, thrombocytopenia, and ototoxicity. Cutaneous hypersensitivity reactions are frequent and may be particularly severe. Several fatal cases of toxic epidermal necrolysis attributed to thiacetazone were recently reported in HIV-co-infected people. Hence it is recommended to avoid this drug in known or suspected HIV positive patients.

OTHER SECOND-LINE AGENTS. In addition to the above-mentioned agents, several less commonly used antituberculous drugs exist. These include para-aminosalicylic acid

(PASA), ethionamide, prothionamide, cycloserine, capreomycin, and kanamycin. All of these agents are less active against MTB and have more side effects than the more frequently used drugs; hence their use is limited to situations of multidrug resistance or other special circumstances.

ADDITIONAL DRUGS WITH ANTITUBERCULOUS ACTIVITY. Several drugs with known antituberculous activity exist but have been less well studied and their role in antituberculous regimens has yet to be determined. These include the quinolones ciprofloxacin, ofloxacin, and sparfloxacin; the rifamycin derivatives rifabutin and rifapentine; beta lactam–beta lactamase inhibitor combinations, e.g., amoxicillin–clavulanic acid; and a drug used in the treatment of *M. leprae*, clofazimine.

Treatment Regimens

There are several treatment regimens that have proven efficacies in excess of 90%. All of them incorporate the basic principle of using multiple antimicrobial agents for prolonged periods of time administered under direct observation. However, they differ in their duration, the specific agents used, and their dosing schedule. Thus, health care providers have several therapeutic options and regimen selection should be tempered by drug availability, the likelihood of the patient's organisms being drug resistant, and the patient's HIV serostatus.

TREATMENT OF PULMONARY TUBERCULOSIS. In developed countries, patients with active pulmonary TB who have no history of previous treatment and who have a low likelihood of harboring a resistant organism should be started on a 2-month intensive phase of daily INH, RIF, and PZA, supplemented with EMB or STM if the prevalence of INH resistance in the community is 4% or higher. Drug susceptibility testing should be performed on all initial isolates, and drugs used in the continuation phase should be guided by these results. If the organism is sensitive to all drugs, INH and RIF, administered three times weekly, should be continued for 4 more months, to complete a 6-month course.

In resource-poor countries a less expensive alternative is a regimen consisting of daily INH, RIF, PZA, and STM for the first 2 months and daily INH and thiacetazone for 6 months, to complete an 8-month course. However, the high incidence of adverse reactions to thiacetazone, particularly in HIV-infected patients, makes the regimen less desirable, especially in settings in which high rates of HIV co-infection can be expected.

In areas where culture facilities are not readily available it is crucial to identify, through detailed questioning, patients who are likely to have received antituberculous drugs, since they may harbor resistant organisms. Whenever possible, a pretreatment sputum specimen from these patients should be obtained for susceptibility testing. Cultures are crucial for patients who remain sputum smear positive at 3 months. If this is not possible, the WHO recommends that patients for whom drug resistance is suspected be treated with an initial daily regimen of INH, RIF, PZA, and EMB for the first 3 months, supplemented with STM for the first 2 months, followed by a 5-month continuation phase consisting of INH, RIF, and EMB administered three times weekly.

Patients with pulmonary TB who are diagnosed on clinical and radiologic grounds and for whom an adequate microbiologic evaluation yields negative cultures can be treated with an abbreviated 4-month course consisting of daily INH, RIF, and PZA for the first 2 months, followed by daily INH and RIF for the next 2 months.

IMMUNOCOMPROMISED PATIENTS. Patients infected with HIV and those immunocompromised for other reasons should receive INH, RIF, PZA, and EMB or STM for the first 2 months and INH and RIF for the next 7 months. Therapy should continue for at least 6 months after sputum smear conversion is documented. Thiacetazone should be avoided in HIV-infected patients, since it is associated with a high incidence of adverse reactions.

PRACTICAL POINTS IN TREATMENT. Although therapy for TB is most often highly effective and well tolerated, special situations are encountered that merit attention.

Adverse Drug Reactions. When adverse drug reaction is suspected, all drugs should be stopped at the same time. Single drugs should never be removed from the therapeutic regimen, because this may lead to inadvertent monotherapy with the consequent risk of development of drug resistance. After the adverse drug reaction subsides, sequential reinstitution of the drug regimen should be undertaken, one drug at a time, beginning with the least likely culprit and proceeding in steps of 3 to 5 days with each drug, until all drugs have been restarted. In the majority of cases, this approach either identifies the culprit or results in no further adverse drug reaction.

Drug Resistance. Drug resistance is increasingly frequent, both in the developed and in the developing world. When resistance to INH, alone or in combination with STM, is encountered, a 9-month regimen of RIF, PZA, and EMB is usually effective. An alternative is a 12-month course of RIF and EMB.

When resistance to RIF alone is encountered, an increasingly recognized problem in HIV-infected individuals, INH and EMB should be used for 18 to 24 months, and STM should be given at least until sputum conversion is documented and perhaps for 2 to 3 months thereafter. The role of PZA in this setting is not well established but it seems prudent to include it in the regimen, at least during the first 2 to 3 months of therapy.

When resistance to INH coexists with EMB resistance, with or without resistance to STM, RIF and PZA should be combined with a quinolone and STM or an aminoglycoside to which the organism is susceptible (kanamycin or amikacin). The aminoglycoside may be dropped if there is good clinical and bacteriologic response, at a dose equivalent to 120 g of STM. The remaining drugs should be continued for at least 6 months after sputum conversion.

When resistance to INH and RIF is encountered, a four-drug regimen, including an aminoglycoside, PZA, EMB, and a quinolone should be used. EMB should be used at the higher end of the dosing spectrum, which may make it a bactericidal drug. This regimen should be continued for at least 18 months after sputum conversion and preferably for 24 months.

Little information is available on the appropriate treatment of cases with more extensive drug resistance, and these should be based on known susceptibility patterns and include several drugs to which the organism is sensitive.

TREATMENT OF EXTRAPULMONARY TUBERCULOSIS. Extrapulmonary TB is, in most cases, treated in the same way as pulmonary disease. Exceptions to this rule include the use of steroids in CNS and pericardial disease and surgical intervention in some situations, as discussed previously.

THERAPEUTIC COMPLIANCE. Because the success of antituberculous therapy depends on adherence to the prescribed regimens, and because noncompliance risks the development of drug-resistant organisms, directly observed therapy should be attempted in every case. Recent reports from China document very high completion rates and very low failure rates in large-scale treatment programs using fully intermittent, directly observed regimens.

Since even under the best circumstances treatment failures

do occur, following completion of therapy surveillance should include sputum smears, and when possible cultures, at 3 months and 6 months after treatment, as well as chest radiographs at the end of treatment and at 1-year follow-up.

RESPONSE TO TREATMENT. The objectives of antituberculous chemotherapy are to rapidly decrease the infectivity of active cases, to reduce morbidity and mortality, and to effect a bacteriologic cure. Evidence from several lines of research supports the assertion that when patients who harbor susceptible organisms comply with current multidrug regimens, they are generally rendered noninfectious within a 2-week period or sooner, making their prolonged isolation unnecessary. This is true although studies have shown that cultures remain positive in 50% of patients at 1 month and in 15% at 2 months. Cultures should be negative in more than 90% of patients at 3 months; positive smears or cultures after 3 months should raise the suspicion of drug resistance or noncompliance, and merit further evaluation.

Clinical response to treatment has been specifically evaluated in several studies and is highly variable, depending on treatment regimen and initial extent of disease. A recent study of the course of fever during treatment of pulmonary TB found that 89% of 161 patients were afebrile at the end of 1 week and 93% after 2 weeks of treatment, which in most patients consisted of INH, RIF, and PZA. Delayed defervescence was associated with alcoholism and advanced disease. Persistence of fever beyond 3 to 4 weeks should prompt consideration of other explanations, including neoplasm, drug hypersensitivity, drug resistance, and noncompliance. Cough, which is associated with both the infectivity of the patient and the extent of disease, should also decrease promptly. In a small study in which the patient's coughing was monitored during the night, a 65% decrease in coughing episodes was shown after 2 weeks of treatment.

Serial radiographic evaluation is neither a sensitive nor efficient way to monitor response to treatment. The chest film appearance lags behind the clinical improvement and only begins to show amelioration 1 to 3 months after treatment is instituted. However, patients who have exacerbation of symptoms, particularly those infected with HIV, should have radiographs repeated, and if symptoms have worsened, they should be evaluated for possible intercurrent illness. In 90% of cases resolution or stabilization of radiographic changes can be expected by the end of 6 months. Whenever possible, an end-of-treatment radiograph should be obtained to document this and establish a new baseline.

■ PREVENTION AND CONTROL

The most actively pursued control strategy for TB in developing countries consists of vigorous case finding and treatment of cases, particularly those that contribute most to disease transmission, i.e., sputum smear positive cases. An integral part of control programs is ensuring adequate treatment completion and cure rates, as determined by the demonstration of two consecutive negative sputum samples: after 4 months of therapy and at the end of treatment. The WHO states that the first and foremost objective of a TB control program is to achieve at least an 85% cure rate in patients with smear-positive pulmonary TB. This strategy is thought to result in a rapid reduction of disease prevalence and its rate of transmission while at the same time reducing the rate of acquired drug resistance. WHO guidelines state that only when the 85% cure rate is achieved should case finding be expanded to include other cases. Because poor compliance is a strong predictor of treatment failure, both at the individual level and at the program level, a major portion of available resources should be mobilized to ensure patient adherence with the treatment regimen. Since one of the most significant barriers to adequate control programs in developing countries is lack of resources, a careful cost-benefit analysis should be conducted before any departures from established guidelines.

Prevention of TB can be approached by immunization with BCG and preventive chemotherapy with INH.

Isoniazid Chemoprophylaxis

Chemoprophylaxis with INH is more accurately viewed as treatment of primary TB infection to prevent later dissemination or reactivation and progression to active disease. The concept is supported by results of several double blind, placebo controlled trials conducted by the U.S. Public Health Service and involving more than 70,000 people. These trials showed an 80% risk reduction in the first year and a greater than 60% overall reduction in TB rates in individuals receiving INH.

IN DEVELOPED COUNTRIES. In these areas the incidence of MTB infection and TB is low, and INH chemoprophylaxis of infected individuals is considered an essential part of TB control programs. In this setting, it is recommended that all patients aged <35 with prior TB infection as evidenced by a positive PPD receive 300 mg of INH daily for at least 6 months. In this age group, the risk of INH-induced hepatitis is very low and is outweighed by the benefit of prevented TB. Patients aged >35 are at increased risk of adverse side effects, hence in this group INH prophylaxis is recommended only for people who are at increased risk of developing TB. These groups include all recently infected individuals as evidenced by a PPD status conversion within the last 2 years, close contacts of active cases, and persons with certain medical conditions increasing their risk of developing TB: diabetes mellitus, end-stage renal disease, prolonged corticosteroid therapy, immunosuppressive therapy, hematologic or reticuloendothelial malignancies, and conditions associated with rapid weight loss or chronic malnutrition. Patients co-infected with MTB and HIV have an annual risk of progression to TB of 5 to 10%. Although the appropriate duration of chemoprophylaxis in these patients has not been adequately established, current recommendations are that they receive INH for at least 12 months.

IN DEVELOPING COUNTRIES. In these areas the majority of the adult population is infected with MTB. Limited resources are focused on finding of active cases and their appropriate treatment. The routine use of INH chemoprophylaxis in this setting is not a strategy recommended by most TB control agencies and is viewed as an impractical measure. Special situations exist, however, that warrant the use of INH chemoprophylaxis regardless of other considerations. Individuals infected with both HIV and MTB have an extremely high risk of developing TB. Controlled studies conducted in Zambia and in Haiti evaluated the effect of 6 and 12 months, respectively of daily INH in HIV-infected individuals. Both studies showed a decrease in the incidence of TB in patients receiving INH. Although the optimal duration of INH preventive therapy in this patient population remains to be determined, current recommendations are for 12 months of therapy. A multicenter trial conducted in the United States, Mexico, Brazil, and Haiti from 1992 to 1998 compared the efficacy of INH for 12 months with that of RIF and PZA for 2 months. Both regimens were self-administered by HIV-infected, PPD-positive individuals. Protection and adverse effects were essentially the same for both arms of the study, and the short course of RIF/PZA was recommended as an alternative to the standard INH regimen.

Whenever INH chemoprophylaxis is considered for a patient, the possibility of active disease should be carefully examined and ruled out by symptom review and chest radiography. If any suspicion of active disease exists, appropriate treatment should be started until disease is adequately ruled out. INH chemotherapy in this setting would amount to monotherapy and would likely result in INH-resistant TB.

BCG Immunization

Immunization with bacille Calmette-Guérin (BCG), an avirulent attenuated form of *M. bovis*, has been a major part of TB control efforts in much of the world. However, in spite of the fact that it is probably the most widely used vaccine in the world, BCG has been the source of great controversy. Controlled clinical trials have shown efficacy for the vaccine in preventing pulmonary TB to range from 0% to more than 70%. Explanations to account for the observed variability in protection conferred by this vaccine include: (1) variability in the potency of the strain of BCG used; (2) regional differences in the prevalence of infection with mycobacteria other than tuberculosis; and (3) differences in handling of the vaccine and vaccine administration techniques. In fact, because of its low impact on the number of cases of pulmonary TB in adults, vaccination with BCG is no longer thought to be an efficient means for decreasing the overall rate of TB in a population. This fact, however, is in contrast with the usefulness of BCG vaccination in infants and young children. In this population, the vaccine prevents the development of disseminated disease and meningitis. It is this evidence that forms the basis of the current WHO recommendation for BCG vaccination in the developing world. It is estimated that approximately 80% of children <2 years of age in developing countries receive BCG. It is clear that a safe, inexpensive, and efficacious vaccine would have a significant impact on TB control efforts worldwide.

■ DISEASE CAUSED BY MYCOBACTERIA OTHER THAN TUBERCULOSIS

Soon after the first description of the tubercle bacillus by Koch, other mycobacterial species began to be identified and were usually classified according to their source. As early as 1885 mycobacteria other than tuberculosis (MOTT) were isolated from human sources, but these were for the most part thought of as commensals or saprophytes. The first such organism was *M. smegmatis*. It was not until the middle of the 20th century that disease caused by these organisms, variously known as "atypical," "anonymous," or "nontuberculous" (NTM) mycobacteria, began to be recognized. Knowledge of their pathogenic potential accumulated between the 1950s and early 1980s, and the spectrum of disease attributable to these organisms broadened. Early in the HIV epidemic it was recognized that organisms of the *M. avium* complex (MAC) were a frequent cause of disseminated infection in severely immunocompromised patients. Although currently the burden of disease caused by MOTTs falls on the HIV-infected population, disease caused by these organisms still occurs in patients with no identifiable immune deficit. Unlike MTB, which is transmitted from person to person, MOTTs are variably distributed in nature and are acquired from the environment. Among the 54 currently named mycobacterial species, less than one third can occasionally cause disease in humans. Disease caused by MOTTs is not nearly as important a public health problem in the developing world as is TB (Table 77–7).

PULMONARY DISEASE. Chronic pulmonary disease is most commonly caused by *M. avium* complex organisms and *M. kansasii*, but may occasionally be caused by a number of other MOTTs (Table 77–7). Before the AIDS epidemic the vast majority of MAC isolates were from the lung and only a minority of these were thought to be the cause of disease.

Clinical Manifestations. Both colonization and disease occur more frequently in persons with underlying lung disease. Infection and disease due to MAC may occur, however, in persons with no previous lung disease. Indeed, during the last two decades, a form of pulmonary MAC disease has been increasingly diagnosed in young women who have no underlying lung disorder. Classically, pulmonary MAC disease presented as upper lobe fibronodular cavitary disease reminiscent of TB in middle-aged and elderly white men, most of whom had underlying chronic obstructive pulmonary disease, pneumoconioses, or previously treated and healed TB. More recently, a more subtle form of the disease has been recognized, presenting as lower lung zone, scat-

TABLE 77–7. Nontuberculous Mycobacteria: Clinical Manifestations

Clinical Disease	Common Etiologic Agents	Rare Etiologic Agents
Chronic pulmonary infection (usually adults)	*M. avium* complex *M. kansasii* *M. abscessus* *M. xenopi* *M. malmoense*	*M. simiae* *M. szulgai* *M. fortuitum/M. peregrinum* *M. chelonae* *M. smegmatis* *M. shimoidei*
Lymphadenitis (usually children <5 yr)	*M. avium* complex *M. malmoense* *M. haemophilum*	*M. scrofulaceum* *M. fortuitum/M. peregrinum* *M. abscessus/M. chelonae*
Skin and soft tissue infections (traumatic or nosocomial)	*M. marinum* *M. fortuitum/M. peregrinum* *M. abscessus/M. chelonae* *M. ulcerans* (tropics)	*M. avium* complex *M. kansasii* *M. terrae* complex *M. haemophilum* (immunosuppression)
Infections of joints, tendon sheaths, bones	*M. marinum* *M. avium* complex *M. terrae* complex	*M. fortuitum/M. peregrinum* *M. abscessus/M. chelonae* *M. kansasii*
Dissemination (usually immunosuppression)	*M. avium* complex *M. genavense* *M. kansasii*	*M. abscessus/M. chelonae* *M. haemophilum*

From Salfinger M: Characteristics of the various species of mycobacteria. *In* Rom WN, Garay SM (eds): Tuberculosis. New York, Little, Brown, 1996.

TABLE 77–8. Suggested Empiric Regimens for the Treatment of Pulmonary *Mycobacterium avium* Complex Disease

Initial phase: first 2 mo	Clarithromycin, 500 mg PO b.i.d. plus Ethambutol, 25 mg/kg PO q.d. plus Clofazimine, 200 mg PO q.d. plus either Streptomycin, 10–12 mg/kg q.d. or Amikacin, 12–15 mg/kg q.d.
Continuation phase: next 22 mo	Clarithromycin, 750 mg PO q.d. plus Ethambutol, 15 mg/kg PO q.d. plus Clofazimine, 50–100 mg PO q.d.

Modified from Iseman MD: *M. avium* complex: An emerging respiratory pathogen. J Respir Dis 16:950, 1995.

tered, subpleural nodulation. Most affected patients are young women and a significant proportion have thoracic scoliosis and narrow anteroposterior chest dimension.

Pulmonary involvement by MAC in AIDS patients may take the form of a localized lung infiltration, diffuse infiltration, or endobronchial disease, sometimes leading to airway obstruction and atelectasis.

Diagnosis. Because MAC may be present as a saprophyte in the lung, its mere isolation is insufficient evidence to implicate this organism as a cause of disease. The American Thoracic Society has published guidelines on the criteria needed for the diagnosis of MAC lung disease. Two or more sputums or bronchial washings should be AFB smear-positive and/or produce moderate to heavy growth on culture in a patient with cavitary infiltrate, and other causes for the process should be excluded. In patients with noncavitary infiltrates, a diagnosis can be made when the above criteria are met and intensive pulmonary cleansing fails to clear the organism from the sputum. In persons with HIV infection, MAC usually causes systemic disease that does not involve the lungs. MAC may be isolated from the sputum of HIV-infected patients whose lung disease is caused by other, more common pathogens, e.g., *Pneumocystis carinii*.

Therapy. Treatment of MAC lung disease is difficult and has not been prospectively evaluated in controlled trials. Treatment usually needs to be continued for 18 to 24 months and includes multiple drugs (Tables 77–8 and 77–9).

LYMPH NODE DISEASE. Lymphadenitis caused by MOTTs is most commonly seen in children <5 years old. MAC is the most frequent culprit, although *M. kansasii* and other organisms can sometimes be found (Table 77–7). In the developing world, lymphadenitis is much more commonly caused by MTB than by MOTTs, whereas the converse is true in industrialized countries. The cervical and submandibular nodes are most frequently involved. Painless, progressive swelling is usually seen, most often without associated constitutional symptoms. Occasional rupture with drainage may occur. Fibrosis and calcification lead to healing. The treatment of choice is surgical excision of the involved nodes, as chemotherapy seems to be of little benefit.

DISSEMINATED DISEASE. Disseminated disease due to MOTTs was rare before the advent of the AIDS epidemic. Since then, however, MAC has been recognized as one of the most common pathogens in patients with advanced AIDS; other nontuberculous mycobacteria also cause illness in patients with HIV infections (Table 77–7). The respiratory and gastrointestinal tracts serve as portals of entry, and with progressive immune suppression, the organism gains access to the blood stream and a chronic bacillemia ensues.

Clinical Manifestations. The infection can involve any organ, but most frequently causes gastrointestinal tract symptoms. Stool acid-fast smears and cultures are frequently positive. Several studies have documented both a decreased survival and reduced quality of life in patients with disseminated MAC.

Therapy. Although the optimal regimen for treating disseminated MAC in patients with AIDS remains to be defined, treatment improves survival and decreases symptoms. Monotherapy with the new macrolides, azithromycin and clarithromycin, has been used with initial improvement, but the mycobacteria frequently develop resistance to these antibiotics. Currently used regimens include two to six drugs (Table 77–8). A regimen of clarithromycin, rifabutin, and ethambutol is better tolerated than, and is as effective as, regimens consisting of four or more drugs. Moreover, selective use of prophylactic regimens in patients with <100 CD4 cells has increased survival.

OTHER CLINICAL SYNDROMES. *M. marinum* and *M. ulcerans* cause disease of the skin and subcutaneous tissues (Chapter 79). *M. chelonei* and *M. fortuitum* are the only rapidly growing mycobacteria associated with human disease, usually in the setting of postsurgical infections, but sometimes

TABLE 77–9. Drugs With Potential Usefulness Against Pulmonary *Mycobacterium avium* Complex (MAC) Disease

Antibiotic	Dosage	Side Effects/Toxicity	Comments
Clarithromycin	500 mg PO b.i.d. 750 mg PO q.d.	Unpleasant taste, GI distress, hepatitis	Very active against MAC
Ethambutol	25 mg/kg PO q.d.	Optic neuritis, GI distress	Monitor vision monthly
Clofazimine	50–200 mg PO q.d.	Skin pigmentation, pruritus, delayed GI distress	Skin changes predictable, revert after drug cessation
Streptomycin or	10–12 mg/kg/day	Renal impairment, hearing loss, vestibular dysfunction	Give early in therapy course, monitor renal and eighth nerve function
Amikacin	12–15 mg/kg/day		
Ciprofloxacin	500 mg PO b.i.d. 750 mg PO q.d.	Agitation, tremor, insomnia, hepatitis, neutropenia	Daily morning doses cause less insomnia
Azithromycin	250–500 mg PO q.d.	Unpleasant taste, GI distress	Less well studied than clarithromycin for MAC
Rifampin*	600 mg PO q.d. 450 mg if < 45 kg	Hepatitis, thrombocytopenia, purpura, flu syndrome	Multiple clinically significant drug interactions
Rifabutin	450 mg PO q.d.	Thrombocytopenia, neutropenia, hepatitis	Drug interaction less potent than with rifampin

*Rifampin induces significant hepatic catabolism of clarithromycin. The combination of these two agents should be avoided.
GI, gastrointestinal.
Modified from Iseman MD: *M. avium* complex: An emerging respiratory pathogen. J Respir Dis 16:950, 1995.

causing disseminated disease. *M. gordonae* and *M. fortuitum* are frequently found in tap water and may contaminate staining reagents and cultures and may give rise to false positive AFB smears. Because of this, the use of sterile water is recommended in the processing of smears.

Bibliography

American Thoracic Society: Diagnosis and treatment of disease caused by nontuberculous mycobacteria. Am Rev Respir Dis 142:940, 1990.

American Thoracic Society: Treatment of tuberculosis and tuberculosis infection in adults and children. Am J Crit Care Med 149:1359, 1994.

Barnes PF, Chan LS, Wong SF: The course of fever during the treatment of pulmonary tuberculosis. Tubercle 68:255, 1987.

Bishai WR, Graham NM, Harrington S, et al: Brief report: Rifampin-resistant tuberculosis in a patient receiving rifabutin prophylaxis. N Engl J Med 334:1593, 1996.

Bloch AB, Cauthen GM, Onorato IM, et al: National survey of drug-resistant tuberculosis in the United States. JAMA 271:665, 1994.

Blower SM, McLean AR, Porco TC, et al: The intrinsic transmission dynamics of tuberculosis epidemics. Nat Med 1:815, 1995.

Blower SM, Small PM, Hopewell PC: Control strategies for tuberculosis epidemics: New models for old problems. Science 273:497, 1996.

Boachie-Adjei O, Squillante RG: Tuberculosis of the spine. Orthop Clin North Am 27:95, 1996.

Carpels G, Fissette K, Limbana V, et al: Drug resistant tuberculosis in sub-Saharan Africa: An estimation of incidence and cost for the year 2000. Tubercle Lung Dis 76:480, 1995.

Cauthen GM, Dooley SW, Onorato IM, et al: Transmission of *Mycobacterium tuberculosis* from tuberculosis patients with HIV infection or AIDS. Am J Epidemiol 144:69, 1996.

Centers for Disease Control and Prevention: Prevention and treatment of tuberculosis among patients infected with human immunodeficiency virus: Principles of therapy and revised recommendations. MMWR 47(RR-20), 1998.

Chaulet P, Boulabal F, Grosset J: Surveillance of drug resistance for tuberculosis control: Why and how? Tubercle Lung Dis 76:487, 1995.

China Tuberculosis Control Collaboration: Results of directly observed short-course chemotherapy in 112,842 Chinese patients with smear-positive tuberculosis. Lancet 347:358, 1996.

Cohn DL, Catlin BJ, Peterson KL, et al: A 62-dose, 6-month therapy for pulmonary and extrapulmonary tuberculosis: A twice weekly, directly observed, and cost effective regimen. Ann Intern Med 112:407, 1990.

Comstock G: Variability of tuberculosis trends in a time of resurgence. Clin Infect Dis 19:1015, 1994.

Coombs DL, O'Brien RJ, Geiter LJ: USPHS tuberculosis short-course chemotherapy trial 21: Effectiveness, toxicity, and acceptability. Ann Intern Med 112:397, 1990.

Dankner WM, Waecker NJ, Mitchell AE, et al: *Mycobacterium bovis* infections in San Diego: A clinicopathologic study of 73 patients and a historical review of a forgotten pathogen. Medicine 72:11, 1993.

De Cock KM, Soro B, Malik Coulibali I, et al: Tuberculosis and HIV infection in sub-Saharan Africa. JAMA 268: 1581, 1992.

Di Perri G, Cazzadori A, Vento S, et al: Comparative histopathological study of pulmonary tuberculosis in human immunodeficiency virus–infected and noninfected patients. Tubercle Lung Dis 77:244, 1996.

Dolin PJ, Raviglione MC, Kochi A: Global tuberculosis incidence and mortality during 1990–2000. Bull WHO 72:213, 1994.

Espinal MA, Reingold AL, Lavandera M: Effect of pregnancy on the risk of developing active tuberculosis. J Infect Dis 173:488, 1996.

Fine PE: Variations in protection by BCG: Implications of and for heterologous immunity. Lancet 346:1339, 1995.

Graham NM, Galai N, Nelson KE, et al: Effect of isoniazid chemoprophylaxis on HIV-related mycobacterial disease. Arch Intern Med 156:889, 1996.

Hopewell PC: Impact of human immunodeficiency virus infection on the epidemiology, clinical features, management and control of tuberculosis. Clin Infect Dis 15:540, 1992.

Horsburgh CR Jr: Tuberculosis without tubercles. Tubercle Lung Dis 77:197, 1996.

Kahn E, Starke J: Diagnosis of tuberculosis in children: Increased need for better methods. Emerging Infect Dis 1:115, 1995.

Kenyon TA, Valway SE, Ihle WW, et al: Transmission of multidrug-resistant tuberculosis during a long airplane flight. N Engl J Med 334:933, 1996.

Kopanoff DE, Snider DE, Caras GI: Isoniazid-related hepatitis: A U.S. Public Health Service cooperative surveillance study. Am Rev Respir Dis 117:991, 1978.

Kushigemachi M, Schneiderman LJ, Barrett-Connor E: Racial differences in susceptibility to tuberculosis: Risk of disease after infection. J Chron Dis 37:853, 1984.

Lingenfelser T, Zak J, Marks IN, et al: Abdominal tuberculosis: Still a potentially lethal disease. Am J Gastroenterol 88:744, 1993.

Mankin HF: Case 9-1996. Vertebral tuberculosis. N Engl J Med 334:784, 1996.

Marshall JB: Tuberculosis of the gastrointestinal tract and peritoneum. Am J Gastroenterol 88:989, 1993.

Munk ME, Emoto M: Functions of T-cell subsets and cytokines in mycobacterial infections. Eur Respir J 20:668S, 1995.

Murray CJ, DeJonghe E, Chum HJ, et al: Cost effectiveness of chemotherapy for pulmonary tuberculosis in three sub-Saharan African countries. Lancet 338:1305, 1991.

Murray CJ, Styblo K, Rouillon A: Tuberculosis in developing countries: Burden, intervention and cost. Bull IUATLD 65:6, 1990.

Murray J, Kielkowski D, Reid P: Occupational disease trends in black South African gold miners: An autopsy-based study. Am J Res Crit Care Med 153:706, 1996.

Nafeh MA, Medhat A, Abdul-Hameed A, et al: Tuberculous peritonitis in Egypt: The value of laparoscopy in diagnosis. Am J Trop Med Hyg 47:470, 1992.

Narain JP, Raviglione MC, Kochi A: HIV-associated tuberculosis in developing countries: Epidemiology and strategies for prevention. Tubercle Lung Dis 73:311, 1992.

Nunn P, Felten M: Surveillance of resistance to antituberculosis drugs in developing countries. Tubercle Lung Dis 75:163, 1995.

O'Reilly LM, Daborn CJ: The epidemiology of *Mycobacterium bovis* infections in animals and man: A review. Tubercle Lung Dis 76 (Suppl 1):1, 1995.

Pesanti EL: The negative tuberculin test: Tuberculin, HIV, and anergy panels. Am J Respir Crit Care Med 149:1699, 1994.

Raviglione MC, Narain JP, Kochi A: HIV-associated tuberculosis in developing countries: Clinical features, diagnosis and treatment. Bull WHO 70:515, 1992.

Sehgal VN: Cutaneous tuberculosis. Derm Clin 12:645, 1994.

Shafer RW, Edlin BR: Tuberculosis in patients infected with human immunodeficiency virus: Perspective on the past decade. Clin Infect Dis 22:683, 1996.

Shafer RW, Singh SP, Larkin C, Small PM: Exogenous reinfection with multidrug-resistant *Mycobacterium tuberculosis* in an immunocompetent patient. Tubercle Lung Dis 76:575, 1995.

Shluger NW, Rom WN: Current approaches to the diagnosis of active pulmonary tuberculosis. Am J Respir Crit Care 149:264, 1994.

Small PM, Hopewell PC, Schecter GF, et al: Evolution of chest radiographs in treated patients with pulmonary tuberculosis and HIV infection. J Thorac Imaging 9:74, 1994.

Small PM, Schecter GF, Goodman PC, et al: Treatment of tuberculosis in patients with advanced human immunodeficiency virus infection. N Engl J Med 324:289, 1991.

Small PM, Shafer RW, Hopewell PC, et al: Exogenous reinfection with multidrug-resistant *Mycobacterium tuberculosis* in patients with advanced HIV infection. N Engl J Med 328:1137, 1993.

Vareldzis BP, Grosset J, De Kantor I, et al: Drug-resistant tuberculosis: Laboratory issues: World Health Organization recommendations. Tubercle Lung Dis 75:1, 1994.

Wilson ME, Fineberg HV, Colditz GA: Geographic latitude and the efficacy of bacillus Calmette-Gúerin vaccine. Clin Infect Dis 20:982, 1995.

Wolinsky E: Mycobacterial disease other than tuberculosis. Clin Infect Dis 15:1, 1992.

World Health Organization: Tuberculosis control and research strategies for the 1990s: Memorandum from a WHO meeting. Bull WHO 70:17, 1992.

World Health Organization: Treatment of tuberculosis: Guidelines for national programmes. Geneva, WHO, 1995.

78 Leprosy*

Wayne M. Meyers

DEFINITION. Leprosy is a chronic disease caused by *Mycobacterium leprae*. It affects the cooler parts of the body principally, especially the skin, upper respiratory tract, anterior segments of the eyes, superficial segments of peripheral nerves, and testes. In 1995, the World Health Organization (WHO) estimated that there were 1.93 million patients with active leprosy in the world.

LEPROSY AND SOCIETY. Comprehending the sources of the stigma of leprosy is essential to understanding the attitudes of society toward this disease and the effect that this stigma has on patients with leprosy. In Western cultures, these attitudes are at least partially attributable to a misunderstanding of what is called leprosy in the Old Testament. Other cultures not influenced by Judaic laws and traditions,

---

*All the illustrations in this chapter are in the public domain.

however, also have a similar tradition. For example, in China, possibly as early as the eighth century B.C., people with a condition later recognized as leprosy were stigmatized.

The Hebrew word *tsara-ath* was rendered *lepra* when the Old Testament was translated into Greek about 200 B.C. In preparing the Latin Vulgate version around 400 A.D., St. Jerome perpetuated the use of the word *lepra*, and Wycliffe, translating from the Vulgate in 1384, changed the word *lepra* to *leprosy*. In the original text, *tsara-ath* was not a specific disease but a group of diseases with obscure identities, and the word referred more generally to ceremonial uncleanliness. Leprosy was common in Europe and Great Britain in the 14th century. To Wycliffe, leprosy in its most severe forms may thus have portrayed the physical image of an unholy and loathsome human condition. Old Testament *tsara-ath*, as described in Leviticus 13 and 14, for example, had none of the distinctive features of leprosy. There is thus no rationale for including *tsara-ath*, as described in the Old Testament, in our understanding and care of patients with leprosy today.

A continuing effort is being made to minimize the stigma peculiarly associated with leprosy. For example, the Fifth International Leprosy Congress in 1948 adopted a resolution to abandon the word *leper* for *leprosy patient*. *Hansen's disease* is preferred by some for leprosy. The U.S. Public Health Service Hospital for the treatment of patients with leprosy at Carville, Louisiana, in 1981 was named the National Hansen's Disease Center and is now called the Gillis W. Long Hansen's Disease Center. Because of the stigma of leprosy, physicians must carefully consider the social implications and assiduously avoid a casual diagnosis of this disease.

ETIOLOGY AND HISTORY. *M. leprae* is a species in the order Actinomycetales and the family Mycobacteriaceae. This bacillus was first seen by Hansen in Bergen, Norway, in 1873 in fresh mounts of scrapings from a leproma from a Norwegian patient with leprosy, and it was the first reported bacterial pathogen of a chronic disease in humans. *M. leprae* is an acid-fast bacillus 0.3 to 0.5 μm wide by 4 to 7 μm long. The acid-fastness is weaker than that of other mycobacteria but, like other mycobacteria, is related to the mycolic acid in the cell wall. Viable undamaged *M. leprae* stain solidly; degenerating organisms first stain irregularly, then become granular, and eventually are fragmented. Serial evaluations of the staining quality thus provide a method for assessing therapeutic efficacy. All claims of in vitro cultivation of *M. leprae* are unsubstantiated. In the absence of successful cultivation of *M. leprae*, identification depends on the results of a series of tests. The criteria for the identification of organisms as *M. leprae* are as follows: (1) Organisms do not grow on routine mycobacteriologic media, (2) organisms infect the footpads of normal laboratory mice in a characteristic manner, (3) acid fastness is extractable with pyridine, (4) suspensions of the bacilli oxidize dopa, (5) organisms invade the nerves of hosts, (6) killed suspensions of the bacilli produce a characteristic pattern of response when injected into the skin of patients with the various clinical forms of leprosy (i.e., tuberculoid patients react strongly and lepromatous patients are nonreactive), (7) produces the species-specific antigen phenolic glycolipid-I (PGL-I), and (8) demonstrates species-specific DNA sequences.

M. leprae organisms multiply slowly in experimental animals, with a generation time of 13 days in the logarithmic growth phase in the mouse footpad. This characteristic may account, at least in part, for the long incubation time of leprosy in humans. Localization of the heaviest infiltrations of leprosy to the cooler parts of the body, selective growth in the footpads of normal mice, and the high susceptibility of the armadillo (central body temperature 32°C to 35°C) to disseminated infections all suggest that the optimal temperature for the growth of *M. leprae* is less than 37°C.

EPIDEMIOLOGY

Distribution and Incidence. There are approximately 6000 cases in the United States, where 136 new cases were reported in 1995. Most of these patients are immigrants, but indigenous leprosy does exist in the United States, primarily in Louisiana, Texas, and Hawaii.

Prevalence rates vary widely. Of all patients, Southeast Asia has 75% (India alone has 65%), Africa 12%, and the Americas 8%.

Transmission. The route or routes of the natural transmission of *M. leprae* are not known. The high frequency of single early lesions in skin that is usually covered by clothing argues against the local inoculation of *M. leprae* at the site of the lesion. Skin-to-skin contact was for many years considered the most important mode of transmission. This concept, although not abandoned, is now being challenged. Intact skin of patients with multibacillary leprosy regularly discharges small numbers of *M. leprae*, but open ulcers can be a source of large numbers of organisms. Thus, infection could take place by skin-to-skin contact or through fomites. The nasal mucosa of untreated lepromatous patients contains large numbers of *M. leprae* that are discharged regularly in the nasal secretions. *M. leprae* released in secretions obtained by noseblowing and dried under ambient conditions remain viable for as long as 1 week; the upper respiratory tract passages are thus a likely source of contagion. The experimental disseminated infections in immunosuppressed mice that follow the inhalation of aerosols containing *M. leprae* support this concept. Breast tissue and milk of mothers with lepromatous leprosy contain *M. leprae*, suggesting that infants could be infected during nursing. Increasing evidence demonstrates placental transmission of leprosy. Sporadic reports describe leprosy in infants as young as 2 1/2 months, and fetal synthesis of antibodies to *M. leprae* has been documented. Natural transmission of leprosy by insects has not been proved.

Animal Reservoirs. With the discovery of naturally acquired leprosy in (1) armadillos in Louisiana and Texas, (2) several chimpanzees from Africa, and (3) a mangabey monkey captured in West Africa, there is reason to believe that leprosy may be a zoonosis. Serologic and molecular biologic techniques demonstrate that as many as 50% of armadillos in some regions of Louisiana have had contact with *M. leprae*, and there are reports of 10% or more of clinical disease in focal surveys of wild armadillos. In all three of these species, the organisms causing the disease could not be distinguished from *M. leprae* of human origin. Although the data are still fragmentary, many authorities believe that infected armadillos transmit leprosy to humans.

Natural History of Infection. The spread of leprosy depends on the dissemination of the bacillus in a susceptible population. The prevalence of clinical disease in most populations rarely exceeds 5%. However, lymphocyte transformation studies in endemic areas demonstrate that approximately half of all close contacts (occupational and household) of leprosy patients are specifically sensitized, suggesting that exposure to *M. leprae* is frequent in these areas. The prevailing concept that repeated exposure is required to contract leprosy does not seem reasonable, because this concept is not valid for other infectious diseases. It may be true, however, that both the numbers of viable *M. leprae* being shed by a patient and the degree of susceptibility of the contact may vary, so that long periods of association would make optimal coincident conditions for transmission in both patient and contact more likely.

Experimental infections can be established in the mouse

footpad by inoculation of a single viable *M. leprae.* Immunologically intact mice are partially resistant to leprosy; therefore, it would be expected that a susceptible person could be infected by a single or only a few viable *M. leprae.*

Geographic, ethnic, and socioeconomic factors may contribute to the spread of leprosy by affecting both the number of untreated or ineffectively treated bacillary-positive patients and the opportunity for exposure. In some Asian populations, 50% or more of all patients with leprosy have the lepromatous form, whereas in Africans this form occurs in only 5 to 10%. Socioeconomic factors are difficult to evaluate, and their relationship to prevalence or clinical severity is unknown. No convincing evidence shows that the prevalence of leprosy is unusually high in chronically malnourished populations, but in special situations nutrition and psychologic trauma may influence the progress of the disease. Studies of patients in leprosaria in Malaysia and China showed that both the severity of leprosy and the mortality were increased in World War II during the occupation.

Improved living conditions have probably had an important role in diminishing the prevalence of leprosy. For instance, no other satisfactory explanation has been offered for the virtual disappearance of leprosy from northern Europe after the Middle Ages and from Scandinavia in the early 20th century, well before the advent of effective chemotherapeutic agents. If transmission is airborne, the construction of dwellings that provide more spacious sleeping quarters could have contributed in a major way to the disappearance of leprosy in these geographic areas. Consistent with this concept is the existence of grossly inadequate housing in all geographic areas where leprosy is highly endemic now.

The widely presumed hypersusceptibility of children is difficult to establish and may represent only an early selection of susceptible individuals and/or increased exposure to contagious patients. The proportion of children in most samples of all detected patients is approximately 20 to 30%. For example, of the 615 leprosy cases diagnosed in Louisiana between 1855 and 1970, 5% of patients had onset at 0 to 9 years and 19% at 10 to 19 years; also, of 2000 children who lived in one leprosarium in the Philippines before the chemotherapeutic era, 23% developed clinical leprosy. Of particular interest in this latter sample was the high proportion (75%) of those with early lesions that healed spontaneously; thus, approximately 6% of all children who were exposed developed active persistent leprosy.

In adults, leprosy is more common in males than in females (2:1 to 3:1), but in children the sex ratio is approximately 1:1. Genetic factors may influence susceptibility and control the form of disease that develops after infection.

PATHOGENESIS AND PATHOLOGY. No toxins have been identified in *M. leprae,* and the pathologic changes are most directly associated with the ability of this bacillus to survive in macrophages or to elicit delayed-type hypersensitivity reactions. If the macrophages of the host digest the bacilli early, either the disease is not detectable or only minor lesions develop. If macrophages are totally incapable of destroying the bacilli, widely disseminated lepromatous leprosy follows. Survival of *M. leprae* in macrophages and the nature of the tissue response to antigens of the organisms depend on the immune response of the individual. Thus, knowledge of immunity to *M. leprae* is essential for understanding the pathologic changes of leprosy.

Immunity

Lepromin Reaction. The potential of an individual to resist leprosy is assessed by the reaction to an intradermal injection of suspensions of killed *M. leprae.* Classically, such suspensions were derived from lepromatous tissue from patients, but infected tissues from armadillos are now a ready and satisfactory source. The reagent is called *lepromin,* and the response, the *lepromin reaction.* This reaction, first studied in Japan by Hayashi and extensively evaluated by Mitsuda in 1919, has two components: an early response called the *Fernandez reaction,* read 48 hours after inoculation, and a late response, the *Mitsuda reaction,* read at 3 or 4 weeks. The Mitsuda reaction correlates most consistently with the immunologic status of the patient and therefore is used by clinicians as an aid in the classification of the form of leprosy and in the prognosis of the disease. Mitsuda reactions are strongly positive (> 5 mm in diameter) in tuberculoid patients, weak or negative (0 to 2 mm) in lepromatous patients, and intermediate (3 to 5 mm) in borderline patients. The reactions are composed of epithelioid cell granulomas and thus are a direct assessment of the level of delayed-type hypersensitivity, or cell-mediated immunity (CMI), to antigens of *M. leprae.* It is important for the clinician and sometimes helpful to the patient to understand that the lepromin reaction is never diagnostic. The primary reason for this is that Mitsuda reactions are positive in more than 90% of most adult normal populations, even in areas nonendemic for leprosy.

Cell-Mediated Immune Responses. Precise mechanisms are still being formulated, but abundant evidence shows that CMI to *M. leprae* is markedly suppressed in lepromatous patients. For example, modifications of the lepromin reaction, using concentrated lepromin, show that macrophages cannot clear *M. leprae* from the skin at the test site in lepromatous patients, whereas in tuberculoid patients the intracellular destruction of leprosy bacilli is highly efficient. Lepromatous patients have various degrees of suppression of reactions to most skin test antigens, but the reactions to *M. leprae* are most consistently and most severely depressed. This suppression is less pronounced in clinical forms of the disease that are progressively more like tuberculoid leprosy.

There is a gradual decrease in the sensitivity of lymphocytes to *M. leprae,* proceeding from the tuberculoid to the lepromatous forms of the disease. Lymphocyte subsets in lesions of tuberculoid leprosy reveal T-helper lymphocytes distributed within the granulomas, with T-suppressor lymphocytes predominating in the mantle of the granuloma. In lepromatous lesions, T-helper cells are diminished markedly throughout the cellular infiltrates. Delayed-type hypersensitivity in the high-resistance forms of leprosy is thought to be conferred by T-helper cells, and cloned T-helper cells recognize several protein antigens of *M. leprae.* Lepromin and the unique antigen of *M. leprae,* PGL-I, have been reported to induce suppressor T-cell activity in lymphocytes from lepromatous patients but not those from tuberculoid patients; however, this finding is controversial. Thus, *M. leprae* contains both immunostimulating and immunosuppressive antigens, and possibly previous sensitization to homologous antigens or cross-reactive mycobacterial antigens determine the reactivity of T cells to *M. leprae* antigens. Interferon-γ stimulates similar responses in macrophages from lepromatous patients and normal subjects, suggesting that the immunologic defect in lepromatous leprosy is not in the response of macrophages but in T lymphocytes. Interferon-γ provokes features of delayed-type hypersensitivity in vivo in lesions of lepromatous leprosy, with apparent decreases in numbers of *M. leprae.* Patients with lepromatous leprosy show defects in interleukin-2 (IL-2), and IL-2 restores T-lymphocyte proliferation in response to specific antigens.

Although HLA genes do not determine susceptibility to leprosy, they do control the form of leprosy in susceptible individuals. The specific influence of a given HLA gene varies among different ethnic groups. Ir genes regulating the immune response to *M. leprae* may code for restriction determinants that restrict and regulate the presentation of antigens of *M. leprae* to T-helper and T-suppressor cells. The majority of restriction determinants are thought to be in the polymorphic areas of HLA-DR molecules.

Immunologic factors in reversal reactions and erythema nodosum leprosum (ENL) differ but are not well delineated. Th-1 cytokines tend to predominate in reversal reactions, whereas Th-2 cytokines are more prominent in ENL. For example, tumor necrosis factor-α (TNF-α) and IL-6 are increased in ENL.

In patients with advanced lepromatous leprosy, the thymus-dependent areas of lymph nodes and the spleen are heavily replaced by infiltrations of bacilli-laden macrophages, impeding the interactions of antigens and subpopulations of lymphocytes and macrophages and the circulation of T lymphocytes through these areas. This would be expected to contribute secondarily to suppression of CMI in such patients.

Immunologic processes involved in damage to nerves are not well understood. Antineural tissue antibodies are common in sera of patients with leprosy, especially in lepromatous forms. Their role, if any, in leprous neuritis is unknown.

Antibody Responses. Immunoglobulin production (IgG, IgA, and IgM) and antibody to mycobacterial antigens are markedly elevated in lepromatous leprosy but only slightly, if at all, in tuberculoid leprosy. These antibodies are not protective but do provide a basis for serologic detection of two *M. leprae*–specific antigens: PGL-I and an epitope of the 36-kd protein. Nearly all untreated patients with multibacillary leprosy have detectable antibody levels. Serologic testing, especially of contacts, may detect leprosy in a preclinical stage, and early treatment of these patients would prevent sequelae and help control the spread of leprosy.

Serologic abnormalities in lepromatous patients include (1) false-positive reactions for syphilis; (2) autoantibodies such as rheumatoid factor, thyroglobulin antibodies, antinuclear antibodies, and cryoglobulinemia; (3) elevated levels of C-reactive protein; and (4) elevated levels of amyloid-related serum protein.

Histopathology. Biopsy specimens should be taken from the active border of well-defined lesions and fixed in neutral buffered 10% formalin or other suitable fixative. The Fite-Faraco staining method best demonstrates *M. leprae* in tissue sections; however, the Ziehl-Neelsen method is not dependable for staining of *M. leprae* in such sections. Histopathologists must never make a diagnosis of leprosy unless the evidence is convincing. The essential features of the histopathologic changes in the skin are summarized in Table 78–1 and pictorially demonstrated in Figures 78–1 and 78–2.

Tissues other than the skin are affected to various degrees in leprosy. The most frequently invaded structures are peripheral nerves, especially at sites where the nerves are near

TABLE 78–1. Criteria for Classification of Leprosy

Group	Clinical Features	Histologic Features	Lepromin Reaction (Mitsuda)	Bacillary Density in Skin
Tuberculoid (TT)	Single or a few anesthetic macules or plaques. Borders well defined. Peripheral nerve involvement common.	Epithelioid-lymphocyte granulomas, with or without giant cells, in skin and nerves. No subepidermal clear zone. Bacilli rarely found in nerves.	Strongly positive	Rare
Borderline tuberculoid (BT)	Lesions similar to TT but more numerous. Borders of lesions less distinct. Satellite lesions sometimes present around larger lesions. Peripheral nerve involvement common.	Granulomas similar to TT. Nerves are infiltrated. Bacilli frequently found in nerves.	Positive	Scanty
Borderline (BB)	More lesions than BT. Borders more vague. Satellite lesions often seen. Peripheral nerve involvement common.	Epithelioid cells and histiocytic infiltrations focalized by lymphocytes. Nerves show increased cellularity. Bacilli readily found in nerves.	Negative or weakly positive	Moderate
Borderline lepromatous (BL)	Lesions are numerous and similar to BB. Some nerve damage.	Histiocytic infiltrations show a tendency to evolve toward both epithelioid cells and foamy cells. Lymphocytes present. Nerves have less cellular infiltration. Bacilli plentiful in nerves.	Negative	Heavy
Lepromatous (LL)	Multiple, nonanesthetic, macular or papular, symmetrically distributed lesions. No neural lesions until late. Late complications of madarosis, leonine facies, testicular damage, etc.	Foamy histiocytes containing large numbers of bacilli. Bacilli in walls of blood vessels and arrector muscles. Few or no lymphocytes. Subepidermal clear zone. Numerous bacilli in nerves and perineurium without significant intraneural cellular infiltration.	Negative	Heavy
Indeterminate (I)	Vaguely defined hypopigmented or erythematous macule.	Often indistinguishable from "chronic dermatitis." Lymphocytes and histiocytes around skin appendages and nerves.	Weakly positive or negative	Rare or scanty

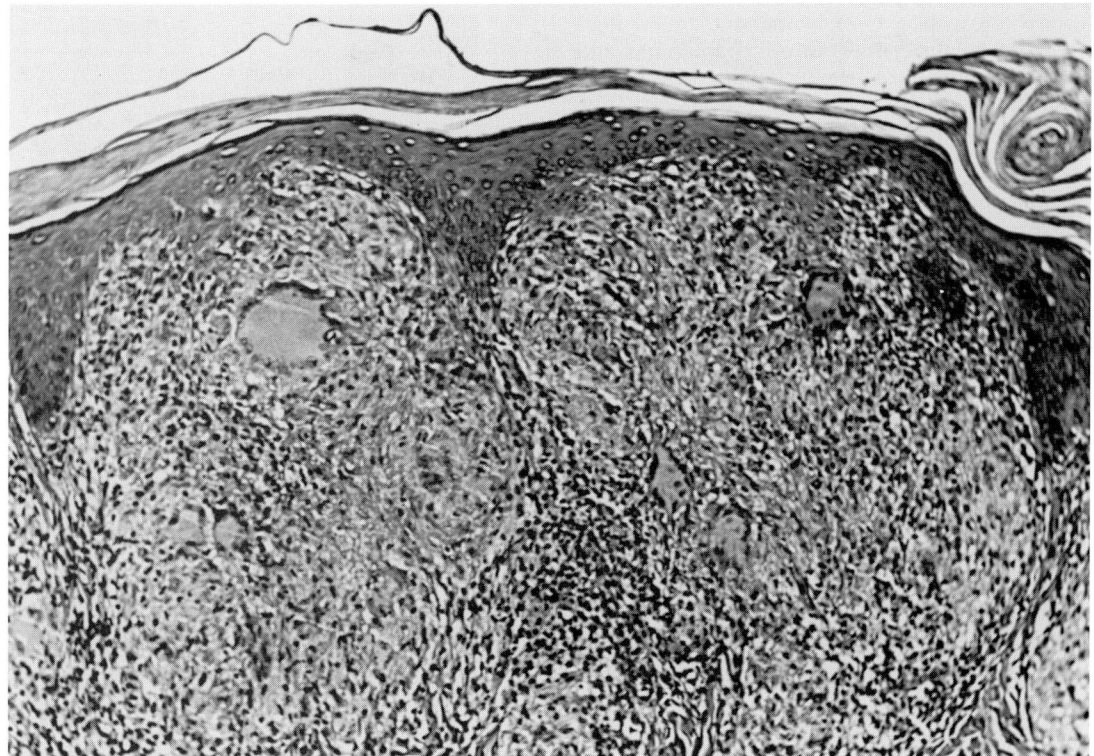

Figure 78–1. Tuberculoid leprosy showing a cellular infiltration of epithelioid cells, giant cells, and lymphocytes in the dermis. The infiltration invades the epidermis. (H&E stain, × 115.) (Courtesy of the Armed Forces Institute of Pathology. Photograph Neg. No. 72-12465.)

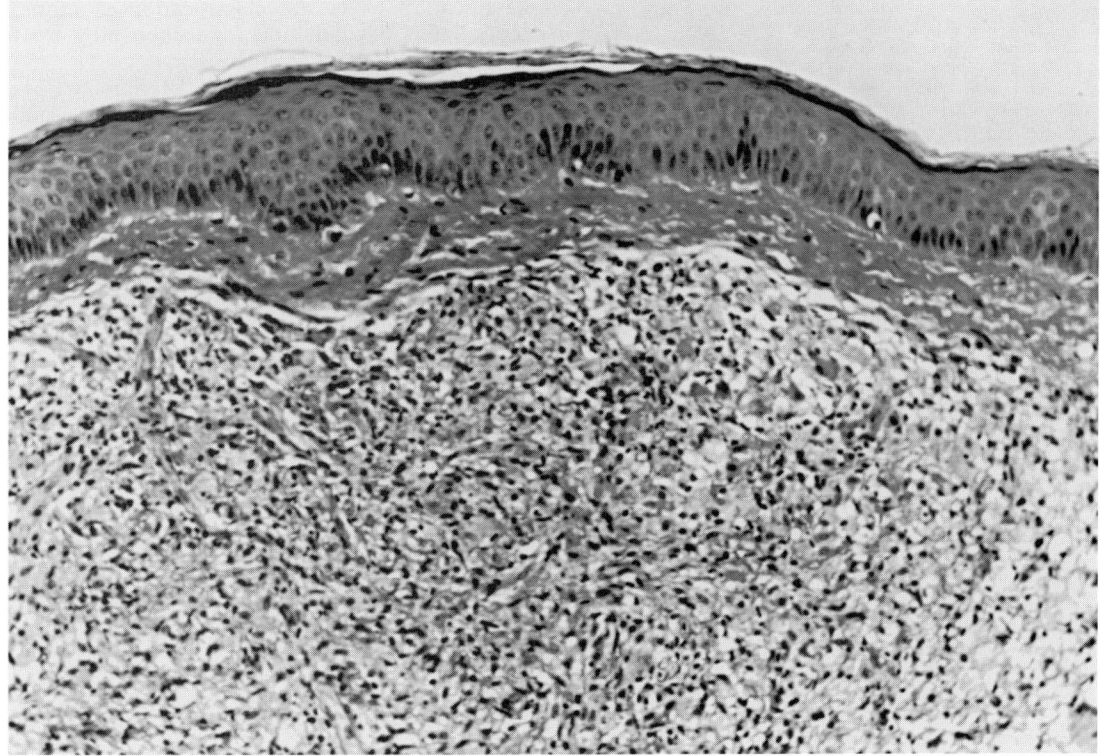

Figure 78–2. Lepromatous leprosy showing nearly complete replacement of the dermis by foamy histiocytes (macrophages), leaving a well-defined subepidermal clear zone. (H&E stain, × 208.) (Courtesy of the Armed Forces Institute of Pathology. Photograph Neg. No. 65-1653.)

the body surface (Fig. 78–3). Lymph nodes in tuberculoid leprosy sometimes contain epithelioid cell granulomas and in lepromatous leprosy may be heavily replaced by bacilli-laden macrophages, especially in the paracortical areas. The liver and spleen may show similar cellular reactions. In addition to these changes, lepromatous infiltrations may invade the following structures: (1) the upper respiratory tract from the nasal mucosa to the larynx; (2) the eye, which may show episcleritis, scleritis, keratitis, iritis, and iridocyclitis; (3) the testis, in which the interstitial tissue and seminiferous tubules may be replaced completely; and (4) bones and joints, causing synovitis, periostitis, and osteitis with replacement of bone marrow by cellular exudates and fibrosis.

CLINICAL MANIFESTATIONS. The incubation period is usually 2 to 5 years but may be as long as 20 years. There are no well-established prodromal symptoms, but some experienced clinicians may recognize focal paresthesias or itching before the appearance of lesions. The nature of the lesions and progress of disease depend on the immune response to *M. leprae*. Only minor strain variations in the etiologic agent have been observed (e.g., growth pattern in the mouse footpad). These strain differences probably do not influence disease patterns, except for those strains that are drug-resistant.

Most clinicians follow the classification schema outlined

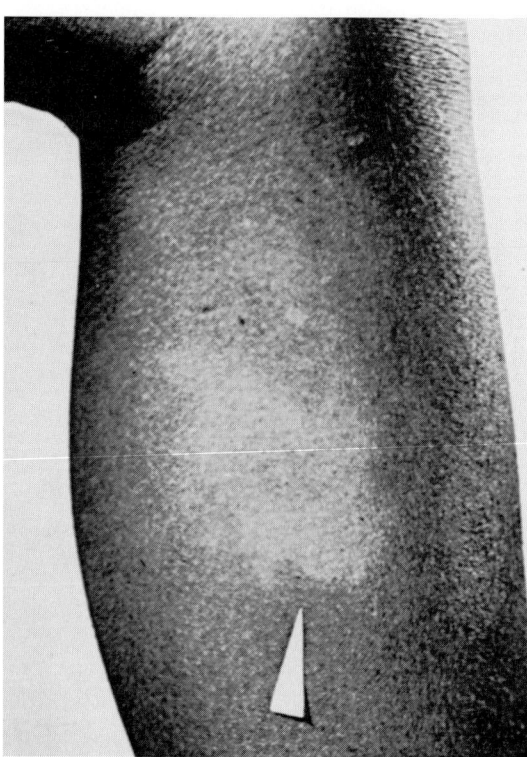

Figure 78–4. Lesion of indeterminate leprosy on calf of a Filipino patient. Note that the lesion is macular and mildly hypopigmented, with vaguely defined borders. (Courtesy of the Armed Forces Institute of Pathology, Photograph Neg. No. 74-9029-1.)

by Ridley and Jopling. Table 78–1 summarizes the criteria for classification. Accurate classification is more than academic—it is fundamental for establishing treatment programs and determining prognosis.

Indeterminate Leprosy. The indeterminate (I) lesion is frequently the earliest manifestation of leprosy and may heal spontaneously, remain unchanged for months or years, or progress toward the tuberculoid or lepromatous forms. Either a single macule or a few poorly defined ones occur in the skin. In more deeply pigmented skin, the macule is mildly hypopigmented (Fig. 78–4) and is slightly erythematous in lighter skin. Skin texture, sensation, and sweating may be slightly altered, but these mild changes may be difficult to detect. Peripheral nerves are normal, and skin smears taken from lesions are either negative or contain only a few bacilli. Diagnosis based only on clinical findings is risky; histopathologic evaluations are advised.

Tuberculoid Leprosy. In tuberculoid leprosy (TT), patients have a single lesion or a few randomly placed hypopigmented or erythematous lesions in the skin (Fig. 78–5). These lesions may arise de novo or develop from indeterminate macules. Lesions may be macular or infiltrated, but the edges are always sharply demarcated from the surrounding normal skin, and the edges frequently are finely papulated. The size of lesions ranges from less than 1 cm to those that cover entire body regions, such as the cheek, thigh, or buttock. Tuberculoid lesions may heal spontaneously or enlarge gradually, leaving a healed, repigmented center.

Within the lesions, sensation is impaired, sweating is diminished, and hair is eventually lost.

Damage to peripheral nerve trunks is common in tuberculoid leprosy, and enlarged cutaneous nerves can sometimes be palpated adjacent to or within lesions (Fig. 78–6). Enlarged

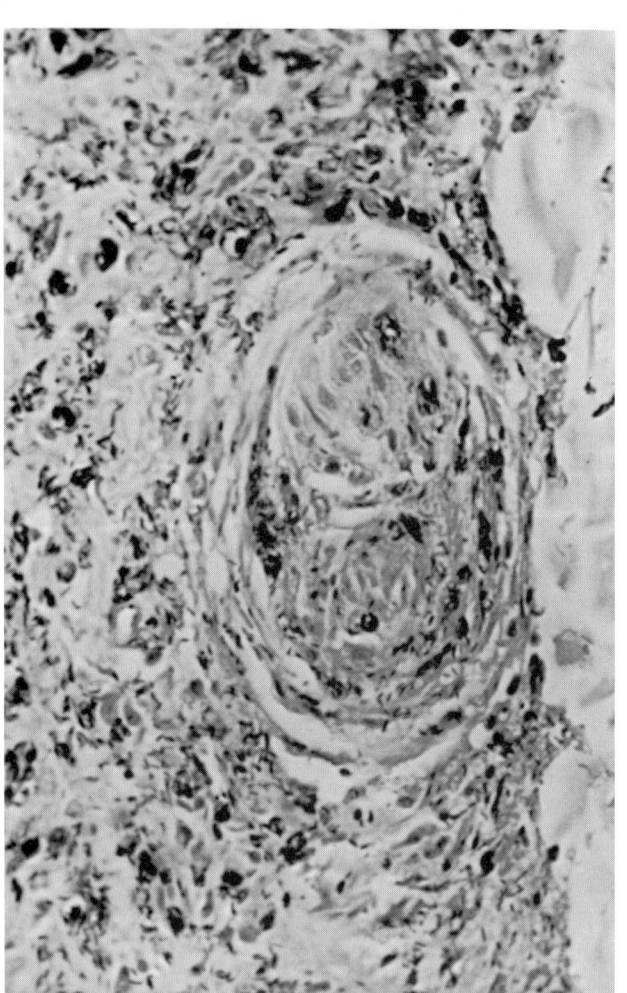

Figure 78–3. In lepromatous leprosy, there are large numbers of acid-fast bacilli *(black clusters)* in histiocytes and within nerves. Note that the dermal nerve is not severely damaged. (Fite-Faraco stain, × 524.) (Courtesy of the Armed Forces Institute of Pathology, Photograph Neg. No. 73-7532.)

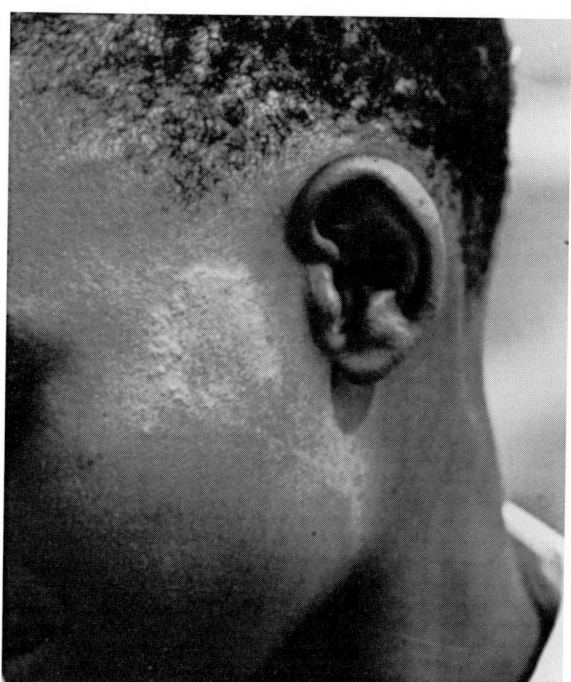

Figure 78-5. Early tuberculoid leprosy in an Angolan boy. The lesion is hypopigmented, and the borders are finely papulated. This was the only lesion. (Courtesy of the Armed Forces Institute of Pathology, Photograph Neg. No. 75-15598.)

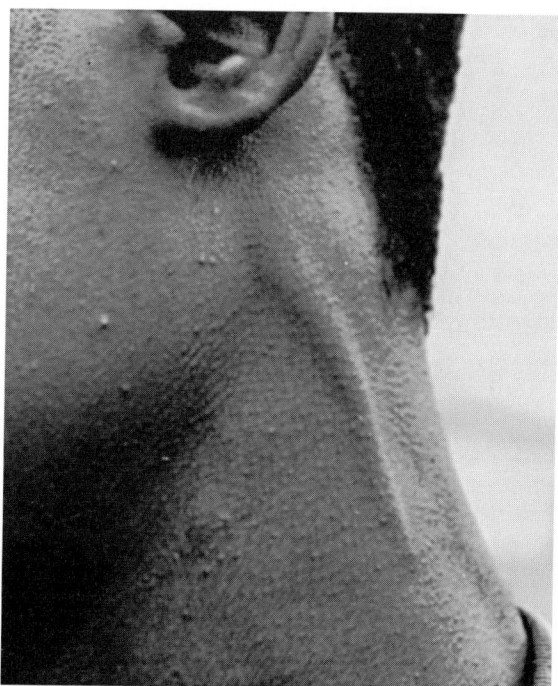

Figure 78-6. Enlarged great auricular nerve in a Congolese with healed lesion of tuberculoid leprosy vaguely visible on adjacent cheek. (Courtesy of the Armed Forces Institute of Pathology, Photograph Neg. No. 77-9359-5.)

or tender nerves should alert a clinician to the possibility of leprosy, particularly in endemic areas. Any readily palpable cutaneous nerve is most likely enlarged, but evaluation of nerve trunk size requires experience because of the wide range of normal sizes.

Borderline Leprosy. Borderline leprosy (BB), sometimes called *dimorphous* or *intermediate leprosy,* has features of both tuberculoid and lepromatous forms (Fig. 78-7). This is an unstable form of the disease that may evolve toward tuberculoid leprosy by reversal reactions or downgrade toward lepromatous leprosy. The salient features of the subgroups of the borderline form are described in Table 78-1.

Borderline patients are particularly prone to major damage to nerves, often early in the disease. These patients frequently consult a physician because of pain in nerves or neurotrophic sensory and/or motor changes such as damaged hands or feet, clawing of the hands (Fig. 78-8), or footdrop. Important nerves most frequently enlarged or tender are the ulnar from the midarm to just distal to the olecranon groove, the median and radial nerves at or above the wrist, and the lateral popliteal just distal to the head of the fibula. Facial palsies frequently lead to exposure keratitis because the eyelids cannot be closed (lagophthalmos), and this is sometimes further aggravated by anesthesia of the cornea if the trigeminal nerve is affected.

Lepromatous Leprosy. The leprosy bacillus multiplies freely in lepromatous patients, and the disease disseminates widely, often before the onset of striking cutaneous manifestations. Lepromatous leprosy (LL) may evolve from indeterminate or borderline leprosy or may be the first recognized form.

Juvenile Leprosy. In its earliest form, lepromatous leprosy presents as "juvenile leprosy," a clinical entity delineated approximately 50 years ago from observations of large numbers of children in homes for children of patients with leprosy in India. This form, also known as *prelepromatous leprosy,*

is difficult to detect and is often unrecognized until a more advanced stage develops. Skin texture is usually not appreciably changed, and the vague macules with indistinct borders are seen only under appropriate lighting, preferably daylight. Patients experience no alterations in sensation or sweating, and acid-fast bacilli are only infrequently seen in smears from their skin. Histopathologic analysis may confirm the

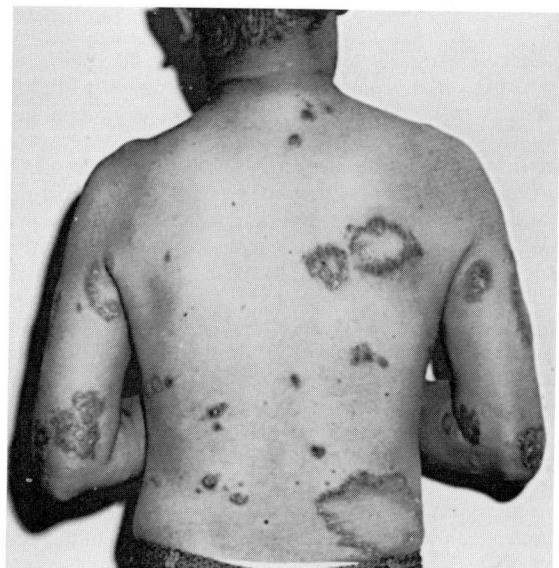

Figure 78-7. Borderline leprosy in a Filipino, with multiple erythematous annular lesions, plaques, and nodules. The lesions are in mild reversal reaction, and peripheral nerves were painful and tender. (Courtesy of the Armed Forces Institute of Pathology, Photograph Neg. No. 74-8485-2.)

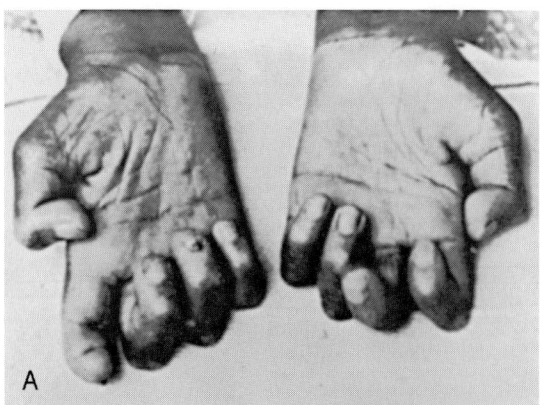

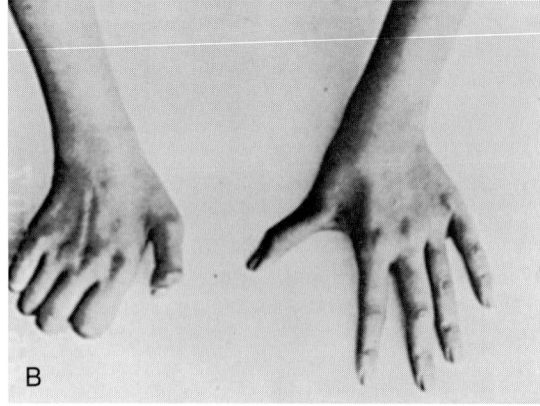

Figure 78–8. Clawing of hands in patients with long-standing borderline leprosy. Note wasting of thenar, hypothenar, and interosseous muscles. (Courtesy of the Armed Forces Institute of Pathology, Photograph Neg. No. 75-15807.)

diagnosis; if not, patients should be closely monitored until an explanation is found for the mild clinical changes. Failure to diagnose and treat leprosy at this stage often condemns patients to the development of gross forms of lepromatous leprosy.

Macular Lesions. Early lepromatous leprosy, like the juvenile form, presents as vaguely hypopigmented or slightly erythematous macules with slight or no sensory changes. These macules are small but may coalesce to cover large areas of skin, even most of the body. Clinical diagnosis is again difficult, but skin smears usually demonstrate acid-fast bacilli, and biopsy specimens are diagnostic.

Nodular Changes. If not treated in the macular stage, infiltrations of the skin gradually increase, and nodules may develop. The heaviest infiltrations are in the cooler areas, such as the ears (pinnae), face, exterior surfaces of the extremities, and buttocks (Fig. 78–9). At this stage, nerves are frequently enlarged, with sensory loss in the hands and feet. Eyebrows begin to thin at the lateral margins and may disappear completely. Pubic, axillary, and other body hair (except that on the scalp) is usually diminished.

The testes become atrophic at a late stage, leading to gynecomastia and sterility. The nasal mucosa is frequently thickened, causing a stuffy nose, and if the larynx is infiltrated, the voice may change. Lepromas may be found in the conjunctiva and sclera. Punctate or interstitial keratitis of the cornea and other ocular changes may be seen by the loupe and slit lamp.

Lucio Leprosy. Patients of Latin-American ancestry, especially those from Mexico, may develop a diffuse lepromatous

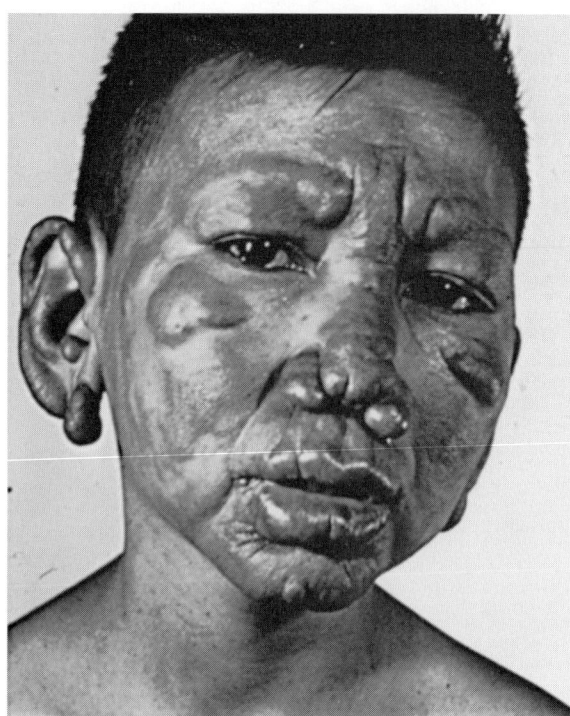

Figure 78–9. Advanced lepromatous leprosy in a Filipino adolescent, with nodular thickening of skin and loss of eyebrows. The heaviest infiltrations are over the central part of the face and ears—the coolest areas. (Courtesy of the Armed Forces Institute of Pathology, Photograph Neg. No. 77-9359-2.)

form called *Lucio leprosy*. This is frequently so diffuse that the disease remains unrecognized until there are sensory changes and the eyebrows and other body hair begin to disappear. Advanced forms of Lucio leprosy are complicated by an obstructive vasculitis in the skin, producing dermal infarcts and irregular ulcers (Lucio phenomenon) (Fig. 78–10). These patients are prone to fatal septicemias.

Neuritic Leprosy. In rare cases, leprosy afflicts one or more major nerve trunks, unaccompanied by lesions of the skin.

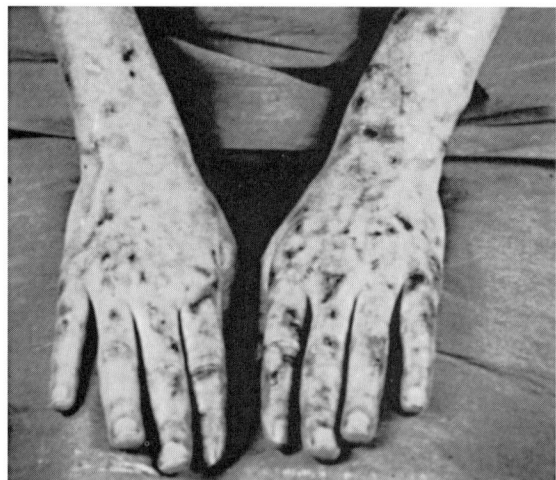

Figure 78–10. Lucio leprosy in a patient of Mexican origin at USPHS Hospital, Carville, LA, showing angular ulcers (Lucio phenomenon). (Courtesy of the Armed Forces Institute of Pathology, Photograph Neg. No. 74-9029-6.)

These patients have pain, anesthesia, paresis, or muscular atrophy in the affected area. Nerve trunks may be enlarged and tender. Histopathologically, this form of leprosy is usually either of the borderline or the tuberculoid form and may be confirmed by carefully taken biopsy specimens of a branch of the affected nerve.

Reactions. The course of leprosy, whether treated or not, is often interrupted by acute reactional episodes. These fall into two general categories: reversal reactions and erythema nodosum leprosum.

Reversal Reactions. Reversal reactions are seen in borderline leprosy and represent delayed-type hypersensitivity reactions with an upgrading of CMI to antigens of *M. leprae*. Lesions become erythematous and edematous, and patients frequently have acute neuritis (see Fig. 78–7). The disease tends to move toward the tuberculoid form. By this mechanism, patients, even with the near-lepromatous form, may be self-healing and produce the classic burned-out leprosy. The neuritis can cause severe sensory loss, and paralytic deformities such as clawhand, footdrop, and lagophthalmos are classic examples (Fig. 78–11). Patients with completely anergic or polar lepromatous leprosy probably never experience reversal reactions spontaneously.

Erythema Nodosum Leprosum. ENL is an immune-complex reaction seen only in lepromatous and borderline lepromatous cases. Approximately half of all lepromatous patients have ENL after a few months of chemotherapy. Tender subcutaneous and intracutaneous nodules have a rapid onset

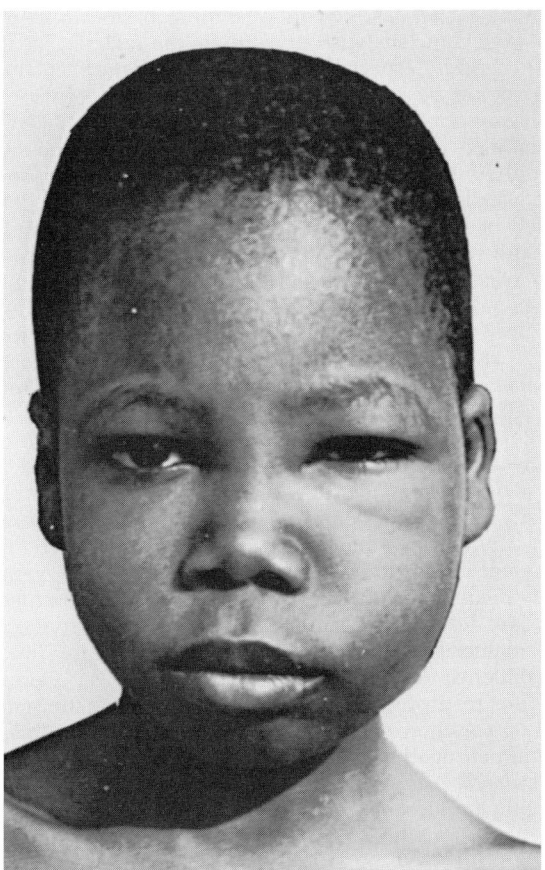

Figure 78–11. Congolese boy with borderline tuberculoid leprosy in reversal reaction. Left side of face is swollen, and there is a mild palsy resulting from damage to facial nerve. Patient responded rapidly to corticosteroid therapy. (Courtesy of the Armed Forces Institute of Pathology, Photograph Neg. No. 77-9359[A]-1.)

and become erythematous (Fig. 78–12). These reactions are accompanied by fever, frequently by iridocyclitis, and sometimes by synovitis. Biopsy specimens of ENL lesions show heavy infiltrations of polymorphonuclear leukocytes and sometimes an intense vasculitis. This reaction frequently leads to extensive ulceration of the skin. Glomerulonephritis sometimes complicates ENL, and secondary amyloidosis is a late sequela in some patients with repeated prolonged episodes.

DIAGNOSIS. Experienced clinicians accurately diagnose most cases with advanced lesions, purely on the physical findings. However, overconfidence may lead to mistaken diagnoses, especially in patients with early lesions. Histopathologic evaluation is strongly recommended for classification and for documentation (see Figs. 78–1 to 78–3 and Table 78–1).

Leprosy occurs in almost all geographic areas; an awareness of this lessens the number of mistaken and delayed diagnoses. In the United States, the average delay between a patient's first visit to a physician and diagnosis is 1 to 2 years.

The history may reveal contact with patients with leprosy or residence in an endemic area, but many patients are unaware of any specific exposure. Footdrop sometimes is the presenting symptom. Lepromatous patients may first consult an otolaryngologist because of a chronic stuffy nose.

Physical Findings. Sensory evaluations of skin lesions must be carefully executed. Regional variations in the richness of the nerve supply to different body areas should be noted. For example, extensive damage to dermal nerves of the face must be identified before sensory changes can be detected by routine testing; on the other hand, the skin over the knees, elbows, and greater trochanters normally is mildly hypoesthetic. A few fibers of cotton or, more quantitatively, graded nylon bristles are used to test light touch, and heat-cold discrimination is tested by using warm and cold water in test tubes. Changes in spontaneous sweating can be observed directly or after induction with pilocarpine. Hair is preserved in early lesions but is lost in advanced lesions.

Main nerve trunks must be palpated for tenderness and enlargement, and the skin in areas of lesions is palpated for enlarged cutaneous nerves (see Fig. 78–6). Leprosy is the most common infectious disease causing peripheral neuropathy in the world.

Skin Smears. Examination of smears for acid-fast bacilli is an important diagnostic procedure. Smears are taken from the edge of macules or plaques, nodules, ear lobes, and nasal mucosa. Smears from skin are made by lightly squeezing and holding a fold of skin between the thumb and forefinger to avoid introducing blood in the smear and making a short, shallow slit in the skin with a razor or scalpel blade. The instrument is next turned at a right angle to the slit, and the edge of the incision is scraped lightly. The cells and fluid thus obtained are spread on a slide, heat fixed, and stained by the routine Ziehl-Neelsen method used to demonstrate mycobacteria. Evaluation of smears is best performed by those experienced in this procedure. An occasional acid-fast bacillus may, for example, be a harmless contaminant or a saprophytic organism.

Differential Diagnosis. The differential diagnosis of leprosy is extensive, and the following partial lists serve only to stimulate clinicians to exercise every diagnostic precaution. Macular changes in pigmentation may be seen in scars, birthmarks, actinic dermatitis, dermatophytosis, and filariasis (especially streptocerciasis). Some infiltrated lesions of the skin that can resemble leprosy are leishmaniasis, granuloma annulare, granuloma multiforme, lupus erythematosus, psoriasis, pityriasis rosea, sarcoidosis, and neurofibromatosis. Peripheral neuropathies that can be confused with leprosy are car-

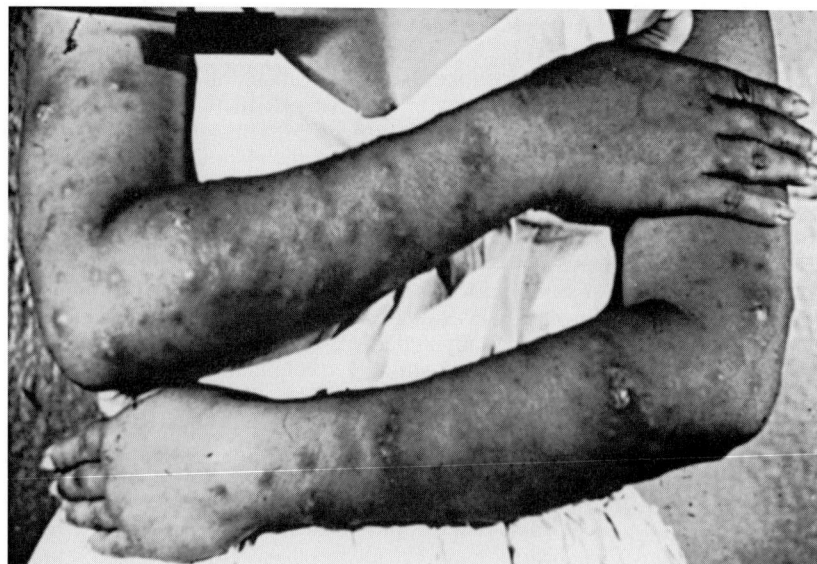

Figure 78–12. Erythema nodosum leprosum in a Filipino girl with lepromatous leprosy. (Courtesy of the Armed Forces Institute of Pathology, Photograph Neg. No. 74-9029-7.)

pal tunnel syndrome, syringomyelia, lead toxicity, diabetes mellitus, primary amyloidosis of nerves, familial hypertrophic neuropathy, and congenital insensitivity to pain.

Serologic and Skin Tests. There are as yet no widely accepted skin or serologic tests for leprosy; however, this is an area of active study. The apparently unique PGL-I of *M. leprae* has been used for developing a specific serologic test for specific antibodies. Results to date, however, suggest that only patients with LL and BL disease regularly have positive results. At least 50% of patients with TT and BT have negative results. Although labor intensive, serial testing of contacts can detect leprosy several years before clinical symptoms of multibacillary disease appear. The lepromin test is useless in the diagnosis of leprosy. Sera from lepromatous patients are often falsely positive for syphilis.

TREATMENT. Treatment of patients with leprosy involves two primary principles: (1) specific chemotherapy for active disease and (2) prevention and correction of deformities or disability. Treatment should be on an outpatient basis. Patients should not be isolated and should be hospitalized only for complications such as severe reactions or correction of deformities.

Chemotherapy. The three most commonly used drugs are dapsone (diaminodiphenylsulfone, or DDS), clofazimine (Lamprene), and rifampin. Until the early 1980s, monotherapy with dapsone was used routinely; however, at that time, dapsone-resistant strains of *M. leprae* were being detected with alarming frequency. Secondary dapsone resistance has been reported in as many as 9.3% of patients at risk and primary resistance in as many as 62.5% of patients presenting for the first time with leprosy.

Multiple Drug Regimens. Multibacillary patients, for the purpose of establishing therapeutic regimens, are defined as those with more than three lesions or with skin smears that are positive for acid-fast bacilli at one or more sites. Paucibacillary patients are those who are skin-smear negative and (1) have three or fewer lesions that (2) are not erythematous or indurated; and (3) do not have neuritis.

Field trials indicate that multiple drug therapy is effective, and relapse rates are at an acceptably low level. Treatment regimens are being changed, and multiple drug therapy is required. The current regimen recommended for adults by a WHO study group is as follows: (1) For multibacillary leprosy (BB, BL, and LL), dapsone 100 mg daily (self-adminis-

tered), clofazimine 50 mg daily (self-administered), clofazimine 300 mg monthly (supervised), and rifampin 600 mg monthly (supervised); and (2) for paucibacillary leprosy (most BT and TT), dapsone 100 mg daily (self-administered) for 6 months and rifampin 600 mg monthly (supervised) for 6 months. The regimen for multibacillary leprosy should be continued for at least 2 years or until skin smears are negative. Many clinicians wish to continue the regimen for much longer periods, especially for LL cases. Paucibacillary patients should be seen every 6 to 12 months to ensure that they have no relapse.

Combined drug therapy should minimize the possibility of drug-resistant strains and perhaps eliminate persisting *M. leprae*. Persisting organisms are viable bacilli that can be isolated in small numbers from patients who are responding to treatment. These persisting organisms are drug sensitive when tested in the mouse footpad and may account for relapses when treatment is discontinued. Persisting *M. leprae* have been detected after as long as 5 years of rifampin, 6 years of clofazimine, and 12 years of dapsone therapy.

Dapsone Regimen. Dapsone monotherapy is never recommended; however, because dapsone is relatively safe, stable, and inexpensive, it will probably continue to be used occasionally as monotherapy in some parts of the world. This drug is bacteriostatic and is given to adults at a dose of 100 mg daily. The effect of dapsone on *M. leprae* is slow, requiring 3 to 6 months' treatment to render bacilli noninfectious for the mouse footpad. The duration of treatment is variable, and there are no guidelines. The suggested duration for paucibacillary leprosy is 18 months after disease activity is no longer detectable. For multibacillary disease, many clinicians treat patients for life. An occasional patient is allergic to dapsone, resulting in a severe desquamating dermatitis. Other uncommon side reactions are anemia, hepatitis, peripheral neuropathy, and psychosis.

Clofazimine (Lamprene). This is a riminophenazine dye that has both antileprosy and anti-inflammatory activity, especially against ENL. When used as monotherapy, the adult dose is 100 to 300 mg daily; however, monotherapy is not recommended. The lesser amounts may be used for maintenance antileprosy therapy, whereas the larger doses may be required in patients with ENL. The major side reactions are hyperpigmentation of the skin and gastrointestinal manifestations. Patients occasionally develop an adynamic ileus.

These side reactions are reversible on discontinuing or lowering the daily dose. Strains of *M. leprae* resistant to clofazimine are rare.

Rifampin. This drug is relatively rapidly bactericidal to *M. leprae*, rendering a highly positive lepromatous patient noninfectious within 1 week; rifampin-resistant *M. leprae* has been described, and thus monotherapy with rifampin is not recommended.

Assessment of Chemotherapy. The efficacy of chemotherapy is readily assessed by serial evaluations of skin smears to determine the morphologic index (MI). The MI is the percentage of acid-fast bacilli uniformly stained by standardized procedures. With effective therapy, the bacilli first are stained irregularly then become granular and finally fragmented. Histopathologic evaluations also demonstrate this phenomenon but in a less quantitative manner.

Physicians unfamiliar with current chemotherapy of leprosy are advised to consult the relevant literature or a specialist in the field because of rapidly changing guidelines based on updated results of trials.

Treatment of Reactions. Reactions in leprosy are medical emergencies; however, early treatment lessens the chances of developing deformities or disability. Patients are hospitalized if the reactions are severe. Specific chemotherapy is not interrupted during reactions.

Reversal Reactions. Reversal reactions in isolated skin lesions, without nerve involvement, are usually of little consequence, but patients should be closely monitored for signs of damage to nerves. Patients with painful, tender nerves should be assessed for impaired function of muscles. Analgesics are given, and the affected part is put at rest. If pain is severe and there is paresis or paralysis of muscles, corticosteroids in high doses must be started (e.g., prednisone 40 to 60 mg daily). After clinical improvement, the drug is tapered to a minimal effective dose until the reaction subsides. Appropriate physiotherapy must be instituted early.

Patients who are first seen with paralytic deformities (e.g., lagophthalmos or footdrop) of relatively recent onset but who are not currently in acute reaction should be given a trial of corticosteroid therapy and physiotherapy. Some of these patients will recover function of the affected part.

Erythema Nodosum Leprosum. Mild ENL is treated with analgesics; more severe reactions require either thalidomide or corticosteroid therapy. Thalidomide is the drug of choice but is teratogenic and must not be administered to women of childbearing age. The initial adult dose of thalidomide is 100 to 400 mg daily, which is then tapered to the minimal effective dose. Corticosteroids, if used, are given as for reversal reactions. If long-term corticosteroid therapy is necessary, some clinicians prescribe an alternate-day regimen to minimize side effects.

Clofazimine is effective against ENL and does not have the disadvantages of either thalidomide or corticosteroids. However, the anti-inflammatory action of clofazimine is not manifested until after 4 to 6 weeks of continuous use. The dose is adjusted to the minimal effective level.

Iridocyclitis often accompanies ENL and requires emergency measures. Topical ophthalmic corticosteroid preparations should be added to the systemic anti-inflammatory regimens and, if possible, ophthalmologic consultation obtained.

Management of Neurotrophic Complications. This is an extensive and complex problem, but several basic principles can be followed: (1) The disease process should be explained to patients so that insensitive hands, feet, and eyes are not unduly exposed to trauma; (2) patients should be taught self-examination of the hands and feet and instructed to report the earliest signs of inflammation or trauma to the physician

for treatment; (3) adequate footwear and gloves or other protective devices should be made available to those with insensitive or deformed feet and hands; (4) appropriate and early physiotherapy must be instituted; and (5) patients should be referred to the appropriate specialist for evaluation and correction of deformity (Chapter 14).

Prognosis. Without chemotherapy, the prognosis is potentially poor, except for those with limited and self-healing disease. Borderline and tuberculoid patients frequently suffer mutilations, and patients with the borderline form can downgrade to the lepromatous form. In lepromatous leprosy, the disease is progressive; patients frequently become debilitated and may die of laryngeal obstruction or renal failure. Blindness may result from exposure keratitis or repeated episodes of iridocyclitis. Patients with deformity are frequently stigmatized and cannot be gainfully employed. With effective chemotherapy and control of reactions, prognosis is good in nearly all patients. If treatment is started early, prognosis is excellent and mutilations can be prevented.

PREVENTION AND CONTROL. The control of leprosy is based on early detection and treatment of patients. Candidate antileprosy vaccines are now under development, and some are being tested under field conditions. These vaccines are composed of (1) either heat-killed *M. leprae* alone or in combination with live BCG or (2) preparations of cultivable mycobacteria (e.g., ICRC bacillus, *Mycobacterium "w,"* or *Mycobacterium vaccae*). Heat-killed *M. leprae* plus BCG is known to increase CMI to *M. leprae* in lepromatous patients and has an immunotherapeutic effect. A highly immunogenic cell wall protein-peptidoglycan complex of *M. leprae* offers promise for a purified vaccinogenic product for leprosy. Initial evaluations of the efficacy of these vaccines for immunoprophylaxis are variable, ranging from no effect to 80% efficacy. Chemoprophylaxis with sulfone may be used for individuals who are at risk; however, wide application is not feasible.

LEPROSY AND AIDS. In contrast to infections with *M. tuberculosis*, *M. avium-intracellulare*, and *M. kansasii*, several observations suggest that there is little or no interaction between leprosy and HIV. In some reports, however, HIV infection posed an overall risk factor of up to 2.2 for leprosy. This question requires continued study of large populations in endemic areas of both diseases.

Bibliography

Becx-Bleuminck M: Operational aspects of multidrug therapy. Int J Lepr 57:540, 1989.

Brennan PJ: The microbiology of *Mycobacterium leprae*, Part II. Reflections on major developments and those responsible for them. Int J Lepr 62:594, 1994.

Brody SN: The Disease of the Soul. Leprosy in Medieval Literature. Ithaca, NY, Cornell University Press, 1974.

Cole ST: The genome of *Mycobacterium leprae*. Int J Lepr 62:122, 1994.

Dietrich M, Gaus W, Kern P, Meyers WM: An international randomized study with long-term follow-up of single versus combination chemotherapy of multibacillary leprosy. Antimicrob Agents Chemother 38:2249, 1994.

Feenstra P: Sustainability of leprosy control services in low-endemic situations. Int J Lepr 62:599, 1994.

Fritschi EP: Reconstructive Surgery in Leprosy. Bristol, England, John Wright & Sons, 1971.

Grosset JH: Progress in the chemotherapy of leprosy. Int J Lepr 62:268, 1994.

Hastings RC (ed): Leprosy, 2nd ed. New York, Churchill Livingstone, 1994.

Noordeen SK: Eliminating leprosy as a public health problem—Is the optimism justified? World Health Forum 17:109, 1996.

Ottenhoff THM: Immunology of leprosy: Lessons from and for leprosy. Int J Lepr 62:108, 1994.

Ridley DS: Skin Biopsy in Leprosy. Historical Interpretation and Clinical Application, 3rd ed. Basel, Documenta Geigy, Ciba-Geigy, 1990.

Ridley DS, Jopling WH: Classification of leprosy according to immunity. A five group system. Int J Lepr 34:255, 1966.

Sansarricq H (ed): La Lèpre. Paris, Ellipses, 1995.

79 Nontuberculous Mycobacterial Skin Infections

Wayne M. Meyers

Paleopathologic findings suggest that mycobacterial infections in humans date to at least the tenth millennium B.C. Some authorities speculate that humans acquired tuberculosis from animals because of closer contact with animals through domestication of livestock in the Neolithic era. Historically, renowned physicians and scientists such as Hippocrates, Sylvius, Laennec, Schöenlein, and Villemin recognized tuberculosis as a specific infectious disease. Robert Koch cultured *Mycobacterium tuberculosis* in vitro in 1882.

There are two major types of infection of the skin by *M. tuberculosis*: primary tuberculosis, such as that noted occasionally in those who perform autopsies on victims of tuberculosis (prosector's paronychia), and reinfection tuberculosis, as characterized by the common lesion of lupus vulgaris. Approximately 75% of patients with lupus vulgaris have tuberculosis of other organs (Chapter 77); therefore, this is a common problem in some developing countries.

In the decades after the identification of *M. tuberculosis*, mycobacteria that differed from *M. tuberculosis* were isolated, and these became known as atypical mycobacteria.

In 1954, Timpe and Runyon first classified atypical mycobacteria into four groups on the basis of their growth characteristics (Table 79–1). Each of the Runyon groups is composed of multiple species. Because of advances in identification of mycobacterial species by cultivation, molecular biologic, and other techniques, this classification has been largely abandoned and specific etiologic agents named.

More than 60 mycobacterial species have now been identified. Approximately one third of these species cause infection in humans. Of these species, the following more common atypical or nontuberculous mycobacteria causing lesions in the skin are discussed in some detail: *M. leprae, M. ulcerans, M. marinum, M. kansasii, M. avium-intracellulare, M. scrofulaceum, M. fortuitum* complex, *M. haemophilum*, and *M. szulgai*.

Leprosy, caused by *M. leprae*, is a common infection of the skin and is discussed in Chapter 78. All of the remaining species in the previous list are mainly environmental organisms; they apparently have no important animal reservoirs

TABLE 79–1. Classification of Atypical Mycobacteria Causing Disease in Skin of Humans

Runyon Group	Pigmentation	Growth Rate	Species
I	Photochromogens*	Slow	M. kansasii M. marinum
II	Scotochromogens†	Slow	M. scrofulaceum M. szulgai
III	Nonphotochromogens‡	Slow	M. avium M. intracellulare
IV	Variable	Rapid	M. fortuitum M. chelonae
Other§		Slow	M. ulcerans

*Pigment produced only on exposure to light.
†Pigment produced in dark or light.
‡Nonpigmented.
§*M. ulcerans* has not been classified in the Runyon system.

and are often resistant to antimycobacterial drugs. Thus, eradication of these pathogens is not currently feasible.

79.1 Mycobacterium ulcerans Infection (Buruli Ulcer)*

DEFINITION AND ETIOLOGY. *M. ulcerans* is a slow-growing mycobacterium that infects the skin and subcutaneous tissues, giving rise to indolent ulcers. *M. ulcerans* grows optimally on routine mycobacteriologic media at 32°C and elaborates a necrotizing immunosuppressive cytotoxin. Large ulcers almost certainly caused by *M. ulcerans* were first described by Cook in Uganda in 1897; however, the etiologic agent was not isolated and characterized until 1948 in Australia by MacCallum and associates.

Mycobacteria biochemically similar to *M. ulcerans* have been isolated from the environment in The Congo, but they are not pathogenic for mice, the usual animal model.

EPIDEMIOLOGY. The source of *M. ulcerans* in nature is not known; however, koalas in southeastern Australia acquire *M. ulcerans* infections naturally. Because all major endemic foci are in swampy terrain or subtropical countries, environmental factors are thought to have an essential role in the survival of the organism. The disease is rarely transmitted from patient to patient. Infection is probably most frequently caused by introduction of *M. ulcerans* from surface-contaminated skin as a result of trauma. The inciting trauma has been as slight as a hypodermic needle puncture or as severe as gunshot or exploding land mine wounds. Individuals of all ages are affected, but the highest frequencies of infection are in those in the second and third decades of life. The largest concentrations of patients are in Uganda and The Congo, but there are significant foci in most countries in central and West Africa, in Southeast Asia, and in Australia, and there are a few patients in Central and South America. Focal outbreaks have followed flooding, human migrations, and manmade topographic modifications such as dams and resorts. Deforestation and increased basic agricultural activities may significantly contribute to the marked increases in incidences of *M. ulcerans* infections. In West Africa, the disease is rapidly emerging.

PATHOGENESIS AND PATHOLOGY. After inoculation into the skin, *M. ulcerans* proliferates and elaborates a toxin that causes necrosis of the dermis, panniculus, and deep fascia. Early lesions are closed, but as the necrosis spreads, the overlying dermis and epidermis become infarcted and eventually ulcerate, leaving undermined edges and a necrotic slough in the base of the ulcer. Histopathologic sections reveal a contiguous coagulation necrosis of the deep dermis and panniculus, with destruction of nerves, appendages, and blood vessels. Interstitial edema is noted. Clumps of extracellular acid-fast bacilli are plentiful and are frequently limited to the base of the ulcer and adjacent necrotic subcutaneous tissue. Bone is occasionally involved. In active lesions, inflammatory cells are conspicuously few, presumably as a result of the immunosuppressive activity of the toxin. With healing, a granulomatous response occurs, and the ulcerated area is eventually replaced by a depressed scar. No evidence shows that HIV infection predisposes to Buruli ulcer or renders infection with *M. ulcerans* more aggressive.

CLINICAL MANIFESTATIONS. Lesions are usually single and begin as firm, painless, nontender, movable, subcutaneous nodules 1 to 2 cm in diameter. Many patients complain of itching in the lesion. In 1 or 2 months, the nodule becomes

---

*All the illustrations in this chapter are in the public domain.

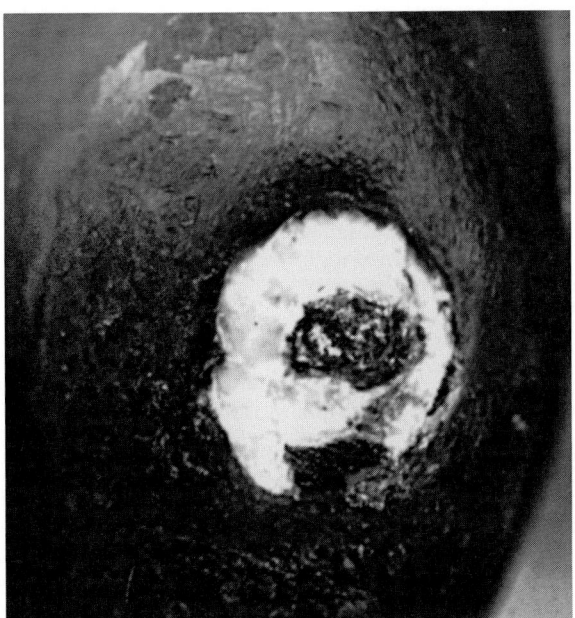

Figure 79–1. *Mycobacterium ulcerans* infection in the deltoid area of a Congolese boy. The patient presented with this lesion 3 months after a hypodermic injection at this site. Note induration of adjacent skin and undermined border of the ulcer with a necrotic base. (Courtesy of the Armed Forces Institute of Pathology, Photograph Neg. No. 76–11034–5.)

fluctuant and ulcerates, leaving an undermined edge that often extends 15 cm or more (Fig. 79–1). The skin adjacent to the lesion, and often that of the entire corresponding limb, may be indurated by edema. Ordinarily, no regional lymphadenopathy or systemic manifestations are noted. Ulcers may remain small and heal without treatment or may spread rapidly, undermining the skin over large areas, even an entire leg, thigh, or arm. Important structures such as the eye, breast, or genitalia are sometimes lost or severely damaged. Most lesions heal spontaneously, but without appropriate therapy, frequently leave extensive scarring, with deformity and lymphedema (Fig. 79–2).

DIAGNOSIS. Smears from the necrotic base of ulcers stained by the Ziehl-Neelsen method usually reveal clumps of acid-fast bacilli. Biopsy specimens that include the necrotic base and the undermined edge of lesions with subcutaneous

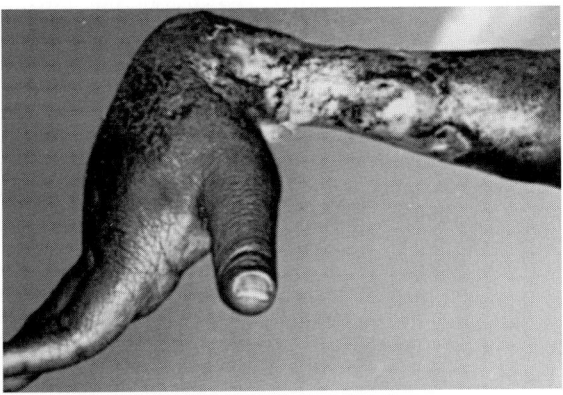

Figure 79–2. Healed *Mycobacterium ulcerans* infection of the forearm and wrist. Scar has caused contraction deformity with subluxation of the wrist and lymphedema of the hand. (Courtesy of the Armed Forces Institute of Pathology, Photograph by Dr. D. M. Connor; Neg. No. 65–2982–1.)

tissue are nearly always diagnostic. *M. ulcerans* can be cultured from a high percentage of lesions, either from exudates or biopsy specimens, but visible growth often requires 6 to 8 weeks of incubation at 32°C. Molecular biologic techniques are often useful in establishing the diagnosis, especially when culture and histopathologic analyses are negative for *M. ulcerans*. There are no specific serologic or skin tests.

TREATMENT. Preulcerative lesions are excised en bloc, and the skin is closed primarily. Ulcers are widely excised, and skin grafts applied. Continuous local heating to 40°C (e.g., by circulating water jackets) promotes healing without excision. Amputation of limbs is rarely necessary. Rifampin promotes healing of preulcerative lesions or early ulcers but is often not effective for extensive lesions. Appropriate physiotherapy is important when contracture deformities are likely to develop.

PREVENTION. No effective prophylactic measures have been demonstrated, but bacille Calmette-Guérin (BCG) vaccination may produce protection or delay onset of lesions for approximately 6 months.

79.2 Mycobacterium marinum *Infection**

DEFINITION AND ETIOLOGY. *M. marinum* was first identified in 1926 in marine fish in an aquarium in Philadelphia but was first isolated as a pathogen of humans from a group of patients who had used a common swimming pool in Sweden in 1954. These lesions are thus often known as swimming pool granulomas. *M. marinum*, also known as *M. balnei*, grows on routine mycobacteriologic media incubated at 30°C to 32°C, but not at 37°C.

EPIDEMIOLOGY. *M. marinum* is presumed to be ubiquitous, and lesions have been reported in many countries. Many patients have been in contaminated swimming pools. The infection is occasionally acquired from tropical fish aquaria or by fishermen or those who work or swim in bayous, rivers, or coastal or brackish water. The organisms are introduced into the skin at sites of trauma. Person-to-person transmission is not known. In nature, water-dwelling animals become infected and shed *M. marinum* into water. The water flea *Daphnia* can serve as a host. Because of the cross-reactivity of *M. marinum* with antigens from many other mycobacteria, epidemiologic studies based on skin testing are not valid.

PATHOGENESIS AND PATHOLOGY. Incubation periods vary slightly but are usually from 1 to 6 weeks. The low-temperature growth requirement limits infection to the skin, usually to the area of inoculation, but regional proximal lymphatic spread resembling that in sporotrichosis occurs occasionally. Rare instances of disseminated infections in immunosuppressed patients have been described. Histopathologically, in early lesions pyogranulomatous infiltrations are seen, but in older lesions tuberculoid granulomas with caseation necrosis are noted. Acid-fast bacilli are few and are usually located in the granulomas.

CLINICAL MANIFESTATIONS. The earliest sign is erythema with tenderness at the inoculation site, followed by a papule or violaceous nodule that ulcerates and drains pus (Fig. 79–3). Older lesions may be verrucous. The cutaneous surfaces of the hands, elbows, and knees are preferred sites, and bursae of the elbows and knees are sometimes invaded. Sporotrichoid spread of lesions is well known. Spontaneous cure in 3 months to several years is the rule, but lesions have persisted for as long as 17 years.

DIAGNOSIS. Histopathologic findings are not specific,

---

*All the illustrations in this chapter are in the public domain.

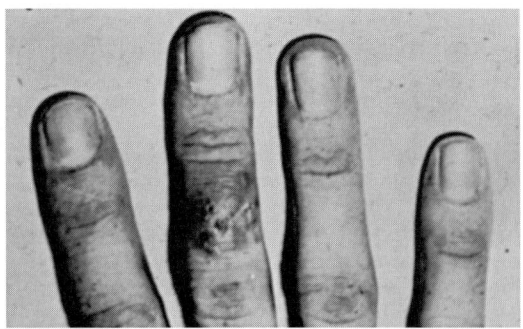

Figure 79–3. *Mycobacterium marinum* infection, "swimming pool granuloma," on the dorsum of the middle finger. There is an ulcer in the center of the nodule. (Courtesy of the Armed Forces Institute of Pathology, Photograph Neg. No. 75–12395.)

even when acid-fast bacilli are seen in tissue sections, making cultivation of the organism necessary for diagnosis. No serologic tests are useful, and skin tests are nonspecific.

TREATMENT. Most lesions heal spontaneously, but because of the protracted course of the disease, many patients seek therapy. When possible, surgical excision or curettage and electrodesiccation have been recommended. Antituberculous drugs, even with multidrug regimens, are not regularly successful. Treatment with tetracycline, 1 to 2 g daily, or minocycline, 100 mg b.i.d. plus sulfamethoxazole, 800 mg b.i.d., and trimethoprim, 60 mg b.i.d., sometimes leads to healing of the cutaneous lesions. Others recommend combined therapy with ethambutol-rifampin, isoniazid-cycloserine, trimethoprim-sulfamethoxazole, or rifampin-ethambutol-amikacin.

PREVENTION. Adequate maintenance of swimming pools interrupts epidemics, but sporadic cases can be prevented only by avoiding potentially contaminated sources.

79.3 Mycobacterium kansasii *Infection**

DEFINITION AND ETIOLOGY. *M. kansasii* commonly infects the lungs (Chapter 77) and only occasionally causes lesions of the skin. *M. kansasii* grows at 37°C.

EPIDEMIOLOGY. In nature, *M. kansasii* is found most frequently in tap water but occasionally in cows and swine. The organism apparently has a worldwide distribution, but in the United States, it is most common in the Midwest and Southwest. Pulmonary infections are acquired by inhalation and are probably transmissible. The mode of primary infection of the skin is unknown but is most likely by direct inoculation.

PATHOGENESIS AND PATHOLOGY. The incubation period is unknown, but one reported lesion developed 1 year after specific trauma. Histopathologic sections show granulomas with caseation, and acid-fast bacilli are usually scarce. Immunosuppressed patients with primary infections elsewhere sometimes have secondary spread to the skin. These lesions show a variable acute and chronic inflammatory response, and acid-fast bacilli may be numerous.

CLINICAL MANIFESTATIONS. The primary lesion in the skin may be a single nodule, or sporotrichoid spread may be noted. Some nodular lesions are preceded by tender erythematous swellings. Lesions have been reported to last as long as 22 years. Patients with disseminated disease with spread

to the skin have erythema, induration, abscesses, cellulitis, and ulcers.

DIAGNOSIS. Diagnosis requires cultivation of *M. kansasii* from exudates or biopsy specimens. No serologic reactions or specific skin tests are useful.

TREATMENT. Chemotherapy should be based on results of in vitro sensitivity tests on the isolated *M. kansasii*. Primary lesions have healed after 4 months of combined therapy with isoniazid, *p*-aminosalicylate, and streptomycin. Use of rifampin in all combined regimens, however, is highly recommended.

PREVENTION. No prophylactic measures are known.

79.4 Infection by "Rapid-Growing" Mycobacteria*

DEFINITION AND ETIOLOGY. This group of mycobacteria grows within 5 days, frequently in 48 hours, even on many of the routine bacteriologic media, at 32°C to 37°C. The nomenclature of the rapid growers is imprecise, and some use the term *M. fortuitum* complex for all members of this group whereas others separate them into two species—*M. fortuitum* and *M. chelonae*. The two species are now divided into five subgroups: *M. fortuitum* into three biovariants and *M. chelonae* into the subspecies *abscessus* and *chelonae*. (Note: *M. chelonae* was formerly spelled *M. chelonei*.)

EPIDEMIOLOGY. These ubiquitous mycobacteria are common saprophytes in soil and water. *M. fortuitum* was first identified as the cause of an injection abscess in 1938 in Brazil. Penetrating wounds of the skin, including surgical incisions and hypodermic injections, are frequent methods of introducing these infectious agents. These organisms may cause disease in amphibians, rodents, and other animals, but no epidemiologic data suggest that these animals are sources of human infection. Infections have been traced to hot tubs and hydrotherapy pools.

PATHOGENESIS AND PATHOLOGY. Incubation periods range from 2 to 7 months. The earliest clinical lesion is a fluctuant abscess that usually forms one or more sinuses that drain pus. A study of specimens in the Registry of Geographic Pathology has shown a striking and unique histopathologic reaction to this group of organisms. The reaction is characterized by a pyogranulomatous response containing clear spaces. These clear spaces are spherical, vary from 20 to 300 μm in diameter, and contain acid-fast bacilli (Fig. 79–4). The bacilli are sometimes clumped and aligned and at other times randomly scattered. The surrounding inflammatory cells are a mixture of neutrophils, epithelioid cells, histiocytes, and Langhans' giant cells. At the perimeter of these inflammatory foci are various amounts of scar tissue with lymphocytes, plasma cells, and Russell bodies. The number of neutrophils varies. In some lesions, they predominate and form abscesses; in other foci, the granulomatous component—epithelioid cells, histiocytes, and Langhans' giant cells—predominates. In larger lesions, many small pyogranulomatous foci appear to coalesce. Although the acid-fast bacilli are concentrated in the clear central vacuoles, occasional bacilli are seen in the adjacent and surrounding histiocytes. The origin and nature of these clear central vacuoles are obscure but may be derived from enlarging phagolysosomes. Most lesions remain localized to the site of inoculation. Spread is rare but has been reported in immunosuppressed patients.

CLINICAL MANIFESTATIONS. Mild local erythema and tenderness develop within a few days at the site of an injection or injury. These changes are usually so minor that pa-

---

*All the illustrations in Chapters 79.3 and 79.4 are in the public domain.

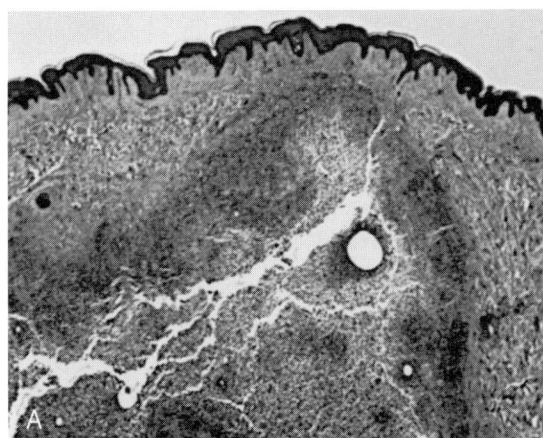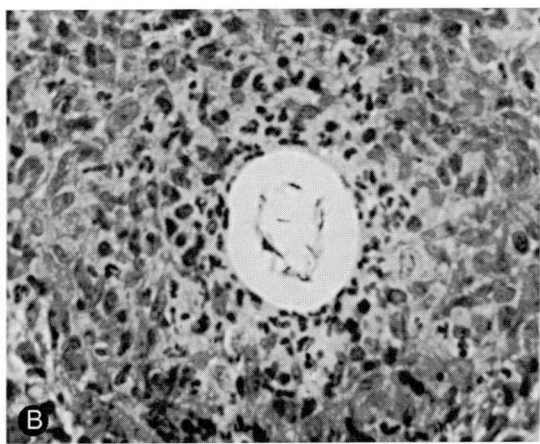

Figure 79–4. Skin from patient with *M. chelonae* infection. *A*, There is a large area of necrosis, suppuration, and granulomatous reaction within the dermis. At this level, the process has not penetrated to the surface of the skin, but in other areas, sinuses have already formed. Within the necrotic area are numerous scattered, circumscribed, spherical vacuoles in which special stains reveal acid-fast bacilli. (H & E stain, × 25.) (Courtesy of the Armed Forces Institute of Pathology, Photograph Neg. No. 81–13874.) *B*, Higher magnification of a vacuole. It is circumscribed and spherical, is surrounded by a mixed suppurative and granulomatous reaction, and contains discrete and clumped acid-fast bacilli in a delicate matrix. (Ziehl-Neelsen stain, × 630.) (Courtesy of the Armed Forces Institute of Pathology, Photograph Neg. No. 81–13871.)

tients do not consult a physician until a subcutaneous nodule, fluctuation, or ulceration occurs, sometimes with associated regional lymphadenopathy. Sites of predilection are the deltoid areas and buttocks (usual sites of injections) (Fig. 79–5). Larger lesions may have numerous sinuses.

DIAGNOSIS. A history of trauma at the site of the lesion is common. Diagnosis depends on cultivation and identification of the etiologic agent. In closed lesions, exudates may be obtained by aspiration. Smears stained by the Ziehl-Neelsen method usually demonstrate acid-fast organisms. Positive cultures are obtained from a high percentage of active lesions.

TREATMENT. Most lesions heal after incision if drainage is maintained. Preulcerative nodules caused by *M. chelonae* have been excised and closed primarily without recurrence. *M. fortuitum* and *M. chelonae* are frequently resistant to antibi-otics and chemotherapy, but in vitro drug sensitivity tests should be performed and appropriate therapy initiated. Successful treatment with amikacin, doxycycline, minocycline, erythromycin, clarithromycin, sulfonamides, and the quinolones has been reported, but the results are variable.

PREVENTION. Infection acquired by hypodermic injection or wound contamination is completely preventable by using sterile equipment and aseptic procedures. Periodic examination of hydrotherapy pools and other water baths for rapid-growing mycobacteria may help control hospital-acquired infections.

79.5 Miscellaneous Mycobacterial Infections*

Of the many mycobacterial species known, increasing evidence shows that, given a large enough inoculum and a sufficiently immunosuppressed host, most species of mycobacteria would be pathogenic. A few are mentioned briefly here.

M. AVIUM-INTRACELLULARE COMPLEX AND M. SCROFULACEUM. *M. avium* and *M. intracellulare* were initially differentiated by animal virulence; however, culture and biochemical properties are so similar that these two distinct species are often classed as the *M. avium* complex, or MAC. In the older literature, *M. scrofulaceum*, because of some antigenic and biochemical likenesses, was grouped with the MAC to form the *M. avium-intracellulare-scrofulaceum* complex, or MAIS complex.

M. scrofulaceum is a common saprophyte and a frequent contaminant in cultures obtained from human tissues; hence, the causal relationship of this organism to lesions must be accepted cautiously. *M. scrofulaceum*, however, is a common cause of cervical lymphadenitis and scrofuloderma in children (Fig. 79–6) but is rarely the etiologic agent of primary lesions in the skin. Combined isoniazid and rifampin therapy has been reported to be successful.

MAC has been reported as the cause of only a few primary skin lesions in immunocompetent patients. One reported pa-

---

*All the illustrations in this chapter are in the public domain.

Figure 79–5. Injection ulcer caused by *Mycobacterium fortuitum* in buttock of Congolese child who had a hypodermic injection at this site 2 months previously. (Courtesy of the Armed Forces Institute of Pathology, Photograph Neg. No. 78–3306.)

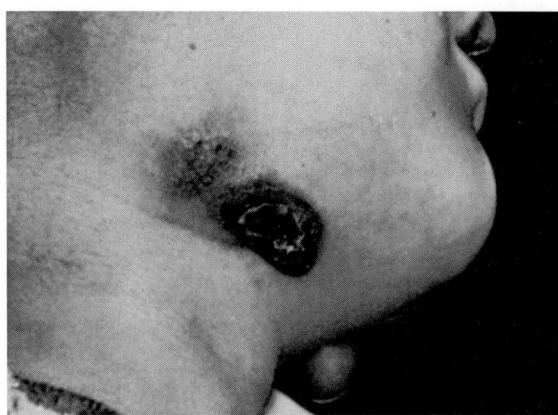

Figure 79–6. Scrofuloderma in a child. The ulcer and sinus tract in the skin communicated with an underlying cervical lymphadenitis. (Courtesy of the Armed Forces Institute of Pathology, Photograph Neg. No. 53–11701.)

tient had extensive ulcerated lesions that developed over 11 years over 20 to 30% of the body surface. Combined therapy with isoniazid, cycloserine, or ethionamide, and streptomycin has been effective. Combination regimens that include the macrolides (clarithromycin or azithromycin) and rifabutin seem to be the most efficacious.

Patients with AIDS have been reported to be unusually susceptible to MAC infections, and cutaneous lesions are becoming more common.

M. SZULGAI. This ubiquitous scotochromogen grows at 25°C to 37°C and was first isolated in 1972. Although mainly a pulmonary pathogen, it is reported to have occasionally caused bursitis, cervical lymphadenitis, and cutaneous lesions. In the skin, these are usually abscesses or cellulitis. Therapy with isoniazid, rifampin, ethambutol, and streptomycin is reported to be effective.

M. HAEMOPHILUM. This slow-growing organism with an optimal growth temperature of 30°C is so named because iron-supplemented media are required for cultivation. An ever-increasing number of patients have cutaneous lesions caused by *M. haemophilum*. Patients usually have numerous nodules, abscesses, or ulcers. While most patients have been immunosuppressed, immunocompetent individuals are susceptible.

OTHER IDENTIFIED MYCOBACTERIA CAUSING CUTANE-

OUS LESIONS. The following mycobacteria are rarely associated with chronic inflammatory lesions of the skin: *M. gordonae*, *M. thermoresistible*, and *M. smegmatis*. Although no standard chemotherapeutic regimen is used, those that contain ciprofloxacin and rifampin are most effective.

LESIONS CAUSED BY UNIDENTIFIED ACID-FAST BACILLI. From 1957 to 1971, a benign disease was observed in 29 patients in the northern central United States and Canada who had indurated erythematous papules (Fig. 79–7), primarily of the limbs, and regional lymphadenopathy. These lesions ulcerated and contained large numbers of acid-fast bacilli that could not be cultured but were not *M. leprae*. The files of the Armed Forces Institute of Pathology contain several similar additional cases, some in immunosuppressed patients. The etiologic agent of these lesions has not been identified, but morphologic features of acid-fast bacilli and histopathologic features suggest *M. haemophilum* may be the cause.

BACILLE CALMETTE-GUÉRIN. Vaccination with BCG (an attenuated *M. bovis*) occasionally causes progressive disease. Large lupus vulgaris–like lesions develop at the inoculation site, accompanied by regional lymphadenopathy. Immunosuppressed patients may rarely develop systemic infections. Most progressive infections caused by BCG respond to isoniazid therapy.

Bibliography

Chapman JS: The Atypical Mycobacteria and Human Mycobacteriosis. New York, Plenum Medical Book Company, 1977.

Connor DH, Meyers WM, Krieg RE: Infection by *Mycobacterium ulcerans*. In Binford CH, Connor DH (eds): Pathology of Tropical and Extraordinary Diseases. An Atlas, Vol 1. Washington, DC, Armed Forces Institute of Pathology, 1976, pp 226–235.

Cox SK, Strausbaugh LJ: Chronic cutaneous infection caused by *Mycobacterium intracellulare*. Arch Dermatol 117:794, 1981.

Cross GM, Guill MA, Aton JK: Cutaneous *Mycobacterium szulgai* infection. Arch Dermatol 121:247, 1985.

Dalovisio JR, Pankey GA, Wallace RJ, et al: Clinical usefulness of amikacin and doxycycline in the treatment of infection due to *Mycobacterium fortuitum* and *Mycobacterium chelonei*. Rev Infect Dis 3:1068, 1981.

Falkinham JO III: Epidemiology of infection by nontuberculous mycobacteria. Clin Microbiol Rev 9:177, 1996.

Feldman RA, Hershfield E: Mycobacterial skin infections by an unidentified species. A report of 29 patients. Ann Intern Med 80:445, 1974.

Gengoux P, Portaels F, Lachapelle JM, et al: Skin granulomas due to *Mycobacterium gordonae*. Int J Dermatol 26:181, 1987.

Heurlin N, Petrini B: Treatment of non-tuberculous mycobacterial infection in patients with AIDS. Scand J Infect Dis 25:619, 1993.

Meyers WM: Mycobacterial infections of the skin (including leprosy, tuberculosis of the skin, Buruli ulcer, and less common mycobacterial infections). In Doerr W, Seifert G (eds): Tropical Dermatology, Vol 8, 2nd ed. Berlin, Springer-Verlag, 1995, pp 291–377.

Meyers WM, Shelly WM, Connor DH: Heat treatment of *Mycobacterium ulcerans* infection without surgical excision. Am J Trop Med Hyg 23:924, 1974.

Meyers WM, Tignokpa N, Priuli GB, Portaels F: *Mycobacterium ulcerans* infection (Buruli ulcer): First reported patients in Togo. Br J Dermatol 134:1116, 1996.

Mitchell PJ, McOrist S, Bilney R: Epidemiology of *Mycobacterium ulcerans* infection in koalas (*Phascolarctas cinereus*) on Raymond Island, southeastern Australia. J Wildlife Dis 23:386, 1987.

Pimsler M, Sponsler TA, Meyers WM: Immunosuppressive properties of the soluble toxin from *Mycobacterium ulcerans*. J Infect Dis 157:577, 1988.

Portaels F: Epidemiology of mycobacterial diseases. Clin Dermatol 13:207, 1995.

Portaels F, Fonteyne PA, de Beenhouwer H, et al: Variability in the 3′ end of the 16S rRNA sequence of *Mycobacterium ulcerans* is related to geographic origin of isolates. J Clin Microbiol 34:962, 1996.

Ratledge C, Stanford J (eds): The Biology of the Mycobacteria, Vols 1 and 2. London, Academic Press, 1982.

Street ML, Umbert-Millet IJ, Robert GD, Su NPD: Nontuberculous mycobacterial infections of the skin. Reports of fourteen cases and review of the literature. J Am Acad Dermatol 24:208, 1991.

Timpe A, Runyon EH: The relationship of "atypical" and acid-fast bacteria to human disease: A preliminary report. J Lab Clin Med 44:202, 1954.

Wayne LG: The "atypical" mycobacteria: Recognition and disease association. CRC Critical Rev Microbiol 12:185, 1985.

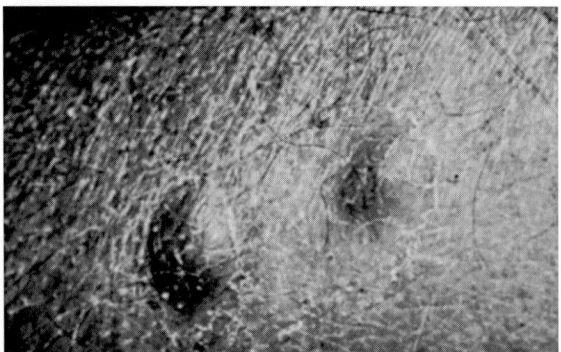

Figure 79–7. Two of many similar papules in skin of 51-year-old American who was under immunosuppressive therapy following an organ transplant. The nodule was caused by an unidentified acid-fast bacillus. (Courtesy of the Armed Forces Institute of Pathology, Photograph Neg. No. 75–12220–1.)

80 *General Principles*

Roderick J. Hay

Mycoses are diseases caused by fungi, which are among the most common microorganisms in man's environment. Fungi are highly successful organisms that have spread widely as saprophytes and parasites and affect humans both indirectly and directly. As agents of spoilage and destruction, they cause serious losses to crops and stored foodstuffs and to a wide range of manufactured materials. Some of the toxins produced by fungi are highly potent, and outbreaks of mycotoxicoses have been reported in the tropics where individuals or communities consume grain or other produce that has become moldy. Many fungi produce airborne spores, sometimes in very large numbers, and these may sensitize atopic subjects, causing symptoms of respiratory allergy after inhalation. Apart from their toxigenic and allergenic potentials, several fungi are capable of causing disease directly, by invasion of external or internal body surfaces. The type of infection caused varies from localized superficial colonization of hair shafts to invasive disease with a high mortality.

DISTRIBUTION AND MEDICAL IMPORTANCE. Some mycoses are restricted to certain geographic areas; others have a worldwide distribution. Their recognition may be comparatively simple but in many instances the full spectrum of investigative diagnostic aids, including microscopy, culture, and serology are required before a fungal etiology can be established. Mycoses are common, particularly in the tropics, where they constitute an important public health problem. Fungi do not rank with parasites or bacteria as causes of mortality, but they are widespread and common causes of morbidity, and individual patients may develop progressively disabling or disseminated disease. Although most fungal infections are acquired exogenously from a source in nature, some mycoses, e.g., candidosis, are initiated by fungi that are a normal part of the human microflora.

MORPHOLOGY. The basic vegetative organization of most pathogenic fungi is filamentous. In substrates supporting their growth, they take the shape of cylindrical, branching chains of cells or hyphae, usually about 3 to 5 μm in diameter. They are bound by a rigid carbohydrate cell wall and may, or may not, have cross walls or septa along their length. Hyphae increase in length only at their tips. Because they frequently send out side branches, new growing tips are constantly formed, and the rate of colonization of host substrate therefore increases rapidly. On artificial media and often in the natural environment this vegetative phase is followed by the development of a reproductive phase in most fungi. Fungi produce an enormous range of spore types which are useful for distinguishing between different species or groups of fungi. Spores are also the means whereby the pathogen may gain access to its host. Many spores (conidia) are dispersed aerially, and infection is therefore commonly established by the respiratory route. Some fungi, e.g., yeasts, are unicellular and reproduce via production of daughter cells by budding. The range of morphologic expression among fungi is wide. In several of the more important pathogenic species, they may assume one form when growing in their natural habitat (e.g., soil, decaying vegetation) or in culture media, and a different form in parasitized tissues. The saprophytic and pathogenic phases in several species, e.g., *Histoplasma capsulatum* and *Blastomyces dermatitidis*, correspond to filamentous (hyphal) and yeastlike (budding) growth, respectively. This phenomenon (dimorphism) is characteristic of some, but not all, pathogenic fungi.

DIAGNOSIS. Isolation and identification of the causal agent are valuable laboratory procedures. Serologic tests may also be helpful, although they sometimes yield equivocal results. Direct microscopy of skin fragments or examination of tissue sections stained with special fungal stains (e.g., methenamine silver Grocott modification or periodic acid–Schiff [PAS]) can provide direct and unequivocal evidence of fungal etiology and identity. A feature of most types of mycoses is the acquisition of hypersensitivity, and in some instances, the development of antibodies. Immunologic tests may therefore be of value in epidemiologic studies (using skin tests to assess previous infection) and in diagnosis (using serologic procedures to detect and quantitate specific antibodies). Direct microscopy is a simple method of demonstrating the presence of fungi in lesions, particularly in superficial infections.

DISEASE CLASSIFICATION. Traditionally, mycoses have been classified according to their route of infection and body site involved.

Superficial Mycoses (see Chapter 81). These mycoses, e.g., pityriasis versicolor, affect only the dead, fully keratinized portions of the epidermis and its appendages. Living tissues are seldom invaded. Some of these mycoses, e.g., tinea, although confined to keratinized parts of the body, may elicit acute or chronic inflammatory changes in the skin, which can be painful, unsightly, or disfiguring. Invasion of nails may result in dystrophy. Superficial mycoses may be acute or chronic, inflammatory or noninflammatory, and—unusual among fungal infections—acquired by contagion.

Subcutaneous Mycoses or Mycoses of Implantation (see Chapter 82). These diseases, e.g., mycetoma, are introduced through the skin surface by a penetrating wound, such as a thorn prick or splinter wound. The agents are usually environmental saprophytes. Once established they provoke an intense and destructive host response. The lesions tend to be localized and progressive, usually without any tendency to heal spontaneously.

Systemic Mycoses (see Chapter 83). Some of these mycoses, which are caused by respiratory pathogens, e.g., histoplasmosis, are acquired by inhalation of airborne spores, and the initial site of multiplication is the lung. Most infections are self-limiting, but serious progressive or disseminated disease occurs in a small proportion of patients, particularly those who are immunocompromised. Opportunistic mycotic infections (see Chapter 83.7), e.g., mucormycosis, owe their origins more to the susceptibility of the host than to the inherent pathogenicity of the infecting fungus. They occur in patients whose normal defenses have been compromised by primary debilitating diseases, e.g., AIDS, leukemia, diabetes, and malnutrition; by defects in the immune system; or by treatment with steroids or broad-spectrum antibiotics.

Bibliography

Baker RD: The Pathologic Anatomy of Mycoses: Human Infections with Fungi, Actinomycetes and Algae. New York, Springer-Verlag, 1971.

Chandler F, Kaplan W, Ajello L: A Color Atlas and Textbook of the Histopathology of Mycotic Diseases. London, Wolfe Medical Publications, 1980.
Emmons CW, Binford CR, Utz JP, et al: Medical Mycology, 3rd ed. Philadelphia, Lea & Febiger, 1977.
Rippon J: Medical Mycology: The Pathogenic Fungi and the Pathogenic Actinomycetes, 3rd ed. Philadelphia, WB Saunders, 1988.

81 Superficial Mycoses

Roderick J. Hay

81.1 Dermatophyte Infections (Ringworm, Tinea)

DEFINITION. The dermatophyte fungi cause infections that are confined to the superficial stratum corneum as well as keratinized structures, e.g., hair or nail arising from skin. Deep invasion occurs only rarely. The infections caused by these organisms are known collectively as ringworm. Alternatively, the word *tinea* followed by the Latin term for the appropriate part of the body involved is used, such as tinea capitis for ringworm of the scalp.

ETIOLOGY. In humans, dermatophyte infections are seen in both tropical and temperate climates, although the predominant pattern of invasion may differ in these areas. For instance, in Europe and the United States, tinea pedis affecting the interdigital spaces on the feet is the most common symptomatic form of ringworm, whereas in the tropics, groin, body, and scalp infections are more prevalent. Infections are derived from three main sources—humans (anthropophilic), animals (zoophilic), and soil (geophilic). Those originating from the soil are not common. Zoophilic infections tend to produce lesions of the scalp or body and are often highly inflammatory. In contrast, the anthropophilic organisms may be found in lesions in any site and often, depending on the species involved and the site of invasion, the inflammatory response is minimal.

The natural course of a human infection is frequently self-limiting, although infections of certain sites, including the toenails, soles, and, in some instances, scalp, or by certain organisms, e.g., *Trichophyton rubrum* or *Trichophyton concentricum*, may be chronic. The condition of the host is also important in determining the course of infection. Atopic subjects are more likely to develop persistent infections.

The organisms that cause dermatophyte infections in humans are confined to three genera, *Trichophyton, Microsporum,* and *Epidermophyton* (Table 81–1). Each has a characteristic pattern of growth and production of spores (macro- or microconidia). Different species can be distinguished on the basis of colonial morphology, spore production, and nutritional requirements in vitro.

EPIDEMIOLOGY. The epidemiology of dermatophyte infections is incompletely understood. However, various trends have emerged over the years. The most common cause of ringworm throughout the world is *Trichophyton rubrum*. In the early part of the century, infections with this organism were most prevalent in the Far East. However, since then considerable spread has taken place and in many areas of the tropics *T. rubrum* is the major cause of groin or body infections. Asymptomatic involvement of the sole may occur also in any climate. Scalp infection caused by this organism

TABLE 81–1. Most Common Dermatophyte Fungi of the Tropics

Genus	Species	Source
Trichophyton	*T. rubrum*	Humans
	T. mentagrophytes	Rodents, cats, dogs
	T. interdigitale	Humans
	T. tonsurans	Humans
	T. concentricum	Humans
	T. schoenleinii	Humans
	T. violaceum	Humans
	T. soudanense	Humans
Microsporum	*M. audouinii*	Humans
	M. canis	Cats, dogs
	M. ferrugineum	Humans
	M. gypseum	Soil
Epidermophyton	*E. floccosum*	Humans

is rare, however. In temperate areas, toenail and toe web invasion are seen often. *Trichophyton violaceum* is an organism that has been isolated predominantly from patients in India and the Far and Middle East. *T. violaceum* also causes ringworm in other sites, including the body.

Ringworm of the Scalp. The distribution of the agents of ringworm of the scalp throughout the tropical world is complex. In some parts of Europe, parts of the United States, and South America, *Microsporum canis*, whose natural host is the cat or dog, is the most important cause of ringworm of the scalp. This contrasts with some areas of the southern United States, inner cities of the United Kingdom, and Mexico, where *Trichophyton tonsurans* is the main agent in this infection. In Africa, there is considerable variation in the main types of scalp ringworm seen. Frequently, small pockets of infection with distinct organisms can be noticed, e.g., *Microsporum audouinii* in Nigeria and *T. violaceum* in North Africa. In India and the Middle East, *T. violaceum* is the major cause of ringworm of the scalp. The factors underlying the occurrence of small endemic foci of ringworm of the scalp include the stability of the population, absence of control measures, and, on occasion, spread via external agents such as hairdressers' equipment.

Favus. *Trichophyton schoenleinii* is the major cause of the scalp infection known as favus, which is characterized by the formation of perifollicular crusts (scutula) that may amalgamate to form a dense mat on the scalp. Favus, once common in Europe, is now found normally in small endemic foci, often involving a single family or a group of families. Such clusters of cases have been described, for instance, in Ethiopia and southern Brazil. However, larger numbers of cases have also been seen in North Africa, South Africa, and parts of the Middle East. The organism is noted for its persistence and may involve all of the female members of one family. Infection acquired in childhood may persist in females into adult life.

Tinea imbricata. *Trichophyton concentricum* is the cause of the infection known as tinea imbricata or tokelau. It is characterized by the appearance of homogeneous sheets or concentric rings of scaling that may cover large areas of the body (Fig. 81–1). Tinea imbricata is best known in the Pacific Islands and Melanesia, but scattered reports of the disease in isolated populations, often living in primitive conditions, have been reported from Malaysia, India, Brazil, and Mexico.

PATHOLOGY AND PATHOGENESIS. In many forms of dermatophytosis, the organisms are confined to the stratum corneum. There is minimal hyperkeratosis and acanthosis and a sparse infiltrate of lymphocytes around upper dermal blood vessels. In severe forms of animal ringworm, a dense

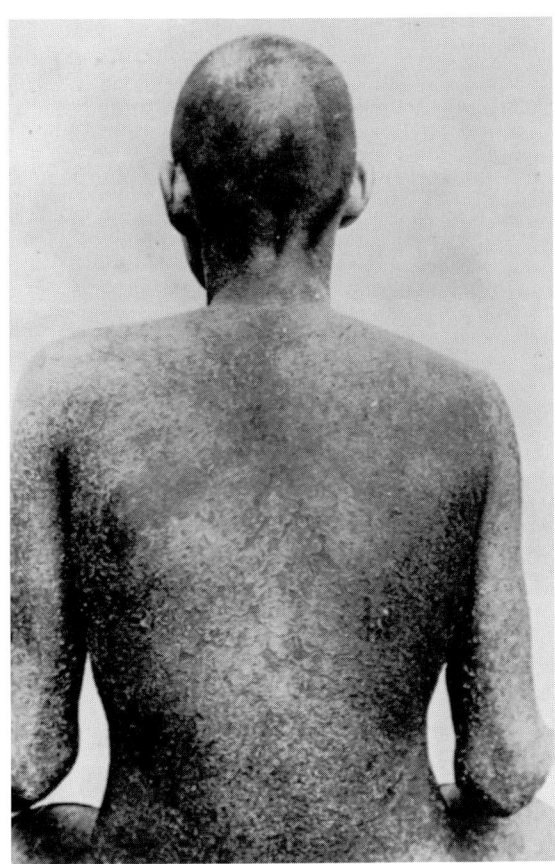

Figure 81–1. Tinea imbricata, caused by *T. concentricum*, is characterized by concentric rings of scales. (Courtesy of the Armed Forces Institute of Pathology, Photograph Neg. No. 39237.)

infiltrate of polymorphonuclear leukocytes and lymphocytes can be found in the upper dermis. In a late stage of this process, lymphocytes and histiocytes predominate in the infiltrate. Resistance to dermatophytosis depends on a number of nonspecific and immunologic factors. Serum from uninfected individuals contains a factor(s) that is inhibitory to the growth of dermatophyte fungi. Unsaturated transferrin, for instance, can inhibit the organisms. Sebaceous material may be inhibitory also. Changes in the fatty acid composition of sebum may explain the common observation that ringworm of the scalp is rare after puberty. When it does occur in adults, it almost always affects women.

The rate of epidermal turnover in an infected area increases, and this may explain the appearance of scaling. It is not clear, however, if this is directly triggered by the organism or involves some immunologic mechanism. The roles of complement and phagocytosis are not well established in dermatophyte infections. Polymorphs, for instance, are not common in the inflammatory response to ringworm except in kerion in the dermis or favus in the epidermis, but they have been shown to destroy dermatophyte hyphae in vitro. The production of antibodies in dermatophytosis is highly variable. Persistent *T. rubrum* infections or favus are more likely to be associated with positive serologic reactions. However, transfer of immune serum in animals is not associated with clearance of lesions. In contrast, the appearance of delayed-type hypersensitivity (DTH) as a measure of T lymphocyte–mediated immunity correlates well with the clearance of lesions in some infections, and immunity can be transferred in mice with sensitized lymphocytes. In addition to these responses, the clearance of infection is affected also by the site of invasion and the organisms. Certain organisms, such as *T. rubrum*, are usually associated with poor lymphocyte transformation responses, although this varies with the site of infection. Some organisms appear to be more prominent than others in chronic infections by virtue of their weak immunogenicity or their ability to modulate immune responses.

CLINICAL MANIFESTATIONS. The main clinical features of dermatophytosis depend on the site of infection. In temperate areas occluded surfaces such as the groin, toe webs, and axillae are most often infected, but in the tropics any site may be involved.

Tinea Pedis. Athlete's foot is a term used to describe scaling and maceration accompanied by itching between the toes, particularly the fourth interdigital space. It is a syndrome that may be caused by *Candida* species, erythrasma, or other bacteria, as well as by dermatophytes. In dermatophyte infections, the cracked area between the toes may be wet or dry and, in some infections, particularly those caused by *Trichophyton interdigitale*, vesicular. The infection is sometimes self-limiting, or it may persist for considerable periods. Involvement of the dorsum of the foot or the sole may occur. *T. rubrum* infection is often responsible for a dry type of invasion over the sole and sides of the foot in a "moccasin type" of distribution. Symptoms may be minimal. Nail invasion, although not common in the tropics, may accompany this type of infection.

Tinea pedis is not the predominant form of dermatophytosis in the tropics; however, it is seen in certain situations. It is more common in people who wear shoes and socks and is therefore associated with urban development in tropical areas. Individuals from temperate climates with intermittently active or persistent tinea pedis nearly always have an exacerbation of their infection in the tropics. The asymptomatic dry form of sole infection caused by *T. rubrum* is also being recognized more frequently in the tropics.

Tinea pedis in tropical areas must be distinguished from other conditions, particularly pompholyx and, less commonly, plantar psoriasis. The possibility of the toe web infections being caused by *Candida, Scytalidium,* or bacteria should be considered. Skin in the interdigital space in these infections is usually wet and soggy. The interplay between bacteria and fungi is poorly understood, but in the tropics secondary gram-negative bacterial infection on top of interdigital dermatophytosis may occur.

Tinea Cruris (Ringworm of the Groin). Dermatophyte infections of the groin are seen frequently in the tropics. A ring of erythema with a scaling margin radiates from the groin down the inner border of the thigh (Fig. 81–2). It is intensely itchy. The eruption may be accompanied by marked folliculitis. Tinea cruris is more common in males and may extend posteriorly to include the natal cleft. In women in tropical areas, an extensive form of ringworm may be found in the waist area that involves a large part of the skin surface around the hip girdle. Coexistent patches of tinea corporis are frequently seen with this type of infection. Common causes of dermatophytosis in this site are *T. rubrum* and *Epidermophyton floccosum*, but *Candida* intertrigo may closely resemble tinea cruris.

Tinea Corporis (Ringworm of the Body). The characteristic lesion of dermatophyte infection on trunk or limbs is an annular plaque with a varying degree of erythema and a prominent edge (Fig. 81–3). Scaling is most prominent at this margin. However, the appearance of this lesion varies with the organism and host. Zoophilic dermatophytes such as *M. canis* may produce highly inflammatory lesions. In their most florid form, inflammatory ringworm plaques on the body or

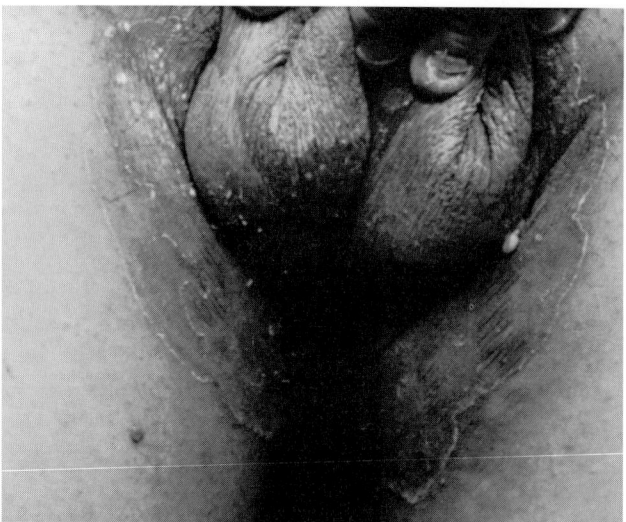

Figure 81–2. Tinea cruris caused by *T. rubrum*. (Courtesy of the St. John's Institute of Dermatology, London.)

scalp become indurated and pustular (kerion). At the other end of the spectrum, inflammation may be minimal, and single or multiple plaques on the body or face may be accompanied by few symptoms. Particularly in the Far East, *T. rubrum* is often associated with persistent and minimally inflammatory tinea corporis. Discoid eczema, impetigo, psoriasis, and discoid lupus erythematosus may all be mistaken for ringworm.

Tinea Capitis (Ringworm of the Scalp). Invasion of scalp hairs is seen in certain dermatophyte infections. They can be divided into three main groups: endothrix infections, in which spores (arthrospores) are formed within the hair matrix; ectothrix infections, in which sporulation occurs around the hair; and favus. All three types of infection are more common in childhood (Fig. 81–4). Those that spread from person to person are likely to occur in overcrowded conditions, including refugee camps, and can spread rapidly to achieve epidemic proportions. Chronically infected patients

may develop some permanent alopecia; persistent infections are much more common with certain organisms, including *T. tonsurans* and *T. schoenleinii*.

Endothrix and Ectothrix Infections. In ectothrix infections, scalp hairs may break at any level, but often this occurs several millimeters above the skin surface. There is often considerable exudation and erythema. In endothrix infections, the onset is often more insidious. Hairs break at scalp level usually, and inflammation may be minimal. However, kerion may develop with either type, although it is more common with the former. The organisms that cause scalp infections have been discussed in the section on epidemiology.

Favus. Favus presents with hair loss accompanied by the formation of crusts or scutula. These tend to coalesce to form a dense mat in patches or large areas of the scalp. The infected scalp has a peculiar musty odor. Atypical forms that are more prevalent in adults may be accompanied by minimal crust formation. In an area where favus is endemic, female patients presenting with cicatricial alopecia, for instance, should be examined for scalp infection. Family infections with favus are often seen. Hairs invaded by *T. schoenleinii* have a characteristic appearance, with air spaces within the infected shaft.

The diagnosis of tinea capitis is facilitated by filtered ultraviolet light examination (Wood's light), although not all organisms fluoresce under these conditions (Table 81–2).

Ringworm of the scalp must be distinguished from seborrheic dermatitis, psoriasis, or cicatricial alopecia. The last may be produced in end-stage favus.

Onychomycosis. Dermatophyte invasion of the nails is more common in temperate areas and the subtropics but is seen with a number of organisms, particularly *T. rubrum*. The nail plate is invaded from the distal border and lateral surfaces, usually from the underside. The affected nail becomes thickened and opaque, with a varying degree of onycholysis. Patients with onychomycosis often have infection of other sites such as the soles or toe webs. In addition to psoriasis, other fungal infections, e.g., candidosis or *Scytalidium* infections, must be differentiated from onychomycosis caused by dermatophytes.

Dermatophytosis of Other Sites. Dermatophyte infection

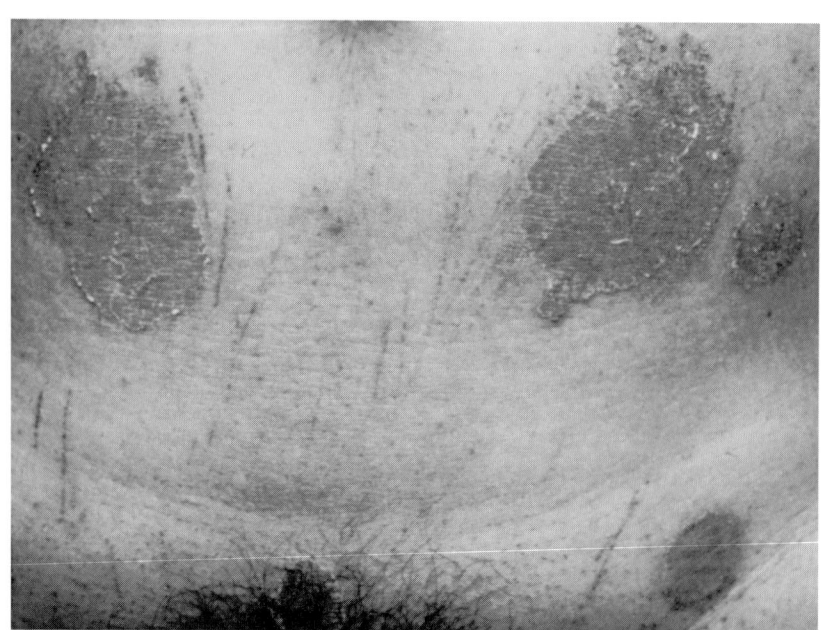

Figure 81–3. Tinea corporis caused by *T. rubrum*. (Courtesy of the St. John's Institute of Dermatology, London.)

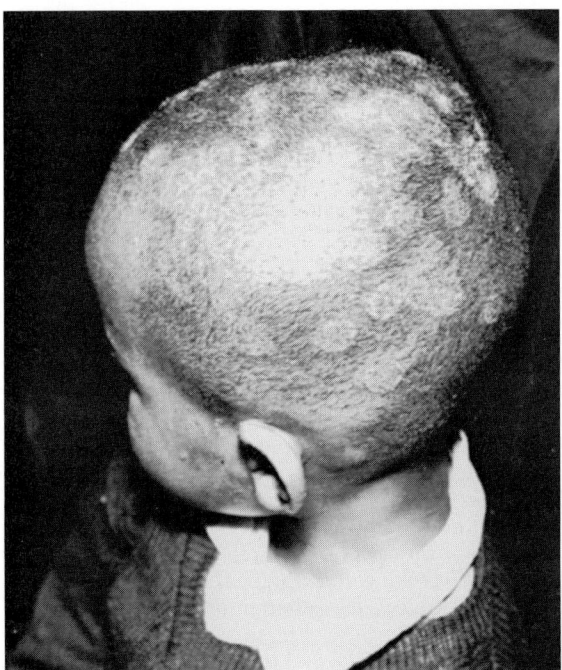

Figure 81–4. Tinea capitis, caused by *Microsporum audouini,* presents as multiple patches of alopecia with scaling in this little boy. (Courtesy of the Armed Forces Institute of Pathology, Photograph Neg. No. 57–6860.)

of the beard area (tinea barbae) may be highly inflammatory and persistent. Involvement of the palms is most commonly seen with *T. rubrum* infection. Often only one hand is involved, and the fingernails on that side may be invaded also. The palm shows mild scaling similar to the dry type of sole infection.

LABORATORY DIAGNOSIS. The laboratory diagnosis of dermatophytosis is entirely dependent on local facilities. However, the identification of the organism, although not absolutely essential, is helpful for several reasons. First, the likely source of the infection can be recognized. Second, certain organisms show different patterns of infection and responses to treatment, and recognition of the organism will assist the physician in determining the likely course of the infection. Finally, appropriate control mechanisms depend on the identification of the organism, particularly in zoophilic infections. There are several methods of laboratory recognition of dermatophyte infections.

Direct Examination. Scrapings can be taken from the lesion using a blunt scalpel and examined with a microscope after being mounted in 10% potassium hydroxide on a glass slide.

TABLE 81–2. Ringworm of the Scalp: Effect of Wood's Light Examination

Hair Usually Fluorescent

   M. canis, M. audouinii, M. ferrugineum, M. distortum

Hair Not Fluorescent

   M. gypseum, T. verrucosum, T. tonsurans, T. violaceum, T. soudanense, T. yaoundei, T. gourvilii

Dull Fluorescence

   T. schoenleinii

The presence of dermatophyte hyphae can be demonstrated in infected material or hairs.

Wood's Light Examination. Examination of infected scalps using a source of filtered ultraviolet radiation is extremely helpful in screening large numbers of potentially infected children, e.g., in schools. Certain, but not all, dermatophytes fluoresce green under Wood's light (Table 81–2).

Culture. Scrapings or hairs may be plated directly onto Sabouraud agar. Colonies develop in 7 to 28 days. Their gross and microscopic appearance, as well as nutritional requirements, can be used in identification.

TREATMENT. Most dermatophyte infections require treatment. However, the advisability of prolonged therapy in nail or sole infection must be weighed against the symptoms experienced by the patient (often minimal) and the low rate of success.

Topical Therapy. Dermatophytoses can be treated topically by a number of different methods. Certain simple compounds, including dyes, are known to have weak antifungal properties that may be sufficient to treat certain types of dermatophytosis, e.g., tinea cruris. Gentian violet and magenta paint are examples. A second therapeutic approach is promotion of the exfoliation of stratum corneum by compounds known as keratolytic agents. Salicylic acid in concentrations of 5 to 20% in ointment base is an effective keratolytic agent. Whitfield's ointment (BPC), which contains 3% salicylic acid and 3% benzoic acid, a weak antifungal agent, is an inexpensive and effective method of treating all dermatophyte infections apart from scalp or nail disease or kerion. It may be prescribed half-strength for sensitive areas. The newer specific antifungal compounds may result in a more rapid response and be less irritative. However, these are more expensive.

Specific Antifungals. The specific antifungal compounds that can be used against dermatophytes include the imidazole compounds (miconazole, clotrimazole, econazole, and tioconazole) as well as a miscellaneous group of antifungal drugs, e.g., tolnaftate and haloprogin. All are available for topical therapy in 1 to 2% concentration. Many are effective against candidosis and pityriasis versicolor. Terbinafine cream produces responses in tinea pedis after as little as a single application. Topical antifungals have no place in the management of tinea capitis.

Systemic Therapy. For nail and scalp disease or severe infections, including kerion, the topical agents have less value, and systemic treatment is required. Griseofulvin is given in a daily dose of 500 to 1000 mg in adults or 10 mg/kg in children. The drug is best prescribed in microcrystalline form and is usually well absorbed when given with a meal. Side effects, e.g., headache, nausea, or urticaria, occur in less than 5% of those treated. Of patients with toenail infections, 20 to 40% respond to courses of griseofulvin given over 1 to 2 years. There is good evidence that for scalp infections effective treatment in large numbers of children can be attained by giving intermittent supervised therapy, e.g., 30 mg/kg at 3-week intervals.

More recently terbinafine (250 mg daily) and itraconazole (100 to 400 mg daily) have been introduced and considerably shorten treatment periods while providing effective therapy. For instance, in nail infections terbinafine 250 mg daily for 6 to 12 weeks or an intermittent (pulsed) regimen using itraconazole 400 mg daily for 1 week every month for 2 to 3 months will produce over 80% recovery rates. Intermittent fluconazole 150 mg weekly is also proposed for a similar indication. These treatments are more effective and more expensive than griseofulvin.

Removal of Infected Tissues. Surgery is occasionally recommended for resistant nail infections. However, an alternative to this is application of a 40% urea ointment to the nail under occlusion for 1 week. The nail can be removed painlessly by excision after this treatment.

Additional Therapy. Systemic corticosteroids are rarely required in dermatophyte infections. In patients with animal ringworm or kerion, however, examination is advisable within 3 to 5 days of starting antifungal therapy, as a severe generalized allergic or dermatophytid reaction may take place. This may require concurrent therapy with topical or systemic corticosteroids.

81.2 Dermatophyte-like Infections Caused by Scytalidium

Two nondermatophyte organisms have been found to cause infections that closely resemble the dry type of palmar or plantar and nail infections caused by *T. rubrum* (Fig. 81–5). Their prevalence in the tropics is unknown, although they have been shown to cause sole infections in the Caribbean and are not uncommon in immigrants from the tropics living in Europe.

ETIOLOGY. *Scytalidium dimidiatum* (*Hendersonula toruloidea*) is a plant pathogen found in many parts of the tropics. It is a black mold without obvious distinguishing features that may easily be mistaken for a laboratory contaminant, and its growth is inhibited by cycloheximide, which is often used in mycologic media. *Scytalidium hyalinum* is similar but is white to gray in color. The laboratory diagnosis depends on culture on cycloheximide-free media.

TREATMENT. The treatment of these infections is extremely difficult, because the organisms are not generally susceptible to any antifungals; Whitfield's ointment may prove useful for plantar infections.

81.3 Superficial Candidosis (Candidiasis)

DEFINITION. Superficial infections caused by species of the genus *Candida* are common in all parts of the world. They include conditions such as thrush and vaginal candidosis as well as interdigital candidosis. The pattern of *Candida* infections in the tropics differs from that seen in temperate areas. This is in part due to different trends in medical therapy and also to differences in the prevalence of underlying disease states, such as diabetes mellitus.

ETIOLOGY AND EPIDEMIOLOGY. *Candida albicans* is the most common organism to be associated with superficial candidosis. However, other species such as *Candida tropicalis* or *Candida guilliermondii* may be involved. *C. albicans* is a common saprophyte on mucosal surfaces, particularly the mouth, gastrointestinal tract, and vagina. Oral colonization may originate early in infancy, although its incidence is increased by a number of factors, including hospitalization and bottle-feeding. However, predisposing conditions in the tropics are largely unexplored. For instance, the effect of malnutrition on oral carriage of *Candida* is unknown. *C. albicans* may be isolated also from the environment, particularly where contact with humans is frequent, e.g., washbasins and drinking bowls.

PATHOGENESIS. *C. albicans* usually causes infection, as opposed to colonization, in individuals with predisposing

factors (Table 81–3). Some of these factors are systemic, and others relate to local conditions on the skin or mucosa. The effect of climate on infection is unknown, although a number of studies have confirmed the high incidence of saprophytic carriage of *Candida* species in the tropics.

CLINICAL MANIFESTATIONS. The clinical manifestations of superficial candidosis vary with the site of infection.

Oral Candidosis (Thrush). This is a common condition, particularly in the elderly, infants, and denture wearers. It may also follow immunosuppression or antibiotic therapy and is an important infection as a marker of AIDS and the progression of human immunodeficiency virus (HIV) infection. Generally the risk of oropharyngeal candidosis in AIDS patients increases with declining CD4 counts. The infection presents with solitary or confluent white plaques on the oral mucosa (pseudomembranous candidosis) (Fig. 81–6). Alternatively, the mucosa may appear glazed and erythematous (erythematous candidosis). Oral candidosis in AIDS patients in the tropics is often accompanied by esophageal infection. Persistent oral candidosis may also be a problem in the elderly. One of the earliest features of oral candidosis is the appearance of cracking at the angles of the mouth, or angular cheilitis. Other causes, e.g., vitamin or iron deficiency, should be considered.

Vaginal Candidosis. Vaginal infection with *Candida* species is common, and although it is particularly associated with diabetes and the third trimester of pregnancy, the majority of those affected have no obvious underlying abnormality. It has been suggested, without objective evidence, that the widespread use of oral contraceptives may also be a predisposing factor. The symptoms of vaginal candidosis are irritation and discomfort associated, in many cases, with a creamy discharge. The rash in the groin is erythematous with a prominent border. Small "satellite" pustules or crusts are often seen outside this border. As with oral infections, the vaginal mucosa may be covered with small white plaques or may become red and friable. This infection must be distinguished from *Trichomonas* infections and gonorrhea.

Paronychia and *Candida* Onychomycosis. Infection of the nail folds by *Candida* species is one cause of paronychia. The periungual skin is raised and painful, and a prominent gap develops between the fold and the nail plate. Pus may be discharged. More rarely, invasion of the nail plate with onycholysis occurs. Certain bacteria, such as *Staphylococcus aureus*, also play a role in the formation of paronychia, and the condition is best regarded as being caused by a number of factors, although women with heavy domestic responsibilities (washing, cooking) seem to be predisposed. Patients with abnormal nail folds associated with skin disease, such

TABLE 81–3. Predisposing Factors in Superficial Candidosis

Infancy, pregnancy, old age
Occlusion of epithelial surfaces, e.g., by dentures, occlusive dressings
Disorders of immune function
Primary, e.g., chronic granulomatous disease
Secondary, e.g., leukemia, corticosteroid therapy
Chemotherapy
Immunosuppressive
Antibiotic
Endocrine disease, e.g., diabetes mellitus
Carcinoma
Miscellaneous, e.g., damaged nail folds

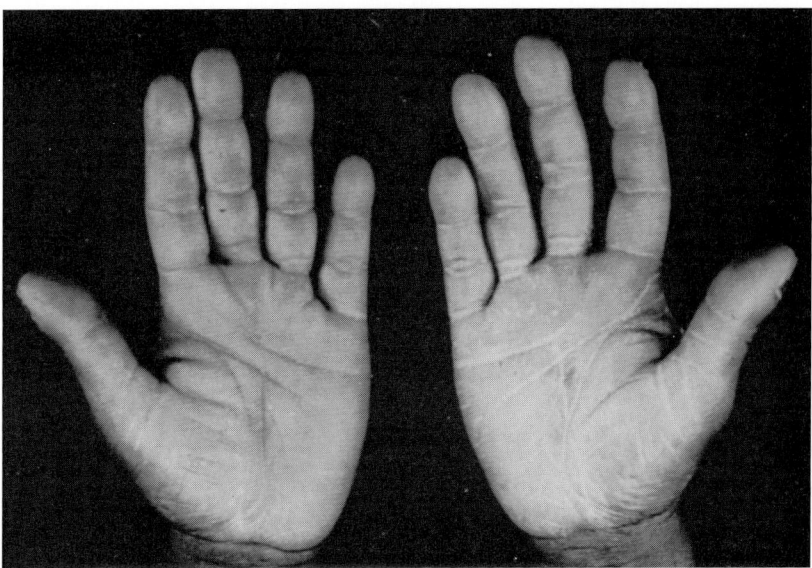

Figure 81–5. *Scytadidium dimidiatum* infection of the palms mimicking a "dry" type of dermatophyte infection. (Courtesy of the St. John's Institute of Dermatology, London.)

as hand eczema or contact dermatitis, may also be infected.

Interdigital Candidosis. *Candida* may cause scaling and maceration between the toes (athlete's foot). In addition, a superficial erosion on the hand between the fingers on the dorsal web space may also be caused by *Candida* infection. This type of interdigital erosion is seen much more frequently in warm climates.

Intertrigo. Intertrigo is the name given to a painful or irritative inflammatory dermatosis confined to body folds to which secondary bacterial or *Candida* infections may contribute. Treatment of *Candida* infection alone rarely produces a cure. The infection is most common in overweight or diabetic individuals.

Diaper rash is mainly a problem of the colder latitudes but may occur elsewhere if diapers are used on infants. Secondary infection with *Candida* may occur in this area on top of an irritative dermatosis caused by urine.

Chronic Candidosis. Chronic *Candida* infections of the mouth, vagina, nails, or other skin surfaces are rare but may persist despite treatment. The most extreme example, chronic mucocutaneous candidosis, is a rare condition that occurs worldwide. It is usually recognized in infancy or childhood, and there are frequently underlying genetic, endocrine, or immunologic features. Severe oral and nail infection as well as widespread infection and granuloma formation on other surfaces may develop. There is some tendency for the condition to improve in adult life if the affected individual does not succumb to intercurrent illness.

LABORATORY DIAGNOSIS. The laboratory diagnosis can be confirmed by demonstration of the *Candida* organism in potassium hydroxide wet mounts. Yeast and hyphal forms are seen in the same area. *Candida* can be cultured on Sabouraud agar.

TREATMENT. Topical treatment with gentian violet is effective in some patients. However, locally applied amphotericin B, nystatin, or an imidazole preparation is preferable. Creams, lozenges, suspensions, or pessaries (vaginal tablets) are available. The systemic treatments for superficial candidosis are fluconazole, itraconazole and ketoconazole. These are best reserved for severe oral or chronic forms of candidosis. AIDS patients with oral candidosis may respond to topical therapy, but in many cases it is necessary to use systemic treatment. Resistance to fluconazole may develop if the drug is employed continuously in the face of clinically unresponsive infection.

Vaginal infections respond to intensive topical therapy given for 3 to 5 days using a combination of cream and pessaries. Amphotericin B, nystatin, or an imidazole such as miconazole is usually successful. If the intitial treatment is unsuccessful, the male partner should be treated as well. Control measures are rarely practicable. However, patients at risk for oral or systemic candidosis such as those with neutropenia or leukemia, may be given fluconazole.

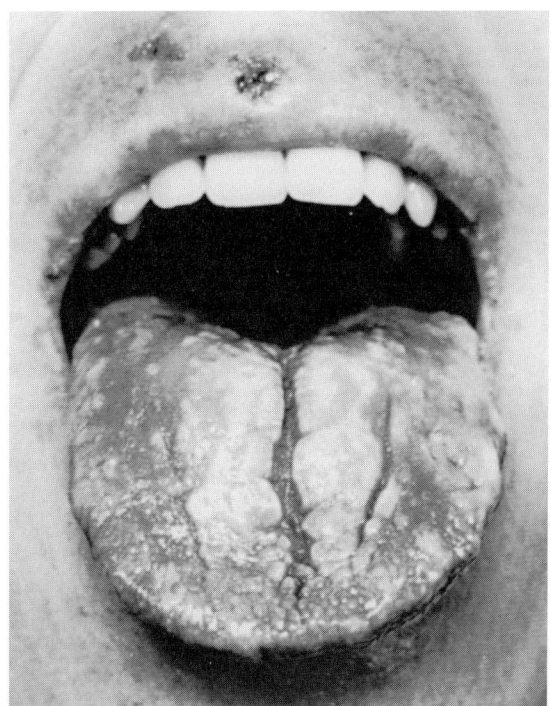

Figure 81–6. Chronic oral candidosis of the tongue. (Courtesy of the St. John's Institute of Dermatology, London.)

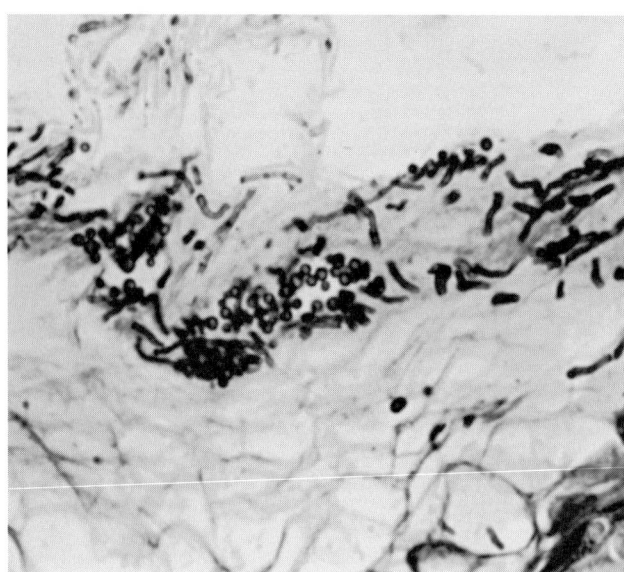

Figure 81–7. Yeasts and pseudohyphae of *Malassezia* in the stratum corneum of a patient with tinea versicolor. (PAS stain, × 633.) (Courtesy of the Armed Forces Institute of Pathology, Photograph Neg. No. 75–5301.)

81.4 *Pityriasis (Tinea) Versicolor*

DEFINITION. This common infection is widespread in the tropics and may affect over 60% of the population in certain areas. It is caused by the lipophilic yeast, *Malassezia*.

ETIOLOGY. *Malassezia* species are present on normal skin, where they exist as saprophytes. There are at least six different *Malassezia* species, recognized only recently. The development of pityriasis versicolor lesions is usually, but not invariably, accompanied by the formation of short, stubby hyphae of these organisms (Fig. 81–7). In temperate areas, pityriasis

versicolor is seen most often in patients returning from an overseas vacation. Rarely, it may occur in immunocompromised individuals, in particular those with Cushing syndrome.

EPIDEMIOLOGY. Pityriasis versicolor occurs throughout the world and is extremely common in the tropics.

PATHOLOGY AND PATHOGENESIS. *Malassezia* normally inhabits the superficial layers of keratin, particularly around the orifices of hair follicles. The sequential development of hyphal forms can be observed during the course of immunosuppressive therapy, which suggests that immune factors play a role in preventing the infection. However, the high prevalence of the disease in normal people in the tropics indicates that other factors are involved. Exposure to sunlight, heat, and humidity as well as locally applied oils have all been cited, but without objective proof.

CLINICAL MANIFESTATIONS. The lesions of pityriasis versicolor are small, scaling macules that are hypopigmented or hyperpigmented. Scaling is rarely prominent but can be elicited by scratching affected areas. This feature is important in distinguishing this infection from other types of macular pigmentary disorders, e.g., vitiligo. Under Wood's light, the patches fluoresce pale yellow, but this sign is often unreliable. The areas most commonly infected are the upper trunk, neck, and upper arms (Fig. 81–8). In the tropics, the infection may extend beyond these areas to involve the face, abdomen, lower arms, and penis. The rash is rarely symptomatic but may cause concern because of its superficial resemblance to certain types of leprosy.

LABORATORY DIAGNOSIS. The appearance of well-defined macules with fine scaling is distinctive usually. However, the diagnosis can be confirmed by demonstration of the clusters of yeasts and pseudo-hyphae in potassium hydroxide mounts (Fig. 81–7). Recognition of the fungi is facilitated by the addition of equal quantities of blue ink (Parker Quink) to the potassium hydroxide.

TREATMENT. Applications of 20% sodium thiosulfate or 2.5% selenium sulfide twice daily for 7 to 10 days are usually effective. The response to a topical imidazole may be more rapid, and a single 400-mg dose of ketoconazole or 5 days of 200 mg itraconazole are also reported to be effective. No control measures are practicable.

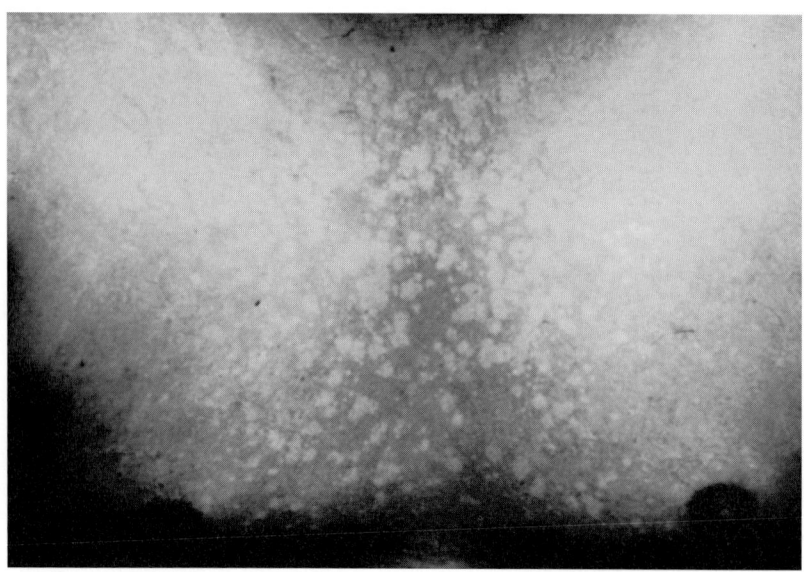

Figure 81–8. Pityriasis (tinea) versicolor on the chest. (Courtesy of the St. John's Institute of Dermatology, London.)

81.5 Miscellaneous Superficial Fungal Infections

BLACK PIEDRA. Black piedra is an uncommon persistent infection confined to hair shafts and is seen in small endemic foci in the tropics, e.g., Latin America or Central Africa. Individual or clusters of cases may occur. The infection is seen most often on the hairs of the scalp. The hallmark of this condition is the presence of small, gritty nodules on the hair shafts. These represent areas of hyphal invasion in which the characteristic spores (ascospores) of the organism *Piedraia hortae* may be found.

WHITE PIEDRA. White piedra is caused by the yeasts *Trichosporon inkin*, *Trichosporon ashasii*, or *Trichosporon mucoides*. The appearances are similar to those of black piedra, although the swellings are "softer" and pale. The infected areas may involve hair on the scalp, groin, or, rarely, the axillae. Infections are not commonly diagnosed but have been recognized in different climates from temperate to tropical areas.

TINEA NIGRA. Tinea nigra is the superficial infection caused by a black yeast, *Phaeoanellomyces werneckii*, which is associated with the appearance of focal areas of hyperpigmentation, usually on the palms or soles. It is seen exclusively in the tropics and subtropics and is never common. The infection has been recognized primarily in Central and South America as well as in the Far East. Patients rarely complain of symptoms directly attributable to the infection. Characteristically, the lesion is a dark brown or black stain that appears on the palms or the soles and, on rare occasions, elsewhere. There is little scaling, and multiple lesions are rare. The diagnosis can be confirmed by demonstration of the characteristic darkly pigmented arthrospores in scrapings. The infection responds well to Whitfield's ointment.

Bibliography

Budimulja U, Kuswadji K, Bramono S, et al: A double-blind randomised stratified controlled study of the treatment of tinea imbricata with oral terbinafen or itraconazole. Br J Dermatol 130 (Suppl 43):29, 1994.

Faergeman J. *Pityrosporum* infections. J Am Acad Dermatol 31:S18, 1994.

Faergemann J, Brabander S: Tinea versicolor and *Pityrosporum orbiculare*: A mycological investigation. Sabouraudia 17:171, 1979.

Frieden IJ, Howard R: Tinea capitis: epidemiology, diagnosis, treatment and control. J Am Acad Dermatol 31:S46, 1994.

Hughes JR, Moore MK, Pembroke AC: Tinea nigra palmaris. Clin Exp Dermatol 18:481, 1993.

Jones RE, Rinehardt JR, Rinaldi MG: Acquired immunity to dermatophytes. Arch Dermatol 109:840, 1974.

Kamalam A, Thambiah AS: Tinea capitis in Madras. Sabouraudia 11:106, 1973.

Kouck P, Ouankou MD: Les epidermomycoses a Yaounde: Aspects cliniques et therapeutiques. Med Afr Noire 25:449, 1978.

McCarthy GM: Host factors associated with HIV related oral candidiasis: A review. Oral Surg Oral Med Oral Pathol 73:181, 1992.

Moore MK: Skin and nail infections by non-dermatophytic filamentous fungi. Mykosen (Suppl 1):128, 1978.

Rebell G, Taplin D: Dermatophytes: Their Recognition and Identification. Miami, Florida, University of Miami Press, 1970.

Rippon JW: Epidemiology and emerging patterns of dermatophyte species. *In* Borges M, Odds FL, Hay RJ (eds): Current Topics in Medical Mycology. New York, Springer-Verlag, 1985, p 208.

Roberts SOB: Treatment of the superficial and subcutaneous mycoses. In Speller DC (ed): Antifungal Chemotherapy. New York, John Wiley and Sons, 1980.

Shrum JP, Millikan LE, Bataireh O: Superficial fungal infection in the tropics. Dermatol Clin 12:687, 1994.

Soyinka F: Epidemiologic study of dermatophyte infections in Nigeria (clinical survey and laboratory investigations). Mycopathologia 63:99, 1978.

Therizol-Ferly M, Kombela M, Gomez de Diaz M, et al: White piedra and *Trichosporon* species in equatorial Africa. 2: Clinical and mycological associations; an analysis of 449 superficial inguinal specimens. Mycoses 37:255, 1994.

82 Subcutaneous Mycoses: General Principles

Roderick J. Hay

DEFINITION. Subcutaneous mycoses are chronic fungal infections resulting from the percutaneous inoculation of the causal agents from an exogenous source. Therefore, they are acquired by implantation rather than by inhalation or contact. The primary site of multiplication is the dermis or subcutis, and although lesions generally remain localized to the site of inoculation, there is usually a slow and inexorable spread to surrounding tissue. As a rule, lesions do not undergo spontaneous remission and, if unchecked, tissue destruction may be severe. Dissemination to distal sites is rare.

ETIOLOGY. The principal forms of subcutaneous mycoses are mycetoma, sporotrichosis, and chromomycosis. Less common are the subcutaneous zygomycoses, i.e., rhinosporidiosis, lobomycosis, and phaeohyphomycosis. Exceptionally, subcutaneous infections have been caused by dermatophyte fungi. Mycetoma, chromomycosis, and phaeohyphomycosis may be caused by a variety of different organisms. In contrast, sporotrichosis and rhinosporidiosis are caused by a single species of pathogenic fungi. The causes of rhinosporidiosis and lobomycosis have not been isolated in culture.

EPIDEMIOLOGY. The normal habitat of the fungi causing subcutaneous mycoses is soil or vegetation. Humans are an accidental and nonessential host, with infection resulting from the incidental introduction of a fungus into the skin. Survival mechanisms that evolved to allow these organisms to withstand harsh natural environments also ensure their survival in the human host.

82.1 Mycetoma (Maduromycosis)

Roderick J. Hay

DEFINITION. Mycetoma is a chronic, localized, slowly progressive, subcutaneous infection caused by species of actinomycetes or fungi. It is characterized by destructive granulomatous and suppurative responses, by the production of tumefaction, by deformity, and by draining sinus tracts that may communicate with each other and with the skin surface. In affected tissues, filaments of the causal agents form compact grains or granules, each of which is often characteristic of the infecting species. The infection follows traumatic implantation of the agent from an exogenous source, often a contaminated thorn. Lesions are localized initially to the inoculation site but spread slowly to involve contiguous tissues, including muscle and bone.

ETIOLOGY. Mycetoma has multiple etiologies, with more than 20 species of fungi or bacteria being commonly implicated. About 60% of infections are caused by actinomycetes (actinomycetoma) and 40% by filamentous fungi (eumycetoma). Predominant causes vary markedly in different parts of the world. Species most prevalent in the tropics include the actinomycetes *Streptomyces somaliensis*, *Actinomadura madurae*, *Actinomadura pelletieri* and *Nocardia brasiliensis* and the fungi *Madurella mycetomatis*, *Madurella grisea*, *Leptosphaeria senegalensis*, *Scedosporium apiospermum*, and species of *Fusarium*, *Acremonium*, and *Aspergillus* (Table 82–1).

HISTORY. The disease was reported initially from India over 300 years ago. It was named "madura foot," in the mid-nineteenth century after the district in which it was prevalent. The preferred name "mycetoma" was introduced in 1861 to distinguish the disease from other tumors. Later reports established the widespread occurrence of mycetoma throughout the world and the wide range of causal organisms.

EPIDEMIOLOGY. Mycetoma is endemic in many tropical countries and is most commonly reported from Africa, Central and South America, India, and the Far East. Although sporadic cases occur in temperate countries, the condition is seen most frequently between latitudes 15 degrees south and 30 degrees north, typically regions with a short rainy season of 4 to 6 months, daily temperature range of 30 to 37°C, and a humidity of 60 to 80%, alternating with a dry season. The geographic distribution of the individual agents causing mycetoma is determined principally by rainfall rather than by other climatic factors. Areas of endemicity are characterized by savannah or forest and the presence of thorny trees or bushes such as Acacia scrub. Many of the agents causing mycetoma have been isolated from soil, or local plants or trees. In some areas, males are more frequently affected than females, but there is no consistent differential sex distribution. The disease can affect all age groups but is most commonly reported in young adults. Many patients are field laborers or herdsmen whose occupation exposes them to minor penetrating wounds.

PATHOGENESIS AND PATHOLOGY. Infection is initiated by traumatic implantation, often by the piercing of skin or mucosal surfaces with thorns or wood splinters. On several occasions, agents of mycetoma have been isolated in culture from thorns and other vegetable matter. Mycetoma may involve any part of the body but is most common on the feet followed by the hands and other parts of the body that come into contact with the soil or vegetation during working, sitting, or lying. Other sites commonly affected include the back, neck, and back of the head.

Once introduced subcutaneously, the agent begins to grow in the tissues, eliciting a suppurative inflammatory response that is predominantly neutrophilic and may be accompanied by a granulomatous reaction with varying proportions of epithelioid cells, plasma cells, lymphocytes, and giant cells. Other pathologic features include fibrosis, local endarteritic changes, and the formation of dense scar tissue. The agent appears in infected tissues as compact grains or granules up to 5 mm in diameter whose appearance may be diagnostic of the species involved. These are often invested with refractile eosinophilic material (Splendore-Hoeppli phenomenon). At the margin of each grain, the intensity of the host-parasite reaction results in local necrosis, multiple abscesses, osteitis, and osteomyelitis, and the formation of sinuses and fistulas that interconnect and erupt onto the skin surface. Different agents induce different pathologic changes of bone. In some, the dominant feature may be bone resorption; in others, osteoblastic activity toward the periphery of the lesion may result in the encasement of grains by bone. In a third type, bone regeneration is incomplete, resulting in spicule formation. The most common and most distinctive radiologic appearance is focal bone destruction with cavity formation. Cavities are generally small and abundant in cases of actinomycetoma and larger and less numerous in eumycetoma.

Regional extension with destruction of deep tissues is slow, inexorable, and, at times, extensive. Spread may occur proximally as well as distally, but the process involves only the lymphatics or the blood stream.

CLINICAL MANIFESTATIONS. In tropical countries, patients most commonly present with long-standing infections. The initial lesion, which appears several months after the traumatic incident, is a small, firm, painless subcutaneous nodule or plaque that increases progressively in size.

Subsequent evolutions of eumycetoma and actinomycetoma may differ. In the former, lesions remain localized and

TABLE 82–1. Macroscopic and Histopathologic Features of Mycetoma Grains

Organisms	Size (mm)	Texture	H&E Section
Eumycetoma			
1. Dark grains			
Madurella mycetomatis	0.2–5.0	Hard, brittle	Cement, compact, vesicles sometimes prominent
M. grisea	0.34–5.0	Soft	Cement lacking, compact outer layer
Leptosphaeria senegalensis	0.44–6.0	Soft	Cement, dark periphery with vesicular center
Exophiala jeanselmei	0.24–3.0	Soft	Cement absent, often hollow
Pyrenochaeta romeroi	0.34–6.0	Soft	Cement lacking, compact outer layer
2. Pale grains			
Fusarium species			
Acremonium species			
Scedosporium apiospermum	0.1–2.0	Soft	Compact, pigment lacking, interwoven fungal filaments
Aspergillus nidulans			
Neotestudina rosatii			
Actinomycetoma			
1. Pale (white to yellow) grains			
Actinomadura madurae	0.14–5.0	Soft	Variegated
Nocardia brasiliensis	0.04–1.0	Soft	Small, pale blue, eosinophilic
2. Yellow to brown grains			
Streptomyces somaliensis	0.24–6.0	Soft	Grains fractured, basophilic
3. Red to pink grains			
Actinomadura pelletieri	0.064–2.0	Soft	Small, basophilic

H&E, hematoxylin and eosin.

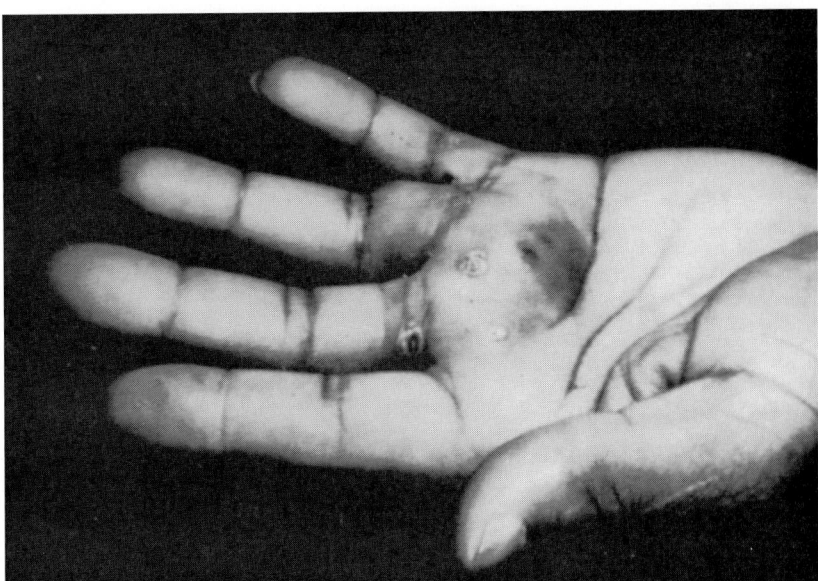

Figure 82–1. Mycetoma (eumycetoma) affecting the palm. (Courtesy of the St John's Institute of Dermatology, London.)

the condition progresses slowly. Neither swelling nor destruction of adjacent anatomic structures is marked until late in the course of the disease. The tumor is usually firm and round but may be soft and lobulated (Fig. 14–10). Skin nodules break down to form ulcerated areas discharging sanguineous, seropurulent, or purulent exudates. As it progresses, the condition is characterized by marked swelling and deformity, and the production of draining sinus tracts through which fungal grains are expelled onto the surface of the skin (Fig. 82–1). In actinomycetoma infections, lesions may have less well defined margins and tend to merge with surrounding tissue. Progression is often more rapid and involvement of bone earlier and more extensive than with eumycetomas (Fig. 82–2).

Most mycetomas are painless, even when well established. Localized sweating over the lesion is common. Although the patient may appear wasted and anemic, this is usually caused by other processes, e.g., malnutrition, unrelated to mycetoma. Mycetoma may result in loss of function of an affected limb and consequent inability to work.

The condition does not remit spontaneously, although temporary improvement is not unknown. Spread tends to follow fascial planes, but nerves and tendons are resistant; hence, neurologic symptoms are lacking. The foot is the most common site involved, with about 70% of infections affecting the lower limbs. Other sites include the buttocks and perineum, hands, back, and scalp, although many other localizations are encountered.

DIAGNOSIS

Histopathology. Grains produced by different agents may be distinctive enough for a definite diagnosis to be made by examination of tissue sections stained with hematoxylin and eosin (Fig. 82–3). Fungal grains have a coarser texture, consisting of a dense mass of interwoven filaments (hyphae) 2 to 5 μm in diameter. Many are pigmented, being permeated by a dark-brown cement-like material, which confers a gritty texture to the grains. In tissue sections, individual hyphae or vesicular swellings can always be distinguished. Actinomycete grains, in contrast, are more finely textured, the hyphae being 1 μm or less in diameter and not individually distinguishable. They are never black. Distinctive macroscopic and histopathologic features of the most common causes of mycetoma are indicated in Table 82–1.

Direct Examination. Exudates should be examined for the

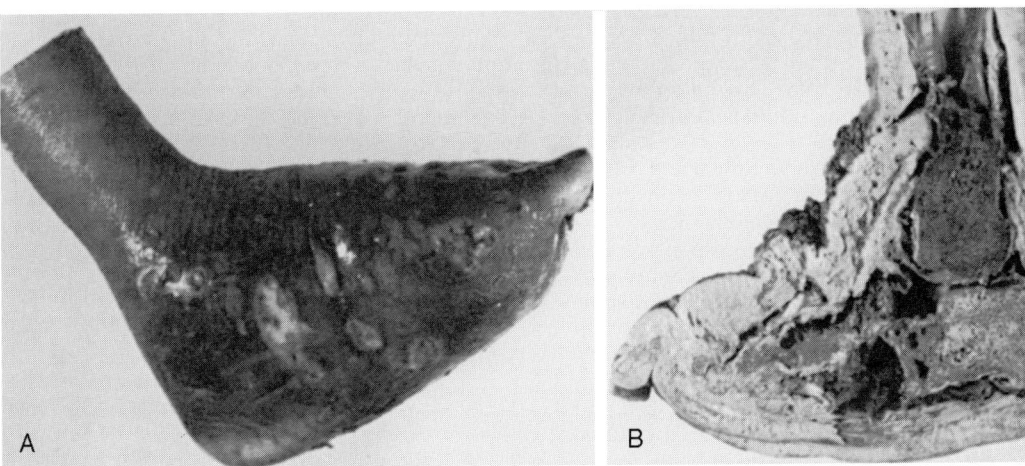

Figure 82–2. *A, Nocardia* actinomycetoma of the foot. *B,* Hemisection of the foot showing advanced destruction of the bones. (Courtesy of the Armed Forces Institute of Pathology, Photograph Neg. No. N-77646.)

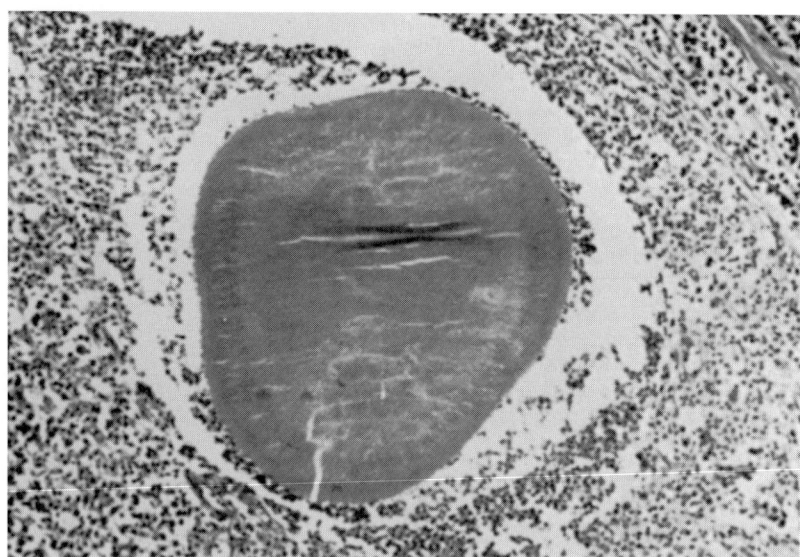

Figure 82–3. Grain of *Streptomyces somaliensis* surrounded by acute inflammatory cells (H&E stain, × 360). (Courtesy of the St John's Institute of Dermatology, London.)

presence of grains. Their size, texture, and color provide clues to the etiology of the infection. Opening a surface pustule over a sinus tract with a sterile needle may reveal the grains. Differentiation of fungal and actinomycete grains is readily achieved by crushing the grain between two glass slides and examining it microscopically for broad (fungal) or narrow (actinomycete) filaments.

Culture. A provisional diagnosis can be made by consideration of the characteristics of the grain in relation to the predominant species for any one geographic area. The definitive diagnosis, however, requires isolation of the agent in culture and its identification. In view of the multiple etiology, a range of culture media and conditions of incubation should be employed. Different genera and species are distinguished by their morphologic and physiologic characteristics.

Serology. Precipitins may be present in the sera of patients with long-standing mycetoma. Their detection requires the services of aspecialized laboratory because of the wide range of potential antigens and their unavailability from commercial sources. Cross-reactions between different fungal species and between actinomycete agents are common.

Differential Diagnosis. Chronic osteomyelitis of bacterial etiology, e.g., syphilitic, actinomycotic, or tuberculous, may resemble mycetoma, particularly in the early stages. Cases of mycetoma lacking sinus tracts may resemble soft tissue tumors such as lipomas, or cystic lesions, e.g., cold abscess or implantation dermoid. Botryomycosis, in which persistent bacterial infection is associated with granule and sinus formation, must be distinguished also. This pattern of infection is seen most often in immunologically deficient individuals.

TREATMENT. The distinction between a fungal and actinomycete etiology is of critical importance because of the different responses of the two conditions to chemotherapy.

Eumycetoma. As a rule, eumycetoma is unresponsive, and management should be directed toward early diagnosis. A trial of chemotherapy may be justified, particularly as some *M. mycetomatis* infections respond to ketoconazole. Other antifungals such as itraconazole or griseofulvin are occasionally successful. Radical surgical removal is an alternative. Because eumycetoma infections are generally well circumscribed and progress rather slowly, excision may be temporarily successful, particularly if there has been no invasion of bone. Arteriography may demonstrate the extent of infection. In advanced cases of eumycetoma, amputation may offer the only

real hope of eradication. All traces of infection have to be removed, otherwise relapse is inevitable; recurrence rates of 80% have been recorded. If the disease is only slowly progressive and if the patient can be reviewed regularly, the decision about surgical intervention can be deferred for several years.

Actinomycetoma. Medical treatment is often effective in cases of actinomycetoma. Good results have been obtained with a combination of dapsone (100 mg twice daily) and streptomycin (1 g daily for 1 month). Perhaps the most effective combination is trimethoprim/sulfamethoxazole (co-trimoxazole) and streptomycin or rifampin. One of the last 2 drugs is usually given for the first 3 to 4 months of therapy. The dapsone regimen is usually preferred because it is inexpensive. The average duration of treatment is about 9 months, and responses to chemotherapy are generally good, even when there has been involvement of bone. Alternatives include amikacin and fusidic acid.

PROGNOSIS. The prognosis in actinomycetoma is usually good but with eumycetoma the outlook is less clear. Apart from the mutilation resulting from amputation in eumycetoma, loss of function can render the afflicted subject unemployable. Moreover, the recurrence rate can be high. When lesions affect the back, abdomen, neck, scalp, or other sites where excision or amputation is impracticable, little practical aid can be offered.

With actinomycetoma, the prognosis is reasonable, with improvement or cure likely in about 70% of patients. Clinical response involves reduction of swelling, closing of sinuses, formation of new bone, and healing of skin abnormalities. If practicable, monitoring of serum precipitin levels provides an objective measure of response to management.

PREVENTION. Unfortunately, preventive measures are impracticable in view of the widespread occurrence of the agents in nature and the frequency with which minor skin wounds occur in endemic areas.

Bibliography

Hay RJ, Mahgoub ES, Leon G, et al: Mycetoma. J Med Vet Mycol 30(Suppl 1):41, 1992.
Mahgoub ES: Medical management of mycetoma. Bull Who 54:303, 1976.
Mahgoub ES, Gumaa SA, El Hassan AM: Immunological status of mycetoma patients. Bull Soc Pathol Exot 70:48, 1977.
Mahgoub ES, Murray IG: Mycetoma. London, William Heinemann, 1973.

Mariat F: Sur la distribution geographique et la repartition des agents des mycetomes. Bull Soc Pathol Exot 56:35, 1963.

Peyron IP, Heroum P, Lesquere C, et al: Interet de la radiologie dans le diagnostic des mycetomes. Med Trop 39:27, 1979.

82.2 *Sporotrichosis*

Roderick J. Hay

DEFINITION. Sporotrichosis is a chronic fungal infection principally affecting the skin, lymphatics, and subcutaneous tissues. Pulmonary and disseminated forms occur less frequently, with involvement of the lungs, osteoarticular and musculoskeletal tissues, viscera, mucous membranes, and central nervous system. Lesions may be nodular, pustular, or ulcerative but exhibit a wide morphologic range.

ETIOLOGY. Sporotrichosis is caused by a single species of fungus, *Sporothrix schenckii*, which is widely distributed throughout the world. It is a common saprophyte which can be readily isolated from soils, particularly those rich in organic matter or vegetable debris, or from a wide range of plants and plant materials. The fungus has a filamentous vegetative organization consisting of fine, branching hyphae on which minute unicellular spores are formed. In common with many other pathogenic fungi, it is dimorphic, existing as a mold in nature and a yeast in infected tissue.

HISTORY. The first description of sporotrichosis and its causal agent was reported in 1898. Many of the earlier reports originated in France, but it is now uncommon there. One of the most remarkable outbreaks occurred in the gold mines of South Africa in the 1940s, when almost 3000 cases were recorded, the source of infection being heavy growth of *S. schenckii* on the surface of timber used as pit props.

EPIDEMIOLOGY. Sporotrichosis occurs worldwide but is most common in warm, temperate, or tropical countries. In temperate countries, infections are sometimes associated with minor gardening trauma from rose thorns or splinters. Most cases are sporadic, but epidemics may occur in hyperendemic areas. In Guatemala, 53 cases were diagnosed during a 3-year period around a single lake. There is no sex, age, or race predilection. The disease affects individuals whose occupation brings them into contact with soil, plants, or plant materials such as straw, wood, or reeds. It is most commonly reported from Central and South America, Africa, and Australasia.

PATHOGENESIS AND PATHOLOGY. Once introduced into the dermis, the fungus provokes a granulomatous response with foci of suppuration and necrosis. Associated with localized lesions are foci of neutrophils, histiocytes, and epithelioid cells. Langerhans giant cells may be present. In some lesions, there are circumscribed microabscesses surrounded by tissue infiltrated with lymphocytes, neutrophils, and plasma cells. In skin lesions, pseudoepitheliomatous hyperplasia associated with a mixed pyogenic-granulomatous reaction may be seen. Rete pegs are elongated and broadened.

Unusual among the mycoses, the causal agent is rarely seen in histopathologic material from primary infections. When present, it is often pleomorphic appearing as a small, round, oval, or cigar-shaped budding yeast cell, 2 to 3 μm wide by 3 to 8 μm long. In some instances, a central fungal cell is surrounded by radiating eosinophilic material (asteroid body).

CLINICAL MANIFESTATIONS. Sporotrichosis has a wide range of clinical expression. It is not contagious and is acquired from the environment, usually by implantation through the skin. Although inhalation with the resultant establishment of a primary pulmonary infection is a recognized mechanism of pathogenesis, the most common route of entry is by minor traumatic subcutaneous inoculation, or via an abrasion. The incubation period usually varies from 1 to 4 weeks, exceptionally up to 6 months. About 75% of infections affect an upper extremity. There is some evidence to suggest that in certain patients self-limited infections may occur.

Cutaneous Sporotrichosis. The most common and familiar form of sporotrichosis is lymphangitic sporotrichosis, in which a small, firm, movable subcutaneous nodule develops at the site of inoculation. The nodule later becomes soft and breaks down to form a persistent friable ulcer or chancre. Subsequently, additional nodules develop along the lymphatics draining the area, which, in turn, progress to ulceration. The lymphatic vessels connecting the nodules may become acutely inflamed or indurated and cordlike. The presence of a persistent ulcer on a finger or hand and a chain of swollen lymph nodes extending up the arm is suspicious, but this may be caused by other organisms. If untreated, the lesions may persist for years. In about a quarter of cutaneous infections, the lesion remains "fixed," without lymphatic spread. Fixed infections are more common in children and in Latin America. Facial lesions also often behave in this way.

Less commonly lesions may present as chronic ulcers, mycetoma-like lesions, or well-defined granulomas. Disseminated cutaneous lesions have been reported in patients with AIDS.

Pulmonary Sporotrichosis. Primary pulmonary infection was originally thought to be rare, but it may not be uncommon in endemic areas. In most cases, it is asymptomatic, but a residual infection may rarely occur in individuals with a low level of immunity and lead to disseminated disease.

Disseminated Sporotrichosis. This is uncommon and is generally seen in subjects with underlying diseases or predisposition such as alcoholism. It is always endogenous, originating by hematogenous spread usually from lung foci. Multiple cutaneous nodules that eventually ulcerate may develop over the body surfaces. Other sites affected include joints, the lungs, bone, mucous membranes, and the central nervous system.

DIAGNOSIS. Classic cutaneous lymphatic sporotrichosis is clinically distinct, but the complexity and variability of other forms of the disease may make the clinical diagnosis difficult. Direct examination of pus or skin scales is seldom helpful, and *S. schenckii* is usually absent or rare in tissue sections. Immunofluorescence may assist in visualizing single fungal cells, but culture and serologic testing are of the greatest value as ancillary diagnostic procedures. *S. schenckii* is readily isolated from clinical material on a variety of culture media. It normally appears 3 to 10 days after inoculation and is identified by the colonial and microscopic morphology and by the demonstration of dimorphism in vitro.

Serology. Serologic procedures may be of value, although they are not always reliable. Antibodies may not be demonstrable in patients with proved infection, and existing serodiagnostic reagents lack specificity. Nevertheless, the demonstration of antibodies to *S. schenckii* by double diffusion, agglutination, or immunofluorescence may provide a valuable clue in deep disseminated sporotrichosis.

Differential Diagnosis. The condition must be distinguished from other mycoses and from a range of infective skin lesions such as tularemia, leishmaniasis, anthrax, tuberculosis, and pyogenic bacterioses. Lymphatic spread similar to that of sporotrichosis may also occur in nontuberculous mycobacterial infections, often those caused by *Mycobacterium marinum*, and some South American forms of leishmaniasis.

TREATMENT. The usual treatment is orally administered potassium iodide (KI) in saturated solution, which usually produces a cure within 3 months. An adult can be given 1 mL of KI three times daily, with drops in incremental increases to a maximum of 4 to 6 mL three times daily after 1 month. To increase palatability, the drug may be administered in milk. Treatment should be continued for 3 to 4 weeks after clinical cure. This form of treatment is most effective for cutaneous sporotrichosis. Alternatives include itraconazole 100 to 200 mg daily or terbinafine 250 mg daily. In cases of disseminated disease amphotericin B is normally used (Chapter 84). An intriguing and apparently effective treatment is the use of externally applied heat.

PROGNOSIS. This is excellent for cutaneous forms of the disease but is less satisfactory for patients with disseminated sporotrichosis, particularly if associated with another severe underlying disease.

PREVENTION. As with other subcutaneous mycoses in which the agent is widely distributed in nature, environmental control is not practicable.

Bibliography

Campos P, Arenas R, Coronado H: Epidemic cutaneous sporotrichosis. Int J Dermatol 33:38, 1994.

Galiana J, Conti-Diaz IA: Healing effects of heat and a rubefacient on nine cases of sporotrichosis. Sabouraudia 3:64, 1963.

Kaplan W, Gonzalez-Ochoa A: Application of the fluorescent antibody technique to the rapid diagnosis of sporotrichosis. J Lab Clin Med 62:835, 1963.

Lurie HI: Sporotrichosis. In Baker RD (ed): Human Infections with Fungi, Actinomycetes and Algae. New York, Springer-Verlag, 1971, pp 614–675.

Mariat F: The epidemiology of sporotrichosis. In Wolstenholme GEW, Porter R (eds): Systemic Mycoses. London, J & A Churchill, 1968, pp 1–159.

Mayorga R, Caceres A, Toriello C, et al: Etude d'une zone d'endemic sporotrichosique au Guatemala. Sabouraudia 16:185, 1978.

82.3 Chromoblastomycosis

Roderick J. Hay

DEFINITION. Chromoblastomycosis (chromomycosis) is a chronic mycosis affecting skin and subcutaneous tissues characterized by the development of slow-growing verrucous nodules that eventually coalesce and form hyperkeratotic masses.

ETIOLOGY. The condition is caused by several species of related fungi, the most common and widespread of which are *Fonsecaea pedrosoi, Fonsecaea compactum, Phialophora verrucosa,* and *Cladosporium carrionii.* Irrespective of the causal species, all have an identical appearance in infected tissues, i.e., single or clustered, rounded or angular, thick-walled, dark-brown bodies ("sclerotic cells"). In culture, considerable variation exists in the types and predominance of spore forms, and they are difficult to distinguish without experience. The organisms are commonly found in soil and wood as saprophytes. The first case was reported from the United States in 1915, but it was subsequently shown to be a disease of tropical and subtropical countries.

EPIDEMIOLOGY. Chromoblastomycosis is diagnosed more commonly in males than in females. Because, in common with other types of subcutaneous mycoses, infection is from an exogenous source, lesions occur most frequently among those whose occupation exposes them to thorn pricks, splinters, and other penetrating wounds. Therefore, the disease is more prevalent in rural than in urban dwellers and among those who walk barefoot rather than those who wear shoes. All races are affected and the condition is uncommon among children. Although experimental infections can be established in animals, they are not normally naturally infected. There are some indications that climate affects the prevalence of different species. In Madagascar infections with *C. carrionii* occurred in areas of low rainfall (50 to 60 cm annually), in contrast to infections caused by *F. pedrosoi,* which occur in areas with a high rainfall (220 to 300 cm annually). The disease has a worldwide distribution and has a particularly high prevalence in Costa Rica (1/21,000 population) and Madagascar (1/30,000 population).

PATHOGENESIS AND PATHOLOGY. In some instances, there is a history of trauma, but usually the patient can remember no specific incident that preceded development of the primary lesion. The sites affected most frequently are the feet and legs, but other exposed parts of the body, e.g., the hands, arms, buttocks, back, neck, and face, may be involved. Early primary lesions are rarely seen or recognized as such, and the patient does not usually seek medical attention until the lesion has been present for a number of years.

Lesions are usually hyperkeratotic and characterized by pseudoepitheliomatous hyperplasia with microabscess formation. Granulomatous nodules are present in the dermis and are composed of epithelioid cells, with occasional giant cells, surrounded by plasma cells, macrophages, eosinophils, and lymphocytes. Fibrosis of the dermis and subcutaneous tissue is a prominent feature. The fungal cells, i.e., muriform cells or sclerotic bodies, are 5 to 12 μm in diamter, common in some tissue sections and rare in others. They may be associated with giant cells. Their distinctive dark-brown color, thick walls, and multiplication by splitting rather than by budding are diagnostic. Secondary bacterial infection is often present.

CLINICAL MANIFESTATIONS. The initial lesion is a warty papule that enlarges slowly to form a verrucous plaque. In some instances, the primary lesion is a pustule, a flat plaque, or an ulcer. As the infection progresses, ulceration and serous exudation can become features (Fig. 82–4). Eventually, the lesion becomes dry and crusted, with a roughened surface and raised margin (Fig. 82–5). Some lesions may be pedunculated. Large hyperkeratotic plaques up to 3 cm thick with central scar formation may be formed. Characteristically, the lesion does not spread peripherally, although there may be spread by autoinoculation and via the lymphatics to adjacent

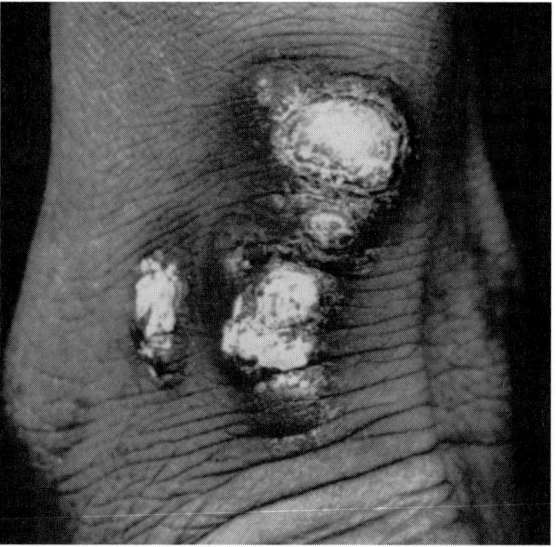

Figure 82–4. Chromomycosis. An early lesion on the ankle. (Courtesy of the St John's Institute of Dermatology, London.)

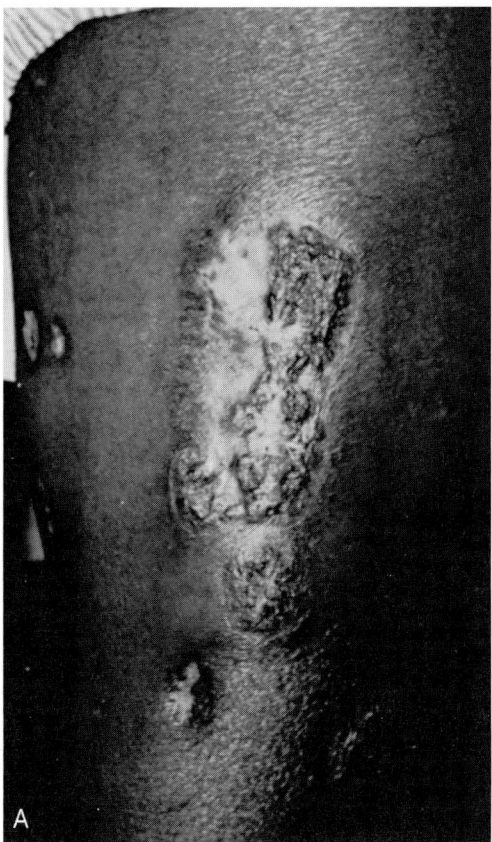

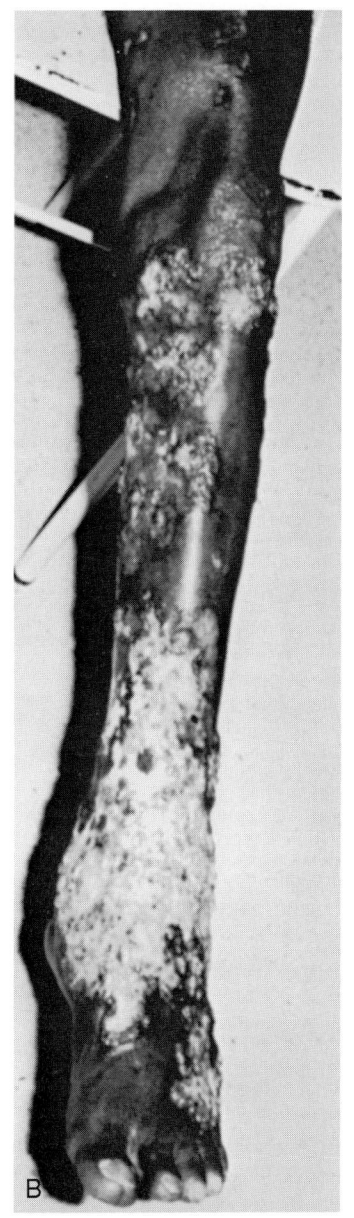

Figure 82–5. Chromomycosis. Scarred verrucous lesions of the thigh *(A)* and leg and foot *(B)* in a 53-year-old Brazilian man. (Courtesy of the Armed Forces Institute of Pathology, Photograph Neg. No. 74–12824.)

areas. The condition is not painful but may itch. Superinfection may be responsible for lymph stasis and resultant elephantiasis, and secondary infected lesions have an unpleasant smell.

Lesions of chromoblastomycosis are almost always confined to the skin and subcutaneous tissues. Rarely chromoblastomycosis organisms have been isolated from the brain, suggesting that hematogenous spread and systemic infection are possible.

DIAGNOSIS. Clinical history and manifestations are often diagnostic. Early or atypical lesions can be recognized by direct microscopy, the distinctive brown fungal cells being readily distinguished in 20% potassium hydroxide mounts of skin scrapings (Fig. 82–6). Cells seen in tissue sections are also diagnostic. Culture and identification of the specific etiologic agent can be time consuming and should always be entrusted to a specialist laboratory, because the polymorphic appearance of many isolates makes their positive identification difficult. Serologic tests have not been reliable indicators of infection. Antibodies are produced during the course of infection, but neither presence nor titer is diagnostic.

Differential Diagnosis. Chromoblastomycosis may resemble blastomycosis, and in parts of the world where the latter is endemic, a differentiation between the two diseases must be made (Chapter 83.3). Other conditions that may simulate chromomycosis include cutaneous tuberculosis and leishmaniasis, syphilis, and yaws.

TREATMENT. No simple antifungal regimen is universally satisfactory, although itraconazole with or without flucytosine has been effective in many cases. Terbinafine is a recently reported alternative and in extensive lesions amphotericin B should be given intravenously (Chapter 84) at the outset of treatment in addition to flucytosine. Local application of heat may also be effective in certain cases. In advanced cases with multiple extensive lesions, amputations are occasionally considered necessary.

PROGNOSIS. Chromoblastomycosis progresses slowly and usually remains localized. Since hematogenous spread is such a rare event, the condition is not life-threatening. Moreover, in contrast to mycetoma, chromoblastomycosis does not invade the deeper tissues with attendant destruction and loss of function. The principal clinical problems relate to the pain,

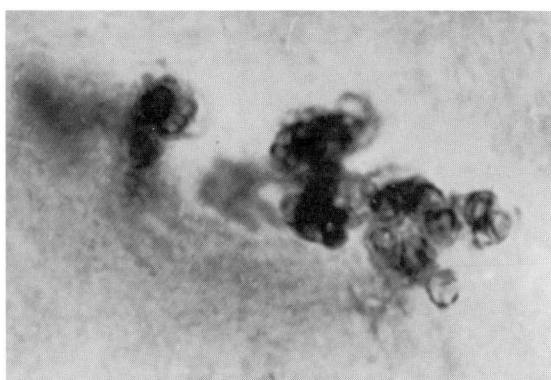

Figure 82–6. Scraping of chromomycosis mounted in 20% potassium hydroxide. Note the thick-walled pigmented fungal cells. (Courtesy of the St John's Institute of Dermatology, London.)

tissue damage, and elephantiasis associated with bacterial superinfection. Cures are rare in patients with advanced disease.

PREVENTION. No preventative measures are available.

Bibliography

Brygoo ER, Segretain G: Etude clinique epidemiologique et mycologique de la chromoblastomycose a Madagascar. Bull Soc Pathol Exot 53:443, 1960.
Cameron HM, Gatei D, Bremner AD: The deep mycoses in Kenya: A histopathological study. 3: Chromomycosis. East Afr Med J 50:406, 1973.
Restrepo A: Treatment of tropical mycoses. J Am Acad Dermatol 31:S91, 1994.
Zaias N: Chromomycosis. J Cutan Pathol 5:155, 1978.

82.4 Rhinosporidiosis

Roderick J. Hay

DEFINITION. Rhinosporidiosis is a chronic, localized granulomatous infection of nasal and other mucosal surfaces, conjunctiva, and skin that is characterized by hyperplasia and development of polyps.

ETIOLOGY. The causal agent is *Rhinosporidium seeberi.* In infected tissues, it forms abundant sporangia up to 350 μm in diameter and containing large numbers of spores. Details of its ecology and life cycle are unknown. It has not been cultivated in vitro, nor have experimental infections of animals been established.

DISTRIBUTION. The disease has been reported from many tropical and temperate countries throughout the world, but 90% of reported cases are from India and Sri Lanka.

PATHOGENESIS AND EPIDEMIOLOGY. The mechanism by which infection is acquired is not known. Rhinosporidiosis is most common in children and young adults, but any age group may be affected. Males are more commonly affected than females (3:1). The disease is not contagious, and infection is thought to be exogenous. The high proportion of patients with a history of long exposure to freshwater suggests that *R. seeberi* may occur naturally in rivers or lakes, possibly as a pathogen of fish or insects, and that humans become infected by continued contact with such contaminated environments. Because of the localized nature of the condition and its presumed exogenous origin, rhinosporidiosis can provisionally be regarded as a mycosis of implantation.

The most common site of rhinosporidiosis is the nose (70% of infections), with sessile or pedunculated polyps affecting one or both nostrils. Lesions may affect the conjunctiva also and, more rarely, the larynx, genitals, and skin. Dissemination has been reported but is exceptional.

PATHOLOGY. Examination of hematoxylin and eosin–stained sections reveals hyperplasia and a chronic inflammatory reaction with neutrophils, lymphocytes, plasma cells and occasional foreign-body giant cells, and abundant globular sporangia of varying sizes and stages of development.

DIAGNOSIS. Polyps of rhinosporidiosis can be recognized by their pink or purple color and friable consistency and by the presence of small, white sporangia on the polyp surface. Diagnosis is confirmed by examination of biopsy sections and the detection of the distinctive sporangia. Culture, serologic tests, and animal inoculation procedures are not helpful in establishing or confirming a diagnosis.

Differential Diagnosis. Rhinosporidiosis must be differentiated from nasal polyps. Lesions in other sites, particularly on the genitalia or anal region, must be distinguished from warts, condylomata, and hemorrhoids.

TREATMENT. Chemotherapy is of little proven value. The treatment of choice is surgical excision, with or without cauterization.

Bibliography

Mohapatra LN: Rhinosporidiosis. *In* Baker RD (ed): Human Infection with Fungi, Actinomycetes and Algae. New York, Springer-Verlag, 1971.

82.5 Subcutaneous Zygomycosis due to Basidiobolus

Roderick J. Hay

DEFINITION. Subcutaneous zygomycosis (subcutaneous phycomycosis, entomophthoromycosis due to *Basidiobolus*) is a localized mycotic infection causing a firm, progressive swelling of the subcutaneous tissues and characterized by eosinophil infiltration and granuloma formation.

ETIOLOGY. The causal fungus is *Basidiobolus haptosporus,* a common saprophyte in decaying vegetation overlying soil. It has also been found in the intestines of frogs, toads, lizards, and other small reptiles.

EPIDEMIOLOGY. The disease was first described in Indonesia in 1956, but it is most commonly reported from Africa. Sporadic cases have also been reported from India, the Middle East, Asia, and Europe. The condition affects children and adolescents rather than adults, and boys rather than girls.

PATHOGENESIS AND PATHOLOGY. The mode of entry of the fungus has not been clearly established but most likely follows implantation from an exogenous source. Once established, the lesion affects mainly subcutaneous tissues, largely replacing fat with fibrous tissue. It is characterized, particularly toward the margins of the tumor, by microabscesses in which eosinophils predominate. Strands of broad 5- to 15-μm thin-walled, branching, and generally nonseptate hyphae are found toward the edge of the lesions, each rounded by a distinctive eosinophilic sheath several micrometers wide (Splendore-Hoeppli phenomenon). In subacute stages, hyphae may be surrounded by epithelioid and plasma cells. Giant cells may also be present together with varying quantities of "fibrinoid" material. In later stages fibrosis and necrosis are prominent, along with a variable cellular infiltration.

CLINICAL MANIFESTATIONS. The subcutaneous swelling is firm, movable, and well-defined; satellite lesions may be palpable at the advancing margins. The masses are disk-shaped, with the consistency of rubber. The overlying skin is usually intact and may be tense, edematous, hyperpigmented, or normal. Ulceration may occur but is uncommon, and regional lymph nodes are rarely affected. Pain and tenderness are usually absent. Any part of the body may be affected, but the most common sites are the limbs, buttocks, trunk, and neck (Fig. 82–7). Penetration of deeper tissues and viscera has been reported but this is uncommon.

DIAGNOSIS. The clinical picture is usually characteristic, but a firm diagnosis requires histopathologic confirmation. The agent can be cultivated readily and has distinctive colonial and microscopic features. Serologic tests are not helpful.

Differential Diagnosis. At presentation, subcutaneous malignant lymphoma may have clinical similarities to subcutaneous zygomycosis, but it is characterized by more rapid growth. Clinical characteristics should serve to distinguish it from sarcoma, mycetoma, or bacterial cellulitis. Lymphatic edema and elephantiasis are differentiated by the absence of a clear margin and by the tendency to affect the extremities.

TREATMENT. The most effective treatment is itraconazole in doses of 100 to 200 mg daily. An alternative is oral potassium iodide (KI), in saturated solution in doses up to 10 mL three times daily for 3 months. Not all patients respond well, although a combination of KI and trimethoprim/sulfamethoxazole (co-trimoxazole), 14 mg/kg of sulfamethoxazole twice daily, has been used with some success. Amphotericin B has been used in patients refractory to treatment.

PROGNOSIS. The infection generally pursues a slow and

benign course, with increasing lateral extension of the initial tumor.

PREVENTION. This is not practicable.

Bibliography

Cameron HM, Gatei D, Bremner AD: The deep mycoses in Kenya: A histopathological study. 2: Phycomycosis. East Afr Med J 50:396, 1973.

Clark BM: The epidemiology of phycomycosis. *In* Wolstenholme GEW, Porter R (eds): Systemic Mycoses. London, I & A Churchill, 1968.

Clark BM, Edington GM: Subcutaneous phycomycosis and rhinoentomophthoromycosis. *In* Baker RD (ed): Human Infection with Fungi, Actinomycetes and Algae. New York, Springer-Verlag, 1971.

82.6 *Subcutaneous Zygomycosis due to* Conidiobolus

Roderick J. Hay

DEFINITION. Subcutaneous infections caused by *Conidiobolus* (rhinoentomophthoromycosis) lead to a chronic, localized, subcutaneous fungal infection affecting tissues of the nose, cheek, and upper lip. It is also called nasofacial phycomycosis.

ETIOLOGY. The condition is caused by *Conidiobolus coronatus*, a ubiquitous saprophyte in tropical rain forest areas. Clark (1968) isolated it most commonly from soil and decaying vegetation in Nigeria during September and October, when rainfall was regular but not excessive. Unlike *Basidiobolus*, no association with reptiles or amphibians has been recognized. The disease was reported initially in 1961, affecting horses. The first reported human cases were by Martinson in 1963 in Nigeria, but the agent was isolated in culture from a patient in the Congo in 1965. Earlier isolated reports in the literature suggest that the condition existed a decade or more earlier but had not been recognized as a new disease entity.

EPIDEMIOLOGY. In contrast to subcutaneous zygomycosis due to *Basidiobolus*, rhinoentomophthoromycosis is a disease of young adults rather than children. Males are more commonly affected than females. Most cases affect men 20 to 40 years old who work outdoors in tropical forest areas. Most infections are reported from West Africa, particularly Nigeria, but cases have been recognized in India and South America. The geographic range is probably explained in part by climatic factors, the agent failing to grow well at temperatures below 15°C.

PATHOGENESIS AND PATHOLOGY. The mode of infection is unknown but is probably inoculation of contaminated soil or vegetable matter through minor trauma or insect bites. The initial site of infection is the region of the inferior turbinates. Epithelium may show transitional or squamous metaplasia, but ulceration is uncommon. The condition affects subepithelial tissue and muscle. Bone is not affected, but radiographs may show evidence of soft tissue swelling. Histopathologic features are identical to those already described for subcutaneous zygomycosis, both in the nature of tissue responses and the appearance of the pathogen.

CLINICAL MANIFESTATIONS. Infection apparently originates in the nasal mucosa, leading to nasal obstruction, which may be unilateral. Tissue swelling becomes pronounced, affecting the nose and nasolabial folds, cheeks, and upper lip and eventually producing gross facial distortion (Fig. 82–8). The infected areas have distinct margins, but the mass is not movable over the underlying tissues. As the condition

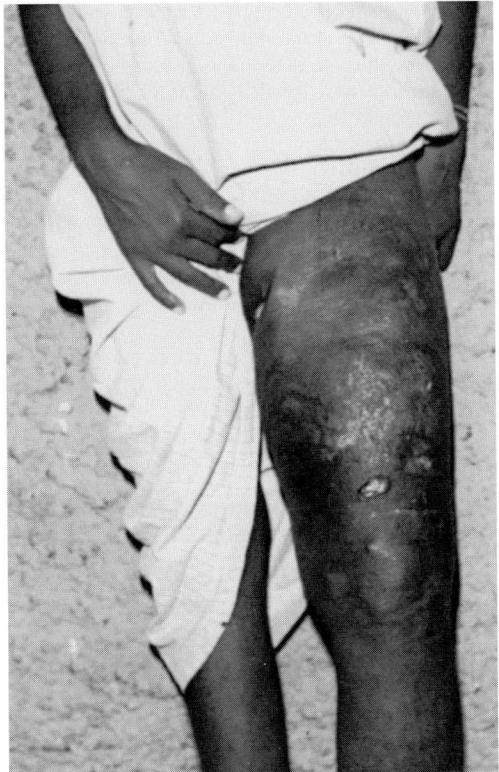

Figure 82–7. Subcutaneous zygomycosis in the thigh of an Ugandan woman. (Courtesy of the Armed Forces Institute of Pathology, Photograph Neg. No. 70–11661.)

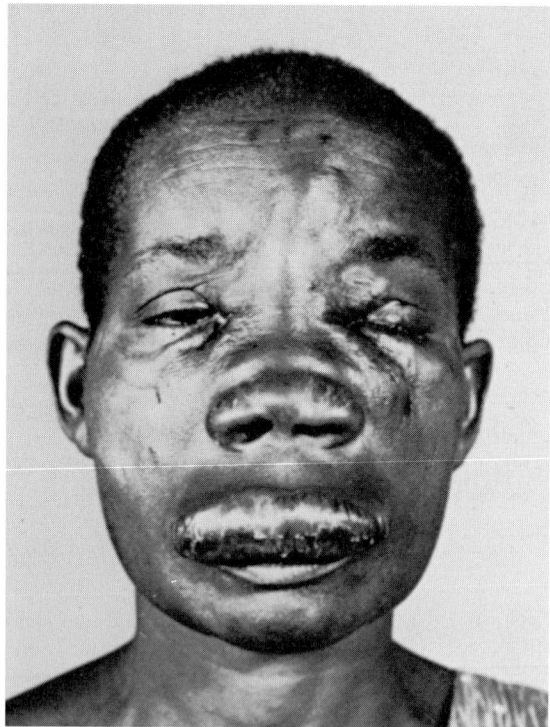

Figure 82–8. Nigerian patient with subcutaneous zygomycosis due to *Conidiobolus*. (Courtesy of the Armed Forces Institute of Pathology, Photograph Neg. No. 76–6165.)

progresses, infection may spread rarely to the paranasal sinuses, palate, and pharynx. Satellite lesions may be detectable at the margins. The overlying skin becomes stretched but does not ulcerate. The reason for the curiously restricted anatomic distribution is unknown. There are few symptoms. Nasal discharge is an early finding, but pain, tenderness, and constitutional upset are rare. Pharyngeal involvement may result in dysphagia. The most serious effect on the patient may result from the severe disfigurement.

DIAGNOSIS. The clinical features are highly distinctive, i.e., localized swelling of the nose and face in tropical countries. Biopsy may be diagnostic when the characteristic hyphae are present and associated with an eosinophilic sheath and eosinophilic granuloma. Positive diagnosis may depend on culture and identification of the etiologic agent. Serologic tests have not been developed.

Differential Diagnosis. *Conidiobolus* and *Basidobolus* infections can be differentiated by the site involved.

TREATMENT. Treatment is the same as for subcutaneous zygomycosis due to *Basidiobolus* (Chapter 82.5).

PROGNOSIS. Spontaneous remission is unknown. Surgical intervention may be required to alleviate nasal obstruction or to reduce gross deformities. The response to therapy is less satisfactory than that in subcutaneous zygomycosis.

PREVENTION. None is practicable.

Bibliography

Clark BM: The epidemiology of phycomycosis. *In* Wolstenholme GEW, Porter R (eds): Systemic Mycoses. London, J & A Churchill, 1968, pp 179–192.

Clark BM, Edington GM: Subcutaneous phycomycosis and rhinoentomophthoromycosis. *In* Baker RD (ed): Human Infection with Fungi, Actinomycetes and Algae. New York, Springer-Verlag, 1971, pp 684–690.

Cockshott WP, Clark BM, Martinson FD: Upper respiratory tract infection due to *Entomophthora coronata*. Radiology 90:1016, 1968.

Martinson RD: Rhinophycomycosis. J Laryngol Otol 77:691, 1963.

82.7 *Other Subcutaneous Mycoses*

Roderick J. Hay

PHAEOHYPHOMYCOSIS

Definition and Etiology. This is a term used to describe infections with dark-pigmented fungi that are distinct clinically and pathologically from chromomycosis or mycetoma and where the organisms are usually present as irregular hyphae in tissue. Within this heterogeneous group is a wide range of uncommon subcutaneous mycoses described in the literature under many disease names. These include cladosporiosis, subcutaneous mycotic cyst, phaeosporotrichosis, and cystic chromomycosis. The range of causal organisms is also a wide one, embracing some 16 genera and almost 30 species. Phaeohyphomycosis is an uncommon disease, and its prevalence in the tropics is unknown.

Clinical Manifestations and Treatment. Lesions are usually solitary and circumscribed, occurring on the feet, legs, hands, and other body sites. As with all subcutaneous mycoses, entry of the pathogen is assumed to occur by a penetrating wound, the site of the injury being contaminated with the pathogen. Over a period of months or years, the lesions may increase in size, producing a crusted or cystic mass that remains localized. Rarely, phaeohyphomycosis may affect the brain, producing symptoms and pathology of cerebral abscesses. Diagnosis depends on the recognition of brown fungal elements by direct microscopy or in tissue sections, which may be filamentous, irregularly swollen, or yeastlike, and by isolation and identification of the agents in a specialist laboratory. The treatment for localized forms of the disease is surgical excision. Recurrence may result from inadequate or careless excision. The prognosis in cerebral forms of the disease is poor.

LOBOMYCOSIS. Lobomycosis or Lobo disease is a chronic, localized mycosis of skin and subcutaneous tissues characterized by keloidal or verrucoid lesions that contain abundant round or lemon-shaped cells. The disease is rare and only recorded in remote and tropical areas of South and Central America. It has also been described in freshwater dolphins. As the causative organism has not been isolated in vitro, its habitat is unknown.

Patients present with circumscribed plaques or keloid-like lesions usually on exposed areas such as the face, ears or trunk (Fig. 82–9). These may slowly increase in size and plaques may cover wide areas of the body. They are usually asymptomatic. The diagnosis is made by biopsy and histopathology of the lesions. The organisms are present as chains of cells each with a short tubelike connection between individual cells. They are usually arranged in lines and can be found within giant cells (Fig. 82–10). There is no place for culture or serology in the diagnosis of lobomycosis. The

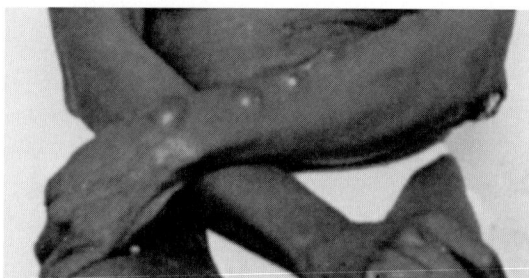

Figure 82–9. Lobo's disease. Nodules on the left forearm that developed 30 years after a local injury. (Courtesy of the Armed Forces Institute of Pathology, Photograph Neg. No. 75–771.)

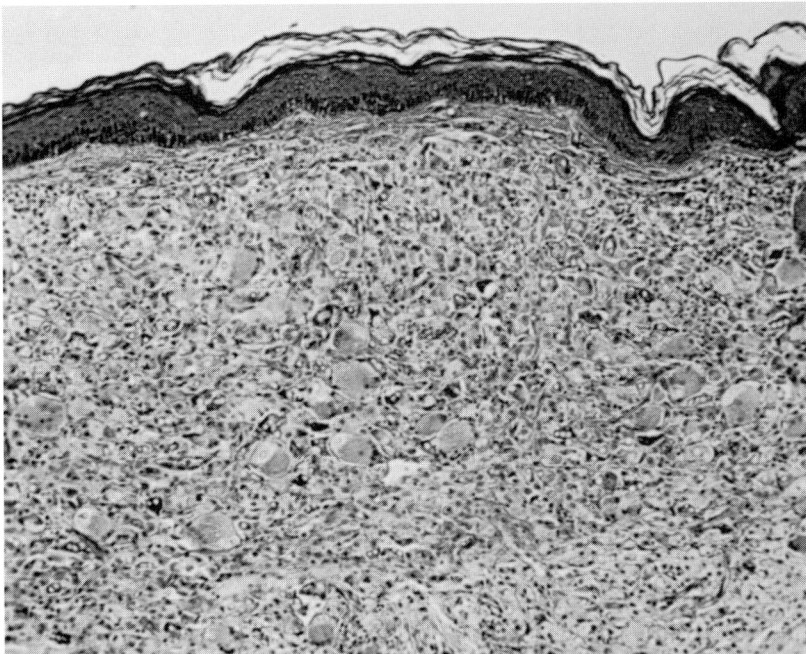

Figure 82-10. Biopsy from a lesion in Figure 82-9 showing giant cells and large numbers of yeast cells in the dermis ($\times$ 70). (Courtesy of the Armed Forces Institute of Pathology, Photograph Neg. No. 61–6506.)

treatment is surgical removal of lesions and there are no studies to suggest that antifungal therapy is effective.

82.8 Protothecosis*

Ann M. Nelson and Ronald C. Neafie

DEFINITION AND DISTRIBUTION. Protothecosis is a rare infection caused by achlorophyllic algae belonging to the genus *Prototheca*. Infections have involved skin, subcutaneous tissue, olecranon bursa, and rarely, lymph nodes or deep organs. Slightly more than 50 cases have been reported in the world literature from temperate and tropical areas of all continents.

ETIOLOGY. The index case of protothecosis in humans (Fig. 82–11) was caused by *Prototheca zopfi*. With one exception, all other infections in humans where the species was determined, have been caused by *Prototheca wickerhamii*. *P. wickerhamii* and *P. zopfi* are ubiquitous achloric algae usually found in soil and contaminated water. Both are spherical unicellular organisms, 3 to 30 μm in diameter with hyaline sporangia and asexual reproduction by internal septation and cytoplasmic cleavage. *Prototheca* are thought to be mutant strains of chlorophyllic (green) algae. *P. wickerhamii* divides to form characteristic morulas (Fig. 82–12), a form described only rarely in *P. zopfii*. Infections by both organisms have been reported in a variety of animals. A third species, *P. stagnora*, is not known to cause disease in humans.

Chlorella is similar to *Prototheca* and must be differentiated in tissue sections. Both *Prototheca* and *Chlorella* are distinct from fungi and bacteria by size, morphology, and type of reproduction. In addition, *Prototheca* and *Chlorella* lack the glucosamine of the fungal cell wall and the muramic acid of bacteria. *Prototheca* do not have chloroplasts, whereas *Chlorella* do. Although infections by *Chlorella* have been described in several animals, there is only one published report involving humans.

CLINICOPATHOLOGIC FEATURES. There are two clinical syndromes associated with *Prototheca* infection: a localized

infection of the olecranon bursa in patients with normal immunity and an eczematoid dermatitis in immunosuppressed individuals. Some infections have been associated with trauma and/or contact with contaminated water. One case each of the following visceral or systemic infections have been reported: an ulcerated mass involving the nasopharynx in a patient with prolonged intubation, hepatobiliary disease, peritonitis, meningitis, algemia, and disseminated infection. There are also recent reports of protothecosis in human immunodeficiency virus (HIV)–infected patients.

Protothecosis of the olecranon bursa develops usually several weeks after injury to the elbow. The lesions are localized to the bursa, but there may be epithelial hyperplasia and underlying sinus tracts. The bursa is thickened, and histopathologic changes include an area of caseation necrosis surrounded by granulation tissue, Langhan giant cells, and fibrosis. *Prototheca* organisms are scattered throughout the areas of necrosis.

In the cutaneous and subcutaneous forms, there are single or multiple lesions on the skin or within the subcutaneous tissue, usually over an exposed portion of the body, such as a limb or the face. The lesions are papulomacular to plaquelike and may have an overlying crust or focal ulceration; they spread slowly often in a centrifugal pattern and do not resolve. The inflammatory response varies from minimal to necrotizing granulomatous reaction and appears related to the depth of the invasion. The organisms may be in any or all layers of the skin and may be single or in clusters, extracellular or within giant cells. These lesions must be differentiated from other chronic granulomatous diseases of the skin.

DIAGNOSIS. Scraping of the skin, biopsy specimen, and aspirates can all be cultured on Sabouraud medium and require 1 to 2 days for growth. Typical sporulating forms can be identified on stained wet mounts. Although the organisms are usually apparent with routine staining by hematoxylin and eosin (H&E), they are much better seen with fungal stains, such as Gomori methenamine-silver (GMS), periodic acid–Schiff (PAS), and Gridley fungus (GF). *Prototheca* species are distinguished from *Cryptococcus, Coccidioides, Blastomyces*, and other fungi by the type of division. Sugar assimilation

---

*All the illustrations in this chapter are in the public domain.

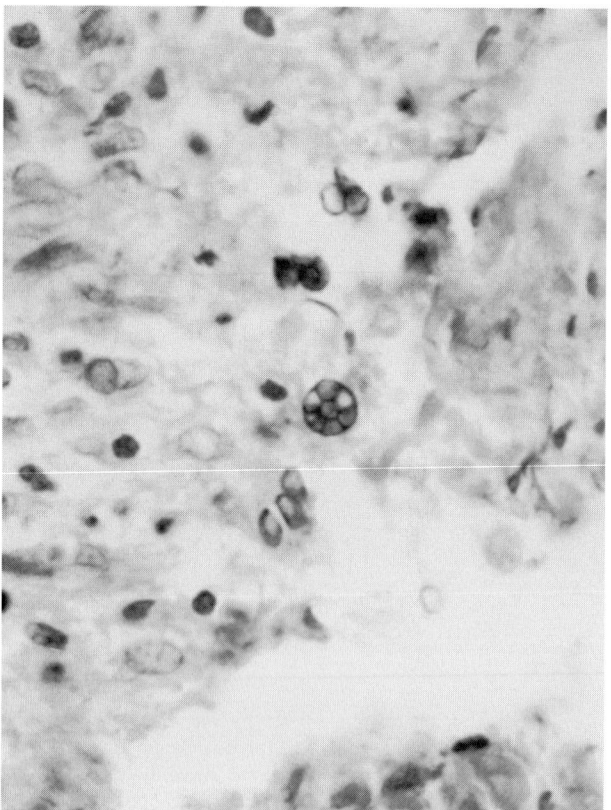

Figure 82–11. Prothecosis of the foot of a rice farmer from Sierra Leone. The lesion began as a papule on the instep 9 years earlier. It now encircles the foot, and there is a satellite lesion. (Armed Forces Institute of Pathology, Neg. No. 75–12872–2. Photograph courtesy of Dr. P. O. Wakelin.)

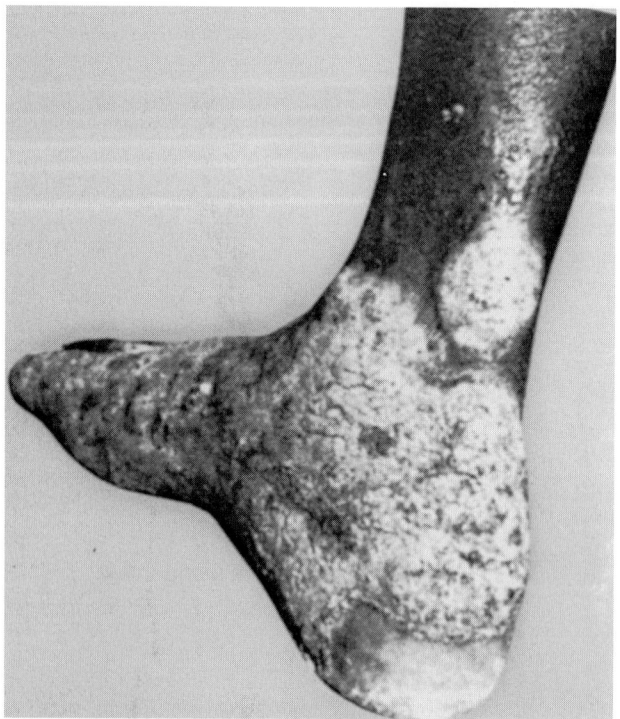

Figure 82–12. Characteristic morula of *P. wickerhamii* in subcutaneous tissue of wrist. (Courtesy of the Armed Forces Institute of Pathology, Photograph Neg. No. 86–7088.)

tests and fluorescent immunoassay aid in species determination. Specific antisera for each of the *Prototheca* species are available and can be used on either fresh or formalin-fixed tissue.

TREATMENT. Simple bursectomy cures protothecosis of the olecranon bursa. The cutaneous lesions in immunosuppressed patients resist treatment and may persist for several years, eventually spreading to other sites. Topical treatments, including Castellani paint, saturated copper sulfate, potassium permanganate, and amphotericin B, as well as systemic griseofulvin, penicillin, emetine hydrochloride, 5-fluorouracil and pentamidine isothionate, have not been effective. In vitro studies have demonstrated sensitivity to amphotericin B, tetracycline, gentamicin, and ketoconazole. Combined therapy with tetracycline and amphotericin B appears to be effective. Isolated cutaneous, bursal, and soft tissue lesions are best treated with local excision and ketoconazole. Infections which are multifocal, visceral, or occur in an immunocompromised host require amphotericin B or combined therapy.

Bibliography

Chandler FW, Watts JC: Protothecosis and infections caused by green algae. *In* Pathologic Diagnosis of Fungal Infections, 2nd ed. Chicago, American Society of Clinical Pathologists, 1987, pp 43–53.

Joubert MF, Ferguson TG, Pankey GA: *Prototheca wickerhamii* algemia (letter). Infect Dis Clin Pract 2:428, 1993.

Kaminski ZC, Kapila R, Sharer LR, et al: Meningitis due to *Prototheca wickerhamii* in a patient with AIDS. Clin Infect Dis 15:704, 1992.

Kuo TT, Hsueh S, Wu JL, et al: Cutaneous protothecosis: A clinicopathologic study. Arch Pathol Lab Med 111:737, 1987.

McAnally T, Parry EL: Cutaneous protothecosis presenting as recurrent chromomycosis. Arch Dermatol 121:1066, 1985.

Naryshkin S, Frank I, Nachamkin I: *Prototheca zopfii* isolated from a patient with olecranon bursitis. Diagn Microbiol Infect Dis 6:171, 1987.

Nelson AM, Neafie RC, Connor DH: Cutaneous protothecosis and chlorellosis: Extraordinary aquatic-borne algal infections. Clin Dermatol 5:76, 1987.

Woolrich A, Koestenblatt E, Don P, et al: Cutaneous protothecosis and AIDS. J Am Acad Dermatol 31:920, 1994.

83 Systemic Mycoses

The systemic mycoses are fungal infections that involve the internal organs, e.g., the lungs or brain. Some are primarily respiratory illnesses caused by organisms that are confined to recognized endemic areas. In some infections, subclinical disease is the most common form, recognized only by the development of a delayed-type skin reaction to an intradermal injection of specific antigen. In contrast, systemic infections caused by the opportunistic mycoses occur predominantly in immuno-compromised individuals. The portal of entry is variable and may involve lung as well as the gastrointestinal tract, skin, or other sites. These infections are worldwide in distribution.

83.1 Histoplasmosis

Eileen E. Navarro, Thomas J. Walsh, and Roderick J. Hay

DEFINITION. Histoplasmosis refers to a common granulomatous infection caused by *Histoplasma capsulatum*, a dimorphic fungus distributed throughout the world. *H. capsulatum* var. *capsulatum*, which is more ubiquitous in its geographic distribution, generally causes a subclinical infection in individuals from an endemic area. Symptomatic disease, referred to as small-form or classic histoplasmosis, however, is dependent on an interplay between the intensity of infection and the hosts' immune status, presenting as a spectrum ranging from chronic progressive pulmonary infection to acute fulminant, or chronic indolent, disseminated histoplasmosis. Infections due to *H. capsulatum* var. *duboisii*, on the other hand, are restricted to West Africa, reflecting this variants' limited ecologic niche. African histoplasmosis, as this disease entity is called, classically presents with cutaneous and skeletal involvement, with very little reticuloendothelial dissemination.

CLASSIC OR SMALL-FORM HISTOPLASMOSIS

Etiologic Agent. *H. capsulatum* grows in its mycelial form at lower temperatures (25° to 30°C). This phase, characterized by hyphae with slender conidiophores and characteristic tuberculate macroconidia, is the saprobic state found in the environment. When incubated at 37°C on enriched medium, the conidia germinate into the yeast phase, which is the phase demonstrated in host tissue. Darling, who first described the pathologic features of histoplasmosis in 1905, named the organism *Histoplasma capsulatum*, because of the appearance of small intracellular yeasts packing the cytoplasm of macrophages, resembling encapsulated parasites.

Epidemiology. The tropical distribution of *H. capsulatum* was established from this initial description of the pulmonary histopathology of construction workers building the Panama Canal, who succumbed to acute histoplasmosis. Skin testing surveys of the native population indicate areas of high prevalence of infection throughout Latin America. No broad population based studies are available from many other areas in the tropics. Nevertheless, given the environmental isolation of *H. capsulatum* in Southeast Asia, the Indian continent, and the Middle East, the adaptation of aggressive immunocompromising medical therapies in the developing world, and the spread of the AIDS pandemic, an increase in symptomatic histoplasmosis in developing areas in the tropics may be anticipated. Furthermore, the mobility of contemporary society no longer restricts the presentation of histoplasmosis to the well-defined endemic areas in the river valleys of the United States and Latin America, with increasing reports of imported infections acquired by travelers.

Modes of Transmission. Histoplasmosis is acquired by the respiratory route; conidia are aerosolized when soil containing bat or bird guano is disturbed and are efficiently distributed by wind. Intense concentrations of conidia are described in endemic areas, as in the Mississippi and Ohio river valleys in the United States, where infections are associated with outdoor activities and exposure to starling roost or soil upheaval. Outside of endemic areas, restricted niches with conditions that support the luxuriant growth of *H. capsulatum* also occur, such as in bat infested caves where exposures to the increased concentrations of conidia in the confined space have resulted in epidemics.

Pathogenesis. Infection with *H. capsulatum* is initiated when aerosolized conidia are inhaled into the alveolar air space. Alveolar macrophages, modulated by T lymphocytes, contain this initial infection, resulting in localized granulomatous inflammation. This self-limiting process produces minimal symptoms, evidenced only by the development of an immune response, manifested by a delayed-type skin reaction and the production of specific precipitins and complement-fixing antibodies, as well as asymptomatic calcifications in the lung, spleen, and mediastinal lymph nodes. A small percentage of these episodes advance to progressive pulmonary infection or disseminated infection, often associated with an immunocompromised state.

Clinical Manifestations. Illness due to histoplasmosis may be classified according to site (pulmonary, extrapulmonary, or disseminated infection), by duration of infection (acute, subacute, and chronic), and by pattern of infection (primary versus reactivation). Most infections in normal hosts are asymptomatic and subclinical and even symptomatic primary infection may be overlooked or underdiagnosed given the brief, mild nature of this illness. Symptomatic infections may present as epidemic acute primary pulmonary infections (APPH), chronic cavitary pulmonary histoplasmosis (CCPH), as well as acute and chronic disseminated infections. An asymptomatic fungemia occurs with the primary infection, as evidenced by splenic calcifications, in addition to the pulmonary calcifications visualized on chest radiographs. This cryptic dissemination to multiple organs permits subsequent reactivation at pulmonary and extrapulmonary sites as the host becomes immunocompromised, resembling the pathogenesis of tuberculosis. Reactivation years later in extrapulmonary tissues, particularly the central nervous system (CNS) and eyes, adrenal glands, mucocutaneous surfaces, and other sites, often occurs in elderly and immunocompromised patients. The protean manifestations of disseminated histoplasmosis may mimic other mycotic infections, tuberculosis, or neoplasms. Acute disseminated disease, in contrast to reactivated disseminated infection, is often reported in young children and infants or, increasingly, in patients with cellular immune deficiency and is a fulminant, often fatal infection.

Pulmonary Histoplasmosis

ACUTE PRIMARY PULMONARY HISTOPLASMOSIS (APPH). This develops in normal, immunocompetent hosts exposed to a heavy inoculum. A history of potential environmental exposure is sought in patients with APPH, and local public health authorities should be notified if a putative source is identified. The symptoms of APPH often resemble those of an influenza-type illness. The sudden onset of fever, erythema nodosum or multiforme, and a brassy cough brought about by airway compression from lymphadenopathy may be accompanied in severe cases by pericarditis, nights sweats, cyanosis, hemoptysis, or even disseminated disease. The chest radiograph in APPH typically demonstrates a diffuse alveolar-interstitial infiltrative or reticulonodular pattern. The presence of hilar lymphadenopathy and a Ghon-like complex may lead to a diagnosis of tuberculosis. These radiographic changes resolve slowly or leave a miliary pattern of pulmonary calcifications. Features that may differentiate this from tuberculosis are the pattern of grouped calcification in paratracheal nodes and the generally larger calcifications (>4 mm in the parenchyma and >1 cm mediastinum) in histoplasmosis. In patients with active pulmonary histoplasmosis, yeast cells of *H. capsulatum* may be observed on direct examination of sputum, often within pulmonary alveolar macrophages.

CHRONIC CAVITARY PULMONARY HISTOPLASMOSIS (CCPH). This is an indolent but progressive respiratory infection of patients with underlying chronic obstructive pulmonary disease that is rarely described in the tropics. As a group, these patients are usually elderly, cigarette-smoking males who suffer from progressive deterioration of pulmonary function, likely due to a combination of both chronic lung disease and histoplasmosis. The symptoms of low-grade fever, weight loss, malaise, and cough, as well as the radiographic features of apical fibrocavitary infiltrates mimic tuberculosis.

Disseminated Histoplasmosis

ACUTE DISSEMINATED HISTOPLASMOSIS. This occurs with primary disease, often in young children or infants, or in the iatrogenically immunosuppressed host with underlying malignancy or inflammatory conditions. Since factors, e.g., the intensity of infection and the immune status of the host, modify expression of this infection, the disease often varies in its severity and is protean in its clinical manifestations and course, from a fulminant, fatal disease marked by shock to the more subacute disease with little systemic inflammation and focal, organ-specific signs and symptoms.

The most severely compromised hosts present with acute progressive disseminated histoplasmosis. Hectic fever, cough, dyspnea, and radiographic evidence of infiltrates and adenopathy highlight the primary pulmonary process, whereas the weight loss, infiltration of organs of the reticuloendothelial system and bone marrow, diffuse cutaneous lesions and CNS involvement attest to the systemic spread of infection. Rapidly fatal overwhelming infections marked by disseminated intravascular coagulation (DIC), adult respiratory distress syndrome (ARDS), bone marrow suppression, and multiorgan failure occur in a minority of patients. Children who present with this syndrome often have marked hepatosplenomegaly, gastrointestinal symptoms including bleeding, and anemia. AIDS patients, on the other hand, present with more lymphadenopathy, CNS manifestations, and various cutaneous lesions. The skin lesions vary from several to multiple erythematous macules, purpura, ulcers, and papules resembling molluscum contagiosum.

CHRONIC PROGRESSIVE DISSEMINATED HISTOPLASMOSIS. Patients with this form of disease have limited constitutional symptoms of wasting and fatigue, with prominent mucosal lesions. The mucosal involvement is characterized by painful nodules on the tongue or gingiva, as well as shallow denuded lesions or crater-like ulcers with heaped up edges in the buccal mucosa or nasal vestibule, which are often mistaken for malignancies. Swelling of the vocal cords and nodules on the larynx have also been described. Biopsies of these lesions reveal abundant yeast forms with inflammation and very little granulomatous reaction. In the more subacute forms of the infection, constitutional symptoms are more prominent, with distinct involvement of the gastrointestinal tract marked by abdominal pain and diarrhea, intestinal masses in the terminal ileum and cecum, bowel obstruction or perforation, and, occasionally, massive bleeding. Chronic basilar leptomeningitis with vasculitis and small cerebral granulomas or ring-enhancing cerebral mass lesions characterize CNS involvement with histoplasmosis. Culture-negative endocarditis with large and friable vegetations of the aortic and mitral valve may also occur. The histopathology of the valvular lesions are unique, such that, in addition to the presence of extracellular yeast, mycelial elements are also seen, and the scant inflammatory response is predominantly histiocytic. Adrenal involvement may occur as a terminal event in untreated disease.

DIAGNOSIS. Histoplasmosis may be identified by direct microscopic examination of specimens, by isolation and characterization of the fungus in cultures, by DNA probing of isolates, or by demonstration of specific exoantigens produced in culture.

Collection and Transport of Specimens. Since the respiratory tract is the most common portal of entry, most diagnostic specimens are sputum, bronchoalveolar lavage, transtracheal aspirates, or lung biopsy. Extrapulmonary specimens may include tissue as well as body fluids. Care must be taken to transport, process, and culture specimens promptly to avoid overgrowth by more rapidly growing bacteria or saprophytic fungi. The conidia of the mycelial form of dimorphic fungi are highly infectious and easily transmissible by aerosolization. When cultures are handled for identification, or sent to reference laboratories, sealing or taping the primary tube or plate must be undertaken to prevent aerosolization of the organisms.

Direct Examination. Direct examination of specimens for *H. capsulatum* is best accomplished with special stains. The budding yeast cells of *H. capsulatum* (2 to 4 μm) in a calcofluor white or potassium hydroxide preparation of sputum may be too small for reliable detection and may be confused with *Torulopsis glabrata*, which is similar in size and shape and which often colonizes the human oropharynx. The small yeast cells of *H. capsulatum* are observed frequently within the cytoplasm of macrophages. In contrast, the yeast cells of *T. glabrata* are seldom found intracellularly.

Bone marrow aspirates, buffy coat smears, and peripheral blood smears are valuable for the early detection of *H. capsulatum* in disseminated histoplasmosis. Giemsa or Wright stain reveals the intracellular yeast within circulating monocytes or tissue macrophages. Staining of a paraffin-embedded clot section of bone marrow aspirate by periodic acid–Schiff (PAS), Gomori methenamine stain (GMS), Giemsa and Wright stains also allows detection of *H. capsulatum* in granulomas. Touch preparations of bone marrow biopsies, lymph nodes, and other tissues are also an efficient means of detecting fungi in these tissues.

Cultures. Primary isolation media used in the diagnosis of systemic mycoses, including *H. capsulatum* should contain antibacterial antibiotics and cycloheximide to inhibit saprophytic fungi sometimes found in sputum. Normally sterile specimens, such as homogenized or minced tissue may be inoculated directly onto blood agar, brain-heart infusion (BHI) agar, Sabouraud glucose agar (SGA), and enriched broth such as BHI broth. All cultures for histoplasmosis should be incubated at 25° to 30°C under humidified, aerobic conditions for 4 to 8 weeks. All plating of specimens and study of cultures should be performed within a biosafety cabinet. If mycologic expertise is unavailable, plates growing a hyaline mold should be shrink sealed in the biosafety cabinet to prevent accidental opening before being forwarded to a reference laboratory.

Culture of specimens infected with *H. capsulatum* at 25° to 30°C reveals a slowly growing colony with aerial mycelium that varies in color from white to buff to brown. During early growth of the mycelial culture, spherical to oval to pyriform microconidia (2 to 5 μm in diameter) are present. With continued growth, the mold develops slender conidiophores and characteristic globose and pyriform, tuberculate and nontuberculate macroconidia (Fig. 83–1) measuring 8 to 16 μm in diameter. Conversion of the mycelial form of *H. capsulatum* to the yeast form is performed by incubating the mycelial culture at 37°C on enriched medium, such as BHI agar with cysteine. Spherical to oval budding yeast cells (2 to 5 μm in diameter) develop in at least 7 to 10 days. Yeast cells also may be isolated directly on blood agar plates or other enriched media incubated at 37°C.

A recent advancement in the identification of *H. capsulatum* from cultures is the development of nucleic acid probes, commercially available in a nonisotopic kit format (AccuProbe, Gen-Probe Inc., San Diego, CA). Isolates of any age, cultured on any medium, may be used successfully with the AccuProbe system. The procedure takes approximately 1 hour and offers the advantages of early testing on very young cultures, rapid processing, easy interpretation of results, and a high level of accuracy.

Tissue Histopathology. Histopathologic examination of paraffin-embedded specimens by hematoxylin and eosin (H&E), GMS, and PAS may reveal large numbers of tiny yeasts within the cytoplasm of macrophages in acute pulmonary or disseminated histoplasmosis (Fig. 83–2). The yeast cells of *H. capsulatum* must be distinguished from cells of the intracellular parasites *Leishmania donovani* and *Toxoplasma gondii*.

Antigen Detection. Detection in serum and urine of a carbohydrate antigen of *H. capsulatum* is a valuable tool in

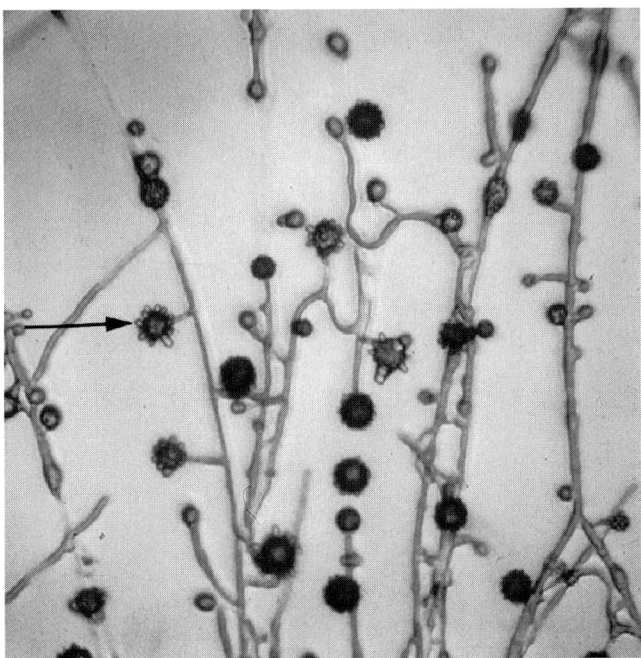

Figure 83–1. *Histoplasma capsulatum.* Slender conidiophore bearing characteristic tuberculate macroconidia *(arrow)* may be mistaken for *Sepedonium* spp. The occurrence of microconidia and the dimorphic nature of *H. capsulatum* differentiates it from *Sepedonium.* (Sabouraud dextrose agar, × 600.)

diagnosis and therapeutic monitoring of disseminated histoplasmosis, particularly in human immunodeficiency virus (HIV)–infected patients. The antigen has also been detected in cerebrospinal fluid in patients with CNS histoplasmosis, as well as in infected tissue. Commercial testing is now available for this antigen by sending specimens to the Histoplasmosis Reference Laboratory, 1001 W. 10th Street, OPN 441, Indianapolis, IN 46202–2897. (Phone: 1-800-HISTODG; Fax: 317-630-7522).

Serology and Skin Testing. Several serologic tests are available for the diagnosis of infection with *H. capsulatum,* with complement fixing antibodies against the yeast phase being the more sensitive, and immunoprecipitating antibodies to the H antigen the more specific, of available assays. Antibodies become positive weeks after infection, and titers generally wane several months after uncomplicated infection, correlate poorly with severity of illness, and are present in low levels in the general population in an endemic area. The utility of skin testing is currently limited to the documentation of prior exposure to *H. capsulatum*; it is not useful in the diagnosis of individual patients.

Differential Diagnosis. Histoplasmosis may resemble tuberculosis, which can simulate both the histopathologic and clinical features of the disease, including pulmonary, gastrointestinal, and CNS manifestations.

Primary pulmonary histoplasmosis can resemble various viral, bacterial, or mycotic infections as well as other granulomatous pulmonary processes such as sarcoidosis. The persistent fever and hepatosplenic involvement in disseminated histoplasmosis can initially resemble many chronic indolent infections, e.g., typhoid fever, or malaria. The cutaneous lesions have been mistaken for molluscum contagiosum, or lesions caused by varicella, *Leishmania, Rochalimea, herpes simplex* or other systemic mycoses such as those due to *Penicillium marneffei,* or *Cryptococcus neoformans.* Lymphadenopathy and mucosal lesions may resemble head and neck malignan-

cies and the gastrointestinal diseases could be mistaken for amebomas, ileal tuberculosis, or actinomycosis. The reticuloendothelial proliferation and bone marrow infiltration may suggest neoplasia, visceral leishmaniasis, brucellosis, or malaria.

Treatment. Treatment of pulmonary histoplasmosis depends on the immune status of the host and extent of disease. While amphotericin B continues to be the drug of choice for severe, refractory or relapsing infections, the azoles, particularly itraconazole, have expanded the treatment alternatives for milder infections and suppressive therapy (Chapter 84). Immunocompetent patients with acute pulmonary histoplasmosis usually have self-limiting disease, which may be managed with supportive care. Patients with acute pulmonary histoplasmosis who are elderly, less than 2 years old, debilitated, or immunocompromised may require systemic antifungal therapy with itraconazole (administered as a loading dose of 400 mg b.i.d. for 3 days followed by 200 mg b.i.d.) or ketoconazole (400 mg PO daily), for 4 to 6 weeks, in addition to oxygen or ventilatory support. Profoundly immunocompromised patients or those with severe pulmonary histoplasmosis with hypoxemia, hypercarbia, or life-threatening extrapulmonary disease are treated with amphotericin B at a dose of 0.7 to 1.0 mg/kg/day. Itraconazole given for 6- to 12-month courses is the preferred agent for chronic cavitary histoplasmosis. The same treatment approach has been successfully implemented in patients with chronic progressive disseminated histoplasmosis.

Patients with acute disseminated histoplasmosis and AIDS should be treated initially with amphotericin B 1 mg/kg/day until stable, followed by itraconazole at 200 mg PO twice a day for prevention of relapse. Patients with AIDS and mild to moderate disseminated histoplasmosis have been treated successfully with itraconazole; ketoconazole in the HIV-infected patient has been associated with frequent failures or relapses. Therapeutic response, particularly in HIV-infected patients who have a high *H. capsulatum* carbohydrate antigen burden, can be monitored by serial urine and serum samples. Histoplasma meningitis may be refractory to treatment, with frequent relapses even with intrathecal amphotericin B. Surgical resection of valves in endocarditis with systemic amphotericin B affords the best chance for cure.

Prevention. There is no effective practicable environmental control, although it is useful to post warning notices in caves known to contain the organism. Spraying contaminated soil with 3% cresol or formalin may eliminate viable organisms.

AFRICAN HISTOPLASMOSIS

Etiology and Epidemiology. As its name suggests, African histoplasmosis is restricted to the African continent and has not been recognized north of the Sahara desert or in countries south of the Zambesi River. It is most prevalent, although still uncommon, in countries of West Africa. The portal of entry is presumed to be respiratory, although cases with pulmonary involvement are rare in African histoplasmosis. It is also not possible to use histoplasmin surveys to estimate the risk of subclinical exposure, because small-form (classic) histoplasmosis can be endemic in the same areas and both organisms are closely related antigenically.

Clinical Manifestations. The most common clinical sites of involvement in African histoplasmosis are skin and bone. Skin lesions present as small papules that often develop an umbilicated center, nodules, abscesses, or ulcers. With larger lesions, underlying bone deposits are common. Solitary skin lesions may also occur. Bone deposits of African histoplasmosis are well circumscribed and lytic. Long bones and the skull are typical sites of invasion. Patients presenting with lesions of African histoplasmosis should be investigated radiologically for occult bone foci. Involvement of other sites, includ-

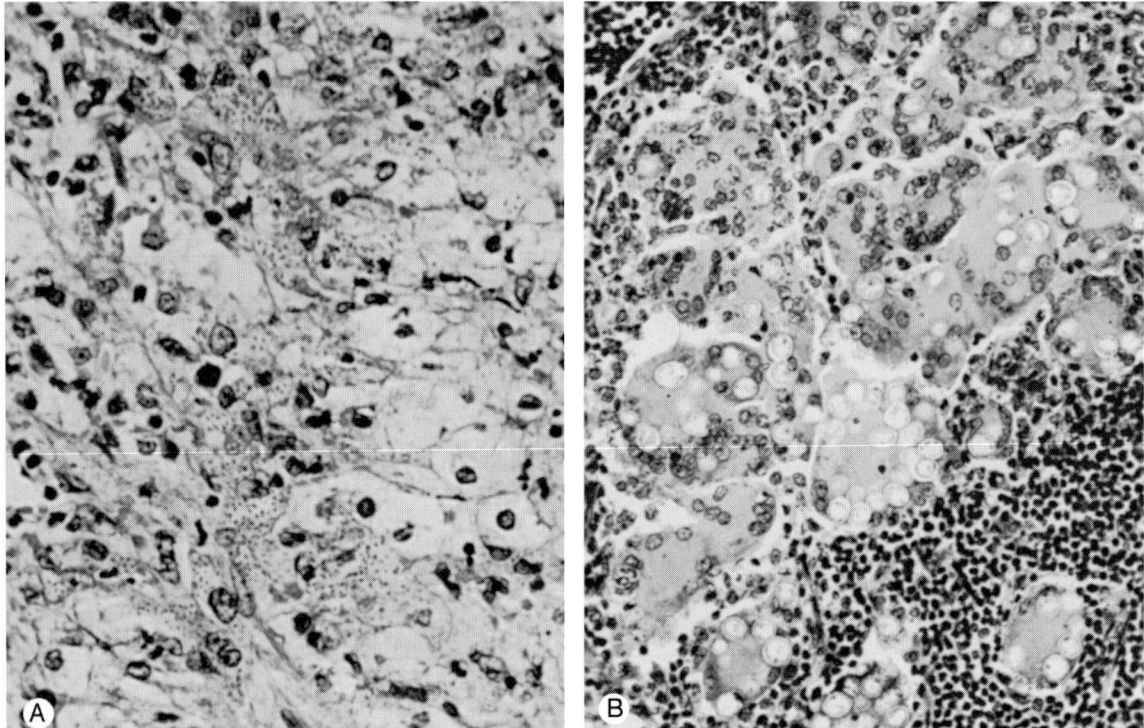

Figure 83–2. *A,* Small intracellular yeasts packed in tissue macrophages from a patient with classic histoplasmosis (*Histoplasma capsulatum.* var. *capsulatum*). (H & E, × 400). *B, H. capsulatum* var. *duboisii* infection, revealing aggregates of giant cells with large ovoid yeast cells. (H&E stain, × 310.) (Courtesy of the Armed Forces Institute of Pathology, Photograph Neg. Nos. 54–17185 and 54–19426, respectively.)

ing the lung, lymph nodes, and gastrointestinal tract, are less common. However, multiorgan invasion occurs rarely and is associated with a poor prognosis.

Diagnosis. The diagnosis is made by biopsy and smears taken from skin or bone lesions. These may also be cultured on Sabouraud agar, although *H. capsulatum* var. *duboisii* cannot be distinguished from var. *capsulatum* by culture. Microscopically, *H. duboisii* appears as numerous large, round or oval, thick-walled yeast cells 8 to 15 μm in diameter, located within giant cells (Fig. 83–2B). These cells are much larger than the *H. capsulatum* cells, which are 2 to 4 μm in diameter. The place of serology in African histoplasmosis has not been clearly established.

Treatment. Solitary cutaneous lesions may be removed surgically and in many cases do not recur. Oral itraconazole (200 to 600 mg daily) is useful in most cases, either on its own or in addition to surgery. However, in widespread infections amphotericin B may be necessary (Chapter 84). Reasonable responses have also been seen with ketoconazole. Relapse after therapy is common.

Bibliography

Ajello L, Manson-Bahr PEC, Moore JC: Amboni caves, Tanganyika, a new epidemic area for *Histoplasma capsulatum.* Am J Trop Med Hyg 9:33, 1960.

Cockshott WP, Lucas AO: *Histoplasma duboisii.* Q J Med 33:223, 1964.

Edwards PQ, Billings EL: Worldwide pattern of skin sensitivity to histoplasmosis. Am J Trop Med Hyg 20:228, 1971.

Goodwin RA, Loyd JE, Des Prez RM: Histoplasmosis in normal hosts. Medicine 60:231, 1981.

Kirsch CM, Ajello L, Kuttin ES, et al: Occurrence of *Histoplasma capsulatum* Darling 1906 in Israel with a review of the current status of histoplasmosis in the Middle East. Am J Trop Med Hygiene 26:140, 1977.

Suzaki A, Kimura M, Kimura S, et al: An outbreak of acute pulmonary histoplasmosis among travelers to a bat inhabited cave in Brazil. J Jpn Assoc Infect Dis 69:444, 1995.

Wang TL, Cheah JS, Holmberg K: Case report and review of disseminated histoplasmosis in South East Asia: Clinical and epidemiological implications. Trop Med Internat Health 1:35, 1996.

Wheat LJ, Connolly-Springfield PA, Baker RL, et al: Disseminated histoplasmosis in the acquired immune deficiency syndrome: Clinical findings, diagnosis, and treatment, and review of the literature. Medicine 69:361, 1990.

Wheat JD, Hafner R, Korzun AH, et al: Itraconazole treatment of disseminated histoplasmosis in patients with the acquired immunodeficiency syndrome. Am J Med 98:336, 1996.

Wheat LJ, Kohler R, Tewari L: Diagnosis of disseminated histoplasmosis by detection of *Histoplasma capsulatum* antigen in serum and urine specimens. N Engl J Med 314:83, 1986.

83.2 Coccidioidomycosis

J. R. Graybill

DEFINITION AND HISTORY. Coccidioidomycosis is a disease discovered in the "tropics" of Latin America but later appreciated much more in the southwestern United States and Mexico. Initially, *Coccidioides immitis* was thought to resemble a protozoan, hence its somewhat misleading name. The first reported patient was an Argentinean soldier who ultimately succumbed with progressive granulomas caused by this organism. Coccidioidomycosis was initially thought to be a rare progressive disfiguring disease, and only with the pioneering work of Smith and colleagues was it appreciated to be a relatively common fungal pathogen within its ecological niche. Smith used skin tests with coccidioidin and serologic tests for complement fixing (IgG) and precipitin (IgM) antibodies to delineate large populations of U.S. subjects at risk for disease.

ETIOLOGY AND DISTRIBUTION. *C. immitis* lives free in nature as a mycelium, residing in warm dry climates with mild winters and spring rains. After the rains the mycelium grows to the surface, where its very fragile structure of intercalating ghost cells and arthroconidia rapidly breaks up in a breeze and can carry miles. Although the organisms can be found throughout the Americas, the most intense zones are the lower Sonoran life zone in the southwestern United States and Mexico, a few dry areas in Venezuela and Colombia, and the pampas of Argentina (Fig. 83–3). In recent years a massive increase in cases of coccidioidomycosis has occurred in California, perhaps a consequence of dry-wet cycles in climate.

TRANSMISSION. Infection is by inhalation of the conidia; the primary group at risk for exposure is agricultural workers. Other occupations in which digging is critical, such as archaeological excavations are high risk as well. Following inhalation, the conidia are ingested by alveolar macrophages, and over the course of several days convert to the round cell parasitic phase. Cells enlarge to form ultimately multicellular structures called spherules (Fig. 83–4). These are 8 to 25 μm in diameter and consist of a thick outer wall containing many endospores. Maturation takes about 3 days, at which time the spherule ruptures and disgorges hundreds of endospores, which repeat the process. Control of the infection is ultimately accomplished by macrophages activated by cell-mediated immunity. This is reflected by the elaboration of multiple proinflammatory cytokines after infection.

PATHOGENESIS AND CLINICAL MANIFESTATIONS. The clinical course of coccidioidomycosis may thus follow a completely asymptomatic path from inhalation of the organism until asymptomatic resolution (up to half of patients); a transient pneumonia characterized by fever, chest pain, and dry cough (up to 45% of patients); or a variety of potentially more serious complications.

Primary Infection. Of these complications, one major group is the hypersensitivity manifestations associated with primary infection. These include a variety of rashes, such as erythema multiforme and erythema nodosum, and also migratory arthralgias. They may be associated with eosinophilia and are the initial and sometimes only clinical manifestations of disease. They are associated with a generally good prognosis. In these patients the skin test is usually strongly positive (a positive is 5+ mm indication at 72 hours). The IgM serologic test may be positive, but the IgG reaction tends to be negative or at a low titer. These allergic reactions may subside over weeks or may blend into the symptoms of invasive pneumonia.

Pulmonary Infection. Pneumonia is manifested clinically by fevers, dry cough, and occasional chest pain. Pneumonia may resolve over the course of a month or more, or may persist as chronic lung disease, or occasionally may take a fulminating course similar to miliary tuberculosis. This more commonly occurs in immunosuppressed patients, e.g., those with AIDS, but this is not necessarily the case. Pulmonary infiltrates that persist more than 3 months are designated chronic pulmonary coccidioidomycosis. This may take the form of asymptomatic nodules, which can persist for years, slowly resolve, or cavitate. Nodules may rapidly cavitate. Cavities may be associated with productive cough and hemoptysis. Cavities may spontaneously rupture into the pleural space or be associated with pleural effusions (Fig. 83–5).

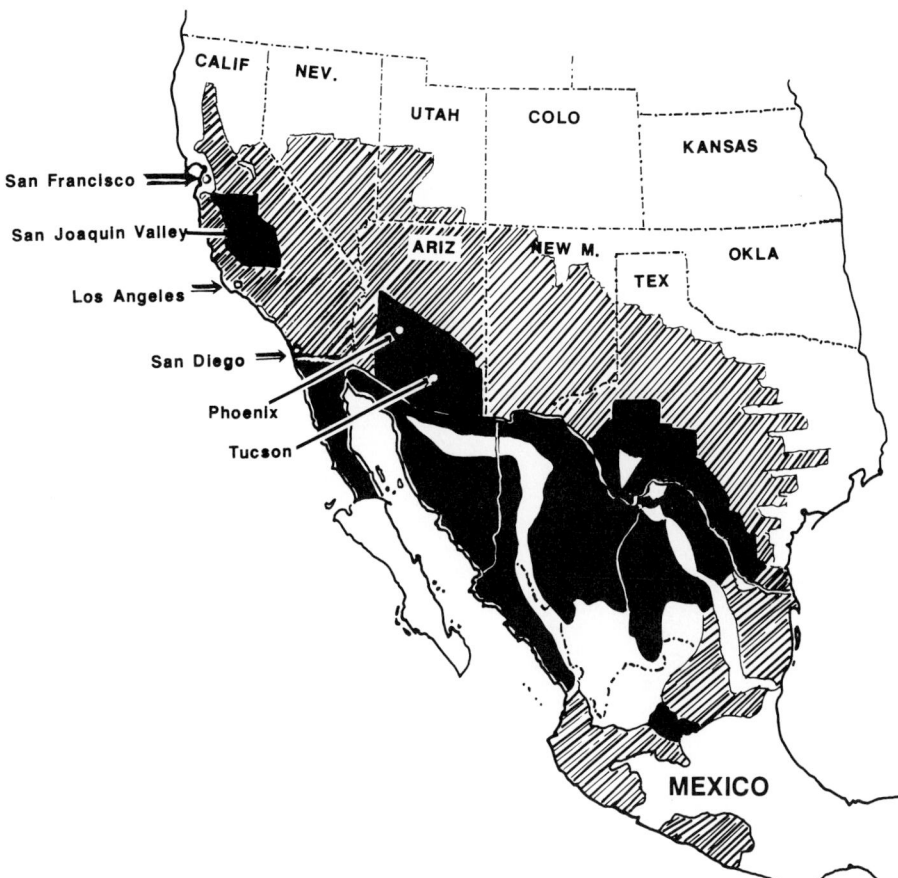

Figure 83–3. Endemic areas of coccidioidomycosis in North America: ■ 30–70% and ▨ 6–30% of the population with positive skin test to coccidioidin.

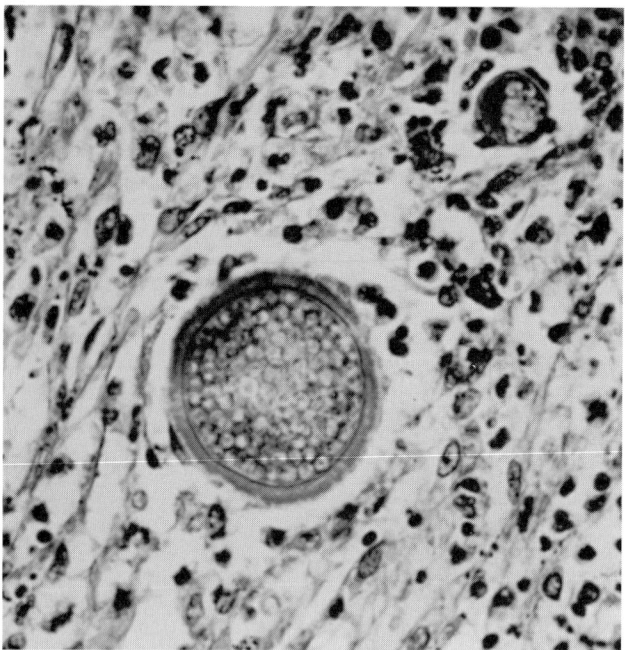

Figure 83–4. Mature *Coccidioides immitis* spherule in the lung. (× 530.) (Courtesy of the Armed Forces Institute of Pathology, Photograph Neg. No. 59–5706.)

Small cavities tend to resolve slowly over the course of months or even up to 2 years, while large ones (> 5 cm in diameter) tend to persist. Cavities may be secondarily infected with *Aspergillus*, coinfected with *Myobacterium tuberculosis*, or be the nidus of secondary bacterial infections. Chronic pulmonary coccidioidomycosis is often a disease of recurring episodes of pulmonary infiltrates, nodules and cavities, cough, fever, and hemoptysis, waxing and waning over years.

Disseminated Coccidioidomycosis. Dissemination of disease may occur in about 20% of nonimmunosuppressed patients. A genetic predisposition includes Filipinos, blacks, Mexican Americans, and Native American Indians. One third or more of patients with disseminated disease develop meningitis, which may occur alone or in association with other foci of extrameningeal disease.

Meningitis. Coccidioidal meningitis is a progressive vasculitic disease that may be reflected as meningismus, headache, personality changes, and a variety of focal lesions including cranial neuropathies or long tract signs. Mortality is >90% if the disease is untreated for a year, and virtually 100% by 2 years. The cerebrospinal fluid is typical of that associated with granulomatous meningitis, namely lymphocytic pleocytosis, hypoglycorrhachia, and elevated protein. Cerebrospinal fluid eosinophilia is one hallmark that should prompt consideration of coccidioidal meningitis.

Skin and Bone Lesions. Extrameningeal involvement can target virtually any organ, but the most common are the skin and osteoarticular sites. Skin disease may range from small granulomas that wax and wane to ulcers and even abscesses draining pus loaded with *C. immitis* spherules (Fig. 83–6). The latter phase is suggestive of poor immune response and uncontrolled disease. Bone and joint disease is more common in the weight-bearing joints, especially the vertebrae, hips, and knees. Paraspinous abscesses are relatively common and may be associated with vertebral disease (Fig. 83–7). The joints are commonly swollen and tender. The spherules are more readily recovered from the synovium than from joint fluid, and diagnoses have been delayed by failure to obtain a synovial biopsy.

Chronic Relapsing Infections. More than any other mycosis, coccidioidomycosis reflects the interplay of the combat between host and fungal pathogen. Disease may relapse and resolve over years. Meningitis is particularly troublesome,

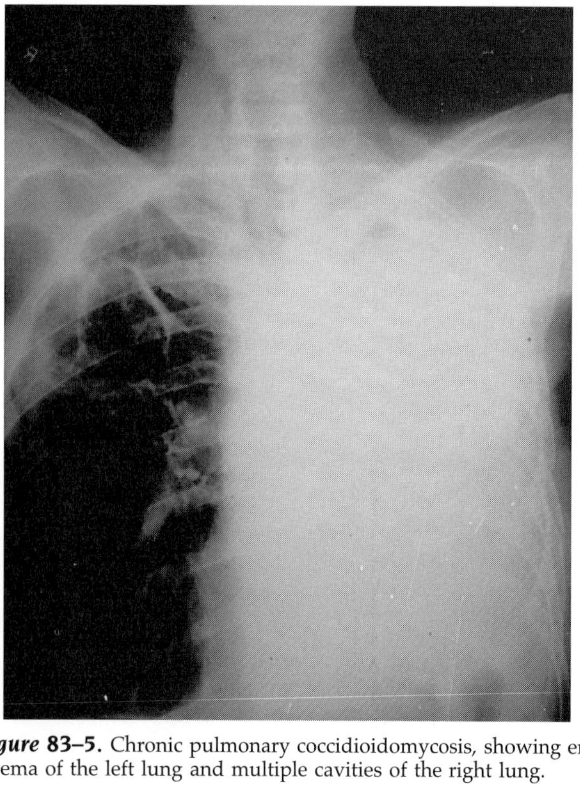

Figure 83–5. Chronic pulmonary coccidioidomycosis, showing empyema of the left lung and multiple cavities of the right lung.

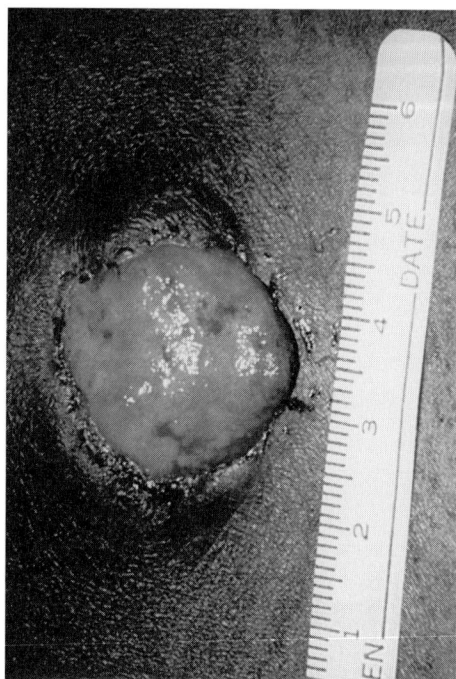

Figure 83–6. Ulcerative skin lesion of disseminated coccidioidomycosis.

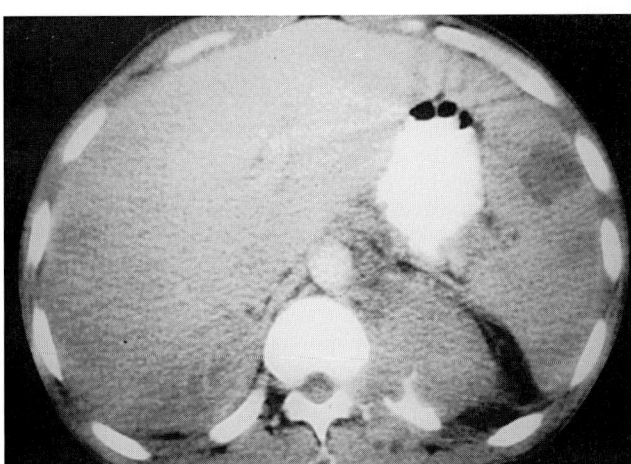

Figure 83–7. CT scan showing right-sided partial vertebral destruction from coccidioidomycosis as well as associated paraspinous abscess.

with a tendency to recur up to a decade after "satisfactory" response to treatment. Skin and lung lesions may enlarge and shrink seemingly unrelated to any antifungal therapy. Dissemination and fatal outcome appear more common in pregnancy. The lifetime course of disease may range from rapid progression to death to years of intermittent relapses.

DIAGNOSIS. Diagnosis of coccidioidomycosis is relatively easy when suspected.

Culture. The organism is not commensal, and any positive culture indicates active disease. *C. immitis* grows readily on most culture media, converting at room temperature to a mold with intercalating ghost cells and arthroconidia. The mold may initially be nondescript, and in this form is not pathognomonic. Conversion in vitro to the spherule form can be attempted in Converse medium incubated at 37° to 40°C.

In routine cultures the mold may take 7 to 10 days to appear. *C. immitis* conidia are extremely infectious, being the most hazardous of the fungal pathogens for laboratory transmission. All fungal cultures should be kept in sealed plates and manipulated only in a microbiologic hood to avoid the problem of accidental transmission. Because it takes some days for spherules to convert to the infectious mycelial form, infected tissues are not hazardous as long as they are fixed or discarded within several days. Of note, transmission from infected bandage material has occurred when the bandages were not promptly autoclaved.

Tissue Samples. The tissue form of the organism is the spherule, which has a pathognomonic appearance. Rarely fat globules or foreign particles can be mistaken for *C. immitis*; however, size, the double-edged thick wall, and the contained endospores should resolve confusion (Fig. 83–3).

Serologic Tests. There are also indirect ways to make the diagnosis. There are a variety of currently used serologic techniques, but the most common are the complement fixation (CF), immunodiffusion–complement fixation (IDCF), precipitin, and immunodiffusion-tube-precipitin (IDTP). The precipitin reaction turns briefly positive in the first weeks of infection, but then reverts to negative. The IDCF commonly does not become positive until a month after infection, but persists much longer, and loosely correlates with severity of disease. As patients worsen titers tend to rise, and as they improve titers tend to fall, but changes are slow and not as reliable indicators of disease activity as once thought. The serology is particularly useful in diagnosis of meningitis, in which cerebrospinal fluid cultures are negative in more than

half of the patients, and in which IDCF antibody titer is diagnostic. Other less specific findings include lymphocytic pleocytosis, hypoglycorrhachia and elevated protein. More recently, detection of circulating coccidioidal antigen has been useful in diagnosis, especially in patients who have no detectable antibodies.

Skin Tests. The coccidioidin (mycelial phase antigen) and spherulin (spherule phase antigen) skin tests may be used to test for prior exposure but do not help diagnose active disease. A positive test in a patient with active disease is thought to suggest a better prognosis than a negative (anergic) test. We have not found the skin test very useful, and rarely perform it.

TREATMENT AND PROGNOSIS. Treatment of coccidioidomycosis is extremely frustrating. Coccidioidomycosis was among the first mycoses treated with amphotericin B, in the late 1950s. Since then reports of amphotericin B therapy have been quite varied, with responses differing depending on the form of disease, the immune competence of the host, and the regimens used. In general, clinical improvement has been associated with falling CF antibody titers and conversion of the skin test to positive, while the reverse has occurred with worsening disease. Despite almost universal susceptibility to multiple antifungal drugs, the overall successes have been limited, with relapses very common. Reports of response rates to amphotericin B are less reliable than those to antifungal azole drugs, in part because uniform criteria were not given for evaluation of response, and adequate follow-up was not done. In general, amphotericin B should be used in patients with very aggressive miliary or disseminated disease, dosing at 0.5 to 1.0 mg/kg/day for the first weeks, then decreasing to 50 mg three times per week in adults, for a total course that is highly variable. In my experience, a cumulative dose for a course of amphotericin B would be as much as 2 to 3 g. For less aggressive disease (Table 83–1), either itraconazole or fluconazole should be used. Of 44 patients treated with itraconazole at 400 mg per day, 57% achieved remission, and only 16% later relapsed. There were fewer relapses with itraconazole than with fluconazole or ketoconazole. However, itraconazole capsules should not be used with antacids or H$_2$ blockers, both of which impair gastric absorption. A new liquid formulation has markedly improved absorption, and the solution is optimally taken in the fasting state. Itraconazole also should not be used together with any agent that increases activity of hepatic drug metabolizing enzymes (e.g., barbiturates, phenytoin, carbamazepine, rifampin, rifabutin). Also, competition for a common route of excretion can cause elevation of coadministered

TABLE 83–1. Response and Relapse Rates for Coccidiodomycosis Using Various Antifungal Regimens*

	AMB	KTZ	ITZ	FLU
Nonmeningeal				
Response	50–70%	29%†	57%	67%
Relapse	20–50%	38%‡	16%	37%
Meningeal				
Response	50%	—	79%	80%
Relapse	50%	All azoles have approximately 75%		

*AMB, amphotericin B; KTZ, ketoconazole; ITZ, itraconazole; FLU, fluconazole.

†Response to initial therapy of 108 subjects randomized to 400 or 800 mg/day. Additional patients responded after their dose was raised, in some to as high as 1600 mg/day.

‡Relapses among totals of 40 patients who achieved remission.

drugs, e.g., astemizole, terfenadine, cyclosporine, digoxin, and others. Fluconazole has fewer of these problems. In a large clinical trial by the Mycoses Study Group (MSG) of fluconazole therapy of 78 patients, responses were 86% of 14 patients with bone and joint disease, 55% of 40 patients with chronic pulmonary disease, and 76% of 21 patients with soft tissue disease. Fluconazole treatment was prolonged, generally between 1 and 2 years of therapy. Although ketoconazole is licensed for treatment of coccidioidomycosis, the response rates are lower and the drug is less well tolerated than either fluconazole or itraconazole.

Duration of treatment is highly variable for the antifungal triazoles. In general, treatment should be continued until the patient has clearly responded, and probably for 6 to 9 months after that time. Clinical evaluation is complex and has been measured by the MSG using criteria such as extent of involvement of lesions, symptoms, cultures, and serologies. Although there have been to date no published comparative trials, the MSG criteria have been used in multiple studies and form a good basis for comparison. Each new drug tested with this system has some selection bias, because about half of the patients in any new drug trial have failed prior therapies and are thus "experienced" with antifungal drugs.

Coccidioidomycosis in AIDS. This has been increasing over recent years and is concentrated in the endemic areas for patients with coccidioidomycosis. Although coccidioidomycosis is not very common in human immunodeficiency virus (HIV) infections, occurring in well under 1% nationwide, in high-risk areas it is a more common pathogen, and in Arizona ultimately developed during a 41-month period in 25% of AIDS patients. The primary risk factor is a CD4 count of <200. Infection can vary from a positive serology unaccompanied by other findings all the way to diffuse pulmonary disease. The most common forms are diffuse lung disease (aggressive course, multilobar infiltrates), focal pulmonary disease, and meningitis. Diffuse lung disease has the lowest CD4 counts, the shortest survival (median 1 month), and the highest mortality (70%), a range of 0 to 17 months. There is no clearly optimal antifungal drug. Focal pulmonary disease responds well to antifungals and is associated with a higher CD4 count and good response to therapy.

Coccidioidal Meningitis. In earlier days this was considered the most severe form of coccidioidomycosis and occurred in one third or more of patients with disseminated disease. The process is a lymphocytic basilar meningitis that does not respond well to intravenous amphotericin B. Brain abscesses and vasculitis with stroke syndrome also occur. Hence for many years the primary regimen was intrathecal amphotericin B, initiated at 0.1 mg/dose and continued on a three times per week basis up to 0.5 mg/dose. Treatment was highly individualized, depending both on clinical response and on drug tolerance. Because amphotericin B is highly irritant, it was almost always given with intrathecal corticosteroids. Even then, progressive arachnoiditis necessitated frequent shifts to lumbar or cisternal administration. Amphotericin B has caused arachnoiditis and occasional anterior vertebral artery thrombosis. As the cerebrospinal fluid glucose slowly increases, the cell count declines, and the protein returns toward normal, the dose interval is lengthened, usually to twice weekly, then once weekly, then once biweekly, and then once monthly. Such regimens often lead to courses of 2 to 4 years before treatment is ultimately terminated. Longer courses may be associated with better response. Even then there may be late relapses.

The advent of antifungal azoles has markedly altered treatment of coccidioidal meningitis. Itraconazole has been used, but the experience is fewer than 20 cases, and the reported response rates are not meaningful. Fluconazole, on the other hand, has been evaluated in a large MSG trial, in which a response rate of 79% was reported. HIV-positive and HIV-negative patients have similar response. Fluconazole in a loading dose of 800 mg/day should be used for the first 3 to 4 days, and then the dose may be reduced to 400 mg/day. Treatment should be continued indefinitely, because more than 75% of patients relapse when treatment is stopped, even after many years. Some suggest that fluconazole doses should be 800 mg/day for a sustained period of months or longer.

PREVENTION. Attempts should be made to reduce inhalation of dust in areas where coccidioidomycosis is endemic. Those working in dusty environments may wear masks, although this has not been shown to be effective. Efforts to vaccinate against *C. immitis* have led to one very large trial with a killed spherule vaccine. Despite some immunologic response, the vaccine was ultimately not successful in preventing disease. Further investigations to develop a protective vaccine are in progress.

Bibliography

Ampel NM, Dols CL, Galgiani JN: Coccidioidomycosis during human immunodeficiency virus infection: Results of a prospective study in a coccidioidal endemic area. Am J Med 94:235, 1993.

Banuelos AE, Williams PL, Johnson RH, et al: Central nervous system abscesses due to *Coccidioides* species. Clin Infect Dis 22:240, 1995.

Catanzaro A, Galgiani JN, Levine BE et al: Fluconazole in the treatment of chronic pulmonary and nonmeningeal disseminated coccidioidomycosis. Am J Med 98:249, 1995.

Como JA, Dismukes WE: Oral azole drugs as systemic antifungal therapy. N Engl J Med 330:263, 1994.

Dewsnup DH, Galgiani JN, Graybill JR, et al: Is it ever safe to stop azole therapy for *Coccidioides immitis* meningitis? Ann Intern Med 124:305, 1996.

Dooley DP, Cox RA, Hestilow KL, et al: Cytokine induction in human coccidioidomycosis. Infect Immun 62:3980, 1994.

Drutz DJ, Catanzaro A: Coccidioidomycosis: State of the art. Part I. Am Rev Respir Dis 117:559, 1978.

Drutz DJ, Hyppert M: Coccidioidomycosis: Factors affecting the host-parasite interaction. J Infect Dis 147:372, 1983.

Einstein HE: Coccidioidomycosis of the central nervous system. Neurology 5:101, 1974.

Fish DG, Ampel NM, Galgiani JN, et al: Coccidioidomycosis during human immunodeficiency virus infection. Medicine 69:394, 1990.

Galgiani JN, Ampel NM: Coccidioidomycosis in human immunodeficiency virus–infected patients. J Infect Dis 162:1165, 1990.

Galgiani JN, Catanzaro A, Cloud GA, et al: Fluconazole therapy for coccidioidal meningitis. Ann Intern Med 119:28, 1993.

Galgiani JN, Grace GM, Lundergan LL: New serologic tests for early detection of coccidioidomycosis. J Infect Dis 163:671, 1991.

Galgiani JN, Stevens DA, Graybill JR: Ketoconazole therapy of progressive coccidioidomycosis: Comparison of 400 and 800 mg doses and observations at higher doses. Am J Med 84:603, 1988.

Graybill JR, Stevens DA, Galgiani JN, et al: Itraconazole treatment of coccidioidomycosis. Am J Med 89:292, 1990.

Jones JL, Gleming PL, Ciesielski CA, et al: Coccidioidomycosis among persons with AIDS in the United States. J Infect Dis 171:961, 1995.

Labadie J, Hamilton RH: Survival improvement in coccidioidal meningitis with high-dose amphotericin B. Arch Intern Med 146:2013, 1986.

Levine HB, Gonzalez-Ochoa A, ten Eyck DR: Dermal sensitivity to *Coccidioides immitis*. Am Rev Respir Dis 107:379, 1973.

Pappagianis D: Evaluation of the protective efficacy of the killed *Coccidioides immitis* spherule vaccine in humans. Am Rev Respir Dis 148:656, 1993.

Pappagianis D: Marked increase in cases of coccidioidomycosis in California: 1991, 1992, and 1993. Clin Infect Dis 19 (Suppl 1):S14, 1994.

Peterson CM, Schupperl K, Kelly PC, Pappagianis D: Coccidioidomycosis and pregnancy. Obstet Gynecol Surv 48:149, 1993.

Ragland AS, Arsura E, Ismail Y, Johnson R: Eosinophilic pleocytosis in coccidioidal meningitis: Frequency and significance. Am J Med 95:254, 1993.

Smith CE, Saito MT, Beard RR, et al: Serologic tests in the diagnosis and prognosis of coccidioidomycosis. Am J Hyg 52:1, 1952.

Smith CE, Saito MT, Simons SA: Pattern of 39,500 serologic tests in coccidioidomycosis. JAMA 160:546, 1956.

Stevens DA: Coccidioidomycosis: A Text. New York, Plenum Press, 1980.

Stevens DA: Current concepts: Coccidioidomycosis. N Engl J Med 332:1077, 1995.

Tucker RM, Denning DW, DuPont B, Stevens DA: Itraconazole therapy for chronic coccidioidal meningitis. Ann Intern Med 112:108, 1990.

Williams PL, Johnson R, Pappagianis D, et al: Vasculitic and encephalitic complications associated with *Coccidioides immitis* infection of the central nervous system in humans: Report of 10 cases and review. Clin Infect Dis 14:673, 1992.

83.3 Blastomycosis

Robert W. Bradsher

DEFINITION. Blastomycosis is the infection caused by the fungus *Blastomyces dermatitidis*. Infection typically presents as either an acute or indolent pneumonia or as a chronic skin lesion. The terminology of "North American blastomycosis" has been abandoned because of increasing reports of this infection from other continents and the acceptance of paracoccidioidomycosis rather than the outdated terminology of "South American blastomycosis" for disease due to *Paracoccidioides brasiliensis*.

ETIOLOGY. *B. dermatitidis* is a dimorphic fungus that grows at room temperature as a mold and at 37° C as a budding, yeastlike cell. The mold grows well, if slowly, on a wide range of culture media, including Sabouraud agar. The white to tan colony is composed of hyphae measuring approximately 2 μm in diameter and smooth, round, or oval microconidia measuring from 2 to 10 μm in diameter. The mold closely resembles *Histoplasma capsulatum*, except for the presence of tuberculate macroconidia and the finely roughened microconidia of *H. capsulatum*. Blastomyces yeastlike cells are multinucleate, round, and 8 to 15 μm in diameter and have broad-based buds between mother and daughter cells. *B. dermatitidis* may exist in one of two mating types. Co-culture of isolates having opposite mating types results in formation of distinctive structures called ascocarps, which contain ascospores. These sexual structures classify the perfect state of this fungus as an ascomycete, called *Ajellomyces dermatitidis*.

EPIDEMIOLOGY. Most reported cases of blastomycosis have been from the United States and central or eastern Canada. Occasional cases have been reported from Africa, Mexico, and Central America. In the United States, endemic areas include states surrounding the Mississippi and Ohio rivers with greatest numbers in Kentucky, Arkansas, Mississippi, North Carolina, Tennessee, Louisiana, Illinois, and Wisconsin. A few common-source outbreaks have been described. Although most investigators have not been successful in recovering the organism from soil, Klein and coworkers provided strong evidence of the location of *B. dermatitidis* in microfoci in soil by isolating the organism in association with an epidemic of infection. There was an association with beaver dams in that epidemic, but the beavers were likely just innocent bystanders; the moist, highly organic soil allowed the organism to grow. Because a majority of patients in that outbreak were not ill, the investigations also supported the concept of subclinical infection as is found frequently in histoplasmosis and coccidioidomycosis. Infection has occurred in animals such as dogs, cats, and cows, but spread to humans has not occurred. The only documented case of person-to-person transmission was that of a man with genitourinary disease causing pelvic blastomycosis in his wife.

Although there is no occupational or medical predisposition to developing blastomycosis, many persons have exposure to soil associated with animals or bodies of water. Whether water or animals are the primary factors for the microfoci in soil or simply represent an area with greater potential for exposure because of occupational or recreational

activities is not yet clear. A review of 1114 cases from the literature revealed that 87% of patients were between 20 and 69 years old. Infection of prepubertal children is rare but well documented. The male-female ratio is approximately 6:1.

Unlike other similar fungal infections, blastomycosis has been reported as a significant pathogen in patients with AIDS in only a relatively small number of cases. When blastomycosis does occur in this setting, it is typically during the last stages of AIDS in association with a very low CD4 lymphocyte count and the disease is rapidly progressive, widely disseminated, and usually fatal. If response to antifungal therapy occurs, lifetime suppression with antifungals should continue.

PATHOGENESIS AND PATHOLOGY. The portal of infection is the lung, although pulmonary infection may cause few symptoms and may heal spontaneously with cure or subsequent signs of infection at distant sites. Presenting signs and symptoms are generally nonspecific but referable to sites of hematogenous seeding in the skin, bone, prostate, epididymis, or other organs. The inflammatory response is a mixture of granulomatous and pyogenic elements. Collections of neutrophils range in size from microscopic to large abscesses (Fig. 83–8). Pseudoepitheliomatous hyperplasia and acanthosis is found in skin and mucous membrane lesions, which has prompted misdiagnosis of squamous cell carcinoma or keratoacanthoma in some patients.

CLINICAL MANIFESTATIONS

Skin Lesions. Approximately one third to one half of patients have skin lesions at the time of diagnosis, making this accessible site the best diagnostic clue. Lesions are often multiple and tend to be located on the face and extremities (Fig. 83–9), and they are typically painless, erythematous, well-circumscribed hyperkeratotic, crusted nodules or plaques that enlarge over weeks; these may ulcerate to leave an undermined edge (Fig. 83–10). Some central healing can occur in chronic cases, forming a hypopigmented, atrophic, fibrotic area. Lesions may occur in the mucous membranes of the nose, lips, larynx, and vagina.

Lung Lesions. Pulmonary findings are present radiologically in half of patients. The infection may either resemble bacterial pneumonia in radiologic appearance in patients who present more acutely (Fig. 83–11), or as a mass lesion in patients with a more indolent course. Chronic pulmonary lesions may show fibrosis and cavitation. Calcification, pleural effusion, or hilar adenopathy is rarely encountered.

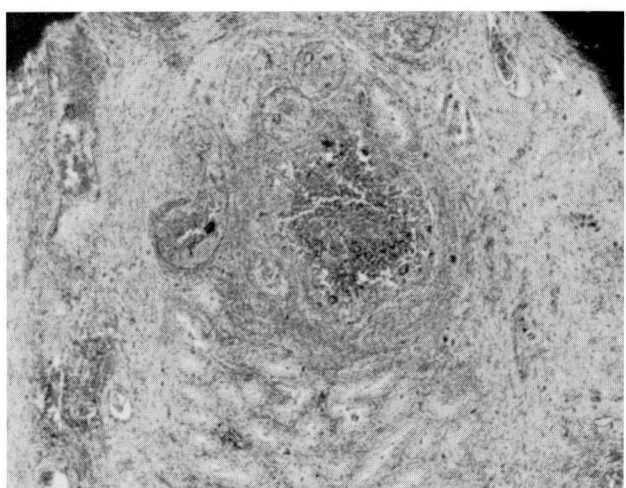

Figure 83–8. Testicular blastomycosis (H & E stain, × 23). Note microscopic abscess surrounded by granulomatous inflammation.

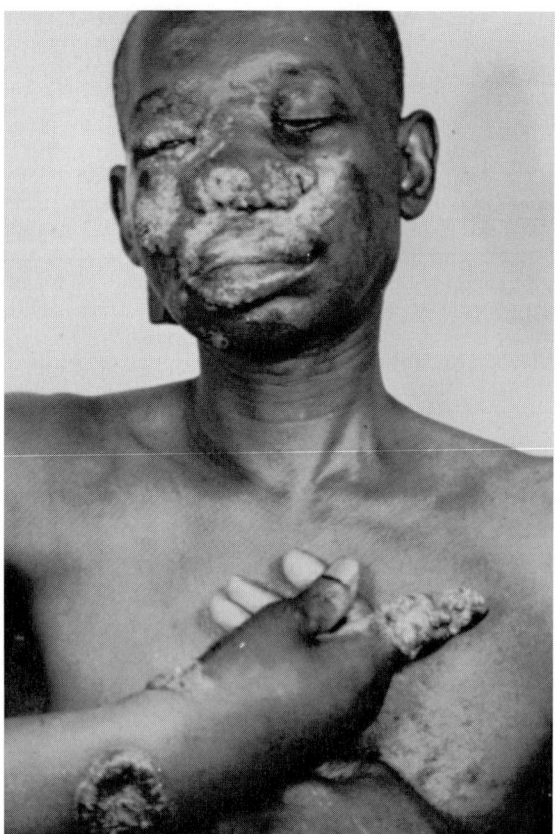

Figure 83–9. Cutaneous blastomycosis in a 50-year-old patient in the USPHS Hospital, New Orleans, LA. No pulmonary lesions were visible radiographically. (Courtesy of the Armed Forces Institute of Pathology, Photograph Neg. No. 75–9748.)

Bone Lesions. Osteomyelitis occurs in one fourth of patients, affecting almost any bone. Osteolytic lesions and an adjacent cold abscess are typical features. Almost every organ has been reported to be infected. In the majority, either concomitant skin or lung infection allows the diagnosis to be made easily.

Systemic Infections. Once infection has progressed beyond the lung, spontaneous remission is rarely observed. After a period ranging from weeks to years, chronic infection may disseminate to multiple organs and cause death. Systemic symptoms of fever and weight loss are mild early in the course but become progressively more severe with extension of the disease.

DIAGNOSIS. Culture for fungus should be performed on sputum, pus, and prostatic secretions or urine. Direct microscopic examination of clinical material following digestion of human tissue with 10% potassium hydroxide added to exudate on the microscope slide is the most rapid and effective means for diagnosis. Cytologic specimens stained by the Papanicolaou method have allowed the diagnosis. Skin lesions can be biopsied for culture and histopathologic section. The best tissue stains are Gomori methenamine silver and periodic acid–Schiff stains. Skin tests are not helpful and are not available. Serologic studies in the past have likewise been unreliable for diagnosis. Better results have been obtained with enzyme immunoassays using better antigens, but the best way to diagnose blastomycosis is to identify the organism in exudate or tissue or by culture.

Differential Diagnosis. Skin lesions may be mistaken for basal or squamous cell carcinoma. Nasal lesions resemble leishmaniasis and paracoccidioidomycosis. Laryngeal lesions mimic epidermoid carcinoma both clinically and pathologically. Pulmonary blastomycosis may suggest bronchogenic carcinoma symptomatically and radiographically.

TREATMENT. The vast majority of patients coming to medical attention will require chemotherapy (Chapter 84). The drug of choice for all patients was amphotericin B in the past, as it continues to be for those with life-threatening blastomycosis or those with central nervous system (CNS) infections. It is given intravenously as 0.5 mg/kg daily or double that dose on alternate days. Eight weeks of therapy is curative in most cases, but cavitary lung lesions and severe multiorgan disease may require 10 to 12 weeks of therapy to prevent relapse. Toxicity often limits the amount of drug that can be given.

Itraconazole has replaced amphotericin B in the majority of patients with blastomycosis because of higher efficacy than ketoconazole and fewer adverse effects than with either amphotericin B or ketoconazole. Cure rates of approximately 95% were achieved in those who took itraconazole for the entire treatment period. At a dose of 200 to 400 mg/day, itraconazole is the drug of choice for compliant patients with less than overwhelming blastomycosis or those with CNS disease. Fluconazole has been found to have a lower success rate in treating blastomycosis and requires much higher doses than itraconazole.

PREVENTION. No means of prevention are known.

Bibliography

Berkowitz I, Diamond TH: Disseminated *Blastomyces dermatitidis* infection in a non-endemic area. S Afr Med J 71:717, 1987.

Bradsher RW: Water and blastomycosis: Don't blame beaver. Am Rev Respir Dis 136:1324, 1987.

Bradsher RW: Histoplasmosis and blastomycosis. Clin Infect Dis 22 (Suppl 2):S102, 1996.

Bradsher RW, Pappas PG: Detection of specific antibodies in human blastomycosis by enzyme immunoassay. South Med J 88:1256, 1995.

Craig MW, Davey WN, Green RA: Conjugal blastomycosis. Am Rev Respir Dis 102:86, 1970.

Dismukes WE, Bradsher RW, Cloud GC, et al: Itraconazole therapy of blastomycosis and histoplasmosis. Am J Med 93:489, 1992.

Furcolow ML, Chick EW, Busey JD, et al: Prevalence and incidence studies of human and canine blastomycosis cases in the United States 1885–1968. Am Rev Respir Dis 102:60, 1970.

Halvorsen RA, Duncan JD, Merten DF, et al: Pulmonary blastomycosis: Radiologic manifestations. Radiology 150:1, 1984.

Klein BS, Vergeront JM, Weeks RJ, et al: Isolation of *B. dermatitidis* in soil associated with a large outbreak of blastomycosis in Wisconsin. N Engl J Med 314:529, 1986.

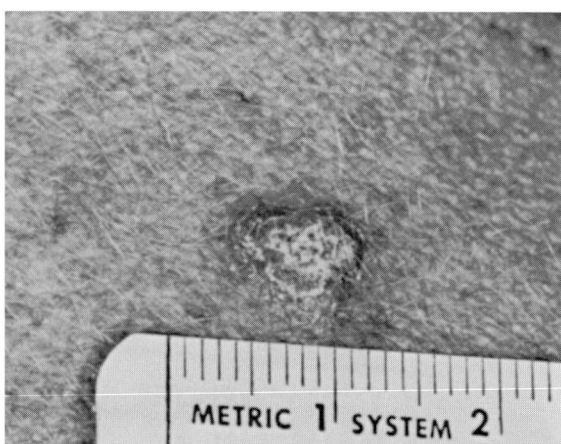

Figure 83–10. Small hyperkeratotic skin lesion of blastomycosis.

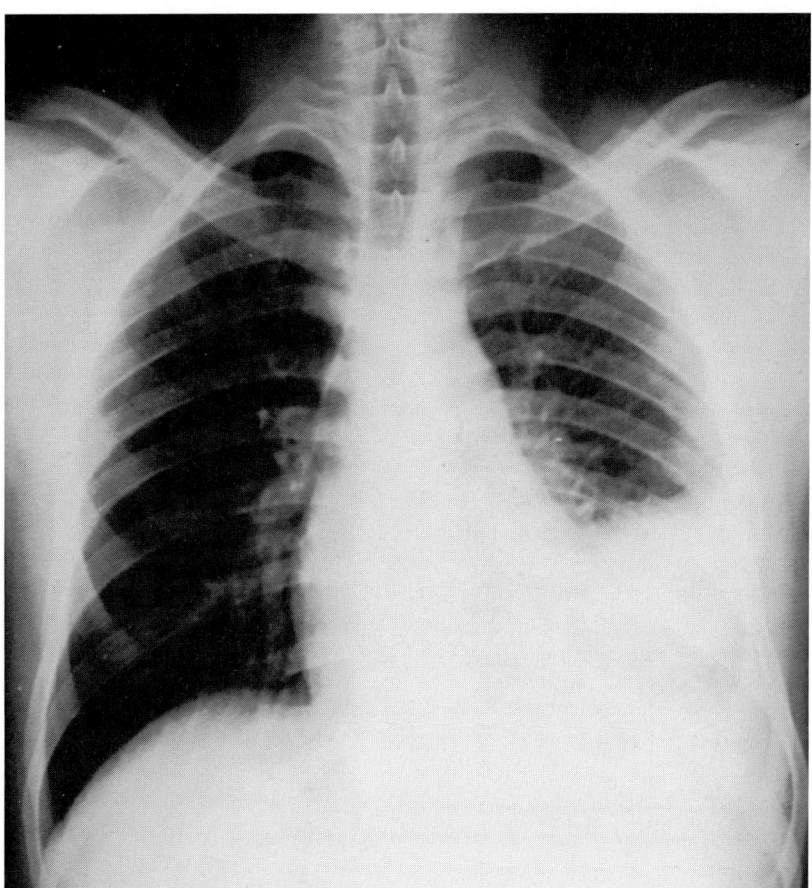

Figure 83–11. Blastomycosis of left lower lobe.

Pappas PG, Pottage JC, Powderly WG, et al: Blastomycosis in patients with the acquired immunodeficiency syndrome. Ann Intern Med 116:847, 1994.
Witorsch P, Utz JP: North American blastomycosis: A study of 40 patients. Medicine 47:169, 1968.

83.4 *Paracoccidioidomycosis*

Ricardo Negroni

DEFINITION. Paracoccidioidomycosis (formerly called South American blastomycosis) is a systemic mycosis limited in geographic distribution to South and Central America that is caused by infection with a dimorphic fungus, *Paracoccidioides brasiliensis.*

ETIOLOGY. *P. brasiliensis* appears in infected tissues as spherical cells of 10 to 40 μm in diameter, with a thick bifringent cell wall and several peripheral buds like a pilot wheel (Fig. 83–12). Mother cells with a single blastoconidium and short chains of three to four budding cells are often found. This yeastlike form grows in vitro in brain-heart infusion agar at 37°C. In Sabouraud dextrose agar at 25°C *P. brasiliensis* grows very slowly and yields cotton-like, whitish colonies that exhibit microscopically branched, septated, and hyaline hyphae with chlamydospores and aleurioconidia.

EPIDEMIOLOGY. Paracoccidioidomycosis is endemic in humid subtropical areas of Latin America, from southern Mexico to 34° South latitude in Argentina and Uruguay. It has a high prevalence in Brazil but it is also frequently reported in Colombia, Venezuela, Argentina, and Paraguay.

The endemic zones have acid soils, rich in organic material, with many streams and rivers and exuberant vegetation. The habitat of *P. brasiliensis* is not well known; it probably lives in soils by rivers or lakes and has been isolated from different sources: soil samples as well as dog food contaminated with soil, bat, and penguin feces. Spontaneous infections of armadillo and squirrel monkey have been reported. Animal-to-human and human-to-human transmission have not been confirmed.

The infection is probably acquired by airborne inhalation of conidia. Direct infection of skin or mucosal surfaces appears very uncommon. Primary pulmonary infection is often asymptomatic and self-limited (i.e., paracoccidioidomycotic infection). The reactivation of latent pulmonary foci or foci in other sites gives way to progressive forms of the infection, which are always severe (i.e., paracoccidioidomycotic disease states). This disease is frequently observed in adult males between 30 to 60 years of age and is more common in rural workers. The juvenile type of paracoccidioidomycosis is less prevalent (only 3% of clinical cases) and attacks both sexes.

PATHOLOGY. Inside the alveolar macrophages, aleurioconidia of *P. brasiliensis* turn into yeastlike budding structures, which cause a nonspecific inflammatory response of polymorphonuclear leukocytes and mononuclear cells. In a few days these inflammatory changes progress to epithelioid cell granuloma with giant cells, plasmocytes, and lymphocytes. Microabscesses are common and caseous necrosis is observed in lymph nodes (Fig. 83–12). Tissue repair is made by collagen fibrosis. Cell-mediated immunity is a very important defense mechanism; antibodies are also produced during progressive disease but their significance in the control of infection is uncertain.

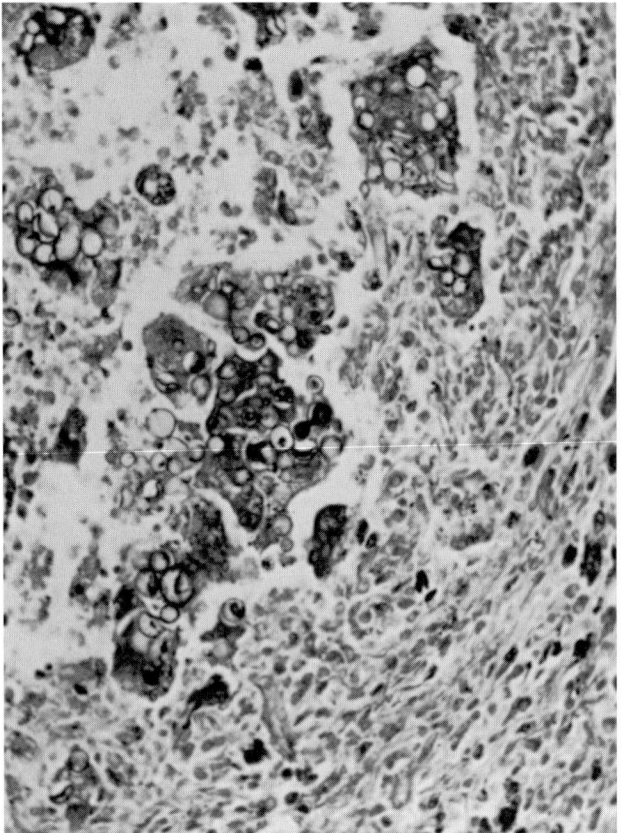

Figure 83–12. Paracoccidioidomycosis of the lung. Clusters of *Paracoccidioides brasiliensis* in giant cells. No peripheral buds are seen. (PAS stain, × 275.) (Courtesy of the Armed Forces Institute of Pathology, Photograph Neg. No. 73–3048.)

CLINICAL MANIFESTATIONS

Nonprogressive Infections. Paracoccidioidomycosis is often asymptomatic or subclinical and self-limited. Symptomatic primary pulmonary infections are rarely diagnosed and clinical and radiologic findings are similar to other acute pulmonary infections of viral or bacterial origin. Calcification in the lungs and lymph nodes is infrequent and 6 to 50% of inhabitants of endemic regions have positive paracoccidioidin skin tests as evidence of a prior subclinical infection.

Disease Types

Subacute Form of Juvenile Type. This clinical form attacks children and adolescents of both sexes and probably results from a rapid dissemination of a primary infection. It has a subacute course, with marked toxemia, septic fever, asthenia, anorexia, loss of weight, subcutaneous abscesses, nodular hypertrophy in multiple locations, hepatosplenomegaly, diarrhea, jaundice, anemia, and leukocytosis with eosinophilia. Radiologic alterations of the lungs and mucous membrane lesions occasionally occur. Acneiform papules of the skin, or scrofuloderma, are produced by suppuration of underlying lymph nodes; osteomyelitis and gastrointestinal involvement are often present. The clinical presentation resembles severe tuberculosis, leukemia, or lymphoma. In moderate cases, the overall general condition is more stable and lesions are usually confined to localized nodules.

Chronic Form of Adult Type. This clinical form usually occurs in adult males. The onset is insidious and the general condition is slowly impaired, with loss of weight, asthenia, and exertional dyspnea being prominent features. Lesions may be unifocal or multifocal.

In 25% of cases, only pulmonary alterations are detected, characterized by low-grade fever, cough, mucopurulent or blood-streaked sputum, and dyspnea. Chest x-ray studies show bilateral and symmetric lesions, generally parahilar in distribution, resembling the wings of a butterfly and formed by infiltrates, micronodules, and linear shadows. Death occurs, after several years, as a result of cachexia or respiratory impairment.

Multifocal presentation is observed in more than 70% of patients; skin, mucous membranes, lungs, lymph nodes, adrenal glands, abdominal organs, and central nervous system (CNS) are often involved. Typical oropharyngeal lesions are ulcers with hemorrhagic granulomatous foci and an infiltrated hard base (mulberry-like stomatitis). A firm red-violet edema is frequently detected in the lips and gingival mucosa (thromboid-like lip). Coalescence of these lesions makes eating and drinking painful. Laryngeal attacks cause dysphonia, dysphagia, and obstructive dyspnea. Skin lesions, more common on the face, include papules, nodules, and ulcers. Ulcers occur over granulomatous changes which become vegetative or papillomatous. Cervical lymph nodes are generally hypertrophic and firm but sometimes they are suppurative or necrotic, opening to the skin by sinus tracts or ulcerations, causing typical scrofuloderma. Adrenal gland involvement occurs in over 15% of patients with the chronic adult form of disease and, in severe cases, causes an Addison-disease syndrome. CNS involvement is observed in 10% of cases; abscessed granulomas located in the posterior fossa and subacute meningoencephalitis have been reported. Other lesions from progressive paracoccidioidomycosis occur in the testicles, epididymis, prostate, bones, liver, and spleen. Death may occur from respiratory failure, malnutrition, or intercurrent infections.

Post-Therapeutic Latency. After effective therapy, clinical cure can be achieved but sometimes lesions remain latent and relapses occasionally occur. The paracoccidioidin skin test is usually positive and serologic tests are negative or are positive at low titers.

DIAGNOSIS.

Microscopy and Culture. Diagnosis is confirmed by finding typical yeastlike elements of *P. brasiliensis* in microscopic examinations of wet preparations of specimens submitted for mycologic studies. Cultures should be done in yeast extract agar, brain-heart infusion agar, and Sabouraud dextrose agar with antibiotics and incubated at 25° and 37°C for 4 weeks. This fungus grows slowly and its isolation is difficult. Clinical specimens can be inoculated intratesticularly in guinea pigs and hamsters; after 2 or 3 weeks, pus from testicular lesions reveals characteristic multiple budding cells of *P. brasiliensis*.

Histology. Histopathologic studies may also assist in the diagnosis of this systemic mycosis. For a better observation of *P. brasiliensis* in histologic section, special stains, e.g., periodic acid–Schiff and Grocott, are required.

Serology. Progressive forms of paracoccidioidomycosis usually have positive serology tests; specific antibodies can be detected by immunodiffusion in agar gel, counterimmunoelectrophoresis, complement fixation, and enzyme-linked immunosorbent assay. Titers are proportionate to severity of the infection; with cure they fall or become negative. A specific glucoprotein antigen of 43 kDa can be used for these tests.

Paracoccidioidin Skin Test. This has little diagnostic value but is a very valuable tool for epidemiologic studies. Most infected persons have positive reactions. However, clinically ill patients with severe progressive disease often have negative skin tests, which revert to positive with clinical improvement.

TREATMENT. Sulfonamides, ketoconazole, itraconazole, and amphotericin B have been successfully used in the treatment of paracoccidioidomycosis. The following treatment schedules are accepted: ketoconazole 200 to 400 mg/day for 12 months or itraconazole 100 mg/day for 6 months. Both drugs are administered only by oral route. Amphotericin B should be used only in severe cases with malabsorption; it is given intravenously at a daily dose of 0.7 to 0.8 mg/kg, up to a maximum total dose of 35 mg/kg (Chapter 84).

Itraconazole is the treatment of choice, being effective in more than 95% of cases, but its absorption requires gastric acidity and its effect is reduced by mesenteric lymph node blockade caused by the infection. It should not be used for patients with tuberculosis under treatment with rifampin.

Co-trimoxazole is still frequently used in Brazil, especially (1) in recently diagnosed patients with no previous therapy; (2) in chronic unifocal progressive disease; and (3) as maintenance after a course of amphotericin B. It is given to adults every 12 hours for 2 to 3 years at a dosage of 80 mg of trimethoprim and 400 mg of sulfamethoxazole.

Paracoccidioidomycosis is always a severe infection that requires prolonged treatment. Relapses are common and cure frequently leaves incapacitating sequelae, e.g., laryngeal and tracheal stenosis, buccal atresia, and pulmonary fibrosis.

CONTROL. No control measures to prevent paracoccidioidomycosis are available and no vaccine has been developed.

Bibliography

Brummer E, Castañeda E, Restrepo A: Paracoccidioidomycosis: An update. Clin Microbiol Rev 6:89, 1993.

Franco MF, Mendes RP, Rezkallah-Iwasso MT, Montenegro MR: Paracoccidioidomycosis. Baillieres Clin Trop Med Commun Dis 4:185, 1989.

Franco M, Lacaz C da S, Restrepo MA, Del Negro G: Paracoccidioidomycosis. Boca Raton, FL, CRC Press, 1994.

Lacaz C da S, Porto E, Costa Martins JE: Paracoccidioidomicose. *In* Lacaz C da S, Porto E, Costa Martins JE (eds): Micología Médica, 8th ed. São Paulo, Brazil, Sarvier, 1991, pp 248–297.

Negroni R: Paracoccidioidomycosis (South American blastomycosis). Int J Dermatol 32:847, 1993.

Negroni R: Azole compounds in the treatment of paracoccidioidomycosis. *In* Van den Bossche H, Odds F, Rinaldi M, Dupont B (eds.): Dimorphic Fungi in Biology and Medicine. New York, Plenum Press, 1993, pp 391–396.

Restrepo MA: Paracoccidioidomycosis. *In* Murphy JW, Friedman H, Bendinelli M (eds): Fungal Infection and Immune Response. New York, Plenum Press, 1993, pp 251–276.

San Blas G: Paracoccidioidomycosis and its etiologic agent *Paracoccidioides brasiliensis.* J Med Vet Mycol 31:99, 1993.

83.5 Cryptococcosis

Françoise Dromer and Bertrand Dupont

DEFINITION. Cryptococcosis is a life-threatening infection caused by the encapsulated yeast *Cryptococcus neoformans.* Rare until the 1980s, it has become a major opportunistic infection in patients with AIDS.

TAXONOMY. Although it was first isolated in 1894, the complete life cycle of *C. neoformans* was not understood until 1975 when Kwon-Chung demonstrated that the fungus reproduces sexually. The teleomorph or sexual stage is *Filobasidiella neoformans* var. *gattii* for serotypes B and C, and var. *neoformans* for serotypes A and D. It is placed in the family Filobasidiaceae of the order Filobasidiales under the phylum Basidiomycota. We usually refer to the fungus by its anamorph (asexual phase), *C. neoformans.*

ECOLOGY. *C. neoformans* var. *neoformans* is found in pigeon and other birds' droppings, in fruits (essentially citrus fruits),

and in soil. The ecological niche of the variety *gattii* has been recently identified in some varieties of eucalyptus trees in Australia and Southern California. Infections due to variety *gattii* are diagnosed only in these areas or as imported cases in temperate climates. Serotyping of the infecting isolates may help to identify the source of infection.

The variety *neoformans* (serotypes A and D) is found worldwide with infections due to serotype D mostly diagnosed in Europe. Variety *gattii* (serotypes B and C) is limited to tropical and subtropical areas. Identification of the variety is based on biochemical differences such as growth on special media. Identification of the serotypes is based on differences in the carbohydrate composition of the capsule, namely the proportion and spatial arrangement of the components of glucuronoxylomannan. Recent reviews of Australian cases have shown that virulence might differ between the varieties, with variety *gattii* being responsible for more chronic infections, for large granulomas requiring surgery, and for poor and slow response to antifungal therapy. Preliminary results suggest also that infections due to serotypes A and D may differ in the susceptibility of the host to each serotype and in the type of infection produced.

EPIDEMIOLOGY. Prior to the AIDS epidemic, cryptococcosis was a rare infection (300 cases recorded worldwide in 1955). AIDS is now a major risk factor for cryptococcosis. It was diagnosed in >80% of the patients in a nationwide study of cryptococcosis in France. Cryptococcosis occurs at a stage of profound immunodeficiency (median of CD4 T-lymphocyte counts <50 /mm³). It is diagnosed in 5 to 25% of AIDS patients depending on the country (<10% in the United States and Europe; >20% in Thailand or Africa). Cryptococcosis is an AIDS-defining illness for a third of the patients. Patients with AIDS are only rarely infected with variety *gattii* (eight cases reported so far) even in areas where non-AIDS patients are still being infected by this type in unchanged proportions.

Cryptococcosis can also occur in human immunodeficiency virus (HIV)–negative individuals. Corticosteroid therapy accounts for >30% of the predisposing factors in this population. Other risk factors are cancer and hematologic malignancies (especially those involving lymphoid tissues), organ transplantation (mostly kidney), various underlying diseases (autoimmune disorders, sarcoidosis, diabetes mellitus, cirrhosis, chronic renal failure, idiopathic CD4 lymphocytopenia, and rarely defects in humoral immunity). Finally, about 25% of patients have no obvious risk factors and, only rarely, exposure to bird droppings.

As with some other systemic mycoses, the incidence of infection among HIV-negative patients is two or three times higher in males than females, a phenomenon attributed to different rates of exposure to environmental sources of the fungus. In AIDS patients, however, the sex ratio is higher in Western countries (5:1 to 100:1) owing to a higher incidence of AIDS among males, and equal in Africa owing to the different epidemiology of HIV infection there. Cryptococcosis is rare in children.

CLINICAL MANIFESTATIONS. The prognosis of cryptococcosis is critically dependent on the involvement of the central nervous system (CNS), but any body site can be infected with *C. neoformans.*

CNS Involvement. Meningoencephalitis is diagnosed in more than 75% of cases, more frequently in HIV-positive patients than in HIV-negative patients. The term meningoencephalitis rather than meningitis is used because of frequent involvement of the brain tissue. Symptoms are rarely acute. More often, patients complain of dizziness, headache, nausea, and loss of memory. Changes in personality and behavior can be noted. Fever is rarely high and is usually intermittent.

As infection progresses, impaired vision or hearing, coma, seizures, and paralysis can occur. Signs of meningeal irritation (nuchal rigidity, Kernig or Brudzinski sign) are often lacking. Brain edema and hydrocephalus are more common, as evidenced by papilledema, ataxia, and cranial nerve palsies. Localizing signs, e.g., hemiplegia are uncommon. Signs of neurologic dysfunction can be present in up to 50% of patients with cryptococcal meningitis and are associated with a poor prognosis in most studies. The interval between the onset of symptoms and consultation may vary from a few days to several months. A short duration of onset (<2 weeks) is usually predictive of a poor response to therapy and, subsequently, death.

The frequency of brain involvement (probably 10% of cases) is unknown since imaging is not always performed. Computed tomography or magnetic resonance scans may detect brain edema, hydrocephalus, and mass lesions known as cryptococcomas (apparently more frequently during infections due to variety *gattii*). Biochemistry and cytology of the cerebrospinal fluid (CSF) are not specific for cryptococcal infection. Pleiocytosis, elevated protein and low glucose levels, associated with elevated pressure, are the most common features, but the CSF findings may be normal in AIDS patients. A limited inflammatory reaction (less than 30 cells/mm^3) has been associated with a poor prognosis.

Cryptococcal Pneumonia. The lung is believed to be the primary site of infection. The risk of spread to other organs justifies the treatment of all immunocompromised patients with cryptococcal pneumonia. Its presence, however, with meningitis is diagnosed in only 15 to 30% of patients. Cryptococcal pneumonia is not distinctive clinically. Symptoms consist of low-grade fever, dull chest pain, and dry cough. Focal infiltrates are the most common signs of infection; cavitation and pleural effusion are rare (Fig. 83–13). Asymptomatic pneumonia or mediastinal lymph nodes can also be detected in previously healthy individuals during a systematic chest x-ray study. Simple colonization of the bronchial tree has been described in patients with pre-existing lung disease. However, this diagnosis should be made with caution in patients with factors predisposing to infection and dissemination.

Cutaneous Infection. Metastatic skin lesions can occur during disseminated cryptococcosis in approximately 5 to 10% of patients irrespective of their HIV status. Lesions can be single or, more often, multiple. The typical lesion is an ulcerated papule producing an exudate rich in cryptococci, an important diagnostic feature if other investigations have been negative for *C. neoformans*. However, almost any kind of skin lesion can occur. Primary infection of the skin is believed to be rare and historically may follow accidental injuries by contaminated needles in the mycology laboratory. Isolated skin infections were present in 30% of HIV-negative patients, and associated with a serotype D isolate in more than 50% of the cases in the French survey.

Involvement of Other Sites. Almost any body site can be infected with *C. neoformans*. In AIDS patients blood cultures are often positive (15 to 30%). Asymptomatic involvement of the urinary tract is frequent (15 to 30%) especially in AIDS patients. The prostate gland is a reservoir of the fungus and this may explain the frequency of recurrent infections after apparently successful therapy. Bones can be infected (vertebra, skull, pelvis, ribs), with osteolytic lesions seen on x-ray studies and the subsequent development of cold abscesses with cryptococcus-rich exudates. Joints may also be involved with symptoms of arthritis. Lymph node involvement is common. Occasional cases of keratitis (after corneal transplantation), retinitis, myocarditis, endocarditis, peritonitis, hepatitis, pyelonephritis, and myositis have also been reported. As noted above, all apparently isolated extrameningeal lesions should be treated as potential manifestations of disseminated disease in immunocompromised patients.

DIAGNOSIS

Differential Diagnosis. None of the clinical features observed during cryptococcal infection is distinctive. Toxoplasmosis, infections due to *Mycobacterium tuberculosis*, *Listeria*, *Histoplasma capsulatum*, *Actinomyces*, *Brucella*, or other pathogens, as well as brain tumors can mimic cryptococcal meningoencephalitis. Pneumonia can be caused by other infections

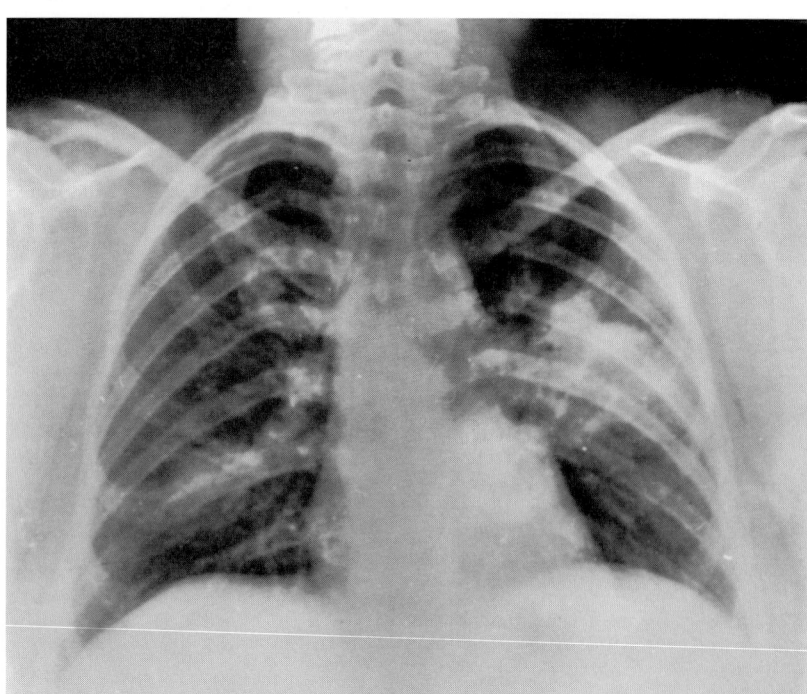

Figure 83–13. Pulmonary cryptococcosis with multiple bilateral pulmonary infiltrates. (Courtesy of Dr. John Bennett.)

such as tuberculosis, aspergillosis, and pneumocystosis. Skin lesions due to *C. neoformans* are not specific either but can be distinguished from other causes by direct examination and culture of skin scrapings or exudates. Low-grade fever, which is a common presentation of cryptococcosis in patients with AIDS, can be a sign of many diseases ranging from lymphoma to other opportunistic bacterial, fungal, viral, or parasitic infections.

Laboratory Diagnosis. The diagnosis of cryptococcosis can be confirmed by direct examination of clinical samples, antigen testing, or culture. Since the prognosis is dependent on the presence of meningitis and dissemination, investigations should include at the least cultures from CSF, urine, and blood as well as sputum or bronchoalveolar lavage samples if there is an abnormal x-ray finding.

India Ink Preparation. Clinicians should keep in mind that the larger the volume of fluid the greater the chance of making a rapid diagnosis. At direct examination, after mounting a drop of sedimented CSF in a drop of India ink, encapsulated yeasts (2 to 10 μm in diameter) can be seen in more than 70% of patients with AIDS and cryptococcal meningitis. Urine, pleural fluid, or bronchoalveolar lavage can be processed the same way.

Culture. Clinical specimens should be plated on Sabouraud agar without cycloheximide and with antibiotics for specimens potentially contaminated with bacteria, and incubated at 30° to 35°C. Although *C. neoformans* is able to grow at 37°C, a lower temperature will improve the growth rate. Use of media such as the Niger seed (*Guizotia abyssinica*) agar medium supplemented with antibiotics can be used to isolate *C. neoformans* from specimens heavily contaminated with other yeasts such as the sputum from AIDS patients with oropharyngeal candidiasis. The majority of isolates of *C. neoformans* produces phenoloxidase thus forming brown melanin–containing colonies on this medium. For blood cultures, the lysis centrifugation method has been the most sensitive.

C. neoformans grows as creamy mucoid colonies. Although most of the plates will show typical colonies in a few days, those with negative cultures should be retained for 3 to 4 weeks, especially those from patients receiving antifungal therapy. Identification of the yeast as *C. neoformans* is made by using commercial test kits.

Antigen Detection. Cryptococcal antigen is detected in serum in more than 90% of patients with cryptococcal meningitis. The diagnosis of cryptococcosis can be based on an isolated positive antigen result in serum or CSF samples from patients at risk for the infection. The reported performances of the commercially available tests are usually excellent with a sensitivity and a specificity above 95%. Causes of false negative results are lack of pronase treatment of the sample (not mentioned in certain kits), limited infections, and the rare (<10%) prozone phenomenon, usually not uncovered by pronase pretreatment. Before the introduction of pronase, the most common cause of false positive results was the presence of rheumatoid factor. False positivity has also been described during disseminated infection due to *Trichosporon beigelii*, meningitis due to the gram-negative bacillus DF-H2, and after technical errors leading to contamination of the sample with bacteria or condensation from agar gels.

Antigen titers vary depending on the infected host's immune status (serum and CSF samples from AIDS patients usually have extremely high titers), the sites of infection (serum samples from patients with extrameningeal infections usually have low, or even negative, titers), and the kit used. There has been no study on the variability of the titer with infecting serotype.

Histopathology. Tissue sections stained with mucicarmine highlight the capsule, whereas other fungal stains will only outline the cell. In this case, cryptococcal cells are often small and surrounded by an empty space for the site of the capsule. Capsules in tissues often appear larger than in body fluids or in culture (Fig. 83–14).

TREATMENT

Cryptococcal Meningitis. All patients with cryptococcal meningitis should receive antifungal therapy, as should all patients with extrameningeal cryptococcosis and an underlying risk factor. The therapeutic approach depends on the host and the type of infection. Reported death rates from cryptococcal meningitis despite treatment still range from 8% to 20% and fatalities can occur even in patients without underlying disease. Death usually occurs early, in the first 2 weeks, and is believed to be due to massive brain edema.

Until the late 1980s, only two drugs were available: amphotericin B, which is still the drug of choice, although its use is often accompanied by renal toxicity and numerous side effects such as fever and chills; and flucytosine, which has a dose-dependent bone marrow toxicity (blood levels should be kept below 100 μm/mL) and the ability to induce resistance among *C. neoformans* isolates when used as sole therapy. Triazoles, e.g., fluconazole and itraconazole, have been introduced more recently for the treatment of cryptococcosis. They are available in oral form and have fewer side effects.

Multicenter studies carried out in the United States on patients with AIDS and cryptococcal meningitis have helped define the best protocols. Primary therapy with amphotericin B (≥ 0.7 mg/kg/day) and flucytosine (100 mg/kg/day) for 2 weeks followed by fluconazole (≥400 mg/day) for an addi-

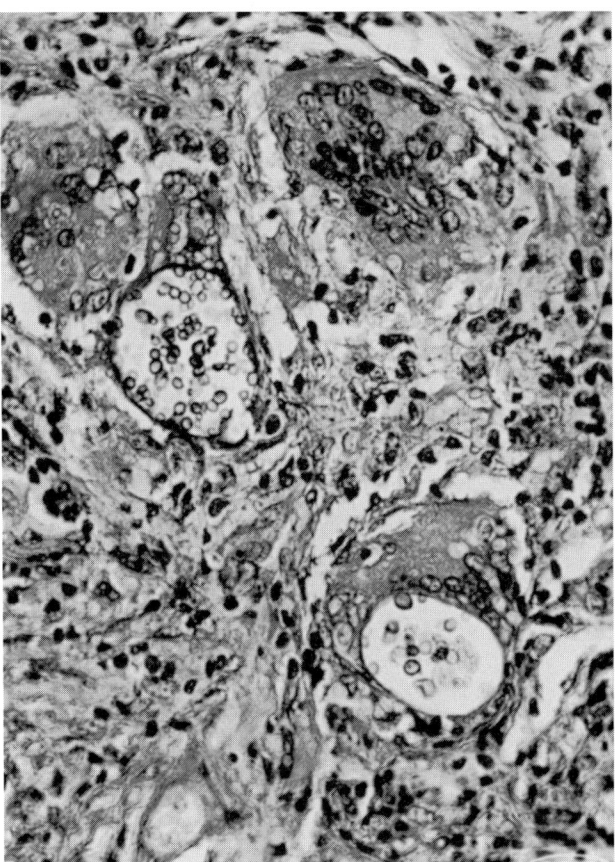

Figure 83–14. Small forms of *Cryptococcus neoformans* in giant cells in a primary pulmonary nodule. These organisms were mucicarmine stain-positive. (× 350.) (Courtesy of the Armed Forces Institute of Pathology, Photograph Neg. No. 61–6700.)

tional 8 to 10 weeks was the best approach in patients with concomitant AIDS. With this regimen the time to sterilization of CSF is shortened and the occurrence of early death and the risk of subsequent relapse is reduced. Lifelong maintenance therapy is mandatory in patients with AIDS to prevent relapses that occur in >50% of the cases. This long-term treatment is best achieved with fluconazole (≥200 mg/day) rather than amphotericin B (1 mg/kg/day once a week). Fluconazole appears to be more effective than itraconazole in preventing relapses. In HIV-negative patients with meningitis, a similar primary regimen is probably appropriate until prospective studies have proved otherwise. It is not certain yet whether HIV-negative patients with sustained immune deficiency such as organ transplant recipients or patients under prolonged corticosteroid therapy benefit from maintenance therapy.

Extrameningeal Infections. In patients with an isolated extrameningeal infection, triazole therapy should be prescribed. Surgery has probably limited value in the treatment of cryptococcosis, although physicians from Australia recently reported a number of surgical excisions for pulmonary mass lesions due to the variety *gattii*. Early ventriculoperitoneal shunting is required in the presence of symptomatic hydrocephalus.

Treatment Outcome. The effectiveness of treatment is determined by sterilization of infected sites. However, sterilization is often delayed especially when azole antifungal agents are used as primary therapy. Encapsulated yeasts can be seen long after sterilization of the CSF and are not necessarily indicative of treatment failure if the patient's clinical state is improving and if cultures remain negative. According to a recent study, alterations in antigen titers in serum are not predictive of treatment responses. However, a rise in antigen titer in CSF was predictive of treatment failure or of relapse after completion of therapy. Another concern is the possibility of antifungal resistance. Amphotericin B resistance has only been reported on occasion. A recent study showed that independent predictors of successful primary treatment with fluconazole were a negative blood culture, combination therapy with flucytosine, and susceptibility of the isolate to fluconazole. It is possible, therefore, that in the future susceptibility testing may be important in following treatment, although, at present, it is not an established practice.

Bibliography

Dismukes WE: Management of cryptococcosis. Clin Infect Dis 17(Suppl 2):507, 1993.

Dromer F, Mathoulin S, Dupont B, et al: Comparison of amphotericin B and fluconazole efficacy in the treatment of cryptococcosis in HIV-negative patients: Retrospective analysis of 83 cases. Clin Infect Dis 22(Suppl 2):154, 1996.

Kwon-Chung KJ, Bennett JE: Cryptococcosis. *In* Kwon-Chung KJ, Bennett JE (eds): Medical Mycology. Philadelphia, Lea & Febiger, 1992, pp 397–446.

Mitchell TG, Perfect JR: Cryptococcosis in the era of AIDS—100 years after the discovery of *Cryptococcus neoformans*. Clin Microbiol Rev 8:515, 1995.

Powderly WG, Cloud GA, Dismukes WE, Saag MS: Measurement of cryptococcal antigen in serum and cerebrospinal fluid: Value in the management of AIDS-associated cryptococcal meningitis. Clin Infect Dis 18:789, 1994.

Speed B, Dunt D: Clinical and host differences between infections with the two varieties of *Cryptococcus neoformans*. Clin Infect Dis 21:28, 1995.

Witt MD, Lewis RJ, Larsen RA, et al: Identification of patients with acute AIDS-associated cryptococcal meningitis who can be effectively treated with fluconazole: The role of antifungal susceptibility testing. Clin Infect Dis 22:322, 1996.

83.6 *Penicilliosis* marneffei

Thira Sirisanthana

DEFINITION. Systemic infection caused by the fungus, *Penicillium marneffei*, is endemic in Southeast Asia, the Guangxi region of China, and Hong Kong. Cases of this disease were rare, but the incidence has increased markedly during the past 5 years. This increase is exclusively due to secondary infection among patients with human immunodeficiency virus (HIV) infection.

HISTORY. *P. marneffei* was first isolated from the liver of a bamboo rat *(Rhizomys sinensis)* in Vietnam in 1956. Segretain reported the first infection in humans in 1959. He accidentally inoculated himself during an experimental study and developed a nodule at the site of inoculation, lymphangitis, and lymph node enlargement. The infection seemed to respond to a high dose of oral nystatin. More than a decade later, the first natural human infection with *P. marneffei* was reported. The patient was a minister who had been in Southeast Asia. He had undergone a splenectomy for the management of Hodgkin disease. The fungus was unexpectedly isolated from his spleen. The second reported case was in 1984. The patient was an American who had traveled in the Far East. He had recurrent episodes of hemoptysis thought to be caused by bronchiectasis. A pneumonectomy revealed a granuloma; tissue section showed yeast cells of *P. marneffei,* and the culture grew *P. marneffei.* Also in 1984, five patients were reported from Bangkok, Thailand. More cases were subsequently reported from the Guangxi region of China and from Hong Kong.

In 1988, the first case of *P. marneffei* infection in an HIV-infected patient was reported. Subsequently, additional cases were reported mainly from Thailand and Hong Kong. The highest incidence was found in northern Thailand. From 1991 to 1996, 920 HIV-infected patients at Chiang Mai University Hospital were found to have penicilliosis marneffei. This figure included 21 cases of children with perinatally acquired HIV infection. Additionally, *P. marneffei* has been recognized in individuals infected with HIV from the United Kingdom, France, Germany, the Netherlands, Switzerland, Italy, the United States, and Australia when they visited an endemic area.

ETIOLOGY. *P. marneffei* is the only dimorphic fungus of the genus *Penicillium.* It grows as a mold on Sabouraud dextrose agar at 25°C. In its mycelial form, the colony is grayish white and downy. During differentiation the color of the colony changes to grayish pink. The reverse side became cerise to brownish red, as a soluble red pigment diffuses into the agar medium. Microscopic examination reveals hyaline, septate branching hyphae with lateral and terminal conidiophores. The conidiophores consist of basal stripes with terminal verticils of three to five metulae, each metula bearing 3 to 7 phialides. The conidia are oval, smooth-walled, measuring approximately 3×2 μm. They are formed basipetally in chains from each phialide (Fig. 83–15). On brain-heart infusion agar at 37°C, rough, glabrous, tan-colored colonies of yeast are seen within a few days. Microscopic examination of this growth reveals unicellular, pleomorphic, ellipsoidal-to-rectangular yeast cells (about 2×6 μm) that divide by fission and not by budding.

EPIDEMIOLOGY AND NATURAL HISTORY. Many features of the epidemiology and natural history of *P. marneffei* infection remain unknown. The organism was first isolated from a species of bamboo rats *(Rhizomys sinensis)* in Vietnam. In the Guangxi region of China, *P. marneffei* has been isolated

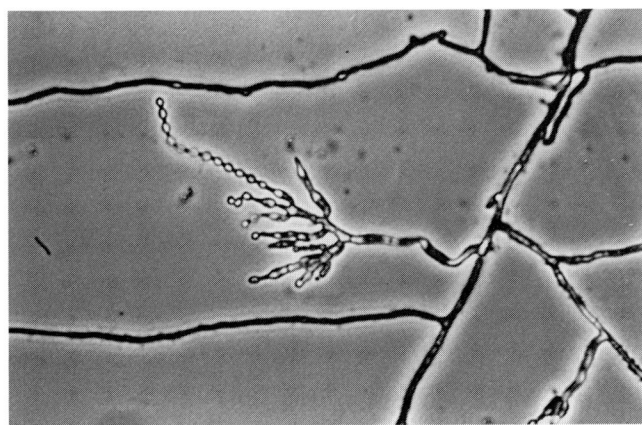

Figure 83–15. Photomicrograph of *Penicillium marneffei* from slide culture, mounted in cotton blue (× 600.)

from the internal organs of more than 90% of another species of bamboo rats (*Rhizomys pruinosus*). It was also isolated from the feces of a few bamboo rats and from soil samples from bamboo rats' burrows. In a recent study from northern Thailand, the fungus was isolated from another two species of bamboo rats, *Rhizomys sumatrensis* and *Cannomys badius*. More than 600 cases of penicilliosis marneffei have been reported. These patients, most of whom were infected with HIV, were natives of Thailand, Malaysia, Hong Kong, and Guangxi or visitors to these areas. Since the bamboo rats usually live near the forest and have limited contact with people living in villages and towns, it is believed that both humans and bamboo rats are infected with *P. marneffei* from a common reservoir, rather than the patients being infected from the rats. The type of exposures leading to infection in humans and the route of entry of *P. marneffei* are unknown. By analogy with other endemic systemic mycoses, such as histoplasmosis and coccidioidomycosis, it seems quite likely that *P. marneffei* conidia may be inhaled from a contaminated reservoir in the environment and subsequently disseminated from the lungs when the infected host experiences immunosuppression. In a study of 550 cases with *P. marneffei* in HIV-infected patients in northern Thailand, it was found that the disease was significantly more likely to occur in the rainy season, suggesting that there might be an expansion of the environmental reservoirs with favorable conditions for growth during these rainy months.

Each clinical case of *P. marneffei* infection might represent the outcome of three possible processes: primary infection, reinfection, or reactivation of latent disease. The natural history after primary infection is varied. Patients have been reported with long periods of asymptomatic *P. marneffei* infection (i.e., several years) prior to presentation with disseminated disease. In other cases, disseminated infections occurred within a few weeks of exposure to the organism. The appearance of *P. marneffei* infections in HIV-infected infants also suggests that the duration between infection and clinical dissemination of the organism sometimes may be brief. Primary infection is an important problem for children who acquire HIV infection perinatally. In adults with disseminated *P. marneffei* infections who live in an area where the organism is endemic, the infection could result from reinfection or reactivation of a latent infection.

PATHOLOGY. The primary site of infection is the reticuloendothelial system. Commonly involved organs include the liver, spleen, lymph node, bone marrow, skin, and lungs. *P. marneffei* invades the histiocytes and survives and multiplies

intracellularly. The cell-mediated response to the fungus leads to formation of histiocytic granulomata. Lymphocytes, plasma cells, epithelioid cells, and multinuclear giant cells participate in the reaction. As the granuloma expands, its center becomes necrotic, the yeast cells are released, and neutrophils accumulate, forming a central abscess. In patients with compromised immune function, the tissue necrosis may occur with little or no granuloma formation. The focal necrosis is surrounded by histiocytes engorged with proliferating yeast cells. Extracellular fungi are abundant. This pathologic picture correlates with a progressive and disseminated infection in the patients.

The yeast cells within the histiocytes are round or ovoid, measuring about 3 μm in diameter. They divide by binary fission. Extracellular organisms may appear more elongate, up to 8 to 13 μm in length, giving them a sausage-like appearance. These sausage-shaped fungi and the crosswalls formed during binary fission are characteristic of *P. marneffei* in pathologic sections. The cells of *P. marneffei* are not stained by hematoxylin and eosin. With Gomori methenamine silver and periodic acid–Schiff, the yeast cells stain well, the crosswall picking up the stain more avidly than the outside wall.

CLINICAL MANIFESTATIONS. Patients with *P. marneffei* infection commonly present with symptoms and signs of infection of the reticuloendothelial system. These include fever with or without chills, lymphadenopathy, hepatomegaly, and splenomegaly. Symptoms and signs of infection of the respiratory system, e.g., cough, dyspnea, thoracic pain, and pulmonary infiltrates are also present in the majority of the cases, reflecting the probable route of acquisition of the fungus. Other presentations, such as cutaneous and subcutaneous lesions, and osteoarticular lesions, are secondary to dissemination of the fungus via the blood stream. Cutaneous and subcutaneous lesions are observed in up to two thirds of patients. Arthritis and osteomyelitis are not uncommon. Pericarditis, peritonitis, and oropharyngeal ulceration have been reported. Constitutional symptoms, such as weight loss, anorexia, and asthenia, may occur even during mild disease. More severe infection may lead to profound cachexia.

Although the clinical signs of penicilliosis marneffei in both HIV-infected and non-HIV-infected patients are similar, the former usually have a more acute onset, higher fever, and more severe respiratory signs. They are more likely to have fungemia and their skin lesions are more numerous and tend to be papules, maculopapular rash, necrotic papules, or acne-like pustules. They are mostly distributed on the head, face, upper body, and upper extremities (Fig. 83–16). Non-HIV-infected patients are more likely to have one or several subcutaneous nodules, which may turn into abscesses and cause skin ulceration. Penicilliosis marneffei occurs late in the course of HIV infection. CD4+ cell counts, determined within 1 month of the diagnosis of *P. marneffei* infection, were consistently less than 50 cells/μL. Cases have been reported in which penicilliosis occurred with other HIV-related infections, such as tuberculosis, cryptococcosis, esophageal candidiasis, *Salmonella* septicemia, toxoplasmosis, and *Pneumocystis carinii* pneumonia. This has led the Ministry of Public Health of Thailand to include penicilliosis marneffei as an AIDS-defining illness.

Biochemical and hematologic laboratory findings are nonspecific and include elevation of liver enzymes and bilirubin, anemia, and leukocytosis or leukopenia. Chest radiographs may show diffuse reticulonodular, localized alveolar, or diffuse alveolar infiltrates.

DIAGNOSIS. In non-HIV-infected persons, *P. marneffei* disease is rare, even in an endemic area. Making the diagnosis depends very much on the physician's and laboratory technician's awareness of the disease. On the other hand, *P.*

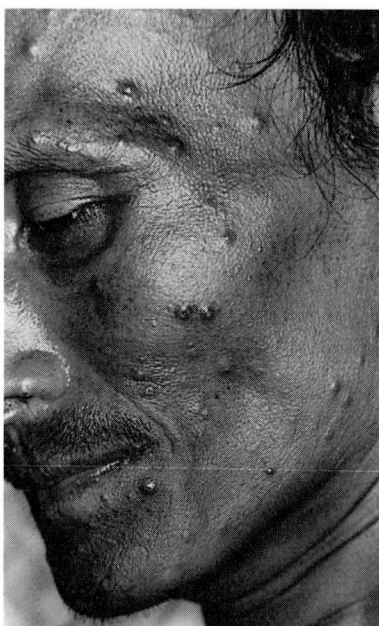

Figure 83–16. Skin lesions in HIV-positive patient with *Penicillium marneffei* infection. Some of the papules had central umbilication resembling lesions of molluscum contagiosum.

marneffei infection should be suspected in HIV-infected patients in or having visited endemic areas who present with fever, hepatosplenomegaly, lymphadenopathy, and skin lesions. A presumptive diagnosis can be established by the microscopic examination of the Wright-stained sample of bone-marrow aspirate and touch smears of the skin biopsy specimen and of the lymph-node biopsy specimen. Many intracellular and extracellular basophilic, spherical, oval, and elliptical yeast cells (3 to 8 μm in diameter) may be seen with this technique. Some of these cells have clear central septation, which is a characteristic feature of *P. marneffei* (Fig. 83–17). It is relatively easy to culture *P. marneffei* from various clinical specimens, such as bone marrow, blood, skin, draining abscesses, lymph nodes, sputum, and bronchoalveolar washings. The differential diagnoses of *P. marneffei* infection are tuberculosis, disseminated histoplasmosis, and disseminated cryptococcosis.

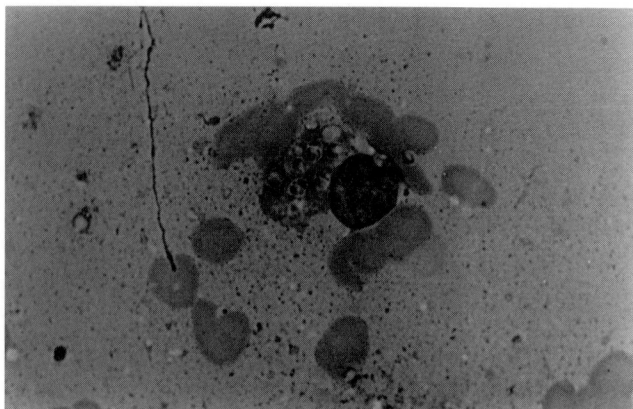

Figure 83–17. Photomicrograph of Wright-stained touch smear of skin biopsy specimen from a patient infected with HIV and *Penicillium marneffei*. Note spherical, oval, and elliptical yeast cells with clear central septation in a macrophage (× 1000).

TREATMENT. The mortality rate of patients infected with *P. marneffei* is very high, regardless of whether the patient is concurrently infected with HIV. This is probably due to failure to make a timely diagnosis. With increased awareness of the disease and prompt diagnosis and treatment the outcome has markedly improved. An initial survival rate of 80% can be expected. In vitro, *P. marneffei* is highly susceptible to miconazole, ketoconazole, and itraconazole, with intermediate susceptibility to amphotericin B (Chapter 84). The recommended treatment regimen is to give amphotericin B intravenously in a dose of 0.6 mg/kg/day for 2 weeks, followed by itraconazole 400 mg/day orally in two divided doses for the next 10 weeks. Most patients respond well, with the resolution of fever and other signs and symptoms within the first 2 weeks. In HIV-infected patients, 200 mg/day of itraconazole should be continued as secondary prophylaxis for life.

Bibliography

Chariyalertsak S, Sirisanthana T, Supparatpinyo K, Nelson KE: Seasonal variation of disseminated *Penicillium marneffei* infections in northern Thailand: A clue to the reservoir? J Infect Dis 173:1490, 1996.

Deng Z, Ribas JL, Gibson DW, Conner DH: Infection caused by *Penicillium marneffei* in China and Southeast Asia: Review of eighteen published cases and report of four more Chinese cases. Rev Infect Dis 10:640, 1988.

Drouhet E: Penicilliosis due to *Penicillium marneffei*: A new emerging systemic mycosis in AIDS patients travelling or living in Southeast Asia; review of 44 cases reported in HIV infected patients during the last 5 years compared to cases of non AIDS patients reported over 20 years. J Mycol Med 4:195, 1993.

Hilmarsdottir I, Meynard JL, Rogeaux O, et al: Disseminated *Penicillium marneffei* infection associated with human immunodeficiency virus: A report of two cases and a review of 35 published cases. J Acquir Immune Defic Syndr 6:466, 1993.

Supparatpinyo K, Khamwan C, Baosoung V, et al: Disseminated *Penicillium marneffei* infection in Southeast Asia. Lancet 344:110, 1994.

83.7 *Other Opportunistic Mycoses*

Roderick J. Hay

Opportunistic organisms are those that cause invasive disease in the presence of some deficiency in host defense. These infections are extremely rare in normal individuals. However, a distinction between these mycoses and those caused by the primary pathogens is one of convenience, and opportunism in the latter group occurs quite frequently. For instance, patients with AIDS are prone to develop the disseminated form of histoplasmosis in an endemic area.

In the United States, Europe, and other temperate areas, opportunistic infections are well recognized in patients under treatment for carcinoma or leukemia as well as in those who have received transplanted organs. The immunosuppressive effects of the underlying disease or its treatment are important in determining the likelihood and occurrence of these infections. In the tropics, the pattern is largely unexplored except in infections in AIDS patients. However, in these areas certain conditions such as diabetes mellitus may be more prevalent, whereas organ transplantation is less frequent. Underlying disease such as malnutrition and tuberculosis may also be associated with systemic fungal infections in the tropics.

Bibliography

Kibbler CC, MacKenzie DWR, Odds FC (eds): Principles and Practice of Clinical Mycology. Chichester, England, John Wiley & Sons, 1996.

Van den Bossche H, MacKenzie DWR, Cauwenbergh G, et al: Mycoses in AIDS patients. New York, Plenum Press, 1990.

Warnock DW, Richardson MD (eds): Fungal Infection in the Compromised Patient. Chichester, England, John Wiley & Sons, 1991.

■ ASPERGILLOSIS

DEFINITION. The term aspergillosis covers a group of infectious and allergic conditions caused by fungi of the genus *Aspergillus*. It includes invasive infections seen in immunocompromised patients, as well as allergic bronchopulmonary aspergillosis, a form of intrinsic allergic asthma, and aspergilloma. These conditions are well recognized in temperate areas but are worldwide in distribution.

ETIOLOGY. Aspergilli are common saprophytic molds readily isolated in the laboratory as contaminants. The species most commonly involved with human infections is *Aspergillus fumigatus*, which has been implicated in invasive and allergic bronchopulmonary aspergillosis as well as aspergilloma. *Aspergillus flavus* is less commonly isolated from cases of invasive disease and aspergilloma, although it is the main cause of the tropical infection paranasal aspergilloma. *Aspergillus niger* is another cause of aspergilloma, as well as otomycosis, in the tropics. Other species of *Aspergillus* are implicated occasionally in these infections.

EPIDEMIOLOGY. The distribution of these organisms is worldwide. However, there are subtle variations. For instance, in Europe *A. fumigatus* is the species most often isolated from sinus washings. In Sudan, the predominant organism is *A. flavus*. Such changes in the predominance of different organisms may possibly influence the distribution of the syndromes that comprise aspergillosis.

PATHOGENESIS, CLINICAL MANIFESTATIONS, AND TREATMENT. The clinical symptoms and subsequent progress of aspergillosis infections depend on the site, method of entry, and underlying condition of the host. In severely ill or compromised patients, invasion and dissemination may occur. However, aspergillosis may also proliferate in large quantities in dilated bronchial airways, lung cavities (aspergilloma), or the external ear. In atopic subjects and some nonatopic subjects, chronic carriage of *Aspergillus* in the bronchial tree leads to an allergic condition associated with considerable edema and peribronchial inflammatory infiltrates. Allergic bronchopulmonary aspergillosis has features of both type I and a type IV hypersensitivity response.

Allergic and Bronchopulmonary Aspergillosis. This is a persistent form of intrinsic asthma associated with chronic carriage of aspergilli within the airways. In early cases, airway obstruction is reversible, although the patient may expectorate mucoid plugs. In chronically affected patients, secondary destructive changes such as bronchiectasis may be found. The condition is diagnosed by demonstration of the characteristic clinical pattern of disease associated with a positive intradermal skin test to *Aspergillus*, eosinophilia, and on occasion, antibodies to the organism.

Treatment is directed toward relief of airway obstruction, using bronchodilators or systemic corticosteroids. The use of antifungal agents has been disappointing because of the frequency of relapse and recolonization.

Aspergilloma. An aspergilloma is a solid mycelial mass caused by the growth of *Aspergillus* species within a cavity, usually within the lung. The latter is most commonly the result of a previous tuberculous infection. Although the patient may be asymptomatic, cough is frequent and severe hemoptysis may occur.

The diagnosis is confirmed by the demonstration of a mobile intracavitary mass on the radiograph. Although cultures are often negative, patients frequently have high titers of antibody to *Aspergillus*.

Treatment is usually conservative. Surgical removal is the only reliable method of curing the aspergilloma although a few cases have responded to itraconazole. Spontaneous expectoration of the fungal mass may occur.

Invasive Aspergillosis. Although it occurs most commonly in immunocompromised neutropenic patients, e.g., those with leukemia, *Aspergillus* can also cause invasive disease following severe concurrent infection or, in children, in association with congenital neutrophil defects. The most common site of infection is the lung (Fig. 83–18), although metastatic brain or kidney abscesses, among others, may develop.

The development of a focal pulmonary lesion with cavitation in an immunosuppressed patient is a typical, but not universal, radiologic feature of invasive aspergillosis. Culture and serologic tests are often negative in this form of disease.

Amphotericin B is given in full dosage (Chapter 84). Alternatives include lipid-associated amphotericin B and itraconazole. In addition, predisposing factors should be relieved when possible, e.g., by leukocyte transfusions or by modification of steroid dosage.

Chronic Necrotizing Pulmonary Aspergillosis. *Aspergillus* may cause an indolent lung infection, usually in patients with pre-existing cavitary or fibrotic lung disease associated with limited invasion of lung parenchyma. The main symptoms are chronic cough, weight loss, and fever, but complications such as aspergillus empyema or aspergilloma may develop. The diagnosis is difficult to establish, but the presence of persistent positive sputum cultures, positive serology, and persistent localized pulmonary shadowing in an ill patient

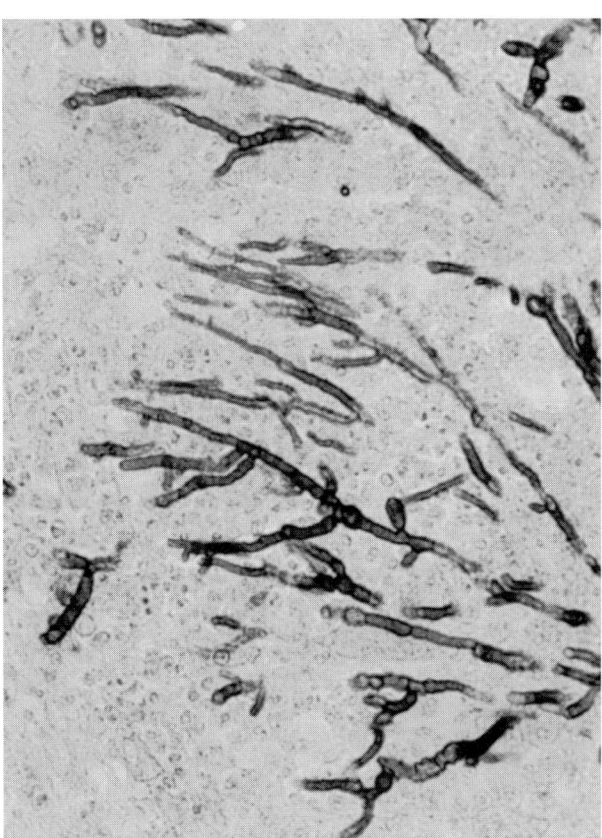

Figure 83–18. *Aspergillus* in lung. Acute infection with dichotomous branching of hyphae. (Gridley fungus stain, × 400.) (Courtesy of the Armed Forces Institute of Pathology, Photograph Neg. No. 61–6516.)

should arouse suspicion. A lung biopsy, if feasible, will confirm the diagnosis. Treatment is difficult but successes have been seen with oral itraconazole or amphotericin B.

Paranasal Aspergillus Granuloma. This is a sclerosing granuloma that originates in the paranasal sinuses. The causative organism is usually *Aspergillus flavus*. The infection is seen in Sudan, India, and the Middle East but may be more widespread in the tropics. Early symptoms include unilateral nasal obstruction and facial pain or headache. Later, proptosis associated with orbital invasion may develop, or more persistent headache with evidence of meningismus may herald central nervous system (CNS) involvement. Subsequently, tumor seedlings may occur within the CNS, giving rise to focal neurologic signs.

Patients presenting in the early phases of this condition are commonly investigated and treated for chronic sinusitis, and the diagnosis is made after biopsy of the sinus lesion. On radiographic examination, opacification of the sinuses may be found. Magnetic resonance imaging shows dense fibrosis. The most frequent site of infection is the maxillary sinus, followed by the ethmoids. There may be considerable periosteal thickening in these areas, and in late lesions lytic zones may be distinguished.

When this diagnosis is suspected the organism is usually readily cultured. Alternatively, the histologic examination of the lesion shows a sclerosing granuloma in which hyphal fragments are sparsely scattered. It is important to combine histologic and cultural investigations, as *A. flavus* can be isolated from sinuses without granuloma formation. Serologic tests for *A. flavus* in infected patients are often positive.

The first line of treatment is surgical removal. The tumor should be removed as completely as possible, with the patient receiving itraconazole or intravenous amphotericin B (Chapter 84). Relapse occurs frequently, and the condition may progress relentlessly to death.

Bibliography

Black JM: Pulmonary aspergillosis. Proc R Soc Med 53:974, 1960.
Kilman JW, Ahn C, Andrews NC, et al: Surgery for pulmonary aspergillosis. J Thorac Cardiovasc Surg 57:642, 1969.
Milošev B, el-Mahgoub S, Aal OA: Primary aspergilloma of paranasal sinuses in the Sudan. Br J Surg 56:132, 1969.
Turner-Warwick M: *Aspergillus fumigatus* and lung disease. Postgrad Med J 55:642, 1979.

■ SYSTEMIC CANDIDA INFECTIONS

DEFINITION. *Candida* species are capable of causing both superficial and deep infections, although the onset of the former only rarely presages the development of the latter. A number of different clinical patterns of systemic infection are seen. Infections may be focal and confined to a body cavity such as the peritoneum or to the cerebrospinal fluid (CSF). Infection of the lower urinary tract may occur also. Alternatively, where blood stream spread develops, the disease may follow a benign self-limiting or progressive invasive course. Endocarditis caused by *Candida* usually follows homograft valve surgery but may occur in drug addicts.

ETIOLOGY. *Candida albicans* is the most common cause of systemic candidosis, but other species may be involved also. *Candida tropicalis*, for instance, is not uncommonly isolated from patients with deep candidosis. *Candida* species other than *C. albicans*, particularly *Candida parapsilosis*, are isolated in almost half of the patients with *Candida* endocarditis.

EPIDEMIOLOGY. Little is known about the distribution and importance of systemic *Candida* infections in the tropics. However, the rate of saprophytic carriage is high, and it is likely that invasive candidosis may contribute to the morbidity and mortality of a number of conditions, from malnutrition to carcinoma.

PATHOLOGY AND PATHOGENESIS. The organisms causing systemic *Candida* infections gain entry via a number of routes. In many instances, blood stream spread follows penetration of the gut wall by organisms within the gastrointestinal tract. Alternative routes of invasion include the bladder, the lung, and intravenous lines. The organisms may be implanted also directly following surgery or the insertion of peritoneal dialysis catheters. The factors affecting invasion are not clear. However, as with superficial infections, deep candidosis is nearly always seen in compromised patients, particularly those with leukemia and those receiving immunosuppressive therapy. Patients with prolonged periods of neutropenia and particularly those who have been receiving systemic antibiotic therapy are prone to infection with *Candida*.

CLINICAL MANIFESTATIONS. There are a number of different clinical varieties of deep candidosis.

Candidemia. Although *Candida* species may be isolated from blood, this finding is not necessarily accompanied by invasion of internal organs or progressive disease. Candidemia may occur in the presence of indwelling intravenous catheters, in postoperative states, or in immunosuppressed patients. Such patients may be managed with amphotericin B or fluconazole and by the removal of intravenous catheters. They should be investigated also for evidence of invasive candidosis. In a substantial proportion of patients, candidemia is transient.

Systemic Candidosis. Deep invasive *Candida* infections, with or without positive blood cultures, are less common than candidemia. Sites of invasion include the kidneys, liver, muscle, skin, brain, and retina. Contrary to a widely held belief, the lung is not a common site for invasive *Candida* infections, and if involved, the radiologic appearance may be unexceptional because of the diffuse nature of the invasive process. Endocarditis is seen more commonly as a distinctive form of the disease.

In many patients with systemic candidosis, there is considerable difficulty in confirming the laboratory or clinical diagnosis unless retinopathy is present or there are lesions accessible for biopsy. Both fungal cultures and serologic tests are negative in a substantial proportion of patients.

Candida Endocarditis. This is seen most frequently following homograft valve surgery or in drug addicts. The mitral or aortic valves are involved most commonly, often producing large vegetations. Emboli from these can obstruct major blood vessels. The diagnosis is confirmed by culture and serologic testing. High titers of antibody may occur in this form of candidosis.

Deep Focal Invasion. This may follow surgery or local injury. The main areas involved are the peritoneum (after peritoneal dialysis or gastrointestinal perforation) and the meninges (following surgery). The infection usually remains localized. *Candida* urinary tract infections are not uncommon and are seen most frequently in patients with urinary tract obstruction, indwelling bladder catheters, and diabetes mellitus. The appearance of *Candida* in the urine is not necessarily an indication for treatment unless the patient experiences symptoms (e.g., pain on urination or frequency), or unless, in severely ill patients, there is risk of dissemination.

TREATMENT. In neutropenic patients amphotericin B is usually given (Chapter 84). Flucytosine can be added in some patients such as those with extensive infections or involvement of the eye or CNS. Fluconazole (400 to 800 mg daily) is an alternative, particularly in non-neutropenic patients. It is not effective in infections due to some *Candida* species such as those caused by *Candida krusei* and *Candida (Torulopsis) glabrata*.

Bibliography

Ellis CA, Spivack ML: The significance of candidemia. Ann Intern Med 67:511, 1967.
Hyun BH, Collier FC: Mycotic endocarditis following intracardiac operations. N Engl J Med 263:1339, 1961.
Kozinn PJ, Hasenclever HF, Taschdjian CL, et al: Problems in the diagnosis and treatment of systemic candidosis. J Infect Dis 126:548, 1972.
Myerowitz RL, Pazin GJ, Allen CM: Disseminated candidosis. Changes in incidence, underlying diseases and pathology. Am J Clin Pathol 68:29, 1977.
Stone HH, Geheber CE, Kolg LD, et al: Alimentary tract colonization by *Candida albicans*. J Surg Res 14:273, 1973.

■ MUCORMYCOSIS

DEFINITION. Mucormycosis (zygomycosis, systemic phycomycosis) is a systemic fungal infection caused by certain Zygomycetes fungi of the genera *Rhizopus*, *Absidia*, or, on rare occasions, *Cunninghamella* and *Saksenaea*.

ETIOLOGY AND PATHOGENESIS. There are a number of sites of primary invasion in mucormycosis, including the paranasal sinuses, skin, lungs, and gastrointestinal tract. The organisms are common environmental saprophytes in most parts of the world. However, they only produce invasive disease in compromised patients, such as those with leukemia, diabetic ketoacidosis, burn injuries, or malnutrition. This infection has not been widely described from the tropics. There are scattered reports of cases in South Africa and the Far East, however, and its distribution is likely to be worldwide.

CLINICAL MANIFESTATIONS. There are a number of different clinical varieties of mucormycosis.

Rhinocerebral Mucormycosis. This form is most often seen in patients with poorly controlled, insulin-dependent diabetes mellitus. The presenting features are most commonly those of an orbital cellulitis, with unilateral facial swelling, proptosis, and orbital pain. Alternatively, palatal perforation may be found. The process is rapidly progressive, and invasion of adjacent structures, including the optic nerve, cranium, and other sinuses, may occur. The infection is accompanied often by extensive infarction, as blood vessel invasion is a prominent feature. Secondary spread to other areas such as the lung may occur.

Pulmonary Mucormycosis. Lung invasion may occur in any affected group but is found most often in immunosuppressed or leukemic patients. Extensive pulmonary infection is associated often with disseminated infection elsewhere.

Other Sites of Invasion. Invasion of burns or postoperative wounds with secondary spread and extensive thrombosis has been described. It has also been recognized that contaminated dressing packs may be associated with this pattern of infection. Severe gastrointestinal hemorrhage or perforation may be the presenting feature of gastrointestinal invasion. The stomach and jejunum are the sites invaded most frequently. This form of mucormycosis has been described in malnourished patients.

DIAGNOSIS. Mucormycosis may be manifested by distinctive clinical features that aid in establishing the diagnosis. However, cultures are frequently negative, and serologic testing is unhelpful. The distinctive broad aseptate hyphae may be seen in biopsy specimens or smears taken from infected areas. Biopsy is normally the best method of establishing the diagnosis and should be performed early in the course of the infection.

TREATMENT. When possible, extensive surgical debridement of infected areas should be performed, combined with administration of amphotericin B or a lipid-associated amphotericin B at high dosage (Chapter 84). Treatment is continued until clinical remission is achieved.

Bibliography

Kahn LR: Gastric mucormycosis: Report of a case with a review of the literature. S Afr Med J 37:1265, 1963.
Lehrer RI, Howard DH, Sypherd PS, et al: Mucormycosis. Ann Intern Med 93:93, 1980.
Meyer RD, Armstrong D: Mucormycosis—changing status. CRC Crit Rev Clin Lab Sci 4:421, 1973.
Tanphaichitra D: Rhinocerebral mucormycosis with emphasis on clinical diagnosis, altered host defence mechanisms and management. Postgrad Med J 55:622, 1979.

84 *Treatment of Systemic Mycoses*

Edward C. Oldfield III

The treatment of the systemic mycoses remains a clinical challenge. The infections are chronic, with a tendency to relapse, and the standard therapy, amphotericin B, has multiple toxicities. From the 1950s until recently, there were few significant new antifungal agents. With the introduction of the azoles, especially the oral agents ketoconazole, fluconazole, and itraconazole, there is the promise of relatively nontoxic long-term therapy. The purpose of this chapter is to discuss the properties and use of the major antifungals: amphotericin B, flucytosine, ketoconazole, fluconazole, and itraconazole. For specific indications to institute therapy for a systemic fungal infection, duration of therapy, and parameters indicating response, refer to the chapter on the particular systemic mycosis.

■ AMPHOTERICIN B

Amphotericin B is a member of the class of antibiotics called macrolide polyenes and is a product of *Streptomyces nodosus*. Despite its formidable and essentially unavoidable toxicities, amphotericin B remains the standard therapeutic agent for many of the deep mycoses.

MECHANISM OF ACTION. The polyene structure of amphotericin B is responsible for both its therapeutic and its toxic properties. All cells susceptible to polyenes contain sterols in their cell membranes. Amphotericin B interacts with membrane sterols, leading to an alteration in the integrity of the cell membrane, with subsequent leakage of intracellular contents. In the fungi, the interaction is with ergosterol and results in inhibition of fungal growth, whereas in human cells, the interaction is with cholesterol, resulting in toxic side effects.

SENSITIVE ORGANISMS. Most of the fungi responsible for systemic mycotic infections are sensitive to amphotericin B. These include *Coccidioides immitis*, *Cryptococcus neoformans*, *Histoplasma capsulatum*, *Blastomyces dermatitidis*, *Candida* species, *Torulopsis glabrata*, *Aspergillus* species, *Paracoccidioides brasiliensis*, and the causative agents of mucormycosis. Activity has been noted also against a number of protozoan pathogens: trichomonads, *Entamoeba*, *Naegleria*, *Leishmania*, and trypanosomes. Isolates of *Pseudallescheria boydii*, *Candida lusitaniae*, *Trichosporon beigelii*, and *Scedosporium inflatum* are commonly resistant. Intrinsic resistance has been reported among other species; however, these data are difficult to interpret because of a lack of standardization among laboratories and the variance between in vitro and clinical results. At present, there seems little to be gained from routine in vitro susceptibility testing or measurement of serum levels of amphotericin B.

The development of acquired resistance during therapy has not been a problem. As a rule, the fungi isolated from patients who have been treated and subsequently relapsed have been as sensitive as the initial isolates.

Synergism of amphotericin B with a number of agents has been noted. This effect has had the most clinical promise with flucytosine and is discussed in the section on that drug. Amphotericin B has been noted to be synergistic with agents not normally believed to have intrinsic antifungal activity, i.e., rifampin, tetracycline, and minocycline. The clinical importance of this interaction remains untested.

PHARMACOLOGIC PROPERTIES. Peak serum concentrations of amphotericin B with standard therapeutic doses are 0.5 to 2.0 μg/mL. The fate of the drug is unknown, and no metabolites have been identified. There is a biphasic excretion of drug from the body, with a rapid elimination half-life of 24 hours, followed by a prolonged terminal half-life of 15 days. Renal excretion accounts for only 3 to 5% of total drug elimination. For this reason, there is no accumulation of amphotericin B in serum during renal failure, and no dosage adjustment is required, even in the anephric patient. A dosage reduction may be needed to avoid further nephrotoxicity, but it should be noted that this will result in decreased serum levels. Amphotericin B is not removed by peritoneal dialysis or hemodialysis. Biliary excretion has been noted to be 19%, but hepatic disease does not necessitate a dosage change.

Cerebrospinal fluid (CSF) penetration has been poor even with inflamed meninges. The levels of amphotericin B in the CSF are 30 to 50 times lower than concomitant serum levels. Urine concentrations are similar to those in serum. Levels in the aqueous humor are about two thirds of those in serum, and poor vitreous humor penetration has been noted. Levels of amphotericin B in pleural, peritoneal, and synovial fluid are also about two thirds of serum levels.

PREPARATIONS. Amphotericin B (Fungizone, Squibb) is available as a sterile powder for intravenous use in vials containing 50 mg of amphotericin B and 41 mg of desoxycholate, which creates a colloidal dispersion of the insoluble antibiotic. It is reconstituted with 10 mL of sterile water without additives and then added to 5% dextrose in water. The addition of even minimal amounts of sodium or chloride will reduce bioactivity and induce the prompt appearance of turbidity in the infusion bottle. Therefore, amphotericin B should not be mixed with electrolytes or acidic solutions.

Amphotericin B is light-sensitive, but during a 24-hour period there is no appreciable loss of activity. Therefore, no special precautions, such as wrapping the bottle with aluminum foil, are necessary.

The drug is poorly absorbed from the gastrointestinal tract; oral doses as high as 5 g result in inadequate serum levels. The oral solution shoul never be used to treat systemic infections; its only use is for candidal infections of the oropharynx.

Three new lipid formulations have been developed in an effort to reduce the nephrotoxicity of the old amphotericin B desoxycholate (ABD) formulation: amphotericin B lipid complex (ABLC), amphotericin B colloidal dispersion (ABCD), and liposomal amphotericin B (AmBisome). All have less nephrotoxicity than the old formulation, similar efficacy (but at higher doses of 2 to 5 mg/kg/day), and similar infusion-related toxicity. The lipid formulations have increased concentration in the spleen, liver, and lung. This uptake in the reticuloendothelial system results in decreased delivery of drugs to the kidneys. Because the cost is 10- to 20-fold greater than the old formulation, their use should be reserved for patients with renal insufficiency or who are otherwise refractory to or intolerant of conventional treatment. Only ABLC and AmBisome were approved by the Food and Drug Administration in 1998. The recommended dose of ABLC is 5.0 mg/kg given as a single daily infusion at an infusion rate of 2.5 mg/kg/hour. If the infusion exceeds 2 hours, shake the infusion bag to mix the contents. Homemade formulations of amphotericin B desoxycholate mixed with intravenous lipids cannot currently be recommended.

THERAPEUTIC USAGE

Intravenous Therapy. Therapy with amphotericin B is initiated with a 1-mg test dose in 5% dextrose in water infused over 20 minutes to evaluate the extent of the commonly encountered febrile response. Vital signs should be monitored closely. Subsequent dosage increments to the full therapeutic dose of 0.3 to 1.0 mg/kg are determined by the severity of the toxic reactions encountered and the severity of the fungal infection. If the toxic reactions are minimal or the fungal infection is fulminating, rapid attainment of a full therapeutic dose can be achieved. If the toxic reactions are severe or the fungal infection is chronic, a more gradual institution of therapy may be desirable. For chronic infections, the dose may be increased daily until the desired level is reached. For instance, the daily dose of amphotericin B may be increased from the 1-mg test dose on the first day to 5-, 10-, 20- and 40-mg doses in 500 mL of 5% dextrose in water on days 2, 3, 4, and 5, respectively. The duration of infusion is commonly 2 to 3 hours, although controlled studies have shown that 1-hour infusions are safe if the creatinine clearance is greater than 25 mL/minute and the dose is less than 1.0 mg/kg. Infusions of less than 1 hour's duration should be avoided, as cardiac arrhythmias have been noted in dogs when rapid infusions are used. In cases in which the fungal disease is more severe, rapid attainment of therapeutic levels is desirable. In this situation, the full therapeutic dose (usually 20 to 50 mg) may be put in 500 mL of 5% dextrose in water. The equivalent of 1 mg is then infused over 20 to 30 minutes. If no severe reactions are encountered, the remainder is infused over 2 to 3 hours, with monitoring of vital signs.

If toxic reactions are noted, hydrocortisone, 25 mg, may be added to the infusion bottle. Hydrocortisone decreases the frequency but not the severity of fever and chills. Increasing the dose of hydrocortisone does not provide additional benefit. Premedication with acetaminophen and diphenhydramine may further ameliorate the toxicity. As the infusions are continued, many patients will develop tolerance to the amphotericin B, and the addition of hydrocortisone may be discontinued. Intravenous meperidine hydrochloride, in an average dose of 45 mg, has been shown to be effective in terminating rigors and chills during an infusion. For patients with severe rigors, the meperidine may be given prophylactically just prior to the amphotericin B infusion. Ibuprofen administered prior to the infusion decreases severe chills. However, there is a potential to enhance the nephrotoxicity of amphotericin B with ibuprofen, which also decreases renal blood flow and has tubular toxicity. Heparin, 500 to 1000 U, is commonly added to the infusion solution to decrease the incidence of phlebitis. Heparin is not needed if the infusion is through a central venous catheter.

The usual recommended maintenance dose is 0.3 to 0.7 mg/kg/day, generally not exceeding 50 mg/day. An exception is the treatment of invasive aspergillosis, which may require daily doses of 1.0 to 1.5 mg/kg. During maintenance therapy, the use of a double dose on alternate days (usually not exceeding 70 mg) has been shown to be as efficacious as daily therapy. The trough concentrations are similar on the off day to those obtained with daily therapy, and the peak concentrations with either regimen tend to reach a plateau at doses exceeding 50 mg. With the alternate-day regimen, prolonged outpatient therapy is greatly facilitated, and the patients feel better on the off day. The renal toxicity is equivalent with either regimen.

During prolonged therapy, toxicity is to be expected but can be monitored with twice-weekly serum creatinine, blood urea nitrogen, potassium, magnesium, and hematocrit determinations. The total duration of therapy is variable and depends on the particular fungus being treated, the anatomic site of involvement, and the clinical response.

Other Routes of Administration. Intrathecal therapy may be required for fungal meningitis because of the poor penetration into cerebrospinal fluid. Only selected cases of cryptococcal and coccidioidal meningitis will require intrathecal therapy. An initial dose of 0.1 mg is followed by increments of 0.1 mg until a total daily dose of 0.5 to 1.0 mg is attained. The dose is usually administered by the lumbar route on a thrice-weekly schedule. Toxic reactions are common and include radicular pain, paresthesias, urinary retention, monoparesis, and acute toxic delirium. Hydrocortisone hemi-succinate (10 to 25 mg) is usually added to the injection to decrease radicular pain.

Intraperitoneal administration has been recommended at a dose of 1 mg of amphotericin B added to 1000 mL of dialysis fluid. Intra-articular use has been reported at doses ranging from 5 to 25 mg per injection. Bladder irrigation may be accomplished with 50 mg in 1000 of sterile water. Ocular penetration is poor with intravenous administration, but direct intravitreal administration in rabbits has led to retinal necrosis and detachment.

TOXICITY. Amphotericin B is noted for its formidable and essentially unavoidable toxicity. However, with appropriate management, most patients can complete a course of therapy and the side effects can be minimized. On occasion, with chronic indolent infections, toxicity may preclude the successful completion of therapy, and alternate therapeutic regimens may be required.

General Toxicity. Toxicity associated with the infusion of amphotericin B has been noted in up to 93% of patients. This includes fever, occasionally in excess of 40°C, rigors, headaches, anorexia, nausea, vomiting, dyspnea, and hypotension.

Nephrotoxicity. The most severe form of toxicity is renal. During the therapeutic use of amphotericin B, it is common for the creatinine level to rise to the range of 2.0 to 3.0 mg/dL. In many patients, the creatinine will reach a plateau at this level and therapy may be continued. However, in others, the creatinine level will continue to rise. Once the creatinine rises above 3.0 mg/dL, it is advisable to reduce the dose or temporarily withhold the infusion to prevent a further decrease in glomerular filtration. In some series, more than 80% of patients developed a significant alteration of renal function. In those patients who receive a total dose of less than 4 g, the renal insufficiency is usually reversible. However, once the total dose exceeds 5 g, most patients will exhibit some degree of persistent renal insufficiency.

The mechanism of renal toxicity appears to be due to a combination of direct tubular damage, primarily distal, and renal artery constriction. Pathologically, there are degenerative changes of the tubules, with intratubular and interstitial calcifications. Glomerular involvement is minimal. Functionally, there are consistent decreases in glomerular filtration rate and renal blood flow. There is also a consistent impairment of distal tubular function, with an increased renal clearance of potassium, and an impairment of renal hydrogen excretion, with the development of renal tubular acidosis. There is usually an absence of red blood cells, red blood cell casts, or significant proteinuria in the urine sediment, but cylindruria is common.

Renal toxicity is enhanced by intravascular volume depletion secondary to low sodium intake, diuretics, vomiting, diarrhea, or cirrhosis with ascites. Correcting volume depletion is essential for successful therapy by rehydration, high salt diet, discontinuation of diuretics, or volume expansion. Infusion of 500 to 1000 mL of normal saline before each dose of amphotericin B has become a common practice and appears to decrease nephrotoxicity. However, the increased sodium load may further increase potassium losses and require increased supplementation. The lipid formulations of amphotericin B have reduced nephrotoxicity and should be considered in those patients who develop progressive declines in renal function despite sodium supplementation.

Hematologic Toxicity. Anemia is a common side effect. A decrease in hematocrit of 10 units can be expected in three fourths of patients, and one third will have a reduction of 15 units or greater. There is no correlation between the total dosage of amphotericin B or degree of azotemia and the magnitude of the anemia. The anemia is normochromic and normocytic, without a reticulocytosis. The hematocrit decreases early in therapy and then stabilizes. Transfusions have not been beneficial, as the hematocrit will return gradually to the pretransfusion level. Thrombocytopenia and neutropenia have been noted rarely.

Hypokalemia. Renal potassium wasting commonly results in decreased levels of serum potassium. Oral supplementation will be necessary in 25% of patients. Hypomagnesemia has also been noted.

Allergic Reactions. Allergic reactions are remarkably absent with amphotericin B. Because well-documented reports of drug eruptions are so rare, when a rash appears during therapy, it can usually be attributed to some other cause.

Hepatotoxicity. Alterations in hepatic function have been extremely rare.

Pregnancy. Amphotericin B has been used in pregnancy without evidence of teratogenesis or persistent toxicity in infants. Treatment of a pregnant woman should not be considered an indication for termination of pregnancy.

THERAPEUTIC INDICATIONS. For specific indications, dosage, duration, and synergism, refer to the chapter on the particular systemic fungal infection.

■ FLUCYTOSINE

Flucytosine (5-fluorocytosine) is a fluorinated pyrimidine that was first synthesized as an antitumor agent in 1957. The drug has a narrow spectrum of activity and is used primarily because of its synergism with amphotericin B against certain fungi.

MECHANISM OF ACTION. Flucytosine is deaminated within the fungal cell to 5-fluorouracil, which is a commonly used antitumor agent. The 5-fluorouracil is then incorporated into fungal RNA as 5-fluorouridine triphosphate and leads to faulty protein synthesis and subsequent growth inhibition. Flucytosine also blocks thymidylate synthetase, leading to a decrease in DNA synthesis.

SENSITIVE ORGANISMS. Flucytosine is active against *Cryptococcus neoformans, Candida albicans,* some other *Candida* species, *Torulopsis glabrata,* and the causative agents of chromomycosis. Primary resistance is rare with *Cryptococcus neoformans* and *Torulopsis glabrata.* The sensitivity of *Candida* *albicans* varies from 50 to 90%, depending on the method used. When flucytosine is used alone, the development of secondary resistance during therapy has been a more serious problem. This is the primary reason why flucytosine is rarely used alone. As many as two thirds of isolates obtained during therapy have been resistant; however, they remained sensitive to amphotericin B.

Synergism with amphotericin B has been noted for *Cryptococcus neoformans* and for *Candida* species. An additive effect is commonly seen with *Candida* even if the isolate exhibits partial in vitro resistance to flucytosine.

PHARMACOKINETICS. Oral absorption of flucytosine is excellent, even in renal failure. Administration with meals does not decrease total absorption. Penetration of tissue is excellent, resulting in levels in the liver, kidneys, spleen, heart, and lungs that are equal to or greater than those in serum. The concentration of flucytosine in CSF averages 75% of simultaneous serum levels. The drug is concentrated in the urine with levels of 1000 to 2000 μg/mL, and lesser but adequate levels are maintained with renal insufficiency.

Excretion is primarily by the kidneys, with only minimal metabolism. The half-life of flucytosine with normal renal function is 3 to 4 hours, but even minor decreases in renal function will lead to prolongation. Both peritoneal dialysis and hemodialysis remove significant amounts of the drug.

DOSAGE AND ADMINISTRATION. Flucytosine (Ancobon, Roche) is manufactured in tablets or capsules of 250- or 500-mg strength. The standard daily dose is 150 mg/kg divided into four equal doses of 37.5 mg/kg. It is critical that the dosage be adjusted in the presence of renal insufficiency, as even mild azotemia may lead to significant increases in serum levels. In order to avoid accumulation of toxic levels in serum, i.e., greater than 100 μg/mL, a number of dosage adjustments have been recommended. One commonly used regimen maintains a normal dose of 37.5 mg/kg but prolongs the interval between doses, with a 12-hour interval for creatinine clearance between 20 and 40 mL/min and a 24-hour interval for creatinine clearance between 10 and 20 mL/min. For patients on hemodialysis, a dose of 37.5 mg/kg after each dialysis may be used.

During treatment, it is essential to monitor serum creatinine, blood urea nitrogen, liver function, and platelet and white blood cell counts. Particular caution must be used when there is pre-existing renal insufficiency, decreased platelet count, neutropenia, or liver disease.

TOXICITY. As a rule, flucytosine is well tolerated. In one large series, 18% of patients experienced gastrointestinal, 7% hepatic, and 18% hematologic complications. The gastrointestinal toxicity usually takes the form of nausea, vomiting, and diarrhea. This is usually not severe; however, severe colitis with multiple colonic perforations may develop. Hepatitis may occur and is usually nonprogressive. The abnormalities usually resolve with discontinuation of the drug.

Neutropenia has been the most common hematologic toxicity. There may also be thrombocytopenia or a combination of the two. The bone marrow toxicity usually resolves with decreased dosage or discontinuation of flucytosine. However, fatal bone marrow suppression has been reported. This hematologic toxicity correlates with serum levels of 100 to 125 μg/mL or greater, usually with associated renal insufficiency. When available, serum levels should be monitored to avoid toxic levels.

Less commonly reported toxicity has included maculopapular rashes and eosinophilia. Flucytosine should be used with caution in women of childbearing age because of teratogenicity noted in experimental animals.

THERAPEUTIC INDICATIONS. The combination of amphotericin B and flucytosine is the treatment of choice for cryptococcal meningitis; it improves cure rates and decreases relapses when compared with therapy with amphotericin B alone. This combination is indicated also in disseminated cryptococcal disease and severe infections with *Candida* species and *Torulopsis*. The combination will allow a decreased dose of amphotericin B (0.3 mg/kg) and, hence, a decrease in renal toxicity. The presence of amphotericin B decreases the emergence of flucytosine resistance but may lead to an increase in flucytosine toxicity.

■ AZOLES

One of the most significant advances in the treatment of the systemic mycoses has been the introduction of the azoles: fluconazole, itraconazole, and ketoconazole. Although there are few direct comparisons with amphotericin B, they are efficacious, less toxic, and more convenient, especially when chronic therapy is indicated.

All of the azoles are synthetic compounds with a five-membered azole ring and are classified as imidazoles (miconazole and ketoconazole) or triazoles (fluconazole and itraconazole).

The azoles are potent inhibitors of ergosterol synthesis, the major membrane sterol of fungi. They block the cytochrome P-450 dependent enzyme C-14 α-demethylase, which is needed to convert lanosterol to ergosterol. Many of the drug interactions and toxic effects of the azoles are related to interaction with human enzymes that are dependent on cytochrome P-450. In general, imidazoles have significantly more affinity and hence interaction with the mammalian enzymes than the triazoles.

SENSITIVE ORGANISMS. All of the azoles have a broad spectrum of activity against the systemic mycoses including the dimorphic fungi, yeasts, and dermatophytes. The azoles are fungistatic and not fungicidal. In general, fluconazole has become the preferred agent for *Coccidioides immitis*, *Cryptococcus neoformans*, and oropharyngeal and esophageal *Candida* infections. Itraconazole has become the preferred agent for *Histoplasma capsulatum*, *Blastomyces dermatitidis*, *Sporothrix schenckii*, *Paracoccidioides brasiliensis*, and *Pseudallescheria boydii*. Itraconazole has proved to be an important advance in the treatment of invasive *Aspergillus* infections.

Although much remains to be defined about the place of azole therapy, it is commonly used for subacute clinical presentations, chronic suppression, and meningitis (especially fluconazole). Amphotericin B is now commonly reserved for more fulminant presentations of the same fungal infections.

Primary resistance among *Candida krusei*, which has been a frequent isolate from patients receiving fluconazole prophylaxis during neutropenic episodes, is common. *Fusarium* and *Zygomycetes* are commonly resistant to all of the azoles. The development of fluconazole resistance among *Candida* isolates during chronic suppressive therapy of oral and esophageal candidiasis has become an increasingly common problem among patients with AIDS. These isolates may be cross-resistant to itraconazole and may only be responsive to amphotericin B.

Substantial efforts are being devoted to the development of reliable in vitro sensitivity testing. Recent data have shown increasing clinical relevance, but as yet sensitivity testing is available only at a few reference centers and is not considered routine practice.

PHARMACOLOGIC PROPERTIES
Ketoconazole. Ketoconazole is supplied as 200-mg tablets for oral use (Nizoral, Janssen Pharmaceuticals). Peak serum concentrations of 2 μg/mL and 3.42 μg/mL occur at 2 to 4

hours after an oral dose of 200 mg and 400 mg, respectively. Ketoconazole is a base which must be converted to the hydrochloride salt before it can be absorbed. Any drugs that decrease gastric activity such as H_2 receptor blockers (ranitidine, cimetidine) or proton pump inhibitors (omeprazole) or antacids can markedly reduce absorption and result in clinical failures. Likewise, persons with AIDS commonly have a gastropathy with low gastric acid secretion, and may have erratic absorption. Ketoconazole is highly lipophilic with high concentrations in fatty tissues, liver, kidney, and skin. Protein binding of ketoconazole is more than 90%; urine concentrations are low (0.4 μg/mL) and CSF concentrations are about 5% of concomitant serum levels. Ketoconazole undergoes extensive hepatic metabolism, and no dosage adjustment is needed with renal insufficiency.

Itraconazole. Itraconazole is supplied as 100-mg capsules (Sporanox, Janssen) and is similar in many respects to ketoconazole: It is highly lipophilic, highly protein bound, achieves low CSF levels, and undergoes extensive hepatic metabolism. Gastric acidity is required for optimal absorption. Itraconazole absorption is increased two- to threefold when taken with food and can be further increased when taken with a cola beverage (pH, 2.5). Because of the extended time to reach steady state (10 to 14 days), itraconazole therapy should be initiated with a loading dose. For serious or life-threatening infections, a loading dose of 200 mg three times a day for 3 days is given. No adjustment of dose is required with renal insufficiency, but caution should be used in patients with hepatic impairment.

Fluconazole. Fluconazole is supplied as 50-, 100-, and 200-mg tablets (Diflucan, Roerig) and as an intravenous preparation and is quite different from the other two azoles. Fluconazole is water soluble and has low protein binding, high levels in the urine, and excellent CSF penetration (70 to 90% of peak plasma concentration). These properties make fluconazole an excellent choice for the treatment of urinary tract infections and meningitis due to susceptible fungal pathogens. Because the time to achieve steady state is 6 to 10 days after treatment is begun, a single loading dose of double the maintenance dose is given on the first day of therapy. Oral and intravenous doses are the same because oral bioavailability is greater than 90%. Unlike the other azoles, there is minimal hepatic metabolism, with 80% of the drug excreted unchanged in the urine. The dose of fluconazole should be reduced by 50 and 75% when the creatinine clearance is less than 50 and 20 mL/min, respectively.

DRUG INTERACTIONS. Because the azoles have an affinity for mammalian cytochrome P-450 enzymes, there are substantial drug interactions. As a result of interference with drug metabolism, itraconazole, ketoconazole, and fluconazole will lead to increased serum concentrations of warfarin, phenytoin, cyclosporine, and tolbutamide as well as other sulfonylureas. Ketoconazole and itraconazole inhibit the metabolism of terfenadine, astemizole, and cisapride, which may result in fatal cardiac arrhythmias; coadministration is contraindicated. Alprazolam and midazolam metabolism is inhibited by ketoconazole and itraconazole and their coadministration is also contraindicated. Further drug interactions reported with fluconazole include increased serum concentrations of theophylline and rifabutin. Itraconazole has been reported to increase digoxin levels.

Rifampin, isoniazid, phenytoin, phenobarbital, and carbamazepine decrease ketoconazole and itraconazole levels. Coadministration has been noted to result in clinical failures or relapse. Conversely, ketoconazole may result in decreased serum concentrations of rifampin and clinical failures in the treatment of *Mycobacterium tuberculosis*.

TOXICITY. The most common side effects of itraconazole and ketoconazole are nausea, vomiting, and abdominal pain. The gastrointestinal toxicity can be decreased by administration of the azoles with a meal. Hepatitis has been noted with all three azoles. A reversible idiosyncratic hepatitis has been reported in about 1 in 800 patients on itraconazole. Asymptomatic elevation of transaminases has been noted in less than 3% of patients. An average of 12% of patients taking ketoconazole develop elevations of hepatic enzymes, but only 1 in 15,000 have been estimated to develop symptomatic hepatitis. Rare fatal cases of hepatitis have been reported with all three azoles. For ketoconazole, monitoring of liver function tests has been recommended every 2 weeks for the first 2 months and then monthly or bimonthly. If there is a rise in transaminases to 3 to 5 times normal or the development of clinical symptoms or jaundice, the azole should be discontinued immediately.

Unlike fluconazole and itraconazole, ketoconazole has significant effects on the endocrine system. Ketoconazole blocks synthesis of testosterone and may lead to oligospermia, decreased libido, impotence, and gynecomastia. At higher doses, ketoconazole can block adrenal steroid synthesis. The cortisol response to adrenocorticotropic hormone has been blunted for 8 hours after an oral dose but returns to normal by 16 hours. Because of the suppressive effects on adrenal steroid synthesis, higher doses of ketoconazole are given as single daily doses to allow recovery of adrenal hormone secretion. All of the endocrine effects are dose dependent and almost always reversible. A syndrome of severe hypokalemia, hypertension, adrenal insufficiency, and rhabdomyolysis has been reported in patients taking itraconazole at doses of 600 mg/day.

All three azoles are tetratogenic, and embryotoxic effects have been noted in animal studies. The azoles are secreted in human milk and are not recommended for nursing mothers.

THERAPEUTIC INDICATIONS. For specific indications, dosage, and duration, refer to the chapter on the particular systemic fungal infection.

Bibliography

Branch RA: Prevention of amphotericin B–induced renal impairment: A review on the use of sodium supplementation. Arch Intern Med 148:2389, 1988.

Burks LC, Aisner J, Fortner CL, Wiernik, PH: Meperidine for the treatment of shaking chills and fever. Arch Intern Med 140:483, 1980.

Como JA, Dismukes WE: Oral azole drugs as systemic antifungal therapy. N Engl J Med 330:263, 1994.

Denning DW, Lee JY, Hostetler JS, et al: NIAID Mycoses Study Group multicenter trial of oral itraconazole therapy for invasive aspergillosis. Am J Med 97:135, 1994.

Galgiani JN: Susceptibility testing of fungi: Current status of the standardization process. Antimicrob Agents Chemother 37:2517, 1993.

Graybill JR: Lipid formulations for amphotericin B: Does the emperor need new clothes? Ann Intern Med 124:921, 1996.

Lewis JH, Zimmerman HJ, Benson GD, Ishak KG: Hepatic injury associated with ketoconazole therapy—Analysis of 33 cases. Gastroenterology 83:503, 1984.

Mauger TF: Havener's Ocular Pharmacology, ed 6. St. Louis, Mosby, 1994, pp 313–319.

Oldfield EC III, Garst PD, Hostettler C, et al: Randomized, double-blind trial of 1- versus 4-hour amphotericin B infusion durations. Antimicrob Agents Chemother 43:1402, 1990.

Rex JH, Rinaldi MG, Pfaller MA: Resistance of *Candida* species to fluconazole. Antimicrob Agents Chemother 39:1, 1995.

Sabra R, Branch RA: Amphotericin B nephrotoxicity. Drug Safety 5:95, 1990.

Sonino N: The use of ketoconazole as an inhibitor of steroid production. N Engl J Med 317:812, 1987.

Systemic Antifungal Drugs. The Medical Letter 39:86, 1997.

Tucker RM, Denning DW, Hanson LH, et al: Interaction of azoles with rifampin, phenytoin, and carbamazepine: In vitro and clinical observations. Clin Infect Dis 14:165, 1992.

Wingard JR, Merz WG, Rinaldi MG, et al: Increase in *Candida krusei* infection among patients with bone marrow transplantation and neutropenia treated prophylactically with fluconazole. N Engl J Med 325:1274, 1991.

85 *General Principles*

G. Thomas Strickland

■ PARASITISM

DEFINITIONS. Parasite comes from the Greek word *parasitos* and is defined as "a plant or an animal which lives upon or within another living organism at whose expense it obtains some advantage." Parasitism is a type of *symbiosis*, in which an intimate and obligatory relationship exists between two heterospecific organisms. The *parasite*, generally the smaller of the two, is usually metabolically dependent on its host. This association may be beneficial to both *(mutualism)*, beneficial to one with little effect on the other *(commensalism)*, or beneficial to one and detrimental to the other *(parasitism)*. The term parasite is generally reserved for animal species of protozoa, helminths, and arthropods.

NATURAL HISTORY

Host. The organism on or within which the parasite lives is called the *host*. The life cycle of the parasite may take place in a single host species (e.g., *Entamoeba histolytica*—man), in two host species (e.g., *Plasmodium vivax*—man and mosquito), or in more than two host species (e.g., *Clonorchis sinensis*—man, snail, and cyprinoid fish).

A *definitive host* (e.g., man for *Taenia saginata*) is one in which a parasite undergoes sexual reproduction. Man may be the only definitive host for some parasites (e.g., *Trichomonas vaginalis*), whereas others may have several definitive hosts (e.g., bushbuck, other game animals, and man for *Trypanosoma brucei rhodesiense*). Animals that harbor a parasite that is pathogenic for other animals are called *reservoir hosts* (e.g., dogs for *Leishmania tropica*). Parasites that have reservoir hosts (e.g., *Brugia malayi*) are more difficult to eradicate than those that do not (e.g., *Wuchereria bancrofti*); the reservoir host serves as an alternate in the life cycle, thus increasing the chance of transmission and survival.

The animal in which the larval or asexual stage habitates (e.g., freshwater snail for *Schistosoma* species) is known as the *intermediate host*. A *transfer or paratenic host* (e.g., large predator fish for *Diphyllobothrium latum*) is not necessary for the completion of the life cycle of the parasite but is utilized as a temporary refuge and vehicle for reaching the obligatory or definitive host. An *incidental host* is one that is accidentally infected and is not required for the parasite's survival or development (e.g., man for *Toxoplasma gondii*).

Vector. A *vector* (from the Latin *vehere*, to carry), usually an arthropod, transfers an infectious agent from one host to another. The parasite may develop or multiply within the body of the vector before becoming infective, in which case the vector is called a *biologic vector*. Biologic vectors are actually hosts—definitive hosts in the case of anopheline mosquitoes for human *Plasmodium* species or intermediate hosts in the case of *Cyclops* species for *Dracunculus medinensis*. A *mechanical vector* carries a parasite from one host to another but is not essential for the parasite's life cycle (e.g., houseflies for *Entamoeba histolytica*).

■ PROTOZOA

DEFINITIONS. *Protozoa*, derived from the Greek words *protos*, meaning first or primary, and *zoon*, meaning animal, is a phylum comprising some of the morphologically simplest organisms of the animal kingdom. Most species are unicellular and are microscopic in size; most are free-living, but some have commensalistic, mutualistic, or parasitic relationships. Approximately 10,000 of the described living species are parasitic. Protozoa infect most vertebrate and invertebrate species and have developed the capacity to adapt to living in most host organs.

The parasitic protozoa, unlike almost all helminths, can replicate (sexually, asexually, or both ways) within the host's body—a phenomenon that largely explains their survival as well as the overwhelming infections that develop from single exposures.

CLASSIFICATION. It remains convenient to divide protozoa pathogenic to man into four phyla or subphyla (or superclasses in the case of the sporozoa) according to their type of locomotion: (1) Sarcodina (amebae); (2) Mastigophora (flagellates); (3) Ciliophora (ciliates); and (4) Sporozoa.

Sarcodina. *Ameboid* movements produce pseudopods in the Sarcodina. Reproduction is almost exclusively asexual, usually by binary fission. Amebae that infect man include *Entamoeba histolytica* (Chapter 86). Other species of Sarcodina that can be either parasitic (e.g., *Naegleria fowleri*, normally a free-living organism) or mutualistic or commensalistic (e.g., *Entamoeba hartmanni* and *Entamoeba coli*) are covered in Chapters 90 and 99. Most are parasites or commensals of the gastrointestinal tract.

Mastigophora. *Flagella* produce a whiplike motion. Most species, like those of the Sarcodina, have both *cysts* (transmission stage) and *trophozoites* (proliferative stage). Flagellates that infect man include *Giardia lamblia* (Chapter 87), *Trichomonas vaginalis* (Chapter 91), *Trypanosoma brucei gambiense*, *T. b. rhodesiense*, and *T. cruzi* (Chapters 93 and 94), and *Leishmania* species (Chapter 95). Species in this group are capable of infecting many different tissues and cells.

Ciliophora. *Cilia* supply the motion in this subphylum. They have two kinds of nuclei, a macronucleus and a micronucleus. Reproduction is by asexual transverse binary fission and sexual conjugation. *Balantidium coli*, the largest intestinal parasite of man, is a ciliate (Chapter 90.1).

Sporozoa. Protozoa in this subphylum typically have no locomotor organs in the adult stage(s) and reproduce alternately by asexual multiplication (schizogony) and sexual multiplication (sporogony). They are exclusively parasitic. Pathogens of man in this group include *Plasmodium* species (Chapter 92), *Toxoplasma gondii* (Chapter 97), *Cryptosporidium parvum* (Chapter 88), *Cyclospora* (Chapter 89), and *Isospora*, *Sarcospora*, *Microspora*, and *Cystoisospora* (Chapters 90.2 and 100). Based upon ribosomal gene analysis, *Pneumocystis carinii* (Chapter 97) is now considered to be a fungus. However, it obviously still remains somewhere between protozoa and fungi and can best be covered in this text among the former.

PHYSIOLOGY. With the exception of the Sarcodina trophozoites, which have an ectoplastic covering, protozoa have cell membranes.

Ectoplasm. Across this membrane, nutrients can be actively transported, phagocytized, or moved by pinocytosis.

Some species have a peristome through which food passes directly into the cytosome and cytopharynx to the endoplasm.

Endoplasm. Protozoa are eukaryotic; some have multiple nuclei. Cytoplasmic inclusions and a variety of organelles are responsible for metabolic, reproductive, and protective functions.

Reproduction. Asexual or binary fission-type reproduction is characteristic of the Sarcodina, Mastigophora, and Ciliophora. In some species, asexual reproduction is more complex. Sexual reproduction in the Sporozoa always takes place in the definitive host (e.g., mosquito for malarial parasites, cat for *T. gondii*); it results in the formation of a zygote. Asexual reproduction occurs in the intermediate host (e.g., man for malarial parasites and for *T. gondii*).

TRANSMISSION

Intestinal Protozoa. These are usually transmitted from host to host by the fecal-oral route via food and water. Many species have a cystic stage that is capable of resisting adverse environmental conditions (e.g., drying, heat, and cold). *Toxoplasma gondii* is also transmitted by ingestion of undercooked meat (contaminated with cysts) or soil, food, or other vehicles contaminated with cat feces (contaminated with oocysts).

Blood and Tissue Protozoa. Most of these have two hosts—vertebrate (man) and an invertebrate vector (arthropod). The parasite is usually transmitted by the vector's bite (e.g., in infections with *Plasmodium* species, *T. b. gambiense* and *T. b. rhodesiense*, *Leishmania* species, or *Babesia* species) or by exposure to contaminated vector feces (e.g., in infections with *T. cruzi*).

MAGNITUDE OF THE HEALTH PROBLEM. Protozoal infections cause man more disease and misery than any other group of infectious agents.

In the Tropics

Malaria. Infections with *Plasmodium* species are one of the greatest causes of mortality and morbidity in the world today, particularly in children under 5 years of age and in pregnant women. The World Health Organization (WHO) has given up the goal of global eradication of malaria and has set a long-term aim of control of transmission with drugs and insecticides in areas where this is feasible, and control of disease with selective chemoprophylaxis and/or chemotherapy where transmission control is not possible (e.g., most of sub-Saharan Africa). Malaria was a greater global medical problem in the 1980s and 1990s than it was in the 1970s and will be even more of a scourge in the 21st century. The continuing development of resistance to insecticides by the anopheline vectors has meant that new chemicals are required, and these are too expensive to be used by those who need them.

Multiple drug–resistant *P. falciparum* has spread from Southeast Asia into the Indian subcontinent, the Western Pacific, and sub-Saharan Africa. It is widespread in most malaria-endemic areas of South America. During the mid-1990s, some strains of *P. vivax* in Indonesia, New Guinea, the Solomon Islands, and northern South America have developed resistance to chloroquine, complicating and increasing the cost of treatment of this species as well.

Estimates of the numbers infected and dying from malaria are totally inaccurate. In endemic areas, most individuals exposed to infectious bites have low levels of parasitemia. Many, frequently children, have high intensity parasitemias that are often associated with illness (Chapter 92). Severe malarial anemia kills the youngest children, whereas older children and sometimes adults die of cerebral malaria. Malaria also causes hypoglycemia, which is often confused with cerebral malaria and may be fatal if not specifically treated.

African Trypanosomiasis. Infection with either *Trypanosoma brucei gambiense* or *T. b. rhodesiense* almost always causes severe human illness. If untreated, it is fatal; fortunately, however, relatively few people are infected. *Trypanosoma brucei brucei*, which is morphologically identical to the subspecies causing human sleeping sickness (Chapter 93), causes infection in cattle (nagana) across much of Central and East Africa. Thus, cattle raising is limited, greatly interfering with economic development and with the nutritional status of the entire area but probably protecting the environment from overgrazing, which has occurred in much of Africa. The prospects for reducing the impact of African trypanosomiasis are slim: (1) Chemotherapeutic agents lack efficacy and safety; (2) control of transmission is difficult because of the habits of the tsetse fly; and (3) vaccine development is hampered by the ability of the parasite to evade the immune response by varying its antigens.

American Trypanosomiasis. *Trypanosoma cruzi* affects as many as 15 million people living in South and Central America. Although acute infections may be fatal, most infections are not detected (Chapter 94). Unfortunately, chronic complications years later often lead to severe disability and death from Chagas' cardiopathy and the "mega" syndromes. The poor who live in crudely built huts infested with the vector, "the kissing bug," contract Chagas' disease. Infection can be transmitted transplacentally from mother to fetus and by blood transfusion, and with increasing immigration from Central and South America to the United States, there is concern regarding the safety of blood transfusions. There are still no efficacious and safe drugs for treating the infection, particularly the chronic form. The large and varied animal reservoirs make transmission control more difficult, and vaccine development remains in the future.

Leishmaniasis. *Leishmania* species infect millions worldwide and cause clinical syndromes varying from a minimal, single, self-healing chronic ulceration (urban oriental sore) to a severe and often fatal generalized febrile illness (kala-azar [Chapter 95]). *Leishmania* species causing these different syndromes appear morphologically identical. Polymorphisms can be detected, however, by using biochemical, immunologic, and genetic techniques that correlate with epidemiologic and clinical differences. Better diagnosis has demonstrated more cases of subclinical and mild infections than of the characteristic diseases. Patients with silent chronic infections with species causing visceral disease, i.e., *L. donovani*, *L. infantum*, or *L. chagasi*, sometimes develop visceral leishmaniasis when they become infected with HIV. Tens of thousands have been infected with *L. donovani*, and thousands have died of visceral leishmaniasis during the past 20 years associated with the civil war and famine in southern Sudan.

In Temperate Climates. All the above noted protozoal infections are potential dangers to travelers to endemic areas from more developed countries (Chapter 142), and all should be suspected in emigrants from developing countries (Chapter 148). Clinical illness due to pneumocystosis, cryptosporidiosis, toxoplasmosis, primary amebic meningoencephalitis, and babesiosis also are more common in patients who have HIV infections or are otherwise immunosuppressed.

Both giardiasis and cryptosporidiosis have caused massive outbreaks of diarrhea when they have contaminated municipal water systems (Chapters 87 and 88). The latter is a particularly difficult problem in patients with HIV infections, since there is no effective curative treatment. Cyclosporidiosis has caused diarrhea in North Americans consuming raspberries imported from Central America (Chapter 89).

Trichomoniasis. *Trichomonas vaginalis* is one of the most common causes of vaginal irritation and discharge among women in temperate climates (Chapter 91). Infection with this organism is very contagious and sexually transmitted and can cause nongonococcal urethritis in both males and females. Nitroimidazole drugs provide the best means of cure. There is no evidence that these compounds cause congenital malformations in pregnant women treated for trichomoniasis; the recommendation that treatment be withheld during pregnancy is not supported.

NEW DEVELOPMENTS. There have been several developments in protozoology since the last edition of this book was published.

Entamoeba dispar. Although morphologically identical, isoenzyme electrophoresis and DNA analyses have clearly shown that there are two separate species of what was formerly called *E. histolytica*: the organism causing invasive amebiasis, *E. histolytica*, and a gut commensal, *E. dispar*. At present there is no clinically available reliable way to separate the pathogenic from the commensal species other than on clinical grounds, the microscopic detection of erythrocytes in trophozoites, or the presence of amebic antibodies in the blood.

Malaria Vaccine. The parasite can evade the immune response by several mechanisms, of which antigenic variation is believed to be one of the most important. The existence of these evasive mechanisms makes malaria vaccine development very difficult. Vaccine candidates are being developed from three stages of the malaria parasites, for both *P. falciparum* and *P. vivax*: (1) the sporozoite stage (to prevent infection); (2) the asexual blood stages (to prevent clinical disease); and (3) the gamete stage (to prevent transmission to the feeding vectors). The workable vaccine will probably be a "cocktail" of several antigens from two or three of the parasite stages. As of 1999, none of the different malaria vaccines has shown efficacy during clinical trials.

Chemotherapy.

Malaria. The spread of multidrug-resistant falciparum malaria has increased the difficulty and the cost of treating and controlling that disease (Chapter 92). Mefloquine is available for treatment and prophylaxis in many areas having multiple drug–resistant *P. falciparum*. However, its use should be limited because of cost (which is considerably more than for chloroquine) and potential for toxicity and for the parasite to develop resistance to its action. The combination of sulfadoxine and pyrimethamine is still effective when used in many areas to treat chloroquine-resistant falciparum malaria and is less costly than mefloquine and the other newer agents. Quinine and a tetracycline are used effectively in many areas

where chloroquine-resistant *P. falciparum* is present. The Chinese-developed herbal drug artemisinin and its derivatives are being extensively used to treat multidrug-resistant *P. falciparum* infections. These agents have a very rapid onset of action but have a high recrudescent rate when used alone. Therefore, they are best used in combination with another antimalarial, e.g., mefloquine.

Other Protozoal Infections. There is still no effective treatment for cryptosporidiosis (Chapter 88) or for babesiosis (Chapter 96). The treatment currently available for African (Chapter 93) and American (Chapter 94) trypanosomiasis has limited effect and is frequently toxic. However, evaluation of potential new therapeutic agents for treating these infections is continuing. WHO-sponsored clinical trials have evaluated 7-day and 14-day courses of eflornithine for treating late stage *T. brucei gambiense* sleeping sickness. Both regimens were more effective than other treatments.

Acquired Immunodeficiency Syndrome (AIDS). Infection with human immunodeficiency virus (HIV) impairs cellular immunity and leads to opportunistic infections (Chapter 22). Some of these are included among the criteria for diagnosing AIDS, and other protozoa that have either rarely or not previously caused infections in humans are being detected in patients with HIV infections (Chapter 100).

Infection Without Illness. Both *Giardia lamblia* (Chapter 87) and *Entamoeba histolytica* (Chapter 86) are commonly found in male homosexuals. However, neither appears to cause increased illness in those who are HIV positive. The immune defects produced by HIV infection do not appear to favor ameba invasion or *Giardia* pathogenicity. Malaria also does not cause illness more frequently in AIDS or in HIV-positive individuals.

Disease Mechanisms. *Pneumocystis carinii*, *Toxoplasma gondii*, and *Leishmania donovani* cause endogenous disease in those who have HIV infections, whereas *Cryptosporidium* and *Isospora* cause exogenous infections of the gastrointestinal tract. An HIV-induced defect in the immune response can interfere with containment of chronic asymptomatic infections. The pathology occurs where the latent stages of the parasite primarily persist: *P. carinii* in the lung, *T. gondii* in the brain, and *L. donovani* in the liver, spleen, and bone marrow.

Opportunistic parasitic infections are not as frequent as expected in developing countries. This may be because many HIV-positive individuals die of more virulent agents causing bacterial septicemias, pneumonias, and meningitis before their immune response is suppressed sufficiently for endogenous opportunistic agents to become pathogenic.

SECTION A   Intestinal and Genital Infections

86 *Amebiasis*

Terry F.H.G. Jackson and Vinodh Gathiram

DEFINITION. Amebiasis is an infection caused by the ameba *Entamoeba histolytica*, which grows in vitro at 37°C and produces quadrinucleated cysts approximately 10 to 15 μ in diameter. *E. histolytica* is a tissue-invasive pathogen.

The disease profile observed relates directly to the extent of invasion and ranges from subclinical to deep tissue invasion. Intestinal amebiasis has a variable clinical picture and may result in acute or chronic symptoms. At one extreme of the clinical spectrum is acute amebic dysentery, which can be life threatening. At the opposite extreme is the asymptomatic cyst passer. The majority (approximately 90%) of those infected with *E. histolytica* have asymptomatic intestinal infections. Some patients present with frequent unformed stools, lower abdominal cramps, fatigue, intermittent constipation and diarrhea, and excessive abdominal distention and gas.

Extensive tissue invasion gives rise to serious complications, which may follow symptomatic or asymptomatic intestinal infection, including amebic liver abscess, pleuropulmonary amebiasis, amebic pericarditis, ameboma or amebic stricture, and, rarely, cerebral, genital, or cutaneous amebiasis.

E. histolytica and *E. dispar* are morphologically identical. These amebae are now documented as separate species. Until recently, however, they were considered to be one species, *E. histolytica*. This distinction has had a major impact on our understanding of amebiasis.

HISTORY

Early Investigations. Since its first discovery in 1875 by Fedor Losch, the causative organism of invasive amebiasis, *E. histolytica*, has been the center of much controversy. Losch described the presence of motile trophozoites in the dysenteric stools of a Saint Petersburg (Russia) laborer. He named the parasites *Amoeba coli*. Losch never attributed etiologic significance to the presence of these amebae in the stool of patients even though he successfully infected four of five dogs per rectum with them and demonstrated identical ulcerative lesions teeming with these *A. coli* in both the dogs and the patients at autopsy. He attributed the dysentery to bacteria and concluded that the amebae merely served to perpetuate the inflammatory reaction.

During the next 16 years, many other researchers confirmed Losch's observation of concomitant infections with bacteria and amebae in dysenteric patients without making the association between the presence of amebae and dysentery. Reporting on their classic study in 1891, Councilman and Lafleur (Baltimore) described the presence of *A. coli* in bacteriologically sterile liver abscess, thereby demonstrating the pathogenic potential of the organism independent of concomitant bacteria. They called the parasite *Amoeba dysenteriae*.

The demonstration of cyst production by these pathogenic amebae enabled Quincke and Roos, 2 years later, to complete the picture of the life cycle of *A. coli*; however, they failed to adequately describe the specific characteristics of the cyst, e.g., the number of nuclei. Interestingly, they described successful infection of cats by both inoculation of trophozoites per rectum and feeding of cysts per os. This is important because many authorities believe to this day that only primates can be successfully infected orally with cysts.

In 1895, healthy individuals were shown to asymptomatically harbor a parasite named *Entamoeba coli* by Casagrandi and Barbagallo. The generic name *Entamoeba* was therefore established by these workers. Schaudinn (1903) reserved the name *E. coli* for the nonpathogenic species and introduced the name *E. histolytica* for the dysentery-producing ameba. During the next few years, various researchers recognized other *Entamoeba* species, e.g., the quadrinucleate *E. tetragena* and the so-called small *E. minuta*. This culminated when Kuenen and Swellengrebel (1913) concluded that the life cycle of *Entamoeba* had three forms: (1) the virulent histolytica stage in dysenteric stools, (2) the avirulent stage in normal and convalescent subjects' stools, and (3) a cystic stage, which was the progeny of only the avirulent forms and was responsible for propagation of the species. According to them, the histolytica phase, therefore, did not have any direct part in the life cycle of the parasite.

The convoluted picture that had developed by this time could have been resolved by the risky but nevertheless classic work of Walker and Sellards, who in 1913 fed cysts and trophozoites of *E. histolytica, E. coli,* and free-living amebae from the Manila water supply to human volunteers. They proved conclusively that both free-living amebae and *E. coli* were nonpathogenic to humans. Of 20 men fed different strains of *E. coli*, 17 became parasitized and none developed

symptoms; they deduced that "*E. coli* is an obligatory parasite . . . and that it is nonpathogenic and consequently plays no role in the etiology of entamoebic dysentery." Furthermore, they stated that *E. tetragena* was identical to *E. histolytica* and that *E. minuta* was the pre-encysted stage of *E. histolytica*. However, the most definitive of their feeding experiments was accomplished by feeding cysts from a carrier convalescing from amebic dysentery to three volunteers. This resulted in two of them developing amebic dysentery while the third was an asymptomatic cyst passer. Cysts obtained from one of the dysenteric subjects colonized but failed to produce dysentery in a further three volunteers. Two other volunteers fed with cysts from the asymptomatic carrier became asymptomatically parasitized, and when cysts from one of these subjects were in turn fed to four other persons, dysentery developed in one, two others were asymptomatically colonized, and the fourth was not successfully colonized. This study proved that *E. histolytica* can give rise to both invasive amebiasis and asymptomatic infection; furthermore, cysts from asymptomatically infected subjects can cause invasive amebiasis. Although this study provided the key to understanding *Entamoeba* spp., insufficient attention was paid to the work, and 70 to 80 contentious years followed before modern biochemical methods were used to reconfirm these findings.

Theories to Explain Relationship Between Infection and Disease. By 1917, it was widely accepted that the quadrinucleate cysts of the tetragena type were those of *E. histolytica*. A gross discrepancy between the prevalence of the parasite and active disease became increasingly apparent; furthermore, it was not possible to predict the appearance of dysentery in asymptomatic infected individuals. In attempting to explain the poor correlation between the prevalence of cyst passers and that of invasive disease, three broad schools of thought developed:

1. *Promethean Theory.* This theory is based on the mythical Greek character Prometheus, who had his tissues devoured all day by an eagle after nocturnal regeneration to compensate for the ravages of the previous day. *E. histolytica* was perceived to be an obligatory tissue parasite that normally survived in equilibrium with its host, causing development of disease in its host only when the host lost the ability to tolerate the parasite. Major concerns with this theory were raised when it was realized that the parasites in in vitro culture could survive on bacteria in the absence of human tissues.

2. *Commensal Theory.* *E. histolytica* was viewed as a gut commensal that was responsible for propagation of the species. Some yet unconfirmed stimulus (e.g., nature of gut flora, dietary implications, rapid passage) caused the ameba to mutate into a tissue-invading form that lost its capability of cyst production and therefore effectively committed suicide because transmission to another host was impossible. This concept was popular with scientists until recent times, even though the hypothetical trigger responsible for the mutation escaped acceptable scientific resolution.

3. *Two-Species Theory.* Emile Brumpt, in 1928, noting the difference in prevalence of invasive amebiasis in tropical climates and temperate areas, put forward the concept that *E. histolytica* comprised two morphologically identical species. The one he named *E. dispar* was nonpathogenic and confined to temperate zones, where despite a relatively high prevalence of asymptomatic carriers, the prevalence of disease was low. The other, *E. dysenteriae*, was the pathogenic species (as its name implies) responsible for invasive amebiasis; in addition, he claimed that

this species was more prevalent in tropical zones where the prevalence of disease was considerably higher. In his opinion, it was possible to have healthy carriers of *E. dysenteriae* with mild tissue invasion, the amebae in such cases feeding predominantly on bacteria. If for some reason the host's defenses were compromised, *E. dysenteriae* invaded the deeper tissues, giving rise to symptoms. Such changes in the host defense mechanisms, however, did not have any effect on the invasive capability of *E. dispar*. *E. dispar* and *E. dysenteriae* had independent life cycles, both producing quadrinucleate cysts that were morphologically identical.

Although Brumpt's hypothesis best described the epidemiology of the parasite and has proved to be closest to current beliefs based on modern scientific analysis of the organism, it was never widely accepted during the following 50 years.

Recent Investigations. Peter Sargeaunt, working from the London School of Hygiene and Tropical Medicine, introduced isoenzyme electrophoresis to study polymorphism in the intestinal protozoa of humans. Between 1978 and 1988, he worked with scientists from Mexico, India, Japan, Australia, Israel, and most extensively South Africa. The outcome after studying approximately 10,000 amebic isolates was the realization that Emile Brumpt had been correct and that there were indeed two morphologically identical species that had up to this stage been grouped together as one organism, *E. histolytica*. As early as 1982, he suggested that we revert to the nomenclature proposed by Emile Brumpt—*E. dispar* and *E. dysenteriae*.

Shortly after this, Egbert Tannich of Bernhard Nocht Institute in Hamburg, Germany, elegantly confirmed the observations by Sargeaunt by means of DNA studies. Louis Diamond of the National Institutes of Health, working with Graham Clark, went on to reconfirm Tannich's observations using riboprinting; they also pointed out that the estimated genetic distance between the two species was as great as that between humans and mice. In a more recent publication, they proposed that these two species be named *E. dispar* and *E. histolytica*. The latter is the causative organism of invasive

amebiasis; the former is widely believed to be a gut commensal. This nomenclature is now in use worldwide.

ETIOLOGY AND LIFE CYCLE. *E. histolytica* is the most important of the intestinal amebae of humans. The three distinct stages in the life cycle (Fig. 86–1) are the trophozoite, precyst, and cyst. The cyst, the infective stage, is ingested by contact with fecally contaminated food, water, or fingers. Both young uninucleate and more mature quadrinucleate cysts are infective. Ingested cysts pass through the stomach, and excystation occurs in the lower small bowel. A metacystic ameba containing the four cystic nuclei emerges from each cyst. Cytoplasmic division occurs, and eight small metacystic trophozoites are formed. These grow to full size. Cysts thus provide for both transmission and reproduction. The uninucleate trophozoite is the actively growing and multiplying stage, having a single nucleus and pseudopods. These pass along the intestinal canal until conditions favorable for colonization are found. This can occur anywhere in the large bowel but happens most frequently in the cecal area. Multiplication is by rapid and repeated binary fission. Depending on various parasite and host factors, trophozoites may invade the tissue of the large intestine, probably by both lytic and physical means, and may also metastasize to the liver and other extraintestinal sites. In the presence of dysentery or diarrhea, trophozoites do not become encysted during their evacuation. However, if bowel passage is not rapid (e.g., occurs with semiformed or formed stools), as trophozoites are carried toward the rectum, they eliminate food vacuoles and other cytoplasmic inclusions and become precysts. The precyst then forms a cyst wall and develops from a uninucleate into a mature quadrinucleate cyst. These cysts facilitate transmission to the next host. Cysts form only in the intestinal lumen, although immature cysts may mature outside the body under favorable conditions.

DISTRIBUTION AND PREVALENCE. *E. histolytica* has a worldwide distribution, being found in arctic, temperate, and tropical climates. It is more prevalent in tropical areas, where invasive disease is frequent and symptoms tend to be severe. This is related to poorer sanitation and nutrition and de-

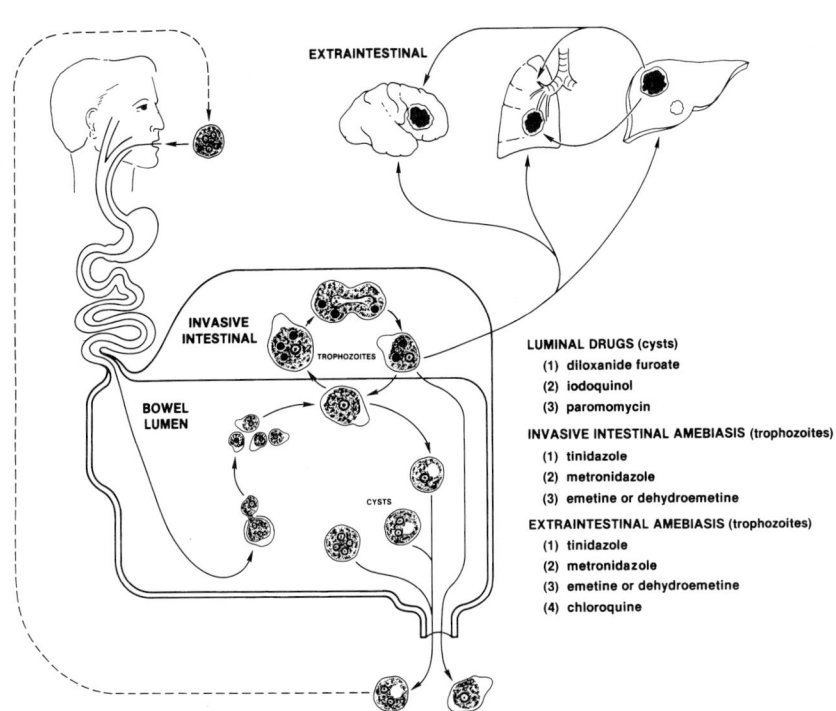

EXTRAINTESTINAL

INVASIVE INTESTINAL

TROPHOZOITES

BOWEL LUMEN

CYSTS

LUMINAL DRUGS (cysts)
(1) diloxanide furoate
(2) iodoquinol
(3) paromomycin

INVASIVE INTESTINAL AMEBIASIS (trophozoites)
(1) tinidazole
(2) metronidazole
(3) emetine or dehydroemetine

EXTRAINTESTINAL AMEBIASIS (trophozoites)
(1) tinidazole
(2) metronidazole
(3) emetine or dehydroemetine
(4) chloroquine

***Figure* 86–1.** Life cycle of *E. histolytica* showing sites of infection and action of chemotherapeutic agents.

creased resistance in those living in tropical climates, as well as other poorly understood factors.

It is difficult to determine accurately the true prevalence of amebiasis. Populations surveyed may differ, and the prevalence in certain groups is higher than in the general population, e.g., in families of infected patients, in male homosexuals, and in persons in mental hospitals, prisons, and institutions for children. Differences in laboratory techniques, competence of laboratory personnel, stool collection methods, and number of specimens examined from each person may lead to either underdiagnosis or overdiagnosis. In some earlier surveys, the now recognized nonpathogen *E. hartmanni* was included with *E. histolytica* in prevalence figures. A difference of opinion about what constitutes amebic disease also clouds attempts at establishing valid geographic prevalence data. Some tend to include all unidentified dysenteries in the amebic category. Walsh has estimated that approximately 10% of the world population carries the parasite, although a much smaller percentage has the disease.

Recognized high-risk areas for acquiring amebiasis include Mexico, the western portion of South America, West Africa, South Africa (particularly in the black population), parts of the Middle East, and southern and Southeast Asia. Invasive disease is more common in these areas. Many of the cases identified in North America and in Europe are imported, but a level of endemicity is present, and occasional waterborne epidemics have occurred. Approximately 40 years ago, it was estimated that 5 to 10% of the population of the United States were passing amebic organisms in their stools. The generally accepted figure now is <3% but is higher in institutionalized individuals, male homosexuals, Native Americans on reservations, and some lower socioeconomic areas of the country.

EPIDEMIOLOGY

Infectious Stage. Motile trophozoites passed with diarrheal or dysenteric stools can survive only briefly outside the body, are destroyed by gastric secretions, and therefore have no role in transmission.

Cysts are relatively hardy and can survive outside the body long enough to be ingested. They are sensitive to desiccation and to temperatures of >40°C or <5°C and are killed almost immediately by boiling. They are relatively resistant to chlorine, not being destroyed by concentrations usually used for water purification. Cysts may remain viable for 1 month at 4°C in both sewage and natural surface water. Viable cysts may be recovered from the intestines and feces of flies and cockroaches. Cysts have survived for as long as 48 hours at 20 to 25°C on foods, e.g., cheese, bread, green salads, and fruits.

Strains of E. *histolytica* and E. *dispar*. *E. histolytica* is unique among the amebae of humans in its ability to invade tissue. *E. dispar*, as discussed earlier, is a morphologically identical species that is nonpathogenic and noninvasive. Sargeaunt has shown that *E. histolytica* and *E. dispar* occur worldwide as a spectrum of zymodemes (strains determined by characteristic isoenzyme patterns). This has been confirmed by Clark and Diamond using riboprinting. Isoenzymes, particularly phosphoglucomutase and hexokinase, allow for consistent differentiation of pathogenic *E. histolytica* from the morphologically identical nonpathogenic species *E. dispar*. It is important to note that *E. histolytica* can give rise to both invasive amebiasis and asymptomatic infection. Longitudinal studies of asymptomatic carriers of *E. histolytica* indicate that 10% develop invasive disease but the majority spontaneously clear their infections. Seroepidemiologic studies have shown that infections with *E. histolytica* give rise to an equivalently strong serologic response whether or not the infected subject displays symptoms; subclinical invasion is implied in the asymptomatic subjects. This information is useful in epidemiologic investigations, because subjects passing typical quadrinucleate cysts in the presence of a strong serologic response are harboring *E. histolytica*, not *E. dispar*. On the other hand, seronegativity in the presence of such cysts indicates an infection with nonpathogenic *E. dispar*. *E. hartmanni*, formerly known as *small race E. histolytica*, is a separate nonpathogenic species that can be differentiated on the basis of its smaller quandrinucleate cysts and distinct isoenzyme patterns (Chapter 90.6).

Transmission. Potential animal reservoirs of *E. histolytica* and *E. dispar* include monkeys, dogs, and pigs, but these have a very minor role in transmission in comparison with humans, the principal reservoir of infection. Infection with cysts usually occurs by either direct person-to-person transmission or contamination of water or food. In institutionalized groups (e.g., in homes for the mentally retarded or the elderly and in prisons), transmission is often by direct fecal contamination of the environment. Daycare centers for young children have been implicated in the transmission of giardiasis (Chapter 87) and, to a lesser extent, amebiasis. High rates of infection with *E. dispar* have been recognized in male homosexuals. Transmission is thought to occur during oral-anal sexual practices and is related to sexual promiscuity.

In underdeveloped areas where supplies of pure water are inadequate and often fecally contaminated, amebiasis and other enteric infections have high prevalences. Remarkable waterborne epidemics of amebiasis have also occurred in the United States. In some areas, contaminated water or sewage is used to grow or freshen vegetables before selling them. Human excreta, or night soil, is used as a fertilizer in growing vegetables, making ingestion of leafy and root vegetables especially hazardous. Contaminated water can be used in making salads and cold drinks, and contamination of cold foods can occur from the fecally soiled fingers of food handlers. The extent of the latter problem is difficult to measure but is thought to be considerable in developing countries and may occur to a lesser extent in the developed countries. Where flies and cockroaches are numerous and have access to feces and then to unprotected foodstuffs, these insects may cause individual or group infections. Persons of all ages are susceptible to infection, but the rate is lower in infants and young children. Females are as likely to be infected as males, but invasive amebiasis is much more common in males. Racial differences in prevalence and pathogenicity appear to be determined less by genetic factors than by socioeconomic status.

PATHOGENESIS AND PATHOLOGY. Excystment occurs in the small intestine; it is influenced by the host's digestive enzymes, the quantity of food ingested, and the velocity of intestinal transit. The resulting small metacystic trophozoites are carried in the fecal stream into the cecum, where various factors allow colonization and tissue invasion by *E. histolytica* strains with virulent capabilities. If trophozoites are abundant, there is an increased chance that some will make contact with the mucosa long enough to grow, multiply, and eventually invade the tissues. Colonization is decreased with bowel hypermotility. Amebae develop only under conditions of very low oxygen tension, as in the colon. A suitable enteric bacterial flora must also be present to lower the oxidation reduction potential and to provide necessary metabolic requirements for amebae remaining outside the tissues on the bowel mucosa or in the glandular crypts.

Characteristics of Virulence. In addition to the pathogenic potential of the strain of ameba, a number of other parasite and host factors influence tissue invasion. The number of amebae ingested is directly related to the frequency and magnitude of intestinal lesions. Pathogenic *E. histolytica* contains surface adhesions that allow attachment to the colonic epithelium. Pathogenic strains of *E. histolytica* have many mechanisms by which they damage tissue and become invasive. These include secreted proteolytic enzymes, release of cell-free cytotoxins, contact-dependent cytolysis, and phagocytosis. Among host factors, the nutritional status of the host is a contributing element, but it is not certain how the host's nutrition influences either the capacity of the parasite to cause tissue damage or the susceptibility of the host to the parasite. Some observations supporting a nutritional role are that invasion is more common in the Bantu of South Africa, whose diet is composed mainly of corn, and that the addition of cholesterol, an important nutritional factor for amebae, to the diet of guinea pigs increases the frequency and size of ulcerous bowel lesions. It is speculated that nutritional deficiencies facilitate disease by means of atrophy of the mucosa, leading to increased susceptibility to lysis and penetration by amebae. Stress may also have a role in the pathogenesis of amebiasis. Thus, asymptomatic female carriers may develop severe amebiasis during pregnancy and the puerperium. Synergism between amebae and the intestinal bacteria might be necessary to produce pathologic effects.

Pathology

Colonic Lesions. Adherence of the parasite to colonic mucins is mediated by a lectin that is inhibited by galactose/N-acetyl-galactosamine. Contact between *E. histolytica* and host cells results in lysis of the target cell. The ameba also contains a number of proteolytic enzymes. The initial lesions of amebic invasion thus begin as small foci of necrosis in the large bowel mucosa. These foci coalesce to form ulcers; some remain small and discrete, whereas others merge to form large ulcers. Polymorphonuclear leukocytes constitute the initial host response to *E. histolytica*. On contact with trophozoites, these neutrophils also undergo lysis, releasing more proteolytic enzymes, which result in further tissue destruction. Inflammatory cells in the lesions are therefore characteristically found at the periphery. Undermining of the ulcer margin and confluence of one or more ulcers lead to sloughing of mucosa and development of broad ulcers with irregular outlines. Amebic ulcers may be disseminated throughout the colon but more frequently are limited to one region, particularly the cecum. Lesions in the terminal ileum rarely occur. The typical amebic ulcer is undermined and is sharply defined, without ragged edges (Fig. 86–2). The crater contains gray necrotic tissue composed of fibrin, cellular debris, and amebic trophozoites. The exudate often raises the undermined mucosa, producing the characteristic flask-shaped ulcer (Fig.

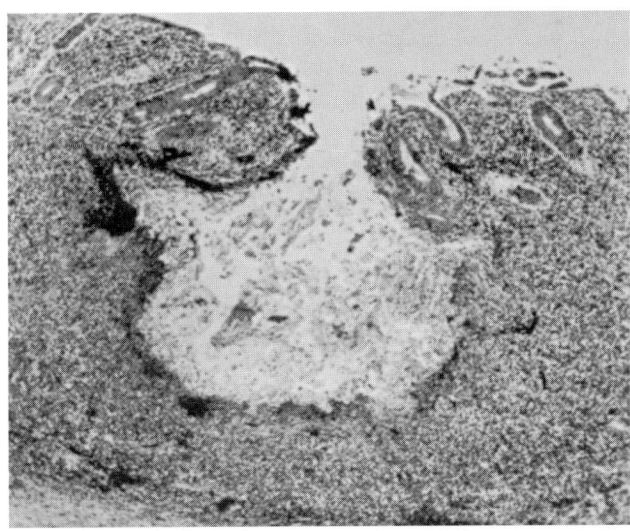

Figure 86–3. Section of colon showing a flask-shaped ulcer involving the mucosa and submucosa. The neutrophilic infiltrate of the border of the lesion suggests secondary bacterial infection. (From Medical Museum Collection, Armed Forces Institute of Pathology.)

86–3). Once deeper tissue invasion has occurred, the amebae invade blood vessels, causing a vasculitis with subsequent thrombosis and infarction, leading to the sharply demarcated lesions of transmural colitis. The mucosa between ulcers may be coated with mucus. Initially there is minimal edema, and the inflammatory response is limited to the margins of the ulcer. As the ulcers widen, however, secondary bacterial infection occurs, leading to accumulation of neutrophils, lymphocytes, histiocytes, plasma cells, and sometimes eosinophils in the ulcer crater and surrounding tissue. If eosinophils are present, Charcot-Leyden crystals may appear in the stool or dysenteric exudate. Trophozoites may be present on the mucosal surface, in the exudate, in the crater, and frequently in the submucosa, muscularis, serosa, and blood vessels (Fig. 86–4). Healing is usually accompanied by fibrosis. Stenosis of the affected colonic segment may occur consequent to healing of a transmural lesion.

Complications of Intestinal Amebiasis. In addition to extraintestinal amebiasis, which originates from initial intestinal involvement, complications of intestinal amebiasis may include perforation with or without peritonitis, intra-abdominal abscess, amebic appendicitis, hemorrhage, ameboma, and amebic stricture.

PERFORATION OF THE INTESTINE. This is the most frequent complication of transmural intestinal amebiasis. It occurs most often in the cecum and next most commonly in the rectosigmoid. Slow leakage into the peritoneal cavity is more common than the more dramatic acute perforation. Peritonitis or intra-abdominal abscess follows either of these situations. In situations where there is a slow leak, the omentum and even healthy bowel may migrate to the area of perforation in an attempt to seal off the affected area, resulting in an abdominal mass. These wraps of omentum and bowel are so effective that signs of visceral perforation are masked. Only when the wraps are disturbed does the patient develop signs of peritonitis and septicemia. Perforation may also occur from the primary involved colon into other hollow organs in the abdominal cavity.

AMEBIC APPENDICITIS. This almost always occurs as a complication of transmural amebic colitis. The amebic appendix is slightly thickened, tends to be gangrenous, and has an apparently intact mucosa except for a gray sanguineous

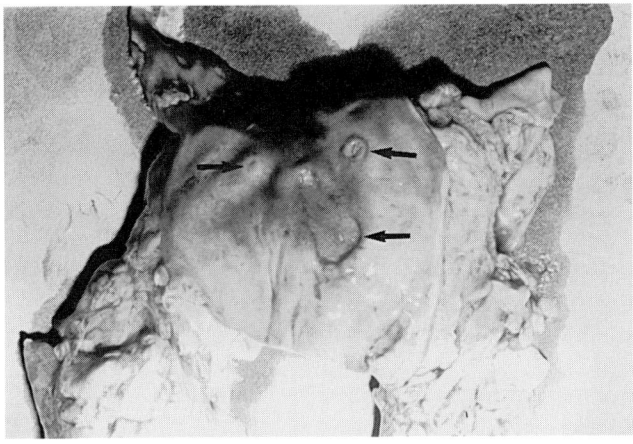

Figure 86–2. Amebic ulcers of the cecum. Note the raised margins *(arrows)* of ulcers. (Courtesy of the Department of Anatomical Pathology, University of Natal Medical School.)

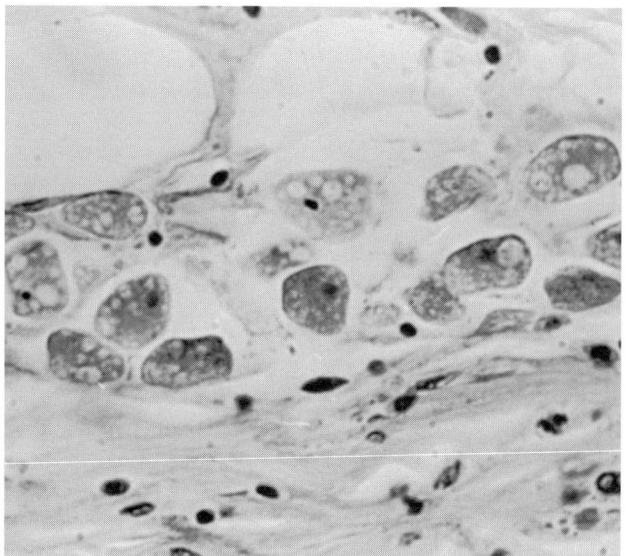

Figure 86–4. Trophozoites of *E. histolytica* in the submucosa of the colon. (Courtesy of the Louisiana State University School of Medicine, New Orleans.)

slough covering irregular superficial ulcers. Microscopic changes resemble those in the colon.

MASSIVE HEMORRHAGE. Fortunately, this is rare. It results from vasculitis involving a large artery. Superficial ulceration may lead to the oozing of numerous small blood vessels in the mucosa.

AMEBOMAS. These are inflammatory thickenings of the bowel wall that are firm, hard, well-defined lesions resembling a carcinoma. They occur in about 1% of patients with colonic amebiasis. Amebomas occur in any area of the colon but are more common in the cecum. They are typical granulomas, consisting of a mass of fibroblasts, collagen, and chronic inflammatory cells, with an obliterating vasculitis, numerous eosinophils and Charcot-Leyden crystals, and relatively few amebae.

AMEBIC STRICTURES. These are also caused by granulation tissue, usually without fibrosis. They are generally single, but occasionally there may be two or more. *E. histolytica* is present in the lesion. Fibrous strictures result after healing of transmural colonic lesions. Strictures are most commonly observed in the anus, rectum, or sigmoid colon.

Hepatic Lesions. Amebic trophozoites may enter the radicles of the portal vein and metastasize to the liver. The liver abscess is an area of liquefactive necrosis caused by a combination of hepatocellular lysis, tissue damage secondary to amebic and neutrophil proteolytic enzymes, and infarction caused by vasculitis and thrombosis.

ABSCESS. One or more of these initial lesions may enlarge into a single abscess or many amebic abscesses (Fig. 86–5). The center of the abscess contains yellow or gray opaque liquid material. This is amorphous and necrotic but does not contain leukocytes as the term *abscess* would suggest. Amebic trophozoites are located in the fibrinous material next to the viable hepatic tissue. The surrounding liver is edematous and may be infiltrated with mixed chronic inflammatory cells. Most abscesses develop in the right lobe of the liver.

Other Extraintestinal Lesions

PLEUROPULMONARY AMEBIASIS. Pleuropulmonary involvement is the next most frequent extraintestinal site after hepatic amebiasis. This is usually a direct extension of a liver abscess through the diaphragm but may, rarely, also develop via hematogenous spread, leading to both pleural and pulmonary involvement. Rupture into the pleural space leads to an amebic empyema or effusion. Rupture into the lung may result in consolidation, abscess formation, or a hepatobronchial fistula. Microscopically, pulmonary amebiasis shows no significant differences from the amebic process in the liver or other organs.

AMEBIC PERICARDITIS. This usually results from extension of a left lobe liver abscess through the diaphragm into the pericardium. More rarely, it may originate from a right lobe abscess or a lung abscess or empyema. A presuppurative phase characterized by either a sympathetic effusion or fibrinous pericarditis may precede actual extension of the infection into the pericardium. Constrictive pericarditis is a rare complication.

CEREBRAL AMEBIASIS. This rare complication develops from hematogenous spread from a liver or lung abscess. Cerebral lesions may be single or multiple and may localize in any area of the brain. Small lesions appear grossly as minute areas of softening with petechial hemorrhages. Larger lesions are necrotic and contain yellowish-green material with hemorrhage.

CUTANEOUS AMEBIASIS. This form, also rare, may develop from a hepatic abscess fistula, by extension of rectal amebiasis to the perianal or genital area, or by infection of the penis during anal intercourse. The ulcers are deep and necrotic and have a raised border.

OTHER LESIONS. Cases of secondary amebic infections of the urinary tract, genital tract, and other organs have very rarely been described.

CLINICAL MANIFESTATIONS. Infection with the nonpathogenic *E. dispar* results in asymptomatic carriage of the parasite. Invasive disease never develops in these patients even in the presence of severe immunosuppression, including AIDS. Mild diarrhea in these patients can usually be attributed to other colonic pathogens. Infection with the pathogenic species, *E. histolytica*, may result in either nondysenteric intestinal amebiasis, with mild to moderate symptoms or asymptomatic cyst passage, or invasive amebiasis.

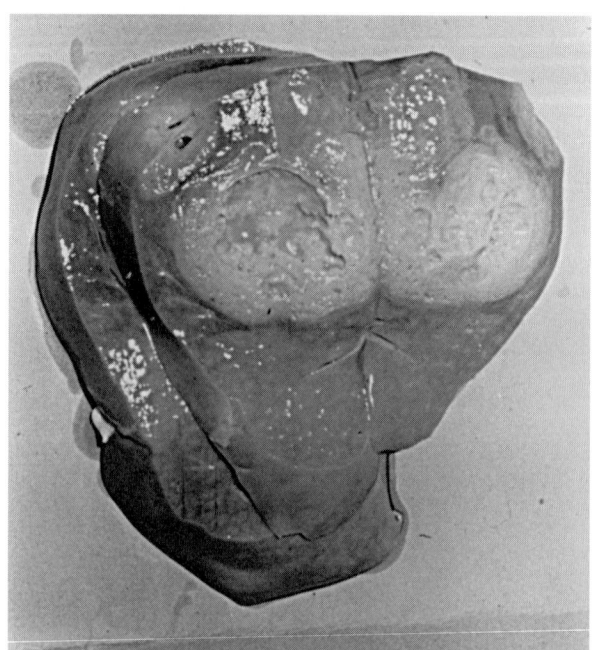

Figure 86–5. Numerous amebic abscesses of the liver. (Courtesy of the Department of Anatomical Pathology, University of Natal Medical School.)

Asymptomatic Cyst Passers. The majority of patients with amebic infections in temperate climates where infection with the nonpathogenic E. *dispar* predominates are asymptomatic cyst passers. This ameba is morphologically indistinguishable from E. *histolytica* but has characteristic isoenzymes and unique surface epitopes that can be recognized by monoclonal antibodies. In tropical areas, however, as many as 10% of asymptomatic cyst passers are infected with E. *histolytica,* which has a pathogenic isoenzyme pattern. The majority of these patients spontaneously clear their infection; the remainder develop invasive amebiasis.

Amebic Dysentery (Acute Amebic Colitis)

Mucosal Disease. This usually presents with dysentery with a gradual onset over 1 to 3 weeks. Individuals who have had long-standing mild symptoms or who have been asymptomatic cyst passers can also begin to pass loose, grossly bloody stools. Typical symptoms and signs also include abdominal cramps, fever, and tenesmus. Dehydration may occur with prolonged diarrhea. The stools are liquid and contain bloody mucus, but leukocytes are not as prevalent as in bacterial dysenteries. The peripheral white blood cell count is often elevated, with a polymorphonuclear leukocytosis. Anemia is not a feature unless disease is long standing.

A less common presentation is a nondysenteric colitis. A spectrum of symptoms is noted. These range from totally asymptomatic individuals to those with increased numbers of soft stools, intermittent constipation, distention, and flatulence. Other individuals do not have frank dysentery but show clinical evidence of some localized invasion of the bowel wall. The latter is manifested by frequent stools, lower abdominal cramps, weight loss, anorexia, and nausea. The white blood cell count and differential count are usually normal.

Transmural Disease. Patients may have extensive colonic involvement with gross colonic destruction. The presentation may be acute, with bacterial peritonitis consequent to intestinal perforation. These patients are usually toxic, febrile, and hypotensive, with profuse bloody mucoid diarrhea. In those patients who develop a slow leak from the site of perforation, the inflamed bowel becomes enveloped by omental wraps in an attempt to seal off the leak. These patients usually present with an abdominal mass. Toxic megacolon and profuse intestinal hemorrhage can also occur from transmural disease, which has a high mortality.

Ulcerative Postdysenteric Colitis. As a sequel to acute amebic dysentery, some patients may develop a postdysenteric colitis. Two forms have been described: (1) that with mild symptoms and no colonic ulceration (i.e., functional postdysenteric colonic irritability) and (2) that with colonic ulceration and more severe symptoms (i.e., ulcerative postdysenteric colitis). Amebic trophozoites are not present, and further antiamebic treatment is of no value. Clinically, it is difficult to differentiate this entity from ulcerative colitis, and the proctoscopic appearance is similar. Treatment with steroids or sulfasalazine is useful in both conditions. It is essential to rule out active amebic infection, which can be exacerbated by these drugs.

Complications of Intestinal Amebiasis

Perforation and Peritonitis. With acute perforation, sudden pain occurs at the perforation site and signs of an acute abdomen are present. Slow leakage does not present as acutely but should be suspected in a seriously ill patient whose condition gradually deteriorates along with the development of increased distention and signs of ileus, or if an abdominal mass develops.

Appendicitis. It is difficult clinically to differentiate amebic from other causes of inflammatory involvement of the appendix. Amebic appendicitis should be considered in the presence of other signs of amebic colitis, and antiamebic drug therapy should then be administered before any surgery.

Ameboma. Amebomas may cause pain, a tender mass, and rarely intussusception. They often occur during the course of proven amebic dysentery, justifying a presumptive diagnosis. When not associated with amebic dysentery or the presence of ulcers, amebomas may easily be confused with adenocarcinoma or annular carcinoma when recognized after barium enema examination or at sigmoidoscopy or colonoscopy.

Amebic Stricture. A stricture either develops during an attack of amebic dysentery or follows transmural colitis that heals by fibrosis. Amebic strictures are often symptomless, although they may produce abdominal or rectal pain, partial obstruction, and constipation.

Cutaneous Amebiasis. Amebic skin lesions grow rapidly and are characteristically painful. With prompt diagnosis and appropriate treatment, the lesions also heal rapidly.

Amebic Liver Abscess. Liver abscess may occur in the presence or absence of intestinal symptoms. It often develops after a latent period following earlier diarrhea or other intestinal disorders, particularly in patients with a history of prior travel to or residence in endemic areas. Only about 20% of patients with amebic liver abscess have E. *histolytica* present on stool examinations. However, the parasite can be isolated on stool culture in as many as 70% of patients. The right lobe is more often involved than the left, in a ratio of about 5:1.

Onset of symptoms can be either insidious or acute. Clinical findings may vary, but pleuritic pain in the right lower anterior chest or right hypochondrium is typical. In the case of left lobe abscess, pain may localize to the epigastrium. In many cases, abscesses extend upward to involve the diaphragm, leading to diaphragmatic elevation and immobility and compression of the right lower lobe of the lung. In these instances, the lower lobe of the lung may be dull to percussion, and patients may have atelectasis, right-sided pleural effusion, cough, dyspnea, and pain referred to the right shoulder. Tenderness over an enlarged liver is a common clinical sign. Other signs may include a visible mass or bulging of the right lower rib cage in patients with a large abscess, intercostal tenderness, and point tenderness over a palpable enlarged liver. Patients usually are febrile, with mild pallor and a nonproductive cough. Chills and profuse sweating may occasionally be present. Jaundice (usually mild) is infrequent and may occur with large abscesses. These symptoms and signs should alert the physician to the possibility of amebic liver abscess; both liver scanning and amebic serologic tests should be promptly performed. The alkaline phosphatase level may be elevated, but liver enzyme values are either normal or only mildly elevated. Often found are a leukocytosis with left shift, an elevated sedimentation rate, and a normochromic normocytic anemia.

Pleuropulmonary Amebiasis. Most patients with this complication complain of pain, cough, hemoptysis, and dyspnea. Pain typically occurs in the lower right area of the chest and may be pleuritic. When extension occurs into the pleural space, the cough is usually nonproductive. If the abscess drains into a bronchus, large amounts of abscess material may be coughed up; this may be reddish-brown, dirty-brown, purulent, or frank amebic pus. Chills, fever, and leukocytosis are frequently present.

Amebic Pericarditis. Amebic pericarditis may present with generalized deterioration in the patient's condition, left-sided or retrosternal chest pain, increasing lethargy, and dyspnea. Examination usually reveals tachycardia with pulsus paradoxus and a pericardial friction rub. Patients may occasionally be hypotensive and have thready pulses. If associated point tenderness of the liver and other signs and symptoms of liver abscess are present, amebic involvement of the pericardium and/or pleuropulmonary space should be seriously suspected.

Amebic Brain Abscess. The onset of symptoms is abrupt, and the course is fulminant, resembling that of a pyogenic brain abscess. Headache, fever, seizures, and coma may be present. Cerebral amebiasis is almost always fatal.

DIAGNOSIS

Intestinal Amebiasis. Definitive diagnosis of invasive intestinal amebiasis is made by demonstration of *E. histolytica* parasites in the stool. These amebae may have ingested red blood cells (hematophagus). A tendency is to overdiagnose intestinal parasites, particularly *E. histolytica,* by mistakenly identifying nonpathogenic amebae, macrophages, or white blood cells as *E. histolytica.* Physicians must be certain that the laboratory is using correct procedures in collecting and examining specimens and that the examinations are performed by experienced parasitology technicians.

Stool Specimen Collection. *E. histolytica* cysts may remain viable for some time in unpreserved stools. Trophozoites, occurring with dysenteric and diarrheal stool specimens, are labile and usually disappear (within 30 minutes of passage) from a fresh stool. Refrigeration, freezing, or incubation at 37°C of liquid or formed stools often has a deleterious effect on both trophozoites and cysts. It is preferable to collect specimens in preservatives, which retain the structure and characteristics of cysts and trophozoites until the specimen can be examined. A number of commercial collection kits are available.

Amebic cysts and trophozoites are passed intermittently in the stool, and the diagnostic yield is better in specimens collected over a period of 3 days or longer; 70 to 90% of infections should be diagnosed by a series of examinations. Therefore, at least three negative results of adequately performed examinations carried out on separate days should be completed before proceeding to more specialized techniques, if warranted by the patient's clinical condition. Many preparations, including antibiotics and antiparasitic drugs, sulfa drugs, antacids, kaolin products, bismuth subsalicylate, most enema products, oily laxatives, and barium, can cause a transient inhibition of multiplication of *E. histolytica* or can interfere with their recognition.

Examination of Specimens. With fresh stools, flecks of mucus, with or without blood staining, should be sought. A particle of mucus is placed on a slide, diluted with saline, covered with a coverslip, and examined. Alternatively, particles of stool are similarly examined. *E. histolytica* trophozoites have glasslike pseudopodia and progressive motility, and they may contain ingested red blood cells if blood is present in the stool (Fig. 86–6). An iodine-stained smear is also made to assist in differentiating *E. histolytica* from nonpathogenic amebic cysts. A concentration test should also be performed; the formalin-ethylacetate method is particularly useful (Chapter 150). Smears of mucus or fecal material can also be made immediately from fresh stool for later permanent staining. Permanent stained smears may be necessary for definite confirmation of *E. histolytica* parasites. Unfortunately, microscopy does not differentiate between the pathogenic *E. histolytica* and the nonpathogenic *E. dispar* because they are morphologically identical. Isoenzyme electrophoresis is available in only a few laboratories. Monoclonal antibodies that distinguish between pathogenic and nonpathogenic species are being used in antigen capture enzyme-linked immunosorbent assays (ELISA) that will be invaluable in clinical laboratories.

Although associated with amebiasis, Charcot-Leyden crystals are not pathognomonic because they may also be present in other colonic diseases and in infections with *Trichuris trichiura* and *Schistosoma* species. Stools from patients with

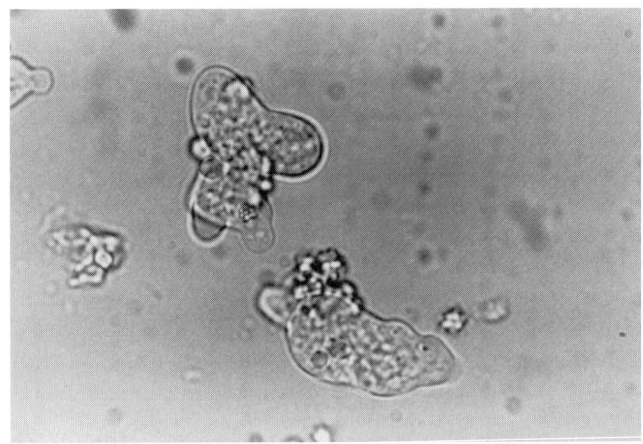

Figure 86–6. Hematophagus trophozoites of *E. histolytica.*

amebic dysentery uncomplicated by secondary bacterial infection seldom contain more than a few leukocytes, in contrast to the sheets of leukocytes usually seen with acute shigellosis and *Campylobacter* infections.

Culture. Laboratories experienced in culture techniques for *E. histolytica* may increase the diagnostic yield by using this supplemental procedure.

Sigmoidoscopic Examination. In dysenteric amebiasis, typical ulcerative lesions are often visualized, and scrapings may be obtained through the sigmoidoscope for immediate examination or fixation for later examination. Cotton swabs are not recommended for this purpose because they absorb liquid material. A glass tube and rubber bulb may be used to aspirate liquid material. Scrapings can be taken with biopsy forceps. Biopsy specimens may be obtained from ulcers or suspected amebomas or amebic strictures. Hematoxylin-eosin slides are prepared, and these should be examined by a pathologist experienced in identifying *E. histolytica* trophozoites in tissue (Figs. 86–3 and 86–4). *E. histolytica* in rectal biopsy samples may be detected more easily in ethanol-fixed tissues stained with either a fluorescent antibody or with periodic acid–Schiff.

Barium X-Ray Examination. This is seldom useful in nondysenteric cases and must not be performed before a sufficient number of stools have been examined or sigmoidoscopy has been performed, because barium interferes with identification of parasites. In acute dysenteric cases, evidence of ulceration, spasm, loss of haustral pattern, or narrowing of the cecum may be seen. When amebic colitis is diffuse, it roentgenographically resembles diffuse inflammatory bowel disease. The risk of perforation from a barium enema must be considered in patients with possible toxic megacolon. Amebomas or amebic strictures, initially recognized by barium enema, must be differentiated from carcinoma by biopsy and serologic tests.

Serologic Tests. Serum antibodies reflect amebic invasion and do not correlate with protective immunity. However, strong seropositivity is usually observed in all persons harboring *E. histolytica,* whether or not they are symptomatic. In patients clinically suspected of having amebic dysentery, liver abscess, pericarditis, ameboma, or other less common forms of invasive amebiasis, a positive serologic response with a reliable, well-evaluated test is strong evidence of an amebic etiology. Conversely, a negative serologic test result makes the diagnosis of amebic liver abscess or ameboma almost untenable and makes the diagnosis of amebic colitis unlikely. Serologic tests are positive in 96% of patients with amebic liver abscess and in about 85% of those with dysen-

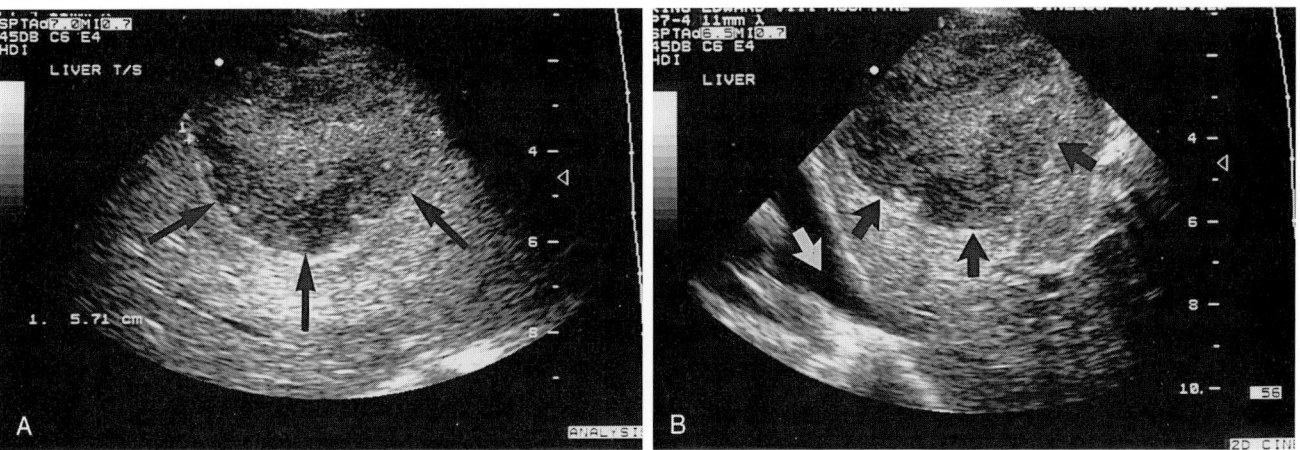

Figure 86–7. *A*, Ultrasound scan of an amebic liver abscess. *B*, Ultrasound scan of a right lobe liver abscess *(black arrows)*. The abscess is lying adjacent to the diaphragm. There is a sympathetic pleural effusion *(white arrow)*.

tery at the time of admission. It is important to note that patients with both amebic liver abscess and dysentery can present clinically before antibody titers are measurable; confirmation of infection can be obtained by repeating the test 7 to 10 days after admission. Serologic tests are particularly useful in the important differential diagnoses between amebic dysentery and inflammatory bowel disease, amebic and pyogenic liver abscess, and ameboma and colonic carcinoma.

Seropositivity, albeit at decreasing titers, persists for 6 months to 3 years, depending on the sensitivity of the test used, after clinical and parasitologic cure of invasive amebiasis in the absence of reinfection. Many serologic tests have been used for the diagnosis of amebiasis, including the immunofluorescence (IF) test, the indirect hemagglutination (IHA) test, the latex agglutination test, the gel diffusion precipitation test, counterimmunoelectrophoresis, and ELISA (Chapter 152). The IHA tests produced in some regions can be too sensitive, resulting in false-positive results. Thus, the titer of the test is needed to assist in clinical decision making. A promising variation of the ELISA technique for detecting antigen to *E. histolytica* in fecal, serum, and abscess samples has been developed in several laboratories (Chapter 152). Polymerase chain reaction tests are being developed for detecting parasite DNA and should become invaluable in the future.

Amebic Liver Abscess. Clinical suspicion of amebic liver abscess can best be confirmed by a positive amebic serologic test result in conjunction with positive results of a radioisotopic, sonographic, or radiologic procedure, followed by a response to specific therapy.

Scans. Noninvasive procedures to demonstrate a hepatic abscess include ultrasonography (Fig. 86–7*A* and *B*), technetium scan (Fig. 86–8), gallium scan, computed tomography (Fig. 86–9), and magnetic resonance imaging. When a technetium scan result is positive, ultrasound scanning can distinguish between cystic and solid lesions. The finding of increased gallium activity (with a ^{67}Ga scan) at the periphery of a large gallium-negative lesion has been described as useful in the diagnosis of an amebic liver abscess, but large neoplasms with central necrosis may also show this feature.

Chest Radiograph. This frequently shows elevation of the right diaphragm and changes of right basal atelectasis. A right pleural effusion is occasionally seen (Fig. 86–10*A* and *B*). These are frequent findings when the abscess is in the superior portion of the right lobe of the liver. Similar left-sided changes may be seen with left lobe abscesses.

Signs of pericardial effusion may also be seen radiologically or sonographically.

Aspiration. Percutaneous diagnostic needle aspiration may be needed to differentiate between amebic and pyogenic abscesses. Aspiration should be carried out using ultrasound guidance or it should be performed at the site of maximal tenderness. Amebic aspirates often resemble anchovy paste or are chocolate colored, reddish, or grayish brown, but they may also be yellowish or white. Amebic abscesses do not have the foul odor of pyogenic abscesses. Amebic trophozoites are rarely present in the central necrotic contents of the abscess cavity itself but can sometimes be seen in the terminal few milliliters of aspirated fluid, which is believed to be from the advancing abscess wall. Ten units of streptodornase

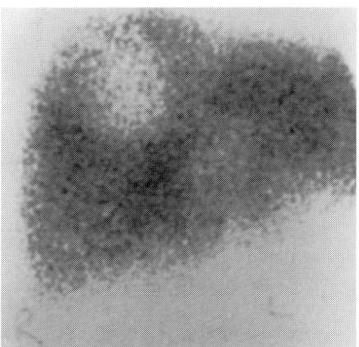

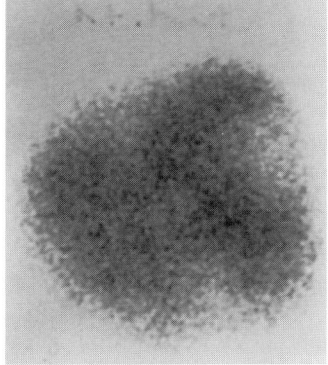

Figure 86–8. Hepatic radioisotope scan of an amebic liver abscess showing a large filling defect in the right lobe.

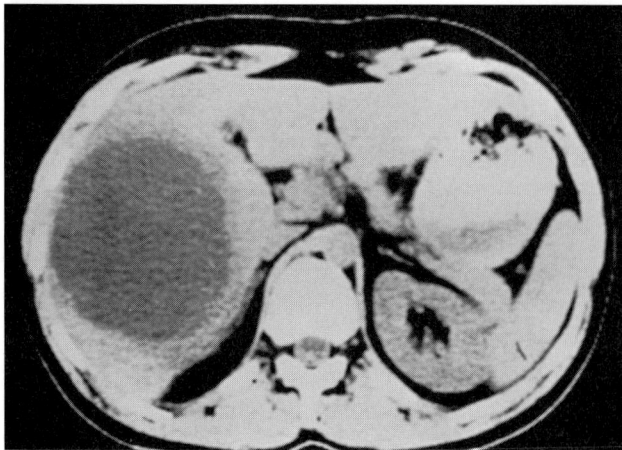

Figure 86–9. Computed tomography scan of the abdomen showing almost complete replacement of the right lobe of the liver by an amebic abscess 10 cm in diameter. (Courtesy of the National Naval Medical Center, Bethesda, MD.)

should be added to each milliliter of fluid to break down the fibrin. This is incubated for 30 minutes at 35°C and examined in saline wet mounts and in stained preparations. Gram stain and aerobic and anaerobic cultures should also be performed on all aspirates to detect a possible bacterial cause of the abscess. Metronidazole is highly effective against invasive amebiasis as well as anaerobic bacteria, a leading cause of bacterial liver abscess. In a patient with suspected liver abscess, treatment with metronidazole can lead to rapid improvement of amebic and anaerobic bacterial abscesses. However, if satisfactory clinical improvement is not obtained in about 3 days, aspiration should be performed.

Blood Tests. A leukocytosis of 12,000 to 20,000/mm³ and normochromic, normocytic anemia are usually present. Eosinophilia is not a feature of either hepatic or intestinal amebiasis. The erythrocyte sedimentation rate is frequently elevated. Alkaline phosphatase is elevated in as many as 75% of patients. Aminotransaminase elevations, when they occur,

are minimal and are present in <50% of patients. Bilirubin levels are seldom elevated, except with large abscess cavities that cause biliary obstruction.

TREATMENT

Drugs. Useful drugs include metronidazole (Flagyl), tinidazole (Fasigyn), chloroquine phosphate, emetine hydrochloride, iodoquinol, and paromomycin (Humatin). Metronidazole, tinidazole, emetine, and dehydroemetine are tissue amebicides that act on bowel, liver, and other sites of invasive amebiasis. Chloroquine is amebicidal in the liver. Iodoquinol, paromomycin, and diloxanide furoate all are poorly absorbed, primarily luminal-acting drugs (Fig. 86–1). Emetine, dehydroemetine, and chloroquine are second-line agents and more toxic than the commonly used metronidazole and tinidazole. They are not used when the nitroimidazoles are available and are not discussed further in this edition. See previous editions of this text for details of their use in treating amebiasis. Tetracycline is indirectly amebicidal in the bowel and has no advantage over other available drugs. Erythromycin has some direct amebicidal action but is not used in the treatment of amebiasis. Adult and pediatric dosages for treatment of various types of amebic disorders are summarized in Table 86–1.

Tissue Amebicides

Metronidazole. This nitroimidazole compound is marketed as tablets and as an intravenous preparation. Metronidazole is amebicidal and is highly effective in invasive amebiasis; it is the usual drug of choice for more severe infections. Because it is so well absorbed, it does not work well as a luminal-acting drug. Common side effects include nausea, headache, and a metallic taste. Dizziness, vomiting, abdominal cramps, and diarrhea are less common. The urine may become dark from a metabolite of the drug. Overgrowth of *Candida* in the mouth, vagina, or intestine may occur. Metronidazole may potentiate the anticoagulant effect of coumarin. It has a disulfiram (Antabuse) effect and should not be used with alcohol. Extensive clinical experience and epidemiologic data show that this drug is not carcinogenic or mutagenic in humans.

For symptomatic nondysenteric intestinal amebiasis, acute amebic dysentery, or amebic liver abscess, adults should re-

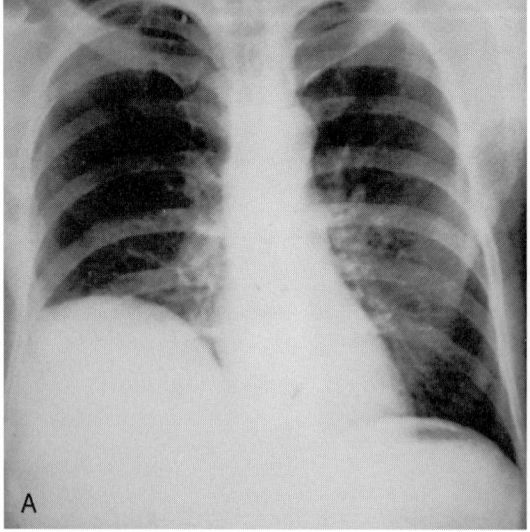
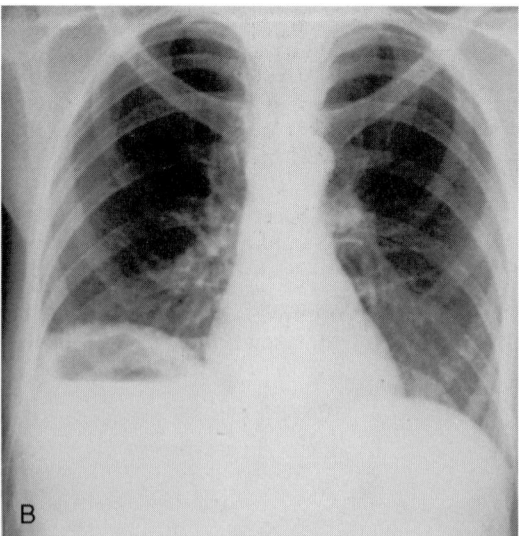

Figure 86–10. Chest radiographs of a patient with amebic liver abscess. *A,* Marked elevation of the right hemidiaphragm. (Courtesy of the Veterans Administration Hospital, New Orleans.) *B,* Outline of the abscess cavity (air injected) with fluid level after closed aspiration. (Courtesy of the Louisiana State University School of Medicine, New Orleans.)

TABLE 86–1. Summary of Drug Treatment of Amebiasis

Drugs	Adult Dose	Pediatric Dose
Asymptomatic Cyst Passer and Mildly Symptomatic Nondysenteric Amebiasis		
paromomycin	500–650 mg t.i.d. × 10 days	30 mg/kg/day in 3 doses × 10 days
or iodoquinol	650 mg t.i.d. × 20 days	40 mg/kg/day in 3 doses × 20 days
or diloxanide furoate	500 mg t.i.d. × 10 days	20 mg/kg/day in 3 doses × 10 days
Moderately Severe Nondysenteric Amebiasis and Amebic Dysentery, Ameboma and Amebic Liver Abscess		
metronidazole	800 mg t.i.d. × 5 days	50 mg/kg/day in 3 doses × 5 days
or tinidazole	800 mg t.i.d. × 5 days	40 mg/kg/day (max 2 g) in single dose × 5 days
To be followed by paromomycin, iodoquinol or diloxanide furoate, as in treating amebic cyst passers		

ceive 800 mg t.i.d. and children 50 mg/kg/day in three divided doses for 5 days. Single daily doses of 2 to 2.4 g for 1 or 2 days have had comparable efficacy. Intravenous metronidazole may be given as a loading dose of 1 g, followed by 500 mg every 6 hr, until oral metronidazole can be taken. To prevent relapses from persistent cysts, metronidazole should be followed by a luminal-acting drug.

Tinidazole (Fasigyn). This synthetic nitroimidazole derivative is marketed as tablets of various formulations. Its action is similar to that of metronidazole. In comparative studies, it has been equally effective in divided or single daily doses for invasive intestinal and hepatic amebiasis. Intestinal amebiasis and amebic liver abscess are treated with 800 mg t.i.d. for 5 days; single daily doses of 2 g have also been used for 2 to 6 days. As with metronidazole, it is prudent to follow these regimens with a luminal amebicide to decrease the possibility of relapse, because tinidazole is also not very active against the cyst stage. Single daily doses for children are 40 mg/kg for 5 days, with a maximum dose of 2 g. Precautions are similar to those for metronidazole.

Luminal Amebicides

Diloxanide Furoate (Furamide). This substituted acetanilid is available as tablets in various formulations. It is poorly absorbed and is effective in asymptomatic cyst passers and with tissue-active amebicides. The only frequently observed side effect is excessive flatulence, although other mild gastrointestinal symptoms occasionally occur. The dosage for adults is 500 mg t.i.d. for 10 days. The pediatric dosage is 20 mg/kg/day divided into 3 doses for 10 days. Diloxanide furoate is not recommended in pregnancy because little is known about possible teratogenic effects.

Iodoquinol. This halogenated oxyquinoline was formerly known as Diodoquin. Iodoquinol acts against amebae in the intestinal lumen only and is ineffective in invasive amebiasis. Because so little of the drug is absorbed, it has only minimal toxicity (e.g., abdominal pain, diarrhea, and rash). It may interfere with results of thyroid function tests for several months and is contraindicated in patients with iodine intolerance or hepatic damage. A related compound, iodochlorhydroxyquin (Entero-vioform) has caused the syndrome of subacute myelo-optic neuropathy and should not be used. In doses recommended for treating intestinal protozoa, iodoquinol does not cause optic atrophy.

Used alone in treatment of asymptomatic amebiasis or used after a tissue-active amebicide in symptomatic amebiasis, the dosage of iodoquinol in adults is 650 mg t.i.d. for 20 days. Children should receive 40 mg/kg/day t.i.d. for 20 days.

Paromomycin (Humatin). This broad-spectrum antibiotic is marketed as a 250-mg capsule and in some countries as a pediatric syrup. Paromomycin is poorly absorbed after oral administration; nearly all of the drug is recoverable in the stool. It is most effective in treating asymptomatic cyst passers and patients with mildly symptomatic intestinal amebiasis. It is equally effective as other luminal-acting drugs in clearing cysts from the lumen in the follow-up to treatment of invasive amebiasis with tissue-active drugs. Nausea, abdominal cramps, and diarrhea may occur. The drug should be used with caution in persons with ulcerative lesions of the bowel. The adult dose is 500–650 mg t.i.d. for 10 days. Children should receive 30 mg/kg/day in 3 divided doses for 10 days. Although this drug has not been used often in the past few years, it is now being given to treat cryptosporidiosis in HIV-positive patients (Chapter 88).

Treatment of Asymptomatic Cyst Passers. Therapy is summarized in Table 86–1. The majority of asymptomatic cyst passers harbor the nonpathogenic *E. dispar* and do not require treatment. However, these amebae are morphologically identical to *E. histolytica,* and a means to differentiate between these parasites is seldom available to medical care providers. Infection with the pathogenic *E. histolytica* is associated with a positive serologic test result, which may be used to augment microscopy to identify infections with *E. histolytica.* Asymptomatic *E. histolytica* cyst passers are a potential public health hazard, and long-term carriage might possibly lead to later acute invasive disease.

Treatment of Nondysenteric Intestinal Amebiasis. Moderately severe symptoms may be present in the absence of blood or mucus in the stool. In this situation, metronidazole or tinidazole should be given initially, followed by a luminal-acting drug (Table 86–1). Those with mildly symptomatic amebiasis may be given paromomycin or diloxanide furoate alone; if this fails, a more vigorous retreatment regimen may be tried (e.g., for moderately severe cases).

Treatment of Amebic Colitis

Mucosal Disease. Initial treatment requires a potent, well-absorbed tissue-active drug (e.g., metronidazole or tinidazole), followed by a luminal-acting drug to prevent relapse (Table 86–1). Severe diarrhea requires correction of water and electrolyte loss.

Transmural Disease. The use of antibiotics as well as amebicidal drugs, is indicated if there is evidence of septic peritonitis or septicemia. Patients must be kept well hydrated. Indications for surgery are signs of peritonitis, air under the diaphragm, an intra-abdominal abscess, and ischemia of the colon on angiography. Other indications for surgery are intestinal hemorrhage consequent to transmural disease and the development of strictures during convalescence. Hemorrhage, a rare occurrence, may require blood transfusion. Gastric suction may be needed.

Reducing the degree of sepsis and controlling blood loss are the prime objectives during surgery. In the early stages of transmural disease, the bowel is easily manageable and does not resemble wet blotting paper. This description refers to the extreme form of transmural disease. Intra-abdominal sepsis is the major preventable factor contributing to mortality. Colonic irrigation can be performed via colostomy because the perforation is often walled off by omentum and surrounding large and small bowel, which permits resection of an empty colon without soiling the abdominal cavity. Attempts to remove the wraps should be avoided because this inevitably leads to perforation and abdominal soiling. The primary anastomosis is not performed at the time of colonic resection. A gentle barium examination can be performed via the colostomy a few weeks later. If there is no sign of a leak, the colostomy is closed.

Acute amebic colitis must be differentiated from ulcerative colitis before administering corticosteroids. In amebiasis, corticosteroids may cause fulminant infection and perforation. Amebomas and amebic strictures are treated similarly to amebic dysentery.

Treatment of Amebic Liver Abscesses. Oral or intravenous metronidazole or tinidazole should lead to rapid clinical improvement of amebic liver abscess. This drug should be followed by a luminal-active drug (Table 86–1).

Aspiration. Percutaneous aspiration, preferably with ultrasound guidance, is reserved for abscesses that may potentially rupture (i.e., an abscess >10 cm in diameter), a left lobe abscess to prevent rupture into the pericardium, or any abscess close to a serosal surface. Aspiration is also indicated for abscesses not responding promptly to drugs alone and for abscesses of uncertain cause. The majority of amebic liver abscesses that are relatively small (<10 cm) usually respond to drug therapy alone.

Serial liver scans and sonograms have shown that most liver abscesses completely heal over 4 to 8 months after chemotherapy. The resolution time may be longer for large abscesses; however, patients usually remain asymptomatic in these cases.

Complications of Amebic Liver Abscess. When extension into the thorax causes hepatobronchial fistula, pleural effusion, empyema, lung abscess, or pulmonary consolidation, treatment with metronidazole or tinidazole is indicated. In addition, aspiration of the liver abscess as well as the pleural effusion should be performed. Amebic pericarditis is treated by adequate drainage of the pericardial sac using needle aspiration and occasionally by surgery, along with a tissue amebicide.

PREVENTION AND CONTROL

Direct and Foodborne Transmission. Education about transmission of amebiasis and methods of avoiding infection is the same as for any fecal-oral transmitted infection. Infected food handlers should be identified and treated. They must also wash their hands after defecation, and appropriate sanitary facilities must be made available. Infected individuals in institutions and daycare centers should be identified and treated. Homosexual males should be made aware of transmission by oral-anal sexual practices and of the relation of infection to sexual promiscuity, and those found to be infected should be treated. Follow-up stool examinations should be performed after treatment to confirm the absence of cyst carriage. Contamination of food by flies may be prevented by screening and the use of insecticides. Travelers to endemic areas should avoid cold foods and salads. Vegetables can be infected from night soil, sewage, or contaminated water; therefore, before eating, they should be washed with

a weak detergent, rinsed in potable water treated with strong concentrations of chlorine or iodine, and then rinsed again with potable water. Fruits in endemic areas should be peeled before eating.

Waterborne Transmission. Water sources should be protected from fecal contamination and made safe by both proper filtration and chlorination. Boiling of water destroys amebic cysts almost immediately. Water can be effectively treated with iodine water purification tablets, tincture of iodine, or liquid chlorine laundry bleach. Only ice prepared from treated water should be used.

Certain antiamebic drugs are recommended by some for prophylactic use. The prophylactic effectiveness of these drugs has never been scientifically proved, and they should not be used for this purpose.

Bibliography

Abd-Alla MD, Jackson TFHG, Gathiram V, et al. Differentiation of pathogenic *Entamoeba histolytica* infections by detection of galactiose inhibitable adherence protein antigen in sera and feces. J Antimicrob Microbiol 31:2845, 1993.

Adams EB, MacLeod IN: Invasive amebiasis. I. Amebic dysentery and its complications. Medicine 56:315, 1977.

Adams EB, MacLeod IN: Invasive amebiasis. II. Amebic liver abscess and its complications. Medicine 56:325, 1977.

Ahmed L, El Rooby A, Kassem MI, et al: Ultrasonography in the diagnosis and management of 52 patients with amebic liver abscess in Cairo. Rev Infect Dis 12:330, 1990.

Ahmed L, Salama ZA, El Rooby A, Strickland GT: Ultrasonographic resolution time for amebic liver abscess. Am J Trop Med Hyg 41:406, 1989.

Delarey Nel J, Simjee AE, Patel A: Indications for aspiration in amoebic liver abscess. South Afr Med J 75:373, 1989.

Gathiram V, Jackson TFHG: Frequency distribution of *Entamoeba histolytica* zymodemes in a rural South African population. Lancet 1:719, 1985.

Gathiram V, Jackson TFHG: Pathogenic zymodemes of *Entamoeba histolytica* remain unchanged throughout their life-cycle. Trans R Soc Trop Med Hyg 84:806, 1990.

Goldman M: *Entamoeba histolytica*-like amoebae occurring in man. Bull WHO:355, 1969.

Ibarra-Perez C: Thoracic complications of amebic abscess of the liver. Report of 501 cases. Chest 79:672, 1981.

Irusen EM, Jackson TFHG, Simjee AE: Asymptomatic intestinal colonisation by pathogenic *Entamoeba histolytica* in amoebic liver abscess: Prevalence, response to therapy and pathogenic potential. Clin Infect Dis 14:889, 1992.

Jackson TFHG: *Entamoeba histolytica* cyst passers—to treat or not to treat? S Afr Med J 72:657, 1987.

Jackson TFHG, Gathiram V, Simjee AE: Seroepidemiological study of antibody responses to the zymodemes of *Entamoeba histolytica*. Lancet 1:716, 1985.

Lamont NMcE, Pooler NR: Hepatic amebiasis. A study of 250 cases. Q J Med 107:389, 1958.

Luvuno FM. Surgery for complicated amoebiasis. Baillieres Clin Trop Med Commun Dis 3:349, 1988.

Patterson M, Healy GR, Shabot JM: Serologic testing for amoebiasis. Gastroenterology 78:136, 1980.

Powell SJ, Wilmot AJ: Ulcerative post-dysenteric colitis. Gut 7:438, 1966.

Ralls PW, Henley DS, Colletti PM, et al: Amebic liver abscess: MR imaging. Radiology 165:801, 1987.

Ravdin JI (ed): Amebiasis: Human Infection by *Entamoeba histolytica*. New York, John Wiley & Sons, 1988.

Simjee AE, Patel A, Gathiram V, et al: Serial ultrasound in amoebic liver abscess. Clin Radiol 36:31, 1985.

Simjee AE, Gathiram V, Jackson TFHG, Khan BFY: A comparative trial of metronidazole and tinidazole in the treatment of amoebic liver abscess. S Afr Med J 68:923, 1985.

Tucker PC, Webster PD, Kilpatrick ZM: Amebic colitis mistaken for inflammatory bowel disease. Arch Intern Med 135:681, 1975.

Walsh JA: Problems in recognition and diagnosis of amebiasis: Estimation of the global magnitude of morbidity and mortality. Rev Infect Dis 8:228, 1986.

Wilmot AJ: Clinical Amoebiasis. Oxford, Blackwell Scientific Publications, 1962.

87 *Giardiasis*

Stephen G. Wright

DEFINITION. Giardiasis is infection of the lumen of the small intestine with the flagellate protozoan *Giardia lamblia*, also called *Lamblia intestinalis*. Many infected persons have no symptoms, whereas a smaller proportion have diarrheal disease that varies in severity.

HISTORY. In the late seventeenth century, Van Leeuwenhoek, using his microscope, saw trophozoites of *G. lamblia* in his own stool. In the nineteenth century, Vilem Lambl found parasites in the stools of children. Giardiasis was recognized as a common cause of diarrhea among troops repatriated from various areas of Europe during World War I and increasing since the 1960s, with the earlier cases in children, particularly those with hypogammaglobulinemia.

INCIDENCE AND DISTRIBUTION. Giardiasis occurs in all parts of the world, temperate and tropical. It is not essentially a disease of warm climates but of poverty where sanitation and sanitary practices are poor, fecal contamination of the environment is common, and there is no clean water for drinking and washing hands and household utensils. It is most common in the tropics and subtropics where prevalence rates range from 10 to 20%, with infection most common in the poorest segments of the population. Children from indigenous populations are most often infected, and symptomatic, but adults too may be affected.

Prevalence is relatively low in the temperate parts of the world although infection in American and Finnish visitors to St. Petersburg in the former USSR indicated its endemicity there and it is also well recognized in other eastern European countries. It is, with *Cryptosporidium*, the most common protozoan parasite reported to the Communicable Diseases Surveillance Centre in Great Britain with 5000 to 6000 cases reported each year. Giardiasis gained attention as a result of symptomatic disease occurring among European travelers to Asia in the late 1960s and 1970s. There have also been infections in holiday visitors to Madeira, Italy, Sardinia, and other areas of the Mediterranean littoral. Water-borne outbreaks have occurred in Aspen, Colorado, Camas in Washington State, and Rome, New York, and in England. Food-borne outbreaks have also been reported from the United States.

TRANSMISSION. Infection follows ingestion of viable cysts of the parasite in contaminated food or water. Cysts may also be transported to the mouth on fingers, particularly of children, as a result of contact with feces on the ground around the home. Person-to-person spread also occurs in children. As few as 100 cysts produced infection in prison volunteers. Volunteer studies have been carried out using two different strains, both derived from human sources with diarrhea. Trophozoites were lavaged directly into the small intestine. One strain infected all 10 volunteers, whereas none of the 5 receiving the other strain became infected. The prepatent period averaged 7.5 days. Cyst excretion showed considerable variation from large numbers to occasional, and on some days, no cysts passed. Half of those infected developed symptoms, with 40% showing the typical clinical features of giardiasis.

Studies of water-borne outbreaks of giardiasis in the United States have usually shown defective water treatment plants with malfunctioning filters that do not retain giardia cysts. The cysts in surface water sources sometimes come from beavers. A variety of mammals, including dogs, can become infected and excrete cysts. These reservoirs may be important in the outbreaks occurring in backpackers and others visiting rural areas. The role of animal reservoirs may be greater in temperate regions where pets live in close proximity to their owners. In the tropics, high levels of environmental contamination are the dominant factor in transmission.

Both sexes seem equally susceptible to infection. In the tropics, children are more often infected than adults, and symptomatic disease is more common among children, although indigenous adults may have diarrhea due to giardiasis. Although there has been an emphasis on *Giardia* as a cause of diarrhea in children and adults, *Giardia* as a cause of diarrhea in the elderly in tropical as well as temperate regions should not be overlooked. In this group there may be relative immune deficiency owing to involution of the immune system.

Parasite Resistance. Heating to 50°C kills the encysted trophozoite; the survival ratio of cysts stored at 37°C in water is low. At 21°C, some cysts remain viable for up to 20 days. A high proportion of cysts stored at 8°C in tap water are viable for up to 5 weeks. Acceptable levels of chlorination in drinking water will kill *Giardia* cysts if the contact time is long enough. However, the occurrence of giardiasis in towns where water is chlorinated but inadequately filtered indicates the fallibility of chemical treatment alone. Higher levels of chlorination in swimming pool water are insufficient to kill encysted trophozoites.

Predisposing Factors. Children who are malnourished may be prone to giardiasis. Children attending day care centers, residents of homes for the mentally retarded, and homosexuals all have an increased risk of giardiasis from person-to-person spread. Reduced gastric acid secretion due to malnutrition, atrophic gastritis, antacid treatment, or surgery predisposes to giardiasis. It is possible that reduced gastric acid secretion in association with *Helicobacter pylori* infection may increase susceptibility to *Giardia* and other causes of persisting diarrhea. Adults and children with hypogammaglobulinemia often have giardiasis as a cause of diarrhea. While *Giardia* is recognized as a cause of diarrhea among those infected with human immunodeficiency virus (HIV), it does not seem to be particularly severe among this group, even following progression to AIDS. There is no association with any particular group of the ABO blood grouping system, but an association between HLA-B12 and giardiasis has been reported.

Parasitology. It is believed that exposure to low gastric pH in the stomach followed by the alkaline duodenal conditions leads to release of trophozoites from ingested cysts. However, this is not likely to be the whole story, as hypochlorhydria is a recognized risk factor for giardiasis. We do not know to what extent excystation is a passive event related to digestive effects on the cyst wall or an active event initiated by the parasite in response to conditions in the gut. The quadrinucleate trophozoite when released divides and then starts to replicate by asexual reproduction, the trophozoite population rising logarithmically.

The work of Filice was critical in separating three species groups of *Giardia: G. agilis, G. muris,* and *G. duodenalis (lamblia)*, based on the morphology of the median bodies. Within each of these presently defined species there is variation over a range of features, e.g., by restriction endonuclease analysis, particularly in *G. lamblia*. These variations are stable in vitro and in vivo. In gerbils, cross-protection between strains is evident.

Morphology. The cyst is oval and measures $8 \times 12 \times 8$ μm. The median body is easily seen, and four nuclei may be identified. Electron microscopy reveals fine detail of the cyst. The pear-shaped trophozoite measures about 15 μm long, 10

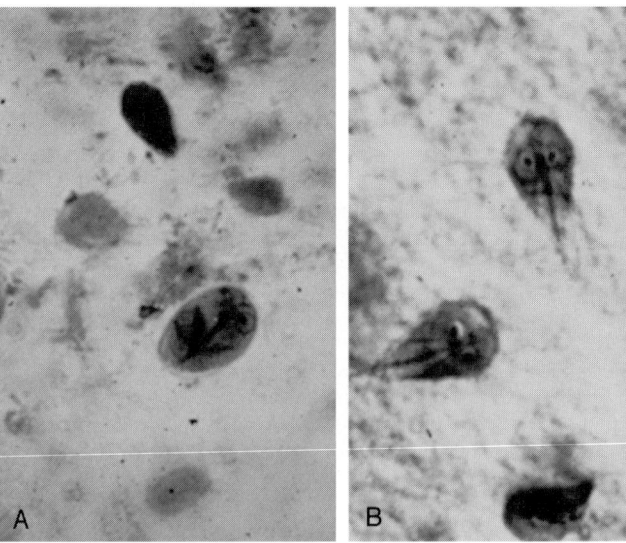

Figure 87–1. *Giardia lamblia. A,* Cyst. *B,* Trophozoite. (From Smith JW, et al: Diagnostic Medical Parasitology: Intestinal Protozoa. Chicago, The American Society of Clinical Pathologists, 1976.)

μm wide, and 2 to 4 μm thick (Figs. 87–1 and 90–10). It has a curved dorsal surface and a concave ventral surface, much of which is taken up by a disk with regular striations termed the sucker disk (Figs. 87–2 and 90–10). Two of the eight flagella emerge near the midline on the ventral surface of the organism, and the others emerge symmetrically around the periphery, three on each side. The beating of the flagella produces the trophozoite's spiraling motion and may cause a suction force that can maintain the trophozoite in a position closely applied to the microvilli of the gut epithelium. The extent of small bowel colonization in humans is not certain. *Giardia muris* colonizes the proximal quarter of the mouse small intestine.

Scanning and transmission electron microscopy confirm the appearances seen on light microscopy but give much clearer definition of parasite fine structure (Fig. 87–2). Studies of the cytoskeleton of *Giardia* have shown that it diverged as a species at an early stage in evolutionary history. Analyses of small subunit ribosomal RNA, which is highly conserved, led some authors to ascribe *Giardia* to an early position in evolutionary terms but these views have been questioned by more recent data. The cytoskeletal proteins, α giardin and β giardin, constitute the microribbons of the ventral sucker disk; they are linked to cross-bridges and microtubules. There are contractile proteins around the edge of the sucker disk. *G. lamblia* in the gerbil and *G. muris* in the mouse leave a cookie cutter–shaped "footprint" of the sucker disk in the microvillous carpet of the enterocytes at sites of attachment. Endosymbionts including a relatively common virus, giardiavirus, have been identified in trophozoites.

Parasite Kinetics. Comparatively little is known about the kinetics of infection in humans, at least as far as trophozoite populations are concerned. Cyst excretion can vary markedly among infected populations, with extreme variations even in the same person. The median duration of infection in children was 2 months, with a range of up to 11 months. Using cultured trophozoites, encystation was induced by increasing concentrations of bile.

Mouse giardiasis (caused by *G. muris*) has been studied extensively. Following infection with 1000 cysts, trophozoite populations rise to peak at about 10^6 organisms 2 weeks after infection. There is a progressive decline in parasite numbers over the next 4 weeks and most strains of mice eradicate the infection in 4 to 8 weeks. The mechanisms are poorly understood, but some strains of mice reduce parasite numbers much more efficiently than others, indicating that genetically determined factors may be important. Nude mice deficient in T cells, mice deficient in mast cells, and C3H/He mice have prolonged infections.

Metabolic Activity. *G. lamblia* is an aerotolerant anaerobe. It uses a range of substrates as energy sources but glucose metabolism by the Embden-Meyerhof pathway, leading to accumulation of acetate, ethanol, and alanine in the culture medium, is the best characterized. Trophozoites will grow, albeit at slower rates, in medium depleted of glucose, indicating that alternative energy sources are available.

Arginine can be a starting point for metabolism and, in vitro, is used during the logarithmic phase of multiplication. Alanine is interesting because it appears to be both an end product of glucose metabolism and a starting point for metabolism. The encysted trophozoite is not inactive and uses more oxygen during the synthetic phase of cyst wall production and less when encystation is complete. *Giardia* cannot synthesize lipids and so it obtains these from the host's gut lumen, particularly from biliary lipids. It also actively takes

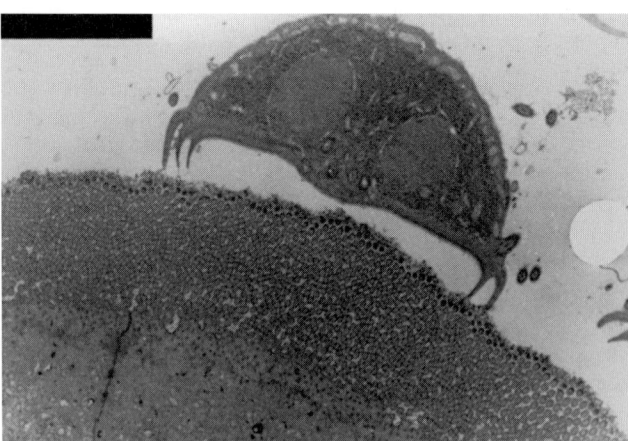

Figure 87–2. A *Giardia* trophozoite close to the microvillous border of a jejunal epithelial cell. The tips of microvilli beneath the trophozoite are more densely stained, probably representing damage to these structures caused by the parasite. (Electron micrograph reproduced by permission of Prof. G. N. Tytgat and Dr. K. Huibregtse, University of Amsterdam.)

up bile salts. This requirement for phospholipid may determine its predilection for the proximal jejunum.

PATHOGENESIS. The sequence of events leading to infection with *G. lamblia* is similar to that described for other intestinal pathogens that cause diarrhea: ingestion, colonization, and adhesion. Strain variation among parasites may contribute to variations in clinical manifestations. However, within one family, presumed to be exposed to a common strain, the whole range of pathogenicity may occur, from asymptomatic to severe diarrhea.

Colonization and Adhesion. On the one hand, acid provides a chemical barrier to the entry of most pathogens, and reduced gastric acid predisposes to *Giardia* and other infections. On the other hand, at least in vitro, exposure to acid is essential for excystation (hydrochloric acid at pH 2.0). A large infecting dose increases the risk of infection, as shown by Rendtorff's volunteer studies. This may also increase the probability of symptomatic infection through more rapid buildup of trophozoite populations. Parasite adhesion has been investigated using cultured trophozoites. There are at least two mechanisms involved. One is mechanical and relates to the beating of the two ventral flagella, perhaps aided by contractile elements in the ventral sucker disk. The other mechanism is mediated by a lectin on the surface of the parasite. The lectin allows mannose-dependent adhesion of parasites to mammalian red blood cells experimentally. The lectin is located intracellularly, where it is in the form of a prolectin, which is modified by host protease when it is expressed on the surface membrane. The nature of the enterocyte receptor is not clear.

Mechanism for Diarrhea. There is no single cause for the absorptive defects observed in giardiasis. Electron microscopic studies show damage at the microvillous border, the site of much terminal digestive and absorptive activity (Fig. 87–2). Absorption of actively transported substrates such as glucose and amino acids is markedly reduced in animals infected with *G. lamblia*. In *G. muris* infections, brush border lactase levels were lowest at the time of peak trophozoite populations before the peak in infiltrate of inflammatory cells or increase in crypt cell mitoses. These findings suggest that microvillous damage is proportional to parasite numbers. When parasites move about on the surface of the small intestine, lectin adhesion to enterocytes is continually being made and broken. Breaking adhesion sites may disrupt enzymes and surface membranes of microvilli. Failure to absorb nutrients may lead to the accumulation of osmotically active molecules in the gut lumen, which would then cause diarrhea.

Luminal events may also affect digestive processes. It is possible that the active uptake of bile salts by trophozoites alters micelle formation sufficiently to cause malabsorption of fat. Alterations in bile salt concentrations may influence the activity of pancreatic lipase to impair fat digestion. Bile salt deconjugation is a recognized cause of fat malabsorption. However, in vitro this does not occur and results of clinical studies have not been consistent. *Giardia* can interfere with the function of pancreatic lipase in vitro, a finding that may have a parallel in humans as indicated by the occurrence of gross steatorrhea in a man with long-standing chronic pancreatitis when he had acute giardiasis. Following eradication of the infection, fat absorption returned to normal suggesting that his reserves of fat-absorbing capacity were just adequate until the additive effects of *Giardia* on lipase occurred. In contrast, six children with giardiasis were studied with a standard test of pancreatic function and all were normal.

There is small bowel overgrowth of bacteria in patients with giardiasis, but the microflora comprises facultative anaerobes and not the obligate anaerobes associated with the bile salt deconjugation of jejunal diverticulosis and intestinal strictures. These organisms secrete enterotoxin and alcohol, which may contribute to intestinal damage. When fat passes into the ileum there is a paradoxical slowing of intestinal transit, which would encourage the persistence of upper small bowel colonization by *Giardia* and the enterobacteria previously noted.

Immunopathology. More severe degrees of functional upset are associated with increasingly severe degrees of morphologic change in the jejunum. Villi are shortened, crypts are deeper, and there is an increase both in interepithelial lymphocyte counts and in the lamina propria infiltrate with lymphocytes and plasma cells (Fig. 87–3). These findings are common to many mucosal diseases of the gut. The significance of the changes in relation to functional impairment is uncertain, but there is increasing evidence that the changes in mucosal architecture relate to the stimulatory effects of T-cell products on the crypt cell population. One or more *Giardia* antigens or food antigens entering through a leaky mucosa may have this stimulatory effect. This would explain the crypt hypertrophy but not the reduction in villous height because stimulatory effects from T cells in the crypts should not cause cytotoxic effects on the villi. Enterocyte damage caused by *Giardia* trophozoites may impair intercellular adhesion and allow increased cell desquamation into the gut lumen. The distribution of *Giardia* trophozoites is predomi-

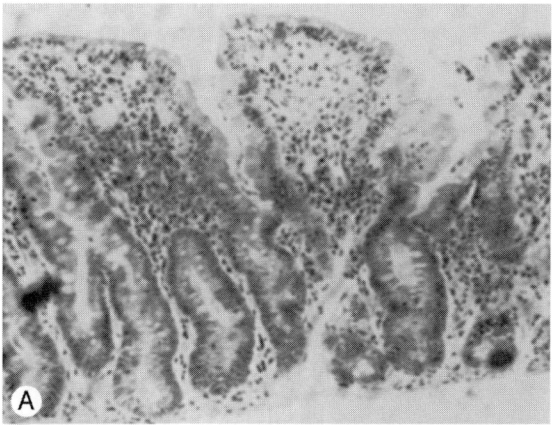
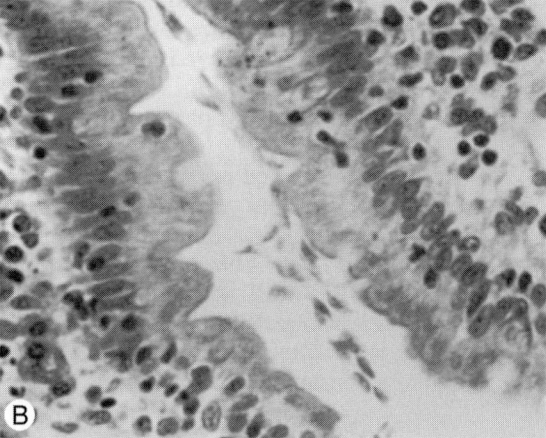

Figure **87–3.** Jejunal biopsy section from a patient with symptomatic giardiasis. *A,* There are definite abnormalities, with shortened villi, deepened crypts, and an increased inflammatory infiltrate in the lamina propria. *Giardia* trophozoites are seen in the intervillous spaces. *B,* With greater magnification, the characteristic morphologic features of the parasites can be seen.

nantly intervillous (Fig. 87–3), and crypts are rarely colonized. Therefore, for *Giardia* antigen to drive this, a secreted or excreted antigen would have to diffuse down into the crypt region.

Protective Immunity. Nonspecific and specific host responses are important in controlling the parasite population. A bile salt–dependent breast milk lipase is toxic to *Giardia* in vitro and may be important in protection before weaning.

Humoral responses are best characterized. Antibody responses to *Giardia* were followed in volunteers infected with trophozoites of one of two strains. Serum antibody was detected in *all* 10 who received the strain producing patent infections but in *none* of the 5 who received the other strain, suggesting that strain variation in infectivity, and not humoral immunity, is important in some cases. All infected subjects had IgM antibody when either of the challenge strains was used as antigen. Most had detectable antibody by day 14. Serum IgG and IgM antibodies were present in 70% and 60% of infected volunteers with a similar time course. Five of 10 had detectable antigiardia IgA in jejunal fluid. IgM antibody titers in serum declined within weeks of effective treatment, unlike IgG antibody, which persisted up to 6 months after treatment.

A range of antigens evoking antibody responses have been identified. A surface antigen with a molecular weight of 82 to 88 kDa has been defined. The giardins, a family of proteins of which two are presently described, are antigenic and are localized to the sucker disk. An interesting surface antigen with a molecular weight of 170 kDa seems to be capable of variable expression.

Attention has recently focused on the phenomenon of surface protein variation. In human volunteers the strain exhibited the original surface variant for the first 14 days but thereafter a new variant appeared. The advantage that expression of new variant surface proteins would give the protozoa is that host secretory IgA would not recognize it, and so harmful immunologic effects would be avoided. These proteins can bind metals, e.g., zinc, which is important for the activity of a number of brush border enzymes and thymidine kinase, and this may contribute to mucosal dysfunction.

In vitro antibody agglutinates trophozoites, immobilizing and killing them by binding to flagella. IgM antibody with complement activation by the classic pathway will kill parasites. Both secretory IgA and IgM could cause these effects in the gut lumen. Antibody-dependent cytotoxicity has also been observed. The absence of a major role for *G. lamblia* in the enteropathy of AIDS suggests that immune responses mediated by CD4+ cells do not have much influence in protection.

PATHOLOGY. Infected persons have a range of severity of functional and morphologic changes. Persons who are asymptomatic usually have normal absorption and normal histologic appearance of the jejunal mucosa. Mild symptoms are usually associated with some reduction in D-xylose absorption and minor histologic abnormalities without reduction of villous height. Impaired absorption of fat, D-xylose, and vitamin B$_{12}$ and hypolactasia are common in those severely affected. There is obvious reduction in villous height, increase in crypt depth with increased numbers of mitotic figures, and an increased infiltrate of plasma cells and lymphocytes in the lamina propria (Fig. 87–3A). Interepithelial lymphocyte counts are increased. *Giardia* trophozoites may be seen in the intervillous spaces and on the microvillous border of epithelial cells (Figs. 87–2 and 87–3). Terminal ileal biopsies showing *Giardia* were examined and found to be normal histologically with no increase in mucosal inflammation irrespective of the numbers of parasite seen.

Severe villous atrophy due to *G. lamblia* alone has been reported, but it is exceptional. When such severe histologic changes are found, celiac disease should be suspected; serial biopsies after eradication of *Giardia*, gluten withdrawal, and gluten challenge are needed to confirm this diagnosis. Giardiasis causes severe diarrhea in those patients whose celiac disease had been covert. Folate deficiency causing macrocytosis and megaloblastic anemia occasionally occurs. Protein-losing enteropathy has been found in giardiasis.

CLINICAL MANIFESTATIONS. Symptoms in acute infections begin after an incubation period of about 2 weeks. Usual symptoms are anorexia, nausea, lassitude, and diarrhea, with frequent passing of offensive yellow stools. Systemic upset does not occur. Abdominal distention and discomfort, a bad taste in the mouth, and flatulence are usual at this stage; weight loss occurs because of the anorexia and diarrhea. These symptoms may persist for several weeks and then start to resolve spontaneously with return of appetite, regaining of weight and resolution of diarrhea.

After infection, a variety of outcomes are possible: (1) an acute diarrheal illness that resolves spontaneously, with eradication of the infection by natural means; (2) continuing diarrhea with weight loss and continuing infection; (3) resolution of diarrhea with continuing cyst excretion.

Complications. A proportion of those infected remain markedly symptomatic with no tendency toward spontaneous resolution. Weight loss in this group suggests malabsorption, confirmed by abnormal tests of absorption. When symptoms have been present for several months, the patient may have glossitis, indicating folate deficiency although this is not common. Instances of food allergy apparently brought on by symptomatic giardiasis have been reported. When the infection is treated, the food allergy disappears. It is possible that the offending allergen enters through a mucosa that is more permeable to macromolecules. Colonization of the biliary tract has been reported in symptomatic patients.

The main complications of giardiasis relate to the effect of the infection on nutritional status of the host. Recurrent symptomatic giardiasis in children can cause failure to thrive and may play a part, with other gastrointestinal infections, in causing overt malnutrition in the tropics. Specific nutritional deficiencies are not as common as they are in tropical sprue.

DIAGNOSIS

Demonstration of the Parasite. This depends on finding the parasite (Fig. 87–1). Cysts are usually found by microscopy of concentrated stool samples (Chapter 150). It may be necessary to examine several samples because of the considerable variations in cyst excretion from day to day. A fecal smear of fluid stools should be examined directly for cysts and trophozoites.

If *Giardia* have not been found in several stools in a symptomatic patient, particularly if there is a clinical suspicion of malabsorption, sampling the upper gastrointestinal tract by intubation, jejunal biopsy, or string test is indicated (Chapter 150). Flecks of mucus adhering to the biopsy fragment or capsule should be mounted in saline for microscopic examination, and mucosal impression smears should be made from the epithelial surface of the biopsy specimen. Trophozoites can be seen on or near the epithelial surface in histologic sections stained with hematoxylin and eosin (Fig. 87–3). When the parasite cannot be found by any of these methods but giardiasis is still suspected on clinical grounds, drug treatment may be indicated.

Antigen Detection. Increasing numbers of studies have demonstrated that this means of detecting parasites works satisfactorily and can be as good as, if not better than, microscopic demonstration of *Giardia*. Enzyme-linked immunosorbent assay (ELISA)–based techniques and monoclonal anti-

TABLE 87–1. Drugs and Dosages Used in Treating Giardiasis

	Metronidazole	Tinidazole	Quinacrine
Adult Dose			
Long course	200–250 mg 3 times daily for 14 days		100 mg 3 times daily for 5–10 days
Short course	2.0 g daily for 3 days	2.0 g once	—
Pediatric Dose			
Long course	10–15 mg/kg/day in 3 divided doses for 14 days		6 mg/kg/day in 3 divided doses for 5–10 days
Short course	35–40 mg/kg daily for 3 days	50 mg/kg once	—

bodies have both been used with good results. Commercial kits are now available. Using an ELISA technique, 76 of 77 positive specimens were correctly identified with no false positive results. Antigen was detected for 2 days after the parasite could no longer be detected by conventional methods following treatment.

Serology. Serum antibodies to *G. lamblia* have been found using indirect fluorescent antibody (IFA) and ELISA techniques, using cyst or, more recently, trophozoite antigens. About 80% of symptomatic patients have detectable antibodies. Antibodies persist in circulation for about 6 months after eradication of the infection. In an area where there is little giardiasis, antibodies in a symptomatic patient may indicate infection and should prompt further diagnostic tests. In an endemic region antibodies may only indicate past infection, although the occurrence of serum IgM responses in symptomatic patients in endemic areas and the relatively rapid decline in titer after eradication may have practical value.

Radiographic Changes. Radiologic changes in an upper gastrointestinal series comprise dilatation of small bowel loops and thickening of mucosal folds. These changes occur in patients with malabsorption from many causes and are not specific for giardiasis.

TREATMENT

Drugs. Metronidazole, tinidazole, and quinacrine are the agents most often used for treatment of giardiasis. Long courses at low dose or short courses at high dose can be used (Table 87–1).

Both metronidazole and tinidazole interact with alcohol like disulfiram; therefore patients should not drink alcohol while taking either drug. Their other side effects include nausea, a metallic taste in the mouth, headache, and drowsiness. These are not usually noticeable at lower dosages and resolve quickly after treatment is completed. Because of occasional drowsiness with high-dose regimens, patients should be advised not to ride a bicycle, drive a car, or operate any dangerous machinery during treatment. Side effects seem to be less marked with tinidazole, which has the advantage of single dosage in the short-course regimen, allowing for a greater likelihood of patient compliance. Metronidazole has been used extensively for many years without any evidence that it is unsafe in pregnancy.

The common side effects of quinacrine include nausea, vomiting, abdominal pain, and temporary yellow staining of the skin. Psychosis also occurs occasionally. Quinacrine is contraindicated in patients with psoriasis. The efficacy of nonabsorbed antibiotics, e.g., bacitracin, neomycin, and bacitracin zinc, has been shown with cure rates of 87.5%, 86.4%, and 87.5%, respectively. Paromomycin is also useful and has the advantage of being safe in pregnancy. Albendazole, 600 or 800 mg in single doses, cured 62% and 75%, respectively over 10 days' follow-up.

Drug Resistance. This has been suspected clinically in those relatively few patients who remain persistently infected de-

spite the use of currently available drugs in optimal dosage. In vitro sensitivity testing has shown variations in drug sensitivity among strains as well as drug-resistant strains.

Response to Therapy. Diarrhea usually stops within 1 to 2 weeks of completing treatment, occasionally within a day or so. Cyst excretion ceases 2 days after initiation of treatment. Abnormalities of intestinal function and morphology resolve within 1 to 2 months of treatment. Persistent symptoms respond, in most cases, to a low-lactose diet and avoidance of alcohol, herbs, and spices. If giardiasis persists, further courses of treatment should be given. Rapid reinfection is very frequent among children in hyperendemic areas.

PREVENTION AND CONTROL. Clean drinking water, proper disposal of excreta, and clean hands would prevent most transmission of giardiasis. Heating drinking water to over 50°C kills cysts. A 2% solution of iodine kills cysts and can be used by travelers to endemic areas to sterilize drinking water. Filters are also available to purify drinking water. Avoiding salads, uncooked foods, and unpeeled fruits is also helpful. Thoroughly cooked foods and boiled water in drinks are safe.

Bibliography

Ament ME, Rubin CE: Relationship of giardiasis to abnormal intestinal structure and function in gastrointestinal immunodeficiency syndromes. Gastroenterology 62:216, 1972.

Belosevic M, Faubert GM, Maclean JD: Disaccharidase activity in the small intestine of gerbils (Meriones unguiculatus) during primary and challenge infections with Giardia lamblia. Gut 30:1213, 1989.

Burtin P, Taddio A, Ariburnu O, et al: Safety of metronidazole in pregnancy: a meta-analysis. Am J Obstet Gynecol 172:525, 1995.

Danciger M, Lopez M: Numbers of Giardia in feces of infected children. Am J Trop Med Hyg 24:237, 1975.

Dykes AC, Juranek DD, Lorenz RA, et al: Municipal waterborne giardiasis: An epidemiologic investigation. Ann Intern Med 92:165, 1980.

Ferguson A, Gillon J, Thamery D: Intestinal abnormalities in murine giardiasis. Trans R Soc Trop Med Hyg 74:445, 1980.

Gilman RE, Marquis GS, Miranda E, et al: Rapid reinfection by Giardia lamblia after treatment in a hyperendemic third world community. Lancet 1:343, 1988.

Green EL, Miles MA, Warhurst DC: Immunodiagnostic detection of Giardia antigen by a rapid visual enzyme-linked immunosorbent assay. Lancet 1:691, 1985.

Keystone JS, Kradjens S, Warren MR: Person to person transmission of Giardia lamblia in day care nurseries. J Can Med Assoc 119:241, 1978.

Meyer EA, Jarroll EL: Giardiasis. Am J Epidemiol 111:1, 1980.

Nash TE: Immunology: The role of the parasite. In Thompson RCA, Reynoldson JA, Lymbery AJ (eds): Giardia from Molecules to Disease. Wallingford, Oxon, CAB International, 1994, pp 139–154.

Nash TE, Herrington DA, Losonsky GA, Levine MM: Experimental human infections with Giardia lamblia. J Infect Dis 156:974, 1987.

Oberhubert G, Stolte M: Histologic detection of Giardia lamblia in the terminal ileum. Scand J Gastroenterol 30:905, 1995.

Peattie DA: The giardins of Giardia lamblia: Genes and proteins with promise. Parasitol Today 6:52, 1990.

Rendtorff RC: The experimental transmission of human intestinal protozoan parasites. II. Giardia lamblia cysts given in capsules. Am J Hyg 59:209, 1954.

Thompson RCA, Reynoldson JA, Mendis AHW: Giardia and giardiasis. Adv Parasitol 32:72, 1993.

Wright SG, Tomkins AM, Ridley DS: Giardiasis: Clinical and therapeutic aspects. Gut 18:343, 1977.

88 Cryptosporidiosis*

Dennis D. Juranek

DEFINITION. Cryptosporidiosis is an intestinal infection with *Cryptosporidium* species—an intracellular protozoan parasite that is found in highest concentration in the jejunum but that may infect any part of the small or large intestine, including secretory ducts that empty into the small intestine. *C. parvum* is the species implicated in human infection and disease; it also infects at least 79 species of mammals. Clinical manifestations vary from a self-limited diarrheal illness of 1 to 2 weeks' duration in immunocompetent persons to severe, life-threatening disease associated with voluminous watery diarrhea, anorexia, and weight loss in immunocompromised persons, especially those with AIDS.

HISTORY. *Cryptosporidium* was first recognized in the stomach and small intestine of asymptomatic mice by Tyzzer in 1907. Since then *Cryptosporidium* species have been identified in more than 170 species of animals, including most animals and fowl found on farms; household pets; and wild rodents, other mammals, birds, fish, and reptiles. The first two reports of a human infection occurred in 1976; one involved a 3-year-old immunocompetent child and the other an immunocompromised adult. From 1976 to 1982, human infections were reported rarely. In 1982, reporting dramatically increased when it was recognized that cryptosporidiosis was a common opportunistic infection in people with AIDS. At first the increased recognition was limited to immunocompromised persons; however, with the aid of better laboratory diagnostic techniques, outbreaks and sporadic infections in immunocompetent people began to be recognized.

INCIDENCE AND DISTRIBUTION. Cryptosporidiosis occurs worldwide. Infection is more prevalent in developing than in developed countries. *C. parvum* oocysts are found in about 2% (range 0.3–22%) of immunocompetent people with diarrhea in developed countries compared with 6% (range 1.4–41%) in developing countries. The prevalence of *Cryptosporidium* infection in people positive for the human immunodeficiency virus (HIV) in developed and developing countries is 14% (range 6–70%) and 24% (range 8.7–48%), respectively. *Cryptosporidium* is also an important cause of acute diarrhea in infants and children, especially in developing countries. In some areas, up to 15% of acute gastroenteritis in children is caused by this organism. Seroprevalence rates in developed countries are generally in the 25 to 35% range. Seroprevalence rates in developing countries are often two to three times higher. Outbreaks of cryptosporidiosis have been associated with drinking water contaminated by human or animal feces, accidental ingestion of lake or pool water, poor diaper changing and hygienic practices in child care centers, exposure to ill persons in hospitals, eating or drinking fecally contaminated food or beverages, and exposure to young infected animals at petting zoos, dairy farms, and veterinary hospitals.

PARASITOLOGY

Taxonomy. *Cryptosporidium* is in the phylum Apicomplexa, one that includes several genera of protozoa commonly referred to as coccidia (class, Coccidea; order, Eucoccidiorida), which complete all stages of development in the gastrointestinal tract of vertebrates. *Cryptosporidium* is the only genus in the family Cryptosporidiidae. It has an apical complex but possesses neither cilia nor flagella. Eight species of *Cryp-*

tosporidium are currently recognized: *C. baileyi* (birds), *C. felis* (domestic cat), *C. meleagridis* (turkey), *C. muris* (mouse, cattle), *C. nasorum* (fish), *C. parvum* (mammals), *C. serpentis* (snakes), and *C. wrairi* (guinea pig). Their oocysts range in size from 4 to 8 μm in diameter. *C. parvum* (4–6 μm) is the least host-specific of the eight species and has been reported in 79 mammalian species. It is the only species believed to infect humans. An infection with *C. baileyi* reported in an immunocompromised human in 1991 was later confirmed as *C. parvum* by DNA analysis. Molecular tools for distinguishing different species, and possibly subspecies, are being rapidly developed and may soon clarify the species-level taxonomy of the genus *Cryptosporidium*.

Life Cycle. The life cycle of *Cryptosporidium* is depicted in Figure 88–1. Photo- and electron micrographs of selected developmental stages of the parasite are shown in Figures 88–2 to 88–5. Although the parasite is located intracellularly, it is extracytoplasmic, lying between the cell membrane and cytoplasm. The sporulated oocyst is the only developmental stage that occurs extracellularly, but this part of the cycle is also completed before the oocyst is excreted in the feces. Thus, oocysts of *Cryptosporidium* spp., unlike many other coccidia, are immediately infectious when they are passed in a stool. Internal autoinfection (a process whereby merozoites resulting from asexual reproduction or sporozoites emerging from newly developed thin-walled oocysts infect more enterocytes) is common and is probably responsible for the chronic nature of the disease in immunocompromised people.

PATHOGENESIS

Infectious Dose. The dose required to produce infection in 50% of healthy human volunteers was estimated in one study to be 132 oocysts; ingestion of as few as 30 oocysts resulted in a 20% infection rate. This study and other data show that no more than a few cysts are needed to cause infection. The infectious dose of *C. parvum* in other animal models is smaller than that demonstrated in the human volunteer study, e.g., infant macaques develop a self-limited illness after inoculation with 10 oocysts, and gnotobiotic lambs have been infected with a single oocyst.

Sites of Infection and Pathology. Most of the information about the pathogenesis of human cryptosporidiosis stems from histologic studies of intestinal biopsy material obtained from infected immunodeficient individuals (usually patients with AIDS) (Figs. 88–1 to 88–4). Developmental stages have been detected in the pharynx, esophagus, stomach, duodenum, jejunum, ileum, appendix, colon, and rectum of humans; at post-mortem examination the jejunum is usually the most severely affected. Infection of the bile duct, gallbladder, liver, pancreatic duct, pancreas, and lungs has also been reported in AIDS patients. Histologic lesions include villous atrophy, an increase in crypt length, and mild to moderate infiltration (usually plasma cells and neutrophils but also macrophages and lymphocytes) in the lamina propria. These abnormalities are similar to those observed in mice, pigs, and lambs as well as germ-free calves that have been experimentally infected with *C. parvum*.

Pathophysiology of Diarrhea and Malabsorption. This is not clear. Although a parasite-produced enterotoxin is suspected, its existence has not been proved. In a piglet model, a loss of the vacuolated villus tip epithelium (constituting about two thirds of the villus surface area), accompanied by a 50% reduction in the glucose-coupled sodium cotransport mechanism, has been demonstrated. The result is a predominance of transitional junctional epithelium, in which increased glutamine metabolism drives a sodium-hydrogen exchange to which is coupled chloride transport. Thus, glutamine is thought to drive neutral sodium chloride absorption in an apparent prostaglandin-inhibited manner in the pig infected with *Cryptosporidium*.

---

*All the material in this chapter is in the public domain, with the exception of any borrowed figures or tables.

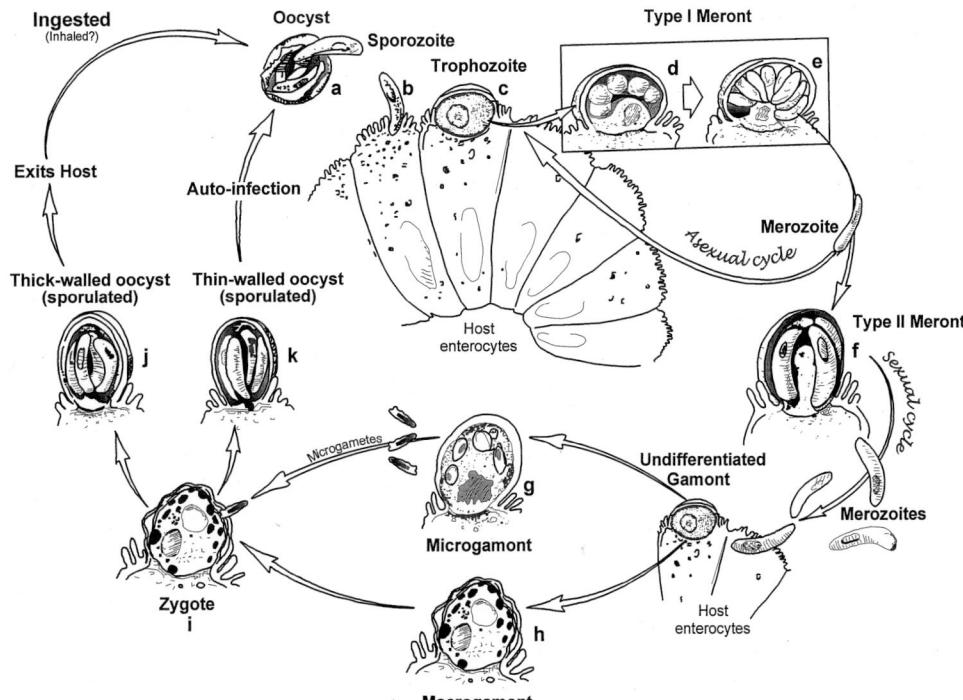

Figure 88–1. Life cycle of *Cryptosporidium parvum*. After ingestion, oocysts excyst in the lumen of the intestine *(a)*; four sporozoites *(b)* emerge from each oocyst, penetrate enterocytes that line the intestine, and develop into trophozoites *(c)*. Trophozoites undergo asexual reproduction (merogony) *(d and e)* to form merozoites. Merozoites emerging from type I meronts can reinfect host cells and either repeat the asexual cycle or infect host cells and develop into type II meronts *(f)*. Type II meronts liberate four merozoites each. It is believed that only merozoites from type II meronts can initiate sexual reproduction. Type II merozoites enter host enterocytes, where they undergo gametogony to form male microgamonts *(g)* or female macrogamonts *(h)*. Microgametes (sperm cell equivalent) emerge from microgamonts to fertilize mature macrogamonts to produce zygotes *(i)* that further develop into thick-walled *(j)* or thin-walled *(k)* oocysts. These oocysts sporulate (develop infective sporozoites) while in the intestinal lumen. Emergence of sporozoites from thin-walled oocysts while still in the intestine results in autoinfection. Thick-walled oocysts are excreted in the host's feces and are immediately infectious to the same or another host if ingested. (Adapted from Current WL, Garcia LS: Clin Microbiol Rev 4:325, 1991.)

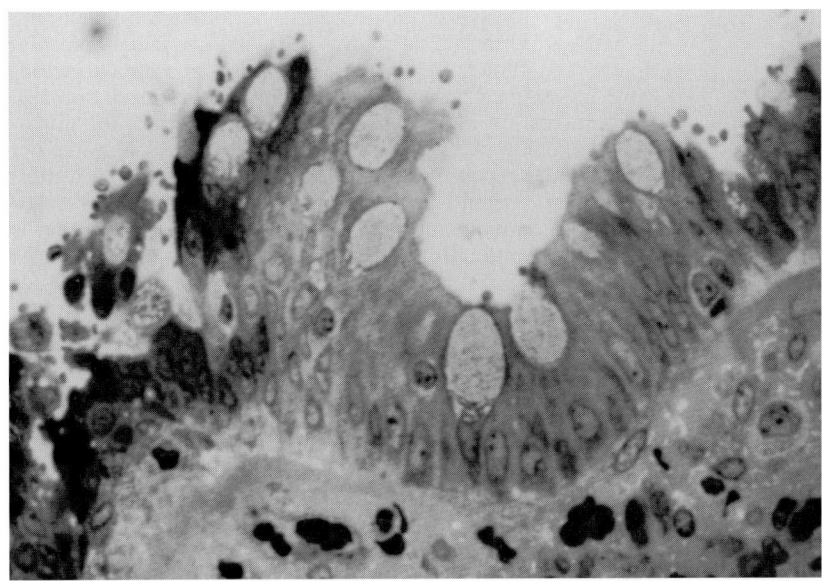

Figure 88–2. Light micrograph of the rectal biopsy specimen from an AIDS patient showing endogenous stages of *Cryptosporidium* sp. Toluidine blue-stained section. (Courtesy of D. P. Casemore.)

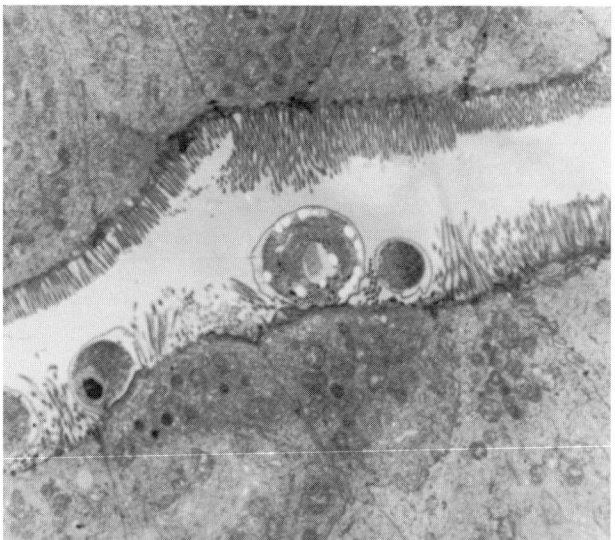

Figure 88–3. Electron micrograph of mouse intestine showing *C. parvum*. A uninucleate meront (trophozoite) with prominent nucleolus within a parasitophorous vacuole is shown with a macrogamete; parts of two other meronts are also present (× 6000). (Courtesy of D. P. Casemore.)

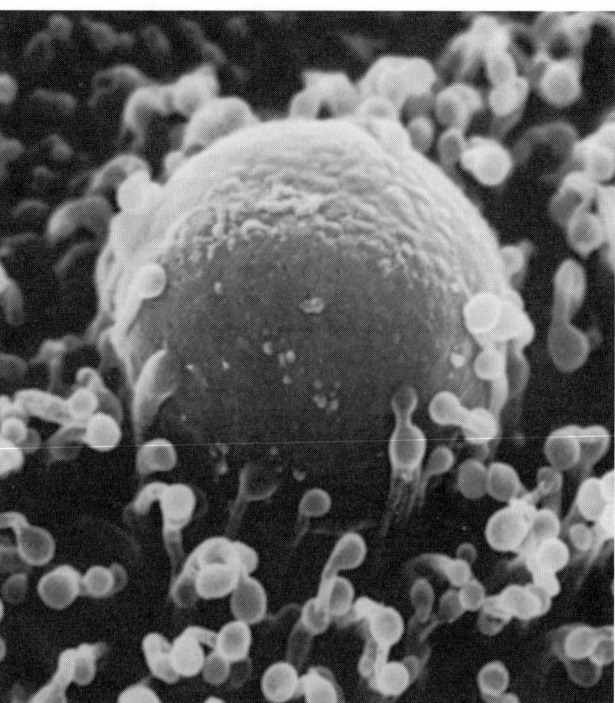

Figure 88–5. Scanning electron micrograph showing oocyst of *Cryptosporidium* sp. surrounded by intestinal microvilli in an AIDS patient infected with HIV-2 (× 40,000). (Courtesy of the Electron Microscopy Laboratory. London School of Hygiene and Tropical Medicine.)

Immunology. Immune competence is an important determinant in the severity and duration of cryptosporidiosis in humans. Whereas cryptosporidiosis is a self-limiting disease of 7 to 14 days' duration in immunocompetent individuals, it can be a chronic, life-threatening illness in severely immunocompromised people, e.g., those with AIDS or hypogammaglobulinemia or those receiving immunosuppressive drugs for cancer or to prevent tissue rejection following organ transplantation. It is probable that both humoral and cell-mediated immunity (CMI) are involved in the body's defense against cryptosporidiosis, although CMI seems to be the more important. Severe and persistent disease in patients

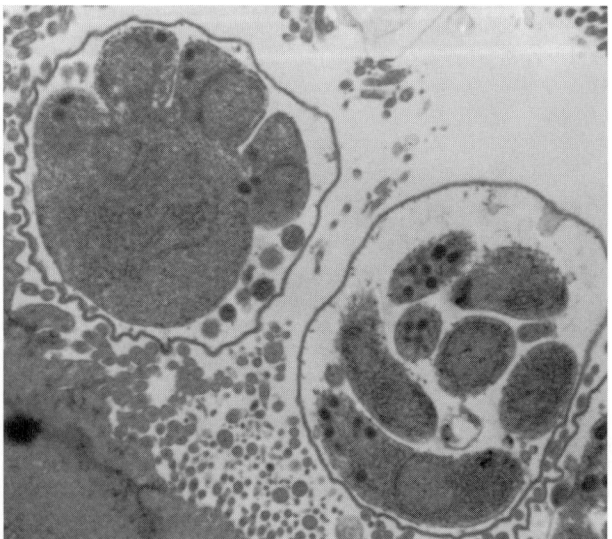

Figure 88–4. Electron micrograph showing schizonts (type I and II meronts [trophozoites]) of *Cryptosporidium sp.*; one contains 4 partly developed, and the other parts of 8 fully developed, merozoites that have budded into the parasitophorous vacuole (× 16,000). (Courtesy of D. P. Casemore.)

with AIDS correlates well with CD4 counts ≤180 cells/mm³. In one study, only 5 (13%) of 39 patients infected with *C. parvum* and with CD4 counts ≤180 cells/mm³ had self-limiting disease, whereas all 8 patients with CD4 counts ≥180 cells/mm³ had infections that cleared and did not relapse during a follow-up period of 1 to 24 months. Normal CD4 cell function has been reported in some patients with hypogammaglobulinemia who had severe infection. Measles (which suppresses CMI) has been implicated as a predisposing factor for symptomatic cryptosporidiosis in developing countries. Humoral responses to *Cryptosporidium* infection have been demonstrated in a wide variety of animals, including immunocompetent and immunocompromised humans. In humans, *Cryptosporidium* primarily parasitizes the microvillous region of the enterocyte (Figs. 88–1 to 88–4), a site not likely to be exposed to serum antibodies. This makes it difficult to understand how serum antibodies can play a major role in acquired immunity. A more plausible explanation is that local antibodies (intestinal immunoglobulins A [IgA] and G [IgG]) coupled with CMI mechanisms are required for parasite clearance from the enterocyte. Short-term resistance to infection in animals experimentally rechallenged with oocysts after recovery from a primary infection has been demonstrated.

Age is an important factor in the development of clinical disease in animals, but it is less important in humans. In most animals, cryptosporidiosis is a diarrheal disease of newborns or those less than 6 months of age. Mature animals generally exhibit no sign of infection or are parasite free. Illness in humans occurs at all ages. The age of ill persons in published reports ranges from a 3-day-old delivered vaginally to a *Cryptosporidium*-infected mother to a 95-year-old. Prevalence surveys usually reveal the highest rates of infection in children less than 2 years of age. Although incomplete protective immunity may explain the high rate of infection in young children, it is likely that children also have more frequent exposure to oocysts, i.e., fecal exposures commonly associated with lack of toilet training, frequent placement of soiled hands and objects in the mouth, intimate child-to-child play, and poor-quality drinking water (especially in developing countries).

EPIDEMIOLOGY. Cryptosporidium infection occurs in people and animals throughout the world. Differences observed in the sex distribution of infected persons in some studies probably reflect differences in exposure rather than a difference in susceptibility to infection with the parasite. Serologic surveys suggest that exposure to *Cryptosporidium* is frequent in both developed and developing countries. In the United States, 17 to 32% of young adults from different states have IgG antibody to *Cryptosporidium*. In contrast, 75% of 11- to 13-year-old children in rural China were found seropositive. In an impoverished area of Brazil, more than 90% of children were seropositive by the age of 1 year. The presence of oocysts in the stool is usually associated with symptoms, but asymptomatic infections have been reported in immunocompetent as well as immunocompromised people.

C. parvum is transmitted by ingestion of oocysts excreted in the feces of infected humans or animals. Infection can therefore be transmitted from person to person, through ingestion of fecally contaminated water or food, from animal to person, or by contact with fecally contaminated environmental surfaces. The pathway by which most people become infected probably varies with age, lifestyle (e.g., use of child care facilities, recreational activities, sexual preferences and practices), living conditions (including sanitation, hygiene, and source of drinking water), and frequency of exposure to livestock (especially calves and lambs).

Fecal-Oral Transmission. Person-to-person spread of *C. parvum* is one of the most common modes of transmission. Children still wearing diapers who attend child care centers are at especially high risk, either through intimate play or because of careless diaper-changing practices. Infections acquired by children in child care or other settings are often transmitted to caregivers as well as to other children and adult family members. Other types of high-risk exposures include direct contact with feces while caring for an infected person (e.g., bathing, changing soiled bedding, or emptying a bedpan) at home or in a medical facility and sexual practices that bring oral contact with the feces of an infected person. Infections and outbreaks attributed to person-to-person spread between medical care staff and patients as well as between patients have been reported.

Food-borne transmission has been implicated in several outbreaks of *Cryptosporidium* infection. Although oocysts do not survive cooking, infected food handlers may unwittingly transmit oocysts from poorly washed hands to beverages, green salads, or other foods that are not cooked or heated after handling. Similarly, raw fruits and vegetables can become contaminated in the field from human or animal feces or from contaminated water. Food products implicated in reported outbreaks include fresh pressed apple cider, unpasteurized milk, potato salad, sausage, and offal.

Water-borne Outbreaks. Many well-documented outbreaks of cryptosporidiosis have been attributed to contamination of municipally treated drinking water, including an outbreak in Milwaukee in 1993 that affected over 400,000 persons. The sources of water used by communities reporting outbreaks include surface water (lakes, rivers, and streams), well water, and spring water. In nearly all the reported waterborne outbreaks in developed countries, the quality of the water after treatment by the water utility met community or state standards for potability. Although some wells and springs may be vulnerable to *Cryptosporidium* oocyst contamination, surface water supplies pose the greatest health risk. Studies in the United States indicate that *Cryptosporidium* oocysts are present in 60 to 97% of the surface waters tested. Concentrations of oocysts found in surface waters have varied from ≤1 to ≥65 oocysts/L water. Oocyst concentrations have been highest near points where wastewater treatment plants discharge treated human sewage into rivers. Because *Cryptosporidium* spp. are highly resistant to chemical disinfectants used in the treatment of water intended for drinking, removal of the parasite from contaminated water by tightly controlled prefiltration and filtration processes is an important component of the water treatment process. Even with this extra attention, the filters most commonly used in large cities (rapid sand or multimedia filters) do not always remove 100% of oocysts. Surveys for the presence of *Cryptosporidium* oocysts in fully treated (disinfected and filtered) municipal water in the United States demonstrated that small numbers of oocysts (mean, 3/100 L) had breached filters and were present in tap water in 27 to 54% of communities evaluated. None of these communities had a recognizable outbreak of cryptosporidiosis. Thus, the health risk (especially for immunocompromised persons) associated with consumption of (filtered or unfiltered) public drinking water contaminated with small numbers of *C. parvum* oocysts is unknown, since current laboratory methods do not determine if these oocysts are viable or infectious.

Controlled laboratory studies indicate that oocysts survive for long periods in water. Some oocysts kept at 4°C in laboratory-quality water or potassium dichromate solution remained infectious up to 1 year; at 15 to 20°C, some oocyst survival was detectable for up to 3 months. Preliminary data indicate that oocysts may die more rapidly in natural bodies of water. Studies using river water indicate that 99.7% of oocysts die within 30 days at 20 to 30°C and that a slightly lower proportion (94%) die within 30 days in cold (4°C) water. In addition to the question of viability, it is not known if the small number of oocysts that are often present in drinking water constitute a sufficient dose to cause illness in humans, whether immunosuppressed persons are more susceptible to small doses of oocysts, or if strains of *C. parvum* vary in infectious dose and virulence.

Infection Associated with Swimming. Several outbreaks of cryptosporidiosis have been traced to accidental ingestion of contaminated water while swimming in pools or lakes and while playing in amusement park wading pools, in wave pools, or on water slides. No obvious fecal accidents were observed in most of these outbreaks. It is suspected that there are sufficient numbers of oocysts on perianal surfaces of infected individuals who do not shower before entering a pool to contaminate the pool water. Several recreational water outbreaks have been traced to individuals who had recently recovered from *Cryptosporidium*-related diarrhea and who were thought to be shedding oocysts at the time. This hypothesis is consistent with data indicating that some children continue to shed oocysts in their stools for more than 30 days after they recover from clinical illness. *Cryptosporidium* is not killed by the 3 to 5 mg/L of chlorine normally used to disinfect swimming pools. Moreover, many types of pool filters do not remove oocysts, and the circulation time of pool water through a filter capable of removing oocysts is too slow to prevent exposure of persons who are in the pool at the time of contamination or who may enter the pool several hours later.

Exposure to Calves. While *C. parvum* is capable of infecting a wide variety of mammals, the calf is most frequently implicated as the source of human infection. Outbreaks have been reported among veterinary students handling ill calves and in children visiting dairy farms or petting zoos. A number of sporadic human infections among laboratory workers also have been attributed to contact with infected calves or calf feces. *Cryptosporidium* infection is especially common in dairy herds. It is estimated that 50% of dairy calves shed oocysts and that the parasite is present on more than 90% of dairy farms in the United States. Seroprevalence of antibodies against *Cryptosporidium* is higher in dairy farmers in Wisconsin than in others in the same community who have no exposure to dairy cattle. Dairy cattle upstream from water treatment plants have been strongly implicated as the source of contamination in several water-borne outbreaks of cryptosporidiosis in England. Cattle have been present in the watersheds of several communities in the United States that have experienced a water-borne outbreak of cryptosporidiosis; however, epidemiologic studies have failed to conclusively link cattle to these outbreaks, since other sources of water contamination (e.g., human sewage) also were present. Lambs also have been documented as a source of human infection. The importance of other domesticated and wild animals as reservoirs of *Cryptosporidium* infection for humans is poorly defined. In contrast to the strong epidemiologic data implicating calves and lambs as important sources of human infection, dogs and cats do not pose a major risk despite reports of infection in these animals.

CLINICAL MANIFESTATIONS. Although cryptosporidiosis is more severe and chronic in immunosuppressed persons, there are many exceptions to this general rule. Asymptomatic and mild infections in AIDS patients and severe diarrhea of several months' duration in immunocompetent persons have been reported. Cryptosporidiosis is primarily a gastrointestinal disease, but illness may occasionally be associated with an ascending infection of the bile or pancreatic ducts, with signs and symptoms of acalculous cholecystitis, sclerosing cholangitis, hepatitis, or pancreatitis. Respiratory infection may be accompanied by cough and shortness of breath. Concurrent infection with other enteric pathogens, e.g., *Giardia* and *Campylobacter* has been reported and may alter the clinical presentation.

Acute Diarrheal Illness. Watery diarrhea is the characteristic complaint of patients with cryptosporidiosis. It may contain mucus, but blood or leukocytes are rarely seen. Other common symptoms include epigastric cramps or pain, nausea, vomiting, and weight loss. Low-grade fever (38°C) is reported by about half of immunocompetent patients but less commonly reported in those with AIDS. In the immunocompetent, the median incubation period is 7 days with a range of 2 to 12 days. Diarrhea in people with an intact immune system is self-limiting with a mean duration of 9 days (range, 2–55 days); the median maximum number of bowel movements reported during a massive outbreak in Milwaukee was 12 per day (Table 88–1). Recurrence of diarrhea after a brief period of improvement has been described. Shedding of oocysts continues for 8 to 50 days (mean, 12–14 days) after clinical symptoms have resolved.

Chronic Diarrheal Illness. The symptom complex in patients with AIDS or hypogammaglobulinemia or those receiving immunosuppressive chemotherapy is similar to that in immunocompetent persons except that illness may begin with only mild symptoms that progressively worsen over time (especially in AIDS patients). Diarrhea in immunocompromised persons is usually protracted (months to years) and frequently severe and may be life-threatening. Diarrheal fluid losses of >20 L/day have been reported. In many patients, diarrhea is accompanied by severe abdominal pain, malabsorption, anorexia, and major weight loss. Whereas AIDS patients rarely experience spontaneous clearance of a *Cryptosporidium* infection, illness in patients with reversible im-

munodeficiencies usually resolves rapidly when the cause of the immunosuppression is removed.

DIAGNOSIS

Oocysts or Antigen in Stool. Failure to recognize *Cryptosporidium* as a cause of human disease until 1976 was in large part associated with the use of inadequate staining techniques to identify oocysts in the feces of humans and animals. An acid-fast stain, e.g., Ziehl-Neelsen or modified Kinyoun carbolfuchsin technique (Chapter 150), is adequate for the diagnosis of most infections. Increased sensitivity can be achieved by the use of a concentration technique, e.g., the formalin-ethylacetate sedimentation or Sheather's sucrose flotation method (Chapter 150), prior to staining. Oocysts are shed intermittently, and multiple stool examinations may be necessary. *C. parvum* oocysts, which are 4 to 6 μm in diameter, stain red with acid-fast stains. Yeasts, many of which are morphologically similar to *Cryptosporidium*, either do not stain or stain the same color as the counterstain. Oocysts remain acid-fast stainable for at least a year if stored cold (4°C) in 2.5% potassium dichromate or 10% formalin. Indirect fluorescent methods that use fluorescein-tagged monoclonal antibody are highly specific and are about ten times more sensitive than acid-fast stains in detecting small numbers of oocysts in stool. Regardless of the procedure used, oocysts are generally easier to detect in the stool of patients with diarrhea than in those with formed or semi-formed stool.

Enzyme immunoassay tests that detect *Cryptosporidium* antigen in stool are also commercially available; they are comparable in sensitivity and specificity to microscopic examination methods, are more expensive, but are faster for processing large numbers of specimens.

Many laboratories do not include *Cryptosporidium* in their testing procedure for stool specimens submitted for "ova and parasite" examination. A national survey in the United States found that only 5% of laboratories routinely provided this service; most performed *Cryptosporidium* testing only when the physician specifically requested it.

Biopsies. Light or electron microscopy can detect the developmental stages of *Cryptosporidium* in jejunal, ileal, or colonic biopsy specimens; these stages can be visualized in the microvillous region of the enterocyte (Fig. 88–1). Other fecal pathogens may be present concurrently, especially in people with AIDS or those living in developing countries. In individuals suspected of having pulmonary cryptosporidiosis, one should try to identify parasite stages in transbronchial or bronchoalveolar lavage specimens or sputum before resorting to tissue biopsy.

Serologic Diagnosis. Serum antibodies to *Cryptosporidium* can be detected by using indirect immunofluorescence (IFA), immunoblot, or enzyme-linked immunosorbent assay (ELISA) techniques. Crude and purified ELISA antigens derived from calf oocysts have been developed for detecting IgG, IgA, and IgM antibodies. Because detectable antibodies against *Cryptosporidium* tend to develop slowly after infection and are rarely present within a week after onset of illness, these diagnostic tools are being developed primarily for use in epidemiologic studies. No serologic tests are currently available commercially.

MANAGEMENT

Chemotherapy. A safe and highly effective chemotherapeutic agent against cryptosporidiosis has not yet been identified. Infection in immunocompetent people is self-limiting and does not require specific treatment, but antimotility drugs and oral rehydration may be useful in the acute phase of the illness. In immunosuppressed persons (e.g., those with AIDS), specific chemotherapy is indicated. Although some drugs reduce the frequency and volume of diarrhea in some patients, none does so consistently, and none eradicates infec-

TABLE 88–1. Clinical Characteristics of Persons With Laboratory-Confirmed and Clinical Cases of *Cryptosporidium* Infection Among Visitors Who Had <48 Hours' Exposure to the Service Area of the Milwaukee Water Works Compared With Laboratory-Confirmed and Clinically Defined Cases Among Residents of the Milwaukee Area

	Visitor Laboratory-Confirmed Cases (n = 54)	Visitor Clinically Defined Cases (n = 40)	Milwaukee Laboratory-Confirmed Cases (n = 285)	Milwaukee Clinically Defined Cases (n = 201)
Clinical Characteristics				
Diarrhea	54 (100%)	40 (100%)*	285 (100%)	201 (100%)*
Watery diarrhea	54 (100%)	40 (100%)*	265 (93%)	201 (100%)*
Abdominal cramps	51 (94%)	34 (85%)	238 (84%)	168 (84%)
Fatigue	50 (93%)	32 (80%)	274 (87%)	145 (72%)
Loss of appetite	41 (76%)	25 (63%)	230 (82%)	147 (73%)
Nausea	34 (63%)	24 (60%)	199 (71%)	119 (59%)
Fever	27 (50%)	18 (45%)	162 (57%)	72 (36%)
Chills	28 (52%)	15 (38%)	65 (64%)†	91 (45%)
Sweats	24 (44%)	13 (33%)	55 (55%)†	83 (41%)
Muscle or joint aches	35 (65%)	25 (63%)	152 (54%)	100 (50%)
Headache	35 (65%)	26 (65%)	53 (51%)†	122 (61%)
Vomiting	17 (32%)	9 (23%)	136 (48%)	37 (18%)
Cough	12 (22%)	2 (5%)	68 (24%)	56 (28%)
Sore throat	9 (17%)	3 (8%)	48 (17%)	35 (17%)
Mean duration of diarrhea	9 days	5 days	12 days	4.5 days
Mean maximum number of stools per day	10	9	19	7.7
Mean maximum temperature	101.2°F	101°F	101°F	100.5°F
Mean duration of vomiting	2.4 days	2.9 days	2.9 days	2.0 days
Mean maximum number of vomiting episodes per day	2.4	2.7	3.9	2.6

*Required to meet the clinical case definition.
†Data from only 101 case-patients.
From Mac Kenzie WR, Schell WL, Blair KA, et al: Clin Infect Dis 21:57, 1995.

tion. Paromomycin, clarithromycin, nitazoxanide, and hyperimmune bovine colostrum are among the current drugs of greatest clinical interest. At least 90 other agents have been tested or administered, including co-trimoxazole, spiramycin, azithromycin, erythromycin, furazolidone plus tetracycline, diloxanide furoate, quinine plus clindamycin, amphotericin B plus flucytosine, α-difluoromethylornithine, interferon-γ, and interleukin-2. Although many initially showed evidence of efficacy, none has lived up to expectations when subjected to larger, controlled studies or to widespread use by physicians in clinical practice. Delay in initiating immunosuppressive chemotherapy until after a mild or subclinical *Cryptosporidium* infection has been eliminated may prevent a life-threatening diarrheal illness. Similarly, in persons who acquire cryptosporidiosis while undergoing immunosuppressive therapy, reducing the dose of immunosuppressive medication often enables them to overcome the infection.

General Measures. Rehydration and symptomatic treatment may be necessary in both immunocompetent and immunosuppressed individuals. Codeine phosphate, diphenoxylate, loperamide, kaoline plus pectin, bismuth subsalicylate, and opiates may be useful. Somatostatin analogues (octreotide and vapreotide) also have been used with some success in AIDS patients with severe, refractory diarrhea. Hyperimmune bovine colostrum (containing IgG antibodies) has been administered orally to immunosuppressed patients with variable results, perhaps related to the variable level of antibodies and other unidentified anti-*Cryptosporidium* factors in the preparations used. Bovine transfer factor has been of value in the management of cryptosporidiosis associated with AIDS. Immunomodulation, or passive transfer of antibodies or lymphocytes, might also have a place in the treatment of *Cryptosporidium* infection in immunodeficient patients.

PREVENTION AND CONTROL

Prevention of Fecal-Oral Transmission. There is no effective vaccine, and there are no drugs for prophylaxis. To prevent person-to-person transmission, including spread in institutional settings, strict attention to personal hygiene (especially hand washing) and environmental sanitation should be emphasized. People should be advised to avoid sexual practices that could result in oral exposure to feces of an infected partner. Standard enteric precautions should be used by individuals in close contact with infected animals or humans. Oocysts are highly resistant to most antiseptics used in medical and other institutions for environmental control of microbes. Only ammonia (5% for 120 minutes or 50% for 30 minutes), formol saline (10% for 120 minutes), hydrogen peroxide (3% [10 vol] for 30 minutes), or chlorine dioxide (0.4 mg/L for 15 minutes) have been reported as effective. Desiccation of oocysts by exposure to dry air for 4 hours also kills them.

Cooking kills *Cryptosporidium* in food. Oocysts may be killed in milk and beverages by pasteurization (71.7°C for 5 sec), heating to 60°C for 30 minutes, or freezing at −70°C for 1 hour. However, oocysts are able to survive for short periods in ice made at temperatures similar to those in home freezers. Oocysts were infectious for mice after being frozen in small cubes of ice at −15°C for more than 24 hours but were not infective after 7 days; they survived freezing for more than 10 days at −10°C. Vegetables and fruits that are to be eaten uncooked should be thoroughly washed with potable water before consumption. No safe and effective chemical disinfectant against *Cryptosporidium* has been identified for decontaminating produce.

Treatment of Drinking Water. Prevention of water-borne disease includes protection of drinking water supplies from human and animal fecal contamination, proper treatment of potentially contaminated water, and safe storage of treated water. Cattle and other ruminants should be kept away from rivers and ponds that serve as community drinking water. Similarly, latrines, septic tanks, and other human waste disposal systems should be located so that they do not contaminate the water supply through underground seepage or surface runoff during rain storms. Concentrations of chlorine (1–2 mg/L) and other chemicals routinely used to disinfect drinking water are not effective against *Cryptosporidium*. Oocysts exposed for 2 hours to full-strength bleach (5.25% sodium hypochlorite ≈ 50,000 mg/L of chlorine) still infected mice. A well-operated conventional water filtration plant that includes prefiltration coagulation and sedimentation can markedly reduce the number of oocysts in community drinking water but may not remove all of them. Membrane-type filters (e.g., reverse osmosis) are capable of removing all oocysts as well as other microbes from community water, but they require a source of low-turbidity water so that they do not immediately plug up with debris. Reverse osmosis systems are available in individual, household, or community sizes that service up to 3000 people. Contaminated water can be purified for personal use by boiling for 1 minute. This is also effective against other water-borne pathogens acquired from drinking water. Personal-use filters having an absolute 1 μm or smaller pore size are effective against *Cryptosporidium*. However, smaller porosity filters (0.1–0.2 μm) or filters impregnated with pentiodide resins are necessary to remove bacterial pathogens as well. In developing countries, use of 3- to 5-gallon plastic water vessels (water containers that have a spigot for dispensing water and a fill lid designed to prevent entry of hands or objects commonly used to scoop out water) has been found effective in preventing recontamination of potable water stored in individual households.

Prevention in Immunocompromised Persons. Because cryptosporidiosis can be life-threatening in the immunocompromised, these individuals should be told about all the ways that *Cryptosporidium* can be transmitted, including possible infection risks that might be considered inconsequential for others. Depending on the setting, extra counseling about the risks posed by exposure to young animals (especially calves and lambs), recreational water, and beverages made from tap water may be warranted. Immunocompromised persons should avoid contact with any animal that has diarrhea. Immunosuppressed persons who wish to assume the small risk of acquiring a puppy or kitten aged <6 months should request that their veterinarian examine the animal's stool for *Cryptosporidium* before they have contact with it. They should be advised of the risk of acquiring infection by accidental ingestion of recreational water: Many lakes, rivers, and salt water beaches as well as some swimming pools and recreational water parks are intermittently contaminated with human or animal waste that contains cryptosporidia. People who are taking special precautions to avoid cryptosporidiosis from drinking tap water should be advised that ice made from contaminated tap water also can be a source of infection. They should also be advised that their risk of acquiring *Cryptosporidium* infection from water or food may increase when traveling in a developing country.

Bibliography

Adal KA, Sterling CS, Guerrant RL: *Cryptosporidium* and related species. *In* Blaser MS, Smith PD, Ravdin JI, et al (eds): Infections of the Gastrointestinal Tract. New York, Raven Press, 1995, pp 1107–1128.

Addiss DG, Juranek DD, Schwartz DA: Cryptosporidiosis. *In* Horsburgh CR Jr, Nelson AM (eds). Emerging Infections: Clinical and Pathologic Update. Washington, American Society for Microbiology, 1997, pp 243–256.

Boyce TG, Pemberton AG, Addiss DG: *Cryptosporidium* testing practices among clinical laboratories in the United States. Pediatr Infect Dis J 15:87, 1996.

Casemore DP, Gardner CA, O'Mahony CO: Cryptosporidial infection with special reference to nosocomial transmission of *Cryptosporidium parvum*: A review. Folia Parasitol 41:17, 1994.

Cook DJ, Kelton JG, Stanisz AM, et al: Somatostatin treatment for cryptosporidial diarrhea in a patient with acquired immunodeficiency syndrome (AIDS). Ann Intern Med 108:708, 1989.

Cordell RL, Addiss DG: Cryptosporidiosis in child care settings: A review of the literature and recommendations for prevention and control. Pediatr Infect Dis J 13:310, 1994.

Current WL, Garcia LS: Cryptosporidiosis. Clin Microbiol Rev 4:325, 1991.

Dupont HL, Chappell CL, Sterling CS, et al: The infectivity of *Cryptosporidium parvum* in healthy volunteers. N Engl J Med 332:855, 1995.

Fayer R (ed): *Cryptosporidium* and Cryptosporidiosis. New York, CRC Press, 1997.

Flanigan TP, Soave R: Cryptosporidiosis. *In* Sun Tsieh (ed): Progress in Clinical Parasitology. New York, Springer-Verlag, 1993, pp 1–20.

Goldstein ST, Juranek DD, Ravenholt O, et al: Cryptosporidiosis: An outbreak associated with drinking water despite state-of-the-art water treatment. Ann Intern Med 124:459, 1996.

Greenberg PD, Cello JP: Treatment of severe diarrhea caused by *Cryptosporidium parvum* with oral bovine immunoglobulin concentrate in patients with AIDS. J Acquir Immune Defic Syndr Hum Retroviral 13:348, 1996.

Guerrant RL: Cryptosporidiosis: An emerging, highly infectious threat. Emerging Infect Dis 3:51, 1997.

Juranek DD: Cryptosporidiosis: Sources of infection and guidelines for control. Clin Infect Dis 21(Suppl 1): S57, 1995.

Juranek DD: Working Group on Waterborne Cryptosporidiosis. *Cryptosporidium* and Water: A Public Health Handbook. Atlanta, Centers for Disease Control and Prevention, 1997.

Kaplan JE, Masuer H, Holmes KK, et al: 1997 USPHS/IDSA guidelines for the prevention of opportunistic infections in persons infected with human immunodeficiency virus. MMWR 46(No. RR-12):1, 1997.

Kehl KS, Cicirello H, Havens PL: Comparison of four different methods for detection of *Cryptosporidium* species. J Clin Microbiol 33:416, 1995.

LeChevallier MW, Norton WD: Giardia and *Cryptosporidium* in raw and finished water. J Am Water Works Assoc 87:54, 1995.

Mac Kenzie WR, Hoxie NJ, Proctor ME, et al: A massive outbreak in Milwaukee of *Cryptosporidium* infection transmitted through the public water supply. N Engl J Med 331:161, 1994.

Meinhardt PL, Casemore DP, Miller KB: Epidemiologic aspects of human cryptosporidiosis and the role of waterborne transmission. Epidemiol Rev 18:118, 1996.

Millard PS, Gensheimer KF, Addiss DG, et al: An outbreak of cryptosporidiosis from fresh-pressed apple cider. JAMA 272:1592, 1994.

O'Donoghue PJ: *Cryptosporidium* and cryptosporidiosis in man and animals. Int J Parasitol 25:139, 1995.

Petersen C: Cryptosporidiosis in patients infected with the human immunodeficiency virus. Clin Infect Dis 15:903, 1992.

Robertson LJ, Campbell AT, Smith HV: Survival of *Cryptosporidium parvum* oocysts under various environmental pressures. Appl Environ Microbiol 58:3494, 1992.

Weber R, Bryan RT, Bishop HS, et al: Threshold of detection of *Cryptosporidium* oocysts in human stool specimens: Evidence for low sensitivity of current diagnostic methods. J Clin Microbiol 29:1323, 1991.

White AC Jr, Chappell CL, Hayat CS, et al: Paromomycin for cryptosporidiosis in AIDS: A prospective, double-blind trial. J Infect Dis 170:419, 1994.

89 *Cyclosporiasis*

Bradley A. Connor and David R. Shlim

DEFINITION. Cyclosporiasis is an intestinal infection with the coccidian organism *Cyclospora*. Infection is associated with diarrhea, fatigue, anorexia, and a prolonged course in the absence of treatment.

HISTORY. *Cyclospora* first came to worldwide attention in 1990–1991, following the publication of three reports. The largest series of cases, and the first clinical description of illness due to this organism, came from Shlim et al. at the Canadian International Water and Energy Consultants (CIWEC) Clinic in Kathmandu. The organism, 8 to 10 μm in diameter and resembling a large *Cryptosporidium*, was associated with an outbreak of prolonged diarrhea, anorexia, fatigue, and weight loss in 55 patients and was not cured by the usual antiparasitic medications.

This agent had a prokaryotic appearance and characteristics of blue-green algae: The internal organelles resembled the photosynthesizing organelles of the blue-green algae, and the particle autofluoresced under ultraviolet epifluorescence. However, other findings were not characteristic of algae, and the organism was referred to as a cyanobacterium-like body, or CLB.

It soon became apparent that this newly described organism, the CLB, had been identified before. Soave in New York described round organisms, 8 to 9 μm in diameter, in the stool of immunocompetent travelers to Mexico and Haiti who presented with gastrointestinal symptoms. She called the organism a "big *Cryptosporidium*." Researchers in Haiti, treating patients with AIDS, noted a similar-appearing organism as early as 1983, and others in Peru studying cryptosporidiosis in Peruvian children first noted a "large cryptosporidium-like organism" in 1985–1987.

The first published report of this organism, however, was made by Ashford, who reported a previously undescribed oocyst-like body in three patients in Papua New Guinea in 1979. The uncertainty surrounding the taxonomic classification of CLB was resolved with the 1993 report of Ortega et al. that the organism sporulated while incubating in a potassium dichromate solution. Two sporozoites were noted, and the organism most closely resembled a previously identified organism known as *Cyclospora*. These researchers proposed the name *Cyclospora cayetanensis* after the university in Lima where this research had been done.

ETIOLOGY. *Cyclospora* appears under the microscope as nonrefractile, double-walled spheres, 8 to 10 μm in diameter. Microscopists familiar with the organism can easily identify it on plain wet mounts (Fig. 89–1). The organism floats in Sheather's sucrose solution. On a modified acid-fast stain *Cyclospora* is variably red; some organisms resist the stain and appear as "ghosts." The organism tends to cling to mucus strands and has an intense blue autofluorescence under ultraviolet light.

Most patients infected with *Cyclospora* have only a few organisms on direct stool examination, and the diagnosis is made after formalin–ethyl acetate concentration (Fig. 89–1; Chapter 150). Specimens preserved in formalin for a few days may resist subsequent attempts at concentration.

Ten to twenty percent of *Cyclospora* organisms incubated in a potassium dichromate solution at temperatures of 25 to 32°C sporulate after 5 days. Complete sporulation, producing

two sporocysts that rupture to reveal two crescent-shaped sporozoites measuring 1.2 by 9.0 μm, occurs after 7 to 12 days in culture. The sporozoites within the sporocyst have a membrane-bound nucleus and micronemes characteristic of coccidia of the phylum Apicomplexa (family Eimeriidae). Molecular phylogenetic analysis has also confirmed that *Cyclospora* is a coccidian closely related to *Eimeria* species and distinct from *Isospora* and *Cryptosporidium*.

EPIDEMIOLOGY

Distribution. Since 1991, *Cyclospora* has been noted in an increasing number of countries throughout the world: United States, Haiti, Peru, Papua New Guinea, Mexico, Puerto Rico, India, Guatemala, Morocco, Pakistan, South Africa, the Dominican Republic, Malaysia, Thailand, Nepal, Cambodia, the Solomon Islands, Vietnam, and Indonesia. The organism is found in both immunocompetent and immunosuppressed individuals.

An outbreak of *Cyclospora* infection affecting approximately 1450 individuals (75% laboratory-confirmed) occurred in the United States and Canada in late spring and early summer 1996. Both event-related and sporadic cases were noted in Ontario, Canada, and in 14 states and the District of Columbia during this period.

Prevalence and Incidence. In Nepal, *Cyclospora* infected approximately 7% of the American Embassy community during the 1992 *Cyclospora* season and accounted for 11% of patients with diarrhea seen at the CIWEC Clinic.

In a review of 6525 stool specimens at Chicago hospitals from 1989 to 1991, 34 were positive for *Cyclospora*. In Massachusetts, in a prospective study of 1042 stool specimens submitted from May to November 1993 from patients with diarrhea, three specimens were positive for *Cyclospora*. These three patients had no history of foreign travel and were not infected with HIV.

Only two surveys have been conducted among indigenous populations. In Peru, Ortega et al. (1993) found *Cyclospora* in 6 and 18% of Peruvian children under age 30 months who underwent weekly stool examinations in two separate studies lasting 18 and 24 months, respectively. In Nepal, Hoge et al. (1995) studied 124 children aged 6 months to 5 years who presented with diarrhea at a local clinic. *Cyclospora* was found in 5% of this group, compared with 2% among 103 control subjects not having diarrhea. The mean age of children with *Cyclospora* infection was 34 months, and no cases were found in children less than 18 months of age, suggesting possible protection from breast-feeding. Among 184 stool samples reviewed at a local hospital in Nepal, six (3%) had *Cyclospora*.

Transmission. The transmission of *Cyclospora* is presumed to be fecal-oral, although there is no clear evidence of person-to-person transmission.

Water-borne Transmission. An outbreak of *Cyclospora* infection among the staff of Cook County Hospital in Chicago in the summer of 1990 implicated the water supply of a hospital building. Water was further implicated in a case-control study in Kathmandu. Patients with *Cyclospora* were more likely than controls to have drunk untreated water in the week before their illness. *Cyclospora* was also detected in drinking water from the home of a patient. Unboiled milk was also implicated in this study, but it is not known whether this was due to actual transmission by the milk or to adulteration with untreated water.

A point-source outbreak was identified in a British Gurkha soldier camp in Pokhara, Nepal, where six confirmed cases of *Cyclospora* infection were noted. The water supply for the camp was routinely chlorinated, and the chlorine levels were monitored daily. Despite adequate chlorination of the water, *Cyclospora* was present in a sample taken from the water storage tank. A patient and three family members in Peru

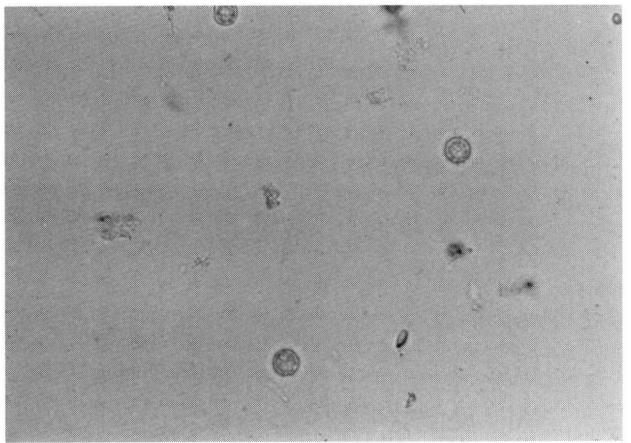

Figure 89–1. *Cyclospora* oocysts, unstained; light microscopy on wet mount of concentrated stool specimen.

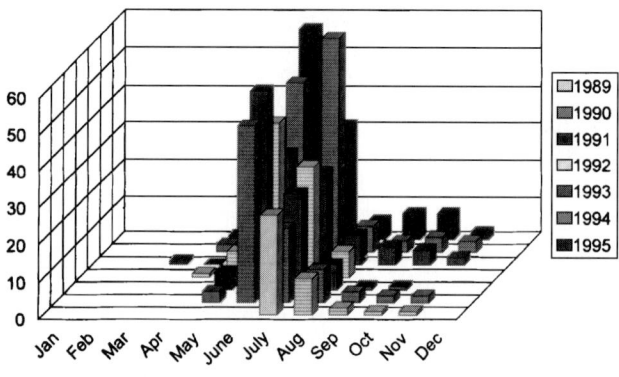

Diagnosed at CIWEC Clinic (Total 515 Cases)

Figure 89–2. Seasonality of *Cyclospora* infections in Nepal 1989–1995.

who drank unchlorinated canal water developed *Cyclospora* diarrhea. Interestingly, *Cyclospora* was also found in the stool of a duck bred by the same family.

Food-Borne Transmission. There is also evidence that *Cyclospora* may be food-borne. It was identified on a head of lettuce in Nepal in 1990. A pilot for an American airline who regularly flew a route to Haiti from New York developed *Cyclospora* diarrhea after eating airline food prepared in a Haitian kitchen. Preliminary investigations of the multistate outbreak of infection in 1996 in the United States and Canada showed a strong association between risk for *Cyclospora* infection and the consumption of raspberries imported from Guatemala.

Seasonality. There is a distinct seasonality in *Cyclospora* outbreaks and cases. In Nepal, the organism has occurred in virtually identical seasonal outbreaks since 1989 (Fig. 89–2). No *Cyclospora* cases are noted in Nepal between December and March each year. They begin in the hot dry season preceding the monsoon rains, and the peak coincides with the maximal rainfall. Infections caused by other enteric pathogens also peak in June each year, but all other enteric pathogens are present in Nepal throughout the year.

In Peru, cases occur from January to July, with a peak from April to June. Of nine cases in travelers to India, Nepal, Pakistan, Cambodia, the Solomon Islands, and Mexico, all travel took place between May and October. Nontravelers with cyclosporiasis are identified at Cornell University Medical College in New York City in the late spring and early summer each year. Community-acquired cases in Massachusetts were noted only in May and June. Two outbreaks in 1995, in Palm Beach County, Florida, and Westchester County, New York, took place in the late spring and early summer. The 1996 North American outbreak occurred during this same season.

PATHOGENICITY. Evidence that *Cyclospora* infections cause diarrhea comes from the following: (1) The initial report from Nepal found the organism present when people were ill and absent when they recovered; and (2) a subsequent case-control study in Nepal reported *Cyclospora* present in 11% of 964 patients with diarrhea but in only 1 of 96 asymptomatic controls; this patient, however, developed diarrhea 3 days later.

Cyclospora has the characteristics of a small bowel pathogen: (1) Upper gastrointestinal symptoms, e.g., nausea, anorexia, and eructation, are predominant, and there is an absence of tenesmus and dysentery; (2) there is invariably malabsorption of D-xylose, and weight loss is almost univer-

sal; and (3) five of the nine *Cyclospora*-infected patients in Nepal undergoing upper GI endoscopy had moderate to marked erythema of the distal duodenum. In addition, duodenal aspirates demonstrated *Cyclospora* adherent to mucus in two of the nine, and histopathology in small bowel biopsies revealed epithelial disarray with acute and chronic inflammation, partial villous atrophy, and crypt hyperplasia (Fig. 89–3). Jejunal biopsies from two patients with *Cyclospora* diarrhea showed pathologic changes similar to those in the Nepal patients and, by electron microscopy, possible intracellular sporozoites.

Little is known about whether individuals can develop immunity to *Cyclospora*. AIDS patients studied in Haiti were noted to have recurrent disease. Hoge et al. (1993) noted *Cyclospora* infections in two successive years in expatriate patients in Nepal. Expatriates with recurrent infections had lived in Nepal for significantly less time than expatriate controls (median 11 months vs. 23 months, p<.0001), suggesting that immunity may develop with repeated exposures. *Cyclospora*-specific antibodies have been detected in the serum of patients.

CLINICAL MANIFESTATIONS. *Cyclospora* infection produces a characteristic illness that can often be recognized clinically. The incubation period is only 2 to 11 days after exposure. As many as 30% of patients report an abrupt onset of fever, vomiting, and a frequent watery diarrhea. This acute phase subsides after a few days, and a characteristic pattern of unusually severe fatigue, anorexia, intermittent diarrhea, and nausea ensues. The symptoms can be consistent from day to day or intermittent, with remissions and exacerbations occurring every few days. Increased upper intestinal belching and bloating are frequently noted. In some patients, diarrhea is not prominent; anorexia and fatigue may be the presenting symptoms. Weight loss is usual, with one study estimating the mean weight loss in untreated infections to be 3.6 kg.

Illness in untreated cases persists for several weeks, the average length of symptoms being 6 or 7 weeks. The organism was detected 8 weeks after the onset of illness in five patients from Chicago.

TREATMENT. *Cyclospora* infections respond to treatment with trimethoprim-sulfamethoxazole (160/800 mg given orally twice daily for 7 days). Patients from Haiti with concomitant cyclosporiasis and AIDS have had their diarrhea

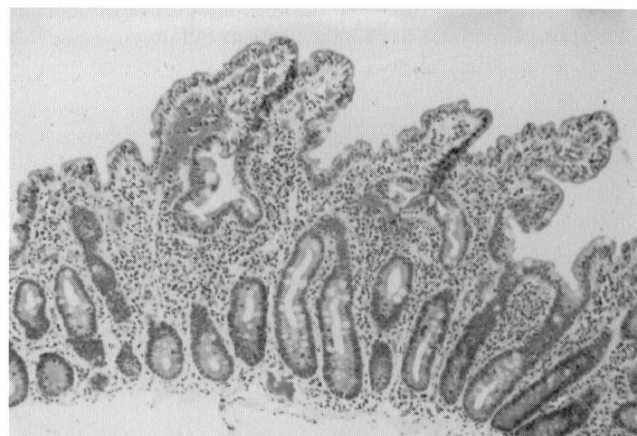

Figure 89–3. Photomicrograph of section of endoscopic duodenal biopsy showing partial atrophy of villi. Elongated hypertrophic crypts (with a villus-to-crypt ratio of 1:1) and chronic inflammation of lamina propria with increased mononuclear cells. (H & E stain; original magnification × 250.)

and abdominal cramps cleared on average 2.5 days after starting the same regimen, which was continued for 10 days. Norfloxacin, metronidazole, tinidazole, quinacrine, and azithromycin, administered to a relatively small number of patients, have not been effective therapy.

PREVENTION. Travelers to *Cyclospora*-endemic areas should be aware of the higher risk during the late spring and summer. Since *Cyclospora*, like *Cryptosporidium*, is not killed by chlorination, drinking water treated only by halogens may not be safe. Boiling kills *Cyclospora*. Therefore, every effort should be made to boil drinking water, to drink tea and coffee, and not to rely on treatment with iodine. Fresh fruits and salads (particularly raspberries and salad greens grown in developing countries) should be carefully washed before eating. Prophylaxis with trimethoprim-sulfamethoxazole has not been evaluated and is not recommended, but an individualized approach is important; e.g., such prophylaxis might be appropriate in an HIV-positive traveler visiting Nepal in the summer.

Bibliography

Centers for Disease Control: Outbreaks of Cyclospora cayetanensis infection—United States 1996. MMWR 45:549, 1996.

Connor BA, Shlim DR, Scholes JV, et al: Pathologic changes in the small bowel in nine patients with diarrhea associated with a coccidia-like body. Ann Intern Med 119:377, 1993.

Hoge CW, Shlim DR, Rajah R, et al: Epidemiology of diarrhoeal illness associated with coccidian-like organism among travellers and foreign residents in Nepal. Lancet 341:1175, 1993.

Hoge CW, Shlim DR, Ghimire M, et al: Placebo-controlled trial of co-trimoxazole for cyclospora infections among travellers and foreign residents in Nepal. Lancet 345:691, 1995.

Ortega YR, Sterling CR, Gilman RH, et al: Cyclospora species: A new protozoan pathogen of humans. N Engl J Med 328:1308, 1993.

Pape JW, Verdier RI, Boncy M, et al: Cyclospora infection in adults infected with HIV. Ann Intern Med 121:654, 1994.

Shlim DR, Cohen MT, Eaton M, et al: An alga-like organism associated with an outbreak of prolonged diarrhea among foreigners in Nepal. Am J Trop Med Hyg 45:383, 1991.

90 Miscellaneous Intestinal Protozoa

Martin S. Wolfe

This chapter covers less common intestinal protozoa that are proven or probable pathogens for humans, as well as other nonpathogenic intestinal protozoa that must be differentiated morphologically from those of medical significance (Table 90–1).

Most of the intestinal protozoa pass through trophozoite and cyst stages. The trophozoites are motile, multiply by binary fission, and actively feed. Cysts are less susceptible to changes of environment, can survive better outside the intestinal tract, and are primarily responsible for transmission of the infection.

Identification of specific protozoa is based on certain characteristics of the cyst (Table 90–2) and trophozoite (Table 90–3). Distinguishing features of the trophozoite include the type of motility, food inclusions, and the number and structure of the nuclei. Cysts are distinguished by size and shape, nuclear number and structure, type of chromatoidal bodies when present, and amount and distribution of glycogen. All these features are best demonstrated by permanently stained

TABLE 90–1. Some Important Intestinal Protozoa of Humans

Organism	Potentially Pathogenic	Stages of Organism	
		Trophozoite	*Cyst*
Amebae			
Entamoeba histolytica	+	+	+
E. hartmanni	−	+	+
E. coli	−	+	+
E. polecki	+	+	+
Iodamoeba bütschlii	−	+	+
Endolimax nana	−	+	+
Flagellates			
*Dientamoeba fragilis**	+	+	−
Chilomastix mesnili	−	+	+
Pentatrichomonas hominis	−	+	−
Giardia lamblia	+	+	+
Retortamonas intestinalis	−	+	+
Enteromonas hominis	−	+	+
Ciliates			
Balantidium coli	+	+	+
Sporozoa			
Isospora belli	+	−	+
Sarcocystis species	+	−	+
Cryptosporidium species	+	−	+
Cyclospora species	+	−	+
Other			
Blastocystis hominis	?	?	?

*Considered an ameba-like flagellate.

fecal smears, which should be performed along with unstained and iodine-stained smears of direct and concentrated stool specimens (Tables 90–2 and 90–3). Certain intestinal protozoa may be isolated and maintained in artificial culture media (Chapter 150).

90.1 Balantidiasis

DEFINITION. Balantidiasis is caused by *Balantidium coli*, a large pathogenic ciliated protozoan that in rare instances infects humans and produces intestinal symptoms.

DISTRIBUTION AND PREVALENCE. *B. coli* has a worldwide distribution. It has most commonly been reported from various parts of Latin America, the Far East, and Pacific Islands, but such reports are rare. Prevalence is highest in areas of poor hygiene and nutrition and where pigs and humans have close contact.

TRANSMISSION AND EPIDEMIOLOGY. *B. coli* is widespread in the animal world. Infection is particularly common in pigs, which tolerate the parasite well and are the main source of transmission to humans. In one review, more than 50% of human cases had contact with pigs. The handling and slaughtering of pigs and the use of pig excrement for fertilizing vegetables favor increased transmission. Person-to-person contact occurs through fecal contamination. Waterborne epidemics have also occurred. Cysts are the infective stage and may remain viable for weeks in moist feces. Excystation occurs in the bowel, and the trophozoites live in the large intestine, where they either remain in the lumen or invade the intestinal mucosa. Encystation occurs either as fecal material is being moved down the bowel or after passage of a semiformed stool.

PATHOGENESIS AND PATHOLOGY. *B. coli* trophozoites can penetrate the mucosa, producing necrosis and ulceration. Masses of *B. coli* trophozoites can then be found in the submucosa, with or without an associated inflammatory reaction (Fig. 90–1). Following mucosal invasion, secondary bacterial invasion may occur, leading to cellular infiltration. Multiplication of balantidia in the tissues leads to ulcers or subsurface abscesses. The ulcers are discrete and round or irregular with undermined edges, and the gross appearance resembles amebic ulceration of the large bowel.

B. coli, like *Entamoeba histolytica*, may exist for a limited period in the lumen of the large bowel without producing symptoms. Without evidence of invasion, the mucous membrane may be hyperemic and show superficial necrosis. Metastatic spread is extremely rare. The appendix may be invaded by balantidia.

CLINICAL MANIFESTATIONS. As in amebiasis, symptomatology ranges from the asymptomatic carrier state; to

TABLE 90–2. Salient Features of Cysts of Some Intestinal Protozoa of Humans

Parasite	Usual Shape	Usual Size (μm)	Number Nuclei	Nuclear Karyosome	Glycogen Mass (in Iodine)	Chromatoidal Bodies	Other Characteristics
Entamoeba histolytica	Round	10–15	1–4	Small granule	Diffuse, brown. In young cysts	Rod-shaped or thick bars	In fresh unstained cyst: nuclei not visible; chromatoids conspicuous when present
E. hartmanni	Round	<10	1–4	Small granule	Similar to *E. histolytica*	Similar to *E. histolytica*	Similar to *E. histolytica*
E. coli	Round	15–20	1–8	Coarser than in *E. histolytica*	Large, deep brown. In young cysts	Splinter-like or filamentous	Nuclei usually visible in unstained cyst; cyst wall heavy
E. polecki	Round	12–14	1; rarely 2	Large, massed	—	Rod-shaped or spherical; ends angular, pointed, or round	Spherical, ovoid, or irregular inclusion body may be present
Iodamoeba bütschlii	Ovoid; round	6–15	1–2	Bulky, round	Large or small, sharply delimited, deep brown	None	Usually granular mass next to karyosome
Endolimax nana	Ovoid; round	7–10 × 6–7	1–4	Eccentric mass	Occasionally present in young cysts	None	Often cytoplasmic volutin granules confused with karyosomes
Chilomastix mesnili	Lemon-shaped	7–9 × 4.5–6	1	Mass at 1 pole	Sometimes present	None	Oral apparatus beside nucleus
Giardia lamblia	Ovoid	8–12 × 6–10	4	Punctiform, central	None	None	Nuclei at anterior pole; fibrils in cytoplasm
Retortamonas intestinalis	Pear-shaped	4–7 × 3–5	1	Slightly eccentric	None	None	Cyst wall appears double in fresh preparations; margin of cytostome may show when stained
Enteromonas hominis	Elongate; ovoid	6–8 × 4–6	1–4	Small; central	None	None	1 or 2 nuclei at each end; well-defined cyst wall
Blastocystis hominis	Round	10–15	1–8	—	None	None	Nuclei marginal between inner and outer wall
Balantidium coli	Round	50–65	1 macronucleus 1 micronucleus	—	None	None	Macronucleus kidney-shaped, large, conspicuous; has contractile vacuole
Sarcocystis spp.	Ovoid	Sporocyst 10 × 15	—	—	None	None	Oocyst wall usually absent; sporocysts single or paired
Isospora belli	Ovoid	Oocyst 12 × 30	—	—	None	None	Oocyst wall present; 2 sporocysts 9 × 11 μm each within oocyst wall
Cryptosporidium spp.	Spherical	Oocyst 5 × 6	—	—	None	None	Phase-contrast microscopy shows 1 to 6 prominent dark granules and numerous fine dark granules; after sporulating, oocysts contain 4 sporozoites and a spherical residium
Cyclospora spp.	Spherical	Oocyst 8 × 10	—	—	None	None	Larger than cryptosporidia
Enterocytozoon bieneusi	Round	Spore 1 × 1.5	—	—	None	None	Smaller than cryptosporidia

TABLE 90–3. Salient Features of Viable Trophozoites of Some Intestinal Protozoa of Humans

Parasite	Size (μm) Living	Normal Motility	Pseudopodia	Stained Nucleus	Other Characteristics
Entamoeba histolytica	10–25 (rounded forms)	Active, progressive, streaming; cytoplasm flows into pseudopod	Tonguelike, explosively formed	Round; minute karyosome; fine chromatic lining of membrane; ringlike	Living nucleus not visible
E. hartmanni	<12		Similar to *E. histolytica*		
E. coli	20–30 (rounded forms)	Sluggish, not progressive	Blunt, hemispherical, semilunar	Round; coarse karyosome; coarse chromatic lining of membrane; ringlike	Living nucleus visible
E. polecki	16–18 (rounded forms)	Usually sluggish	Rounded, extruded slowly, occasionally 2 or more	Round; karyosome usually small; nuclear membrane thin; ringlike	Living nucleus occasionally seen
Iodamoeba bütschlii	9–13 (rounded forms)	Like *E. coli*	Like *E. coli*	Round; large round karyosome	
Endolimax nana	8–12 (rounded forms)	Usually nonmotile; occasionally slightly progressive	Round, budlike	Round; large irregular karyosome	
Dientamoeba fragilis	5–20 (rounded forms)	Usually sluggish or nonmotile	Triangular (tentlike), rectangular, veil-like, cloverleaf	2 (or 1) nuclei, with mass of chromatin granules embedded in clear matrix	
Chilomastix mesnili	13–24 × 6–11	Flagellate; spiral; body rigid	—	Round; small eccentric or central karyosome	Body pear-shaped; buccal structures prominent; spiral twist in body
Pentatrichomonas hominis	10–15 × 5–8	Flagellate; continuous, jerky, wobbly; body plastic	—	Round or oval; karyosome more or less central	3–5 anterior flagella; undulating membrane and axostyle present
Giardia lamblia	9–21 × 5–15	Active; tumbling and turning like falling leaves; spinning	—	Right and left nuclei; ovoid with prominent irregular karyosomes	Has sucking disk, 8 flagella
Retortamonas intestinalis	4–9 × 3–4	Flagellate; jerky and progressive	—	Round; membrane delicate; karyosome eccentric	2 anterior flagella and 2 blepharoplasts near nucleus
Enteromonas hominis	4–10 × 3–6	Similar to *R. intestinalis*	—	Ovoid; membrane delicate; karyosome large	Body pear-shaped; 3 anterior flagella and 1 along flattened surface and extending free posteriorly
Balantidium coli	50–70 × 30–60	Ciliate; strong progressive swimmer; rapid, gliding	—	Macronucleus sausage-shaped; micronucleus ovoid or round	V-shaped peristome; anus at posterior end

chronic symptoms with intermittent diarrhea and constipation, abdominal pain, and weight loss; to a dysenteric form with blood and mucus in the stool, anorexia, nausea, tenderness over the colon, weight loss, and weakness. Fulminating dysentery, although rare, may lead to intestinal perforation, hemorrhage, and shock. Chronic symptoms may persist for many years. A characteristic fetid breath odor has been noted in some patients, resembling that of a pigpen.

DIAGNOSIS. Diagnosis depends on demonstrating *B. coli* in the stool by direct or concentration examinations. Large trophozoites (Fig. 90–2) have been found in about 90% of cases, with cysts being seen only infrequently (Fig. 90–8). *B. coli* trophozoites can be cultured with bacteria in media used for *E. histolytica*.

TREATMENT. The treatments of choice are tetracycline, 500 mg four times a day for 10 days, or iodoquinol, 650 mg three

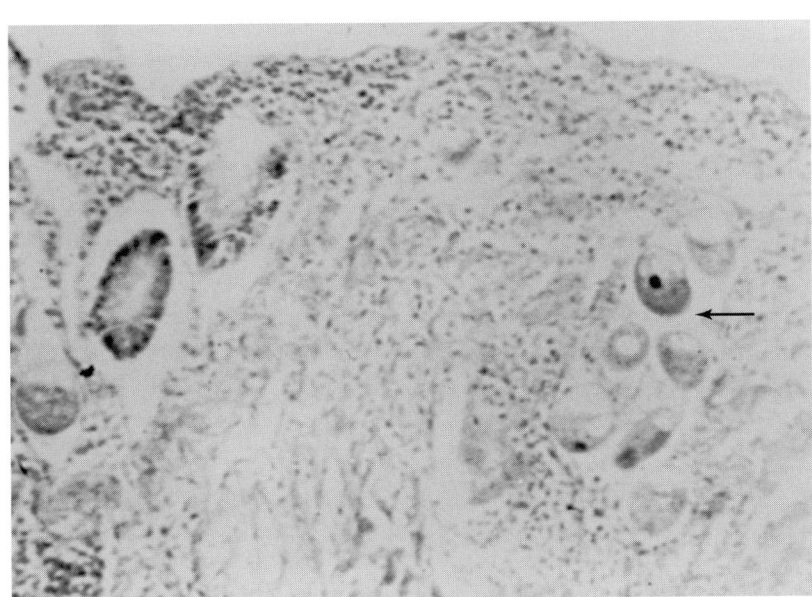

***Figure* 90–1.** *Balantidium coli.* Tissue section of colon biopsy specimen showing ulcer with inflammatory response, necrosis, and *B. coli* trophozoites *(arrow).* (H & E stain.)

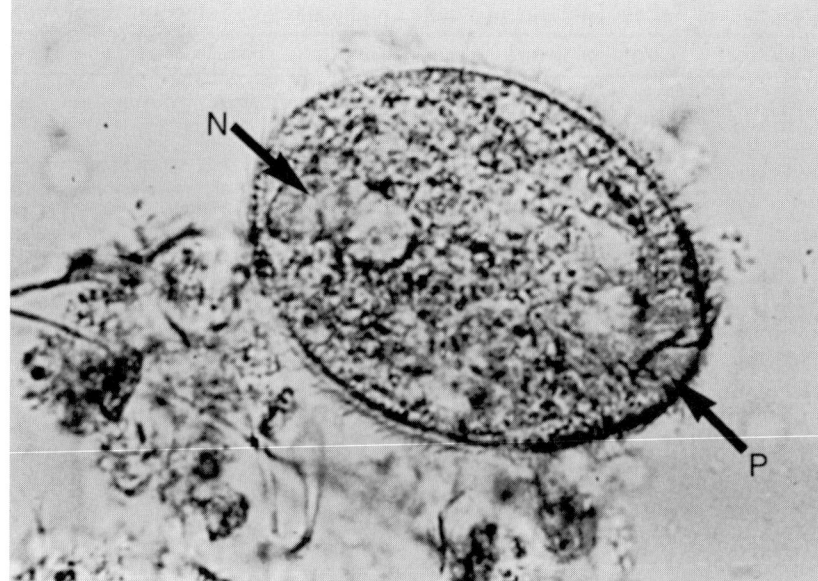

Figure 90–2. *Balantidium coli* trophozoite in stool. Note peristome *(P)*, kidney-shaped macronucleus *(N)*, and cilia. (× 400.) (From Smith W, et al: Diagnostic Medical Parasitology: Intestinal Protozoa. Chicago, The American Society of Clinical Pathologists, 1976.)

times a day for 20 days. Mixed results have been reported with metronidazole.

Bibliography

Arias VM, Koppisch E: Balantidiasis: A review and report of cases. Am J Pathol 32:1089, 1956.
Baskerville L, Ahmed Y, Ramchard S: Balantidium colitis: Report of a case. Am J Dig Dis 15:727, 1970.
Swartzwelder JC: Balantidiasis. Am J Dig Dis 17:173, 1950.

90.2 Isosporiasis

DEFINITION. Isosporiasis is caused by *Isospora belli*, a protozoan of the subphylum Sporozoa, which has alternating generations, one sexual (sporogony) and one asexual (schizogony), in the small bowel mucosa. *Isospora hominis*, formerly grouped together with *I. belli*, is now recognized as a *Sarcocystis* species.

DISTRIBUTION AND PREVALENCE. *I. belli* has a worldwide distribution, but is rarely reported in humans. It is most prevalent in South America and Africa and is usually reported in residents of or returnees from these and other tropical areas. In recent years, *I. belli* has been increasingly recognized as an opportunistic infection in immunosuppressed male homosexuals in the United States. It is also being found more frequently in those from Haiti and Africa with chronic diarrhea associated with AIDS (Chapter 22).

TRANSMISSION AND EPIDEMIOLOGY. Infection occurs from oral ingestion of mature oocysts. The oocyst is ovoid, has a thin, translucent cyst wall, and contains two spherical sporocysts, which in turn each contain four crescent-shaped uninucleate sporozoites (Fig. 90–3). Following ingestion, excystation of these sporulated oocysts occurs in the proximal small intestine. The released sporozoites invade epithelial cells and become round trophozoites. These forms enter the asexual stage, schizogony, and enlarge into mature schizonts containing merozoites. The host cell then ruptures, releasing the merozoites, which invade other epithelial cells. This process may continue for weeks or months and, rarely, for many years. Some merozoites may become sexual gameto-cytes, either multicellular male microgametocytes or unicellular female macrogametocytes. Male microgametocytes rupture and release flagellated microgametes that fertilize the female macrogametocytes. The fertilized macrogametocytes become unsporulated oocysts that are liberated into the bowel lumen and eliminated in the feces. Stool oocysts usually mature within 48 hours following evacuation from the body, and are then infective.

Infection occurs from ingestion of food or water contaminated with feces containing mature oocysts. In experimental infections in humans, symptoms developed in 1 week and oocysts were recovered 9 to 15 days after ingestion. There is no evidence of an animal reservoir of *I. belli*.

PATHOGENESIS AND PATHOLOGY. The mechanism by which the invading parasites produce mucosal lesions is unclear. Pathologic changes have been best described in the biopsy specimens of six patients studied by Brandborg and associates. The pathology of the small bowel mucosa varied, but none of the patients had a normal mucosa. The two most severely ill patients, both of whom died, had a flat mucosa.

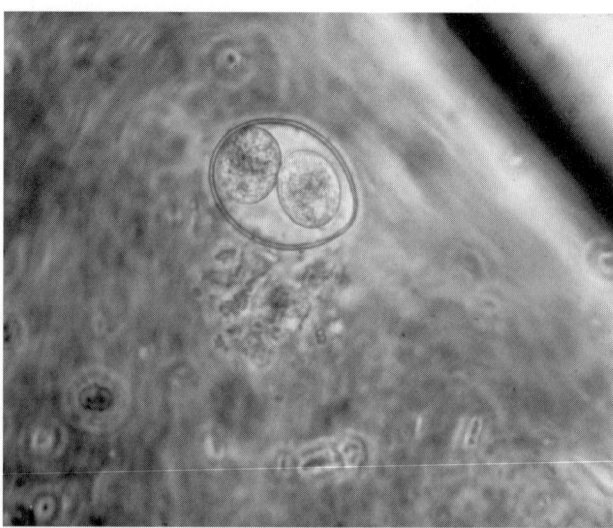

Figure 90–3. *Isospora belli* oocyst with two sporocysts in stool.

Another had elongated crypts with stubby residual villi, and yet another had tall villi with focal fusion and flattening. The least severely ill patient had a patchy abnormality, with some biopsies showing only a mild nonspecific abnormality. The epithelium in all six patients was often normal, except that all the specimens had foci of vacuolization not necessarily related to the parasites. The parasitized cells were destroyed, but the adjacent cells often appeared normal. The lamina propria contained increased numbers of lymphocytes, plasma cells, and eosinophils. The mucosa was sufficiently damaged to account for the diarrhea and steatorrhea, which are often found in patients infected with *I. belli*.

Little is known of host susceptibility in *I. belli* infections, but immunologic deficiency predisposes to enteritis. Isosporiasis with diarrhea persisting for longer than 1 month indicates AIDS in an HIV–positive individual.

CLINICAL MANIFESTATIONS. Some *I. belli* infections are asymptomatic, but others may lead to significant disease. Symptoms include diarrhea, abdominal colic, flatulence, malaise, anorexia, weight loss, and low-grade fever. The clinical picture resembles giardiasis, cryptosporidiosis, or cyclosporiasis. The stools are often pale and may contain undigested food, mucus, and Charcot-Leyden crystals. In normal hosts, the majority of those infected have a self-limited illness, with resolution after several weeks. Some immunosuppressed patients, particularly those with AIDS, may be ill for months or years. Peripheral eosinophilia may be present.

DIAGNOSIS. Oocysts are usually scanty in the stool. Zinc sulfate or sugar flotation is the most sensitive stool concentration technique. The best method for staining stool smears is a modified acid-fast stain (Chapter 150). Duodenal drainage and intestinal mucosal biopsy may detect some infections not found by stool examinations. It is often necessary to examine multiple serial biopsy sections to find organisms, which may be in both sexual and asexual stages.

TREATMENT. No effective drug treatment was available until recent years, when combined therapy with pyrimethamine and sulfadiazine for 7 weeks was found curative. Subsequently, trimethoprim (160 mg)–sulfamethoxazole (800 mg), every 6 hours for 10 days, then twice a day for 3 weeks, was found curative. In patients allergic to sulfonamides, pyrimethamine alone (50 to 75 mg daily) has cured infections. In immunosuppressed patients with recurrent or persistent infection, the above therapy must be continued indefinitely.

Bibliography

Brandborg LL, Goldberg SB, Breidenbach WC: Human coccidiosis—a possible cause of malabsorption. The life cycle in small-bowel mucosal biopsies as a diagnostic feature. N Engl J Med 283:1306, 1970.

Pape JW, Johnson WD: *Isospora belli* infections. *In* Sun TC (ed): Progress in Clinical Parasitology, Vol 2. New York, Field & Wood Medical Publishers, 1991, p 11.9.

Pape JW, Verdier R-I, Johnson WD: Treatment and prophylaxis of *Isospora belli* infection in patients with the acquired immunodeficiency syndrome. N Engl J Med 320:1044, 1989.

Trier JS, Moxey PC, Schimmel EM, et al: Chronic intestinal coccidiosis in man: Intestinal morphology and response to treatment. Gastroenterology 66:923, 1974.

90.3 Dientamoeba fragilis Infection

DEFINITION. *Dientamoeba fragilis*, formerly thought to be an ameba occurring only in a labile trophozoite form, has more recently been considered an ameba-like flagellate more closely related to the genera *Histomonas* and *Trichomonas*.

DISTRIBUTION AND PREVALENCE. *D. fragilis* has a worldwide distribution. When only fresh stool examinations are performed, it is generally considered a rare parasite. Its prevalence is higher in surveys employing preserved stool specimens, permanently stained fecal smears, and multiple stool examinations. The highest prevalence figures have been reported from residents of mental institutions and some missionary groups in the tropics. In recent years *D. fragilis* has become a more commonly recognized parasite in the general American population.

TRANSMISSION AND EPIDEMIOLOGY. The mode of transmission remains uncertain. There is some epidemiologic evidence of water-borne and person-to-person transmission. A close correlation has been found between the incidence of *Enterobius vermicularis* and *D. fragilis* infections. The combination of these two parasites observed in a study in Canada was about nine times higher than expected on the basis of random distribution. It has therefore been postulated that pinworm eggs or larvae may be a transmitting agent of *D. fragilis*.

PATHOGENESIS AND PATHOLOGY. The ability of *D. fragilis* to invade the host has not been demonstrated; it appears that irritation of the colonic mucosa is the most likely cause of the symptoms found in infected individuals. Fibrosis was present in appendices infected with *D. fragilis*, and it was postulated that the parasite released an irritant responsible for this. In some cases the parasite has been found in bile ducts.

CLINICAL MANIFESTATIONS. *D. fragilis* has been considered a nonpathogen by some, and many of those infected are asymptomatic. Symptoms present in others include intermittent diarrhea, abdominal pain, anorexia, and fatigue. Symptoms reported less commonly include fever, irritability, weight loss, and vomiting. A number of workers have reported a low-grade eosinophilia in infected individuals in the absence of associated pinworm or other helminthic infections; particularly striking was a 50% incidence of eosinophilia in 28 infected children in California. Generalized tenderness to abdominal palpation is present in some infected individuals, but physical examination is otherwise usually unremarkable.

DIAGNOSIS. *D. fragilis* is diagnosed by finding trophozoites in the stool (Fig. 90–4). The presence of the labile trophozoite will often be missed if only fresh stool specimens are examined. Collection into various preservatives immediately on passage of a stool and the preparation and careful examination of stained fecal smears will lead to higher recovery rates (Chapter 150). Some workers report that examination of a purged stool is more productive. *D. fragilis* may also be isolated by culture techniques. Examination of multiple specimens passed on alternate days has also been found useful, as the excretion of parasites may fluctuate markedly from day to day.

TREATMENT. Tetracycline and iodoquinol, alone or in combination in doses used for amebiasis, are often mentioned as the drugs of choice, but careful scrutiny of the literature indicates that cure rates are not high with these drugs. Paro-

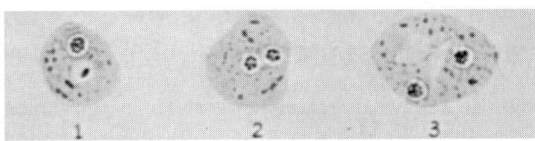

Figure 90–4. *Dientamoeba fragilis.* 1, Uninucleate. 2 and 3, Binucleate. (After Dobell and O'Connor. From Craig CF: Amebiasis and Amebic Dysentery. Springfield, IL, Charles C Thomas, 1934.)

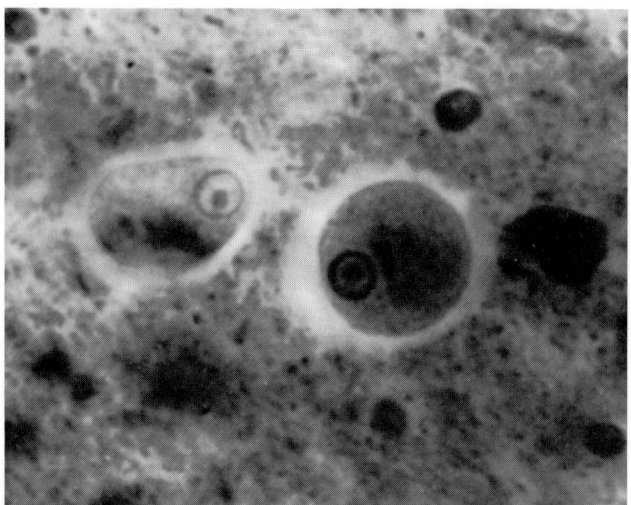

Figure 90–5. *Entamoeba polecki.* Uninucleate cysts in stool. Note prominent karyosome and nuclear membrane. (12 × 14 μm.)

momycin, in a dosage of 500 mg three times a day for 7 days, appears to be more effective. Metronidazole, furazolidone, and diloxanide furoate deserve further evaluation against *D. fragilis.*

Bibliography

Kean BH, Malloch CL: The neglected ameba: *Dientamoeba fragilis:* A report of 100 "pure" infections. Am J Dig Dis 11:735, 1966.
Ockert G: Symptomatology, pathology, epidemiology, and diagnosis of *Dientamoeba fragilis. In* Honigberg BM (ed): Trichomonads Parasitic in Man. New York, Springer-Verlag, 1990, pp 394–410.
Simon M, Shookhoff HB, Terner H, et al: Paromomycin in the treatment of intestinal amebiasis: A short course of therapy. Am J Gastroenterol 48:504, 1967.
Yang J, Scholten TH: *Dientamoeba fragilis:* A review with notes on its epidemiology, pathogenicity, mode of transmission, and diagnosis. Am J Trop Med Hyg 26:16, 1977.

90.4 Entamoeba polecki *Infection*

DEFINITION. *Entamoeba polecki* is an ameba common in the intestine of pigs and monkeys but is rarely reported in humans. It is usually, but not always, nonpathogenic.

DISTRIBUTION AND PREVALENCE. The majority of cases reported in humans have been found in Papua New Guinea, but the distribution appears to be worldwide. It is likely that *E. polecki* is not infrequently mistaken for the much more common and similar-appearing *Entamoeba histolytica,* unless careful examination of permanently stained fecal smears is performed.

TRANSMISSION AND EPIDEMIOLOGY. *E. polecki* occurs in both trophozoite and cyst forms. The most likely source of infection is transmission via cysts from pigs and monkeys to humans, although human-to-human transmission may also occur.

CLINICAL MANIFESTATIONS. The great majority of recognized cases have been asymptomatic. However, at least three patients with heavy infections had intestinal symptoms, including anorexia, diarrhea, mucoid stools, abdominal cramps, malaise, and eosinophilia.

DIAGNOSIS. *E. polecki* cysts are the usual form found in stool examinations (Fig. 90–5). The cysts are consistently uni-

nucleate, and the persistence of uninucleate cysts in multiple stool examinations should raise a strong suspicion of *E. polecki.* Differentiating characteristics in permanently stained fecal smears are described in Tables 90–2 and 90–3.

TREATMENT. Numerous antiamebic drugs are ineffective against *E. polecki,* but a symptomatic case was cured with metronidazole, 750 mg three times a day for 10 days, followed by diloxanide furoate, 500 mg three times a day for 10 days. Another study reported six of eight patients successfully treated with a single course of metronidazole in a regimen similar to that used for *E. histolytica.*

Bibliography

Gay JD, Abell TL, Thompson JH, et al: *Entamoeba polecki* infection in Southeast Asian refugees: Multiple cases of a rarely reported parasite. Mayo Clin Proc 60:523, 1985.
Salaki JS, Shirey JL, Strickland GT: Successful treatment of symptomatic *Entamoeba polecki* infection. Am J Trop Med Hyg 28:190, 1979.

90.5 Blastocystis hominis *Infection*

Blastocystis hominis is a common inhabitant of the human intestinal tract. In some stool surveys it has been reported in 10 to 15% of subjects. For many years, most workers regarded *B. hominis* as a harmless yeast. Studies by Zierdt offer convincing evidence that it is a protozoan. A number of reports in recent years have attributed pathogenicity to *B. hominis,* particularly when the number of organisms present is consistently more than 5 per oil immersion field (Fig. 90–6; Fig. 90–8). When the organism is present in numbers less than this, Zierdt disregards it as a possible agent of disease; in these instances the organism appears uniformly small.

Reported symptoms associated with heavy *B. hominis* infection, in the absence of other recognized pathogenic organisms, include mild diarrhea, nausea, anorexia, and fatigue. It remains unclear whether *B. hominis* itself is the cause of these

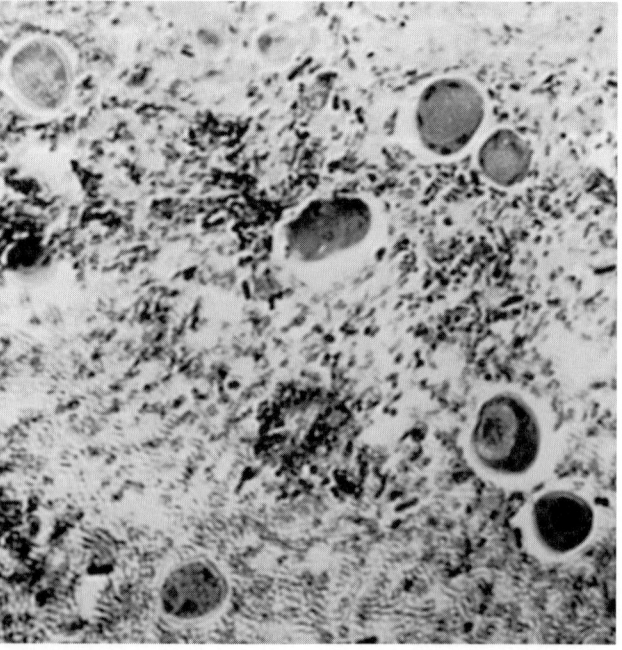

Figure 90–6. *Blastocystis hominis.* Stool smear from patient with diarrhea. (H & E stain, × 800.) (Courtesy of Dr. C. H. Zierdt.)

symptoms or if it is only a marker of some other unidentified pathogen. Markell and Udkow have given an interesting perspective to the controversy over the pathogenicity of *B. hominis*. In 32 subjects initially found with *B. hominis* alone, or in combination with nonpathogenic protozoa, an additional series of stool specimens up to a total of six were examined. In 27 of these 32 patients, at least one known pathogen, in addition to *B. hominis*, was found. *B. hominis* persisted, but symptoms improved in all 27 patients treated specifically for these other pathogens. They concluded that *B. hominis* was not a pathogen and that treatment with common antiprotozoal drugs does not eliminate it from the stool; that "symptomatic blastocystosis" was attributable to either an undetected parasite or parasites in some patients or functional bowel problems in others.

On the basis of these findings, it is recommended that symptomatic patients with heavy infection with *B. hominis* have repeated stool specimens tested by concentration and thorough stained slide examination. With this extra effort, one of the recognized pathogenic protozoa may be found. However, because it remains possible that heavy *B. hominis* infections alone could cause symptoms, an alternative is to treat with one of the antiprotozoal drugs that have been used with mixed results in *B. hominis* (i.e., iodoquinol, metronidazole, tinidazole, or furazolidone). However, it must be recog-

nized that a symptomatic response could represent the elimination of some other undetected pathogen.

Bibliography

Editorial: *Blastocystis hominis*: Commensal or pathogen? Lancet 337:521, 1991.
Markell EK, Udkow MP: *Blastocystis hominis*: Pathogen or fellow traveler? Am J Trop Med Hyg 35:1023, 1986.
Shlem DR, Hoge CH, Rajah R, et al: Is *Blastocystis hominis* a cause of diarrhea in travelers? A prospective controlled study in Nepal. Clin Infect Dis 21:97, 1995.
Zierdt CH: *Blastocystis hominis*—past and future. Clin Microbiol Rev 4:61, 1991.

90.6 *Nonpathogenic Intestinal Protozoa*

A number of nonpathogenic amebae (Fig. 90–7) and flagellates (Fig. 90–8) are frequently found on stool examination, indicating fecal contamination by the host. If intestinal symptoms are present, further search should be made for recognized pathogens.

AMEBAE

Entamoeba hartmanni. Formerly known as "small race" *Entamoeba histolytica*, this organism is morphologically identi-

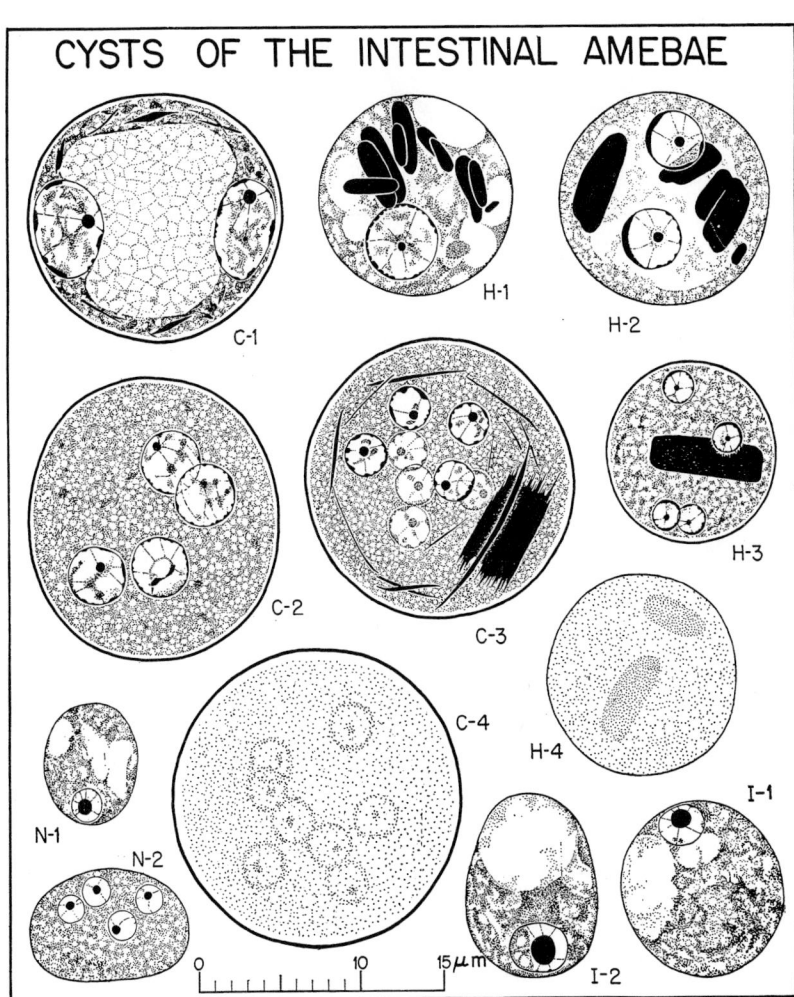

Figure 90–7. *C-1,* Iron-hematoxylin–stained binucleate cyst of *Entamoeba coli. C-2,* Iron-hematoxylin-stained quadrinucleate cyst of *E. coli. C-3,* Iron-hematoxylin-stained mature cyst of *E. coli. C-4,* Unstained mature cyst of *E. coli. H-1,* Iron-hematoxylin–stained uninucleate cyst of *Entamoeba histolytica. H-2,* Iron-hematoxylin–stained binucleate cysts of *E. histolytica. H-3,* Iron-hematoxylin–stained mature cyst of *E. histolytica. H-4,* Unstained cyst of *E. histolytica* showing chromatoidal bars. *N-1,* Iron-hematoxylin–stained uninucleate cyst of *Endolimax nana. N-2,* Iron-hematoxylin–stained mature cysts of *E. nana. I-1* and *I-2,* Iron-hematoxylin–stained mature cysts of *Iodamoeba bütschlii.*

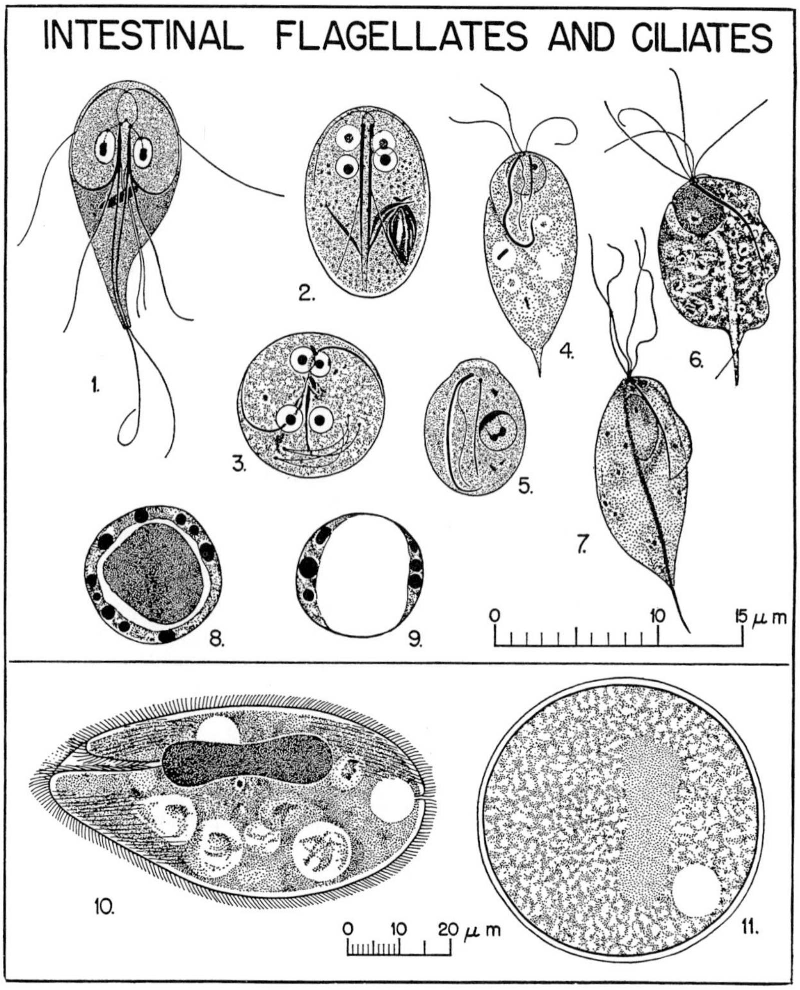

INTESTINAL FLAGELLATES AND CILIATES

Figure 90–8. *1,* Iron-hematoxylin–stained trophozoite of *Giardia lamblia. 2,* Iron-hematoxylin–stained cyst of *G. lamblia. 3,* End view of iron-hematoxylin–stained cyst of *G. lamblia. 4,* Iron-hematoxylin–stained trophozoite of *Chilomastix mesnili. 5,* Iron-hematoxylin–stained cyst of *C. mesnili. 6,* Iron-hematoxylin–stained trophozoite of *Pentatrichomonas hominis. 7,* Iron-hematoxylin–stained trophozoite of *Trichomonas vaginalis.* (*T. vaginalis* dwells in the genitourinary tract and cannot survive in the alimentary canal.) *8,* Iron-hematoxylin–stained *Blastocystis hominis. 9,* Unstained *B. hominis. 10,* Trophozoite of *Balantidium coli. 11,* Unstained cyst of *B. coli.*

cal to *E. histolytica* and is differentiated primarily on the basis of size (Tables 90–2 and 90–3). Trophozoites in wet preparations measure less than 12 μm and cysts less than 10 μm; on permanent stained smears, trophozoites measure less than 11 μm and cysts measure less than 9 μm.

Entamoeba coli. This is a rather common intestinal protozoan; young cysts can sometimes be difficult to distinguish from *E. histolytica.* Most mature cysts will have at least five nuclei visible and be about 15 μm in diameter (Table 90–2 and Fig. 90–7). *E. coli* and *E. histolytica* trophozoites may also pose some difficulty in differentiation (Table 90–3). *E. coli* usually do not have progressive motility nor contain ingested red blood cells.

Endolimax nana. This is perhaps the most common intestinal protozoan. *E. nana* trophozoite and cyst stages are smaller than *E. histolytica,* and the nuclear structure is characteristic (Tables 90–2 and 90–3 and Fig. 90–7).

Iodamoeba bütschlii. This organism is primarily distinguished by the highly vacuolated cytoplasm of the trophozoite and the large glycogen vacuole of the cyst (Tables 90–2 and 90–3 and Fig. 90–7).

FLAGELLATES. The commonly seen flagellate *Chilomastix mesnili* can be differentiated from *Giardia lamblia* by its pear or lemon shape and single nucleus (Tables 90–2 and 90–3 and Fig. 90–8). *Pentatrichomonas hominis,* another flagellate, occurs only in the trophozoite stage and has a single nucleus (Table 90–3 and Fig. 90–8). *Enteromonas hominis* and *Retorta-*

monas intestinalis are uncommon flagellates and are often overlooked when present. They are usually identified by "ruling out" everything else (Tables 90–2 and 90–3).

Bibliography

Garcia LS, Voge M: Diagnostic clinical parasitology. II. Identification of the intestinal protozoa. Am J Med Technol 46:821, 1980.

91 Trichomoniasis

Michael F. Rein and Jonathan Zenilman

DEFINITION. Trichomoniasis is a specific genitourinary tract infection with *Trichomonas vaginalis.* The organism is highly site specific, and the clinical syndromes are vaginitis and, in men, urethritis. *T. tenax* is sometimes found in the mouth, often in association with gingivitis, and *Pentatrichomonas hominis* is sometimes isolated from the colon of patients with diarrhea, but the pathogenicity of neither organism is established. Trichomoniasis is defined by the presence of the organism whether or not the patient is symptomatic.

HISTORY. Donné described the organism in 1836, making it the first sexually transmitted pathogen to be specifically recognized. However, the organism was for a long time regarded as a harmless commensal. Its pathogenicity was established early in the 20th century through inoculation studies. Therapy was inadequate until the development of metronidazole in the 1960s.

ETIOLOGY. The organism is generally oval and 10 to 20 μm wide and can be easily visualized by light microscopy. Its characteristic twitching motility is provided by four anterior flagella and a recurrent flagellum embedded in an undulating membrane, which runs along two thirds of the cell (Figs. 90–8[7] and 91–1). The organism has a large single nucleus and a highly developed Golgi complex. An axostyle, composed of microtubules, projects from the anterior end. Hydrogenosomes replace the mitochondria found in most other organisms. The organism is actively phagocytic, is hemolytic, intermittently dependent on phase of its growth cycle, and optimal growth occurs under moderately anaerobic conditions. *T. vaginalis* reproduces by binary fission; cysts are not formed. Individual strains vary in surface antigens and vary in virulence both in vitro and in vivo.

DISTRIBUTION AND INCIDENCE. Trichomoniasis occurs worldwide, in both urban and rural settings. Because it is not reportable, data on incidence and prevalence are unreliable and are subject to selection biases. The Centers for Disease Control estimates that some 3 million infections are acquired annually in the United States. The prevalence of trichomoniasis among women in sexually transmitted disease clinics ranges from 7 to 32% and up to 80% in some prostitutes. Studies of men in Africa have shown that as many as one third of cases of nongonococcal urethritis may be caused by *Trichomonas*.

The prevalence of infection is significantly associated with nonuse of barrier contraceptives.

Information on the incidence and prevalence of infection in men is essentially nonexistent. The disease is frequently self-limited in men.

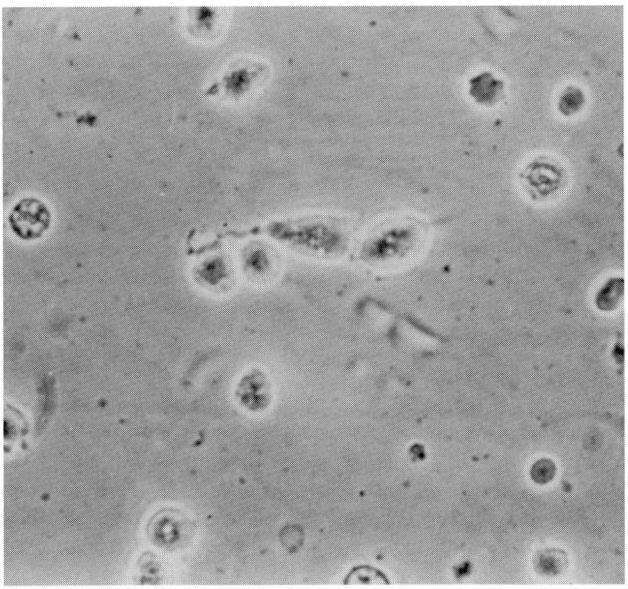

Figure 91–1. Trichomoniasis. Wet mount of vaginal discharge showing several round polymorphonuclear neutrophils and two ovoid trichomonads. Anterior flagella are visible. (Phase contrast, × 1000.)

TRANSMISSION AND EPIDEMIOLOGY. The venereal nature of trichomoniasis is supported by (1) high prevalence among the sexual partners of infected individuals (90 to 100% of women; 30 to 70% of men); (2) highest prevalence among groups with high level of sexual activity; (3) established coprevalence with other sexually transmitted diseases (e.g., the prevalence of gonorrhea among women with trichomoniasis is twice as high as the prevalence of gonorrhea among women without trichomoniasis in the same groups); (4) an increased cure rate if sexual partners are treated simultaneously; and (5) failure, with few exceptions, of the disease to appear in household contacts who are not sexual partners. Recognizing the sexually transmitted nature of the infection is extremely important because patients with trichomoniasis should be screened for other sexually transmitted diseases that may be clinically silent but of greater eventual medical significance.

The organism can survive for several hours in a suitably moist environment, and the possibility of nonvenereal transmission is often raised. Nonvenereal acquisition of *T. vaginalis* by adults is extremely rare. Perinatal acquisition of disease, however, is reported in about 5% of female babies vaginally delivered by infected mothers.

PATHOGENESIS AND PATHOLOGY. The mechanisms by which *T. vaginalis* causes disease are not well understood. The organism is isolated from the vagina in >95% of infected women and from the urinary tract alone in <5%. Squamous but not columnar epithelium is infected, and organisms are rarely isolated from the endocervix. The urethra is, however, involved in 90% of cases, and organisms have been isolated from bladder urine. In men, trichomonads have been recovered from the epididymis and identified in the prostate.

Trichomoniasis in women ranges from asymptomatic carriage to severe inflammation. Initially asymptomatic disease frequently becomes symptomatic, supporting the need to treat asymptomatic carriers. In men, trichomoniasis is often asymptomatic. Clinical disease presents as urethritis, but only a minority of patients actually develop symptoms.

Trichomonal vaginitis elicits vaginal discharge containing large numbers of polymorphonuclear neutrophils (PMNs). Organisms are found free in the vaginal cavity or adhering to the epithelium. Tissue invasion does not occur. Colposcopy reveals microscopic hemorrhages in about 50% of cases, but these are visible to the naked eye in only 1 to 2% of cases.

In vitro, trichomonads destroy epithelial cells with which they make direct contact. In biopsy specimens of human infection, microulcerations are observed under clumps of trichomonads.

Low titers of serum antibody are detected in infections, but the humoral response cannot be used for diagnosis. Local IgA is detected in most infections. Delayed hypersensitivity can be demonstrated by skin testing in many infected women. PMNs and macrophages are capable of killing *Trichomonas*.

CLINICAL FEATURES

Disease in Women. In various series, 50 to 90% of women with trichomoniasis have symptoms, but this observation depends on the way in which the series are collected. Lower genital tract symptoms in women are also nonspecific. Many women with trichomoniasis have other sexually transmitted infections, and it is sometimes difficult to attribute specific clinical features to trichomoniasis alone. For example, in our clinic, 24 to 30% of women with gonorrhea have trichomonas coinfection. Vaginal discharge is described by 50 to 75% of infected women, but the discharge is considered malodorous by only 10%. One quarter to one half of infected women note vulvar irritation or pruritus, and as many as 50% suffer dyspareunia. Dysuria, usually "internal," is sometimes present but usually mild.

Lower abdominal discomfort is described by only 10% of women, and its presence, particularly if accompanied by adnexal tenderness on bimanual examination, should suggest the possibility of coincident salpingitis of a different cause.

Some women report that symptoms began or were exacerbated immediately after a menstrual period. In experimentally induced infection, the incubation period reportedly ranges from 3 to 28 days.

The vulva is erythematous in fewer than one third of patients. On speculum examination, excessive discharge is noted in 50 to 75% of infected women. A yellow vaginal discharge suggests trichomoniasis, but the classically yellow or green frothy discharge is seen in only a minority of patients. Indeed, bubbles are present in only 8 to 50% of infected women in various series, and bubbles are also seen in bacterial vaginosis, so their presence is nonspecific.

Vaginal wall erythema is observed in 20 to 75% of cases. Punctate hemorrhages are occasionally seen on the cervix (strawberry cervix), but this sign is not sensitive or specific.

Disease in Men. Most infected men are asymptomatic and come to treatment as sexual contacts of infected women. *T. vaginalis* causes some cases of nongonococcal urethritis (NGU), which are usually recognized because they fail to respond to standard therapies for gonorrhea and *Chlamydia*. When symptomatic, such infections resemble NGU due to other causes. Rarely, involvement of the epididymis and prostate is encountered.

Nongenital Sites of Infection. Trichomoniasis at nongenital sites of sexual exposure (e.g., anus, oral cavity) are uncommon, even in populations with high levels of exposure.

Disease in Children. Perhaps 5% of babies born to infected women contract trichomoniasis. Infected children may be febrile and fussy. Trichomoniasis in older children may indicate sexual abuse.

COMPLICATIONS. In the vast majority of cases, trichomoniasis is a benign disease. In pregnant women, however, it has been increasingly associated with premature rupture of membranes, consequent early childbirth, and fetal complications. Therefore, this infection should be diagnosed and treated during pregnancy. Studies have linked pelvic inflammatory disease with trichomoniasis. Trichomoniasis may alter the vaginal-cervical microenvironment, thereby enabling ascent of vaginal flora to the upper genital tract.

Trichomonas infection may be associated with enhanced sexual transmission of HIV (seroconversion), especially in developing countries. This has been a difficult area to study, however, because of the high prevalence of trichomonas in the population and because of the high coinfection rate with other sexually transmitted diseases (e.g., gonorrhea and *Chlamydia*).

DIAGNOSIS. Definitive diagnosis of trichomoniasis rests on demonstration of the parasite (Fig. 91–1). Clinicians are often confronted with symptomatic women who present for evaluation of some combination of vaginal discharge, vulvar irritation, or odor. A history of contact with a new partner supports the diagnosis of sexually transmitted vaginitis. The presence of odor without much irritation is somewhat more consistent with bacterial vaginosis than with trichomoniasis, in which irritation is more prominent.

Physical Examination. Women are examined in the lithotomy position. The vulva should be carefully evaluated for lesions of other sexually transmitted diseases. The presence of *satellite lesions*, small papulopustules beyond an area of erythema, suggests vulvovaginal candidiasis.

Some women with trichomoniasis are sufficiently tender so that the speculum cannot be inserted without undue discomfort. In such women, a swab gently inserted into the vagina can be used to recover material for evaluation. If the diagnosis of trichomoniasis is thereby made, such women should be asked to return for re-evaluation after the infection has resolved, so that coincident sexually transmitted diseases can be sought.

On insertion of the speculum, the vaginal walls may be erythematous and edematous. Vaginal wall inflammation is seen with trichomoniasis and candidiasis but not with bacterial vaginosis. The amount and nature of vaginal discharge are noted. A frankly yellow discharge supports a diagnosis of trichomoniasis, but bubbles are also seen with bacterial vaginosis. It is important to examine the cervix for evidence of cervicitis and purulent or mucopurulent discharge. Cervical discharge is dumped into the vaginal pool. After wiping off the exocervix, cervical material is recovered for appropriate laboratory examination. Vaginal discharge is then obtained by swabbing the vaginal fornices. For vaginal wet mount examination, the specimen can be transferred directly to a microscope slide, or (preferably) the swab may be agitated in a tube containing about 1 mL of saline.

Laboratory Evaluation. *T. vaginalis* can be cultured in various media. The most commonly used formulation is Diamond's medium. Newer culture techniques have been developed to simplify culture diagnosis. The In-Pouch® system is a selective medium that comes in a prepared small plastic pouch, and it is stable at room temperature. The pouch is inoculated with a vaginal specimen at the time of the examination and is then incubated. These systems are widely available but may be too costly for routine implementation in developing countries.

Trichomoniasis can also be diagnosed on Pap smear (cytology), which should be performed annually in sexually active young women. Sensitivity is thought to be only 50 to 60%, but the specificity is high, thereby warranting treatment when the organisms are observed.

After completing the physical examination, it is useful to determine the pH of vaginal secretions. This is conveniently accomplished by inserting a strip of indicator paper into the vaginal discharge pooled in the lower lip of the speculum. Normal vaginal pH of 4.5 or less is maintained in most patients with vulvovaginal candidiasis. Vaginal pH is elevated above 4.5 in three fourths or more of women with trichomoniasis. An elevated pH is also found in most women with bacterial vaginosis and is not specific. The pH of vaginal material may be artifactually elevated if contaminated with cervical discharge, which has an elevated pH. Recent coitus can elevate the apparent pH because semen is considerably more alkaline than normal vaginal secretions.

After the pH has been determined, several drops of 10 to 20% potassium hydroxide should be added to the discharge in the speculum. The clinician then seeks the elaboration of a pungent, fishy, amine-like odor. This positive result of the whiff test is manifested by 75% of women with trichomoniasis but also by most women with bacterial vaginosis. The whiff test is not positive in vulvovaginal candidiasis.

Microscopic Evaluation. Bedside techniques tend to separate infectious vaginitides into either (1) candidiasis or (2) trichomoniasis or bacterial vaginosis. Final differentiation is based on microscopic examination of the vaginal discharge. A drop of the wet mount preparation is examined microscopically under a coverslip, with the substage condenser racked down and the substage diaphragm closed to increase contrast.

In bacterial vaginosis, the normal flora of rods is replaced by clumps of coccobacilli. Few PMNs are observed, with one PMN per epithelial cell being considered normal. The epithelial cells are encrusted with coccobacilli, so-called clue cells.

In trichomoniasis, on the other hand, the flora consists of rods or coccobacilli. The epithelial cells are clean (unless bacterial vaginosis is coincidentally present), and larger numbers of PMNs are usually seen. Motile trichomonads are seen in 40 to 80% of infected women, with most studies yielding a sensitivity of approximately 67%. The organisms are best recognized by their characteristic twitching motility, but this motility decreases in older, cooled preparations.

Stains. Trichomonads may be detected in genital discharge with various stains. The Giemsa stain is approximately 50% sensitive, and an acridine orange stain detects organisms in about 60% of cases. New fluorescent antibody techniques have a sensitivity of 80 to 90% compared with culture. The routine Papanicolaou stain of a cervical specimen is said to detect organisms in 60 to 70% of cases. The Gram stain is useless.

Culture. Culture techniques appreciably increase the detection of trichomoniasis. Trichomonads grow best in anaerobic environment at about 37°C; the addition of antibiotics allows for selective growth. Several media are used, and cultures are usually read daily for 7 days before being discarded as negative. The sensitivity of the culture exceeds 95%. As described earlier, the In-Pouch® technique has simplified this procedure.

DNA-Based Diagnosis. Polymerase chain reaction techniques for diagnosis have been described but are not commercially available.

Serodiagnosis. Although serum antibodies can be detected in many infected patients, serologic diagnosis is experimental and adds nothing to the management of the individual case.

Presumptive Diagnosis. Trichomonads are not recognized in the vaginal discharge of about one third of infected women. In sexually active women, presumptive evidence of trichomonal infection can be based on the presence of an abnormal discharge, particularly if it is yellow; an elevated vaginal pH; a positive whiff test result; and excess PMNs in the wet mount (assuming the patient does not have a purulent cervical discharge). On the other hand, clue cells and the absence of PMNs argue for a diagnosis of bacterial vaginosis.

Diagnosis in Men. Trichomonal infection is difficult to diagnose in men. The wet mount of urethral discharge occasionally reveals motile organisms. The most effective way to make the diagnosis is by a combination of a urethral and first voided urine cultures. A recent study estimated each site yielded 60% sensitivity; when combined, sensitivity was >95%, in the research setting. Most men are "epidemiologically" treated for trichomoniasis because they have had sexual contact with infected women.

TREATMENT. The treatment of trichomoniasis was revolutionized by the development of the 5-nitroimidazoles. *T. vaginalis* is not susceptible to many other antimicrobial agents.

Susceptibility testing of trichomonads is not standardized. Still, >98% strains of *T. vaginalis* are highly susceptible to metronidazole and related drugs, with minimal inhibitory concentrations of 1 μg/mL or less. Minimum trichomonacidal concentrations range from 0.25 to 16 μg/mL. Isolates of *T. vaginalis* with high levels of resistance (>100 μg/mL) to metronidazole have been obtained from patients who were not cured by repeated courses of the drug. Testing under aerobic conditions enhances the difference between susceptible and resistant organisms. Resistance should be considered a possible explanation for repeated treatment failures.

The recommended treatment of trichomoniasis in women consists of 2.0 g of metronidazole administered as a single oral dose (or another 5-nitroimidazole in equivalent dose). This regimen cures about 85% of infected women; if sexual partners are treated simultaneously, the cure rate exceeds 95%. Intravaginal metronidazole preparations have become available but are not as effective as oral treatment.

The 7-day regimen is highly effective in curing men, but the single-dose regimen, although probably effective, has not been extensively evaluated. Asymptomatic male sexual partners of infected women should be treated.

In pregnancy, the treatment approach is similar, although many clinicians defer treatment during the first trimester. The consensus is that the teratogenic risks of metronidazole, especially single-dose therapy, are negligible and are outweighed by the benefits of treatment.

Side effects of metronidazole include nausea and vomiting. When taken with alcohol, metronidazole may produce a disulfiram-like effect manifested as flushing, headache, nausea, vomiting, vertigo, dyspnea, and tachycardia. Some treated women subsequently develop candidiasis. Metronidazole and similar drugs potentiate the effects of anticonvulsants and warfarin. Reversible neutropenia is sometimes observed.

Because they have been associated with unacceptably high failure rates, the wide variety of topical therapies proposed over the years are not considered effective primary therapy for this infection.

PROGNOSIS. Severe complications of trichomoniasis are essentially unreported.

PREVENTION AND CONTROL. Nonoxynol 9, a spermaticide found in many vaginal preparations, is trichomonacidal. The degree of actual protection provided by such preparations is undefined. Appropriately used condoms, including the female condom, prevent the transmission of trichomoniasis. No effective vaccine strategy has been developed.

Bibliography

Draper D, Parker R, Patterson E, et al: Detection of *Trichomonas vaginalis* in pregnant women with the In Pouch TV culture system. J Clin Microbiol 31:1016, 1993.

Honigberg BM (ed): Trichomonads Parasitic in Humans. New York, Springer-Verlag, 1989.

Krieger JN: Trichomoniasis in men: Old issues and new data. Sex Transm Dis 22:83, 1995.

Muller M, Lossick JG, Gorrell TE: In vitro susceptibility of *Trichomoniasis vaginalis* to metronidazole and treatment outcome in vaginal trichomoniasis. Sex Transm Dis 15:17, 1988.

Rein MD, Muller M: *Trichomonas vaginalis. In* Holmes KK, Mardh PA, Sparling PF, et al (eds): Sexually Transmitted Diseases, 2nd ed. New York, McGraw-Hill, 1990, pp 481–492.

Schwebke JR: Metronidazole: Utilization in the obstetric and gynecologic patient. Sex Transm Dis 22:370, 1995.

Soper DE, Shoupe D, Shargold GA, et al: Prevention of vaginal trichomoniasis by compliant use of the female condom. Sex Transm Dis 20:137, 1993.

Wolner-Hanssen P, Krieger JN, Stevens CE, et al: Clinical manifestations of vaginal trichomoniasis: Implications for strategies for diagnosis and of the infection. JAMA 264:571, 1989.

92 *Malaria*

Terrie E. Taylor and G. Thomas Strickland

DEFINITION. Malaria is an acute and chronic disease caused by obligate intracellular protozoa of the genus *Plasmodium*. Four species of *Plasmodium* are capable of infecting humans: *P. malariae* (Laveran, 1881), *P. vivax* (Grassi and Feletti, 1890), *P. falciparum* (Welch, 1897) and *P. ovale* (Stephens, 1922). The parasites are transmitted to humans by female *Anopheles* mosquitoes. The illness that ensues is highly variable but is generally characterized by paroxysms of fever and chills, anemia, and splenomegaly. *P. falciparum* is the species most commonly associated with severe and complicated disease.

ETIOLOGY. The zoologic family *Plasmodiidae* contains protozoan parasites found in the blood of birds, reptiles, and mammals. These organisms undergo two cycles of asexual division (schizogony, or merogony) in the vertebrate host and a single sexual reproductive cycle (sporogony) in the mosquito host. In the genus *Plasmodium*, one cycle of (exoerythrocytic) schizogony occurs in liver parenchymal cells of the vertebrate host; the second (erythrocytic) cycle occurs in the host erythrocytes.

There are more than 100 species of plasmodia, including 82 that infect birds and reptiles and 22 infecting nonhuman primates. Some of the latter are closely related to human plasmodia and can produce disease in humans under both natural and experimental conditions. However, such infections are rare and thus are of little epidemiologic significance.

HISTORY. Few diseases have had a greater impact on human social and economic development than malaria. The disease probably originated in Africa and affected prehistoric humans. Fossil mosquitoes have been found in geologic strata 30 million years old. The infection appears to have been widespread throughout warmer regions of the globe.

The disease was finally named by the Italians in the 18th century *mal aria* (foul air), but the first references to periodic fevers can be found in early Hindu and Chinese writings. In the fifth century B.C., the Greek physician Hippocrates described the clinical manifestations and some of the complications of malaria. He also related the appearance of the disease to the seasons of the year and to the locales in which his patients lived. The association of periodic fevers with stagnant water and swamps led the Greeks and later the Romans to undertake various methods of drainage—an approach to malaria control that is still in use. In the early 17th century, the bark of the Peruvian guina-guina (cinchona) tree was successfully used for treatment of intermittent fever. However, the active ingredient (the alkaloid quinine) was not isolated until 1820 in France (Pelletier and Caventou).

The first major breakthrough in understanding the etiology of the disease was in 1880, when Laveran, a French army surgeon in Algeria, first described exflagellated gametocytes of *P. falciparum* in a fresh blood film from a patient with malaria. Five years later, Golgi reported in detail the asexual forms of *P. vivax* and *P. malariae*. The polychrome staining method developed by Romanowsky in 1891 permitted more detailed morphologic studies.

Transmission remained a mystery until the 1880s, when Patrick Manson discovered that filariasis was transmitted by mosquitoes and postulated that malaria might also be vector-borne. In 1897, Ronald Ross, a British army surgeon in India, found a developing form of the malaria parasite in the gut of a mosquito that had fed on a malarious patient. In 1898, Ross conclusively established the major features of the life cycle of plasmodia by a careful series of experiments in naturally infected sparrows. The complex cycle of development was confirmed by Bignami, Bastianelli and Grassi in Italy in 1898 and 1899, and by Manson and his colleagues in London and Rome in 1900. The exoerythrocytic cycle of *P. cynomolgi* was described by Shortt and Garnham in 1948. In 1980, Krotoski and Garnham demonstrated a dormant liver stage in *P. cynomolgi*, the hypnozoite, which is responsible for the late relapses characteristic of *P. vivax* and *P. ovale* human infections.

During the 20th century, progress has been made in vector control technology and in the development of potent synthetic antimalarial compounds. Larvicides (oil, Paris green) were introduced and these, along with other antimosquito measures, proved useful in controlling malaria and yellow fever in Panama and Cuba. In the late 1930s, Paul Muller in Switzerland discovered the potent insecticidal activity of dichlorodiphenyltrichloroethane (DDT). From 1942 to 1946, new synthetic residual insecticides, e.g., hexachlorocyclohexane (BHC), dieldrin, and chlordane were developed.

Quinine was the drug of choice for treating malaria, but the difficulties involved in procuring it during World Wars I and II stimulated research on synthetic antimalarial compounds. These efforts produced a plethora of drugs: pamaquine (1924), quinacrine (1930), chloroquine (1934), chlorguanide (1945), amodiaquine (1946), primaquine (1950), and pyrimethamine (1951).

In 1955, encouraged by the high potency, low toxicity, ease of administration, and low cost of DDT and other residual insectides, the World Health Assembly adopted the concept of the global eradication of malaria. Two years later, the World Health Organization (WHO) launched a worldwide program of malaria eradication. This program was hindered by the development of DDT resistance in the mosquito populations and by the development of chloroquine resistance in some strains of *P. falciparum*. In 1969, WHO revised the eradication strategy, emphasizing the need for more research and for greater involvement of general health services. During the last 20 years, there has been an increase of malaria in many areas. In 1978, the World Health Assembly endorsed a strategy of malaria control based on the assessment of localized control potential. This ranged from reducing morbidity and mortality with chemotherapy to comprehensive campaigns stressing personal protection and vector control to community-based bioenvironmental interventions. In recognition of the enormous variability in malaria throughout the world, the goals of malaria control were broadened during a Ministerial Conference on Malaria in 1992 and became the prevention of mortality, and the reduction of morbidity and social and economic losses through the progressive improvement and strengthening of local and national capabilities. The four basic technical elements of the current WHO strategy are to provide early diagnosis and prompt treatment; to plan and implement selective and sustainable preventive measures (including vector control); to detect, contain, or prevent early epidemics; and to strengthen local capacities in basic and applied research in order to permit and promote regular assessments of a country's malaria situation, with particular emphasis on the ecological, social, and economic determinants of disease.

DISTRIBUTION AND INCIDENCE. Malaria transmission occurs in more than 100 countries throughout Africa, Asia, and Latin America and on certain Caribbean and Pacific islands (Fig. 92–1). More than 2 billion inhabitants of these areas are at risk of malaria infection. The estimated annual global incidence of malaria is 300 to 500 million clinical cases although many others are not seen by health care providers. In sub-Saharan Africa alone, there are more than 100 million cases each year, with an estimated 1 million deaths, mostly in infants and young children.

Malaria transmission has been interrupted in the United States and Canada, most of the Caribbean, Europe (including the former USSR), parts of South America, Israel, Lebanon, Réunion, Singapore, Hong Kong, Japan, Korea, Taiwan, Brunei, and Australia. However, many cases are imported into these countries; on average, 1000 cases are reported to the U.S. Centers for Disease Control and Prevention (CDC) annually.

P. falciparum is the predominant species in Africa, Haiti, and the Dominican Republic; *P. malariae* exists in the same areas but its prevalence is much lower. *P. vivax* and *P. falciparum* are both present in Mexico, Central and South America, the Indian subcontinent, Southeast Asia, and Oceania. *P. ovale* occurs mainly in Africa, with rare cases reported from other continents. *P. vivax* is rare in Africa because most Africans lack the Duffy blood group antigen necessary for parasite invasion.

■ TRANSMISSION

Malaria is transmitted during the bite of an infected female *Anopheles* mosquito or, more rarely, through the direct inoculation of infected red blood cells (i.e., congenital malaria, transfusion malaria, and malaria from contaminated needles).

LIFE CYCLE. The life cycle of malaria is complex (Fig. 92–2), and there are differences between the *Plasmodium* species (Table 92–1). The infective stage, *sporozoites* (Fig. 92–3) are injected along with saliva into subcutaneous capillaries as the female mosquito prepares to take a blood meal. They are present in the peripheral blood for a very short period of time, typically less than 30 minutes.

Human Phase

Exoerythrocytic Phase. Some sporozoites are destroyed by phagocytes, but many enter liver parenchymal cells (hepatocytes), where they multiply asexually in a process known as *exoerythrocytic schizogony/merogony* (Fig. 92–4A and B in color section). The nucleus undergoes repeated division, resulting in the formation of thousands of uninucleate *merozoites*, each measuring 0.7 to 1.8 μm in diameter. The nucleus of the liver cell is displaced, but there is no inflammatory reaction in the surrounding liver tissue and the host is asymptomatic.

Within 6 to 16 days of initial infection, the hepatic cells containing the tissue schizonts/meronts rupture, and merozoites enter circulating red blood cells. In *P. falciparum* and *P. malariae* infections, the tissue schizonts/meronts rupture at about the same time, and none persist in the liver. By contrast, *P. vivax* and *P. ovale* have two types of exoerythrocytic forms. A primary type develops and ruptures within 6 to 9 days. The secondary type, the hypnozoite, may remain dormant in the liver for weeks, months, or up to 5 years before developing and causing *relapses* of erythrocytic infection. The first hypnozoites identified were those of *P. cynomolgi*, a simian parasite resembling *P. vivax* (Fig. 92–4A and B [color section]).

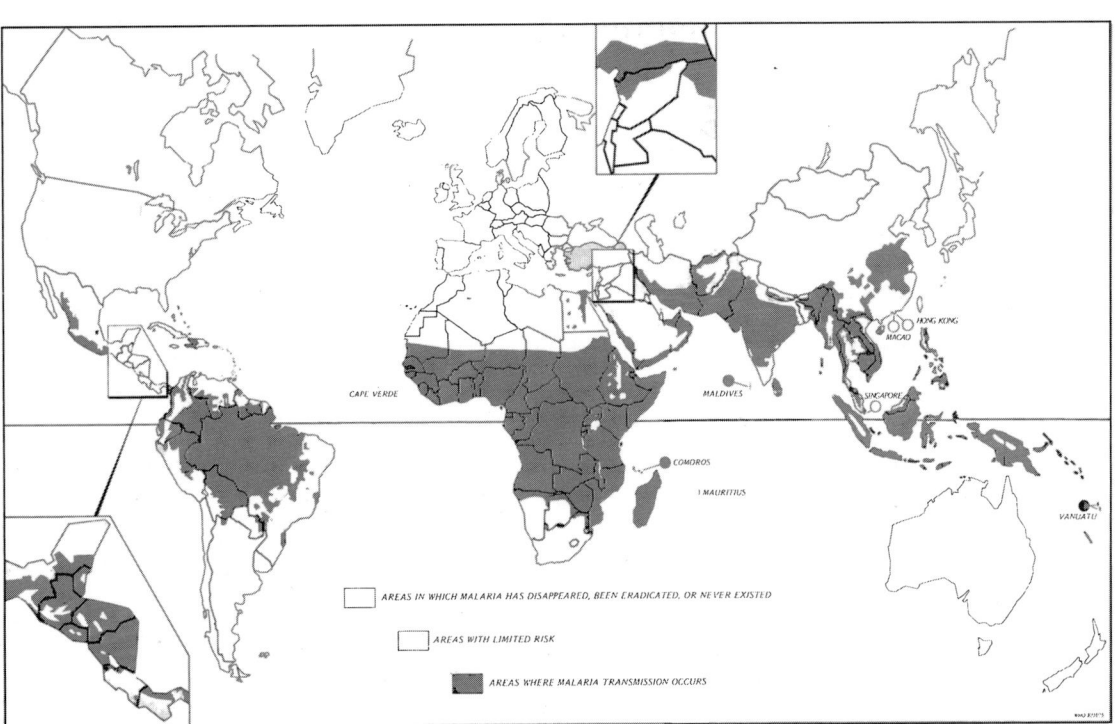

Figure 92–1. Epidemiologic assessment of status of malaria. Reproduced with permission of WHO. (Courtesy of the Director General and Joachim H.-G. Hempel. Epidemiological Methodology and Evaluation, Malaria Action Programme.)

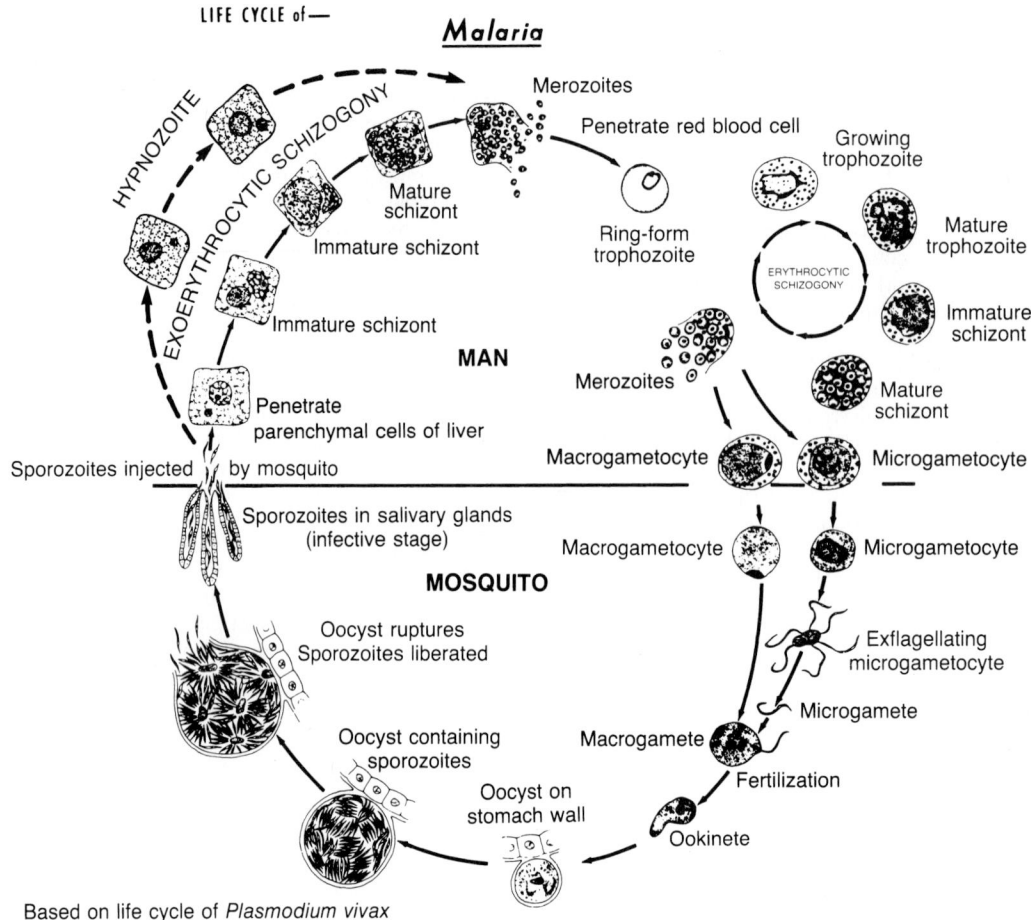

Figure 92–2. Life cycle of malaria (based on cycle for *Plasmodium vivax*). The dormant hypnozoite stage is present in *P. vivax* and *P. ovale* and is responsible for relapsing infections. (Modified from Melvin DM, et al: Common Blood and Tissue Parasites of Man. Life Cycle Charts. Atlanta, Georgia, Centers for Disease Control, 1979.)

TABLE 92–1. Selected Characteristics of Four Species of Human Malaria

	P. falciparum	*P. vivax*	*P. ovale*	*P. malariae*
Exoerythrocytic cycle (days)	5½–7	6–8	9	12–16
Erythrocytic cycle (hr)	48	42–48	49–50	72
Prepatent period (days)	9–10	11–13	10–14	15
Usual incubation period in days (range)*	12 (9–14)	13 (12–17) or longer	17 (16–18) or longer	28 (18–40) or longer
Earliest appearance of gametocytes (days)	10	3	?	?
Secondary exoerythrocytic cycle	none	present	present	none
Average merozoites per tissue schizont	40,000	10,000	15,000	2000
Size of tissue schizont	60 μm	45 μm	70 μm	45 μm
Duration of untreated infection (yr)	1–2	1½–4	1½–4	3–50
Average parasitemia (per mm)†	20,000 or greater	10,000	9000	6000
Minimum duration (and range) of sporogony cycle in mosquito in days‡	9 (9–22)	8 (8–16)	12 (12–14)	16 (16–35)
Severity of primary attack†	severe in nonimmune	mild to severe	mild	mild
Usual periodicity of febrile attacks (hr)	none	48	48	72
Duration of febrile paroxysm (hr)	16–36 or longer	8–12	8–12	8–10

*Patterns in different strains vary.
†Influenced by level of immunity.
‡Temperature dependent.
Modified from Bruce-Chwatt LJ: Essential Malariology. London, William Heinemann Medical Books Ltd., 1980.

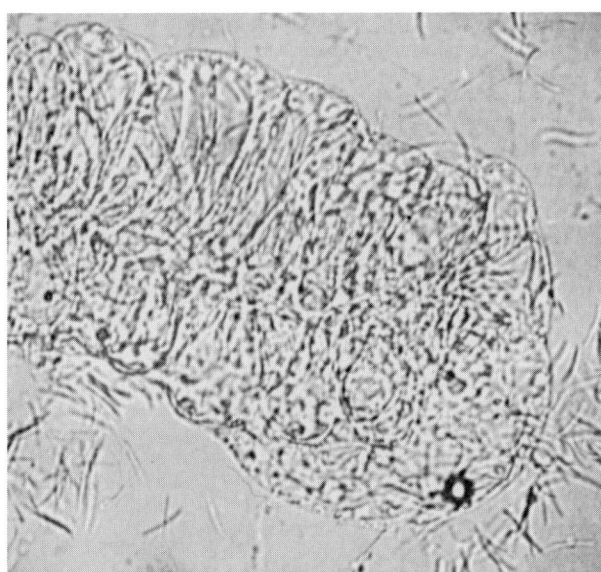

Figure 92–3. Sporozoites.

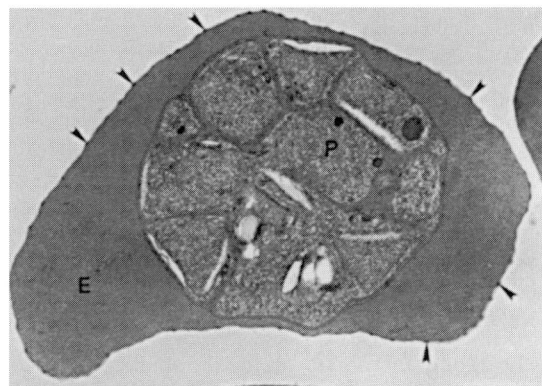

Figure 92–6. Segmenting schizont of *Plasmodium falciparum* (P) in an erythrocyte (E). The surface of the erythrocyte has been altered by the parasite, resulting in dense structures or "knobs" *(arrows)*. The bar represents 1 μm. (Courtesy of Susan G. Langreth.)

P. falciparum and *P. malariae* have no persistent exoerythrocytic phase, and therefore relapses do not occur in infections with these species; recurrent parasitemia is due to proliferation of persistent erythrocytic forms and is known as *recrudescence.* The prolonged, delayed recrudescences occasionally seen with *P. malariae* are due to erythrocytic parasites that have persisted in the circulation.

Erythrocytic Phase. Merozoites released from tissue schizonts invade red blood cells. Following an initial collision and adherence, mediated in part by glycophorins on the red cell surface, the adherent merozoite reorients, bringing its apical end into apposition with the erythrocyte surface. An invagination develops opposite the apex of the parasite, defined by an electron-dense annular junction. Internal parasite organelles (rhoptries and micronemes) discharge their contents and the merozoite begins to move into the invagination. Once inside the red cell, the parasite is sheathed in the parasitophorous vacuole membrane.

Asexual Stages. The youngest stages in the blood are small, rounded trophozoites, known as *ring forms* (Figs. 92–4C, D, and H [color section] and 92–5, row 1 [color section]). As the parasites grow, they become more irregular and ameboid (Figs. 92–4D–G [color section] and 92–5, rows 2 and 3 [color section]). During development, the parasites consume hemoglobin, leaving as the product of digestion an iron-containing pigment, hematin or hemozoin, which is visible in the cytoplasm of the parasite as dark granules. The schizont/meront stage (Figs. 92–4G [color section] and 92–5, row 4 [color section] and 92–6) begins when the parasite undergoes nuclear division and culminates in segmentation to form *merozoites.* This process of asexual multiplication is called *erythrocytic schizogony/merogony.* The infected erythrocytes rupture, liberating merozoites, which must then invade uninfected red cells. The erythrocytic cycle of schizogony is repeated until it is contained by the host's own immunity, antimalarial drugs, or a combination of both. The periodicity of schizogony is different in the four *Plasmodium* species that infect humans (Table 92–1).

Sexual Stages. The parasite life cycle continues when subpopulations of merozoites differentiate into sexual forms known as *gametocytes.* Female macrogametocytes (Figs. 92–4I [color section] and 92–5, row 5 [color section]) and male microgametocytes (Figs. 92–4I [color section] and 92–5, row 6 [color section]) usually appear within 3 to 15 days of the onset of symptoms. The duration of gametocytogony is assumed to be 4 days in *P. vivax* infections and 10 or more days in *P. falciparum* infections.

Vector Phase

Exflagellation. While feeding on an infected human, the female anopheline mosquito (Fig. 92–7) may ingest gametocytes. If so, they undergo further development in the stomach of the mosquito. The nucleus of the male gametocyte divides into 4 to 8 nuclei, each of which combines with cytoplasm to form a long threadlike flagellum, measuring 20 to 25 μm in length. These exflagellated *microgametes* shoot out from the original cell, lash about, and then break free. This process takes only a few minutes at the appropriate temperature. The microgametes move actively toward and through small projections that form on the female parasites, now known as *macrogametes,* and mitosis takes place. The zygotes elongate within 18 to 24 hours and become motile *ookinetes,* between 18 to 24 μm long.

Sporogony. The ookinete forces its way between the epithelial cells to the outer surface of the stomach (midgut) and

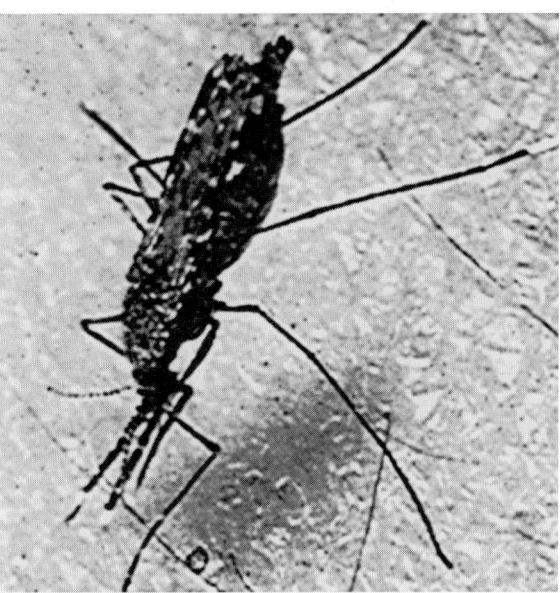

Figure 92–7. Feeding female anopheline mosquito.

rounds up to a small sphere within an elastic membrane; at this point it is called an *oocyst*. The number of oocysts on the stomach of an infected *Anopheles* mosquito may vary between a few and several hundred (Fig. 92–8).

The oocyst is a semitransparent globular body that grows to 40 to 80 μm in size and contains grains of pigment whose distribution, size, and color are characteristic for each species of *Plasmodia*. The oocyst enlarges progressively as the nucleus divides over and over. It may achieve a diameter of 500 μm, and the pigment may become obscured. The divided nuclei form finger-like processes, at the periphery of which develop large numbers of elongated, fusiform *sporozoites*. All plasmodial sporozoites have the same structure. The oocyst ruptures, liberating thousands of motile sporozoites into the body cavity, from which they migrate to the salivary glands (Fig. 92–3). The female mosquito is now infective.

Sporogony, the progress of the malaria parasite in the mosquito from gametocyte maturation through the attainment of sporozoite infectivity, varies from 8 to 35 days depending on external temperatures and on the species (Table 92–1).

■ EPIDEMIOLOGY

Malaria transmission involves the interaction between the malaria parasite, the human host, and the anopheline vector

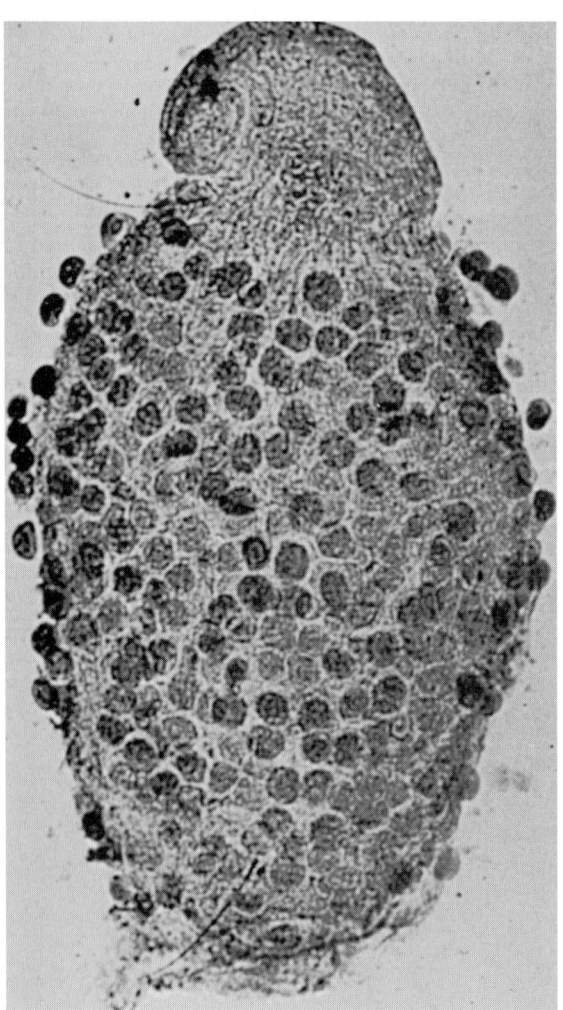

***Figure* 92–8.** Many oocysts on the stomach of a heavily infected mosquito.

and the environment (physical, biologic, and socioeconomic). The level of transmission is determined by (1) the seasonal incidence and prevalence of infection in the reservoir host (human); (2) characteristics of the local vector mosquitoes, including their relative abundance, feeding and resting behaviors, susceptibility to infection, and effectiveness as a vector; (3) the susceptibility of the local human population to infection; and (4) local climatic and environmental features that affect vector breeding and sporogony rates. In many endemic areas, there is a predictable seasonality related to annual variations in temperature, humidity, and rainfall. However, malaria transmission also has fluctuations that cannot be predicted or explained.

The Parasite

The parasite must be present in the blood long enough to produce viable gametocytes at a time when environmental conditions are suitable for transmission. In addition, the parasite must be adapted to a vector capable of transmitting the infection.

Most of the severe morbidity and mortality in malaria is caused by *P. falciparum*. When compared with the three other species infecting humans (Table 92–1), the incubation period is shortest, the exoerythrocytic schizonts release 2.5 to 20 times as many merozoites, and the duration of untreated infections is the least. By contrast, *P. malariae* has the longest duration of untreated infection and sometimes is almost a commensal infection in adults.

The age of erythrocytes is an important determinant of parasitemia. *P. vivax* and *P. ovale* tend to invade only young red cells (reticulocytes). *P. malariae* invades primarily aging erythrocytes. Parasitemias in these species are generally less than 2%. By contrast, *P. falciparum* can invade all erythrocytes, and can produce higher parasitemias.

Each species of human plasmodia consists of a number of different strains that are indistinguishable morphologically but have different features. Some may infect local vectors but not vectors from other areas. They may respond differently to various antimalarial drugs or to cytokine-inducing stimuli. Relapse patterns of *P. vivax* strains from various regions differ and reflect adaptation to local environmental conditions. Long incubation periods for vivax malaria occur in temperate climates where the transmission season is short; prolonged latency enhances the chance that a particular strain of parasite will survive lengthy periods of no transmission.

THE HOST. Sex and age probably do not affect the incidence or severity of malaria infection and disease per se, but because they are often related to frequency of exposure (via occupation, social behavior, and migration) and thus the development of immunity, they can be important host factors.

Immunity. In general, populations in endemic areas continuously exposed to infected mosquitoes develop immunity to malaria illness and, to a lesser degree, to malaria infection. Clinical manifestations, asexual parasitemia, and the production of gametocytes are all reduced by acquired immunity. In endemic areas, malaria prevalence and gametocyte production are highest among infants and young children, the groups with the least acquired immunity. Adults in these areas may still become infected, but the parasitemias are generally less. Individuals with fever and other clinical manifestations are not necessarily those most responsible for transmission. Asymptomatic individuals with gametocytemia are also reservoirs of infection for feeding mosquitoes. Acquired immunity may diminish during pregnancy, and in holo- and hyperendemic areas, pregnant women are the adults at greatest risk of developing severe and complicated disease. In the many areas where malaria transmission is seasonal and/or much lower than in sub-Saharan Africa, the entire population is at risk for malaria infection and disease. In fact, in some areas, e.g., the Philippines, young adult males are at greatest risk of acquiring malaria because of their exposures to forest dwelling vectors. The development of acquired immunity is undisputed, particularly in areas with intense transmission, but its immunologic basis remains elusive.

Genetic Factors. Individuals who are heterozygous for sickle hemoglobin have less severe falciparum malaria infections and they do not die from sickle cell disease. The relative protection conferred against malaria in heterozygotes living in malaria-endemic areas has ensured the survival of a gene that is generally fatal in homozygotes. Balanced polymorphism involving hemoglobin S in certain parts of Africa is due to the selective advantage of the heterozygotes (Fig. 6–2). Epidemiologic evidence exists to support a similar argument for hereditary ovalocytosis (Fig. 6–11). However, the possible protective effects of β-thalassemia (Fig. 6–7), persistence of fetal hemoglobin (HbF), and glucose-6-phosphate dehydrogenase (G6PD) deficiency (Fig. 6–10) against malaria have not been confirmed.

Individuals lacking the Duffy a and b (Fy^a and Fy^b) blood group determinants (Duffy-negative blood type) are resistant to infection with *P. vivax* because the specific receptors for invasion of vivax merozoites are absent. The low incidence of *P. vivax* malaria in Africa is explained by the fact that most Africans are Duffy negative.

Two human leukocyte antigens are present in higher-than-expected concentrations in West Africans and may confer protection against severe malaria. The class I antigen HLA-Bw53 has been associated with protection against cerebral malaria in Gambian children, and in the same population, the class II antigen HLA-DRB1*1302 was associated with protection against severe malarial anemia.

Nutritional Factors. Contrary to what might be expected, most of the available data suggest that nutritional deficiencies protect the host from severe and complicated malaria infection. Famines can blunt malaria epidemics, the establishment of feeding centers for refugee populations can spark outbreaks of malaria, and severe malaria is rare in children with marasmus and/or kwashiorkor. Malnutrition may be antagonistic to the growth of malaria parasites.

THE VECTOR. The effectiveness of a vector in transmitting malaria depends on (1) its presence in adequate numbers in or near human habitation; (2) its preference for human blood (*anthropophilic*) rather than animal blood (*zoophilic*); (3) sufficient longevity to complete sporogony and transmit the infection; and (4) its behavior regarding feeding and resting indoors (*endophilic*) vs. outdoors (*exophilic*). Temperature and humidity greatly affect the rate of parasite development in the vector and the mosquito's longevity.

There are about 400 species of anophelines, of which approximately 80 are proven vectors. However, only 27 are considered effective. Anophelines that are excellent vectors of a malaria strain from one area may not transmit strains from another, and in each area often only 1, and usually not more than 2 or 3, species are important vectors.

THE ENVIRONMENT. Malaria transmission is profoundly influenced by climate. The optimal conditions occur when the temperature is between 20° and 30°C and the mean relative humidity is at least 60%. Sporogony does not occur at temperatures below 16°C or at temperatures higher than 33°C. Water temperatures regulate the duration of the aquatic breeding cycle of the mosquito vector. A high relative humidity increases mosquito longevity and therefore increases the probability that an infected mosquito will survive long enough to become infective. Malaria infections and malaria illness are often more common during rainy seasons because the number of breeding sites is increased and because female anophelines survive longer when the humidity is high. However, too much rainfall can be deleterious to vector larvae and pupae by washing them away, thus decreasing transmission; and prolonged droughts may be associated with increased transmission if they reduce the size and flow rates of large rivers sufficiently to produce suitable breeding sites.

The proximity of human habitation to breeding sites directly influences vector–human contact and, therefore, transmission. The stability of breeding sites is influenced by water supply, soil, vegetation, etc. Irrigation schemes, dams, and other manmade changes can radically alter stable patterns of malaria transmission.

EPIDEMIOLOGIC TERMINOLOGY. *Stable endemic malaria* is present when natural transmission occurs over many years and there is a predictable incidence of illness and prevalence of infection. Transmission is generally high and epidemics are unlikely. *Unstable malaria* occurs in settings where transmission rates vary from year to year and collective immunity is low. Epidemics are more likely in this setting. *Autochthonous (indigenous) malaria* is contracted locally. Secondary cases are those derived from imported cases and are referred to as *introduced malaria*. Malaria infections acquired by blood transfusion, shared needles, intentional inoculation, or laboratory accident are all known as *induced malaria*. *Cryptic malaria* cases are those that occur in isolation and are not associated with secondary cases.

A number of parameters are commonly used to classify malaria in an area. Care must be taken to distinguish between malaria infection (patent parasitemia) and malaria illness. Descriptive terms include:

Malaria incidence: Number of new infections or cases detected per time unit (e.g., annually) per unit of population (e.g., per 1000).

Malaria prevalence: Total number of cases or infections at one point in time, per unit of population. When the measure used is microscopically proven parasitemia, malaria prevalence and *parasite rate* are synonymous.

Entomologic inoculation rate: Number of sporozoite positive bites per person per time unit.

Annual parasite incidence: Number of new parasitologically confirmed cases per 1000 population per year.

Infant conversion rate: Fraction of parasitologically negative infants becoming positive per time unit.

Spleen rate: Proportion of individuals in a stated age range with enlarged spleens.

The degree of endemic malaria is determined by examination of a statistically significant sample of a population and is assessed and classified as follows:

Hypoendemic: Spleen rate or parasite rate of 0 to 10% in children between the ages of 2 and 9.

Mesoendemic: Spleen rate or parasite rate of 11 to 50% in children between the ages of 2 and 9.

Hyperendemic: Spleen rate or parasite rate consistently over 50% in children between the ages of 2 and 9. Adult spleen rate is also high.

Holoendemic: Spleen rate or parasite rate consistently over 75% in children between the ages of 2 and 9. Adult spleen rate is low and the transmission index is high.

Mathematical models have been applied to malaria but none generate predictions accurate enough on which policy decisions can be based. Social conditions, in particular, are subject to wide variation and rapid change.

EPIDEMICS. Epidemics of malaria with high mortality rates are less frequent now than in the past. However, the epidemic potential continues to exist. An epidemic occurs when an unexpected increase in the number of cases occurs in an area. The genesis of epidemics involves one or more of the following situations: (1) an increase in susceptibility of the population; (2) the introduction of a new vector or a new strain of parasite; (3) changes in the pattern of vector–human contact; and/or (4) increased effectiveness of the local vector in transmitting the disease.

Increased susceptibility of populations generally occurs when a large number of nonimmune individuals move into a malarious area, e.g., as occurred when transmigrants moved from Java to Irian Jaya or gold miners begun digging in the Amazonian rain forest. Inadvertent introduction of a more efficient vector, e.g., the importation of *Anopheles gambiae* into Brazil in the 1930s by a ship sailing from Africa, can produce explosive epidemics. Manmade dams, irrigation schemes, and artisanal gold mining can, by creating more breeding sites, increase the density of local vectors. Finally, a decrease in the number of animals in an area can force a previously predominantly zoophilic mosquito to use humans as the primary source of blood meals, thus increasing transmission.

IMPORTED MALARIA. Increased international air travel has escalated the incidence of imported malaria (and other infectious diseases) to nonendemic areas. Tourists often travel during the incubation period and do not become ill until after they return home. Delays in diagnosis, misdiagnosis, and inappropriate treatment can occur and may cause unnecessary morbidity and mortality. Physicians and public health officials must remain aware of the possibility of imported malaria infections. Over 1000 cases of imported malaria have been reported in the United States annually during the 1990s. Many of these have been in immigrants, some of whom were infected while returning to their native country for visits; also at risk are business and pleasure travelers.

AUTOCHTHONOUS MALARIA. Malaria was endemic throughout much of the United States and Western Europe up until the middle of the 20th century. Most infections were due to *P. vivax* which was transmitted during the warmer seasons in the south central and southeastern United States and in the warmer humid areas in the West. The mosquito vectors, primarily *Anopheles quadrimaculatus*, east of the Rocky Mountains, and *Anopheles freeborni*, west of the mountains, are still present and locally transmitted cases of malaria are occurring with increasing frequency each summer. These are mostly due to *P. vivax* but a few have been caused by *P. malariae* and *P. falciparum*. Most of these occurred when migrant laborers from malaria-endemic countries infected mosquitoes which in turn infected local inhabitants. California has had the most outbreaks of locally acquired malaria, but recently cases have been reported as far north as Michigan, New York City, and New Jersey. The risk of autochthonous malaria transmission in the United States is increasing during the 1990s because the large immigrant population provides sources of infectious gametocytes to feeding anopheline mosquitoes and warm, humid weather allows completion of the sporogenic cycle.

■ PATHOPHYSIOLOGY

Pathophysiologic changes in malaria involve many different organ systems and stem from a number of different parasite-derived stimuli. Blood-stage parasites are the main source of these various stimuli; exoerythrocytic stages, gametocytes, and sporozoites do not induce pathophysiologic changes.

ETIOLOGY. The pathophysiology of malarial illnesses is multifactorial.

Erythrocyte Destruction. Red blood cells are destroyed when parasitized cells rupture, but there is accelerated destruction of uninfected erythrocytes also. Severe anemia, with its hemodynamic consequences, can develop. With severe intravascular hemolysis ("blackwater fever"), hemoglobinuria can precipitate acute renal failure. Hematopoiesis is suppressed during the acute infection, but resumes in iron-replete individuals once they become aparasitemic.

Cytokines. A mediator that has yet to be completely identified or described, but which is known to be released at the time of schizont rupture, stimulates local macrophages, and is associated with the production of cytokines. The most well studied of these is tumor necrosis factor (TNF). TNF, a monokine, has been detected in the circulation of humans and animals infected with malaria parasites. TNF concentrations are higher in patients with more severe disease, and remain elevated longer in patients who die compared with those who recover. Recombinant TNF, when administered to nonmalarious subjects, produces a clinical syndrome with findings typical of malaria: fever, hypoglycemia and adult respiratory distress syndrome (ARDS). Anti-TNF antibodies infused into malaria patients has a dose-related effect on fever. TNF can also kill *P. falciparum* parasites in vitro and may, by upregulating the expression of adhesion molecules on endothelial cell surfaces, enhance the sequestration of mature infected red cells to vascular endothelium. Different strains of *P. falciparum* evoke different TNF responses in vitro and there is evidence to suggest that individuals with a TNF promotor genotype associated with an enhanced response to standard stimuli are more likely to develop severe disease. It may be that TNF is a necessary, but not sufficient in itself, cause of severe and complicated malaria. Some patients with uncomplicated *P. vivax* malaria have plasma TNF concentrations as high or higher than those observed in patients with complicated falciparum infections.

Nitric Oxide. TNF may contribute to the pathogenesis of malaria by stimulating the intravascular synthesis of nitric oxide, an evanescent neurotransmitter. Nitric oxide would, according to this hypothesis, diffuse through the blood-brain barrier and disrupt neurotransmission. The effect would cease as soon as the stimulus (TNF) is no longer present, and patients could recover with very little permanent damage to the central nervous system (CNS). This cascade is intriguing because many malaria patients with severe CNS dysfunction survive with no discernible neurologic deficits. Few of the other theories of malaria pathogenesis have such a tidy explanation for the reversibility of the observed symptoms. Indirect measurements of nitric oxide tend to show a positive correlation with disease severity, and in sequential studies, also a correlation with parasite clearance and clinical cure rates. These findings suggest that nitric oxide, like TNF, may have both harmful and beneficial effects during the course of a malaria infection.

Sequestration of Infected Erythrocytes. *P. falciparum* is distinguished from the other three human species of malaria parasites because its mature forms (schizonts) are rarely identified in peripheral blood films. These late-stage parasites "sequester" in capillaries and venules of various tissues and are thus effectively invisible when parasitemias are assessed by a peripheral blood film. Although it is possible to estimate roughly the biomass of the sequestered parasites based on the proportion of life-cycle stages observed in the peripheral film, no precise measure of these hidden parasites exists at this time. These late-stage parasites are very active metabolically, consuming up to 75 times more glucose than earlier ring stages and generating lactate as an end product. They adhere to capillary endothelial cells and may be present in such large numbers that blood flow is impaired.

It has long been hypothesized that the sequestration of parasitized red blood cells (PRBC) is the primary pathogenetic event in *P. falciparum* infections, and much research has been directed toward elucidating the details of putative endothelial receptors and PRBC ligands. If sequestration proves to be a critical contributor to morbidity and mortality in falciparum malaria, then disrupting it may be beneficial to the host.

The putative infected red cell receptors (CD36, intercellular adhesion molecule 1 [ICAM-1], vascular cell adhesion molecule 1 [VCAM-1], E-selectin, thrombospondin, chondroitin sulfate) were detected largely on the basis of in vitro binding assays and verified using competitive inhibition assays. Each of these receptors has also been identified in association with *P. falciparum* schizont-infected red cells in vivo, but clinicopathologic correlates have not been made. Recent data from Kenya demonstrated that PRBC isolated from the placentae of primigravidae adhered exclusively to chondroitin sulfate; parasites isolated from the peripheral blood of primigravidae adhered to either CD36 or chondroitin sulfate, whereas those isolated from the peripheral blood of nonpregnant women adhered preferentially to CD36. These findings suggest that organ-specific cytoadherence could be contributing to clinical symptomatology.

The adhesive moieties on the surface of the PRBC have not been conclusively identified either, but the leading candidates are members of a large family of strain-specific, high molecular weight proteins, *P. falciparum* erythrocyte membrane protein 1 (PfEMP-1). Recent data suggest that a superfamily of *var* genes, scattered across and making up about 6% of the *P. falciparum* genome, encode these proteins. Antigenic switching rates and modulation of the adherence phenotype may be as high as 2% per generation, even in the absence of immune pressure, and this could be an effective technique for eluding the host immune system. Other possible ligands are motifs present in human band 3, a native protein which is presumed to be altered as a result of *P. falciparum* infection; peptides patterned on these motifs blocked cytoadherence in vitro, and reversed cytoadherence in *Aotus* and *Saimiri* monkeys.

BIOCHEMICAL AND ELECTROLYTE CHANGES

Hypoglycemia. Because of its deleterious effects on the CNS, and because of the necessity of treatment with exogenous glucose, this is the most important of the biochemical aberrations described to date. Hypoglycemia (blood glucose concentrations <40 mg/dL or 2.2 mmol/L) can develop, prior to any antimalarial treatment, in up to 20% of children with severe *P. falciparum* malaria. Plasma insulin levels are low and gluconeogenic precursors and adrenal hormones are present in high concentrations in the blood, so parasite consumption of glucose and/or inadequate hepatic gluconeogenesis are the most likely etiologies for pretreatment hypoglycemia. It is not possible to detect hypoglycemia on clinical grounds in these patients, so in situations where the blood glucose cannot be measured, immediate treatment with 50% dextrose is recommended. Patients who present with pretreatment hypoglycemia have a worse prognosis than those who do not.

Antimalarial treatment can precipitate hypoglycemia. Rapid infusions of quinine (≥10 mg/kg/hr) can stimulate pancreatic insulin secretion; pregnant women appear to be especially susceptible to this complication of treatment. Also, hypoglycemia can develop after several days of quinine treatment when the reduced tissue sensitivity to insulin, a feature of acute malaria, begins to resolve.

Acid-Base Changes. Metabolic acidosis is now recognized as an important marker of severity in falciparum malaria infections, and "acidotic breathing" alone was associated with a 19% mortality rate in Kenyan children. In this population, the mortality rate in children with impaired consciousness uncomplicated by acidotic breathing was 12%; in children with acidotic breathing and impaired consciousness, the mortality rate was 32% (Fig. 92–9). Elevated plasma and cerebrospinal fluid lactate levels are also associated with a poor outcome but few studies have examined both pH and lactate, so although they are likely to be highly correlated, the precise relationship is not known. Acidosis and hypoglycemia are strongly associated, suggesting parasite and/or host metabolism may be contributing to both. Circulatory shock is rarely a feature of severe and complicated malaria,

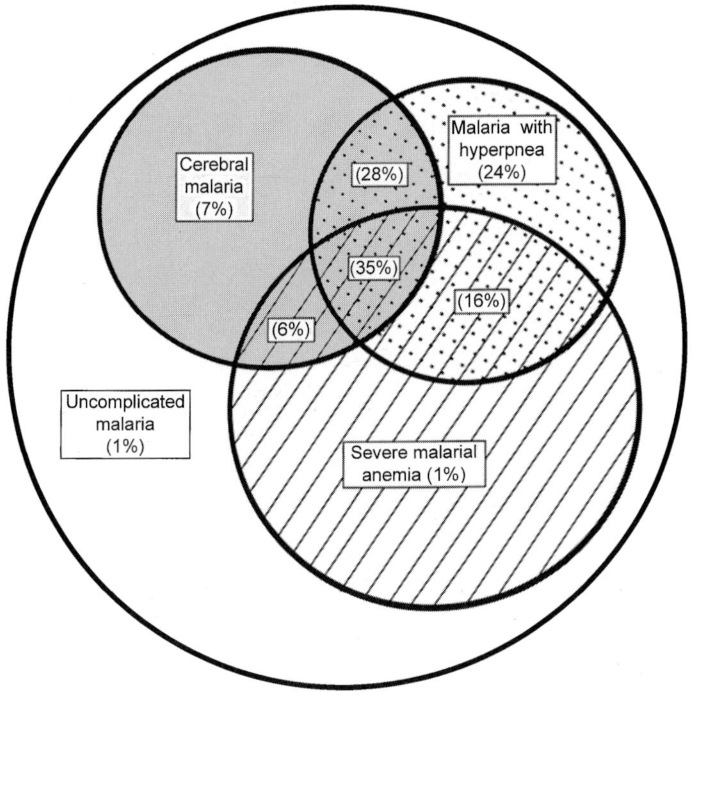

Figure 92–9. Mortality rates for major clinical syndromes of severe pediatric malaria. (Adapted by AY Cook from Marsh K, Forster D, Wairuiru C, et al: Indicators of life-threatening malaria in African children. N Engl J Med 332:1399, 1995.)

so impaired perfusion is unlikely to be a cause of the metabolic acidosis of malaria. This acidosis generally improves rapidly, once treatment with intravenous (IV) fluids and an effective antimalarial drug is started. The transient nature of the acidosis is consistent with the possibility that seizures are contributing factors. Convulsions are common in malaria, grand mal seizures alone can cause an acute lactic acidosis, and there is an association between seizures and acidosis in pediatric malaria patients. Acidosis persists longer in those patients who die and is also associated with a slower respiratory rate; this suggests that the usual centrally mediated respiratory response to metabolic acidosis is compromised in these patients.

Hyponatremia. Low serum sodium concentrations have been observed in a significant proportion of patients, both adults and children, with *P. falciparum* malaria. In children, hyponatremia seems to be associated with less dehydration and with appropriate concentrations of antidiuretic hormone (ADH). Up to 50% of adults may have inappropriately high concentrations of ADH. In these patients, enthusiastic rehydration has been counterproductive and caused respiratory complications.

HEMATOLOGIC CHANGES. Anemia, leukopenia and thrombocytopenia are common, and often prominent, features of acute malaria infections. PRBC are lysed as part of the malaria life cycle, but "innocent bystander" red cells are lysed also. There is a hidden mass of sequestered PRBC, and hematopoiesis is suppressed while there are circulating parasites, so the actual anemia that develops may be greater than anticipated on the basis of the initial peripheral parasitemia. Hematologic recovery, marked by an increase in the reticulocyte count, generally ensues within 7 to 10 days of complete parasite clearance. Until then, iron sequestration, erythrophagocytosis, and dyserythropoiesis occur. Maturation defects are usually present in the bone marrow, and the serum iron is reduced. Bone marrow cellularity and the myeloid:erythroid ratio are initially normal, but both usually fall during recovery in association with the reticulocytosis.

GASTROINTESTINAL CHANGES. PRBC sequester in the intestinal vasculature causing small bowel malabsorption (D-xylose, vitamin B_{12}, and various fats).

PULMONARY CHANGES. ARDS, noncardiogenic pulmonary edema, is a common feature of complicated malaria in adults, but only rarely develops in children. The specific cause of this syndrome in malaria patients has yet to be identified.

NEUROLOGIC CHANGES. In cases of fatal falciparum malaria, the brain is usually the most heavily parasitized organ; more venules contain sequestered PRBC, and there often is an increased density of sequestered cells in the brain compared with other organs. CNS dysfunction is the hallmark of cerebral malaria and symptoms can be focal (e.g., conjugate gaze deviation, focal convulsions) or generalized (e.g., coma, decerebrate or decorticate posturing). Many of the CNS symptoms are readily reversible; 90% of children who recover from cerebral malaria have no neurological sequel, and 90% of those with sequelae improve significantly within a month of their discharge from the hospital.

RENAL CHANGES. Mild renal abnormalities, including slightly elevated urea nitrogen and creatinine levels, proteinuria, and an abnormal urinary sediment, are common in malaria. Acute renal failure is a common complication of severe malaria, particularly in adults. As in cerebral malaria, the insult often resolves, and many patients do not require long-term dialysis.

■ PATHOLOGY

Death from malaria is almost always due to infection by *P. falciparum*. Vivax, ovale, and quartan malaria are seldom fa-

tal. The presence of malaria pigment (hemozoin) in many organs is often grossly visible; these organs appear dark gray or brown, and the pigment is evident in tissue sections. Most of the autopsies in fatal falciparum infections have been conducted on adults, a large proportion of whom have been nonimmune. The possibility that findings in the population most severely affected by this disease, African children, are different should be borne in mind.

CENTRAL NERVOUS SYSTEM. Brains of patients dying of cerebral malaria are often edematous, with broadened and flattened gyri. The cut surface may show congestion and petechiae in the white matter. Histologically, venules and capillaries are often full of PRBC (Fig. 92–10 [in color section]), and ring hemorrhages can be seen (Fig. 92–11). In older hemorrhages, midzonal necrosis is surrounded by proliferating glial cells (Durck granuloma). The degree of cerebral sequestration is generally higher in patients dying of cerebral malaria than in patients dying without CNS symptoms. In some cases, where parasite clearance has preceded death, there are only a few or no parasites at all detectable in brain tissue (Fig. 92–11).

BONE MARROW. During the acute infection, the bone marrow is often hyperemic, with PRBC and hemozoin in the reticuloendothelial cells. Many of the marrow sinusoids appear blocked by parasitized erythrocytes attached to endothelial cells. A normoblastic or megaloblastic hyperplasia occurs, even in the absence of reticulocytes in the peripheral blood.

SPLEEN. The spleen is often enlarged and tense, and the cut surface can be slate gray with prominent malpighian corpuscles. The blood vessels, Billroth cords, and sinusoids are commonly engorged with PRBC. There is reticuloendothelial hyperplasia, and the macrophages lining the sinusoids contain malaria pigment, parasitized and unparasitized red cells. Hemorrhages and infarcts may be present. The organ is often friable; rarely it ruptures, causing death.

LIVER. The liver is also often enlarged and slate gray. During the acute infection, Kupffer cells may increase in both number and size. They contain hemozoin, parasites, parasitized and unparasitized erythrocytes (Fig. 92–12). Lymphocytic infiltrations are common in the portal tracts.

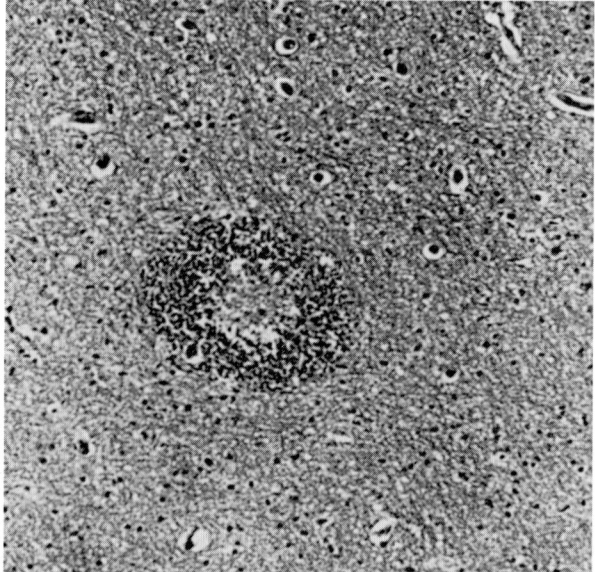

Figure 92–11. Acute falciparum malaria. Patient dying of cerebral malaria has ring hemorrhage surrounding obstructed arteriole (H& E stain, × 130.) (Courtesy of the Armed Forces Institute of Pathology, Photograph Neg. No. 66–2329.)

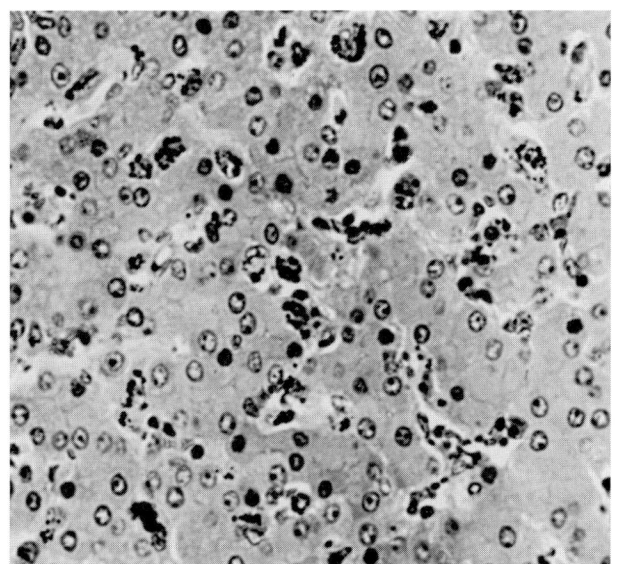

Figure 92–12. Acute falciparum malaria. Kupffer cells of liver contain grains of malaria pigment (darker spots). (H&E stain, × 395.) (Courtesy of the Armed Forces Institute of Pathology, Photograph Neg. No. 66–1426.)

KIDNEYS. The kidneys are usually slightly enlarged and congested. Punctate hemorrhages may be present in the pelvis, cortex, or medulla. Malaria pigment is in the glomeruli, and the capillaries often contain PRBC. Monocytes and lymphocytes may collect in the small vessels of the medulla (Fig. 92–13). The kidneys of patients dying of massive hemoglobinuria ("blackwater fever") are dark, enlarged, and edematous. The cut surface is pale and shows cortical swelling, hemorrhages, and medullar congestion. The striking microscopic change is tubular necrosis with hemoglobin casts and an interstitial lymphocytic infiltration.

LUNGS. The lungs are frequently congested and edema-tous, with PRBC within pulmonary capillaries. Mononuclear cells may be present in thickened alveolar walls. Alveolar septal edema in association with damaged capillary endothelia may be present. More severe changes include hyaline membrane formation and focal intra-alveolar hemorrhage (Fig. 92–14).

HEART. Cardiac changes are usually minimal. Capillaries may be congested and occluded with PRBC. Occasionally, edema and a mononuclear cell infiltrate of the interstitial tissues are present.

GASTROINTESTINAL TRACT. The intestinal mucosa may be edematous and congested; the small vessels often contain PRBC (Fig. 92–15).

PLACENTA. PRBC are commonly observed on the maternal side of the placenta, but are rarely present on the fetal side. In contrast with other tissues, in which mature stages are most commonly observed in tissue sections, all stages of the erythrocytic cycle of *P. falciparum* can be observed. Pigmented maternal monocytes are often present in the intervillous spaces. Inflammatory masses of pigmented red cells, free pigment, monocytes, and fibrin are also characteristic findings. Trophoblastic basement membranes are thickened, and cytotrophoblastic proliferation may be present.

■ IMMUNE RESPONSE

ACQUIRED IMMUNITY. This develops as a result of natural infections and can be sustained over time. Syphilitic patients treated with *P. vivax* (the resulting hyperpyrexia was thought to be detrimental to *T. pallidum*) developed strain-specific immunity. Individuals living in endemic areas develop an "antitoxic immunity" called *premunition*; although they continue to become infected with malaria, they no longer develop severe, life-threatening illnesses. Continued exposure to the bites of infected mosquitoes is necessary to sustain this immunity, however. This perpetual "boosting" is the entomologic and immunologic basis of the epidemiologic category of stable malaria. Immunization with irradiated spo-

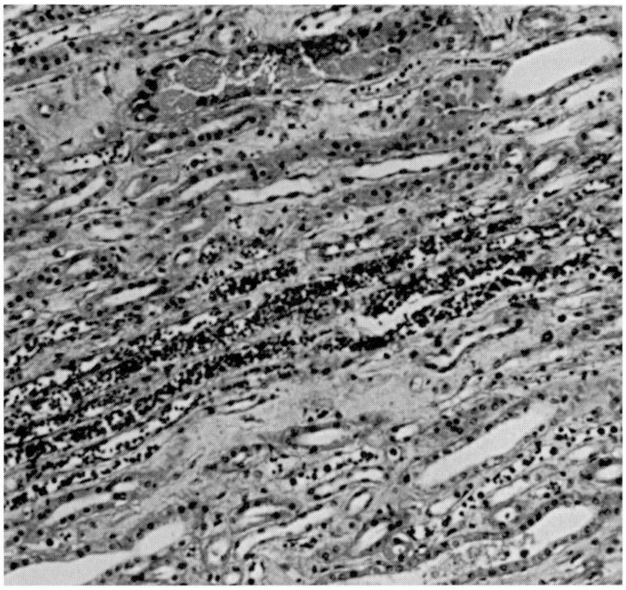

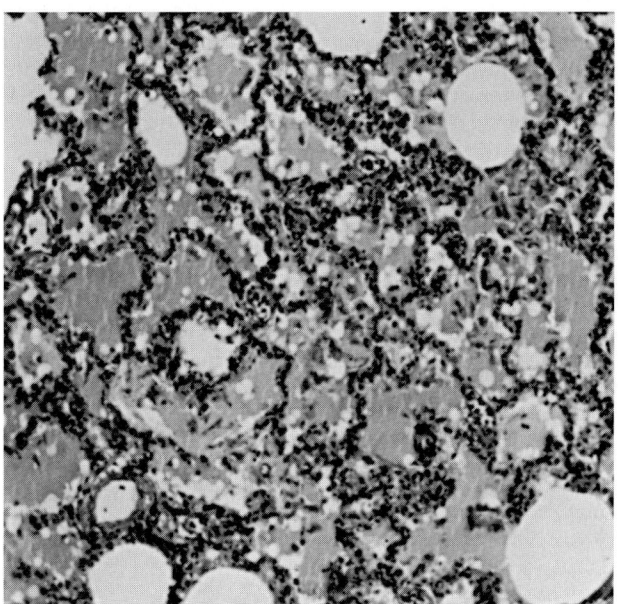

Figure 92–13. Acute falciparum malaria. Patient died with renal failure with acute tubular necrosis. Note the monocytic and lymphocytic collections in the medulla. (H&E stain, × 130.) (Courtesy of the Armed Forces Institute of Pathology, Photograph Neg. No. 67–2239.)

Figure 92–14. Acute falciparum malaria. Patient died with pulmonary edema with chronic inflammatory cells and parasitized erythrocytes in thickened aveolar walls. (H&E stain, × 95.) (Courtesy of the Armed Forces Institute of Pathology, Photograph Neg. No. 66–7186.)

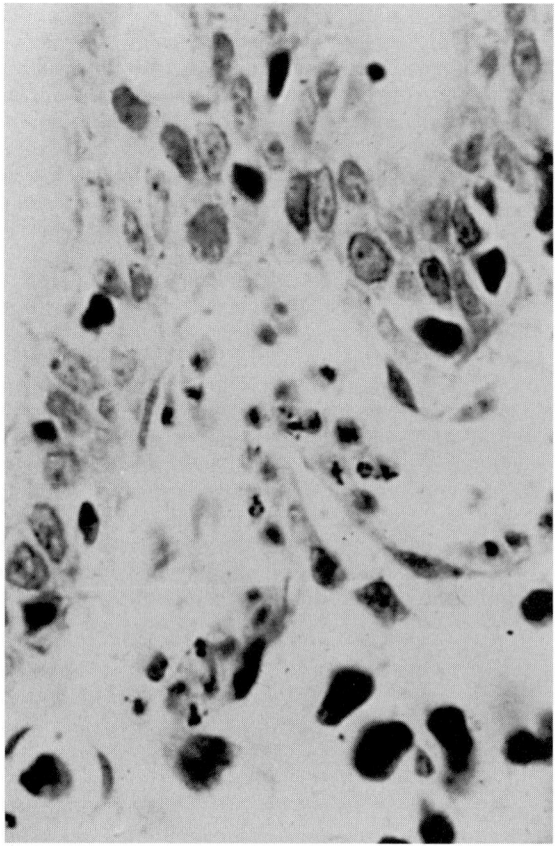

Figure 92–15. Acute falciparum malaria. Jejunal biopsy specimen demonstrating edema and capillaries packed with schizont-infected erythrocytes in the lamina propria. (Courtesy of Walter Karney.)

rozoites protects humans against challenge with viable sporozoites, thus demonstrating that stage-specific as well as strain-specific and antitoxic immunities can be elicited.

Describing the immunologic correlates of acquired immunity to malaria has proved to be very difficult; it is not possible to measure acquired immunity. Attempts to induce this in exposed populations with a vaccine have not succeeded, despite enormous efforts over many years. Both cell-mediated and humoral responses appear important in acquired immunity, but the relative contribution of each is not known. Except for very brief periods, the malaria parasite is an intracellular organism, and human red cells lack both MHC class I and class II molecules. The role of antibodies has been demonstrated in classic passive transfer experiments, in which immune serum from adults reduced or eliminated parasitemia in children with acute infections. Infants in endemic areas are protected from cerebral malaria (but not from severe anemia), presumably due to the passive transfer of antibodies from the mother.

Successful animal experiments in the 1970s and 1980s producing protective immunity with irradiated sporozoites have sustained studies of liver-stage antigens as potential vaccine targets. The technique of reverse immunogenetics was employed to discern the basis of the protective association between HLA-B53 and cerebral malaria; HLA-B53–restricted cytotoxic T cells recognize a conserved peptide from the exoerythrocytic, liver-stage parasite (LSA-1).

ANTIDISEASE IMMUNITY. Antitoxic immunity may be elicited by the parasite "toxin" which stimulates macrophages to produce cytokines. The toxin released by *P. falci-*

parum at the time of schizont rupture is likely to be a phospholipid. IgM antibody to this toxin, which blocks the induction of TNF in vitro, has been found in the serum of patients with malaria, although it disappeared 4 weeks after parasite clearance. This finding, supported by more detailed studies in mice, suggests that the toxin itself, or an epitope, might be a suitable immunologic target for preventing (or treating) severe malaria. An immunogen capable of inducing antibodies that could disrupt cytoadherence and sequestration might also have a significant antidisease effect.

VACCINE DEVELOPMENT. The in vitro cultivation of *P. falciparum* by Trager and Jensen in 1976 and advances in genetic engineering and monoclonal antibody technology have improved the potential for development of a malaria vaccine. Current research is directed at three developmental stages of the parasite—the sporozoite, the merozoite, and the gamete—and at elucidating the nature of "antidisease" immunity. A sporozoite vaccine is expected to prevent infection; less than 100% efficacy might be effective, particularly in an already partially immune population. Merozoite vaccines would prevent the invasion of red cells by merozoites, thereby reducing levels of parasitemia and ameliorating disease severity and duration. Antibodies to antigens found on the surface of *P. falciparum* gametes can completely block transmission by interfering with the development of the sexual stages of the parasite in the mosquito. Such a vaccine would not, on its own, confer advantage to the immunized individual; its effect would be to decrease transmission at the community or population level. "Antidisease" immunity could be elicited against a parasite-derived, disease-producing toxin or against a mediator further along the pathogenetic cascade.

The requirements of a malaria vaccine will vary with the target population. Multiple-component vaccines may be possible. One vaccine might, by reducing morbidity and mortality, work best in individuals chronically exposed to high levels of transmission, while others might be more useful in inducing short-term, high-level protection for travelers.

Pre-erythrocytic (Infection-Blocking) Vaccines. The success of irradiated sporozoite vaccines is the theoretical underpinning of this approach, but since it is not feasible to produce a vaccine by irradiating infected mosquitoes, research has concentrated on developing a subunit vaccine. An epitope of the major circumsporozoite antigen (Asn-Ala-Asn-Pro, or NANP) was chosen because it is highly conserved between geographic isolates, has a protective effect in animal models, and its demonstrated ability to inhibit the invasion of hepatocytes has an in vitro correlate, the circumsporozoite precipitation (CSP) reaction. Two major controlled trials of CSP have been conducted in human volunteers, one using (NANP)$_3$ linked to tetanus toxoid, the other using a fusion protein containing 32 NANP repeats fused to 32 amino acids of the tetracycline resistance protein of the expression plasmid. The results were sobering, in that only 1 of 15 and 1 of 34 volunteers, respectively, were fully protected. The latter version of the vaccine was also tested in Burkina Faso, and no differences in malaria incidence or disease severity were observed between vaccine recipients and controls. It may well be that other immune mechanisms (e.g., cytotoxic T cells) are involved, even though the immunogen is located on the sporozoite.

Blood Stage (Disease-Modifying) Vaccines. SPf66 is the first blood-stage vaccine to undergo extensive field trials. It consists of three merozoite-specific peptides (33 kDa, 55 kDa, and 83 kDa) hybridized into a 45-amino-acid peptide with a tetrapeptide sequence from the CS protein and then polymerized to form a synthetic vaccine. The only significant protective efficacy was demonstrated in Colombian patients; after three doses of the vaccine, there was a crude protective efficacy of 34% (95% confidence interval [CI], 19 to 46%) against a malaria episode (the association of clinical signs or symptoms possibly related to malaria, together with a microscopic identification of asexual forms of either *P. falciparum* or *P. vivax* in peripheral blood). Results of field trials of the same vaccine in sub-Saharan Africa were less compelling: among Tanzanian children aged 1 to 5 years, the estimated vaccine efficacy was 31% (95% CI, 0 to 52%), and in Gambian infants, the protective efficacy was 8% (95% CI, 18 to 29%). Another double-blinded clinical trial demonstrated that immunizing children living in northwestern Thailand with three doses of SPf66 provided no more protection, i.e., an SPf66 efficacy of −9% (95% CI, −33 to 14), against falciparum malaria than three doses of recombinant hepatitis B vaccine.

Sexual Stage (Transmission-Blocking) Vaccines. The major emphasis of the development of transmission-blocking vaccines is on eliciting a specific antibody response to transmission-blocking target antigens. Significant challenges to this process have been the relatively poor immunogenicity of naturally occurring gametocyte antigens and their inherent antigenic diversity and variation. Gamete (zygote/ookinete) target antigens are probably not expressed while in the human host, so the challenges posed by gametocyte antigens should not exist. Two postfertilization target antigens have been characterized, and one, Pfs25, is present in *P. falciparum*. Recombinant Pfs25 induces antibodies that can completely block transmission, and field studies of this vaccine candidate should begin soon.

Antidisease Vaccines. These vaccines are more theoretical than real, but as knowledge of malaria pathogenesis (e.g., cytoadherence, cytokine induction) becomes better understood, mechanisms to block the induction of pathology may emerge.

■ CLINICAL MANIFESTATIONS

GENERAL FINDINGS. Clinical signs and symptoms of malaria are associated with (1) schizont rupture and events emanating from that and (2) the inevitable destruction of parasitized and unparasitized red cells. Semi-immune patients are less likely to develop severe and complicated disease when they are infected.

PRODROMAL SYMPTOMS. Some patients have vague prodromal symptoms before parasitemia is at a level that can be detected by the usual microscopic techniques. These manifestations (malaise, myalgia, headache, anorexia, fever) may persist for 2 to 3 days before an acute paroxysm begins. The incubation period, or time from exposure to onset of symptoms, can be prolonged by partial immunity and/or by chemoprophylaxis.

PERIODICITY. In primary attacks, several days are required before the periodicity predicted by the lengths of various parasite life cycles is established. Often, in patients with "asynchronous" infections, this periodicity is never clinically apparent. After 5 to 7 days, *P. vivax*, *P. malariae*, and *P. ovale* infections can become synchronous and cause periodic febrile paroxysms (Figs. 92–16 and 145–2C). In vivax and falciparum malaria, schizonts mature and rupture with tertian periodicity, i.e., every 48 hours; vivax has been referred to as *benign tertian malaria* and falciparum as *malignant tertian malaria*. *P. malariae* schizonts rupture at 72-hour intervals, causing a quartan periodicity.

The typical paroxysm has an abrupt onset with a feeling of coldness and a chill. The patient's teeth may chatter prompting the need for warmth or cover. Within 30 to 60 minutes, the patient feels hot and has profuse sweating, usually accompanied by a headache, malaise, and myalgia. Nausea, vomiting, and cough may also add to the general misery. Temperatures of 40° to 41°C (104° to 106°F) are usual in primary falciparum infections, but peak fevers in infections with the other three species of plasmodia are usually lower, i.e., 39° to 40°C (102° to 104°F). The hot stage lasts from 2 to 6 hours. The sweating stage, in which the patient's temperature falls rapidly, lasts 2 to 3 hours. The entire paroxysm, which often begins in the early afternoon, averages 9 to 10 hours. In between paroxysms, the patient may feel well.

SYMPTOMS. Generalized constitutional symptoms include fever, chills, dizziness, backache, myalgia, malaise, and fatigue (frequently summarized as "total body pain" by endemic-area adults). Gastrointestinal symptoms (i.e., anorexia, nausea, vomiting, abdominal pain, and diarrhea) can be prominent, causing confusion with gastroenteritis. Patients may have nonproductive cough and dyspnea, consistent with acute respiratory infections. Young children and semi-immune adults may present with only fever and headache.

SIGNS. Physical examination usually reveals a fever, tachycardia, and warm, flushed skin. The spleen is often palpable,

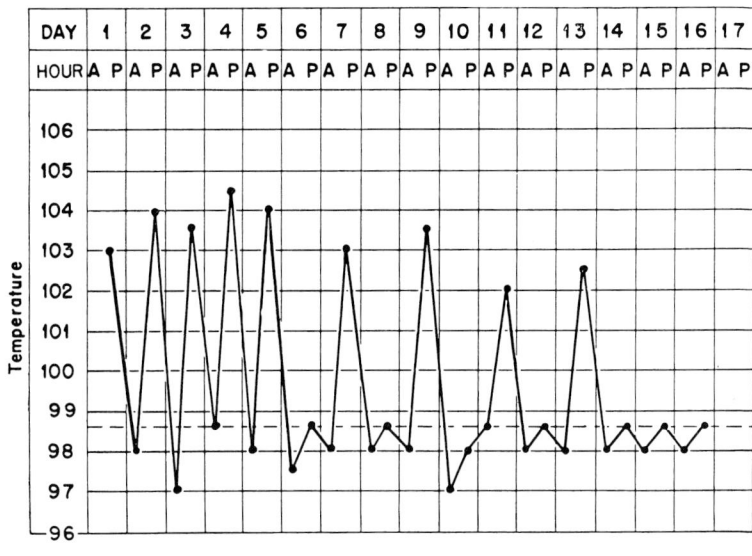

Figure 92–16. Fever chart in a *P. vivax* infection showing an initial quotidian tendency becoming tertian. No specific therapy. (A = A.M.; P = P.M.) (From Russell, West, Manwell, et al: Practical Malariology, 2nd ed. London, Oxford University Press, 1963.)

usually soft, and occasionally tender. The liver is frequently enlarged and sometimes tender. Orthostatic hypotension may occur. Mental confusion, tachypnea, and jaundice are not unusual. Some patients have recurrent herpes simplex infections ("fever blisters").

LABORATORY FINDINGS. Anemia, leukopenia, and thrombocytopenia are usual. The reticulocyte count is normal or depressed, despite the hemolysis, and becomes elevated only after the parasitemia has cleared. Urinalysis reveals albuminuria and urobilinogen; increased conjugated bilirubin is present in many patients.

Abnormalities in liver function tests may cause diagnostic confusion with viral hepatitis. Serum transaminases, e.g., alanine aminotransferase (ALT) and aspartate transaminase (AST), are usually elevated. Both the direct and the indirect bilirubin can be elevated. Prothrombin times can be prolonged. Serum albumin is frequently depressed, and globulins, particularly in repeat infections, can be elevated. There is a polyclonal increase in immunoglobulins, both IgM (in acute attacks) and IgG. This is associated with a rapid appearance of specific antimalarial antibodies and reduced complement levels. False positive serologic tests for syphilis (VDRL), rheumatoid factor, heterophil agglutinins, and cold agglutinins may be present.

Hyponatremia is not uncommon; in some patients, the clinical picture is consistent with inappropriate secretion of ADH, but this is not a universal finding. Increases in serum creatinine and blood urea nitrogen may be transient, or they may presage acute renal failure. Hypoglycemia frequently complicates falciparum malaria and can occur both before treatment and as a result of quinine therapy.

VIVAX AND OVALE MALARIA. Clinically, infections with these two species are very similar. Both can be found alone or in conjunction with *P. falciparum* infections. In nonimmune individuals, the incubation period is usually 12 to 18 days, but occasionally, with certain strains, it can be much longer, i.e., 6 to 18 months. Relapses are common within 6 months, unless specific treatment to eradicate hypnozoites is given. Parasitemia rates are usually lower than in falciparum malaria. Fatalities are rare, but deaths have been reported occasionally following rupture of an enlarged spleen, either spontaneously or after trauma.

In the initial phase of illness, the fever can be erratic or continuous. If the infection continues for 5 to 7 days, a synchronous cycle may develop with temperature elevations approximately every 48 hours, the classic benign tertian periodicity (Figs. 92–16 and 145–2C). The fever can be as high as 40°C (104°F), and the patient often feels worse than a patient with uncomplicated falciparum malaria. Physical findings usually include an enlarged, tender spleen by the second week of infection and a palpable liver. Anemia is common in chronic infections.

QUARTAN MALARIA. *P. malariae* malaria is the mildest and most chronic of all the human malaria infections. Older erythrocytes are favored for invasion, so parasitemias are lower, anemia is less pronounced, and diagnosis may be difficult. However, *P. malariae* can cause relatively severe acute illness and may be associated with persistent ill health with recurrent attacks of fever, malaise, headaches, fatigue, and sweating. The incubation period can be as short as 18 days, but is often many weeks. Recrudescences can occur even after 30 to 50 years, sometimes associated with some stressful situation, e.g., a surgical procedure, and the infection has been transmitted by blood transfusion from donors with subpatent infections. The patient may have several febrile paroxysms before parasites are seen in the peripheral blood. As in vivax and ovale malaria, the paroxysms commonly occur during the day, usually in the afternoon, but in quartan malaria, as the name implies, they are classically separated by intervals of 72 hours. Splenomegaly is common.

FALCIPARUM MALARIA. *P. falciparum* causes the most severe form of malaria infection. It can kill up to 25% of nonimmune adults within 2 weeks of a primary attack unless appropriate treatment is given. The initial attack often follows mild prodromal symptoms. The incubation period is usually 10 to 14 days, but may be longer. The fever is irregular at first, but usually occurs daily. Paroxysms are also irregular, and the fever spikes are often dramatically high (39° to 40°C or 102° to 104°F). Multisystem organ involvement is more common in falciparum malaria than in the other human malarias and can present as confusion, drowsiness, cough, dyspnea, vomiting, and diarrhea.

Physical examination often reveals hepatosplenomegaly and pallor. Some patients have basilar pulmonary rales. The pulse may be rapid (100 to 120 beats/min) and in adults, the blood pressure may be low (e.g., 90 to 100 mmHg, systolic). Orthostatic changes are also common in adults. The patient may complain of lightheadedness. Abdominal tenderness, especially in the right and left upper quadrants, is frequently present. Jaundice is associated with hyperparasitemia. Semi-immune patients have milder, sometimes asymptomatic infections.

MIXED INFECTIONS. Mixed infections, usually with *P. falciparum* and another species, are common in certain endemic areas. Management should focus on the parasite posing the most severe threat; treatment to prevent relapses from the persistent hepatic forms of *P. vivax* and *P. ovale* must also be given.

MALARIA IN CHILDREN. In nonimmune children, falciparum infections embrace the entire spectrum from uncomplicated disease (characterized by fever, headache, nausea) to life-threatening infections (most commonly cerebral malaria, acidosis, and/or severe anemia). Only a small proportion of children develop life-threatening disease and the determinants of these susceptibilities are not known. The age peak for severe malarial anemia is generally <2 years of age in holo- and hyperendemic areas; cerebral malaria afflicts older children (mean age 3.5 years) in these areas.

MALARIA IN PREGNANCY

Malaria in the Mother. Recrudescences and relapses of malaria are frequent during the second half of pregnancy, probably because of the immunosuppression associated with pregnancy; as with acquired immunity, the immunologic correlates of this immunosuppression have not yet been described. Malaria can potentiate the expected anemia of pregnancy. Acute renal insufficiency and hypoglycemia can complicate falciparum malaria in pregnant women.

Low birth weight has been associated with placental malaria infections, particularly in primigravidae living in endemic areas. In communities at risk for epidemic malaria, epidemics can be an important cause of abortions, miscarriages, stillbirths, and neonatal deaths.

Congenital Malaria. Congenital malaria can occur with all four species causing human infections. The incubation period is between 2 and 8 weeks. Symptomatic congenital malaria is rare in areas with stable malaria, presumably because of the transplacental transfer of protective antimalarial IgG antibodies. The signs and symptoms can be subtle; the classic malaria paroxysm of chills, fever, and sweats is absent, although fever is usual. The infant feeds poorly and is restless and drowsy. Hepatomegaly, splenomegaly, and anemia are common; anorexia and lethargy are prominent symptoms. Because there are no exoerythrocytic stages in congenital *P. vivax* and *P. ovale* infections, radical cure with primaquine is not necessary.

TRANSFUSION MALARIA. Any of the four species of hu-

TABLE 92–2. Indicators of Severe and Complicated Malaria

Cerebral malaria: Unrousable coma not attributable to other cause in a patient with falciparum malaria. Coma should persist for at least 30 minutes after a generalized convulsion.

Severe anemia: Hematocrit < 15% or hemoglobin < 5 g/dL in the presence of parasitemia > 10,000/μL.

Renal failure: Urine output < 400 mL/24 hr in adults, or 12 mL/kg/24 hr in children, and a serum creatinine > 3.0 mg/dL.

Pulmonary edema or adult respiratory distress syndrome.

Hypoglycemia: Whole blood glucose concentration < 2.2 mmol/L, or 40 mg/dL.

Circulatory collapse, or shock: Systolic blood pressure < 50 mmHg in children aged 1–5 years, or < 70 mmHg in patients >5 years of age, with cold clammy skin or a core skin temperature difference >10°C.

Spontaneous bleeding from gums, nose, gastrointestinal tract, or laboratory evidence of DIC.

Repeated generalized convulsions: More than two observed within 24 hr.

Acidemia: Arterial pH < 7.25, or acidosis defined as a plasma bicarbonate <15 mmol/L.

Macroscopic hemoglobinuria: Unrelated to hemolysis secondary to G6PD deficiency.

Other manifestations that do not define "severe and complicated malaria" but which are features of severe disease include:
    Any impairment of consciousness
    Prostration (inability to sit or walk)
    Hyperparasitemia (>2% in nonimmune persons; >10% in others)
    Jaundice (evident clinically, or serum bilirubin >3.0 mg/dL)
    Hyperpyrexia (rectal temperature >40°C)

DIC, disseminated intravascular coagulation; G6PD, glucose-6-phosphate dehydrogenase.

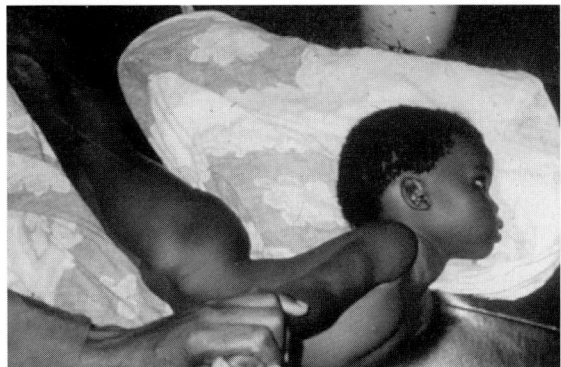

Figure 92–17. Malawian child with opisthotonos due to cerebral malaria. (Photograph by T. Taylor.)

man malaria can be transmitted directly from a blood donor, from accidental infection by a contaminated needle, or from drug users sharing needles. The incubation period following the injection is as short as a few days for *P. falciparum,* but can be up to 40 days or longer for *P. malariae.* As in congenital malaria, radical cure to prevent relapses is not necessary.

■ COMPLICATIONS

Most life-threatening complications occur in nonimmune patients with falciparum malaria infections and involve the CNS (cerebral malaria), the pulmonary system (respiratory failure secondary to ARDS), the renal system (acute renal failure), and/or the hematopoietic system (severe anemia) (Table 92–2). Metabolic acidosis and hypoglycemia are the most common systemic complications. As any of these can develop rapidly, it is prudent to treat falciparum infections in nonimmune persons as a potential medical emergency and ensure frequent observations are made, focusing on the organ systems at highest risk.

CEREBRAL MALARIA. Generally defined as altered consciousness in a patient with *P. falciparum* parasitemia and no other obvious cause of altered consciousness, cerebral malaria is a common complication. In research settings, a score of 2 or less on the Blantyre Coma Scale (for children) (Table 92–3) or 8 or less on the Glasgow Coma Scale (for adults) is added to the definition for external standardization purposes. In patients meeting the definition of cerebral malaria, mortality rates are typically between 15 to 25% (Fig. 92–9); most survivors recover completely, but 10% are discharged with neurologic sequelae. Cerebral malaria is by far the most common complication of falciparum infection in children; multiorgan system involvement characterizes severe and complicated adult disease.

The neurologic findings are highly variable. Patients may be deeply comatose (unresponsive to painful stimuli). They exhibit a variety of postures (opisthotonos, decerebrate rigidity, decorticate rigidity) (Fig. 92–17), respiratory patterns (acidotic breathing, Cheyne-Stokes respirations), and focal findings (conjugate gaze deviation, nystagmus). Convulsions (focal and generalized) are very common, particularly in children. Intracranial pressure is often elevated in children with cerebral malaria and deaths consistent with various herniation syndromes have been described, but no significant associations between intracranial pressure and outcome or response to specific treatment with mannitol have been observed.

Among patients who survive, the recovery is relatively rapid; most children who survive an episode of cerebral malaria have regained full consciousness within 48 hours. The rapid evolution and reversibility of the dramatic neurologic features of cerebral malaria are among the most intriguing aspects of the disease.

HYPOGLYCEMIA. The presence of pretreatment hypoglycemia is a poor prognostic feature; children with cerebral malaria who are hypoglycemic (blood glucose ≤2.2 mmol/L or

TABLE 92–3. Blantyre Coma Scale for Assessing Level of Consciousness in Children with Malaria

Best Motor Response*	Score	Best Verbal Response*	Score	Eye Movements	Score
Localizes	2	Normal cry, or speaks	2	Follows, watches	1
Withdraws	1	Weak, abnormal cry	1	Does not follow	0
Extends, or nil	0	Nil	0		
Sum findings from all three categories. A total score of 5 is "fully conscious," a sum of 0 is "completely unresponsive."					

*To painful stimuli, e.g., pressure on a nail bed, on the sternum, or on a supraorbital ridge.

40 mg/dL) are significantly more likely to die or to recover with neurologic sequelae. Hypoglycemia can result from rapid infusions of IV quinine, a potent insulin secretagogue, or from prolonged treatment with quinine. The relative insulin resistance of acute malaria subsides within 3 to 4 days, rendering patients on sustained quinine treatment vulnerable to this complication. Prompt recognition and treatment with intravenous 50% dextrose will usually restore the blood glucose concentration, but may not have an effect on the level of consciousness.

METABOLIC ACIDOSIS. Capillary blood pH <7.3 or plasma lactate concentrations >5 mmol/L are both strongly associated with severe disease and with poor outcomes. Acidosis, manifested as abnormally deep breathing or documented chest recession, has recently been recognized as a poor prognostic feature in parasitemic children with no neurologic compromise, in addition to those who also have cerebral malaria (Fig. 92–9). Whether specific interventions targeted at acid-base status would prove useful in reducing mortality is currently under investigation.

SEVERE ANEMIA. Life-threatening anemia can develop rapidly; children who have adjusted to a low hemoglobin or hematocrit can rapidly decompensate when challenged by a febrile illness such as malaria (Fig. 92–9). Decisions regarding blood transfusion are difficult, particularly in malaria-endemic areas where human immunodeficiency virus (HIV) infection is common. Children with severe anemia and respiratory distress will need transfusions which may be lifesaving. However, less severely anemic children who are clinically stable may be treated conservatively with transfusion reserved for those who develop signs of clinical deterioration. Malaria prophylaxis is useful to prevent early reinfection. Recent studies have shown that iron supplementation for infants living in malaria-endemic areas protects them against severe anemia. This complication usually affects younger children (<3 years old) than those who generally have cerebral malaria (3 to 6 years old), but the actual peak ages vary with the exposure to infection.

RESPIRATORY FAILURE. Respiratory failure associated with ARDS is much more commonly a complication of falciparum malaria in adults than in children. This complication can develop rapidly; clinically it is indistinguishable from the ARDS that develops as a result of septicemia, toxic inhalants, or other causes. Patients become hypoxemic and may require mechanically assisted ventilation. There are few studies describing the response to this aggressive treatment in malaria patients, but when it is available, it should be used, because patients do make impressive recoveries.

ALGID MALARIA. The majority of patients with severe malaria remain well perfused, but a small proportion develop algid malaria: their blood pressure is low, extremities are cold and clammy, and hypoglycemia and acidosis are common. In some cases, this represents septic shock, and pathogens are cultured from the blood. The judicious administration of fluids and inotropes is recommended for this small group of patients.

ACUTE RENAL FAILURE. Mild proteinura, azotemia, and oliguria occur frequently in otherwise uncomplicated *P. falciparum* infections. Acute renal failure is another complication that is far more common among adults than among children; it is also more common in patients with hemoglobinuria ("blackwater fever"). Acute renal failure can also result from acute tubular necrosis, a sequelae of reduced renal perfusion. Anuria is a poor prognostic sign, and renal or peritoneal dialysis are often necessary, if they are available. Few data exist to describe the proportion of patients on dialysis who recover renal function, but as in cerebral malaria, many of these abnormalities are reversible and patients supported through the crucial period often enjoy full recoveries.

POSTMALARIA NEUROLOGIC SYNDROME. This is a rare transient neurologic syndrome occurring within 2 months after acute severe falciparum malaria. It is self-limiting with a median duration of 60 hours. The most common manifestations are an acute confusional state or psychosis and generalized convulsions. Although some patients have been febrile during the episode, none were parasitemic. Mefloquine given following treatment for the acute malaria is a risk factor for the syndrome but is not the only one.

■ DIAGNOSIS

The diagnosis of malaria infection is more straightforward than the diagnosis of malaria illness. Because semi-immune individuals can sustain asymptomatic parasitemias, a proportion of semi-immune individuals with incidental parasitemias will have symptoms that are unrelated to the parasites within their blood cells. Without exhaustive, expensive testing to exclude other common etiologies of fever, headache, myalgia and malaise, it is difficult to ascertain the precise relationship between symptoms and parasitemia in semi-immune patients in endemic areas. Furthermore, because *P. falciparum* is absent from the peripheral blood for a portion of its life cycle, and because symptomatic parasitemias are sometimes below the limits of microscopic detection, it is possible for individuals to be aparasitemic and to have a malaria illness. Thus, the limits of the parasitologic diagnosis of malaria should be appreciated: a single negative blood film may not exclude the diagnosis of a malaria illness, and a positive blood film may not necessarily prove the diagnosis.

BLOOD FILMS. The gold standard of malaria diagnosis remains the blood film, even with the caveats noted above. For detecting parasites, a thick blood film is superior, because it concentrates the red cells by a factor of 20 to 40 (Figs. 92–4C and D [in color section]). Identifying species on thick films may be difficult because the red cells have lysed, and the morphologic features of the parasites have been altered. Species identifications are made more easily using thin blood films (Figs. 92–4E–I and 92–5 [in color section]). Thick and thin films can be prepared on the same slide, although they are processed differently (thin films must be fixed in methanol before they are stained). Symptoms may precede detectable parasitemia by 1 to 2 days, and timing blood films with respect to fever spikes is less important than repeating several films daily in order to make a diagnosis. Quantitating parasitemias is useful prognostically, for predicting whether the illness is caused by malaria and the need for blood transfusion and for following response to antimalarial treatment; parasites can be counted as a percentage of red cells on a thin film, or against white blood cells on a thick film, and if the total red cell or white cell counts are known, the parasite densities can be calculated. Blood can be stained with Giemsa, Leishman, Field, or Wright's stains (Chapter 151).

The most important initial distinction is to determine whether malaria parasites are present. Species identification is more difficult and may require an expert opinion. *P. falciparum* parasites can be recognized by the presence of mostly small ring forms (Fig. 92–4C and H and 92–5 [in color section]), their banana-shaped gametocytes (Fig. 92–4I and 92–5 [in color section]), the greater probability of parasitemias exceeding 2% of red cells, and for multiple-infected red cells (Fig. 92–4H [in color section]), and the absence of schizonts (Fig. 92–4C [in color section] and Table 92–4).

TABLE 92–4. Differential Characteristics of Human Malarial Parasites in Stained Thin Blood Films

Characteristics	P. falciparum	P. vivax	P. ovale	P. malariae
Infected erythrocyte enlarged	−	+	±	−
Infected erythrocyte fimbriated* and/or oval	rare	rare	frequent	rare
Infected erythrocyte decolorized	−	+	+	−
Infected erythrocyte with Schüffner dots*	−	+	+	−
Infected erythrocyte with Maurer dots*	+	−	−	−
Multiple parasites in a single erythrocyte*	+	rare	−	−
Parasite, all forms in peripheral blood	−	+	+	+
Parasite, large coarse rings	−	+	+	+
Parasite, double chromatin dots*	+	rare	−	−
Parasite, accolé forms*	+	rare	−	−
Parasite, band forms*	−	−	−	+
Parasite, sausage-shaped gametocytes	+	−	−	−
Number of merozoites in erythrocytic schizont	8–24	12–24	8–12	6–12

*Not invariable but suggestive when seen.

Malaria pigment (hemozoin) in monocytes or leukocytes suggests a current or recent malaria infection, even in the absence of a patent parasitemia. Parasites may also be demonstrated in a bone marrow specimen, but this is rarely required.

DIAGNOSTIC ALTERNATIVES. Blood films are not readily affordable for routine diagnostic purposes in clinics and laboratories in many endemic areas, and they require an expertise which is often lacking in many developed country laboratories. Alternative diagnostic methods have been developed to cope with these deficiencies. However, these techniques are still too costly for general use in malaria-endemic areas.

Antigen Detection Techniques. A dipstick antigen-capture assay has been developed, based on qualitative detection of *P. falciparum* histidine-rich protein 2 (PfHPR-2) in peripheral blood for the diagnosis of *P. falciparum* infection. The technique is feasible in the field and sensitivities and specificities range between 75 and 95% in various settings. A microscope is not required, and the assay becomes negative within a week of effective antimalarial treatment. Similar assays are not available for detecting the other three species of plasmodia although a *P. vivax* dipstick is being evaluated.

Fluorescent Staining of Parasite Nuclei. When blood is collected in microhematocrit tubes coated with acridine orange, the nuclei of any malaria parasites present will be stained and are easily visualized by fluorescence microscopy. The technique is rapid, and is substantially faster than a blood film when the parasitemia is low. False positive results are rare, and this technique can detect parasites at concentrations below the threshold of routine microscopic detection. A centrifuge is required, along with capillary tubes coated with acridine orange, and a 60× oil-immersion objective capable of transmitting ultraviolet light, or a lens system with a fiberoptic cable.

Another approach involves direct staining of thin blood films with acridine orange, followed by fluorescence microscopy using a standard microscope fitted with interference filters. Screening these films requires less time at the microscope than is required to interpret either standard thin films or the microhematocrit method. The concordance between this technique and a standard thin film is 100% for parasitemias >1%; at parasitemias <1%, the sensitivities of the microhematocrit fluorescence and the direct fluorescent staining drop significantly, but the direct approach is the superior technique. Neither of the fluorescent techniques contributes to species diagnoses.

Polymerase Chain Reaction (PCR)–Based Assays. Fingerprick (capillary) blood samples, spotted onto filter paper, provide sufficient genetic material for PCR-based assays. Spe-cies-specific probes can be used; the technique is highly sensitive and specific, and although the samples are easily collected and stored, sophisticated laboratory support is required for their analysis. This approach offers significant advantages when large numbers of samples are involved and can be batched. It is less useful for individual patient diagnoses, requires very careful laboratory technique to prevent sample and reagent contamination which can give false positive results, and is expensive.

MALARIAL ANTIBODY TESTS. Although having limited usefulness in endemic areas since the presence of specific malarial antibodies in the blood cannot separate current infection from past exposure, there are a few situations in which antibody testing may be helpful (Chapter 152). Antibody testing has provided useful epidemiologic information on community-wide exposures to malaria, particularly in areas with low levels of transmission, for evaluating the effectiveness of control programs. On rare occasions, malaria antibody testing helps in diagnosing an individual patient. A negative malaria antibody test helps to rule out malaria in an individual having possible exposure to infectious vectors, whereas a positive test supports the diagnosis of malaria in someone with a potential exposure, e.g., visit to a malaria endemic country.

DIFFERENTIAL DIAGNOSIS. The clinical diagnosis of malaria is difficult. Early symptoms may mimic influenza, acute upper respiratory tract infections, and gastroenteritis. Malaria may be confused with other febrile illnesses, including visceral leishmaniasis, hepatitis, amebic liver abscess, relapsing fever, yellow fever, typhoid fever, tuberculosis, brucellosis, endocarditis, pyelonephritis, trypanosomiasis, blood disorders, poliomyelitis, dengue, and the prerash stage of other viral infections. In endemic areas, clinical judgment is often required to distinguish between infection and disease.

PROGNOSIS. Prognosis is excellent for complete recovery from primary attacks of *P. vivax*, *P. ovale* and *P. malariae*. Falciparum malaria carries a good prognosis if diagnosed rapidly and treated appropriately, although mortality may still occur. If *P. falciparum* infections are untreated, or if appropriate management is delayed, mortality can be high. The prognosis of individual patients with *P. falciparum* infections is related to the density of parasitemia and the presence of various clinical features that have been shown to be associated with a poor outcome (Table 92–2, Fig. 92–9).

◼ SYNDROMES ASSOCIATED WITH CHRONIC MALARIA

Repeated attacks of malaria can contribute to a chronic state of ill health in endemic areas; the effects of malaria infection on cognitive development have not been investigated. Recent studies in which parasitemia was assessed by PCR suggest the extent of malaria infections may have been severely underestimated in the past. If so, our understanding of the contributions of chronic malaria infections to ill health may need to be revised.

HYPERACTIVE MALARIAL SPLENOMEGALY

Definition and Etiology. Hyperreactive malarial splenomegaly (HMS), formerly called tropical splenomegaly syndrome (TSS), is an immunologic disorder related to chronic malaria. The diagnosis is based on the presence of massive splenomegaly (Fig. 92–18), high circulating titers of malaria antibodies, elevated IgM concentrations, lymphocytic infiltration of the hepatic sinusoids (Fig. 92–19), hematologic findings of hypersplenism, and the exclusion of other diagnostic possibilities. The pathogenesis is unknown but appears to involve genetic susceptibility and chronic exposure to malaria.

Distribution and Incidence. Although HMS may be widespread in the tropics, most investigations of idiopathic splenomegaly have been carried out in Uganda, Zambia, Nigeria and New Guinea. In these studies, the reported incidence of HMS varied from 0.5 to 80% of the adult population. There is a close geographic association between HMS and malaria endemicity, although genetic and tribal factors within a given area affect the incidence.

Immunologic Findings. Patients with HMS have a polyclonal macroglobulinemia, circulating immune complexes, and autoantibodies, including isohemagglutinins, rheumatoid factor, antinuclear factor, cold agglutininins, and cryoprotein. High-titer IgM antimalaria antibodies are present, and a correlation between IgM levels and spleen size has been described. IgM levels fall promptly following splenectomy or more gradually following malaria chemoprophylaxis. Patients with HMS do not have defects in cell-mediated immunity. However, antibody response following certain immunizations, e.g., *Salmonella adelaide* flagellin or monovalent influenza vaccine, is depressed.

Pathogenesis and Pathology. In areas where HMS occurs, splenomegaly fails to regress in a proportion of children as immunity to malaria develops. Hypertrophy of the reticuloendothelial elements in the liver and spleen progresses with exposure to malaria. It has been hypothesized that HMS is the result of chronic stimulation of the splenic and hepatic reticuloendothelial system by circulating antigen-antibody complexes that are triggered by a nonspecific mitogen from the malaria parasite. Both a complement-fixing lymphocytotoxin in the sera and a reduction in the number of suppressor T lymphocytes in the blood have been described in patients with HMS. Immunoglobulin gene arrangements have been demonstrated in some patients with HMS, suggesting that HMS may be a premalignant condition.

On microscopic section, the spleen has normal architecture, with dilated sinusoids containing erythrocytes and lymphocytes. Large macrophages ingesting erythrocytes and granulocytes are in abundance. Malaria parasites and pigment are absent. There is lymphocytic infiltration of the hepatic sinusoids (Fig. 92–19). Kupffer cells are hyperplastic and hypertrophied.

Clinical Manifestations. Most patients have huge spleens (to the level of the umbilicus or below) and complain of a dragging left-sided abdominal pain (Fig. 92–18). Anemia with an increased reticulocyte count is universal. Thrombocytopenia is usual, but patients seldom have a tendency to bleed. The liver is also enlarged and smooth. There may be an increased susceptibility to bacterial infections, but other clinical complications are unusual. Neutropenia may be present. Occasionally, life-threatening episodes of hemolytic ane-

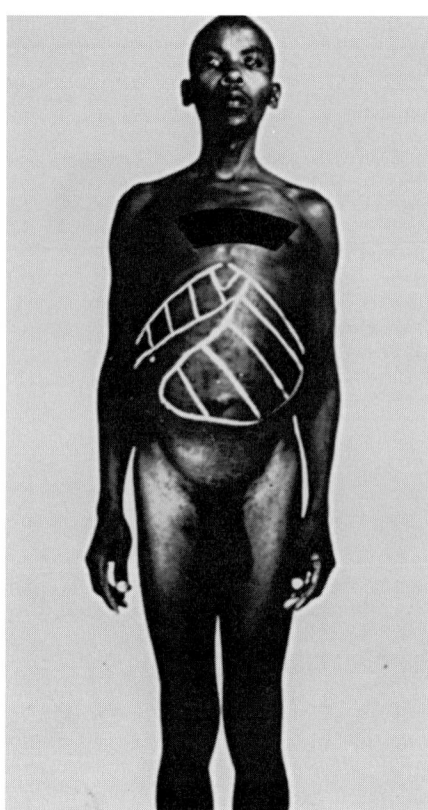

Figure 92–18. Ugandan patient with hyperreactive malarial syndrome with a very large spleen and liver. (Courtesy of Dr. Patrick Hamilton.)

mia occur in HMS, particularly in pregnant or lactating women. The bone marrow shows hypercellularity with hyperplasia of both the erythroid and the myeloid series. Splenic sequestration of erythrocytes as well as a greatly expanded plasma volume has been demonstrated.

Treatment and Prognosis. Chronic (lifelong) antimalarial prophylaxis is the treatment of choice for HMS; splenectomy is no longer recommended. Long-term follow-up of patients treated with splenectomy demonstrates a compensatory hepatomegaly and an increased susceptibility to severe infections, including malaria itself. Following appropriate treatment, hepatosplenomegaly and elevated IgM concentrations regress.

NEPHROTIC SYNDROME (Chapter 7)

Definition and Etiology. The high incidence of nephrotic syndrome (NS) occurring in some tropical areas has been attributed to quartan malaria. NS is more common in areas where malaria is endemic, and patients with NS have increased infection rates with *P. malariae*. Induced infections with *P. malariae* in humans and monkeys have produced NS.

Distribution and Incidence. Detailed studies have described NS associated with quartan malaria in Uganda, Nigeria, Ivory Coast, Senegal, and Papua New Guinea. In the past, the association was reported in Southeast Asia, India, and Guyana. The entity has since disappeared in areas where *P. malariae* was eradicated (e.g., Guyana).

Pathology and Pathogenesis. Pathologic lesions are variable. A common lesion in children consists of localized or diffuse thickening in the capillary wall of the glomerular tuft, with periodic acid–Schiff (PAS)-positive material, segmented sclerosis of peripheral capillary loops, and increased mesangial cells (Fig. 7–2). Progression to total glomerular sclerosis

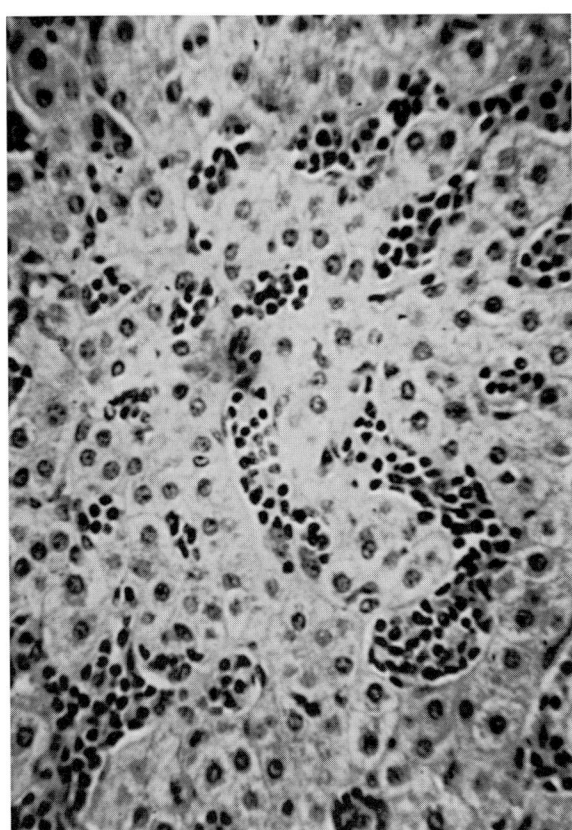

Figure 92–19. Hyperreactive malarial syndrome. Hypertrophy of Kupffer cells and increased chronic inflammatory cells in the hepatic sinusoids. (H&E stain.) (Courtesy of Dr. Michael Hutt.)

and secondary tubular atrophy may occur. A proliferative glomerulonephritis has been described in adults. Immunofluorescence studies of biopsy specimens taken early during the disease demonstrate granular deposits of IgG and IgM in virtually all glomeruli, C3 component of complement in two thirds of the glomeruli, and *P. malariae* antigens in one fourth. Specific *P. malariae* antibodies were confirmed in most samples. Biopsy specimens taken >3 months after the onset of renal symptoms usually still had antibodies and complement but not *P. malariae* antigens. The depositions vary from a coarse to a fine granular pattern. The coarse granular pattern correlates with the presence of electron-dense material localized within the glomerular basement membrane (Fig. 7–3).

Clinical Manifestations. Approximately half of those with quartan malaria NS have their first symptoms before the age of 15. The classic findings of NS, including persistent heavy proteinuria, hypoalbuminemia, edema and ascites, are usually present (Fig. 7–1). Hypertension, azotemia, and hematuria are rare in children, although the first two are not uncommon in adults. Most patients have poorly selective proteinuria. Blood smears in children, but not adults, are likely to demonstrate *P. malariae*. The most common clinical course includes transient remissions, persistent symptomless proteinuria, and slowly progressive deterioration of renal function and hypertension, with renal failure developing within 3 to 5 years.

Treatment and Prognosis. Patients with quartan malaria NS do not respond to malarial chemotherapy. The response to corticosteroids, cyclophosphamide, and azathioprine is variable. Remission of abnormalities with treatment occurs almost exclusively in those with only mild proliferative changes on the initial renal biopsy.

BURKITT'S LYMPHOMA. Endemic cases of Burkitt lymphoma, a B-cell lymphoma, are geographically associated with Epstein-Barr virus (EBV) infections (Chapters 12 and 24). There is also a strong epidemiologic association between EBV infections and malaria; both are widespread in the tropics, particularly at lower altitudes. The progression of EBV infections is generally controlled by virus-specific cytotoxic T cells. The concentration of these T cells is significantly reduced during symptomatic malaria illness, thus permitting increased proliferation of EBV-infected lymphocytes, and increasing the chances that a malignant transformation to Burkitt lymphoma may occur.

ENDOMYOCARDIAL FIBROSIS. Exposure to malaria has been associated with this cardiomyopathy (Chapter 3).

■ TREATMENT

GENERAL PRINCIPLES. The aims of antimalarial drug use vary with the epidemiologic situation (treatment of clinical illness, interruption of transmission, prevention of infection). The choice of specific drugs and drug regimens is determined by the *Plasmodium* species causing the infection, drug sensitivities of the infecting parasites, and by the economic realities of the particular situation.

DEFINITIONS. Antimalarial drugs act selectively on different stages of the parasite life cycle. *Blood schizonticides* is the traditional term for drugs that destroy asexual parasites (trophozoites) in red blood cells; these drugs are effective in treating symptomatic patients. In fact, none of the antimalarial drugs is effective against meronts (schizonts), so this term is slightly misleading. *Tissue schizonticides* act on the exoerythrocytic stages to prevent relapses of *P. vivax* and *P. ovale* infections. Some antimalarials prevent transmission: *gametocides* destroy the sexual stages, and *sporontocides* inhibit the development of oocysts on the gut wall of the mosquito. Blood schizonticides alone eradicate *P. falciparum* and *P. malariae* infections, but for complete (radical) cure of vivax and ovale malaria, a tissue schizonticide is necessary as well.

Certain drugs act in a prophylactic capacity by preventing infection or by abrogating clinical symptoms. *Causal prophylactics* act on hepatic stages of malaria parasites. *Suppressive (clinical) prophylactics* prevent clinical symptoms by destroying malaria parasites as they initially invade red cells; all blood schizonticides can be considered suppressive prophylactics. Some antimalarial drugs exert more than one effect and can thus be put to several uses. No single antimalarial encompasses all of these actions.

ANTIMALARIAL COMPOUNDS. The most important antimalarial drugs are arranged into those in current use and those under active development. The following compounds are in current use:

Artemisinine (qinghaosu), artemether, and artesunate (artemisinins)
Atovaquone (hydroxynaphthoquinone)
Chloroquine and amodiaquine (4-aminoquinolines)
Halofantrine (phenanthrene-methanol)
Mefloquine (4-quinoline-carbinolamines)
Primaquine (8-aminoquinolines)
Proguanil (biguanides)
Pyrimethamine (diaminopyrimidine)
Quinine, quinidine (cinchona alkaloids)
Sulfadoxine (sulfonamides, sulfones)
Tetracyline, doxycycline (tetracyclines)

The following compounds are under development:

Artemether (sesquiterpene lactone) and artemisinin derivatives

Benflumetol (fluoremethanol)
Pyronaridine (2-methoxy-7-chloro-10-3'-, 5'-bis(pyrrolidino-
1-methyl)-4'-hydroxyanilinobenzo-(b)-1,5-naphthyridine)
Short half-life combination antifolates
WR238-605, 80/53 (8-aminoquinolines)
Proteinase inhibitors

Antimalarial Pharmacology—Drugs in Current Use

ARTEMISININS. Artemisinin (qinghaosu) is a sesquiterpene lactone extracted in 1972 at the Chinese Institute of
Materia Medica from a medicinal herb (*Artemisia annua*),
sweet wormwood. It has a very rapid onset of action, but a
rather high recrudescence rate when used alone. The parent
compound and two artemisinin derivatives are currently in
use: artemether, most commonly administered by intramuscular injection, and artesunate, which can be administered
by mouth, by intravenous infusion, or by rectal suppository.
Another derivative, arteether, is in the late stages of development. Artesunate suppositories are particularly useful for
treating moderately to severely ill patients in places where
parenteral therapy is not available.

Antimalarial Actions. This class of drugs has stage-specific
antimalarial effects. Late-stage ring parasites and trophozoites are more susceptible than are schizonts (meronts) or
small rings. They are also gametocidal and thus may reduce
transmission. Liver stages of *P. vivax* and *P. ovale* are not
affected. These drugs may kill malaria parasites by becoming
free radicals in a reaction catalyzed by iron. These reactive
species could then react with and damage specific membrane-associated proteins.

Pharmacology and Metabolism. Pharmacokinetic studies
have been hampered by the difficulties encountered in developing a reproducible assay for the primary drugs and their
metabolites. After oral administration, peak concentrations
of artemisinin in the blood occur from 0.5 to 2 hours, and
are associated with a half-life of 2 to 2.5 hours. Intravenous
artesunate is converted almost immediately into dihydroartemisinin, which is then eliminated from the plasma with a
half-life of 45 minutes. Intramuscular (IM) administration is
associated with the slowest elimination because the drugs
are dissolved in oil and are released slowly. Artemether concentrations peak 5 to 6 hours after intramuscular administration and disappear with a half-life of 8 to 11 hours. There are
no data describing the pharmacokinetics of the artemisinin
derivatives in malaria patients; given the rapid uptake of
these drugs in PRBC and their binding to acute-phase proteins, the pharmacokinetics might be different in patients
than in normal volunteers.

Toxicity. These drugs have been used safely in many patients in uncontrolled settings but high doses of the artemisinin derivatives are neurotoxic in vitro and in experimental
animals. Since limited data on potential toxicities from clinical trials are available, some caution in their use is advised.
They are fetotoxic and thus are not recommended for use
during pregnancy.

Uses. Parasite clearance times are consistently more rapid
in patients treated with the artemisinin drugs than in patients
treated with other antimalarials. However, these rapid parasite clearance times have not been associated with statistically
significant decreases in mortality. These drugs are extremely
useful in settings where *P. falciparum* has developed multidrug resistance. Because recrudescence is common when
these drugs are employed as single agents, and because resistance may be more likely to develop when they are used
alone, combination chemotherapy with longer half-life drugs
(e.g., mefloquine) is the current approach in areas where
multidrug-resistant falciparum parasites predominate. Using

artemisinin derivatives formulated as suppositories is a
promising, but still unproven, alternative for the treatment
of severe disease in peripheral settings. Artesunate suppositories have been effective (in combination with oral mefloquine) in treating severe malaria in Thai adults.

CHLOROQUINE. This drug is marketed for oral administration as a diphosphate or sulfate salt and for IM or IV injection
as the dihydrochloride. The spread of chloroquine-resistant
P. falciparum and *P. vivax* parasites has limited the usefulness
of this drug, particularly in the treatment of severe and
complicated disease.

Antimalarial Actions. Chloroquine is a 4-aminoquinoline
with marked, rapid blood schizonticidal activity against susceptible strains of malaria parasites; it is most active against
late ring stages and mature trophozoites. The drug is not
effective against exoerythrocytic forms in the liver. Chloroquine is gametocidal against *P. vivax*, *P. ovale*, and *P. malariae*, and is effective against immature, but not mature, gametocytes of *P. falciparum*. The action of chloroquine is rapid,
with parasitemia disappearing in 48 to 72 hours after the
standard regimen has been administered, assuming the parasites are sensitive to the drug.

Pharmacology and Metabolism. The drug is rapidly and
almost completely absorbed from the gastrointestinal tract,
following which it is localized in the tissues. It is metabolized
by alkylation in the liver and excreted slowly by the kidneys,
with a half-life of from 3 to 7 days in a normal healthy adult.
Following daily administration of chloroquine, about 10%
appears in the feces, and about 60% in the urine, of which
about two thirds is the parent compound. With therapeutic
doses given orally, an effective blood concentration is usually
reached within minutes. Acidification of urine increases renal
excretion.

Toxicity. At doses used for suppression and treatment of
malaria, toxic effects are rare. Minor reported side effects
include nausea, vomiting, dizziness, headache, blurred vision, fatigue, diarrhea, and convulsions. Gastrointestinal
symptoms may be reduced by taking the drug after meals.
Pruritus is sometimes a problem in individuals, particularly
blacks. In prolonged high daily doses, e.g., as those in the
treatment of patients with rheumatoid arthritis, chloroquine
may cause a severe, often irreversible retinopathy characterized by loss of central visual acuity, pigmentation of the
macula, and retinal artery constrictions. Cumulative doses
exceeding 100 g are associated with an increased risk of
retinopathy when chloroquine is used prophlactically. However, retinopathy has not been reported following treatment
for malaria infection at recommended doses.

There are no reports of teratogenic effects in humans when
chloroquine has been used as an antimalarial drug; therefore,
it may be administered during pregnancy. Hypotension,
acute circulatory failure, and cardiopulmonary arrest have
been reported following the parenteral administration of
chloroquine, particularly in infants and young children. Transient high blood concentrations induce hypotension and
sometimes sudden death. Therefore, IV chloroquine should
always be given slowly; IM or subcutaneous chloroquine
should be given in small frequent doses. The lethal single
oral dose is estimated to be 1 g in children and 4 g in
adults. Intensive care support with mechanical ventilation,
diazepam, and epinephrine are recommended for individuals
with acute chloroquine toxicity. Dose reduction may be required in patients with severe renal and hepatic disease,
although some authorities recommend a standard therapeutic regimen for these patients.

Uses. Chloroquine is the drug of choice for treatment or
prevention of infections with *P. ovale* and *P. malariae* and for
sensitive *P. falciparum* and *P. vivax* parasites.

AMODIAQUINE. This drug is marketed as the dihydrochloride dihydrate. The efficacy, side effects, recommendations, and precautions for amodiaquine are essentially the same as those for chloroquine, with a few exceptions.

Pharmacology and Metabolism. Amodiaquine is also a 4-aminoquinoline. There is no parenteral preparation for amodiaquine. There are in vivo and in vitro data suggesting that amodiaquine is more active than chloroquine against some strains of *P. falciparum* resistant to chloroquine.

Toxicity. Amodiaquine has side effects similar to those of chloroquine. It also has been associated with hepatotoxicity and agranulocytosis, with a risk of death of 0.01% when used for chemoprophylaxis of malaria. Amodiaquine is not licensed or marketed in the United States.

Uses. Amodiaquine has been used as an alternative to chloroquine in the first-line treatment of uncomplicated *P. falciparum* malaria in areas with a high level of chloroquine resistance. However, *P. falciparum* in these areas is almost always resistant to amodiaquine as well.

HALOFANTRINE. Halofantrine hydrochloride is a 9-phenanthrene-methanol; the drug exists as a racemic mixture and both stereoisomers have equal antimalarial activity. Like mefloquine, it was initially developed by the Walter Reed Army Institute of Research (WRAIR).

Antimalarial Actions. This drug is a blood schizonticide; its mechanism of action is unknown. It has no effect against the hepatic stages of the parasite.

Pharmacology and Metabolism. Absorption of the oral preparation is incomplete and variable; the drug is lipophilic, and absorption is enhanced if the drug is administered with, or shortly after, a fatty meal. Peak plasma levels of the parent drug occur in 6 hours; the principal metabolite, desbutylhalofantrine, which also has antimalarial activity, peaks at 12 hours. Excretion is primarily in the feces. Pharmacokinetic parameters in patients differ significantly from those in healthy volunteers; there is extensive interindividual variation; absorption is slower in patients with uncomplicated malaria than in volunteers, as is elimination. The desbutyl metabolite has a terminal half-life longer than that of the parent drug, and this may contribute to the antimalarial effect of the compounds. There is no parenteral formulation of the drug.

Toxicity. Halofantrine is generally well tolerated. It exerts a significant, dose- and concentration-related effect on prolongation of the QT interval, and has been associated with cardiac arrhythmias and sudden death, particularly in individuals with pre-existing QT prolongation on their electrocardiograms. This effect is more pronounced following the second 24 mg/kg dose. It is embryotoxic and is excreted in the milk of animals, and is therefore not recommended for treatment during pregnancy or breast-feeding. Abdominal pain, diarrhea, pruritus, skin rash, and elevated transaminases have been reported in some individuals taking the drug.

Uses. Clinical trials report that 500 mg of halofantrine (8 mg/kg) every 6 hours for three doses cured 85 to 95% of those infected with any of the four species of *Plasmodium*. Because of a high recrudescence rate after the first treatment, two treatments with a 7-day interval are recommended. *P. falciparum* was less responsive in areas where mefloquine-resistant parasites are common, but a 3-fold increase in dose was effective. There is a higher risk of complications associated with QT prolongation at this dose, however. Fever and parasitemia clear rapidly, both usually responding within 2 to 3 days of the initiation of effective treatment. The recommended pediatric dose is 8 mg/kg three times at 6-hour intervals. The drug is available as a suspension (100 mg/5 mL) and as a 250-mg tablet. It is useful in areas where

multidrug-resistant strains of *P. falciparum* are present, but the increased doses required to treat mefloquine-resistant parasites may be associated with an unacceptably high risk of cardiotoxicity.

MEFLOQUINE. This 4-quinoline-carbinolamine was a major advance in the treatment of multidrug-resistant *P. falciparum* infections; unfortunately, resistance to mefloquine has developed rapidly in areas where it is widely used.

Antimalarial Actions. The exact mechanism of action of mefloquine is not known, but it destroys early trophozoites and therefore acts earlier than sulfadoxine-pyrimethamine, but later than the artemisinin derivatives. It is not effective against the exoerythrocytic stages; its gametocidal and sporonticidal activities are not known.

Pharmacology and Metabolism. Mefloquine is structurally related to quinine. After a single dose, peak plasma levels occur within 2 to 12 hours. The drug binds extensively to plasma proteins. It is metabolized primarily to one component that has no antimalarial activity. It has a long but variable elimination half-life, ranging from 13 to 24 days.

Toxicity. Single oral doses of 15 mg/kg, and split doses of 25 mg/kg (15 mg/kg, followed by 10 mg/kg 8 to 12 hours later) are well tolerated and well absorbed, even in unconscious patients receiving the drug via nasogastric tube. The most common adverse effects are mild: anorexia, nausea, vomiting, dizziness, and sleep disorders. Higher doses are associated with early vomiting, which can reduce bioavailability and thus decrease efficacy. Children are also more likely to vomit after receiving mefloquine treatment than are adults. Neurologic and psychiatric side effects have been reported following the therapeutic and prophylactic use of mefloquine both alone and in combination with other antimalarials. The more serious reactions have included severe depression with suicidal tendencies, anxiety neurosis, hallucinations, acute psychosis, seizures, mutism, manic behavior, delirium, and altered consciousness (stupor, coma). Controlled trials of mefloquine as prophylaxis and treatment have generated estimates of the risk of serious neurotoxicity of about 1 in 15,000 and 57 per 100,000, respectively.

Uses. Mefloquine has been effective in the treatment (1000 to 1250 mg/adult treatment) and prevention (250 mg/wk) of multidrug-resistant *P. falciparum*. Mefloquine is also active against *P. vivax* and *P. malariae*. The drug is not recommended for persons involved with activity requiring fine coordination and special performance (e.g., airplane crews, operators of heavy or dangerous equipment), or for children weighing less than 15 kg. It should not be administered concurrently with quinine or quinidine. If these drugs are used in the initial treatment of malaria, mefloquine administration should be delayed for at least 12 hours after the last dose. There is limited experience with the drug in the first trimester of pregnancy; its use for prophylaxis and treatment during the second and third trimesters has not been associated with an increased incidence of poor birth outcomes. The drug is poorly soluble and is not formulated for parenteral administration.

PRIMAQUINE. Primaquine tablets contain the diphosphate salt.

Antimalarial Actions. Primaquine is an 8-aminoquinoline derivative. The drug is gametocidal and sporontocidal for all species of human malaria. It is a poor blood schizonticide, but is effective against exoerythrocytic hypnozoites and will usually prevent relapses due to *P. vivax* and *P. ovale*. Unfortunately, primaquine fails to prevent relapses in individuals infected with some strains of *P. vivax*; 26 (43%) of 60 American soldiers contracting vivax malaria in Somalia relapsed despite receiving the recommended course of 15 mg base daily for 14 days.

Pharmacology and Metabolism. The drug is rapidly absorbed and excreted after oral administration. Peak plasma levels occur within 30 to 60 minutes and fall rapidly. The half-life is about 4 hours. It is metabolized to a more polar metabolite; it is not known which of these is responsible for the observed antimalarial activity. Very little drug concentrates in tissues.

Toxicity. There are two major types of side effects. The more important, intravascular hemolysis, is a complication in individuals with G6PD deficiency. Gastrointestinal tract side effects include anorexia, nausea, epigastric pain and, sometimes, severe abdominal cramps. G6PD deficiency is an inherited X-linked trait occurring most frequently in blacks and persons of Mediterranean and Asian extraction (Chapter 6). Intravascular hemolysis occurs when red blood cells are exposed to oxidant stress. The severity of hemolysis depends on which genetic variant of G6PD deficiency the patient has. In most blacks, hemolysis is self-limited, even when drug administration is continued. In the Mediterranean variant and the Canton variant present in some persons of Chinese ancestry, however, hemolysis is more severe and often is not self-limited, sometimes continuing after the drug is withdrawn. Therefore, it is generally recommended that a test for G6PD deficiency be performed before administering the drug in full therapeutic doses. Other very rare untoward effects from primaquine include methemoglobinemia, hemoglobinuria, and, rarely, agranulocytosis, granulocytopenia, and leukopenia. Primaquine should not be administered to pregnant women because its safety in pregnancy has not been established.

Uses. Primaquine is used to prevent relapses of *P. vivax* and *P. ovale* infections. Its excellent gametocidal and sporontocidal action against all four plasmodia species makes it potentially useful in combination with a blood schizonticide to prevent transmission in endemic areas.

PROGUANIL. Proguanil is formulated in tablets of the hydrochloride salt.

Antimalarial Actions. Proguanil has a slow schizonticidal action on erythrocytic forms. It is also effective against the primary tissue phase of *P. falciparum*. Thus, it provides excellent causal prophylaxis against *P. falciparum* and is sporonticidal against this species. Proguanil is less active against *P. vivax,* and some patients on proguanil prophylaxis develop vivax malaria after the drug is discontinued.

Pharmacology and Metabolism. The drug is rapidly absorbed following oral ingestion. Its antimalarial action is accounted for by its rapid conversion to cycloguanil; proguanil is eliminated slowly, mainly in the urine and feces, in which about 40% appears as the parent compound. The half-life of cycloguanil is much shorter than that of proguanil itself. Cycloguanil is a powerful inhibitor of dihydrofolate reductase, and like pyrimethamine, the binding affinity of cycloguanil is much greater for the parasitic enzyme than for the mammalian homologue. Approximately 3% of Caucasian and African populations and up to 20% of Asian populations fail to convert the parent compounds to the active metabolite.

Toxicity. The advantage of this drug is its safety. Even at high doses, the only reported adverse effects are mouth ulcers, abdominal discomfort, loss of appetite, vomiting, hair loss, diarrhea and rarely, hematuria.

Uses. Proguanil is used for causal prophylaxis of falciparum malaria, particularly in combination with chloroquine. Resistance to pyrimethamine and proguanil frequently coexists because of the similar modes of action of these drugs. Clinical responses in established infections are slow when proguanil is used alone for treatment. Combinations of proguanil with dapsone or short-acting sulfonamides are being evaluated as treatment regimens. In combination with atovaquone it has an excellent cure rate in treating uncomplicated *P. falciparum* infections.

PYRIMETHAMINE. This dihydrofolate reductase inhibitor is a 2,4-diaminopyrimidine.

Antimalarial Actions. The drug is a slow but effective blood schizonticide. It is also active against the primary tissue forms of *P. falciparum* and, to a lesser extent, to *P. vivax* and is an excellent sporonticidal agent. It is not effective for radical cure of vivax and ovale malaria because it is inactive against latent exoerythrocytic stages. Resistance develops rapidly when it is used as a single agent, and it is most commonly deployed in a fixed combination with sulfadoxine.

Pharmacology and Metabolism. Pyrimethamine has a half-life of about 92 hours. It is slowly but completely absorbed from the intestinal tract and then firmly bound to proteins in the tissues. Pyrimethamine localizes in the liver, spleen, kidneys, and lungs. It is excreted in the urine and gives stable and prolonged plasma levels following single doses. The drug is excreted in the milk of nursing mothers. Pyrimethamine is a selective inhibitor of the plasmodial enzyme dihydrofolate reductase and therefore interferes with nucleic acid metabolism.

Toxicity. When given for malaria chemoprophylaxis or treatment, no significant toxic effects have been reported for pyrimethamine. Teratogenic effects were noted in animal studies, but it has not been associated with any adverse pregnancy outcomes despite extensive use in endemic areas.

Uses. Pyrimethamine is not indicated for treatment of acute malaria infections except in combination with sulfonamides and sulfones.

QUININE. This drug has been a traditional antimalarial compound for centuries. It is customarily isolated from the bark of the cinchona tree; it can be synthesized, but with difficulty. It is available in oral formulations, but it can be administered intravenously or intramuscularly when necessary.

Antimalarial Actions. Quinine is active against mature asexual erythrocytic stages of all forms of human malaria parasites. The drug does not affect exoerythrocytic forms. The gametocytes of *P. vivax, P. ovale,* and *P. malariae* and immature gametocytes of *P. falciparum* are sensitive to quinine. Mature gametocytes of *P. falciparum* are not susceptible. Quinine is regarded by many experienced clinicians as the drug of first choice for treatment of severe cases of falciparum malaria.

Pharmacology and Metabolism. Quinine is quickly and almost completely absorbed from the intestinal tract and following IM injections. Peak plasma concentrations occur within 4 hours. Most of the drug is bound to plasma proteins, 80% is eliminated by hepatic biotransformation, and the remaining 20% is excreted as quinine by the kidneys. The volume of distribution and systemic clearance rates are reduced in proportion to disease severity; as a result, the highest plasma concentrations are in patients with severe malaria. The drug binds strongly to acute-phase proteins and these are increased in proportion to the severity of disease. Despite the discrepancies in plasma quinine concentrations in healthy normal volunteers, patients with uncomplicated malaria and patients with severe infections, there is a rough equivalence in free quinine concentrations, and toxic effects are few. The therapeutic range has not been well defined and varies with local parasite sensitivities. It is probably between 8 to 15 mg/L, and toxic effects are rare when concentrations are less than 20 mg/L (free quinine <2 mg/L). There is no accumulation in the tissues, even with continued administration. Quinine readily crosses the placenta, but cerebrospinal fluid levels are 1/20 to 1/50 of those in plasma. Acidification of urine increases renal excretion.

Toxicity. Quinine has a bitter taste. A common syndrome known as *cinchonism* (tinnitus, headache, nausea, abdominal pain, minor visual disturbances, transient loss of hearing, and tremors) occurs in many patients taking the drug. These symptoms may appear during the first 1 to 3 days of therapy and subside quickly when the drug is stopped. With the recommended doses, serious adverse effects are very rare. Rapid infusion rates and prolonged treatment are associated with hypoglycemia. The more serious, and probably idiosyncratic, toxic effects include urticaria, "asthma" attacks in susceptible individuals, angioedema of the face, mucous membranes and lungs, deafness, blindness, hemolytic anemia, and agranulocytosis. Severe poisoning results in convulsions, delirium, depressed respiration, coma, circulatory failure, and death. Quinine is a local irritant, sometimes causing gastric pain, nausea, and vomiting when given orally. Blackwater fever (hemoglobinuria) seems to be associated with quinine use, but the underlying mechanism is obscure.

There are reports of a limited risk of premature labor associated with quinine, but these have not been borne out in careful studies. Pregnant women may be susceptible to acute hemolytic anemia, thrombocytopenia, and hypoglycemia due to the drug.

Uses. Its major use is for the treatment of patients with severe and complicated malaria. The dihydrochloride salt of quinine is used for parenteral therapy while the sulfate, bisulfate, hydrochloride, ethylcarbonate, hydrobromide, and dihydrochloride salts are available in a variety of oral formulations. IM and IV administrations of quinine dihydrochloride achieve satisfactory plasma concentrations. In order to achieve therapeutic levels rapidly, without precipitating hypoglycemia, the IV loading dose (20 mg/kg) should be infused over 3 to 4 hours, and the IM loading dose can be split into two doses of 10 mg/kg, diluted 1:3 to 1:5, administered 4 hours apart.

QUINIDINE. This drug, the dextrorotary optical isomer of quinine, is also effective against *P. falciparum*. Its use is particularly important in settings where IV quinine is not readily available. Most developed country hospitals keep stocks of quinidine for the IV treatment of cardiac arrhythmias.

Antimalarial Actions. These are similar to those described for quinine.

Pharmacology and Metabolism. Absorption and distribution are similar to quinine. Mean plasma levels are slightly lower than with equivalent doses of quinine. Peak plasma level after a single oral dose occurs within 4 hours. Food decreases the rate but not the extent of absorption and may reduce side effects. Quinidine is 80 to 90% bound to plasma proteins, but protein binding may be decreased in patients with impaired hepatic function. It is present in breast milk in quinidine-treated mothers. Metabolism and elimination are primarily (60 to 85%) hepatic, but 15 to 40% appears in the urine as unchanged drug. The elimination half-life is not prolonged in nonmalarious patients with renal failure. Severe malaria may delay metabolism and elimination.

Toxicity. This is similar to quinine and is dose related; QT prolongation is four-fold greater with quinidine than with quinine, and cardiac monitoring is recommended, especially when quinidine is given parenterally. Severe hypotension due to peripheral vasodilation may occur after rapid parenteral administration; the hypotension should be treated with volume replacement and administration of vasopressor amines. Large doses of quinidine depress myocardial contractility and aggravate or induce heart failure. Quinidine may produce AV block. Syncopal episodes and sudden death during quinidine therapy may be due to ventricular fibrillation, probably as a result of a markedly prolonged QT interval.

Hypotension and disturbances in cardiac conduction are related to serum concentrations. Therefore, when it is used intravenously, quinidine should be given with careful monitoring, preferably in the hospital. It is best to determine the serum quinidine levels after the initial loading dose and at least daily.

Uses. Quinidine can be used either intravenously or orally to treat chloroquine-resistant *P. falciparum*. It is particularly useful when parenteral preparations of quinine are not available.

SULFONAMIDES AND SULFONES. Sulfonamides and sulfones inhibit plasmodial dihydropteroate synthetase, an earlier step in the folate pathway than that affected by pyrimethamine.

Antimalarial Actions. These are highly effective blood schizonticides for *P. falciparum* but are less active against the asexual blood forms of other malaria parasite species. Like pyrimethamine, they are too slow to be used as single agents; the sulfonamides and sulfones are used in combination with pyrimethamine or proguanil for the treatment of malaria.

Pharmacology and Metabolism. There is considerable variation in the rates of absorption and excretion of different compounds. They are excreted in the urine mainly as metabolites. The estimated half-lives of those frequently used as antimalarials are as follows: sulfadoxine, 100 to 200 hours; sulfalene, 65 hours; and dapsone, 28 hours. Failures with sulfonamides may be due to host differences in ability to acetylate the drug rather than to drug-resistant parasites.

Toxicity. These drugs are generally well tolerated. The sulfonamides may occasionally cause urticaria, Stevens-Johnson syndromes, and other hypersensitivity reactions. Hepatitis occurs, but is rare. Both sulfonamides and sulfones may precipitate hemolysis in persons with G6PD deficiency and methemoglobinemia in patients with hereditary NAD methemoglobinemia reductase deficiency. Acute hemolytic anemia may be produced in otherwise healthy persons, particularly black individuals. These compounds are contraindicated in persons with a previous history of hypersensitivity and in premature infants. Because of the danger of kernicterus, sulfones and sulfonamides are contraindicated for pregnant women near term and for infants in the first month of life.

Uses. Sulfonamides and sulfones are used in combination with other drugs for the treatment of chloroquine-resistant *P. falciparum* infections.

TETRACYCLINE. Tetracycline is manufactured as the hydrochloride salt for oral use.

Antimalarial Actions. Tetracycline has a very slow blood schizonticidal activity in man. Activity against tissue schizonts of chloroquine-resistant *P. falciparum* has also been demonstrated. Doxycycline and minocycline are as effective as tetracycline and have the advantage of once-daily dosage regimens.

Toxicity. Major side effects of tetracycline include permanent discoloration of teeth, hypoplasia of tooth enamel, and impaired bone growth in children <8 years of age. For these reasons, tetracycline should not be used in young children or pregnant women. Gastrointestinal complaints, including nausea, vomiting, abdominal pain, and diarrhea are common with the use of this drug. Overgrowth of *Candida* in the mouth, gut, vagina, or skin is a frequent problem in those taking tetracyclines. Doxycycline can also cause photosensitivity, which is not a trivial concern in tropical areas.

Uses. Tetracycline and doxycycline are used for treatment of, and prophylaxis for, chloroquine- and pyrimethamine-sulfonamide–resistant *P. falciparum* infections. Resistance by the parasites to tetracyclines has never been demonstrated. Since the action of these drugs against *P. falciparum* is so slow, they should always be used in combination with a rapidly acting blood schizonticide, e.g., quinine.

COMBINATION DRUGS. When a sulfonamide or sulfone is given together with a dihydrofolate reductase inhibitor, a potentiating effect against malaria parasites is observed. The synergy is often so marked that the combination is effective against strains of *Plasmodium* resistant to the individual component drugs. The potentiating effect occurs because the drugs block sequential steps in the biosynthesis of purines and pyrimidines. Mammalian cells are permeable to folate and can use preformed folate, whereas bacteria and protozoa cannot.

Sulfadoxine-Pyrimethamine (S-P). This combination is marketed in tablets containing 500 mg of sulfadoxine and 25 mg of pyrimethamine. Toxic manifestations are rare and are usually attributable to the sulfadoxine component. Severe cutaneous reactions (erythema multiforme, Stevens-Johnson syndrome, and toxic epidermal necrolysis) have been reported in individuals using this particular combination on a weekly basis for chemoprophylaxis. Fatalities occurred in 1 to 11,000 to 25,000 users, an unacceptably high incidence, and so the recommendation for use in malaria prophylaxis was withdrawn. However, this combination is highly recommended in chloroquine-resistant areas where *P. falciparum* is not yet resistant to S-P as single-dose treatment of malaria and for treatment of febrile travelers taking other malaria prophylactic regimens. The safety of the combination in pregnancy has not been established, but the drug has been used to treat large numbers of pregnant women. No apparent adverse effects were noted, and the incidence of placental malaria infections was significantly less than when less effective drugs were used. Symptomatic improvement may be delayed in patients treated with S-P.

Pyrimethamine-Sulfalene. This drug is considered equivalent to S-P in efficacy and toxicity. Each tablet contains 25 mg of pyrimethamine and 500 mg of sulfalene.

Pyrimethamine-Dapsone. This combination, which contains 12.5 mg of pyrimethamine and 100 mg of dapsone, is used for causal prophylaxis. Other drug regimens are recommended for this purpose and there are no data addressing the relative efficacy of this combination versus any of the other regimens.

Mefloquine-Pyrimethamine-Sulfadoxine. This fixed combination contains 250 mg of mefloquine hydrochloride, 500 mg of sulfadoxine, and 25 mg of pyrimethamine. The rationale for the combination was to retard the development of mefloquine-resistant parasites. Unfortunately, resistance to the various components has developed, and the indications for the combination have dwindled.

COMPOUNDS UNDER DEVELOPMENT

Arteether. The development of an injectable formulation of arteether has been supported by a partnership between the WHO, the WRAIR, and the Dutch government. The drug appears very similar in terms of efficacy and toxicity to arteether; it is in phase II trials in 1998.

Research is focusing on investigating artemisinin derivatives with slower metabolic breakdown and which bypass generation of dihydroartemisinin since these may be less neurotoxic and have better activity against both chloroquine-sensitive and -resistant strains of *P. falciparum* than the parent compound. Synthetic trioxanes and tetroxanes with much greater in vitro activity against *P. falciparum* than artemisinin have been prepared. These compounds are easily prepared from inexpensive, accessible starting compounds.

Atovaquone. This hydroxynaphthoquinone has broad spectrum antiprotozoal activity and was originally developed and licensed as a treatment for *Pneumocystis carinii* pneumonia and cerebral toxoplasmosis. It is active against both the primary liver stages and the erythrocytic stages of *P. falciparum,* and it has a novel mode of action: it inhibits electron transport. It appears to be very safe and well tolerated. When used as a single agent, resistant parasites emerge rapidly; recrudescence rates average around 30%. It is synergistic with proguanil and is being used clinically in a fixed-dose combination (500 mg of atovaquone, 200 mg of proguanil); cure rates of this dose, administered twice daily for 3 days, have been 85 to 100% in clinical trials.

Benflumetol. This fluoromethanol was synthesized by the Institute of Military Medical Sciences in Beijing, and registered for use in China in 1987. At present, there is little experience with this drug outside of China. It is a blood schizonticide, and while it is poorly soluble in water or oil, it dissolves readily in unsaturated fatty acids and is formulated in linoleic acid. It has been co-administered orally with artemether in China, and preclinical trials of this combination are underway.

Pyronaridine. This is another compound that has emerged from the Chinese antimalarial drug development effort. It is a blood schizonticide used in China since the 1970s. There has been little experience with the drug outside China, but it cleared *P. falciparum* parasites in 40 of 40 Cameroonian patients and was associated with very few adverse effects. It has potential as a replacement for chloroquine (i.e., an oral formulation for the treatment of uncomplicated malaria); studies are underway to generate the pharmacokinetic and clinical data that will help to determine its role.

Short Half-Life Antifolates. The antifolate combinations in use now have long elimination half-lives. The advantages of single-dose treatment and a prophylactic effect are balanced by the disadvantage of enhanced selection of resistant parasites and the increased incidence of adverse effects. Alternative antifolate combinations, using compounds with short half-lives, are being studied. These include the biguanides and triazines and the short-acting sulfonamides and sulfones. The combination of the biguanide, chlorproguanil, with dapsone has potential for treatment of uncomplicated malaria and is being evaluated in clinical trials.

WR238 605. This 8-aminoquinoline is being developed by the WRAIR as a primaquine replacement. It is much more active than primaquine against the persistent liver forms of *P. vivax* and *P. ovale,* and it also has blood schizonticidal activity. Although it was originally designed as a causal prophylactic and radical curative drug, it may have clinical utility as treatment of uncomplicated falciparum malaria.

Proteinase Inhibitors. This group of drugs has recently provided an exciting breakthrough in treating HIV infections and will yield therapeutic options for other viral infections. Proteinases have been identified in *Plasmodia* that degrade hemoglobin as a principal source of amino acids for protein synthesis. These and other *Plasmodia* proteinases are novel targets for antimalarial chemotherapy.

Therapeutic Regimens

The recommended treatment for malaria is outlined in Table 92–5 and the dosages of antimalarial drugs are given in Table 92–6. Managing a patient with malaria requires (1) establishing the diagnosis, (2) identifying the species of malaria parasite, (3) estimating the parasitemia, (4) determining the immune status of the patient, (5) ascertaining the likely geographic origin of the infecting parasite(s), and (6) appreciating the severity of the clinical illness. Species identification helps in deciding on specific drugs, and is best accomplished by examining a well-stained thin blood film. Determining where infection is likely to have occurred helps to predict drug response by identifying the possibility of drug resis-

TABLE 92–5. Recommended Drugs for Treatment of Malaria

Type	Parasitemia Clinical Illness	Recommended Drugs (Route)	Alternative Drugs (Route)
A. *P. falciparum*			
1. Exposure in areas where chloroquine resistance is established *or*	severe[b]	quinine or quinidine (IV) *plus* pyrimethamine-sulfadoxine[d] (PO)	quinine or quinidine (IV) *plus* tetracycline[e] (PO) *or* mefloquine (PO)
Infection known to be chloroquine-resistant[a]	not severe[c]	quinine or quinidine (PO) *plus* pyrimethamine-sulfadoxine[d] (PO)	quinine or quinidine (PO) *plus* tetracycline[e] (PO) *or* mefloquine (PO) *or* artemisinin derivative (PO, IM or IV) *plus* mefloquine (PO)
2. Exposure only in areas without known chloroquine resistance	severe[b] not severe[c]	quinine or quinidine (IV) *followed by* chloroquine (PO) chloroquine (PO)	chloroquine (IV or IM[g]) *followed by* chloroquine (PO) amodiaquine (PO)
3. Exposure in areas with known chloroquine and pyrimethamine sulfadoxine resistance *or*	severe[b]	quinine or quinidine (IV) *plus* tetracycline[e] (PO)	quinine or quinidine (IV) *followed by* mefloquine (PO)
Infection known to be resistant to both drugs[h]	not severe[c]	quinine or quinidine (PO) *plus* tetracycline[e] (PO)	mefloquine (PO) *or* artemisinin derivative (PO, IM or IV) *plus* mefloquine (PO)
4. Exposure area unknown		as in section A, no. 3	as in section A, no. 3
B. *P. malariae*		chloroquine[f] (PO)	amodiaquine[f] (PO)
C. *P. vivax* and *P. ovale*		chloroquine[f] (PO) *followed by* primaquine (PO)	amodiaquine[f] (PO) *followed by* primaquine (PO)
D. Species unknown	severe[b] not severe[c]	Treat as if *P. falciparum*, as outlined in section A.	
E. Mixed infections with two or more species	severe[b] not severe[c]	Initiate treatment for *P. falciparum*, as outlined in section A. Then treat other species as necessary.	

[a]Chloroquine prophylaxis treatment failure.
[b]Parasitemia ≥1% and/or clinical manifestations severe and/or complications present, or if patient is unable to take oral medication.
[c]Parasitemia <1%, clinical manifestations not severe, and no complications present.
[d]Pyrimethamine-sulfalene considered equivalent to pyrimethamine-sulfadoxine.
[e]Doxycycline can be used instead.
[f]If illness is life-threatening, if there are complications, or if the patient is unable to take oral medication, IV quinine or quinidine is preferred. Otherwise, oral chloroquine or amodiaquine can be given.
[g]Intramuscular (IM) or slow IV drip route preferred. Parenteral chloroquine can cause severe toxicity in infants and young children.
[h]Prophylaxis or treatment failure with both drugs.

tance. The severity of the illness determines which drugs are selected and by which route they are administered. The initial assessment of parasitemia is useful because there is an association between level of parasitemia and disease severity. Serial assessments of parasitemia are useful in determining treatment efficacy, and the need for blood transfusion can often be predicted on the basis of the initial parasitemia and hematocrit/hemoglobin. If a patient has any markers of severe and complicated malaria, or if he or she is unable to tolerate oral medications, drugs should be administered intravenously.

TREATMENT OF FALCIPARUM MALARIA. The chemotherapy of falciparum malaria is complicated by the problem of drug-resistant parasites. Any *P. falciparum* infection in a nonimmune individual should be considered a potential medical emergency. The patient should be hospitalized and observed carefully for any complications (Table 92–2). Serial blood films every 6 to 8 hours should be made to assess the therapeutic response. Failure of a drug to reduce parasitemia within 48 hours indicates the possibility of drug failure.

Uncomplicated P. *falciparum* with Exposure in Areas Where Resistance to 4-Aminoquinolines is Established. These areas include South America, the Indian subcontinent, Southeast Asia, Indonesia, China, some islands in the Pacific (including New Guinea and the Philippines) and sub-Saharan Africa (Chapter 149). The recommended treatment for uncomplicated chloroquine-resistant malaria is sulfadoxine-pyrimethamine (Table 92–5). However, resistance to this combination is already common in Southeast Asia and Brazil and is rapidly increasing. Alternative first-line treatments for uncomplicated disease include quinine, mefloquine, and halofantrine and, in settings where resistance is developing to all of these drugs, quinine plus tetracycline or mefloquine plus one of the artemisinin derivatives.

Uncomplicated Chloroquine-Sensitive P. *falciparum* Infections. Falciparum malaria contracted in areas with no reported chloroquine resistance should be treated initially with chloroquine unless the IV route is required (Table 92–5). Asexual parasites should be eradicated from the blood within 4 to 5 days of starting treatment; persistence implies treatment failure. Gametocytes may persist in the blood for weeks after successful treatment.

Complicated P. *falciparum* Infections. Any of the indicators of severe disease (Table 92–2) is sufficient to place a patient in the category of "severe and complicated malaria," and mandates administration of IV antimalarial drugs (Table 92–5). Patients can deteriorate and new complications can develop rapidly even after treatment has started, so continued close observations of renal, pulmonary, glycemic, acid-base, hematologic, and neurologic status are important.

Quinine. IV quinine is the drug of choice, unless an artemisinin is available. When given parenterally, a loading dose of 20 mg/kg of quinine dihydrochloride is diluted and administered slowly over 3 to 4 hours. Maintenance doses of 10 mg/kg are given every 8 to 12 hours, each being administered over 2 to 3 hours (Table 92–6). The volume of the infusate can be calibrated to the patient's hydration status; normal saline, with 5 or 10% dextrose, or half-strength Darrow's/5% dextrose are all satisfactory infusion fluids. In settings where IV infusions are not possible, IM injections of quinine (diluted 1:3 to 1:5) have been safe and effective. Therapeutic plasma concentrations of quinine are achieved during the initial loading dose and can be maintained with the regimen outlined above. Little is known, however, about the relative sensitivities of parasites from different regions. It is possible that lower doses might be sufficient in certain parts of the world. However, few adverse effects have been attributed to the quinine regimen described above; it seems reasonably safe, particularly when compared with the dangers of an inadequately treated falciparum infection.

Once the patient has improved and can take medications by mouth, oral formulations of quinine can be given for a total of 7 days. Many patients prefer to take a single dose of sulfadoxine-pyrimethamine, and this, too, is acceptable, providing that the local parasites are sensitive to this combination.

Quinidine. When quinine is not available to treat severe and complicated *P. falciparum* malaria, quinidine is an acceptable alternative (Table 92–6). A loading dose of quinidine gluconate, 15 mg/kg, infused over 4 hours is followed by 7.5 mg/kg over 4 hours, at 8-hour intervals. Continuous electrocardiographic monitoring is advised, with particular attention paid to QT interval prolongation. Indications for temporarily slowing or stopping quinidine include a QT interval >0.6 second, a QRS complex wider than 50% of baseline, hypotension unresponsive to fluid challenge, or a serum quinidine level above 7 μg/L (21 μmol/L).

Chloroquine. Chloroquine dihydrochloride may be used parenterally to treat infections from the few remaining areas where *P. falciparum* isolates are known to be sensitive to this drug (Table 92–6). If close monitoring is possible, chloroquine (10 mg base/kg) can be infused intravenously over 8 hours, followed by a constant rate infusion of 15 mg base/kg over 24 hours. Alternatively, when possible, a continuous rate infusion of 0.83 mg base/kg/hr for 30 hours can be given. In more remote settings, chloroquine can be given as IM or subcutaneous injections (3.5 mg base/kg every 6 hours or 2.5 mg base/kg every 4 hours for a total dose of 25 mg base/kg, respectively). Chloroquine is well absorbed from the gastrointestinal tract, even in comatose patients; so if necessary, it can be given by nasogastric tube.

Supportive Care. Serial assessments of the organ systems prone to malaria complications allow any developing complications to be addressed quickly. Accordingly, repeated measures of blood glucose, lactate, and pH are necessary to monitor these metabolic variables. Hypoglycemia can be treated with IV infusions of 50% dextrose; whether acidosis requires specific treatment is an open question at present, but acidosis per se is very strongly associated with disease severity and as such, is a useful indicator of clinical status. Pulmonary status can be assessed by physical examination, the patient's subjective sense of dyspnea, pulse oximetry, chest x-rays, and blood gases. Frequent neurologic examinations and use of a numeric coma score (Table 92–3) are helpful in following neurologic status. The renal system can be monitored by following urinary output, blood urea nitrogen, and creatinine concentrations. Serial blood counts can observe the evolution of the inevitable anemia and the thrombocytopenia that occurs in more severe malaria. Vigorous supportive care should be instituted when necessary, because many of the deteriorations seen in malaria patients are reversible. The need for blood transfusion should be determined on clinical grounds. Treatment of the rare coagulopathy is controversial.

In hyperparasitemic (>5% of red cells parasitized) patients, exchange blood transfusion has been successful. A proportion of the patient's PRBC are removed and replaced with uninfected red blood cells. This therapeutic approach is often impractical in malaria endemic areas since the medical expertise and equipment required to prepare the blood and to monitor the fluid and electrolyte status of the patient is often not available. Exchange transfusion has not been subjected to a prospective trial but has proven effective in severely ill patients.

TREATMENT OF MALARIA DUE TO P. vivax, P. ovale, AND P. malariae. Chloroquine-resistant *P. vivax* has recently been reported from Papua New Guinea, the Solomon Islands, Indonesia, Brazil, and Colombia (Chapter 149); but in general, these species are sensitive to chloroquine and most patients can be treated with oral preparations as outpatients (Table 92–5). The clinical response is generally rapid. Quinine or sulfadoxine-pyrimethamine have been used successfully to treat patients with chloroquine-resistant vivax infections.

Patients with *P. vivax* and *P. ovale* infections transmitted by mosquitoes should be given primaquine to prevent relapses from persistent exoerythrocytic stages in the liver (Table 92–5). Resistance to terminal prophylaxis with primaquine is widespread in strains of *P. vivax* from the western Pacific and Southeast Asia and it has been reported from Somalia and Central America. Primaquine has no effect on the erythrocytic stages. It can cause hemolytic anemia in individuals with G6PD deficiency (Chapter 6). At standard doses, hemolysis is usually subclinical in blacks with G6PD deficiency because the destruction is limited to older red cells. Patients with the more severe Mediterranean and Canton variants of G6PD deficiency should be treated with chloroquine for each relapse. The incidence of side effects is lower with weekly, compared to daily, dosages. Primaquine is not required for *P. malariae* and *P. falciparum* infections because these species do not have hypnozoite stages. In addition, patients infected with *P. vivax* and *P. ovale* congenitally or by direct blood inoculation do not require primaquine since they do not have exoerythrocytic stages of these parasites.

TREATMENT OF MALARIA WHEN SPECIES AND/OR EXPOSURE AREA IS UNKNOWN. If the species of malaria parasite is unknown, or cannot be rapidly and reliably determined, or if its likely origin is not known, the patient should be treated as though he or she is infected with multidrug-resistant *P. falciparum* (Table 92–5).

TREATMENT OF MIXED INFECTIONS. In mixed infections, therapy for *P. falciparum* should be initiated first; the other species can then be treated as necessary (Table 92–5).

TREATMENT OF MALARIA IN CHILDREN. In general, the treatment of malaria infections in children is essentially the same as that for adults (Table 92–5). The diagnosis can be difficult as the disease resembles other common pediatric infections. Children may have salicylate poisoning, which contributes to the development of metabolic acidosis and hypoglycemia as well as severe malaria. Malaria often presents as a medical emergency, especially in endemic areas when travel to a health care facility is difficult and time-

TABLE 92–6. Dosages for Antimalarial Drugs

Drug	Adult Dose				Pediatric Dose			
	Treatment	Route	Prophylaxis[a]	Route	Treatment	Route	Prophylaxis[a]	Route
Amodiaquine dihydrochloride[b]	600 mg of *base* initially, then either 400 mg of *base* at 24 and 48 hr, or 300 mg of *base* at 6, 24, and 48 hr	PO	see text		10 mg/kg of *base* initially, then 5 mg/kg of *base* at 6, 24, and 48 hr	PO	see text	PO
Artemisinin derivatives	Artemether, 3.2 mg/kg, then 1.6 mg/kg at 24-hr intervals for 5 days	IM	not indicated		as for adults			
	or							
	Artesunate, 2 mg/kg, then 1 mg/kg at 4 hr and 24 hr, then 1 mg/kg daily, total of 7 days	IV	not indicated		as for adults			
	or							
	Artesunate, 5 mg/kg on day 1, followed by 2.5 mg/kg on days 2 and 3 in combination with mefloquine (15–25 mg/kg) on day 2	PO	not indicated		as for adults			
Chloroquine phosphate *or* Chloroquine sulfate *or* Hydroxychloroquine sulfate	600 mg of *base* initially, then 300 mg of *base* at 6, 24, and 48 hr	PO	300 mg of *base* weekly (heavier individuals could be given drug every 5 or 6 days)	PO	10 mg/kg of *base* initially, then 5 mg/kg of *base* at 6, 24, and 48 hr	PO	5 mg/kg of *base* weekly	PO
Chloroquine dihydrochloride	300 mg of *base* every 8 to 12 hr	IM	not indicated		3.5 mg/kg of *base* every 6 hr,[d] to total of 25 mg/kg	IM or SC	not indicated	
Doxycycline	100 mg twice daily for 7 days	PO	100 mg once daily	PO	2 mg/kg twice daily for 7 days	PO	2 mg/kg once daily for those >8 yr of age	PO
Halofantrine	500 mg every 6 hr for 3 doses; repeat in 7 days	PO	not indicated		8 mg/kg every 6 hr for 3 doses; repeat in 7 days	PO	not indicated	
Mefloquine	750 to 1250 mg in a single dose	PO	250 mg weekly	PO	15 mg/kg in a single dose	PO	<1 yr = 31 mg 1–4 yr = 62 mg 5–12 yr = 125 mg (all given weekly)	PO
Pyrimethamine-sulfadoxine	3 tablets in a single dose (each tablet contains 25 mg of pyrimethamine plus 500 mg of sulfadoxine)	PO	see text		0.5–4 yr = ½ tablet 5–8 yr = 1 tablet 9–14 yr = 2 tablets (in a single dose)	PO	see text	

Drug	Treatment (Adult)	Prophylaxis (Adult)	Treatment (Pediatric)	Prophylaxis (Pediatric)
Pyrimethamine-sulfalene	PO — 3 tablets in a single dose (each tablet contains 25 mg of pyrimethamine plus 500 mg of sulfalene)	PO — see text	PO — as with pyrimethamine-sulfadoxine	PO — see text
Primaquine	PO — 15 mg of *base* daily for 14 days *or* 45 mg of *base* weekly for 8 wk	PO — as in treatment[f]	PO — 0.25 mg/kg of *base* daily for 14 days *or* 0.75 mg/kg of *base* weekly for 8 weeks	PO — as in treatment[f]
Proguanil	not indicated	PO — 200 mg daily	not indicated	PO — <2 yr = 50 mg daily; 2–6 yr = 100 mg daily; 7–10 yr = 150 mg daily; >10 yr = 200 mg daily
Quinidine sulfate *or* Quinidine gluconate	PO — 600–650 mg of base 3 times daily for 3 to 7 days[g]	not indicated	PO — 10 mg/kg 3 times daily for 3 to 7 days[g]	not indicated
Quinidine gluconate	IV — 10–15 mg/kg (salt) loading dose in 500 mL of isotonic saline with glucose over 1–2 hr; then 1.0 to 1.5 mg/kg per hr by constant infusion for a maximum of 72 hr[d]	IV — not indicated	IV — same as adult dose	IV — not indicated
Quinine dihydrochloride	IV — 20 mg/kg over 4 hr, followed by 10 mg/kg every 8–12 hr[d]	IV — not indicated	IV — 20 mg/kg over 4 hr, followed by 10 mg/kg every 8–12 hr[d]	IV — not indicated
Quinine sulfate	PO — 650 mg 3 times daily for 3 to 7 days[g]	PO — not indicated	PO — 10 mg/kg 3 times daily for 3 to 7 days[g]	PO — not indicated
Tetracycline	PO — 250 or 500 mg 4 times daily for 7 days[e]	PO — not indicated	PO — 10 mg/kg 4 times daily for 7 days[e]	PO — not indicated

[a] Except for primaquine, chemoprophylactic regimens are begun prior to entering, continued during, and for 4 weeks after leaving a malarious area. The drug should be taken on the same day each week.

[b] Amodiaquine dosage varies because some tablets contain 150 mg of *base* and others 200 mg of *base*.

[c] Dose for 4-aminoquinolines, amodiaquine, and chloroquine is expressed as *base*, not the salt. Ensure that correct amount of *base* is given.

[d] Switch to oral medication as soon as possible. Reduce dose by one third if used parenterally for more than 72 hours. Parenteral chloroquine may be given with care intramuscularly, subcutaneously, or intravenously by slow constant infusion (see text).

[e] Tetracyclines should be used only in combination with quinine or quinidine to treat severe *P. falciparum* infections in those ≥8 years of age who were infected in areas where resistance to both chloroquine and pyrimethamine-sulfadoxine is present. They are toxic to younger children.

[f] Terminal prophylaxis with primaquine is to be given with last 2 weeks of chemoprophylaxis after leaving the malarious area.

[g] Duration of quinine and quinidine treatment is shorter if they are given with another drug (e.g., doxycycline) or if the patient has partial immunity to malaria. They act rapidly and are administered for initial 2 to 4 days of combined therapy.

consuming. Oral drugs should be used whenever possible; quinine is the drug of choice when parenteral treatment is required; artesunate suppositories can be used in severely ill children whenever appropriate parenteral therapy is not available. Doses can be calculated quickly and safely on body weight.

Chemoprophylaxis

This is given to nonimmune persons entering malaria-endemic areas. Anyone traveling to malarious areas, even for brief visits, is at risk of acquiring malaria. Chemoprophylaxis reduces but does not totally prevent this risk. For this reason, travelers and others at risk of contracting malaria should be encouraged to carry with them effective treatment for malaria. If symptoms develop in a setting where diagnostic and treatment facilities are lacking, effective antimalarial chemotherapy can be started without delay. The choice of the optimal "standby" drug depends on local parasite drug sensitivities. Chemoprophylaxis may also be appropriate for certain high-risk groups living in endemic areas, e.g., infants, young children, and pregnant women.

Drug prophylaxis does not prevent infection, but aborts or modifies the clinical attack. Thus, an individual may acquire malaria even if he or she is following a recommended regimen. If taken for a sufficient period of time after the individual leaves an endemic area, chemoprophylaxis may produce, in effect, a radical cure, because the medication exhausts the duration of the exoerythrocytic stage of the malaria parasite.

Selection of a particular drug for chemoprophylaxis depends on the distribution and intensity of transmission, the pattern of drug resistance, and the planned duration of residence in the area. Special problems include prophylaxis for infants, very young children, and pregnant women and the balance between short-term individual protection and long-term community welfare.

AREAS WHERE ONLY CHLOROQUINE-SENSITIVE MALARIA IS PRESENT

Suppressive Prophylaxis. Chloroquine phosphate is highly effective for suppression of infections caused by *P. vivax* (most strains), *P. ovale*, and *P. malariae*, and chloroquine-sensitive strains of *P. falciparum*. Administration should be initiated before entering a malarious area and should be continued for 6 weeks after leaving the area (Table 92–6).

Chloroquine can cause ophthalmic toxicity. Severe, irreversible retinopathy has been described in individuals taking high daily doses for prolonged periods for treatment of non-parasitic diseases. However, a large number of people have used chloroquine as malaria chemoprophylaxis for many years without complication. Periodic ophthalmologic examinations have been advised after a total cumulative chloroquine dose exceeding 100 g of base, which would be attained after 6.5 years of prophylaxis at the recommended dose. Chloroquine is safe in pregnancy and for young children. Alternative drugs are the antifolates, proguanil or pyrimethamine (Table 92–6). These drugs have no significant toxicity in prophylactic doses, but their use is limited by the high incidence of parasite resistance to them.

Terminal Prophylaxis. Relapses of *P. vivax* and *P. ovale* infections can be prevented by single daily doses of primaquine during the last 2 weeks of, or just following, a course of suppressive therapy with chloroquine or a comparable drug (Table 92–6). Primaquine should be given for terminal prophylaxis only after the individual has left the endemic area. Terminal prophylaxis with primaquine is not indicated for all travelers. The decision should be made on an individual basis, taking into account the intensity and duration of the exposure to *P. vivax* and *P. ovale* and the patient's G6PD status.

AREAS WHERE CHLOROQUINE-RESISTANT STRAINS OF *P. falciparum* ARE PRESENT. For suppression of chloroquine-resistant *P. falciparum* malaria in adults, the recommended drug is mefloquine, 250 mg (one tablet) weekly. Alternatives are doxycycline, 100 mg daily, or the combination of chloroquine, 300 mg base weekly, and proguanil, 200 mg daily (Table 92–6).

■ PREVENTION AND CONTROL

FOR INDIVIDUALS. There is no single method to prevent malaria infection. However, a number of precautions can be taken to reduce the risk. Malaria transmission usually occurs between dusk and dawn. The chance of being infected is reduced by remaining in well-screened areas during these hours and by sleeping under mosquito netting. A very effective means of preventing malaria infection is to sleep under a bednet that has been dipped in pyrethroids (e.g., permethrin). Outdoor exposure to mosquito bites can be reduced by wearing clothing that covers the arms and legs and by applying mosquito repellent to thick clothing and exposed areas of the skin. The most effective repellents are *N,N*, diethyltoluamide (DEET) and dimethylphthalate (DIMP), ingredients in many commercially available insect repellents.

FOR POPULATIONS. During the 1970s, following the failed attempt at malaria eradication, the WHO adopted a revised strategy of malaria control based on a realistic assessment of an individual country's epidemiologic conditions and potential for effective control. Unlike eradication, a malaria control program is of indefinite duration and has recurring costs. It attempts to reduce, not eliminate, transmission. An integrated control program involves the simultaneous use of several control methods based on the epidemiologic characteristics of transmission in the area involved and the availability of resources.

Insecticide-Impregnated Mosquito Nets. This intervention, which reduces transmission by erecting a barrier that simultaneously protects humans from mosquitoes and exposes mosquitoes to a potent insecticide, has been evaluated in a number of different epidemiologic settings and has been effective in reducing not only malaria-associated morbidity, but all-cause mortality in children as well. It has a greater effect on reducing malaria disease than on reducing malaria infection. Thus, community prevalence of malaria infection may remain unchanged while fewer children are becoming sick and dying from malaria. Its effectiveness when applied as a means for controlling malaria in communities is likely to be different than efficacy measures made during the course of clinical trials. There have as yet been no definitive studies on the effect of impregnated mosquito nets on the acquisition of antimalarial immunity, and this is an important question; merely postponing malaria mortality would not be desirable.

Use of bednets treated with a biodegradable pyrethroid insecticide for reducing malaria morbidity and mortality is very cost effective. WHO estimates a program to purchase and distribute nets (at US$5 each) and insecticide (annual cost of US$0.5 to 1.0) would cost as little as US$10 to 20 per year of life saved.

MEASURES FOR PREVENTION OF MALARIA IN INDIVIDUALS AND FOR LARGE-SCALE CONTROL OF DISEASE. These measures can be divided according to a modified classification of that proposed by Russell in 1952:

1. Measures to prevent mosquitoes from feeding on humans (insecticide-treated nets, protective clothing, repellents, screening, appropriate housing construction style and sites).

2. Measures to prevent or reduce the breeding of mosquitoes by eliminating collections of water or altering the

environment at breeding sites (source reduction, drainage, filling).

3. Measures to destroy mosquito larvae (larvicides, larvicidal oil, increasing or decreasing the degree of salinity, shading, introduction of pathogens or predators).
4. Measures to destroy adult mosquitoes (residual and space spray insecticides, use of insecticide-treated bednets, release of genetically altered mosquitoes).
5. Measures to eliminate the malaria parasites in the human host or to prevent transmission to mosquitoes (mass drug therapy campaigns, diagnosis and early treatment of cases, therapy based on symptoms, use of gametocidal and sporontocidal drugs).
6. Measures to protect the susceptible host (chemoprophylaxis, immunoprophylaxis).

Malaria control should integrate available technology with knowledge about the epidemiology of each area, and should include the capacity to evaluate the impact of various interventions on the local malaria threat.

MALARIA IMMUNIZATION. This is discussed in the Immune Response section.

Bibliography

General

Facer CA, Playfair JHL: Malaria, Epstein-Barr virus and the genesis of lymphomas. Adv Cancer Res 53:33, 1989.
Giles HM, Warrell DA: Bruce-Chwatt's Essential Malariology, 3rd ed. Boston, Little Brown, 1993.
Olliaro P, Cattani J, Wirth D: Malaria, the submerged disease. JAMA 275:230, 1996.
Strickland GT, Hoffman SL: Strategies for the control of malaria. Scient Am Sci Med 1:24, 1994.
Wallace MR, Sharp TW, Smoak B, et al: Malaria among United States troops in Somalia. Am J Med 100:49, 1996.

Ecology and Epidemiology

Greenwood BM, Bradley AK, Greenwood AM, et al: Mortality and morbidity from malaria among children in a rural area of The Gambia, West Africa. Trans R Soc Trop Med Hyg 81:478, 1987.
Krotoski WA, Bray RS, Garnham PCC, et al: Observations on early and late post-sporozoite tissue stages in primate malaria. I. Discovery of a new latent form of Plasmodium cynomolgi (the hypnozoite), and failure to detect hepatic forms within the first 24 hours after infection. Am J Trop Med Hyg 21:24, 1982.
Miller LH, Mason SJ, Clyde DR, et al: The resistance factor to Plasmodium vivax in blacks: The Duffy-blood group genotype, FyFy. N Engl J Med 295:302, 1976.
Zucker JR: Changing patterns of autochthonous malaria transmission in the United States: A review of recent outbreaks. Emerg Infect Dis 2:37, 1996.

Pathophysiology

Brooks MH, Malloy JP, Bartelloni PJ, et al: Pathophysiology of acute malaria. 1. Correlation of clinical and biochemical abnormalities. Am J Med 43:735, 1967.
Clark IA, Rockett KA, Cowden WB: Proposed link between cytokines, nitric oxide and human cerebral malaria. Parasitol Today 7:205, 1991.
English M, Waruiru C, Amukoye E, et al: Deep breathing in children with severe malaria: Indicator of metabolic acidosis and poor outcome. Am J Trop Med Hyg 55:521, 1996.
Fried M, Duffy PE: Adherence of Plasmodium falciparum to chondroitin sulfate A in the human placenta. Science 272:1502, 1996.
Grau GE, Taylor TE, Molyneux ME, et al: Tumor necrosis factor and disease severity in children with falciparum malaria. N Engl J Med 320:1586, 1989.
Hill AVS, Elvin J, Willis AC, et al: Molecular analysis of the association of HLA-B53 and resistance to severe malaria. Nature 360:434, 1992.
Holst FGE, Hmeer CJ, Kern P, Dietrich M: Inappropriate secretion of antidiuretic hormone and hyponatremia in severe falciparum malaria. Am J Trop Med Hyg 50:602, 1994.
Kremnser PG, Winkler S, Wildling E, et al: High levels of nitrogen oxides are associated with severe disease and correlate with rapid parasitological and clinical cure in Plasmodium falciparum malaria. Trans R Soc Trop Med Hyg 90:44, 1996.
Krishna S, Waller DW, ter Kuile F, et al: Lactic acidosis and hypoglycaemia in children with severe malaria: Pathophysiological and prognostic significance. Trans R Soc Trop Med Hyg 88:67, 1994.

Lam KMC, Syed N, Whittle H, Crawford DH: Circulating Epstein-Barr virus–carrying B cells in adult malaria. Lancet 337:876, 1991.
Larkin GL, Thuma PE: Congenital malaria in a hyperendemic area. Am J Trop Med Hyg 45:587, 1991.
Looareesuwan S, Davis TME, Pukrittayakamee S, et al: Erythrocyte survival in severe falciparum malaria. Acta Trop 48:263, 1991.
Luzzatto L: Genetics of red cells and susceptibility to malaria. Blood 54:961, 1979.
MacPherson GG, Warrell MJ, White NJ: Human cerebral malaria: A quantitative ultrastructural analysis of parasitized erythrocyte sequestration. Am J Pathol 119:385, 1985.
Miller LH, Good MF, Milon G: Malaria pathogenesis. Science 264:1878, 1994.
Molyneux ME, Looareesuwan S, Menzies IS, et al: Reduced hepatic blood flow and intestinal malabsorption in severe falciparum malaria. Am J Trop Med Hyg 40:470, 1989.
Newton CRJC, Kirkham FJ, Winstanley PA, et al: Intracranial pressure in African children with cerebral malaria. Lancet 337:573, 1991.
Newton CRJC, Peshu N, Kendall B, et al: Brain swelling and ischaemia in Kenyans with cerebral malaria. Arch Dis Child 70:281, 1990.
Phillips RE, Looareesuwan S, Warrell DA, et al: The importance of anaemia in cerebral and uncomplicated falciparum malaria: Role of complications, dyserythropoiesis and iron sequestration. Am J Med 58:305, 1986.
Turner GDH, Morrison H, Jones M, et al: An immunohistochemical study of the pathology of fatal malaria. Am J Pathol 145:1057, 1994.

Clinical Manifestations

English MC, Waruiru C, Lightowler C, et al: Hyponatremia and dehydration in severe malaria. Arch Dis Child 74:201, 1996.
Hulbert TV: Congenital malaria in the United States: Report of a case and review. Clin Infect Dis 14:922, 1992.
Karney WW, Tong MJ: Malabsorption in Plasmodium falciparum malaria. Am J Trop Med Hyg 21:1, 1972.
Marsh K, Forster D, Waruiru C, et al: Indicators of life-threatening malaria in African children. N Engl J Med 332:1399, 1995.
Molyneux ME, Taylor TE, Wirima JJ, Borgstein A: Clinical features and prognostic indicators in pediatric cerebral malaria: A study of 131 comatose Malawian children. Q J Med 71:441, 1989.
Taylor TE, Molyneux ME, Wirima JJ, et al: Blood glucose levels in Malawian children before and during the administration of intravenous quinine for severe falciparum malaria. N Engl J Med 319:1040, 1988.
Taylor TE, Borgstein A, Molyneux ME: Acid-base status in paediatric Plasmodium falciparum malaria. Q J Med 86:99, 1993.
Waller D, Krishna S, Crawley J, et al: Clinical features and outcome of severe malaria in Gambian children. Clin Infect Dis 21:577, 1995.
White NJ, Miller KD, Marsh K, et al: Hypoglycemia in African children with severe malaria. Lancet 1:708, 1987.
White NJ, Warrell DA, Chanthavanich P, et al: Severe hypoglycemia and hyperinsulinemia in falciparum malaria. N Engl J Med 309:61, 1983.
World Health Organization: Severe and complicated malaria. Trans R Soc Trop Med Hyg 80 (Suppl 2):1, 1990.

Chronic Manifestations

Bates I, Bedu-Addo G, Bevan DH, Rutherford TR: Use of immunoglobulin gene arrangements to show clonal lymphoproliferation in hyper-reactive malarial splenomegaly. Lancet 337:505, 1991.
Bottius E, Guanqirolli A, Trape J-F, et al: Malaria: Even more chronic in nature than previously thought; evidence for subpatent parasitemia detectable by the polymerase chain reaction. Trans R Soc Trop Med Hyg 90:15, 1996.
Hendrickse RG, Adeniyi A, Edington GM, et al: Quartan malarial nephrotic syndrome. Lancet 1:1143, 1972.
Hoffman SL, Piessens WF, Ratiwayanto MS, et al: Reduction of suppressor T lymphocytes in the tropical splenomegaly syndrome. N Engl J Med 310:335, 1984.
Nguyen TH, Day NP, Ly VC, et al: Post-malaria neurological syndrome. Lancet 348:917, 1996.
Stuiver PC, Ziegler JL, Wood JB, et al: Clinical trial of malaria prophylaxis in tropical splenomegaly syndrome. Br Med J 1:426, 1971.
Whittle HC, Brown J, Marsh K, et al: T-cell control of Epstein-Barr virus-infected B cells is lost during P. falciparum malaria. Nature 312:448, 1984.
Wing AJ, Hutt MSR, Kibukamusoke JW: Progression and remission in the nephrotic syndrome associated with quartan malaria in Uganda. Q J Med 16:273, 1972.

Diagnosis

Barker RH, Banchongaksorn T, Courval JM: A simple method to detect Plasmodium falciparum directly from blood samples using the polymerase chain reaction. Am J Trop Med Hyg 46:416, 1992.
Beadle C, Long GW, Weiss WR, et al: Diagnosis of malaria by detection of Plasmodium falciparum HRP-2 antigen with a rapid dipstick antigen-capture assay. Lancet 343:564, 1994.
Lowe BS, Jeffa NK, New L, et al: Acridine orange fluorescence techniques as alternatives to traditional Giemsa staining for the diagnosis of malaria in developing countries. Trans R Soc Trop Med Hyg 90:34, 1996.

Clinical Management

Bojang KA, Palmer A, Boele van Hensbroek M, et al: Management of severe malarial anemia in Gambian children. Trans R Soc Trop Med Hyg 91:557, 1977.

English M, Wairuiru C, Marsh K: Transfusion for respiratory distress in life-threatening malaria. Am J Trop Med Hyg 55:525, 1996.

Menendez C, Kahigwa E, Hirt R, et al: Randomised placebo-controlled trial of iron supplementation and malaria chemoprophylaxis for prevention of severe anaemia and malaria in Tanzanian infants. Lancet 350:844, 1997.

Chemotherapy

Bloland PB, Lackritz EM, Kazembe PN, et al: Beyond chloroquine: Implication of drug resistance for evaluating malaria therapy efficacy and treatment policy in Africa. J Infect Dis 167:932, 1993.

Boele van Hensbroek M, Onyiorah E, Jaffar S, et al: A trial of artemether or quinine in children with cerebral malaria. N Engl J Med 335:69, 1996.

Bryson HM, Goa KL: Halofantrine: A review of its antimalarial activity, pharmacokinetic properties and therapeutic potential. Drugs 43:236, 1992.

Hennequin C, Bouree P, Bazin N, et al: Severe psychiatric side effects observed during prophylaxis and treatment with mefloquine. Arch Intern Med 154:2360, 1994.

Hien TT, Day NPJ, Phy NH, et al: A controlled trial of artemether or quinine in Vietnamese adults with severe falciparum malaria. N Engl J Med 335:76, 1996.

Lange WR, Frankenfiled DL, Moriarty-Sheehan M, et al: No evidence for chloroquine-associated retinopathy among missionaries on long-term malaria chemoprophylaxis. Am J Trop Med Hyg 51:389, 1994.

Looareesuwan S, Wilairatana P, Vanijanonta S, Viravan C: Efficacy and tolerability of sequential, artesunate suppository plus mefloquine, treatment of severe falciparum malaria. Ann Trop Med Parasitol 89:469, 1995.

Miller KD, Greenberg AE, Campbell CC, et al: Treatment of severe malaria in the United States with a continuous infusion of quinidine gluconate and exchange transfusion. N Engl J Med 321:65, 1989.

Monlun E, Le Metayer P, Szwandt S, et al: Cardiac complications of halofantrine: A prospective study of 20 patients. Trans R Soc Trop Med Hyg 89:430, 1995.

Muller O, Boele van Hensbroek M, Jaffar S, et al: A randomized trial of chloroquine, amodiaquine and pyrimethamine-sulphadoxine in Gambian children with uncomplicated malaria. Trop Med Int Health 1:124, 1996.

Murphy GS, Basri H, Purnomo, et al: Vivax malaria resistant to treatment and prophylaxis with chloroquine. Lancet 341:96, 1993.

Olliaro P, Nevill C, LeBras J, et al: Systemic review of amodiaquine treatment in uncomplicated malaria. Lancet 348:1196, 1996.

Olliaro PL, Trigg PI: Status of antimalaria drugs under development. Bull WHO 75:565, 1995.

Phillips RE, Warrell DA, White NJ, et al: Intravenous quinidine for the treatment of severe falciparum malaria: Clinical and pharmacokinetic studies. N Engl J Med 312:1273, 1985.

Price RN, Nosten F, Luxemburger C, et al: Artesunate versus artemether in combination with mefloquine for the treatment of multidrug-resistant falciparum malaria. Trans R Soc Trop Med Hyg 89:523, 1995.

Price RN, Nosten F, Luxemberger C, et al: Artesunate/mefloquine treatment of multi-drug resistant falciparum malaria. Trans R Soc Trop Med Hyg 91:574, 1997.

Ringwald P, Bickii J, Basco L: Randomised trial of pyronaridine versus chloroquine for acute uncomplicated falciparum malaria in Africa. Lancet 347:24, 1996.

Riou B, Barriot P, Rimailho A, Baud FJ: Treatment of severe chloroquine poisoning. N Engl J Med 318:1, 1988.

Schapira A, Solomon T, Julien M, et al: Comparison of intramuscular and intravenous quinine for the treatment of severe and complicated malaria in children. Trans R Soc Trop Med Hyg 87:299, 1993.

Smoak BL, DeFraites RF, Magill AJ, et al: Plasmodium vivax infections in U.S. Army troops: Failure of primaquine to prevent relapse in studies from Somalia. Am J Trop Med Hyg 56:231, 1997.

Ter Kuile FO, Nosten F, Luxemburger C, et al: Mefloquine treatment of acute falciparum malaria: A prospective study of non-serious adverse effects in 3673 patients. Bull WHO 73:631, 1995.

Touze JE, Bernard J, Keundjian A, et al: Electrocardiographic changes and halofantrine plasma level during acute falciparum malaria. Am J Trop Med Hyg 54:225, 1996.

Tran TH, Day NP, Nguyen HP, et al: A controlled trial of artemether or quinine in Vietnamese adults with falciparum malaria. N Engl J Med 335:76, 1996.

Watkins WM, Lury JD, Kariuki D, et al: Efficacy of multiple-dose halofantrine in treatment of chloroquine-resistant falciparum malaria in children in Kenya. Lancet 2:247, 1988.

White NJ: The treatment of malaria. N Engl J Med 335:800, 1996.

White NJ, Miller KD, Churchill FC, et al: Chloroquine treatment of severe malaria in children: Pharmacokinetics, toxicity and new dosage recommendations. N Engl J Med 319:1493, 1988.

Winstanley P, Newton C, Watkins W, et al: Toward optimal regimens of parenteral quinine for young African children with cerebral malaria: The importance of unbound quinine concentrations. Trans R Soc Trop Med Hyg 87:201, 1993.

Prevention and Control

Alonso P, Linsay SW, Armstrong JRM, et al: The effect of insecticide-treated bed nets on mortality in Gambian children. Lancet 337:1499, 1991.

Beck HP, Feiger I, Huber W, et al: Analysis of multiple Plasmodium falciparum infections in Tanzanian children during the phase III trial of the malaria vaccine SPf66. J Infect Dis 175:921, 1997.

Binka FN, Kubaje A, Adjuik M, et al: Impact of permethrin impregnated bednets on child mortality in Kassena-Nankana district, Ghana: A randomized controlled trial. Trop Med Int Health 1:147, 1996.

D'Allesandro U, Olaleye BO, McGuire W, et al: Mortality and morbidity from malaria in Gambian children after introduction of an impregnated bednet programme. Lancet 345:479, 1995.

Hoffman SL, Wistar R, Ballou WR, et al: Immunity to malaria and naturally acquired antibodies to the circumsporozoite protein of Plasmodium falciparum. N Engl J Med 315:601, 1986.

Kroeger A, Mancheno N, Alarcon J, Pesse K: Insecticide-impregnated bed nets for malaria control: Varying experiences from Ecuador, Colombia, and Peru concerning acceptability and effectiveness. Am J Trop Med Hyg 53:313, 1995.

Lobel HO, Miani M, Eng T, et al: Long-term malaria prophylaxis with weekly mefloquine. Lancet 341:848, 1993.

Nevill CG, Some ES, Mung'ala VO, et al: Insecticide-treated bednets reduce mortality and severe morbidity from malaria among children on the Kenyan coast. Trop Med Int Health 1:139, 1996.

Nosten F, Luxemburger C, Kyle DE, et al: Randomised double-blind placebo-controlled trial of SPf66 malaria vaccine in children in northwestern Thailand. Lancet 348:701, 1996.

Price RN, Nosten F, Luxemburger C, et al: Effects of artemisinin derivatives on malaria transmissibility. Lancet 447:1654, 1996.

Snow RW, Rowan KM, Greenwood BM, et al: A trial of permethrin treated bednets in the prevention of malaria in Gambian children. Trans R Soc Trop Med Hyg 81:563, 1987.

Steffen R, Fuchs E, Schildknecht J, et al: Mefloquine compared with other malaria chemoprophylaxis regimens in tourists visiting East Africa. Lancet 341:1299, 1993.

93 African Trypanosomiasis

Jacques Pépin

DEFINITION. Members of the family Trypanosomatidae, genus *Trypanosoma*, include the etiologic agents of American trypanosomiasis (Chagas disease), endemic in Central and South America, and of human African trypanosomiasis (HAT), also known as *sleeping sickness*, endemic in sub-Saharan Africa. *Trypanosoma brucei gambiense* and *Trypanosoma brucei rhodesiense* are the etiologic agents of HAT. These morphologically identical subspecies, cyclically transmitted by various species of tsetse flies, cause, respectively, Gambian and Rhodesian HAT (Table 93–1). A third subspecies, *Trypanosoma brucei brucei*, can infect only animals. HAT is an acute (*rhodesiense*) or chronic (*gambiense*) disease characterized by an early stage lasting weeks (*rhodesiense*) or months (*gambiense*), during which trypanosomes are found in the blood and/or lymph node aspirates of patients with nonspecific symptoms, followed by a late stage of central nervous system (CNS) invasion lasting weeks (*rhodesiense*) or months (*gambiense*) when trypanosomes are found in the cerebrospinal fluid (CSF) of patients with neurologic symptoms, mostly somnolence progressing, if untreated, to coma and death.

HISTORY. In 1880, Griffith Evans discovered that trypanosomes might be pathogens by finding them in the blood of animals. Fifteen years later, David Bruce showed that trypanosomes caused the cattle disease *nagana*. The new species was named *T. brucei* a few years later. The first scientific evidence of human trypanosomiasis came in 1902, when Dutton and Forde recognized trypanosomes in the blood of a British sailor returning from The Gambia, hence the name *T. gambiense*.

The etiology of sleeping sickness had been under investiga-

TABLE 93–1. Differences Between Gambian and Rhodesian Sleeping Sickness

	Gambian	Rhodesian
Agent	*T. b. gambiense*	*T. b. rhodesiense*
Main vectors	*G. palpalis* group (riverine tsetse)	*G. morsitans* (savanna tsetse)
Distribution	Western and central Africa	Eastern and southern Africa
Highest incidence countries	The Congo, Angola, Sudan, Uganda, Congo-Brazaville	Uganda, Tanzania, Mozambique, Zambia
Location	Around water holes and rivers	Savanna, recently cleared bush
Main reservoir	Humans	Antelope and cattle
Disease	Chronic, late CNS invasion	Acute, early CNS invasion
Duration	Months to years	Weeks to months
Parasitemia	Low	High
Diagnosis	Lymph node aspirate, CSF examination	Peripheral blood examination, CSF examination
Serology	CATT	None
Treatment		
Early stage	Pentamidine	Suramin
Late stage	Melarsoprol or eflornithine	Melarsoprol
Late stage, relapses	Eflornithine	Melarsoprol
Control	Active case finding	Tsetse trapping

CNS, central nervous system; CSF, cerebrospinal fluid; CATT, Card Agglutination Test for Trypanosomiasis.

tion for a few years when Castellani, in 1903, documented the presence of trypanosomes in the CSF of patients in Uganda. In 1909, Kleine proved that trypanosomes had to undergo a cycle of development in the tsetse fly vector to be infective. The following year, Stephens and Fantham identified *T. rhodesiense* as a separate species on the basis of higher parasitemias, the occurrence of posteronuclear forms, and a more acute infection in humans.

When Europeans began to penetrate inland Africa in the late 19th century, huge epidemics of sleeping sickness, to a large extent caused by population migrations, devastated many regions of the continent and were a major obstacle to the exploitation of Africa's resources. An epidemic in the Congo between 1896 and 1906 was said to have killed 500,000 people; another one in Uganda, along the shores of Lake Victoria, killed two thirds of the population. Institutes of tropical medicine were created to overcome this problem.

After the cause of sleeping sickness was identified, research focused on treatment, and Paul Erlich made major contributions. In the early 1940s, Ernst Friedheim, a physician and chemist, developed melarsoprol, from its synthesis to clinical trials in Africa.

Trypanosomiasis control was the first large-scale public health intervention in Africa. The concept of mobile teams, specialized in HAT case finding and treatment, was first developed in Cameroon by Jamot in the 1920s and rapidly adopted by other endemic countries. At that time, many African countries reported tens of thousands of cases per year, and in some regions HAT caused almost half of the overall mortality. Mobile teams proved highly successful, with important reductions in incidence during the next few decades, effectively complemented by massive campaigns of pentamidine chemoprophylaxis after World War II.

Today, the importance of HAT as a public health issue

lies not in its annual incidence but in the potential for the development of explosive epidemics where case finding is neglected, as in Uganda in the 1970s and in The Congo currently. Trypanosomiasis in cattle has been a major obstacle to economic development in Africa but may at the same time provide some protection for the environment.

BIOLOGY. Trypanosomes are digenetic parasites whose life cycle involves two hosts: a definitive mammalian host and an intermediate arthropod host, the vector that transmits the infection to a new vertebrate.

Parasitic Stages. Normally, the blood stream forms ingested by the vector while feeding undergo a cycle of development in the intermediate host. The cycle culminates in the production of infective forms, the metacyclic trypanosomes, which then can be transmitted to a new mammalian host during the vector's next blood meal.

Classification and Structure. Trypanosomes have been classified according to the localization of their development in the vector and other characteristics. The subgenus *Trypanozoon* includes the human-infecting polymorphic salivarian species, whose developmental cycle in the tsetse fly vector is completed in the salivary glands and whose transmission is by inoculation through the hypopharynx. Because it is unclear if the two agents of HAT are in fact different species, they are often considered as nosodemes of the "*brucei* complex" and referred to as the subspecies *T. brucei gambiense* and *T. brucei rhodesiense*. The third morphologically identical subspecies of the *brucei* complex, *T. brucei brucei*, causes the animal disease nagana but is not pathogenic for humans because it is destroyed by a lytic factor shown to consist of two lipoproteins: a human haptoglobin-related protein and paraoxonase-arylesterase. Trypanosomes are characterized at some stage in their life cycle by the presence of a free flagellum arising from the kinetoplast, an organelle containing DNA and associated with the mitochondrion. During development, these organisms multiply and pass through a number of different stages (Fig. 93–1) in which they resemble

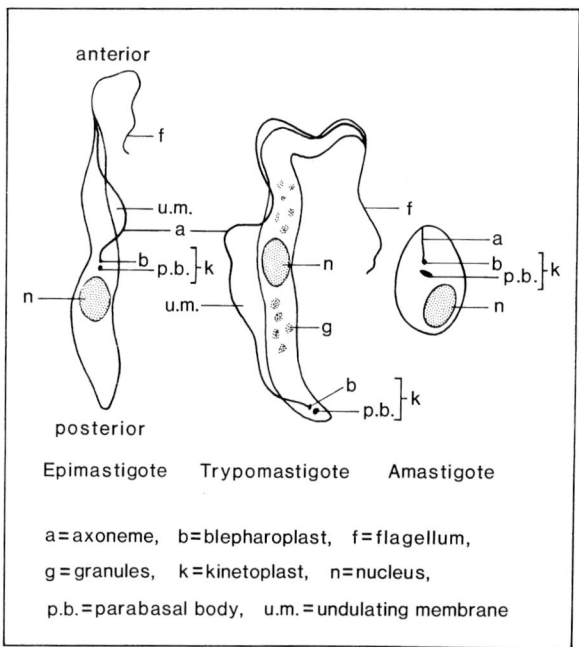

Figure **93–1.** Morphologic stages of trypanosomes. Amastigote stage does not occur in African trypanosomiasis. (Modified from Ash LR, Orihel TC: Atlas of Human Parasitology, 2nd ed. Chicago, American Society of Clinical Pathologists, 1984.)

other genera of the family, e.g., *Leishmania*. The flagellum and undulating membrane give motility to trypanosomes, and locomotion is usually in the direction of the free flagellum. Multiplication occurs by longitudinal binary fission. The kinetoplast and the nucleus divide before the cytoplasm. The flagellum does not divide, but a new one rapidly develops from the new kinetoplast.

Epimastigote. This stage occurs in the insect vector. This form is slender and elongated and has a central vesicular nucleus. The kinetoplast is close but anterior to the nucleus. The flagellum passes along the border of a short, undulating membrane to the anterior end of the parasite, where it becomes free. The epimastigote is not infective for humans but changes in the anterior or posterior station to infective, metacyclic trypanosome, which is short and stumpy and has a centrally placed nucleus and a posterior kinetoplast. It is considered a form of young trypomastigote.

Trypomastigote. This stage is the long, slender form (17 to 30 μm in length) found in the blood of mammalian hosts. The nucleus is centrally located, and the kinetoplast is subterminal. The flagellum initially is contiguous to the body of the parasite and helps to form the undulating membrane. The free flagellum lies anteriorly. Polymorphic trypomastigotes may be present, particularly associated with high parasitemia. These forms exhibit morphologic differences and vary with respect to size, position of the nucleus, and length of the flagellum. The slender form actively divides every 5 to 10 hours, whereas the shorter, stumpy form does not divide but is more infective to the vector. Unlike *T. cruzi*, the etiologic agent of American trypanosomiasis, *T. b. rhodesiense* and *T. b. gambiense* have no amastigote intracellular stage.

Life Cycle. The trypanosomes are transmitted cyclically by blood-sucking flies of the genus *Glossina* (Fig. 93–2). Trypomastigotes are ingested during the blood meal. In the midgut of the fly, the ingested blood forms lose their surface antigenic coat and begin to multiply. Long, slender forms are produced and move to the salivary glands and form epimastigotes. In turn, these epimastigotes change into short, stumpy, infective, metacyclic trypanosomes, which enter the bite wound through the hypopharynx. Flies become infective 18 to 35 days after feeding on an infected host, depending on temperature and humidity. The intratsetse cycle is complex and is completed probably <10% of the time. Congenital transmission has been reported with *T. b. gambiense* but is rare. Transmission through blood transfusions is even more unusual.

VECTOR. The genus *Glossina* (Fig. 93–3) contains more than 22 species of tsetse fly, all restricted to Africa, of which only a few are important in the transmission of sleeping sickness. Both sexes feed on mammalian blood and inflict painful bites. Tsetse flies are viviparous and produce mature larvae that pupate after burrowing into sandy soil. They live in hot, dark, moist places in different ecologic habitats that relate to epidemiologic differences in the two types of HAT. Tsetses are active only during short periods separated by long intervals of rest. They can disperse randomly for up to 5 km from a point of release and can travel as far as 2 km within a day. Fewer than 1% of flies are naturally infected in an endemic area, with no more than 5% in epidemic foci. A fly remains infective for its life, which lasts a few months. Infected flies are less active than uninfected ones and need more frequent blood meals.

The common vectors of *T. b. gambiense* are the riverine tsetse flies of the *palpalis* group: *Glossina palpalis, G. tachinoides,* and *G. fuscipes*. Their principal habitat is dense vegetation along rivers and forests, where proper conditions of temperature, moisture, and light are combined with the availability of blood meals. Their distribution is focal. Hu-

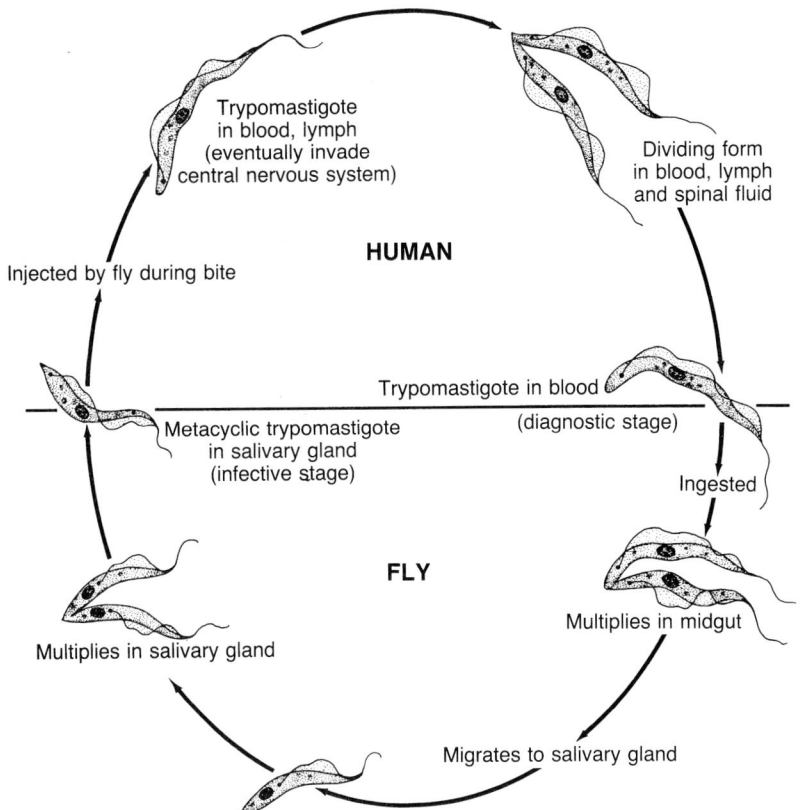

HUMAN

Trypomastigote in blood, lymph (eventually invade central nervous system)

Dividing form in blood, lymph and spinal fluid

Injected by fly during bite

Trypomastigote in blood (diagnostic stage)

Metacyclic trypomastigote in salivary gland (infective stage)

Ingested

Multiplies in midgut

Multiplies in salivary gland

FLY

Migrates to salivary gland

Epimastigote stage in salivary gland

Figure 93–2. Life cycle of *Trypanosoma brucei gambiense* and *T.b. rhodesiense*. (Modified from Melvin DM, et al: Common Blood and Tissue Parasites of Man. Life Cycle Charts. Atlanta, GA, Centers for Disease Control, 1979.)

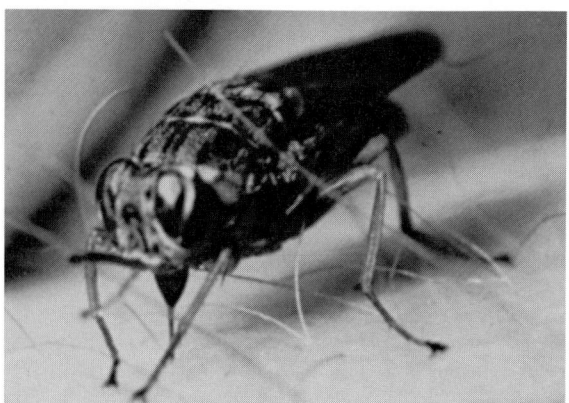

Figure 93–3. Tsetse fly biting. (Courtesy of Dr. J. Patana and the Wellcome Museum of Medical Science.)

mans are a variable source of blood meals (8 to 40%) and are frequently bitten at water sites, especially during the dry season. *T. b. rhodesiense* is transmitted by tsetse flies of the morsitans group: *G. morsitans*, *G. pallidipes*, and *G. swynnertoni*. These tsetse flies, widely distributed through the woodland and thickets of eastern African lakes and savanna, are zoophilic and less flexible in their choice of blood meals than the *G. palpalis* group. *G. fuscipes* can be a vector during epidemics.

EPIDEMIOLOGY

Distribution. HAT exists only in subSaharan Africa, where its vector is found. Between 7 and 10 million km² are infested with tsetse flies. Animal trypanosomiases, especially of cattle, also have an important economic impact in some parts of Africa. Uganda is the only country where both *T. b. gambiense* and *T. b. rhodesiense* are endemic, but the former is found in the northwestern and the latter in the southeastern part of the country, with a clear demarcation between the two endemic areas. Gambian HAT corresponds generally to western

and central Africa, Rhodesian HAT to eastern and southern Africa (Fig. 93–4).

Prevalence and Incidence. The population at risk is 55 million, most of whom are at relatively low risk of contracting the disease. HAT distribution is patchy within a given country, with areas where the vector is present but where transmission does not occur. Underdiagnosis and underreporting are such that routine national health information systems do not give reliable figures, especially because resurgence of Gambian HAT has occurred mostly in countries where civil war or strife makes active case finding impossible. The World Bank estimated in its 1993 World Development Report that each year HAT causes 55,000 deaths and a loss of 1,780,000 disability-adjusted life years, a modest figure compared with malaria and AIDS but in the same range as other tropical diseases such as onchocerciasis, lymphatic filariasis, and leishmaniasis.

The country with by far the highest incidence of Gambian HAT is The Congo, where 19,340 new cases were reported in 1994. The true incidence is at least twice that number, maybe much more, because many mobile case-finding teams have been paralyzed owing to political instability and insufficient funding. Epidemics are occurring in southern Sudan and northern Angola, where surveillance and control are impossible because of war. More than 1500 cases per year are identified in northwestern Uganda. Most other endemic countries in western and central Africa report fewer than 500 cases per year. Rhodesian HAT is better controlled, now that the 1970s to 1980s epidemic in southeastern Uganda has subsided (< 500 cases in 1994), with only residual endemicity in Kenya, Mozambique, Zambia, Tanzania, and Malawi.

Transmission. Human-fly contact is the major determinant of the epidemiology of HAT, but the quality of passive and active case finding is also having a major impact on its incidence. In regions where both the vector and the parasite are present, only a few years of insufficient case finding are necessary for an epidemic to appear, and it may then require 15 to 20 years to be controlled. Several factors can enhance human-fly contact: increased tsetse populations (for climatic

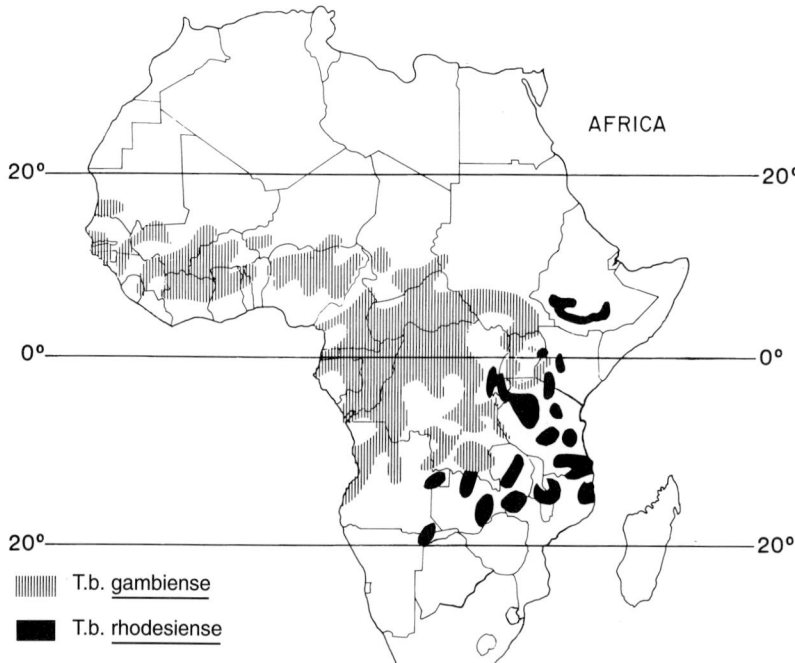

Figure 93–4. Distribution of *Trypanosoma brucei gambiense* and *T.b. rhodesiense* human African trypanosomiasis.

or ecologic reasons), changes in tsetse feeding habits (e.g., if an alternative animal source of blood meal is destroyed by an epidemic), or human behavior that brings people closer to tsetses (e.g., using a new water source where tsetse flies are abundant, migrations provoked by war). The incidence of the disease is determined by exposure and not by sex or age. Poor case finding allows transmission to occur more easily: The size of the human reservoir slowly increases, and infected humans remain infectious for longer periods, so that the proportion of infectious tsetses increases until an epidemic develops. In active foci, the annual incidence of HAT is often > 10 per 1000 and can reach staggering figures if nothing is done (several foci in The Congo now have annual incidence rates of > 100 per 1000). HAT is essentially a rural disease, and tourists are rarely infected.

Gambian Trypanosomiasis. For *T. b. gambiense*, the long incubation period and the chronicity of the disease reflect a high degree of parasite adaptation to the human host and have a major role in the dynamics of infection (Table 93–1). Infected individuals are asymptomatic for many months. They are ambulant, lead normal lives, are repeatedly bitten by flies, and are primarily responsible for spreading the parasite. Once the disease progresses to CNS involvement, parasites are found less frequently in the blood stream, and the treatment of such individuals has little impact on transmission.

A recent study showed that immunity appears after adequate treatment of a first episode of HAT, giving a protection of approximately 85%, a surprising phenomenon considering the antigenic variation of trypanosomes. This immunity may to some extent explain the recent resurgence of HAT in exactly the same foci as in the 1930s: After many years of high incidence, a large proportion of the adults may become immune, and only after new generations of immunologically naive individuals have appeared is an epidemic possible. Familial clustering of cases is also noted, the risk of HAT in a child being strongly correlated with a past history of HAT in the mother but not in the father.

The existence of an animal reservoir of *T. b. gambiense* has been debated for many years. Various animals have been found to be infected with *T. b. gambiense*: pigs, goats, dogs, sheep, cattle, and chickens. However, these animal infections are relatively rare and short lived and have a low-level parasitemia. The extent that tsetses feed on both infected animals and humans is unknown. The near eradication of Gambian HAT in some countries through control programs that focused only on the human reservoir suggest that infected animals do not have a significant role in sustaining the human disease.

Rhodesian Trypanosomiasis. *T. b. rhodesiense* trypanosomiasis is, however, a zoonosis, and in endemic situations humans are only incidental hosts (Table 93–1). Antelopes, particularly bushbuck and hartebeest, are important reservoirs. Cattle are the only proven domestic reservoirs. Many other animals can become infected but are not effective reservoirs because either parasitemia is transient or the animal quickly succumbs to the disease. *T. b. rhodesiense* HAT is, to some extent, an occupational disease, mainly of adult men, being more frequent in fishermen, hunters, game wardens, and so forth. Sporadic cases are the rule, and the disease sometimes occurs in visitors to the game parks of eastern Africa. When an epidemic develops (e.g., the recent one in southeastern Uganda), the incidence is similar for both sexes and all age groups.

IMMUNE RESPONSE, PATHOGENESIS, AND PATHOLOGY

Antigenic Variation. The major protein on the surface of blood stream trypanosomes is the variant surface glycoprotein (VSG). Approximately 10^7 copies of a single VSG are normally found on the surface, protecting invariant constituents of the parasite outer membrane from the immune system. Antibodies are continually produced against this VSG, until individual parasites switch from the expression of one VSG to another, against which new antibodies must be directed. This antigenic variation enables the population of trypanosomes to escape the immune response. The VSG switch rate varies from 10^{-2} to 10^{-6} per parasite per doubling time, and a single clone can produce >100 different VSGs, expressing only one at a time. HAT is thus characterized by recurring parasitemia, each new wave of parasites representing the selection of an immunologically distinct antigenic variant.

Polyclonal Activation of B Cells. Pronounced immunologic changes occur during the course of HAT. In the early stage, there is marked reactivity of the lymphoid tissue with predominant plasma cells. Polyclonal activation of B cells with hypergammaglobulinemia, especially increased IgM, is a striking and constant feature. Little of this IgM is a specific antitrypanosome antibody, however, and the activation is thus not entirely induced by the continually changing VSGs. Heterophile antibodies, rheumatoid factor–like substance, and anti-DNA autoantibodies are also produced. Later on, the immune system becomes depleted of lymphocytes and plasma cells, which are replaced by histiocytes. A relative immunosuppression develops, with impairment of both cellular and humoral immunity not severe enough to expose patients to opportunistic infections.

Immunopathology. Our understanding of the pathogenesis of sleeping sickness remains inadequate. Most theories implicate immunopathologic processes. Immune complexes formed between variant antigens and antibodies frequently associated with complement have been demonstrated both in the circulation and deposited in target organs. Anemia, sometimes severe, is partly due to immune complexes–induced hemolysis. Autoantibodies directed against antigenic components of erythrocytes, brain, and heart may contribute to tissue damage. The urticaria and pruritus sometimes seen in HAT could be caused by a type I immediate hypersensitivity reaction toward the trypanosomes. However, the classic clinical and pathologic features of HAT cannot be readily explained by any of the four types of immunopathologic reactions. A direct role for a toxin produced by trypanosomes has not been proved. One theory is that polyclonal proliferation of B lymphocytes in lymph nodes, brain, and meninges could lead to tissue damage through an unknown mechanism.

The dominant pathologic changes of HAT are present in the lymphatic, cardiac, and central nervous systems. In the early stage, lymphocytic and histiocytic proliferation occurs in the spleen and lymph nodes, which are enlarged and contain trypanosomes. Later, fibrosis may occur. Leukocytes contain cellular debris, erythrocytes, and trypanosomes. Cellular degeneration is found in association with a marked infiltration of monocytes, macrophages, lymphocytes, large lymphoid cells, and plasma cells. In the late stage, an endarteritis appears, with endothelial proliferation involving small vessels accompanied by perivascular infiltration of plasma cells and lymphocytes. Vascular permeability is increased, and trypanosomes infiltrate the interstitial spaces and lymphatic system, where they multiply. The liver shows Kupffer cell hyperplasia, portal tract infiltrates, and fatty degeneration. Glomerulonephritis has been noted. Cardiac involvement and polyserositis are prominent features of *rhodesiense* disease. A pancarditis involving all layers has been described, including mural and valvular endocardium, the myocardium and its conduction system, and the epicardium with the autonomic nervous system. The pathologic changes observed have consisted of marked cellular infiltration, including plasma and morular cells, as well as myocytolysis and fibrosis. The pancarditis may cause death of patients with *rhodesiense* HAT before major CNS damage has developed.

Central Nervous System Pathology. CNS involvement results in meningoencephalitis or meningomyelitis. Perivascular infiltration associated with prominent neuroglial proliferation is present and is most marked in the pia-arachnoid of the brain and spinal cord.

Edema, hemorrhages, and granulomatous lesions are present in the brain. Thrombosis as a result of endarteritis is a major cause of cerebral degeneration. Demyelinization is minimal. Two cytotoxic abnormalities suggestive of HAT may be found: lymphophagocytosis and the morular or Mott cells (Fig. 93–5), which are plasma cells with large eosinophilic inclusions. These cells may have an important role in the local production of IgM in the CSF.

CLINICAL MANIFESTATIONS AND COMPLICATIONS

T. b. gambiense. *T. b. gambiense* trypanosomiasis is characterized by a long period of asymptomatic infection, followed by an early febrile stage during which trypanosomes are found only in the blood or lymph node aspirates, without parasitologic or cytologic evidence of CNS involvement, and then by a late neurologic stage during which trypanosomes are present in the CSF.

The duration of the incubation is difficult to delineate in individuals who spend their whole life in endemic areas; anecdotal data from patients who lived in such areas for only short periods suggest that this asymptomatic phase lasts in general several months, sometimes as long as a few years. About half of these asymptomatically infected subjects have cervical lymphadenopathy.

Early Stage Illness. At some point in this process, patients start having nonspecific symptoms corresponding to early stage HAT: intermittent fever not responding to antimalarials, headaches, myalgias, malaise, and fatigue. The cyclic nature of these symptoms, not always reported by patients, corresponds to fluctuations in the degree of parasitemia, possibly related to antigenic variation allowing the parasite to escape successive waves of antibodies produced by the host. Most of these patients have cervical lymphadenopathy, a minority (10 to 20%) have splenomegaly, and hepatomegaly is rare. The classic Winterbottom's posterior cervical lymphadenopathies (Fig. 93–6) are seen in as many as 85% of hospitalized patients. They are 1 to 2 cm in diameter, soft, nontender, mobile, and usually numerous. However, less typical lymphadenopathy is seen (e.g., smaller nodes or supraclavicular lymphadenopathy). At this stage, it is only the

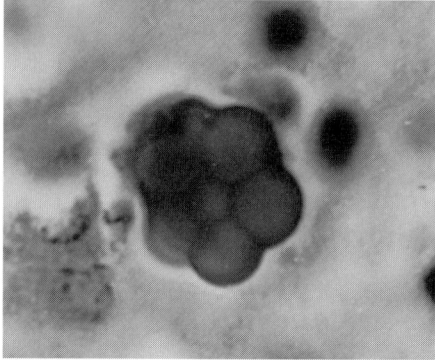

Figure 93–5. Morular cell of Mott (× 2000). (Courtesy of the Wellcome Museum of Medical Science.)

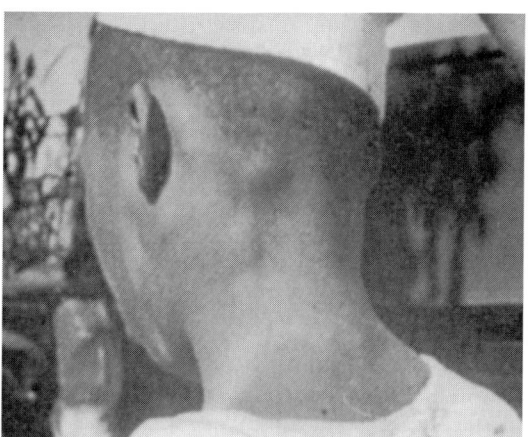

Figure 93–6. Enlargement of posterior cervical lymph nodes—Winterbottom's sign. (Courtesy of Dr. James R. Busvine, London School of Hygiene and Tropical Medicine.)

lymphadenopathy, the notion that a patient comes from an endemic area, and the lack of other explanations for the fever that lead a clinician to consider the diagnosis. Pruritus and transient edemas (mostly of the face) are seen in <10% of patients but should alert a clinician to possible HAT.

Late-Stage Illness. After a few months of this nonspecific syndrome, patients progress toward late stage CNS involvement. Weight loss can be important, patients being no longer able to carry out normal tasks. Headaches become constant and unresponsive to analgesics. Somnolence appears and progressively worsens; nighttime insomnia is the exception. The frequency and severity of somnolence vary in parallel with the CSF leukocyte count: uncommon if <50/mm³ and almost universal and often debilitating if >100/mm³. These patients are difficult to arouse, even to eat or drink; they talk less and less until, if untreated, they become comatose. Behavior changes, mania, or frank psychosis occur in <10% of cases, but in an endemic area all patients with a recent onset of serious psychiatric disorders should be investigated for HAT, including having a lumbar puncture (LP). Convulsions are rare in adults. On physical examination, substantial wasting is noted. The lymphadenopathies are less prominent than in the early stage, and neck stiffness is rare, except in patients with a CSF leukocytosis of >300/mm³. Generally no focal signs are found on neurologic examination, but in an endemic area any new neurologic syndrome such as extrapyramidal signs (tremors, increased tonicity, or muscular rigidity), cerebellar ataxia, or even hemiparesis should raise the possibility of HAT. The hand-chin reflex can be elicited in 50% of patients but is nonspecific. Deep hyperesthesia (Kerandel's sign) is uncommon in Africans and results in delayed, intense pain when soft tissues are compressed. Cutaneous lesions (trypanids) are seen only in Caucasians as an irregular, circinate, evanescent rash on the trunk, shoulders, and thighs, with erythematous areas 7 to 10 cm in diameter and clear centers. In late stage disease, the diagnosis is usually obvious after taking the patient's history. The physical examination adds little, and the LP confirms the diagnosis. If left untreated, sleeping sickness is ultimately fatal in all patients, an intercurrent infection such as aspiration pneumonia often being the terminal event.

Infection in Children. In children, progression to late stage is more rapid than in adults. Virtually all patients with congenital trypanosomiasis have severe anomalies of the CSF when the diagnosis is made in these irritable and febrile infants born of women usually just diagnosed with HAT.

Before 5 years of age, HAT is characterized more by retardation in psychomotor development, walking, and talking than by somnolence. Convulsions occur in 20 to 30% of cases. In older children, the clinical syndrome is comparable to that of adults.

T. b. rhodesiense. This is a much more acute infection: The incubation phase, the early stage, and the late stage with CNS involvement all develop over a matter of weeks. An inoculation chancre, 5 to 15 days after the bite, is more common than in Gambian HAT but remains unusual in Africans. It is a painful, circumscribed, rubbery, indurated, dusky-red papule 2 to 5 cm in diameter, which disappears after 2 to 3 weeks. Regional lymphadenopathy or adjacent cellulitis occurs. Fever and parasitemia appear hours to days later or, in the absence of a chancre, within 1 to 3 weeks of the infective bite. Cervical lymphadenopathy is less common than in Gambian HAT, but submandibular, axillary, or inguinal lymph nodes can be enlarged. Symptoms and signs of CNS involvement are the same as in *gambiense* infection but progress more rapidly, and without treatment the disease is fatal within 1 to 3 months. Myocarditis is an uncommon complication, but patients occasionally die of arrhythmias or heart failure before they have overt neurologic disease.

DIAGNOSIS

Nonspecific Laboratory Anomalies. The main laboratory abnormalities associated with HAT are anemia, hypergammaglobulinemia, an increased sedimentation rate, and thrombocytopenia. Coagulation abnormalities, features of disseminated intravascular coagulation, and liver function test anomalies are uncommon and more marked in *rhodesiense* than *gambiense* infections. No eosinophilia is seen. Elevated serum (and eventually CSF) total IgM levels, to more than four times the normal value, are frequent in Gambian HAT and have been used in some centers as a screening tool. In late stage HAT, mononuclear cells in the CSF are increased but the CSF remains clear and Mott cells are rarely present. CSF protein levels are elevated (0.4 to 1.0 g/L).

Parasitologic Assays. The classic parasitologic assays are the lymph node aspirate and the wet and thick smears of blood.

Lymph Node Aspirate. In the lymph node aspirate, which is especially useful for the diagnosis of Gambian HAT, lymph node fluid is aspirated from enlarged nodes with a syringe and placed on a slide, where it is examined immediately at high dry magnification ($\times$ 400). The trypanosomes are mobile for 15 to 20 minutes and tend to concentrate on the edges of the coverslip.

Blood Smears. In the wet smear, a drop of unstained blood is examined immediately after sampling between slide and coverslip. Thick smears of blood are examined after Giemsa staining as in malaria diagnosis (Wright's and Leishman's stains are inferior; Fig. 93–7). In Gambian HAT, parasitemia fluctuates and is low; repeated examinations over a few days may be necessary before a trypanosome is documented. More sensitive assays are the hematocrit centrifugation technique for examination of the buffy coat layer and, the current gold standard, the miniature anion-exchange centrifugation technique in which blood is filtered through a resin that retains blood cells but not trypanosomes, the eluate being then centrifuged and examined in a viewing chamber (available from PRCT, BP 1425, Daloa, Côte d'Ivoire). The lower limits for number of trypanosomes detectable are 10^4/mL for the wet smear, 5×10^3/mL for the thick smear, 5×10^2/mL for the hematocrit centrifugation technique, and 10^2/mL for the miniature anion-exchange centrifugation technique. The quantitative buffy coat technique using acridine orange is promising; it is possibly as sensitive as the latter method but easier to perform. Animal inoculation has been abandoned.

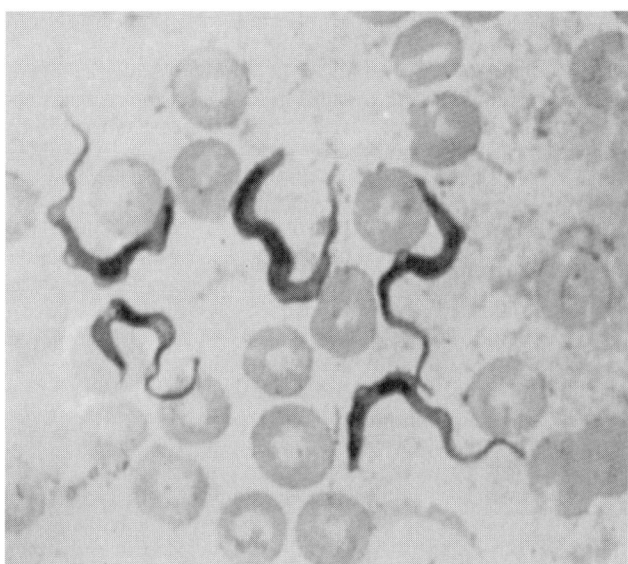

Figure 93–7. *Trypanosoma brucei gambiense* in stained blood film.

Rhodesian trypanosomiasis. In *T. b. rhodesiense* HAT, the same techniques are used; the lymph node aspirate is less often performed or diagnostic, and examination of the blood is more likely to show trypanosomes. Trypanosomes may be found in the inoculation chancre before their appearance in the peripheral blood; the chancre is punctured, and a drop of the exudate is examined as in a wet preparation.

Cerebrospinal Fluid. As the disease progresses, trypanosomes become more difficult to find in the blood or lymph nodes and easier to find in the CSF. For some patients, only the CSF examination reveals trypanosomes. For patients with trypanosomes in the blood or lymph nodes, LP must always be performed for a leukocyte count and trypanosome detection, to select appropriate therapy. Double centrifugation is the most sensitive method for detection of CSF trypanosomes: 6 to 8 mL of CSF is centrifuged; the sediment is drawn in a capillary tube and centrifuged again before being examined as the tube is held between slide and coverslide. The frequency of CSF trypanosomes being detected increases in parallel with the CSF pleocytosis, but trypanosomes are occasionally found despite a normal CSF cell count, further proof that CNS involvement occurs early.

Serology. The purpose of serology is to identify suspected cases for concentration on the performance of labor-intensive parasitologic assays. The Card Agglutination Test for Trypanosomiasis (CATT, available from the Laboratory of Serology of the Institute of Tropical Medicine, Antwerp, Belgium) is the only serologic assay currently used for *T. b. gambiense*. Many others were developed but are seldom used because they generally require laboratory facilities unavailable in endemic areas. The CATT can be performed in the field, without electricity, and results are available within 10 minutes. Its 96% sensitivity is adequate; its specificity is unfortunately not as good, owing to cross-reactivity with animal trypanosomes. The positive predictive value is excellent (66 to 89%) when the CATT is used in a hospital for passive case finding among individuals with symptoms and signs compatible with HAT, but it is only 15 to 30% when used in active case-finding surveys in endemic foci, where only 1 to 10% of the population tested is infected with *T. b. gambiense*. Performing the CATT on diluted serum (1:10) rather than whole blood increases specificity but decreases sensitivity. Despite its shortcomings, the CATT is very useful for case-finding teams and doubles the number of infected individuals detected when compared with surveys using only parasitologic assays. It can be performed, with similar results, using a micromethod on filter paper or diluted blood, reducing three-fold the cost of screening. In active foci, the cost of the CATT is more than compensated over a few years by the savings generated by better control of HAT. The CATT is currently underused. No serologic assay can detect antibodies against *T. b. rhodesiense*. Its usefulness would be doubtful, the short incubation period and the high degree of parasitemia in Rhodesian HAT being such that parasitologic diagnosis is generally not difficult. An experimental antigen detection assay has been developed, with a 91.5% sensitivity compared with parasitologic examinations of blood.

Clinical Diagnosis. In endemic areas, some patients (<5% of cases if the laboratory is adequate) in whom no trypanosomes can be documented are treated on the basis of a presumptive diagnosis. They come from an endemic focus and have neurologic symptoms compatible with HAT, their CSF white cell count is at least moderately elevated, and their CATT result, if available, is positive. Short- and long-term improvement with melarsoprol or eflornithine almost always confirms the diagnosis.

Differential Diagnosis. In early-stage HAT, other causes of protracted febrile illness should be considered, such as drug-resistant malaria, typhoid fever, and miliary tuberculosis. The prominent lymphadenopathy can be suggestive of mononucleosis, HIV-associated persistent generalized lymphadenopathy (Chapter 22), or tuberculous lymphadenitis (Chapter 77). In late-stage HAT, the differential diagnosis is that of chronic lymphocytic meningitis: tuberculous meningitis, syphilis, and HIV-associated cryptococcal meningitis. The epidemiologic argument (residence in or travel to an endemic area) often is the determinant in raising the index of suspicion and making the diagnosis.

TREATMENT. The treatment of HAT varies according to whether the disease is caused by *T. b. gambiense* or *T. b. rhodesiense* (the latter being more resistant to some trypanocidal drugs) and whether or not a patient has neurologic involvement, in which case penetration of the drug in the CNS is crucial. Both subspecies being morphologically identical, the first question is usually addressed on geographic grounds, by assessing the probable site where the infection took place (Table 93–1). For the exceptional patient who has traveled to areas endemic for both *T. b. gambiense* and *T. b. rhodesiense*, only research tools (e.g., trypanosome lysis assays) can distinguish between the two subspecies. The second question implies that LP must be performed on all patients, even those without neurologic symptoms. By definition, any patient with CSF trypanosomes and/or a CSF pleocytosis >5/mm^3 is in late stage, even in the absence of neurologic symptoms. CNS involvement occurs earlier than generally thought; many patients without any neurologic symptoms have a slightly elevated (6 to 50/mm^3) CSF white cell count, and if treated with pentamidine or suramin, most are not cured. Melarsoprol and suramin are not licensed for use in the United States but can be obtained through the Parasitic Disease Drug Service of the Centers for Disease Control and Prevention (404-639-3670). Information on current availability of eflornithine in the United States can also be obtained from the Parasitic Drug Service. Eflornithine can also be obtained from the Division of Control of Tropical Diseases of the World Health Organization (WHO) (41–22–791–3868).

T. b. gambiense: Early Stage. Pentamidine, an aromatic diamidine, is the standard treatment. Suramin is thought to be less effective, and melarsoprol, which would be curative, is best avoided in these patients because of its toxicity.

Pentamidine. Pentamidine, provided at a reduced price by the manufacturer through WHO, is now available only as the isethionate salt (Pentacarinat, May and Baker). Its half-life is 22 to 47 hours, and it does not sufficiently penetrate the CSF to be curative for late stage cases. It can be given IM or IV at 4 mg/kg daily for 7 days. Its cure rate (93%) is remarkably uniform throughout Africa and has not decreased despite decades of widespread use. The IM injections are extremely painful and may cause sterile abscesses. More serious adverse effects are hypotension (especially if given IV), hypocalcemia, hyperkalemia, renal failure, neutropenia, ventricular arrhythmias, hypoglycemia (during treatment), and diabetes (after treatment). In Africa, 1% of patients die during or shortly after a course of pentamidine, but it is usually difficult to identify a precise cause.

Other Drugs. Diminazene, also a diamidine, widely used throughout Africa for animal trypanosomiases, has been used for both Gambian and Rhodesian early stage HAT. It has never been licensed for human use, however, and no clinical trials have compared its efficacy and toxicity with that of pentamidine. In some animal models, diminazene induced severe neurologic toxicity, and some neurologic adverse effects have been reported in humans. Limited data suggest that its failure rate (at 7 mg/kg IM every 48 hours for three injections) is twice that of pentamidine. A combination of suramin (2 IV injections) and pentamidine (6 IM injections), used in The Congo for more than 3 decades, has never been compared with pentamidine monotherapy, and there is no evidence that the combination is superior to pentamidine alone.

T. b. gambiense: Late Stage.

Eflornithine. Eflornithine (Ornidyl, Hoechst Marion Roussel) is the drug of choice for neurologic involvement. An inhibitor of ornithine decarboxylase and thus of polyamines synthesis, eflornithine is as effective as melarsoprol and is much less toxic. Unfortunately, it is too expensive for endemic countries, at $600 for 14 days. Its administration is cumbersome (large volumes have to be given IV for many days), and it is unclear whether it will remain available in the future. At 100 mg/kg IV every 6 hours for 14 days, it cures 90% of late stage new cases and 98% of relapsing cases. Only 2% of patients die during eflornithine treatment, most of them as a result of advanced HAT. Bone marrow toxicity (anemia, leukopenia, and thrombocytopenia) occurs in >50% of patients, but without clinical consequences. Convulsions (4 to 8%) are related to high CSF eflornithine levels; they subside when the drug is discontinued for a few days and do not recur when it is resumed. Oral eflornithine is less effective than IV administration. Its bioavailability is 55%, and osmotic diarrhea precludes giving higher doses. Once a patient has received 2 weeks of IV eflornithine, adding a few weeks of oral eflornithine does not increase the cure rate. No pretreatment with other trypanocidal drugs needs to be given when eflornithine is used. Limited data suggest that eflornithine is less effective in HIV-infected patients, who should be treated with melarsoprol, and in children, who should be given higher doses (150 mg/kg every 6 hours for 14 days).

Melarsoprol. Melarsoprol (Arsobal, Rhone Poulenc Rorer) remains the standard treatment of late stage Gambian HAT in most rural hospitals of Africa. This trivalent arsenical drug is very effective (cure rate, 94 to 97%) but also very toxic (death rate, 4 to 6%). Its efficacy is more related to its excellent trypanocidal activity than to good CSF penetration, estimated to be <1%. As for pentamidine, there is no evidence of increasing resistance to melarsoprol despite large-scale use of the drug for 50 years.

TREATMENT REGIMENS. Patients with CSF leukocyte counts of 6 to 19/mm^3 are given two series of three daily injections

(3.6 mg/kg, up to 180 mg, with the full dose being given from the first injection) separated by a 1-week drug-free interval. Those with a CSF white cell count ≥ 20/mm³ receive three such series (same interval between second and third series). Giving more than nine injections increases toxicity without improving efficacy.

COMPLICATIONS. Reactive encephalopathy, secondary to some autoimmune phenomenon rather than arsenic toxicity, is a dramatic complication of melarsoprol treatment. It occurs in 4 to 8% of late stage cases, more often if there are trypanosomes in the CSF or if white cell count is >100/mm³. Patients who appeared well a few hours earlier develop grand mal seizures, coma (or more rarely just behavior changes), and sometimes neurogenic pulmonary edema; the case-fatality rate is >60%. Reactive encephalopathy usually occurs at the end of the first series, during the first interval, or at the beginning of the second series. Prednisolone given during melarsoprol treatment halves the mortality and reduces by two thirds the frequency of encephalopathy, without increasing the risk of treatment failure. It should be administered to all patients at 1 mg/kg, up to 40 mg/day, started 1 to 2 days before melarsoprol, continued during the two to three series and the intervals between, and rapidly tapered over 3 days after the last injection of melarsoprol. If an encephalopathy occurs, the patient should receive an anticonvulsant (phenobarbital, diazepam, or phenytoin), dexamethasone (or hydrocortisone) to reduce cerebral edema, and subcutaneous epinephrine (1 mg every 2 hours for 6 hours, then every 4 hours until improvement). Dimercaprol, a heavy metal chelator, should not be given to treat encephalopathy. If available, eflornithine is usually given to complete the treatment of a patient who developed melarsoprol-induced encephalopathy; if unavailable, melarsoprol can be resumed once the patient has recovered to complete the standard regimen, and it never induces a second bout of encephalopathy.

Polyneuropathy is the other important (10%) adverse effect of melarsoprol. If the patient complains of paresthesias, melarsoprol should be withheld until improvement, while thiamine (100 mg t.i.d.) is given. In the absence of such precautions, paraplegia or even quadriplegia can occur. Cutaneous reactions are uncommon. Phlebitis at the injection sites is frequent because the propylene glycol solvent is irritating to veins; extravasation induces a chemical cellulitis. Fever in the first days of treatment can be secondary to trypanosomes lysis, but bacterial superinfections, especially pneumonia, must be suspected. Tremors can appear during treatment, are not predictive of encephalopathy, and respond well to β-blockers. Patients given prednisolone should also receive thiabendazole if *Strongyloides stercoralis* is found in their stools to avoid disseminated strongyloidiasis. Antimalarials are routinely administered at the beginning of treatment, and promethazine (25 mg b.i.d.) is given on the same days as melarsoprol; whether or not it prevents "allergic" reactions is doubtful, but at least it sedates patients who are usually nervous about receiving melarsoprol. Anthelmintics and antimalarials can be omitted if the absence of parasitic coinfections can be documented in a reliable laboratory. Pretreatment with suramin and pentamidine has been advocated for decades to reduce the level of parasitemia before melarsoprol is administered in the hope of reducing antigen release, which is thought to be important in the pathogenesis of reactive encephalopathy. Its efficacy has never been demonstrated, but it is still used by many treatment centers (pentamidine, 1 to 2 doses of 4 mg/kg 24 to 72 hours before first injection of melarsoprol).

T. *b. gambiense*: Follow-up and Treatment of Relapses.
After treatment, patients with both early stage and late stage disease should be monitored for 2 years, with LP performed every 6 months (it is useless to perform LP during treatment). Early stage cases, with initial CSF by definition normal, should be considered as relapsing if a follow-up LP shows a CSF white cell count of 20/mm³ or more (trypanosomes are rarely found in such patients). Patients with equivocal results (6 to 19/mm³) should be retested after 1 to 2 months. Patients relapsing after treatment of early stage Gambian HAT with pentamidine (or suramin or diminazene) should be given the standard regimen of either melarsoprol or eflornithine, which cures most of them.

Late stage cases can have an increased CSF leukocyte count at the first LP despite being cured. Therefore, the trend of the CSF white cell count is more important than the absolute value. For late stage cases initially treated with melarsoprol or eflornithine, a relapse is certain if trypanosomes are found in CSF (one fourth of relapses) or in blood/lymph node aspirate (rarely). Most relapses are diagnosed on the basis of a CSF pleocytosis. A relapse is likely if the CSF leukocyte count is ≥ 50/mm³ and higher than the previous determination, or 20 to 49/mm³ and higher than the previous one with recurrence of symptoms. When in doubt, it is preferable not to treat and to repeat the LP 1 to 2 months later. Most cases relapsing after melarsoprol treatment of late-stage HAT are not cured by a second course of melarsoprol. Such patients should be treated with eflornithine, for them, truly the "resurrection drug." Eflornithine is even more effective in postmelarsoprol relapses than in new cases because of higher CSF drug levels in the former, presumably a consequence of chronic meningitis with impairment of the blood–brain barrier. Ongoing trials suggest that in postmelarsoprol relapses, a 7-day course of eflornithine (same daily dosage) is as effective as the standard 14-day regimen, reducing the cost by half. This should not yet be extrapolated to new cases. Patients suffering relapse after having initially received eflornithine should be re-treated with melarsoprol. For the rare patient who suffers relapse twice, after having received melarsoprol once and eflornithine once, simultaneous administration of both drugs (same dosage as usual) should be considered. The other alternative is high-dose nifurtimox, a drug used in the treatment of acute Chagas' disease, which needs to be given at a higher (25 to 30 mg/kg/day for 30 days) and toxic (confusion, tremors, anorexia) dose, with a cure rate of approximately 65%.

Patients who do not suffer relapse after a first treatment with melarsoprol or eflornithine have remarkably few sequelae, even if stuporous when admitted to hospital. Children have more frequent sequelae, especially poor school performance. Patients with many relapses have impaired cognitive functions and sometimes choreoathetotic movements.

T. *b. rhodesiense*: Early Stage. Although published studies show wide variations in the frequency of treatment failures (0 to 31%), suramin (Bayer 205, Bayer) is thought to be more effective than pentamidine for such patients. Again, melarsoprol would be very effective but cannot be recommended because of the risk of encephalopathy. Suramin should be given as five IV injections of 20 mg/kg (up to 1.5 g) on days 1, 3, 6, 14, and 21. Although anaphylaxis is very rare (1/20,000), a 200-mg test dose is usually given before the full dose. Adverse effects are fever, proteinuria (which is reversible), paresthesias, and urticaria. Pruritus is more frequent with concomitant filariasis. Because suramin binds to many proteins, its CSF penetration is very poor and its half-life extremely long (44 to 54 days).

T. *b. rhodesiense*: Late Stage. Eflornithine, even at twice the usual dose (800 mg/kg/day), is ineffective for such patients. Melarsoprol is the only curative drug, with success in 95% of cases. Encephalopathy is more common (5 to 18%) than in *gambiense* disease, and mortality during treatment is higher (3 to 12%). To avoid this complication, experienced clinicians have recommended starting with small doses of melarsoprol and increasing progressively. Although this has never been compared with a regimen with the full dose from the first injection, the WHO-recommended regimen is 0.36 mg/kg (day 1), 0.72 (day 2), 1.1 (day 3), 1.8 (days 10, 11, and 12), 2.2 (day 19), 2.9 (day 20), and 3.6 mg/kg (up to 180 mg) on days 21, 28, 29, and 30. Adjuvant drugs should be given as in Gambian HAT (promethazine, antimalarials, anthelmintics). Pretreatment with two to three doses of IV suramin (5, 10, 20 mg/kg over 3 to 5 days) is usually given; however, its usefulness is unproven.

T. b. rhodesiense: Follow-up and Treatment of Relapses. Patients should be monitored as in Gambian HAT, except that LP should be performed every 3 months during the first year. Criteria for diagnosing a relapse should be the same as for Gambian HAT. Patients who suffer relapse after suramin treatment should be given melarsoprol (same regimen as earlier). Patients suffering relapse after melarsoprol treatment of late stage Rhodesian HAT should be given a second course of melarsoprol (3.6 mg/kg up to 180 mg daily for all injections of four series of three injections), which is curative for most. For those who suffer relapse after a second course of melarsoprol, empirical recommendations are either a combination of high-dose eflornithine (200 mg/kg IV every 6 hours for 14 days) plus melarsoprol (12 injections of the full dose) in the hope of some synergism, or nifurtimox (25 to 30 mg/kg/day/30 days PO).

PREVENTION AND CONTROL. The cornerstone of Gambian trypanosomiasis control is detecting and treating mostly asymptomatic infected individuals who represent the human reservoir of the parasite. By the time CNS involvement becomes obvious, most patients are no longer parasitemic. Treatment of passively detected, symptomatic individuals in whom trypanosomes have been found only in the CSF has no impact on transmission of the parasite. Therefore, identifying and treating asymptomatic persons is the only way to alter the transmission dynamics of HAT. Classically, this has been carried out through regular half-yearly screening of populations for cervical lymphadenopathy in recognized foci. During the colonial era, people had no choice but to attend such sessions; participation rates were >90%, and this classic method of examining aspirates from those with lymphadenopathy for trypanosomes gave excellent results. Nowadays, with participation rarely >50%, the classic method does not achieve control. Whether health education can improve participation is doubtful.

Screening Populations in Endemic Areas. Case finding among those who attend screening sessions can be improved through a field-adapted serologic assay, the CATT, with results available within minutes. The case-finding team can concentrate its efforts on CATT-positive individuals, from whom they obtain not only lymph node aspirates but also thin and thick smears of blood. If all assays yield negative results, the miniature anion-exchange centrifugation technique is used. In general, using the CATT for identifying those without cervical lymphadenopathy who have HAT doubles the number of parasitologically proven cases detected and leads to a decrease in HAT incidence. Only patients in whom trypanosomes have been detected should be treated, because during active case finding many CATT positives are false positives, and administration of toxic drugs to such persons would be difficult to justify. An experiment in The Congo showed that rapid control of an epidemic with minimal drug toxicity could be achieved when CATT-positive/parasitology-negative/normal-CSF individuals were treated with a single injection of diminazene, in addition to treatment of CATT-positive/parasitology-positive individuals with standard regimens of pentamidine or melarsoprol, and melarsoprol treatment of CATT-positive/parasitology-negative individuals with a white cell count >5/mm³. Primary health care centers can contribute to passive case finding if their staff is properly trained, but this has little impact on transmission because most patients they diagnose have late-stage disease without parasitemia.

Glossina Control. Tsetse fly trapping is a useful adjuvant to active case finding of Gambian HAT. Because of its cost (traps deteriorate rapidly and need to be replaced every 6 months), it should be considered only for foci with an annual incidence of >10 per 1000. Very important (>99%) and sustained reduction in tsetse densities can be achieved rapidly. However, because of the long incubation period of Gambian trypanosomiasis, this does not have an immediate effect on incidence.

Tsetse trapping has been used with success in the recent *T. b. rhodesiense* epidemic in Uganda. Case finding by sleeping sickness orderlies was also promoted to identify infected individuals earlier, which allowed for more effective and less toxic therapy. Because of the much shorter incubation period, it is generally thought that active case finding is less important in Rhodesian HAT control, and trapping should be given high priority.

Prevention in Travelers. At the individual level, little needs to be done for a traveler visiting an endemic area. HAT is rare among tourists and long-term expatriates because their lifestyle is generally associated with a low exposure to infectious tsetse flies. Chemoprophylaxis is no longer recommended. Long-term expatriates who lived in an endemic area must provide this information to their physicians, should they consult them for a febrile illness.

Bibliography

Bailey JW, Smith DH: The quantitative buffy coat for the diagnosis of trypanosomes. Trop Doct 24:54, 1994.

Borst P, Rudenko G: Antigenic variation in African trypanosomes. Science 264:1872, 1994.

Cattand P, Miézan BT, de Raadt P: Human African trypanosomiasis: Use of double centrifugation of CSF to detect trypanosomes. Bull WHO 66:83, 1988.

Ekwanzala M, Pépin J, Khonde N, et al: In the heart of darkness: Sleeping sickness in Zaire. Lancet 348:1427, 1996.

Fairlamb AH: Novel approaches to the chemotherapy of trypanosomiasis. Trans R Soc Trop Med Hyg 84:613, 1990.

Greenwood BM, Whittle HC: The pathogenesis of sleeping sickness. Trans R Soc Trop Med Hyg 74:716, 1980.

Jennings FW: Combination therapy and African trypanosomiasis. Trans R Soc Trop Med Hyg 84:618, 1990.

Khonde N, Pépin J, Niyonsenga T, et al: Epidemiological evidence for immunity following *T. b. gambiense* sleeping sickness. Trans R Soc Trop Med Hyg 89:607, 1995.

Méda HA, Doua F, Laveissière C, et al: Human immunodeficiency virus infection and human African trypanosomiasis: A case-control study in Côte d'Ivoire. Trans R Soc Trop Med Hyg 89:639, 1995.

Miézan T, Doua F, Cattand P, et al: Evaluation du Testryp CATT appliqué au sang prélevé sur papier filtre et au sang dilué, dans le foyer de trypanosomiase à *Trypanosoma brucei gambiense* en Côte d'Ivoire. Bull WHO 69:603, 1991.

Milord F, Loko L, Ethier L, et al: Eflornithine concentrations in serum and cerebrospinal fluid of 63 patients treated for *T. b. gambiense* sleeping sickness. Trans R Soc Trop Med Hyg 87:473, 1993.

Milord F, Pépin J, Loko L, et al: Efficacy and toxicity of eflornithine for treatment of *T. b. gambiense* sleeping sickness. Lancet 340:652, 1992.

Mulligan HW, Potts WH (eds): The African Trypanosomiases. London, George Allen and Unwin, 1970.

Noireau F, Lemesre JL, Nzoukoudi MY, et al: Serodiagnosis of sleeping sickness in the Republic of Congo: Comparison of indirect immunofluorescent antibody test and card agglutination test. Trans R Soc Trop Med Hyg 82:237, 1988.

Pépin J, Milord F: The treatment of human African trypanosomiasis. Adv Parasitol 33:1, 1994.

Pépin J, Ethier L, Kazadi C, et al: The impact of HIV infection on the epidemiology and treatment of *T. b. gambiense* sleeping sickness in Nioki, Zaire. Am J Trop Med Hyg 47:133, 1992.

Pépin J, Milord F, Guern C, et al: Trial of prednisolone for prevention of melarsoprol-induced encephalopathy in *gambiense* sleeping sickness. Lancet 333:1246, 1989.

Pépin J, Milord F, Khonde N, et al: Gambiense trypanosomiasis: Frequency of, and risk factors for, failure of melarsoprol therapy. Trans R Soc Trop Med Hyg 88:447, 1994.

Pépin J, Milord F, Khonde N, et al: Risk factors for encephalopathy and mortality during melarsoprol treatment of *T. b. gambiense* sleeping sickness. Trans R Soc Trop Med Hyg 89:92, 1995.

Smith AB, Esko JD, Hadjuk SL: Killing of trypanosomes by the human haptoglobin-related protein. Science 268:284, 1995.

World Bank: World Development Report 1993: Investing in Health. New York, Oxford University Press, 1993, p 218.

World Health Organization: Epidemiology and control of African trypanosomiasis. Report of a WHO expert committee. World Health Organ Tech Rep Ser 739, 1986.

94 American Trypanosomiasis

Alan J. Magill and Steven G. Reed

DEFINITION. American trypanosomiasis, or Chagas' disease, is caused by infection with the flagellate protozoan parasite, *Trypanosoma cruzi*. *T. cruzi* is an anthropozoonotic parasite infecting many vertebrates and is transmitted by triatomine insects, the reduviid bugs. Human infection with *T. cruzi* leads to an acute phase lasting several weeks characterized by relatively high parasitemia followed by a chronic phase characterized by positive serology and very low parasitemia that is lifelong. Many years following the initial infec-

tion, chronic cardiomyopathy develops in 20 to 30%, gastrointestinal megasyndromes develop in <10%, and peripheral nerve involvement occurs in a few percent of infected individuals. The risk of developing late stage complications depends on the geographic origin of the infecting strains. Like mucosal leishmaniasis, severe disease is more frequent as one moves south from Texas to central Brazil.

HISTORY. In 1909, a gifted Brazilian scientist, Carlos Chagas, discovered the etiologic agent, described the clinical picture of disease, and documented the insect vectors and reservoir hosts. In the 1930s, Mazza of Argentina published a long series of observations that confirmed Chagas' earlier findings and aroused new interest in the disease. In an epidemiologic study conducted in Bambui, Minas Gerais, Brazil, in 1943, Emmanuel Dias demonstrated that spraying houses with the residual insecticide benzene hexachloride was an effective way to control bug populations and suppress transmission. In the 1960s, Fritz Koberle and his group clarified that the gut "megasyndromes" (megaesophagus and megacolon) were due to aperistalsis as the result of parasympathetic denervation. The past 2 decades have seen a remarkable increase in research on Chagas' disease, particularly in its immunology and molecular biology. The Southern Cone Initiative was launched in 1991 with the goal of elimination of the transmission of Chagas' disease. The program expanded to include the Andean and Central American countries in 1997. As a result of the success of this program, Uruguay was certified free of vectorial and transfusional transmission of Chagas' disease in 1997.

BIOLOGY OF THE ORGANISM AND LIFE CYCLE. *T. cruzi* is a polymorphic trypanosome with an indirect life cycle (Fig.

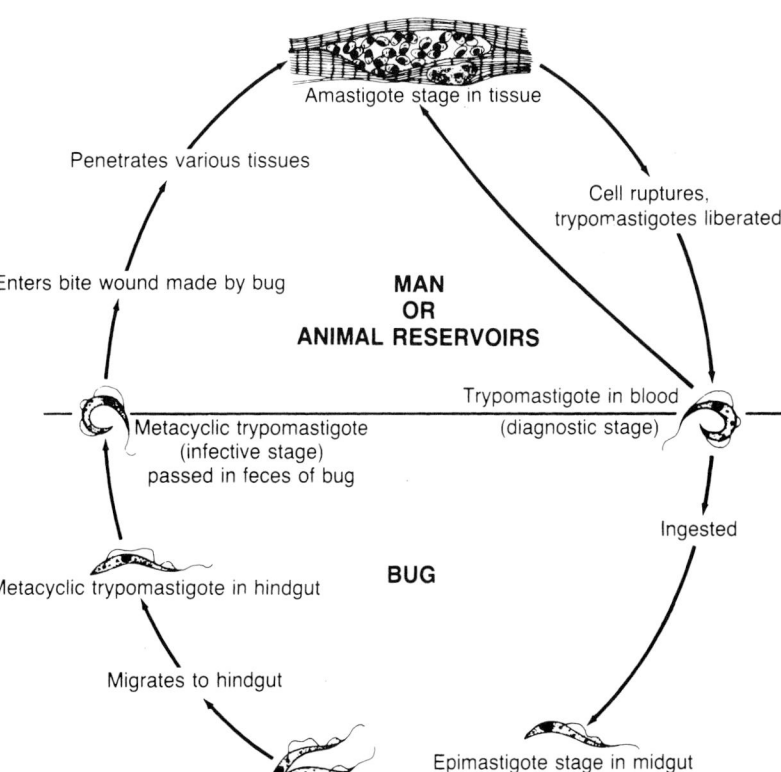

Figure 94–1. Life cycle of *Trypanosoma cruzi*. (Modified from Melvin DM, et al: Common Blood and Tissue Parasites of Man. Life Cycle Charts. Atlanta, GA, Centers for Disease Control, 1979.)

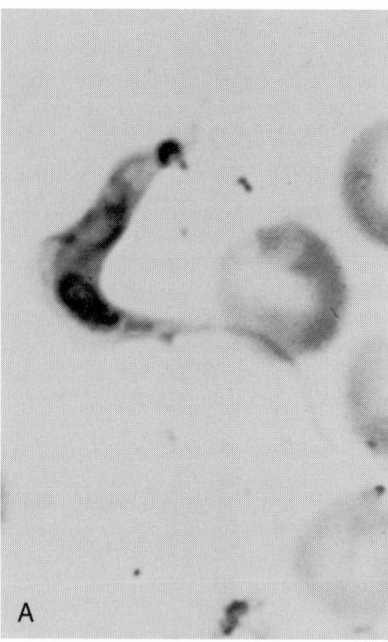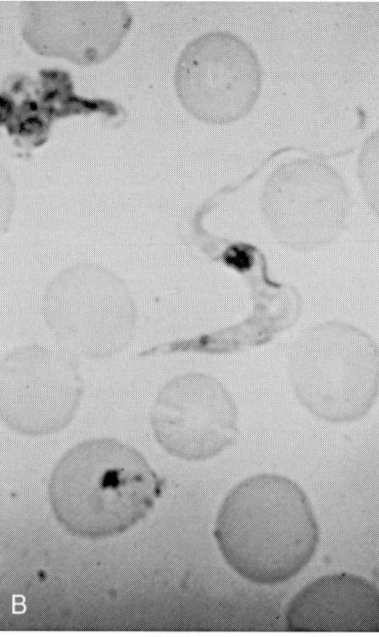

Figure 94–2. *A,* Giemsa-stained trypomastigote of *Trypanosoma cruzi* showing large kinetoplast. *B,* Giemsa-stained trypomastigote of *Trypanosoma rangeli* showing a small kinetoplast (× 1200).

94–1). The two developmental stages in the vertebrate host are infective trypomastigotes found in the blood stream and dividing amastigotes found in tissue (Figs. 94–2*A* and 94–3*A*). Trypomastigotes are flagellated forms measuring 15 to 20 μm in length with a very large posterior kinetoplast. They circulate in the blood and are infective to muscle, nerve, and other host cells. They attach and enter host cells by specific receptors. Once inside the host cell, they transform into oval amastigotes about 3 μm in diameter. As intracellular parasites, they multiply by binary fission and daughter amastigotes develop into trypomastigotes, which are released on rupture of the host cell and enter the circulation. The time from trypomastigote penetration of a cell to its rupture is thought to be about 5 days, but it varies according to cell size and strain differences. Amastigote multiplication in the tissues and trypomastigote dissemination continues indefinitely.

Triatomine bugs, the insect vectors, are obligate blood feeders measuring 5 to 45 mm in length, depending on the species (Figs. 94–4 and 139–9). They aspirate blood directly from capillaries and are infected by ingestion of circulating trypomastigotes (Fig. 94–2*A*). In the insect, trypomastigotes transform into epimastigotes, flagellated forms measuring 20 μm in length with an anterior kinetoplast near the nucleus. The epimastigotes divide in the midgut by binary fission. Daughter epimastigotes migrate to the hindgut where they develop into metacyclic trypomastigotes, the infective form for humans, which are then excreted in bug feces (Fig. 94–1). Metacyclic trypomastigotes appear as early as 20 days after ingestion of contaminated blood. Bugs usually remain infective for life and can transmit *T. cruzi* for several years (Chapter 138).

Humans are usually infected by contamination of the skin from bugs that defecated during or shortly after feeding.

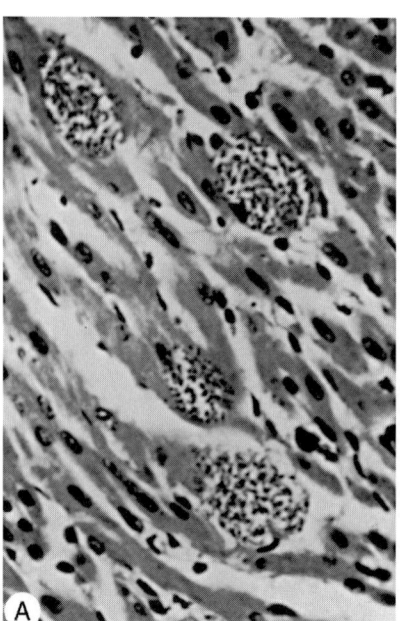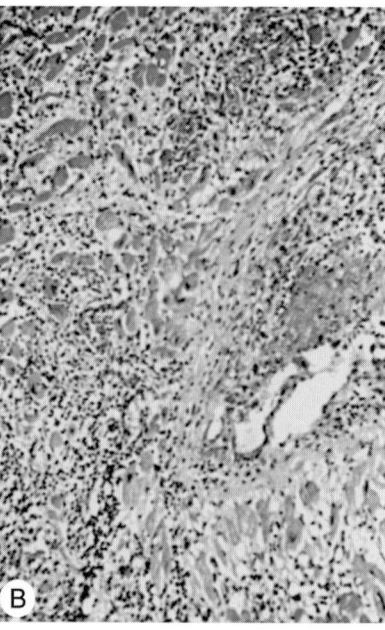

Figure 94–3. *A,* Myocardium in the acute phase of infection showing pseudocysts containing many amastigotes without inflammatory response (× 400). *B,* Chronic chagasic myocarditis with extensive inflammatory cell infiltrate, fragmentation of muscle fibers, and hemorrhage but no visible parasites (× 250).

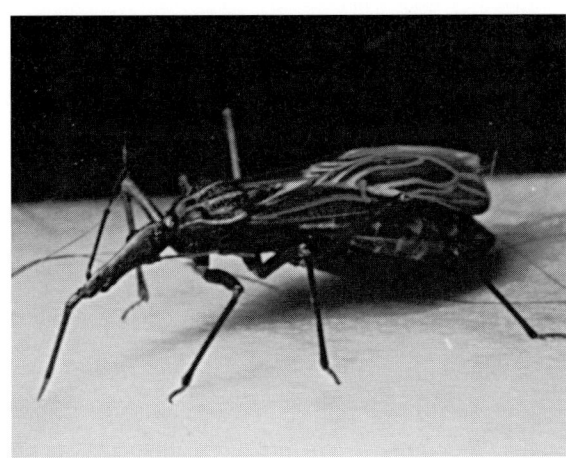

Figure **94–4.** An adult reduviid bug—*Rhodnius prolixus* (× 2). (Courtesy of Dr. Robert Wirtz, Walter Reed Army Institute of Research.)

Infective metacyclic trypomastigotes in the feces penetrate the slightest break in the skin or intact mucosal tissue to infect local tissue histiocytes. Intracellular amastigotes develop and multiply within tissue macrophages, giving rise to nests of infected cells that rupture and disseminate blood trypomastigotes into the circulation to invade other tissue cells. Amastigotes are already present in the heart by the time blood trypomastigotes reach detectable levels.

EPIDEMIOLOGY

Geographic Distribution. Human Chagas' disease is found in all countries of the Americas from the southwestern United States to Argentina and Chile. Human cases in the island nations of the Caribbean and in the dense neotropical rain forests of the Amazon region are nonexistent or rare, although sylvatic transmission cycles have been identified. Currently, Bolivia has the highest rural seroprevalence rate of about 20%, but the majority of cases are reported from central and southern Brazil.

There is a marked difference in the geographic distribution of pathogenic *T. cruzi* isolates, the frequency of chagasic cardiomyopathy and megasyndromes, and the response of patients to specific chemotherapy with nifurtimox or benznidazole. In general, *T. cruzi* isolates from North and Central America are much less pathogenic in experimental animals than those from Brazil. Megasyndromes are rare outside of Brazil, Chile, and Argentina. Cardiomyopathy is more common in central and southern Brazil but is seen throughout the Americas.

Human Infections. In endemic areas the prevalence of human infection with *T. cruzi*, as measured by serologic tests, is often high, whereas clinically detectable disease is infrequent. In Latin America, there are an estimated 16 to 18 million seropositive people, representing 4 to 5% of the population. About a quarter of the population of Latin America (up to 100 million people) are considered at risk. In earlier years, infected people were typically poor subsistence farmers residing in remote rural homesteads who rarely traveled outside their locale. However, successful rural control programs and migration of seropositive people to nonendemic urban centers of both Latin America and North America have changed this distribution pattern.

Laboratory accidents and imported cases of acute infection account for the small number of persons treated in the United States for acute infection. Human Chagas' disease caused by autochthonous vector transmission is rare in the southern and southwestern United States where *T. cruzi* usually circulates between opossums and armadillos. Human infections are infrequent because the local bugs rarely enter high-quality American homes, vector density is very low, and people do not infringe on the sylvan cycle. Additionally, the absence of positive serology in animal trappers from Louisiana suggests that northern strains of *T. cruzi* are less infective for humans.

During the 1980s and 1990s millions of people emigrated to the United States from regions of Central America where *T. cruzi* infection is common. Seroprevalence studies of selected populations yield estimates of up to 100,000 infected persons currently living in the United States.

The risk of vector transmission of *T. cruzi* infections in short-term travelers to endemic areas is extremely low. Only one symptomatic case has been reported in a traveler returning to Europe following a 2-week stay in Colombia where she stayed in primitive housing. It is possible that asymptomatic infections occasionally occur and the risk of infection with the current popularity of adventure travel destinations and itineraries should be considered.

Reservoir Hosts. *T. cruzi* has been found in more than 100 species of mammals, representing 24 families of the following orders: Marsupialia, Edentata, Chiroptera, Carnivora, Lagomorpha, Rodentia, and Primates. Domestic animals are frequently infected, and typical prevalence rates may reach 80% for dogs, 60% for cats, and 60% for guinea pigs. Peridomiciliary rodents also have a high infection rate, up to 90% for mice and 60% for rats. In view of the wide host specificity and broad geographic distribution of *T. cruzi* in the Americas, eradication of the parasite is impossible.

Dogs constitute an important reservoir for human infection because they live in close contact with humans and sleep around the house at night when the bugs are actively feeding. Cases of acute Chagas' disease are periodically seen in domestic hunting dogs in the United States. Infection is thought to occur by ingestion of contaminated bugs or sylvatic animals. The role of cats in human transmission is not clear because they are rarely indoors at night when bugs feed. Perhaps *T. cruzi* is passed from infected bugs via mice to cats by the food chain. Goats (Argentina) and guinea pigs (Peru and Bolivia) are also important reservoirs in certain situations.

Vector. More than a hundred of the known triatomine species exist in Central and South America (Fig. 139–9). A few species, because of their adaptation to houses, are important vectors and determine the distribution of human *T. cruzi* infections (Chapter 138). *Triatoma infestans* is the most important species because of its preference for infesting cracks in the walls of poor housing and its ability to dislocate other triatomine occupants. It is the principal vector in Chile, Argentina, Brazil, Paraguay, Uruguay, Bolivia, and Peru. *Panstrongylus megistus* is also an efficient vector in Brazil. In Venezuela, Colombia, and parts of Central America, *Rhodnius prolixus* (Fig. 94–4) is the principal triatomine involved in transmission. *R. prolixus* also frequently transmits *Trypanosoma rangeli*, which is infective but not pathogenic for humans. Wild-caught bugs may contain both *T. cruzi* and *T. rangeli*, which can be distinguished by the site of multiplication in the bug and by flagellate morphology (Fig. 94–2). Other species are regionally important vectors, e.g., *Triatoma dimidiata* in Ecuador and *Rhodnius pallescens* in Panama.

Each of the five growth stages (instars) of juvenile triatomines requires a blood meal to molt, and adults feed several times. Any of the developmental stages can be infected with and transmit *T. cruzi*. However, to be important vectors of human disease the bugs must colonize houses and prefer human blood. The period that the trypomastigotes survive on the skin depends on the rate of desiccation of the fecal drop. Humid conditions allow more time to scratch the bite site and spread contaminated feces to the mucosa or the puncture wound that remains in the skin after withdrawal of the bug's proboscis. Human vectors frequently feed on the face, facilitating transmission via the mucosa when the awaking person rubs bug feces into his or her eye.

Sylvan and Domestic Cycles. Sylvan transmission usually occurs independently of humans. However, people become at risk for infection when they enter the sylvan cycle, and the sylvan cycle of *T. cruzi* serves as a source of infection for domestic transmission. The opossum, which has a high tolerance to infection, may be an important reservoir host that bridges the sylvan and domestic cycles because it is a peridomiciliary nester and enters houses in search of food. Similarly, synanthropic rodents invade the domestic environment.

Triatomine bugs have become domiciliated as a result of humans' impact on their environment with destruction of their natural habitats by deforestation and cultivation. As natural habitats disappear, a few species of bugs, e.g., *T. infestans, R. prolixus,* and *P. megistus* "move in" with humans. Often, a transitory step for a bug to enter the domestic environment is the initial colonization of small sheds harboring chickens and other domestic animals. These colonization events explain why Chagas' disease was largely a disease of poor, rural, subsistence farmers.

The center of domestic transmission is the house where bugs hide during the day and find frequent blood meals at night (Fig. 94–5). Bugs prefer houses constructed of mud and wattle with cracked walls and thatched roofs, which provide ideal hiding places during the day. At night, the bugs prey on their human hosts and their domestic animals. If a convenient blood source is available, the bugs will remain in the wall fabric near that source resulting in a patchy distribution throughout the house.

Direct Transmission. Although transmission by triatomine bugs accounts for most human infections, there are other modes of transmission.

Blood Transfusions. Transfusion-associated Chagas' disease (TA-CD) is a significant problem in endemic areas and a growing problem in nonendemic areas. Risk of infection depends on the amount of blood transfused, parasite concentration in the infected blood, and immune status of the recipient. The estimated risk for transmission is 13 to 23% for each unit of contaminated blood transfused. However, incidence of new TA-CD infections in endemic areas is declining because of donor education, screening for infected persons by questionnaires, increased use of serologic testing, and parasite

inactivation in donor blood. Donor seropositivity reported in urban centers varies widely from 1.7% in São Paulo, Brazil to 53% in Santa Cruz, Bolivia. However, the prevalence of seropositivity also depends on the type of volunteers used and the serologic method used for screening. In any case, the prevalence of *T. cruzi* infected blood is higher than that for human immunodeficiency virus (HIV) or hepatitis B and C in some areas.

TA-CD has been rarely reported in the United States and Canada. The few reported cases occurred in immunosuppressed patients having fulminant disease. TA-CD leading to milder, unrecognized illnesses or asymptomatic infection in immunocompetent persons undoubtedly occurs. Serosurveys of blood donors in southern California have found about 1 in 1000 seropositive donors. A seroprevalence survey in the Washington, D.C. area showed 5% of 205 Salvadoran and Nicaraguan immigrants were infected. With increasing immigration from endemic areas of Central and South America, it is possible that the TA-CD in the United States will increase.

Person to Person. Congenital transmission occurs in about 1% of deliveries of serologically positive mothers. Infants can also be infected through breast-feeding. *T. cruzi* has also been transmitted by organ transplantation.

Ingestion. Transmission by ingestion of contaminated food has also been recorded. In Brazil, 58 people were infected in four outbreaks linked to cold soup and sugar cane contaminated with animal urine and feces from bugs. In the state of Nayarit, Mexico, *Triatoma phyllosoma* is eaten for its supposed aphrodisiac properties.

Occupational. More than 50 laboratory infections in research workers have occurred, usually from pipetting suspensions of *T. cruzi* by mouth or from accidental injection while inoculating animals.

PATHOGENESIS. A number of mechanisms have been postulated for the pathogenesis of Chagas' disease. These depend on various factors that qualitatively and quantitatively interfere with the development of *T. cruzi* infection. In general, these factors are parasite dependent (i.e., polymorphism, cell tropism, virulence, antigenicity, size of inoculum) and host dependent (i.e., genetics, sex, age, route of infection, immune response, reinfection, nutrition).

Parasite Factors. Isolates of *T. cruzi* parasites from patients can be characterized by isoenzyme analysis into at least five groups, called zymodemes. Analysis of kinetoplast DNA reveals many variants, or strains, within zymodemes. *T. cruzi* strain differences probably explain geographic morphologic polymorphism and geographic differences in the frequencies of "megasyndromes," tissue tropisms, virulence in animal hosts, and chemotherapeutic responses.

T. cruzi infecting humans can be classified into three main zymodemes (Z1, Z2, and Z3) based on isoenzyme data from Brazil, Bolivia, Chile, Venezuela, Colombia, Peru, Paraguay, French Guiana, and Central America. With one exception, zymodeme Z2 has only been reported south of the Amazon basin, and multiple-banded Z2 patterns are especially common in southern regions of South America (Bolivia, Chile, Paraguay, Peru). The correlation between biochemical differences and variation in virulence is not well understood. There is tremendous variation in pathogenicity of laboratory strains for experimental animal infections, but molecular markers of virulence have not yet been identified.

Immune Response. Research has focused on mechanisms by which trypomastigotes and amastigotes avoid the immune response and persist for years in their vertebrate hosts. Both metacyclic trypomastigotes from the bug and circulating trypomastigotes from the vertebrate host resist serum killing by the alternate complement pathway. These trypomastigotes shed a glycoprotein that inhibits the formation of comple-

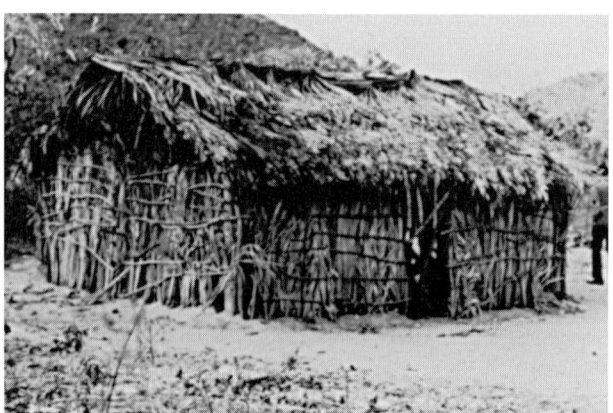

Figure 94–5. A palm thatch house in Mambai Goiás, Brazil, which at demolition contained over 1000 *Triatoma infestans.*

ment C3 convertases and accelerates their decay. Presumably, this inhibitory glycoprotein blocks trypomastigote lysis by the alternate complement pathway. However, host antibodies are eventually generated that neutralize this protective glycoprotein, exposing the trypomastigotes to complement-mediated lysis. These antibodies probably play an important role in the suppression of circulating trypomastigotes in patients with chronic infections.

After entering the circulation, trypomastigotes must identify and infect susceptible host cells. This probably occurs through receptor-ligand–mediated endocytosis. Macrophages and monocytes, as well as trypomastigotes, have fibronectin receptors; this molecule enhances both parasite-cell binding and parasite uptake. The receptor-ligand system that facilitates infection of cardiac muscle, nerve cells, and other cells is not known.

As intracellular parasites, the trypomastigotes must evade intracellular killing mechanisms, particularly the lethal effects of the oxidative burst. A proportion of trypomastigotes pass through the phagosomal membrane to infect the cytoplasm, a privileged site free from lysosomal enzymes. In heart and nerve cells, trypomastigotes develop into amastigotes that multiply. Differentiation of amastigotes into trypomastigotes in the host cells occurs about 24 hours before cell rupture, but many parasites do not achieve full differentiation and are killed by the surrounding inflammatory cells, neutrophils, eosinophils, monocytes, and macrophages. Parasite transmission from cell to cell usually involves the transformation of the daughter amastigotes into infective trypomastigotes, which are able to successfully infect other cells. However, amastigotes are also capable of infecting macrophages directly.

In experimental models, both CD4 and CD8 T cells have been shown to be important for resistance to T. cruzi. Lysis of infected macrophages by CD8-positive, cytotoxic T cells (CTL) may also be an important mechanism of host defense. CD4 T cells are also necessary to generate the specific antibody that contributes to parasite clearance. Both types of T cells produce cytokines, principally interferon gamma (IFN-γ) capable of activating macrophages to kill intracellular amastigotes. IFN-γ in animal models is very effective at inhibiting parasite replication in macrophages and can prevent acute disease in mice. Furthermore, in vivo neutralization of IFN-γ using monoclonal antibody greatly increases host susceptibility, further demonstrating the importance of this cytokine in controlling disease.

More recently, the pathogenicity of experimental T. cruzi infections has been linked to the induction of immunosuppressive cytokines (predominantly transforming growth factor beta [TGF-β] and interleukin 10 [IL-10]) by the parasite following infection. These cytokines inhibit the macrophage activating capability of IFN-γ. In fact, studies have shown that an increase in these suppressive cytokines, rather than a decrease in IFN-γ, is responsible for disease progression. It is logical that an organism so well adapted for intracellular survival should have the ability to increase macrophage cytokines that prevent its destruction.

The pathogenesis of end-organ destruction in Chagas' disease is not completely understood. The infrequent finding of tissue-dwelling amastigotes in the sectioned heart leads some to argue that amastigotes are sequestered in tissues other than the heart and gut. For example, smooth muscle in the wall of the suprarenal vein, which carries a high concentration of corticoids, is a site of amastigote proliferation. It is also not clear if continued presence of T. cruzi amastigotes or parasite DNA is required for tissue destruction; however, several studies have shown T. cruzi DNA is present in cardiac tissue and may even be integrated into the host genome.

Others believe that infection with T. cruzi stimulates autoimmunity, which results in chronic pathologic changes in the absence of parasites. Autoimmune lymphocytes and autoantibodies against endocardium, interstitium of striated muscle, and blood vessels have been detected in chagasic patients. T. cruzi shares common antigens with heart tissue, and it has been speculated that these parasite antigens stimulate an autoimmune response by molecular mimicry.

Recent studies support this hypothesis by defining antigens shared by the parasite and host. The best characterized example is the family of ribosomal proteins known as P (or phospho) proteins, which are highly antigenic. The genes have been cloned for both mammalian and T. cruzi P proteins. One member, P0, displays remarkable conservation between the human and parasite but the T. cruzi protein has unique regions that make it very immunogenic. Infected individuals have antibodies not only to the parasite P0 but also to human P0, perhaps due to a phenomenon known as epitope spreading. Human anti-P0 autoantibody has been observed in another autoimmune disease, systemic lupus erythematosus, at a rate of approximately 25%. In contrast, up to 85% of individuals with T. cruzi infection have P0 autoantibody.

PATHOLOGY

Acute Phase. Rapid parasite multiplication occurs inside cells producing a cystlike structure that ruptures to release daughter amastigotes. Early in the infection the intracellular parasites promote little inflammatory reaction (Fig. 94–3A). However, after the first generation of amastigotes, immunologically competent lymphocyte and plasma cells rapidly make their appearance. As the infection progresses, parasites are more difficult to find and inflammatory cells become common (Fig. 94–3B). Amastigotes can be found in almost every organ during the acute phase, but the most marked pathology occurs in the heart, brain, and liver.

The heart is enlarged and dilated with focal hemorrhage. Excess serous fluid and congested organs are seen according to the degree of heart failure. Microscopically, myofibers contain enormous numbers of amastigotes that are released into the interstitium when the myofiber ruptures. The acute myocardial inflammatory changes in Chagas' disease are probably the most severe of all known forms of myocarditis. Focal inflammatory reactions against these parasites and disrupted tissues also destroy nearby normal tissue, including the cardiac conducting system. There are perivascular collections of lymphocytes and plasma cells. Muscle fibers exhibit hyaline degeneration and often appear separated and fragmented with large nests of parasites between them. The epicardium and pericardium are likewise involved.

In severe cases of acute disease, the brain and meninges are congested and contain petechiae. Scattered, small inflammatory foci, occasionally with parasites, are often seen in the brain. The liver is usually enlarged with fatty degeneration. Parasites are only seen in the Kupffer cells. The spleen and peripheral lymph nodes are also enlarged, congested, and infiltrated with inflammatory cells, but parasites are rarely seen.

The lesions of the esophagus and gastrointestinal tract are predominantly located in the muscle layers and in the intramural nerve plexus. As in the heart, focal myositis is observed around degenerated amastigotes in the interstitium. The lesions of the sympathetic and parasympathetic nervous systems include perigangliionitis, ganglionitis, neuritis, perineuritis, chromatolysis, and death and necrosis of nerve fibers.

Chronic Phase. The severe myocarditis associated with Chagas' disease leads to chronic chagasic cardiomyopathy. Grossly, the chagasic heart is thin-walled, enlarged, and flabby with a prominent right ventricular outflow tract. The heart valves are not involved, but there is dilatation of the valve rings and enlargement and fibrosis of the atrial walls. Ventricular apical walls are thin and fibrotic with aneurysm formation that may contain mural thrombi.

Microscopically, there is chronic myocarditis with focal endocarditis, myocarditis and pericarditis with infiltration of chronic inflammatory cells, fibrosis, and atrophy. Inflammation, fibrosis, and atrophy also occur in the intracardiac conduction system. No other type of cardiopathy develops fibrosis so intensely as chronic Chagas' disease.

There is a characteristic and marked thinning of the visceral wall seen in gastrointestinal megasyndromes. Variable amounts of inflammation and fibrosis are seen, most commonly in the esophagus and sigmoid colon. Microscopically, there is a marked decrease in the ganglion cells of the myenteric plexus.

CLINICAL MANIFESTATIONS

Acute Illness. Acute illness can follow natural transmission, congenital infection, blood transfusion, oral transmission, or laboratory accident. The clinical severity of acute illness can vary widely. Most infections are asymptomatic, 10 to 20% have a mild undifferentiated febrile syndrome, and less than 5% have a severe illness associated with acute heart failure or meningoencephalitis. Death is uncommon but is usually due to acute cardiac failure when it occurs. More severe illness is seen in very young children. The incubation period is 7 to 14 days with the onset of high continuous fever in severe cases and low grade fever in less severe cases. An elastic, nonpitting edema may extend from the face to involve the whole body. Hepatosplenomegaly and peripheral adenopathy are frequent. Following resolution of the acute illness after 4 to 8 weeks, infected individuals enter the indeterminate phase.

An inoculation granuloma ("chagoma") is seen in about half the patients. A chagoma begins as a small, tender, erythematous papule that enlarges over 7 to 10 days to a dusky, erythematous, indurated lesion several centimeters in size, covered with scaling skin. Motile trypomastigotes can often be demonstrated in wet mount preparations of needle aspirates taken from chagomas. The chagoma resolves over about a month and leaves a hyperpigmented scar.

Contamination of the conjunctiva occurs when infected bug feces are rubbed into the eye. Inflammation of the conjunctiva, in response to proliferating parasites, produces a visible edematous reaction, commonly called Romaña's sign (Fig. 94–6). It is characterized by bipalpebral, unilateral, chronic edema and may be associated with local lymph gland enlargement. Occasionally, trypomastigotes are found in tears. The edema associated with Romaña's sign lasts for several days to weeks, differentiating it from most other causes of unilateral bipalpebral edema.

Anemia, lymphocytosis, and modest elevations in liver and muscle enzymes are common in the acute illness. Nonspecific electrocardiographic (ECG) changes are seen in many patients; more severe cases have changes consistent with myocarditis and first-degree atrioventricular block. On x-ray studies, varying degrees of cardiomegaly may be detected, and heart failure (a sign of poor prognosis) may be present.

Indeterminate Phase. Patients in the indeterminate phase remain asymptomatic and do not develop clinical illness unless they become immunocompromised. They have antibodies to multiple *T. cruzi* antigens and very low (subpatent) levels of circulating parasites. Xenodiagnosis is positive in about 50% of those with positive serology. However, 10 to 30% of patients in the indeterminate phase will progress over the ensuing decades and develop signs and symptoms of end-organ dysfunction due to chronic Chagas' disease.

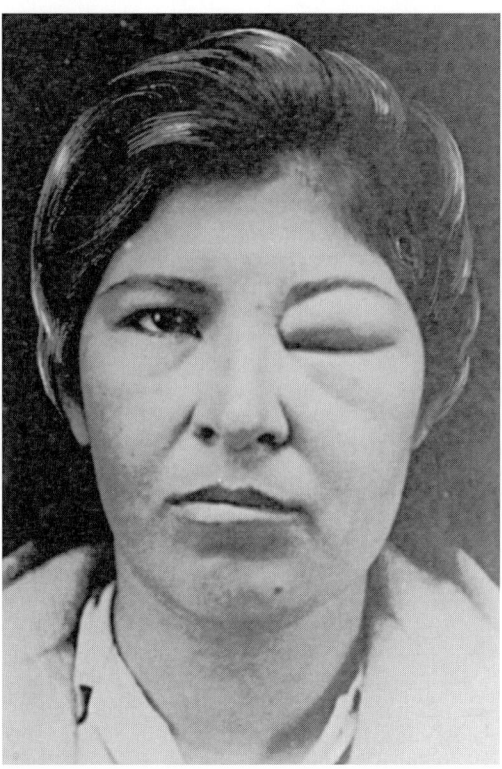

Figure 94–6. Unilateral orbital edema. (Romaña's sign in acute Chagas' disease). (Courtesy of Dr. Ramon S. Freire, Chaco, Argentina.)

Chronic Disease

Cardiomyopathy. The natural history of chagasic cardiomyopathy has been studied in a series of longitudinal, epidemiologic studies in endemic areas. In a rural area of Brazil, 141 seropositive children were compared to 282 matched seronegative controls. There was a prevalence of ECG abnormalities in 11.3% of the seropositive patients and 3.5% of the seronegative controls. In the 3-year period of follow-up, five new cases of complete right bundle branch block (CRBBB) were detected in the seropositive group. This study, along with others, suggests significant progression early in the course of infection in some individuals.

ECG changes are often the first sign of dysfunction but are usually not identified because patients are asymptomatic. Ventricular extrasystoles and first-degree heart block are common and CRBBB, with or without left anterior hemiblock, is considered a very specific abnormality associated with Chagas' disease. Atrial fibrillation and left bundle branch block are uncommon abnormalities. Progression of the damage to Purkinje fibers may lead eventually to complete heart block with Stokes-Adams attacks. Cardiomyopathy with an enlarged heart (Fig. 94–7) usually appears in the second or third decade following initial infection. It is more common in males, possibly because of increased cardiac work. Although cases cluster in families, no single risk factor predicts individual or population risk (Chapter 3).

Chagasic cardiomyopathy often develops insidiously. The presenting manifestations of 42 definite or probable cases of Chagas' heart disease reported in immigrants (mostly from Central America) living in southern California were symptomatic AV block, congestive heart failure, anginal chest pain, conduction abnormalities on ECG, sudden death averted by resuscitation, sustained ventricular tachycardia, and pulmonary or systemic emboli from an intracardiac mural thrombo-

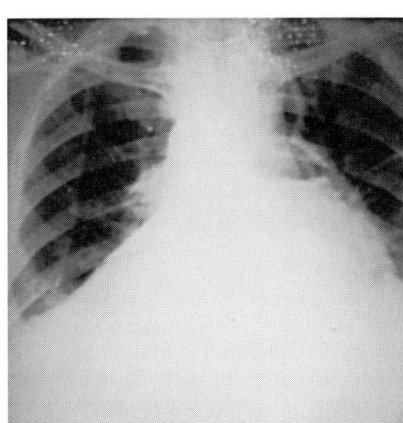

Figure 94–7. Anteroposterior radiograph of the chest showing a generally enlarged heart and a fluid level in a megaesophagus behind the heart in a patient with chronic Chagas' disease.

sis. Over 70% had received treatment for other presumed cardiac diagnoses (coronary artery disease or idiopathic dilated cardiomyopathy) for periods up to 9 years (mean, 20 ± 33 months). Interestingly, none of these patients could recall an illness compatible with acute Chagas' disease. A left ventricular aneurysm was found in 14 of 25 with definite Chagas' heart disease. These findings also suggest that Chagas' heart disease is more common in the United States than currently reported.

Megasyndromes. Megasyndromes are late stage manifestations due to the dilation of the esophagus or sigmoid colon (Fig. 94–8). Destruction of submucosal parasympathetic ganglion cells leads to aperistalsis, retention of solid residues, and dilation of the viscous organs. Although rarely fatal, megasyndromes cause significant morbidity in those affected

due to difficulty in swallowing (megaesophagus) or constipation (megacolon). Megasyndromes have not been described north of the equator and are uncommon outside of Brazil. They are seen in 15 to 50% of seropositive patients in Brazil, but the frequency varies greatly with the region under consideration.

MEGAESOPHAGUS. The characteristic presentation of megaesophagus is progressive difficulty in swallowing, especially of dry foods, and may reach a point at which solid food cannot be ingested. Improvement of dysphagia following intake of water is characteristic. Based on barium contrast radiologic studies, four grades of esophageal enlargement are described. Grade 1 has a transverse esophageal diameter of <4 cm, grade 2 is 4 to 7 cm, grade 3 is 7 to 10 cm, and grade 4 is >10 cm. Grade 4 is dolichomegaesophagus, which appears as an enormous viscus on top of the diaphragm. Pressure at the gastroesophageal sphincter is increased, and there is no relaxation after swallowing. Manometry is also useful showing absence of primary peristaltic waves, disorganized activity in grades 1 to 2, and no peristalsis in grades 3 to 4. In advanced cases, esophagitis is common, and reflux may lead to frequent aspiration and pulmonary infections. This is aggravated by pressure on the lungs from the dilated viscus' interfering with lung drainage. Frequently, to provide saliva for lubrication, the parotid gland hypertrophies. This, coupled with wasting due to malnutrition, is responsible for the "cat facies" seen in advanced megaesophagus (Fig. 94–9). Esophageal carcinoma is more common in patients with Chagas' megaesophagus than in the nonchagasic population.

MEGACOLON. The characteristic presentation of megacolon is progressive constipation associated with abdominal distention and marked tympanism. Obstipation, fecal impaction, and pseudodiarrhea due to passage of liquid stools around impacted feces are seen in severe cases. Anorexia, anemia, and asthenia are common. The two main complications are volvulus of the sigmoid colon, which may present as an acute surgical emergency, and fecaloma in severely obstipated patients.

Megasyndromes of other organs occur but usually are not detected clinically. In one study, a concomitant chagasic

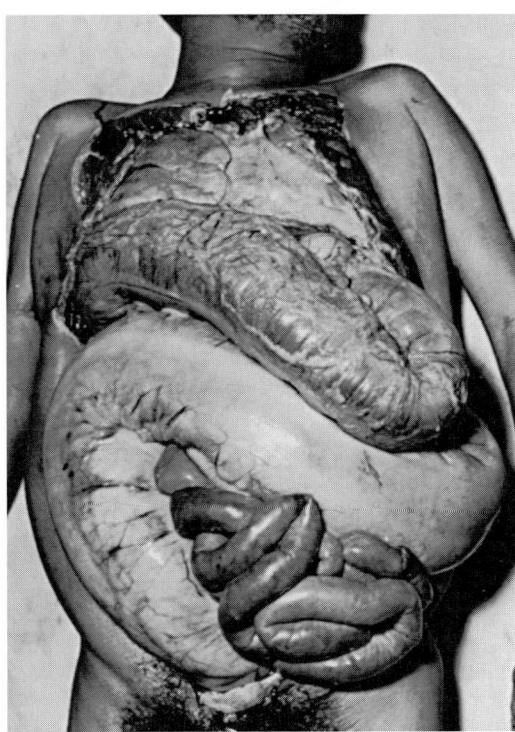

Figure 94–8. Megacolon in chronic Chagas' disease. (Courtesy of Dr. Fritz Köberle, São Paulo, Brazil.)

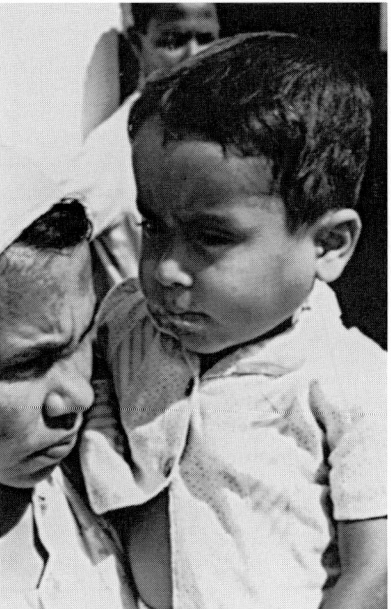

Figure 94–9. Child with advanced megaesophagus. Note the parotid enlargement producing the so-called cat facies.

chronic cardiopathy was observed in 50% of the cases displaying esophageal dysperistalsis.

Other Lesions. Myositis also occurs in skeletal muscles, and dysfunction of the motor end plate and the lower motor neuron pathway is demonstrated by absent knee and ankle deep tendon reflexes. Animal studies show a diminution in the number of anterior horn cells of the spinal cord. There is some evidence for exocrine and endocrine gland dysfunction in chronic infections, as well as an abnormal hormonal regulation of gut function.

Congenital Infections. The prevalence of *T. cruzi* infection among pregnant women living in endemic areas of Latin America ranges from 2 to 51% (urban) and 23 to 81% (rural). Up to 10% of pregnant women in nonendemic areas are seropositive. Congenital infection is documented in 1 to 10% of pregnancies, mostly from women with chronic infection.

Prompt diagnosis of congenital infection is desirable in order to initiate specific treatment in the infant early in the course of infection. Parasitologic tests are more often positive in the first 6 months of life, as parasitemia is higher early in the course of infection. The microhematocrit test is clinically useful in this population.

Congenital Chagas' disease may cause spontaneous abortion, premature birth, intrauterine growth retardation, and stillbirth. The clinical spectrum of congenital infection is similar to acute Chagas' disease and varies from asymptomatic infection to severe compromise. Between 50 and 75% have no signs or symptoms of disease. Infection is detected only by an active search among children born to seropositive mothers. A mild illness is more common and hepatosplenomegaly is the most common syndrome (15 to 20%). Pneumonitis, meningoencephalitis, and diffuse dermal granulomas of the newborn can be seen. The most severe cases have hemorrhagic symptoms (e.g., petechiae, ecchymosis, bleeding). Some infants die during the first week of life and others show meningoencephalitic symptoms (from slight tremor to generalized convulsions). A few infants have jaundice, or disseminated chagomas (hemorrhagic and even necrotic lesions of the skin and mucous membranes). Occasionally, metaphysitis, intracranial calcifications, and ocular lesions have been described.

T. cruzi as an Opportunistic Infection in the Immunocompromised. Recrudescence of chronic infection is seen in seropositive patients undergoing chemotherapy for hematologic malignancies, receiving chronic steroid therapy, and following organ transplantation. Clinical disease, even severe, can be seen in this group. Seronegative, immunosuppressed patients receiving contaminated blood are also at risk of fulminant disease. Cutaneous eruptions that resemble bacterial cellulitis have been described in several patients with reactivation following cardiac transplantation. These lesions are described as large, irregular-shaped, erythematous, indurated plaques within which were areas of normal-appearing skin and necrotic eschars. Diagnosis is confirmed by visualizing amastigotes in tissue obtained by punch biopsy.

Co-infection With HIV. In the past decade, several cases of acute Chagas' disease have been described in individuals co-infected with HIV. Most of these cases have been reported from urban centers in Brazil. When reported, CD4 counts have been low, ranging from <50 to 382 per mL.

The most common (75%) presentation is meningoencephalitis (unifocal and multifocal) with fever, headache, seizures, vomiting, and focal neurologic findings. Cerebrospinal fluid (CSF) analysis shows mild lymphocyte predominant pleocytosis (<100 cells per mL), increased protein, and occasionally trypomastigotes. Parasites are often seen in peripheral blood by direct methods as well. CT imaging of the brain shows single or multiple hypodense subcortical lesions, with and without ring enhancement. The subcortical location is helpful in differentiating reactivated Chagas' disease from toxoplasmosis, which is more common in the thalamus and basal ganglia. The second most common site of involvement is the heart (50%) with clinical manifestations of heart failure and arrhythmias.

DIAGNOSIS. A definitive diagnosis of infection with *T. cruzi* is made by detecting parasites in blood or tissues (parasitologic diagnosis) or by detecting antibodies to *T. cruzi* antigens in the blood (serologic diagnosis).

Parasitologic Diagnosis. Parasitologic methods include direct microscopy with and without concentration techniques, xenodiagnosis, in vitro culture, in vivo culture, and detection of *T. cruzi* DNA. The optimal method depends on the level of parasitemia (phase of the disease). In chronically infected persons, parasitemia may also be intermittent partially accounting for the decreased sensitivity of parasitologic methods in this group.

Microscopy. When the immunocompetent patient is febrile during the acute illness, motile trypomastigotes can be detected by relatively insensitive methods, e.g., direct examination of wet preparations of anticoagulated blood or buffy coat. Examination of Giemsa-stained thin and thick blood films is also useful. Parasites rapidly disappear as fever and edema resolve. Blood concentration techniques such as centrifugation after clot retraction at 640XG (Strout concentration) or the microhematocrit method (Chapter 151) increase sensitivity. Trypomastigotes can be identified in other specimens, e.g., CSF, pericardial fluid, mass lesions, bone marrow, and organ biopsies in the immunocompromised patient. The trypomastigotes of *T. cruzi* are distinguished morphologically from those of *T. rangeli* by microscopic examination of Giemsa-stained blood films (Fig. 94–2). Criteria for the morphologic differentiation of *T. rangeli* from *T. cruzi* are reviewed in Chapter 94.1.

During the indeterminate and chronic phase, parasitemia is subpatent and a parasitologic diagnosis requires more sensitive methods. Unfortunately, these methods take several weeks to yield a final result and so are not useful to the clinician who wants to initiate specific therapy based on parasitologic confirmation.

Chagas' disease can also be diagnosed from histologic sections of infected tissue, but this method is insensitive. Typically, clusters of amastigotes are seen in muscle cells surrounded by no, acute or chronic inflammation (Figs. 94–3*A* and *B*).

Xenodiagnosis. Xenodiagnosis refers to a technique in which clean, laboratory-reared juvenile bugs are fed on the seropositive patient. A month later their feces and hindgut contents are examined for infection with flagellates. In competent hands xenodiagnosis is very specific for the diagnosis of *T. cruzi* infection, but the sensitivity may be no greater than 50% in chronic patients with a positive serology. The level of parasitemia in the patient, species of bug, method of examination, and frequency of bug examination determine the sensitivity of the test. Triatomine bugs (Fig. 94–4) are extremely susceptible to infection and this characteristic makes them valuable in xenodiagnosis. Xenodiagnosis is useful in confirmation of infection, isolation of strains, and the evaluation of chemotherapy. In areas with sympatric *T. rangeli*, the parasites can be distinguished by the site of multiplication in the bug and by the morphology of the epimastigote stage. Facilities for xenodiagnosis are frequently not available outside Latin America.

In Vitro Culture. In vitro culture using biphasic media (e.g., NNM, Warren, or LIT) can detect circulating parasites, but is not as sensitive as xenodiagnosis. Cultures should be inoculated at 26°C and examined weekly for 4 weeks for epimastigotes.

Animal Inoculation. Blood from patients can be inoculated into susceptible laboratory animals, which become patent with circulating trypomastigotes between 5 and 15 days.

T. cruzi DNA. Although the number of circulating parasites is very low in persons with chronic infection, *T. cruzi* has highly repetitive nuclear and kinetoplast DNA sequences that can be used as targets for amplification with the polymerase chain reaction (PCR). Assays are in development by several groups but the technique is not routinely available.

Serologic Diagnosis. Antibodies appear during the acute illness and persist for life. However, the isotype, affinity, and avidity of these antibodies to multiple parasite determinants evolve throughout the course of infection. Patients in the indeterminate phase are usually detected serologically during blood bank or epidemiologic screening. The clinician is largely dependent on serology for a presumptive diagnosis of chronic infection with *T. cruzi* and there are a wide variety of commercially available assays in Latin America with high sensitivity including the indirect hemagglutination assay (IHA), the indirect fluorescence assay (IFA), the complement fixation test (CF), and enzyme-linked immunosorbent assay (ELISA). Tests using crude epimastigote lysates or whole parasites as the capture antigen have lower specificity. Sera from patients with leishmaniasis, syphilis, malaria, infection with *T. rangeli*, and collagen vascular diseases cross react in these Chagas' assays. Therefore, clinicians in endemic areas must be aware of the performance characteristics of the particular tests being used.

In the United States, there are currently (1999) three qualitative, ELISA-based assays commercially available and cleared by the U.S. Food and Drug Administration for the presumptive diagnosis of Chagas' disease: Abbott Chagas Antibody EIA (Abbott Laboratories, Abbott Park, IL), Hemagen Chagas Kit (Hemagen Diagnostics, Waltham, MA), and the Chagas IgG ELISA (Gull Laboratories, Inc., Salt Lake City, Utah). Each manufacturer performs a partial purification of a crude lysate of culture-derived epimastigotes as the source of capture antigen. They measure human IgG antibodies that bind to the antigen. Sensitivity and specificity are quoted at 95 to 100% for the assays, but may be lower depending on the definition of a true positive used as the gold standard. Limited testing of sera from patients with other diseases show cross reactions in those with recent influenza vaccine immunization. These assays represent a significant advance toward the standardization of serology for *T. cruzi* infection. The ELISA serologic assays should be considered screening assays and confirmed with a more specific assay, e.g., the radioimmune precipitation assay, if available. Serologic results are best used in conjunction with clinical and epidemiologic findings.

Clinicians in the United States can also send specimens through their local health department to the Division of Parasitic Diseases at the Centers for Disease Control and Prevention, Atlanta, GA (770-488-4475) for IFA serologic testing and in vitro culture. An IFA titer >1:32 is considered diagnostic for human infection.

Most recently, the introduction of defined and specific *T. cruzi* antigens, such as synthetic peptides synthesized from cloned genes of the parasite, promise a new generation of assays with remarkable specificity and sensitivity. In many cases, these peptides consist of repetitive sequences with an extremely high avidity for specific antibody. These peptides can readily be synthesized on a large scale and readily lend themselves to the development of standardized reagents specific for *T. cruzi* infections.

Serologic Testing in Nonendemic Areas. Serologic screening should be considered in persons at increased risk of Chagas' disease. Patient groups that may benefit from serologic testing include pregnant women and persons who have acquired or iatrogenic immunosuppression. Screening of pregnant women allows infants at risk of congenital infection to be monitored with appropriate parasitologic studies and specific treatment given if transmission occurred. Persons who will receive immunosuppressive drugs as part of therapy for a disease process or organ transplantation may benefit from knowledge of their serologic status prior to initiation of therapy. Persons with acquired immunocompromise, in particular those with early HIV infection, may benefit from serologic testing to assess risk of *T. cruzi* as an opportunistic infection. In addition, all who are infected may benefit from ECG monitoring, although the cost benefit of this strategy has not been assessed.

Selection of Diagnostic Tests in Different Clinical Situations. Parasitologic tests should be used in acute illness following natural vector transmission, congenital infection, receipt of contaminated blood, accidental laboratory infection, and reactivation illness in the immunocompromised. The first step should be the examination of anticoagulated, unstained blood or buffy coat by direct microscopy looking for motile trypomastigotes accompanied by examination of Giemsa-stained thin and thick films to morphologically confirm the diagnosis of *T. cruzi*. If these procedures fail to identify parasites, then concentration of peripheral blood should be attempted. If parasites are still not identifiable, then more sensitive techniques (in vitro or in vivo culture, xenodiagnosis, and PCR) can be used if they are available and the clinical situation warrants; however, results may be delayed by several weeks. Empirical therapy may be warranted depending on the clinical condition and circumstances of exposure. In immunocompromised patients, any clinically involved tissue or specimen in addition to peripheral blood should be examined for parasites.

Following resolution of the acute illness, serologic tests are the best method of confirming infection. The choice of assay is dependent on what is locally available. When congenital infection is suspected, serologic tests cannot be used in the infant during the first 6 months because of transplacentally acquired IgG antibodies from the infected mother. Serial determinations of IgM antibodies have not proved reliable, and diagnosis in the first 6 months is based on parasitologic tests and conventional serology after the first 6 months.

DIFFERENTIAL DIAGNOSIS

Acute Infections. Acute Chagas' disease must be considered together with typhoid fever, kala-azar, schistosomiasis, brucellosis, infectious mononucleosis, toxoplasmosis, malaria, and glomerulonephritis as a cause for undifferentiated fever with or without signs of a portal of entry in an endemic area. Romaña's sign must be differentiated from local allergic edema, e.g., that due to insect bite, which resolves much more rapidly. Other ocular alterations, e.g., severe conjunctivitis or trauma, must also be considered.

Cardiomyopathy. Cardiac failure in Chagas' disease is biventricular without acute pulmonary edema. The dilated heart promotes functional tricuspid incompetence. Myocarditis and pericarditis may be due to other causes, e.g., rheumatic fever or viral myocarditis. Endomyocardial fibrosis may closely mimic chagasic cardiomyopathy, but serology is negative. Other forms of cardiomyopathy, particularly alcoholic, must be considered.

TREATMENT

Criteria of Cure. The effect of specific therapy on acute disease is measured by clinical cure (the remission of signs and symptoms of disease), parasitologic cure (the reduction or elimination of parasitemia), and serologic cure (negative seroconversion). The known differences in virulence and sensitivity of parasite isolates from different geographic areas complicates interpretation of efficacy. Results from one area may not be predictive of other areas. Also, the definition of serologic cure is very dependent on the type of serologic assay used. Antibodies detected by conventional techniques (IFA, IHA, CF) using crude antigens are not useful in the evaluation of treatment. Antibodies detected against living trypomastigotes by complement-mediated lysis or antibodies to defined antigens may be a more reliable marker of ongoing infections. Negative seroconversion is thought to indicate parasitologic cure.

Specific Chemotherapy. Two drugs are available for specific treatment, nifurtimox (Lampit, Bayer 2502) and benznidazole (Rochagan, Roche 7-1051, Radamil). Neither of these drugs is licensed in the United States or Europe. Nifurtimox is available for domestic use within the United States (not available for export outside the United States) through a compassionate use investigational new drug (IND) protocol from the Parasitic Disease Drug Service of the CDC, Atlanta, GA (404-639-3356). Strains of *T. cruzi* from Argentina and Chile are reported to be more sensitive to nifurtimox than Brazilian strains.

A significant incidence of lymphomas is seen in rabbits treated with both agents. Although of concern, there are no reports of increased incidence in lymphomas in immunocompetent patients from endemic areas where both drugs have been in use for years.

Nifurtimox. Nifurtimox is a nitrofuran that is active against both trypomastigotes and amastigotes. It interferes with the parasite's carbohydrate metabolism by inhibiting pyruvic acid synthesis. It is given to adults in an oral dose of 8 to 10 mg/kg/day in 3 divided doses, after meals. Children tolerate the drug better than adults, and some recommend a higher dose of 15 mg/kg/day in 3 divided doses, after meals, for children. The peak plasma concentration occurs 1 to 3 hours after treatment. The concentration of the drug in tissues and urine is low. Recommended duration of treatment varies from a minimum of 30 days up to 120 days. Therapy must be given under strict medical supervision because serious side effects may occur. Tremors, excitation, insomnia, anorexia, and weight loss are frequent. Peripheral neuritis, psychosis, and hemolytic anemia associated with glucose-6-phosphate dehydrogenase deficiency are dose-dependent and appear near the end of treatment. Polyneuropathy, the most serious adverse effect, usually resolves when treatment is stopped.

Benznidazole. This nitroimidazole derivative is more trypanocidal than nifurtimox and also acts against the amastigote stage. More than 40% of the drug binds to protein and more than 70% of the metabolites are excreted in the urine. The drug is rapidly absorbed and distributed throughout the body. It is given to both adults and children orally at 5 to 10 mg/kg body weight daily in 2 doses. As with nifurtimox, children tolerate the drug better and receive the higher dose. Therapy is given for 30 to 60 days under strict medical supervision. About half of the patients develop light-sensitive rashes that can rarely progress to exfoliative dermatitis. Peripheral neuritis, anorexia, weight loss, and hematologic alterations (neutropenia, agranulocytosis, thrombocytopenia), are also common complications. Benznidazole was well tolerated in children during several large clinical trials. In South America, especially Brazil, this drug is the first choice for specific therapy and is widely available in local pharmacies.

Treatment During the Acute Illness. There is a consensus that specific treatment is beneficial in acute cases, shortening the time to clinical cure and reducing the level of tissue parasitization. However, carefully controlled studies with re-

peated xenodiagnosis show that parasitologic cure is achieved in only about half the cases in central Brazil.

Treatment During the Indeterminate Phase. Specific treatment in the indeterminate phase is controversial because of the difficulty in assessing therapeutic efficacy. Patients lack clinical findings, have very low grade parasitemias, have persistent serologic positivity, and require long periods of follow-up to assess any difference in treatment arms. However, recent studies support the use of specific treatment in indeterminate-phase patients. In one study of 131 patients treated with benznidazole at 5 mg/kg/day for 30 days versus 70 untreated patients, treated patients had a lower incidence of ECG changes (4 vs. 30%) during the 8-year average follow-up and a lower rate of clinical deterioration (2 vs. 17%). Serologic titers in the treated group also declined relative to the untreated group (19 vs. 6%). In another study of 64 asymptomatic Brazilian school-age children treated with benznidazole (7.5 mg/kg/day for 60 days) versus 65 untreated children, 58% of the treated children became seronegative versus 3% of the untreated children (56% efficacy [95% confidence interval, 41 to 67%]) over a 3-year follow-up period. Those without negative seroconversion all had a significant decrease in antibody titers compared with the untreated group. Benznidazole was well tolerated in this trial with only 5% of all participants complaining of minor adverse effects. Cutaneous maculopapular rash and pruritus were more common in the benznidazole group. A third study from Argentina randomized 55 children to benznidazole (5 mg/kg/day for 60 days) vs. 51 untreated children. After 48 months of follow-up, 5% of the benznidazole group was parasitologically positive by xenodiagnosis vs. 51% of the placebo group. In addition, about 60% of the treated group became seronegative. These recent data support the use of specific treatment with benznidazole, particularly for infected children or in adults up to a few years after infection. Treatment may improve prognosis by minimizing parasite invasion of vital tissues and diminishing inflammatory responses that damage the heart muscle and the peripheral autonomic nervous system. The goal is to prevent the development of chronic chagasic cardiomyopathy or megasyndromes. There are fewer data on which to base recommendations for the use of nifurtimox during the indeterminate phase.

Treatment for Patients With Chronic Disease. Specific treatment with benznidazole or nifurtimox is usually not recommended for patients who are symptomatic with overt anatomic evidence of cardiomyopathy or megasyndromes.

Chagasic cardiomyopathy. Chronic chagasic cardiomyopathy is a panmyocarditis that leads to heart failure and arrhythmias. Standard treatments are used although β-blocking agents are contraindicated. Optimal antiarrhythmic therapy is individualized for patients based on objective studies. Complete heart block causing bradycardia and low cardiac output responds to a pacemaker, which may allow the patient to return to normal activity. However, patients with large hearts, indicating dilation and thinning of ventricular muscle, do poorly with pacemakers. The presence of minor ECG abnormalities is related to an increased risk of disease progression, and these individuals should be followed closely. Use of specific treatment in these patients is controversial, but current and planned trials may resolve the issue. Prophylaxis of thromboembolic phenomena with anticoagulant therapy should be considered.

Heart transplantation for end-stage chagasic cardiomyopathy is controversial. Some experts feel strongly that cardiac transplantation should not be performed in this group. Recrudescence of parasitemia, despite benznidazole prophylaxis, associated with febrile illness and myocarditis is a major problem. Skin lesions were seen in many of these patients after transplantation. A report of 10 patients showed a life expectancy of 78% for the second year and 65% for the third year. Recurrent parasitemias in this group were successfully treated with benznidazole, and there was no sign of disease recurrence in the allograft. A higher incidence of malignant neoplasia has been reported in chagasic patients after transplantation when compared to those with other diseases associated with the use of benznidazole, a known mutagenic agent. Therefore, long-term use of benznidazole for suppression of parasitemia is not advised.

Megasyndromes. Relief of the functional obstruction at the lower esophageal sphincter is the primary goal of treatment for megaesophagus. Grade 1 and early grade 2 disease can be managed initially with balloon dilation. There is a 50% recurrence after 5 years. Grade 2 disease is best managed surgically with a Heller extramucosal cardiomyotomy or a Thal procedure. Grade 3 and 4 disease is usually managed with total esophagectomy and replacement with a segment of intestine. Local injection of botulinum toxin to reduce lower esophageal pressure has also been employed successfully in a few patients. Periodic esophagoscopy is recommended for surveillance of esophageal carcinoma.

Mild chagasic megacolon is managed with high dietary fiber and stool softeners. More advanced disease requires regular use of laxatives and enemas. Severe cases are best managed surgically with resection of the involved colon. Volvulus without ischemic complications can be reduced by nonsurgical means, but any suspicion of ischemic necrosis should lead to urgent laparotomy.

Treatment for Immunocompromised Patients, Including AIDS. Benznidazole has been given to immunocompromised patients with reactivation Chagas' disease. In AIDS patients with a reactivation illness, the initial dose, duration of therapy, and the need for maintenance therapy are not known. Standard regimens have been used. Prophylactic use of specific treatment has not been established. Immune system reconstitution with highly active antiretroviral therapy (HAART) may be the best alternative if feasible.

Alternative Treatments. Allopurinol and itraconazole are reported to be useful in the treatment of chronic Chagas' disease. Definitive recommendations concerning use of these agents awaits further clinical evaluation. Recombinant INF-γ in combination with nifurtimox or benznidazole has been reported as well. The use of such immunomodulating agents, especially in immunocompromised patients, is potentially useful.

Evaluation and Treatment of Seropositive Patients in Nonendemic Areas. The asymptomatic patient who is referred for clinical evaluation following a positive serologic test will likely be more common in the future. Clinicians should be aware of the nature of the screening assay and seek confirmatory testing and expert assistance as available. These patients should have a thorough epidemiologic history that includes birth or residence in an endemic country, living in a domicile where vector transmission is likely, history of Chagas' disease in persons living in the same domicile, history of blood transfusions, and prior occupational exposure. If possible, determination of the geographic location and approximate time period of infection may help in assessing risk of late-stage complications. An individual clinical history should focus on cardiac and gastrointestinal symptoms. An ECG should be performed and repeated at periodic intervals to detect conduction abnormalities and arrhythmias. Additional studies e.g., echocardiography, are dictated by the initial findings. Esophageal and colonic complaints may be evaluated by radiographic studies.

PROGNOSIS. Mortality in the acute phase is <5% in untreated patients. Specific treatment essentially prevents death.

The natural history of infection following the resolution of the acute phase likely depends on many variables, including the size and mix of parasite strains in the initial inoculum, the genetic background of the host, the possibility of superinfection with different strains, and the effect of specific treatment in the acute phase.

Complete data are also not available to formulate an accurate prognosis for patients with chronic infections. Usually, 70 to 90% of those infected with *T. cruzi* having lifelong positive serology never develop clinically manifest chronic Chagas' disease. Approximately 25% of the seroreactors develop ECG abnormalities, and 1% may develop detectable megaesophagus between 20 and 50 years of age.

Congestive heart failure at presentation, global left ventricular dysfunction, and presence of an apical left ventricular aneurysm are strong predictors of cardiac death. Four-year survival is <50% with one of these risk factors. Life expectancy after the onset of heart failure is <2 years.

CONTROL. In the absence of a vaccine or inexpensive and risk-free specific therapy, the only way to control Chagas' disease is to prevent its transmission. Prevention focuses on the elimination of domiciliated bugs in houses, elimination of infected blood in blood banks, and reduction of congenital transmission.

Vector Control. The principles of vector control are based on the behavior of the domiciliated bugs (Chapter 139). Natural infection occurs in the house and bugs tend to remain in the same house as long as it is inhabited. Under the cover of darkness, the bugs leave their refuge and travel across the surface of the walls to reach their human prey. It is during this walk that the bugs make contact with residual insecticides sprayed on the walls. Benzene hexachloride, dieldrin, and malathion have been used extensively in the past because they are inexpensive and kill bugs up to 3 to 4 months after application. The new generation of insecticides, the synthetic pyrethroids (deltamethrin and cypermethrin), are more expensive, but they are applied in low concentrations and last up to 9 months. Insecticide resistance in bugs has been reported only for dieldrin in Venezuela.

Improved Housing. The long-term solution is elimination of the habitat of domiciliated bugs through improved housing. Durable bricks can be produced with local materials at an acceptable price. However, political decisions must be made to place this cottage industry in endemic areas. Finally, there is a need for public health education to convince local residents of the value of bug-proof architecture. In one area of Venezuela, local residents preferred to live in their traditional mud huts (Fig. 94–5) rather than in modern brick houses provided free by the government.

Small changes in human behavior can also reduce transmission. Sleeping in a hammock under a mosquito net with a cloth roof will reduce the chances of contact with bugs and their feces. However, bugs congregate near the retaining hooks in the wall and run along the net. Bugs do not like light and night illumination is a deterrent. Better hygiene and, particularly, the banishment of all animals (e.g., chickens and dogs) from the house will diminish the risk of bug invasion.

National Control Programs. National control programs include three operational phases. During the preparatory phase, seroprevalence is determined and each house is examined for bug infestation. This information is used to estimate required resources: money, personnel, insecticide, equipment, and transport. During the attack phase, insecticide is sprayed on the inside and outside walls, roof, and furniture of all houses and outhouses. The effective dose of insecticide depends on factors, e.g., climate, sunlight, porosity of the sprayed surface, and the method of application. Sprays are not completely effective because they do not kill eggs or well-fed bugs hiding deep in the walls and do not prevent reinvasion from the peridomicile. To maintain vector suppression, house-to-house searches for bugs are conducted to find houses with persistent infestations for repeat spraying. This "evaluation-spray cycle" is repeated until the frequency of infested houses is reduced to ≤5%. During the vigilance phase, the responsibility for detecting bug-infested houses is passed to the community. Public health teams teach the residents to identify and capture bugs and to take them to the local health post where their identification is confirmed by an expert. Houses with persistent infestation often require structural improvement, including the plastering of walls to eliminate bug hiding places. Without public health education and community participation, the prospects of permanent control are bleak. Results from the national control programs in Brazil show that the seroprevalence of schoolchildren has been reduced from 20 to 40% to 0 to 2% in many endemic areas.

Multinational Control Programs. The Southern Cone Initiative, a multinational effort to eliminate vector transmission, was launched in 1991 by Argentina, Bolivia, Brazil, Chile, Paraguay, and Uruguay. The goal is to interrupt the transmission of Chagas' disease by elimination of domiciliary populations of the principal vector, *Triatoma infestans*, using residual formulations of pyrethroid insecticides and by improved screening of blood donors. Striking reductions in the rate of infections in the 0- to 14-year-old age cohort has been documented between 1985 and 1996 in Southern Cone countries. In 1985, there were 169,000 new infections reported in Brazil. The 1996 estimate was 7000, a 96% reduction. Similar marked reductions in house infestations by *T. infestans* have been documented throughout the region as well. The spectacular success of this program has led to its expansion to the rest of South and Central America in 1997.

Control in Blood Banks. The prevention of transmission of *T. cruzi* in blood banks requires an effective screening process to detect infected donors and a method of killing the trypanosomes in infected blood. The technology is now in hand to implement screening using synthetic antigens in blood banks of both developing and developed countries. Standardized peptide reagents, due largely to their stability, also permit the development of simple and inexpensive assays for use in field or rural blood bank settings. In the absence of effective screening the usual practice in endemic areas is to treat all blood with gentian violet at a concentration of 0.25 g/L for 24 hours in the refrigerator before use. Although this procedure is safe, the quality of the blood is often questioned by the patient because of its purple color. The development of colorless compounds as blood sterilants would be helpful.

Preventing Vertical Transmission. Women with acute infections must not nurse until they have been treated with benznidazole. For many mothers with chronic infections, there is little recourse because of the risk of neonatal malnutrition and death. Children nursing from infected mothers should be monitored for infection.

Future Developments. The control of Chagas' disease should be an attainable goal with the knowledge, methodologies, and materials at hand. Intensive efforts to eliminate vectors from houses and then improved screening of blood donors will be the areas of emphasis. Interruption of transmission for Argentina and Brazil is predicted for the year 2000.

Bibliography

Brashear RJ, Winkler MA, Schur JD, et al: Detection of antibodies to *Trypanosoma cruzi* among blood donors in the southwestern and western United States. Transfusion 35:213, 1995.
Brener Z, Gazzinelli RT: Immunological control of *Trypanosoma cruzi* infection and pathogenesis of Chagas' disease. Int Arch Allergy Immunol 114:103, 1997.
Brenner RR, Stoka AM: Chagas' Disease Vectors: Vol I, Taxonomic, Ecological and Epidemiological Aspects. Vol 2, Anatomic and Physiological Aspects. Vol 3, Biochemical Aspects and Control. Boca Raton, FL, CRC Press, 1987.
Carmona MA, Ferreira EAB, Cohen RV, et al: Advanced achalasia of the esophagus. Postgrad Gen Surg 5:185, 1993.
Castro JA, Diaz de Torzano EG: Toxic effects of nifurtimox and benznidazole, two drugs used against American trypanosomiasis (Chagas' disease). Biomed Environ Sci 1:19, 1988.
Chagas C: American trypanosomiasis: Study of the parasite and of the transmitting insect. Proc Inst Med Chicago 3:220, 1993.
Cutait DE, Cutait R: Surgery of chagasic megacolon. World J Surg 15:188, 1991.
de Andrade AL, Zicker F, Oliveira RM, et al: Randomized trial of efficacy of benznidazole in the treatment of early *Trypanosoma cruzi* infections. Lancet 348:1407, 1996.
de Andrade AL, Zicker F, Rassi A, et al: Early electrocardiographic abnormalities in *Trypanosoma cruzi*–seropositive children. Am J Trop Med Hyg 59:530, 1998.
de Carvalho VB, Sousa FL, Vila JHA, et al: Heart transplantation in Chagas' disease: 10 years after the initial experience. Circulation 94:1815, 1996.
de Oliveira RB, Troncon LE, Dantas Ro, et al: Gastrointestinal manifestations of Chagas' disease. Am J Gastroenterol 93:884, 1998.
Ferreira MS, Nishioka SA, Silvestre MTA, et al: Reactivation of Chagas' disease in patients with AIDS: Report of three cases and review of the literature. Clin Infect Dis 25:1397, 1997.
Freilij H, Atlcheh J: Congenital Chagas' disease: Diagnostic and clinical aspects. Clin Infect Dis 21:551, 1995.
Gomes YM: PCR and sero-diagnosis of chronic Chagas' disease: Biotechnological advances. Appl Biochem Biotechnol 66:107, 1997.
Grant I, Gold JWH, Wittner M, et al: Transfusion-associated acute Chagas' disease acquired in the United States. Ann Intern Med 111:849, 1989.
Hagar JM, Rahimtoola SH: Chagas' heart disease in the United States. N Engl J Med 325:763, 1991.
Hagar JM, Rahimtoola SH: Chagas' heart disease. Curr Probl Cardiol 20:825, 1995.
Herwaldt BL, Juranek DD: Laboratory acquired malaria, leishmaniasis, trypanosomiasis, and toxoplasmosis. Am J Trop Med Hyg 48:313, 1993.
Koberle F: Chagas' disease and Chagas' syndromes: The pathology of American trypanosomiasis. Adv Parasitol 6:63, 1968.
Mattoso LF, Reeder MM: Radiological diagnosis of Chagas' disease (American trypanosomiasis). Semin Roentgenol 33:26, 1998.
Prata A: Chagas' disease. Infect Dis Clin North Am 8:61, 1994.
Reed SG: Immunology of *Trypanosoma cruzi* infections. Chem Immunol 70:124, 1998.
Ribeiro AL, Rocha MO: Indeterminate form of Chagas' disease: Considerations about diagnosis and prognosis. Rev Soc Bras Med Trop 31:301, 1998.
Sosa SE, Segura EL, Ruiz AM, et al: Efficacy of chemotherapy with benznidazole in children in the indeterminate phase of Chagas' disease. Am J Trop Med Hyg 59:526, 1998.
Viotti R, Vigliano C, Armenti H, et al: Treatment of chronic Chagas' disease with benznidazole: Clinical and serologic evolution of patients with long term follow-up. Am Heart J 127:151, 1994.
Wendel S: Transfusion-transmitted Chagas' disease. Curr Opin Hematol 5:406, 1998.

94.1 Trypanosoma rangeli *Infections**

Alan J. Magill

ETIOLOGY, HISTORY, AND DISTRIBUTION. In 1920 Tejera found flagellates in the intestinal contents of the triatomine bug, *Rhodnius prolixus*, in Venezuela. The long epimastigotes with a small kinetoplast were morphologically different from *Trypanosoma cruzi* epimastigotes. In 1942 a trypomastigote, with a small subterminal kinetoplast, was found in the blood of Guatemalan children. Both of these were forms of *Trypanosoma rangeli*, which has been reported from most countries of South and Central America. Its distribution is restricted to the New World along with the triatomine bugs, the natural vectors.

TRANSMISSION AND LIFE CYCLE. The transmission of infective metacyclic trypomastigotes of *T. rangeli* to humans and animals is by bite of the bug rather than through excreta. The mode of multiplication in the vertebrate host is probably

---

*All the material in this chapter is in the public domain, with the exception of any borrowed figures or tables.

TABLE 94–1. Morphologic Differences Between *Trypanosoma rangeli* and *Trypanosoma cruzi* Trypomastigotes

	T. rangeli	*T. cruzi*
Morphology	Slender, elongate, better developed undulating membrane	Fatter, C-shaped
Length (including free flagellum)	30 μm (25–37 μm)	20 μm (12–30 μm)
Location of nucleus	More anterior	Central
Kinetoplast	Small, round, subterminal	Large, subterminal

by binary fission of the slender epimastigote. No amastigote form is known. Members of the genus *Rhodnius* are the usual vectors. Flagellates in the bug's intestine invade the hemolymph and then escape into the salivary glands. The presence of flagellates in an anterior dissection of a triatomine bug indicates *T. rangeli* infection. It is often pathogenic for triatomine bugs, causing a shortened life span. *T. rangeli*–like trypanosomes have been isolated in sylvatic animals from many South American countries, but their taxonomic status is unclear.

CLINICAL MANIFESTATIONS AND DIAGNOSIS. *T. rangeli* does not produce clinical illness in humans or in wild or domestic animals. Persistent infection is possible as demonstrated in two experimentally infected human volunteers. Parasitemia continued in these individuals episodically for years; however, parasites were detected only by xenodiagnosis late in the infection.

For clinicians, infection with *T. rangeli* has two implications: diagnostic confusion with *T. cruzi* in the individual patient and possible cross reactions with serologic tests for *T. cruzi*. Concurrent infections in humans have been described. Most of these occur in poor, rural endemic populations living in houses where triatomine bugs are found. Infection has not been described in travelers or other nonendemic populations.

The differentiation of *T. rangeli* from *T. cruzi* is based on morphology in blood smears, hemoculture, xenodiagnosis, behavior of the flagellates in susceptible triatomine bugs, the vector host in different geographic areas, and modern genetic-based methodologies. However, many of these techniques are not available to clinicians. Table 94–1 and Figure 94–2 highlight the morphologic differences between the trypomastigotes of *T. rangeli* and *T. cruzi* as seen in a Giemsa-stained blood film.

Occult infection with *T. rangeli* may lead to a false-positive serologic test result for *T. cruzi*. The great variability in sensitivity and specificity of serologic tests for Chagas' disease has never allowed this question to be resolved. Serologic tests for Chagas' disease based on crude antigens may lead to higher false positive results, as *T. rangeli* and *T. cruzi* share common antigens. Numerous methods to differentiate the two parasites, e.g., specific monoclonal antibodies and species-specific PCR-based assays, have been published but are not routinely available. There have been no reports of *T. rangeli* as an opportunistic infection in immunocompromised patients.

Bibliography

D'Alessandra-Bacigalupo A, Saravia NG: *Trypanosoma rangeli*. In Kreier JP, Baker JR (eds): Parasitic Protozoa. San Diego, Academic Press, 1992.

Vallejo GA, Chiari E, Macedo AM, Pena SDJ: A simple method for distinguishing between *Trypanosoma cruzi* and *Trypanosoma rangeli*. Trans R Soc Trop Med Hyg 87:165, 1993.

95 *Leishmaniasis*

Alan J. Magill

95.1 *Leishmaniasis: General Principles**

DEFINITION. The leishmaniases are a diverse group of clinical syndromes caused by protozoan parasites of the genus *Leishmania*. The parasites are transmitted by sandflies of the genera *Phlebotomus* (Old World leishmaniasis) and *Lutzomyia* (New World leishmaniasis).

HISTORY. Increasingly precise descriptions of parasites from lesions of cutaneous leishmaniasis were made by Cunningham (1885), Borovsky (1898), and Wright (1903). The organism in visceral leishmaniasis was first described in 1903 by Leishman, who examined the spleen of a British soldier with kala-azar who had been stationed at Dum Dum near Calcutta (hence, the name "Dumdum fever"). Later the same year, Donovan also identified the parasite in splenic tissue, and the organism is often called a Leishman-Donovan (LD) body. In 1904, Rogers observed the conversion of amastigotes to promastigotes in culture, and promastigotes were found in sandflies by Adler and Theodor in 1925. Transmission of Oriental sore by infected sandfly bite was achieved by Wenyon in Baghdad (1911) and Sergent in Algeria (1921). The leishmanin skin test was described by Montenegro in 1926, and in 1942, the British Commission in India experimentally transmitted kala-azar to human volunteers by sandfly bite.

ETIOLOGY

Life Cycle. *Leishmania* organisms have a relatively simple life cycle (Fig. 95–1). Promastigotes in the proboscis of a female sandfly are introduced into the skin of a vertebrate host during a blood meal. The promastigotes invade reticuloendothelial cells, transform into amastigotes, multiply within phagolysosomes, and invade other reticuloendothelial cells. Sandflies feeding on infected individuals ingest parasitized cells, and the amastigotes transform into promastigotes, which multiply in the gut and migrate to the proboscis, completing the cycle.

The Organism

Amastigote Stage. The amastigote, found within reticuloendothelial cells in the vertebrate host, is a round or oval organism measuring 2 to 5 μm in greatest diameter (Figs. 95–2 and 95–3 [see in color section], and 95–4). In Wright's- or Giemsa-stained preparations, the pale blue cytoplasm is surrounded by a plasma membrane and contains a large dark-purple nucleus and a small, purple, rod-shaped structure, the kinetoplast. A delicate thread connects the kinetoplast to a dotlike basal body, from which an axoneme arises and extends to the anterior end of the organism. Multiplication is by binary fission, and mitotically dividing forms may be seen in spleen smears.

Promastigote Stage. The promastigote, found in the sandfly digestive tract, measures 1.5 to 3.5 by 15 to 20 μm and has a single free flagellum 15 to 28 μm long (Fig. 95–5). Old cultures may contain short, broad forms and rounded forms 4 to 5 μm in diameter with long flagella centrally directed to form rosettes. Ultrastructurally, the organism is surrounded by a trilaminar plasma membrane, beneath which is a row of microtubules. The cytoplasm contains a large central nucleus, ribosomes, rough and smooth endoplasmic reticulum, a Golgi apparatus, various vesicles, and a single mitochondrion. The kinetoplast is a complex body and appears as an electron-dense granular band with a distinct fibrillar pattern,

---

*All the material in this chapter is in the public domain, with the exception of any borrowed figures or tables.

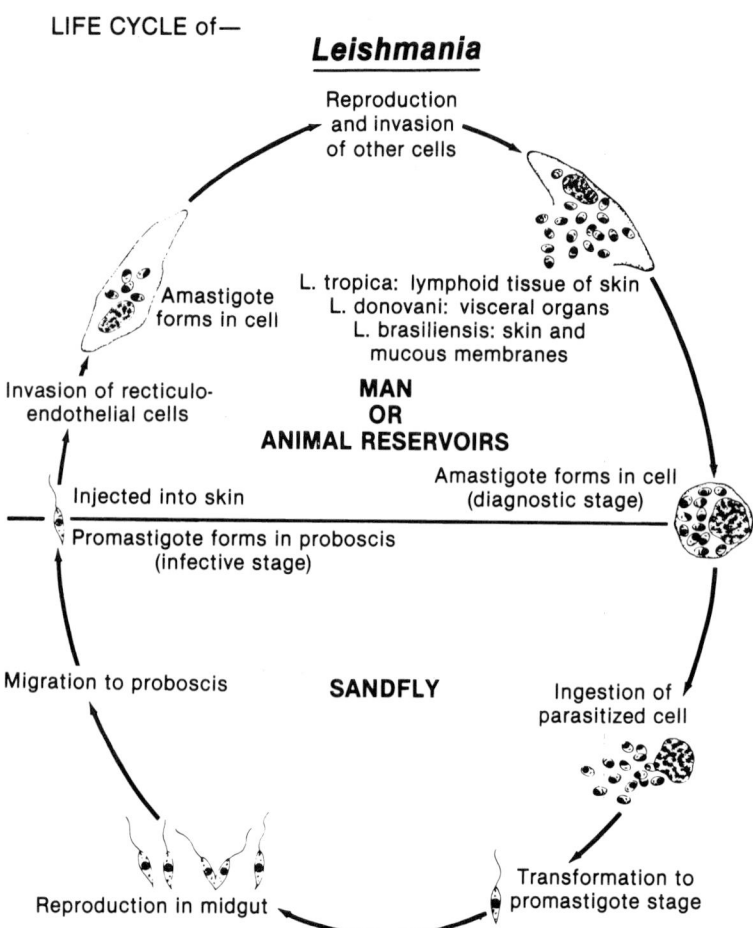

LIFE CYCLE of—

Figure 95–1. The life cycle of *Leishmania.* (Modified from Melvin DM, et al: Common Blood and Tissue Parasites of Man. Life Cycle Charts. Atlanta, GA, Centers for Disease Control, 1979.)

lying within an extension of the mitochondrion. The axoneme, which arises from the basal body, and a paraxial rod are contained within the flagellar sheath.

Culture and Animal Inoculation. Promastigotes can be grown in a variety of media at 22° to 25°C. A biphasic medium, e.g., Nicolle's modification of Novy and MacNeal's medium (NNM) is often used. Schneider's *Drosophila* medium supplemented with fetal bovine serum is often more effective in primary isolation from New World cutaneous lesions. When animal or human specimens are being cultured, penicillin and streptomycin should be added with the inoculum to prevent bacterial overgrowth. 5-Fluorocytosine can be used to inhibit fungal contamination, but amphotericin B should not be added because it may inhibit growth of *Leishmania.* Promastigotes are generally found 2 to 7 days after inoculation of amastigotes into Schneider's medium and after 7 to 21 days in NNN medium. The golden hamster (*Mesocricetus auratus*) is susceptible to infection with *Leishmania donovani* amastigotes, and after intraperitoneal inoculation, the parasites multiply exponentially until the death of the animal usually within 6 months. Hamster inoculation can detect small numbers of parasites in aspirates and tissues.

Taxonomy. The taxonomy of *Leishmania* is confusing, and there is no single, generally agreed-on classification. One taxonomic classification is presented in Figure 95–6. Although subtle differences in size and ultrastucture are reported, the species that infect humans are difficult to distinguish morphologically. Isolates have usually been assigned to species and subspecies based on their geographic origin, the clinical syndrome they produce, and ecologic characteristics. Traditionally, promastigotes derived from in vitro culture are analyzed by protein electrophoresis and the pattern of isoenzymes obtained is compared with reference standards. In addition, parasites of the *L. mexicana* complex have been differentiated from those of the *L. braziliensis* complex by the

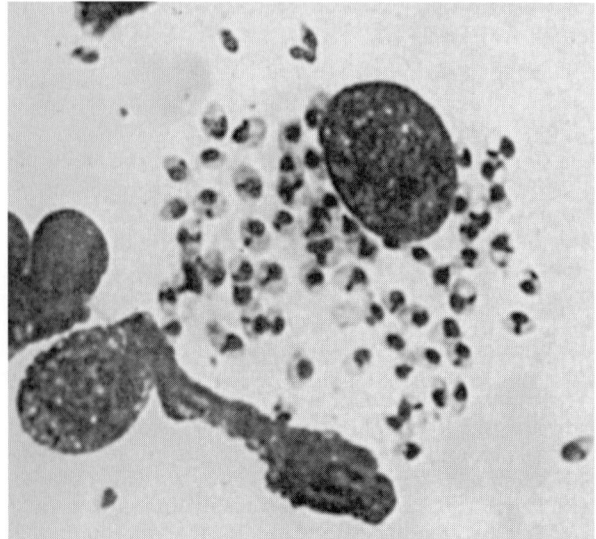

Figure 95–4. Amastigotes of *Leishmania donovani* in a splenic aspirate smear.

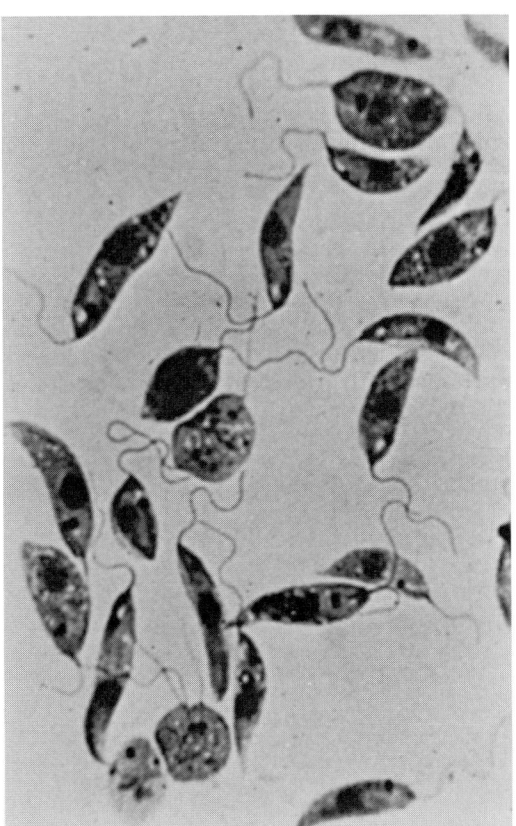

Figure 95–5. Promastigotes of *Leishmania donovani* from culture.

location at which they develop in the sandfly, their growth in culture, and the pattern of disease produced in hamsters. More recently, the use of molecular methods to characterize nuclear and kinetoplast DNA from cultured isolates has been used.

Serologic and Biochemical Classification. A variety of serologic and biochemical tests have also been studied as potential aids in speciating *Leishmania* isolates, including agglutination tests, serotyping of factors excreted into culture media, fluorescent staining with monoclonal antibodies, measuring buoyant density of nuclear and kinetoplast DNA in cesium chloride gradients, identifying parasite isoenzymes, and characterizing parasite metabolism by radiorespirometry.

Clinical Classification. A simplified clinical classification separates the leishmaniases into three major syndromes: (1) visceral leishmaniasis (VL), (2) cutaneous leishmaniasis (CL), and (3) mucosal leishmaniasis (ML). VL is characterized clinically by fever, wasting, pancytopenia, hepatosplenomegaly (especially splenomegaly), and hypergammaglobulinemia. "Incomplete" syndromes, in which one or more of these clinical features are missing, are common. VL is usually caused by parasites of the *L. donovani* complex. CL is characterized clinically by ulcerative skin lesions and caused by parasites from the *L. tropica*, *L. mexicana*, or *L. braziliensis* complexes. Less common CL lesions include nodular, psoriaform, and verrucous forms. Other uncommon cutaneous syndromes include diffuse cutaneous leishmaniasis (DCL) and leishmaniasis recidivans (LR), also known as "lupoid" leishmaniasis. In the New World, ML is most often associated with *L. braziliensis braziliensis* and characterized by a primary cutaneous lesion that may be followed months to years later by destructive nasopharyngeal lesions ("espundia"). In the Old World, ML-like syndromes associated with *L. major*

have rarely been reported. Table 95–1 summarizes the recognized clinical syndromes, associated species, geographic distribution, major reservoirs, and major vectors.

Another clinically useful classification is to describe clinical syndromes in terms of the parasite burden. For example, polyparasitic syndromes, such as VL and DCL, are characterized by very large numbers of parasites in the host. Oligoparasitic syndromes, such as ML, CL, and LR, have relatively fewer parasites. This has implications for the clinician in choosing the best technique for diagnosis and determining optimal treatment.

TRANSMISSION AND EPIDEMIOLOGY

The Vector. The phlebotomine sandflies that transmit *Leishmania* parasites are small (1.5 to 2.5 mm), hairy flies that are recognized by their characteristic hopping movement and the position of their wings, which are held in a nearly erect V configuration over the body (Fig. 95–7). Less than 10% of the 600 known species of sandflies are thought to be involved in the transmission of human leishmaniasis. The female requires one or more blood meals for each batch of eggs to mature. Males feed on fruit juices and do not suck blood. Sandflies are generally inactive in daylight, seeking shelter in dark, moist places. They breed in dark, damp places rich in organic matter, e.g., leaf litter in tropical rain forests, rubble and loose earth, caves, and rock holes. Eggs are laid in batches of 15 to 80. The four wormlike larval instars feed on particulate organic matter and require high humidity. Pupation occurs in a drier environment. Soon after adult emergence, males become sexually active and are capable of inseminating females, who store sufficient sperm to fertilize eggs at intervals throughout their lives. Under favorable conditions, the life cycle is completed in 2 to 3 months. Female sandflies feed on a variety of warm- and cold-blooded hosts, including humans, cats, dogs, rodents, cattle, bats, birds, and lizards. They can acquire *Leishmania* with their first blood meal and are capable of disease transmission 7 to 10 days later. They then remain infective throughout adult life, which is usually only a few weeks. *Leishmania*-infected sandflies have abnormal feeding behavior, probing more while attempting to take a blood meal. This behavior may facilitate transmission to the vertebrate host.

Sandfly saliva contains maxadilan, a potent vasodilatory peptide. The presence and relative abundance of maxadilan has been correlated with the course of human infection. For example, sandflies of the *Lutzomyia longipalpis* complex transmit *Leishmania chagasi* in the New World. VL caused by *L. chagasi* is common in Brazil but rare in Costa Rica, whereas nonulcerative CL caused by *L. chagasi* is found in Costa Rica but not in Brazil. Costa Rican sandfly saliva has a negligible content of salivary maxadilan, induces very little erythema but enhances cutaneous proliferation, whereas Brazilian sandfly saliva has more maxadilan, induces moderate to marked erythema, but does not exacerbate cutaneous infections. Substances in sandfly saliva are at least partly responsible for the tropism observed in *Leishmania* isolates.

The Reservoir. *Leishmania* organisms that infect humans usually have canine or rodent reservoirs in which they may cause inapparent or mild infections, cutaneous lesions only, or severe visceral disease. They are generally zoonotic, occurring in completely wild or peridomestic situations. The epidemiology of various forms of leishmaniasis is discussed in Chapters 95.2, 95.3, and 95.4.

IMMUNOLOGY. The protective immune response to leishmaniasis is primarily cell-mediated. High titers of antibodies detected in VL appear to play no part in defense against the parasite, and naturally occurring antibodies that cause complement-mediated lysis of promastigotes in vitro do not prevent acquisition of disease. In contrast, a positive leish-

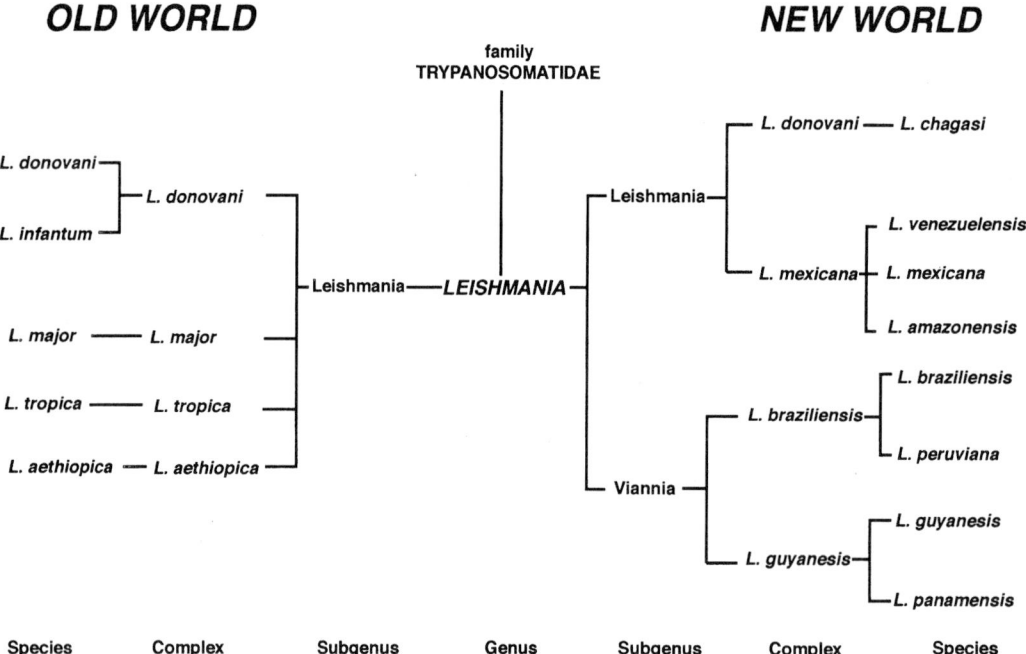

Figure 95–6. Taxonomic classification, based on isoenzyme characterization, of *Leishmania* parasites pathogenic for humans. Animal parasites of the Old World (*L. arabica*, *L. turanica*, and *L. gerbilli*) and New World (*L. aristedesi*, *L. enrietti*, *L. deanei*, *L. equatorensis*, and *L. hertigi*) are not shown. Likewise, newly described human parasites of the New World (*L. colombiensis*, *L. naiffi*, *L. shawi*, and *L. lainsoni*) are not shown. (Adapted from Control of the Leishmaniases. WHO Technical Report Series No. 793. Geneva, World Health Organization, 1990.)

manin skin test correlates with resistance to leishmaniasis. It is negative during active VL, becoming positive after recovery. In addition, some patients with subclinical, self-curing VL have had positive leishmanin skin tests associated with well-developed tuberculoid granulomas demonstrated in liver biopsies. Cell-mediated immunity (CMI) is not entirely beneficial, as it also causes tissue destruction. The onset of ulceration correlates with the development of a positive leishmanin skin test in CL. In ML, the reaction to the leishmanin skin test is much larger in individuals with more severe mucosal damage. T-helper lymphocyte subsets associated with resistance and susceptibility have been identified in mouse models of leishmaniasis. It is unclear if the immuno-logic insights gained in mouse models will be clinically useful in human infections and whether this can be exploited to develop vaccines or immunotherapy.

Spectrum of Clinical Disease. In all forms of leishmaniasis, there is a spectrum of clinical disease similar to that observed in leprosy. In CL, the spectrum varies from a nonhealing infection (DCL) to the exaggerated hypersensitivity seen in ML and LR, in which severe tissue damage is mediated by the immune response (ML and LR). In VL, many infections are subclinical and self-healing, although they can be activated by malnutrition or an immunosuppressive process. In those who develop the syndrome of VL, delayed hypersensitivity is suppressed specifically to leishmanial antigens and nonspecifically to tuberculin and other unrelated antigens; there is proliferation of reticuloendothelial cells and an exaggerated humoral immune response with the production of polyclonal, nonprotective immunoglobulins. Defective CMI in patients with leishmaniasis has been associated with increased suppressor cell activity and defective production of interferon gamma (IFN-γ), interleukin-1, and interleukin-2 by peripheral blood mononuclear cells.

Diagnostic Testing. It is important to remember that there is not a single diagnostic test that will give a definitive answer in all clinical settings. It is always preferable to perform more than one parasitologic assay. For example, smears, cultures, and a polymerase chain reaction (PCR) can be employed in the confirmation of parasites from a bone marrow or splenic aspirate. Obtaining the appropriate specimen requires an invasive procedure, so all available resources should be used to maximize the diagnostic yield.

The Leishmanin Skin Test. Injection of killed promastigotes (Montenegro test) or preparations made from killed promastigotes will induce a delayed-type hypersensitivity (DTH) reaction in individuals with prior exposure to *Leishmania*. In most leishmanin skin test (LST) preparations currently in use, cultured promastigotes are washed in 0.5%

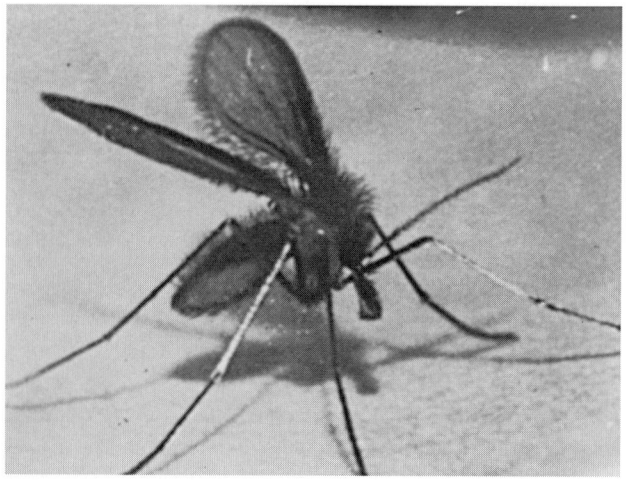

Figure 95–7. A sandfly, *Phlebotomus longipes*. (Courtesy of Dr. Gemetchu, Geneva.)

TABLE 95–1. Leishmania Infecting Humans

Clinical Syndrome	Geographic Distribution	Major Reservoirs	Major Vectors
Visceral Leishmaniasis			
Classic Old World Kala-azar			
L. donovani	Bangladesh, China, India, Nepal, Pakistan	Humans	*Phlebotomus argentipes*
L. tropica (rare)	Sub-Saharan Africa, East Africa India, Israel, Kenya, Saudi Arabia	Rodent, dog, ? humans	*P. orientalis, P. martini*
Infantile visceral leishmaniasis			
L. infantum	Mediterranean littoral	Dog, fox	*P. perniciosus, P. ariasi*
	Central Asia, China, Middle East	Fox, jackal, dog	*P. caucasicus, P. ariasi*
American visceral leishmaniasis			
L. chagasi	South and Central America	Dog, fox, opossum	*Lutzomyia longipalpis*
Atypical visceral disease			
L. tropica	India, Israel, Kenya, Saudi Arabia		
L. amazonensis	Brazil	Rodent	
Post–Kala-azar Leishmaniasis (PKDL)			
L. donovani	Bangladesh, India, Nepal, Ethiopia, Kenya, Sudan		
Typical Cutaneous Leishmaniasis (CL)*			
Old World			
L. tropica (dry or urban Oriental sore)	Mediterranean littoral, Middle East, southwest Asia	Dog, humans	*P. sergenti*
L. major (moist or rural Oriental sore)	Central Asia, Middle East, southwest Asia, sub-Saharan Africa	Rodent	*P. papatasi, P. dubosqi*
L. aethiopica	Ethiopia, Kenya	Hyrax	*P. longipes, P. pedifer*
L. infantum (uncommon)	Central Asia, Iran, Mediterranean littoral		
New World			
L. mexicana (chiclero ulcer)	Central America, Mexico, Texas	Rodent	*Lu. olmeca*
L. guyanensis (Pian bois)	Brazil, Colombia, French Guiana, Guyana, Surinam	Sloth, anteater	*Lu. umbratilis*
L. amazonensis	Amazon basin	Rodent, marsupial	*Lu. flaviscutellata*
L. peruviana (uta)	Peru, Argentina	Dog	*Lu. peruensis, Lu. verrucarum*
L. venezuelensis	Venezuela		*Lh. olmeca bicolor*
L. braziliensis	Brazil, Bolivia, Colombia, Ecuador, Paraguay, Peru, Venezuela	Rodent	*Lu. wellcomei*
L. panamensis	Costa Rica, Colombia, Panama	Sloth, dog	*Lu. trapidoi*
L. chagasi	Honduras, Costa Rica		
Mucosal Leishmaniasis ("Espundia")			
L. braziliensis	Argentina, Brazil, Bolivia, Ecuador, Paraguay, Peru		
L. panamensis (rare)	Colombia		
L. guyanensis (rare)	Colombia, Brazil		
L. major, L. aethiopica (rare)	Sudan		
Diffuse Cutaneous Leishmaniasis (DCL)			
L. aethiopica	Ethiopia, Kenya, Namibia, Yemen	Hyrax, rat	
L. venezuelensis	Venezuela	Rodent	
L. mexicana	Dominican Republic, Mexico, Texas	Rodent	*Lu. christophei*
L. amazonensis	Amazon basin	Rodent	
Leishmaniasis Recidivans			
L. tropica	Middle East	Unknown	*P. sergenti, P. papatasi*

*Typical CL refers to the classic chronic ulcerative disease, nodular forms (10% in New World), and uncommon atypical forms, e.g., plaques, verrucous, and psoriaform lesions.

phenol saline, diluted to 1×10^6/mL, and 0.1 mL is injected intradermally. Another method is to disrupt a promastigote pellet via sonication or microfluidization. The resulting material is filtered to remove particulates and the crude, soluble solution is standardized by protein content. The injection site is examined 48 hours later, and induration of ≥5 mm is considered a positive test. A positive LST denotes present or past infection with *Leishmania*. The LST is generally positive when the lesions of CL and ML are present, but negative in active VL. Although *Leishmania* share common antigens with mycobacteria and trypanosomes, the LST is not positive in pulmonary tuberculosis, leprosy, African trypanosomiasis, or Chagas' disease. Occasional false positive reactions have been noted in patients with glandular tuberculosis and systemic fungal infections, but rigorous studies have not been done.

Although there are many different LST preparations in use

worldwide, there are no preparations approved for use in the United States (1999). Sensitivity, specificity, and appropriate dose-ranging studies in different geographic settings with standardized products have not been performed. It is not advisable to assume that performance characteristics obtained in one area are applicable to another. For example, a study in Brazil comparing LSTs made from New World antigens to LSTs made from Old World antigens showed markedly different results in individuals with confirmed CL and VL. The Old World LST, containing *L. major*, detected only 19% of prior CL cases, whereas the New World LST, containing a mixture of New World parasites, detected 100% of the prior CL cases. In addition, a soluble antigen from New World *L. chagasi* detected 96% of cases of prior VL, whereas an Old World LST, made from *L. infantum*, detected 71% of cases.

PRINCIPLES OF TREATMENT

Definition of Cure. Cure is defined as clinical, parasitologic, or immunologic. It is important to understand these terms in order to interpret the literature and decide on optimal therapy for the individual patient. Clinical cure is the resolution of the signs and symptoms of disease within a defined time period. For example, resolution of fever within a week of therapy in VL, resolution of anemia and splenomegaly within 6 to 8 weeks in VL, or the complete epithelialization of an ulcer of CL within 6 weeks of the start of therapy. Parasitologic cure refers to the absence of parasites by smear or culture within a defined time period. For example, a splenic aspiration may be 3+ prior to therapy and smear-negative at the end of therapy, indicating parasitologic cure. Many (if not most) individuals are clinically cured but are not parasitologically cured following therapy. Finally, immunologic cure is defined as the decrease in antibody titers following therapy and the conversion from a negative LST to a positive LST in resolved VL.

Persistence of Viable Parasites. Successful chemotherapy leading to clinical or parasitologic "cure" does not eradicate parasites from the host. For example, viable parasites can be obtained from healed scars of New World CL patients years after successful therapy. As in tuberculosis, reactivation of overt disease following immunosuppression results from old foci of infection that were controlled by an immune response. The lack of efficacy of pentavalent antimonials in experimental animal models of immunosuppression and in patients with AIDS supports the fact that an intact immune system is required for the resolution of disease.

Variability of Treatment Regimens. *Leishmania* are a diverse group of protozoan parasites found in many different geographic regions of the tropical and subtropical world. Each parasite "species" exists within a unique zoonotic or anthroponotic cycle. Some of these parasites infect humans and lead to a wide variety of systemic, cutaneous, and mucosal clinical syndromes. Each geographic region has a unique combination of parasite strains, sandfly vectors, mammalian reservoirs, and human hosts of different genetic backgrounds. A treatment regimen that is efficacious in one area may not be efficacious in another. For example, what works best for VL in the Sudan may not be optimal for Brazil. Therefore, it is not possible or desirable to recommend a single treatment regimen that would be safe and effective for all forms of the disease in all geographic regions.

Bibliography

Abramson MA, Dietze R, Frucht DM, et al: Comparison of New and Old World leishmanins in an endemic region of Brazil. Clin Infect Dis 20:1292, 1995.

Ashford RW, Desjeux P, deRaadt P: Estimation of population at risk of infection and number of cases of leishmaniasis. Parasitol Today 8:104, 1992.

Desjeux P: Human leishmaniases: Epidemiology and public health aspects. World Health Stat Q 45:267, 1992.

Kar K: Serodiagnosis of leishmaniasis. Crit Rev Microbiol 21:123, 1995.

Killick-Kendrick R: Phlebotomine vectors of the leishmaniases: A review. Med Vet Entomol 4:1, 1990.

Magill AJ: Epidemiology of the leishmaniases. Derm Clin 13:505, 1995.

Pearson RD, de Queiroz Sousa A: Clinical spectrum of leishmaniasis. Clin Infect Dis 22:1, 1996.

Peters W, Killick-Kendrick R (eds): The Leishmaniases in Biology and Medicine. London, Academic Press, 1987.

Warburg A, Saravia E, Lanzaro GC, et al: Saliva of *Lutzomyia longipalpis* sibling species differs in its composition and capacity to enhance leishmaniasis. Philos Trans R Soc Lond B Biol Sci 345:223, 194.

World Health Organization: control of the leishmaniases: Report of a WHO Expert Committee. WHO Tech Rep Series No. 793, 1990.

95.2 Visceral Leishmaniasis (Kala-azar)*

DEFINITION. VL is a chronic infectious disease caused by parasites of the *Leishmania donovani* complex and characterized by irregular fever, enlargement of the spleen and liver, weight loss, pancytopenia, and hypergammaglobulinemia. The disease is also known as kala-azar (Hindi for black sickness).

ETIOLOGY. VL is most often caused by one of three species of the *L. donovani* complex (Table 95–1) that occur in different parts of the world: (1) *L. donovani* (Indian subcontinent); (2) *L. infantum* (Mediterranean littoral, Middle East, Africa, China); and (3) *L. chagasi* (South America). Biochemical studies indicate that *L. chagasi* and *L. infantum* are very similar (if not identical), and it is possible that the organism was brought to the New World by the dogs of the conquistadors and early settlers. There are no clinically useful morphologic or serologic methods for distinguishing the species, but there are differences between *L. donovani* and *L. infantum* or *L. chagasi* infections in biochemical characteristics, epidemiology, clinical features, and response to treatment that suggest distinct species are involved. Organisms with biochemical characteristics of *L. tropica* have occasionally been isolated from bone marrow cultures of patients with VL and "viscerotropic leishmaniasis" in Kenya, the Middle East, and India.

DISTRIBUTION AND INCIDENCE. Mediterranean or infantile kala-azar is found in Portugal, Spain, France, Italy, Greece, Yugoslavia, North Africa, the Mediterranean islands, Lebanon, Iraq, Iran, Saudi Arabia, Yemen, southern Russia, cental Asia, and northern China (Fig. 95–8). Indian kala-azar occurs in the eastern part of India (Assam, Bengal, Bihar, Uttar Pradesh, Madras, Sikkim), Nepal, and Bangladesh. African kala-azar is common in Kenya, Ethiopia, and the Sudan, but sporadic cases occur in Chad, Upper Volta, the Central African Republic, Uganda, the Democratic Republic of the Congo, Zambia, and Somalia. American kala-azar occurs in northeastern Brazil, Paraguay, Argentina, Venezuela, Colombia, Guatemala, El Salvador, Honduras, and Mexico (Fig. 95–9). Precise incidence figures are not available, but in 1992 the worldwide incidence of VL was estimated to be at least 100,000 per year.

TRANSMISSION AND EPIDEMIOLOGY. *L. donovani* is transmitted by phlebotomine sandflies (Fig. 95–7) of the genera *Phlebotomus* in the Old World and *Lutzomyia* in the New World (Table 95–1). The epidemiology depends on the interaction of sandflies, reservoir hosts, and susceptible humans. The Ganges river basin and the southern Sudan, the two major epidemic areas, both demonstrate astonishingly high prevalence rates of infection and tens of thousands of deaths over the 1990s. Population movement, poor nutrition, and desperate poverty characterize both areas.

---

*All the material in this chapter is in the public domain, with the exception of any borrowed figures or tables.

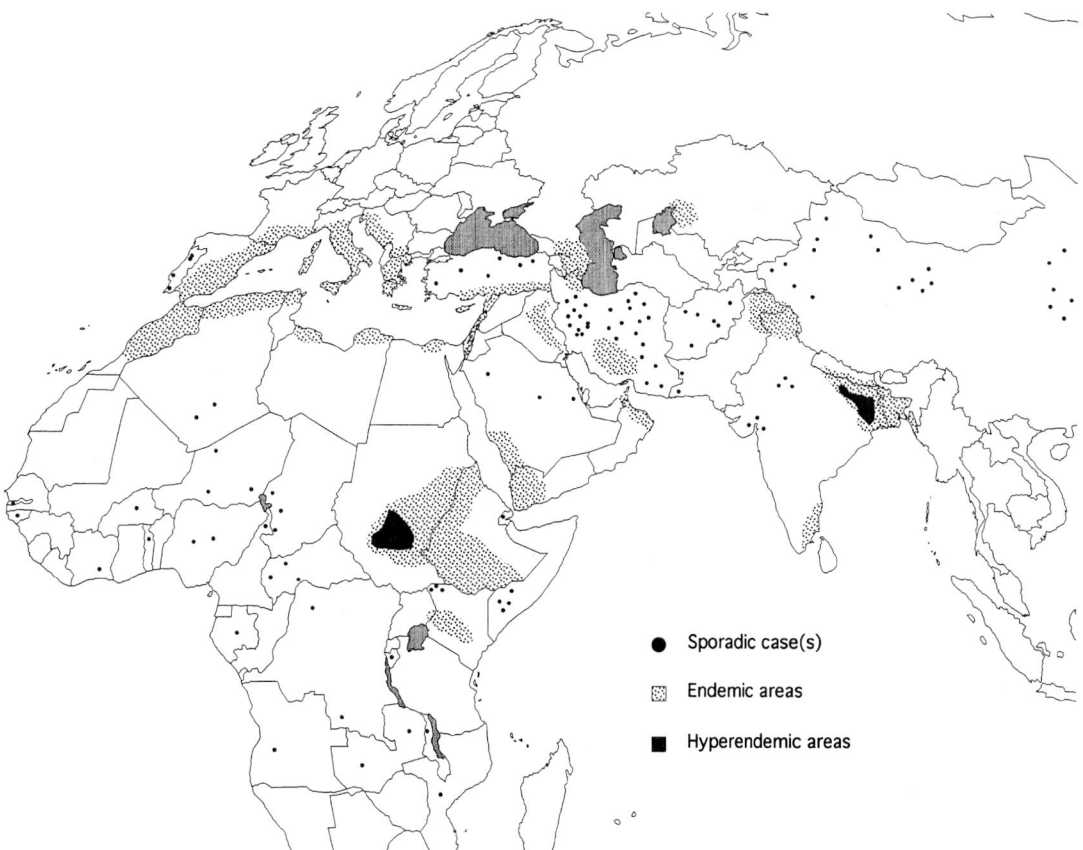

Figure 95–8. Geographic distribution of Old World visceralizing *Leishmania*. *L. infantum* is the predominant species in the Mediterranean basin. It is also found throughout the Middle East, Caucasus, Central Asia, northwest China, and in sporadic cases from Africa. *L. donovani* is the predominant organism on the Indian subcontinent. It is also found in Africa, China, and Iraq. (From Magill AJ: The epidemiology of the leishmaniases. Dermatol Clin 13:505, 1995.)

Reservoir Hosts

Humans. In India, where the domestic sandfly vector *Phlebotomus argentipes* feeds solely on humans, people appear to be the only reservoir, and large epidemics occur that can be traced to migration of an infected individual into a new locality. The possibility of an animal reservoir that maintains the cycle in interepidemic periods has not been excluded.

Dogs. Around the Mediterranean, dogs are the main reservoir and the disease is urban and periurban, transmitted by *P. perniciosus*, *P. major*, *P. simici*, and *P. longicuspis*. Non–HIV associated disease in this area usually occurs in infants and young children. Young dogs and certain breeds (foxhounds and beagles) are especially susceptible to infection with *L. infantum* and develop overt disease that is often fatal. Dogs are also important reservoirs in China, where the main vector is *P. crisis*, and in South America, where the main vector is *Lu. longipalpis*.

Wild Canines. In southern France and central Italy, foxes with inapparent infection are the reservoir, *P. ariasi* and *P. perfiliewi* are the vectors, and VL is primarily a rural disease affecting older children and adults. Foxes are also reservoirs in Brazil (Fig. 135–3), and jackals are probably an important source of the sporadic, mainly rural cases that occur in the Middle East and central Asia.

Multiple Hosts, Rodents. The epidemiology of VL in Africa is incompletely understood. In Kenya, where *P. martini* is the probable vector, epidemics of VL occurred in the 1950s and 1970s, suggesting a human reservoir, but domestic dogs have occasionally been found infected with *L. donovani*. In the Sudan, between the epidemics in the 1950s and the current ongoing one, VL usually occurs sporadically in nomads who occupy temporary villages in the dry season near patches of scrub that harbor the vector *P. orientalis*. *L. donovani* has been isolated from *Arvicanthis niloticus* and other rodents in the Sudan, and rodents are probably important in maintaining enzootic foci in interepidemic periods. Parasite isolates from the Sudan, Ethiopia, and Kenya are more closely related biochemically to *L. donovani* than to *L. infantum*.

Unusual Routes of Transmission. *Leishmania* can be transmitted by means other than sandfly bite, e.g., blood transfusion, sexual contact, congenital transmission, and occupational exposure, but these events occur rarely. Organisms have been demonstrated in nasal mucus of patients with VL, but it is unlikely that direct transmission occurs. Animals can become infected after eating infected carcasses. Experimentally, humans can develop VL following intradermal inoculation of *L. donovani* promastigotes.

PATHOGENESIS AND PATHOLOGY. Following inoculation by the sandfly, promastigotes enter reticuloendothelial cells and multiply. At the site of inoculation, a granuloma develops, consisting of histiocytes filled with amastigotes and surrounded initially by epithelioid cells and later in addition by giant cells. Parasites spread to local lymph nodes and then, hematogenously within macrophages, to the liver, spleen, and bone marrow where they stimulate a granulomatous CMI response that results in subclinical disease and spontaneous resolution or where they multiply further and cause the clinical syndrome of VL.

Spleen. Patients with progressive disease develop marked splenomegaly due to hyperplasia of reticuloendothelial cells that are filled with parasites, and splenic infarcts are common. In acute cases, the spleen is smooth and friable, but in the more usual chronic cases it is firm.

Liver. The liver is usually enlarged and contains numerous amastigote-laden Kupffer cells with little or no cellular reaction (Fig. 95–10). In subclinical cases, noncaseating granulomas with few parasites are scattered throughout the liver.

Lymph Nodes. Lymph nodes may be enlarged and contain macrophages filled with amastigotes, usually with few surrounding lymphocytes. Tonsillar lymphoid tissue may also contain *Leishmania*. In subclinical cases or in lymphatic leishmaniasis, there is a granulomatous and giant cell reaction closely resembling tuberculosis but without caseation.

Mouth and Nasopharynx. In the Sudan, East Africa, and India, VL is sometimes associated with oral and nasopharyngeal lesions. The histologic appearance of these lesions varies from numerous parasitized histiocytes to granulomas with few parasites. Parasites are more abundant in oral lesions than in nasopharyngeal ones but may be demonstrated in nasal and pharyngeal secretions.

Gastrointestinal Tract. In the gastrointestinal tract, there is proliferation of reticuloendothelial cells in the duodenum and jejunum, infiltration of the submucosa with parasitized cells, and sometimes, villous atrophy with hyperplasia of crypt cells. Small ulcerations may occur in which parasites can be demonstrated.

Other Organs. The bone marrow usually contains numerous parasite-laden macrophages. The skin may contain *Leishmania*, and in fatal cases, all levels beneath the epidermis are often heavily infiltrated, with masses of parasitized cells concentrated around the sweat glands and arterioles. Para-

sites have also been identified in heart muscle, the adrenal glands, and the parotid glands. The kidneys may show an interstitial nephritis or a mild proliferative glomerulonephritis and may contain immune complexes. Renal amyloidosis is an uncommon late complication.

CLINICAL MANIFESTATIONS

Symptoms. The incubation period is generally 2 to 6 months, although disease occasionally occurs many years after the patient has left an endemic area. The patient usually does not recall a primary skin lesion. The onset of the disease in naive adults (migrants, soldiers, and visitors to an endemic area) is frequently acute with high fever, chills, and malaise. This syndrome, initially described early in the 20th century in India, is often mistaken for malaria; however, early clinicians commented that VL patients did not appear as "toxic" as malaria patients. In endemic areas, the disease progression is described as more gradual, with intermittent fever, progressive enlargement of the spleen and liver, and vague abdominal discomfort. The initial acute illness may not be recognized. Other common symptoms include weight loss, epistaxis, diarrhea, and nonproductive cough.

Signs. The patient is often weak and emaciated. The abdomen is usually distended by a markedly enlarged spleen and a moderately enlarged liver (Fig. 95–11). In acute VL, the spleen may not be palpably enlarged. Femoral and inguinal lymphadenopathy is often noted, especially in African VL, and generalized lymphadenopathy is a feature of lymphatic leishmaniasis. Trophic changes of the hair (thinning, dryness, hypopigmentation, and loss of curl) and of the skin on the lower legs are common. Heart murmurs are often present, and edema of the legs, jaundice, petechiae, and purpura may sometimes be noted.

Skin. Cutaneous abnormalities are common. Many pa-

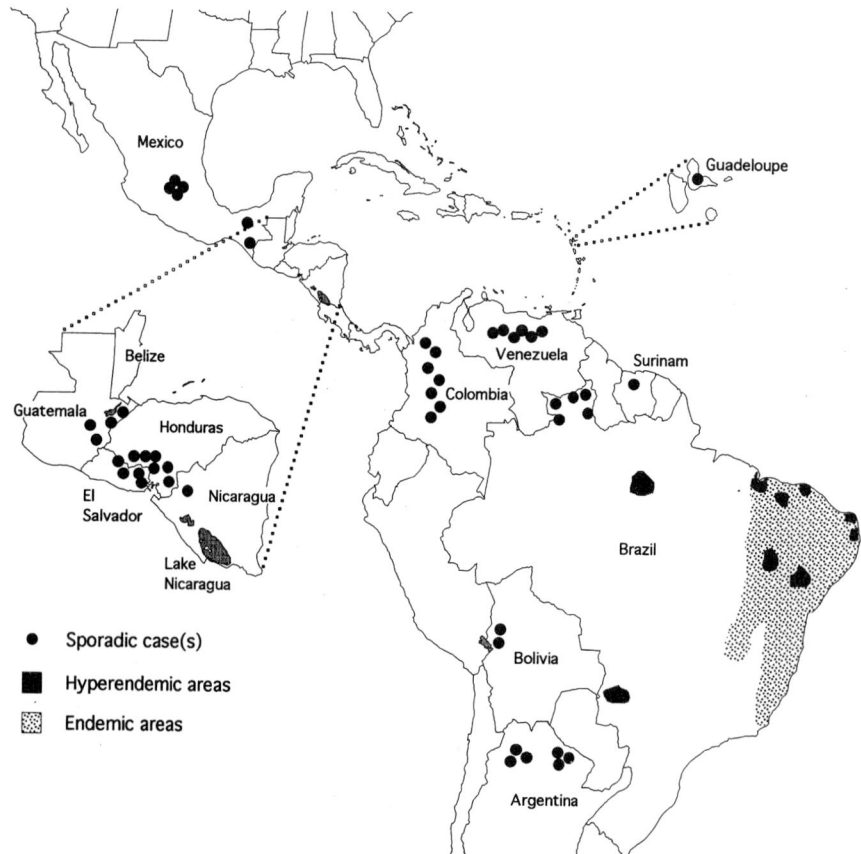

Figure 95–9. Geographic distribution of New World visceralizing *Leishmania* (American visceral leishmaniasis) caused by *L. chagasi* and *L. amazonensis*. (From Magill AJ: The epidemiology of the leishmaniases. Dermatol Clin 13:505, 1995.)

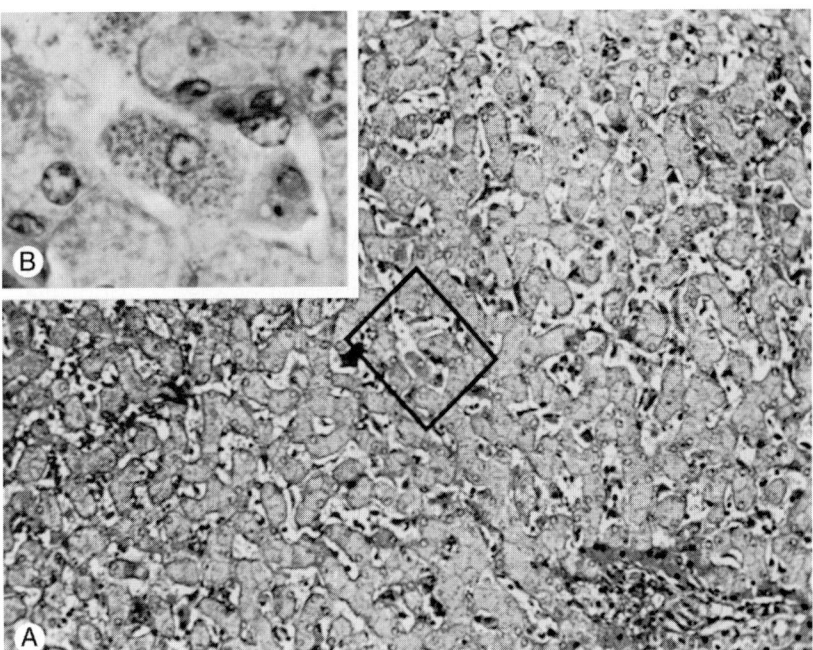

Figure 95–10. Visceral leishmaniasis. *A,* Section of liver showing dilated sinusoids and greatly enlarged Kupffer cells (×165). (Courtesy of the Armed Forces Institute of Pathology, Photograph Neg. No. 70-7723.) *B,* Kupffer cell in *A* magnified to ×1800. The cytoplasm contains numerous *Leishmania* amastigotes. (Courtesy of The Armed Forces Institute of Pathology, Photograph Neg. No. 70-7722.)

tients, especially in India, acquire an earth-gray color of the skin, which gave rise to the name kala-azar (black sickness). The primary lesion at the site of inoculation appears as a small papule or a cutaneous ulcer that may be mistaken for a basal cell epithelioma, although this has almost always resolved by the time the patient seeks medical care. Especially in Africa, skin lesions may accompany VL. Such lesions are polymorphic, although often they appear as diffuse, warty, nonulcerated lesions in which variable numbers of parasites are found. Lesions of post–kala-azar dermal leishmaniasis (PKDL) are usually not present during active visceral infection.

Oral and Nasopharyngeal Lesions. Mucosal lesions are

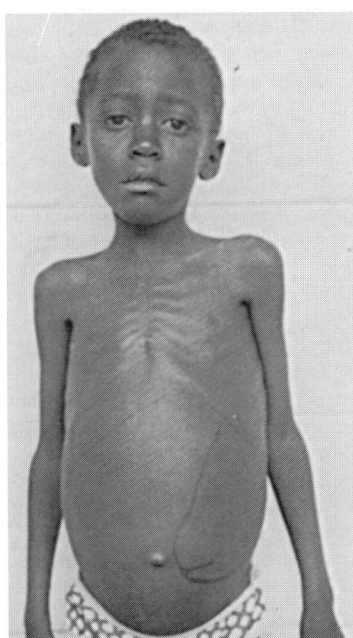

Figure 95–11. A young Kenyan girl with visceral leishmaniasis.

occasionally seen in patients with VL in the Sudan and rarely in patients from East Africa and India. Oral lesions appear as nodules or ulcers of the gum, palate, tongue, or lip. Lesions of the nasal mucosa may cause perforation of the septum. Nasopharyngeal and laryngeal lesions present with mucosal swelling and hoarseness. These lesions may be associated with active visceral infections or with PKDL. They respond well to antimony therapy and may be due to an exaggerated nonhealing immune response.

Other Systemic Manifestations. Uncommon presenting syndromes, which precede the development of overt VL, include bacteremia, acute hepatitis, and Guillain-Barré syndrome. Only after the classic signs and symptoms of VL develop are these unusual (or uncommonly recognized) manifestations of VL associated with *Leishmania* infection. In addition, uncommon systemic manifestations associated with overt VL include retinal hemorrhages, massive hepatic necrosis, pancytopenia without splenomegaly, cholecystitis, and distal extremity paresthesias. Lymphatic leishmaniasis also occurs not infrequently. Both generalized and regional adenopathy with and without systemic symptoms may occur. The diagnosis of lymphatic leishmaniasis is made by finding noncaseating granulomas and amastigotes in a lymph node biopsy specimen.

Laboratory Abnormalities

Hematologic. Hemoglobin concentrations of 5 to 9 g/dL, white blood cell (WBC) counts of 2000 to 4000/mm³ and platelet counts of 50,000 to 200,000/mm³ are typical, although much lower counts are sometimes seen in advanced disease. The anemia is multifactorial. Erthrocyte survival time is shortened owing to hypersplenism and possibly autoimmune mechanisms. Bone marrow depression is indicated by a reticulocytosis lower than expected for the degree of anemia. Coexistent iron deficiency may be present. The Coombs test is usually positive, with both C3 and IgG present on red blood cells, but does not correlate with the severity of the anemia. The neutrophil survival time is shortened, and the WBC differential demonstrates neutropenia, relative lymphocytosis, and an almost complete absence of eosinophils. Agranulocytosis is rare.

Other. Liver transaminases (alanine transaminase [ALT]

more than aspartate transaminase [AST]) are mildly elevated in the majority of patients, but elevations of serum bilirubin are uncommon. The prothrombin time is usually 2 to 4 seconds longer than that in controls, and serum albumin is generally less than 3 g/dL. A polyclonal hypergammaglobulinemia of 5 to 10 g/dL, most of which is IgG, is usual. In some reports, albuminuria is common, but in others the urinalysis is normal, as are tests of renal function.

Complications. Bacterial pneumonia may be present on admission or may develop during treatment. Pulmonary tuberculosis is a common co-infection, and it should be suspected in any patient responding poorly to therapy. Cancrum oris, a necrotizing oral infection, occurs late in the course when neutropenia is severe. Hepatic cirrhosis is an uncommon sequela of VL, and portal hypertension may cause persistent splenomegaly despite successful treatment of kala-azar. Post–kala-azar anterior uveitis can occur after treatment for VL. Patients present with deteriorating visual acuity, and slit lamp examination shows irregular nodules in the iris. Other rare ocular complications reported are retinal hemorrhages, keratitis, central retinal vein thrombosis, papillitis, and iritis. Disseminated intravascular coagulation, immune complex–mediated glomerulonephritis, and renal amyloidosis presenting with a nephrotic syndrome are also rarely seen. Death in patients with VL is often associated with, and perhaps caused by, concurrent infections, e.g., tuberculosis, dysentery, measles, and bacterial pneumonias. Deaths due to cardiac failure in severely anemic persons also occur.

Subclinical or Oligosymptomatic Infections. In areas endemic for VL, many inhabitants develop a positive LST without a history of overt clinical disease, and such individuals appear to be resistant to naturally occurring and experimental infection with *L. donovani*. The difference between true asymptomatic infection and oligosymptomatic disease is difficult to establish in most endemic areas because nonspecific illness is rarely diagnosed and does not warrant evaluation in the context of the culture and health care infrastructure. For example, in a prospective study in Brazil, 28 of 86 children with antibodies to *L. donovani* developed classic VL within a few weeks to 15 months after seroconversion. Twenty others remained asymptomatic during observation for up to 5 years, and 38 had a prolonged "subclinical" illness, manifested by mild constitutional symptoms and intermittent hepatomegaly that resolved without antileishmanial treatment after an average of 35 months.

Other reports of nonspecific, chronic illness associated with "viscerotropic" *Leishmania* infection have come from India and Italy. Most recently, nine cases of a mild, nonspecific illness characterized by cough, malaise, chronic fatigue, abdominal pain, and intermittent fevers and diarrhea were documented in returning U.S. veterans of Operation Desert Storm. All were parasitologically confirmed from bone marrow or lymph node aspirates, and 6 of the 9 isolates were characterized as *L. tropica* by isoenzyme analysis. All acquired their infection in the Eastern province of Saudi Arabia, an area not previously known to be endemic for *L. tropica* and not endemic for classic VL. One of the soldiers presented more than 2 years after the last possible exposure. It is possible that similar "viscerotropic" syndromes are more common than currently believed.

The reports from Brazil and the Operation Desert Storm experience indicate that nonspecific mild disease associated with *Leishmania* infection may be more common than previously thought. Therefore, "viscerotropic" leishmaniasis should be considered in individuals with unexplained constitutional complaints in endemic areas or in travelers with a history of exposure.

Infections in Immunocompromised Hosts. In the past decade, *Leishmania* has emerged as a significant opportunistic infection (OI) in patients with human immunodeficiency virus (HIV) infection (Chapter 22). Co-infection with *Leishmania* and HIV is a recognized problem in France, Italy, Portugal, and Spain and has been reported in 20 other countries. Well over a thousand cases have been reported. In the Mediterranean countries, it is estimated that up to 70% of adult cases of VL are now associated with HIV, and about 10% of people with AIDS have newly acquired or reactivated VL. As the incidence of HIV infection increases in India, Brazil, and East Africa, the numbers of people at risk of co-infection will also increase dramatically.

Clinical signs and symptoms of VL usually occur as a late-stage manifestation in patients with AIDS. CD4 T-lymphocyte counts, when reported, are usually less than 50 mm³ and are almost always less than 200 mm³. In general, patients with overt disease associated with VL have very high parasite burdens but seem to tolerate the parasite co-infection reasonably well. Many clinicians believe that *Leishmania* does not cause severe symptoms in these patients but rather is just one more of the many OIs that plague patients with severely depressed CD4 counts. Numerous viscerotropic, dermotropic, and novel *L. infantum* zymodemes have been isolated from co-infected patients in Europe.

The clinical presentation of VL in AIDS patients is believed to be similar to the presentation in non-HIV infected hosts. Fever, splenomegaly, and pancytopenia are common. Involvement of the gastrointestinal tract is more common in AIDS patients. Abundant parasite-laden macrophages are found in the submucosa from the esophagus to the rectum. Co-infected patients may have atypical presentations that include a variety of pulmonary syndromes, e.g., pleural effusion, pulmonary nodules. Afebrile patients with minimal splenomegaly have been reported as well.

The principles of diagnosis in co-infected patients are not different. The parasite burden tends to be higher and serologic tests may be negative; therfore, classic parasitologic methods are preferable. Even buffy coat smear of peripheral blood was 53% and 67% positive in two studies from Spain. Fever or hepatosplenomegaly in an HIV-infected patient who has resided in or visited an area endemic for VL should prompt an examination of the bone marrow with both smears and cultures for *Leishmania*.

Response to initial treatment with pentavalent antimony is only 50%, whereas response to liposomal amphotericin B is near 100%. However, relapse is common after both drugs. The optimal induction therapeutic regimen, including choice of drug, dose, and duration for different infecting parasites is not known. Optimal intermittent maintenance regimens are likewise unknown. Currently, immune system reconstitution through highly active antiretrovial therapy (HAART) may be the optimal therapy where feasible. It is reasonable to recommend an initial course of induction therapy using liposomal amphotericin B to decrease the patasite burden closely followed by HAART to raise the CD4 cell count.

VL may also occur as an OI in solid organ (renal, heart) transplant recipients, persons receiving immunosuppressive therapy (cancer chemotherapy, chronic corticosteroids), and with other immunosuppressive diseases. VL characterized by fever, splenomegaly, and cytopenias occurs several months following transplantation. Standard parasitologic diagnostic methods are satisfactory. The problem is almost always a failure to consider the diagnosis.

Post–Kala-azar Dermal Leishmaniasis. PKDL was first described in India using the term *dermal leishmanoid*. It occurs in up to 20% of patients with VL in India and is rare in China. Prior to the current epidemic of VL in the Sudan, PKDL was thought to be uncommon (approximately 2%) in

East Africa; however, PKDL has been reported in over 50% of Sudanese VL patients treated in the current epidemic.

In India, skin lesions usually appear 2 to 10 years after successful treatment of VL, but in East Africa they often appear within a few months of treatment. In the Sudan, onset of PKDL was reported to occur at a mean of 56 days (range, 0 to 180 days). Macules and papules first occur around the mouth and spread to the rest of the face and to a lesser extent on the extensor surfaces of the arms, the trunk, and occasionally the legs. Initially, they appear as small hypopigmented patches, which enlarge and may progress to nodules that sometimes resemble leprosy (Fig. 95–12).

Histologically, there is a spectrum of cellular response, varying from numerous parasites with few inflammatory cells to a granulomatous reaction containing few parasites. Occasionally, a xanthomatous form occurs, with raised, orange-colored, nonulcerated plaques. Parasites isolated from patients with PKDL are serologically and biochemically identical to *L. donovani* isolated from patients with VL. Because the lesions of PKDL may persist for up to 20 years, such patients may act as a chronic reservoir of infection.

DIAGNOSIS. A clinical diagnosis of VL is often made with varying degrees of certainty depending on the local epidemiologic factors and clinical presentation. Parasitologic diagnosis refers to the demonstration of amastigotes in tissues or clinical specimens, visualizing promastigotes in in vitro cultures, the detection of parasite genetic material, or antigen detection. Immunologic diagnosis refers to the detection of an antibody or DTH response in the host to *Leishmania* antigens.

Clinical Diagnosis. The positive predictive value of a clinical diagnosis of late-stage VL, with classic signs and symptoms, in an endemic area is likely to be very high. Serologic tests do not change the likelihood of disease. A confirmatory parasitologic diagnosis, always preferable, is frequently difficult because of the invasive nature of the procedures and the requirement for expert microscopy. Clinical improvement in response to appropriate therapy virtually confirms the clinical diagnosis. A clinical diagnosis early in the course of infection when the classic features of disease are not yet established is much less certain.

Demonstration of Parasites. Splenic aspiration is the surest

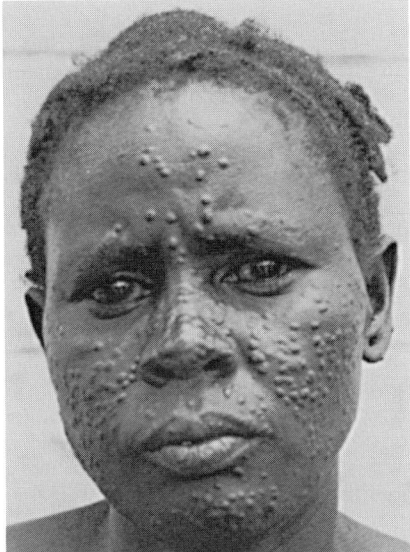

Figure 95–12. Nodular lesions of post-kala-azar dermal leishmaniasis in a Kenyan woman.

method of confirming the diagnosis. However, deaths have occurred after splenic aspiration, presumably owing to splenic laceration, and careful observation after the procedure is mandatory. In experience in Kenya with more than 3000 splenic aspirations in more than 400 patients, 3 patients developed shock and died with 24 hours after splenic aspiration, and intra-abdominal bleeding was diagnosed in another 4 patients who recovered with conservative, nonsurgical therapy. Contraindications to splenic aspiration are a soft spleen in acute disease, a prothrombin time ≥5 seconds compared with the normal control, or a platelet count below 40,000/mm^3. In patients <5 years old, splenic aspiration should be performed only by a physician fully experienced with the procedure. The procedure uses a 21-gauge needle attached to a 5-mL syringe, which is inserted just under the skin over the middle of the spleen. As suction is applied, the needle is rapidly inserted into the spleen and withdrawn, with the needle remaining in the spleen only a fraction of a second. The small amount of splenic tissue and blood in the needle is expressed into culture medium and onto slides for thin smears. Splenic smears stained with Giemsa or Leishman's stain demonstrate amastigotes in 98% of cases and can give the diagnosis within an hour (Fig. 95–4). Splenic smears are often quantitated by the method of Chulay and Bryceson to assist in response to therapy. Promastigotes are generally found after incubation at 25°C for 2 to 7 days in Schneider's medium or 7 to 21 days in NNM medium.

Bone marrow aspiration is preferred in many areas because of concern about the hazards of splenic aspiration and unfamiliarity with the technique. Bone marrow smears usually contain relatively fewer amastigotes, and parasites are found in only 80 to 85% of cases (Fig. 95–2 [see in color section]). Amastigotes are frequently found in aspirates or biopsies of liver specimens (Fig. 95–10) or lymph nodes. Buffy coat smears can demonstrate amastigotes in Indian and Kenyan kala-azar, but it is unusual to make the diagnosis by this method.

The confirmation of VL is usually not difficult, as it is a polyparasitic syndrome. Therefore, more sensitive parasitologic tests are often not required. However, if the diagnosis could be confirmed by a noninvasive test, this would prove to be a great advantage. Antigen detection assays using whole blood and PCR amplification of *Leishmania* DNA from the peripheral blood have both been reported, but sensitivity is lower compared with splenic or bone marrow aspiration.

Nodular lesions of PKDL usually have abundant parasites easily seen on smears, papules have fewer parasites, and macules and hypopigmented lesions have the fewest parasites.

Serologic Tests. A variety of serologic tests are used worldwide. Tests are often specific to the geographic region and employed by local investigators. Few have seen wide use and so the test performance characteristics (sensitivity, specificity, etc.) are not comparable. In general, current serologic tests for VL have sensitivities >90% but with lower specificities. False positive results are seen in some other infectious diseases, following treatment for VL, as antibodies may persist for many months, and in some asymptomatic cases.

The formol-gel test detects high levels of IgG or IgM from any cause. It is of limited value because it becomes positive late in the course of VL, and false positive tests are common. It may be useful in field situations or rural health centers where other serologic tests are unavailable. The complement fixation test, using antigen prepared from *L. donovani* or from the cross reactive *Mycobacterium phlei* (Kedrowsky bacillus), has also been replaced by tests with greater sensitivity and specificity.

The indirect fluorescent antibody test (IFA) is positive in more than 95% of patients with visceral leishmaniasis, generally with titers above 1:256. These are readily distinguishable from the low-titer positive that occur occasionally in malaria, typhoid fever, and other diseases. Whole, culture-derived promastigotes, usually *L. donovani*, are fixed in wells of a special glass slide. Serum at different dilutions is applied to the wells. Antibodies in the serum that bind to surface antigens on the promastigotes are then detected by an antibody to the Ig molecule conjugated to a fluorescent marker. A microscopist reports a titer (the reciprocal of the dilution) that corresponds to a certain percentage of parasites that fluoresce. IFA testing is somewhat subjective and requires rigorous technique and relatively expensive equipment.

The enzyme-linked immunosorbent assay (ELISA) test using whole or soluble promastigote antigens appears to be as sensitive and specific as the IFA, and because of economy and technical practicality, it is especially useful for large-scale epidemiologic studies of human and canine leishmaniasis. Both the IFA and ELISA can be performed on sera eluted from filter papers impregnated with 50 µL of capillary blood. The specificity of serologic tests for visceral leishmaniasis can be improved by using a competitive binding assay, in which the binding of *L. donovani*–specific monoclonal antibodies is inhibited by antibodies present in the sera of patients with VL, or by using specific leishmanial proteins purified from parasites or recombinant DNA expression systems. The direct agglutination test (DAT) is widely available. Sensitivity of 92% and specificity of 100% was reported in 50 Sudanese VL patients.

The recombinant protein rK39 is used as the antigen in an ELISA to detect antibodies in the serum of patients with VL. It has sensitivities of 95 to 100% for classic VL, and specificity is also very high with only a handful of reported false positives. Titers to rK39 also decrease following successful chemotherapy and tend to rise in cases of relapse, making it useful for the recognition of treatment failures. Antigen rK39 has also been used in rapid "dipstick" assays. The antigen is striped onto nitrocellulose paper and a drop of whole blood is placed onto a sample pad with immunolabeled gold. Human IgG binds to the labeled gold and migrates up the strip. If antibodies to rK389 are present in the serum, they bind to the rK389 antigen stripe giving a visual positive test result. Sensitivity in a large trial in India was 100% and specificity was 98%.

Western blot analysis using promastigote antigens has proved to be sensitive and specific for the diagnosis of Mediterranean VL. Antibodies in patient serum recognize several antigens with a sensitivity of 60 to 90%. Several groups have reported that these immunoblots are specific tests that allow differentiation of VL from other diseases that cause fever, splenomegaly, and pancytopenia. None is commercially available.

Leishmanin Skin Test. The Montenegro test is almost uniformly negative in active VL but becomes positive in 90% of patients 6 weeks to 1 year after recovery. Tuberculin sensitivity usually is similarly depressed during active kala-azar, indicating a broad defect in CMI. In vitro lymphocyte blastogenesis responses to leishmanin and tuberculin are also depressed.

Differential Diagnosis. The differential diagnosis of late-stage VL is limited to hematologic and lymphatic malignancies. Disseminated histoplasmosis and hepatosplenic schistomiasis have rarely been reported to mimic late-stage VL. Early disease has a much broader differential that includes malaria, African trypanosomiasis, brucellosis, enteric fevers, bacterial endocarditis, generalized histoplasmosis, chronic myelocytic leukemia, Hodgkin disease and other lympho-

mas, sarcoidosis, hepatic cirrhosis, and tuberculosis. Tropical splenomegaly syndrome is especially difficult to differentiate, although high titers of antimalarial antibodies and a characteristic histologic appearance of the liver suggest this disease. Patients with multiple myeloma and Waldenström's macroglobulinemia have monoclonal hypergammaglobulinemia.

TREATMENT

Nonspecific or Supportive Care. Patients should receive a nutritious diet. Antimicrobial agents are given when concurrent pneumonia, tuberculosis, or other bacterial infections are present. Patients with chronic disease generally tolerate anemia well, but blood transfusion may be needed if the hemoglobin level falls below 6 g/dL. Coexistent iron or vitamin deficiency requires specific treatment.

Specific Antileishmanial Therapy. Pentavalent antimony compounds (SbV) have been the drugs of choice for the treatment of VL worldwide since the mid-1930s. Reports of primary treatment failures with SbV in India became more prevalent in the mid-1990s leading to trials of lipid-associated amphotericin B compounds as initial therapy for both Mediterranean and Indian VL. Currently, many favor the use of lipid-associated amphotericin B as first-line therapy for VL. Reports from the Sudan suggest that sodium stibogluconate when given at appropriate doses is still very effective (almost 98% cure rate).

Pentavalent Antimonials. Sodium stibogluconate (SSG) and sodium antimony gluconate are made by several different manufacturers in India and China. SSG (Pentostam), made by Glaxo-Wellcome, London, is also widely used in Asia, much of Europe, and English-speaking parts of Africa. It is not known how these different preparations compare with each other in terms of safety and efficacy, as no comparative trials have ever been performed. However, it is unwise to assume one preparation will perform the same as another. Another SbV preparation, meglumine antimoniate (Glucantime, Rhone Poulenc, Paris), is used in Latin America and French-speaking parts of Africa and Europe. SbV can be administered intravenously or intramuscularly. There is variation in the total antimony (Sb) content, the proportion of SbV to trivalent Sb (trivalent Sb is much more toxic than SbV), and the physical and chemical characteristics of different lots of SbV from the same manufacturer and between preparations from different manufacturers. Many investigators believe these lot variations are responsible for the different safety and efficacy profiles observed in treated patients. Recently, several cardiac deaths in India were associated with use of a SbV preparation with high osmolarity. In addition, SbV dissociates or polymerizes over time, so storage conditions and shelf life are important considerations. Storage at 4°C in the dark is optimal.

SSG (Pentostam) is available as a solution containing 100 mg of antimony (Sb) per mL. In the United States, Pentostam is available from the Centers for Disease Control and Prevention under an investigational new drug (IND) application. Studies of VL in India and Kenya have demonstrated that higher doses (20 mg of Sb/kg/day vs. 10 mg of Sb/kg/day) and longer courses of therapy (28 days in Kenya and 40 days in India vs. 20 days) increase the rate of initial response to chemotherapy and decrease the rate of relapse. Currently, the recommended treatment regimen for primary disease is 20 mg of Sb/kg/day for 28 days. Longer durations should be considered for those slow to respond and disease acquired in India. Formerly, 850 mg per day was considered to be the upper limit of a safe daily dose. Experience gained over the last decade supports the safety and higher efficacy of the full 20 mg/kg daily dose without an upper limit.

Intramuscular injections are moderately painful. Undiluted intravenous injections should be given slowly through a 23-

to 26-gauge needle. When feasible, dilution of the daily dose at least 1:10 with 5% D/W, is preferable to reduce the incidence of local thrombosis.

SSG (Pentostam) is a safe drug, although with a poorly tolerated side effect profile. Nausea, anorexia, abdominal pain, malaise, headache, arthralgias, myalgias, and lethargy are frequent, beginning about 7 to 10 days into therapy. These side effects are more noticeable in CL and ML patients, as they do not have systemic symptoms associated with their disease. In general, VL patients seem to tolerate SbV better than CL or ML patients. Arthralgias in particular can be quite problematic. Fortunately, these symptoms resolve shortly after therapy is complete. Recent observations have shown that nearly 100% of patients treated with SbV preparations develop elevations in serum amylase and serum lipase (lipase greater than amylase). Although 50% are asymptomatic, many develop some degree of anorexia, nausea, and midepigastric pain consistent with pancreatitis. A few deaths attributed to pancreatic necrosis have been reported in patients receiving SbV; therefore, monitoring of serum amylase and lipase in patients receiving SSG is recommended whenever feasible. The increase in serum amylase and lipase occurs shortly after beginning therapy and peaks at 7 to 14 days. Values return to normal despite continuing the drug. When patients develop symptoms or signs of pancreatitis, it is recommended that SSG be temporarily halted for a few days. Serum amylase and lipase rapidly return to normal, and the regimen can then usually be completed without another interruption. Even in asymptomatic patients, it is reasonable to temporarily interrupt therapy for significant elevations of serum amylase or lipase. Reasonable guidelines for interrupting therapy are fivefold elevation of amylase and a 15-fold elevation of lipase.

Anemia, neutropenia, and thrombocytopenia associated with hypoplasia of the bone marrow have all been seen during SbV therapy, occasionally severe enough to interrupt therapy. Abnormalities reverse on discontinuation of the drug. Again, baseline values prior to treatment and monitoring during therapy are recommended if feasible. Transient increases in serum transaminases are also seen in the majority of patients during treatment. AST levels rise threefold to fourfold above the upper limit of normal between days 7 and 14 but decline despite continued therapy. Renal tubular acidosis and acute renal failure associated with SbV have been reported. SSG causes lymphopenia that has been associated with occasional cases of herpes zoster occurring during the course of treatment.

Electrocardiographic (ECG) abnormalities, including nonspecific ST- and T-wave changes and T-wave flattening or inversion, occur in more than one half of patients receiving SSG, and the frequency of these changes is proportional to the total daily dose and the duration of therapy. One patient treated in Kenya with SSG at a dosage of 20 mg of Sb/kg 3 times daily for disease unresponsive to lower doses, developed a prolonged QT interval after 2 weeks of treatment and died suddenly on treatment day 23. Torsades de pointes with prolonged QT interval and syncopal episodes has also been reported. An ECG should be obtained prior to therapy and repeated weekly for standard doses; if doses above 20 mg of kg/day are considered, more frequent ECG monitoring should be considered. Treatment should be suspended if the corrected QT interval (the measured QT interval divided by the square root of the RR interval) becomes prolonged beyond 0.50 second. T-wave flattening or inversion, the most common ECG abnormality during antimony adminstration, is not an indication to stop treatment.

Meglumine antimoniate is provided as a solution containing 85 mg of Sb per ml. The recommended dosage is the same as for SSG, 20 mg of Sb/kg/day for at least 28 days. The side effects of meglumine antimoniate are similar to those of SSG.

Amphotericin B. Amphotericin B deoxycholate has also been used successfully in cases of VL resistant to other medications. Traditionally, it is administered by slow intravenous infusion over 4 to 6 hours, starting at 0.1 mg/kg daily and gradually increasing to 1 mg/kg every 2 days, until a total dose of about 20 mg/kg has been given. The need for incremental escalation of doses in Indian VL was addressed in a clinical trial of 120 patients. There was no difference in infusion-related side effects between those receiving the incremental dose and those receiving 1 mg/kg from day 1. Cure rates in VL clinically resistant to SbV and pentamidine (see later) approach 100%. The widespread use of amphotericin B deoxycholate has been hindered because of the well-known infusion-related side effects of fever, chills, and thrombophlebitis; long-term problems of renal insufficiency, anemia, and hypokalemia; and poor tolerability (anorexia, nausea) (Chapter 84). Also, amphotericin B deoxycholate should be used with caution in those previously receiving SbV. Sudden cardiac death has been reported following the first dose of amphotericin B deoxycholate in these patients. It is thought the ECG abnormalities associated with SbV therapy predispose to cardiac events. It seems prudent to recommend that a baseline ECG be obtained and a rest period be observed until the ECG normalizes, usually within 10 days of the end of SbV therapy, before starting amphotericin B deoxycholate.

The desire to develop less toxic and more effective preparations of amphotericin B to treat systemic mycoses led to the introduction of lipid-associated amphotericin B preparations in the mid-1990s. There are currently three agents available: liposomal amphotericin B (AmBisome, Fujisawa USA, Inc., Deerfield, IL); amphotericin B cholesterol dispersion (Amphotec, Sequus, Menlo Park, CA; and amphotericin B lipid complex (Abelcet, Liposome Co., Princeton, NJ). All three drugs are approved for indications other than VL and are available in the United States. Liposomal amphotericin B (AmBisome) was approved in August 1997 by the U.S. Food and Drug Administration (FDA) for the treatment of VL.

Lipsomal amphotericin B (AmBisome) has been shown in a series of trials to be a very effective and safe drug for the treatment of VL acquired in Brazil, India, Kenya, and the Mediterranean. The current FDA-approved regimen for immunocompetent patients, based on data from the Mediterranean and Brazil, is 3 mg/kg daily on days 1 to 5, a sixth dose on day 14, and a seventh dose on day 21 (total dose with this regimen is 21 mg/kg). Overall success rate with this dose regimen is practically 100%. Lower dose regimens have been effective in trials from Brazil, India, and Kenya. A dose of 3 to 4 mg/kg daily on days 1 to 5 with a sixth dose on day 10 is probably adequate for VL acquired in the Mediterranean and Brazil, and a dose of 2 to 3 mg/kg daily on days 1 to 5 and a sixth dose on day 10 for VL acquired in East Africa and India. It should be recognized that the use of a lower dose regimen may have a somewhat lower efficacy than the near 100% reported with the higher dose regimen, but the cost savings and decreased potential for infusion-related side effects may make a lower dose regimen optimal for some geographic regions. The current FDA-approved regimen for immunosuppressed patients is a higher dose regimen of 4 mg/kg daily on days 1 to 5, 10, 17, 24, 31, and 38 (total dose of 40 mg/kg). Even with the higher total dose, relapse is common. All regimens have a low rate of infusion-related side effects and uncommonly lead to renal insufficiency.

Although both amphotericin B cholesterol dispersion and amphotericin B lipid complex have been used in patients with VL, there is less experience with these drugs and an apparently higher incidence of infusion-related side effects. The lipid-associated amphotericin B preparations do not appear to be more effective than amphotericin B deoxycholate, but they can be given in higher daily doses with less toxicity, thereby reducing the duration of treatment. These agents are more expensive than amphotericin B deoxycholate, so their use in endemic areas may be limited. For the rare case of VL treated in the United States, liposomal amphotericin B (AmBisome) is the only FDA-approved drug and should be used unless contraindicated.

Pentamidine. Pentamidine (as the isethionate or methane sulfonate salt) is provided as a sterile powder that must be dissolved in sterile water and administered by intramuscular or slow intravenous injection. In patients unresponsive to SbV, treatment with pentamidine is an option. The recommended dose for VL is 4 mg/kg daily three times per week for at least 24 injections (8 weeks). Longer durations of 4 to 6 months have been used as well. Experience in Kenya indicates that it is often effective with little risk of serious toxicity. Common side effects include pain, induration, and sterile abscesses at the injection sites, as well as immediate hypotensive reactions if the drug is given too rapidly intravenously. Both hypoglycemia and diabetes may occur. Resistance to pentamidine in India is now common, as the 99% cure rates associated with shorter course regimens in the 1980s have been replaced by a lower initial rate and a relapse rate of 20% or more with a 9-week regimen. Addition of SbV to pentamidine does not appear to increase the cure rate significantly in studies from India. High-dose, long-duration therapy with pentamidine is more toxic than SbV and amphotericin B; therefore, it has a limited role in the treatment of VL.

Aminosidine. Aminosidine (paromomycin) is an aminoglycoside with broad antiparasitic activity. Parenteral aminosidine, used as monotherapy in Kenyan VL at 15 mg/kg/day for a mean of 19 days, cured 15 of 19 (79%) patients. When used at the higher dose of 20 mg/kg/day for 21 days in India, 29 to 30 (97%) patients were cured at 6 months' follow-up. A lower dose of 16 mg/kg/day was 93% effective. Aminosidine can be considered an acceptable monotherapy in Indian VL at a dose of at least 16 mg/kg/day for 21 days. When used in combination with standard doses of SbV for a shorter duration (17 to 20 days) in Kenyan, Sudanese, and Indian VL, cure rates of 82 to 90% were observed. Aminosidine has a favorable side effect profile. Therefore, aminosidine in conjunction with SbV for the treatment of VL allows the use of a shorter regimen of SbV.

Allopurinol. Because allopurinol inhibits *L. donovani* in vitro, it has been used in patients with visceral leishmaniasis. Cures were not achieved when allopurinol was used alone in previously untreated patients, and a controlled trial in Kenya of SSG alone (20 mg of Sb/kg/day) versus SSG plus allopurinol (21 mg/kg/day), each given for 30 days, demonstrated no advantage of the combination. Allopurinol has apparently been useful when used in combination with pentavalent antimonials in a few patients whose disease had relapsed.

Other Drugs. Ketoconazole has been used in Kenyan and Indian VL, both as monotherapy and in combination with SbV, with very limited success. Its use in VL is not recommended.

Immunotherapy. Intramuscular IFN-γ has been used as both monotherapy and adjunct therapy in SbV-resistant and primary VL in Kenya, Brazil, and India. As monotherapy, IFN-γ was only partially effective in the primary treatment of 5 of 9 patients with Indian VL. IFN-γ (100 μ/M² body surface area) plus meglumine antimoniate (20 mg/kg/day) for 10 to 60 days was first reported to be effective in 6 of 8 Brazilian patients with VL unresponsive to multiple courses of SbV alone. Subsequent trials in Brazil, Kenya, and India showed a faster elimination of parasites from tissues and a higher cure rate when IFN-γ is used in combination with SbV. Currently, IFN-γ should be considered when faced with SbV-resistant VL and in selected cases of relapse. IFN-γ has a significant side effect profile consisting of fever, chills, myalgias, fatigue, headache, and depression. It is also expensive, which restricts its use to selected locations and patients.

Treatment of Relapses. Relapse usually occurs within 6 months of the end of treatment, often within 2 months. Persistent splenomegaly and thrombocytopenia are useful prognostic indicators. Co-infection with tuberculosis and HIV should be considered in those who fail to respond or relapse. Treatment of coexisting tuberculosis usually results in response of the VL to SbV. Patients who fail to respond or relapse after initial therapy often respond to additional treatment with SbV. However, if they are treated with the same regimen used to treat initially, they have a high risk of treatment failure and develop resistance to SbV. Relapses should therefore be treated with SbV in higher doses (20 to 30 mg of Sb/kg/day) for longer periods of time (60 to 90 days). If doses higher than 20 mg/kg/day are given, caution and frequent ECG monitoring are recommended. There are case reports of response to one SbV preparation after failure with another SbV (e.g., success with Glucantime following failure with Pentostam or vice versa), but in general, this practice is not recommended. Where avaliable, lipid-associated amphotericin B and aminosidine should be used in place of SbV for a second round of therapy.

Splenectomy. Splenectomy is occasionally employed in patients with VL who are resistant to other forms of treatment. There is usually a prompt rise in hemoglobin levels and WBC and platelet counts after splenectomy, but additional chemotherapy is necessary, or cure is unlikely. Splenectomized patients are at increased risk of overwhelming sepsis due to penumococci and other encapsulated bacteria and should receive antipneumococcal vaccination before splenectomy. Because malaria is often fatal in splenectomized individuals, lifelong antimalarial prophylaxis is essential in countries where malaria occurs.

Post–kala-azar Dermal Leishmaniasis. Treatment of PKDL with a 20 mg/kg daily dose of SbV usually leads to improvement in the skin lesions, although pigmentary changes may persist indefinitely. The duration of therapy is usually longer than in VL, with courses of 120 days or longer sometimes used. In Africa, PKDL often clears without treatment.

PROGNOSIS. Infection with *L. donovani* comprises a spectrum of diseases, and spontaneous cure of inapparent infection is more common than was formerly realized. In contrast, the established syndrome of VL is almost always fatal in the absence of specific chemotherapy. The death rate with specific therapy (historically, almost always SbV) is low, even in desperate conditions. For example, there were 589 deaths recorded in 54,650 cases (1%) of VL cases in 1990 in Bihar, India. In one of the most difficult treatment environments imaginable, the epidemic of VL in the war-torn southern Sudan, the death rate was reported at 336 of 3076 cases (11%). Failure to respond to initial SbV therapy is uncommon in previously untreated, immunocompetent patients outside of India.

Response to treatment should be monitored by daily assessment of temperature, weekly assessment of hemoglobin levels and spleen size, and splenic or bone marrow aspirate smear and culture at the end of treatment. In most patients, the fever disappears within 7 days, the hemoglobin level rises, the patient feels much better, the spleen becomes smaller within 2 weeks (although return to baseline size does not occur until months after therapy), and the parasites disappear by the end of treatment. When fever persists and the general condition does not improve during treatment, concomitant tuberculosis should be suspected. Within 6 to 12 months, the spleen usually becomes nonpalpable, and elevated immunoglobulin levels and serologic tests become normal. Persistent splenomegaly after otherwise successful treatment may be due to portal hypertension.

Follow-up examination is important for the early detection and treatment of relapses. Relapse is suggested by an increase in spleen size, a fall in hemoglobin levels, and a decrease in eosinophil counts to fewer than $50/mm^3$ and should be confirmed by the demonstration of parasites. Depending on the regimen used, relapse occurs in 3 to 7% of patients in China, 0.5 to 13% in India, and 5 to 30% in Kenya. Relapses are most common during the first 2 to 6 months after finishing treatment, but occasionally, they occur several years later, particularly in patients who become immunocompromised by disease or medication.

PREVENTION AND CONTROL

Treatment of Cases. In epidemics of VL in which humans are the reservoir (India and perhaps Kenya and the Sudan), case finding and treatment may help interrupt the epidemic.

Reservoir Control. Conventional wisdom states that identification and destruction of infected dogs reduces the incidence of VL in areas where the dog is the reservoir (the Mediterranean, China, and South America). However, an interventional trial in Brazil failed to support that hypothesis. Infected dogs were eliminated from two intervention valleys and dogs in a third control valley were untouched. Human seroprevalence rates were determined by dot-ELISA in all three areas over the 12-month study period. Prevalence and seroconversion increased the same amount in each valley.

Vector Control. In India during the early part of the twentieth century, houses known to be microfoci were burned. During the malaria eradication campaigns, VL virtually disappeared from India, but since spraying of DDT has stopped, the incidence of VL has again increased to high levels.

Vaccines. A variety of vaccine preparations, including killed promastigotes with and without adjuvants, parasite fractions, recombinant antigens, and genetically engineered "avirulent" live parasites, are in various stages of development and clinical trials. None are licensed or commercially available at this time.

Bibliography

Alvar J, Canavate C, Gutierrez-Solar B, et al: *Leishmania* and human immunodeficiency virus co-infection: The first 10 years. Clin Microbiol Rev 10:298, 1997.

Badaro R, Jones TC, Carvalho EM, et al: New perspectives on a subclinical form of visceral leishmaniasis. J Infect Dis 154:1003, 1986.

Badaro R, Jones TC, Lorenco R, et al: A prospective study of visceral leishmaniasis in an endemic area of Brazil. J Infect Dis 154:639, 1986.

Berenguer J, Gomez-Campdera F, Padilla B, et al: Visceral leishmaniasis (kala-azar) in transplant recipients: Case report and review. Transplantation 65:1401, 1998.

Berman JD: Human leishmaniasis: Clinical, diagnostic, and chemotherapeutic developments in the last 10 years. Clin Infect Dis 24:684, 1997.

Berman JD: U.S. Food and Drug Administration approval of AmBisome (Liposomal amphotericin B) for the treatment of visceral leishmaniasis (Editorial response). Clin Infect Dis 28:49, 1999.

Berman JD, Badaro R, Thakur CP, et al: Efficacy and safety of liposomal amphotericin B (AmBisome) for visceral leishmaniasis in endemic developing countries. Bull WHO 76:25, 1998.

Bryceson ADM: Therapy in man. *In* Killick-Kendrick R, Peters W (eds): The Leishmaniases in Biology and Medicine. London, Academic Press, 1987, p 847.

Bryceson ADM, Chulay J, Mugambi M, et al: Visceral leishmaniasis unresponsive to antimonial drugs, II: Response to high dosage sodium stibogluconate or prolonged treatment with pentamidine. Trans R Soc Trop Med Hyg 79:705, 1985.

Chulay JD, Bryceson ADM: Quantitation of amastigotes of *Leishmania donovani* in smears of splenic aspirates from patients with visceral leishmaniasis. Am J Trop Med Hyg 32:475, 1983.

Chulay JD, Spencer HC, Mugambi M: Electrocardiographic changes during treatment of leishmaniasis with pentavalent antimony (sodium stibogluconate). Am J Trop Med Hyg 34:702, 1985.

Davidson RN, Di Martino L, Gradoni L, et al: Liposomal amphotericin B (AmBisome) in Mediterranean visceral leishmaniasis: A multi-center trial. Q J Med 87:75, 1994.

Gasser RA Jr, Magill AJ, Oster CN, et al: Pancreatitis induced by pentavalent antimonial agents during treatment of leishmaniasis. Clin Infect Dis 18:83, 1994.

Hashim FA, Ali MS, Satti M, et al: An outbreak of acute kala-azar in a nomadic tribe in western Sudan: Features of the disease in a previously non-immune population. Trans R Soc Trop Med Hyg 88:431, 1994.

Herwaldt BL, Berman JD: Recommendations for treating leishmaniasis with sodium stibogluconate (Pentostam) and review of pertinent clinical studies. Am J Trop Med Hyg 46:296, 1992.

Magill AJ, Grogl M, Gasser RA Jr, et al: Visceral infection due to *Leishmania tropica* in veterans of Operation Desert Storm. N Engl J Med 328:1383, 1993.

Meleney HE: The histopathology of kala-azar in the hamster, monkey and man. Am J Pathol 1:147, 1925.

Meredith SEO, Kroon NCM, Sondrop E, et al: Leish-KIT, stable direct agglutination test based on freeze-dried antigen for serodiagnosis of visceral leishmaniasis. J Clin Microbiol 33:1742, 1995.

Meyerhof A: U.S. Food and Drug Administration approval of AmBisome (liposomal amphotericin B) for treatment of visceral leishmaniasis. Clin Infect Dis 28:42, 1999.

Modabber F: Vaccines against leishmaniasis. Ann Trop Med Parasitol 89 (Suppl 1):83, 1995.

Ramesh V, Mukherjee A: Post–kala-azar dermal leishmaniasis. Int J Dermatol 34:85, 1995.

Seaman J, Mercer AJ, Sondorp HE, Herwaldt BL: Epidemic visceral leishmaniasis in southern Sudan: Treatment of severely debilitated patients under wartime conditions and with limited resources. Ann Intern Med 124:664, 1996.

Singh S, Gilman-Sachs A, Chang KP, et al: Diagnostic and prognostic value of k39 recombinant antigen in Indian leishmaniasis. J Parasitol 81:1000, 1995.

Sundar S, Reed SG, Singh VP, et al: Rapid accurate field diagnosis of Indian visceral leishmaniasis. Lancet 351:563, 1998.

Sundar S, Sinha PR, Agarwal NK, et al: A cluster of cases of severe cardiotoxicity among kala-azar patients treated with a high-osmolarity lot of sodium antimony gluconate. Am J Trop Med Hyg 59:139, 1998.

Thakur CP, Bhowmick S, Dolfi L, et al: Aminosidine plus sodium stibogluconate for the treatment of Indian kala-azar: A randomized dose-finding clinical trial. Trans R Soc Trop Med Hyg 89:219, 1995.

Zijlstra EE, El-Hassan AM, Ismael A: Endemic kala-azar in Eastern Sudan: Post kala-azar dermal leishmaniasis. Am J Trop Med Hyg 52:299, 1995.

95.3 *Cutaneous Leishmaniasis of the Old World**

DEFINITION. CL of the Old World is an infection characterized by nodular and ulcerative skin lesions caused by *Leishmania tropica, L. major, L. aethiopica,* and rarely, *L. infantum* (Fig. 95–6). Local names for this disease include Oriental sore, Baghdad boil, Delhi boil, Biskra button, and Aleppo evil.

ETIOLOGY. *L. tropica* is a heterogeneous species complex with strains that can be distinguished on ecologic, biochemical, and serologic grounds (Table 95–1). *L. major* (also known as *L. tropica major* in older literature) is a parasite of desert rodents that occasionally infects humans as a rural zoonosis. *L. tropica* (*L. tropica minor* or *L. tropica tropica*) is a parasite of dogs and humans that occurs in an urban environment. *L. aethiopica* (*L. tropica aethiopica*) is a parasite of the hyrax, found in the Rift Valley of Ethiopia and Kenya, which infects people when they encroach on the environment after deforestation of mountain slopes. *L. major* strains isolated from West Africa, Sudan, and Ethiopia have a common excreted factor serotype that differs from that of Middle Eastern strains. (See Chapter 95.1 for a detailed description of the parasite.) *L. infantum,* the usual cause of Mediterranean VL, has been isolated from cutaneous lesions as well.

DISTRIBUTION AND EPIDEMIOLOGY (Fig. 95–13)

***Leishmania major* Infections.** *L. major* is primarily an infection of desert rodents. The giant or great gerbil (*Rhombomys*

---

*All the material in this chapter is in the public domain, with the exception of any borrowed figures or tables.

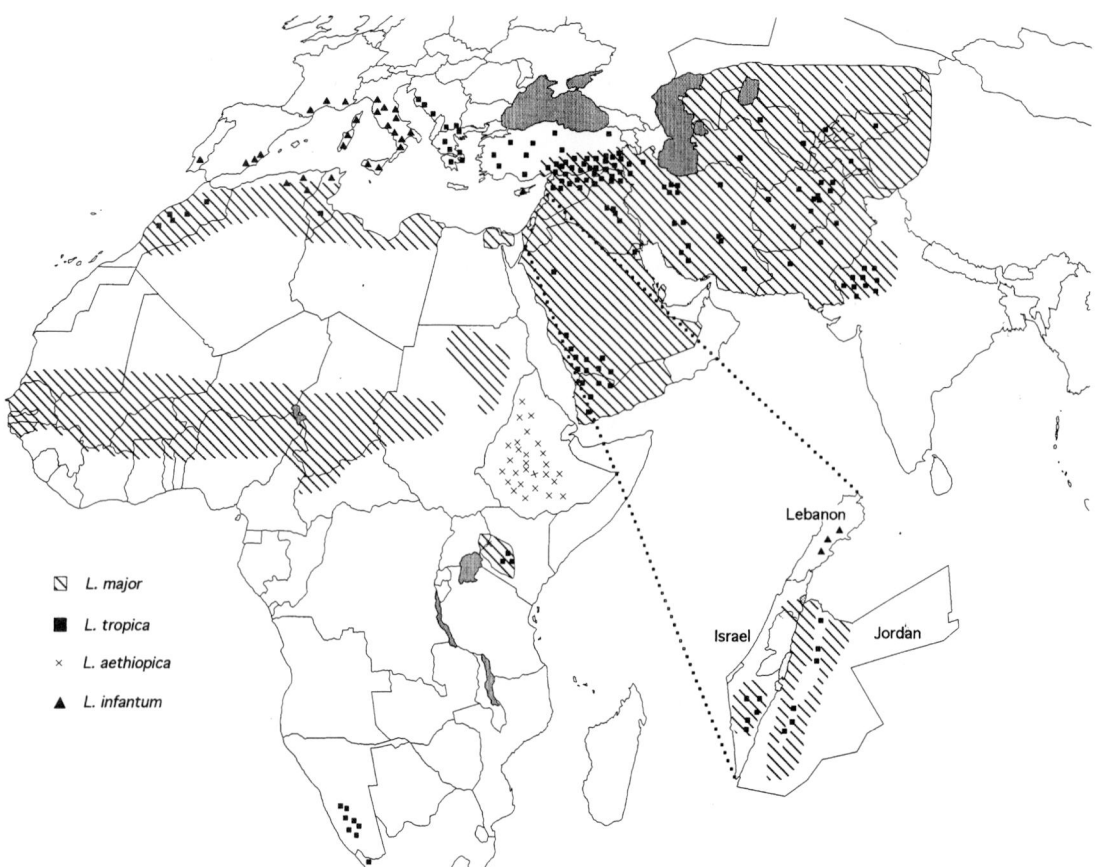

Figure 95–13. Geographic distribution of Old World cutaneous *Leishmania*. (From Magill AJ: The epidemiology of the leishmaniases. Dermatol Clin 13:505, 1995.)

opimus) lives in dry desert areas of central Asia, in southern Russia, throughout Iran and Pakistan, and in parts of Iraq and northwestern India and China. These gerbils may have an infection rate of 30%, with cutaneous lesions on relatively hairless parts of the body, chiefly the head, ears, and base of the tail (Fig. 95–14). Other rodents in these areas play a secondary role in maintaining the infection. In Libya, Saudi Arabia, and Israel, the fat rat (*Psammomys obesus*) is an important host. Infection in all these areas is maintained by *Phlebotomus caucasicus* and *P. papatasi*, although only the latter transmits the infection to humans. Other vectors of lesser importance are *P. mongolensis*, *P. alexanderi*, and *P. ansarii*. Inhabitants of villages near gerbil burrows may have infection prevalence rates of 100%, and other groups of people who enter the ecosystem, e.g., travelers, hunters, and military

patrols, may also have high attack rates. The peak incidence of disease occurs in late summer and autumn, and most children in endemic areas acquire a sore between 2 and 3 years of age, rarely reaching maturity without a scar.

CL caused by *L. major* is also found in a wide area of sub-Saharan Africa between the 10th and 13th parallels north, from Senegal in the West to the Sudan and Kenya in the East. The Nile rat (*Arvicanthis niloticus*) is a major host, although infection has been demonstrated in other rodents. Human disease is a rural zoonosis, and the main vector is *P. papatasi* in Sudan and *P. duboscqi* elsewhere.

Leishmania aethiopica Infections. *L. aethiopica* is found in mountain valleys of the Rift Valley in Ethiopia and Kenya. It infects the rock hyrax (*Procavia habessinica*) and the tree hyrax (*Heterohyrax brucei*), and humans are infected when their homesteads encroach on deforested mountain slopes. The vectors are the high-altitude sandflies *P. longipes* (Ethiopia) and *P. pedifer* (Kenya). Human disease caused by *L. aethiopica* is usually self-healing, but a small percentage of infected individuals develop nonhealing DCL. The situation in Namibia superficially resembles that in Ethiopia and Kenya because sporadic human cases of CL occur and *Leishmania* have been isolated from hyrax and from *P. rossi* near hyrax burrows. However, the parasites from humans and *P. rossi*, although identical, were biochemically different from parasites isolated from hyrax, and both parasites were different from *L. aethiopica*.

Leishmania tropica Infections. *L. tropica* has been demonstrated in cutaneous lesions on the ears, lips, nose, and inner canthus of the eyes of dogs in Iran, Iraq, and India, and in Morocco where it is transmitted by *P. sergenti*. In southern

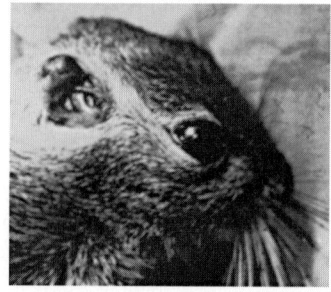

Figure 95–14. Lesion of *Leishmania major* on the ear of a gerbil (*Rhombomys opimus*).

France, Italy, and some Mediterranean islands, *P. papatasi* is the vector. The infection was formerly common in many large cities of the Middle East (Baghdad, Teheran, Aleppo, and Damascus) leading to it being known as "urban" CL. It is also found in southern Italy, Greece, Pakistan, and northwestern India. In the first half of the 20th century, 40 to 70% of Europeans living in Delhi became infected. With residual insecticide spraying for malaria control, there was a marked decrease in the sandfly populations and a concomitant decline in the incidence of urban CL. However, a major epidemic of anthroponotic CL due to *L. tropica* has occurred in war-ravaged Kabul, Afghanistan with thousands of cases identified.

Leishmania infantum **Infections.** *L. infantum* has been isolated from cutaneous lesions in countries throughout the Mediterranan littoral, Iran, and the Caucasus. Isoenzyme analysis shows that some isolates are more commonly found in cutaneous lesions. These "dermotropic" strains have also been isolated from visceral sites in AIDS patients.

PATHOLOGY AND PATHOGENESIS. At the site of inoculation, parasites enter macrophages and induce a cell-mediated immune response. A varying histologic appearance results from the interplay of host and parasites. In a typical case, lymphocytes, plasma cells, and large mononuclear cells surround the infected macrophages in a poorly organized granulomatous reaction. As the parasites are eliminated, epithelioid and giant cells appear, usually associated with tissue necrosis. Healing occurs with fibrosis. Small granulomas with central fibrinoid necrosis containing numerous parasites may be found, principally when disease is acquired in countries bordering the Mediterranean or in West Africa. In rural CL caused by *L. major*, granulomas may be found in nodules along the lymphatics or in local lymph nodes.

Nonhealing Forms. In LR, there is healing with fibrosis in the center of the lesion but failure to heal peripherally where a granulomatous reaction without caseation is seen. Parasites are scanty, and the histologic changes are similar to those of lupus vulgaris. In DCL, there is a defect in the CMI response, and numerous macrophages filled with amastigotes are seen with no cellular reaction or only a few surrounding lymphocytes. Although *Leishmania* have been found in the peripheral blood of a few patients infected with *L. major*, visceral lesions do not occur in this disease. Recently, an immunocompetent male patient with a chronic nonulcerative skin rash, mild splenomegaly, and leukopenia for 15 years was reported. Amastigotes were visualized on touch preparations from a biopsy of the skin rash, and the isolate obtained from culture was characterized as *L. infantum*. He most likely acquired male infection in southern Europe while on holiday, as he had never traveled outside of Europe. This remarkable case clearly demonstrates the capability of *Leishmania* to cause chronic, oligosymptomatic illness for years.

CLINICAL MANIFESTATIONS. After experimental inoculation of human volunteers, the incubation period of CL is generally 2 to 8 weeks, but in exceptional cases, the incubation period may be as long as 3 years. Different forms of CL vary in some of their clinical features. The lesions of rural disease caused by *L. major* tend to be multiple and are accompanied by marked inflammation and crusting. They mature rapidly and heal relatively quickly, lasting a few months. The lesions of urban disease caused by *L. tropica* tend to be single, develop more slowly, and persist for a year or more. The lesions of CL caused by *L. aethiopica* are the least inflamed and most chronic, generally lasting several years. The clinical appearance of the lesions reflects the degree of the host's immune response and may vary from small papules to nonulcerated plaques to large ulcers with well-defined, raised, indurated margins. When multiple lesions are present, they are usually similar in appearance and enlarge and heal together (isophasic reaction). The lesion begins as a small, often pruritic papule that enlarges with an infiltrated border. It may persist as a flattened plaque or may progress after a few days or weeks, with the surface becoming covered with fine, papery scales (Fig. 95–15), which are white and dry at first but later become moist and adherent, uncovering a shallow ulcer as they fall off. As the ulcer enlarges, it oozes serous fluid and may become covered with a thick crust. The edge of the ulcer is surrounded by a raised, indurated area with a characteristic dusky discoloration. Satellite lesions are common and may ultimately merge with the parent lesion. After a few months to more than a year, healing begins with central granulation tissue that spreads peripherally. The resultant depressed white or pink scar is often cosmetically disfiguring, especially when on the face. *L. major* infections may be associated with severe scarring, which can cause disability if located at critical sites, e.g., the wrist or elbow.

Multiple lesions are common, especially in rural CL, and occasionally, more than 100 lesions may be counted on an individual patient. Lesions usually occur on exposed parts of the body, e.g., face, hands, feet, arms, and legs, but rarely on the trunk and never on the palms or soles or hairy scalp. Uncommon sites of ulcers include the ears, tongue, and eyelids. Fever has occasionally preceded the appearance of multiple nodules. Lymphatic spread may occur in *L. major* infections, with subcutaneous nodules in a linear distribution and regional lymphadenopathy. When the primary lesion is on the hand, this may resemble sporotrichosis. Secondary bacterial infection of an ulcer is unusual. It may cause pain and, rarely, bacteremia.

Leishmaniasis Recidivans. Also known as lupoid leishmaniasis, LR is an unusual chronic form of CL that is found primarily in Iran and Iraq and may persist for 20 to 40 years. The lesion often begins on the face and enlarges relentlessly, healing in the center and advancing at the periphery, analogous to some forms of cutaneous tuberculosis. Mucous membrane involvement may lead to nasal destruction. The dense scar tissue in the center of the lesion contains small granulomas, whereas the nodules and papules at the periphery resemble the "apple jelly" nodules of lupus vulgaris. Organisms are extremely difficult to demonstrate in biopsy specimens but can more often be isolated by culture or animal inoculation. The LST is strongly positive.

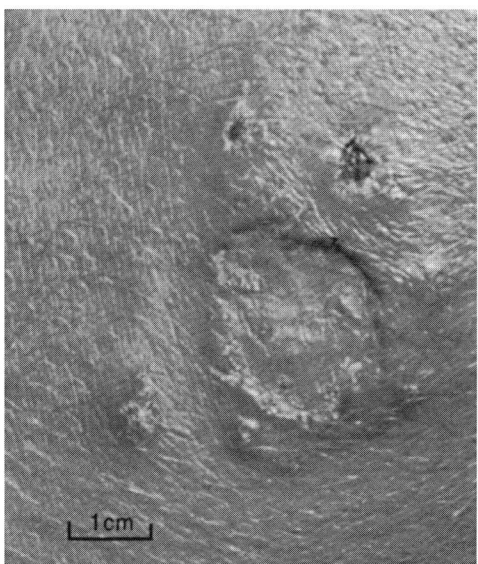

Figure 95–15. Oriental sore caused by *Leishmania major*. Note the satellite lesions.

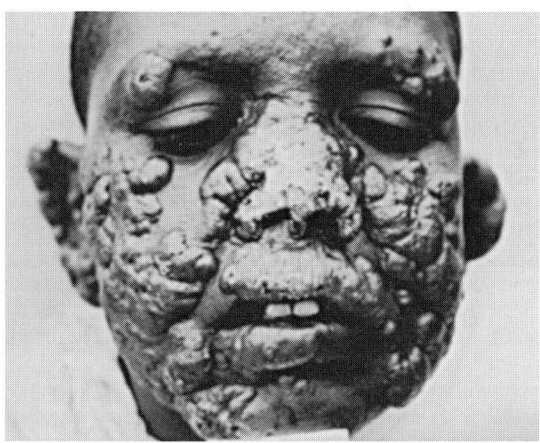

Figure 95–16. Nodular lesions of diffuse cutaneous leishmaniasis caused by *Leishmania aethiopica*. (Courtesy of Dr. A. D. M. Bryceson.)

Diffuse Cutaneous Leishmaniasis. DCL is an uncommon result of infection with *L. aethiopica* in Ethiopia and Kenya. Patients with DCL lack specific CMI responses to leishmanial antigens, although delayed hypersensitivity to tuberculin and other antigens appears normal. This is similar to the specific anergy that occurs in lepromatous leprosy. DCL usually begins as a single, nodular, nonulcerating lesion, often on the face, which enlarges and is followed by multiple similar lesions scattered over the entire body, especially on the face and nose, limbs, and buttocks (Fig. 95–16). The nodules of DCL are often described as soft and fleshy, whereas the nodules of lepromatous leprosy are often more indurated. The lesions do not ulcerate and may coalesce to form plaques. *Leishmania* have been recovered rarely from blood and bone marrow, but visceral lesions do not develop. The LST is persistently negative unless and until recovery occurs.

DIAGNOSIS

Demonstration of the Organism. Organisms can sometimes be identified in slit skin smears prepared as for diagnosing leprosy. The margin of the lesion is squeezed between the thumb and forefinger until bloodless; a scalpel blade is used to make a small incision; the cut edge of the incision is scraped with the blade; and the tissue juice on the blade is spread on a clean glass slide and stained with Giemsa or Leishman's stain. Alternatively, a small biopsy specimen may be removed from the edge of the lesion and an impression smear made by pressing the cut surface lightly against a slide. A portion of the biopsy specimen is macerated and cultured in NNM or Schneider's medium, and the remainder is fixed for pathologic examination. Varying numbers of organisms can be identified in histologic sections according to the immune status of the individual. Amastigotes in sections must be differentiated from yeast cells and the intracellular forms of *Histoplasma capsulatum* and *Toxoplasma gondii*. Organisms are especially difficult to find in biopsy specimens of LR, and culture of biopsy specimens must be undertaken in suspected cases. Tissue juice aspirated from the margin of lesions can also be cultured. Cultures generally become positive within 2 to 7 days in Schneider's medium but may take longer (up to 21 days) to grow in NNM medium.

Skin Test. The LST becomes positive within 3 months of the onset of skin lesions and remains positive for life. Skin test–positive individuals may have skin lesions for which the etiology is not leishmaniasis. The skin test is strongly positive in leishmaniasis recidivans but remains negative in DCL.

Serologic Tests. Immunoglobulin levels are normal in CL. Low titers of antileishmanial antibodies are detected in more

than half of patients with cutaneous leishmaniasis, but these tests are generally of little diagnostic help.

Differential Diagnosis. On clinical grounds, the lesions of CL must be distinguished from diphtheritic or veldt sores, tropical ulcer, tertiary syphilis, yaws, lupus vulgaris, blastomycosis, basal cell carcinoma, squamous cell carcinoma, and other causes of chronic nodules and ulcers. Although the LST is sometimes helpful, definitive diagnosis depends on demonstration or isolation of the organism.

TREATMENT

Typical Old World Cutaneous Leishmaniasis. The majority of Old World CL lesions are self-healing, requiring a few months to a few years to heal completely. In general, specific chemotherapy, especially systemic administration, is less commonly employed in Old World disease compared with New World disease.

Chemotherapy. Antileishmanial drugs should be given to patients with large or multiple lesions, especially if they are secondarily infected, and to patients with lesions in functionally or cosmetically important areas, e.g., the wrist or face. Pentavalent antimonials (SbV; sodium stibogluconate and meglumine antimoniate) are usually effective if given in adequate doses for an adequate duration. Treatment with 10 to 20 mg of Sb/kg/day for 2 to 4 weeks or longer may be needed. Toxicity is unusual with this treatment regimen (Chapter 95.2). Various other drugs have been used to treat CL, but the lack of controlled trials makes evaluation of their efficacy impossible. Local infiltration of 0.3 to 0.8 mL of sodium stibogluconate has been used with success and merits consideration, especially for early nonulcerated lesions. The use of toxic or unusual drugs in the treatment of Old World CL is seldom indicated. Ketoconazole is not effective in the treatment of *L. tropica* infections. Itraconazole is not effective in the treatment of *L. major* infections in Iran, but efficacy was seen in a small study of Indian CL (unknown species).

Local Therapy. Because members of the *L. tropica* species complex do not survive at temperatures above 37°C, local heat therapy may be useful in treating unresponsive lesions. This can be accomplished with an ordinary infrared heating lamp or by using a specially fitted prosthesis that can be molded to fit closely against the lesion. The intralesional temperature should be raised to 40° to 42°C for 12 hours at a time to achieve a rapid response.

Intralesional SbV has been used extensively for Old World CL. Each lesion is injected individually, dividing the dose into four quadrants if possible. Reported number of injections and the daily dose used vary widely, but efficacy is similar to intramuscular administration.

A topical formulation of 15% paromomycin with 12% methylbenzethonium chloride in soft white paraffin (P ointment or the "El-On" preparation) developed in Israel was shown to decrease the healing time in treated *L. major* lesions (100% cure at 21 to 30 days) compared with untreated lesions (100% cure at 51 to 60 days) on the same patient. This product is marketed in Israel. Because this preparation causes significant local reactions consisting of pruritus, paresthesias, and vesicle formation in about 25% of patients, other preparations have been developed. A 10% paromomycin/10% urea formulation used twice daily for 14 days was no better than placebo in controlled trials in Iran and Tunisia. A longer regimen (up to 12 weeks) of 12 to 15% paromomycin/10% urea applied daily cured 23 of 27 patients at the Hospital for Tropical Diseases in London in a mean of 6.7 weeks and was reported as nontoxic. None of the topical agents are effective against CL caused by *L. tropica*. Currently, paromomycin-based formulations appear quite promising, but the best formulation and optimal dose regimen are not yet determined.

It is likely that the optimal dose regimens will have to be determined for each major geographic area. Topical miconazole and co-trimoxazole have not been effective in Old World CL acquired in Saudi Arabia.

Leishmaniasis Recidivans. The lesions of LR respond to the higher doses of SbV used for VL. Local heat therapy and intralesional injections of SbV are commonly used in the Middle East.

Diffuse Cutaneous Leishmaniasis. DCL in Ethiopia responds poorly to treatment with SbV. The addition to SSG of aminosidine sulfate at 14 mg/kg/day given intravenously has led to long-lasting clinical and parasitologic cures. Pentamidine has been helpful in many patients, although it must be administered for many months and lesions usually reappear when the drug is stopped. Pentamidine, given as a single weekly injection of 4 mg/kg for at least 4 months longer than it takes to eliminate parasites from slit skin smears, appears to offer the best compromise between maximal efficacy and minimal toxicity. Diabetes has developed in 10% of Ethiopian patients with DCL treated with pentamidine. (See Chapter 95.2 for additional details about pentamidine toxicity.)

PREVENTION AND CONTROL

Vector Control. Reducing the vector population can decrease the incidence of CL. Improved general sanitation and removal of refuse and rubble in which sandflies breed reduce the incidence of urban CL. Residual spraying with DDT for malaria control had eliminated CL in many areas, although it has returned with the cessation of spraying.

Reservoir Control. In the central Asian republics of the former Soviet Union, disease incidence has been reduced by poisoning gerbil burrows with picrotoxin or by deep plowing on irrigation projects to destroy burrows and eliminate gerbils from the area.

Immunization. Vaccination against CL was used for many years in Russia, Israel, Iran, Iraq, and Jordan. Live, attenuated *L. major* promastigotes are inoculated intracutaneously ("leishmanization"), and a lesion is allowed to develop and run its natural course. This results in a single scar in a cosmetically acceptable location, and the immunity that develops is comparable to that following a natural infection. There is a small risk of developing a CL lesion requiring treatment or the development of LR at the site of immunization.

Bibliography

Bryceson ADM: Diffuse cutaneous leishmaniasis in Ethiopia. I. The clinical and histological features. Trans R Soc Trop Med Hyg 63:708, 1969.

Bryceson ADM: Diffuse cutaneous leishmaniasis in Ethiopia. II. Treatment. Trans R Soc Trop Med Hyg 64:369, 1970.

Dowlati Y: Treatment of cutaneous leishmaniasis (Old World). Clin Derm 14:513, 1996.

Ridley DS, Ridley MJ: The evolution of the lesion in cutaneous leishmaniasis. J Pathol 141:83, 1983.

Samady JA, Schwartz RA: Old World cutaneous leishmaniasis. Int J Dermatol 36:161, 1997.

Sharquie KE, Al-Talib KK, Chu AC: Intralesional therapy of cutaneous leishmaniasis with sodium stibogluconate antimony. Br J Dermatol 119:53, 1988.

95.4 *Cutaneous Leishmaniasis of the New World**

DEFINITION. CL of the New World is a zoonosis caused by parasites of the species complexes *Leishmania mexicana* and *L. braziliensis*, transmitted by sandflies, and characterized by ulcerative skin lesions (Fig. 95–6). Some persons with

---

*All the material in this chapter is in the public domain, with the exception of any borrowed figures or tables.

L. braziliensis infection develop destructive oral, nasal, or pharyngeal lesions, called mucosal leishmaniasis or "espundia." Local names for New World CL include uta (Peru), chiclero ulcer or bay sore (Mexico), dicera de Baurid (Brazil), and pian bois, or forest yaws (Guyana). Collectively, these diseases are also referred to as American CL.

ETIOLOGY. There are currently three organisms in the *L. mexicana* complex and four in the *L. braziliensis* complex that are known to infect humans (Table 95–1). Members of the *L. mexicana* complex develop only in the midgut and foregut of their sandfly vectors, whereas members of the *L. braziliensis* complex develop in the hindgut as well as the midgut and foregut. *L. chagasi* has also been isolated from lesions of CL on rare occasions. (See Chapter 95.1 for a detailed description of the parasite.)

DISTRIBUTION AND EPIDEMIOLOGY. The geographic distribution of New World CL is shown in Figure 95–17. New World CL is an uncommon disease in returning U.S. travelers but should be considered when evaluating an ulcerative lesion in persons with an exposure or travel history. The CDC released SSG (Pentostam) for 59 civilian U.S. travelers between 1985 and 1990. Most acquired their disease in forested areas of Mexico or Central America. Those conducting field studies were at highest risk, but casual tourists with brief exposures also became infected.

Leishmania mexicana Infections. The parasite causing chiclero ulcer is common throughout southern Mexico, Belize, and Guatemala and causes the rare cases of CL acquired in the southern United States. It is transmitted among forest rodents by *Lutzomyia olmeca*, which is not highly attracted to humans. However, the prolonged exposure of "chicleros," who live for many months in the forest collecting chewing gum latex from chicle trees, explains the high incidence of infection in these workers, i.e., 30% during the first year of employment. Timber cutters, road builders, and agricultural workers are also commonly infected. In south Texas, the southern plains wood rat, *Neotoma micropus* is the reservoir and *Lu. anthophora* the primary vector of the enzootic cycle.

Leishmania amazonensis Infections. This parasite occurs in the Amazon region of Brazil and neighboring countries. It is primarily a disease of forest rodents, but marsupials and foxes can be secondary hosts. Infection rates of 20% occur in some rodent species in Brazil, but human disease is uncommon because the vector *Lu. flaviscutellata* is nocturnal, is not very anthropophilic, and lives in swampy areas of the forest seldom frequented by people.

Leishmania venezuelensis Infections. This parasite has been isolated only from humans with CL in Venezuela. Similar to other members of the *L. mexicana* complex, it grows rapidly in hamsters and develops in the hindgut of sandflies. It is atypical, however, in its poor long-term growth in blood agar medium. *Lu. olmeca bicolor* is the probable vector. The mammalian host has not yet been discovered.

Leishmania v. braziliensis Infections. *L. braziliensis*, which primarily causes infection of forest rodents, causes cutaneous and mucosal leishmaniasis in humans. Human infection occurs in Brazil, Guatemala, Belize, Honduras, Nicaragua, Peru, Ecuador, Bolivia, Costa Rica, Panama, Colombia, Venezuela, Paraguay, and Argentina. The major vector, *Lu. wellcomei*, avidly bites humans and rodents and, unlike most sandflies, feeds during daylight hours. The other vectors, *Lu. intermedius* and *Lu. pessoai*, are also anthropophilic. Disease is common among persons living in farming communities in newly cleared forest areas and in road construction and mining workers.

Leishmania v. panamensis Infections. This parasite is found in Panama and adjacent areas of Central America and Colombia. The principal reservoir is the sloth, *Choloepus*

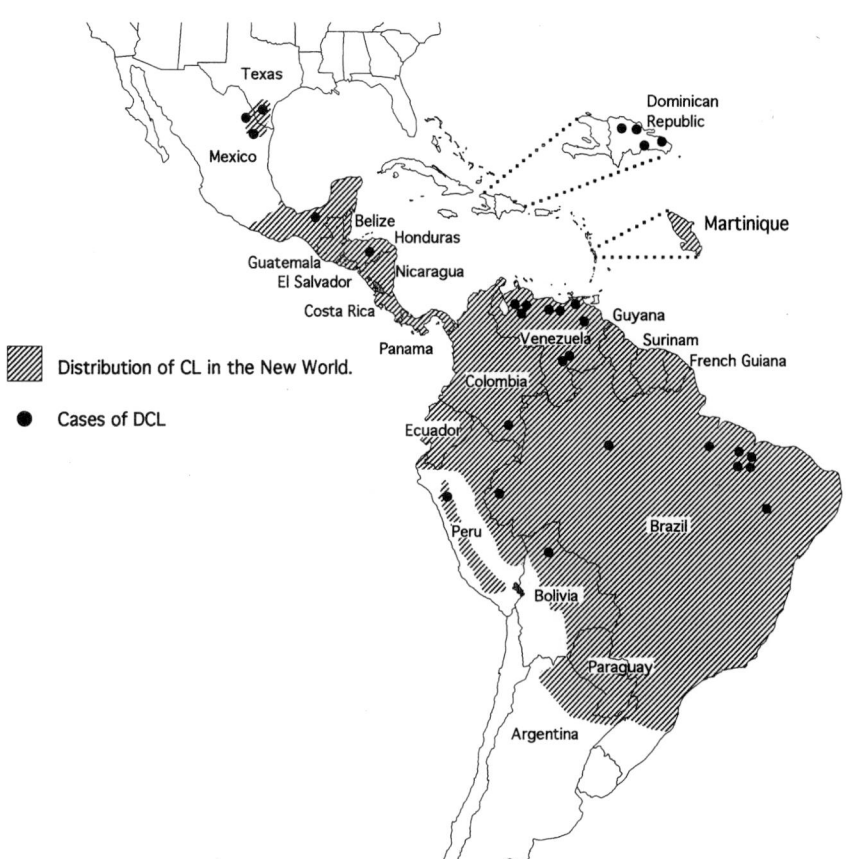

Distribution of CL in the New World.

● Cases of DCL

Figure 95–17. Geographic distribution of New World cutaneous *Leishmania*. *L. braziliensis* is found from Mexico to Argentina. *L. peruviana* is found on the Western slopes of the Peruvian Andes. *L. guyanensis* is found north of the Amazon river in Brazil, Guyana, Surinam, French Guiana, Venezuela, Colombia, and Ecuador. *L. panamensis* is found in Honduras, Nicaragua, Costa Rica, Panama, Colombia, Ecuador, and Venezuela. *L. amazonensis* is found in Brazil. *L. mexicana* is found in Texas, Mexico, Belize, Guatemala, the Dominican Republic, Honduras, Costa Rica, Panama, Colombia, and Venezuela. *L. venezuelensis* is found in Venezuela. (From Magill AJ: The epidemiology of the leishmaniases. Dermatol Clin 13:505, 1995.)

hoffmanni. Other sloths, procyonids, and forest primates are secondary hosts. The major vector, *Lu. trapidoi,* usually lives in the forest canopy in close contact with the known reservoirs. However, at certain times of the year, when rainfall is moderate, it can be found close to the ground where it can bite humans. Human disease is common in rural agricultural workers, especially in the first year after settlement before deforestation is complete, and in military personnel participating in jungle warfare maneuvers.

Leishmania v. guyanensis Infections. Pian bois or forest yaws, the human disease caused by *L. guyanensis* occurs in the Guyanas and northern Brazil. Because the principal vector, *Lu. umbratilis,* has a high infection rate (up to 7%) and readily bites humans in the daytime when disturbed from its resting sites on tree trunks, disease is common among forest workers. The major reservoirs of *L. guyanensis* are the two-toed sloth, *Choloepus didactylus,* and the lesser anteater, *Tamandua tetradactyla.*

Leishmania v. peruviana Infections. *L. peruviana* is found only at 900 to 3000 M above sea level in the Peruvian Andes and the highlands of Argentina, where dogs with inapparent infection are the reservoir hosts. Human disease (uta) is contracted in and around the home, and in some villages 90% of people are infected or scarred. *Lu. verrucarum* and *Lu. peruensis* are the probable vectors.

Infections Caused by Other Leishmania Species. Parasites have been cultured from lesions of CL in various parts of South America that have isoenzyme patterns and growth characteristics in culture and laboratory animals that are different from those of known species of *Leishmania.* The parasites isolated from persons with DCL in the Dominican Republic are also biochemically distinct. Species names have not yet been proposed for these parasites. *L. pifanoi,* suggested as

a name for the parasite causing DCL in Venezuela, seems to be very similar to *L. amazonensis. L. chagasi* causes nonulcerative CL in Honduras and Costa Rica.

PATHOLOGY. Lesions of American CL demonstrate a variety of pathologic changes. Early skin lesions generally show hyperplasia of the epidermis and necrosis of the dermis, with scattered neutrophils, eosinophils, and mononuclear cells. As the disease progresses, there is heavy infiltration with plasma cells and lymphocytes, followed later by epithelioid cells and Langhans giant cells. Long-standing lesions usually contain well-formed granulomas. Variable numbers of parasites are found within macrophages and free in the tissues (Fig. 95–3 [see in color section]). Mucosal lesions show necrotizing granulomatous inflammation with a paucity of organisms. In contrast, the lesions of DCL contain large numbers of amastigote-laden macrophages but very few lymphocytes.

CLINICAL MANIFESTATIONS

Cutaneous Disease. The lesions of New World CL are generally similar to those of Old World disease. A few weeks to several months after infection, an erythematous, often pruritic papule develops at the site of inoculation. In a group of U.S. military personnel, cutaneous lesions were noted a median interval of 17 days (range, 2 to 78 days) after exposure to *L. panamensis.* The initial papule may become scaly or gradually enlarge, developing a raised indurated margin with central ulceration (Fig. 95–18). Verrucous and acneiform lesions are uncommon, but nodular lesions are seen in about 10%. Ulcerative lesions are usually painless, unless secondarily infected. The natural history varies, depending on the infecting species, location of the lesion, and host immunity. *L. mexicana* infections generally have one or a few lesions, which heal spontaneously within 6 months. In Guatemala, 22 of 25 lesions caused by *L. mexicana* (88%) completely

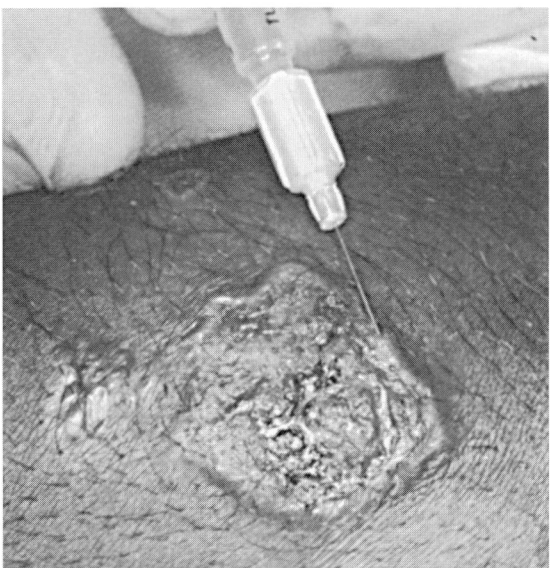

***Figure* 95–18.** Cutaneous leishmaniasis due to *Leishmania panamensis*. Note the elevated margin and the satellite lesion. The picture also demonstrates the technique of aspirating tissue fluid for parasite culture. (Courtesy of Dr. L. D. Hendricks, Walter Reed Army Institute of Research, Washington, DC.)

reepithelialized by a median lesion age of 14 weeks (range, 6 to 44 weeks), and 17 (68%) were classified as cured 6 months later. However, lesions on the ear occur in 40% of patients and are chronic, lasting many years (Fig. 95–19). Simple cutaneous lesions caused by parasites of the *L. braziliensis* complex generally require 6 to 18 months for spontaneous healing but sometimes persist much longer. In addition, enlargement of the lymph nodes draining the bite site commonly accompanies or precedes the ulcer in *L. braziliensis* infections. Multiple skin lesions due to metastatic spread

along lymphatics are common with *L. guyanensis* infections, and subcutaneous lymphatic nodules resembling sporotrichosis are often seen in *L. panamensis* infections.

Trauma to uninvolved skin can lead to the formation of lesions caused by *Leishmania* (Koebner phenomenon). Persons living in endemic areas note the ulcers of CL develop along machete cuts or other such blunt and sharp trauma. Postoperative granulomas caused by *Leishmania* have been reported as postsurgical complications as well.

Mucosal Disease. Of persons infected with *L. braziliensis* 1 to 3% develop metastatic spread of disease to the nasal, pharyngeal, and buccal mucosa, known as espundia. ML is more common in southern latitudes and is much less common in northern South America and Central America. Mucosal lesions appear several months to many years after the initial cutaneous lesion, which has usually healed. Erythema and edema of the involved mucosa are followed by ulcerations covered with a mucopurulent exudate. There is often mutilating destruction of the nasal septum (Fig. 95–20), palate, lips, pharynx, and larynx. The lesions are chronic and progressive, and death can be caused by aspiration or inanition. Mucosal lesions occur rarely in *L. panamensis* and *L. guyanensis* infections. The nasal mucosa is the first site involved. Patients may complain of stuffiness, difficulty in breathing through their nose, and occasional bleeding as their first symptoms. Hoarseness should prompt evaluation of the vocal cords for laryngeal involvement.

There are no known clinical, serologic, or skin test reaction responses that predict the development of ML in a person with primary CL. However, a significant genetic component for the risk of developing ML has long been suspected. Recently, an association between HLA loci and the presence of ML has been demonstrated. In a study in Brazil comparing 43 patients with ML to 111 matched controls, there was a significant decrease in frequency of HLA-DR2 as well as a significant increase in HLA-DQw3 in patients as compared with controls. In addition, polymorphisms in the tumor necrosis factor alpha (TNF-α) and beta (TNF-β) genes associated with high circulating levels of TNF-α has been demonstrated in Venezuelan patients with ML. Therefore, susceptibility to ML may be directly associated with regulatory polymorphisms associated with TNF-α production.

Diffuse Cutaneous Leishmaniasis (DCL). In Venezuela, Bra-

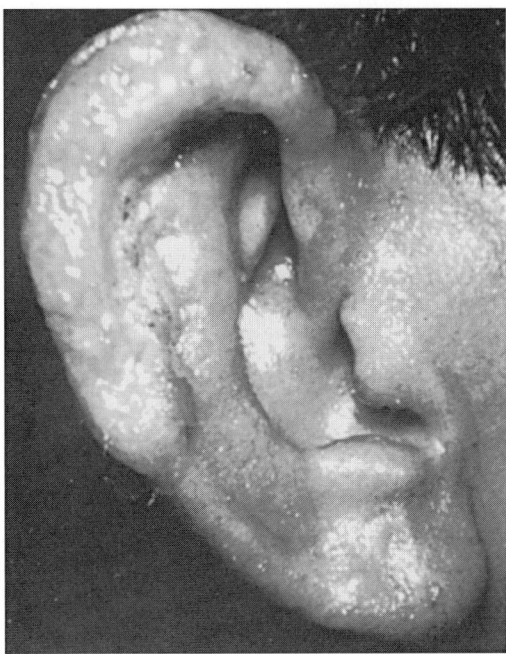

***Figure* 95–19.** Chiclero ulcer. (Courtesy of the Louisiana State University School of Medicine, New Orleans.)

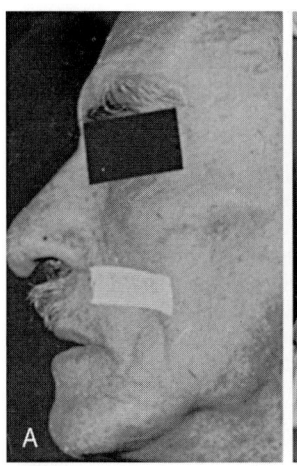
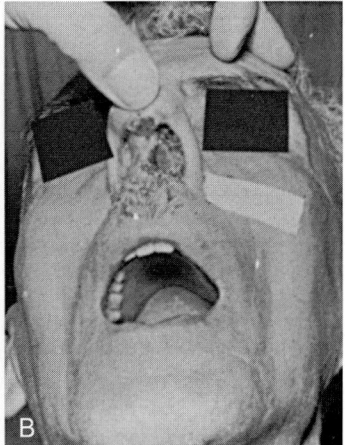

***Figure* 95–20.** Mucocutaneous leishmaniasis in a Costa Rican patient who had the disease for more than 15 years. *A*, Lateral view showing the tapir nose. *B*, Destruction of the nasal septum. (Courtesy of the Louisiana State University School of Medicine, New Orleans.)

zil, Mexico, and the Dominican Republic, a diffuse form of cutaneous leishmaniasis occurs that is similar to DCL in Ethiopia (Fig. 95–16). The initial lesion is usually a macule, papule, or nodule (rarely an ulcer). Because of an immunologic defect in the host, the parasite spreads locally and hematogenously to cause generalized nodular lesions consisting of heavily parasitized macrophages. The nasal mucosa and laryngopharynx are sometimes involved, but visceral lesions do not occur. As in patients with DCL in Ethiopia, there is specific anergy to leishmanin but not to unrelated antigens, e.g., tuberculin.

DIAGNOSIS

Demonstration of the Organism. As in other forms of leishmaniasis, definitive diagnosis requires demonstration of the parasite. The methods are the same as those for diagnosis of CL of the Old World (Chapter 95.3). Studies in Guatemala and Colombia show that yield of parasites is similar whether the aspirate is collected from the edge of the lesion or from the ulcer base. It is important to completely debride the crusted material from the ulcer before trying to aspirate. Wet-to-dry gauze pads and a scalpel are often required for adequate debridement. This can be quite painful to the patient, and local anesthesia with injectable 1% lidocaine is recommended if available. The sensitivity of culture can also be improved by 20 to 25% if 3 to 5 cultures per ulcerative lesion are obtained. In practice, if the only goal is to demonstrate parasites prior to instituting therapy, then several smears can be made and examined before resorting to culture. Organisms are generally numerous in smears and biopsy specimens (Fig. 95–3 [see in color section]) of lesions of DCL and cutaneous leishmaniasis caused by *L. mexicana* but are often scanty in *L. braziliensis* infection of both the skin and mucous membranes, especially in long-standing disease. Cultures of tissue juice aspirated from the indurated margin of a skin lesion (Fig. 95–18) or cultures or hamster inoculation of biopsy specimens of skin or mucosal lesions are more likely to confirm *L. braziliensis* infection.

The use of monoclonal antibodies to detect amastigotes in tissue smears of CL of the New World increases sensitivity, but the technique requires an experienced observer and expensive equipment. The use of the polymerase chain reaction (PCR) to amplify *Leishmania* DNA targets has had mixed results. Assay performance is laboratory dependent and the general availability is poor. Although PCR may be useful for ML in particular, it is unlikely that the technology will greatly impact the ability to diagnose patients in endemic areas.

Skin Test. The LST is positive in almost all patients with active CL and ML, although it may be negative during the first few months. Treatment is occasionally justified despite the failure to demonstrate parasites in persons with typical lesions and a positive skin test, especially in those with espundia. In DCL, the skin test is uniformly negative.

Serologic Tests. Standard serologic tests are not useful for the diagnosis of New World CL or ML. Assays using crude antigen preparations are positive at low titer in only 70 to 80% of cases and are especially likely to be negative early in the course of the disease when a diagnosis is most desired. Serial measurement of antibody may be helpful in evaluating the response to treatment in patients who have a positive test initially. The use of recombinant proteins instead of crude antigen improves sensitivity and specificity.

Differential Diagnosis. New World CL must be distinguished from sporotrichosis, blastomycosis, yaws, syphilis, cutaneous tuberculosis, *Mycobacterium marinum* infection, and dermatologic cancers. Diseases that may resemble espundia include paracoccidioidomycosis, histoplasmosis, tuberculosis, syphilis, malignant tumors, and lethal midline granu-

loma. Nodular DCL must be differentiated from lepromatous leprosy.

TREATMENT

Typical New World Cutaneous Leishmaniasis. Systemic chemotherapy is generally indicated in New World CL in contrast to Old World CL. Indications include the multiplicity of lesions (*L. guyanensis* infection), the chronicity of untreated disease (*L. mexicana* ear lesions and *L. braziliensis* complex infections), or progression of mucosal disease in the absence of chemotherapy.

Pentavalent Antimonials. SbV is the treatment of choice for all forms of New World CL. In Latin America, Glucantime is used because Pentostam (SSG) is not generally available. In the United States, SSG is available under an IND application from the Centers for Disease Control. A randomized controlled trial in patients with *L. panamensis* infections showed that treatment with SSG at a dosage of 20 mg of Sb/kg/day for 20 days gave a significantly higher cure rate than did a dosage of 10 mg of Sb/kg/day for 20 days. This dosage and duration are also recommended for other forms of simple New World CL. Lower doses and shorter regimens may be effective in certain geographic regions. Toxicity of SSG is discussed in Chapter 95.2. If toxicity does occur at the higher doses, the drug should be withheld for a few days until side effects resolve and treatment can then usually be resumed at the same dose.

Other Drugs. In patients unresponsive to SbV, amphotericin B deoxycholate is sometimes effective. It is administered by slow IV infusion in gradually increasing doses to 1 mg/kg, at which level it should be given on alternate days. Prolonged treatment to a total of 2 to 3 g is generally required. There is insufficient information on which to make confident recommendations for the lipid-associated amphotericin B compounds, although there are case reports of failure.

Pentamidine should also be considered as an alternative to SbV and in patients unresponsive to SbV. Recent trials in Colombia have shown that 2 mg/kg given IM every other day for 7 doses or 3 mg/kg given IM every other day for 4 doses cured 72 of 75 (96%) evaluable patients. The injections were well tolerated and no significant side effects were noted.

Ketoconazole at a dosage of 600 mg once daily for 28 days appears to be as effective (70% cure rate) as a low dosage of SSG (10 mg of Sb/kg/day) in patients with CL caused by *L. panamensis*. Ketoconazole is less effective for *L. braziliensis* infections, curing only 7 of 23 (30%) infections. Because it can be given orally, ketoconazole may thus have a role in some patients for whom parenteral therapy is not possible.

Allopurinol has been used frequently for the treatment of New World CL. However, in a recently completed, randomized, placebo-controlled, double-blinded study conducted in Colombia, allopurinol given at 20 mg/kg daily for 28 days was no better than placebo in the treatment of ulcerative CL caused by *L. panamensis*. Therefore, based on this study and other uncontrolled studies, allopurinol is not recommended as monotherapy for New World CL. Its use in combination with SbV in cases of relapsed CL remains an option, as there are reports of success with this combination.

Aminosidine as a single agent is not considered effective in New World CL, but may have some utility as adjunctive therapy. Mefloquine has not been shown to be effective when evaluated in a comparative trial. Currently, there is no oral regimen that can be recommended as primary monotherapy for New World CL. Oral agents in combination with parenteral SbV and oral agents alone for long-term maintenance therapy in immunosuppressed patients may have some utility in selected clinical situations.

Local Agents. Intralesional injections of SbV, accepted therapy for disease in the Old World, have not seen wide use in the Americas. There are no large comparative trials on which to base recommendations.

Topical application of paromomycin formulations has been evaluated in Ecuador and Colombia. In Ecuador, an open, nonrandomized trial of 15% paromomycin with 12% methylbenzethonium chloride in white paraffin (the Israeli "El-On preparation"; Chapter 95.3) cured 90% of 52 patients. In Colombia, another open, nonrandomized trial of 15% paromomycin with 5% methylbenzethonium chloride combined with parenteral Glucantime at 20 mg/kg daily for 7 days cured 18 of 20 (90%) patients. The true efficacy remains to be determined in controlled trials, but topical paromomycin formulations may have a role in combination with SbV to decrease the number of injections required for cure.

Mucosal Leishmaniasis. In patients with advanced ML, adequate nutrition must be ensured, and destructive or obstructive lesions may require ventilatory support or treatment, as in aspiration pneumonia. Plastic surgery may be required after parasitologic cure in patients with extensive tissue destruction from espundia.

It is unclear if specific chemotherapy of primary *L. braziliensis* ulcerative lesions decreases the risk of subsequent mucosal disease. Many experienced clinicians in endemic areas believe that treatment with SbV does not affect the natural history of ML. Several well-documented case reports of mucosal lesions developing in individuals despite appropriate therapy with SbV support this conclusion.

Espundia usually responds to treatment with SbV, but relapse is common unless dosages of 20 mg of Sb/kg/day are administered for at least 30 days or longer. Relapses have been successfully treated with 20 mg of Sb/kg/day for 60 to 90 days. Early disease responds better than late disease. Liposomal amphoterin B (AmBisome) has been used with success in cases unresponsive to SbV. There is no benefit to the addition of allopurinol to SbV in the treatment of ML.

Diffuse Cutaneous Leishmaniasis. In contrast to Ethiopian DCL, Venezuelan DCL usually improves after initial treatment with SbV, although relapse is invariable and patients who relapse often do not respond to additional SbV treatment. Although untested, it would seem reasonable to treat newly diagnosed DCL patients with 10 to 20 mg of Sb/kg once or twice daily until apparent clinical and parasitologic cure is achieved and for several months thereafter.

Immunotherapy. Subcutaneous INF-γ (100 μg/M² of body surface area) has been successfully used in combination with low-dose SbV (10 mg of Sb/kg daily) to treat CL and ML patients who failed a first course of standard SbV therapy.

Studies in Venezuela have shown that treatment with three injections of heat-killed *L. amazonensis* promastigotes mixed with viable bacille Calmette-Guérin (BCG) given intradermally every 6 to 8 weeks is as effective as Glucantime in achieving clinical cures of localized CL caused by *L. braziliensis*, and either of these treatments is more effective than BCG alone. Treatment with chemotherapy plus combined immunotherapy was also variably effective in 8 of 9 patients with DCL.

PROGNOSIS. Cutaneous lesions usually heal within 1 month after initiation of treatment with SbVs, although large ulcers may require longer. In a study of ulcerative CL caused by *L. braziliensis*, 32% of lesions had re-epithelialized at the end of a 3-week treatment course, 60% at 6 weeks, and 90% at 13 weeks. Mucosal disease caused by *L. braziliensis*, which may appear many years after the primary cutaneous lesion has resolved, is progressive unless treated. The risk of espundia may be reduced in persons whose primary cutaneous lesions are treated with adequate dosages of SbV. DCL is characteristically a relapsing or chronically progressive disease.

PREVENTION AND CONTROL. Vaccines and chemoprophylactic drugs are not available. Because of the forest location of vectors and reservoirs, control of American CL and ML is not possible. The only exception is uta, which, because of its domiciliary nature, can be controlled by spraying houses with insecticides. Insect repellents, long-sleeved shirts, and fine-mesh bed netting may reduce the risk of infection for individuals. Permethrin-impregnated clothing is also effective. In a study of Colombian military personnel in an endemic area for 6.6 weeks and followed for an additional 12 weeks, 4 of 143 (3%) soldiers wearing permethrin-impregnated uniforms acquired disease, whereas 18 of 143 (18%) soldiers who did not wear impregnated uniforms acquired disease ($P = 0.002$).

Bibliography

Ballou WR, McClain JB, Gordon DM, et al: Safety and efficacy of high-dose sodium stibogluconate therapy of American cutaneous leishmaniasis. Lancet 2:13, 1987.

Cerf B, Reed SG, Netto EM, et al: Epidemiology of American cutaneous leishmaniasis due to *Leishmania braziliensis braziliensis*. J Infect Dis 156:73, 1987.

Convit J, Castellanos PL, Ulrich M, et al: Immunotherapy of localized, intermediate, and diffuse forms of American cutaneous leishmaniasis. J Infect Dis 160:104, 1989.

Falcoff E, Taranto NJ, Remondegui CE, et al: Clinical healing of antimony-resistant cutaneous or mucocutaneous leishmaniasis following the combined administration of interferon γ and pentavalent antimonial compounds. Trans R Soc Trop Med Hyg 88:95, 1994.

Franke ED, Llanos-Cuentas A, Echevarria J, et al: Efficacy of 28 day and 40 day regimens of sodium stibogluconate (Pentostam) in the treatment of mucosal leishmaniasis. Am J Trop Med Hyg 51:77, 1994.

Grimaldi G Jr, Tesh RB: Leishmaniasis of the New World: Current concepts and implications for future research. Clin Microbiol Rev 6:230, 1993.

Grimaldi G Jr, Tesh RB, McMahon-Pratt D: A review of the geographic distribution and epidemiology of leishmaniasis in the New World. Am J Trop Med Hyg 41:687,1989.

Herwaldt BL, Arana BA, Navin TR: The natural history of cutaneous leishmaniasis in Guatemala. J Infect Dis 165:518,1992.

Herwaldt BL, Stokes SL, Juranek DD: American cutaneous leishmaniasis in U.S. travelers. Ann Intern Med 118:779, 1993.

Marsden PD: Mucosal leishmaniasis ("espundia" Escomel, 1911). Trans R Soc Trop Med Hyg 80:859, 1986.

Navin TR, Arana BA, Arana FE, et al: Placebo-controlled clinical trial of sodium-stibogluconate (Pentostam) versus ketoconazole for treating cutaneous leishmaniasis in Guatemala. J Infect Dis 165:528, 1992.

Navin TR, Arana FE, de Merida, et al: Cutaneous leishmaniasis in Guatemala: Comparison of diagnostic methods. Am J Trop Med Hyg 42:36,1990.

Netto EM, Marsen PD, Llanos-Cuentas EA, et al: Long-term follow-up of patients with *Leishmania (Viannia) braziliensis* infection and treated with Glucantime. Trans R Soc Med Hyg 84:367, 1990.

Ridley DS, Marsden PD, Cuba CC, et al: A histological classification of mucocutaneous leishmaniasis in Brazil and its clinical evaluation. Trans R Soc Trop Med Hyg 74:508, 1980.

Shaw JJ, Lainson R: Ecology and epidemiology: New World. *In* Peters W, Killick-Kendrick R (eds): The Leishmaniases in Biology and Medicine. London, Academic Press, 1987, p 291.

Soto J, Buffet P, Grogl M, et al: Successful treatment of Colombian cutaneous leishmaniasis with four injections of pentamidine. Am J Trop Med Hyg 50:107,1994.

Soto J, Medina F, Dember N, et al: Efficacy of permethrin-impregnated uniforms in the prevention of malaria and leishmaniasis in Colombian soldiers. Clin Infect Dis 21:599, 1995.

Weigle KA, de Davalos M, Heredia P, et al: Diagnosis of cutaneous and mucocutaneous leishmaniasis in Columbia: A comparison of seven methods. Am J Trop Med Hyg 36:489, 1987.

96 *Babesiosis* *

Barbara L. Herwaldt

DEFINITION. Babesiosis is caused by intra-erythrocytic protozoa (order Piroplasmidora, family Babesiidae, genus *Babesia*) transmitted in nature by ticks. Various wild and domestic animals serve as reservoir hosts, and humans are incidental hosts. In humans, babesiosis is characterized by malaria-like symptoms and hemolytic anemia. Most reported zoonotic cases have been acquired in the United States and to a lesser extent in Europe, where babesiosis is primarily a veterinary problem in cattle. Current issues related to babesiosis in the United States include the increasing number and size of babesiosis-endemic areas; recognition of additional zoonotic species; interrelationships between babesiosis and other tick-borne diseases as well as with AIDS; and transmission by blood transfusion.

HISTORY. Babesiosis was named after Viktor Babes, who in 1888 reported noting intra-erythrocytic organisms, which he thought were bacteria, while studying cattle that had febrile hemoglobinuria. In 1893, Theobald Smith and F. L. Kilbourne reported that *Babesia bigemina*, the etiologic agent of Texas cattle fever, is tick-borne; they thus were the first to demonstrate transmission of an organism by an arthropod. The first reported human cases of babesiosis in Europe and the United States occurred in 1956 (Yugoslavia) and 1966 (California); the first in the northeastern United States occurred in 1969 (Nantucket Island, Massachusetts).

ETIOLOGY AND GEOGRAPHIC DISTRIBUTION. More than 100 *Babesia* species that infect mammals have been described, but some may be synonymous. Taxonomy has traditionally been based primarily on morphology and host specificity, which are inadequate criteria for definitive species identification. In Europe (e.g., Ireland, the British Isles, France), most of the sporadically reported human cases of babesiosis have been caused by the bovine parasite *Babesia divergens* (Table 96–1).

In the United States, which does not have a national surveillance system for babesiosis, most of the hundreds of reported cases have been caused by the rodent parasite *Babesia microti* (Table 96–1). The major focus of transmission is in the Northeast. It now includes not only offshore islands (e.g., Nantucket Island, Martha's Vineyard, Block Island, eastern Long Island, Shelter Island) but also some mainland areas (e.g., Connecticut); the state with the most cases is probably New York. Transmission also occurs in the upper Midwest, particularly in northwestern Wisconsin.

In the western United States (Washington and California), WA1-type piroplasms have caused cases of babesiosis diagnosed thus far in the 1990s (Table 96–1). These organisms are phylogenetically more closely related to piroplasms of the genus *Theileria*, which cause lymphoproliferative disease in cattle in Africa and Eurasia, than to *B. microti* and *B. divergens*. Two cases of babesiosis were acquired in California in 1966 and 1979, but the infecting species was not definitively identified for either case. The one reported case of babesiosis acquired in Missouri in 1992 was caused by a piroplasm (MO1; Table 96–1) that probably is distinct from but shares morphologic, antigenic, and molecular characteristics with *B. divergens*, which is not thought to be present in the United States.

Only a few human cases of babesiosis have been reported from outside the United States and Europe; typically, the etiologic agent was not identified. However, results of serosurveys suggest that piroplasms are transmitted elsewhere. The relative paucity of reported cases may result in part from restricted ranges of vectors and reservoir hosts, underdiagnosis of babesiosis, and misidentification as cases of malaria.

TRANSMISSION, EPIDEMIOLOGY, AND ECOLOGY. *B. divergens* and *B. microti* are transmitted by the bite of infected ixodid (hard-bodied) ticks; the vectors of WA1-type parasites and MO1 have not yet been identified. The epidemiology and ecology of *B. microti* are much better understood than those of *B. divergens*, which is transmitted by *Ixodes ricinus*.

Tick-Borne Transmission. *B. microti* is transmitted by the deer tick (*Ixodes scapularis*), in which it multiplies both sexually and asexually. This tick also transmits *Borrelia burgdorferi*, the causative agent of Lyme disease and the agent of human granulocytic ehrlichiosis; ticks and persons co-infected with *B. microti* and *B. burgdorferi* have been identified. The larval and nymphal stages of *I. scapularis* feed on various small mammals, which serve as reservoir hosts for *B. microti*; the major host is the white-footed mouse (*Peromyscus leucopus*). Infection is passed trans-stadially from larvae (unengorged length, ~0.8 mm) to nymphs (~1.5 mm) and, less efficiently, to adults (~5 mm).

---

*All the material in this chapter is in the public domain, with the exception of any borrowed figures or tables.

TABLE 96–1. Piroplasms Known to Infect Humans*

Organism	Geographic Distribution†	Animal Reservoir	Tick Vector	No. of Reported Human Cases‡	Year First Reported Human Case Was Acquired
Babesia divergens§	Europe	Cattle	*Ixodes ricinus*	24* (0)	1956
Babesia microti	Northeastern and upper midwestern United States	*Peromyscus leucopus* and other small mammals	*Ixodes scapularis*	Hundreds (>20)	1969
MO1	Missouri	?	?	1‖ (0)	1992
WA1-type piroplasms	Washington California	?	?	5¶ (1)	1991

*Two European cases of babesiosis that have been attributed to *Babesia bovis* are thought by some authorities to have been caused by *B. divergens* and are counted as such in this table.

†Geographic distributions are not static and may be much more widespread than shown here. For example: reactivity to WA1 antigen has been found in serum specimens from persons who have not been in the western United States, and zoonotic *Babesia microti* infection has been reported elsewhere (e.g., in Europe).

‡Only symptomatic cases are counted. Numbers of reported tick-borne and transfusion-transmitted cases are shown outside and inside the parentheses.

§Countries include France, the British Isles, Russia, Spain, Sweden, and the former Yugoslavia.

‖The case was fatal and occurred in a 73-year-old splenectomized man.

¶The five symptomatic tick-borne cases of infection caused by WA1-type parasites (all acquired in the 1990s) include four cases (one fatal) in splenectomized persons in California and one case in an apparently immunocompetent, normosplenic, 41-year-old man in Washington. Previously, two cases "of babesiosis" in asplenic persons were acquired in California (infecting species not characterized).

The adult tick feeds on white-tailed deer (*Odocoileus virginianus*). Although deer are incompetent reservoir hosts, proliferation of deer permits ticks to increase in abundance (the female tick lays ~2,000 eggs after feeding on deer) and to be transported to previously uninfested areas. *B. microti* most commonly is transmitted to humans by nymphs and less commonly by larvae (rarely infected) and adult ticks. Because the adult tick is relatively large, it is more apt to be noticed and removed from the skin before transmission occurs. In addition, whereas nymphs are most abundant in spring and summer, the adult tick feeds during winter months, when the relatively few persons outdoors typically have little exposed skin.

Factors influencing the risk of tick-borne transmission of piroplasms to humans include the frequency with which persons enter the ecosystem where transmission occurs; the abundance and relative proximity of the vector and its sources of blood meals, including reservoir (e.g., mice) and nonreservoir (e.g., deer) hosts; tick infection rates (e.g., on Nantucket Island in June, about 40% of *I. scapularis* nymphs may have the infective sporozoite stage of *B. microti* in their salivary glands); and local ecologic conditions. Reforestation, expanding deer populations, and increasing recreational use of babesiosis-endemic habitats have contributed to the emergence of zoonotic babesiosis in the northeastern United States.

Blood-Borne Transmission. Transmission of *B. microti* and WA1-type parasites, which can cause protracted asymptomatic parasitemia, has occurred during blood transfusion (Table 96–1). Both erythrocytes (liquid-stored and frozen-deglycerolized) and platelet concentrates (because of residual erythrocytes) can be infectious. In addition, a case of *B. microti* infection apparently was transplacentally or perinatally acquired.

PARASITE-HOST INTERACTION. After introduction into the blood stream, the parasite invades erythrocytes, where it multiplies asynchronously by asexual budding (rather than by schizogony, as malaria parasites do) to produce two merozoites (daughter cells). Occasionally, four merozoites, joined by thin cytoplasmic strands, are formed, thus generating the pathognomonic tetrad form ("Maltese cross") (Fig. 96–1 in color section). Lysis of infected erythrocytes liberates merozoites, which then infect other erythrocytes. Although complement apparently facilitates the invasion of erythrocytes by *Babesia rodhaini* (isolated from a tree rat in Africa), the role of complement in erythrocyte invasion by the zoonotic *Babesia* species has not been defined. Although sporozoites inoculated by ticks are thought to infect erythrocytes directly, the possibility that the zoonotic *Babesia* species have exoerythrocytic forms (e.g., in lymphocytes), as do the *Theileria* species and *Babesia equi* (infects horses), is being explored.

The host's defense is critically dependent on having a spleen with adequate filtering and phagocytic capacity for infected or otherwise deformed erythrocytes; production of antibody by the spleen may facilitate phagocytosis. T cell–mediated cellular immunity (e.g., various macrophage-produced factors) is key; complement and other host defense mechanisms may also be important.

CLINICAL MANIFESTATIONS. The incubation period for tick-borne cases typically ranges from 1 to several weeks, but most patients do not recall having been bitten. For cases acquired by blood transfusion, the incubation period has ranged from 17 days to several months. The clinical manifestations cover the spectrum from asymptomatic infection to fatal disease. The combination of fever and hemolytic anemia should suggest the possibility of babesiosis, especially for persons who have been in babesiosis-endemic areas or who have undergone transfusion.

In Europe, the reported symptomatic cases of *B. divergens* infection have been in asplenic persons, about half of whom have died. In contrast, in the United States, *B. microti* commonly infects spleen-intact persons, most of whom remain asymptomatic or develop mild to moderate flulike symptoms. Not surprisingly, *B. microti* infection is underdiagnosed in all age groups, including childhood. However, asplenia and other causes of immunosuppression (e.g., AIDS, corticosteroid therapy) as well as advanced age are risk factors for clinical illness. Although WA1-type parasites and MO1 have caused severe, even fatal, disease, too few cases have been reported to draw conclusions about their virulence in the human host.

Many clinical manifestations and laboratory findings associated with babesiosis result from intravascular hemolysis, but even low-level parasitemias can be associated with severe disease. Manifestations of babesiosis commonly include irregular fever (temperature may reach 40°C), chills, sweats, malaise, fatigue, weakness, headache, and myalgia. Arthralgia, nausea, vomiting, anorexia, abdominal pain, depression, emotional lability, hyperesthesias, and dark urine (because of hemoglobinuria) may also be present. The physical examination may be unremarkable or may detect fever, petechiae, jaundice (particularly with *B. divergens* infection), and mild hepatosplenomegaly. *B. microti* infection has been associated with infarcts of the nerve fiber layer of the retina.

Laboratory abnormalities commonly include evidence of hemolytic anemia (e.g., decreased hematocrit and serum haptoglobin level and increased reticulocyte count, and lactate dehydrogenase and indirect [unconjugated] bilirubin) levels, as well as thrombocytopenia. Hemoglobinuria, proteinuria, renal insufficiency, a positive direct Coombs test, a mildly decreased leukocyte count, atypical lymphocytosis, hemophagocytosis, and mildly elevated serum transaminase values can also be noted.

DIAGNOSIS. The techniques for diagnosing babesiosis include examination of blood smears and experimental inoculation of animals as well as various molecular and serologic methods. Epidemiologic (e.g., geographic area of acquisition of infection), morphologic, host specificity, and antigenic characteristics can provide clues for species identification, but molecular taxonomic methods are more specific.

Examination of Stained Blood Film. The first step for diagnosing babesiosis is to examine a Giemsa- or Wright-stained thin blood smear for intra-erythrocytic ring forms (see Fig. 96–1 in color section). False positive smears result from mistaking nonparasitic intra-erythrocytic inclusions (e.g., Pappenheimer bodies in asplenic patients) or debris overlying erythrocytes (e.g., precipitated stain, platelets) for ring forms. On the other hand, if the parasitemia level is low or if only automated blood analyzers are used, the parasite can easily be overlooked. Parasitemia levels typically range from <1 to 10% but can be >50% in asplenic patients.

Piroplasms of different species can look similar (e.g., *B. microti* and WA1 are morphologically indistinguishable by light microscopy), and piroplasms of the same species can look dissimilar in different hosts (e.g., *B. divergens* ring forms are located peripherally in bovine but not in human erythrocytes). Morphologic differentiation of *Babesia* and *Plasmodium* (especially *P. falciparum*) ring forms can be very difficult, especially if only rare ring forms are noted. Tetrad forms (Fig. 96–1) are diagnostic of babesiosis but are rarely noted in *B. microti* infection. In addition, *Babesia* ring forms tend to be somewhat more pleomorphic than those of *P. falciparum*.

Animal Inoculation. This can be used to amplify low-level or subpatent parasitemia. Jirds (Mongolian gerbils [*Meriones unguiculatus*]) are good experimental hosts for *B. divergens*, as are splenectomized calves. Jirds and hamsters (*Mesocricetus* *auratus*) can be inoculated to amplify *B. microti*; the sensitivity of hamster inoculation is about 3×10^2 parasites/mL of inoculum (vs. about 1×10^5/mL for blood smear examination). Although isolates of WA1-type piroplasms have been obtained by inoculating jirds and hamsters with blood from persons infected in Washington State, attempts with blood from persons infected in California have been unsuccessful. Similarly, no animal host for MO1 has been identified. In contrast to *B. microti*, *B. divergens* and WA1 (isolated from the index case in Washington) can be grown in stationary erythrocyte cultures.

PCR Analysis. Like animal inoculation, polymerase chain reaction (PCR) analysis is useful for detecting low-level parasitemia. In contrast to animal inoculation, which can require weeks of postinoculation monitoring, PCR rapidly establishes the diagnosis. In addition, PCR can be used for broad-range detection of the zoonotic *Babesia* species as well as *Theileria* species or, by using species-specific primers, for species identification.

Serology. Although the diagnosis of babesiosis should be parasitologically confirmed whenever possible, serologic testing for anti-*Babesia* antibody can provide supportive evidence for current or prior infection; indirect immunofluorescent antibody testing is available through the Division of Parasitic Diseases of the Centers for Disease Control and Prevention (770-488-4431). Serologic testing is relatively species-specific. For example, if the antigen source for the assay is *B. microti*, serum from patients infected with other *Babesia* (or *Plasmodium*) species will react minimally, if at all.

TREATMENT AND PROGNOSIS. Therapy for babesiosis traditionally has been reserved for patients who have or are at risk for moderate or severe illness. However, preliminary data suggest that treatment may decrease the duration of parasitemia and benefit even mildly ill patients.

Chemotherapy. Standard therapy currently consists of a 7- to 10-day course of the combination of clindamycin (up to 1.2 g twice daily or 600 mg four times daily, parenterally, or 600 mg thrice daily, orally; children: 20–40 mg/kg/day) and quinine (650 mg thrice daily, orally; children: 25 mg/kg/day). The effectiveness of this regimen, which was first reported in 1982, was noted when it was used to treat a patient infected with *B. microti* who was initially thought to be infected with chloroquine-resistant *P. falciparum*. Therapy with quinine is frequently associated with cinchonism (tinnitus, headache, nausea, visual disturbance). IV quinidine in place of oral quinine should be considered for use in patients who require parenteral therapy. However, the interchangeability of these two antimalarial drugs, which are dextrostereoisomers, in the treatment of babesiosis has not been systematically investigated.

Exchange Transfusion. If indicated by the patient's parasitemia level (e.g., >10%) or clinical status, an exchange transfusion should be performed to decrease the parasite load expeditiously and to prevent massive hemolysis. Patients having *B. divergens* infections with rapidly rising parasitemia levels should be promptly treated with exchange transfusion, followed by chemotherapy.

Other Therapeutic Issues. Therapeutic alternatives are needed for patients who have persistent or relapsing infection or who do not tolerate clindamycin or quinine. Preliminary data suggest that the combination of atovaquone suspension (750 mg twice daily for adults) and azithromycin (500–1000 mg daily for adults) may be effective, as may the combination of quinine and either atovaquone or azithromycin. Anecdotal reports support the use of such drugs as

doxycycline, pentamidine, and trimethoprim-sulfamethoxazole, but no convincing data are available. Severely immunocompromised patients (e.g., those with AIDS) can have remitting-relapsing clinical courses and may benefit from maintenance antibabesial therapy (which, however, has not yet been defined).

Complications. During treatment, the patient's clinical status (e.g., temperature) and laboratory values (e.g., hematologic values, parasitemia levels) should be monitored closely. If hemolysis persists or worsens despite therapy, the possibility of autoimmune or drug-induced hemolysis should be ruled out. In addition, potentially life-threatening complications of babesiosis and of the patient's underlying diseases may develop. Complications can include myocardial infarction, noncardiogenic pulmonary edema, disseminated intravascular coagulation, renal failure, and death. The pathophysiology of noncardiogenic pulmonary edema, which can occur despite a decreasing parasitemia level, probably is multifactorial. Contributing factors may include decreased deformability and increased cytoadherence of infected erythrocytes in capillaries and venules, increased vascular permeability and capillary leakage, increased production of cytokines (e.g., tumor necrosis factor, interleukin-1), elevated levels of endotoxin, complement activation, and immune complex deposition. Recovery from babesiosis may be delayed by prolonged malaise, which may be more common if the patient also has Lyme disease.

PREVENTION AND CONTROL. Prevention of babesiosis is particularly important for persons at high risk for severe illness (e.g., the asplenic). If these individuals cannot avoid babesiosis-endemic areas during periods of intense transmission, they should use personal tick-protective measures (e.g., wear long sleeves and pants; tuck shirt into pants and pants into socks; impregnate clothing with permethrin-containing acaricides; apply N,N-diethylmetatoluamide [DEET]–containing repellent to exposed skin). After potential exposures, they should inspect their body for ticks and promptly remove attached ticks by grasping them with tweezers near their point of attachment, withdrawing gently and applying even pressure. Transmission of piroplasms typically is relatively inefficient, requiring attachment of the tick for >24 hours. Measures to control the populations of ticks and reservoir hosts may have a role in some settings. Prevention of transfusion-transmitted babesiosis currently depends on donor questioning about a history of babesiosis and assessment of hematocrit and temperature.

Bibliography

Herwaldt BL, Persing DH, Précigout EA, et al: A fatal case of babesiosis in Missouri: Identification of another piroplasm that infects humans. Ann Intern Med 124:543, 1996.

Herwaldt BL, Springs FE, Roberts PP, et al: Babesiosis in Wisconsin: A potentially fatal disease. Am J Trop Med Hyg 53:146, 1995.

Krause PJ, Feder HM: Lyme disease and babesiosis. Adv Pediatr Infect Dis 9:183, 1994.

Krause PJ, Spielman A, Telford SR, et al: Persistent parasitemia after acute babesiosis. N Engl J Med 339:160, 1998.

Meldrum SC, Birkhead GS, White DJ, et al: Human babesiosis in New York State: An epidemiological description of 136 cases. Clin Infect Dis 15:1019, 1992.

Persing DH, Herwaldt BL, Glaser C, et al: Infection with a Babesia-like organism in northern California. N Engl J Med 332:298, 1995.

Spielman A, Wilson ML, Levine JF, et al: Ecology of *Ixodes dammini*–borne human babesiosis and Lyme disease. Annu Rev Entomol 30:439, 1985.

Telford SR 3rd, Gorenflot A, Brasseur P, et al: Babesial infections in humans and wildlife. Parasitic Protozoa 5:1, 1993.

97 *Toxoplasmosis*

Jacob K. Frenkel and James L. Fishback

DEFINITION. Toxoplasmosis is a generalized infection of animals and humans. It is caused by the sporozoan *Toxoplasma gondii*. The infection may be asymptomatic or may be accompanied by fever or symptoms of lung, liver, heart, brain, lymph node, or eye involvement; during pregnancy, fetal infection may result. Immunity is associated with chronic infection, which may recrudesce when a patient is immunosuppressed, particularly causing encephalitis in patients with AIDS. Death may result from acute or recrudescent infection. The infection is transmitted by oocysts shed in the feces of cats, the definitive host, usually via contaminated soil, by tissue cysts from infected meat, and rarely, by tachyzoites in blood.

ETIOLOGY AND HISTORY

Discovery of the Organism. *Toxoplasma* was discovered first in laboratory animals and simultaneously in two tropical countries in 1908 long before it was appreciated as a pathogen of humans and domestic animals. Charles Nicolle and Louis Manceaux described a *Leishmania*-like parasite in the gondi, a small North African rodent used in research on leishmaniasis and typhus fever at the Pasteur Institute in Tunisia. Alfonso Splendore described it from laboratory rabbits at the Portuguese hospital in São Paulo, Brazil. The name *Toxoplasma gondii* was given to the parasite by Nicolle and Manceaux in 1909 after they differentiated this new tissue parasite from *Leishmania* and *Piroplasma*.

Human Disease. The first well-documented human case of toxoplasmosis was described in 1923 by Josef Janku in Prague in a congenitally infected baby with retinochoroiditis due to what was believed to be *Encephalitozoon* (Chapter 100.2). Toxoplasmosis became recognized as a human disease through the clinical and pathologic descriptions of babies with the congenital infection by Abner Wolf, David Cowan, and Beryl Paige from New York, together with the isolation of *Toxoplasma*. The first adult case of toxoplasmosis was diagnosed in 1940 by Henry Pinkerton and David Weinman in a Peruvian patient with concomitant bartonellosis. The development of diagnostic tests, especially the dye test by Albert Sabin and Harry Feldman in 1948, was an important milestone. The recognition of ocular toxoplasmosis in humans was aided by the development of the skin test.

Life Cycle. Numerous animals were found infected, e.g., dogs, cats, sheep, pigs, rats, pigeons, and zoo animals. It became clear that ingestion of raw or undercooked meat could lead to infection, but it remained a mystery how herbivorous "meat animals" became infected. Attempts at transmission of *Toxoplasma* through arthropods were not successful. There was no evidence of sexually transmitted infection. In 1967, William Hutchison showed that cats that had eaten *Toxoplasma*-infected mice shed an infectious stage in their feces. Although first associated with eggs of the nematode *Toxocara cati*, this transmission hypothesis was soon "dewormed" and linked to a new stage, the *Toxoplasma* oocyst, in 1970.

Parasite Stages. Recognition of the coccidian oocyst in the

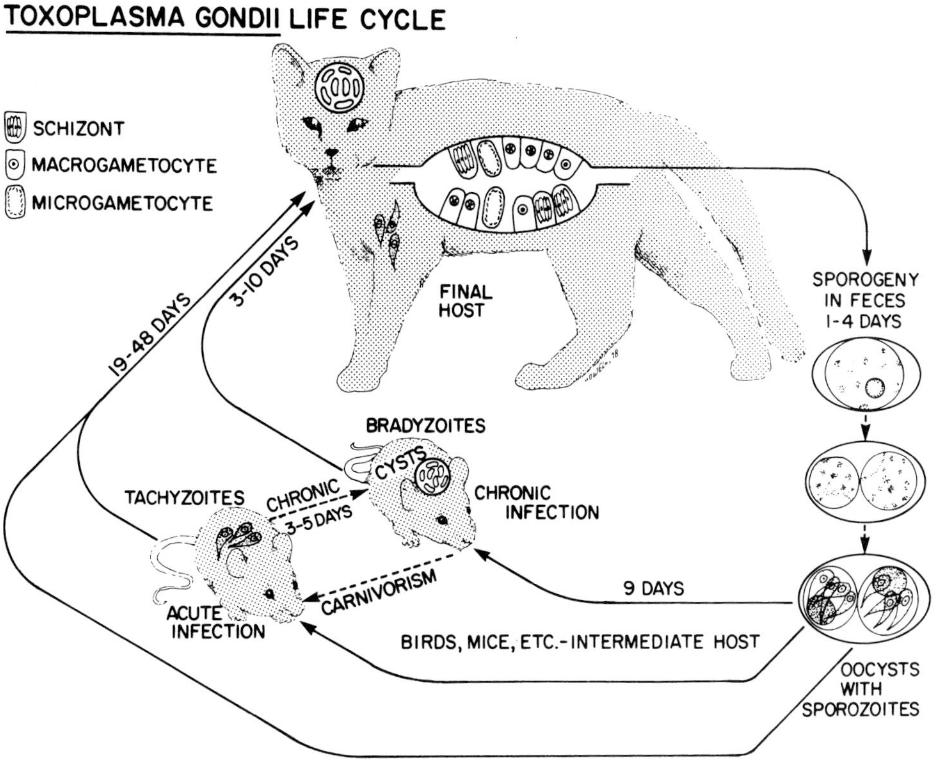

Figure 97–1. Life cycle of *Toxoplasma gondii*; details in text. (From Frenkel JK: *In* Montali RJ, Migaki G (eds): The Comparative Pathology of Zoo Animals. Washington, DC, Smithsonian Institution Press, 1980, pp 329–342.)

TOXOPLASMA GONDII LIFE CYCLE

SCHIZONT
MACROGAMETOCYTE
MICROGAMETOCYTE

FINAL HOST

SPOROGENY IN FECES 1-4 DAYS

19-48 DAYS

3-10 DAYS

BRADYZOITES

CYSTS

CHRONIC INFECTION

TACHYZOITES

CHRONIC 3-5 DAYS

ACUTE INFECTION

CARNIVORISM

9 DAYS

BIRDS, MICE, ETC.-INTERMEDIATE HOST

OOCYSTS WITH SPOROZOITES

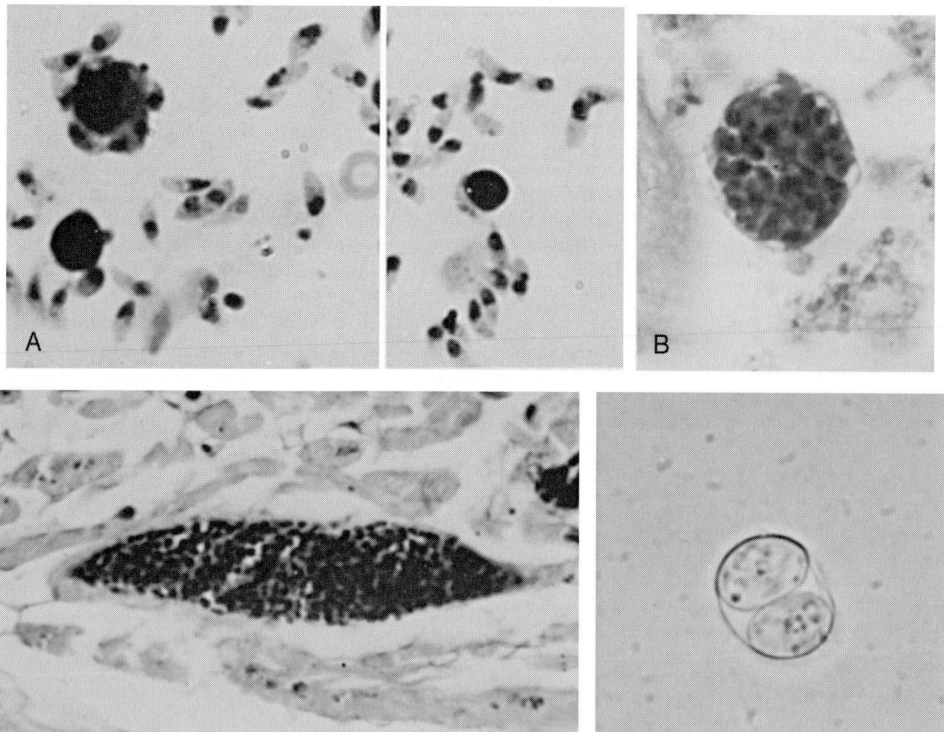

Figure 97–2. *A,* Tachyzoites of *Toxoplasma* in mouse peritoneal fluid (× 1000). (Courtesy of The Louisiana State University School of Medicine, New Orleans.) *B,* Tissue cyst of *T. gondii* containing bradyzoites in section of brain. (Courtesy of Dr. Paul A. McGarry, Louisiana State University School of Medicine, New Orleans.) *C,* Tissue cyst of *T. gondii* containing bradyzoites in heart muscle (periodic acid–Schiff, hematoxylin stain, × 700). (From Marcial-Rojas RA: Pathology of Protozoal and Helminthic Diseases, Baltimore, Williams & Wilkins, 1971.) *D,* Oocyst of *T. gondii* from feces of cat, containing two sporocysts with four sporozoites in each (unstained, × 1500).

life cycle of *Toxoplasma* explained its transmission to herbivores. It also led to the recognition of the two-host coccidian life cycle (Fig. 97–1). An enteroepithelial cycle was identified in the intestine of cats. The cycle has five multiplicative stages, followed by the development of macrogametocytes and microgametocytes, gametogony, and oocysts, which are shed in the feces. The oocyst is ovoid and measures 9 × 13 μm (Fig. 97–2*D*). It sporulates in the feces or soil, differentiating into two sporocysts, each with four sporozoites.

Previously, two tissue forms had been known. The tachyzoites are 2 to 4 μm × 6 to 7 μm ovoid organisms that multiply rapidly during the acute infection (Fig. 97–2*A*). The bradyzoites in tissue cysts are found during chronic infection, principally in muscles and brain (Fig. 97–2*B* and *C*). Tachyzoites and tissue cysts occur in all animals now recognized as intermediate hosts and in cats, the final host, which may be regarded as a complete host (Fig. 97–1).

The incubation, or prepatent, period in cats until oocyst shedding, varies with the infecting stage. After infection with tissue cysts, almost 100% of cats shed oocysts, and the prepatent period is 3 to 10 days. However, after the ingestion of oocysts or tachyzoites, only 16 to 20% of cats shed oocysts, and the prepatent period ranges from 19 to 48 days. The cyst stage, defined as giving rise to a short prepatent period, is reached 3 to 5 days after infection with tachyzoites, 7 days after infection with cysts, and 9 days after infection with sporozoites. It takes even longer for bradyzoites and cysts to become resistant to pepsin or for cysts to become morphologically recognizable by their cyst wall or by the presence of large periodic acid–Schiff–positive cytoplasmic inclusions.

DISTRIBUTION AND PREVALENCE. *Toxoplasma* is spread worldwide principally by the millions of oocysts shed by cats. Theoretically, birds can carry *Toxoplasma* to an area lacking cats, such as islands; however, purely carnivorous transmission to one or a few predators at a time is unlikely to maintain the infection.

The incidence of *Toxoplasma* infection in humans varies widely, and as shown by Feldman, the prevalence increases with age. Prevalence rates in individuals 15 to 25 years old are 14% in the United States, 50% in Colombia, 56% in Brazil, 61% in Costa Rica, 27% in New York City and London, 81% in French Parisians, but only 53% in Spanish, North African, and Portuguese persons living in Paris. Other ethnic differences have been found by Wallace in Hawaii. Within the United States, rates were highest in the eastern and central areas (18 to 20%) and lowest in the mountain and Pacific areas (3 to 8%). Dryness limits the survival of oocysts in soil. Low prevalence rates may also result from a low density of cats and intermediate hosts, giving rise to great variations from one locality to another. In a survey of settlements of Alaskan Eskimos and Indians by Donald R. Peterson and associates, prevalence rates were found to vary between 5 and 50%, and cats were found in as many as 50% of habitations. The high antibody prevalence rates found in France and Germany probably stem from local customs of eating undercooked meat, especially mutton. Prevalence rates of infection in humans and other mammals can generally be estimated serologically, because antibody persists for years and possibly for life.

TRANSMISSION. The modes of transmission recognized and the stages involved were, first, transplacental transmission by tachyzoites, followed by carnivorism via tissue cysts, and then, in 1970, fecal-oral spread by oocysts. However, the biologic frequency and importance of those modes follow the reverse order.

Oral Transmission

Oocysts. A cat that has eaten a single infected bird or mouse may shed millions of oocysts capable of infecting theoretically a similar number of intermediate hosts; transplacental or carnivorous transmission can infect only one or few animals at a time. Oocysts persist in moist soil for weeks and months. Deposits of infected cat feces remained infectious to mice for a year in Costa Rica and for 18 months in Kansas. Rain, earthworms, dung beetles, and cockroaches may be instrumental in slightly spreading the oocysts from where the feces have been deposited. After 2 weeks, oocyst-contaminated moist soil cannot be recognized, except by inoculation into susceptible animals. Therefore, humans, especially children, can become infected with oocysts from seemingly clean soil (Fig. 97–3). Outbreaks of toxoplasmosis in a riding stable in Atlanta, Georgia, in the municipal water supply of Victoria, Canada, and in a group of soldiers in jungle warfare training in Panama have been circumstantially traced to oocyst contamination of soil and water, respectively. A recent study in Panama suggested that some dogs that have the habit of rolling in cat feces may serve as mechanical vectors for oocysts to children.

Tissue Cysts. Most intermediate hosts, though infected by oocysts, transmit the infection with their tissue cysts when eaten by a carnivore. Ground-feeding birds and rodents are probably the most important intermediate hosts, because they in turn transmit the infection to cats, thereby closing the natural transmission chain. Sheep and pigs transmit the infection to humans, who are essentially a dead-end host (Fig. 97–3).

Carnivorism is the manner by which cats are infected naturally. Kittens may be infected by prey brought by their mothers. Other carnivores also become infected but are of little importance in the transmission chain because they are rarely preyed on and do not shed oocysts. Meat-related outbreaks have been attributed to mutton, hamburgers, and steak tartare. In northern Germany, raw pork (Hackepeter) is a favorite repast, made possible by the eradication of *Trichinella*. In parts of the Arab world, ground lamb mixed with spices (kibbe) is eaten as a delicacy. Undercooked pork has

also been recently incriminated as a cause of toxoplasmosis in the United States.

Transplacental Transmission. Transplacental infection occurs in humans, sheep, and goats when first infection occurred during pregnancy. Only in mice and goats has transmission in successive pregnancies been recognized. However, transplacental transmission during chronic infection has been observed in immunosuppressed women. Infection-immunity or premunition prevents transmission to the fetus by immunocompetent mothers.

Congenital transmission to the fetus occurs in 30 to 40% of women first infected during pregnancy. This is statistically most likely when infection rates average 3% per year; with higher infection rates, more women are immune by the time they become pregnant; with lower infection rates, few contract infection during pregnancy. High infection rates have been found in infants of immigrants from North Africa, an area of low incidence, to France, who acquire local habits of eating undercooked meat, especially mutton and steak tartare.

Uncommon Types of Transmission. Leukocyte transfusions with blood from immunosuppressed leukemic donors have served to transmit the infection, and *T. gondii* has been isolated from peripheral blood of symptomatic patients. However, blood from asymptomatic carriers is generally safe. Transplanted hearts of seropositive donors transmit toxoplasmosis because *Toxoplasma* cysts are common in the heart. These cysts are rare in the kidneys.

EPIDEMIOLOGY. Epidemiologic studies are generally based on serologic tests that show increasing prevalence rates with age. In humans and practically all animals studied, these antibody prevalence rates are cumulative, although the titers generally decline. Only in cattle is antibody prevalence

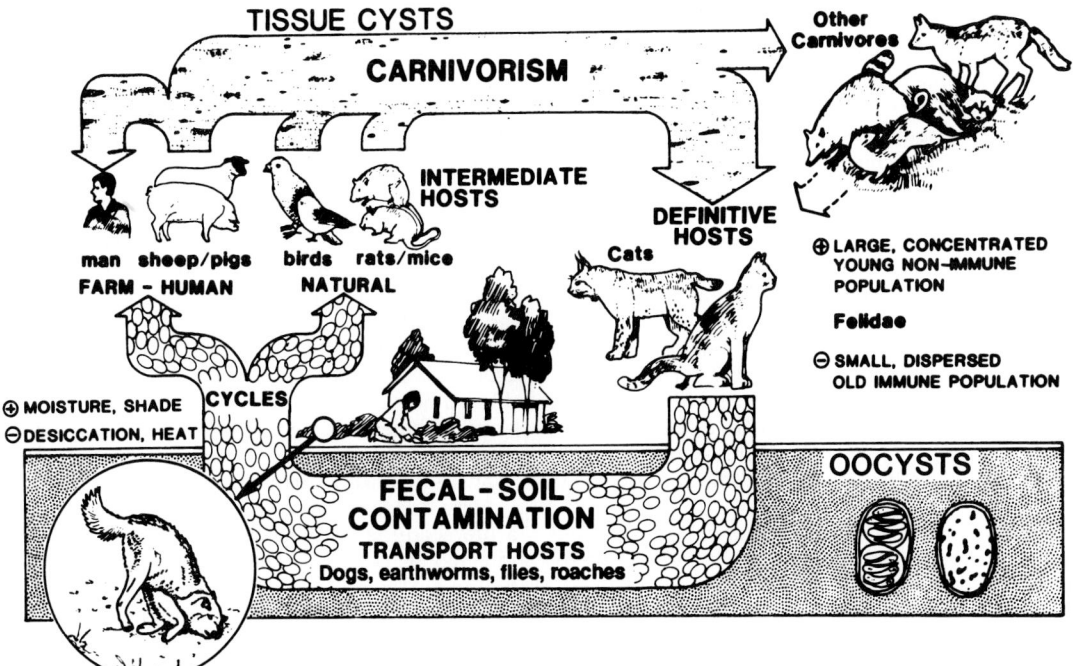

Figure 97–3. Transmission of toxoplasmosis. The three important reservoirs are cats, soil, and intermediate hosts. Oocysts from cats, the final host, feed the soil reservoir. Ground-feeding birds and rodents constitute the intermediate hosts of the natural cycle; sheep, pigs, and humans are the intermediate hosts of the farm-human cycle. Tissue cysts of bradyzoites are found in all intermediate hosts as well as in cats. Cats become infected from the tissue cysts of the intermediate hosts and close the cycle by shedding oocysts. Other carnivores become infected but are dead-end hosts, as are humans. Dogs may serve as mechanical vectors. (Modified from Frenkel JK, Ruiz A: Am J Epidemiol 113:254, 1981.)

not cumulative, because infections are short lived. Also, the indirect fluorescent antibody (IFA) test result has become negative in humans after 40 years and may be misleading because infection persists.

Tropics and Subtropics. In much of the tropics, where the highest incidence of infection is during childhood, oocysts in contaminated soil around the house are believed to be the major sources of infection. For example, in Costa Rica, as many as 30% of children have been infected before 5 years of age during their crawling and dirt-eating stages, and there is a 61% prevalence of infection at age 25. Ingestion of undercooked eggs and meat could be excluded as a major cause of acquiring infection. Toxoplasmosis is also commonly acquired in childhood in Hawaii and other Pacific Islands studied by Wallace, in Japan, tropical Africa, Tahiti, Brazil, Colombia, and Panama, from where detailed studies are available.

Developed Countries. In North America, seroconversion rates are generally lower, with seroconversion either being evenly distributed by age or occurring predominantly during adulthood. Although the exact sources of infection cannot be stated definitively, the ingestion of infective meat as a source can be circumstantially inferred. Eating undercooked meat is a habit that is individually acquired. Contact with contaminated soil appears to be less important during childhood or adult life in the United States.

In part of Europe, undercooked meat (often mutton) is consumed, and the juice of raw meat is sometimes given to children for its supposed nutritional qualities. This combination of factors is believed to account for the high incidence rates of toxoplasmosis in French children. Although cats may also be numerous in developed countries, young children spend more time indoors there than in tropical areas.

PATHOGENESIS AND PATHOLOGY. *Toxoplasma* is generally acquired by ingestion and causes enteritis in experimental animals infected with large doses of oocysts or tissue cysts. In humans, the usual dose of infection is low, and the enteric phase of infection is either asymptomatic or unrecognized. From the gut, tachyzoites disseminate via lymphatics to regional lymph nodes and by blood to the liver, lungs, and rest of the body. Antibody usually develops in a week or two, so that by the time lesions and clinical symptoms are produced, a proportion of extracellular *Toxoplasma* are destroyed in the blood stream. Much of the dissemination is from cell to cell or hematogenously inside monocytes and granulocytes. Four pathogenetic mechanisms can be recognized: necrosis of individual cells, delayed hypersensitivity, antigen-antibody reaction, and infarction.

Active Infection. Tachyzoites multiply probably in all nucleated cell types and destroy their host cells, entering adjacent cells, and eventually give rise to focal necrosis. The organisms divide every 5 to 12 hours, and 16 to 32 organisms are sufficient to destroy most cells; therefore, significant cell destruction may take place before effective immunity can be acquired.

Autopsies of adults show interstitial pneumonia, focal hepatitis, myocarditis, myositis, and encephalitis associated with tachyzoites and a few cysts. Biopsy specimens of enlarged lymph nodes show preservation of architecture, reticular cell hyperplasia, prominent histiocytes infiltrating the germinal center, absence of necrosis, slight periadenitis, and a paucity of *Toxoplasma* organisms; cysts have occasionally been found in serial tissue sections, and the organism has been isolated by inoculation into mice. Placental lesions are usually microscopic in humans, but macroscopic necrosis has been reported in animals.

Recrudescent lesions in the brain and lungs in immunosuppressed patients show huge numbers of tachyzoites in target-like focal lesions, usually only in one organ (e.g., the brain, retina, or lung), where cellular immunity is most compromised. Hematogenous dissemination is probably inhibited by circulating antibody.

Chronic Infection. Bradyzoites persist in tissue cysts during chronic infection, mainly in the brain, retina, and skeletal and cardiac muscle. Because delayed-type hypersensitivity is usually acquired with immunity, rupture of these cysts with liberation of bradyzoites is characterized by tissue necrosis and chronic inflammation. This is clinically important in the retina, where function is highly concentrated, or it may lead to focal encephalitis or myositis, which is self-limited. Antibody and cellular immunity are usually sufficient to destroy the released bradyzoites; however, in immunosuppressed patients, there is renewed proliferation of tachyzoites, as mentioned previously.

Congenital Infection. At autopsy in congenitally infected infants, either generalized or central nervous system (CNS) lesions predominate. Pneumonia, hepatitis, and myocarditis are usually most severe, with mononuclear inflammatory reaction and tachyzoites at the periphery of the lesions. Generalized lesions later subside, leaving areas of fibrosis. However, active encephalitis persists as a consequence of the reduced immunity in the brain, with necrosis of infected cells, microglial nodules, small scattered infarcts, and periventricular necrosis.

The third mechanism of pathogenesis results in the periventricular zone of necrosis seen in babies with congenital toxoplasmosis. A spread of *Toxoplasma* to the brain eventually leads to infection of ependymal cells and to dissemination within the ventricular system. Ependymitis in the aqueduct leads to aqueductal obstruction and the accumulation of *Toxoplasma* antigen in the lateral and third ventricles. Seepage of this *Toxoplasma* antigen through ependymal ulcerations is accompanied by vasculitis and thrombosis, resulting in infarction necrosis of periventricular tissues. This has been interpreted as an antigen-antibody reaction. The high titers of intravascular antibody are transferred from the mother and in part elaborated by the infants themselves. This vasculitis and periventricular necrosis was not encountered in ten babies with congenital toxoplasmosis in Costa Rica, and it is possible that their antibody titer, because of malnutrition, was not elevated.

A fourth pathogenic mechanism is infarction necrosis, resulting from vascular thrombosis adjacent to foci of *Toxoplasma* infection in the brain, spleen, and other areas where a single arterial supply with few anastomoses and end arteries are found.

CLINICAL MANIFESTATIONS AND COMPLICATIONS. Although it is usually asymptomatic, toxoplasmosis can produce illness. This is discussed under four headings: acute acquired infection, neonatal toxoplasmosis, ocular toxoplasmosis, and infection in immunocompromised hosts.

Acute Acquired Toxoplasmosis

Signs and Symptoms. The range of signs and symptoms of acute acquired toxoplasmosis is best illustrated by persons infected in outbreaks. The following symptoms were reported by Teutsch and associates in an outbreak involving 37 patrons of a riding stable in Atlanta, Georgia, which was attributed to the ingestion of oocysts: 89% of the individuals had fever, 84% had headache and lymphadenopathy (usually, the cervical lymph nodes were enlarged, firm, and discrete but not markedly tender), 60% had myalgia (occasionally diagnosed as polymyositis), 54% had stiff neck and/or anorexia, and 20% had a macular or urticarial rash (generally accompanied by fever and confusion). Arthralgia (24%) and hepatitis (11%) were less common findings. In all, 95% of those acquiring infection were symptomatic. Although 25 of the 37 individuals visited a physician, only 3 were diagnosed as having toxoplasmosis. Miller and coworkers reported the development of *Toxoplasma* antibody in laboratory workers after they began to work with oocysts. In this group of scientists, only three of seven reported symptoms: swelling of midcervical lymph nodes, which persisted for 4 months, a mild influenza-like episode, and fatigue and malaise without more specific symptoms.

After infection with tissue cysts, the incubation period could also be determined. Of five students reported by Kean and colleagues with common exposure to undercooked hamburger in New York, all had headache, fever, and myalgia, with enlarged lymph nodes persisting for 3 months. Three had a fleeting erythematous macular rash of limited distribution during the first week, and three had splenomegaly for as long as 4 months. The incubation period was 10 to 12 days. In another meat-related outbreak, reported by Masur, the incubation period was 7 to 17 days, with five of seven individuals being symptomatic and one developing retinochoroiditis.

There are sporadic reports of patients, some of whom died, with symptoms of myocarditis, encephalitis, hepatitis, and pneumonia. The manner of their infection is unknown.

Lymphadenopathy. This most commonly follows acute infection, whether accompanied by symptoms or not. It is three times as common in women as in men and is usually located in the neck. This lymphadenopathy, which coincides with the appearance of immunity, is accompanied by high titers of IgG and IgM antibody. In biopsy specimens, reticular cell hyperplasia is seen, and occasionally a *Toxoplasma* cyst.

Laboratory Tests. These show normal or slightly reduced leukocyte counts, often with lymphocytosis or monocytosis with rare atypical cells. The early hematocrit is normal, but prolonged illness may be accompanied by anemia. Chest films appear normal or show interstitial pneumonia. Serum aminotransferase levels may be slightly elevated. Heterophil tests are negative. Antibody titers to *Toxoplasma*, both IgG and IgM, are high or rising.

Neonatal Toxoplasmosis. As many as 60% of babies infected in utero are asymptomatic at birth, as shown in a large prospective study of Desmonts and Couvreur in Paris. Other infected babies may be aborted or stillborn. Many are born prematurely. Eichenwald classified 152 babies with symptomatic toxoplasmosis into 44 with predominantly generalized illness and 108 with predominantly neurologic illness. In the former group, the most frequent findings were splenomegaly (90%), jaundice (80%), fever (77%), anemia (77%), hepatomegaly (77%), lymphadenopathy (68%), pneumonia (40%), and rash (25%). All reflect generalized infection, contracted via the umbilical vein. Associated findings were abnormal spinal fluid (84%), retinochoroiditis (66%), hypothermia (20%), and convulsions (18%), indicating early CNS involvement. Babies with prominent neurologic involvement showed retinochoroiditis (95%), abnormal spinal fluid (55%), anemia (50%), convulsions (50%), intracranial calcifications (50%) (Fig. 97–4), internal hydrocephalus (28%), fever (25%), splenomegaly (21%), lymphadenopathy (16%), hepatomegaly (16%), and microcephaly (30%). The mortality rate was about 12%, and the sequelae observed during a 4-year period (100 patients) included mental retardation (86%), convulsions (81%), spasticity and palsies (70%), severely impaired sight (63%), hydrocephalus or microcephaly (42%), and deafness (16%); only 11% of the children were considered normal. Most of Eichenwald's patients were referred to him for illness; therefore, the more severe aspects of the disease are represented.

Alford, Stagno, and Reynolds observed the mildest symptoms in a prospective study on intrauterine infection. They found 10 infected infants among 7500 live births screened at

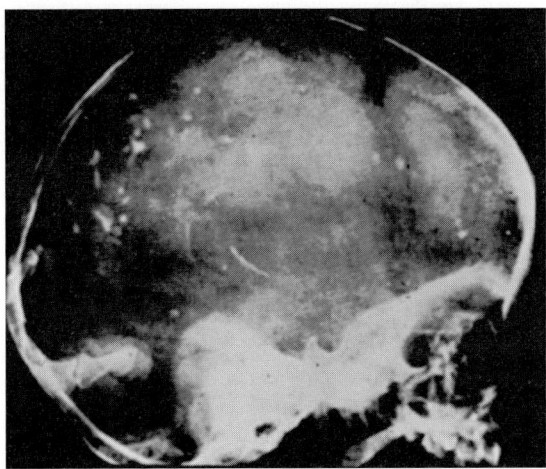

Figure 97–4. Cerebral calcifications in a radiograph of a 7-week-old baby who died with congenital toxoplasmosis. (Courtesy of Dr. Jack Beverley, University of Sheffield Medical School, Sheffield, England.)

the University of Alabama Medical Centers. Findings of interest for the diagnosis of milder illness were gestational prematurity (five), intrauterine growth retardation (two), abnormal spinal fluid (eight), IgM elevations (nine), and IgM antibody (ten). Follow-up studies of this group and some others for as long as 11 years showed that retinochoroiditis developed in about 75% of the children.

In babies with clinically active congenital toxoplasmosis, the retinal lesions are usually bilateral and usually involve the macular area, although often obscured by the intense vitreous inflammatory exudate. The lesion appears as a fuzzy white area, the size of the disc or larger, surrounded by an orange, normal-appearing fundus. Because the maculae are involved in about two thirds of these infants, visual impairment is great. In neonates infected in the second trimester, trophic cataracts and microphthalmia, nystagmus, and cerebral calcification are commonly found (Fig. 97–4); IgG and IgM antibody titers are generally high.

Ocular Toxoplasmosis. Retinochoroiditis found in children or adults is usually a unilateral, painless, focally necrotic retinal lesion with fuzzy outlines (Fig. 97–5). It is accompanied by a whitish vitreous exudate that sometimes obscures

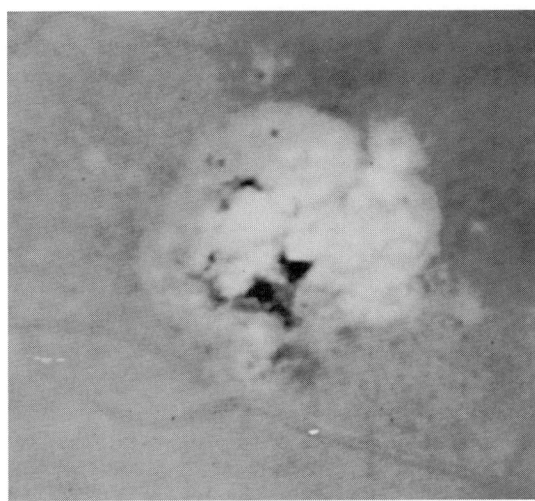

Figure 97–5. Presumed toxoplasmic retinochoroiditis. (Courtesy of the University of Florida College of Medicine, Gainesville.)

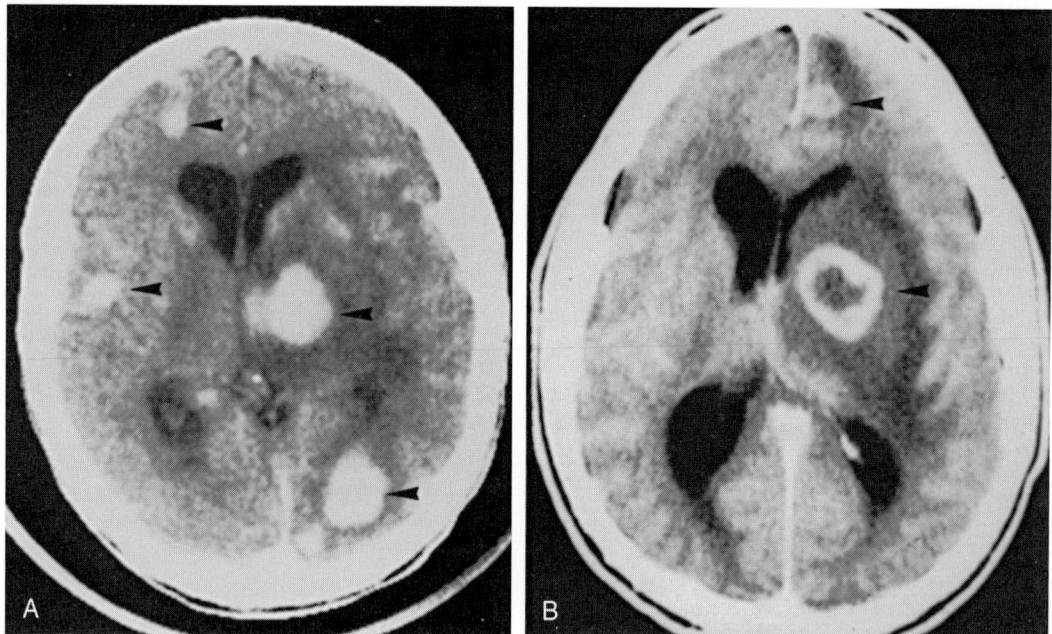

Figure 97–6. Recrudescent toxoplasmic encephalitis in two patients with AIDS. *A*, CT scan of brain with multiple enhancing lesions in right and left cerebral hemispheres and cerebellum. There is extensive edema with subfalcial herniation and left to right shift of the midline and left ventricle. (Courtesy of Dr. George Hensley, University of Miami School of Medicine.) *B*, CT scan of brain with a more advanced ring-enhancing lesion, indicating central necrosis in the right basal ganglia. There is compression of the right lateral ventricle and a shift to the left. A smaller lesion is present in the frontal lobe. Generalized edema is present. (Courtesy of Dr. Charles Poser, Harvard University Medical School.)

the lesion and causes marked blurring of vision. Circumscribed white or pigmented healed scars are often present in either eye. A new lesion sometimes arises from the edge of an old one. Because the organisms and the lesions are in the retina, retinochoroiditis is the proper designation. Most of these patients have stable low IgG titers, suggesting that these may be late sequelae of congenital or pediatric infection. In rare instances, however, these lesions are preceded by symptoms of generalized illness, in which case antibody titers are high compared with those in the general population. The lesions are often recurrent, but the majority are of limited duration. With clearing of the vitreous exudate, visual acuity may return to what it was before if the lesion is away from the macula. However, prolonged smoldering lesions have been described; they occasionally follow treatment with corticosteroids that is not covered by antitoxoplasmal therapy, and others are in patients with lymphomas. Progressive lesions may result in blindness and glaucoma.

Associated with retinochoroiditis may be edema of the retina and optic nerve, optic neuritis, iridocyclitis, and, in rare instances, panuveitis.

Toxoplasmosis in Immunocompromised Hosts. Two types of infection are seen—recrudescent chronic infections, occurring in about one quarter of patients with *Toxoplasma* antibody and AIDS, and severe primary infections. With relapse, encephalitis is most common (Figs. 97–6 and 97–7), and retinochoroiditis, myocarditis, and focal pneumonia are rare manifestations. Most cases are relapses of chronic infection caused by AIDS or immunosuppressive drugs that impair cellular immunity, especially corticosteroids and cyclophosphamide. The lesions are characteristically focal and often simulate an abscess or tumor, although they may be multicentric. IgM antibody is rarely present. IgG antibody titers are elevated and tend to be stable.

Primary infections occur in immunosuppressed patients by

natural routes, by heart transplant, or by leukocyte transfusion. They are generalized and involve many organs, as described for acute acquired toxoplasmosis, but tend to be more severe. The usual predisposing factors are that the patient has been receiving immunosuppressive drugs, and rarely, early undiagnosed leukemia, lymphoma, or AIDS is present. IgG antibody titers are elevated and rising, or stable, and IgM titers are usually high.

DIAGNOSIS. Diagnostic techniques consist of identification of *Toxoplasma*, histopathologic examination, tests for antibody, and tests for antigen and for delayed-type hypersensitivity.

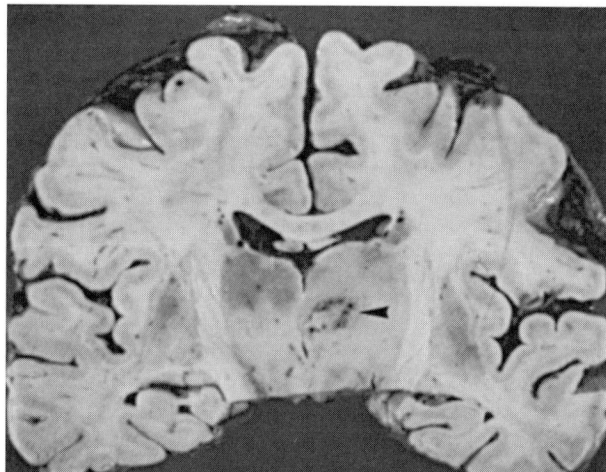

Figure 97–7. Recrudescent toxoplasmic encephalitis. In this cross section of the brain, a spherical necrotic lesion surrounded by hemorrhage is seen in the right thalamus. (Courtesy of Dr. George Hensley, University of Miami School of Medicine.)

Identification of the Parasite. *Toxoplasma* tachyzoites (Fig. 97–2A) can be demonstrated on tissue imprints that are dried, fixed with methanol, and stained with Giemsa as 7 × 3-μm ovoid organisms possessing a red nucleus and a blue cytoplasm. In tissue sections, tachyzoites are best demonstrated by hematoxylin and eosin stain, are ovoid or rounded, and measure 3 to 4 μm. Bradyzoites are of similar size but are more closely packed, and hence, their size is not easily determined in tissue sections (Fig. 97–2B and C). They are distinguished by containing a form of glycogen. Therefore, they stain prominently with the periodic acid–Schiff (PAS) technique. On tissue imprints, they are well stained with Giemsa. Whereas the finding of cell or tissue necrosis with tachyzoites (and cysts) establishes the presence of active infection, the presence of only cysts would indicate only chronic infection, except in the placenta and the newborn. Staining with specific antibody marked with fluorescein or enzyme and the ultrastructural features demonstrated by electron microscopy facilitate identification of the organisms.

Parasite Isolation. Ventricular fluid, placenta, biopsy or autopsy tissues, or the buffy coat of a centrifuged blood specimen may be inoculated intraperitoneally into mice (if possible, athymic, nude mice), hamsters, or cell culture. Contaminated material may be mixed with penicillin (1000 units/mL) and streptomycin (100 μg/mL) for half an hour before SC injection. Identification of tachyzoites in the peritoneal fluid is sometimes possible after 4 to 8 days (Fig. 97–2A). If the animals survive, they are examined after 4 to 6 weeks for the presence of tissue cysts in the brain, using stained tissue imprints (Giemsa) or tissue sections (PAS) (Fig. 97–2B), and for the development of *Toxoplasma* antibody, which should be absent in uninoculated control mice. The cells of inoculated cultures can be stained, or the supernatants are spun down and the Giemsa-stained sediment examined for tachyzoites (Fig. 97–2A).

Serology

Interpretation of Results. When seeking a serologic diagnosis, it is important to distinguish pre-existing antibody and passively transferred antibody from antibody related to the illness. Although numerous techniques for measurement for *Toxoplasma* antibody have been described, it is best to become familiar with one or two available tests. Most diagnoses can be made with one test for IgG, and almost all diagnoses can be made with an additional test for IgM. IgM antibody is developed first during infection and persists for 6 months in the conventional test but as long as 6 years in the capture test. IgM is not transferred by the intact placenta and, if leaking across a break, has a half-life of 3 to 5 days. Determination of the IgM fraction is therefore useful to separate lower antibody titers of early infection (in which IgM would be present) from those of late chronic infection (in which IgM would be absent) and to distinguish actively acquired antibody (IgM present) from passively transferred antibody (IgM absent) in a baby.

Serologic diagnosis may be based on demonstration of a rise in antibody titers (IgG) between two or more specimens tested in the same test run (Table 97–1). The presence of elevated IgM titers can be considered presumptive evidence of recent infection. To support the diagnosis of acute febrile toxoplasmosis, a four-tube antibody rise is required. If the specimens are taken during the late illness or for the presence of lymphadenopathy, titers in excess of 1:1000 should be present. In many tropical areas, such titers are common in the normal population, presumably because of frequent reinfections. Stable antibody titers are usually associated with immunity and when found during the first trimester of pregnancy would predict protection of the fetus (Fig. 97–8A).

For the diagnosis of congenital toxoplasmosis, a titer of > 1:1000 can be considered tentatively diagnostic, subject to confirmation by findings of antibody in the IgM fraction, the exclusion of rheumatoid factor and antinuclear antibody, and the isolation of *Toxoplasma*, if possible. Passively transferred antibody shows a tenfold decay every 3 months, whereas in the presence of infection, high antibody titers are stable or increase. An international standard has been prepared and is used by some laboratories. International units are approximately one fourth of the reciprocal of the titers expressed here as fractions (Fig. 97–8C).

TABLE 97–1. Guide to Interpretation of Serologic Tests for Toxoplasmosis (Dye Test or Indirect Fluorescent Antibody Test for IgG)

Clinical Problem	Titer				
	0	1:2–1:16	1:32–1:128	1:256–1:512	1:1024+
None (asymptomatic)	Susceptible to infection	Remote infection, probably immune			Recent infection or reinfection
Pregnancy	Susceptible to infection	Remote infection, probably immune			Need to monitor neonate for infection
Newborn, asymptomatic or with jaundice	Incompatible	Incompatible	Unlikely (can be found in babies treated for toxoplasmosis)	Unlikely	Possible*
Newborn with encephalitis	Incompatible	Incompatible	Incompatible	Unlikely	Likely if titer is stable or rises*
Lymphadenopathy	Incompatible	Incompatible	Incompatible	Unlikely	Possible
Fever with pneumonia, myocarditis, or hepatitis	Incompatible	Incompatible	Unlikely	Unlikely	Possible*
Retinochoroiditis	Incompatible	Possible	Possible	Possible	Possible
Encephalitis	Incompatible	Incompatible	Unlikely	Unlikely	Possible*
Encephalitis in patient who is immunosuppressed	Nondiagnostic	Unlikely (possibly transfused)	Possible	Possible	Likely*

*Tests for *Toxoplasma* antibody in the IgM fraction may be informative.
Incompatible: With such a titer, toxoplasmosis should not be diagnosed.
Unlikely: The lowest titers found in typical forms of the syndrome.
Possible: A characteristic titer, but not necessarily diagnostic.
Modified from Frenkel KJ: *In* Prier JE, Friedman H (eds): Opportunistic Pathogens. Baltimore, University Park Press, 1974.

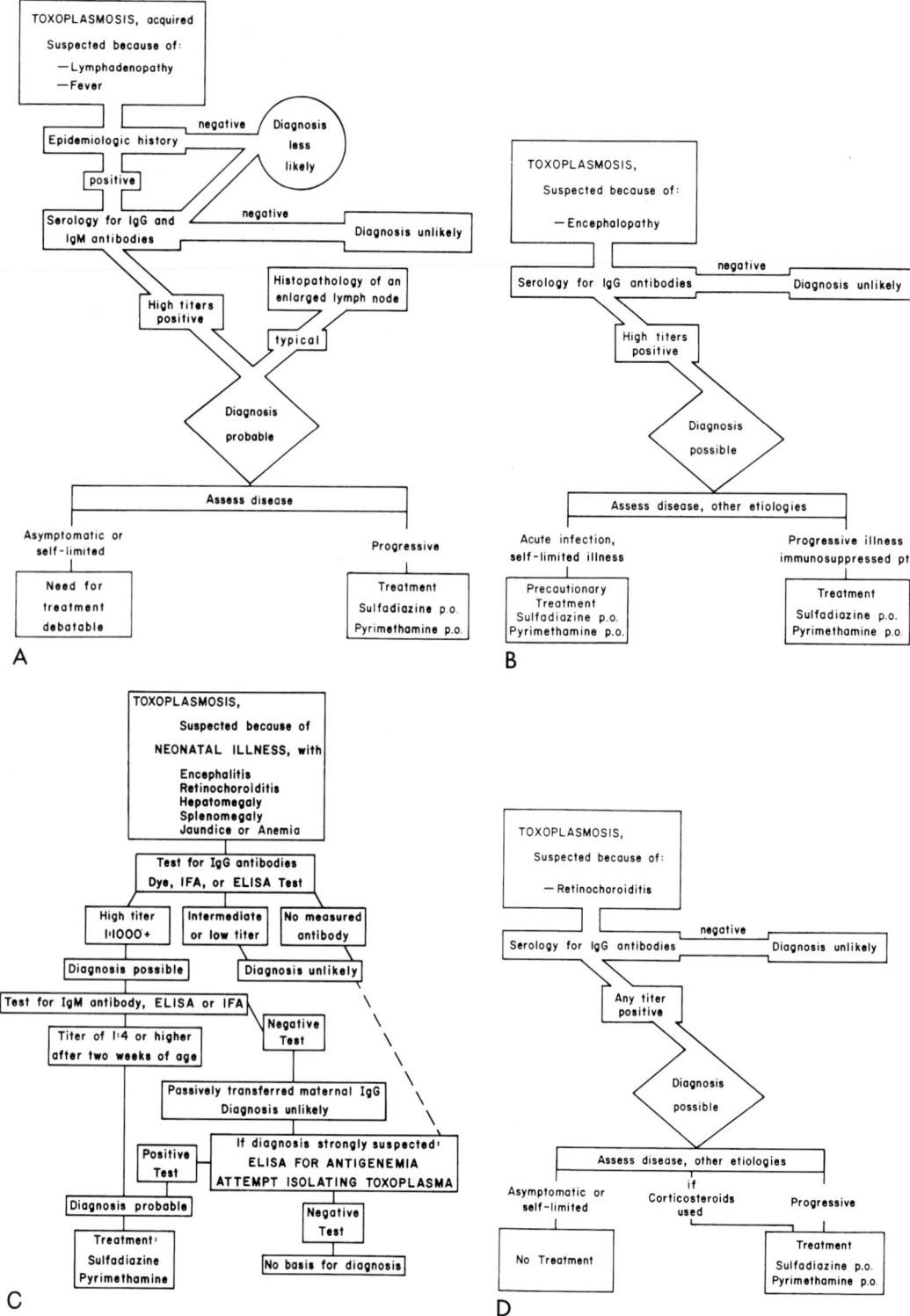

***Figure* 97–8.** Algorithms for the diagnosis and treatment of toxoplasmosis: *A,* In the presence of fever or lymphadenopathy. *B,* In the presence of encephalopathy. *C,* In the presence of neonatal illness. *D,* In the presence of retinochoroiditis. (Modified from Mahmoud AAF, Warren KS: J Infect Dis 135:493, 1977.)

Toxoplasmic retinochoroiditis, which is usually a manifestation of chronic toxoplasmosis, generally is accompanied by stable low antibody titers. Any titer, even in undiluted serum, is sufficient to support a presumptive diagnosis with a compatible lesion. However, in areas of high antibody prevalence, such serologic support becomes correspondingly less certain (Fig. 97–8D).

Recrudescent toxoplasmosis may be accompanied by high, low, and, rarely absent antibody titers. The possibility of antibodies having been transfused must be kept in mind.

Diagnostic help should be sought from biopsy and isolation. The cerebrospinal fluid of patients with toxoplasmic encephalitis often contains antibody, which is helpful diagnostically.

Serologic Tests. IgG and IgM antibodies can be determined by means of antihuman IgG and antihuman IgM, labeled with either fluorescein (IFA) or an enzyme that later colors an added substrate (enzyme immunoassay [EIA]). In conventional tests, *Toxoplasma* tachyzoites on a slide are overlaid with the patient's serum, followed by antihuman IgG or IgM, depending on what one wishes to measure. The result of an IgM titer may be falsely positive with presence of antinuclear antibody or rheumatoid factor. These test results may be negative when large quantities of IgG compete for binding with IgM, and rarely vice versa. These problems are avoided by the IgM capture test. Antihuman IgM attached to wells of a test plate or to test tubes when overlaid with a patient's serum captures the patient's total IgM. The content of *Toxoplasma* antibody is then measured by the amount of *Toxoplasma* antigen the captured IgM binds. The *Toxoplasma* antigen can be supplied in several forms: whole tachyzoites or soluble antigen (either free or attached to latex beads or red blood cells). In the double sandwich IgM-EIA, the *Toxoplasma* antigen is identified by means of anti-*Toxoplasma* serum linked to alkaline phosphatase, which imparts color to an added substrate. In the reverse IgM-EIA, the *Toxoplasma* antigen itself is labeled with enzyme, and only the appropriate substrate is added. In the immunosorbent agglutination assay (ISAgA or the IgM-ISA), *Toxoplasma* tachyzoites are agglutinated in a distinctive carpet-like pattern. In the latex IgM-ISA, soluble *Toxoplasma* antigen-coated latex particles are also agglutinated in a carpet-like pattern. In the HA IgM-ISA, red blood cells coated with soluble *Toxoplasma* antigen are agglutinated.

The dye test of Sabin and Feldman depends on lysis of *Toxoplasma* by the patient's antibody in the presence of complement, simulating the presumed mechanisms of humoral immunity in the body. It is highly specific and is particularly useful when testing sera of many species of animals, because no species-specific antiglobulin is required. However, the dye test requires living *Toxoplasma*, and it does not separate IgG from IgM. The antigens for the indirect hemagglutination test (IHA) (using *Toxoplasma* antigen-coated red blood cells), the latex agglutination test (LAT), and the direct agglutination of *Toxoplasma* (HA) may be available in kits. The usefulness of complement fixation and precipitin tests is limited.

DNA *Determination by Polymerase Chain Reaction* (PCR). This depends generally on a laboratory that routinely performs PCR tests because of substantial interlaboratory variability, even with more commonly ordered assays. Several primers for *Toxoplasma* are available. DNA extraction and analysis of PCR products by electrophoresis gel must be done in physically separate rooms from where amplification is performed to minimize false-positive reactions. Adequate controls and positive displacement pipettes (to reduce aerosols), as well as other methods to reduce contamination, must be ritually used by the selected laboratory. PCR has been successfully used with serum, cerebrospinal fluid, amniotic fluid, aqueous fluid, and bronchoalveolar lavage fluid. PCR may also detect chronic infection in tissue, and thus biopsy material is not suitable for the diagnosis of acute toxoplasmosis by PCR, unless confirmed by histologic examination of and immunohistochemistry to detect tachyzoites. In situ DNA hybridization can be performed on the involved tissues.

Skin Tests. Delayed-type hypersensitivity responses are positive in a majority of people with antibody. The skin test is useful for population surveys and can be used to support a clinical diagnosis of toxoplasmic retinochoroiditis when no serologic tests are available. Skin test positivity is used in some countries to identify pregnant women who are immune and who need not be concerned about contracting infection during pregnancy.

Differential Diagnosis. The signs and symptoms of toxoplasmosis are usually so nonspecific that they are not diagnosed. Most illnesses are mild and often are not recorded. In the study by Teutsch and colleagues, if any days of work or school were missed, they were not ascertained, and none of the five students in Kean and associates' study became ill enough to be incapacitated. However, patients have been recorded to have a temperature up to 39.5°C and marked malaise lasting for 2 months, sometimes with myalgia and sore throat, suggesting infectious mononucleosis or cytomegalovirus infections, which must be excluded. The persistent lymphadenopathy, sometimes with splenomegaly and a Coombs test–negative hemolytic anemia, may suggest a lymphoma; lymph node biopsy is diagnostic. The algorithms presented in Figure 97–8 outline diagnostic steps to be followed with several presenting symptoms.

Although retinochoroiditis is often due to *Toxoplasma*, isolated anterior ocular segment inflammatory disease is unlikely to be due to toxoplasmosis. The differential diagnosis includes cytomegalovirus infection, syphilis, brucellosis, leptospirosis, tuberculosis, visceral larva migrans, and retinoblastoma.

TREATMENT. Indications for treatment are diagnosed clinical illness, active lesions (e.g., in the eye), congenital infection (whether the infant is symptomatic or not), and symptoms and signs compatible with toxoplasmosis in immunosuppressed patients. Prophylaxis against a relapse of toxoplasmic encephalitisis is used in severely immunosuppressed patients who are serologically positive. Treatment of an immunocompetent pregnant woman who acquired the infection during pregnancy is complicated by the fact that only a third of the babies become infected and because of possible toxic drug effects on the fetus. The mere presence of a high antibody titer is *not* an indication for treatment.

Chemotherapy and Prophylaxis (Table 97–2)

Sulfonamides and Pyrimethamine. The most effective treatment for toxoplasmosis consists of sulfadiazine and pyrimethamine because the considerable individual inhibitory effects of each drug act synergistically in combination. In the combined treatment regimen, sulfadiazine (or sulfamerazine, sulfamethazine, sulfapyrazine, sulfalene, or sulfadoxine) is given to adults in 500-mg doses q.i.d. and to children in doses of 25 to 35 mg/kg q.i.d. For pyrimethamine, a dihydro-

TABLE 97–2. Chemotherapy for Toxoplasmosis— Daily Drug Doses

Drug	First 3 Days		Fourth Day Onward	
	Adult	*Child*	*Adult*	*Child*
Pyrimethamine (once daily)	75 mg	2 mg/kg	25 mg	1 mg/kg
Sulfadiazine* (4 times daily)	500 mg	25 mg/kg	500 mg	25 mg/kg
Antagonists†				
Folinic acid (leucovorin), or baker's yeast			3–10 mg 5–10 g	1 mg 100 mg

*Certain other sulfonamides, as mentioned in the text, may be substituted.
†To be given if platelet counts are <100,000/mm³ or if twice weekly platelet counts are not feasible. Antagonists of toxicity may be given prophylactically with the treatment.

folic reductase inhibitor (Daraprim, Chloridin, Malocide), the adult dose is 75 mg daily for 3 days, followed by 25 to 50 mg/day. Children are given 1 mg/kg/day with meals, and if they are asymptomatic, the dose can be reduced to half that after 3 days.

The sulfadiazine-pyrimethamine combination is effective principally on the actively multiplying tachyzoites. Chronic infections with bradyzoites probably persist in most instances unless treatment is maintained for several months. It is important to continue treatment until circumstantial evidence shows that the patient has developed immunity and can control chronic infection. No drug-resistant strains of *Toxoplasma* have been encountered while testing 44 isolates against sulfadiazine in mice. The striking effectiveness of treatment of congenitally infected babies has been demonstrated.

Folinic Acid. Toxicity of the sulfadiazine-pyrimethamine combination consists of bone marrow depression, first manifested by thrombocytopenia and leukopenia. This is relieved by *folinic acid* or yeast without impairing their chemotherapeutic effect, because *Toxoplasma* fails to incorporate the vitamin.

Platelet and white blood cell counts should be performed weekly, if possible. When this is not possible or with the decline of platelets to < 100,000/mm^3, folinic acid (leucovorin calcium) is administered in a dose of 3 to 10 mg PO daily for adults and 1 mg daily for children, together with sulfadiazine-pyrimethamine. When folinic acid is not available, fresh baker's or brewer's yeast can be substituted; 5 to 10 g daily for adults or 100 mg daily for children is mixed with food or formula. *Folic acid should not be substituted.*

Drug Reactions. Patients with AIDS often develop manifestations of hypersensitivity to sulfonamides and need to be treated with high doses of pyrimethamine alone or with an alternate drug combination. If pyrimethamine induces vomiting, one of the mentioned sulfonamides can be given alone for a few days.

Other Antitoxoplasmal Agents. The *sulfamethoxazole-trimethoprim* combination (co-trimoxazole, Bactrim, Septra, Septrin) has been used successfully in humans, although effectiveness has been shown experimentally only for sulfamethoxazole. This combination can be used for both treatment and prophylaxis when sulfadiazine and pyrimethamine are not available.

Dapsone-pyrimethamine (200 mg/75 mg) has been used once weekly as prophylaxis of toxoplasmic encephalitis in patients with AIDS.

Clindamycin is effective against *Toxoplasma* but does not penetrate well into the CNS, except in the presence of encephalitis. It has been useful together with pyrimethamine in the treatment of toxoplasmic encephalitis in patients who did not tolerate sulfonamides.

Atovaquone, a hydroxyquinone inhibiting the mitochondrial respiratory chain, has been used in 750-mg doses q.i.d. and is given with meals to increase its absorption. It has fewer side effects than standard treatment and appears to have a static as well as killing effect on *Toxoplasma* tachyzoites and bradyzoites. It should be used together with the dihydrofolic acid reductase inhibitors and one of the sulfonamides.

Spiramycin, a macrolide, relative of erythromycin, has been used in Europe to treat women infected during pregnancy because of potentially lesser toxicity to the fetus. Spiramycin (Rovamycin) is given in a dose of 500 to 750 mg q.i.d. for adults or 50 to 100 mg/kg b.i.d. for children. Treatment for 4 to 6 weeks has been advised. This drug is said to be concentrated in the placenta but not to cross it freely, and drug levels in neonates are low. Spiramycin has been used in congenitally infected infants every other month, alternating with sulfadiazine-pyrimethamme treatment. Newer macro-lides (i.e., clarithromycin, azithromycin, and roxithromnycin) have also been used with pyrimethamine to treat toxoplasmosis.

Experimental drugs being tested are arprinocid, a purine analogue, which had been used as an anticoccidial agent in chickens; trimetrexate, a pyrimethamine analogue used in tumor chemotherapy; and polyether ionophores, e.g., monensin and lasalocid, which are effective in cats' intestines but not in tissue infections because they are not appreciably absorbed. Rifapentine, rifabutin, other 6,7-di-substituted 2,4-diaminopteridines, and epiroprim have shown some promise in experimental animals. 2',3'-Dideoxydinosine (didanosine, ddI), a nucleoside analogue reverse transcriptase inhibitor used in the treatment of HIV infection, has also been shown to kill *Toxoplasma* in cell culture and in chronically infected mice. This raises the possibility that patients with AIDS treated with ddI might be protected against reactivation of chronic *Toxoplasma* infection.

Corticosteroids. Anti-inflammatory corticosteroids may be used to inhibit manifestations of hypersensitivity e.g., retinochoroiditis. Because anti-inflammatory doses are also immunosuppressive, corticosteroids should always be used with the sulfadiazine-pyrimethamine combination. Prednisone, 50 to 75 mg/day, is given until signs of acute vitreous inflammation have started to diminish, usually after 5 to 10 days. The dose is then tapered by 5 mg/day to 0, whereas sulfadiazine-pyrimethamine is continued for a total of 4 to 6 weeks.

PROGNOSIS. The outlook for immunocompetent patients with acute toxoplasmosis is good. However, acute infection, especially in a fetus or young child, may be followed by single or repeated attacks of retinochoroiditis. Prolonged treatment for several months appears to reduce the frequency of these attacks.

Neonatal Toxoplasmosis. The risks that both toxoplasmosis and treatment pose to a fetus suggest that abortion should be considered when a woman acquires acute toxoplasmosis early during pregnancy as indicated by rising IgM titers. However, the presence of high IgG titers by EIA or IFA tests or dye test titers in the second month of pregnancy generally indicates that infection had occurred before pregnancy, in which case the risk of the fetus' acquiring toxoplasmosis is virtually nil. Babies born subsequently can be expected to be free from congenital toxoplasmosis except when the mother has AIDS.

Chronic Toxoplasmosis. Chronic asymptomatic *Toxoplasma* infection, as indicated by a persistent antibody titer, prevalent in many populations, is generally benign and accompanied by immunity. However, if such individuals are immunosuppressed, recrudescent toxoplasmosis must be anticipated and should be mitigated by chemoprophylaxis. However, relapsing toxoplasmosis is rare when compared with the frequency of recurrence of cytomegalovirus infection.

PREVENTION AND CONTROL

Soil Transmission. *Toxoplasma* oocysts remain viable in moist and shaded soil for a year or longer. Oocysts are ingested by geophagia, whether compulsive (pica) or inadvertent, similar to ingestion of *Ascaris* eggs. Hands should therefore be washed after contact with soil potentially contaminated by cat feces. Oocysts are destroyed by exposure to heat over 60°C, but the usual chemical disinfectants are ineffective.

Meat Transmission. Tissue cysts that have persisted for months or years in the animal remain viable in pork, mutton, and other meat for several days at room or refrigeration temperatures. Most of the organisms are destroyed when meat is frozen and thawed; however, they are destroyed more effectively when it is heated to 60°C, indicated by a change in the color of the meat. Hands should be washed after contact with raw meat. Soap and water, alcohol, and chemical disinfectants inactivate bradyzoites from tissue cysts on the skin.

Neonatal Transmission. Prevention of *Toxoplasma* infection is most important during pregnancy and early childhood, when the consequences of infection tend to be more severe. The admonition to wash hands after contact with cats, soil, and raw meat and before eating or touching the face and to cook meat thoroughly should be incorporated into the general instructions for pregnant women. Work gloves should be used when handling soil potentially contaminated by cat feces.

Because infection of older children, especially young girls, is of value for immunization and the risk of appreciable illness is small, prevention becomes less important in this group. A vaccine to protect seronegative women during pregnancy is under investigation. This vaccine would also be useful to protect seronegative heart transplant candidates, to prevent a primary infection, transferred with the heart, from occurring during a period of immunosuppression. Many specialists are offering chemoprophylaxis to those with HIV infection who have *Toxoplasma* antibodies.

Cats. Only control of the spread of oocysts by cats would ultimately reduce transmission to fewer animals and humans (Fig. 97–3). To interrupt the natural cycle in wild and stray cats would be impractical at present. The opportunities for intervention in the farm–human cycle depend to a large degree on local conditions and beliefs. Where cats are pets, it may sometimes be possible to keep them indoors and to control their diet, feeding them only dry, canned, or cooked food. A vaccine that immunizes cats without oocyst shedding has been developed, and vaccination of cats is theoretically feasible. Whatever opportunities exist locally should be used to separate stray cats from human habitation and to control infection of meat animals, especially when their meat is eaten undercooked or raw (e.g., carpaccio, churrasco, Hackepeter, kibbe, Schabefleisch, and steak tartare).

Bibliography

Benenson MW, Takafuji ET, Lemon SM, et al: Oocyst-transmitted toxoplasmosis associated with ingestion of contaminated water. N Engl J Med 307:666, 1982.

Bertoli F, Espino Arosemena JR, Fishback JL, et al: A spectrum in the pathology of toxoplasmosis in patients with acquired immunodeficiency syndrome. Arch Pathol Lab Med 119:214, 1995.

Bowie WR, King AS, Werker DH, et al: Outbreak of toxoplasmosis associated with municipal drinking water. Lancet 350:173, 1997.

Dannemann BR, McCutchan JA, Israelski D, et al: Treatment of toxoplasmic encephalitis in patients with AIDS. A randomized trial comparing pyrimethamine plus clindamycin to pyrimethamine plus sulfadiazine. Ann Intern Med 116:33, 1992.

Desmonts G, Couvreur J: Congenital toxoplasmosis. A prospective study of 378 pregnancies. N Engl J Med 290:1110, 1974.

Frenkel JK, Hassanein KM, Hassanein RS, et al: Transmission of *Toxoplasma gondii* in Panama City, Panama: A five-year prospective cohort study of children, cats, rodents, birds and soil. Am J Trop Med Hyg 53:458, 1995.

Frenkel JK, Ruiz A: Endemicity of toxoplasmosis in Costa Rica. Transmission between cats, soil, intermediate hosts and humans. Am J Epidemiol 113:254, 1981.

Guerina NG, Hsu HW, Meissner HC, et al: Neonatal serologic screening and early treatment for congenital *Toxoplasma gondii* infection. N Engl J Med 330:1858, 1994.

Kean BH, Kimball AC, Christensen WN: An epidemic of acute toxoplasmosis. JAMA 208:1002, 1969.

Luft BJ, Remington JS: Toxoplasmic encephalitis. J Infect Dis 157:1, 1988.

Masur H, Jones TC, Lempert JA, et al: Outbreak of toxoplasmosis in a family and documentation of acquired retinochoroiditis. Am J Med 64:396, 1978.

Mcauley J, Boyer KM, Patel D, et al: Early and longitudinal evaluations of treated infants and children and untreated historical patients with congenital toxoplasmosis—the Chicago collaborative treatment trial. Clin Infect Dis 18:38, 1994.

Mets MB, Holfels E, Boyer KM, et al: Eye manifestations of congenital ocular toxoplasmosis. Am J Ophthalmol 122:309, 1996.

Miller NL, Frenkel JK, Dubey JP: Oral infections with *Toxoplasma* cysts and oocysts in felines, other mammals, and in birds. J Parasitol 58:928, 1972.

Mitchell CD, Erlich SS, Mastrucci MT, et al: Congenital toxoplasmosis occurring in infants perinatally infected with human immunodeficiency virus 1. Pediatr Infect Dis J 9:512, 1990.

Opravil M, Hirschel B, Lazzarin A, et al: Once weekly administration of dapsone/pyrimethamine vs. aerosolized pentamidine as combined prophylaxis for *Pneumocystis carinii* pneumonia and toxoplasmic encephalitis in human immunodeficiency virus–infected patients. Clin Infect Dis 20:531, 1995.

Podzamczer D, Miro JM, Bolao F, et al: Twice-weekly maintenance therapy with sulfadiazine-pyrimethamine to prevent recurrent toxoplasmic encephalitis in patients with AIDS. Ann Intern Med 123:175, 1995.

Roizen N, Swisher CN, Stein MA, et al: Neurologic and developmental outcome in treated congenital toxoplasmosis. Pediatrics 95:11, 1995.

Sarciron ME, Lawton P, Saccharin C, et al: Effects of 2'3'-dideoxydinosine on *Toxoplasma gondii* cysts in mice. Antimicrob Agents Chemother 41:1531, 1997.

Sousa OK, Saenz RE, Frenkel JK: Toxoplasmosis in Panama. A 10 year study. Am J Trop Med Hyg 38:315, 1988.

Spencer CM, Goa KL: Atovaquone: A review of its pharmacologic properties and therapeutic efficacy in opportunistic infections. Drugs 50:176, 1995.

Teutsch SM, Juranek DD, Sulzer A, et al: Epidemic toxoplasmosis associated with infected cats. N Engl J Med 300:695, 1979.

Wallace GD: The role of the cat in the natural history of *Toxoplasma gondii*. Am J Trop Med Hyg 22:313, 1973.

Welch PC, Masur H, Jones TC, et al: Serologic diagnosis of acute lymphadenopathic toxoplasmosis. J Infect Dis 142:256, 1980.

Wilson CB, Remington JS, Stagno S, et al: Development of adverse sequelae in children born with subclinical congenital *Toxoplasma* infection. Pediatrics 66:767, 1980.

98 Pneumocystosis

Walter T. Hughes

DEFINITION. Pneumocystosis is an acute pneumonitis caused by the protozoan/fungus-like microbe *Pneumocystis carinii*. With rare exception, the organism and the disease it causes remain localized to the lungs.

ETIOLOGY AND HISTORY. The taxonomy for *P. carinii* has not been clearly established. When first discovered, it was believed to be a form of *Trypanosoma cruzi*; however, recognition as a separate entity soon followed. Recent data suggest it is phylogenetically more closely related to fungi than to protozoa. The organism is found in infected tissue as cystic and extracystic forms. The cyst is 4 to 6 μm in diameter (Fig. 98–1) and may contain as many as eight intracystic cells (referred to as *sporozoites*). These intracystic structures are pleomorphic nucleated cells measuring 1 to 2 μm in diameter (Fig. 98–2). The extracystic cell is a thin-walled, round to crescent-shaped, nucleated structure measuring about 1.5 to 4 μm in diameter (referred to as a *trophozoite*). The trophozoite is believed to be an excysted sporozoite.

DISTRIBUTION AND INCIDENCE. *P. carinii* has been identified in the lungs of humans and animals from most countries of the world. The latent organisms may be sparsely dispersed as foci in the alveoli without causing clinical manifestations. This asymptomatic form is recognized only in biopsy or autopsy specimens of the lung. In unselected autopsy studies in the United States, *P. carinii* has been found in 0.2 to 4.0% of cases. Serologic surveys in the United States and the Netherlands indicate that 75% of children have acquired antibody to *P. carinii* by approximately 4 years of age.

Overt pneumonitis occurs almost exclusively in debilitated and malnourished infants, children with congenital immune deficiency disorders, individuals with cancer, patients receiving immunosuppressive drugs, those with AIDS, and those with severe protein-calorie malnutrition. In addition, 7% of

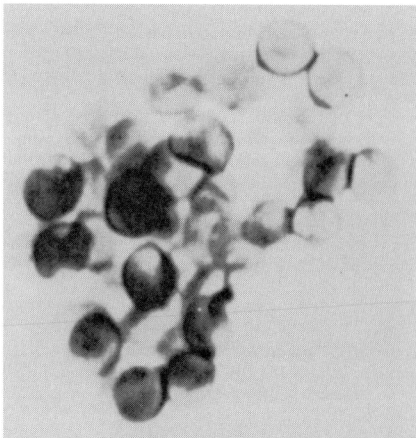

Figure 98–1. A toluidine blue O stain of specimens obtained from needle aspirate of infected lung. Only the cyst form of *P. carinii* is seen as a structure 4 to 6 μm in diameter.

African children with kwashiorkor have been found to have foci of *P. carinii* in the lungs. The impact of *P. carinii* pneumonitis on undernourished populations has not been studied. However, from 60 to 80% of children with marasmus, marasmus-kwashiorkor, or kwashiorkor have evidence of impaired cell-mediated immunity, indicating susceptibility to infections such as *P. carinii*. There are no data to compare attack rates between tropical and nontropical populations.

Although *P. carinii* has been discovered in various animals, the species have been limited to wild and domesticated mammals, especially rodents.

TRANSMISSION AND EPIDEMIOLOGY. The natural habitat and mode of transmission of *P. carinii* are unknown. Person-to-person and animal-to-person transmission have not been precisely documented. Animal-to-animal transmission by the airborne route has been demonstrated in laboratory experiments. Endemics and epidemics of *P. carinii* pneumonitis have been described in nurseries and nursling homes for debilitated infants in Europe. A few reports of clustering of

cases in cancer hospitals further suggest a contagion pattern for humans.

PATHOGENESIS AND PATHOLOGY. In some asymptomatic individuals, small numbers of *P. carinii* may persist as latent forms in the lung. Either single isolated cysts or small clusters of the organism are encountered with careful searching through lung sections. Although it has been believed that pneumonitis from *P. carinii* is caused by latent organisms acquired early in life, some recent studies suggest that newly acquired organisms may also have a role in immunosuppressed hosts. The organisms are located on the alveolar septal wall, which shows little or no evidence of inflammatory reaction. Some cysts are in the cytoplasm of alveolar macrophages undergoing various stages of digestion.

As clinical manifestations of *P. carinii* infection evolve, the number of organisms increases, causing massive infestation. In immunosuppressed children and adults, the lungs become noncompliant and liver-like. There is desquamation of alveolar cells into the lumina, where large numbers of organisms exist (Fig. 98–3). With extensive disease, mononuclear cells infiltrate the alveolar septa. In the infantile type, seen in certain European outbreaks, the histopathologic response is that of a pronounced interstitial plasma cell infiltration. The thickness of the alveolar septa may be increased to five to ten times the normal size. Hyaline membranes are sometimes seen.

Only with rare exception are *P. carinii* organisms found at

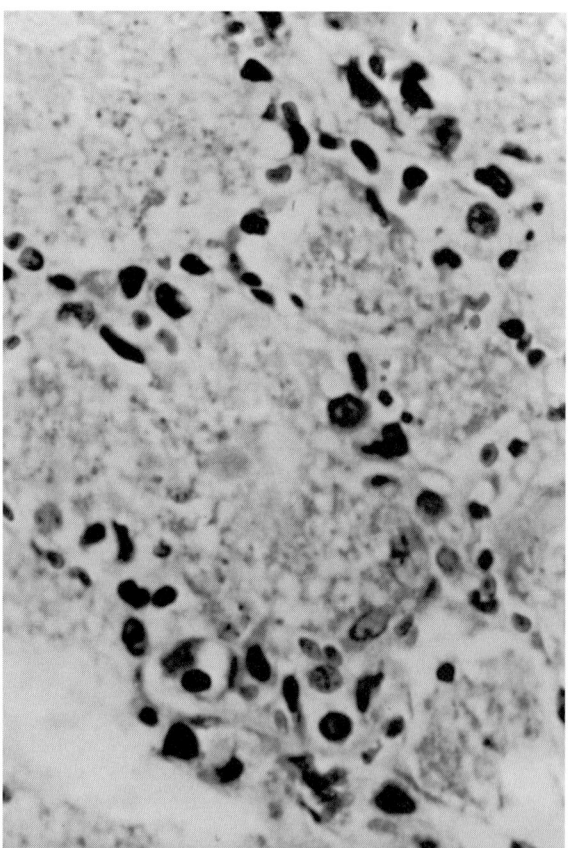

Figure 98–3. A lung section from a fatal case of *P. carinii* pneumonitis of the child and adult type. The hematoxylin and eosin-stained section shows the extensive desquamative alveolopathy, with alveoli filled with the characteristic foamy "proteinaceous"-like material. *P. carinii* is not visible with this stain but requires special stains, such as those shown in Figures 98–1 and 98–2, to be recognized.

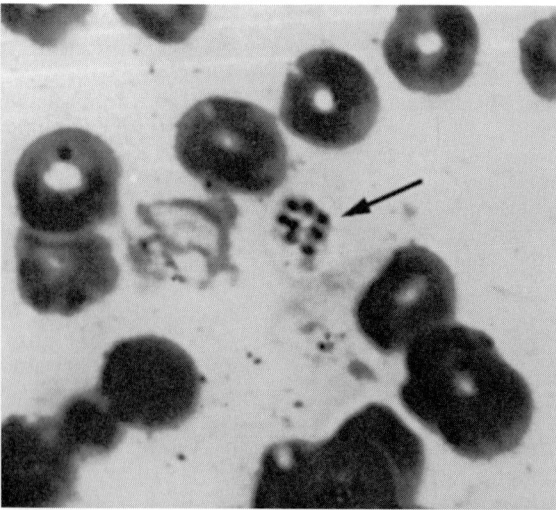

Figure 98–2. A Giemsa stain of a needle aspirate specimen from an infected lung showing the intracystic structures (sporozoites) of *P. carinii (arrow)*. The cyst wall is unstained. Comparison for size can be made with adjacent red blood cells.

extrapulmonary sites. Even in fatal cases, the organisms and the disease remain localized to the lungs.

CLINICAL MANIFESTATIONS AND COMPLICATIONS. The clinical features of the pneumonitis in immunosuppressed children and adults are remarkably uniform. The onset is usually abrupt. Fever is usually present early in the course, and tachypnea is pronounced. Cough is dry and nonproductive. Intercostal retractions, flaring of the nasal alae, and cyanosis occur in severe cases. Rales are usually absent. In the infantile type, affecting children from 2 to 6 months of age, the onset is insidious. Tachypnea becomes increasingly pronounced, fever is usually absent, and crepitant rales can usually be heard. Diarrhea may precede the pneumonitis in some cases. *P. carinii* pneumonitis in both adults and children may present with either an acute fulminating onset or the more subtle onset of the infantile type.

The chest radiograph reveals a bilateral diffuse pneumonitis usually more intense in the mid and lower lung fields than in the upper portions. Air bronchograms may reveal further evidence of disease (Fig. 98–4).

The arterial oxygen tension (PaO_2) is reduced, the carbon dioxide level is usually normal, and the arterial pH is normal or increased. The alveolar-arterial gradient is usually increased and serves as a reliable indicator for the extent of the disease.

Either the child-adult or the infantile type may occur in malnourished individuals, and the clinical features are related more to age than to the cause of immunocompromise.

DIAGNOSIS. A definitive diagnosis requires identification of *P. carinii* in specimens obtained directly from the lung. Samples of secretions obtained by tracheal aspiration, expectorated sputum, hypopharyngeal swabs, and gastric aspiration may sometimes yield the organism, but these are not dependable approaches to diagnosis. Invasive techniques such as lung biopsy, fiberoptic bronchoscopy with bronchoalveolar lavage, or needle aspiration of the lung are the most precise methods for diagnosis. If invasive diagnostic techniques are not feasible or not available, the diagnosis can be suspected on the basis of clinical features alone when other causes of pneumonitis are not apparent. Under these circumstances, the relatively nontoxic agent trimethoprim-sulfamethoxazole can be used, and patients should be observed for a cause-effect response. However, certain bacterial and chlamydial infections may also respond to this therapy.

After specimens are obtained, several staining procedures are available. Each specimen should preferably be examined by at least three methods: the Gomori-Grocott methenamine-silver nitrate stain, toluidine blue O stain, and Giemsa stain. The Gomori stain provides the easiest preparation for locating *P. carinii* cysts. The cyst stains brownish black, and background tissues are green. Only the cyst forms are stained, and the trophozoites and intracystic structures are not visible. The 4- to 6-µm cyst may appear cup-shaped, round, oval, or crescent shaped. Toluidine blue O staining is quickly and simply done, and the organism appears similar to the Gomori-stained cyst, except that it is lavender or blue rather than brownish black (Fig. 98–1). The Giemsa stain reveals the organism more fully than the other two stains (Fig. 98–2). This polychrome stain does not identify the cyst wall but does stain the intracystic structures (sporozoites) and trophozoites. A fluorescein-labeled antibody method to identify cysts is commercially available and is highly sensitive.

Serologic tests are of little diagnostic help in *P. carinii* pneumonitis. An indirect immunofluorescent antibody test and complement fixation tests have been used but are hampered by the high proportion of normal children and adults who have detectable antibody, presumably from subclinical infection early in life.

TREATMENT. Four drugs have been approved by the Food and Drug Administration (FDA) for the treatment of *P. carinii* pneumonitis: trimethoprim-sulfamethoxazole, parenteral pentamidine isethionate, atovaquone, and trimetrexate-leucovorin. Of these, trimethoprim-sulfamethoxazole is the drug of choice. This is given orally in the dosage of trimethoprim 20 mg/kg/day and sulfamethoxazole 100 mg/kg/day. The total daily dose is divided by four and administered at 6-hour intervals. An intravenous preparation is available in most countries and can be given to those who cannot take the oral tablet or suspension. The parenteral dosage is trimethoprim 15 mg/kg/day and sulfamethoxazole 75 mg/kg/day in four divided doses. A course of 14 to 21 days is usually adequate. The adverse effects are essentially those of sulfonamides.

The doses of other drugs are listed in Table 98–1. Pentamidine is as effective as trimethoprim-sulfamethoxazole, but its use is associated with a higher rate of more serious side effects. When given, the intravenous route is preferred. No oral formulations are available for pentamidine and trimetrexate. Aerosolized pentamidine does not provide effective treatment for the pneumonitis.

Atovaquone is a relatively new drug available only as an oral suspension. Its efficacy is close to that of trimethoprim-sulfamethoxazole and pentamidine, and it is remarkably free of significant adverse effects. This drug also has activity against malaria, toxoplasmosis, and babesiosis.

Several other drugs and drug combinations have been adequately studied in clinical trials to prove their efficacy in the treatment of *P. carinii* pneumonitis. These may be considered as alternatives to trimethoprim-sulfamethoxazole. They include dapsone-trimethoprim and clindamycin-primaquine.

Supportive Therapy. Oxygen should be administered as needed to maintain the PaO_2 at >70 mmHg. However, care should be taken to avoid oxygen toxicity by keeping the fraction of inspired oxygen below 50% as long as possible.

Recent studies of patients with AIDS suggest the use of

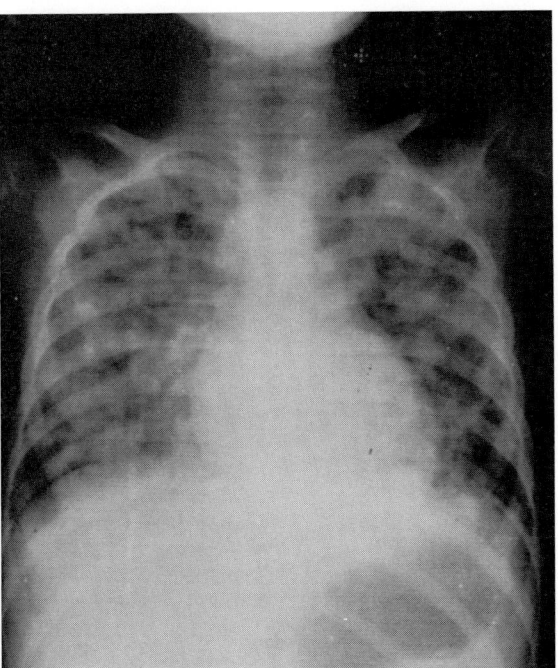

Figure 98–4. Chest radiograph of a patient with extensive *P. carinii* pneumonitis. Bilateral diffuse alveolopathy is evident with air bronchogram.

TABLE 98–1. Drugs With Demonstrated Efficacy for the Treatment of *P. carinii* Pneumonia

Drug*	Route of Administration	Dose
Trimethoprim-sulfamethoxzole (drug of choice)	PO (tablet or suspension)	20 mg trimethoprim/100 mg sulfamethoxzole per kg/day in four divided doses. The adult dose is 1280 mg trimethoprim and 6400 mg sulfamethoxazole per day in four divided doses.
	IV	15 mg trimethoprim and 75 mg sulfamethoxazole per kg/day in four divided doses. There is no need to exceed the adult dose mentioned above.
Pentamidine isethionate	IV or IM	4.0 mg/kg/day as a single dose. The IV route is preferred. The total dose should not exceed 56 mg/day.
Atovaquone	PO (suspension)	750 mg t.i.d.
Trimetrexate-gluconate	IV	Trimetrexate 45 mg/m^2 given as a single daily infusion over 60–90 minutes, plus leucovorin 20 mg/m^2 over 5 to 10 minutes q 6 hr (total daily dose = 80 mg/m^2). Leucovorin may be given orally at the same dosage.
Dapsone-trimethoprim	PO (tablet)	Dapsone 2.0 mg/kg/day, not to exceed a total daily dose of 100 mg. The dose may be divided into two or three doses per day. Trimethoprim 20 mg/kg/day, not to exceed a total dose of 1280 mg. The dose may be given in two or three divided doses.
Clindamycin-primaquine	PO (tablets, capsules) (IV and suspension for clindamycin)	Clindamycin 1800 mg PO in three divided doses daily (adult). Primaquine 30 mg PO once daily (adult).

*Note: Clindamycin, trimethoprim, and primaquine given alone are ineffective.

corticosteroids within the first 3 days of therapy may enhance survival of patients with PaO$_2$ values of 70 mmHg and lower. Adults may be given prednisone 40 mg b.i.d. during the first 5 days of treatment, then 40 mg daily for days 6 through 10. If needed, the drug may be continued at 20 mg daily for an additional 10 days. Careful attention should be given to adverse events related to the corticosteroid immunosuppression.

Because bacterial, viral, or fungal infections sometimes accompany *P. carinii* pneumonitis, efforts should be made to identify and treat these infections.

Prognosis. Without treatment, the pneumonitis is usually fatal in compromised hosts. With either trimethoprim-sulfamethoxazole or pentamidine, the mortality rate has been reduced to as low as 10% in experienced tertiary care centers. After treatment is begun, fever, tachypnea, and pulmonary infiltrates usually persist unchanged for 4 to 6 days. If no improvement is apparent after 1 week of treatment, the alternative drug should be used and a search made for an associated infection.

After recovery, if an immunodeficiency exists, recurrence can be expected at a later date in at least 10 to 15% of cases. In patients with AIDS, recurrence can be expected in >30% of cases if no prophylaxis is given.

PREVENTION AND CONTROL. *P. carinii* pneumonitis can be prevented by administration of trimethoprim-sulfamethoxazole. The prophylactic dose is trimethoprim 5 mg/kg/day and sulfamethoxazole 25 mg/kg/day in two divided doses. Studies show that this drug combination given only 3 consecutive days per week is as effective as daily doses, provided compliance in administration is sound. Protection is afforded only as long as the patient receives the drug. Such a regimen is recommended for individuals who are at unusually high risk for the disease. Severely malnourished patients whose dietary deficits might not be restored could benefit from this prophylaxis. However, correction of the nutritional state should receive first priority. Aerosolized pentamidine has been approved by the FDA for adults with AIDS, but studies of children have not been reported. The adult dose is 300 mg of pentamidine administered by a Respirgard II nebulizer once monthly.

Efficacy has been demonstrated for dapsone, either alone or in combination with trimethoprim or pyrimethamine. The following scheme has been recommended for the prevention of *P. carinii* pneumonia in AIDS. The approach is applicable to other immunocompromised hosts at risk of the infection.

1. Trimethoprim-sulfamethoxazole is the preferred drug at any of the following schedules:
   • Trimethoprim 160 mg plus sulfamethoxazole 800 mg once or twice a day to adults either daily or 3 days per week
   • Trimethoprim 5 mg/kg/day plus sulfamethoxazole 25 mg/kg/day given daily or 3 days per week to infants and children, not to exceed the adult dose
2. For patients who cannot tolerate trimethoprim-sulfamethoxazole, any of the following regimens may be selected:
   • Dapsone 100 mg as a single or divided dose daily. The dose for children is 2 mg/kg/day
   • Dapsone 50 mg/day plus pyrimethamine 50 mg and leucovorin 25 mg/week; also provides prophylaxis for *Toxoplasma* encephalitis
   • Dapsone 200 mg plus pyrimethamine 75 mg plus leucovorin 25 mg once per week
   • Aerosolized pentamidine 300 mg delivered by nebulizer once per month

Some physicians prefer dapsone with or without pyrimethamine to aerosolized pentamidine because of low cost and ease of administration of dapsone and because of the option to expand prophylaxis for *Toxoplasma* encephalitis with the addition of pyrimethamine. Prophylaxis must be maintained until the host is no longer immunocompromised.

Several experimental drugs are in various stages of development for the treatment and prevention of *P. carinii* pneumonitis.

Bibliography

Centers for Disease Control: 1995 revised guidelines for prophylaxis against *Pneumocystis carinii* pneumonia for children infected with or perinatally exposed to human immunodeficiency virus. MMWR 44(RR-4):1, 1995.

Centers for Disease Control: 1997 USPHS/IDSA guidelines for the prevention of opportunistic infections in persons with human immunodeficiency virus. MMWR 46(RR-12)1, 1997.

Hughes WT: *Pneumocystis carinii. In* Scholassberg D (ed): Current Therapy for Infectious Diseases. Chicago, Mosby-Year Book, 1996, pp 570–571.

Masur H, Kovacs JA: Treatment and prophylaxis of *Pneumocystis carinii* pneumonia. Infect Dis Clin North Am 2:419, 1988.

Opravil M, Hirschel B, Lazzarin AL, et al: Once-weekly administration of dapsone/pyrimethamine vs. aerosolized pentamidine as combined prophylaxis for *Pneumocystis carinii* pneumonia and toxoplasmic encephalitis in human immunodeficiency virus–infected patients. Clin Infect Dis 20:531, 1995.

99 *Free-Living Amebic Infections*

Joseph J. Drabick

DEFINITION. Infections of humans due to free-living amebae (FLA) are relatively uncommon. FLA are distinct from other pathogenic amebae (e.g., *Entamoeba histolytica*) by virtue of their general free-living existence and ubiquity in nature. They are responsible for three distinct clinical syndromes in human hosts: primary amebic meningoencephalitis (PAM), granulomatous amebic encephalitis (GAE), and amebic (acanthamoebic) keratitis (AK). Sinopulmonary, cutaneous, and otic infections have also been rarely reported, frequently in association with GAE.

ETIOLOGY. Of all the species of FLA, two genera, *Naegleria* and *Acanthamoeba*, have caused most reported human disease. *Naegleria fowleri* causes most cases of PAM. This ameba has a flagellated phase that can be induced by exposing the ameboid trophozoite to distilled water. The trophozoites range in size from 10 to 30 μm and possess a clear nucleus with a prominant dense central nucleolus. The trophozoites form spherical, smooth, single-layered cysts approximately 10 μm in diameter. The organism is aerobic and usually subsists on bacteria, but when it invades a human host it consumes blood cells and cellular debris. The ameba is thermophilic and thrives in temperatures up to 45°C.

GAE is caused primarily by several species of *Acanthamoeba* (*A. astonyxis*, *A. castellani*, *A. culbertsoni*, *A. polyphaga*, *A. palestinensis*, and *A. healyi*) and by recently described amebae of the order Leptomyxida. The implicated leptomyxid amebae have been ascribed to the species *Balmuthia mandrillaris*. *Acanthamoeba* spp. lack a flagellated phase, and the trophozoites are larger (20 to 40 μm) and much more sluggish than those of *Naegleria* in wet mount. The surface is distinguished by the presence of fine projections called *acanthopodia*, which arise from the cell membrane. The nuclear structure is similar to that of *Naegleria*. Its cysts possess a double wall, are more angular (polyhedral), and measure roughly 15 μm in diameter. Cyst morphology is used in differentiating the species of *Acanthamoeba*. The leptomyxid amebae are morphologically similar to those in the *Acanthamoeba* group.

AK is also caused by *Acanthamoeba* spp. (*A. polyphaga* and *A. castellani* in particular), as are cutaneous, otic, and sinopulmonary disease.

EPIDEMIOLOGY. FLA are ubiquious, with a worldwide distribution; they have been isolated from diverse environmental sources including soil and water (both natural and man-made sources). Their cysts are even found suspended in air. *Naegleria* has a more limited ecologic niche, favoring warm bodies of water.

Primary Amebic Meningoencephalitis. PAM classically is a disease of healthy, usually male children or teenagers, although all ages and both sexes have been affected. Patients usually have a history of having swum in or being otherwise exposed to warm stagnant bodies of water in hot summer months. Thermophilic *N. fowleri* thrive in such conditions. Thermal pollution associated with power plants has also been shown to facilitate growth of the organism. The first human case was described in 1965 in Australia, and most cases today are reported from Australia and the United States, probably because of the ability to establish a diagnosis. Cases in Europe, Africa, and Central America have also been reported. Although many people are exposed to the ameba, only a very small fraction develop disease, and the factors involved in this selection are unclear. Seroprevalence studies have shown that the majority of adults from endemic areas for PAM (e.g., the southern United States) have significant antibody titers, suggesting that exposure is common.

Granulomatous Amebic Encephalitis. As opposed to PAM, GAE is a disease of immunosuppressed or otherwise debilitated individuals. AIDS, chronic liver disease, chronic steroid use, diabetes, and allogenic organ transplantation are associated with this entity. The mode of acquisition of the infective acanthamoebae is not as clear cut as with *Naegleria* infections owing to their wide ecologic distribution. Acanthamoebae are occasionally observed as commensals in the upper respiratory tracts of normal people, and serosurveys support common exposure to these protozoans. GAE in most cases then appears to be an opportunistic infection in a person with compromised natural immunity. The leptomyxid amebae have an epidemiology similar to that of the acanthamoebae.

Amebic (Acanthamoebic) Keratitis. The first reported case of AK occurred in 1972 in a farmer who stuck his eye with some straw. The few other cases of this entity described in the ensuing decade all were associated with minor ocular trauma. In the mid-1980s, a marked increase in the number of cases was reported. The majority of these cases were associated with contact lens use. Soaking lenses in homemade saline solution and wearing contact lenses while swimming were determined to be significant risk factors in the cases. It has been postulated that coincidental bacterial contamination assists proliferation of the amebae by acting as food for them in the contact lens storage container. The number of cases of AK has decreased in recent years, probably because of better contact lens hygiene after the FDA and the Contact Lens Association of Ophthalmologists made public statements about the infection.

PATHOLOGY, PATHOGENESIS, AND IMMUNITY

Primary Amebic Meningoencephalitis. In PAM, warm contaminated water sniffed into the nasopharynx introduces the amebae. From there they can invade the olfactory mucosa, go through the cribiform plate into the olfactory nerve, and finally enter the brain. Invasion proceeds into the subarachnoid space and then into the Virchow-Robin space. The infection results in a rapidly progressive, purulent, hemorrhagic necrosis of the cortex, beginning with the olfactory bulbs. The inflammation is polymorphonuclear, and the pathology is similar to that of purulent bacterial meningitis, although the inflammatory exudate tends to be exclusively basilar (Fig. 99–1). *Naegleria* trophozoites are found predominantly in the olfactory nerves and perivascular spaces of small arteries and arterioles. No cysts can be demonstrated, although trophozoites can be readily demonstrated in the cerebrospinal fluid (CSF). The amebae are readily stained with hematoxylin and eosin or iron hematoxylin.

Granulomatous Amebic Encephalitis. In contrast to *Naegleria*, the acanthamoebae associated with GAE appear to gain access to the central nervous system (CNS) by a hematogenous route. Primary foci in the lungs and skin have been described. Cutaneous abscesses due to acanthamoebae have recently been identified in patients with AIDS. The brain involvement is patchy but tends to involve the thala-

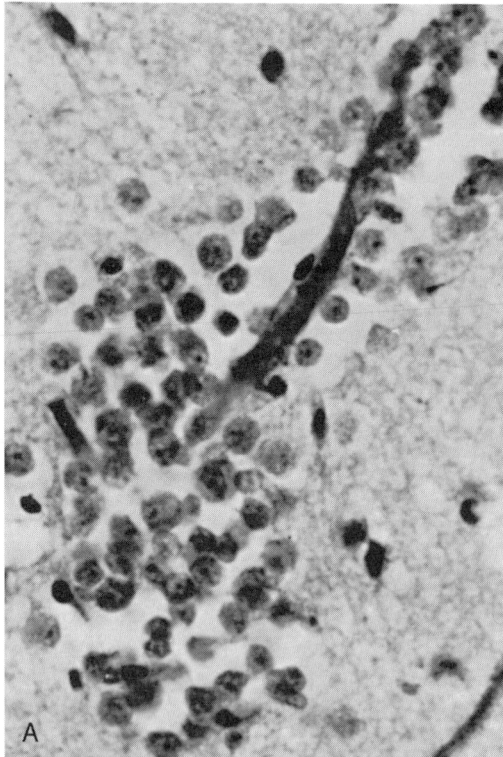

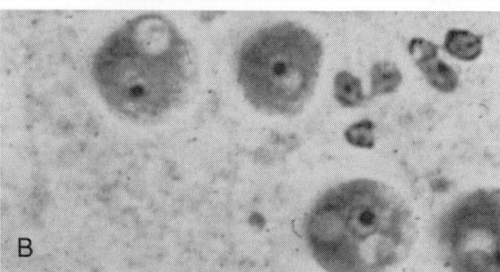

Figure 99–1. *A,* Cluster of amebae in perivascular space of formalin-fixed brain of patient with PAM; note rounding up of amebae (× 400). *B,* Higher magnification of same amebae. Note the single contractile vacuole and characteristic nucleus with a large, dark karyosome surrounded by a clear halo and a fine nuclear rim (× 1000). Cultures and fluorescent antibody tests were positive for *N. fowleri.*

mus, diencephalon, brain stem, and posterior fossa structures. Within the lesions, both trophozoites and cysts may be observed, and the inflammatory response is chronic, with a granulomatous response characterized by the presence of multinucleated giant cells. This immunologic response may be altered in some individuals, depending on the degree and nature of their immune impairment.

Amebic (Acanthamoebic) Keratitis. In AK, the acanthamoebae in a contaminated contact lens storage container are thought to adhere to the contact lens, from which they can penetrate minor corneal abrasions resulting from wearing the contact lens. The victims of AK are usually healthy, myopic people. The microscopic pathology is similar to that observed for GAE, in that both trophozoites and cysts are found with a mixed inflammatory infiltrate. As the disease progresses, more polymorphonuclear cells are drawn to the area chemotactically by immune complexes, resulting in a corneal ring-like infiltrate. The disease can evolve to destroy the cornea altogether.

Virulence Factors. FLA have several attributes that can

contribute to virulence, including the ability to adhere to epithelium, migrate through tissues, and elaborate several cytopathic enzymes including broadly acting elastase and collagenase to aid in invasion. FLA can also ingest erythrocytes and defensive leukocytes.

Immune Responses. Host immunity is complex and involves both humoral and cell-mediated immunity. The major mechanism of immunity against these amebae is through the activation of phagocytic cells, in particular polymorphonuclear cells. Activation is through elaborated cytokines and through opsonization of the amebae by specific antibody. The prevalence of antiamebic antibodies may be the basis for natural antiamebic immunity. In animal models, active immunization with killed or processed *Naegleria* or *Acanthamoeba* is strongly protective against subsequent challenges with live amebae. Administration of antinaeglerial antiserum was useful in rabbits inoculated intracisternally with the amebae. These findings suggest that passive immunotherapy could have a role in the treatment of this infection.

CLINICAL MANIFESTATIONS

Primary Amebic Meningoencephalitis. PAM is a rapid, fulminant illness with an incubation period of a few days to 2 weeks. Patients occasionally complain of distortions in taste and smell at the onset of the illness, reflective of the mode of entry of the pathogen, but rapidly develop clinical signs of acute meningitis including fever, vomiting, headache, and neck stiffness. Obtundation progresses to deep coma. Convulsions can occur. Patients generally die within a week of the onset of symptoms.

Granulomatous Amebic Encephalitis. GAE has a more insidious onset in individuals at risk for this opportunistic disease. Patients present with changes in mental status, focal neurologic deficits, seizures, headache, fever, and visual abnormalities. The presenting signs and symptoms depend on the location of the CNS lesions. The duration of illness varies considerably but averages approximately 1 month. The disease may result from an antecedent site of primary infection on the skin or in the lungs.

Amebic (Acanthamoebic) Keratitis. Patients with AK initially complain of a foreign body sensation in the affected eye in association with tearing, photophobia, and ocular pain. As the disease progresses, patients experience blurring of vision, blepharospasm, and conjunctival injection. The course tends to wax and wane, and this can lead to delay in diagnosis. Iritis is marked, and the ocular pain is quite severe, sometimes out of concert with the clinical findings. Seen in the early phase of the illness is a dendriform keratitis, but as the disease progresses, a characteristic ring infiltrate occurs in approximately 80% of patients. Severe cases can be marked by a hypopyon, elevated intraocular pressure, and anterior nodular scleritis.

Cutaneous Lesions. The cutaneous lesions associated with acanthamoebae are tender papulonodular lesions, which can evolve to ulceration. The lesions tend to be scattered on the trunk and extremities.

DIAGNOSIS. The key to diagnosis for all FLA infections is direct demonstration of the organism. Serologic tests are of value only in prevalence studies.

CSF obtained from patients with PAM demonstrates high white blood cell counts with a predominance of polymorphonuclear cells, as in acute bacterial meningitis. CSF glucose level is low, and protein elevated. On Gram stain, the trophozoites are not seen easily; therefore, in patients with a potential water exposure and a purulent but apparently aseptic CSF, a wet mount of the CSF should be prepared and examined for motile trophozoites, which are usually apparent on careful inspection.

Patients with GAE usually have an imaging study such

as computed tomography (CT) performed to evaluate their neurologic signs and symptoms. On CT, multiple nonenhancing lesions are usually observed. In GAE, in contrast to naeglerial PAM, the CSF does not contain amebae, and lumbar puncture is generally contraindicated because of the presence of space-occupying lesions on CT. GAE is usually diagnosed post mortem at autopsy. A diagnosis in life can be made only by directed brain biopsy of the lesions seen on CT. If a patient has concurrent skin lesions, these can be examined by biopsy instead to make the diagnosis indirectly.

AK is frequently misdiagnosed as being herpetic, bacterial, or fungal in origin. The diagnosis should be suspected early in contact lens wearers or individuals with a history of minor ocular trauma. Corneal scrapings should be examined under wet mount for motile trophozoites as well as cysts. Spray-fixed slides can be stained with Giemsa or periodic acid–Schiff stain and examined for stained organisms.

Calcofluor white can stain both cysts and trophozoites. Indirect fluoromicroscopy with species-specific labeled antibody can render an etiologic diagnosis on both prepared smears of tissue or culture as well as tissue sections. Amebae can be cultured by inoculating fresh biopsy material onto a non-nutrient agar plate overlaid with *Escherichia coli* (or similar bacterial strain to act as food for the amebae). Culture can increase the diagnostic yield of biopsy or corneal scrapings. In patients with suspected AK, the contact lens and its storage system can also be evaluated for the presence of amebae.

TREATMENT. Most cases (>95%) of PAM have been fatal. In the few patients who survived, high-dose systemic amphotericin B with intrathecal amphotericin was used. Adjunctive therapies have included rifampin, miconazole, and sulfisoxazole, but whether these provide additional benefit is unknown. Because azoles have in vitro activity, fluconazole may be of benefit, at least in theory, by virtue of its ability to cross the blood–brain barrier.

As with PAM, GAE is nearly uniformly fatal. In vitro drug testing against the causative *Acanthamoeba* species has demonstrated that drugs of the diamidine class such as pentamidine and propamidine have the greatest activity. Other drugs with activity include the azole antifungals and some aminoglycosides (neomycin, paromomycin). Amphotericin B has less activity against these organisms than against *Naegleria*. There is a report of a single patient who responded to high-dose pentamidine therapy. In theory, fluconazole may be of value.

If detected early, AK can be successfully cured. Affected areas of the cornea should be debrided, and intense medical therapy should commence with topical propamidine 0.1% as the key drug, along with topical neosporin and miconzole. Patients should apply drops at a minimum of each hour for the first several days. Therapy should be individualized, but a minimum course of about a month is generally required. Topical steroids should be avoided. The propamidine can itself cause a keratopathy, which is reversible but can be confused with persistent or recurrent infection. For refractory cases, topical polyhexamethylene biguanide treatment is effective. Penetrating keratoplasty is required for severe cases in which a delay in diagnosis had occurred.

PREVENTION. PAM and GAE are very rare conditions, and thus it is difficult to comment on public health measures for control. Because of wide evidence of seroprevalence and natural immunity, a vaccine, although theoretically possible to prepare, would be impractical. Small clusters of PAM have occurred in association with environmental exposure to warm water in which *Naegleria* would be expected to flourish. In such cases, it is probably prudent to avoid water

sports in the implicated bodies of water, especially those that could involve forcing water into the nasopharynx.

AK can be prevented by attentive contact lens hygiene such as performing appropriate sterilization with heat or benzylkonium-preserved saline and not using homemade saline solutions. Likewise, lenses should not be worn while swimming. These measures have already contributed to a decline in cases of AK since the mid-1980s.

Bibliography

Asbell PA: *Acanthamoeba* keratitis: There and back again. Mt Sinai J Med 60:279, 1993.

Bottone EJ: Free-living amebas of the genera *Acanthamoeba* and *Naegleria*: An overview and basic microbiologic correlates. Mt Sinai J Med 60:260, 1993.

Brown RL: Successful treatment of primary amebic meningoencephalitis. Arch Intern Med 151:1201, 1991.

Ferrante A: Free-living amoebae: Pathogenicity and immunity. Parasite Immunol 13:31, 1991.

Larkin DF, Kilvington S, Dart JK: Treatment of acanthamoeba keratitis with polyhexamethylene biguanide. Ophthalmology 99:185, 1992.

Martinez AJ: Free-Living Amebas: Natural History, Prevention, Diagnosis, Pathology and Treatment of Diseases. Boca Raton, FL, CRC Press, 1985.

Martinez AJ: Free-living amebas: Infection of the central nervous system. Mt Sinai J Med 60:271, 1993.

Seidel JS, Harmatz P, Visvesvara GS, et al: Successful treatment of primary amebic meningoencephalitis. N Engl J Med 306:346, 1982.

Visvesvara GS: Epidemiology of infections with free-living amebas and laboratory diagnosis of microsporidiosis. Mt Sinai J Med 60:283, 1993.

Visvevara GS, Schuster FL, Martinez AJ: *Balmuthia mandrillaris*. N g, N Sp, agent of amebic meningoencephalitis in humans and other animals. J Eukaryot Microbiol 40:504, 1993.

100 Other Tissue Protozoan Infections

100.1 Sarcosporidiosis

Jacob K. Frenkel

DEFINITION. *Sarcocystis* organisms are obligatory two-host coccidians. They form muscle cysts containing bradyzoites in the intermediate host, or host of prey, and undergo sporogony in the intestine of a definitive or predatory host. Humans are definitive hosts for some *Sarcocystis* species, which give rise to enteritis and to sporocysts in the feces. Humans act as intermediate hosts for others, which form muscle cysts, causing myositis when they disintegrate.

ETIOLOGY AND HISTORY. *Sarcocystis* infections were first described in the 19th century with the finding of sporozoan cysts in heart or skeletal muscle of animals and humans. Transmission remained obscure because the infection could not be reproduced by passage. During the mid-1970s, the coccidian affinities of *Sarcocystis* were recognized, and the transmission cycles in several animal species were shown to involve two hosts. More than 100 *Sarcocystis* species have been found in the skeletal muscle and heart of various animals, but the definitive hosts generally remain to be identified, except for some domestic species (Fig. 100–1).

TRANSMISSION AND EPIDEMIOLOGY. Humans serve as an accidental intermediate host for several *Sarcocystis* species and as a regular definitive host for at least two species (Fig. 100–2). Humans with muscle sarcocysts are an aberrant host for species of *Sarcocystis* that normally live in the muscle of prey animals (e.g., monkeys), transmitted by unidentified

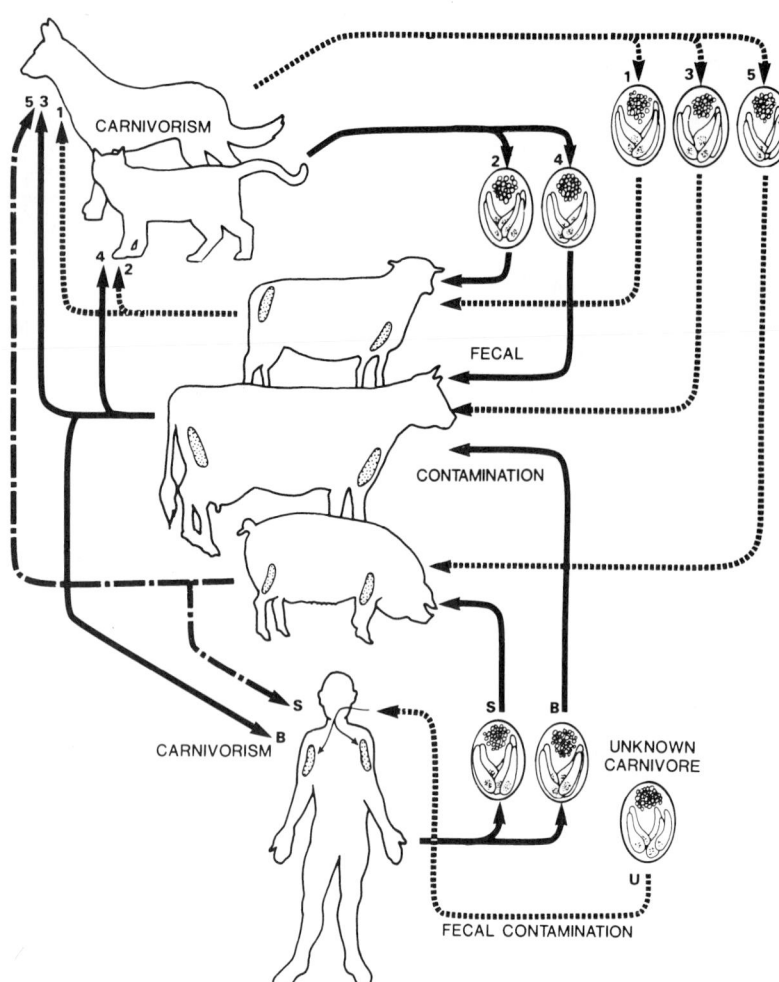

Figure 100–1. *Sarcocystis* transmission cycles involving humans and some domestic animals. Humans are the definitive host of *S. bovihominis (B)* and *S. suihominis (S)*, the two intestinal sarcosporidia. Humans are the accidental intermediate host with *Sarcocystis* of unknown species *(U)*, where skeletal and heart muscles are parasitized. Also indicated are the cycles of *S. ovicanis (1)*, *S. ovifelis (2)*, *S. bovicanis (3)*, *S. bovifelis (4)*, and *S. suicanis (5)*. (From Frenkel JK: *In* Mehlhorn H [ed]: Parasitology in Focus. Berlin, Springer, 1988, p 549.)

predatory carnivores (e.g., pythons). Humans are presumably infected by ingesting sporocysts from the feces of the carnivore, usually with contaminated soil. One or two proliferative generations probably occur in blood vessel walls, liver, or muscle, after which muscle sarcocysts are formed.

Humans are the regular definitive host of certain *Sarcocystis* species of cattle and pigs. Acquired by ingestion of raw or undercooked meat, the liberated bradyzoites enter the intestinal mucosa and develop into gametes, which after fertilization develop into oocysts. Unlike those in the one-host coccidia, the oocysts or sarcocysts sporulate in the mucosa, so that *S. bovihominis* and *S. suihominis* are shed as sporulated sporocysts. These sporocysts were formerly called *Isospora hominis* when they were believed to be one-host coccidia (see Chapter 90.2) of a single species.

DISTRIBUTION AND INCIDENCE. The ease with which the cycle is maintained determines distribution and incidence. For example, *S. bovicanis* (Fig. 100–1) is distributed worldwide because cattle and dogs live in close proximity, dogs are fed slaughter wastes, and cattle eat dog feces. *S. bovihominis* and *S. suihominis* (Fig. 100–1) occur where people eat raw or undercooked beef, pork, or venison and where human feces are accessible to cattle or pigs.

Sarcocystis in skeletal muscle of humans has been described so rarely and sporadically as to suggest accidental parasitism. Beaver and colleagues analyzed the morphology of sarcocysts and their location in cardiac or skeletal muscle in about 40 human cases and found four morphologic types of organisms that resembled species commonly found in local mon-

keys. The organisms of 13 infections probably acquired in Southeast Asia resembled a *Sarcocystis* species found in *Macaca fascicularis*; in 8 infections probably acquired in India, the organism resembled *Sarcocystis* species found in *Macaca mulatta*; and in 1 of 4 infections probably acquired in Africa or Europe, the organism resembled the *Sarcocystis* found in *Cercopithicus talapoin*. Among three types of cysts found in human hearts, the organism of one resembled *S. bovicanis*. The causative organism of three infections acquired in the United States could not be identified. One of these was in a Kansas farmer who had a hobby of keeping exotic animals. *Sarcocystis lindemanni* is of doubtful validity because it apparently describes a nonparasitic artifact.

PATHOGENESIS AND PATHOLOGY. Intact sarcocysts in skeletal or cardiac muscle of humans measure up to 100 μm in diameter and 325 μm in length and generally are not accompanied by inflammatory reaction (Fig. 100–2). Each sarcocyst contains numerous bradyzoites measuring 7 to 16 μm in length, depending on the species. Inflammation follows disintegration of these cysts and death of the intracystic bradyzoites, probably from antibody and complement, neutrophils, and eosinophils; lymphocytes accumulate, followed by plasma cells and, later, focal fibrosis. Vasculitis is commonly present in the muscle and subcutaneous tissues. This may stem from an earlier phase of intravascular schizogony, which has been observed in experimental animals but not in humans, or from nearby inflammation. Histopathologic diagnoses are myositis with vasculitis and sometimes myonecrosis.

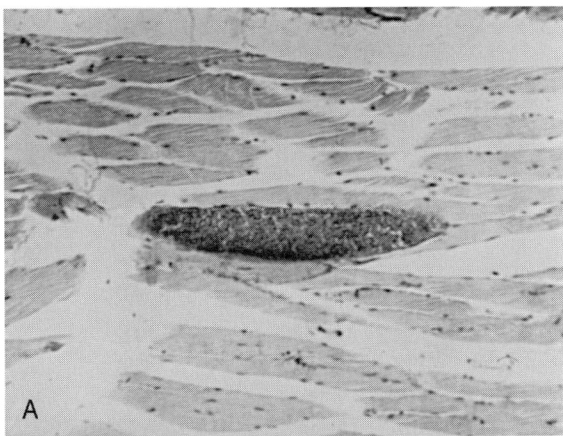
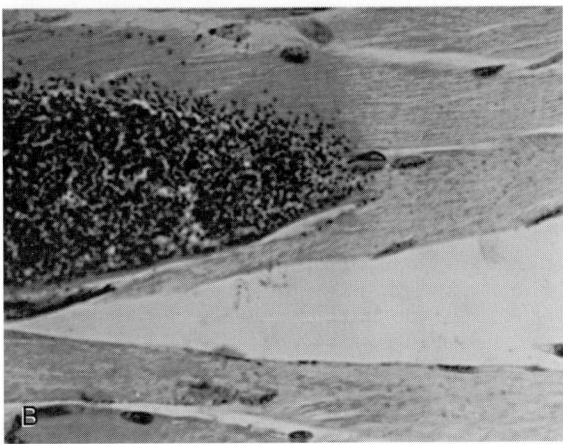

Figure 100–2. Sarcocyst in human skeletal muscle (PAS stain, × 150 [A] and × 600 [B]).

The finding of sporulated oocysts or sporocysts, probably *S. bovihominis*, in the lamina propria of the small intestine was observed in six resected specimens of segmental eosinophilic necrotizing enteritis in Thailand. Although in five patients the focally obstructive inflammatory lesions were possibly related to the numerous gram-positive bacilli present, the intense tissue eosinophilia in four patients, one of whom demonstrated no evidence of bacteria, strongly suggests a relationship to the sporocysts of *Sarcocystis*.

CLINICAL MANIFESTATIONS

Muscle Infection. Painful muscle swellings, measuring 1 to 3 cm in diameter, initially associated with erythema of the overlying skin in various parts of the body, occur episodically and last for 2 days to 2 weeks. These present in most of the patients. In some, these lesions were accompanied by fever, diffuse myalgia, muscle tenderness, weakness, eosinophilia, and bronchospasm. No clinical findings had been noted in patients in whom myocardial *Sarcocystis* infection was found accidentally by autopsy.

Enteric Infection. After ingestion of pork containing *S. suihominis*, volunteers developed diarrhea, vomiting, chills, and diaphoresis, starting 6 to 24 hours after ingestion and continuing for 12 to 24 hours. Sporocysts were shed between 11 and 71 days after the meal. Consumption of beef containing *S. bovihominis* was followed by abdominal discomfort and, in some volunteers, by nausea and diarrhea; sporocyst shedding started between 13 and 39 days after the meal and continued for 9 to 179 days. Eosinophilic enteritis and ulcerative obstructive enterocolitis may be occasional complications. Cases of enteritis after eating venison have been described in Europe.

DIAGNOSIS. Diagnosis of *Sarcocystis* myositis is by muscle biopsy (Fig. 100–2). Other cyst-forming organisms (e.g., *Toxoplasma gondii* and *Trypanosoma cruzi*) must be differentiated. Sarcocysts are often septate, and the cyst wall is distinct ultrastructurally. Bradyzoites of *Sarcocystis* and *Toxoplasma* are periodic acid–Schiff positive, but *T. cruzi* is not. Serologic reactions have not been investigated in detail. They appear to be specific for the genus but nonspecific as to species.

Intestinal sarcosporidiosis is diagnosed by finding already sporulated sporocysts, each containing four sporozoites, in freshly voided stool specimens with the aid of flotation procedures. Eosinophilia is often present.

TREATMENT AND PROGNOSIS. Because *Sarcocystis* organisms in muscle and intestine are fully formed terminal stages in that host and no new cells are parasitized, specific treatment of the muscle and enteric infection is unsatisfactory. However, corticosteroids should palliate the allergic inflammatory reactions episodically occurring after cyst rupture. Because the intracystic bradyzoites are not capable of infecting new cells in the host, there is no risk of recrudescence.

PREVENTION. Muscle involvement can be prevented by avoiding food and water that are potentially contaminated with feces of predatory carnivores. Enteric infection can be prevented by avoiding ingestion of raw beef and pork; most frozen (− 20°C) and well-cooked meats are safe, however.

Bibliography

Beaver PC, Gadgil RK, Morera P: Sarcocystis in man: A review and report of five cases. Am J Trop Med Hyg 28:819, 1979.

Bunyaratvej S, Bunyawongwiroj P, Nitiyanant P: Human intestinal sarcosporidiosis—report of 6 cases. Am J Trop Med Hyg 31:36, 1982.

Dubey JP, Speer CS, Fayer R: Sarcocystosis of Animals and Man. Boca Raton, FL, CRC Press, 1988, pp 1–215.

McLeod R, Hirabayashi RN, Rothman W, et al: Necrotizing vasculitis and Sarcocystis: A cause-and-effect relationship. South Med J 73:1380, 1980.

Mehlhorn H, Heydorn AO: The Sarcosporidia. Life cycle and fine structure. Adv Parasitol 16:43, 1978.

Wong KT, Pathmanathan R: High prevalence of human skeletal muscle sarcocystosis in Southeast Asia. Tran R Soc Trop Med Hyg 86:631, 1992.

Wong KT, Pathmanathan R: Scanning electronmicroscopy of the human muscular sarcocyst. Parasitol Res 81:359, 1995.

100.2 Microsporidiosis

Louis M. Weiss

DEFINITION. Microsporidia are primitive eukaryotic obligate intracellular protozoan parasites infecting every major animal group. They are classified in a separate phylum, the Microspora, consisting of approximately 120 genera and more than 900 species. Sprague's classification is commonly used, although molecular analysis of rRNA genes will likely modify it.

ETIOLOGY AND HISTORY. These organisms were first recognized by Nageli in 1857 as silkworm parasites, which he named *Nosema bombycis*. Within their hosts, the majority infect the digestive tract, but reproductive, respiratory, muscle, excretory, and nervous system infections are well documented. In fact, microsporidia have been found in every tissue and organ, and spores are common in environmental sources such as ditch water. Microsporidia are increasingly recognized as pathogens in the setting of immunodeficiencies (especially in AIDS). It is likely that microsporidia commonly infect humans but are self-limited or asymptomatic in immunocompetent hosts. The spectrum of disease due to the different microsporidia that infect humans includes diarrhea, keratoconjunctivitis, disseminated disease, hepatitis, myositis, kidney and urogenital infection, ascites, cholangitis, and asymptomatic carriage.

Several microsporidian genera have been associated with human disease: *Nosema* (although *N. corneum* was recently renamed *Vittaforma corneae*), generally found in insects; *Pleistophora*, a pathogen of fish and insects; *Encephalitozoon*, found in many mammals; *Enterocytozoon*, found in patients with AIDS and in several species of fish; and *Septata* and *Trachipleistophora*, found in patients with AIDS. Studies of small subunit rRNA have shown that *S. intestinalis* is closely related to *Enc. hellem* and *Enc. cuniculi*, consistent with its placement on morphologic analysis in the family Encephalitozoonidae, and its status as a separate genus has been challenged, with the organism being renamed *Encephalitozoon intestinalis*. The genus *Microsporidium* has been used to designate microsporidia of uncertain taxonomic status.

BIOLOGIC CHARACTERISTICS. Microsporidia are eukaryotes but share several prokaryotic features, lacking eukaryotic ribosomal characteristics, mitochondria, and peroxisomes. The spore is characteristic of the phylum in that it is unicellular, with a resistant spore wall, one nucleus or two abutted nuclei, (diplokaryon) sporoplasm, an anchoring disk, and an extrusion apparatus consisting of a single polar tube with an anterior attachment complex. Although spores are environmentally resistant, they may be killed by exposure for 30 minutes to 70% ethanol, 1% formaldehyde, or 1% hydrogen peroxide or by autoclaving at 120°C for 10 minutes. In general, spores range in size from 1 to 12 μm. The spore coat consists of an electron-dense proteinaceous exospore, an electron-lucent endospore composed of chitin and protein, and an inner membrane or plasmalemma. The extrusion apparatus consists of a long polar tube (filament), which is attached to the inside of the anterior end of the spore by an anchoring disk and forms from 4 to approximately 30 coils around the sporoplasm in the spore, depending on the species. During infection (germination), the polar tube rapidly everts out of the spore, piercing an adjacent host cell and thereby inoculating the sporoplasm directly into that cell, functioning essentially as a hypodermic needle. Of the microsporidia that infect humans, Encephalitozoonidae (*Enc. hellem, Enc. cuniculi, Enc. [S.] intestinalis*), *Trachipleistophora hominis*, and *Vittaforma corneae* have been cultured in vitro. Only limited replication in vitro has thus far been reported for *Enterocytozoon bieneusi*.

CLINICAL DISEASE AND PATHOLOGY

Infections in Patients Without AIDS. Conclusive evidence that microsporidia could be associated with human disease was not available until 1973, when a 4-month-old athymic boy died with severe diarrhea and malabsorption (Fig. 100–3). At autopsy, a disseminating infection due to microsporidia classified by transmission electron microscopy (TEM) as *Nosema connori* was identified. In another case, a 3-year-old Colombian boy with seizures and hepatomegaly had 1.5 × 2.5 μm gram-positive organisms in his urinary sediment. Serologic analyses identified IgG and IgM antibodies against *Enc. cuniculi*. *Pleistophora*, previously thought to be limited to fish and insects, was identified in 1985 in the skeletal muscle of an HIV-negative patient with myositis. *Ent. bieneusi* has also been identified as a cause of self-limited diarrhea in several immunocompetent hosts and in a liver transplant recipient.

Corneal Infections. In 1973 and 1981, two cases with corneal involvement were documented in immunocompetent patients from Botswana and Sri Lanka. These organisms were described as *Microsporidium ceylonesis* and *M. africanus*. Two additional cases of microsporidian interstitial keratitis have been identified in immunocompetent hosts and identified as *N. ocularum* and *N. corneum* (now called *V. corneae*). Histologic

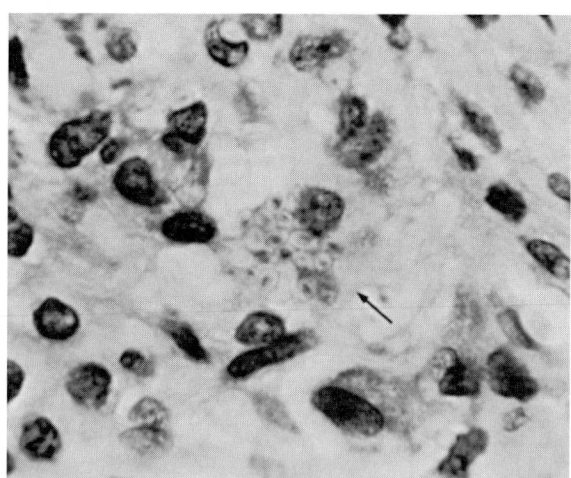

Figure 100–3. Microsporidia *(arrow)* *(Nosema connori)* in a human infant (× 1260). (Courtesy of Drs. Daniel Connor and Ann Cali and the Armed Forces Institute of Pathology, Photograph Neg. No. 71–5882.)

sections have revealed findings ranging from intact stromal lamellae with a paucity of inflammatory cells to frank necrotizing keratitis. Highly refractile organisms of 3.5 to 4.5 μm by 1.5 to 3 μm are found within macrophages or lying free between corneal lamellae but not within superficial epithelial cells, as is seen in patients with AIDS. Furthermore, TEM demonstrated that these organisms were larger, binucleate, and lacking in parasitophorous vacuoles, consistent with their classification as being *Nosema*-like. One patient required enucleation, one underwent unsuccessful penetrating keratoplasty, one was successfully treated with a corneal transplant, and the last was maintained on various topical agents without effect until keratoplasty.

Infections in Patients With AIDS. The majority of patients with AIDS and microsporidiosis have had diarrhea; however, cases of keratoconjunctivitis, hepatitis, myositis, sinusitis, kidney and urogenital infection, ascites, cholangitis, disseminated infections, and asymptomatic carriage have been described. Members of the family Encephalitozoonidae are capable of disseminated infection, and these microsporidia have been identified in all tissues on autopsy.

Ocular Involvement. AIDS-related ocular microsporidial infection has been restricted to the superficial epithelium of the cornea and conjunctiva (i.e., superficial keratoconjunctivitis). This keratitis rarely progresses to corneal ulceration. Most patients present with bilateral coarse punctate epithelial keratopathy and conjunctival inflammation resulting in redness, foreign body sensation, photophobia, and changes in visual acuity. Biopsy specimens examined with TEM have revealed numerous microsporidian spores within the corneal and conjunctival epithelium. Of the reports in the literature of microsporidian keratitis due to Encephalitozoonidae, all but three have been attributed to *Enc. hellem*, including three cases originally classified as *Enc. cuniculi*. *T. hominis* has also been associated with keratoconjunctivitis in patients with AIDS.

Muscle Involvement. Myositis has been associated with *Plesitophora*, *T. hominis*, and a *Nosema*-like microsporidian. Although *Pleistophora* and the *Nosema*-like microsporidia have only been described in muscle, *T. hominis* has been associated with disseminated disease, sinusitis, and keratoconjunctivitis.

Gastrointestinal Involvement. The major syndrome associated with microsporidiosis in AIDS is diarrhea and wasting. This is usually due to *Ent. bieneusi* (> 90% of cases in the

United States) and occasionally *Enc. (S.) intestinalis*, although in Europe this organism may be a more frequent cause of diarrhea. In HIV-infected patients evaluated for diarrhea, the prevalence has ranged from 10 to 40%. Kotler and Orenstein, in a study of patients presenting to a gastroenterology clinic, found that 39% of patients with HIV and diarrhea had microsporidosis and that the presence of microsporidia was associated with wasting, a mean CD4 count of $28/mm^3$, and an abnormal D-xylose test result. In contrast, only 2.6% of HIV-infected patients without diarrhea had microsporidiosis. Coyle and colleagues, using a polymerase chain reaction (PCR) employing primers to the small subunit rRNA gene of *Ent. bieneusi*, also found a significant association between the presence of diarrhea and microsporidia in patients with AIDS.

Ent. bieneusi infection is limited to the gastrointestinal tract, and disseminated disease has not been described. In intestinal biopsy specimens, *Ent. bieneusi* is found only on the apical surface, whereas *Enc. (S.) intestinalis* is found on both the apical and basal surface of enterocytes and in the lamina propria (Fig. 100–4). Besides diarrhea, *Ent. bieneusi* has been associated with cholangitis.

DIAGNOSIS. Serologic testing is commercially used for testing rabbits to ensure *Encephalitozoon*-free animals. The sensitivity and specificity of these tests are unknown, however, because serologic cross-reactivity among microsporidia has been demonstrated by both immunofluorescence and Western blotting. Nonetheless, human serologic data related to *Enc. cuniculi* are intriguing. In one study, 6 of 69 healthy adults in England, 38 of 89 Nigerians with tuberculosis, 13 of 70 Malaysians with filariasis, and 33 of 92 Ghanians with malaria had positive findings on microsporidia serology. In other studies, 14 of 115 travelers returning from the tropics and 10 of 30 HIV-positive men (all had traveled to the tropics) were seropositive, but none of 48 nontravelers were. These data suggest that microsporidia are as common in humans as they are in other mammals, and are associated with travel or residence in the tropics or developing nations.

Definitive species diagnosis of microsporidiosis currently requires TEM visualization of spore ultrastructure (Fig. 100–5) and developmental stages; however, species-specific PCR rRNA primers have been described. In patients with enteric microsporidiosis undergoing endoscopy, the small in-

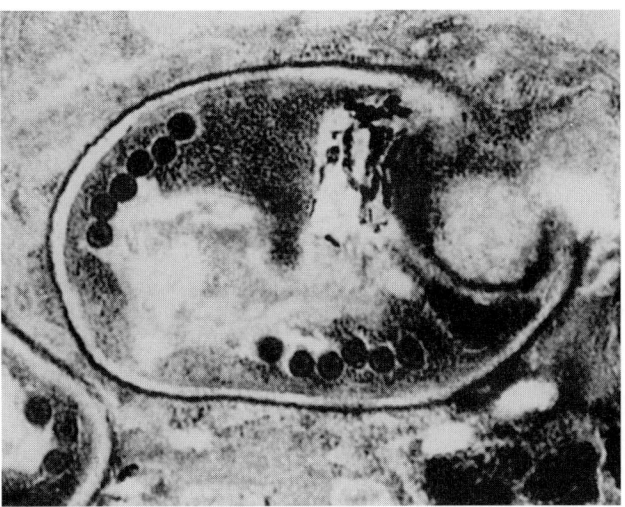

***Figure* 100–5.** Transmission electron micrograph of a spore of *Enc. hellem* from a patient with keratoconjunctivitis. The characteristic coiled polar tube is present in cross section.

testine has provided the highest diagnostic yield, but organisms have been seen in colon biopsy material. In tissue sections (Figs. 100–3 and 100–4), touch preparations, or corneal scrapings, microsporidia are discernible with hematoxylin-eosin, Giemsa, tissue Gram, or chromotrope 2R stains. Microsporidia have been demonstrated in stool specimens by a modified trichrome stain (chromotrope 2R), Uvitex 2B, and calcofluor white. The sensitivity and specificity of these techniques are under evaluation. Polyclonal sera prepared to Encephalitzoonidae have been used for immunofluorescence. PCR reactions for Encephalitozoonidae (*Enc. cuniculi, Enc. hellem,* and *Enc. (S.) intestinalis*) and *Ent. bieneusi* based on cloned rRNA genes from these organisms have been described.

TREATMENT. Albendazole, a benzimidazole that binds to β tubulin, is effective against many helminths and protozoa. It has recently become evident that in patients with AIDS, diarrhea, and *Enc. (S.) intestinalis*, treatment with albendazole 400 mg PO b.i.d. results in resolution of the diarrhea and elimination of the organism. In vitro, albendazole has activity against all of the Encephalitozoonidae at concentrations of < 0.1 μg/mL. Clinical and radiographic improvement was seen in a case of chronic sinusitis due to *Enc. hellem* treated with albendazole 400 mg b.i.d. In addition, marked clinical improvement with albendazole 200 mg b.i.d. occurred in a patient with disseminated infection due to *Enc. cuniculi* involving the conjunctiva, sinuses, kidneys, and lungs. Resolution of myositis was noted in patients infected with a *Nosema*-like microsporidian and in a case of disseminated infection with myositis due to *T. hominis*. Albendazole treatment results in amelioration of symptoms in as many as 50% of patients with *Ent. bieneusi*. Albendazole as a systemic agent is indicated if the organism is demonstrated in the urine or in nasal smears of patients with keratoconjunctivitis.

Fumagillin has also demonstrated consistent activity against microsporidia both in vitro and in vivo. Fumagillin is a water-insoluble antibiotic produced by *Aspergillus fumigatus*. It is used for the treatment of *Entamoeba histolytica* in humans, and its water-soluble derivative, Fumidil B, has been used to treat microsporidosis of honeybees caused by *Nosema apis*. The soluble salt Fumidil B (fumagillin bicylohexylammonium) is toxic to mammals and should not be ingested; however, solutions of Fumadil B applied topically are

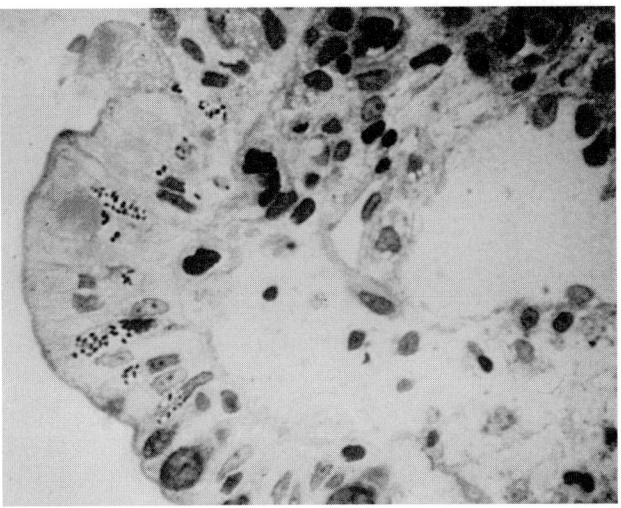

***Figure* 100–4.** Intestinal biopsy from a patient with *Enc. (S.) intestinalis* stained with Chromotrope 2R. Microsporidia are present on the apical and basal surface of the enterocytes and in the lamina propria. (Courtesy of Drs. Donald P. Kotler and Jan M. Orensten.)

not toxic to the cornea. In vitro fumagillin inhibits the growth of Encephalitozoonidae as well as many other microsporidia. This agent causes stasis of growth, not death of organisms, and relapses of infection on discontinuation of fumagillin have occurred.

The efficacy of imidazole compounds on microsporidiosis is variable. Sulfa drugs have had variable results in vitro and in vivo and are not recommended for treatment. In vitro testing suggests that chloroquine and sparfloxacin have some activity against Encephalitozoonidae.

PREVENTION. Although the epidemiology of the microsporida that infect humans is unknown, it is likely these are food- or waterborne pathogens, and the usual sanitary measures that prevent contamination of food and water with the urine and feces of animals should decrease the chance for infection. In addition, handwashing and general hygienic habits probably reduce the chance for contamination of the conjunctiva and cornea.

Bibliography

Coyle CM, Wittner M, Kotler DP, et al: Prevalence of microsporidiosis *(Enterocytozoon bieneusi* and *Encephalitozoon [Septata] intestinalis)* in AIDS related diarrhea as determined by the polymerase chain reaction to microsporidian small subunit ribosomal RNA. Clin Infect Dis 23:1002, 1996.

Dieterich DT, Lew EA, Kotler KP, et al: Treatment with albendazole for intestinal disease due to *Enterocytozoon bieneusi* in patients with AIDS. J Infect Dis 169:178, 1994.

Hollister WS, Canning EU, Weidner E, et al: Development and ultrastructure of *Trachipleistophora hominis* n.g., n.sp. after in vitro isolation from an AIDS patient and inoculation into athymic mice. Parasitology 112:143, 1996.

Kotler DP, Orenstein JM: Prevalence of intestinal microsporidiosis in HIV infected individuals referred for gastroenterological evaluation. Am J Gastroenterol 89:1998, 1994.

Molina JM, Oksenhendler E, Beauvais B, et al: Disseminated microsporidiosis due to *Septata intestinalis* in patients with AIDS: Clinical features and response to albendazole therapy. J Infect Dis 171:245, 1995.

Rastrelli PD, Didier ES, Yee RW: Microsporidial keratitis. Ophthalmol Clin North Am 7:617, 1994.

Sprague V, Becnel JJ, Hazard EI: Taxonomy of the phylum Microspora. Crit Rev Microbiol 18:285, 1992.

Weber R, Bryan RT, Schwartz DA, Owen RL: Human microsporidial infections. Clin Microbiol 7:426, 1994.

Weiss LM, Cali A, Tanowitz HB, Wittner M: Utility of microsporidian rRNA in diagnosis and phylogeny: A review. Folia Parasitol (Praha) 41:81, 1994.

Wittner M, Tanowitz HB, Weiss LM: Parasitic infection in AIDS patients: Cryptosporidiosis, isosporiasis, microsporidiosis, cyclosporiasis. Infect Dis Clin North Am 7:569, 1993.

100.3 *Cystoisosporidiosis*

Jacob K. Frenkel

Isospora belli has been considered to undergo only a classic coccidian cycle, with schizogony and gametogony in the small intestinal epithelium (see Chapter 90.2). However, a

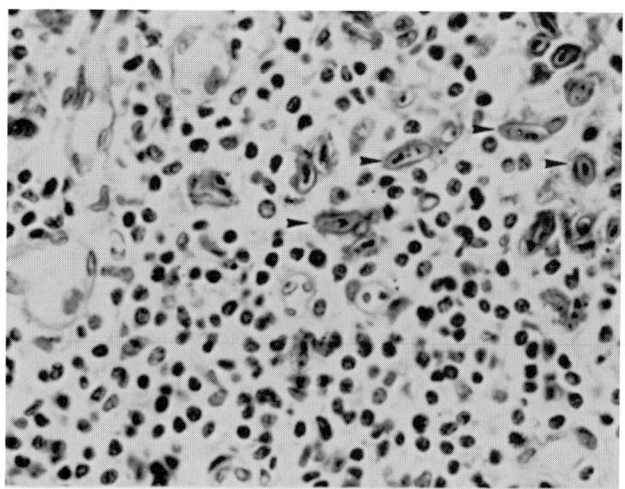

Figure 100–6. Unizoic cysts of *Cystoisospora belli* in mesenteric lymph node *(arrowheads)* of an AIDS patient ($\times$ 600, periodic acid-Schiff hematoxylin). (Courtesy of Dr. Carlos Restrepo.)

new stage, individual encysted zoites, so-called hypnozoites (Fig. 100–6), was identified at autopsy of two patients with AIDS who had chronic watery diarrhea with malabsorption and who shed *I. belli* oocysts in their feces. These unicellular cysts were present in the lamina propria and lymph nodes of both patients and in the liver and spleen of one. Ultrastructurally, they have the typical coccidian morphology, as well as a crystalline body. Similar cysts had previously been found in rodents capable of serving as intermediate hosts that were experimentally infected with feline isosporiasis. The genus *Cystoisospora* was created for such two-host coccidia with hypnozoites, previously classified in the genus *Isospora*. The presence of unizoic cysts indicates that the human *I. belli* would better be classified as *Cystoisospora belli*. Humans can acquire infection either from oocysts or from an intermediary host carrying hypnozoites. The hypnozoites in these immunodeficient patients suggest that humans act as intermediate hosts, and they may have resulted from either autoinfection or reinfection, with oocysts. An intense inflammatory reaction, including plasma cells, lymphocytes, neutrophils, and eosinophils, accompanied the tissue cysts in gut and lymph nodes (Fig. 100–6).

Bibliography

Dubey JP: Critical comment. Pathol Res Pract 190:1094, 1994.

Michiels JF, Hofman P, Bernard E, et al: Intestinal and extraintestinal *Isospora belli* infection in an AIDS patient. Pathol Res Pract 190:1089, 1994.

Restrepo C, Macher AM, Radany EH: Disseminated intestinal isosporiasis in a patient with the acquired immune deficiency syndrome. Am J Clin Pathol 87:40, 1987.

PART VI
Helminthic Infections

---

101 General Principles

G. Thomas Strickland

DEFINITIONS. *Helminth* is derived from the Greek word *helmins* and means worm. As usually interpreted, the word denotes several groups of parasitic worms. In contrast to the small unicellular protozoa, the helminths are large multicellular organisms with complex tissues and organs.

CLASSIFICATION. There are three groups of helminths that parasitize humans: (1) annelids (segmented worms), (2) nematodes (roundworms), and (3) platyhelminths (flatworms).

Annelida. Hirudinea (leeches [Chapter 126.2]) is the only class of annelids of medical importance.

Nematoda. Members of this phylum are nonsegmented roundworms. They are characterized by longitudinally oriented muscles and by a triradiate esophagus. They are bilaterally symmetrical and have a complete digestive tract, and the sexes are usually distinct. Most species are free-living and inhabit soil and water. Most of the 80,000 species parasitic to vertebrates have developed a biologic dependence on a single host (Chapters 102–116). The word nematode is derived from the Greek *nema* for thread and *eidos* for form.

It is useful to divide nematodes into groups according to the body organ of humans in which they reside.

Adults That Reside in the Gut. This group includes human parasites of the following species: *Ascaris lumbricoides* (Chapter 104), *Ancylostoma duodenale* and *Necator americanus* (Chapter 105.1), *Trichuris trichiura* (Chapter 103.2), *Enterobius vermicularis* (Chapter 103.1), *Strongyloides stercoralis* (Chapter 105.2), *Capillaria philippinensis* (this nematode has apparently recently adapted to parasitizing humans) (Chapter 103.3), and *Trichostrongylus orientalis* (Chapter 103.4).

Adults That Reside in the Blood or Lymphatic or Subcutaneous Tissues. This group includes human parasites of the following species: *Wuchereria bancrofti* (Chapter 106.1), *Brugia malayi* (Chapter 106.2), *Brugia timori* (Chapter 106.3), *Loa loa* (Chapter 107), *Onchocerca volvulus* (Chapter 108), *Mansonella ozzardi*, *M. perstans*, and *M. streptocerca* (Chapter 109), and *Dracunculus medinensis* (Chapter 110).

Larval Stages That Cause Human Pathologic Conditions in Various Tissues. These, with the exception of *Trichinella spiralis*, are nonhuman parasites that are unable to develop to adults in humans, an aberrant host. In general, these nematodes follow the same migration pattern here as in their definitive host, except that it is interrupted.

INFECTIONS THAT ARE USUALLY LIMITED TO THE SKIN AND SUBCUTANEOUS TISSUES. Creeping eruption is primarily caused by the dog and cat hookworms (i.e., *Ancylostoma braziliense*, *A. caninum*, and *Uncinaria stenocephala* [Chapter 115]) as well as other rare animal parasites that infect by skin penetration. Skin penetration by human hookworms (Chapter 105.1) and *Strongyloides* (Chapter 105.2) sometimes causes similar findings. Some *Dirofilaria* parasites of various animals (Chapter 109.4) cause subcutaneous nodules in man.

INFECTIONS PRIMARILY INVOLVING THE MUSCLES. The larvae of *Trichinella spiralis* can migrate through many tissues, including the heart and brain, before encysting in muscle (Chapter 111).

INFECTIONS CAUSING A VISCERAL LARVA MIGRANS SYNDROME. The larval stages of the dog and cat ascarids, *Toxocara canis* and *T. cati*, and *Capillaria hepatica* (Chapter 112) commonly cause lesions in multiple organs, principally the liver, brain, lungs, and eye.

Angiostrongylus costaricensis (Chapter 114.2) and marine ascarids (e.g., the anisakids and eustrongylids) (Chapter 116) primarily cause abdominal lesions.

Angiostrongylus cantonensis, the rat lungworm, causes eosinophilic meningitis (Chapter 114.1). *Gnathostoma spinigerum*, a stomach worm of domestic and wild cats and dogs, can cause a creeping eruption, an abdominopulmonary hypereosinophilia syndrome, and an eosinophilic myeloencephalitis (Chapter 113).

The dog heartworm, *Dirofilaria immitis*, sometimes causes pulmonary nodules in humans following bites from infectious mosquitoes (Chapter 109.4). A pulmonary hypereosinophilia syndrome can be caused by migrating human ascarid (Chapter 104), hookworm (Chapter 105.1) and *Strongyloides* (Chapter 105.2) larvae and microfilariae of *W. bancrofti*, *B. malayi*, and various animal filariae (Chapter 106).

Platyhelminthes. Flatworms are usually dorsoventrally flattened, are bilaterally symmetrical, and have three body layers lacking a body cavity. They include the trematodes and cestodes. The word is derived from the Greek *platys*, meaning broad, and *helmins*, meaning worm.

Trematoda. This class includes the flukes that are parasitic to humans and animals. They are usually hermaphroditic, and a digestive canal is present except in the sporocyst stage of digenetic species. Trematode eggs are excreted in the stool, urine, or sputum of the definitive host. All flukes require a mollusk as their first intermediate host. The larval stage that escapes from the mollusk may then enter a second intermediate host (fish, crustacean), encyst on vegetation, or penetrate directly into the skin of the definitive host. Infection generally results from the ingestion of insufficiently cooked fish, crustaceans, and vegetation (Fig. 117–1).

The important trematodes of humans belong to the following genera: (1) adults that live in the venous system—*Schistosoma* (Chapter 118); (2) adults that live in the intestines—*Fasciolopsis*, *Echinostoma*, *Heterophyes*, *Gastrodiscoides*, and *Metagonimus* (Chapter 119); (3) adults that live in the biliary system—*Clonorchis*, *Opisthorchis*, *Fasciola*, and *Dicrocoelium* (Chapter 120); and (4) adults that live in the bronchi—*Paragonimus* (Chapter 121).

Cestoda. This is a subclass of Cestoidea comprising the true tapeworms, which have a head (scolex) and segments (proglottids). Adults are all parasitic and hermaphroditic and live in the intestinal lumen of vertebrate hosts. Those that can infect humans include *Diphyllobothrium latum* and *D. pacificum* (Chapter 123.1), *Taenia saginata* and *T. solium* (Chapter 123.2), *Hymenolepis nana* and *H. diminuta* (Chapter 123.3), and *Dipylidium caninum* (Chapter 123.4). Their larval stages (hydatid, cysticercus, sparganum, coenurus) may be found in various organs and tissues of humans and other intermediate hosts (Chapter 124).

ANATOMY AND PHYSIOLOGY. Helminths are complicated multicellular organisms. Those infecting humans range in length from 0.3 mm (e.g., *T. canis* [Chapter 112] and *A. braziliense* [Chapter 115] larvae) to 12 m (e.g., adult *T. saginata* [Chapter 123.2]). They are round (nematodes) or flat (flukes and tapeworms). They all have an outer coating, the cuticle, which provides protection and is involved in active transport of water, electrolytes, and other substances.

Almost all helminths are unable to multiply in their host. The reproductive organs make up a large portion of the body cavities. The nematodes are sexually distinct, with separate males and females. The trematodes and cestodes are both diecious (schistosomes) and monoecious (other flukes and the tapeworms). The monoecious trematodes reproduce by self-fertilization or by cross-fertilization. Among the tapeworms, each proglottid possesses both male and female sex organs. Usually, sperm is transferred between adjacent mature proglottids of the worm.

TRANSMISSION. Parasitic worms infect humans in almost all regions of the world, but there is a particular abundance in the tropics of both parasite species and infected individuals. This is the result of climatic and sociologic factors. Many of these parasites require special conditions of temperature and humidity for survival and multiplication. Others require particular vertebrate or invertebrate hosts, e.g., fish, snails, crustaceans, or insects, for the completion of their life cycles. The intermediate hosts, particularly insect vectors, gain ready access to humans in tropical regions owing to the lack of preventive measures by the indigenous populations.

Oral Transmission. The distribution of intestinal nematodes whose eggs are passed in human feces (Chapters 102 to 105) is affected by climatic conditions (e.g., rainfall, temperature, and humidity) as well as sanitary practices. The customs in many regions of using human excreta (night soil) for fertilizer and of indiscriminate defecation result in widespread pollution of soil, water supplies, and foods (particularly vegetables). This results in a high prevalence of fecally transmitted nematodes in most of the tropics and subtropics.

Eating habits account for the transmission of other helminths. Ingestion of undercooked or raw meat (*T. spiralis* [Chapter 111], *Taenia* species [Chapter 123.2]) or fish (anisakid larvae [Chapter 116], *D. latum* [Chapter 123.1], and *Clonorchis sinensis* and *Opisthorchis* species [Chapter 120.1 and 120.2]) infected with larval stages of the parasite transmits some helminths. Other helminthic infections follow the ingestion of larvae-contaminated water (*D. medinensis* [Chapter 110]), raw snails (*Angiostrongylus* species [Chapter 114]), raw or undercooked crabs (*Paragonimus westermani* [Chapter 121], and aquatic plants (*Fasciola hepatica* [Chapter 120.3] and *Fasciolopsis buski* [Chapter 119.1]).

People are infected with *Toxocara canis* (Chapter 112) and *Echinococcus granulosus* (Chapter 124.2) following the ingestion of substances contaminated with dog feces containing the helminth eggs.

Transmission by Skin Penetration. Larval stages of hookworm parasites (Chapter 105.1) and *S. stercoralis* (Chapter 105.2) in the soil cause infection when they penetrate the intact skin. Third-stage larvae of dog and cat hookworms can penetrate unbroken skin but cannot develop fully in humans. They cause a creeping eruption (Chapter 115). Cercariae of *Schistosoma* species penetrate the skin of those exposed to contaminated water (Chapter 118). Those species not capable of developing in humans cause a rash, called swimmer's itch.

Transmission by Bite of a Vector. The filarial parasites (Chapters 106 to 109) develop within the biologic vector, which is also an intermediate host. These can be mosquitoes (*W. bancrofti* [Chapter 106.1] or *B. malaya* [Chapter 106.2]), black flies (*O. volvulus* [Chapter 108]), or *Chrysops* flies (*Loa loa* [Chapter 107]).

MAGNITUDE OF THE HEALTH PROBLEM
In The Tropics and Subtropics
Prevalence of Infection. Because many people are infected with more than one species of helminth, there are more

different species of helminths infecting people than there are people in the world. The numbers infected with hookworms, *Ascaris*, *Trichuris*, pinworm, schistosomes, onchocerca, and filariae are each in the hundreds of millions. A common trinity of intestinal helminthiasis includes ascariasis, hookworm infection, and trichuriasis.

Intensity of Infection. Some helminth infections (e.g., schistosomiasis, hookworm disease, and onchocerciasis) are among those medical conditions that cause major human suffering in the world. It is difficult to document morbidity in the vast majority of those infected with these parasites and with other helminth infections (e.g., clonorchiasis, taeniasis, ascariasis, trichuriasis, enterobiasis, and filariasis).

The magnitude of disease caused by helminths is related to the intensity of infection. Individuals with light infections have a tendency to have few or no abnormal findings, whereas those with heavy and prolonged infections often have clinical symptoms and signs and develop complications. This is well documented in schistosomiasis, hookworm disease (versus infection), onchocerciasis, and filariasis.

HOOKWORM DISEASE. The major cause of death in Puerto Rico prior to Bailey K. Ashford's treatment campaign during the first decade of the twentieth century was anemia from hookworm disease (Chapter 6). Hookworm disease is still a major cause of iron deficiency anemia in children and pregnant and lactating women in the tropics and subtropics (Chapter 105.1). Iron deficiency is still one of the major nutritional problems in these areas (Chapter 132.1). Even *Trichuris trichiura* can cause anemia, malnutrition, and diarrhea in children with heavy infections (Chapter 103.2).

SCHISTOSOMIASIS. It has been said that it is difficult to demonstrate increased morbidity or mortality due to schistosomiasis (Chapter 118), and in endemic areas, where praziquantel therapy is widely used, schistosomal disease has been markedly reduced. Even though re-infections occur frequently, repeated courses of chemotherapy reduce the intensity of infection, which reduces the burden of disease.

Abdominal ultrasonography is an excellent means of detecting morbidity in schistosomiasis, not only in individuals in hospitals and clinics, but also in groups examined in their communities. The technique is inexpensive and noninvasive. It can accurately detect hepatosplenomegaly, urinary tract obstruction, hepatic periportal fibrosis, and bladder polyps and masses. Sonography is showing that many individuals, even those with a paucity of symptoms, have detectable schistosomal morbidity.

ONCHOCERCIASIS. It is estimated that 20 million people are infected with *O. volvulus* (Chapter 108). The majority of those infected have dermatitis and lesions involving the subcutaneous tissues, which cause considerable discomfort, interfering with their ability to work. Moreover, 340,000 are blind from this parasite, and more have eye lesions that have not yet progressed to blindness. Often, those blinded are young adult males—fathers and former providers for the family. Those who are afflicted with onchocerciasis are often illiterate subsistence farmers who frequently live in isolated communities. The parasite does not normally infect city dwellers and is not transmitted in developed countries, nor is it much of a threat to travelers.

Although there are no good cost-effective means to control transmission by the vector, there is an excellent drug, ivermectin, that can reduce both morbidity and transmission.

Cysticercosis. During 1972 and 1973, medical officers working in West Irian (New Guinea) began seeing an epidemic of severe burns from rolling into open fires. This had not previously been a medical problem. In 1971, the natives had received a gift of pigs from the Indonesian government. Unlike the native pigs of New Guinea, these gift pigs from

Bali were heavily infected with the larval stage of *T. solium* (*Cysticercus cellulosae*). The New Guinea tribesmen became infected from eating the undercooked pork, following their habitual way of preparing the meat. The resultant adult tapeworms caused no symptoms (Chapter 123.2), but the eggs passed in the feces infected pigs and humans alike with the larval stage of the parasite, causing cysticercosis in both (Chapter 124.1). Infection was related to heavy contamination of the environment with human feces and was expedited by heavy rains with standing ground water. Many people were heavily infected with multiple cerebral cysticerci (Fig. 124–2), and they and others frequently had multiple subcutaneous cysticercus nodules. Epileptic seizures occurring at night while sleeping near open fires caused the epidemic of severe burns. Those having seizures would roll into the fires and, being unconscious, would not be able to move out of the flames.

This is an example of a disease that caused a severe epidemic when first brought into a community. (Intestinal capillariasis [Chapter 103.3] appeared in a similar manner in the Ilocos Norte district of the Philippines in the late 1960s.) The epilepsy caused by cysticercosis in New Guinea occurred during the acute invasive phase of infection, unlike the epilepsy of chronic cysticercosis, common in Mexico, with which patients frequently have calcified cerebral cysts.

In the Arctic. Trichinosis has been reported frequently in the Eskimo populations of Canada, the United States, and Greenland. Infection is acquired by eating raw or undercooked polar bears or walruses. The arctic form of *Trichinella* is referred to as *T. nativa* (Chapter 111). It has some different biologic characteristics from *Trichinella* in more southern climates and it is more enteropathogenic and less muscle invasive. Prolonged diarrhea is the most important clinical manifestation.

In Temperate Climates. Prior to the middle of the twentieth century, the helminthiases were a significant cause of morbidity in the United States. Infections with the intestinal nematodes were particularly common in the Southeast.

In Natives

INTESTINAL NEMATODE INFECTIONS. Pinworm is still common in the United States (Chapter 103.1). Infections with other intestinal nematodes are unusual, except in such populations as poor rural people in the South, inhabitants of Indian reservations, those in institutions for the mentally retarded, recent immigrants and migrant laborers from developing countries, and long-term residents (e.g., missionaries and Peace Corps volunteers) in developing countries.

The principal exception to the association of infection with residence in the tropics during the past few years is *S. stercoralis* (Chapter 105.2). This intestinal nematode can replicate in humans (i.e., has the potential to cause autoinfection). Therefore, infections can persist for many years. Strongyloidiasis continues to be diagnosed in the United States and Great Britain in former Far Eastern prisoners of war. In addition, the strongyloidiasis hyperinfection syndrome can occur in immunosuppressed and malnourished individuals, including those infected with HIV. All patients infected with this helminth should be treated.

TRICHINOSIS. This infection is becoming less common in domestic pigs, but epidemics associated with eating undercooked bear and wild boar have been reported during the past few years (Chapter 111). Certain ethnic groups, e.g., Vietnamese and Central Europeans, often prefer cured but undercooked pork sausage. Several epidemics have followed consumption of sausage prepared in this manner from infected pigs. The increasing use of microwave ovens, which do not always heat meat evenly throughout, may cause an increase in the incidence of trichinosis.

FISH-TRANSMITTED HELMINTHIASES. Diphyllobothriasis (Chapter 123.1) and anisakiasis (Chapter 116) are being recognized with increasing frequency in the United States. Fluke infections occur in people who ingest raw, inadequately cooked, or improperly salted or pickled freshwater or brackish-water fish: heterophyasis and metagoniomiasis (Chapter 119), clonorchiasis (Chapter 120.2), and opisthorchiasis (Chapter 120.1).

A digenetic trematode, *Nanophyetus salmincola*, has been reported to infect people in the Pacific Northwest of the United States who ingested incompletely cooked or home-smoked salmon or steelhead trout. About half of the patients with nanophyetiasis had abdominal pain or discomfort, loose stools or diarrhea and excessive bloating and gas, and/or eosinophilia. Clinical manifestations in other patients from Siberia with nanophyetiasis were dose related, i.e., those with heavier infection had greater symptoms. Praziquantel, 60 mg/kg body weight given in 3 divided doses in a single day, was curative. The life cycle of this parasite is similar to that of the other intestinal trematodes, *Heterophyes* and *Metagonimus*, and involves a mollusk, fish, and fish-eating definitive host. This zoonosis must be added to the list of potential infections associated with the habit of eating raw fish.

In Immigrants and Travelers. Many helminths are found in immigrants to the more developed countries from the tropics (Chapter 148) and in those who have lived for prolonged periods in less developed countries. The usual intestinal nematodes as well as the liver flukes (*C. sinensis* and *Opisthorchis viverrini*), the lung fluke (*P. westermani*), and *Schistosoma mekongi* and *S. japonicum* (Chapter 118) are sometimes found in emigrants from Southeast Asia. Those from the Caribbean may have intestinal nematode and *S. mansoni* (Chapter 118) infections. Those from Mexico and Central America may have intestinal nematodes. Epilepsy can be caused by cerebral cysticercosis, which is particularly common in Mexico (Chapter 124.1). Emigrants and visitors from Africa can have a multitude of helminth infections, including those with the intestinal nematodes, *S. mansoni* and *S. haematobium*, *T. saginata* (Chapter 123.2), *W. bancrofti* (Chapter 106.1), and *O. volvulus* (Chapter 108).

Acquired Immunodeficiency Syndrome. Because helminths, with rare exceptions, do not multiply within the human host, they do not cause opportunistic infections in patients with AIDS. The exception could be *Strongyloides*, which has the capability to autoinfect, causing long-lasting infections (Chapter 105.2). In the normal host it produces chronic gastrointestinal disease, which is often undetected. In immunocompromised individuals, e.g., those receiving corticosteroids and/or chemotherapy for malignancies, *Strongyloides* can produce a hyperinfection syndrome with rampant multiplication and dissemination of larvae throughout the lungs and other organs.

Other helminths, including schistosomes, ascarides, hookworms, flukes, and tapeworms, are not more frequent or more pathogenic in those with HIV infections.

CHEMOTHERAPY

Praziquantel. The introduction of effective and safe drugs to treat schistosomiasis has been a major achievement in the past years; metrifonate (for treating *Schistosoma haematobium*) and oxamniquine (for *S. mansoni*) have been replaced by praziquantel (for treating all *Schistosoma* species) (Chapter 118). Praziquantel gives high cure rates and usually requires only a single dose. Fortunately, the cost of this important drug has been decreasing as countrywide control programs are obtaining it in bulk and parasite resistance to the drug remains rare.

Praziquantel is also effective in treating other fluke infections, with the exception of *F. hepatica* (Chapters 119 to 121), and the tapeworms (Chapter 123). Most importantly, it has provided a specific agent to treat cerebral cysticercosis (Chapter 124.1).

Broad-Spectrum Anthelmintics. There are several excellent broad-spectrum anthelmintics available for treating intestinal nematode infections (Table 102–2). Thiabendazole is still the drug of choice for strongyloidiasis, although some recent investigations have shown that ivermectin can also cure this infection.

Mebendazole, in prolonged and high doses, followed by albendazole, which is better absorbed following oral ingestion, has been effective in treating some patients with hydatid disease (Chapters 124.2 and 124.3).

Ivermectin. This drug has been used as a single oral dose to treat and control onchocerciasis (Chapter 108). Commu-nity-based control programs in *Onchocerca*-endemic areas using mass semiannual and annual therapy with ivermectin have reduced community prevalence of microfilariae to levels that have lowered the infectious reservoir and disrupted transmission of onchocerciasis.

Ivermectin is also used for treating filariasis. As used in treating *O. volvulus*, ivermectin kills microfilariae but not the adult worms (Chapter 106). Combinations of ivermectin with diethylcarbamazine (DEC) or with albendazole, all given as single doses, may be more efficacious than any of these drugs alone. However, the mainstay of therapy for filariasis remains DEC. Ivermectin is also used in veterinary practice for treating and preventing canine heartworm and onchocerciasis in cattle. This drug has some therapeutic benefit against most nematodes, including intestinal parasites in humans.

SECTION A **Intestinal Nematode Infections**

102 *General Principles*

G. Thomas Strickland

MAGNITUDE OF THE PROBLEM. Intestinal nematode infections constitute by far the most common parasitic infections in humans, with one or more species infecting the intestinal tracts of well over one fourth of the world's population. *Ascaris* and *Enterobius* (pinworm) species infect 1 billion people each; *Trichuris* species and hookworm infect more than a half billion each; and including numerous transient pinworm infections, there are estimated to be over 25 million helminthic infections in the United States. In endemic areas where indiscriminate defecation is common, the prevalence of intestinal nematodes and protozoa may reach 85%, often with individuals being infected with more than one intestinal parasite.

Few enteric nematodes multiply in their human hosts. Infections thus tend to be self-limited over weeks or months to a few years if the individual is no longer subjected to repeated exposure from the environment. However, important exceptions exist, as with *Strongyloides stercoralis*, which may persist by autoinfection for more than 40 years. *Strongyloides* is also the only nematode infecting humans that has a free-living, as well as parasitic, generation in its life cycle. *Capillaria philippinesis* is the other nematode that may cause progressive "autoinfection." Like *Strongyloides*, *Trichuris* may rarely cause overwhelming superinfection in immunocompromised hosts. Systemic tissue migration is often associated with eosinophilia, another characteristic of nematode infections.

GENERAL MORPHOLOGY. The general structure of nematodes is diagrammed in Figure 102–1. Intestinal nematodes range in size from microscopic (*Trichinella*, *Strongyloides*, and *Capillaria*) to 30 to 35 cm or more (*Ascaris*). The elongated, cylindrical, unsegmented bodies are covered with a secreted, non-nucleated glistening *cuticula* with cephalic or caudal sensory papillae (amphids and phasmids). A muscular layer with the excretory system and longitudinal nerve trunks lies beneath the subcuticular secretory cells. The simple tubular alimentary canal includes an anterior buccal cavity (sometimes with teeth or cutting plates), a muscular esophagus, valve, midgut, rectum, and ventral cloaca. The smaller male has a single tubular reproductive system with testis, vas

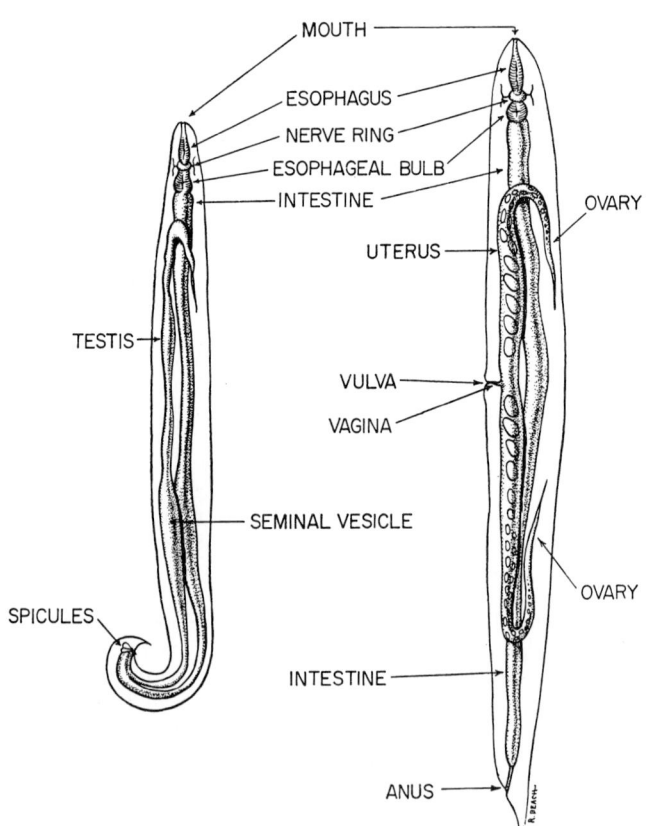

Figure 102–1. Morphology of a typical nematode.

deferens, seminal vesicle and ejaculatory duct with copulatory spicules, gubernaculum, and extremity. The larger female has a threadlike, tubular ovary, oviduct, seminal receptacle, uterus, and vaginal opening that may be single (*Trichuris*), double (pinworm), or multiple (others). Ova have a vitelline membrane in a chitinous shell with yolk granules and fertilized cell that may embryonate or have larval development when passed, as in hookworm and pinworm ova (Fig. 102–2).

TYPES OF INTESTINAL NEMATODE INFECTIONS. Intestinal nematode infections are best approached according to their types of life cycles in the human host and environment (Table 102–1).

Nematodes Limited to the Intestinal Tract (Chapter 103). Those nematodes that have life cycles that are limited to the gastrointestinal tract include pinworm (*Enterobius vermicularis*) (Chapter 103.1) and whipworm (*Trichuris trichiura*) (Chapter 103.2), as well as *Trichostrongylus* spp. and *C. philippinensis*. Pinworms and whipworms require no intermediate host, and development from larvae to adult worms is completed in the human gut. Embryonated pinworm eggs become infective as early as a few hours after deposition at 37°C, whereas whipworm eggs require a few days for the development of infective larvae within the shell. Although less well understood, *C. philippinensis* (Chapter 103.3) and *Trichostrongylus orientalis* (Chapter 103.4) are ingested as larvae (in raw fish or plants, respectively) that mature and remain localized in the human small bowel. Like *Strongyloides*, adult female *Capillaria* produce infectious larvae that may cause progressive, life-threatening autoinfections.

Unlike the other common intestinal nematodes, this group of nematodes do not migrate through the lung or the liver. Instead, eggs or larvae are ingested, usually from fecally contaminated hands, food, or water, and the larvae mature to adults in the intestinal tract. The adults then reside in the upper small bowel (*C. philippinensis*), cecum (*E. vermicularis*), or colon (*T. trichiura*) for 2 to 4 weeks (*E. vermicularis*) up to 20 years (*T. trichiura*). Adults measure from 2 mm to 5 cm and lay up to 10,000 eggs per day, which are usually shed in the stool (*E. vermicularis* are shed as adult worms) to complete the life cycle. With only rare exceptions, the adult worms remain in the intestinal lumen or wall and cause disease by local mucosal or perianal irritation and inflammation.

Nematodes That Migrate Through Lungs (Chapter 104). These have a more complex life cycle. Humans ingest embryonated *Ascaris* eggs that have matured for 1 to 2 weeks in the environment; these hatch in the small intestine. The larvae penetrate the bowel wall and migrate via the venous blood stream through the heart to the lungs, muscle, or meninges (Fig. 104–1). In the lungs, *Ascaris* larvae break into alveoli and move or are coughed up the trachea to be swallowed and mature into adult worms in the intestine. Adult female worms measuring up to 30 to 35 cm may then lay up to 200,000 eggs per day. This entire cycle takes approximately 3 months. Adult worms live about 1 year. *Ascaris lumbricoides* may infect one fourth of the world's population. Symptoms are caused by allergic reactions to the systemically migrating parasite, by mechanical obstruction, or by irritation from adult worms in the intestine.

The related ascarids, *Toxocara* and *Anisakis*, primarily cause infections in domestic animals (dogs and cats) and marine mammals (seals, dolphins, whales), which are the definitive hosts. Only the larval stages cause limited disease in humans, in whom the life cycle is not completed. Visceral larva migrans results from infection of children with larval dog or cat ascarids (Chapter 112), whereas superficial intestinal irri-

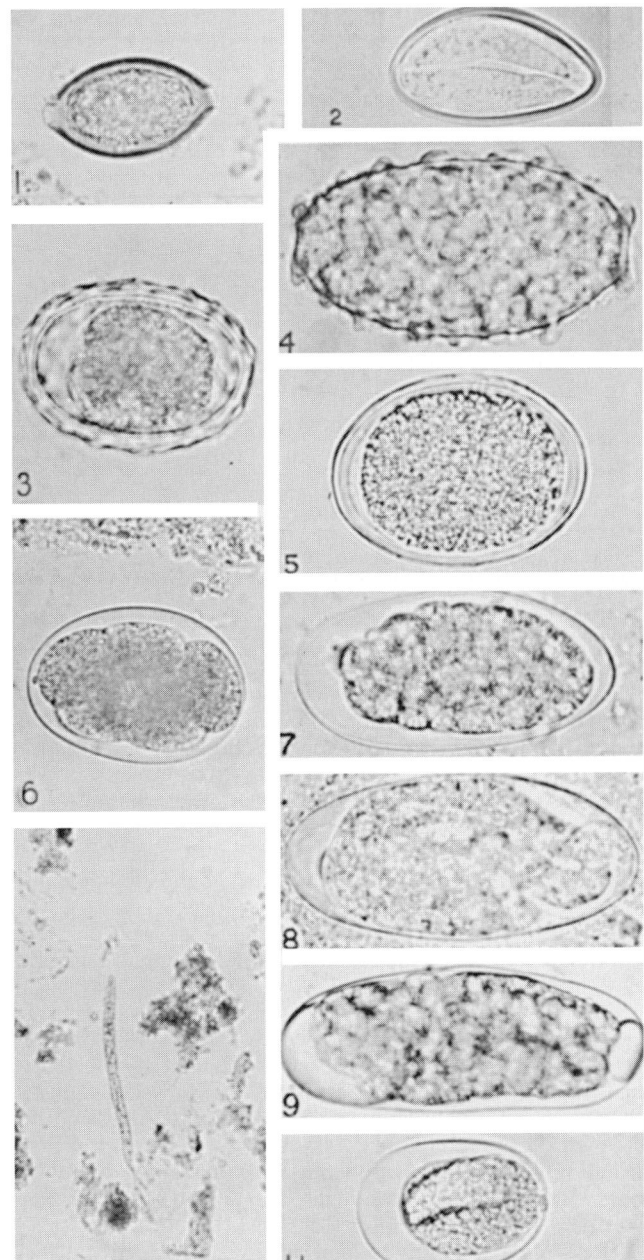

Figure 102–2. Some common nematode eggs; *(1)* whipworm, *Trichuris trichiura; (2)* pinworm, *Enterobius vermicularis; (3)* large roundworm, *Ascaris lumbricoides,* fertilized egg; *(4) A. lumbricoides,* unfertilized egg; *(5) A. lumbricoides,* decorticated egg; *(6)* hookworm egg; *(7)* immature egg of *Trichostrongylus orientalis; (8)* embryonated egg of *T. orientalis; (9)* egg of *Meloidogne javanica,* a plant nematode, which sometimes is found in stools; *(10)* rhabditiform larva of *Strongyloides stercoralis,* the stage usually found in the stool; *(11)* egg of *S. stercoralis,* rarely seen in the stool. All figures x 500 except *(10)* × 75.

tation or ulceration may follow ingestion of *Anisakis* larvae in raw fish (Chapter 116).

Nematodes That Migrate Through Skin and Lungs (Chapter 105). This cycle is the most complex: penetration of the skin by larvae that migrate through the venous blood to the lungs, into alveoli, and up the trachea and are swallowed. Adults develop in the intestine and produce eggs that are shed in the stool or hatch in the bowel (Figs. 105–2 and

TABLE 102–1. Types of Life Cycles of Enteric Nematodes

Host Tissue Involved	Infective Stage	Mode of Transmission	Parasites* Common Name	Parasites* Scientific Name
Intestine only	Eggs	Direct oral	Pinworm	*Enterobius vermicularis*
	Eggs		Whipworm	*Trichuris trichiura*
	Larvae		*Capillaria*	*Capillaria philippinensis*
	Larvae		*Trichostrongylus*	*Trichostrongylus orientalis*
	Larvae		Anisakis	(*Anisakis* spp)
Intestine and lung	Eggs	Direct oral	Roundworm	*Ascaris lumbricoides*
	Eggs		Visceral larva migrans	(*Toxocara canis* and *T. cati*)
	Larvae		Trichinosis	*Trichinella spiralis*
	Larvae		Eosinophilic meningitis	(*Angiostrongylus cantonensis*)
	Larvae		Eosinophilic gastroenteritis	(*Angiostrongylus costaricensis*)
Skin, lung, and intestine	Larvae	Skin	Hookworm	*Ancylostoma duodenale* and *Necator americanus*
	Larvae		Cutaneous larva migrans	(*Ancylostoma braziliense*)
	Larvae		Threadworm	*Strongyloides stercoralis*
	Larvae	?Arthropod	Pseudohookworm	*Ternidens diminutus*

*In parentheses are related parasites that complete their life cycles in animal hosts; *Toxocara* (dog and cat ascarids that cause visceral larva migrans in children) and *Ancylostoma braziliense* (dog hookworms that cause cutaneous larva migrans) are discussed in detail in separate chapters, as is trichinosis and *Anisakis*.

105–4). Intestinal nematodes transmitted in this manner probably cause greater morbidity and mortality than the others. Hookworm causes potentially severe anemia on a global scale (Chapter 105.1). Hookworm infections are usually limited to within 2 to 5 years after the last exposure. In contrast, *Strongyloides stercoralis* is capable of completing its life cycle in the same human host and can persist by "autoinfection" for 40 to 50 years (Chapter 105.2). In immunocompromised individuals, *S. stercoralis* may produce a life-threatening clinical syndrome of "hyperinfection."

The canine hookworms that cause cutaneous larva migrans in humans remain in the skin and fail to complete their life cycle in humans (Chapter 115).

CONTROL. General control measures include community-based education (about hygienic practices), socioeconomic development (with improved sanitary facilities, water supplies, and food handling), and individual or selected mass chemotherapy. Although many nematodes are eradicated by broad-spectrum agents, e.g., mebendazole, most clinicians would reserve therapy in endemic areas to a targeted population with heavy or symptomatic infections, especially after the characteristic peak transmission season for that area.

TREATMENT. A number of relatively safe, effective drugs are available for the treatment of the intestinal nematodes (Table 102–2). Mebendazole and albendazole have broad ranges of activity and are effective against hookworms, *A. lumbricoides*, *T. trichiura*, and *E. vermicularis*. Pyrantel pamoate has activity against all of these common intestinal nematodes

except for *T. trichiura*. Other drugs, e.g., bephenium hydroxy-naphthoate, pyrvinium pamoate, piperazine, and levamisole, have more restricted spectrums of activity and, in several instances, are more toxic but less expensive than mebendazole, albendazole, or pyrantel pamoate. Thiabendazole is the treatment of choice for *S. stercoralis*. The pharmacology and untoward effects of these drugs are reviewed below. Specific details of therapy are covered separately in the sections on individual nematodes.

Mebendazole (Vermox). Mebendazole, a benzimidazole, is highly effective for the treatment of disease due to *A. lumbricoides*, hookworms, *T. trichiura*, and *E. vermicularis*. It is also used for the treatment of *C. philippinensis*, *Angiostrongylus cantonensis*, and *Trichinella spiralis* infections and for other conditions, e.g., echinococcal cysts and *Mansonella perstans* infection.

Mebendazole inhibits microtubule assembly and blocks glucose uptake by nematodes. Immobilization and death of susceptible nematodes follow, but it can take several days for nematodes to be cleared from the gastrointestinal tract. Mebendazole also inhibits the development of the ova of hookworms and *T. trichiura*.

Mebendazole is available in 100-mg chewable tablets. It is poorly absorbed orally and extremely well tolerated at the dosages used to treat intestinal nematode infections. Transient abdominal pain and diarrhea occur in some persons. Occasionally, *A. lumbricoides* will migrate to the pharynx during mebendazole therapy, but this is not a contraindication to its use. Rarely, mebendazole causes leukopenia, agranulocytosis, or hypospermia. These untoward effects are more likely when prolonged, high-dose therapy is used, as in the treatment of echinococcosis.

Albendazole (Zentel) and Flubendazole. Albendazole has a spectrum of anthelmintic activity similar to that of mebendazole, but albendazole has the advantage of being effective when administered as a single dose for the treatment of *T. trichiura*, *A. lumbricoides*, and the hookworms. Albendazole is consequently better suited for mass treatment programs. Albendazole is also better absorbed than mebendazole from the gastrointestinal tract, and its primary metabolite, albendazole sulfoxide, is scolicidal for echinococcal cysts. Albendazole has replaced mebendazole for the treatment of echinococcal cysts, and it is also effective for the treatment of neurocysticercosis.

TABLE 102–2. Efficacy of Broad-Spectrum Anthelminthics

Infection	Mebendazole	Albendazole	Pyrantel Pamoate	Thiabendazole
Pinworm	+ + +	+ + +	+ + +	+
Roundworm	+ + +	+ + +	+ + +	+ +
Hookworm	+ + +	+ + +	+ +	+ +
Whipworm	+ +	+ +	−	−
Threadworm	−	+	−	+ +

−	Less than 30% cured.
+	30 to 60% cured.
+ +	60 to 85% cured.
+ + +	Greater than 85% cured.

Albendazole is formulated in 200-mg tablets and as a 2% oral solution. It is usually well tolerated when administered as a single dose for the treatment of intestinal nematode infections. High-dose, prolonged therapy for echinococcal disease has been complicated by hepatitis and obstructive jaundice in a few patients.

Flubendazole, the parafluoro analogue of mebendazole, also has a range of activity similar to that of mebendazole.

Thiabendazole (Mintezol). Thiabendazole, also a benzimidazole, is one of the most potent anthelmintic drugs, but a high frequency of untoward effects has limited its use primarily to infections with *Strongyloides stercoralis* and *S. fuelleborni*, *Trichostrongylus* species, and *Angiostrongylus costaricensis*; cutaneous larva migrans; visceral larva migrans; and trichinosis. It has been used as an alternative drug for *C. philippinensis* and *Dracunculus medinensis*.

Thiabendazole is available in 500-mg tablets and as an oral suspension of 500 mg/5 ml. It is rapidly absorbed after oral administration. No parenteral preparation is available. This is a potentially important limitation in patients with disseminated *S. stercoralis* infection. The precise mechanism of action is unknown.

Side effects are experienced by approximately half of the persons treated with thiabendazole. The most frequent are nausea, vomiting, anorexia, and dizziness. Less common are diarrhea, epigastric pain, pruritus, drowsiness, giddiness, headache, hallucinations, leukopenia, crystalluria, olfactory disturbances, and allergic manifestations, including rash, erythema multiforme, and Stevens-Johnson syndrome. The release of helminthic antigens probably is responsible for some of the allergic reactions. Activities requiring alertness should be avoided during therapy. Thiabendazole should be given with caution to persons with hepatic disease or dysfunction, and it is relatively contraindicated in pregnancy.

Pyrantel Pamoate (Antiminth). Pyrantel pamoate is effective for the treatment of *E. vermicularis*, *A. lumbricoides*, and hookworms, but not *T. trichiura*.

Pyrantel pamoate is available in tablets with 125 mg of pyrantel base and as a suspension with 50 mg of base/ml. Pyrantel and its analogues are depolarizing neuromuscular blocking agents in susceptible helminths. They result in nicotinic activation and spastic paralysis of worms. Pyrantel also inhibits acetylcholinesterases.

Pyrantel has minimal toxicity at the dosages used to treat intestinal helminths. Mild gastrointestinal side effects, including anorexia, nausea, vomiting, and abdominal discomfort, are experienced by some persons. Headache, dizziness, rash, or fever occur on occasion. Pyrantel should not be used with piperazine, which produces hyperpolarization in helminths. The two appear to be mutually antagonistic.

Bephenium hydroxynaphthoate (Alcopar). This drug is used for the treatment of hookworm infections in some areas. It is more effective against *Ancylostoma duodenale* than against *Necator americanus*; a single dose of 5 gm of the salt (2.5 gm of base) is effective for the former, whereas five daily 5-gm doses are needed for the latter. Bephenium hydroxynaphthoate also has some activity against *A. lumbricoides*, and it has been used to treat persons with mixed hookworm and *Ascaris* infections. The drug is dispensed in small granules and is administered with water on an empty stomach, usually before breakfast. Bephenium is generally well tolerated, but nausea and vomiting occur on occasion.

Piperazine (Piperazine Citrate). Piperazine is effective for the treatment of *A. lumbricoides* and *E. vermicularis*, but it has largely been replaced by mebendazole or pyrantel pamoate, which are less toxic. In a few developing areas, piperazine is still used because it is inexpensive.

Piperazine salts are available as 500-mg tablets and as syrups or suspensions containing 100 mg/ml. The drug is well absorbed orally and is usually well tolerated. On occasion, there are gastrointestinal disturbances, transient neurologic side effects, or urticarial reactions. Visual disturbances, ataxia, and hypotonia occur rarely. Epileptic activity may be exaggerated, and piperazine should not be given to persons with a history of seizures. Neurotoxicity has also been observed in persons with impaired renal function.

103 Nematodes Limited to the Intestinal Tract (Enterobius vermicularis, Trichuris trichiura, *and* Capillaria philippinensis)

Donald A. P. Bundy and Edward Cooper

103.1 Enteriobiasis

DEFINITION. Enterobiasis is due to the intestinal nematode *Enterobius vermicularis*, the pinworm. *E. vermicularis* is an ancient parasite of humans; eggs of *E. vermicularis* in a coprolite from western Utah have been radiocarbon dated to 7837 B.C.

DISTRIBUTION. *E. vermicularis* is found worldwide in both temperate and tropical areas. It is the most common helminthic infection in the United States and Western Europe. The prevalence is greatest among young school-aged children living under conditions of high population density and indoor conditions.

ETIOLOGY. *E. vermicularis* was discovered by Linnaeus in 1758 and originally named *Oxyuris vermicularis*. The disease was referred to as *oxyuriasis* for many years. *E. vermicularis* infects only humans, although related pinworm species infect animals.

Morphology. Adult females are 8 to 13 mm long and up to 0.5 mm wide. The anterior extremity lacks a true buccal capsule. It is characterized by three labia and, laterally, by a pair of cephalic, winglike alae. The muscular esophagus terminates in a distinct bulb (Figs. 103–1*B* and 103–2*B*). The posterior tip of the female is distinctly attenuated and constitutes the posterior third of the worm (Fig. 103–1*A*). The reproductive system is T shaped. The vulva opens at the base of the T near the junction of the anterior and middle thirds of the body. The long, clear, pointed end of the female, the clear cephalic alae, and typical eggs within the uteri are demonstrated in Fig. 103–1. In cross section, adult females are characterized by their bilateral crests and characteristic eggs within (Fig. 103–2*A*). Males have a ventrally curved tail with caudal alae and a single large copulatory spicule. They are smaller than the females, with a length of 2 to 5 mm.

Life Cycle. Approximately 11,000 eggs are produced by each gravid female. The eggs are ovoid, 50 to 60 mm by 20 to 30 mm, and asymmetrically flattened on one side (Fig. 102–2). The shell consists of a thick outer albuminous layer, which has a role in adherence to objects in the environment; a thin inner hyaline layer; and the embryonic membrane.

At the time of oviposition, eggs contain larvae, which must undergo further maturation before they become infective. Atmospheric oxygen acts as a stimulus to development. At

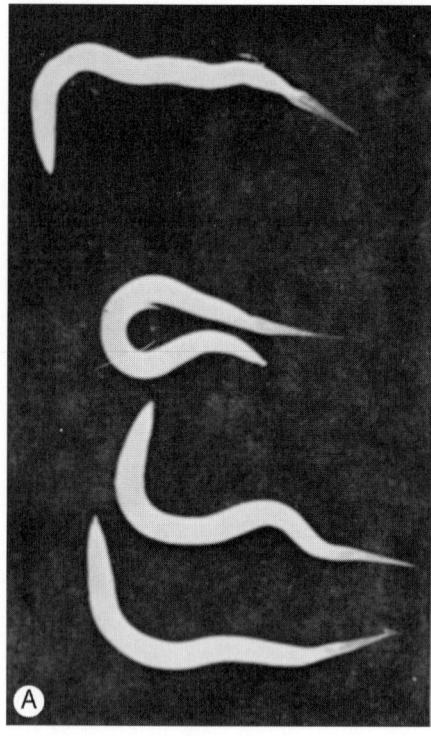

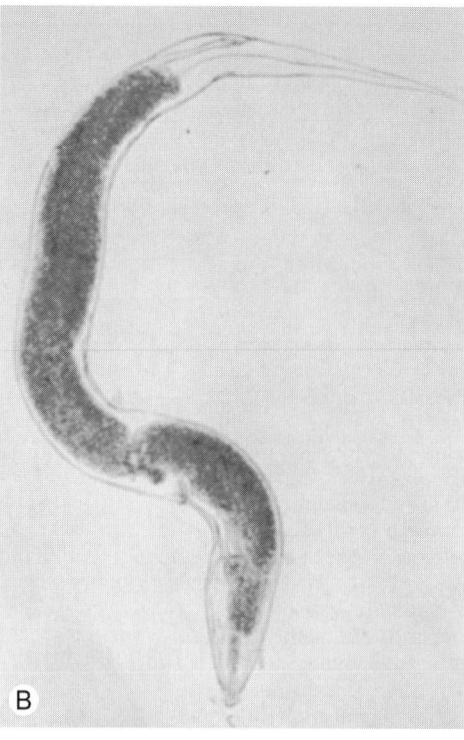

Figure **103–1.** *Enterobius vermicularis* adult female worms. *A,* Note shapes and the clear, attenuated, and pointed posterior end. *B,* Note cephalic alae, bulb behind esophagus, vulva, egg mass, anus, and pointed posterior end. (Courtesy of the Louisiana State University School of Medicine, New Orleans.)

body temperature, eggs can become infective within 6 hours. They begin to lose infectivity after 1 or 2 days under warm, dry environmental conditions. Egg survival is greatest under conditions of lower temperature and higher humidity. Eggs usually remain viable for <2 weeks; the maximum length of survival is reportedly 19 weeks.

After being ingested, eggs hatch in the upper small intestine, liberating larvae, which are 140 to 150 μm long. The larvae migrate to the region of the ileum, molting twice along the way to become adults. Copulation takes place in the lower small intestine. Adult females finally settle in the cecum, appendix, or adjacent areas of the ascending colon. Adult females live up to 13 weeks and males for approximately 7 weeks. The earliest that oviposition is observed is 5 weeks. Most patients have a few to several hundred adult worms.

At the time of oviposition, the gravid female leaves the colon and migrates out through the anus to lay her eggs while transversing the perianal or perineal skin. Female worms have been observed to move 2.5 inches in 30 minutes. Eggs are expelled by uterine contraction, death and disintegration of the worm, or disruption during scratching.

EPIDEMIOLOGY. *E. vermicularis* is found in children of all socioeconomic classes; males and females are equally susceptible. Infestation follows ingestion of eggs, which usually reach the mouth on soiled hands or contaminated food. The mechanical stimulation of migrating worms and the local irritation caused by the worms or deposited eggs often produce pruritus ani. Scratching results in contamination of the fingers and thereby contributes to autoinfection and spread to the environment.

In children, enterobiasis is most prevalent among school-

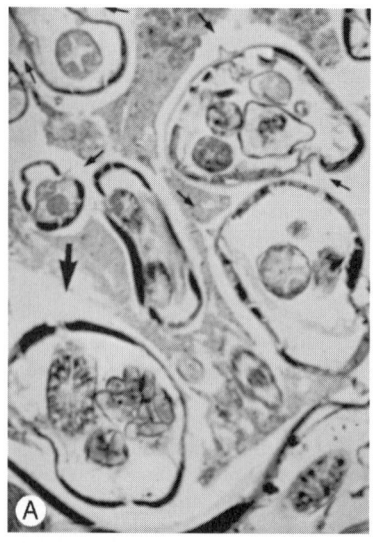

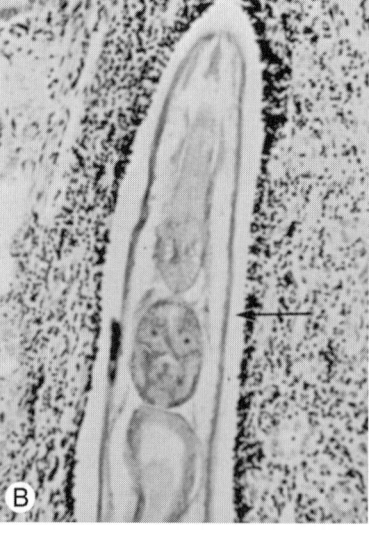

Figure **103–2.** *E. vermicularis* in appendix. *A,* Cross section of adult pinworms in lumen shows bilateral crests *(narrow arrows);* one worm contains eggs *(wide arrow). B,* Longitudinal section of adult worm in lymphatic nodule shows prominent esophageal bulb *(arrow).* (Courtesy of the Louisiana State University School of Medicine, New Orleans.)

aged children between the ages of 5 and 10 years; it is relatively uncommon in children <2 years. Poor personal hygiene and exposure to infected peers in the classroom are contributing factors. It has been postulated that as many as 20 to 30% of elementary school students in the United States are infected. The prevalence among children living in crowded conditions, e.g., summer camps or institutions has been as high as 80 to 90% in some reports. Transmission of *E. vermicularis* is also common within families of infected children. Anyone who handles children's clothing or bedding is at increased risk. Contrary to some previous reports, enterobiasis occurs commonly in tropical regions of the world and in both rural and urban populations. Enterobiasis has also been reported among male homosexuals, who may become infected through the practice of anilingus.

PATHOLOGY. The most important consequence of *E. vermicularis* is cutaneous irritation in the perianal region. The associated pruritus results in scratching and self-induced trauma to the skin. Perianal eczematous dermatitis with secondary bacterial infection results in some children. Folliculitis has been reported with enterobiasis in adults. The eosinophil count in persons with *E. vermicularis* infection is usually normal.

Vulvovaginitis occurs in some girls when worms migrate to the vagina. An association between *E. vermicularis* infestation and urinary tract infection in young girls has also been suggested. It has been postulated that perineal irritation due to *E. vermicularis* with associated scratching results in introital colonization with coliforms and thereby predisposes to urinary tract infection.

E. vermicularis does not produce significant intestinal pathologic changes. Worms are occasionally found in the appendix after surgical excision (Fig. 103–2A), but they do not cause acute appendicitis. On rare occasions, adult worms reach the peritoneum by traversing the female genital tract or migrating through a perforation in the bowel caused by appendicitis, diverticulitis, or intestinal malignancy. Granulomatous reactions to dead worms or eggs have been found in the vaginal wall, cervix, endometrium, salpinx, ovary, and peritoneum. On gross examination of the peritoneum, these appear as white or yellowish nodules, which may be confused with tuberculosis or metastatic neoplasms. Seen microscopically are granulomas with eosinophils and giant cells. Ova often remain well preserved even after worms are no longer identifiable. *E. vermicularis* has on rare occasions been found in other ectopic sites, e.g., the conjunctival sac and the external auditory canal. Eggs presumably were delivered there by soiled fingers.

CLINICAL CHARACTERISTICS. *E. vermicularis* infection can result in perianal or perineal pruritus, but the majority of those infected never come to clinical attention. In one large study in New England, anal pruritus and perianal skin lesions were only slightly more common among the infected cases than in controls. Nonetheless, there are certainly instances in which intense perianal or perineal pruritus is associated with *E. vermicularis* and responds to appropriate anthelmintic chemotherapy. On some occasions, enterobiasis is complicated by secondary bacterial dermatitis or folliculitis.

Local symptoms vary from a mild tickling sensation to acute pain. Symptoms tend to be most troublesome at night and may produce sleep disturbances, restlessness, and insomnia. No evidence shows that enterobiasis is responsible for nail biting or thumb sucking. Infection may be associated with a colitis that is reversible by anthelmintic therapy. It is unclear whether this is a rare event or one that has been overlooked previously. The psychologic impact on parents who learn that their child has "worms" can be distressing.

E. vermicularis is a well-recognized cause of vulvovaginitis in prepubertal girls. It has also been incriminated as a potential cause of secondary enuresis and urinary tract infection. In a few cases, peritoneal granulomas secondary to migrating *E. vermicularis* have been associated with abdominal pain in adult women. More commonly, peritoneal nodules are found incidently at the time of laparotomy (Fig. 103–2B).

DIAGNOSIS. The diagnosis of enterobiasis depends on the identification of adult worms or ova. Adult female worms are small, whitish, and pin shaped (Fig. 103–1A). They are occasionally seen in the perianal area or vagina of infected persons. The most successful diagnostic approach, however, makes use of a strip of transparent tape, which is held with the adhesive side out affixed to a tongue depressor. Before the person defecates or bathes on arising in the morning, the buttocks are spread and the tape is pressed against the anal or perianal skin several times. The strip is then transferred to a microscope slide with adhesive side down. Debris can be cleared by adding a drop of toluene. Eggs are prominent at low power. Examination of one smear detects approximately 50% of infections. Six consecutive negative swabs on separate days are necessary to exclude the diagnosis, but 90% of infections can be detected with three swabs. Parents can be taught the adhesive tape technique to obtain samples early in the morning. Other swab systems using glass or wooden applicators or cellophane have been used with similar efficacy.

Some physicians advocate a digital rectal examination to obtain anal material for analysis when the adhesive tape technique fails. Fecal material from the gloved finger is mixed with normal saline and examined under a coverslip. In contrast, routine stool examination for ova and parasites is positive in only 10 to 15% of infected persons. On rare occasions, *E. vermicularis* eggs are found incidentally in Papanicolaou-stained vaginal smears or in the urine sediment.

TREATMENT. *E. vermicularis* is susceptible to a number of anthelmintic drugs, with cure rates of >90%. Mebendazole is administered in a dose of 100 mg PO, repeated once or twice 2 to 4 weeks later. Pyrantel embonate is used in a single dose of 10 mg/kg, also repeated once or twice 2 to 4 weeks later. Albendazole is given as a single 400-mg dose to adults and children >2 years, repeated after 7 days. Children <2 years are given 100 mg in a single dose, also repeated after 7 days. Piperazine 50 mg/kg is effective, provided that this dose is taken on each of 7 successive days and repeated after 2 to 4 weeks. Because many members of the family are usually infected, treatment for the entire family is recommended. Benzimidazoles should not be given during the first trimester of pregnancy.

PREVENTION AND CONTROL. General and specific hygienic measures, including handwashing, particularly after bowel movements, are important. Simple laundering of clothes and linen is adequate to disinfect them. Linen and clothing should not be shaken because this can disseminate infective eggs. Extensive house cleaning is not necessary, but frequent vacuuming around beds, curtains, and other potentially contaminated areas is advised. Food should be covered to limit exposure to dust-borne eggs. Anthelmintic treatment of the entire household may be necessary to interrupt transmission in families with several small children.

Bibliography

Cram EB: Studies on oxyuriasis. XXVIII. Studies and conclusions. Am J Dis Child 65:46, 1943.

Haswell-Elkins MR, Elkins DB, Manjula K, et al: The distribution and abundance of *Enterobius vermicularis* in a South Indian fishing community. Parasitology 95:339, 1987.

Jones JJ: Pinworms. Am Fam Physician 38:159, 1988.

Liu LX, Chi J, Upton MP, Ash LR: Eosinophilic colitis associated with the larvae of the pinworm *Enterobius vermicularis*. Lancet 346:410, 1995.

Symmers E St C: Pathology of oxyuriasis. Arch Pathol Lab Med [Chicago] 50:475, 1950.

103.2 *Trichuriasis*

DEFINITION. *Trichuris trichiura* is among the most common of human helminths. Estimates suggest that there are around 900 million infections globally, about the same number as for hookworm and only slightly fewer than for *Ascaris*. Although this infection was traditionally thought to be benign, it is now recognized that intense infection is associated with colitis and a dysentery syndrome and that even moderate infection can impair development in childhood. The infection often occurs concurrently with ascariasis.

ETIOLOGY. *T. trichiura* infects humans as its primary host, but numerous members of the genus *Trichuris* infect domestic animals. *T. suis* is a morphologically identical parasite that rarely and abortively infects humans. *T. vulpis* of dogs has also been reported occasionally in humans, based on the larger size of its eggs, although this may not always be a reliable criterion. The name *whipworm* derives from the morphology of the 3- to 5-cm adult. The anterior three fifths of the worm is threadlike, and the posterior two fifths is more substantial, containing the reproductive organs.

Life Cycle. The life cycle of the parasite (Fig. 103–3) begins with ingestion of the embryonated egg. The often cited descriptions of larvae hatching in and penetrating the duodenum appear to have been based on a misinterpretation of experimental infections. Larvae are now recognized to emerge in the cecum, where they penetrate the crypts of Lieberkühn and migrate within the mucosal epithelium. On moulting to the adult, the posterior end is projected out of the epithelium, leaving the threadlike anterior portion embedded in a syncytium created from epithelial cells. In contrast to most other helminths of humans, *T. trichiura* has no transient tissue migration at the larval stage; instead, the adult worm maintains intimate "intracellular" tissue contact throughout life. The mature female produces 2000 to 6000 eggs per day. The eggs are passed in feces, where they must mature in soil for a period that varies with temperature but is at least 10 to 14 days. About 3 months is required for a patent infection to be produced from the ingestion of eggs. Adult worms may persist for years.

EPIDEMIOLOGY AND DISTRIBUTION. *Trichuris* is distributed worldwide. It is prevalent generally in the same distribution as *Ascaris*, wherever fecal contamination of moist soils allows maturation of eggs. The egg is less resistant to low temperatures and drying than the eggs of *Ascaris*, and so trichuriasis is relatively more common in areas where warm, moist soil and shade prevail. In many areas of the developing world, where latrines have been installed, the incidence of soil-transmitted nematodes is still high because of the practice of using untreated fecal matter as fertilizer (night soil). *Trichuris* eggs are commonly found on vegetables that have been fertilized with night soil. As with other helminths, the intensity of infection in communities is uneven, with most individuals harboring few worms and a few individuals harboring disproportionately large numbers. Thus, in a community where the average worm burden is 100 worms, some individuals harbor several thousand. These individuals appear to be predisposed to intense infection, for immunologic or ecologic reasons, and tend to reacquire infections of above average intensity even after successful treatment. The intensity of infection is age related, with the most intense infections typically occurring in children of school age. Treatment of this age group has been advocated as a cost-effective

LIFE CYCLE of —

Trichuris trichiura

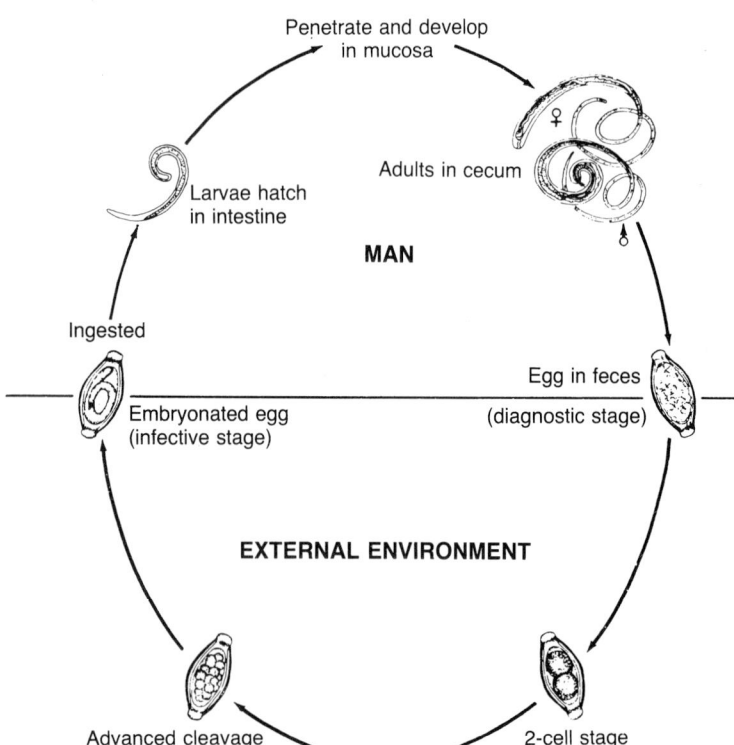

Figure 103–3. Life cycle of *Trichuris trichiura*. (From Melvin DM, Brooke MM, Sadun EH: Common Intestinal Helminths of Man. Atlanta, Centers for Disease Control. DHEW Publication No. [CDC] 75–8286, 1964.)

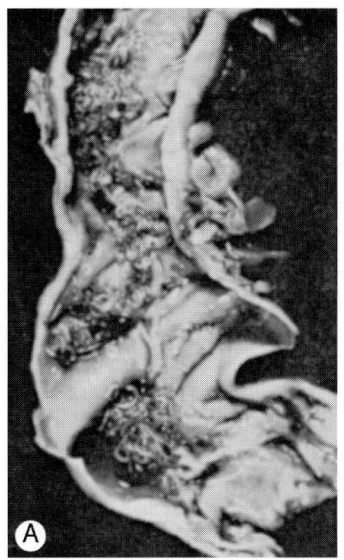
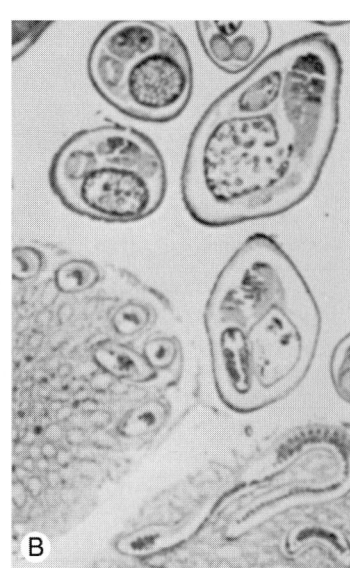

Figure 103–4. *A*, Masses of *T. trichiura* (whipworms) in colon of a child. *B*, Section of large intestine showing adult whipworms (natural infection of *T. vulpis* in dog). Thin anterior portions of worms are embedded and threaded in the mucosa; broader posterior parts of worms, containing eggs, are in lumen. (Courtesy of the Louisiana State University School of Medicine, New Orleans.)

approach to community-wide control because treatment of this group reduces transmission to the rest of the population.

PATHOLOGY AND CLINICAL MANIFESTATIONS. Infection results in a well-defined humoral immune response and an IgE-mediated local anaphylaxis, but a cell-mediated inflammatory response is conspicuously absent from the infected mucosa. Local eosinophilic infiltration is present in the submucosa, and in heavy infection the bowel wall may be edematous and friable. Under these circumstances, the mucosa may bleed easily, but the worms do not actively suck blood. Blood loss from inflamed mucosa may be important in persons with marginal iron intake (Chapter 132.1). Heavy infection (Fig. 103–4) may be manifested by abdominal pain and chronic diarrhea. Rectal prolapse (Fig. 103–5) is described in patients with heavy infection. The clinical picture of trichuriasis has been divided into two descriptions, the classic dysenteric form (trichuris dysentery syndrome, massive infantile trichuriasis) and the more recently recognized milder form, chronic *Trichuris* colitis with growth retardation. The latter is not sharply demarcated from the former, but affected children are more likely to be brought to medical attention because of short stature or pica rather than because of chronic diarrhea. Finger clubbing and rectal prolapse with chronic

diarrhea in children are considered pathognomonic of trichuriasis in endemic areas. Recent studies suggest that infection not only may impair physical growth but also may affect cognitive ability. Given the occurrence of the most intense infections in children of school age, it has been suggested that infection may compromise education.

DIAGNOSIS, TREATMENT, AND PREVENTION. The diagnosis is made by finding the characteristic barrel-shaped eggs with their polar hyaline plugs in a stool specimen (Figs. 102–2[1] and 103–7). The eggs are usually about 50 × 20 μm but may be larger or abnormal in shape when the patient has been treated. Charcot-Leyden crystals are often present in stool, and eosinophilia (up to 15%) may be seen in peripheral blood.

Therapy of trichuriasis is more difficult than that of infections with other soil-transmitted nematodes. A 3-day course of either mebendazole 100 mg b.i.d. or albendazole 400 mg once a day is usually curative in heavy infections. A single dose of mebendazole 500 mg or albendazole 400 mg may be effective in mild to moderate infections and is appropriate for community treatment. Although high priority should be given to the treatment of pregnant women, these drugs should not be administered during the first trimester. Note

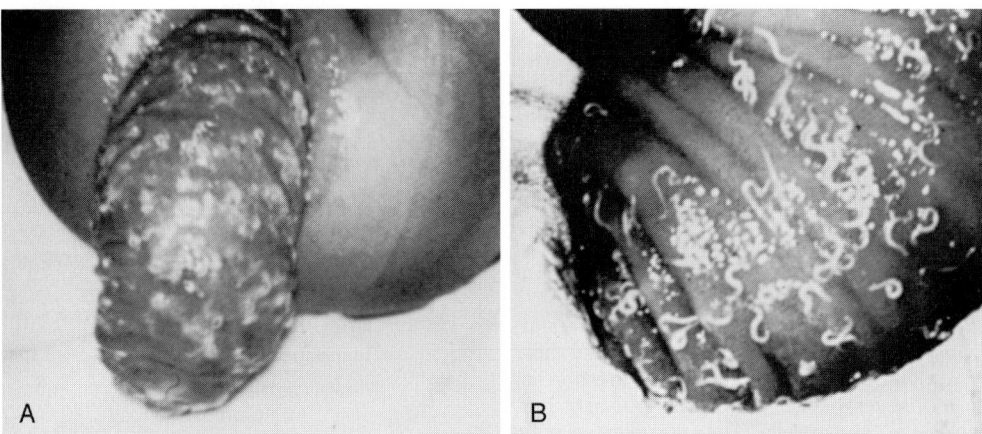

Figure 103–5. *A*, Prolapse of rectum in a heavy infection with *T. trichiura*. *B*, Adult *T. trichiura* attached to prolapsed bowel. (Both figures courtesy of Drs. P. C. Beaver and R. V. Platou, Tulane University School of Medicine, New Orleans.)

that all treatment regimens for trichuriasis are even more efficacious against ascariasis, which often occurs concurrently.

Bibliography

Abadi K: Single dose mebendazole therapy for soil-transmitted nematodes. Am J Trop Med Hyg 34:129, 1985.

Albonico M, Smith PG, Ercole E, et al: Rate of reinfection with intestinal nematodes after treatment of children with mebendazole or albendazole in a highly endemic area. Trans R Soc Trop Med Hyg 89:538, 1995.

Bundy DA: Epidemiological aspects of *Trichuris* and trichuriasis in Caribbean communities. Trans R Soc Trop Med Hyg, 80:706, 1986.

Bundy DA, Cooper ES, Thompson DE, et al: Age-related prevalence and intensity of *Trichuris trichiura* infection in a St Lucian community. Trans R Soc Trop Med Hyg 81:85, 1987.

Bundy DA, Cooper ES, Thompson DE, et al: Epidemiology and population dynamics of *Ascaris lumbricoides* and *Trichuris trichiura* infection in the same community. Trans R Soc Trop Med Hyg, 81:987, 1987.

Bundy DAP, Cooper ES: *Trichuris* and trichuriasis in humans. Adv Parasitol 28:107, 1989.

Bundy DA, Thompson DE, Golden MHN, et al: Population distribution of *Trichuris trichiura* is a community of Jamaican children. Trans R Soc Trop Med Hyg 79:232, 1985.

Cooper ES, Spencer JM, Whyte-Alleng CAM, et al: Immediate hypersensitivity in the colon of children with *Trichuris* dysentery. Lancet 338:1104, 1991.

de Silva DG, Lionel ND, Jayatilleka SM: Flubendazole in the treatment of *Ascaris lumbricoides* and *Trichuris trichiura*: A comparison of two different regimens with single-dose. Ceylon Med J 29:199, 1984.

Finzi-Smith J, Cooper E, Bennett F: Intestinal permeability, diet and growth. Lancet 338:1404, 1991.

Fishman JA, Perrone TL: Colonic obstruction and perforation due to *Trichuris trichiura*. Am J Med 77:154, 1984.

Forrester JE, Scott ME, Bundy DA, Golden MH: Clustering of *Ascaris lumbricoides* and *Trichuris trichiura* infections within households. Trans R Soc Trop Med Hyg 82:282, 1988.

Gilman RH, Chong YH, David C, et al: The adverse consequences of heavy *Trichuris* infection. Trans R Soc Trop Med Hyg, 77:432, 1983.

Kan SP: The anthelmintic effects of flubendazole on *Trichuris trichiura* and *Ascaris lumbricoides*. Trans R Soc Trop Med Hyg 77:668, 1983.

Lillywhite JE, Bundy DAP, Didier JM, et al: Humoral immune responses in human infection with the whipworm *Trichuris trichiura*. Parasite Immunol 13:491, 1991.

MacDonald TT, Choy MY, Spencer J, et al: The histopathology and immunohistochemistry of the caecum in children with the *Trichuris* dysentery syndrome. J Clin Pathol 44:194, 1991.

Nokes C, Bundy DAP: Does helminth infection affect mental processing and educational achievement? Parasitol Today 10:14, 1994.

Ramalingam S, Sinniah B, Krishnan U: Albendazole, an effective single dose broad spectrum anthelmintic drug. Am J Trop Med Hyg 32:984, 1983.

Ramdath DD, Simeon DT, Wong MS, Grantham-McGregor SM: Iron status of schoolchildren with varying intensities of *Trichuris trichuria* infection. Parasitology 110:347, 1995.

103.3 Intestinal Capillariasis

DEFINITION. A small intestinal nematode related to *Trichuris trichiura* causes serious infections in areas of the Philippines and Thailand. *Capillaria philippinensis*, in the order Enoplida, superfamily Trichuroidea, is capable of autoinfection and therefore may cause extensive pathologic change of the small intestine after a relatively light exposure.

ETIOLOGY. The 2- to 4-mm adults are threadlike; the female has an esophagus in the anterior half of the body and reproductive organs in the posterior half, which may contain both eggs and the free larvae that are responsible for autoinfection and multiplication. The adults are in the mucosa of the small bowel and cause a syndrome of chronic diarrhea and wasting that may be fatal if untreated. The infection is spread by ingestion of several species of freshwater fish that have infectious larvae within muscle. The natural reservoir host has not been identified, but fish-eating water birds are probable. Monkeys can be experimentally infected but have not been found to be infected in the wild. The custom of

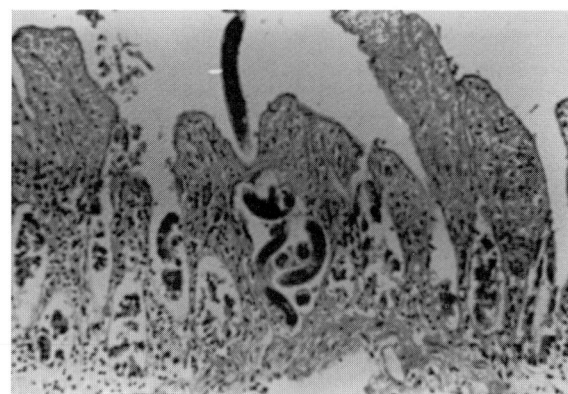

Figure 103–6. *Capillaria philippinensis.* Three transverse sections of larval *C. philippinensis* embedded in intestinal glands (× 100). (Courtesy of Armed Forces Institute of Pathology, Photograph Neg. No. 69–1065.)

eating raw fish probably determines the transmission of infection. Outbreaks have occurred when fecal contamination of freshwater lagoons has allowed eggs from infected patients to be disseminated in large numbers to a local source of fish.

EPIDEMIOLOGY AND GEOGRAPHIC DISTRIBUTION. Most cases have been recognized in the Philippines, where the infection was first noted in the 1960s. Endemic areas are recognized in several provinces; both sporadic cases and outbreaks occur. A few cases have been reported from Thailand and may be expected in other areas of Southeast Asia where freshwater fish are eaten without cooking. There have been two case reports from Egypt.

PATHOLOGY, CLINICAL MANIFESTATIONS, AND DIAGNOSIS. Larvae from infected fish can invade the small bowel on

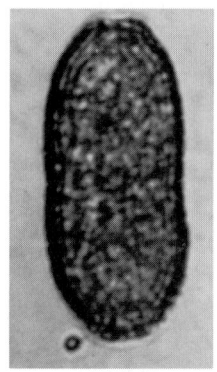
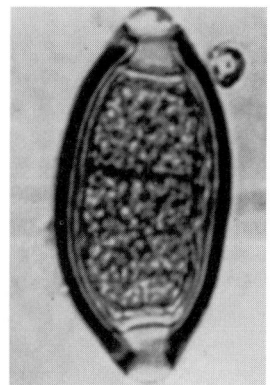

	CAPILLARIA PHILIPPINENSIS	TRICHURIS TRICHIURA
Size:	45 X 21 μm	52 X 26 μm
Shape:	peanut	ellipse
Plugs:	bipolar not protuberant	bipolar protuberant
Shell:	pitted	smooth

Figure 103–7. Comparison of *C. philippinensis* and *T. trichiura* eggs. (From Whalen GE, et al.: Lancet 1:13, 1969.)

ingestion and cause a chronic malabsorption-diarrhea syndrome characterized by induration and villous atrophy, which is most prominent in the jejunum (Fig. 103–6). The adults invade the mucosa and lamina propria. Inflammation is not prominent around parasites, but chronic inflammation is noted within the lamina propria. The small intestine may contain thousands of parasites because of the ability of the adult females to produce infectious larvae. The chronic diarrhea, which is usually watery, leads to electrolyte and protein abnormalities. Muscle wasting and myocardial degeneration ensue terminally. Death has been attributed to hypokalemic or metabolic cardiomyopathy or to secondary infection of debilitated patients.

The diagnosis is made by finding the characteristic eggs in the stool (Fig. 103–7); larvae may also be seen. Repeated examinations may have to be made because shedding of diagnostic stages may be infrequent or sporadic.

TREATMENT AND PREVENTION. Because autoinfection may lead to multiplication and clinical deterioration, infection with *Capillaria* should be promptly treated with mebendazole 100 mg b.i.d. or 200 mg once daily for 20 days. Albendazole is also effective at 400 mg daily in two divided doses for 10 days. Failure to complete the course usually results in relapse. Supportive fluid, electrolyte, and nutritional therapy may also be necessary. Cooking of fish prevents infection.

Bibliography

Alcantara AK, Uylangco CV, Cross JH: An obstinate case of intestinal capillariasis. Southeast Asian J Trop Med Public Health 16:410, 1985.
Cross JH, Basaca-Sevilla V: Albendazole in the treatment of intestinal capillariasis. Southeast Asian J Trop Med Public Health 18:507, 1987.

103.4 Trichostrongyliasis

DEFINITION. Trichostrongyliasis is an infection caused by any of several *Trichostrongylus* species. These nematodes are primarily parasites of herbivorous animals (e.g., sheep or cattle). Humans become infected when they ingest food or water contaminated by the feces of infected animals or humans. *Trichostrongylus* adults reside in the duodenum or the upper jejunum with their heads embedded in the mucosa.

DISTRIBUTION. *Trichostrongylus* species have been reported with variable frequencies from many areas of the world. Human infections appear to be most prevalent in the Middle East and Asia. The most thorough investigations have been carried out in Iran, where nine *Trichostrongylus* species have been identified in humans. In general, *T. colubriformis* is the species most frequently encountered in the Near and Middle East, whereas *T. orientalis* is the principal species in Asia.

ETIOLOGY

Morphology. *Trichostrongylus* adults are small, hairlike, reddish-brown roundworms. The males measure 4 to 6 mm in length, and the females, 5 to 8 mm. The head, which is unarmed, lies embedded in the mucosa of the small intestine. A distinct buccal capsule is absent, but there is a definite notch where the excretory pore opens. The males are characterized by a copulatory bursa with rays and spicules that are diagnostic for each species. In females, the paired reproductive system opens through a common vulva. The eggs are elongated and oval, possess a transparent hyaline shell, and resemble those of hookworms, except that they are larger (85 to 115 μm) and slightly more pointed at one or both ends.

When found in the feces, *Trichostrongylus* eggs are usually in the morula stage (Fig. 102–2 [7,8]). *Trichostrongylus* species cannot be differentiated from one another on the basis of the morphologic characteristics of their ova.

Life Cycle. Under favorable conditions of humidity and temperature, ova hatch within 24 to 36 hours. They are remarkably resistant to long periods of cold and desiccation. The hatched larvae pass through three free-living stages, reaching the infective stage in 60 hours or more. Eggs and larvae flourish in areas with shade, high humidity, and grass or carpet vegetation. Infection usually follows ingestion of larvae in contaminated food or water, although larvae can enter through unbroken skin. Unlike *Strongyloides stercoralis* and the hookworms, *Trichostrongylus* species do not need to migrate through the lungs for completion of the life cycle.

EPIDEMIOLOGY. *Trichostrongylus* species and related genera are common parasites of herbivorous animals, including cattle, sheep, donkeys, goats, deer, and rabbits. The use of sheep or cow manure as fertilizer contributes to the spread of infection in farming communities. Humans are often incidental hosts and vary in their susceptibility to various *Trichostrongylus* species. The prevalence of human infection may be as high as 1 or 2% in endemic areas. The use of night soil in Asia creates conditions favorable to the spread of *T. orientalis*, which appears to be spread primarily from humans to humans.

PATHOLOGY AND CLINICAL MANIFESTATIONS. Little is known about the pathology of human trichostrongyliasis. The usual site of infection is the duodenum or the upper jejunum. Adult worms are thought to suck blood at times and to damage the mucosa of the small intestine at or near their sites of attachment. Shortened villi have been observed in the small intestine of experimentally infected rabbits.

Most human infections are mild and asymptomatic, but epigastric pain, diarrhea, and flatulence have been observed in some. Rarely, anemia and emaciation have been associated with heavy infections. Eosinophilia is present in a minority of those infected, and on rare occasions, the percentage of eosinophils may exceed 25%.

DIAGNOSIS. The diagnosis of trichostrongyliasis depends on the identification of ova in the stool. Concentration techniques are often necessary to find the rare ova in the usual, light infection. Care should be taken to differentiate *Trichostrongylus* eggs, which are larger and more pointed on one or both ends, from those of the hookworms (Fig. 102–2). The diagnosis is occasionally made by finding *Trichostrongylus* larvae in duodenal aspirates. Identification of infecting *Trichostrongylus* species requires examination of adult worms, especially males.

TREATMENT. Thiabendazole 25 mg/kg b.i.d. (maximal daily dose of 3 g) for 2 days is recommended, but thiabendazole-resistant *Trichostrongylus* strains have been identified and thiabendazole is frequently associated with side effects. Pyrantel pamoate 11 mg/kg once (maximal dose 1 g) has been used as an alternative, with better results reported from Japan and Korea than from Iran. Mebendazole 100 mg b.i.d. for 3 days or a single dose of albendazole 400 mg is also effective.

PROPHYLAXIS. Effective prophylaxis against trichostrongylus involves sanitary disposal of human excreta and prevention of fecal contamination of the topsoil by infected animals. The treatment of infected herd animals, such as cattle or sheep, may also reduce the risk to humans. Potentially contaminated vegetables should be thoroughly cooked and water boiled before ingestion.

Bibliography

Ghadirian E: Human infection with *Trichostrongylus lerouxi* (Biocca, Chabaud, and Ghadirian, 1974) in Iran. Am J Trop Med Hyg 26:1212, 1977.

Hoste H, Kerboeuf D, Parodi AL: *Trichostrongylus colubriformis*: Effects on villi and crypts along the whole small intestine in infected rabbits. Exp Parasitol 67:39, 1988.

Markell EK: Pseudohookworm infection—trichostrongyliasis. N Engl J Med 278:831, 1968.

104 Intestinal Nematodes That Migrate Through Lungs (Ascariasis)

Donald A.P. Bundy and Nilanthi DeSilva

DEFINITION. Infection by *Ascaris lumbricoides*, the largest of the intestinal nematodes, is more prevalent worldwide than infection with any other helminth. It is estimated that the worldwide prevalence of human ascariasis is in excess of 1 billion. This is because the female worm produces a prodigious number of eggs that are relatively resistant to drying or to extremes of temperatures. *Ascaris* eggs in the soil are available to infect enormous numbers of people. The adult worms usually remain in the small intestine; passage of the larvae through the lungs is accompanied by pneumonitis, which is usually subclinical.

ETIOLOGY

Adult Worms and Ova. The cylindrical pink or cream-colored adult worm tapers at both ends. The male is smaller (120 to 250 mm by 3 to 4 mm) than the female (200 to 400 mm by 5 to 6 mm), and the male's posterior end is frequently slightly coiled or recurved. Females produce up to 200,000 fertilized or unfertilized eggs per day, which they deposit in the intestinal lumen. The 40 by 60 μm eggs have a characteristic mamillated outer coat and thick hyaline shell (Fig. 102–2[3–5]). *A. lumbricoides* has no important animal reservoir, although the morphologically similar *A. suum* may occasionally infect humans and *A. lumbricoides* may infect pigs. Isoenzyme electrophoresis and genetic studies have indicated, however, that even in communities where humans and pigs live in close proximity, the ascarids of humans and pigs form two closely related but separate species. Dog and cat ascarids of the genus *Toxocara* may infect but do not develop to sexual maturity in humans. The tissue-invasive larvae of these ascarids are responsible for the syndrome of visceral larva migrans (Chapter 112).

Development. The life cycle of *Ascaris* begins with the production of eggs by adult female worms in the human distal small intestine; these are excreted in feces (Fig. 104–1). The mamillated outer coat of the egg may be important in survival, in that it may cause soil particles to adhere to the egg, providing protection against complete desiccation. Under advantageous conditions of warm, moist, shaded soils, the embryo molts within the eggshell; the infectious stage is a second-stage larva. The period of development in the soil is temperature dependent and may range from 2 weeks to several months. The eggs are infectious by ingestion or possibly by inhalation of contaminated dust, but larvae do not hatch in soil and do not invade the skin. The larvae hatch in the jejunum, penetrate the intestinal wall, and migrate by way of the hepatic venules to the right side of the heart and the pulmonary circulation, where they break into the alveolar spaces and undergo two further molts. Most

LIFE CYCLE of—

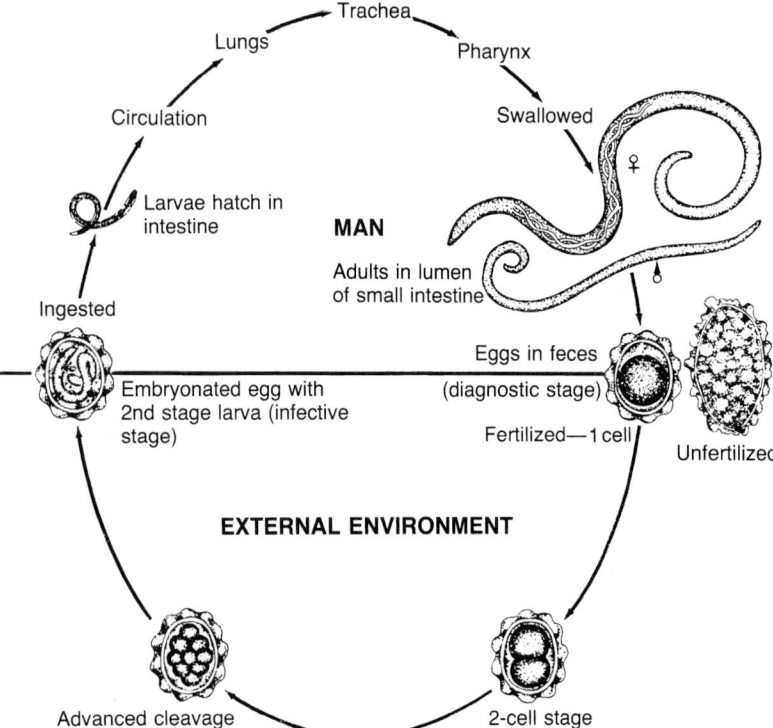

Ascaris lumbricoides

Figure 104–1. Life cycle of *Ascaris lumbricoides*. (From Melvin DM, Brooke MM, Sadun EH: Common Intestinal Helminths of Man. Atlanta, Centers for Disease Control, DHEW Publication No. [CDC] 75–8286, 1964.)

larvae will have reached the lungs by 2 weeks after ingestion of eggs. From the alveoli, the 1.5-mm-long larvae ascend to the trachea and are swallowed, undergo a last molt in the intestine, and develop to adults. Development from ingestion of eggs to the production of eggs may take from 10 to 12 weeks (Fig. 104–1). The number of adult worms per infected person may vary widely in an infected population; egg production per female worm decreases as the worm burden increases, and thus egg counts may not linearly reflect intensity of infection. Infections consisting only of female worms produce infertile eggs, which do not develop to the infectious stage. Occasional male-only infections result in no eggs in stool. Adults live for approximately a year.

EPIDEMIOLOGY. *A. lumbricoides* is distributed worldwide; an estimated 1.3 billion persons are infected. The infectious eggs are found in soil, where they remain viable for years. In the tropics, where moist, shaded soils afford perfect conditions, transmission of *Ascaris* is continuous. In regions where periods of aridity or temperature fluctuations may temporarily decrease the number of infectious eggs in soil, transmission of *Ascaris* may be seasonal. Clay soils favor *Ascaris* egg survival by retaining water around coated eggs and allowing them to withstand desiccation. Eggs may also be more efficiently spread from clay soil; rain may spatter them onto vegetables, and eggs mixed with clay may adhere to persons and clothing, increasing the chances for ingestion or inhalation. *Ascaris* eggs can withstand freezing, and therefore, the infection is common even in northern temperate zones. Pawlowski has estimated that 9×10^{14} eggs per day contaminate the world's soil, which is a tribute to the enormous egg production of the worm and the general inadequacy of sanitation.

The prevalence of infection varies geographically. Approximately 71% of all infections have been estimated to occur in Asia (especially in China, India, and Southeast Asia), 13% in Latin America and the Caribbean, and 8% in sub-Saharan Africa. Areas of sporadic transmission may have small localized areas of high transmission. Only cold, arid climates are free of infection. Even in areas of high prevalence, the intensity of infection in the population is not uniform. A small proportion of the population usually harbors the majority of worms, and this subset of heavily infected persons is concentrated in children <10 years. In addition, both individuals and families are predisposed to a high or low intensity of infection, such that the size of the worm burden reacquired after successful treatment is positively associated with the intensity of infection before treatment. Factors that determine predisposition probably include both differences in exposure to infection and variations in individual susceptibility.

PATHOLOGY. Most infected persons are asymptomatic. However, because so many individuals have infections, the overall morbidity caused by ascariasis is considerable.

Pulmonary Phase. Larvae migrating through the lungs may induce pulmonary hypersensitivity or inflammation in sensitized hosts, which can be manifested as asthma. This is especially likely to occur in localities where transmission is seasonal or sporadic, e.g., in Saudi Arabia. The reaction to migration of larvae in tissue may be severe. Eosinophilic inflammation and granulomatous reaction may be seen in the lungs, and local hypersensitivity may cause hypersecretion of mucus, bronchiolar inflammation, and serous exudate. In severe instances, vasculitis with perivascular granulomatous reactions may occur in conjunction with degenerating larvae. This spectrum of eosinophilic inflammation fits into the clinical entity referred to as Löffler's syndrome. Sputum containing eosinophils or Charcot-Leyden crystals may be produced, and larvae can sometimes be recovered from the sputum or gastric aspirate.

Other allergic manifestations to migrating larvae are also encountered, including episodes of urticaria, which are more common at the end of the pulmonary phase.

Intestinal Phase. The intestinal phase of the infection is generally asymptomatic, but it is now widely accepted that even moderately heavy infections can affect the health, growth, and physical fitness of children. *Ascaris* infection produces disturbances in the absorption of several nutrients including lactose, nitrogen, and vitamin A, all of which could contribute to growth faltering. Recent research also indicates that moderate to heavy worm burdens may adversely affect cognitive development in schoolchildren and that even light worm burdens may have a marked impact on the health of younger children.

Heavy worm burdens can cause much more serious complications; the most frequently reported, especially in children <10 years old, is obstruction of the terminal ileum by a bolus of worms (Fig. 104–2). Rarely, the section of intestine containing the bolus of worms may act as a fixed point on which the rest of the bowel twists, thus causing a volvulus. Ileocecal intussusception as well as solitary intestinal perforation has been attributed to *Ascaris*, but the causative role of *Ascaris* in these cases is not always clear.

Migrating Adult Worms. Other complications of ascariasis result from the tendency of the adult worms to migrate. Numerous stimuli have been held responsible for worm migration, including fever, medication, anesthesia, and diet. Some drugs used to treat other parasitic infections may not kill *Ascaris* and stimulate migration. Male worms are thought to be more prone to migrate and be expelled, which may explain the frequency of female-only infections. Worms migrate up or sometimes down the gastrointestinal (GI) tract and may cause bile duct obstruction (Fig. 104–3) or bile duct perforation with bile peritonitis or liver abscess. Appendicitis (Fig. 104–4) and pancreatic duct obstruction with peritonitis are rarely reported. These occur infrequently (about 1 to 2 cases per 1000 *Ascaris* infections) in an individual who is infected. However, with >1 billion people infected with *Ascaris*, complications associated with worm movement commonly occur in those living in endemic areas. When they do occur, the complications of ascariasis are associated with a case-fatality rate of about 5%. The possibility of *Ascaris* infection should be kept in mind before treating patients with medicines or anesthetics that may induce migration and increase the chance of obstruction or perforation.

IMMUNE RESPONSE. Although cross-sectional studies of communities infected with *Ascaris* often show features consistent with the development of immunity to the parasite, examination of antibody responses to *A. lumbricoides* has not shown humoral immunity to have a role in limiting infection. Antibodies to both adult and larval *Ascaris* antigens simply reflect the intensity of infection and do not protect against heavy infections.

CLINICAL MANIFESTATIONS AND COMPLICATIONS

Pulmonary Migration. *Ascaris* larvae usually cause few symptoms along their migratory path, but in sensitized hosts, pulmonary manifestations may be noted starting within 1 week after ingestion of eggs of either *A. lumbricoides* or *A. suum*. Fever, cough, wheezing, and dyspnea can be accompanied by sputum production, sometimes with small amounts of blood; chest pain and cyanosis are noted in the most severe cases. Chest film examination may show various unilateral or bilateral abnormalities, ranging from nodular densities to diffuse interstitial patterns. The illness may persist as long as larvae continue to pass through the lungs but usually is limited to several weeks. Leukocytosis is frequently associated, and there may be marked eosinophilia, fulfilling the picture of Löffler's syndrome. Severe pulmonary inflamma-

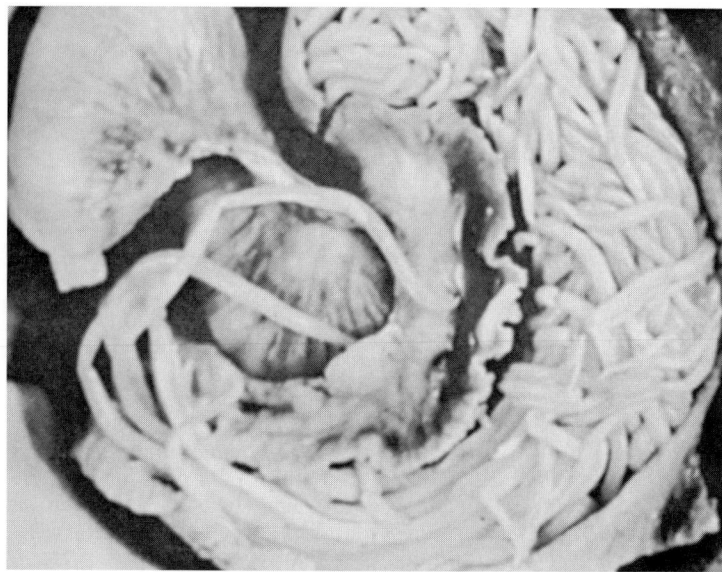

Figure 104–2. Terminal part of ileum opened, showing obstructing bolus of ascarids. (Courtesy of Drs. D. W. Aiken and F. N. Dickman. From JAMA 164:1317, 1957.)

tion associated with ascariasis has progressed to death, but this is rare.

Intestinal Infections. Adult worms probably cause few symptoms, except in heavy infections and unusual circumstances. It is difficult to know how frequently abdominal discomfort, nausea, anorexia, and diarrhea are attributable to ascariasis, although these symptoms are common in patients who are harboring *Ascaris*. The more serious complications of ascariasis, resulting from migration of the adult worms, are unquestionably associated with symptoms. Migrating worms may reach the upper GI tract and be vomited or may be passed per rectum. A number of worms may intertwine

and form a bolus, which can cause partial or complete intestinal obstruction, with abdominal pain, vomiting, and occasionally a palpable abdominal mass (Fig. 104–2). Rarely, such a mass of worms may cause volvulus or lead to perforation of the small intestine. More frequently the migrating worms enter ducts or diverticuli, where they may perforate or cause obstruction. The common bile duct is perhaps the most often obstructed, causing biliary colic or cholangitis (Fig. 104–3). A worm that ascends higher in the biliary tree may result in

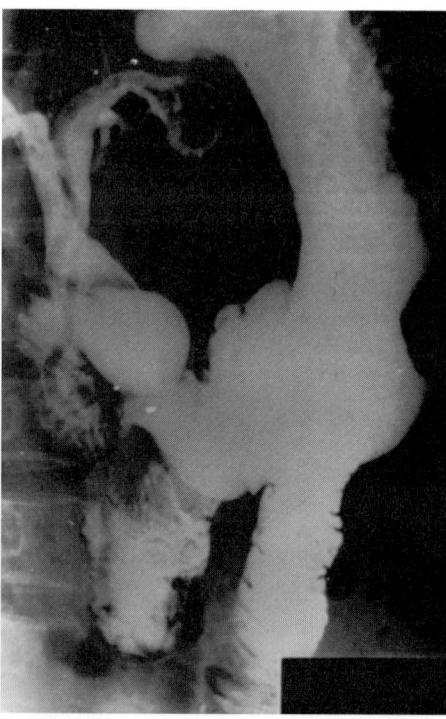

Figure 104–3. Ascariasis. Adult worms (linear lucencies) enter the bile ducts through the ampulla of Vater as well as through a surgically created choledochoduodenostomy. Barium was given orally.

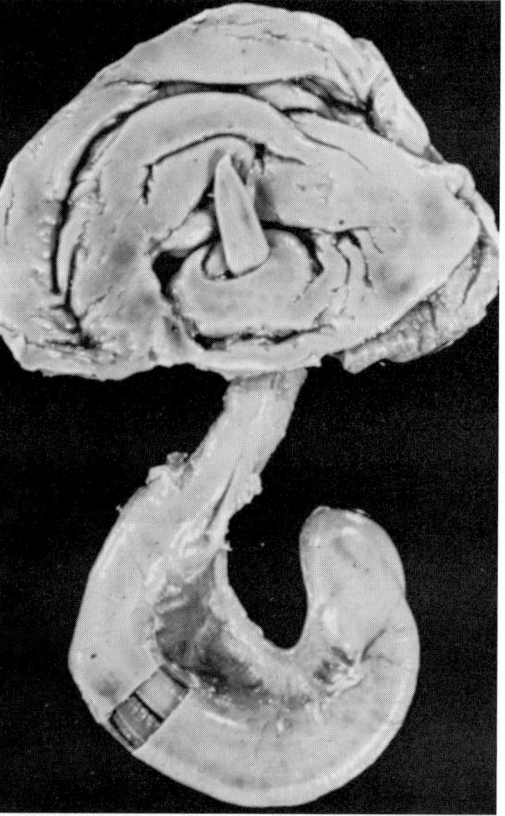

Figure 104–4. Adult *A. lumbricoides* in appendix. (Courtesy of the Louisiana State University School of Medicine, New Orleans.)

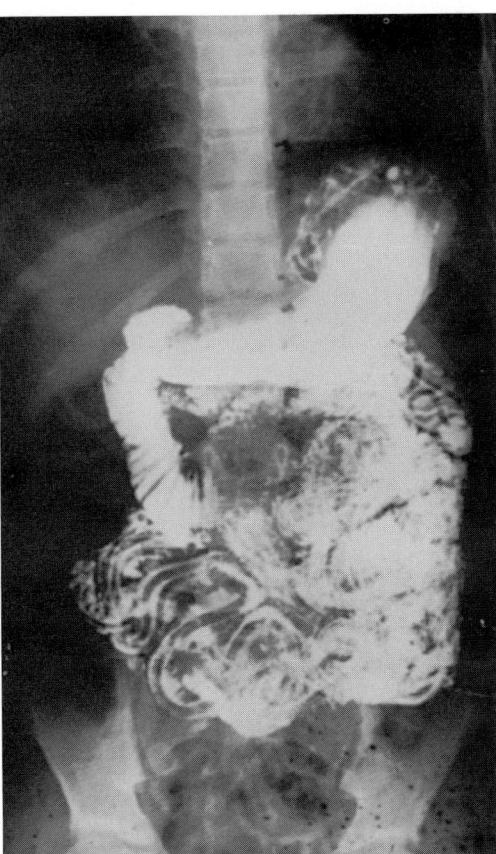

Figure 104–5. Adult *A. lumbricoides* visualized in small intestine by x-ray following barium. Ascarids may be detected at times without barium, by air contrast, but are less distinct. (Courtesy of Louisiana State University School of Medicine and the Charity Hospital of New Orleans.)

liver abscess or may penetrate the bile duct and lead to bile peritonitis. Pigmented calcium stones may occasionally form around a nidus of *Ascaris* eggs or fragments of dead adult worm. The pancreatic duct may also be obstructed and lead to pancreatitis of various degrees of severity. Appendicitis may be triggered by *Ascaris* obstructing the appendix (Fig. 104–4). Perforation of the bowel has been reported, usually with a history of acute abdominal pain followed by symptoms of peritonitis or localized abscess, but the role of *Ascaris* in causing the perforation is unclear. Intestinal obstruction is occasionally caused by adhesions attributable to extraintestinal *Ascaris*.

DIAGNOSIS. The diagnosis of ascariasis usually is easily made by stool examination. Characteristic eggs (55 to 75 μm by 35 to 50 μm) may be seen on direct examination or may be concentrated by centrifugation techniques (Fig. 102–2[3]). Unfertilized eggs may be somewhat more difficult to recognize because of their atypical size and appearance (Fig. 102–2[4]). Decorticate eggs lacking the outer mamillated covering are sometimes produced (Fig. 102–2[5]), and these may be confused with the eggs of other nematodes; the thick hyaline shell is typical of *Ascaris*. Infections consisting of only male worms produce no eggs; if such infections are symptomatic, the worms may sometimes be detected radiologically as linear filling defects outlined by contrast media (Fig. 104–5). Intestinal worms may sometimes ingest barium and be seen as thin, curved linear densities after the barium meal has passed the portion of the intestine in which the worm resides. In cases of suspected biliary ascariasis or pancreatitis, duode-

noscopy with retrograde cholangiopancreatography can be very useful both in establishing a diagnosis and in providing a nonsurgical means of removing the worms from the biliary or pancreatic ducts. Ultrasonography is also a useful tool in the diagnosis of biliary ascariasis but is of less value in cases of pancreatitis.

TREATMENT

Chemotherapy. The treatment of ascariasis can be accomplished by several effective drugs. Pyrantel pamoate (10 mg/kg up to a maximum of 1 g) can be given as a single dose. Adverse effects include occasional GI disturbances, headaches, dizziness, rash, and fever. Mebendazole given at a dosage of 100 mg b.i.d. for 3 days or as a single dose of 500 mg is highly effective against ascariasis. Albendazole, a benzimidazole derivative with a broad spectrum of action like mebendazole, also has a similar efficacy: A single dose of 400 mg is sufficient to eliminate most infections. Transient GI discomfort and headache have been reported with both drugs. Neither drug should be administered during the first trimester of pregnancy because animal experiments have shown teratogenic potential. Albendazole is not licensed for general use in the United States. Piperazine in a single dose of 75 mg/kg (to a maximum of 3.5 g for adults and children >12 years old and a maximum of 2.5 g for children between the ages of 2 and 12) is also very effective. It has occasionally caused urticarial reactions, GI disturbances, and dizziness and on rare occasions may exacerbate epilepsy or cause ataxia, muscle weakness, and visual disturbances. It should be used only if any of the previously named alternatives are not available.

Supportive Therapy. The therapy of complications of ascariasis depends on the presentation. Intestinal obstruction may necessitate surgery, although patients who are clinically stable and well hydrated are often successfully managed conservatively with nasogastric suction, intravenous hydration, and antispasmodics followed by anthelmintics given by nasogastric tube once the obstruction has subsided. This is done to avoid paralyzing the worms in the ileum, where the paralyzed tangled mass could precipitate complete obstruction. Most affected patients respond to this course of management by passing numerous worms rectally. Obstruction of the bile or pancreatic ducts must be relieved endoscopically or surgically, but conservative therapy may be appropriate in simple biliary colic.

PREVENTION. Uncomplicated ascariasis in individual patients is relatively easy to treat. The more difficult problem is preventing reinfections, because the eggs may be stable in the environment for years. Soil treatments have been tried but are generally impractical, and sanitation must be adequate to prevent all untreated human waste from reaching the soil. However, chemotherapy targeted at school-age children or community-based mass chemotherapy is now considered a feasible and effective approach to worm control, because single oral dose treatment with mebendazole or albendazole is very effective, safe, and inexpensive. By targeting school-age children for repeated chemotherapy, the worm burden in the community can be reduced, thus alleviating morbidity and perhaps even reducing transmission.

Bibliography

Albonico M, Smith P, Hall A, et al: A randomized controlled trial comparing mebendazole and albendazole against *Ascaris, Trichuris* and hookworm infections. Trans R Soc Trop Med Hyg 88:585, 1994.

Bundy D, Medley G: Immuno-epidemiology of human geohelminthiasis: Ecological and immunological determinants of worm burden. Parasitology 104:S105, 1992.

Chan M, Medley G, Jamison D, Bundy D: The evaluation of potential global mortality attributable to intestinal nematode infections. Parasitology 109:373, 1994.

Crompton D, Nesheim M, Pawlowski Z: Ascariasis and its prevention and control. London, Taylor & Francis, 1989.

Elkins DB, Haswell-Elkins M, Anderson RM: The epidemiology and control of intestinal helminths in the Pulicat Lake region of Southern India. I. Study design and pre- and post-treatment observations on *Ascaris lumbricoides* infection. Trans R Soc Trop Med Hyg 80:774, 1986.

Elkins DB, Haswell-Elkins M, Anderson RM: The importance of host age and sex to patterns of reinfection with *Ascaris lumbricoides* following mass anthelmintic treatment in a South Indian fishing community. Parasitology 96:171, 1988.

Farthing M, Keusch G, Wakelin D: Enteric Infection 2. Intestinal Helminths. London, Chapman & Hall Medical, 1995.

Guyatt H, Chan M, Medley G, Bundy D: Control of *Ascaris* infection by chemotherapy: Which is the most cost-effective option? Trans R Soc Trop Med Hyg 89:16, 1995.

Khuroo M, Zargar S, Mahajan R: Hepatobiliary and pancreatic ascariasis in India. Lancet 335:1503, 1990.

Lord WD, Bullock WL: Swine ascaris in humans. N Engl J Med 306:113, 1982.

Pawlowski ZS: Ascariasis. Clin Trop Med Comm Dis 2:595, 1987.

Savioli L, Bundy D, Tomkins A: Intestinal parasitic infections: A soluble public health problem. Trans R Soc Trop Med Hyg 86:353, 1992.

Schulman A: Intrahepatic biliary stones: Imaging features and a possible relationship with *Ascaris lumbricoides*. Clin Radiol 47:325, 1993.

Stephenson L, Latham M, Adams E, et al: Weight gain of Kenyan school children infected with hookworm, *Trichuris trichiura* and *Ascaris lumbricoides* is improved following once- or twice-yearly treatment with albendazole. J Nutr 123:656, 1993.

Stephenson L, Latham M, Adams E, et al: Physical fitness, growth and appetite of Kenyan schoolboys with hookworm, *Trichuris trichiura* and *Ascaris lumbricoides* infections are improved four months after a single dose of albendazole. J Nutr 123:1036, 1993.

Thein-Hlaing, Myat-Lay-Kyin, Hlaing-Mya, Maung-Maung: Role of ascariasis in surgical abdominal emergencies in the Rangoon Children's Hospital, Burma. Ann Trop Paediatr 10:53, 1990.

WHO Model Prescribing Information—Drugs used in parasitic diseases. Geneva, WHO, 1995.

105 Intestinal Nematodes That Migrate Through Skin and Lung

Robert H. Gilman

105.1 Hookworm Infections

DEFINITION. Human hookworm disease (ancylostomiasis) is caused by *Necator americanus* and *Ancylostoma duodenale*. In addition, *Ancylostoma ceylonicum*, which infects a number of animals, is occasionally found in humans in restricted geographic areas. Hookworms have a complex life cycle of entering the skin, migrating through the lungs, and residing in the small intestine. The hallmark of hookworm disease is iron deficiency anemia due to chronic blood loss.

DISTRIBUTION. Hookworms are among the most important helminthic pathogens of humans. Both *A. duodenale* and *N. americanus* are widely distributed in tropical and subtropical Asia and Africa, but *A. duodenale* occurs in the Middle East, North Africa, and southern Europe. *N. americanus* is the predominant species in the New World, but focal sites of *A. duodenale* are in the Caribbean islands and in Central and South America. *N. americanus* is found sporadically in the southeastern United States. Human infection with *A. ceylonicum* has been reported in the Philippines and in Calcutta, India.

ETIOLOGY
Morphology

Adults. Adult hookworms are small, cylindrical, creamy-white nematodes. Males measure 5 to 11 mm long and 0.3 to 0.45 mm wide. The females are 9 to 13 mm long and 0.35 to 0.6 mm wide. Males and females of *A. duodenale* are slightly larger than those of *N. americanus.* The anterior end of *N. americanus* is sharply curved in a direction opposite to the curve of the rest of the body, giving the worm a hooklike appearance. The head of *A. duodenale* continues in the same direction as the curvature of the body.

Identification of hookworm species is based on the length, the number and arrangement of the teeth or cutting plates (Fig. 105–1), the length of the esophagus, the morphology of the bursa of the male, the position of the vulva in the female, and the size of the eggs. These points are summarized in tabular form for *A. duodenale* and *N. americanus* and for two closely related hookworm species in Table 105–1.

The posterior tip of male hookworms is expanded to form a typical copulatory bursa supported by fleshy rays with a pattern that is characteristic of the species. The alimentary canal and genital ducts open into this bursa. A pair of long copulatory spicules is regulated by an accessory copulatory device, the gubernaculum.

Females have a subterminal ventrally located anus on the conical posterior extremity. The reproductive system is double, the tubules of the ovary being coiled intricately over the alimentary canal and confined to the posterior two thirds of the body. The vulva is located ventrally at the junction of the anterior third and the middle of the body of *N. americanus* and at the beginning of the posterior third of the body of *A. duodenale.* During copulation, the copulatory bursa of the male surrounds the vulva, thus giving the spermatozoa access to the reproductive system of the female. After mating, the male becomes detached. Fertilization takes place in the upper portion of the uterus or in the seminal receptacle.

Ova. *N. americanus* produces an estimated 10,000 to 20,000 eggs per female per day, and *A. duodenale,* 10,000 to 25,000. The eggs of the two species are almost indistinguishable, differing only in size. *N. americanus* is 64 to 76 μm by 36 to 40 μm, and *A. duodenale* is 56 to 60 μm by 36 to 40 μm. The eggs are eliminated in feces in two- to eight-celled stages of cleavage. A clear space is present between the cells and the shell (Fig. 102–2*[6]*).

Host Virulence Factors. Filiform larvae of the L3 stage, the stage when larvae enter the skin, are stimulated to increased metabolic activity and feeding by various substances (e.g., human serum and reduced glutathione). This restimulation is necessary because the larvae are often in a state of reduced activity until they enter the human host. The reduction in activity probably permits an increase in their survival in the environment under relatively hostile conditions until they can find and enter a suitable host. These stimulated worms produce a polypeptide ASP-1, which is immunogenic and in preliminary studies in mice is a useful vaccine for inhibiting hookworm infection.

During skin penetration, infective hookworm larvae encounter hyaluronic acid as they migrate between epidermal keratinocytes and through the ground substance of the dermis. Hookworm larvae have a potent hyaluronidase that facilitates their passage through the epidermis and dermis during larval invasion.

In the intestine, and possibly before, the worms elaborate a number of substances to assist their survival. To resist the acute inflammatory response, they elaborate a glycoprotein that is a potent neutrophil inhibitory factor (NIF). This blocks the adhesion of activated human neutrophils to vascular endothelial cells as well as the release of hydrogen peroxide from activated neutrophils and the ingestion of serum opsonized particles by specifically inhibiting neutrophil binding to the integrin receptor CD11b/CD18.

In the intestine, hookworms produce a potent anticoagulant peptide (ACAP-1) that inhibits human coagulation factor XA. This anticoagulant is poorly immunogenic, permitting it

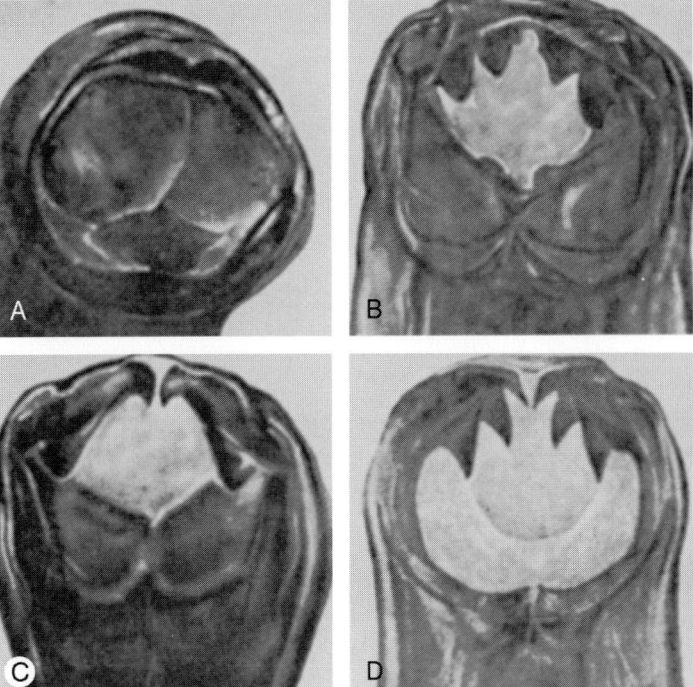

Figure 105–1. *A,* Mouthparts of *Necator americanus.* Note two pairs of chitinized cutting plates characteristic of this species. *B,* Mouthparts of *Ancylostoma duodenale.* Note two large pairs of teeth, each of the medial pair bearing a small accessory process. *C,* Mouthparts of *A. braziliense.* Note two pairs of teeth, a large outer pair and a small inner pair without accessory processes. *D,* Mouthparts of *A. caninum.* Note three well-developed pairs of teeth.

to act for prolonged periods without interference from the host immune response. In addition, platelet aggregation is inhibited and platelet-dense granules are decreased in number. Finally, fibrinolysis is stimulated by hookworm excretory-secretory products.

Other excretory-secretory products such as glutathione-*S*-transferase, an anti-IgG enzyme, and an acetylcholinesterase prevent the parasite from being expelled by inhibiting the host inflammatory and immune response.

The previous mechanisms not only permit hookworms to enter and feed effectively but also sustain chronic infections. Hookworm-infected individuals have detectable antibody to hookworm antigens; however, these antibodies do not protect individuals from new or repeated infections. Hookworm-infected individuals who receive treatment and remain in an endemic area usually become reinfected at the same intensity.

Development

Soil Stage. Hookworm ova are passed in the feces and develop in the soil (Fig. 105–2). Under optimal conditions of moisture and temperature (23 to 33°C), eggs hatch in 1 to 2 days. Each one liberates a rhabditiform larva, which is 250 to 300 μm long. The anterior end is bluntly rounded and characterized by a long, narrow buccal cavity. The larvae feed actively on bacteria and organic debris, gradually double in

TABLE 105–1. Differential Characteristics of Common Hookworms

	Necator Americanus	Ancylostoma Duodenale	Ancylostoma Braziliense	Ancylostoma Caninum
Shape	Head curved opposite to curvature of body, giving hooked appearance to anterior end	Head continues in same direction as curvature of body	Similar to *A. duodenale*	Similar to *A. duodenale*
Length				
Female (mm)	9–11 × 0.35	10–13 × 0.60	9–10.5 × 0.38	14 × 0.6
Male (mm)	5–9 × 0.30	8–11 × 0.45	8–8.5 × 0.35	10 × 0.4
Buccal capsule	A pair of dorsal and ventral semilunar cutting plates	Two pairs of curved ventral teeth of nearly the same size, rudimentary inner pair	Two pairs of ventral teeth, inner smaller	3 pairs of ventral teeth, inner smallest
Length of esophagus	0.5–0.8 mm in length. Opening small, oval, long axis dorsoventral	1.3 mm long. Opening oval, long axis transverse	Opening very small, long axis dorsoventral	Opening large, oval, long axis dorsoventral
Bursa of male	Long, wide and rounded, dorsal ray small, bipartite	Broader than long, dorsal ray tripartite	Small, almost as broad as long, with short stubby rays	Large and flaring, with long, slender rays
Caudal spine in female	Absent	Present	Present	Present
Vulva	Anterior third to middle of body	Posterior to middle of body	Posterior to middle of body	Posterior to middle of body
Size of eggs (μm)	64–76 × 35–40	50–60 × 35–40	55–60 × 34–40	60–75 × 38–45

Adapted from Belding DL: Textbook of Parasitology, 3rd ed. New York, Appleton-Century-Crofts, 1965, p 426.

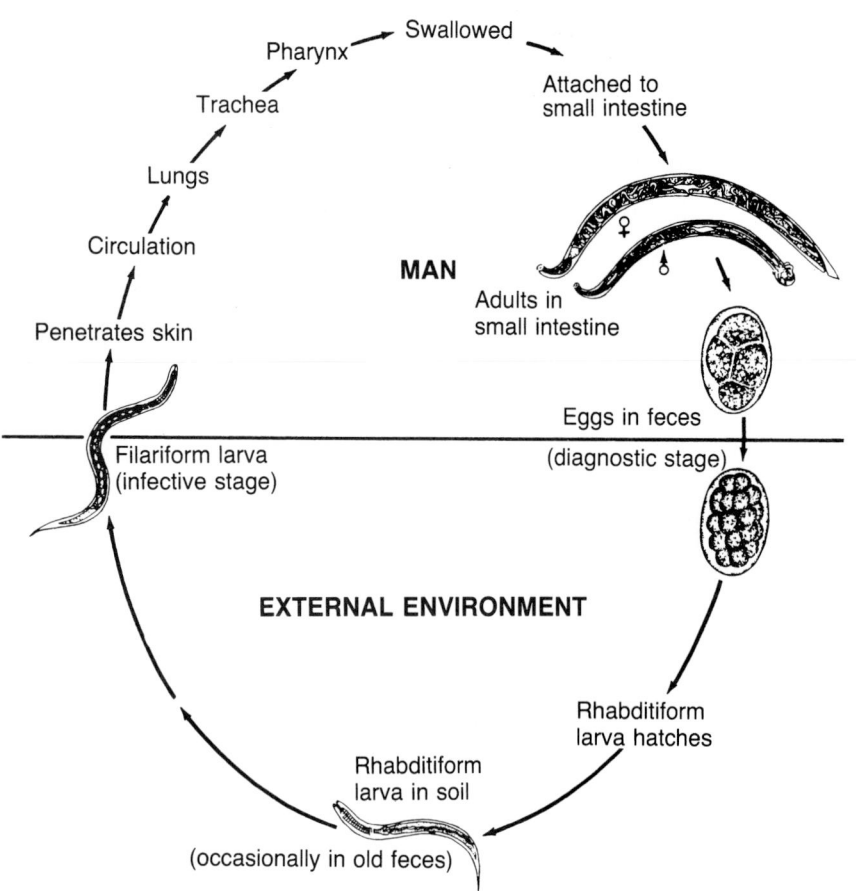

Figure 105–2. Life cycle of hookworm. (From Melvin DM, Brooke MM, Sadun EH: Common Intestinal Helminths of Man. Atlanta, Centers for Disease Control, DHEW Publication No. [CDC] 75–8286, 1964.)

size, and molt twice to become slender, nonfeeding, infectious third-stage or filariform larvae. Development from eggs to filariform larvae requires 5 to 10 days under favorable conditions.

Filariform larvae live in the top one-half inch of soil, with their ends projecting upward from the surface. They spend their lives within a few inches of where eggs were deposited. Under optimal conditions, the larvae may remain infective for several months; however, the death rate is highest in the first 10 days, and under tropical conditions, 90% of the larvae die in the first 3 weeks. Larvae survive best in light soil that is protected from drying or excessive water.

A. duodenale worms, faced with inclement seasonal conditions, have evolved a protective mechanism by which the hookworm larvae may remain dormant, a phase indicated by a subsequent decrease in total output of eggs. In Bengal, larvae acquired during the rainy season of 1 year remain dormant until just before the monsoon of the following year, when they resume development and mature. This phenomenon was further corroborated by the unusually prolonged prepatent periods (from initial infection until commencement of ova production) in volunteers given *A. duodenale* infection. Why *N. americanus* cannot respond to seasonal adversity by arrested development is not known.

Host Stage. Filariform larvae can migrate vertically through the soil to a potential host in response to contact (thigmotropism), carbon dioxide, or warmth. When contact is made with human skin, the larvae use discontinuities in the epidermis of the host, e.g., fissures or hair follicles, to penetrate the skin. They exsheathe as they enter the host. The usual site of entrance is the dorsum of bare feet or between the toes. Miners and farmers may acquire infection through the interdigital spaces of the hand.

The larvae gain access to the venous circulation and are carried to the lungs, where they break out into the alveoli and move through the respiratory tree to the pharynx. They are swallowed, pass through the esophagus and stomach, and arrive in the small intestine before molting to become adults.

Although infection is principally acquired through the skin, *A. duodenale* can enter by the oral route when larvae are present on vegetables grown in soil contaminated with feces. Maturation then occurs entirely in the intestine without tissue invasion. *A. duodenale* migrates to and remains dormant within the muscle of pigs, calves, rabbits, and other animals. Experimental models suggest that infection may result if meat of such a paratenic host is eaten uncooked, but whether this results in human infection is uncertain. Finally, transmammary transmission of *Ancylostoma caninum* is well documented in dogs. Circumstantial evidence from China shows that transmammary infection may occur in humans with *A. duodenale*.

Eggs first appear in the stool 5 weeks or more after invasion of the skin by filariform larvae. Maximal egg production occurs at 12 to 18 months. *A. duodenale* adults can live up to 6 to 7 years. *N. americanus* usually live 5 to 6 years but in one case persisted for as long as 15 years. In general, the worm burden begins to decline within 1 to 3 years in the absence of reinfection.

EPIDEMIOLOGY. Several factors favor the spread of hookworm infection: poor sanitary practices in which infected individuals defecate in areas frequented by others; shaded sandy or loamy soil; a warm, moist climate; and a population that does not wear shoes. Special habits or customs of a region are often important factors in transmission. In some regions, adults use certain defecation areas. These spots often provide the proper environment for the development of infective hookworm larvae. Adults revisit these sites daily, thus exposing themselves to infection and reinfection. Young children often defecate close to their houses in areas in which they play.

Cultural differences in attitude toward human excrement also contribute to the prevalence and intensity of infection. For example, the heavy infections attributable to the use of night soil as fertilizer in China contrast to the generally light infections found in India, where Hindu culture limits the use of human feces as manure.

Temperatures ranging between 26.7 and 32.2°C (80 and 90°F) are optimal for larval development. Larvae are readily killed by desiccation or freezing. Hookworm infection is also limited to those tropical and subtropical areas where the rainfall averages 50 inches or more per year.

Sex-associated differences in the prevalence or severity of infection have been observed in some populations but are probably due to occupational activities that result in different degrees of exposure. In the past, hookworm infection was common among underground workers who were exposed in mines or tunnels that lacked sanitary facilities. In hyperendemic areas, the prevalence of infection increases with age during childhood but plateaus during the second to fifth decade, suggesting that partial immunity may develop.

Hookworm infections were once common in the southern United States. A large survey commissioned by the Rockefeller Foundation in 1910 revealed a prevalence of 42% in some areas of the South. The treatment and control measures that followed led to a dramatic reduction in the disease. For example, in eastern counties of Kentucky, the prevalence dropped from 37% in 1914 to 4% in 1963. As the prevalence diminished, so did the intensity of infections and the frequency of symptomatic disease. Severe anemia due to hookworm disease is now extremely rare in the United States.

PATHOLOGY

Larvae. Penetration of the skin by infectious filariform larvae of *N. americanus* often causes local dermatitis, which is associated with edema, erythema, and a vesicular or papular eruption. These changes subside spontaneously in approximately 2 weeks unless secondary bacterial infections occur. Cutaneous reactions are less common with *A. duodenale.*

As the migrating larvae leave the capillaries of the lungs and penetrate into the alveoli, minute hemorrhagic lesions are produced. These are numerous in heavy infection and may be accompanied by an infiltrate with eosinophils and mononuclear cells. In general, the pulmonary reaction is mild.

Adults. Adult hookworms inhabit the upper half of the small intestine, where they attach and suck blood (Fig. 105–3). Transient injury to the intestinal mucosa results from the mechanical and lytic destruction of tissue at the point of attachment. Blood loss is due to bleeding at the site of attachment as well as to the blood removed by the worms. Less than half of the erythrocytes sucked into the worm are destroyed during passage through the worm's gut; the remainder enter the host's intestinal tract.

N. americanus seems to be more benign than *A. duodenale.* Blood loss is on the order of 0.03 mL/day per *N. americanus* adult and from 0.15 to 0.26 mL/day per *A. duodenale* adult. Hypoproteinemia frequently accompanies hookworm disease, but no evidence shows that hookworms themselves cause malabsorption or result in permanent damage to the intestinal mucosa.

CLINICAL MANIFESTATIONS. The clinical features of hookworm infection correspond to the life cycle of the organism and the intensity of infection.

Cutaneous Larva Migrans. Also called *ground itch* or *dew itch,* cutaneous larva migrans is associated with the penetration of the skin by filiform larvae. It most commonly affects travelers. It is associated with intense itching, and in some instances erythematous, pruritic papules develop at the penetration site as well as raised, reddened, serpiginous tracks that mark the migration of the worm. They are the most frequent on the lower extremities, followed by the buttocks and anogenital area, although both the trunk and upper extremities may also be affected. Only a minority of patients have eosinophilia. The skin lesions are easy to recognize and

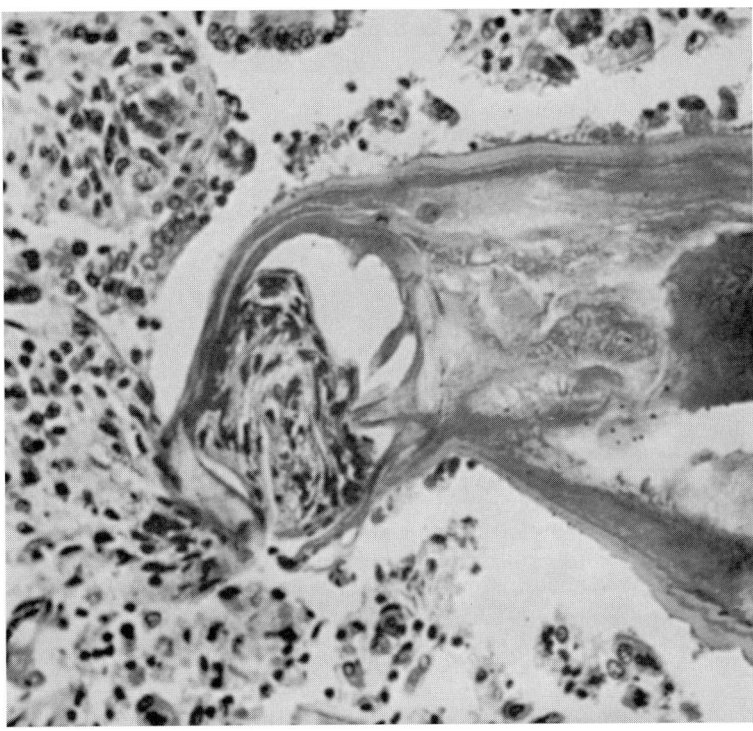

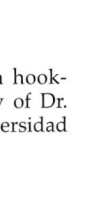

***Figure* 105–3.** Longitudinal section through hookworm attached to intestinal mucosa. (Courtesy of Dr. Pedro Morera, Facultad de Microbiologia, Universidad de Costa Rica.)

disappear rapidly, in nearly all cases, if appropriately treated. Skin lesions left untreated clear in weeks to several months.

Pulmonary Manifestations. As larvae pass through the lungs, patients may complain of cough and wheezing. In a small percentage of patients, infiltrates may appear on the chest film in conjunction with eosinophilia. This can lead to the diagnosis of Löffler's syndrome, but in general, the pulmonary manifestations are relatively mild.

Gastrointestinal Manifestations. Epigastric pain, flatulence, and tenderness occur early in the intestinal phase of infection. In experimentally induced human *N. americanus* infections, abdominal pain and flatulence appeared 35 to 40 days after exposure to filariform larvae; eosinophilia (1350 to 3828/mm³) peaked between 38 and 64 days; and eggs first appeared in the stool during the sixth week. The abdominal pain with hookworm infection may be severe enough to suggest peptic ulcer disease. On occasion, it is accompanied by diarrhea with blood and mucus. Rarely, massive exposure to filariform larvae results in acute gastrointestinal hemorrhage with uncompensated blood loss, a condition that is severe and potentially life threatening. This is most likely to occur in young children with heavy primary infections.

Anemia. The hallmark of chronic hookworm disease is iron deficiency anemia, the development of which depends on the number and species of infecting hookworm, the iron reserves and requirements of the host, and the availability of iron in the diet. Iron loss is due to bleeding at the site of hookworm attachment as well as to blood sucked into the worm. In areas where iron intake is high, even relatively heavy hookworm infections may not cause anemia. However, if the iron content of the diet is low, even moderate worm burdens can result in severe iron deficiency (Chapter 132.1).

Clinical Findings. The anemia of hookworm disease is usually chronic and may be severe, with hemoglobin levels in the range of 3 to 8 g/dL (Chapter 6). Lassitude, weakness, apathy, and depression are characteristic of anemia. On physical examination, the mucous membranes, conjunctivae, and skin appear pale. Iron deficiency has also been associated with koilonychia and angular stomatitis. In blacks, the skin may appear depigmented. A yellowish-green hue (chlorosis) was once commonly observed in Caucasians with severe hookworm disease but is now extremely rare.

Complications. Severe cases of anemia and hypoalbuminemia are accompanied by cardiovascular changes. Dyspnea, palpitations, and sinus tachycardia are common. The physical findings suggest a high-output state with widened pulse pressure, peripheral arterial bruits, a systolic flow murmur usually best heard in the pulmonic area, elevated jugular venous pressure, and cardiomegaly. Peripheral edema may be a manifestation of congestive heart failure and/or hypoalbuminemia. Cardiomegaly may be observed on the chest radiograph, and nonspecific ST-T wave changes may be present on the electrocardiogram. The effects of hookworm disease can be particularly severe in growing children and during pregnancy. Severe anemia is thought to stunt physical and intellectual growth and to contribute to increased maternal and neonatal mortality.

Eosinophilic Enteritis. The zoonotic hookworm, *A. caninum*, induces human eosinophilic enteritis by inducing allergic responses to its secretions. In Australia, this condition is not uncommon and patients are usually infected by single, sexually immature adult dog hookworms. Pathologically, these patients demonstrate edema and eosinophilic infiltration of the gut wall, ascites, and regional lymphadenopathy, as well as submucosa and lymph node granulomas with central eosinophil degranulation and degradation products. Ulcerations may develop around the hookworm bite site. Because *A. caninum* has an almost worldwide distribution, it

is probable that *A. caninum*–induced eosinophilic enteritis occurs outside Australia. Anisakiasis and enterobiasis, both of which can cause the same condition, must be excluded in the differential diagnosis.

Laboratory Findings. Erythrocytes are hypochromic and microcytic in patients with hookworm disease, and the reticulocyte count is low. The serum ferritin and iron levels are low, and the iron-binding capacity (transferrin) is elevated. The bone marrow iron stores are depleted. Eosinophilia is common, but the total white blood cell count is usually normal. Of note, hookworm infection was the most common explanation for eosinophilia among Southeast Asian refugees referred for evaluation of eosinophilia at one center. Low levels of parasite-specific IgG and IgE can be detected in serum. Hookworms do not produce malabsorption, but in some areas, iron deficiency due to hookworms may be present concurrently with folic acid deficiency due to other causes, e.g., tropical sprue. The effects of folic acid deficiency may become overt only after iron repletion.

Hypoalbuminemia often accompanies hookworm infection and generally correlates with the degree of anemia. The relative contributions of worm-induced intestinal protein loss, diminished protein intake, and decreased albumin synthesis in malnourished persons have not been determined, but in general, hookworm-infected patients are no more malnourished than uninfected subjects living in the same geographic area.

DIAGNOSIS. Hookworm disease should be considered in any patient from an endemic area who presents with anemia. The diagnosis is confirmed by identifying hookworm ova in the stool (Fig. 102–2[6]). It is not easy or necessary to differentiate between eggs of *N. americanus* and those of *A. duodenale*. Direct fecal examination in saline or an iodine solution is suitable for detection of clinically significant infections. This technique identifies persons with more than 1200 eggs per gram of stool. Zinc sulfate flotation or formalin-ether concentration techniques can be used to identify persons with lighter infections.

In stool specimens that have not been examined for several days, it may be necessary to distinguish between the rhabditiform larvae of hookworms and those of *Strongyloides stercoralis* (Fig. 105–5; Table 105–2). In contrast to *S. stercoralis*, a rhabditiform hookworm larva has a long buccal tube extending from its mouth to its esophagus. The presence of embryonated eggs and rhabditiform larvae in the same stool is suggestive of hookworm infection or a mixed infection with hookworm and *S. stercoralis*. If only rhabditiform larvae are present, *S. stercoralis* should be suspected, but it must be borne in mind that mixed infections are common. On rare occasion, it may be necessary to differentiate hookworm larvae from those of *Trichostrongylus* species, which are larger and more pointed at one end (Fig. 105–5).

TREATMENT

Infection Therapy. The therapy of hookworm disease consists of iron repletion and anthelmintic medications. The benzimidazoles, albendazole and mebendazole; pyrantel pamoate; and bephenium hydroxynaphthoate are effective against hookworms and generally well tolerated.

Unless there are mitigating circumstances, treatment of light, asymptomatic infections is not necessary in endemic areas where reinfection is likely. Persons with heavy infections or iron deficiency should be treated. Discretion should be used in the treatment of light, asymptomatic infections in travelers returning to the United States or Europe who will not have further exposure. Only rarely do they develop anemia, but most are treated because safe, effective medications are available.

Mebendazole and Albendazole. Mebendazole is effective

against both hookworm species; the standard dosage is 100 mg b.i.d. for 3 days. This regimen results in a cure rate of 76 to 95% and in reduction of mean egg counts by 84 to 99%. Mebendazole is also effective against *Ascaris lumbricoides* and *Trichuris trichiura* and is the drug of choice for persons concurrently infected with hookworm and these intestinal nematodes. Mebendazole is usually well tolerated, but it should not be used during pregnancy because of evidence of teratogenicity in animal studies. Albendazole is a newer benzimidazole. It has a spectrum of activity and toxicity similar to those of mebendazole but, in studies to date, has been effective when given as a single dose. Albendazole thus is ideal for mass treatment programs. It is not licensed for use in the United States.

Pyrantel Pamoate. This drug is more active against *A. duodenale* than against *N. americanus*. It is given as a single dose of 11 mg of pyrantel base/kg body weight (maximal dose 1 g) PO. Pyrantel is usually well tolerated but, on occasion, causes mild gastrointestinal side effects, headache, dizziness, or drowsiness. Transient elevations of liver enzymes have also been reported.

Bephenium Hydroxynaphthoate. This drug is also more active against *A. duodenale* than against *N. americanus*. The standard treatment regimen for *A. duodenale* is a single dose of 5 g of the salt (2.5 g of base). For *N. americanus* infections, three single daily doses of 5 g are needed to ensure a high cure rate. The drug is dispensed in small granules and is usually given with water on an empty stomach before breakfast. Bephenium can excite ascarides and cause their migration; mebendazole and albendazole are better choices when persons are concurrently infected with hookworm and *A. lumbricoides*.

Anemia Therapy. Rapid correction of anemia is best accomplished by administration of ferrous sulfate. Iron replacement is continued for 3 months after normal hemoglobin values are achieved to replete iron stores. Anemia can be corrected even without anthelmintic therapy. During pregnancy, anemia is treated with ferrous sulfate alone and anthelmintic treatment is delayed until after delivery because of the potential teratogenicity of the anthelmintic drugs.

Chronic anemia due to hookworm infection is usually well tolerated, even if severe, and blood transfusion is seldom indicated. If required, blood should be given carefully because it may lead to hypervolemia and precipitate congestive heart failure. The use of packed red blood cells, administration of diuretics, and monitoring of central venous pressure have been recommended when transfusions are given to minimize these risks. The potential for HIV infection is another reason to limit transfusions.

CONTROL. The transmission dynamics and morbidity associated with the major helminth infections (*A. lumbricoides*, *T. trichiura*, and the hookworms) depend on the size of the worm burdens. Thus, the important parameter for evaluating the impact of control on morbidity and transmission is the intensity of infection, which is measured by estimating the mean number of eggs excreted in a gram of stool. Worm burdens are not evenly distributed in infected individuals, but rather most individuals tend to have few worms while a relatively small percentage of people are heavily infected. This overdispersion of the intensity of infection has the effect that prevalence estimates, the most commonly used measures of infection in communities, can seriously mislead. The distribution of hookworm infection is independent of those of *Ascaris* and *Trichuris* infection, which frequently have a similar distribution.

Hookworm was rampant in the southeastern United States in the early 1900s but now has been eradicated owing to improved sanitation and the use of footwear. In developing countries, such an approach also would work but is blocked by poverty and the low priority that most governments give to installing the infrastructure necessary for clean water supplies and sewage disposal.

Therapy for children with hookworm and other nematodes has given mixed results in studies. In some, no long-term advantage has been found. However, especially in areas where hookworm infection is intense, such therapy produces benefits in growth rates, hemoglobin levels, appetite, and ability to perform physical tasks. Cognitive improvement, especially in terms of ability to do repetitive tasks, and intellectual concentration have also been demonstrated. Whether most of these effects are just due to the reversal of anemia is still open to question. In experimental models, hookworms not only affect the absorption of iron but produce malabsorption of carbohydrates and a protein-losing enteropathy. These latter two effects would not be ameliorated by just giving iron and raising the hemoglobin level.

Periodic deworming keeps the worm burden low, and increasing iron stores reverses iron deficiency anemia. Unfortunately, periodic worm therapy requires a well-organized health system to be sustainable and competes with other needs for limited health funds. Iron therapy to replace lost iron can be done by giving iron tablets, but these are unpleasant to take and are associated with gastric upset and poor compliance. Supplementation of staple foods with iron has also begun in many countries and is a simple and cost-effective method for reducing iron deficiency anemia caused by either hookworm or physiologic blood loss in women. Earlier fears that iron supplementation would increase the burden of infection associated with tuberculosis and malaria are not justified. Iron may decrease the absorption of zinc, which is an important detriment to iron supplementation of food.

Control of hookworm and its effects differ, depending on the level of development in the country, the intensity and geographic extension of infection, the rapidity of reinfection, and the frequency of anemia.

Bibliography

Crosby WH: The deadly hookworm: Why did the Puerto Ricans die? Arch Intern Med 147:577, 1987.

Farid Z, Nichols JH, Bassily S, Schulert AR: Blood loss in pure *Ancylostoma duodenale* infection in Egyptian farmers. Am J Trop Med Hyg 14:375, 1965.

Furmidge BA, Horn LA, Pritchard DI: The anti-haemostatic strategies of the hookworm, *Necator americanus*. Parasitology 112:81, 1995.

Gilles HM, Williams EJW, Ball PAJ: Hookworm infection and anaemia: An epidemiological, clinical, and laboratory study. Q J Med 33:1, 1964.

Gilman RH: Hookworm disease: Host-pathogen biology. Rev Infect Dis 4:824, 1982.

Holzer BR, Frey FJ: Differential efficacy of mebendazole and albendazole against *Necator americanus* but not for *Trichuris trichiura* infestations. Eur J Clin Pharmacol 32:635, 1987.

Hotez P, Capello M, Hawdon J, et al: Hyaluronidases of the gastrointestinal invasive nematodes *Ancylostoma caninum* and *Anisakis simplex*: Their possible function in the pathogenesis of human zoonoses. J Infect Dis 170:918, 1994.

Hotez PJ, Cerami A: Secretion of a proteolytic anticoagulant by *Ancylostoma* hookworms. J Exp Med 157:1594, 1983.

Hotez PJ, Pritchard DI: Hookworm infection. Sci Am 272:42, 1995.

Martinez-Torres C, Ojeda A, Roche M, Layrisse M: Hookworm infection and intestinal blood loss. Trans R Soc Trop Med Hyg 61:373, 1967.

Maxwell C, Hussain R, Nutman TB, et al: The clinical and immunologic responses of normal human volunteers to low dose hookworm (*Necator americanus*) infection. Am J Trop Med Hyg 37:126, 1987.

Migasena S, Gilles HM: Hookworm infection. Clin Trop Med Comm Dis 2:617, 1987.

Miller TA: Hookworm infection in man. Adv Parasitol 17:315, 1979.

Moyle M, Foster DL, McGarth DR, et al: A hookworm glycoprotein that inhibits neutrophil function is a ligand of the integrin CD11b/CD18. J Biol Chem 269:10008, 1994.

Nutman TB, Ottesen EA, Ieng S, et al: Eosinophilia in southeast Asian refugees: Evaluation at a referral center. J Infect Dis 155:309, 1987.

Pugh RNH, Teesdale CH, Burnham GM: Albendazole in children with hookworm infection. Ann Trop Med Hyg Parasitol 80:565, 1986.

Roche M, Layrisse M: The nature and causes of "hookworm anemia." Am J Trop Med Hyg 15:1030, 1966.

Schad GA, Chowdhury AB, Dean CG, et al: Arrested development in human hookworm infections: An adaptation to a seasonally unfavorable external environment. Science 180:502, 1973.

Variyam EP, Banwell JG: Hookworm disease: Nutritional implications. Rev Infect Dis 4:830, 1982.

105.2 *Strongyloides Infections*

DEFINITION. Strongyloidiasis, threadworm infection, results from infection by *Strongyloides stercoralis*, the female of which is usually embedded in the mucosa of the small intestine. *S. stercoralis* is less common than hookworm but may cause more severe, life-threatening illness. It is unusual among helminths in its ability to multiply within the host individual and maintain persisting infection for many years. Recognized since 1876, when Normand described the larvae in stools of French soldiers in Southeast Asia with Cochin-China diarrhea, *S. stercoralis* has a complex life cycle of entering the skin, migrating through the lungs, and residing in the small bowel (Fig. 105–4). Symptoms of chronic infection, which may persist for many years after exposure, are primarily episodic creeping urticaria (larva currens), epigastric or cramping abdominal pain, and diarrhea. The capacity of *S. stercoralis* to mature and multiply indirectly outside the host (heterogonic development) and its ability to overwhelm immunocompromised hosts with autoinfection are well recognized.

Although almost all *Strongyloides* infections are with *S. stercoralis*, the primate parasite *S. fulleborni* is recognized in humans in Africa and in Papua New Guinea.

ETIOLOGY AND DEVELOPMENT. As illustrated in Figure 105–4, the life cycle of *S. stercoralis* is complex. Like other intestinal nematodes, it may involve both host and soil stages. However, unlike most other helminths, the complete life cycle can also occur completely in the soil (free-living cycle) or completely in the host (internal or external autoinfection). The free-living cycle rarely extends beyond a single generation. Conversely, the autoinfection cycle is the basis of both persistence of infections for many years and the overwhelming hyperinfection syndrome. These three types of cycles thus involve (1) host and soil, (2) soil only (free-living or indirect cycle), and (3) internal or external autoinfection.

Host Stage. Human infection begins with exposure of the skin to filariform (third-stage) larvae that reside in fecally contaminated, moist soil for days to weeks (Fig. 105–4). These larvae are 400 to 500 μm long by 15 μm wide and have slender bodies, straight intestinal tracts, notched tails, and no visible genital primordium. Filariform larvae migrate through the venous blood stream to the lungs, where they penetrate into the alveoli and ascend the airways to the trachea and glottis before being swallowed to complete their life cycle in the small intestine. There, after two molts, adult females emerge and penetrate and reside in the superficial mucosa of the duodenum and jejunum. Adult females measure 2.2 mm long by 0.04 mm wide and have a delicate striated cuticula, elongated esophagus (less than one third of the body length), and paired ovaries, oviducts, and uteri. The evidence for the existence of male worms is controversial, and reproduction is believed to be parthenogenetic (c.f., *S.*

LIFE CYCLE of—

Strongyloides stercoralis

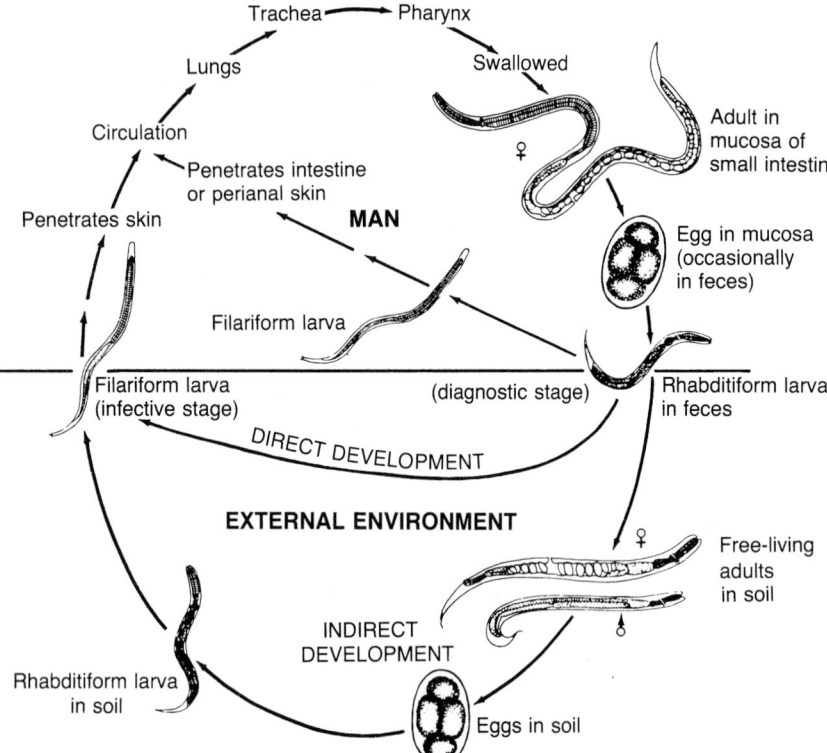

Figure 105–4. Life cycle of *Strongyloides stercoralis*. (From Melvin DM, Brooke MM, Sadun EH: Common Intestinal Helminths of Man. Atlanta, Centers for Disease Control, DHEW Publication No. [CDC] 75–8286, 1964.)

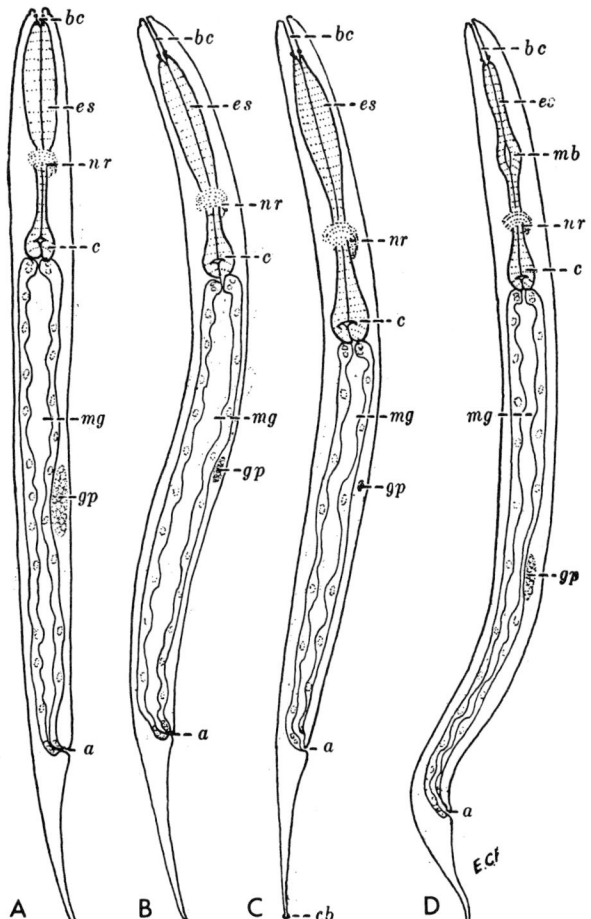

Figure 105–5. Figures of typical rhabditiform larval stages of: *A, Strongyloides; B,* hookworm; *C. Trichostrongylus;* and *D, Rhabditis* (ca. × 400). Explanation of labels: *a,* anus; *bc,* buccal chamber; *c,* cardiac bulb of esophagus; *cb,* beadlike swelling of caudal tip; *es,* esophagus; *gp,* genital primordia; *mb,* midesophageal bulb; *mg,* midgut; *nr,* nerve ring. (Drawing by E. C. Faust. From Beaver PC, Jung RC, Cupp EW: Clinical Parasitology, 9th ed. Philadelphia, Lea & Febiger, 1984.)

ratti in rats). Nearly 1 month after initial infection, the adult female begins to lay oval, thin-shelled, embryonated eggs (32 by 55 μm) that closely resemble hookworm eggs but are usually not seen because they rapidly hatch in the intestinal mucosa to produce first-stage, noninfectious rhabditiform larvae (Fig. 105–5). It is this rhabditiform larval stage that is characteristically found in the stool or the upper small bowel. The time from infection to the shedding of the larvae is usually 3 to 5 weeks. Rhabditiform larvae are shorter (200 to 250 μm) and wider (15 to 30 μm) than the infective filariform larvae and have a shorter buccal chamber and more prominent genital primordium when compared with the closely similar rhabditiform larvae of hookworm (Table 105–2). Un-

TABLE 105–2. Rhabditiform Larvae

Characteristics	Strongyloides	Hookworm
Size, average	225 × 16 μm	275 × 17 μm
Posterior tip	Blunter	Sharper
Buccal chamber	Short or absent	Long
Genital primordia	Larger	Smaller

der favorable soil conditions, rhabditiform larvae can transform into infected filariform larvae within 24 hours after fecal passage, a process that may also occur in the perianal region after defecation.

Soil Stage. Once passed into the soil, rhabditiform larvae may undergo two molts and mature over several days into infective filariform larvae (direct, homogonic cycle) that may survive for several weeks under moist conditions (Fig. 105–4). Alternatively, if conditions of light, warmth, oxygen, and moisture are optimal, noninfective rhabditiform larvae may develop into worms that are usually about half the size of the adults seen in the intestine (females about 1 mm and males about 0.75 mm long). Males are commonly found in free-living populations where meiosis is also demonstrable. Indeed, sexual reproduction may be the main purpose of this phase, which rarely lasts beyond a single generation and so has little role in the persistence of the parasite outside the host.

Autoinfection. Autoinfection may occur by rapid transformation of rhabditiform larvae to infectious dwarf filariform larvae in the gut lumen, where they penetrate the intestinal mucosa (*internal autoinfection*) to proceed via the lungs to maintain infection in humans (Fig. 105–4). Alternatively, the filariform larvae may develop in the colorectal area and penetrate the perianal skin (with resultant pruritic creeping eruption or *larva currens* and *external autoinfection*) before migrating through the lungs back to the small intestine.

EPIDEMIOLOGY

Distribution. Strongyloidiasis has a patchy, widespread distribution through warm, wet tropical and subtropical areas, and in temperate regions, it is encountered in institutions where sanitary facilities are poor or in moist conditions such as mines or tunnels. Some have conservatively estimated that 50 to 100 million people are infected. *Strongyloides* infections are endemic in tropical Asia, Africa, and Latin America as well as in the southern United States and southern and eastern Europe. Although infection is widespread, the prevalence is typically low (<10%) and often exhibits a slow increase with age. Some areas (e.g., Zanzibar, Amazonia) show higher local prevalences equivalent to other intestinal helminthiases, but these are anomalous. Prevalence is reportedly elevated in older HTLV-1–affected patients in regions where this virus is endemic (e.g., Japan, Caribbean).

Immigrants, travelers, or veterans from endemic areas, e.g., southern Asia may have prolonged infections. The latter are primarily older males, veterans with prior histories of having lived in endemic tropical areas, and those with underlying malignant, metabolic, pulmonary, or renal disease who may be chronically infected and have mild to moderate relapsing symptoms. A prospective study in rural Tennessee revealed *S. stercoralis* in 6.1% of 229 hospitalized patients and 2.6% of 346 domiciliary patients at the Johnson City Veterans Administration Hospital. One third of these patients had never traveled abroad. *S. stercoralis* was also found in 3% of schoolchildren in a prospective survey conducted in Clay County, Kentucky, an area where 24% of children harbored intestinal parasites (*Ascaris* 14%; *Trichuris* 13%; *Giardia* 3%). Although *S. stercoralis* and other species may be found in dogs, cats, or monkeys, humans are the principal reservoir. Because infection can be maintained for 40 years or more, and because effective therapy (thiabendazole) has been available only since 1967, many persons, e.g., military personnel who were in the South Pacific in World War II, the Korean War, or the Vietnam War, may remain infected and at risk for episodic symptoms of chronic infection or overwhelming hyperinfection if they become immunosuppressed.

Transmission. It is now recognized that the free-living cycle is of very short duration and has a limited role in maintaining transmission. This implies that transmission required proximity to an infected individual. A recent study in Jamaica showed a significant and sequential decline in the probability of infection depending on whether an individual shared a bed, house, communal yard, or neighborhood with an index case; clustering of infection within households is commonly observed. This may also explain the patterns of prevalent infection in institutional settings. Vertical transmission is suggested by reports of *Strongyloides* sp. larvae in human breast milk in Africa, but the observed age profiles of infection are difficult to reconcile with transmammary passage.

PATHOGENESIS AND PATHOLOGY. Although the specific host and parasite factors that are responsible in the pathogenesis of strongyloidiasis are poorly understood, the capacity of *S. stercoralis* to persist despite normal host defenses characterizes the delicate balance of chronic infection. Intact cellular immunity appears to keep the tissue migration, as well as the development of the parasite in the intestine, under control with only intermittent symptoms. Any illness that results in loss of cellular immunity or corticosteroid therapy may lead to uncontrolled parasite multiplication and dissemination in the patient and the hyperinfection syndrome.

Migration Phase. The characteristic pruritic urticarial skin eruption and occasional eosinophilic pulmonary infiltrates or wheezing (Löffler's syndrome) are related to immediate hypersensitivity reactions to the migrating larvae. Alveolar hemorrhage and cellular reaction in the lungs and peripheral eosinophilia and increased IgE levels are often noted.

Intestinal Phase. In the intestine, adult female worms, eggs, and larvae are found in the superficial submucosa and in the mucosal crypts, causing mechanical trauma, mucous discharge, and microscopic ulceration but usually minimal inflammation. Increased epithelial cell turnover from the small bowel has been described in heavy infection and may cause malnutrition and hypoproteinemia. Granulomas may occasionally form. Progressive involvement may lead to edema, flattened villi, malabsorption, and even ulceration, enteritis, and secondary bacterial invasion. Rarely, larvae are seen in the biliary or pancreatic ducts, liver, urine, or inflammatory exudates. Particularly in the hyperinfection syndrome, both direct filariform larval damage and secondary polymicrobial infection may be found in virtually any organ. The usual sites of larval reinvasion are the ileum, appendix, and colon, where a granulomatous colitis may be noted along with steatorrhea, hypocalcemia, and hypoproteinemia.

CLINICAL MANIFESTATIONS. The clinical manifestations of *S. stercoralis* infection are acute infection, chronic persisting infection, and the disseminated hyperinfection syndrome in immunosuppressed hosts. The latter two syndromes are the best characterized.

Acute Infection. Clinical manifestations of acute strongyloidiasis reflect the intensity of the infection and are likely related to the three stages of infection, with: (1) skin penetration by filariform larvae, (2) pulmonary migration of larvae, and (3) intestinal penetration by adult worms. Although an estimated one third of individuals may remain asymptomatic, an initial pruritic maculopapular rash or rapidly migrating linear urticaria called *larva currens*, which may move 10 cm/day, is well described at the site of skin penetration by the infectious filariform larvae. Larva currens is usually seen on the buttocks area with external autoinfection. Although infrequent, cough, shortness of breath, wheezing, fever, transient pulmonary infiltrates, and eosinophilia (Löffler's syndrome) may be encountered with the migration of larvae through the lungs. Finally, when adult worms develop and penetrate the mucosa in the small bowel, nonspecific aching or epigastric abdominal pain and diarrhea may

develop. With heavy infections in the upper small bowel, vomiting, malabsorption (of iron and other nutrients), steatorrhea, weight loss, edema, or even small bowel obstruction may occur. Obstruction may be due to paralytic ileus with edema in the small bowel wall.

Chronic, Persisting Infection. Best described in veterans or in former prisoners of war who have returned from endemic, tropical areas in Asia or in the South Pacific, a syndrome of chronic strongyloidiasis with intermittent cutaneous and enteric symptoms has been documented. Rates of infection determined by careful laboratory examinations of fecal specimens among former British, Australian, and American prisoners of war who had worked on the Burma-Thailand railroad during World War II were found 30 to 40 years later to be 21 to 37%. Although one third of documented infections were asymptomatic, two thirds of the patients had recurring episodic symptoms. The classically recognized triad of symptoms is urticaria, abdominal pain, and diarrhea. By far the most common was episodic, rapidly moving, creeping urticarial skin eruptions, most often on the buttocks or perianal area (at irregular intervals lasting 1 to 2 days), in 85 to 100% of symptomatic, infected individuals. Second in frequency were abdominal symptoms, led by intermittent epigastric pain, indigestion, or heartburn (65 to 67%), and watery diarrhea or cramping abdominal pain (42 to 67%). These symptoms were significantly reduced after treatment with thiabendazole 25 mg/kg b.i.d. for 2 days, a course that was repeated once after 1 week. Symptoms of shortness of breath, wheezing, chest pain, and cough (35 to 52%) suggested pulmonary involvement, and eosinophilia and elevated serum IgE concentrations were common but not universal. Immune complexes may rarely be associated with a reactive arthritis.

Further studies of chronic endemic infections in the United States have come from southeastern Kentucky, where infection with *S. stercoralis* is the most commonly diagnosed parasitic infection (in 2.5% of fecal specimens examined) at the University of Kentucky Medical Center. These endemic cases most commonly involved white men who were older than 50 years, who were from lower socioeconomic backgrounds, and who often had a chronic or debilitating illness. The characteristic syndrome was one of mild to moderate chronic relapsing diarrhea, nausea, vomiting, and abdominal pain and tenderness, often with eosinophilia (in 85% of cases) and occasional hypoalbuminemia (in 20% of cases). In the prospective rural Tennessee study, *Strongyloides* infection was associated with abdominal bloating, eosinophilia, and guaiac-positive stools, as well as with taking steroids, cimetidine, or antacid medications.

Hyperinfection Syndrome. When the critical host-parasite balance is upset in an individual chronically infected with *Strongyloides* by any drug or illness that compromises the host's immune status, a severe, life-threatening hyperinfection syndrome may result. Widely recognized since 1966, 89 of 103 cases of disseminated strongyloidiasis in one report were in patients immunocompromised by recognized malignancies (especially lymphoma or leukemia) and/or corticosteroid therapy (for asthma, malignancy, lymphoma, leukemia, systemic lupus erythematosus, renal transplantation, ulcerative colitis, and so forth). Severe strongyloidiasis has also been reported in at least 30 cases following renal transplantation as well as with cimetidine therapy. In a review of autopsies from sub-Saharan Africa and Washington, DC, in addition to the association with hematologic malignancies and corticosteroid therapy, several cases of disseminated strongyloidiasis were described in persons with protein-calorie malnutrition, lepromatous leprosy, and other severe infections, e.g., tuberculosis and syphilis. It is apparent that loss of intact cellular immunity is associated with conversion of rhabditiform larvae to filariform larvae followed by uncontrolled, widespread dissemination of the filariform larvae via the blood stream to involve virtually any organ. Extraintestinal infections most often involve the lung, with associated bronchospasm, focal or diffuse infiltrates, and even cavitation. In addition, abdominal lymph nodes, liver, spleen, pancreas, thyroid, endocardium, kidney, brain, and meninges may be involved. Intestinal symptoms with hyperinfection include profound diarrhea, malabsorption, and electrolyte abnormalities. Remarkably absent are cellular immune responses to migrating larvae. Thymic T-lymphocyte depletion and loss of the eosinophilia typify disseminated hyperinfection in immunocompromised hosts. Of special concern is the 86% mortality associated with the hyperinfection syndrome, often with bacterial infection secondary to extensive larval spread from the intestine. Sepsis, meningitis, peritonitis, or endocarditis was documented in 45% of cases studied. It is somewhat surprising that despite the severity of cryptosporidial and *Isospora* infections in patients with AIDS, extraintestinal strongyloidiasis has *not* yet been associated with AIDS in areas of Africa highly endemic for *S. stercoralis* (Chapter 22).

DIAGNOSIS. The important aspects of diagnosing *Strongyloides* infections include a high index of clinical suspicion in patients with histories of exposure and characteristic skin and intestinal symptoms. Second, an experienced person may have to search extremely diligently in fecal specimens, even with formalin-ether concentration, to find the characteristic rhabditiform larvae (Fig. 102–2[10]). It is important to recognize that *Strongyloides* larvae do not typically float in hypertonic saline solutions, which are often used to concentrate other parasites. Several researchers have described the distinct advantages, particularly in endemic areas, of the Baermann funnel gauze method of concentrating *Strongyloides* larvae in fecal specimens, using warm water and larval sedimentation in the neck of the funnel (Chapter 150). Substantially improved yields of greater than fourfold have been described over other traditional methods, and some investigators have reported that this technique is superior to duodenal aspiration or the string capsule method (Enterotest) for obtaining duodenal fluid (Chapter 150). In vitro culture of fecal specimens facilitates the development of filariform larvae and eventually causes multiplication through the heterogonic cycle. Culture on damp charcoal (where the larvae migrate to the surface for collection) or Harada-Mori culture on vertical strips of damp filter paper (where the larvae migrate down) are among the most successful of traditional methods. However, culture on nutrient agar plates into which the larvae make characteristic burrows is now emerging as the method of choice. Culture methods require handling an infectious agent and the differential diagnosis of the larval stage (particularly from hookworm species) and are most appropriate for specialist diagnostic laboratories.

Although previous serologic tests were complicated by lack of sensitivity and specificity, an improved immunofluorescence antibody assay using *Strongyloides* antigen has been described and may be helpful. Improved enzyme-linked immunosorbent assay also gives excellent specificity and sensitivity, particularly if combined with Western blot. All immunodiagnostic methods are complicated by cross-reactivity with filarial antigen, which may result in false positives in areas where *Onchocerca*, *Wuchereria*, or *Brugia* are coendemic with *Strongyloides*. *S. stercoralis* antigen is not yet widely available for routine diagnostic use.

Great diagnostic problems may arise in persons who have traveled to endemic areas (even many years before) and then become immunocompromised by an underlying disease or are given corticosteroids for any reason. A careful search for larvae is required in stool or small bowel aspirates. Rarely, filariform larvae may be seen in the sputum, spinal fluid, or urine. In immunosuppressed patients, the clue of peripheral eosinophilia is lost, and indeed, <7% eosinophils was noted in three fourths of the 58 patients reviewed by Igra-Siegman and coworkers; these 43 patients had an 84% mortality (in contrast to the 27% mortality if >8% eosinophils were present).

TREATMENT. Because of the potential for chronic symptomatic infection, autoinfection over many years, and the hyperinfection syndrome, all individuals who are infected with *S. stercoralis* should be treated. The traditional form of treatment is thiabendazole 25 mg/kg PO b.i.d. for 2 or 3 days. Because of the difficulty in confirming eradication of the infection, many experts prefer to repeat a 2-day course of therapy 1 week after the initial course, with careful follow-up for persisting symptoms or infection. Fifteen percent of patients suffered relapse after therapy in a prospective rural Tennessee study. Immunocompromised patients suspected of having a life-threatening, hyperinfection syndrome warrant this daily dose for a longer period, probably 5 to 14 days. Because a parenteral preparation of thiabendazole is not available, intermittent administration via a nasogastric tube may be required for patients with intestinal obstruction. Schumaker and coworkers have described administration of thiabendazole for patients undergoing hemodialysis.

Toxicity of thiabendazole, even in lower doses, includes nausea, vomiting, malaise, dizziness, and smelly urine (Chapter 102). Albendazole 400 mg daily for 3 days is less efficacious than thiabendazole but has few side effects. Ivermectin 200 µg/kg appears to give excellent cure rates with few side effects but is currently registered for this indication only in France.

PREVENTION. As with most other enteric infections, critical to the prevention of strongyloidiasis is an improved standard of living, with particular reference to personal hygiene and improved sanitary and waste disposal facilities. Because the prevalence of infection is relatively low in most endemic areas and transmission is highly correlated with proximity to infected individuals, treatment of individuals is likely to be particularly effective as a preventive measure.

Regarding the prevention of the hyperinfection syndrome, most important is an adequate awareness of the symptoms of chronic *Strongyloides* infection so that it can be treated. This is particularly important in any immunocompromised patient or person given corticosteroids, especially with a history of exposure to an endemic area.

STRONGYLOIDES FULLEBORNI INFECTION. Throughout several areas of equatorial Africa, widespread infection with *S. fulleborni* has been described in several species of Old World monkeys and other primates. Similar to *S. stercoralis* in morphology and life cycle, *S. fulleborni* may also cause cutaneous, pulmonary, and intestinal symptoms, as well as eosinophilia in humans in central and eastern Africa, in Zambia, and along the Fly River in the Kuringa region of Papua New Guinea, where nonhuman primates have not been found to be infected as in Africa. Although *S. fulleborni* has been associated with abdominal distention, respiratory distress, generalized edema, and a fatal outcome in infants, the capacity of *S. fulleborni* to cause prolonged autoinfection or the hyperinfection syndrome is not established. Also in contrast to *S. stercoralis*, *S. fulleborni* is diagnosed by finding characteristic 55 by 35 µm thin-shelled ovoid, embryonated eggs, rather than rhabditiform larvae, in the stool.

Bibliography

Ashford RW, Barnish G: Strongyloidiasis in Papua New Guinea. Clin Trop Med Comm Dis 2:765, 1987.

Badaro R, Carvalho EM, Santos RB, et al: Parasite-specific humoral responses in different clinical forms of strongyloidiasis. Trans R Soc Trop Med Hyg 81:149, 1987.

Bartholomew C, Butler AK, Bhaskar AG, Jankey N: Pseudo-obstruction, and a spure-like syndrome from strongyloidiasis. Postgrad Med J 53:139, 1977.

Beal CB, Viens P, Grant RGL, Hughes JM: A new technique for sampling duodenal contents: Demonstration of upper small-bowel pathogens. Am J Trop Med Hyg 19:349, 1970.

Berk SL, Verghese A, Alvarez S, et al: Clinical and epidemiologic features of strongyloidiasis: A prospective study in rural Tennessee. Arch Intern Med 147:1257, 1987.

Berry AJ, Long EG, Smith JH, et al: Chronic relapsing colitis due to *Strongyloides stercoralis*. Am J Trop Med Hyg 32:1289, 1983.

Brown RC, Girardeau MHF: Transmammary passage of *Strongyloides* sp. larvae in the human host. Am J Trop Med Hyg 26:215, 1977.

Bundy DAP, Guyatt HL: Anthelmintic chemotherapy: The individual and the community. Curr Opin Infect Dis 8:466, 1995.

Conway DJ, Lindo JF, Robinson RD, Bundy DAP: Towards effective control of *Strongyloides stercoralis*. Parasitol Today 11:420, 1995.

Cruz T, Reboucas G, Rocha H: Fatal strongyloidiasis in patients receiving corticosteroids. N Engl J Med 275:1093, 1966.

Da Costa LR: Small-intestinal cell turnover in patients with parasitic infections. BMJ 3:281, 1971.

Faust EC, De Groat A: Internal autoinfection in human strongyloidiasis. Am J Trop Med 20:359, 1940.

Genta RM: Strongyloidiasis. Clin Trop Med Comm Dis 2:645, 1987.

Gill GV, Bell DR: *Strongyloides stercoralis* infection in former Far East prisoners of war. BMJ 2:572, 1979.

Grove DI: Strongyloidiasis in Allied ex-prisoners of war in Southeast Asia. BMJ 280:598, 1980.

Grove DI: Treatment of strongyloidiasis with thiabendazole: An analysis of toxicity and effectiveness. Trans R Soc Trop Med Hyg 76:114, 1982.

Grove DI, Blair AJ: Diagnosis of human strongyloidiasis by immunofluorescence using *Strongyloides ratti* and *S. stercoralis* larvae. Am J Trop Hyg 30:344, 1981.

Hira PR, Patel BG: Human strongyloidiasis due to the primate species *Strongyloides fulleborni*. Trop Geogr Med 32:23, 1980.

Lima JP, Delgado PG: Diagnosis of strongyloidiasis: Importance of Baermann's method. Am J Dig Dis 6:899, 1961.

Lindo JF, Conway DJ, Atkins NS, et al: Prospective evaluation of enzyme-linked immunosorbent assay and immunoblot methods for the diagnosis of endemic *Strongyloides stercoralis* infection. Am J Trop Med Hyg 51:175, 1994.

Lindo JF, Robinson RD, Terry SI, et al: Age-prevalence and household clustering of *Strongyloides stercoralis* infection in Jamaica. Parasitology 110:97, 1995.

Milder JE, Walzer PD, Kilgore G, et al: Clinical features of *Strongyloides stercoralis* infection in an endemic area of the United States. Gastroenterology 80:1481, 1981.

Milner PF, Irvine RA, Barton CJ, et al: Intestinal malabsorption in *Strongyloides stercoralis* infestation. Gut 6:574, 1965.

Morgan JS, Schaffner W, Stone WJ: Opportunistic strongyloidiasis in renal transplant recipients. Transplantation 42:518, 1986.

Pampiglione S, Ricciardi ML: Experimental infection with human strain *Strongyloides fulleborni* in man. Lancet 1:663, 1972.

Pelletier LL Jr: Chronic strongyloidiasis in World War II Far East exprisoners of war. Am J Trop Med Hyg 33:55, 1984.

Pelletier LL Jr, Gabre-Kidan T: Chronic strongyloidiasis in Vietnam veterans. Am J Med 78:139, 1985.

Petithory JC, Derouin F: AIDS and strongyloidiasis in Africa. Lancet 1:921, 1987.

Scowden EB, Schaffner W, Stone WJ: Overwhelming strongyloidiasis: An unappreciated opportunistic infection. Medicine 57:527, 1978.

Smith JD, Goette DK, Odom RB: Larva currens: Cutaneous strongyloidiasis. Arch Dermatol 112:1161, 1976.

Vince JD, Ashford RW, Gratten MJ, et al: *Strongyloides* species infestation in young infants at Papua New Guinea: Association with generalized oedema. Papua New Guinea Med J 22:120, 1979.

Walzer PD, Milder JE, Banwell JG, et al: Epidemiologic features of *Strongyloides stercoralis* infection in an endemic area of the United States. Am J Trop Med Hyg 31:313, 1982.

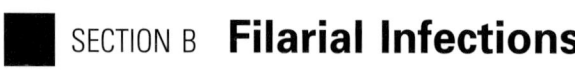

SECTION B **Filarial Infections**

---

106 *Filariasis*

Christopher L. King and David O. Freedman

General Principles

ETIOLOGY AND BIOLOGY. The filariases are a group of vector-borne parasitic diseases of humans, caused by long threadlike nematodes that, in their mature adult stage, reside in the lymphatics or in connective tissue (Fig. 106–1). With some types of filarial infection, the adult parasite itself, during a lifetime that may span decades, may provoke impressive and chronic inflammatory reactions in tissues. Adult females continuously produce huge numbers of larvae, called microfilariae, which in some types of filarial infection can cause significant, debilitating, and long-term chronic pathology. Because the efficacy of each antifilarial drug differs for different life-cycle stages of the same parasite, treatment of the individual patient should first target that stage of that specific parasite that is associated with morbidity. Complete eradication of adult worms is always desirable but is not necessarily part of control programs or treatment of the individual patient.

Disease expression varies with species of filaria. A common theme, however, is that newly exposed individuals characteristically have manifestations of acute symptomatology that is often much exaggerated when compared with natives of the endemic area. For example, in onchocerciasis, traditional clinical descriptions include keratitis, chorioretinitis, dermatitis, and the presence of subcutaneous nodules. These descriptions are based on observations made in individuals with a lifetime of exposure to, and thus a lifetime of immunologic experience with, the etiologic agent of onchocerciasis, *Onchocerca volvulus*. With the recent increases in travel to onchocerciasis endemic areas by the immunologically naive, descriptions of a different syndrome consisting of an evanescent papular dermatitis without ocular involvement are emerging. Not only is there an immunologic heterogeneity between endemic and nonendemic individuals, but short-term residents are typically lightly infected. In addition, they are more likely to seek medical care earlier.

An asymptomatic incubation period that is at minimum 6 months and can be as long as 3 years significantly lessens the chance of the relevant travel history being elicited from an individual who presents much later with nonspecific symptoms. For this reason, some clinicians advocate routine post-travel serologic screening for filariasis in any individual with a year or more of exposure in an area endemic for any of the filarial parasites.

The mechanisms of microfilarial periodicity that have baffled investigators for many years continue to be elusive. Nocturnally periodic microfilariae (Table 106–1) are those that circulate in the peripheral circulation between 9 P.M. and 2 A.M. and are usually undetectable at other times. Subperiodic microfilariae circulate at all times during the day but

TABLE 106–1. Different Species of Human Filariasis

Species	Periodicity	Distribution	Vector	Location of Adult	Location of MF
Wuchereria bancrofti	Nocturnal	Cosmopolitan; mainly India China, Indonesia	*Culex Anopheles Aedes* (mosquitoes)	Lymphatic	Blood
	Subperiodic	Eastern pacific	*Aedes* (mosquitoes)	Lymphatic	Blood
Brugia malayi	Nocturnal	Southeast Asia, Indonesia, India	*Mansonia Anopheles* (mosquitoes)	Lymphatic	Blood
	Subperiodic	Indonesia, Southeast Asia	*Coquilletidia Mansonia* (mosquitoes)	Lymphatic	Blood
Loa loa	Diurnal	West and central Africa	*Chrysops* (deer fly)	Subcutaneous	Blood
Mansonella ozzardi	None	South and Central America, Caribbean	*Culicoides* (biting midge) *Simulium* (black fly)	Unclear	Blood
Mansonella perstans	None	South and Central America, Africa	*Culicoides* (biting midge)	Body cavities, mesentery, perirenal	Blood
Onchocerca volvulus	None	South and Central America, Africa	*Simulium* (black fly)	Subcutaneous	Skin
Mansonella streptocerca	None	West and central Africa	*Culicoides* (biting midge)	Subcutaneous	Skin

peak in intensity late in the afternoon if they are diurnally subperiodic or at night if they are nocturnally subperiodic. These cycles are apparently a highly evolved host adaptation to the feeding habits of the vector in the particular area. Parasites of the same species (e.g., *Wuchereria bancrofti*) that have no other detectable biologic differences will exhibit differing periodicities depending on geographic location and vector species. The skin-dwelling microfilariae and some of the blood-borne microfilariae do not have a periodicity.

LIFE CYCLES. All the human filarial parasites have the same basic life cycle with five larval stages of development: three in the intermediate arthropod vector and two in the human host (Fig. 106–1). Infection begins with the bite of an infected arthropod vector. Infective larvae (L3 stage) are deposited into the skin or blood, where at least 6 to 12 months are required until sexual maturity. During this period the parasite undergoes two rapid (a few days) molts. At maturity the adult female produces L1 larvae called microfilariae. Each molt consists of the shedding of the current nematode cuticle to allow for further growth. The short-lived L3 and L4 stages are thought not to be associated with any of the pathologic manifestations of disease. Once the microfilariae are ingested by the vector, maturation through two molts to the infective larval (L3) stage takes from 1 to 3 weeks. For L1 microfilariae to mature to L5 adults, obligatory passage through the arthropod intermediate host is necessary. Thus, there is no multiplication of the adult filarial worms in humans. Adult worm load is proportional to the number of infective L3 larvae acquired. Therefore, if the infected individual is no longer exposed to infected vectors, no further increase in parasite burden occurs. Also, there is no multiplication of the filariae in the insect vector; only maturation occurs.

SPECTRUM OF HUMAN PATHOGENS. There are eight filarial species in which humans are the definitive hosts, six of which are thought to be pathogenic: *Wuchereria bancrofti* (Chapter 106.1), *Brugia malayi* (Chapter 106.2), *B. timori* (all causing lymphatic filariasis), *Onchocerca volvulus* (causing dermatitis and eye lesions) (Chapter 108), *Loa loa* (causing

Calabar swellings and allergic manifestations (Chapter 107), *Mansonella streptocerca* (causing skin disease) (Chapter 109.3), *M. perstans* (Chapter 109.2), and *M. ozzardi* (Chapter 109.1). *W. bancrofti*, *B. malayi*, and *O. volvulus* are responsible for the majority of human filarial disease. Except for subperiodic *B. malayi* in primates and domestic animals in Indonesia there is little evidence for any clinically important nonhuman reservoir.

Several animal filariae, namely, *Dirofilaria immitis* and *D. repens* in dogs, *D. tenuis* in raccoons, and zoonotic species of *Brugia* can, uncommonly, infect humans. The parasites die in the larval stages before reaching maturity and cause few symptoms. Localization is to the lungs in *D. immitis* infection (appearing as coin lesions) or to the subcutaneous tissues and lymph nodes in the other filariae species (Chapter 109.4).

PRINCIPLES OF DRUG TREATMENT. Two drugs, diethylcarbamazine (DEC) and ivermectin, are the mainstays of antifilarial treatment. Treatment regimens differ according to whether the aim is treatment of an individual patient or community-based interruption of transmission by suppression of microfilariae available to vectors. DEC has substantial adulticidal effects against *L. loa* and the lymphatic filariases. Intensive efforts at repeated courses of adulticidal therapy are clearly more important in those nonendemic individuals who will not be re-exposed to infective vectors. DEC is microfilaricidal to all species of human filaria except *M. ozzardi* and *M. perstans*, and suppression of microfilaremia may vary from weeks to months. DEC is contraindicated in onchocerciasis because of its toxicity. Ivermectin is microfilaricidal to *O. volvulus*, *W. bancrofti*, *Brugia* sp., and perhaps *M. ozzardi*. It is established first-line therapy for treatment and control of onchocerciasis but in lymphatic filariasis has a drawback in treating individual patients because unlike DEC, it has no macrofilaricidal effect. In lymphatic filariasis control programs aimed at breaking the transmission cycle, annual DEC/ivermectin combination therapy may be the most effective regimen. Early removal of infected nonendemic persons from the area of transmission tends to hasten the clinical recovery.

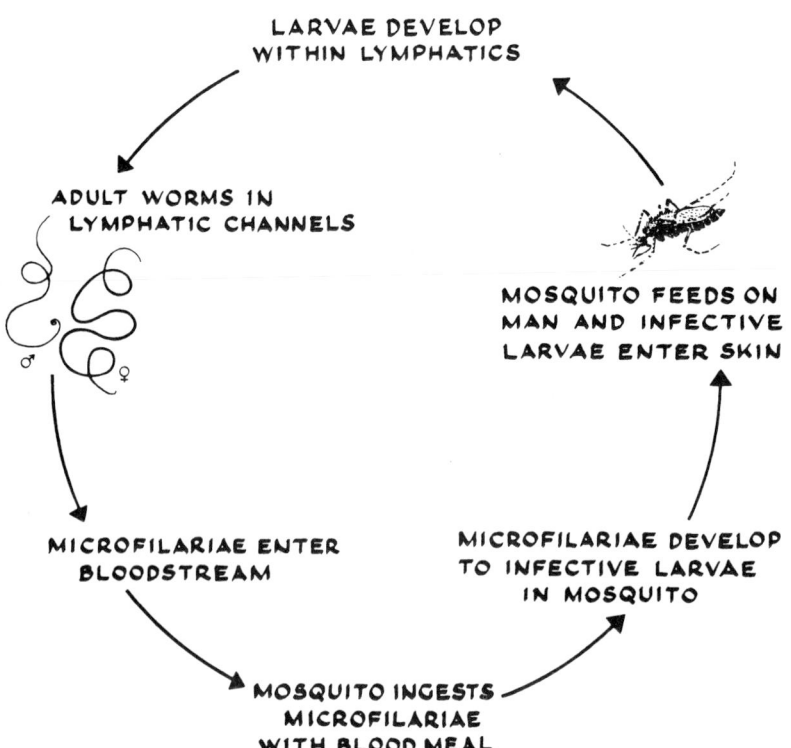

Figure 106–1. Life cycle of lymphatic-dwelling filariae of humans. In addition to the elements illustrated, subperiodic *Brugia malayi* has a zoonotic cycle.

PRINCIPLE OF DIAGNOSIS. Outside of research settings, definitive diagnosis of any of the filarial infections is dependent upon the demonstration of the 130 to 360 μm long microfilariae in blood or skin snips. The presence or absence of a sheath, the arrangement of the nuclei in the tail, and the tissue of origin are usually sufficient to differentiate the species (Fig. 106–2). Diagnostic sampling must always take into account the periodicity of every possible filarial parasite that is epidemiologically possible in the particular patient. In well-equipped clinical settings, biopsy or ultrasound demonstration of adult parasites can be diagnostic. Serologic testing for antifilarial IgG, generally by ELISA, is not widely avail-

able and, when done, usually utilizes a crude heterologous antigenic preparation. Standardization is often poor; a positive result, at best, cannot differentiate between the eight filarial species and, at worst, may cross-react with other helminthic infections, e.g. strongyloidiasis. Despite the lack of specificity, sensitivity of this type of serology is almost 100%. Most individuals resident in endemic areas will have antibodies whether they are currently infected or not. Thus, serologic evaluation in filarial disease is helpful only in two situations: (1) in individuals from nonendemic areas exposed to or infected with filarial parasites who are presumably seronegative initially; and (2) to detect a quantitative decrease in antibody levels that may occur as a response to definitive therapy.

INCIDENCE AND DISTRIBUTION. The filariases, although not ubiquitous, are distributed essentially throughout the tropics with extensive overlap between the species (Fig. 106–3). An estimated 300 million people, mostly in India, Southeast Asia, and sub-Saharan Africa, live in areas endemic for lymphatic filariasis, with approximately 130 million actually infected. No proper data for the prevalence and distribution of bancroftian filariasis in Africa exist, so many more people are likely to be infected; 30 million people are constantly exposed to onchocerciasis; and the best current estimates are that approximately 18 million people are infected, 270,000 of whom are blind.

CONTROL PROGRAMS. The Onchocerciasis Control Program (OCP) has been ongoing for over 15 years in an area of West Africa most affected by the blinding savanna strain of *O. volvulus*. A strategy of aggressive vector control using aerial insecticiding of rivers where black fly larvae breed has essentially interrupted transmission in the area under control. The program has cost US$360 million to date and is slated to end in the year 2002. Because infected black flies will invade from around the perimeter of the controlled region, residual control efforts costing several million dollars per year would be necessary to sustain the effect of the program. National

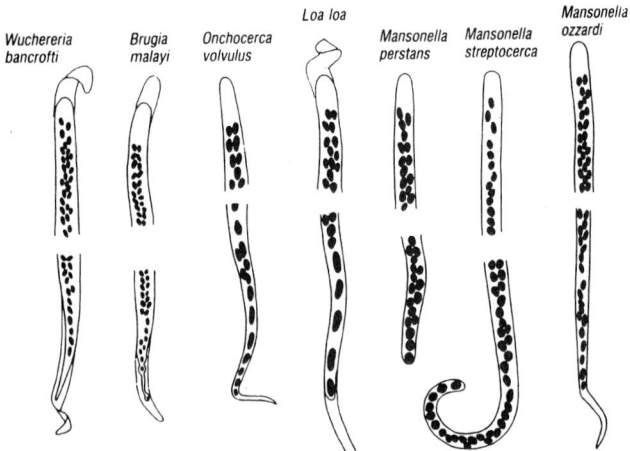

Wuchereria bancrofti   *Brugia malayi*   *Onchocerca volvulus*   *Loa loa*   *Mansonella perstans*   *Mansonella streptocerca*   *Mansonella ozzardi*

Figure 106–2. Microfilariae of seven filaria-infected humans as seen in Giemsa-stained blood films. They can be differentiated by the characteristics of their nuclei in their heads *(top)* or tails *(bottom)*, the presence or absence of a sheath, and whether they were detected in the blood or in skin snips.

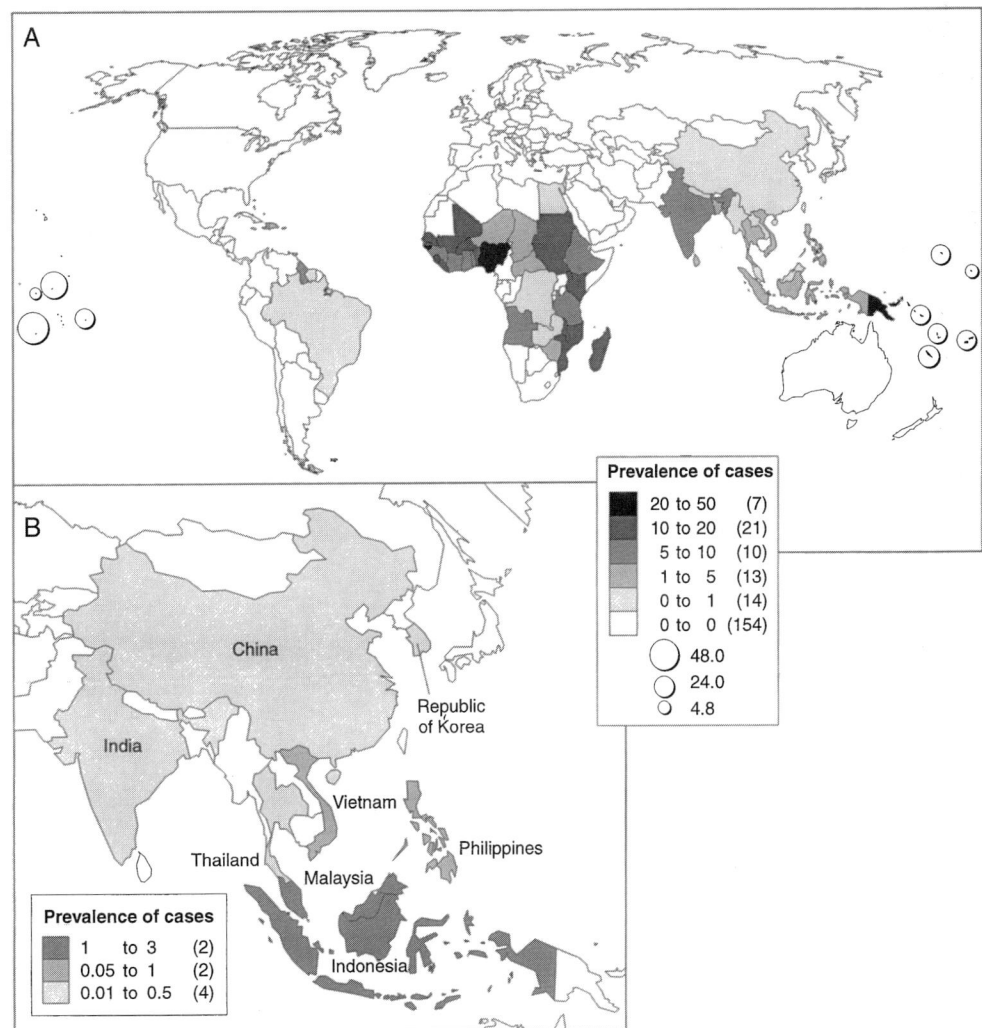

Figure 106–3. Geographic distribution of bancroftian *(a)* and brugian *(b)* filariasis case prevalences. Circles denote the corresponding prevalences (%) estimated for various Pacific islands and vary in size proportionately with the prevalence on each island. The figures in brackets indicate the number of countries. (From Michael E, Bundy DAP: Global mapping of lymphatic filariasis. Parasitol Today 13:472, 1997.)

governments in the region may be unable or unwilling to sustain this effort.

Building a sustainable infrastructure for the mass community-based distribution of the microfilaricide ivermectin has become the primary control strategy on a global basis for both onchocerciasis and lymphatic filariasis. Annual mass treatment of an affected community with ivermectin, which is available free from the manufacturer, should break the transmission cycle within 10 to 15 years. APOC (African Program for Onchocerciasis Control), to run from 1997 to 2007, will assist all 16 affected African countries outside the OCP to establish sustainable national programs for ivermectin distribution. Owing to the more widespread distribution of lymphatic filariasis and the huge numbers of people affected, plans for a similar program for control of that disease are still very much in the embryonic stage.

106.1 *Bancroftian Filariasis*

DEFINITION. Bancroftian filariasis is caused by the mosquito-borne nematode, *Wuchereria bancrofti.* The adult worms, males and females, live in lymphatic vessels and nodes of the human host, where the females produce first-stage larva called microfilariae that circulate in the blood. The infection

is most often clinically unapparent, but it is now clear that even these asymptomatic individuals almost always have underlying lymphatic damage caused by local mechanical damage by the highly motile adult worms. With progressive infection, inflammatory immune damage to lymphatics results in a wide spectrum of clinical manifestations that depend on the part affected. Humans are the only natural host for *W. bancrofti.* The lack of an experimental laboratory animal model has severely hampered research into the clinical, biochemical, and genetic determinants of the disease process.

HISTORY. Descriptions of elephantiasis are found in early Indian, Egyptian, and Persian writings and drew the attention of medical observers in Africa and the South Pacific in the 17th and 18th centuries. The worldwide distribution of elephantiasis in tropical and subtropical areas and the epidemiologic association of elephantiasis with hydrocele, chylocele, and chyluria were established by the middle of the 19th century. Their common etiology, however, remained a mystery until discoveries were made of microfilariae in hydrocele fluid (Demarquay, 1863), chylous urine (Wucherer, 1868), and blood (Lewis, 1872) and of the adult worm in a lymphatic abscess (Bancroft, 1877). Manson's great contribution was his description, while working in Amoy, China between 1875 and 1879, of the uptake of microfilariae by *Culex* mosquitoes and their maturation to infective forms. This is the first description of the mosquito as a vector of any of the parasitic diseases. Manson also made the association of endemic microfilaremia with elephantiasis and other lymphatic disease. Effective drug therapy awaited the description of the microfilaricidal effects of the piperazine derivative diethylcarbamazine (Hewitt, 1947) and, more recently, ivermectin. The adulticidal effects of DEC have been appreciated in the last decade.

ETIOLOGY. *W. bancrofti* (Cobbold, 1877) reaches sexual maturity in lymphatic vessels and nodes of humans. The adults are white, threadlike worms that are convoluted in lymph nodes but have been shown by ultrasound to be almost completely extended in lymph vessels. The female, which is about twice the size of the male, measures between 80 and 100 mm in length and 0.2 to 0.3 mm in width. Thousands of developing embryos may be found within the gravid paired uteri of the female, each enclosed within translucent hyaline membranes that elongate to become the sheaths of the microfilariae once they are released. When examined in stained blood films a microfilaria has a length of 240 to 300 μm and a width of 7 to 9 μm and is covered by a translucent sheath. It usually assumes a graceful curved position, differential features are shown in Fig. 106–2. In Asia and the Pacific, *W. kalimantani,* a filariid infecting only animals, has infective-stage larvae and microfilariae that are morphologically indistinguishable from those of *W. bancrofti.*

The human *W. bancrofti* parasites have diversified into a large number of strains, as is clear from the different periodicities of the microfilaremias that they cause. Each strain has established a particular transmission equilibrium with the natural vector(s). The nocturnally periodic microfilariae, adapted to culicine and anopheline vectors, reach peak densities between 9 P.M. and 2 A.M. and disappear completely from the circulation soon thereafter. The rapidity with which the levels taper off depends on peak intensity. Less commonly and predominantly in the South Pacific, *Aedes*-adapted microfilariae have a subperiodic cycle.

DEVELOPMENT AND LIFE CYCLE. The infective L3 larvae escape from the proboscis of the mosquito at the time of feeding and penetrate the skin at the puncture wound (Fig. 106–1). The routes by which the L3s home to lymph nodes and vessels remain elusive. At least 6 to 12 months are required for two rapid (a few days each) molts and the slower development of the sexually mature adult female (L5 stage) capable of producing L1 larvae called microfilariae. Even in the absence of reinfection microfilaremia may persist for 10 years or more. Once the microfilariae are taken up in the blood meal of mosquitoes and within hours of arrival in the midgut, the microfilariae shed their sheaths, penetrate the wall of the gut, and find their way to the muscles of the thorax. In the thorax, over a period of 7 to 21 days, two molts occur; the development of infective L3 larvae signals the readiness to begin the cycle anew.

EPIDEMIOLOGY AND NATURAL HISTORY

Distribution. *W. bancrofti* is the most abundant and widespread of the human filarial infections, occurring throughout much of the tropical and subtropical regions of the world (Table 106–2). It infects an estimated 115 million individuals worldwide. However, the use of assays that detect infection by measuring adult worm–derived antigens in the circulation has indicated that infection rates in endemic areas may be twice that estimated from prevalence of microfilaria in blood samples. Most infections occur in south Asia and tropical sub-Saharan Africa (Fig. 106–3). In Asia, the parasite is endemic in both urban and rural areas in the Indian subcontinent, the island of Sri Lanka, and Burma. Infections predominate in scattered rural foci in Thailand and Indochina; extensively in the south and eastern alluvial plains of China; among aboriginal and proto-Malay peoples in the hill forest of the Malay Peninsula and northern Borneo; and in many forested and agricultural regions of the Philippines. Most of the cities in these regions are spared infections. In Indonesia the parasite occurs focally with low prevalences in low-lying hill forests of Sumatra, Kalimantan, and Sulawesi and more intensely along coastal fringes of small islands east of Lombok. Bancroftian filariasis is transmitted in urban areas along the northern coast of Java, particularly in the cities of Jakarta and Semarang. Overall, the South Pacific continues to be highly endemic for filariasis, particularly in coastal and low-lying hills in Papua New Guinea and Iran Jaya and in many islands of Melanesia, Micronesia, and Polynesia. The parasite is diurnally subperiodic throughout Polynesia, New Caledonia, and the Loyalty Islands.

In sub-Saharan Africa, the nocturnally periodic, anopheline-borne rural strains of *W. bancrofti* are found in patchy distribution throughout a wide belt from 25 degrees north to 20 degrees south. In East Africa, *Culex* species as well as anophelines transmit *W. bancrofti* all along the coastal regions and offshore islands of the Indian Ocean, particularly in Kenya, Tanzania, and Madagascar, where transmission occurs in both urban and rural areas. The other areas of high prevalence of filariasis extend from Senegal to southern Sudan and low-lying areas of western Ethiopia, with populous Nigeria being one of the more intensely affected African countries. In Egypt, the parasite occurs mostly in the Nile delta and is transmitted mainly by *Culex* mosquitoes. Within the past two decades the prevalence of bancroftian filariasis has increased markedly in these foci and spread to urban

TABLE 106–2. Global Burden of Disease (GBD) Estimates of the Number of Cases and Prevalence of Filariasis (Infection and Chronic Disease Combined) by Endemic Regions[a]

Region	Population (millions)	Total No. of cases (millions) *Wuchereria bancrofti*	Prevalence (%)
Sub-Saharan Africa[b]	564	50.6	9.0
Asia[c]	2770	62.3	2.3
Pacific Islands[d]	6	1.8	29.1
Latin America[e]	441	0.4	0.1
World	3781	115.1	3.0[f]

[a]Data are modified and updated for sub-Saharan Africa by incorporating new estimates made for Ghana, Ethiopia, Sudan, Sierra Leone, Seychelles, and Democratic Republic of the Congo. Figures are for both sexes combined.

[b]Includes Egypt.

[c]Includes India and China.

[d]Includes Cook Islands, Fiji, French Polynesia, Guam, Kiribati, Marshall Islands, Micronesia, Nauru, New Calendonia, Niue, Palau Islands, Papua New Guinea, Solomon Islands, Tonga, Tuvalu, Vanuatu, and Western Samoa.

[e]Includes the Caribbean nations.

Adapted from Michael E, Bundy DA: Global mapping of lymphatic filariasis. Parasitol Today 13: 472, 1997.

areas in Egypt. Filariasis is no longer found around the Mediterranean or in the Middle East.

Bancroftian filariasis was introduced to the Western Hemisphere from Africa with the slave trade. The disease has been greatly reduced in the Americas, with only Haiti and the Dominican Republic remaining important foci in the Caribbean. In South America filariasis occurs only along the eastern tropical coast extending from Guyana to Salvador, Brazil, primarily around urban and semiurban areas, particularly Recife.

DETERMINING FACTORS. The prevalence and intensity of filariasis in an endemic area depends on the intensity of transmission. This relationship arises from the fact that, unlike protozoal or bacterial infections, helminths do not multiply in their human host. Therefore, infection levels relate directly to the number infective larvae to which humans are exposed. As a consequence, bancroftian filariasis is a highly focal disease. Studies show a remarkable heterogeneity of transmission of infection, even among communities within a few kilometers of each other. This probably accounts for the focality of bancroftian filariasis infection. Local ecologic factors that favor the breeding of mosquito vectors, and the fact that flight distance of many mosquito species is limited, contribute to the marked spatial variation of transmission. As might be expected, communities with the most intense transmission within an endemic area have the greatest microfilarial loads and prevalence of lymphatic pathology of the lower extremities and male genitalia. However, among endemic areas this association with transmission intensity and infection and disease may be modified by differences in genetic susceptibility, prior treatment, and co-infections.

Different species of mosquito vectors have variable susceptibility to filariasis and the capacity to transmit the infection to the host. All strains of *W. bancrofti* are thought to be maintained by interhuman transmission, and there is no evidence of a natural animal reservoir. However, monkeys of genus *Presbytis* and some species of the genus *Macaca* can be experimentally infected. The leaf monkey, *Presbytis cristatus*, is a natural host of a closely related species, *W. kalamantani*, found in Indonesia.

The frequency of disease and infection in an endemic population may also be influenced by immunologic tolerance either by exposure of the fetus to parasite antigens from infected mothers during gestation or by repeated exposure of children to infective larvae and/or persistent microfilaremia. When individuals move from nonendemic areas to places having *W. bancrofti* transmission, they develop severe allergic hypersensitivity disease not observed among endemic residents.

The Vector. The major factor in determining the geographic distribution of filariasis is the adaptability of the parasite to local vectors (Chapter 138). Three genera of mosquitoes transmit *W. bancrofti*: *Anopheles*, *Culex*, and *Aedes*. In general, less intense transmission is needed to produce a given prevalence of infection and disease in sub-Saharan Africa than in Asia and Oceania, and the genus *Anopheles* (Fig. 139–4) appears to produce infection and disease more efficiently than the other two genera. *Anopheles* species transmit much of the bancroftian filariasis in rural areas. Adaptation to the day-biting *Aedes* mosquitoes (Fig. 139–5) of the Pacific has depended on the evolution of a strain of *W. bancrofti* with diurnal periodicity. Transmission by sewage-breeding *Culex* species (Fig. 139–6) allowed the establishment of infection within urban and semiurban populations.

The vectoral capacity of mosquitoes for transmitting filariasis depends on a number of factors. These include (1) human-biting density, (2) the proportion of feedings obtained from humans (human-biting index), (3) the amount of blood ingested, (4) the ability of the parasites to be ingested by the mosquito, (5) the timing of feeding as related to the periodicity in the levels of microfilariae within the host, (6) the survivability of the vector, (7) the efficiency of the mosquito in supporting development of microfilariae into the infective stage of the parasite, and (8) its ability to deliver the parasite to humans. All these variables are summarized in the annual transmission potential (ATP), which is the estimated number of bites that an individual receives by mosquitoes with infective-stage larvae (L3) during 1 year. However, estimates of ATP may be similar between different endemic populations, e.g., India and Papua New Guinea, yet result in strikingly different infection levels. Some of these differences probably result from variations in the techniques to determine ATP but may also point to the fact that ATP represents only the risk of infection and not actual transmission.

The Parasite. Surprisingly little is known about the biology of the parasite and its relationship to transmission within a population. No good animal model of *W. bancrofti* exists, which has made studying this parasite particularly difficult. Strain differences occur in the periodicity of microfilariae in the blood to match the feeding behavior of the mosquitoes. In the eastern Pacific, where the day-biting *Aedes* mosquitoes are the major vector, microfilariae are present in the blood during the day and show less periodicity. In the remaining area of its distribution, where nocturnal biting vectors, *Culex* and *Anopheles* mosquitoes, predominate, the parasite is nocturnally periodic. The biologic significance of this periodicity of microfilariae in the circulation remains a puzzle, especially when many other species of blood-borne nematode parasites remain in the circulation throughout the day. It may prolong survival of the microfilariae in the circulation, which is estimated to be 6 months or more.

Marked differences in the level of endemicity and transmission potential required to maintain transmission are noted in different parts of the world. This may occur, in part, as a consequence of vector competency but may also result from parasite variation that affects such parameters as (1) the proportion of infective larvae gaining access to lymphatics and the proportion of those reaching fecundity; (2) parasite longevity; (3) the density of microfilariae in peripheral blood at the times of vector feeding; (4) the ability of microfilariae to congregate at the site of vector feeding; and (5) the success with which microfilariae develop to infective larvae (taking into account rates of maturation and effects of the parasite on survivability of the vectors). In Papua New Guinea, for example, levels of microfilaremia may reach 10,000/mL of peripheral blood, with virtually all adults in some communities having infection. In contrast, although transmission potentials are reported to be similar in Calcutta, India, the prevalence and intensity of infection are much lower.

Host Factors

Age. Infection is slowly acquired with age such that the oldest individuals have the highest prevalence and intensity of infection. Patent infections have been reported in infants less than 1 year of age. However, even in intense areas of transmission, e.g., Papua New Guinea, infections are not usually seen until 3 to 4 years of age and then prevalence increases from ages of about 5 to 20 years. In areas of light to moderate transmission, e.g., in East Africa and India, the prevalence increases more gradually or plateaus in adulthood. Microfilaremia rates in these area rarely exceed 40%. This led to the suggestion that partial concomitant immunity may develop. The use of assays that detect circulating adult worm derived–antigens indicates that infections are much more common than initially thought based on the microfilaremia rate. Moreover, prevalence based on circulating antigen assays continues to increase with age. This suggests that microfilariae may be cleared from the blood more rapidly in adults, perhaps by acquisition of partial stage-specific immunity or loss of immune tolerance to microfilariae. However, in populations with intense transmission, prevalence and intensity of infection continue to rise with the result that almost all adults in certain communities are infected based upon the presence of circulative antigen. Microfilaremia carrier rates in these same communities often exceed 50%. Whether partial acquired immunity to bancroftian filariasis exists remains uncertain.

Clinical illness also tends to increase with age. First signs and symptoms of disease include acute adenolymphadenitis that is followed by chronic lymphedema of the extremities and the appearance of genital lesions in the second and third decades of life. These signs generally show a steady increase in frequency and severity with age.

Sex. The role of gender in susceptibility to infection and disease remains poorly understood. This has arisen, in part, from difficulties in separating levels of exposure between the sexes because of occupation and other behavioral factors. Men generally have higher microfilaremia levels and clinical disease. This greater prevalence of clinically apparent disease in men is a consequence of hydrocele. This is the most common clinical manifestation of *W. bancrofti*. This occurs because lymphatics of the testis, epididymis, and spermatic cord have limited drainage. Chronic lymphedema, especially of the lower extremities, and acute adenolymphangitis have been reported to be more common in women.

Exposure. Exposure can also have an impact on community-specific microfilarial loads and the development of both acute and chronic disease. For example, the frequency of chronic lymphedema, microfilaremia rates, and geometric mean microfilaremia density in the community showed a direct positive correlation with transmission intensity (ranging from approximately 30 to almost 3000 infective larvae per person per year) in villages located within a 15 km radius of each other in Papua New Guinea.

Occupation and socioeconomic status are important risk factors for infections. Filariasis primarily affects persons of the lowest socioeconomic levels, owing to inadequate protection from mosquitoes and to environmental conditions favorable to breeding of vectors. Certain occupations lead to a higher risk for filariasis. Well-known examples include work in abaca plantations in the Philippines and in coconut plantations in Polynesia, as breeding of the *Aedes* vectors occurs in axils of the abaca plant and within discarded coconut husks and tree holes.

Transmission of bancroftian filariasis is quite inefficient and nonresidents who move into endemic areas, e.g., missionaries or volunteers, rarely develop patent infections. However, they may occasionally develop symptoms of acute disease.

Genetics. The genetic background of the human host influences the outcome of most infections. Ethnic differences may be important in susceptibility and development of lymphatic filariasis. For example, indigenous people of the east coast of the Indian subcontinent live adjacent to people who migrated from the Ganges River over 600 years ago. Virtually no intermarriage has occurred between the two groups because of the caste system. Although both groups have similar microfilaremia rates, most of the acute and chronic pathology occurs in the nonindigenous peoples. Similar observations have been made with respect to more recent transmigrants from nonendemic to endemic regions for filariasis in Indonesia and Africa. However, no formal studies of the relationship of genetic difference and disease among these groups have been undertaken. Only a few reports have addressed the relationship between different HLA alleles and chronic lym-

phatic disease. In one study no relationship was observed with elephantiasis and HLA status. Other studies have shown associations of HLA-B15, B27, and the class II antigens DQ5 with elephantiasis. DR3 and 2B3 were negatively associated with chronic pathology. Studies remain to be performed focusing on genome scans using polymorphic microsatellite markers.

Immune Responses. The immunologic hallmark of infections with filarial parasites is induction of allergic-type responses. Typically this produces peripheral eosinophilia and elevated levels of polyclonal and parasite-specific IgE. Although filarial-specific subclasses are present, IgG4 is most prominently elevated. Since IgG4 and IgE are often directed to the same antigenic determinants, it has been suggested that IgG4 may act to block IgE-mediated immediate hypersensitivity responses. Indeed, an increased ratio of parasite IgG4 to IgE is more prominent in asymptomatic microfilaremic individuals than in microfilaremic or amicrofilaremic individuals with chronic pathology, suggesting parasite-specific IgE may participate in acquired immunity but at the same time promote disease. The elevated levels of IgE and IgG4 indicate increased production of interleukin 4 (IL-4) which specifically regulates production of these two isotypes. IL-4 is also acutely upregulated in experimental animals after exposure to filarial antigens.

Cellular immune responses to filarial antigens produce a wide range of CD-dependent immune responses among humans residing in endemic areas for filariasis. This variation may partially account for the spectrum of clinical manifestations and participate in development of partial acquired immunity. Particular focus has been on the complex immune mechanisms that actively participate in modulating the host immune response. Some infected individuals show an impaired filarial antigen–specific T and B cell immunity, which is thought to lead to a microfilaremic state and suppress clinically apparent chronic pathology. This diminished immune response results from a selective impairment of filarial Ag–driven IFN-γ and IL-2 with maintenance of filarial Ag-driven IL-4, IL-5, and IL-10 secreting lymphocytes. Interleukin 10 and TGF-β suppress parasite antigen–specific IFN-γ and IL-2 production. However, recent studies indicate that impaired immune responses correlate better with infection status than with clinical disease. This is based on newer diagnostic assays using circulating antigens that had eluded detection previously. Uninfected individuals living in endemic areas tend to have greater lymphocyte reactivity to both adult worm and microfilarial antigens. Whether this increased reactivity to the parasite antigens correlates with development of protective immunity or whether the absence of active infection fails to generate a state of peripheral tolerance remains uncertain. Heavy exposure to infective-stage parasites may cause filarial antigen–specific immunosuppression and, if sufficiently intense, generalized immunosuppression.

Studies that have examined associations of immune responses with pathogenesis fail to account for the impact of patent infections acquired over many years, the cumulative parasite burden, treatment, and exposure to developing parasites. One emerging hypothesis is that neonates can become sensitized to helminth antigens in utero to produce a range of cytokine responses. In some individuals, under the appropriate conditions, in utero exposure produces a primarily IL-4, IL-5, and IL-10 dominated cytokine response, which can lead to filarial antigen–specific suppression of IFN-γ with IL-2 production. With subsequent patent infections in childhood, most individuals maintain a modulated or tolerant immune response to the parasite. However, with repeated infection and progressive death of parasites, the host is exposed to additional antigens. These broaden the repertoire of immune responses such that clinically apparent lymphatic pathology develops with increasing age, even though microfilaremia may persist in some individuals. However, there is no direct evidence that an ordered or preferential progression occurs from one clinical manifestation to another. Studies of filarial immunity are complicated by the fact that a broad array of immune responses to different antigenic components of various stages of the parasite contribute to the diverse clinical and pathologic signs of filariasis. This is most clearly defined for tropical eosinophilia, which appears to be a disease of hyperreactivity to microfilariae.

PATHOLOGY AND PATHOGENESIS. Adult worms reside within lymphatic channels, most frequently within dilated vessels of the parenchyma or the capsule of inguinal, epitrochlear, and axillary lymph nodes; within major lymphatics distal to these nodes; and within the lymphatics of testis, epididymis, and spermatic cords. High-frequency ultrasound can directly visualize adult worms in the dilated lymphatics. The highly motile worms are often clustered together. Adult worms are also found in the abdominal cavity and retroperitoneal regions of the abdomen. Early in the disease, affected vessels begin to dilate, followed by subsequent inflammation in, and around, the lymph nodes and vessels harboring the developing adult worms. Recent evidence suggests up-regulation of endothelial ligands; e.g., vascular cell adhesion molecule 1 (VCAM1) participates in development of lymphatic pathology. In addition to cytokines, e.g., IL-1 produced by sensitized T cells, mechanical damage to lymph vessels by the whip-like action of the constantly motile adult worm or by its excretory secretory products may participate in the endothelial activation. Additional cells are recruited to the lesion, resulting in endothelial thickening with an infiltrate of lymphocytes, particularly CD8 cells, histiocytes, plasma cells, and eosinophils that accumulate around the parasite and adjacent tissues (Fig. 106–4). Further proliferation of endothelial cells and connective tissue cells may lead to obliterative lymphangitis with scarred, cordlike vessels (Fig. 106–5). The most severe reactions occur around dead or dying adult worms that produce infiltrates of polymorphonuclear cells and histiocytes. This can progress to local necrosis (pus) and marked edema of surrounding tissue (Fig. 106–6). Granulomatous changes may supervene, characterized by the presence of epithelioid and giant cells, and the parasite may be enveloped by coagulated lymph or caseous material. Dead worms lyse or become calcified and surrounded by concentric fibrosis (Fig. 106–4).

Living microfilariae do not generally produce lesions. Dead microfilariae cleared by the reticuloendothelial tissue, cause capillary congestion, edema, and collections of lymphocytes, plasma cells, and eosinophils. The gross pathologic sequelae of repeated inflammatory reactions result in obstruction to normal lymphatic flow, dilation of lymphatic vessels, valvular incompetence of the afferent lymphatic channels, dermal backflow of lymph, and ultimately total lymphatic obstruction (Fig. 106–7). This leads to lymph varices, hydrocele, and elephantiasis, most often of the scrotum, legs, arms, and breast. The skin can become greatly thickened in elephantiasis, which is characterized by markedly increased hyperplasia of the connective tissues, edema, and diffuse infiltrations of plasma cells, eosinophils, and monocytes.

CLINICAL MANIFESTATIONS. The signs and symptoms of bancroftian filariasis differ widely from one endemic area to another. These differences may reflect the relative intensity of exposure to infected vectors between endemic areas.

Asymptomatic Amicrofilaremia. In all endemic areas there exist asymptomatic individuals who are infected with live adult worms as indicated by the presence of circulating filar-

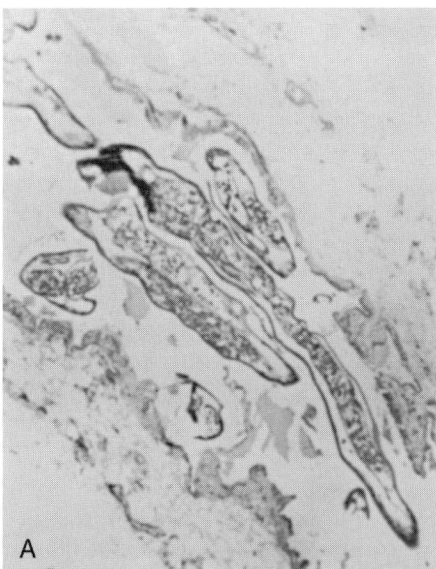

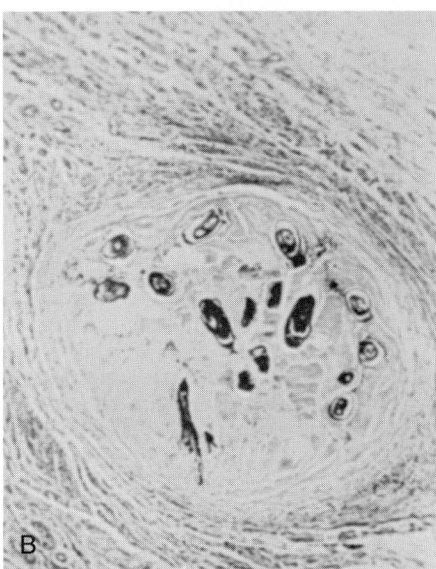

Figure 106–4. *A,* Longitudinal section of intact filarial worm in a lymph vessel. *B,* Granuloma containing a partially calcified filarial worm. (From Galindo L, von Lichtenberg F, Baldizón C: Am J Trop Med Hyg 11:739, 1962.)

ial antigen but who are amicrofilaremic, at least by currently available parasitologic techniques.

Asymptomatic Microfilaremia. Although images of severe end-stage deformity predominate in the literature, clinically asymptomatic microfilaremia is the most common manifestation of bancroftian filariasis, and in all endemic areas a proportion of the infected individuals never become symptomatic. The long-held tenet that these individuals had infection but not disease has been disproved by biopsy and lymphatic imaging studies demonstrating subclinical immune-mediated damage to lymphatics in the majority of asymptomatic individuals (Fig. 106–8).

Acute Manifestations. Acute attacks of retrograde adenolymphangitis, accompanied by fever, chills, and malaise and lasting 3 to 15 days each, occur several times per year and are typical presenting manifestations of disease. Patients usually give a clear history of pain, erythema, and tenderness in the affected lymph node region for hours or a day prior to

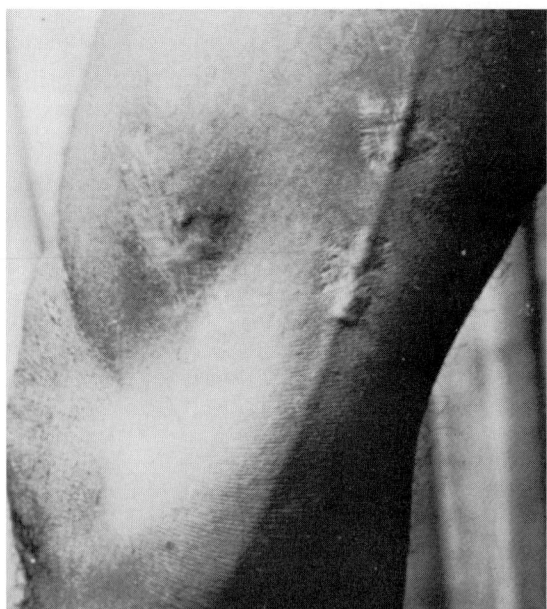

Figure 106–5. Filarial scars overlying a cordlike sclerotic lymphatic vessel. (Courtesy of Dr. David Dennis.)

the onset of lymphangitis. Some individuals may have only one or a few attacks in a lifetime. The patients, however, are likely to have had asymptomatic microfilaremia and subclinical disease for a number of years prior to any acute manifestation. Adenolymphangitis most often affects the groin and, in males, the lymphatics of the genitalia, leading to funiculitis, orchitis, and epididymitis, but essentially any lymph node group may be involved. Localized inflammatory nodules in breast, scrotum, or subcutaneous tissues have been reported as acute manifestations of infection. In some parts of the world, infected superficial nodes, usually inguinal, may suppurate and form sterile abscesses that often leak lymph before rapidly healing with a characteristic scar (Figs. 106–5 and 106–9).

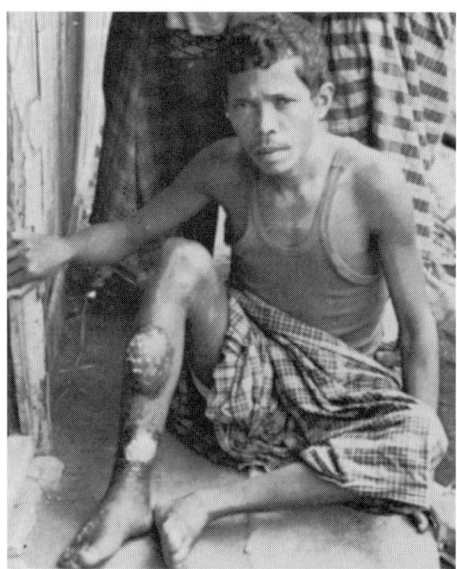

Figure 106–6. Filarial abscesses developing in the lower leg with acute lymphedema distally. The abscesses are covered by a locally prepared poultice.

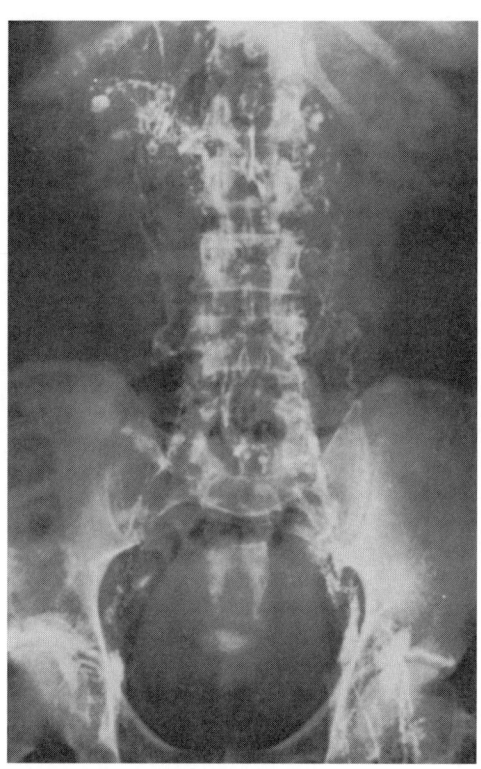

Figure 106–7. Bilateral lower extremity lymphangiogram of a patient infected with *W. bancrofti* demonstrates dilated and tortuous varicosed lymphatics and distended and distorted femoral, inguinal, and retroperitoneal lymph nodes. Obstruction to cephalad flow of lymph produced retrograde filling of the renal pericaliceal lymphatics and rapid excretion of the contrast material in the urine. (Note the faintly opacified distended bladder in the pelvis.) This explains the pathophysiology of chyluria in filariasis.

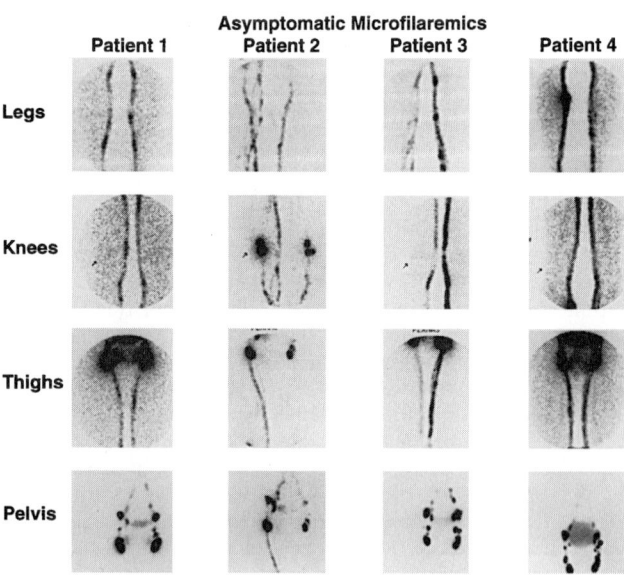

Figure 106–8. Lymphoscintigraphic images 4 hours post injection of isotope into the foot. Each panel shows a face-on view of both lower limbs at the same time. Normal lymph vessels are discrete and continuous and of uniform caliber and density. The majority of asymptomatic microfilaremic individuals have subclinical abnormalities, including dilated tortuous discontinuous vessels, collateral vessel formation around obstructed lymph vessels, and nonvisualization of vessels. Grossly enlarged lymph nodes, e.g., in the popliteal region in Patient 2, are not seen in normal subjects.

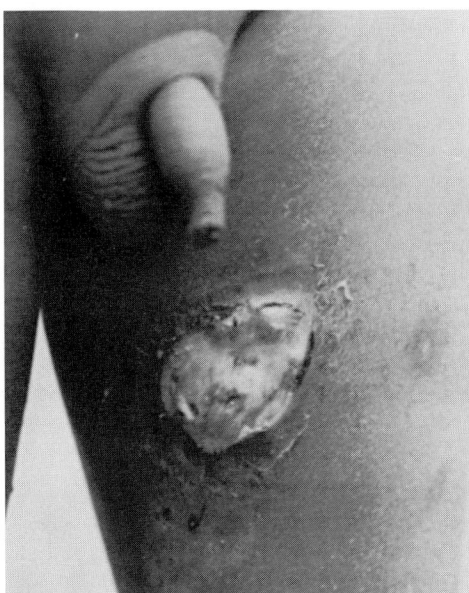

Figure 106–9. Clean-based ulcer resulting from the rupture of a filarial abscess. (Courtesy of Dr. David Dennis.)

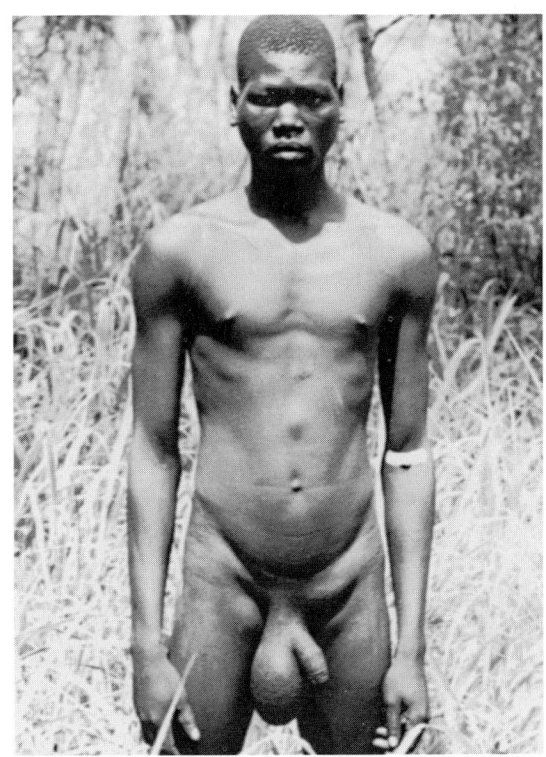

Figure 106–10. Nilotic tribesman of lowland western Ethiopia with bilateral filarial hydrocele and inguinal lymphatic varices progressing toward "hanging-groin." (Courtesy of Dr. David Dennis.)

Chronic Manifestations. Months to years of acute episodes ranging from very mild to severe are followed by development of chronic obstructive disease due to lymphatic insufficiency, disease onset is sometimes rapid but often insidious. The incidence of the main clinical manifestations (hydrocele, lymphedema, elephantiasis, and chyluria) increases with age.

Genital Manifestations. In many areas, by far the most common chronic manifestation is hydrocele (Fig. 106–10). Many patients give no history of recurrent attacks of epididymoorchitis, emphasizing the need for disrobing all male patients in an appropriate setting in order to carry out a complete genital examination. As a result of blockage of draining lymphatics, straw-colored hydrocele fluid accumulates, sometimes in huge volumes, in the closed peritoneal sac surrounding the testicle (Fig. 106–11). The fluid rapidly reaccumulates after any surgical drainage procedure. Chronic epididymitis, funiculitis, and edematous thickening of scrotal skin are also chronic manifestations of disease. Females may occasionally have lymphedema of the vulva, but lesions of the ovary or fallopian tubes are not reported.

Lymphedema and Elephantiasis of Extremities. Reversible episodes of lymphedema of the extremities progress to elephantiasis in the distribution of the affected lymphatics over a period of years. Lower extremities are affected more often than upper. In *W. bancrofti* infection the thighs as well as the lower legs are affected, in contrast to *B. malayi* infection, in which only the lower leg is affected.

The progressive phases of filarial lymphedema are often graded according to the WHO classification, as follows:

Grade 1 lymphedema: mostly pitting edema; spontaneously reversible on elevation.
Grade II lymphedema: mostly nonpitting edema; not spontaneously reversible on elevation.
Grade III lymphedema (elephantiasis): gross increase in volume in a grade II lymphedema, with dermatosclerosis and papillomatous lesions.

Attacks of acute lymphangitis often continue even in those with grade III disease. In these individuals with dermatosclerosis and advanced verrucous skin changes (Fig. 106–12), a role for chronic *secondary* bacterial superinfection originating

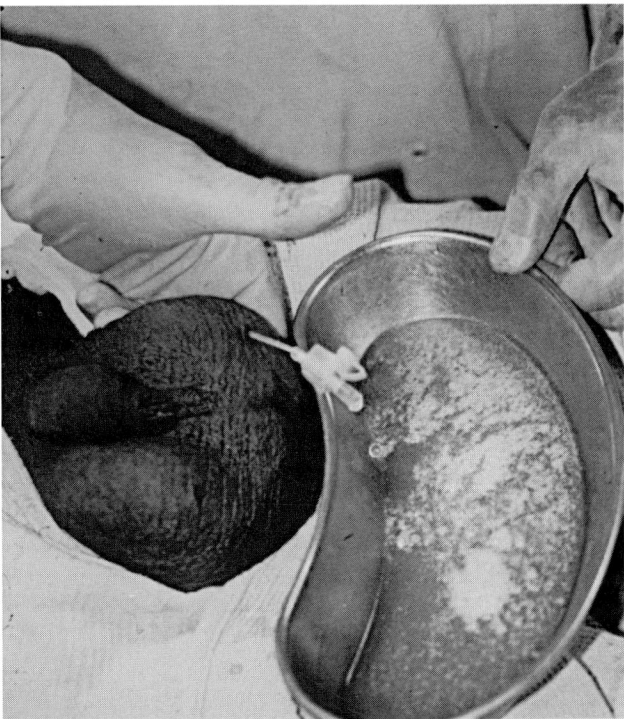

Figure 106–11. Hydrocele is the most common manifestation of clinical filariasis in males, necessitating mandatory genital examination in all patients. Straw-colored hydrocele fluid is noninflammatory and generally without microfilariae. Therapeutic drainage is discouraged, as fluid rapidly reaccumulates.

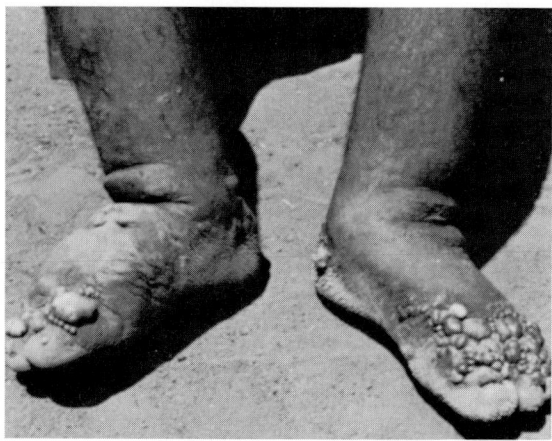

Figure 106–12. Filarial elephantiasis showing nodular and verrucous changes of the skin. Note the characteristic skin folds at the junction of the foot and ankle.

in breaks in the epidermis is clear-cut. The hypothesis that the clinical evolution of the lymphatic insufficiency occurs from repeated bacterial infections superimposed on other processes plays an etiologic role in progression of chronic lymphatic pathology is contested by two points: (1) in limbs with no obvious portal of entry no histologic evidence has been found to support this suggestion: and (2) in none of the animal models of filarial disease is there any pathologic evidence for a primary role for bacteria in filarial inflammation.

Chyluria. Chyluria, a rare event, occurs when increased pressure in obstructed renal lymphatics causes rupture into the urinary collecting system and reflux of intestinal chyle into the urinary tract (Fig. 106–7). As a result of loss of this milky chlyle, which contains important amounts of dietary lipids, proteins, and vitamins, weight loss and malnutrition often ensue. The condition is painless, and microfilaremia may or may not occur in these individuals.

Other Clinical Manifestations. Conditions for which an association with bancroftian filariasis have been suggested include hematuria, glomerulonephritis, monoarthritis of the knee joint, nerve palsies, and tenosynovitis.

Features in Newly Exposed Individuals. Newly exposed individuals characteristically manifest typical acute inflammatory symptoms with more rapid progression to chronic or irreversible disease than do natives of the endemic area. Prolonged severe episodes of adenolymphangitis, often with genital involvement, may lead to development of lymphedema and elephantiasis within 6 to 12 months of arrival. Disease abates quickly with removal of the patient from the endemic area. These individuals are almost always amicrofilaremic.

Natural History of Lymphatic Filariasis. Although the psychosocial morbidity associated with this deforming disease is profound, there is little mortality associated with bancroftian filariasis. Untreated individuals remaining in endemic areas often end up with lymphedema and elephantiasis, but many other remain asymptomatic.

DIAGNOSIS. While most infected individuals in an endemic area are clinically asymptomatic, a clinical diagnosis of lymphatic filariasis may be made in those with the appropriate pattern of acute episodic adenolymphangitis, acute inflammation of scrotal contents, or irreversible lymphedema. Eosinophilia is an inconstant finding in individuals with long-standing exposure and infection.

Parasitologic Diagnosis. Outside of research settings, de-finitive diagnosis often depends on the parasitologic demonstration of the 250 to 320 μm long microfilariae (Fig. 106–13 in color section). Diagnostic sampling must take into account the nocturnal periodicity of *W. bancrofti* in most endemic areas and the subperiodic cycle in the South Pacific. While a Giemsa-stained thick blood smear, performed as for the diagnosis of malaria, may be sufficient for the diagnosis of a heavily infected individual, this technique, sampling only 20 to 60 μL of blood, is not sensitive enough to detect microfilaremias of less than 100 mf/mL of blood. A wet preparation in which fresh finger-prick blood is diluted in a small amount of 3% acetic acid, placed in a hemocytometer counting chamber, and examined for motile microfilariae has greater sensitivity. While finger-prick blood smears may be all that is available in the field, one of three commonly used concentration procedures that sample larger amounts of blood is mandatory to rule out microfilaremia or to detect low-level infection.

The most sensitive technique is to collect 1 to 10 mL of anticoagulated (EDTA or heparin) blood in a syringe and pass it through a 5 μm polycarbonate Nuclepore membrane in a Swinney adapter; 50 mL of water is then passed through the membrane to lyse red cells. The membrane is then removed from the holder and placed on a microscope slide to be examined wet; alternatively, it may be air-dried, fixed with methanol, and stained with Giemsa or hematoxylin. Because of the high cost of the individual membranes, the technique is not practical for extensive use in the tropics.

A useful procedure is that of Knott, in which 1 mL of anticoagulated blood is placed in a conical centrifuge tube with 9 mL of 2% formalin. The tube is then centrifuged at 1500 rpm for 1 minute or left to stand overnight. After the supernatant is decanted and the sediment spread on a slide to air-dry, the slide is fixed with methanol and stained with Giemsa (1:40) or hematoxylin.

A sheathed microfilaria in which the caudal nuclei do not reach the end of the tail is characteristic of *W. bancrofti* isolated from blood (Fig. 106–2 and Fig. 106–13 in color section). Some parasitologists prefer the hematoxylin stain, as it distinctly stains the sheath of all sheathed species a light purple; Giemsa stains the sheaths of *W. bancrofti* and *B. malayi* a faint pink, but it fails to stain that of *L. loa*. Wright's stain should not be used. Microfilariae on filters may not always be suitable for morphologic study no matter which stain is used. A minimum of two each of daytime and nighttime blood samples is necessary in areas where nocturnally periodic filariae coexist with nonperiodic or diurnally periodic forms. The microfilariae remain alive in anticoagulated blood kept at room temperature for at least 2 days, so that immediate examination is not necessary.

A single dose of diethylcarbamazine (DEC) can in many cases provoke daytime microfilaremia in nocturnally periodic disease, but this practice is discouraged outside of mass surveys, as it is less sensitive and can result in drug reactions in heavily microfilaremic persons.

Microfilariae of *W. bancrofti* have also been found in the urine of the occasional asymptomatic, amicrofilaremic patient but are usually not present in chyluric patients. Chyle in urine can be confirmed by xylene or ether, which dissolves the top floating, creamy layer after the specimen is shaken. Incidental findings of microfilariae of *W. bancrofti* have been made in cytologic preparations of cervix, vagina, and gastric brushings. This presumably represents blood contaminating the specimen. A highly experienced pathologist would be needed to identify the sections of adult worms that are found from time to time in specimens of diverse human body tissues (Fig. 106–4).

Serology. Serologic and other immunodiagnostic procedures (including skin testing and in vitro tests of parasite-specific cell-mediated immunity) have not been particularly useful as diagnostic tools because the majority of individuals from endemic regions have developed antibodies against the filarial parasite.

Currently, serologic tests for filaria-specific antibody are immunoassays using crude antigens derived from either adult worms of *B. malayi* or the dog filarid *D. immitis*. None of these assays can distinguish among the eight filarial parasites that commonly infect humans; nor can they distinguish among actively infected patients, those merely exposed (but not microfilaremic), or patients successfully treated. More recently research assays have been developed that have the ability to detect circulating *W. bancrofti* parasite antigen even in the daytime blood of those with nocturnally periodic microfilariae. Two tests are now commercially available, one from TropBioMed (Townsville, Australia). The serum-based assay is probably the most sensitive and specific test currently available; however the filter-based assay remains to be refined. A rapid card test using a different monoclonal antibody that measures circulating antigens (ICT test) and utilizes finger-prick blood is accurate, rapid, and easily used in population-based studies.

Differential Diagnosis. Bacterial infection, thrombophlebitis, or trauma may be mistaken for acute filarial adenolymphangitis. Tuberculosis, leprosy, sarcoidosis, and other systemic granulomatous diseases may be confused with filarial disease. Filarial lymphangitis is retrograde, which helps differentiate it from bacterial lymphangitis. The long incubation period and prolonged exposure necessary to acquire filarial disease should be kept in mind. Chronic lymphedema may be caused by malignancy, postoperative changes, congenital malformations, or a hereditary form of lymphostasis (Milroy's disease) as well as renal or cardiac failure. Physical examination cannot distinguish a filarial from a nonfilarial cause of lymphedema or elephantiasis. A foreign body reaction to silica dust introduced into traumatized legs accounts for elephantiasis in some parts of the world. Patients with filarial lymphedema are often amicrofilaremic, so that diagnosis depends on the clinical history as well as the physical examination and may be supported by positive serology. In cases of orchitis and epididymitis the sexually transmitted diseases including gonococcal infections must be considered as a possible diagnosis.

TREATMENT. The mainstay of treatment for lymphatic filariasis has been DEC, a piperazine derivative. DEC (Hetrazan, Banocide, Notezine, Filarizan) rapidly kills microfilariae and can kill some, but not all adults of both *Wuchereria* and *Brugia*. DEC is not active in vitro against Brugia spp., suggesting that the drug works through the host's immune response. The standard dosage is 6 mg/kg administered over a period of 10 to 14 days (for a total cumulative dose of 72 mg/kg), which reduces microfilaremia levels by approximately 80 to 90% in several days. Microfilaria levels may remain low for more than 6 to 12 months, but they subsequently increase. The overall effect on adult worms appears to be related to the total dose given, with spaced doses (e.g., weekly or monthly for many months or years) probably being superior to a more concentrated course of treatment (e.g., daily for 12 days). Initially, a lower dose can be given, 1 to 3 mg/kg once a day for 2 or 3 days, prior to advancing to a higher twice-daily dose. This has the effect of slowly removing some of the microfilariae and reducing side effects of the drug, especially in individuals with heavy parasite burdens.

Side effects, including fever, headache, myalgia, vomiting, weakness, and asthma, usually result from rapid destruction of microfilariae and perhaps adult worms, especially in heavily infected individuals. These symptoms develop within the first 2 days, often within 12 hours, after initiation of treatment, and may persist for 3 or 4 days. Abscesses have been reported in the scrotum and groin after treatment, presumably from a reaction to a dead worm (Fig. 106–9). DEC is not recommended for treatment during pregnancy, although no teratogenic effects of drug have been reported. Special care should be taken for treatment of individuals residing in areas where onchocerciasis and loiasis are prevalent. Both these organisms are also sensitive to DEC, and their death can cause severe reactions. Peripheral eosinophilia often accompanies infection with this parasite, and if treatment is effective this should resolve. There is usually a transient increase in peripheral eosinophilia with treatment coincident with killing of parasites. If peripherial eosinophilia and/or clinical symptoms persist after treatment the peripheral blood should be re-examined for microfilaremia and/or circulating antigen. The drug is rapidly excreted and nontoxic; repeat treatment may be safely given 1 month following completion of the first course. Treatment usually reduces or eliminates episodes of acute lymphatic inflammation and prevents further progression of obstructive lesions. Reduction or elimination of hydroceles is one of the more dramatic effects of treatment, even with a single dose. In some cases chronic lymphedema actually regresses. However, treatment generally fails to improve advanced elephantiasis.

Reactions to DEC treatment are usually most severe in infections with *B. malayi* and *B. timori*, and the incidence of side effects is directly related to the microfilarial density and worm burdens.

Two additional drugs are effective against lymphatic filariasis; ivermection (Mectizan) and albendazole. Ivermectin appears to kill only microfilariae but can be given as a single dose of 400 µg/kg. Although ivermectin leads to a more rapid and complete clearance of microfilariae, sustained reductions 6 months or longer after treatment are equivalent or better with a single 6 mg/kg dose of DEC. This is consistent with DEC having a greater effect upon adult worms. When ivermectin is used in combination with DEC as single dose, microfilariae are more rapidly cleared, but more importantly, recrudescence is delayed. Recent studies suggest that albendazole (given in combination with ivermectin) as single dose of 400 mg is more effective in clearing microfilariae than ivermectin alone.

PREVENTION AND CONTROL. The WHO has now set a goal of eradication of filariasis worldwide in the next 10 years. Mass treatment of affected populations with DEC medicated salts or repeated annual doses of ivermection and/or DEC produces significant reductions in *W. bancrofti* microfilaremia that can be sustained for a year or longer. These control programs, even after a single year of treatment, have produced marked reductions or interruptions of transmission. This approach has proved to be a much more cost-effective method of control than vector elimination programs alone. Theoretically, annual mass treatment will be effective if given for at least 5 years, the estimated median life span of adult *W. bancrofti* worms, and could eliminate the parasite in the community. Albendazole, added to this combination therapy, might enhance the efficacy of the DEC and ivermection. In addition, albendazole and ivermection have the advantage that they are effective against most intestinal helminth infections such that control programs directed toward lymphatic filariasis have the added benefit of reducing intestinal helminthic infections within a community. Such programs have become increasingly feasible, since DEC is very inexpensive and is extremely stable. It can even withstand cooking. Ivermectin and albendazole have been generously donated by their manufacturers for control purposes.

Control programs have been highly successful. In some areas, however, reluctance of patients to cooperate has presented problems, especially in areas with *Brugia* infections. Administration of repeated annual treatment have been well accepted by the local populations, especially with the additional benefits that ivermectin has in treating scabies, and the ability of albendazole to eliminate intestinal helminths. Reduction in hydroceles produces readily observable benefits. Treatment of populations with DEC-medicated salts over prolonged periods has produced some notable successes, particularly in China.

Bibliography

Amaral F, Dreyer G, Figueredo-Silva J, et al: Live adult worms detected by ultrasonography in human Bancroftian filariasis. Am J Trop Med Hyg 50:753, 1994.

Bockarie MJ, Alexander N, Hyun P, et al: Randomized community-based trial of annual single-dose diethylcarbamazine with or without ivermectin against *Wuchereria bancrofti* infection in human beings and mosquitoes. Lancet 351:162, 1998.

Bundy DA, Grenfell BT, Rajagopalan PK: Immunoepidemiology of lymphatic filariasis: The relationship between infection and disease. Immunol Today 12:A71, 1991.

Freedman DO, de Almeida Filho PJ, Besh S, et al: Lymphoscintigraphic analysis of lymphatic abnormalities in symptomatic and asymptomatic human filariasis. J Infect Dis 170:927, 1994.

Kazura JW, Bockarie M, Alexander N, et al: Transmission intensity and its relationship to infection and disease due to *Wuchereria bancrofti* in Papua New Guinea. J Infect Dis 176:242, 1997.

Michael E, Bundy DA: Global mapping of lymphatic filariasis. Parasitol Today 13:472, 1997.

Michael E, Grenfell BT, Bundy DA: The association between microfilaraemia and disease in lymphatic filariasis. Proc R Soc Lond B Biol Sci 256:33, 1994.

More SJ, Copeman DB: A highly specific and sensitive monoclonal antibody–based ELISA for the detection of circulating antigen in bancroftian filariasis. Trop Med Parasitol 41:403, 1990.

Ottesen EA: Efficacy of diethylcarbamazine in eradication of infection with the lymphatic dwelling filariae of humans. Rev Infect Dis 7:341, 1985.

Wartman WB, King BG: Filariasis in American armed forces in WWII. Medicine 26:334, 1947.

Weil GJ, Wammie PJ, Weiss N: The ICT filariasis test: A rapid format antigen test for diagnosis of Bancroftian filariasis. Parasitol Today 13:401, 1997.

World Health Organization: Lymphatic filariasis: The disease and its control. Fifth report of the WHO Expert Committee on Filariasis. World Health Organ Tech Rep Ser 821:1, 1992.

106.2 *Brugian Filariasis*

DEFINITION. Brugian filariasis denotes human infection with *B. malayi* and *B. timori*. Although the parasite is closely related to *Wuchereria bancrofti* and was not assigned to a separate genus until 1958 by Buckley, important differences in biology, epidemiology, and, especially, clinical manifestations exist. Unlike *W. bancrofti*, which has no animal reservoir, the subperiodic form of *B. malayi* is a zoonosis with an important reservoir in monkeys and cats. In contrast to *W. bancrofti*, the repeated episodes of adenolymphangitis caused by the lymphatic-dwelling *Brugia* adults eventually result in elephantiasis of only the distal extremities. Chronic genital disease does not occur.

ETIOLOGY

Morphology. *B. malayi* (Brug, 1927) is similar to *W. bancrofti* in morphology. The adult worms are about half the size of those of *W. bancrofti* and have distinguishing features of male genitalia and adjacent papillae. The sheathed microfilariae are 200 to 275 μm by 4 to 7 μm and have an ungraceful and kinked appearance, a long cephalic space, a packed nuclear column in which the cells are overlapping, and, most importantly for differentiation from *W. bancrofti*, two discrete terminal nuclei that reach the tip of the tail (Fig. 106–2 and

Fig. 106–13 in color section). Although there is overlap, periodic microfilariae have a greater total length than the subperiodic microfilariae. The pink-staining sheath (Giemsa or hematoxylin) is absent in 50% of periodic microfilariae but in only 5% of the subperiodic form. When compared with *B. malayi*, the microfilariae of *B. timori* (Partono, 1977) have a longer total length (up to 310 μm), a longer cephalic space, and a sheath that does not stain with Giemsa. Morphologic differentiation of the two human *Brugia* species requires experience and well-stained specimens. DNA analysis has confirmed that the species are distinct.

DEVELOPMENT AND LIFE CYCLE. With the exception of the differences in the arthropod vector species, the development and life cycle of the parasite are essentially the same as that of *W. bancrofti* (Fig. 106–1). However, *Brugia* has a shorter developmental time in the vector mosquitoes and a prepatent period (time from infection to appearance of microfilariae) that may be as short as 3 1/2 months as compared with 6 to 12 months for *W. bancrofti*.

EPIDEMIOLOGY

Brugia malayi. *B. malayi* is found only in Asia, from India in the west to Korea in the northeast and Indonesia in the south (Fig. 106–3B). An estimated 13 million are infected with brugian filariasis as compared with 106 million for bancroftian filariasis. Brugian filariasis in India is found mostly in Kerala, but scattered foci of low prevalence are reported in Orissa, Assam, Madhya Pradesh, Andhra Pradesh, and Tamil Nadu. In Indonesia, *B. malayi* foci are found in Sumatra, Kalimantan, Sulawesi, Burunia, and Iran Jaya. Vietnam and the Philippines report significant numbers of cases. In Malaysia, only scattered foci remain in the peninsular part, but there are moderately endemic foci in Sabah and Sarawak. Infection that had been highly endemic throughout southeastern China, has been nearly eradicated, owing to control campaigns over the past decade.

As an adaptation to different vector species in different biogeographic zones, two major forms of *B. malayi* are distinguished: the nocturnally periodic and the nocturnally subperiodic. The periodic form, which has no animal reservoir, is transmitted by *Mansonia* and *Anopheles* species of open swamp and wet rice cultivation areas and by anophelines in hill-forest regions. Only the nocturnally periodic form exists in India, Sulawesi, Vietnam, and China. The subperiodic form, which is transmitted by *Mansonia* species in riverine swamp forest ecosystems is found along with periodic forms in Malaysia and Indonesia.

Brugia timori. *B. timori* is limited in distribution to the small volcanic islands of eastern Indonesia that include Timor, Alor, Flores, Sumba, Roti, and Savu. It is especially endemic in low-lying riverine valleys of foothills and in coastal areas. It is nocturnally periodic with an anopheline vector.

Other *Brugia* Species. In addition to the two *Brugia* species infecting humans, at least eight species that parasitize animals are known. These filariae share the same mosquito vectors and the L3s and microfilariae are often morphologically very similar to those of *B. malayi*. This leads to difficulty in trying to implicate some of the non-*malayi* species as possible zoonoses capable of infecting humans. *B. pahangi*, the most often implicated, is capable of naturally infecting humans.

CLINICAL MANIFESTATIONS. The symptomatology of brugian filariasis (both *B. malayi* and *B. timori*) is significantly different from that of *W. bancrofti* infection. It is more distinct, more dramatic, and more destructive. In brugian filariasis, episodes of prolonged fever (5 to 15 days), adenolymphangitis, abscesses of affected lymph nodes, and local residual scarring occur frequently in infected individuals. These classic acute symptoms are usually restricted to involvement of

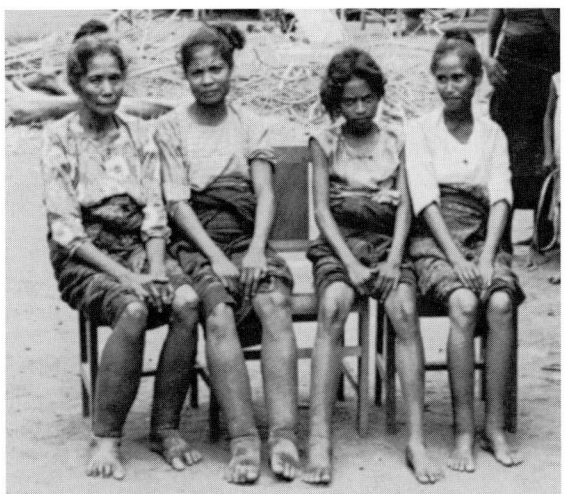

Figure 106–14. Elephantiasis in Timorian filariasis showing the "water-bag" deformity and fissuring at ankles.

a single lymph node at a time, most often in the inguinal area but sometimes in the axillae. Extension of the acute episode, when it occurs, is due to a characteristic retrograde lymphangitis. Insidious onset of chronic lymphedema or elephantiasis, as may occur in bancroftian filariasis, is uncommon. With recurrent episodes, progression to elephantiasis occurs in a small proportion of cases (Fig. 106–14). The swelling is restricted to distal extremities beyond the knee or elbow (Fig. 106–15). Sclerotic cordlike lymphatics and enlarged firm nodes of the arms and legs are usual (Fig. 106–5). Urogenital disease and chyluria do not occur.

DIAGNOSIS. Diagnostic methods are the same as for *W. bancrofti* (Chapter 106.1). Differences in microfilariae can be visualized in stained blood films (Fig. 106–2 and Fig. 106–13 in color section).

TREATMENT AND CONTROL. Treatment is essentially the same as for *W. bancrofti*. The microfilaricidal response to a single 200 μg/kg dose of ivermectin is qualitatively different from the rapid response seen in *W. bancrofti* infection. A gradual decrease in microfilariae to 15 to 20% of pretreatment levels occurs over several weeks and is sustained for at least 6 months.

Bibliography

Denham DA, McGreevy PB: Brugian filariasis: Epidemiological and experimental studies. Adv Parasitol 16:243, 1977.

Mak JW, Navaratnam V, Grewel JS, et al: Treatment of subperiodic *Brugia malayi* infection with a single dose of ivermectin. Am J Trop Med Hyg 48:591, 1993.

Michael E, Bundy DAP, Grenfell BT: Reassessing the global prevalence and distribution of lymphatic filariasis. Parasitology 112:409, 1996.

Partono F: The spectrum of disease in lymphatic filariasis. Ciba Found Symp 127:15, 1987.

Partono F, Dennis DT, Atmosoedjono S, et al: *Brugia timori* sp. n. (Nematoda: filarioidea) from Flores Island, Indonesia. J Parasitol 63:540, 1977.

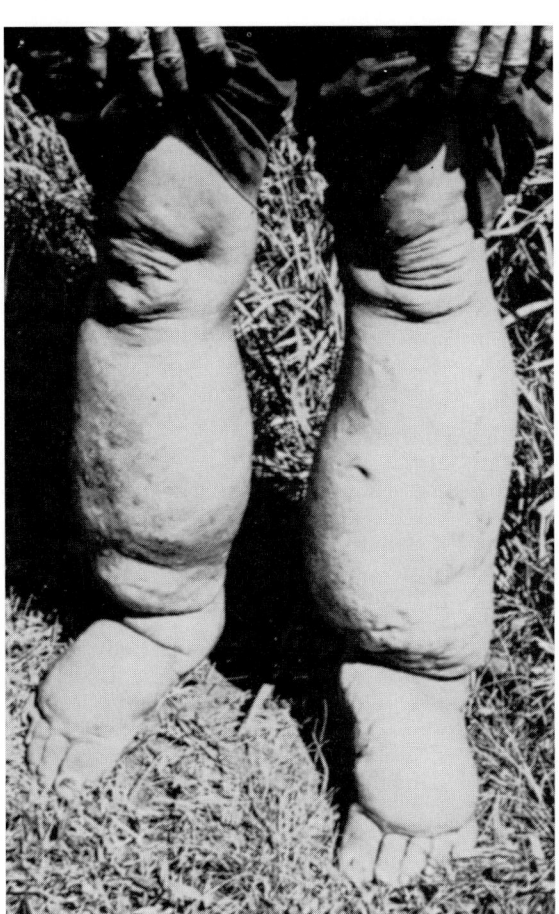

Figure 106–15. The so-called water-bag deformity of elephantiasis due to *Brugia* infection. The swelling does not often extend above the knee.

106.3 Tropical Pulmonary Eosinophilia

ETIOLOGY. Tropical pulmonary eosinophilia (TPE) results from *W. bancrofti* or *B. malayi* infection. These infections can cause diffuse pulmonary infiltrates with marked local and systemic eosinophilia. The pathogenesis of TPE is postulated to result from an intense inflammatory response to microfilariae as they migrate through the pulmonary blood vessels. This produces an exaggerated allergic type hypersensitivity response characterized by marked peripheral and pulmonary eosinophilia as well as strikingly high levels of polyclonal and parasite-specific IgE. The basic pathology relates to the apparent role of the eosinophil in causing local tissue damage and alterations in pulmonary physiology. Activated eosinophils release toxic oxygen products (hydrogen peroxide and hydroxyl radicals), lipid mediators (leukotriene C_4), and granular proteins (eosinophil cationic protein and major basic protein) that affect pulmonary respiratory epithelium and smooth muscle function.

EPIDEMIOLOGY. Little is known about the epidemiology of TPE, in part because of its infrequent occurrence and failure to consistently distinguish it from other causes of pulmonary eosinophilia. It occurs in long-time residents of endemic areas, but not in travelers or individuals who live in endemic areas for only a couple of years. TPE may also develop in susceptible individuals who leave endemic areas, even months to years after their departure. Most reported cases have been from South India; TPE may be more common there relative to other endemic areas in the world.

PATHOLOGY AND PHYSIOLOGY. Pulmonary function tests in individuals with TPE show primarily restrictive abnormalities with a minor obstructive component as demonstrated by decreased forced expiratory volume (FEV_1). Arterial oxygen saturation may also be diminished. A severe alveolitis develops with acute or subacute TPE with activated eosinophils constituting more than 50% of total cells recovered by bronchoalveolar lavage. Increased concentrations of filarial-specific IgE and IgG4 are also present in bronchial washings.

Earlier studies of TPE, before the filarial etiology was clearly defined, contained detailed pathologic studies of lung biopsies from affected individuals. These studies showed numerous granulomas within the lungs, some which contained remnants of microfilariae and adult worms; this suggests that trapping of these parasites in the lung elicits the marked alveolitis. Because of the absence of blood-borne microfilariae in TPE patients it has been hypothesized that TPE results from an intense inflammatory response to microfilariae as they migrate through the pulmonary blood vessels. Why this occurs in only a small proportion of individuals living in filarial endemic areas remains uncertain. Attempts to find a genetic association with TPE have so far been unsuccessful.

CLINICAL MANIFESTATIONS

Symptomotology. Tropical pulmonary eosinophilia most often occurs in young adult males (male : female ratio 4:1) in their twenties and thirties. Signs and symptoms usually begin slowly, progressing over a period of months. Typically, individuals complain of a nonproductive cough, wheezing, fever, generalized malaise, fatigue, and weight loss. One clue that these symptoms may be associated with TPE is the propensity for their occurrence at night. Although unproven, this could result from the nocturnal release of microfilariae that become trapped in the lungs. Signs include rales and rhonchi detected during auscultation of the chest and hepatosplenomegaly accompanied by generalized lymph node enlargement in children; these latter findings are uncommon in adults.

LABORATORY AND RADIOGRAPHIC FINDINGS. Marked peripheral eosinophilia and very elevated serum levels of polyclonal and filarial-specific IgE are the hallmarks of TPE. The absolute eosinophil count usually exceeds 3000/μL of blood, and the total serum IgE is greater than 10,000 ng/mL, which exceeds levels observed in individuals with other clinical manifestations of filariasis and most other helminthic infections. The absence of microfilaremia is characteristic of all TPE patients and should be confirmed by evaluating night blood samples.

The chest radiograph of individuals with TPE usually shows diffuse small (1 to 3 mm in diameter) interstitial or reticulonodular infiltrates with increased bronchovascular markings. Hilar lymphadenopathy and pleural effusion are usually not present. In advanced, untreated cases, diffuse interstitial fibrosis may be present on the chest radiograph.

DIAGNOSIS. The diagnosis rests upon a constellation of clinical, epidemiologic, and laboratory features that are consistent with TPE. But probably the most important feature is successful resolution of symptoms with DEC treatment. The potentially affected individual should have a history of long-term residence in a filarial endemic area, most often South India. Elevated peripheral eosinophilia >3000 μl/mL of blood and >10,000 ng/mL of serum IgE coincident with an absence of peripheral microfilaremia should be present to support the diagnosis of TPE.

Failure to respond to DEC treatment should suggest alternative diagnoses. A diverse array of illness can also cause pulmonary infiltrates with eosinophilia. These include Churg-Strauss syndrome (allergic granulomatosis with angiitis), vasculitides, e.g., Wegener's granulomatosis and periarteritis nodosa, allergic bronchopulmonary aspergillosis, idiopathic hypereosinophilic syndrome, and severe asthma associated with environmental allergens.

TREATMENT. The mainstay of treatment is with DEC, which is given in the same dosage schedule as for bancroftian filariasis (Chapter 106.1). Clinical improvement usually occurs within 2 to 5 days after treatment is initiated and is rarely associated with side effects. Patients may require repeated treatments, since in many individuals pulmonary disease persists. The failure of pulmonary findings to completely resolve in many patients raises some interesting questions. DEC treatment may fail to completely eliminate the filarial infection. Alternatively, the allergic hyperresponsiveness may activate immunologic processes to such an extent as to induce a hyperresponsiveness to other allergens even after all parasites are eliminated. Thus, in some circumstances, it may be appropriate to treat patients with corticosteroids.

Bibliography

Ottesen EA, Neva FA, Paranjape RS, et al: Specific allergic sensitization to filarial antigens in tropical eosinophilia syndrome. Lancet 1:1158, 1979.

Pinkston P, Vijyayan VK, Nutman T, et al: Acute tropical pulmonary eosinophilia: Characterization of the lower respiratory tract inflammation and its response to therapy. J Clin Invest 80:216, 1987.

Udwadia FE: Tropical eosinophilia: A correlation of clinical histopathologic and lung function studies. Dis Chest 52:531, 1967.

Udwadia FE: Tropical eosinophilia: A review. Respir Med 87:17, 1993.

107 Loiasis

Amy Klion

DEFINITION. Loiasis is caused by infection with the filarial nematode *Loa loa*. The adult worms migrate through the subcutaneous tissues causing intermittent "Calabar swellings" and sometimes migrate beneath the conjunctiva (hence, the popular name *eye worm*). Microfilariae are found in the peripheral blood during the day.

DISTRIBUTION. Loiasis is endemic to the rain forests of Central and West Africa, including Democratic Republic of Congo, Northwest Angola, Gabon, Central African Republic, Cameroon, Nigeria, Chad, southwest Sudan, Benin, and Equatorial Guinea. Isolated cases have also been reported in Uganda, Malawi, Zambia, and Ethiopia, and in the region from Ghana to Guinea.

TRANSMISSION

Vectors. A generic life cycle of filarial nematodes is covered in Chapter 106. The vectors are large tabanid flies of the genus *Chrysops*, known in Africa as red flies. The species *C. silacea* and *C. dimidiata* are the most important. Day-biting females pick up the microfilariae of *Loa* in their blood meals. The ingested microfilariae lose their sheaths, penetrate the gut wall, and migrate to the cells of the fat body, where they molt twice. The infective filariform larvae develop in 10 to 12 days and move to the proboscis. Many larvae (up to 100) can develop in a single fly. When the fly bites a new host, larvae are injected and develop into adult worms over the course of 6 to 12 months.

Adult Worms. Adult *Loa* are thin transparent worms that migrate through the subcutaneous tissues at rates of up to 1 cm/min. Females measure 50 to 70 × 0.5 mm, and males 30 to 35 × 0.3 to 0.4 mm. The cuticle of the middle region in both sexes has numerous small bosses that aid in identifying portions of worms removed at biopsy. Adult worms may survive for 4 to 17 years.

Microfilariae. In bisexual infections, microfilariae are released into the blood stream, where they are most plentiful between 10 A.M. and 2 P.M. It is this diurnal periodicity, their size (approximately 290 by 7.5 μm), the presence of a sheath, and three or more terminal nuclei that distinguish the microfilariae of *Loa loa* from the blood-borne microfilariae of *Wuchereria bancrofti* and *Mansonella perstans*, other filarial pathogens of humans whose geographic distribution overlaps that of *Loa loa*.

EPIDEMIOLOGY. It has been estimated that *Loa loa* infects 3 to 13 million people in West and Central Africa. The distribution of the disease is determined by that of the vectors, which breed in wet mud on the edge of shaded streams beneath the high-canopied rain forest in which the adult *Chrysops* live. Flies are attracted by the movement of people or vehicles or by rising wood smoke. Particularly favorable vector-host conditions are created by rubber plantations, which form a dense canopy 30 to 50 feet above ground level. Infection rates are usually higher in adults, particularly males, than in children, probably because of an increased exposure to biting flies. Flies are most common during the rainy season and will enter houses only if they are well lit inside.

Reservoirs. Nonhuman primates, especially the drill (*Mandrillus leucophaeus*), harbor a form of *Loa*, but the microfilariae of this form are nocturnally periodic and the vectors are night-biting *C. langi* and *C. centurionis*. Although the simian and human strains have been hybridized experimentally, it is unlikely that nonhuman primates act as reservoir hosts, because the nocturnal *Chrysops* species do not usually bite humans.

CLINICAL MANIFESTATIONS. As is true of the other filarial infections of humans, the clinical spectrum of loiasis is quite broad, ranging from asymptomatic infection to life-threatening complications, including encephalitis, cardiomyopathy, and renal failure. With the exception of eye worm (see below), clinical signs and symptoms are more common in visitors to *Loa*-endemic areas than in persons native to these areas and reflect a heightened immune response to the parasite. Conversely, microfilariae are detectable in the peripheral blood of most endemic individuals with loiasis but are rare in infected visitors.

Calabar Swellings. Recurrent episodes of localized angioedema, or Calabar swellings (Fig. 107–1), are one of the

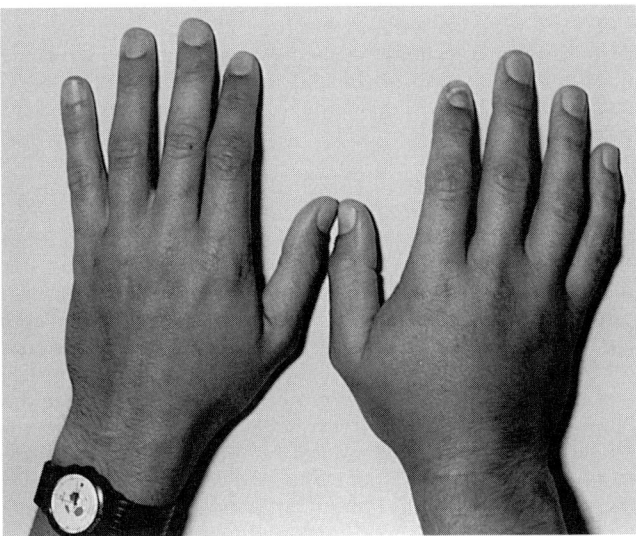

Figure 107–1. Calabar swelling of the right hand in a nonendemic patient with loiasis.

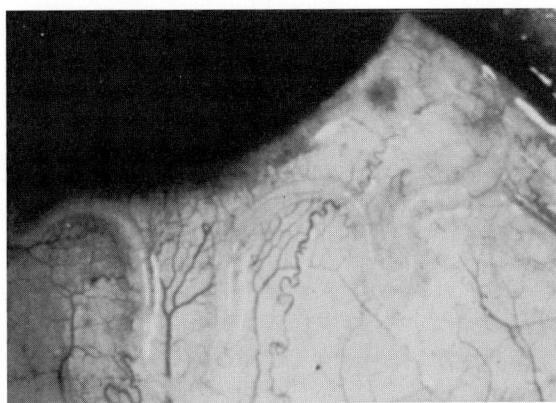

Figure 107–2. Adult *Loa* worm migrating beneath conjunctiva. (Courtesy of Dr. J. Anderson.)

characteristic manifestations of loiasis. Although their precise etiology is unproved, Calabar swellings are thought to be a hypersensitivity response to antigenic material released by a migrating, developing or adult worm. They are most common on the face and extremities and may occur in response to local trauma. Typically, an area of pain or itching develops followed within hours by the development of a 10- to 20-cm area of nonpitting edema. The edema lasts from a few days to several weeks and is usually painless, except when the location of the swelling causes restriction of joint movement or nerve compression. Peripheral nerve compression is most common in the region of the carpal tunnel and may be transiently exacerbated by diethylcarbamazine (DEC) treatment. In severe cases, the deficit may be permanent.

Eye Worm. Subconjunctival migration of the adult worm, eye worm (Fig. 107–2), is generally accompanied by transient swelling of the lid and intense conjunctivitis. Although most episodes resolve spontaneously and completely, rare cases of retinal artery occlusion and macular retinopathy due to aberrant migration of the adult parasite have been reported.

Other Symptoms. Nonspecific systemic symptoms including pruritus, urticaria, myalgia, arthralgia, fatigue, and malaise are common. Eosinophilia is marked in most infected individuals and may exceed 70% (or 20,000 cells/mm³).

Complications

Central Nervous System. The most serious complication of *Loa loa* infection is meningoencephalitis, which occurs predominantly in patients with high numbers of circulating microfilariae, particularly in the setting of treatment with DEC. The severity of central nervous system involvement ranges from mild headache and meningismus to coma and death. Occasionally, microfilariae are found in the cerebrospinal fluid, and, in fatal cases, degenerating microfilariae have been seen in necrotizing granulomas in the brain.

Renal. Hematuria and proteinuria are commonly seen in loiasis and may be due to immune complex glomerulonephritis or mechanical trauma resulting from the filtration of large numbers of microfilariae. The urinary sediment is usually unremarkable, except for the occasional detection of microfilariae. Transient worsening may occur following DEC treatment; most cases resolve completely with treatment, however, and progression to chronic renal insufficiency is unusual.

Endomyocardial Fibrosis. Loiasis has been implicated in the etiology of some cases of endomyocardial fibrosis (EMF) in equatorial Africa based on the higher prevalence of EMF in *Loa*-endemic areas than in other regions in Africa and high levels of antifilarial antibodies detected in some individuals with EMF (Chapter 3). Although clinical resolution of biopsy-proven EMF with antifilarial therapy has been documented in one patient with concomitant loiasis, the relationship between these two clinical entities remains ill-defined.

Other Complications. Transient pulmonary infiltrates and pleural effusion responsive to antifilarial therapy have been reported in patients with loiasis. Other uncommon manifestations of loiasis include arthritis, lymphangitis, and hydrocele.

DIAGNOSIS. Loiasis should be considered in any individual with a compatible travel history who presents with unexplained eosinophilia, Calabar swellings, or an adult worm migrating under the skin or across the eye. Sometimes, the diagnosis is suggested by dead calcified worms seen on a roentgenogram.

Microscopic Identification. Demonstration of sheathed microfilariae with nuclei extending to the tip of the tail in a daytime blood specimen or identification of an adult worm removed from the subcutaneous tissue is diagnostic. Although microfilariae are sometimes seen in thick blood smears stained with Giemsa or Wright's stain, concentration techniques, including Knott's concentration, saponin lysis, and filtration of anticoagulated blood through a 5 μm Nuclepore filter, are useful in patients with low numbers of circulating microfilariae.

Serology. Immunodiagnostic tests are available commercially and at some academic centers and may be useful in confirming the diagnosis of filariasis in travelers from endemic areas who have characteristic clinical symptoms or unexplained eosinophilia but no detectable microfilariae in blood or tissue specimens. However, currently available immunodiagnostic tests do not distinguish between the various human filarial infections, including lymphatic filariasis and onchocerciasis, which have similar clinical presentations and overlapping geographic distributions with loiasis. The high prevalence of antifilarial antibodies in native populations of *Loa*-endemic areas limits the utility of serologic tests in this group.

TREATMENT

Diethylcarbamazine. In patients with few or no circulating microfilariae, DEC at a dose of 8 to 10 mg/kg/day for 21 days is the drug of choice. The drug is not directly toxic to the parasites but rather works in conjunction with the host immune responses to kill microfilariae and adult worms. DEC is curative in most cases, although multiple courses of therapy are often necessary and relapses have been documented as late as 8 years after treatment.

Side Effects of Therapy and Their Management. Mild side effects, including Calabar swellings, urticaria, arthralgias, fever, and right upper quadrant tenderness, are common during the first few days of therapy and generally respond to antihistamines or a short course of corticosteroids. DEC should not be used in patients with concomitant onchocerciasis, because of the risk of severe cutaneous and ocular reactions in these individuals.

Serious complications of DEC treatment, including meningoencephalitis and renal failure, are most common in patients with high numbers of circulating microfilariae (>2500/mL) and are thought to be due to the massive release of antigens from dying microfilariae. Although advocated in the past, neither a gradual increase in DEC dose nor pretreatment with corticosteroids is completely effective in preventing encephalitis in such patients. Consequently, if therapy is indicated in a patient with high numbers of circulating microfilariae, cytapheresis should be used to reduce the microfilarial load prior to the initiation of DEC and corticosteroid therapy. In a recent study, albendazole, at a dose of 200 mg twice daily for 3 weeks, reduced *Loa* microfilaremia slowly over the course of several months without adverse effects. Like

other benzimidazoles, albendazole is thought to have a primary effect on the adult parasites by inhibiting microtubular function and glucose uptake.

CONTROL AND PREVENTION

Vector Control. Elimination of insect vectors using larval insecticides has been hampered by the inaccessibility of vector breeding sites. The clearance of forest around dwellings, screening of houses for mosquitoes, and use of protective clothing can effectively reduce personal exposure to *Chrysops* in endemic areas.

Prophylaxis. DEC at a dose of 300 mg weekly is effective in preventing loiasis in long-term travelers to endemic areas.

Bibliography

Carme B, Boulesteix J, Boutes H, et al: Five cases of encephalitis during treatment of loiasis with diethylcarbamazine. Am J Trop Med Hyg 44:684, 1991.

Chandenier J, Pillier-Loriette C, Datry A et al: Value of cytapheresis in the treatment of loaiasis with high blood microfilaria levels. Results in 7 cases. Bull Soc Pathol Exot 80:624, 1987.

Duke BOL: Behavioural aspects of the life cycle of Loa. *In* Canning EU, Wright CA (eds): Behavioural Aspects of Parasite Transmission. London, Academic Press, 1972, pp 97–108.

Klion AD, Massougbodji A, Sadeler B-C, et al: Loiasis in endemic and nonendemic populations: Immunologically mediated differences in clinical presentation. J Infect Dis 163:1318, 1991.

Klion AD, Massougbodji A, Horton J, et al: Albendazole in human loiasis: Results of a double-blind, placebo-controlled trial. J Infect Dis 168:202, 1993.

Klion AD, Ottesen EA, Nutman TB: Effectiveness of diethylcarbamazine in treating loiasis acquired by expatriate visitors to endemic regions: Long-term follow-up. J Infect Dis 169:604, 1994.

Nutman TB, Miller KD, Mulligan M, et al: Diethylcarbamazine prophylaxis for human loiasis. Results of a double-blind study. N Engl J Med 319:752, 1988.

108 Onchocerciasis

Philip J. Cooper and Thomas B. Nutman

DEFINITION. Onchocerciasis (also known as *river blindness* and *enfermedad de Robles*) is an infection of humans caused by the filarial nematode *Onchocerca volvulus*. The parasite is transmitted by the bite of black flies of the genus *Simulium*. Infection may be without obvious clinical sequelae, but chronic heavy infections are generally associated with disease affecting the skin and eyes and in severe cases may cause significant disfigurement of the skin and visual impairment or blindness.

EPIDEMIOLOGY

Distribution. Onchocerciasis has a worldwide distribution and is found in 37 countries in Central Africa and the northern part of South America, and the Arabian peninsula (Fig. 108–1). An estimated 17.8 million people are infected; of these, approximately 336,400 are blind and 500,000 are severely visually impaired. An estimated 85.6 million people are thought to be at risk of infection worldwide. Onchocerciasis is most prevalent in sub-Saharan Africa (Fig. 108–1A) and is a major public health problem along rivers where the black fly vectors breed from Senegal, Guinea, and Sierra Leone in the west to southern Sudan and the Ethiopian Highlands in the east. The other African countries affected include parts of Angola, Benin, Burkina Faso, Burundi, Cameroon, the Central African Republic, Chad, Equatorial Guinea, Gabon, Ghana, Guinea-Bissau, Ivory Coast, Liberia, Malawi, Mali, Niger, Nigeria, Tanzania, Togo, Uganda, Upper

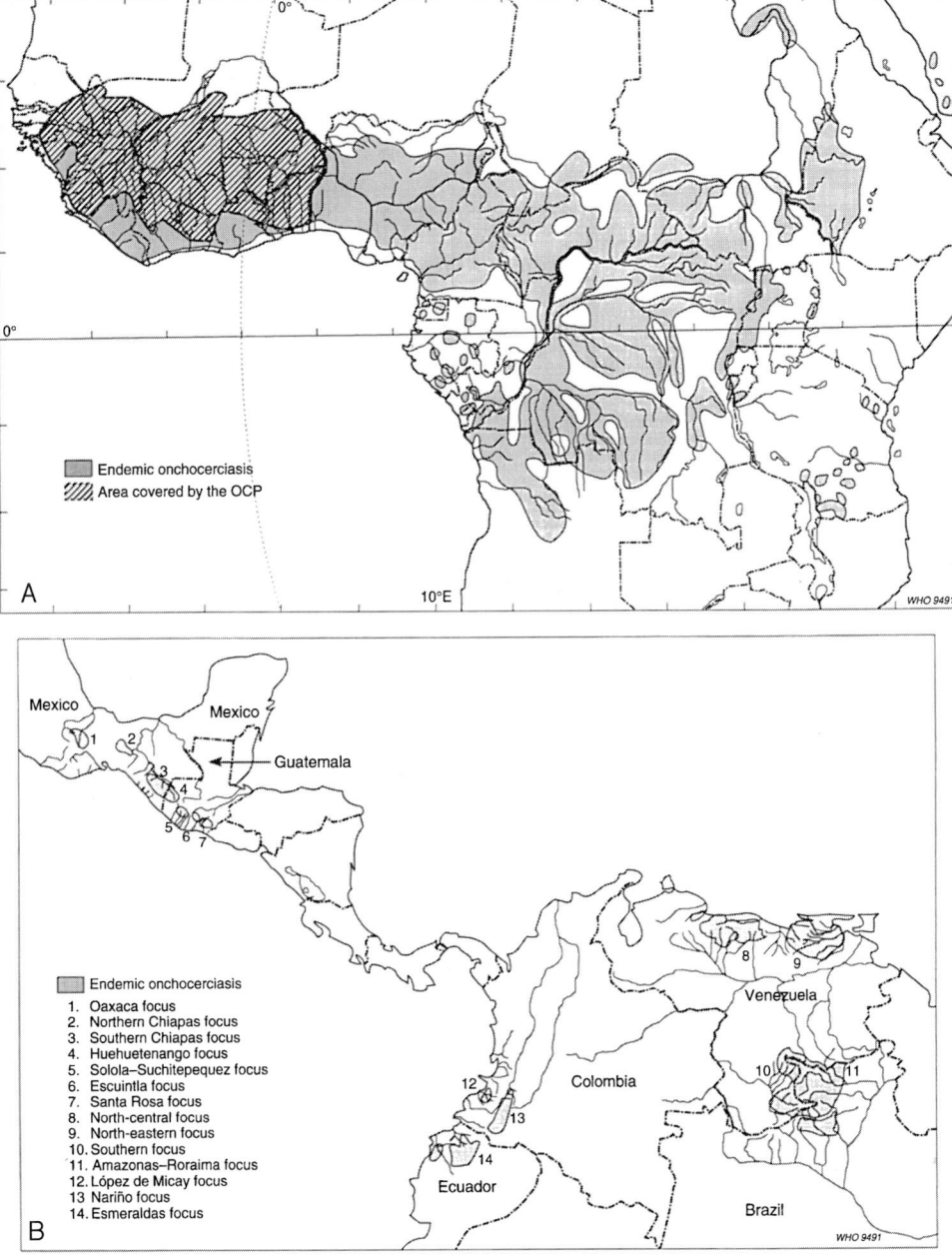

Figure 108–1. Maps showing the distribution of onchocerciasis. *A*, Africa and the Arabian Peninsula; *B*, Central and South America. (By permission of the World Health Organization.)

Volta, and the Democratic Republic of Congo. Onchocerciasis was formerly endemic in western Kenya, but a larvicide spraying campaign in the 1960s led to elimination of the disease from that country. In the Americas, isolated foci have been described in Mexico, Guatemala, Colombia, Ecuador, Venezuela, and Brazil (Fig. 108–1*B*). It is likely that onchocerciasis in the Americas was imported at the time of African slavery. Onchocerciasis is also found in Yemen, and it is likely that the cases reported in Saudi Arabia are imported, because transmission in that country has not been confirmed. *O. volvulus* has no known important animal reservoirs, although natural infection has been detected in gorillas in Africa.

Onchocerciasis foci have been classified epidemiologically into hyperendemic, mesoendemic, and hypoendemic according to disease prevalence: >60%, 30 to 60%, and <30%,

respectively. In hyperendemic areas, the disease is acquired early in life, and by the age of 20 years, >90% of inhabitants may be infected. In hyperendemic areas, microfilarial densities tend to be greater and the risk of developing severe pathologic sequelae is greatly increased. Communities with a low prevalence and low community microfilarial densities may show little evidence of clinical disease attributable to onchocerciasis. Blinding disease in highly endemic communities in the savanna of West Africa may affect up to 30% of the population, whereas in rain forest foci the prevalence of blindness tends to be less, although blindness rates of 15 to 20% are not uncommon.

Transmission and Life Cycle

The Parasite. The female adult is long and thin (up to 50 cm long and approximately 0.3 mm wide). Females are typically found coiled in subcutaneous nodules or onchocercomas.

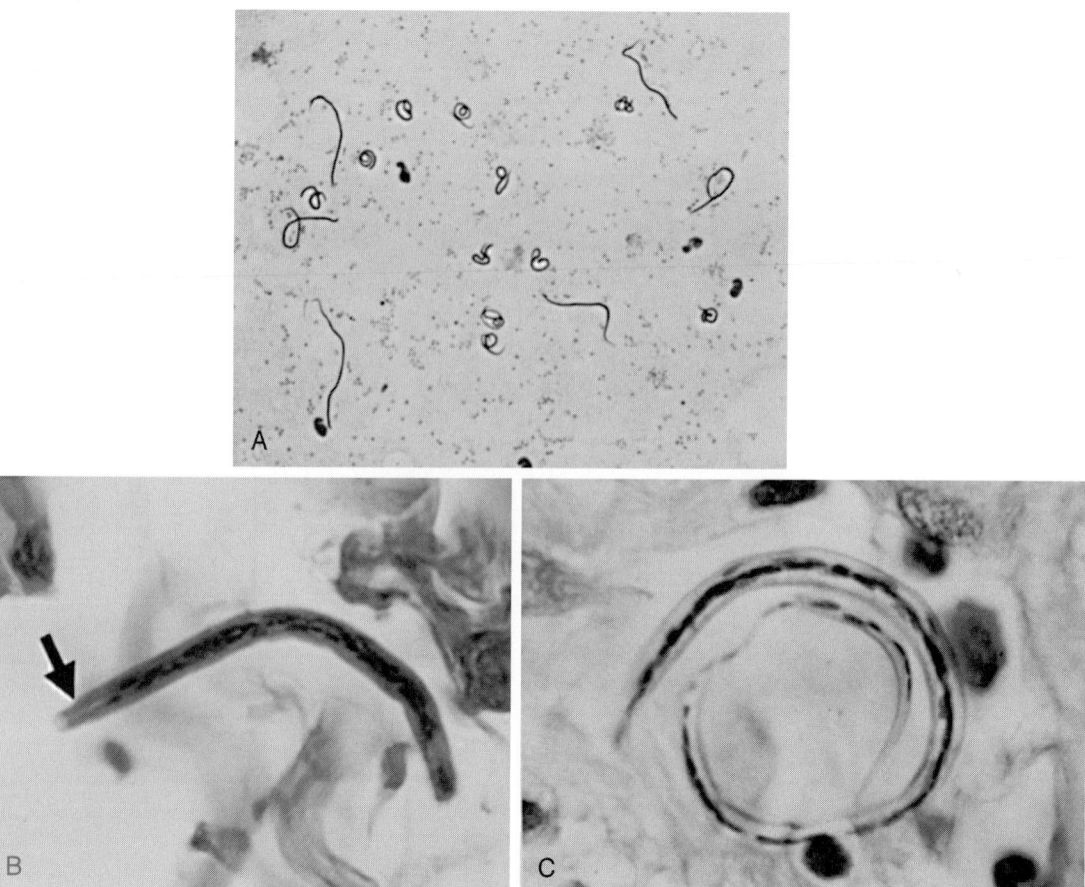

Figure 108–2. Microfilariae of *Onchocerca volvulus*. *A,* Touch smear preparation from dissected onchocercal nodule on iliac crest of patient in The Congo. Coiled and extended microfilariae at different stages of development were released from the uteri of gravid female worms during dissection (Giemsa stain, × 100). (Courtesy of the Armed Forces Institute of Pathology, Photograph Neg. No. 72–507.) *B,* Anterior end of a microfilaria of *O. volvulus* in skin. There is a characteristic cephalic clear space of about 9 μm before the first nucleus *(arrow)* (H&E stain, × 1080). (Courtesy of the Armed Forces Institute of Pathology, Photograph Neg. No. 72–3238.) *C,* Posterior end of a microfilaria of *O. volvulus* in dermal collagen. There is a caudal clear space of about 12 μm from the elongated terminal nucleus to the tip (H&E stain, × 1080). (Courtesy of the Armed Forces Institute of Pathology, Photograph Neg. No. 71–100072.)

Males may also be found in nodules and are 2.5 to 5 cm long and approximately 125 to 200 μm wide. Microfilariae, produced by gravid females, invade the subcutaneous tissues, skin, and eyes. They vary from 220 to 360 μm in length by 5 to 9 μm in width (Fig. 108–2*A*). *O. volvulus* microfilariae are unsheathed and can be identified by the following features: a cephalic space (7 to 13 μm long) and anterior nuclei that are side by side (Fig. 108–2*B*); a caudal space (9 to 15 μm long) with elongated terminal nuclei; and a tail that tapers to a fine point (Fig. 108–2*C*). It is important to distinguish *O. volvulus* microfilariae from those of *Mansonella ozzardi* (which live in the superficial capillaries of the skin) and *M. streptocerca* (which are also found in dermal tissues), with which they can be easily confused.

Parasite strain differences between the savanna and the rain forest of West Africa have been identified by biochemical and DNA-based techniques.

The Vector. The infection is transmitted by black flies of the genus *Simulium* (Figs. 108–3 and 139–15). Black flies are pool feeders, and the saliva of the fly has anticoagulant properties and probably also acts as a chemoattractant to skin-dwelling microfilariae, which may be ingested in large quantities. The microfilariae migrate to the flight muscles, and after a period of 6 to 12 days, infective L3 stage larvae emerge and migrate into the proboscis, where they are transmitted at the next

blood meal. Black flies breed in well-oxygenated water in fast-flowing rivers and streams. They usually do not fly more than 2 km from their breeding sites, although they may be carried by wind for hundreds of kilometers. Female black flies require blood meals for ovulation, and it is during these that the fly receives and transmits *O. volvulus* microfilariae and L3-stage larvae, respectively (Fig. 108–4). The relationship between the location of breeding sites and human communities, the opportunities for transmission, and the efficiency and biting habits of the vector determine the epidemiology of the disease.

Vector species vary geographically between endemic regions. The main vectors, *Simulium damnosum, S. neavei, S. metallicum,* and *S. exiguum,* are complexes of sibling species. In Africa and the southern Arabian peninsula, onchocerciasis is associated mainly with members of the *S. damnosum* complex and to a lesser extent with the *S. neavei* group. The vectors of onchocerciasis in Central America and Venezuela belong to the *S. ochraceum* and *S. metallicum* species complexes. In Colombia and Ecuador, the vectors are *S. exiguum* and *S. quadrivittatum,* and *S. oyapockense* and *S. guianense* on the Brazil-Venezuela border. The vector distribution determines that of the disease in Africa, whereas in Latin America the vectors have a much wider distribution than does the disease, and this is likely to have led to disease expansion in

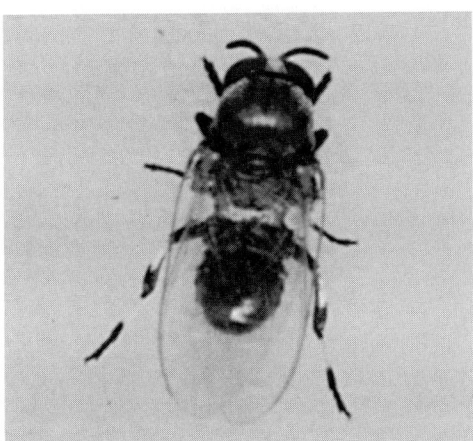

Figure 108–3. One of the black flies in the *Simulium damnosum* complex, feeding on a person. The length of the fly is about 3.5 mm (× 14.8). (Courtesy of the Armed Forces Institute of Pathology, Photograph Neg. No. 72–4519E.)

some foci due to migration of infected groups to previously unaffected areas.

The Infected Host. The infective larvae undergo two more molts in the following 12 months before they become mature adult worms. Female worms become encapsulated in host-derived fibrous nodules and are fertilized by peripatetic adult males, which are thought to migrate between nodules (Fig.

108–4). Gravid females produce thousands of tissue-invasive microfilariae daily, starting from 10 to 15 months after infection. Microfilariae, which have a life span of about 6 to 24 months, may be found in the skin, eyes, and lymph nodes. Adult worms usually live for about 10 years but may survive for up to 15 years.

An estimate of the risk of infection is the annual transmission potential (ATP), which is the calculated number of infective larvae transmitted to a person who is continuously exposed to black flies for 1 year. The ATP may be as high as 90,000 in some areas, and an ATP of ≥ 1500 is associated with a high prevalence of blindness.

PATHOLOGY. Onchocercomas are innocuous and cause discomfort only where they overlie bony prominences or interfere with movement of joints (Figs. 108–5 and 108–6). Tissue pathology is caused by severe inflammatory reactions where microfilariae die and degenerate. Onchocerciasis is a chronic disease, the severe clinical features of which result from cumulative episodes of acute and subacute inflammation and the scarring that results.

Nodules. Most adult female worms become encapsulated in fibrous nodules (Fig. 108–7*A* and *B*) in the deep dermis or subcutaneous tissues or in deeper sites in muscles and near joints. It is likely that worms elicit a host inflammatory response that immobilizes them and leads to their incarceration. Nodules are composed of a fibrous capsule, an inflammatory cellular infiltrate, and one or several enclosed coiled adult worms. Nodules often have their own vascular sheath composed of vessels, nerves, and lymphatics, and the adult worms inside are bathed in an extensive capillary network.

Figure 108–4. Life cycle of *O. volvulus*. (From Melvin DM, Brooke MM, Healy GR, et al: Common Blood and Tissue Parasites. Life Cycle Charts. Atlanta, Centers for Disease Control, 1961.)

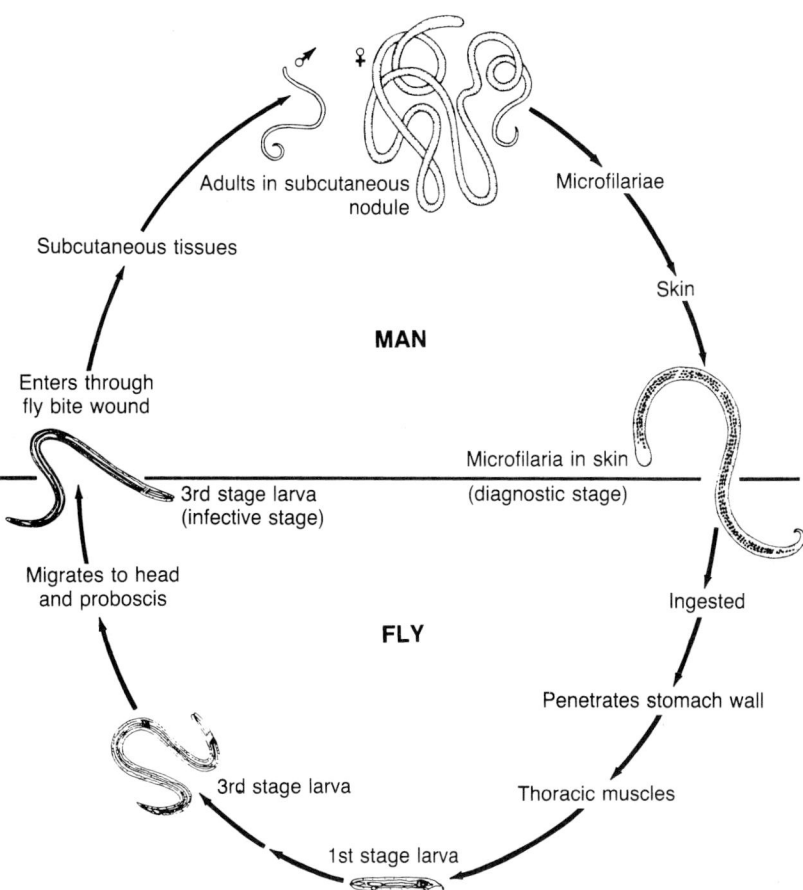

Onchocerca volvulus

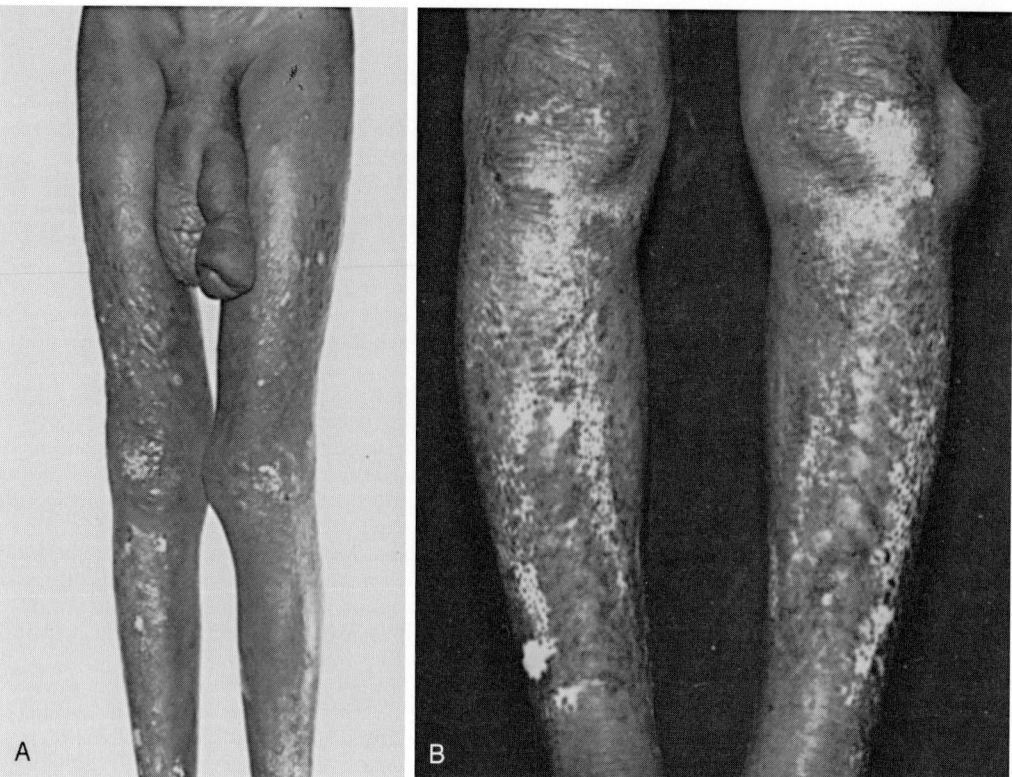

Figure 108–5. *A,* This 11-year-old boy in the Ubangi Territory of northern Congo has onchocercal nodules over his knees and ribs; severe dermatitis with depigmentation, papules, wrinkling, and thickening; and inguinal lymphadenopathy with elephantoid changes of the penis and scrotum. (Courtesy of the Armed Forces Institute of Pathology, Photograph Neg. No. 68–7912–1.) *B,* This 48-year-old man in the rain forest of Cameroon has a cluster of onchocercal nodules over his left knee and "leopard skin" of the knees and shins. (Courtesy of the Armed Forces Institute of Pathology, Photograph Neg. No. 72–17223.)

The undramatic inflammatory reaction to adult worms consists of a few inflammatory cells composed of lymphocytes, macrophages, eosinophils, and plasma cells scattered sparsely through the fibrous nodular tissue. Young nodules may have a granulomatous component characterized by foamy histiocytes, epithelioid cells, and foreign body giant cells, which gradually matures to form the hyalinized capsule. Giant cells apposed to the parasite surface are highly suggestive of parasite death. Nodules also contain microfilariae, which migrate through the nodular tissue to invade the surrounding skin. The male worms may be found either in close apposition to the females or on the outer surface of nodules. Nodules are often closely aggregated like clusters of grapes, and new nodules often form as satellites around older ones, even at the sites where older nodules have previously been removed surgically. The fibrous nodules may protect adult worms from mechanical damage and provide a more easily regulated immune environment for the survival of adult worms.

Cutaneous Lesions. The presence and/or degeneration of skin-dwelling microfilariae causes damage to the skin. Live microfilariae secrete enzymes, e.g., collagenase during their migration, and these may cause long-term damage to dermal collagen and elastin, leading to the loss of skin elasticity and early aging characteristic of long-standing onchocerciasis. Microfilariae are seen histologically at the dermoepidermal junction (Fig. 108–8), and live, intact microfilariae are generally observed free of inflammatory cells. Dead and degenerating microfilariae attract eosinophils and/or neutrophils, which accumulate around the larvae. Associated changes are local edema, hyperemia, and the deposition of helminthotoxic eosinophil-derived granules, e.g., major basic protein (MBP)

and eosinophil cationic protein (ECP). Granulomatous inflammation characterized by the presence of histiocytes, epithelioid cells, and giant cells follows. The inflammatory changes, concentrated around vessels and appendages, in the upper dermis include edema and fibrosis. Acute papules

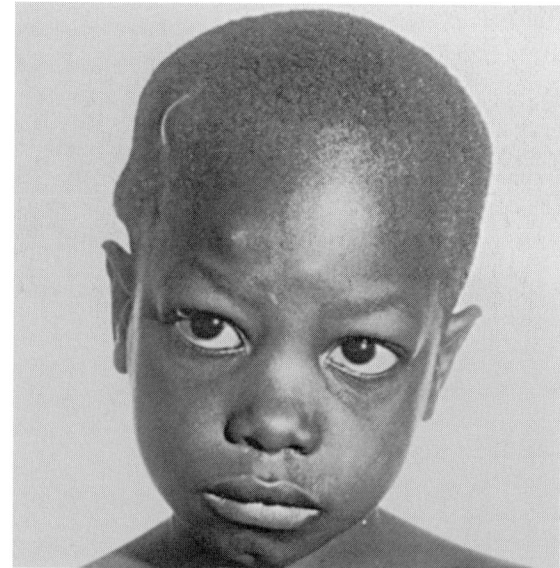

Figure 108–6. Young boy in Ubangi Territory of The Congo, who has three onchocercal nodules on his forehead and skull. (Courtesy of the Armed Forces Institute of Pathology, Photograph Neg. No. 69–3619.)

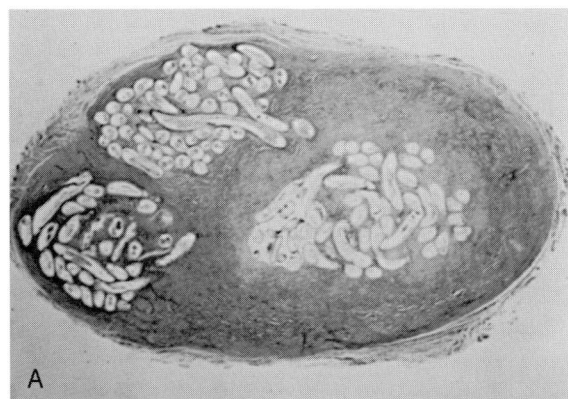

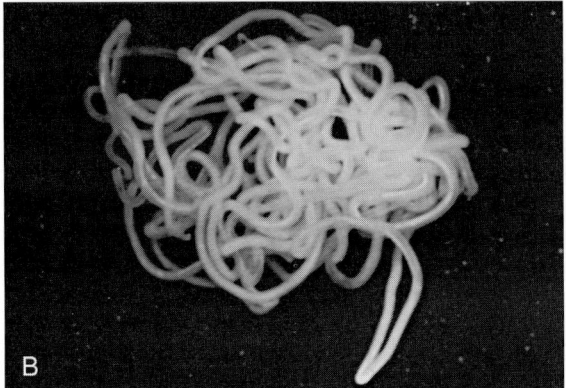

Figure 108–7. Adult worms of *O. volvulus*. *A,* Microscopic section through an onchocercal nodule (1.3 × 0.7 cm), showing several coiled adult worms (mostly gravid females). The worms are surrounded and incarcerated by hyalinized scar (Russell-Movat, × 8.2). (Courtesy of the Armed Forces Institute of Pathology, Photograph Neg. No. 69–3639.) *B,* Entangled adult worms, after collagenase digestion of an onchocercal nodule. The cluster measures about 1.1 × 0.9 cm. The individual worms are up to 0.5 mm across and 50 cm long (× 6.9). (Courtesy of the Armed Forces Institute of Pathology, Photograph Neg. No. 80–12068.)

have intraepidermal microabscesses with dead or degenerating microfilariae surrounded by eosinophils and neutrophils (Fig. 108–8). A variable perivascular infiltrate composed of lymphohistiocytic cells may also be seen.

In long-standing disease, histologic features may include hyperkeratosis, parakeratosis, acanthosis, pigmentary incontinence, dilation of dermal lymphatics, loss of melanin from basal cells, loss of elastic fibers in the dermis, and atrophy of the dermis with loss of rete ridges. Dermal collagen may be disrupted by deposition of large amounts of eosinophil-derived MBP and mucin ground substance. With more advanced changes, microfilariae may be found only in the deeper dermis. Onchocercal dermatitis is often present around the buttocks and pelvic girdle area, with lymphadenitis and fibrosis of the inguinal and femoral nodes. Histologic study of these lymph nodes shows atrophic follicles and lymphoid tissue almost completely replaced with fibrous material.

Lichenified onchodermatitis (LOD) (also known as *localized onchocerciasis* and *sowda*) is characterized by enlarged soft regional lymph nodes associated with localized skin changes (Fig. 108–9C). A hyper-reactive inflammatory cell infiltrate of the dermis is accompanied by sclerosis and edema. Very few microfilariae are detectable, and other histologic changes may include phagocytosed melanin in the dermis, hyperkeratosis,

acanthosis, dermal fibrosis, and a perivascular infiltrate that contains plasma cells.

Scarring in lymph nodes may lead to regional lymphedema, hanging groin (Fig. 108–9F), or elephantiasis. Histologically, the lymph nodes draining areas of onchodermatitis show capsular fibrosis, atrophic follicles, and dilatation of the subcapsular sinusoids and lymphatics. Microfilariae and microfilarial debris may be present in a chronic granulomatous inflammatory infiltrate. After treatment with microfilaricidal drugs, including ivermectin and diethylcarbamazine (DEC), a transient reactive lymphadenopathy occurs. After ivermectin treatment, the lymph nodes seem to be the primary site of microfilarial death, and many thousands of dead and degenerating larvae are present in lymph node sections and are surrounded by a predominantly eosinophil inflammatory infiltrate with deposition of MBP and ECP. Regional lymphedema may result from degranulation of eosinophils in the skin or from lymphatic insufficiency following the inflammatory engorgement of the regional lymph nodes where microfilariae are being destroyed.

Ocular Lesions. Lesions in the eye are caused by localized death of microfilariae. Microfilariae may enter the eye through the bulbar conjunctiva, along the sheaths of the scleral vessels and nerves, or by embolization in the choroidal or ciliary capillaries. Relatively few eyes have been examined histopathologically, and most of these have had end-stage disease that would have obscured earlier changes. Undamaged microfilariae may be found histologically in both anterior and posterior segments. As in the skin, live microfilariae elicit little reaction, and pathology results only when they die.

Corneal Lesions. Punctate keratitic opacities, also known as *snowflake* or *fluffy opacities* (see Fig. 108–10A in color section), are observed clinically in the corneal stroma and resolve without scarring. These are characterized by focal accumula-

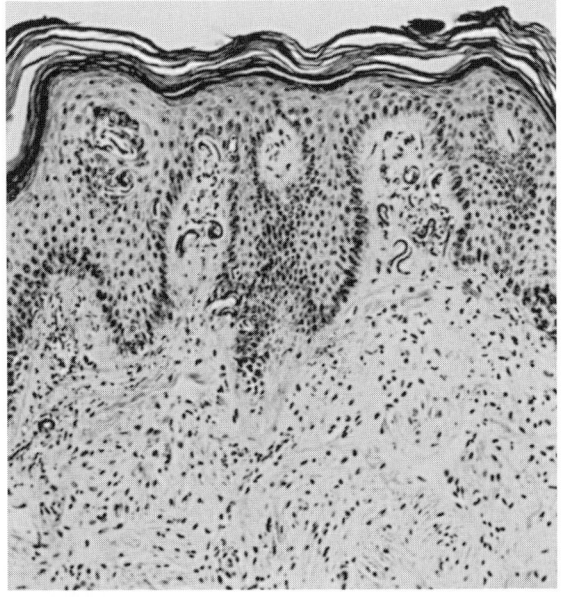

Figure 108–8. Post-treatment skin of the buttocks of a patient in Cameroon, after two oral doses of diethylcarbamazine (DEC). There are many microfilariae in the dermal papillae, with some migrating into the epidermis as a result of the treatment. Other features characteristic of onchocercal dermatitis include edema, dilated lymphatics, hyperkeratosis, and acanthosis with elongation of rete ridges (H&E stain, × 125). (Courtesy of the Armed Forces Institute of Pathology, Photograph Neg. No. 73–5681.)

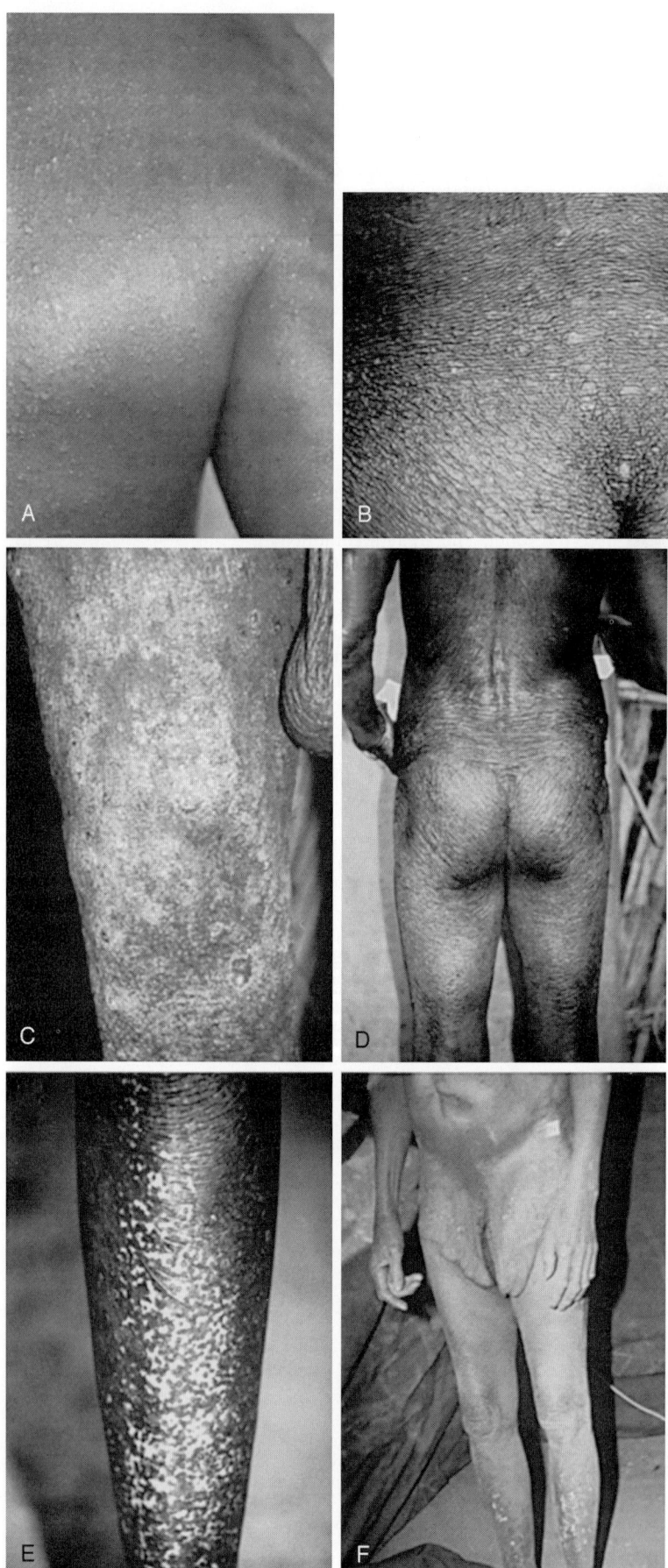

Figure 108–9. Skin changes in onchocerciasis. *A,* Acute papular onchodermatitis. *B,* Chronic papular onchodermatitis. *C,* Lichenified onchodermatitis. *D,* Onchocercal atrophy confined to the buttocks. *E,* Depigmentation or "leopard skin." *F,* Hanging groin, with redundant folds of atrophic skin. (Courtesy of Dr. M. Murdoch.)

tions of lymphocytes and eosinophils and edema around degenerating microfilariae. Sclerosing keratitis (see Fig. 108–10B in color section) is a progressive fibrovascular pannus and inflammatory infiltrate composed mainly of lymphocytes and eosinophils that starts at the level of Bowman's membrane.

Uveitis. Mild chronic nongranulomatous uveitis is common with heavy microfilarial invasion. More severe uveitis with secondary sequelae (anterior or posterior synechiae, seclusio- or occlusio-pupillae, secondary cataract, and secondary glaucoma) is rarer. Chronic granulomatous anterior uveitis also occurs and causes loss of the iris pigment frill and a pumice-stone appearance of the iris. Mild uveitis has been associated with microfilarial invasion of the iris, whereas more severe granulomatous uveitis may be due to invasion of the ciliary body.

Chorioretinal Lesions. The severity and extent of chorioretinal changes vary. The retinal pigment epithelium (RPE) may show signs of migration, clumping, atrophy, or focal hyperplasia. Chronic nongranulomatous chorioretinitis consists of an infiltrate of lymphocytes, plasma cells, and eosinophils with secondary degenerative changes in the overlying RPE and neuroretina. Loss of the photoreceptors and outer layers of the retina may be due to inflammatory damage to the RPE and choriocapillaris. This is followed by consecutive loss of the inner neuroretina, ganglion cells, and nerve fibers. Profound chorioretinal atrophy with loss of almost all the retina and choroid may follow. Optic atrophy is common in the more advanced stages of ocular onchocerciasis and may be associated with a large glaucomatous cup.

Immune-Mediated Pathology. Pathology is caused by the inflammatory reactions associated with the death and degeneration of microfilariae. The clinical spectrum of disease may be associated with variation of individual host responses to the parasite. Tissue pathology in onchocerciasis may be caused (1) directly by invading microfilariae through the secretion of tissue-damaging enzymes such as collagenase; (2) by the host response to microfilariae, including the secretion of toxic products by granulocytes, particularly eosinophils; (3) by the deposition of immune complexes in the tissues; or (4) by a number of other immunologic mechanisms including autoimmunity.

Infected persons demonstrate specific cellular immune recognition of *O. volvulus* antigens. They have increased circulating levels of parasite-specific immunoglobulins. Polyclonal activation of B cells and hypergammaglobulinemia (IgG and IgM) are a common finding. This may result from chronic antigen stimulation or from concurrent helminth or protozoal infections. Polyclonal IgE and IgG4 elevation is found in the majority of patients. Levels of IgG4 seem to correlate closely with parasite burden and decline after treatment as the parasites are destroyed. A protective role for parasite-specific antibodies has not been proved, although serum from infected patients is able to enhance granulocyte-mediated killing of microfilariae in vitro.

Cellular responses to parasite antigens are often less in infected patients than in noninfected control groups, and this immunosuppression may affect the responses of infected patients to other nonparasite antigens, e.g., tuberculin, streptococcal antigens, and tetanus toxoid. Although an increased incidence of other infectious diseases, e.g., tuberculosis, has not been demonstrated in endemic areas, the prevalence of lepromatous leprosy has been reported to be much greater in a hyperendemic region than in other nearby areas in West Africa.

The causes of this immunosuppression might include direct subversion of the immune response by the parasite to protect itself or downregulation of the immune response by the host to prevent tissue-damaging pathology. It has also been suggested that in utero and perinatal exposure to parasite antigens might lead to tolerance. CD4+ T-helper cells have been subdivided into two principal groups, depending on the pattern of cytokine secretion: Th1 T-helper cells tend to secrete interleukin-2 (IL-2) and interferon-γ (IFN-γ) and are important in delayed-type hypersensitivity reactions and the production of IgG1, whereas Th2 cytokines produce IL-4, IL-5, IL-10, and IL-13, which promote eosinophilia and the production of IgG4 and IgE. Parasite antigen-stimulated T cells from patients with onchocerciasis typically secrete Th2-type cytokines. IL-10 is produced in large amounts in such cultures and downregulates antigen presentation and lymphocyte proliferation. The cross-regulatory cytokines, IL-4 and transforming growth factor-β, may also have a role in this process.

Most patients complain of episodes of acute dermal or corneal changes, which are associated histologically with microfilarial killing, but whether this is attributable to acquired immunity, innate immunity, or a combination of both is not clear. Patients may have high levels of dermal microfilariae but show relatively little dermal and ocular disease. However, it is likely that most patients with high microfilarial burdens will eventually develop clinical disease, and strong epidemiologic evidence shows that those with higher microfilarial burdens are more likely to develop severe ocular disease.

Eosinophils probably have a central role in microfilarial killing. In vitro studies demonstrate activated and degranulating eosinophils in close apposition to dying and degenerating microfilariae. This is best illustrated after treatment with the microfilaricidal drugs DEC and ivermectin. After treatment there is an active sequestration of eosinophils into the skin and lymph nodes, where they surround and degranulate in the vicinity of dying microfilariae. The eosinophil granule protein, MBP, has been shown to be toxic to microfilariae in vitro. Neutrophils are also capable of killing microfilariae in vitro, but there is little evidence for a significant role of these granulocytes in vivo. Within 2 weeks of treatment with ivermectin, circulating levels of eosinophils decline to 50 to 75% of pretreatment levels, indicating that the presence of microfilariae is a major stimulus to eosinophilia. After ivermectin treatment, the levels of both polyclonal and parasite-specific antibodies decrease, but there is a transient reversal of cellular hyporesponsiveness, which is maintained if ivermectin is administered regularly.

Immune complexes are present in the serum of infected individuals, although the functional significance of these is unclear. Immune complex–mediated disease may contribute to the immunopathology of onchocerciasis, and associations between circulating immune complexes and disease manifestations have been demonstrated in some studies but not in others.

A role for autoimmunity has been proposed in the pathogenesis of a number of the clinical findings including chorioretinopathy, onchodermatitis, and rheumatic symptoms. This has followed the identification of cross reactivity between human and parasite antigens and the demonstration of autoantibodies that recognize self antigens in human infection sera. The significance of these findings is not clear, because parasite antigens are known to activate both B and T cells polyclonally and represent an epiphenomenon related to excessive immune stimulation.

Little is known about the immunopathogenesis of ocular lesions. The pathogenesis of punctate opacities of the cornea is likely to be similar to that of acute papular onchodermatitis. Histologically, punctate opacities are composed of aggregates of mononuclear cells and eosinophils surrounding degenerate microfilariae in the corneal stroma. A number of mechanisms have been put forward to explain the pathogenesis of posterior segment lesions, including inflammatory reactions to dead microfilariae, eosinophil-derived toxic effector molecules, immune complex disease, toxic secretory/excretory products of microfilariae, and autoimmunity. Current evidence favors a central role for microfilariae in the retina and choroid in the initiation of disease though self-perpetuating autoimmune phenomena that then extends existing disease. This could explain why onchocercal chorioretinopathy tends to continue to evolve despite effective chemotherapy.

CLINICAL MANIFESTATIONS AND COMPLICATIONS. In areas of high endemicity, onchocerciasis may cause severe morbidity from unsightly and troublesome skin disease and visual loss and blindness. The severity of clinical disease depends on the intensity of infection and duration of exposure and infection. The differences in clinical manifestations between patients probably are largely determined by parasite burden, history of infection, and immune status. Individuals with light infections, e.g., expatriates or temporary visitors to endemic areas, usually complain of pruritus, which may be severe, and have a localized rash but very rarely have nodules or eye lesions.

Skin Disease. The earliest symptom of onchocercal skin involvement is itching. This is also the most common complaint in endemic communities. In Africa, this is most severe over the lower trunk, pelvis, buttocks, and thighs in a distribution that mirrors the sites of highest infection density. The skin changes attributable to onchocerciasis have recently been graded into a standardized classification system. Acute skin changes include papular, maculopapular, and urticarial rashes. Acute papular onchodermatitis (APOD) consists of small, widely scattered pruritic papules (Fig. 108–9A), which progress to vesicles and pustules in more severe cases. Erythema and edema may also be noted to affect a single limb or area of the trunk or face. A similar pattern is seen after treatment with microfilaricidal drugs, e.g., DEC or ivermectin. Scratching of pruritic lesions may lead to secondary bacterial infection and ulceration. Secondary infections with mycoses and scabies have been associated with onchocercal skin disease.

Chronic papular onchodermatitis (CPOD) consists of flat-topped papules (Fig. 108–9B) that vary greatly in size (from approximately 3 to 9 mm) and height above the skin surface (some lesions may be macular, others are elevated up to 5 mm). Itching may occur but is not invariable, and postinflammatory hyperpigmentation is characteristic. Individuals with CPOD may also have acute lesions.

LOD or sowda (Fig. 108–9C) is classically seen in Yemen and parts of the Sudan but can occur elsewhere. LOD typically affects teenagers and young adults and is characterized by pruritic, hyperpigmented, hyperkeratotic plaques. With increasing severity, the plaques become confluent. The distribution is usually asymmetric, often involving one limb, and is associated with regional lymphadenopathy. In later stages, the skin is grossly lichenified, but this may resolve with or without treatment. Itching is very intense in the acute stage, and this condition may coexist with APOD or CPOD. Dermal microfilariae tend to be absent or scanty in patients with LOD and are found only in the affected area.

Atrophy is relatively common in areas of high endemicity. Atrophic skin adopts many of the characteristics of aging, such as loss of elasticity and contours, and the skin appears excessively wrinkled (Figs. 108–5 and 108–9D). Hairs may be lost, and sweating may be reduced. The wrinkled skin usually is extremely thin and has little subcutaneous tissue.

Onchocercal depigmentation is often described as *leopard skin*. Patches of complete pigment loss are seen, with islands or spots of normally pigmented skin centered around hair follicles (Figs. 108–5 and 108–9E). The skin sometimes is not fully depigmented and is seen as yellow-brown areas on black skin.

In Guatemala and Mexico, chronic skin lesions attributable to onchocerciasis are not as prevalent as in many parts of Africa. A number of skin lesions peculiar to the Central American region have been reported, including *erisipela de la costa*, characterized by a macular rash and edema of the face, and *mal morado*, associated with reddish-mauve discoloration, particularly on the trunk and upper limbs.

Dermal onchocerciasis is seen frequently in expatriates or visitors from nonendemic areas with a brief exposure history in an endemic area. Microfilarial counts may be low or undetectable, and a localized papular or urticarial rash is often observed. This may be associated with localized swelling or edema.

Nodules. Nodules or onchocercomas may be clinically palpable over bony prominences (Fig. 108–5 and 108–6). In Africa, nodules are found predominantly in the pelvic region, localized to the iliac crest, trochanter, and sacrum. In Guatemala and Mexico, a greater proportion of nodules are found in the upper thorax and head.

Some nodules are too deep to be palpable, although very small ones can be located by infected patients. A typical nodule containing viable worms is firm, round, nontender, mobile, and attached to the underlying tissues. In long-standing infections, large conglomerations of up to 50 nodules may be found in a single sack. Nodules may vary from 0.5 cm in diameter to >10 cm when aggregated.

Lymphadenitis. Lymph node changes are commonly noted where the nodes drain areas of onchodermatitis. The nodes usually are only slightly enlarged, firm, and nontender. Acute regional lymphadenopathy may accompany acute papular eruptions and lymphedema, but lymph node pathology usually is clinically silent. A rare manifestation of onchocercal lymph node involvement is hanging groin or adenolymphocele (Fig. 108–9F). This consists of a pouch of lymphedematous tissue in which hang atrophic inguinal or femoral nodes. Extensive regional pathology of nodes may lead to elephantiasis of the limbs or genitalia (Fig. 108–5A).

Ocular Changes. Ocular disease generally follows chronic and heavy infections, and the prevalence of ocular lesions increases with increasing endemicity of infection. Ocular involvement is rare in individuals with a brief exposure history and in light infections.

Punctate Keratitis. The earliest sign of ocular involvement is the appearance of punctate corneal opacities or snowflake opacities in the corneal stroma (see Fig. 108–10A in color section). These can be seen by the naked eye but are more reliably visualized using a direct ophthalmoscope or slit lamp. Live microfilariae may be seen coiled up in the corneal stroma. As they die, they straighten out and become surrounded by a mixed cellular infiltrate and circumscribed edema. The microfilariae disintegrate until only a gray blurred lesion is present; this eventually heals completely without scarring within days to a few weeks. Dead microfilariae may be seen within the opacity. These measure about 0.5 mm in diameter. Punctate opacities were commonly seen after treatment with older microfilaricidal drugs, particularly DEC.

Intraocular Microfilariae. The finding of intraocular microfilariae generally follows the appearance of punctate opacities, although the two lesions are not invariably associated. Ocular microfilariae can be detected by slit lamp examination by retroillumination of the iris. Microfilariae in the anterior chamber are seen as small wriggling worms that float in the convection currents of the aqueous humor. Live microfilariae in the cornea are transparent and coiled up. Dead and live microfilariae may also be seen attached to the posterior surface of the cornea to Descemet's membrane, in the lens capsule, in the vitreous, and, with careful biomicroscopic examination, in the retina.

Conjunctivitis and Limbitis. Affected eyes often have some degree of conjunctival hyperemia and occasionally chemosis. Epiphora and limbitis may be seen, most commonly after chemotherapy.

Sclerosing Keratitis. Sclerosing keratitis is an irreversible corneal lesion (Fig. 108–10B in color section). It is the result of prolonged massive invasion of the cornea by microfilariae, giving rise to corneal damage. Sclerosing keratitis usually starts medially and laterally in the limbal zone of the cornea and is seen initially as an area of translucence or haze in the peripheral cornea. With time, the limbal haze opacifies and the keratitis progresses, forming two tongues that tend to become a confluent zone involving the whole of the lower limbus. The sclerosed area may finally extend up to the pupillary area, causing blindness. Sclerosing keratitis may progress until the entire cornea is opaque and vascularized. Sclerosing keratitis is seen more commonly in the savanna than rain forest areas of West Africa and was described frequently in Mexico and Guatemala.

Anterior Uveitis. Acute episodes of iritis may be encountered, but a more common presentation is the changes of chronic iritis or iridocyclitis, reflecting a more insidious process. Usually noted is a mild anterior uveitis with a faint flare and a few cells. The eye may at times remain uninflamed despite heavy infestation with microfilariae. Severe anterior uveitis may occur, with development of posterior synechiae and a pear-shaped deformity of the pupil. Extensive synechiae may cause seclusio- and occlusio-pupillae, secondary cataracts, and secondary glaucoma. Sequelae of anterior uveitis are probably the main causes of onchocerciasis-related blindness in Central America.

Chorioretinal Disease. Chorioretinitis or chorioretinopathy in onchocerciasis is a slowly progressive and insidious condition, and visual loss may not be evident for many years. Acute inflammatory chorioretinitis is rarely seen, although occasionally it follows chemotherapy with microfilaricidal agents. *Chorioretinopathy* is therefore probably a more appropriate term to describe the findings commonly seen: RPE atrophy and chorioretinal scarring. Chorioretinopathy in onchocerciasis has a characteristic distribution and pattern of progression. It is first seen clinically as a loss of pigment lateral to the macula (see Fig. 108–10C and D in color section) or nasal to the optic disc. This occurs at the level of the RPE, where pigment loss is seen clinically as a gray-yellow mottling. RPE loss progresses in an arc around the macula. RPE mottling eventually may become confluent, producing areas of geographic atrophy (see Fig. 108–10F in color section). Extensive atrophy may be accompanied by pigment clumping, choriocapillary atrophy (the choroidal vessels become exposed) (see Fig. 108–10F in color section), and subretinal fibrosis, which appears as well-defined plaquelike white areas. Rarely, new vessels may develop in areas of subretinal fibrosis. The macula is often preserved until relatively late in the course of disease. Mild forms of RPE atrophy may be revealed only by fluorescein angiography. Active inflammation can be seen as areas of posterior retinal edema or as pale, ill-defined areas of swelling in the choroid. Fundal changes are usually symmetric.

White intraretinal dots and shiny deposits are commonly described. Shiny deposits are commonly seen in rain forest foci and tend to remain unchanged. Much more common are white punctate discrete dots that resolve without obvious long-term sequelae and may represent focal sites of microfi-

larial death, rather like punctate corneal opacities. An increase in intraretinal pigment is often noted, particularly adjacent to areas of RPE atrophy. This becomes more marked with more severe disease but disappears as the retina atrophies in advanced chorioretinopathy. Retinal abnormalities indicative of active uveitis—namely, intraretinal hemorrhages, retinitis, retinal vasculitis, and cotton-wool spots—are sometimes present.

Vitreoretinal abnormalities, particularly posterior vitreous detachments, may also occur. Other abnormalities, e.g., macular hole and epiretinal membranes, have been described and may have a higher incidence in patients with onchocercal chorioretinal disease.

Optic Nerve Disease. Acute papillitis may occur, but postneuritic optic atrophy more often is evident (see Fig. 108–10E in color section). This is likely to reflect previously undocumented periods of active inflammation. Onchocercal optic atrophy may present as consecutive, postneuritic, or primary. Consecutive atrophy follows extensive destruction of the retina, whereas postneuritic atrophy follows previous episodes of active inflammation of the optic nerve. Both these forms are associated with peripapillary hyperpigmentation and sheathing of the central retinal vessels. Primary optic atrophy is not associated with either chorioretinal lesions or signs of previous inflammation of the optic nerve head and thus presents the most difficult diagnostic dilemma. All three types have been linked epidemiologically to onchocerciasis. Microfilariae may be found within the optic nerve and its sheaths, and the death of these microfilariae could initiate an inflammatory response with later atrophic changes. Optic atrophy has been reported to occur after treatment with DEC and suramin.

Glaucoma. The association between onchocerciasis and glaucoma is variable. Intraocular pressure can be elevated during onchocerciasis-induced anterior uveitis, and severe secondary glaucoma may occur from extensive synechiae formation. Chronic angle-open glaucoma has also been described in patients with onchocerciasis. More commonly, however, intraocular pressures are low in endemic populations.

Geographic Differences in Clinical Disease. Differences have been reported in the clinical presentation of onchocerciasis in the savanna versus the rain forest regions in West Africa. In savanna populations, few palpable nodules are found, dermal infection intensities are high, and lesions of the skin and lymph nodes are few; in rain forest areas, numerous palpable nodules, moderate skin infection intensities, and gross lesions of the skin and lymph nodes are noted. The pattern of ocular disease also differs between the two bioclimatic zones. Blindness is more prevalent in the savanna, and much of this is accounted for by sclerosing keratitis, which is less common in rain forest regions. Chorioretinal lesions, an important cause of visual loss in rain forest areas, are probably equally common in savanna regions but may be obscured by severe anterior segment disease. Differences in clinical disease have been reported from different foci in the Americas. In Central America, the parasites are more highly concentrated in the upper parts of the body, occasionally producing leonine facies, mal morado, and erisipela de la costa. These features have not been described in other geographic areas. Ocular disease in Guatemala is characterized by severe anterior segment disease, particularly sclerosing keratitis and iritis, which account for most cases of blindness, and relatively few posterior segment lesions. In contrast, in Ecuador, the pattern of disease resembles that in forest foci of West Africa, with few severe anterior segment lesions and most visual loss attributable to disease in the posterior segment.

Reasons given to explain the geographic variation in disease include differences in environment, infection intensity, parasite strains, or host genetic differences. Genetic (DNA) and biologic parasite strain differences between the savanna and forest regions of West Africa have been demonstrated, with savanna microfilariae being more pathogenic for the rabbit cornea than forest-derived microfilariae.

Other Complications. Microfilariae may invade many tissues and have been found in the peripheral blood, urine, sputum, cerebrospinal fluid, and cervical mucus. A form of dwarfism, Nakalanga dwarfism, has been attributed to pituitary involvement in this disease in the Mabira forest of Uganda. An association with epilepsy has been reported but remains unproven. Acute arthritis and tensosynovitis are occasionally reported after chemotherapy. Rheumatism and muscle pains are particularly common in endemic regions. Other abnormalities include an increased prevalence of abdominal hernias (particularly direct inguinal), gynecomastia, and reproductive abnormalities including secondary amennorrhea, spontaneous abortion, and both male and female infertility. Anecdotal evidence suggests that congenital transmission of onchocerciasis may occur, and a number of studies report the presence of microfilariae and/or nodules in neonates and infants.

Interactions With Other Infectious Diseases. The prevalence of lepromatous leprosy, which is associated with an impaired response to *Mycobacterium leprae*, has been reported to be increased in hyperendemic areas for onchocerciasis. Interactions with HIV have not been noted in early asymptomatic infection, but few data are available on patients with advanced HIV disease. Antibody responses to the parasite are increasingly impaired as CD4 counts decline. Caution must be exercised in the treatment of patients who have onchocerciasis and who are from areas coendemic for loiasis. Severe and occasionally fatal encephalitis, due to the death of intracerebral *Loa loa* microfilariae, may follow treatment with ivermectin.

DIAGNOSIS. Everyone living in or traveling through endemic regions is at risk, and the chances of acquiring infection increase with greater exposure time. A presumptive diagnosis can be made on the basis of a history of exposure in an endemic area, the presence of subcutaneous nodules, or typical skin and ocular signs. Definitive diagnosis depends on the identification of microfilariae in skin snips.

Skin Snip. This is the most commonly used procedure for diagnosis. Typically, a small crease of skin is lifted with the point of a needle and a small circular disk-shaped slice of epidermis and superficial dermis is obtained with a razor or scalpel blade. A simpler method is to snip a small skin biopsy specimen using a corneoscleral punch. This allows snips of approximately uniform size to be taken and is particularly useful in surveys. Care must be taken to sterilize the biopsy punch (in glutaraldehyde) between patients because of the theoretic risk of transmitting hepatitis B, HIV, and other similarly transmissible agents. The snip should include the tips of the dermal papillae and should be bloodless, although blood tends to well up at the site of the wound after biopsy. The snip is placed into normal saline on a slide or in the well of a microtiter plate and examined at least 1 hour later (preferably 3 hours to 24 hours). Incubation for 1 hour or more should allow the emergence of 80 to 90% of microfilariae. Counting after 24 hours must follow the addition of a drop of 10% formaldehyde in saline to prevent bacterial contamination. Snips are usually taken from one or more standard sites: the iliac crest, buttock, calf, scapula, and outer canthus of the eye. The site depends on the clinical signs for individual diagnosis and on the known microfilarial distribution, which may vary between different geographic locations, for surveys. In epidemiologic surveys or chemotherapeutic trials, the snips are usually weighed to obtain the number of microfilariae per milligram of skin.

The emergence of microfilariae from skin snips confirms the diagnosis. The microfilariae of *O. volvulus* must be distinguished from other filarial microfilariae, particularly those of *M. ozzardi* and *M. streptocerca*. If in doubt, slides should be prepared and stained.

In heavily infected individuals, microfilariae may appear in the blood and urine, although the prevalence of microfilaremia varies geographically. After therapy with DEC, microfilariae have been reported in the blood, urine, lacrimal fluid, sputum, and cerebrospinal fluid.

Nodules. Diagnosis may be confirmed by surgical removal of subcutaneous nodules or aspiration of nodule contents and the demonstration of typical adult worms. Ultrasonography is a noninvasive technique that can distinguish onchocercomas from lymph nodes, lipomas, fibromas, and foreign body granulomas. A typical nodule appears as a central, relatively homogeneous echogenic area containing echodense particles with a lateral acoustic shadow. The latter is absent in very small nodules. Ultrasound can also detect impalpable nodules.

Slit Lamp Examination. This allows demonstration of intraocular microfilariae. Patients are asked to place their head between their knees for about 10 minutes. When they sit up, the microfilariae become concentrated behind the central cornea and are easier to visualize and count. Microfilariae in the anterior chamber can be visualized with a slit lamp or with an ophthalmoscope set at +20 diopters by looking against the red fundal reflex. Although more difficult to see, microfilariae in the cornea can be found by retroillumination against the red reflex through the dilated pupil. Slit lamp examination of the fundus with a 90 diopter lens can be used to identify intraretinal microfilariae. These are generally seen close to retinal vessels as small, motile, and highly refractile objects.

The Mazzotti Test. The use of skin snips is a relatively insensitive technique for detecting low infection levels. The Mazzotti test may be used when skin snips have not revealed microfilariae but *O. volvulus* infection is still suspected clinically. The Mazzotti test might precipitate severe reactions in those with heavy microfilarial burdens or might cause ocular damage in those with microfilariae in the eyes. For this reason, the test should be performed only after skin snips and ocular examination have revealed no microfilariae. Patients are given a single dose of 25 to 50 mg PO of DEC. Infected individuals develop intense pruritus within a few hours. The itching is maximal in areas where microfilariae are most numerous and may be accompanied by erythema, edema, and papules. The itching subsides in 2 to 3 days. The presence of *M. streptocerca* may cause false-positive reactions.

The topical application of DEC under an occlusive dressing, the DEC patch test, is a new, sensitive method of diagnosis in light or early infections. The presence of a localized inflammatory reaction at the site of the patch indicates a positive test.

Serology. Although no assay has superseded skin snips, important advances have been made in serologic diagnosis of this disease in the past decade. Traditional serologic tests were unreliable because the antigens cross reacted with those of other helminths. More recently, an enzyme-linked immunosorbent assay (ELISA) using a cocktail of *O. volvulus*–derived recombinant antigens has been developed and is highly sensitive and specific. Serology cannot, however, distinguish between current and past infection and is most useful for detecting infection in specific patient groups: (1) expatriates with a brief exposure history, (2) in areas where the disease has been under long-term control to detect disease transmission among children, and (3) in surveys of new areas where disease transmission is suspected and microfilarial levels are low.

DNA Probes. Highly specific and sensitive polymerase chain reaction–based assays have been developed for the detection of *O. volvulus* DNA in microscopically negative skin snips or scrapings. This has proved useful in detecting very low infection levels but requires expensive equipment and reagents, as well as rigorous training and quality control. This method has also been successfully used to detect infected flies in studies of disease transmission.

Differential Diagnosis. Early onchodermatitis is rarely diagnosed correctly and must be distinguished from atopic dermatitis, food allergies, contact dermatitis, insect bites, and scabies. The exposure history should suggest the diagnosis. The chronic skin lesions may be mistaken for severe chronic eczema, malnutrition, and presbydermia. "Leopard skin" must be distinguished from other causes of hypochromia including vitiligo, leprosy, streptocerciasis, and the endemic treponematoses.

TREATMENT AND PROGNOSIS. The most effective drug currently available is ivermectin. Ivermectin has proved vastly superior to older drugs, e.g., DEC (a microfilaricide) and suramin (a macrofilaricide), both of which were associated with severe and frequently dangerous adverse reactions. In many ways, ivermectin, which is distributed as Mectizan or Stromectol (Merck & Co.), has revolutionized treatment and control strategies for the disease in the 1990s. Ivermectin is highly effective, well tolerated, microfilaricidal, and able to suppress microfilarial levels in the skin for at least 6 months, after which levels start to rise again. Because the drug is thought to have no or minimal macrofilaricidal effects, it should be given every 6 months or annually for the lifetime of adult worms, which may be for 12 or more years.

Adverse reactions occur with ivermectin but are less frequent and severe than those reported with DEC and suramin. Ivermectin is safe and effective in large-scale field trials and can be administered at a community level without medical supervision. Ivermectin treatment leads to improvement or resolution of anterior segment lesions including punctate keratitis, sclerosing keratitis, and iritis and has reduced the incidence of optic nerve disease in the mesoendemic savanna of northern Nigeria. However, ivermectin seems to have no impact on the evolution of chorioretinopathy in individuals having this lesion at the time of treatment, although it reduces incidence of new lesions in previously unaffected eyes.

Onchocerciasis-induced blindness is associated with an increased mortality rate, which is probably due to lack of economic and nutritional support for the blind in endemic areas, which tend to be rural and economically deprived.

Nodulectomy. Nodulectomy has been a popular method of control in Guatemala, Mexico, and Ecuador, where head nodules are common. In Guatemala, prolonged nodulectomy campaigns may have reduced the incidence of blindness, whereas in Ecuador, removal of all palpable nodules has reduced the load of microfilariae in the skin and eyes. In Africa, nodulectomy has never been widely practiced, because the nodules tend to be deeper and are more difficult to remove. Furthermore, nodulectomy in Africa has not been shown to reduce microfilarial counts or to be practical. However, the benefit of removing head nodules in terms of the development of ocular disease has been demonstrated and is recommended.

CHEMOTHERAPY

Ivermectin. Ivermectin is the drug of choice for the treatment of onchocerciasis and has been used extensively since 1987. It is a semisynthetic macrocyclic lactone, used with great success against a wide range of veterinary parasites. It causes a spastic paralysis of *O. volvulus* microfilariae in vitro by modulation of γ-aminobutyric acid–mediated neurotransmission. Ivermectin has little direct microfilaricidal effect in vitro, and an intact host immune response seems to be important for its microfilaricidal effects in vivo. The impact of ivermectin on adult worms is not clear. The long-term suppression of microfilariae may be due to a block in the release of mature microfilariae from adult females, once the uteri become clogged with degenerate microfilarial debris after treatment. It may take 3 to 9 months for this necrotic debris to be cleared and for normal embryogenesis to resume. Further, with repeated ivermectin treatments there is a reduction in the fecundity of viable females, a reduction in the proportion of inseminated females, an increase in the death rate of adult females, and a reduction in the number of adult males per nodule. Ivermectin, by reducing the reservoir of microfilariae in endemic populations, also reduces the uptake of microfilariae by black flies and the transmission of infective larvae.

Ivermectin is rapidly effective in reducing microfilarial burdens and causes little or no adverse reaction or Mazzotti reaction. After treatment, microfilariae usually disappear from the skin within 1 week and from the eyes within 2 to 3 months. The drug is administered at 150 μg/kg (usually two tablets of 6 mg for an 80-kg adult). After 2 years of semiannual treatments, there is no apparent difference between further semiannual or annual treatments as the microfilariae counts continue to fall.

It has been recommended that the drug not be given to children <5 years old or weighing <15 kg, to pregnant women, to mothers in the first week of lactation, to those who are otherwise seriously ill, or during outbreaks of meningitis. However, evidence from large community trials shows that the drug can be administered safely to the first 3 exclusion groups, although it is not yet licensed for use in these groups. Tablets of 3 mg are available for the treatment of small children. Great caution, however, should be used in administering the drug in areas where loiasis is endemic. The death of *L. loa* microfilariae may cause severe or even fatal encephalitis. In these situations, heavy infections with *L. loa* should be excluded using thin blood films.

A mild Mazzotti reaction occurs in 10 to 15% of patients receiving a first dose of ivermectin, and a severe reaction may occur in 1 to 5%. Most reactions occur on the second day after treatment (e.g., 36 to 48 hours after dosing). During subsequent treatments, the frequency and severity of adverse reactions are considerably reduced. No fatal reactions have been directly attributable to ivermectin. Typical reactions include pruritus, rash, fever, lymphedema, and occasionally, severe postural hypotension. European expatriates complain of pruritus and skin reactions more commonly than inhabitants of endemic areas. Mild reactions generally require no treatment, and menthol ointment is as effective as any other medication for pruritus. Severe reactions may be treated with intramuscular steroids. Antihistamines and antipyretics have no demonstrable impact on the course of the post-treatment reaction, although they may ameliorate some of the symptoms of mild reactions.

Ivermectin is now being administered on a community level as the primary control strategy in many endemic countries. Community compliance is probably aided by the other effects of ivermectin, which include the expulsion of intestinal worms and treatment of ectoparasitic infections, e.g., scabies. By 1996, >20 million doses of ivermectin had been distributed, and approximately 1.2 million doses are currently being administered every month. The drug is supplied free by the manufacturer, Merck & Co., for the treatment of all patients with onchocerciasis. Drug distribution is coordinated for the World Health Organization (WHO) by the Mectizan Expert Committee at the Carter Center, Atlanta, Georgia.

Diethylcarbamazine. This microfilaricidal drug has now been completely replaced by ivermectin, and there is currently no justifiable use for this drug in the treatment of onchocerciasis. DEC (banocide, Hetrazan, Notezine) is rapidly microfilaricidal but has no macrofilaricidal effects. However, microfilarial levels often return to pretreatment levels within 1 year of a single course, and its benefit in patients with serious ocular disease is doubtful. DEC was frequently associated with often severe and occasionally fatal post-treatment reactions. This was similar to that already described as following ivermectin but tended to be more severe, with pruritus, rash, fever, swollen and tender lymph nodes, facial and periorbital edema, arthralgia, and postural hypotension, followed occasionally by death. DEC is also associated with the development and deterioration of optic nerve disease and chorioretinopathy. The severity of the reaction was greater in patients with higher microfilarial burdens. A small single dose of DEC still has a role in diagnosing occult infections although it should be reserved only for those in whom no skin-dwelling microfilariae can be detected.

Suramin. Suramin (Bayer 205, Germanin, Moranyl, Antrypol) is a complex water-soluble urea derivative with both macrofilaricidal and microfilaricidal effects. It is currently the only recommended macrofilaricidal drug, but its administration is associated with severe toxicity. There remains a limited role for this drug in symptomatic patients who have left an endemic area and for treating severe onchodermatitis that fails to respond to ivermectin. The drug should be administered under medical supervision, and patients should be healthy and well nourished.

A fresh 10% solution is injected IV, commencing with a test dose of 100 mg given slowly over 2 minutes to test for hypersensitivity. A total course should be given in the following weekly doses: 0.2 g (3.3 mg/kg), 0.4 g (6.7 mg/kg), 0.6 g (10.0 mg/kg), 0.8 g (13.3 mg/kg), 1.0 g (16.7 mg/kg), and 1.0 g (16.7 mg/kg). The doses can be reduced proportionally for those weighing less than 60 kg.

This regimen minimizes the risk of toxic reactions and kills most adult worms and microfilariae in the skin and eyes. The microfilaricidal effect of suramin is delayed, and patients may complain of a Mazzotti reaction up to 6 weeks after the first dose. However, there is still the danger of occasionally fatal reactions and deterioration in eye disease, particularly iridocyclitis and optic nerve disease. Direct toxicity includes tenderness of the palms and soles, polyuria with proteinuria and granular casts in the urine, fatigue, anorexia, malaise, and sometimes ulceration of the mouth, diarrhea, and prostration. Reactions to adult worms include urticaria and swelling around dying worms, tenderness and swelling of nodules, and sterile abscesses. The most serious complications are exfoliative dermatitis and a fatal progressive wasting syndrome. Reactions may be ameliorated by concurrent administration of corticosteroids or depletion of microfilarial loads by administering ivermectin before suramin.

Amocarzine. Amocarzine (Ciba-Geigy) is a macrofilaricide with microfilaricidal effects. The drug is not currently commercially available. It is an amoscanate derivative and is administered postprandially at a dosage of 3 mg/kg PO b.i.d. for 3 days. Amocarzine has been shown to be effective and relatively well tolerated in community-based studies in Guatemala and Ecuador, although recent studies in Ghana have cast doubt on a useful role for this drug. After amocarzine treatment, dermal microfilarial levels fall rapidly owing to its microfilaricidal effect and more gradually owing to the de-

layed macrofilaricidal effect. The drug may cause a mild post-treatment reaction characterized by fever, pruritus, and rash, and it may cause transient dizziness and a positive Romberg sign. It has advantages over suramin but requires further evaluation.

Drugs Under Development. The benzimidazole derivative UMF 078 has been shown to have macrofilaricidal activity in animal models after both PO and IM administration and is currently entering the preclinical toxicology phase of development.

PREVENTION AND CONTROL. There are no effective prophylactic drugs or vaccines. People are best protected by avoiding areas of maximal biting, wearing protective clothing, and using insect repellents. The overall objective of onchocerciasis control is to achieve a reduction in the infection as a public health and socioeconomic problem. The primary public health problem associated with the disease is visual loss and blindness, but onchocercal skin and lymphatic disease also cause considerable disability. Thus, the primary objective of most control strategies is morbidity control by reducing community microfilarial burdens to levels where clinical disease is absent or very rare, rather than disease eradication, which is an unrealistic goal in most foci of infection.

As with all vector-borne parasitic diseases, there are 3 principal methods of control: (1) reduce transmission by attacking the vector, (2) reduce the parasite reservoir in the community by mass chemotherapy, and (3) change human behavior to reduce exposure to the vector. The choice of control strategy depends on the accessibility of breeding sites to aerial spraying and the flight range of the vector. The highly successful Onchocerciasis Control Programme (OCP) in West Africa has reduced disease transmission in many West African countries owing to aerial spraying with larvicides. Vector control has not been performed in many other endemic African countries and in the American foci. In these areas, control strategies now rely on reducing the parasite reservoir by long-term distribution of ivermectin.

Vector Control. The success of any program based on vector control depends on the flight range or dispersal of the vector and the degree of isolation of the endemic area. In Kenya, where the flight range of *S. neavei* was only a few miles, the vector and parasite were totally eliminated by treating the rivers with DDT. Continual vigilance was necessary because it took 15 years for transmission to be interrupted. The foci in West Africa are much more extensive, and complete eradication of the vector, members of the *S. damnosum* complex, has not been attempted because reinvasion from nontreated areas occurs rapidly. The OCP, with financing from the World Bank and management from the WHO, has been highly successful in controlling disease in OCP countries. The program was initiated in 1974 by WHO in the Volta River Basin of West Africa and now involves 11 countries and 50,000 km of rivers. The aim of the program was to eliminate onchocerciasis as a public health problem by reducing the ATP to <200 infective larvae per person per year. After 15 years of control, using aerial spraying of breeding sites with temephos (Abate) and *Bacillus thuringiensis* (Bt 14), it is estimated that 30 million people have been protected from infection, 10 million children have been born into areas free of disease transmission, and between 125,000 and 200,000 have been prevented from going blind. Although the OCP has been a very expensive program to finance, it has been regarded as highly cost effective, with a rate of return on investment of about 20%, because many areas that were previously uninhabitable have been repopulated and agricultural production has increased markedly. However, attempts in the future will increasingly be made to devolve the responsibilities of the OCP to national governments, nongovernment organizations, and local organizations.

Mass Therapy With Ivermectin. Vector control is considered unrealistic in most endemic countries owing to the inaccessibility of breeding sites. Control in these countries depends on mass distribution of ivermectin. The two possible strategies for ivermectin control are large-scale distribution to inhabitants of infected communities and passive drug distribution to patients reporting to local health facilities. The first strategy is most appropriate in highly endemic areas (e.g., prevalence >40%), whereas the second is recommended for low-risk communities (e.g., where community microfilarial levels are low and there is no excess risk of blindness). Attempts to eliminate the parasite reservoir using mass distribution with ivermectin have had mixed success. A community-based control program using semiannual ivermectin treatments during a 5-year period in a hyperendemic focus in Ecuador has reduced community microfilarial prevalence to negligible levels and probably resulted in interruption of transmission. However, to achieve this, a population coverage of >90% was required at each survey. The success and long-term sustainability of ivermectin distribution programs require education of inhabitants of endemic communities about the disease and the benefits of treatment, as well as participation of the entire community in drug delivery.

In countries where vector control programs are well advanced, mass distribution of ivermectin is likely to prevent recrudescence of infection and to control disease where vector control temporarily breaks down. However, it is unlikely that mass ivermectin distribution will replace vector control or even shorten the period for which vector control is required.

Protective Immunity and Vaccine Development. Limited evidence supports the presence of a protective immune response in endemic areas: (1) Age-prevalence profiles show a peak in early adulthood followed by a gradual decline, suggesting the possible development of an age-acquired immunity; (2) resistance to reinfection with new infectious L3-stage larvae has been documented despite ongoing infection (concomitant immunity); and (3) small groups of individuals having no evidence of infection despite continuous exposure have been identified in endemic areas. The latter, who have been termed *putatively immune*, have distinct immunologic responses that differentiate them from infected subjects: (1) lower parasite-specific antibody levels, (2) increased cellular responses to parasite antigen, and (3) a relative increase in the production of the Th1 cytokine, IFN-γ. However, putatively immune individuals constitute a very small proportion of endemic populations, and it is impossible to determine exposure history with any certainty.

Progress in the development of a vaccine against onchocerciasis has been disappointing. A protective immune response can be induced in experimental animals inoculated with irradiated L3-stage larvae, and some degree of protection has been demonstrated using a number of *O. volvulus*–derived recombinant antigens. Despite the large number of antigens developed as potential vaccine candidates using modern recombinant techniques, none is promising enough in 1998 to be considered for testing in human populations.

Bibliography

Anderson J, Fuglsang H: Ocular onchocerciasis. Trop Dis Bull 74:257, 1977.
Awadzi K, Hero M, Opoku NO, et al: The chemotherapy of onchocerciasis. XVIII. Aspects of treatment with suramin. Trop Med Parasitol 46:19, 1995.
Cupp EW, Bernado MJ, Kuszewski AE, et al: The effects of ivermectin on transmission of Onchocerca volvulus. Science 231:740, 1986.
Eberhard ML, Lammie PJ: Laboratory diagnosis of filariasis. Clin Lab Med 11:977, 1991.
Greene BM, Taylor HR, Cupp EW, et al: Comparison of ivermectin and diethyl-

carbamazine in the treatment of human onchocerciasis. N Engl J Med 313:133, 1985.
McCarthy J, Ottesen EA, Nutman TB: Onchocerciasis in endemic and nonendemic populations: Differences in clinical presentation and immunologic findings. J Infect Dis 170:736, 1994.
Murdoch ME, Hay RJ, Mackenzie CD, et al: A clinical classification and grading system of the cutaneous changes in onchocerciasis. Br J Dermatol 129:260, 1993.
Ottesen EA, Campbell WC: Ivermectin in human medicine. J Antimicrob Chemother 34:195, 1994.
Ottesen EA: Immune responsiveness and the pathogenesis of human onchocerciasis. J Infect Dis 171:659, 1995.
Poltera AA, Zea-Flores G, Guderian R, et al: Onchocercacidal effects of amocarzine (CGP 6140) in Latin America. Lancet 337:583, 1991.
Rodger FC: The pathogenesis and pathology of ocular onchocerciasis: I-V. Am J Ophthalmol 49:104, 1960.
World Health Organization: Onchocerciasis and its control. Report of a WHO Expert Committee on onchocerciasis control. World Health Organ Tech Rep Ser 852, 1995.

109 *Miscellaneous Filarial Infections*

109.1 Mansonella ozzardi *Infection**

Wayne M. Meyers and Ronald C. Neafie

DEFINITION. For many years, the disease mansonelliasis (or mansonellosis) was thought of as uniquely infection by the filaria *Mansonella ozzardi*. Today mansonelliasis includes infection by the following three species of *Mansonella*: *M. ozzardi*, *M. perstans*, and *M. streptocerca*.

ETIOLOGY AND HISTORY. In 1897, Manson first described microfilariae of *M. ozzardi* in the blood of Amerindians in Guyana. The species was named for Ozzard, who obtained the specimens Manson later studied. Faust, in 1929, described fragments of adult worms obtained by Daniels from patients in Guyana and named the new genus *Mansonella*. Orihel and Eberhard, in 1982, redescribed adult worms from patas monkeys (*Erythrocebus patas*) experimentally infected with this filaria and expanded the genus *Mansonella* to include filariae formerly classified as *Dipetalonema perstans* and *Dipetalonema streptocerca*.

M. ozzardi adult females recovered from humans measure 65 to 81 mm in length and 210 to 250 μm in diameter. Only one fragment of a male worm from humans has been described. This fragment was of the posterior end of the worm and measured 38 mm in length and 200 μm in maximum diameter. Adult worms recovered from experimentally infected monkeys are considerably shorter and smaller in diameter than those collected from humans. The cuticle is smooth. Microfilariae are unsheathed and measure 170 to 240 μm by 3.5 μm with a cephalic space 2 to 6 μm long, and the anterior two or three nuclei either overlap or are side by side. Caudal space is 3 to 8 μm long, and the terminal nuclei oval (Fig. 109–1).

DISTRIBUTION AND EPIDEMIOLOGY. *M. ozzardi* prevails in Caribbean islands and in Central and South America, perhaps as far south as Argentina. Several species of *Culicoides* dipterans and the black fly *Simulium amazonicum* transmit *M. ozzardi*. Larvae develop within the thoracic musculature of these insects. Although monkeys are susceptible to

---

*All the material in this chapter is in the public domain, with the exception of any borrowed figures or tables.

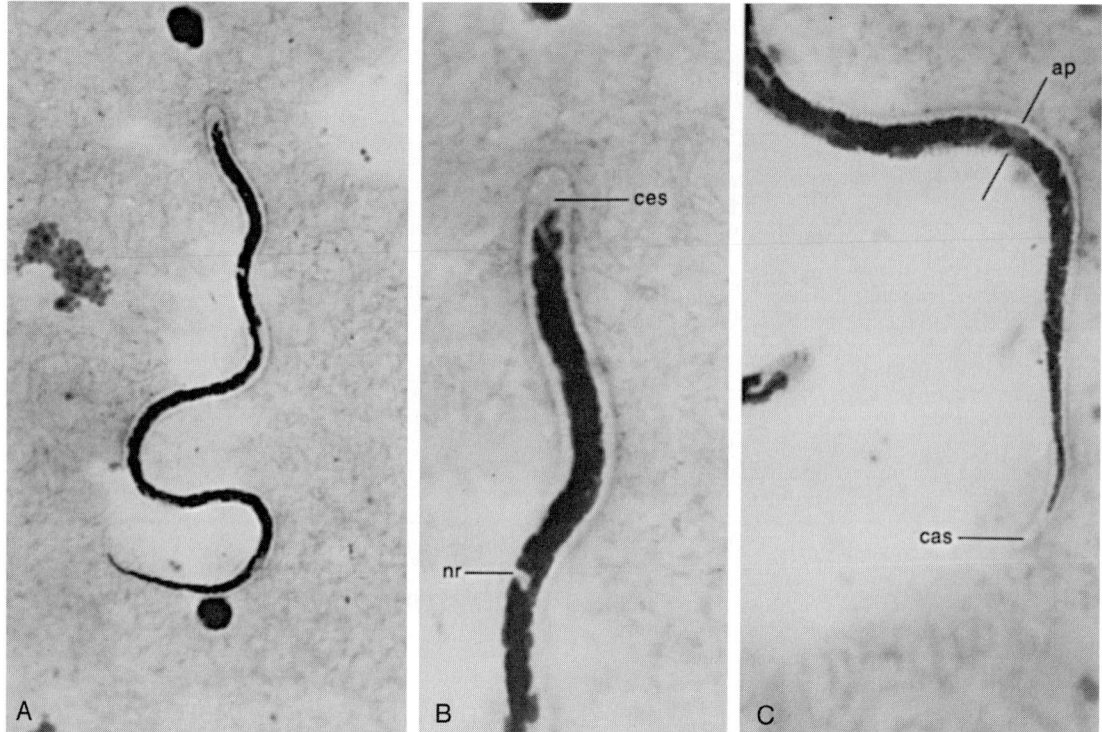

Figure 109–1. Thick blood film, *Mansonella ozzardi* microfilaria (Giemsa stain). *A*, × 820. (Courtesy of the Armed Forces Institute of Pathology, Photograph Neg. No. 74-19692.) *B*, Anterior end, cephalic space (ces), nerve ring (nr), × 1620. *C*, Posterior end, anal pore (ap), caudal space (cas), × 1620.

experimental infection, humans are the only known natural definitive host. Prevalence increases with age, and both sexes are equally affected. Focally, infection rates may reach 70%.

PATHOGENESIS AND CLINICAL MANIFESTATIONS. Adult worms in humans appear to favor the thoracic and peritoneal cavities but may enter lymphatics. *M. ozzardi* is a well-adapted parasite, usually provoking no inflammatory response. In the Amazon region in Brazil, however, Amerindians who are heavily infected complain of varices of the lower extremities, pain in the knees and ankles, erythematous pruritic cutaneous plaques, inguinal lymphadenopathy, fever, headache, and vertigo. Histopathologically, the microfilariae are in small blood vessels of the skin and subcutaneous tissue and may provoke perivascular infiltrates of lymphocytes and plasma cells. A peripheral eosinophilia is often noted.

DIAGNOSIS. Diagnosis depends on demonstration of characteristic microfilariae in peripheral blood films, skin snips, or biopsy specimens. Adult *M. ozzardi* organisms are rarely encountered. Nuclepore filtration of peripheral blood requires a pore size of <5 μm to demonstrate microfilariae of *M. ozzardi*.

TREATMENT. Because the symptoms most patients experience are mild and varied, efficacy of treatment is difficult to assess. Reports on the effect of diethylcarbamazine vary, and ivermectin has not been evaluated.

Bibliography

Buckley JJ: On the development, in *Culicoides furens* Poey, of *Filaria* (= *Mansonella*) *ozzardi* Manson, 1897. J Helminthol 12:99, 1934.

Macfie JWS, Corson JF: A new species of filarial larva in the skin of natives of the Gold Coast. Ann Trop Med Parasitol 16:465, 1922.

Marinkelle CJ, German E: Mansonelliasis in the Comisaria del Vaupes of Colombia. Trop Geogr Med 22:101, 1970.

Nelson GS, Davies JB: Observations on *Mansonella ozzardi* in Trinidad. Trans R Soc Trop Med Hyg 70:16, 1976.

Orihel TC, Eberhard ML: *Mansonella ozzardi*: A redescription with comments on its taxonomic relationships. Am J Trop Med Hyg 31:1142, 1982.

109.2 Mansonella perstans Infection*

Ronald C. Neafie and Wayne M. Meyers

DEFINITION. *Mansonella perstans* infection is limited to the disease caused by the filarial nematode *Mansonella perstans*. This filaria has many synonyms, including *Dipetalonema perstans* and *Acanthocheilonema perstans*, and is also known as the Ugandan or Kampala *eye worm*. Manson first described microfilariae of *M. perstans* in 1891, and Daniels discovered the adult worms in 1898.

ETIOLOGY AND EPIDEMIOLOGY. Adult worms inhabit the pleural, peritoneal, and pericardial cavities, the mesentery, and perirenal and retroperitoneal tissues, but they are rarely available for study. The female worm is 60 to 80 mm by 100 to 150 μm, and males are 35 to 45 mm by 50 to 70 μm. The adult female at midbody contains an intestine and two uteri (Fig. 109–2). In both sexes, the cuticle is 1 to 2 μm thick. Microfilariae of *M. perstans* are nonperiodic, measure 100 to 200 μm by 3.5 to 4.5 μm, and are unsheathed. The round terminal nucleus is at the tip of the tail (Fig. 109–3). Biting midges *(Culicoides)* transmit *M. perstans*.

M. perstans is endemic throughout much of tropical Africa, especially in the region from Senegal east to Uganda and south to Zimbabwe. In South America, *M. perstans* prevails along the Atlantic coast from Panama to Argentina. The parasite has been reported in New Guinea. Infection rates of >50% have been reported.

---

*All the material in this chapter is in the public domain, with the exception of any borrowed figures or tables.

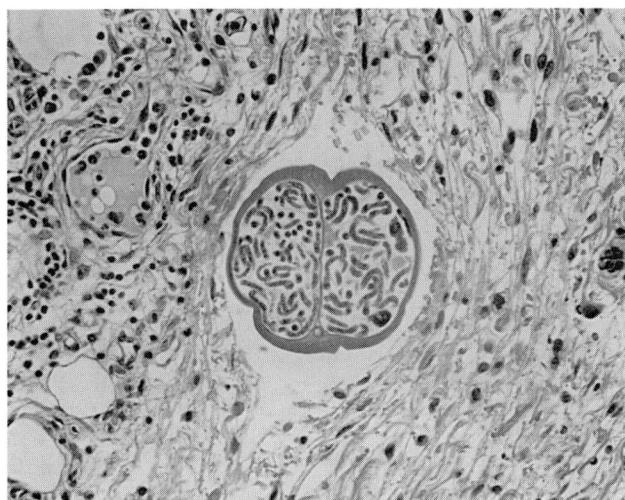

Figure 109–2. Gravid female *Mansonella perstans* in connective tissue of spermatic cord. The worm is 115 μm in diameter. (Courtesy of the Armed Forces Institute of Pathology, Photograph Neg. No. 96-5853.)

PATHOGENESIS AND CLINICAL MANIFESTATIONS. Most patients have no readily discernible symptoms. Expatriates tend to report symptoms most often. Symptoms frequently associated with infection by *M. perstans* include subcutaneous swellings on the arms, shoulders, and face (Calabar swellings), abdominal pain, pruritus, pleuritis, arthralgia, and fatigue. Death of one patient was attributed to fibropurulent pericarditis associated with *M. perstans* adults and microfilariae in the pericardium. Pleural effusion and chronic lymphedema have been reported. Periorbital edema and conjunctival pruritus may develop in both natives and expatriates. Irritative granulomatous nodules in the conjunctiva and acute periorbital inflammation surrounding dead *M. perstans* worms are called *bung-eye* and *bulge-eye* in Uganda, where these manifestations seem to be more common. Inflammatory lesions caused by *M. perstans* in and around the eyes have been reported from Nigeria and the Sudan. Thus, worms dying naturally or as a result of treatment cause various symptoms, depending on their anatomic location.

DIAGNOSIS AND TREATMENT. Diagnosis is made by identifying characteristic microfilariae of *M. perstans* in peripheral

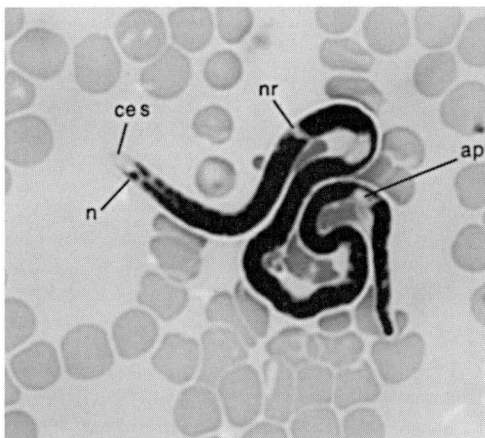

Figure 109–3. Thin blood film. *Mansonella perstans* microfilaria (Giemsa stain, × 890); cephalic space (ces), nucleus (n), nerve ring (nr), anal pore (ap). (Courtesy of the Armed Forces Institute of Pathology, Photograph Neg. No. 74-5605.)

blood or, uncommonly, in cerebrospinal fluid and urine. Concentration techniques may be necessary to detect light infections. Microfilariae are frequently an incidental finding in biopsy specimens of tissue and can be readily identified by their morphologic features. Rarely, adult *M. perstans* organisms are recovered intact or appear in histologic sections. Their identification requires demonstration of specific morphologic features.

Diethylcarbamazine (DEC) consistently eliminates microfilariae of *M. perstans* from the blood stream after prolonged therapy (2 mg base/kg body weight q.i.d. for eight periods of 10 days each, with 3-week intervals between periods). The slow clearing of microfilariae suggests a lethal or sterilizing effect of DEC on the adult worms and little or no direct effect on the microfilariae. Patients complaining of the usually vague symptoms often report immediate improvement with DEC therapy. A series of patients in Sweden responded favorably to mebendazole (100 mg b.i.d. for 4 to 7 weeks), two of them after therapeutic failure of DEC. Single-dose therapy with ivermectin has not proved effective.

Bibliography

Adolphi PE, Kagan IG, McQuay RM: Diagnosis and treatment of *Acanthocheilonema perstans* filariasis. Am J Trop Med Hyg 11:76, 1962.
Baird JK, Neafie RC, Connor DH: Bung-eye, bulge-eye, and nodules in the conjunctiva caused by *Mansonella perstans*. Am J Trop Med Hyg 38:553, 1988.
Baird JK, Neafie RC, Lanoie L, Connor DH: *Mansonella perstans* in the abdominal cavity of nine Africans. Am J Trop Med Hyg 37:578, 1987.
Foster DG: Filariasis—a rare cause of pericarditis. J Trop Med Hyg 59:212, 1956.
Maertens K, Wery M: Effect of mebendazole and levamisole on *Onchocerca volvulus* and *Dipetalonema perstans*. Trans R Soc Trop Med Hyg 69:355, 1975.
Orihel TC: "Cerebral filariasis" in Rhodesia—a zoonotic infection? Am J Trop Med Hyg 22:596, 1973.
Owen HB, Hennessey RSF: A note on some ocular manifestations of helminthic origin occurring in natives of Uganda. Trans R Soc Trop Med Hyg 25:267, 1932.
Van den Enden E, Van Gompel A, Van der Stuft P, et al: Treatment failure of a single high dose of ivermectin for *Mansonella perstans* filariasis. Trans R Soc Trop Med Hyg 87:90, 1993.
Wahlgren M, Frolov I: Correspondence: Treatment of *Dipetalonema perstans* infections with mebendazole. Trans R Soc Trop Med Hyg 71:422, 1983.

109.3 *Streptocerciasis**

Wayne M. Meyers and Ronald C. Neafie

DEFINITION. Streptocerciasis is an infection caused by the filarial nematode *Mansonella streptocerca* (Macfie and Corson, 1922). Before 1982, the genus of this filaria was designated variously as *Dipetalonema, Acanthocheilonema,* and *Tetrapetalonema.*

ETIOLOGY AND HISTORY. In the course of their studies on onchocerciasis in the Gold Coast (Ghana), Macfie and Corson in 1922 described microfilariae in skin snips that they recognized to be distinct from other known microfilariae that infect humans. Adult filariae presumed to be *M. streptocerca* were first seen in chimpanzees in 1946 and in the tissues of humans in 1972. Adult female *M. streptocerca* organisms are approximately 27 by 0.085 mm, and the adult male is 17 by 0.05 mm. The cuticle is thin and smooth, and the lateral chords are inconspicuous. The microfilariae are 180 to 240 μm by 2.5 to 5.0 μm and are unsheathed; sharp curving of the posterior end frequently gives them a characteristic shepherd's crook configuration (Fig. 109–4). In fresh mounts, they swim less actively than do microfilariae of *Onchocerca volvulus.* The cephalic clear space is 3 to 5 μm long, and the first four nuclei are oval, occur in single file, and are followed

---

*All the material in this chapter is in the public domain, with the exception of any borrowed figures or tables.

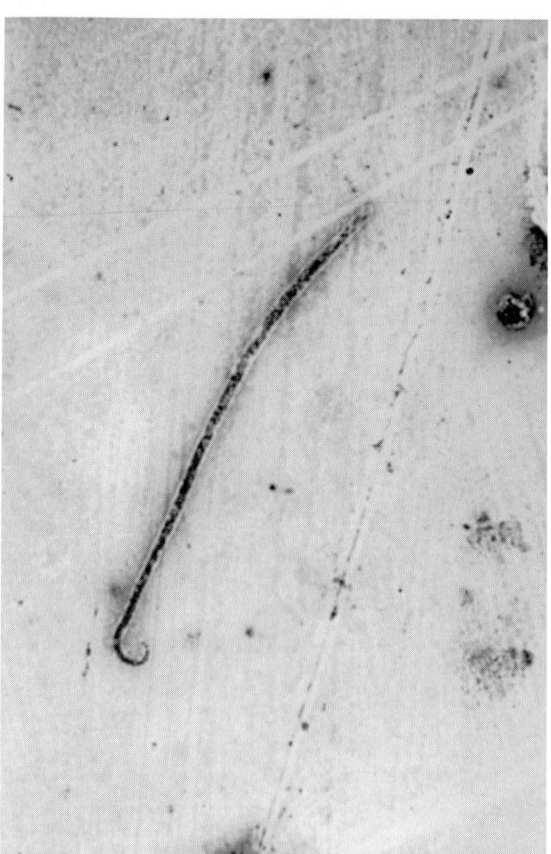

Figure 109–4. Whole microfilaria of *Mansonella streptocerca* obtained from skin snip. Note the "shepherd's crook" configuration (Giemsa stain, × 350). (Courtesy of the Armed Forces Institute of Pathology, Photograph Neg. No. 70-7193.)

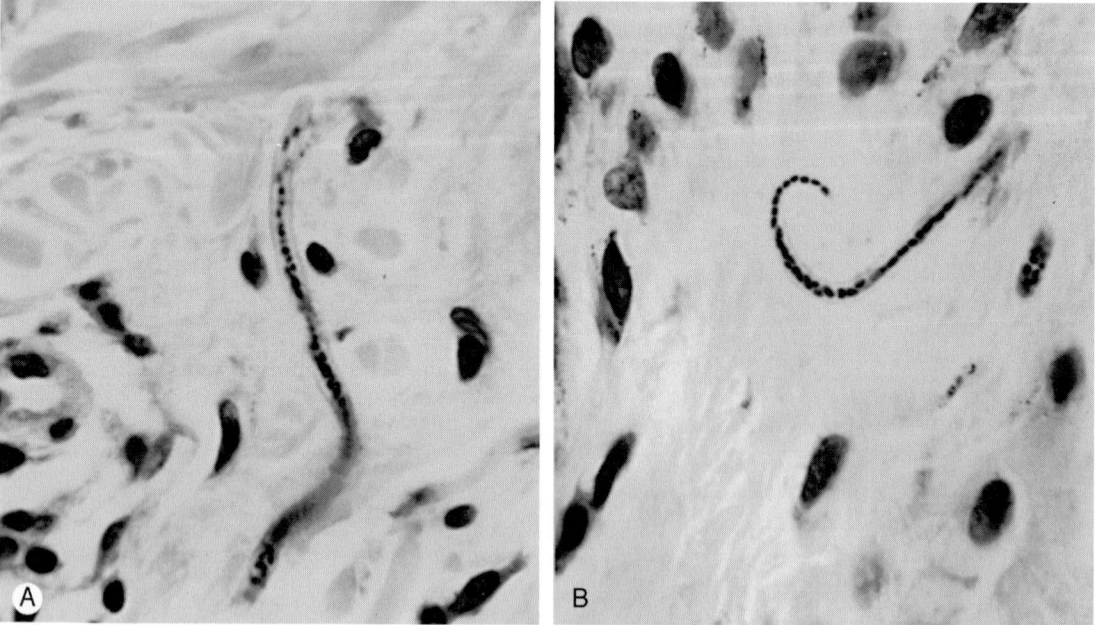

Figure 109–5. Diagnostic features of microfilariae of *Mansonella streptocerca* in sections of skin. The microfilariae are extravascular in the dermal collagen. *A,* Anterior end, showing cephalic space and nuclei (× 1080). (Courtesy of the Armed Forces Institute of Pathology, Photograph Neg. No. 71-10075.) *B,* Posterior end with "shepherd's crook" configuration and nuclei that reach nearly to the tip (× 1080). (Courtesy of the Armed Forces Institute of Pathology, Photograph Neg. No. 71-10074.)

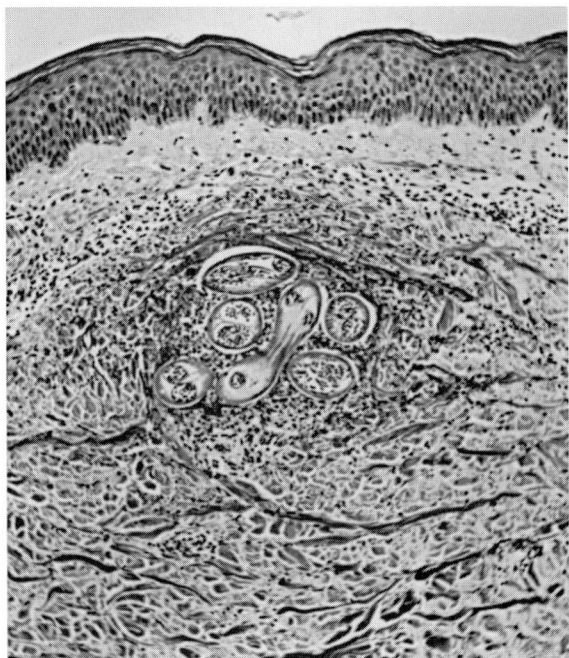

Figure 109–6. Section of skin containing multiple cross sections of gravid female *Mansonella streptocerca*. Biopsy specimen was from a papule that formed within 18 hours after ingestion of diethylcarbamazine. Note cellular exudate surrounding the coiled worm (× 110). (Courtesy of the Armed Forces Institute of Pathology, Photograph Neg. No. 73-1230.)

by seven to ten smaller, more rounded nuclei (Fig. 109–5*A*). The terminal nucleus is oval or round, and the caudal space is 1 μm long (Fig. 109–5*B*).

EPIDEMIOLOGY AND DISTRIBUTION. Streptocerciasis is limited to western and central Africa and is most abundant

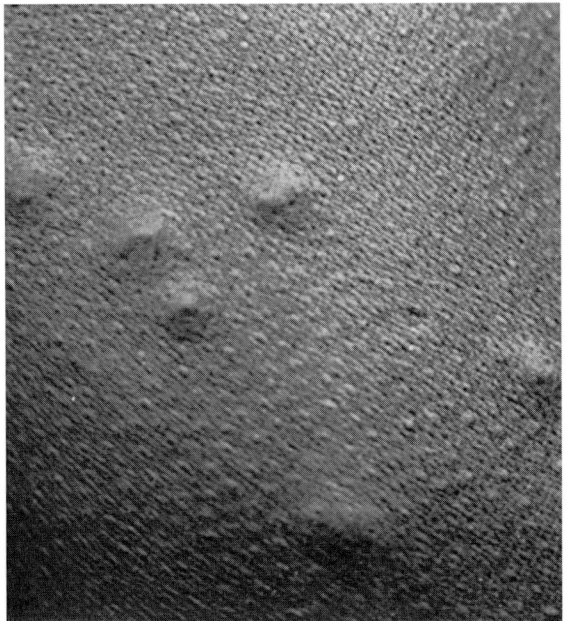

Figure 109–7. Multiple papules on the chest of a Congolese man with streptocerciasis. Papules developed within 18 hours after ingestion of 50 mg of diethylcarbamazine. (Courtesy of the Armed Forces Institute of Pathology, Photograph Neg. No. 77-5005.)

in the tropical rain forest, where it is transmitted by the biting midge *Culicoides grahami*. Prevalence rates vary widely. In The Congo, as many as 90% of the inhabitants of limited geographic areas are infected. Whether or not streptocerciasis is a zoonosis has not been established, but morphologically identical parasites found in chimpanzees suggest this possibility.

PATHOGENESIS AND PATHOLOGY. All adult filariae thus far observed (in approximately 100 patients) have been found in the dermis of long-term residents of endemic areas; thus, the length of the incubation period is unknown. Most worms inhabit the skin of the upper trunk and shoulder girdle. Live worms appear to glide readily between the dermal collagen bundles, provoking no reaction, but when worms die, an intense cellular response develops. Microfilariae are extravascular and have been observed between collagen fibers in the dermis and, rarely, in lymph nodes. Microscopic changes in the skin resemble those of onchocerciasis but are less intense. No evidence yet shows that the eye is affected by *M. streptocerca*. With diethylcarbamazine (DEC) therapy, a marked increase in the cellular exudates and edema occurs, especially around microfilariae. DEC kills adult worms, and a cellular exudate forms around the coiled dead worms (Fig. 109–6). Lymph nodes are diffusely fibrotic, and the lymphatics are dilated. Whether or not these changes can cause elephantiasis is unknown.

CLINICAL MANIFESTATIONS. Many patients are asymptomatic, but the most consistent complaint is a chronic itching dermatitis, most pronounced over the thorax and shoulder girdle. The skin is thickened, hypopigmented macules develop, and one or a few papules are sometimes present. Axillary and inguinal lymphadenopathy is common. The macules in the skin are frequently confused with lesions of leprosy, and many patients with streptocerciasis are misdiagnosed and treated for leprosy for long periods. Macules of streptocerciasis are not hypesthetic, but many clinicians prefer to rely on the results of histopathologic studies for diagnosis, because sensory changes in early leprosy are often difficult to detect.

DEC at an initial dose of as little as 50 mg provokes a response analogous to the Mazzotti reaction. There is exacerbation of itching with cutaneous edema and the formation of papules around killed adult worms (Fig. 109–7). The severity of this reaction occasionally requires interruption of therapy and administration of antihistamines.

DIAGNOSIS. Rapid diagnosis in most patients is made by demonstrating microfilariae in wet mounts of skin snips, usually obtained from skin over the scapulae (Fig. 109–4). In contrast with those of *O. volvulus*, the microfilariae of *M. streptocerca* are sluggish and when immobile assume the shepherd's crook configuration (Figs. 109–4 and 109–5*B*). Diagnosis is frequently made by histopathologic identification of microfilariae of *M. streptocerca* (Fig. 109–5).

TREATMENT. DEC kills the microfilariae and adults of *M. streptocerca*. Optimal doses have not been established, but the drug is usually given at the same dose as for onchocerciasis. Because DEC kills the adult worms, repeated courses of therapy may be curative for patients who do not dwell in endemic areas. The usefulness of ivermectin has not been adequately evaluated. Prognosis is excellent.

Bibliography

Gardiner CH, Meyers WM, Lanoie LO: Recovery of intact male and female *Dipetalonema streptocerca* from man. Am J Trop Med Hyg 28:49, 1979.
Macfie JWS, Corson JF: A new species of filaria larva found in the skin of natives in the Gold Coast. Ann Trop Med Parasitol 16:465, 1922.
Meyers WM, Connor DH, Harman LE, et al: Human streptocerciasis. A clinico-

pathologic study of 40 Africans (Zairians) including identification of the adult filaria. Am J Trop Med Hyg 21:528, 1972.

Meyers WM, Moris R, Neafie RC, et al: Streptocerciasis: Degeneration of adult *Dipetalonema streptocerca* in man following diethylcarbamazine therapy. Am J Trop Med Hyg 27:1137, 1978.

Meyers WM, Neafie RC, Moris R, Bourland J: Streptocerciasis: Observation of adult male *Dipetalonema streptocerca* in man. Am J Trop Med Hyg 26:153, 1977.

Neafie RC, Connor DH, Meyers WM: *Dipetalonema streptocerca* (Macfie and Corson, 1922): Description of the adult female. Am J Trop Med Hyg 24:264, 1975.

109.4 Dirofilariasis*

Ronald C. Neafie and Wayne M. Meyers

DEFINITION. Dirofilariasis is an infection caused by filarial nematodes of the genus *Dirofilaria*. The two forms of dirofilariasis are (1) pulmonary dirofilariasis caused by *Dirofilaria immitis*, the dog heartworm, and (2) subcutaneous dirofilariasis caused by *D. tenuis* (*Dirofilaria conjunctivae*), *D. repens*, *D. striata*, and *D. ursi*–like worms.

PULMONARY DIROFILARIASIS

Morphology. Only immature *D. immitis* nematodes have been found in the lungs of humans. The worms are 100 to 350 μm in diameter. The cuticle is thick and multilayered and projects inward at the lateral cords to form prominent internal longitudinal ridges (Fig. 109–8). Lateral cords usually are poorly preserved, whereas somatic musculature is usually abundant. Internal organs consist of an intestine and two reproductive tubes in females and an intestine and a single reproductive tube in males.

Epidemiology

Distribution. Pulmonary dirofilariasis has been reported from Japan, Australia, and the United States (especially the southern and eastern states). Human infection rates are largely determined by the prevalence of canine dirofilariasis and the extent to which humans are exposed to bites by the mosquito vectors.

Life Cycle. Although *D. immitis* infects the cat, fox, wolf, coyote, sea lion, and other mammals, the dog is by far the most important reservoir host. Coiled masses of adult worms inhabit the right ventricle of the definitive host, and their microfilariae circulate in the peripheral blood. The parasite is transmitted by many species of mosquitoes, which probably also transmit the parasite to humans, a dead-end host. Para-

*All the material in this chapter is in the public domain, with the exception of any borrowed figures or tables.

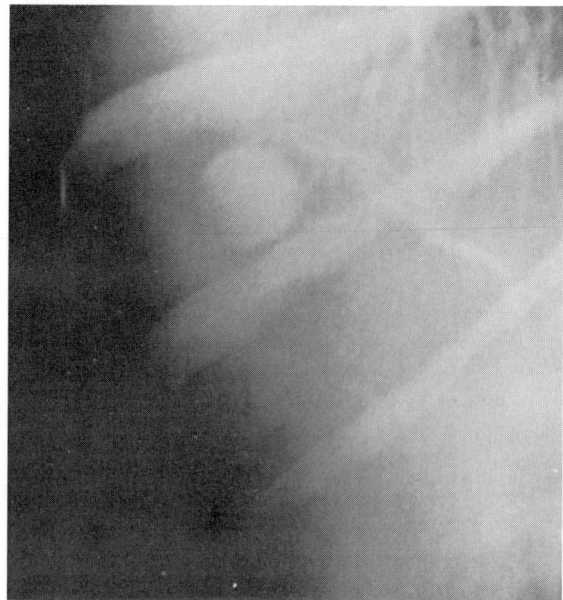

Figure 109–9. Roentgenogram of "coin lesion," 2.5 by 2.0 cm, in right lung. (Courtesy of the Armed Forces Institute of Pathology, Photograph Neg. No. 72-10156.)

sites probably develop partially in the right ventricle before dying and being swept into small pulmonary arteries. Neither mature worms nor microfilariae have been found in humans.

Pathology. Lesions are usually limited to the periphery of the lung and are sharply defined. They have a central area of necrosis surrounded by a zone of granulomatous inflammation and a fibrous wall. A single coiled, usually necrotic, and occasionally calcified worm is found in the lumen of an artery within the area of necrosis. Multiple lesions are rare.

Clinical Manifestations. Most patients are asymptomatic; coin lesions detected during routine radiographic examinations of the chest are the most common presentation (Fig. 109–9). These lesions are 1 to 3 cm in diameter and well circumscribed. Clinical symptoms, when present, include chest pain, cough, hemoptysis, fever, chills, and malaise. Clinical differential diagnoses of coin lesions include carcinoma, tuberculosis, fungal infection, and hamartoma.

Diagnosis. Diagnosis is made by identifying the worm in

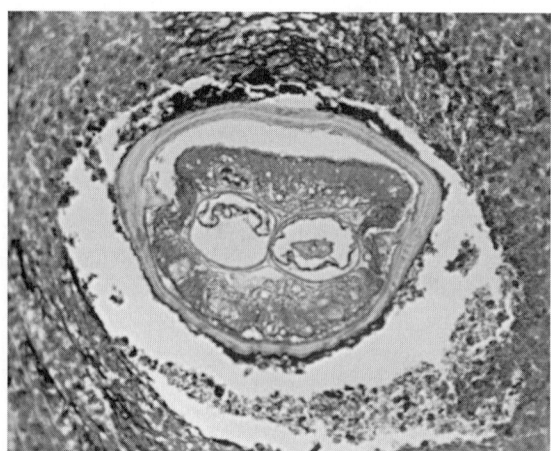

Figure 109–8. Transverse section of immature female *Dirofilaria immitis* in lung (Movat stain, × 275). (Courtesy of the Armed Forces Institute of Pathology, Photograph Neg. No. 71-1045.)

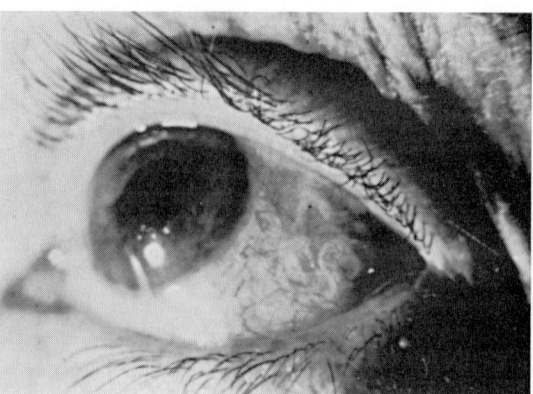

Figure 109–10. Female *Dirofilaria tenuis* in conjunctiva of left eye. (Courtesy of the Armed Forces Institute of Pathology, Photograph Neg. No. 74-6351-2.)

biopsy or autopsy specimens. Serologic tests are available but are not specific for dirofilariasis.

Treatment. No chemotherapeutic agents are effective. The lesions are frequently removed because the coin lesion is mistaken for cancer.

SUBCUTANEOUS DIROFILARIASIS

Etiology, Epidemiology, and Life Cycle. In 1957, Faust reviewed 37 known cases of dirofilariasis in humans. Most patients had worms in the skin and lived in the southern United States. Most infections previously attributed to *D. conjunctivae* are probably due to *D. tenuis*, a parasite of the subcutaneous tissue of the raccoon. *D. repens*, a parasite of the subcutaneous tissue of dogs and cats in Europe, Africa, and Asia, causes lesions in humans. Mosquitoes transmit both *D. tenuis* and *D. repens* to natural hosts and probably transmit the parasite from animals to humans. Subcutaneous dirofilariasis has been reported from the United States, Africa, Asia, Europe, and South America. Rarely, gravid *D. tenuis* nematodes are reported in humans. Although *D. repens* can reach sexual maturity in human tissue, gravid worms have not been described.

Morphology. *D. tenuis* females are 80 to 130 mm by 260 to 360 μm, and males are 40 to 48 mm by 190 to 260 μm. The cuticle is thick and multilayered and contains external and internal longitudinal ridges. Other morphologic characteristics are the same as for *D. immitis*. *D. repens* is greater in diameter than *D. tenuis*.

Pathology. Humans are an abnormal host, and although the parasites may reach maturity in humans, no microfilariae are seen in tissues surrounding the worm or in the circulation. Early lesions consist of a coiled, degenerating worm

in an abscess in subcutaneous tissue. Chronic lesions are granulomatous and contain epithelioid cells, foreign body giant cells, histiocytes, and eosinophils.

Clinical Manifestations. Lesions caused by *D. tenuis* and *D. repens* develop in many parts of the body but most commonly are found in the conjunctiva (Fig. 109–10), eyelid, scrotum, breast, arm, and leg. The lesion develops over a period of several weeks into a subcutaneous nodule that may be tender, painful, erythematous, and occasionally migratory.

Diagnosis. Diagnosis is usually made by identifying the worm in the biopsy specimen. Worms are occasionally extracted from the lesion and identified by gross examination. As in pulmonary dirofilariasis, no serologic tests are specific for subcutaneous dirofilariasis.

Treatment. The only known treatment is surgical removal of the worm.

Bibliography

Baird JK, Neafie RC, Marty AM: Parasitic infections. *In* Dail DH, Hammar SP (eds): Pulmonary Pathology. New York, Springer-Verlag, 1994, pp 491–536.

Beaver PC, Orihel TC: Human infection with filariae of animals in the United States. Am J Trop Med Hyg 14:1010, 1965.

Beaver PC, Wolfson JS, Waldron MA, et al: *Dirofilaria ursi*–like parasites acquired by humans in the northern United States and Canada: Report of two cases and brief review. Am J Trop Med Hyg 37:357, 1987.

Dayal Y, Neafie RC: Human pulmonary dirofilariasis: A case report and review of the literature. Am Rev Respir Dis 112:437, 1975.

Font RL, Neafie RC, Perry HD: Subcutaneous dirofilariasis of the eyelid and ocular adnexa; report of six cases. Arch Ophthalmol 98:1079, 1980.

MacDougall LT, Magoon CC, Fritsche TR: *Dirofilaria repens* manifesting as a breast nodule. Diagnostic problems and epidemiologic considerations. Am J Clin Pathol 97:625, 1992.

Orihel TC, Isbey EK Jr: *Dirofilaria striata* infection in a North Carolina child. Am J Trop Med Hyg 42:124, 1990.

SECTION C Other Tissue Nematode Infections

110 *Dracunculiasis*

Arif R. Sarwari

DEFINITION. Dracunculiasis (dracontiasis, guinea worm disease) is a painful, incapacitating disease caused by the parasite *Dracunculus medinensis* and transmitted by drinking water containing cyclopoid copepods, freshwater microcrustaceans that harbor infective larvae. This nematode lives in the connective and subcutaneous tissues of humans until the female worm emerges through the skin to discharge its larvae into water. The clinical course is characterized by allergic prodromal symptoms, cutaneous ulceration, and frequently severe disability. Dracunculiasis can be eliminated completely by the provision of safe drinking water, and in 1986 the World Health Organization (WHO) targeted it as the next disease to be eradicated after smallpox.

HISTORY. Guinea worm disease has been recognized since antiquity. Some believe it to be the "fiery serpent" referred to by Moses. Galen coined the term *dracontiasis*, and famous Roman and Greek physicians such as Plutarch and Pliny described the parasite in recognizable terms. Dracunculiasis

was known to Persian and Arabic physicians including Avicenna, who first described its clinical symptoms and called the disease *Medina sickness* because it was common in Medina. The contemporary term *guinea worm disease* derives from a European explorer who named the disease for the geographic region where he found it, along the western African coast. The staff of Aesculapius, Roman god of medicine, may have originated from the ancient, still valid practice of removing the adult guinea worm by slowly winding it around a stick.

The role of the copepod intermediate host was first described by Aleksei Fedchenko in the early 1870s. He was the first to recognize that the life cycle of a human parasite required an arthropod as an intermediate host. Linnaeus gave the parasite its modern scientific name of *Dracunculus medinensis* in his *Systema Naturae*, published in 1758.

ETIOLOGY. The family Dracunculoidea includes parasites of birds and mammals. Dracunceloidea are nematodes characterized by extreme sexual dimorphism. Only one species, *D. medinensis*, is found in humans.

Morphology and Physiology. The adult female worm appears as a creamy white, slender, translucent cord and is one of the longest nematodes known. It measures 60 to 80 cm (2 to 2.5 ft) and is only 1.7 to 2.0 mm wide. Worms 120 cm long have been recorded. A double uterus occupies most of the

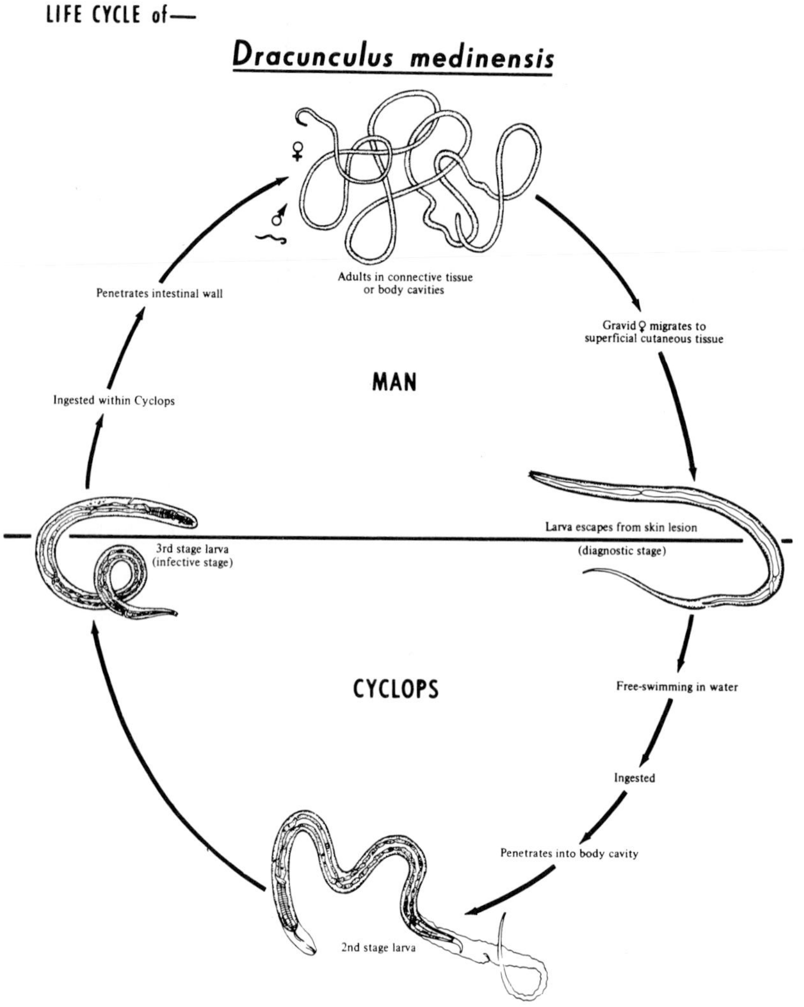

LIFE CYCLE of—

Dracunculus medinensis

Figure 110–1. Life cycle of *Dracunculus medinensis*. (From Melvin DM, Brooke MM, Healy GR, et al.: Common Blood and Tissue Parasites of Man. Life Cycle Charts. Atlanta, Georgia, Centers for Disease Control, 1979.)

body cavity and contains millions of eggs, embryos, and first-stage larvae. Adult males are rarely seen because they do not live long after mating. They are also much smaller, only 12 to 29 mm long and 0.4 mm wide. The rhabditiform larvae are 500 to 700 μm long and are flat. Little is known of how the worms subsist in the body.

Life Cycle (Fig. 110–1). After an incubation period of 10 to 14 months, the female worm migrates to the subcutaneous tissue, usually at the feet or legs, where a painful blister appears. When the affected part is immersed in water, the blister bursts, and the female worm protrudes through the skin and expels thousands of larvae into the water by contracting its uterus. The uterus may contain as many as 3 million larvae. On first immersion, approximately 500,000 to 600,000 larvae are released. The adult female continues to release larvae on subsequent contact with water, but the number decreases substantially.

Intermediate Host. Larvae are actively motile until they are ingested by the copepod intermediate host, a species of *Cyclops* (Fig. 110–2). These carnivorous microcrustaceans, barely visible to the naked eye, are 1 to 3 mm long. On reaching the midintestine of the copepod, the larvae break through the soft wall and enter the hemocoelom, where they remain. Larvae remain active in pond water for 4 to 7 days, but the ability to infect *Cyclops* decreases after 3 days.

The development of *D. medinensis* larvae in the copepod is temperature dependent and species specific but at optimal temperatures (25 to 30°C) is approximately 2 to 3 weeks. The larvae molt twice. Third-stage larvae are 240 to 608 μm long by 12 to 23 μm wide. Naturally infected adult copepods usually harbor only one infective larva; multiple infections are rare and may kill the copepod.

Definitive Host. Humans become infected with guinea worm by drinking water containing cyclops infected with third-stage larvae. The copepods are killed by gastric juices. The liberated larvae penetrate the intestinal tract wall and migrate into the abdominal or thoracic cavity, where they develop into mature adults. Mating occurs at about 3 months. The female worm continues to mature until its body consists almost entirely of a coiled distended uterus containing millions of rhabditoid larvae. Sometime during maturation, the female begins an extensive migration that ends at the site of emergence.

EPIDEMIOLOGY

Distribution. More than 120 million rural people in Africa and 20 million in Asia (Fig. 110–3) are considered at risk of infection with guinea worm. The number of reported cases worldwide fell from 3.5 million in 1986 to just 120,000 in 1995. In Asia, the disease is present in parts of India and Pakistan. Residual disease may also be present in Yemen and Saudi Arabia. Dracunculiasis does not occur south of the equator in Africa. Endemic disease exists in 17 African countries. In western and central Africa, these include Benin, Burkina Faso, Cameroon, Central African Republic, Chad,

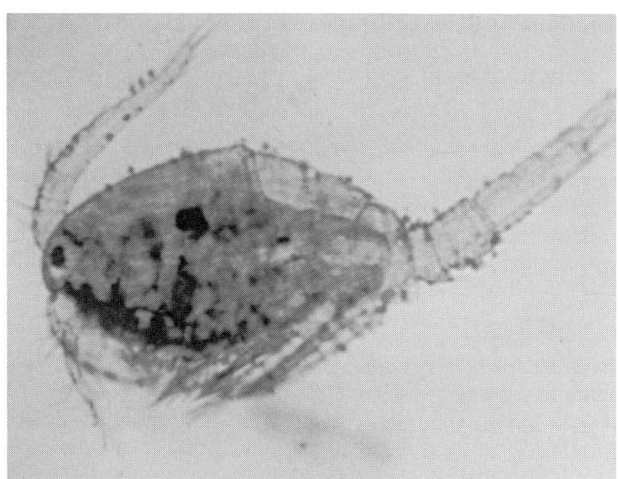

Figure 110–2. Lateral view of a cyclopoid copepod, the microcrustaceans that serve as the intermediate host of the guinea worm.

Ghana, Cote d'lvoire, Mali, Mauritania, Niger, Nigeria, Senegal, and Togo. In eastern Africa, dracunculiasis is endemic in Ethiopia, Sudan, and northern Uganda. There is a small focus of the disease in northwestern Kenya. Two African countries, The Gambia and Guinea, may have eradicated the infection, but documentation is lacking.

Accurate estimates of prevalence and morbidity of guinea worm disease were not readily available until implementation of the Guinea Worm Eradication Programs in the early

1990s. Dracunculiasis is typically a disease of rural communities far from health centers and therefore from normal case-finding mechanisms. Few patients seek medical help, because there is no effective treatment. Furthermore, dracunculiasis is a disabling disease; those infected cannot travel long distances without help. In rural endemic areas, infected persons often remain at home while recuperating.

Transmission. Dracunculiasis is a focal disease that occurs seasonally. It has two general seasonal patterns. In semiarid areas e.g., the Sahel of western Africa and parts of India and Pakistan, contaminated surface sources of drinking water are present only during the brief rainy season, and transmission coincides with the rains. In endemic areas with surface sources of water throughout the year but distinct rainy and dry seasons, transmission occurs usually during the dry season, when surface water sources are scanty and polluted. Severe drought, if sustained in semiarid areas, may interrupt transmission of the parasite because people are forced to use drinking water from sources other than surface sources and because infection does not persist for > 1 to 2 years. These conditions existed in the Sind region of Pakistan in the 1930s and the Nara region of Mali in the 1970s.

A temperature of at least 15°C is required for complete development of the larvae in the copepod, and optimal temperatures are 25 to 30°C. *D. medinensis* larvae cannot penetrate cyclops; therefore, only predatory cyclops species that ingest larvae serve as intermediate hosts (vectors). The copepod intermediate host flourishes only in standing surface water, as is found in ponds and large open wells (Fig. 110–4). Guinea worm disease is uncommon in communities where people obtain their drinking water from flowing rivers or streams.

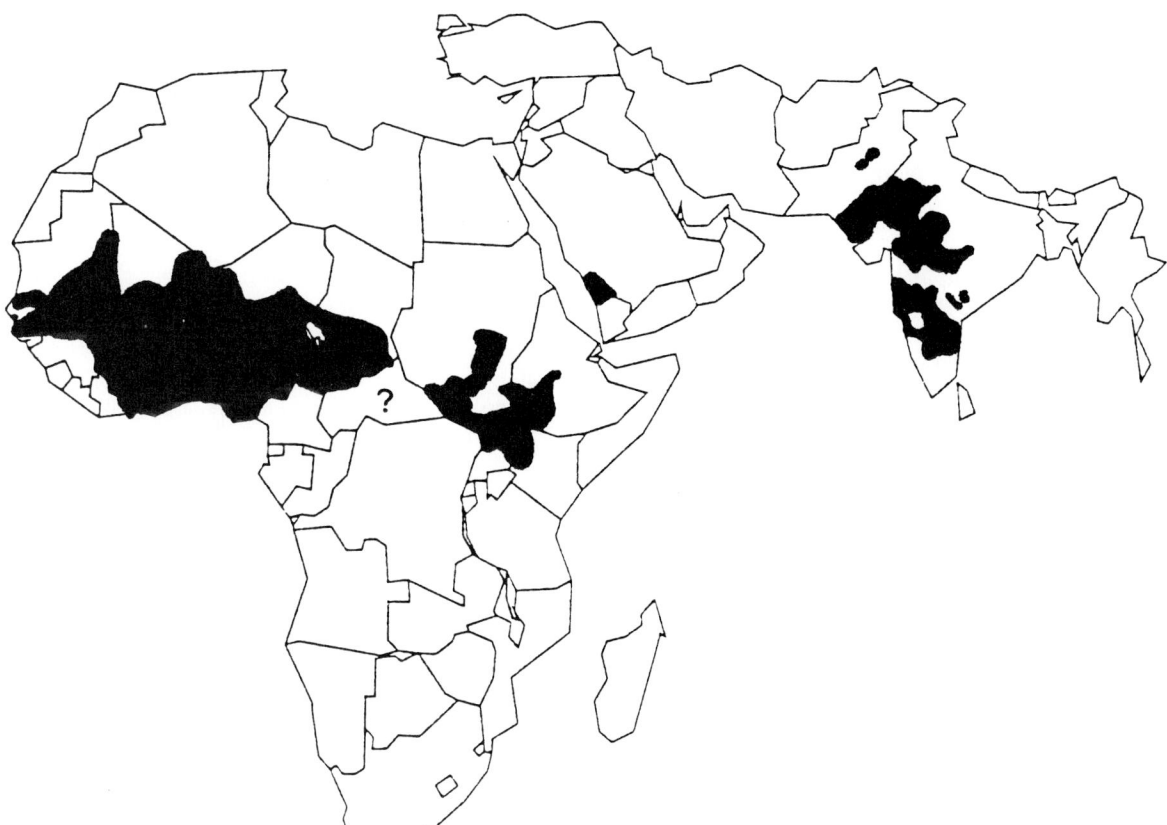

Figure 110–3. Distribution of *Dracunculus medinensis*. Endemic areas are in black. Guinea worm is not present in the New World.

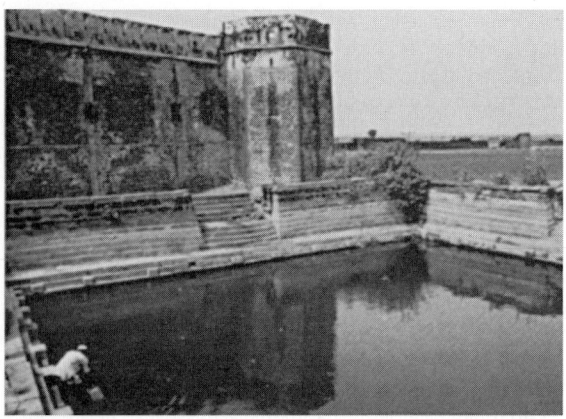

Figure 110–4. A step well in Maharashtra State, India. These large open wells, which also collect rainwater, provide ideal conditions for breeding of *Cyclops* and for contamination of the water by larvae.

Humans are the only known host of *D. medinensis*. A wide range of mammals from many parts of the world have been reported to be infected, but the species of *Dracunculus* has not always been clear. The occasional cases of dracunculiasis reported in animals (usually dogs) are probably isolated accidental infections with *D. medinensis* from humans. The failure of the disease to reappear in areas, e.g., southern Russia, where it has been eradicated from humans, is regarded as evidence for an apparent absence of zoonotic transmission.

Socioeconomic Factors. The epidemiologic pattern of infection in a community is related to exposure, as influenced by occupation and water consumption habits. No evidence shows the development of acquired immune protection or resistance to infection due to gender or age. Many people experience recurrent infections. A proportion of a population at risk never becomes infected; this has been attributed to killing of larvae by high gastric acidity. However, radiographs show calcified worms in some supposedly uninfected people.

Dracunculiasis affects adults more frequently than children (Fig. 110–5). The highest infection rates usually occur in the age group from 15 to 45 years, the most economically productive segment of society. Rural farmers are at particular risk because they may drink comparatively large amounts of water from ponds or other contaminated water sources near their work. Children <5 years and adults >55 years are rarely infected. The male:female infection rates are inconstant and relate to the degree of exposure to *D. medinensis* as determined by occupation and water consumption habits.

Guinea worm is a disabling and economically crippling disease. A large portion of a village labor force may be affected simultaneously. Worms take an average of 3 to 8 weeks to emerge fully; the reported period of incapacitation averages 3 months but may be >9 months. During this time, infected persons may be unable to walk or move about easily. Permanent crippling by dracunculiasis has been very rare. The disease is a major economic burden because of agricultural work loss; peak case rates often coincide with major agricultural activities of clearing land, planting, or harvesting. In one fertile area of 1.6 million inhabitants in Nigeria, estimated losses in rice production alone due to high dracunculiasis infection rates were $20 million per year. Dracunculiasis has an adverse effect on the ability of mothers to care for themselves and their children and to contribute to family income. School absenteeism increases during the guinea worm season. Although some schoolchildren are themselves infected, others must remain at home to carry out critical agricultural activities that infected adults are unable to perform.

CLINICAL MANIFESTATIONS. Infected persons are asymptomatic during most of the 10- to 14-month incubation period. Symptoms begin just before a worm emerges. About one third of patients detect the serpiginous form of the worm or can palpate it just beneath the skin, usually a few days but occasionally as long as a month before the worm emerges.

Allergic Manifestations. A few hours before the development of the local cutaneous lesion, 30 to 80% of patients have pronounced systemic symptoms (e.g., erythema, urticarial rash, intense pruritus, nausea, vomiting, diarrhea, dizziness, syncope, and occasional fever). Suborbital edema may be noted. Urticaria may appear up to 8 days before the worm begins to emerge.

Local Lesion. In most patients, the first physical sign is formation of a large reddish papule 2 to 7 cm in diameter with a vesicular center and an indurated margin. This is where the cephalic end of the worm is approaching the skin. Within 1 to 3 days, the papule changes into a blister due to the production of necrotizing secretions by the adult worm. Formation of the blister is accompanied by local pruritus and an intense burning pain that induces the patient to immerse the affected body part in water for relief. The blister fluid is bacteriologically sterile and at first contains predominantly polymorphonuclear leukocytes, followed by increasing numbers of lymphocytes, eosinophils, and macrophages. Larvae are always present in the fluid, and white blood cells adhere to them. Ninety-five percent of the lesions occur on the lower extremities, particularly on the feet and ankles, but they may be found anywhere on the body, including the hand, arm, trunk, buttocks, scrotum, knee joints, calf, thigh, shoulders, or even the angle of the jaw.

After 3 to 5 days, the blister ruptures and discloses a small superficial ulcer, 1.2 to 1.8 cm in diameter. At the center of the erosion, which sometimes heals quickly and spontaneously, is a minute hole large enough to admit a probe. The head of the worm occasionally protrudes through the hole, but the worm usually is not visible (Fig. 110–6). In response

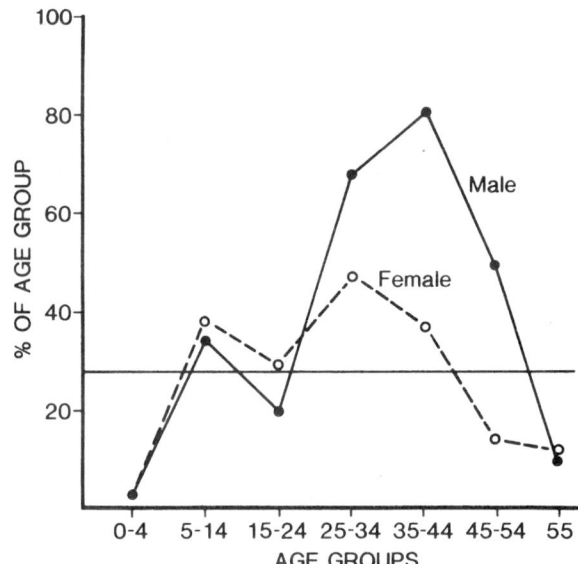

Figure 110–5. Guinea worm attack rate by age and sex in Ghana. (From Belcher DW, Wurapa FK, Ward WB, Lourie IM: Guinea worm in southern Ghana: Its epidemiology and impact on agricultural productivity. Am J Trop Med Hyg 24:246, 1975. Reprinted by permission.)

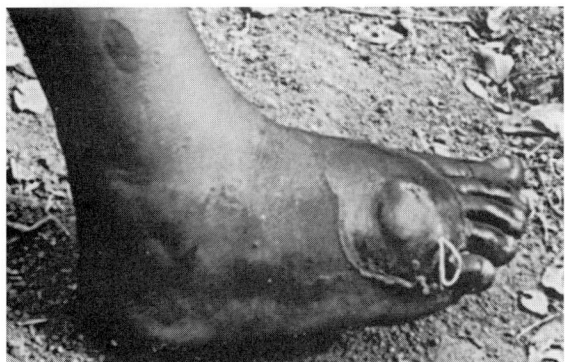

Figure 110–6. Large suppurating blister on the foot of a 6-year-old girl. A portion of a female *Dracunculus* is being extruded.

to contact with fresh water, a loop of uterus prolapsed through a ruptured anterior part of the body or through the mouth of the worm is projected through the hole. When the uterus has projected about 2.5 cm, it suddenly bursts and discharges an opaque whitish material containing motile, first-stage rhabditoid larvae. The process is repeated on subsequent exposure to water until the entire uterus is freed and all the larvae discharged. The act of prolapsing the uterus and releasing the larvae results in death of the worm.

In general, only one to two worms emerge per year; however, massive infections have been reported. In one instance, 56 adult worms emerged from one person in the same year. Severe local reactions may occur if the worm becomes injured or lacerated while lying in the subcutaneous tissues. The extremity may become extremely painful, inflamed, and edematous, and the patient is unable to walk.

Complications. Worms that fail to emerge usually die, become calcified, and cause no symptoms. They may be detected by radiography or felt as hard, convoluted cords under the skin. Nonemergent or aberrant worms may, however, cause abscesses. Worms have been found in an abscess cavity in the pericardium of a 35-year-old man with constrictive pericarditis, in the subconjunctival space, and in extradural abscesses.

The principal complication of guinea worm disease is secondary bacterial infection. Depending on the site of emergence, acute abscesses, cellulitis, arthritis, synovitis, epididymo-orchitis, bubo, chronic ulcerations, or fibrous ankylosis of joints and contractures of tendons may occur. Approximately 40% of patients are totally incapacitated for about 6 weeks. Worms may rupture in the tissues, leading to the formation of large abscesses. Intra-articular infections with acute arthritis, usually of the knee or ankle joints, may occur. Tetanus is a potentially lethal complication.

DIAGNOSIS. Diagnosis of guinea worm disease requires either a demonstration or a documented history of worm emergence. Guinea worm is distinctive (Fig. 110–6). Once the blister has broken, the diagnosis can be confirmed by placing cold water on the ulcer or ethyl chloride near it. This results in release of actively mobile larvae that can be viewed through a microscope under low power.

On occasion, a worm can be palpated in the subcutaneous tissues or its outline seen by reflected light. In doubtful cases, cold water placed over the site may cause the worm to emerge or to move. Worms that fail to emerge may become calcified and produce a characteristic radiologic picture. Cutaneous larvae migrans may be confused with a serpiginous guinea worm beneath the skin (Chapter 115). However, the former is caused by abortive infections with dog or cat hookworms, which are much shorter than guinea worms. Eosino-

philia is often present during worm emergence, with values usually between 13 and 18% although possibly >30%. Although eosinophilia occurs before worm emergence and in cryptic infections, its presence is not useful for diagnosis.

Serologic tests are not useful in routine diagnosis. None has proved sufficiently sensitive and specific. Cross reactivity with other nematode infections such as onchocerciasis poses a problem.

TREATMENT. Winding each emerging worm onto a small stick a few centimeters per day, as has been done for centuries, is useful provided it begins when the worm just emerges (Fig. 110–7). Precautions, such as sterile dressings and antiseptics, are used to prevent secondary infection. The process can be facilitated by plunging the affected body part into cold water. This causes the worm's uterus to contract and expel larvae; then, the anterior portion of the worm becomes flaccid.

Drugs. Four benzimidazole compounds are reported to have an effect on the emerging adult female worms: metronidazole (400 mg for an adult, given daily for 10 to 20 days), niridazole (25 mg/kg of body weight given daily for 10 days), thiabendazole (50 mg/kg of body weight given daily for 3 days), and mebendazole (400 to 800 mg for an adult, given daily for 6 days). All appear to act similarly; they provide symptomatic relief and facilitate removal of worms. These compounds have marked anti-inflammatory properties and thus reduce the intense tissue reaction that develops around the worm once it begins to emerge from the skin. However, they have no effect on pre-emergent worms or on the larvae. In a placebo-controlled clinical trial, ivermectin was also not found to have any effect on pre-emergent worms. The development of a ferret model of dracunculiasis is currently being used to explore further treatment options.

Surgery. Surgical removal of pre-emergent female worms, after administration of a local anesthetic, is sometimes practiced in India. If the outline of the worm can be seen or palpated, the whole parasite can be easily extracted intact after making a small incision. However, complete removal is difficult if the worm is in the deep fascia or wound around tendons or if the surface has been damaged and the worm is adherent to the surrounding tissue.

PREVENTION AND CONTROL. Guinea worm disease is acquired only by drinking water contaminated with infected copepods. Therefore, it is the only communicable disease

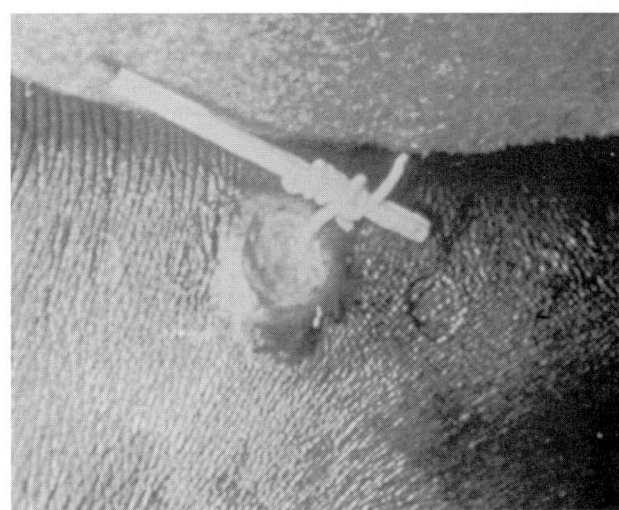

Figure 110–7. Traditional method of winding emerging guinea worm onto a small stick a few centimeters each day.

that could be eradicated completely if populations living in endemic areas were provided with and used safe drinking water. In Kwara State, Nigeria, the provision of protected water supplies in the form of boreholes reduced the prevalence of dracunculiasis in affected communities from 50% or more to near zero within 3 years of intervention. The epidemiology of guinea worm disease suggests that it can be eradicated, and a global effort to eradicate dracunculiasis is currently under way. The disease is focal, and its geographic range is limited. Infection is obvious, and infectivity is low. Humans are the only host for *D. medinensis*. The fragility of the guinea worm transmission cycle is attested to by the eradication of the disease from areas once endemic for dracunculiasis in Asia, the Middle East, parts of Africa, and a small focus in the Americas. Cameroon, Ghana, India, Nigeria, and Pakistan have recently pioneered surveillance methods as part of their Guinea Worm Eradication Programs.

There is no effective vaccine or treatment for dracunculiasis. However, health education alone or with the provision of new or improved sources of drinking water, filtration of drinking water, and/or chemical treatment of drinking water sources can significantly reduce the incidence of the disease.

Improvement of Water Supplies. Introduction and use of safe water supplies virtually eliminates guinea worm disease in a community within 1 to 2 years. Piped water supplies are ideal. When cases continue to occur in urban centers with piped water, it is because patients are infected elsewhere. For example, guinea worm disease persisted in Ibadan, Nigeria, after piped water was installed because many inhabitants had land in the surrounding areas that they farmed about 1 month each year. During that time, they often drank contaminated pond water. When technically and economically feasible, boreholes and tube wells can provide safe water.

Filtering household or individual drinking water is also an effective way to prevent guinea worm infection. A cloth filter is placed over the neck of a vessel from which drinking water is poured. Cheap, durable, efficient nylon filters have been developed. A pore size of 100 μm removes all copepod stages capable of ingesting and nurturing larvae but allows free flow of water. When synthetic filters are too costly, water can be filtered effectively through locally available cotton cloth double or triple folded.

Chemical Treatment of Ponds and Wells. Numerous chemical disinfectants and pesticides have been shown to control cyclops when applied to sources of drinking water. However, temefos (Abate) is considered the compound of choice because of its effectiveness, low toxicity, and safety for the environment. The WHO Expert Committee on Pesticides has declared temefos to be safe for use in drinking water at a target dose of 1 mg/L. That concentration eliminates copepods from a water source for 4 to 7 weeks.

Many factors must be considered when using temefos. Chemical treatment is expensive and less permanent than provision of safe water. Depending on the formulation used, temefos may give an unpleasant odor and taste to water. Repeated applications are necessary. The cost greatly escalates if many large water sources must be treated. Timing of application to coincide with transmission is crucial. Temefos is best applied when water sources are few and well defined and when transmission is highly seasonal.

Health Education. Ignorance of the etiology and mode of transmission of guinea worm is widespread. Health education is vital to acceptance and use of control measures, such as filters. In Burkina Faso, health education to promote filtration of drinking water through a nylon cloth reduced prevalence rates from as high as 54% to zero in only two transmission seasons. Health education may be critical to whether people choose safe drinking water when many sources of water are available. Health education also can change behavior so that persons with emerging worms do not place the affected part in water. This simple change in behavior would result in eradication.

Bibliography

Adamson PB: Dracontiasis in antiquity. Med Hist 32:204, 1988.
Belcher DW, Wurapa FK, Wand WB, et al: Guinea worm in southern Ghana: Its epidemiology and impact on agricultural productivity. Am J Trop Med Hyg 24:243, 1975.
Edungbol LD, Watts SJ: Epidemiological assessment of the distribution and endemicity of guinea worm infection in Asa, Kwara State, Nigeria. Trop Geogr Med 37:22, 1985.
Edungbola LD, Watts SJ, Alabi TO, et al: The impact of a UNICEF assisted rural water project on the prevalence of guinea worm disease in Asa, Kwara State, Nigeria. Am J Trop Med Hyg 39:79, 1988.
Hopkins DR, Ruiz-Tiben E: Surveillance for dracunculiasis, 1981–1991. MMWR CDC Surveill Summ 41:1, 1992.
Muller R: Guinea worm disease: Epidemiology, control and treatment. Bull WHO 57:683, 1979.
Reddy CRRM, Devi CS, Reddy M, et al: Dracontiasis. Review of surgical problems and treatment. Int Surg 52:481, 1969.
Reddy CRRM, Narasaiah IL, Parvath G: Epidemiological studies on guinea worm infection. Bull WHO 40:521, 1969.
Sullivan JJ, Long EG: Synthetic-fibre filters for preventing dracunculiasis, 100 vs 200 micrometers pore size. Trans R Soc Trop Med Hyg 82:465, 1988.
World Health Organization: Dracunculiasis: Global surveillance summary—1986. Wkly Epidemiol Rec 62:337, 1987.

111 *Trichinosis**

K. Darwin Murrell

DEFINITION. Trichinosis (trichinellosis) is a disease caused by parasites of the genus *Trichinella* (Owen, 1835) that humans acquire from eating the muscles of wild or domestic animals. The severity is usually proportional to the number of larvae ingested, and the disease is characterized by fever, gastrointestinal symptoms, myositis, swollen eyelids, and eosinophilia.

HISTORY. Some authorities believe the disease syndrome was recognized in Biblical times and was responsible for the Mosaic proscription of pork. This is questioned by Old Testament scholars, however, who believe the admonition was against beasts of prey and animals with obnoxious habits. The encysted larval stage of *Trichinella spiralis* was first examined microscopically in 1835 by James Paget, a British medical student who was studying muscle tissue from a cadaver. Sir Richard Owen confirmed Paget's findings and published the first description and scientific designation for this parasite. Joseph Leidy of Philadelphia demonstrated the parasite in swine muscle in 1844, and Zenker related human trichinosis to the ingestion of infected pork in 1860. The essentials of the life cycle of *T. spiralis* were clarified during the 1850s by Leuckhart and Virchow. By the early 20th century, trichinosis was recognized as an important public health problem. Despite improvements in many countries, notably in Western Europe, it remains a problem in Eastern Europe, the United States, Mexico, and South American countries and is increasing in significance in certain tropical regions, including Thailand, Kenya, Tanzania, and Senegal. Studies on isolates of *Trichinella* indicate major differences in the genetic and biologic properties of parasites of arctic, temperate, and tropical regions. As discussed later, it is now widely accepted that the genus is polytypic.

---

*All the material in this chapter is in the public domain, with the exception of any borrowed figures or tables.

ETIOLOGY. Infection occurs by ingestion of meat containing infective, encysted larvae. The most severe manifestations of the disease or infection are usually due to the larval offspring of the viviparous female worms rather than to the adult worms. Extensive invasion of the striated muscles and the epithelial lining of the small intestine stimulates a pronounced inflammatory response to the worm and its released antigens; it is this defensive response of the host that produces illness and sometimes death.

Biology. *Trichinella* is nearly unique among helminthic parasites in that all stages of development occur within a single host; >100 species of mammals have been reported to be susceptible to infection. The infective encysted larvae may remain viable in the host's musculature for many years; they may also survive long periods in decaying and putrefying muscle. These attributes confer a high probability of successful transmission.

Morphology. The adult worms are small and slender, with slightly tapered anterior ends, a common feature of the superfamily Trichuroidea (Fig. 111–1*A*). The males measure 1.4

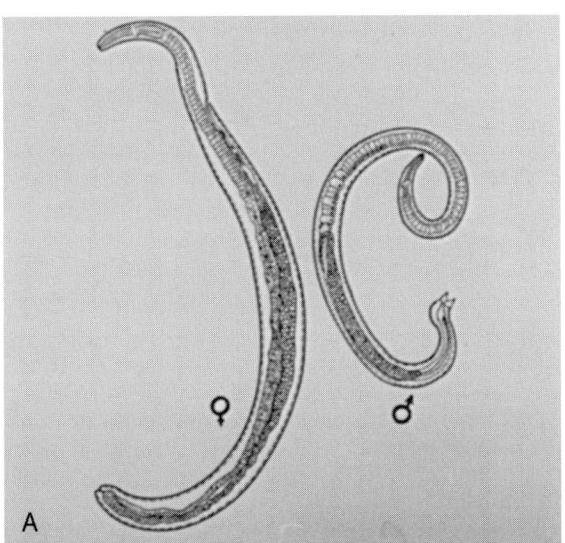

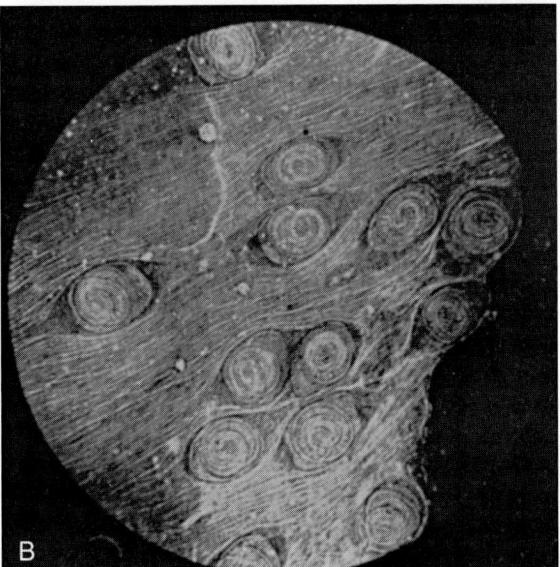

Figure 111–1. *A,* Morphology of adult male and female *Trichinella spiralis. B,* Compression of hog diaphragm muscle showing encysted trichinae.

to 1.6 mm in length by 40 to 60 μm in transverse diameter. The male has two pseudobursal flaps at the posterior end, with two pairs of papillae between the flaps; the pseudobursae aid in embracing the female during coitus. The female is a little more than twice as long as the male, 2.2 to 3.6 mm, and about one and a half times as broad. The vulva is situated near the middle of the esophageal region. A column of cells called *stichocytes* is associated with the capillary-like esophagus; the secretions of these cells contain potent antigens that are important in the host's response to the parasite.

LIFE CYCLE. When humans consume raw or rare flesh infected with cysts of *Trichinella* (Fig. 111–2), the cysts are digested out of the muscle in the stomach; the larvae (L₁, or first stage) are resistant to gastric juice. After passage to the small intestine, the larvae burrow beneath the columnar epithelium and lie just above the lamina propria, completely enveloped by tissue. There they undergo four molts within about 36 hours and develop into adult worms. Still within the tissue, the male and female worms mate. After fertilization, the females begin to discharge live larvae (as early as 4 to 7 days after infection). Production of larvae may continue for 4 to 16 weeks or more, depending on host species, until the worms are finally expelled from the intestine; the longevity of adult worms in the human intestine is not known with certainty.

Each newborn larva (about 100 μm long by 6 μm in diameter) makes its way into the lamina propria, where it enters a draining lymph node or blood vessel and is carried to the arterial circulation via the thoracic duct. Newborn larvae are capable of invading nearly any tissue but can survive only in a striated skeletal muscle cell. Invasion of the muscle cell induces changes that culminate in a new host unit termed the *nurse cell* except for *T. pseudospiralis.* The larvae begin to coil, and the nurse cell completes the formation of the cyst around the larvae by 17 to 21 days after infection (Fig. 111–1*B*). The cyst size in humans averages 400 by 260 μm; the encysted larvae have grown to 800 to 1000 μm in length and are now fully infective. Unusual for nematodes of this group, these larvae can be typed as to sex after artificial excystation. In humans, calcification of the cyst may begin within 6 months to a year, a process that eventually leads to death of the encysted larvae.

EPIDEMIOLOGY AND DISTRIBUTION. *Trichinella* is widespread among wild mammals, especially carnivores, wild pigs, and other species that are cannibalistic or eat carrion. Formerly, infected pork was considered the only important source of infection for humans, who infected their domestic pigs through the practice of feeding them garbage containing meat scraps. Horse meat is increasingly a source of infection, especially in France and Italy, where >2000 cases have been reported since the early 1980s. Instances of infected cattle and sheep have been reported from China, but the importance of these hosts in human transmission is unknown. On a worldwide basis, pork is decreasing in importance as a source of trichinosis, whereas wild animal meat is increasing in importance (Table 111–1). For instance, in 1986, infected bear meat accounted for 38% of traceable human cases in the United States. In the former Soviet Union, >90% of trichinosis cases are attributed to eating bear and wild boar meat. In tropical Africa, trichinosis is primarily sylvatic, and humans are infected by ingesting improperly cooked bush pigs and wart hogs. Trichinosis also occurs in Egypt and Lebanon, where pork appears to be the main source of infection. Sylvatic infections in wild animals are also reported from Asia, although direct transmission to humans rarely occurs except in Thailand and China. Most human infections in Central and South America have been traced to domesticated pigs, but too few wild animals have been examined to be certain

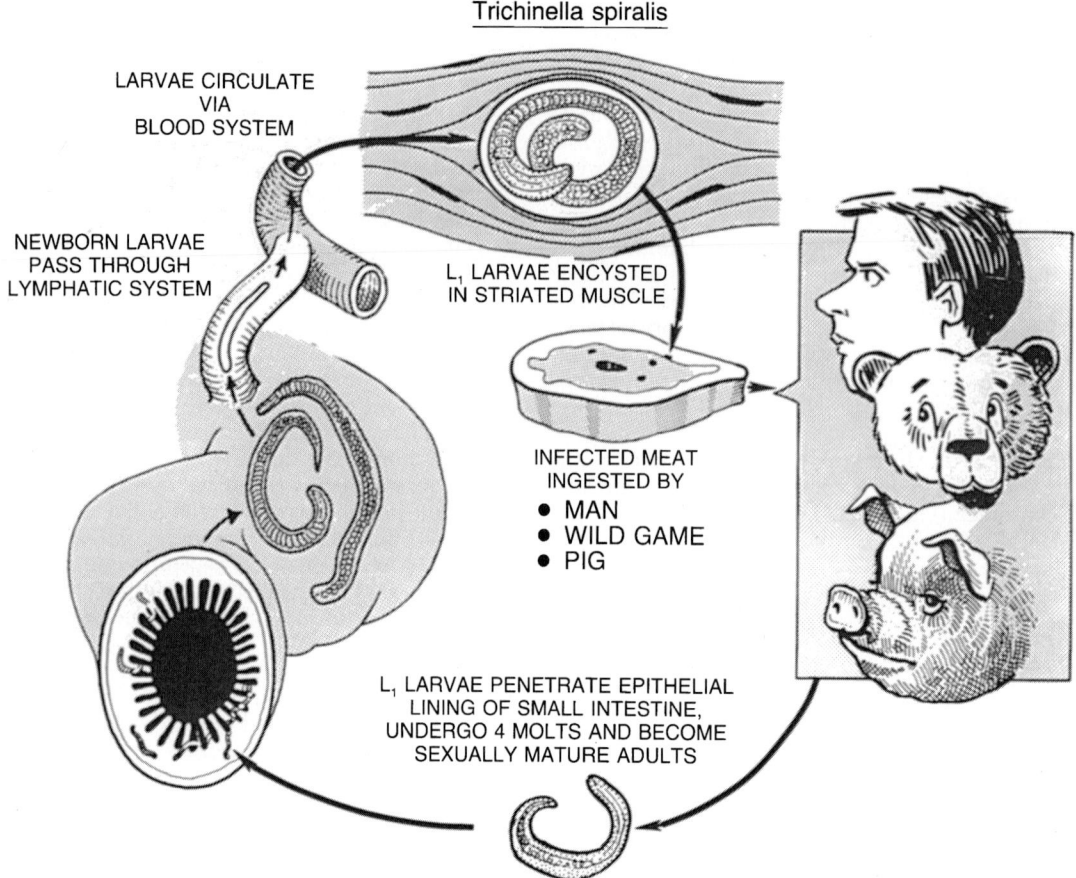

Figure 111-2. Life cycle of *Trichinella spiralis* showing stages and locations of development.

that there is no indigenous cycle in wild animals in this region. The number of human trichinosis cases from all sources in the United States declined from 129 in 1990 to 16 in 1993 and 35 in 1994.

Species and Strains of *Trichinella*. The natural maintenance cycle of *Trichinella* is among carrion-feeding or cannibalistic carnivores. Domestic pigs and rats are secondary hosts, although domestic pigs have been the main source of human infections in most developed and agricultural societies (Fig. 111-3). The relative importance of both domestic pigs (synanthropic) and wild animals (sylvatic) as potential sources of human infection must be considered carefully in designing control programs. Not all wild animal infections are directly transmissible to swine; pigs are more resistant to sylvatic *Trichinella* than humans are.

Isolates from different hosts of geographic localities should not be considered identical; *Trichinella* is a complex of at least five species, all of which are nearly distinguishable morphologically. Alloenzyme and DNA analytic techniques have provided molecular support for the biologic differences among the distinct types. These data, coupled with other comparative biological factors (e.g., host range, parasite fecundity, resistance to temperature extremes, nurse cell development dynamics), have yielded a new taxonomy for the genus (Table 111-2). This taxonomy includes five species and is an extension of the earlier taxonomy proposed by Britov and Boev (see Murrell and Bruschi, 1994); the additional species, *T. britovi*, was named in honor of that distinguished Soviet scientist. The establishment of *T. britovi* resolves much of the confusion about the identity of the type reported from the temperate zone of the Palearctic region (i.e., Europe and the former eastern Soviet Union). It has been isolated from various carnivores and pigs in that region.

It is now clear that *Trichinella* species can no longer be identified on the basis of host species or geographic locale. This taxonomy also recognizes that differences often reported in clinical syndromes from infections with different species are possible (Table 111-2).

Studies have demonstrated that the domestic pig species, *T. spiralis*, has been introduced into wild animal populations,

TABLE 111-1. Examples of Recent Outbreaks of Human Trichinosis

Country	Date	No. of Cases	Source
United States	1990	105	Pork
Argentina	1992	151	Pork
Lebanon	1982	1000	Pork
Egypt	1975	51	Pork
Ethiopia	1990	20	Wild boar
China			
Yunnan province	1983	5558	Pork, bear, other?
Henan province	1992	167	Pork
Heilongjiang	1981	147	Mutton?
	1985	1073	Horse meat
Italy	1985	100	Wild boar
Lithuania	1992	819	Pork, wild boar
Slovakia	1980	77	Wild boar

From Murrell KD: Foodborne parasites. Int J Environ Health Res 5:63, 1995.

increasing the importance of a sylvatic reservoir of *Trichinella* to the domestic cycle. An important difference between *T. nativa* parasites and the *T. spiralis* of domestic pigs is the remarkable resistance to freezing shown by the former.

Swine. The high incidence of human trichinosis previously reported in the United States and Europe was caused primarily by failure to control the disease in swine. A strong association between garbage feeding and swine trichinosis was apparent from prevalence data obtained on market hogs. In the United States in the 1950s, the prevalence rate of trichinosis in garbage-fed hogs was about 11%, whereas only 1% of grain-fed hogs were found to be infected. With the introduction of garbage-cooking laws to prevent the transmission of vesicular exanthema and hog cholera in swine, the rates for garbage-fed hogs fell to about 0.05 to 0.1% by the 1990s. The use of frozen foods undoubtedly also had an important role in this decrease. In Europe, a major factor in reducing the incidence of swine trichinosis has been the adaptation of routine inspection procedures at the slaughter plants. In Germany, for example, the reported prevalence of swine trichinosis is <0.00003%. It is 0.0008% in the former Soviet Union and 0.0% in Denmark.

Rats have traditionally been assigned an important role in the transmission of *T. spiralis* to hogs. Rats obtain their infections from the same sources as hogs and represent only one of several important sources of infection. The fact remains, though, that hogs will eat rats when they are available; thus, the opportunity for direct transmission of *T. spiralis* to hogs by infected rats must be considered significant in any epidemiologic investigation.

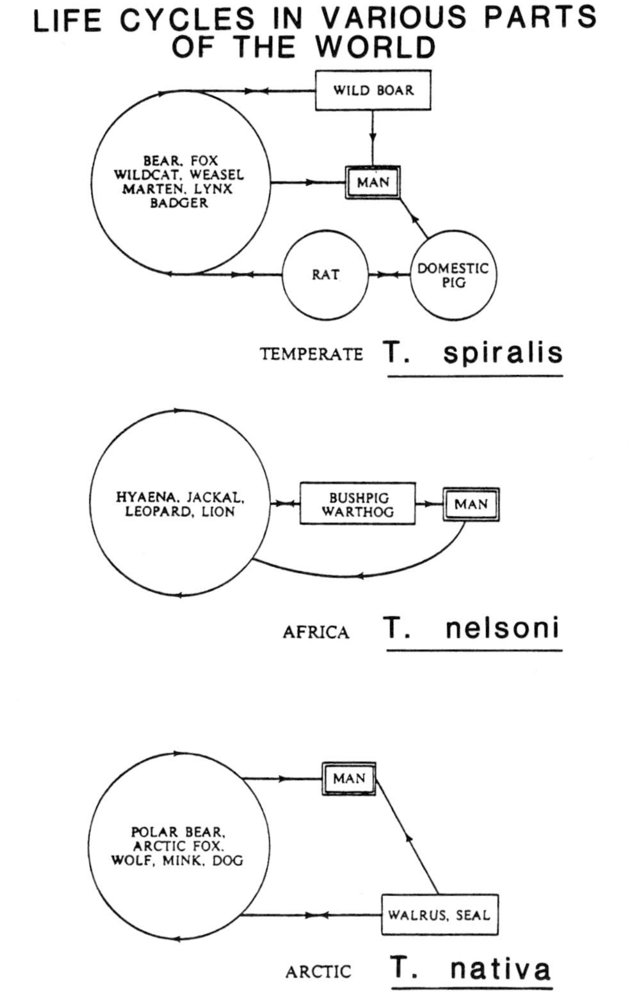

Ethnic Eating Habits. Certain eating customs have an important role in perpetuating human trichinosis. For example, ethnic groups of central European and Southeast Asian origin prefer the taste of raw pork; others may be infected by tasting raw sausages to check the flavor of seasonings. In the past, in the United States, persons of German and Italian extraction had an infection rate at autopsy of nearly 2½ times the national average because of their affinity for cured but uncooked sausage products. Large outbreaks of trichinosis among Indochinese immigrants have occurred. Investigation revealed that they had cooked locally purchased pigs for community celebrations according to their practice in their homeland, an area with apparently low or nonexistent incidence of swine infections. The widespread adoption of fast cooking methods using microwave ovens may become an increasing problem owing to uneven heat distribution.

PATHOGENESIS AND CLINICAL MANIFESTATIONS. The level of infection generally determines the symptoms of trichinosis, although a patient's resistance, size, age, and general health are important variables. The degree of illness is usually related to the number of larvae per gram of muscle: light infection, probably subclinical, up to 10 larvae; moderate infection, 50 to 500 larvae; and severe, life-threatening infection, 1000 or more larvae. Species of *Trichinella* may also be an important variable because infections with the Kenyan and the southern European types appear to be less clinically severe.

Most human infections with *Trichinella* have been attributed to *T. spiralis*. Now that it is possible to type the parasite genetically, a more precise characterization of the pathogenicity of the various species is possible, and some of the confusion and inconsistencies reported for the clinical course of trichinosis will eventually be clarified. Table 111–3 presents the incidence rate for the various symptoms observed during the horse meat–derived trichinosis outbreaks caused by different *Trichinella* species and demonstrates that differences in clinical manifestations can be related to parasite species.

The symptoms of trichinosis can be separated into two primary components, an *early phase* related to the presence of the parasite and a *later phase* associated with the inflammatory and allergic responses caused by muscle invasion. It is possible to distinguish an incubation period, ranging from 5 to 51 days, with a mean of 7, 16, 21, and 30 days in severe, moderate, mild, and abortive trichinosis, respectively. When the incubation period is brief, the course of infection is more severe, although mortality is sometimes associated with a longer incubation period. During this period, gastrointestinal symptoms occur.

The incubation period ends when the acute infection phase begins and is characterized by the presence of fever, myalgia, periorbital edema, and eosinophilia (i.e., the so-called trichinotic syndrome or general trichinosis syndrome). Acute infection lasts 1 to 8 weeks, and it may have a mild, moderate, or severe course, depending on the fever severity and length, the intensity of symptoms, the time taken to recover from disease, and the presence of complications.

Intestinal Phase. The initial consequences of infection occur within the first week after ingestion of infected meat, during the intestinal phase (Table 111–4); this period is associated with the development of worms to the adult stage within the small intestine. The symptoms reflect mucosal irritation and include nausea, abdominal aches or cramps, loss of appetite, vomiting, mild fever, and either mild diarrhea or constipation. Patients may complain of frontal headaches, dizziness, and weakness. These symptoms are easily confused with flu, especially in light to moderate infections.

LIFE CYCLES IN VARIOUS PARTS OF THE WORLD

TEMPERATE **T. spiralis**

AFRICA **T. nelsoni**

ARCTIC **T. nativa**

Figure 111–3. Major transmission pattern of *T. spiralis*, *T. nelsoni*, and *T. nativa* in endemic regions.

TABLE 111–2. Biologic and Zoogeographic Characteristics of the Species of *Trichinella*

	T. spiralis	*T. nativa*	*T. nelsoni*	*T. britovi*	*T. pseudospiralis*
Infectivity for:					
Humans	High	High	High	Moderate	Moderate
Swine	High	Low	Low	Low	Low
Rats	High	Low	Low	Low	Moderate
Mice (Mus)	High	Low	Low	Low	Moderate
Chickens	No	No	No	No	Yes
Pathogenicity for humans	High	High	Low	Moderate	Low–moderate
Resistance to freezing	Low	High	Low	Low	Low
Nurse cell development (in days)	16–37	20–30	34–60	24–42	Absent (no capsule forms around L_1)
Distribution	Cosmopolitan	Arctic	Equatorial Africa	Temperate	Cosmopolitan
Major host reservoirs	Suidae	Ursidae	Hyaenidae		Mammals
	Rattus	Canidae	Felidae	Canidae	Birds
Availability of diagnostic DNA probes	Yes	Yes	Yes	Yes	Yes
Unique alloenzyme markers	6	2	4	1	12

From Murrell KD, Bruschi F: Trichinellosis. *In* Sun T (ed): Progress in Clinical Parasitology, Vol 4. Boca Raton, FL, CRC Press, 1994, pp 116–150.

Severe diarrhea, persisting for weeks, sometimes occurs in patients with heavy infections. Infected Innuit Indians in North America experience an unusually high frequency of diarrhea and a low frequency of myalgia. This may reflect chronic exposure and the development of intestinal immunity.

Muscle Invasion Phase. This stage, beginning as early as 9 to 10 days after exposure, is associated with penetration of the newborn larvae into muscle cells, initiating a strong inflammatory response, especially in the extraocular muscles; masseters; muscles of the larynx, tongue, diaphragm, and neck; intercostals; and muscular attachments to tendons and joints. The fibers become edematous and enlarged. Inflammation is attended by an infiltration of neutrophils, eosinophils, lymphocytes, and tissue histiocytes; this process reaches its peak at about 5 to 6 weeks of infection and diminishes when the encapsulation process ends. Early symptoms of this stage are swelling of the eyelids and facial edema. After this, muscle swelling, tenderness, pain on movement, and fever usually develop. Headache, fainting, urticaria, splinter hemorrhages beneath the fingernails and toenails, conjunctivitis, loss of appetite, hoarseness, dysphagia, dyspnea, and edema of the legs may also occur. Fever can be delayed until several weeks after infection, but temperature may eventually reach 104°F for a week or more in heavy infections. Pain is noticed at about the time facial edema appears. It is most severe between the second and fourth weeks of infection but may persist for a longer period and can be intense enough to make chewing, talking, and swallowing difficult. Respiratory symptoms, including dyspnea, result from involvement of respiratory muscles, and myocarditis may also result from unsuccessful attempts by the larvae to invade the heart.

Neurologic Complications. Neurologic symptoms may accompany migration of the larvae through central nervous system tissue; the resulting intracerebral hemorrhage and marked meningeal irritation may stimulate meningitis. Patients may exhibit dizziness, ataxia, hysteria, and psychotic disturbances. Seizures, monoparesis, and eventually coma can accompany severe infections. Larvae cannot successfully encyst in the nervous system.

Myocardial Complications. Myocarditis is a frequent serious complication of trichinosis and may lead to acute congestive heart failure, usually 4 to 8 weeks after infection. Larvae migrate through the myocardium between the second and fifth weeks, producing at least two clinical patterns: (1) sudden death, presumably from dysrhythmia, or (2) in the majority of patients, a prolonged illness associated with tachycardia, hypotension, elevated venous pressure, and peripheral edema. Pericardial effusion is common in the absence of echocardiographic evidence of ventricular dilation or impaired systolic function. Although most patients who survive trichinosis recover completely, a few continue to have chronic cardiac manifestations. Focal granulomas are eventually replaced by interstitial fibrosis. Larvae cannot successfully encyst in heart muscle.

TABLE 111–3. Incidence of Symptoms and Physical Signs Reported in Horse Meat Trichinosis Outbreaks

Outbreak	Italy, 1975 *T. britovi*	France, 1976 *T. spiralis* (?)	France, 1985 *T. nativa*	France, 1985 *T. spiralis*	Italy, 1986 *T. britovi*
No. of cases studied	89	125	343	396	161
Fever	+	65%	90%	85%	70%
Myalgia	+	59%	93%	88%	67%
Asthenia		NE	87%	77%	NE
Facial edema	+	57%	58%	84%	62%
Diarrhea	+	16%	50%	41%	21%
Vomiting		8%	NE	NE	9%
Headache		60%	58%	51%	66%
Rash		5%	44%	11%	4%
Ocular involvement		31%	28%	34%	26%
Mortality rate	0%	0%	0%	0.4%	0%

NE, not evaluated.
From Murrell KD, Bruschi F: Trichinellosis. *In* Sun T (ed): Progress in Clinical Parasitology, Vol 4. Boca Raton, FL, CRC Press, 1994, pp 116–150.

TABLE 111–4. Pathogenesis of Trichinosis

Days After Infection	Developmental Phase	Symptoms and Signs (Heavy Infections)
2 to 7	Intestinal	Gastrointestinal signs, i.e., nausea, abdominal pain; headache
9 to 28	Muscle	Muscular pain, facial edema, fever, chills, eosinophilia, tachycardia, coma, respiratory difficulties
14+	Encystment or chronic	Mental apathy, neurotoxic symptoms, possible myocarditis, anemia, muscular swelling

Convalescent Phase. The third, or chronic, period, the convalescent phase, is associated with a decrease in muscular symptoms beginning in the second month after infection. Fever and itching subside also. At this time, evidence of congestive heart failure may appear, especially if the patient becomes active too soon. Larvae remain alive in the cysts for many years, even after the cyst wall becomes calcified. These larvae release antigens that cause a continuing low to moderate eosinophilia, circulating antibody, and immediate and delayed hypersensitivity responses to skin test antigens.

Fatal outcome is infrequent in trichinosis, normally occurring only in massive infections, and is most frequently associated with myocarditis, encephalitis, and pneumonitis. About 2% of cases in the United States have ended in death.

DIAGNOSIS. Guidelines for the diagnosis of infection have been recommended by the International Commission on Trichinellosis (www.krenet.it/ICT). Diagnosis may be made by either a direct or an indirect demonstration of infection. Eosinophilia, leukocytosis, elevated levels of muscle enzymes, and increased immunoglobulin levels, especially total IgE, are the most characteristic laboratory findings of this disease. Very specific immunodiagnostic tests are now available.

Direct Demonstration

Enteral Phase. Adult *Trichinella* can sometimes be recovered from the intestinal mucosa at post-mortem examination and could theoretically, but not practicably, be recovered from a living patient by duodenal aspiration or biopsy.

Parenteral Phase. (1) Dissemination stage: Newborn larvae are transported via the blood stream and are disseminated to various parts of the body. Experimentally, they can be filtered from the blood by means of a 3-μm-pore filter, but this method is unlikely to be useful in routine diagnosis because of the relatively small number of newborn larvae in the blood.

(2) Muscle stage: This stage offers the best chance for direct demonstration of the organism. The larvae may be found by examination of a biopsy specimen taken from a superficial skeletal muscle. A specimen measuring approximately 1 cm^3 should be taken, preferably from either the deltoid or gastrocnemius muscles. A portion of the specimen is fixed and examined histologically. The remainder is handled in either one or both of the following ways: (1) compression between glass slides, followed by microscopic examination (Fig. 111–1B), and/or (2) digestion in 1% pepsin and 1% hydrochloric acid, with agitation, followed by microscopic examination of a filtrate or washed sediment of the digested specimen. The digestion time required for liberation of any larvae depends on the size of the muscle fragments and the volume of digestive fluid, but under most circumstances, digestion for a few hours is sufficient for the detection of any larvae that may be present. Larvae that have reached the musculature within the first 3 weeks of infection are more readily detected

by the compression and histologic techniques; otherwise, digestion of muscle tissue is the preferred method.

Indirect Demonstration. A nondiagnostic biopsy does not exclude the possibility of infection, however. Circulating antibody can be detected even in lightly infected patients 3 to 4 weeks after infection and as early as 2 weeks in heavily infected individuals. Various serologic tests can be used, but the bentonite flocculation test (BFT), fluorescent antibody test, and enzyme-linked immunosorbent assay (ELISA) have proved most useful. With the BFT, titers of 1:5 are considered positive; titers generally fall markedly after 1 or 2 years, so that a rise and fall in titer generally indicates recent infection. ELISA is more sensitive and can also detect a rise and fall in titer (Table 111–5). However, some problems in specificity have been observed when these tests are used with crude antigen extracts. Considerable effort has been made to produce more refined antigens. Stichosome antigens derived either from the larva's excretions and secretions during in vitro culture or by somatic extraction have proved superior to crude extracts. Skin tests lack specificity and are further handicapped by the persistence of reactivity in patients as long as 10 years after initial infection.

Differential Diagnosis. Trichinosis can mimic a wide variety of diseases. Most mild cases are misdiagnosed as influenza or other viral fevers unless the clinician recognizes a history of recent ingestion of pork or game, febrile myalgia, periorbital edema, and rising eosinophilia (to 50% or higher) and takes steps to confirm the diagnosis by either serologic tests or muscle biopsy. Similar symptoms among others who dined on the same occasion reflect a common source of infection and further substantiate the diagnosis.

TREATMENT. The treatment regimens for trichinosis are presented in Table 111–6 according to the method of Pawlowski (1991). Factors such as *Trichinella* species involved, intensity and length of infection, and host response characteristics, especially immunocompetence and/or premunition, should help dictate the treatment.

Campbell distinguishes between a symptomatic treatment in which the drugs of choice are corticosteroids, especially in severe infections, and a specific therapy for intestinal stages (prepatent and patent infections) and the muscle stage. In the very early infection phase, the objective is to reduce the number of larvae that invade the muscles; when the larvae are already in the muscle tissue, the anthelmintic must reduce muscle damage, the major determinant of clinical manifestations. Particular attention should be paid to maintaining therapeutic plasma levels of the drug for an appropriate period; this is preferable to obtaining high levels for short periods.

PREVENTION AND CONTROL. Because infection in humans is by consumption of meat containing encysted larvae, direct prevention should be directed at preparing pork or game so that any larvae present are uninfective. In contrast to some countries in Europe, government inspection of pork is not practiced in the United States or in most of Asia, Africa, and South and Central America. Consumers should cook all pork to at least 60°C for about 4 minutes. Pork less than 6 inches thick can also be rendered safe if frozen to 5°F (−15°C) for 20 days, −10°F (−23°C) for 10 days, or −20°F (−29°C) for 6 days. However, *T. nativa* larvae in bear meat are reported to survive freezing for a year or longer.

In those areas where pork is the primary source of infection, it is important to prevent infection of pigs. Control of trichinosis in swine herds depends on appropriate management. The practices most effective in preventing transmission include (1) strict adherence to garbage-feeding regulations, particularly cooking requirements (212°F for 30 minutes); (2) stringent rodent control; (3) avoidance of exposure of pigs to dead animal carcasses, including other pigs; (4) proper dis-

TABLE 111–5. Detection of Specific Antibodies by Different Immunologic Techniques in Trichinosis Outbreaks

	Germany 1977	Hong Kong 1981	Germany 1982	France 1985	Yugoslavia 1985	Italy 1986
No. of cases studied	58	18	51–107*	40	48	110
Approximate period of infection	1 month	2 weeks	2 months	2 months	2 months	2 months
Test:						
IIF-IgG	95% tt†	ND	ND	85% tt	98% tt	82% tt
ELISA-IgG	100% ce‡	94% ce	99% ce	84% ce	100% es§	78% ce
ELISA-IgM	86% ce	100% ce	100% ce	82% ce	95% es	78% ce
ELISA-IgE	7% ce	100% ce	19% ce	13% ce	46% es	80% ce‖
ELISA-IgA	62% ce	ND	ND	13% ce	69% es	ND

*Depending on test used.
†Test tube whole fixed L_1 larvae.
‡Crude extract *T. spiralis* L_1 larvae antigen.
§Excretory/secretory *T. spiralis* L_1 larvae antigen.
‖Obtained with an amplified ELISA.
ND, not done.
From Murrell KD, Bruschi F: Trichinellosis. *In* Sun T (ed): Progress in Clinical Parasitology, Vol 4. Boca Raton, FL, CRC Press, 1994, pp 116–150.

posal of pig and other animal carcasses (e.g., burial, incineration, or rendering), which would minimize infection risk for commensal wild animals; and (5) construction of effective barriers between pigs and wild animals and domestic pets. Furthermore, the education of farmers, meat processors, hunters, and trappers about the potential dangers of feeding wild game to swine should be promoted. Identification and elimination of infected hogs would have the effect of reducing transmission of *T. spiralis* to other swine and would eventually lower the transmission level below the threshold required to maintain the domestic pig–human cycle.

In many countries, a major control strategy is inspection of pork for human consumption. The European Union members, Eastern European countries, and the former members of the Soviet Union require direct inspection of pork at slaughter, either by microscopic examination (trichinoscope) or by a pooled sample digestion method; both techniques use pig diaphragm muscle samples. The U.S. Department of Agriculture (USDA) requires commercial establishments to meet stringent standards for freezing, cooking, or curing pork.

An important technologic advancement is the development of an immunodiagnostic test for use in slaughterhouse inspection of pork. A large field trial of this test has been carried out by the USDA. The results were excellent, and a ruling permitting its use for pork inspection has been issued.

This test has also proved highly effective for the diagnosis of human infections.

It is clear from the experience of European countries that mandatory inspection of pork is highly effective for the control of trichinosis, particularly when coupled with trace-back procedures to identify farms with problems. Subsequent institution of careful management practices and long-term monitoring is highly important for permanent control. Those countries relying on postslaughter control strategies (advice to consumers, regulation of commercial processes) can also achieve effective control, but such measures may have less effect on reducing the risk of transmission to pigs at the farm. This, then, makes it important that veterinary services institute a program of surveillance of pig farms (by serologic or tissue inspection means) to identify those farms needing remediation. Trichinosis is a food-borne disease of low prevalence and, because of its focal nature, is a candidate for eradication from domestic pigs. The effectiveness and practicality of whole hog carcass gamma irradiation to kill larvae have been demonstrated; 30 kilorads has been shown to be completely effective in sterilizing the encysted larvae.

Transmission to humans from wild game may remain a problem; however it is subject to control by the institution of game meat inspection, as is carried out in many European countries.

TABLE 111–6. Treatment of Trichinosis

	Drugs of Choice	Length of Treatment	Precautions
Gastrointestinal phase	Pyrantel 10 mg/kg/day or mebendazole 200 mg/day or albendazole 400 mg/day	5 days 5 days 3 days	
Acute severe infection	Prednisolone 40–60 mg/day and mebendazole 5 mg/kg/day or albendazole 400–800 mg/day	Until fever and allergic signs recede	Bed rest; specific treatment of complications when present
Moderate or mild infection	Prednisolone 20–40 mg/day		Treatment of eventual hypoalbuminemia and hypokalemia
Late phase	No treatment except in rare cases with active infection at biopsy, when mebendazole or albendazole and corticosteroids are the choice		Symptomatic treatment; mental and physical rehabilitation

From Murrell KD, Bruschi F: Trichinellosis. *In* Sun T (ed): Progress in Clinical Parasitology, Vol 4. Boca Raton, FL, CRC Press, 1994, pp 116–150.

Bibliography

Campbell WC: History of trichinosis: Paget, Owen and the discovery of *Trichinella spiralis*. Bull Hist Med 53:520, 1979.

Gould SE: Anatomic pathology. *In* Gould SE (ed): Trichinosis in Man and Animals. Springfield, IL, Charles C Thomas, 1970, pp 147–189.

Murrell KD: Strategies for the control of human trichinosis transmitted by pork. Food Technol 39:65, 1985.

Murrell KD: Foodborne parasites. Int J Environ Health Res 5:63, 1995.

Murrell KD, Bruschi F: Trichinellosis. *In* Sun T (ed): Progress in Clinical Parasitology, Vol 4. Boca Raton, FL, CRC Press, 1994, pp 116–150.

Pawlowski Z: Trichinellosis. *In* Rakel RE (ed): Conn's Current Therapy 1991. Philadelphia, WB Saunders, 1991, pp 118–119.

Pozio E, La Rosa G, Murrell KD, Lichtenfels R: Taxonomic revision of the genus *Trichinella*. J Parasitol 78:654, 1992.

112 *Toxocariasis**

Peter M. Schantz

DEFINITION. Toxocariasis in humans is caused by infection with embryonated eggs of the dog ascarid, *Toxocara canis*, and less commonly those of the cat, *T. cati*. These roundworms are not able to complete their life cycles in humans, and they cause a spectrum of disease ranging from no symptoms to eosinophilia, visceral larva migrans (VLM), or ocular larva migrans (OLM).

ETIOLOGY AND EPIDEMIOLOGY

Life Cycle. Adult *T. canis* and *T. cati* live in the intestines of dogs and cats, respectively (Fig. 112–1). Puppies are commonly infected by vertical transfer of larvae from their dams prenatally or early postnatally (transplacental or lactogenic transmission, respectively); egg shedding in puppies' feces may begin as early as 2 weeks of age. In cats, lactogenic but not transplacental transmission from dams to kittens occurs. Young pups and kittens lose these infections spontaneously between 3 and 6 months of age; new infections in older animals are acquired from ingestion of eggs in the soil environment or by ingestion of larvae in infected rodents, birds, or other paratenic hosts. Eggs are shed in the feces and require 2 to 3 weeks in moist soil at temperatures of ≥27°C to embryonate and become infective. Transmission of this parasite to humans occurs through ingestion of embryonated eggs from the soil directly or from contaminated hands (Fig. 112–1). The eggs hatch and release larvae in the proximal small intestine, where they penetrate the mucosa and are carried to the liver by the portal circulation. Some larvae remain in the liver, causing granuloma to form; others are carried to the lungs, and some then enter the systemic circulation and are carried to various parts of the body until they reach a vessel too small for passage. There the larvae penetrate the vessel and migrate into the surrounding tissue.

Transmission. Humans are infected mainly through ingestion of embryonated eggs (Fig. 112–1); however, infection may also occur following ingestion of larvae in liver, meat, or other tissues of transport hosts. Studies of soil samples where dogs have access in most areas of the world have shown embryonated eggs of *Toxocara* species. Playing in contaminated environments or putting fingers, toys, or other objects into the mouth after they were in contact with contaminated soil is an obvious means of infection, which explains the predominance of toxocariasis in childhood. Serologic surveys show a higher prevalence of antibody titers in children up to 10 years of age than in other groups. Most infections are asymptomatic or are unrecognized. VLM is more common in younger children (mean age of 3), whereas OLM is more likely to occur in older children (mean age of 8).

HISTORY. In the first half of this century, several parasitologists speculated that certain animal parasites might cause disease in humans. However, it was not until 1952 that Beaver and colleagues described larvae of *T. canis* in the tissues of children with eosinophilia-hepatomegaly, which was a common clinical syndrome of previously unknown cause. The investigators proposed the term *visceral larva migrans* to describe the syndrome. Wilder observed nematode larvae in 24 of 46 eyes that had been enucleated, in most instances after a clinical diagnosis of retinoblastoma. She identified the worms as third-stage hookworm larvae, but Nichols reexamined the species and identified the larvae as *T. canis*. The concept of larva migrans was redefined by Beaver to describe the prolonged migration and long persistence of larvae whose behavior reflects the behavior of paratenic hosts. Subsequently, Sprent described the complex life cycles of *Toxocara* spp. The development of a sensitive and specific serologic test greatly stimulated clinical and epidemiologic research. *Toxocara* larva migrans syndromes are now recognized as common zoonotic infections in all countries. In developed countries, toxocariasis ranks with pinworm infection among the most frequent human helminth infections.

DISTRIBUTION. *T. canis* in dogs and infection of humans with its larvae have a worldwide distribution. Many studies performed in the United States, Great Britain, Canada, Brazil, Africa, and the Middle East have revealed the prevalence of infection in dogs to be from 2 to 90%. In general, the highest infection rates are in pups as a result of transmission from their dams; after 6 months of age, prevalence in dogs is usually <10%.

The prevalence of eggs in soil has been widely investigated. Numerous surveys demonstrate that infective *Toxocara* eggs are commonly found in soil samples taken from urban and suburban parks and other public places; these sites provide a potential source of infection for children and adults who do not have dogs or cats in their households.

PATHOGENESIS AND PATHOLOGY. In humans, the infective process begins when embryonated eggs are swallowed; in the intestine, the shell is digested partially, and the contained larva escapes. The 16- to 20-mm larvae enter the vascular system, and those that pass through the liver and the lungs into the systemic circulation eventually reach capillaries and are arrested. They may burrow then into the tissue, causing hemorrhage, necrosis, and secondary inflammation. Larvae migrate extensively through the body and have been found in every tissue and organ system, including the liver, lungs, heart, and brain. Some larvae die and some become dormant for years before again becoming active. The distribution and survival of larvae are determined by the size of the inoculum and the frequency of reinfection. Granulomas, 1 to 2 mm in diameter, usually form around the larvae. These have a preponderance of eosinophils (Fig. 112–2). Later, fibrosis and possible calcification occur. The remarkable capacity of *Toxocara* larvae to survive and continue migrating in host tissues despite vigorous immunologic response seems to be associated with the larvae's capacity to shield themselves from host antibody and cells by producing and shedding substances from the larval surface.

CLINICAL MANIFESTATIONS. The clinical manifestations depend on the number of invading larvae and the part(s) of the body affected. In many cases, infection is asymptomatic; in all cases, however, infection is potentially capable of causing severe disease. Two syndromes caused by *Toxocara* infection, VLM and OLM, are well defined.

Visceral Larva Migrans. VLM, usually diagnosed in quite young children (average age 2 years), is a marked inflamma-

---

*All the material in this chapter is in the public domain, with the exception of any borrowed figures or tables.

LIFE CYCLE of—

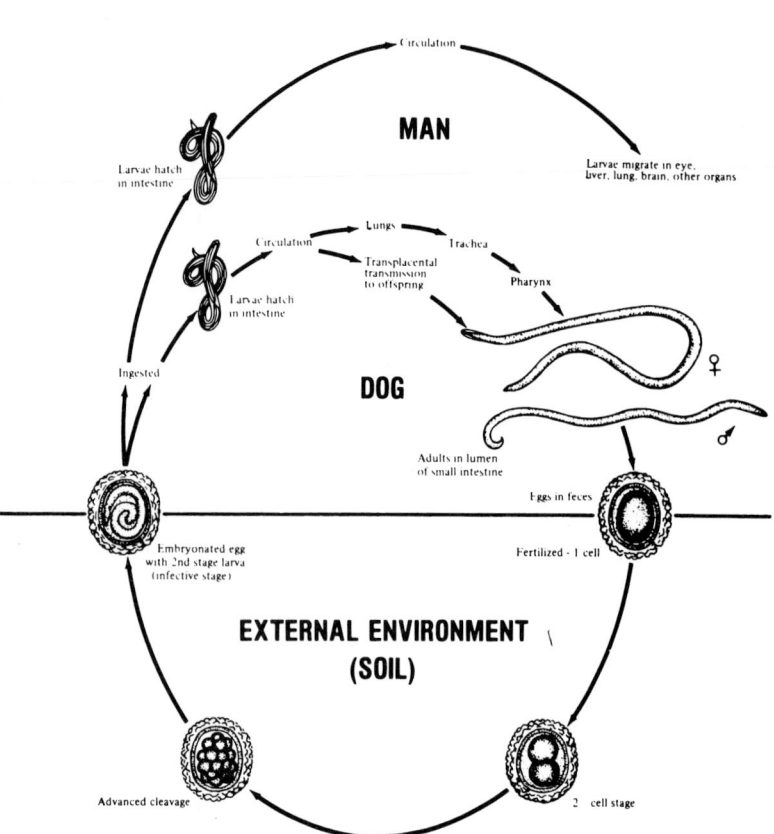

Figure 112–1. Life cycle of *Toxocara canis*. (From Melvin DM, Brooke MM, Healey GR, et al.: Common Blood and Tissue Parasites of Man. Life Cycle Charts. Atlanta, Georgia, Centers for Disease Control, 1961.)

tory immune response to numerous larvae migrating in the liver and other tissues. VLM is characterized by persistent eosinophilia, leukocytosis, fever, hepatomegaly, hypergammaglobulinemia, and elevated titers of blood group isohemagglutinins. Clinical signs often include wheezing or coughing, and pulmonary infiltration is evident in one third of patients. Asthma and recurrent bronchitis have been asso-

ciated with *Toxocara* antibody reactivity. Neurologic manifestations, including focal or generalized seizures and behavior disorders, have been reported in as many as 28% of patients with VLM. The term *covert toxocariasis* has been suggested to describe the signs and symptoms in patients with clinical features that singly are nonspecific but together form a recognizable symptom complex. Such signs and symptoms include abdominal pain, anorexia, sleep and behavior disturbances, cervical adenitis, wheezing, limb pains, and fever. VLM is ordinarily self-resolving once patients are prevented from reinfecting themselves. Rare fatal cases have resulted from larval migration through the myocardium or the central nervous system.

Ocular Larva Migrans. Ocular involvement is more common in older children and adults. It is believed that with fewer infecting larvae, the immune response is less and the eye is invaded randomly several months after infection. Loss of vision in one eye in a child may not be recognized immediately. Disuse of the affected eye commonly leads to strabismus, and the parents may note that a squint has developed. In other individuals, routine examination may reveal poor or absent sight in one eye, and ophthalmoscopy demonstrates a retinal scar or, if invasion of the eye has been recent, a tumor formed by the granuloma. Some vitreous haze is common; a cataract sometimes develops. Prior scar formation with consequent flattening, a tumor-like lesion of the fundus of one eye, and eosinophilia are highly suspicious signs of the presence of ophthalmic toxocariasis. Rarely, patients have periorbital swelling caused by a subcutaneous granuloma containing toxocaral larva. They seldom have the VLM syn-

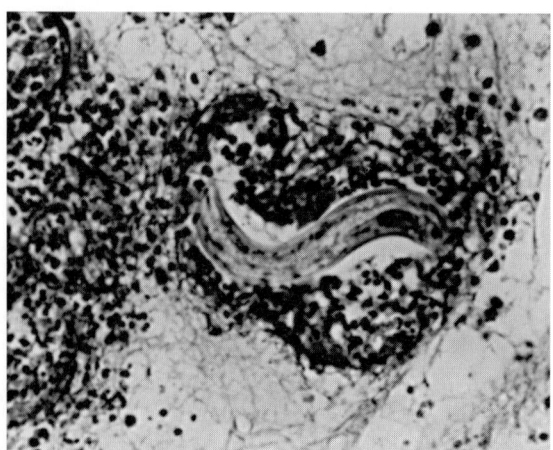

Figure 112–2. A portion of a *T. canis* larva is surrounded by inflammatory cells in a preretinal mass (× 220). (Courtesy of the Armed Forces Institute of Pathology, Photograph Neg. No. 298563-29081.)

drome. At one time it was thought that toxocaral larvae had a special predilection to invade the eye, but ophthalmic lesions are found in a minority of patients with toxocaral infection. However, larvae in the eye usually cause symptoms and are detected more readily than are those in other organs.

Laboratory Findings. Eosinophilia is common in active infections, but its duration is inconsistent and is probably related to the quantity and recency of the infecting dose and the frequency of reinfection. In OLM, peripheral eosinophilia may be absent and evaluation of aqueous humor reveals eosinophils and normal levels of lactic dehydrogenase and phosphoglucose isomerase.

DIAGNOSIS. The diagnosis of toxocaral VLM should be considered in any person with persistent hypereosinophilia. A history of geophagia and association with dogs or cats is helpful. The clinical and laboratory findings (other than serologic tests) are nondiagnostic and do not help to differentiate VLM from other conditions associated with eosinophilia. Because the parasite does not mature beyond the larval stage in human tissues, adult worms do not develop in the intestine and diagnosis by egg detection in feces is not possible.

OLM should be considered in any patients who have raised, unilateral, whitish or gray lesions in the fundus.

Identification of larvae in biopsy tissue permits definitive diagnosis of *Toxocara* infection (Fig. 112–2); other larval nematodes can be differentiated on the basis of characteristic morphologic features. Biopsy is often unrewarding because, unless the infection is massive, biopsy specimens may not yield larvae.

Serologic Tests. Enzyme-linked immunosorbent assay (ELISA), using excretory-secretory antigens from infective-stage larvae, is the best diagnostic test for VLM and OLM. In patients whose clinical signs and history suggest VLM, a positive toxocaral ELISA titer is strong presumptive evidence of *Toxocara* infection. A rising or a falling titer of at least twofold in a recently ill patient is consistent with VLM infection. Because toxocaral antibody titers may remain elevated for years after infection, a measurable titer is not proof of a causative relationship between *T. canis* and the current illness. Surveys have shown that as many as 1 to 10% of asymptomatic children have ELISA titers of 1:32 or more. In patients with ocular lesions compatible with OLM, positive ELISA titers support the diagnosis but do not rule out retinoblastoma. Toxocaral ELISA testing is available at the Centers for Disease Control and Prevention and several other clinical laboratories in the United States.

Differential Diagnosis. Toxocaral VLM must be differentiated from signs and symptoms caused by other tissue-migrating helminths (ascarids, hookworm, filiarie, *Strongyloides stercoralis*, and *Trichinella spiralis*) and hypereosinophilic syndromes. Ocular disease may be confused with retinoblastoma, ocular tumors, developmental anomalies, exudative retinitis (Coats disease), trauma, and other childhood uveitides.

Hepatic capillariasis can be confused with toxocariasis involving the liver. Patients have hepatomegaly, eosinophilia, and abnormal results of liver function tests. A liver biopsy may demonstrate eggs of *Capillaria* species within a hepatic granuloma (Fig. 112–3).

TREATMENT AND PROGNOSIS. Asymptomatic toxocariasis does not require institution of anthelmintic therapy. Although there are isolated reports of ocular disease occurring years after an episode of VLM, available data suggest that asymptomatic individuals have spontaneous resolution of their eosinophilia and seroreactivity without adverse sequelae.

Treatment of patients with symptoms of VLM is primarily

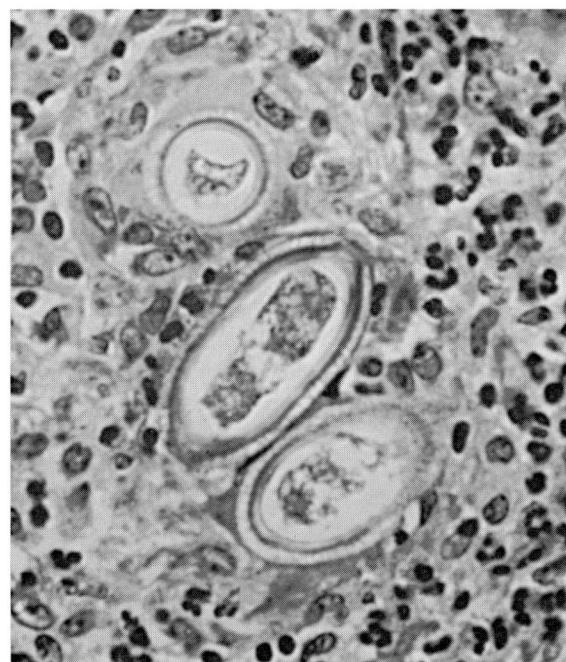

Figure 112–3. Focus of granulomatous reaction around three eggs of *Capillaria* species (H&E stain, × 450). (Courtesy of Dr. V. M. Areán, University of Florida College of Medicine.)

supportive. Anthelmintics, diethylcarbamazine 50 to 150 mg PO t.i.d. for 1 to 3 weeks and thiabendazole 25 to 50 mg/kg/day PO for 1 to 3 weeks, have been used in the management of VLM but have not been consistently effective. The newer benzimidazole compounds, albendazole (10 mg/kg/day PO for 5 days) and mebendazole (20 to 25 mg/kg/day PO for 21 days), are preferable to other anthelmintics because of their greater safety, although the efficacy of treatment remains controversial. Severe pulmonary, myocardial, or central nervous system involvement may warrant corticosteroid therapy.

Treatment of acute ocular toxocariasis is directed toward suppressing the inflammatory response associated with larval migration or worm death. Systemic and intraocular corticosteroids (prednisone 30 to 60 mg PO each day for 2 to 4 weeks; triamcinolone acetonide 40 mg sub-tenon weekly for 2 weeks; or topical prednisolone acetate) are the most consistently effective form of intervention if instituted within the first 4 weeks of illness. Concurrent use of anthelmintic drugs has not provided additive benefit in managing OLM. If visualization of the nematode is made possible by clearing of the vitreal inflammatory reaction, laser photocoagulation becomes an effective means of destroying the migrating larva.

Treatment of patients with long-standing ocular *Toxocara* infection (>8 weeks) is also problematic. Corticosteroids may be effective in treating exacerbations of ocular inflammation; however, relapse and progression of ocular disease are common. Intraocular fibrous adhesions, retinal traction and detachment, retrolental plaques, and chronic vitreal inflammation are most effectively managed by surgical intervention. Commonly used procedures include pars plana vitrectomy and scleral buckling.

PROGNOSIS. The prognosis following treatment is good in terms of limiting further damage. For OLM with severe symptoms, subtotal pars planus vitrectomy has produced good therapeutic results.

PREVENTION. Most cases of human toxocariasis can be

prevented by simple measures, such as careful personal hygiene, elimination of intestinal parasites from pets, and not allowing children to play in potentially contaminated environments. Efforts must be directed at increasing awareness, especially among pet owners, about potential zoonotic hazards and how to minimize them. Veterinarians are uniquely suited to provide pet owners with sound advice. They have the knowledge and have established rapport with clients, and a high proportion of pet owners use veterinary services.

All pet dogs and cats should receive anthelmintics periodically to prevent dissemination of infectious eggs. It is particularly important to treat puppies and bitches shortly after whelping and several times during the first year to prevent passage of infectious eggs. Laws prohibiting puppies and dogs from running free and defecating in public areas, particularly areas used by children, may not be strictly enforced. Therefore, parents should not allow children, especially those with pica, to play unattended outdoors where they are likely to have access to infectious eggs.

Bibliography

Badley JE, Grieve RB, Rockey JH, Glickman LT: Immune-mediated adherence of eosinophils to *Toxocara canis* infective larvae: The role of excretory-secretory antigens. Parasite Immunol 9:133, 1987.

Bass JL, Mehta KA, Glickman LT, et al: Asymptomatic toxocariasis in children. Clin Pediatr 26:441, 1987.

Beaver PC: The nature of visceral larval migrans. J Parasitol 55:3, 1969.

Beaver PC, Snyder MD, Carrera GM, et al: Chronic eosinophilia due to visceral larva migrans. Pediatrics 9:7, 1952.

Buijs J, Borsboom G, van Gemond JJ, et al: *Toxocara* seroprevalence in 5-year-old elementary school children: Relation with allergic asthma. Am J Epidemiol 140:839, 1994.

Glickman LT, Schantz PM: Epidemiology and pathogenesis of zoonotic toxocariasis. Epidemiol Rev 3:230, 1981.

Glickman LT, Schantz PM, Grieve RB: Toxocariasis. *In* Walls KW, Schantz PM (eds): Immunodiagnosis of Parasitic Diseases, Vol 1, Helminthic Diseases. New York, Academic Press, 1986, pp 201–231.

Hagler WS, Pollard ZF, Jarrett WH, Donnelly EH: Results of surgery for ocular *Toxocara canis*. Ophthalmology 88:1081, 1981.

Magnaval J-F: Comparative efficacy of diethylcarbamazine and mebendazole for the treatment of human toxocariasis. Parasitology 110:529, 1995.

Nichols RL: The etiology of visceral larva migrans. 1. The diagnostic morphology of infective second-stage *Toxocara* larvae. J Parasitol 42:349, 1956.

Schantz PM: Toxocaral larva migrans now. Am J Trop Med Hyg 41(Suppl):21, 1989.

Shields JA: Ocular toxocariasis: A review. Surv Ophthalmol 28:361, 1984.

Sturchler DK, Schubarth P, Gualzata M, et al: Thiabendazole vs. albendazole in treatment of toxocariasis: A clinical trial. Ann Trop Med Parasitol 83:473, 1989.

Taylor MRH, Keane CT, O'Connor P, et al: The expanded spectrum of toxocaral disease. Lancet 1:692, 1988.

113 Gnathostomiasis

Thanongsak Bunnag

DEFINITION. Human gnathostomiasis, also called *eosinophilic myeloencephalitis*, *Tau-cheed* (Thailand), *Yangtze River edema* and *Shanghai's rheumatism* (China), *Rangoon tumor* (Burma), *Woodbury bug* (Australia), *Chokofishi* (Japan), and *nodular eosinophilic panniculitis* (Ecuador), is caused by the tissue nematode *Gnathostoma spinigerum* (Owen, 1836). The disease typically causes intermittent subcutaneous migratory swelling and less commonly involves internal organs. Immature adult worms have been recovered from the subcutaneous tissues, internal organs, and central nervous system (CNS).

ETIOLOGY

Morphology. The adult worm is a reddish, slightly transparent nematode with a globular cephalic bulb. The cuticle of the head bulb is armed with 8 to 11 transverse rows of minute hooklets. Only the anterior half of the body below the cervical region constriction is spinous (Fig. 113–1). Males are 10 to 25 mm long and females 25 to 54 mm long. The 65 to 70 μm by 38 to 40 μm eggs are ovoid, unsegmented, and greenish and have a mucoid plug at one end.

Life Cycle. The adult worm lies coiled in a tumor mass in the stomach wall of the definitive hosts—cats, dogs, and several wild carnivores (Fig. 113–2). Eggs are extruded from the lesions and evacuated in the feces. They hatch 10 to 12 days after reaching water, where they release cylindrical, ensheathed first-stage rhabditiform larvae. After ingestion by a freshwater copepod (*Cyclops*), they develop into second-stage larvae in the body cavity within 2 weeks (Fig. 113–3). Encystation of the third-stage larvae occurs in the flesh of the host when an infected copepod is eaten by any of many intermediate hosts, including fish, amphibians, reptiles, birds, and mammals. On ingestion by the definitive host, the parasites become localized in the stomach wall, where they mature in 3 to 12 months.

EPIDEMIOLOGY

Geographic Distribution. Twelve species of the genus have been reported from different animals in various localities. *Gnathostoma spinigerum* is the species causing almost all cases of human gnathostomiasis. A few cases caused by *G. hispidum* (Fedchenko, 1872), *G. doleresi* (Tubangui, 1925), and *G. nipponicum* (Yamaguti, 1941) were recently reported from Japan in humans who consumed infected loaches imported from China.

Gnathostomiasis is primarily an Asian infection, with most

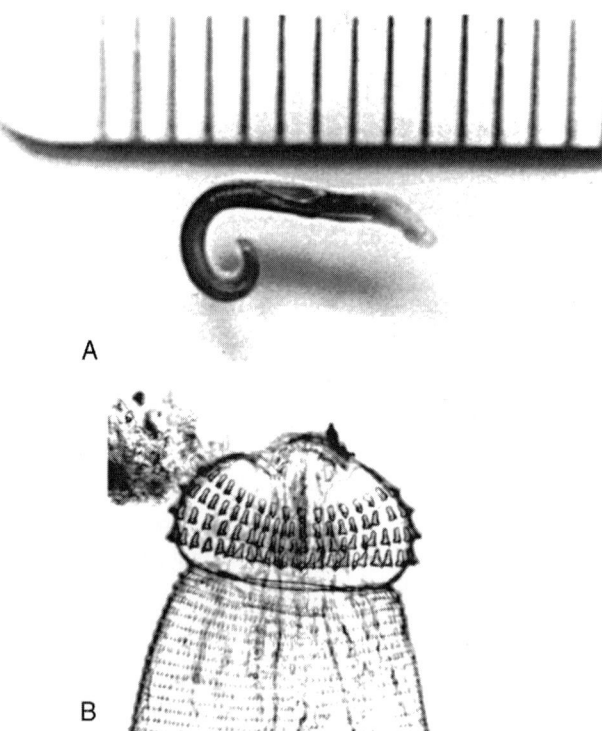

Figure 113–1. *A*, A living immature adult *Gnathostoma spinigerum* recovered from the brain of a patient. *B*, Head bulb with four rows of hooklets and minute cuticular spines on the anterior half of the body.

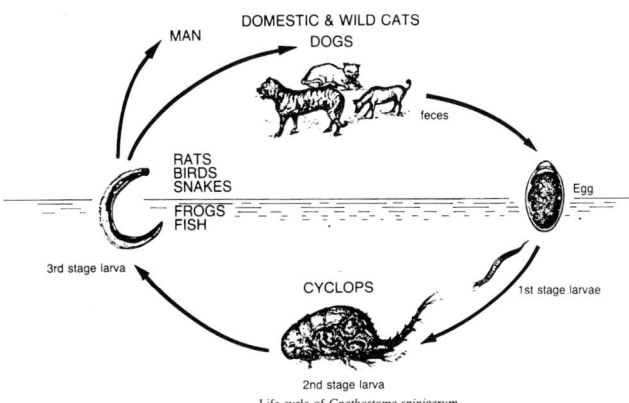

Figure 113–2. Life cycle of *Gnathostoma spinigerum*.

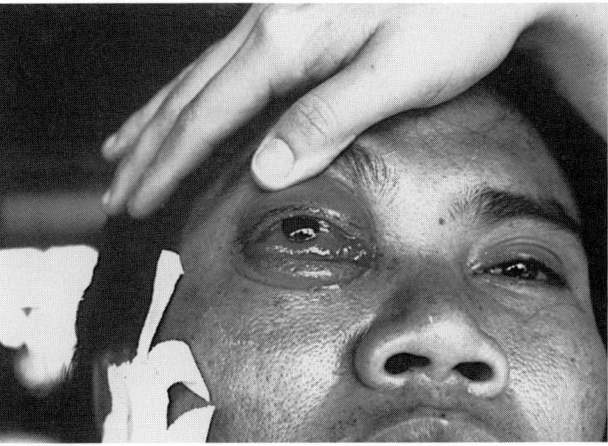

Figure 113–4. Subconjunctival edema and hemorrhage caused by *Gnathostoma spinigerum*.

cases reported from Thailand and Japan. Human infections have also occurred in Australia, Bangladesh, Burma, Cambodia, China, Ecuador, India, Indonesia, Laos, Malaysia, Mexico, the Philippines, and Vietnam. Infected animals have been found in the United States, Zimbabwe, Palestine, and the former Soviet Union. Domestic cats and dogs are key hosts in China, Japan, and Thailand; prevalence rates of 26 to 30% have been found in rural areas. *G. spinigerum* has low host specificity; 44 species of vertebrates (including 16 species of freshwater fish, 2 of frog, 11 of reptiles, 11 of birds, and 4 of mammals) can serve as intermediate hosts.

Humans usually acquire infection by consuming undercooked flesh of transport hosts containing third-stage infective larvae. Common sources of infection are salted fermented freshwater fish (called *somfuk* in Thailand) and raw freshwater fish eaten with rice (sasemi) in Japan. Infections acquired by drinking water contaminated with infected copepods are less common. Three cases of parasitologically proven gnathostomiasis in neonates have been reported. The infections were presumably transmitted prenatally or perinatally from mother to infant. All age groups are susceptible to gnathostomiasis, and there is no sex preference.

PATHOGENESIS AND PATHOLOGY. The worm is unable to complete its normal life cycle in humans. The migrating worm causes pathology by mechanical injury to tissues, by an immunologic response, and by toxic parasite products. Lesions occur along the worm's migratory routes and consist of tracklike necrosis and/or various degrees of hemorrhage. Acute inflammation with diffuse eosinophilic infiltration is prominent in edematous skin lesions and is accompanied by peripheral hypereosinophilia. Unilateral ocular invasion

occurs occasionally and causes subconjunctival edema, hemorrhage, and occasionally retinal damage (Fig. 113–4). The neuropathology of cerebral gnathostomiasis consists of numerous large areas and tracks of hematoma and/or necrosis. *G. spinigerum* has been recovered from the brain, spinal cord, and choroid plexus.

CLINICAL MANIFESTATIONS. The incubation period is unknown in most cases. Patients usually present with either of two distinct clinical forms: larval gnathostomiasis or eosinophilic myeloencephalitis.

Larval Gnathostomiasis. An early manifestation of abdominopulmonary hypereosinophilic syndrome consists of low-grade fever, right upper quadrant abdominal pain, an enlarged and tender liver, pleuritis or pneumonitis, malaise, and hypereosinophilia. This form of gnathostomiasis may be mild and remain unrecognized, or it may be severe and last for >6 weeks. Creeping eruption, with the serpentine track similar to but bigger than that produced by animal hookworm larvae, is rare (Fig. 113–5). Intermittent subcutaneous swellings are due to migration of an immature adult worm.

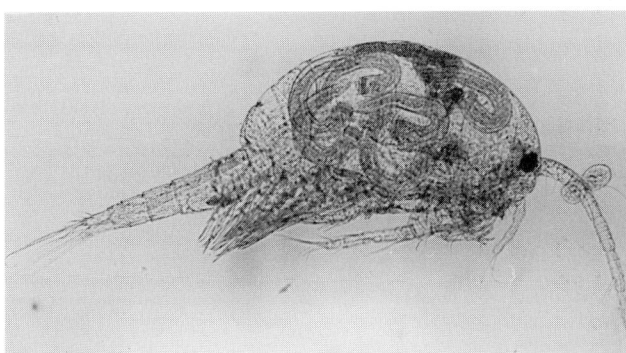

Figure 113–3. Second-stage larvae of *Gnathostoma spinigerum* in the hemocele of *Cyclops*.

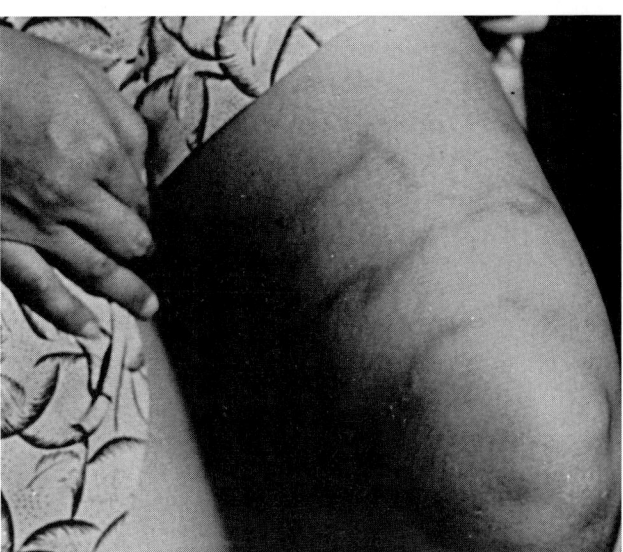

Figure 113–5. *Gnathostoma* creeping eruption is large and serpiginous and has a transient pruritic track. (Courtesy of Professor Manoon Bhaibulaya.)

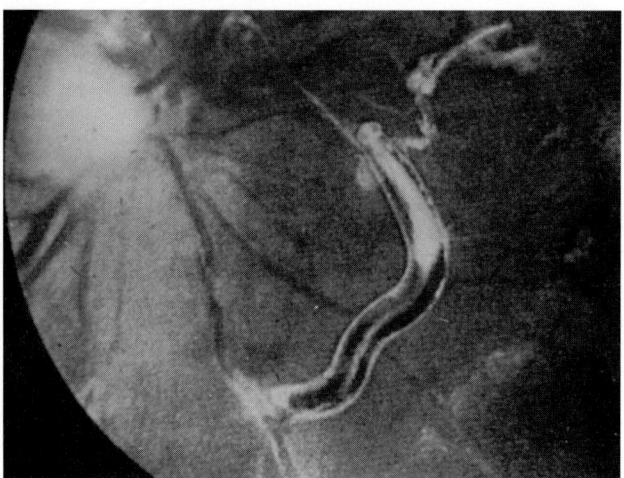

Figure 113–6. *Gnathostoma spinigerum* larva in the vitreous humor of a Thai patient. It causes hemorrhage, retinal detachment, and, later, blindness.

It usually is a painless swelling with local inflammatory reaction, edema, intense pruritus, and leukocytosis with a relatively high eosinophilia. The swelling often occurs in the eyelid. Chemosis, conjunctival edema, and/or hemorrhage may be observed in ocular gnathostomiasis (Fig. 113–4), and in a few cases a nematode can be found in the anterior chamber, the vitreous humor, or the retina (Fig. 113–6). Visual impairment is due to inflammation, hemorrhage, and occasionally to retinal detachment. Blindness due to larval gnathostomiasis has been reported.

Rapidly occurring subcutaneous swelling without a regional lymphadenitis or fever may recur near to or distant from the original site and lasts about 1 week. The interval between episodes of swelling varies from days to months. Other symptoms depend on the internal organs involved, imitating an acute abdomen or an abdominal tumor or causing spontaneous pneumothorax, hemoptysis, pneumonitis, hematuria, or leukorrhea.

Eosinophilic Myeloencephalitis. The neurologic manifestations of gnathostomiasis are a unique symptom complex called *eosinophilic myeloencephalitis*. The worm migrates along a large nerve trunk into the CNS, commonly producing agonizing nerve root pain, followed by paralysis of the extremities with urinary retention and, rarely, quadriplegia. Sudden severe headache and sensorial impairment, followed by coma, occurs in a few cases, suggesting a cerebrovascular accident. In rare instances, neurologic episodes occur in association with cutaneous migratory swelling. In endemic areas, cerebral gnathostomiasis should be considered a cause of cerebral hemorrhage, especially in younger individuals.

Laboratory Findings. A peripheral blood leukocytosis with relative hypereosinophilia occurs in acute cases. The degree of eosinophilia, sometimes as high as 90%, does not correlate with clinical severity. In cerebral gnathostomiasis, the cerebrospinal fluid (CSF) is usually bloody or xanthochromic and has a pleocytosis. In two thirds of cases, the CSF cell count is <500 cells/mm.[3] The predominant cells may be either lymphocytes or neutrophils; eosinophilia is usually >20%. Other investigations (e.g., electroencephalograms, cerebral angiography, computed tomography) are not diagnostically helpful. The results of intradermal skin and various serologic tests are inconclusive. Currently enzyme immunoassay (EIA) for IgG antibody against an aqueous extract of the third-stage larvae of *G. spinigerum* appears to be the most promising serodiagnostic test.

DIAGNOSIS. The diagnosis of larval gnathostomiasis is frequently difficult. Epidemiologic circumstances suggestive of gnathostoma infection include a history of travel to an endemic area, a positive dietary history, and characteristic clinical findings. Other eosinophilic syndromes, including tropical pulmonary eosinophilia (Chapter 106.3) and toxocariasis (Chapter 112), can sometimes be confused with larval gnathostomiasis. Painless, recurrent migratory subcutaneous swellings and eosinophilic leukocytosis must be differentiated from other larval helminthic infections, e.g., ectopic fascioliasis, paragonimiasis, and sparganosis (Chapter 124.5). Calabar swellings (caused by *Loa loa*) associated with microfilariae in the blood in central Africa and the bilateral periorbital edema of acute trichinellosis can usually be differentiated by epidemiologic and clinical findings (Chapter 107). Gnathostoma creeping eruptions are most likely to be confused with those caused by dog and cat hookworms (Chapter 115). The former is rather large and serpiginous and has a transient pruritic, sometimes hemorrhagic track (Fig. 115–1).

Eosinophilic myeloencephalitis differs clinically from eosinophilic meningitis caused by *Angiostrongylus cantonensis* (Chapter 114.1). It should be suspected if the patient develops paralysis of the extremities after severe nerve root pain of the involved extremities or impairment of sensorium with hemorrhage and xanthochromic CSF with an eosinophilic pleocytosis. Definitive diagnosis of gnathostomiasis relies on identification of the worm from surgical specimens or from sputum, urine, vaginal discharge, or other secretions.

TREATMENT. Surgical removal of the worm is the only specific and effective treatment for gnathostomiasis. A combination of supportive, symptomatic, and anti-inflammatory treatments are preferable, however. Albendazole 400 mg once daily for 3 weeks may be an effective tissue larvicidal for cutaneous gnathostomiasis. Therapeutic ultrasound may give symptomatic relief of superficial swelling. Intensive neurologic care is important in critical cases. High-potency analgesics, e.g., morphine hydrochloride, are required to relieve the pain of severe radiculitis.

PROGNOSIS. Subcutaneous swelling, migratory or stationary, recurs intermittently for months or years without apparent damage. Blindness and impaired vision of various degrees are usual in ocular gnathostomiasis. Permanent neurologic sequelae, such as paraplegia, are the most prominent morbidity. The fatality rate in cerebral gnathostomiasis has been estimated to be as high as 40% in Thailand but is in reality much lower because either many milder cases are not diagnosed or medical advice is not sought.

PREVENTION. In endemic areas, the disease can be prevented by adequately cooking freshwater fish, chicken, frogs, snakes, eels, and other intermediate or transport hosts. Untreated groundwater is potentially infectious because it can contain infected copepods.

Bibliography

Bunnag T, Comer DS, Punyagupta S: Eosinophilic myeloencephalitis caused by *Gnathostoma spinigerum*. Neuropathology of nine cases. J Neurol Sci 10:419, 1970.

Kraivichian P, Kulkumthorn M, Yingyourd P, et al: Albendazole for the treatment of human gnathostomiasis. Trans R Soc Trop Med Hyg 86:418, 1992.

Nawa Y: Historical review and current status of gnathostomiasis in Asia. Southeast Asian J Trop Med Public Health 22(Suppl):217, 1991.

Punyagupta S: Recent knowledge on clinical gnathostomiasis. J Med Assoc Thai 50:686, 1957.

Punyagupta S, Bunnag T, Juttijudata P: Eosinophilic meningitis in Thailand. Clinical and epidemiological characteristics of 162 patients with myeloencephalitis probably caused by *Gnathostoma spinigerum*. J Neurol Sci 96:241, 1990.

Punyagupta S, Juttijudata P, Bunnag T, et al: Two fatal cases of eosinophilic myeloencephalitis. A newly recognized disease caused by *Gnathostoma spinigerum*. Trans R Soc Trop Med Hyg 62:801, 1968.

Punyagupta S, Limtrakul C, Vichipanthu P, et al: Nine cases of radiculomyeloencephalitis associated with eosinophilic pleocytosis. Am J Trop Med Hyg 17:551, 1968.
Suntharasamai P, Desakorn V, Migasena S, et al: ELISA for immunodiagnosis of human gnathostomiasis. Southeast Asian J Trop Med Public Health 16:274, 1985.

114 Angiostrongyliasis

114.1 *Angiostrongylus Meningitis*

Thanongsak Bunnag

DEFINITION. Eosinophilic meningitis (eosinophilic meningoencephalitis, cerebral angiostrongyliasis) is a zoonosis characterized by central nervous system (CNS) involvement and an eosinophilic pleocytosis of the cerebrospinal fluid (CSF). *Angiostrongylus cantonensis*, a rat lungworm, has been recognized as the causative agent, and immature parasites have been recovered from the eye chamber, brain, and CSF of humans.

ETIOLOGY

Morphology. *A. cantonensis* is a small nematode of the superfamily *Metastrongyloidea*, first described by Chen (1935) in the lungs of rats. Its life cycle was elucidated by Mackerras and Sandars (1955). Both male and female adult parasites are filiform and taper slightly at both ends. The cephalic tip is transparent and has a smooth cuticle with transverse striae. Fully mature females average about 25 mm in length. They are characterized by their milky white uterine tubules, which wind spirally around the blood-filled intestine, giving a "barber's pole" appearance. Fully developed males average 18 mm in length and possess well-developed caudal bursa copulatrix. Third-stage infective larvae are about 500 μm in length.

Life Cycle. *A. cantonensis* is a neurotropic parasite that requires a period of development in the CNS of its definitive vertebrate hosts. Mature adults inhabit the pulmonary arteries of a wide variety of rodents of the genuses *Rattus* and *Bandicota* (Fig. 114–1). Eggs laid by the female lodge in the pulmonary arteries, where they hatch. The first-stage larvae enter the alveolar space, migrate up the trachea and down the alimentary tract, and are excreted in the rodent's feces. Terrestrial snails, slugs, and aquatic snails serve as intermediate hosts either by being penetrated by first-stage larvae or by ingesting rodent feces containing the larvae. Two further stages of development take place in the mollusk, where the parasites become third-stage larvae in about 2 weeks. When ingested by rodents, infective third-stage larvae migrate via the circulation to the brain, where they undergo two further stages of development, becoming young adults within 4 weeks. They then go to the subarachnoid space, enter the venous system, and arrive in the pulmonary arteries, where, after 2 more weeks, sexual maturity is attained. Humans are an accidental host, and survival of fifth-stage larvae is not certain; some die in the brain and spinal cord; some reach the eye chamber; and only a few reach the lungs.

A. cantonensis shows little host specificity; a wide variety of terrestrial slugs and snails as well as freshwater species can transmit infection. Some of the major natural host species are the slugs *Veronicella alte* and *V. siamensis*; the terrestrial snails *Achatina fulica* and *Bradybaena similaris*; and the freshwater snails *Pila ampulacea, P. polita, P. scutata,* and *Viviparus* spp. *Pila* spp. and *Achatina fulica* are (proven) important sources of human infection in Thailand and Taiwan (Chapter 136). Suitable paratenic hosts of *A. cantonensis* include fish, amphibians, reptiles, crustaceans, land planarians, and possibly vegetables contaminated with larvae.

EPIDEMIOLOGY

Geographic Distribution. Eosinophilic meningitis occurs widely in the tropics from 23°N to 23°S. Transmission requires a warm climate, moderate to heavy rainfall, and an abundance of vegetation suitable for the propagation of both the rodent vertebrate hosts and the mollusk intermediate hosts. The parasite was first recognized in the rat in Canton in 1935 and in humans in Taiwan in 1944. Cerebral angiostrongyliasis is more common in Southeast Asia than in the Pacific Islands. Human infection occurs in Australia, American Samoa, mainland China, the Cook Islands, the Caroline Islands, Cuba, Egypt, Hawaii, Hong Kong, Indonesia, Ivory Coast, Malaysia, Okinawa, Papua New Guinea, the Philippines, Taiwan, Thailand, and Vietnam. In addition, the parasite has been found in the Malagasy Republic, Sri Lanka, India, and all Southeast Asian countries where the giant African snail *A. fulica* has been imported.

Southeast Asian cases occur mainly during the rainy season, when the invertebrate hosts are active. Elsewhere the disease is sporadic, varying with local customs. There have been dozens of parasitologically proven cases and thousands of clinically diagnosed cases, with occasional reports of fatalities.

Transmission. Humans accidentally acquire infection by consuming the tissues of infected mollusks—either by ingesting improperly cooked intermediate hosts (snails and slugs) or raw paratenic hosts (e.g., freshwater shrimp, *Macrobrachium lar*) or by eating food (e.g., salad greens) contaminated by slugs or snails. A group of 12 serious cases with 1 fatality was reported from Thailand, where *A. cantonensis* had been acquired by eating undercooked monitor lizards. Drinking water containing third-stage larvae liberated from dead mollusks is difficult to validate as a source of infection. The

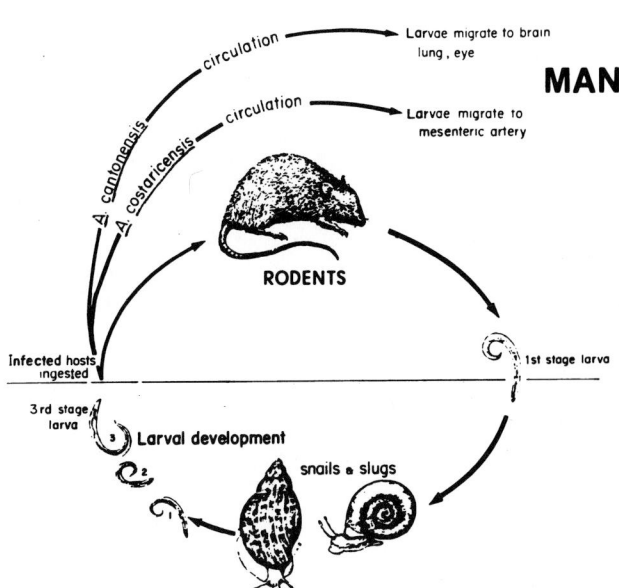

Figure 114–1. Life cycle of *Angiostrongylus cantonensis* and *A. costaricensis.*

disease is prevalent in adults in Thailand and the Pacific Islands but is more common among children in Taiwan. Twice as many males as females are infected in Thailand, but a sex preference has not been observed in other areas.

PATHOLOGY AND PATHOGENESIS. The neuropathology of human angiostrongyliasis has been well described, with brain congestion and inflammation of the leptomeninges. Gross hemorrhage is unusual, and living larvae of *A. cantonensis* are often seen on the surface of the brain and spinal cord. The development and movement of living parasites as well as dead and degenerating worms in brain tissue and the subarachnoid space provoke the inflammatory reaction.

Microscopic changes are characterized by a marked cellular infiltration of lymphocytes, plasma cells, macrophages, and eosinophils in the meninges and by granulomas surrounding dead worms. Invariably noted are numerous tracks or microcavities representing the passage of migrating worms through the brain and spinal cord. Older tracks contain debris, glitter cells, and Charcot-Leyden crystals; newer tracks show disruption of brain tissue with or without microscopic hemorrhage. Venous engorgement with necrosis of vessel walls and perivascular hemorrhage has been noted. Sections of *A. cantonensis* larvae are easily recognized in the brain, in meninges, and sometimes in blood vessels (Fig. 114–2). The lungs can be involved; in a few instances mature worms, alive or dead, have been found in the pulmonary artery. Living worms have been removed frequently from human eyes without apparent eye pathology.

CLINICAL MANIFESTATIONS. The disease is generally benign and self-limiting, but occasionally there is severe illness with lasting neurologic sequelae or even death. The number of infecting larvae ranges from a few to hundreds and the larval load correlates with disease severity.

Symptoms and Signs. The usual incubation period is 2 weeks but ranges from 3 to 36 days. Nausea, vomiting, and abdominal discomfort are seen in some cases soon after ingestion of infected food. Severe headache of insidious onset is the chief complaint in 96% of cases in Thailand; in Taiwan, however, 78% have an abrupt onset of headache. The headache is intermittent, intractable, bitemporal, or occipital and continues throughout the clinical illness. Nausea, vomiting, and moderate stiffness of the neck and/or back are frequent during the early stage of disease. Paresthesias of the trunk and extremities commonly manifest as exaggerated sensitivity to touch and may persist for several weeks or months.

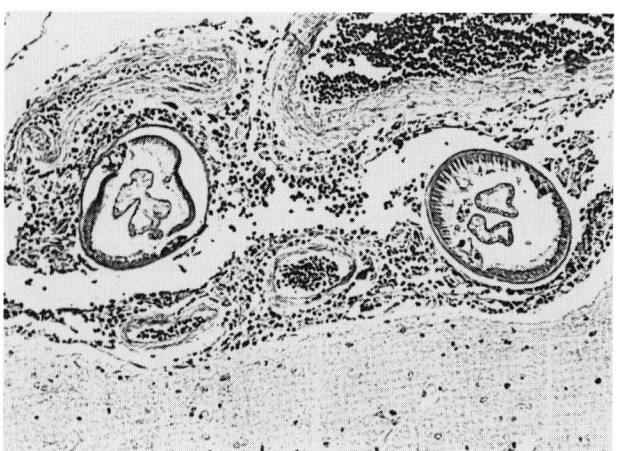

Figure 114–2. Cross section of *Angiostrongylus cantonensis* larvae in the meninges with lymphocytes and eosinophils.

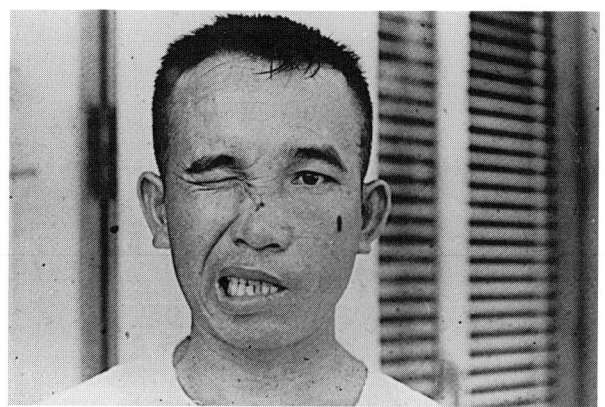

Figure 114–3. Unilateral facial paralysis of the lower motor neuron type in a patient with Angiostrongylus meningitis.

Altered consciousness, ranging from somnolence to coma, has been reported in 5% of Thai cases but in 82% of those from Taiwan. Generalized weakness and flaccid paralysis of the extremities associated with coma occur in a few severe cases. Low-grade pyrexia or no fever is usual, except in those with severe symptoms and in children.

Cranial nerves are sometimes affected, particularly the optic, facial, and abducens nerves. Visual impairment occurs, and from 12 to 25% of patients have abnormal funduscopic findings. Diplopia, reduced visual fields, optic atrophy, and periorbital edema are present occasionally. Living young adult parasites have been recovered from the eye chambers in a dozen cases. Retinal hemorrhage and detachment are serious complications of ocular angiostrongyliasis. Unilateral facial paralysis of the lower motor neuron type and lateral abducens paralysis occur in less than 5% of patients (Fig. 114–3). Pulmonary symptoms and abnormal findings on chest films have occurred in severe cases, and *A. cantonensis* adults have been demonstrated in histologic sections of pulmonary arteries.

Laboratory Findings. Elevation of the initial CSF pressure above 200 mm of water (in some cases over 500 mm of water) with grossly opalescent or turbid, but not purulent, fluid occurs in 88% of cases in Thailand. The CSF contains between 500 and 2000 leucocytes/mm^3 with a relatively high percentage of eosinophils, typically 25 to 75%. The eosinophilic pleocytosis reaches a peak around the twelfth day of illness and gradually resolves over several months. In occasional cases, both the CSF pleocytosis and the symptoms reappear after 2 or 3 months. Mild xanthochromia can occur in severe cases. CSF protein is elevated in approximately two thirds of patients, but CSF glucose is usually normal.

Peripheral eosinophilia ranging from 15 to 50% persists for about 3 months. There is no correlation between the degree of eosinophilia in the peripheral blood and the percentage of eosinophils in the CSF. Serum biochemistry, electroencephalography, and cerebral angiography results are usually normal.

DIAGNOSIS. Cerebral angiostrongyliasis is usually diagnosed on the basis of residence in, or travel to, an endemic area, consumption of undercooked food potentially containing larvae, and compatible clinical and CSF findings. Computed axial tomography (CAT scan) of the brain may be abnormal. EIA using fourth-stage larvae as antigen is the most promising test for detecting antibodies to *A. cantonensis* but is not readily available. A definitive diagnosis is made only rarely by recovering *A. cantonensis* larvae from the CSF or ocular chamber or at autopsy (Fig. 114–2).

Differential Diagnosis. In endemic areas, eosinophilic pleocytosis associated with neurologic involvement has been found in other helminthic diseases, including infections with *Gnathostoma spinigerum*, *Paragonimus westermani*, *P. heterotrema*, *Schistosoma japonicum*, and *Taenia solium* cysticerci. Of these, cerebral gnathostomiasis is encountered most frequently and should be suspected if a patient with hemorrhagic or xanthochromic spinal fluid and eosinophilic pleocytosis develops paralysis of the extremities following severe radiculitis or sensory loss.

TREATMENT. Analgesics and sedatives give only minimal relief. Headache usually subsides dramatically, but temporarily, following lumbar puncture. Careful removal of CSF at intervals of 3 to 7 days is therefore recommended until there is definite clinical and laboratory improvement. In more critical cases, corticosteroids may be employed to reduce cerebral pressure or to treat those with cranial nerve involvement. Corticosteroids do not appear to benefit mild cases.

A. cantonensis is susceptible to broad-spectrum anthelmintics, e.g., thiabendazole, mebendazole, albendazole, and ivermectin. However, these drugs should not be used—clinical deterioration or death can result from a reaction to dead or dying worms in the brain. Emergency surgical removal of *Angiostrongylus* larvae is required for patients with ocular involvement. In cases of intravitreal angiostrongyliasis, removal of the worm after it has been immobilized using an intravitreal cryoprobe is recommended to avoid complications.

PROGNOSIS. The disease is usually self-limiting. Clinical symptoms persist for 2 to 4 weeks and generally are much reduced within a few days of initial treatment. In about 40% of cases, headache persists longer than 1 month; the neurologic deficit may last longer. The fatality rate is low: 3% in Taiwan, 0.5% in Thailand, and no deaths reported from Tahiti. Those who die do so in coma between 2 and 4 weeks after infection.

PREVENTION. Control methods include health education about the nature and source of the disease, proper cooking of mollusks or paratenic hosts, and proper washing of vegetables. Freezing of mollusks and crustaceans at −15°C for 12 hours will destroy infective larvae of *A. cantonensis*. Community control measures include the control of mollusks and land planarians, but the most effective measure is rodent eradication.

Bibliography

Bunnag T, Benjapong W, Noeypatimanond S, et al: The recovery of *Angiostrongylus cantonensis* in the cerebrospinal fluid in a case of eosinophilic meningitis. J Med Assoc Thai 52:665, 1969.

Jaroonvesama N, Charoenlarp K, Buranasin P, et al: ELISA testing in cases of clinical angiostrongyliasis in Thailand. Southeast Asian J Trop Med Public Health 16:110, 1985.

Punyagupta S, Bunnag T, Juttijudata P, et al: Eosinophilic meningitis in Thailand. Epidemiologic studies of 484 typical cases and the etiologic role of *Angiostrongylus cantonensis*. Am J Trop Med Hyg 19:950, 1970.

Punyagupta S, Juttijudata P, Bunnag T, et al: Eosinophilic meningitis in Thailand. Clinical studies of 484 typical cases probably caused by *Angiostrongylus cantonensis*. Am J Trop Med Hyg 24:921, 1975.

Rosen L, Loison G, Laigret J, et al: Studies on eosinophilic meningitis: III. Epidemiology and clinical observations on Pacific islands and the possible etiologic role of *Angiostrongylus cantonensis*. Am J Epidemiol 85:17, 1967.

Singalavanija A, Wangspa S, Teschareon S: Intravitreal angiostrongyliasis. Aust NZ Ophthalmol 14:381, 1986.

Sonakul DS: Pathological findings in four cases of human angiostrongyliasis. Southeast Asian J Trop Med Public Health 9:220, 1978.

Yii CY: Clinical observations on eosinophilic meningitis and meningoencephalitis caused by *Angiostrongylus cantonensis* in Taiwan. Am J Trop Med Hyg 25:233, 1976.

114.2 *Abdominal Angiostrongyliasis*

Pedro Morera

DEFINITION AND HISTORY. Abdominal angiostrongyliasis is a granulomatous inflammatory reaction with heavy eosinophilic infiltration of the intestinal wall, especially of the ileocecal region, caused by *Angiostrongylus costaricensis* Morera and Cespedes, 1971 (= *Morerastrongylus costaricensis* Chabaud, 1972). This disease has been observed in Costa Rican children since 1952; since 1971 it has been reported from other sites in Central and South America. In addition, cotton rats naturally infected with the parasite have been found in the United States.

ETIOLOGY

Morphology. *A. costaricensis* is a filiform nematode normally living within the mesenteric arteries of the definitive host. The female is 33 mm long, with vulva and anus located near the caudal end; the male is 20 mm long, with a copulatory bursa and two spicules approximately 300 μm in length.

Development. Eggs are oviposited within the mesenteric arteries and carried by the blood into the intestinal wall, where they embryonate (Fig. 114–1). First-stage larvae hatch, migrate through the intestinal wall, and, by excretion in the rat feces, reach the soil, where they are eaten by the intermediate host, usually slugs. Two molts take place in the mollusk, and after 18 days the infective third-stage larva matures. The definitive host, a rodent, usually the cotton rat, becomes infected by eating the mollusk. The prepatent period lasts 24 days.

DISTRIBUTION AND INCIDENCE. The disease has been reported from the United States to Argentina, including some Caribbean islands. In addition, one human case has been reported from Africa. In Costa Rica its distribution is universal, from sea level to an altitude of 2000 M; 20 to 60 cases were reported annually from the first recognition of *A. costaricensis* until the mid-1980s. However, since that time, owing to better identification of the disease by medical personnel, the annual incidence has increased to 600 cases per year (20 per 100,000 inhabitants).

TRANSMISSION AND EPIDEMIOLOGY. In Costa Rica the cotton rat, *Sigmodon hispidus*, is the most important definitive host, and at least 12 different species of rats and 1 coati have been found naturally infected with the parasite. Also, marmosets and two rodents have been found naturally infected with *A. costaricensis* in eastern Peru and southern Brazil, respectively.

Although several mollusks are naturally infected with *A. costaricensis*, veronicellid slugs are considered the main intermediate hosts (Chapter 136). There is no evidence that people intentionally eat slugs; however, small ones deeply hidden in salad greens could be finely chopped and inadvertently eaten raw. In addition, several cases have followed ingestion of these mollusks by infants. Most human infections are probably caused by ingestion of the infective larvae shed in the mollusk's secretions (Fig. 114–1). Slugs have been found in ripe fruits that have fallen to the ground. Characteristic mucous trails left by the mollusks can be observed throughout the endemic areas. The propensity for small children to put things in their mouths could explain why they have the highest infection rates.

At least two species of veronicellid slugs in Costa Rica (*Sarasinula plebeia* and *Diplosolenodes occidentalis*) and one in Brazil (*Phyllocaulis variegatus*) are naturally infected with *A. costaricensis*; 50% of 6025 slugs from 20 Costa Rican localities, from sea level to an altitude of 2000 M, were found infected

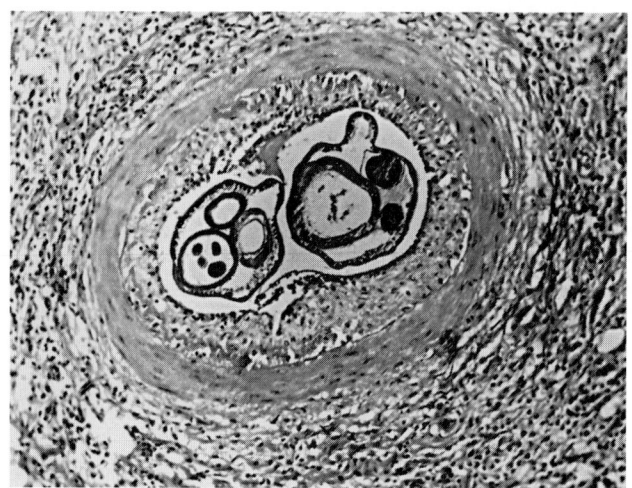

Figure 114–4. Adults of *Angiostrongylus costaricensis* within a mesenteric artery. The intima is swollen, and the endothelium is damaged.

and more than 16,000 infective larvae were counted in a single specimen.

PATHOLOGY. In most cases, the lesions are located in the iliocecal region of the intestinal tract. They also occur in the hepatic flexure and descending colon, regional lymph nodes, liver, and testicles. Two major pathogenic mechanisms are present in infections caused by *A. costaricensis:* (1) The adult worms living within the mesenteric arteries (Fig. 114–4) damage the endothelium, inducing thrombosis and, consequently, necrosis of the tissues perfused by the vessel; and (2) eggs, embryos, and larvae as well as excretion-secretion products cause inflammatory reactions. Combinations of these as well as the patient's susceptibility and the number and localization of parasites determine the pathophysiology of the infection.

Intestinal Lesions. The gross pathologic examination shows a hardened and thickened intestinal wall with yellowish foci in the serosal surface of the intestine. The intestinal lumen is reduced, sometimes causing partial or complete obstruction. Necrotic areas may perforate. In many cases, the surgeon detects cecal lesions during an appendectomy.

Histopathology demonstrates granulomatous inflammatory reactions (Fig. 114–5A) with heavy eosinophilic infiltration, especially in the intestinal mucosa and submucosa; the serosa and muscular layers are often involved to a lesser

degree. Eggs (Fig. 114–5B), embryos, and larvae are in small cavities lined by endothelium. Unfertilized eggs usually degenerate and are difficult to recognize. These structures as well as the excretion-secretion antigens are easily identified by immunochemical techniques. Large areas of necrosis are caused by arterial thrombosis.

Extraintestinal Lesions. Eggs and embryos are present in the mesenteric lymph nodes, which also show reticuloendothelial hyperplasia and eosinophilic infiltration. Hepatic lesions caused by *A. costaricensis* are similar to those caused by *Toxocara canis* (Chapter 112). However, the finding of eggs (Fig. 114–5C), embryos, and even adult worms in the hepatic parenchyma establishes the diagnosis. In excised necrotic testicles, histologically showing extensive parenchymal hemorrhagic necrosis, worms have been observed obstructing the arteries of the spermatic cord.

CLINICAL MANIFESTATIONS. Abdominal angiostrongyliasis affects children predominantly. Among 116 patients studied in a pediatric hospital, half were of school age, 40% were of preschool age, 10% were infants, two thirds were male.

Symptoms and Signs. When the worms are located in the iliocecal region, most patients complain of pain in the right iliac fossa and the right flank. Palpation in this area often causes pain. Rectal examination is also painful in about one half of patients, and most patients present with fever of 38 to 38.5°C, rarely accompanied by chills. In chronic cases, a mild fever may persist for several weeks. Anorexia, vomiting, and constipation are also present in about half the patients. An important finding is a tumor-like mass, which, if present, can be palpated in the lower right quadrant and may be confused with a malignancy.

Laboratory Findings. Although a few patients have no hematologic abnormalities, leukocytosis and eosinophilia are usually present. White blood cell counts usually range between 15,000 and 50,000/mm³ and eosinophilia from 20 to 50%. The leukocytosis has been as high as 169,000/mm³, with a 91% eosinophilia. Radiologic changes are localized in the terminal ileum, cecum appendix, and ascending colon. Studies using contrast medium show incomplete filling and irritability of the involved areas. The lumen is reduced by the thickening of the intestinal wall (Fig. 114–6).

Extraintestinal Findings. Sometimes the patient complains of pain in the right upper quadrant. In these cases, the liver is almost always enlarged and tender to palpation. At laparoscopy, small yellowish spots (granulomas) are seen on the surface of the liver. Most patients have hepatic involvement along with intestinal angiostrongyliasis.

When the testicle is involved, the most remarkable finding is acute pain, accompanied by redness that later changes to

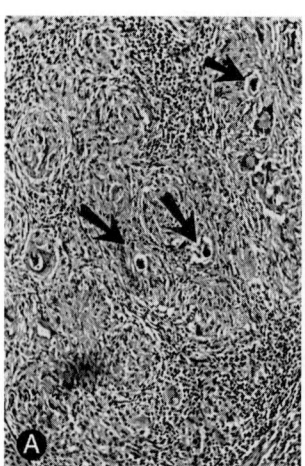
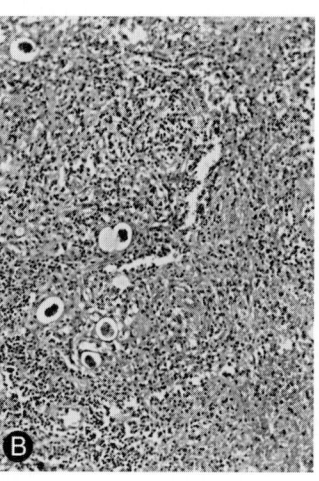
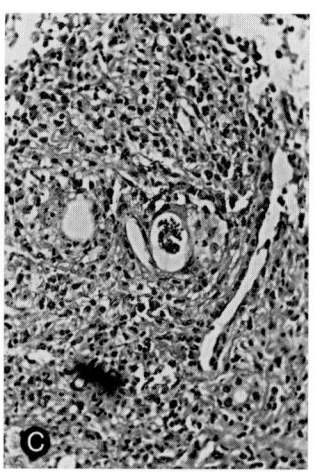

Figure 114–5. *Angiostrongylus costaricensis* ova in tissues. *A,* Section of intestine showing several granulomas and giant cells: Eggs (*arrows*) are scattered in the tissue. *B,* Eggs in the cecum wall surrounded by inflammatory cells (eosinophils). *C,* Embryonated egg in the liver.

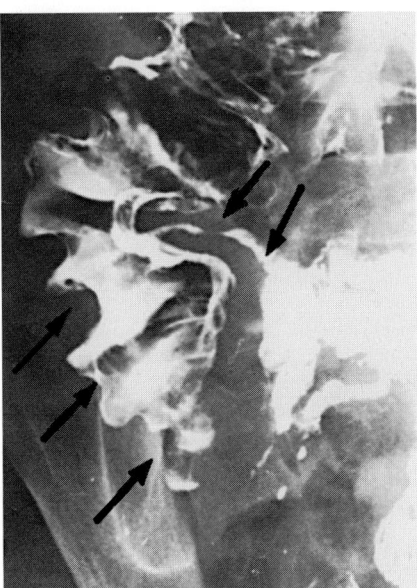

Figure 114–6. Radiograph after barium enema showing filling defect of the ileocecal region and ascending colon. The external wall of the colon shows festooned aspect of the mucosa.

purple. Eosinophilia and leukocytosis are also conspicuous. All patients with testicular necrosis have been misdiagnosed as having testicular torsion, the correct diagnosis being made only following surgery.

DIAGNOSIS. The clinical diagnosis is based on the characteristic features. The symptoms and findings can be confused with those of appendicitis, and the appendix is frequently involved in the process. The diagnosis is often made at surgery. Barium enema examination can show filling defects in the colon (Fig. 114–6) that often resemble colon carcinoma. A latex test and enzyme-linked immunosorbent assay (ELISA) have been used for serodiagnosis. Eggs and larvae do not appear in the stool.

TREATMENT. Surgery is sometimes required for abdominal angiostrongyliasis. However, as knowledge of this often self-limiting disease increases, more cases have been followed without surgery. Two drugs, diethylcarbamazine and thiabendazole, have been used, with remission of symptoms reported. However, no clinical trials have proved the efficacy of these drugs. In fact, in vitro and in vivo trials in experimentally infected rats demonstrate that parasites are excited, rather than killed, by the drugs, causing erratic migrations and worsening of the lesions. Thus, chemotherapy is not recommended until experimental studies demonstrate a more efficacious drug.

Bibliography

Graeff-Teixeira C, Avila-Pires FC, Machado R, et al: Identificacão de roedores silvestres como hospedeiros do Angiostrongylus costaricensis no sul do Brazil. Rev Inst Med Trop Sao Paulo, 32:147, 1990.

Loria-Cortes R, Lobo-Sibaja HF: Clinical abdominal angiostrongyliasis. A study of 116 children with intestinal eosinophilic granuloma caused by Angiostrongylus costaricensis. Am J Trop Med Hyg 29:538, 1980.

Morera P: Life history and redescription of Angiostrongylus costaricensis (Morera and Cespedes, 1971). Am J Trop Med Hyg 22:613, 1973.

Morera P: Abdominal angiostrongyliasis. Clin Trop Med Comm Dis 2:747, 1980.

Morera P, Cespedes R: Angiostrongylus costaricensis n. sp. (Nematoda: Metastrongyloidea), a new lungworm occurring in man in Costa Rica. Rev Biol Trop 18:173, 1971.

Morera P, Perez F, Mora F, et al: Visceral larva migrans–like syndrome caused by Angiostrongylus costaricensis. Am J Trop Med Hyg 31:67, 1982.

115 *Cutaneous Larva Migrans**

Ronald C. Neafie and Wayne M. Meyers

DEFINITION. Cutaneous larva migrans is the dermatitis caused by invasion of the skin by larval nematodes. The filariform larvae of the dog and cat hookworm, *Ancylostoma braziliense,* account for most infections, but several other larval nematodes can cause the disease also (Table 115–1). The major emphasis of this chapter, however, is on hookworm larvae that cannot or rarely do complete their life cycle in humans. Synonymous terms include creeping eruption, sandworm, plumber's itch, duck hunter's itch, and epidermitis linearis migrans.

ETIOLOGY

Morphology. Infective filariform larvae (third stage) of *Ancylostoma braziliense* are 850 μm long and 35 μm in diameter. In processed tissue sections, they are only about 20 μm in diameter. They have minute double lateral alae that extend most of the length of the larva. All hookworm larvae that cause cutaneous larva migrans in humans and those of *Strongyloides stercoralis* are similar morphologically. In contrast, the larvae of *Gnathostoma spinigerum* are several hundred micrometers in diameter and can be readily identified by their numerous cuticular spines.

Life Cycle. The general life cycles of hookworms, threadworms, and *Gnanthostoma* have been described in Chapters 105.1, 105.2, and 113. Adult *A. braziliense* and *A. caninum* organisms inhabit the intestines of dogs and cats. Embryonated eggs passed in the stool, under appropriate conditions of temperature and humidity, hatch and release rhabditiform larvae within 1 or 2 days. After feeding, growing, and molting, they become infective filariform larvae, usually in about a week. Humans are an aberrant host of these hookworms; thus, these larvae invade the skin of humans but ordinarily penetrate no deeper than the epidermis.

GEOGRAPHIC DISTRIBUTION AND EPIDEMIOLOGY. Cutaneous larva migrans occurs wherever bare skin contacts contaminated soil containing the infective larvae of dog or cat hookworms. Thus, the disease is most common in warmer tropical or subtropical regions. It is especially prevalent in southeastern United States and is most frequent during the warm and rainy seasons. Children are more likely to acquire the infection because of their frequent contact with contaminated soil, e.g., in sand piles. People who frequent beaches (hence the synonym *sandworm*) are at increased risk. *Plumber's itch* came into use because the disease is often acquired while repairing plumbing underneath houses.

PATHOLOGY. The larvae are limited to the epidermis, where they wander about, producing serpiginous tunnels or tracks (Fig. 115–1). They are located in burrows in the deeper layers of the epidermis (Fig. 115–2) and are most likely found in biopsy specimens taken just ahead of the clinically evident track. The specimen usually does not contain the larva but reveals only an infiltration of lymphocytes and eosinophils in the upper dermis. Exact identification of the larva often is impossible. It is not known why the larvae are unable to complete the life cycle. Some believe the larvae lack the specific collagenase needed for penetration of human dermis.

CLINICAL MANIFESTATIONS. Within a few hours after the skin is penetrated by a larva, an itching red papule develops. A serpiginous track arises from the papule as the worm wanders aimlessly, creating tunnels within the epidermis. The surrounding tissues are edematous and acutely inflamed, and the unoccupied portion of the track dries and becomes

---

*All the illustrations in this chapter are in the public domain.

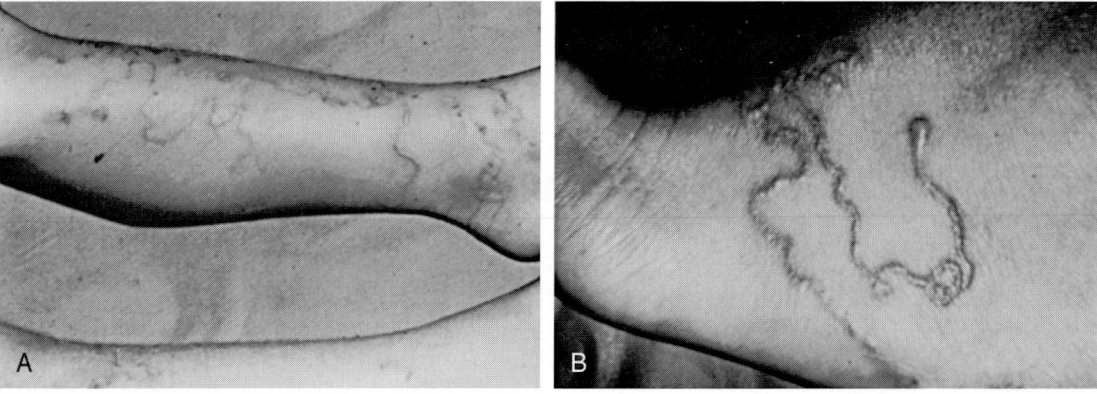

Figure 115–1. *A* and *B*, Creeping eruption caused by the larva of *Ancylostoma braziliense.*

TABLE 115–1. Causes of Cutaneous Larva Migrans

	Common Name	Incidence	Clinical Characteristics
Ancylostoma braziliense	Cat, dog hookworm	Most common	Threadlike linear burrows, highly pruritic, moves 1–2 cm/day, may persist for months
Ancylostoma caninum	Dog hookworm	Common	Papular, rarely linear burrows, clears spontaneously in 1–3 weeks
Ancylostoma duodenale	Human hookworm	Common	Papulovesicular, pruritic, minimal migration in the skin, clears within 2 weeks
Necator americanus	Human hookworm	Common	Same as for *A. duodenale*
Uncinaria stenocephala	European dog hookworm	Rare	Threadlike linear burrows, pruritic, moves 1–2 cm/day, may persist for months
Gnathostoma spinigerum	Cat, dog nematode	Rare	Deep, wide burrows, furunculoid, may persist for years
Bunostomum phlebotomum	Cattle hookworm	Rare	Papular lesion, minimal migration, clears within 2 weeks
Strongyloides stercoralis (larva currens)	Human threadworm	Rare	Perianal band of urticaria and pruritic induration extends up to several cm/day around anus, may persist for weeks, recurrent owing to autoinfection
Strongyloides myopotami	Nutria strongylid	Rare	Papular or linear threadlike, serpiginous, pruritic lesion

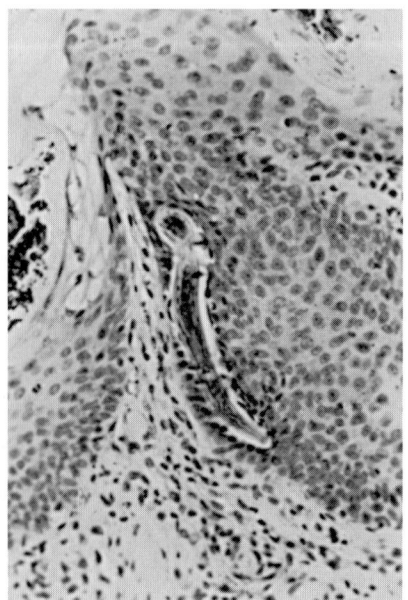

Figure 115–2. Longitudinal section of a larva of *Ancylostoma* species in epidermis. (H&E stain, × 175.) (Courtesy of the Armed Forces Institute of Pathology, Photograph Neg. No. 76-888.)

encrusted and scarred. The larva may migrate several centimeters a day. This migration is associated with severe pruritus that leads to scratching and frequently to secondary infection. In severe infections, itching may be so intense that patients suffer intolerably, cannot sleep, and may even become psychotic. The larvae can live for several months if untreated.

DIAGNOSIS. Diagnosis is usually made on the basis of the clinical history and the appearance of the characteristic serpiginous track. Biopsy is not recommended, because the larva is usually beyond the obvious lesion and is rarely seen in the specimen.

PREVENTION AND TREATMENT. Avoiding contact of exposed skin with contaminated soil (e.g., by wearing shoes and using a beach towel when lying on the sand) is the most appropriate preventive measure. Periodic deworming of domestic cats and dogs reduces soil contamination. Sandboxes and other similar facilities where children frequently play should be protected from dogs and cats, especially cats that may use them as defecation sites.

Thiabendazole taken orally or applied topically in an ointment or cream is effective and has generally replaced local freezing with ethyl chloride or carbon dioxide. Thiabendazole can be administered in a dosage of 25 mg/kg b.i.d. for 2 or 3 days. If lesions persist, this regimen should be repeated in 3 to 7 days. Topical thiabendazole should be given as a 10% suspension overlaid with 0.1% dexamethasone cream for 3 days. Comparison of single-dose ivermectin (12 mg) and albendazole (400 mg) reveals ivermectin to be superior to albendazole and less toxic. Penicillin or other appropriate antibiotics should be given for secondary bacterial infections.

Bibliography

Caumes E, Carriere J, Datry A, et al: A randomized trial of ivermectin versus albendazole for the treatment of cutaneous larva migrans. Am J Trop Med Hyg 49:641, 1993.

Davis CM, Israel RM: Treatment of creeping eruption with topical thiabendazole. Arch Dermatol 97:325, 1968.

Edelglass JW, Douglass MC, Stiefler R, et al: Cutaneous larva migrans in northern climates. A souvenir of your dream vacation. Am Acad Dermatol 7:353, 1982.

Katz R, Ziegler J, Blank H: Natural course of creeping eruption and treatment with thiabendazole. Arch Dermatol 91:420, 1965.

116 *Anisakidosis*

Robert H. Sudduth

DEFINITION. Anisakidosis is the disease caused by the larval nematodes belonging to the subfamily Anisakinae through the consumption of raw or inadequately cooked marine fish or squid. It is commonly called herring worm or codworm disease.

ETIOLOGY. The disease is usually caused by infection with the third-stage larvae of *Anisakis simplex* and *Pseudoterranova decipiens*; occasionally other *Anisakis* larvae are involved. *A. simplex* larvae are 19 to 36 mm in length and 0.3 to 0.6 mm in width and white or milky in color with a long stomach, an intestine with no cecum, and a blunt tail with mucron (type I larva). Rarely, another type of *Anisakis* larvae with a shorter stomach and attenuated tails (type II larva) causes human infection. *P. decipiens* larvae are 25 to 50 mm in length

and 0.3 to 1.2 mm in width and yellowish or brownish in color; they have an anteriorly projected cecum.

DISTRIBUTION AND TRANSMISSION. Anisakidosis occurs mainly in Japan, and less frequently in the Hawaiian islands and coastal areas of North America and northern Europe, where people consume raw or inadequately cooked saltwater fish or squid. Humans are usually infected by eating raw herring, salmon, cod, mackerel, flatfish, greenling, red snapper, and squid in which the infectious larvae are present. As of 1990 there have been more than 12,000 cases in Japan and only 519 cases in 19 countries outside of Japan. Fifty-one cases have been reported in the United States, where the disease is underdiagnosed and underreported. With the increased popularity of sushi and sashimi in the United States, the incidence is expected to increase.

Life Cycle. The primary hosts of *Anisakis* are dolphin, porpoise, and whale; those of *Pseudoterranova* are seal, fur seal, walrus, and sea lion. These sea mammals ingest third-stage larvae, which penetrate the gastric mucosa and develop into adult male and female worms. The worms live in clusters with their anterior ends embedded in the gastric wall, and from there they discharge their eggs into the sea (Fig. 116–1). Eggs develop and hatch in the cold water of the polar seas. Swimming second-stage larvae are ingested by small marine crustacea, e.g., krills, and develop to the third stage in their haemocoels. Third-stage larvae are transferred from krills to squid or fish and further from squid to fish or fish to fish by the predatory food chain. More than 150 species of fish become transport hosts of third-stage larvae. In general, third-stage larvae are concentrated in fish viscera; relatively few fish harbor larvae in their muscle. Among numerous trans-

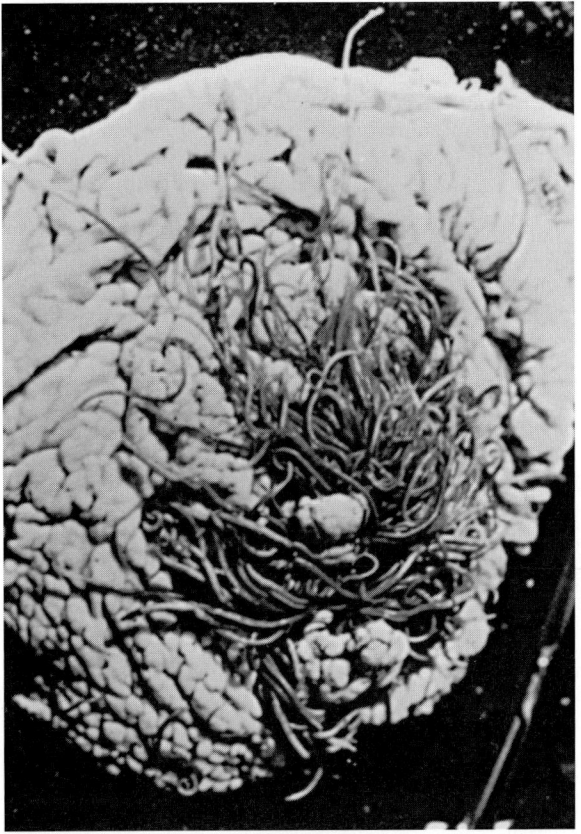

Figure 116–1. *Anisakis simplex* adult worms attached to the first stomach of a blue-white dolphin. (Courtesy of the Armed Forces Institute of Pathology. Photograph Neg. No. 76-2114.)

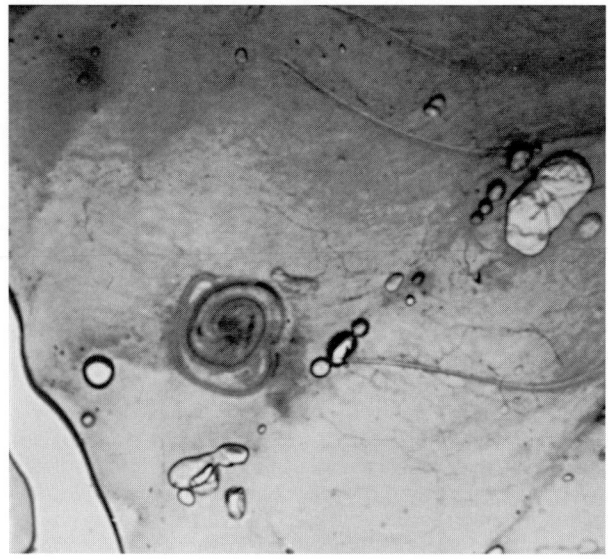

Figure 116–2. *Anisakis simplex* third-state larva in salmon fillet.

port hosts only the fish that have larvae in their flesh (Fig. 116–2) are important infectious sources for human anisakidosis. Herring, salmon, common mackerel, cod, and squid can transmit *Anisakis* infection, whereas cod, halibut, flatfish, greenling, and red snapper can transmit *Pseudoterranova* infection.

PATHOGENESIS AND PATHOLOGY. When humans consume raw or inadequately cooked infectious fish or squid, the larvae invade the submucosa of the stomach or intestine. The site of invasion is swollen and becomes hemorrhagic; larvae in the submucosa are surrounded by inflammatory cells, mostly eosinophils (Fig. 116–3). Occasionally, ecdysis occurs; however, the larvae die within 10 days and the exudative inflammation gradually subsides. Larvae can detach and be eliminated from the digestive tract, or if sufficient penetration has occurred, an eosinophilic granuloma develops around the dead worm, frequently forming a tumor-like nodule and prolonging the inflammatory response. With chronic anisakidosis, abscesses composed of numerous eosinophils, neutrophils, macrophages, and lymphocytes may form. There is evidence, both clinical and experimental, that the clinically

acute presentation is an Arthus-type allergic reaction, caused by reinfection in a sensitized host. Intestinal lesions are much more exudative and acute than stomach lesions.

CLINICAL MANIFESTATIONS. The clinical manifestations of anisakidosis are varied and depend largely on the site of penetration. In Japan, the stomach is involved in 94% of cases, the small intestine in 5%, and ectopic sites in 1%. In other countries, intestinal anisakidosis accounts for 75%, gastric 10%, and ectopic sites 15%. The reason for this difference is unclear. The disease may present acutely with severe abdominal pain, nausea, vomiting, diarrhea and urticaria, or occasionally it may have a chronic, indolent course with vague symptoms and intermittent abdominal pain. Rarely the larvae penetrate through the thickness of the gastrointestinal wall and migrate to various sites, causing symptoms that depend on the location. The *Pseudoterranova* larva appears to be less invasive than the *A. simplex* larva, and the most severe cases are thus due to the latter. *Pseudoterranova* is more frequently expelled by vomiting, terminating the disease.

Gastric Anisakidosis. The acute gastric presentation, presumably arising in a previously sensitized host, is the most commonly recognized clinical presentation. This usually begins 1 to 12 hours after eating the fish or squid. Most patients complain of severe epigastric pain with nausea and vomiting. After a few days, the acute symptoms subside and a vague epigastric pain remains with intermittent nausea and vomiting for several weeks or months. Mild fever and leukocytosis are usually present, and eosinophilia develops after 24 hours if the worms are not removed.

Intestinal Anisakidosis. This is caused by *A. simplex* larvae or (rarely) by *Pseudoterranova* larvae. They usually invade the distal ileum. The symptoms can again be acute, even presenting with peritonitis, or the disease can be mild and chronic. Some cases have been found only incidentally at laparotomy. Usually 1 to 5 days after the infecting meal, the patient has the sudden onset of abdominal pain with nausea and vomiting. Slight or no fever and a mild leukocytosis with eosinophilia are observed, and peritoneal fluid may be present. The inflammatory changes can lead to narrowing of the intestinal lumen and produce abdominal pain from obstruction. The inflammation generally slowly resolves. Usually, inflammation is limited to the intestine, and the parietal peritoneum is not involved.

Ectopic Anisakidosis. Ectopic anisakidosis refers to cases in which the larvae are found outside of their usual location

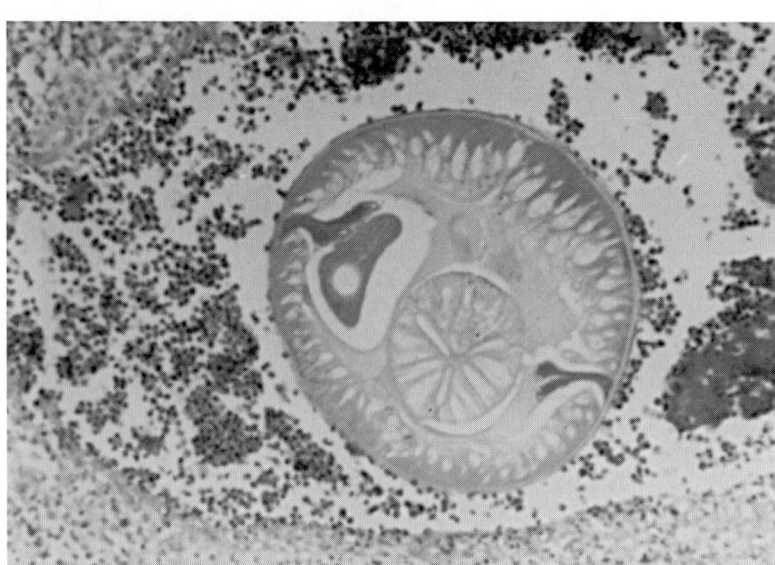

Figure 116–3. Intestinal anisakidosis with extensive infiltration of eosinophils surrounding an intact larva.

in the stomach or distal small bowel. These sites are most commonly elsewhere in the gastrointestinal tract, including the oropharynx, the esophagus, various small bowel locations, and the colon. In North America one of the most common presentations is the "tingling throat syndrome," in which the patient may actually feel the worm in the oropharynx or proximal esophagus; this syndrome is usually due to *Pseudoterranova* larvae, and it is most often terminated by the patient coughing up the worm.

True extragastrointestinal anisakidosis occurs when the larva penetrates the full thickness of the stomach or intestine and migrate to various sites. The condition is rare: only 45 cases have been reported in Japan. The most common site has been the abdominal cavity, but has also included the mesentery, liver, pancreas, ovary, lymph node, subcutaneous tissue, and pleural cavity. These sites are usually associated with mild clinical symptoms, and the larvae are occasionally found incidentally at operation.

DIAGNOSIS. A history of consumption of raw or inadequately prepared fish or squid shortly before the onset of the disease is an important clue. In the case of gastric anisakidosis, symptoms most commonly mimic peptic ulcer disease, cholecystitis, gastroenteritis, or an acute abdomen; endoscopy is the most useful method for diagnosis. Larvae invading the stomach wall are recognized easily and can be removed for morphologic identification of the worm. Usually only one larva is involved, although multiple larvae have occasionally been found. The most common endoscopic finding is a fairly severe edema on the greater curvature of the stomach, but any site may be involved. Other findings may include erythema, erosions, a tumor-like nodule, and occasional ulcers. If endoscopy is delayed and the worm is no longer present, the thickened gastric folds may suggest the diagnosis of lymphoma or gastric carcinoma, whereas a biopsy showing eosinophils could suggest idiopathic eosinophilic gastritis. The acute onset, history of raw fish ingestion, and resolution with time help resolve the dilemma. An upper gastrointestinal series can reveal most of the same findings, but has the disadvantage of not allowing worm removal or directed biopsies. If endoscopic ultrasonography is performed, a thickened gastric wall involving largely the submucosa is found, with a heterogenic echo pattern in this layer.

Generally, intestinal anisakidosis is difficult to diagnose. Symptoms of an acute abdomen following consumption of raw fish strongly suggest intestinal anisakidosis. However, it mimics appendicitis, Crohn's disease, intestinal obstruction, and diverticulitis, and patients often undergo laparotomy. A characteristic history combined with no or slight fever, mild leukocytosis with eosinophilia, and peritoneal fluid is key to the diagnosis. Barium studies are helpful when they show luminal narrowing of the terminal ileum with proximal dilatation. Serodiagnosis has the potential to be helpful in intestinal and extragastrointestinal cases. Enzyme-linked immunosorbent assays and radioallergosorbent tests have been developed and appear sensitive and specific for *A. simplex*, but are not commercially available.

TREATMENT. The patient may regurgitate the worm, thereby terminating the illness. Endoscopic removal of the larvae is the best treatment for gastric anisakidosis. Endoscopy needs to be performed early before the larva becomes embedded in the submucosa, since the symptoms may persist until the larva is resorbed. Larvae invading the stomach wall are removed easily by the forceps of an endoscope. After removal, symptom resolution is usually prompt and dramatic. Eosinophilic granuloma present in chronic gastric anisakidosis requires no surgery; only symptomatic conservative treatment is recommended. Intestinal anisakidosis, if correctly diagnosed, also needs no surgery and should be treated conservatively with fluids and nutritional therapy. Effective drugs are not yet established. Corticosteroids were believed to hasten clinical resolution in one case. This has some appeal given the presumed allergic nature of the process; however, there are no controlled trials.

PREVENTION. Distribution of anisakid worms is worldwide, and the contamination of marine fish and squid with anisakid larvae is widespread. Salmon and Pacific rockfish (red snapper) are implicated most often in the transmission of anisakidosis in the United States. The best prevention is not to consume raw or inadequately cooked, salted, or marinated fish or squid. The Food and Drug Administration recommends that all fish intended for raw (including marinated or partly cooked) consumption be blast-frozen to $-35°C$ ($-31°F$) or below for 15 hours, or be regularly frozen to $-23°C$ ($-10°F$) or below for 7 days. However, sushi served in professional sushi bars are rarely responsible for *Anisakis* infection. Professional chefs do not usually use fish, e.g., salmon, cod, mackerel, herring, whiting, haddock, which are infected with anisakid larvae for preparation of sushi.

INFECTION BY LARVAL EUSTRONGYLIDS. Three fishermen in Baltimore, MD, developed severe abdominal pain after swallowing live freshwater minnows. Laparotomy demonstrated roundworms penetrating the cecum and ecchymosis of the transverse colon in one patient and perforation of the cecum in a second. The third parient, who developed similar symptoms, recovered 4 days later without surgery. Roundworms were found in the abdominal cavity of both patients who had surgery. Minnows collected in East Baltimore waters were infected with roundworms identical to those recovered from the two patients at surgery. These worms were identified as fourth-stage larval nematodes of the genus *Eustrongylides*. They were 80 to 120 mm long and 1 to 2 mm in diameter.

A 24-year old man from New York City developed eustrongylidiasis from eating sushi. He had right lower abdominal pain with exquisite tenderness, guarding, and rebound tenderness. An appendectomy was performed. The appendix and distal ileum appeared normal, but a 4.2 cm pinkish red fourth-stage larva of the genus *Eustrongylides* was detected moving on the surgical drapes.

Nematodes of the genus *Eustrongylides* lack phasmids and belong to the subclass Adenophorea, order Enoplida, and superfamily Dioctophymatoidea. Adult eustrongylids are parasites of the gastrointestinal tract of fish-eating birds, and their larvae are found in the connective tissue or body cavity of freshwater fish. Amphibians, reptiles, and, rarely, mammals may become infected with larval eustrongylids and may be paratenic hosts.

Bibliography

Centers for Disease Control: Intestinal perforation by larval *Eustrongylides*—Maryland. MMWR 31:383, 1982.
Ikeda K, Kamashiro R, Kifune T: Nine cases of acute gastric anisakiasis. Gastrointest Endosc 35:304, 1989.
Ishikura H, Kikuchi K, Nagasawa K, et al: Anisakidae and anisakidosis. Prog Clin Parasitol 3:43, 1993.
Kakizoe S, Kakizoe H, Kakizoe K, et al: Endoscopic findings and clinical manifestations of gastric anisakiasis. Am J Gastroenterol 90:761, 1995.
Kliks MM: Anisakis in the western United States: Four new case reports from California. Am J Trop Med Hyg 32:526, 1983.
Oshima T: Anisakiasis—Is sushi bar guilty? Parasitol Today 3:44, 1987.
Oshima T, Kliks M: Effect of marine mammal parasites on human health. Int J Parasitol 17:415, 1987.
Sakai K, Ohtani A, Muta H, et al: Endoscopic ultrasonography findings in acute gastric anisakiasis. Am J Gastroenterol 87:1618, 1992.
Sakanari JA, McKerrow JH: Anisakiasis. Clin Microbiol Rev 2:278, 1989.
Wittner M, Turner JW, Jacquette G, et al: Eustrongyloidiasis—A parasitic infection acquired by eating sushi. N Engl J Med 320:1124, 1989.

117 *General Principles*

John H. Cross

The phylum Platyhelminthes (flatworms) contains three classes of animals. The classes Trematoda and Cestoidea contain only parasitic forms, whereas the class Turbellaria contains chiefly free-living species. Animals belonging to the Platyhelminthes characteristically have a flattened, bilaterally symmetric body, without a body cavity or coelom. Generally, flatworms are hermaphroditic and most are symbionts, living on or in the body of their hosts.

Most trematode (fluke) species are parasites of vertebrates and undergo initial development in snails through a series of multiplying larval stages. The trematodes display marked host specificity toward their snail host but less so toward the vertebrate host. Many flukes that primarily infect other animals are found sporadically as human parasites, whereas those considered to be primary human parasites may have either domestic or wild animals as important reservoir hosts (Tables 117–1 to 117–3).

TREMATODES OF HUMANS EXCLUSIVE OF THE SCHISTOSOMES. The trematodes of humans, exclusive of the schistosomes, are hermaphroditic, generally flat and leaf shaped as adults, and range in length from a few millimeters to several centimeters. A representative life cycle, that of the lung fluke *Paragonimus*, is shown in Figure 117–1. Adult worms have both oral and ventral suckers, a digestive tract that bifurcates a short distance below the oral sucker and ends blindly, and complete sets of male and female organs. Two testes are located usually in the posterior part of the body. A single ovary anterior to the testes connects with a system of laterally placed glands that produce the eggshell materials and with a uterus that coils to a genital pore located near the ventral sucker (Fig. 117–1). Eggs are usually passed in host feces (Fig. 117–2). In all species, the eggs possess an operculum (a lidlike covering or escape hatch) at one end of

the shell through which the larva escapes. Generally, free-swimming ciliated miracidia are released and penetrate the first intermediate host, a freshwater snail. In some species, however, the egg must be ingested by an appropriate snail host before emergence of the miracidium. Within the snail, a complex developmental cycle results in liberation, after several weeks, of large numbers of the free-swimming larval stage, the cercariae. After a brief period of independent existence, the larvae encyst in or on a second intermediate host, which (depending on the trematode species involved) may be another mollusk, a fish, a crab or other crustacean, or a plant. The encysted metacercaria (actually an immature adult worm) cannot undergo further development until ingested by humans or another suitable definitive (vertebrate) host. In such a host, after excystation is facilitated by the digestive process, the worms develop in a relatively simple way to adulthood, although some worms that do not parasitize the intestinal tract may migrate through the body.

The importance of human trematode infections as public health problems was recognized at an international conference on food-borne parasitic zoonoses held in Thailand in 1990, and in 1993 a World Health Organization Study Group convened in the Philippines to carry out in-depth discussions specifically on food-borne trematodiases. An estimated 40

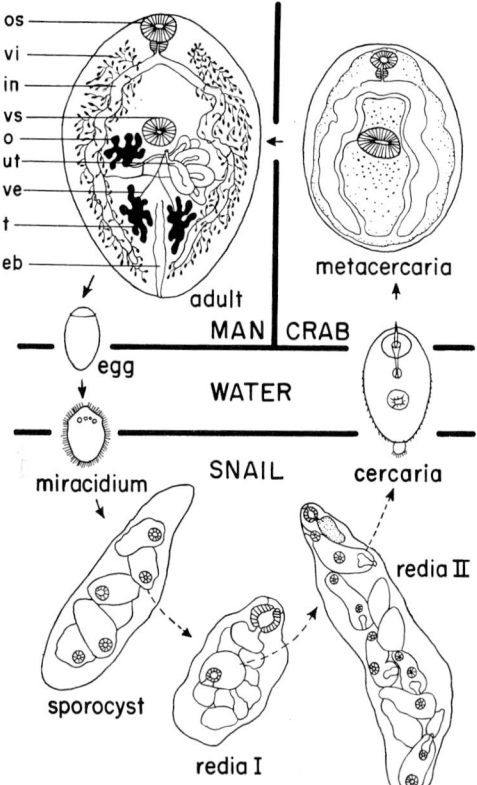

Figure 117–1. *Paragonimus,* an example of a trematode life cycle: *eb,* excretory bladder; *in,* intestinal caeca; *o,* ovary; *os,* oral sucker; *t,* testis; *ut,* uterus; *ve,* vas efferens; *vi,* vitellaria; *vs,* ventral sucker. (From Markell EK, Voge M: Medical Parasitology, 5th ed. Philadelphia, WB Saunders, 1981.)

TABLE 117–1. Reservoirs of Some Intestinal Flukes

Species of Trematode	Host	Typical Location in Host
Fasciolopsis buski	Pigs, occasionally dogs, rabbits, and humans	Duodenum, jejunum
Echinostoma ilocanum	Dogs, rats, mice, and humans	Small intestine
Echinochasmus perfoliatus	Dogs, cats, pigs, foxes, and humans	Small intestine
Heterophyes heterophyes	Cats, dogs, foxes, other piscivorous mammals, and humans	Small intestine
Metagonimus yokogawai	Piscivorous mammals, mice (experimental infection), pelicans, and humans	Small intestine
Gastrodiscoides hominis	Pigs, "mouse deer" (*Tragulus napu*), rats (*Rattus brevicaudatus*), and humans	Cecum, colon

TABLE 117–2. Reservoirs of Some Liver Flukes

Species of Trematode	Host	Typical Location in Host
Clonorchis sinensis	Dogs, cats, and humans	Biliary passages
Opisthorchis felineus	Dogs, cats, foxes, pigs, rats, martens, wolverines, beavers, rabbits, seals, and humans	Biliary and pancreatic passages
Opisthorchis viverrini	Dogs, cats, civet cats, piscivorous mammals, and humans	Biliary passages
Fasciola hepatica	Sheep, cattle, wild rabbits, hares, other herbivorous and omnivorous mammals, and humans	Liver and biliary passages
Fasciola gigantica	Cattle, water buffalo, other herbivorous mammals, and humans	Biliary passages
Dicrocoelium dendriticum	Sheep, goats, deer, other herbivorous and omnivorous mammals, and humans	Biliary passages

TABLE 117–3. Reservoirs of Some Lung Flukes

Species of Trematode	Host	Typical Location in Host
Paragonimus westermani	Tigers, cattle, many crab- or crayfish-eating mammals, and humans	Lungs
Paragonimus kellicotti	Mink, many other crayfish-eating mammals, and humans	Lungs
Paragonimus africanus	Mongooses (two species), civet cats, dogs, and humans	Lungs
Paragonimus miyazakii	Weasels, yellow martens, dogs, wild boars, and experimentally in rats, cats, dogs, rabbits, and humans	Lungs

million people of 750 million at risk are infected with one or more of 100 different species of flukes. Infections with trematodes are more common in humans worldwide than are infections with any other group of helminths. Unfortunately, these parasitoses are being ignored by public health authorities.

SCHISTOSOMES OF HUMANS. The schistosome species that infect humans differ in several ways from other trematodes. They are diecious organisms (separate sexes) that live in the mesenteric or vesicular veins; infection results from skin invasion by free-swimming cercariae in fresh water. The schistosome species differ from each other in internal and external morphology of the adults (Fig. 118–2), in shape of their eggs (especially the form and location of the single spine on the shell) (Fig. 118–3), in the snails that serve as intermediate hosts (Fig. 118–5), and in the range of mammalian hosts they parasitize.

The body of the male has a short preacetabular portion and a wide, flattened postacetabular portion, whereas the female (up to 2.6 by 0.03 cm) is filiform, is round in transverse section, and has a thinner but longer body. Adults have

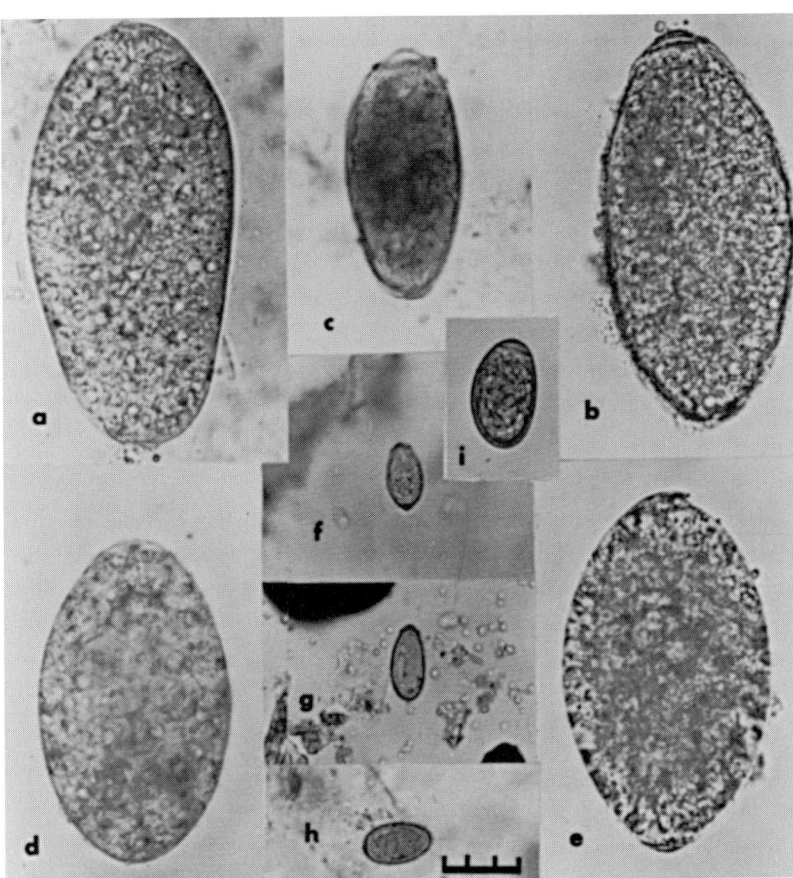

Figure 117–2. Some trematode eggs. *a, Fasciola gigantica; b, Fasciola hepatica; c, Paragonimus westermani; d, Fasciolopsis buski; e, Echinostoma* species; *f, Opisthorchis viverrini; g, Clonorchis sinensis; h, Metagonimus yokogawai; i, Dicrocoelium dendriticum.* (Eggs of *O. viverrini, M. yokogawai,* and *D. dendriticum* kindly supplied by Dr. Lawrence Ash.) All eggs photographed at same magnification: whole scale equals 30 µm.

a glandular anterior end and a ventral sucker (acetabulum) on the ventral surface. The alimentary system is an oral cavity that leads to the esophagus and then to the gut, which bifurcates into two ceca that reunite posteriorly to form a single posterior stem that ends blindly. The male reproductive system includes a number of testes dorsal and posterior to the ventral sucker, the number and arrangement varying according to species. Females have an elongated ovary in their posterior half, the location of which also varies with the species. The male worm possesses a ventral longitudinal cleft, the gynecophoric canal, in which a female is enclosed. Nonoperculated eggs are passed in host feces, except for one species, *Schistosoma haematobium*, in which they are passed in host urine. On reaching fresh water, the eggs hatch by rupture, releasing miracidia (Fig. 118–4) that swim in search of an appropriate snail host. After penetrating the snail, the miracidia undergo polyembryonic multiplication that gives rise to and release of large numbers of infective cercariae. The life cycle is completed when the free-swimming cercariae penetrate the skin of the human or animal definitive host and complete their development in the liver and then in the mesenteric or vesicular blood vessels (Fig. 118–6).

Bibliography

Beaver PC, Jung RC, Cupp EW (eds): Clinical Parasitology, 9th ed. Philadelphia, Lea & Febiger, 1984.

Binford CH, Connor DH (eds): Pathology of Tropical and Extraordinary Diseases. An Atlas. Washington, DC, Armed Forces Institute of Pathology, 1976.

Cross JH (ed): Emerging problems in food-borne parasitic zoonoses: Impact on agriculture and public health. Proceedings of the 33rd SEAMEO-TROPMED Regional Seminar. Southeast Asian J Trop Med Public Health 22(Suppl):395, 1991.

Malek EA (ed): Snail-Transmitted Parasitic Diseases Vol 1 & 2. Boca Raton, Florida, CRC Press, 1980.

Rollinson D, Simpson AJG (eds): The Biology of Schistosomes. From Genes to Latrines. San Diego, Academic Press, 1987.

World Health Organization: Control of foodborne trematode infections. Report of a WHO Study Group. World Health Organ Tech Rep Ser 849:157, 1995.

118 *Schistosomiasis*

G. Thomas Strickland and Bernadette L. Ramirez

DEFINITION. Schistosomiasis is a parasitic disease with a wide range of clinical manifestations that affects more than 200 million people in 77 countries. Infection with *Schistosoma japonicum, S. mansoni,* or *S. haematobium* and several other species of the digenetic trematode *Schistosoma* results in schistosomiasis, also known as snail fever. Infection takes place when cercariae, shed into fresh water by snail intermediate hosts, penetrate the skin of an individual exposed to this water. After multiorgan migration, adult worms abide in intestinal and bladder venules. Human disease is primarily associated with the host's granulomatous response to eggs retained in the tissues.

The public health importance of schistosomiasis is often underrated for several reasons. First, like all helminthic infections, the distribution of worms in any community is extensive but uneven, i.e., a minority have heavy infections and severe disease, while the majority have lighter infections and fewer symptoms. Second, severe disease usually follows after numerous years of silent or mildly symptomatic infection. Only 10% of infected individuals have severe clinical disease;

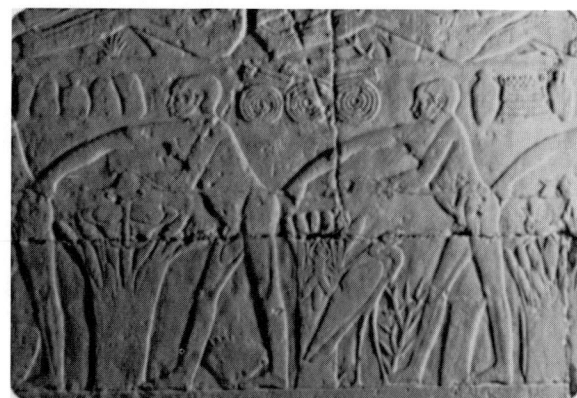

***Figure* 118–1.** Photograph of Nineteenth Dynasty Egyptian Pharaonic temple mural showing a boatman with ascites and scrotal edema said to be the result of hepatosplenic schistosomiasis. (Courtesy of Mr. Abdel Aziz Salah, U.S. Naval Medical Research Unit No. 3. Cairo, Egypt.)

this still represents 20 million seriously ill people worldwide. Of the remaining 180 million infected people, half are estimated also to have symptoms, a public health problem of immense scope.

HISTORY. The probable biologic origin of *S. japonicum* was the Yangtze River Valley; that of *S. mansoni* was the upper Nile River basin; and that of *S. haematobium* was the lake plateau of Africa. Ancient Egyptian papyri refer to hematuria in males, and Nineteenth Dynasty Pharonic temple murals depict men with probable ascites and scrotal edema, commonly thought to be the result of hepatosplenic schistosomiasis (Fig. 118–1). This dates the African clinical disease as early as 1500 B.C. Other clinical descriptions have been found in Babylonian inscriptions, medieval Arabic literature, and Napoleonic remembrances of the "menstruating males of Egypt." Furthermore, calcified *Schistosoma* eggs have been identified in Egyptian mummy tissue from the Twentieth Dynasty (1200 to 1090 B.C.). In China, there are records of schistosomiasis of comparable antiquity. *Schistosoma* infections in the New World are more recent in origin, probably beginning with African slave trade to the Americas during the 16th and 17th centuries.

In 1851, Theodore Bilharz, whose name became synonymous with the clinical human disease (bilharziasis), first identified the etiologic agent of Egyptian endemic hematuria as the worm *Distomum haematobium* (later *Schistosoma haematobium*) during an autopsy of a patient in Cairo, Egypt. He later described the underlying pathology of the bladder. Sir Patrick Manson did not note the differentiation of the three major disease-causing species until the early 20th century. The complete life cycle of the parasite and the role of the snail intermediate host were defined in 1913 by Miyairi and were confirmed experimentally by Leiper in 1915. McDonough introduced the first effective chemotherapy using tartar emetic in 1918. The association of chronic liver disease, characterized by hepatomegaly and splenomegaly, with *S. mansoni*, and by inference, *S. japonicum*, was not apparent until Symmers' description of clay pipestem fibrosis in Egypt in 1904 and Say's report on splenomegaly in 1924. Interest in schistosomiasis remained limited until World War II, when tropical parasitology became more important as military troops became exposed to infection. For instance, General MacArthur's successful reinvasion of the Philippines in 1944 started on the island of Leyte, which is a major center of transmission of *S. japonicum* infection. During the late 1950s, a mouse model of *S. mansoni* infection with hepatosplenomegaly, portal hypertension, and esophageal varices was developed. It was also during this time that the pathology was determined to be due to schistosome eggs trapped in the presinusoidal venules of the liver. In the 1960s, the immunologic complexities of the host's granulomatous response to the schistosome egg and the mechanisms of concomitant protective immunity began to be defined by Kenneth Warren and others. It was further determined in the 1970s that chronic disease often takes decades to develop and is associated with heavy worm burdens. Along with the renewed interest in schistosomiasis have come focal control programs, successfully carried out in Japan and Puerto Rico, as well as less toxic and more effective antischistosomal drugs.

ETIOLOGY

Parasite Species. *Schistosoma*, the only bisexual genus of the class Trematoda, constitutes a large group of helminth parasites that differ from other human flukes by (1) living in blood vessels, (2) having nonoperculated eggs, and (3) lacking an encysted metacercarial stage. The human is a definitive host for *S. japonicum*, *S. mansoni*, and *S. haematobium*; *S. mekongi* and *S. malayi* (the latter two being separate disease-causing schistosomes similar to *S. japonicum*); and *S. intercalatum*. *S. mattheei*, which causes natural infections in sheep, cattle and horses, also causes human infections and pathology. *S. bovis*, *S. rodhaini*, *S. margrebowiei*, *S. spindale*, and *S. incognitum* eggs or worms have been found in humans without evidence of significant pathophysiology. The cercariae of approximately 20 species of nonhuman schistosomes, mostly infecting birds or small mammals, penetrate human skin, die without migration or maturation, and produce a dermatitis.

Biology of Parasite Stages

Adult Worms. These are barely visible without using magnification, being from 12 to 26 mm in length and from 0.3 to 0.6 mm in width. The adult male worm is shorter and thicker than the longer, slender female. The male has a longitudinal body cleft, the gynecophoral canal or schist, in which the female lies in a folded fashion most of her life (Fig. 118–2). Both sexes have rudimentary attachment structures, the oral and ventral suckers. The former surrounds the mouth. The alimentary canal passes from the oral cavity into an esophagus, dividing just anterior to the ventral sucker and forming two intestinal canals that fuse near the middle of the worm to form a single trunk. This tubular structure ends in a blind

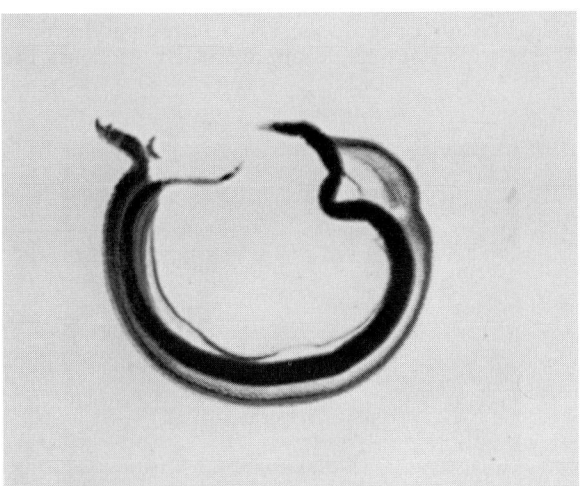

***Figure* 118–2.** *Schistosoma mansoni.* Adult male with female in gynecophoral canal (× 10). The black color in the female is due to pigment in ingested erythrocytes. (Courtesy of the Armed Forces Institute of Pathology, Photograph Neg. No. 56–3334.)

terminus near the posterior end of the worm. The male tegumental surface may be tuberculated or smooth, depending on the species; the surface of the female worm is smooth in all species.

The reproductive organs vary slightly in number and location among the major schistosome species. In general, those in male worms consist of several testes, a number of vasa deferentia joining to form a vesicula seminalis, an ejaculatory duct, and a genital pore situated posterior to the ventral sucker. The female reproductive system is composed of a single elongated ovary, an oviduct, vitelline glands, shell glands, and an ootype in the central canal that passes forward to the uterus. The straight or slightly sinuous tubule-shaped uterus leads to the genital pore just behind the ventral sucker. The rudimentary excretory system consists of a few special function cells joined in a series of collecting tubules.

The worms take up nutrients by way of their intestine and integument. The energy metabolism of the adult worm is nearly totally dependent on energy-inefficient anaerobic glycolysis. Only egg production requires oxygen and aerobic metabolism. The adult schistosome uses one fifth of its dry body weight of glucose per hour, converting 80% to lactic acid. Adult worms contain a proteolytic enzyme, hemoglobin protease, which breaks down hemoglobin, and the ingestion of red blood cells is important to their nutrition. As the gut terminates blindly, the insoluble hematin-like pigment is regurgitated. This pigment is phagocytized by the nearby hepatic reticuloendothelial cells and results in pigmentation of the host's liver. The high metabolic rate of the schistosome is due to the female worm's continuous high output of eggs.

Adult worms mate in the small vasculature of the liver and make a paired migration against the flow of venous blood to the predistined venous plexus. When the vessel caliber impedes further paired migration, the female progresses further alone and lays her eggs. The favored eventual location of the adult worm and, consequently, egg deposition varies according to species; *S. haematobium* is concentrated near the bladder, *S. mansoni* in the inferior mesenteric vessels of the large intestine, and *S. japonicum* in the superior mesenteric vessels of the large and small intestine. Studies of transmigrated populations suggest that 3 to 7 years, and up to 30 years in exceptional cases, is the usual life span of adult worms.

Ova. Schistosome eggs are round or oval with one spiny appendage (Fig. 118–3). Size and shape vary according to species. Each fertilized female worm releases many eggs each day; notably, adult *S. japonicum* female worms lay as many as 3500 eggs daily (Table 118–1). The eggs of *S. mansoni* are released singly, whereas those of *S. japonicum* and *S. haematobium* are deposited in groups. Clusters of *S. japonicum* eggs have a greater predilection for calcification. Each egg contains a single miracidium, a ciliated larval stage, which matures over 6 to 10 days and may remain alive up to 3 weeks after oviposition. Most eggs desiccate and die if they do not come into contact with fresh water soon after leaving the host. However, mature *S. japonicum* eggs may survive outside the body for up to 80 days under moist winter conditions, e.g., in China and Japan, where they hatch and infect snails the following spring. It is likely that the spiny appendage of the egg serves as an anchor against blood flow. All schistosome eggs absorb nutrients and secrete histiolytic enzymes, which facilitate their teleologic passage through tissue into the environment. Approximately 50% of released schistosome eggs are excreted into the environment in a viable state.

Miracidia. Human schistosome eggs, housing the miracidia, are viable only in fresh water. The hatching and survival

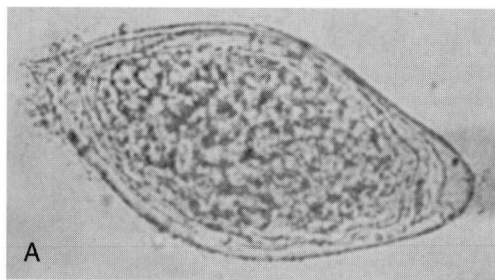

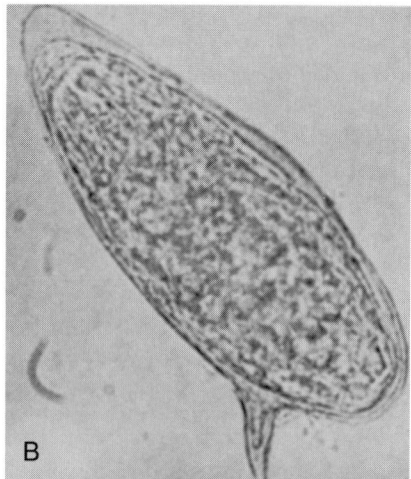

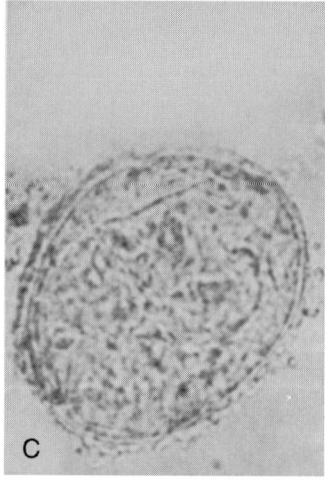

Figure 118–3. Ova of schistosomes commonly infecting humans. *A, S. haematobium* with terminal spine, taken from urine (× 500). *B, S. mansoni* with prominent lateral spine, taken from feces (× 500). *C, S. japonicum* taken from feces (× 500). (Courtesy of Dr. R. L. Roudabush. Ward's Natural Science Establishment, Rochester, NY.)

gonadal tissue of the snail. Cercariae metamorphose from germinal cells in the daughter sporocysts, migrate through the vascular sinuses, and exit from the edge of the snail's mantle. Sporocysts may regenerate and produce more cercariae. During this 4- to 6-week asexual stage in the snail, as many as 100,000 cercariae may be produced by each snail. Snail life expectancy is reduced by schistosome infection because of damage to hepatic and gonadal tissue.

Cercariae. The infective larva emerges from the snail intermediate host under specific conditions of light and temperature. Maximum stimulants for shedding of *S. mansoni* and *S. haematobium* cercariae are provided by bright, direct sunlight and water temperatures of 24° to 30°C, leading to higher rates of transmission during the summer months in the subtropics. *S. japonicum* cercariae are shed at night. Snails may be infected by multiple miracidia, but the mean daily output of a snail singly infected with *S. mansoni* or *S. haematobium* is 500 to 2000 cercariae/day. Snails infected with *S. japonicum* yield only 2 to 20 cercariae/day.

Cercariae are unisexual fishlike organisms with a pear-shaped head and a forked tail, measuring 400 to 600 μm in length. The head contains oral and ventral suckers, flame cells, a primitive nervous system, and a nonfunctional gut. Cercariae may survive in fresh water up to 72 hours but gradually begin to lose infectivity after 12 hours. Although all species of cercariae are similar in appearance, their activity in water varies with the species: *S. mansoni* and *S. haematobium* cercariae move vertically, alternating between active movement toward the surface and slow sinking; *S. japonicum* cercariae attach themselves to the water surface film, where they tend to remain at rest unless disturbed. In contrast to schistosomula and adult worms, cercariae use aerobic metabolism. Cercariae attach themselves to the skin of the definitive host by their ventral or oral suckers, assisted by mucoid secretions from the postacetabular glands. Vertical, vibratory movements of the cercarial body and lytic secretions from the preacetabular penetration glands accomplish penetration of the skin, usually complete within 3 to 5 minutes. Only about 40% of cercariae that penetrate the skin eventually become viable adult worms. Survival is inversely related to the host's acquired immunity to schistosomiasis.

Schistosomula. The schistosomulum is the tail-less cercarial body that has undergone dramatic outer membrane modification. The trilaminar cercarial membrane becomes heptalaminar and is now tolerant to a saline environment. Metabolism shifts from an efficient tricarboxylic acid cycle to the less efficient anaerobic glycolysis. The schistosomulum remains in the subcutaneous tissue approximately 48 hours before

of the miracidia are dependent on freshwater contact at a temperature between 20° and 30°C. Miracidia are ovoid and about 160 μm long and are propelled by flagellating cilia on four rows of epidermal plates (Fig. 118–4). Miracidia demonstrate negative geotaxis and positive phototaxis. At a rate of about 700 cm/minute, miracidia swim to and attach to the soft part of the appropriate snail intermediate host. Lytic substances secreted from miracidial glands aid penetration.

Sporocysts. After snail penetration, the miracidium loses its cilia and becomes a nonmotile sac, the mother sporocyst. Over the next 10 to 15 days, germinal cells in the mother sporocyst differentiate into motile daughter sporocysts. The daughter sporocysts migrate to and grow in the hepatic and

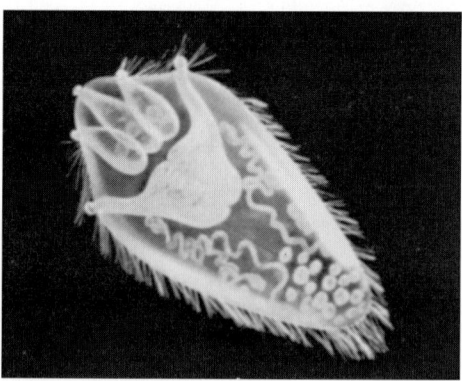

Figure 118–4. Miracidium of *S. japonicum* (darkfield, × 1000). (Courtesy of the Armed Forces Institute of Pathology, Photograph Neg. No. 218934–42.)

TABLE 118–1. Characteristics of Schistosomal Eggs

Species	Shape	Dimensions (μm)	Intrauterine Eggs	Eggs Produced/ Female Worm/Day
S. japonicum	Round, small lateral hook	70–100 × 50–65	30–50	500–3500
S. mansoni	Oval, prominent lateral spine	115–175 × 45–70	1–5	100–300
S. haematobium	Oval, terminal spine	110–170 × 40–70	20–100	20–200

beginning the 3- to 6-day migration to the lungs. Transition of the schistosomulum into an adult worm occurs between 1 to 4 weeks after skin penetration and is marked by the previously described anatomic developments. However, its most striking change is the development of an immunologically tolerant tegumental membrane.

Intermediate Host

Morphology and Biology. The snail intermediate hosts of *S. mansoni* and *S. haematobium* belong to the same family, *Planorbidae*, class Gastropoda (Table 136–1). These freshwater, nonoperculate, hermaphroditic snails have lungs and have hemoglobin in their blood, which gives them a characteristic pink or red color. The subfamily *Bulinidae* are the major intermediate hosts for *S. haematobium* and *S. intercalatum* and are distinguishable by their ovate shells (Figs. 118–5*A* and 136–2); the genus *Biomphalaria* serves as the intermediate host for *S. mansoni* and is characterized by its disk- or lens-shaped shells (Fig. 118–5*B* and 136–2).

The snail intermediate hosts of *S. japonicum* are members of *Oncomelania hupensis* species. They are unisexual, have gills instead of lungs, and are operculate freshwater snails with conical or turriculate shells that are adapted to live on land and tend to be confined to stable marshy habitats with constant high humidity (Table 136–1 and Figs. 118–5*C* and 136–1). *Oncomelania* species are amphibious rather than purely aquatic, a feature that complicates mollusciciding efforts in endemic regions. There are six geographic strains of *Oncomelania*: *O. hupensis* from China, *O. hupensis quadrasi* from the Philippines, *O. hupensis nosophora* from Japan, *O. hupensis lindoensis* from Indonesia, *O. hupensis formosana*, and *O. hupensis chiui* from Taiwan.

The freshwater mollusks that serve as intermediate hosts for incomplete avian schistosome infections (causing cercarial dermatitis) include species of *Lymnaea, Physa, Polypylis, Gyraulus, Segmentina, Stagnicola,* and *Chilina* (Table 136–1). Some of the saltwater molluscan hosts include representatives of *Nassrius, Littorina, Haminoea, Ceritthidea,* and *Batillaria.*

Life Cycle. The life cycle of the schistosome is complex and alternates between sexual (vertebrate host) and asexual (invertebrate host) generations. However, as seen by the survival of the schistosome from antiquity, the life cycle is obviously functional (Fig. 118–6).

Vertebrate Host. Following cercarial contact with skin for as little as 5 minutes, penetration takes place. The now tail-less schistosomula find their way into the microcirculation, to the heart, then to the lungs, and eventually (e.g., 5 to 10 days) to the small vessels of the liver. Histologic studies show that schistosomula are able to stretch the capillaries between the arterioles and venules of the lungs and thus remain within the circulation during this most hazardous stage of their migration. Those schistosomula not reaching the hepatic portal system on the first pass may return to the heart-lung circulation to restart the circuit. It is unlikely that any schistosomula running this gauntlet three times and not reaching the portal system survive. Over the next 2 to 3 weeks, following settling in the liver, schistosomula become mature unisexual worms, which, if they mate, begin laying eggs about 4 to 6 weeks after their initial cercarial skin penetration.

In the mesenteric venous plexus of the human host, the shorter, thicker male worm mates with the longer, thinner female worm in the male gynecophoral canal (Figs. 118–2 and 118–7). The female leaves the male after successful mating and migrates against the flow of blood to the small venules of the intestine or bladder, depending on the species. Incompletely embryonated eggs are laid, with approximately half being swept upstream, where they become lodged in the microvasculature of the liver and other organs, and 50% becoming attached to and embedded in the mesenteric venule wall. By a process not completely understood, but includes the release of lytic enzymes from the egg and assisted by host muscular contractions, the egg penetrates the lumen of the host organ, i.e., the intestine or bladder. The penetration process takes approximately 8 to 12 days, coincident with egg maturation. The process of penetration is arrested in a certain percentage of eggs, whereupon a granuloma is formed and the egg dies, calcifies, and is eventually absorbed by the host. Eggs that reach the lumen of the intestine or bladder are passed out in the stool or urine.

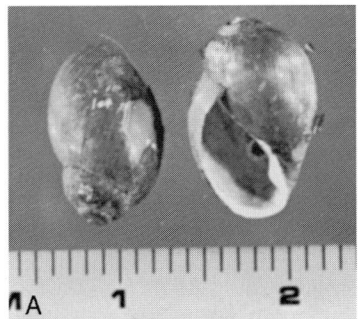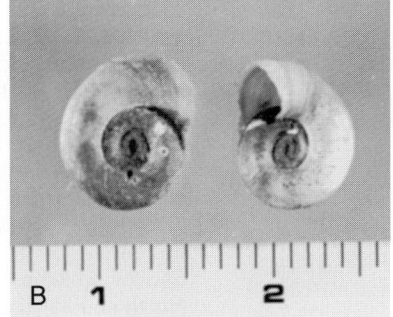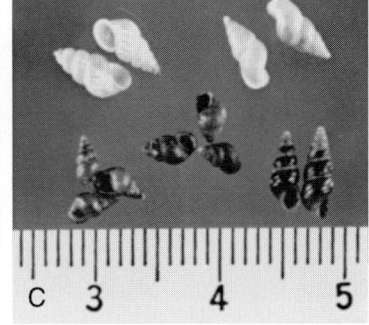

Figure 118–5. *A,* Both sides of an empty shell of a typical *Bulinus* species, the intermediate hosts of *S. haematobium* (× 5.7). (Courtesy of the Armed Forces Institute of Pathology, Photograph Neg. No. 70–11816–22.) *B,* Both sides of an empty shell of a typical *Biomphalaria* species, the intermediate hosts of *S. mansoni* (× 6.1). (Courtesy of the Armed Forces Institute of Pathology, Photograph Neg. No. 70–11816–21.) *C,* Empty shells of species of the genus *Oncomelania,* the intermediate hosts of *S. japonicum* (× 5). (Courtesy of the Armed Forces Institute of Pathology, Photograph Neg. No. 70–11816–18.)

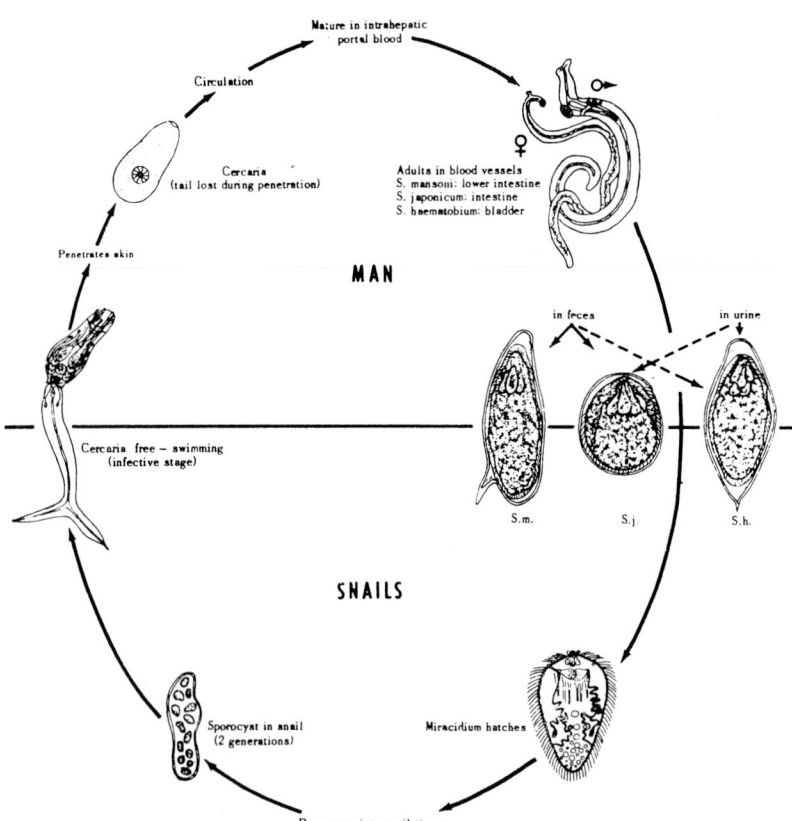

Figure 118–6. Life cycle of schistosomes in human infection. (From Melvin DM, Brooke MM, Sadun EH: Common Intestinal Helminths of Man. Life Cycle Charts. Atlanta, Georgia, Centers for Disease Control, 1964.)

Invertebrate Host. With satisfactory environment conditions, each mature egg that reaches fresh water hatches a single ciliated miracidium, which then seeks out its own regionally specific freshwater intermediate snail host. Fortunate miracidia penetrate the snail, lose their cilia, and metamorphose into two generations of sporocysts, which migrate to the digestive gland of the snail and mature into hundreds of fork-tailed cercariae. The intermediate host phase takes 3 to 5 weeks.

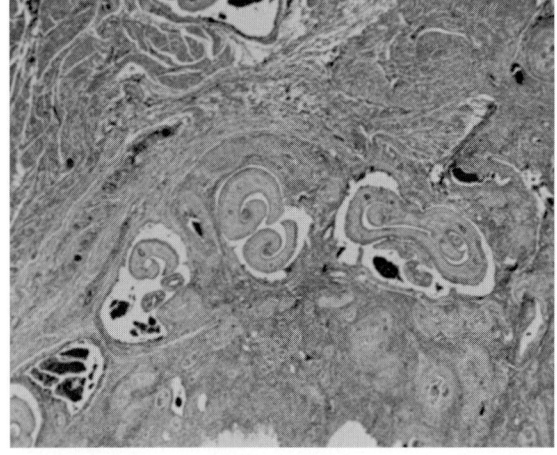

Figure 118–7. Biopsy sample from bladder wall showing worm pair(s) of *Schistosoma mansoni* within veins. The dark material is schistosomal pigment within the female. Note also the multiple granulomas and ulceration in the bladder mucosa and submucosa that is caused by the parasite ova. (× 25.) (Courtesy of the Armed Forces Institute of Pathology, Photograph Neg. No. 83–5186.)

At full maturity, cercariae emerge from the snail and swim tail first near the water surface in a teleologic search for a human host. Without successful host contact, the cercariae die within 48 to 72 hours.

Variations in Parasite and Snail Strains. Differences in schistosome distribution are linked to the locations of the intermediate snail hosts and their congeniality to different parasite strains. Studies of isoenzymes and random amplification of polymorphic DNA (RAPD) have provided mechanisms for the identification of parasite and snail strains. This has significant relevance to immunologic studies as well as to surveillance of schistosomiasis. These methods are being applied to studies of the schistosomes of the *S. haematobium* group and their intermediate hosts in Mali, Senegal, and Zambia. Molecular techniques had also established the existence of four different strains of *S. japonicum* in China. Already the assumption that all schistosome parasites of one species are the same is no longer tenable.

EPIDEMIOLOGY

Distribution. Schistosomiasis is increasing in prevalence, largely because of increased exposure to contaminated water associated with (1) greater use of irrigation for agricultural development; (2) increase and redistribution of world population (from hunter/nomad to farmer); and (3) inadequate control measures. An estimated 500 to 700 million people in 77 countries are believed exposed to infection and about 200 million are believed to be infected. The geographic distribution of schistosomiasis is confined to an area between 36° North and 34° South latitude, where freshwater temperatures average 25° to 30°C. In general, this includes (1) *S. japonicum*, which is transmitted only in China, Indonesia, and the Philippines by *Oncomelania hupensis* (Fig. 118–8); (2) *S. mansoni*, which is transmitted by members of the *Biomphalaria* genus in 53 countries from the Arabian peninsula, much of Africa,

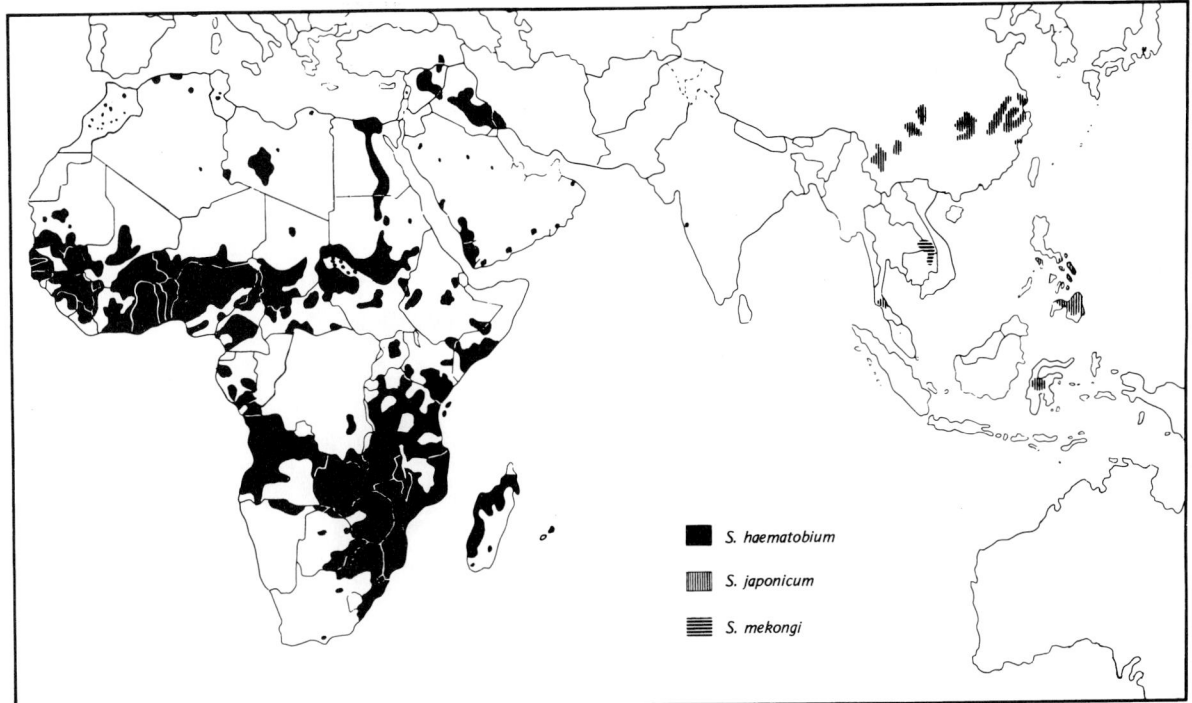

Figure 118–8. Global distribution of schistosomiasis due to *Schistosoma haematobium, S. japonicum,* and *S. mekongi.* (From The control of schistosomiasis: Report of a WHO Expert Committee. Geneva, World Health Organization, 1985. WHO Technical Report Series, No. 728, 1985, pp. 17–18. Reprinted by permission.)

Brazil, Suriname, Venezuela, and some Caribbean islands (Fig. 118–9); and (3) *S. haematobium,* which is transmitted by members of the *Bulinus africanus* group in 52 countries in sub-Saharan Africa, by tetraploid members of the *B. tropicus/truncatus* complex in the Mediterranean region and Southwest Asia, by members of *B. forskalii* group in Arabia and Mauritius, and by all three snail groups in West Africa (Fig. 118–8); and (4) less common species of human and animal schistosomes that occasionally infect humans. Incomplete infections with avian schistosomes, causing cercarial dermatitis, occur in fresh water throughout the Americas (particularly around the Great Lakes of the United States), Europe, Africa, Japan, and Malaysia.

Endemic Infection

Prevalence. Endemic populations show human infection beginning as early as 6 months of age. The peak intensity and prevalence of infection, as measured by egg excretion, usually occur between 8 to 12 years of age in heavily infected communities and somewhat later in lightly infected areas. In most communities, both the intensity and prevalence of ova excretion decrease after the preadolescent/adolescent peak. Infants usually first become infected while being bathed in the local irrigation canal, river, or lake. People, particularly children, in tropical and subtropical regions frequently use the same water source for defecation and urination, swimming, and bathing. The greatest cercarial exposure usually occurs in boys aged 5 to 10 years. Adolescents usually have less recreational time in the water but have more potential exposure during vocational activities, e.g., agricultural activities for males and some females and washing dishes and clothes and bathing younger siblings for females. Adults often have considerable exposure to cercariae-infested waters. The lower prevalence and intensity of infection among them reflects a partial acquired immunity, as well as less recreational exposure to the water. Many endemic rural pop-

ulations have a 30 to 50% prevalence rate of schistosome egg excretion at any one time; but almost everyone (i.e., 90%) has had an infection sometime during his or her life and many have repeated infections. These estimates, superimposed on the 500 to 700 million humans living in schistosome endemic areas, easily qualify schistosomiasis as one of the major public health problems in the world.

Morbidity. The distribution of infection intensity within a population is best described by a negative binomial curve, with a majority of infected community members harboring a small number of worms and only a small proportion having heavy worm burdens. Because the morbidity of schistosomiasis correlates with the worm burden, as determined by fecal and urinary egg counts, a large proportion of the infected community is asymptomatic during a single cross-sectional observation.

The precise morbidity of a schistosome infection can best be estimated by performing abdominal ultrasonography on random samples of members of communities. The toll taken by hepatosplenic disease with incapacitating ascites or fatal hematemesis or renal failure from chronic urinary obstruction and pyelonephritis is dramatic and important but undoubtedly reflects only a fraction of the schistosome burden in an endemic community. More difficult to measure is the impact of chronic mild diarrhea, anemia, hypoproteinemia, hematuria, bacteriuria, or other more subtle schistosome-associated symptoms and secondary diseases on the socioeconomic output of a population.

Schistosomiasis in Nonendemic Countries. Owing to the absence of an appropriate snail population and the presence of sanitation systems, schistosomiasis is not transmitted in North America and Europe. However, because of a large immigrant population from endemic areas, physicians in California, England, and France (large African, Middle East and Far East immigrant populations) and in New York and Flor-

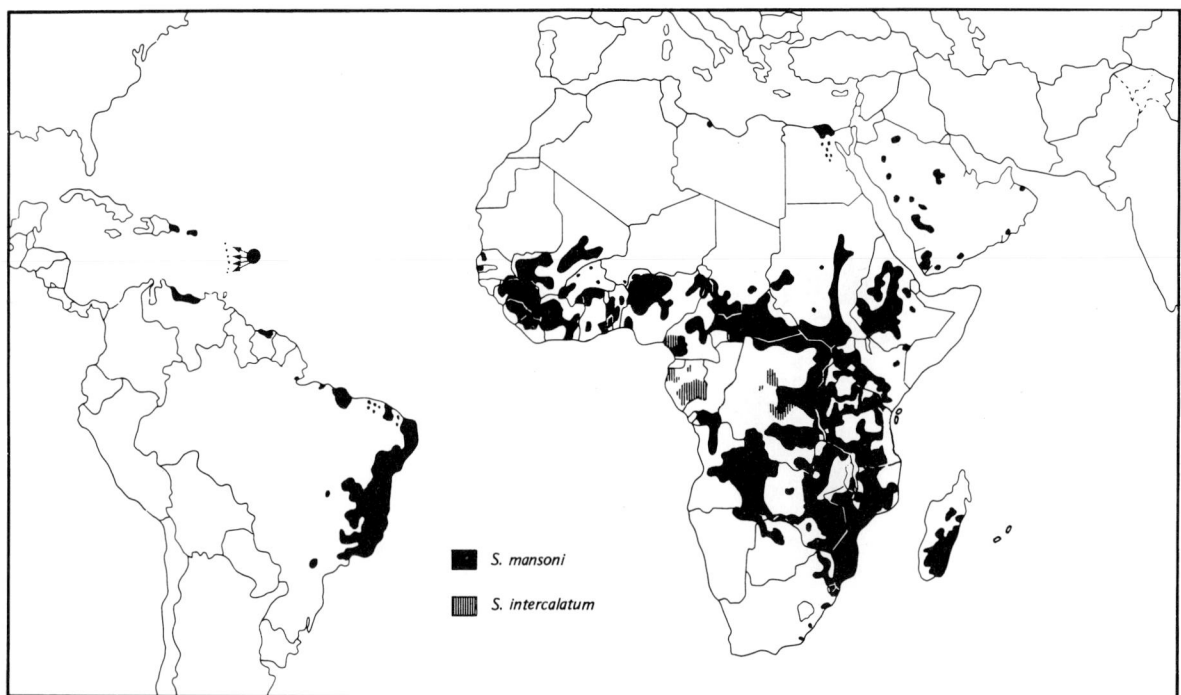

Figure 118–9. Global distribution of schistosomiasis due to *Schistosoma mansoni* and *S. intercalatum.* (From The control of schistosomiasis: Report of a WHO Expert Committee. Geneva, World Health Organization, 1985. WHO Technical Report Series, No. 728, 1985, pp. 17–18. Reprinted by permission.)

ida (large Caribbean immigrant populations) as well as university physicians (foreign students) through the developed world are increasingly being called on to diagnose and treat schistosomiasis. Also, in recent years, worldwide travel to other countries for business and pleasure has significantly increased. This sometimes results in exposure of immunologically naive individuals to schistosomiasis during their sojourn in endemic areas. Although the problem of transmission does not exist on the return of travelers to their nonendemic home countries, the diagnosis of schistosomiasis may not be straightforward, particularly when the patient presents with clinical manifestations that may be confused with other diseases.

Ecology
Snails. Endemic human schistosomiasis is ecologically most dependent on the presence of the snail intermediate host and the deposition of human and reservoir host excreta into its warm freshwater habitat. These snails are *Schistosoma* species–specific and frequently geographically specific (Table 136–1). For instance, *Oncomelania hupensis*, the snail hosts for *S. japonicum*, are not compatible with the similar species, *S. mekongi*, and the snail host for the latter, *Neotricula aperta*, cannot be infected with *S. japonicum*.

The aquatic snails important to the transmission of *S. mansoni* and *S. haematobium* live in lightly shaded, slow-flowing (15 M/minute), shallow (<2 M) waters, whereas the amphibious intermediate host of *S. japonicum* spends much of its time out of water, preferring moist soil at the edge of slow-flowing streams or irrigation canals. The infective dynamics of the intermediate host are such that low percentages of snails (e.g., 0.2 to 2%) are infected at any one time in an area highly endemic for schistosomiasis; even though a single snail may shed thousands of cercariae, the numbers detectable in an infested body of water are vanishingly small. Furthermore, snail cercarial shedding is seasonal in many areas.

Reservoir Hosts. There has been no identified functional reservoir host for *S. mansoni* and *S. haematobium.* However, *S. mansoni* infections have been found in rodents, baboons, and insectivores in Africa and South America. *S. haematobium* has been found in animals, but rarely. In marked contrast, reservoir hosts play a very important role in the transmission of *S. japonicum* infections. Natural infections have been demonstrated in 31 mammalian species, including dogs, cats, cattle, water buffaloes, pigs, horses, sheep, and goats. A few wild rodents have been found to be heavily infected. On the island of Taiwan, a strain of *S. japonicum* is infectious to water buffaloes and other animals but not to humans.

PATHOGENESIS AND PATHOLOGY. The pathogenesis and pathology of schistosomiasis are largely ones of host reaction to a foreign body, e.g., the different stages of the schistosome parasite. During the migratory larval stage, mild transient foreign body reactions are seen. However, most pathology results from the granulomatous response to the schistosome egg and is directly related to the intensity of infection. In chronic schistosomiasis, increased collagen synthesis occurs in the granuloma. Schistosomal fibrosis is caused by an imbalance between collagen synthesis and degradation.

Migratory Phase
Dermatitis. Cercariae penetrate the skin by opening the epidermis with lytic enzymes and wiggling into the epidermis (Fig. 118–10). Careful examination reveals mild erythema at the point of entry, but this usually goes unnoticed. This reaction is rarely seen on primary exposure to schistosomes since it requires prior exposures to cercariae. However, with prior cercarial humoral and cell-mediated immune (CMI) sensitization, schistosome dermatitis, a pruritic papular rash, may result. Pathologically, each focal lesion demonstrates edema and heavy dermal and epidermal eosinophil and mononuclear cell infiltrates. The greatest pathologic responses occur following exposure to avian schistosomes, probably because of subcutaneous cercarial death shortly

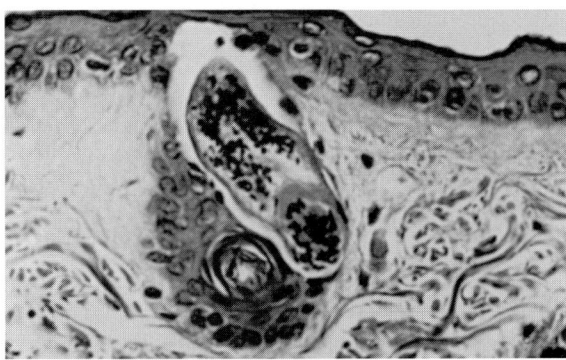

Figure 118–10. *S. mansoni* schistosomulum in dermis immediately after skin penetration in biopsy sample taken from a primate with experimental infection (× 255). (Courtesy of the Armed Forces Institute of Pathology, Photograph Neg. No. 74–9470.)

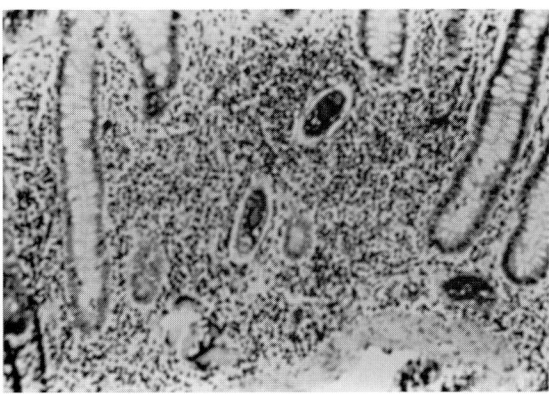

Figure 118–11. *S. mansoni* ova in the colon causing a heavy mononuclear cellular infiltrate in the submucosa. (Courtesy of U.S. Naval Medical Research Unit No. 3, Cairo, Egypt.)

after skin penetration. Lesser pathology is seen with *S. mansoni* and *S. haematobium*, and cercarial dermatitis is unusual with *S. japonicum*. Cercarial dermatitis resolves in 7 to 10 days without permanent tissue damage or scarring. Avian schistosomiasis is common in the Great Lakes and Delaware Bay regions in the United States and in Lake Geneva.

Pulmonary Lesions. The metamorphosed cercariae, the schistosomula, migrate via the hemolymphatic system through the heart to the lungs, usually without recognizable pathology. In heavy infections, schistosomula may produce a pneumonitis akin to hookworm pneumonitis. This pathogenic state is histologically undocumented but is logically one of eosinophil-dominated acute inflammatory response to a helminthic foreign body.

Hepatic Stage. The schistosomula next appear in the liver, by way of the vascular system, where they develop into adult worms without causing overt hepatic pathology. Adult worms migrate to the mesenteric and vesicular microvasculature, also without host damage. While living in the mesenteric vessels the adult worm is nonpathogenic.

Acute Schistosomiasis. Approximately 4 to 7 weeks after initial infection, at the time of first egg release, acute systemic schistosomiasis, also called Katayama fever, may occur. It is more common in *S. japonicum* infections but has been reported in infections with *S. mansoni* as well. This rarely fatal serum sickness–like disease results from the release of large numbers of schistosome eggs that antigenically cross react with an antibody to a shared cercariae-schistosomula-adult worm antigen. This results in an antigen:antibody ratio that leads to large-sized immune complexes that must be cleared by reticuloendothelial cells, causing hypertrophy of lymphoreticular tissue. The prototypic Katayama syndrome has been rarely seen in recent years, and thus the pathology remains incompletely defined.

Chronic Schistosomiasis. The pathogenesis of chronic schistosomiasis is almost exclusively explained by the host's granulomatous response to schistosome eggs deposited in tissues.

Egg Granuloma

HISTOPATHOLOGY. Eggs trapped in tissues release enzymes and other antigenic substances that sensitize local host lymphocytes. These lymphocytes secrete lymphokines, which recruit other immune cells (Fig. 118–11). Eventually, macrophages, lymphocytes, eosinophils, and fibroblasts make up a compact cellular infiltrate, the egg granuloma (Fig. 118–12). Schistosome egg granulomas are similar for all species, although in *S. japonicum* infections granulomas usually show a greater amount of necrosis, perhaps owing to egg clustering

at the site of inflammation and greater amounts of diffusible egg toxins. Early, acute granulomas are usually composed of eosinophils and neutrophils as well as mononuclear cells. Macrophages, lymphocytes, fibroblasts, and multinucleated giant cells dominate the chronic granuloma. The acute granuloma is large and diffuse, whereas the more chronic granuloma is smaller and better circumscribed. The dynamics of the evolving egg granuloma are based on the concept of immune modulation. Collagen deposition and fibrosis are integral features of the chronic granuloma and account for most of the irreversible pathology.

The egg granuloma is protective as well as pathologic. Animal studies using athymic or otherwise lymphocyte-depleted mice incapable of generating a granulomatous response show hepatocellular necrosis in the area surrounding the schistosome egg. The same is true in other tissues and most authors agree that the granuloma reduces or confines this tissue necrosis.

IMMUNE RESPONSE. Induction of granulomatous inflammation is attributed to CD4+ T-helper lymphocytes. In the murine model, a variety of lymphokines and cytokines serve as mediators of the granulomatous inflammatory response. In the synchronous pulmonary granuloma model generated around intravenously injected eggs in naive mice, interleukin (IL)-1 mRNA expression and IL-1 production were detectable within the first 4 days of granuloma growth; 4 to 6 days

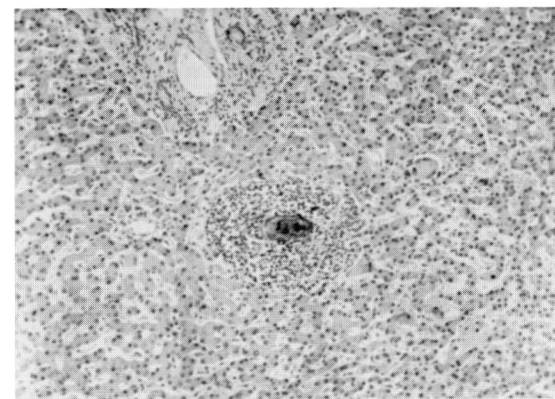

Figure 118–12. Egg of *S. mansoni* within hepatic lobule. Mixed leukocytic infiltrate around eggs may occur anywhere in the hepatic substance. (× 175.) (Courtesy of the Armed Forces Institute of Pathology, Photograph Neg. No. N–7661.)

afterward, tumor necrosis factor alpha (TNF-α) mRNA message appeared and cytokine production was observed. With the aging of the granuloma, production of both cytokines diminished. Thus, these cytokines are considered to be the primary recruiters of cellular aggregation in granuloma growth. The participation of TNF-α in granuloma formation was also confirmed in infected mice. While treatment of animals with anti-TNF-α antiserum decreased hepatic granuloma size, repeated injection of murine rTNF-α into chronically infected mice enhanced the downmodulated granuloma response. With the administration of specific antilymphokine monoclonal antibodies and recombinant murine lymphokines, as well as serial assays of lymphokine production by granuloma lymphocytes of infected mice, the role of γ-INF, IL-2, and IL-4 was delineated. γ-Interferon was found to be produced very early at the inception of the liver granulomatous response. By the time granulomas reached maximal size at 8 weeks after infection, the production declined. Concurrently IL-2 and IL-4 production peaked with maximal granuloma growth and declined with the onset of the immune modulation of the inflammation. Whereas these latter lymphokines appear to play a proinflammatory role, γ-IFN when administered in large doses diminished granulomatous inflammation, and thus regulates the maintenance of the granulomatous response. The T-helper cell population of the granulomas may also influence the lymphokine profile of the developing granuloma. So far precursor type Th0, and Th2 subset of helper cells have been cloned from liver granulomas. The former secreted both IL-2, IL-4 and γ-IFN lymphokines and adoptively transferred the granulomatous response.

Granuloma induced by the schistosome egg is an inflammatory reaction that is tightly controlled by the interaction of T-helper cell type 1 (Th1) and Th2 cytokines produced locally. Th2 cytokines play a primary role in granuloma formation, whereas the Th1-associated lymphokines may act as an endogenous downregulator of the response.

Intestinal Schistosomiasis. As egg-laying worms may be found in the microvasculature of both the superior (*S. japonicum*) and inferior (*S. mansoni*) mesenteric venous distribution, all areas of the small and large intestines may be involved (Fig. 118–11). Colonoscopic or sigmoidoscopic examinations of *S. mansoni* or *S. japonicum* infected patients often show small petechiae in otherwise normal rectal mucosa, dull patches with sandpaper-like appearance, superficial erosions, stellate superficial ulcers and hyperemic, easy-bleeding areas. An important complication of the hepatointestinal form of *S. japonicum* infection is appendicitis caused by the extension of lesions into the vermiform appendix in the form of nodular tubercles.

INTESTINAL POLYPOSIS. The large intestine usually demonstrates the most severe pathology. Multiple focal granulomatous lesions can be extensive and, in severe cases, coalesce to form a large hemorrhagic granuloma, denuded of all normal mucosa. In some cases, the granulomatous lesions become polyploid. The polyps are usually friable and on biopsy show acute and chronic inflammatory reaction and large numbers of schistosome eggs. Polyp formation results from deposition of ova in the superficial layers of the submucosa where the connective tissue is loose, thus permitting greater accumulations of granuloma tissue. Subsequently, the muscularis mucosa becomes involved, and the overlying mucosa undergoes hyperplastic changes. The protein-losing enteropathies and malabsorption-type anemias of schistosomiasis are likely the results of this phenomenon.

OTHER COMPLICATIONS. Severe and long-standing large bowel granulomatous lesions may become fibrotic and constrict the normal bowel caliber. These large granulomatous

and later fibrotic lesions begin usually as microperforations of extensive bowel wall granulomas. Frank bowel perforation is rarely found.

Hepatosplenic Schistosomiasis

HEPATOMEGALY. In *S. mansoni* and *S. japonicum* infections, the major hepatic pathology of egg granulomas results from simple physical obstruction and tissue compression. Portal presinusoidal egg granulomas of the liver (Fig. 118–12) result in hepatomegaly and portal fibrosis with little primary hepatocellular damage. Portal hypertension follows with the shifting of hepatic blood flow from mainly portal to arterial sources. Hepatomegaly may be detected in the midsternal line due to a disproportionate enlargement of the left lobe of the liver. This is frequently seen in early hepatosplenic disease and may reflect a preferential egg flow distribution.

SPLENOMEGALY. Increased hepatic presinusoidal venous pressures lead to increased splenic vein pressures and vessel tortuosity. Intrasplenic venous pressures are also increased, with resultant congestive splenomegaly. A second factor contributing to splenomegaly is splenic hyperplasia. Cell proliferation in the red pulp and germinal centers of lymphoid follicles occurs early in infection. Later, at a time when serum immunoglobulins are elevated, basophil proliferation may be seen. Histologic sections of the spleen show distended venous sinuses and dense splenic cords, reflecting changes from both portal hypertension and hypercellularity. Giant follicular lymphoma has been reported in association with schistosomal hypersplenism.

VARICES AND ASCITES. Severe long-standing hepatosplenic schistosomiasis leads to esophageal varices and ascites. This "collateralization" of the abdominal venous system may enable schistosome eggs to bypass the liver and reach areas of the body not normally accessible, e.g., the lungs and central nervous system (CNS).

SYMMERS' PIPESTEM FIBROSIS. This is a periportal fibrosis without bridging, nodular formation, or significant hepatocellular destruction and is undoubtedly a result of egg-induced chronic presinusoidal inflammation leading to the deposition of fibrous material. These fibrotic changes cause a broadening and lengthening of the portal areas so that they resemble a clay "pipe stem" on anatomic cross section (Fig. 118–13).

More information is known about liver fibrosis in schistosomiasis than in any other liver disease. Products of schistosome eggs, inflammatory cells, and stimulating factors from these cells all promote fibroblast activity. This leads to a proliferation of collagen-synthesizing cells, increased peptide synthesis, and increased turnover of collagen. The balance between collagen formation and degradation is critical for determining whether the schistosome-infected liver returns

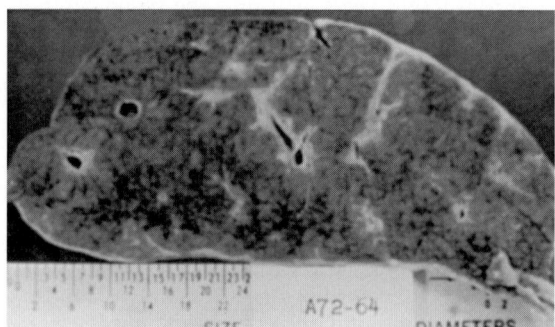

Figure 118–13. Cut surface of the liver showing Symmers' clay pipe-stem fibrosis in a patient infected with *Schistosoma mansoni*. (Courtesy of U.S. Naval Medical Research Unit No. 3, Cairo, Egypt.)

to normal structure or becomes fibrotic. Tissue collagenases, mainly of macrophage origin, are greatly increased in the schistosome-infected liver. A predominance of collagenolysis over collagen synthesis, demonstrated in experimental animals infected with *Schistosoma*, explains the reversal of fibrosis that occurs clinically after chemotherapy.

Urinary Tract Schistosomiasis. The pathogenesis of urinary schistosomiasis *(S. haematobium)* relates to the mucosal and submucosal granulomatous lesions of the ureters and bladder. As in the intestine, granulomatous lesions occur throughout the urinary tract and are prone to the same hemorrhagic, polyploid, and fibrotic complications.

OBSTRUCTIVE UROPATHY. Obstructive uropathy occurs when egg granulomas are located in the ureteral mucosa or in the bladder mucosa near the ureteral inlet or when massive bladder granulomas and/or polyploid lesions obstruct the ureteral inlet (Fig. 7–4). The pathogenesis of chronic bacteriuria relates in part to bladder and ureteral obstruction with resultant urine stasis and probably in part to the disruption of the normal bacteriostatic mechanisms of the intact bladder mucosa.

BLADDER CANCER. Bladder carcinoma is associated with chronic urinary schistosomiasis (Chapter 12). The cell type is usually squamous, and the early in situ stages are found near bladder granulomas. It usually spreads laterally and from the mucosa through the bladder wall into contiguous tissues. Lymphatic spread to the para-aortic lymph nodes is common.

Epidemiologic studies comparing populations highly endemic for urinary schistosomiasis and those without *S. haematobium* infection show (1) a dramatic, multifold rate increase in bladder cancer; (2) an abnormal age distribution of bladder cancer, following the pattern of heaviest endemic urinary schistosomiasis; and (3) a predominance of an unusual cancer cell type, squamous cell, suspected as in other circumstances (i.e., lung cancer, cervical cancer) to be a result of chronic irritation.

Three pathogenic mechanisms have been suggested to explain the association of bladder cancer and urinary schistosomiasis:

1. Prolonged irritation of bladder epithelium resulting from long-standing egg granulomas leads to a constant reparative process that progresses to hyperplasia and then to malignancy.
2. Localized bladder obstruction leads to urine stasis, local sepsis, and consequent alkalinity of an inflamed schistosomal bladder, which induces malignancy. This mechanism is supported by the frequent autopsy observation of schistosomal fibrotic stenosis below the site of the neoplasm.
3. Carcinogens have been found in the urine of patients with schistosomal bladder cancer. Large amounts of the enzyme glucuronidase are found regularly. In the presence of urinary stasis, secondary bacterial infection, and alkaline urine, this enzyme may release carcinogenic substances from their harmless conjugated forms. Furthermore, carcinogenic metabolites of trytophan occur in high levels in patients with schistosomal bladder cancer. These metabolites are reduced by the administration of vitamin B_6, which is needed for the growth, maturation, and oviposition of schistosomes. Perhaps a schistosome-induced vitamin B_6 deficiency results in carcinogenic tryptophan metabolites. In addition, schistosomiasis was treated for many years with parenteral antimony drugs, much of which was excreted in the urine. Antimony has been shown to be a potent carcinogen.

Renal Schistosomiasis

GLOMERULONEPHRITIS. Although common in schistosomiasis mansoni, glomerulonephritis is usually asymptomatic and clinically insignificant. Renal biopsies of patients with *S. mansoni* infection without clinical renal disease showed a high prevalence of histopathologic glomerulonephritis with schistosome antigen-antibody immune complex deposits in the glomeruli. This finding is not unexpected, because circulating schistosome immune complexes are found frequently in *S. mansoni* infections, and an immune complex syndrome, Katayama fever, occurs.

NEPHROTIC SYNDROME. This is seen occasionally in patients with *S. mansoni* and/or *S. haematobium* infections. There remains some controversy as to the precise infectious cause of nephrotic syndrome in this setting, as many reported cases also have had associated chronic *Salmonella* bacteremia and/or *Salmonella* bacteriuria. The few renal biopsy specimens available from such patients have shown minimal-change disease and only schistosome immune complex deposits.

AMYLOID. Deposits of amyloid have been detected in renal biopsy samples from patients with chronic schistosomiasis haematobia and mansoni who have no other long-standing infection. The pathogenic mechanism is undefined but is presumed to be the same as that of other chronic infection states and is hypothesized to be the result of an aberrant immunoregulatory condition.

Cardiopulmonary Schistosomiasis

PNEUMONITIS. The pathogenesis of larval pneumonitis, seen shortly after heavy schistosome infection, and the Löffler-like pneumonitis, seen soon after antischistosome chemotherapy for heavy infections, is undoubtedly based on a local allergic reaction, although specimens for pathologic study are rarely available. In the case of larval pneumonitis, there is an allergic reaction to the migratory schistosome larvae as they congregate in the pulmonary microvasculature on their way to the liver. The post-treatment pneumonitis is hypothesized to be the allergic response to the abrupt release of common antigen(s) from the dying adult worms. The pulmonary focus of this response may be due to sensitization of local immune cells by larvae or perhaps to the fact that the lungs happen to be the most visible organ of a systemic immune complex phenomenon (although generalized lymphadenopathy is not found). Peripheral eosinophilia, a marker of a reaginic allergic response, is much more prominent in larval pneumonitis than in the Löffler-like syndrome.

SCHISTOSOMAL COR PULMONALE. Cor pulmonale, seen infrequently in schistosome infections, manifests pathologically as three groups of vascular changes: (1) organic changes produced by multiple schistosome egg tubercles; (2) toxic-allergic changes leading to arteritis; and (3) medial hypertrophy, diffuse intimal arteriolar proliferation, and premature atheroma of the pulmonary artery.

These changes occur after prolonged deposition of large numbers of schistosome eggs in the prearteriolar pulmonary circulation. The resulting obliterative arteritis leads to pulmonary hypertension, increased right ventricular pressure, pulmonary artery and right atrial dilatation, and right ventricular hypertrophy (Figs. 2–6 and 2–7). Histologic sections of the lung demonstrate rather characteristic dumbbell-shaped interarterial and para-arterial granulomas. Cor pulmonale is more common in schistosomiasis mansoni than in infections with the other species and is closely associated with the presence and severity of portal hypertension and the resulting propensity for ova to bypass the portal venous system and reach the systemic venous system, from which they are trapped as they pass through the lungs.

Central Nervous System Schistosomiasis. CNS schistosomiasis is usually the result of embolic egg deposition within the cranial or spinal cord vasculature, resulting in infarctions and/or granulomatous lesions. All three species can produce such lesions, although *S. japonicum* is responsible for most of the brain lesions, and *S. mansoni* infection is the most common cause of spinal cord lesions (i.e., transverse myelitis). In rare cases, the aberrant location of an adult worm can cause focal deposition of ova or can obstruct the anterior spinal artery and cause local spinal cord necrosis. It is estimated the frequency of the cerebral form of schistosomiasis japonica is about 1 person per 1000 infected individuals, although it may be much higher in lightly infected individuals. Cerebral schistosomiasis japonica is an important cause of focal epilepsy in endemic areas of the Far East.

Speculations as to the probable route of migration of eggs from the site of oviposition to the brain are varied. Evidence for local or direct oviposition by aberrant worms has been presented based on the finding of nests or clusters of eggs in the brain but mature worms have never been found in the brain in any case of human cerebral schistosomiasis. Another possibility may be the maturation of circulating cercariae in the brain itself but this appears to be less likely. The more probable route, however, may be via venous anastomosis between systemic and hemorrhoidal veins, which is believed to facilitate access to the dural sinus by the adult worms. The parent worms in the mesenteric veins, during periods of increased intra-abdominal pressure, may enter the Batson intercommunicating plexus, which drains into the internal jugular vein and thence upward into the dural sinuses draining the brain. Thus, the mature worms or their ova may reach the brain directly from the abdominal cavity without going by way of the heart or lungs. However, infection with portal collaterals and portal hypertension does not necessarily favor the formation of ectopic cerebral lesions. Apparently, other mechanisms still unknown may influence ectopic deposition of ova and consequent development of cerebral lesions.

Two types of lesions have been recognized in the cerebral form of *S. japonicum* infection. These are (1) diffuse lesions of the brain that may be asymptomatic or may cause seizures. On contrast radiography, this group may not present a discrete mass but on autopsy has diffuse small lesions of the gray and white matter. This is supportive of the embolic mechanism of egg dissemination; and (2) a predominantly solitary lesion consisting of large irregular granulomas containing schistosome ova in fairly large aggregations. This type of lesion suggests local oviposition by aberrant worms.

On histologic examination, the lesion in cerebral schistosomiasis is essentially that of a chronic granulomatous infiltration with or without caseation. Morphologically, it is not easily distinguishable from other granulomas of the brain, particularly a tuberculoma, which are encountered in *S. japonicum* endemic areas. Lymphocytes, plasma cells, and eosinophils are scattered around the periphery of the granulomas but eosinophil infiltration may be minimal. The schistosome egg may be surrounded either by giant cells or collagenous fibers, both of which are embedded in necrosis. These pseudotubercles are distinct from the tubercles of tuberculosis by the lighter staining of the giant cell nuclei and ova and the regular shape of the giant cells. The smaller veins and arteries may exhibit perivascular round cell cuffing consisting of lymphocytes, eosinophils, and plasma cells.

Association of Schistosomiasis and Other Infections

CHRONIC *SALMONELLA* INFECTIONS. Chronic persistent *Salmonella* bacteremia occurs with increased frequency in patients infected with the three major human schistosomes. Among intracellular bacteria, only *Salmonella* has been found to be associated with greater frequency with schistosomiasis. Likewise, other nonintracellular gram-negative or gram-positive bacteria, commonly causing bacteremia in other groups with hepatic abnormalities, are not frequent causes of infection in chronic schistosomiasis. *Salmonella* species specificity is a prominent feature of this syndrome, as is the absence of mortality from this gram-negative bacteremia.

Attempts to explain the pathogenesis of chronic *Salmonella* infections in schistosomiasis has spawned two major hypotheses: (1) an immunologic tolerance caused by schistosomiasis that allows *Salmonella* organisms to survive and persist; and (2) the physical attachment and proliferation of *Salmonella* bacteria on the integumentum or in the intestinal tract of the adult schistosome worm with persistent release of bacteria into the blood stream.

The physical attachment hypothesis began with the in vitro observations that both gram-positive and gram-negative bacteria could colonize the intestine of the adult schistosome worm. Later, it was shown that *Salmonella paratyphi A* would firmly attach to *S. mansoni* adult worms taken from a schistosome-infected patient. The integumental attachment was randomly distributed over the surface of the worm and was probably related to somatic antigen and bacterial pili.

The immunologic tolerance hypothesis is based on shared antigens between the schistosome adult worm and *Salmonella*. By using large numbers of adult schistosome worms, *Salmonella* antibody may be adsorbed out of serum from patients with typhoid fever, turning their serum from Widal positive (1:640 titer) to negative. Conversely, it could be further demonstrated that rabbit serum became Widal positive after immunizing the rabbit with the insoluble fraction of macerated adult schistosome worms. Research using in vitro spleen cell cultures has shown a reduced antibody response to *Salmonella* lipopolysaccharide antigen in mice with chronic schistosomiasis but a normal response to other gram-negative lipopolysaccharide antigens. Further dissection of this specific immune defect indicated a B-lymphocyte origin, independent of macrophages and T lymphocytes. These data suggest that the antigenic associations between the schistosome and *Salmonella* may provide partial immune tolerance for *Salmonella* bacteria along with the immunologic tolerance to the adult worm.

HEPATITIS VIRUS INFECTIONS. Hepatitis B and/or C infections are usually common in populations with endemic schistosomiasis. Patients with hepatosplenic schistosomiasis have hepatitis B surface antigen (HBsAg) rates significantly greater than those of noninfected controls, as well as schistosome-infected patients with less evidence of hepatic involvement. Patients with chronic schistosomiasis mansoni when infected with hepatitis B and/or C viruses are prone to have clinically more severe infections, to develop persistent hepatosplenomegaly, and to be chronic carriers of hepatitis B and/or C. In addition, a history of prior parenteral treatment for schistosomiasis has been associated with serologic evidence for hepatitis B and/or C infections showing that this has been a cause of transmission of these viruses in the past. Many patients with decompensated liver disease have evidence of active infections with both agents. It appears that in many cases chronic active hepatitis and/or cirrhosis caused by hepatitis B and/or C viruses leads to hepatic decompensation with ascites, portal hypertension, and bleeding esophageal varices in a patient with chronic schistosomiasis mansoni.

Effect on Growth and Development, Nutritional Status, and Work Ability.

In both Filippino and Chinese children the intensity of *S. japonicum* infection was significantly related to reduced stature, weight, arm muscle area, and skinfold thickness. It was further observed that the growth retarding effects of schistosomiasis japonica were independent of other parasites, notably hookworm. It was suggested that work productivity may be affected by the magnitude of the schistosomiasis-associated growth differences in adolescence. The anthropometric reductions during childhood and adolescence caused by schistosomiasis japonica suggest a strong independent effect of infection on malnutrition and growth and development (Chapter 133.2). Recent epidemiologic studies in China confirmed that splenomegaly and higher intensities of *S. japonicum* infection were the leading risk factors for reduced work ability in the population studied.

Previous studies to establish an association between nutritional status and *S. mansoni* infection or morbidity in Kenyan and Brazilian children had shown that the relationship between intensity of infection and nutritional indices, although significant, was complex. However, it was noted that intensity of infection correlated with hepatomegaly, a condition more clearly related to nutritional status. Children with hepatomegaly were significantly more stunted and/or wasted than those without hepatomegaly, and had less variety in their diet. It was suggested that schistosome-associated morbidity leads to a subsequent nutritional defect.

IMMUNOLOGY. The host's acute and chronic immunologic response to the different parasite stages (i.e., cercaria, schistosomulum, adult worm, and schistosome egg) is extremely complex and has been studied extensively in both human and animal models over the past years. Drawing from this wide range of experimental evidence, the immunologic response may be categorized as: (1) protective immunity (e.g., antibody production and cell cytotoxicity); (2) morbid immunity (e.g., granuloma formation and fibrosis leading to bladder lesions and obstructive uropathy or hepatosplenomegaly and portal hypertension); (3) age-related resistance to reinfection; and (4) antiembryonation responses.

Protective Immunity. In nature, protective immunity seems limited to a reduction in the rate of survival of reinfecting schistosomula, without effect on the worms that have reached the adult stage. This protective response is maintained while a living adult worm remains in the host, and consequently, has been called concomitant immunity. Studies in the mouse model indicate that there are two distinct mechanisms: (1) an early elimination phase, while schistosomula are still in the skin, and (2) a later fatality of schistosomula as they pass from the lung to the liver.

Immunity During Skin Penetration. Immunologic processes triggered by adult worms attack schistosomula. Protective immunity during the early skin-penetration stage involves two separate and probably complementary mechanisms:

EOSINOPHILS AND IgG. In vitro studies have shown that eosinophils mediated by an antibody-dependent cell-mediated cytotoxicity play an important role in protective immunity. The Fc portions of IgG antischistosome antibodies attach to the Fc receptors of eosinophils to bring the schistosomula and the eosinophils together, whereupon degranulation with the release of eosinophil major basic protein leads to irreversible binding of the eosinophils to the schistosomula. This is followed by (1) eosinophil release of lytic agents, (2) schistosomula membrane damage, and (3) parasite death. Activated eosinophils, irrespective of the specificity of the activation stimulus, were more efficient at killing schistosomula than nonactivated eosinophils. Some authors suggest that by arming the effector eosinophil the mast cell is important in this eosinophilic antibody-dependent cell-mediated cytotoxicity.

MACROPHAGES AND IgE IMMUNE COMPLEXES. The second cytotoxic system involved in the early skin-penetration stage of reinfection immunity involves IgE immune complexes and is mediated by the macrophage. Specifically, antischistosomal IgE, in aggregate form, binds to a receptor site on the surface of the schistosomulum attached to a macrophage. This triggers the release of lysosomal enzymes, resulting in the death of the schistosomulum.

Immunity During Migration. Schistosomula are killed also during passage from the lung to the liver. The mechanism is unknown, but it has been associated with the advent of mature egg laying during primary infection.

Schistosomule Immune Evasion. The migrating schistosomules attempt to evade immunologic destruction by at least two mechanisms. There is a continuous turnover of surface membranes that leads to a loss of antigenic components that could be recognized by antibodies. Also, as the young schistosomula mature, their surfaces become covered with or converted to hostlike antigen such that by day 4 to 5, the aforementioned antischistosome antibody-mediated protective immune responses are no longer functional.

Immunity to Adult Worms. There appears to be no effective protective immunologic response against the adult worm, although specific adult worm antibodies and lymphocyte responses can be detected and have been modestly useful as a diagnostic assay. Conversely, the adult worm is responsible for no significant immunopathology.

Morbid Immunity. The immunopathology of schistosomiasis can be divided into early and late disorders.

Schistosome Dermatitis. The first immunopathology seen is the allergic dermatitis occurring after exposure to skin-penetrating cercariae and is more protective than morbid. Both humoral and CMI responses to cercarial antigens have been demonstrated in infected humans and experimental animals.

Katayama Fever. This occurs 5 to 7 weeks after heavy initial schistosome infection. It has been associated with two immunologic abnormalities: (1) depression in CMI to nonschistosome antigens and (2) demonstrable circulating large immune complex formation. Both of these occur at a time when a high schistosome egg antigen load is being presented to the host. The suggested immune mechanism for Katayama fever is one of an antibody-excess immune complex phenomenon, as seen in serum sickness, in which excess antibody in relation to antigen forms lattice structures. It is well known that larger immune complexes, when cleared by the reticuloendothelial system, activate the complement scheme, generating chemotactic factors that produce an inflammatory response at the site of complex entrapment.

Immune Complex Lesions. Other more chronic immune complex lesions in schistosomiasis have been demonstrated; however, their clinical and pathologic significance is uncertain. For example, biopsy of subclinical glomerulonephritis has shown schistosome immune complex deposits on the glomerular basement membrane, and circulating immune complexes of schistosome origin have been demonstrated regularly in the serum of experimental animals and humans. However, circulating antigens and antigen-antibody complexes may play a beneficial role in the regulation of concomitant immunity and in the protective modulation of the granuloma formation.

Egg Granuloma Formation. During the chronic stages of infection, egg granuloma formation, with the accompanying immune modulation, is the dominant immunologic phenomenon. CMI responses are almost exclusively the cause of granuloma formation around *S. mansoni* and *S. haematobium* eggs. Humoral immune responses appear to play a more important role in the granulomas around *S. japonicum* ova. This granulomatous reaction protects the host from diffusible parasite toxin and appears to be required for normal transmission of parasite eggs from the host to the environment.

Immunologic Modulation. The importance of immune modulation is derived from its teleologic necessity (i.e., granulomas are protective but must be modulated or they will cause host mortality and loss of parasite perpetuation) and because the chronic egg granuloma stage is the most prevalent form of human schistosomiasis. The acute florid granulomatous response to the schistosome egg results in a large-volume granuloma that causes a severe obstructive state in the affected organ. Only in the immune-modulated state, as in chronic schistosomiasis, when the granulomas are smaller but still protective, does the host's immunologic response and the disease state maintain an acceptable balance.

The most complete information collected about this important immune response has been gathered using the *S. mansoni*–infected mouse model, in which immune modulation begins around the 12th week after cercarial penetration and reaches its maximum at age 16 to 24 weeks after infection. During this time, the schistosome egg granuloma decreases in volume and changes in cellular composition. With the reduction in granuloma volume comes some relief of the vascular obstruction, resulting in reduced organ size and pathology. Associated with the downward modulation of granuloma size is an inversely proportional increase in humoral responses to schistosome antigens. With immune modulation comes a marked increase in serum antibody levels to the schistosome major serologic antigen (MSA), soluble egg antigen (SEA), and soluble worm antigen preparation (SWAP). In the spleens of mice with chronic schistosome infection, this parallels the relative decrease in the T-lymphocyte population and the relative and absolute increase in B-lymphocyte populations. Examination with direct fluorescent antibody techniques of liver biopsy specimens and colon biopsy specimens of polyps from patients has shown that the lymphocytes surrounding *S. mansoni* ova granulomas secrete considerable antibody. Studies with *S. mansoni*–infected mice have shown, as expected, that IgM is predominant during the first few weeks. After about 8 to 12 weeks, IgG becomes predominant. The role of localized antibody or immune complexes in this immunologic modulation is intriguing.

This unique and protective granulomatous immune modulation response can be transferred adoptively by spleen or lymph node cells from mice with chronic schistosome infection only, not from those with acute infection. Nor can it be transferred with immune serum. The reduction in granuloma size after spleen cell transfer is specific for schistosome egg granulomas and does not affect the granulomatous response to nonschistosomal agents. Granulomatous modulation is abrogated after T-lymphocyte depletion of transferred spleen cells by anti-Thy 1.2 serum but is maintained in macrophage-depleted, B-lymphocyte–depleted, or unfractionated transferred spleen cells. Schistosome immune modulation does not take place in athymic, genetically T-lymphocyte–deficient or otherwise T-cell–depleted mice. Splenic suppressor T lymphocytes have been implicated as being responsible for immune modulation.

Cell-Mediated Immunity. Concurrent with granulomatous immune modulation, mice with chronic schistosome infection demonstrated a depressed lymphocyte proliferation response to SEA, MSA, and SWAP. This same immunosuppression to specific schistosome antigens is also seen in chronic human schistosomiasis. Other T-lymphocyte–dependent responses were depressed in chronic murine schistosomiasis. In addition, a progressive loss of T-helper cell activity directed at TNP-schistosomula has been demonstrated.

In humans, where controlled schistosome infections are not possible, the picture is less clear. For instance, serum and adherent peripheral blood mononuclear cells, in addition to the T lymphocyte, have been implicated as suppressive agents. Several investigators have shown evidence of a suppressive serum factor in chronic human schistosomiasis. Schistosome immune complexes are suspected as the sup-

pressor factor in the serum, although their exact mechanisms of action are open to speculation. Adherent peripheral blood mononuclear cells also have been found responsible for depressed response to schistosome-specific antigens in patients with chronic, but not acute, schistosomiasis.

Age-Related Resistance to Reinfection. It has been recognized for many years that a variety of experimental hosts develop an acquired immunity to schistosome infection after either a natural primary infection or immunization with irradiated larvae or with isolated antigens. Evidence from epidemiologic studies in endemic communities demonstrate the development with age of a resistance to infection, or to reinfection after treatment, with *S. mansoni* or *S. haematobium*. Reinfection studies uniformly support the existence of a strong resistance to (re)infection with schistosomes in adults. However, available epidemiologic evidence suggests that this age-related type of resistance may not be due to slowly developing immunity acquired during a childhood of exposure, as generally assumed, but that factors inherent in age itself may be (co)determinant. Age appears to be more important than experience, and age-related resistance a more accurate label than acquired immunity.

ANTIBODIES. Studies in Kenyan schoolchildren of resistance, reflected by low levels of reinfection after treatment of *S. mansoni* infections, observed positive correlations between intensities of reinfection and the presence of antibodies of the IgM and IgG2 isotypes that recognized carbohydrate epitopes present in both the egg and schistosomulum antigens. The levels of such antibodies predicted susceptibility to reinfection, rather than simply reflecting pretreatment intensities of infection, and it was suggested that they served to block the binding and action of antibodies of other, protective isotypes, and hence prevented the expression of immunity in young children. Further progress came with the observation in The Gambia of a negative association between intensities of reinfection with *S. haematobium* and the levels of IgE antibodies against adult worm antigens, indicating the involvement of such antibodies in protection. Similar results were obtained for *S. mansoni* in studies in Brazil and Kenya and are consistent with previous experimental demonstrations of a protective effect of IgE, both in a rat model of schistosome immunity and as a mediator of human eosinophil–dependent killing of schistosomula in vitro. It was further shown that the expression of resistance is dependent on the balance between protective IgE and blocking IgG4 antibodies to larval antigens, whereas the blocking effect of IgG2 antibodies acts independently. In addition to IgE, evidence is also accumulating for a positive correlation between IgA and resistance. The conclusion at this stage, therefore, is that a key feature of the expression of human immunity is not so much the presence or absence of an antibody response but rather the balance between different antibody isotypes.

CYTOKINES. Experiments in the mouse model of schistosome immunity have consistently demonstrated a predominant role in protection for Th1 cell responses with γ-IFN production. This might not be the case in humans; instead Th2 cell responses (which enhance both IgE production through IL-4 and eosinophil numbers and activity through IL-5, and which are generally induced by helminth infection) might be more important. Although this is not yet definite, evidence supporting this hypothesis is beginning to accumulate. In several studies, an association has emerged between high levels of lymphocyte proliferation to adult worm or larval antigens and low levels of infection or of reinfection after treatment; this association remains significant after adjusting for age. Although the participation of individual T-cell subsets in such responses has proved more difficult to test, it is generally found that γ-IFN production to schistosome antigen is low, whereas IL-5 production is substantial. In one of these studies there was a significant association between IL-5 production in response to egg antigens and low levels of subsequent reinfection, although statistical significance was lost after adjusting for age.

Antiembryonation Responses. The hypothesis that granuloma modulation and disease abatement in chronic infection with *S. japonicum* could be ascribed to antibody-mediated effects on egg maturation and egg viability, arose from studies performed with mice in the Philippines. This novel hypothesis has received little additional attention and the phenomenon might be confined to *S. japonicum*, even the *S. japonicum* Philippine strain.

CLINICAL MANIFESTATIONS AND MANAGEMENT

Schistosome Cercarial Dermatitis. Cercarial dermatitis results from incomplete infection by small mammal or avian schistosomes and occurs in immune populations from endemic areas following heavy re-exposure to *S. mansoni* and *S. haematobium*; *S. japonicum* rarely causes dermatitis. Depending on the circumstance under which the disease is acquired, it has been variously designated as "swimmer's itch," "schistosome dermatitis," "clam digger's itch," "sawah itch," or "koganbyo." In all cases, it involves the association of humans and cercariae-shedding intermediate snail hosts.

Unsensitized and sensitized individuals respond with marked differences to the penetration of the skin by cercariae. Initial exposures to these cercariae produce only mild, transient reactions that often pass unnoticed or cause a prickling sensation as the water evaporated and the parasites penetrate the skin. Macules usually appear within 12 hours and, in nonsensitized individuals, soon disappear. However, in persons sensitized by previous exposures to these cercariae, the macules will be followed by papules, possibly accompanied by erythema, vesicle formation, edema, and pruritus, which may persist for 7 to 10 days (Fig. 118–14). Reactions vary markedly, not only because of differences in host susceptibility but also because human and nonhuman schistosome cercariae differ in their ability to produce the skin rash.

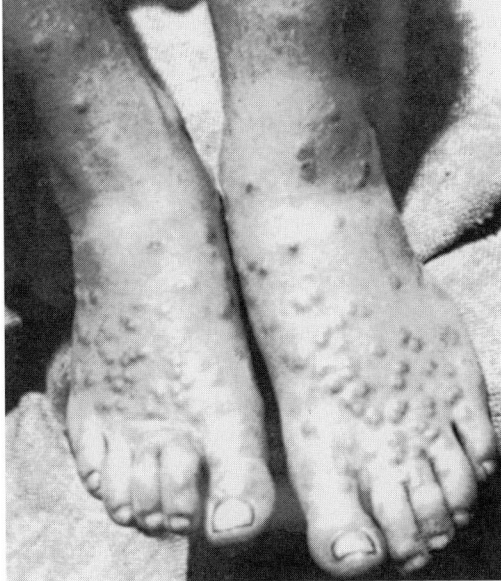

Figure 118–14. Marked reaction in sensitized amateur fisherman about 4 days after fishing in a brackish-water lagoon near Sydney, Australia. The infection was caused by cercariae of *Austrobilharzia terrigalensis*. (Courtesy of Dr. A. J. Bearup, School of Public Health and Tropical Medicine, University of Sydney, N.S.W., Australia.)

Treatment is usually not needed. Palliative topical agents, e.g., corticosteroid creams, can be applied, and in severe cases, oral or parenteral antihistamines can be administered.

Katayama Fever. This distinct syndrome has been reported after initial heavy infection with the three common human schistosome species. However, the name is derived from an area endemic for *S. japonicum*, and the disease is seen most often in those infected with that species. It also occurs following infection of nonimmune individuals with *S. mansoni*. In Egypt, where the syndrome is being reported more frequently, acute schistosomiasis is rarely occurring in those with chronic schistosomiasis haematobia who are being infected with *S. mansoni* for the first time.

Katayama fever became known after 19th-century reports from the Katayama River Valley in Japan (an area previously hyperendemic for schistosomiasis japonica) detailed a clinical syndrome of abrupt onset of fever, chills, abdominal pain, diarrhea, nausea, vomiting, cough, headache, urticaria, hepatosplenomegaly, and lymphadenopathy. There is marked eosinophilia and usually marked elevations in levels of IgE and IgG. This illness may last from several days to weeks and may cause significant mortality. It was seen most often in immigrants to the Katayama River Valley and was said to have led to the prohibition of marriage between people in this area and outsiders because of illness and deaths among new spouses. With the advent of schistosomal chemotherapy and control and the reduction in the intensity of infections, Katayama fever has become less common in recent decades. The clinical syndrome most resembles serum sickness and usually occurs 5 to 7 weeks after heavy initial infection—when the first schistosome egg production and release would be expected.

In nonendemic countries, it would most likely be seen in tourists who had wandered into heavily cercariae-infested waters and returned home within a month of exposure. Thus, a history of water contact in a schistosome-endemic area, perhaps with a history of mild swimmer's itch, in a patient with a serum sickness–like disease would provide the clues necessary to search for schistosomal eggs or antibodies. Anti-inflammatory therapy with salicylates, other analgesics or corticosteroids may be used for those with a moderate level of symptoms. In life-threatening disease, corticosteroids are recommended.

Chronic Schistosomiasis. Chronic schistosomiasis is the most prevalent form of this disease; most clinicians and laypersons refer to this when they indicate that a patient "has schistosomiasis." All forms of chronic schistosomiasis share the basic pathogenic mechanism of long-standing egg granuloma formation in an organ or organ system. This form of disease is rarely brought to the physician's attention before 6 months after the initial infection. Because of the different selective places of egg laying among schistosome species dwelling in the venous circulation of the abdomen, two basic patterns of disease are easily distinguishable: gastrointestinal (*S. mansoni* and *S. japonicum*) and urinary (*S. haematobium*). However, the clinician must be aware of significant overlap between these two categories.

Onset of Illness. Patients would likely first present with lethargy, chronic mild mucohemorrhagic diarrhea with mild cramping abdominal pain, and minimal hepatomegaly (gastrointestinal) or with lethargy, dysuria, and terminal hematuria (urinary). The differential diagnoses of these insidious and nonspecific signs and symptoms are myriad, and unless the physician takes a travel history and is clinically alert, schistosomiasis is unlikely to even be considered.

Endemic populations usually accept these early signs and symptoms as normal. Only as the heavier infections progress does schistosomiasis become a specifically recognizable clinical disease, and even then, the differential diagnosis can be confused by other complicating factors, e.g., concomitant viral hepatitis infection.

Intestinal Schistosomiasis. This is common in *S. mansoni* and *S. japonicum* infections but is much less common in *S. haematobium* infection. The entire intestinal tract may be diseased; however, the large intestine is usually involved more often and more severely.

Mild to moderate infections result in colonic irritative bowel habits, manifested as malaise, mild mucohemorrhagic diarrhea, and sometimes cramping abdominal pains. Physical examination may be normal or may show moderate abdominal distention, diffuse mild abdominal tenderness, and hyperactive bowel sounds. In general, the signs and symptoms are those of focal granulomatous large bowel disease. Sigmoidoscopy may show areas of granular inflammation with hyperemic pinpoint elevations, shallow ulcerations, or small hemorrhages. Patients rarely present with both severe bowel disease and severe hepatosplenomegaly; in nearly all cases, one or the other syndrome is dominant.

INTESTINAL GRANULOMATOSIS AND/OR POLYPOSIS. This is found in 10 to 15% of some Middle Eastern symptomatic *S. mansoni*–infected populations requiring hospitalization and is usually accompanied by a protein-losing enteropathy manifesting as chronic severe mucohemorrhagic diarrhea with weight loss and anemia. Physical examination reveals a distended abdomen with diffuse tenderness or localized tenderness in the area of the transverse and descending colon. Lesions in the descending colon are recognized most frequently, and this area is usually most heavily involved. Barium enema, sigmoidoscopy, and colonoscopy have demonstrated over 100 pedunculated and sessile polyps in some cases (Fig. 118–15). Some large, severe, long-standing granulomatous or polypous lesions may result in partial or complete lower bowel obstruction. These patients frequently have a palpable, tender, sausage-like mass in an area corresponding to one of the colonic segments. Overt large bowel perforation rarely occurs. Usually, the obstructive lesions are at least partially reversible with chemotherapy. However, residual fibrotic scarring may lead to permanent partial bowel obstruction or bowel wall deformation.

COMPLICATIONS. Localized bowel granulomas may also serve as the focal point for intussusception. Reduction of this lesion by barium enema must be undertaken with extreme care to avoid perforation. Rectal prolapse occurs rarely in intestinal disease of this extent and is usually slowly reversible with chemotherapy. Anorectal fistulas and perianal abscess formation are common. An increased incidence of colonic carcinoma has never been documented in association with severe intestinal schistosomiasis.

Many of the manifestations and complications of schistosomal intestinal granulomas and/or polyp disease are the same as those of inflammatory bowel disease (Crohn disease and ulcerative colitis). Disastrous errors in medical management have occurred when this was mistaken for other granulomatous bowel diseases or mass lesions with resultant surgical and/or corticosteroid therapy.

HYPERTROPHIC OSTEOARTHROPATHY. This clinical complex occurs very rarely in a few patients with severe schistosomal bowel disease. Patients present usually with mucohemorrhagic diarrhea, arthritis in several large joints, and clubbing of the digits. Periosteal inflammation with new bone formation is seen on the radiograph. This syndrome is associated most often with severe intestinal polyposis and heavy *S. mansoni* infection. Pulmonary symptoms or findings on the chest radiographs usually seen with other forms of hypertrophic osteoarthropathy are absent. It is reversible with treatment of the underlying schistosome infection, although

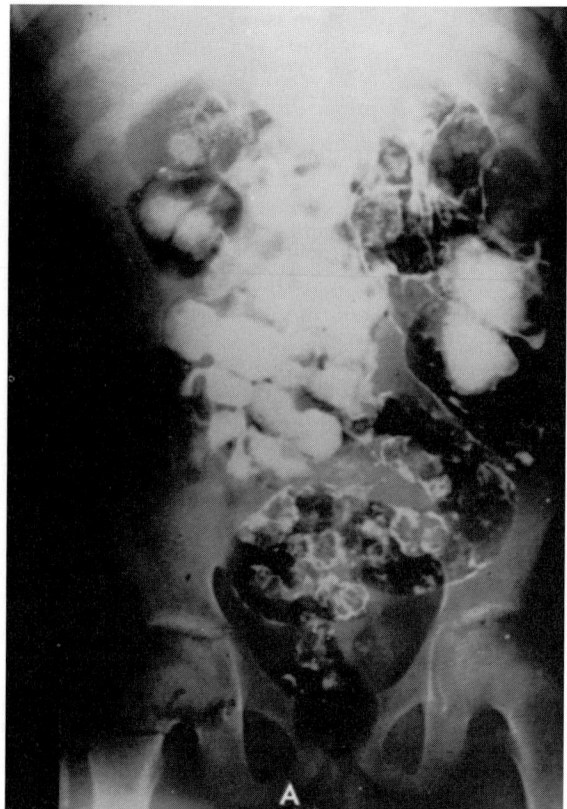

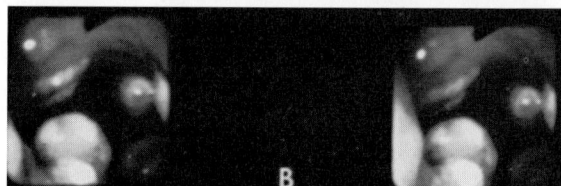

Figure 118–15. Colonic polyposis. *A,* Radiograph after air contrast barium enema demonstrates multiple rectosigmoid polyps in a patient heavily infected with *S. mansoni. B,* Colonoscopic view of polyps. (Courtesy of U.S. Naval Medical Research Unit No. 3, Cairo, Egypt.)

symptomatic treatment with corticosteroid anti-inflammatory agents may bring more immediate relief to the patient.

Hepatosplenic Schistosomiasis. This usually results from chronic *S. mansoni* or *S. japonicum* infections. Heavy infection and consequent egg burden are thought to be largely responsible for this manifestation of schistosomiasis, although limited studies of human leukocyte antigen (HLA) typing have suggested a genetic predisposition to the hepatosplenic syndrome. On clinical examination, patients have grossly enlarged livers, with the left lobe sometimes disproportionately enlarged (Fig. 118–16). The liver is firm, finely nodular, and nontender. Jaundice is characteristically absent, and liver cell function is usually normal until the terminal stages.

HYPERSPLENISM. The spleen is invariably palpable and, in many cases, massively enlarged. It is firm, without sharp edges, and nontender. Usually, splenomegaly is moderate and tolerable to the patient, although hypersplenism with mild hemolytic anemia and increased red cell destruction may be present. A small group of patients with massive hypersplenism complain of severe abdominal discomfort and have on occasion undergone splenectomy.

PORTAL HYPERTENSION. The major clinical findings beyond

with the rationale that the irreversible disease state might be arrested. The best results obtained in treatment of portal hypertension were esophagogastric devascularization and splenectomy (EGDS), although risk of rebleeding persists; classic (proximal) splenorenal shunt (SRS) should be abandoned; distal splenorenal shunt may complicate with hepatic encephalopathy, although later and in a lower percentage than in SRS.

Urinary Tract Schistosomiasis. *S. haematobium* has a predilection for the urinary tract venous plexus. Most infections are mild and asymptomatic.

Onset of Illness. Dysuria, urinary frequency, and terminal hematuria of an insidious onset are the earliest symptoms and signs. Physical examination is usually normal, but urinalysis reveals many red blood cells and a few white blood cells on microscopic examination and hematuria and proteinuria by chemical reagent strips. Symptoms and laboratory

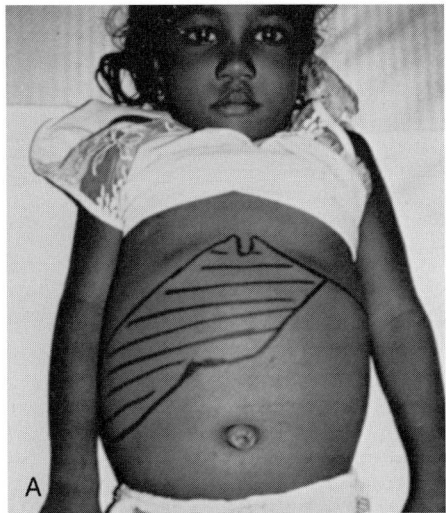
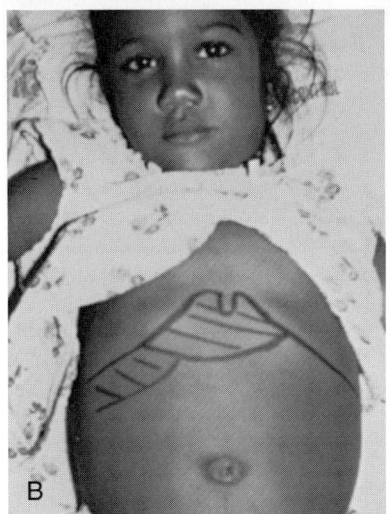

Figure 118–16. *Schistosoma mansoni* infection. Four-year-old girl with a distended abdomen with hepatomegaly. *A,* Before therapy. *B,* Two months after therapy. (Courtesy of Dr. Joseph Cook.)

hepatosplenomegaly are a direct result of portal hypertension. Patients with more advanced disease have splenomegaly but the liver may be normal or diminished in size. Esophageal varices are present and fatal hemorrhage is not uncommon. However, patients with schistosomiasis tolerate variceal bleeding episodes better than patients with alcoholic or hepatitic causes of hepatic portal hypertension, because the parenchymal cells and the resulting hepatic function remain intact. End-stage hepatosplenic schistosomiasis is heralded by massive ascites. Although ascites may predate death by years, it is generally refractory to medical treatment and pathologically irreversible.

Sigmoidoscopy shows mild to moderate focal granulomatous bowel disease. Radiographs taken after a barium swallow frequently demonstrate esophageal varices, but studies after a barium enema and upper gastrointestinal radiographs are usually normal. Sonography of the liver is an excellent noninvasive technique to demonstrate the pathognomonic periportal fibrosis (Figs. 5–1 and 118–17) and can estimate the degree of portal hypertension by measuring the distention of the portal vein.

Chemotherapy for *Schistosoma* infection is warranted even in severe disease if an active infection can be demonstrated,

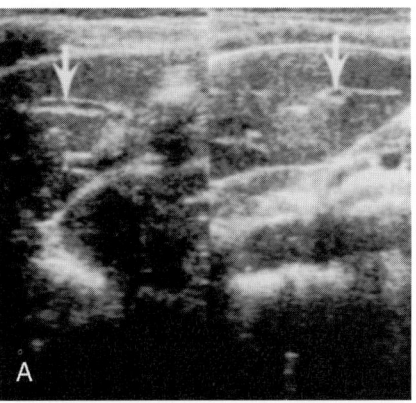
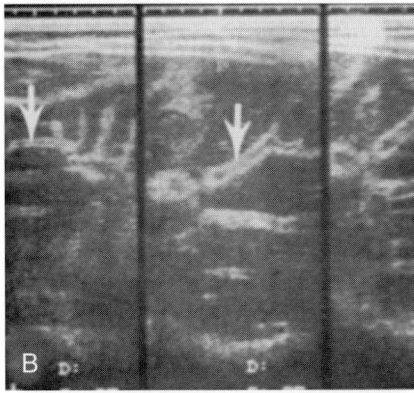
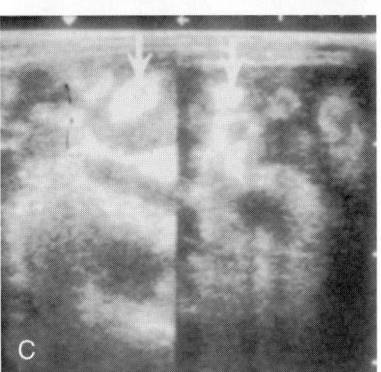

Figure 118–17. Examples of minimal *(A)*, moderate *(B)*, and extensive *(C)* periportal fibrosis of the liver demonstrated by ultrasonography. The arrows point to typical lesions.

findings are related directly to intensity of infection and are often reversible with appropriate chemotherapy. Chronic infection may lead to four major disease manifestations: obstructive uropathy, chronic bacteriuria, carcinoma of the bladder, and bladder calcification.

Obstructive Uropathy. Hydronephrosis, hydroureter, pyelonephritis, and renal failure is often silent clinically but can be demonstrated by intravenous pyelogram (Fig. 118–18), by ultrasonography, or by renogram function testing in patients with *S. haematobium* infection. Most lesions occur in the lower third of the ureter or in the bladder (Figs. 118–19 and 118–20).

PYELONEPHRITIS. Pyelonephritis secondary to obstruction and leading to gram-negative septicemia is not uncommon and may be the presenting manifestation as well as a leading cause of mortality in urinary schistosomiasis.

RENAL FAILURE. Renal failure secondary to any of the complications of schistosomal obstructive uropathy is also a common cause of fatal schistosomiasis. Unfortunately, because obstructive disease is associated with heavy and extensive infection, bilateral ureteral obstruction occurs more commonly than would be predicted. Therefore, the bilaterality of the human urinary tract offers minimal protection in this disease. Renal failure may be the direct result of prolonged ureteral obstruction, chronic pyelonephritis, or severe ureterovesicular urinary reflux, each a complication of severe urinary schistosomiasis. Because of the clinically silent nature of many of these early obstructive lesions, all patients with documented urinary schistosomiasis should have an intravenous pyelogram or ultrasonography.

Chronic Bacteriuria. Epidemiologic surveys in endemic

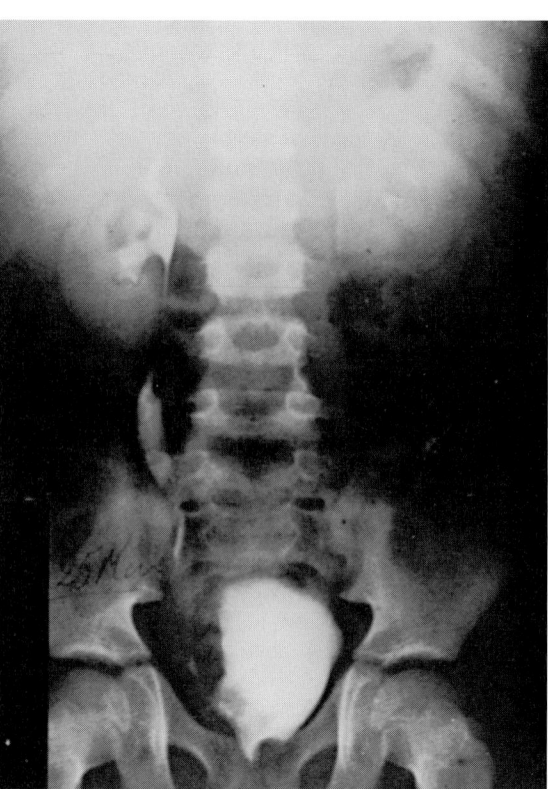

Figure 118–19. Intravenous pyelogram showing a large bladder filling defect caused by granulomatous polyp formation in a patient infected with *S. haematobium*. Early right hydronephrosis and hydroureter may also be seen. (Courtesy of U.S. Naval Medical Research Unit No. 3, Cairo, Egypt.)

populations have demonstrated bacteriuria rates of up to 5% in school boys with *S. haematobium* infection. Several species of coliform bacteria have been identified as the causative organism, although a *Salmonella* species was the most frequent cause. Antibiotic treatment of bacteriuria is usually unsuccessful unless it follows antischistosomal treatment and elimination of the underlying schistosomal mucosal lesions.

Bladder Carcinoma. Bladder carcinoma is an epidemiologically important complication of chronic *S. haematobium* infection. The presenting signs and symptoms of bladder irritation, gross hematuria, weight loss, and metastasis (particularly to inguinal, femoral, and retroperitoneal lymph

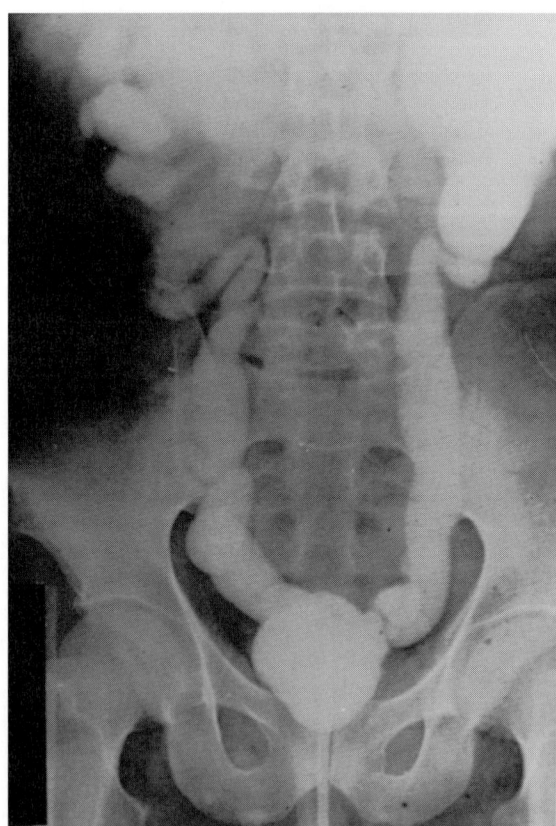

Figure 118–18. Severe obstructive uropathy with severe bilateral hydronephrosis and hydroureter in a patient with chronic *S. haematobium* infection. (Courtesy of U.S. Naval Medical Research Unit No. 3, Cairo, Egypt.)

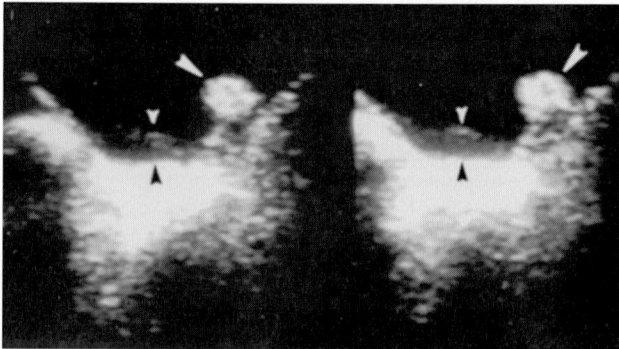

Figure 118–20. Ultrasonographic view of bladder of patient with schistosomiasis caused by *S. haematobium*. Thickening and irregularity of the bladder wall *(small arrows)* and a large polyp *(large arrow)* are present.

nodes) usually lag 10 to 20 years behind the peak *S. haematobium* infection age. Most bladder cancer is diagnosed in the third and fourth decades of life. Diagnosis is by biopsy, although urine lactate dehydrogenase (LDH) levels and urinary cytologic studies are sometimes helpful.

Bladder Calcification. The "fetal head" sign (Fig. 118–21) is seen in abdominal radiographs and reflects calcium deposits around myriads of schistosome eggs in the bladder and ureteral walls. Sonography can also demonstrate the calcification in the bladder wall. Although the *S. haematobium*–infected bladder frequently loses distensibility and contractibility because of thickened fibrotic walls, it does not become as rigid as it would appear on radiograph. Schistosome bladder calcification resolves over years if the patient remains free of schistosome infection.

Renal Disease. Nephrotic syndrome is occasionally related to *S. mansoni* infections. In Egypt, schistosome nephrotic syndrome is accompanied often by *Salmonella* bacteriuria and/or bacteremia. The characteristic findings of edema, hypoalbuminemia, massive proteinuria, and hyperlipidemia are evident. As with other forms of infection associated with nephrotic syndrome, management is relatively easy, and fatal renal disease is rare. Resolution, although slow, is nearly 100% after treatment with antischistosomal and antibacterial agents (Chapter 7).

Cardiopulmonary Schistosomiasis. This is a complex of primary pulmonary pathologic conditions, some of which secondarily affect the heart after exposure to chronic abnormal pressure gradients. All three human schistosomes participate in these disease states.

Larval Pneumonitis. Larval pneumonitis, similar to other helminth larval migrations (e.g., hookworm), occurs days to weeks after heavy cercarial exposure and is marked by low-

grade fever of gradual onset and mild cough. Basilar crepitations and scattered wheezing may be heard on examining the chest, and radiographs reveal basilar mottling. These symptoms last 2 to 4 weeks and are associated with marked eosinophilia and spontaneous resolution. Embolic worms are thought to cause a similar, more localized disease and may develop into mass lesions of the lung.

Reactionary Pneumonitis. This Löffler-like syndrome is commonly seen in patients carefully observed during chemotherapy of heavy infections. The clinical and laboratory findings are similar to those of larval pneumonitis, except that spontaneous resolution is usually more rapid and eosinophilia less striking. Marked reactionary pneumonitis is an indication to temporarily discontinue chemotherapy.

Schistosomal Cor Pulmonale. This uncommon presentation of chronic schistosomiasis is seen in all schistosome endemic areas of the world, although most often reported in *S. mansoni* infections from Egypt and Brazil, usually in patients having hepatosplenic schistosomiasis mansoni with portal hypertension, which allows shunting of eggs through portosystemic collaterals to the lungs.

Hallmarks of this disease are easy fatigability, palpitations, dyspnea on exertion, cough with occasional hemoptysis, right ventricular hypertrophy, and dilation of the pulmonary artery (Fig. 3–7). The electrocardiogram may show right ventricular hypertrophy and strain (Fig. 3–6), and occasional patients develop large aneurysms of the pulmonary arteries. Lesser degrees of these features are seen more commonly. Antischistosomal therapy usually provides no improvement but it is given to prevent further progression of disease.

Central Nervous System Schistosomiasis. Clinical presentation relates to the location of egg granulomas. Clinical diagnosis of all nervous system schistosomiasis is invariably presumptive. Only occasional autopsy or surgical findings firmly support the diagnosis.

Cerebral Schistosomiasis. Focal and generalized seizures are the most common presenting symptom of cerebral schistosomiasis, with headache, optic field defects, and speech abnormalities also being reported. Diagnosis is difficult and may be heralded only by papilledema, focal encephalographic (EEG) changes, or a cerebrospinal fluid examination showing slightly increased pressure, a mild increase in protein, and the presence of a few lymphocytes. Isotopic brain scans and CT scans can localize the lesions.

The vast majority of cases of cerebral schistosomiasis are seen in *S. japonicum* and occur in 2 to 4% of diagnosed cases. The greater number and smaller size of eggs laid by *S. japonicum* compared with *S. mansoni* is considered responsible for the greater incidence of ectopic deposits of *S. japonicum* ova in the brain as well as for the more rapid development of acute cerebral and systemic symptomatology. *S. japonicum* likewise shows a tendency toward the development of large intracranial granulomas which may cause so much pressure as to necessitate surgical intervention in contrast to the small granulomas produced by *S. mansoni* or *S. haematobium* in the spinal cord. The acute phase, which occurs within months after exposure, may be accompanied by fever, urticaria, absolute eosinophilia, and angioneurotic edema suggesting an allergic encephalopathy. There may be delirium, confusion, personality changes, incontinence, coma, nuchal rigidity, pyramidal tract signs, and cerebellar symptoms. The acute phase may merge into a chronic phase, which could either be asymptomatic or may mimic intracranial neoplasm.

Seizures secondary to brain schistosomiasis may be motor, sensory, and psychomotor. Psychomotor and motor involvement are the more predominant forms of neurologic disturbances. The majority of the motor disturbances are grand

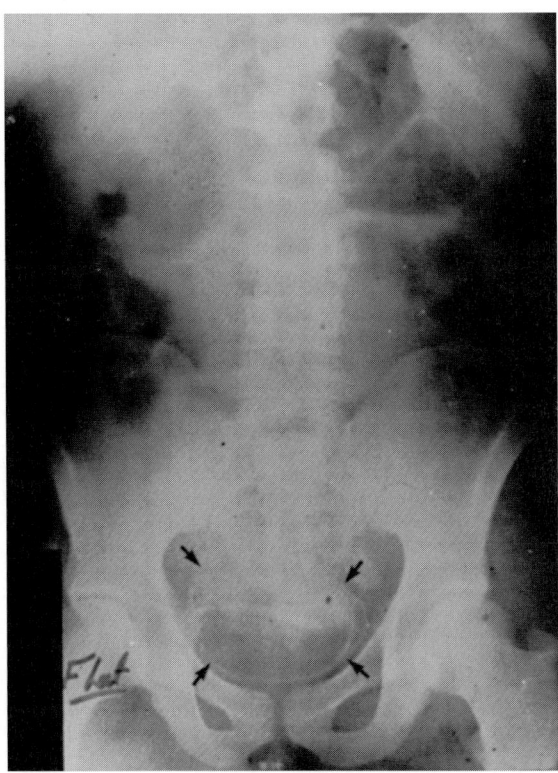

Figure 118–21. "Fetal head" bladder calcification may be seen (*arrows*) in this plain radiograph of the abdomen of a patient with chronic *S. haematobium* infection. (Courtesy of U.S. Naval Medical Research Unit No. 3, Cairo, Egypt.)

mal or jacksonian epileptic seizures. The most common site of the lesion is the parietal lobe. The eosinophil count is increased in most cases. EEG studies of patients with chronic *S. japonicum* infection with subjective symptoms of fatigue, mild headache, and dizziness revealed abnormal findings in about half of the subjects.

Treatment with antischistosomal drugs has been reported to result in improvement with disappearance of seizures in almost all patients.

Spinal Schistosomiasis. Most often seen in *S. mansoni* infections, but also in infections with *S. haematobium*, spinal schistosomiasis usually presents as a transverse myelitis of variable degrees with attendant localizing neurologic signs (i.e., paraplegia and loss of bladder and anal sphincter control). There may be a rash around the body effecting the dermatome at the level of the spinal cord lesion. This complication, usually caused by aberrant adult worms or ova in the anterior spinal artery, has been reported among American and European expatriates exposed to infection in freshwater African lakes, particularly Lake Malawi. It appears not to occur in natives of endemic areas who have had previous exposures to schistosomiasis. The lesions are often reversible. Therefore, antischistosomal chemotherapy is indicated. As with other space-occupying lesions in the CNS, corticosteroid anti-inflammatory therapy must also be considered.

Other Schistosome Lesions. Ectopic lesions in schistosomiasis, the result of the aberrant location of either worm or egg, are not common, are frequently asymptomatic or undiagnosed, and may span all organ systems and tissues of the body. *S. haematobium* egg granulomas have occurred in extraocular spaces and on the globe, resulting in proptosis, reduction of extraocular movements, and visual disturbances. Perigenital subcutaneous egg granulomas have been reported, as have granulomas in the spermatic cord, epididymis, testes, prostate, seminal vesicle, uterine cervix, ovary, and urethra, causing local clinical disease. Pancreatic, gallbladder, omental, peritoneal, and stomach egg granulomas have also been documented and are thought to be responsible for local pathology. Egg granulomas have also been found incidentally in the heart, kidney, and adrenal glands at postmortem examination without recognized clinical manifestations.

Association of Schistosomiasis and Other Infections

Salmonella-Schistosome Syndrome. Chronic persistent *Salmonella* bacteremia has been described in association with *S. mansoni*, *S. haematobium*, and *S. japonicum* infections in patients from many endemic areas of the world. The most common characteristics of the clinical syndrome are (1) a long history (from several weeks to 1 year) of an indolent febrile disease; (2) a frequent, sometimes daily, bacteremia with one of many species of the genus *Salmonella*; and (3) chronic active schistosomiasis. Patients complain of fatigue, malaise, weight loss, and fever. Some authors have described the clinical features as being "more like kala-azar than typhoid fever." The clinical disease bears no resemblance to clinical typhoid fever. Prostration and delirium never occur, and only rarely are salmonella isolated from the stool. A petechial rash on the lower extremities is common, but the classic abdominal rose spots are rarely seen. Localized infections, as are found in the osteomyelitis of sickle cell disease, chronic cholecystitis, or abscess formation, do not occur. In Egypt, where *S. mansoni* and the urinary tract–associated *S. haematobium* are both endemic, chronic *Salmonella* bacteriuria is a common clinical problem.

Chronic persistent *Salmonella* bacteremia is not the result of end-stage or moribund schistosomiasis. It occurs most commonly in males between the ages of 15 and 30 years. Mortality is rare, and the response to antibiotic therapy is

dramatic. However, recurrent *Salmonella* bacteremia is common if the underlying schistosome disease is not treated.

Hepatitis B and C Infection. Recent clinical studies have demonstrated an association between hepatosplenic schistosomiasis and hepatitis B or C infection. The greatest clinical relevance lies in the knowledge that in severe hepatosplenic disease the clinician may be dealing with two infections. Patients with this dual infection more often develop jaundice, intractable ascites, and hepatic failure. Mild to moderate elevations in hepatocellular liver function test results occur commonly, as does the demonstration of HbsAg and/or antibodies to hepatitis C. In fact, patients with chronic schistosomiasis who have elevations in serum alanine aminotransferase (ALT) or aspartate transaminase (AST) have a high probability of having comcomitant hepatitis B and/or C infections. Proper precautions for dealing with potentially infected blood products should be taken. The clinical management is more complicated and the prognosis more guarded than for chronic hepatosplenic schistosomiasis alone.

DIAGNOSIS. Residence or travel history is of utmost importance. History and physical examination may also supply one of the rare specific features, "swimmer's itch" (Fig. 118–14). Other aspects of clinical history and findings on physical examination, although important and supportive, are usually nonspecific and of minimal assistance in the diagnosis of schistosome infections. The most specific symptomology for diagnosis of schistosomiasis haematobia is hematuria, whereas loose stools with blood and mucus should suggest a possible infection with *S. mansoni* or *S. japonicum* in someone with a history of exposure to infection.

Laboratory Findings

Schistosome Egg Identification. Egg identification is the appropriate method of establishing the diagnosis (Fig. 118–3). Egg quantitation is also important in the assessment of clinical disease and its epidemiologic impact, as is egg viability. The Kato thick smear technique is described. Other methods are described in detail elsewhere (Chapter 150).

KATO THICK SMEAR. A 50-mg sample of feces (an amount about the size of a garden pea) is pressed through a 105-mesh steel sieve onto a glass slide. This sample is covered with a cellophane coverslip impregnated with glycerin and is then inverted and pressed onto a bed of filter paper. The slide is turned so that the coverslip is facing up and is left for 24 to 48 hours while the fecal matter clears. Then, all eggs on the slide are counted using $100\times$ magnification. Multiplying by 20 gives the number of ova per gram of stool. The daily ova excretion can be calculated if the day's stool weight is known.

The Kato thick smear (Fig. 118–22) involves no equipment beyond the simple microscope. However, the test requires an amount of expertise by the laboratory medical technologist in the correct identification and counting of the parasite ova. Moreover, a major limitation of the test is that formed stools are desirable. In the case wherein the patient has diarrheic stools, the sensitivity of the test is greatly affected. The Kato thick smear is quantitative and useful for special clinically and epidemiologically based studies. However, because of the small volume of stool examined, it has low sensitivity and will not detect some light infections. A single stool examination, for instance, results in missing from 10–15% of cases lightly infected. Repeated Kato thick smear examinations of stool samples increase the sensitivity of the test. However, collection of repeated stool samples is not always convenient for the individual patient and is not practical in community-based control programs.

RECTAL BIOPSY OR BLADDER MUCOSAL BIOPSY. These are valuable when stool samples are difficult to obtain or are negative, as is often the case in light or partially treated infections.

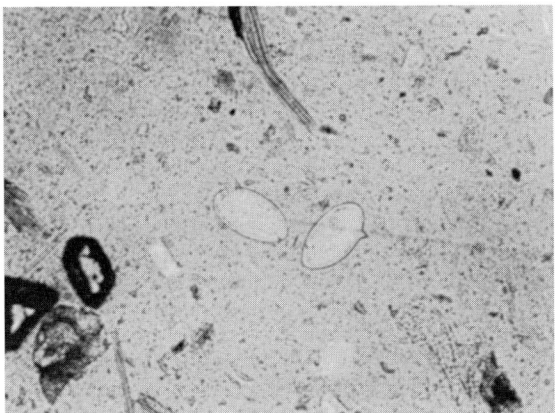

Figure 118–22. *S. mansoni* eggs in feces (Kato preparation, × 125). (Courtesy of the Armed Forces Institute of Pathology, Photograph Neg. No. 76–2406.)

These biopsies may be performed easily during proctoscopy, sigmoidoscopy, or cystoscopy by taking 1 to 3 small mucosal samples from inflamed or granulomatous lesions or from random areas of apparently normal mucosa. The mucosal sample is pressed between a coverslip and a glass slide until it becomes transparent; and eggs, if present, may be seen with low-power microscopy (Fig. 118–23). Schistosome eggs are seen sometimes in biopsy samples from the small bowel in patients with *S. mansoni* and *S. japonicum* infections, but this is not advocated as a primary diagnostic procedure. A portion of the biopsy sample should be fixed in formalin and processed for histologic examination.

URINE SPECIMENS. Eggs in the urine, as in the case of infection with *S. haematobium*, may be detected by simple centrifuge sedimentation or micropore urine filtrates and microscopic examination (Chapter 150). The excretion of schistosome eggs into the urine is not uniform over a 24-hour period, and samples collected between 10 A.M. and 2 P.M. are more likely to be positive.

Egg Quantitation. This clinically important examination is usually measured over 24 hours by collecting an entire day's urine or stool sample, homogenizing the entire sample, and then counting the eggs in a measured aliquot (Chapter 150). Twenty-four-hour stool and urine egg counts of <100 eggs per gram (epg) are considered light infection; counts of 100

to 400 epg are considered moderate infection; and those >400 epg are considered heavy infection.

Egg Viability. Egg viability is also important in determining the activity of schistosome infections, especially in areas where antischistosomal drugs are readily available. Schistosome eggs are excreted in the urine and stool long (e.g., months) after a patient has been treated successfully. Eggs passed more than 1 week after treatment are usually not viable. Egg viability testing is accomplished by two methods: (1) careful examination of single viable eggs shows a living ovum as clear and transparent. Under high magnification, living ova may show the moving organelles (flame cells) of the miracidium; and (2) a more reliable but more difficult method is induced egg hatching. It is performed by diluting a small amount of urine or stool sediment in distilled water at room temperature and exposing it to light for 15 to 20 minutes. Examination with a hand lens reveals swimming miracidia (Chapter 150).

Antibody Detection Tests. Serologic tests are not helpful in the diagnosis of many patients because they (1) become positive too late after infection; (2) become negative too long after cure; or (3) occasionally cross react with other helminths.

The circumoval precipitin test (COPT), the cercaria-Hullen reaction, the miracidia immobilization test, and the cercarial fluorescent antibody test are reasonably accurate but rarely practical because of the need for viable schistosome eggs, cercariae, or miracidia, respectively. The hemagglutination test detects high levels of antischistosome antibody, but the sensitivity and specificity are highly variable because of the wide range of type and purity of schistosome antigens used. With the advent of hybridoma technology, allowing for antigen purification and standardization, sensitive and specific assays (e.g., enzyme-linked immunosorbent assay [ELISA]) have provided useful serologic tests for detecting both schistosomal antibodies and antigens (Chapter 152).

As with other infectious diseases, serologic tests are most useful in epidemiologic studies of endemic populations, in specific diagnoses in nonendemic populations, and in the assessment of individual response to treatment. Serologic tests to detect antischistosome antibodies are useful if stool and urine samples are negative for parasite ova and the diagnosis of schistosomiasis is still strongly suspected, as, e.g., in cerebral schistosomiasis. Antibody titers may remain elevated for prolonged periods of time in individuals from endemic countries with a history of remote infection. Serology, in contrast, may be quite helpful in travelers from nonendemic countries in which the diagnosis is suspected.

Antigen Detection Tests. Assays based on the detection of antigens circulating in the serum and/or excreted in the urine, are now becoming clinically available. During epidemiologic surveys antibody detection suffices in eradicated or controlled areas with low expected prevalence, but detection of ova in stools or urine or circulating antigens is needed for assessment of the incidence of infection or reinfection.

An important recent development is circulating anodic antigen (CAA) and circulating cathodic antigen (CCA) detection assays in various epidemiologic situations and their use in development of field-applicable assays. A new dipstick assay based on the anti-CCA sandwich ELISA, on a nitrocellulose format, is able to detect CCA in urine of patients infected with *S. mansoni* with a sensitivity of 92%. The results were qualitatively as good as those obtained by ELISA or by fecal examination by the Kato thick smear method. The simplicity and speed of the antigen dipstick may ultimately lead to its more extensive application in screening programs. Circulating antigen assays potentially have great value in monitoring large-scale interventions, e.g., chemotherapy and vaccination programs.

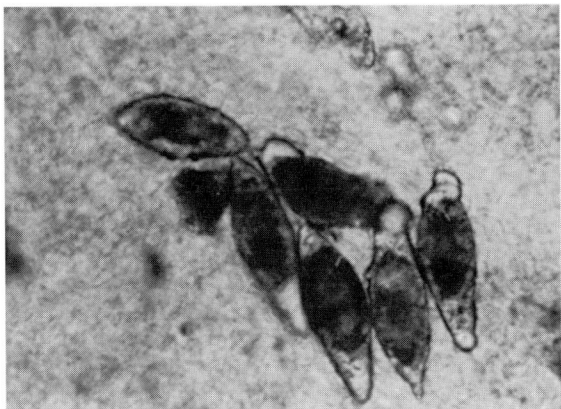

Figure 118–23. Calcified *S. haematobium* eggs in a crushed piece of bladder mucosa from an Egyptian patient (unstained, × 316). (Courtesy of the Armed Forces Institute of Pathology, Photograph Neg. No. 76–2408.)

Associated Clinical Laboratory Findings. Mild anemia is a common finding associated with schistosomiasis. It has several etiologies resulting from the malabsorptive complications of intestinal disease, the iron loss of chronic mucohemorrhagic diarrhea or hematuria, the hemolysis of hypersplenism, or any combination of these. Hypoalbuminemia is common and may be caused by intestinal malabsorption or chronic infection. Normal liver function tests are the rule, except for an elevation in alkaline phosphatase. Hypergammaglobulinemia is common. Mild albuminuria and red cells in the urine sediment are consistent findings in *S. haematobium* infections.

Screening for Hematuria and/or Proteinuria. During the 1990s there have been numerous studies evaluating the efficacy of chemical reagent strips detecting blood and/or protein in the urine for screening for infection with *S. haematobium* in endemic communities. Reagent strip screening is cost effective in some circumstances. Screening for blood is more useful than for protein. The best positive predictive values and posttest probabilities were obtained in communities with high prevalence of infections, in males, and in children. However, reagent strip screening for blood is not very reliable for detecting *S. haematobium* infection in older persons, particularly women, in communities with low or modest (i.e., <20% prevalence) infection rates with *S. haematobium*. The observation of blood in urine or stool should suggest the diagnosis of schistosomiasis in endemic areas.

X-Rays and Scans. X-ray examinations, e.g., barium enema (Fig. 118–15A), barium swallow, and intravenous pyelogram (Figs. 118–18, 118–19, and 118–24) frequently document pathology but are not diagnostic, the one exception being the "fetal head" bladder calcification (Fig. 118–21) seen in chronic urinary schistosomiasis. Sonography also documents a thickened bladder wall, hydronephrosis and hydroureter, and bladder polyps or calcification (Fig. 118–20). It can demon-strate the thickened fibrosed portal tracts, which are characteristic of Symmers' pipestem fibrosis (Figs. 5–1 and 118–17), and the enlargement of the portal vein, which correlates with increased portal venous pressure. Esophagoscopy documents esophageal varices but does not establish their etiology. Sigmoidoscopy, colonoscopy (Fig. 118–15B), and cytoscopy document granulomatous or polyp disease but are of greatest value in providing access to biopsy specimens for tissue egg identification. Liver biopsy may also demonstrate granuloma egg remnants but more typically shows the characteristic periportal fibrosis. The most definitive way to diagnose liver disease due to schistosomiasis is through a wedge biopsy. This approach provides sufficient tissue to determine the presence of characteristic clay pipestem fibrosis or granulomas due to schistosomiasis.

TREATMENT. After active infection is confirmed by the demonstration of viable egg excretion, chemotherapy is indicated. Three nontoxic and efficacious drugs are now available (praziquantel, oxamniquine, and metrifonate), and two others are in developmental phase holding pattern (amoscanate and oltipraz).

Chemotherapeutic Agents

Praziquantel. This is the most important drug for treating schistosomiasis. It is effective orally in a single dose against all species of schistosomes infecting humans. Praziquantel is a mixture of stereoisomers of pyrazinoisoquinoline ring structures. It is active not only against the digenetic trematodes but against many cestodes (e.g., *Diphyllobothrium latum*, *Taenia saginata*, and *Hymenolepis nana*) and other flukes (e.g., *Clonorchis sinensis* and *Paragonimus westermani*). Although the mode of action is unknown, a strong tetanic contraction of the helminth's musculature occurs within a few minutes of administration of the drug.

Host immune responses enhance the effects of praziquantel. The evidence derives mainly from experiments on *S.*

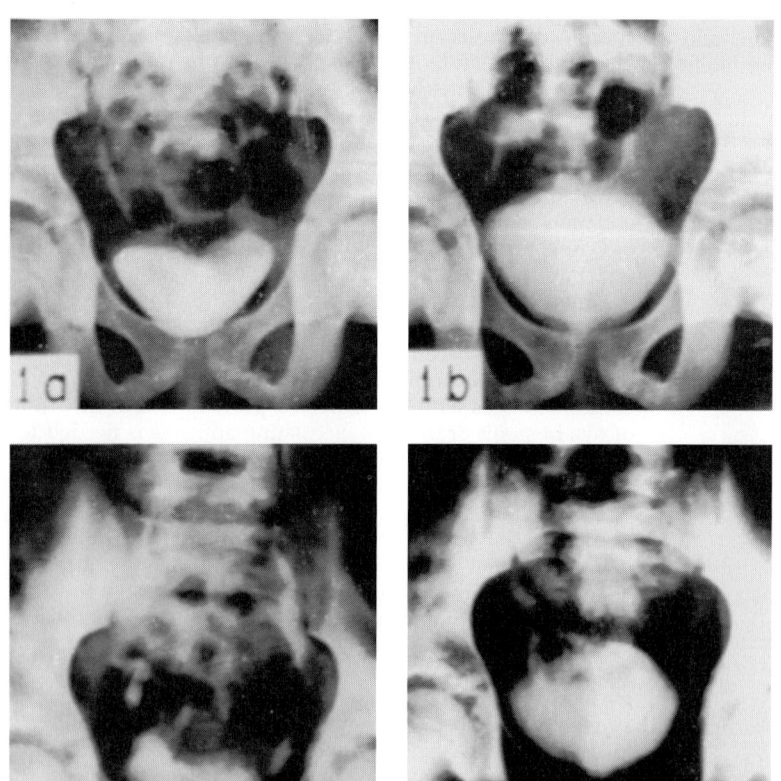

***Figure* 118–24.** Intravenous pyelograms demonstrating bladder masses due to *S. haematobium* infection in two Egyptian patients *(1a and 2a)*. These abnormalities were reversible following praziquantel therapy *(1b and 2b)*.

mansoni infections in the mouse. Electron microscopy and indirect immunofluorescence indicate that praziquantel disrupts the integrity of the surface membranes of *S. mansoni*, particularly those covering the dorsal tubercles of adult male worms, and this causes antigens which are targets of antibody attack to be revealed. Two *S. mansoni* antigens in particular are implicated in the immune-dependent action of praziquantel: a 200-kDa glycoprotein and a 27-kDa antigen with nonspecific esterase activity. Consistent with the involvement of the latter antigen, increased nonspecific esterase activity was demonstrated histochemically on the surface of intact praziquantel-treated male worms. However, patients who have depressed immune responses (i.e., concomitant human immunodeficiency virus [HIV] infection) respond as well to praziquantel as others who only have schistosomiasis mansoni.

DOSAGE AND TOXICITY. Single doses of 40 mg/kg of body weight have resulted in 70 to 95% cure rates in both *S. mansoni* and *S. haematobium* infections. Patients having light infections have better cure rates than those with high ova counts. Furthermore, the intensity of infection is reduced in those who are not cured with praziquantel. Side effects (e.g., nausea, abdominal pain, and vomiting), usually of short duration, beginning a few hours after treatment, and disappearing spontaneously within 48 hours, have been reported. The drug has been well tolerated in community control efforts. Treatment of *S. japonicum* has generally required a higher dose, the most efficacious being a total dose of 60 mg/kg (i.e., 2 doses of 30 mg/kg of body weight given within 6 to 24 hours). This higher dose can also be used in infections with *S. mekongi*, and *S. malayi*, two species of schistosome transmitted in Southeast Asia which are very similar to *S. japonicum*.

Oxamniquine. This tetrahydroquinoline compound is effective against *S. mansoni*, especially the strains in the Americas and West Africa. It is well absorbed from the gastrointestinal tract; its metabolites are excreted in the urine. The site of metabolism and the mechanism of action are unknown.

DOSAGE AND TOXICITY. Oxamniquine is effective in a single oral dose of 15 mg/kg in strains from the Caribbean and South America. A dose of 20 mg/kg has been more efficacious in children in several studies. North and East African strains of *S. mansoni* are less sensitive to this compound, and doses of up to 60 mg/kg given over 2 or 3 days have been required to achieve the same results as 15 mg/kg with strains in the Western Hemisphere. Side effects, usually mild, are decreased by the administration of a single dose after a meal and late in the day. Drowsiness and dizziness are the most commonly reported (7 to 15%) side effects. Fever on day 3 or 4 after initiation of therapy has been noted in carefully monitored patients and appears to be related to worm death and their shift to the liver but is of little clinical importance. This drug has been used successfully in Africa and in Brazil, where a countrywide control effort was based on community chemotherapy with oxamniquine.

The drug is relatively expensive, making it difficult to use in control programs in which the higher dosage is needed (i.e., in Egypt, Sudan, and Kenya).

Metrifonate. This organophosphate compound is metabolized slowly to dichlorvos. It is an anticholinesterase and presumably acts by blocking the worm's acetylcholinesterase, thereby causing paralysis of the worm. It is active only against *S. haematobium*, and the paralysis may be only temporary. Other worms (e.g., *S. japonicum* and *S. mansoni*) in the mesenteric plexus are only swept into the portal vein, where they survive and later migrate back to their usual habitat. (The same may happen to *S. haematobium* worm pairs in the mesenteric plexus.) Egg laying may be temporarily interrupted, but the disease state is not affected in this case. However, *S. haematobium* worms, when temporarily paralyzed, are swept from the vesicular plexus into the vena cava and onto the pulmonary vasculature where they are unable to return to their habitat and are destroyed by the immune response.

DOSAGE AND TOXICITY. Clinical tolerance to this drug is generally good. Nausea, vomiting, and bronchospasm have been reported but are rare. Plasma cholinesterase activity drops to less than 5% of pretreatment levels within 6 hours but quickly returns to normal, whereas erythrocyte cholinesterase is inhibited to 50% of pretreatment values and takes 8 to 10 weeks to resume normal levels. The usual dose is 7.5 to 10 mg/kg of body weight given in 3 doses at 2-week intervals. Cure rates have been 40 to 50% after 2 doses and 70 to 80% following the full course. There are no contraindications to retreatment.

Amoscanate. This lipophilic compound with a reactive isothiocyanate group has shown efficacy in treating *S. haematobium*, *S. mansoni*, and *S. japonicum*. A smaller particle formulation has caused less toxicity than earlier large particle size formulations that produced erratic therapeutic results and liver and CNS reactions. Amoscanate induces a rapid hepatic shift of *S. mansoni* in rodents and causes damage to the tegument and female reproductive organs of schistosomes. As long as praziquantel remains effective therapy for schistosomiasis, amoscanate's history of toxicity could prevent further development of this compound.

Oltipraz. This 1,2-dithiole chemically synthesized antischistosomal compound has efficacy against human *S. mansoni*, *S. haematobium*, and *S. intercalatum*. Clinical evaluation was suspended in 1984 because of late-onset toxicity. It has a slow onset of antischistosomal action that is believed to be related to the parasite's glutathione metabolism. Its activity is greater against mature worms than against immature forms. In small groups of patients, oltipraz has produced cure rates of 86 to 92% with *S. haematobium* infection. However, this drug may be too toxic for clinical use and is currently not scheduled for further development.

General Side Effects. In addition to the chemical side effects of the chemotherapeutic agents, worm death, relocation, and degeneration may also result in pathology. Most drugs cause worm paralysis or mechanical dysfunction, which results in release from attachment to the venule wall. Worms are then swept away by blood flow, usually lodging in the liver, lungs, or, in rare cases, the CNS. This results in large focal granuloma formation with the expected complications. Beyond this local response to a large foreign body, the degeneration of the adult worm undoubtedly releases large amounts of soluble or small particulate antigens over a relatively short period of time. This antigenic release is probably responsible for the fever and the Löffler-like pneumonitis commonly seen 2 or 3 days after initiation of chemotherapy. Usually, these generalized side effects are mildly symptomatic or subclinical, but in heavy infections, they may be severe. Severe generalized side effects of this type usually have an immunologic basis and may be treated with a short course of corticosteroids.

Drug Resistance. Resistance is usually defined as a genetically transmitted loss of sensitivity in a parasite population that was previously sensitive to a given drug. The largest amount of information on drug resistance in schistosomiasis is concerned with drugs of the hycanthone/oxamniquine family. Development of resistance to hycanthone was first reported in 1973 following isolation of a strain of *S. mansoni* from a treated uncured Brazilian patient. During the following years, several other cases were reported in Brazil and Kenya. As a general rule, all hycanthone-resistant strains are also resistant to oxamniquine, while usually retaining their sensitivity to other drugs. Resistance to praziquantel, the current drug of choice for human schistosomiasis, had recently been reported following induction of resistance by drug pressure of the parasite in *S. mansoni*–infected mice. However, human cases of resistance to praziquantel are rare. Monitoring of endemic populations for praziquantel resistance is important to identify drug resistance at its early stages and to design strategies to control its spread.

Evaluation of Therapy. Definitive parasitologic cure has occurred only when there is total disappearance of viable eggs from the excreta for at least 6 months after treatment, in the absence of exposure to reinfection. Not infrequently, adult worms are incapacitated only temporarily by chemo-

therapy. In this case, egg release is interrupted only to begin again a few weeks later. Final laboratory evaluation should include examination of excreta on 3 consecutive days and, if negative for viable eggs, this may be followed by examination of a rectal mucosa biopsy. In epidemiologic studies and antischistosomal drug trials in endemic areas, these rigid criteria for cure are impractical and not pertinent. Percentage of egg reduction is another way of assessing the incomplete early effects of chemotherapy. The early cure rates and egg reduction measurements are undoubtedly representative of the positive impact of the drug on the infection, but they must not be confused with complete cure.

Management of the Individual Patient. Because of the wide range of clinical disease presentation, the multiorgan

TABLE 118–2. Management of Schistosomiasis

Schistosome Dermatitis	Self-limited and usually not diagnosed
	Topical corticosteroids and parenteral antihistamines reduce symptoms in severe cases
Katayama Fever	Nonsteroidal anti-inflammatory therapy for mild or moderate disease
	Corticosteroids for life-threatening disease
	Antischistosome therapy according to species
Gastrointestinal Schistosomiasis	
S. mansoni	Praziquantel, 40 mg/kg in a single dose or
	Oxamniquine, 15 mg/kg in a single dose for adults (20 mg/kg for children), except in North and East Africa, where the dose is 60 mg/kg over 2 or 3 days, given in 3 or 4 equally divided doses;
S. japonicum	Praziquantel, 60 mg/kg in 2 or 3 doses given in one day
Hepatosplenic Disease	
S. mansoni	Praziquantel or oxamniquine
	Ultrasonography to establish extent of disease
S. japonicum	Praziquantel; ultrasonography to establish extent of disease
Ascites	Low-salt diet and diuretics
Bleeding esophageal varices	Esophagoscopy to establish diagnosis. Usually can be managed conservatively with transfusion and esophageal sclerotherapy
	Surgical shunt procedures for portal hypertension may be considered in severe cases (after repeated hemorrhage). A selective shunt operation that decompresses the splenic venous compartment without interfering with portal venous perfusion of the liver gives best long-term results
Colonic polyposis	Colonoscopy to establish extent of disease
	Chemotherapy usually shrinks polyps; pedunculated polyps may be removed at colonoscopy; surgical bowel resection if permanent fibrotic obstructive bowel lesion
	For intussusception, barium enema treatment must be performed with great care to avoid perforation
	For rectal prolapse, chemotherapy only
	For anorectal fistulas and abscess, surgical drainage and antibiotic therapy
Urinary Schistosomiasis	Praziquantel, 40 mg/kg in single dose or metrifonate, 7.5–10 mg/kg biweekly × 3
Uncomplicated	Ultrasonograpy or intravenous pyelogram in all patients to detect silent obstructive disease
Obstructive uropathy	Often responds to chemotherapy; may require surgery if permanent obstructive fibrotic lesion is present
Urinary tract infection	Bacteriuria will not be eradicated with antibiotic unless accompanied by antischistosomal therapy
	Pyelonephritis may be life-threatening and requires parenteral antibiotics
Renal failure	Hemodialysis or renal transplant
Bladder cancer	Radical surgery and cancer chemotherapy are usually only palliative
Cardiopulmonary Schistosomiasis	
Larval pneumonitis	Self-limited disease
	Short-course steroid therapy if there is respiratory distress
Reactionary pneumonitis	Interrupt antischistosomal chemotherapy until resolution
	Short-course steroid therapy if respiratory distress is present
Cor pulmonale	Antischistosomal therapy to arrest further progression of disease; symptomatic therapy
CNS Schistosomiasis	Antischistosomal therapy with praziquantel
	Steroid therapy is recommended to reduce inflammation and size of space-occupying lesions
Other	
Salmonella-schistosome syndrome	Simultaneous antischistosomal and antibiotic therapy
	Re-treatment with both may be necessary
Hepatitis B or C schistosome disease	Antischistosomal therapy
	Precautions to prevent transmission of hepatitis B or C to hospital and laboratory staff and patient's contacts

involvement of complications, and the variation in antischistosomal chemotherapy according to infecting species and strain, a simplified standard management regimen for schistosomiasis cannot be devised. Patient care must be individualized. Table 118–2 offers broad guidelines for the management of the more common presentations of schistosomiasis.

Prognosis. Heavy urinary schistosomiasis often leads to obstructive uropathy and/or pyelonephritis with gram-negative bacteremia and resultant renal failure. Bladder cancer is a long-term potential consequence of chronic heavy S. haematobium infection. If untreated, long-standing hepatosplenic schistosomiasis may eventually result in intractable portal hypertension with recurrent esophageal variceal bleeding and ascites. Hepatic failure with associated hepatitis B or C infections can be a terminal event also.

Certain local fibrotic changes of schistosomal granulomatosis (e.g., of the ureter, intestine, or liver) may remain after complete eradication of infection and may cause permanent and potentially fatal disease. However, with the advent of the newer efficacious and less toxic chemotherapeutic agents, the prognosis in most schistosomal infections is excellent, providing reinfection can be prevented and end-stage irreversible disease has not yet been established (Fig. 118–24).

PREVENTION AND CONTROL. Schistosomiasis cannot be eradicated on a worldwide scale at present, although certain foci have been cleared successfully. To date, all successful focal eradication programs have been multifaceted in approach, and this undoubtedly is the direction for future attempts at worldwide eradication of schistosomiasis.

Schistosomiasis control is the realistic goal of the present and the near future. Control logically falls into two parallel interdependent strategies: control of population morbidity and control of transmission, which incorporate five general methods (Table 118–3).

Chemotherapy. This is the most cost-effective form of control and the only one that reduces both the transmission of the biologic cycle (by reducing the number of ova in the excreta) and the disease morbidity (by reducing the number of ova retained in the body). Both effects can be obtained by lowering the body burden of parasites; complete cure is not essential. Earlier drugs available for treating schistosomiasis were not sufficiently efficacious and were too toxic for routine use in control programs. However, newer antischistosomal drugs given safely in single (or only a few) doses, cure at least 75% of those infected, and reduce ova excretion by 90 to 95% in those not cured: oxamniquine (for S. mansoni infections), metrifonate (for S. haematobium infections), and praziquantel (for all schistosoma infections). These drugs may be applied in two ways—mass treatment chemotherapy or targeted population chemotherapy. Chemotherapy, either mass or targeted, is the linchpin of control and should be an integral part of every program.

Mass Chemotherapy. This is most appropriate in a defined, medically manageable population with high prevalence rates, i.e., >30%. It is performed by giving all members of the population drug treatment with no attempt at individual diagnosis or evaluation of cure. The rationale is that the savings in time, effort, and money to diagnose and to evaluate cure in individual patients outweight the cost and relatively small risk of a safe drug being administered to the noninfected community members. Overall population morbidity and transmission would be reduced, and with the addition of other control methods, the reduction of eggs excreted into the environment might break the transmission cycle.

Targeted Population Chemotherapy. This approach relies on the identification of individual moderate to heavy egg excretors followed by specific treatment and evaluation of cure.

TABLE 118–3. Schistosomiasis Control Methods

1. Chemotherapy
   a. Mass
   b. Targeted population
2. Snail control
   a. Mollusciciding
   b. Biologic control
   c. Environmental modification
3. Reduction of water contact and contamination
   a. Provision of domestic water supplies
   b. Provision for sanitary disposal of excreta
4. Vaccination
5. Improved living standards

This method is more medically aesthetic (e.g., noninfected persons are not given an unnecessary drug), and drug costs may be reduced considerably. However, it requires more time, technology, and equipment. A cost-effective method to detect those in the community who may be infected with S. haematobium is to screen for hematuria and proteinuria using chemical reagent strips. Many community-based studies have shown that both hematuria and proteinuria correlate with S. haematobium infection but the positive predictive value of these tests (reagent strip testing for hematuria being the best) is much less valuable in older people, particularly women, in communities with infection rates <15%.

Snail Control. Although snail control is a rapid and effective means of reducing transmission, it requires a prolonged effort (Chapter 136). The snails almost always return in significant numbers, and, if they are infected by schistosome miracidia, the biologic cycle is resumed. Therefore, snail control should be used in combination with other approaches.

Mollusciciding. This is the usual method of snail control. Niclosamide is the most frequently used chemical and is most cost-effective when a small body of water is to be treated. It is well suited to arid areas where transmission is seasonal and confined to relatively small habitats. It also can be targeted to focal areas to kill infected snails, as was done in the Cul-de-Sac Valley and elsewhere in St. Lucia and areas of Puerto Rico. These projects show that routine focal control of snails is as effective as areawide control and is less expensive. The long-term effects of molluscicides on the ecology of fresh water is not clear. Furthermore, there is a particular problem with the *Oncomelania* snails that transmit S. japonicum in that they are amphibious and a significant number of them tend to be out of the water at any given time. A report on the prolonged use of niclosamide (14 years at 3-monthly intervals) as a molluscicide against *Biomphalara glabrata* for the control of S. mansoni had shown that the snail population reestablished itself within 3 months of molluscicide application. Therefore, the continual use of niclosamide as the only method of control of schistosomiasis is not effective.

Biologic Control. This is an alternate method of snail control. This method uses the natural predators and parasites of snails (e.g., ducks, fish, turtles, and fungi), other species of snails that compete with the schistosome carriers, and bacteria and viruses. In Puerto Rico, a competitive species of snail, *Marisa cornuarietis*, has been effective in reducing the transmission of S. mansoni by B. glabrata in some habitats. Although some of these methods have had some local usefulness, they have not been demonstrated to be feasible on a mass level.

Environmental Modification. Perhaps of more importance than killing snails are measures designed to prevent or reduce their breeding, and site modification to produce conditions detrimental to the intermediate host may prove comparatively simple and inexpensive in localized sites. The burying of snails by digging out irrigation ditches was an effective but labor-intensive method of *Oncomelania* snail control in China. Other methods of environmental modification, e.g., cementing over or enclosing irrigation ditches, not only reduced the snail habitat but reduced human exposure to water. Although planning for site modification requires a multidisciplinary approach, this strategy of snail control is most feasible particularly when community participation is encouraged and when the local government units are involved in finding solutions to their local problems. Engineering methods, e.g., increasing the rate of water flow in irrigation canals and cementing of canals, can also be used.

Reduction of Water Contact and Contamination. The provision of clean water supplies to infected populations not only reduces exposure to cercariae but also reduces other waterborne infections. However, sociocultural habits are difficult to modify, and frequently the population continues to use the nearby contaminated stream or irrigation canal. Likewise, the provision of indoor or outdoor latrines has not always reduced the transmission of schistosomiasis. A successful program requires that the provision of clean water and sanitary excreta disposal be combined with health education and other methods of control. Those living in endemic areas must understand how to prevent the biologic transmission of schistosomiasis and must have the incentive and the tools to participate in its control.

Improved Living Standards. As living standards improve, e.g., in Puerto Rico and Japan, it becomes much easier to control and, eventually eradicate schistosomiasis. A more educated population, supplied with indoor water and toilets and working in offices or factories or farming with tools and equipment that reduce water contact, is less likely to be infected with schistosomes. Communities with improved living standards are also more likely to have satisfactory diagnostic and therapeutic facilities available for detecting and treating schistosomiasis.

Vaccination. Control and even eradication of schistosomiasis have been achieved in some countries using integrated measures but this disease remains endemic in >75 countries. The application of control measures, particularly population-based chemotherapy, has in many countries greatly reduced the incidence of serious disease manifestations, but vaccines are urgently needed to supplement existing control measures.

Mounting evidence for acquired immunity to schistosomiasis supports the case for immunologic intervention. On the other hand, rapid reinfection poses a threat to younger age groups due to the slow maturation of natural resistance. However, rational approaches, based on advances in immunology and molecular biology, have substantially increased the odds of producing an effective vaccine. Since the parasite cannot replicate in the human host and serious morbidity generally occurs only after a relatively long period of heavy worm burden, complete protection against infection is not essential. The chances of success would increase if more than one of the various host-parasite interphases were targeted, e.g., reducing morbidity through decreased worm loads as well as through suppression of egg production. Several promising schistosome antigens have now reached an advanced phase of development and are currently undergoing independent confirmatory testing according to a standardized protocol. Since schistosomiasis cannot realistically be controlled by a single approach, vaccination is envisaged to be implemented in conjunction with other means of control, notably chemotherapy.

Anti-Infection Vaccination. A vaccine to prevent or attenuate infection with schistosomes would be the most important control method and would provide a tool for eradication of schistosomiasis. Vaccination with radiation-attenuated cercariae confers the highest levels of resistance to challenge infection in experimental schistosomiasis and requires antigen-specific T cells. There are currently several schistosome antigens that have been characterized and are important candidates for a defined antischistosomal vaccine: paromyosin, heat shock protein 70, triosephosphate isomerase, glutathione-S-transferase (GST), and the integral membrane protein Sm23.

Anti-Morbidity Vaccination. Fibrosis in schistosomiasis is associated with the granulomatous response to parasite eggs trapped in the liver. In experimental animals injection of IL-12 peritoneally with eggs prevents subsequent pulmonary granuloma formation on intravenous challenge with eggs. In addition, sensitization with eggs plus IL-12 partly inhibits granuloma formation and dramatically reduces the tissue fibrosis induced by natural infection with *S. mansoni* worms.

These results are an example of a vaccine against parasites, which acts by preventing pathology rather than infection. IL-12 is known to favor the priming of Th1 rather than Th2 cells, and the effects on fibrosis are accompanied by replacement of the Th2-dominated pattern of cytokine expression characteristic of *S. mansoni* infection with one dominated by Th1 cytokines. Elevated Th2 cytokine expression and fibrosis are common manifestations of a wide variety of infectious diseases and atopic disorders which might be ameliorated by vaccination with antigen and IL-12.

Antifecundity Vaccination. Immunization of mice with recombinant 26-kDa GST (reSjc26GST) induces a pronounced antifecundity effect after experimental infection with Chinese *S. japonicum*. A similar vaccination trial carried out on pigs, important reservoirs for schistosomiasis japonica, showed that immunization with reSjc26GST can reduce worm burden following exposure of pigs to reinfection with *S. japonicum*. In addition, reSjc26GST can induce an antifecundity effect, thereby reducing pathology, coupled with a delay or interruption of the development of immature to mature eggs. As a consequence, vaccination with reSjc26GST would also affect the transmission of schistosomiasis japonica.

■ OTHER HUMAN SCHISTOSOME INFECTIONS

Schistosomiasis intercalatum

DEFINITION. Schistosomiasis intercalatum is an endemic intestinal disease with blood and mucus in the stool, abdominal pain, diarrhea, and other gastrointestinal symptoms that are caused by the blood fluke *Schistosoma intercalatum*.

ETIOLOGY
Adult Morphology. The dimensions of the adult parasites may vary with the host and may be confused with other species of schistosomes. The males range in length from 115 to 145 mm and in breadth (with the gynecophoral canal folded) from 3 to 5 mm. The testes vary in number from 2 to 7, but most of these parasites have 4. The ventral, lateral, and dorsal surfaces of the male are spinose, and the cuticle is tuberculate from the area of the testes posteriorly. Adult female worms range from 130 to 240 mm in length by 3 mm in breadth. The ovary lies between the intestinal ceca and, in many specimens, is spirally twisted.

Ova. The intrauterine eggs measure 140 to 180 μm in length by 30 to 50 μm in breadth. After 80 days, the number of eggs passed from an experimental infected host averages between 25 and 60 per worm. A terminal spine that is usually slightly bent characterizes eggs that occur in the feces. The eggshells are Ziehl-Neelsen positive, i.e., acid-fast, when fixed in Bouin's solution; frequently, the contained miracidium appears to be hourglass-shaped.

Intermediate Hosts. The proven intermediate hosts consist of *Bulinus forskalii* in Cameroon and Gabon and *B. africanus* group in parts of Zaire.

UNIQUE BIOLOGIC CHARACTERISTICS. The best criteria for considering *S. intercalatum* as a separate species and distinguishing it from other schistosomes lie in a number of biologic characteristics. The most distinctive features are (1) the Ziehl-Neelsen–positive staining reaction of the eggshell in histologic sections; (2) the behavioral pattern of the cercariae, which tend to congregate near or at the water surface (as do those of *S. japonicum*); (3) the tendency of the cercariae to adhere to objects; (4) the cercarial glandular secretions that take the form of granular strings; and (5) it is the sole species found in most of its known transmission foci (in a few places *S. intercalatum* coexists with *S. mansoni*; it coexists with *S. haematobium* only in Cameroon.

Natural hybrids between *S. haematobium* and *S. intercalatum* are found in Loum, Cameroon. Over a 10-year period the number of cases of intestinal schistosomiasis caused by *S. intercalatum* has markedly decreased, while the cases of urinary schistosomiasis caused by *S. haematobium* and the hybrid parasite have increased. *S. haematobium* and *S. intercalatum* hybrids raised in the laboratory exhibit heterosis by their enhanced infectivity to both snail hosts and experimental animals as well as by an increased growth rate and reproductive potential.

EPIDEMIOLOGY. The epidemiology of *S. intercalatum* is essentially similar to that of *S. mansoni*, and the ranges of the two parasites overlap in a few areas.

Distribution and Incidence. This distinctly African disease is endemic in parts of Cameroon, Gabon, and north and east to the Democratic Republic of the Congo, and possibly other parts of Central and West Africa (Fig. 118–9). The disease is spread to new foci by migrant African laborers as well as by the regular seasonal migration of nomads between the southern and northern Cameroon, especially because potential snail vector species are widely disseminated throughout Central Africa. Surveys made in endemic regions reveal a prevalence rate for *S. intercalatum* of between 5 and 25%.

Animal Reservoirs. Two natural infections have been found in *Hybomys univittatus*, the one-striped mouse. However, more potential hosts need to be examined in endemic foci. Laboratory infections have been produced in hamsters, gerbils, rats, mice, guinea pigs, rabbits, goats, sheep, and rhesus monkeys. Other species of monkeys and the American opossum have also been infected.

PATHOLOGY. Lesions occur when the often bent, terminal-spined eggs of *S. intercalatum* are deposited in the mesenteric venules and break through to the lumen of the intestine, where they are passed in the feces. The infection causes less tissue reaction than do the other human schistosomes, for undefined reasons. Hepatomegaly may occur frequently and may be severe; liver biopsies reveal perioval granulomas.

CLINICAL MANIFESTATIONS. Rectal bleeding is the most common finding. The clinical symptomatology may include episodes of pain in the left iliac fossa with tenesmus. Anorexia, nausea, abdominal pain, and diarrhea occur frequently, and blood and mucus may be present in the stool. Endoscopy may reveal hyperplasia of the mucosa near the rectal valves, inflammation of the intestinal wall, ulcers, and sometimes polyposis. These conditions are usually relieved following adequate treatment. There may be alterations in the results of liver function tests and complications include severe rectal or genital lesions, e.g., salpingitis with secondary sterility.

DIAGNOSIS. The diagnosis rests on the demonstration of the characteristic bent, terminal-spined eggs. These may be documented in the feces or in mucosal snips from the rectum or, less frequently, in the urine sediment. The eggs are Ziehl-Neelsen positive, whereas those of the other species with terminal-spined eggs, *S. haematobium*, are not. The contained miracidium is often narrowed in the middle, giving it an hourglass shape.

TREATMENT. The treatment of choice is praziquantel, which gives high cure rates when used in a single dosage of 40 mg/kg.

Schistosomiasis Mekongi amd Schistosomiasis Malayi

DEFINITION. Schistosomiasis mekongi and schistosomiasis malayi occur in the lower Mekong River Basin in Laos and Kampuchea, and in Malaysia and Thailand and are caused by *S. japonicum*–like schistosomes, *S. mekongi* and *S. malayi*, respectively. Clinical disease has gastrointestinal manifestations and may be severe.

ETIOLOGY

Adult Worm. The morphologic characteristics of the adult worms are similar to those of *S. japonicum*, although some worms are slightly larger and have more testes and larger ovaries and other more subtle anatomic differences.

Ova. The eggs are round, with a mean diameter of 57 to 66 μm, and have a small knob-like appendage. They are similar in appearance to *S. japonicum* ova but are more rounded and slightly smaller.

Intermediate Host. The strongest evidence for separate speciation of *S. mekongi* and *S. malayi* rests with their intermediate hosts. The miracidium of the Mekong schistosome will develop only in the aquatic *Neotricula aperta* and the Malaysian schistosome only develops in *Robertsiella kaporensis*. *Oncomelania* snails, the intermediate host of *S. japonicum*, cannot be infected by either *S. mekongi* or *S. malayi* miracidia.

EPIDEMIOLOGY

Distribution and Incidence. *S. mekongi* infection was first described on Khong Island, the largest island in the Mekong River, and in the Lower Mekong Basin region in Cambodia and Laos, while *S. malayi* has been found focally in Thailand and Malaysia (Fig. 118–8). Population studies indicate a prevalence rate of 15 to 50% with schoolchildren to age 15 years being most heavily and most frequently infected.

Reservoir Hosts. Dogs are the only known reservoir host for *S. mekongi*, and their role in the maintenance of the disease cycle is yet to be determined.

PATHOGENESIS AND PATHOLOGY. Because of the small population infected with *S. mekongi* or *S. malayi* and the few clinical or pathologic studies, little information is available about the pathogenesis and pathology. However, the disease most resembles schistosomiasis japonica. Animal model experiments indicate that the pathology is identical to that of the Philippine strain of *S. japonicum*. Pathogenesis is likewise, similar, except for delayed oviposition in mice and the inability to infect rabbits.

CLINICAL MANIFESTATIONS. Clinically, schistosomiasis mekongi mirrors *S. japonicum* infection. Presenting complaints include generalized weakness, mild diarrhea, and "thong darn," or abdominal distress. A clinical study found hepatomegaly in 44% and splenomegaly in 18% of infected patients. Two of 25 patients with hepatosplenomegaly had portal hypertension with ascites. CNS or cardiopulmonary complications have not been reported.

DIAGNOSIS. Demonstration of eggs in the stool establishes the diagnosis. Other clinical laboratory findings are normal or unhelpful; however, as noted in other forms of schistosomiasis, alkaline phosphatase levels are markedly elevated.

TREATMENT. Praziquantel (60 mg/kg) is the treatment of choice for schistosomiasis mekongi, based on clinical trials.

TABLE 118–4. Geographic Distribution and Hosts of the Zoonotic Mammalian Schistosomes

Schistosome	Geographic Distribution	Snail Intermediate Hosts	Natural Definitive Hosts
Schistosomatium douthitti	Northern United States (including Alaska), Canada	*Stagnicola pabistris* *Lymnaea stagnalis*	Muskrats, meadow mice
Heterobilharzia americana	United States: Florida, Georgia, Texas, Louisiana, North Carolina and South Carolina	*Lymnaea cubensis* *Pseudosuccinea columella*	Bobcats, raccoons, dogs, nutria, white-tailed deer, rabbits, opossums
Schistosoma spindale	Malaya, Sumatra, and India	*Indoplanorbis exustus*	Cattle, buffaloes, goats
	South Africa, Zambia, and Rhodesia	*Bulinus tropicus*	Cattle, reedbucks, other antelopes
Schistosoma bovis	Southern Europe	*Planorbarius metidjensis*	Sheep, goats, cattle, equines, camels, humans
	Northern Africa and south-western Asia	*Bulinus (Bulinus) truncatus*	
	East Africa	*B. forskalii*	
	West Africa	*B. senegalensis*	
	South Africa	*B. (Ph.) africanus*	
	Central Africa	*B. ugandae*	
Schistosoma mattheei	South Africa, Zaire	*B. (Ph.) globosus*	Cattle, sheep, goats, zebras, impalas, humans
Schistosoma margrebowiei	Zambia, South Africa		Equines, cattle, sheep, antelopes, humans
Schistosoma rodhaini	Zaire, Uganda	*Biomphalaria sudanica* *B. pfeifferi*	Rodents, dogs, humans
Schistosoma incognitum	Indonesia	*Radix rubiginosa*	Rodents

Schistosomiasis Mattheei

DEFINITION. Schistosomiasis mattheei is a natural schistosome infection of sheep, cattle, and horses that also infects humans in South Africa, causing mild gastrointestinal disease.

ETIOLOGY

Adult Worm. Adult worms most resemble *S. intercalatum.* The female worm is able to produce eggs parthenogenetically and is perhaps carried by excess males of other species. It was once thought that *S. intercalatum* was a hybrid of *S. mattheei* and *S. haematobium.*

Ova. *S. mattheei* eggs may be found in urine or feces, measure 120 to 180 μm in length, have a terminal spine, and resemble *S. intercalatum* eggs in general configuration.

EPIDEMIOLOGY. Sheep, cattle, horses, and antelope are the natural hosts of *S. mattheei*; humans are only a secondary host. In humans, *S. mattheei* infection has invariably been found in association with *S. haematobium* or *S. mansoni* and has been seen in up to 30% of some populations in South Africa. Because of the mild disease it causes, *S. mattheei* infection in humans does not constitute a serious public health problem; its veterinary importance is significant, however.

PATHOGENESIS AND PATHOLOGY. The pathogenesis and pathology of human *S. mattheei* infection are thought to be similar to those of other human intestinal schistosome infections. Egg granulomas have been found in the large intestine and liver and are responsible for mild hepatosplenomegaly and granulomatous bowel disease. Because of the invariable coinfection with *S. mansoni* or *S. haematobium*, the overall pathologic impact of *S. mattheei* is difficult to assess.

CLINICAL MANIFESTATIONS. Human *S. mattheei* infections are associated with schistosomal bowel disease. Patients most often present with mild blood-containing mucoid diarrhea, diffuse intermittent cramping abdominal pain, and general malaise. However, as in other schistosome infections, the majority of infected patients are asymptomatic. Mild hepatosplenomegaly may be found on physical examination, and sigmoidoscopy reveals mucosal granulomatous lesions. Severe gastrointestinal disease and cardiopulmonary or CNS complications have not been reported.

DIAGNOSIS. Clinical diagnosis rests with finding *S. mattheei* eggs in the stool or, occasionally, in the urine and is supported by the known epidemiologic distribution of disease.

TREATMENT. Clinical drug trials have not been performed in *S. mattheei* infections. Praziquantel should be efficacious.

Some Potential Human Schistosomes

Several other species of schistosomes, normally parasites of mammals, may occasionally infect humans. Experiments with monkeys suggest that nonpatent visceral schistosomiasis may be produced in humans as a result of infection with the cercariae of *Schistosomatium douthitti, Heterobilharzia americana,* and *Schistosoma spindale.* Young preadult worms were recovered from livers of rhesus monkeys exposed to these schistosomes, but later the worms were lost. However, in South American monkeys, cebus, and squirrel, *Heterobilharzia americana* produces a patent infection with the deposition of large numbers of eggs in the tissues and their excretion in the feces. Other zoonotic species of *Schistosoma* include *S. bovis, S. margrebowiei,* and *S. rodhaini.* These produce a patent infection in humans, with passage of viable eggs in the stools or urine. *S. incognitum,* commonly found in rodents in Indonesia, is suspected to occasionally infect humans. The geographic distribution and hosts of these mammalian schistosomes are indicated in Table 118–4.

Bibliography

General

Abdel-Wahab MF: Schistosomiasis in Egypt. Boca Raton, FL, CRC Press, 1982.
Abdel-Wahab MF: *Schistosomiasis mansoni* in Egypt. Clin Trop Communic Dis 2:371, 1987.
Brindley PJ, Ramirez B, Tiu W: Networking schistosomiasis japonica. Parasitol Today 11:163, 1995.
Hagan P, Gryseels B: A perspective on schistosomiasis research. Parasitol Today 10:166, 1994.
Harinasuta C: Epidemiology and control of schistosomiasis in Southeast Asia. Southeast Asian J Trop Med Public Health 15:431, 1984.
Sturrock RF: Biology and ecology of human schistosomes. Clin Trop Med Communic Dis 2:249, 1987.

Epidemiology

Coutinho EM, Abath FG, Barbosa CS, et al: Factors involved in *Schistosoma mansoni* infection in rural areas of northeast Brazil. Mem Inst Oswaldo Cruz 92:707, 1997.

El-Khoby T, Galal N, Fenwick A, et al: The epidemiology of schistosomiasis in Egypt: Summary findings in nine governorates. Am J Trop Med Hyg (In press).

Hammad TA, Gabr NS, Hussein MH, et al: Determinants of infection with schistosomiasis haematobia using logistic regression. Am J Trop Med Hyg 57:464, 1997.

He YX, Hu YQ, Yu QF, et al: Review: Strain complex of *Schistosoma japonicum* in the mainland of China. Southeast Asia J Trop Med Public Health 25:232, 1994.

Tchuem Tchuente LA, Southgate VR, Njiokou F, et al: The evolution of schistosomiasis at Loum, Cameroon: Replacement of *Schistosoma intercalatum* by *S. haematobium* through introgressive hybridization. Trans R Soc Trop Med Hyg 91:664, 1997.

World Health Organization: Atlas of the Global Distribution of Schistosomiasis. Parasitic Diseases Programme. Geneva, World Health Organization, 1987.

Pathology/Pathophysiology

Andrade ZA, Cheever AW: Alterations of intrahepatic vasculature in hepatosplenic schistosomiasis mansoni. Am J Trop Med Hyg 20:425, 1971.

Andrade ZA, Andrade SG: Pathogenesis of pulmonary arteritis. Am J Trop Med Hyg 19:305, 1970.

Bassily S, Farid Z, Baroum RS, et al: Renal biopsy of *Schistosoma-Salmonella* associated nephrotic syndrome. J Trop Med Hyg 79:256, 1976.

Biempica L, Dunn MA, Kamel IA, et al: Liver collagen-type characterization in human schistosomiasis. Am J Trop Med Hyg 32:316, 1983.

Cheever AW: Differential regulation of granuloma size and hepatic fibrosis in schistosome infections. Mem Inst Oswaldo Cruz 92:689, 1997.

Cheever AW, Kamel IA, Elwi AM, et al: *Schistosoma mansoni* and *S. haematobium* in Egypt. IV: Hepatic lesions. Am J Trop Med Hyg 27:939, 1978.

Corbett EL, Butterworth AE, Fulford AJ, et al: Nutritional status of children with schistosomiasis mansoni in two different areas of Machakos District, Kenya. Trans R Soc Trop Med Hyg 86:266, 1992.

Da Silva LC: Review: Portal hypertension in schistosomiasis: Pathophysiology and treatment. Mem Inst Oswaldo Cruz 87 (suppl 4):183, 1992.

Dunn MA, Kamel R: Hepatic schistosomiasis. Hepatology 1:653, 1981.

Li Y, Li Y, Yu D, et al: A multivariate analysis of the relationship between work ability and *S. japonicum* infection in Dongting Lake region, in China. Rev Inst Med Trop Sao Paulo 35:347, 1993.

LoVerde PT, Amento C, Higashi GI: Parasite-parasite interaction of *Salmonella typhimurium* and *Schistosoma*. J Infect Dis 141:177, 1980.

McGarvey ST, Aligui G, Daniel BL, et al: Child growth and schistosomiasis japonica in northeastern Leyte, the Philippines: Cross-sectional results. Am J Trop Med Hyg 46:571, 1992.

McGarvey ST, Wu G, Zhang S, et al: Child growth, nutritional status, and schistosomiasis japonica in Jiangxi, People's Republic of China. Am J Trop Med Hyg 48:547, 1993.

Schwartz DA: Helminths in the induction of cancer. II: *Schistosoma haematobium* and bladder cancer. Trop Geogr Med 33:1, 1981.

Smith JH, Kamel TA, Elwi A, et al: A quantitative post mortem analysis of urinary schistosomiasis in Egypt. I: Pathology and pathogenesis. Am J Trop Med Hyg 23:1054, 1974.

Warren KS: Determinants of disease in human schistosomiasis. Clin Trop Med Communic Dis 2:301, 1987.

Immunology

Barral-Netto W, Hoffstetter M, Cheever AW, et al: Specificity of antibody and cellular immune responses in human schistosomiasis. Am J Trop Med Hyg 32:106, 1983.

Boros DL: The role of cytokines in the formation of the schistosome egg granuloma. Immunobiology 191:441, 1994.

Butterworth AE: Human immunity to schistosomes: Some questions. Parasitol Today 10:378, 1994.

Butterworth AE, Dunne DW, Fulford AJ, et al: Human immunity to *Schistosoma mansoni*: Observations on mechanisms, and implications for control. Immunol Invest 21:391, 1992.

Capron A, Dessaint JP, Capron M, et al: Schistosomiasis: From effector and regulation mechanisms in rodents to vaccine strategies in humans. Immunol Invest 21:409, 1992.

David JR, Butterworth AE, Vadas MA: Mechanism of the interaction mediating killing of *Schistosoma mansoni* by human eosinophils. Am J Trop Med Hyg 29:842, 1980.

Dunne DW, Butterworth AE, Fulford AJ, et al: Immunity after treatment of human schistosomiasis mansoni: Association between IgE antibodies and adult worm antigens and resistance to infection. Eur J Immunol 22:1483, 1992.

Fulford AJ, Butterworth AE, Sturrock RF, et al: On the use of age-intensity data to detect immunity to parasitic infections, with special reference to *Schistosoma mansoni* in Kenya. Parasitology 105:219, 1992.

Grogan JL, Kremsner PG, Deelder AM, Yazdanbakhsh M: Antigen-specific proliferation and interferon-gamma and interleukin-5 production are down-regulated during *Schistosoma haematobium* infection. J Infect Dis 177:1433, 1998.

Hagan P: Reinfection, exposure and immunity in human schistosomiasis. Parasitol Today 8:12, 1992.

Kaplan MH, Whitfield JR, Boros DL, Grusby MJ: Th2 cells are required for the *Schistosoma mansoni* egg-induced granulomatous response. J Immunol 160:1850, 1998.

Kresina TF, Guan XH, Posner M, et al: Comparison of immune repertoires of Chinese and Philippine patients infected with *Schistosoma japonicum*. Infect Immun 59:4698, 1991.

Liu SX, Song GC, Xu YX, et al: Anti-fecundity immunity induced in pigs vaccinated with recombinant *Schistosoma japonicum* 26kDa glutathione-S-transferase. Parasit Immunol 17:355, 1995.

McKerrow JH: Cytokine induction and exploitation in schistosome infections. Parasitology 115 (Suppl): S107, 1997.

Medhat A, Shehata M, Bucci K, et al: Increased interleukin-4 and interleukin-5 production in response to *Schistosoma haematobium* adult worm antigens correlates with lack of reinfection after treatment. J Infect Dis 178:512, 1998.

Mutapi F, Ndhlovu PD, Hagan P, et al: Chemotherapy accelerates the development of acquired immune responses to *Schistosoma haematobium* infection. J Infect Dis 178:289, 1998.

Mwatha JK, Kimani G, Kamau T, et al: High levels of TNF, soluble TNF receptors, soluble ICAM-1, and IFN-gamma, but low levels of IL-5, are associated with hepatosplenic disease in human schistosomiasis mansoni. J Immunol 160:1992, 1998.

Olds GR, Olveda R, Wu G, et al: Immunity and morbidity in schistosomiasis japonicum infection. Am J Trop Med Hyg 55:121, 1996.

Ramirez BL, Kurtis JD, Wiest PM, et al: Paromyosin: A candidate vaccine antigen against *Schistosoma japonicum*. Parasit Immunol 18:49, 1996.

Roberts M, Butterworth AE, Kimani G, et al: Immunity after treatment of human schistosomiasis: Association between cellular responses and resistance to reinfection. Infect Immun 61:4984, 1993.

Webster M, Ramirez B, Aligui G, et al: The influence of sex and age on antibody isotype responses to *Schistosoma mansoni* and *Schistosoma japonicum* in human populations in Kenya and the Philippines. Parasitology 114:383, 1997.

Wynn TA, Cheever AW, Jankovic D, et al: An IL-12-based vaccination method for preventing fibrosis induced by schistosome infection. Nature 376:594, 1995.

Wynn TA, Cheever AW: Review: Cytokine regulation of granuloma formation in schistosomiasis. Curr Opin Immunol 7:505, 1995.

Clinical

Ariizum M: Cerebral schistosomiasis japonica: Report of one operated case and fifty clinical cases. Am J Trop Med Hyg 12:40, 1963.

Baltazar RF, Adapon B, Borromeo V, et al: Cerebral schistosomiasis: Clinical features and angiographic findings. Philipp J Intern Med 8:67, 1970.

Browning MD, Narooz SI, Strickland GT, et al: Clinical characteristics and response to therapy in Egyptian children infected with *Schistosoma haematobium*. J Infect Dis 149:998, 1984.

Hofstetter M, Nash TE, Cheever AW, et al: Infection with *Schistosoma mekongi* in Southeast Asian refugees. J Infect Dis 144:420, 1981.

Laughlin LW, Farid Z, Bassily S, et al: Intestinal protein loss in schistosomal polyposis of the colon. Gastroenterology 59:433, 1970.

Lehman JS, Farid Z, Smith JH, et al: Urinary schistosomiasis in Egypt: Clinical, radiological, bacteriological and parasitological correlations. Trans R Soc Trop Med Hyg 67:384, 1973.

Nebel OT, El Massry NA, Castell DO, et al: Schistosomiasis disease of the colon: A reversible form of polyposis. Gastroenterology 67:939, 1974.

Olveda RM, Domingo EO: Schistosomiasis japonica. Clin Trop Med Communic Dis 2:397, 1987.

Prata A: Schistosomiasis mansoni in Brazil. Clin Trop Med Communic Dis 2:349, 1987.

Queiroz FP, Brito E, Martinelli R, et al: Nephrotic syndrome in patients with *Schistosoma mansoni* infection. Am J Trop Med Hyg 22:622, 1973.

Rocha H, Cruz T, Brito E, et al: Renal involvement in patients with hepatosplenic schistosomiasis mansoni. Am J Trop Med Hyg 25:108, 1976.

Sadigursky M, Andrade ZA: Pulmonary changes in schistosomal cor pulmonale. Am J Trop Med Hyg 31:779, 1982.

Scrimgeour EM, Gajdusek DC: Involvement of the central nervous system in *Schistosoma mansoni* and *S. haematobium* infection: A review. Brain 108:1023, 1985.

Strickland GT, Merritt W, El-Sahly A, et al: Clinical characteristics and response to therapy in Egyptian children heavily infected with *Schistosoma mansoni*. J Infect Dis 146:20, 1982.

Strickland GT: Leading article: Tropical infection of the gastrointestinal tract and liver series. Gastrointestinal manifestations of schistosomiasis. Gut 35:1334, 1994.

Wilkins A, Gilles H: Schistosomiasis haematobia. Clin Trop Med Communic Dis 2:333, 1987.

Wittes R, MacLean JD, Law C, Lough JO: Three cases of schistosomiasis mekongi from northern Laos. Am J Trop Med Hyg 33:1159, 1984.

Diagnosis

Abdel-Wahab MF, Esmat G, Milad M, et al: Characteristic sonographic pattern of schistosomal hepatic fibrosis. Am J Trop Med Hyg 40:72, 1989.

Abdel-Wahab MF, Esmat G, Farrag A, et al: Grading of hepatic schistosomiasis by the use of ultrasonography. Am J Trop Med Hyg 46:403, 1992.

Abdel-Wahab MF, Ramzy I, Esmat G, et al: Ultrasound for detecting *Schistosoma haematobium* urinary tract complications: Comparison with radiographic procedures. J Urol 148:346, 1992.

Abdel-Wahab MF, Strickland GT: Abdominal ultrasonography for assessing morbidity from schistosomiasis. 2: Hospital studies. Trans R Soc Trop Med Hyg 87:135, 1993.

Bergquist NR: Review: Present aspects of immunodiagnosis of schistosomiasis. Mem Inst Oswaldo Cruz 87 (Suppl 4):29, 1992.

Hammad TA, Gabr NS, Talaat MH, et al: Hematuria and proteinuria as predictors of *S. haematobium* infection: An epidemiological appraisal. Am J Trop Med Hyg 57:363, 1997.

Medhat A, Zarzour A, Nafeh M, et al: Evaluation of an ultrasonographic score for urinary bladder morbidity in *S. haematobium* infection. Am J Trop Med Hyg 57:16, 1997.

Peters PAS, Kazura JW: Update on diagnostic methods for schistosomiasis. Clin Trop Med Communic Dis 2:419, 1987.

Rabello A: Diagnosing schistosomiasis. Mem Inst Oswaldo Cruz 92:669, 1997.

Strickland GT, Abdel-Wahab MF: Abdominal ultrasonography for assessing morbidity from schistosomiasis. 1: Community studies. Trans R Soc Trop Med Hyg 87:132, 1993.

Treatment

Bella H, Rahim AGA, Mustafa MD, et al: Oltipraz—antischistosomal efficacy in Sudanese infected with *Schistosoma mansoni*. Am J Trop Med Hyg 31:775, 1982.

Cioli D, Pica-Mattocia L, Archer S: Drug resistance in schistosomes. Parasitol Today 9:162, 1993.

Day TA, Bennett JL, Pax RA: Praziquantel: The enigmatic antiparasitic. Parasitol Today 8:342, 1992.

Fallon PG, Cooper RO, Probert AJ, et al: Immune-dependent chemotherapy of schistosomiasis. Parasitology 105(suppl):S41, 1992.

Fallon PG, Doenhoff MJ: Drug-resistant schistosomiasis: Resistance to praziquantel and oxamniquine induced in *Schistosoma mansoni* in mice is drug specific. Am J Trop Med Hyg 51:83, 1994.

Keittivuti B, Keittivuti A, O'Rourke T, D'Agnes T: Treatment of *Schistosoma mekongi* with praziquantel in Cambodian refugees in holding centres in Prachinburi Province, Thailand. Trans R Soc Trop Med Hyg 78:477, 1984.

King CH, Mahmoud AF: Drugs five years later: Praziquantel. Ann Intern Med 110:290, 1989.

Nash TE, Hofstetter M, Cheever AW, Ottesen EA: Treatment of *Schistosoma mekongi* with praziquantel: A double-blind study. Am J Trop Med Hyg 31:977, 1982.

Omer AHS, Teesdale CH: Metrifonate trial in treatment of various presentations of *Schistosoma haematobium* and *S. mansoni* infections in the Sudan. Ann Trop Med Parasitol 72:145, 1978.

Raia S, da Silva LC, Gayotto LC, et al: Portal hypertension in schistosomiasis: A long-term follow-up of a randomized trial comparing three types of surgery. Hepatology 20:398, 1994.

Control

Butterworth AE, Sturrock RF, Ouma JH, et al: Comparison of different chemotherapy strategies against *Schistosoma mansoni* in Machakos District, Kenya: Effects on human infection and morbidity. Parasitology 103:339, 1991.

Capron A, Riveau G, Grzych JM, et al: Development of a vaccine strategy against human and bovine schistosomiasis: Background and update. Trop Geogr Med 46:242, 1994.

Cook JA: Strategies for control of human schistosomiasis. Clin Trop Med Communic Dis 2:449, 1987.

Coura-Filho P, Mendes NM, de Souza CP, et al: The prolonged use of niclosamide as a molluscicide for the control of *Schistosoma mansoni*. Rev Inst Med Trop Sao Paulo 34:427, 1992.

Jordan P, Cool JA, Bartholomew RK, et al: Schistosomiasis mansoni control in Cul de Sac Valley, Saint Lucia. II: Chemotherapy as a supplement to a focal molluscicidng programme. Trans R Soc Trop Med Hyg 74:493, 1980.

Jordan P, Bartholomew RK, Grist E, et al: Evaluation of chemotherapy in the control of *Schistosoma mansoni* in Marquis Valley, Saint Lucia. I: Results in humans. Am J Trop Med Hyg 31:103, 1982.

Olveda RM, Daniels B, Ramirez R, et al: Schistosomiasis japonica in the Philippines: The long-term impact of population-based chemotherapy on infection, transmission, and morbidity. J Infect Dis 174:163, 1996.

Prentice MA, Jordan P, Bartholomew RK, et al: Reduction in transmission of *Schistosoma mansoni* by a four-year focal mollusciciding programme against *Biomphalaria glabrata* in Saint Lucia. Trans R Soc Trop Med Hyg 75:789, 1981.

Sleigh AC, Hoff R, Mott KE, et al: Manson's schistosomiasis in Brazil: 11-year evaluation of successful disease control with oxamniquine. Lancet 1:635, 1986.

Strickland GT: The prevention and control of schistosomiasis. Rev Infect Dis 4:951, 1982.

Wiest PM, Wu G, Zhong S, et al: Impact of annual screening and chemotherapy with praziquantel on schistosomiasis japonica on Jishan Island, People's Republic of China. Am J Trop Med Hyg 51:162, 1994.

World Health Organization: The control of schistosomiasis. WHO Tech Rep Ser 728, 1985, pp 113.

119 Intestinal Fluke Infections

Danai Bunnag, John H. Cross, and Thanongsak Bunnag

Intestinal trematode (fluke) infections have been reported from Southeast Asia, the Far East, the Middle East, and North Africa. More than 70 species infect an estimated 50 million persons, but only a few cause disease. These species include the families Fasciolidae, Echinostomatidae, Heterophyidae, and to a lesser extent the Gastrodiscidae, Lecithodendriidae, Plagiorchiidae, Microphallidae, and Diplostomatidae. Many species have been identified after anthelmintic treatment and recovery of the adult worms, but the full distribution of fluke infections and their public health importance are not known.

Bibliography

Cross JH: Parasites of the small intestine. *In* Surawicz C, Owen RL (eds): Gastrointestinal and Hepatic Infections. Philadelphia, WB Saunders, 1995.

Harinasuta T, Bunnag D, Radomyos P: Intestinal fluke infections. Bailliere's Clin Trop Med Comm Dis 2:695, 1987.

Radomyos P, Bunnag D, Harinasuta T: Worms recovered in stools following praziquantel treatment. Arzneimittelforschung/Drug Res 34:1186, 1984.

WHO Study Group: Control of Foodborne Trematode Infections. World Health Organ Techn Rep Ser No. 849, 1995.

119.1 Fasciolopsiasis

DEFINITION. Fasciolopsiasis buski is an infection by the giant intestinal fluke, *Fasciolopsis buski*. In general, it causes only mild or no symptoms, but individuals with heavy worm loads may have intestinal symptoms, toxemic and allergic manifestations, and malabsorption. Rarely death occurs.

GEOGRAPHIC DISTRIBUTION. *F. buski* is a common intestinal parasite of humans and pigs in central and south China, Taiwan, Vietnam, Thailand, Laos, Kampuchea, Bangladesh, India, and Indonesia. The distribution of infection within these countries is limited, and prevalence rates are low. Human infections have also been reported from Japan, Malaysia, the Philippines, a number of Western countries, and in some instances in immigrants from endemic areas.

ETIOLOGY

Morphology. *F. buski* is the largest of the intestinal trematodes and attaches to the duodenal and jejunal walls. It has a fleshy, reddish beef color, is generally elongate-ovoid, has no cephalic cone, and is 20 to 75 mm long, 8 to 20 mm wide, and 0.5 to 3 mm thick (Fig. 119–1A). Its large egg is hen's egg shaped and yellowish-brown. It has a clear, thin shell with a small operculum at one end, measures 130 to 140 μm by 80 to 85 μm, and is unembryonated when laid (Fig. 119–1B). In appearance, the egg is nearly identical to those of *F. hepatica* and *F. gigantica* (Fig. 117–2).

Life Cycle. The adult flukes live in the small intestine of pigs and humans. Eggs are passed with feces. When the eggs reach fresh water, miracidia develop in 3 to 7 weeks at warm temperatures, hatch, and enter the snail, the first intermediate

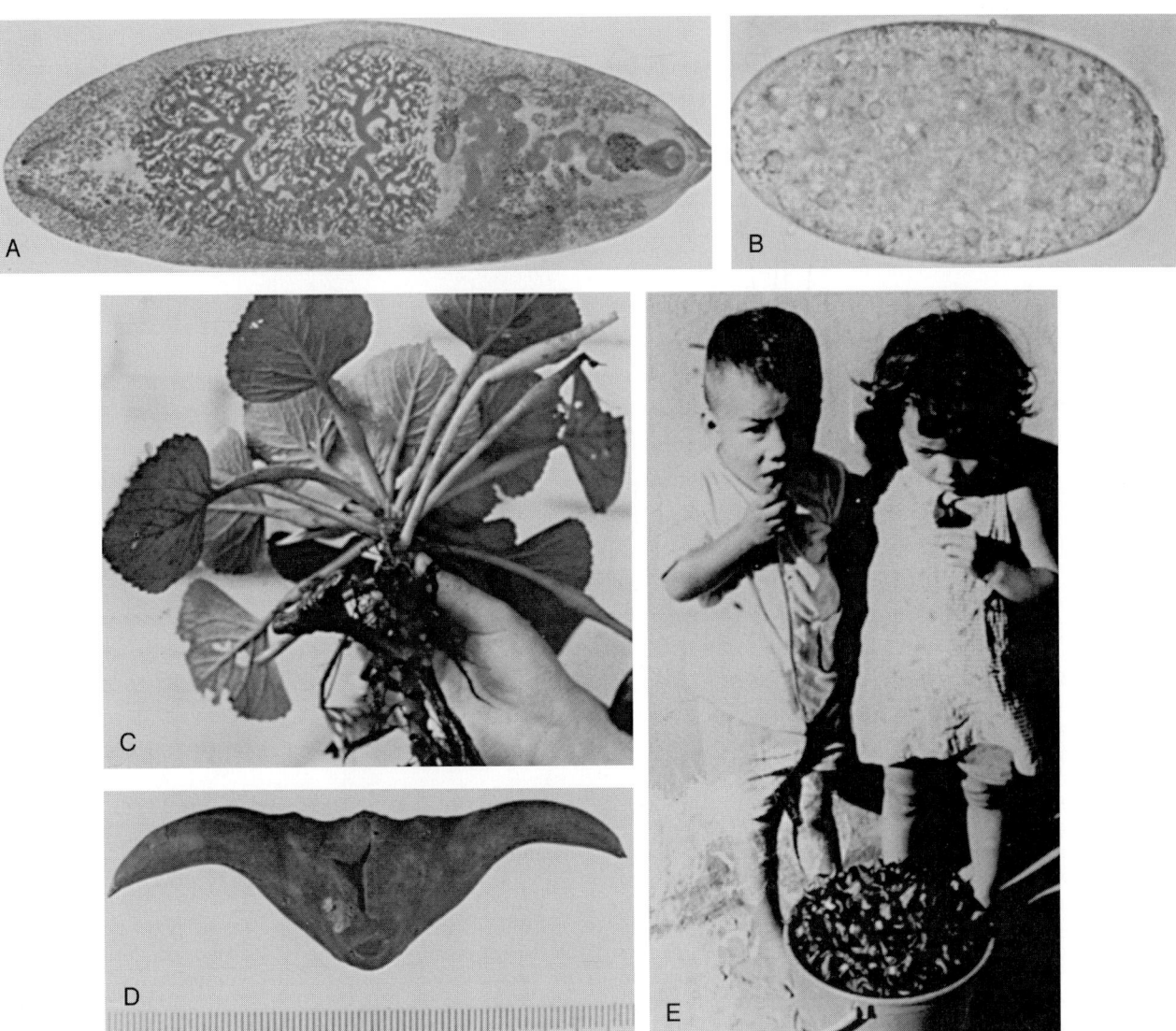

Figure 119–1. *A,* Adult *Fasciolopsis buski* (7 cm). *B,* Egg with a relatively small operculum (130 to 140 μm × 80 to 85 μm). *C* and *D,* Water caltrop *Trapa bicornis* with fruit seed. *E,* Children get infected by peeling with their teeth the outer layers of the fruit seed, where the metacercariae are encysted. (Courtesy of Professor Prayong Radomyos, Faculty of Tropical Medicine, Mahidol University, Bangkok, Thailand.)

host; they then form sporocysts, rediae, and then cercariae. The cercariae swim about and encyst on various freshwater plants, where they develop into metacercariae in approximately 4 weeks. When pigs or humans ingest freshwater plants, the metacercariae excyst in the duodenum, attach to the mucosa, and develop into adult worms in about 3 months. The life span of the fluke is about 1 year (Fig. 119–2).

F. buski is distributed widely among several planorbid snail hosts. In mainland China, Vietnam, and Taiwan, the snail hosts include *Segmentina hemisphaerula, Hippeutis cantori,* and *Gyraulus* species. In India (Assam), Bangladesh, and Thailand, *Segmentina (Trochorbis) trochoideus* is a host. The metacercariae encyst on the seed pods of the water caltrop (*Trapa natans* in China and *T. bicornis* in Thailand and Bengal) (Figs. 119–1C, D), the bulb of the water chestnut (*Eliocharis tuberosa*) and water lily shoots in Bangladesh, and other edible aquatic vegetation, including water morning glory (*Ipomoea aquatica*), water bamboo (*Zizania aquatica*), and watercress (*Neptunia oleracea*).

EPIDEMIOLOGY. Information on the distribution of fascio-

lopsiasis is limited. It is distributed focally in endemic areas, with reported prevalence rates that range from 5% in parts of China to 50% in Assam, Bangladesh, and Thailand. The infection seems restricted to areas where people raise pigs and water plants, and to populations that commonly eat freshwater plants. On many farms, pigs are kept near the ponds where water plants are grown. Pig excreta are washed into ponds that have abundant snail intermediate hosts. The cycle is continued when water plants are fed to pigs.

Humans are infected by consuming raw edible water plants, the stems, bulbs, tubers, and seed pods of which are often peeled with the teeth. In central Thailand and rural Bangladesh, where water caltrop and water lilies are cultivated in canals along the roadside, there is a high prevalence of fasciolopsiasis in children 5 to 14 years old. On their way to school, they pick water caltrop and eat it fresh (Fig. 119–1E). After age 7, females are infected more often than males.

PATHOGENESIS AND PATHOLOGY. The flukes normally attach to the duodenal and jejunal mucosa, but in heavy infections they may be found in the pylorus, ileum, and

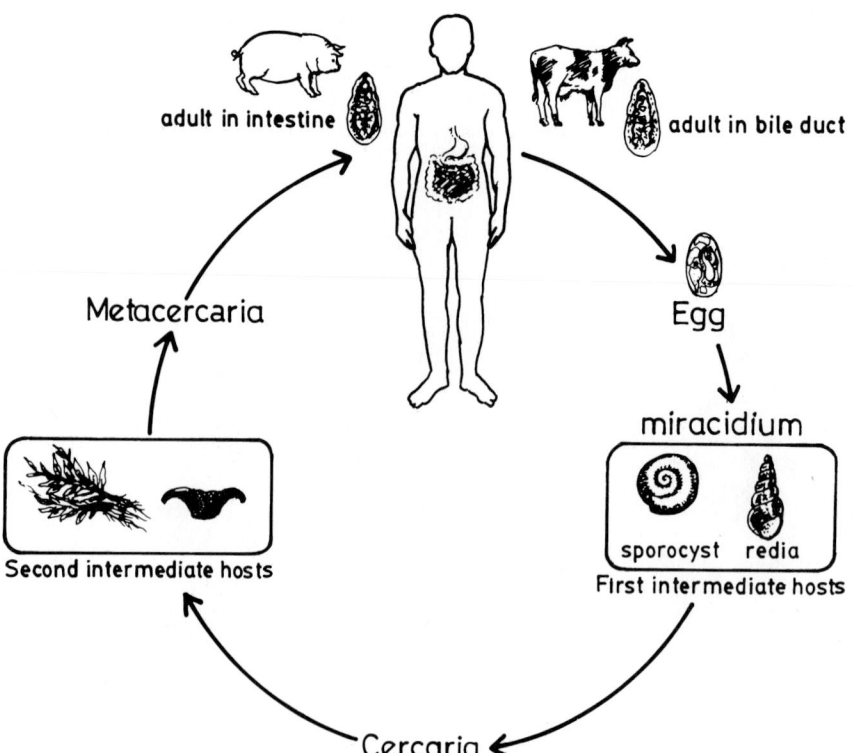

Figure 119–2. Life cycle of the Fasciolidae: *Fasciolopsis buski* (pig) and *Fasciola hepatica* and *gigantica* (cattle).

colon. Localized inflammation, mucous secretion, and ulceration occur at attachment sites and may be followed by deep erosions and hemorrhage. Heavy worm burdens may result in intestinal obstruction. Severe cases in children are marked by profound intoxication and sensitization from absorption of fluke metabolites. Hypoalbuminemia secondary to malabsorption or protein-losing enteropathy may result in edema of the face and extremities. Impaired vitamin B_{12} absorption and reduced serum vitamin B_{12} levels are occasional findings.

CLINICAL MANIFESTATIONS. Most infections are light and asymptomatic. In heavy infections, diarrhea occurs and is accompanied by hunger pain that may simulate a peptic ulcer. The diarrhea initially alternates with constipation but later may be persistent. The stool is greenish yellow and foul smelling and contains undigested food. The appetite is usually normal or even excessive, but some patients have anorexia, nausea, and vomiting. In severe cases, anasarca and ascites develop and the skin becomes dry and rough. Death is rare, associated with extreme cachexia and prostration.

DIAGNOSIS. Specific diagnosis is by demonstrating the characteristic eggs (Fig. 119–1B) or adult flukes in feces and vomitus. The eggs must be distinguished from those of various echinostomes and *Fasciola* species. Leukocytosis with relative eosinophilia is common.

The symptoms associated with heavy infections may be confused with those of giardiasis or peptic ulcer or with other causes of bowel obstruction. Generalized edema may mimic nephrotic syndrome and other causes of hypoproteinemia.

TREATMENT. Three drugs are recommended in treatment. *Praziquantel* is the drug of choice, as a single 15 mg/kg dose given after the evening meal or before retiring to bed. The flukes are expelled the next day, and 100% cure rates are achieved. Side effects, which include headache, dizziness, abdominal pain, drowsiness, nausea, pruritus, and myalgia, are minimal and generally disappear within 48 hours.

Niclosamide 40 mg/kg/day (up to a maximum of 4 g) is given for 1 or 2 days. *Tetrachloroethylene* 0.1 mL/kg (up to a maximum of 5 mL) given once only is less effective, as is albendazole.

PREVENTION. In endemic areas, freshwater plants should be cooked before being eaten. Health education, prohibition of use of night soil and pig excreta as pond fertilizer, mass treatment of infected humans and pigs, modern methods of pig husbandry (i.e., pigs fed on commercial feeds rather than water plants), snail destruction when practical, and ecologic modification through urbanization and industrialization have resulted in reduced prevalence rates in some endemic areas in Thailand and Taiwan and eradication of some foci of infection.

Bibliography

Bunnag D, Radomyos P, Harinasuta T: Field trial of the treatment of fasciolopsiasis with praziquantel. Southeast Asian J Trop Med Public Health 14:216, 1983.
Gilman RH, Mondal G, Maksud M, et al: Endemic focus of *Fasciolopsis buski* infection in Bangladesh. Am J Trop Med Hyg 31:796, 1982.
WHO Study Group: Control of foodborne trematode infections. World Health Organ Tech Rep Ser No. 849, 1995.

119.2 Echinostomiasis

DEFINITION. Echinostomiasis is an infection by trematodes of the family Echinostomatidae and related genera.

ETIOLOGY. There are as many as 30 genera in the family Echinostomatidae, mostly parasites of birds, dogs, cats, and other mammals. Of 12 species reported in humans, the most common are *Echinostoma ilocanum*, *E. malayanum*, *E. revolutum*, and *Hypoderaeum conoideum*. Less common are *E. lindoense*, *E. recurvatum*, *E. jassyense* (*E. melis*), *E. macrorchis*, *E.*

cinetorchis, Echinochasmus perfoliatus, Paraphostomum sufrarty-fex, and *Himasthla meuhlensi.*

Morphology. In general, the echinostome flukes have either a characteristic horseshoe-shaped collar or one or two rows of straight spines that surround the dorsal and lateral sides of the oral sucker (Fig. 119–3*I*). The flukes are elongated and small, measuring 5 to 15 mm long and 1 to 2 mm wide, with slightly tapering rounded ends (Fig. 119–3*A, C, F*). The cuticle of the anterior portion of the body is covered by minute scalelike spines that vary by species.

The eggs are large, yellow to yellowish brown, thin shelled, operculated, ovoid, and unembryonated when laid. They vary in size from 83 to 154 μm by 53 to 95 μm (Fig. 119–3*B, D, E*).

Life Cycle. The adult worms live attached to the intestinal wall of birds, mammals, and sometimes humans. Eggs are passed in the feces. When the eggs reach water, miracidia develop, hatch, and penetrate snails (the first intermediate host); then, over 6 to 7 weeks, they develop into sporocysts, mother rediae, daughter rediae, and cercariae. The cercariae escape from the snails to encyst either in freshwater snails (e.g., *Pila, Viviparus, Lymnaea*), fish, tadpoles, or possibly in vegetation. Humans and definitive hosts become infected if they ingest the raw or undercooked second intermediate host.

EPIDEMIOLOGY. Human echinostomiasis is common in Indonesia, the Philippines, Taiwan, and Thailand. In some endemic areas in northeastern Thailand, the prevalence rate is about 50%. A few cases have also been reported in Malaysia, Japan, and some Western countries.

High prevalence of infection in reservoir hosts, the wide range of definitive and intermediate hosts, the lack of sanitary facilities, unhygienic health practices, and the custom of eating raw or undercooked freshwater animals all are important in transmission of the infection to humans.

Echinostoma ilocanum (Fig. 119–3*C, D*) is highly endemic in Luzon, Mindanao, and Leyte in the Philippines, where local prevalence rates have ranged from 1 to 44%. Human infections have also been reported from Indonesia and northeastern Thailand. In China, only enzootic foci have been found (14% in dogs).

The collar of the *E. ilocanum* organism has 49 to 51 spines. The planorbid snails *Gyraulus convexiusculus* (Philippines, Indonesia), *Hippeutis umbilicus* (Philippines), and *G. prashdi* (India) are first intermediate hosts. Any freshwater snail, such as *Pila conica* (Philippines) and *Viviparus javanicus* (Indonesia), is a source of infection.

Echinostoma malayanum (Fig. 119–3*A, B*) is enzootic-endemic in northeastern and northern Thailand. In Malaysia and Indonesia, human infection is rare because freshwater snails are usually well cooked before eaten. The adult worms possess 43 crown spines and inhabit the small intestine of reservoir hosts (e.g., rats, dogs). Various freshwater snails, e.g., *Indoplanorbis exustus* (Thailand) and *Lymnaea leuteola* (India), are first intermediate hosts. Metacercariae are found in *I. exustus, L. (Radix) rubiginosa, G. convexiusculus* and in tadpoles in Thailand and *V. javanicus* and *Pila scutata* in Malaysia and Indonesia.

Echinostoma revolutum is normally a parasite of ducks, geese, and rats. The worm has 37 circumoral spines. The worm was first recognized in Taiwan, where human infection is estimated at 3 to 7%. The northeastern provinces of Thailand are also endemic-enzootic areas, but the prevalence is unknown. A few cases have been recorded in Indonesia also. In addition to the first intermediate snail hosts, *I. exustus* and *L. (Radix) rubiginosa* in Thailand and *Physa* species (*Segmentina* species and *Helisoma* species) in Taiwan, a second mollusk host or tadpole in Thailand and clams (*Corbicula producta*) in Taiwan are required for encystment of the meta-cercariae.

Hypoderaeum conoideum is a common intestinal parasite (Fig. 119–3*E, F*) of ducks, other fowl, rats, and humans in northeastern Thailand, where a 55% prevalence rate was found in 1965. The body of the fluke is elongated and tapered posteriorly; the head collar has two rows of 45 to 53 spines. Intermediate hosts are freshwater snails, including *I. exustus, L. (Radix) rubiginosa,* and tadpoles.

E. lindoense was highly endemic a few decades ago among humans and animals in the remote Lindu Valley in Central Sulawesi, Indonesia. The infection has since disappeared, probably as a result of biologic competition between the snail hosts in Lindu lake and *Tilapia mossambica* fish, introduced in 1951.

PATHOLOGY AND CLINICAL MANIFESTATIONS. The pathology and clinical manifestations of echinostomiasis have not been well studied. The flukes attach to the small intestine mucosa and produce shallow ulcers and a mild inflammatory response with cellular infiltration. Heavy infections may result in local necrosis.

Apparently, mild infections produce little morbidity. With heavy infections, patients have diarrhea and vague abdominal complaints of flatulence and intestinal colic. In children, symptoms similar to those of Fasciolopsiasis buski, including diarrhea, abdominal pain, anemia, and edema, have been reported.

DIAGNOSIS. Diagnosis is by recovery of eggs (Fig. 119–3*B, D, E*) in the feces; the eggs must be differentiated from those of other trematodes such as *Fasciola hepatica, F. gigantica,* and *F. buski* (Fig. 119–2). Definitive identification depends on the morphology of adult worms (Fig. 119–3*A, C, F, I*) recovered in feces after anthelmintic therapy or at autopsy.

TREATMENT. Praziquantel in a single dose of 40 mg/kg at bedtime or albendazole 400 mg b.i.d. for 3 days is effective.

PREVENTION. Echinostomiasis can be prevented by ensuring that snails and other aquatic animals are cooked adequately before being eaten.

Bibliography

Bhaibulaya M, Charoenlarp P, Harinasuta C: Report of cases of *Echinostoma malayanum* and *Hypoderaeum concideum* in Thailand. J Med Assoc Thai 47:720, 1964.
Carney WP: Echinostomiasis—a snail-borne intestinal trematode zoonosis. Southeast Asian J Trop Med Public Health 22(Suppl):206, 1991.
Carney WP, Sodoma M, Purnomo: Echinostomiasis. A disease that disappeared. Trop Geogr Med 32:101, 1980.
Cross JH, Basaca-Sevilla V: Studies on *Echinostoma ilocanum* in the Philippines. Southeast Asian J Trop Med Public Health 17:23, 1986.

119.3 *Heterophyiasis*

DEFINITION. Heterophyiasis is an infection by the minute intestinal flukes of the genus *Heterophyes* or related members of the family Heterophyidae, which sometimes cause abdominal colic and mucous diarrhea.

■ HETEROPHYIASIS DUE TO *HETEROPHYES HETEROPHYES*

GEOGRAPHIC DISTRIBUTION. More than ten heterophyid species have been found in humans, of which *Heterophyes heterophyes* and *Metagonimus yokogawai* are the most important. Human infection is common in the Nile delta of

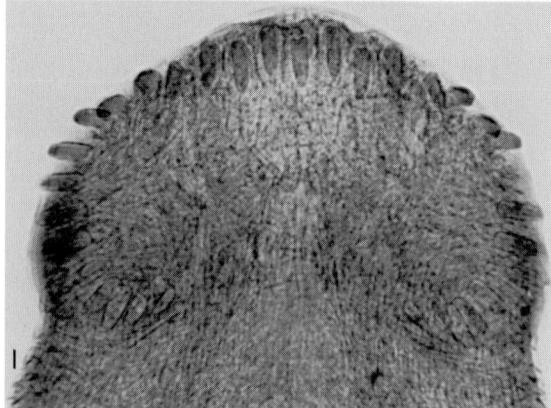

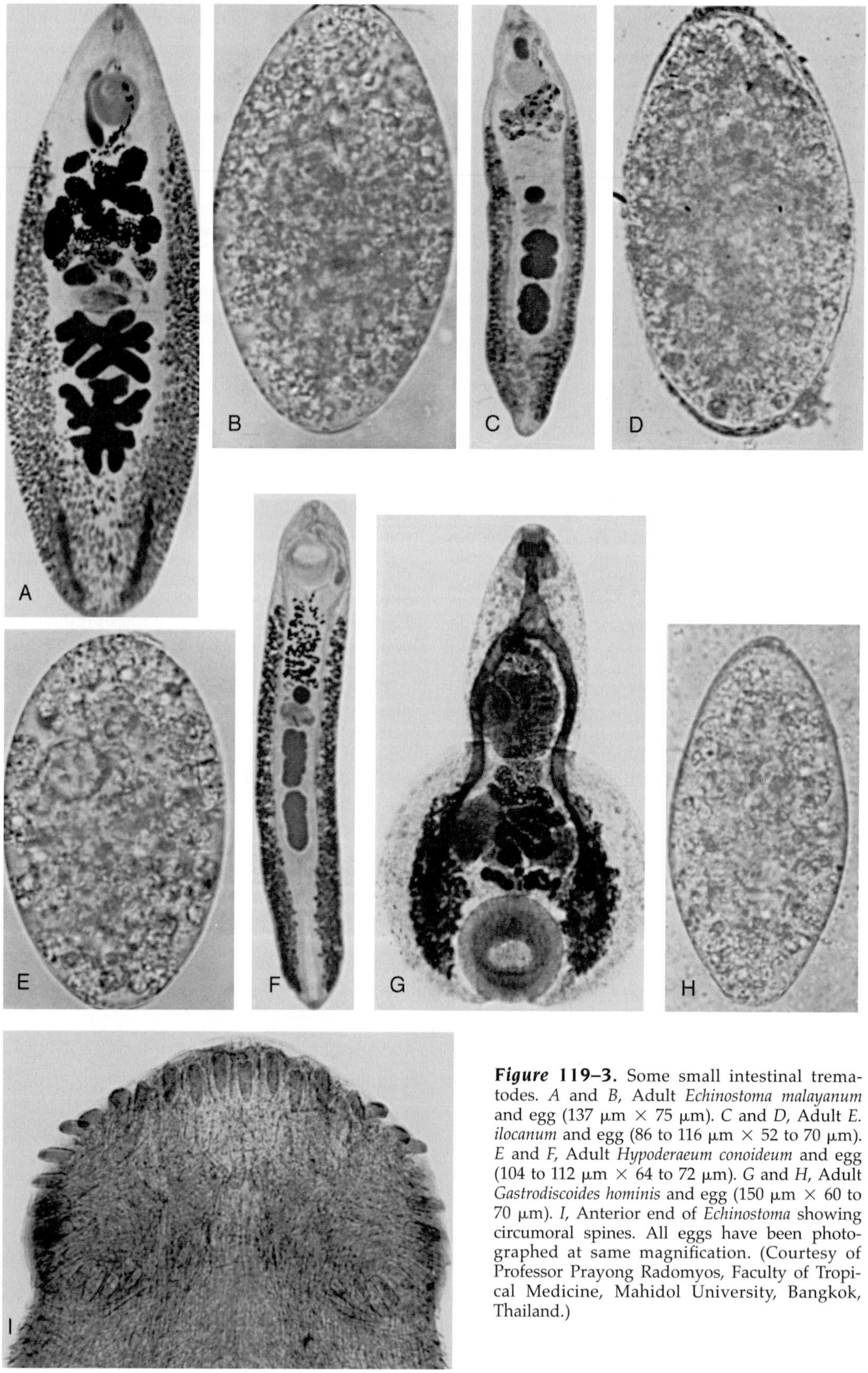

Figure 119–3. Some small intestinal trematodes. *A* and *B*, Adult *Echinostoma malayanum* and egg (137 μm × 75 μm). *C* and *D*, Adult *E. ilocanum* and egg (86 to 116 μm × 52 to 70 μm). *E* and *F*, Adult *Hypoderaeum conoideum* and egg (104 to 112 μm × 64 to 72 μm). *G* and *H*, Adult *Gastrodiscoides hominis* and egg (150 μm × 60 to 70 μm). *I*, Anterior end of *Echinostoma* showing circumoral spines. All eggs have been photographed at same magnification. (Courtesy of Professor Prayong Radomyos, Faculty of Tropical Medicine, Mahidol University, Bangkok, Thailand.)

Egypt and in Iran, Tunisia, and Turkey. In Asia, foci have been reported in Japan, Korea, Taiwan, mainland China, the Philippines, and Indonesia. Possibly the infection occurs throughout Southeast Asia. In India, infection is found in dogs.

ETIOLOGY

Morphology. *H. heterophyes* is a pyriform, gray, minute fluke 1.0 to 1.8 mm by 0.3 to 0.7 mm with a broadly rounded posterior end. Its tegument scales are closely set and most numerous in the anterior portion of the body. The oral sucker is subterminal and one-third the size of the ventral sucker. The eggs are ovoid, light brown, operculated, and 28 to 30 μm by 15 to 17 μm. They are the same size as other heterophyid and opisthorchid eggs but differ from *M. yokogawai* in having a thicker shell.

Life Cycle. Adult *H. heterophyes* organisms attach to the intestinal mucosa of the jejunum and upper ileum of fish-eating mammals. Eggs are passed in feces but hatch only after ingestion by brackish or freshwater snails, the first intermediate hosts, in which they undergo development through one or two generations of sporocysts. Resulting cercariae emerge from the snails and encyst in brackish or freshwater fish, the second intermediate host, in which they become infective metacercariae.

Proven snail hosts are *Perinella conica* in Egypt and *Cerithedea cingulata* (syn. *Tymphonotonus microptera*) in Japan. Fish hosts in Egypt are mullet species *Mugil cephalus* and *M. capito*, *Tilapia nilotica*, and *Aphanius fasciatus*; hosts in Japan are the minnow *Gambusia affinis* and *Acanthogobius* species.

Dogs, cats, foxes, birds, and other fish-eating mammals are reservoir hosts.

EPIDEMIOLOGY. Humans become infected when parasitized fish are eaten raw, cooked inadequately, or pickled or salted improperly. Metacercariae are capable of living up to 7 days in salted fish. The brackish-water fish, *Mugil capito*, caught off the coast of Israel, have been found heavily infected, some with 2300 to 6000 metacercariae per gram of fish.

PATHOLOGY. The flukes attach to the small bowel mucosa and may cause shallow ulcers, mild inflammation, or superficial necrosis. Ova and sometimes adult flukes may enter blood vessels and embolize to the heart and central nervous system.

CLINICAL MANIFESTATIONS. After ingestion of infective metacercariae and a prepatent period (average, 9 days), clinical findings may include mild and intermittent mucous diarrhea, dyspepsia, and abdominal colic. Eosinophilia may be present. Eggs that filter through the mesenteric lymphatics may result in (1) a myocarditis that can lead to chronic congestive cardiac failure or death or (2) embolisms to the brain with findings similar to cerebral hemorrhage. In the Philippines, severe cardiac damage due to vessel occlusion by the ova has been described.

DIAGNOSIS. Diagnosis is generally based on recovery of characteristic eggs in feces. They may be difficult to differentiate, however, from those of other *Heterophyes* or from *Clonorchis* or *Opisthorchis* (Fig. 117–2). The specific diagnosis can be made only by morphologic identification of adult worms recovered after anthelmintic therapy or at autopsy. Geographic and epidemiologic information may aid in diagnosis. *Heterophyes* and *Metagonimus* infection can be excluded in persons who have not eaten potentially infectious fish for 1 year, because both flukes have relatively short lives. This is not true for *Opisthorchis*, however, which has a longer life span >25 years.

TREATMENT. The drug of choice is praziquantel as a single 15 to 25 mg/kg dose taken at bedtime.

PREVENTION AND CONTROL. Efforts must focus on health education to inform about the danger of eating raw, undercooked, or improperly salted or pickled fish, as well as on reduction of infection in the reservoir hosts.

■ METAGONIMIASIS

DEFINITION. Metagonimiasis is infection by the minute trematode *Metagonimus yokogawai*, a species closely related to *H. heterophyes*.

ETIOLOGY

Morphology. *M. yokogawai*, which resembles *H. heterophyes* in size and shape, is 1.0 to 2.5 mm by 0.4 to 0.75 mm and is wider posteriorly than anteriorly. The ventral sucker is located to the right of the midline. The eggs are 26 to 28 μm by 15 to 17 μm, fully mature when laid, and difficult to distinguish from those of *H. heterophyes* (Figs. 117–2 and 119–4F).

Life Cycle. The life cycle is similar to *H. heterophyes*. The first intermediate host is the snail *Semisulcospira libertina* and related species. The second intermediate hosts are several species of freshwater fish, particularly Cyprinidae: trout (*Plectoglossus altivelis* and *Odontobulis obscurus*) and salmon (*Salmo perryi* and *Tribolodon hakonensis*). The cercariae encyst under the scales in the tissue of the gills, fins, and tail.

Dogs, cats, pigs, and pelicans are important reservoirs.

GEOGRAPHIC DISTRIBUTION AND EPIDEMIOLOGY. The parasite is probably the most common intestinal fluke infection in the Far East. It is endemic in parts of China, Japan, Korea, Taiwan, the Philippines, and Indonesia. Prevalence is particularly high in Japan, Korea, and Taiwan, with rates of 2 to 50% reported from Japan. Infections have also been reported from Siberia, the Balkans, Spain, and Israel.

Humans are infected by eating raw or undercooked fish. The prevalence rate of metagonimiasis is difficult to estimate in endemic areas where clonorchids and other heterophyids are also present, because the eggs are similar (Fig. 117–2).

PATHOLOGY. The flukes invade the mucosa of the small intestine, duodenum, or jejunum, causing inflammation, granulomatous infiltration, and ulcerations. They ultimately become encapsulated. On rare occasions, eggs deposited in the tissue are carried by the blood stream and embolized in other organs, as in heterophyiasis.

CLINICAL MANIFESTATIONS. The disease caused by *M. yokogawai* is similar to that by *H. heterophyes*. Mucous diarrhea is the usual finding, but serious manifestations may result from massive embolization of eggs to vessels in the heart or brain.

DIAGNOSIS. Diagnosis is by demonstrating eggs in the feces (Figs. 117–2h and 119–4F) or finding adult flukes after an anthelmintic or at autopsy. The eggs resemble those of *H. heterophyes*.

TREATMENT. Treatment is as for heterophyiasis.

PROGNOSIS. The prognosis is good except when there are ectopic lesions in the brain or heart.

PREVENTION. Abstinence from eating raw or inadequately cooked freshwater fish prevents infection.

■ OTHER HETEROPHYID INFECTIONS IN HUMANS

Infections by other Heterophyidae species occur in areas of Asia where people eat raw or partially cooked freshwater fish. The flukes are minute, usually <1 mm long. The reservoir hosts are fish-eating birds and mammals. The following species have been reported from humans: *Centrocestus formosanus* from Taiwan and mainland China; *Haplorchis pumilio* (Fig. 119–4G), *H. yokogawai*, and *H. taichui* (Fig. 119–4C, H)

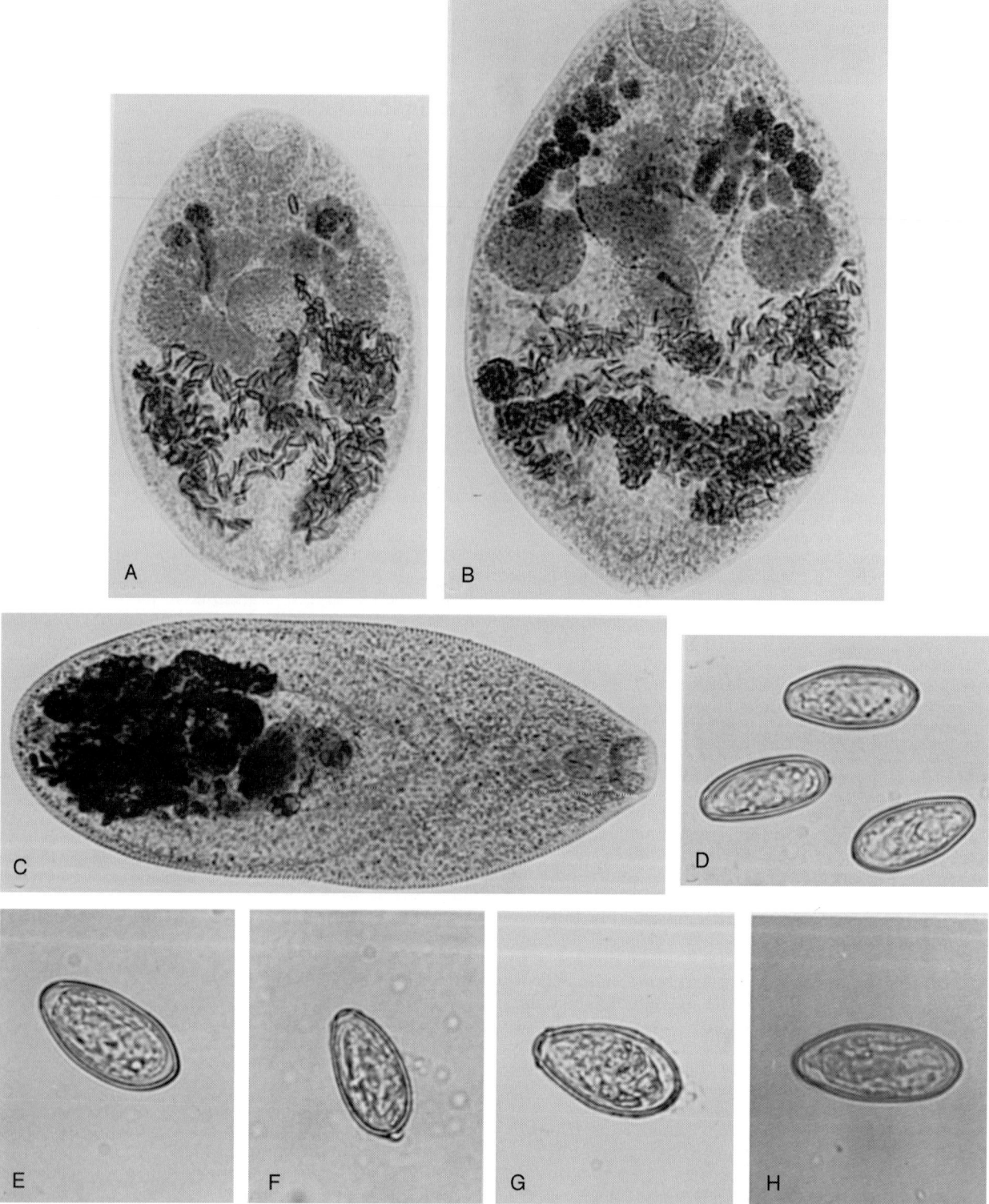

Figure 119–4. Some minute intestinal trematodes. *A*, Adult *Phaneropsolus bonnei. B*, Adult *Prosthodendrium molenkempi. C*, Adult *Haplorchis taichui. D*, Eggs of *P. molenkempi. E, P. bonnei. F, Metagonimus yokogawai. G, Haplorchis pumillo. H, H. taichui.* All eggs were photographed at the same magnification. (Courtesy of Professor Prayong Radomyos, Faculty of Tropical Medicine, Mahidol University, Bangkok, Thailand.)

from Taiwan, the Philippines, Indonesia, and Thailand; *Metagonimus minutus, Diorchitrema formosanum*, and *D. amplicaecale* from Taiwan; *Procerovum calderoni* from the Philippines and China; *Stellantchasmus falcatus* from Hawaii (from eating raw mullet), Japan, the Philippines, and Thailand; and *Pygidiopsis*

summa from Korea (up to 4000 worms have been recovered from individuals).

The intestinal lesions produced by these flukes are similar to those described for *H. heterophyes* and *M. yokogawai*. At autopsy, eggs of *Haplorchis yokogawai, H. pumilio*, and *H.*

taichui have been found in cardiac lesions but rarely cause vascular occlusion. Treatment with a single dose of 15 to 25 mg/kg of praziquantel is effective.

Bibliography

Chai JY, Lee SH: Intestinal trematodes infecting humans in Korea. Southeast Asian J Trop Med Public Health 17:163, 1991.
WHO Study Group: Control of foodborne trematode infections. World Health Organ Tech Rep Ser No. 849, 1995.

119.4 Gastrodisciasis

DEFINITION. Gastrodisciasis is an infection by the small amphistome trematode *Gastrodiscoides hominis*, which inhabits the cecum and ascending colon.

ETIOLOGY

Morphology. The adult worm, 5 to 14 mm long by 4 to 6 mm wide, is bright pink and pyriform with a conical anterior. The ventral surface of the discoid posterior portion has a large acetabulum that bears a characteristic notch (Fig. 119–3G). The eggs are greenish brown, operculated, immature when laid, and 150 μm by 60 to 70 μm (Fig. 119–3H).

Life Cycle. The complete life cycle is unknown but is probably similar to that of the amphistomes.

EPIDEMIOLOGY. *G. hominis* is a relatively common human parasite in Asia. It has been reported from Assam, Bihar, and Orissa in India; Vietnam, Burma, China, the Philippines, Thailand, Kazakhstan, and Guyana. In India, a 41% prevalence was found in one survey in which pigs were the reservoir host. Other known reservoirs are the deer mouse (*Tragulus napu*) in Malaysia and rats in Indonesia, Japan, and Thailand.

PATHOLOGY. Adult *G. hominis* organisms attach to the mucosa of the cecum and ascending colon, where they may produce lesions similar to those described in pigs. At the attachment site, papular lesions with minute surface desquamation may progress to necrosis. Lymphocytes, plasma cells, and eosinophils infiltrate the mucosa and submucosa.

CLINICAL MANIFESTATIONS. The flukes live in the cecum and ascending colon but usually produce no symptoms. However, mucous diarrhea has been reported.

DIAGNOSIS. Diagnosis is by finding characteristic eggs or the adult fluke after an anthelmintic. The eggs resemble those of *F. buski* but are narrower and greenish brown (Fig. 119–3H).

TREATMENT. Praziquantel at the same dosage used in fasciolopsiasis is effective.

Bibliography

Ahluwalia SS: *Gastrodiscoides hominis* (Lewis and McConnell) Leiper, 1913. The amphistome parasite of man and pigs. Indian J Med Res 48:315, 1960.
Surinthrangkul B, Gonthian S, Pradatsundarasar A: *Gastrodiscoides hominis* from man in Thailand. J Med Assoc Thai 48:96, 1965.

119.5 Miscellaneous Intestinal Fluke Infections

■ LECITHODENDRIIDAE FLUKE INFECTIONS

DEFINITION. *Phaneropsolus bonnei* and *Prosthodendrium molenkempi* are two minute trematodes in the Lecithodendriidae that infect humans.

ETIOLOGY

Morphology. *P. bonnei* is small, ovoid, and 0.48 to 0.78 mm long by 0.22 to 0.35 mm wide (Fig. 119–4A). Its cuticular spines are long at the posterior end. The eggs are small, 23 to 33 μm by 13 to 18 μm, oval, thin shelled with an indistinct operculum, dark colored, and unembryonated when laid (Fig. 119–4E).

P. molenkempi is small, 0.4 to 0.8 mm long by 0.4 to 0.6 mm wide (Fig. 119–4B). The body is round and covered with cuticular spines. The subterminal oral sucker and the acetabulum are in the middle third of the body. The eggs are 24 to 26 μm by 8 to 10 μm, operculated, oval, dark brown, and unembryonated when laid (Fig. 119–4D).

Life Cycle. The life cycles of *P. bonnei* and *P. molenkempi* are not completely understood. Natural infections in reservoir hosts have been found in monkeys (*Macaca iris* and *Nycticebus coucang* in Malaysia, *Macaca mulatta* in India, and *Macaca fuscicularis* in Thailand), in insectivorous bats (*Scotophilus kuhlii* and *Taphozons melanopogon*), and in rats (*Rattus rattus*) in Thailand. It is highly probable that *Bithynia goniomphalus* is the snail intermediate host and that dragonflies and damselflies (*Crocothemis servilia, Orthetrum sabina, Trithemis pallidinervis, Brachythemis contaminata*) act as the second intermediate hosts.

GEOGRAPHY AND EPIDEMIOLOGY. Both flukes were recognized initially at autopsy in Indonesia and subsequently after anthelmintic treatment and during surveys. Both flukes are endemic among rural populations of northeastern Thailand and adjacent Laos, and in some areas prevalence rates are 10 to 40%. Infections with both species have sometimes been found in the same individuals. Infection from both flukes results from consumption of raw or inadequately cooked small fish contaminated with infected naiads (water nymphs of dragonflies). Manning and Lertprasert have suggested, however, that *P. bonnei* and *P. molenkempi* are present in a sylvatic cycle throughout Southeast Asia but that humans are only accidentally infected when they eat infected naiads collected with freshwater fish.

PATHOLOGY AND CLINICAL MANIFESTATIONS. Although large numbers of flukes (4356 *P. bonnei* and 1339 *P. molenkempi*) have been recovered after treatment, there are no established intestinal pathologic or clinical findings. It has been difficult to separate clinical symptoms caused by the lecithodendriids from those caused by other parasites in northeastern Thailand and Laos, where polyparasitism is common.

DIAGNOSIS. The diagnosis is based on finding the characteristic eggs and adult worms in feces or at autopsy. It is difficult to differentiate the eggs of *P. bonnei* and *P. molenkempi* from each other and from *Opisthorchis viverrini* and other heterophyid eggs (Figs. 117–2 and 119–4D–H).

TREATMENT AND PREVENTION. A single dose of 40 mg/kg of praziquantel is effective. Prevention is by not eating raw freshwater fish or naiads.

■ MICROPHALLIDAE FLUKE INFECTION

The members of this trematode group are minute intestinal parasites of a wide range of vertebrates. Morphologically they resemble the Heterophyidae; their life cycle resembles that of the Plagiorchiidae.

Spelotrema brevicaeca has been reported on several occasions in humans in the Philippines. The eggs are suspected of causing lesions in the heart, brain, and spinal cord of patients dying of acute cardiac dilation. The complete life cycle is unknown. The encysted metacercarial stage has been found in the crab *Cararius maenas*, which is the source of infection for Filipinos. The adult worms are small, pyriform, 0.5 to 0.7 mm by 0.3 to 0.4 mm, and have a spinose cuticle. The eggs are operculated, yellowish, and 15 to 16 μm by 9 to 10 μm. Diagnosis is based on finding the eggs in stools or in tissue or by recovery of adult worms after anthelmintic treatment.

■ PLAGIORCHIIDAE FLUKE INFECTION

Three species of *Plagiorchis* infect humans in the Philippines, Indonesia, Japan, and Thailand.

P. philippinensis was recovered at autopsy in Ilocanos, Philippines. The infection is acquired by eating larvae of certain insects, the second intermediate host. *P. javensis* was found once in an Indonesian, and *P. muris* once in Japan.

Human infections by these species may be misdiagnosed, because the fluke eggs are small and similar to those of *O. viverrini* and *Clonorchis sinensis*.

■ DIPLOSTOMATIDAE FLUKE INFECTION

Flukes in this family are intestinal parasites of birds and mammals. In humans, the disease results from eating raw or inadequately cooked flesh of frogs or snakes that contain the larval stage mesocercariae.

■ ALARIASIS

In North America, the adults of various species of *Alaria* inhabit the intestine of wild carnivores (e.g., wolves, foxes, raccoons, bobcats, and skunks). Eggs in feces hatch in water and invade freshwater snails of the genus *Helisoma*, from which cercariae emerge and infect frog tadpoles. A fatal case of *Alaria americana* infection reported from Ontario, Canada, is assumed to have resulted from eating inadequately cooked frogs' legs. Autopsy revealed numerous mesocercariae in the ascitic fluid, lungs, liver, heart, kidneys, pancreas, spleen, brain, and spinal cord. Eye infections are also reported.

■ NEODIPLOSTOMUMIASIS

Neodiplostomum seoulense is the only diplostomatid fluke known to infect humans in Korea and has been reported among snake eaters. The parasite is enzootic among house rats, frogs and their tadpoles, and several terrestrial snakes. Epigastric discomfort or pain, diarrhea, fever, and eosinophilia have been noted in humans. Eggs from the feces are readily differentiated from those of *Paragonimus*, *Echinostoma*, or *Fasciola*. They are 81 to 102 μm long by 51 to 63 μm wide and are golden brown, bilaterally asymmetric with an oblique opercular margin, and immature when laid.

Almost 100% of persons treated with praziquantel (20 mg/kg in a single dose) have been cured.

Bibliography

Freeman RS, Stuart PF, Cullen JB, et al: Fatal human infection with mesocercariae of the trematode *Alaria americana*. Am J Trop Med Hyg 25:803, 1976.
Hong ST, Cho TK, Hong SJ, et al: Fifteen human cases of *Fibricola seoulensis*. Korean J Parasitol 22:61, 1984.
Hong ST, Shoop WL: *Neodiplostomum seoulense*, the amended name for *Fibricola seoulensis*. Korean J Parasitol 33:399, 1995.
Manning GS, Lertprasert P: Studies on the life cycle of *Planeropsolus bonnei* and *Prosthodendrium molenkempi* in Thailand. Ann Trop Med Parasitol 67:361, 1973.
McDonald HR, Kazacos KR, Schatz H, Johnson RN: Two cases of intraocular infection with *Alaria* mesocercaria (Trematoda). Am J Ophthalmol 117:447, 1994.

120 Liver Fluke Infections

Danai Bunnag, John H. Cross, and Thanongsak Bunnag

Seven species of flukes in three distomate families—Opisthorchiidae, Fasciolidae, and Dicrocoelidae—infect the liver, more specifically, the biliary tract of humans. Some are found worldwide, whereas others are limited in geographic distribution. The major liver flukes that cause disease in humans are *Opisthorchis viverrini*, *O. felineus*, and *Clonorchis sinensis*. Of less importance and with sporadic occurrence are *Fasciola hepatica*, *F. gigantica*, *Dicrocoelium dendriticum*, and *Eurytrema pancreaticum*.

120.1 Opisthorchiasis

DEFINITION. Opisthorchiasis is infection of the intrahepatic biliary tract by *Opisthorchis viverrini* and *O. felineus* (the cat liver fluke). Most infections in humans are asymptomatic. Clinical manifestations include abdominal discomfort or pain, hepatomegaly, an enlarged gallbladder, and relapsing cholangitis. Occasional complications are gallstones and obstructive jaundice; cholangiocarcinoma is associated with opisthorchiasis.

GEOGRAPHIC DISTRIBUTION. *O. viverrini* is endemic in northern and northeastern Thailand and in Laos and Kampuchea. Up to 10 million persons may be infected; the overall prevalence rate in these endemic areas is 35% but in some areas is >90%. *O. felineus* has been reported from Poland, Germany, the Russian Federation, and Kazakhstan, with the largest endemic area in western Siberia. About 1.6 million people may be infected, with focal prevalence rates as high as 95%.

ETIOLOGY

Morphology. Living *O. viverrini* and *O. felineus* are transparent, have a leaf-like shape, and are 8 to 12 mm long (Fig. 120–1B). The length-to-width ratio of *O. viverrini* is approximately 2:1 and thus resembles *C. sinensis* (Fig. 120–1A), whereas that of *O. felineus* is about 3:1. Their eggs are yellowish brown and oval and have an operculum that rests on shoulders with or without a tubercle-like knob at the abopercular end (Figs. 117–2F and 120–1B). The eggs average 28 μm by 16 μm and contain a miracidium when laid.

TRANSMISSION AND EPIDEMIOLOGY

Life Cycle. The life cycles of *Opisthorchis* and *Clonorchis* are similar (Fig. 120–2). The adult worms live in the distal biliary ducts and sometimes in the gallbladder and pancreatic duct. Eggs are released into the bile and pass to the feces. On reaching water, the eggs are eaten by appropriate species of snails, the first intermediate host. Within the snails, the miracidia hatch and develop sequentially as sporocysts, rediae, and cercariae. In 4 to 6 weeks, mature cercariae are released into the water and penetrate the muscle of susceptible freshwater scaly fish to develop into metacercariae. The metacercariae mature and become infective in 6 weeks. Consumption of infected fish is the source of infection for the definitive hosts, humans or other fish-eating mammals. The metacercariae excyst in the duodenum or jejunum and migrate through the ampulla of Vater and the common bile duct to the bile ducts, where they mature within 4 weeks and begin to produce eggs. The life span of the flukes is >20 years. This natural cycle continues almost year round; snail infection

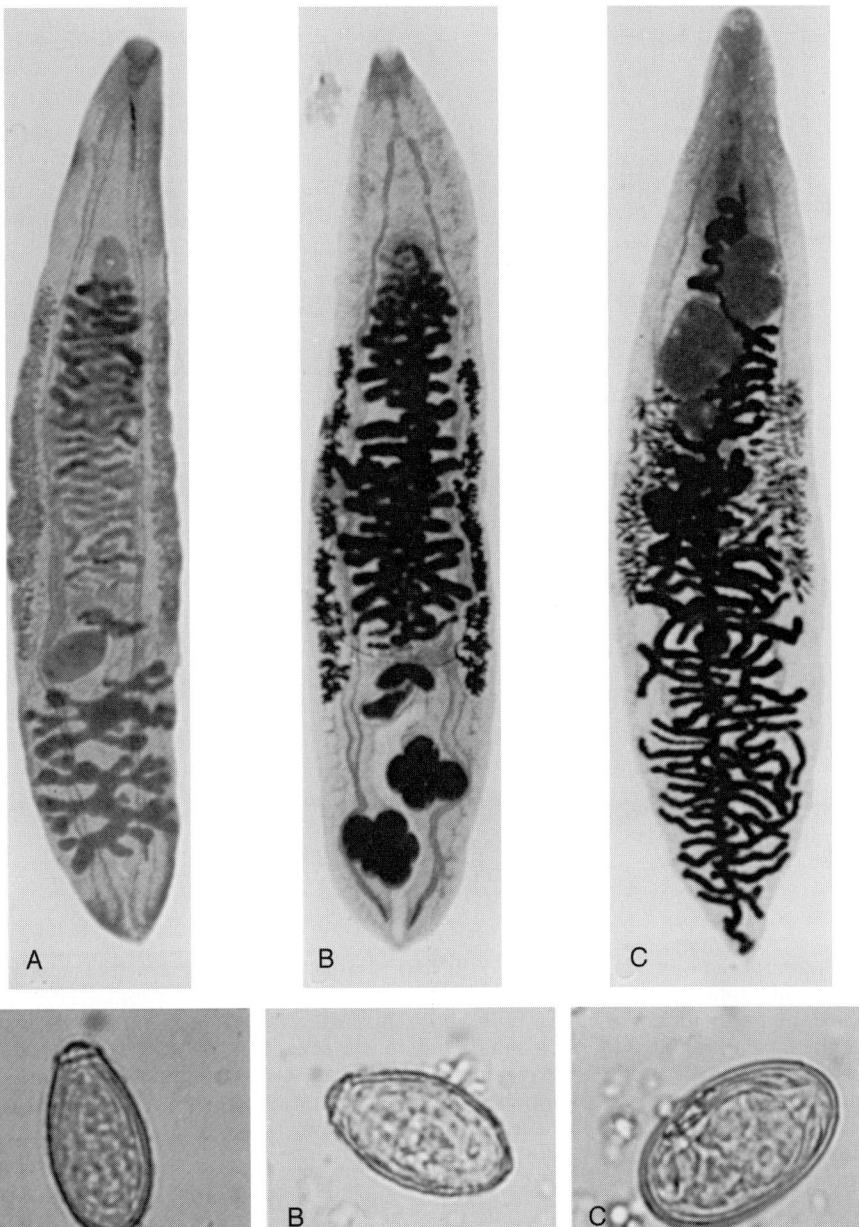

Figure 120–1. Small liver flukes. *A,* Adult *Clonorchis sinensis* and egg. *B,* Adult *Opisthorchis viverrini* and egg. *C,* Adult *Dicrocoelium dendriticum* and egg. All eggs photographed at same magnification. (Courtesy of Professor Prayong Radomyos, Faculty of Tropical Medicine, Mahidol University, Bangkok, Thailand.)

rates are generally <0.1%, and cercarial output averages 280 per snail.

INTERMEDIATE HOSTS. The snail intermediate hosts for *O. viverrini* are *Bithynia siamensis goniomphalos, B. (Digoniostoma) funiculata,* and *B. siamensis siamensis;* hosts for *O. felineus* are *Codiella leachi* and *C. infata.* Second intermediate hosts for *O. viverrini* are many species of cyprinoid fish or carp: *Cyclocheilicthys apogon (Pla Kua Na), Puntius leiacanthys (Pla Tapein Sai),* and *Hampala dispar (Pla Suud);* infection rates in the fish are commonly over 95%. In central, eastern, and southern Europe and in Siberia, the metacercariae of *O. felineus* are found in several freshwater fish (e.g., *Leuciscus rutilus, Blicca bjorkna, Tinca tinca,* and *Barbus barbus*).

In hyperendemic-enzootic areas, domestic cats, dogs, and many fish-eating mammals are definitive hosts.

O. viverrini Infection. The high prevalence in northeastern Thailand is explained by lack of hygienic knowledge and facilities, increasing development of water reservoirs and irrigation systems, flourishing snail and fish intermediate

host populations, and the popular practice of consuming raw fish such as *Koi Pla,* a dish prepared from chopped raw cyprinoid fish. Prevalence of infection in some villages is >90%. Intensity of infection generally increases with age owing to continuing new infections, lack of protective immunity, and the long life span of the flukes. In older age groups, the worm burden in males is twice that in females.

O. felineus Infection. In western Siberia, people consume raw freshwater fish and 1-day-old slightly salted, frozen, or poorly cooked fish. Newly arrived immigrants acquire the infection during their first year of residence.

PATHOLOGY AND PATHOGENESIS. The pathologic changes induced by the worms are apparently the result of mechanical irritation caused by the worm suckers, toxic metabolic substances, immunologic response of the host, and secondary bacterial infection. These effects increase with intensity and duration of infection; as many as 20,000 worms have been found at autopsy. Early changes are mild, with excessive mucin production, desquamation, and adenoma-

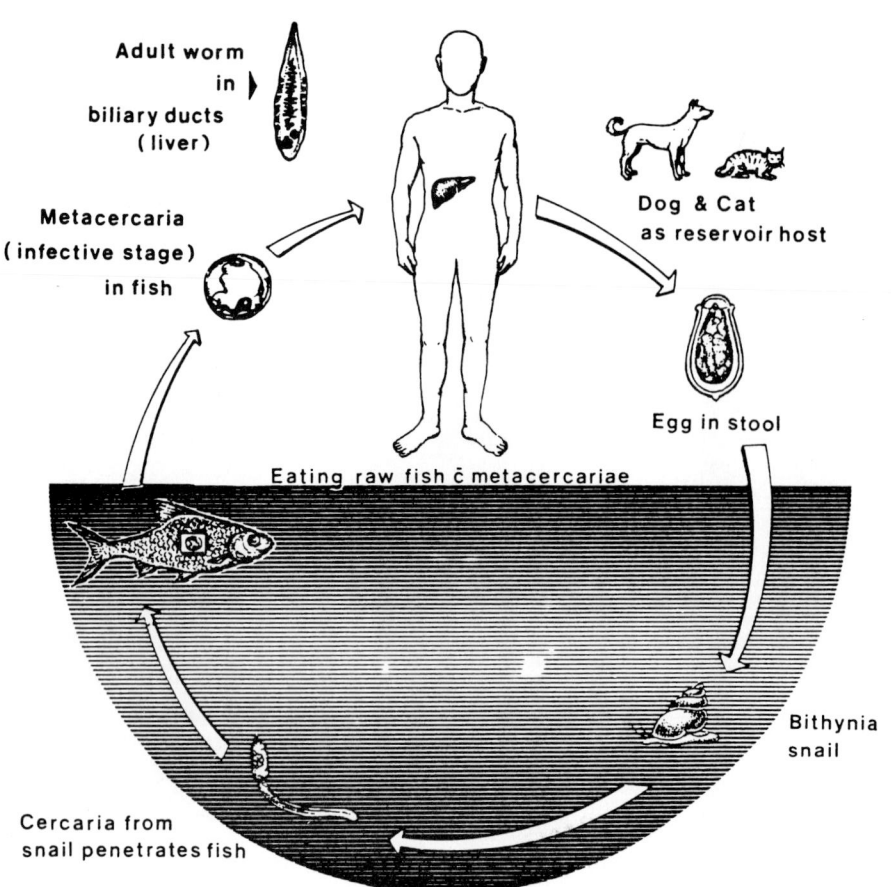

Adult worm
in
biliary ducts
(liver)

Metacercaria
(infective stage)
in fish

Dog & Cat
as reservoir host

Egg in stool

Eating raw fish c̄ metacercariae

Figure 120–2. Life cycle of *Opisthorchis viverrini.*

Bithynia
snail

Cercaria from
snail penetrates fish

tous hyperplasia of duct epithelium. With progression, glandular proliferations project into the lumen. Heavy and severe infections are marked by biliary obstruction, bile retention, periductal infiltration with eosinophils and round cells, fibrosis, and necrosis and atrophy of surrounding hepatic cells (Fig. 120–3). Dilatation of the intrahepatic bile ducts is uniform, accompanied by distal clubbing or cyst formation. The gallbladder is frequently nonfunctional, contains white or muddy bile, and enlarges to 10 to 20 cm in length.

Severe opisthorchiasis has been associated with cirrhosis,

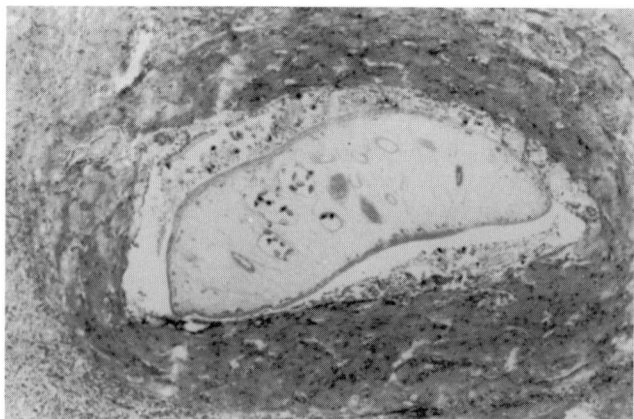

Figure 120–3. The bile duct shows marked dilation and glandular hyperplasia of duct epithelium, and a cross-section of *Opisthorchis viverrini* in the lumen. (Courtesy of Dr. M. Riganti, Faculty of Tropical Medicine, Mahidol University, Bangkok, Thailand.)

obstructive jaundice, cholangitis, pancreatitis, and cholangiocarcinoma. High levels of *N*-nitrosamines in food may be associated with cholangiocarcinoma.

CLINICAL MANIFESTATIONS. The signs and symptoms are similar for the three liver fluke infections: *Opisthorchis viverrini, Opisthorchis felineus,* and *Clonorchis sinensis.* In endemic areas, although infection begins early in life, most patients are asymptomatic, have a benign infection, and are diagnosed only on routine stool examination. If symptoms occur, they usually start in the third decade of life or later.

Acute symptoms starting shortly after exposure have been reported only for *C. sinensis* and *O. felineus* infections. They may resemble serum sickness or Katayama fever; after a 2- to 3-week prepatent period, patients have irregular high fever, lymph node enlargement, myalgia, arthralgia, rash, and eosinophilia. Facial edema occurs occasionally; an allergic hepatitis has been observed in severe cases.

An early symptom is dull pain or discomfort in the right upper abdominal quadrant that may radiate to the epigastrium and left hypochondrium; it typically appears in the late afternoon and lasts 1 to 3 hours. The pain may return in days or weeks, or intermittent remissions may last for months or years. With progression, the pain may limit patients' physical activities. Other symptoms are lassitude, anorexia, flatulence, occasional loose stools, poor appetite, low-grade fever, and hepatomegaly. With associated malnutrition, weight loss and slight pedal edema are common. A peculiar hot cutaneous sensation felt over the upper abdomen or the back is characteristic of opisthorchiasis. It bears no anatomic relation to somatic nerves.

Complications. In the advanced stage of infection, the liver is enlarged, and the gallbladder is palpable and functions poorly. Some patients develop intermittent fever and jaundice from relapsing cholangitis or pyogenic cholangitis.

Cholangiocarcinoma is commonly observed in association with opisthorchiasis. Deterioration is rapid and the outcome fatal.

DIAGNOSIS AND DIFFERENTIAL DIAGNOSIS. Diagnosis is by finding *Opisthorchis* eggs in feces (Figs. 117–2*F* and 120–1*B*); in patients with biliary obstruction, however, the eggs can be recovered only in bile by needle aspiration or at surgery or autopsy. The eggs are difficult to differentiate from those of the small intestinal flukes, *Metagonimus yokogawai*, *Heterophyes heterophyes*, *Phaneropsolus bonnei*, *Prosthodendrium molenkampi*, *Haplorchis taichui*, *Metorchis conjunctis*, and *Opisthorchis guayaquiliensis* (Figs. 117–2 and 119–4*D–H*). Geographic distribution of the parasites may assist in diagnosis. Definitive diagnosis is by identification of adult worms recovered after anthelmintic treatment, at operation, or at autopsy (Fig. 120–2*B*).

In patients with biliary obstruction, the condition must be differentiated from other causes and from enlarged gallbladder, cholangitis with jaundice, carcinoma of the liver, and cholangiocarcinoma. Cholangiography, ultrasonography, and liver scanning can often show lesions compatible with the infection. Immunodiagnosis by enzyme-linked immunosorbent assay (ELISA) using crude somatic extracts of *O. viverrini* is available in a few laboratories and may assist in establishing the diagnosis. Antigen detection–monoclonal antibody–ELISA test may be of value in diagnosis but is not readily available.

TREATMENT AND PROGNOSIS. Praziquantel is highly effective and safe. In asymptomatic and mild to moderate cases, a 1-day regimen of 25 mg/kg three times after meals or a single dose of 40 mg/kg yielded 100% and 90% cure rates, respectively. In heavy infection, a single dose of 50 mg/kg gave a cure rate of 97%. Eggs disappear from the feces in 1 week; clinical symptoms and a dysfunctioning enlarged gallbladder take several months to return to normal. Drug side effects are mild and transient; they include headache, dizziness, sleepiness, nausea, and vomiting. Administration of the drug at bedtime, if the single-dose regimen is used, minimizes side effects.

Mebendazole 30 mg/kg/day for 3- and 4-week periods gave cure rates of 89% and 94%, respectively. No flukes were recovered after treatment.

Albendazole at a dosage of 400 mg b.i.d. for 3 and 7 days gave cure rates of 40% and 63%, and egg excretion was reduced by 92% after each regimen. Most of the flukes were expelled within 3 days of treatment.

Relapsing cholangitis and obstructive jaundice should also be treated with antimicrobials because only 5 to 10% of cases are relieved with praziquantel alone. Palliative surgery may be required in complicated cases with obstructive jaundice.

The prognosis is good for persons with light infections. Death is rare in patients with heavy, long-standing infections that progress to cholangitis and septic shock. Cholangiocarcinoma associated with opisthorchiasis has a poor prognosis.

PREVENTION AND CONTROL. In endemic areas, infection can be prevented by cooking freshwater fish. Extensive health education in concert with local primary health care programs can successfully change local eating habits, improve sanitation, and stop the use of night soil as fertilizer in fish ponds. Mass treatment of infected populations is recommended with praziquantel as a single 40 to 50 mg/kg dose at bedtime. Currently, molluscicide application is impractical and expensive.

Bibliography

Bunnag D, Harinasuta T: Studies of the chemotherapy of human opisthorchiasis in Thailand: III. Minimum effective dose of praziquantel. Southeast Asia J Trop Med Public Health 12:413, 1981.

Haswell-Elkins MR, Mairiang E, Mairiang P, et al: Cross-sectional study of *Opisthorchis viverrini* infection and cholangiocarcinoma in communities within a high risk area in northeast Thailand. Int J Cancer 59:505, 1994.

Mairiang E, Haswell-Elkins MR, Mairiang P, et al: Reversal of biliary tract abnormalities associated with *Opisthorchis viverrini* infection following praziquantel treatment. Trans R Soc Trop Med Hyg 87:194, 1993.

Mott KE, Nuttall I, Desjeux P, Cattand P: New geographical approaches to control of some parasitic zoonoses. Bull WHO 73:247, 1995.

Pungpak S, Riganti M, Bunnag D, Harinasuta T: Clinical features in severe opisthorchiasis viverrini. Southeast Asian J Trop Med Public Health 16:405, 1985.

Srivatanakul P, Parkin M, Sukarayoudhin S, Masathien C: Cholangiocarcinoma: Association of *Opisthorchis viverrini* and CA-19 antigen. Thai Cancer J 16:35, 1990.

120.2 *Clonorchiasis*

DEFINITION. Clonorchiasis is an infection of the biliary tract by *Clonorchis sinensis*, the Chinese liver fluke. The scientific name of the species is *Opisthorchis sinensis*, but because the genus *Clonorchis* is well established, the name is retained.

ETIOLOGY

Morphology. *C. sinensis*, 10 to 25 mm long and 3 to 5 mm wide, is larger than *O. felineus* and *O. viverrini* (Fig. 120–1*A*). The eggs are small, 20 to 30 μm long and 15 to 17 μm wide; they resemble those of *O. viverrini* but are broader than those of *O. felineus* (Figs. 117–2*G* and 120–1*A*).

Life Cycle. The life cycle of *C. sinensis* is similar to that of *Opisthorchis* (Fig. 120–2). The first intermediate hosts for *C. sinensis* are hydrobiid snails: *Parafossarulus manchouricus*, *Bithynia fuchsianus*, *Alocinma longicornis* in most endemic areas; and *Thiara granifera*, *Semisulcospira libertina*, and *Melanoid tuberculata* in other areas. The snails live in fish-culturing ponds, lakes, and slow-moving waters. Infection rates in the snails are usually low. More than 100 species of freshwater fish belong to 13 families that are known to serve as second intermediate hosts of *C. sinensis*. The most important fish species are *Pseudorasbora parva*, *Ctenopharyngodon idellus*, *Hemiculter* spp., *Cyprinus carpo*, and *Carassius* spp. Reservoir hosts include dogs, cats, pigs, mink, rats, and other fish-eating mammals.

EPIDEMIOLOGY. Human clonorchiasis is mainly endemic in Japan, Korea, China, Taiwan, and Vietnam, where the first and second intermediate hosts are found and where the populations are accustomed to consuming raw fish, e.g., sashimi and pickled fish in vinegar (sunomono) in Japan, fish covered with pounded chili paste in Korea, and raw fish congee (*Yu shun chuk*) in Hong Kong. In most endemic areas, fish are raised in ponds fertilized with night soil from human or animal feces. However, the many cases reported from Hong Kong (where neither the snail nor fish intermediate hosts are indigenous) are due to importation of infected fish from China.

More than 7 million people are estimated to be infected, with 4.7 million in China and close to 1 million in Korea. A reduction in prevalence has occurred in Japan and is attributed to industrialization, insecticide pollution of water, land reclamation, and health education, all of which have contributed to a decrease in the snail population. Higher infection rates and a more intensive worm burden have occurred in men in Taiwan. A high prevalence is noted in the Hakkanese ethnic group. In recent years, clonorchiasis has been reported frequently in the United States, Canada, France, Australia, and other countries, all in refugee immigrants from endemic areas.

PATHOLOGY AND PATHOGENESIS. The pathogenesis and pathologic changes in clonorchiasis are similar to those in opisthorchiasis (Chapter 120.1).

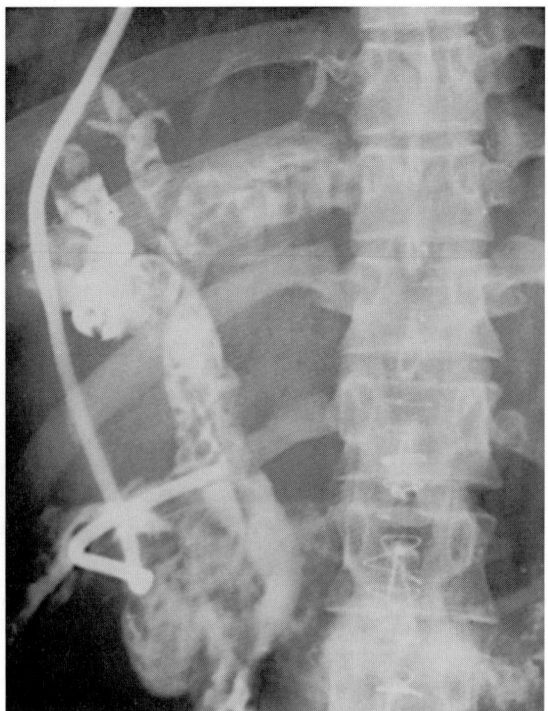

Figure 120–4. Clonorchiasis, T-tube cholangiogram demonstrating dilated bile ducts filled with flukes. (Courtesy of the Armed Forces Institute of Pathology, Photograph Neg. No. 69–5522–3.)

CLINICAL MANIFESTATIONS. Clinical manifestations are similar to findings in opisthorchiasis (Chapter 120.1). On rare occasions, acute symptoms have been noted in visitors to endemic areas: chills and fever, anorexia, pain in the right upper quadrant, generalized abdominal pain and abdominal distention, occasional urticaria, jaundice, and even ascites. Leukocytosis with eosinophilia occurs at times. These findings start 10 to 26 days after consumption of inadequately cooked, massively infected fish and last 2 to 4 weeks. The acute symptoms may persist into the chronic stage; however, many chronic infections are asymptomatic. Heavy chronic infections may be marked by symptoms of weakness, dizziness, weight loss, epigastric discomfort, abdominal fullness, diarrhea, anemia, and edema. Cholangitis, cholelithiasis, pancreatitis, and cholangiocarcinoma are common complications of chronic infection and can be fatal.

DIAGNOSIS. Diagnosis of clonorchiasis is as for opisthorchiasis (Chapter 120.1).

TREATMENT. The drug of choice is praziquantel, 25 mg/kg after meals three times for 1 or 2 days. These regimens yielded cure rates of 85% and 100%, respectively.

PROGNOSIS. The majority of patients do well, except for those who suffer from pyogenic cholangitis, obstructive jaundice (Fig. 120–4), or cholangiocarcinoma.

PREVENTION AND CONTROL. Prevention is by thorough cooking or freezing of freshwater fish. Educational efforts should be directed toward changing eating habits and improving sanitation. The use of night soil or feces from reservoir hosts for fertilizing fish ponds should be prevented; alternatively, storage of night soil is recommended, because eggs of *C. sinensis* die within 2 days at 26°C.

Bibliography

Chen MG, Lu Y, Hua X, Mott KE: Progress in assessment of morbidity due to *Clonorchis sinensis*: A review of the literature. Trop Dis Bull 91:R7, 1994.
Cross JH: Changing pattern of some trematode infections in Asia. Arzneimit-telforschung 34:1224, 1984.
Mott KE, Nuttall I, Desjeux P: New geographical approaches to control of some parasitic zoonoses. Bull WHO 73:247, 1995.
Rim HJ: Therapy of some fluke infections in the past. Arzneimittelforschung 34:1127, 1984.

120.3 *Fascioliasis*

DEFINITION. Fascioliasis (sheep liver fluke disease) is infection by one of two species: *Fasciola hepatica* or *F. gigantica*. The former occurs principally in temperate climates, the latter in the tropics. Both are common hepatic flukes of sheep and other domestic livestock. In humans, both occasionally infect the bile ducts and the gallbladder but more commonly extrahepatic sites.

■ FASCIOLA HEPATICA INFECTION

ETIOLOGY

Morphology. *F. hepatica* is relatively flat, leaflike, and fleshy. It is 20 to 30 mm by 8 to 13 mm, and its broader, anterior portion is covered with scalelike spines. A distinct cephalic cone gives a characteristic shouldered appearance (Fig. 120–5A). The eggs are large, ovoid with an inconspicuous operculum, light yellowish brown, 130 to 150 μm by 60 to 90 μm, and unsegmented when laid (Figs. 117–2B and 120–5A).

Life Cycle. The adult parasites live in the large biliary ducts. Eggs passed in host feces require 9 to 15 days for the miracidia to develop and hatch in water of optimal temperatures of 22 to 26°C. The miracidia penetrate various lymnaeid snails, the first intermediate hosts, and develop (within 4 to 7 weeks) from sporocysts, rediae, and daughter rediae to cercariae. The mature cercariae emerge from the snail and encyst within hours as minute white spherules on various kinds of aquatic vegetation; a few sink to the bottom, where they develop into metacercariae.

When metacercariae are ingested, they excyst in the duodenum, migrate through the intestinal wall into the peritoneal cavity, subsequently leave through Glisson's capsule, and then traverse the liver parenchyma into the bile ducts, where they grow to maturity. The prepatent period in humans may take 3 to 4 months. Although the life span of the flukes in humans is not known, it is estimated to be 9 to 13 years.

Numerous species of amphibious snails of the genus *Lymnaea* serve as intermediate hosts. *L. truncatula* is the most important and widespread host in Europe, Africa, and north Asia; *L. bulimoides* is the principal host in North America and *L. tomentosa* in Australia.

The most important definitive hosts are sheep, but other herbivores, including goats, cattle, horses, camels, hogs, vicuna, rabbits, and deer, are commonly infected.

EPIDEMIOLOGY. *F. hepatica* has a cosmopolitan distribution, being prevalent in most sheep-raising areas. More than 2 million people may be infected. Sporadic human fascioliasis hepatica has been reported from mainland United States and Hawaii, South America (Venezuela, Uruguay, Argentina, Chile, Colombia, Bolivia, Ecuador, Mexico, Cuba, Puerto Rico, Costa Rica, Brazil, Peru), Europe (Portugal, France, England, Poland, the former Soviet Union, Italy, Corsica, Spain, Hungary, Romania, Turkey), Africa (Egypt, Somalia, Algeria, Tunisia, Morocco, South Africa), Asia (Thailand, Indonesia, Malaysia, Japan, China, Philippines, Korea), and the Middle East (Iran, Iraq, Saudi Arabia, Syria, Lebanon).

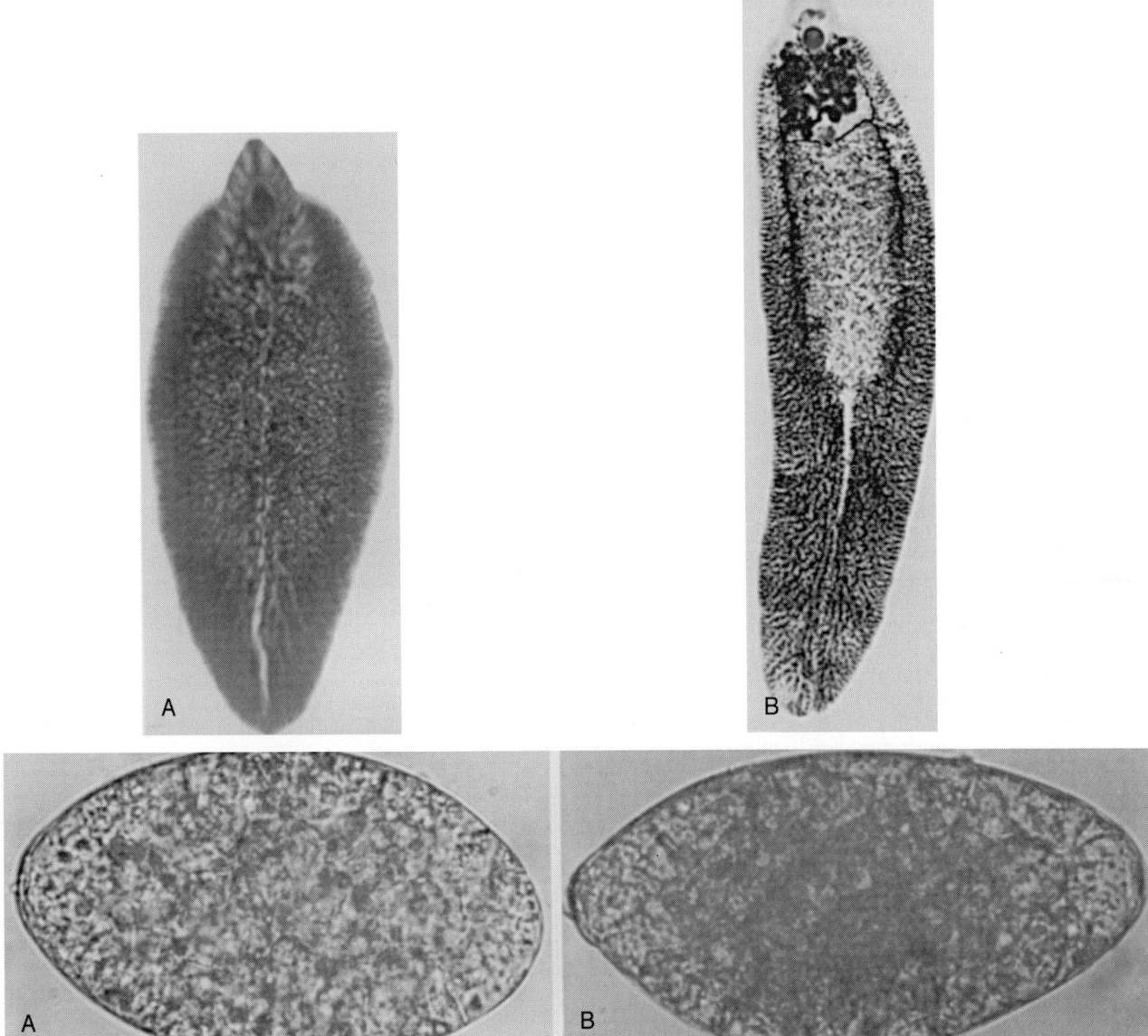

Figure 120–5. Large liver flukes. *A,* Adult *Fasciola hepatica* (3 cm) and egg (130 to 150 μm × 60 to 90 μm). *B,* Adult *Fasciola gigantica* (7 cm) and egg (160 to 190 μm × 70 to 90 μm). (Courtesy of Professor Prayong Radomyos, Faculty of Tropical Medicine, Mahidol University, Bangkok, Thailand.)

Human infection is usually acquired by eating watercress grown in sheep-raising areas.

PATHOGENESIS AND PATHOLOGY. Experimental animal studies indicate that migrating metacercariae cause local hepatic parenchymal destruction, necrosis, and abscess formation. Adult flukes may cause hyperplasia, desquamation, thickening, and dilatation of the bile ducts. Fibrotic changes in the bile ducts may be related to proline produced by adult worms. Sheep heavily infected with *F. hepatica* develop "liver rot." The amount of tissue damage is correlated with the worm load; 600 flukes cause death. Although infection in humans is usually mild, rarely, in heavy infections extensive liver parenchymal necrosis sometimes results in internal hemorrhage. Ectopic fascioliasis is common.

The fluke's antigens provoke various types of complement-fixing, precipitating, and hemagglutinating antibodies.

CLINICAL MANIFESTATIONS. Clinical findings relate to the phase of infection.

Acute Phase. Acute symptoms may persist for several weeks to months. They occur during the period in which the larval flukes migrate through the liver and stop when the larvae penetrate the bile ducts. Patients may develop acute dyspepsia, anorexia, nausea, vomiting, prolonged high fever, abdominal pain in the right hypochondrium, and, sometimes, hepatomegaly, hepatic tenderness, and urticaria with marked eosinophilia. Severe illness with prostration and jaundice is unusual. Asymptomatic acute infection has been reported and seems to be common in Peru.

Chronic Phase. Most patients have few or no symptoms after the flukes have lodged in the biliary passages. Some patients, however, have pain in the epigastrium and right hypochondrium, diarrhea, nausea, vomiting, hepatomegaly, and jaundice. If the flukes lodge in the extrahepatic biliary ducts, symptoms may be those of cholelithiasis. Abnormal liver function and eosinophilia are common.

Ectopic Infection Sites. Infections at aberrant sites (e.g., lungs, intestinal wall, heart, brain, skin) are observed frequently. Manifestations are visceral larval migrans–like, including vague abdominal migratory pain to severe colic when the biliary tract is involved. Exploratory abdominal surgery may be needed to make the diagnosis.

Halzoun. In endemic areas, acute nasopharyngitis known as *halzoun* in Lebanon or *marrara* in Sudan is caused by eating raw infected liver of sheep or goats. Young flukes emerge from the ingested liver and attach to mucosa in the laryngopharyngeal region, where they induce irritation and edema that results in discomfort, dysphagia, and dyspnea.

Laboratory Findings. These may include leukocytosis with relative hypereosinophilia, anemia, increased erythrocyte sedimentation rate, hypergammaglobulinemia, abnormal results of liver function tests, and eosinophilic hyperplasia of the bone marrow.

DIAGNOSIS. In enzootic areas, fascioliasis is suspected in patients who are suffering from fever, hepatomegaly, and eosinophilia and who have a history of consuming raw freshwater plants. Serologic tests (indirect hemagglutination, complement fixation, counterimmunoelectrophoresis, ELISA) are particularly useful for diagnosing ectopic disease and in the early acute phase when the flukes are young and eggs have not yet appeared in the feces. Liver biopsy tissue sometimes demonstrates the flukes or compatible lesions. Abdominal ultrasonography (Fig. 5–3) and cholangiography can demonstrate the flukes in the bile ducts and gallbladder.

Definitive diagnosis is by finding the eggs in feces or sometimes by duodenal aspiration. Spurious infection must be ruled out. Because the eggs of *F. hepatica* (Fig. 120–5*A*), *F. gigantica* (Fig. 120–5*B*), and *F. buski* (Fig. 119–1*B*) are similar and difficult to distinguish from each other (Fig. 117–2), recovery of adult flukes at surgery, autopsy (Fig. 120–5*A*), or after anthelmintics confirms the diagnosis.

TREATMENT. In biliary infection, praziquantel is sometimes effective at a dosage of 25 mg/kg t.i.d. after meals for 2 days. In Egypt, praziquantel has not been effective. Treatment with potentially toxic drugs, such as emetine hydrochloride, or extended treatment with chloroquine has been of little value. Triclabendazole, an imidazole derivative, at dosages of 10 to 12 mg/kg for 1 or 2 days is now the drug of choice but is not yet readily available.

PREVENTION AND CONTROL. Prevention is by not eating watercress salad in endemic areas and by thoroughly cooking sheep and goat livers. In endemic-enzootic areas, control measures are elimination of snail intermediate hosts by adequate drainage of pastures, application of effective molluscicides (e.g., copper sulfate and frescon), and adequate therapy of definitive herbivorous animal hosts (e.g., with Niclofolan).

■ FASCIOLA GIGANTICA INFECTION

Fasciola gigantica is a species closely related to *F. hepatica*; it infects domestic livestock in tropical and subtropical areas and sometimes infects humans.

GEOGRAPHIC DISTRIBUTION. *F. gigantica* is the common liver fluke of herbivorous mammals, particularly cattle in Africa, southern Europe, southern United States and Hawaii, the former Soviet Union, the Middle East, and Southest Asia. Mixed *F. gigantica* and *F. hepatica* infections have been reported from highland areas of Pakistan.

ETIOLOGY

Morphology. *F. gigantica* resembles *F. hepatica* and may attain a length of 7.5 cm; it is more lanceolate, however, and has a less distinct cephalic cone (Fig. 120–5*B*). Its eggs are larger, measuring 160 to 190 μm by 70 to 90 μm (Figs. 117–2*A* and 120–5*B*).

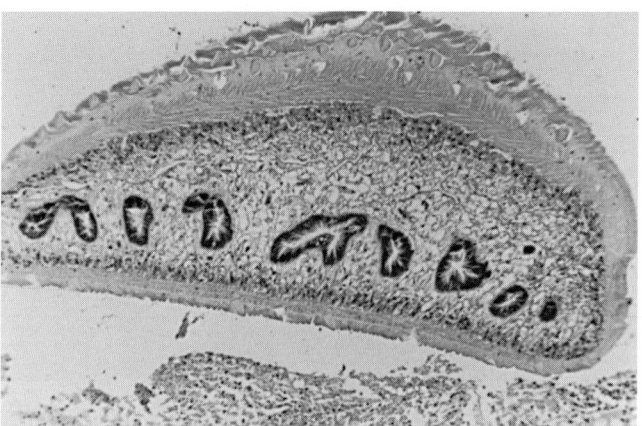

Figure 120–6. Histologic section of *Fasciola gigantica* from a Thai patient, showing necrotic and hemorrhagic areas of liver parenchyma.

EPIDEMIOLOGY. Infection develops in a wide range of susceptible mammals, the definitive hosts, when they ingest infected aquatic vegetation or water containing encysted metacercariae (white spherules). Infection rates in herbivorous mammals may be high in endemic areas: in China, cattle (50%), goats (45%), and water buffalo (33%); in Iraq, water buffalo (71%) and cattle (27%); and in northeastern Thailand, cattle (60%). Human fascioliasis gigantica has occasionally been reported from Zimbabwe, Uganda, Tashkent, Iraq, Vietnam, Hawaii, and Thailand, areas in which infection in animals is not common.

The snail hosts of *F. gigantica* belong to the *Lymnaea (Radix) auricularia* complex: *L. auricularia rufescens* in the Indian subcontinent, *L. auricularia rubiginosa* in Malaysia and Thailand, and *L. natalensis* in Africa.

CLINICAL MANIFESTATIONS, DIAGNOSIS, AND TREATMENT. The life cycle, pathology, and clinical manifestations of *F. gigantica* are similar to those of *F. hepatica*. The prepatent period in the definitive host, from infection until the worms complete liver migration and reach the bile ducts, is 9 to 12 weeks. Patients may have fever, abdominal pain, nausea, vomiting, hepatomegaly, hepatic tenderness, and eosinophilia; unrecognized milder manifestations undoubtedly exist. *F. gigantica* has been observed frequently in ectopic locations. In some cases, *F. gigantica* has induced an abscess or tumor-like reaction either in subcutaneous tissue or in the liver (Fig. 120–6).

Eggs are often absent from the stool. Serodiagnosis is inconclusive, but fascioliasis gigantica can sometimes be excluded on geographic grounds. Recovery of adult flukes by surgical exploration confirms the diagnosis.

Treatment and preventive measures are similar to those for *F. hepatica*.

Bibliography

Apt W, Aguilera X, Vega F, et al: Treatment of human chronic fascioliasis with triclabendazole: Drug efficacy and serologic response. Am J Trop Med Hyg 52:532, 1995.

Chen MG, Mott KE: Progress in assessment of morbidity due to *Fasciola hepatica* infection; a review of the literature. Trop Dis Bull 87:R1, 1990.

Hillyer GV: Fascioliasis in developed countries: Review of classic and aberrant forms of the disease. Medicine 74:13, 1995.

Shaheen H, al Khafif M, Farag RM, Kamal KA: Serodifferentiation of human fascioliasis from schistosomiasis. Trop Geogr Med 46:326, 1994.

WHO: Control of foodborne trematode infections. Report of a WHO study group. World Health Organ Tech Rep Ser No. 849, 1995.

120.4 *Dicrocoeliasis and Eurytremiasis*

DEFINITION. Dicrocoeliasis and eurytremiasis are infections of the bile ducts and pancreatic ducts of herbivorous animals by trematodes of the genus *Dicrocoelium dendriticum* and *Eurytrema pancreaticum*. The parasites rarely infect humans; when they do, however, they are more commonly spurious infections due to ingestion of infected animal livers.

ETIOLOGY

Morphology. The dicrocoeliid fluke is transparent, flat, and lanceolate and measures 5 to 15 mm by 1.5 to 2.5 mm (Fig. 120–1C). Its eggs are dark brown, 38 to 45 μm by 22 to 30 μm, operculated, thick shelled, and fully embryonated when laid (Figs. 117–2I and 120–1C). *E. pancreaticum* (8 to 16 mm by 5 to 9 mm) is more ovate and broader than *D. dendriticum*. Eggs of the two species are indistinguishable.

Life Cycle. The life cycle of the two trematodes are similar and require two intermediate hosts, a snail and an insect. The adult flukes live in the biliary and pancreatic passages of the herbivore. Eggs are passed in the feces and ingested by land snails, which are the first intermediate host. The snail hosts of *D. denriticum* are *Zebrina detrita* and *Helicella candidula* in Europe, *Cionella lubrica* in North America, and *Bradybaena similaris* in Malaysia. Two generations of sporocysts develop in the snail. Cercariae are released in slime balls shed by the snail on vegetation as it crawls along. The cercariae develop into infective metacercariae only if ingested by ants, the second intermediate hosts: *Formica fusca* in the United States and Germany, *F. gigantis* or *F. rufibarbis* in the Middle East, and *F. cinerea* and *F. picea* in the former Soviet Union. Snail hosts for *E. pancreaticum* in China are *Ganesella* species. For second intermediate hosts, *E. pancreaticum* uses grasshoppers (*Conocephalus maculatus*) in Malaysia and tree crickets (*Oecanthus longicaudus*) in the former Soviet Union. The life cycle is completed when the infected insects are eaten by grazing herbivores. The metacercariae excyst and migrate to the biliary passage for *D. dendriticum* and to the pancreatic ducts for *E. pancreaticum*, where they develop into adults.

Humans become infected when they accidentally eat infected ants or grasshoppers.

GEOGRAPHIC DISTRIBUTION AND EPIDEMIOLOGY. *D. dendriticum* is a common parasite in the bile ducts of sheep, deer, water buffalo, and cattle. Its enzootic distribution is reported from Europe, Turkey, northern Africa, and parts of the Far East. Most reported human cases were spurious infections; a few genuine human cases have rarely been reported from Europe, Egypt, Iran, Nigeria, Ivory Coast, and China.

E. pancreaticum is a common parasite of pancreatic ducts and rarely of the bile ducts of herbivorous mammals (cattle, sheep, goats, monkeys, and camels). Eurytremiasis has been reported in humans in Hong Kong, Kiangsu province in China, and at least six times in Japan, twice at autopsy.

CLINICAL MANIFESTATIONS. Dicrocoeliasis and eurytremiasis usually cause mild symptoms. Heavy infections, however, may be marked by vague biliary and gastrointestinal disturbances, including abdominal distress, flatulence, biliary colic, vomiting, and diarrhea or constipation. Jaundice, an enlarged liver, and systemic symptoms are reported occasionally. Eosinophilia is rare.

DIAGNOSIS. Diagnosis is made by finding the characteristic eggs in feces, bile, or duodenal fluid (Fig. 120–1C). Spurious infection must be ruled out by repeated fecal examination. Definitive diagnosis is by recovery of adult flukes at surgery or autopsy (Fig. 120–1C).

TREATMENT. Praziquantel is recommended at the same dose as for opisthorchiasis. Triclabendazole, an imidazole derivative, may be effective.

PREVENTION AND CONTROL. Because infection in humans is generally accidental, no preventive measures are effective.

Bibliography

Drabick JJ, Egan JE, Brown SL, et al: Dicrocoeliasis (lancet fluke disease) in an HIV seropositive man. JAMA 259:567, 1988.

El-Shiekh-Mohamed AR, Mummery Y: Human dicrocoeliasis. Report of 208 cases from Saudia Arabia. Trop Geogr Med 42:1, 1990.

Ishii Y, Koga M, Fujino T. et al: Human infection with the pancreas fluke *Eurytrema pancreaticum*. Am J Trop Med Hyg 32:1019, 1983.

121 *Lung Fluke Infections: Paragonimiasis*

Danai Bunnag, John H. Cross, and Thanongsak Bunnag

DEFINITION. Paragonimiasis is infection by lung flukes of the genus *Paragonimus*, the most common of which is the oriental lung fluke, *P. westermani*. The adult worms usually live encapsulated in pockets in the lungs but may be found also in extrapulmonary locations.

ETIOLOGY. About 48 species and subspecies of *Paragonimus* have been described, some of which may not be valid. In carnivorous animal hosts, they appear to be widely distributed; in humans, seven species are known to cause disease. *Paragonimus* species are distinguishable by their cuticular spines, ovarian shape, relative size of oral and ventral suckers, ova characteristics, chromosomes, and migration route in tissues.

Morphology. The living adult parasites are reddish brown, ovoid or coffee-bean shaped, and have a broad anterior end. They are 7 to 16 mm long, 4 to 8 mm wide, and 2 to 5 mm thick. The tegument is covered with cuticular spines (Fig. 121–1A). The eggs are golden brown, are asymmetrically ovoid with a thick shell, have a relatively flattened operculum, measure 80 to 120 μm by 50 to 65 μm, and are immature when deposited (Fig. 121–1B).

Life Cycle. The adult flukes live in and lay eggs within a pulmonary cyst (Fig. 121–2). The eggs are passed along a tunnel that connects to a large bronchus and are expectorated with sputum or swallowed and passed in feces. On reaching water, they embryonate and hatch in about 3 weeks into miracidia that invade the tissues of appropriate snails (the first intermediate host), in which they undergo asexual transformation into sporocysts, rediae, and daughter rediae. Cercariae emerge from the snails in 3 to 5 months and penetrate crustaceans (crabs or crayfish) (the second intermediate host), in which they develop to become infective-stage metacercariae in 6 to 8 weeks. However, some crabs acquire infection by eating infected snails. When infected crustaceans are eaten raw by a mammalian host (the definitive host), the metacercariae excyst in the duodenum, penetrate the intestinal wall into the abdominal cavity, and then migrate through the abdominal wall, where they grow to young flukes after about a week. The flukes then penetrate the diaphragm to enter the lung tissue, where, enclosed in a pseudocapsule, they grow to adult worms in 5 to 6 weeks. Eggs are produced and

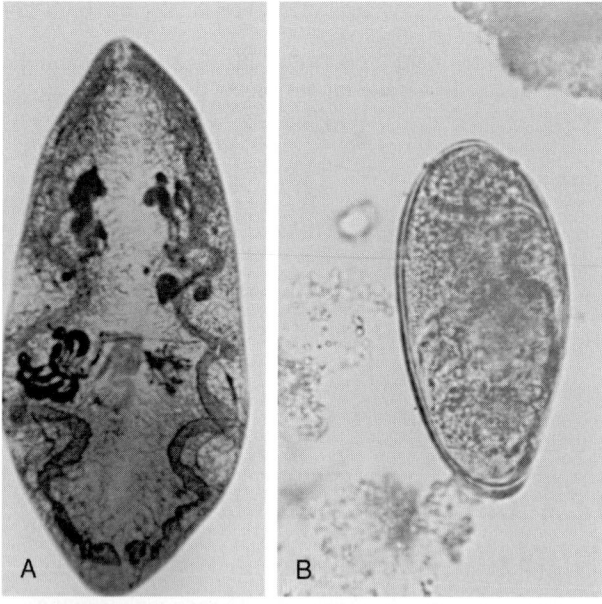

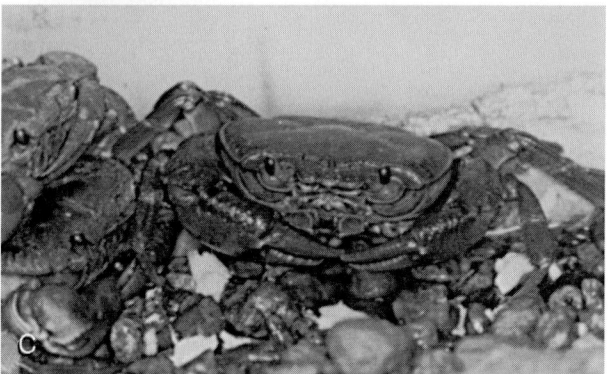

Figure 121–1. Adult *Paragonimus heterotremus (A)* and egg *(B)*. Mountainous stream crab *Larnaudia beusekomae* (Tawaripotamon) *(C)* is an important second intermediate host of paragonimiasis in Thailand. (Courtesy of Professor Prayong Radomyos, Faculty of Tropical Medicine, Mahidol University, Bangkok, Thailand.)

appear in the sputum or feces as early as 8 to 10 weeks after infection. In humans, flukes have been known to live for >20 years.

INTERMEDIATE HOSTS. About 20 species of freshwater snails serve as hosts, mainly members of the families Thiaridae, Pleuroceridae, and Pomatiopsidae. Important snail hosts in China, Japan, Korea, and Taiwan are the pleurocerid *Semisulcospira (Melania) libertina* and *Tricular gregoriana,* and the thiarid *Thiara (Tarebia) granifera;* in the Philippines, *Brotia asperata;* in Malaysia, *B. costula episcopalis* and other melanoid-allied species. Crustacean intermediate hosts are several kinds of freshwater crabs: in China, Japan, and Taiwan, they are *Eriocheir japonicus, Potamon dehaani,* and *P. rathburni;* in Thailand, *Larnaudia (Tawaripotamon) buesekomae* (Fig. 121–1C); in the Philippines, *Sundathelphusa philippina;* and in Korea, the crayfish *Cambaroides similis.* The freshwater shrimp, *Macrobrachium nipponensis* and *Caridina* species, are of less importance as secondary intermediate hosts in Japan, Korea, and China; other crustacean species are hosts elsewhere in the world. In endemic areas of Japan, some mammals (e.g., rat, mouse, pig, and wild boar) serve as paratenic hosts and as sources of human infection when they carry the immature fluke in their muscles (Fig. 121–2).

EPIDEMIOLOGY. Paragonimiasis is essentially a zoonotic disease among carnivorous animals throughout the world, but the three main endemic foci of human paragonimiasis are in Asia, Africa, and Central and South America.

Geographic Distribution. Nearly 200 million people worldwide are at risk, and an estimated 21 million are infected; infection is particularly prevalent in Korea, China, Japan, and Taiwan but also occurs in India, Sri Lanka, Malaysia, Papua New Guinea, Thailand, Laos, Vietnam, and the Philippines. Of the approximately 25 zoonotic species of *Paragonimus* in Asia and Oceania, 4 cause infections of humans: *P. westermani, P. (szechuanensis) skrjabini, P. miyazakii,* and *P. (tuanshanensis) heterotrema.*

In Africa, where *P. africanus* and *P. uterobilateralis* have been identified in humans and animals, paragonimiasis is endemic in eastern Nigeria, Cameroon, Liberia, Guinea, and The Gambia. In Central and South America, where *P. mexicanus* is the principal species in humans and animals, human infections have been reported in Mexico, Guatemala, Panama, Colombia, Peru, Ecuador, Costa Rica, Honduras, Venezuela, El Salvador, and Nicaragua.

Transmission. Contributing factors responsible for transmission of infection to humans include the presence of a large number of reservoir hosts (human and animals), abundance of first and second intermediate hosts, and social customs among certain Asian populations of eating raw or inadequately cooked crabs, crayfish, or shrimp. Infection results from such dishes as "drunken crab" (immersion of live crabs in wine for 12 hours), raw crab sauce or jam, and crayfish-curd in China; in Thailand, *Kung Ten* (raw shrimp salad) and *Nam Prik Poo* (crab sauce); in the Philippines, *Sinugba* (roasted crab) and *Kinilao* (raw crab); and in Korea, *Ke Jang* (crab immersed in soy sauce). In Korea and Japan, raw juice of crabs or crayfish is used in traditional medicine in treatment of measles, diarrhea, and urticaria. Another source of infection is contamination of utensils, chopping blocks, and cloths used during food preparation. In Africa, some women have the local custom of eating raw crustaceans to increase fertility. In Kyushu, Japan, humans have been infected by eating raw infected wild boar meat, a paratenic host.

After assessment by intradermal test in 21 provinces of China, it was estimated that there were 20 million infections; although 6 million are at risk in South Korea, only an estimated 1000 persons harbor active infections.

PATHOLOGY AND PATHOGENESIS. The wide variation in pathologic findings depends on the number of infecting worms, duration of infection, and tissues affected. Toxic and allergic factors may be involved also.

Pulmonary Lesions. Migrating larval flukes in the lungs (and frequently in other tissues) induce local necrosis, hemorrhage, and inflammatory exudate, which are followed by fibrous encapsulation into a worm cyst (Fig. 121–3). In the lungs, initial lesions are usually located a few centimeters beneath the pleural surface, near bronchioles or bronchi. Pathology includes bronchopneumonia, interstitial pneumonia, bronchitis, bronchiectasis, atelectasis, fibrosis, pleural thickening, pleural effusion, angiitis obliterans, and periphlebitis.

Macroscopically, the worm cysts are generally 1 to 4 cm, distended, grayish-white nodules. In cross section, they have irregular outlines and cavities; within are generally one to two worms, uncommonly three to four or none. The total number of cysts in the lungs is usually <20, with the larger proportion located in the right lung.

Microscopically, the cyst wall consists of granulation tissue with fibroblasts, lymphoid cells, mononuclear cells, plasma cells, and eosinophils. Within the cavity are numerous Charcot-Leyden crystals, *Paragonimus* eggs, and necrotic material.

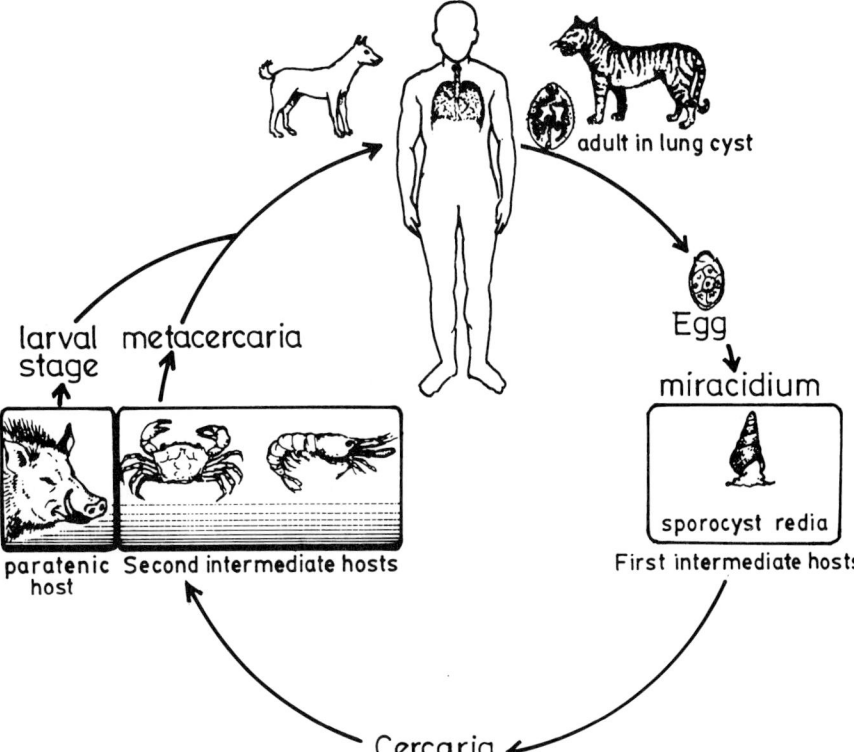

Figure 121–2. Life cycle of *Paragonimus heterotremus*.

In the vicinity of the cysts are tunnels, burrows, egg tubercles, and calcified eggs.

Ectopic Lesions. Though uncommon, young or even mature flukes may migrate from the lungs and reach almost any organ, including the psoas muscle, testes, scrotum, spermatic cord, liver, gut wall, other abdominal viscera, uterine and vaginal wall, and spinal cord. In the ectopic site, the flukes reach sexual maturity. Cysts, granulomas, or abscess may then form around the flukes or their eggs. Some immature flukes migrate from the lungs through the jugular or carotid

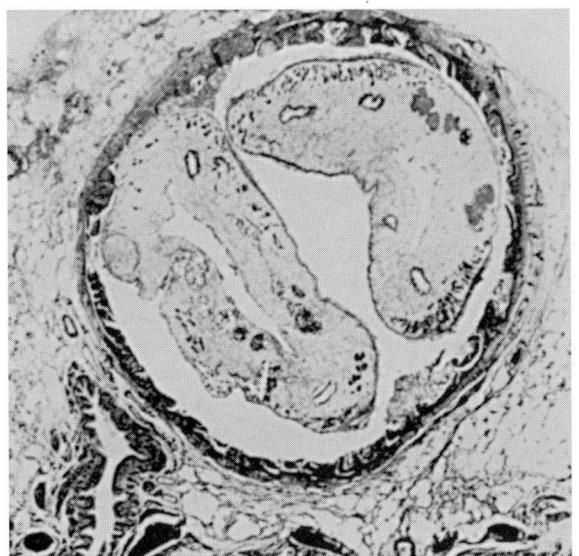

Figure 121–3. *Paragonimus westermani* in the lung of a Bengal tiger. (Courtesy of Dr. T. W. M. Cameron, Macdonald College of McGill University.)

foramen at the base of the skull to reach the temporal and occipital lobes of the brain, where they produce necrosis and eosinophilic granulomatous reactions. In China, migratory subcutaneous swellings are particularly common with *P. skrjabini* (or *Pagumogonimus skrjabini*) infection, and ova have been found at the centers of small eosinophilic granulomas in such aberrant sites as the pericardium, meninges, and liver.

CLINICAL MANIFESTATIONS. In light infections, the majority of patients are asymptomatic. In heavy infections, patients may have few symptoms and appear well despite severe pathology.

Acute Stage. This stage corresponds to the period of invasion and migration of the young flukes. Although this stage often passes undiagnosed, findings may include diarrhea, abdominal pain, urticaria, and eosinophilia, followed by fever, chest pain, cough, dyspnea, malaise, and night sweats.

Pulmonary Paragonimiasis. The incubation period is about 6 months (range, 1 to 27 months). Cough, sputum, and chest discomfort increase gradually and are similar to those in chronic bronchitis. The cough is spasmodic, usually occurs on walking or after exertion, and is productive of a characteristic gelatinous, tenacious, rusty-brown or golden-flake sputum. About half of the patients complain of breathlessness on exertion and some of wheezing. Mild fever may be present. Episodic pleuritic pain and frank hemoptysis are common; the latter is usually induced by heavy work and rarely is severe and life-threatening. Physical signs in the chest are not distinct; digital clubbing may be seen. Pulmonary tuberculosis may coexist; secondary bronchopneumonia and lung abscess are complications.

Laboratory tests show normal hemoglobin value with relative eosinophilic leukocytosis. Chest radiographs in the early stage show ill-defined opacities (Fig. 121–4). Later radiographic findings include cysts (that may have a ring shadow with a crescent-shaped opacity along one side) (Fig. 121–5), extensive infiltration (nodular, exudative, or linear), calcified

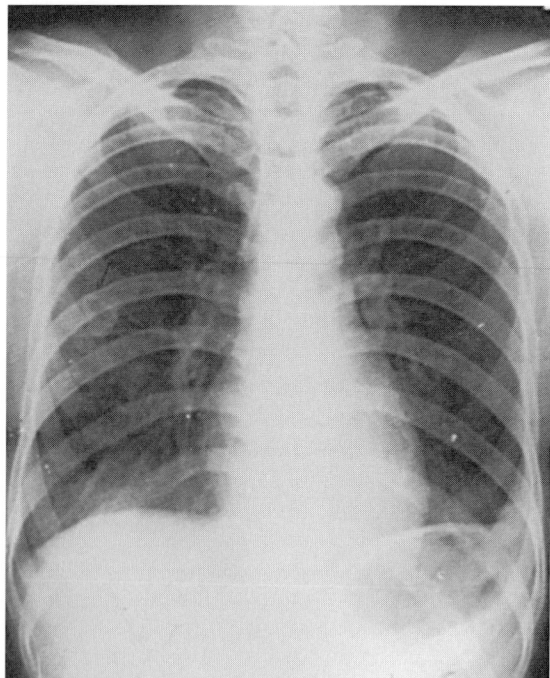

Figure 121–4. Pulmonary paragonimiasis. Chest roentgenogram shows thick-walled cystic lesion in the right upper lobe with pericystic fibrosis and thickening of the interlobular septum on both lower lobes. (Courtesy of Professor Sirivan Vanijanonda, Faculty of Tropical Medicine, Mahidol University, Bangkok, Thailand.)

foci, pleural thickening, loculated pleural effusions, multilocular cavities, and hilar enlargement.

Cerebral and Spinal Paragonimiasis. In endemic areas of Asia, 25% of hospitalized cases are due to brain invasion. Eighty percent of these patients are <10 years old, and most are males. Cerebral disease is particularly prevalent in rural South Korea, where it is the most common cause of cerebral tumor. As many as ten round or oval cysts, a few millimeters to 10 cm in diameter, are found in the temporal and occipital lobes, near the jugular foramen.

In the acute phase, manifestations may resemble meningoencephalitis. Patients suffer headache, vomiting, fever, and visual disturbances. With progression, patients may have papilledema, bitemporal hemianopsia, facial palsy, hemiplegia, paraplegia, jacksonian seizures, and coma. Death during the acute attack is not uncommon. In nonfatal cases, spontaneous remission occurs in 1 to 2 months, but recurrence may follow within 2 years.

Pleocytosis of the cerebrospinal fluid with a high eosinophil count is common. Plain skull radiographs show signs of increased intracranial pressure or cerebral calcification. Cysts can be demonstrated by computed tomography or angiography.

Rarely, spinal cord involvement presents as paraplegia or monoplegia, with weakness of the extremities and disturbance in sensation.

Abdominal Paragonimiasis. Findings may include abdominal pain and tenderness, bloody diarrhea, nausea, vomiting, palpable nodules, and abscess formation in the liver, spleen, or abdominal cavity. These may simulate a bacterial infection. In some instances, cyst rupture into the intestinal lumen releases *Paragonimus* eggs that can be recovered in the feces.

Migratory Subcutaneous Paragonimiasis. Migratory subcutaneous nodules occur in 20 to 60% of patients with *P. skrjabini* and 10% of those with *P. westermani* infections. They

are firm, slightly mobile, tender, a few millimeters to 10 cm in diameter, and they often are mildly irritating. The most common sites are the lower abdomen, inguinal region, and thigh; nodules up to 6 cm in diameter have also been seen behind the ear lobe.

In China, *P. skrjabini* is unable to develop to maturity in the lungs. Instead of findings of hemoptysis and ova in the sputum, the striking feature is trematode larva migrans, associated with migratory subcutaneous nodules accompanied by marked eosinophilic leukocytosis as well as necrotic liver lesions. In many cases, the nodules contain juvenile flukes. Brain involvement with subarachnoid hemorrhage is common. Ectopic infections are also reported with *P. heterotrema, P. mexicanus,* and occasionally *P. westermani.*

DIAGNOSIS. A presumptive diagnosis can be made in a patient who has a history of chronic bronchitis, blood-streaked sputum, and occasional hemoptysis and who lives in an endemic area and has eaten raw crustaceans. Confirmation is by finding characteristic eggs in sputum, stool, pleural effusion, or cerebrospinal fluid (Fig. 121–1*B*), or adult flukes in subcutaneous nodules, in other surgical specimens, or rarely in sputum (Fig. 121–1*A*).

Immunodiagnosis by complement fixation, countercurrent immunoelectrophoresis, and enzyme-linked immunosorbent assay, especially in extrapulmonary disease, can help establish the diagnosis. Immunoblot and monoclonal antibody antigen detection techniques have also been developed. Most treated patients become seronegative after about 6 months. Intradermal tests have been used in screening in epidemiologic surveys and positive responses evaluated further by complement fixation tests.

Differential diagnosis of pulmonary paragonimiasis includes pulmonary tuberculosis, lung abscess, chronic pulmonary infection of other causes, and primary and metastatic pulmonary carcinoma. Cerebral and spinal paragonimiasis must be differentiated from abscess, tuberculoma, and other

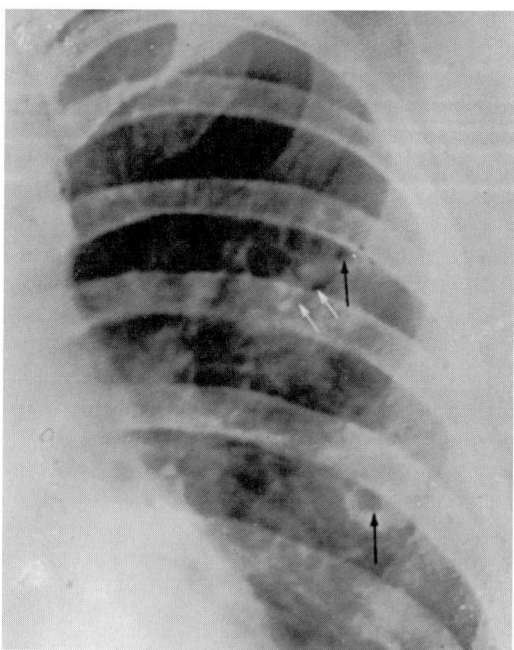

Figure 121–5. Pulmonary paragonimiasis with ring shadows *(black arrows)* and linear lucency *(white arrows)* representing burrow tract. (Courtesy of R. Suwanik Dhonburi, Thailand.) (From Markell EK, Voge M, John DT: Medical Parasitology. 7th ed. Philadelphia, WB Saunders, 1992.)

helminthic infections, including fascioliasis, schistosomiasis japonica, cysticercosis, hydatid disease, angiostrongyliasis, and gnathostomiasis.

Abdominal symptoms mimic many acute conditions, including appendicitis and amebic liver abscess. Subcutaneous paragonimiasis may be confused with gnathostomiasis, sparganosis, onchocerciasis, and cysticercosis.

TREATMENT. The drug of choice is praziquantel 25 mg/kg three times at 4-hour intervals after meals for 3 days. The cure rate is almost 100%; only a few patients with heavy infections need a second course of treatment. Symptoms improve rapidly and disappear within a few months. Eggs clear from the sputum in a few weeks, whereas the radiologic pulmonary lesions take some months to clear, depending on duration and severity of the disease. Drug side effects, including drowsiness and headaches, are mild and transient. The dosage in cerebral paragonimiasis is often higher and must be adjusted according to the clinical response. Because convulsions and coma have been observed, treatment should proceed with caution in the hospital and corticosteroids should be given as in certain cases of cerebral cysticercosis treated with praziquantel (Chapter 124.1).

PROGNOSIS. Pulmonary paragonimiasis is rarely fatal; even without treatment, flukes die or disappear within 10 to 20 years. Most cases of cerebral disease are associated with chronic morbidity due to epilepsy, dementia, and other neurologic sequelae; 5% of the patients die owing to hemorrhage, and usually in the first 2 years of the disease.

PREVENTION AND CONTROL. Health education, especially for young schoolchildren, is needed to change the dietary customs of eating raw or undercooked crab or crayfish. Mass treatment with bithionol in some endemic areas in Korea proved effective in reducing the prevalence of paragonimiasis. Mollusciciding is at present impractical.

Bibliography

Chung PR: Review and problem on *Paragonimus* and paragonimiasis with special reference to its intermediate and natural final hosts. Yonsei Rep Trop Med 14:44, 1983.

Cross JH: Paragonimus. *In* Hoeprich PD, Jordan MC, Ronald AR (eds): Infectious Diseases. Philadelphia, JB Lippincott, 1994, pp 553–557.

Indrawati I, Chaicumpa W, Setasuban P, Ruangkunaporn Y: Studies on immunodiagnosis of human paragonimiasis and specific antigen of *Paragonimus heterotremous*. Int J Parasitol 21:395, 1991.

Oliver G, Boussinesq M, Albaret JL, et al: Epidemiological study of *Paragonimus* sp. in south Cameroon. Bull Soc Pathol Exot 88:164, 1995.

Saborio P, Lanzas R, Arrieta G, Arguedas A: *Paragonimus mexicanus*: Report of two cases and review of the literature. J Trop Med Hyg 98:316, 1995.

Singh TS, Mutum S, Razaque MA, et al: Paragonimiasis in Maipur. Indian J Med Res 97:247, 1993.

Slemenda SB, Maddison SE, Jong EC, Moore DD: Diagnosis of paragonimiasis by immunoblot. Am J Trop Med Hyg 39:469, 1988.

Toscano C, Yu SH, Nunn P, Mott KE: Paragonimiasis and tuberculosis. Diagnostic confusion. Trop Dis Bull 92:R1, 1995.

Vanijanonda S, Bunnag D, Harinasuta T: Radiological findings in pulmonary paragonimiasis heterotremus. Southeast Asian J Trop Med Pub Hlth 15:122, 1984.

Zhang Z, Zhang Y, Shi Z, et al: Diagnosis of active *Paragonimus westermani* infections with a monoclonal antibody-based antigen detection assay. Am J Trop Med Hyg 49:329, 1993.

■ SECTION E **Cestode Infections**

---

122 *General Principles*

Peter M. Schantz, Herbert B. Tanowitz, and Murray Wittner

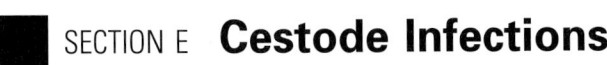

Infection with tapeworms is one of the oldest recognized afflictions of humankind. Their huge size and, at times, untimely egress from the body could hardly go unnoticed. The Cestoda, or tapeworms, are a class of the phylum Platyhelminthes and are exclusively parasitic. In addition to the Cestoda, other classes of Platyhelminthes are the Turbellaria, almost all of which are free living, and the Trematoda, or flukes, which are exclusively parasitic (Chapters 117 to 121). Tapeworms are flattened and do not possess a body cavity. They infect members of all vertebrate classes, whereas their larvae may infect both vertebrates and invertebrates.

CLASSIFICATION. Of the four main groups of cestodes, only two are important as parasites of humans and domestic animals. The order Pseudophyllidea is characterized by the presence of a scolex, or attachment organ, containing two sucking grooves. Examples of this group are members of the genus *Diphyllobothrium* (Chapter 123.1) and worms that infect humans only at the larval stage, e.g., the sparganum (Chapter 124.5). The order Cyclophyllidea, to which all other tapeworms that parasitize humans belong, is characterized by a scolex with four suckers. This group includes those belonging

to the genus *Taenia*, examples of which are the beef and pork tapeworms (Chapter 123.2). The life cycles of the Pseudophyllidea involve a minimum of three hosts. Those of the Cyclophyllidea generally require two, although in some cases the definitive host can also serve as the intermediate host. Adult tapeworms that are medically important range in size from the minute (<1 cm) *Echinococcus* (Chapter 124.2), which has a scolex and three segments, to *Taenia saginata*, reported at times to reach 10 m in length.

MORPHOLOGY

Adult. Adult tapeworms typically possess a scolex or head that may be modified or adorned with structures or organelles that serve as holdfast organs for attachment to the small intestinal mucosa. In the Pseudophyllidea, the structures that function for attachment are termed *bothria*, which are two shallow sucking grooves on the sides of a spatulate scolex (Fig. 122–1A). Some species of Cyclophyllidea, in addition to having four sucking cups or acetabula (Fig. 122–1B), possess hooklets that may form a ring at the top of the scolex or be mounted on a protrusion known as the *rostellum* (Fig. 122–1C). The distal portion of the scolex is termed the *neck*, an area of intense metabolic activity, which is the zone from which new segments or proglottids proliferate and form the strobila. Clinically, the scolex is highly significant, because therapy is aimed at its destruction or elimination, inasmuch as failure to do so results in regrowth of the entire tapeworm. The most proximal proglottids usually are immature. When stained, they contain only the earliest rudiments of the or-

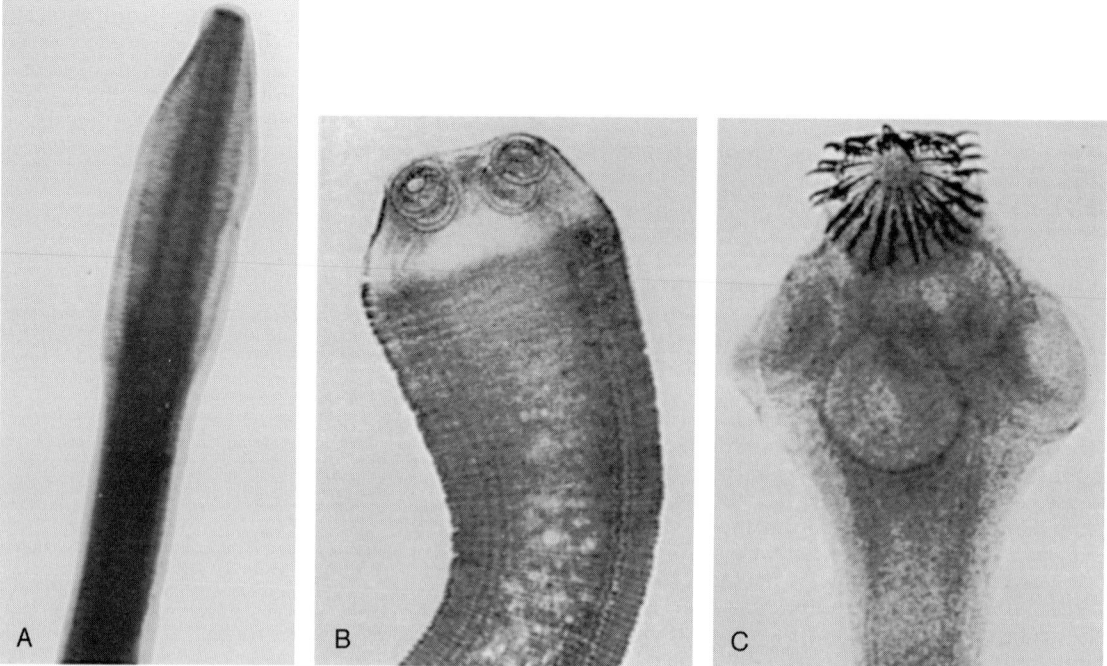

Figure 122–1. Scoleces of various tapeworms. *A, Diphyllobothrium latum. B, Taenia saginata. C, Taenia solium.* (Photomicrographs by Zane Price.) (From Markell EK, Voge M, John DT: Medical Parasitology, 6th ed. Philadelphia, WB Saunders, 1986.)

gans that develop in mature proglottids in the middle of the strobila. Those further distal become mature proglottids and contain one set, and in some species two complete sets, of male and female sex organs (i.e., they are hermaphroditic). The most distal segments are filled with eggs and are termed *gravid proglottids.* In cyclophyllidean cestodes, the sex organs have atrophied, leaving the segment occupied largely by a uterus filled with eggs.

The surface epithelium or tegument is actually a syncytium composed of an anucleate ectocytoplasm that covers the body of the tapeworm and an underlying layer containing nucleated cell bodies or perikarya. The ectocytoplasm has a prominent brush border composed of modified microvilli or microtriches. These structures are cytoplasmic extensions supported by a microfilamentous core. This cestode tegumental brush border increases the absorptive surface and may assist in motility and anchoring. Because cestodes lack a digestive system or alimentary canal, all of their nutriment

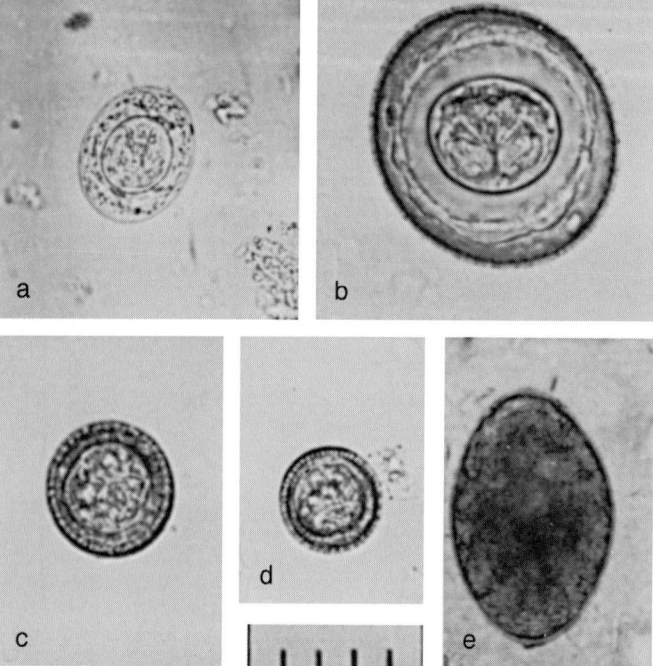

Figure 122–2. Cestode eggs. *a, Hymenolepis nana; b, Hymenolepis diminuta; c, d, Taenia species; e, Diphyllobothrium latum.* All eggs photographed at same magnification; scale equals 50 μm. (From Markell EK, Voge M, John DT: Medical Parasitology, 6th ed. Philadelphia, WB Saunders, 1986.)

is obtained by absorption across this highly organized surface tegument, which also serves to protect the worm from its environment (i.e., host digestive enzymes). Small molecules and carbohydrates are absorbed directly from the lumen of the small intestine.

The nervous system present in the scolex consists of ganglia with connecting commissures. Lateral nerve trunks extend distally and serve to coordinate movement of the chain of proglottids or strobila. The excretory system is developed primitively.

Eggs. The eggs of the tapeworms are characteristic (Fig. 122–2). In members of the genus *Diphyllobothrium,* eggs are discharged through a muscular uterine pore and, therefore, they are found regularly in the feces. In many Cyclophyllidea, however, the gravid proglottids split and the eggs are released through the rents in the proglottids. The eggs of the smaller tapeworms, such as *Hymenolepis nana* and *H. diminuta,* are found in the stool after the disintegration of the gravid proglottids, whereas often those of the genus *Taenia* are not found in the stool because they are passed out in intact segments. In fact, a cellophane tape preparation applied to the perianal area, similar to that used for the diagnosis of pinworm infection, is more reliable in finding *Taenia* eggs. Eggs of the diphyllobothriid tapeworms are operculate (Fig. 122–2*E*), resembling those of many trematodes, and hatch in water to release a free-swimming larva, the coracidium. Cyclophyllidean tapeworm eggs all contain a fully developed hexacanth (six hooked) embryo, the oncosphere. The embryonic envelope that surrounds this oncosphere constitutes what is generally referred to as the *eggshell,* and its morphology is often diagnostic of the species (Fig. 122–2).

LIFE CYCLE. With the single exception of *H. nana,* tapeworms that infect humans require one or more intermediate hosts to complete their life histories. The life cycle of diphyllobothriid cestodes involves two or more intermediate hosts. Coracidia, ingested by water flies or copepods, develop in the body cavity of these hosts into procercoid larvae, which, while retaining the embryonic six hooklets, show evidence of developing bothria. When infected copepods are ingested by the appropriate piscine hosts, the procercoid larva enters the tissues of the fish, where it becomes a plerocercoid or sparganum larva (Fig. 123–1).

Interestingly, the latter may have a number of transport or paratenic hosts. Thus, a plerocercoid that has developed in a minnow may next parasitize a somewhat larger fish and may even pass through a series of such transitory domiciliary relationships until its final piscine host is ingested by a suitable mammal, in which it develops to the adult stage.

Some cestodes only infect humans in the larval stage, e.g., the plerocercoid (sparganum) of *Spirometra mansonoides* (Chapter 124.5), whereas others infect humans in both the adult and larval stages, e.g., *Taenia solium* (Chapters 123.2 and 124.1). In the genera *Multiceps* (Chapter 124.6) and *Echinococcus* (Chapters 124.2–124.4), larval development results in considerable multiplication. Therefore, when they are ingested by a suitable host, large numbers of adult worms may be produced.

CLINICAL MANIFESTATIONS. The clinical manifestations of tapeworm infection may be due to infection with the adult or larval stage. Adult tapeworm infection may persist for many years. During this period, it may be relatively asymptomatic or may cause persistent symptoms. In contrast to infection with the adult stage, infection with the larval stage of a tapeworm often causes serious or fatal disease and can be of great economic consequences.

TREATMENT. Treatment of intestinal cestodes has been greatly improved and simplified in recent decades; the development of efficient taeniacidal drugs, first niclosamide and,

later, praziquantel, have made most older anthelmintics obsolete.

Niclosamide, a chlorinated salicylanilide, was introduced into human and veterinary medicine about 1960 and was shown to be effective against a wide variety of tapeworms and well tolerated, a "worm cure without tears." At a dose of 2 g for adults and about half this amount for children, it was widely concluded that the drug gave a cure rate of about 90% for taeniosis and had somewhat lesser efficacy for diphyllobothriosis. Subsequent experience in many countries, however, led to reports of variable efficacy, and some batches of the drug were less effective than expected, possibly because of variations in particle size. The strong cestocidal activity of praziquantel, a new type of acylated isoquinolinepyrazine, was first reported in 1975. Although the mode of action of praziquantel against cestodes is not fully understood, it causes immobilization and contraction of the worms, followed by vacuolation and disruption of the tapeworm tegument, presumably making them vulnerable to attack by the lytic effect of intestinal enzymes. Clinical trials and long experience have shown that at taeniacidal doses, there are no contraindications to the use of praziquantel in healthy persons. Precautions must be observed, however, in populations in which *T. solium* is endemic; a recent report from Mexico indicated that mass treatment of a population at a dose of 10 mg/kg may have activated a case of latent cerebral cysticercosis. Praziquantel is highly efficacious (>95%) against taeniosis, diphyllobothriosis, and most other intestinal cestodes when given as a single dose of 5 to 10 mg/kg. For *H. nana* infection, a single dose of 25 mg/kg body weight achieves similar high cure rates (>95%) as five daily doses of niclosamide.

After treatment with niclosamide and praziquantel, the proximal part of the large tapeworms, *Taenia* and *Diphyllobothrium* spp., usually disintegrates. Therefore, although most of the strobila is often evacuated within a few hours, it is difficult to find and confirm removal of the scolex. Passage of intact or disintegrating segments and of eggs continues for several days after treatment. Treatment can be considered successful if no eggs reappear in several stool specimens examined at sufficient intervals after treatment to allow regrowth of worms: 3 months for *Taenia* spp. and 1 month for *Hymenolepis, Diphyllobothrium,* and other species. Because *H. nana* has the ability to renew its population through internal autoinfection and because rates of reinfection are high among some populations of children, certain patients may appear to remain infected despite repeated treatments. Nevertheless, drug therapy nearly always reduces worm burdens to tolerable levels, and infections in children are usually lost spontaneously in adolescence.

Bibliography

Campbell WC, Rew RS: Chemotherapy of Parasitic Diseases. New York, Plenum Press, 1986.
Groll E: Praziquantel for cestode infections in man. Acta Trop 37:293, 1980.
Schantz PM: Tapeworms (Cestodiasis). Gastroenterol Clin North Am 25:637, 1996.

123 *Tapeworm Infections*

Peter M. Schantz, Herbert B. Tanowitz, and Murray Wittner

123.1 *Diphyllobothriasis*

ETIOLOGY AND LIFE CYCLE. Diphyllobothriasis is infection of the intestinal tract by the fish tapeworms *Diphyllobothrium* spp. At least 13 species are described in the genus; *D. latum* and *D. dendriticum* are the most prevalent, but most of the others can infect humans. Diphyllobothriids of other genera, including *Diplogonoporus*, a parasite of whales, may also infect humans. Adult *D. latum* ranges in length from less than 1 M to 12 M or more; the largest worms have thousands of proglottids. Some other *Diphyllobothrium* spp., e.g., *D. dentriticum*, are smaller, rarely more than 1 M long. The scolex is finger-shaped and has dorsal and ventral sucking grooves (Fig. 122–1A). Proglottids are usually wider than they are long. In the center of the mature proglottid is a characteristic dark rosette, i.e., the egg-filled uterus (Fig. 123–1), that aids in its recognition. The uterus consists of short loops and extends from the ovary to a midventral uterine pore from which eggs are continuously discharged. The characteristic ovoid eggs measure 42 to 50 μm × 59 to 75 μm and have a lidlike operculum at one end and a small knob on the other (Fig. 122–2E).

Maintenance of the life cycle of *Diphyllobothrium* species requires that feces of infected hosts be discharged into fresh or brackish water that contains susceptible crustaceans and fish and that the infected fish be eaten raw by definitive hosts. The three required hosts can be supplemented by additional predacious fish serving as paratenic hosts that ultimately infect humans and other fish-eating hosts. After the egg hatches, the motile embryo (coracidium) is ingested by minute crustacea, "water fleas" (*Cyclops* and *Diaptomus*), in which the first-stage larva (procercoid) develops. When the procercoid is ingested by the second intermediate host—a fish—further development leads to the plerocercoid or "sparganum" larva, which is infective for the final host. The site of localization of the plerocercoid in fish differs with species of *Diphyllobothrium* and, to some extent, with species of fish. However, when the final host ingests the *Diphyllobothrium* plerocercoid, the worm remains in the gut, the larval portion of the body is shed, and the adult worm develops to maturity in the small intestine (Fig. 123–2). Within 3 to 5 weeks, egg production is initiated; a million or more eggs may be passed daily. Adult *Diphyllobothrium* may survive 10 years or more.

DISTRIBUTION AND EPIDEMIOLOGY. *D. latum* causes a common human infection in northern Europe (Finland, East Prussia, Russian Karelia). In North America, *D. latum* infec-

tions have been reported in Eskimos in western Alaska, where the infection was apparently introduced by Russians during their occupation of that region. *D. latum* may have been introduced to the Great Lakes region by settlers from Scandinavia; however, the absence of recent reports suggests that it may no longer occur there. Tapeworms identified as *D. latum* have also been reported from Canada, Africa, Japan, Taiwan, Manchuria, Siberia, Papua New Guinea, Australia, South America, and elsewhere; however, some of these reports may represent erroneous identifications of other *Diphyllobothrium* species. In Alaska, at least six species of *Diphyllobothrium* are known to exist, and all of them occasionally infect humans.

Humans become infected by ingesting *Diphyllobothrium* plerocercoid larvae in fish or fish roe or liver that is raw or incompletely cooked. A variety of freshwater as well as some marine fishes are sources of infection. Among the most common freshwater fish are pike, perch, and turbot; anadromous fish, e.g., salmon and their predators, may also be infected. Salmon has been reported to be responsible for transmission in Japan and the west coast of the United States.

Diphyllobothrium spp. are not very host-specific. Although humans may be the most important final hosts for *D. latum*, bears, dogs, cats, and other carnivores often permit normal development of adult worms. Other *Diphyllobothrium* spp. are maintained primarily in wild animal hosts and only incidentally infect humans. For example, *D. dendriticum* occurs widely in fish-eating birds and mammals in the Northern Hemisphere and is not uncommon in certain human populations in Alaska. *D. ursi* is a common parasite of bears but has also been reported in humans in Alaska and Canada. *D. pacificum*, a parasite of pinnipeds off the coast of Peru, occasionally infects people who eat contaminated marine fish.

The dietary preferences of certain populations and the practice of discarding human excreta into ponds and rivers facilitate the transmission of *D. latum* and *Diphyllobothrium* spp. In Japan and the Scandinavian countries, the strong cultural preferences for eating raw fish dishes have favored high rates of transmission in the past. Earlier in this century, infection was relatively common among Jewish women who prepared gefilte fish (spiced, minced fish meat) and tasted it for flavor prior to cooking. In general, the incidence of fish tapeworm in humans seems to be declining; in the United States, however, the growing popularity of raw fish dishes, e.g., Japanese sushi and sashimi and Latin American ceviche, is placing consumers at continued risk of infection.

CLINICAL MANIFESTATIONS AND PATHOLOGY. Most patients are asymptomatic or mildly symptomatic, but a small proportion may develop megaloblastic anemia. A single *D. latum* is usually present, but infection with multiple worms can occur. The worm is not invasive, and there is little pathologic damage associated with the infection other than that related to competition between host and parasite for absorption of vitamin B_{12}.

Most infections are asymptomatic. In one large clinical study that compared the frequency of complaints between nonanemic carriers and noninfected persons, only fatigue, diarrhea, dizziness, weakness, numbness of extremities, and a sensation of hunger were reported more frequently in infected persons. No difference was found in the incidence of abdominal pains. Although there is no regular discharge of individual proglottids, such as occurs with *Taenia* spp., a length of the tapeworm is sometimes evacuated or vomited.

Megaloblastic Anemia. *D. latum* has a marked affinity for vitamin B_{12}; in some individuals, depletion of B_{12} produces a megaloblastic anemia that resembles pernicious anemia both clinically and hematologically. This requires that the tapeworm be in the proximal part of the intestine and probably

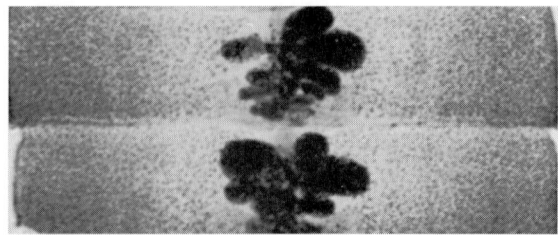

Figure 123–1. Gravid proglottids of *Diphyllobothrium latum*. (Photomicrograph by Zane Price from material furnished by Dr. Justus F. Mueller.) (From Markell EK, Voge M, John DT: Medical Parasitology, 6th ed. Philadelphia, WB Saunders, 1986.)

LIFE CYCLE of —

Diphyllobothrium latum

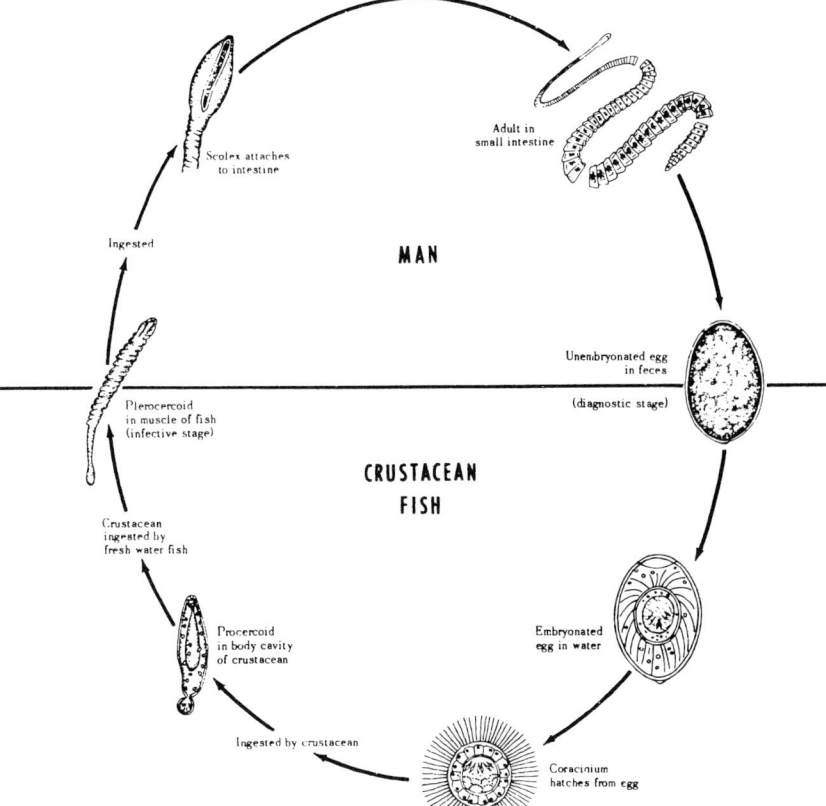

Figure 123–2. Life cycle of *Diphyllobothrium latum.* (From Melvin DM, Brooke MM, Sadun EH: Common Intestinal Helminths of Man. Atlanta, Centers for Disease Control, DHEW Publications No. [CDC] 75–8286, 1964.)

that the host be defective in intrinsic factor secretion with diminished capacity to absorb B_{12}. Only *D. latum* is known to be associated with macrocytic anemia. Among persons harboring the worm, approximately 40% have reduced B_{12} levels, but less than 2% develop anemia. When fully manifest the anemia resembles pernicious anemia, i.e., hyperchromic, macrocytic, and megaloblastic, with thrombocytopenia and mild leukopenia. For unknown reasons, its occurrence is generally limited to Scandinavian countries. The anemia is usually moderate but can become severe, with findings of pallor, glossitis, dyspnea, and tachycardia. There may be neurologic findings, including weakness, numbness, paresthesia, disturbance of movement and coordination, and impairment of deep sensibilities, in the absence of hematologic abnormalities. The anemia and the neurologic manifestations respond to vitamin B_{12} and do not return after the worm has been expelled. Severe anemia associated with diphyllobothriasis has not been reported for several decades, possibly as a result of improved levels of general nutrition.

DIAGNOSIS. Diagnosis requires demonstration of the characteristic eggs (Fig. 122–2*E*); this is usually readily accomplished by either direct or concentration methods because egg production is very high. Segments of proglottids are occasionally passed with feces or vomited, and, if they are intact, their internal morphology is diagnostic for the genus. *Diphyllobothrium* spp. eggs are morphologically similar and cannot be speciated by microscopy. Furthermore, *Diphyllobothrium* eggs are similar to those of a trematode, *Nanophyetus*

salmincola, that occurs widely in the Pacific Northwest region of the United States and in eastern Siberia. If differential diagnosis of the eggs is difficult, a saline purge may provide proglottids for examination. Discrimination of *Diphyllobothrium* spp. is based on examination of scoleces, strobila, and eggs and requires expert assistance. No satisfactory serologic or coproantigen test for *Diphyllobothrium* infection is available.

In tapeworm-induced anemia, free hydrochloric acid may be present in the gastric juice, whereas true pernicious anemia is invariably associated with achlorhydria. Vitamin B_{12} levels may be diminished.

TREATMENT. The treatment of choice is praziquantel. A single dose of 10 mg/kg body weight for both adults and children is curative in nearly all cases (> 90%). Niclosamide is also safe and highly effective, although not so widely available as praziquantel. It is given as a single dose of four tablets (2 g), chewed thoroughly. A single dose of 1 g (two tablets) is recommended for children weighing 11 to 34 kg and a single dose of 1.5 g (three tablets) for those weighing more than 34 kg.

PREVENTION. Careful cooking of fish eliminates all possibility of human infection. Heating to a temperature of 56°C will kill plerocercoids. If a thermometer is not available the fish should be cooked until it loses its translucency and flakes easily with a fork. The sale of fish originating in heavily infected lakes should be regulated. Freezing at −18°C for 24 hours kills the plerocercoid larvae. In the United States, smoked salmon is usually brined before smoking and is not considered a source of infection. Other control measures include educating cooks to avoid sampling of raw fish during preparation. Discontinuation of dumping raw sewage into freshwater lakes prevents viable eggs from contaminating various intermediate hosts. In highly endemic areas, human infection should be detected by survey and treated; pet dogs should be dewormed several times a year.

Bibliography

Adams A, Rausch RL: Diphyllobothriasis. *In* Connor DH, Manz H, Lack EE (eds): Pathology of Infectious Diseases. East Norwalk, CT, Appleton & Lange, 1997.

Centers for Disease Control: Diphyllobothriasis associated with salmon—United States. MMWR 30:331, 1981.

Von Bondsorff B: Diphyllobothriasis in Man. London, Academic Press, 1977.

123.2 *Taeniasis*

ETIOLOGY AND LIFE CYCLE. The pork tapeworm, *Taenia solium*, and the beef tapeworm, *Taenia saginata*, are the common tapeworm parasites of humans. These infections have been known since ancient times and occur whenever infected insufficiently cooked beef or pork is consumed. Human infection caused by larvae of *T. solium*, known as cysticercosis, is covered in Chapter 124.1.

A third form of *Taenia* infectious to humans is widespread in Asia. It is morphologically and genetically distinct but is closely related to *T. saginata*. The larval form occurs in the liver and other tissues of swine. It has been commonly referred to as Taiwan or Asian *Taenia*; however, both subspecies (*T. saginata asiaticus*) and separate species (*T. asiaticus*) status have been proposed.

Adult *T. saginata* organisms vary in size from 4 to 12 M and may be composed of 1000 to 2000 proglottids. In multiple infections with either *T. saginata* or *T. solium*, however, a "crowding effect" is noted so that each worm is usually smaller. As proglottids mature and become gravid, the testes and other reproductive organs first appear and finally disappear, giving place to the enlarging uterus. The proglottids have no uterine pore; instead, eggs are released into the feces or onto the perineum through a longitudinal ventral split in the distended gravid segments (Fig. 123–3). The scolex of *T. saginata* is distinctive, being about 1.5 to 2 mm wide and possessing four sucking disks. It lacks a crown or rostellum with hooks and is said to be an "unarmed" scolex (Fig. 122–1B).

T. solium is somewhat smaller, varying from 1.5 to 8 M with a total of about 1000 proglottids. The characteristic scolex is about 1 mm and possesses a well-developed crown or rostellum upon which are a double row of 22 to 32 large and small hooklets, i.e., an "armed" scolex (Fig. 122–1C).

The adult Asian *Taenia* is similar morphologically to *T. saginata*, although smaller; it varies in length from 4 to 8 M and consists of 300 to 1000 proglottids. Other minor morphologic differences (from *T. saginata*) include a rostellum on the adult scolex, vestigial hooklets on the larval scolex, and wartlike protuberances on the cysticercal surface (Fig. 123–4).

Adult taeniae of these species are found only in humans and generally are attached in the jejunum. The worm is not fixed in position but moves frequently even against the peristaltic stream. Gravid proglottids hold tens of thousands of eggs. The spherical, thick-walled egg is striated radially and contains a mature six-hooked (hexacanth) embryo, termed an oncosphere. The eggs are 30 to 40 µm in diameter and are similar in all members of the genus (Fig. 122–2C and D).

Cattle or pigs become infected by ingesting eggs, contaminating low-lying pastures or barnyards. The action by gastric juice, intestinal enzymes, and bile has been shown necessary to stimulate hatching. Embryos that then penetrate the intestinal mucosa of cattle or pigs enter the circulation and are transported throughout the body. Encystment usually occurs in striated muscle, and within 7 to 12 weeks the larvae, termed *Cysticercus cellulosae* in pigs or *Cysticercus bovis* in cattle, are infectious. Cysticerci measure 1.5 to 3.5 mm × 2 to 9 mm. They are ellipsoidal, white, translucent bladder-like cysts into which an inverted scolex has developed.

Cysticerci of the Asian *Taenia* develop in the liver of swine, cattle, and goats. By 4 weeks the mature cysticercus measures approximately 0.5 to 1.7 × 0.5 to 2.0 mm, considerably smaller than *T. saginata* or *T. solium*. The protoscolex is armed, although the hooklets are lost as the tapeworm matures in the human final host.

Upon consumption of infected raw or inadequately cooked beef or pork, the cysticercus is activated by gastric juices, and surface active agents, e.g., bile salts, stimulate evagination of the scolex. Then, it attaches to the jejunal wall, becoming a mature tapeworm in 10 to 12 weeks in the case of *T. saginata* and Asian *Taenia* and in 5 to 12 weeks with *T. solium*. The adult tapeworm may live as long as 25 years (Figs. 123–5 and 123–6), but average longevity is considerably shorter.

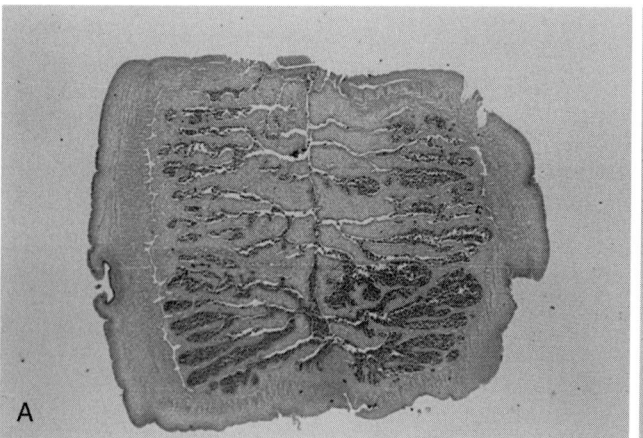
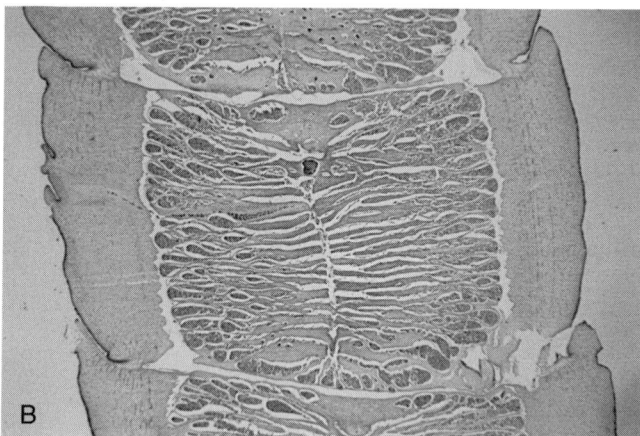

Figure 123–3. H&E stained sections of proglottids that easily distinguish the two species of *Taenia* commonly infecting humans. *Taenia solium* (*A*) has <13 branches of the uterus, while *T. saginata* (*B*) has >15 branches. (Courtesy of Angela Talley, Juan Jimenez, and Robert Gilman.)

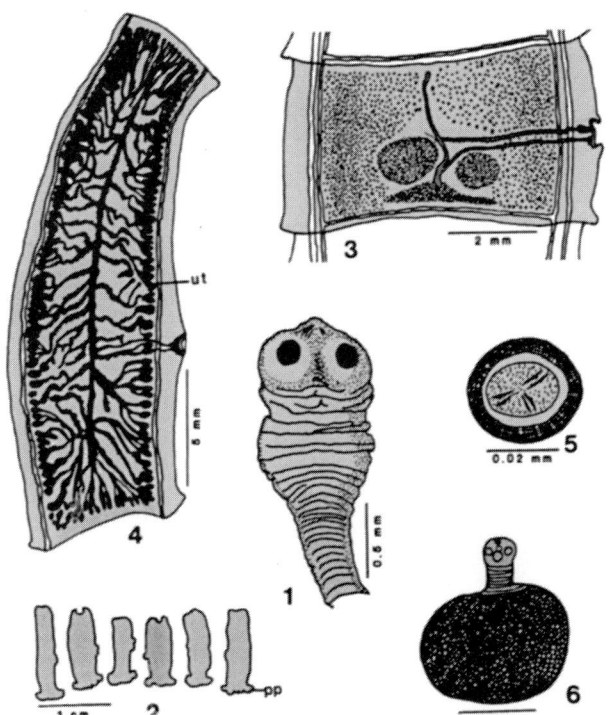

Figure 123–4. Asian *Taenia saginata* or *T. asiatica*. 1. Scolex with rostellum. 2. Gravid proglottid (unpressed); pp = posterior protuberance. 3. Mature proglottid. 4. Gravid proglottid (pressed); ut = uterine twigs. 5. Egg. 6. Cysticercus with wartlike formations on bladder surface. (From Eom KS, Rim H-JL: Morphologic descriptions of *Taenia asiatica* spin. Korean J Parasitol 31:1, 1993.)

EPIDEMIOLOGY AND DISTRIBUTION. Occurrence and prevalence of *T. saginata* and *T. solium* infection are related to local habits of eating raw or undercooked beef or pork, respectively. *T. saginata* is a cosmopolitan parasite, with regions of high endemicity in Latin America, Africa, the Middle East, and Central Asia; in some populations sampled in East Africa prevalence exceeded 50%. Beef tapeworm prevalence is moderate in Europe, South Asia, Japan, and the Philippines and low in Australia and North America. In the United States *T. saginata* cysticercosis is sporadic and at low prevalence in cattle. *Taenia* eggs were found in less than 0.1% of 216,000 stool specimens examined at state health laboratories in 1988.

T. solium also occurs in much of the world but is generally less common and more focal than *T. saginata*. The tapeworm is relatively prevalent in most of Latin America, the Slavic countries, Africa, Southeast Asia, India, and China. Prevalence is low or the parasite infection rate is declining in parts of northwestern Europe. In the United States and Canada, locally acquired *T. solium* is rare or absent, although increasing numbers of imported cases of both taeniasis and cysticercosis have been reported.

The Asian *Taenia* has been reported in Taiwan, Korea, Indonesia, Thailand, and the Philippines. Prevalences of 10 to 20% have been reported in indigenous populations in Taiwan, who commonly ingest meat and viscera of pigs.

Persons of all ages and both sexes are susceptible to taeniasis and age of exposure is mainly determined by the age at which raw meat consumption begins; in Mexican rural communities *T. solium* taeniasis is reported with similar frequency in all age groups older than 2 years. In some communities women are infected more commonly than men. Human fecal contamination of the environment is a necessary factor in sustaining the life cycles of *Taenia* spp. Cattle become infected with *T. saginata* by grazing on ground or ingesting water or roughage contaminated with eggs from human feces. Indirect contamination of pasture by insufficiently processed human sewage may also be important. Pigs become infected with *T. solium* or Asian *Taenia*, often massively, because of their coprophagic habits.

T. saginata larval infection may also occur in other domesticated bovines, including the water buffalo and yak, but it rarely occurs in other ungulates. The Asian *Taenia*, considered closely related to *T. saginata*, most commonly affects pigs, but experimental studies have demonstrated that cattle, goats, and some species of monkey are also susceptible. *T. solium* larval infection occurs typically in pigs but can also infect domestic dogs and cats.

CLINICAL MANIFESTATIONS AND PATHOLOGY. *Taenia* spp. reside loosely within the intestinal lumen; usually only one worm is present, but infections with multiple worms can occur. Other than minor local mucosal inflammation at the site of attachment of the scolex there is little physiopathologic alteration of the gut. Adult taeniae are weakly immunogenic and may induce a moderate eosinophilia and increased levels of serum IgE. Rare acute complications may occur, more commonly with *T. saginata* than with *T. solium* or Asian *Taenia*, following migration of proglottids to unusual sites such as the appendix or pancreatic and bile ducts.

Many, perhaps most, tapeworm carriers are asymptomatic and become aware of the infection only as they notice proglottids passed with feces or the disconcerting sensation caused by the spontaneous movement of *T. saginata* segments through the anus. Mild gastrointestinal symptoms may occur in some patients, including nausea and vague epigastric or periumbilical pain. Other clinical findings occasionally attributed to the worms include anorexia (or increased appetite), weight loss, headaches, convulsions, and allergic symptoms (urticaria, pruritus, other skin disorders), but these symptoms may be associated with concomitant infection with other intestinal parasites or other potential causes.

Cysticercosis, infection with the larval form of *T. solium*, is a potentially serious complication of *T. solium* infection (Chapter 124.1).

DIAGNOSIS. In many cases, especially of *T. saginata* infection, the patient recognizes infection incidental to elimination in the feces of individual or short chains of motile tapeworm segments. The patient's description is usually sufficient for a tentative diagnosis of taeniasis, but confirmation of species is advisable for evaluation of the possible risk of cysticercosis. Proglottids eliminated spontaneously or following treatment should be collected in water or saline solution, using strict precautions to avoid contamination. The standard method for differentiating the species is to count the number of primary uterine branches in gravid proglottids: *T. saginata* has 12 or more; *T. solium* has 10 or less (Fig. 123–3). The uterine structure is usually well visualized by pressing the gravid proglottid between two microscope slides; however, India ink injected into the lateral genital opening further distinguishes the uterine branches (Chapter 150). In the absence of gravid proglottids, stained mature proglottids show two differences: a three-lobed ovary in *T. solium* and a vaginal sphincter in *T. saginata*.

The lack of sensitive methods for diagnosis of intestinal *Taenia* infections has been a major risk factor in limiting clinical and epidemiologic studies. Microscopy is known to be a relatively insensitive technique, as eggs are periodically absent from feces during infection. Egg concentration techniques are generally considered to be the most sensitive coproparasitologic test, although few definitive comparative studies of egg detection methods have been carried out

LIFE CYCLE of—

Taenia saginata

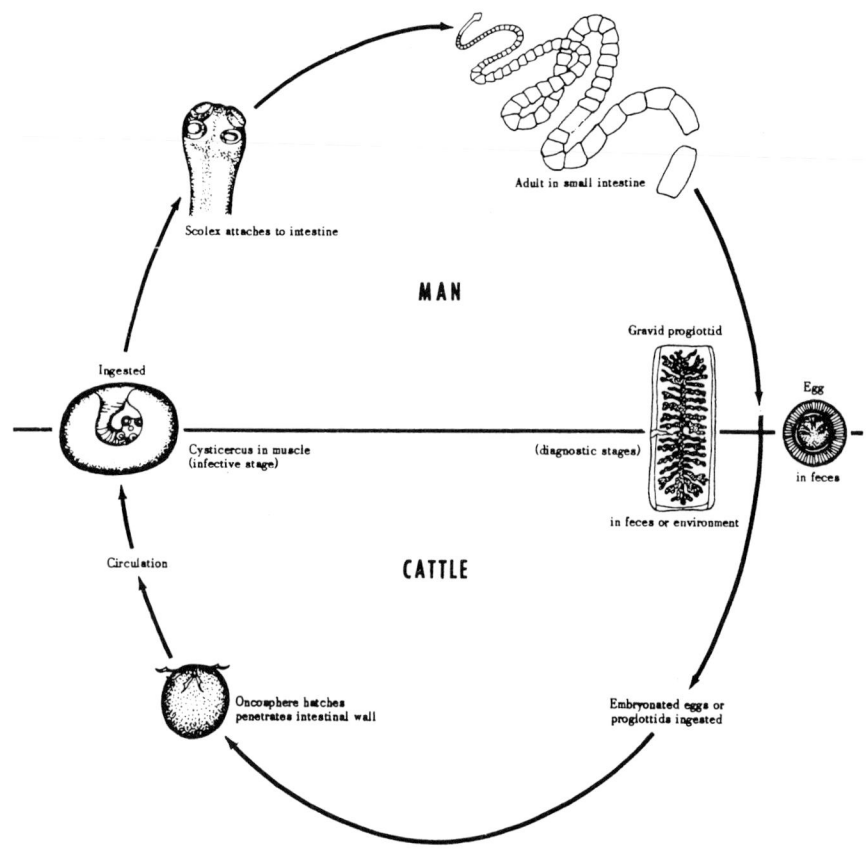

Figure 123–5. Life cycle of *Taenia saginata*. (From Melvin DM, Brooke MM, Sadun EH: Common Intestinal Helminths of Man. Atlanta, Centers for Disease Control, DHEW Publication No. [CDC] 72–8286, 1964.)

LIFE CYCLE of—

Taenia solium

Figure 123–6. Life cycle of *Taenia solium*. (From Melvin DM, Brooke MM, Sadun EH: Common Intestinal Helminths of Man. Atlanta, Centers for Disease Control, DHEW Publication No. [CDC] 72–8286, 1964.)

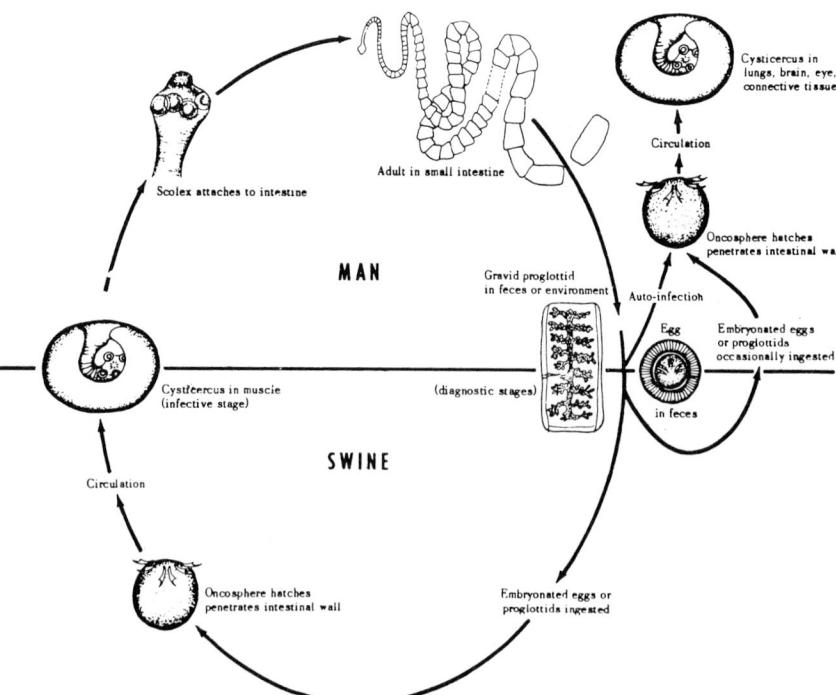

(Chapter 150). Visual demonstration of *Taenia* eggs in feces is not specific because *T. solium* and *T. saginata* eggs appear identical under the light microscope. Microscopic diagnosis can be supplemented with questioning of individuals to determine whether they are aware of passing proglottids; however, false positive and false negative reports of infection occur. Molecular techniques e.g., protein analysis of proglottids and DNA probes for eggs or other worm material have been developed to differentiate the species of *Taenia* present in an infection; the periodic absence of eggs or proglottids from feces limits sensitivity, however. Detection of *Taenia*-specific antigens in host feces may be the most sensitive diagnostic technique. Coproantigen (CoAg) assays are based on capture type ELISAs with polyclonal antisera raised against either worm somatic or excretory-secretory products. Diagnosis by CoAg assay of individuals from egg-negative fecal samples has been demonstrated, as have high levels of specificity, at least to genus level. Extensive field studies in Mexico, Guatemala, and China have shown that a CoAg test detects up to 2.5 times as many cases of taeniasis as microscopy. Unfortunately, CoAg assays are still not widely available for clinical use.

TREATMENT. The treatment of both tapeworm infections is similar. Praziquantel or niclosamide in the same dosage schedule as for *D. latum* is given (Chapter 123.1). In the treatment of *T. solium* infections, precautions should be taken to prevent autoinfection or dissemination. Drugs that induce vomiting should be avoided, because retrograde peristalsis might bring gravid proglottids into the gastroduodenal area, resulting in their subsequent digestion followed by egg hatching, penetration, and cysticercosis. In addition, since niclosamide and praziquantel kill the worm but not the eggs released from the disintegrating gravid segments, cysticercosis is theoretically possible following treatment. However, no cases of cysticercosis are known to have occurred by this mechanism, and there are theoretical reasons to believe that most *Taenia* carriers are immune to invasion by the larval stages by the time taeniasis is diagnosed. As a precaution, however, some clinicians advise that a purge be given 2 hours after treatment of *T. solium* infections to eliminate all mature segments before eggs can be released. The patient should be followed to ensure prompt evacuation. Treatment is successful if no eggs reappear in several stool specimens examined at sufficient intervals post treatment to allow regrowth of worms: 2 months for *T. solium* and 3 months for *T. saginata* and Asian *Taenia*.

PREVENTION. The prevention of beef and pork tapeworm infection can be accomplished by adequate cooking or freezing of these meats or, in the case of Asian *Taenia*, of pig liver. Cysticerci of all species are killed when the internal temperature of the product is below $-5°C$ (23°F) for at least 4 days or around $-20°C$ for at least 12 hours. Cysticerci are killed by cooking meat or other infected tissues until it loses its pink color.

Meat inspection, when performed thoroughly and routinely, reduces the numbers of infected meat products that reach the market; however, inspection procedures lack sufficient sensitivity to be truly effective in eliminating transmission through ingestion of infected meat or meat products. Treatment of all infected individuals would eliminate the source of soil and sewage pollution with *Taenia* eggs.

Bibliography

Allan JC, Craig PS, Garcia NJ, et al: Coproantigen detection for the immunodiagnosis of echinococcosis and taeniasis in dogs and humans. Parasitology 104:347, 1992.

Bowles J, McManus DP: Genetic characterization of the Asian *Taenia*, a newly described taeniid cestode of humans. Am J Trop Med Hyg 50:33, 1994.

Eom KS, Rim H-J: Morphologic descriptions of *Taenia asiatica* sp.n. Korean J Parasitol 31:1, 1993.

Fan PC: Taiwan *Taenia* and taeniasis. Parasitol Today 4:86, 1988.

Pawlowski Z, Schultz MG: Taeniasis and cysticerosis (*Taenia saginata*). Adv Parasitol 10:269, 1972.

123.3 Hymenolepiasis

Two species of small tapeworms of the genus *Hymenolepis* infect humans. The dwarf tapeworm, *Hymenolepis nana*, is a common infection, especially of children, throughout the world and can be passed directly from person to person. In moderate to heavy infections it may cause a variety of abdominal and neurologic symptoms. *Hymenolepis diminuta* is primarily a parasite of rodents and also, infrequently, of humans.

Hymenolepis Nana *Infection*

ETIOLOGY AND LIFE CYCLE. *H. nana* is the smallest adult tapeworm to infect humans regularly, measuring about 25 to 30 mm long by about 0.8 to 1.0 mm wide (Fig. 123–7). The entire chain of proglottids from the anterior immature to the distal gravid segments often consists of no more than 175 to 220 segments. However, there may be considerably fewer proglottids per worm if many worms are present at one time, i.e., the "crowding effect." The minute rounded scolex (3 mm in diameter) possesses four sucking disks and a short-armed retractable rostellum. The infective eggs (Fig. 122–2A), liberated when the distalmost proglottids disintegrate, are most characteristic, measuring 35 to 52 μm in diameter; they contain a hexacanth embryo or oncosphere that resides within an inner membrane. The latter possesses two polar thickenings from which there arise typically four to eight polar filaments. These eggs are released by the gradual disintegration of the terminal gravid proglottids and are infective immediately when passed in the feces. Unlike most other tapeworms that infect humans, no intermediate host is required. Therefore, if the egg is ingested by another or the same host, the oncosphere is liberated in the small intestine and penetrates the villi, where it becomes a cysticercoid larva (a small larva that has a single scolex but does not have a bladder characteristic of a cysticercus) (Fig. 123–8). In about

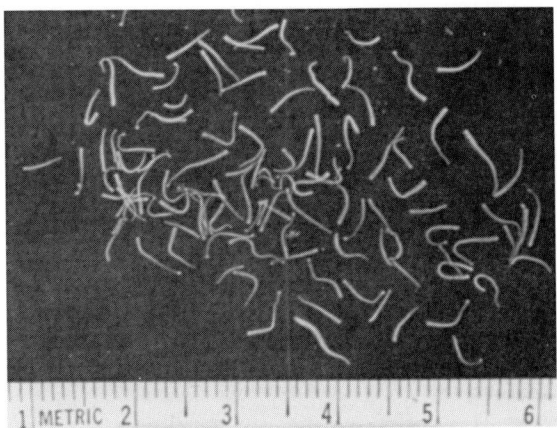

Figure 123–7. *Hymenolepis nana*, dwarf tapeworm, adults. (Courtesy of Dr. Francisco J. Aguilar, Guatemala.)

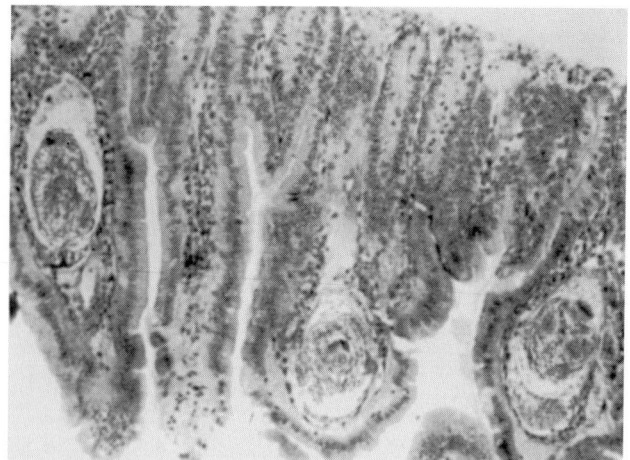

Figure 123–8. *Hymenolepis nana* cysticercoid larvae in the small intestinal villi. (Courtesy of Herman Zaiman, M.D.)

96 hours, the larva re-enters the lumen and attaches to a small intestinal villus by its scolex, usually at a more distal location. In about 10 to 20 days, it matures, and eggs may be found in the feces.

There is evidence that hyper- or autoinfection occurs when ova liberated in the small intestine spontaneously hatch and immediately penetrate a villus to undergo a new cycle. Individual worms live for about a year. However, as a result of hyperinfection, individuals may have a large worm burden for many years. In experimental animals, the worm burden

is limited by the development of immunity, and immunosuppression can cause hyperinfection. In addition, experimental evidence suggests that certain strains of *H. nana* undergo larval or cysticercoid development in various fleas and mealworms. Subsequently, the larvae have been found to develop to adult tapeworms in mice. Human infection with these murine strains is regarded as rare.

EPIDEMIOLOGY AND DISTRIBUTION. Infection with this parasite is worldwide in distribution; millions of people are infected. It is commonly regarded as a hand-to-mouth infection and, as a result, is encountered most frequently in children and in inhabitants of institutions for the mentally retarded and chronic care psychiatric hospitals.

H. nana infection is most common in rural communities in the southeastern portion of the United States, where it has been reported to infect almost 1% of young schoolchildren. Higher infection rates are reported in South and Central American countries, Puerto Rico, and Mexico, where conditions of overcrowding and poor personal and environmental hygiene are present. Families from Latin America who have emigrated recently to urban areas are often heavily parasitized. The infection is also common throughout southern Europe, the Middle East, the Soviet Union, and the Indian subcontinent.

Humans are the natural reservoir for the parasite, and transmission is generally direct from human to human by ingestion of eggs from feces of infected individuals. Although transmission may occur by fomites, water, and food, this is less common, because the eggs succumb quickly outside the host. Larvae of fleas and grain beetles can become infected after ingesting *H. nana* eggs and develop cysticercoids in their hemocoeles. However, probably these insects are seldom of

LIFE CYCLE of— *Hymenolepis diminuta*

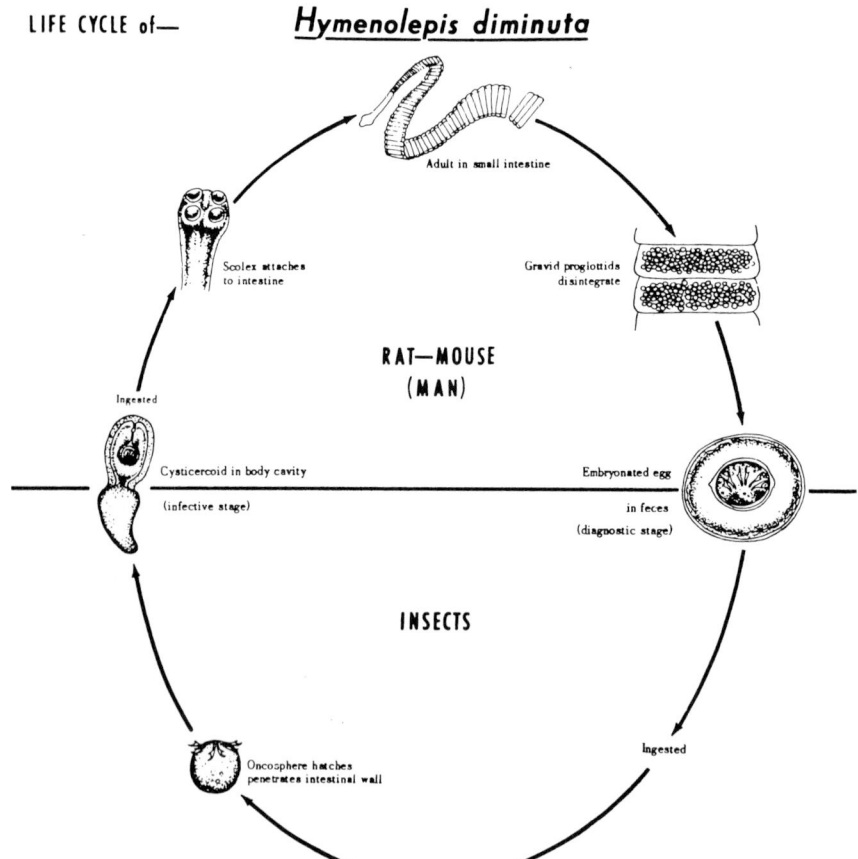

Figure 123–9. Life cycle of *Hymenolepis diminuta*. (From Melvin DM, Brooke MM, Sadun EH: Common Intestinal Helminths of Man. Atlanta, Centers for Disease Control, DHEW Publication No. [CDC] 75–8286, 1964.)

importance as intermediate hosts in human infection. Some murine strains are infectious for humans. Thus, infected pet mice, rats, and hamsters are potential sources of infection.

CLINICAL MANIFESTATIONS, PATHOLOGY, AND DIAGNOSIS. Necrosis and desquamation of intestinal epithelial cells have been observed at the site of attachment of the mature worm. Light infections generally cause no significant mucosal damage and are either asymptomatic or cause vague abdominal complaints. Even heavy parasitism is usually well tolerated. It is believed that many of the clinical symptoms are immunologically mediated. Young children, especially when they are infected with many worms, may have loose bowel movements or occasionally frank diarrhea with mucus. Bloody diarrhea is rare. Diffuse persistent abdominal pain is the most common complaint. Pruritus ani and nasi and urticaria are encountered occasionally. Many children have headaches, dizziness, and sleep and behavioral disturbances, which clear after successful therapy. Serious neurologic disturbances, such as seizures, have been reported. Many patients with hymenolepiasis have a moderate eosinophilia of 5 to 10%.

The diagnosis is made by identifying the characteristic ova in a fecal specimen (Fig. 122–2A). Proglottids are usually not found because they degenerate before passage.

TREATMENT. Successful therapy depends upon understanding the life history of this infection and, therefore, one should recall that the larval stage or cysticercoid is buried in the intestinal mucosa (Fig. 123–8) and presumably is not as easily killed by the drugs employed for treating other tapeworm infections. The treatment of choice is praziquantel inasmuch as it is lethal to the cysticercoid stage within the tissue as well as the worm in the lumen. The recommended dose for adults and children is 25 mg/kg in a single dose.

Treatment can be considered successful if no eggs reappear in several stool specimens examined at 1 month post treatment. Since *H. nana* has the ability to renew its population through internal autoinfection and since rates of reinfection are high among some populations of children, certain patients may appear to remain infected despite repeated treatments. Nevertheless, drug therapy nearly always reduces worm burdens to tolerable levels, and infections in children are usually lost spontaneously in adolescence.

PREVENTION. Control depends on improved personal and environmental hygiene. Although rodents are not an important source of infection to humans, the possibility of murine infection should be considered when the patient has close contact with rodents, pets, or laboratory animals.

Hymenolepis Diminuta *Infection*

The definitive hosts for this tapeworm are primarily rats, mice, and other murine species. It is closely related to *H. nana* and infrequently infects humans. Over 200 human cases have been reported and most frequently occur in children under 3 years of age. The adult worm is 10 to 60 cm × 3 to 5 mm; larger than *H. nana*, it has 800 to 1000 proglottids. The scolex is club-shaped and has a rudimentary apical unarmed rostellum and four small suckers. The mature proglottids resemble *H. nana*. The eggs are spherical and 60 to 86 μm in diameter; their thin, yellowish outer membrane is separated from the inner embryonic envelope by a clear area that, in contrast to the eggs of *H. nana*, contains no polar filaments (Fig. 122–2B). Development of this tapeworm requires an intermediate host. Presumably, rat fleas (*Nosopsyllus, Xenopsyllus*) and mealworms infected with larvae are ingested accidentally, and mature adults develop in about 3 weeks. Cockroaches may serve as intermediate hosts also. These insects become infected by ingesting eggs passed in rodent feces.

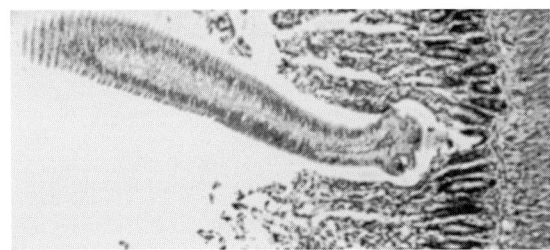

Figure 123–10. *Hymenolepis diminuta* attached to intestinal mucosa of rat.

The eggs develop into cysticercoids in the hemacoele of the insect; when ingested, the cysticercoids are infectious to rodents or humans (Fig. 123–9). Human infection probably occurs by accidental ingestion of mealworms or grain beetles found in dry grains, cereals, flour, and dried fruits.

The adult tapeworms attach to duodenal or jejunal mucosa (Fig. 123–10). Human infections are light, and the life span in humans is short. The diagnosis is made by finding ova in the stool (Fig. 122–2B). Treatment is with praziquantel in a single dose of 5 to 10 mg/kg body weight.

Bibliography

Arai HP (ed): Biology of the Tapeworm *Hymenolepis diminuta*. New York, Academic Press, 1980.

Biswash H, Arora RR, Sehgal S: Epidemiology of *Hymenolepis nana* infections in a selected rural community. J Commun Dis 10:170, 1978.

Schenone H: Praziquantel in the treatment of *Hymenolepis nana* infections in children. Am J Trop Med Hyg 20:320, 1980.

123.4 *Dipylidiasis*

ETIOLOGY AND LIFE CYCLE (Fig. 123–11). *Dipylidium caninum* is a cestode of dogs, cats, and wild Carnivora that occasionally infects humans. Adult tapeworms inhabit the small intestine and measure 15 to 20 cm in length. The worm usually contains 60 to 175 proglottids. *D. caninum* has a characteristic rhomboidal scolex with four oval suckers and an armed retractible conical rostellum containing 30 to 150 thorn-shaped hooks arranged in transverse rows. The vase-shaped proglottids possess a double set of reproductive organs with genital pores midway on each lateral margin. The gravid proglottids are packed with capsules, each containing 15 to 25 eggs (Fig. 123–12). Each egg is 35 to 60 μm in diameter and contains an onchosphere with six hooklets.

Strobila are capable of moving several inches per hour and pass out of the anus or are passed in the feces. Eggs are expelled by contraction of the proglottids or disintegration of the proglottids outside of the intestine on the perianal region.

The intermediate hosts of *Dipylidium* are larval dog, cat, and human fleas. Those cysticercoid larvae that survive metamorphosis of the larval flea are ingested by the definitive host. The larvae are liberated in the small intestine and become adults in about 20 days (Fig. 123–11).

EPIDEMIOLOGY. Most of the infections have occurred in children under 8 years of age, with one third occurring in infants under 6 months. Transmission is thought to be due to accidental swallowing of infected adult fleas, most likely due to the close association between children and dogs and

Dipylidium caninum

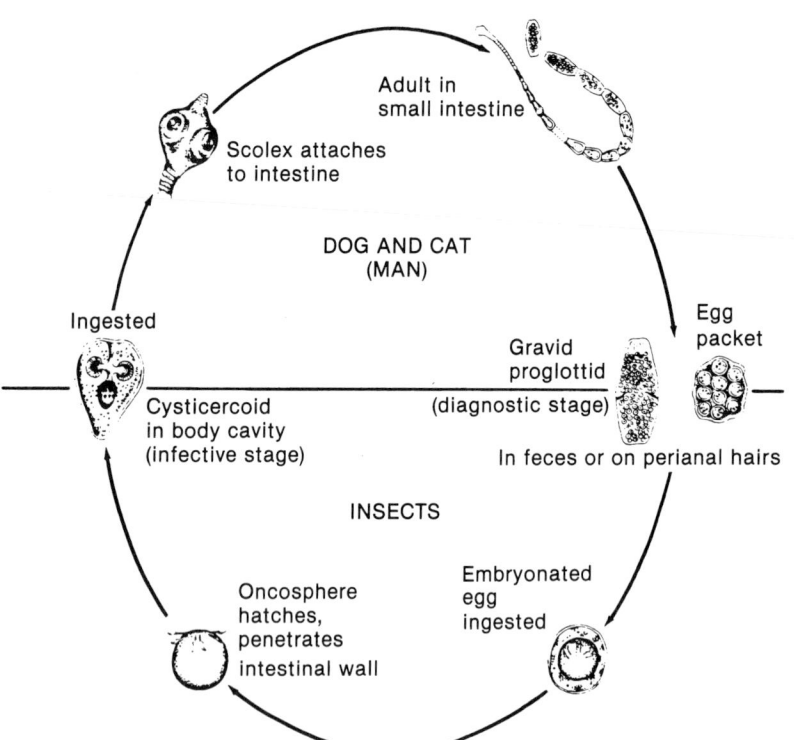

Figure 123–11. Life cycle of *Dipylidium caninum.* (From Melvin DM, Brooke MM, Sadun EH: Common Intestinal Helminths of Man. Atlanta, Centers for Disease Control, DHEW Publication No. [CDC] 75–8286, 1964.)

cats. In addition, transmission may occur as a result of hand-to-mouth contamination.

CLINICAL MANIFESTATIONS AND DIAGNOSIS. Most patients are asymptomatic, but clinical findings attributed to *D. caninum* include abdominal pain, diarrhea, urticaria, and pruritus ani. Diagnosis is often made by parents who observe proglottids moving in their child's stool. Examination for eggs may be unreliable, because proglottids usually do not release eggs within the intestines. There may be moderate eosinophilia.

TREATMENT. Treatment is the same as for *D. latum* infec-

tions. Household pets should be treated with anthelmintics, and insecticides should be used to remove pet ectoparasites and to disinfect their sleeping areas.

Bibliography

Jones WE: Niclosamide as a treatment for *Hymenolepis diminuta* and *Dipylidium caninum* infection in man. Am J Trop Med Hyg 28:300, 1979.
Wijesundera M de S: The use of praziquantel in human infection with *Dipylidium*. Trans R Soc Trop Med Hyg 83:383, 1989.

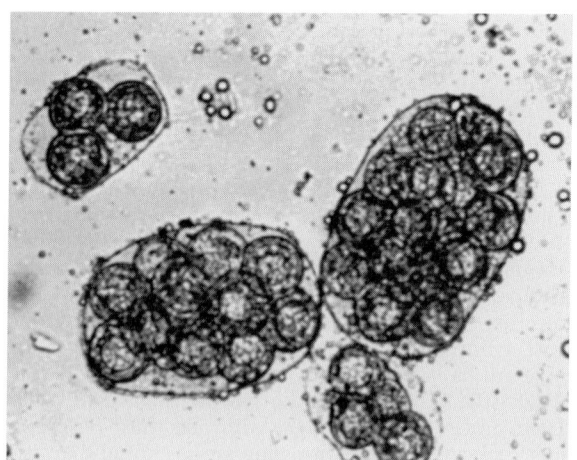

Figure 123–12. Egg capsules of *Dipylidium caninum*. (Photograph by H.J. Griffiths. From Zaiman H (ed): A Pictorial Presentation of Parasites.)

124 Larval Cestode Infections

124.1 Cysticercosis

Carlton A. W. Evans, Hector H. Garcia, and Robert H. Gilman

DEFINITION. Cysticercosis is infection of human tissues with larvae of the pork tapeworm, *Taenia solium.*

ETIOLOGY AND HISTORY

Definitive Host: Human Tapeworm Infection. The adult *T. solium* tapeworm infects the human small bowel. It may live as long as 20 years, usually growing to 2 to 8 m in length (Chapter 123.2). Each tapeworm intermittently produces thousands of eggs when the most distal tapeworm segments (proglottids) are released. These gravid tapeworm segments may be passed intact or may rupture, allowing parasite eggs to disperse in the feces. The eggs are highly infectious and remain viable within the environment for many months.

Intermediate Host: Porcine Cysticercosis. Known since antiquity, porcine cysticercosis was described by Aristotle. Pigs are infected when they ingest material contaminated with human feces containing tapeworm eggs. Within the pig bowel, the eggs hatch, releasing activated oncospheres that penetrate the bowel wall and are then carried by the blood stream to the host tissues. Within 3 months, the oncospheres develop into fluid-filled cysticerci, usually ovoid and 5 to 10 mm long. Each cysticercus contains a 2-mm-long, living larval tapeworm scolex. When humans ingest undercooked, cysticercotic (measly) pork, cysticerci are digested within the bowel, releasing tapeworm larvae that attach to the wall of the jejunum and grow into adult tapeworms, completing the parasitic life cycle (Fig. 123–5). The relationship between cysticerci and the adult intestinal tapeworm was proved in 1853 by feeding condemned convicts with raw measly pork and, after execution, demonstrating the presence of young tapeworms within the human bowel.

Human Cysticercosis. Human cysticercosis is acquired through the fecal-oral route. When humans ingest tapeworm eggs, they develop cysticerci within their tissues in the same way that pigs do (Fig. 124–1). Cysticercosis is therefore contracted from ingesting material contaminated by human feces containing tapeworm eggs, not from eating infected pork containing cysticerci. Strict vegetarians and people who have never eaten pork may develop cysticercosis, although they are not at risk for intestinal tapeworm infection. Humans are an incidental intermediate host and represent a dead end for the parasite. Humans harboring an intestinal tapeworm can infect themselves with cysticercosis (anus-hand-mouth) or others directly through unhygienic food preparation. However, most patients with cysticercosis do not harbor an adult tapeworm within their bowel, and most people infected with a tapeworm do not develop symptomatic cysticercosis. Indeed, it is not known what proportion of tapeworm carriers will develop cysticercosis over time.

EPIDEMIOLOGY. Neurocysticercosis is estimated to be the most common parasitic infection of the brain and the most common cause of adult-onset epilepsy worldwide. Cysticercosis is endemic on all continents except Australasia and is common in non-Muslim developing countries including much of South and Central America, Asia, and Africa. Prevalence varies greatly depending on the prevalence and type of animal husbandry, hygiene, and dietary practices. Autopsy studies have revealed cysticercosis in 0.1 to 3.5% of people in Mexico, although as many as 80% of these infections were apparently asymptomatic and the infection was unrelated to the cause of death. In Peru, 12% of patients with epilepsy are seropositive, compared with about 1% of the general population. In industrialized countries, meat inspection and sewage disposal prevent infection of pigs and propagation of the parasite life cycle, but immigration from developing countries and increasing travel to endemic regions leads to sporadic cases of cysticercosis. For example, cysticercosis accounts for as many as 2% of neurologic/neurosurgical admissions in southern California, and immigrant cooks with tapeworms caused an outbreak of cysticercosis in Orthodox Jews in New York City.

PATHOGENESIS. Living cysticerci actively evade and suppress immune recognition, especially within immunologically privileged sites such as the brain and the eyes. Histopathologic examination of living cysticerci excised from human tissues reveals minimal host inflammation. Only rarely do living cysticerci induce symptoms by causing obstruction to the flow of cerebrospinal fluid (CSF) or pressure on adjacent tissues. Symptoms most commonly result from the inflammation due to death of cysticerci. This explains the usual delay between the formation of cysticerci, which occurs within 3 months of infection, and the development of symptoms several years later. English soldiers returning from India and remaining in Great Britain, a nonendemic area, developed seizures caused by cysticercosis after a median of 7 years.

Inflammation around dying cysticerci may be asymptomatic or it may lead to acute symptoms that can prove fatal. Lymphocytes and plasma cells usually outnumber giant multinuclear cells and foamy macrophages. Eosinophils are conspicuous. Adjacent necrosis and perivascular infiltration of mononuclear lymphoid cells may be followed by formation of a granuloma, fibrous scar, or calcification. Several classification systems define neurocysticercosis as active if living or degenerating cysticerci are present and inactive if there are calcifications or fibrosis. However, cysticerci at different sites may be viable or at various stages of degeneration, and in some studies most patients had both types of lesions.

In the brain, two forms of cysticerci are found. Cysticerci located in the brain parenchyma and/or floating freely in the ventricles most commonly are ovoid 5- to 10-mm structures, each of which contains a scolex (Fig. 124–2). A second, uncommon form called *racemose* (bunches of grapes) cysticerci are large lobulated vesicular structures that lack a scolex and are usually found in the basal cisternal spaces. Racemose cysticerci are not usually present in pediatric cases and may be either a degenerative form or a response to a different anatomic location. In general, parenchymal cysticercosis fol-

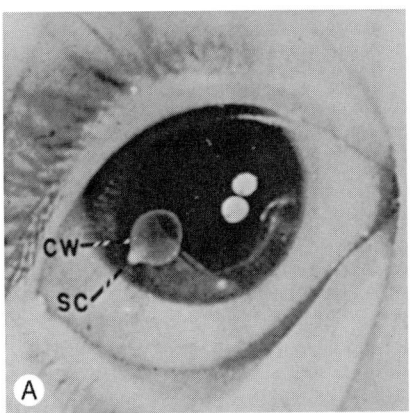

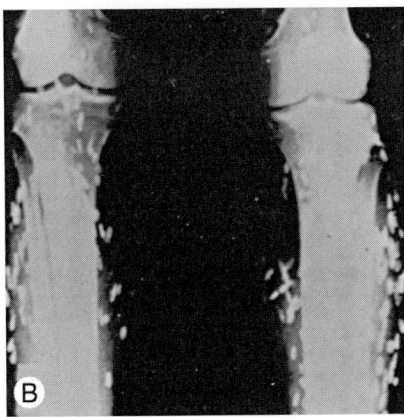

Figure 124–1. Cysticercosis. *A,* Viable cysticercus of *Taenia solium* in human eye showing scolex (sc) and cyst wall (cw). (Courtesy of Dr. A. Trejos, Costa Rica.) *B,* Radiograph of legs showing calcified cysticerci. (Courtesy of Dr. M. Campagna.)

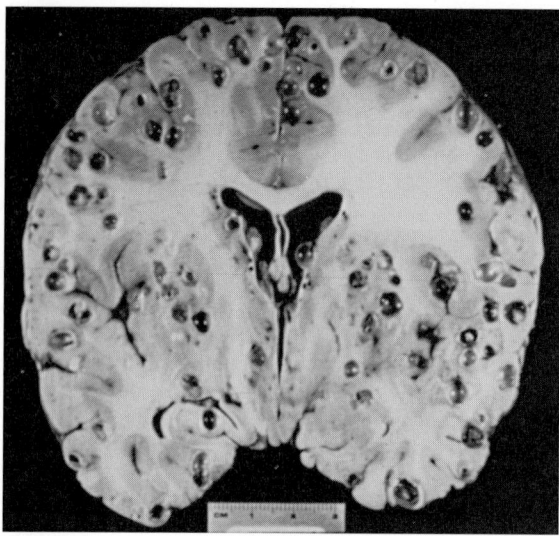

Figure 124–2. Sagittal section of brain of a 13-year-old Ekari girl who died from a massive infection with cerebral cysticercosis. (Courtesy of Dr. D. C. Gajdusek of the National Institutes of Health, and Dr. S. C. Bauserman of the Armed Forces Institute of Pathology; Papua New Guinea Med J 21:329, 1978.)

lows a benign course, whereas racemose cysticercosis often proves fatal.

CLINICAL MANIFESTATIONS. The clinical features of cysticercosis are variable, depending on the inflammatory response around cysticerci and their number, size, and location. Although cysticerci can infect any tissue, most clinically relevant lesions affect the brain and spinal cord (neurocysticercosis), the eye, muscles, and skin.

Neurocysticercosis. The most frequent symptom of cysticercosis is epilepsy. Focal seizures with secondary generalization are most common, but any type of epilepsy may occur. Single or multiple cysticerci are usually present within the brain parenchyma and may be surrounded by focal encephalitis and edema. Raised intracranial pressure may cause headache and vomiting. Cysticerci occasionally may also cause dementia or psychiatric illness, often in association with hydrocephalus. Cysticerci degenerating in or near the meninges cause chronic meningitis. When the base of the brain is affected, the resultant basal arachnoiditis is often particularly severe and may cause cranial nerve palsies and potentially fatal raised intracranial pressure. Intraventricular or basal cysticercosis is a cause of obstructive hydrocephalus. This is rarely intermittent or positional, depending on the location of a free-floating cysticercus. Cysticerci degenerating in any part of the brain may cause vasculitis and cerebral infarcts, most commonly when the base of the brain is infected. The encephalitic form of cysticercosis occurs predominantly in children and young females and consists of massive infection of the brain. Lesions are similar in size, are in the same phase of development, and are associated with an excessive immune reaction causing severe brain edema (Fig. 124–2). These patients have clinical symptoms of intracranial hypertension, seizures that are difficult to control, and reduced level of consciousness. Spinal cysticercosis, although uncommon, is often associated with severe symptoms due to increased pressure either directly from the cysticercus or secondarily from the inflammatory reaction. Cervical spinal cysticercosis is usually associated with racemose cysticercosis of the posterior fossa.

Ophthalmic Cysticercosis. Cysticerci infecting the eye are most commonly retinal or subretinal but may float freely in the vitreous or aqueous humors (see Fig. 124–1A). Light during ophthalmoscopy may induce movement and even evagination of a living parasite. Inflammation around degenerating cysticerci usually threatens vision by causing chorioretinitis, retinal detachment, or vasculitis.

Muscular and Subcutaneous Cysticercosis. Some patients with cysticercosis have characteristic subcutaneous cysticerci palpable as pealike nodules. These are usually asymptomatic, although transient local pain and tenderness may occur as cysticerci degenerate. The frequency of subcutaneous nodules varies considerably by geographic area, with <5% of patients in South America and >20% of patients in Asia having subcutaneous nodules. These lesions are easy to sample by biopsy and thus can provide histopathologic proof of disease. Large numbers of cysticerci may infect the muscles, and rare cases of massive muscular pseudohypertrophy have been reported. The enormous number of cysticerci present in the muscle are associated with an increase in the size of the muscles, although patients are quite weak. These patients may also have many cysticerci in the brain, pleura, heart, and tongue, and as in the encephalitic type of infection, the prognosis is poor.

PROGNOSIS AND NATURAL HISTORY. The natural history of cysticercosis is poorly defined because most infections are asymptomatic. In many rural pig-raising Third World communities, >10% of the population have antibodies to *T. solium* but nearly all are asymptomatic. Because of the lack of longitudinal community studies, the risk of symptomatic disease developing in asymptomatic individuals who have intracranial cysticerci is not known. Also, it is not clear how often symptomatic patients spontaneously recover. Symptomatic cysticercosis is a serious disease that may be progressive and may have fatal consequences. In general, more numerous intracranial cysticerci are associated with more severe disease that is less likely to respond to treatment. The location of cysticerci is also important: Patients with <20 cysticerci with a predominantly parenchymal location and the absence of hydrocephalus have a better prognosis than those who have numerous basal or ventricular lesions, especially if associated with hydrocephalus.

DIAGNOSIS. Neurocysticercosis can cause a wide variety of symptoms. It should be actively excluded in endemic countries and in patients with a history of travel to such an area. Patients should be asked whether they have passed tapeworm segments, even decades previously, and stool specimens should be examined for tapeworm eggs because some cases of cysticercosis result from autoinfection. An enzyme-linked immunosorbent assay (ELISA) for the detection of tapeworm antigen in stool has recently been developed and tested, with promising results. *T. solium* eggs in the feces cannot be macroscopically differentiated from other tapeworm eggs, and only *T. solium* eggs cause human cysticercosis. Treatment with an antihelmintic agent causes the worm to be passed in the feces, allowing definitive identification of the tapeworm species (Fig. 123–3).

Biopsy. A search should be made for subcutaneous cysticerci, excision or biopsy of which confirms the diagnosis of cysticercosis. The gross biopsy specimen is a white, fluid-filled, semiopaque bladder typically 5 to 10 mm in diameter but rarely up to 70 mm. The bladder contains a solid, 2-mm-long larval tapeworm scolex. In live specimens, independent movement of the scolex may be seen after excision. Microscopic examination reveals four suckers and a double row of hooks on the scolex. These are the appartus with which an ingested scolex attaches to the human intestinal wall.

Radiology. Plain radiographs of the thighs or other muscles may reveal numerous calcifications along the fascial plains formed by degenerated cysticerci (see Fig. 124–1B), and plain

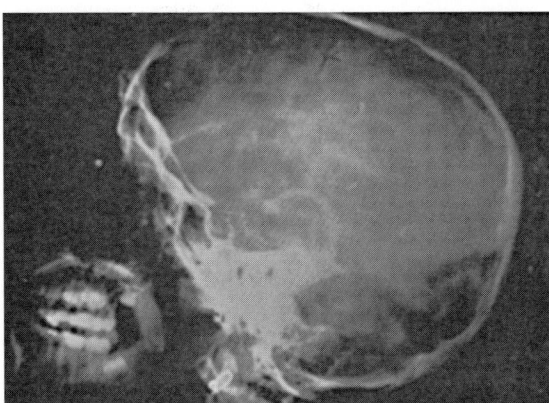

Figure 124–3. Cysticercosis. Skull film showing multiple target-like calcifications in the brain of a child infected with the cysticerci of *Taenia solium*.

radiographs of the skull may reveal intracranial calcifications (Fig. 124–3). Computed tomography (CT) has revolutionized the ante-mortem diagnosis of neurocysticercosis. Living cysticerci are visible as 5 to 10-mm hypodense lesions that do not enhance with intravenous contrast (Fig. 124–4). High-resolution scans reveal the small, hyperdense scolex within each living cysticercus. Degenerating cysticerci, which are more likely to be associated with symptoms, are surrounded by edema with ring or nodular enhancement after administration of intravenous contrast. End-stage calcified cysticerci are seen as hyperdense lesions. Magnetic resonance imaging (MRI) provides more detailed images of living and degenerating cysticerci. MRI frequently demonstrates cysticerci that may not be seen on CT, especially those located in the posterior fossa. However, MRI often does not demonstrate calcifications as clearly as CT.

Serology and Cerebrospinal Fluid Examination. Several different types of serologic tests have been used to diagnose cysticercosis. An enzyme-linked immunoelectrotransfer blot (EITB) has been evaluated in several endemic and nonendemic countries and yields >98% sensitivity and specificity except for 50 to 80% sensitivity for single ring-enhancing lesions. This test uses a group of lentil-lectin purified glyco-protein antigens in an immunoblot format to detect infection-specific antibodies in serum or CSF samples. One of its advantages is its equal sensitivity in serum or CSF, so a lumbar puncture is not required for accurate serologic diagnosis. Despite the reliability of this assay, results must be interpreted with caution in patients from endemic regions, where approximately 1% of the healthy urban population and 10% of rural villagers in pig-raising areas may be seropositive. However, patients with clinical symptoms tend to have more specific bands than those who are asymptomatic, and patients with six or more specific EITB bands have more intracranial lesions than those with fewer bands. The cysticercosis EITB has largely superseded less sensitive ELISA assays.

CSF findings may be normal, and even when abnormal, there are no characteristic features. Moderate CSF pleocystosis and elevated protein concentration may be noted. Eosinophils are also found in approximately one quarter of patients with cysticercosis.

Differential Diagnosis. The heterogeneous clinical features of cysticercosis make diagnosis difficult, but the combination of radioimaging and reliable serology greatly facilitates antemortem diagnosis. A single ring-enhancing intracranial lesion may present a difficult differential diagnosis, because 20 to 50% of patients with these kinds of lesions may not have a positive EITB result. Other possible causes of this lesion are tuberculosis, a neoplasm, or brain abscess caused by bacteria, fungi, or *Toxoplasma gondii*. The differential diagnosis of cystic images other than cysticercosis are subarachnoid or porencephalic cysts, hydatid cysts, and cystic astrocytomas. Intracranial calcifications may also be caused by tuberculosis, toxoplasmosis, tuberous sclerosis, and cytomegalovirus. Cysticerci outside the central nervous system are easier to identify, but subcutaneous cysticerci may be clinically mistaken for multiple subcutaneous lipomas.

TREATMENT. The treatment of cysticercosis is controversial. Drug therapy with either praziquantel (50 to 75 mg/kg/day PO for 2 weeks) or albendazole (15 mg/kg PO for 8 to 15 days) is effective in killing live cysticerci. However, the extent to which this is accompanied by clinical benefits is not clear. Albendazole is currently the drug of choice because of slightly greater efficacy and lower cost. Recently, a short course of three doses of 75–100 mg/kg of praziquantel in the same day has been reported to be efficacious. Between the second and the fifth days of anticysticercal therapy, patients usually have an exacerbation of neurologic symptoms, attributed to local inflammation due to the death of the larvae. For this reason, albendazole or praziquantel is generally given simultaneously with corticosteroids to control edema and intracranial hypertension. Most clinicians treat patients with neurocysticercosis in a hospital to ensure that these adverse effects can be detected and dealt with swiftly. Coadministration of corticosteroids reduces the blood levels of praziquantel; however, this is not thought to be clinically relevant.

Although the weight of clinical opinion is that treatment with praziquantel or albendazole is useful for symptomatic cysticercosis, two placebo-controlled trials did not demonstrate a benefit from this therapy. Most reports of efficacy of treatment with praziquantel or albendazole have been retrospecific or unblinded. Nevertheless, most clinicians prefer to administer one of these drugs to patients with cysticercosis because evidence shows that live cysticerci are effectively killed by these regimens.

Asymptomatic Neurocysticercosis. In most cases, viable cysticerci living within the human brain are asymptomatic, but they may occasionally be discovered by imaging studies performed for other reasons. If the cysticerci are not causing symptoms and are not associated with radiologic evidence of inflammation, the parasites may be assumed to be alive and successfully evading immune-mediated inflammation. In

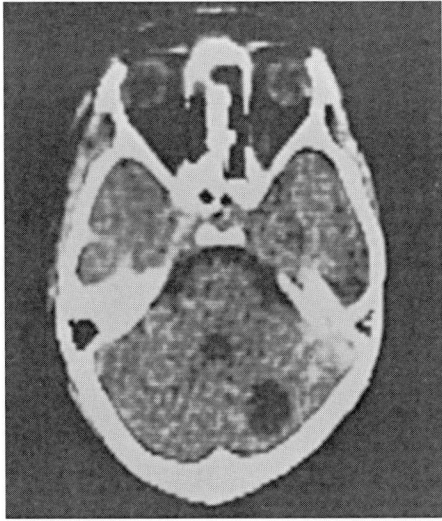

Figure 124–4. Cysticercosis. Cerebral lesion in the brain demonstrated by CT scan. The lesion was not seen on the radiograph because it was not calcified.

such cases, cestocidal treatment would kill the parasites and allow prophylactic or prompt therapeutic administration of corticosteroids if treatment causes symptoms. However, cysticerci infecting the brain often resolve without symptoms, and thus an alternative choice is not to treat but to advise patients to seek medical help if neurologic symptoms develop.

Symptomatic Neurocysticercosis. Anticonvulsant drugs should always be administered as for any other cause of epilepsy. Raised intracranial pressure, with or without associated arachnoiditis, usually responds to oral corticosteroids, which may be required long term in occasional cases of persistent intracranial inflammation. Insertion of a ventriculoperitoneal shunt for hydrocephalus is beneficial in the short term, but shunt blockage is common when the CSF protein concentration is elevated. Concomitant use of corticosteroids in patients with ventriculoperitoneal shunts has been reported to improve prognosis.

A viable cysticercus producing mass effect should be treated with anticysticercal drugs. In the case of patients with epilepsy and viable cysticerci, the role of drug therapy is unclear. However, if epilepsy or other symptoms are caused by one or more cysticerci that are seen on neuroimaging studies to be degenerating, cestocidal therapy is unlikely to be of any benefit. In such cases, an expectant policy has been followed in parts of India, with no intervention during a 6- to 12-week period unless there is clinical deterioration. Repeat CT scan after this period usually shows reduction in size or disappearance of a degenerating cysticercus. In some cases, differentiating a tuberculoma from a cysticercal granuloma may be difficult, often necessitating empirical therapy for tuberculosis.

Ophthalmic Cysticercosis. The inflammation associated with a degenerating intraocular cysticercus is sufficiently severe to require both local and systemic corticosteroids, but permanent loss of vision in the affected eye may still occur. Reports of successful treatment with cestocidal drugs, cryotherapy, and photocoagulation await confirmation, but ocular cysticercosis is usually treated surgically. Excision of a living cysticercus before the onset of significant intraocular inflammation has a good prognosis.

Muscular and Subcutaneous Cysticercosis. Asymptomatic subcutaneous or intramuscular cysticerci do not require treatment, but imaging studies should be performed to preclude the presence of neurologic infection. Cysticerci causing symptoms through local pressure may be excised or treated with cestocidal drugs. Transient symptomatic inflammation around degenerating cysticerci is ameliorated by corticosteroid or nonsteroidal anti-inflammatory drugs.

PREVENTION AND CONTROL. Transmission of cysticercosis depends on the presence of tapeworm carriers. Human infection with intestinal tapeworms is prevented by destruction, freezing, or adequate cooking of cysticercotic (measly) pork. In contrast, human cysticercosis results from fecal-oral contamination with material containing *T. solium* eggs, and basic hygiene and sanitation prevent this disease.

Community Monitoring. Establishing the intensity of cysticercosis in the community and monitoring the effect of cysticercosis control interventions require the use of simple epidemiologic indicators. The age-stratified curve of the prevalence of human cysticercosis infection, as documented by serologic studies, is useful but cannot demonstrate changes in infection patterns because antibodies to cysticercosis persist for many years, even after successful treatment. Studies in Peru have shown that serologic monitoring of infection in pigs is a useful indicator because the prevalence of porcine infection correlates with the prevalence of human cysticercosis. Pigs are kept for <1 year, so changes in infection intensity may be detected rapidly. Also, the rate of infection that occurs in uninfected (sentinel) pigs reflects the intensity of *T. solium* tapeworm infection and fecal contamination in the community. These indicators of porcine infection can therefore be used to monitor the effect of control programs in communities.

Community Interventions. The control of cysticercosis in endemic regions is complex. Control programs using education or the administration of human anthelmintic drugs to eliminate intestinal tapeworms have generally had limited and unsustained effects. Mass simultaneous anthelmintic treatment of both pigs and humans is being tried in some communities. However, endemic cysticercosis has disappeared from many developed countries as a result of improvements in sanitary conditions and changes in pig-raising practices. In areas where these simple measures are not yet attainable, development of an effective vaccine against porcine cysticercosis would provide a potential tool for eradicating the disease.

Bibliography

Allan JC, Craig PS, Garcia Noval J, et al: Coproantigen detection for the immunodiagnosis of echinococcosis and taeniasis in dogs and humans. Parasitology 104:347, 1992.

Camacho SPD, Ruiz AC, Peraza VS, et al: Epidemiologic study and control of *Taenia solium* infections with praziquantel in a rural village of Mexico. Am J Trop Med Hyg 145:522, 1991.

Carpio A, Santillin, Lein P, et al: Is the course of neurocysticercosis modified by treatment with antihelminthic agents? Arch Intern Med 155:1982, 1995.

Cruz M, Davis A, Dixon H, et al: Operational studies on the control of *Taenia solium* taeniasis/cysticercosis in Ecuador. Bull WHO 67:401, 1989.

Cysticercosis Working Group in Peru: The marketing of cysticercotic pigs in the Sierra of Peru. Bull WHO 71:223, 1993.

Diaz F, Garcia HH, Gilman RH, et al: Epidemiology of taeniasis and cysticercosis in a Peruvian village. Am J Epidemiol 135:875, 1992.

Evans CAW, Gonzalez AE, Gilman RH, et al: Immunotherapy for porcine cysticercosis: Implications for prevention of human disease. Am J Trop Med Hyg 56:33, 1997.

Flisser A: Neurocysticercosis in Mexico. Parasitol Today 4:131, 1988.

Garcia HH, Gilman RH, Catacora M, et al: Serological evolution of neurocysticercosis patients after antiparasitic therapy. J Infect Dis 175:486, 1997.

Garcia HH, Gilman R, Martinez M, et al: Cysticercosis as a major cause of epilepsy in Peru. Lancet 341:197, 1993.

Garcia HH, Herrera G, Gilman RH, et al: Discrepancies between cerebral computed tomography and Western blot in the diagnosis of neurocysticercosis. Am J Trop Med Hyg 50:152, 1994.

Gonzales AE, Garcia HH, Gilman RH, et al: Effective, single dose treatment of porcine cysticercosis with oxfendazole. Am J Trop Med Hyg 54:391, 1996.

Gonzalez AE, Gilman R, Garcia HH, et al: Use of sentinel pigs to monitor environmental *Taenia solium* contamination. Am J Trop Med Hyg 51:847, 1994.

Rangel R, Torres B, Del Brutto O, Sotelo J: Cysticercotic encephalitis: A severe form in young females. Am J Trop Med Hyg 36:387, 1987.

Sarti E, Schantz PM, Plancarte A, et al: Prevalence and risk factors for *Taenia solium* taeniasis and cysticercosis in humans and pigs in a village in Morelos, Mexico. Am J Trop Med Hyg 46:677, 1992.

Schantz PM, Moore AC, Munoz JL, et al: Neurocysticercosis in an Orthodox Jewish community in New York City. N Engl J Med 327:692, 1992.

Schantz PM, Sarti E, Plancarte A, et al: Community-based epidemiological investigations of cysticercosis due to *Taenia solium*: Comparison of serological screening tests and clinical findings in two populations in Mexico. Clin Infect Dis 18:879, 1994.

Sotelo J, Del Brutto OH, Penagos P, et al: Comparison of therapeutic regimen of anticysticercal drugs for parenchymal brain cysticercosis. J Neurol 237:69, 1990.

Tsang VC, Brand JA, Boyer AE: An enzyme-linked immunoelectrotransfer blot assay and glycoprotein antigens for diagnosing human cysticercosis (*Taenia solium*). J Infect Dis 159:50, 1989.

Vasquez V, Sotelo J: The course of seizures after treatment for cerebral cysticercosis. N Engl J Med 327:696, 1992.

124.2 Cystic Hydatid Disease

Pedro L. Moro, Armando E. Gonzalez, and Robert H. Gilman

DEFINITION. Cystic hydatid disease is a zoonotic disease in humans and in diverse mammalian species. It is caused by the larval stage (hydatidosis) of a canine tapeworm, *Echinococcus granulosus*.

ETIOLOGY

Definitive Host. The adult tapeworm of *E. granulosus* parasitizes a wide variety of carnivores (e.g., domestic dogs, foxes, wolves, and dingoes). It is 2 to 11 mm long (Fig. 124–5) and usually has only three proglottids; the mature segment is the penultimate one, and the gravid one is the last segment. The scolex has two rows of hooklets, one large and one small, with four suckers. Proglottids may contain from 100 to 1500 eggs, which are spherical and range from 30 to 50 μm. The embryophore is the principal layer; it protects the embryo or oncosphere. The embryophore is thick and impermeable and consists of keratin-like proteins that make the eggs extremely resistant. Eggs can withstand a wide range of temperatures.

Intermediate Hosts. Intermediate hosts are usually farm animals (e.g., sheep, cattle, swine, or horses), which acquire the infection by ingestion of infectious eggs in the pasture (Fig. 124–5). The oncosphere is released by the action of gastric and intestinal enzymes, penetrates the intestinal wall, and is transported by the blood stream to the liver or other organs. Once the oncosphere reaches its final location, it develops into a hydatid cyst. Humans are normally accidental hosts. However, in certain regions of Africa where human hydatid disease is hyperendemic, they may be intermediate hosts.

Two biologic forms of *E. granulosus* have been recognized on the basis of differences in host specificity in the larval stage, the northern and European forms. The former is indigenous to holoarctic zones of tundra and boreal forest, or taiga (North America and Eurasia). The larval stage occurs almost exclusively in ungulates of the family Cervidae (e.g., moose, elk, reindeer), and the definitive host is usually the wolf (*Canis lupus*) and sometimes dogs and wild canids (e.g., coyotes and foxes). The European form involves a synanthropic or domestic cycle that includes domestic animals, generally sheep, as the main intermediate host and domestic dogs as the definitive host. Other domestic farm animals, (e.g., cattle, goats, swine, horses, and camels) can act as intermediate hosts, and their importance varies according to geographic regions. Wild carnivores, (e.g., foxes), may have a role in transmission to domestic intermediate hosts. The existence of certain strains of *E. granulosus* that are more likely to affect certain intermediate hosts has been recognized.

EPIDEMIOLOGY

Distribution. Echinococcal infection is widely prevalent in those regions of the world where dogs are used to care for large flocks of sheep. Hydatid infection is widely distributed in South America, the areas bordering the Mediterranean Sea, southern and central Russia, central Asia, Australia, and Africa. In South America, hydatidosis is endemic in Uruguay, Argentina, Chile, southern Brazil, and Peru.

Prevalence. Mass radiographic screening of the lungs during the 1960s revealed a prevalence of 143 to 150 hydatid cysts per 100,000 population in Uruguay and in Rio Negro province in Argentina. Another survey in an endemic area of the Peruvian highlands demonstrated a 3% prevalence of pulmonary hydatid disease.

Use of an immunoblot assay in Tupac Amaru, a highly endemic area in the central Andes of Peru, demonstrated 1.9% seroprevalence. A recent study in the same area using portable ultrasonography, chest radiography, and an enzyme-

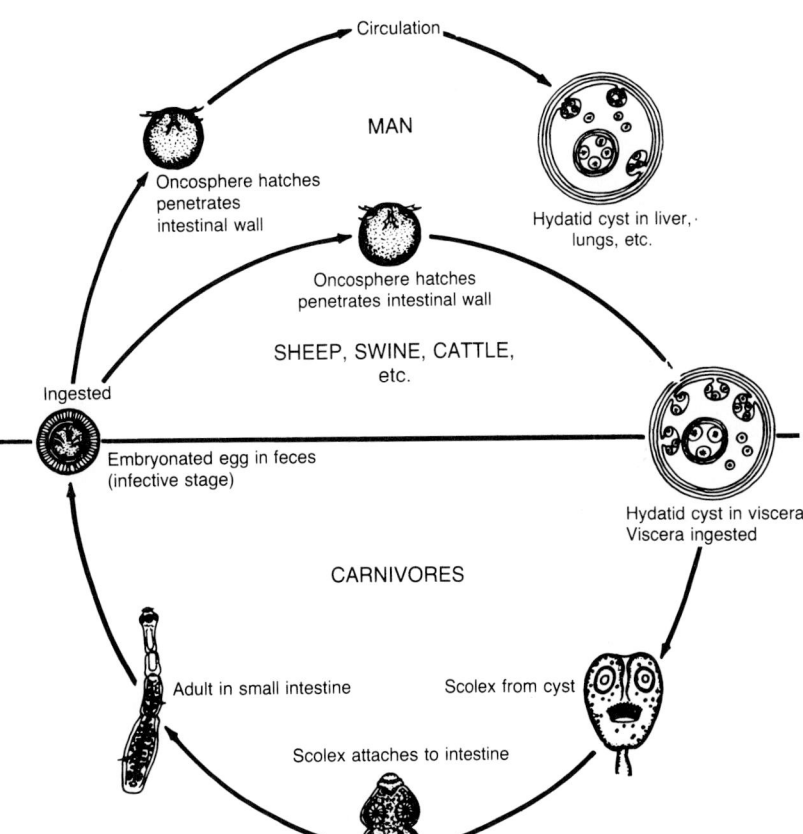

Figure 124–5. Life cycle of *Echinococcus granulosus*. (Modified from Melvin DM, et al.: Common Blood and Tissue Parasites of Man. Life Cycle Charts. Atlanta, Centers for Disease Control, 1979.)

linked immunoelectrotransfer blot (EITB) assay showed that 6% of the population had hydatid cysts and 9% had either cysts or serologic evidence of infection. The infection rates were 32% in dogs and 89% in sheep in the same area. The highest incidence of surgical disease has been reported in northwest Turkana, Kenya, with 198 cases per 100,000 people. Use of portable abdominal ultrasonography demonstrated 5.6% of the tribe had hepatic hydatid cysts. In Libya, prevalence rates of 2% were found when using portable ultrasound scanners and serologic testing. Autochthonous cases of human hydatid disease are rare in the United States.

Transmission. Hydatid disease can be highly endemic in rural areas where sheep are the major farm animals raised and dogs are used to care for large flocks of animals. In the United States, hydatid disease was associated with sheep ranching by farmers of Basque descent who grazed sheep on leased pastures, cropped-over land, and government-owned deserts and forests in Utah and California. A similar sheep-raising practice has been associated with transmission of *E. granulosus* to Indians living on the Navajo and Zuni reservations of New Mexico and Arizona.

The risk of infection is highly influenced by the extent and nature of human association with dogs. Populations at most risk use dogs to herd sheep but also keep them as house pets. Higher risk among Polynesian Maoris than New Zealanders of European extraction are due to the fact that the former have a closer association with their dogs than do the latter. The higher incidence of hydatid disease among Lebanese Christians than Moslems parallels their respective association with dogs. The Turkana of Kenya, who have the highest infection rate in the world, live very closely with dogs (Fig. 124–6A). They maintain a large number of dogs and sleep with them to keep warm in the desert. Dogs lick infants clean after they defecate or vomit. In South American countries where hydatid disease is endemic, dogs are also highly valued.

In addition to this close association between humans and dogs, certain beliefs or lack of them may contribute to maintaining transmission of *E. granulosus*. The Turkana (and in the past Cypriot pastoralists) believe hydatid cysts in their animals are physiologic storage devices for water in times of drought and therefore desirable. In a sheep-raising region of Peru, endemic for hydatidosis, individuals who knew how hydatidosis was transmitted were less likely to be infected with *E. granulosus* than were those who lacked this knowledge.

In endemic regions of the world, the prevalent practice of giving raw infected viscera of slaughtered livestock to dogs facilitates transmission of *E. granulosus*. In urban areas, hydatid disease occurs with greater frequency among abattoir workers, who have greater exposures than the general population.

CLINICAL MANIFESTATIONS AND PATHOLOGY. Signs and symptoms of hydatid disease depend on the organ involved and the size of the cyst. The onset of symptoms varies from months to several years and results from pressure exerted by the growing cyst. Cysts grow at varying rates. A slow rate of cyst growth has been reported in infections in Alaska, whereas in Turkana, Kenya, cysts 5 to 10 cm in diameter have been observed in children 3 to 5 years old.

Cysts occur more frequently in the liver (52 to 77%; Fig. 124–6A and B), followed by the lungs (9 to 44%; Fig. 124–7), and other locations (13 to 19%).

Liver Cysts. Liver cysts occur more frequently in the right lobe, and most individuals with hepatic hydatid cysts are asymptomatic. Physical examination may reveal abdominal distention (Fig. 124–6A) and a palpable mass in the upper right quadrant of the abdomen, with or without hepatomegaly. Only when the cyst has reached large dimensions do complications usually occur. Cysts sometimes become infected with bacteria and may clinically resemble an abscess of the liver. Acute signs and symptoms follow rupture of a

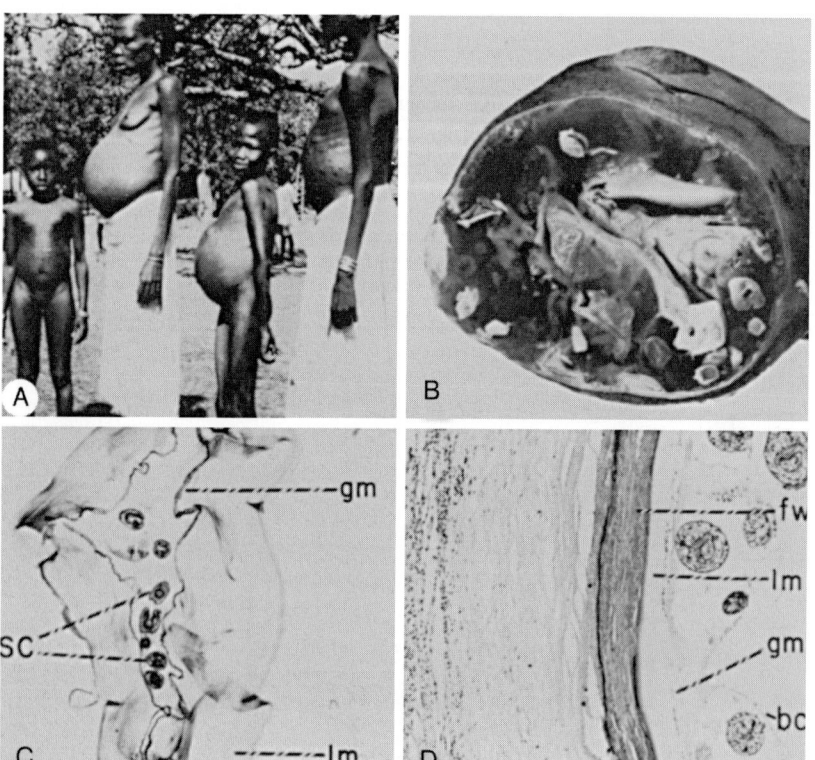

Figure 124–6. Cystic hydatid disease. *A,* Abdominal distention from hydatid cysts in Turkana, Kenya. (From Muller R: Worms and Disease. London, William Heinemann Medical Books, 1975.) *B,* Unilocular hydatid cyst in human liver containing hydatid sand consisting of daughter cysts and free scoleces in the cyst fluid. (Courtesy of the Armed Forces Institute of Pathology, Photograph Neg. No. N–31977.) *C,* Histologic section showing external laminated membrane (lm), internal germinal membrane (gm), and scoleces (SC). (Courtesy of the Armed Forces Institute of Pathology, Photograph Neg. No. 706612.) *D,* Histologic section showing brood capsules (bc) attached to the germinal membrane (gm). Fibrous wall of the host (fw) and laminated membrane of the parasite (lm) are also shown. (Courtesy of the Armed Forces Institute of Pathology, Photograph Neg. No. N–74378.)

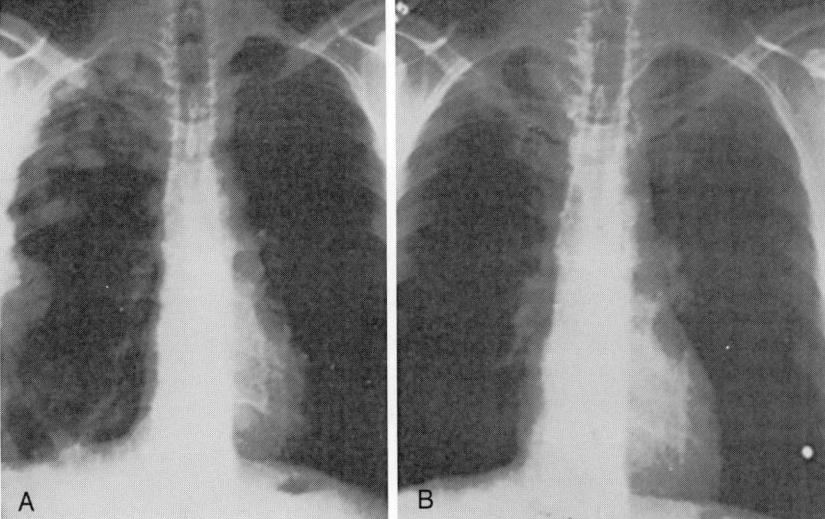

Figure 124–7. Echinococcosis. *A,* Chest radiograph of a young Italian carpenter with multiple cysts in the right upper lung fields and a large cyst on the right lateral chest wall. *B,* Chest radiograph almost 4 years later following a prolonged course of mebendazole therapy. No lesions are present on the radiograph.

cyst, which may occur spontaneously, secondary to a traumatic event, or during surgery. Rupture may occur into a bile duct, resulting in obstructive jaundice and colic-like pain followed by bacterial overgrowth. Rupture into the peritoneal cavity usually leads to secondary formation of numerous peritoneal cysts from hydatid sand and in rare occasions to peritonitis. Rupture and leakage of cyst fluid may also lead to an erythematous rash or an anaphylactic reaction and, rarely, death within a few minutes. Other rare complications may be rupture into the inferior vena cava or suprahepatic veins and portal hypertension.

Lung Cysts. Noncomplicated lung cysts rarely produce symptoms and are usually found accidentally after a routine chest radiograph (Fig. 124–7). In those patients who are symptomatic, chest pain with fever, cough, dyspnea, and hemoptysis are often the presenting symptoms, and the illness may be confused with pulmonary tuberculosis. Complete or partial rupture of a cyst often leads to expectoration of hydatid fluid and/or membranes, followed by bacterial overgrowth and a lung abscess. Physical examination may reveal dullness with absence of breath sounds. Often no pulmonary signs are present. Rupture into the lung may cause pneumothorax and empyema, allergic reactions (e.g., pruritus, urticaria), and rarely anaphylactic shock. Rupture into the pleural space with secondary formation of hydatid cysts occurs very rarely.

Other Sites. The spleen is the next most common abdominal organ affected, accounting for 3 to 5% of all abdominal cysts. Heart or cerebral cysts each has been reported in 1 to 1.5% of patients. Hydatid cysts have been rarely reported in almost any organ. Procedures to detect hepatic and pulmonary cysts should be undertaken if a hydatid cyst is identified at another site.

DIAGNOSIS. Previous exposure to sheepdogs in endemic areas and the presence of an enlarged liver and/or a palpable mass in the upper right quadrant of the abdomen or a cannon ball–appearing lesion on chest radiographs supports the clinical diagnosis of hydatidosis. A patient coming from an endemic area who gives a history of expectoration of a salty-tasting fluid with hemoptysis has a high probability of having a pulmonary hydatid cyst.

Differential Diagnosis. Hepatic hydatid cysts may be confused with any space-occupying lesion, including congenital liver cysts, choledochal cysts, amebic or bacterial liver abscess, and primary and secondary hepatic tumors. Symptoms caused by lung cysts may be similar to those of pulmonary

tuberculosis. Congenital cysts, bronchogenic cysts, and lung abscesses may also be confused with pulmonary hydatid cysts.

Radiography. Abdominal ultrasonography and computed tomography are the methods of choice for detecting abdominal cysts (Fig. 124–8). Sometimes the cyst may be calcified and demonstrated by a plain radiograph (Fig. 124–9). Portable ultrasound scanners now permit population-based field studies to be performed in rural endemic areas. Cysts may appear as solitary lesions with echoes within them or multiloculated cysts with daughter cysts (Fig. 124–8). The honeycomb appearance has been considered pathognomonic of hydatid liver disease, but most do not show this characteristic. A collapsed cyst may produce an irregular, solid echo pattern. A posteroanterior chest radiograph is the method of choice for diagnosis of lung cysts (Fig. 124–7). Unruptured, noncomplicated cysts are well defined and round. Ruptured cysts may produce various signs; air between the laminated membrane and the pericyst wall appears as a thin, lucent crescent in the upper part of the cyst, the crescent or meniscus sign. When the cyst collapses, the crumpled endocyst floats in the pericyst cavity, producing the iceberg, water lily, or camalote sign.

Serology. A wide variety of serologic assays have been developed with varying sensitivities and specificities (Chapter 152). The EITB assay is the method of choice, but the double diffusion test for arc 5 (DD5) is also highly useful when the EITB assay is not available. A positive serologic result provides immunologic confirmation of the disease or prior exposure. A problem with serologic assays for hydatid disease is their lack of sensitivity, which is especially true in the case of pulmonary cysts. Antigen detection assays have been developed and have relative success but are available in only a few sites.

Results of hematologic and biochemical tests are usually normal and nonspecific and offer little help in diagnosis. Eosinophilia may be found in patients with ruptured hydatid cysts, and levels of alkaline phosphatase enzymes may be elevated in a few patients.

Parasitology. Parasitologic examination of expectorated or aspirated fluid may reveal protoscolices and/or hooklets (Fig. 124–10). Hydatid membranes may also be expectorated.

TREATMENT. Completely calcified cysts need not be treated.

Chemotherapy. Albendazole is sometimes effective against hydatid disease (Fig. 124–7). Its use has been indicated for

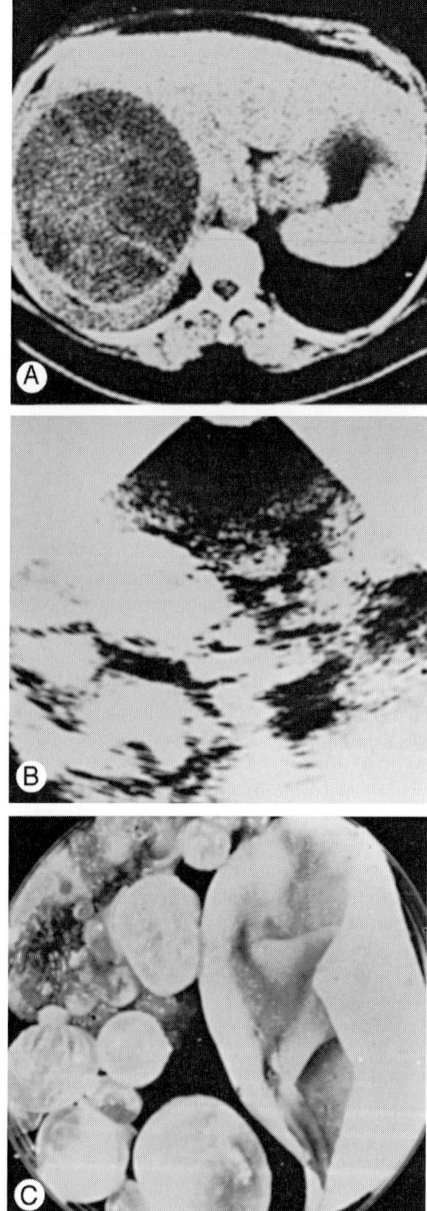

Figure 124–8. Cystic hydatid disease. *A,* CT scan showing septate densities within the 12-cm cyst. *B,* Sonogram of the same cyst showing the septate densities. *C,* Daughter cysts removed from the same cyst. (Courtesy of the Armed Forces Institute of Pathology.)

(1) treatment of inoperable disease and (2) presurgical and postsurgical treatment to prevent or reduce the risk of recurrence after cyst spillage during operation. The dosage used is 10 to 15 mg/kg, or fixed doses of 400 mg b.i.d. in adults, in cycles of 28 days with 14-day periods of rest. The number of cycles is variable and depends on how a patient responds; 3 to 12 cycles have been used, with variable response rates, but in some cases complete cure has been attained. Albendazole is also given both before and after percutaneous drainage of hydatid cysts. Most common side effects are elevated levels of hepatic enzymes (AST and ALT) and abdominal pain. Headache, abdominal distention, and alopecia are rare complications.

Percutaneous Aspiration of Hepatic Cysts Under Ultraso-

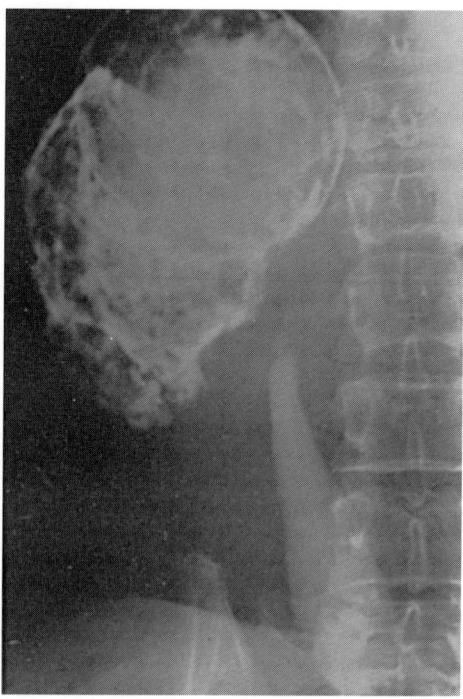

Figure 124–9. Echinococcosis. Plain film of the abdomen demonstrating a calcified mass in the liver. Serologic testing was positive for *Echinococcus.* The patient, being elderly and asymptomatic, was not treated.

nographic Guidance. Recent application of percutaneous aspiration of hydatid cysts under ultrasonographic guidance in conjunction with albendazole therapy has been used with good results and offers an alternative and more cost-effective approach to surgery. The method has a lower rate of complications, shorter (or no) hospitalization period, and lower costs than does surgical removal and is the method of choice for the treatment of hepatic cysts in centers having experience in using this technique.

Percutaneous drainage should be performed with monitor-

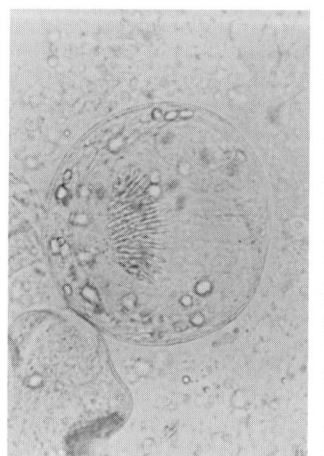
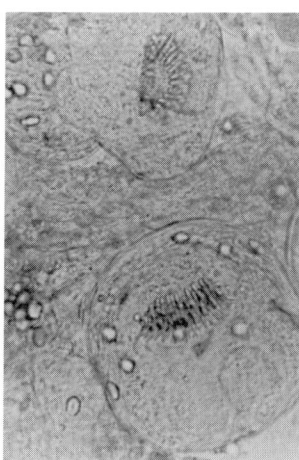

Figure 124–10. Hydatid scoleces in fresh unstained smear *(left)* and iodine-stained smear *(right)* from a hepatic cyst (× 400). (From Salama H, Farid-Abdel Wahab MF, Strickland GT: Diagnosis and treatment of hepatic hydatid cysts with the aid of echo-guided percutaneous cyst puncture. Clin Infect Dis 21:1372, 1995.)

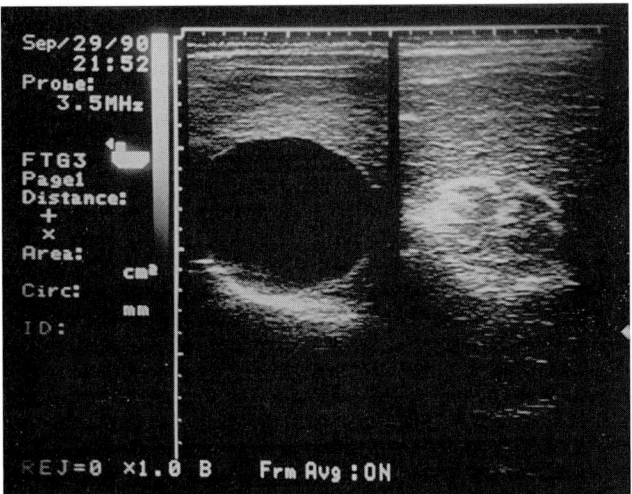

Figure 124–11. Hepatic hydatid cyst visualized by abdominal ultrasonography before *(left)* and after *(right)* complete echo-guided percutaneous aspiration. (From Salama H, et al: Clin Infect Dis 21:1372, 1995.)

ing to treat complications such as anaphylaxis, asthma, or laryngeal edema. The procedure is done under local anesthesia and with ultrasonographic guidance. The cyst is punctured using a transhepatic catheter or a cholangiography needle. Cyst contents are aspirated, and the cavity is filled with an equal volume of hypertonic saline (20 to 30%), which is left in place for 20 minutes before reaspiration (Fig. 124–11). Complications are rare but may consist of urticaria, cyst infection, fever, abnormal results of liver function tests, or recurrence of cyst. To avoid possible cyst infection, some practitioners use prophylactic antibiotic therapy. Combined use of albendazole (10 mg/kg/day for 8 weeks) and percutaneous aspiration has been shown to be more effective than either treatment alone.

Surgery. Surgical removal depends on whether the cyst can be percutaneously aspirated, requires removal, and can be surgically removed. Perioperative use of steroids is recommended owing to the possibility of accidental cyst rupture during operation. Hypertonic saline is the scolicidal agent of choice. Formalin should not be used because of reports of complications and death. When the situation permits, some surgeons use a metal cone to remove the cyst in order to avoid leakage of fluid. The procedure usually followed is aspiration of cyst fluid, after which the cavity is filled with an equal volume of hypertonic saline or other scolicide and then left for 5 to 10 minutes. The contents are once again aspirated, and the procedure is repeated. Finally the contents are reaspirated completely, the cyst is opened, and parasite membranes are removed, followed by closure of the remaining cavity. Infected hydatid cysts are treated by drainage as for a liver abscess, and the residual cavity plugged with greater omentum.

For lung cysts, internal suture in unruptured and recently ruptured cysts has been recommended. This technique often fails in cysts ruptured >10 days previously, and in these cases segmental resection is recommended. Major complications of surgical treatment are hydatid recurrence in 10 to 30%. Anaphylaxis sometimes occurs when cyst fluid is spilled during surgery. The mortality rate associated with first-time surgery is 2 to 3%.

CONTROL. Periodic treatment of dogs with praziquantel, avoiding giving raw infected viscera to dogs, and adequate inspection of abattoirs, as well as educational measures to change human practices that facilitate hydatid disease transmission, have been effective in controlling echinococcosis. Praziquantel given to dogs in eight treatment regimens per year (every 45 days) is highly effective at reducing the number of infections in dogs. In addition, adequate visceral disposal facilities and educational measures have been applied, with reduction of canine and livestock echinococcosis in New Zealand, Tasmania, Cyprus, Argentina, and Chile.

Hydatid disease was controlled in Cyprus mainly as a result of an intensive campaign to shoot all stray dogs.

Bibliography

Araujo FP, Schwabe CW, Sawyer JC, Davis WC: Hydatid disease transmission in California: A study of the Basque connection. Am J Epidemiol 102:291, 1975.

Coltorti EA, Varela Diaz VM: Detection of antibodies against *Echinococcus granulosus* arc 5 antigens by double diffusion test. Trans R Soc Trop Med Hyg 72:226, 1978.

Craig PS, Zeyhle E, Romig T: Hydatid disease: Research and control in Turkana II: The role of immunological techniques for the diagnosis of hydatid disease. Trans R Soc Trop Med Hyg 80:183, 1986.

Davis A, Pawloski ZS, Dixon H: Multicentre clinical trials of benzimidazolecarbonates in human echinococcosis. Bull WHO 64:383, 1986.

French CM, Nelson GS. Hydatid disease in the Turkana District of Kenya. II. A study in medical geography. Ann Trop Med Parasitol 76:439, 1982.

Gill-Grande LA, Rodriguez-Caabeiro F, Prieto JG, et al: Randomized controlled trial of efficacy of albendazole in intraabdominal hydatid disease. Lancet 342:1269, 1993.

Horton RJ: Chemotherapy of *Echinococcus* infection in man with albendazole. Trans R Soc Trop Med Hyg 83:97, 1989.

Khuroo MS, Dar MY, Yatton GN, et al: Percutaneous drainage versus albendazole therapy in hepatic hydatidosis: A prospective, randomized study. Gastroenterology 104:1452, 1993.

Khuroo MS, Wani NA, Javid G, et al: Percutaneous drainage compared with surgery for hepatic hydatid cysts. N Engl J Med 337:881, 1997.

Macpherson CNL: An active intermediate host role for man in the life cycle of *Echinococcus granulosus* in Turkana, Kenya. Am J Trop Med Hyg 32:397, 1983.

Macpherson CNL, Spoerry A, Zeyhle E, et al: Pastoralists and hydatid disease: An ultrasound scanning prevalence survey in East Africa. Trans R Soc Trop Med Hyg 83:243, 1989.

Macpherson CNL, Zeyhle E, Romig T, et al: Portable ultrasound scanner versus serology in screening for hydatid cysts in a nomadic population. Lancet 2:259, 1987.

Moro PL, Guevara A, Verastegui M, et al: Distribution of hydatidosis and cysticercosis in different Peruvian populations as demonstrated by an enzyme-linked immunoelectrotransfer blot (EITB) assay. Am J Trop Med Hyg 51:851, 1994.

Moro PL, McDonald J, Gilman RH, et al: Epidemiology of *Echinococcus granulosus* in the central Peruvian Andes. Bull WHO 75:553, 1997.

Purriel P, Schantz PM, Beovide H, Mendoza G: Human echinococcosis (hydatidosis) in Uruguay: A comparison of indices of morbidity and mortality, 1962–1971. Bull WHO 49:395, 1973.

Rogan MT, Craig PS, Zeyhle E, et al: Evaluation of a rapid dot-ELISA as field test for the diagnosis of cystic hydatid disease. Trans R Soc Trop Med Hyg 85:773, 1991.

Salama H, Abdel-Wahab MF, Strickland GT: Diagnosis and treatment of hepatic hydatid cysts with the aid of echo-guided percutaneous cyst puncture. Clin Infect Dis 21:1372, 1995.

Schantz PM, von Reyn CF, Welty T, et al: Epidemiologic investigation of echinococcosis in American Indians living in Arizona and New Mexico. Am J Trop Med Hyg 26:121, 1977.

Schantz PM, Williams JF, Riva Posse C: The epidemiology of hydatid disease in southern Argentina. Comparison of morbidity indices, evaluation of immunodiagnostic tests and factors affecting transmission in southern Rio Negro province. Am J Trop Med Hyg 22:629, 1973.

Shambesh MK, Macpherson CNL, Beasley WN, et al: Prevalence of human hydatid disease in northwestern Libya: A cross-sectional ultrasound study. Ann Trop Med Parasitol 86:381, 1992.

Thompson RCA, Limbery AT, Constantine CC: Variation in Echinococcus: Towards a taxonomic revision of the genus. Adv Parasitol 35:145, 1995.

Verastegui M, Moro P, Guevara A, et al: Enzyme-linked immunoelectrotransfer blot test for diagnosis of human hydatid disease. J Clin Microbiol 30:1557, 1992.

Wilson JF, Diddams AC, Rausch RL: Cystic hydatid disease in Alaska—a review of 101 autochthonous cases of *Echinococcus granulosus* infection. Am Rev Respir Dis 98:1, 1968.

124.3 *Alveolar Hydatid Disease*

Robert H. Gilman and Ben H. Lee

DEFINITION. Alveolar hydatid disease is one of the most lethal of the helminthic diseases. It is a zoonotic disease caused by infection with the larval stage of the canine tapeworm *Echinococcus multilocularis,* which is manifested as multilocular hydatid cysts in visceral organs. Echinococcosis is infection of humans with the cystic larval stage of *E. granulosus* or *E. vogeli,* which gives rise to hydatid (i.e., unilocular) cyst disease, or that of *E. multilocularis,* which gives rise to alveolar cyst disease. Both types of echinococcosis typically present primarily with hepatic cysts.

HISTORY. Some cases of human hydatid disease were noted to have hepatic cysts that failed to develop a restricting laminated membrane, thus allowing the parasite to invade the parenchyma in an alveoli-like pattern—hence the term *alveolar* or *malignant hydatid cyst.* In the 1950s, the findings of Vogel in Germany, Rausch and colleagues in Alaska, and Lukashenko in the former Soviet Union distinguished *E. multilocularis* as a separate species from *E. granulosus.*

ETIOLOGY. Humans are abnormal, accidental, dead-end hosts of *E. multilocularis.* They acquire alveolar hydatid disease by ingesting the eggs shed from its final host, typically foxes. The primary lesion in alveolar hydatid disease is always in the liver (Fig. 124–12*A* and *B*).

The oncosphere (embryo) hatches from the egg in the small intestine and is transported via the portal circulation to the liver. After hepatic localization, oncospheres undergo larval development, forming multilocular hydatid cysts. These cysts grow slowly, reproducing asexually by lateral budding, and spread through the liver (Fig. 124–12) and contiguous organs to produce chronic space-occupying, tumor-like lesions. The cysts occasionally metastasize, typically to the lungs and brain.

The rate of cyst growth varies among individuals, and cases of spontaneous larval death in people infected with the cestode have been reported. A recent study suggests that individuals expressing HLA-DR13 are more susceptible to disease progression after infection with *E. multilocularis* than those who do not express this class II antigen.

DISTRIBUTION AND PREVALENCE. *E. multilocularis* is enzootic in the Northern Hemisphere, where foxes and small rodents serve as hosts in its natural life cycle.

In North America, it is predominantly distributed throughout a central portion of the United States–Canadian border that contiguously includes three Canadian provinces and 12 of the United States: Alberta, Saskatchewan, Manitoba, Montana, Wyoming, North and South Dakota, Nebraska, Minnesota, Iowa, Wisconsin, Illinois, Indiana, Michigan, and Ohio. However, imported red foxes from the endemic Northwest to the southeastern seaboard of the United States for fox-hunting enclosures have been found to be infected with *E. multilocularis.* This has raised strong concerns that the cestode may have established itself among indigenous mammals of the southeastern coastal states, although infection among indigenous rodents has not been reported.

E. multilocularis is found in central Europe, including Switzerland, which has an annual morbidity rate of 0.18 cases of alveolar hydatid disease per 100,000. Similar rates have been

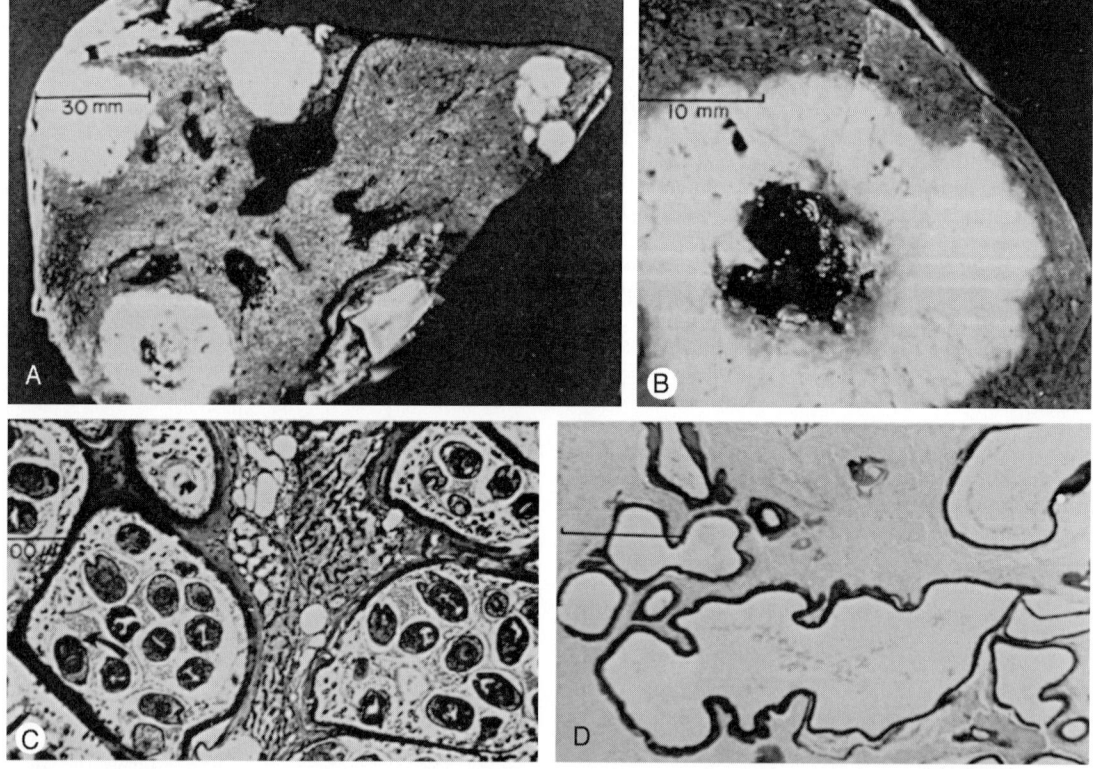

Figure 124–12. Multilocular hydatid disease. *A,* Multiple primary lesions in human liver. *B,* Enlargement of one of the lesions seen in *A* showing central necrosis. *C,* Histologic section of cyst from a vole, the normal host, stained with hematoxylin and eosin showing abundant scoleces *(large arrow)* and calcareous corpuscles *(small arrow). D,* Histologic section of a cyst from a man, an abnormal host, stained by the periodic acid-Schiff technique showing the intensely stained laminated membrane surrounding vesicles void of scoleces and calcareous corpuscles. (From Wilson JF, Rausch RL: Am J Trop Med Hyg 29:1340, 1980.)

documented in France, Germany, and Austria. In Asia, it is distributed throughout much of the former Soviet Union and some parts of Siberia, where the prevalence reaches 0.09 per 100,000 inhabitants. It is also found in the northern islands of Japan and in western and northern China.

EPIDEMIOLOGY. Foxes are the primary definitive host of *E. multilocularis*, but wolves, coyotes, cats, and dogs can also serve as final hosts for the cestode. The adult tapeworm lives in the small intestine, and its eggs are voided in feces. Intermediate hosts such as voles, lemmings, shrews, and mice ingest the eggs, which undergo larval development and are in turn ingested by the final hosts.

E. multilocularis is an arctic and alpine parasite, and its life cycle is efficient and well suited to these harsh environments; the adult tapeworm survives the winter in the intestines of canids, and the cyst survives in hibernating rodents with low body temperatures. The parasite eggs also resist cold climates and accumulate in the environment for transmission to rodents at the spring thaw. The multilocular cysts grow quickly in the natural rodent hosts, with scoleces developing in 2 to 4 months. Because scoleces number 100 to 200/mg of tissue, the biotic potential of the cysts is high (Fig. 124–12C). Additionally, the cysts produce massive infections in canids—100,000 to 160,000 worms per dog. Each gravid segment contains approximately 100 eggs, which develop 30 to 35 days after infection. This resulting environmental contamination is optimal for continued transmission.

E. multilocularis is classically maintained in a fox-rodent cycle. Thus, hunters and fur traders are at increased risk of infection. Domestic cycles can also become established in rural communities with the dog/cat-rodent cycle. Arctic villages are particularly susceptible to domestic transmission because of large populations of sled dogs and the lack of preventive measures for environmental and food contamination with dog feces infested with eggs of *E. multilocularis*.

PATHOLOGY. Contrary to the term *cyst*, the lesions caused by *E. multilocularis* appear as one or more firm, solid, yellow-gray cancer-like masses that are always primarily in the liver. The lesions can occupy any area of the liver with multiple foci, including the surface (Fig. 124–12A and B). The outer layer of the cyst has an ill-defined margin that diffuses into the host tissue. Larval exogenous proliferation is most active at the periphery of the lesion. In advanced cases, the central deeper portions of lesions often undergo extensive hepatic degeneration with central necrosis and calcification, presenting as a large, pus-filled cavity. This central abscess, filled with pea soup–like fluid, has a firm wall several millimeters thick and can occupy as much as half the organ; one patient in Alaska was reported to have a central abscess containing 7 to 8 L of pus. The lesions spread by direct extension into surrounding viscera and can metastasize via lymphatic or hematogenous routes.

Seen microscopically are numerous convoluted vesicles of various sizes. These are lined with the external laminated membrane of the parasite (Fig. 124–12D), thus giving rise to the term *alveolar* hydatid disease. This hyaline membrane is much thinner than that in the cyst of *E. granulosus* and is best visualized by the periodic acid–Schiff technique. Because humans are an abnormal host, brood capsules, scoleces, and calcareous corpuscles rarely develop as they do in normal hosts. The larger vesicles represent older portions of the cyst, and they give rise to the smaller microcysts by asexual lateral budding reproduction of the germinal membrane. The vesicles are usually surrounded by a dense layer of scar tissue 3 to 15 mm thick. Inflammatory cells consisting of histiocytes and eosinophils are typically distributed around the proliferating vesicles at the periphery of the cyst.

CLINICAL MANIFESTATIONS. The most common physical examination findings of alveolar hydatid disease are right upper quadrant pain, a palpable hepatic mass, and hepatomegaly; other findings include jaundice, shortness of breath, and central nervous system symptoms from brain metastases. The multilocular cyst grows slowly in humans, and a person may be infected for 30 years before symptoms appear.

The larval tissue mass biologically functions as a malignant tumor. It causes massive hepatic lesions and can directly invade surrounding viscera such as the inferior vena cava (IVC), portal vein, and common bile duct. The mass effect of the larval mass typically progresses to cause portal hypertension, compression/occlusion of the IVC, thrombocytopenia, esophageal variceal bleeding, cholestatic jaundice, cholangitis, liver abscesses, and Budd-Chiari syndrome. Portal hypertension and cholestatis complications are more likely to occur with hilar involvement. Superinfection of central abscesses in advanced larval masses from ascending biliary tract infections can be associated with fever, malaise, and toxicity. Pieces of the germinal membrane can metastasize to distant organs in 2% of patients to infect the brain, lungs, and mediastinum.

Without treatment, alveolar hydatid disease ultimately leads to death of the patient. The 10-year survival rate of untreated disease is <10%. To emphasize the importance of early diagnosis, treated disease carries a much better prognosis, with a 10-year survival rate approximating 90%.

DIAGNOSIS. Alveolar hydatid disease is usually diagnosed in persons who are 50 years of age or older and have a history of living in an endemic area. Patients are evaluated by history and physical examination, ultrasonography and computed tomography (CT), and serologic tests. Radiographs reveal diffuse space-occupying lesions that permeate the liver, resembling carcinomas or sarcomas. Diffuse mineralization of dead cyst material can occasionally be visualized. Completely calcified hepatic lesions <2 cm in diameter in hyperendemic regions should be considered nonviable *E. multilocularis* larval infections; hepatic lesions with mixed density patterns on CT, however, must be considered as active infection.

Confirmation of the diagnosis is established histologically by demonstrating the multilaminar cyst membrane using the periodic acid–Schiff technique (Fig. 124–12D). The extent of disease is usually determined during exploratory laparotomy.

Serology. Serologic tests are helpful in supporting the diagnosis if the findings on history and physical examination are compatible with alveolar hydatid disease (see Chapter 152). The indirect hemagglutination test, also used for *E. granulosus* diagnosis, yields positive results in 90% of patients with alveolar hydatid disease, and the titers are much higher than those found in patients with cystic hydatid disease. Em2 enzyme-linked immunosorbent assay (ELISA) testing, introduced in 1985, is a highly specific and reliable method for differentiating alveolar from cystic hydatid disease. Em2 ELISA can also be used to verify the success for complete versus incomplete cyst resection; however, it is an unreliable marker for monitoring the progression or regression of alveolar hydatid disease, and it cannot differentiate between active or spontaneously inactive cicatrized cysts. Western blot analyses based on humoral responses against the Em16 and especially Em18 *E. multilocularis* antigens have been shown to be reliable indicators of active alveolar hydatid disease. A reasonable serologic protocol is the use of Em2 ELISA as the primary screening tool in endemic populations, followed by Em18 ELISA to identify patients with active alveolar hydatid disease, who would then be referred for immediate treatment.

TREATMENT
Surgical Resection. Surgical resection of the primary cyst is the therapy of choice for alveolar hydatid disease. In con-

trast to the unilocular cyst of *E. granulosus*, which is a well-defined sphere contained in a fibrotic pericyst, the multilocular cyst is pleomorphic and infiltrates the organ in all directions. It is impossible to separate the cyst from host tissue. Thus, resection must include the cyst, diseased tissue, and surrounding normal tissue. Early detection of echinococcosis is imperative because screening programs using ultrasonography and serologic tests increase the resectability rate from 20% to 80%. Postoperative chemotherapy with albendazole is recommended, as well as preoperative chemotherapy, when applicable (e.g., incidental finding on exploratory laparotomy versus planned cyst resection). When partial hepatectomy is feasible, the cure rate of cyst resection is excellent.

For patients who have extensive disease or who are high-risk surgical candidates, chemotherapy should be considered as an alternative to surgery. Complications of disease can also be surgically treated, e.g., sclerotherapy for esophageal varices, biliary stenting for cholestatic disease, and Roux-en-Y to drain central abscesses with bacterial superinfection.

Postoperative follow-up should be provided with regular CT or ultrasound imaging and serologic testing. After complete resection of the lesion, patients rapidly seroconvert to negative. If any residual lesions remain (e.g., unresectable disease, incomplete resection), serologic results can remain positive for several years, even with chemotherapy. Residual larval tissue may occasionally be controlled and inactivated by natural host defenses. The results of any case should be reported in literature.

Chemotherapy. Long-term chemotherapy, with either albendazole (10 mg/kg/day) or mebendazole (40 mg/kg/day), is the treatment of choice for nonresectable alveolar hydatid disease. It is not certain whether the observed effect of chemotherapy is parasitostatic or parasiticidal, nor have the optimal dose and duration of therapy been definitively established.

The 10-year survival rate of alveolar hydatid disease approaches 90% with long-term chemotherapy. A recent study found that among patients with nonresectable alveolar echinococcosis taking long-term (5 to 7 years) albendazole or mebendazole chemotherapy, almost half experienced larval tissue mass regression and an additional 38% had static larval masses; the cysts in the remaining cases continued to grow despite chemotherapy. Reactivated disease has been reported to occur with discontinuation of long-term chemotherapy.

Severe late complications of chemotherapy include cholestatic disease (e.g., cholangitis, liver abscess, cholestatic jaundice) and esophageal variceal bleeding, likely from post-therapy hilar fibrosis. Other side effects of long-term high-dose treatment with mebendazole include febrile reactions, reversible leukopenias, and reversible alopecia. Fewer side effects have been reported with the less toxic drug albendazole. Additionally, therapeutic serum levels are more rapidly reached with albendazole than with mebendazole.

Liver Transplantation. Orthotopic liver transplantation is an alternative therapy for cases in which the organ has been extensively invaded by the larval cestode. The 6-year survival rate of liver transplantation therapy is 66%. Follow-up serology for recurrence of disease after transplantation is best done with anti-Eg IgG studies versus the more specific anti-Em2 IgG, which is more useful in follow-up of patients with surgical resection. However, in occasional reported cases, true recurrence of alveolar echinococcosis developed after transplantation, presumably by hematogenous and/or direct spread in conjunction with post-transplantation immunosuppression treatment.

CONTROL. Control of alveolar hydatid disease in communities relies on education to improve hygienic practices, mass treatment of village dogs with praziquantel, and encouragement of the elimination of surplus dogs in enzootic areas.

Bibliography

Ammann RW, Ilitsch N, Marincek B, et al: Effect of chemotherapy on the larval mass and the long-term course of aleolar echinococcosis. Hepatology 19:735, 1994.

Bresson-Hadni S, Miguiet FP, Mantion G, et al: Orthopic liver transplantation for incurable alveolar echinococcis of the liver, report of 17 cases. Hepatology 13:1061, 1991.

Davidson WR, Appel MJ, Doster GL, et al: Diseases and parasites of red foxes, gray foxes and coyotes from commercial sources selling to fox-chasing enclosures. J Wildl Dis 28:581, 1992.

Gemmell MA, Eckert J, Soulsby EJL: FAO/UNEP/WHO Guidelines for Surveillance, Prevention and Control of Echinococcosis/Hydatidosis. Geneva, World Health Organization, 1981.

Gottstein G, Bettens F: Association between HLA-DR13 and susceptibility to alveolar echinococcosis. J Infect Dis 169:1416, 1994.

Ito A, Wang XG, Liu YH: Differential serodiagnosis of alveolar and cystic hydatid disease in the People's Republic of China. Am J Trop Med Hyg 49:208, 1993.

Rausch RL, Wilson JF, Scantz PM, et al: Spontaneous death of *Echinococcus multilocularis* cases diagnosed serologically (by EM2 ELISA) and clinical significance. Am J Trop Med Hyg 36:576, 1987.

Wilson JF, Rausch RL, Wilson FR: Alveolar hydatid disease: Review of the surgical experience in 42 cases of active disease among Alaskan Eskimos. Ann Surg 221:315, 1995.

124.4 Polycystic Hydatid Disease*

Peter M. Schantz

DEFINITION. Polycystic hydatid disease (PHD) is a zoonotic disease of humans. It is caused by infection with the larval stages of *Echinococcus vogeli* and, less commonly, *E. oligarthrus*. The cestodes that cause PHD are indigenous to the humid tropical forests in Central and northern South America. Humans become infected after accidental ingestion of eggs passed in the feces of final hosts.

ETIOLOGY AND EPIDEMIOLOGY. The natural hosts of *E. vogeli* are the bush dog, *Speothos venaticus*, and the paca, *Cuniculus paca*. The larval stage occurs occasionally in rodents of other species, including the agouti and spiny rat. Bush dogs are wary and rarely seen animals that are an unlikely source of infection for humans. The intermediate host, the paca, is widely hunted for food in northern South America, and local hunters routinely feed the viscera of pacas to their dogs; thus, infected dogs may be the primary source of infection for humans.

The definitive hosts of *E. oligarthrus* are felids including jaguarundi, ocelots, and pumas; the intermediate hosts are the same as for *E. vogeli*. Although the hydatid cysts of both species are similar macroscopically, differentiation of *E. vogeli* and *E. oligarthrus* (as well as other species of *Echinococcus*) can be made on the basis of the length and proportions of the rostellar hooks. Human infection with *E. oligarthrus* is extremely rare; only three human cases are documented. The remote behavior of the definitive hosts presumably limits human exposure.

DISTRIBUTION AND PREVALENCE. About 80 human cases of PHD have been recorded, mainly (>85%) from Brazil, Colombia, Ecuador, and Argentina. The natural hosts of *E. vogeli* range throughout neotropical areas of Central and South America, and as local awareness and availability of diagnostic capability increase, it is probable that increasing numbers of cases will be recorded. The known range of *E. oligarthrus* extends from northern Mexico to southern Argentina; the three confirmed cases of human disease caused by this species have been reported from Venezuela and Brazil.

*All the material in this chapter is in the public domain, with the exception of any borrowed figures or tables.

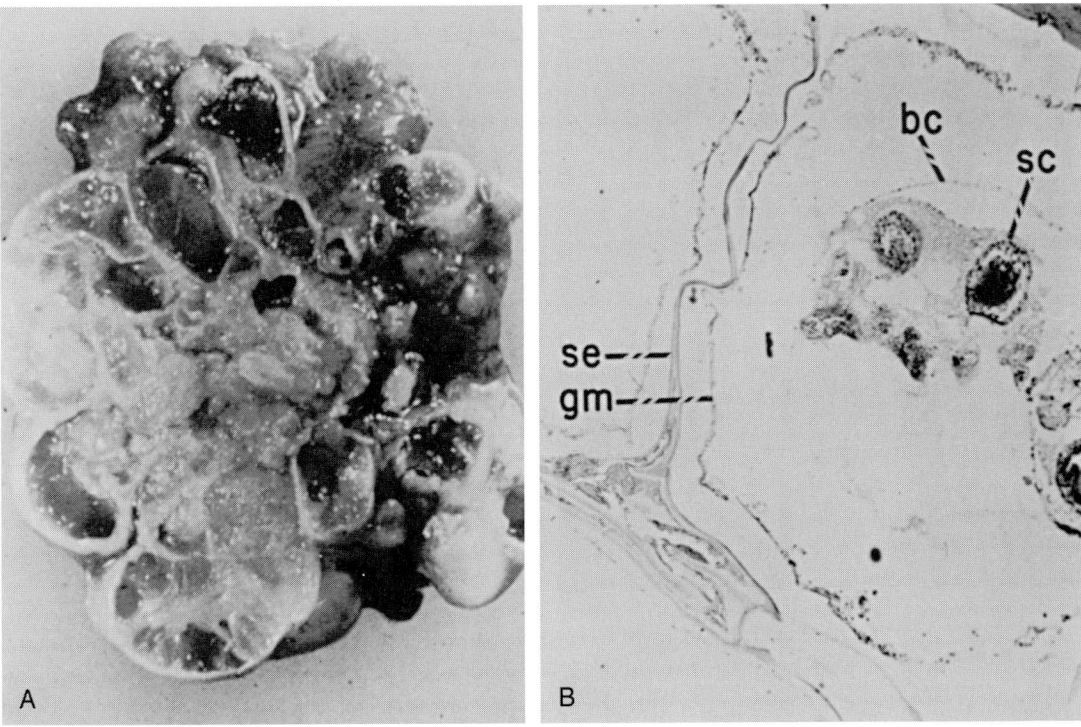

***Figure* 124–13.** Polycystic hydatid disease. *A,* Frontal section of a human heart showing a polycystic hydatid cyst of *Echinococcus vogeli. B,* Histologic section of a portion of a cyst showing internal septa (se), germinal membrane (gm), brood capsules (bc), and necrotic scoleces (sc). (From D'Alessandro A, et al.: Am J Trop Med Hyg 28:303, 1979.)

CLINICAL MANIFESTATIONS AND PATHOLOGY. Patients' ages at diagnosis have ranged from 6 to 78 years (median 44), and the most common signs at presentation were hepatomegaly, palpable peritoneal masses, and jaundice. PHD has characteristics intermediate between the cystic and alveolar forms. Of cases in which the causative agent was speciated, the ratio of *E. vogeli* to *E. oligarthrus* was approximately 10:1. The primary localization of *E. vogeli* infections is the liver, but cysts often invade contiguous sites. Hepatomegaly or tumor-like masses in the liver have been typical findings. The lungs are involved in about 15% of cases. The three known cases of *E. oligarthrus* infection have involved the eyes (two cases) and the heart. The prognosis in PHD is poor; approximately 14% of patients die of complications of biliary obstruction and portal hypertension.

At laparotomy, the larva of *E. vogeli* appears as a whitish-gray polycystic structure that contains a yellow fluid or gel (Fig. 124–13*A*). The entire cyst may be only 10 mm in diameter or may form vesicular aggregates that replace most of the liver. The scolex with its four circular suckers and rostellum with hooks can be seen in wet mount preparations and tissue sections. The large hooks are 38 to 46 μm long, and the small hooks are 30 to 37 μm.

Seen microscopically are numerous vesicles, varying in size from a few millimeters to centimeters (Fig. 124–13*B*). The vesicles are partitioned by septa formed from the hyaline laminated membrane, which is 8 to 65 μm thick and stains intensely by the periodic acid–Schiff technique. The internal surface of the septa is lined with a germinal membrane that is 3 to 13 μm thick and contains calcareous corpuscles. The brood capsules bud internally from the germinal epithelium. Externally, the cyst is surrounded by fibrous tissue, with only slight cellular infiltration. Portions of these cysts are frequently necrotic and mineralized, and the only remains of *Echinococcus* are the hooks and calcareous corpuscles.

DIAGNOSIS. The diagnosis of PHD should be considered in patients who present with abdominal masses and who reside or previously resided in rural Central or South American regions where the cestode agents are known to occur. Radiologic imaging (x-ray films, ultrasonography, or computed tomography) is very useful for demonstrating polycystic structures and diffuse mineralization in the liver or other sites. Serologic tests are often but not invariably useful for confirming the diagnosis. Specific *E. vogeli* antigens may differentiate hydatid disease due to *E. vogeli* from that caused by *E. granulosus;* however, tests using specific antigens are not widely available.

TREATMENT. The principles of management of cystic and alveolar echinococcosis also apply to polycystic echinococcosis. Because the lesions are so extensive, surgical resection may be difficult and usually is incomplete. A combination of surgery with albendazole is most likely to be successful.

Bibliography

D'Alessandro A: Polycystic echinococcosis in tropical America: *Echinococcus vogeli* and *E. oligarthrus.* Acta Trop 67:43, 1997.

D'Alessandro A, Ramirez LE, Chapadeiro E, et al: Second recorded case of human infections by *Echinococcus oligarthrus.* Am J Trop Med Hyg 52:29, 1995.

Gottstein B, D'Alessandro A, Rausch RL: Immunodiagnosis of polycystic hydatid disease/polycystic echinococcosis due to *Echinococcus vogeli.* Am J Trop Med Hyg 53:558, 1995.

Lopera RD, Melendez RD, Fernandez I, et al: Orbital hydatid cyst of *Echinococcus oligarthrus* in a human in Venezuela. J Parasitol 75:467, 1989.

Meneghelli UG, Martinelli ALC, Llorach Velludo MAS, et al: Polycystic hydatid disease *(Echinococcus vogeli).* Clinical, laboratory and morphologic findings in nine Brazilian patients. J Hepatol 14:203, 1992.

Rausch RL, D'Alessandro A, Rausch VR: Characteristics of the larval *Echinococcus vogeli,* Rausch and Bernstein, 1972 in the natural intermediate host, the paca, *Cuniculus paca* L. (Rodentia: Dasyproctidae). Am J Trop Med Hyg 30:1043, 1981.

World Health Organization Informal Working Group on Echinococcosis. Guidelines for treatment of cystic and alveolar echinococcoses in humans. Bull WHO 74:231, 1996.

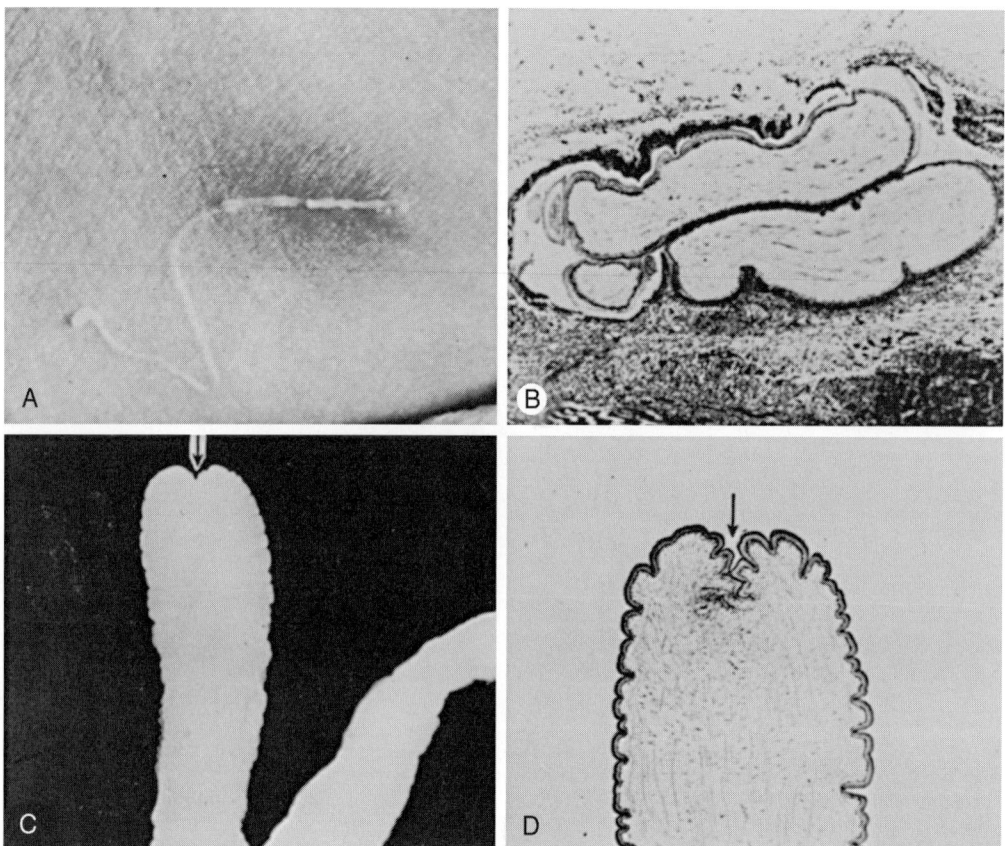

Figure 124–14. Sparganosis. *A*, Sparganum of *Spirometra* species from incised lesion on the chest. (Courtesy of Drs. J. H. Miller and S. H. Abadie, Louisiana State University School of Medicine.) *B*, Histologic section of sparganum showing inflammation. (Courtesy of Dr. J. F. Mueller, State University of New York Medical Center, Syracuse.) *C*, Flattened anterior end of a sparganum demonstrating the invaginated slit of the head (arrow) and pseudosegmentation. (Courtesy of the Armed Forces Institute of Pathology, Photograph Neg. No. 70–7390.) *D*, Histologic section showing head and pseudosegmentation. (Courtesy of the Armed Forces Institute of Pathology, Photograph Neg. No. 70–7310.)

124.5 *Sparganosis*

J. Fernando Diaz and Robert H. Gilman

DEFINITION. Sparganosis is caused by infection with spargana, which are second-stage larvae (plerocercoids) of diphyllobothrid tapeworms of the genus *Spirometra*.

ETIOLOGY. Many species of *Spirometra* have been described, but they are morphologically similar and taxonomically confusing. It is usual to refer to the parasite in Southeast Asia as *Spirometra mansoni* and that in North America as *Spirometra mansonoides*. The adult tapeworms occur in domestic and wild carnivores and are similar to *Diphyllobothrium* (Chapter 123.1). They are distinguished by the characteristic compact uterine coils and mature proglottids. The life cycles also differ, as *Spirometra* usually use amphibians, reptiles, and mammals as second intermediate hosts, whereas *Diphyllobothrium* use fish (Fig. 123–4). The adult parasite does not develop in humans, but humans can be infected with the larval stages by ingesting the procercoid in the first intermediate host, *Cyclops*, when drinking contaminated water. Humans may also act as a paratenic host by ingesting the plerocercoid in second intermediate hosts such as frogs or mammals. Another route of infection in Southeast Asia is from poultices prepared from frogs infected with plerocercoids that are applied directly to ulcers, sores, and inflamed eyes.

DISTRIBUTION AND PREVALENCE. Humans are a rare incidental host of these zoonotic parasites that are prevalent in cats, dogs, and wild carnivores in many parts of the world. Human infections are most common in Southeast Asia, but infections have been recorded in East Africa and North America.

CLINICAL MANIFESTATIONS AND PATHOLOGY. Spargana cause little reaction in the normal host, but in humans they usually migrate to the subcutaneous tissues, where they become encapsulated in inflammatory nodules that may develop into abscesses. Under these circumstances, the parasite is discharged (Fig.124–14*A*). The parasite may be viable for ≤19 years. In the subconjunctival tissues, the larvae provoke a more acute inflammation with conjunctivitis and periorbital edema. Sparganosis may also infect the central nervous system (CNS), breast, lungs, epididymis, bladder, heart, and kidneys. Although CNS involvement is rare, spargana has been reported as causing brain abscesses, intradural spinal canal infection, and extradural spinal cord infection. In these cases, sparganosis may produce seizures, headache, hemiparesis, paresthesias, memory loss, and confusion.

The inflammation consists of lymphocytes, histiocytes, plasma cells, and neutrophils; eosinophils may be abundant or absent (Fig. 124–14*B*). The parasites can usually be extracted alive, and they may be several centimeters in length. They are glistening white, opaque worms with a typical undulating cestode movement (Fig. 124–14*A* and *C*).

DIAGNOSIS. If the intact parasite is extracted, it can be recognized by the head with the characteristic deep invagination (Fig. 124–14C and D). Histologic sections of the worm show the typical features of cestode larvae (Fig. 124–14D). The wormlike appearance and the solid body of the spargana along with the absence of suckers and hooks usually distinguish them from the cystic stages of other cestodes that occur in subcutaneous tissues. Differential diagnosis of parasite-induced cerebral mass lesions includes infection with *Echinococcus, Multiceps, Toxoplasma,* cysticerci, and *Paragonimus.*

Recent enzyme-linked immunosorbent assay (ELISA) techniques have shown high sensitivity, although in a small number of patients. Computed tomography scan findings show multifocal areas of low density within white matter. Magnetic resonance imaging findings, which include widespread white matter degeneration and cortical atrophy, are not specific.

TREATMENT AND CONTROL. Surgical excision is usually possible, but in patients with many infections, supplementary treatment with praziquantel might be advisable (Chapter 124.2). In endemic areas, the local population should be discouraged from drinking "raw" water from natural ponds. The archaic use of frog poultices should be discouraged.

SPARGANUM PROLIFERUM. This is a rare larval cestode found in the skin, muscles, viscera, and brain of humans. These larvae are cylindrical or slightly flattened and can be 20 cm long and 2 mm wide; they proliferate by lateral budding to produce massive infections.

Bibliography

Griffin MP, Tompkins KJ, Ryan MT: Cutaneous sparganosis. Am J Dermatopathol 18:70, 1996.

Holodniy M, Almenoff J, Loutit J, et al: Cerebral sparganosis: Case report and review. Rev Infect Dis 13:155, 1991.

Nishiyama T, Ide T, Himes SR, et al: Immunodiagnosis of human sparganosis mansoni by microchemiluminescence enzyme-linked immunosorbent assay. Trans R Soc Trop Med Hyg 88:663, 1994.

124.6 Coenuriasis

J. Fernando Diaz and Robert H. Gilman

DEFINITION. Coenuriasis is a zoonotic disease of humans caused by infection with the larval stage (coenurus) of *Taenia (Multiceps)* species.

ETIOLOGY, DISTRIBUTION, AND EPIDEMIOLOGY. Adult tapeworms are found in the small intestine of canids, usually dogs. Gravid proglottids are passed at defecation. The proglottids eventually disintegrate to free the eggs, which disperse throughout the environment. When ingested by susceptible herbivores or humans, the eggs develop into coenuri in the subcutaneous muscles and central nervous system.

The taxonomy of coenuri is confusing, but the anatomic location of the coenuri may relate to the species. *Taenia (Multiceps) multiceps* has a wide distribution in temperate areas, where it usually circulates in a domestic cycle between dogs and herbivorous mammals, including sheep, goats, cattle, and horses. Coenuri infect the brain and spinal cord of the intermediate host and cause a common disease of sheep known as *gid* or *staggers.* Human neurocoenuriasis is rare but has been reported from the United States, England, France, Africa, and Brazil.

Taenia (Multiceps) serialis is also a parasite of temperate areas with wide distribution. Coenuri are usually found in intermuscular connective tissue of lagomorphs and rodents, including the rabbit, squirrel, and nutria. *T. serialis* is rare in humans and has been found in Canada, the United States, France, and Africa.

Taenia (Multiceps) brauni is a tropical tapeworm of eastern Africa with a sylvatic life cycle, including the dog, fox, jackal, and genet as definitive hosts and rodents such as the swamp rat, porcupine, and gerbil as intermediate hosts. The coenuri infect subcutaneous tissue of the intermediate hosts. There are <100 reports of *T. brauni* in humans.

Taenia (Multiceps) glomeratus has been found in subcutaneous tissue of humans in Nigeria.

CLINICAL MANIFESTATIONS AND PATHOLOGY. Patients with coenuriasis usually have a space-occupying lesion caused by a single cyst 2 to 6 cm in diameter. Neural coenuri have been found in the cerebrum, ventricles, posterior horn of the lateral ventricle, brain stem, and spinal cord and among the cranial nerves. The clinical manifestations of neurocoenuriasis are similar to those of neurocysticercosis (Chapter 124.2). Subcutaneous coenuri are commonly found in the intercostal region and anterior abdominal wall. These cysts may be confused with a lipoma, ganglion, and neurofibroma. Ocular coenuri have been recorded from the vitreous, anterior chamber, and conjunctiva.

DIAGNOSIS. Space-occupying lesions in the deep organs

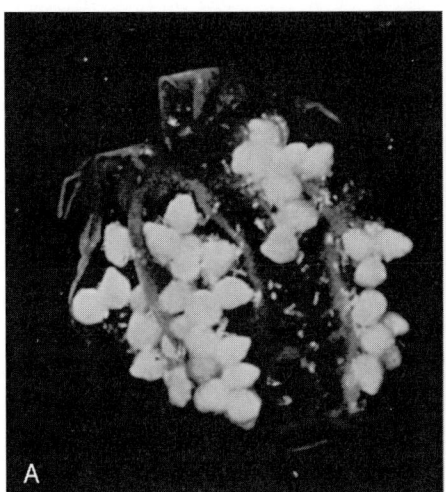
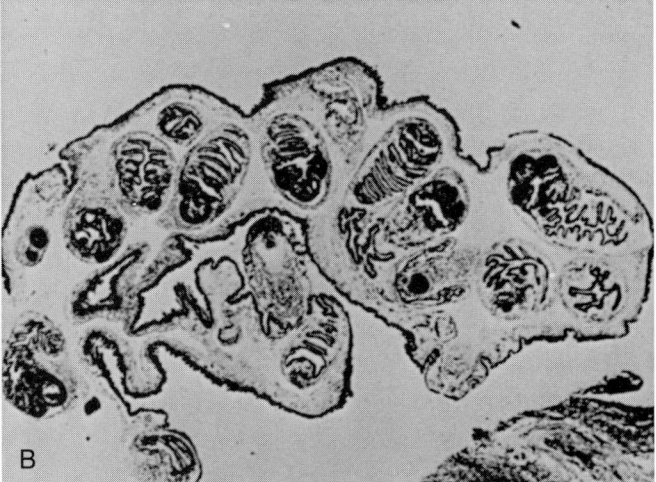

Figure 124–15. Coenuriasis. *A,* Coenurus from subcutaneous tissue of a man showing scoleces attached to cyst wall. (Courtesy of the Armed Forces Institute of Pathology, Photograph Neg. No. 70–4295.) *B,* Section of coenurus showing thin cyst wall and numerous scoleces developing from the germinal membrane. (Courtesy of the Armed Forces Institute of Pathology, Photograph Neg. No. 69–4736.)

are visualized with radiographic techniques such as x-ray films, radioisotopic scans, computed tomography scans, and ultrasonograms. Subcutaneous coenuri may be palpated, and ocular coenuri may be observed directly by endoscopic examination. Definitive diagnosis rests on surgical excision and parasitologic identification. The coenurus has a thin wall surrounding a single cavity that contains a clear fluid (Fig. 124–15A and B). Numerous scoleces 3 mm in diameter attach to the cyst wall, and no brood capsules are found as in the unilocular hydatid cyst of *E. granulosus*. Each scolex has four circular suckers and two rows of hooks on a rostellum. There are large and small hooks. The hook lengths for *T. multiceps* are 150 to 170 μm and 90 to 130 μm; those for *T. serialis* are 135 to 175 μm and 68 to 120 μm; those for *T. brauni* are 95 to 140 μm and 70 to 90 μm; and those for *T. glomeratus* are 90 to 100 μm and 65 to 70 μm.

TREATMENT AND CONTROL. Surgical excision is the usual treatment, although both praziquantel and albendazole are likely to be as effective as in the treatment of cysticercosis. However, praziquantel can produce toxic endophthalmitis and loss of vision in intraocular coenurosis. The best treatment of an intravitreal cestode cystic larva is its removal through a closed vitrectomy. Preventive measures include hygienic practices to reduce contact with dogs and to break the transmission of eggs from dog feces to humans. Elimination of adult worms with praziquantel or niclosamide reduces environmental contamination with eggs.

Bibliography

Benger A, Rennie RP, Roberts JT, et al: A human coenurus infection in Canada. Am J Trop Med Hyg 30:638, 1981.

Ibechukwu BI, Onwukeme KE: Intraocular coenurosis: A case report. Br J Ophthalmol 75:430, 1991.

Malomo A, Ogunniyi J, Ogunniyi A, et al: Coenurosis of the central nervous system in a Nigerian. Trop Geogr Med 42:280, 1990.

Templeton AC: Anatomical and geographical location of human coenurus infection. Trop Geogr Med 23:105, 1971.

125 Poisonous Plants and Fish

William A. Sodeman, Jr.

Toxic and poisonous plants and animals exist in all environments. The numerical richness of tropical flora and fauna increases the relative number of toxic species. Poisonings are increasing in frequency. This increase is related directly to increased exposure. Several factors are involved in this increase. Indigenous populations receive some protection from the tradition and folklore that serve as a repository for prior experience concerning foodstuffs that are toxic at any given time. Development of natural resources in the tropics has opened vast areas to immigration, which exposes a naive population to new toxins and poisons. This same development, coupled with technological progress in processing and transportation of foodstuffs, permits wide dissemination of occasionally toxic foods, usually fish or shellfish. Distribution occurs often before their toxicity can be recognized. Finally, the ease of travel has opened previously remote areas to tourism. The resultant increase in populations at risk is followed by an increase in numbers of poisonings.

125.1 Shellfish Poisoning

Clinically, three types of shellfish poisoning may be recognized.

GASTROINTESTINAL SHELLFISH POISONING. The onset of symptoms, i.e., nausea, vomiting, diarrhea, and abdominal pain, is 8 to 12 hours after ingestion. Bacterial contamination of the shellfish is believed to be the cause.

ALLERGIC SHELLFISH POISONING. The onset of symptoms occurs 30 minutes to 6 hours after ingestion. In this type, symptoms include skin rash and itching, nasal congestion, dryness of the throat, and edema of the tongue, causing potentially fatal respiratory distress. It is thought to be due to individual sensitivity to the shellfish.

PARALYTIC SHELLFISH POISONING. This is also called dinoflagellate poisoning and saxitoxin poisoning.

Etiology and Pathophysiology. This is an acute poisoning due to saxitoxin, a powerful curare-like neurotoxin that is produced by toxic species of planktonic dinoflagellates (*Protogonyautax catenella* and *Protogonyautax tamarensis*) and concentrated in filter-feeding mollusks (clams, oysters, scallops, mussels). The principal action of the toxin occurs centrally on the respiratory and vasomotor centers and peripherally at the neuromuscular junctions and the sensory nerve endings and the mechanism involves blocking of sodium channels. The toxin is absorbed through the gastrointestinal tract and excreted by the kidneys. Toxins derived from other species, such as the cyanobacterium *Anabaena circinalis*, may contribute neurotoxins that can be concentrated in shellfish. Toxins of this sort may accumulate in freshwater as well as saltwater species.

Clinical Manifestations and Prognosis. The onset of symptoms, which are usually neuromotor in nature, is usually 30 minutes following ingestion of the shellfish. Paresthesia starts in the lips and tip of the tongue and spreads to involve the face, scalp, neck, and extremities. This may be accompanied by weakness of the limbs, ataxia, incoherent speech, aphonia, tightness of the throat and chest, and increased salivation. The pulse is thready; superficial reflexes may be lost, whereas deep reflexes are depressed. If the patient survives the first 12 hours, the prognosis is good. However, the mortality rate is 1 to 7%, with death usually occurring from respiratory paralysis within 24 hours.

NEUROTOXIC SHELLFISH POISONING. This acute poisoning is produced by a toxin elaborated by the dinoflagellate *Ptychodiscus brevis* and is concentrated in filter-feeding mollusks. Paresthesia begins in the circumoral area but progresses to involve the extremities. Cerebellar dysfunction with ataxia occurs as well. Seizures may occur. Treatment is supportive and recovery expected.

***Pfiesteria piscicidia* Poisoning.** This toxic dinoflagellate is commonly associated with fish kills. Although it can be concentrated in shellfish or finfish, toxic exposure in humans is more likely to be by direct contact with the toxin. The toxin is an exotoxin elaborated into the water. It is lipid soluble, and thus may be directly absorbed through the skin or from aerosols. Concentrations sufficient to cause illness in humans are likely only in the presence of fish kills, although there is evidence that lower-level exposures can cause skin lesions in humans and fish.

This has become a major environmental problem in the coastal waters of North Carolina, Virginia, and Maryland in the late 1990s. Phosphate- and nitrogen-rich runoff from fertilization of crops and pork and poultry production facilities and from fields where their waste was used for fertilization into the streams and rivers feeding into coastal sounds and the Chesapeake Bay have been proposed as the cause of huge overgrowth of *P. piscicidia* during the summer season. This is believed to be the etiology of ulcerative lesions on fish, high fish kills, and vague (but consistent) acute and chronic symptoms in some people exposed to these waterways.

The onset after heavy exposure is rapid, occurring in an hour or less. The presentation may include headache, nausea, vomiting, and abdominal cramps but not diarrhea. Redness and watering of the eyes develops rapidly. Skin lesions manifest as poorly healing ulcers. Many of these are in association with cuts from handling fish or shellfish but ulcers may develop on intact skin as well. Neurologic and neuropsychiatric symptoms predominate. Narcosis and an altered mental state come on rapidly. Numbness and tingling in the hands and feet is described. Perceptual difficulties such as the inability to know where one's feet are cause difficulty walking. Impaired concentration and mentation is described. The impairment in memory may be profound enough to cause difficulty with speech and language. Spatial impairment may make driving hazardous. Marked personality change is also described. Most of these changes remarkably improve with cessation of contact with the toxin. However, chronic memory impairment may persist for years.

The nature of the toxin is not clear. There is no direct treatment except avoidance. Supportive therapy is required. The skin ulcerations rapidly become secondarily infected and may require antibiotic therapy.

TREATMENT. As no specific antidote is known, treatment is symptomatic and supportive. In the gastrointestinal type of shellfish poisoning, reports indicate that in most cases the signs and symptoms responded to the administration of a broad-spectrum antibiotic, diphenoxylate hydrochloride with atropine sulfate (Lomotil), and rehydration (intravenously when indicated). Antihistamines, epinephrine, and corticosteroids have been used to good effect in the allergic type of shellfish poisoning. The paralytic type of poisoning, however, often requires treatment of respiratory and circulatory collapse by means of intravenous infusions and cardiotonic drugs, as well as drugs to control the arrhythmias. In some cases, assisted ventilation is needed.

125.2 Fish Poisoning

There are 500 species of known toxic fish; most are reef fish. Some are toxic at all times; others are toxic only during certain seasons. In some fish, all the tissues are toxic; in others, only the tissues of certain organs are toxic.

CIGUATERA POISONING

Etiology. From the medical and economic standpoints, this is the most important type of poisoning. Three hundred species of fish have been incriminated in a wide geographic distribution from the West Indies to the Pacific. Although cold water species have generally not been susceptible to bioaccumulation of this toxin, there has been at least one report of poisoning by farm-raised salmon, nominally a cold water species. The ciguatoxic fish cannot be recognized by external appearance. Species that are toxic in one locality may be nontoxic in another. The origin of the toxin is the dinoflagellate *Gamberdiscus toxicus* and possibly others. At least three toxins have been identified. The toxins are tasteless and odorless. They are lipid soluble and heat stable. The latter is a feature of importance which permits the toxin to survive the cooking process. The effect of the toxin on membranes results in opening of sodium channels. There is one report of a ciguatera toxin variant that blocks rather than opens sodium channels. An ionotropic effect on the heart is described, which may underlie the bradycardia and arrhythmia that occurs in some patients. As isolation techniques have developed, it now appears that several toxins may accumulate in the fish and the resulting clinical syndrome may vary in its presentation and severity depending on the various concentrations and the mix of toxins present. The toxin is transferred by transvection via the food chain through herbivorous reef fish to carnivorous tropical reef fish (groupers, snappers, dolphins, barracuda) where it is concentrated. It is harmless to the fish themselves.

Clinical Manifestations and Prognosis. In the United States, the disease occurs most frequently during the late spring and summer. The onset of clinical manifestations of poisoning occurs 4 to 30 hours after ingestion. In the main, the manifestations are gastrointestinal and neurologic, with nausea (and, on occasion, a metallic taste in the mouth), vomiting and diarrhea, abdominal pain and cramps, paresthesia around the mouth (and in some cases the fingers and toes), cold-to-hot sensory reversal dysesthesia, increased salivation, dilatation of the pupils, strabismus, ptosis, weakness, myalgia of the legs, incoordination, and even paralysis. Pruritus of the soles of the feet and palms of the hands may be present. Difficulties with temperature differentiation (hot from cold) and a sensation that one's teeth are loose are highly correlated with ciguatera intoxication when present but these findings occur irregularly. Coma has rarely been

reported. The mortality rate is as high as 10%. Usually, death occurs from respiratory failure or hypovolemic shock.

Treatment. Treatment is supportive and symptomatic. A wide variety of pharmacologic agents have been used both experimentally and clinically. Emesis should be induced, a cathartic given, 10% calcium gluconate given intravenously (to relieve neurologic symptoms), sedation for convulsions, e.g., diazepam or paraldehyde, and nikethamide for respiratory depression. Atropine sulfate has been used in patients in whom there is excessive production of mucus, but it tends to make aspiration of secretions more difficult. Amitriptyline hydrochloride, an antidepressant with some sedative effects, gives relief from neurologic symptoms in some patients. The mechanism of action is not elucidated. Intravenous administration of mannitol has also been effective in relieving most symptoms of ciguatera poisoning. It is administered in doses of 0.5 to 1.0 g/kg as a 20% solution over 30 minutes. Mannitol is now probably the treatment of choice, although its mechanism of action is unknown. Patients with laryngeal obstruction will require intubation or tracheostomy. In patients severely affected, the myalgia, paresthesias of the hands and feet, and pruritus may recur intermittently for as long as 6 months to 2 years after the initial attack. Coffee, tea, and chocolate may exacerbate the symptoms. A rapid immunoassay for toxin in fish tissue has been developed but has only limited availability. This offers promise in prevention of poisoning.

TETRAODON POISONING

Etiology. Tetraodontoxin, a neurotoxin, is widely distributed among the order Tetraodontoidea (Plectognathi). This includes puffers (blowfish, toadfish, fugu), ocean sunfish, and porcupine fish. They are characterized by having very small scales. The toxin concentrates mainly in the liver, ovaries, intestine, and skin of the fish. Puffer musculature is nonpoisonous. Toxicity is related to the reproductive cycle, being highest just before spawning in late spring or early summer.

Clinical Manifestations and Prognosis. The clinical features of tetraodon poisoning are characterized by the rapid onset, within 5 to 30 minutes, of weakness; dizziness; paresthesias of the lips, tongue, throat, and, later, the limbs; nausea (but usually no vomiting or diarrhea), and abdominal pain. Pallor, sweating, and increased salivation may be present. There is a tachycardia, hypotension, and increasing difficulty with breathing, which may be complicated by a general flaccid ascending paralysis, leading to respiratory failure, convulsions, and death in 6 to 24 hours. Usually, consciousness is retained throughout. The mortality rate was as high as 60% in Japanese outbreaks.

Treatment. Treatment is symptomatic and supportive because there is no specific therapy or antidote. It should include induced emesis (but in patients in whom there is evidence of increasing paralysis only when there is a cuffed endotracheal tube in place), and administration of a cathartic and 10% intravenous calcium gluconate to combat neurologic symptoms. Respiratory and cardiac stimulants and assisted respiration are indicated in many cases.

SCOMBROID POISONING

Etiology. Scombrotoxic poisoning follows ingestion of contaminated, imperfectly refrigerated fish of the tuna and mackerel families and, occasionally, sprats and pilchards. Bacterial contaminants (*Proteus, Salmonella, Clostridium,* and *Escherichia coli*) break down the histidine of fish muscles to saurine, a histamine-like substance. Victims often complain that the fish has a peppery taste.

Clinical Manifestations and Treatment. Signs and symptoms resemble those of a histamine poisoning. The onset occurs about 3 hours after ingestion of the fish, and the findings are of an acute allergic or histamine-like reaction, with headache; flushing of the head and upper trunk; generalized urticaria; swelling of the eyelids, periorbital tissue, lips, tongue, and throat; muscular weakness; myalgia; and diarrhea. Recovery usually occurs in 3 to 16 hours, although occasional deaths have been reported. Antihistamines are effective with or without emesis or gastric lavage.

OTHER FISH POISONING

Elasmobranch Poisoning. This occurs after ingestion of the liver or skeletal muscles of sharks and rays. The onset of symptoms usually occurs after 30 minutes. These are usually mild following ingestion of the musculature and include some abdominal pain but mainly diarrhea. Symptoms are more severe after ingestion of the liver and include, in addition to diarrhea and abdominal pain, nausea, vomiting, headache, tingling around the mouth, and a burning sensation of the tongue. In severe cases, this may progress to ataxia, visual disturbances, difficulty with breathing, coma, and death. Most patients, however, recover completely in 5 to 20 days.

Two lipid-soluble toxins, carchatoxin-A and carchatoxin-B, have been reported as the cause of fatal mass poisoning following the ingestion of meat and liver from *Carcharhinus leucas*. The toxins have a high degree of toxicity with rapid onset of effects within 5 to 10 hours. The toxins occurred in freshly killed shark. They were heat stable and present in cooked meals. All individuals eating shark were affected.

The clinical presentation began with periorbital burning and numbness in the extremities. Ataxia occurred and in many patients progressed rapidly to coma and death. A total of 180 people were affected, with 50 deaths. A few patients had evidence of gastrointestinal irritation. Cardiovascular symptoms including shock and bradycardia were occasionally noted.

Isolation of the two toxins and their partial characterization permitted their distinction from other known ichthyosarcotoxins. No environmental source for the toxin was identified. Sharks are near-ultimate predators and a food-chain amplification is suspected.

Hallucinatory Fish Poisoning. This may occur after ingestion of certain species of mullet. Signs and symptoms begin about 2 hours after ingestion of the fish and are all neurologic, e.g., incoordination, nightmares, ataxia, and hallucinations. No fatalities have been recorded, and cathartics are recommended in treatment.

Miscellaneous. Other intoxications have been described, e.g., fish roe poisoning, fish blood poisoning, and fish liver poisoning. Treatment is symptomatic.

The contamination of the sea and its fauna by metallic wastes, particularly mercury, has been described in Japan, i.e., Minamata disease (Chapter 20).

Bibliography

Banner AH: Hazardous marine animals. *In* Tedeschi CG, Eckert WG, Tedeschi LG (eds): Forensic Medicine. Vol. 3, Environmental Hazards. Philadelphia, WB Saunders, 1977.

Barton ED, Tanner P, Teuchen SG, et al: Ciguatera fish poisoning: A Southern California epidemic. West Med J 163:31, 1995.

Boisier P, Ranaivoson G, Rasolofonirina N, et al: Fatal mass poisoning in Madagascar following ingestion of a shark *(Carcahrhinus leucas)*: Clinical and epidemiological aspects and isolation of toxins. Toxicon 33:1359, 1995.

DeFusco DJ, O'Dowd P, Hokama Y, et al: Coma due to ciguatera poisoning in Rhode Island. Am J Med 95:240, 1993.

DiNubile MJ, Hokama Y: The ciguatera poisoning syndrome from farm raised salmon. Ann Intern Med 122:113, 1995.

Glasgow HP Jr, Burkholder JM, Schmechel DE, et al: Insidious effects of a toxic estuarine dinoflagellate on fish survival and human health. J Toxicol Environ Health 46:501, 1995.

Lawrence DN: Ciguatera fish poisoning in Miami. JAMA 244:254, 1980.

Negri AP, Jones GJ: Bioaccumulation of paralytic shellfish poisoning (PSP) toxins from the cyanobacterium *Anabaena circinalis* by the freshwater mussel *Alathyria condola*. Toxicon 33:667, 1995.

Russel FE: Poisonous Marine Animals. London, TFH Publications, and Academic Press (London), 1971.

125.3 Mushroom Poisoning

DEFINITION AND ETIOLOGY. Hundreds of toxin-containing mushroom species are known worldwide. They represent about 10% of mushrooms, and only 10% of known mushroom species are considered edible. A small but significant percentage of toxic mushrooms can produce fatal poisoning. Most poisonings are accidental, as a result of either culinary error or ingestion by small children. Mushrooms of certain species are abused as hallucinogens, and there are suicide attempts by mushroom ingestion.

Mushroom toxicity is highly variable. Toxin content may vary with season, geographic origin, maturity of the fungus, and method of preparation. Some mushrooms are toxic when raw but not when cooked. A few are toxic when fresh but safe when dried. Individual human sensitivity to some toxins is variable. Other food eaten with mushrooms modifies toxicity. Alcohol may modify toxicity as well. Although it is not well characterized, there is individual variability in susceptibility to some of the toxins. Often only one person joining in a mushroom meal will fall ill. Edible mushrooms, as with any fresh produce, may spoil and cause illness because of the spoilage rather than the presence of a toxin.

CLINICAL CLASSIFICATION. The taxonomy of fungi is complex and not without controversy. For clinical purposes it is more useful to separate the mushrooms into six groups on the basis of the toxin that they harbor, with a seventh catchall group for those fungi in which the toxin is poorly characterized.

The Cyclopeptide Group. This group of toxins, often referred to as amanitins, produces toxic effects in liver and kidney. The onset is rapid, often within 24 hours. Early symptoms of toxicity are gastrointestinal and visual. Fatality is a result of damage to liver and kidney. Many but not all species of *Amanita* contain this class of toxin.

The Monomethylhydrazine Group. This toxin, which is derived from gyromitrin, damages liver. It has a rapid onset of under 3 hours. The acute intoxication produces both gastrointestinal symptoms and ataxia. The toxin is carcinogenic as well as toxic. The genus *Gyromitra* is the principal offender.

The Coprine Group. Coprine requires the presence of alcohol in the blood stream for its toxic effect. Its action is rapid in onset, often in 2 hours or less. Gastrointestinal upset, flushing, and chest pain are described.

The Muscarine Group. Muscarine produces cholinergic-like effects when ingested. The onset is rapid, customarily within several hours. Lacrimation, salivation, perspiration, and abdominal cramps occur. There may be bradycardia and a fall in blood pressure to shock levels. A number of genera contain muscarine.

The Ibotinic Acid/Mucimol Group. The onset of action is rapid, often within 3 hours. The effects are primarily neurologic with confusion, discoordination, dizziness, and convulsions. Nausea and vomiting is described. The mortality is low. Several of the genus *Amanita* are involved.

The Psilocybin/Psilocin Group. These toxins are known primarily for their hallucinogenic effect. They also cause fever, headaches, and convulsions. Mortality is very low.

Miscellaneous. There are many other toxic mushrooms but the toxins are too poorly characterized to classify. Most give rise to gastrointestinal symptoms and headache.

CLINICAL MANIFESTATIONS AND MANAGEMENT. Manifestations of toxicity may be immediate or may be delayed for up to 17 days. Outcome in any individual case is heavily dependent on the nature and dose of toxin.

Identification of the suspect mushroom in a case of poisoning is often not possible. Species abound, toxic effects may be delayed long after ingestion, and mistaken identification as an edible mushroom is often the problem in the first place. The recognition of a characteristic syndrome plus a history of recent ingestion of wild mushrooms should prompt clinical intervention, especially when the syndrome has lethal implications.

Mushroom intoxications may be classified by the species involved, by the toxin involved, or by the clinical presentation. For the nonmycologist physician it is the clinical presentation that proves most useful. There are three basic patterns of clinical presentation: gastrointestinal symptoms, renal symptoms, and neuropsychiatric symptoms. These in turn may be subdivided into more specific presentations.

Gastrointestinal Symptoms. The key criterion that separates the various gastrointestinal syndromes is the duration of the latent period between ingestion of the mushroom and the onset of signs and symptoms.

Rapid Onset. Many different genera and species have toxins that affect the gastrointestinal tract and have a rapid, almost immediate, onset of action. These tend not to be fatal intoxications. Generally, the toxins induce nausea, vomiting, and/or diarrhea. Symptoms can persist for days and become clinically important as a result of dehydration and acid-base imbalance. In patients with limited tolerance for dehydration and electrolyte abnormality, e.g., patients on cardioactive drugs, the very old or very young, or patients with other intercurrent diseases, e.g., diabetes, special attention must be paid to early intervention and management.

The mechanism of toxin action is not well understood. One exception is the ingestion of *Coprinus atramentarius*, the Inky Cap. This mushroom produces coprine, which after metabolic conversion to cyclopropanone hydrate, inhibits acetaldehyde dehydrogenase. This causes a disulfiram-like effect following the ingestion of alcohol. The mushroom is not toxic in the nonalcohol drinker. Alcohol ingestion produces headache, nausea, and vomiting. Diarrhea does not occur. The sensitization to alcohol may last up to 72 hours. Several other species of *Coprinus* in Europe and Africa have been implicated as causing this syndrome as well as *Clitocybe clavipes* in Japan.

Delayed Onset—6 Hours. Ingestion of *Gyromitra esculenta* produces gastrointestinal symptoms after a latent interval of about 6 hours. The toxin involved is gyromitrin or monomethylhydrazine. This can be found in other species of *Gyromitra* as well. The toxin causes vomiting, headache, abdominal cramping, diarrhea and, when severe, neurologic symptoms and evidence of liver damage. The most prominent sign is the emesis, which may be persistent enough to cause metabolic alkalosis. The demonstration of methemoglobin in the circulation is evidence of ingestion of *Gyromitra*. The management is largely that of treating the dehydration and electrolyte abnormalities. Pyridoxine will reverse some of the toxicity. It should be administered IV in a dose of 25 mg/kg, adjusting the dose to the patient's symptoms. Severe intoxication requires the management of the liver damage and coma.

The toxin is water soluble and volatile. It can be leached out of the mushroom by parboiling or volatilized by drying. Detoxifying is common practice in Europe. Toxin-containing vapor from cooking fresh mushrooms can itself be toxic if inhaled.

Delayed Onset—12 Hours. *Amanita phalloides* and other ama-toxin-containing mushrooms (in at least four genera) can cause fatal intoxication, which occurs with delayed onset of symptoms. Amatoxins act directly on the intestine to produce acute gastroenteritis. The usual latent interval is 12 hours. The gastrointestinal response is nausea and vomiting, cramping abdominal pain, and diarrhea. This runs a short course of about 8 hours, and then the patient experiences a symptom-free interval of 3 to 5 days. Following this interval, the character of the illness changes, and there is the development of hepatic insufficiency. Clinically the picture is that of severe viral hepatitis. There is elevation of hepatocellular enzymes, falling levels of liver-produced coagulation factors, and finally hypoglycemia. Amatoxins also have an affinity for the proximal convoluted tubule of the kidney and can produce acute tubular necrosis with renal failure.

Amatoxins are cyclic octapeptides that are hepato-selective. They interfere with the activity of RNA polymerase and eventuate in cell death. They are not destroyed by drying or leached by parboiling. Treatment is a complex process that varies with the stage of development of the intoxication. If the ingestion is recognized early (within 6 hours) as in a culinary error, a suicide attempt, or inadvertent ingestion by a child, the stomach should be evacuated by induced emesis or lavage. The fatal dose for an adult is 5 to 10 mg of toxin, an amount that could be found in a single large cap. Vigorous attempts to lower the dose are proper. Amatoxin binds strongly with activated charcoal, and once the stomach has been cleaned, administration of a slurry of activated charcoal in water may bind some of the toxin in the intestinal lumen.

The acute gastroenteritis is treated symptomatically with fluid and electrolyte replacement. Even if recognition of toxin ingestion is delayed, administration of activated charcoal may help break the enterohepatic cycle of the toxin by binding it in the lumen. A forced diuresis may speed the excretion of the toxin and lessen its stay within the kidney. Once liver or renal failure supervenes, these are managed by standard approaches.

Renal Syndromes. In addition to the amatoxin-containing mushrooms described above, which can cause acute tubular necrosis, some species of *Cortinarius* can cause renal failure also. Several toxins are known in this genus, but the one responsible for the renal failure and its mechanism of action is not known. This mushroom species has great variability in toxicity. Some species seem safe if eaten raw but toxic if cooked. The latent interval may be long, 3 to 17 days.

The initial manifestation of the renal toxicity is the appearance of polydipsia and polyuria. There may be associated chills, headache, and muscular pain. In some patients there are gastrointestinal symptoms. The renal failure develops as a result of acute tubular necrosis. Fatalities do occur. The management is that of acute renal failure. Dialysis over XAD-4 Amberlite may remove toxin.

Neuropsychiatric Syndromes. Several distinct neuropsychiatric syndromes occur following toxic mushroom ingestion. These may present as muscarine toxicity, coma, or hallucinations.

Muscarine Toxicity. Mushrooms of the genera *Clitocybe* and *Inocybe* contain muscarine. This compound, even in small doses, acts as a parasympathetic stimulant and can produce sweating, abdominal pain, and miosis. The effect is temporary, and atropine in full doses can reverse most of the symptoms.

Coma Producers. *Amanita muscaria* and *Amanita pantherina* contain ibotenic acid. This is metabolized to muscimol, which is a γ-aminobutyric acid agonist in the central nervous system. Patients become drowsy and then comatose, but this is interrupted by periods of delirium and excitement. It is fatal in heavy doses.

TABLE 125–1. Genera With Psilocybin- and/or Psilocin-Containing Species

Amanita	Naematoloma
Boletus	Panaeolus
Clitocybe	Pluteus
Conocybe	Psathyrella
Copelandia	Psilocybe
Gymnopilus	Russula
Lycoperdon	Stropharia

Compiled from Lincoff and Mitchel, 1977; Lampe and McCann, 1985.

Hallucinogens. Many mushrooms are known and abused for their effect as hallucinogens. The active toxin is psilocybin. Mushrooms of many genera (Table 125–1) have been implicated. The effect is that of alcohol intoxication with hallucinations. Responses vary with chronic use. In children, particularly with high doses, severe reactions occur with hyperthermia and convulsions. Treatment is symptomatic for mild intoxications. In the long-term abuser, specific management for substance abuse may be in order. Severe intoxication requires specific management of the hyperthermia and the seizures.

Bibliography

Campbell GR: An Illustrated Guide to Some Poisonous Plants and Animals of Florida. Englewood, FL, Pineapple Press, 1983.

Hardin JW, Arena JM: Human Poisoning from Native and Cultivated Plants. Durham, NC, Duke University Press, 1974.

Huffman DM, Tiffany LH, Knaphus G: Mushrooms and Other Fungi of the Midcontinental United States. Ames, Iowa State University Press, 1989.

Lampe KF, McCann MA: Handbook of Poisonous and Injurious Plants. Chicago, American Medical Association, 1985.

Lincoff G, Mitchel DH: Toxic and Hallucinogenic Mushroom Poisoning. New York, Van Nostrand Reinhold, 1977.

125.4 Plant Poisoning

DEFINITION AND ETIOLOGY. Many plants have responded to the challenge for survival by evolving chemical toxins and irritants to fend off browsing animals. Many of these compounds are extracted and purified for use as drugs in combating human disease, e.g., digitalis, belladonna, and curare. Many of these compounds also cause disease as a result of inadvertent ingestion or contact. The numbers are so large that only the most common can be listed (Table 125–2) and these with limited detail. Generally plant toxins pose the greatest hazard for young children and visitors new to an environment. Most native residents have absorbed a body of folklore that identifies hazardous plants.

The outcome of most plant poisonings is dose related. Toxin concentrations vary with season, the maturity of the plant, and geographic origin. Not all parts of a plant need be toxic. In many areas methods of food preparation have been evolved to detoxify the plant material. The processing of bitter manioc, *Manihot utilissima*, is one example. Rapid, inexpensive transportation of fresh foodstuffs, coupled with a keen interest in culinary experimentation, has greatly enhanced the possible exposure to toxic plants.

In addition to plant toxins, mycotoxins and external and internal environmental contaminants can cause disease. Pesticide residues pose the most common hazard, but other adulterants are known.

CLINICAL MANAGEMENT. There is a great individual variability in response to some plant toxins. Also, some reactions are allergic and depend on individual development of hypersensitivity. Hayfever and *Rhus* dermatitis (poison ivy sensitivity) are perhaps the most common examples. This too, has changed with the sophistication of food delivery systems and the palate. A new generation of grocery store check-out clerks has discovered mango sensitivity dermatitis.

The range of toxins present in various plants is so great that there are no really useful general rules concerning the management of plant poisonings except that prevention is always more effective than treatment.

The most useful clinical separations of plant poisonings are those due to plant toxins causing contact dermatitis, those causing allergic sensitivity, and those responsible for internal or systemic poisoning.

MYCOTOXINS

Aspergillus flavus. Aflatoxins resulting from contamination of peanuts with this fungus are believed to be a cause of the high incidence of primary cancer of the liver in the indigenous inhabitants of Africa and Asia (Chapter 12). Prevention of ingestion of this toxin is the only "treatment" available.

Claviceps purpurea. This fungus, which infects rye, wheat, and other grains, produces ergotism. Its lysergic acid diethylamide–like fraction may produce hallucinogenic visions, whereas other alkaloids produce contraction of smooth muscle. Symptoms of toxicity include vomiting, diarrhea, abdominal pain, cold extremities, claudication, ischemic peripheral

Text continued on page 889

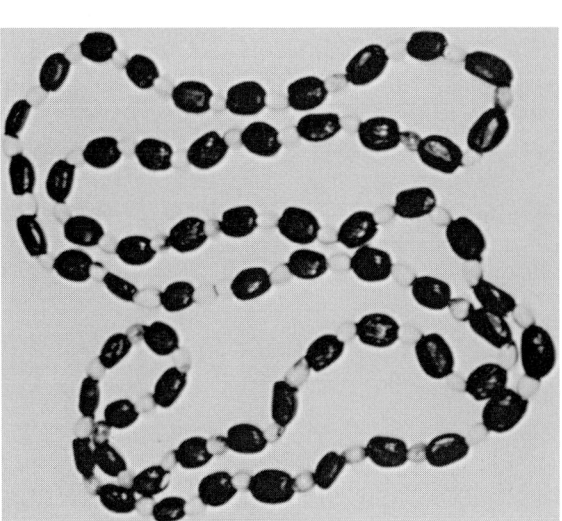

Figure 125–1. Necklace made from the toxic castor bean (*Ricinus communis*) (small, light-colored bean) and Job's tears (*Coix lacryma-jobi*) seeds, which are nontoxic. (Courtesy of Julia Morton.)

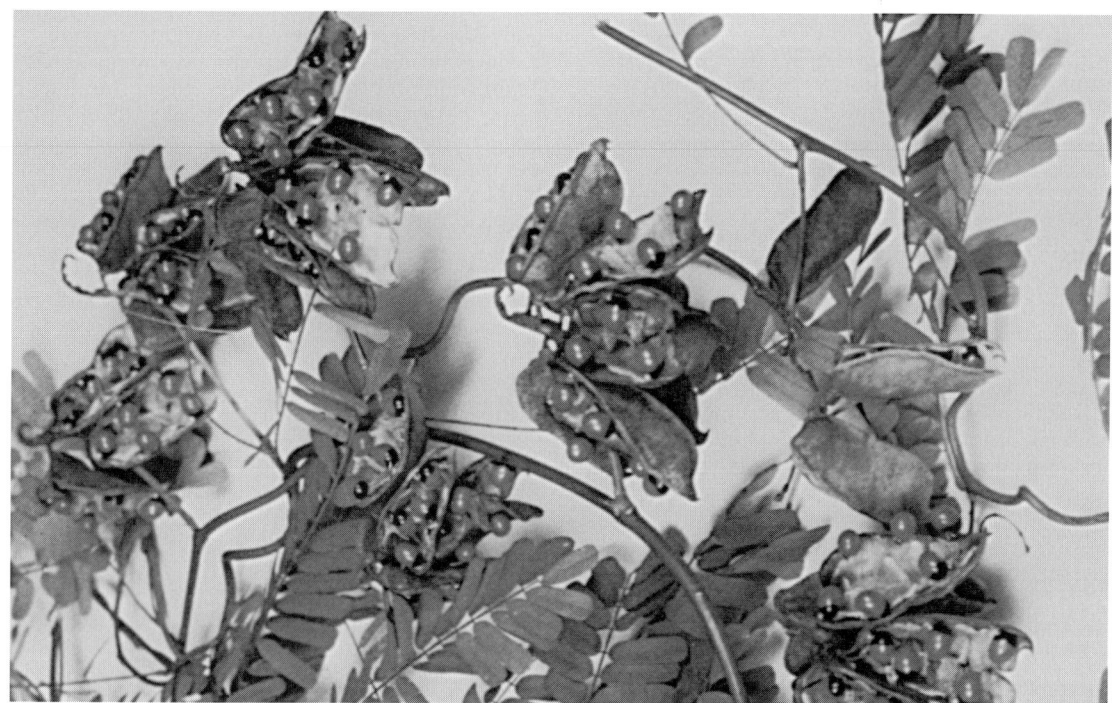

Figure 125–2. Rosary pea *(Abrus precatorius)* is toxic when ingested. (Courtesy of Julia Morton.)

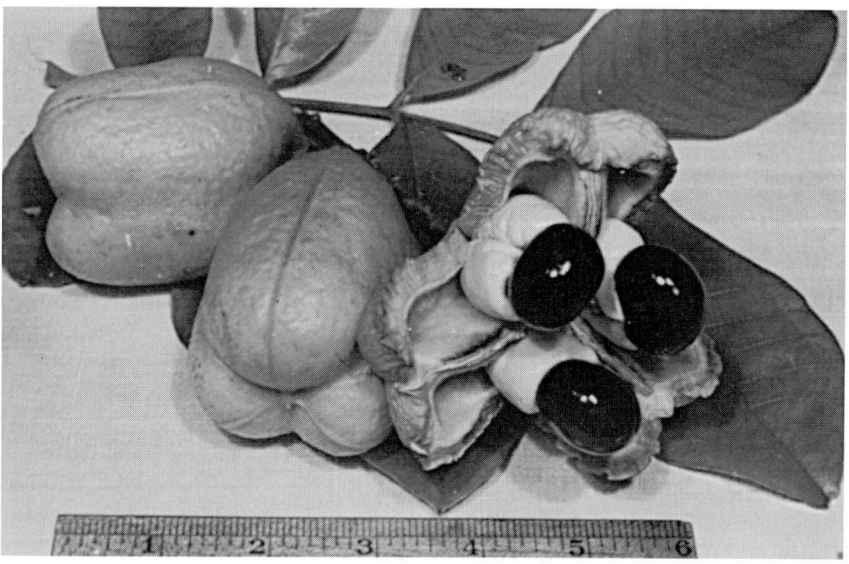

Figure 125–3. Akee *(Blighia sapida).* (From Morton K, Morton J: Fifty Tropical Fruits of Nassau. Text House, FL, 1946. By permission.)

TABLE 125–2. Table of Common Toxic Plants

Toxic Plants	Clinical Manifestations	Guidelines for Therapy
Dermatitis-Producing Plants—Examples Include:		
Mechanical Injury		
Yucca (Spanish bayonet)		
Zygophyllaceae		
Tribulus terrestris (puncture vine)		
Irritants and Allergens—Examples Include:		
Anacardaceae		
Anacardium occidentale (cashew nut)	Irritation and vesiculation as well as purgative effect if ingested.	Corticosteroid creams and lotions.
Nut shell oil contains cardol, cardanol, anacardic acid		
Mangifera indica (mango)	Irritant and allergic—*mango dermatitis*.	Corticosteroid creams and lotions.
Foliage, sap, and skin of the unripe fruit contain cardanol-like compound		
Rhus (Toxicodendron) radicans (poison ivy)	Irritation and vesiculation.	Corticosteroid creams and lotions.
Leaves and stem contain substance similar to cardanol		
Other *Rhus* species		
Araceae		
Dieffenbachia species	Irritation of the skin. If ingested, burning of the mouth and swelling of the tongue. In severe poisoning, convulsions, coma, and death from uremia.	If ingested, gastric lavage or emesis and symptomatic treatment.
All parts except fruit contain calcium oxalate and other toxic principles		Corticosteroid creams and lotions; antihistamines orally.
Related genera that may cause less severe injury:		
Philodendron species		
Alocasia (elephant ear) species		
Monstera (Swiss cheese) species		
Euphorbiaceae		
Euphorbia species, e.g., *Euphorbia pulcherrima* (poinsettia)	Dermatitis and blistering, swelling of the face, rash, and burning eyes (if rubbed into the eye, may cause keratoconjunctivitis or uveitis).	Corticosteroid creams and lotions; antihistamines orally.
Latex in all parts		
Hippomane mancinella (manchineel)	Similar to above.	
All parts containing latex		
Hura polyandra (devil tree)	Dermatitis, keratoconjunctivitis.	
All parts containing sap		
Ricinus communis (castor bean)	Dermatitis (in sensitive individuals), in addition to other toxic effects if ingested.	
Entire plant is poisonous (Fig. 125–1)		
Photosensitization (inflammation of any exposed, highly vascularized area of the skin)		
Verbenaceae		
Lantana camara (wild sage)	Photosensitization, in addition to clinical features of atropine-like poisoning if ingested (see Neuromuscular Poisons).	
Narcotic Poisons—Examples Include:		
Amaryllidaceae		
Boophone disticha (gifbol)	*Buphanine poisoning.* This presents as acute drunkenness. There is rapid onset of ataxia, giddiness, and mydriasis. Patient is initially talkative and later subdued, becoming stuporous, and coma supervenes. Death occurs from respiratory failure.	Gastric lavage with activated charcoal added to the water. Symptomatic treatment.
Bulb contains alkaloid buphanine (like hyoscine)		
Celastraceae		
Catha edulis (khat, wild tea)	*Khat poisoning.* Leaves are chewed or infused and are an inebriant narcotic. Effects are initially stimulative and later depressive. Subject is often excessively polite but later becomes divorced from reality and deteriorates mentally.	Treatment of drug addiction.
Leaves contain cathine, cathinine, and cathidine		
Cannabaceae		
Cannabis sativa (cannabinol, cannabidiol)	Causes cerebral stimulation, later depression, and in some cases, delirious rages. Intoxication may cause death from cardiac failure.	Treatment of drug addiction.
Leaves at top of plant		
Solanaceae		
Datura stramonium (jimsonweed, thorn apple)	Mydriasis, thirst, dry mouth, headache, rapid pulse, high blood pressure, hallucinations, delirium, coma, and death.	Gastric lavage with activated charcoal, emesis, pilocarpine, and sedation.
Unripe seed pods contain alkaloids hyoscyamine and scopolamine		

Table continued on following page

TABLE 125–2. Table of Common Toxic Plants *Continued*

Toxic Plants	Clinical Manifestations	Guidelines for Therapy
Narcotic Poisons—Examples Include:		
Nicotiana species (tobacco) Nicotine	Poisoning has occurred through use of nicotine-containing insecticide. Manifestations include vomiting, diarrhea, muscular weakness, irregular pulse, palpitations, and death from respiratory paralysis.	Gastric lavage with potassium permanganate added. Tannin (which binds nicotine by forming nicotine tannate).
Rivea corymbusa, Ipomoea, morning glory seeds	Hallucinogen similar to LSD but not as potent.	Treatment of addiction.
Solanum species (including potato skin not covered by earth and immature sprouting) Potatoes contain solanine	Manifestations of intoxication are nausea and vomiting, ataxia, hallucinations, drowsiness, and dilatation of the pupils.	Gastric lavage with addition of activated charcoal. Symptomatic treatment.
Neuromuscular Poisons—Examples Include:		

Leguminosae
  Lathyrus sativus (pea)
    Seeds contain alkaloid
	Lathyrism. Onset is slow, suggesting that the toxin is cumulative. Outbreaks have been described in India and elsewhere. Larger-than-usual amounts of the pea consumed over a period of 6 mo lead to abrupt or insidious onset of spastic paralysis in the lower limbs of (usually) young males. Signs are thought to be due to damage to pyramidal tracts and motor nerves.	Cumulative poison—neurologic changes are irreversible.

Loganiaceae
  Gelsemium sempervirens (yellow jessamine)
    All parts, especially root and nectar, contain alkaloids that depress and paralyze motor nerve endings
	Mydriasis, sweating, weakness, impaired speech, ataxia, asphyxia, and death.	Gastric lavage, atropine, and supportive treatment.

Strychnos nux-vomica All parts contain alkaloids	Signs of strychnine poisoning; constriction of the throat, chest, and abdomen; involuntary muscle spasms; miosis; convulsions; asphyxia; and death.	Gastric lavage with activated charcoal and symptomatic treatment.

Meliaceae
  Melia azedarach (chinaberry or syringa)
    Alkaloids in fruit and bark
	Vomiting and diarrhea, excitement, sweating, mydriasis, paralysis, and asphyxiation.	Gastric lavage and symptomatic treatment.

Ranunculaceae
  Aconitum napellus (monkshood)
    All parts (especially roots and seeds)
	Nausea and vomiting, burning of the mouth and pharynx, numbness, paralysis, difficulty with breathing, convulsions, and death.	Atropine and symptomatic treatment.

Verbenaceae
  Lantana camara (wild sage)
    All parts, especially unripe beans
	Produce symptoms of atropine-like poisoning, vomiting and diarrhea, dilatation (later constriction) of pupils, muscular weakness, coma, and death; photosensitization dermatitis.	Gastric lavage (or emesis) and symptomatic and supportive treatment.

Toxins Producing Purgation and Later Systemic Effects		

Ericaceae
  Rhododendron (azaleas) species
    All parts toxic; andromedotoxin
	Salivation, lacrimation, vomiting, hypotension, slowing of pulse, paralysis, and convulsions.	Gastric lavage with activated charcoal, atropine, and antihypotensive drugs.

Euphorbiaceae
  Euphorbia species
    All parts contain latex euphorbon
	Dermatitis and, if ingested, diarrhea, vomiting, coma, and death.	Gastric lavage and symptomatic treatment.

Hippomane mancinella (manchineel) All parts are toxic, especially fruit; toxic principle resembles alkaloid physostigmine	Abdominal pain, vomiting, diarrhea, and reportedly death.	Gastric lavage with activated charcoal; symptomatic and supportive treatment.
Hura polyandra (devil tree) All parts, particularly seeds and sap, contain hitrine, crepitine, and hurin	Ingested seeds produce nausea, vomiting, abdominal pain, bloody diarrhea, coma, convulsions, and death.	Same as above.
Jatropha curcas (Barbados nut) Contains curcin and oil	Nausea, vomiting, abdominal pain, bloody diarrhea, coma, convulsions, and even death.	Same as above.
Ricinus communis (castor bean) Whole plant toxic, ricin (highest in seeds), an allergen, and purgative oil (seeds)	Allergic dermatitis. Ingested seeds, if chewed, produce nausea, vomiting, diarrhea (bloody), mydriasis, convulsions, and death in uremia and/or jaundice in 3 to 7 days.	Same as above.

TABLE 125–2. Table of Common Toxic Plants *Continued*

Toxic Plants	Clinical Manifestations	Guidelines for Therapy
Leguminosae		
Abrus precatorius (rosary pea, black-eyed Susan) (Fig. 125–2) Seeds contain abrin, abrine, hemagglutinin, and abralin (a glycoside)	If bitten or drilled (as in necklaces), seeds, when ingested, may after a latent period produce nausea, vomiting, diarrhea, weakness, abdominal pain, rapid pulse, and rectal bleeding or other evidence of a bleeding diathesis, as well as hemolytic anemia, oliguria, and uremia.	Gastric lavage with activated charcoal, symptomatic and supportive treatment. Blood transfusion and dialysis when indicated.
Laburnum species All parts, particularly seeds and bark, contain alkaloid cytisine	Abdominal pain, diarrhea and vomiting, excitement, mydriasis, incoordination, convulsions, respiratory depression, and death.	Gastric lavage with activated charcoal or emesis.
Wisteria sinensis (wisteria) Pods contain resin and glycoside wisterin	Severe diarrhea, vomiting, and collapse.	Gastric lavage or emesis, and symptomatic treatment.
Liliaceae		
Colchicum autumnale (autumn crocus) Whole plant contains alkaloid colchicine	Thirst, mydriasis, nausea and vomiting, diarrhea (bloody), oliguria, weakness, difficulty with breathing, and death.	Gastric lavage with activated charcoal; symptomatic and supportive treatment (assisted respiration and dialysis when indicated).
Phytolaccaceae		
Phytolacca americana (pokeweed) Mature leaves, stems, roots, and seeds contain alkaloid and saponin	Vomiting and diarrhea, abdominal pain, salivation, respiratory paralysis, and death.	Gastric lavage with activated charcoal; symptomatic treatment.
Umbelliferae		
Cicuta maculata (water hemlock) Often mistaken for parsnips; roots contain resin and cicutoxins	Abdominal pain, vomiting, convulsions, respiratory paralysis, and death.	Gastric lavage or emesis, and symptomatic treatment.
Conium maculatum (poison parsley) All parts contain alkaloid coniine	Abdominal pain, vomiting, diarrhea, muscular weakness, respiratory depression, convulsions, and death.	Gastric lavage or emesis, and symptomatic treatment.
Toxins Producing Systemic Effects		
Cardiac		
Apocyanaceae		
Nerium oleander (oleander) All parts contain glycosides resembling digitalis, oleandrin, and neriin	Dermatitis and, if ingested, dilated pupils, nausea, vomiting, bloody diarrhea, cardiac irregularity, labored respiration, coma, paralysis, and death.	Gastric lavage; emesis; in the main, symptomatic, and supportive treatment with drugs to combat irregularity of cardiac rhythm.
Thevetia peruviana (yellow oleander) All parts, particularly the seed, contain cardiac glycosides thevetin, thevetoxin, neriifolin, peruvoside, and ruvoside	Clinical manifestations are similar to those with *Nerium.*	Same as above.
Papaveraceae		
Argemone mexicana Seeds contain a glycoside, sanguinarine	*Epidemic dropsy.* This is seen in India (Bengal) and also in Mauritius, Fiji, and South Africa. Seeds may contaminate mustard seed oil. Toxin causes dilatation and increased permeability of capillaries and interferes with pyruvic acid oxidation. Characteristics of the disease are edema; dilatation of vessels in skin, subcutaneous tissues, and uveal tract (glaucoma); cardiac insufficiency; and liver abnormalities. Mortality rate may be 5–44%.	Bed rest, high-protein diet, vitamin supplements, and digitalis (but its action is variable); glaucoma may require surgical intervention.
Scrophulariaceae		
Digitalis purpurea Leaves, stem, and flowers contain glycoside	*Digitalis poisoning.* Leaves used medicinally, also in herbal tea. Manifestations of toxicity include nausea, psychiatric disturbances, cardiac arrhythmias, paresthesia, sometimes facial neuralgia, and death from cardiac arrhythmias and refractory hyperkalemia.	Gastric lavage or emesis, treatment of arrhythmias, and supportive treatment.

Table continued on following page

TABLE 125–2. Table of Common Toxic Plants *Continued*

Toxic Plants	Clinical Manifestations	Guidelines for Therapy
Liver and Pancreas		
Compositae		
Senecio burchelli (ragwort) All parts contain pyrrolizidine alkaloids	Seeds often contaminate wheat. Manifestations of toxicity may produce veno-occlusive disease of the liver, which has been described in Jamaica, Israel, Egypt, India, and South Africa. The acute stage of the disease is characterized by the sudden onset of abdominal distention with slight tenderness over the liver, which is smooth and slightly enlarged, acute ascites, and ankle edema. In the later stages, there is progressive liver failure, hematemesis (portal hypertension), and death. At autopsy, the liver shows centrilobular thrombosis, congestion, and nonportal fibrosis.	Admission to hospital for evaluation; "treatment" is prevention.
Euphorbiaceae		
Manihot esculenta (bitter cassava, manihot, tapioca) Root contains cyanogenic glucosides (normally leached out by boiling the root) *Prunus armemiaca* (apricot pits)	Possibly pancreatic calcification and goiter. *Manihot* is a pest-resistant high-yield crop that forms the staple diet for 10% of global caloric needs. It is in the areas where this plant forms the staple diet that the incidence of pancreatic calcification is highest. It has been incriminated as a cause of goiter and tropical ataxic neuropathy. Manifestations of acute toxicity (which might occur if cooking water is ingested) include convulsions, respiratory difficulty, and death from depression of cardiac and respiratory centers.	"Treatment" is prevention—adequate processing of food. In acute cases, gastric lavage with potassium permanganate (to neutralize hydrocyanic acid) and glucose (to retard the liberation of further acid).
Leguminosae		
Crotalaria fulva All parts contain alkaloid	Veno-occlusive disease of liver and lungs.	
Sapindaceae		
Blighia sapida (akee) Unripe fruit contains hypoglycine and hypoglycine A (Fig. 125–3)	*Vomiting sickness of Jamaica.* Six to 48 hours after ingestion, there is vomiting, followed by a period of drowsiness or sleep, after which the vomiting recurs. There is hypoglycemia (due to blocking of gluconeogenesis), often with coma and death. It is particularly severe in young children, in whom the speed of recognition and treatment often determines the outcome.	Emetic and intravenous glucose.
Abortifacients		
Euphorbiaceae		
Euphorbia species *Jatropha curcas* (purging nut)	May be inserted into the vagina. Nut is ingested.	Treatment of acute poisoning, as indicated above.
Leguminosone		
Abrus precatorius (rosary pea, black-eyed Susan) (see Toxins Producing Purgation)	A paste is made of the seeds, applied to a stick, and inserted into the vagina. (Subcutaneous administration can kill an animal or human in a few hours.)	Complications of an abortion and/or intoxication (e.g., renal shutdown) will require appropriate medical and gynecologic treatment.

gangrene, hypotension, compensatory bradycardia, headache, convulsions, and coma. Treatment is largely symptomatic and includes the use of analgesics and vasodilators.

Fusarium Species. These grow on grain stored in open fields in winter and produce the toxins responsible for toxic alimentary aleukia. The disease is characterized by necrotic rashes on the skin, leukopenia, agranulocytosis, necrosis, hemorrhages, and, ultimately, death.

Bibliography

Morton JF: Poisonous and injurious higher plants and fungi. *In* Tedeschi CG, Eckert WB, Tedeschi LG (eds): Forensic Medicine. Vol. 3, Environmental Hazards. Philadelphia, WB Saunders, 1977.
Mushroom poisoning (editorial). Lancet 2:351, 1980.
North P: Poisonous Plants and Fungi. London, Blandford Press, 1967.
Short ALK, Watling R, MacDonald MK, et al: Poisoning by *Cortinarius speciosissimus*. Lancet 2:942, 1980.
Watt JM, Breyer-Brandwijk MG: The Medicinal and Poisonous Plants of Southern and Eastern Africa. Edinburgh, Churchill Livingstone, 1962.

126 Animals Hazardous to Humans

General Principles

William A. Sodeman, Jr.

Humans' interaction with the rest of the animal kingdom has always been fraught with the possibilities of injury from either direct trauma or by venoms. The process of urbanization and cultivation had for many years reduced the opportunities for untoward interaction between humans and animals. Two circumstances have led to a resurgence of injury related to animals. The first, erratic in occurrence but not uncommon, is the temporary stress caused by natural cataclysm. Natural catastrophes, e.g., floods, storms, and droughts, tend to press humans and animals into uncommon juxtaposition. The second feature is the popularity of recreational visits to the diminishing natural environments. The numbers of people who engage in caving, diving, wilderness hiking, bird watching, photo safaris, and the like have undergone a remarkable increase, and with this comes increased exposure and increased numbers of untoward incidents. Previously uncommon or rare hazards have emerged as significant health problems.

126.1 Venomous Marine Animals

William A. Sodeman, Jr.

Venomous marine animals range worldwide. Relative numbers and varieties are greater in the warm waters of tropical and subtropical seas. Their clinical importance has undergone a recent and rather unexpected escalation. In the past, human exposure was limited by geography, because many venomous marine animals are abundant only in less populated areas. The predominant exposure had been occupational, usually among fishermen and professional divers.

There was a relatively limited recreational exposure. Currently professional and recreational diving has undergone a greater than geometric expansion in popularity, vastly increasing the exposure.

Much of the recreational diving focuses on marine reef environments rich in venomous species. A second feature is the change in access with easy travel opportunities to previously remote areas also rich in venomous marine species. The consequence is a greatly increased incidence of injury and fatality from venomous marine animals.

Toxin-containing marine protozoans abound, but because their expression is as a food chain poisoning they are discussed in Chapter 125.1 under shellfish poisoning, ciguatera poisoning, and other poisonings.

INVERTEBRATES. Venomous invertebrates are found in five phyla: the Porifera, the Coelenterata, the Mollusca, the Annelida, and the Echinodermata. Relatively few of the many thousands of species in these five phyla pose a hazard to humans.

Sponges, Porifera. Sponges produce a number of toxins that may be retained on the surface of the sponge or released into the water. These prove an effective defense, and few sponges are eaten by higher forms. Toxic sponges are widespread and not necessarily tropical. The most common toxic sponges and their distribution are listed in Table 126–1. Human exposure is a result of handling or otherwise contacting the sponge with abraded skin. Russell reports a case with both local and systemic symptoms after handling sponges. Local symptoms include pain, pruritus, and swelling of the skin. The papules may go on to vesiculate. Left untreated, the dermatitis may be unusually persistent. Systemic complaints include malaise, weakness, and syncope. Nausea and paresthesia are described also.

Sponge fisherman's disease, an occupational problem among Mediterranean fishermen, is associated with a coelenterate living in close association with the sponges rather than a Porifera toxin.

Coelenterates, Coelenterata. Three classes, the Hydrozoa (fire coral, the Portuguese man-of-war, and the stinging hydroids), Scyphozoa (true jellyfish), and Anthozoa (the true corals and sea anemones) all have venomous forms. Injuries are produced by nematocysts, individual stinging units, which when triggered inject minute quantities of venom into the integument of an intruder. The severity and the consequences of coelenterate stings depend primarily on the species involved in the sting but also vary with the anatomic site of the sting, the total number of nematocysts involved,

TABLE 126–1. Toxic Marine Sponges

Name	Common Name	Distribution
Fibulia nolitangere (Duchassaing and Michelotti)	Do-Not-Touch-Me sponge	West Indies
Microciona prolifera (Ellis and Solander)	Red moss, oyster sponge	Cape Cod to North Florida
Haliclona viridis (Duchassaing and Michelotti)	Green sponge	West Indies
Tedania ignis (Duchassaing and Michelotti)	Fire sponge	West Indies
Tedania nigrescens (Schmidt)		West Indies
Neofibularia mordens Hartman	Australia stinging sponge	Australia

Compiled from Russell, 1971; Campbell, 1983; Halstead, 1988.

and the duration of contact. Nematocysts are located frequently on the tentacles, and one approach to clinical measurement of the exposure is the length of the tentacles involved in the contact.

Hydrozoa. *Aglaophenia cupressina* Lamouroux, *Lytocarpus philippinus* (Kirchenpauer), and *Rhizophysa eysenhardti* Gegenbaur are seaweed-like organisms with, collectively, a worldwide distribution (Table 126–2). Skin contact produces a painful papulovesicular dermatitis that may last for days.

Millepora alcornis (Linnaeus), *Millepora dichotoma* (Forskål), and *Millepora complanata* (Lamarck) are referred to commonly as fire corals. The various species are found in tropical waters worldwide (Table 126–2). They produce primarily skin irritation with painful pruritic papules.

Physalia physalis (Linnaeus), the Portuguese man-of-war, is a colonial hydroid often mistaken for a true jellyfish. It has a wide geographic distribution in the Atlantic Ocean and the Mediterranean Sea, and a related species, *Physalia utriculus* (La Martinière), has an equally wide Indo-Pacific distribution (Table 126–2). They are more plentiful in the tropics, but they can be found as far north as Canada, the Hebrides, and Japan. *Gonionemus vertens* (Agassiz) and *Olindioides formosa* Goto (Table 126–2) are toxic jellyfish-like hydroids. Envenomation causes painful cutaneous lesions and in some cases systemic reactions. Contact with the tentacles produces lines of papules, which are extremely painful. These may vesiculate and heal with pigmentation. Muscle spasms and pain may appear in the involved extremity.

With extensive exposure, systemic reactions may occur. Nausea, vomiting, headaches, vertigo, and weakness are all described. Pain and muscle spasm, particularly in the back, occur but are less frequent. Lacrimation, rhinorrhea, pain on respiration, and arrhythmia may occur. Neurotoxins are suspected to be involved.

Treatment of stings involves three separate steps. The first goal is to arrest the envenomation by inactivation and/or removal of the nematocysts. Next is to treat the local reaction, pain, and swelling. The third step, when necessary, is the treatment of systemic reactions. Prompt removal of any adhering tentacles will reduce envenomation. These should be lifted away rather than brushed across the skin, with care that the rescuing finger does not get stung. A seawater rinse, not a scrub, may wash away loose nematocysts. Prompt application of vinegar or dilute (3 to 10%) acetic acid will inactivate the nematocysts. Methyl alcohol or ethyl alcohol, which in the past has been the recommended treatment, should be avoided. Alcohol has now been shown to stimulate nematocyst discharge. Freshwater is also a stimulant for nematocyst discharge. Removal of adherent nematocysts is a problem with a number of possible solutions that often have to be adapted to available resources. Rubbing the affected area with wet sand, a cloth, or vigorous washing is likely to cause further discharge of nematocysts and, thus, should be avoided. Dusting the area with fine sand, baking soda, powder, or flour and then scraping the caked powder off with the dull back edge of a knife has proven effective and safe. Application of aerosol shaving cream, then shaving the nematocysts off with a safety razor, is a handy alternative method of removal. A host of other agents are part of the folklore of treatment, including papain, ammonia, lime juice, and boric acid. None have had any systematic study.

Relief of pain and swelling may be facilitated with topical application of steroid cream and/or anesthetic creams or aerosols. Antihistamines in some cases will reduce the swelling. Occasionally the pain will be severe enough to require narcotic analgesics. Secondary infection may follow vesiculation, particularly if the sting has occurred in a grossly contaminated environment. Topical or systemic antibiotics may

TABLE 126–2. Venomous Coelenterates (Representative List)

Name	Common Name	Distribution
Hydroids		
Aglaophenia cupressinia Lamouroux	Stinging hydroid	Indian Ocean
Lytocarpus philippinus (Kirchenpauer)	Feather hydroid	Tropical Pacific, Indian, and Atlantic oceans, Mediterranean Sea
Rhizophysa eysenhardti		Tropical oceans
Millepora alcornis Linnaeus	Fire coral	Caribbean Sea
Millepora dichotoma Forskål	Fire coral	Red Sea, Indo-Pacific
Millepora complanata Lamarck	Fire coral	West Indies
Physalia physalis (Linnaeus)	Portuguese man-of-war	Tropical Atlantic Ocean, Mediterranean Sea
Physalia utriculus (La Martinière)	Portuguese man-of-war	Indo-Pacific
Gonionemus vertens (Agassiz)	Orange-striped jellyfish	Temperate Pacific and Atlantic oceans, Mediterranean Sea
Olindioides formosa Goto	Stinging medusa	Japan
Jellyfish		
Chironex fleckeri Southcott	Deadly sea wasp	Northeastern Australia
Chiropsalmus quadrigatus Haeckel	Sea wasp	Northern Australia, Indian Ocean, Philippine Islands
Chiropsalmus quadrumanus (Müller)	Sea wasp	North Australia, Indian Ocean, Atlantic Coast—Carolina to Brazil
Carukia barnesi Southcott		Australia—Queensland coast
Carybdea rastoni Haacke	Sea wasp	Tropical Pacific Ocean—Southern Japan to Australia
Carybdea alata Reynaud	Sea wasp	Tropical Indian, Pacific, and Atlantic oceans
Cyanea capillata (Linnaeus)	Giant jellyfish	Atlantic and Pacific basins—arctic to tropics
Cassiopea xamachana Bigelow	Upside down jellyfish	Caribbean Basin, Gulf of Mexico
Anthozoa		
Acropora palmata (Lamarck)	Elk horn coral	Florida, Bahamas, West Indies
Various sea anemones in the families: Actiniidae Actinodendronidae Actinodiscidae Aliciidae Hormathiidae Renillidae Sagartiidae Stoichactiidae Zoanthidae		

Compiled from Russell, 1971; Campbell, 1983; Halstead, 1988.

be in order. Muscle spasms can be alleviated with intravenous calcium gluconate, 10 mL of a 10% solution. Evidence of toxicity affecting the cardiovascular system or the pulmonary system may require the use of epinephrine or intervention with cardiopulmonary resuscitation (CPR).

Scyphozoa. Several of the true jellyfish are distinguished as

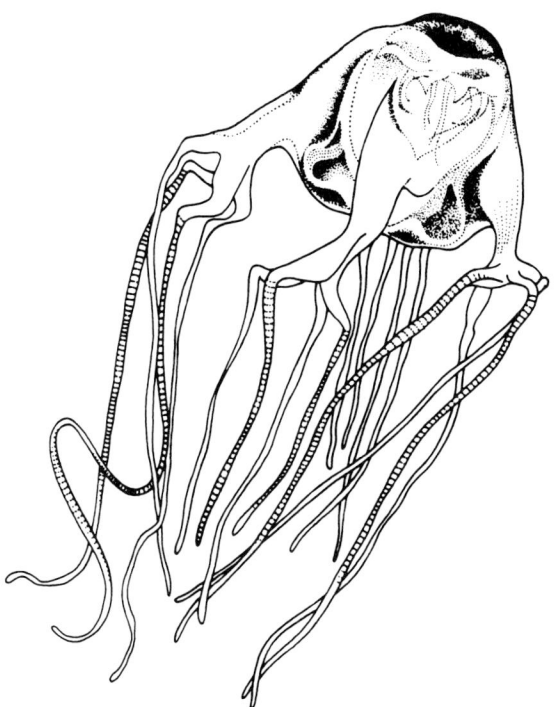

Figure 126–1. *Chironex fleckeri*, although usually associated with the north coast of Australia, can be found in the Atlantic Ocean, the Gulf of Mexico, and Caribbean Sea as well. (Courtesy of A. A. Fischer, M.D.: Atlas of Aquatic Dermatology. Copyright 1978 American Cyanamid Company, Lederle Laboratories Division. Reproduced by permission.)

lethal for humans. Many others, although not lethal, cause painful skin lesions and disturbing systemic reactions. *Chironex fleckeri* Southcott, the deadly sea wasp (Fig. 126–1), is distributed on the Australian coastline. Other sea wasps, *Carybdea rastoni* Haacke and several species of *Chiropsalmus*, are found in all tropical oceans. *Cassiopea* species are found in the Caribbean Sea and the Gulf of Mexico. *Cyanea capillata* (Linnaeus), which grows to giant proportions, may be found in arctic as well as tropical waters in both ocean basins. A number of other stinging species are known (Table 126–2).

Chironex fleckeri Southcott is a small, up to 5 inches in length, undistinguished jellyfish with lethal potential (Fig. 126–1). *Chiropsalmus quadrigatus* Haeckel and *Chiropsalmus quadrumanus* (Müller) are only slightly less dangerous and far more widespread in distribution. The sting is followed by almost immediate pain, then swelling, which proceeds to vesiculation and then to necrosis with further breakdown. The pain is agonizing. There can be rapid progression through muscle spasm, pulmonary edema, vascular collapse, and respiratory failure with death. Although patients may survive as long as 2 to 3 hours, death can be rapid—1 minute or less. An antivenin is manufactured in Australia and, if available, can be lifesaving. Otherwise, treatment follows that outlined above.

Carukia barnesi Southcott is responsible for the Irukandji syndrome, a severe but not fatal envenomation, that is reported from Australia. The sting appears as an erythematous patch with localized pain that increases in severity and spreads to involve the back and extremities. There may be systemic symptoms with fever and tachycardia. Respiratory symptoms with cough, tightness, mucoid sputum, and hemoptysis are distinguishing features.

Many jellyfish stings remain unidentified as to causative organism. Repeated stings can give rise to hypersensitivity with the possibility of anaphylaxis.

Anthozoa. This class includes the true corals, sea anemones, and sea pansies. Many species are toxic, and the geographic distribution collectively spares no marine environment (Table 126–2).

The toxicity associated with coral cuts is poorly characterized. Cuts are associated frequently with a stinging sensation. These cuts break down frequently to form painful ulcerations that are slow to heal and tend to recur. Treatment is scrupulous care of the sort that would be applied to any laceration.

Sea anemones and sea pansies are highly variable in their toxicity, and many cause only mild stinging. Severe reactions do occur, with local edema and necrosis that result in slow-healing ulcers. Relatively nonspecific systemic symptoms are reported. Treatment is careful cleansing, protection of the affected area, and specific treatment of secondary infection.

Echinoderms, Echinodermata. Venomous echinoderms are found among the Asteroidea (starfishes), Echinoidea (sea urchins), and Holothuroidea (sea cucumbers). Whereas many creatures in this phylum have proven toxic on ingestion, relatively few are venomous for humans.

Asteroidea. Only one starfish, *Acanthaster planci* (Linnaeus) (Table 126–3) has proven venomous, although several other species have produced dermatitis on contact. This starfish, commonly known as the crown of thorns, grows to a large size. It is covered with large spines that in turn are covered by an integument containing venom-producing glands. Envenomation is a result of wounding by contact with the spines. Wounds are painful with associated swelling and erythema. Systemic reactions include nausea, vomiting, numbness, and paralysis. There is no specific antidote, and treatment is first aid and supportive care.

Echinoidea. Many sea urchins are known for their venomous stings (Table 126–3). There are two venom delivery systems. The first involves the long needle-like spines of the

TABLE 126–3. Venomous Echinoderms (Representative List)

Name	Common Name	Distribution
Starfish		
Acanthaster planci (Linnaeus)	Crown of thorns starfish	Indo-Pacific
Sea Urchins		
Diadema antillarum Philippi	Black urchin	West Indies
Diadema setosum (Leske)	Black sea urchin	Indo-Pacific, China, Japan
Paracentrotus lividus Lamarck	Sea urchin	Atlantic coast of Europe and West Africa
Araeosoma thetidis (Clark)	Tam o'shanter urchin	Australia, New Zealand
Toxopneustes pileolus (Lamarck)	Sea urchin	Indo-Pacific, Japan
Tripneustes ventricosus (Lamarck)	White sea urchin	West Indies, Tropical South Atlantic Ocean
Sea Cucumbers		
Cucumaria echinata Von Marenzeller		Japan
Holothuria argus (Jaeger)	Tiger fish	Indo-Pacific
Euapta lappa (Müller)		West Indies

Compiled from Russell, 1971; Campbell, 1983; Halstead, 1988.

families Diadematidea, Echinidea, and Echinothuridae. These spines can contain venom that is released after the spine penetrates the integument. The second method of venom delivery involves pedicellariae. These are seizing organs found scattered among the spines on the surface of the urchin. They come in many varieties and are utilized in taxonomic classification of urchins. The jaws of the pedicellariae clamp onto prey and maintain their hold even if broken free from the urchin. Venomous pedicellariae continue envenomation even when broken off and must be removed promptly.

Penetration of spines is associated with the release of a colored fluid (violet-purple) that stains the wound and is a good clinical marker of possible envenomation. With an envenomating sting, another diagnostic sign is pain, which develops quickly, and is out of proportion to the trauma of the sting. Pain is followed by the development of edematous swelling and redness. In addition to local reactions, partial paralysis of an involved extremity, facial edema, and arrhythmia have been reported. Generally the pain will subside after several hours, although the staining of the wound may persist for days. Secondary infection does occur and may require debridement, drainage, and/or antibiotics.

Pedicellarial stings have been associated with local complaints of pain and somewhat more frightening systemic reactions, including paralysis, aphonia, respiratory distress, and occasionally death. The pain will subside in about 1 hour, but paralysis persists often for several hours longer.

Treatment is largely symptomatic. There are no specific antidotes. Two therapeutic features specific to sea urchins are the need to inspect the bite carefully and promptly remove any adherent pedicellariae to terminate the envenomation. Spines may break off in the wound also. There is much folklore concerning the need or lack of need for their removal. Unlike pedicellariae, there is no apparent need for urgent extraction of spines, but they may require surgical removal at a later date.

Holothuroidea. Sea cucumbers are spineless echinoderms that are wormlike in appearance. Several species (Table 126–3) are equipped for defense with organs of Cuvier. These tubules, derived from the respiratory tree, are filled with the toxin holothurin. The organs can be extruded from the body of the sea cucumber to cause release of holothurin into the water. Skin contact with this venom has caused dermatitis, and corneal contact has caused blindness in humans. The treatment is symptomatic.

Mollusca. Of the five classes of Mollusca only the gastropods and cephalopods harbor species venomous for humans. Shellfish are a common food item, and many more are poisonous than venomous. Some families, particularly the Muricidae, have well-developed poison glands but lack a mechanism for delivery of the venom. A number of species of the family Aplysiidae, nudibranchs or sea hares, feed on coelenterates and carry undischarged nematocysts, which they use for defense and predation. Contact with these animals can produce the coelenterate stings discussed above.

Conidae. Cone shells are much sought after gastropod mollusks. More than 400 species are described, and they are found worldwide in warm water oceans and seas. They are carnivorous predators with highly developed venom delivery systems used in hunting and defense. Eight species are lethal for humans (Table 126–4). Many of the remaining species are capable of inflicting painful stings.

Venom is delivered by injection through a modified radular tooth, which is hollow, barbed, and carries an attached venom sac (Fig. 126–2). The cone shell is a desirable collector's item, and stings are associated usually with handling during collection. The best characterized component of venom is a neurotoxin that has an effect on the neuromuscu-

TABLE 126–4. Venomous Mollusks

Name	Common Name	Distribution
Cone Shells		
Conus aulicus Linnaeus	Court cone	Polynesia
Conus geographus Linnaeus	Geographer cone	Indo-Pacific
Conus gloriamaris Hwass	Glory-of-the-sea	Philippines, Malaysia
Conus magus Linnaeus		Indo-Pacific
Conus marmoreus Linnaeus	Marbled cone	Polynesia
Conus striatus Linnaeus	Striated cone	Indo-Pacific
Conus textile Linnaeus	Textile cone	Indo-Pacific
Conus tulipa Linnaeus	Tulip cone	Indo-Pacific
Pteropod		
Creseis acicula Rang	Sea butterfly	Atlantic and Pacific oceans
Cephalopods		
Octopus maculosus Hoyle	Blue-ringed octopus	Indo-Pacific, Japan

Compiled from Russell, 1971; Campbell, 1983; Halstead, 1988.

lar junction and causes paralysis of skeletal muscle. There are other venom components that vary from species to species.

The sting results in prompt pain at the site of puncture. There is associated swelling and erythema. The perception of the pain is highly variable from person to person. Neurologic symptoms appear promptly. Sensory symptoms include numbness and paresthesias. Motor symptoms include incoordination and muscular paralysis. In mild envenomation only weakness may be manifest as a motor change. In the case of severe envenomation paralysis will progress to become generalized. Deep tendon reflexes will disappear. Aphonia, dysphagia, diplopia, and blurred vision all may occur. Fatal cases proceed to coma and death from cardiac or respiratory failure. Nausea is an early complaint, but there is little else in the way of smooth muscle dysfunction. Recovery is slow and in the cases of serious envenomation may take weeks before the return of full muscular function without fatigue.

Whereas most of the attention has focused on the eight cones that are lethal for humans, i.e., *Conus aulicus* Linnaeus, *C. geographus* Linnaeus, *C. gloriamaris* Hwass, *C. magus* Linnaeus, *C. marmoreus* Linnaeus, *C. striatus* Linnaeus, *C. textile* Linnaeus, and *C. tulipa* Linnaeus, the other cones are capable of producing a limited systemic reaction with nausea, weakness, and limited paralysis. Should these reactions occur while diving to collect shells, they can cause death by drowning. All live cone shells should be treated with care and respect as venomous animals.

Treatment is largely symptomatic. The curare-like effect of the neurotoxin may respond to the use of neostigmine. Maintenance of airway and provision of artificial ventilation may be required.

Pteropoda. The pteropod *Creseis acicula* Rang (Table 126–4) is a gastropod commonly called a sea butterfly. Contact with its needle-like shell has caused stings associated with a self-limited maculopapular dermatitis. Little is known concerning possible toxins in this organism. Treatment is symptomatic.

Cephalopoda. The cephalopods include cuttlefish, squid, and octopi, all of which utilize venom in the predation for food. Only the octopus is associated with envenomation in humans (Table 126–4). Fatalities and near-fatal serious envenomations have been associated only with *Octopus maculosus* Hoyle, the Australian blue-ringed octopus, in Australian waters. There is some taxonomic confusion, and several other

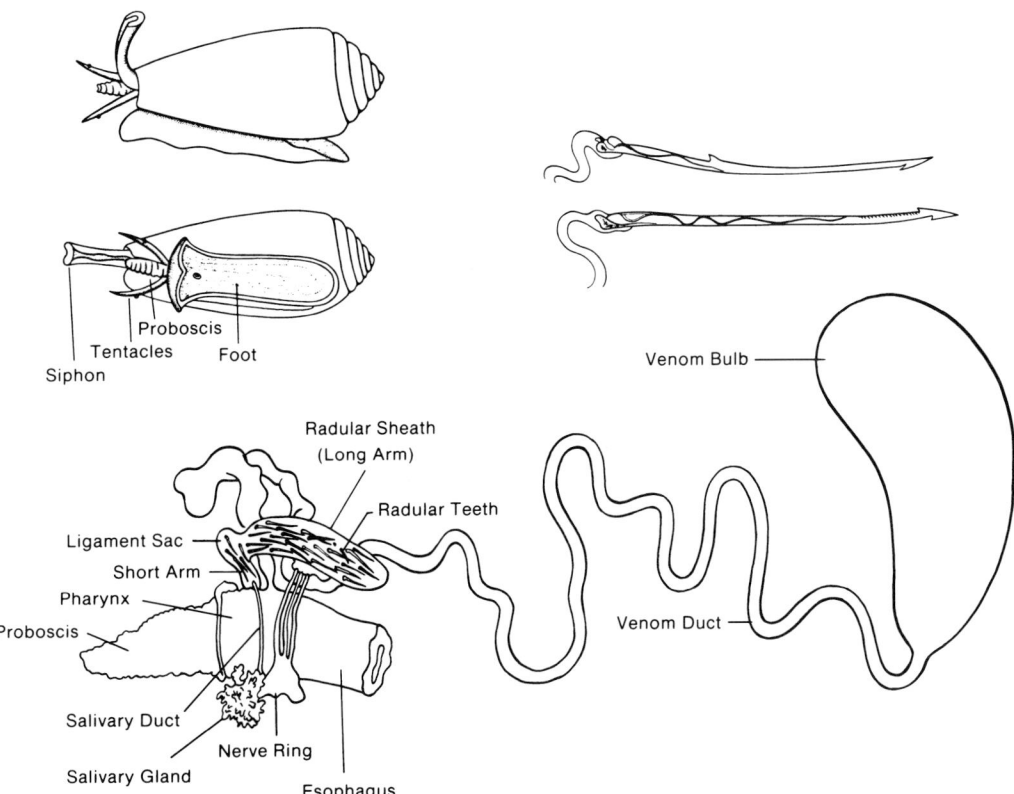

Figure 126–2. This general representation of the venom apparatus of *Conidae* is applicable to all species, whether or not toxic for humans. The armed, barbed tooth is held in the proboscis and thrust into the integument of prey or an attacker. (Courtesy of Bruce W. Halstead, M.D.: Poisonous and Venomous Marine Animals of the World, 2nd ed. Princeton, NJ, The Darwin Press, 1988.)

spotted octopi may be implicated also. There are a few reports of envenomation by other octopi, but none have been well studied.

Envenomation in humans is associated with a bite. The jaws of the octopus are beaklike and produce two puncture wounds. These bites bleed freely. Envenomation is associated with a rapidly spreading burning sensation. The wound site becomes edematous and erythematous. If the envenomation is severe, neurologic symptoms may occur. These may be both motor and sensory. Paralysis, difficulty with swallowing, and loss of equilibrium are described. In a well-documented fatality reported by Mabbet, the patient developed respiratory distress and was placed in a respirator, but died despite the treatment.

Treatment is symptomatic. Mild envenomations are self-limited. CPR measures may be lifesaving to permit severely bitten patients to reach medical facilities. Most envenomations are a result of handling the octopus, and caution is advised.

Flatworms, Platyhelminthes. The nemertean *Amphiporus lactifloreus* (Johnston), the ribbon worm, has a true venom apparatus, but human envenomation has not been described.

Roundworms, Annelida. Several polychaetes of the family Amphinomidea, the bristle worms (Table 126–5), have venom-containing setae, or bristles, which can extend and contract and are capable of penetrating skin (Fig. 126–3). The resulting painful dermatitis may be associated with secondary infection and gangrene. Treatment is symptomatic but must include the removal of any retained setae.

Several species of the family Glyceridae have biting jaws associated with venom glands. The bite of *Glycera dibranchiata*

Ehlers produces pain, swelling, and erythema. The wound heals over several days with gradual subsidence of symptoms.

VERTEBRATES

Fishes. There are over 200 species of marine fish known to be venomous, mainly shallow-water reef fish or inshore fish (Table 126–6). Many species are found off the coasts of California and Florida and in the Gulf of Mexico and the Caribbean. They include stingrays, scorpion fish, zebra fish, stonefish, weevers, toadfish, stargazers, certain sharks, catfish, and surgeon-fish. Ill effects result from puncture of the skin by spines and inoculation of venom, as occurs in the case of stingrays, scorpion fish, stonefish, stargazers, and various

TABLE 126–5. Venomous Roundworms

Name	Common Name	Distribution
Bristle Worms		
Chloeia flava (Pallas)	Sea-mouse	Indo-Pacific, Japan
Chloeia viridis Schmarda	Red-tipped bristle worm	Both coasts of tropical America
Eurythoë complanata (Pallas)	Orange bristle worm	Tropical worldwide
Glycera dibranchiata Ehlers	Blood worm	Canada to Carolina
Hermodice carunculata (Pallas)	Green bristle worm	West Indies, Florida

Compiled from Russell, 1971; Campbell, 1983; Halstead, 1988.

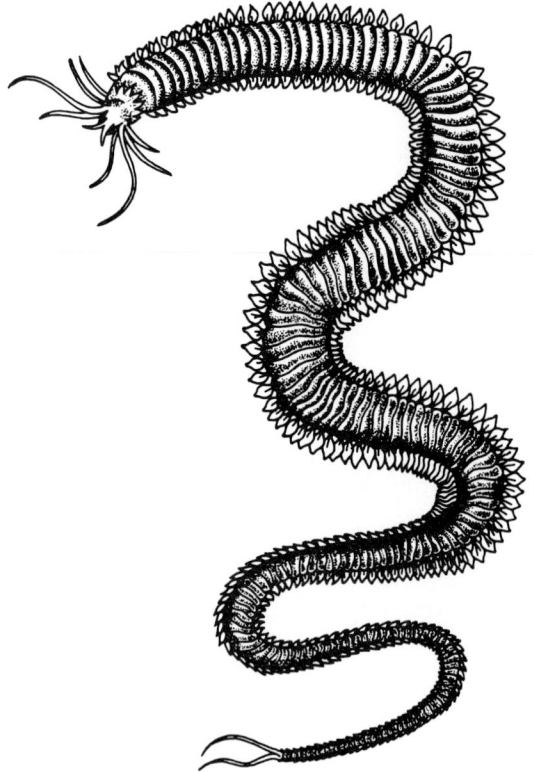

Figure 126–3. The bristle worm can cause cutaneous envenomation, with the development of dermatitis, as a result of contact with the bristles. (Courtesy of A. A. Fischer, M.D.: Atlas of Aquatic Dermatology. Copyright, 1978 American Cyanamid Company, Lederle Laboratories Division. Reproduced by permission.)

sharks, or from eating fish eggs or blood of certain fish (the toxic substance in this case being intrinsic, i.e., originating in a gland or other structure).

Rajiformes, Stingrays, and Skates. These are bottom feeders (Table 126–6). When stepped on, the muscular tail with its barb is wielded vigorously and may cause extensive wounds, and even death from hemorrhage. The venom affects the cardiovascular system, causing peripheral vasoconstriction or dilatation and cardiac arrythmias (including asystole). It can cause depression of respiration (mediated by the medullary centers) and convulsions as well. Other symptoms include nausea, vomiting, diarrhea, and weakness. Pain at the site of injury is immediate and intense, spreading and intensifying over a period of 30 to 90 minutes and then gradually diminishing over the next 6 to 48 hours.

Treatment is common to all wounds inflicted by venomous fish. It should be directed at (1) relief of pain, (2) neutralization of the effects of the venom, and (3) prevention of secondary infection. The pain results from the inoculation of the venom, the traumatization by the spine, and probably the introduction of other foreign bodies. Wounds should be irrigated, therefore, with saline solution. If the puncture wound is small, it should be excised and then irrigated. Opinions vary on the use of tourniquets. Heat treatment, i.e., soaking the limb in hot water (48.8°C) for 30 minutes to 1 hour, is efficacious. Stingray venom is destroyed by heat. Intravenous administration of calcium gluconate (to relieve muscle spasms) and local infiltration of 0.5 to 2% procaine give some relief of pain. Occasionally, however, meperidine hydrochloride may be necessary. Debridement and suturing (with or without a drain) are usually necessary. Tetanus toxoid and

an antibiotic to combat secondary infection should be given. Secondary shock may occur as a result of the direct action of the venom on the cardiovascular system and requires prompt and vigorous therapy. Cardiovascular and respiratory stimulants, as well as assisted ventilation, may be indicated.

Electric rays, members of the family Torpedinidae, can produce a discharge of up to 220 volts, which can temporarily disable a swimmer.

Scorpion Fish and Zebra Fish (Table 126–6). These are becoming popular with tropical marine aquarium enthusiasts. They have venomous spines which, on penetration, produce immediate and intense local pain that radiates along the course of lymphatics. This pain may last 16 to 24 hours. The surrounding tissues become swollen, discolored, and even gangrenous. General symptoms include shock, nausea, vomiting, diarrhea, hypotension, respiratory distress, convulsions, and, occasionally, death. Treatment is supportive and symptomatic, similar to that used to treat stingray wounds.

Stonefish (Table 126–6). These are found only in the tropical Indo-Pacific and are the most dangerous of the venomous fish, particularly because of their camouflaged appearance. Injury causes immediate pain, which is moderately severe to excruciating in intensity, with the victim often rapidly losing consciousness. The pain may last for hours or days. At the site of the injury, there is swelling and, in many instances, ischemia, which leads to subsequent necrosis and sloughing. General signs and symptoms include shock, respiratory distress, and, sometimes, death, probably as a result of direct action of the toxin on the heart. Treatment is symptomatic and supportive, although procaine and morphine are said to do little to alleviate the intense pain. Heat treatment reportedly produces some relief. Antivenom should be used if available.

Weever Fish. These perchlike marine fish are distributed on the Atlantic and Mediterranean coasts of Europe and North Africa (Table 126–6). The venom of these fish has effects similar to those of stingray venom. Victims are usually fishermen (fish being caught in nets) or bathers (fish being stepped on in the sand). Pain in the immediate area is instantaneous, spreading in the first half-hour and then gradually

TABLE 126–6. Venomous Fish Families

Families	Common Name	Distribution
Dasyatidae	Stingrays	Collectively worldwide in temperate and tropical waters
Gymnuridae	Butterflyrays	Same as stingrays
Myliobatidae	Bat stingrays	Same as stingrays
Urolophidae	Round stingrays	Pacific and Indian oceans
Rajidae	Skates	North and South Atlantic
Torpedinidae	Electric rays	Atlantic and Indian oceans, Mediterranean Sea
Chimaeridae	Catfish	North Atlantic, North Pacific, Australia
Heterodontidae	Hornshark	California coast
Squalidae	Dogfish	Atlantic and Pacific oceans
Ariidae	Marine catfish	Worldwide
Trachinidae	Weever fish	European coast
Scorpaenidae	Scorpion fish	Indo-Pacific
Batrachoididae	Toadfish	Worldwide
Acanthuridae	Surgeon-fish	Indo-Pacific
Uranoscopidae	Stargazers	Indo-Pacific

Compiled from Russell, 1971; Campbell, 1983; Halstead, 1988.

subsiding and disappearing over the next 2 to 24 hours. Rarely, envenomation has been fatal. Swelling, which involves the wound and the regional lymph glands, may last for days. Treatment should include opening of the wound with a knife and suction and irrigation with cold water or sterile saline solution to remove as much poison as possible. It is of interest to note that weevers can cause wounds even when dead.

Catfish. Both freshwater (North American) and marine catfish can cause injuries. The marine variety is a shore fish and is commonly found in muddy waters around boat slips. On envenomation, the victim experiences sharp pain. This lasts 30 minutes to 48 hours. The area surrounding the wound (and possibly the entire limb) becomes ischemic; later, it becomes cyanotic and edematous. Numbness and localized gangrene occur in some cases, and the complications of shock and respiratory distress may occur also in severe injuries. Treatment is symptomatic and supportive and follows the general principles indicated previously for the treatment of other venomous fish stings.

126.2 Leeches

William A. Sodeman, Jr.

Leeches belong to the phylum Annelida of the class Hirudinea. They occur mainly in Southeast Asia, India, tropical Australia, and parts of South America. The blood-sucking species of medical importance are either terrestrial or live in freshwater.

Leeches have two suckers, one anteriorly (containing the mouth and cutting parts) and one posteriorly. The leech attaches to the skin of animals, including humans, by means of the cutting plate, rapidly perforates the skin, and secretes an anticoagulant, hirudin, into the wound. With the sucker, it then draws blood from the victim. If present in large numbers, leeches may cause considerable blood loss, as well as psychological trauma. If ingested, they may become attached to the buccal mucosa, pharynx, or larynx, producing hemorrhage and signs of obstruction. Leeches attached to the skin may be fairly easily detached by rubbing them with salt or by burning them with a match. Those attached internally have been removed endoscopically with a snare, but some may require surgical removal. All wounds should be irrigated and dressed. Antibiotics may be indicated in the event of secondary infection. Prophylaxis includes the use of protective clothing and repellent creams (particularly those containing diethyltoluamide).

126.3 Fish

William A. Sodeman, Jr.

SHARKS. Only about 30 of 350 species of sharks have been identified in attacks on humans. Sharks tend to inhabit waters between latitude 47° South and 46° North, with a slight preponderance in the Southern Hemisphere and where water temperature is above 20°C. Attacks usually occur in the late afternoon and night, when sharks normally feed, or whenever there is food or blood in the water.

Sharks use vision as the primary sensory organ at distances of 50 feet or less; their visual acuity for color and moving objects is better than previously thought. At distances greater than 50 feet, other sensory organs are used. These include (in some species) visual adaptations for sight under low light conditions, a highly developed olfactory sense, chemoreceptors in the skin that detect water movement and changes in salinity, and "hearing" sense. Sharks have the ability to detect low-frequency vibrations at great distances in the water (bathers and other fish), as well as electrical fields of infinitesimal energy, by means of electroreceptors located in the head.

Sharks are unpredictable, and there does not appear to be any uniform attack approach. Attacks may be provoked or unprovoked. Bright colors or patterns may attract sharks. The fatality rate of shark attacks based on records of a series of 1165 attacks was 35%.

Attack prevention is not absolute, but a few precautionary measures should be observed. Swim in groups; if water is shark-infested, stay out; do not enter or remain in water with a bleeding wound; avoid turbid or polluted water; and wear dark protective clothing. Shark repellents and nets in beach areas have been used effectively.

The bites of sharks will generally produce severe, ragged wounds. Initial first aid is of the greatest importance. A pressure bandage or tourniquet should be used to control hemorrhage; analgesics should be given and transfusions started to combat shock. Some advocate that these measures should be instituted on the beach and that undue haste in removing the patient to a hospital decreases the chances of survival. In any event, when conditions permit, the patient should be hospitalized for more complete evaluation and definitive treatment.

GIANT DEVILFISH OR MANTA RAY. The manta ray is not aggressive but is dangerous because of its large size, measuring up to 5 m across. The coarse dermal tentacles may cause skin abrasions and may interfere with divers' air lines.

BARRACUDA. There are about 20 species of barracuda, which vary in aggressiveness. The great barracuda can be exceedingly pugnacious. It can measure up to 8 feet in length and is usually found in the Caribbean, off the coast of Brazil, and in the Indo-Pacific.

The barracuda relies almost entirely on sight and is attracted to bright colors, shiny reflections, or injured fish. It will follow divers without attacking. If it does attack, it usually does so only once, but this may be fatal. Bites (which are straight cuts as opposed to the curved cuts of shark bites) should be treated similarly to shark bites.

MORAY EELS. These eels are notoriously powerful biters, but attacks are usually provoked by poking into crevices between rocks. Wounds produced by the bite are ragged, and treatment of victims should follow the same principles as for treatment of shark bites.

NEEDLEFISH. Needlefish are found in tropical waters, bays, and inshore areas. They are attracted by light and may leap out of the water toward the light, impaling anyone in the way, especially if the victim happens to be light fishing at night. Puncture wounds may be severe, even fatal, if vital organs are penetrated. Wounds require prompt surgical attention.

GIANT GROUPERS OR SEA BASS. These fish may bite or cause injury by their very size (up to 3.6 m in length and weighing up to 360 kg).

Bibliography

Banner AM: Hazardous marine animals. *In* Tedeschi CG, Eckert WG, Tedeschi LG (eds): Forensic Medicine. Vol 3, Environmental Hazards. Philadelphia, WB Saunders, 1977.

Campbell GR: An Illustrated Guide to Some Poisonous Plants and Animals of Florida. Englewood, FL, Pineapple Press, 1983.

Clark E: Sharks: Magnificent and misunderstood. National Geographic 160:138, 1981.

Halstead BW: Dangerous Marine Animals That Bite, Sting, Shock and Are Nonedible. Centerville, MD, Cornell Maritime Press, 1980.

Halstead BW: Poisonous and Venomous Marine Animals of the World, ed 2. Princeton, NJ, The Darwin Press, 1988.

Iverson ES, Skinner RH: How to Cope with Dangerous Sea Life. Miami, Windward Publishing, 1977.

Mabbet H: Death of a skin diver. Australia Skin Diving and Spear-Fishing Digest. December:13, 1954.

Russell FE: Poisonous Marine Animals. London, TFH Publications, and Academic Press (London), 1971.

Southcott RV: The neurologic effects of noxious marine creatures. *In* Hornabrook RW (ed): Topics of Tropical Neurology. Philadelphia, FA Davis, 1975.

126.4 Lizards

William A. Sodeman, Jr.

There is one genus of poisonous lizards, *Heloderma*, which has two species: *H. suspectum* (Gila monsters) and *H. horridum* (Mexican beaded lizards). They inhabit the desert areas of Mexico and Arizona and are easily recognizable, being heavy and yellow or pink in color.

The actual venom of the Gila monster is as poisonous as that of the rattlesnake, but the mechanism for venom transfer is poorly developed. Submaxillary glands secrete poison that is passed along ducts to grooved teeth, and the victim is envenomated by the chewing action of the powerful jaws. The venom has its effect on the central nervous system, causing paralysis, dyspnea, and convulsions. Treatment is symptomatic and supportive.

Some of the large lizards, turtles, and crocodiles are capable of producing severe injury by biting.

126.5 Snakes

David A. Warrell

The four families of venomous snakes, Atractaspididae, Elapidae, Hydrophiidae, and Viperidae, contain some 500 species, whereas the fifth family, the Colubridae, once considered nonvenomous, contains at least 40 species venomous to humans. Less than 200 species have caused clinically severe envenoming, ending in death or permanent disability (Table 126–7).

DISTRIBUTION OF VENOMOUS SNAKES. Venomous species are widely distributed, except at altitudes above 5000 m, in polar regions, and in most islands of the western Mediterranean, Atlantic, Caribbean, and Pacific, and in Madagascar, New Caledonia, New Zealand, Hawaii, Ireland, Iceland, and Chile. The range of *Vipera berus* extends into the Arctic Circle. Sea snakes exist in the Indian and Pacific oceans and in estuaries, rivers (New Guinea), and freshwater lakes (Philippines, Cambodia).

CLASSIFICATION. Medically important snakes always possess one or more pairs of enlarged teeth in the upper jaw, the fangs, which penetrate the skin of their victim and conduct venom into the tissues along a groove or through a lumen.

Colubridae. The fangs of colubrids are relatively short, are situated at the posterior end of the maxilla, and are capable only of restricted movement. Three species found in Africa, the boomslang *(Dispholidus typus)* and the vine, twig, or

TABLE 126–7. Glossary of English and Latin Names of Snakes Mentioned in This Chapter

Latin Name	English Name
Acanthophis	Death adders
Agkistrodon blomhoffii brevicaudus	Pallas's viper, mamushi
Atractaspis engaddensis	Israeli burrowing asp or mole adder or viper
Bitis arietans	Puff adders
Bothrops asper	Terciopelo, caissaca
B. atropos	Berg adder
B. gabonica	Gaboon viper
B. nasicornis	Rhinoceros viper or River Jack
Bothrops atrox	Fer-de-lance, barba amarilla, caissaca
B. jararaca	Jararaca
Bungarus caeruleus	Common Indian krait
B. candidus	Malayan krait
B. fasciatus	Banded krait
B. multicinctus	Chinese krait
Calloselasma (Agkistrodon) rhodostoma	Malayan pit viper
Causus	Night adders
Crotalus adamanteus	Eastern diamondback rattlesnake
C. atrox	Western diamondback rattlesnake
C. durissus durissus	Central American rattlesnake
C. durissus terrificus	South American rattlesnake
C. horridus	Timber rattlesnake
C. scutulatus	Mojave rattlesnake
C. viridis	Western rattlesnake
C. viridis helleri	Southern Pacific rattlesnake
Daboia russelli russelli	Russell's viper (Western)
D. russelli siamensis	Russell's viper (Eastern)
Dendroaspis polylepis	Black mamba
D. viridis	Western green mamba
Dispholidus typus	Boomslang
Echis carinatus *E. ocellatus*	Saw-scaled or carpet vipers
Enhydrina schistosa	Beaked sea snake
Hemachatus haemachatus	Ringhals
Lachesis muta	Bushmaster
Microides *Micrurus*	American coral snakes
Naja atra	Chinese cobra
N. nekaouthia	Monocellate cobra
N. melanoleuca	Black or forest cobra
N. mossambica	Mozambique cobra
N. naja	Indian cobra
N. nigricollis	Black-necked or spitting cobra
N. siamensis	Indochinese spitting cobra
Notechis scutatus	Tiger snake
Ophiophagus hannah	King cobra
Oxyuranus scutellatus	Taipan
Pseudonaja textilis	Eastern brown snake
Rhabdophis subminiatus	Red-necked keelback
R. tigrinus	Japanese keelback or yamakagashi
Thelotornis capensis *Th. kirtlandii*	Bird, twig, or vine snake
Trimeresurus flavoviridis	Japanese habu
T. mucrosquamatus	Chinese habu
Vipera berus	European adder or viper
V. lebetina	Levantine viper
V. palaestinae	Palestine viper

bird snake *(Thelotornis kirtlandii* and *T. capensis)*, have been responsible for the deaths of a few people who handled them injudiciously. Over the last 60 years, the Japanese yamakagashi *(Rhabdophis tigrinus)* has caused at least 20 cases of coagulopathy with two deaths, whereas the related Southeast

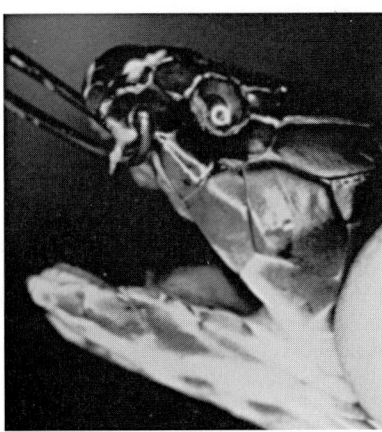

Figure 126–4. Short fixed front fang of an elapid snake (Indochinese spitting cobra *Naja siamensis*).

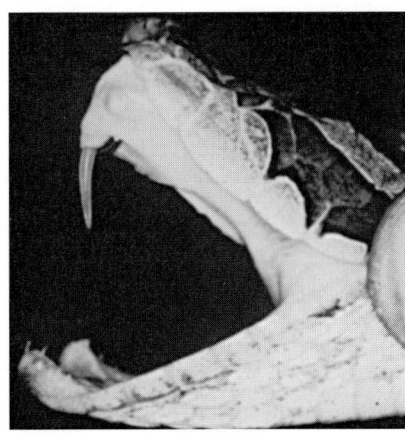

Figure 126–6. Long hinged front fang of Malayan pit viper (*Calloselasma rhodostoma*).

Asian red-necked keelback *(R. subminiatus)* has been responsible for cases of severe envenoming.

Atractaspididae. The burrowing asps, also known as burrowing or mole vipers or adders and stiletto snakes, have long front fangs and strike sideways.

Elapidae. This family includes cobras, kraits, mambas, coral snakes, and Australasian terrestrial venomous snakes (sometimes classified with Hydrophiidae). The relatively short anterior fangs of these snakes are permanently erect and capable of little movement (Fig. 126–4). In the ringhals, and African and Asian spitting cobras, the venom channel opens forward before it reaches the tip of the fang, allowing venom to be ejected as a fine spray for a distance of several meters into the eyes of an aggressor.

Hydrophiidae. The fangs of sea snakes are short, placed anteriorly, and have limited movement (Fig. 126–5).

Viperidae. The fangs are situated anteriorly, are long, curved, and capable of a wide range of movement (Fig. 126–6). Members of the subfamily Crotalinae—rattlesnakes, moccasins, South American lance-headed vipers, and Asian pit vipers—possess a heat-sensitive pit organ behind the nostril (Fig. 126–7). The Old World vipers, subfamily Viperinae, include the European, African, and Asian vipers and adders.

MEDICALLY IMPORTANT VENOMOUS SPECIES. Table 126–8 lists some species that commonly cause human deaths and serious disability (usually resulting from local necrosis). Some species, e.g., the night adders (genus *Causus* of Africa)

and green pit vipers (genus *Trimeresurus* of Asia), frequently bite, but the effects are usually trivial.

INCIDENCE AND IMPORTANCE OF SNAKEBITE. Snakebite is largely a problem of the rural tropics, and as a result, reliable data for incidence, morbidity, and mortality are scarce. The following examples probably represent underestimates of the true incidence of mortality resulting from snakebite. In India, the reported annual mortality has exceeded 20,000 during the last 100 years, and in Maharashtra State alone, there are more than 1000 deaths each year. In Burma, where Russell's viper is the most important species, snakebite has been the fifth most common cause of death and is currently responsible for more than 1000 deaths each year (approximately 3.3/100,000 population). In Sri Lanka, where kraits and Russell's viper are important, the annual death rate exceeds 800 (6/100,000 population). In parts of West Africa (northeastern Nigeria, central Benin) the incidence of snakebite, mainly by *Echis ocellatus*, exceeds 400/100,000 population/year with a case fatality of up to 12%. Snakebite is common in parts of Latin America. In Brazil there are an estimated 20,000 snakebites each year, attributable to *Bothrops* species and *Crotalus terrificus*, but with less than 100 reported deaths.

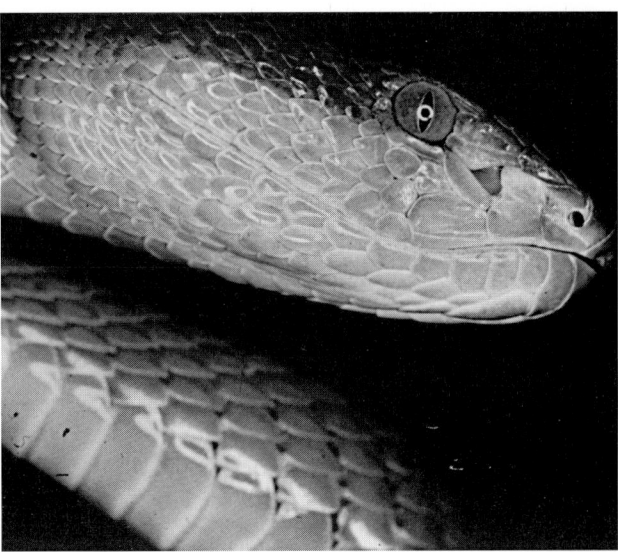

Figure 126–7. Heat-sensitive pit organ of white-lipped green pit viper (*Trimeresurus albolabris*).

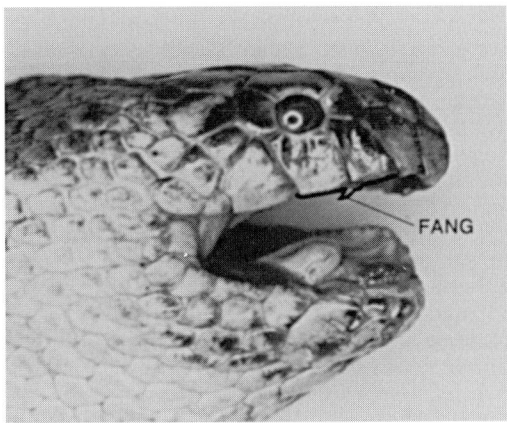

Figure 126–5. Small fixed front fang of sea snake (*Lapemis curtus*).

TABLE 126–8. Species Responsible for Most Deaths and Morbidity Resulting From Snakebite

Area of Distribution	Latin Name*	English Name
North America	*Crotalus adamanteus*	Eastern diamondback rattlesnake
	C. atrox	Western diamondback rattlesnake
	C. viridis	Western rattlesnake
Central America	*C. durissus durissus*	Central American rattlesnake
	Bothrops asper	Terciopelo, caissaca
South America	*B. atrox*	Fer-de-lance, barba amarilla
	B. asper	Terciopelo
	B. jararaca	Jararaca
	Crotalus durissus terrificus	South American rattlesnake
Europe	*Vipera berus*	Viper, adder
	V. ammodytes	Long-nosed viper
Africa	*Echis* species	Saw-scaled or carpet viper
	Bitis arietans	Puff adder
	Naja nigricollis, N. mossambica, etc.	African spitting cobras
	N. haje	Egyptian cobra
	Dendroaspis species	Mambas
Asia, Middle East	*Echis* species	Saw-scaled or carpet vipers
	Vipera lebetina	Levantine viper
	V. palaestinae	Palestine viper
Southeast Asia, India	*Naja* species	Asian cobras
	Bungarus caeruleus	Indian krait
	Daboia russelli	Russell's viper
	Echis species	Saw-scaled or carpet vipers
	Calloselasma (Agkistrodon) rhodostoma	Malayan pit viper
	Trimeresurus species	Green pit vipers
Far East	*N. atra*	Chinese cobra
	B. multicinctus	Chinese krait
	Agkistrodon species	Mamushi
	Trimeresurus flavoviridis	Habu
	T. mucrosquamatus	Chinese habu
Australasia	*Acanthophis* species	Death adder
	Notechis scutatus	Tiger snake
	Oxyuranus scutellatus	Taipan
	Pseudonaja textilis	Eastern brown snake

*Scientific (Latin) names are important because they are used internationally to describe the range of specificity of antivenoms.

The highest number of snakebite mortalities has been reported in certain hunter-gatherer tribes. Among the Yanomamo of Amazonian Venezuela, snakebite is responsible for 2% of adult deaths; among the Waorani of Ecuador, for 5% of all deaths; and among the Kaxinawa of Acre, Brazil, for more than 20% of adult deaths. The Phi Tong Luang of northeastern Thailand, the Hadza of Tanzania, some tribal groups in Papua New Guinea, and the aborigines of central Australia have suffered a high mortality from snakebite.

In the United States, there are approximately 45,000 bites/year, 7000 of which are caused by venomous species, with 9 to 14 deaths/year.

EPIDEMIOLOGY. Most snakebites occur on the lower limbs of farmers, herdsmen, and hunters in the rural tropics. The incidence of bites by a particular species in a particular geographic area depends on the size of human and snake populations, the snake's irritability (its inclination to bite when trodden on or disturbed) and diurnal rhythm, and the extent to which human activities encroach on its chosen habitat. There are few convincing reports of unprovoked aggression by snakes, and, in the tropics at least, snakebite is always the result of an inadvertent tread or touch. Many bites happen when the snake is trodden on in the dark. However, most cases of spitting cobra (*Naja nigricollis*) bite in West Africa and krait bite in Southern Asia (*Bungarus caeruleus, B. candidus, B. multicinctus*) occur while the victims are asleep in their homes. These commensal species enter houses in search of their prey—rodents, toads, lizards, and other snakes. In developed countries, snakes inspire curiosity and are popular pets, and most bites occur on the hands as a result of the snake's being picked up. In the United States, 25% of bites result from snakes being attacked or handled. Irritable species that strike readily when disturbed include *Echis* species, the Malayan pit viper (*Calloselasma rhodostoma*, formerly known as *Agkistrodon rhodostoma*), and most species of rattlesnake (*Crotalus*), lance-headed vipers (*Bothrops*), and cobras (*Naja*), whereas the Gabon (*Bitis gabonica*) and rhinoceros (*B. nasicornis*) vipers and the banded krait (*Bungarus fasciatus*) seem relatively reluctant to bite. Serious bites by back-fanged (colubrid) snakes have been confined to professional and amateur herpetologists who were handling the snakes. Seasonal variation in the incidence of snakebite is attributed to farming activity in relation to rainfall and to the yearly reproductive cycle of the snake. Severe flooding, by flushing out and concentrating the snake population, has given rise to epidemics of snakebite in Colombia, Pakistan, India, and Burma. Development of jungle areas for highways and irrigation or hydroelectric schemes have resulted in an increased incidence of snakebite in Brazil and Sri Lanka. On rare occasions, snakebite or injection of snake venom has been used for suicide or murder.

VENOM APPARATUS. The venom glands are surrounded by compressor muscles and are situated behind or below the eye. The venom duct opens within a sheath at the base of the fang, and venom is conducted toward the tip in a partially or completely closed groove or fang canal (Fig. 126–8). Venomous snakes can inject doses of venom lethal to their natural prey at each of up to 10 or more consecutive strikes; the quantity of venom injected is highly variable, with no convincing evidence that it can be adjusted according to the size of the prey or the intention of the snake. The high proportion of bites without envenoming reported for species such as *C. rhodostoma* is more likely to be the result of mechanical inefficiency than to voluntary control by the snake, and the concept of a defensive bite may not be valid. Of a group of 824 patients bitten by venomous species, 53% showed only trivial or no evidence of envenoming. There is no support for the popular belief that snakes are less dangerous after they have eaten. It is most important to emphasize that the snake uses only a fraction of the content of its venom gland at each strike.

VENOM COMPOSITION. Snake venoms may contain 20 or more components, so their effects cannot be attributed to single toxins. Dried venom is more than 90% protein, consisting of a variety of enzymes, nonenzymatic polypeptide toxins, and nontoxic proteins. Metals such as zinc are associated with some of the enzymes, such as ecarin, the procoagulant enzyme of *E. carinatus* venom, which activates prothrombin. Carbohydrate is present in glycoproteins, such as the serine protease ancrod (Arvin), the procoagulant of *C. rhodostoma* venom, which cleaves fibrinopeptide A from fibrinogen and has been used to treat thrombotic disorders. Biogenic amines such as histamine and 5-hydroxytryptamine may be partly responsible for the pain of snakebite; they are found

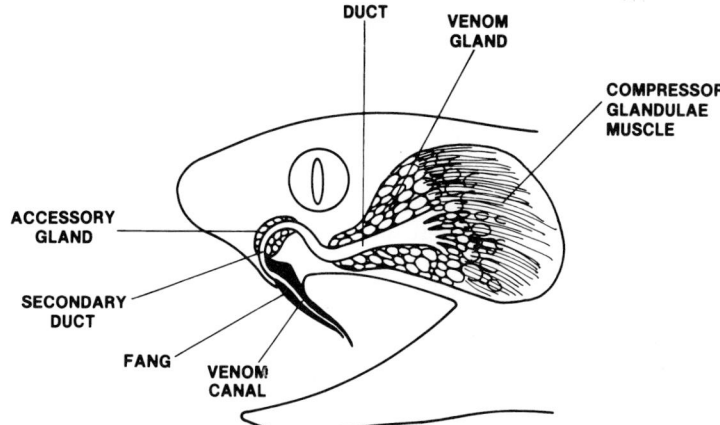

Figure 126–8. Venom apparatus of a viperine snake.

in greater quantity and variety in venoms of Viperidae than in those of Elapidae or Hydrophiidae. Many snake venoms contain phospholipase A₂, which is responsible for presynaptic neurotoxic activity, rhabdomyolysis, vascular endothelial damage, and hemolysis. The bright yellow color of some Viperidae venoms is attributable to L-amino acid oxidase, which has a riboflavin prosthetic group. Other venom enzymes include phosphoesterases, monoesterases, diesterases, acetylcholinesterase, proteolytic enzymes, and hyaluronidase. The role of these enzymes in human envenoming is uncertain.

Polypeptide Toxins (Neurotoxins). These low molecular weight proteins are found in elapid, hydrophiid, and several viperid venoms. Postsynaptic (α-) neurotoxins, such as α-bungarotoxin and cobrotoxin, contain 60 to 62 "short chain" or 67 to 74 "long chain" amino acids and bind to acetylcholine receptors on the motor end-plate. Presynaptic (β-) neurotoxins, such as β-bungarotoxin, crotoxin, taipoxin, and notexin, are phospholipases A₂ consisting of approximately 120 amino acids; they prevent release of acetylcholine at the neuromuscular junction by blocking voltage-gated potassium channels. Other neurotoxins of doubtful clinical significance interfere with ionic fluxes and stimulate release of acetylcholine from nerve endings.

Antihemostatic Factors. Hemorrhagin activity is found mainly in Viperidae venoms and is responsible for spontaneous hemorrhage by damaging vascular endothelium. Procoagulant venom factors (enzymes) act at various points of the clotting cascade (Fig. 126–9), while fibrinolytic factors may act directly or by activating plasminogen. Defibrination and associated platelet abnormalities result in persistent bleeding from vessels damaged by hemorrhagin, venipuncture, or other trauma but do not cause spontaneous hemorrhage in the absence of hemorrhagin.

Local Cytotoxicity. Local swelling, blistering, and necrosis, prominent features of envenoming by Viperidae and some cobras, are caused by primary effects of cytotoxic venom components, e.g., proteases and the 60 or 62 amino acid polypeptides misleadingly known as "cardiotoxins," in *Naja* and *Hemachatus* venoms, and by the release of endogenous substances that increase capillary permeability.

Autopharmacologic Effects. These actions of venoms, mainly of Viperidae, include the release and potentiation of bradykinin, histamine, 5-hydroxytryptamine, and adenosine triphosphate from platelets and inhibition of angiotensinase. In humans, presynaptic neurotoxins of Hydrophiidae, several Australasian Elapidae, and a few species of Viperidae (e.g. *Crotalus durissus terrificus* and Sri Lankan *Daboia russelli*) produce systemic rhabdomyolysis. A number of other venoms

cause myonecrosis at the site of local injection. Sarafotoxins, highly homologous to endothelins, have been isolated from the venom of the Israeli burrowing asp *(Atractaspis engaddensis).*

Variation in Venom Composition. The diversity of clinical manifestations of snakebite is explained by the variation of venom composition from species to species. There may also be considerable variation in venom composition within a single species throughout its geographic range, at different seasons of the year, and as a result of aging.

Pharmacology. The toxic polypeptides of Elapidae and Hydrophiidae venoms are relatively small molecules that are absorbed rapidly into the blood stream, whereas the much larger molecules of Viperidae venoms are taken up more slowly through lymphatics. The distribution of venoms from the site of inoculation is affected also by their binding to tissues, the production of local thrombosis and vasoconstriction, and the presence of spreading factors such as hyaluronidase. Some venoms, notably of the Viperidae, break down permeability barriers leading to extravasation and edema. Most venoms are concentrated and bound in the kidney,

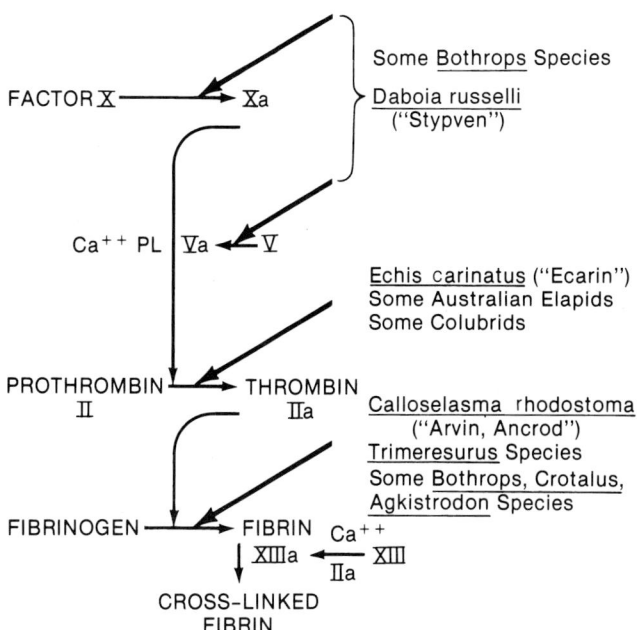

Figure 126–9. Sites of action of some snake venom procoagulants on the clotting cascade.

and some components are eliminated in the urine, whereas crotaline venoms are selectively bound in the lungs, concentrated in the liver, and excreted in bile.

CLINICAL MANIFESTATIONS. The patient who has been bitten by a snake may present with symptoms resulting from fear, from prehospital treatment, and from effects of the venom itself. A snakebite is a terrifying experience, especially for those who believe that all bites are rapidly fatal. Physiologic manifestations of anxiety, and even frank hysteria, may confuse the clinical picture. Thus, patients who are bitten but not envenomed may feel flushed, dizzy, and breathless, with constriction of the chest, and may notice a thumping pulse, palpitations, sweating, and effects of hyperventilation. Such symptoms dominate many accounts of snakebites written by the victims and are falsely attributed to neurotoxicity. Misguided prehospital treatment can result in congestion and ischemia of a limb whose circulation is occluded by a tourniquet, bleeding or sensory loss resulting from local incisions, and vomiting and other side effects caused by ingested herbal remedies. Rarely, the terror of snakebite may precipitate angina pectoris, myocardial infarction, or cardiac arrhythmia.

General Symptoms and Signs. The evolution of symptoms and signs of envenoming depends on the nature of the venom, the dose, and the site of injection.

The earliest symptom is pain, which is usually felt immediately. Local swelling may start within minutes, and total defibrination can develop in half an hour (*C. rhodostoma* and *Echis* species). Rarely, death may occur as soon as 15 minutes after an elapid (e.g., *N. naja* or *Dendroaspis* species) or viper (e.g., *D. russelli*) bite. Usually, however, death comes hours after an elapid or sea snake bite and days after a viper bite.

Local Effects. This is characteristic of bites by the Viperidae, including the pit vipers of the subfamily Crotalinae, African spitting cobras (e.g., *N. mossambica, N. nigricollis*) and Asian cobras (e.g., *N. naja, N. kaouthia,* and *N. siamensis*). Tender swelling spreads from the site of the bite, and there is early tender enlargement of lymph nodes draining the bitten area. Within a few hours, serosanguineous bullae may appear under the epidermis (Fig. 126–10). With elapid bites, blistering is nearly always followed by tissue necrosis, usually superficial, which may extend up the fascial planes of the limb (Fig. 126–11). Bullae caused by Viperidae bites frequently dry up and slough without the development of ne-

crosis. A pale, anesthetic, demarcated area of skin with a characteristic odor of putrefaction signals the appearance of necrosis. This is an effect of the venom, but the necrotic tissue is vulnerable to secondary infection by bacteria, including anaerobes.

An important result of massive swelling of the bitten limb is loss of circulating volume; a swollen limb can accommodate several liters of blood. The result may be hypotension due to hypovolemia. Envenoming by rattlesnakes (*Crotalus*) produces local pain with swelling that appears within 15 minutes of the bite and may spread rapidly. Bruising along the path of lymphatics, bullae, and local necrosis may develop. Paresthesias of the tongue and lips and an abnormal metallic taste are common early symptoms following bites by western (*C. viridis*), eastern diamondback (*C. adamanteus*), western diamondback (*C. atrox*), and timber (*C. horridus*) rattlesnakes. Other symptoms include weakness, rigors, sweating, fasciculation, spontaneous bleeding, neurotoxic effects (*C. adamanteus, C. scutulatus*) and gastrointestinal symptoms. Bites by the Mojave rattlesnake (*C. scutulatus*) and *C. durissus terrificus* may produce little or no local swelling but severe systemic signs.

Bleeding and Clotting Disturbances. This combination is characteristic of vipers such as *D. russelli* and *Echis* species, pit vipers such as *C. rhodostoma, C. viridis, Trimeresurus* and *Bothrops* species, and some Australian snakes such as the eastern brown snake (*Pseudonaja textilis*), tiger snake (*Notechis scutatus*) and taipan (*Oxyuranus scutellatus*). Spontaneous bleeding is most frequently detected in the gingival sulci (Fig. 126–12). The most dangerous forms of hemorrhage are intracerebral, gastrointestinal, and retroperitoneal. Incoagulable blood is suggested by oozing from venipuncture sites or other sites of recent trauma.

Hypotension and Shock. Early syncope can occur as part of the autopharmacologic syndrome after bites by *Vipera*, Australasian elapids, and *Atractaspis*. More common causes of hypotension are hypovolemia resulting from massive hemorrhage or local or systemic leakage from the vascular compartment (Fig. 126–13), vasodilatation, and a direct action on the myocardium. Acute pituitary adrenal insufficiency may cause shock within the first 10 days of bites by *D. russelli* and *Bothrops* species.

Neurotoxicity. This is a feature of envenoming by elapids, Australian snakes, and sea snakes. A few species of Viperidae

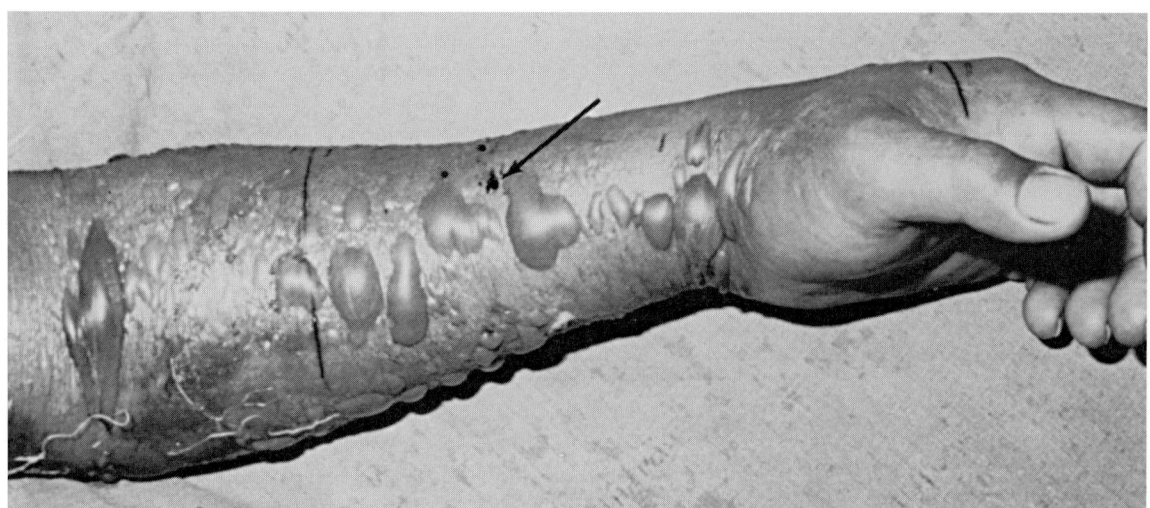

Figure 126–10. Intense edema, bruising, and formation of bullae 24 hours after a bite on the forearm *(arrow)* by a Malayan pit viper *(Calloselasma rhodostoma).*

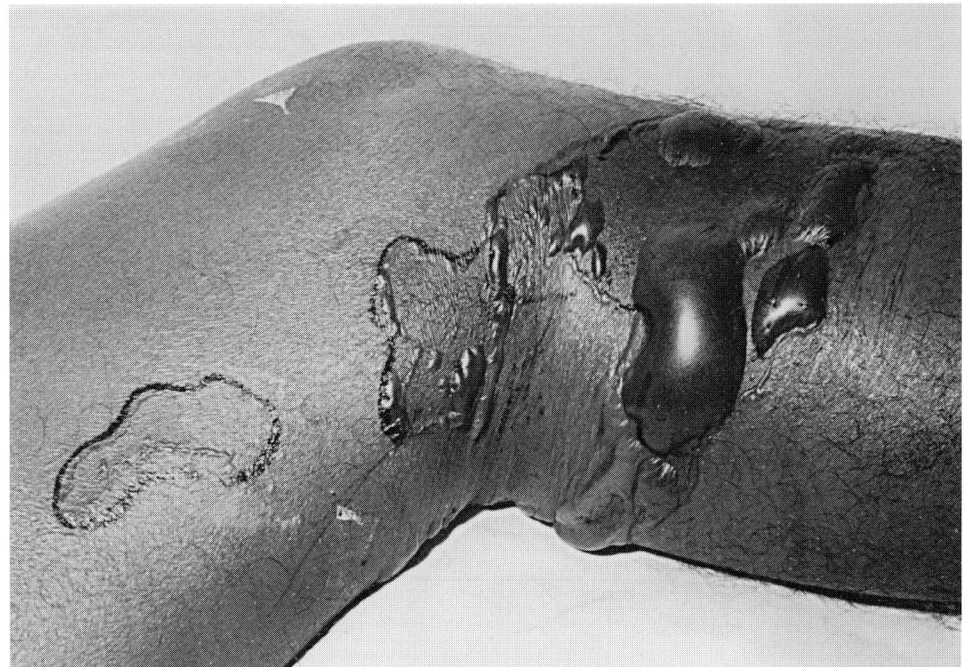

Figure 126–11. Blistering with necrosis of skin and subcutaneous tissue 5 days after a bite on the shin by a Sri Lankan cobra (*Naja naja*).

also produce neurotoxic effects. These include *C. durissus terrificus*, Pallas's pit viper (*Agkistrodon blomhoffii brevicaudus*), *B. atropos*, and *D. russelli* (apparently only in Sri Lanka). Typically, neurotoxic symptoms develop early, but after krait bite there may be a delay of 10 or more hours. Symptoms include vomiting, headache, paresthesia, drowsiness, apathy or euphoria, hyperacusis, diplopia, blurred vision, heaviness of the eyelids, and difficulty in speaking.

The levator palpebrae superioris and extraocular muscles are the most sensitive to neuromuscular blockade, and in some patients, the only feature of envenoming is ptosis and ophthalmoplegia. More serious effects are paralysis of the palate, jaws, tongue, vocal cords, neck muscles, and muscles of deglutition and respiration (Fig. 126–14). The intercostal muscles are affected before the diaphragm and limbs. The patient appears to be curarized. Objective sensory impairment is unusual. It is unlikely that neurotoxic venoms have

any effect on the central nervous system in humans. Paralyzed patients are fully conscious unless they are hypoxemic (respiratory failure) or hypotensive (circulatory failure). Ptosis and fatigue may be misinterpreted as coma. Neurotoxicity is completely reversible; in some cases there is a rapid response to specific antivenom or anticholinesterase, and in others there is slow, spontaneous resolution. With no specific antivenom, patients supported by artificial ventilation recover sufficient diaphragmatic movement to breathe adequately in 1 to 4 days. The ocular muscles recover in 2 to 4 days, and there is usually full recovery of motor function in 3 to 7 days. Upper airway obstruction by the tongue or inhaled vomitus may precipitate respiratory arrest.

Rhabdomyolysis. This must be distinguished from local muscle necrosis caused by cytotoxic venoms. The neurotoxins of sea snakes. Australasian elapids, *C. durissus terrificus* and *D. russelli* in Sri Lanka produce systemic rhabdomyolysis. The symptoms are muscle pain and stiffness, with trismus and respiratory muscle paralysis. Myoglobinemia, myoglobinuria, hyperkalemia, and renal failure may result.

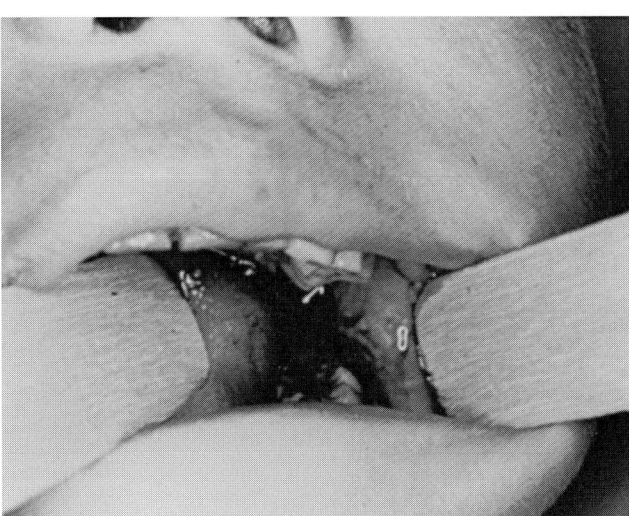

Figure 126–12. Extensive spontaneous bleeding from gingival sulci 1 hour after a bite by a Malayan pit viper (*Calloselasma rhodostoma*).

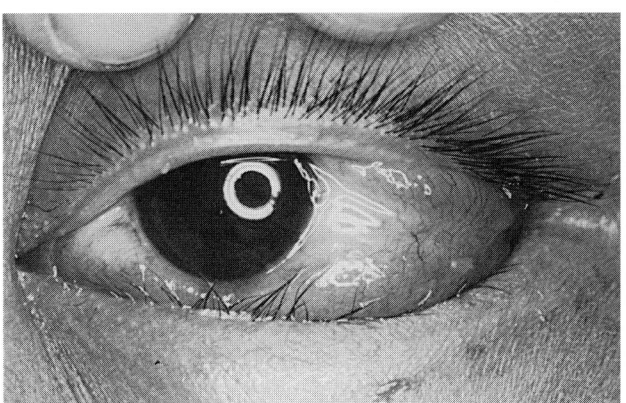

Figure 126–13. Clinical evidence of increased systemic vascular permeability: chemosis (edema of the conjunctiva) 48 hours after a bite by Russell's viper (*Daboia russelli siamensis*) in Burma.

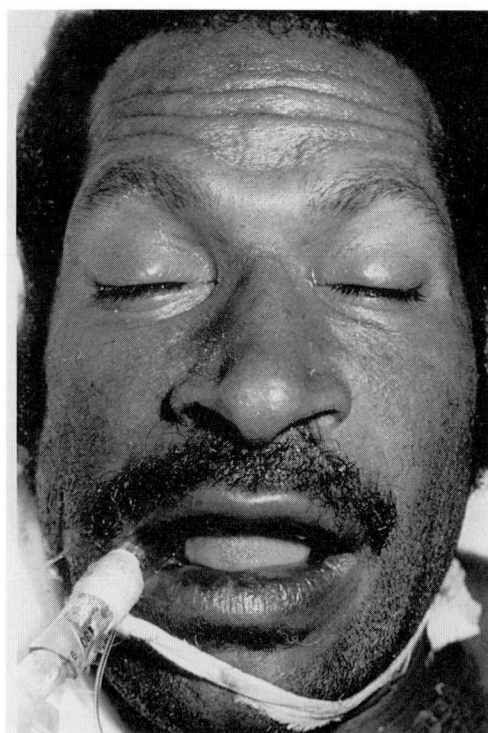

Figure 126–14. Neurotoxic envenoming after a bite by a Papuan taipan (*Oxyuranus scutellatus canni*). Note complete bilateral ptosis (the patient is attempting to open his eyes by contracting the frontalis muscle), inability to open the mouth, protrude the tongue, and breathe spontaneously (mechanical intubation via endotracheal tube).

Renal Failure. Renal failure can complicate almost any severe case of snakebite, but it is the major cause of death in victims of *D. russelli*, sea snakes, and *C. durissus terrificus*. Mechanisms of renal damage include ischemia (from hypotension, renal vasoconstriction, or disseminated intravascular coagulation), hemorrhage, direct nephrotoxicity or pigment nephropathy associated with massive intravascular hemolysis, generalized rhabdomyolysis, and associated electrolyte disturbances. Antivenom may cause immune complex nephritis as part of the late reactions occurring 7 days or more after treatment.

Autopharmacologic Effects and Venom Hypersensitivity Reactions. Patients bitten by the Palestine viper (*V. palaestinae*) commonly develop abdominal colic, persistent diarrhea, sweating, hypotension, and angioneurotic edema of the tongue and lips and may collapse within minutes of the bite. Similar symptoms have been described, less commonly, in patients bitten by *V. berus* and other European vipers, the bushmaster (*Lachesis muta*), the Israeli burrowing viper (*Atractaspis engaddensis*), and some Australasian snakes, and strongly suggest release by the venom of endogenous amines, e.g., histamine or activation of kinins, known properties of many snake venoms. Another possible explanation, in those previously exposed to the same venom, is hypersensitivity. Laboratory workers who habitually handle venoms are prone to become sensitized. They may develop conjunctivitis, rhinitis, asthma, and dermatitis on re-exposure.

Venom Ophthalmia Caused by Spitting Cobras. The ringhals (*Hemachatus haemachatus*) and spitting cobras of Africa (e.g., *N. nigricollis, N. mossambica*) and of Thailand, Indochina, Malaysia, Indonesia, and the Philippines (e.g., *N. siamensis, N. sumatrana, N. sputatrix*) can eject venom in a fine stream from the tips of the fangs for a distance of a few meters. If venom enters the eye, there is intense local pain, leukorrhea, blepharospasm, and palpebral edema. Because most patients make an uneventful recovery, these injuries used to be thought trivial, but slit lamp examination reveals corneal erosions in more than half of the cases. There is the same risk of secondary infection as with other corneal injuries (Fig. 126–15), leading to permanent blindness in some cases. The venom may be absorbed also into the anterior chamber, resulting in anterior uveitis with hypopyon.

PATHOLOGY. Patients who died from predominantly neurotoxic envenomation show no postmortem abnormalities except those attributable to terminal hypoxia. Those who died from the action of venoms with predominant hemorrhagin and procoagulant activity may show extensive hemorrhages in the bitten limb, body cavities, gastrointestinal tract, retroperitoneal tissues, renal tract, and brain. Hemorrhagic infarction of the anterior pituitary may complicate bites by *D. russelli* in Burma and southern India (Fig. 126–16). Sea snake venom causes scattered and discrete death of skeletal muscle fibers, clogging of the renal tubules with myoglobin, and myoglobinuria. The commonest renal lesion in patients dying with acute renal failure is tubular necrosis. Fibrin thrombi may be found in renal arterioles (Fig. 126–17). A variety of histologic changes have been described in survivors. In some cases these may be attributable to pre-existing renal disease and in others to serum sickness induced by antivenom. In patients dying of an unknown cause, the discovery of fang marks with or without local changes should raise the possibility of snakebite, which can be confirmed by immunodiagnostic and other tests (see Detection of Venoms in Snakebite Victims).

LABORATORY INVESTIGATIONS. The peripheral white blood cell count is raised in patients severely envenomed by many species of snakes. Anemia is the result of bleeding or, much more rarely, hemolysis. Venoms of *D. russelli* in India and Sri Lanka and some colubrids cause intravascular hemolysis. Venoms containing procoagulant often produce thrombocytopenia; this is common following bites by *D. russelli, Trimeresurus, Bothrops, C. rhodostoma*, and the Pacific rattlesnake (*Crotalus viridis helleri*) but is relatively rare after an *Echis* bite. Important simple tests for venom-induced defibrination are the simple whole blood clotting test and clot quality test. A few milliliters of blood are placed in a new, clean, dry glass test tube, left undisturbed for 20 minutes, and then tipped once to check for clotting. Serum potassium is elevated by the generalized rhabdomyolysis of sea snake envenoming. Serum enzymes, such as aspartate and alanine aminotransferases and creatine kinase, are mildly elevated in patients with local tissue damage but are grossly raised in

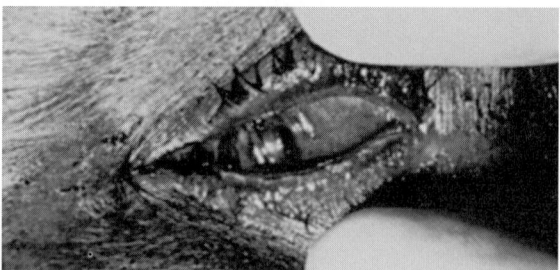

Figure 126–15. Severe venom ophthalmia that led to blindness in a patient "spat at" by a black-necked spitting cobra *Naja nigricollis* in Nigeria. Failure to treat with a local antimicrobial agent may allow secondary infection of corneal abrasions with these disastrous results (panophthalmitis requiring enucleation).

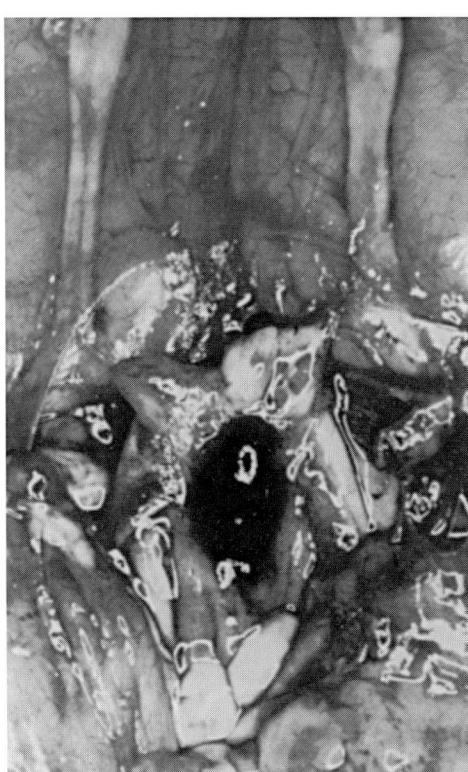

Figure 126–16. Hemorrhagic anterior pituitary stump in a patient who died 36 hours after a bite by Russell's viper *(Daboia russelli siamensis)* in Burma.

victims of sea snake bite. Electrocardiographic changes, such as inverted T waves, raised ST segments, prolonged Q-Tc intervals, and arrhythmias, have been reported in patients bitten by vipers and pit vipers. The urine of snakebite victims commonly contains red and white blood cells and granular casts. Dark urine should be tested for hemoglobin and myoglobin.

DETECTION OF VENOMS IN SNAKEBITE VICTIMS; IMMUNODIAGNOSIS. Specific snake venom antigens have been detected in wound aspirate, blood, urine, cerebrospinal fluid, and other body fluids by a variety of techniques, including immunodiffusion, countercurrent immunoelectrophoresis (CIE), passive hemagglutination, radioimmunoassay, and enzyme immunoassay (EIA). EIA is the simplest and most sensitive technique. The Commonwealth Serum Laboratories (CSL) in Australia have issued venom detection kits based on this principle. In some cases, the EIA may give results in time to guide clinical management, but main value is in the investigation of the pathophysiology and epidemiology of snakebite and, for forensic purposes, in confirming the cause of deaths suspected to have been caused by snakebite. Venom antibody is also detectable by EIA and may persist for many years after the bite.

MANAGEMENT OF SNAKEBITE. Snakebite is a rare emergency in most parts of the world, and because its management is thought to require specialized knowledge, many clinicians close their minds to the simple therapeutic principles that could prevent morbidity and mortality. Management starts with first aid by relatives, friends, or fellow workers of the snakebite victim who happen to be present when the bite occurs. Therefore, first aid principles should be a priority subject for community health education in schools, at clinics, and via the media.

First Aid Treatment. Most snakebite victims are terrified and require reassurance. The bitten limb should be immobilized, if possible, with a splint or sling and the patient quickly moved to the nearest treatment facility. Pain can be treated with oral acetaminophen or intravenous meperidine. Aspirin should not be used, as it may lead to persistent gastric bleeding in patients with incoagulable blood. Local incisions and suction are more likely to introduce infection and cause persistent bleeding than to remove significant amounts of venom from the wound. In one study of viper bites in Jammu, India, 94% of patients who had received incisions

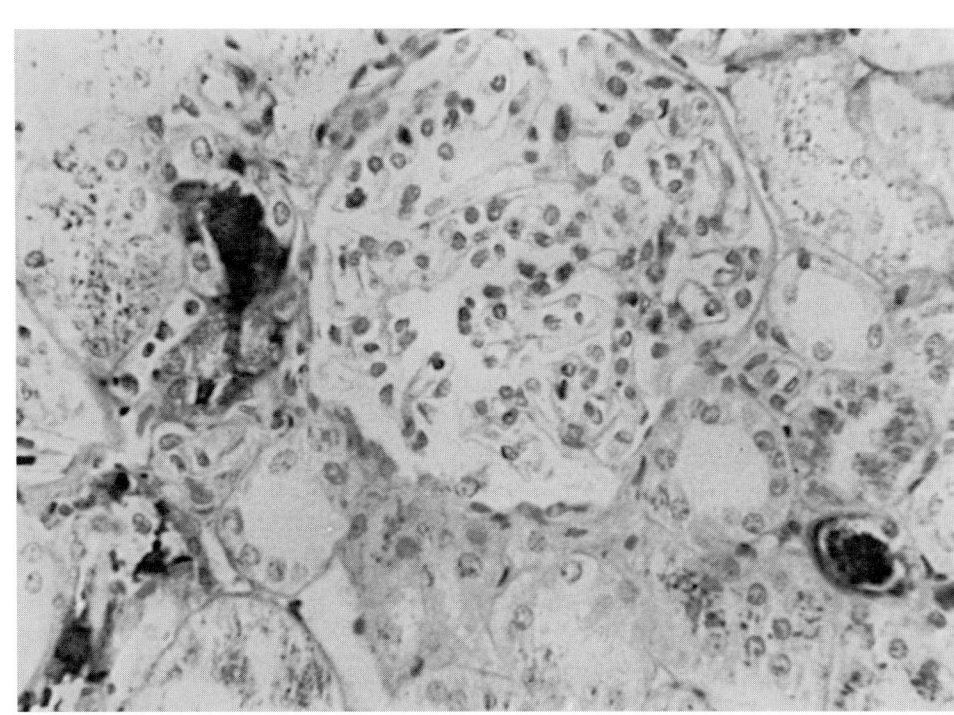

Figure 126–17. Kidney of a patient who died 15 hours after being bitten by Russell's viper *(Daboia russelli siamensis)* in Burma. The glomerulus is congested, and there is granular material in the tubules. Arterioles contain fibrin (dark staining). (Anti-human fibrinogen PAP method × 512.) (Courtesy of Dr. Nicholas Francis.)

developed local infection, compared with none in the group without incisions. Vacuum extractors have not yet been adequately tested. Potassium permanganate instillation and ice packs can cause local necrosis. Electric shock treatment is potentially dangerous and of unproven value.

Tourniquets. A broad, firm (but not tight), constricting band may temporarily delay the spread of viper venoms along lymphatics and superficial veins, but this effect has not been proved to be clinically useful and may lead to congestion and edema of the limb—confusing signs that suggest envenoming where there may be none. A tight (arterial-occlusive) tourniquet is effective in preventing venous return from the occluded limb and delays death in animals given elapid and Australasian snake venoms. However, such tourniquets have also been responsible for gangrenous limbs; peripheral nerve damage; and increased fibrinolytic activity, bleeding, and local effects of venom. Recent studies in restrained monkeys have shown that crepe bandaging and splinting of the injected limb are effective in delaying the spread of snake and spider venoms. A firmly applied crepe bandage (with splint) or the much more painful and dangerous arterial tourniquet is justified only in the case of bites by dangerously neurotoxic elapids, sea snakes, and Australasian snakes when the delay in reaching medical care is likely to be more than 30 minutes but less than 2 hours. In these particular circumstances, compression may delay the development of respiratory paralysis or cardiovascular collapse until medical help is available. The arterial tourniquet must be released for 15 seconds every 30 minutes and should not be applied for more than 2 hours. Compression may exaggerate the local effects of necrotic venoms. A local pressure pad applied over the bite wound has been advocated for Russell's viper bites in Burma.

Early Complications. Problems that may arise on the way to a medical facility include the following: (1) Vomiting may occur; therefore, patients should lie on their side to avoid aspiration. Persistent vomiting can be treated with chlorpromazine (25 mg for adults, 1 mg/kg for children), by injection. (2) Anaphylactic shock with angioedema and diarrhea should be treated with epinephrine 0.1% by intramuscular injection (adult dose, 0.5 mg; children, 0.01 mg/kg [see below]) followed by antihistamines, such as chlorpheniramine maleate (10 mg for adults, 0.2 mg/kg for children) and hydrocortisone (adult dose, 100 mg; children, 2 mg/kg) by intravenous injection. (3) Respiratory or cardiac arrest should be treated by mouth-to-mouth respiration and external cardiac massage. (4) Airway obstruction due to paralysis of the jaw and tongue should be treated by laying the patient on his or her side, inserting an oropharyngeal airway, and raising the jaw. (5) Intramuscular injections can lead to large hematomas in patients with defibrinated blood; therefore, oral or intravenous routes should be used whenever possible. A pressure pad should be applied to venipuncture sites.

If possible, the snake should be brought to the hospital for identification, provided no risk of further bites is involved. Snakes, even those that appear dead, and severed heads should not be handled but should be carried on a stick or maneuvered into a container.

Treatment by Medically Trained Personnel in Hospital or Dispensary. Because of the uncertainties about the type, quantity, and quality of venom injected and the variable time course for development of signs of envenoming, all victims of snakebite should be hospitalized and observed for at least 24 hours. Frequent observations of the level of consciousness, blood pressure, pulse rate, respiratory rate, and new signs, such as ptosis, should be made. Any ligatures should be released, preferably after starting administration of antivenom (see Antivenom Treatment). Physical examination should include assessment of local swelling, almost invari-

ably present within 15 minutes of significant pit viper envenoming and within 2 hours of viper envenoming but absent in patients bitten by some neurotoxic species (especially kraits, sea snakes, and coral snakes). Tender enlargement of regional lymph nodes draining the bitten area is an early sign of envenoming by Viperidae and Australasian elapids. Spontaneous bleeding is most often detected in the gingival sulci (Fig. 126–12), and from the nose, gastrointestinal tract, and genitourinary tract. Hypotension is an important sign of hypovolemia or cardiotoxicity in patients bitten by vipers, pit vipers, and cobras. Ptosis is the earliest sign of neurotoxic envenoming (Fig. 126–14). Respiratory muscle power should be assessed objectively, e.g., by measuring vital capacity. If a procoagulant venom is suspected, hemostasis should be checked at the bedside by the 20-minute whole blood clotting test, or by laboratory tests of hemostasis, if they can be performed rapidly.

Antivenom Treatment. The only specific treatment for envenoming is antivenom, also known as antivenin and antisnakebite serum, which is usually raised in horses. Most commercial antivenoms are now pepsin-digested, ammonium sulfate–precipitated $F(ab')_2$ fragments of equine IgG, but still carry a risk of serum reactions. Recently, ovine, papain-digested, Fab fragment antivenom has been developed. Unfortunately, the clinical testing of antivenoms has been neglected, and consequently, the indications, dosage, and assessment of the activity of most antivenoms in patients remain uncertain. Theakston and Warrell (1991) and Meier and White (1995) list the antivenoms available worldwide and their range of activity.

Indications. Because of their high cost and the inherent danger of reactions, antivenoms should not be used indiscriminantly. Antivenom is indicated if there is systemic envenoming evidenced by hypotension or other signs of cardiovascular toxicity, signs of neurotoxicity or generalized myotoxicity, impaired consciousness, spontaneous systemic bleeding, and incoagulable blood. Supporting evidence of severe envenoming is provided by a peripheral leukocytosis of more than $20,000/mm^3$, electrocardiographic abnormalities, elevated serum enzymes, hemoglobinuria, myoglobinuria, severe anemia or hemoconcentration, uremia, and oliguria. In the absence of systemic envenoming, massive local swelling (involving more than half of the bitten limb), bites on fingers, and rapidly progressive swelling following bites by species known to cause necrosis are indications for antivenom.

Special Indications. In the case of rattlesnake envenoming, especially by the most dangerous species (*C. atrox, C. adamanteus, C. durissus* subspecies, *C. scutulatus, C. viridis* subspecies, and *C. horridus*), it is recommended that antivenom be given early, before systemic envenoming has become obvious. In this case, the rapid spread of local swelling is considered an indication for antivenom. Similarly, with bites by several species of North American coral snake (genera *Micrurus* and *Micruroides*), antivenom is recommended following definite bites in which there is immediate pain and any other symptom or sign of envenoming. In Australia, the Commonwealth Serum Laboratories (CSL) recommend that antivenom be given for any proved or suspected snakebite if there are tender regional lymph nodes or other evidence of systemic spread of venom, as well as for any bite by an identified highly venomous snake.

Contraindications. There is no absolute contraindication to antivenom, but because of the increased danger of severe reactions, atopic individuals and those known to be hypersensitive to equine serum should be pretreated with epinephrine, hydrocortisone, and antihistamine (doses above) and watched carefully for at least 2 hours after completion of antivenom administration.

Timing of Antivenom Treatment. Antivenom should be given as soon as indicated, but it is almost never too late. For example, sea snake envenoming has been reversed up to 2 days after the bite, and blood coagulability has been restored in victims of *Echis* bite 10 days or more after the bite.

Administration of Antivenom. The expiration date stated on ampules of antivenom is too early if storage has been at 4°C, but opaque solutions should always be rejected, as precipitation of protein indicates loss of activity and increased risk of antivenom reactions. Only specific antivenom, i.e., antivenom whose range of specificity includes the biting species, should be given. Some antivenoms raised against the venom of one or two species have wide paraspecific activity. For example, the Australian CSL "Tiger-Sea-Snake Antivenom" raised against the venoms of *Notechis scutatus* and *Enhydrina schistosa* neutralizes at least 12 different sea snake venoms.

Ideally, antivenom should be diluted in an appropriate volume of fluid and given by "push" injection over 10 to 15 minutes or by IV infusion over 30 minutes. The incidence and severity of reactions are the same with both techniques, but where equipment and supervision are available, administration is controlled more easily by infusion. Epinephrine 0.1% solution, 0.5 ml for adults or 0.01 ml/kg for children, must be ready for intramuscular injection, in case of early anaphylactoid reactions during the infusion. The patient must be watched carefully while antivenom is being given and for at least 1 hour afterward. At the first sign of a reaction, administration of antivenom should be stopped and epinephrine should be given by subcutaneous injection. Once the symptoms of the reaction have subsided, antivenom infusion can be continued slowly if the patient's condition still warrants it. Intravenous chlorpheniramine maleate (10 mg in adults, 0.2 mg/kg in children) and hydrocortisone (100 mg in adults, 2 mg/kg in children) can be given later to prevent recurrent urticaria and to calm the patient. Corticosteroids are not indicated, except for the treatment of serum sickness-type reactions.

Antivenom reactions are not predicted reliably by conjunctival or intradermal tests. In patients known to be hypersensitive to equine serum, pretreatment with epinephrine and antihistamine may be partially effective in preventing reactions. "Rapid desensitization" is not recommended.

The appropriate initial dose has been established for only a few antivenoms. Assessment of antivenom dose will remain a matter of clinical judgment. Antivenom potencies based on animal protection tests may be highly misleading for calculating the dose required in human victims. Approximate initial starting doses of a selected group of antivenoms for bites by some of the most important species are presented in Table 126–9. *The dose of antivenom for children and adults should be the same.*

Response to antivenom may be dramatic. Patients often feel indefinably better soon after the infusion has started. In patients with shock, the blood pressure may rise to normal within a few minutes. Rapid recovery from respiratory paralysis in patients with neurotoxic envenomation is rare but has occasionally been described, e.g., in bite victims of the Australian and Papuan death adder (genus *Acanthophis*) and Asian cobras (genus *Naja*). Spontaneous systemic bleeding usually stops within 15 to 30 minutes of initiating antivenom therapy in the case of *E. carinatus* and *C. rhodostoma* bites, and blood clotting is usually restored within 1 to 6 hours if an adequate neutralizing dose of antivenom has been given. Further antivenom should be given if severe signs of enven-

TABLE 126–9. A Guide to Initial Dosage of Selected Important Antivenoms

Species		Manufacturer, Antivenom	Approximate Initial Dose
Latin Name	*English Name*		
Acanthophis species	Death adder	CSL,* monospecific	3000–6000 U
Bitis arietans	Puff adder	Behringwerke, SAIMR,† polyspecific	80 mL
Bothrops atrox *B. jararaca*	Lance-headed vipers	South American Institutes, *Bothrops*, polyspecific	40 mL
Bungarus caeruleus	Indian krait	Haffkine, polyspecific	100 mL
Calloselasma (Agkistrodon) rhodostoma	Malayan pit viper	Thai Red Cross (Saovabha), Bangkok, monospecific	100 mL
		Thai Government Pharmaceutical Organization, monospecific	50 mL
Crotalus adamanteus	Eastern diamondback rattlesnakes		
C. atrox	Western diamondback rattlesnakes	Wyeth, Crotalidae polyspecific	30–100 mL
C. viridis subspecies	Western rattlesnakes	Therapeutic antibodies "Crotab"	4 vials
Daboia russelli	Russell's viper	Myanmar Pharmaceutical Industry, monospecific	40 mL
		Therapeutic antibodies "Polongatab"	20 ml
		Haffkine, polyspecific	100 mL
Echis species	Saw-scaled or carpet vipers	SAIMR, *Echis*, monospecific Therapeutic antibodies "Echitab"	20 mL
		Behringwerke, *Bitis-Echis-Naja*, polyspecific	100 mL
Hydrophiidae	Sea snakes	CSL, *Enhydrina schistosa*	1000 U
Naja kaouthia	Monocellate Thai cobra	Thai Red Cross, monospecific	100 mL
N. naja	Indian cobra	Haffkine, Kasauli, polyspecific	100 mL
Notechis scutatus	Tiger snake	CSL, monospecific	3000–6000 U
Pseudonaja textilis	Eastern brown snake		
Trimeresurus albolabris	Green pit viper	Thai Red Cross, monospecific	100 mL
Vipera species	European adders	Imunoloski Zavod-Zagreb, *Vipera*, polyspecific	10 mL
		Therapeutic antibodies "Vipertab"	100–200 mg
V. palaestinae	Palestine viper	Rogoff Medical Research Institute, Tel Aviv, Palestine viper, monospecific	50–80 mL

*Commonwealth Serum Laboratories, Australia.
†South African Institute for Medical Research.

omation persist after 1 to 2 hours or if blood coagulability is not restored within about 6 hours. Some effects of envenoming, such as local necrosis, nephrotoxicity following Russell's viper bites, and presynaptic neurotoxicity, are unlikely to be reversed by antivenom.

Antivenom Reactions. There are three types of antivenom reaction.

Early (anaphylactoid) reactions usually develop within 10 to 20 minutes of IV injection of antivenom or within 30 minutes to 3 hours of starting IV infusion of diluted antivenom. Premonitory symptoms include restlessness, cough, itching of the scalp, nausea, vomiting, a feeling of heat, or an increase in pulse rate. Later, there is diffuse and confluent urticaria, generalized pruritus, fever, tachycardia, autonomic manifestations, and, in a few patients, severe hypotension, airflow obstruction, and angioedema. The incidence of early reactions is greatest when large doses of relatively unrefined antivenom are given by intravenous injection. The original assumption that all of these reactions resulted from immediate (IgE-mediated type I) hypersensitivity to equine serum was not correct. The mechanism is complement activation by IgG aggregates or residual Fc fragments. Mortality from antivenom reactions is low if appropriate treatment is given.

Pyrogenic reactions, which may be nonspecific and nonimmunologic, may occur within 1 or 2 hours of antivenom treatment and can precipitate febrile convulsions in children.

Late reactions of the serum sickness type may develop 5 to 10 days after antivenom treatment. A high incidence of these reactions, related to the dose of antivenom given, has been reported in North America. Clinical features include fever, pruritus, urticaria, subcutaneous and periarticular swellings, polyarthritis, lymphadenopathy, mononeuritis multiplex and other neurologic symptoms, and proteinuria.

Supportive Treatment

Neurotoxic Envenoming. Many patients, unable to swallow their secretions, aspirate, develop upper airway obstruction, and die. Others die of respiratory paralysis. Endotracheal intubation should be performed at an early stage, when pooling of secretions in the pharynx becomes evident, before obstruction or respiratory arrest has developed. If respiratory muscle power is inadequate, ventilation must be assisted by mouth-to-tube respiration, Ambu bag, or respirator. Patients have recovered from respiratory paralysis after being manually ventilated by relays of relatives or nurses for up to 30 days and after mechanical ventilation for up to 10 weeks. All effects of neurotoxic envenomation are fully reversible; therefore, artificial ventilation should always be attempted.

Circulatory Collapse. This may be a direct effect of the venom on the heart and vasculature, the result of hypovolemia or autopharmacologic effects of the venom. In all cases, antivenom, followed by plasma expanders, is indicated. Clinical observation of jugular venous pressure or measurement of central venous pressure or pulmonary wedge pressure (via a Swan-Ganz catheter) helps to prevent fluid overload and precipitation of pulmonary edema. If hypotension persists despite restoration of central venous pressure to +10 to 15 cm H_2O, an infusion of dopamine should be started at an initial dose of 2 μg/kg/minute through the central catheter.

Occlusion of Major Arteries. This usually occurs in tensely swollen limbs and could result from compression in fascial compartments or from high local concentrations of venom procoagulant. It may be difficult to diagnose vascular occlusion in an edematous limb that is cold and has impalpable pulses. Arteriography could be used in patients with no coagulation disturbance, or blood flow could be detected by the Doppler ultrasound method.

Local Necrosis. Once definite signs of necrosis have appeared, surgical debridement, immediate split-skin grafting, and antibiotic prophylaxis, to include coverage for anaerobic organisms, are necessary. Occasionally, thrombosis of a major vessel or neglected local necrosis may necessitate amputation of a limb. This is usually the result of inadequate initial antivenom treatment, prolonged application of a tight tourniquet, or inadvisable treatment such as cryotherapy. On rare occasions, increased pressure within tight fascial compartments, e.g., in the digits and anterior tibial compartment, may contribute to ischemic necrosis. In view of the great dangers of decompression by fasciotomy in patients with incoagulable blood, objective evidence of a high compartmental pressure or vascular occlusion should be obtained before surgery is considered and surgery should not be embarked on before hemostasis has been restored with antivenom, clotting factors, and platelets. Fasciotomy is rarely, if ever, indicated in snakebite victims.

Renal Failure. Some snakebite victims admitted with oliguria and elevated blood urea nitrogen and creatinine levels are simply hypovolemic. Acute tubular necrosis resulting from hypotension is the most common cause of renal failure after snakebite. Urine output, specific gravity, and sodium concentration should be followed, and the patient should be treated conservatively by strict fluid balance or, if necessary, by peritoneal dialysis or hemodialysis. In patients bitten by sea snakes and the other species whose venoms cause generalized rhabdomyolysis, alkaline diuresis should be initiated with mannitol, sodium bicarbonate, and furosemide to prevent renal damage from myoglobin. Hyperkalemia should be corrected by the usual methods.

Other Drugs. Heparin, antifibrinolytic agents, e.g., ε-aminocaproic acid, corticosteroids, antihistamines, and a large range of herbal and other remedies, have been advocated for treatment of snakebite. There is no adequate evidence, based on controlled trials, that any of these agents is other than harmful. In particular, heparin has exaggerated bleeding and contributed to the death of snakebite victims.

Anticholinesterases have a variable but sometimes useful effect in patients with neurotoxic envenoming. It is worth giving to any patient with neurotoxic envenoming a test dose of edrophonium chloride by intravenous injection (for adults 2 mg followed after 45 seconds by 8 mg if there is no response) as in the Tensilon test for myasthenia gravis. Atropine 0.6 mg should be given first by IV injection to block the unpleasant muscarinic effects of edrophonium. The effects should be assessed objectively, and if convincing, neostigmine methylsulfate and atropine should be given at least every 4 hours or by continuous infusion. The dose of neostigmine is 50 to 100 μg/kg every 4 hours. Anticholinesterases have proved most effective in cases of bites by Asian *Naja* species and Australian death adder (*Acanthophis*), but there are also reports of benefit after bites by green mamba (*Dendroaspis viridis*), forest cobra (*Naja melanoleuca*), and Malayan and Indian kraits (*Bungarus candidus* and *B. caeruleus*).

Management of Snake Venom Ophthalmia. First aid consists of immediate generous irrigation of the affected eye or mucous membrane with water or any other plentiful bland liquid. At the hospital or dispensary, the eye should be examined by fluorescein staining or with slit lamp. Unless the possibility of corneal abrasions can be excluded, topical antimicrobials should be applied and the eye closed with a dressing pad.

PREVENTION OF SNAKEBITE. To reduce the risk of bites, snakes should never be disturbed, attacked, or handled, even if they are said to be harmless species or appear to be dead. In snake-infested areas, boots, socks, and long trousers should be worn for walks in undergrowth or deep sand. A light should always be carried at night. Particularly dangerous activities are collecting firewood; dislodging logs and boulders with the bare hands; pushing sticks into burrows, holes, or crevices; and climbing rocks and trees covered with dense foliage. Unlit paths and roads are especially dangerous after heavy rains.

It is pointless and undesirable to attempt to exterminate dangerous species of snakes.

Bibliography

Bücherl W, Buckley EE, Deulofeu V (eds): Venomous Animals and Their Venoms, Vols I and II. New York, Academic Press, 1971.

Cardoso JLC, Fan HW, Franca FOS, et al: Randomized comparative trial of three antivenoms in the treatment of envenoming by lance-headed vipers (Bothrops jararaca) in São Paulo, Brazil. Q J Med 86:315, 1993.

Gopalakrishnakone P (ed): Sea Snake Toxinology. Singapore, National University, 1994.

Hutton RA, Warrell DA: Action of snake venom components on the haemostatic system. Blood Rev 7:176, 1993.

Junghanss T, Bodio M: Notfall-Handbuch Giftiere. Stuttgart, Georg Thieme Verlag, 1996.

Lalloo DG, Trevett AJ, Korinhona A, et al: Snakebites by the Papuan taipan Oxyuranus scutellatus canni): Paralysis, hemostatic and electrocardiographic abnormalities and effects of antivenom. Am J Trop Med Hyg 52:525, 1995.

Lee CY: Snake Venoms. Handbook of Experimental Pharmacology. Vol. 52. New York, Springer-Verlag, 1979.

Meier J, White J (eds): Clinical Toxicology of Animal Venoms. Boca Raton, FL, CRC Press, 1995.

Myint-Lwin, Warrell DA, Phillips RE, et al: Bites by Russell's viper (Vipera russelli siamensis) in Burma: Haemostatic, vascular and renal disturbances and response to treatment. Lancet 2:1259, 1985.

Reid HA, Thean PC, Chan KE, et al: Clinical effects of bites by Malayan viper (Ancistrodon rhodostoma). Lancet 1:617, 1963.

Russell FE: Snake Venom Poisoning. Philadelphia, JB Lippincott, 1980.

Spawls S, Branch B: The Dangerous Snakes of Africa. London, Blandford, 1995.

Sutherland SK: Australian Animal Toxins: The Creatures, Their Toxins and Care of the Poisoned Patient. Melbourne, Oxford University Press, 1983.

Sutherland SK, Coulter AR, Harris RD: Rationalisation of first-aid measures for elapid snake bite. Lancet 1:183, 1979.

Theakston RDG, Warrell DA: Antivenoms: A list of hyperimmune sera currently available for the treatment of envenoming by bites and stings. Toxicon 29:1419, 1991.

Warrell DA: Injuries, envenoming, poisoning and allergic reactions caused by animals. In Weatherall DJ, Ledingham JGG, Warrell DA (eds): Oxford Textbook of Medicine, 3rd ed. Oxford, England, Oxford University Press, 1996, pp 1124–1151.

Warrell DA, Davidson NM, Greenwood BM, et al: Poisoning by bites of the saw-scaled or carpet viper (Echis carinatus) in Nigeria. Q J Med 46:33, 1977.

Warrell DA, Greenwood BM, Davidson NM, et al: Necrosis, haemorrhage and complement depletion following bites by the spitting cobra (Naja nigricollis). Q J Med 45:1, 1976.

Watt G, Theakston RDG, Hayes CG, et al: Positive response to edrophonium in patients with neurotoxic envenoming by cobras (Naja naja philippinensis). A placebo-controlled study. N Engl J Med 315:1444, 1986.

126.6 Bats

William A. Sodeman, Jr.

Bats are of medical importance because they transmit disease to humans and in some cases are direct agents of injury. In addition, bat roosts provide an environment highly suited to the transmission of some fungal diseases to humans. The role of bats in the direct transmission of diseases to humans has been characterized best for the viral infections, rabies, and Venezuelan equine encephalomyelitis. Many other viral, bacterial, fungal, and parasitic organisms have been described as associated with bats (Table 126–10), but the human risk is not well characterized. Vampire bats cause direct injury during feeding. Secondary infections or parasitization of these open lesions by fly larvae, particularly screwworm, can be serious health problems at times. Histoplasma capsulatum often contaminates guano deposits and has caused human infection. Several other fungi are associated with bats, but transmission to humans has not been established.

TABLE 126–10. Viruses, Bacteria, Fungi, and Parasites Associated With Bats

Organism	Location
Venezuelan equine encephalomyelitis	Mexico, Guatemala, Ecuador, Panama, USA, Colombia
Rabies	USA, Mexico, Colombia, Venezuela, Guyana, Brazil, Peru, Bolivia, El Salvador, Trinidad, Canada, Guatemala, Panama, Argentina, Germany, Turkey, Yugoslavia, India, Thailand, South Africa
Yellow fever	Ethiopia
Rio Bravo virus	USA, Mexico, Trinidad, Guatemala
Tamana bat virus	Trinidad
St. Louis encephalitis	USA, Guatemala
Tacaribe virus	Trinidad, Guatemala
Nepuyo virus	Honduras, Trinidad
Catu virus	Brazil
Bimiti virus	Trinidad
Guama virus	Trinidad
Japanese encephalitis virus	Japan
Leptospira	Brazil, Trinidad
Brucella	Brazil
Histoplasma capsulatum	Panama, Mexico, Colombia, Trinidad, USA
Scopulariopsis	Mexico, Colombia
Trypanosoma evansi	Mexico, Central and South America

Almost all of the direct transmission and injury related to bats is in association with the New World vampire bats. The three species, Desmodus rotundus (Geoffroy), Diphylla ecaudata Spix, and Diaemus youngi (Jentinck), have a wide distribution in Central and South America. These bats have a great economic impact as a result of injury to, or transmission of, infection to livestock.

Vampire bats feed primarily on blood. These bats will prey on mammals, birds, and reptiles. Domesticated animals are the preferred target. The incisor and canine teeth are modified to permit painless incision. The bat laps blood with its tongue. A plasminogen activator, desmokinase, has been isolated from Desmodus, and a similar substance has been demonstrated in Diaemus. Saliva flows down a groove on the dorsal surface of the tongue, and blood returns up paired ventral grooves. The anticoagulant and the mechanical licking combine to maintain blood flow. Bats are nocturnal feeders.

RABIES. Most bat rabies in humans is transmitted by the vampire bats, but bat rabies does occur in many other genera of bats (Chapter 30.1). There are regular reports of transmission to humans by frugivorous or insectivorous bats, but these are rare. When this does occur, the bats may be driven to attack by furious rabies with transmission of the virus in saliva associated with a bite. A bite is not essential, and virus can be transmitted by licking an open wound or by direct contact with intact mucous membrane. The possibility of transmission from bats to other animals to humans also exists.

Rabies virus seems to undergo compartmentalization in bats. It is possible to derive the likely animal of origin by typing the rabies virus strain. Human infections in the United States have most commonly been with the virus associated with Lasionycteris noctivagans (the silver-haired bat). The strain associated with vampire bats produces paralytic rather than furious rabies.

Bats infected with rabies generally develop paralytic disease. Death is a result of inanition because of the paralysis. It is possible some bats survive, but a healthy carrier state does not seem to occur. The virus is transmitted in saliva. Several cases of apparent infection of humans exposed to aerosolized saliva, but not to bites, have been reported.

Bat rabies in humans has been reported from many countries in all continents except Australia (Table 126–10). Immunization against rabies offers the best protection. Sleeping in bat-proof lodgings affords protection also. Environmental control to eliminate bat roosts is difficult to implement. Any contact with an aggressive bat is suspect for possibility of transmission. Bats behaving unusually are similarly suspect. Even the examination of a dead bat has been associated with transmission. Aerosolization of virus containing secretion can occur when a bat colony is disturbed and has been associated with transmission as well. Bat rabies in livestock causes considerable economic loss in the tropics. The disease is called derriengue or limping illness, emphasizing its paralytic nature. Treatment of cattle with controlled doses of warfarin will cause death of a feeding vampire from hemorrhage.

VENEZUELAN EQUINE ENCEPHALOMYELITIS (VEE). Epidemic VEE in horses has been associated with the presence of virus-infected vampire bats (Chapter 30.2). Bats may be responsible for mechanical transmission of the virus under such circumstances, but this would be a minor route of dissemination.

OTHER VIRUSES. Many other viruses have been shown to occur naturally in bats: yellow fever virus, Montana myotis leukoencephalitis virus, Rio Bravo virus, Tamana bat virus, Nepuyo virus, St. Louis encephalitis virus, Catu virus, Tacaribe virus, Mount Elgan virus, and Entebbe virus. The role of bats in the natural history and transmission of these viruses is not clear.

BACTERIAL INFECTIONS. *Leptospira* and *Brucella* have both been reported to occur naturally in bats. *Leptospira*-infected bats are found in Asia and Europe as well as the Americas (Chapter 72). *Brucella* infection has been found in vampire bats in Brazil (Chapter 64). There is no evidence yet for transmission from bats to humans.

HISTOPLASMOSIS. Bat guano provides a rich medium for the growth of *Histoplasma capsulatum* (Chapter 83.1). The environment in the bat roost fosters this growth. Humans exposed to dried guano have suffered massive infection and death by inhalation.

OTHER FUNGI. Many other fungi have been found in association with bat roosts, including *Candida* and *Scopulariopsis*, which can infect humans. The involvement of bats seems limited to the provision of a rich environment in the roost to foster the growth of these organisms.

PARASITES. *Trypanosoma evansi*, the causative agent of surra in domestic animals, has been demonstrated in vampire bats. These bats can mechanically transmit the trypanosome from host to host. *Trypanosoma cruzi* has been reported also, but evidence for transmission to humans is lacking.

Bibliography

Baer GM (ed): The Natural History of Rabies. New York, Academic Press, 1975.

Crespo RF, Fernández SS, López DA, et al: Intramuscular inoculation of cattle with warfarin: A new technique for control of vampire bats. Bull Pan Am Health Organ 13:147, 1979.

Greenhall AM, Schmidt U (eds): Natural History of Vampire Bats. Boca Raton, FL, CRC Press, 1988.

Meredith CD, Standing E: Lagos bat virus in South Africa. Lancet 1:832, 1981.

Price JL: Serological evidence of infection of Tacaribe virus and arboviruses in Trinidadian bats. Am J Trop Med Hyg 27:162, 1978.

Warrell MJ: Human deaths from cryptic bat rabies in the USA. Lancet 346:65, 1995.

Winkler WG: Airborne rabies. *In* Baer GM (ed): The Natural History of Rabies, Vol II. New York, Academic Press, 1975, pp 115–121.

127 *Pentastomiasis**

Joseph J. Drabick

DEFINITION. Pentastomiasis is a parasitic zoonosis of humans caused by pentasomes, a group of peculiar endoparasites with characteristics of both arthropods and annelids currently delegated their own phylum but recently shown to be highly related to crustaceans. Synonymous terms are tongue worm infection, porocephaliasis, and linguatuliasis.

ETIOLOGY. Adult pentastomes generally parasitize the respiratory tracts of reptiles or carnivorous mammals in whom they are well tolerated. Usual intermediate hosts are herbivorous mammals but many classes of animals have been infected depending on the infecting pentastome. Humans can act as an intermediate host or a temporary definitive host. The disease was first described in 1847, making it one of the earliest described zoonoses.

CLASSIFICATION. This group of parasites is old; it is speculated that adult pentastomes probably parasitized carnivorous dinosaurs in Mesozoic times. Recent fossil evidence places the group as early as the Cambrian Period. The phylogenetic relationships of the pentastomes have been argued for years but recent molecular studies have verified that they are close kins of crustaceans (Phylum Arthropoda) which through evolution have been highly adapted for their endoparasitic lifestyle. The Pentastomida is divided into two orders: Porocephalida and Cephalobaenida, the latter considered more primitive. Ninety-nine percent of human infection is caused by two species within the first order: *Armillifer armillatus* and *Linguatula serrata*. Infection has been ascribed anecdotally to *Armillifer moniliformis*, *Armillifer grandis*, *Leiperia cincinnalis*, *Sebekia* spp., and *Raillietiella hemidactyli*. Only the latter species is a member of the Cephalobaenida.

MORPHOLOGY. Pentastomes range from a few millimeters to more than 15 cm in length, dependent on the species. The sexes are separate; the males are much smaller than females. They tend to be colorless and transparent and possess two pairs of hooks on either side of a projection that bears the true mouth. Because of this arrangement, the group was misnamed pentastome (five-mouthed). The integument is composed of chitin. External pseudoannulation can give a corkscrew or string-of-beads appearance in some species. Others (Linguatulidae) are flattened and resemble tongues, hence their name. Superficially, adults resemble helminths and are frequently mistaken for them; however the first larval stage in all forms superficially resembles a mite (Fig. 127–1).

EPIDEMIOLOGY

Life Cycle. Adult parasites exist in the respiratory tract of the definitive host, where they attach themselves by means of their hooks and suck epithelial cells, blood, lymph, and mucus into their digestive tract (Fig. 127–1). Like many helminthic parasites, female pentastomids are prodigious egg-producers. After copulation and internal fertilization, the embryonated eggs pass into the environment in nasal secretions, saliva, and feces where the eggs are well adapted to an aqueous environment; hence, water as well as wet vegetation may be sources of infection for the intermediate host. After ingestion, the first-stage larvae hatch and tunnel through the tissues of the host until it finally encysts. After a series of molts the larvae become infectious for the definitive host. The death of the intermediate host may trigger the mature

---

*All material in this chapter is in the public domain, with the exception of any figures or tables.

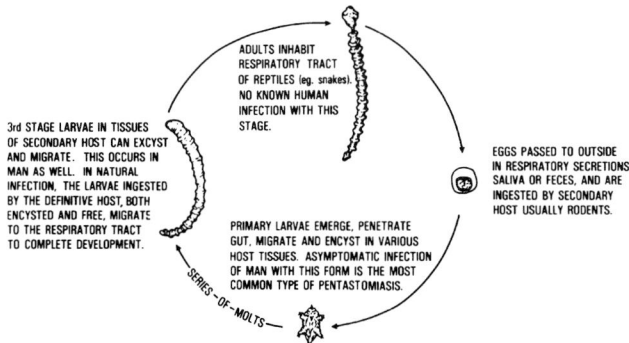

Figure 127–1. Lifecycle of *Armillifer*. (From Drabick JJ: Rev Inf Dis 9:1087, 1987.)

infective larvae to excyst and migrate to the outside. Apparently, this behavior facilitates the likelihood of ingestion by the definitive host. With ingestion of the intermediate host by the carnivorous definitive host, the third-stage larvae migrate up the esophagus to the lungs and/or nasopharynx. After several more molts they mature, mate, and lay eggs, completing the life cycle. Both encysted and migrating third-stage larvae are infectious for the definitive host.

Distribution. Pentastomes are cosmopolitan, with a concentration in tropical and subtropical areas. Most cases of pentastomiasis have been reported from equatorial Africa, the Middle East, and Southeast Asia. Sporadic cases have been noted in the Americas and Europe. Eating habits and lifestyles are the primary factors in determining the rates and severity of infection. Most cases of human pentastomiasis are subclinical and thus comments on prevalence are difficult to make. Human infection with *L. serrata* may be fairly common in the Middle East given the fact that approximately 50% of dogs from various sites have been shown to be infected and the infection can be transmitted by food or hands contaminated by a sneezing dog. Recently, a new species of pentastome, *Linguatula arctica*, has been described in reindeer and caribou of far Northern Europe. This species has an anomalous life cycle in that the ruminants are themselves the definitive hosts; human infection with this species has not been demonstrated to date.

PATHOLOGY AND PATHOGENESIS. In humans there is minimal to moderate immune response to the parasite. Most encysted larvae eventually die and leave fibrotic nodules that may calcify, appearing as radiopaque densities on radiographs. Lesions are found most commonly in the liver (Fig. 127–2), but can also involve the intestinal wall, mesentery, peritoneum, and lung. Systemic eosinophilia is not a feature of pentastomiasis. It has been discovered that pentastomes secrete a lipid-containing substance onto their surfaces from specialized glands which help the parasite evade immune detection.

CLINICAL MANIFESTATIONS. An individual becomes a secondary host for *A. armillatus* by ingesting eggs in contaminated food or drink or by intimate contact with the definitive reptilian host in the preparation of food or harvesting of skins. Likewise, an individual can be infected as a secondary host by *L. serrata* by exposure to canine nasal secretions or feces containing eggs. Humans are highly tolerant to this form of pentastomiasis. The vast majority of cases are asymptomatic, manifested only as an incidental finding at autopsy, surgery, or radiologic examination (Fig. 127–2). Problems can arise when the encysted larvae enlarge during molting, causing pressure on vital organs or rarely when migrating larvae perforate organs. Hypersensitivity reactions probably occur

as well. Anecdotal cases of pneumonitis, atelectasis, intestinal obstruction, bile duct blockage, and pericarditis have been reported. Eye involvement occasionally associated with acute glaucoma has been reported, including some cases in the southern United States.

Halzoun. The other form of clinical pentastomiasis is found in the Middle East and is caused by ingested third-stage larvae found in the raw liver or lymph nodes of sheep or goats. In this instance, humans are infected as temporary definitive hosts. The infection is called halzoun and occurs when such foods are consumed. In Sudan, the syndrome is called *marrara* after the dish that causes it. The syndrome is characterized as an acute, self-limited nasopharyngitis associated with coughing, sneezing, dysphagia, hoarseness, and facial edema. Symptoms usually last less than a week, resolving spontaneously, but airway obstruction and pyogenic complications can occur. Third-stage larvae can be demonstrated in nasal discharge, sputum, and vomitus and are described as small living worms, 5 to 10 mm in length. Persistent infection with adult pentastomes has only rarely been reported in the literature.

Subcutaneous Pentastomiasis. Cases of subcutaneous infection with *R. hemidactyli*, called creeping or crawling disease, has been described in Southeast Asia among tribes that swallow small live lizards as a folk remedy. A case of a cutaneous larva migrans–like lesion was recently described in Costa Rica due to a *Sebekia* species. The mode of acquisition in this case was unclear.

DIAGNOSIS AND TREATMENT. The diagnosis of pentastomiasis is usually made by demonstrating the presence of

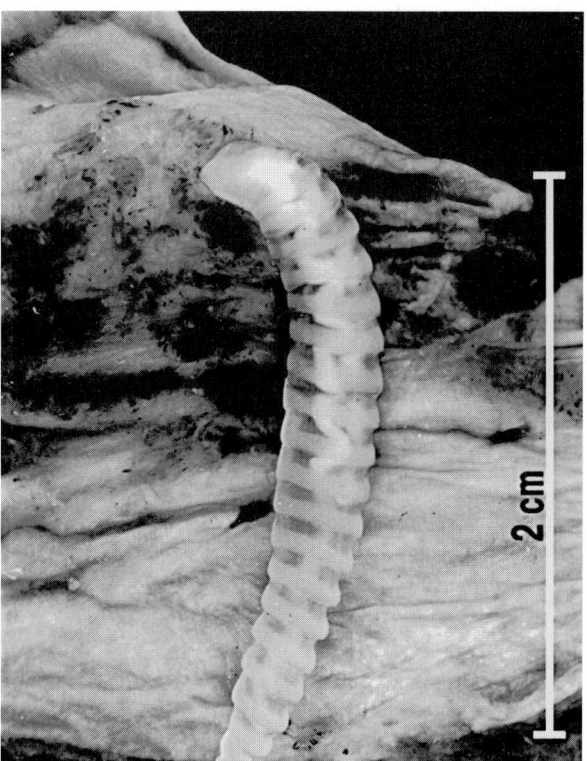

Figure 127–2. *Armillifer armillatus* excysted third-stage larva. This specimen had emerged from its cyst and was found crawling over the abdominal surface of the diaphragm of a man from the Congo necropsied 18 hours after an accidental death. Several other specimens were found free and motile in the abdominal cavity. (Courtesy of Armed Forces Institute of Pathology, Photograph Neg. No. 72–4558.)

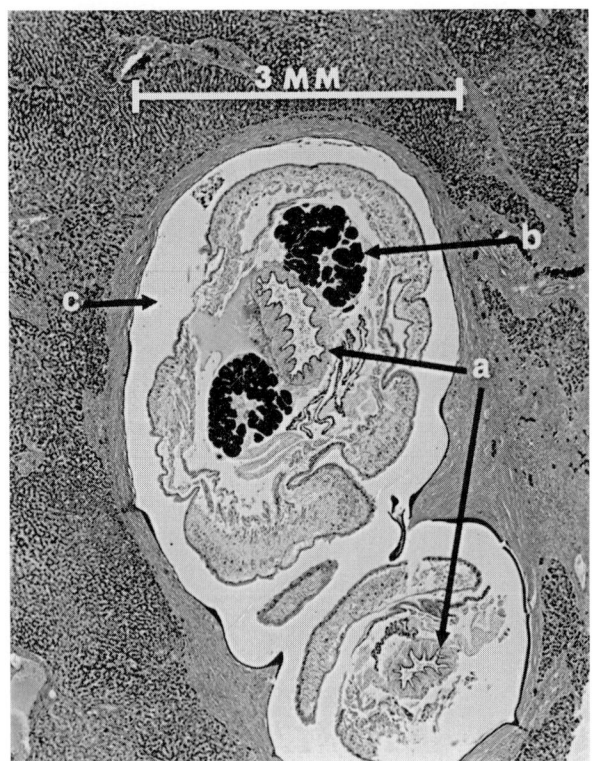

Figure 127–3. *Armillifer armillatus* larval pentastomid cyst in human liver. The intestine (*a*) and acidophilic glands (*b*) are apparent. There is a space (*c*) between the current cuticle and that of a former molt. The host reaction is predominantly fibrosis. (Courtesy of Armed Forces Institute of Pathology, Photograph Neg. No. 75–2703.)

the parasite in tissues at autopsy, biopsy, or surgery (Figs. 127–2 and 127–3). The typical radiographic lesion is a C-shaped or "cashew nut" opacity less than 1 cm in diameter with lesions predominantly in the liver and hila of the lungs. Serologic tests for pentastome infections have been developed but their role in diagnosis is unclear. Most recently an enzyme-linked immunosorbent assay based on a 48-kDa metalloproteinase isolated from the frontal glands of a pentastome has been developed and shows promise as a potential tool for seroprevalence studies.

Treatment of larval pentastomiasis is unnecessary except in rare instances in which symptoms arise owing to pressure effects, in which case surgery is indicated for removal. Halzoun is usually self-limited, but airway protection may be required in cases with severe laryngeal edema. Antibiotic and surgical therapy may be required for secondary pyogenic complications. Antihistamines and steroids are indicated in the event of hypersensitivity reactions. There are few data on the chemotherapy of veterinary infections (reptiles in zoos) but diethylcarbamazine has been reported to be active against linguatuliasis. Since pentastomes are arthropodian, ivermectin may also be theoretically active given its known activity against ectoparasitic mites like *Sarcoptes scabiei*.

PREVENTION. As with so many tropical diseases, control of pentastomiasis would best be realized with more effective water and food sanitation. As in the cases of other parasitic infections, the eating of uncooked exotic meats can cause infection.

Bibliography

Drabick JJ: Pentastomiasis. Rev Infect Dis 9:1087, 1987.
Haugerund RE: Human pentastomiasis. Tidsskr Nor Laegeforen 108:28, 1988.
Jones DAC, Henderson RJ, Riley J: Preliminary characterization of the lipid and protein components of the protective surface membranes of a pentastomid *Porocephalus crotali*. Parasitology 104:469, 1992.
Jones DAC, Riley J: An ELISA for the detection of pentastomid infections in the rat. Parasitology 103:331, 1991.
Mairena H, Solano M, Venegas W: Human dermatitis caused by a nymph of *Sebekia*. Am J Trop Med Hyg 41:352, 1989.
Riley J: The biology of pentastomids. Adv Parasitol 25:45, 1986.
Self JT, Kuntz RE: Host-parasite relations in some Pentastomida. J Parasitol 53:202, 1967.

128 Injurious Arthropods

Robert A. Wirtz and Abdu F. Azad

Contact with arthropods and their products can result in adverse reactions in humans that range from mild seasonal annoyance to anaphylactic shock and death. The severity of these reactions is dependent on the way in which the arthropod or its products is encountered, the type and composition of the allergen, and the prior history of exposure.

The most common modes of exposure are through arthropod bites or stings (envenomization) and direct contact, ingestion, or inhalation of venoms or allergens. Stinging arthropods (e.g., wasps, bees, ants, scorpions) actively inject venom mixtures through specialized structures. Biting arthropods (e.g., spiders, flies, bugs, mites, ticks) inject digestive or salivary secretions and venoms through piercing mouthparts or modified appendages (e.g., fangs). Biting arthropods can be grouped according to duration of host contact, i.e., transient versus prolonged (Fig. 128–1). Passive envenomation is the release of venom in or onto the surface of the skin; this includes defensive irritants and vesicants (e.g., blister beetles, millipedes, cockroaches) and venom-containing hollow spines (e.g., caterpillars). Some arthropods may forcibly release toxins from some distance (millimeters to over 1 meter). Potent allergens and toxic secretory products, e.g., defensive secretions, dried feces (frass), wing scales, other exoskeleton fragments, and whole arthropods (e.g., mites, thrips, aphids), are often ingested or inhaled.

Venoms and salivary secretions are also capable of eliciting an allergic reaction. These are usually mild; however, in sensitized individuals they can be life-threatening. Allergic reactions to stings cause more deaths than any other type of arthropod injury, and hypersensitive individuals often die before supportive therapy can be given.

In general, important determinants of the envenomation effect of arthropod bites relate to the arthropod, its toxin, and the human host. The species of arthropod, the effectiveness of toxin delivery, and the number of arthropods making the attack will all influence the medical outcome. Likewise, the volume and nature of the toxin will be important. Finally, the status of the victim with regard to age, size, weight, and the nature of the immune response will be critical. Arthropod injury is one of the most common causes of lesions of the human integument. Although winter brings some relief from flying insects in temperate climates, the ectoparasites persist. In the tropics, the densities of biting insects can reach remarkable proportions. In developed countries, the widespread use of insecticides has reduced insect populations.

Biting and envenoming arthropods from many orders and families are commonly involved in producing similar dermatologic conditions. Different species within the same genus, however, can produce remarkably different effects. Further-

BITING ARTHROPODS

TRANSIENT HOST CONTACT

Mosquitoes

Flies

LONG-TERM HOST CONTACT

Ectoparasites

Endoparasites

Fleas

Lice

Fleas

Fly Larvae

True Bugs

Soft ticks

Hard Ticks

Mites

Fleas

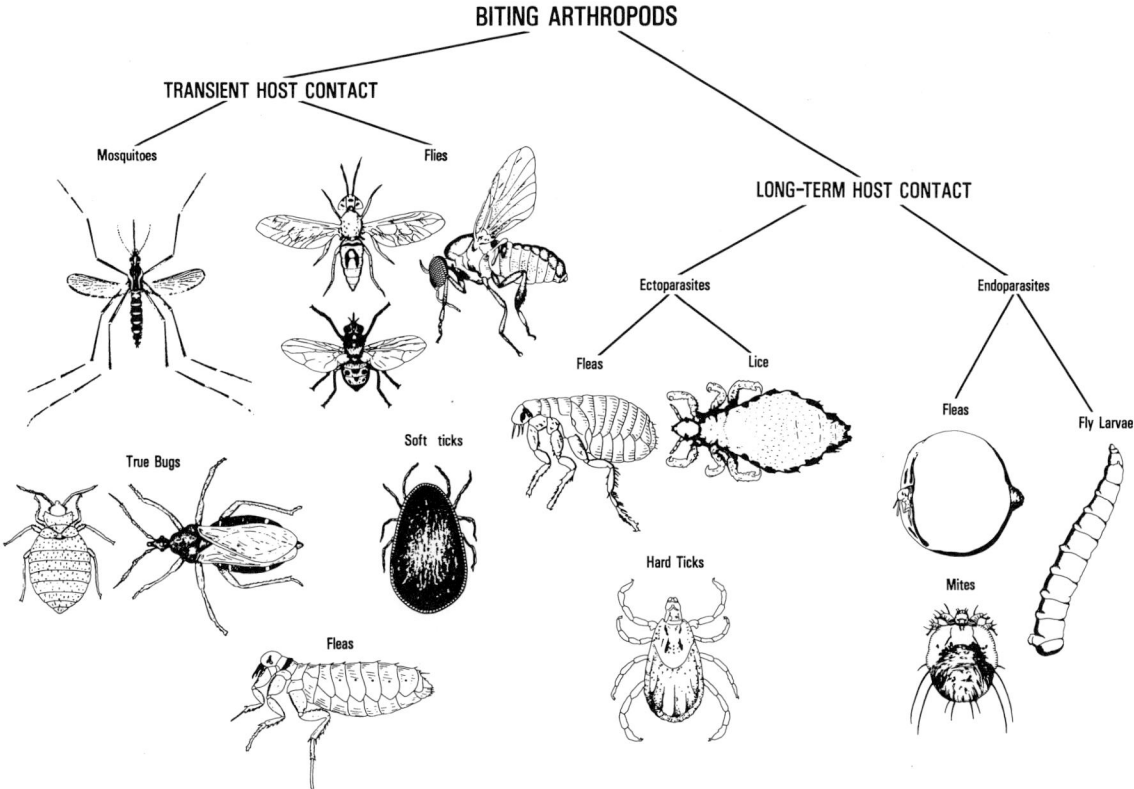

Figure 128–1. Biting arthropods can be broadly grouped into categories based on the length of contact with humans.

more, a given arthropod may produce different symptoms in different people.

Delusory parasitosis is an emotional disorder in which the individual has an unwarranted belief that he or she is infested with live organisms, usually mites or other small arthropods. Excoriation and gouging may be seen as a result of desperate scratching and cleansing. This disease can become intractable and induce a consuming anxiety in the patient and family. Victims can be well educated and appear rational and sensible about other matters not pertaining to their obsession. Delusory parasitosis has occasionally been misdiagnosed owing to the small size of many arthropods. An adequate search for parasites on the patient, pets, and in the immediate work and home environment should be made before symptoms are labeled as delusional. "Sick building syndrome" and "cable mite dermatitis" exemplify cases in which symptoms initially attributed to arthropod infestations or diagnosed as psychoneurotic were later associated with physical irritants found in the work or home environment.

Entomophobia (acarophobia), often used in referring to delusory parasitosis, is an unfounded fear of insects. Greater understanding of—and familiarity with—insects generally lessens this fear.

128.1 *Allergy*

Allergies to arthropods are recognized as a significant health threat worldwide. The tremendous diversity of arthropods and their products and the large biomass represented by this phylum present a continuing, complex array of potent allergens to the immune system.

Chronological exposure to arthropod allergens usually results in a sequence of reactions. Initially, there is no discernible response; this is followed by the appearance of only a delayed reaction. Both immediate and delayed reactions usually occur with further exposure. Many individuals remain at this stage, whereas others progress to only an immediate response, and finally to a point at which no reaction is observed with exposure. It may be difficult to determine when clinical symptoms are attributable to reaginic hypersensitivity and IgE antibodies and when the reactions are due to the nonallergenic components of arthropod products. Development of an arthropod allergy is dependent on the genetic predisposition of the individual, the species of arthropod and size of infestations, and the type of allergens as well as the duration of exposure. Cross reactivity among different arthropod allergens exists, so that once sensitized, a subject may react to a variety of species. Potent arthropod allergens can promote two very different types of reaction—immediate and delayed. The immediate reaction may advance to a state of hypersensitivity in some individuals.

REAGINIC HYPERSENSITIVITY. In the immediate (within 6 hours) anaphylactic (type I) response, reaginic IgE antibodies formed on previous exposure to the allergen are fixed to tissue mast cells. When the antigen is reintroduced into the host, it binds with the antibody attached to the cell surface, triggering the release of histamine and other substances. Local anaphylaxis in the skin, a urticarial or bullous response, is the immediate reaction to an insect bite. In generalized anaphylaxis, e.g., that seen after a bee sting in a sensitized person, a massive release of histamine and other mediators results in life-threatening complications, e.g., cardiovascular shock or laryngeal edema.

DELAYED HYPERSENSITIVITY. Papular urticaria was the name applied to insect bites before their true origin was determined. These nodules represent the delayed reactions. They are common in children whose experience of exposure is limited. Because the skin is irritated by bites, scratching with subsequent secondary infection often modifies their appearance. Bites on the lower leg often show greater reaction owing to relative circulatory stasis. The bite marks of fleas, mosquitoes, black flies, midges, or assassin bugs frequently have the same appearance. Treatment is usually limited to calamine lotions and the prevention of secondary infection.

Delayed hypersensitivity reactions to insect bites are mainly the result of a type IV reaction, in which the allergen may be different from that responsible for type I reactions. In the type IV reaction, mononuclear cells respond to the allergen at the site of introduction, producing an intense cellular infiltration that results in a nodule. Histologic studies of insect bites show that immediate macular wheal reactions, which may be associated with an erythematous flare, have prominent eosinophilic infiltration. This is in contrast to a delayed response, in which lymphocytes and plasma cells predominate.

TESTS FOR HYPERSENSITIVITY. Hypersensitivity is an exaggerated type I immediate response. The division into local and systemic response is somewhat artificial because a sufficient stimulus will result in a generalized reaction.

Skin Tests. Skin testing is the initial method used to determine sensitivity. Within minutes of introduction of the allergen, histamine release from skin mast cells causes vasodilation (erythema), localized edema from increased vascular permeability (wheal), and itching. Many antigens are available commercially in cutaneous and intracutaneous skin test kits.

Blood Tests. Two more sensitive techniques are sometimes available in specialized laboratories. The histamine release assay is a technique that requires the incubation of a patient's leukocytes with the relevant allergen. If the basophils are coated with specific IgE, histamine release can be measured. The radioallergosorbent test (RAST) measures the amount of specific IgE antibody present in the serum and is sensitive to 0.0001 μg of antibody. Although these in vitro methods avoid the risk of sensitizing the patient, they are not as sensitive as skin testing, and their correlations with the clinical history are 85% and 70%, respectively. In addition, they are more time-consuming and more expensive than skin tests.

CONTACT, AIRBORNE, AND INGESTED ALLERGENS. Disorders resulting from inhalation or ingestion of arthropod parts and products, or from direct contact, are separated from those resulting from envenomization. The pathogenic mechanisms include hypersensitivity reactions (allergies) from arthropod allergens and irritant effects from the physical structure of spines, setae, and other materials. Inhalation and physical contact with airborne materials are the mechanisms most pertinent to these allergies. Whole arthropods, body parts, secretions, and excretions can become airborne. Symptoms are often seasonal, with the frequency of exposure increasing as arthropod populations burgeon, or are occupational in nature. Symptoms can range from mild dermal irritation to anaphylaxis.

House dust mites and cockroaches are the most prevalent sources of inhalation allergies in a domestic environment. Notable examples of seasonal variation in public health or occupational exposure include reactions to mayflies (Ephemeroptera), caddis flies (Trichoptera), midges (Diptera), larval and adult moths (Lepidoptera), dermestid and carpet beetle larvae, and adult staphylinid and blister beetles (Coleoptera) (Fig. 128–2).

Mite Allergies. House dust allergy, in which several species of *Dermatophagoides* mites and other arthropods are sources of the inhalation and contact allergens, is estimated to affect

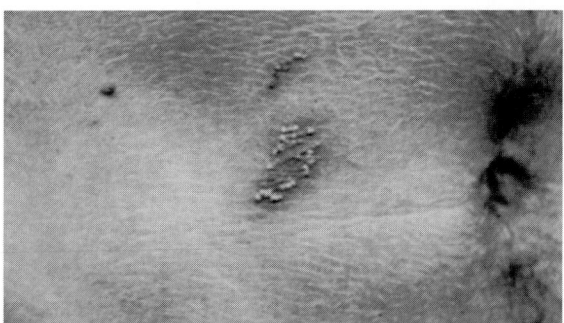

Figure **128–2.** Contact dermatitis from staphylinid beetle (*Paederus* species) on the body of an adult in Ethiopia. (Courtesy of the Armed Forces Institute of Pathology, Photograph Neg. No. 75–5784.)

4% of the United States population and is a significant public health problem worldwide. Mites breed best at relatively high temperatures and humidity, and studies have shown enormous volumes of mites and mite products in living areas. Using extracts of mite cultures for skin testing, over 50% of asthmatic and nonasthmatic atopic individuals have exhibited positive tests. Most allergens in mite cultures are present in fecal particles, and potent glycoprotein fractions of low molecular weight have been isolated. Diagnosis and immunotherapy of the house dust mite allergy is currently based on crude mite preparations. Molecular cloning of mite allergens is being investigated to circumvent the limitations of the small and variable quantities present in these extracts.

Treatment of the house dust mite allergies by hyposensitization with *Dermatophagoides* extracts has yielded variable results, possibly because of the use of relatively crude preparations and the possible involvement of other allergens. Reduction of exposure by using specially designed vacuum cleaners, laundering bed sheets, and enclosing mattresses in plastic covers may have some long-term effect.

Most instances of mite-induced occupational dermatitis are observed in individuals whose work brings them in contact with infested materials. The majority of mites infesting stored and processed foods belong to the families Acaridae, Carpoglyphidae, Glyciphagidae, and Pyroglyphidae. A specific type of product usually harbors a given species; the common terms applied to mite-induced skin inflammations reflect the respective industries (e.g., baker's itch, grain itch, straw itch).

Cockroach Allergies. Hypersensitivity to cockroach allergens is worldwide. Only approximately 50 of the 4000 species of cockroaches are pestiferous, and fewer than a dozen substantially affect health and welfare. Individuals living in environments heavily infested with cockroaches have a higher prevalence of positive skin tests (59%) than do those in areas with lower infestation rates (5%). Over 50% of asthmatics have positive skin scratch tests, while the incidence among nonasthmatic atopics approaches 35%. Over 12% of individuals without a history of allergy also exhibit cockroach hypersensitivity. These data suggest that 10 to 15 million North Americans are allergic to cockroaches; studies in Asia showed similar prevalences.

Other Arthropod Allergies. Lepidopterism is the general term for the ill effects that larval and adult moths and butterflies have on humans. Included are problems associated with inhalation, ingestion, dermal contact, and tissue penetration by products or structures from any life-cycle stage. The urticating hairs or nettling setae (macrotrichia) of caterpillars can be a source of contact dermatitis in an occupational environment and in some instances a significant public health problem. Barbed setae of some species can be difficult to extract. If these enter the eye, fragments may embed in the eyelid, scratching the conjunctiva or cornea, or even penetrate into the interior, resulting in loss of vision.

The barbed setae of adult female *Hylesia* spp. are responsible for serious outbreaks of urticating rashes and upper respiratory tract complications in South America, most notably in Brazil and Peru, where cases may number in the thousands. Symptoms usually occur seasonally, often when moths are attracted to lights in inhabited areas.

Periodic increases in the moth population have resulted in public health problems affecting thousands of individuals in the United States. Both the gypsy moth, *Lymantria dispar*, and the puss moth, *Megalopyge opercularis*, have been implicated. An estimated 500,000 individuals were affected by wind-blown hairs of the mulberry tussock moth, *Euproctis similis*, near Shanghai, China. Last-instars larvae carry over 2 million urticating setae per caterpillar. The Oriental tussock moth, *Euproctis flava*, also was associated with symptoms affecting an estimated 250,000 persons on Honshu Island, Japan, in 1956. Areas throughout the Far East are routinely affected by these moths.

The mass emergence of nonbiting midges (Diptera: Chironomidae) along the Nile in northern Sudan results in allergic symptoms, especially bronchial asthma and rhinitis. Low molecular weight hemoglobins appear to be the primary allergens. Larval populations can reach 100,000/m², and the adult midges at times reach levels that hinder or prevent work and recreation for thousands of individuals. Palliative measures include the use of strong decoy lights to attract midges away from populated areas, which are illuminated by weak reddish lights.

DESENSITIZATION. The clearest indication for desensitization is a patient who has had a life-threatening anaphylactic episode and shows marked skin sensitivity to insect venom. Mixed venom preparations are available containing bee, wasp, and vespid (yellow jacket, yellow hornet, and white-faced hornet) components. Purified venom antigens are preferable to whole-body extracts, which promote many nonspecific immunoglobulins. Because systemic reactions may occur during the course of treatment, therapy is best given in special clinics. The duration of treatment necessary to achieve persistent blocking immunity to stings is unknown. Many allergists advise that treatment be discontinued after 5 years, or sooner if RAST or skin tests become negative. Both IgE and IgG levels may rise during immunotherapy, and modified forms of the type I reaction may be seen. A serum sickness syndrome has been reported with whole-body extract. There is some evidence that factors other than venom-specific IgE may contribute to clinical anaphylaxis. In desensitization to salivary allergens, whole-body extracts are used because salivary antigens are not usually available.

There are few studies on the immunotherapy of patients with allergic respiratory diseases due to inhalation of insect allergens. The recommended treatment follows methods used for patients with asthma caused by plant pollens and molds.

128.2 *Biting Arthropods*

Transient Host Contact

Most arthropods that bite humans have only transient host contact (Fig. 128–1). Hematophagous insects are frequently winged and highly mobile. This accounts for their ability to quickly attack and escape capture or detection. Some arthropods hide in structures close to the host and feed only when the host is nearby. Other arthropods that bite man may have no intention to attack, bites being stimulated by various conditions, i.e., defense, attractive odors, or erroneous food selection.

Penetration or irritation of skin can be caused by bites of some members of the phylum Arthropoda in the classes Chilopoda, Insecta, and Arachnida. Adults, larvae, or nymphs, both terrestrial and aquatic, of many different arthropods can bite humans. Biting mouth parts are generally classified into chewing (mandibulate) and sucking (haustellate). Mandibulate mouth parts are generally not structurally adapted for biting humans, although various members of the orders Coleoptera (beetles), Neuroptera (aphis lions and dobson flies), Hymenoptera (wasps, bees, and ants), and Odonata (damselflies and dragonflies) may use their mouth parts for breaking the skin. Bites often become infected with bacteria, usually pathogenic cocci, present on the human skin or on contaminated arthropod mouth parts. Cockroaches (Dictyoptera) do not usually attack humans but will eat dried or fresh blood, skin, and fingernails of incapacitated individuals. This scavenger behavior suggests a source of direct injury and possible contamination.

HEMATOPHAGOUS ARTHROPODS. These arthropods normally feed on warm-blooded vertebrates (including humans) for blood that is both life-supporting and necessary for growth and gonotropic development. Therefore, their mouth parts are designed for probing and sucking blood and tissue fluids. In general, the term "biting arthropod" implies piercing and sucking mechanisms. Hematophagous arthropods have to pierce the host's skin to obtain blood. Since injury to skin triggers a series of repair reactions in the host (e.g., blood clotting, platelet aggregation, increased vascular permeability, and leukocyte chemotaxis), to obtain blood, hematophagous arthropods must modify or antagonize some of these adverse reactions. Arthropod saliva contains pharmacologic substances (e.g., proteases, carbohydrases, anticoagulants, and antiplatelet, anticomplement, and vasodilatory prostaglandins) that counteract host hemostasis.

The arthropod mouth parts are highly variable in morphology. The adults of the order Diptera have the most diverse mouth part types. Only females of the lower Diptera (i.e., mosquitoes, black flies, biting midges, horse flies, and snipe flies) are hematophagous. Males and females of the higher muscid Diptera (i.e., tsetse flies, biting house flies, and stable flies) are blood feeders. Although the goal of acquiring blood is the same, the structure and function of mouth parts of these distinct groups differ. Consequently, the damage to human tissue caused by these mouth parts is different.

Diptera. Diptera (flies and mosquitoes and their relatives) is a large order, containing over 100 families. They develop by complete metamorphosis (egg-larva-pupa-adult).

Mosquitoes have mouth parts composed of six united stylets, which can be seen as only a single filament-like structure with the unaided eye. The major part of the food channel is formed by the labrum-epipharynx, the mandibles, and the hypopharynx; the last is also used for injection of salivary fluids. A pair of maxillae and mandibles serve to penetrate surface capillaries. Although mosquitoes are considered solenophageous (vessel blood feeders), some evidence suggests that they are telmophageous (pool blood feeders).

The mouth parts of horse flies (Tabanidae), black flies (Simuliidae), biting midges (Ceratopogonidae), phlebotomine sand flies (Psychodidae), and some snipe flies (Rhagionidae) have six short bladelike structures. Cutting and penetration are accomplished by a pair of mandibles that act as scissors and a pair of maxillae that may aid in piercing and thrusting into the tissues (some horse flies) or be used for anchoring mouth parts in the tissues (some black flies, biting flies, and sand flies). The labium, which ensheaths the blades, has a labellum that is used for sponging and lapping blood. Frequently, flies that feed in this manner leave spots or streams of blood (Fig. 128–3). These bites can be very painful and produce local lesions that persist for hours or days. Sensitized individuals develop allergic reactions. The very minute biting midges cause pain inverse to their size, and frequently, much larger insects, i.e., mosquitoes or black flies, are blamed for the discomfort.

Some mosquitoes and flies (i.e., some biting midges and sand flies) bite at various times of the day and night. Black flies, horse flies, snipe flies, some mosquitoes (especially those of the genus *Aedes*), some biting midges, and many sand flies are daytime feeders. On the eastern and southern coastal areas of the United States, the salt-marsh mosquito, *Aedes sollicitans*, attacks humans and other animals at the rate of thousands per 15 minutes of exposure time. Similarly, synchronous emergence of black flies in large numbers, especially in temperate climates, renders certain areas uninhabitable for humans, livestock, and even wild animals.

The mouth parts of stable flies (Muscidae) and tsetse flies (Glossinidae) have a labrum-epipharynx for the food canal and a hypopharynx with the salivary duct. The haustellum has tissue-cutting denticles on the tip of the labellum. The tsetse fly has a thinner haustellum that can probe deep into the skin, whereas the stable fly has a thicker, shorter proboscis. The stable fly and tsetse fly are daytime blood feeders. They cut through tissues and capillaries while probing for blood. Salivary fluids are inoculated in the process of pooling blood for ingestion. The stable fly, *Stomoxys calcitrans*, is a serious biting pest; it resembles a house fly in general appearance, but the stable fly possesses a prominent proboscis, which both sexes use for sucking blood. When ready to feed, it quickly redirects the proboscis downward. The tsetse fly (*Glossina* species) has a similar proboscis. The fly may lower the mouth parts to probe a number of times before settling down to feed. Each time the fly probes, intense pain can be felt (Fig. 128–4).

Diptera Larvae. Mouth parts of Diptera larvae are neither used in the same way nor morphologically similar to the mouth parts of adults. In general, the larvae are found within special habitats. Mouth hooks of some maggots are attached to a cephalopharyngeal sclerite. The hooks act to lacerate

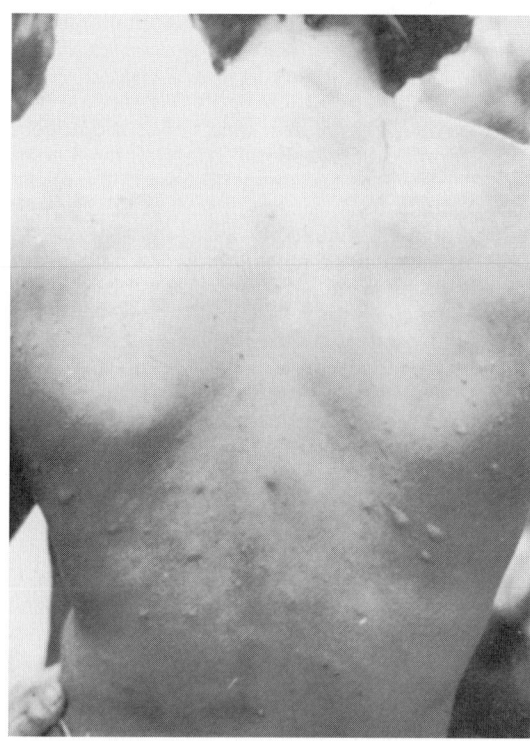

Figure 128–4. Tsetse fly (*Glossina fuscipes*) bites on the back of an adult male in Ethiopia. (Courtesy of the Armed Forces Institute of Pathology, Photograph Neg. No. 75–5783.)

tissue. A few larvae can bite on a short-term basis. The bite of a predatory tabanid larva can be quite painful. A hole is punched in the dermis, and salivary toxins can be inoculated; blood can be drawn but is not usually ingested. In equatorial Africa, the Congo floor maggot, *Auchmeromyia luteola*, is a hematophagous larva that feeds at night and hides in the walls of houses during the day. In these respects, it resembles the South American *Triatoma* species. However, the Congo floor maggot does not transmit disease. It is restricted to feeding at floor level; thus, a bed or hammock solves the problem of bites in humans.

True Bugs. The piercing and sucking mouth parts of blood-sucking Hemiptera of the families Reduviidae (assassin bugs) and Cimicidae (bedbugs) have four fascicles to penetrate the skin and blood vessels. There are over 2500 species of Reduviidae, of which the subfamily Triatominae (or cone-nose bugs) (14 genera, 111 species) is hematophagous. Some of the species are vectors of Chagas disease (i.e., *Triatoma infestans*, *Triatoma dimidiata*, *Rhodnius prolixus*, *Panstrongylus megistus*). In cone-nose bugs, the maxillae penetrate the skin and blood vessels, and the mandibles anchor into the skin.

Of the 74 species of cimicids, only two have well-known associations with humans. The bedbugs are cosmopolitan in distribution. The common bedbug, *Cimex lectularius*, is widespread throughout the temperate and tropical regions, whereas the distribution of the Indian bedbug, *C. hemipterus*, is restricted to tropical and subtropical climates. Bedbugs use both mandibles and maxillae for feeding from blood vessels. Bites of males, females, and nymphs from both species occur at night or under subdued light on people in bed. Ingestion of blood and engorgement may require only a few minutes. Little pain may be associated with their bites. Reactions to bites are variable, depending on the allergic response. The insects hide in the cracks and crevices of walls and beds

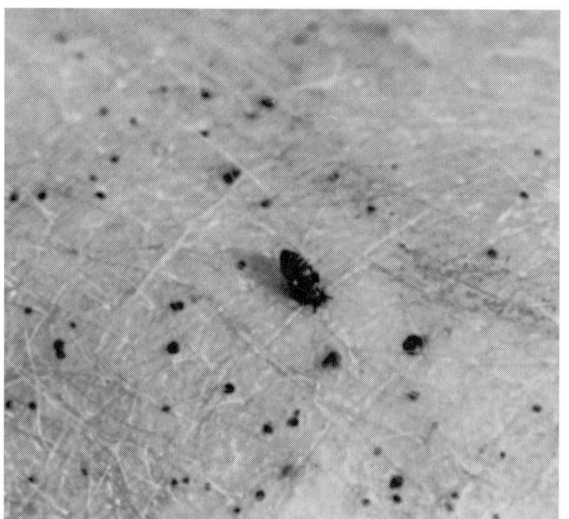

Figure 128–3. Blood-encrusted lesions following *Simulium* bites. A simulium is seen feeding. (Courtesy of Dr. Harold Trapido, Louisiana State University School of Medicine, New Orleans.)

during the day. The foul odor of the feces of bedbugs is pungent in heavily infested houses.

Fleas. Adult fleas are obligate parasites of warm-blooded vertebrates. Bladelike structures called maxillary stylets and the epipharynx can quickly penetrate capillaries. The cat flea (*Ctenocephalides felis*), a very common pest of dogs, can cause severe bite reactions. The nonparasitic eggs, larvae, and pupae are found in pet resting areas, e.g., on rugs, in dog bedding, and under furniture in the home. Other species of fleas that attack humans are the Oriental rat flea (*Xenopsylla cheopis*) and the human flea (*Pulex irritans*). Fleas readily bite humans when they are starved and can prove very annoying.

Soft Ticks. Argasidae (order Acarina) can produce painful bites. Species of the genus *Ornithodoros* are found in both hemispheres. They are usually associated with wild animal resting areas. The mouth parts of soft ticks have teeth on the chelicerae for cutting tissues and a hypostome for collecting pooled blood and tissues. These ticks feed quickly and are different from the hard ticks that anchor into the dermis.

NONHEMATOPHAGOUS ARTHROPODS. Occasionally, bites by non-bloodsucking insects can be as painful or even more excruciating than those by bloodsucking insects. The rasping mouth parts of minute thrips (order Thysanoptera) can be surprisingly painful, but little reaction occurs except in sensitive individuals. Other plant-eating insects and predators of other insects have mouth parts just as capable of penetrating human skin as of entering the epidermis of a leaf or the chitinous membranes of insects. Blood can be ingested by some in this process. Many species of centipede (Chilopoda), and spiders (Araneida) occasionally bite humans if they are touched. Such bites may include transitory pain, swelling, necrotic lesions, systemic reactions (vomiting, headache, cardiac arrhythmias, and convulsions), or even death. Predatory assassin bugs (e.g., Platymeris) inoculate enzyme-rich saliva with trypsin, hyaluronidase, and phospholipase, causing severe, persistent pain. Some arthropods that cannot inject salivary fluid may deposit the fluid on the skin surface and thus cause a reaction. Millipedes will not bite, and many of the known species are harmless. However, their exuded secretions may cause intense burning if they enter the eyes or may produce blisters on the skin.

Long-term Host Contact

Some biting arthropods require considerable time on the host to complete a normal life cycle (Fig. 128–1). The continuous availability of food from one host reduces the necessity for these arthropods to seek another. Depending on the species, only one life stage may be found on the host for an extended time. If development and reproduction occur on the host, the extent of the damage to the host may be correlated with the length of stay and arthropod population size. In most cases, their sedentary parasitologic role allows more potential for secondary dermal infection.

ECTOPARASITES

Fleas. Fleas were mentioned earlier as transient biters of humans. Hundreds of adult fleas can infest the body and head hairs, a problem that may have originated from an animal pet. For example, the sticktight flea, *Echidnophaga gallinacea*, and the cat flea, *Ctenocephalides felis*, may remain and feed on the same host for a long time, if undisturbed. The fleas, protected by the head hair and body warmth, have a continuous food supply. Pyrethrum soaps and shampoos are effective in control.

Hard Ticks. These maintain contact with the human host for several days while feeding on blood cells and tissue fluids. The bite of hard ticks is not usually detected during feeding. The discovery of a tick on the body or head may be

well after the tick is fully engorged, even as large as 2 cm. The larvae, called seed ticks, may occur in large numbers, whereas usually fewer nymphs and adults are found on the body. Ticks that enter the ear canal can cause complications due to their engorged size, which makes it difficult to remove them intact.

Removal. Contact is rendered more certain by the depth of hypostomal (mouth part) penetration and the recurved denticles of the hypostome. In some genera that have shorter hypostomes, the secretion of a cementing substance aids in anchoring the tick, making removal more difficult. If the tick is forcibly pulled off, the mouth parts may remain in the tissues and promote a chronic granulomatous reaction. The accepted method for removing ticks is with forceps (lift the abdomen of the tick upward and forward over the front of the tick, grasping very near the point of attachment (not the skin), and pull outward and forward). Formamidine derivatives are effective in causing ticks to detach.

Tick Paralysis. Ticks can cause a more serious condition, paralysis, which occurs worldwide and resembles acute poliomyelitis. More than 40 species of soft and hard ticks secrete salivary toxins that are responsible for paralysis in humans and some animals. In the United States, the Rocky Mountain wood tick, *Dermacentor andersoni*, and the American dog tick, *Dermacentor variabilis*, are implicated. Five or 6 days after attachment of the tick, the patient becomes restless and irritable and may have numbness or tingling of the extremities, lips, throat, and face. Difficulty in walking is followed by an inability to stand. Rapidly progressive ascending flaccid paralysis, which can reach the bulbar centers, causing dysphagia, slurred speech, and diplopia, may occur. Death may result from respiratory failure or aspiration pneumonia.

Ticks responsible for this condition, which is more common in children, are often concealed in long hair at the nape of the neck, particularly in girls. Provided that the paralysis is not too far advanced, rapid and complete recovery follows removal of the tick. Diagnosis depends on the clinical history and recovery of the tick.

Lice. Sucking lice (Phthiraptera) closely associated with humans are the head louse (*Pediculus humanus capitis*), the body louse (*Pediculus humanus corporis*), and the crab louse (*Phthirus pubis*). The lice are flattened dorsoventrally and have legs adapted for clinging to hair. The bite is accomplished with three stylets that are pushed into the skin from within the head of the louse. The paired maxillae form a food duct, and the hypopharynx forms the salivary channel. The mouth is held in place by a circlet of teeth at the end of the proboscis. Nymphs and adults require blood for survival. Lice must feed daily to survive. The names of the lice give some indication as to where they might be found on humans.

Head and Body Lice. The head louse is about 3 mm long. Nymphs are difficult to see on the head because they blend in color and size with flakes of the scalp; hence, the name "mechanical dandruff" has been used. The lice move surprisingly fast in the hairy environment, but the eggs (nits) remain as telltale signs. The female louse lays individual eggs or nits (approximately 0.6 mm in length) and attaches them to hairs of the host. Nits are so strongly glued on the hairs that they remain long after the lice are controlled. Infestation of head lice occurs on other parts of the body. Morphologic characteristics for the identification and separation of body and head lice overlap.

Lice are found in all socioeconomic groups but occur more frequently among the poor because of infrequent washing and overcrowding. Infestations have been common in military troops during wartime. Epidemics occur in many schools. Head lice appear to be most common in tropical South America, whereas body lice occur mainly in colder areas (e.g., in the Andes), a difference probably related to the amount of clothing worn. Body lice are more apt to be found in areas where clothing comes into close contact with the body, with nits being laid in the seams of clothes and rarely attached to hairs.

Bites of the lice cause pinpoint macules and pigmentation of the skin. Intense itching is the usual characteristic of heavy infestation. Pediculosis is associated with itching and rash and may be followed by irritability and depression. On the head, enlarged postauricular lymph nodes and scalp infection may result from scratching. Hemorrhagic macules or papules develop at the sites of feeding lice, and vertical excoriations due to scratching may be present. The condition of postinflammatory skin thickening and pigmentation in people continuously exposed to lice has been called vagabond's disease.

Crab Lice. The crab louse, as the French name *papillon d'amour* implies, is usually acquired by sexual contact or contact with infested objects, e.g., blankets or articles of clothing. The normal habitat of this louse is the pubic hair, which it scales by means of its crablike claws. It sometimes can be found on eyebrows and eyelashes or on the axillary hairs. These somewhat sedentary lice cause irritating papules in the groin. Pruritus occurs at the feeding sites, and with continued feeding, bluish macules mark the skin.

Treatment. Lotions or shampoos that incorporate insecticides, e.g., pyrethrins, are used to control lice. The compound should be applied only to the infested areas. Reapplication 1 week later may be necessary to control those nymphs that emerge following treatment. Clothing and bedding of infested individuals should be laundered at 55°C for 20 minutes or dry-cleaned to destroy nits and lice.

ENDOPARASITES

Tungiasis. This is caused by the very small (1 mm) female *Tunga penetrans* (chigoe flea, jigger flea), a highly specialized flea that burrows into the skin, feeds on tissue fluids, and grows to about 1 cm within 2 weeks of infestation as eggs develop beneath the dermis. In the skin, the flea is oriented with its head farthest from the dermal surface. Close inspection reveals a black dot in the center of the lesion, locating the female's posterior end, from which she respires and discharges excrement and eggs. After the eggs are extruded, the carcass of the flea collapses and sloughs along with the covering keratin. The eggs hatch, and the larvae develop to become adult fleas in about 3 weeks. After copulation the female flea begins a pattern of jumping that persists until she dies or attaches and burrows into the skin of a warm-blooded animal. Infestations usually occur on the feet and legs; fleas tend to concentrate on the ankles, the instep, and between the toes but generally avoid the weight-bearing portion of the soles (Fig. 128–5). Fleas may attack any portion of the body, including the trunk, limbs, head, face and even eyelids, of individuals who lie on the ground. Fleas beneath the nails are especially painful and have given rise to the sailor's oath, "Well, I'll be jiggered." Patients with leprosy, who have reduced sensation in their feet, are especially prone to severe and recurrent infestation.

Although tungiasis is usually innocuous, secondary infections, including tetanus and gas gangrene, kill some patients in tropical Africa.

Pigs are natural hosts of these fleas, which prefer sandy soil; close contact with pigs predisposes to infestation. The flea evolved in the tropical and subtropical Americas, spread to Africa in the late 1800s, and has since expanded its range into the Indian subcontinent.

Treatment involves removal of the chigoe by widening the cavity with a sterile needle so that the flea can be extracted intact. The usual care should be taken to dress the cavities and prevent secondary infection.

Myiasis. Human myiasis is the invasion or infestation of the human body and tissues by Diptera larvae or maggots. The families of flies commonly involved are very diverse (i.e., Muscidae, Calliphoridae, Sarcophagidae, Piophilidae, Stratiomyidae, Syrphidae, Oestridae, Gasterophilidae, and Cuterebridae). Myiasis can be divided into primary and secondary types: Primary myiasis implies a breach in the skin made by the larva itself; in secondary myiasis, open devitalized tissues, i.e., wounds, infections, or burns, are parasitized. Although certain species of flies are obligate parasites and require living tissue for their development, some other species are facultative and require either live or dead tissues for their development. Some members of the family Piophilidae (cheese skippers), Stratiomyidae (soldier fly larvae), and Syrphidae (rat-tailed larvae) can cause accidental gastrointestinal myiasis. The classification adopted by James (1947) is probably most useful to the clinician because it is based on the part of the body affected. Except for the various types of skin myiasis (i.e., furuncular, creeping dermal myiasis, and wound infection), myiasis (of the nose, mouth, ear, eye, gastrointestinal tract, anal or sexual orifices, and urinary passages) is treated on an individual basis.

Traumatic (Wound) Myiasis. Although the wounds through

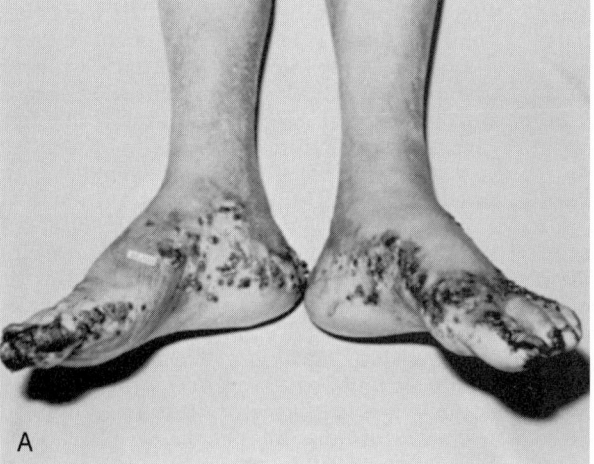 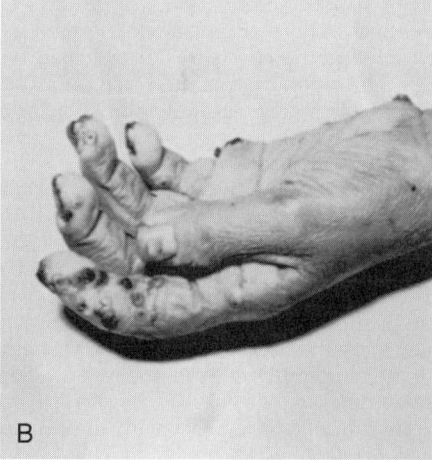

A   **B**

Figure **128–5.** Tungiasis. Lesions due to *Tunga penetrans*, the chigoe or burrowing flea. (Courtesy of Dr. Rodolfo Cespedes. Hospital San Juan de Dios, San José, Costa Rica.)

which the larvae enter are usually sizable, a minor injury can be the portal of entry. The female fly, often attracted by blood or pus, lays her eggs near the lesion. The quickly hatching maggots have easy access to the wound. Skin breaches due to disease, e.g., leprosy, treponematoses, leishmaniasis, or cancer, or to wounds can also be parasitized in this way. Often the maggots remain superficial, but they can penetrate deep, causing meningitis or even necessitating amputation of a limb. Female flesh flies (Sarcophagidae) deposit freshly hatched first-stage larvae directly in wounds, ulcers, or even unbroken skin.

The dominant fly species involved vary with the geographic location. In southern Europe, Russia, Africa, and the Middle East, *Wohlfahrtia magnifica* is the most common species. The Old World screwworm (*Chrysomyia bezziana*) is a major cause of myiasis in Asia and sub-Saharan Africa. In the Americas, the primary screwworm, *Cochliomyia hominivorax*, is well known to livestock farmers as a serious pest. Eggs laid in batches of 10 to 300 hatch within 24 hours. The larvae penetrating the tissues in a head-down position are gregarious and form a pocket-like wound. The female fly prefers clean, fresh wounds for oviposition. Because she mates only once, an extensive program of sterile male release was effective in controlling the problem in livestock in the United States, and in eradicating it from Curaçao, although it has since started to return. Before this control program, in 1935 in Texas, 12 million livestock cases and 55 human cases of myiasis were recorded. In the northern part of the United States, *Wohlfahrtia vigil* is an important agent of myiasis.

Many other fly species may infest wounds but stay on the surface of the lesion. In the 1930s, before the advent of antibiotics, some species of blowfly maggots were used in medicine to debride suppurating wounds.

Furuncular Myiasis. In subcutaneous myiasis, the skin lesion can be mistaken for a staphylococcal boil—hence the name. Although the lesion is often complicated by a secondary bacterial infection, close inspection reveals a maggot with its posterior spiracles visible in the wound (Fig. 128–6). Two species of obligatory myiasis producers are responsible: *Dermatobia hominis* in South and Central America and *Cordylobia arthropophaga* in Africa. No previous skin lesion is necessary for the larva to effect penetration. *Dermatobia hominis* (berne, tórsalo) is named the human botfly, even though it principally infests cattle and other animals and is responsible for great economic losses in hides and milk and meat production. The mechanism of infection is unique because the fecund female fly catches mosquitoes or flies during flight. She glues her eggs to the undersurface of the captured insect and then releases it. When this insect comes into contact with a mammalian host, the eggs hatch with a spring-lid mechanism at the operculum, and the larvae burrow into the skin. Scalp infections are common in humans, but lesions may occur on any exposed skin. The growing larvae assume a bottle shape, with the narrow posterior end juxtaposed to the skin surface, thus making removal more difficult. The larvae mature in about 4 weeks and then leave the host to pupate in the soil.

The adult female *Cordylobia anthropophaga* (Tumbu fly) deposits over 100 eggs, usually on urine- or feces-contaminated sand, soil, or clothing (e.g., clothes hung out to dry, soiled bedding). Within 2 days, larvae emerge; they can remain alive for 2 weeks without feeding, but on contact with skin, they penetrate. Because larvae mature within 9 days, skin tumors form rapidly. The erythema is more marked and secondary infection less common than in myiasis caused by the human botfly. The larva is easier to extract, but a large number of lesions may be present.

Creeping Dermal Myiasis. This is strictly a form of larva migrans and as such must be distinguished from subdermal migrating eruptions caused by helminths, e.g., *Ancylostoma braziliense* (Chapter 115), *Strongyloides stercoralis* (Chapter 105.2), and *Gnathostoma spinigerum* (Chapter 113). Creeping dermal myiasis involves humans as an accidental host of botflies. *Gasterophilus intestinalis*, a natural parasite in horses, produces narrow, raised lines in the skin because the first-stage larva is incapable of developing beyond the first stage in humans and migrates about in the dermis. Itching is the accompanying symptom. In contrast, the galleries of *Hypoderma lineatum*, the common cattle grub, are deeper and wider because *Hypoderma* larvae can complete development in humans. Typical tumor-like warbles containing mature larvae may form, e.g., those seen in cattle. The deep tissue migration is accompanied by pain; severe complications may ensue.

Myiasis of the Nose, Mouth, Ear, and Accessory Sinuses. This is usually caused by the same species responsible for wound myiasis and may be a complication when the wound is on the head. Debilitated or comatose patients are especially at risk because oviposition is easier. Pain, edema, and purulent discharge are often associated with maggot growth in cases restricted by bone and cartilage. Destruction and erosion of the nose or mouth can be caused by maggots (Fig. 128–7). Movement of maggots to the base of the brain can result in meningitis and death. In aural myiasis, pain and discomfort are accompanied by deafness and tinnitus. Infection and penetration of the tympanum can ensue. Larvae of the obligatory myiasis producer flies, such as the old world screwfly (*Chrysomyia bezziana*), sheep nasal botfly (*Oestrus ovis*), and Russian gadfly (*Rhinoestrus purpureus*), are most commonly the cause of nasal myiasis.

Ocular Myiasis. Although some maggots may destroy the eye by spreading from a contiguous wound, there are other types of ocular myiasis. For example, external ophthalmomyiasis, an acute catarrhal or parasitic conjunctivitis, is caused by first-stage larvae of *Oestrus ovis*, the sheep botfly. Close inspection of the inflamed conjunctival area will reveal a wriggling mass of tiny larvae, a sequel to an opportunistic deposition of the larvae during a fly strike by the female *Oestrus*. This type of myiasis is most common among those working with sheep and goats. Internal ophthalmomyiasis is

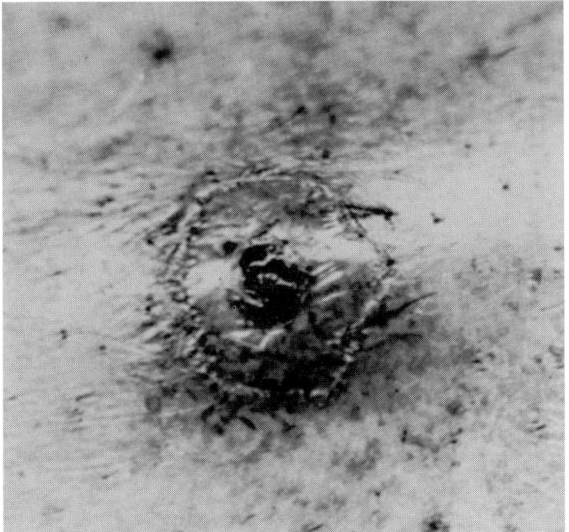

***Figure* 128–6.** Myiasis. The posterior end of the warble *Dermatobia hominis* can be seen, with the shiny black spiracles in the center of the dermal lesion. (Courtesy of the Armed Forces Institute of Pathology, Photograph Neg. No. N-49503.)

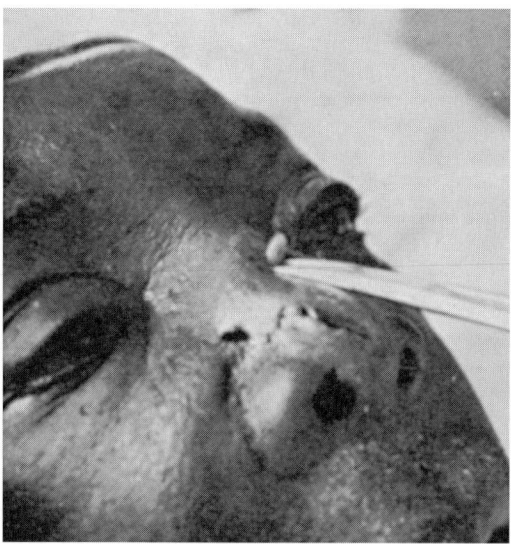

Figure 128–7. Infection with *Cochliomyia hominivorax*. Over 230 screwworm larvae were removed from this patient's nasal passages. (Courtesy of Dr. W. E. Dove and associates, Bureau of Entomology and Plant Quarantine, U.S. Department of Agriculture.)

produced by deep migrating larvae of a species such as *Hypoderma lineatum*. If the maggot is in the anterior chamber, it can be seen moving, and there is a chance of extraction. Posterior chamber involvement may cause retinal detachment or optic nerve invasion, with resultant blindness.

Myiasis of the Anal Region and Vagina. Secretions and excretions from these areas are highly attractive to many species of flies. Deposition of large numbers of eggs from filth flies and flesh flies can result in large numbers of larvae in as few as 8 to 12 hours. Poorly cared for and exposed children or adults can become victims. This is especially true in areas with high fly populations, such as the tropics.

Myiasis of the Bladder and Urinary Passages. The preceding explanation applies to this location as well. Newly hatched larvae at the urinary meatus migrate up the urethra only to be subsequently passed in the urine. Bladder and urethral pain may be associated with dysuria. Priapism may occur, but it is rare. Small flies of the genus *Fannia*, which resemble house flies, are most frequently implicated. Members of the genera *Psychoda*, *Musca*, *Calliphora*, and *Sarcophaga* are also implicated in urinary myiasis. Care must be taken to confirm that the urine specimen was not passed into a receptacle already containing contaminating maggots.

Enteric Myiasis. Pseudomyiasis due to maggot contamination of passed feces must be included in this discussion, even though it is still debated whether real development occurs in the human enteron. In most cases, ingested fly eggs or larvae that were deposited on foodstuff may pass intact through the intestinal tract. Acute enteritis has been described, and many cases have been documented. The ingestion of fly larvae in food is the obvious route of infection. Maggots from the genera *Musca*, *Fannia*, and *Sarcophaga* have been recovered. One species often recovered from stools is the aquatic rat-tailed maggot *Eristalis tenax*.

Treatment. Although species of many different genera and families are implicated in human myiasis, it is worthwhile attempting a specific identification of the maggot. The chitinous spiracular plates of mature larvae have different configurations that often allow identification of the genus. The maggots should be preserved in 70% alcohol and sent to

a reference laboratory. If possible, live maggots should be furnished to a local medical entomologist; some maggots can be reared to adults for more precise identification.

Treatment entails extraction of the maggots. In furuncular myiasis, the application of petroleum jelly to the lesion suffocates the maggots, which may come wriggling out backward, e.g., the African tumbu fly. *Dermatobia hominis* is more difficult to remove, and incision under local anesthesia is usually necessary. Maggots in orifices, tissues, and organs are best removed individually, but if they are lodged in the nose, this may require endoscopy and even a general anesthetic. There are no medications that will dislodge maggots. When exposed to any chemical insult, maggots tend to retract, making it more difficult to find and remove them.

Acariasis

Scabies. Infestation of the epidermis by *Sarcoptes scabiei hominis* is responsible for one of the most common itching dermatoses in the world. It is usually associated with crowded conditions. Transmission is from person to person by close body contact and through sharing the same bed and clothing. Often transmission of scabies occurs during sexual encounters. The newly fertilized female mite burrows into the epidermis and lays 2 to 3 eggs a day for 30 days. The larvae hatch in 3 to 4 days and migrate to the skin surface. Maturation from eggs to adults takes about 10 to 14 days. The females feed on cells of the stratum corneum, and it is their secretions and excretions that sensitize the host and produce the familiar irritation. Typical infection usually involves less than 20 mites.

CLINICAL MANIFESTATIONS. Newly infested persons may have large populations before the infestation is noticed. There is a period of about a month before sensitization and symptoms develop. Within 100 days from the arrival of a single fertilized female mite, several hundred females can develop; mite mortality is high, however, because scratching kills them. Although the mite may burrow anywhere on the skin (Fig. 128–8), there are certain sites that are more commonly affected, i.e., the hands and wrists (Fig. 128–9), the female breast, the penis, the natal cleft, and, in children, the feet. Scratching and secondary infection often cause puzzling skin lesions. The more classic sign of a run or burrow is seldom seen. This appears as a short, wavy, reddish line. A tiny blister at the distal extremity contains the female mite, which

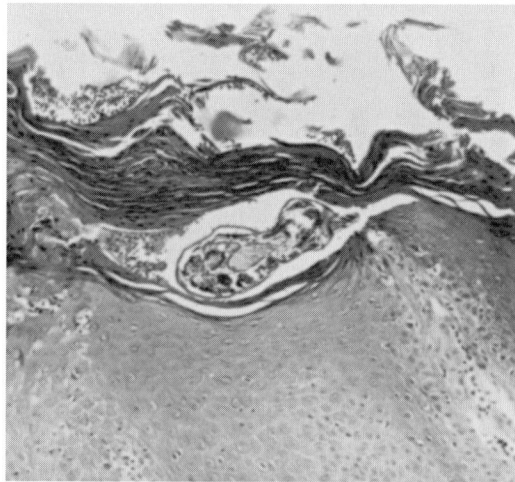

Figure 128–8. An adult *Sarcoptes scabiei hominis* in a burrow. Note the spinose walls. (Courtesy of the Louisiana State University School of Medicine. New Orleans.)

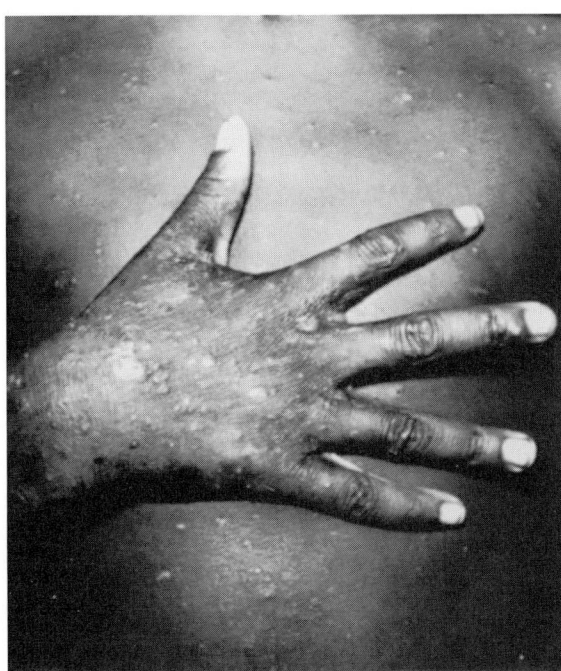

Figure **128–9.** Advanced scabies infestation on the hand, thorax, and abdomen in a Zairean child. (Courtesy of the Armed Forces Institute of Pathology, Photograph Neg. No. 68–7834–20.)

can be extracted with a pin and identified under the microscope. Erythematous itching papules are common lesions, and these may turn to pustules as a result of secondary staphylococcal infection. An eczematous reaction may occur, or, in long-standing infections, erythematous nodules may develop.

COMPLICATIONS. Epidemics of acute glomerulonephritis associated with pyoderma and scabies have been documented in Trinidad. Hyperinfestation of the epidermis with the skin honeycombed with mite burrows is sometimes referred to as Norwegian scabies. This situation results from hyperinfestation with thousands to a million mites. Clinically, this often appears as crusted psoriasiform lesions on the hands and feet and is highly contagious because of the large numbers of loosely attached, easily transferred mites present in the exfoliating skin. Itching is absent in many patients, suggesting that failure of the immune response has allowed the mites to multiply unchecked. Hyperinfection has been observed in patients immunosuppressed after renal transplant or in those using topical corticosteroids for a long period. In addition, this type of scabies occurs in demented and paralyzed patients who do not scratch.

DIAGNOSIS AND TREATMENT. Diagnosis, especially in the tropics, is based on the clinical appearance. Although ideally the identification of a mite is desirable, it is often impossible or too time-consuming. Treatment instructions should be precise. The patient should take a bath and discard his or her clothes, and bed linens should be laundered. The scabicide should be thinly applied with a swab over the entire body, sparing only the face. In children, the scalp may be affected. After donning fresh clothes, the patient should not bathe for 48 hours. A second successive treatment may be recommended. Worldwide, benzylbenzoate emulsion (20% to 35%) is the most common scabicide, but there are other effective preparations. Many are eye irritants, however. In the United States, gamma benzene hexachloride (lindane) in cream or

lotion form is most frequently used. It is left on for only 12 hours to minimize percutaneous absorption. Secondary skin sepsis may be so marked as to require prior treatment with antibiotics. Simultaneous treatment of all affected family members is important. It is common to see a mother nursing a scratching child, and both have scabies.

Mite-Induced Dermatitis. Many species of mites that feed on humans actually do not burrow into the skin, but tissue swelling around them gives the appearance of dermal penetration. Most instances of mite-induced dermatitis are observed in individuals whose occupations bring them into contact with mite-infested materials. Several species of mesostigmatid, prostigmatid, and astigmatid mites can attack humans and cause irritating rashes (Table 128–1). Among mesostigmatid mites, members of the families Dermanyssidae, Macronyssidae, and Laelapidae are known to attack and bite humans. In rodent-infested buildings it is not uncommon for people to be bitten by the tropical rat mite *(Ornithonyssus bacoti)* and the house mite *(Liponyssoides sanguineus)*. Other species such as the chicken mite *(O. sylviarum)* frequently attack humans and their pets. The severity of dermatitis resulting from the bites of these mites varies with the sensitivity of the individual. The bite causes small urticarial wheals and papules that may be associated with pruritus. Many species of mites that commonly parasitize poultry, wild birds, commensal and wild rodents, and household pets may also cause dermatitis in humans and their pets. The family Sarcoptidae contains important parasitic species that cause scabies in humans and mange and other skin diseases in domestic and wild animals. *Sarcoptes scabiei canis* causes sarcoptic mange in dogs, and dog owners may become infested and develop sensitivity. This mite can penetrate the skin, but it does not multiply on the human host. Irritating papular lesions are similar to those with infestation by *S. scabiei hominis*. The families Acaridae, Glycyphagidae, and Pyroglyphidae contain many of the "stored product mites" that attack humans and occasionally cause the severe dermatitis known as grocer's itch *(Glycyphagus domesticus)*, baker's itch *(Acarus siro)*, and copra itch *(Tyrophagus putrescentiae)* (Table 128–1). Among prostigmatid mites, the straw itch mite *(Pymotes tritici)* and cheyletid mite *(Cheyletiella yasguri* and *Cheyletiella blakei)* are common nuisances to humans, causing multiple lesions. Dermatitis associated with *P. tritici* is commonly known as straw, hay, or grain itch.

Chiggers. In many parts of the world, trombiculid mite larvae (chiggers) can cause severe skin irritation. In Europe *Trombicula autumnalis* (the harvester mite) and in the United States *T. alfreddugesi* and *T. splendens* are examples of the chiggers that cause much itching distress in humans. Chiggers neither feed on blood nor burrow into the skin. The secretions of the mite and host reaction to the saliva and mouth parts combine to form a feeding tube (stylostome). At this stage, the mite is strongly anchored to the skin, frequently in hair follicles and pores, for the ingestion of tissue fluids and predigested cells. Some blood cells are ingested. Red maculopapular lesions develop within 24 hours. A tiny dot in the center may be the larva, just barely visible. Again, welts and swelling around the mite may make it appear as though the chigger burrowed into the skin. After the mite is replete, it leaves the host, but itching may continue.

The natural environments of chiggers are grassy, rodent-infested areas. Persons walking through such areas should use insect repellent, e.g., diethyltoluamide, or should wear permethrin-treated clothing. Antiseptics applied to the welts will usually kill the chiggers. Temporary relief from itching is obtained with a combination of benzocaine (5%), methyl salicylate (2%), salicylic acid (0.5%), ethyl alcohol (73%), and water (19.5%).

TABLE 128–1. Example of Mites That Are Implicated in Dermatitis and House Dust Allergies

Mite Species	Geographic Distribution	Hosts	Usual Habitat
Ornithonyssus bacoti*	Worldwide	Mice, rats, chickens, wild rodents, carnivores, wild birds, humans	Nest-acquired mites, rodent burrows, cracks in buildings
Ornithonyssus sylviarum*	Worldwide (temperate zones)	Mice, rats, chickens, pigeons, wild rodents, humans	Cracks and crevices in buildings; skin, feathers
Dermanyssus gallinae	Worldwide	Chickens, wild birds, pigeons, rats, rabbits, humans	Nests of chickens and other birds; rodent burrows
Liponyssoides sanguineus*	Worldwide	Mice, rats, wild rodents, humans	Cracks and crevices in buildings; rodent burrows
Pyemotes tritici*	Worldwide	Parasites of stored grain; insects, humans	Straw, grain, straw mattresses
Cheyletiella yasguri*	Worldwide	Dog, humans	Skin, pelage, floors, furniture, mattresses
Cheyletiella parasitovorax*	Worldwide	Rabbit, cat, humans	Skin, pelage
Demodex folliculorum*	Worldwide	Humans	Sebaceous glands, hair follicles
Eutrombicula alfreddugesi*	North and South America	Wide range of domestic animals, wild birds, humans	Grass, skin of host
Eutrombicula batatas	Central and South America, southwest United States	Chicken, wild birds, rodents, domestic animals, humans*	Grass and weeds, skin of host
Neotrombicula autumnalis*	Europe	Dog, horse, rabbit, various birds, humans	Grass, skin of host
Sarcoptes scabiei*	Worldwide	Domestic animals, humans	Skin
Notoedres cati	Worldwide	Cats, rabbits, dogs, humans	Skin
Acarus siro	Worldwide	Pests of stored foods and vegetable products*†	Stored hay and grain, house dust
Tyrophagus putrescentiae	Worldwide	*†	House dust, pests of stored food products
Lepidoglyphus destructor	Worldwide	*†	Grain dust, barn dust, surface of mattresses, stored hay and grain
Dermatophagoides farinae	Worldwide	*†	House dust: surface of mattresses, blankets, pillows, floors, pets
Dermatophagoides pteronyssinus	Worldwide	*†	House dust: surface of mattresses, blankets, pillows, floors, pets, bedding and cages
Euroglyphus maynei	Worldwide	*†	House dust: surface of mattresses, blankets, pillows, floors, pets, bedding and cages

*Discussed in text.
†Free-living mites.

128.3 Envenomation

The number of people seeking medical assistance because of bites is far fewer than those seeking attention because of stings of bees, wasps, hornets, and ants. A 1971 survey of physicians in Mississippi revealed that they were consulted in about 2381 cases of bee, wasp, and ant stings; 499 spider bites; and 387 unidentified bites or stings. An earlier nationwide survey by Parrish showed that from 1950 to 1959, of 460 deaths due to venomous animals, 50% were caused by hymenopterans, 14% by spiders, 1.7% by scorpions, and 30% by snakes.

Active Envenomation

Envenomation by arthropods is commonly the result of the injection of a toxin used in defense or to subdue prey. (The main types of venomous arthropods are shown in Figure 128–10). Active envenomation usually requires movement of the arthropod to inflict the injury. The mechanism of delivery of the toxin can be anteriorly stationed (i.e., mouth parts or modified front legs) or posteriorly stationed (i.e., stinging apparatus or venoms). Various mechanisms of muscular contraction serve to actively inoculate venom.

ANTERIORLY STATIONED VENOM

Spiders. The morbidity and mortality caused by spiders (class Arachnida) are usually rare, yet they are highly publicized. Fortunately, very few of the 100,000 species are dangerous to humans. Spiders have fangs on the end of the chelicerae, with venom stored in glands located in the cephalothorax or chelicerae. Almost all spiders have venom for the purpose of paralyzing or killing insects or small animals for food. Although humans are not part of their diet, they can be victimized by some spiders that have fangs large enough to penetrate the dermis. Even the more toxic spiders, in the immature stages, may not be able to break the skin. Usually, they are not aggressive, but some will bite to defend themselves or their egg masses. Venoms of spiders can be very toxic, even in small quantities (0.2 to 5.0 mg of dry weight), with mouse LD_{50}, in mg/kg of body weight of 0.34 intravenously to 62.5 subcutaneously. Biochemicals found in spider venoms of several toxic species have been analyzed and have been found to be consistent intraspecifically but to vary between species. Amines, amino acids, proteins, and proteolytic enzymes are commonly pooled into potent complexes, causing variable medical abnormalities. Human fatalities have occurred after the bites of species from the genera *Latrodectus*, *Loxosceles*, *Phoneutria*, and *Atrax*.

Latrodectus Species. Several species of *Latrodectus* are found worldwide, primarily in warmer climates. The female

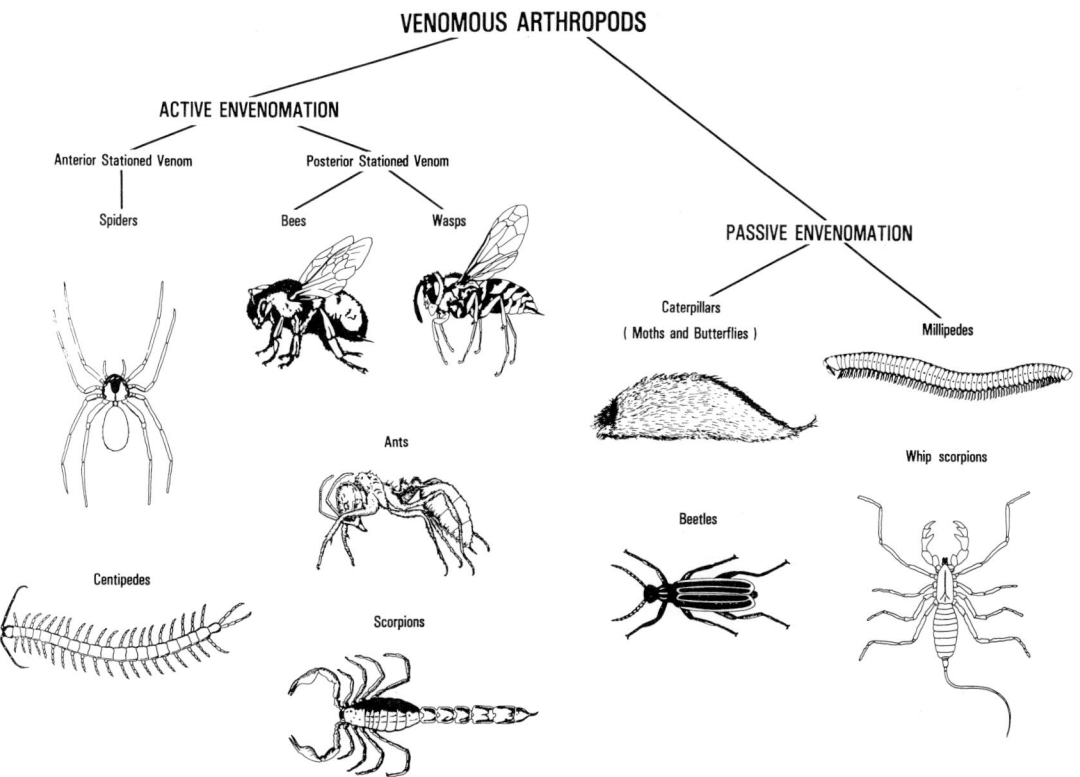

Figure 128–10. Venomous arthropods can be broadly categorized under active envenomation and passive envenomation.

black widow, *Latrodectus mactans*, is well known by its large, glossy black abdomen with a red, hourglass-shaped marking on the ventral side. The mature female is about 30 mm long with legs extended. The spider spends her time in an irregularly patterned web, usually in the shadows of plants, woodpiles, and old buildings. Bites commonly occur on the hands. However, many people are bitten on the buttocks and genitals while using privies and outhouses.

The bite may pass unnoticed; two tiny red spots may be seen at the site, or a severe local reaction may occur. The neurotoxic fraction in the venom is a protein of low molecular weight that affects the spinal cord and nerve endings. Absorption is accompanied by pain and numbness in the affected part. In 15 minutes to a few hours, generalized agonizing muscular pains appear, together with symptoms of shock. The blood pressure falls, and there is marked sweating, a feeling of weakness and nausea, and labored respiration. The marked rigidity of the muscles of the abdominal wall may simulate tetanus or an acute abdomen. Rarely, if paralysis and coma ensue, they may be followed by cardiac or respiratory failure.

Loxosceles Spiders. These spiders occur in the Americas. They are usually light brown with a darker violin-shaped mark on the cephalothorax. The body length of the adult is about 1 to 1.5 cm. They are commonly called fiddleback spiders or brown recluse spiders. The name "recluse" is appropriate, because they are secretive, shy spiders that hunt at night for silverfish and other insects. Their webs are not distinctive. In the central United States, *Loxosceles reclusa* can be collected in many homes. People are bitten indoors, often while sleeping or while donning clothing stored in closets or laid on the floor. *L. reclusa* can produce severe bites, but they are not as severe as those of *Loxosceles laeta* of South America.

The venom of *Loxosceles* is cytotoxic; it produces marked local necrosis that is slow to heal. The bite is associated with intense pain and local vasoconstriction and is followed by edema, erythema, blistering, and hemorrhage, with eventual frank necrosis and tissue loss (Fig. 128–11). Serious complications are acute hemolysis, pulmonary edema, and renal insufficiency.

Phoneutria Species. The wandering spider or bird spider of South America, *Phoneutria nigriventer*, has one of the most pharmacologically active venoms of all spiders. The dose in mg/kg of body weight for killing 20-g mice was 0.006 intravenously and 0.013 subcutaneously. The mean quantity of venom obtained by electric extraction was 1.25 mg of dry weight. In humans, the venom is neurotoxic, affecting the central nervous system. There is intense local pain caused by the high serotonin content of the venom. In children, muscle spasms and convulsions may be followed by death in a matter of hours. *Phoneutria* spiders are hunting spiders with no apparent web for entrapping prey. They are large, having a body length of 3 cm, and very aggressive, usually hiding during the day and hunting between dusk and dawn. They are sometimes found in boxed fruit, particularly bananas. Other species of *Phoneutria* are also found in South and Central America.

Lycosidae Species. The venom of wolf spiders can cause marked local cytotoxic effects but little systemic illness. Local edema and necrosis are followed by crusting and scarring. There may be very little pain, although the resultant keloid scars are often painful. These spiders, which vary in size, are agile predators during the day and night. They usually run from humans. Other members of this and other spider families have also been responsible for bites of varying degrees of severity.

Centipedes. Members of the class Chilopoda are also venomous because of a pair of strong hollow-tipped claws with

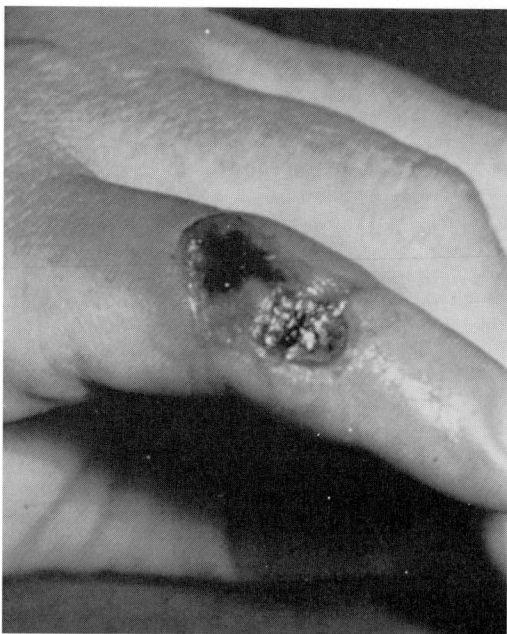

Figure 128–11. Local necrosis of a finger following the bite of the brown recluse spider *Loxosceles reclusa*. (From Dillaha CJ, Jansen GT, Honeycutt WM, et al: JAMA 188:33, 1964. Reprinted by permission.)

venom glands located on the first body segment behind the head. Although centipedes are carnivorous, hunting prey at night, most species are harmless. Humans are not usually bitten. Centipedes can be quite large, measuring from 10 cm long in the southern United States to over 25 cm long in the tropics. Members of the genus *Scoloperdra* can cause severe local pain and occasional skin necrosis, but no human deaths have been reported as a result of their bites.

POSTERIORLY STATIONED VENOM

Bees, Wasps, and Hornets. The venoms of the insect order Hymenoptera are some of the most studied and characterized of all venoms. The venoms of bees and wasps have active toxic components that result in similar sting reactions.

Stings. A modified ovipositor, the stinging apparatus, penetrates the skin, and venom is injected by muscular action. The stinging apparatus is similar in structure in honeybees, wasps, hornets, and bumblebees. Honeybees, bumblebees, and vespids are social insects that use their venom for defense. Near a nest, multiple stings might be expected. The aggressiveness of bees usually increases near the hives, but there is some variability according to species. Stings from the varieties of honeybee, primarily *Apis mellifera mellifera, A. m. ligustica,* and *A. m. scutellata* (killer honeybee), are dangerous essentially for those individuals who are at risk. Systemic toxic reactions from stings may occur with multiple stings (≥50). Toxic reactions may include vomiting, diarrhea, shock, and renal failure. Most fatalities due to bee stings have followed the occurrence of more than 500 stings. Despite the dramatic reports about the African killer bee (*A. m. scutellata*) stings, killer bee venom is less lethal to animals than the European bee. Moreover, *A. m. scutellata* has considerably less venom in its venom reservoirs. The highly developed colony-defensive behaviors of *A. m. scutellata* makes it much more aggressive and unpredictable than the other subspecies.

Toxins. The polypeptide melittin, which constitutes 50% of honeybee venom, damages erythrocytes, leukocytes, and lysosomes, with the subsequent release of enzymes. Melittin stimulates the activity of endogenous phospholipase A, which then affects guanylate cyclase activity. Phospholipase

A, 12% of honeybee venom, directly attacks phospholipids and tissue thromboplastin. Exogenous histamine (0.1% to 1.5% of bee venom) and melittin appear to be responsible for the pain associated with the inoculation, but the antigenicity of the bee venom is primarily associated with phospholipase A. Hyaluronidase, composing 1% to 3% of bee venom, is a spreading factor that has some antigenicity. Apamin, composing about 2% of bee venom, has a neurotoxic effect. Mast cell peptide, composing 1% to 2% of bee venom, causes the destruction of mast cells (MCD).

Components of wasp and hornet venoms are histamine, hyaluronidase, serotonin, phospholipases A and B, kinins (one for wasps and another for hornets), and acetylcholine (hornets only). The kinins, apparently in the presence of trypsin, result in the formation of a kind of bradykinin. Interestingly, serotonin is part of wasp venom, and a secondarily derived compound from the hemolytic activity of melittin in bee venom. Acetylcholine is not often a common chemical in the venom of other stinging arthropods.

Ants. Ant stings are common in the southern United States. The imported fire ants, *Solenopsis richteri* and *S. invicta,* and the native United States fire ants, *S. geminata* and *S. xyloni,* cause stings that result in sharp pain similar to that of a bee sting, although less intense (Fig. 128–12).

Stings. The sting causes an immediate erythematous rash, followed by a wheal (up to 10 mm in diameter). After a few hours, a vesicle containing clear fluid forms. Within 24 hours, the vesicle becomes turgid and pustulated. The pustule will remain for several days to more than a week before rupturing or resolving to a scab formation. Inconspicuous, small fibrotic nodules or small pigmented areas can result.

Large numbers of stings on the extremities may occur in young children and in any unsuspecting person. Hundreds of fire ants can boil up the foot of a person who steps into the dirt mound nest. The stinging mechanism for some ants, e.g., fire ants and harvester ants, is to use the mandibles to hold onto the skin, to arch the back at the thread waist

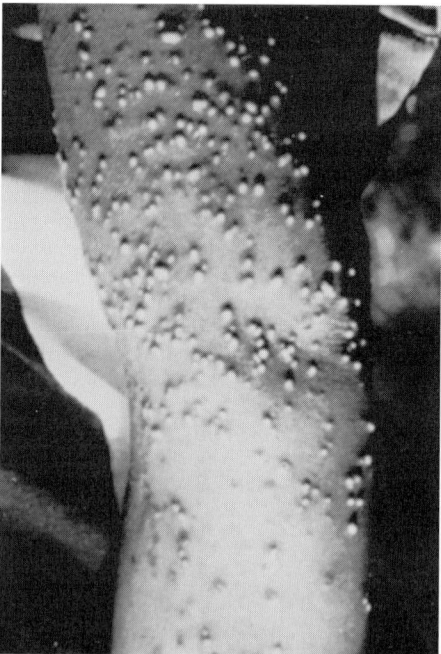

Figure 128–12. Fire ant stings. Severe reaction to multiple stings from *Solenopsis invicta* on the arm of a male in Mississippi. (Courtesy of the Armed Forces Institute of Pathology, Photograph Neg. No. 75–14977.)

(peduncle), and to project the stinger from the posterior of the globular abdomen into the victim. Anaphylaxis can be caused by these and other species of ants, although much less frequently than with other Hymenoptera.

Toxins. Venoms of fire ants are primarily 2,6-dialkylpiperidines (99%), which apparently cause the toxic effects. Only 0.1% of the venom is protein, containing three fractions with estimated molecular weights of 2000, 5000, and 10,000. Phospholipase A and hyaluronidase are also venom components.

More primitive ants, e.g., myrmecine and ponerine, have venoms that are more proteinaceous. Fractionation of these venoms resulted in isolation of histamines, hyaluronidase, kinin-like material, hemolytic proteins, and biochemicals that might resemble honeybee melittin.

The more advanced formicine ants have a reduced stinging apparatus and more developed anal glands for defensive and alarm secretions. Examples of compounds found in these glands are formic acid, terpenes, and ketones. Most of these seem to be used for communication between the ants themselves and other arthropods. However, the mandibles of some ants break the dermis and release a concentrated solution of formic acid into the wound. Formic acid, which is very cytotoxic, and a carrier compound, i.e., N-undecane, which aids penetration, are effective chemical combinations against human intruders.

Scorpions. These are nocturnally active arachnids; they can be easily recognized by having a pair of pincers in the front of a segmented body that ends in a five-segment tail armed with a terminal stinger. They have eight legs in addition to the pincers. Discovery of scorpions during the daytime is usually made by removing their protective shelter in the field (e.g., loose bark, piles of debris, rocks), in the house (e.g., in footwear, storage rooms and boxes, cabinets, clothing on the floor), and in other places somewhat protected from light. Usually, scorpions can be found immobile with the stinger laying flat or coiled next to the body. Although they may appear sluggish, the disturbance of removing their protection can cause a flurry of activity. The stinger or telson is raised above the abdomen in a defensive posture. Alternatively, they will run to other cover with the terminal segments flattened straight behind the body. The stinger is usually used to kill other arthropods. The method of striking its prey or victim (in attack or defense) is to thrust the telson over the back and head to the front. The pincers are used to hold the prey in attack, but in defense, the telson can be quickly thrust forward a number of times without the pincers being used. This is usually the case when a hand or bare foot finds the scorpion's hiding place. Unfortunately, children are often struck, possibly because of their exploratory nature.

Distribution. The distribution of dangerous scorpions is quite broad throughout the world. There are about 650 species. The most dangerous family of scorpions is Buthidae. In South America, there are four species of the genus *Tityus* (*T. serrulatus, T. bahensis, T. trinitatis,* and *T. trivittatus*) that are highly toxic to humans. The genus *Centruroides* has about 25 species found in Mexico, Central America, and the southern United States that are considered important. In the Old World, the family Buthidae includes dangerous species in the genera *Androctonus, Buthacus, Leiurus, Buthus, Parabuthus,* and *Butheolus*. In the same region, the family Scorpionidae has perilous species in the genera *Heterometrus, Pandinus, Scorpio, Opisthophthalmus,* and *Hadogenes*.

Venom. A pair of venom glands found within the bulbous telson synthesize and store venoms of varying toxicity, depending on the species of scorpion. Consequently, information about the potentially hazardous species in a given geographic area is important. The biochemical components of the venoms of scorpions of some species are currently being studied, but little information is available as yet. In general, scorpions produce two types of venoms, hemolytic and neurotoxic. Proteins and enzyme toxins of some species cause only local reactions, whereas those of others may be highly toxic.

The local pain of some scorpion stings is sometimes caused by the presence of 5-hydroxytryptamine (serotonin). Hyaluronidase has also been found in the venoms of some scorpions.

Clinical Manifestations. The effects of envenomation vary with the species. No severe reactions are produced by some scorpions; high mortality rates in children are caused by others. In addition to species differences, toxicity is probably based on a dose/weight relationship. Severe pain may occur at the site of the sting, with radiation into the affected limbs. Chills with abundant cold sweats may be associated with severe thirst and vomiting. Venoms may have neurotoxic effects with paralysis and convulsions or cardiovascular effects with myocarditis and tachycardia or may cause intravascular hemolysis. Death is often due to respiratory paralysis. Pancreatitis and defibrination syndromes have been described, with widespread hemorrhages present in most organs at autopsy. Stings by scorpions with neurotoxic venom may produce little local reaction.

TREATMENT OF ACTIVE ENVENOMATION

Anaphylaxis. Anaphylactic shock in people sensitized to venom components requires urgent treatment. The release of histamine and other mediators causes vasodilation and increased capillary permeability, with a sudden fall in blood pressure, edema of entire extremities, and bronchospasm. A fall in cardiac output may produce secondary myocardial and tissue hypoxia, arrhythmias, and metabolic acidosis. Intramuscular administration of epinephrine is immediately indicated in a dose of 0.5 mL of 1:1000. This dose should be repeated every 15 minutes until improvement occurs. Epinephrine causes constriction of the peripheral vasculature and bronchodilation. It may also inhibit further histamine release. Another treatment scheme, presented in Table 128–2, combines epinephrine with an intravenous antihistamine. Antihistamines are effective in the management of angioedema, pruritus, and urticaria (Table 128–3). Intravenous hydrocortisone sodium succinate may have a long-term beneficial effect. Circulatory collapse may require fluid replacements. In bronchospasm resistant to epinephrine, IV aminophylline, oxygen, and assisted respiration may be indicated. Acute laryngeal edema may require an emergency tracheostomy.

Symptoms occur so rapidly in sensitized persons that they should carry an emergency kit of two syringes containing epinephrine and an antihistamine. Approximately 100 deaths a year occur in the United States as a result of bee or wasp stings.

Local Reactions. Large local reactions of the skin, i.e., urticaria, may be IgE-mediated. If the stinger is present (which frequently occurs in honeybee stings), it should be removed. Cold compresses are a useful first aid measure in hymenopteran sting treatment. Although antihistamines are invariably prescribed, there is no good evidence that they are beneficial. Superimposed infections such as cellulitis or septicemia require antibiotic therapy.

Ant Stings. In ant stings, medical treatment does not alter pustule formation. In fire ant stings in rabbits, no benefit is shown from treatment with topical or systemic steroids, antihistamines, sympathomimetics, local abrasion, topical povidone-iodine solution, or pustule aspiration. Care should be taken to avoid secondary infection.

Spider Bites. Rest and immobilization of a bitten limb are necessary. A firm compression with a bandage on the bite

TABLE 128–2. Treatment of Anaphylaxis

Reaction	Immediate Treatment	Mild Reaction Treatment	Severe Reaction Treatment

Conjunctivitis
Rhinitis
Urticaria/angioedema
Pruritus
	Epinephrine HCl (1:1000)
	  0.3–0.5 mL SC (adults)
	  0.15–0.3 mL SC (children)
		Terfenadine 60 mg PO q 12 hr	

Erythema	Diphenhydramine HCl 25–50 mg PO or terfenadine 60 mg PO		

Laryngeal edema	Epinephrine HCl (1:1000) 0.3–0.5
	  mL SC
	Epinephrine (racemic) via nebulizer
	  0.5–0.75 mL in 3.0 mL total
	  volume
	Diphenhydramine HCl, 50 mg IV
	  or IM
		Epinephrine HCl (1:1000) 0.3–0.5
		  mL SC q 20–60 min
		Epinephrine (racemic) via
		  inhalation q 20–60 min
		Terfenadine 60 mg PO q 12 hr
			Oxygen
			Monitor blood gases
			Hydrocortisone or methylprednisolone IV
			Nebulized racemic epinephrine (0.5–0.75
			  mL in 3.0 mL) q 20–60 min
			Tracheostomy

Bronchospasm	Epinephrine hydrochloride (1:1000)
	  0.3–0.5 mL SC
	Diphenhydramine HCl 50 mg IV
	Albuterol, isoetharine, or
	  metaproterenol nebulizer solution
	  0.3–0.5 mL in 3.0 mL total
	  volume
		Albuterol (up to 0.5 mL) *or*
		Metaproterenol (up to 0.3 mL) *or*
		Isoetharine (up to 0.3 mL)
		  diluted to 3.0 mL in saline
		  and nebulized q 20–60 min
			Oxygen
			Intravenous fluids
			Monitor blood gases
			Observe for respiratory failure
			Methyl prednisolone 60–125 mg IV q 4–6 hr
			Nebulized β-agonists q 20–60 min
			Aminophylline 5–6 mg/kg IV over 30
			  min if not on theophylline

Hypotension	Epinephrine HCl (1:1000) 0.3–0.5
	  mL SC
	Diphenhydramine HCl 50 mg IV
	Cimetidine, 300 mg IV
		Intravenous fluids
		Epinephrine (1:1000) 0.3–0.5 mL
		  SC q 20–30 min
		Methyl prednisolone 60–125 mg
		  IV
			Oxygen
			Military antishock trousers
			Hydrocortisone or methylprednisolone IV
			Cimetidine 300 mg IV q 4–6 hr
			Diphenhydramine HCl, 50 mL IV q 5–6 hr
			Metaraminol bitartrate, 100 mg in 500 mL
			  5% D/W drip

Modified with the assistance of Dr. Gary B. Carpenter, Chief of Allergy and Immunology, Walter Reed Medical Center, from a table used in the seventh edition.

may reduce toxin dissemination, and ice packs are recommended for treating bites from *Latrodectus* species. If systemic signs occur following a bite by this species, an ampule of antivenom (Lyovac) can be given by slow intravenous injection in 50 mL of saline solution after skin testing for hypersensitivity. Pain requires analgesics and may be sufficiently intense to justify the administration of meperidine (Demerol) or morphine. For muscle spasms, 10 mL of 10% calcium gluconate every 4 hours can be used, as can other muscle relaxants, e.g., methocarbamol. There is no clear indication for corticosteroids or antihistamines. Necrotizing bites of South American *Loxosceles* spiders can be treated by locally

TABLE 128–3. Antihistamines

Group	Generic Name	Trade Name	Average Oral Dose		Sedation
			Adult	**Child**	
H₁ Antagonists					
Ethanolamines	Diphenhydramine HCl	Benadryl	25–50 mg q 4–6 hr	12.5–25 mg q 4–6 hr	+ + + +
	Dimenhydrinate		50 mg q 4 hr	25 mg q 4 hr	+ + + +
Ethylenediamines	Tripelennamine HCl	Pyribenzamine, PBZ	50 mg q 4–6 hr	25 mg q 4–6 hr	+ + +
Alkylamines	Chlorpheniramine maleate	Chlor-Trimeton, CTM	4 mg q 6 hr	2 mg q 6 hr	+ + +
	Brompheniramine maleate	Dimetane	8 mg q 6 hr	4 mg q 6 hr	+ +
	Triprolidine HCl	Actidil	2.5 mg q 6 hr	1.25 mg q 6–12 hr	+ +
Cyclizines	Hydroxyzine HCl	Atarax	25–100 mg q 6–12 hr	10–25 mg q 6–12 hr	+ +
Phenothiazines	Promethazine HCl	Phenergan	25–50 mg q 6–8 hr	12.5–25 mg q 6–8 hr	+ + + +
Miscellaneous	Cyproheptadine HCl	Periactin	4 mg q 6 hr	2 mg q 6 hr	+ + +
	Astemizole	Hismanal	10 mg q 24 hr	5 mg q 24 hr	0
	Cetirazine	Zyrtec	10 mg q 24 hr	5 mg q 24 hr	±
	Loratadine	Claritin	10 mg q 24 hr	5 mg q 24 hr	0
H₂ Antagonists*					
	Cimetidine HCl	Tagamet	300–400 mg q 6 hr	20–40 mg/kg/day	0
	Rantidine	Zantac	150 mg q 12 hr		0
	Famotidine	Pepcid	20 mg q 12 hr or 40 mg at bedtime		0

*Although primarily anti–peptic ulcer and reflux medications, H₂ antagonists may be used in conjunction with classic (anti-H₁) antihistamines for the treatment of chronic urticaria or severe systemic anaphylaxis with hypotension.

Modified, with the assistance of Dr. Gary B. Carpenter, Chief of Allergy and Immunology, Walter Reed Army Medical Center, from a table used in the seventh edition.

available antivenom. In other areas, treatment of bites consists of supportive care and 40 mg of dexamethasone given every 6 hours for the first 48 hours. Application of local antiseptic to open ulcers is necessary. In the healing phase, skin grafting may be indicated.

Centipede Bites. The pain of a centipede bite can be relieved by infiltrating the affected area with 1% lidocaine (Xylocaine).

Scorpion Stings. Immediate treatment of a scorpion sting is directed toward delaying absorption of the venom. A constricting band is applied to the limb and is released every 20 to 30 minutes. If available, ice packs should be applied to the site, and the patient should be kept at rest. Specific antiserum is available in some countries, e.g., Mexico and Brazil, and should be given if signs occur that the central nervous system is being affected.

Passive Envenomation

Some stinging arthropods play a more passive role. Specialized cells and morphologic structures, i.e., setae and spines, synthesize toxins and irritating chemicals to repel an offending animal. Humans themselves often provide the force necessary to introduce the venom.

CATERPILLARS. Irritant hairs or spines present on caterpillars (order Lepidoptera) cause dermatitis on skin contact. In Brazil, five families of nocturnal moths and the Morphidae family of butterflies have larvae with such structures. The spines are of two general types, either a simple linear shaft of a spinous hair that may be branched with a detachable cap. Both types have a simple poison gland at their hollow base. These urticating hairs may be distributed over the entire body of the caterpillar. The venoms are poorly characterized, but symptoms of itching papules or urticaria, often associated with transient edema, are well known. The puss caterpillars (*Megalopyge* species) in the United States and elsewhere are very hairy, with hidden spines. They should be avoided but are frequently brushed against by accident. Sticky cellophane tape applied to the skin will often pick up the spines, which can be seen microscopically. Calamine lotion is often sufficient to relieve itching. Stinging and irritation can also have an allergic basis, resulting in other medical complications.

BEETLES. Two families of beetles (order Coleoptera) have urticating substances causing skin reaction in humans. The Staphylinidae contain a genus of small beetles, *Paederus*. When accidentally crushed on the skin, a vesicant in the hemolymph of *Paederus* causes painful erythema and blistering (Fig. 128–2). In the Amazon region of Brazil, reactions to these beetles may persist for several weeks and leave a pigmented scar. Another species in Kenya causes the Nairobi eye, conjunctival contamination by the beetle resulting in a unilateral conjunctivitis and orbital edema. The Meloidae (blister and oil beetles) are larger and often brightly colored and are attracted to artificial light at night. Hemolymph exuded through integumental membranes or expelled on crushing contains cantharidin, a vesicant that often causes large blisters. Topical treatment of the blisters with magnesium sulfate or methyl alcohol has been recommended.

MILLIPEDES AND OTHERS. Secretions from a number of other arthropods can also irritate the eyes, nose, and skin. Millipedes (class Diplopoda) are scavengers living on decayed vegetation; some species can forcibly release a defensive, odoriferous fluid from segmental glands. Dermatitis

may be followed by bullae and, occasionally, necrosis. The giant whip scorpion or vinegarroon (*Mastigoproctus giganteus*), and night-hunting arachnid, can directionally eject secretions of acetic acid and caprylic acid. Some beetles (e.g., Carabidae and Tenebrionidae) and true bugs (e.g., Coreidae and Pentatomidae) can also release obnoxious secretions. These are usually gaseous and are repugnant to humans.

Bibliography

Beard RB: Insect toxins and insect venoms. Annu Rev Entomol 8:1, 1963.
Bettini S (ed): Arthropod Venoms. Handbook of Experimental Pharmacology. Vol. 48. New York, Springer-Verlag, 1978.
Biery TS: Venomous Arthropod Handbook. Washington, DC, U.S. Government Printing Office, 1977, AFP 191–243.
Blum MS: Biochemical defenses of insects. *In* Rockstein M (ed): Biochemistry of Insects. New York, Academic Press, 1978, pp. 465–513.
Bousquet J, Müller UR, Dreborg S, et al: Immunotherapy with Hymenoptera venoms. Allergy 42:401, 1987.
Bücherl W, Buckley E (eds.): Venomous Animals and Their Venoms. Vol. III. Venomous Invertebrates. New York, Academic Press, 1971.
Centers for Disease Control and Prevention: Necrotic arachnidism—Pacific Northwest, 1988–1996. MMWR 45:433, 1996.
Delori P, Rietschoten JV, Rochat H: Scorpion venoms and neurotoxins: an immunological study. Toxicon 19:393, 1981.
Ebeling W: Urban Entomology. Davis, University of California, Division of Agricultural Sciences, 1978.
Feingold BF, Benjamini E, Michael D: The allergic responses to insect bites. Annu Rev Entomol 13:137, 1968.
Frazier CA, Brown FK: Insects and Allergy and What To Do About Them. Norman, University of Oklahoma Press, 1980.
Habermann E: Bee and wasp venoms. Science 177:314, 1972.
Harwood RF, James MT: Entomology in Human and Animal Health. New York, Macmillan, 1979.
Keegan HL: Venomous bites and stings in Mississippi. J Miss State Med Assoc 8:495, 1972.
Le Mao J, Dandeu JP, Rabillon J, et al: Antigens and allergens in *Dermatophagoides farinae* mite. Immunology 44:239, 1981.
Minton SA: Venom Disease. Springfield, IL, Charles C Thomas, 1974.
Mueller HL, Schmid WH, Ribiniztain R: Stinging insect hypersensitivity: A 20 year study of immunological treatment. Pediatrics 55:530, 1975.
Nelson WA, Bell JF, Clifford CM, et al: Interaction of ectoparasites and their hosts. J Med Entomol 13:389, 1977.
Ori M: Biology and poisonings by spiders. *In* Tu AT (ed): Insect Poisons, Allergens, and Other Invertebrate Venoms. New York, Marcel Dekker, 1984, pp 397–440.
Orkin M, Maibach HI, Parish LC, et al: Scabies and Pediculosis. Philadelphia, JB Lippincott, 1977.
Owen S, Morganstern M, Hepworth J, Woodcock A: Control of dust mite antigen in bedding. Lancet 335:396, 1990.
Parrish HM: Analysis of 460 fatalities from venomous animals in the United States. Am J Med Sci 245:129, 1963.
Reisman RE, Lazell M, Doerr J: Insect venom allergy: A prospective case study showing lack of correlation between immunologic reactivity and clinical sensitivity. J Allergy Clin Immunol 68:406, 1981.
Riebeiro JMC, Makoul GT, Levine J, et al: Antihemostatic, antiinflamatory, and immunosuppressive properties of saliva of a tick, *Ixodes dammini*. J Exp Med 161:332, 1985.
Rosenstreich DL, Eggleston P, Kattan M, et al: The role of cockroach allergy and exposure to cockroach allergen in causing morbidity among inner-city children with asthma. N Engl J Med 336:1356, 1997.
Schmidt JO: Biochemistry of insect venoms. Annu Rev Entomol 27:339, 1982.
Schumacher MJ, Schmidt JO, Egen NB, Lowry JE: Quality, analysis, and lethality of European and Africanized honey bee venoms. Am J Trop Med Hyg 43:79, 1990.
Smith KGV (ed): Insects and Other Arthropods of Medical Importance. London, British Museum, 1973, Publication No. 720.
Tovey ER, Chapman MD, Platts-Mills TAE: Mite feces are a major source of house dust allergens. Nature 289:592, 1981.
Treatment of anaphylactic shock. BMJ 282:1011, 1981.
Van Bronswijk JEMH, Sinha RN: Pyroglyphid mites (Acari) and house dust allergy. J Allergy 47:31, 1971.
Wikel SK: Immune responses to arthropods and their products. Ann Rev Entomol 27:21, 1982.
Wirtz RA: Allergic and toxic reactions to non-stinging arthropods. Annu Rev Entomol 69:47, 1984.
Yunginger JW: Advances in the diagnosis and treatment of stinging insect allergy. Pediatrics 67:325, 1981.

129 *General Principles*

Benjamin Caballero

Nutritional problems in tropical areas are almost always associated with deficiency states, with protein-energy malnutrition, hypovitaminosis A, and iron and iodine deficiencies being the most prevalent. According to UN organizations' data, around 20% of the world population consumes amounts of foods insufficient to sustain health and an active and productive life. One of every three children exhibits growth delay, and more than 40% of women are anemic. The vast majority of these populations are found in tropical and other developing regions.

Although acute food shortages caused by civil war, drought, or natural disasters periodically and recurrently affect millions of people, particularly in Africa, the number of individuals taking in insufficient amounts of dietary energy has declined over the past 15 years, from 1 billion in 1975 to less than 800 million in 1990. Most of the improvement reflects advances in South Asia, because trends have worsened in the African continent.

Insufficient dietary intake of protein, energy, and/or micronutrients is only one factor leading to nutritional diseases in the tropics. The unsanitary environment leads to frequent infections of the gastrointestinal tract, which, even if relatively minor, cause malabsorption of essential nutrients. A child living in an unsanitary environment can have as many as ten or more episodes of acute gastroenteritis in a year. Each episode leads to a negative balance between intake and losses, with consequent weight loss and delay in longitudinal growth. Children who survive recurring illnesses early in life may never recover from their growth delay, becoming permanently stunted adults. Conversely, an impaired nutritional status increases the risk of infection by affecting the immune system, facilitating bacterial colonization, or increasing the frequency and severity of infectious illnesses.

Many children living in a highly contaminated environment exhibit a state of chronic immune stimulation, characterized by increased production of acute-phase reactants, e.g., C-reactive protein, fibrinogen, acid α-glycoprotein, and others. The nutritional cost of mounting such a response has been the focus of interest. The need for certain essential amino acids to synthesize these acute-phase proteins may result in an increased breakdown of skeletal muscle protein, further impairing growth.

A second factor adversely affecting the utilization of dietary nutrients is the composition of the typical diet in many developing countries. Diets based on cereals and grains tend to have a high content of substances such as phytate, which inhibit the absorption of essential minerals. Some vegetable-based diets may also contain antithyroid factors or other elements interfering with the metabolism and utilization of essential nutrients.

Some of the classic manifestations of vitamin deficiencies can still be identified in refugee camps and in extreme conditions of food scarcity. Outbreaks of beriberi, scurvy, and pellagra have occurred among populations displaced by civil war. Iron deficiency constitutes the most common single-nutrient deficiency in the world and, along with the deficiency of vitamin B_{12} and folic acid, is responsible for the widespread occurrence of anemia in children and pregnant women.

A special section is dedicated to the important issue of the interaction between nutrition and infection. Also, the unique characteristics of the tropical neuropathies, many of them associated with vitamin deficiencies, are discussed in a separate chapter. The nervous system is extremely sensitive to the supply of certain vitamins, and their absence or severe depletion in the diet may lead to rapid damage of the central and peripheral nervous systems' components, which sometimes can be irreversible.

Although nutritional deficiencies are by far the most common in developing countries, there is an increasing trend, particularly in urban areas, toward diseases commonly associated with excess—such as obesity, diabetes, and cardiovascular disease. The rapid migration to the cities produces drastic changes in lifestyle and food choices in children and adults. Energy expenditure for physical activity is reduced owing to a more sedentary way of life, and more "empty" calories and processed foods are consumed; although the diet may still be marginal in certain nutrients, it is likely to contain more calories from fat, including more saturated fats. As a consequence, stunting in linear growth and excess body fat can be observed in many children in the poor slums of large urban areas in developing countries. The long-term impact of these transitional conditions is unclear, but their increasing prevalence will pose a challenge to the primary health care system, which has been historically focused on the management of nutritional deficiencies.

References

Report on the World Nutrition Situation. ACC/SCN, United Nations, 1992.
Solomons NW, Mazariegos M, Vettorazzi C, et al: Growth faltering, protein metabolism and immunostimulation. *In* Protein and Energy Metabolism in Malnourished Populations of Developing Countries. Vienna, International Atomic Energy Agency, 1993, pp 115–126.
The State of the World's Children. UNICEF, 1997.

130 *Protein-Energy Malnutrition*

Benjamin Torun

Protein-energy malnutrition (PEM) is the most important nutritional disease in developing countries because of its high prevalence and its relationship with child mortality rates, impaired growth and development, decreased work capacity, and inadequate social and economic improvement. Fifty-six percent of deaths among children 6 to 59 months old in 53 developing countries have been attributed to malnutrition's potentiating effects in infectious diseases, and mild and moderate malnutrition were involved in 83% of those deaths.

PEM results when the body's needs for protein, energy

fuels (calories), or both cannot be satisfied by the diet. It is usually associated with mineral and vitamin deficits, but the clinical and metabolic alterations of energy and/or protein deficiency predominate. PEM covers the severe clinical syndromes of kwashiorkor (edematous, predominant protein deficiency), marasmus (nonedematous, predominant energy deficiency) or marasmic kwashiorkor (edematous combination of chronic energy deficiency and acute or chronic protein deficit), and the much more numerous mild and moderate cases. The term *malnutrition* is usually used in lay language for PEM.

PEM can be primary in origin, when it is the direct result of inadequate food intake, or secondary, when it is the result of other diseases that lead to low food ingestion, inadequate nutrient absorption or utilization, increased nutritional requirements, and/or increased nutrient losses. Although PEM is mainly a problem in early childhood, it can occur in older children and adults, but severe degrees of primary PEM are rare outside early childhood, except in famine conditions.

HISTORY. The cause of edematous PEM was not understood for a long time because it could be found among children who were not starving and among families in good socioeconomic position. It was initially believed to be caused by tropical parasites or vitamin deficiencies, because of the skin lesions. The real nature of the disease was studied more carefully after Cicely Williams' descriptions in the mid-1930s of kwashiorkor. This term, used by the Ga tribe in the Gold Coast (now Ghana) for "the sickness the older child gets when the next baby is born," already suggested that the disease could be associated with an inadequate diet during the weaning period. Pediatricians who worked in tropical countries showed that the edematous disease could be cured by feeding milk or other high-protein foods. In the 1940s, researchers showed that most patients had low concentrations of serum proteins and that this could also be related to the quality of dietary proteins. By the 1950s, more than 40 names had been given to this clinical syndrome. Some of them, e.g., *infantile pluricarential syndrome*, indicated that young children were mainly affected and that a deficit of various nutrients was involved. Others, e.g., *Mehlnährschade* ("damage by cereal flours"), *starch edema*, and *sugar babies*, indicated that it was caused by the intake of foods with high carbohydrate and low protein contents. Today, the more comprehensive term of *protein-energy* (or *protein-calorie*) *malnutrition* is universally accepted, with edematous and nonedematous manifestations of its severe forms. In the past 30 years, it has been shown that marasmus and kwashiorkor have distinct metabolic features; that some manifestations, e.g., anemia and reduced physical activity, are partly a result of adaptive mechanisms; that the immune response of severely malnourished patients is impaired; and that physical and emotional stimulation are important elements in treating malnourished children. These findings form the basis for current therapeutic approaches.

ETIOLOGY

Biologic Factors

Maternal Malnutrition. This can lead to intrauterine malnutrition and low birth weight (Chapter 15). Lack of sufficient food to satisfy an infant's needs for catch-up results in infantile PEM. Diets with low concentrations of proteins and energy, e.g., overdiluted milk formulas and bulky vegetable foods, can lead to PEM in young children, whose gastric capacity limits the amount of food they can ingest, and in elderly persons with anorexia or difficulty in eating without assistance. Diets poor in protein and rich in carbohydrates are particularly likely to produce kwashiorkor.

Infectious Diseases. These are major contributing and precipitating factors in PEM (Chapter 133.1). Diarrheal disease,

measles, AIDS, tuberculosis, malaria, and other infections frequently result in negative protein and energy balance owing to poor appetite, vomiting, impaired absorption, and increased catabolic processes. Intestinal parasites have little or no effect unless the infection is extensive and causes anemia or diarrhea (Chapter 133.2).

Social and Economic Factors. Poverty is frequently associated with PEM because of low food availability, overcrowded and unsanitary living conditions, and improper child care. *Ignorance* leads to poor child-rearing practices, misconceptions about the use of certain foods, inadequate feeding procedures during illnesses, and improper food distribution within the family members. A decline in the practice and duration of breast-feeding, combined with inadequate weaning practices, is related to increasing rates of infantile PEM.

Social problems e.g., child abuse, maternal deprivation, abandonment of the elderly, alcoholism, and drug addiction can result in PEM. Cultural and social practices that impose food taboos, some food and diet fads, and the migration from traditional rural settings to urban slums also contribute to the appearance of PEM.

Environmental Factors. Overcrowded and/or unsanitary living conditions lead to frequent infections. Droughts, floods, wars, and forced migrations lead to cyclic, sudden, or prolonged food scarcities and can cause PEM among whole populations (Chapter 19). Postharvest losses of food due to bad storage conditions and inadequate food distribution systems contribute to PEM, even after periods of agricultural plenty.

EPIDEMIOLOGY. There are about 840 million undernourished people in the world, most of them in developing countries: about 30% each in southern and eastern Asia, 25% in sub-Saharan Africa, and 8% in Latin America and the Caribbean. Because of this, 36% (210 million) of the children <5 years old in the developing world are underweight (low weight for age), 43% (250 million) are stunted (low height for age), and 9% (52 million) are wasted (low weight for height). This prevalence ranges from 12% underweight, 22% stunted, and 3% wasted in Latin America and the Middle East to 62% underweight, 61% stunted, and 17% wasted in southern Asia. When countries are not disturbed by natural and manmade disasters, e.g., droughts, land wastage, wars, and economic crisis, the trend is for a gradual improvement in the prevalence of child malnutrition.

In industralized countries, primary PEM is encountered mainly among young children of the lower socioeconomic groups, the elderly who live alone, and adults addicted to alcohol and drugs.

Age and Physiologic Conditions

Infants and Young Children. PEM is more frequent among infants and young children because growth increases their nutritional requirements, they cannot obtain food by their own means, and, when living under poor hygienic conditions, they frequently become ill with diarrhea and other infections. Infants who are weaned prematurely from the breast or who are breast-fed for a prolonged time without adequate complementary feeding practices become malnourished for lack of adequate energy and protein intake.

Prolonged intake of insufficient food can result in marasmus, which is the most common form of severe PEM before 1 year of age. Kwashiorkor, the edematous form of the disease, is more frequent after 18 months of age and typically occurs in children with diets consisting of starchy gruels, diluted cereal-based beverages, and vegetable foods rich in carbohydrates but almost devoid of proteins of good nutritional quality (i.e., lacking one or more essential amino acids). Most often, the severe protein deficit is associated with chronic dietary energy deficit and results in a combined form of marasmic kwashiorkor. The appearance of edema is frequently preceded or accompanied by acute diarrhea or another infectious disease.

Older Children and Adults at High Risk. These usually have milder forms of PEM because they can cope better with social and food availability constraints. Infections and other precipitating factors become less severe, and early survival may imply a natural selection of the more fit. Pregnant and lactating women can also have PEM as a result of the increases in their nutritional requirements. However, the consequences of the dietary deficiencies affect mainly the growth, nutritional status, and survival rates of their fetuses, newborn babies, and infants. Elderly persons who are unable to care properly for themselves tend to suffer from PEM. Gastrointestinal alterations can be an important contributing factor.

Adolescents, adult men, and nonpregnant, nonlactating women usually have the lowest prevalence and the mildest forms of the disease because of greater opportunities to obtain food and cultural practices that protect the productive members of the family. Severe primary PEM occurs among them in conditions of extreme privation and famine and in situations of social or chemical dependence without adequate nutritional support, as may be the case with patients with mental disabilities, prisoners, alcoholic individuals, and those addicted to drugs. Severe PEM is seen more frequently in adults as secondary to other illnesses, e.g., chronic infections, cancer, AIDS, malabsorption, and liver and endocrine diseases. In such cases, both the malnutrition and the underlying cause must be treated.

PATHOPHYSIOLOGY AND ADAPTIVE RESPONSES. PEM develops gradually in weeks or months, allowing for metabolic and behavioral adjustments. This results in decreased nutrient demands and a nutritional equilibrium compatible with a lower level of cellular nutrient availability. If the supply of nutrients becomes persistently lower, patients can no longer adapt and may even die. Metabolic disruptions can be due to severe nutrient deficit, complications (e.g., infections), or inadequate treatment (e.g., abrupt administration of large amounts of dietary energy or protein). Patients whose PEM develops slowly—as is usually the case in marasmus—are better adapted to their current nutritional status and maintain a less fragile metabolic equilibrium than those with more acute PEM, as in kwashiorkor of rapid onset.

Energy Mobilization and Expenditure. A decrease in energy intake is followed by a decrease in energy expenditure, accounting for shorter periods of play and physical activity in children and for longer rest periods and less physical work in adults. When the decrease in energy expenditure cannot compensate for the insufficient intake, body fat is mobilized, with a decrease in adiposity and weight loss. Lean body mass diminishes at a slower rate. As the cumulative energy deficit becomes more severe, subcutaneous fat is markedly reduced and protein catabolism leads to muscle wasting.

Protein Metabolism. Metabolic adaptations tend to spare visceral protein and preserve essential protein-dependent functions, more so in marasmus than in kwashiorkor. Enzymatic changes favor muscle protein breakdown and liver protein synthesis, as well as energy mobilization from fat depots. Some visceral protein is lost in the early development of PEM but then becomes stable until the nonessential tissue proteins are depleted; the loss of visceral protein then increases, and death may be imminent unless nutritional therapy is successfully instituted.

The half-life of albumin increases, and a shift from the extravascular to the intravascular pool assists in maintaining adequate levels of circulating albumin. When protein depletion becomes too severe or is complicated by a systemic infection, the adaptive mechanisms fail and the concentration of serum proteins, especially albumin, decreases. The ensuing reduction in intravascular oncotic pressure and the outflow of water into the extravascular space contribute to the development of the edema of kwashiorkor.

Endocrine Functions. In severe PEM there is a marked decrease in activity of hormones involved in building body reserves, increasing metabolism and enhancing nonvital growth-related functions, e.g., insulin, IGF-1, thyroid hormones, and gonadotropin. There is a normal or increased activity of glucocorticoids, which favor muscle protein catabolism, lipolysis, and gluconeogenesis. The functional capacities of the hypothalamic-pituitary axis and adrenal medulla are preserved, thus allowing endocrine and metabolic responses to stress conditions. Some investigators have postulated that the evolution of PEM into either kwashiorkor or marasmus may be partly related to differences in adrenocortical response, in which the better response preserves visceral proteins more efficiently and leads to the better-adapted syndrome of marasmus.

Hematology and Oxygen Transport. The reduction in lean body mass and the lower physical activity of malnourished patients lead to lower oxygen demands. The simultaneous decrease in dietary amino acids results in reduced hematopoietic activity, which spares amino acids for synthesis of other more necessary body proteins. As long as the tissues' needs for oxygen are satisfied by the existing capacity for oxygen transport, the reduction in hemoglobin concentration should be considered an adaptive response and not a functional anemia (i.e., with tissue hypoxia). Although the level of circulating hemoglobin is usually low, severely malnourished patients may have relatively high body iron stores and may retain the ability to produce erythropoietin and reticulocytes in response to acute hypoxia. Nevertheless, these patients are prone to develop functional, severe anemia if they have a superimposed dietary deficiency of iron or folic acid or chronic blood loss, as in hookworm infection.

When tissue synthesis, lean body mass, and physical activity begin improving with dietary treatment, a rise in oxygen demands follows, calling for accelerated hematopoiesis. If iron (Chapter 132.1), folic acid, and vitamin B_{12} (Chapter 131.7) are not available in sufficient amounts, functional anemia with tissue hypoxia develops. On the other hand, administration of hematinics to severely malnourished patients induces a hematopoietic response only after dietary treatment produces an increase in lean body mass (Fig. 130–1).

Cardiovascular and Renal Functions. Central circulation takes precedence over peripheral circulation, which accounts for the cool hands and feet in severe PEM. Cardiac output and blood pressure decrease, and cardiovascular reflexes are altered, leading to postural hypotension and diminished venous return. Hemodynamic compensation results mainly from tachycardia. In severe PEM, peripheral circulatory failure comparable to hypovolemic shock may occur. Renal plasma flow and glomerular filtration rates may be reduced as a consequence of the decreased cardiac output, but water clearance and the ability to concentrate and acidify urine are not impaired.

Immune System and Monokine Metabolism. Malnourished patients have a greater predisposition to infections, which tend to be more prolonged and severe than in well-nourished individuals (Chapter 133.1). In severe PEM there is a decrease in T lymphocytes and in complement and opsonic activities, thus explaining the high susceptibility to gram-negative bacterial sepsis. The synthesis and activity of interleukin-1 are depressed, and this decrement contributes to the poor febrile response and low leukocyte count in infection. On the other hand, cachectin or tumor necrosis factor increases, and this

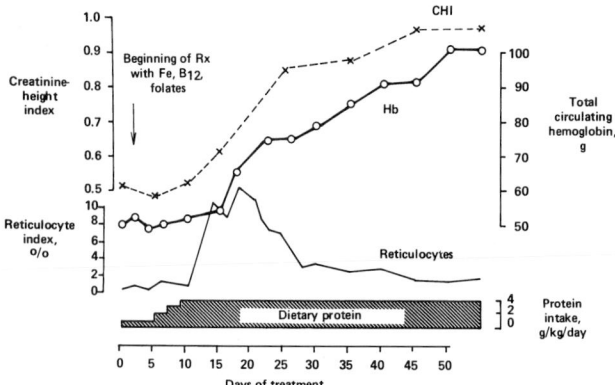

Figure 130–1. Hematologic response of a child with severe protein-energy malnutrition. Treatment with iron, folic acid, and vitamin B_{12} began at an unnecessarily early time, on day 2; dietary energy and proteins were increased gradually to 150 kcal (630 KJ) and 4 g protein/kg/day on day 9. Reticulocyte and hemoglobin response occurred until lean body mass began increasing, as assessed by the creatinine-height index (CHI). (From Torun B, Chew F: *In* Shils ME, Olson JA, Shike M [eds]: Modern Nutrition in Health and Disease, 8th ed. Philadelphia, Lea & Febiger, 1994.)

increase could contribute to the anorexia, muscle wasting, and lipid abnormalities of severe PEM.

Electrolytes. The cellular exchange of sodium and potassium is altered in severe PEM, leading to potassium loss and increased intracellular sodium. The latter may lead to intracellular overhydration. Total body potassium decreases because of the reduction in muscle proteins and loss of intracellular potassium. These alterations contribute to the increased fatigability and reduced strength of skeletal muscle and to the reduced motility of intestinal muscle.

Gastrointestinal Functions. In severe PEM there is a decrease in disaccharidase activity, in gastric and pancreatic secretions, and in bile production, which impair digestion and absorption of carbohydrates, lipids, and amino acids. However, ingestion of nutrients in high therapeutic amounts usually allows for their uptake in sufficient quantity to permit nutritional recovery. Nevertheless, malnourished persons are prone to diarrhea because of these alterations and because of irregular intestinal motility and gastrointestinal bacterial overgrowth. This tends to disappear with nutritional recovery. Normal intestinal absorption is also restored with nutritional recovery, unless there is an underlying food or nutrient intolerance unrelated to primary PEM.

Central and Peripheral Nervous System. Severe PEM at an early age may reduce or delay brain growth, nerve myelination, neurotransmitter production, and velocity of nervous conduction. The long-term functional implications of these alterations have not been clearly demonstrated in humans, because it is impossible to separate nutrition from other factors that can affect motor skills, intelligence, and behavior. The quality of nutritional rehabilitation and psychosocial support, the degree of stimulation by family members, and other environmental factors influence the developmental outcome of a malnourished child.

Other Factors Leading to Kwashiorkor. In addition to a diet deficient in proteins and with a low protein:energy ratio and to the hypothesis related to differences in adrenocortical response, other theories involve the production and disposal of free radicals, metabolic shunts due to infection, and aflatoxin poisoning. The toxic effects of free radicals would be responsible for cell damage leading to edema, fatty liver, and skin lesions. Among the factors that may increase free radi-

cals are infections, toxins, and excessive exposure to iron. Their formation is decreased by the antioxidant function of vitamins A (or beta-carotene), C, and E and by the proteins ceruloplasmin and transferrin, which bind free iron and favor its oxidation. Free radicals and the peroxides they generate are removed through reactions catalyzed by enzymes that contain Cu, Zn, Mn, or Se. However, none of these theories has been proved. Furthermore, the pathogenesis of edematous PEM may not be a single entity, and its causes may differ in accordance with the age of the patients, multiple nutritional deficiencies, and other concomitant conditions.

Disruption of Adaptation. Severe energy deficiency can lead to a serious decompensation causing hypoglycemia, hypothermia, impaired circulatory and renal functions, acidosis, coma, and death. Metabolic decompensation due to severe protein deficiency produces loss of visceral protein and function, hemorrhagic diathesis, jaundice, impaired cardiac and renal functions, water and sodium retention, pulmonary congestion, increased susceptibility to pulmonary infections, coma, and death.

Inadequate dietary management of severely malnourished patients can cause serious metabolic disruption with fatal consequences. This includes premature introduction of a high-energy or high-protein diet. Abrupt administration of too much protein to patients, especially with edematous PEM, as well as large or rapid transfusions of blood or plasma, can result in a swift increase in intravascular protein concentration and entry of extracellular fluid into the vascular compartment, leading to heart failure and pulmonary edema.

Infections can produce serious metabolic disruptions due to enhanced protein catabolism and nitrogen losses, diversion of nitrogen metabolism to the synthesis of acute phase proteins, impaired energy metabolism, and/or production of free radicals.

DIAGNOSIS AND CLINICAL MANIFESTATIONS. Weight loss and delayed growth are the only practical diagnostic indicators in the early stages of PEM. Other clinical manifestations usually do not appear until the disease is well advanced, and they vary according to the severity of the disease, the patient's age, the presence of other nutritional deficits or infection, and the predominance of energy or protein deficiency. Some functional indicators, e.g., decrease in physical activity, immunologic alterations, and behavioral changes, appear early, but their quantitative assessment is not yet well standardized or is too complex for routine use. Dietary history of individual patients, dietary surveys in population groups, and information on dietary habits and food availability help to appraise the risk of PEM and to interpret anthropometric and clinical findings.

Anthropometric Measurements. Several anthropometric measurements and indexes have been used to diagnose and classify PEM. The choice of measurement depends on simplicity, accuracy, and sensitivity, as well as on the availability of measuring instruments and the existence of reference standards for interpretation.

The best assessment is based on measurements of (1) weight and height or length, to calculate weight for height of infants and young children, and body mass index (BMI = weight in kg/height² in meters) of school-age children, adolescents, and adults, as indexes of current nutritional status; and (2) records of age, to calculate height for age, as an index of past nutritional history. When the exact age is not known, assessment of reasonably reliable information may be attempted by constructing a local events calendar.

Those indexes can be interpreted by comparing them with data derived from the U.S. National Center for Health Statistics, as recommended by the World Health Organization

TABLE 130–1. Classification of Current (Wasting) and Past or Chronic (Stunting) PEM in Infants and Children, Based on Weight for Height and Height for Age*

	Normal	Mild	Moderate	Severe
Weight for height (deficit = wasting)	±1 Z (91–110%)	−1.1 to −2 Z (81–90%)	−2.1 to −3 Z (76–80%)	< −3 Z (<76%) or with edema
Height for age (deficit = stunting)	≥−1 Z (≥96%)†	−1.1 to −2 Z (91–95%)	−2.1 to −3 Z (86–90%)	< −3 Z (<86%)

*Standard deviations from the NCHS/WHO median, or Z scores. Percent ranges in relation to the median (in parentheses) were rounded to the multiple of 5 that approximates the corresponding Z scores for children between 6 months and 5 years old.
†Upper normal limits of height for age have not been established.

(WHO). The advantages of using this universal reference outweigh its disadvantages and the limitations of reliable normal local references. The term *wasting* is used for a deficit in weight for height or BMI, and *stunting* for a deficit in height for age. Patients may then fall into four categories: (1) normal, (2) wasted but not stunted (suffering from acute PEM), (3) wasted and stunted (suffering from acute and past or chronic PEM), and (4) stunted but not wasted (past PEM with present adequate nutrition, or nutritional dwarfs).

The severity of wasting and stunting can be graded by calculating weight as a percentage of the reference median weight for height, and height as a percentage of the reference median height for age, as follows:

$$\text{% wt for ht} \atop \text{(or ht for age)} = \frac{\text{observed wt (or ht)}}{\text{reference wt for patient's ht}\atop\text{(or ht for patient's age)}} \times 100$$

Percent deviations from the median are easier to understand by the general public and to calculate by fieldworkers, although standard deviations from the median (Z scores) and centiles are statistically more adequate. The classification shown in Table 130–1 is suggested for most countries, although some might find it convenient to use different cutoff points for specific groups. For example, <95% of the reference height for age might be acceptable in populations that are genetically short. Color-coded charts and graphs, e.g., those devised by Nabarro and McNab, can simplify the measurement and interpretation of weight for height in infants and children.

Weight for age is useful for epidemiologic purposes, but in clinical use it does not differentiate between a truly underweight child (current PEM) and one who is short in stature but well proportioned in weight (past PEM).

Table 130–2 shows the classification of adult PEM based on BMI. For simplicity, the same BMI criteria are suggested to classify males and females. For adolescents, interpretation of BMI must take into account age and sexual maturation. If age- and maturation-specific references are not available, it is suggested that the diagnosis of PEM in adolescent boys and girls be based on a BMI <15.0 at ages 11 to 13 years,

TABLE 130–2. Classification of Protein-Energy Malnutrition in Adult Men and Women

Body Mass Index (BMI)*	PEM
≥18.5	Normal
17.0–18.4	Mild
16.0–16.9	Moderate
<16.0	Severe

*BMI = weight (kg)/height² (m).

and <16.5 at ages 14 to 17 years. The corresponding values for severe PEM would be <13.0 and <14.5, respectively.

Measurement of upper arm circumference has been advocated under field conditions without access to a weighing scale. It is not a sensitive index, but it allows identifying the more severely malnourished children who require urgent treatment.

Mild and Moderate PEM. The main feature is weight loss. Leanness with reduction in subcutaneous adipose tissue may be clinically evident in children and adults. As described earlier, weight for height and BMI are lower than the reference standards. Repeated measurements show a flattening of the weight-for-age curve or weight gains that follow a channel below the lower limit accepted for well-nourished children. This can also be seen in anthropometric community surveys. When PEM is chronic or endemic, children also show slower growth in height and they are stunted.

Children may become more sedentary, and capacity for prolonged physical work is reduced in adolescents and adults. Other nonspecific manifestations, especially among children, may include pallor, apathy, lack of liveliness, short attention span, and frequent episodes of diarrhea. Clinical laboratory tests are not helpful in diagnosing mild or moderate PEM.

Severe PEM. In addition to clinical features, dietary and clinical history are important for diagnosis. Marasmus is usually associated with severe food shortage, prolonged semistarvation, early weaning, or infrequent feeding of infants. Kwashiorkor is often associated with poor protein intake, late weaning, and present or recent episodes of acute diarrhea or measles. Chronic or recurrent diarrhea and infections are common features.

Marasmus. Generalized muscle wasting and absence of subcutaneous fat give patients with severe, nonedematous PEM a skin-and-bones appearance (Fig. 130–2). Marasmic patients frequently have 60% or less of the weight expected for their height, and children are markedly stunted. The hair is sparse, thin, and dry, without its normal sheen. The skin is dry and thin, with little elasticity, and it wrinkles easily. Patients are apathetic but usually aware and have a look of sadness or anxiety on their face. These features and the sunken cheeks caused by disappearance of subcutaneous fat give a marasmic child's face the appearance of a monkey's or an old person's face.

Some patients have no appetite, whereas others are ravenously hungry, but they seldom tolerate large amounts of food and they vomit easily. Weakness is marked, and children frequently cannot stand without help. Blood pressure and body temperature may be low, but tachycardia may be noted. Hypoglycemia can occur, especially after fasting for 6 or more hours, and is often accompanied by hypothermia of 35.5°C or less. The viscera are usually small. Abdominal distention may be present. The lymph nodes are easily palpable.

Common complicating features are acute gastroenteritis,

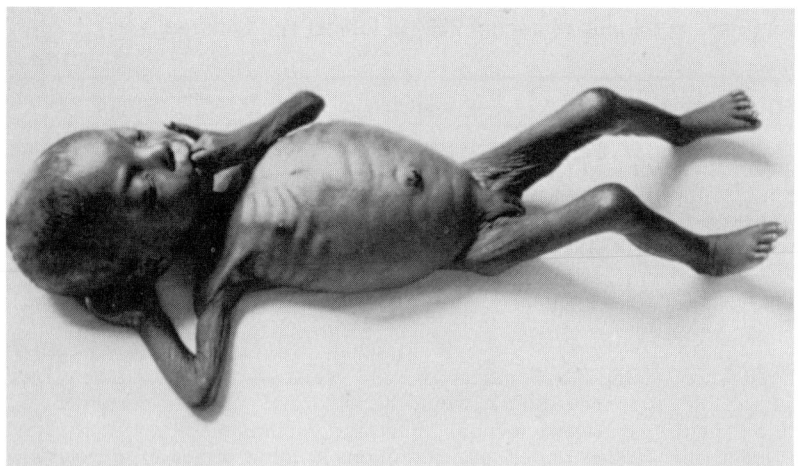

Figure **130–2.** Marasmus in a 5-month-old baby (West Indies). Note the generalized muscle wasting and absence of subcutaneous fat, the growth retardation, and the sparse hair.

dehydration, respiratory infections, and eye lesions due to hypovitaminosis A (Chapter 131.1). Systemic infections lead to septic shock or intravascular clotting with high mortality rates. Dietary history has an important role in the differential diagnosis from the secondary PEM of AIDS, tuberculosis, cancer, and other body-wasting diseases.

Kwashiorkor. The predominant feature is soft, pitting, painless edema, usually in the feet and legs but extending to the perineum, upper extremities, and face in severe cases (Fig. 130–3). Many patients have skin lesions, often confused with pellagra, in the areas of edema, continuous pressure (e.g., at the buttocks and back), or frequent irritation (e.g., in the perineum and thighs). The skin may be erythematous, and it glistens in the edematous regions with zones of dryness, hyperkeratosis, and hyperpigmentation, which tend to become confluent. The epidermis peels off in large scales, exposing underlying tissues that are easily infected. Subcutaneous fat is preserved, and there may be some muscle wasting. Weight deficit, after accounting for the weight of edema, is usually not as severe as in marasmus. Children may be stunted or of normal height, depending on the chronicity of the current episode and on past nutritional history.

Patients may be pale, with cold and cyanotic extremities. They are apathetic and irritable, cry easily, and have an expression of misery and sadness. Anorexia (sometimes necessitating nasogastric tube feeding), postprandial vomiting, and diarrhea are common. These conditions usually improve as nutritional recovery progresses, without specific gastrointestinal treatment. Hepatomegaly with a soft, round edge caused by severe fatty infiltration is often present. The abdomen is frequently protruding because of a distended stomach and intestinal loops. Peristalsis is irregular and frequently slow. Muscle tone and strength are greatly reduced. Tachycardia is common. Both hypothermia and hypoglycemia can occur after short periods of fasting.

The hair is dry, brittle, and without its normal sheen, and it can be pulled out easily without pain. Curly hair becomes straight, and the pigmentation usually changes to dull brown, red, or yellowish white. Alternating periods of poor and relatively good protein intake can produce bands of depigmented and normal hair, termed the *flag sign.*

The same complications occur as in marasmus, but diarrhea and respiratory and skin infections are more frequent and severe. Infections may occur without fever, tachycardia, respiratory distress, or leukocytosis. The most common causes of death are pulmonary edema with bronchopneumonia, septicemia, gastroenteritis, and water and electrolyte imbalances. Differential diagnosis must include other causes of

edema and hypoproteinemia and secondary PEM due to impairment in protein absorption or metabolism.

Marasmic Kwashiorkor. This form of edematous PEM combines clinical characteristics of kwashiorkor and marasmus. The main features are the edema of kwashiorkor, with or

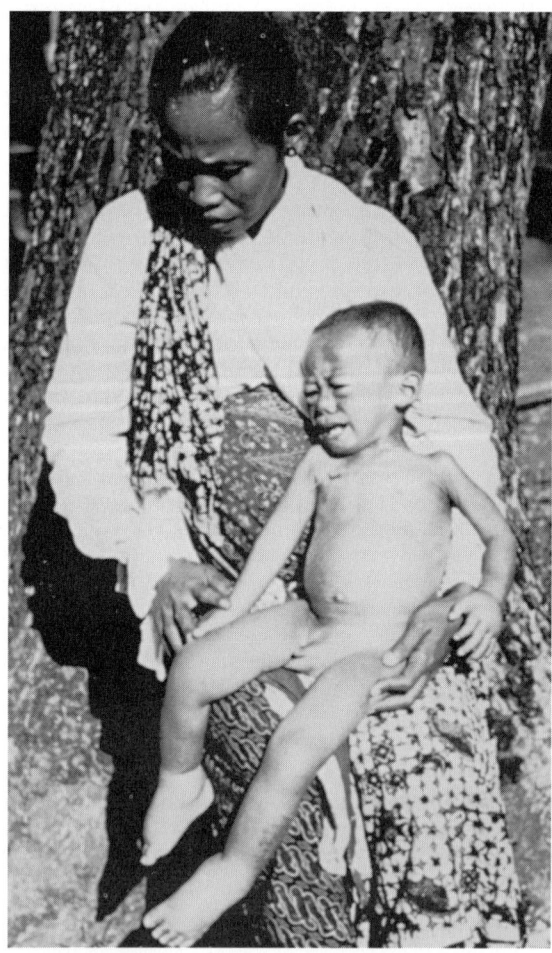

Figure **130–3.** Kwashiorkor in an 18-month-old child (Indonesia). Note the edema in the lower limbs, the wasted muscles with some subcutaneous fat present, the light sparse hair, the flaky dermatosis in the lower legs, and skin pallor (compared with mother). (Courtesy of the late Dr. H. A. P. C. Oomen.)

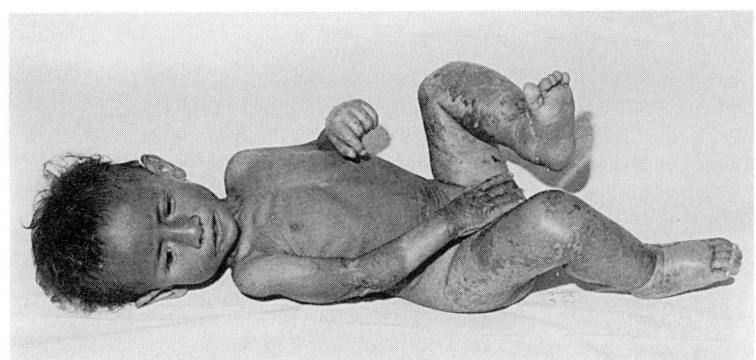

Figure 130–4. Marasmic kwashiorkor in a 22-month-old child (Guatemala). Note the edema in the lower part of the body, the emaciated upper part, the marked stunting, and the skin lesions. (From Torun B, Viteri FE: *In* Warren KS, Mahmoud AAF [eds]: Tropical and Geographic Medicine, 2nd ed. New York, McGraw-Hill, 1990.)

without its skin lesions, and the muscle wasting and decreased subcutaneous fat of marasmus (Fig. 130–4). When edema disappears during early treatment, the patient's appearance resembles that of marasmus. Biochemical features of both marasmus and kwashiorkor are seen, but the alterations of severe protein deficiency usually predominate.

BIOCHEMICAL AND HISTOPATHOLOGIC FEATURES OF SEVERE PEM. These allow better understanding of the pathophysiology but have little practical importance in diagnosing the disease. *Treatment of severe PEM must not be delayed while awaiting laboratory results.*

Biochemical Abnormalities. The most common biochemical findings are as follows: (1) Serum concentrations of total proteins, especially albumin, are markedly reduced in edematous PEM and normal or moderately low in marasmus. (2) Hemoglobin and hematocrit are usually low, more so in kwashiorkor than in marasmus. (3) The ratio of nonessential to essential amino acids in plasma is elevated in kwashiorkor and usually normal in marasmus. (4) Serum levels of free fatty acids are elevated, particularly in kwashiorkor. (5) Blood glucose level is normal, but it may be low after fasting 6 or more hours. (6) Urinary excretions of creatinine, hydroxyproline, 3-methylhistidine, and urea nitrogen are low. Edematous children have markedly reduced urinary creatinine excretion in relation to their height, leading to a low creatinine-height index, whereas marasmic children may have a normal or somewhat low index.

Plasma levels of other nutrients vary and tend to be moderately low. They do not necessarily reflect the body stores. For example, serum iron and retinol levels may be normal with almost depleted body stores, or in kwashiorkor they may be relatively low with adequate stores because of alterations in the transport proteins, transferrin, and retinol-binding protein.

Histopathologic Findings. Histopathologic studies show nonspecific atrophy, mainly in tissues with greater cell turnover rates, e.g., intestinal mucosa, red bone marrow, and testicular epithelium; intestinal villi are flattened, and enterocytes lose their columnar appearance. Marasmus is associated with generalized atrophy of skeletal muscle. The skin changes consist of dermal atrophy, ecchymosis, ulcerations, and hyperkeratotic desquamation, seen primarily in areas subjected to irritation and not necessarily restricted to exposed areas, as in the case of pellagra. The liver in patients with kwashiorkor is enlarged, with fatty infiltration; periportal fat appears first and advances centripetally as severity increases. Special staining techniques and electron microscopy reveal generalized tissue atrophy and other alterations that are not specific to primary PEM. Lesions due to superimposed infections and other nutrient deficiencies often are evident macroscopically and on histopathologic examination. These changes usually revert to normal with nutritional re-

covery, although some residual lesions may persist for some time.

PROGNOSIS AND RISK OF MORTALITY. Weight for height can be restored with adequate treatment, but children's catch-up growth in height may take a long time or might never be achieved. These children have been deprived not only of food but also of opportunities for development, and they may have missed the critical periods for harmonic physical, mental, and social maturation. Many severely malnourished children appear to have residual behavioral and mental problems in terms of creativity, learning ability, and social interaction. This can be partially a result of a poor living environment, however, and the damage may be corrected with adequate care and stimulation.

Mortality rates among children with severe PEM are associated with the quality of treatment. Worldwide, median case fatality has remained unchanged at 20 to 30% for the past 50 years, with levels as high as 40 to 60% among those with edematous PEM as a result of outmoded and faulty management. Low mortality is attainable with adequate treatment, and in some centers it is as low as 4 to 6% for both edematous and nonedematous forms. Table 130–3 lists the characteristics that generally indicate a poor prognosis and demand close surveillance.

TREATMENT

Severe PEM. Whenever possible, patients with uncomplicated PEM should be treated outside the hospital to avoid

TABLE 130–3. Characteristics That Indicate Poor Prognosis in Patients With PEM

· Age <6 months
· Deficit in weight for height >30%, or in weight for age >40%
· Signs of circulatory collapse: cold hands and feet, weak radial pulse, diminished consciousness
· Stupor, coma, or other alterations in awareness
· Infections, particularly bronchopneumonia or measles
· Petechiae or hemorrhagic tendencies (purpura is usually associated with septicemia or a viral infection)
· Dehydration and electrolyte disturbances, particularly hypokalemia, hypernatremia, and severe acidosis
· Persistent tachycardia, signs of heart failure or respiratory difficulty
· Total serum proteins <30 g/L
· Severe anemia (<4gHb/dL) or clinical signs of hypoxia
· Clinical jaundice or elevated serum bilirubin level
· Extensive exudative or exfoliative cutaneous lesions or deep decubitus ulcerations
· Hypoglycemia
· Hypothermia

From Torun B, Chew F: Protein-energy malnutrition. *In* Shils ME, Olson JA, Shike M (eds): Modern Nutrition in Health and Disease, 8th ed. Philadelphia, Lea & Febiger, 1994, p 966.

the risk of cross infections and of increased apathy and anorexia in children due to the unfamiliar setting. Severely malnourished patients with signs of a poor prognosis (Table 130–3) or other life-threatening complications and those who live under deplorable social conditions that do not permit adequate medical and nutritional treatment as outpatients must be hospitalized. Treatment of all forms of severe PEM is similar and consists of (1) resolving life-threatening conditions, (2) initial dietary treatment without disrupting homeostasis, and (3) ensuring full rehabilitation.

Resolving Life-threatening Conditions

FLUID AND ELECTROLYTE DISTURBANCES. Useful indicators of dehydration in severe PEM include a history of watery diarrhea or vomiting, thirst, low urinary output, weak and rapid pulse, low blood pressure, cool and moist extremities, and a declining state of consciousness. Sunken eyeballs and decreased skin turgor are frequently found in well-hydrated patients, whereas hypovolemia may coexist with subcutaneous edema. Treatment differs from that of well-nourished patients, because patients with severe PEM usually have hypo-osmolality with moderate hyponatremia; mild to moderate metabolic acidosis, which disappears when patients receive energy (calories) with the diet and oral or intravenous rehydration solutions; high tolerance to hypocalcemia; decreased body potassium without hypokalemia; and decreased body magnesium, with or without hypomagnesemia.

Whenever possible, oral or nasogastric rehydration should be used. Many clinicians report good results with the oral rehydration salts (ORS) promoted by WHO for children who are not severely malnourished (Chapter 16). Recent WHO recommendations for the management of severe malnutrition advocate the use of solutions that provide more potassium, magnesium, and, especially for edematous PEM, less sodium (30 to 60 instead of 90 mmol/L). A practical approach is the preparation of a mineral mix to complement the diet; this can be combined with WHO's regular ORS and sucrose to prepare a modified ORS solution for patients with severe PEM. Table 130–4 shows the composition of the mineral mix, and Table 130–5 shows the composition of the modified ORS prepared by diluting one standard WHO ORS packet, two 3.12-g packets of mineral mix (or 40 mL of concentrated mineral mix solution), and 50 g of sucrose in 2 L of water.

ORS solution should be given at a slower rate than for better-nourished children: 70 to 100 mL/kg body weight over a period of 12 hours, starting with about 10 mL/kg/hr dur-

TABLE 130–5. Composition of *Modified* Oral Rehydration Solution for Severely Malnourished Patients*

Component	Concentration (mmol/L†)
Glucose	125
Sodium	45
Potassium	40
Chloride	76
Citrate	7
Magnesium	3
Zinc	0.3
Copper	0.04
Osmolarity	300

*Prepared by diluting *one* standard WHO ORS packet, *two* 3.12-g packets of mineral mix (described in Table 130–4), and *50 g* sucrose in 2 L of water, as suggested in Briend A, Golden MHN: Treatment of severe child malnutrition in refugee camps. Eur J Clin Nutr 47:750, 1993.

†1 mmol glucose = 180 mg; 1 mmol Na = 23.0 mg; 1 mmol K = 39.1 mg; 1 mmol Cl = 35.5 mg; 1 mmol citrate = 207.1 mg; 1 mmol Mg = 24.3 mg; 1 mmol Zn = 65.4 mg; 1 mmol Cu = 63.5 mg.

ing the first 2 hours for children with mild to moderate dehydration and up to 30 mL/kg/hr for severe dehydration. An additional 50 to 100 mL ORS solution should be given after each loose stool to children <2 years old, and twice as much to older children. Breast-feeding must continue approximately every half hour. Patients must be evaluated every hour. When patients improve, usually 4 to 6 hours after beginning rehydration, small amounts of liquid dietary formula with potassium, calcium, magnesium, and other electrolytes should be offered every 2 to 3 hours. If signs of dehydration are still present after 12 hours but the condition is improving, another 70 to 100 mL ORS/kg can be given over the next 12 hours. Fluid repletion should allow a diuresis of at least 200 mL in 24 hours in children and 500 mL in adults, or micturition every 2 to 3 hours. When signs of overhydration occur, e.g., when the eyelids become puffy, edema increases, the jugular veins become full, or respiratory rate increases, only breast milk or liquid diet should be given instead of ORS.

Children who vomit frequently or cannot be fed orally must be rehydrated by nasogastric tube, giving ORS solution 3 to 4 mL/kg slowly or drop by drop every half hour. If vomiting persists or abdominal distention increases, ORS should be given at a slower rate. If hydration does not improve after 4 hours, intravenous solutions must be started. When vomiting ceases and hydration improves, ORS should be given by mouth. The nasogastric tube can be removed when the patient tolerates oral solutions for 2 hours.

Intravenous fluids must be used for patients with repeated vomiting or persistent abdominal distention and in severe dehydration with hypovolemia and impending shock. Hypo-osmolar solutions (200 to 280 mOsm/L) must be used. Potassium (when urinating) and sodium should not exceed 6 and 3 mmol/kg/day, respectively, and glucose must provide at least 63 to 126 KJ (15 to 30 kcal)/kg/day. Solutions that have been successfully used include a 1:1 mixture of 10% dextrose in water (D/W) either with isotonic saline (i.e., 5% glucose in 0.5 N saline) or with Darrow's solution; a 1:2:3 mixture of 0.17 sodium lactate-isotonic saline-10% D/W; or Hartmann's solution (lactated Ringer's solution). One of these should be infused during the first hour at a rate of 10 to 30 mL/kg, depending on the patient's condition. After that, 5% glucose in 0.2 N saline (800 mL of 5% D/W, 20 mL of 50% D/W, and 200 mL of isotonic saline), or a 1:2:6 mixture of lactate-isotonic saline-5% glucose, with 50 mL of 50% D/W added

TABLE 130–4. Mineral Mix for Preparation of Modified Oral Rehydration Salt (ORS) Solution and to Complement Liquid Foods

Salt	Amount (g)	mmol* in 1 g	mmol in 3.71 g
Potassium chloride	89.5	6.47 K	24 K
Tripotassium citrate	32.4	1.62 K	6 K
Magnesium chloride · 6H$_2$O	30.5	0.81 Mg^{+2}	3 Mg
Zinc acetate · 2H$_2$O	3.3	0.081 Zn^{+2}	0.300 Zn
Copper sulfate · 7H$_2$O	0.56	0.011 Cu^{+2}	0.040 Cu
Total	156.26†		

*1 mmol K = 39.1 mg; 1 mmol Mg = 24.3 mg; 1 mmol Zn = 65.4 mg; 1 mmol Cu = 63.5 mg.

†Divide the 156.26 g into 50 packets with 3.12 g of dry mineral mix, or dissolve 156.26 g in 1 L of water to prepare a concentrated mineral mix solution that can be stored at room temperature. Add one packet or 20 mL of the concentrated solution to each liter of modified ORS solution or of liquid food.

Based on suggestions in Briend A, Golden MHN: Treatment of severe child malnutrition in refugee camps. Eur J Clin Nutr 47:750, 1993.

to each 500 mL, should be infused at a rate of 5 to 10 mL/kg/hr, based on hourly evaluations of the patient, until oral therapy is initiated. When the patient is urinating, 2 g KCl (27 mmol K) is added to each liter of the infusion solution.

Patients with severe hypoproteinemia (<30 g/L), anuria, and signs of hypovolemia or impending circulatory collapse should be given plasma 10 mL/kg in 1 to 2 hours, followed by 20 mL/kg/hr of a mixture of two parts of 5% dextrose and one part of isotonic saline for 1 or 2 hours. This increases plasma protein concentration by about 5 to 10 g/L and helps prevent the rapid exit of water from the intravascular compartment. If diuresis does not improve, the dose of plasma can be repeated 2 hours later. Further treatment is similar to that of well-nourished patients. Unless the patient is at risk of imminent death, only plasma tested to be negative for human immunodeficiency virus (HIV), hepatitis B (HBV) and C (HCV) should be used.

Increases in pulse and respiratory rate with weight loss, low urine output, and continuing losses from diarrhea and vomiting suggest insufficient fluid therapy. Increases in pulse and respiratory rate with weight gain after accounting for weight of excreta, pulmonary rales, and appearance or exacerbation of edema indicate overhydration.

Hypocalcemia may occur secondary to magnesium deficiency. When a patient has symptoms of hypocalcemia and serum magnesium determinations are not available, it is essential to give not only Ca but also Mg IV or IM. When the symptoms of hypocalcemia disappear, calcium infusion may be discontinued. IM or PO Mg should follow the initial parenteral dosage. As a general therapeutic guideline, a 50% solution of magnesium sulfate can be given in doses of 0.5, 1, and 1.5 mL for patients who weigh <7, 7 to 10, and >10 kg, respectively. The dose can be repeated every 12 hours until there is no recurrence of the hypocalcemic symptoms or until laboratory analysis indicates maintenance of normal serum Mg concentration. Oral Mg supplementation can then continue at a dose of 0.25 to 0.5 mmol (0.5 to 1 mEq)/kg/day.

INFECTIONS. Infections are frequently the immediate cause of death in severe PEM (Chapter 133.1). Clinical manifestations may be mild, and the classic signs of fever, tachycardia, and leukocytosis may be absent. Antigen-antibody reactions are often impaired, and skin tests e.g., tuberculin, often give falsely negative results. Thus, when patients cannot be closely monitored by experienced personnel, it is safer to assume that all ill and severely malnourished patients have a bacterial infection and to treat them immediately with antibiotics, even before obtaining the results of microbiologic cultures, to cover both gram-positive and gram-negative microorganisms; the latter are particularly common in PEM. The choice of drug varies with the suspected etiologic agent, the severity of the disease, and the pattern of drug resistance in the area. When septicemia is suspected, a broad-spectrum antibiotic or a combination e.g., ampicillin and gentamicin is usually given IV. Other supportive treatment may also be necessary, e.g., treatment for respiratory distress, hypothermia, and hypoglycemia.

Drug metabolism may be altered and detoxification mechanisms may be compromised in severe PEM. To decrease the risks of potential toxicity, including the possibility of absorbing drugs normally not absorbed by a healthy intestine, treatment for intestinal parasites, which is rarely urgent, should be deferred until nutritional rehabilitation is under way.

Because of the high mortality rates associated with measles in severe PEM, patients should be vaccinated on the first day (Chapter 25.1). Because seroconversion may be impaired at this early stage of treatment, a second dose of vaccine should be given before discharge.

HEMODYNAMIC ALTERATIONS. Cardiac failure leading to pulmonary edema and frequent secondary pulmonary infection may develop when there is severe anemia, during or after administration of IV fluids, or shortly after the introduction of high-protein and high-energy feedings or of a diet with high sodium content. Diuretics should be given (e.g., furosemide 10 mg IV or IM, repeated as necessary), and other supportive measures should be taken. Many clinicians advocate the use of digoxin (0.03 mg/kg IV every 6 to 8 hours). *The use of diuretics merely to accelerate the disappearance of edema in kwashiorkor is contraindicated.*

SEVERE ANEMIA. Routine use of blood transfusions endangers patients. Hemoglobin levels improve with proper dietary treatment supplemented with hematinics (Chapter 6). Therefore, blood transfusions should be given only in cases of severe anemia with either <40 g hemoglobin/L, <12% packed cell volume (hematocrit), or clinical signs of hypoxia or impending cardiac failure. When there are no resources for screening the blood supply for HIV, HBV, or HCV, transfusion should be used only in life-threatening situations. Whole blood (10 mL/kg) can be used in marasmic patients, but it is better to use packed red blood cells (6 mL/kg) in edematous PEM. The transfusion should be given slowly, over 2 to 3 hours, and repeated if necessary after 12 to 24 hours. If there are signs of heart failure, 2.5 mL blood/kg should be withdrawn before the transfusion is started and at hourly intervals, so that the total volume of blood transfused equals the volume of anemic blood removed.

HYPOTHERMIA AND HYPOGLYCEMIA. Asymptomatic hypoglycemia can be prevented and treated by feeding small volumes of glucose- or sucrose-containing diets and solutions every 2 to 3 hours, day and night. Severe symptomatic hypoglycemia must be treated intravenously with 10 to 20 mL of 20% glucose solution followed by oral or nasogastric administration of 25 to 50 mL of 10% glucose solution at 2-hour intervals for 24 to 48 hours.

Body temperature usually rises in hypothermic patients given frequent feedings of glucose-containing diets or solutions. Patients must be closely monitored when external heat sources e.g., heavy clothing, heat lamps, and radiators are used to reduce the loss of body heat, because they may rapidly become hyperthermic. It is best to keep patients seminude in an ambient temperature of 30 to 33°C.

SEVERE VITAMIN A DEFICIENCY. A large dose of vitamin A should be given on admission, because severe PEM is often associated with vitamin A deficiency, and ocular lesions can develop as a result of increased demands for retinol when adequate protein and energy feeding begins (Chapter 131.1). Water-miscible retinol should be given PO or IM on the first day at a dose of 52 to 105 μmol (15,000 to 30,000 μg or 50,000 to 100,000 IU) for infants and preschool children, or 105 to 210 μmol (30,000 to 60,000 μg or 100,000 to 200,000 IU) for older children and adults, followed by 5.2 μmol (1500 μg or 5000 IU) PO each day for the duration of treatment. The initial dose should be repeated for 2 more days in symptomatic patients. Corneal ulcerations should be treated with ophthalmic drops of 1% atropine solution and antibiotic ointments or drops until the ulcerations heal.

Initial Dietary Treatment. As soon as the measures to manage the life-threatening conditions have been established, nutritional treatment must begin. This must be gradual and at a relatively slow pace, to avoid deleterious metabolic disruptions. The diet must initially provide energy (calories) and protein in amounts below or near daily maintenance requirements for 2 days, followed by gradual increments every 2 or 3 days, as described later. It is best to begin with a liquid formula fed orally or by nasogastric tube, divided equally into 6 to 12 feedings per day, depending on the patient's age and general condition. This frequent feeding of small volumes must be given around the clock to avoid fasting for more than 4 hours and to prevent vomiting, hypoglycemia, and hypothermia. For older children and adults with good appetites, the liquid formula can be partly substituted with solid foods that have a high concentration of good-quality, easily digestible nutrients. Intravenous alimentation is rarely justified in primary PEM and can increase mortality rates.

The same diet can be used to treat marasmic and edematous patients, although marasmic patients may require larger amounts of dietary energy after 1 or 2 weeks of dietary treatment. This can be provided by adding more oil or fat to the diet. Diets with as much as 60 to 75% of their energy from fats are usually well tolerated, even if they cause some degree of steatorrhea.

The protein source must be of high biologic value and easily digested. Cow's milk usually is well tolerated and assimilated by severely malnourished children, as are goat's, ewe's, buffalo's, and camel's milk. Human, mare's, and ass's milk, however, have low protein concentrations. Dried skimmed cow's milk has very low energy density, which must be restored by adding sugar and/or vegetable oil. The latter also provides essential fatty acids. Eggs, meat, fish, soy isolates, and some vegetable protein mixtures are also sources of good protein. Most vegetable mixtures have protein digestibility 10 to 20% lower than animal proteins, making it necessary to feed larger amounts. Their bulk might pose a problem in feeding small children.

The diet must be supplemented to provide daily about 5 to 8 mmol K and 0.5 to 1 mmol Mg (1 to 2 mEq)/kg of body weight, and 150 to 300 μmol Zn and 40 to 50 μmol Cu. Sodium content should be low, especially for patients with edematous PEM. This can be accomplished by adding to the diet appropriate amounts of a mineral mix, e.g., that shown in Table 130–4. Additional supplements should include daily doses of 5.2 μmol (1500 μg or 5000 IU) vitamin A, 1.2 mmol (0.3 mg) folic acid, and other vitamins and trace elements in the doses provided by most commercial preparations; these should be higher than the daily recommended allowances for well-nourished persons. Supplemental calcium to provide about 15 mmol (600 mg) daily should be given when nondairy diets are used. Administration of supplemental iron (1 to 2.1 mmol or 60 to 120 mg daily) should begin 1 week after starting dietary therapy. Earlier administration of iron will not elicit a hematologic response (Fig. 130–1), it might facilitate bacterial growth in the organism, and it might produce metabolic disturbances, according to the free-radical theory.

A practical dietary regimen that avoids the danger of initial excessive intakes of protein and energy by hungry patients is based on the preparation of a basic liquid food with high protein concentration and high energy density, as in the examples shown in Table 130–6. Delivery of proteins and energy is gradually increased using different concentrations of the basic food, as shown for infants and preschool children in Table 130–7. The addition of sugar compensates for the dilution of dietary energy. Vegetable oil is added at 5- to 7-day intervals to the diet of marasmic patients who are not gaining weight at an adequate rate (an average of at least 5 g/kg/day) by the second week. The liquid preparations must be limited in the first week to 100 mL/kg/day, offering additional water during or between feedings in order to provide at least 1 mL of total fluids per kilocalorie in the daily diet. After day 8, patients can be fed to satiety (ad libitum).

Another option, which is particularly useful for conditions of relief, consists of preparing a liquid formula from an industrially prepared food, usually based on cow's milk,

TABLE 130–6. Examples of High-Protein, High-Energy Liquid Foods that Provide 3 to 4 g Protein and 135 to 145 kcal/100 mL

Food Used as Protein Source	Amount (g or mL)	Cereal flour or sugar (g)*	Sugar (g)	Oil (mL)†	Water (mL)
Cow's milk, dried, whole	130	50	50	40	1000
Cow's milk, dried, skim	100	50	50	70	1000
Cow's, goat's, or camel's milk, fluid	1000	50	50	40	—
Buffalo's or ewe's (sheep's) milk, fluid	650	50	50	40	350
Yogurt (from cow's or goat's milk, whole)	1000	50	50	40	—
Eggs, soft- or hard-boiled, liquefied	300‡	—	200	60	750
Vegetable mix, flour§	140	—	100	55	1000
Commercial soy protein formulas, powder	250	—	—	10	1000

*First choice: precooked rice, corn, or other cereal flour or heat-popped ground rice. If not available, substitute with either 50 g sugar or 20 mL vegetable oil; this will diminish total protein concentration by about 0.5 g/100 mL.

†When cereal flour is used, one half the vegetable oil can be substituted with isoenergetic amounts of sugar, where 1 mL oil = 2.2 g sugar.

‡About 6 medium-sized chicken eggs.

§High-protein quality mix, such as Incaparina (developed by INCAP: 58% corn flour + 38% cottonseed flour + 4% mixture of vitamins, minerals, and lysine), which provides 1360 kJ (325 kcal) and 27.5 g protein per 100 g of dry flour.

cereal flour, sugar, oil, vitamins, and minerals, which initially provides about 1 g protein and 75 kcal (315 KJ)/100 mL. One week later, a more concentrated formulation is used to provide 2 to 2.5 g protein and 100 to 120 kcal (420 to 500 KJ). Tables 130–8 and 130–9 show options for preparation of equivalent formulas with locally available ingredients. Volumes are limited initially to 100 to 120 mL/kg/day for young children and gradually fed to satiety (ad libitum) when steady weight gain is established. Additional water is offered between feedings.

The liquid diets described for infants and young children can be given to older children and adults, especially to weak, anorexic, and elderly patients. However, adolescents and adults are often reluctant to eat anything other than habitual foods, and liquid diets must be prescribed as a medicine rather than as a food. When appetite improves, a diet based on nutritious traditional foods should be given but with added sugar and oil to increase energy density, plus vitamins and minerals; the liquid diet should be given between meals and at night. A wide variety of foods should be provided in amounts to satisfy appetite, taking into account the patient's inclinations and taboos.

Treatment must initially satisfy average energy and protein requirements, adjusted for age and sex (about 45 kcal and 0.75 g protein/kg/day for adolescents, and 35 to 40 kcal and 0.6 g protein/kg/day for adults), followed by a gradual increase to about 1.5 times the energy and 3 to 4 times the protein requirements by the seventh day. Minerals and vitamins must be provided in amounts at least twice greater

TABLE 130–7. Example of a Dietary Therapeutic Regimen for Children (based on gradually decreasing dilutions of the high-protein, high-energy liquid foods shown in Table 130–6*)

Days from Beginning of Treatment	Proportions of Foods Shown in Table 130–6 + Water		Additional Sugar (g/100 mL)	Additional Oil (mL/100 mL)	Food Volume per Meal (mL/kg/meal)		100 mL Provides	
	Proportions	Volume (mL)			Every 2 hr	Every 3 hr	Protein (g)	Energy (kcal)
1–2	1 + 2	33 + 67	10	—	8.3	12.5	1–1.3	75–85
3–4	1 + 1	50 + 50	10	—	8.3	12.5	1.5–2	105–115
5–6	3 + 1	75 + 25	5	—	8.3	12.5	2.3–3	120–130
7–8	Undiluted	100 + 0	—	—	8.3	12.5	3–4	135–145
For Marasmic Patients Without Adequate Weight Gain†								
13–17	Undiluted	100 + 0	—	2.5	ad libitum		3–4	160–170
18–22	Undiluted	100 + 0	—	5	ad libitum		3–4	185–195
23–27	Undiluted	100 + 0	—	7.5	ad libitum		3–4	210–220
28–32, etc.	Undiluted	100 + 0	—	10, etc.	ad libitum		3–4	235, etc.

*Formulas should initially be fed at a volume of 100 mL/kg/day. They must be supplemented by appropriate amounts of vitamins, minerals, and electrolytes or by adding to each liter of diet 20 mL (or one packet) of the mineral mix in Table 130–4 and a vitamin mix. After 8 days, the undiluted formula can be fed to satiety (ad libitum). **Additional water must be given** after or between feedings, to provide each day at least 1 mL of total fluids/kcal in the diet.
†Marasmic patients may require more dietary energy when weight gain is <5 g/kg/day. Half a teaspoonful (2.5 mL) of vegetable oil should be added for every 100 mL of liquid diet at 5-day intervals.

than the recommended daily allowances, following the same schedule as for young children. Except for pregnant women, a single dose of 210 μmol (60,000 μg or 200,000 IU) retinol should be given.

The attitude of the person who feeds the patient is important in overcoming the lack of appetite. Patience and loving care are needed to gently coax a child to eat all the diet. The appearance, color, and flavor of the foods also have a role in appetite and food acceptance. An adequate response to the diet results in disappearance of clinical signs of severe PEM accompanied or followed by weight gain, which in children can be at a rate 8 to 15 (or as high as 25) times that of a normal child of the same age. Some patients show only a fourfold or fivefold increase in catch-up. This is most often associated with insufficient energy intakes (e.g., because of inadequately prepared formula, insufficient amounts of formula given at each feeding, too few feedings per day, anorexia, or lack of patience shown by the person who feeds the child) or with overt or asymptomatic infections; urinary infections and tuberculosis are the most commonly seen asymptomatic diseases.

Ensuring Full Rehabilitation. This last stage of treatment begins when a patient is without serious complications, eating satisfactorily and gaining weight, usually 2 to 3 weeks after admission. It may start in the hospital and continue on an outpatient basis, preferably at a nutrition rehabilitation center or similar facility that gives daytime care. When there is no such facility, the hospital must continue to provide care until a patient is ready for discharge. The importance of continuing the high-energy, high-protein diet until full recov-

TABLE 130–8. Examples of Formulas to Prepare 1 L of a Liquid Food to Provide Around 75 kcal and 1.3 g Protein/100 mL During the First Week of Initial Dietary Treatment

Food Used as Protein Source	Amount (g or mL)	Cereal Flour (e.g., rice, corn) g*	Sugar (g)	Oil (mL)	Water (mL)	Mineral Mix (mL)†	Vitamin Mix (mg)‡
Cow's milk, dried, whole	35	50	50	20	1000	20	150
Cow's milk, dried, skim§	25	50	50	30	1000	20	150
Cow's, goat's, or camel's milk, fluid	250	50	50	20	750	20	150
Buffalo's or ewe's (sheep's) milk, fluid	175	50	50	20	825	20	150
Yogurt (from cow's or goat's milk, whole)	275	50	50	20	725	20	150
Eggs, soft- or hard-boiled, liquefied	100‖	—	100	20	950	20	150
Vegetable mix, flour¶	50	—	100	20	1000	20	150
Commercial soy protein formulas, powder	85	—	50	10	1000	20	150

*If precooked flour and heat-popped ground rice are not available, add 50% more of the food protein source (for example, 52 g instead of 35 g of whole dried milk) plus an additional 25 g sugar *or* 10 mL vegetable oil; when more fluid milk or yogurt is used, the volume of additional water must be reduced by the same amount to make a total volume of 1000 mL.
†See Table 130–4.
‡Can be substituted for with a commercial multivitamin product at the dosage recommended by the manufacturer.
§Similar to the F-75 formula in WHO *Manual for the Management of Severe Malnutrition.* Geneva, World Health Organization. In press.
‖About 2 medium-sized chicken eggs.
¶High-protein quality mix, such as Incaparina (developed by INCAP: 58% corn flour + 38% cottonseed flour + 4% mixture of vitamins, minerals, and lysine), which provides 1360 kJ (325 kcal) and 27.5 g protein per 100 g of dry flour.

TABLE 130–9. Examples of Formulas to Prepare 1 L of a Liquid Food to Provide Around 100 kcal and 2.8 g Protein/100 mL After the First Week of Dietary Treatment

Food Used as Protein Source	Amount (g or mL)	Cereal Flour (e.g., rice, corn) g*	Sugar (g)	Oil (mL)	Water (mL)	Mineral Mix (mL)†	Vitamin Mix (mg‡
Cow's milk, dried, whole	90	50	50	20	20	150	1000
Cow's milk, dried, skim§	70	50	50	40	20	150	1000
Cow's, goat's, or camel's milk, fluid	700	50	50	20	20	150	300
Buffalo's or ewe's (sheep's) milk, fluid	450	50	50	20	20	150	550
Yogurt (from cow's or goat's milk, whole)	800	50	50	15	20	150	200
Eggs, soft- or hard-boiled, liquefied	250‖	—	100	25	20	150	800
Vegetable mix, flour¶	100	—	100	30	20	150	1000
Commercial soy protein formulas, powder	190	—	—	—	20	150	1000

*If precooked flour and heat-popped ground rice are not available, add 20% more of the food protein source (for example, 108 g instead of 90 g of whole dried milk) plus an additional 25 g sugar *or* 10 mL vegetable oil; when more fluid milk or yogurt is used, the volume of additional water must be reduced by the same amount to make a total volume of 1000 mL.

†See Table 130–4. All formulas satisfy calcium requirements, except for the egg-based preparations.

‡Can be substituted with a commercial multivitamin product at the dosage recommended by the manufacturer.

§Similar to the F-100 formula in WHO *Manual for the Management of Severe Malnutrition.* Geneva, World Health Organization. In press.

‖About 5 medium-sized chicken eggs.

¶High-protein quality mix, such as Incaparina (developed by INCAP: 58% corn flour + 38% cottonseed flour + 4% mixture of vitamins, minerals, and lysine), which provides 1360 kJ (325 kcal) and 27.5 g protein/100 g dry flour.

ery has taken place must be clearly explained to the child's mother or caretaker. If this can be done at home, the patient can continue treatment there with regular follow-up in a nutrition clinic or its equivalent or with home visits by trained personnel.

INTRODUCTION OF TRADITIONAL FOODS. When edema has disappeared, the skin lesions are notably improved, patients become active and interact with the environment, appetite is restored, and adequate rates of catch-up growth have been achieved, other foods, especially those available at home, are gradually introduced into the diet in addition to the high-energy, high-protein formula. For children, a daily minimum intake of 3 to 4 g of protein and 500 to 625 KJ (120 to 150 kcal)/kg of body weight (or more in marasmus) must be ensured. To achieve this, the energy density of solid foods must be increased with oil, and protein concentration and quality must be high, using animal proteins, soybean protein preparations, and appropriate vegetable protein mixtures. For example, (1) one part of a dry pulse or its flour (e.g., black beans, soybeans, kidney beans, cowpeas) may be combined with three parts of a dry cereal or flour (e.g., corn, rice, wheat); fat or oil should be added to the mashed or strained pulse during or after cooking in amounts equal to the weight of the dry pulse or flour, and to the cereal preparations in amounts of 10 to 30 mL oil per 100 g dry cereal product, depending on the type of preparation. (2) Four parts of dry rice may be combined with one part of fresh or dry fish; fat or oil should be added in amounts equal to 20 to 40% of the dry weights. The food can be served as separate dishes, or the parts can be mashed or blended and fed as paps to infants and young children. The diet must be supplemented with minerals and vitamins as described for the initial dietary treatment until full nutritional rehabilitation is achieved.

EMOTIONAL AND PHYSICAL STIMULATION. Malnourished children need affection and tender care from the beginning of treatment. This requires patience and understanding by the hospital staff and the relatives. Involvement of parents or relatives must be encouraged. Hospital wards should be brightly colored and cheerful, preferably with music. As soon

as children can move without assistance and are willing to interact with the staff and other children, they must be encouraged to explore, to play, and to participate in activities that involve body movements. Relatively small increments in physical activity through active play during the course of nutritional rehabilitation result in faster linear (height) growth and accretion of lean body tissues. Parents should be encouraged to stimulate and teach their children by playing and talking. Toys and play materials can often be made from discarded local articles.

Adult patients should exercise regularly, with gradual increments in cardiorespiratory workload.

TREATMENT OF DIARRHEA AND OTHER HEALTH PROBLEMS. Mild diarrhea often disappears without specific treatment as nutritional status improves. However, persistent or recurrent diarrhea can contribute to the development of a new episode of PEM. Treatment is determined by the underlying cause of diarrhea, usually repeated intestinal infections, excessive bacterial flora in the upper gut that ferment food substrates and deconjugate bile salts, intestinal parasites (particularly giardiasis, cryptosporidiosis, and trichiuriasis), and intolerance to food components (Chapter 133.2). The apparent high prevalence of lactose malabsorption and intolerance in PEM is often founded on inadequate diagnostic procedures. When intolerance to milk or other food is suspected, the diet should be modified, taking care to preserve its nutritional quality and density. Before branding a patient intolerant to a given food, the food should be reintroduced into the diet and adequate diagnostic tests should be performed to confirm the diagnosis.

Other minor complications, e.g., intestinal parasites, must be treated. Children should be vaccinated against infectious diseases.

CRITERIA FOR RECOVERY. Premature termination of treatment increases the risk of a recurrence of malnutrition. The most practical criterion for recovery is catch-up in weight, and almost all fully recovered patients should reach the weight expected for their height or a normal BMI. Repletion of body protein is best assessed through body composition indices, e.g., the creatinine-height index, which in children requires urine collection for 48 to 72 hours. When body composition cannot be assessed, as a general guideline dietary therapy should continue for 1 month after the patient reaches a normal weight (Tables 130–1 and 130–2) without clinical signs of edematous PEM, or for 15 days after the marasmic patient reaches that weight. Some patients, however, apparently remain underweight because they are in the lower end of the normal distribution curves of weight for height or BMI. If they continue growing at a normal rate and have no functional impairments, treatment can be terminated after 1 month of adequate dietary intake and weight gain (or, in adults, weight stabilization). Specific treatment of other nutritional problems (e.g., iron deficiency) sometimes must be prolonged beyond discharge for PEM.

Before being discharged, patients or their parents must be taught about the causes of PEM, emphasizing rational and nutritious use of household foods, personal and environmental hygiene, appropriate immunizations, and early treatment—including dietary management—of diarrhea and other diseases.

MILD AND MODERATE PEM. Ambulatory treatment must be provided, supplementing the home diet with easily digested foods that contain proteins of high biologic value, a high energy density, and adequate amounts of micronutrients. In some instances, nutritional rehabilitation is achieved merely by instructing mothers in improved child-feeding practices and in more nutritious culinary habits or by instructing adult patients about adequate eating habits and better use of food resources. In most instances, however, it is necessary to provide both nutritious food supplements and instructions for their use.

As a general guideline, patients should have an intake of at least twice the protein and 1.5 times the energy requirements. For preschool children, this would signify a daily intake of about 2 to 2.5 g of high-quality protein and 500 to 625 KJ (120 to 150 kcal)/kg of body weight, and for infants <1 year, about 3.5 g protein and 625 KJ (150 kcal)/kg/day.

This is more likely to be achieved if the diet is appetizing to both the child and the mother, if it is ready made or easy to prepare, if enough is available or provided to feed other children in the same household, and if donated food has no important commercial value outside the home that would make it easy and profitable for the family to sell the item for cash. A substitution effect on the home diet (i.e., a decrease in the usual food intake) is almost always unavoidable, but it can be reduced by using low-bulk supplements with high protein and energy concentrations. Special attention should be given to avoid a decrease in breast-feeding. The supplements for breast-fed infants should be paps or solid foods that do not quench an infant's thirst and thus do not change an infant's demand for nursing or a mother's attitude toward lactation.

Adequate amounts of vitamins and minerals must be provided, although mild deficiencies can be overcome by the micronutrients in the food or by use of fortified vehicles, such as bread enriched with iron or sugar fortified with retinol.

PREVENTION AND CONTROL. Special attention must be given to the availability and rational use of nutritious foods, the control and reduction of infections, and health and nutrition education programs for the individual, the family, and the community. The physician, nutritionist, public health worker, and educator can and must have an active role. However, at a national or regional level, control and prevention of PEM can be achieved only through short- and long-term political commitments and effective actions to eradicate the underlying causes of malnutrition.

When limited resources allow attention to only those more susceptible to PEM, a profile of risk factors is useful. The most likely victims are children <2 years of age and from low socioeconomic strata, whose parents have misconceptions about the use of foods, who come from broken or unstable families, whose families have a high prevalence of alcoholism, who live under poor sanitary conditions in urban slums or in rural areas frequently subject to droughts or floods, and whose societal beliefs prohibit the use of many nutritious foods.

The presence of a malnourished child in a family indicates something amiss in that household and suggests that other members might also be at risk of PEM. Therefore, nutritional and health education must not be restricted to rehabilitation of the index case but should include prevention of nutritional deterioration of other family members, especially siblings and pregnant and lactating women. Similarly, a high prevalence of children with malnutrition or growth retardation indicates that the entire community is at some risk of impaired nutrition. Consequently, education programs must be devised for community leaders, civic action groups, and the community as a whole. Such programs must emphasize promotion of breast-feeding, appropriate use of weaning foods, nutritional alternatives using traditional foods, personal and environmental hygiene, feeding practices during illness and convalescence, and early treatment of diarrhea and other diseases. Personal and communal involvement should be pursued through commitments to apply the recommendations. Toward this aim, it is important that all educational programs incorporate the community's own assessment of their nutritional deficiencies and their feelings toward personal participation in solving these problems.

Bibliography

Briend A, Golden MHN: Treatment of severe child malnutrition in refugee camps. Eur J Clin Nutr 47:750, 1993.

De Onis M, Monteiro C, Akre J, Clugston G: The worldwide magnitude of protein-energy malnutrition: An overview from the WHO Global Database on Child Growth. Bull World Health Organ 71:703, 1993.

Dewey KG, Beaton G, Fjeld C, et al: Protein requirements of infants and children. Eur J Clin Nutr 50(Suppl 1):S119, 1996.

Nabarro D, McNab S: A simple new technique for identifying thin children: A description of a wallchart which enables minimally trained health workers to identify children who are so thin, or wasted, that they require immediate nutritional help. J Trop Med Hyg 83:21, 1980.

Pelletier DL, Frongillo EA, Schroeder DG, Habicht JP: The effects of malnutrition on child mortality in developing countries. Bull World Health Organ 73:443–448, 1995.

Schofield C, Ashworth A: Why have mortality rates for severe malnutrition remained so high? Bull World Health Organ 74:223, 1996.

Suskind RM, Lewinter-Suskind L (eds): The Malnourished Child. Nestlé Nutrition Workshop Series, Vol 19. New York, Raven Press, 1990.

Torun B: Short and long-term effects of low or restricted energy intakes on the activity of infants and children. In Schurch B, Scrimshaw NS (eds): Activity, Energy Expenditure and Energy Requirements of Infants and Children. Lausanne, International Dietary Energy Consultancy Group, 1990, pp 335–359.

Torun B: Influence of malnutrition on physical activity of children and adults. In Wahlqvist ML, Truswell AS, Smith R, Nestel PJ (eds): Nutrition in a Sustainable Environment. Proceedings of the XV International Congress of Nutrition. London, Smith-Gordon & Co, 1994, pp 651–654.

Torun B, Davies PSW, Livingstone MBE, et al: Energy requirements and dietary energy recommendations for children and adolescents 1 to 18 years old. Eur J Clin Nutr 50(Suppl 1):S37, 1996.

Torun B, Viteri FE: Influence of exercise on linear growth. Eur J Clin Nutr 48(Suppl 1):S186, 1994.

Ulijaszek SJ, Allen LH, Prentice A, et al: Malnutrition, growth retardation and stunting. In Westerterp-Plantenga MS, Fredrix EWHM (eds): Food and the Human Condition. Heerlen, The Netherlands, Open Universiteit, 1994, pp 19–53.

Viteri FE, Alvarado J: The creatinine height index: Its use in the estimation of the degree of protein depletion and repletion in protein calorie malnourished children. Pediatrics 46:696, 1970.

Waterlow JC. Protein Energy Malnutrition. London, Edward Arnold, 1992.

World Health Organization (WHO): Physical Status: The Use and Interpretation of Anthropometry. World Health Organ Tech Rep Ser 854:452, 1995.
WHO: Management of the Child with Severe Malnutrition: A Manual for Physicians and Other Senior Health Workers. Geneva, World Health Organization (In press).

131 Vitamin Deficiencies

131.1 Vitamin A Deficiency and Xerophthalmia

Alfred Sommer

DEFINITION. Vitamin A deficiency affects a wide variety of bodily functions. The most obvious and dramatic involve the eye (xerophthalmia). Other, earlier effects include pronounced interference in systemic functions, particularly the ability to contain infectious diseases, especially diarrhea and measles, resulting in increased case severity, morbidity, and mortality. By definition, vitamin A deficiency exists when there is inadequate vitamin A available to target tissues. There are no practical methods to detect directly this deficit, although a variety of surrogates, primarily serum retinol and/or its variants, is an adequate index, particularly on a population level. In general, in the absence of an infectious disease (since acute-phase reactants affect serum levels), retinol levels above 20 μg/dL are considered "normal," although higher levels, 30 μg/dL or greater, are compatible with milder forms of xerophthalmia and systemic consequences (e.g., iron deficiency anemia and childhood mortality).

ETIOLOGY
Sources and Functions. Vitamin A (retinol) is a lipid-soluble essential micronutrient required for a wide variety of important bodily functions. Its most important effects are on cellular differentiation, whether resulting in development of mucous-secreting epithelium (e.g., covering the eye, lining the respiratory and genitourinary tracts) or the immune system. Vitamin A is available from the diet as the preformed vitamin (retinyl ester) or from provitamin A carotenoids (vegetable and plant sources), which are converted in the gut to vitamin A. The vitamin is stored in the liver, which has 90% of the body's stores. It is transported through the blood stream, tightly bound to retinol-binding protein (RBP), to target tissues. Cellular receptors bind the vitamin A–RBP complex, incorporating the retinol into the cell, where it is metabolized to its active form, retinoic acid, which binds to nuclear receptors, regulating gene expression. Another role for vitamin A metabolism is clinically relevant: as an essential component of visual pigments involved in vision, particularly under low levels of illumination.

Risk Factors for Deficiency. Vitamin A deficiency arises primarily from an imbalance between dietary intake and metabolic need. Metabolic needs are increased during growth, infectious diseases, and pregnancy, the latter two helping to explain the higher prevalence of deficiency in developing countries.

The most important determinant is dietary intake, and it is here where differences between developed and developing countries are most apparent. In developed countries, most dietary intake is of the preformed vitamin, either from artifi-cially fortified dietary constituents or from animal food products (e.g., milk and other dairy products, egg yolks, liver and liver oils). By contrast, people in developing countries, particularly children, generally lack access to the preformed vitamin, often receiving vitamin A–depleted skim milk formulas (the nonfortified product loses its lipid-soluble vitamin A when the lipid is skimmed off). Instead, they depend on vegetable sources of provitamin A–rich carotenoids (red palm oil, colored fruits [e.g., mango and papaya], and dark green leafy vegetables). Pure β-carotene is readily converted to vitamin A. Dietary sources, however, bind β-carotene closely, making conversion inefficient. Recent studies in Indonesia and elsewhere suggest that pure dark green leafy vegetables and similar products have a conversion rate of only 5% to 15%, even when cooked and sieved. Given the constraints on busy mothers, the low levels of conversion, and the dislike of dark green, leafy vegetables by young children, it is surprising that vitamin A deficiency is not even more severe and widespread.

Requirements. Vitamin A requirements, largely extrapolated from the needs of healthy adults, are 300 retinol equivalents (RE) daily for infants, and 750 RE for adults. One RE is equivalent to 1 μg of retinol and to 6 μg of β-carotene; however, in most instances the equivalent amount of dietary carotene should be considerably higher. Poor children in developing countries having intestinal parasites and other frequent, chronic, and endemic infections have an increased requirement for vitamin A.

EPIDEMIOLOGY. Clinically significant vitamin A deficiency is only rarely encountered in wealthier, Western countries, where it is largely confined to individuals on highly restricted diets, or with end-stage liver disease or severe malabsorption syndrome (e.g., cystic fibrosis).

The great magnitude of disease occurs among children, and to a lesser degree, pregnant women in poor, often tropical countries. Although the number of children with marginal deficiency is unknown, an estimated 5 to 10 million children develop xerophthalmia, while half a million go blind from the condition every year. One to 3 million children die from the deficiency annually. The problem is sufficiently widespread that over 60 countries recognize the existence of vitamin A deficiency as a public health problem and have launched, or planned, large-scale, population-wide control programs.

Deficiency is most widespread and severe in young children, particularly those who did not benefit from prolonged breast-feeding (the best early dietary source of vitamin A and a practice that reduces the risk of infection). Young children, particularly those between 1 and 4 years of age, are also at increased risk because of their limited dietary choices and high rates of childhood infection. Childhood exanthemous diseases can have a particularly dramatic impact on vitamin A status.

Vitamin A deficiency is characterized by "clustering." Children (and mothers) living in the vicinity of a case of xerophthalmia are far more likely to be deficient than those living in a more distant family or compound. Presumably this reflects communal dietary practices and hygiene, and shared risks of protein malnutrition and infection. As children grow older, their dietary tastes change, they forage more widely, and they are at lower intrinsic risk of infectious morbidity and mortality. Most recognized clinical diseases (and deficiency) exist in south and Southeast Asia (India, Indonesia, Pakistan, Bangladesh, Thailand, Philippines) and most of Africa.

PATHOPHYSIOLOGY
Causes for Deficiency. Prolonged vitamin A intake inadequate to meet bodily demands eventually leads to a decline in liver stores, followed by a fall in serum levels, and finally

to inadequate delivery of the vitamin to its target cells. It is important to remember that many factors affect each link in this chain of events. Dietary intake, particularly its quantity and constituents, probably plays the paramount role. However, intestinal worm infections and diarrhea reduce absorption of the vitamin; hepatitis and cirrhosis reduce ability to store the vitamin in the liver, where 90% of the body's vitamin A is stored; protein malnutrition and liver disease reduce production of RBP, precluding release of biologically active holo-RBP from the liver for transport to target cells; and systemic infection and inflammation dramatically increases metabolic demands for vitamin A. For example, respiratory infections result in a massive outpouring of vitamin A in the urine. Measles, by raising metabolic rates, reducing food intake (stomatitis and anorexia), and causing desquamation of epithelial cells, can result in either acute decompensation in a child with previously unrecognized borderline deficiency, or begin the vicious downhill course ("the infection-malnutrition" spiral) which results, 1 to 3 months later, in vitamin A–related mortality or blindness.

Similarly, it's not yet clear the degree to which cellular versus humoral immunity impact on infectious morbidity and mortality in vitamin A deficiency, but both seem to be affected by vitamin A status. Nor is it known the degree to which bodily linings (normally composed of mucous or ciliary-mucous membranes) have their barrier resistance to overwhelming sepsis compromised by squamous metaplasia.

CLINICAL MANIFESTATIONS. Because of its dramatic, classic appearance, ocular changes (xerophthalmia) have, until recently, dominated clinical thinking. In fact, vitamin A deficiency results in profound, but unnoticed systemic effects long before the incident ocular manifestations appear (Fig. 131–1).

Systemic Effects of Vitamin A Deficiency

Infections. The most profound systemic effects represent the way in which the body deals with infection, particularly with measles and diarrhea. Although the exact mechanisms await delineation, it appears that vitamin A status has little impact on the incidence of infection but enormous influence on its severity. Studies in Ghana designed specifically for this purpose demonstrated that mildly deficient children supplemented periodically with large-dose vitamin A were far less

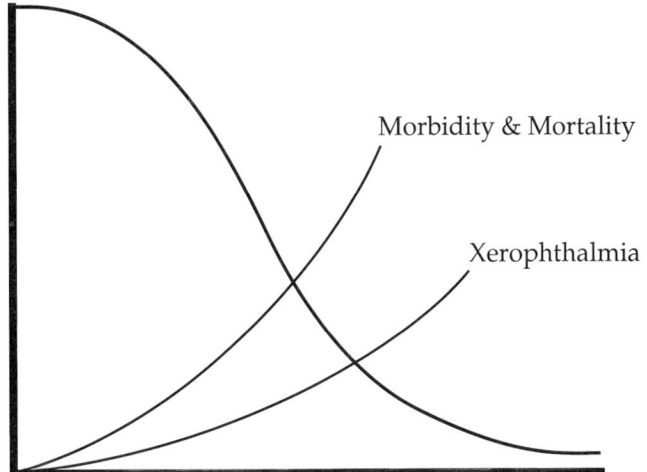

Figure 131–1. As vitamin A status declines, systemic consequences (infectious morbidity and mortality, anemia, and potentially other consequences) begin to rise before ocular signs and symptoms of xerophthalmia become evident.

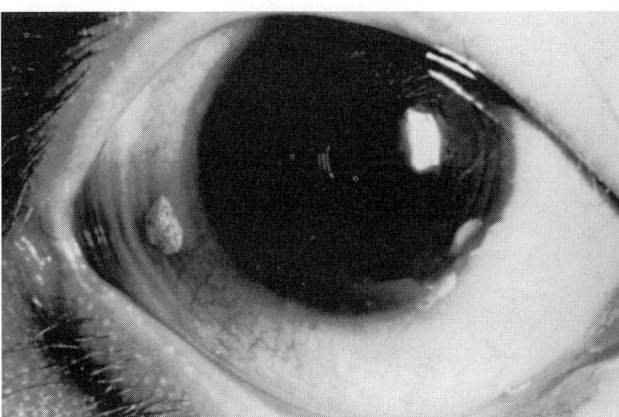

Figure 131–2. Temporal Bitot's spot (X1B). (From Sommer A: Field Guide to Detection and Control of Xerophthalmia. Geneva, World Health Organization, 1978.)

likely to require clinic visits or hospitalization for "all causes," and had far less severe and sustained diarrhea.

Studies in London (1932), Tanzania (1987), and South Africa (1990) all demonstrate that administration of high-dose vitamin A after onset of severe measles reduces case fatality by 50%, as well as reducing the severity of secondary complications (particularly tracheobronchopulmonary disease). Subsequent studies indicate that vitamin A–supplemented children have a significantly higher antimeasles antibody response, validating earlier studies in Indonesia, which indicated that vitamin A deficiency dampens immune competence. Although we do not yet know all types of infections affected by vitamin A status, eight large controlled clinical trials indicate that supplemental administration of preformed vitamin A (from fortifying a common condiment) to weekly doses equivalent to seven required dietary allowances (RDA) or larger doses (100,000 to 200,000 IU, depending on age) once every 4 to 6 months reduced overall preschool childhood mortality by one third or more.

Anemia and Growth. Several well-designed studies have also demonstrated that vitamin A status plays a significant role in iron metabolism, and can contribute to iron deficiency anemia. Other aspects of vitamin A status and health and disease are tangible but less definite: growth, other forms of infection, and vertical transmission of human immunodeficiency virus from mother to child.

Ocular (Xerophthalmia) Effects of Vitamin A Deficiency. The first, clinically apparent ocular change is nightblindness (XN), a symptom often readily elicited from a parent or guardian using a locally appropriate term. This represents an inadequate supply of vitamin A to form normal levels of rhodopsin. The first clinical sign, usually indicating more severe deficiency, is a Bitot spot (X1B) (Fig. 131–2), a manifestation of keratinizing metaplasia of the entire conjunctiva (X1A) magnified, by local production, of diphtheroid bacteria. These first appear temporal to the cornea but with increasing deficiency can spread nasally. Temporal lesions often persist for years despite vitamin A therapy. More severe deficiency leads to keratinization of the corneal surface (corneal xerosis, X2). This and all previous complications are entirely reversible with vitamin A treatment, leaving no significant sequelae.

With more severe deficiency (serum retinol almost invariably falls below 15 µg/dL), corneal necrosis begins, first as one or more localized ulcers (X3A) (Fig. 131–3), which if promptly treated with systemic vitamin A, can resolve to relatively small peripheral scars, thereby preserving the vi-

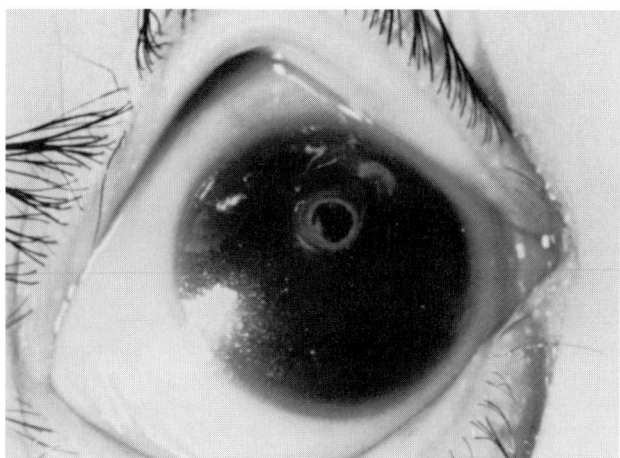

Figure **131–3.** Typical xerophthalmic ulcer (X3A). (From Sommer A, Sugana T: Corneal xerophthalmia and keratomalacia. Arch Ophthalmol 100:404, 1982.)

sual axis. Alternatively, if untreated they can spread rapidly, resulting in localized or limbus-to-limbus corneal necrosis (X3B) (Fig. 131–4). Localized necroses can, if quickly and appropriately treated, result in a large, localized scar. Limbal-to-limbal necrosis (keratomalacia) invariably leads to loss of the eye. Even in these severe instances, however, prompt, massive vitamin A therapy is indicated. The opposite eye, often less severely affected, may yet be saved, as might the child's life. Many children presenting with X3 disease suffer severe, accompanying systemic disturbances (e.g., pneumonia, tuberculosis, severe diarrhea, dehydration, and protein energy malnutrition). Vitamin A alone, however, if promptly administered, can often make the difference between life and death, sight and blindness.

Although the severity of ocular manifestations reflects the severity of vitamin A deficiency, children do not necessarily proceed systematically from one manifestation to another. In some instances, measles being the outstanding example, children with "borderline" vitamin A status (at least as it relates to xerophthalmia) may present with corneal ulcers or keratomalacia without prior evidence of nightblindness or Bitot spots. In most instances, this reflects severe, acute decompensation of their vitamin A status brought on by mea-

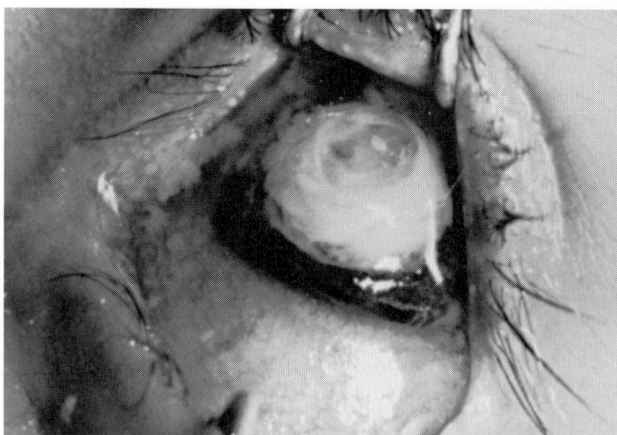

Figure **131–4.** Total necrosis (keratomalacia) (X3B). (From Sommer A, Sugana T: Corneal xerophthalmia and keratomalacia. Arch Ophthalmol 100:404, 1982.)

sles, the cornea responding more rapidly (and dramatically) than the conjunctiva.

DIAGNOSIS

Individual Patients. The diagnosis of an individual case of xerophthalmia is readily made on the basis of the clinical appearance. A history of nightblindness (often translated, in the vernacular, as "chicken eyes" or the like—since chickens cannot see after dusk) from a responsible observer is a highly specific and sensitive symptom. Bitot spots through corneal ulceration and keratomalacia require prompt therapy (see below). Treatment is inexpensive and urgent and should not await costly laboratory confirmation. All forms of otherwise unexplained corneal ulceration, especially those associated with measles, should be treated with vitamin A on the presumption that vitamin A deficiency is the underlying cause, especially in populations where vitamin A deficiency is known to exist, or in special populations, usually immigrants, in the United States.

The value of "diagnosis" is more appropriate for monitoring vitamin A status of an individual suffering severe malabsorption (e.g., cystic fibrosis), in which case sequential measurements of serum retinol are probably the most practical approach.

Population Screening. Diagnosis is also particularly appropriate for establishing the vitamin A status of the pediatric population. The most widely employed technique is surveys establishing the prevalence of different manifestations of xerophthalmia. These require large samples of children and trained observers. In other instances, surveys requiring fewer subjects study the distribution of serum retinol, or more sophisticated but less practical biochemical surrogates of liver stores. These require sensitive collection, transport, and laboratory facilities. New physiologic tests, including conjunctival impression cytology, and even more practical and promising, the pupillary response to threshold levels of illumination, may have the virtues of both simplicity and small sample size, but require further testing and refinement.

TREATMENT. Two conditions requiring immediate high-dose vitamin A therapy are xerophthalmia and measles. Vitamin A deficiency is the cause of xerophthalmia; high-dose vitamin A (200,000 IU PO on 2 successive days; half that dose for children under 1 year of age) will halt and reverse the condition in viable tissue. Since xerophthalmic children are, by definition, vitamin A deficient, it will also increase their chance of survival.

Measles is not caused by vitamin A deficiency, but its complications and sequelae are modulated by vitamin A status: not only does measles interfere with vitamin A metabolism, causing acute decompensation and resulting keratomalacia, but improving vitamin A status using the recommended dosage schedule halves measles case fatality, even among children without any apparent ocular complications.

A third dose of vitamin A, of the same size as the two initial doses, is usually administered 2 to 4 weeks later to help rebuild liver stores as prophylaxis against future deficiency.

PREVENTION. Since vitamin A deficiency causes significant systemic morbidity and mortality before the appearance of its pathognomonic clinical signs (e.g., xerophthalmia), prevention lies in identifying populations in which vitamin A deficiency is prevalent and instituting programs to improve vitamin A status, particularly among preschool-age children. Indonesia represents a remarkable example of what a national program can accomplish. Although vitamin A deficiency per se still exists, the rate of xerophthalmia, nationwide, has declined by over 90% in response to vigorous intervention measures.

There are three basic approaches to improving vitamin A

status in populations. To be effective, it is critical that each reach the group at greatest risk.

Periodic Supplementation. Periodically administering a large dose of preformed vitamin A can increase vitamin A stores in the liver. The commonest preparation, distributed by the United Nations Children's Fund (formerly UNICEF) and other major donors, is 200,000 IU (for children ≥1 year of age) or 100,000 IU (for children <1 year of age) administered every 3 to 6 months. Countries are experimenting with smaller doses among younger children given more frequently as a component of the World Health Organization's Expanded Program for Immunization (EPI). Some studies reported that combining EPI with 25,000 to 50,000 IU vitamin A results in increased incidence of bulging fontanelle. Further studies, however, have suggested this is uncommon, not associated with an increase in intracranial pressure, is transient (lasting no more than 1 to 2 days), and leaves no lasting sequelae. An advantage of combining vitamin A supplementation with the EPI program is that each dose is very inexpensive (US $0.02 to $0.04), but distribution as a free-standing activity is expensive.

It is also advisable to give a mother 200,000 to 300,000 IU early in the postpartum period. Dosing the mother improves her own status, which increases vitamin A content of her breast milk, improving the vitamin A intake of the newborn as well. It is also useful to provide a newborn child with 50,000 IU shortly after birth.

Fortification. Most wealthy Western nations have eliminated micronutrient deficiency, including vitamin A deficiency, by fortifying commonly consumed food products. Small-scale demonstration projects in Indonesia and the Philippines fortifying monosodium glutamate with vitamin A and in Central America, particularly Guatemala, fortifying sugar with vitamin A are proving the effectiveness of this approach.

Increased Vitamin A/β-Carotene–Rich Diet. In theory, consuming a diet rich in vitamin A is the logical, long-term solution to the problem. Unfortunately, there is little in the way of practical experience in successfully changing people's diet, nor is there evidence that it accomplishes its purpose. It was not a change in diet, but fortification, that rid the developed countries of micronutrient deficiencies. Recent studies have demonstrated that β-carotene–rich diets may be poorly converted to vitamin A and do little to improve vitamin A stores and status. In contrast, increasing the intake of foods rich in preformed vitamin A does improve body vitamin A stores, but foods rich in vitamin A are scarce and expensive. Improvement in socioeconomic status, with its attendant change in diet, can reduce vitamin A deficiency. Whether this can occur on its own, from a stand-alone program, remains to be determined.

Bibliography

Beaton GH, Martorell R, L'Abbe KA, et al: Effectiveness of vitamin A supplementation in the control of young child morbidity and mortality in developing countries: Summary Report to CIDA. Toronto: International Nutrition Program, University of Toronto, 1992.

Hussey GD, Klein M: A randomized, controlled trial of vitamin A in children with severe measles. N Engl J Med 323:160, 1990.

Sommer A: Nutritional Blindness: Xerophthalmia and Keratomalacia. New York, Oxford University Press, 1982.

Sommer A: Vitamin A Deficiency and Its Consequences: A Field Guide to Detection and Control, 3rd ed. Geneva, World Health Organization, 1995.

Sommer A, Tarwotjo I, Djunaedi E, et al: Impact of vitamin A supplementation on childhood mortality: A randomised controlled community trial. Lancet 1:1169, 1986.

Sommer A, Tarwotjo I, Hussaini G, et al: Increased mortality in children with mild vitamin A deficiency. Lancet 2:585, 1983.

Sommer A, West KP: Vitamin A Deficiency: Health, Survival, and Vision. New York, Oxford University Press, 1996.

West KP Jr, Pokhrel RP, Katz J, et al: Efficacy of vitamin A in reducing preschool child mortality in Nepal. Lancet 338:67, 1991.

WHO/UNICEF/IVACG Task Force: Vitamin A supplements: A guide to their use in the treatment and prevention of vitamin A deficiency and xerophthalmia. Geneva, World Health Organization, 1997.

131.2 Beriberi

Benjamin Caballero

Beriberi is caused by deficiency of vitamin B₁, thiamine. Primary deficiency was widespread in regions where rice was the main staple, and is classically described in two forms: wet beriberi, in which edema and cardiac insufficiency are prominent features, and dry beriberi, a polyneuropathy. Thiamine deficiency in alcoholics constitutes a third clinical form, Wernicke-Korsakoff encephalopathy.

Etiology and Epidemiology. Beriberi develops after prolonged consumption of thiamine-deficient diets. Most commonly these include rice as their main constituent, but the deficiency has also been reported in people consuming highly milled (refined) wheat. Thiamine is quite unstable, and is easily destroyed during storage, processing, or cooking of cereals. Modern production usually includes fortification of cereals to restore or enhance their thiamine content. Although the extensive endemic areas of beriberi have disappeared, the disease continues to affect small isolated groups in Africa and Asia, usually secondary to consumption of locally produced unfortified rice. In certain cases, the development of deficiency in some of these groups has been attributed to the use of tea or other herbs containing thiamine antagonists. Infantile beriberi can be precipitated in a breast-fed child from a mother consuming a thiamine-deficient diet.

Thiamine is an essential cofactor for a number of enzymes. Its main active form, thiamine pyrophosphate (TPP), is involved in decarboxylation reactions, including those essential for the degradation of branched chain amino acids and for pyruvate metabolism. TPP is also an essential cofactor in the pentose metabolic pathway, which provides substrates for nucleic acid and fatty acid syntheses.

CLINICAL MANIFESTATIONS. Onset of both forms may be similar, consisting of fatigue, anorexia, and weakness of the extremities. Complaints of difficulty in walking, tenderness of calf muscles, and numbness of the limbs are also present.

Dry Beriberi. The progression to the dry form is characterized by increasing difficulty in walking, wasting of peripheral muscles, and overt signs of chronic polyneuropathy: paresthesias, burning sensation in legs and feet, and loss of tendon reflexes. Patients with severe muscle atrophy become bedridden, which, along with the overall state of malnutrition, leads to an increased susceptibility to infections.

Wet Beriberi. The central manifestation of wet beriberi is edema, associated with progressive congestive heart failure. The edema is frequently present not only in the lower extremities but also in the trunk and face. Ascites and pleural effusion may also be present. Other signs of congestive heart failure may be present, such as distended cervical veins, decreased diastolic blood pressure, displacement of the cardiac apex, and dyspnea. Severe anorexia is common, leading to cachexia and death.

Wernicke-Korsakoff Encephalopathy. Thiamine deficiency has specific effects on the central nervous system, leading to Wernicke encephalopathy and to Korsakoff dementia. The former is characterized by ataxia, ophthalmoplegia, psychosis, and coma. Korsakoff dementia is a severe amnesic disorder, almost always associated with Wernicke encephalopathy (the Wernicke-Korsakoff syndrome).

Infantile Beriberi. In contrast to the chronic course of adult beriberi, the infantile form may be of acute onset, usually in infants of 2 to 6 months of age. Although the disease is caused by low thiamine content of breast milk, the mother may not necessarily present clinical signs of beriberi, although her diet would be deficient in the vitamin. Acute manifestations in the infant are centered in signs of cardiac failure: irritability, edema, oliguria, dyspnea, and tachycardia. The course may be fulminant, with death caused by cardiorespiratory failure ensuing in 1 or 2 days. A much less common subacute or chronic presentation is characterized by gastrointestinal manifestations (particularly vomiting) of irregular course, leading eventually to overt signs of congestive heart failure, as in the acute form.

DIAGNOSIS. Thiamine status can be assessed by measuring the activity of the TPP-dependent enzyme, transketolase in red blood cells. The test is done by comparing the activity of this enzyme in two identical samples of erythrocyte hemolysate, with or without added TPP. In a thiamine-deficient person, the sample with added thiamine cofactor will exhibit a higher enzyme activity than the other sample. In practice, deficiency is defined by an increase of 10% or more in enzyme activity after addition of the thiamine cofactor.

Urinary thiamine excretion is indicative of recent intake of the vitamin. The urinary excretion of thiamine 4 hours after a standard, 5-mg dose has also been used to detect deficiency states, with <20 μg used as the cutoff point (Finglass). Blood thiamine levels have not been used routinely to assess deficiency, primarily due to technical difficulties with existing assays and very low free thiamine concentrations. The development of sensitive high-performance chromatography methods to measure free thiamine in red cells has expanded the use of this indicator for diagnosis of deficiency states. The concentration of the free form of the vitamin parallels the response of transketolase activity.

TREATMENT AND PREVENTION. Beriberi is treated by administration of parenteral thiamine (20 mg IM twice daily) for 3 days. Therapy usually continues with oral doses of 30 mg/day until normalization of clinical and laboratory signs of deficiency.

Thiamine stores are limited, and adequate thiamine status is dependent on regular dietary consumption of the vitamin. The recommended intake is related to caloric intake, and is currently 0.5 mg/1000 kcal. In practice, this is approximately equivalent to 1 to 1.5 mg/day, accounting for losses during cooking. Grains are the most common source of thiamine in human diet. The requirement that thiamine losses during processing of foods be replaced by addition of thiamine may exist in some countries but not in others.

Bibliography

Bayliss RM, Brookes R, McCulloch J, et al: Urinary thiamine excretion after oral physiological doses of the vitamin. Int J Vitamin Nutr Res 54:161, 1984.

Finglass PM: Thiamine. Int J Vitamin Nutr Res 63:270, 1994.

Naidoo DP: Beriberi heart disease in Durban: A retrospective study. South Afr Med J 72:241, 1987.

Reuler JB, Girard DE, Cooney TG: Wernike's encephalopathy. N Engl J Med 312:1035, 1985.

Van der Westhuyzen J, Davis RE, Icke GC, et al: Thiamine status and biochemical indices of malnutrition and alcoholism in settled communities of Kung San. J Trop Med Hyg 90:283, 1987.

Ziporin ZZ, Nune WT, Powell RC, et al: Excretion of thiamine and its metabolites in the urine of young adult males receiving restricted intakes of the vitamin. J Nutr 85:287, 1965.

131.3 Scurvy

Benjamin Caballero

Scurvy is caused by a deficiency of vitamin C (ascorbic acid). The disease was probably known since ancient times, but the first systematic description of its clinical manifestations was provided by James Lind in 1753, who also suggested means to prevent it by consumption of fresh fruits.

ETIOLOGY. Humans, monkeys, and guinea pigs are among the few species that cannot synthesize vitamin C from glucose, and must therefore obtain it from their diet. The active form of vitamin C, ascorbate, is a cofactor in eight well-established enzymatic reactions. The most important are those involved in the hydroxylation of the amino acids proline and lysine. This hydroxylation occurs after these amino acids have been incorporated into the collagen protein chain, and are essential for integrity and function of collagen tissue throughout the body. Other ascorbic acid–dependent enzymes catalyze the synthesis of the neurotransmitter norepinephrine from dopamine, the stabilization of peptide hormones (cholecystokinin, adrenocorticotropic hormone, oxytocin), and the biosynthesia of carnitine. Ascorbic acid plays an important role in cellular antioxidant mechanisms. It also keeps iron in its reduced form, enhancing its absorption.

EPIDEMIOLOGY. Diets potentially leading to vitamin C deficiency are those lacking fresh fruits and vegetables. If such a diet is instituted in an otherwise normal individual, it may require about 3 months for signs of scurvy to develop. Good sources of the vitamin are citrus fruits, tomato, mango, guava, and fortified drinks. Ascorbic acid is heat labile, and may be destroyed to a variable degree depending on the duration of cooking.

Endemic scurvy no longer exists. The disease appears sporadically in persons following extremely rigid macrobiotic diets, which may be based solely on grains and exclude all fruits. Other populations at risk of vitamin C deficiency include alcoholics, older persons who are socially isolated and consuming unbalanced diets, and chronically ill individuals unable to consume an adequate diet. Similarly, vitamin C deficiency may develop secondary to gastrointestinal disorders, including inflammatory bowel disease and Whipple disease. Human milk is a good source of vitamin C for the first 4 to 6 months of life, but weaning is a period of increased risk for inadequate intake, particularly in developing countries. In affluent societies, infant formulas and weaning foods are usually fortified with vitamin C.

CLINICAL MANIFESTATIONS

Adult Scurvy. The dominant clinical picture of scurvy is related to impaired connective tissue formation. Early signs include weakness and fatigue, follicular hyperkeratosis, and petechial hemorrhage. Gingival inflammation and bleeding are also frequent. Ecchymosis after minor skin trauma becomes common, and as the disease progresses, bleeding may occur into joints and in the peritoneal and pericardial cavities. In advanced stages the patient is bedridden, hypotensive, and has severe edema. Anemia secondary to blood loss or concurrent deficient dietary iron intake is also common.

The mechanisms of the hemorrhagic manifestations of scurvy have not been clearly elucidated. The coagulation system is normal, and it is presumed that an impaired vascular integrity owing to defective collagen production is a major etiologic factor.

Infantile Scurvy. Bone lesions are the dominant component of the infantile form. The infant may cry when the legs or arms are touched due to tenderness of the limb bones, and may avoid using his or her limbs for standing or crawling.

Pain is caused primarily by subperiosteal hemorrhages in limb bones. Impaired bone growth and ossification become evident as the child grows. Hemorrhagic manifestations include epistaxis, retrobulbar hemorrhage, hematuria, and purpura. Bleeding at the rib's osteochondral junction may produce beading akin to that seen in rickets. Anemia is more frequent than in the adult form, probably because of the more prominent hematuria and higher iron requirements.

DIAGNOSIS. The most practical means of assessing vitamin C status is by measuring plasma and leukocyte ascorbic acid concentrations. Both variables correlate well with dietary vitamin C intake, plasma level being more indicative of recent intake, whereas leukocyte level is reflective of tissue content and body ascorbate pool. Plasma levels are easier to measure and require less blood for the sample. Normal range for plasma ascorbate is 23 to 84 μmol/L (0.4 to 1.5 mg/dL). Levels below 11 μmol/L (<0.2 mg/dL) are indicative of deficiency. Normal concentrations in mixed leukocytes range from 142 to 250 nmol/10^8 cells (25 to 44 μg/10^8 cells).

Urinary ascorbic acid excretion can be used only to confirm overt deficiency if it is less than 10 mg/day, but is not a useful indicator to differentiate between normal and marginally depleted individuals.

In children, radiologic signs of typical scorbutic bone lesions can aid in the diagnosis. Capillary fragility is also easy to document, but not specific.

PREVENTION AND TREATMENT. Persons with clinical manifestations of scurvy should receive 0.5 to 1 g/day of ascorbic acid orally, until clinical signs and leukocyte ascorbic acid levels are normalized. Prevention of scurvy in infants should focus on ensuring an adequate vitamin C intake during pregnancy and on use of vitamin C–rich weaning foods, natural or fortified. Premature infants should receive vitamin C supplementation as part of their routine care. It is also recommended that infants over 4 to 6 months of age receive additional vitamin C as supplements. Although at that age it would be possible to provide adequate vitamin C intake from juices, excessive use of these low-energy dense foods may lead to an inadequate intake of total calories or of other nutrients.

Toxicity. Use of large vitamin C doses, of up to 15 g/day (over 200 times the daily requirement), is common in the United States. Documented adverse effects are rare, suggesting that the vitamin is quite safe. It has been proposed that persons consuming large doses of vitamin C are at higher risk of developing kidney stones because of excess oxalate production. However, although oxalic acid is a product of ascorbate metabolism, most of the excess ascorbic acid is eliminated in the urine unchanged. One related issue is that high concentrations of vitamin C in urine may interfere with the results of laboratory tests based on oxidation-reduction reactions. The same is true for some tests using plasma, such as cholesterol and glucose quantitation. Iron overload has also been reported, presumably facilitated by the enhanced absorption caused by large doses of vitamin C.

Bibliography

Carpenter KJ: The History of Scurvy and Vitamin C. Cambridge, England, Cambridge University Press, 1986.

Ellis CE, Vanderveen EE, Ramussen JE: Scurvy: A case caused by peculiar dietary habits. Arch Dermatol 120:1212, 1984.

Hodges RE, Baker EM, Hood J, et al: Experimental scurvy in man. Am J Clin Nutr 22:535, 1969.

Hodges RE, Hood J, Canham JE, et al: Clinical manifestations of ascorbic acid deficiency in man. Am J Clin Nutr 24:432, 1971.

Jacob RA, Skala JH, Omaye ST: Biochemical indices of human vitamin C status. Am J Clin Nutr 46:818, 1987.

131.4 Rickets and Osteomalacia

Kimberly O. O'Brien

DEFINITION. Although the incidence of rickets and osteomalacia has substantially declined, these two conditions of vitamin D insufficiency and inadequate bone mineralization still occur in many parts of the world. Rickets is characterized by inadequate mineralization of the bone matrix and osteoid in growing bone, prior to the fusion of the epiphyses. It involves both the growth plate and the newly formed trabecular and cortical bone. Osteomalacia describes inadequate bone mineralization following the fusion of the epiphyses.

Rickets and osteomalacia can result from either inadequate endogenous synthesis and dietary intake of vitamin D or from inadequate mineral intake. In addition to the nutritional aspects associated with these conditions, several rare genetic disorders and numerous medical conditions have been implicated in the development of rickets and osteomalacia.

ETIOLOGY. Glisson, DeBoot, and Whistler independently described rickets in the 1600s due to the substantial prevalence of this disease (referred to as English disease) in both Great Britain and Northern Europe. It took nearly 200 years before recognition of its relationship to sunlight exposure. Following fortification of milk with vitamin D and irradiation of food, the incidence of rickets and osteomalacia was substantially reduced in the developed countries.

Dermal Synthesis. Vitamin D does not meet the true definition of a vitamin because it does not have to be obtained from the diet. In fact, vitamin D is a prohormone that can be produced endogenously in the skin. During exposure to sunlight, ultraviolet B (UVB) radiation between the wavelengths of 290 to 320 nm convert 7-dehydrocholesterol in the skin into previtamin D_3. This compound undergoes a thermal isomerization into vitamin D_3 (cholecalciferol), which diffuses through the skin and is transported in the circulation bound to vitamin D binding protein. The dermal production of vitamin D is influenced by the amount of melanin in the skin. Although darker skin tones have the same capacity to produce vitamin D_3, they require longer exposure times to make comparable amounts of previtamin D_3 due to the competition of melanin for the UVB photons. Prolonged exposure to sunlight, as may occur in tropical regions, does not lead to vitamin D intoxication because previtamin D_3 undergoes additional reversible photoisomerizations into two inactive compounds: tachysterol and lumisterol. In addition to lumisterol and tachysterol, vitamin D_3 can also be reversibly photolyzed into a minimum of three other products: suprasterol I and II and 5,6-transvitamin D_3.

Dermal synthesis of vitamin D_3 is affected by the time of day, latitude, and season. Furthermore, endogenous production of vitamin D is completely blocked with the use of sunscreens with sun protection factor of ≥ 8. The capacity to produce vitamin D in the skin is also decreased in the elderly as a result of a decrease in the dermal concentration of provitamin D_3 (7-dehydrocholesterol) with aging. In industrialized cities, ozone air pollution can also absorb the UVB photons and reduce the dermal synthesis of vitamin D.

Dietary Intake. Although the predominant mechanism by which vitamin D is obtained is via casual exposure to sunlight, at some latitudes dietary sources of vitamin D become particularly important because the UVB radiation required for endogenous production of vitamin D may not be present throughout the year. Unless fortified milk or other fortified dairy products are available, very few additional dietary sources are rich in vitamin D except for fish liver oils, egg yolks, and fatty fish. Small amounts of vitamin D in the diet can also be obtained from plant sterols in the form of ergocalciferol (vitamin D_2). Vitamin D_2 is similar to vitamin D_3 except for the presence of an additional double bond and methyl group in the side chain.

Vitamin D Metabolism. Once vitamin D is produced in the skin or obtained from the diet, it must undergo two hydroxylations before becoming biologically active. The first hydroxylation is accomplished using a hepatic 25-hydroxylase to produce 25-hydroxyvitamin D (25(OH)D). This conversion is not tightly regulated and as such, 25(OH)D is often used as an indicator of vitamin D status. Circulating levels of this metabolite normally range between 8 and 60 ng/mL. Levels below 10 ng/mL are often used to define vitamin D deficiency.

Before 25(OH)D becomes biologically active, it undergoes a second hydroxylation in the kidney to form 1,25-dihydroxyvitamin D (1,25(OH)$_2$D). The kidney and placenta are the major sources of the 1α-hydroxylase required for the final hydroxylation of 25(OH)D into this active form of vitamin D. Unlike 25(OH)D, formation of 1,25(OH)$_2$D is tightly regulated and circulating levels of this metabolite (16 to 60 pg/mL) are approximately three orders of magnitude lower than those of its precursor. The active form of vitamin D has both nongenomic and genomic effects. To illicit the genomic actions of this hormone, 1,25(OH)$_2$D must first bind to an intracellular vitamin D receptor.

DISTRIBUTION
Sunlight Exposure
Effects of Latitude. In tropical regions, sunlight exposure is the predominant mechanism by which vitamin D is obtained. However, rickets and osteomalacia are still present in tropical regions despite the presence of adequate UVB radiation required for endogenous vitamin D synthesis. Several contributing factors are responsible for this finding.

Even within a country, variations in UVB exposure can affect the incidence of rickets and osteomalacia. The impact of latitude on vitamin D synthesis has been recently demonstrated in Argentina. At the end of the winter months in Southern Argentina (Ushuaia), over half of the children had values of 25(OH)D below 8 ng/mL, whereas only 12% of the Buenos Aires population were vitamin D deficient. These differences can be explained by a shorter period of UVB exposure in Southern Argentina due to the latitude.

Effects of Clotting. Certain cultural customs can increase the prevalence of rickets and osteomalacia. Osteomalacia is still found in Bedouin women of the Negev as a result of the combination of low dietary vitamin D intake and inadequate sunlight exposure from the traditional clothing that covers almost all exposed skin. Furthermore, darker skin tones make dermal synthesis less efficient, so that longer exposure times are required. Similar findings have been reported in Saudi Arabian populations and in veiled Kuwaiti women.

Nutrition Induced
Infants. Cultural habits that limit sunlight exposure may be of special concern in pregnant and lactating women, as low levels of vitamin D in pregnant women can influence the vitamin D status of the infant. Case reports have observed congenital rickets in infants born to severely vitamin D–deficient mothers. Breast-fed infants with low vitamin D status and little sunlight exposure are also at risk for developing rickets because breast milk contains limited amounts of vitamin D even in well-nourished mothers. Darker-skinned infants are more prone to rickets due to the longer sunlight exposure required in order to synthesize sufficient vitamin D. Rickets is still reported in South African black children due to either calcium and/or vitamin D deficiency.

Nutritional rickets can be evident in premature infants despite normal serum levels of 25(OH)D. In these situations, rickets occurs as a result of an insufficient intake of the phosphorus and calcium required to supply the demands of the substantially elevated rates of bone mineralization that occur in premature infants.

Elderly. In adults, institutionalization can lead to osteomalacia owing to the lack of sunlight exposure. Osteomalacia and osteoporosis are common in elderly adults in nursing homes in the United States and it has been estimated that otherwise healthy elderly individuals with no sunlight exposure may require four times (800 IU) the typical required dietary allowance (RDA) of vitamin D in order to maintain vitamin D status and avoid osteomalacia and osteoporosis.

Vegetarians. Certain dietary practices may also predispose an individual to vitamin D deficiency. Vegetarian diets and those with high contents of whole-meal flour may impair calcium absorption and lead to an increased utilization and degradation of vitamin D. The vegetarian diet and limited sunlight exposure is thought to be responsible for the increased prevalence of osteomalacia among Asian immigrants to England.

Drug Induced. Medications that alter the metabolism or degradation of vitamin D can indirectly cause rickets or osteomalacia. Osteomalacia has been described in individuals on anticonvulsant therapy (e.g., phenobarbital, phenytoin) due to increased hepatic catabolism of vitamin D and inhibition of intestinal calcium absorption. Osteomalacia has also been described in individuals receiving glucocorticoids due to their ability to inhibit vitamin D and calcium transport. Aluminum intoxication caused from total parenteral nutrition or renal disease can be a causal factor in osteomalacia, as aluminum can be deposited in bone and inhibit osteoblast function and hydroxyapatite crystal formation.

Medical Conditions. Illnesses that impair fat absorption, including biliary obstruction, cystic fibrosis, celiac disease, pancreatitis, short gut syndrome and gastrectomy, can lead to malabsorption of vitamin D, as it is a fat-soluble compound. Other diseases associated with fat malabsorption, such as idiopathic steatorrhea, nontropical sprue, regional enteritis, lactose intolerance and small bowel resections, are also implicated in the etiology of osteomalacia. Medical conditions linked to disturbances in phosphate metabolism such as renal failure and various neoplasms are also causal factors in the development of osteomalacia.

Genetic Errors of Metabolism
Vitamin D–Resistant Rickets. Two rare genetic defects in vitamin D metabolism lead to inadequate bone mineralization. The first, vitamin D–resistant rickets (VDRR) type I, is caused by a hydroxylation defect in the renal 25(OH)D 1α-hydroxylase enzyme leading to very low serum levels of 1,25(OH)$_2$D. The defective bone mineralization which ensues can be effectively treated with 0.25 to 1 μg/day of 1,25(OH)$_2$D. VDRR type II is due to a genetic defect in the intracellular 1,25(OH)$_2$D receptor-effector system. This form of VDRR is characterized by elevated circulating levels of 1,25(OH)$_2$D and two thirds of the patients with VDRR type II have alopecia. High doses (up to 60 μg/day) of 1,25-dihydroxy vitamin D_3 (1,25(OH)$_2$D$_3$) and 3 g of elemental calcium may be used to treat this defect. Individuals with either of these disorders exhibit hypocalcemia and hypophosphatemia as well as the other clinical and radiographic stigmata of rickets.

Familial X-Linked Hypophosphatemic Rickets. This is a primary inborn error in renal tubular reabsorption of phosphate and reduced renal synthesis of 1,25(OH)$_2$D. Unlike hypocalcemic rickets, hypophosphatemic rickets is characterized by depressed 1,25(OH)$_2$D relative to the hypophosphatemia and renal urinary phosphate wasting. Large amounts of supplemental phosphorus are used to treat the rickets associated with this disease and supraphysiologic doses of 1,25(OH)$_2$D are also administered to offset the secondary hyperparathyroidism.

Hypophosphatasia. Rickets and osteomalacia can also occur as a result of hypophosphatasia, a rare heritable metabolic bone disease characterized by a deficiency of the tissue-nonspecific alkaline phosphatase isoenzyme. The onset occurs during either the perinatal, infantile, childhood, or adult age period. In this disease, low serum alkaline phosphatase activity is present, and normal or elevated serum levels of calcium and phosphorus are observed. Serum levels of 25(OH)D and 1,25(OH)$_2$D as well as parathyroid hormone are typically normal. Glucocorticoid therapy and/or restriction of dietary calcium may help in the treatment of this disease.

CLINICAL MANIFESTATIONS

Rickets. *Symptoms and Signs.* Clinical signs of rickets include hypotonia, muscle weakness, and in advanced conditions, severe tetany. Hypotonia in infants with rickets may lead to a protuberant abdomen and umbilical hernia. Because of the deformations and softening of the rib cage, defective ventilation may ensue resulting in respiratory obstruction and infection. The clinical and radiologic manifestations of rickets are most apparent in the areas of rapid bone growth, e.g., the long bone epiphyses and the costochondral junctions. Florid rickets is characterized by visible knobby enlargements of the long bones and costochondral junctions. The long bone manifestations are due to expanded epiphyses and are most often observed at the wrists (Fig. 131–5) and ankles. The enlargements at the costochondral junctions are evident along both sides of the thorax and are referred to as the "rachitic rosary" (Fig. 131–6). After weight bearing begins, tibial and femoral bowing may be apparent (Fig. 131–7).

In addition to the long bone manifestations, there may also be deformations of the skull including a softened calvarium, occipital or parietal flattening, and frontal bossing (Fig. 131–8). Rickets can also lead to dental alterations, including numerous caries, enamel hypoplasia, and delayed eruption of the teeth. Under conditions of long-standing rickets, the permanent teeth may be affected.

Radiologic Findings. On radiographic examination, several signs of the defective mineralization may be evident. During the early stages of rickets, the radiologic signs may be most apparent in the wrist (Fig. 131–9) and in a frontal x-ray film of the knee. A widened radiolucent space between the end of the long bone shafts is often observed and the normally dense metaphyseal lines may not be well defined and may appear irregular, frayed, fringed, or hollowed (cupping). In

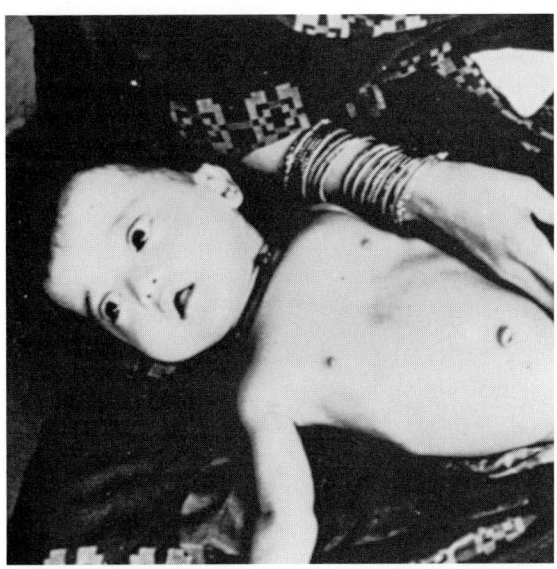

Figure 131–6. Infant with rickets showing rachitic beading. (Courtesy of the National Institute of Nutrition, Indian Council of Medical Research, Hyderabad, India.)

more progressive rickets, the ossification centers can be pale and irregular and have a delayed appearance. The shafts of the long bones may also have a diminished density and a thinning of the cortices.

Osteomalacia. In osteomalacia, reported symptoms include muscle pain, weakness, and bone pain. A waddling

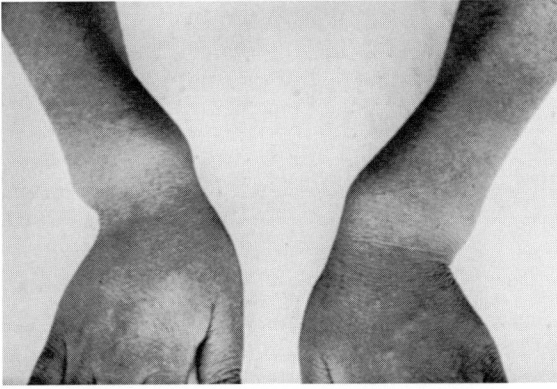

Figure 131–5. Widened epiphyses at the wrist in a child with active rickets. (Courtesy of the National Institute of Nutrition, Indian Council of Medical Research, Hyderabad, India.)

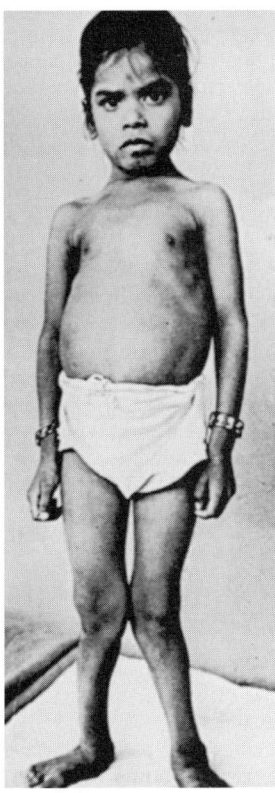

Figure 131–7. Girl with genu valgum due to rickets. (Courtesy of the National Institute of Nutrition, Indian Council of Medical Research, Hyderabad, India.)

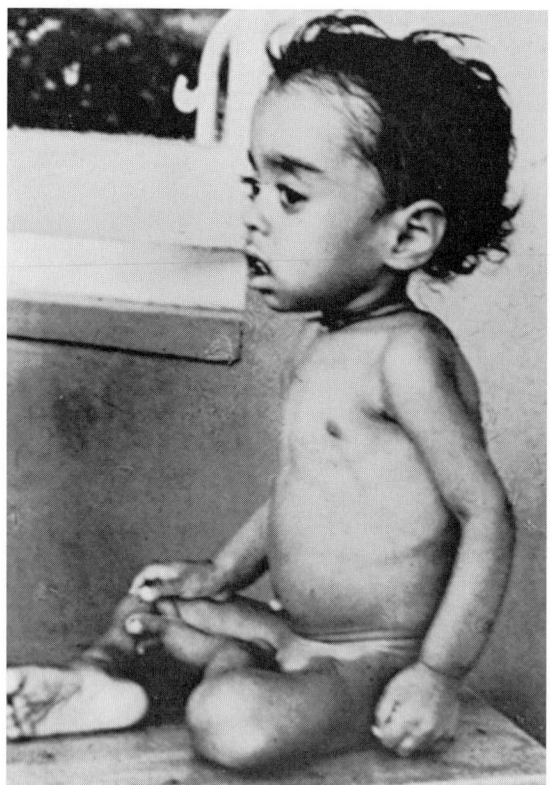

Figure 131–8. Child with active rickets showing bossing of the skull bones and enlarged costochondral junctions (beading). (Courtesy of the National Institute of Nutrition, Indian Council of Medical Research, Hyderabad, India.)

supplementation of vitamin D or periodic supplementation with larger doses. The optimal treatment strategy will be dependent on the anticipated compliance of the subject population, available resources, and practical and economical feasibility. Daily oral doses of 400 IU of vitamin D have been used to treat rickets over an extended period. Larger periodic doses can also be used (2000 IU daily for 6 months or 5000 IU daily for 2 months). Weekly doses of 50,000 IU of vitamin D_2 over an 8-week period have also been used to treat vitamin D insufficiency in adults. Optimal calcium intakes of 800 mg/day in infants and children and 1000 mg/day in adults should be provided to ensure adequate substrate for bone mineralization. If the osteomalacia has occurred due to a malabsorption disorder, initial doses of 50,000 IU/day of vitamin D and 1500 mg of calcium should be administered. The dose should be monitored and adjusted in relation to its therapeutic effects. Once osteomalacia is healed, vitamin D status should be maintained by daily vitamin D intakes of 400 IU per day and additional calcium should be supplied only if the dietary intake is inadequate.

PREVENTION. Adequate sunlight exposure is the easiest means of avoiding vitamin D–deficiency rickets or osteomalacia. Under conditions where this is not possible, increased intake or supplementation of vitamin D should be advocated in populations at risk for these disorders. In some European and African countries, periodic large doses of vitamin D are administered to children prophylactically during visits to the health care provider. Food fortification is another means of ensuring that some food sources are available to supply the vitamin D needs of the population. Most countries routinely fortify milk with vitamin D, although this may not be feasible in relation to the cost and food habits of all population groups. Given adequate sunlight exposure, supplemental vitamin D intake is not required during pregnancy or lactation.

gait may be apparent when pelvic deformities are present. Radiographic examinations of individuals with osteomalacia may exhibit pseudofractures at right angles to the bone shaft most often affecting the pelvis and the ribs (Looser zones). Loss of trabeculae and inadequate calcification in the vertebral bodies can lead to concave or "cod fish" vertebrae. Secondary hyperparathyroidism can lead to subperiosteal resorption of the phalanges and resorption of the distal ends of the long bones often evident in the clavicle and humerus. Radiographs may also exhibit abnormal amounts of osteoid (inadequately mineralized bone matrix coating the trabeculae and the lining of the haversian canals in the cortex). There may also be an increase in the number and width of the osteoid seams. At some sites, e.g., at the vertebral bodies and pelvis, osteoid may be deposited in excess although it remains relatively mineral deficient, which results in local areas of increased radiographic density.

BIOCHEMICAL FINDINGS. Vitamin D–deficient rickets and osteomalacia are both characterized by serum levels of 25(OH)D that are generally well below the normal range. Serum levels of 1,25(OH)₂D are typically normal or slightly below normal although they occasionally are elevated. Serum calcium levels are normal or decreased dependent on the stage of the condition. If decreased serum calcium is observed, serum parathyroid hormone is often elevated. Serum levels of phosphorus are decreased and alkaline phosphatase is substantially elevated.

TREATMENT. Rickets and osteomalacia of nutritional origin should be treated with both vitamin D supplementation and sufficient calcium intake. Restoring vitamin D status can be accomplished in several fashions using either daily

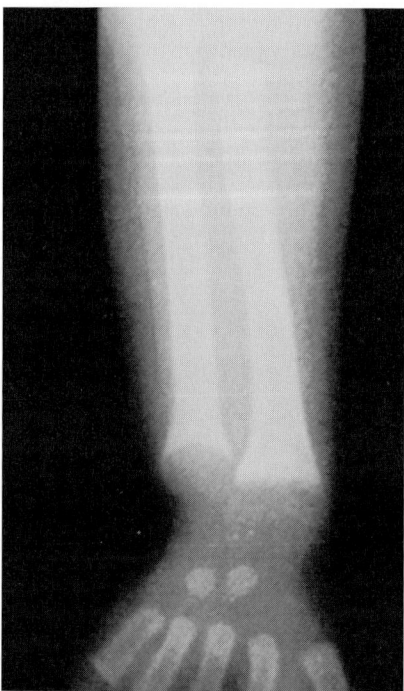

Figure 131–9. Radiograph of the wrist of a child with active rickets showing typical cupping and fraying of the epiphyses. (Courtesy of the National Institute of Nutrition, Indian Council of Medical Research, Hyderabad, India.)

Infants and children in the first year of life who are not obtaining any vitamin D from sunlight exposure should be provided with 200 IU of vitamin D daily.

Bibliography

Bhattacharyya AK: Nutritional rickets in the tropics. World Rev Nutr Diet 67:140, 1992.

Bhimma R, Pettifor JM, Coovadia HM, et al: Rickets in black children beyond infancy in Natal. S Afr Med J 85:668, 1995.

Dawson-Hughes B, Harris SS, Krall EA, et al: Rates of bone loss in postmenopausal women randomly assigned to one of two dosages of vitamin D. Am J Clin Nutr 61:1140, 1995.

El-Sonbaty MR, Abdul-Ghaffar NU: Vitamin D deficiency in veiled Kuwaiti women. Eur J Clin Nutr 50:315, 1996.

Finch PJ, Ang L, Eastwood JB, Maxwell JD: Clinical and histological spectrum of osteomalacia among Asians in South London. Q J Med [New Series] 83:439, 1992.

Holick MF: Environmental factors that influence the cutaneous production of vitamin D. Am J Clin Nutr 61(Suppl):638S, 1995.

Ladizesky M, Lu Z, Oliveri B, et al: Solar ultraviolet B radiation and photoproduction of vitamin D_3 in central and southern areas of Argentina. J Bone Min Res 10:545, 1995.

Liberman UA, Marx SJ: Vitamin D dependent rickets. In Favus MJ (ed): Primer on the Metabolic Bone Diseases and Disorders of Mineral Metabolism, 2nd ed. Philadelphia, Lippincott-Raven, 1993, p 274.

Lowenthal MN, Shany S: Osteomalacia in Bedouin women of the Negev. Isr J Med Sci 30:520, 1994.

131.5 Pellagra

Benjamin Caballero

Pellagra is caused by deficiency of the vitamin niacin. The name is derived from the Italian terms describing the salient clinical features of the disease, *pelle* (skin) and *agra* (rough). The condition developed in the 18th century when maize was introduced as a source of protein, and was endemic in several areas of the world where maize and millet were the main staples. It was also widespread in the southern United States early in this century. This association between pellagra and a maize-based diet was firmly established by Goldberger in 1920. Presently the disease appears recurrently in a few areas where subsistence farming leads to consumption of unfortified maize, or in refugee camps. It is also a nutritional complication of alcoholism.

ETIOLOGY. Niacin is essential for the synthesis of nicotinamide adenine dinucleotide (NAD) and nicotinamide adenine dinucleotide phosphate (NADP), cofactors of a large number of enzymes. In those reactions, NAD/NADP usually acts as an electron acceptor or hydrogen donor, and therefore plays a major role in oxidative reactions. Among the most important NAD/NADP-dependent enzymes are several dehydrogenases: glyceraldehyde-3-phosphate, lactate, pyruvate, and alcohol. NADP is also an essential cofactor for fatty acid synthesis. Humans do not depend exclusively on dietary niacin: the vitamin can be endogenously synthesized, in the liver and kidney, from the amino acid tryptophan. This amino acid, however, must be provided by the diet, since it belongs to the group of essential amino acids. Under normal conditions, it is assumed 60 mg of dietary tryptophan can provide 1 mg of niacin, and from this formula the requirements of niacin may be expressed as niacin equivalents. It should be noted that the conversion of tryptophan to niacin depends in turn on an adequate supply of two other vitamins, B_6 and riboflavin, which are involved in the metabolic reactions of niacin synthesis from tryptophan.

Animal protein (milk, meat, liver) is an excellent source of tryptophan. Vegetable sources contain less, and in addition it may be in a form not readily available for absorption. Maize is low in tryptophan, and its niacin content, although not particularly low, has poor bioavailability. Treating maize with lime, a practice common in Central America and Mexico, releases bound niacin and increases its bioavailability.

Causes of pellagra not directly related to dietary deficiency include liver disease (impaired synthesis and storage); treatment with the antituberculosis drug isoniazid, which inhibits vitamin B_6 (blocking the conversion of tryptophan to niacin); and genetic disorders of tryptophan or niacin metabolism. Chronic exposure to mycotoxins may also cause niacin deficiency by irreversible consumption of nicotinamide during continuing DNA repair. It has also been proposed that a high leucine intake (another essential amino acid) may predispose to niacin deficiency by competitive inhibition of transport and oxidative metabolism of tryptophan.

CLINICAL MANIFESTATIONS. Pellagra has been called the disease of the 4 D's: dermatitis, diarrhea, dementia, and death.

Dermatitis. The dermatitis affects areas of skin exposed to sunlight or at areas of pressure such as elbow or wrists, and has the initial appearance of severe sunburn. Eventually the skin becomes thick, rough and dry, and may acquire a brown pigmentation (Figs. 131–10 and 131–11). The collar of Casal, a ring of dermatitis around the neck, is typical of the disease. The mechanism causing these lesions is not known, but it has been suggested that an impairment in the metabolism of the amino acid histidine may render the skin excessively sensitive to ultraviolet light.

Diarrhea. This is a common but not constant feature of the disease, and usually appears at later stages than the skin lesions. It is most likely a secondary effect of protein malnutrition, resulting in atrophy of the intestinal mucosa.

Dementia. As the condition advances, neuropsychological manifestations appear, ranging from occasional hallucinations to severe dementia. Motor impairment, epileptiform seizures, and anxiety attacks are also frequent. These central nervous system manifestations are most likely caused by deficiency of the neurotransmitter 5-hydroxytryptamine (serotonin), which is synthesized from tryptophan in specific brain regions. Death may result from complications of severe cachexia, or occasionally by suicide.

DIAGNOSIS. The clinical diagnosis can be made from the characteristic appearance and distribution of skin lesions observed in at-risk individuals. The other manifestations of the disease may not be present at early stages. Laboratory diagnosis can be made by measuring the urinary excretion of the niacin metabolite, N'-methyl-nicotinamide. Normal values are >1.5 and <5 mg/g of creatinine, with values <0.5 mg/g of creatinine clearly indicative of deficiency. Pregnant women normally exhibit lower values, and the threshold of deficiency during pregnancy has been set at 0.5, 0.6, and 0.7 mg/g of creatinine for the first, second, and third trimester of pregnancy, respectively. Plasma niacin concentrations are usually very low, and their use for assessing niacin status is questionable. On the other hand, erythrocyte NAD concentrations are sensitive to niacin depletion. The ratio of erythrocyte NAD:NADP concentrations has been proposed as an early index of niacin deficiency.

The differential diagnosis of pellagra may include phototoxic dermatitis caused by drugs or plant toxins. Ariboflavinosis may present a similar dermatologic picture, but skin lesions usually predominate in flexures and skinfolds. In children, the skin manifestation of kwashiorkor may mimic many of the features of pellagra, but it is not confined to skin areas exposed to sunlight, and there is the typical presence of edema.

PREVENTION AND TREATMENT. The recommended daily intake of niacin is related to caloric intake, and ranges from

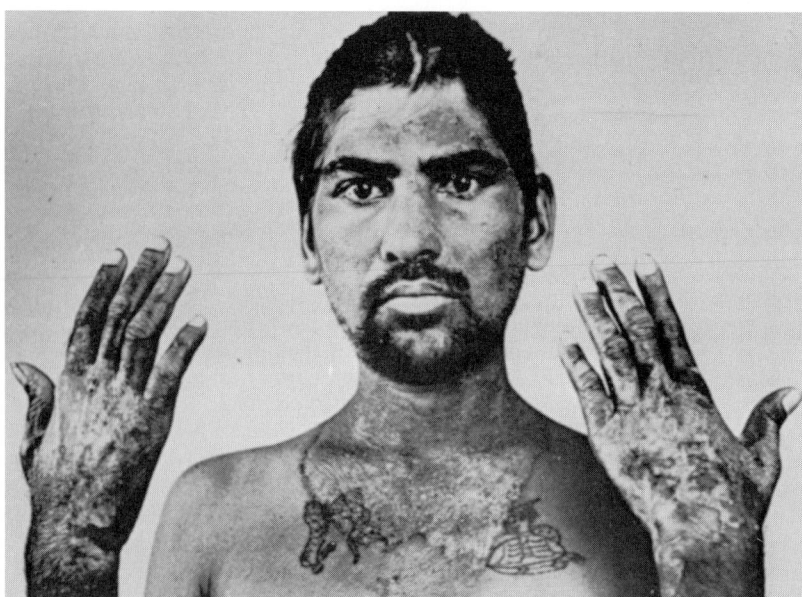

Figure **131–10.** Pellagra showing the characteristic bilateral symmetric dermatitis on the dorsum of both hands and on the exposed part of the neck and chest. The patient has seborrheic dermatitis on the face. (Courtesy of the National Institute of Nutrition, Indian Council of Medical Research, Hyderabad, India.)

15 mg in women to 20 mg in men. Needs can be met by preformed niacin or by dietary tryptophan, at the equivalency of 1 mg niacin = 60 mg of the amino acid. Infants and children require 5 to 12 mg/day. Pregnant and lactating women should consume an additional 3 to 5 mg/day. Prevention focuses on ensuring an adequate intake of niacin-rich foods, primarily animal protein or fortified cereals.

Besides dietary inadequacy, niacin deficiency may develop after prolonged treatment with the antituberculosis drug isoniazid, an inhibitor of the niacin metabolism pathway, and in Hartnup disease, a genetic defect of tryptophan absorption. Treatment with 50 to 250 mg/day of nicotinamide results in rapid reversal of clinical manifestations.

Bibliography

Dillon JC, Malfait P, Demaux G, Foldihope C: Urinary metabolites of nicotinamide during pellagra. Ann Nutr Metab 36:181, 1992.

Jacob RA, Swendseid ME, McKee RW, et al: Biochemical markers for assessment of niacin status in young men: urinary and blood levels of niacin metabolites. J Nutr 119:591, 1989.

Malfait P, Moren A, Dillon JC, et al: An outbreak of pellagra related to changes in dietary niacin among Mozambican refugees in Malawi. Int J Epidemiol 22:504, 1993.

Roe DA: A Plague of Corn: The Social History of Pellagra. Ithaca, NY, Cornell University Press, 1976, pp 1–7.

Spies TD, Cooper C, Blankenhorn MA: The use of nicotinic acid in the treatment of pellagra. JAMA 110:622, 1938.

Swendseid MAE, Jacob RA: Niacin. In Shils ME, Olson JA, Shike M (eds): Modern Nutrition in Health and Diseases. Philadelphia, Lea & Febiger, 1994, pp 376–382.

131.6 Ariboflavinosis

Benjamin Caballero

DEFINITION. Ariboflavinosis is caused by deficiency of the B vitamin riboflavin. The typical clinical manifestations are seborrheic dermatitis, glossitis, and angular stomatitis. Riboflavin deficiency is commonly seen associated with other vitamin deficiencies, usually in populations whose diet contains little animal protein or dairy products.

ETIOLOGY. The major biologic role of riboflavin is as precursor for the synthesis of the enzyme cofactors flavin adenine dinucleotide (FAD) and riboflavin-5′-phosphate (FMN). These cofactors participate in key oxidation-reduction reactions, the most important perhaps being the respiratory chain (FAD), central to adenosine triphosphate synthesis and the

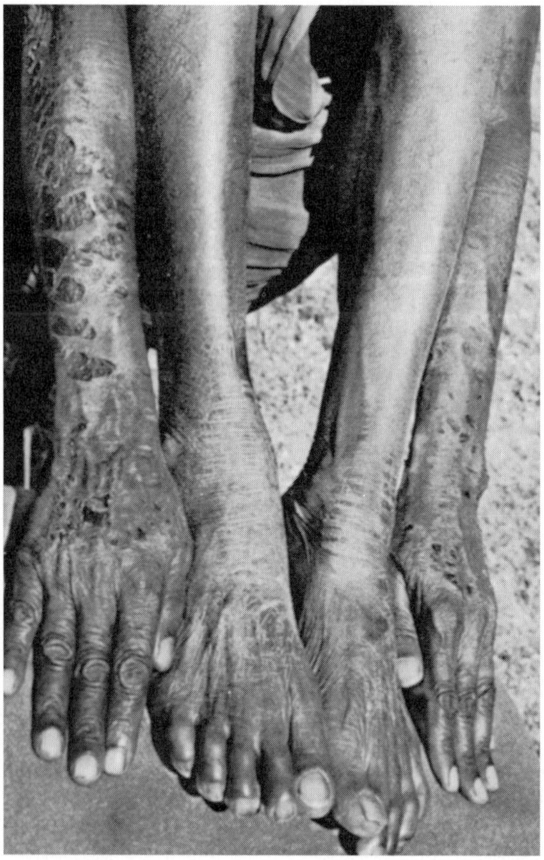

Figure **131–11.** Pellagrous dermatitis on both arms and legs. (Courtesy of the National Institute of Nutrition, Indian Council of Medical Research, Hyderabad, India.)

production of energy. Riboflavin cofactors are also essential for drug metabolism and detoxification involving the cytochrome P450 system. The vitamin also has antioxidant activity, by its role in the glutathione reductase reaction.

Dietary sources of riboflavin are primarily of animal origin, including eggs, fish, meat, and dairy products. Reasonable vegetable sources include broccoli, spinach and asparagus, and fortified cereals. The vitamin is stable to heat and is not destroyed by normal high-temperature heating of milk. It is, however, sensitive to light, and may undergo significant degradation if exposed to sunlight for prolonged periods of time, as is done for sun-drying of foods.

EPIDEMIOLOGY. Poor populations who consume few animal products or milk are at risk of riboflavin and other deficiencies. Thus, the condition is widespread around the world, particularly in areas where food scarcity is the norm. Infants are at risk of riboflavin deficiency during weaning if milk or other fortified products are not introduced. The condition is also seen as a nutritional complication of alcoholism. Thyroid and adrenal insufficiency also impair the synthesis of riboflavin cofactors and may precipitate a deficiency state. Drugs that also interfere with riboflavin metabolism include the antiparasitic quinacrine, and chlorpromazine, imipramine, amitriptyline, and other psychotropic drugs.

CLINICAL MANIFESTATIONS. Isolated primary deficiency is uncommon. Manifestations of deficiency may initially be nonspecific, such as fatigue and weakness. Other common symptoms include itching of the eyes, and soreness in the tongue and mouth. Cheilosis, angular stomatitis, and a dermatitis of the seborrheic type are typical manifestations of established deficiency (Figs. 131–12 and 131–13). The dermatitis is usually located in the face (nasolabial folds, eyes), in flexure areas of the extremities, and in the genital area. Advanced cases may have photophobia, corneal vascularization, anemia (usually normochromic), and brain dysfunction with personality changes.

DIAGNOSIS. The most useful test of riboflavin status is the measurement of the activity of the FAD-requiring enzyme glutathione reductase in red blood cells. The activity of the enzyme is measured in vitro before and after the addition of the FAD cofactor. Individuals with riboflavin deficiency will exhibit a higher degree of response to addition of the cofactor than normal persons. An enzyme activity ratio (after/before FAD addition) above 1.3 is indicative of riboflavin depletion. The urinary excretion of riboflavin is correlated with recent

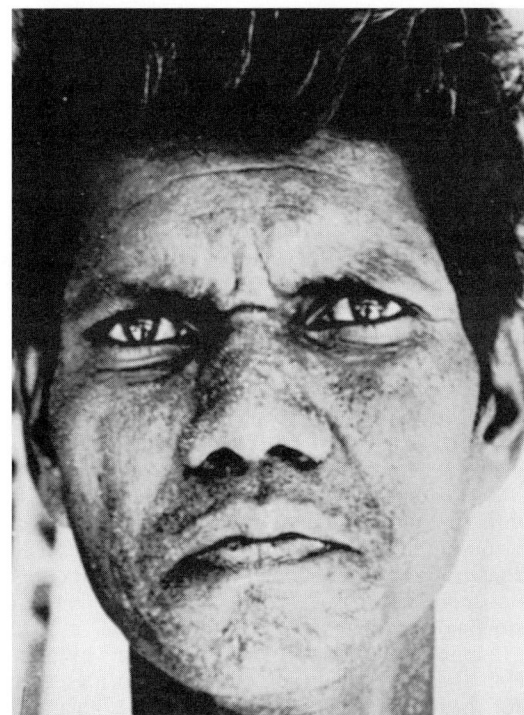

Figure 131–13. Seborrheic dermatitis due to riboflavin deficiency. Whitish sebaceous plugs can be seen on the nose. They have a characteristic fatty acid odor. (Courtesy of the National Institute of Nutrition, Indian Council of Medical Research, Hyderabad, India.)

intake of the vitamin rather than with established tissue depletion. Low values (e.g., <30 μg/g of creatinine) in 24-hour urine collections, however, are consistent with a deficient dietary intake.

Differential diagnosis of riboflavin deficiency may include the dermatosis of zinc deficiency, which also involves the face. Zinc dermatosis, however, is usually perioral, and may extend to extremities and trunk, and is associated with the other manifestations of zinc deficiency, including altered immunity and impaired taste.

PREVENTION AND TREATMENT. A mixed diet that includes dairy products will prevent ariboflavinosis in otherwise normal individuals. The current recommendations of 1.7 mg/day may require consumption of 2 to 3 12-oz glasses of milk per day, which may not be realistic in many areas of the world. Cereal fortification may be another alternative. Requirements during pregnancy increase to 2.5 to 3.0 mg/day.

Deficiency can be treated by administration of 5 to 10 mg of riboflavin daily, until signs of deficiency subside and red cell glutathione reductase activity reaches normal levels.

Bibliography

Brun TA, Chen J, Campbell TC, et al: Urinary riboflavin excretion after a load test in rural China as a measure of possible riboflavin deficiency. Eur J Clin Nutr 44:195, 1990.

Cooperman JM, Lopez R: Riboflavin. In Machlin LJ (ed): Handbook of Vitamins: Nutritional, Biochemical and Clinical Aspects. New York, Marcel Dekker, 1984, pp 299–327.

Dutta P: Disturbances in glutathione metabolism and resistance to malaria: current understanding and new concepts. J Soc Pharm Chem 2:11, 1993.

Goldsmith GA: Riboflavin deficiency. In Rivlin R (ed): Riboflavin. New York, Plenum Press, 1975, pp 221–242.

Roe DA: Current etiologies and cutaneous signs of vitamin deficiencies. In Roe DA (ed): Nutrition and the Skin. New York, Alan R. Liss, 1986, pp 81–98.

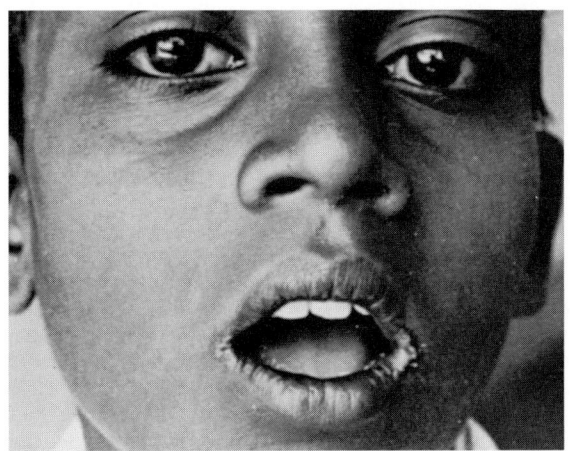

Figure 131–12. Angular stomatitis in a child caused by riboflavin deficiency. The lesion is an acute one. The sharp fissures at the angle of the mouth are evident. (Courtesy of the National Institute of Nutrition, Indian Council of Medical Research, Hyderabad, India.)

131.7 Nutritional Macrocytic (Megaloblastic) Anemia

Nadia M. F. Trugo

DEFINITION. Megaloblastic macrocytic anemia is characterized by the presence of abnormal erythrocyte precursors (megaloblasts) in the bone marrow and macro-ovalocytic erythrocytes in blood, which are the morphologic manifestations of deranged DNA synthesis due to various underlying causes. Nutritional megaloblastic anemia refers to the anemia that is caused by folate and/or cobalamin deficiencies, mainly the former, since nutritional deficiency is far more common for folate than for cobalamin.

PATHOGENESIS AND ETIOLOGY. Folate and cobalamin deficiencies are the most common causes of megaloblastic anemia. Megaloblastic anemia that is unresponsive to one or both of these vitamins may be caused by defective enzymes of DNA biosynthesis and cytotoxic drugs, e.g., nitrous oxide and drugs used for chemotherapy of various cancers or for immunosuppression.

Metabolic Processes. Folate is an essential cofactor involved in many single-carbon transfer reactions in intermediary metabolism, including the synthesis of purines, thymidylate, and methionine. An adequate supply of folate is thus required for DNA synthesis and S-adenosylmethionine-dependent methylation reactions. Both folate and cobalamin are necessary cofactors for homocysteine conversion to methionine. In this reaction methyltetrahydrofolate is demethylated. Impairment of this conversion by cobalamin deficiency causes a decrease in the availability of folate for the synthesis of DNA bases, by trapping methyltetrahydrofolate or by affecting the supply of formyltetrahydrofolate. Therefore, deficiency of either vitamin affects DNA replication and consequently cell division, especially in rapidly proliferating tissues, producing morphologically indistinguishable anemia. Besides the hematopoietic system, the epithelial cell surfaces and the gonads are also affected. In the bone marrow, the impaired DNA replication results in asynchronous maturation of the nucleus and cytoplasm, with cytoplasmic components being synthetized in excessive amounts during the delay between cell divisions, leading to enlargement of cells in the erythroid and myeloid series. Deficiencies of cobalamin or folate may result from inadequate intake, increased requirements, and/or impaired utilization.

Causes of Cobalamin Deficiency. Cobalamin deficiency due to insufficient dietary intake is rare, but may occur in strict vegetarians, since cobalamin is supplied primarily by foods of animal origin. Recommended daily intakes of cobalamin are in the range of 1 to 2 μg for adults. An omnivorous diet usually provides an excess of the cobalamin requirements, and cobalamin body stores represent a further protection, with an efficient conservation through the enterohepatic circulation. The most common cause of cobalamin deficiency is intestinal malabsorption due to decreased production or lack of gastric intrinsic factor, a protein required for cobalamin absorption, as occurs in pernicious anemia, atrophic gastritis, and gastrectomy. Cobalamin malabsorption also occurs in other conditions such as pancreatic disease, overgrowth of intestinal bacteria in intestinal stasis, ileal resection, regional enteritis, and fish tapeworm infection.

Causes of Folate Insufficiency. Differently from cobalamin, dietary inadequacy is a common cause of folate deficiency, since folate intake is not usually in great excess of nutritional requirements and the body reserves are meager. Recommended daily intakes of folate are in the range of 0.15 to 0.20 mg for adults, and twice these values for pregnant women. Diets poor in folate are characterized by a predominance of starches and grains, e.g., white bread, white maize meal, polished rice, and overcooked vegetables, and an insufficient amount of foods of animal origin, dark green vegetables, fresh or lightly cooked, and fruits, a diet that occurs in some parts of Africa and India. In temperate areas, nutritional folate deficiency has been found in elderly persons living on a marginal subsistence diet. Intestinal malabsorption is also a common cause of folate deficiency and is associated with subtotal gastrectomy, extensive intestinal resection, tropical sprue, gluten-sensitive enteropathy, chronic giardiasis, and drugs, e.g., anticonvulsants (phenytoin and phenobarbital). Drugs that are folate antagonists are also implicated in folate deficiency: antiprotozoal (pyrimethamine), antibacterial (trimethoprim, pentamidine), and those used for cancer chemotherapy (methotrexate). Alcoholism may cause folate deficiency, not only because of the reduced folate intake, but also due to altered folate metabolism and interference with the folate enterohepatic cycle. Increased requirements of folate due to diseases such as hemolytic anemia, malignant metastatic tumors, leukemias, and malaria contribute to folate deficiency. Due to the high folate requirements in periods of intense cell proliferation, pregnancy and growth may predispose to folate deficiency.

EPIDEMIOLOGY. Recent and comprehensive worldwide epidemiolgic data on subclinical and clinical (megaloblastic anemia) folate and cobalamin deficiencies, especially in tropical and developing countries, where they affect the most people, are scarce. Most data concerning prevalence and distribution of these deficiencies were obtained more than two decades ago.

Folate Deficiency. Those earlier studies showed that nutritional folate deficiency had a worldwide distribution, differing greatly in severity, with the subclinical, nonanemic forms being predominant, and was, in general, a primary cause of megaloblastic anemia. It affected mainly pregnant women, since their increased folate requirements may be difficult to achieve through the habitual diet, especially in low socioeconomic groups. Megaloblastic anemia due to dietary folate deficiency was reported to be highly prevalent in tropical areas such as India, Burma, Singapore, Malaysia, and Africa, affecting up to 25% of nonsupplemented pregnancies in certain parts of Asia, Africa, and Latin America, and 2.5 to 5% in developed countries. These values were higher (up to 60% in developing countries) when bone marrow aspirates were used for the diagnosis, and subclinical folate deficiency was estimated to affect up to one third of pregnant women on a global scale. The widespread use of iron-folate supplements substantially reduced prevalence of folate deficiencies during pregnancy. Presently, the patterns of folate deficiency may still be the same, but scattered data indicate a decline in the incidence and prevalence of megaloblastic anemia, with a relative increase of subclinical deficiencies. In Brazil, megaloblastic anemia is rare during pregnancy, but 20% of nonsupplemented pregnant women in Rio de Janeiro, and from 22 to 79% in different cities of the Amazon region, have low erythrocyte folate.

Cobalamin Deficiency. This is common in strict Hindus from the Indian subcontinent and is due to inadequate intake. Recent studies suggest that cobalamin deficiency may be more prevalent in other countries than formerly believed, but it is mostly due to malabsorption. In Zimbabwe, 86% of patients with megaloblastic anemia had cobalamin deficiency, mainly in the form of pernicious anemia, suggesting that cobalamin and not folate deficiency may be a main cause of megaloblastic anemia in southern Africa. In rural Mexico, a high prevalence of low levels of cobalamin in plasma of preschool-age children and in plasma and milk of lactating anemic women has been reported. In developed countries, malabsorption of cobalamin affects mainly elderly populations.

CLINICAL MANIFESTATIONS

Symptoms, Signs, and Complications. The clinical features of folate and cobalamin deficiencies are megaloblastic anemia and megaloblastic changes in mucosal cells, leading to pallor, weakness, glossites, anorexia, and diarrhea. Homocysteinemia, which is an independent risk factor for coronary heart disease, occurs in both folate and cobalamin deficiencies. Cobalamin deficiency also results in a complex neurologic syndrome, manifested independently or with megaloblastic anemia, involving peripheral nerves and the central nervous system, leading to paresthesias, problems of balance, and neuropsychiatric changes. Subclinical folate deficiency has been associated with increased risk for various cancers, e.g., in the uterine cervix, bronchus, and colon, as a result of impaired chromosome repair or altered DNA methylation.

Effects on Pregnant Women and Fetus. Risks from folate deficiency during pregnancy include poor pregnancy outcome, prematurity and low birth weight, and an increased prevalence of neural tube defects (NTD), e.g., congenital birth defects, spina bifida, and anencephalus in the fetus. Although NTD have multiple etiologies, maternal folate supplementation during the periconceptional period can reduce both their occurrence and recurrence. The first 3 weeks after conception represent a crucial period because closure of the neural tube occurs about the 23rd day. Although the underlying mechanism for the folate role in prevention of NTD is not known, there are indications that in the vast majority of cases the problem is not of maternal dietary deficiency, and may be due to a maternal and/or fetal defect in folate metabolism or transport into the cells, which can be overcome by maternal supplementation.

LABORATORY DIAGNOSIS

Hematology. Megaloblastic anemia is characterized by marked macro-ovalocytosis, hypersegmentation of neutrophilic leukocytes, increased mean cell volume, and decreased erythrocyte, reticulocyte, leukocyte, and platelet counts in peripheral blood. The decrease in erythrocyte counts leads to low hemoglobin values. In pregnancy, a combination of macrocytosis, a normal finding in this period, and microcytosis caused by a concurrent and more severe iron deficiency, which is common in pregnant women, results in a normal mean cell volume. Examination of the bone marrow can provide a more conclusive diagnosis of megaloblastic anemia in this period. In the marrow, megaloblastosis of erythrocyte precursors is a prominent feature, and large leukocyte precursors are also found, particularly giant metamyelocytes.

Biochemistry. A range of laboratory tests are used to ascertain whether megaloblastic anemia is due to folate or cobalamin deficiency. Biochemical indicators of either vitamin status, corresponding to different degrees of depletion, are used for this purpose and can also be useful for diagnosis of subclinical deficiencies, in the absence of anemia, despite the problems in establishing cutoff levels. Serum (or plasma) cobalamin may be a poor indicator of tissue levels, but levels <150 pg/mL probably indicate a deficiency state. Low serum folate (<3 ng/mL) is an indicator of negative balance that, if persistent, can result in tissue depletion, which is assessed by determining the levels of erythrocyte folate. Values of <160 ng/mL are indicative of folate deficiency. These three indicators are the most widely used to assess cobalamin and folate status.

Other tests provide valuable information regarding the nutritional status of these vitamins and the underlying causes of deficiency but most are not readily available, even in developed countries. Determination of serum holohaptocorrin, the cobalamin storage glycoprotein, can be used to assess body stores. The increase of urinary and serum methylmalonic acid concentrations indicates intracellular cobalamin deficiency. Serum homocysteine is a sensitive indicator of intracellular folate and cobalamin, and it is increased when depletion of either vitamin occurs. The deoxyuridine suppression test in bone marrow leukocytes assays the ability of nonradioactive deoxyuridine to suppress the incorporation of radiolabeled thymidine into DNA via a pathway that is impaired in folate and cobalamin deficiency. The Schilling test can detect cobalamin malabsorption, through measurement of urinary excretion of radiolabeled cobalamin, following a large parenteral dose of nonradioactive cobalamin and an oral dose of the labeled vitamin.

TREATMENT. Folate-deficiency megaloblastic anemia is usually treated with oral folic acid supplements (1 to 2 mg/day). A brisk reticulocytosis is observed 3 to 5 days after beginning the treatment, conversion from megaloblastic to normoblastic bone marrow is complete within 48 to 72 hours, and the hematologic picture normalizes in 2 months. The therapy of cobalamin deficiency is usually done with 0.2 to 1.0 mg of cyanocobalamin or hydroxocobalamin given IM daily for 1 to 2 weeks, once or twice weekly for an additional 4 weeks or until the hematocrit is normal, and then monthly for life (when the cause is due to pernicious anemia). The response is similar to that seen in the treatment of folate deficiency. For patients with neurologic manifestations, 1 mg every 2 weeks for 6 months is recommended. Treatment of cobalamin deficiency with folate accelerates the development of neurologic abnormalities.

PREVENTION AND CONTROL. Owing to the overall high incidence of folate deficiency in unsupplemented women with inadequate diets, it is advisable to give folate supplements (0.2 to 0.4 mg/day) in the latter half of pregnancy.

Comprehensive studies demonstrated that 4 mg/day of folic acid used by women who had a previous NTD-affected pregnancy reduced the risk of having a subsequent NTD by 70%, and that 0.36 to 0.8 mg resulted in significant reductions in the risk of first occurrences of NTD. In developed countries, e.g., the United States, Canada, the United Kingdom and Australia, it is recommended that all women of childbearing age consume 0.4 mg/day of folic acid. This is approximately twice the dietary intake recommended for nonpregnant women. For women with a previous confirmed or suspected NTD-affected pregnancy, a supplement of 4 mg of folic acid is recommended, beginning 2 months before conception and through the first trimester of pregnancy. Possible public health strategies for supplying women with folate in the periconceptional period are the use of supplements by all women of childbearing age, changes in food habits, and food fortification with folate. This last alternative, however, has raised concern since a higher folate intake through fortified foods by the general population could be detrimental to individuals with cobalamin deficiency, especially the elderly.

Bibliography

Allen LH, Rosado JL, Casterline JE, et al: Vitamin B-12 deficiency and malabsorption are highly prevalent in rural Mexican communities. Am J Clin Nutr 62:1013, 1995.

Beck WS: Diagnosis of megaloblastic anemia. Annu Rev Med 42:311, 1991.

Chanarin I: Folate and cobalamin. Clin Hematol 14:641, 1985.

Herbert V: The Herman Award Lecture. Nutrition science as a continually unfolding story: the folate and vitamin B-12 paradigm. Am J Clin Nutr 46:387, 1987.

Lehti KK: Stillbirth rates and folic acid and zinc status in low-socioeconomic pregnant women of Brazilian Amazon. Nutrition 9:156, 1993.

Rayburn WF, Stanley JR, Garret E: Periconceptional folate intake and neural tube defects. J Am Coll Nutr 15:121, 1996.

Savage D, Gangaidzo I, Lindebaum J, et al: Vitamin B-12 deficiency is the primary cause of megaloblastic anaemia in Zimbabwe. Br J Haematol 86:844, 1994.

Trugo NMF, Donangelo CM, Seyfarth BSP, et al: Folate and iron status of non-anemic women during pregnancy: effect of routine folate and iron supplementation and relation of erythrocyte folate with iron stores. Nutr Res 16:1267, 1996.

132 Mineral Deficiencies

132.1 Iron Deficiency

Ray Yip

DEFINITION. Iron deficiency is the result of a long-term negative iron balance whereby absorbed iron does not meet the requirements stemming from normal iron loss and growth. Anemia, the commonly used clinical marker for iron deficiency, represents the most severe form of iron deficiency when the shortage of iron leads to underproduction of hemoglobin or red blood cells. The two most vulnerable periods for iron deficiency during the life cycle are early childhood and the childbearing years for women, especially during pregnancy.

PREVALENCE. Iron deficiency is one of the most common nutrition deficiencies worldwide. In addition to affecting a large proportion of children and women in the developing world, iron deficiency is the only nutrient deficiency of significant prevalence in virtually all developed nations as well. Using anemia as an indicator, the World Health Organization estimated that in developing countries half of both children under 5 years of age and pregnant women, and up to a quarter of nonpregnant women are iron deficient. Comparatively, among children and women in developed countries, the estimated prevalence of iron deficiency is 7 to 12%.

IRON REQUIREMENT AND VULNERABLE PERIOD FOR IRON DEFICIENCY. Factors affecting the three major aspects of iron metabolism—intake, storage, and loss—determine iron requirements and the risk for iron deficiency. For adult men, the daily iron need is about 1.0 mg to make up for the normal turnover of intestinal mucosa with limited blood loss, regarded as physiologic loss. The iron requirement for nonpregnant women is about 1.5 mg. The additional iron is needed in order to make up for the monthly menstrual blood loss. During pregnancy, extra iron is needed to account for blood volume expansion, as well as for fetal and maternal tissue growth, thereby elevating the average daily requirement to about 4.5 mg. To meet the iron needs resulting from rapid physical growth, an infant between 4 and 12 months of age typically requires about 0.8 mg of iron each day, almost as high as the requirement of adult men.

Infancy and Childhood. Infants are born with an endowment of iron stores that can be mobilized to meet their iron requirement during the first few months of life. The amount of iron in storage is proportional to birth weight or size. Even when a mother is iron deficient, sufficient iron will be acquired by the fetus. For full-term infants, iron stores usually become depleted by 6 months of age. Preterm and low birth weight infants usually deplete their iron stores by 2 or 3 months of age. After an infant exhausts his or her initial iron stores, it is difficult to maintain substantial iron stores, even when iron intake is adequate. This is due to the high iron requirement for rapid growth, as reflected by the tripling of birth weight by 1 year of age. Despite the fact that infants have a similar iron requirement as adult men, they consume far less energy than adults and the iron content and bioavailability of most infant diets are lower than that of an adult diet. For this reason, unless specific provision is made to provide extra iron in food or as a supplement, iron deficiency often occurs at about 1 year of age. After age 2, as growth velocity is reduced to a lower baseline level, iron stores can begin to accumulate if dietary iron is sufficient and the risk for iron deficiency declines.

Women of Childbearing Age. Menstrual blood loss results in an average of 50% higher iron requirement for women than for men. For the subset of women with heavy menstrual periods and greater blood loss than average, it is more difficult to meet their iron requirement (Fig. 132–1). This is true even when consuming a diet with relatively high iron bioavailability, as is the case in Western Europe. The use of oral contraceptives is associated with reduced menstrual blood loss, and the use of an intrauterine device is associated with increased menstrual blood loss. In many developing countries low bioavailable iron in the diet is related to infrequent consumption of food from animal sources, making it difficult to meet iron requirements and resulting in a high prevalence of iron deficiency anemia among nonpregnant women. During pregnancy, increased iron absorption can partially compensate for the greater iron need. However, because very few women can meet this high iron requirement from their diet or existing iron stores, routine iron supplementation during pregnancy has been the standard practice in many countries to prevent the development of iron deficiency anemia during pregnancy.

IRON METABOLISM AND FACTORS AFFECTING IRON BALANCE. Iron in the body exists in two major forms: functional iron and stored iron. The majority of functional iron is in the form of heme iron as hemoglobin and myoglobin. There are also a number of enzymes that require iron, but these account for less than 1% of total body iron. Iron intake and loss determine the body's iron balance. The stored iron in the form of ferritin and hemosiderin accumulates when

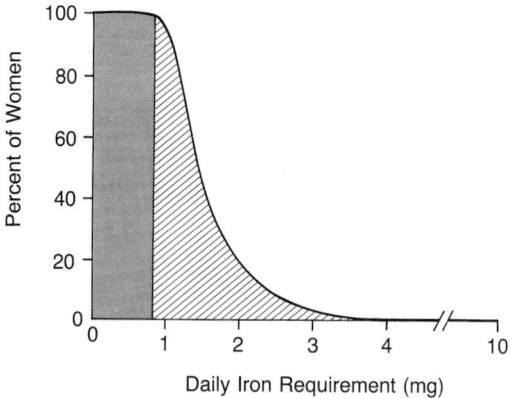

Figure 132–1. Cumulative frequency of daily iron requirements in normal women as calculated from the sum of their basal obligatory losses (dotted area) and loss due to menstruation (cross-hatched area). (From Iron Deficiency in Women. A Report of the International Nutritional Anemia Consultative Group [INACG], 1981. After Hallberg L, et al.: Variation in iron loss in women. *In* Occurrence, Causes, and Prevention of Nutritional Anemias, Symposia of the Swedish Nutrition Foundation VI, 1967. Stockholm, Almqvist and Wiksell, 1968.)

TABLE 132–1. Foods Rich in Ascorbic Acid

West Indian cherry	Cabbage
Guava	Akee
Papaya	Alfalfa shoots
Citrus fruit	Broccoli
Spinach	Cauliflower
Peas	Parsley
Sweet potato	Collard greens
White potato	Cashew (raw fruit pulp)
Beet greens	Lychee
Turnips and turnip tops	Mango
Amaranth leaves	Pineapple
Bean sprouts	Baobab (monkey bread)
Green and red peppers	Longan

there is a positive iron balance which can be mobilized to meet iron needs.

Iron Intake and Dietary Factors. The dietary source of iron strongly influences the efficiency of its absorption. For infants, the iron content of milk consumed is a major determinant of iron status. The iron content of breast milk is low, similar to that of cow's milk. However, 50% of the iron in breast milk can be absorbed in contrast to less than 10% from cow's milk. The better absorption efficiency of breast milk does not entirely make up for the relatively low iron content. After 6 months of age, breast-fed infants require an additional source of iron from the diet to meet their iron requirement. Unfortunately, in most settings complementary food is low in iron content and availability. The amount of iron absorption from a variety of foods ranges from less than 1% to more than 20%. Foods of vegetable origin are at the lower end of the range, dairy products are in the middle, and meat is at the upper end. Meat is a good source of iron because most iron is in the form of heme iron which has an absorption efficiency of 10 to 20%, which is two to three times greater than for nonheme iron (2 to 7%). Nonheme iron found in plant foods and fortified food products is not only less well absorbed, the absorption is strongly influenced by the other foods ingested at the same meal. Ascorbic acid and meat protein are among the most potent enhancers of nonheme iron absorption (Table 132–1). Tannin in tea and phytic acid in grain fibers are the better known inhibitors of nonheme iron absorption.

Iron Loss. The normal turnover of intestinal mucosa with some blood loss can be regarded as physiologic, an amount accounted for in the daily iron requirement. Normal menstrual blood loss is also an obligatory or physiologic loss. The most common reason for abnormal blood loss in infants and younger children is the sensitivity of some children to the protein in cow's milk, resulting in increased acute gastrointestinal blood loss. In many tropical communities where hygienic conditions are less than adequate, hookworm infection is a major cause of gastrointestinal blood loss for older children and adults (Chapter 105.1). Hookworms cause bleeding in the upper intestine, and the severity of blood loss as measured by the hemoglobin content in feces is proportional to the intensity of hookworm infection. Recent studies in endemic areas show that upward of 40% of the iron deficiency anemia and majority of the severe anemia can be attributed to hookworm infections. There are two common forms of hookworm: *Necator americanus* and *Ancylostoma duodenale* and, for the same worm load, *N. americanus* causes a greater amount of bleeding. *Trichuris trichiura*, found in the colon, can also contribute to blood loss, but to a much lesser extent than hookworm (Chapter 103.2).

CONSEQUENCES OF IRON DEFICIENCY. Manifestations of iron deficiency are related to its effect on various tissues. Hematopoietic tissue requires two thirds of the body's iron, and iron deficiency leads to anemia, by far the best known consequence (Chapter 6). Even though iron deficiency is the most common cause of anemia, there are many other causes for anemia other than iron deficiency.

Anemia. The manifestations of iron deficiency anemia are usually subtle unless the anemia is severe. Mild anemia itself is of little health consequence. However, when anemia becomes severe (hemoglobin <8 g/dL), blood oxygen carrying capacity is significantly compromised. Very severe anemia (hemoglobin <4 g/dL), which can be the result of iron deficiency in combination with other conditions, e.g., malaria, is associated with increased childhood and maternal mortality. Deaths associated with severe anemia generally occur at times of increased physiologic stress, i.e., during an acute febrile illness, or peripartum, when oxygen delivery and cardiovascular function are further compromised by a decreasing hemoglobin level due to acute blood loss.

Blood transfusion is a common therapy for severe anemia and this practice in itself can involve significant risk. One of these is related to the high-output cardiac failure from the extra fluid from the transfusion when anemia is very severe. To avoid transfusion-related heart failure, the more severe the anemia, the slower the rate of transfusion must be. Another potential lethal consequence related to transfusion is human immunodeficiency virus (HIV) infection. In areas where HIV is highly endemic, resources are poor, and/or where routine testing of donated blood for HIV is not feasible, transfusion carries substantial risk for HIV infection.

Work Performance. Animal and human studies have demonstrated that anemia due to iron deficiency causes a substantial reduction in an individual's work capacity. This has been studied among workers in rubber and tea plantations in Indonesia and Sri Lanka. In these investigations, the productivity of iron-deficient individuals was significantly lower than that of workers with normal hemoglobin concentrations. After supplementation with iron, the performance of the iron-deficient subjects improved.

Behavior and Intellectual Performance. There is strong evidence that iron deficiency anemia is associated with impaired child development and cognitive functioning among infants and young children. Consistently, children with iron deficiency anemia test less well in psychomotor performance compared to iron-sufficient children. When various developmental test scores are standardized, the magnitude of the deficit associated with iron deficiency anemia is approximately 1 SD. This represents a deficit comparable to that observed for mild childhood lead poisoning or moderate iodine deficiency. Although short-term iron treatment can reverse some aspects of the cognitive deficit, a few long-term studies suggest that part of the deficit cannot be fully reversed. For this reason, control of childhood iron deficiency anemia should be based on primary prevention, rather than relying on the detection of anemic children after significant iron deficiency has occurred.

Immunity and Resistance to Infections. Laboratory evidence suggests that iron deficiency is related to decreased resistance to infection. Iron-deficient children may have abnormalities in the function of lymphocytes and neutrophils. Despite numerous studies that show an impaired resistance to infection under laboratory conditions, there is no conclusive evidence for an increased morbidity related to iron deficiency. Iron deficiency anemia and infections are both common among poor populations. However, a cause-and-effect relationship, although plausible, has not been established. Other studies suggest that iron supplementation of an iron-deficient population may increase their risk for malaria and other forms of infections. This may be related to the fact that subclinical malaria can become clinical due to new red blood cell production, favored by the parasites. There is also clear laboratory evidence that both lactoferrin in the gut and transferrin in blood have bacteriostatic properties. When these iron-binding proteins become saturated with iron, the bacteriostatic property is reduced. Existing clinical and epidemiologic evidence does not support the concept of maintaining iron deficiency in order to protect against infections. The more appropriate interpretation of these findings on iron and infections is that infections must be monitored and treated in those receiving iron for correction of their deficiency.

Enhanced Absorption of Heavy Metals. Both animal and human studies have demonstrated that capacity for lead absorption increased with iron deficiency. An epidemiologic study of iron-deficient children under 5 years old in the United States found that the risk of an elevated blood lead level is three to four times higher among iron-deficient children than nondeficient children. This is likely the result of increased efficiency of iron absorption among iron-deficient individuals which, unfortunately, also enhances the absorption of heavy metals e.g., lead and cadmium.

Adverse Pregnancy Outcomes. Several studies from developed countries have found an association between anemia during pregnancy with preterm delivery, low birth weight, and fetal death. Thus far, only one study has found that the increased risk of preterm births is associated specifically with iron deficiency anemia rather than anemia itself. Since these studies were conducted in developed countries where severe iron deficiency anemia during pregnancy is rare, it is possible there is an even stronger relationship in developing countries where severe anemia during pregnancy is more common.

DIAGNOSIS OF IRON DEFICIENCY. The spectrum of iron status ranges from severe iron deficiency with considerable anemia to severe iron overload with evidence of damage to multiple organs. A number of hematologic and biochemical tests enable characterization of iron status (Fig. 132–2). In general, iron deficiency is defined by conducting one or more iron biochemistry tests that result in measurements falling within ranges comparable with iron deficiency (Table 132–2). Iron deficiency anemia is defined as meeting the criteria for both iron deficiency and anemia based on hemoglobin testing. Even though all iron-related tests respond to changes in iron status, each test reflects different aspects of iron metabolism. For this reason, the tests are of different utility, and results of one test may not always agree with another test.

The Meaning of Anemia. Anemia, as measured by low hemoglobin or low hematocrit, is by far the most commonly used indicator for detecting iron deficiency. Even though there are a number of other causes of anemia in addition to iron deficiency, in areas where anemia prevalence is higher than 20%, the majority of anemia can be attributed to iron deficiency. Common causes of anemia other than iron deficiency include hereditary hemoglobinopathies or red cell production defects e.g., thalassemia minor; recent or current infections; and any chronic conditions with inflammatory response (Chapter 6). Because anemia caused by iron deficiency represents the more severe form of iron deficiency, it cannot be used to detect those with milder forms of iron deficiency (iron deficiency without anemia). Iron deficiency anemia can be diagnosed based on the presence of anemia and other abnormal iron tests e.g., low serum ferritin. Since it is not feasible to perform iron biochemistry tests in many settings, hemoglobin response to iron treatment is a common approach for diagnosing iron deficiency. An increase of 1 or more g/dL of hemoglobin from a course of oral iron for those with anemia is indicative of iron deficiency. For population-based assessment or monitoring, prevalence of anemia

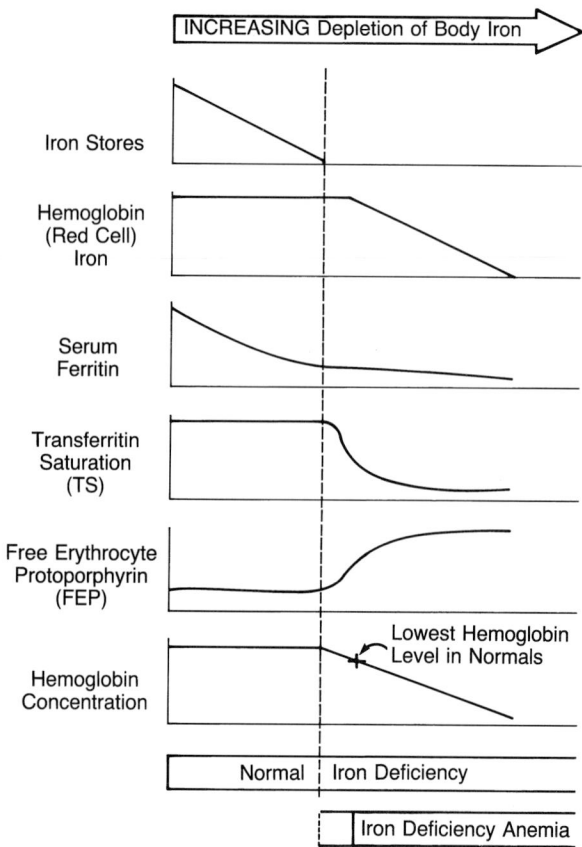

Figure 132–2. Changes in body iron compartments and laboratory parameters of iron status during development of iron deficiency due to a continuous negative iron balance. (From Guidelines for the Eradication of Iron Deficiency. A Report of the International Nutritional Anemia Consultative Group [INACG], 1977.)

is a useful indicator to define the severity of iron deficiency in the community. One common reason for the misdiagnosis of anemia is inadequate laboratory procedures for hemoglobin determination because of capillary blood sampling or due to inaccurate laboratory methods or procedures.

Detection of Anemia by Clinical Examination. In resource-poor settings, where it is not feasible to detect anemia by hemoglobin or hematocrit testing, clinical examination has been widely used to detect those with severe anemia. Clinical evidence regarding pallor of skin, conjunctiva, tongue, and palms is used to formulate an impression. In one study for the detection of severe anemia (hemoglobin <7 g/dL), the sensitivity of clinical detection reached the range of 50 to 60% with 90% specificity.

Biochemistry Testing for Iron Deficiency. For normal individuals, serum ferritin is a good indicator of body iron stores and is useful in assessing the amount of total body iron. Based on quantitative phlebotomy studies, 1 μg/L of serum ferritin is equivalent to 10 mg of stored iron for an average-size adult. Among the multiple tests available for determining iron status, low serum ferritin is the most specific test for iron deficiency (Figs. 132–2 and 132–3). However, low serum ferritin, per se, without other abnormal iron test results indicates only *depleted iron stores.* Low iron stores is a necessary, but not a sufficient, condition for iron deficiency. One major limitation of serum ferritin in defining the extent of body iron stores is the fact that serum ferritin is also an acute-phase reactant and becomes elevated in chronic inflamma-

TABLE 132–2. Definitions Related to Iron Nutritional Status

	Definition	Qualification
Anemia	Hemoglobin below the 5th percentile value of the hemoglobin distribution of healthy individuals of the same sex, age, race, and stage of pregnancy.	A. Iron deficiency is common cause of anemia; conditions other than iron deficiency can result in anemia. B. Baseline prevalence of anemia is 5% when there is no iron deficiency and disease.
Depleted Iron Stores	Low or absent iron stores, but not affecting function and production of iron-dependent cellular components.	A. Low serum ferritin is a criterion. B. Depleted iron stores without other laboratory evidence of iron deficiency is sufficient for diagnosis.
Iron Deficiency	Insufficient iron supply for the proper function and production of iron-dependent cellular components or tissue and physiologic functions.	A. Often characterized by having one or more abnormal tests beyond depleted iron stores, or positive response to iron treatment. B. Anemia not essential for the diagnosis of iron deficiency. C. Iron deficiency without anemia represents milder form of iron deficiency.
Iron Deficiency Anemia	Most severe form of iron deficiency. Hemoglobin production is impaired and criteria for anemia met.	Anemia together with additional laboratory indicators of iron depletion and/or iron deficiency.

tory conditions or acute infections. Transferrin saturation is an indicator of iron transport in plasma. When transferrin saturation is low (<16%), it is often associated with iron deficiency. Elevated transferrin saturation (>55% for women and >60% for men) is a good screening indicator for iron overload due to hereditary hemochromatosis. Besides low serum ferritin, there are other conditions that can cause depressed or elevated transferrin saturation beyond abnormal iron status. Infections and inflammatory conditions often cause depression of serum iron levels, lowering the transferrin saturation value. Serum iron is also sensitive to recent dietary iron intake and there is a diurnal variation, with higher values in the morning and lower values at night. Serum transferrin receptor concentration is also a useful test for iron deficiency. Transferrin receptors on the surface of the red blood cell precursor increase when there is an inadequate supply of iron for the production of hemoglobin. Other than iron deficiency, any condition that results in a high rate of red cell turnover, or increased erythropoiesis, e.g., hemolytic anemia, can also cause the transferrin receptors level to be elevated. The advantage of serum transferrin receptor concentration as an index of iron status is that it is unaffected by infection, inflammation, or anemia of chronic disease. Erythrocyte protoporphyrin, the immediate precursor of hemoglobin, becomes elevated when there is insufficient iron supply for hemoglobin production or when lead is present to interfere with this process. In the United States, this test has been adapted as an outpatient screening for childhood lead poisoning (with an easy-to-operate device known as the hematoflorameter) and appears to be an earlier marker than hemoglobin for iron deficiency. Both infection and inflammatory conditions can cause the erythrocyte protoporphyrin level to be elevated.

MAJOR APPROACHES FOR THE PREVENTION AND CONTROL OF IRON DEFICIENCY. Despite the fact that the general strategy for improving iron nutrition is similar for infants and adult women (i.e., increasing dietary iron intake), the lack of overlap between infant and adult diet requires that separate approaches for intervention be considered. The three general strategies are supplementation through the primary

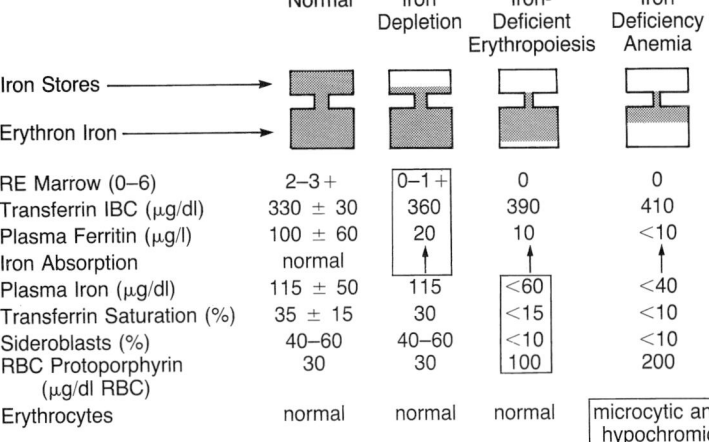

Sequential Changes in the Development of Iron Deficiency

	Normal	Iron Depletion	Iron-Deficient Erythropoiesis	Iron Deficiency Anemia
RE Marrow (0–6)	2–3+	0–1+	0	0
Transferrin IBC (μg/dl)	330 ± 30	360	390	410
Plasma Ferritin (μg/l)	100 ± 60	20	10	<10
Iron Absorption	normal			
Plasma Iron (μg/dl)	115 ± 50	115	<60	<40
Transferrin Saturation (%)	35 ± 15	30	<15	<10
Sideroblasts (%)	40–60	40–60	<10	<10
RBC Protoporphyrin (μg/dl RBC)	30	30	100	200
Erythrocytes	normal	normal	normal	microcytic and hypochromic

Figure 132–3. The sequence of changes induced by gradual reduction in the iron content of the body. (From Bothwell TH, et al.: Iron Metabolism in Man. Oxford, Blackwell Scientific Publications, 1979.)

health care system; food-based approaches, including nutrition education and promotion (dietary selection) (Tables 132–1 and 132–2); and iron fortification through industry-based food processing. These major approaches are not mutually exclusive, and in various settings different approaches would be of greater importance.

Primary Health Care–based Approach—Iron Supplementation and Control of Intestinal Helminth Infection. There are two general approaches to iron supplementation through the primary health care system. One is appropriate for areas where the prevalence of iron deficiency anemia is relatively low, i.e., <10 to 15%, and includes screening for anemia and the provision of iron supplements only to those found to be anemic. The dosage of iron treatment is 3 mg/kg of elemental iron for children under age 5, or 60 mg elemental iron daily for adults for 3 months. The other approach is to provide universal supplementation where the prevalence of iron deficiency anemia is high and where the majority of the population is affected by iron deficiency. For practical purposes, the former approach is suitable for developed areas, and the latter approach is suitable for less developed areas. In most developing countries there is a general lack of adequate iron in the infant diet, and as a result the prevalence of anemia often exceeds 50% by 1 year of age, indicating that the majority of the children are iron deficient. Currently, the United Nations Children's Fund (UNICEF) recommends a daily dose of 12.5 mg of elemental iron for infants 6 to 12 months of age for such purpose. Because there is a lack of low-cost preparation or drops for distribution in developing countries and lack of experience for large-scale supplementation, further evaluation of the feasibility of this approach is indicated. The formulation of iron supplements must take into consideration other nutrients e.g., zinc and vitamin A, which are also likely to be deficient in many developing countries (Chapters 131.1 and 132.3).

By and large, routine iron supplementation is the current cornerstone of efforts to reduce iron deficiency anemia during pregnancy. One major limitation of the iron supplementation approach is the need to establish a system for supply and distribution of iron tablets through the primary health care system. As with any system in which there are multiple steps involved before getting supplies to a target population (iron tablets reaching the hands of women), it is not uncommon to have breakdowns along the supply chain. Poor compliance is another common problem for any medication required over a long period of time by asymptomatic individuals. At higher doses of iron (i.e., >60 mg of elemental iron), gastrointestinal side effects are frequent and contribute to the lack of compliance. To overcome these problems, proper education on the importance of the supplement and its potential side effects is needed as part of the program.

Recent studies from Zanzibar and Vietnam found that the role of hookworm infection can explain up to 40% of the iron deficiency anemia in high endemic areas (Chapter 105.1). In such settings, the potential impact of deworming can be justified as part of the anemia control program. It is safe to deworm women after the first trimester of pregnancy, and the decision for deworming all children and women can be based on local prevalence of the infection, since individual-based screening and treatment may not be feasible.

Nutrition Promotion and an Education-Based Approach—Dietary Diversification and Selection. Among various micronutrients of interest, iron is by far the nutrient with the most advanced knowledge concerning bioavailability from various food items. Factors that can either enhance or inhibit iron absorption have been well studied. Thus far, limited evidence suggests that dietary selection is not an effective approach, mainly because iron-rich food is relatively expensive. Nutrition education can lead to improved feeding patterns and iron status among infants and younger children if iron-fortified food items, e.g., infant cereal, are commonly available. In most developing countries, complementary foods are mainly local items with low iron content and low bioavailability, which can interfere with the absorption of the limited amount of iron in breast milk. Promotion of exclusive breast-feeding can help protect the absorption of iron from breast milk. Promotion of earlier introduction of meat-based complementary foods can also be helpful. In the Middle East and Northern Africa, tea is often introduced during infancy. Education efforts to delay the age of introduction of tea, and avoiding drinking tea near meal times, should be part of the education-based approach.

Industry-Based Approach—Iron Fortification During Food Processing. Iron fortification of commonly consumed food items (in settings where it is feasible) is the most cost-effective option. One of the best examples of the effectiveness in prevention of iron deficiency anemia was demonstrated via the iron and vitamin C fortification of milk powder distributed to lower income families in Chile. For school-age children in Chile, there was also a successful demonstration of the improvement of iron status by providing heme iron–fortified cookies in schools. Iron fortification of common food items, e.g., flour, will affect the iron intake of all segments of the population except for infants. Even though this approach is not specific for women of childbearing age, they stand to gain the most. There are concerns that iron fortification can harm the few who are at risk for iron overload due to various diseases that cause excess iron accumulation. Evidence, thus far, does not support the concept of keeping iron low in a population's food supply as part of the therapy for those with iron overload problems. The more reasonable approach for the few with iron overload disease is through case finding and management.

Bibliography

Bothwell TH, Charlton RW: Iron deficiency in women: A report of the International Nutritional Anemia Consultative Group (INACG). Washington, DC, The Nutrition Foundation, 1981.

Dallman PR, Siimes MA, Stekel A: Iron deficiency in infancy and childhood. Am J Clin Nutr 33:86, 1980.

Pawlowski ZS, Schad GA, Stott GJ: Hookworm infection and anemia: An approach to prevention and control. Geneva, The World Health Organization, 1991.

Yip R: Iron deficiency: Contemporary scientific issues and international programmatic approaches. J Nutr 124:1479S, 1994.

Yip R, Dallman PR: Iron. *In* Filer J, Ziegler E (eds): Current Knowledge in Nutrition, 7th ed. Washington, DC, International Life Science Institute/Nutrition Foundation, 1997.

132.2 Iodine Deficiency Disorders

John T. Dunn

DEFINITION. Iodine deficiency disorders include goiter, hypothyroidism, mental retardation, and iodine-induced hyperthyroidism. All result from inadequate amounts of iodine for the synthesis of thyroid hormones.

NEED FOR IODINE. Iodine is an essential component of the thyroid hormones, thyroxine (T_4) and triiodothyronine (T_3), contributing respectively 64% and 59% of their molecular mass. Inadequate iodine causes insufficient production of thyroid hormone, an important regulator of many metabolic processes, particularly protein synthesis. The minimum daily iodine need for adult humans with normal thyroids is about

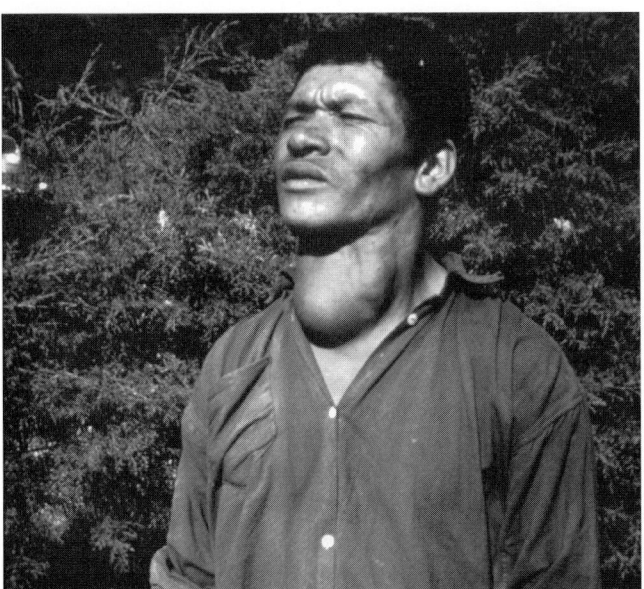

Figure 132–4. A large goiter in a man living in an iodine-deficient area of Bolivia.

75 µg. Children and pregnant women require relatively more. To allow a safe margin, international organizations recommend daily intakes of 150 µg for adults, 50 µg for the first year of life, 90 µg for ages 1 to 7 years, 120 µg for ages 7 to 12 years, and 200 µg for pregnant and lactating women.

Most iodine enters the body as food or water. Seafood is a good source, as are milk, meat, and eggs if they come from iodine-sufficient animals. Industrialized countries have many exogenous sources of iodine including medicines (e.g., amiodarone, vitamin preparations, disinfectants), and prepared foods (e.g., food coloring, bread conditioners). These sources may provide "silent prophylaxis" against iodine deficiency.

The ocean contains about 5 µg iodine/L, but geographic distribution of iodine over the land is quite uneven. New mountains, e.g., the Himalayas, Alps and Andes, and flood plains frequently have iodine-deficient soil. The iodine content may also be quite low in other inland areas, e.g., Central Africa, Central Asia, and the U.S. Great Lakes region. The World Health Organization has estimated that 1.6 billion people live in deficient areas. Iodine deficiency has been effectively eliminated in only a few countries, e.g., the United States, Japan, Canada, United Kingdom, the Scandinavian countries, Switzerland, Austria, and Australia. Most others have significant iodine deficiency in at least part of their territory. The problem is not limited to developing countries; parts of Germany, France, Italy, and Belgium, among others, are also affected. An important conceptual advance was the designation of this topic as "iodine deficiency disorders" rather than confining it to "endemic goiter," because the latter focused attention on one of the mildest consequences of iodine deficiency and was frequently dismissed in favor of other public health problems that appeared more pressing.

CONSEQUENCES OF IODINE DEFICIENCY

Goiter (Fig. 132–4). The pituitary responds to inadequate production of thyroid hormone by increasing its secretion of thyroid-stimulating hormone (TSH: thyrotropin). The net impact is to increase thyroid hormone synthesis and release and to favor T_3 production over that of T_4. The goiter represents an adaptation to iodine deficiency and, if successful, may be the only apparent manifestation, but it has a health importance of its own. Initially, the iodine-deficient thyroid is hyperplastic, but over time becomes nodular and eventually may lead to neck compression, follicular thyroid cancer, or iodine-induced hyperthyroidism.

Hypothyroidism. If the compensation from increased TSH secretion is insufficient, hypothyroidism occurs, typically manifested by slowed metabolism. Thyroid hormone is essential to the proper maturation of the central nervous system, particularly its myelination, and hypothyroidism during early life, including that from iodine deficiency, produces varying degrees of brain damage, particularly mental retardation. Frequently, the more subtle features of this damage escape recognition, but they may have a profound impact on the intellectual vigor of the affected community. Correction of iodine deficiency in such areas improves school performance and scores on intelligence and motor tests. Iodine deficiency affects the brain both by damaging its development and by the effects of hypothyroidism on mentation. The former effects are irreversible but the latter may be corrected by providing adequate iodine for thyroid hormone synthesis or by treating directly with thyroid hormone.

Cretinism (Fig. 132–5). Cretinism is the extreme consequence of iodine deficiency on the developing brain. Cretins have gross mental retardation, and variable degrees of deaf mutism, short stature, squint, and gait disturbances. They have been frequently subcategorized into *neurologic* and *myxedematous* types. Both have severe mental retardation, but neurologic cretins may have normal stature and be clinically euthyroid, whereas the myxedematous have short stature and severe hypothyroidism. Considerable overlap exists between these two subcategories, and the existence of a real distinction is debated. The major damage to the brain in cretinism appears to occur in the second trimester. Myxedematous cretins may, in addition, have exhaustion atrophy of the thyroid and permanent hypothyroidism.

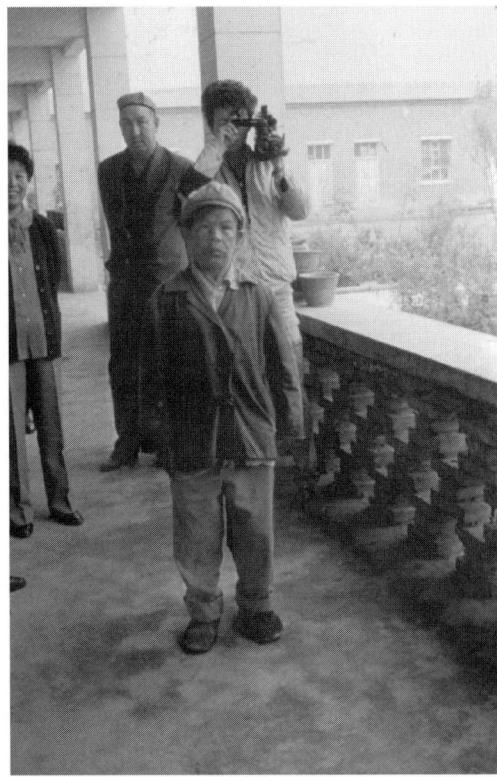

Figure 132–5. A cretin, from western China, with mental retardation, short stature, deaf mutism, and gait disturbance.

Iodine-Induced Hyperthyroidism. Iodine deficiency initially produces a goiter with diffuse hyperplasia, but over time, usually years, autonomous thyroid nodules develop, with the capacity to synthesize thyroid hormone independent of TSH control. Autonomous nodules may produce excessive thyroid hormone when presented with a sudden increase in iodine availability, and hyperthyroidism ensues. Typically this occurs in older subjects and is usually transient. The most severe clinical manifestations are cardiovascular, and when these are not recognized and treated promptly, significant morbidity and death can occur. Iodine-induced hyperthyroidism cannot be prevented entirely, but its morbidity can be minimized with awareness and appropriate treatment. Its public health impact is greatly outweighed by the benefits for the population as a whole from correcting iodine deficiency. The rise in incidence of hyperthyroidism after achieving iodine sufficiency in a population may last one or more years, and then decline to a level lower than that existing before the iodine increase.

Other Consequences. These stem largely from the hypothyroidism. Reproductive loss is a general feature of hypothyroidism and frequently occurs with iodine deficiency. Childhood and neonatal survival also decrease with iodine deficiency. Scattered reports suggest impaired immune tolerance with iodine deficiency, presumably from hypothyroidism. Economic consequences follow from lower intellectual capacity, lower physical stamina, and poorer educability. Iodine deficiency affects domestic animals by lowering production of meat, eggs, wool, and increasing abortions, thus further damaging the economy.

ASSESSMENT OF IODINE DEFICIENCY

Goiter. The size of large thyroids can be adequately estimated by neck palpation. An older scheme defined a goiter as a thyroid each of whose lobes is larger than the terminal phalanx of the subject's thumb. *Grade 1,* or *palpable goiter,* describes thyroid enlargement that is palpable but not visible. *Grade II,* or *visible goiter* refers to enlargement that is visible when the neck is in a normal position. This system gives useful qualitative information when goiters are fairly large, but is inaccurate with smaller thyroids. Ultrasonography provides quantitative information about thyroid size, and allows comparison with measurements from iodine-sufficient areas. Compact instruments can be used in communities for several hundred examinations in a day. Thyroid size, when quantified, is a sensitive and reliable measure for iodine deficiency. Normative data for iodine-sufficient subjects are available, permitting a quantitative definition of enlargement as >2SD from the mean for iodine-sufficient individuals. School-age children are the recommended group for survey because they can be easily assembled and their thyroids reflect recent rather than remote community iodine nutrition. Conditions other than iodine deficiency can cause goiter, but a prevalence greater than 5% usually indicates iodine deficiency. Current guidelines propose the iodine deficiency to be *mild* if the goiter prevalence is 5.0% to 19.9%, *moderate* if 20.0% to 29.9%, and *severe* if 30% or greater.

Urinary Iodine Concentration. Usually 90% or more of ingested iodine eventually reaches the urine, so urinary iodine excretion reflects iodine intake. Community-based investigations have established the median concentration of iodine in casual samples of urine for gauging the level of iodine deficiency. It is much simpler than relating it to creatinine excretion or attempting 24-hour collections. Current guidelines define iodine sufficiency as greater than 100 μg/L urinary iodine, *mild* deficiency as 50 to 99 μg/L, *moderate* deficiency as 25 to 49 μg/L, and *severe* deficiency as below 25 μg/L. Simple chemical methods make this determination feasible in most laboratories, including those in developing countries. Samples may be conveniently collected by a team surveying schoolchildren for goiter.

Serum Thyroid-Related Hormones. A high serum TSH concentration indicates hypothyroidism. Subjects in areas with iodine deficiency typically have a higher median serum TSH concentration than that of iodine-sufficient groups, but it may still be within the normal range. Thus, the serum TSH value has low discriminatory power unless gross hypothyroidism is prevalent. An exception is the neonatal period. Transient hypothyroidism frequently occurs in newborns in areas of iodine deficiency and is detected by transient elevations in neonatal screening with TSH. Such screening is already widely used in the United States, Canada, most Western countries, and Japan to detect congenital hypothyroidism, which occurs approximately once in every 4000 births. The incidence of TSH elevations in newborns may rise to 3% to 5% in areas with iodine deficiency. Thus, this screening provides a sensitive monitoring tool for iodine deficiency. However, to be useful it must be applied to all children born in the country, including those in the most remote impoverished areas.

The serum T_4 concentration is typically low with iodine deficiency and the serum T_3 concentration may be normal or high, but these changes are not sufficiently sensitive to justify the routine use of these measurements. The serum thyroglobulin concentration is a promising test because it reflects hyperplasia and correlates with the degree of iodine deficiency. It is a more reliable indicator than the serum TSH for assessment of older children and adults. The technology is similar to that for TSH and other hormone assays, and commercial kits are available for routine testing.

PREVENTION AND TREATMENT. Iodized salt is the preferred method for correcting iodine deficiency. Salt is a daily dietary necessity, its sources are usually limited and easy to control, and the technology is simple and inexpensive. Potassium iodate is the recommended supplement because it is more stable than potassium iodide. The optimal level of addition can be calculated from the estimated dietary iodine from other sources, the mean daily salt intake, and losses between iodization plant and consumption. For most countries this supplement will be from 20 to 50 mg iodine/kg salt. Alternatively, a single IM injection of iodized vegetable oil, containing 480 mg iodine/mL (Lipiodol), provides coverage for 2 to 3 years, and a single oral administration gives 6 to 12 months of coverage. Another iodization vehicle is drinking water. Iodine supplementation approaches for drinking water include porous polymer baskets that slowly release iodide on immersion in wells, diversion of water through a canister containing iodine crystals, simple addition of an iodine solution daily by dropper into drinking water in schools and homes, or addition of iodine to irrigation water. Bread, sugar, candy, and tea have also been occasionally used as iodization vehicles. Tablets of potassium iodide and Lugol solution can also be used for individuals. The usual choice is iodized salt as a permanent solution, and iodized oil, iodized water, or iodide tablets for urgent correction or for circumstances in which iodized salt is impractical.

Correction of iodine deficiency requires not only a delivery system but a program to support it. Key components include effective introduction of the iodization step into the existing salt trade, education at all levels, and a sound monitoring system. The latter should include regular quality assurance for iodized salt and also periodic surveillance of representative communities, usually by assessing goiter prevalence and median urinary iodine concentrations. Instructive examples from many countries, particularly in Latin America, show that laws requiring iodized salt are not enough by themselves, and initially successful programs can soon fail if not supported by a regular and permanent monitoring system.

The 1990 World Summit for Children pledged the virtual elimination of iodine deficiency by the year 2000. Enormous progress has taken place since then, particularly toward universal salt iodization. In addition to implementing effective prophylaxis measures, attention must constantly be directed to their sustainability.

Bibliography

Delange F: The disorders induced by iodine deficiency. Thyroid 4:107, 1994.

Dunn JT: Seven deadly sins in confronting endemic iodine deficiency, and how to avoid them. J Clin Endocrinol Metab 81:1332, 1996.

Dunn JT, van der Haar F: A Practical Guide to the Correction of Iodine Deficiency. International Council for Control of Iodine Deficiency Disorders, Wageningen, Netherlands, 1990.

Hetzel BS, Dunn JT: The Iodine Deficiency Disorders: Their Nature and Prevention. Annu Rev Nutr 9:21, 1989.

Hetzel BS, Dunn JT, Stanbury JB (eds): The Prevention and Control of Iodine Deficiency Disorders. New York, Elsevier, 1987.

Stanbury JB (ed): The Damaged Brain of Iodine Deficiency. New York, Cognizant Communication Corporation, 1994.

132.3 Zinc and Other Trace Mineral Deficiencies and Excesses

Noel W. Solomons

NUTRITIONAL AND TOXICOLOGIC SCOPE. Trace elements are those that contribute less than 0.01% to the weight of an individual. Essential nutrients are those that predispose to a syndrome of clinical deficiency when the chemical is withdrawn from the diet. Clinical deficiency of iron (Chapter 132.1), iodine (Chapter 132.2), zinc, copper, selenium, chromium, manganese, and molybdenum has been recognized in humans. Fluorine (fluoride) is considered to be a beneficial nutrient. A series of other elements, including lithium, vanadium, boron, strontium, and nickel, are essential in other mammalian species, and are possibly required in human nutrition. Inorganic elements can also accumulate in excess, such that toxicity syndromes are caused by all of the aforementioned trace elements, as well as by tin, cadmium, lead, and mercury.

Assessment of Trace Element Status. Trace element status is difficult to assess, and nutritional deficiencies are hard to detect. There are two general approaches to assessing trace element nutritional status: (1) by static measurements and (2) by functional measures. The former assays the element's concentration in body fluids or tissues. The latter examines the consequences of a contracted supply of the nutrient for cellular, organ, or whole-organism function.

The conventional static measure is the plasma concentration. Circulating levels of zinc, copper, selenium, and chromium are not ideal measures. Functional measures of nutritional status are usually more reliable and valuable, especially in ascertaining the status of a specific patient.

Dietary Sources of Trace Elements. Trace elements are present in higher amounts and are more efficiently absorbed from organ meats or flesh than from seeds, tubers, fruits, or leaves. Since large sections of populations in tropical and subtropical countries have diets predominantly of foods of plant origin, rather than from animal proteins, many are at risk for trace element deficiency.

Interactions With Infection and Other Nutrients. Because of a high prevalence of protein-energy malnutrition, especially the severe, edematous form of kwashiorkor, several trace elements are important in lesser developed countries. Infection can alter the nutritional status with respect to at least one of the trace elements (zinc), and variation in trace element status can affect the response to infection (Chapter 133.1).

◾ ZINC

DEFINITION. Zinc, second to iron as the most abundant trace element in the human body, is an essential nutrient. Of special relevance to developing countries, in which stunting and short stature is pandemic, is the requirement of this element for growth and development. Much of the 2 to 3 g in the normal adult is in bone and skeletal muscle. Organs with a high, specific concentration of zinc include the retina, pancreas, and gonads. The liver is the active metabolic center. Unlike iron, however, zinc does not have a body storage pool, and hence humans are dependent on a constant supply of the mineral. Its major excretion route is from the pancreas and intestine into the feces, with only about 1/20 as much zinc lost in the urine; however, acute infections, renal and hepatic disease, and other pathologic states produce nutritionally significant renal losses.

ZINC PHYSIOLOGY. The best-known metabolic role for zinc is as a component of zinc metalloenzymes, i.e., proteins that require the covalent union with one or more atoms of zinc for their structure, catalytic function, or both. Carbonic anhydrase, alkaline phosphatase, and Zn-Cu superoxide dismutase are among the several hundred zinc metalloenzymes identified in mammalian systems. Some of these are involved in metabolic functions, whereas others have roles in translation and transcription of genetic information for protein synthesis, cell differentiation, and cell division. Additional roles for zinc in these same cellular processes include its action in the stabilization of ribosomes and in forming part of the "zinc-finger" domains of chromatin proteins when a corresponding portion of the DNA strand in the nucleus is in translational activity. Metallothionein (MT) is a binding protein related to the intracellular storage and distribution of zinc. Specific MTs expressed in cells may regulate the metabolism of zinc during cell growth, differentiation, and proliferation. Zinc also plays a role in stabilizing cellular and organellar membranes. In addition to functions in protein synthesis and cellular growth and turnover, zinc has a role in vision in dim light (dark adaptation), in taste and smell acuity, in diverse immune functions, and in reproduction.

DIETARY SOURCES OF ZINC. Zinc is an essential nutrient for plants. Years of cultivation and/or mismanagement of soils can deplete zinc in the soil; both crop yields and zinc content in seeds are reduced. This can have a cascade effect along the food chain.

Oysters of Atlantic Ocean origin and North Sea herring, neither of which is relevant to tropical countries, are the foods richest in zinc. Relatively good sources of zinc, with densities of 12 to 100/1000 kcal, are beef, lamb, organ meats, crustaceans, and some vegetables. Zinc content of fish, fruits, refined cereals, tubers, pastries and baked goods, fats, oils, sweets, and most beverages is low or exceptionally low. However, only among the inhabitants of the Amazon basin have calculations for the nutrient density of a diet suggested zinc to be the most limiting micronutrient. The problem, in addition to a low intake, however, is a low efficiency of zinc's absorption from foods. Dietary fiber and phytic acid, components of unrefined grain and legumes, inhibit zinc uptake, as do the oxalates of green leaves, the tannins in coffee and tea, and the calcium in dairy products.

ZINC REQUIREMENTS AND RECOMMENDED INTAKES.

The United States Committee on Recommended Dietary Allowances (RDA) has recommended the following daily RDA intakes (in mg/day): 5 mg in infants, 10 mg in children <10 years of age, 12 mg for adult women, and 15 mg for adult men. The World Health Organization (WHO) Panel on Trace Elements in Human Health and Nutrition in 1995 took a different tack, providing data for the *mean* zinc intake of population groups which would be compatible with meeting the zinc requirements by all members of the specific group. They outlined two classes of requirement: basal (to prevent deficiencies and adverse consequences) and normative (to maintain desirable tissue levels). They also modeled three possible levels of bioavailability of zinc in the diet: high (50 to 55%); moderate (30 to 35%); and low (15%). For infants on exclusive breast-feeding (high availability), the population daily requirement is 1.5 mg, but up to 8 mg for those on vegetable-based infant formula and weaning foods. The WHO recommendation for a mean intake for basal requirements for 6- to 10-year-old children on a diet of low availability is 10.7 mg and for normative intake requirements, 15 mg. For adult women with a similar diet, the respective basal and normative population mean intakes are 14.6 and 20.6 mg. For adult men, these are set, respectively, at 13.4 and 18.7 mg.

CAUSES AND EFFECTS OF ZINC DEFICIENCY

Infancy. In early infancy, when children are dependent exclusively on breast milk, its zinc content and bioavailability could be a determinant of zinc status and the infant's growth. A WHO survey of trace element breast-milk composition in three industrialized and three developing countries showed in some instances that milk zinc concentrations were greater in poorer countries than in the wealthier ones, and greater in rural milk samples as compared with urban ones. Typically, intakes of zinc from human milk are 1/5 to 1/10 of the RDA for infants, but zinc in this food is very biologically available, appearing to compensate for the low intakes. Attempts to enhance breast-milk zinc by orally supplementing mothers have shown equivocal and inconsistent results in terms of milk zinc and no effect on zinc status of the infant. Several nutrients may be limiting for growth in exclusively breast-fed children; total energy and zinc are two of them. Unless weaning foods are given, the amount of zinc in human milk may not provide for adequate infant growth after 5 months of age.

Pregnancy and the Fetus. The fetus is also vulnerable to zinc deficiency. Compromised zinc nutriture or metabolism in the mother can lead to anatomic anomalies, including defects of development of the neural tube. Higher rates of delivery complications and poor birth outcomes have also been documented in mothers. Iron supplements in prenatal nutrient pills depress circulating zinc levels. The combination of marginal, preconception zinc status, increased zinc demands of pregnancy, and its reduced absorption due to the interference from pharmacologic doses of iron could increase the teratologic and adverse pregnancy outcomes associated with gestational zinc deficiency.

Magnitude of Zinc Deficiency. Given the consequences of low zinc status for fetus, infant, and mother, there is scientific interest in determining whether zinc deficiency is widely endemic in lesser developed countries, or restricted to certain narrow regions and to clinical situations. Zinc intervention trials have evaluated whether acceleration of linear growth occurs following supplementation. In these circumstances, it is assumed that a trophic response to supplemental zinc is evidence for existence of an endemic background of deficiency. To date, positive responses have been limited to the toddler and preschool groups, and this only in certain geographic regions. However, the design of most of these zinc supplementation trials leaves open the possibility that *simultaneous* deficiency of other growth-limiting nutrients masked or attenuated any benefits from zinc.

Zinc Deficiency in Acquired Immunodeficiency Syndrome. A special interest in zinc nutrition in human immunodeficiency (HIV) infection has emerged in the wake of the AIDS pandemic. Nutritional status indicators of zinc, vitamin B_6, and other vitamins are altered in HIV-positive individuals, and the oral intakes (food plus supplements) needed to achieve normal levels require multiples of the RDA established for healthy individuals. Increased requirements, reduced absorption, and/or increased wastage may be operating in patients with AIDS (Chapter 23). Modulation of the immune response may result from a lowered zinc status. Whether this works in favor—or to the detriment—of the function, well-being, and viral progression in HIV infection, however, is not known.

Zinc Deficiency During Diarrheal Illness. Episodes of acute diarrhea increase the excretion of zinc. This has increased interest in providing small amounts of zinc in oral rehydration solutions to replace diarrheal losses. Oral zinc may be *therapeutic* and beneficial in acute diarrhea when administered in dosages of 20 mg of elemental zinc. Moreover, zinc supplementation trials in Mexico and Guatemala have shown a prophylactic effect in lowering the incidence of diarrheal episodes. Whether it works via the nutritional status of the host or by a local, antiseptic effect on the gut flora has not been determined. Finally, there is preliminary evidence of an association of low zinc status and giardiasis (see Chapter 87). It is not known whether low zinc status predisposes to giardiasis or infections with *Giardia lamblia* deplete body levels of zinc.

Zinc and Lathyrism. Lathyrism is one of the oldest neurotoxic diseases known to humankind. It is related to the grass pea (genus *Lathyrus*) and the neurotoxin, 3-oxalyl-L-2,3-diaminopropanoic acid, and is manifested by paresthesias, tremors, and spastic paralysis (Chapter 133.3). It is endemic in regions in which legumes in general, and grass peas in particular, are consumed. It has been suggested that zinc deficiency in the soil leads to a greater expression of the neurotoxin in the seeds, thus increasing the toxic hazards from consuming this food.

ASSESSMENT OF ZINC STATUS. No reliable indices of zinc nutriture are available for assessment of zinc in both clinical situations and at the population level. A number of factors are recognized as being responsible for the lack of accuracy and precision in assessment of zinc status.

Types of Nutrient Deficiencies. Golden has classified nutrient deficiencies into two classes: type I and type II.

Type I Deficiency. This is the classic situation in which restriction in the diet and/or loss from the body will result in a depletion of nutrient stores and a desaturation from tissues. Iron, vitamin A, and vitamin B_{12} deficiencies follow this model. Hence, any marker in body fluids or biopsy material that parallels tissue concentrations or body stores can differentiate nutritional states and classify an individual as deficient, marginal, or adequate in particular nutrient status.

Type II Deficiency. This occurs among those nutrients not having an appreciable storage pool in the body, including nitrogen, magnesium, chloride, sodium, potassium, and zinc. Fluctuations in either circulating or intracellular concentrations of these nutrients are not easily tolerated. Faced with restriction or involuntary wastage, the body reacts by reducing turnover and conserving the total-body supply by reduced output via the physiologic excretion routes. In the case of growing children there is an immediate cessation of growth to further protect critical concentrations.

DIAGNOSTIC MEASUREMENTS

Zinc Measurement. Zinc levels in plasma and tissue are the most commonly sought indices of zinc status, but its concentration in all cellular elements of the blood (red blood cells, white blood cells, platelets) has also been used. The latter are less susceptible to acute redistribution but the large samples of blood required and the tedious differential preparative separation of the cells make this impractical for most laboratories in developing countries. For assessment of a population, the mean and distribution of circulating zinc is generally valid.

Functional Indicators. Indices of physiologic functions of the mineral, e.g., growth, taste, acuity, night vision, immune function, and gonadal function, have been applied to assess zinc status in populations. These indicators, however, are nonspecific and generally require a trial of zinc supplementation to confirm the linkage of dysfunction to zinc deficiency.

Other Procedures. The gold standard for determining zinc nutriture in the individual is isotopic dilution and turnover studies, but these are impractical in the clinical setting. Recently, two novel approaches have been suggested for individual assessment of zinc status: determination of messenger RNA for specific MTs and the in vitro dynamics of zinc uptake by blood cells in serum.

POPULATION-BASED STRATEGIES TO IMPROVE ZINC STATUS. Supplementation, fortification, and food-based strategies constitute the generic approaches to increasing the intakes of nutrients. For a nutrient that is poorly stored, such as zinc, supplementation is likely to be inappropriate except in the context of therapy for zinc depletion. Finding an appropriate vehicle, e.g., water, salt, sugar, or staple (cereal, flour or bread), that will consistently and predictably reach those with marginal zinc status is difficult in a population-based fortification approach. In addition, there is no good mechanism for adding zinc salts to a diet, although zinc is inorganic, nonoxidizing, and stable. Food-based strategies focus on getting more zinc-rich foods into the diet, or getting more zinc into zinc-poor foods. Combined with more zinc in fertilizers, a richer zinc content in the diet would be possible.

Since interfering substances in the diet play such an important role in zinc absorption, measures aimed more at enhancing uptake of zinc than at increasing its intake should be considered. No external enhancer, such as ascorbic acid for iron, is known to improve zinc's absorbability. The reduction of the content of phytate in grains and reduction in fiber content of plant foods are theoretical considerations. The challenge of potential pockets of endemic zinc deficiency should motivate an investigation into new technology for enhancing zinc intake (or uptake) from diets, and promote effectiveness trials in affected populations.

ZINC EXCESS AND TOXICITY. Excessive zinc can represent a hazard to the environment and to human health. The Environmental Protection Agency has recommended that oral exposure to the metal not exceed 21 mg/day. The WHO (1995) presented recommendations based on mean intakes for a population. As a group, the mean upper safe limits for the population of infants would be 13 mg/day; for adult women, 35 mg/day; and for adult men, 45 mg/day. Nutrient supplements possibly represent the most common form for the occurrence of excessive zinc intakes across the world.

The adverse consequences of excessive oral intake of zinc are largely gastrointestinal and nutritional. High intakes of zinc salts produce an unpleasant metallic taste and can produce gastric irritation and hemorrhagic erosions of the stomach. Oral zinc in doses of 100 to 150 mg/day can control accumulation of copper in Wilson disease, and it has been implicated in provoking copper deficiency in normal persons when consumed in doses of >50 mg/day. The two elements need not be consumed simultaneously to produce this interference. High-dose zinc interferes with the absorption of iron, generally when consumed concurrently. Zinc taken with meals may represent an additional contributing factor to the low bioavailability for inorganic iron. Intakes of supplemental zinc of >300 mg/day are also associated with hypercholesterolemia and a depressed immune response.

High, acute influxes of zinc by a parenteral route occur only under unusual situations, e.g., with an unlicensed, injectable medicinal preparation; poorly formulated dialysis baths in hemodialysis; or inadvertent overdose in the mineral admixtures for parenteral alimentation. The consequence of a high parenteral dose of zinc is a hyperamylasemia and fulminating pancreatitis, often with a fatal outcome.

■ COPPER

DEFINITION. Copper is essential by virtue of its role in enzymes that have oxidation-reduction functions involving molecular oxygen and oxygen reactive substances. Body content of copper is from 80 to 120 mg in the adult. The majority of the body's copper is found in the liver. Ceruloplasmin is the physiologic transport protein for copper. Copper is efficiently absorbed from the diet in the absence of specific inhibiting substances. Excretion of copper is through the bile into the fecal stream. There is little reabsorption of biliary copper.

DIETARY SOURCES OF COPPER. Copper is abundant in organ meats and green leafy herbs, and is found in very low amounts in rice, milk, and dairy items. Breast milk is especially poor in this element. Prematurity is also a factor, as the liver content of copper and capability of the fetus to handle this nutrient develop late in the final trimester.

COPPER REQUIREMENTS AND RECOMMENDED INTAKES. The estimated dietary requirement levels for copper are available from two sources: (1) the National Research Council's RDA Committee in its *Recommended Dietary Allowances* (1989) recommends an estimated safe and adequate daily dietary intake (ESADDI) for copper of 1.5 to 3.0 mg for adults. Infants should ingest between 0.4 and 0.7 mg daily. For children ages 7 to 10 years, the recommended range is 1 to 2 mg. (2) The WHO Expert Panel in *Trace Elements in Human Health and Nutrition* (1996) recommends a mean daily intake of copper of at least 1.15 mg for adult women and 1.35 mg for adult men. Formula-fed infants as a group should ingest from 0.3 to 0.6 mg daily, whereas 0.75 mg represents the recommended mean level for children ages 6 to 10 years. These intake levels are not individual recommendations, but rather they represent the bases to evaluate the risk of suboptimal or excess copper intake in populations.

CAUSES AND EFFECTS OF COPPER DEFICIENCY. Copper deficiency is most common in infants. It is especially common in preterm infants, as the majority of in utero transfer of copper to the fetus occurs in the last trimester. The low content of copper in both bovine and maternal milk is a contributing factor. Overt copper deficiency after infancy is seen almost exclusively as an iatrogenic condition, either with total parenteral nutrition or overprescription of oral zinc. It results in a hypochromic anemia, neutropenia, and osseous and connective tissue abnormalities. Hypopigmentation and hypothermia are additional manifestations of copper deficiency.

High intakes of ascorbic acid, iron, zinc, sucrose, and fructose decrease the biologic availability of copper. Acute and persistent diarrheal episodes are associated with excessive losses of copper in watery stools.

Magnitude of Copper Deficiency. Copper deficiency in

early life is associated with prematurity, deprivation, and malnutrition. In Chile, children hospitalized with protein-energy malnutrition were more likely to be copper deficient than zinc deficient and supplementation with 2 mg of copper daily produced enhanced growth and improved immune indices (Chapter 130). Marginal copper deficiency is suspected in children and adults with its consequence reflected in chronic disease, e.g., cardiovascular disease and osteoporosis.

ASSESSMENT OF COPPER STATUS. Overt copper deficiency can be diagnosed based on its clinical and radiologic manifestations. Copper toxicity also presents symptoms and biochemical abnormalities. Milder, marginal forms of copper imbalance are difficult to assess.

Copper deficiency occurs in three settings: (1) in premature children born in disadvantaged conditions and fed milk and rice diets; (2) in protein-energy malnourished children rehabilitated with an unsupplemented, milk-based diet; and (3) in total parenteral alimentation. The former two are relevant to tropical populations. Immune deficiencies are documented in copper-deficient individuals, and recovery from protein-energy malnutrition is enhanced by supplementation of the rehabilitation diets with copper. Also, marginal copper status of the mother has been postulated as a contributor to the idiopathic teratogenesis responsible for many birth defects in the developing world.

Diagnostic Measurements. The serum copper and copper binding proteins, notably ceruloplasmin, can be measured in many clinical chemistry laboratories. However, inflammation, infection, pregnancy, and other hormonal changes can elevate ceruloplasmin, a situation that might mask an underlying nutritional deficiency. In vitro tests to measure the activity of specific cuproenzymes represent another approach, which is seldom clinically available to assess the status of copper.

POPULATION-BASED STRATEGIES TO IMPROVE COPPER STATUS. Supplementation, fortification, and food-based strategies constitute the generic approaches to increasing the intakes of nutrients. For those at specific risk, such as premature infants and malnourished children, copper supplementation of liquid formulas is important.

COPPER EXCESS AND TOXICITY. Excessive copper can represent a hazard to the environment and to human health. Acute intoxication with copper salts can cause fulminant and fatal hepatic necrosis and hemolytic anemia. Taking copper-laden herbicides is a favored form of suicide in certain regions of the world. In smaller amounts (>3 mg), copper salts are an emetic producing nausea and vomiting.

Wilson disease is a hereditary disease of copper accumulation leading to hepatic cirrhosis and neurologic and renal abnormalities. Indian childhood cirrhosis, a juvenile form of progressive hepatic fibrosis, most commonly found in—but not restricted to—the Indian subcontinent, has been related to excessive exposure to environmental copper (Chapter 5). Specifically, in high-caste Hindu families, milk was boiled in copper alloy (brass) vessels. A prevention campaign in the mass media to avoid copper cookware has reduced the incidence of this infirmity in recent years.

■ FLUORINE

DEFINITION. Fluorine, most commonly referred to as fluoride for its monovalent anion form in solution, is a halogen related chemically to chlorine, bromine, and iodine. Early epidemiologic studies showed that dental caries was reduced with consumption of water with a high fluorine content. This element converts the more amorphous osteocalcium phosphate into hydroxyapatite crystals in hard tissues, e.g., bone and teeth.

DIETARY SOURCES. Fluorine is found in both water and diversely in foods. It is 90% absorbable from the former and 30 to 60% is absorbed from the diet. A typical potable-water concentration is 1 part per million (1 mg/L), and the usual fluorine intake ranges from 0.5 to 2 mg/day in adults from both water and diet. For infants, breast milk can be the sole source of the element, with intakes ranging from 5 to 70 μg/day.

RECOMMENDED INTAKES OF FLUORINE. Since fluorine is desirable—but not *essential*—few expert bodies have specified a requirement level. Maximal water concentrations and maximal daily intakes to avoid dental mottling from fluorosis have been elaborated.

Magnitude of Fluoride Scarcity. Low fluorine intakes are seen where water content is less than 0.3 parts per million, and it relates to the geochemical properties of the soils that are leached into the water supply. Low fluorine intakes are associated with higher incidences of dental caries.

ASSESSMENT OF FLUORIDE STATUS. No indices of fluoride status that assess total-body fluoride are commonly available. Moreover, no functional tests of fluoride nutriture have been developed.

Diagnostic Measurements. Blood fluoride has been used to assess the status of this element; normal levels are 0.4 μg/dL and levels in excess of 5 μg/dL occur in areas of endemic, clinical fluorosis. Urinary concentrations of fluoride are indicative of recent oral intake, as 80% of the element ingested is excreted by the kidneys. Urinary concentrations of >1 mg/24 hours are compatible with excessive intakes.

For fluorosis, the characteristic mottling of teeth in a population, confirmed by a high environmental exposure, is diagnostic.

POPULATION-BASED STRATEGIES TO IMPROVE FLUORINE STATUS. Supplementation, fortification, and food-based strategies constitute the generic approaches to increasing intake of nutrients. Adding fluoride to natural water reservoirs or artificial water-holding areas has been the strategy to reduce dental caries rates in low-fluorine regions. Fluoride fortification of foods could be an alternative but greater inconsistency of intake throughout the population occurs.

FLUORINE EXCESS AND TOXICITY. There is only a narrow range of fluoride intake compatible with optimal health. Generally, intakes of fluoride from water <1.5 mg/day have been considered safe for adults and older children, and not conducive to mottling. For infants this daily limit is 0.5 mg, and for toddlers, it is 1.0 mg. Daily intakes of 5 mg of fluorides are associated with skeletal deformities in adults.

Excessive fluorine as fluoride leads to dental mottling (fluorosis) and dental destruction. Excess fluoride intake produces alterations in skeletal mineralization and bone accretion, collagen formation, and reactive hyperparathyroidism. In areas of high environmental fluorine, with intakes of 5 to 40 mg/day, vertebral curvature and deformities of other joints, notably the knees, may occur. When the intake of fluoride from birth to adolescence is over 10 mg/day, endemic genu valgum (bow-leggedness) can occur, as seen in India, Kenya, and Tanzania (Chapter 14). The combination of high fluorine and low calcium intake leads to a form of osteomalacia, due to inhibition of calcium insertion into bone osteoid.

Two possible approaches to prevention and control of fluorosis are (1) reducing the fluoride content of water (defluoridation); and (2) obtaining alternative water sources for the population. Both of these options run into severe constraints. The removal of fluoride from water sources is prohibitively expensive, more costly than most affected populations can afford. Given the pressures on all water sources from growing populations, there is little likelihood that a nearby, unexploited water supply would be available for use by a fluorosis-exposed population.

■ SELENIUM

DEFINITION. Selenium is an essential element related chemically to sulfur on the periodic table. It is a component of glutathione peroxidase, an enzyme involved in the antioxidant system which reduces hydrogen peroxide to oxygen and water, such that more dangerous oxygen-reactive species, e.g., the hydroxyl radical, are not generated. Recently other selenoproteins with specific metabolic functions have been identified. The body contains 6 to 10 mg of selenium. It can metabolize and use inorganic selenium, and seleno amino acids. In tissue proteins, selenium exists as a substitution of sulfur on cysteine.

DIETARY SOURCES OF SELENIUM. Seafood and fish are leading sources of selenium. The ocean waters have relatively abundant amounts of the element. The amount in the terrestrial food-chain depends on the content of the soil. Selenium is not an essential nutrient for plants, and the amount incorporated is a passive consequence of the soil concentration. In plant tissue, selenomethionine is the primary organified form. Selenium from game and livestock is dependent on its amount in the animals' diets. In animal tissue, selenocysteine is the chemical form of the dietary element. Milk and infant formulas are two foods that are notably poor in selenium.

SELENIUM REQUIREMENTS AND RECOMMENDED INTAKES. The National Research Council's RDA Committee in its *Recommended Dietary Allowances* (1989) recommended a daily intake of selenium of 70 μg/day for adult men and 55 μg/day for adult women. For newborn infants, 10 μg of the element is required daily, whereas for school-age children it is 30 μg. The WHO Expert Panel in *Trace Elements in Human Health and Nutrition* (1996) recommends a daily mean intake of selenium of 30 μg/day for adult women and 40 μg/day for adult men. Their average group level recommendation for infants is 6 to 9 μg/day, whereas 25 μg represents the average adequate selenium intake for children ages 6 to 10 years.

CAUSES AND EFFECTS OF SELENIUM DEFICIENCY. Clinical manifestations of selenium deficiency are myositic myopathies and hemolysis. In the former, both skeletal and cardiac muscles are involved with a degenerative process; the cardiomyopathy can be fatal. Characteristic dyspigmentation and structural changes in hair (pseudoalbinism) and nails have been noted in selenium deficiency in children.

Interactions with Protein-Energy Malnutrition. Golden and Ramath proposed that antioxidants impact on the pathogenesis of the edematous form of protein-energy malnutrition (Chapter 130). Selenium, through its role in the control of peroxides, and other antioxidant nutrients are believed to be cofactors in the edematous form of kwashiorkor.

Enzymes that function in the metabolism of iodine to thyroid hormones are selenium dependent. Hence, full expression of adequate iodine nutriture cannot occur in the presence of selenium deficiency. Knowledge about the synergistic interaction of selenium and iodine deficiencies has led to speculation that it is the *selenium* ecology of a region that determines whether endemic cretinism will be of the myxedematous type, as seen in central Africa, or of the neurologic and sensory-deficit variety. In The Democratic Republic of the Congo, which has both types of cretinism, a rough correlation of hyposeleniferous soils and myxedematous cretinism has fostered credence for this theory.

Keshan Disease. Two endemic diseases of central and eastern Asia are believed to involve low environmental selenium levels, limited amounts of the element in the food chain, and consequently marginal selenium status in the human population. One of these is Keshan disease, named for a province in China. It manifests as a severe, progressively fatal cardiomyopathy associated with congestive heart failure; it is common in preschool and young schoolchildren. Populations where this disease is endemic have glutathione peroxidase levels 43% lower than that of well-nourished controls. Supplementation with sodium selenite pills has reduced the incidence of Keshan disease.

Kashin-Beck Disease. The environmental, dietary, and nutritional aspects of selenium have also been implicated in the endemicity of Kashin-Beck disease, an osteoarthropathy affecting children and adolescents, which is prevalent in China, Siberia, and Korea.

ASSESSMENT OF SELENIUM STATUS. Selenium levels in plasma and whole blood have been used as indices of status of the mineral, but their reliability is unproved. Selenoprotein P, the primary transport protein, has been used as a correlate of body selenium status. A functional test, based on the activity of glutathione peroxidase, is considered the most valid for assessing selenium status and its response to changes. Its levels in platelets are more sensitive than those in red blood cells.

As an index of dietary selenium intake in populations that wear shoes, the selenium content in toenails has been measured. Hair selenium has been less useful as a nutritional indicator since the advent of selenium-containing antidandruff shampoos. Measuring selenium in hen's eggs, particularly the selenium content of the yolk, is a good index of the element in the soil.

POPULATION-BASED STRATEGIES TO IMPROVE SELENIUM STATUS. Most approaches to alleviating hyposelenosis in populations have involved adding it into the food chain. In New Zealand and Australia this has taken the form of supplementing edible livestock such as sheep and cattle with selenite in the feed. Over a decade ago, in Finland, a nationwide campaign to place selenium directly into the soil via fertilizers was begun. Evaluation of foodstuffs and the population indicates successful improvement in selenium nutriture using these techniques. In China, in areas endemic for Keshan disease, mass distribution of sodium selenite tablets reduced the high incidence of this malady.

SELENIUM EXCESS AND TOXICITY. Excessive zinc can represent a hazard to the environment and to human health. The WHO recommends 400 μg/day as the upper safe range of adult population mean intakes of selenium. *Hyper*seleniferous areas, with high soil concentrations of selenium, are present, most extensively in Venezuela and China. Daily intakes of up to 7 mg/day of selenium have been documented in areas of China in which seleniferous coal has lost its selenium into the soil. Selenium toxicosis occurs following high intakes due to hyperseleniferous soils or from industrial exposures to both inorganic and organic forms of the element. The manifestations of selenosis include changes in the morphology of the fingernails and loss of hair. With established accumulation, the garlic-smelling breath of dimethylselenides is detectable. Nonspecific constitutional symptoms include fatigue and listlessness.

■ CHROMIUM

DEFINITION. Chromium is found in many valence states but the chromic (III) and chromate (IV) forms are the most stable and most ubiquitous. It is an essential nutrient. Chromium is suspected to function in a complexed form in the chromic (trivalent) oxidation state as the "glucose-tolerance factor" participating in the regulation of insulin.

Chromium is poorly absorbed, with uptake varying from 0.5 to 2% in the range of usual dietary intakes. Type I diabetic patients have an adaptation by which they absorb 2 to 4 times as much chromium from the diet as normal individuals at any given intake level.

Chromium is transported in the circulation on one of the two binding sites of transferrin. In iron overload states, e.g., acquired hemosiderosis (transfusion), African-type (genetic) siderosis, or hemochromatosis where the transferrin saturation is >50%, transport capacity from chromium is reduced and retention in the body is impaired. Excretion is primarily through the urine in proportion to intake.

DIETARY SOURCES OF CHROMIUM. The richest food source is brewer's yeast. Meat and whole grains are also good sources, as are fermented alcoholic beverages, e.g., beer and wine. Milled flours, fruits, vegetables, and milk (including breast milk) are poor sources. Adventitial contamination of the diet by chromium leached from stainless (chrome) steel alloys, in the presence of acidic foods and beverages, often contributes more chromium to the diet than the intrinsic element in the foods themselves.

RECOMMENDED INTAKES OF CHROMIUM. The National Research Council's RDA Committee in its *Recommended Dietary Allowances* (1989) has established an ESADDI for chromium of 50 to 200 μg for all individuals over the age of 7 years. For infants and young children the daily intake should be 10 to 40 μg. Studies in the United States have shown usual intakes from men and women to be 25 and 33 μg, respectively, which are chronically below the lower limit of the ESADDI for that nation. Individuals with glucose intolerance and diabetes have higher chromium requirements.

CAUSES AND EFFECTS OF CHROMIUM DEFICIENCY. Overt chromium deficiency has been described in patients undergoing total parenteral nutrition without supplementation. The manifestations are severe hyperglycemia and neuropathy. Milder syndromes, including fasting hyperglycemia, growth impairment, hyperlipidemia, glaucoma, and excessive body fat in the elderly and diabetics, respond to external chromium supplementation.

Studies from the Middle East and Africa in the late 1960s reported that glucose intolerance in patients with kwashiorkor or milder forms of protein-energy malnutrition responded to exogenous administration of chromium.

ASSESSMENT OF CHROMIUM STATUS. No static index of chromium is able to assess individual status of the nutrient. Only the serial monitoring of glucose, insulin, and lipids before and during supplementation with the element can provide a reliable individual diagnosis. Low urinary excretion of chromium on a *population* basis might be used for epidemiologic assessment.

CHROMIUM EXCESS AND TOXICITY. Chromium has a high tolerance of intake. A 350-fold excess over the ESADDI level is considered to be safe when the element is in the *trivalent* (chromic) state. The hexavalent (chromate) form is found in industrial settings and in paints. This is internalized through the lung membranes in fumes or in particulate form in foods. It is an order of magnitude more toxic than the chromic variety.

▪ MANGANESE, MOLYBDENUM, AND THE ULTRATRACE ELEMENTS

In animal models, deprivation of molybdenum, manganese, lithium, vanadium, boron, and nickel have all resulted in deficiency manifestations. Human syndromes associated with deficiency of manganese and molybdenum have been described, but only under very special circumstances.

MANGANESE. This has an essential role in the post-transcriptional addition of the sugar moieties to glycoproteins in mucus. It is also part of the manganoenzymes: Mn superoxide dismutase and pyruvate carboxylase. Although deficiency of manganese is virtually unknown in humans, indicators of manganese status decline in persons on exclusive parenteral feeding. The estimated dietary requirement level for manganese has been established for adults as 2 to 5 mg. Manganese excess has caused illness. Industrial exposures produce a parkinson-like neuropathy due to selective accumulation of the metal in the basal ganglia. Since manganese is excreted in the bile, its excess accumulation occurs with cholestatic conditions, and could be a consideration in patients with obstructive jaundice due to drinking noxious herbal infusions (bush teas).

MOLYBDENUM. This element is a component of the molybdenum cofactor in the enzymes xanthine oxidase, sulfite oxidase, and aldehyde oxidase. Congenital deficiency of the molybdenum cofactor sulfite oxidase causes abnormal disposal of sulfur from sulfur amino acids, which produces mental retardation and dislocation of the ocular lenses. No dietary deficiency of molybdenum has been documented. Intake requirement has been estimated to be around 25 μg/day for a healthy adult. The body regulates the molybdenum pool by intestinal and renal mechanisms and it is probable that individuals can tolerate both lower and higher customary intakes without diverse consequences. In ruminant animals, certain fodder as well as the combination of high levels of copper and marginal levels of molybdenum causes a deficiency syndrome of agroindustrial importance.

Bibliography

Allen LH: Nutritional influences on linear growth: a general review. Eur J Clin Nutr 48(Suppl 1):S75, 1994.

Cousins RJ: Zinc. *In* Filer JL, Ziegler E (eds): Present Knowledge in Nutrition, chap 29. Washington, DC, International Life Sciences Institute, 1996, pp 297–306.

Golden MHN: Diagnosis of zinc deficiency. *In* Mills CF (ed): Zinc in Human Biology. London, Springer-Verlag, 1989, pp 323–332.

Golden MHN, Ramath D: Free radicals in the pathogenesis of kwashiorkor. Proc Nutr Soc 46:53, 1987.

Kohrle J, Oertel M, Gross M: Selenium supply regulates thyroid function, thyroid hormone synthesis and metabolism by altering the expression of the selenoenzymes Type I 5'-deiodinase and glutathione peroxidase. Thyroidol Clin Exp 4:17, 1992.

Lambein F, Haque R, Khan JK, et al: From soil to brain: Zinc deficiency increases the neurotoxicity of *Lathyrus sativus*, and may affect the susceptibility for the motor neurone disease, neurolathyrism. Toxicon 32:461, 1994.

Levander OA: A global view of human selenium nutrition. Annu Rev Nutr 7:227, 1987.

Mertz W: The essential trace elements. Science 18:1332, 1981.

National Research Council: Recommended Dietary Allowances, 9th ed. Washington, National Academy of Science Press, 1989.

Nielsen FH: Ultratrace elements of possible importance to human health: An update. Progress Clin Biol Res 380:355, 1993.

Ruz M, Solomons NW: Fecal excretion of endogenous zinc during oral rehydration therapy for acute diarrhea: nutritional implications. J Trace Elem Exp Med 7:89, 1995.

Sazawai S, Black RE, Bhan MK, et al: Zinc supplementation in young children with acute diarrhoeas in India. N Engl J Med 333:839, 1995.

Shrimpton R: Zinc deficiency—is it widespread but under-recognized. SCN News 9:24, 1993.

Solomons NW: Biological, ecological and social origins of trace element deficiencies in developing countries. *In* Wahlqvist ML, Truswell AS, Smith R, Nestel PJ (eds): Nutrition in a Sustainable Environment. Proceedings of the XV International Congress of Nutrition. London, Smith-Gordon, 1994, pp 299–302.

Turnlund JR, Keyes WR, Peiffer GL, Chiang G: Molybdenum absorption, excretion, and retention studied with stable isotopes in young men during depletion and repletion. Am J Clin Nutr 62:790, 1995.

Walsh CT, Sandstead HH, Prasad AS, et al: Zinc: Health effects and research priorities for the 1990s. Environ Health Perspect 102(Suppl 2):5, 1994.

World Health Organization: Trace Elements in Human Health and Nutrition. Geneva, WHO, 1996.

Xia Y, Hill KE, Burk RF: Biochemical studies of a selenium-deficient population in China: Measurement of selenium, glutathione peroxidase, and other oxidant defense indices in the blood. J Nutr 119:1318, 1989.

133 Other Nutrition-Related Disorders

133.1 Interactions Between Nutrition and Infection

William R. Beisel

Nutrition interacts with generalized infectious diseases in many ways. The combination of infection and malnutrition is the world's most lethal threat to humans, especially the infants and children and expectant and nursing mothers of tropical lands. Fever and other infection-induced reactions cause sizable losses of body nutrients. Malnutrition, in turn, influences susceptibility, severity, and duration of generalized infections.

EFFECTS OF INFECTION ON BODY NUTRITION. Losses of body nutrients during generalized febrile infections are induced by proinflammatory cytokines (i.e., interleukins-1, -6, and -8, tumor necrosis factor, and interferon gamma) and the acute phase reactions they initiate. Cytokine-induced acute phase reactions cause the signs and symptoms of illness: fever, malaise, myalgias and arthralgias, anorexia, nausea and vomiting, somnolence, plus a wide assortment of metabolic, physiologic, and endocrinologic responses. Metabolic and nutritional changes develop in a relatively stereotyped longitudinal, organism-independent progression during all febrile infections. (Fig. 133–1.)

Although acute phase reactions help defend the body, they incur large nutritional costs, which include

1. Loss of weight, muscle mass, nitrogen and other intra-cellular elements (e.g., potassium, phosphorus, magnesium, zinc, sulfur).
2. Intensified expenditure of energy.
3. A diminished intake and intestinal absorption of nutrients.
4. Augmented metabolic degradation (or direct loss) of vitamins, amino acids, and lipids.

Weeks or months of convalescent refeeding may be required before infection-induced losses of body nitrogen and minerals are fully restored. Atrophy of lymphoid tissues induced by malnutrition cannot be corrected completely without restoration of body zinc. Failure to replete body potassium may result in prolonged metabolic alkalosis, manifested by abnormally high concentrations of plasma bicarbonate. Vitamin deficiencies induced by infection may lead to beriberi, pellagra, scurvy, and ocular pathologies caused by vitamin A deficiency.

Cytokine-Induced Malnutrition. Whenever invading microorganisms activate macrophages and other cells, proinflammatory cytokines are released. Cytokines seek out appropriate cell-surface receptors in diverse organs and tissues throughout the body. Wide varieties of cellular responses are thereby initiated.

In the central nervous system, the temperature regulating center creates fever, while other centers induce anorexia, somnolence, and the release (or suppression) of pituitary hormones. In skeletal muscle, contractile proteins are degraded, and their amino acids released. In the liver, albumin production is slowed, but other proteins are made: enzymes, acute phase reactant plasma proteins (e.g., C-reactive protein, haptoglobin, orosomucoid, amyloid, fibrinogen, and ceruloplasmin), lipoproteins, and metallothionein. The liver also increases its production of glucose, glycogen, and fatty acids. Simultaneously, lymphocytes are stimulated, and phagocytic cells are synthesized.

Endocrine responses stimulate additional metabolic, biochemical, and physiologic activities; adrenocorticotropic hormone, cortisol, aldosterone, growth hormone, and antidiuretic hormone are all produced in excess. Pancreatic islets also increase their secretion of insulin and glucagon. In contrast, production of thyroid hormones and sexual steroids is repressed.

Fever causes metabolic rates to increase about 7% per

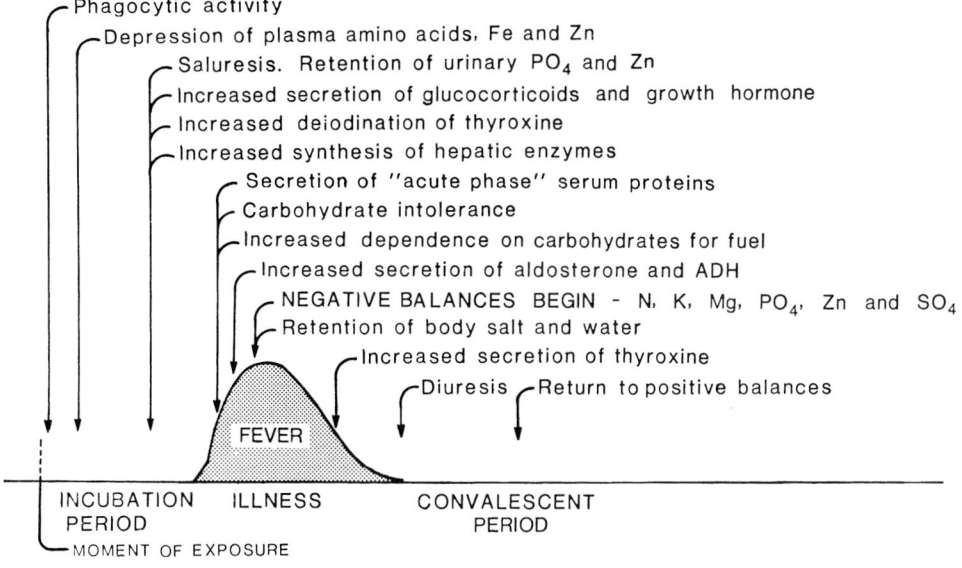

Figure 133–1. The longitudinal progression of physiologic, metabolic, and nutritional events during acute generalized infectious illnesses. These data were acquired in research volunteers exposed to different infectious organisms. ADH, antidiuretic hormone. (From Beisel WR: Magnitude of the host nutritional responses to infection. Am J Clin Nutr 30, 1237, 1977.)

Phagocytic activity
Depression of plasma amino acids, Fe and Zn
Saluresis. Retention of urinary PO_4 and Zn
Increased secretion of glucocorticoids and growth hormone
Increased deiodination of thyroxine
Increased synthesis of hepatic enzymes
Secretion of "acute phase" serum proteins
Carbohydrate intolerance
Increased dependence on carbohydrates for fuel
Increased secretion of aldosterone and ADH
NEGATIVE BALANCES BEGIN - N, K, Mg, PO_4, Zn and SO_4
Retention of body salt and water
Increased secretion of thyroxine
Diuresis   Return to positive balances
FEVER
INCUBATION PERIOD   ILLNESS   CONVALESCENT PERIOD
MOMENT OF EXPOSURE

degree (Fahrenheit). Bodywide hypermetabolism heightens the consumption and/or degradation of nutrients.

Body responses and nutritional losses during cytokine-induced malnutrition differ from those due to starvation alone (Table 133–1). Recurrent infections and the malnutrition they induce can generate a vicious downhill cycle that may ultimately be lethal. Although starvation occurs frequently in tropical countries, infection-induced (i.e., cytokine-induced) losses of body nutrients are a far more important cause of malnutrition.

Direct, Organism-Induced Losses of Body Nutrients. In addition to secondary (indirect) cytokine-induced depletion of body nutrients, microorganisms or their toxins can cause direct losses. Losses of water and electrolytes occur during diarrhea or dysentery. If induced by *Vibrio cholerae* or toxigenic *Escherischia coli*, acute salt and water losses can be massive and rapidly fatal. Nutrients are also lost in purulent exudates, sputum, and blood. Urinary losses of vitamin A are increased during acute phase reactions. Intestinal nutrients may be consumed by competing parasites, especially large roundworms and tapeworms (Chapter 133.2). Hookworms produce sizable direct losses of blood.

TABLE 133–1. Differences in Pathogenesis and Body Composition: Starvation-Induced Malnutrition Versus Infection-Induced (i.e., Cytokine-Induced) Malnutrition

Malnutrition Induced by Uncomplicated Starvation*	Malnutrition Induced by Proinflammatory Cytokines
Body metabolism slowed	Hypermetabolism induced
Oxygen consumption diminished	Oxygen consumption increased
Body temperature depressed	Body temperature elevated
Hunger intense	Anorexia and nausea common
Nitrogen excretion reduced	Nitrogen losses increased
Urea production minimized	Synthesis of urea/NO enhanced
Conservation of body protein maximized	Skeletal muscle degraded; acute phase proteins/ other defensive proteins synthesized
Glucose synthesis and consumption maximally reduced	Glucose synthesis/ consumption stimulated
Ketogenesis stimulated; ketones become important fuel for CNS and other tissues	Ketogenesis minimized
Fatty acids from body fat depots remain major fuel	Hepatic fatty acid synthesis persists/may be enhanced
Triglyceride plasma concentrations decline	Triglyceride synthesis enhanced; fat droplets in liver cells; plasma triglycerides accumulate
Iron and zinc plasma concentrations unaltered	Plasma iron/zinc undergo abrupt cytokine-induced sequestration
Resistance to infection well maintained	Prolonged/recurrent infections common
Immunity well maintained	Immunity severely compromised
Inanition usual cause of death	Infection, septic shock, multiorgan failure usual causes of death

*Because of frequent infections and immature immune systems, uncomplicated starvation is rarely seen in infants and small children.
NO, nitric oxide; CNS, central nervous system.

EFFECTS OF MALNUTRITION ON INFECTIOUS ILLNESSES. Malnutrition, whether generalized or caused by deficiencies of single micronutrients, induces dysfunctions of the immune system and nonspecific host defense mechanisms. These dysfunctions can alter susceptibility to infectious diseases, as well as the severity and duration of infections.

Nutritionally acquired immune deficiency syndrome (NAIDS), in combination with various infections, kills more than 25,000 infants and children every day, mostly in impoverished tropical lands. NAIDS, however, is unlike human immunodeficiency virus–induced AIDS, in that NAIDS can rapidly be reversed by nutritional rehabilitation. NAIDS ensues whenever patients develop symptomatic AIDS, and the interactions are intensely synergistic and rapidly fatal in the absence of antiviral therapy.

Synergistic Versus Antagonistic Interactions. If infection is made worse by malnutrition, the relationship is termed synergistic. Generalized protein-energy malnutrition (PEM), or deficiencies of essential micronutrients, e.g., vitamin A, produce synergistic responses, especially during bacterial infections. But in some infections, illness appears less severe, making for an *antagonistic interaction*. These are seen most often in viral infections, because viral replication is dependent upon nutrients derived from host cells. Nutritionally deprived cells make poor hosts for intracellular pathogens. Despite this, some viral infections (e.g., measles and AIDS) show synergistic responses with malnutrition, rather than antagonistic ones.

Infections in severely malnourished patients may fail to produce fever, inflammatory responses, or leukocytosis, but the absence of these clinical signs does not mean that the infection itself is less severe. And in some infections, no evidence for synergism or antagonism becomes evident in malnourished patients.

Nutritionally Acquired Immune Deficiency Syndromes Caused by PEM. Generalized PEM is frequently seen in tropical countries (Chapter 130). Although PEM is often classified as marasmus (i.e., dry cachexia, in which a shriveled, apathetic child can be described as "nothing but skin and bones") or kwashiorkor (i.e., wet cachexia, in which infection-induced hormonal changes cause severe retention of salt and water), both clinical forms of cachexia generate NAIDS.

PEM-induced NAIDS is severe and life-threatening. All lymphoid tissues (including the thymus, spleen, tonsils, and lymph nodes) undergo severe atrophy, especially in the T-cell areas. Blood lymphocyte counts are reduced, and cultured lymphocytes respond poorly to mitogens. Functions of natural killer lymphocytes are reduced, and the body may lose its ability to identify and destroy grafts of incompatible tissues. Delayed dermal hypersensitivity tests are severely compromised. Immunologic protection against both ongoing and newly acquired infections is greatly reduced. On the other hand, severe PEM may cause a patient to become free of allergies and allergic diseases.

In contrast to overwhelming evidence for dysfunctions of cell-mediated immunity (CMI), which depend on T cells, humoral immunity and B-cell functions are largely maintained during PEM. Immunoglobulins are still produced, and paradoxically, total plasma immunoglobulin concentrations in children with severe PEM are often increased. However, secretory IgA production is diminished.

Despite dysfunctions of CMI, measurable responses to vaccines can still be expected, especially when antigens are T-cell–independent or are combined with adjuvants. However, resultant antibodies may show diminished affinity or lower titers than in healthy controls.

In addition to dysfunctions involving the immune system

itself, many innate, nonspecific forms of host defense are impaired by severe PEM. Malnutrition-induced lesions of the skin and mucous membranes disrupt the integrity of tissue barriers. Abnormal function of bronchial cilia and impaired secretion of bronchial mucus allow respiratory pathogens to gain an access. Mucus-clogged nasal passages and painful pharyngitis inhibit eating. Failure of the malnourished stomach to secrete HCl removes an important defensive mechanism that normally prevents a variety of pathogenic bacteria from gaining access to the intestine; and severe atrophy of intestinal mucosa diminishes nutrient absorption, compromising this natural barrier against pathogen invasion. During PEM, synthesis of protective plasma proteins, e.g., lysosome, transferin and lactoferin, interferon and other cytokines, and complement system components, is reduced.

Phagocytic cell functions become severely impaired during PEM, reducing their ability to migrate to attack microbial invaders. Thus, localizing inflammatory reactions may fail to develop, permitting pathogens to disseminate widely. Malnourished phagocytes also lose their ability to ingest and kill microorganisms, to process antigens, and to secrete cytokines and other antibacterial proteins.

ESSENTIAL MICRONUTRIENT DEFICIENCIES. Deficiencies of single micronutrients usually coexist with generalized PEM, although they may occur as isolated problems. Diarrhea-induced losses of water and electrolytes are of the greatest clinical importance, and can become life-threatening within a few hours. Longer-standing deficiencies of vitamin A, iron, and zinc are also of major gravity because of their frequency in the tropics, as well as their adverse effects on both antigen-specific immunity and generalized host defenses. Although seldom recognized clinically, deficiencies of other essential micronutrients, including B-group vitamins, certain amino acids, polyunsaturated fatty acids, copper, and selenium, can also impact unfavorably on host defenses.

Micronutrient deficiencies can impair body defenses against pathogens by causing atrophic changes in immune system tissues, or by impairing the function of white blood cells. Micronutrient-induced NAIDS is often similar to that caused by PEM, but in addition, each individual micronutrient plays its own specific role in maintaining host defenses at optimal levels (Table 133–2).

Vitamin A (Retinol). Along with vital functions in ocular tissues, vitamin A (once known as the anti-infection vitamin) contributes to immune system activities (Chapter 131.1). Although uncertainty continues to exist about exact mechanisms by which vitamin A combats infection, vitamin A therapy is beneficial for children who develop measles, diarrheas, and other infections.

Infectious illnesses cause vitamin A concentrations to decline in tissues and plasma, and vitamin A is lost in the urine. In combination, hypermetabolic consumption and direct losses of vitamin A can precipitate xerophthalmia, and as an even greater effect, can lead to the deaths of as many as 5000 infants and children each day. These deaths can be prevented by prophylactic or therapeutic vitamin A administration.

A major precursor of vitamin A, beta-carotene, contributes to host resistance by mechanisms somewhat different than vitamin A. Beta-carotene provides antioxidant properties and greater support for the immune system.

Zinc. Because of its function in scores of metalloenzymes, including those essential for nucleic acid metabolism, and its essential role in thymic hormone activity, zinc is needed for the replication and function of lymphocytes, phagocytes, and other cells (Chapter 132.3). Zinc deficiency causes lymphoid tissue atrophy, dysfunctions of T cells and cell-mediated immunity and impaired competence of mucocutaneous surfaces.

Although zinc deficiency can be an isolated problem, it is a consistent component of PEM. Because the body lacks storage depots for zinc, subtle deficiencies are difficult to detect in individual patients. Zinc supplementation of children in low socioeconomic tropical areas has reduced the incidence of weanling diarrhea, persistent diarrhea, and dysentery.

Iron. Because of its role in myeloperoxidase enzymes of phagocytic cells, iron is essential for bactericidal activity (Chapter 132.1). Iron also contributes to immunologic functions. On the other hand, iron is needed by bacteria and intracellular parasites for growth and replication. During generalized infections, cytokine-induced binding proteins cause plasma iron to become sequestered in tissue depots,

TABLE 133–2. Dysfunctions of the Immune System and Other Nonspecific Host Defense Measures Caused by Different Forms of Malnutrition

Host Defensive Mechanisms	PEM	Vitamin Deficiencies							Mineral Deficiencies			
		A	B_{1–3}	B₆	Folate	B₁₂	C	E	Fe	Zn	Cu	Se
Lymphoid tissue atrophy	X	X		X	x					X		x
Lymphopenia	X	X		X	x		X		X	X		
Lymphocyte response to mitogens	X	X		x	X	X		X	X	X	x	x
DTH responses	X	X		X	X	X		X		X	x	
Graft-vs.-host responses	X			X			x					
Response to new antigens	X	X	x	X	x			x	X	X	x	x
Antibody production		X	x	X	x			x	X	X	x	x
Secretory IgA production	X											
NK cell functions	X							x	X	X		x
Thymic hormone dysfunctions	X			x						X		
Phagocyte mobility	X						X	X		X		
Phagocytosis						X	X	X	X	X		
Phagocyte microbicidal functions	X				X	X	X	X	X		x	x
Dermal/mucosal lesions	X	X	X	X						X		
Achlorhydria	X											
Has antioxidant functions		X					X	X				X

X, clinically confirmed; x, experimentally confirmed; PEM, protein-energy malnutrition; IgA, immunoglobulin A; NK, natural killer.
Note: Blank spaces = normal, or no data available. Vitamin A data include beta-carotene.

perhaps as a mechanism that helps deprive pathogens of iron. But infection-induced anemia can result.

Iron status thus becomes a two-edged sword, as best illustrated by its role in malaria. Iron, used to treat anemia in children with subclinical parasitemia, has led to the explosive appearance of lethal cerebral malaria. Nonetheless, oral iron can be given safely to parasitemic children if they are receiving appropriate antimalarial therapy. Midway between these two extremes, iron chelation therapy (administered in an attempt to diminish iron availability to reproducing plasmodia) increases the value of even the most effective antimalarial drugs.

Other Single Nutrients. Because of its necessity for phagocyte mobility and immune functions, vitamin C (ascorbic acid) is essential for host defenses. Epidemic infections were once highly lethal in populations where scurvy was rampant (Chapter 131.3). However, clinical scurvy is rare in most of the world today, generally being confined to areas of urban poverty. Vitamin C, vitamin E, and selenium have additional protective roles because of their antioxidant properties.

At present, deficiencies of B-complex vitamins are also clinical rarities. Of these, deficiencies of vitamin B_6 (pyridoxine) (Chapter 131.6), folate, or vitamin B_{12} (cobalamin) (Chapter 131.7) have the greatest effects on immune system functions. Deficiencies of certain amino acids (e.g., arginine and glutamine), polyunsaturated fatty acids, and essential ultratrace minerals can also have adverse immunologic consequences.

USEFUL CLINICAL POINTS

1. Because infection-induced losses of body nutrients are proportional to disease severity and duration, prompt use of appropriate antimicrobial therapy is a nutritional must! Control of *high* fevers also reduces nutritional losses.
2. Because nutritional rehabilitation requires much time, refeedings should be started without delay after cessation of nausea and anorexia. Postinfection hyperphagia is a welcome sign. Children should be given plentiful feedings of highly nutritious foods, in hope of achieving catch-up growth.
3. Prophylactic supplementation (or therapy) with vitamin A and zinc can reduce morbidity and mortality of infections, even in children with PEM.
4. Possible dangers of therapeutic iron are magnified by severe malnutrition. Treatment of infections, including subclinical ones, should be initiated before oral iron therapy is introduced. If possible, total iron-binding capacity of plasma should be normalized by adequate protein and energy refeedings prior to iron therapy.
5. Immunologic evaluations are expensive, complex, and lengthy, especially under field conditions in the tropics. A rapid, easy, and effective screening alternative in children is to evaluate tonsil size. Tonsils are normally quite large in young children, but with malnutrition-induced atrophy, tonsils may seem to be absent. This tonsillar sign is evidence for severe immune system dysfunction.
6. Dire consequences of infection-induced NAIDS can be reduced quickly by nutritional support, even before nutritional rehabilitation is fully complete.

Bibliography

Beisel WR: Single nutrients and immunity. Am J Clin Nutr 35 (Suppl):417, 1982.
Beisel WR: Nutrition and infection. *In* Linder MC (ed): Nutritional Biochemistry and Metabolism, 2nd ed. New York, Elsevier, 1991, pp 507–542.
Kjolhede C, Beisel WR: Vitamin A and the immune function: A symposium. J Nutr Immunol 4:1, 1995.
Raiten DJ, Talbot JM (eds): Nutrition in pediatric HIV infection: Setting the research agenda. Proceedings of a workshop. J Nutr 126(Suppl):2611S, 1996.

Sazawal S, Black RE, Bhan MK, et al: Zinc supplementation reduces the incidence of persistent diarrhea and dysentery among low socioeconomic children in India. J Nutr 126:443, 1996.
Scrimshaw NS, Taylor CE, Gordon JE: Interactions of Nutrition and Infection. Monograph No. 57. Geneva, World Health Organization, 1968.
Sommer A, West KP Jr: Vitamin A Deficiency. New York, Oxford University Press, 1996.
van Hensbroek MB, Morris-Jones S, Meisner S, et al: Iron, but not folic acid, combined with effective antimalarial therapy promotes haematological recovery in African children after acute falciparum malaria. Trans R Soc Trop Med Hyg 89:672, 1995.
Wyler DJ: Bark, weeds, and iron chelators—drugs for malaria. N Engl J Med 327:1519, 1992.

133.2 The Impact of Parasitic Infections on Nutrition

Rebecca J. Stoltzfus

Since the seminal studies of Mata in the 1960s, the important role of infectious illness as a cause of malnutrition and growth retardation has been recognized. Most of the attention in this area has focused on acute illnesses, especially measles, diarrhea, and respiratory infections, because of their high incidence among children in developing countries and because they may precipitate dramatic forms of malnutrition, e.g., marasmus, kwashiorkor, and xerophthalmia. The impact of parasitic infections on human nutrition is more insidious but merits attention for several reasons. First, these infections are usually subclinical, and therefore are frequently undetected or ignored by both patient and clinician. Second, these infections are usually of very long duration. In many tropical environments, it is common for an individual to be infected with hookworms or *Trichuris trichiura* in early childhood and remain infected for decades. Thus, the impact of the disease on the nutritional status of an individual has many years to take its toll. Third, the prevalence of parasitic infections is extremely high. For instance, about one fourth of the world's population is infected with geohelminths.

NUTRITIONAL IMPACT OF COMMON PARASITIC INFECTIONS. Some general nutrition-related effects are common to all parasitic infections. Intestinal parasites frequently cause gastrointestinal irritation, which may manifest in pain, flatulence, tenderness, or loose stools. It is impossible to say how many worm-infected children have stomachaches that affect their desire to eat. This may contribute to poor appetite in children in tropical countries, a complaint often expressed by mothers. It is also possible that helminth infections may suppress appetite through a chemical mechanism; tumor necrosis factor has been proposed. Another general effect of chronic parasitic infection is the nutritional cost of the cytokine-mediated host responses (Chapter 133.1). These responses may add to the nutrient requirements (especially protein demands) of the host over a long span of time.

Hookworms. The hookworms (*Ancylostoma duodenale* and *Necator americanus*) cause intestinal blood loss by feeding on the intestinal mucosa (Chapter 105.1). After the worm ingests a mucus plug consisting of gastrointestinal epithelium, blood flows from the host capillary bed into the worm, which extracts the blood by sucking motions. The blood flow is facilitated by the secretion of an anticoagulant by the worm. Worms stay attached to one site for 4 to 6 hours, then migrate to a new site. Of the blood ingested, most of the red cells are excreted by the worm. This heme iron is then available for reabsorption by the human host, but a significant proportion is excreted in the feces. The blood loss per day per worm has been estimated by isotopic studies to be on the order of

0.03 mL in the case of *N. americanus*, and 0.15 mL in the case of *A. duodenale*. Because infection intensity is usually measured in eggs per gram of feces, not number of worms, a more practical figure is a daily blood loss of around 2 mL/1000 eggs/g feces for *N. americanus* and 5 mL/1000 eggs/g feces for *A. duodenale*. Hookworm-related blood loss is directly proportional to the intensity of infection, (Fig. 133–2).

The blood loss from a moderate infection of *N. americanus* (2000 eggs/g feces) thus amounts to about 4 mL per day, or about 1.5 mg of iron in a person with normal hemoglobin concentration. This compares with the physiologic daily iron requirement of 1 mg for an adult man, 1.25 mg for an adult woman, or 0.56 mg for a preschool child (Chapter 132.1). It also represents about three times the blood loss typically caused by menstruation. When hookworm blood loss is added to the high-iron physiologic iron requirement of pregnancy, the probability of pregnancy anemia becomes very high, and the anemia is more likely to be severe.

Whether hookworm infection results in anemia depends on whether the individual's dietary iron absorption is high enough to compensate for iron loss. If dietary iron absorption is high, or if a person is given supplemental iron, anemia can be prevented despite chronic hookworm infection. If iron intake is low, even a light or moderate hookworm infection results in significant anemia. The iron loss in heavy hookworm infection is practically impossible to compensate through diet alone, and hookworm anemia eventually results if the worm burden is not decreased. In these cases, anemia eventually becomes severe and life-threatening, and is usually accompanied by hypoalbuminemia and weight loss (Fig. 133–3). General nutritional rehabilitation (i.e., more than iron tablets) may be required to restore health.

Although the usual route of hookworm infection is transdermal, vertical transmission can occur, as evidenced by cases of hookworm infection in young infants. The incidence of vertical transmission, which appears to occur with *A. duodenale* but not *N. americanus*, has not been determined but is probably low. However, even a small number of *A. duodenale* is sufficient to cause severe anemia in an infant. Because of the severity of blood loss and the high iron requirements of young children, it is virtually impossible to prevent anemia in a young child with ankylostomiasis, even with oral iron supplementation.

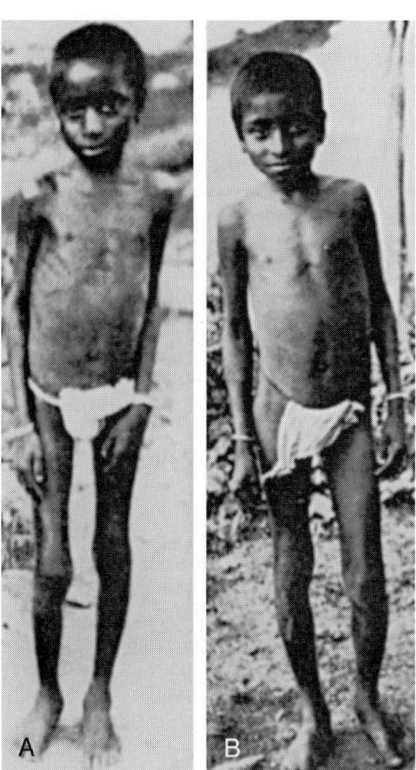

Figure 133–3. *A,* An Indian boy with malnutrition, severe wasting, and anemia. *B,* The same child 6 months after treatment for hookworm.

Schistosomiasis. Schistosomiasis also has serious nutritional consequences (Chapter 118). Intestinal schistosomiasis (*Schistosoma mansoni* or *S. japonicum* infection) causes lesions throughout the intestines, resulting in generalized malabsorption, protein losses, and anemia. If the lesions become severe, significant intestinal blood loss can result. Urinary schistosomiasis (*S. haematobium* infection) causes similar lesions in the bladder and urinary tract, resulting in urinary blood loss. Like hookworm infection, the nutritional impact is dependent on the intensity of infection. Less intense infections may not produce acute malnutrition but may contribute to anemia and growth retardation. Severe infections may precipitate severe anemia, wasting, or both.

Strongyloidiasis. The clinical manifestations of strongyloidiasis (notably abdominal pain and diarrhea) have obvious nutritional consequences, but the contribution of these infections to malnutrition in tropical countries is largely undocumented (Chapter 105.2). The intestinal symptoms of hyperinfection with *Strongyloides* are profound, with severe diarrhea and malabsorption leading to wasting malnutrition. The relative lack of knowledge about strongyloidiasis and its nutritional consequences is not because the infection is uncommon, but rather because it is difficult to diagnose and to characterize epidemiologically.

Trichuriasis and Ascariasis. These are the most common of human infections, but their impact on human nutrition remains a controversy. Trichuriasis can cause blood loss from the colon and rectum (Chapter 103.2). However, the relatively small number of studies available suggest that significant blood loss occurs only in heavy infection. This apparent threshold relationship is quite different from the linear, intensity-dependent relationship of hookworm infection to blood loss. In heavy *T. trichuria* infection, anemia and wasting are common findings.

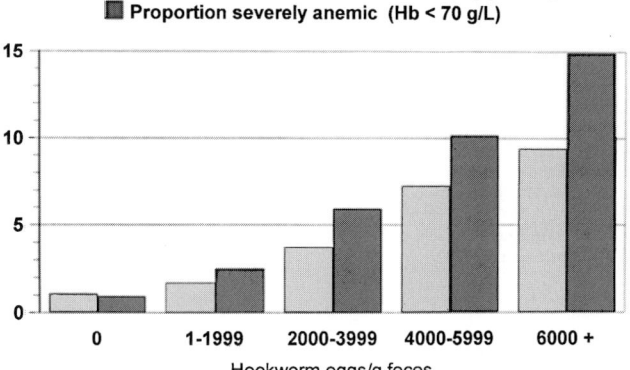

Figure 133–2. Relationship of hookworm infection intensity to fecal heme excretion and the prevalence of severe anemia in Zanzibari schoolchildren. Hookworm eggs per gram of feces and anemia were assessed in 3428 children in primary school grades 1 to 4. Fecal heme concentration was measured in a subsample of 203 children. (Data from Stoltzfus RJ, et al: Am J Trop Med Hygiene 55:399, 1996; and Stoltzfus RJ, et al: Am J Clin Nutr 65:153, 1997.)

Ascaris lumbricoides infection may cause malabsorption of some substances, and the parasite itself metabolizes vitamin A (Chapter 104). Ascariasis is associated with growth retardation, vitamin A deficiency and mild anemia in population studies, but it is not clear whether the association is caused by specific nutritional mechanisms of the parasite or from a general association between poor hygiene and poor diet. Because the prevalence of ascariasis in young children in many areas of the tropics and subtropics is extremely high, treatment of this infection, which is safe, simple, and effective, might improve child nutrition.

Malaria. Malaria, especially *Plasmodium falciparum* infection has several effects on nutrition that are often overlooked because of the dramatic and complex clinical manifestations of this disease (Chapter 92). The anemia of malaria is typically hypochromic and microcytic, but malaria does not cause iron deficiency in the sense of depleted body iron stores. Significant body iron losses do not occur during malaria, except in cases of blackwater fever (hemoglobinuria), which is rare today. Rather, anemia is caused by rapid hemolysis and, especially in chronic malaria, is exacerbated by a suppression of erythropoiesis. The iron content of the lysed red cells is recovered but may remain in the reticuloendothelial system instead of being mobilized for red cell synthesis, even in the presence of anemia. Nonetheless, it is good practice to give oral iron-folate supplements in combination with antimalarial drugs, as a preexisting iron deficiency is likely in most malaria-endemic areas, and iron supplementation facilitates erythropoiesis during convalescence.

Following a bout of malaria, the erythroid hyperplasia required to recover from anemia increases the folate requirement, and this may cause folate deficiency (Chapters 6 and 130.7). This is especially likely if malaria occurs during pregnancy, a time when folate requirements are already increased. Oral iron-folate supplementation also helps to prevent or correct folate deficiency.

In individuals with marginal energy intakes and reserves, as is the case for many children, and pregnant and lactating women in malaria-endemic areas, malaria may contribute to protein-energy malnutrition (PEM) because of the caloric costs of febrile episodes, and the vomiting and anorexia that often accompany the disease (Chapter 130). Individuals at risk for PEM should be provided a calorie-rich diet during the convalescent period.

Malaria in the pregnant woman contributes to malnutrition in the fetus (Chapter 15). Pregnant women, particularly primiparous women, have a higher susceptibility to malaria. The parasites are frequently in the placenta, compromising nutrient flow to the fetus and increasing the risk of low birthweight. In a developing country setting, the risks of malnutrition, morbidity, and mortality for a low-birthweight infant are very high.

IMPLICATIONS FOR CLINICAL CARE

Chemotherapy. When treating clinical anemia, parasitic causes should be investigated or, in some settings, treated presumptively. The most likely parasitic causes are malaria, hookworm, or urinary schistosomiasis, although strongyloides infection or intestinal schistosomiasis might also be a cause. Where hookworm infection is known to be endemic, it is almost always more cost-effective to treat presumptively than to make a diagnosis, and the anthelmintics are so safe that this is justified (Chapter 105.1). Presumptive treatment for hookworm is recommended for children with severe anemia ≥2 years of age in endemic areas. If anemia improves with iron supplementation but reappears rapidly in a child ≤2 years of age, infection with *A. duodenale* should be considered. Schistosomiasis is most likely to cause severe anemia in older children or other groups exposed to infected water

(Chapter 118), whereas malaria is most likely to cause severe anemia in young children and primiparous women (Chapter 92).

Similarly, when treating individuals with PEM, parasitic diseases should be considered as a contributing cause. This is especially important when wasting malnutrition is found in individuals ≥2 or 3 years of age. Below this age, marasmus and kwashiorkor are very likely related to poor feeding practices combined with measles, diarrhea, or respiratory infections. Parasitic infections are more likely to be a cause of clinical malnutrition in older children or adults.

Prophylaxis. In the context of antenatal care, malaria and hookworms may require treatment or prophylaxis. Malaria prophylaxis is most cost-effective when reserved for primiparous women in areas holoendemic for *P. falciparum*. In areas where hookworm infection is prevalent, it is recommended that an anthelmintic drug be given after the first trimester of pregnancy in combination with iron-folate tablets.

IMPLICATIONS FOR COMMUNITY HEALTH PROGRAMS.
Parasite control at the community level can help prevent anemia and PEM in certain population groups. School-based deworming is recommended when the prevalence of helminth infections exceeds 50% and, where hookworms are prevalent, school-based deworming reduces anemia in older children. The benefits of community-based deworming to younger children or women of reproductive age are yet unproved. Where schistosomiasis is prevalent, school-based treatment programs may also improve growth and iron status of children. Helminth control is most sustainable if anthelmintic drugs are combined with community education and development. For controlling malarial transmission in communities, the recommended strategy is the use of insecticide-treated bednets. Where this has been effective, the growth of young children has improved and anemia rates have fallen. Efforts to control these highly prevalent parasites at the community level can alleviate mild to moderate malnutrition and its insidious effects in a large number of people, while reducing the number of cases of acute malnutrition and parasitic disease.

Bibliography

Fleming AF: Haematological manifestations of malaria and other parasitic diseases. Clin Haematol 10:983, 1981.

Garner P, Brabin B: A review of randomized controlled trials of routine antimalarial drug prophylaxis during pregnancy in endemic malarious areas. Bull WHO 72:89, 1994.

Savioli L, Bundy D, Tomkins A: Intestinal parasitic infections: A soluble public health problem. Trans R Soc Trop Med Hyg 86:353, 1992.

Shiff C, Checkley W, Winch P, et al: Changes in weight gain and anaemia attributable to malaria in Tanzanian children living under holoendemic conditions. Trans R Soc Trop Med Hyg 90:262, 1996.

Stephenson LS: Impact of Helminth Infections on Human Nutrition. London, Taylor & Francis, 1987.

Stoltzfus RJ, Albonico M, Chwaya HM, et al: Hemoquant determination of hookworm-related blood loss and its role in iron deficiency in African children. Am J Trop Med Hyg 55:399, 1996.

Stoltzfus RJ, Stoltzfus HM, Tielsch JM, et al: Epidemiology of iron deficiency anemia in Zanzibari school children: The importance of hookworms. Am J Clin Nutr 65:153, 1997.

133.3 Nutritional Neuropathies

Gustavo C. Román

Peripheral neuropathies are relatively common in the tropics. These are usually caused by diabetes, genetic factors, alcoholism, neurotoxins, and micronutrient deficiencies, often combined with consumption of cyanide-producing tropical foodstuffs, e.g., cassava. Usually, a toxic-nutritional component is also present in alcoholic neuropathy and tobacco-alcohol amblyopia. Nutritional neuropathies may occur as epidemic outbreaks or as problems endemic to a particular geographic area. Experimentally, a deficiency of micronutrients, in particular the B-complex vitamins and vitamin E, has been associated with predominantly axonal neuropathies. However, these specific deficits seldom present in isolation because they are usually due to overall dietary deficiency or malabsorption. In individuals with modest dietary reduction of micronutrients, tropical malabsorption, often resulting from recurrent intestinal infections, decreases the availability of vitamins. In most instances, exact diagnosis is not feasible because laboratory determinations of micronutrients and toxins, clinical neurophysiology, and nerve biopsy studies are not available. The etiologic diagnosis usually relies on epidemiologic data and the therapeutic response to multivitamin supplementation and dietary support.

Nutritional neuropathies may be found in endemic form among populations in Africa, Asia, and Latin America with chronically deficient diets and widespread malnutrition. However, the number of individuals seeking medical attention is relatively low. In these populations, a precarious equilibrium is maintained until an added factor precipitates the clinically asymptomatic deficits. These factors include pregnancy and lactation, infections such as malaria and diarrhea, tobacco and alcohol use, as well as increased metabolic requirements for thiamine due to increased carbohydrate intake and intense physical activity under hot and humid weather conditions. Neurologic signs, therefore, occur relatively late as the combination of factors finally leads to deficiency of essential nutrients severe enough to injure the nervous system or when protective nutrients, e.g., sulfur-containing amino acids and antioxidant carotenoids, e.g., lycopene, become unavailable. The most sensitive neural elements, e.g., dorsal root ganglia, large myelinated distal axons, bipolar retinal neurons, and cochlear neurons, are the first to suffer damage and manifest symptoms earliest.

STRACHAN SYNDROME. First recognized by Strachan in Jamaica in the 19th century this syndrome is characterized by orogenital dermatitis, painful sensory neuropathy, amblyopia, and deafness. The syndrome was also observed in prisoners of war in tropical camps during World War II under conditions of dietary restriction. With regional variations, Strachan syndrome has been reported in Africa (Dakar, Senegal; Abidjan, Ivory Coast), India, and the Caribbean.

Patients in Africa with nutritional neuromyelopathies present with sensory ataxia, sensorimotor polyneuropathies, dorsolateral myelopathy, and spastic paraparesis. One fifth have visual deficits, hearing loss, or both. Patients are relatively young (mean age, 35 years) and from very low socioeconomic environments in sub-Saharan Africa. In one fourth malnutrition is evident, with frequent skin and mucosal pellagroid changes. Most cases occur in women, and pregnancy is a precipitating factor in one third. Intestinal problems are frequent, including chronic diarrhea, gastric achlorhydria or hypochlorhydria, and abnormal liver biopsy. Cerebrospinal fluid is usually normal. Abnormal peroneal nerve conduction velocities are found in all patients and sural nerve biopsies show changes consistent with axonal neuropathy. With parenteral vitamin B complex treatment, 65% of the patients improved. The syndrome is attributed to a nutritional deficit resulting from a combination of poor dietary intake and tropical malabsorption.

In India, patients present with a predominantly sensory neuropathy, chronic malnutrition, alcohol abuse, and pellagra and have low blood levels of thiamine, riboflavin, nicotinic acid, pantothenic acid, pyridoxine, and folic acid. Absorption and levels of vitamin B_{12} are normal. Withdrawal of alcohol, balanced diet, and treatment with vitamin B complex resulted in improvement of symptoms and signs of peripheral neuropathy. Traditionally, the neuropathy and myelopathy due to vitamin B_{12} deficiency, as well as to pernicious anemia, have been considered to be rare in the tropics, even among strict vegetarians. Most probably these conditions are under-diagnosed, because most vegan Indian patients with megaloblastic anemia studied in England had dietary vitamin B_{12} deficiency and some had pernicious anemia.

EPIDEMIC NEUROPATHY IN CUBA. A cluster of nutritional neuropathies was recently observed in Cuba and Colombia. The epidemic of neuropathy in Cuba affected 50,862 patients during 1992 and 1993 (incidence rate of 462 per 100,000). Children, adolescents, pregnant women, and the elderly are rarely affected. Most cases occur in those between ages 25 and 64 years. The highest rates are found in the tobacco-growing province of Pinar del Río. Clinical manifestations include retrobulbar optic neuropathy, sensorineural deafness, predominantly sensory and autonomic neuropathy, and dorsolateral myelopathy. Less often dysphonia, dysphagia, and spastic paraparesis are present. Mixed forms are frequent. Neurologic symptoms are preceded by weight loss, anorexia, chronic fatigue, lack of energy, irritability, sleep disturbances, and difficulties with concentration and memory.

Optic Neuropathy. This is characterized by blurred vision, photophobia, central and cecocentral scotomas, deficit of color vision for red and green, and loss of axons in the maculopapillary bundle with temporal disc pallor in advanced cases. Approximately one third of the patients present with concomitant skin and mucous membrane lesions, and evidence of peripheral nerve and spinal cord involvement; 20% have hearing loss. Marked improvement of vision was obtained with parenteral therapy with vitamin B complex and folic acid.

Peripheral Neuropathy. These symptoms include painful dysesthesias in the soles and palms, mainly burning feet, numbness, cramps, and paresthesias. Nerves are sensitive to pressure. Motor involvement is minimal. Objective signs are often mild and include loss or decreased perception of vibration, light touch, and pinprick distally in the limbs in a stocking-glove pattern. Achilles tendon reflexes are decreased or absent. Motor nerve conduction velocities are normal and sensory nerve potential amplitudes are decreased only in severe cases. Some patients have a sensation of body heat with excessive sweating, as well as coldness and hyperhidrosis of hands and feet. Sural nerve biopsies show an axonal neuropathy with predominant loss of myelinated, large-caliber fibers.

Dorsolateral Myelopathy. Some patients presenting with similar sensory peripheral neuropathy symptoms also have complaints of leg muscle weakness, increased urinary frequency, impotence in males, and difficulty walking. These cases often have brisk knee reflexes with crossed adductor responses contrasting with decreased ankle reflexes. Spasticity and Babinski signs are usually absent. Proximal motor weakness is present in one third of these cases. A decrease in position sense in the feet and a positive Romberg sign are often present. Severe cases have sensory gait ataxia.

Sensorineural Deafness. Patients also have high-pitch tinnitus and deafness. Pure tone audiometry demonstrate high frequency (4 to 8 kHz) hearing loss, bilateral and usually symmetric. There are no associated vestibular symptoms.

Etiology. Patients are farmers, with lower income and less education than healthy controls. Possible etiologies excluded were toxic, i.e., organophosphorus pesticides, chronic cyanide, trichloroethylene; genetic, i.e., mitochondrial mutations of Leber hereditary optic neuropathy; and infectious causes, i.e., retroviruses (human immunodeficiency virus and human T-lymphotropic virus types I and II) and coxsackievirus. Factors associated with greater risk of optic neuropathy are use of tobacco, in particular cigar smoking: those who smoked ≥4 cigars per day had the highest risk. Other important risk factors include lack of food for several days, eating lunch <5 days per week, and eating breakfast <1 day per week. Protective factors include having relatives overseas (probably because with US dollars it was possible to buy supplementary food in the black market) and raising chickens at home (perhaps because of the nutritional value of eggs in terms of B-complex vitamins and sulfur-containing amino acids). High levels of lycopene (a non–vitamin A carotenoid antioxidant found in tomatoes, guavas, watermelons, and other red fruits) provide the strongest association with protection. Consumption of riboflavin, an antioxidant, is also protective.

Despite the absence of overt malnutrition in Cuba, a deficit of B-complex vitamins, mainly cobalamin and thiamine, compounded by lack of essential sulfur amino acids in the diet, appears to have been the cause of the outbreak. Cuba had eliminated childhood malnutrition, and nutritional supplementation programs for children, pregnant women, and the elderly had been maintained. This explains the absence of this illness in these groups, which are so often affected by nutritional neuromyelopathies in the tropics.

BERIBERI. Until early in this century, beriberi was a major public health problem in the Far East, among populations depending on polished rice for their staple diet (China, Japan, Indonesia, the Philippines), but it also occurred in Africa and tropical South America. In the Japanese Navy, from 1878 until 1883, beriberi affected annually between 23 and 40% of the total force of about 5000 men with an average mortality of 5%. Admiral Kanehiro Takaki practically eliminated beriberi in Japanese ships by lowering the carbohydrate content of the diet and increasing the amount of protein. Food supplementation with thiamine practically eliminated beriberi around the world. Most cases are currently observed in alcoholic patients. However, beriberi continues to occur in the tropics when the conditions of low thiamine intake, high carbohydrate, and high energy expenditure are met (Chapter 131.2). Recently (1991–1993), an outbreak of epidemic neuropathy occurred in a military garrison in Colombia. It was characterized clinically by edema of the feet, dysesthesias, frequent footdrop, and a high case-fatality rate. The diagnosis of wet beriberi due to thiamine deficiency was confirmed by the presence of typical lesions in the heart in two fatal cases (myocardial edema, central necrosis of muscle fibers, and mitochondrial lesions), with presence of an axonal neuropathy on sural nerve biopsies, low serum levels of thiamine, and relative deficiency of thiamine in the diet. The enormous energy expenditure of soldiers in training in the humidity of the tropics and the possible presence of fish thiaminase in the diet probably contributed to this outbreak. There is no effective body storage of thiamine, and dietary deficiency leads to symptoms in 1 or 2 months. Thiamine plays a central role in energy production, and thiamine requirements depend on the metabolic rate of the body. Beriberi responds rapidly to parenteral thiamine, but it carries a high mortality if the diagnosis is not suspected.

NEUROLOGIC PROBLEMS ASSOCIATED WITH DIETARY CYANIDE INTOXICATION. A number of staple foods in the tropics contain large amounts of cyanogenic glycosides. These plants include cassava (*Manihot esculenta* Crantz; Spanish, yuca; French, *manioc*), yam, sweet potato, corn, millet (*Sorghum* sp.), bamboo shoots, and beans, e.g., *Phaseolus vulgaris*, particularly lima beans and the small black lima beans that grow wild in Puerto Rico and Central America. Tobacco

smoke (*Nicotiana tabacum*) also contains considerable amounts of cyanide (150 to 300 μg per cigarette). Cyanide, sometimes used for extracting gold, contaminates the environment in some gold mining operations. Hydrolysis of plant glycosides releases cyanide as hydrocyanic acid. Intoxication occurs by rapid cyanide absorption through the gastrointestinal tract or the lungs. Detoxification is mainly to thiocyanate in a reaction mediated by rhodanase, a sulfur-transferase that converts thiosulfate into thiocyanate and sulfite. Thiocyanate is a goitrogenic agent that may be responsible for endemic cretinism in some tropical areas. The sulfur-containing essential amino acids, e.g., cystine, cysteine, and methionine, provide the sulfur for these detoxification reactions. Also important is vitamin B_{12} with conversion of hydroxocobalamin to cyanocobalamin.

Cassava is a root crop consumed in large quantities throughout the tropics and constitutes the major source of calories for some 300 million people. In Africa, cassava is the staple diet in western Nigeria, the Democratic Republic of the Congo (DRC), Tanzania, Senegal, Uganda, and Mozambique. In these countries, a number of neurologic disorders have been associated with high dietary intake of cyanogenic glycosides in association with depletion of sulfur-containing amino acids. However, it should be noted that these problems are not common in Latin America, even though the cassava consumption in countries such as Brazil is among the highest in the world. The clinical syndromes associated with chronic cyanide intoxication include tropical ataxic neuropathy, a form of spastic paraparesis known as *konzo*, tropical amblyopia, and nerve deafness.

Tropical Ataxic Neuropathy. In Nigeria, tropical ataxic neuropathy (TAN) has been observed in areas where the diet depends almost exclusively on cassava with an estimated prevalence of 18 to 26 per 1000, equal sex distribution, and onset usually in the third and fourth decades. TAN is a chronic and slowly progressive syndrome characterized by predominantly sensory polyneuropathy, posterior column involvement, optic atrophy, and sensorineural deafness. Onset is slow with painful paresthesias in the legs, numbness, "burning feet," and cramps. On examination there is impaired vibratory perception distally in the feet, loss of knee and ankle reflexes, incoordination of the legs, and broad-based ataxic gait in two thirds of patients. Weakness and atrophy of distal leg muscles, mainly the peroneals, may also occur. Other symptoms include blurring of vision with eventual bilateral optic atrophy (81%), and tinnitus followed by bilateral nerve deafness (36%). A few patients have pyramidal signs. About 40% of patients present with skin and mucosal lesions suggestive of vitamin deficits. In other African countries, e.g., Senegal, similar syndromes have been observed, although not necessarily in association with high cassava intake. The frequency of visual loss (19%), deafness (13%), and mucocutaneous lesions (15%) is much lower in these patients than in those from Nigeria.

Konzo. This is the traditional name given in Kwango, DRC to a form of epidemic spastic paraparesis described during times of drought and famine in cassava-staple areas. Epidemics have occurred in rural areas of Mozambique, Tanzania, DRC, and the Central African Republic. The disease predominates in children (63%) and lactating women, with prevalences ranging from 29 to 34 per 1000. Women and children eat raw and sun-dried, uncooked bitter cassava, whereas men normally eat well-cooked cassava. Traditional methods of cassava preparation in Africa, e.g., soaking, fermentation, and sun-drying, leave substantial amounts of cyanogenic glycosides in the cassava meal.

Signs of acute cyanide intoxication are present followed by sudden onset of nonprogressive spastic paraparesis with flexion contractures of hamstrings and Achilles tendons developing later. Scissoring gait and toe walking are frequently present and patients require one or two sticks to walk. Increased tone in the lower limbs, hyperreflexia, ankle clonus, and Babinski sign are usually present. There is no sensory loss to light touch or pinprick. Impairment of rapid movements and hyperreflexia in the upper limbs are also present. Nystagmus and dysarthria may occur. There is minimal recovery with a nutritious diet and vitamin therapy.

Tropical Amblyopia. A condition variously known as tobacco amblyopia, West Indian amblyopia, Jamaican optic neuropathy, and tropical amblyopia was initially described in Cuba in 1898 by Mádan. Cases similar to those observed in Cuba have been reported in Tanzania in association with peripheral neuropathy. All these conditions are probably clinically identical to the retrobulbar neuropathy of pernicious anemia, tobacco-alcohol amblyopia, and nutritional amblyopia. The common element is the underlying deficit of micronutrients, in particular B-complex vitamins, folic acid, and sulfur amino acids. For these reasons, the term *nutritional* or *deficiency amblyopia* is preferred. Differential diagnosis should include methyl alcohol intoxication, a common cause of epidemic blindness in the tropics resulting from consumption of adulterated alcohol.

Sensorineural Deafness. Patients in Nigeria often present with sensorineural deafness in association with cassava intake and micronutrient deficiencies. This deficit is probably nutritional in origin because similar cases were observed in prisoners of war and in Cuba during epidemic outbreaks of neuropathy.

Bibliography

Borrajero I, Pérez JL, Domínguez C, et al: Epidemic neuropathy in Cuba: Morphological characterization of peripheral nerve lesions in sural nerve biopsies. J Neurol Sci 127:68–76, 1994.

Centers for Disease Control and Prevention. Epidemic neuropathy–Cuba, 1991–1994. MMWR 43:183–192, 1994.

Cuba Neuropathy Field Investigation Team: Epidemic optic neuropathy in Cuba: Clinical characterization and risk factors. N Engl J Med 333:1176, 1995.

Lincoff NS, Odel G, Hirano M: "Outbreak" of optic and peripheral neuropathy in Cuba? JAMA 270:511, 1993.

Newman NJ, Torroni A, Brown D, et al: Epidemic neuropathy in Cuba not associated with mitochondrial DNA mutations found in Leber's hereditary optic neuropathy patients. Am J Ophthalmol 118:158, 1994.

Osuntokun BO: An ataxic neuropathy in Nigeria: A clinical, biochemical and electrophysiological study. Brain 91:215, 1968.

Osuntokun BO, Osuntokun O: Tropical amblyopia in Nigerians. Am J Ophthalmol 71:708, 1971.

Plant GT, Mtanda AT, Arden GB, Johnson GJ: An epidemic of optic neuropathy in Tanzania: Characterization of the visual disorder and associated peripheral neuropathy. J Neurol Sci 145:127, 1997.

Román GC, Spencer PS, Schoenberg BS: Tropical myeloneuropathies: The hidden endemias. Neurology 35:1158, 1985.

Román GC: Epidemic neuropathy of Jamaica. Trans Studies Coll Phys Phila Med Hist 7:261, 1985.

Román GC: An epidemic in Cuba of optic neuropathy, sensorineural deafness, peripheral sensory neuropathy and dorsolateral myeloneuropathy. J Neurol Sci 127:11, 1994.

Román GC: Epidemic neuropathy in Cuba: A plea to end the United States economic embargo on a humanitarian basis. Neurology 44:1784, 1994.

Román GC: On politics and health: An epidemic of neurologic disease in Cuba. Ann Intern Med 122:530, 1995.

Román GC: Tropical neuropathies. Bailliéres Clin Neurol 4:469, 1995.

Román GC: Tropical myeloneuropathies revisited. Curr Opin Neurol 11:539, 1998.

Sadun AA, Martone JF, Muci-Mendoza R, et al: Epidemic optic neuropathy in Cuba: Eye findings. Arch Ophthalmol 112:691, 1994.

134 *General Principles of Infectious Disease Transmission*

G. Thomas Strickland and Trenton K. Ruebush II

Disease is produced by an interaction between a causative agent and a susceptible host. The basic principles of disease transmission apply equally well to diseases caused by infections, chemical and physical agents, and nutritional deficiencies or excesses.

In most cases of infectious disease, the causative agent, an infectious organism, is transmitted to the host from an external source *(exogenous infection)*. Less frequently, owing to a change in the host-agent relationship that favors the infective agent, disease is produced by an organism that is normally carried by the host without signs or symptoms of disease *(endogenous infection)*. The interrelationship among an infectious agent, its host, and the route by which the agent is transmitted from host to host has been termed the chain of infection. Environmental factors may affect all three links in the chain of infection.

INFECTIOUS AGENT

Pathogenicity and Virulence. The infectious agent may be a virus, bacterium, fungus, protozoan, or helminth. The ability of an infectious organism to cause disease in a susceptible host is termed *pathogenicity*. Rabies virus and smallpox virus are examples of highly pathogenic organisms; all infected persons develop clinically apparent illnesses. In contrast, *Staphylococcus epidermidis* rarely causes disease, although it is commonly found colonizing the skin.

The term *virulence* is used to characterize the severity of disease produced by an infectious organism. Rabies virus is highly virulent; only a few patients have ever recovered from such infections. In contrast, *Dientamoeba fragilis* rarely produces symptoms in infected patients. The virulence of most infectious agents varies, depending on the susceptibility of the host. Although *Toxoplasma gondii* usually causes asymptomatic or mild illnesses in normal hosts, infections during the first trimester of pregnancy may lead to severe birth defects, and in immunosuppressed patients, a fatal encephalitis may result.

Host Specificity. Several properties of an infectious agent may influence its pathogenicity and virulence. Host specificity refers to the preference of an infectious agent for a given host. Some organisms have very strict host specificities, e.g., *Treponema pallidum* and *Neisseria gonorrhoeae*, which are pathogenic only for man. In contrast, *Salmonella* species and *Trypanosoma cruzi* infect human beings as well as a wide variety of nonhuman animals. Different strains or developmental stages of an organism may also differ in their pathogenicity and virulence. The larval stages of most helminths are much less host-specific than the adult stages. Cutaneous and visceral larva migrans, for example, are usually caused by helminths that are incapable of developing into adults in man.

Invasiveness. The ability of an infectious agent to penetrate and spread through the host's tissues is referred to as invasiveness. *Vibrio cholerae* does not invade the intestinal mucosa. Instead, it produces its effects by the elaboration of a potent toxin. *Shigella dysenteriae*, however, in addition to producing a toxin, can invade and multiply within mucosal epithelial cells, causing cell death, leading to ulcers in the terminal ileum and colon. With most highly invasive organisms, e.g., *Streptococcus*, the production of lytic enzymes promotes the rapid spread of infection.

Infective Dose. The number of organisms necessary to cause infection also plays a role in the pathogenicity and virulence of infectious diseases. Neutralization of gastric acidity greatly reduces the number of enteric bacteria necessary to produce infection. A similar relationship between infective dose and severity of infection occurs in most helminthic infections. When the worm burden is low, patients usually have few or no symptoms, but heavy infections can result in severe disease.

Additional Factors. The longevity of an infectious agent, its resistance to antimicrobial agents, and the production of toxins are additional factors to be considered in the pathogenicity and virulence of an infectious agent.

Source and Reservoir. In considering programs for the control of infectious diseases, it is important that a distinction be made between the source of an infectious agent and its reservoir. The *source* of an infectious agent is the person, animal, object, or substance from which the organism passes directly to a susceptible host. The *reservoir* is the person, animal, arthropod, plant, or inanimate organic material in which an infectious agent normally lives and multiplies and on which it depends for its survival. The reservoir and source of an organism may be identical, as with *Salmonella typhi* infections. In contrast, with one of the hepatitis viruses, the reservoir is usually man, but the source may be contaminated food, water, blood, or biologic products.

HOST

Site of Entrance of Infection. Infectious agents may enter a host via the skin, mucous membranes, respiratory tract, gastrointestinal tract, or genitourinary tract. *Schistosoma* and *Leptospira* are examples of organisms that can penetrate intact skin. Most other infectious agents require a break in the integrity of the skin due to trauma, surgical wounds or instrumentation, or the bite of an arthropod vector to invade a host and produce disease.

The site of entrance of infectious agents that are deposited in the respiratory tract depends primarily on the size of the organism. Particles smaller than 5 μm in diameter are usually carried to the terminal alveoli, where they may be transported across the alveolar membrane by macrophages. Larger particles are deposited in the bronchioles, bronchi, trachea, or nares.

Infection via the gastrointestinal tract in contaminated food or drink is the usual means of entrance of enteric bacteria and intestinal protozoa and helminths. Entrance to the genitourinary tract may occur during catheterization, instrumentation, or sexual intercourse. Infectious agents may also be transferred transplacentally to the developing fetus, as in the case of rubella and *Toxoplasma*.

Host Defenses. The response of a host to an infectious agent depends on the pathogenicity and virulence of the organism as well as on the host's susceptibility and defenses. The host response may range from inapparent or subclinical infection to severe or even fatal illness. Host factors that may influence susceptibility to an infectious agent and the severity

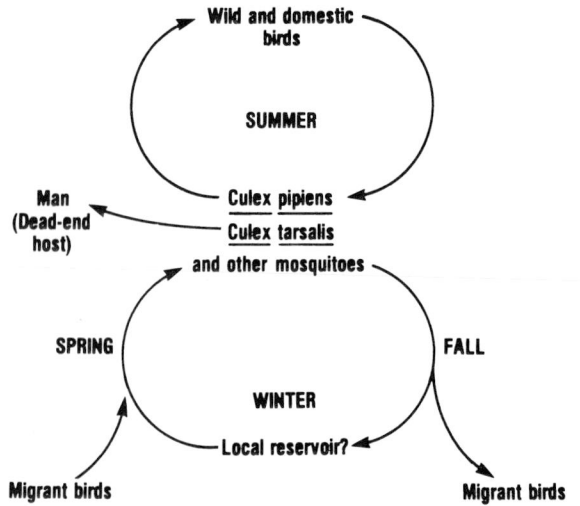

Figure 134–1. St. Louis encephalitis virus transmission cycle in the United States.

ROUTE OF INFECTION. There are four basic routes of transmission of infectious agents from a source to a susceptible host: contact, common-vehicle, airborne, and vector-borne. In many cases, infectious agents are transmitted by more than one of these routes; however, before specific control measures can be considered, the route of transmission must be identified.

Contact Transmission. Three types of contact transmission are recognized: *Direct-contact transmission* requires direct physical contact between an infected person or animal and a susceptible host, such as occurs with syphilis or gonorrhea. *Indirect-contact transmission* results from the contact between a susceptible host and a contaminated inanimate object, as in pinworm infections, which may be transmitted by clothing, bedding, and other articles contaminated with infective eggs. *Droplet spread* involves transmission of infection over short distances via large droplets that contain the infectious agent. The common cold and measles are examples of transmission by this route.

Common-Vehicle Transmission. In this situation, the infectious agent is spread to multiple hosts from a single inanimate source. The vehicle may be water (as in the case of giardiasis or hepatitis A and E), food (as with botulism and trichinosis), milk (as with brucellosis), or biologic substances e.g., blood, blood products (as in the case of hepatitis B and C and malaria), or intravenous fluids.

Airborne Transmission. Dust particles or droplet nuclei that contain an infectious agent are responsible for disease transmission by the airborne route. These particles are much smaller than those involved in direct-contact transmission by droplets and may remain suspended in the air for considerable periods of time. Airborne infectious agents may arise from human, animal, or inanimate sources. Tuberculosis is an example of a disease transmitted by airborne spread from an infected patient. In ornithosis, airborne transmission results from infected birds, whereas Q fever may be transmitted by aerosols from inanimate sources.

Vector-borne Spread. Transmission of an infectious agent to a vertebrate host by an arthropod may be either mechanical or biologic. *Mechanical transmission* includes simple mechanical carriage of an infectious agent on the vector's body or within its intestinal tract, as in flies harboring *Shigella*, as well as the carriage of organisms on the mouth parts of biting insects, such as occurs with African trypanosomiasis. In *biologic transmission*, the infectious agent multiplies within the arthropod vector, and a finite period, known as the extrinsic incubation period, is required before the arthropod becomes infective for another vertebrate host (Fig. 134–1).

Arthropod-borne infectious agents may enter the host by

of clinical manifestations include age, sex, race, ethnic group and other hereditary factors, nutritional and physiologic status, previous or concurrent diseases, and prior immunologic experience.

Carrier State. The carrier state, a form of inapparent infection in which a person harbors an infectious agent in the absence of clinical disease, is extremely important epidemiologically. Prolonged urinary or fecal excretors of *Salmonella typhi* and asymptomatic malaria gametocyte carriers play crucial roles in the transmission of these diseases and their maintenance during unfavorable periods.

Nonspecific and Specific Protection. Host defense mechanisms are of two types: nonspecific and specific. The barrier presented by the intact skin and mucous membranes, tears, saliva, and respiratory, gastrointestinal, and genitourinary secretions are examples of *nonspecific* defenses. The *specific* defense mechanisms of the host are natural and artificial immunity. *Natural immunity* develops following the natural occurrence of an infection. It may be short-lived, as with most viral respiratory illnesses, or essentially lifelong, as with rubella and poliomyelitis. Artificial immunity is of two kinds. *Active artificial immunity* results from vaccination with live, attenuated, or killed vaccines. *Passive artificial immunity* is produced by the administration of immunoglobulin or antitoxins or by the transplacental passage of antibody.

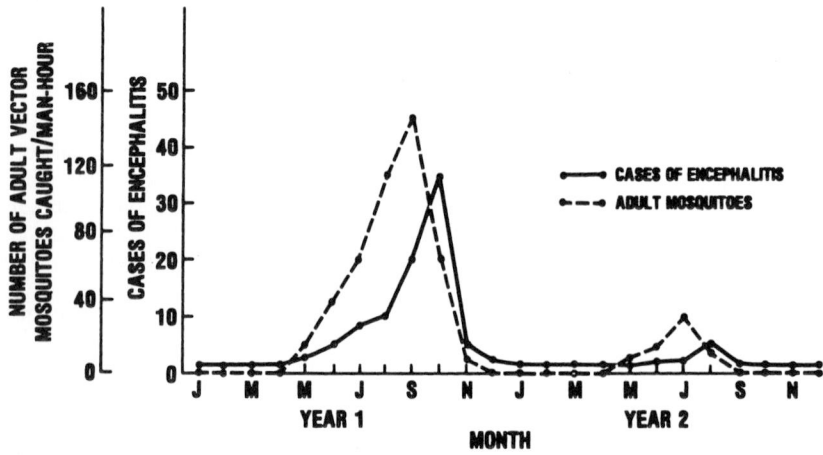

Figure 134–2. Mosquito-borne viral encephalitis. Outbreak in Year 1, before mosquito control program started, shows the occurrence of disease primarily during the summer months and the rise and peak of human cases following the rise in the mosquito population. Regular spraying with insecticide was initiated in Year 2, and no outbreak occurred.

several routes. With malaria, dengue, and yellow fever, the infectious agent is injected directly into the subcutaneous tissues or the blood stream. With plague, the intestinal tract of the flea vector becomes blocked by large masses of bacilli, and when the flea attempts to feed, organisms are regurgitated into the bite wound. Infectious agents may also gain entrance to the host through contamination of the skin or mucous membranes. Rickettsiae of epidemic typhus and trypanosomes of Chagas' disease are discharged in the vector's feces and may be rubbed or scratched into the wound after the vector has fed. Relapsing fever spirochetes, present within the body fluids of infected body lice, may enter the bite wound when the lice are accidentally or purposely crushed.

A variety of factors influence the capability of an arthropod to serve as an efficient vector of human disease. These include the susceptibility of the vector to the infectious agent, the vector's ability to transmit the organism to man, the degree of association between the vector and man and its willingness to bite man, and the vector's population density and survival rate (Fig. 134–2).

Many infectious agents may be transmitted by several different routes. Rabies virus, for example, is most frequently transmitted by direct contact with an infected canine but also may be spread by the airborne route in caves inhabited by infected bats. Anthrax is usually spread by direct contact with contaminated tissues or products of infected animals, but it can also be transmitted by the airborne or common-vehicle route.

ENVIRONMENT. The environment, including its physical, biologic, and socioeconomic components, may influence any of the three major links in the chain of transmission so as to promote or limit the development of infection. *Physical factors*, e.g., cold, heat, rainfall, humidity, and velocity of air currents, may affect both the host's susceptibility to infection and the viability of the infectious agent. These physical factors are particularly important in the case of vector-borne diseases. *Biologic factors*, including human population density and availability of food sources for vertebrate reservoir hosts and vectors, may also influence the transmission of infection. Finally, *socioeconomic and behavioral factors*, e.g., occupation, sanitary conditions, hygienic habits, cultural and religious practices, and catastrophes, (e.g., wars, floods, and famines), may affect the susceptibility of a host and the risk of acquiring infection.

135 *Zoonoses*

James E. Childs and G. Thomas Strickland

DEFINITION. Zoonoses are diseases and infections transmitted naturally between animals and humans. Typically, zoonotic infections include diseases transmitted from vertebrate animals to humans as well as those that are common to animals and humans, but for which animals may not play an essential role in the life cycle. The routes of dissemination include direct, vector, or vehicle transmission, and the pathogens involved vary from the largest macroparasites (e.g., helminths) to the microparasites (e.g., viruses, bacteria, and protozoa). Zoonoses have been classified by both the mechanism (type of maintenance cycle) and direction of transmission (human to animal vs. animal to human; Table 135–1).

HISTORY AND ECOLOGY. In evolutionary terms, all infections of humans and other animals share common origins. Many of the most ancient of well-chronicled human diseases are zoonoses. For example, descriptions of human and animal rabies can be found in the Eshmuna Code of Babylon, dating from the 23rd century B.C. The Latin word "virus," meaning poison or slimy liquid, was used to describe the saliva of rabid dogs, which was identified as an infectious material centuries ago.

Zoonoses also have played a critical role in the development of human societies and the course of history. From the 14th and 15th centuries the Black Death, caused by the pneumonic transmission of the plague bacillus, *Yersinia pestis,* which has an enzootic cycle between rats and their fleas, decimated human populations of Europe, North Africa, and Asia Minor. Zoonoses and vector-borne diseases have profoundly altered the outcome of wars and sent more soldiers to the hospital than has armed conflict.

The reason for the early recognition and description of zoonotic disease relates to both the severity of some of these infections and that, during most of humankind's existence, most important infections were acquired from animals. The highly communicable diseases that became totally dependent on a human reservoir have emerged only within the last 10,000 years or so as human populations achieved a critical size. Pathogens that became totally dependent on a human host, e.g., measles and smallpox viruses, were established and coevolved with humans only since our sociocultural infrastructure developed to the point at which the population size provided a renewable, yet constantly consumed, susceptible population. As infected individuals graduated into the immune population, recovered to become infected again, or died from their disease, a critical population size and birth rate resulted in sufficient numbers of susceptible newborns for propagating infection and transmission. Prior to the development of sustainable agriculture, the domestication of animals, and urban development, it is likely that only agents that cause chronic, persistent infection (e.g., herpesvirus infections) were pathogens uniquely adapted to humans.

Zoonotic agents are dependent primarily on factors that influence the dynamics of animal or vector populations, although many agents (e.g., the cyclozoonotic macroparasite taeniasis with an obligatory human development stage) are dependent on human hosts. The intermediate or reservoir host produces a buffering effect whereby zoonotic agents can persist even when the human population is small or widely dispersed. However, the human risk for infection with a zoonotic agent is strongly influenced by factors that dictate the type and frequency of human encounters with a reservoir or vector of the agent; for this reason, new zoonoses are constantly being recognized and the range of environments they inhabit increase.

Frequently, humans are dead-end hosts for zoonoses, only rarely passing infection back to the animal source. Barriers to the ready establishment of interspecies infections usually limit the human-to-human transmission of a zoonotic disease. For example, monkeypox virus has been transmitted through four generations of human-to-human contact but has not yet become an established human parasite. Ebola and Lassa fever viruses are readily transmitted in hospital settings through infectious blood or excreta and may be passed on through several generations of human-to-human transmission, yet are not continuously propagated by this route (Fig. 135–1). However, important exceptions exist; examples are pneumonic plague (Fig. 61–2) and urban yellow fever, which can become contagious or sustainable, respectively, by vector transmission independent of sylvatic life-cycle constraints once introduced into the human population.

TABLE 135–1. Classification of Zoonoses by Type of Maintenance Cycle*

Maintenance Cycle	Characteristics	Examples
Direct (orthozoonoses)	Maintenance can be achieved by a single vertebrate species. Transmission from an infected to a susceptible host by direct contact, contact with fomite, or by mechanical vector.	Rabies, leptospirosis, anthrax
Cyclozoonoses	Maintenance requires more than one vertebrate host.	Echinococcosis, human taeniases
Metazoonoses	Maintenance cycle requires vertebrates and invertebrates. Agent multiplies or undergoes development in the invertebrate.	Yellow fever, schistosomiasis, plague
Saprozoonoses	Maintenance cycle includes vertebrate and nonanimal sites or reservoirs. Nonanimal includes organic matter (including food), soil, and plants.	Visceral larva migrans, histoplasmosis

*Zoonoses can also be typed by direction of transmission.
After Schwabe CS: Veterinary Medicine and Human Health, 3rd ed. Baltimore, Williams & Wilkins, 1984, p 680.

Yellow fever virus has a forest or sylvatic cycle and is transmitted among canopy-dwelling primates by *Haemagogus* (South America) or canopy-dwelling *Aedes* (Africa) mosquitoes. However, when a human is infected in the forest, this disease can become epidemic and self-perpetuating if the individual reenters a densely populated human environment where urban breeding species of *Aedes* mosquitoes (mainly *Aedes aegypti*) act as competent vectors (Fig. 135–2). When zoonotic agents successfully cross over to infect humans and encounter conditions suitable for their sustained transmission in human populations, their impact can be profound. Historical examples include measles, smallpox, and human immunodeficiency (HIV) viruses.

Zoonoses have altered history. If the recent past is any indication of what the future holds, new agents will continue to be discovered or emerge in rapid succession. In the United States alone, numerous zoonotic diseases have been described since 1970: Lyme disease, the two forms of human ehrlichiosis, and hantavirus pulmonary syndrome (HPS) are only a few examples. Many factors contribute to emergence of disease; however, according to an Institute of Medicine report, "The significance of zoonoses in the emergence of human infections cannot be overstated." When the next devastating infectious disease emerges to threaten humankind, it very likely will be a viral zoonosis transmitted by the respiratory route. The recognition of a *Morbillivirus* capable

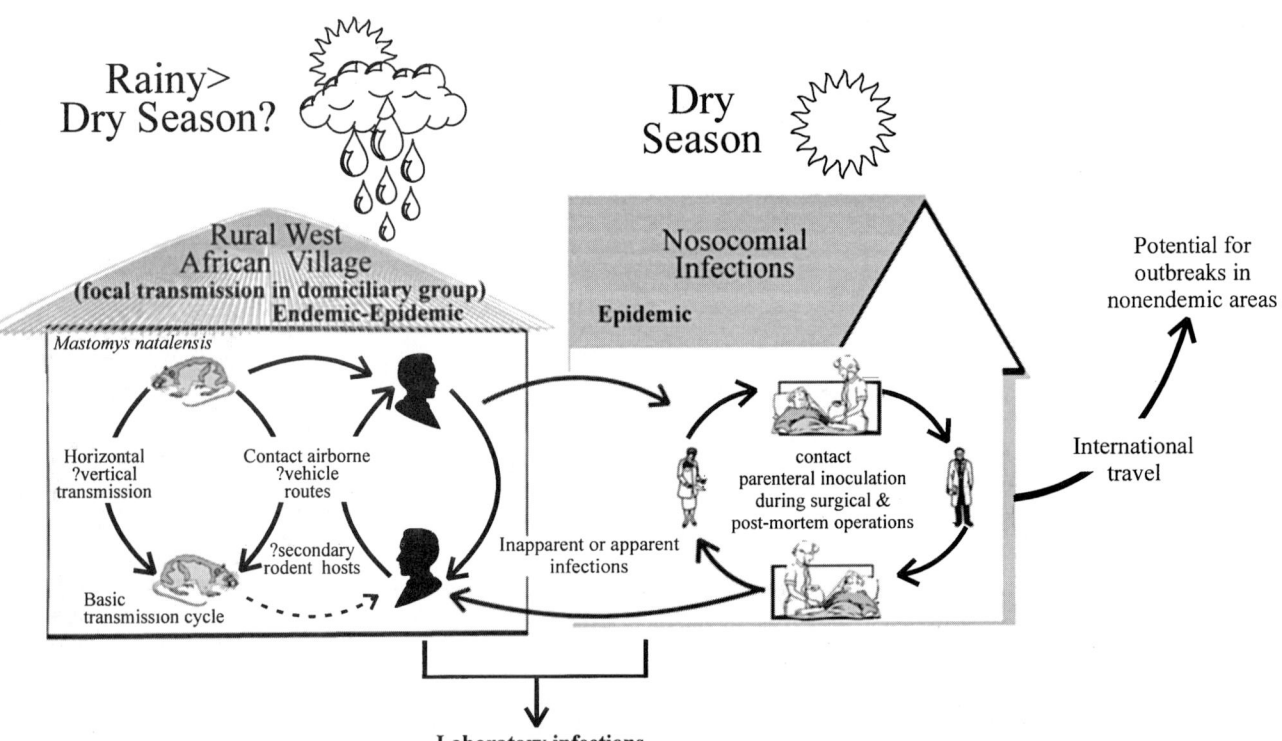

Figure 135–1. Transmission of Lassa virus in West Africa can occur through contact with infected rodent hosts in a village or with blood-contaminated materials in a hospital setting. Major epidemics of Lassa fever are typically identified only after a patient is treated in a hospital without proper barrier nursing precautions and infection spreads by the nosocomial route. A similar epidemiologic pattern may occur with Ebola virus, although the animal reservoirs/vectors are not currently known. (Reproduced, with slight modifications, from Monath, TP: Lassa fever: Review of epidemiology and epizootiology. Bull WHO 1975; 52:577–591.)

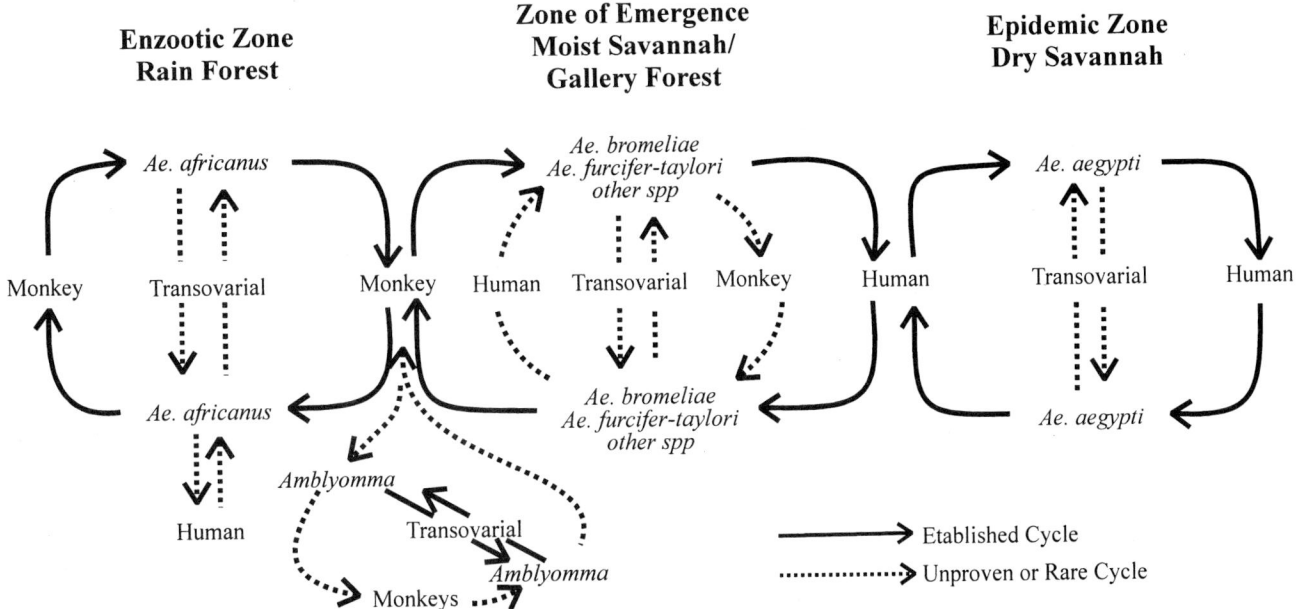

Enzootic Zone
Rain Forest

Zone of Emergence
Moist Savannah/
Gallery Forest

Epidemic Zone
Dry Savannah

Ae. africanus

Ae. bromeliae
Ae. furcifer-taylori
other spp

Ae. aegypti

Monkey   Transovarial   Monkey   Human   Transovarial   Monkey   Human   Transovarial   Human

Ae. africanus

Ae. bromeliae
Ae. furcifer-taylori
other spp

Ae. aegypti

Human

Amblyomma

Transovarial

Amblyomma

Monkeys

————————▶ Etablished Cycle
··············▶ Unproven or Rare Cycle

Figure 135–2. Transmission cycle of sylvatic and urban yellow fever. (Reproduced, with slight modifications, from Monath TP [ed]: The Arboviruses: Epidemiology and Ecology. Boca Raton, FL, CRC Press, 1988.)

of causing fatal disease in both horses and humans in 1994 is a chilling reminder that such evolutionary leaps are genuine and ongoing threats.

EPIDEMIOLOGY. As zoonotic agents are at some point in their life cycle maintained and/or transmitted among nonhuman vertebrates and/or invertebrate intermediates, an understanding of their epidemiology requires knowledge of the factors that influence the natural maintenance of the organisms. This requirement necessitates an appreciation and understanding of animal ecology and behavior. In addition to agent, vector, reservoir host, and environmental factors, issues related to human demography and behavior greatly influence the risk of acquiring zoonotic infections.

Agent and Host Specificity. Zoonotic agents are extremely variable in their host specificity and their impact on individuals and host populations. Even a single species of parasite may display dramatically different host specificities or affinities during different life stages. The tissue-cyst form (bradyzoite) of the protozoan *Toxoplasma gondii*, which develops as a result of ingesting sporulated oocysts produced by an infected felid or by ingesting tissue-cysts from another infected intermediate host, are present in a wide range of mammals and birds that may act as the source of human infection when their inadequately cooked or raw flesh is eaten. On the other hand, the sexual form of this protozoan develops only in felids, most notably the domestic cat, and all oocysts are produced by this single host (Figs. 97–1 and 97–3). Variants of rabies viruses, identified by monoclonal antibodies and genetic sequencing, can now be associated with specific reservoir hosts, typically single species in the mammalian orders Carnivora (e.g., dogs, foxes) and Chiroptera (i.e., bats). The geographic distribution and spread of regional epizootics can be traced to particular virus variants and a principal reservoir species. However, as all mammals appear susceptible to rabies infection, regardless of the exact variant, rabies virus spreads from a principal reservoir to a large number of susceptible species (known as virus "spillover"). However, sustained epizootics do not readily develop among other species, and how unique species-adapted variants arise remains unclear (Chapter 30.1).

Vectors of zoonotic agents may acquire their infections during certain life stages when blood-feeding preferences and vertebrate competency for a given agent are compatible. A major tick vector of the spirochete that causes Lyme disease, *Borrelia burgdorferi*, is *Ixodes scapularis*, which typically acquires infection in the northeastern United States as a larva or nymph while feeding on infected white-footed mice (*Peromyscus leucopus*). Adult ticks obtain their blood meals from medium- to large-sized mammals that may not, as in the case of the white-tailed deer (*Odocoileus virginianus*), be competent reservoirs for the spirochete but may be essential hosts for life stages of the vector. Thus, hosts essential for sustaining transmission cycles of a pathogen may constitute only a subset of those hosts essential for maintaining the life cycle of the vector (Fig. 73–1).

Disease Virulence. The pathologic effects of zoonotic agents on a reservoir host range from inconsequential to fatal. This range of disease outcomes is consistent with evolutionary theory. However, agents that kill their hosts should not always be regarded as "poorly adapted" or indicative of a newly emerged evolutionary partnership, and a benign host-parasite relationship is not a necessary requirement for an evolutionary stable association. Many arenaviruses and hantaviruses establish a carrier state in their rodent hosts that is characterized by persistent viral shedding from the infected host, frequently with no overt pathologic signs. Similarly, *Bartonella henselae*, the agent of cat-scratch disease and other human diseases, causes a high-titered bacteremia in infected cats that can persist for months with no clinical signs (Chapter 60.2).

At the other extreme, rabies virus routinely kills animal hosts essential for its maintenance. Many zoonoses have a profound effect on human health through the morbidity and mortality they cause in domestic animals or wildlife, in addition to diseases caused in humans. For example, the bacterial agents that cause brucellosis, anthrax, and bovine tuberculosis are responsible for serious veterinary health problems as well as being potential sources of human disease. The loss of food and work animals lead to human health consequences (protein-calorie malnutrition) far beyond the obvious zoonotic disease problems.

Molecular Epidemiology. The development of molecular biologic techniques to detect and characterize agents that are difficult to isolate by culturing methods has provided a tremendous impetus to our understanding of zoonotic agents. The use of polymerase chain reaction (PCR) and sequence analysis first indicated that the causative agent of bacillary angiomatosis (BA), a severe vasoproliferative disease in AIDS patients, was closely related to the louse-borne agent of trench fever, *Bartonella quintana* (Chapter 60.3). The subsequent isolation of *B. henselae* and its identification as both the etiologic agent of BA in AIDS patients and the long-sought etiologic agent of cat-scratch disease (Chapter 60.2) have rekindled scientific inquiry and public health appreciation of this formerly obscure group of pathogens. Other pathogens, e.g., hantaviruses, which are notoriously difficult to isolate in cell culture, have been identified and characterized solely on the basis of genetic analyses. The comparison of sequence information obtained from virus in autopsy material from fatal cases of HPS with that of virus obtained from trapped rodents enabled important epidemiologic deductions to be made about the location where infection occurred (Chapter 31.6).

TRANSMISSION. Transmission of zoonotic agents runs the gamut of complex cycles involving multiple life stages and hosts (e.g., Lyme disease) to direct transmission involving contact, e.g., through bite or trauma (rabies virus). Increasingly, common vehicle routes of transmission, e.g., with *Cryptosporidium parvum* disseminated in water and *Salmonella enteritidis* in poultry products, have been involved in large outbreaks in the United States. These events are influencing our treatment of water and food. In these latter examples, the ultimate source of the agent is distinct from the mechanism by which it is disseminated, and clarifying these relationships is crucial to the planning of effective prevention or eradication programs. Many agents can be transmitted by more than one route. The rickettsia responsible for Q fever, *Coxiella burnetii*, can be transmitted by the bite of an infected tick among nonhuman vertebrates, by aerosol, or by contact with contaminated tissues or soil. Rift Valley fever virus can be transmitted to humans by the bite of a mosquito vector or through contact with viremic blood from infected livestock.

Many zoonotic agents are not communicable or transmitted continuously once infection is established in humans. Other agents, e.g., Lassa virus and Ebola virus, can initiate explosive epidemics by direct contact with blood, vomitus, or excreta, once an index patient (presumably infected by contact with a reservoir or vector involved in natural maintenance cycles) is admitted to hospitals not having proper barrier nursing precautions (Fig. 135–1).

Finally, the route of transmission among natural hosts may be different from the route of transmission from reservoir or vector to humans. Viruses that cause hemorrhagic fever in humans through inhalation of small droplet aerosols (e.g., hantaviruses and arenaviruses) may be transmitted by bite or direct contact among their rodent hosts. Some agents transmitted to humans by arthropod vectors (e.g., *Rickettsia rickettsii*, the agent of Rocky Mountain spotted fever, and numerous arboviruses) are maintained at varying efficiency by transovarial transmission within vector populations, without the absolute requirement for amplification within vertebrates. Transovarial transmission can result in extremely high prevalence of an organism among vector populations and may play an important role in overwintering of pathogens in temperate climates and survival of pathogens during seasonal weather extremes in the tropics.

Range, Environment, and Climate. Zoonoses dependent on specific vertebrate or invertebrate vectors obviously are limited by the natural evolutionary or historical geographic ranges of these species. These natural limits are constantly being challenged as humans translocate infected vertebrate and invertebrate reservoirs, and this translocation can ignite new foci of disease or enlarge the geographic areas where particular diseases are enzootic. In addition, the rapid transport of humans incubating disease has caused considerable concern, especially with viral hemorrhagic fevers, e.g., Lassa fever.

Climatic Changes. Within their natural range, vectors and hosts of zoonotic agents are subject to fluctuations in population density as climatic and environmental parameters vary, and these population changes can influence the incidence of human infections. In sub-Saharan Africa, the emergence of epizootic Rift Valley fever virus is associated with above-average rainfall and the periodic flooding of seasonal ponds or depressions that result in a hatch of transovarially infected *Aedes* mosquito eggs. Epizootics of this virus can result in a high incidence of abortion in livestock and occasional outbreaks of severe disease in humans (Chapter 29.10). In the southwestern United States, a mild winter with unusually high rainfall, influenced by an El Niño event in the Pacific, may have contributed to abundant food resources, increased overwinter survival, and resultant high population densities of deer mice (*Peromyscus maniculatus*) in the spring of 1993. These rodents are the primary reservoir for Sin Nombre virus (genus *Hantavirus*), which causes HPS, and risk for human disease was increased with this increase in rodent abundance.

Climatic conditions may directly result in increased human disease, without the intermediate step of amplifying vector or host populations. An outbreak of leptospirosis in Nicaragua in 1995 was associated with heavy rainfall after an extremely severe hurricane season; soil contaminated by animal urine that contained spirochetes was the presumed source of infection. The dependence of many diseases, especially those transmitted by an arthropod vector, on climatic constraints has engendered considerable debate over the impact global warming will have on the future distribution and incidence of infectious diseases.

Demographic Factors. One of the most illustrative examples of how humankind's migration into sylvatic areas is increasing human exposure to zoonotic infections is the epidemiology of American visceral leishmaniasis in Amazonian Brazil (Fig. 135–3). *Leishmania chagasi* is transmitted in the rain forest between native foxes by a sylvatic sandfly species. Gold miners and other migrants settle in the forest and bring in domestic animals, including dogs and chickens. Foxes are naturally attracted to these peridomestic habitats, bringing with them their infectious sandflies, and naturally infected *Lutzomyia longipalpis* have no problems adapting from a wooded habitat to a peridomestic one created by deforestation and construction of rural huts and shacks. They readily feed on chicken, dog, and human blood. Thus, the deforestation of the Amazon is establishing new foci of human transmission of visceral leishmaniasis.

Human Factors. The history of human development from a nomadic, pastoral, hunter-gatherer existence to the increasing urbanization in the 1900s has profoundly influenced the types of zoonotic diseases that are public health concerns. In the urban centers of the United States, diseases that may be directly disseminated through public water supplies, e.g., cryptosporidiosis, pose significant threats. Sporocysts of this protozoan shed by bovids or other mammals are washed into surface water reservoirs, where usual treatment procedures are inadequate to kill them. Epidemics of this disease have involved hundreds of thousands of residents in cities of the United States (Chapter 88). In less-developed countries, disease challenges posed by population growth and increas-

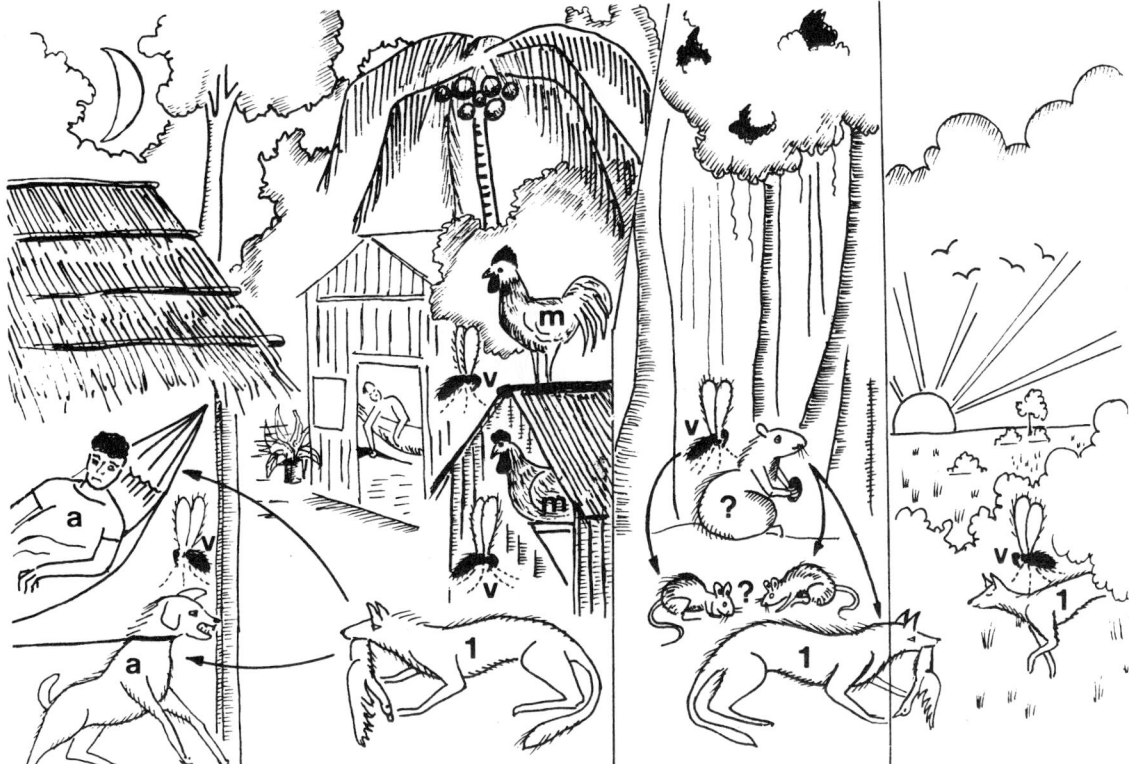

Figure 135–3. The epidemiology of American visceral leishmaniasis due to *L. chagasi*, in Amazonian Brazil. In the sylvatic situation, a transmission cycle occurs among foxes (1) *(Cerdocyon thous)*, probably maintained by a sylvatic population of *Lu. longipalpis* (v and arrows), but possibly with another vector involved (?). Sylvatic *Lu. longipalpis* invade the peridomestic situation in newly established villages, where they concentrate in animal shelters, particularly chicken houses (m). Infection may reach villages by two routes: marauding foxes may be fed on by the peridomestic *Lu. longipalpis* population, which in turn transmits to dogs (a) and man (a). As *Lu. longipalpis* is more attracted to dogs, canine infection is most frequent, and the dog becomes the principal source of infection for man. Alternatively, dogs (and possibly man) may become infected by the bites of infected flies that have been attracted to the lights of houses, directly from the sylvatic cycle. (Modified from Lanson R: Demographic changes and their influence on the epidemiology of American leishmaniasis. *In* Service MW [ed]: Demography and Vector-Borne Diseases. Boca Raton, FL, CRC Press, 1989.)

ing urbanization include arboviral infections. Mosquitoes breeding in water containers and waste materials provide a critical element for the transmission of dengue fever in urban areas, making its zoonotic or sylvatic maintenance cycle much less important in the past 20 or 30 years.

Food Production and Distribution. In developed countries, human dependence on mass centralized food-animal production of chickens or cattle may facilitate dissemination of organisms, e.g., *S. enteritidis* or *Escherichia coli* O157:H7, to a huge population through multiple retail and commercial sources.

Domestic Animals. The domestication and geographic spread of companion and food animals have profoundly influenced the frequency and distribution of zoonotic diseases. Although any species could serve as an example, a brief examination of "man's best friend," the domestic dog, provides valuable lessons. The history of rabies as a major cause of human disease is closely linked to the domestication and translocation of the dog. Although other carnivores, e.g., raccoons and foxes, can serve as important wildlife reservoirs, only the dog has assumed a central role in maintaining and transmitting rabies virus to humans. Genetic analyses of rabies viruses associated with dogs from throughout the New World and many regions of Africa have shown that the virus that causes dog rabies in the 1990s was imported by colonialists from Europe centuries ago. The long incubation period of rabies allowed the successful transport of dogs that were incubating the infection. Most of the world is still af-

fected by the repercussions of this early transportation of animals.

CONTROL. Zoonoses present special challenges for control, since frequently the targets for these efforts are reservoir hosts (both wild and domestic) or vectors. This is not to say that traditional public health measures, e.g., vaccination, do not play a role. Effective human vaccines exist for many zoonotic agents. In some situations, vaccination of domestic animals not only protects the animal but provides an essential barrier to transmission of zoonotic agents to humans and other domestic animals (e.g., rabies vaccination of dogs and cats and Venezuelan equine encephalitis vaccination of horses). In other situations vaccination of wildlife reservoirs may be used to effectively control transmission. The vaccination of red foxes against rabies virus in Europe by using oral baits containing liver or recombinant rabies virus vaccine has eliminated rabies from both domestic and wildlife populations throughout much of the continent.

Frequently, however, control of zoonoses depends on attempts to reduce vector populations or limit contact with reservoir species (Chapter 139). The importance and public health impact of direct chemical interventions. e.g., use of insecticides to control vectors, cannot be overstated, and vector control activities are constantly in need of new, safe, and effective products. In most instances, these control efforts require environmental or human behavioral modification in addition to direct efforts at vector population reduction. Control and surveillance efforts integrating advanced technologies, e.g., remote satellite imaging for forecasting epizootic activity of Rift Valley fever in Africa based on rainfall patterns, hold some promise, but the link to appropriate local control capabilities must be clearly defined and maintained if they are to have any use in developing countries.

Other zoonoses transmitted through contact with food-animal products may be effectively controlled through animal inspection, culling of herds, appropriate treatment of products, and back-tracking of contaminated products to the source for targeted interventions. Frequently, the tracking of contaminated products to their source, e.g., chicken eggs contaminated with *S. enteritidis* or meat infected with *E. coli* O157:H7, is difficult or impossible. Paradoxically, the problem of bacterial contamination of food products also has been exacerbated by the practice of adding antibiotics to animal feed to promote growth.

Zoonoses transmitted directly from animals to humans through inhalation of infected aerosols, e.g., hantaviruses and arenaviruses, may be susceptible to prevention only in certain circumstances. If exposure is occurring in occupational settings (e.g., to farm workers in rural settings) control may be impossible, as it necessitates population reduction of reservoir species over very large areas. If exposure is occurring within the home, other options exist to limit contact with potentially infected reservoir species. These recommendations range from population reduction by using traps or rodenticides to environmental modification geared toward reducing harborage suitable for rodents. In the case of control of hantavirus infections, messages describing how to avoid rodent-infested, seasonally occupied dwellings until proper and safe cleaning has been achieved, or how to safely dispose of rodent carcasses or excreta are important.

Many programs directed at controlling human infectious diseases use surveillance at the local and national level to guide and assess prevention efforts. Most zoonoses, with the exception of animal rabies, are not monitored by national surveillance systems at the level of animal host. Instead, reports of human disease are analyzed to obtain clues as to trends in the prevalence of etiologic agents among natural populations and the geographic distribution of infection. Currently, the capacity to maintain surveillance for zoonoses in both the United States and for tropical diseases through U.S.-supported overseas laboratories is severely limited. Recent attempts to formulate a prevention strategy for emerging infections have emphasized the need for strengthening surveillance programs that monitor vector-borne and zoonotic diseases.

Bibliography

Acha PN, Szyfries B: Zoonoses and Communicable Diseases Common to Man and Animal, 2nd ed. Washington, DC, Pan American Health Organization, 1987.

Black FL: Infectious diseases in primitive societies. Science 187:515, 1975.

Centers for Disease Control and Prevention: Addressing Emerging Infectious Disease Threats: A Prevention Strategy for the United States. Atlanta, US Department of Health and Human Services, Public Health Service, 1994.

Lederberg J, Shope RE, Oaks SC Jr (eds): Emerging Infections: Microbial Threats to Health in the United States. Washington, DC, National Academy Press, 1992.

McNeill WH: Plagues and Peoples. New York, Anchor/Doubleday, 1976.

Monath TP (ed): The Arboviruses: Epidemiology and Ecology. Boca Raton, FL, CRC Press, 1988.

Murray K, Selleck P, Hooper P, et al: A morbillivirus that caused fatal disease in horses and humans. Science 268:94, 1995.

Nichol ST, Spiropoulou CF, Morzunov S, et al: Genetic identification of a hantavirus associated with an outbreak of acute respiratory illness. Science 262:914, 1993.

Relman DA, Loutit JS, Schmidt TM, et al: The agent of bacillary angiomatosis: An approach to the identification of uncultured pathogens. N Engl J Med 323:1573, 1990.

Schwabe CS: Veterinary Medicine and Human Health, 3rd ed. Baltimore, Williams & Wilkins, 1984.

Service MW (ed): Demography and Vector-Borne Diseases. Boca Raton, FL, CRC Press, 1989.

Smith JS, Seidel HD: Rabies: A new look at an old disease. Prog Med Virol 40:82, 1993.

Spielman A, Wilson ML, Levine JF, et al: Ecology of *Ixodes dammini*–borne human babesiosis and Lyme disease. Annu Rev Entomol 30:439, 1985.

Steele JH, Fernandez PJ: History of rabies and global aspects. In Baer GM (ed): The Natural History of Rabies, 2nd ed. Boca Raton, FL, CRC Press, 1991.

136 Mollusks Involved in Disease Transmission

William A. Sodeman, Jr.

Most mollusks have no relationship to humans beyond their collection either as objects of beauty or as food. A few figure in the transmission of disease. Some mollusks transmit infection when eaten because of bacteria or viruses concentrated by filter feeding, such as the bivalves, oysters, mussels, and clams. Many parasites use snails as a first and/or second intermediate host for their larval stages. Transmission to humans can occur with ingestion of raw or poorly cooked snails (Fig. 114–1), but most often the parasite leaves the snail and penetrates the skin of the host (Fig. 118–6) or encysts on another food item that is eaten raw (Figs. 120–1 and 120–2).

This chapter is designed to serve as a guide for physicians practicing in an area endemic for snail-transmitted diseases. Table 136–1 lists the principal snail-transmitted diseases, their mollusk intermediate host, and their geographic distribution. The list is long, but fortunately, in most areas the numbers of snails are limited, and once the species have been determined by expert identification, further field identification is feasible and practical.

Snail identification primarily depends on morphology, including distinctive shells, radula (tooth) patterns, and soft-part anatomy, principally the anatomic variations of the genital apparatus. In a few cases, biochemical, immunologic, or cytogenetic characteristics must be ascertained to distinguish between morphologically similar, closely related species.

Shell morphology is often helpful in separating potential intermediate hosts from the many unsuitable mollusks. There are many areas where shell morphology alone can serve as an adequate guide to the presence or absence of suitable intermediate-host snails, but in some circumstances, the definitive species identification requires at least the study of soft-part anatomy and radular structure.

■ CLASSIFICATION OF MEDICALLY IMPORTANT GASTROPOD MOLLUSKS

The class Gastropoda is divided into two subclasses: Streptoneura, readily identifiable by the presence of an operculum, and the Euthyneura, of which the freshwater pulmonates are the primary concern.

SUBCLASS STREPTONEURA. Snails within the subclass Streptoneura are operculate, with the operculum, a trap door covering the aperture of the shell, fixed to the top of the foot behind the aperture. The operculum may be calcified, but in most freshwater families it is made of an organic noncalcified material. Soft-part anatomy shows a characteristic figure-eight twist to the visceral nerve and, in the aquatic forms,

TABLE 136–1. Principal Mollusk-Transmitted Infections of Humans

Disease	Pathogen	Mollusk (Genus and Species)	Geographic Range as Host
Clonorchiasis (Chapter 120.2)	*Clonorchis sinensis*	*Bithynia (Parafossarulus) manchourica*	China, Korea, Taiwan, Japan
		Bithynia fuchsiana	North China
		Bithynia chaperi	China
		Alocinma longicornis	China
		Semisulcospira amurensis	China
		Gabbia misella	Korea
Fascioliasis (Chapter 120.3)	*Fasciola hepatica*	*Lymnaea (Fossaria) truncatula*	Europe, Africa, Middle East, Asia
		Lymnaea viatrix	Argentina
		Lymnaea rubiginosa	Malaysia
		Lymnaea philippensis	Philippines
		Lymnaea swinhoe	Philippines
		Lymnaea tomentosa	Australia
		Lymnaea japonicum	Japan
		Lymnaea pervia	Japan
		Lymnaea columella	North and South America, Africa, Hawaiian Islands
		Fossaria bulimoides	United States
		Fossaria cubensis	United States
	Fasciola gigantica	*Lymnaea columella*	Africa
		Lymnaea rubiginosa	Malaysia
		Lymnaea acuminata	India
		Lymnaea auricularia	India
		Lymnaea natalensis	Africa
		Biomphalaria alexandrina	Egypt
		Fossaria ollula	Hawaii
Fasciolopsiasis (Chapter 119.1)	*Fasciolopis buski*	*Hippeutis umbilicalis*	India, Asia
		Hippeutis cantori	India, Asia
		Segmentina hemisphaerula	India, Asia
		Segmentina trochoideus	India, Asia
Gastrodisciasis (Chapter 119.4)	*Gastrodiscoides hominis*	*Helicorbis coenosus*	India, China
Heterophyiasis (Chapter 119.3)	*Heterophyes heterophyes*	*Cerithidea cingulata*	Japan
		Pirenella conica	Egypt, Oman
Metagonimiasis (Chapter 119.3)	*Metagonimus yokogawai*	*Thiara granifera*	Asia
		Semisulcospira libertina	Russia
		Semisulcospira laevigata	Russia
		Semisulcospira cancellata	Russia
Nanophyetiasis	*Nanophyetus salmincola schikhobalowi*	*Semisulcospira libertina*	Siberia
		Semisulcospira cancellata	Siberia
Opisthorchiasis (Chapter 120.1)	*Opisthorchis felineus*	*Bithynia leachii*	Europe, Siberia
	Opisthorchis viverrini	*Bithynia laevis*	Thailand, Laos, Malaysia
		Bithynia goniomphalus	Thailand, Laos, Malaysia
		Bithynia funiculata	Thailand, Laos, Malaysia
		Bithynia siamensis	Thailand, Laos, Malaysia
Paragonimiasis (Chapter 121)	*Paragonimus westermani*	*Semisulcospira libertina*	Japan, Taiwan, China, Korea
		Semisulcospira amurensis	North China, Korea
		Thiara tuberculata	Africa, Asia
		Brotia asperata	Philippines
		Brotia costula	Malaysia
	Paragonimus africanus	*Potadoma freethi*	Cameroon, Liberia, Nigeria, The Congo
	Paragonimus skrjabini	*Tricula microstoma*	China
		Tricula fujianesis	China
		Tricula minutoides	China
		Tricula humida	China
	Paragonimus heterotremus	*Tricula gregorina*	China
	Paragonimus caliensis	*Aroapyrgus columbiensis*	Central and South America
	Paragonimus mexicanus	*Aroapyrgus costaricensis*	Central and South America
Schistosomiasis (Chapter 118)	*Schistosoma japonicum*	*Oncomelania hupensis formosana*	Taiwan
		Oncomelania hupensis hupensis	China
		Oncomelania hupensis fausti	China
		Oncomelania hupensis tangi	China
		Oncomelania hupensis robertsoni	China
		Oncomelania hupensis guangxiensis	China
		Oncomelania hupensis lindoensis	Sulawesi
		Oncomelania hupensis nosophora	Japan
		Oncomelania hupensis quadrasi	Philippines
	Schistosoma mekongi	*Tricula aperta*	Thailand, Laos, Cambodia
	Schistosoma malayi	*Robertsiella gismani*	Malaysia
		Robertsiella kaporensis	Malaysia

Table continued on following page

TABLE 136–1. Principal Mollusk-Transmitted Infections of Humans *Continued*

Disease	Pathogen	Mollusk (Genus and Species)	Geographic Range as Host
	Schistosoma haematobium	*Bulinus beccarii*	Southwestern Arabia
		Bulinus camerunensis	Cameroon
		Bulinus cernicus	Mauritius
		Bulinus senegalensis	The Gambia
		Bulinus wrighti	Saudi Arabia, Yemen, Oman
		Bulinus guernei	The Gambia
		Bulinus rohlfsi	West Africa
		Bulinus truncatus	Eastern and western North Africa
		Bulinus abyssinicus	Ethiopia, Somalia
		Bulinus africanus	Eastern South Africa
		Bulinus jousseaumei	The Gambia
		Bulinus obtusispira	Madagascar
		Bulinus globosus	Sub-Saharan Africa
		Bulinus nasutus	East Africa
		Planorbarius metidjensis	Portugal
		Ferrissia tenuis	India
	Schistosoma intercalatum	*Bulinus forskalii*	Cameroon, Gabon
	Schistosoma mattheei	*Bulinus globosus*	South Africa
	Schistosoma mansoni	*Biomphalaria glabrata*	Venezuela, Greater and Lesser Antilles, Guyana, Surinam, French Guiana, Brazil
		Biomphalaria tenagophila	Brazil, Argentina
		Biomphalaria straminea	Brazil, Martinique
		Biomphalaria pfeifferi	North Africa, sub-Saharan Africa
		Biomphalaria choanomphala	Uganda, Tanzania
		Biomphalaria alexandrina	Egypt, Sudan
		Biomphalaria camerunensis	The Congo, Cameroon
		Biomphalaria sudanica	East Africa, Uganda, Sudan

anterior gills. There are three orders, one of which, the Mesogastropoda, contains snails of medical importance.

Order Mesogastropoda. Snails of the order Mesogastropoda are responsible, as intermediate hosts, for transmission of an extraordinary collection of trematodes that can produce disease in humans. Eight families are of medical importance. These are the Ampullariidae (= Pilidae), Viviparidae, Pomatiopsidae, Bithyniidae, Thiaridae, Pleuroceridae, Potatimididae, and Littorinidae.

Family Viviparidae. The families Ampullariidae and Viviparidae can be distinguished by the appearance of the operculum, which grows with a concentric rather than a spiral pattern. Viviparidae are large, globular snails (Fig. 136–1) that are ovoviviparous (bear live young). They are widespread in lakes and rivers. A single species, *Viviparus javanicus*, serves as a second intermediate host for *Echinostoma ilocanum* in Java. Transmission is by ingestion of the raw snail. This snail can also serve as the intermediate host for the rat lungworm, *Angiostrongylus cantonensis*.

Family Ampullariidae. Ampullariidae are also large, globular, egg-laying snails that have a worldwide distribution. Five of the many genera in this family are of medical significance. *Pila luzonica* and *P. conica* serve as second intermediate hosts for *E. ilocanum* on the Philippine island of Luzon. *P. polita* and *P. ampullacea* are the intermediate hosts for this parasite and for the nematode parasite *A. cantonensis* in Thailand. *P. scutata* serves as intermediate host for the latter in Indonesia and Malaysia. *Marisa cornuarietis* (Fig. 136–1) is an aquatic carnivorous snail that has been used in the attempted biologic control of *Biomphalaria* species that can transmit *Schistosoma mansoni* in South America and the Antilles. It does not serve in the transmission of human infection. It is flat in shape rather than globular but differs from planorbids because of its small red-brown operculum. Its shell is marked with reddish bands. It may be found in a broad range of freshwater habitats.

All the remaining families of Mesogastropoda of medical importance have an operculum with a spiral growth pattern.

Family Thiaridae. Although these snails have a worldwide distribution, their medical importance is principally in the Orient and Southeast Asia. One African genus is involved in the transmission of disease. The genus *Thiara* have tall, turreted shells measuring 2.5 to 5 cm as adults. There is a prominent axial beaded sculpture. *Thiara granifera* (Fig. 136–1) in Taiwan and the islands of Southeast Asia and now introduced in Central America, the Antilles, and the United States; *Thiara (Melanoides) tuberculata* in both Africa and Asia; *Brotia costula* Rafinesque in Malaysia and *Brotia asperata* in the Philippines all are reported to serve as first intermediate hosts for the lung fluke *Paragonimus westermani*. Subsequent evaluation suggests that *T. granifera* is not a first intermediate host for *P. westermani*. *T. granifera*, however, has served as an effective competitor in the biologic control of *Biomphalaria glabrata*, an intermediate host for *S. mansoni*. *T. granifera* is a first intermediate host of the intestinal fluke *Metagonimus yokogawai*.

In Africa, *Potadoma freethi* (Greer) (Fig. 136–1) has been identified as a first intermediate host of the lung fluke *Paragonimus africanus*. This snail is found in rivers and large streams. The snail intermediate host for *P. uterobilateralis*, another African lung fluke, has not been identified.

Family Pleuroceridae. This family contains two genera of medical importance: *Oxytrema* in the United States (Table 136–2) and *Semisulcospira* in the Orient.

The genus *Semisulcospira* is widespread throughout the Orient, where various species serve as hosts for *Clonorchis sinensis*, *M. yokogawai*, *P. westermani*, and *Nanophyetus salmincola schikhobalowi*. *Semisulcospira libertina* (Fig. 136–1) serves as a first intermediate host of *M. yokogawai* in Japan, while *S. laevigata* and *S. cancellata* fill this role in Russia. Possible snail hosts in Spain and the Balkans have not been identified. *S. libertina* serves as the intermediate host for the lung fluke *P.*

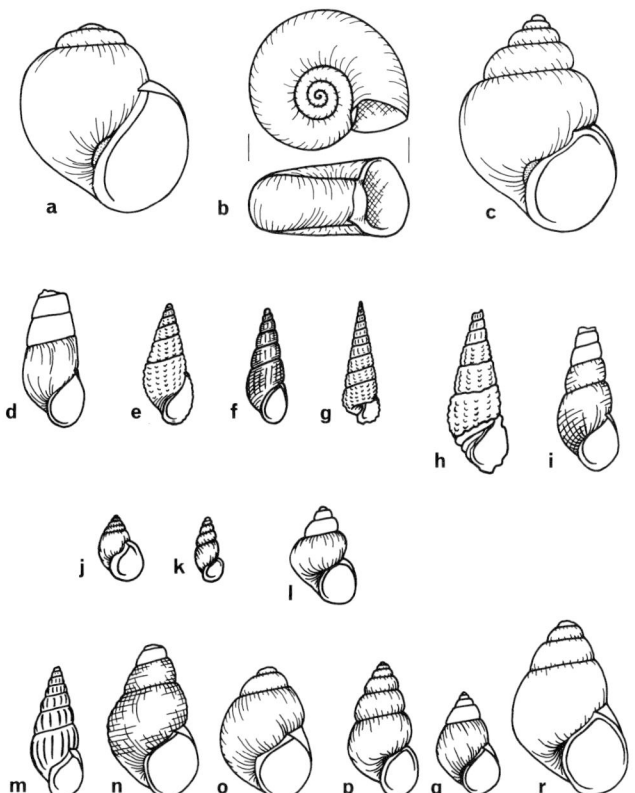

Figure 136–1. a, *Pila luzonica.* b, *Marisa cornuarietis.* c, Viviparidae: *Cipangopaludina chinenesis.* d, *Potadoma freethii.* e, *Thiara granifera.* f, *Melanoides tuberculata.* g, *Pirenella conica.* h, *Semisulcospira amurensis.* i, *Semisulcospira libertina.* j, *Neotricula aperta.* k, *Robertsiella kaporensis.* l, *Bithynia leachii.* m, *Oncomelania hupensis.* n, *Parafossarulus manchouricus.* o, *Bithynia (Gabbia) longicornus.* p, *Pomatiopsis lapidaria.* q, *Bithynia fuchsiana.* r, *Bithynia goniomphalus.* (Scale line: a = 44 mm; a-i to scale; j = 4 mm; j-r to scale. Drawings by Susan Trammell. Produced by George M. Davis, using collections of the Academy of Natural Sciences of Philadelphia.)

westermani in Japan, Taiwan, China, and Korea; *S. amurensis* is the host for this fluke in northern China and Korea. *S. amurensis* also serves as the first intermediate host for *C. sinensis* infection in China.

All these snails are large, up to 5 cm long, with high spires. *S. libertina* is found in the muddy bottoms of canals. *S. amurensis* frequents free-flowing streams. In the past, classifications have included many subgroups and races, with a resultant confusion in the literature.

Family Bithyniidae. This family contains three genera that can transmit disease, *Alocinma*, *Gabbia*, and *Bithynia*. These snails are 1.5 cm or less in length and ovate without a pointed spire. They are deeply sutured. The operculum is calcareous, with a small spiral nucleus that gives way to concentric development.

GENUS BITHYNIA (= BULIMUS). *Bithynia leachii* is the first intermediate host of *Opisthorchis felineus* in Central and Eastern Europe and in Russia as far east as Siberia. This globular snail has wide distribution in ponds in northern Europe and the United States.

Four other species, *B. laevis*, *B. goniomphalus* (Fig. 136–1), *B. siamensis*, and *B. funiculata*, serve as first intermediate hosts of *Opisthorchis viverrini* in Thailand, Laos, and Malaysia. These tiny snails favor muddy canals as habitats. *B. (Parafossarulus) manchouricus* is widespread in the Orient, both on the mainland, including Korea, and on Taiwan and Japan.

It is the host for *Echinochasmus perfoliatus*, an unusual and incidental parasite in humans, and it is an important intermediate host for *C. sinensis* throughout its geographic range. This small snail is globular but has a spire and pronounced ridge sculpture. It is found in sluggish water, including swamps, canals, ponds, and rivers.

B. fuchsiana in northern China and *B. chaperi* act as first intermediate hosts in the transmission of *C. sinensis* in their respective distributions.

GENUS ALOCINMA. The second genus of medical importance in this family includes one species, *Alocinma longicornis* (Fig. 136–1), which also serves as a first intermediate host in the transmission of *C. sinensis* in China. The snail is small, <10 mm, and globular, with a blunter spire than *Bithynia*. It, too, is prevalent in ponds and canal bottoms.

GENUS GABBIA. *Gabbia misella*, a small globular snail with a pronounced spire, has been identified as an intermediate host of *C. sinensis* in Korea.

Family Hydrobiidae. There are two subfamilies.

SUBFAMILY TRICULINAE. This subfamily contains 11 genera, of which two are hosts of human schistosomiasis; one genus also harbors intermediate hosts of *Paragonimus heterotremus* and *P. skrjabini*. *Neotricula aperta* (Temcharoen) (Fig. 136–1), a tiny, globular, operculate snail found in Thailand, Laos, and Cambodia, is the only known host for *Schistosoma mekongi*. *Robertsiella kaporensis* (Davis and Greer) and *R. gismani* (Davis and Greer) (Fig. 136–1) act as intermediate hosts for the newly named species, *Schistosoma malayi* (Chapter 118). Both these hosts are aquatic. *Tricula microstoma* Yue-ying, Wen-zhen, and Yao-xian; *T. fujianesis* Yue-ying, Wen-zhen, and Yao-xian; *T. minutoides*; and *T. humida* all serve as first intermediate hosts for *P. skrjabini* in China. *T. gregorina* serves as the first intermediate host for *P. heterotremus* in China and Thailand.

SUBFAMILY POMATIOPSINAE. This subfamily contains eight genera, one of which, *Oncomelania,*, is of importance in human disease. One species, *Oncomelania hupensis* (Fig. 136–1), is responsible for the transmission of *S. japonicum* throughout Asia. There are a number of subspecies of *O. hupensis*, which are geographically isolated and include *O. h. chiui* and *O. h. formosana* from Taiwan, *O. h. hupensis* from China, *O. h. fausti*, *O. h. tangi*, *O. h. robertsoni*, *O. h. guangxiensis*, *O. h. lindoensis*, from Sulawesi, *O. h. nosophora* from Japan, and *O. h. quadrasi* from the Philippines. All of these except *O. h. chiui* transmit human schistosomes. These various subspecies hybridize. There are remarkable differences in cross-susceptibility to infection with *S. japonicum* from various geographic areas.

Oncomelania are tiny, high-spired operculates that are amphibious. They favor rotting vegetation along river banks, where the mud is moist, as well as rice paddies. The complex relationships among subspecies, races, and susceptibility to infection make specific identification difficult.

Family Potamididae (= Cerithiidae). These have brackish and seawater as well as freshwater representatives of minor medical importance. *Cerithidea cingulata* in Japan and *Pirenella conica* (Blaurville) (Fig. 136–1) in Egypt and Oman serve as hosts of the intestinal fluke *Heterophyes heterophyes*.

GENUS AROAPYRGUS. This neotropical hydrobiid genus contains several species that serve as first intermediate hosts for several species of American paragonimiases. *Aroapyrgus columbiensis* has been identified as the first intermediate host for *P. caliensis. A. costaricensis* is the first intermediate host for *P. mexicanus*. Many other species of *Aroapyrgus* are suspected of serving as first intermediate hosts for *Paragonimus* species. Considerable controversy remains about the speciation of these parasites in the Americas.

SUBCLASS EUTHYNEURA. This subclass is separated into four orders, three of which—the Basommatophora, the Sty-

TABLE 136–2. Incidental or Rare Mollusk-Transmitted Infections of Humans

Disease	Pathogen	Mollusk (Genus and Species)	Geographic Range as Host
Echinostomiasis (Chapter 119.2)	Echinostoma ilocanum	First intermediate host:	
		Gyraulus convexiusculus	Philippines, Japan
		Hippeutis umbilicalis	Philippines
		Second intermediate host:	
		Pila luzonica	Philippines
		Pila conica	Philippines
		Pila polita	Thailand
		Pila ampullacea	Thailand
		Viviparus javanicus	Java
	Echinostoma malayanum	First intermediate host:	
		Lymnaea luteola	India
		Second intermediate host:	
		Indoplanorbis exustus	India
		Gyraulus convexiusculus	India
	Echinostoma macrordis	Gyraulus chinensis	Taiwan
Eosinophilic meningitis (Chapter 114.1)	Angiostrongylus cantonensis	Lymnaea (R.) rubigenosa	Indonesia
		Pila scutata	Indonesia, Malaysia
		Pila polita	Thailand
		Pila ampullacea	Thailand
Salmon poisoning	Nanophyetus salmincola	Oxytrema silicula	Northwestern United States
Schistosomiasis (Chapter 118)	Schistosoma bovis	Bulinus forskalii	East Africa
		Bulinus senegalensis	The Gambia
		Bulinus scalaris	The Gambia
		Bulinus truncatus	Middle East
		Bulinus africanus	South Africa
		Bulinus ugandae	Sudan, Uganda
		Planorbarius metidjensis	Spain
	Schistosoma rodhaini	Biomphalaria sudanica	The Congo
		Biomphalaria pfeifferi	Uganda, The Congo
Swimmers' itch (cercarial dermatitis) (Chapter 118)	Ornithobilharzia canaliculata	Batillaria minima	Florida
	Gigantobilharzia gyrauli	Gyraulus parvus	United States
	Gigantobilharzia huronensis	Physa gyrina	United States
	Gigantobilharzia huttoni	Haminoae antillarum	Florida
	Gigantobilharzia sturniae	Segmentina hemisphaerula	Japan
	Austrobilharzia penneri	Cerithidea scalariformis	Florida
	Austrobilharzia varigalandis	Littorina planaxis	California
		Littorina pintado	Hawaii
	Trichobilharzia ocellata	Lymnaea stagnalis	United States and Europe
	Trichobilharzia physellae	Physa parkeri	United States
		Physa anatina	United States
	Trichobilharzia yokogawai	Lymnaea swinhoe	Japan

lommatophora, and the Systellommatophora—have representatives of medical importance.

Order Basommatophora. This order has 4 families with genera of medical importance, all for their role as intermediate hosts of trematodes. These are the families Ancylidae, Lymnaeidae, Physidae, and Planorbidae.

Family Ancylidae. A single genus of the Ancylidae, *Ferrissia tenuis*, has been implicated as the intermediate host for *Schistosoma haematobium* in India.

Family Lymnaeidae. This family is large and geographically widespread. The liver flukes *Fasciola hepatica* and *Fasciola gigantica* use genera of this family as intermediate hosts. Several species of *Trichobilharzia* that can cause schistosome dermatitis in humans also use Lymnaeidae as hosts. Nine species of *Lymnaea* serve as intermediate hosts of *F. hepatica*.

These include *Lymnaea (Fossaria) truncatula* (Fig. 136–2) in Europe, Africa, the Middle East, and Asia; *L. viatrix* in Argentina; *L. rubiginosa* in Malaysia; *L. (Austropeplea) philippensis* and *L. swinhoe* in the Philippines; *L. tomentosa* in Australia; and *L. japonica* and *L. pervia* in Japan. *L. columella* (Fig. 136–2) is now widespread in North and South America, Africa, and the Hawaiian Islands. Five species, *L. rubiginosa* in Malaysia, *L. acuminata* and *L. auricularia* in India, and *L. natalensis* (Fig. 136–2) and *L. columella* in Africa, are intermediate hosts for *F. gigantica*. *Lymnaea (Radix) a. rubigenosa* serves as an intermediate host for *A. cantonensis* in Indonesia.

Two species of *Fossaria*, *F. bulimoides* and *F. cubensis*, act as intermediate hosts for *F. hepatica* in the United States. *F. ollula* transmits *F. gigantica* in Hawaii.

Family Planorbidae. Many species are medically important.

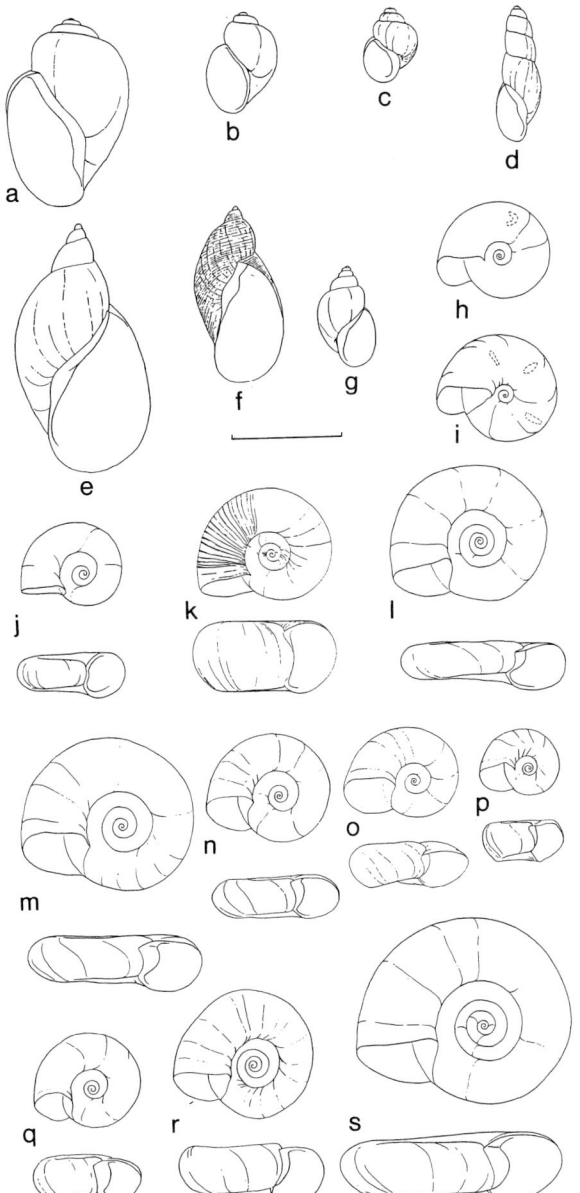

Figure 136–2. a, *Bulinus globosus*. b, *Bulinus truncatus*. c, *Bulinus wrighti*. d, *Bulinus senegalensis*. e, *Lymnaea natalensis*. f, *Lymnaea columella*. g, *Lymnaea truncatula*. h, *Hippeutis umbilicalis*. i, *Segmentina hemisphaerula*. j, *Planorbarius metidjensis*. k, *Indoplanorbis exustus*. l, *Biomphalaria sudanica*. m, *Biomphalaria camerunensis*. n, *Biomphalaria alexandrina*. o, *Biomphalaria pfeifferi*. p, *Biomphalaria choanomphala*. q, *Biomphalaria straminea*. r, *Biomphalaria tenagophila*. s, *Biomphalaria glabrata*. (Scale line = 1 cm or 0.5 cm in [h] and [i] only.) (Drawn by Dr. David S. Brown, Department of Zoology. The Natural History Museum, London.)

The family is separated into two subfamilies, Planorbinae and Bulininae. Snails of the subfamily Planorbinae are discoidal and usually small, although some may reach as much as 4 cm in diameter.

SUBFAMILY PLANORBINAE. *Gyraulus convexiusculus* acts as the first intermediate host of the intestinal trematode *Echinostoma ilocanum* in the Philippines and Java and as the second intermediate host of *Echinostoma malayanum* in India. *Gyraulus chinesis* serves as intermediate host for *Echinostoma macrordis* in Taiwan.

Hippeutis umbilicalis (Fig. 136–2) also acts as a first intermediate host of *E. ilocanum* in the Philippines. This snail and *Hippeutis cantori*, *Segmentina trochoideus*, and *S. hemisphaerula* (Fig. 136–2) act as intermediate hosts of *Fasciolopsis buski* in India and the Orient. Infection is by ingestion of metacercarial cysts on plants such as water chestnuts.

The snail *Helicorbis coenosus* is an intermediate host of the intestinal fluke *Gastrodiscoides hominis* in India and China, and in India it acts as intermediate host of *F. buski*.

The genus *Biomphalaria* lies within the subfamily Planorbinae. This large genus contains all of the intermediate hosts of *S. mansoni* in Africa, Southwest Asia, and the Western Hemisphere. (Chapter 118). Eight of the 31 recognized species act as intermediate hosts of *S. mansoni*. In the Western Hemisphere, these include *Biomphalaria glabrata*, *B. tenagophila*, and *B. straminea* (Fig. 136–2). *B. glabrata* serves as a host throughout its range in the islands of the Caribbean as well as in the coastal strip from Venezuela to southern Brazil. *B. tenagophila* is a host in a much more restricted range in the southernmost part of Brazil and Argentina. *B. straminea* has a much broader geographic range through North, South, and Central America as well as the Antilles. It has been found infected only in Brazil and Martinique. Six of the 16 remaining species of Western Hemisphere *Biomphalaria* have proved to be susceptible to *S. mansoni* infection in the laboratory, but none serves as a host in nature.

There are five established intermediate hosts for *S. mansoni* in Africa and the Middle East. These are *B. pfeifferi*, *B. choanomphala*, *B. alexandrina*, *B. camerunensis*, and *B. sudanica* (Fig. 136–2). Terminologic complexity in the past concerning African *Biomphalaria* has now been greatly simplified. *B. pfeifferi* is the most widespread host, prevalent all over sub-Saharan Africa, with a few additional North African foci. Eight previously identified species and subspecies are now recognized as *B. pfeifferi*. In addition to *S. mansoni*, *B. pfeifferi* in Central Africa is the intermediate host for the rodent schistosome *S. rodhaini*, which rarely infects humans.

B. choanomphala acts as the intermediate host for *S. mansoni* in Uganda and Tanzania. *B. alexandrina* is the intermediate host for *S. mansoni* in the highly endemic area of the Nile delta as well as in the Sudan. *B. camerunensis* serves as an intermediate host for *S. mansoni* in the Congo and the Cameroon. *B. sudanica* is the most important intermediate host of *S. mansoni* in East Africa as well as in Uganda and the southern Sudan. It also acts as an intermediate host for *S. rodhaini* in the Congo.

The relationships between many of the *Biomphalaria* are close, and species identification is often difficult. In many areas, however, only one species can be found, thus simplifying the problems of field identification for control purposes.

B. alexandrina has been found an intermediate host for *F. gigantica* in Egypt.

The remaining genus and species of medical importance in this subfamily is *Planorbarius metidjensis*. This snail is found in Morocco and Algiers as well as in Spain and Portugal and has been the host for *S. haematobium* in Portugal and *Schistosoma bovis* in Spain.

SUBFAMILY BULININAE. The genus *Bulinus* serves as the principal host for *S. haematobium* in Africa and the Middle East (Chapter 118). This genus in turn is divided into two subgenera, *Bulinus* proper and *Physopsis*. There are 37 recognized species in these two subgenera, which are further divided into four groups. Fourteen of these serve as hosts for *S. haematobium* in nature (Table 136–1). The *Bulinus forskalii* group contains four susceptible snails: *Bulinus beccarii* in southwestern Arabia, *Bulinus camerunensis* in Cameroon, *Bulinus cernicus* on Mauritius, and *Bulinus senegalensis* (Fig.

136–2) in The Gambia. In addition, *B. forskalii* acts as the intermediate host for *Schistosoma intercalatum* in Cameroon and Gabon and for *S. bovis* in East Africa. *B. senegalensis* and *B. scalaris* also serve as the intermediate hosts of *S. bovis* in Gambia. All of these snails are small, high-spired stream dwellers.

The Reticulatus group includes *Bulinus wrighti* (Fig. 136–2), which serves as an intermediate host of *S. haematobium* in Saudia Arabia, Yemen, and Oman.

The Tropicus/Truncatus subgroup has three *S. haematobium* vectors: *Bulinus guernei* in The Gambia, *B. rohlfsi* in West Africa, and *B. truncatus* (Fig. 136–2) in both eastern and western North Africa. *B. truncatus* also functions as the principal host for *S. bovis* in the Middle East.

The Africanus subgroup comprises the subgenus *Physopsis*. *Bulinus abyssinicus* serves as an intermediate host for *S. haematobium* in Ethiopia and Somalia, while *B. africanus* is a widespread intermediate host for both *S. haematobium* and *S. bovis* in eastern South Africa. *Bulinus jousseaumei* is a host for *S. haematobium* in The Gambia, and *Bulinus obtusispira* has the same role in Madagascar. *Bulinus globosus* (Fig. 136–2) is widespread in sub-Saharan Africa, where it is confined mainly to the lowland areas. It is a host for *S. haematobium* and *S. mattheei*. *Bulinus nasutus* is an East African intermediate host for *S. haematobium*. *Bulinus ugandae* is a natural host for *S. bovis* in the Sudan and Uganda.

Another genus in the subfamily is *Indoplanorbis*. *I. exustus* is an intermediate host for *Echinostoma malayanum*, an intestinal fluke reportedly infecting humans in Southeast Asia. This snail can also serve as an intermediate host for the nematode *A. cantonensis* in Malaysia.

Orders Stylommatophora and Systellommatophora. The former order contains terrestrial snails and some slugs, and the latter comprises only tropical slugs. Many terrestrial snails and slugs are involved as intermediate hosts in the transmission of four parasites that may infect humans. Two are nematodes: the rat lungworm *A. cantonensis* (Chapter 114.1) and the related American parasite *Moreostrongylus costaricensis* (Chapter 114.2). The other two parasites are the related liver flukes *Dicrocoelium dendriticum* and *Dicrocoelium hospes* that infect herbivores (Chapter 120.4). Infections in humans by all four of these parasites have been reported but are rare.

A. cantonensis does not seem to be terribly fastidious or, for that matter, very demanding about its intermediate host. It uses slugs of both orders as well as many terrestrial and aquatic snails. The parasite was originally identified in China and is now reported from the islands of the West and South Pacific, Cuba, Puerto Rico, and Louisiana. The intermediate host range in Cuba includes many terrestrial snails and slugs. Transmission is by accidental ingestion of a mollusk or by ingestion of poorly cooked snails and slugs.

M. costaricensis commonly uses veronicellid slugs as the intermediate host, but in Costa Rica, many terrestrial and aquatic mollusks are naturally infected. These include *Helisoma trivolvus*, *Succineidae* sp., and *Bulimus* sp. Again, transmission is by accidental ingestion of the slug or slug mucus containing larvae.

Dicrocoelium dendriticum is a fluke that normally parasitizes the biliary tree of sheep and other herbivores. Its distribution includes both North and South America, Europe, the Middle East, India, and China. The fluke uses various terrestrial snails as first intermediate hosts. Many genera of a number of families are involved. Infection may be quite localized in a given area despite widespread distribution of snails. Infection is acquired by accidental ingestion of infected ants, the second intermediate host. *D. hospes* has a much more limited distribution in Africa. It, too, is rare in humans. The only

identified host snails are in the genus *Limicolaria* and include *Limicolaria aurora* as well as other species.

■ CONTROL

One obvious means of eliminating snail-related diseases is to control the intermediate host. The success of control measures is variable, and many factors affect their use. As a consequence, there is no simple protocol for control measures. Each attempt at control needs to consider the host, intermediate host, infecting agents, and physical setting, as well as the relationships among these four variables, if a workable approach is to be identified.

Control methods take the form of protection from exposure to the definitive host and the intermediate host, as well as antisnail measures.

EXPOSURE CONTROL. Logical approaches to controlling mollusk-transmitted diseases include restriction of human exposure to the mollusk and/or restriction of exposure of the mollusk to infecting organisms. Control of human contact with infected mollusks is largely accomplished by quarantine and posting of infected waters. This is effective, realistically, only in dealing with commercial food-processing operations. Regulation of shellfish beds is effective in the control of oyster- and clam-transmitted viral hepatitis and in control of transmission of cholera and *Salmonella* infection. In cases in which water contact is an important feature of disease transmission, particularly the skin-penetrating trematodes, wearing boots and other protective aids can be effective. Most of these are voluntary measures and, for this reason, are only modestly effective. Continuing attention to public health education shows slow progress in this important control mechanism.

ANTISNAIL MEASURES. Four mechanisms for direct snail control may be used. These include snail removal by mechanical or manual means, snail control by environmental manipulation, the use of molluscicides, and the use of biologic control.

Snail Removal by Mechanical Means. This is largely a measure of the past. No selective mechanisms currently exist to concentrate snails for removal.

Environmental Manipulation. This has proved to be a useful tool in snail control, but costs as well as local engineering problems severely limit its application. Where transmission of infection involves irrigation schemes or fish farms, it is often possible to plan for intervals of desiccation. Although some snails can estivate and survive dry periods by burrowing into moist, muddy bottoms, the snail population does tend to be held down by these measures.

Where desiccation is impossible, some control of snail population size is possible by the use of rapid flow in canals and channels. Many host snails are adapted only to slow-moving or stagnant habitats. There has been success, particularly in Japan, with cement lining of canals to create a habitat unsuitable for amphibious snails. Although these measures are effective, costs inhibit their extensive use.

Molluscicides. The use of molluscicides is limited by the cost and the water dynamics, which control achievable concentrations of the compounds. A concern is that some of these compounds may damage the environment. Four compounds are currently used in chemical control of mollusks. These compounds have been subjected to extensive trial and are commonly available in quantity.

Copper Sulfate. This compound has been used the longest and is effective only against aquatic snails. Its effect is considerably reduced by organic matter in the environment, and it currently has limited application.

Sodium Pentachlorophenate (NaPCP). This compound is available in many formulations, some of which have slow-release residual capability. NaPCP is absorbed by mud and is broken down by sunlight. It is a toxic substance and must be used with attention to the safety of workers.

Niclosamide. Niclosamide (Bayluscid) is effective at a much lower concentration than NaPCP. It may be applied as a powder or an emulsion and is effective against amphibious snails.

N-Tritylmorpholine. N-tritylmorpholine (Frescon) is available in many forms, including bait. It is less soluble than the other compounds mentioned. It has excellent stability in the environment and is effective in low concentration.

Molluscicides of Plant Origin. The only such molluscicide to receive extensive field trial is Euclod (*Phytolacca dodecundra*) in Ethiopia. Several other plants, including *Swartzia madagascariensis*, *Tetrapleura tetrapleura*, and *Warburgia salcitaris*, have shown promise but have not been subjected to extensive field trial. The ability to incorporate the use of such natural compounds into self-help programs offsets the comparative inefficiency of the compounds.

Biologic Control. Biologic control measures take two forms.

Competitive Species. The first is the introduction of competitive species that displace the snail intermediate hosts. The most successful has been the thiarid snail *T. granifera* in Puerto Rico, where, in some locations, it has displaced *B. glabrata*, the *S. mansoni* host. This snail has spread to Haiti, where it has displaced planorbids from a number of streams in the southern region. *Thiara tuberculata* has been introduced in a controlled trial on the Caribbean island of St. Lucia, with an initial report of success in the suppression of *B. glabrata*. Follow-up studies have not shown a continuing benefit from this approach to control. Additional species used for competitive snail control include *Marisa cornuarietis*, *Helisoma duyri* for both *Bulinus* and *Biomphalaria*, and *Melanopsis praemorusa* and *Potamorygus jenkinsi* for *Bulinus* species.

Predator Species. The other approach to biologic control has been the use of predators or parasites to reduce snail populations. A number of parasites harmful to snails have been identified, but no extensive scientific evaluation of parasites has been performed.

Predators have been used with variable success in snail control. The use of the predatory snails *Marisa cornuarietis* in Puerto Rico and *Pomacea haustrum* in Brazil has been partially successful in controlling *B. glabrata*, the host for *S. mansoni*, in these areas. The use of the sciomyzid fly, the larvae of which attack snails, has been field tested in Hawaii. There the fly *Sepeolon macropus* has been used against *Lymnaea ollula*, the host for *F. gigantica*. The difficulty of successful introduction of this fly into new enviornments limits the application of this measure.

A number of fish, including *Tilapia melanopleura* (Nile perch), as well as several species of chichlids that normally include snails in their diet, have proved useful, particularly in the control of snails in fish-farm tanks. The Louisiana crawfish, *Procambarus clarkii*, has been introduced in fish-farming programs in eastern Africa. Introduction is associated with reduction, in some cases disappearance, of *Biomphalaria* and *Bulinus* from the affected environment.

The combined problem of the introduction of new, potentially environment-damaging species, plus the difficulty of this introduction, markedly limits the use of this mechanism of control.

■ COLLECTION METHODS

The two most important aspects of snail collection are the collection site and preservation of the snails. How the snails are picked up, whether by scoop, dredge, forceps, or spoon, is important only in quantitative studies. The method of collection should safeguard collectors from exposure to infectious material and should not damage the snails. Quantitative collection methods are useful in evaluations, particularly related to control programs, but these are not necessary for a casual survey.

SITE RECORD. This should include locations, preferably with reference points that can be identified on a map, the date and time, and a habitat description.

PRESERVED SPECIMENS. Ideally, both the shell and the soft parts should be preserved. Although the shell is useful to the taxonomist, soft parts are usually essential to complete species identification. Soft-part dissection as well as measurement is simplified if the snail is relaxed and extended when fixed. Two preservation protocols are recommended.

Alcohol Fixation. This is the simplest fixation method. Extended snails may be obtained as follows: A live snail is picked up with forceps and held until it is extended. With the aperture facing up, it is carefully lowered to the level of the aperture into water with a temperature of 65 to 70°C for 15 seconds. With care, the snail remains extended and dies, after which it can be plunged into the water for an additional 20 seconds. A temperature of 65 to 70°C produces thermal death without cooking the snail or coagulating its hemolymph.

Obtaining extended specimens is somewhat easier if the snail is narcotized. Solutions of rapid-acting barbiturates, such as 0.2% Nembutal, do this. The same effect can be achieved by placing the snail in a vial or dish with several menthol crystals added to the water. In either case, narcotization takes 4 to 6 hours. Slugs may be relaxed by overnight refrigeration.

After the relaxed snails are killed, large specimens can usually be removed from the shell by holding the snail in cool water and gently tugging the snail out of its shell by pulling on the foot with forceps. The snail is then placed in fixative, and the shell dried. In this fashion, body and shell are preserved for study. Tiny snails or snails with internal lamellae in the shell usually cannot be withdrawn from the shell undamaged and must be dropped directly into a fixative.

Alcohol diluted to 70% is a suitable fixative for field work. The addition of glycerin 1:10 by volume also helps preservation. Alcohol fixation does produce some hardening and friability of tissues after long preservation.

Railliet-Henry Fixative. A better fixative for long-term preservation of dissectable material is Railliet-Henry fixative. This is made as follows:

Distilled water 930 mL
NaCl 6 g
Formalin 50 mL
Glacial acetic acid 20 mL

These reagents are readily available in most clinical laboratories. Snails preserved in this fixative remain soft for many years. When shells are added to this acid fixative, carbon dioxide evolves, and care must be taken to prevent the tops from blowing off the vials.

With both fixation methods, a single change of fixative after 24 hours improves preservation. Preserved specimens must be clearly marked with all identifying information.

Bibliography

Ansari N: Epidemiology and Control of Schistosomiasis (Bilharziasis). Baltimore, University Park Press, 1973.
Boray JC: Studies on the relative susceptibility of some lymnaeids to infection

with *Fasciola hepatica* and *F. gigantica* and on the adaptation of *Fasciola* spp. Ann Trop Med Parasitol 60:114, 1966.

Brown DS: Freshwater Snails of Africa and Their Medical Importance, 2nd ed. London, Taylor & Francis, 1994.

Bruce JI, Sornmani S: The Mekong schistosome. Malacol Rev (Suppl 2), 1980.

Burch JB: A guide to freshwater snails of the Philippines. Malacol Rev 13:123, 1980.

Davis GM: The Origin and Evolution of the Gastropod Family Pomatiopsidae, with Emphasis on the Mekong River Triculinae. Monograph 20. Philadelphia, Academy of Natural Sciences, 1979.

Davis GM, Ruff MD: *Oncomelania hupensis* (Gastropoda: Hydrobiidae): Hybridization, genetics and transmission of *Schistosoma japonicum*. Malacol Rev 6:181, 1974.

de Souza CP, Cunha R de C, Andrade ZA: Development of *Schistosoma mansoni* in *Biomphalaria tenagophila*, *Biomphalaria straminea* and *Biomphalaria glabrata*. Rev Inst Med Trop Sao Paulo 3:201, 1995.

de Souza CP, Jannotti-Passos LK, de Freitas JR: Degree of host-parasite compatibility between *Schistosoma mansoni* and their intermediate molluscan hosts in Brazil. Mem Inst Oswaldo Cruz 90:5, 1995.

Frag HF, El Sayad MH: *Biomphalaria alexandrina* naturally infected with *Fasciola gigantica* in Egypt. Trans R Soc Trop Med Hyg 89:36, 1995.

Frandsen F, McCullough F, Madsen H: A practical guide to the identification of African freshwater snails. Malacol Rev 13:95, 1980.

Kendall SB: Relationships between species of *Fasciola* and their molluscan hosts. Adv Parasitol 3:59, 1965.

Kitikoon V: Studies on *Tricula aperta* and related taxa, the snail intermediate hosts of *Schistosoma mekongi*. III. Susceptibility studies. Malacol Rev 14:37, 1981.

Lo CT: *Echinostoma macrorchis*: Life history, population dynamics of intramolluscan stages, and first and second intermediate hosts. J Parasitol 81:569, 1995.

Malek EA: Studies on "tropicorbid" snails (Biomphalaria:Planorbidae) from the Caribbean and Gulf of Mexico areas, including the southern United States. Malacol Int J Malacol 7:183, 1969.

Malek EA: Snail-Transmitted Parasitic Diseases, Vols I and II. Boca Raton, FL, CRC Press, 1980.

Malek EA: Snail Hosts of Schistosomiasis and Other Snail-transmitted Diseases in Tropical America: A Manual. Scientific publication No. 478. Washington, DC, Pan American Health Organization, 1985.

Mandahl-Barth G: Intermediate Hosts of Schistosoma African Biomphalaria and Bulinus. WHO Monograph Series No. 37. Geneva, World Health Organization, 1958.

Pace GL: The freshwater snails of Taiwan (Formosa). Malacol Rev (Suppl 1), 1973.

Pan American Health Organization: A Guide for the Identification of the Snail Intermediate Hosts of Schistosomiasis in the Americas. Washington, DC, Pan American Health Organization, 1968.

Perera G, Yong M, Rodriguez J, Gálvez D: Cuban endemic molluscs infected with *Angiostrongylus cantonensis*. Malacol Rev 16:87, 1983.

Rosewater J: The family Littorinidae in the Indo-Pacific. Indo-Pacific Mollusca 2:417, 1970.

Sodeman WA Jr: *Thiara (Tarebia) gramfera* (Lamarck): An agent for biological control of *Biomphalaria*. *In* National Research Council: Aquaculture and Schistosomiasis. Proceedings of a Network Meeting Held in Manila, Philippines, August 6–10, 1991. Washington, DC, National Academy Press, 1992.

Tropmed Technical Group: Snails of medical importance in Southeast Asia. Seamo-Tropmed Technical Meeting 17:282, 1986.

Tze-kong L, Yue-ying L, Wen-zhen Z, Yao-xian W: A discussion on the classification of *Oncomelania* (Mollusca). Sinozoologia 3:97, 1982.

Yue-ying L, Tze-kong L, Yao-xian W, Wen-zhen Z: Subspecific deafferentation of Oncomelaniid snails. Acta Zootaxon Sinica 6:253, 1981.

Yue-ying L, Wen-zhen Z, Yao-xian W: Studies on *Tricula* (Prosobranchia:Hydrobiidae) from China. Acta Zootaxon Sinica 8:135, 1983.

137 *Ticks and Mites in Disease Transmission*

Daniel E. Sonenshine and Abdu F. Azad

■ GENERAL PRINCIPLES

Ticks and mites are members of the subclass Acari, one of the dominant subclasses of the Class Arachnida (Subphylum Chelicerata). Arachnids appeared during the late Archeozoic or early Paleozoic eras, i.e., during the period of proliferation of bottom feeding invertebrates (e.g., trilobites). Adaptive radiation followed colonization of the terrestrial environment, with explosive multiplication of new life forms. Virtually all of the arachnid taxa, including the Acari, are believed to have evolved during this warm, moist period.

Arachnids, including ticks and mites, are distinguished from insects by lack of a clearly defined head, by chelicerae instead of mandibles, by the absence of antennae, and by the presence of 4 pairs of walking legs (except in larvae of the Acari, which have only 3). The body is subdivided into the anterior prosoma, bearing the appendages, and the posterior opisthosoma (the so-called abdominal region). The Acari are readily distinguished from other arachnids by the virtual absence of obvious segmentation, so that the prosoma and the opisthosoma are fused in ticks and most mites. They can also be recognized by the presence of the gnathosoma (termed capitulum in ticks), a unique structure at or near the anteriormost end of the body that bears the mouthparts. The gnathosoma or capitulum consists of a ring of cuticle that surrounds the chelicerae and supports the paired pedipalps. It is formed by the fusion of the ancestral pedipalp coxae. The ring of cuticle projects the remaining segments of the pedipalps forward so they lie lateral to, instead of behind, the chelicerae. This allows these two pairs of appendages to work together during feeding. Also present on the gnathosoma is an unpaired appendage, the hypostome, located on the ventromedial surface between the palps. In the capitulum of ticks, the hypostome is prominent and, with rare exceptions, is covered ventrally with numerous recurved teeth. The remainder of the highly fused body, termed idiosoma, is divided into two regions, the anterior podosoma, bearing the walking legs, and the posterior opisthosoma, or "abdominal" region, located behind it. However, the opisthosoma is not a true abdomen and this unsegmented body region cannot be considered homologous with the abdomen of other arachnid taxa. Thus, tremendous fusion has taken place in the Acari and, except during embryonic development, little evidence of body segmentation can be found in these organisms.

The Acari make up a vast assemblage of species that have become established in virtually every known terrestrial and fresh or brackish water habitat. Many are free living as herbivores, fungivores, and predators; others are parasitic, including both ectoparasites and endoparasites. The specialized adaptations of the parasitic species contribute to their harmful effects on human and animal health. Mites and ticks also are important as vectors of many pathogenic diseases. Indeed, ticks transmit a greater variety of disease-causing pathogens than any other arthropod disease vector. Aside from the microbial pathogens they transmit, some tick species also can paralyze their hosts or cause violent allergic and even toxic effects. As a result, the biology and disease relationships of the Acari are of intense interest to biologists, physicians, veterinarians, and public health officials.

137.1 *Ticks (Suborder Ixodida)*

Characterization

All ticks are obligate blood-sucking ectoparasites, i.e., they attach themselves to the external surface of the host body. Most ticks are relatively large as adults, i.e., 5 to 15 mm long, as compared with mites, which usually measure <1 mm in length. There is a single pair of respiratory pores or spiracles (also known as stigmata). The hypostome is prominent and covered ventrally with retrorse teeth that help in anchoring

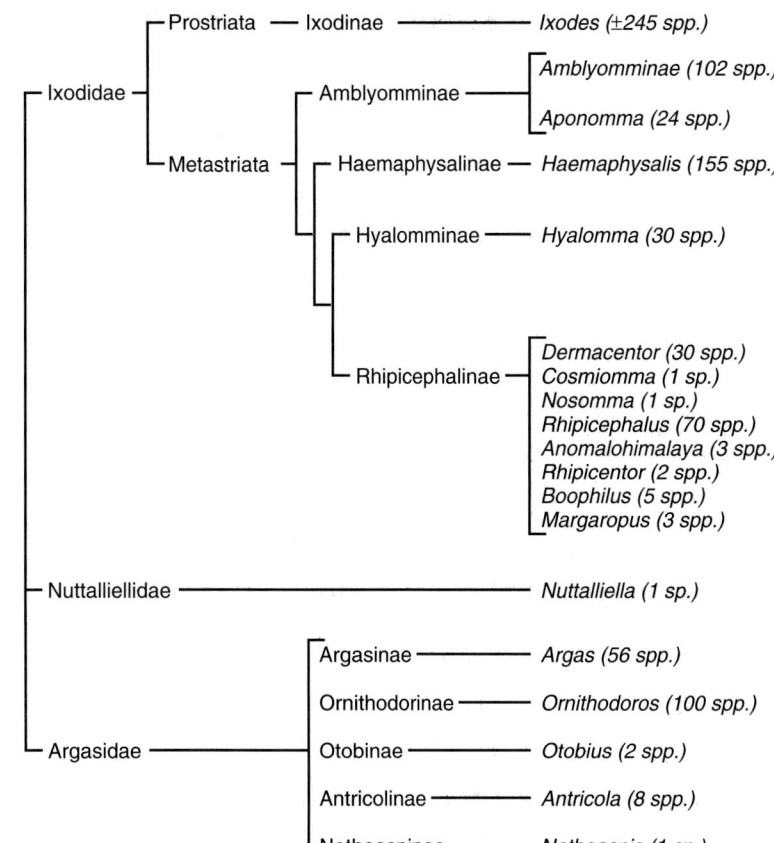

Figure 137–1. Diagram illustrating systematic and evolutionary relationship in ticks.

the tick to its host. Contrary to a popular misconception, ticks do not truly "bite" their hosts. Rather, using their hypostomes, they attach themselves to the skin where they remain for long periods, from hours to even days, while sucking blood. In ixodids, copious quantities of cement are secreted into the wound during the first few hours of attachment, penetrating and surrounding the hypostome and chelicerae. The cement quickly hardens to bond the tick firmly to the host skin. The chelicerae are extended and used to cut into the skin. The terminal ends of the chelicerae, termed digits, bear prominent laterally oriented cutting denticles that rip and tear host tissue, thereby permitting the entry of the tick's mouthparts into the skin. Skin penetration by the chelicerae also cuts small blood vessels, thereby forming a feeding pool. Feeding proceeds by sucking the oozing blood into a channel on the dorsal surface of the hypostome, the preoral canal. This channel directs pooled blood from the wound into the mouth, located at the hypostome base and into the powerful sucking pharynx. The four-segmented tarsi bear sensory sensilla on their terminal segments, believed to provide chemical recognition signals that facilitate host recognition and feeding site selection.

Classification

The subclass Acari is divided into two major orders, the order Parasitiformes, and the order Acariformes. Ticks constitute the suborder Ixodida (Metastigmata of some authors), a suborder of the Parasitiformes. This suborder comprises three families: (1) the Ixodidae, (2) the Argasidae, and (3) the Nuttalliellidae, the latter represented by a single species, *Nuttalliella namaqua*. The family Ixodidae, or hard ticks, is the largest and economically most important family, with 14

genera and approximately 670 species. The family is further subdivided into the Prostriata, containing the genus *Ixodes*, and the Metastriata containing the remaining 13 genera. The family Argasidae, or soft ticks, comprises five genera and approximately 170 species (Fig. 137–1).

FAMILY IXODIDAE

The Ixodidae (hard ticks) have a tough, sclerotized scutum, which covers the anterior part of the dorsum (entire dorsum in males) (Fig. 137–2). Elsewhere, the body cuticle is characterized by innumerable tiny surface folds, except in males of some species in which it is covered by sclerotized ventral plates. Eyes, when present, occur on the posterolateral margins of the scutum. Also present in the middle of the dorsal surface of metastriate ticks are a pair of tiny pore clusters, the foveal pores. The foveal pores are most prominent in females in which they serve as the release sites of the female sex pheromone, 2,6-dichlorophenol. The palps have 4 segments (also termed articles), but the terminal fourth segment is retractable and is recessed into segment 3. Females bear a pair of porose areas and a pair of remarkable, eversible sacs termed Gené organ. These sacs emerge during oviposition and add a protective waxy coating to the eggs. The spiracles are located posterior to coxa IV and are situated within a prominent spiracular plate. On the tarsi of the walking legs, padlike pulvilli occur adjacent to the claws in all life stages, enabling these ticks to climb virtually any surface. The nymphal and larval stages resemble the adults but lack the external genital pores and porose areas. Sexual dimorphism is pronounced in the adults, especially in the size of the scutum which covers the entire dorsum of the male (and limits expansion during feeding) but only the anterior half of the body in the female. Sexual dimorphism is absent in the immature forms. Larvae bear only three pairs of walking legs.

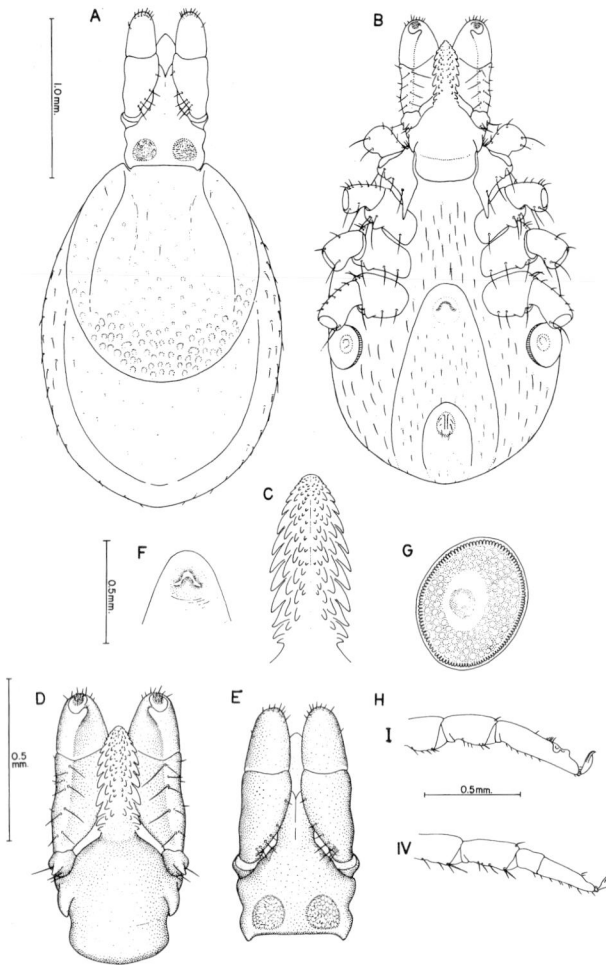

Figure 137–2. The structure of a representative ixodid tick, a female of the bird tick, *Ixodes dentatus. A,* Entire tick, dorsal aspect. *B,* Entire tick, ventral aspect. *C,* Hypostome. *D,* Capitulum, showing the relationships of the palps, hypostome, and the basis capituli; ventral aspect. *E,* Capitulum, dorsal aspect. *F,* Genital pore. *G,* Spiracular plate. *H,* Tarsal segments of legs I and IV; tarsus I bears Haller's organ.

Genus Ixodes. This is the largest genus of hard ticks, with approximately 245 species (Fig. 137–3). The genus is worldwide in distribution. These ticks are readily recognized by the anal groove, which curves anterior to and encloses the anus. In the males, the ventral surface is covered by sclerotized ventral plates. Most species of the genus are nest- or burrow-inhabiting (i.e., nidicolous) parasites with cryptic, nonfeeding males. Several species are non-nidicolous and are distributed widely throughout wooded or grassy environments. All are three-host ticks; each life stage drops off after feeding to molt on the ground or in the nest. Important species include (1) *I. persulcatus,* an important vector of Russian spring-summer encephalitis (RSSE; tick-borne encephalitis) (Chapter 30.5) and Lyme borreliosis (Chapter 73); in the former Soviet Union (2) *I. ricinus,* the major European vector of tick-borne encephalitis, as well as Lyme borreliosis, louping ill, babesiosis, and tick pyemia; (3) *I. scapularis* (same as *I. dammini),* the primary vector of Lyme borreliosis in the eastern United States and eastern Canada, as well as human granulocytic ehrlichiosis (Chapter 70) and human babesiosis (Chapter 96), (4) *I. pacificus,* the primary vector of Lyme borreliosis to humans in the western United States; (5) *I.*

petaurista and *I. ceylonensis,* vectors of Kyasanur Forest disease in India (Chapter 31.7); and (6) *I. holocyclus,* responsible for severe or fatal tick paralysis in Australia.

Genus Dermacentor. Species of this genus typically have an ornate scutum with eyes (absent in *D. dissimile)* and short, thick palps. All are three-host ticks. The genus is widespread, with species in many localities throughout the world. The distribution is Holarctic, Asian, and African. Important species include *D. variabilis* (American dog tick), the predominant vector of Rocky Mountain spotted fever (RMSF) in the eastern United States (Chapter 67.1) and *D. andersoni* (Rocky Mountain wood tick), the vector of RMSF and Colorado tick fever in the Rocky Mountain region.

Genus Haemaphysalis. According to Hoogstraal and Aeschlimann, this large and varied genus contains about 155 species. These ticks are easily recognized by their characteristic lateral projections of palpal article II, the sides of which extend well beyond the lateral margins of the basis capituli. All are three-host ticks. Although found in many regions of the world, the distribution is predominantly Old World, with only five species in the Nearctic and Neotropical regions. Hosts include mammals and birds. *H. spinigera* and other species in India transmit Kyasanur Forest disease. In the former Soviet Union, *H. longicornis* has been reported to transmit fatal meningoencephalitis and RSSE. An unusual association occurs in India, where *H. intermedia* and *H. wellingtoni* transmit Ganjam virus, an agent identical with that causing Nairobi sheep disease in East Africa. In North America, an important species is *H. leporispalustris,* which transmits *Rickettsia rickettsii* among wild lagomorphs and thereby contributes to the maintenance of RMSF in its natural environment.

Genus Amblyomma. This is one of the largest of the ixodid tick genera, found mostly in tropical and humid subtropical regions of the world. These ticks parasitize a wide variety of hosts, including reptiles, birds, mammals, and even amphibians. These ticks are easily recognized by their remarkably ornate multicolored scuta and their unusually long mouthparts, particularly palpal segment 2, which is about twice as long as segment 3 (Fig. 137–4). All species are three-host ticks. In Africa, *A. hebraeum* and *A. variegatum* are important vectors of animal disease, especially heartwater, and are also important as pests of livestock. Crimean-Congo hemorrhagic fever (CCHF) also has been recovered from *A. variegatum* on many occasions, and specimens also have been found infected with the yellow fever virus. In the United States, *A. americanum,* an important pest of livestock, deer, and humans, is a known vector of *Rickettsia rickettsii,* the causative agent of RMSF. It also has been implicated in the transmission of *Ehrlichia chafeensis,* the causative agent of human monocytic ehrlichiosis (Chapter 70).

Genus Hyalomma. These ornamented medium-sized to large ticks have festoons (rectangular demarcations along the posterior end of the body), eyes, and elongated palps. The males have distinctive adanal shields. *Hyalomma* species frequently parasitize a diversity of wild and domesticated mammals and birds. They are found almost entirely in savanna, semiarid or arid deserts, and grassy steppes in southern and southeastern Europe, Asia, and Africa. The most important human disease transmitted by these ticks is CCHF (Chapter 31.5). Other pathogens include tick-borne arboviruses carried by bird-infesting *Hyalomma* ticks and spread during the spring and fall migrations when vast flocks of birds migrate between southern Eurasia and Africa. *H. dromedarii* and *H. anatolicum excavatum,* vectors of the deadly tropical theileriosis of livestock (caused by *Theileria annulata)* are adapted to extremely dry environments and survive for long periods in the sand and dust along camel paths and caravansaries.

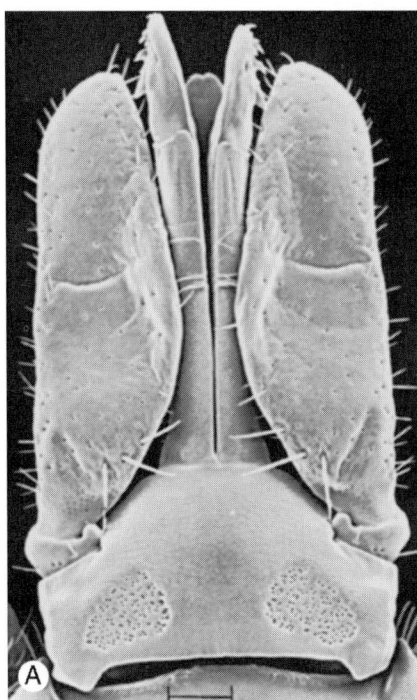
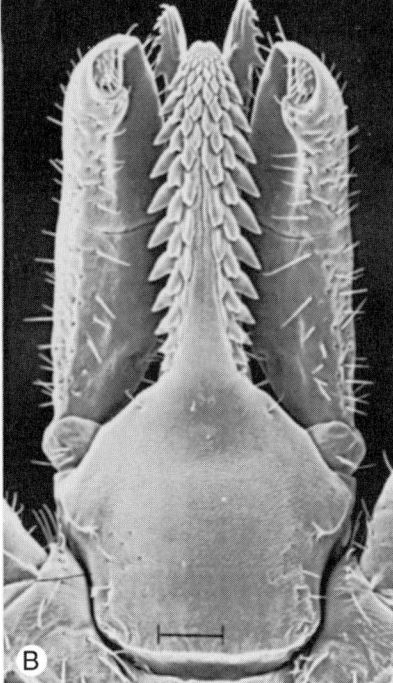
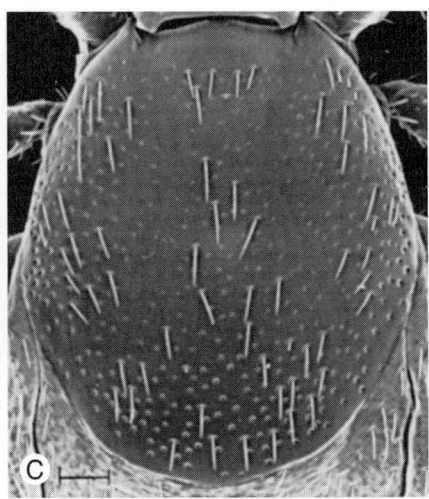

Figure 137–3. Scanning electron micrographs illustrating the mouthparts and scutum of a female deer tick, *Ixodes scapularis*. *A,* Capitulum, dorsal aspect. *B,* Capitulum, ventral aspect. *C,* Scutum, dorsal aspect. (Measurement bars 200 μm. Photos prepared by Drs. Richard Robbins and James E, Keirans, U.S. Public Health Service.)

Genus *Rhipicephalus.* These inornate ticks are easily recognized by the distinctive protruding, pointed lateral margins of the basis capituli, giving it a hexagonal shape when viewed from above (dorsal aspect). Males have adanal shields. The genus contains 70 species. These ticks are widely distributed throughout Africa, Asia, and Europe. The genus includes the brown dog tick, *R. sanguineus,* which has also spread to North America and Australia, and is now a major pest of pet animals in many homes. *R. sanguineus* is an important vector of *Ehrlichia canis,* the causative agent of the often fatal canine ehrlichiosis of dogs and other carnivores. It also transmits *Rickettsia conorii,* which causes boutonneuse fever (fièvre boutonneuse, Mediterranean spotted fever), a rickettsial disease similar to RMSF, in the Mediterranean region and throughout large areas of Africa and western Asia (Chapter 67.2). In southern and southeastern Africa, the brown ear tick, *R. appendiculatus,* is notorious as the primary vector of the deadly East Coast Fever, a highly fatal disease of cattle in that region. *Rhipicephalus* ticks are almost entirely parasites of mammals and are rarely found on birds or reptiles.

FAMILY ARGASIDAE

The Argasidae (soft ticks) have a tough, leathery integument (except in the larval stage, which has a minutely folded cuticle reminiscent of ixodids) (Fig. 137–5). There is no scutum, but a pseudoscutum is present in the obscure bat ticks of the genus *Nothoaspis.* A dorsal shield occurs in the larva (not a true scutum). The capitulum is ventral, near the anterior end, and not visible from the dorsal aspect. Eyes, when present, occur on the ventral surface of the body, usually on the ventrolateral folds. The spiracles occur on the ventrolateral folds between the coxae of legs III and IV, but never on large plates as in the Ixodidae. Coxal pores, the openings of the coxal glands, are located between the paired coxae of legs I and II. The walking legs of nymphs and adults lack prominent padlike pulvilli. Sexual dimorphism is absent in the immature stages and expressed in the adults only by differences in the appearance of the genital aperture.

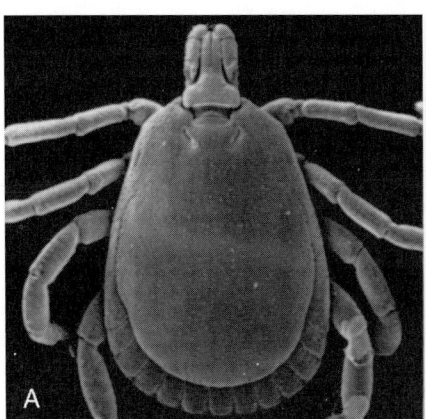
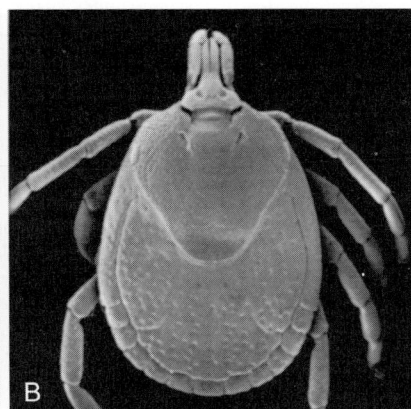
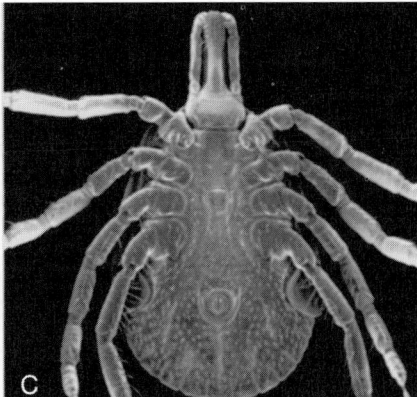

Figure 137–4. Scanning electron micrographs illustrating the characteristic features of the genus *Amblyomma* (*A. americanum*). *A,* Male, dorsal aspect. Note 11 festoons visible beyond the scutum. *B,* Female, dorsal aspect. *C,* Female, ventral aspect.

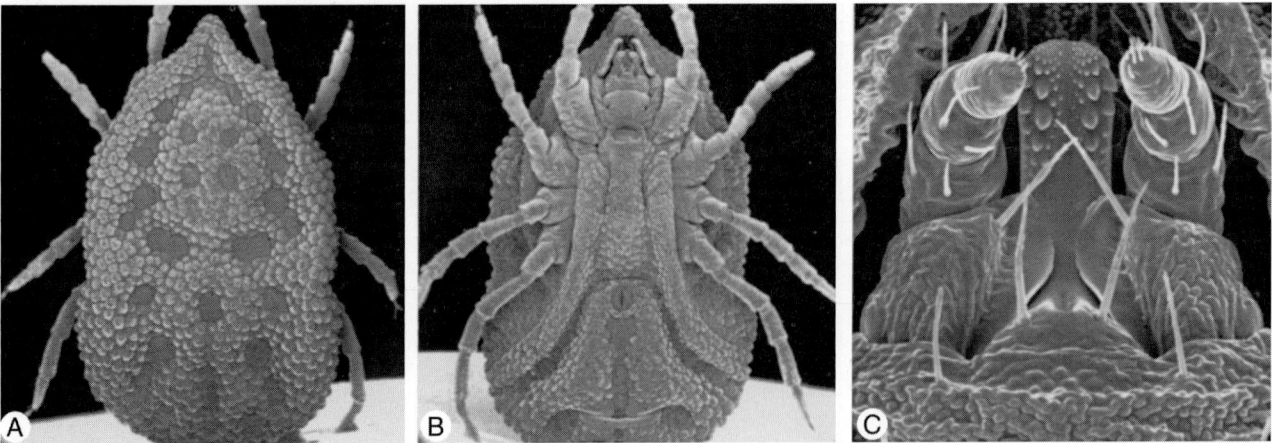

Figure 137–5. Scanning electron micrographs illustrating the characteristics of the genus *Ornithodoros* (*O. capensis*). *A*, Male, dorsal aspect. *B*, Male, ventral aspect. *C*, Male, ventral aspect. Enlargement showing detail of the capitulum recessed in the camerostomal cavity and the adjacent cheeks.

Genus Argas. Ticks of the genus *Argas* are recognized by the flattened body margin; a sutural line separating the dorsal and ventral margins; and a leathery, folded cuticle. There are distinct marginal plates and marginal striae. The flattened margins are evident even when the tick has fed. The many small integumental folds usually have a small button-like appearance, each with a pit on its top. Eyes are absent in the ticks of this genus. At least 56 species are known at present. Although some species parasitize mammals, most are parasites of bats or birds. The genus is worldwide in distribution. Several of these ticks have been incriminated in the transmission of disease, e.g., *Aegyptianella* spp., a rickettsia transmitted by *Argas persicus*, *A. walkerae*, and *A. pullorum*. Severe allergic reactions to the bites of the pigeon tick, *A. reflexus* have been reported in many countries of Europe. Many species of bird- or bat-infesting *Argas* ticks transmit viral encephalitides and other infectious viral agents.

Genus Ornithodoros. In the ticks of this genus, the nymphs and adults have a leathery cuticle with innumerable tiny wrinkles termed mammillae and a rounded body margin; there is no lateral sutural line (Fig. 137–5). The body margin may appear rounded or flattened, but never marginated and lacks marginal plates or striae. Mammillae are smaller and more numerous than the broader integumental folds found in *Argas*. Typically, the anterior end of the body is more or less pointed and hoodlike in appearance. The genus contains 100 species. The host range of these ticks is very diverse and includes reptiles, birds, and mammals. The genus is worldwide in distribution. Most *Ornithodoros* species shelter in dry caves, rodent burrows, bird's nests and rookeries, or human-constructed shelters. Aside from a few species that are parasitic on bats or tortoises in humid areas, most *Ornithodoros* species occur in dry climates. Several species of this genus, e.g., the North American *O. hermsi* and the African tampan, *O. moubata* (sensu strictu) are vectors of tick-borne relapsing fever (Chapter 71). Others have been implicated in the transmission of African swine fever, which has been responsible for enormous losses in swine. The pajaroello tick, *O. coriaceus* is the vector of bovine epizootic abortion and is also feared because of the severity of its bites. Other *Ornithodoros* spp. that parasitize birds and bats have been found to transmit viral encephalitides and can even cause severe allergic responses in humans.

Genus Otobius. In the genus *Otobius*, the nymphs have a spinose integument. The adults do not feed and the hypostome is vestigial. The integument of the adults is granu-lated. There are only two nymphal stages. The genus contains three species. *O. megnini*, the spinose ear tick, is an important pest of livestock but also infests deer, coyotes, rabbits, and various other wildlife.

Life Cycle and Feeding Habits

The life cycle of all ticks includes the egg, the larva, one or more nymphal stages, and the adult. Metamorphosis is incomplete (i.e., the immature stages resemble the adults). The larval and nymphal stages resemble the adults, although larvae have only three pairs of legs. The life cycle of ixodid ticks is compressed, with only 1 nymphal stage, but extended in argasid ticks, with 2 or more nymphal stages. The life cycle of nuttalliellid ticks is unknown. All ticks are obligate blood-sucking parasites. They must feed on blood during some or all stages in their life cycle. All species are oviparous. In most species, larvae attack hosts, feed, drop, and develop in sheltered microenvironments where they molt into nymphs. Nymphs emerge and seek hosts again, feed, drop from their hosts, and molt into adults or, in the case of the argasid ticks, into later-stage nymphs. In a few species, the ticks remain and complete their development on the same host. Adult ticks seek hosts, feed, and the engorged females drop off to lay their eggs. In contrast to most hematophagous arthropods, ticks are remarkably long-lived. Many are able to survive for one or more years without feeding. Tick life cycles vary greatly, with the greatest differences evident between the Ixodidae and Argasidae.

IXODID LIFE CYCLES. Ixodid ticks have only a single nymphal stage. In most species, larvae, nymphs, and adults feed and drop off to molt in the natural environment, but nonfeeding males occur in a few cases. Each instar feeds on a separate host. Such species are known as three-host ticks. In some other species, immature-stage ticks remain and molt on the same host, reattaching to feed again. Such species are known as two-host ticks when the nymphs drop off after feeding (e.g., *Hyalomma dromedarii*) and one-host ticks when both immatures and adults feed on the same host (e.g., *Boophilus microplus*). All life stages feed slowly over a period of several days to more than a week while synthesizing new cuticle. New cuticle is needed to accommodate the enormous blood meal, up to 100 times (or more) than the tick's prefeeding weight. Following contact with the host, the ticks use their chelicerae to establish the feeding site, while they anchor themselves in the skin with their hypostomes. Attachment is reinforced by secretion of cement substances with the saliva into and around the wound site. To concentrate the blood meal, the salivary glands extract excess water and secrete it back into the host. Digestion proceeds relatively slowly when compared with that of blood-feeding insects. Digestion is almost entirely intracellular, an unusual phenomenon that allows pathogenic organisms greater opportunities for survival and may, perhaps, contribute to the remarkable diversity of tick-borne disease agents. As adults, females feed only once. Mating, guided by sex pheromones, takes place on the host, except in species of the genus *Ixodes* where it may occur in the nest, in vegetation, or on the host. Following mating, the females suck blood rapidly and swell enormously. Replete, mated females fall from their hosts, find a sheltered location, and deposit hundreds to thousands of eggs. For example, engorged females of the common American dog tick, *Dermacentor variabilis*, lay approximately 5380 eggs. The largest number of eggs reported from a single female was 22,891, from an *Amblyomma nuttalli* female. All of the eggs are deposited in a single, continuous stream over many days or weeks, i.e., there is only one gonotrophic cycle. When egg laying is complete, the females die. Males swell only slightly during feeding. However, they can remain on their hosts, feed repeatedly, and inseminate several females. Except in *Ixodes* species, males and females require a blood meal to stimulate oogenesis and spermatogenesis. Most of the life cycle is spent off the host. In most ticks, each life stage must find a host, feed, drop off, and molt to the next stage. Molting occurs off the host in most species, usually in some sheltered microenvironment, e.g., in the soil, under leaf litter, or in nests of associated hosts. Because of their extended feeding periods, species that attach to wide-ranging hosts may spread rapidly, providing a mechanism for dissemination of disease to distant foci.

The duration of the life cycle depends on the regional temperatures and opportunities for feeding. In tropical climates with frequent rainfall, development times are relatively short and several generations may occur each year. In colder temperate or subarctic climates, development is slower and the ticks diapause (i.e., cease feeding or developmental activity) during the colder months, extending the life cycle to 2 or more years. In Europe, the life cycle of the sheep tick (or castor bean tick), *Ixodes ricinus*, may require up to 4 years in the northern parts of its range.

ARGASID LIFE CYCLES. In most species, the argasid life cycle is very different from its ixodid relatives. Most argasid ticks have two or more nymphal stages in their life cycle, each of which must take a blood meal; 2 to 4 are common, but as many as 6 or 7 instars have been recorded in some species. This pattern is termed the *multihost* life cycle. Virtually all argasid ticks are multihost parasites, but there are notable exceptions, e.g, the two-host tick *Ornithodoros lahorensis* and the one-host ticks *Otobius megnini* and *Otobius lagophilus*. Most argasid ticks feed rapidly, often completing their blood meal within as little as 15 to 30 min, although some individuals may require 1 or 2 hr. The integument is deeply folded, allowing the body the opportunity for extensive stretching without additional cuticle growth. Nevertheless, the ticks can consume several times their unfed body weight at each feeding. The blood meal is concentrated rapidly by elimination of water via the coxal glands (coxal fluid), often visible while the tick is feeding or shortly afterward. In some argasid species, the larvae remain attached for several days, similar to the feeding behavior of ixodid ticks. Following feeding, the ticks drop and seek shelter in nearby cracks, crevices, in the dust, or in tiny openings in or near their host's nests. Molting occurs off the host, except in those few species noted earlier. In contrast with the ixodids, female

argasids take smaller blood meals, lay small clutches of eggs (typically, only several hundred eggs are deposited), and survive to feed again. This is termed the multiple gonotrophic cycle. Adults are ready to feed within several months after their previous meal. As many as six gonotrophic cycles have been reported in some species. Mating usually occurs off the host, in the sheltered microenvironments in or near the host's nest, occasionally during feeding. Because of the multiple nymphal stages, argasid ticks often live for many years. In addition, these ticks are highly resistant to starvation, extending the range of their life cycle even further. In some species that feed on migratory bats or birds, diapause serves to delay oviposition or development during the seasonal periods when hosts are absent. The implications of the remarkable longevity of these ticks for human and animal health are obvious. Pathogens transmitted by these vectors may survive unnoticed for years or even decades, emerging periodically in isolated foci when humans or animals encounter the ticks.

Behavior and Host Range

HABITATS. Most ixodid ticks are found widely dispersed in vegetation in forests, brushy habitats, meadows, or other grassy environments. Others occur in deserts or semidesert environments where the ticks survive in sand, in gravel, or under shale and rocks. While questing for hosts, ticks climb emergent stems, blades of grass, branches of low bushes, or other vegetative supports and wait for passing hosts. This is the "ambush" mode of host-seeking behavior favored by non-nidicolous ticks. When desiccated, they retreat toward the ground and seek shelter at the base of the vegetation or other protected moist microhabitats. Here the relative humidity is at or near saturation, which enables the ticks to take up water by direct sorption from the hydrating atmosphere. Atmospheric water condenses on hygroscopic salt solutions secreted by the ticks onto their hypostomes, whereupon the diluted salt solutions are imbibed, restoring the tick to its normally hydrated state. In all but the nest-inhabiting species of the genus *Ixodes*, host-seeking behavior is seasonal and is usually limited to the warmer periods of the year. Day length (i.e., photoperiod) and incident solar radiation are important factors influencing the onset and termination of this activity. At other times, one or more life stages remain in diapause, and the ticks survive from one year to the next until stimulated to commence the next seasonal cycle of host-seeking activity.

Argasid ticks and most species of the genus *Ixodes* are nidicoles, living in the nest, burrows, or other shelters made by their hosts. These ticks depend on the return of their hosts to the nest or burrow to feed. Nest-, burrow-, or cave-inhabiting argasids avoid bright light and settle in the more humid zones of their microenvironments. These behavioral attributes prevent the ticks from wandering from these shelters. Argasids adapted to migratory birds or bats may exhibit ovipositional diapause, delaying egg deposition and hatching until the hosts return and commence the nesting season. These patterns of periodic host-seeking activity interspersed with diapause ensure the coincidence of tick population expansion with the periods when host population and weather conditions are most favorable for species survival.

HOST RANGE. Host range varies greatly among the different species of ixodid ticks. Most species have a well-defined, restricted range of hosts. According to Hoogstraal and Aeschlimann, host specificity is an important factor contributing to confining tick species within narrow ecological niches and geographic ranges. For example, the American dog tick, *Dermacentor variabilis*, the major vector of RMSF, occurs primarily in areas of the eastern and central United States dominated by deciduous forest communities. Immatures of this species feed almost exclusively on small mammals, whereas the adults feed on larger mammals, especially medium-sized carnivores. Other species, e.g., the Lone Star tick, *Amblyomma americanum*, are opportunistic and attack a wide range of terrestrial vertebrate hosts. Argasid ticks typically exhibit well-defined host-selection patterns. Many feed exclusively on the bats or birds that inhabit the nests that they infest. A few species are less discriminating and attack virtually any warm-blooded vertebrate that enters the niche. In general, the opportunistic species are more likely to attack humans than those tick species with a highly restricted host range.

Medical and Veterinary Importance of Ticks

Ticks transmit a greater diversity of disease-causing agents than any other group of arthropod vectors. These include protozoan parasites, e.g., *Babesia* spp. and *Theileria* spp. affecting livestock, pets, and wildlife, bacterial agents such as *Borrelia* spp., numerous rickettsiae, and an even greater number of arboviruses. In addition, some ticks cause severe toxemias and fatal paralysis of their hosts.

DISEASE RELATIONSHIPS OF THE IXODIDAE (HARD TICKS)

Lyme Disease. Lyme borreliosis (Chapter 73) is the most prevalent vector-borne disease in the United States. This disease is caused by at least three species of spirochetes. In the United States and Canada, the spirochete is *Borrelia burgdorferi* (sensu latu) and is transmitted by certain species of the genus *Ixodes*. In Europe and northern Asia, Lyme disease may be caused by *Borrelia afzelli* and *Borrelia garinii*, as well as *B. burgdorferi*. Approximately 15,000 cases were reported by the U.S. Centers for Disease Control and Prevention in 1996, mostly in the Northeast. Other foci of Lyme disease occur in the midwestern region near the Great Lakes (especially Wisconsin and Minnesota) and on the Pacific Coast. In the eastern and central United States, the vector is the black-legged tick (also known as the deer tick), *Ixodes scapularis* (Fig. 137–3). In the Pacific coast region, the vector to humans is *Ixodes pacificus*, but the spirochetes can be disseminated among wild animal reservoirs by other species of this genus. *I. scapularis* ticks acquire the spirochetes when the larvae feed on spirochetemic small mammals, e.g., mice, shrews, and others. The white-footed mouse, *Peromyscus leucopus*, is the most important small mammal reservoir in most of the region where Lyme borreliosis is prevalent. Fed larvae molt, whereupon the hungry, spirochete-infected nymphs are ready to feed again. *I. scapularis* nymphs frequently attack large animals, including humans, as well as mice (Fig. 73–3). At first, when the nymphs attach to the skin of their hosts, spirochetes are present only in the tick's digestive tract, but the influx of fresh, warm blood excites their multiplication and migration. Within 2 or 3 days, they access the tick's salivary glands and are transmitted when saliva is injected into the feeding pool. Thus, the tiny nymph is the primary vector of the disease to humans and other animals. Adult ticks that acquired spirochetes during the nymphal blood meal also transmit these bacteria, but their much larger body size makes it easier to observe and remove them. The incidence of infection in the tick population is remarkably high; in some localities in New York state, 25% of the nymphs and 50% of the adult *I. scapularis* were found infected with spirochetes. In the eastern and central United States, the tick population is highly dependent on white-tailed deer (*Odocoileus virginiana*). Adult deer ticks feed mostly on these animals. Although ticks transmit *B. burgdorferi* to white-tailed

deer, the bacteria cannot survive in these animals, i.e., deer are not competent reservoir hosts. However, white-tailed deer are the preferred hosts for adult ticks, which feed by the thousands on the deer herds during the fall months. Each fully fed (replete) female tick can lay about 1500 eggs. Consequently, deer are considered to be the amplifying hosts for the *I. scapularis* population. In summary, the major contributing factors that enhance the epizootics of Lyme borreliosis are: (1) it is a zoonosis, with transmission of the disease-causing bacteria between ticks and wild vertebrates, especially small mammals; (2) transmission within the tick population is trans-stadial (i.e., from one life stage to the next) rather than transovarial (i.e., from the female parent to her progeny); (3) small mammals, especially mice, occasionally other vertebrates, are the reservoir-competent hosts; (4) the zoonosis is most common where deer and suitable small mammal reservoirs are abundant. Migratory birds also contribute to the dissemination of Lyme borreliosis, but their role in the epidemiology of the disease has not been thoroughly explored. Several other species of ticks, e.g., *Ixodes neotomae*, *Ixodes spinipalpus*, and *Ixodes dentatus*, which rarely if ever bite humans, disseminate the infection in wildlife and help to maintain this zoonosis even when the primary vectors are absent or not abundant.

Lyme disease also is prevalent is Europe, especially in northern Europe and northern Asia. The tick vector in most of the European continent is the castor bean tick (sheep tick), *Ixodes ricinus*. Like its North American cousin, *I. ricinus* attacks numerous different vertebrate species. The immatures feed mostly on small mammals, birds and lizards, whereas the adults attack deer, sheep, and other large animals. In northeastern Europe and northern Asia, the tick vector is *Ixodes persulcatus*. Both tick species readily bite man.

Domestic animals, especially dogs, are also affected by Lyme disease. In Lyme disease endemic regions, many dogs develop arthritis, loss of appetite, fever, and may even become lame; some also show neurologic symptoms.

Rocky Mountain Spotted Fever. Despite its name, most cases of RMSF occur in the eastern United States and Canada (Chapter 67.1). In recent years, about 700 to 800 cases per year were reported in the United States; North Carolina, South Carolina, Tennessee, and Oklahoma accounted for half of all reported cases. RMSF is caused by *Rickettsia rickettsii*, a small, entirely intracellular bacteria.

The primary vector to humans is a tick, the American dog tick, *Dermacentor variabilis* in the eastern United States and *Dermacentor andersoni* in the western part of the country. Several other tick species can also transmit *R. rickettsii* and help maintain the zoonosis in wildlife. Ticks serve as the reservoir host and the organism persists in the tick population from generation to generation by transovarial transmission. Small mammals, especially mice and voles, serve as the amplifier hosts as well as hosts for feeding the immature stages. Thus, rickettsia-infected ticks introduce the pathogens into mice, voles, squirrels, and other small mammals on which they feed. Subsequently, other ticks acquire the rickettsiae when they feed on these same animals, serving as a common infectious blood pool. Rickettsiae multiply in their tick hosts and infect the tick's organs, including the salivary glands. Infected adults attack large mammals, including humans, and transmit the rickettsiae when they inject saliva as they feed.

Boutonneuse Fever. Known also as Mediterranean spotted fever and by other names, this disease is similar in its clinical symptoms to RMSF (Chapter 67.2). In addition, a small, dark ulcer or eschar, resembling a button, usually appears at the site of the tick bite. The causative agent is *Rickettsia conorii*, transmitted principally by the brown dog tick, *Rhipicephalus* *sanguineus*. Other species of ticks, e.g., *Ixodes ricinus*, are also capable of transmitting the pathogen. The disease occurs in most of the countries bordering the Mediterrean Sea, as well as in large areas of Africa and Asia.

Ehrlichiosis. Although known mostly in domestic animals, two species of *Ehrlichia*, *E. chafeensis* and an as yet unnamed species, have been identified as the causative agents of disease in humans (Chapter 70). *E. chafeensis* causes a disease known as human monocytic ehrlichiosis, with symptoms superficially resembling RMSF. Cases have been reported primarily from the southeastern, mid-Atlantic, and south central United States. The primary vector is believed to be the Lone Star tick, *Amblyomma americanum* (Fig. 137–4), and the primary reservoir host is the white-tailed deer. A similar disease, known as human granulocytic ehrlichiosis, was identified in people with febrile illness in the north central United States. Thus far, only *Ixodes scapularis* has been implicated as the vector of the *Ehrlichia* spp. causing this disease.

Crimean-Congo Hemorrhagic Fever. CCHF is a true tick-borne arbovirus, because it passes trans-stadially and trans-ovarially within the tick population and survives interseasonally in these vectors (Chapter 31.5). The virus is a member of the genus *Nairovirus* (Family Bunyaviridae). The geographic distribution is immense, including most of Africa, southeastern Europe, and Asia. At least 31 tick species, including 2 argasid tick species in 2 different genera and 29 ixodid tick species comprising 7 different genera have been reported as vectors of this virus. The two-host vectors *Hyalomma marginatum rufipes* and other subspecies are especially important because the immatures feed on migratory birds as well as hares and hedgehogs, whereas the adults select artiodactyls and, when available, humans. Thus, these ticks are important in disseminating the virus intercontinentally along the routes followed by birds. The vast numbers in these flocks ensure repeated inundation of host populations along the bird flyways with virus-infected ticks. The *H. marginatum* complex and other human-biting *Hyalomma* species contribute to the periodic epidemics and epizootics of CCHF because of their aggressiveness in attacking human hosts and their large numbers. These ticks serve as the reservoirs as well as the vectors of the pathogens. The immature ticks, especially *H. marginatum rufipes*, readily feed on migratory birds, providing a means of long-range dispersal of the virus between Eurasia and Africa. Nevertheless, few bird species show antibodies and no virus has been isolated from wild birds. Small mammals, especially hedgehogs and hares, serve as the primary reservoir-competent hosts for infecting the immature ticks.

Major epidemics of CCHF have occurred in the recent past. One of the most notable of these outbreaks occurred in the Crimea (former Soviet Union) from 1944 to 1945, when hundreds of Soviet soldiers were infected while assisting the war-devastated population of the region. The case-fatality rate in that epidemic was approximately 10% and even higher rates have been reported in more recent episodes.

Omsk Hemorrhagic Fever. OHF is an acute, febrile disease with a distinct hemorrhagic syndrome. It is caused by the genus *Flavivirus*, family Togaviridae. This virus is in the same category as the causative agents of the closely related tick-borne encephalitis (TBE), Powassan virus, louping ill virus, Kyasanur Forest disease, and other tick-borne Togaviridae. These agents were formerly known as group B viruses. Clinically, the disease is similar to CCHF, but much milder with low mortality (<1%). Typical OHF foci are lowland steppe forest and grassland communities in western Siberia (former Soviet Union). Ticks, especially *Ixodes persulcatus* and *Ixodes apronophorus*, maintain the virus in nature, whereas *Dermacentor reticulatus* is regarded as primarily responsible for spread of the agent (amplification) within the wild host community and to humans.

Tick Paralysis. Although notorious primarily because of the disease-causing microbes they transmit, ticks also may cause illness by secreting noxious substances that cause paralysis, allergic reactions, or toxemia (Chapter 128). Tick paralysis has been reported from all of the world's habitable continents. *Ixodes holocyclus* in Australia, *Ixodes rubicundus* in South Africa, and *Dermacentor andersoni* and *Dermacentor variabilis* in North America are the tick species responsible for the majority of the cases of this disease. Paralysis results from the introduction with tick saliva of a protein, termed holocyclin in *I. holocyclus*. Except in *I. rubicundus* where transmission was found with nymphs, the female tick appears to be the vector of the paralyzing toxin. A single tick is sufficient to cause illness and death. Tick paralysis is completely reversible if the tick is found in time and removed. In Australia, where sudden removal of *I. holocyclus* can exacerbate the symptoms, administration of antitoxin is the preferred treatment.

DISEASE RELATIONSHIPS OF THE ARGASIDAE (SOFT TICKS)

Species of *Argas* and *Ornithodoros* are important as vectors of several viral and bacterial diseases. Several argasid tick species may also cause paralytic symptoms and tick toxicoses.

Quaranfil Virus Disease. This is found in Egypt and, possibly, adjacent countries where the heron tick, *Argas arboreus*, infests herons and similar roosting birds. The virus is circulated among the nestling birds in the heron rookeries and is transmitted from bird to bird by the nest-infesting ticks. Occasionally, humans become infected, resulting in severe illness. However, these ticks rarely if ever bite humans; thus, the route of infection to people is enigmatic.

Relapsing Fever. Relapsing fever is the best known and, in terms of numbers of human cases, the most important human disease transmitted by argasid ticks. Tick-borne relapsing fever is caused by at least 14 highly vector-specific *Borrelia* species, each transmitted by a specific *Ornithodoros* species (Chapter 71). Relapsing fever can also be caused by antigenically different spirochetes transmitted by lice (louse-borne relapsing fever), resulting in a severe and, when untreated, often fatal disease. Ticks transmit the spirochetes when they emit coxal fluid during feeding.

In the western United States, several outbreaks of tick-borne relapsing fever have occurred when people entered woodland shelters, e.g., hunting cabins infested with *Ornithodoros hermsi*, especially after house cleaning that drove out nesting rodents. Other vectors in the western United States and Mexico include *Ornithodoros turicata*, *Ornithodoros parkeri*, and possibly *Ornithodoros coriaceus*. The latter, the so-called "pajaroello" tick, is greatly feared in the western United States and Mexico because of its vicious bites as well as its ability to transmit epizootic bovine abortion, a viral pathogen that causes abortions in livestock and wild ruminants. In eastern and southern Africa, relapsing fever is transmitted by species of the *Ornithodoros moubata* complex (sensu Walton 1962). These ticks live in the primitive mud and thatch huts commonly used by the indigenous people, where they survive in cracks and crevices in the walls, roof and other locations.

137.2 *Mites*

Characterization

In contrast to the ticks, mites exhibit much greater diversity in their body structure and biology. Most mites are smaller than ticks although a few reach sizes as great as 7 mm in length. This assemblage of tiny arthropods consists of more than 200 families and over 30,000 species; thousands, perhaps tens of thousands, more species remain to be described. In contrast to the ticks, the chelicerae of mites are quite variable but usually scissor-like, with their cutting edges most often located on the medial facets. Mites lack Haller organ, although various types of leg sensilla are present, and the hypostome, when present, is small and lacks retrorse teeth. The genital pore is located in the podosomal region in the parasitiform mites but in the opisthosomal region in the acariform mites (Figs. 137–7 and 137–9).

Classification

Mites are subdivided into two main taxonomic groupings, the order Parasitiformes and the order Acariformes. The dendrogram (Fig. 137–6) illustrates this divergence and the suborders associated with these two orders. Parasitiform mites have 1 to 4 pairs of stigmata posterior to coxae II; the coxae are distinct and freely movable; the setae are not birefringent and are characterized as not optically active, i.e., isotropic. Acariform mites usually have propodosomal sensory organs and podocephalic canals; the coxae are fused with the body wall. Often, there is a distinct separation between the propodosomal (body region bearing the first 2 pairs of walking legs) and the metapodal portions (body region bearing the last 2 pairs of walking legs) of the body. Typically, the setae are anisotropic (optically active) and birefringent.

TETRASTIGMATID MITES (SUBORDER TETRASTIGMATA [ALSO HOLOTHYROIDEA]). These are relatively large (2 to 7 mm long), heavily sclerotized mites. There is a pair of stigmata lateral to coxae III and another on the lateral margins of the dorsal shield posterior to the ventral stigmata. These mites are believed to be carnivorous. Although not known to be responsible for transmission of any known disease agents, some mites of this group have been reported to cause ill effects when swallowed.

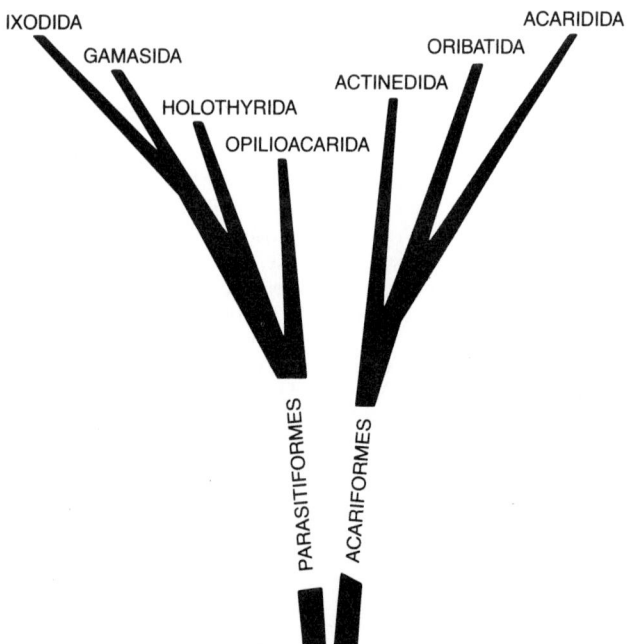

Figure 137–6. The systematic and evolutionary relationships among the orders and suborders of the subclass Acari. (From Krantz GW: A Manual of Acarology. Corvallis, Oregon State University Press, 1978.)

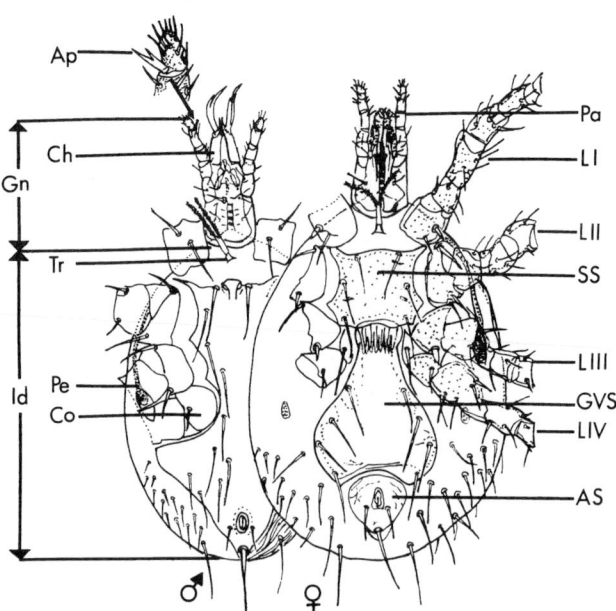

Figure 137–7. The major body structures of a representative mesostigmatid mite, as found in *Laelaps echidninus*. The male and female are shown in ventral view. Ap, Apotele; AS, anal shield; Ch, chelicera; Co, coxa (of leg IV); Gn, gnathosoma; GVS, genitoventral shield; Id, idiosoma; L, leg (I–IV); Pa, palp; Pe, peritreme; Tr, tritosternum; SS, sternal shield. (Redrawn from various sources, including Azad AF, 1986.)

MESOSTIGMATID MITES (SUBORDER MESOSTIGMATA [ALSO GAMASIDA]). This suborder contains numerous species that transmit diseases to humans and animals. These mites are closest to the ticks in general appearance. Mesostigmatid mites are generally robust, with sclerotized body plates. They have a single pair of stigmata located just posterior to and adjacent to coxae III (Fig. 137–7). Extending anteriorly from each stigmatal opening is a curved tube, the peritreme, of uncertain function. The chelae of the chelicerae are normally chelate-dentate, but many modifications occur; in males of some species, the chelae may be modified for spermatophore transfer (the spermatodactyl). The pedipalps have five distinct segments and an apotele with a two- to four-tined seta-like structure on the medial surface of the tarsal segment. An elongated bristle-like structure, the tritosternum, occurs on the ventral surface of the gnathosoma. The body bears a prominent peritreme on either side. Most mesostigmatid mites are free living, especially in soil and on the ground. Many are parasitic, either on insects or on vertebrates. An example is the tropical rat mite, *Ornithonyssus bacoti*, which parasitizes rodents and birds throughout the world. These mites are intermittent feeders, sucking blood within minutes when exposed to a host. Females produce up to 100 eggs, which hatch into nonfeeding larvae and molt into protonymphs. The protonymphs feed, molt to nonfeeding deutonymphs, and then molt to adults.

PROSTIGMATID MITES (SUBORDER PROSTIGMATA [ALSO ACTINEIDA]). This is a large, diverse group of mites, including many species that transmit (or cause) human and animal diseases. The group is characterized by the presence of a pair of stigmata at the base of the chelicerae. The chelicerae show many modifications, including modification into piercing stylets, hooklike structures, or even fusion. The pedipalps are simple and may also have fangs or claws. Genital suckers occur in both sexes. A tracheal system occurs in the majority of families. Typically, prostigmatid mites are only

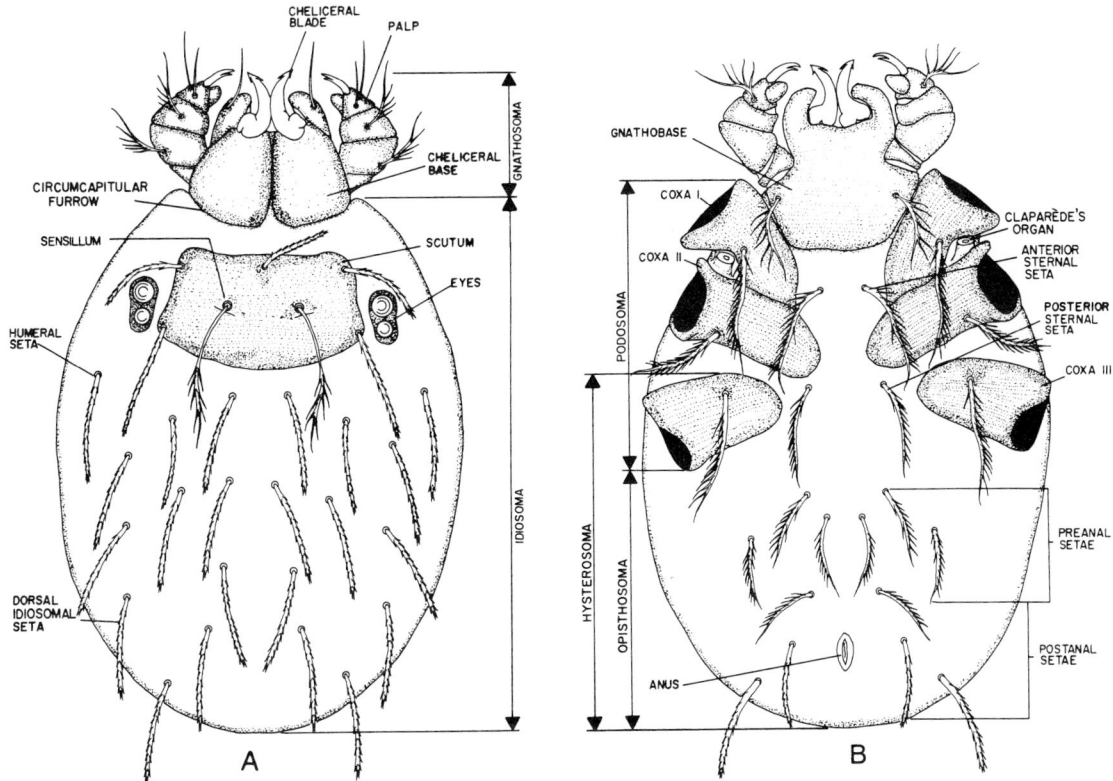

Figure 137–8. The idiosoma and gnathosoma of a representative chigger mite (larva of the Trombiculidae), *Eutrombicula alfreddugesi*. *A*, Dorsal aspect; *B*, ventral aspect. (From Goff ML, et al: J Med Entomol 19:221, 1982.)

weakly and incompletely sclerotized. This group includes several disease-transmitting species, especially those that include the chigger mites (Family Trombiculidae) responsible for transmission of scrub typhus (caused by *Rickettsia tsutsugamushi*) (Figs. 137–8 and 137–9).

ASTIGMATA (SUBORDER ASTIGMATA [ALSO ACARIDIDA]). These are mostly small (i.e., <1 mm), slow-moving mites. Many are fungivorous; others are saprophagous or feed on detritus. Few are predaceous. Several species are exclusively parasitic. The body is soft, with little or no sclerotization. The palpi are distinct, though small, with only two segments. True claws are lacking on the walking legs, al-

though a terminal clawlike spine may be present. Females have a terminal or posterodorsal bursa copulatrix, whereas males frequently have anal suckers. As in other Acariformes, the idiosoma is subdivided by a furrow into an anterior propodosoma and a posterior hysterosoma. This group includes many disease-causing or disease-transmitting mites, especially (1) skin-infesting *Sarcoptes scabiei*; (2) the allergy-causing house dust mites, *Dermatophagoides farinae* (Fig. 137–10), *Dermatophagoides pteronyssinus*, and others; (3) the dog mange mite, *Demodex canis*, which is similar to the human follicle mite, *Demodex folliculorum*; and (4) the straw itch mite, *Pyemotes tritici*, and many others.

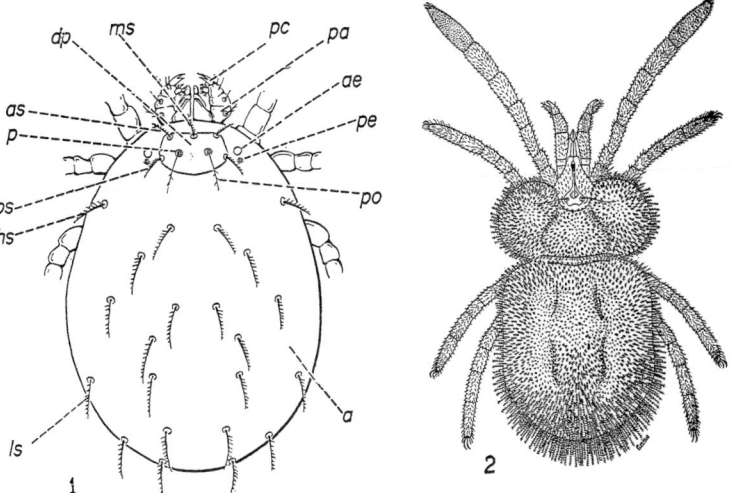

Figure 137–9. *Eutrombicula alfreddugesi*. *1*, Larva (North American chigger), greatly enlarged (a, abdomen; ae, anterior eye; as, anterolateral seta; dp, dorsal plate; hs, humeral seta; ls, lateral seta; ms, median seta; p, pseudostigma; pa, palpus; pc, palpal claw; pe, posterior eye; po, pseudostigmatic organ; ps, posterolateral seta). *2*, Adult.

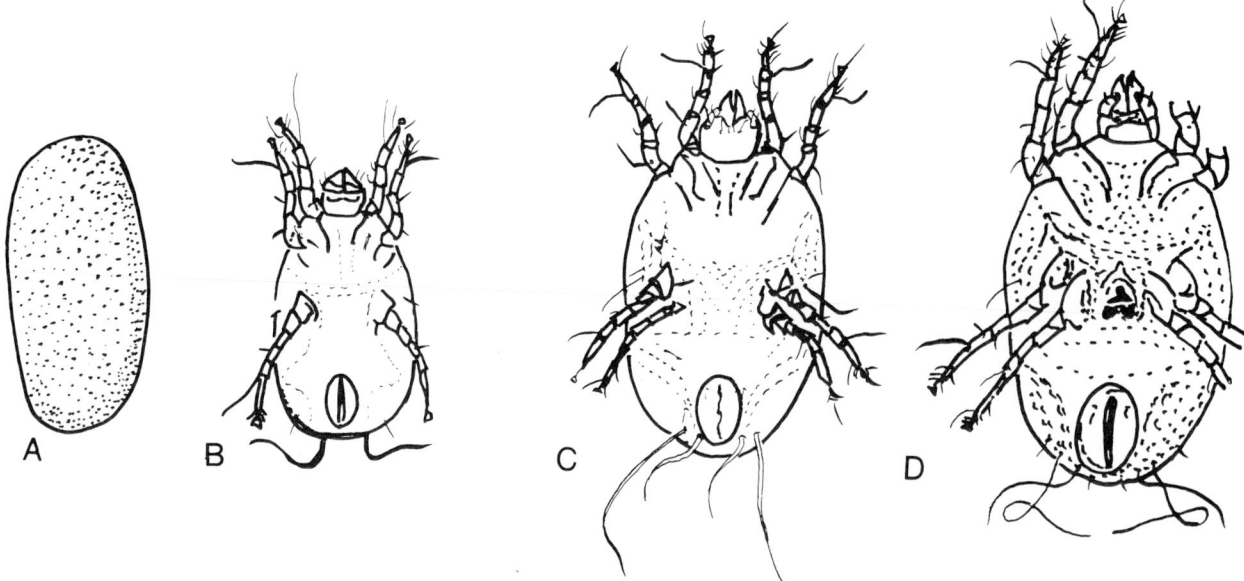

Figure 137–10. The developmental stages of the house dust mite, *Dermatophagoides farinae. A,* Egg; *B,* larva; *C,* nymphal stage (protonymph-tritonymph); *D,* adult. (Modified from Wharton GW: J Med Entomol 12:577, 1976.)

Habitats and Life Cycle

Mites occupy an exceptionally diverse array of habitats. Numerous species live entirely in the soil, feeding on fungi, bacteria and other microorganisms, or on decomposing organic matter. Others live on the ground, especially in the upper layers of the soil, at the interface with the duff, detritus, and/or the leafy layer that characterizes the top of the root zone of vegetation. These may include predaceous species, dung-feeding species, and others feeding on vegetation. Numerous species are phytophagous, feeding on a variety of plants or stored foods. Many of these mites are parasitic, including some that have obligate parasitic life cycles. Many are parasitic on insects, whereas other parasitize vertebrates. Some, such as the itch mite, *Sarcoptes scabiei,* live their entire lives in the tissues of their host (Chapter 128.2). Although most of these mites are classified as ectoparasites, living in the skin, feathers, or fur of their hosts, others such as the nasal mites (Family Halarachnidae) are endoparasitic, living in the nasal passages of seals and walruses or in the lungs, bronchi, tracheas, or sinuses of various mammalian hosts.

The typical life cycle includes the egg, protonymph, deutonymph, tritonymph, and the adult. Often, one or more of the immature stages is omitted as development is accelerated. In the insect-parasitizing hay-itch mite, *Pyemotes ventricosus,* the female does not lay eggs but reproduces viviparously. The opisthosomal region of the female swells during feeding, forming a balloon-like structure. Young mites develop within this sac and emerge when they are sexually mature adults.

Behavior and Host Range

The enormous diversity of disease-causing and disease-transmitting mites makes it difficult to generalize regarding their behavior and host range. In the Mesostigmata (Gamasida), most of the parasitic mites are nidicoles, living in the nest or burrow environment of the mammal or bird hosts. Typically, they are intermittent feeders, attacking hosts when present, feeding for brief periods, and returning to the shelter of the nest material to molt or lay eggs. The chicken mite, *Dermanyssus gallinae,* is an example of this parasitic habit. These mites live in cracks, crevices, detritus, or fibrous material and

usually leave their shelters only at night. Others are permanent ectoparasites, e.g., *Ornithonyssus sylviarum,* which lives out its entire life cycle on the host. A closely related parasite, *Ornithonyssus bursa,* has a similar parasitic habit but leaves its host to lay eggs. Many parasitic mites are true hematophages, piercing the host skin and sucking blood. Others, such as the spiny rat mite, *Echinolaelaps echidninus,* feed on bloody exudates from abrasions and skin lesions; they cannot penetrate the unbroken skin. Although numerous mesostigmatid mites are opportunistic, i.e., feeding on virtually any hosts that they encounter, other species exhibit varying degrees of host specificity, e.g., the snake mite, *Ophionyssus natricis.* Examples of parasitism are also numerous among the acariform mites. Among the prostigmatid mites, one of the most important parasites is the chigger mite (Family Trombiculidae). In these species, only the larva is parasitic. The larval mite burrows into the skin, forming a cavity (stylostome) in which it feeds and shelters, causing inflammation and severe irritation that the host cannot relieve by grooming. When satiated, the mite escapes to continue its development on the ground, much to the relief of the host. The nymphs and adults are predaceous. Other prostigmatid mites are obligate parasites in all stages, spending their entire lives on the same host, e.g., feather mites such as *Syringophilus bipectinatus.* These tiny mites live inside the quill feathers, feeding on desquamated cells and sebaceous secretions from which they derive necessary nutrients. Not only are these mites highly species specific, they are even specialized for specific feather groups. Among the astigmatids, one finds similar examples of highly adapted obligate ectoparasitic life cycles. Thus, fur mites spend their entire lives on and among the hairs of their mammalian hosts, mostly on rodents. These mites bear special adaptations for this habitat, e.g., a somewhat laterally compressed body and modification of the palps and legs to form claspers for clinging to the hairs. In *Listrophorus* spp., the endites of the palpal coxae form an apparatus for attaching to hair. As a result of these adaptations, these mites are relatively host specific.

Medical and Veterinary Importance of Mites

MESOSTIGMATID MITES. These mites transmit a variety of human and animal diseases. The human-biting *Liponyssus* *sanguineus*, found occasionally in rodent-infested households, transmits the agent of rickettsial pox, caused by *Rickettsia akari* (Chapter 67.3). An eschar (skin ulcer) appears at or near the site of inoculation. Some mesostigmatid mites are serious pests of domestic fowl, e.g., the chicken mite, *Dermanyssus gallinae*; the northern fowl mite, *Ornithonyssus sylviarum*; and the tropical fowl mite, *Ornithonyssus bursa*, which is a serious pest of chickens, turkeys, and other domestic fowl in various parts of the world. In infested buildings, these mites may proliferate in such enormous numbers that they kill many of the birds. Other parasitized birds become extremely irritable, their skin becomes inflamed and scabby, and the birds become progressively anemic and emaciated; as might be expected, weight gain and egg production diminish precipitously. *O. sylviarum* also bites humans, resulting in erythema, induration, and pruritus around the wound sites. *D. gallinae* may also bite humans, leading to painful urticaria.

Rodent mites may also constitute a problem. *Ornithonyssus bacoti*, the tropical rat mite, parasitizes small mammals and occasionally other vertebrates. It may also attack humans, with severe and painful dermatitis resulting from these bites. In contrast to these ectoparasitic mites, some mesostigmatid mites are endoparasitic, e.g., species of the genus *Halarachne*, which lives in the respiratory system of seals, or the nasal mite, *Pneumonyssus caninum*, which inhabits the nasal passages and sinuses of dogs. Mite-infested dogs develop inflammation of the nasal passages, excessive production of mucus, rhinitis, sinusitis, sneezing, and violent head-shaking behavior.

PROSTIGMATID MITES. These include chigger mites, the vectors of scrub typhus. This disease, caused by *Rickettsia tsutsugamushi* (Chapter 69), is prevalent in eastern Asia, especially Japan, eastern China, Taiwan, Vietnam, India, the Philippines and many islands in the South Pacific, and even parts of Australia. It does not occur in the Americas, Europe or Africa, because *R. tsutsugamushi* is highly host specific and cannot infect the species of trombiculid mites (i.e., chigger mites) in these regions. However, even where they do not carry disease, the attacks of chigger mites are serious and often cause intense itching and severe dermatitis; in highly sensitized individuals, this may even lead to hospitalization to control the condition (Fig. 137–9).

ASTIGMATID MITES. These include many species that are serious pests or causative agents of disease, including allergies. Among the best known are the mange mites, especially the families Psoroptidae, Sarcoptidae, and Demodicidae. Species of *Psoroptes* pierce the skin and suck fluids, which congeal to induce scabbing and related growths; the scab provides shelter for the mites, which reproduce rapidly in this protected environment. In rabbits, the rabbit ear mite, *Psoroptes cuniculi* proliferates deep in the ear canal and can penetrate into the brain; the mites eventually kill these animals unless they are treated early enough to prevent penetration by mites into the inner ear. In humans, females of the human itch mite, *Sarcoptes scabiei*, tunnel into the stratum corneum of the skin (Fig. 128–8). These burrows fill with eggs, hatched larvae, excrement, ecdysial cuticles and other debris, all of which induce an intense irritation in the affected host (Fig. 128–9). Transmission occurs by direct physical contact between infected and uninfected individuals. In addition, transfer experiments show that canine mites can infect humans. Fortunately, human and animal cross-infestations are self-limiting.

DUST MITE ALLERGY. An increasingly recognized mite-associated illness is dust mite allergy. Proteins in mite feces, rather than the mites themselves, are regarded as the primary allergen responsible for the allergic reactions (Chapter 128.1). In the United States, after pollen or hay fever, house dust is the most common cause of allergic reactions in humans. The problem may be seasonal in northern temperate climates, declining during the heating season when mites are killed by low indoor humidities, but year-round in humid tropical or subtropical climates. Common symptoms resemble allergies to pollen and other dustlike substances, with upper respiratory distress, swelling of nasal membranes and sinuses, sneezing, tearing, and related symptoms. Dust mite allergies occur worldwide but are most prevalent in regions with a warm, humid climate. In households, mattresses, pillows, stuffed furniture, carpets, and other household objects where human or animal dander can accumulate in large quantities may provide the optimal microenvironments where the mites feed and develop.

Bibliography

Anderson, BE, Sims KG, Olson, JG, et al: *Amblyomma americanum*: A potential vector of human ehrlichiosis. Am J Trop Med Hyg 49: 239, 1993.
Arthur DR: Ticks and Disease. Oxford, England, Pergamon Press, 1962.
Azad AF: Mites of public health importance and their control. WHO Publication VBC/86.931. Geneva, World Health Organization, 1986.
Burgdorfer W: The enlarging spectrum of tick-borne spirochetoses: R.R. Parker memorial address. Rev Infect Dis 8:932, 1986.
Daniels TJ, Falco RC, Schwartz, I, et al: Deer ticks (*Ixodes scapularis*) and the agents of Lyme disease and human granulocytic ehrlichiosis in a New York City park. Emerg Infect Dis 3:353, 1997.
Des Vignes F, Fish D: Transmission of the agent of human granulocytic ehrlichiosis by host-seeking *Ixodes scapularis* (Acari: Ixodidae) in southern New York state. J Med Entomol 34:379, 1997.
Galun R, Obenchain FD (eds): Physiology of Ticks. Oxford, England, Pergamon Press, 1982.
Gregson JD: Tick paralysis: An appraisal of natural and experimental data. Monograph No. 9, Canada Department of Agriculture. Ottawa, 1973.
Griffiths DA, Bowman CE (eds): Acarology, Vol I. Chichester, England, Ellis Horwood, 1984.
Hoogstraal H: Argasid and nuttalliellid ticks as parasites and vectors. Adv Parasitol 24: 135, 1985.
Hoogstraal H, Aeschlimann A: Tick-host specificity. Bull Soc Entomol Suisse 55:5, 1982.
Krantz GW: A Manual of Acarology. Corvallis, Oregon State University, 1978.
Lockhart JM, Davidson WR, Stallknecht, DE, et al: Isolation of *Ehrlichia chafeensis* from wild white-tailed deer (*Odocoileus virginianus*) confirms their role as natural reservoir hosts. J Clin Microbiol 35:1681, 1997.
Oliver JH Jr: Chromosomes, genetic variance and reproductive strategies among mites and ticks. Bull Entomol Soc Am 29:9, 1983.
Oliver JH Jr, Owsley MR, Hutcheson HJ, et al: Conspecificity of the ticks *Ixodes scapularis* and *I. dammini* (Acari: Ixodidae). J Med Entomol 30:54, 1993.
Savory T: Arachnida. New York, Academic Press, 1977.
Sonenshine DE: Biology of Ticks. New York, Oxford University Press, 1991.
Sonenshine DE, Mather TN: Ecological Dynamics of Tick-Borne Zoonoses. New York, Oxford University Press, 1994.

138 Insects in Disease Transmission

Duane J. Gubler

HISTORY. Although early scholars recognized a relationship between certain arthropods and illness in humans and animals, the concept of disease transmission by insects is relatively new. The first actual demonstration that a parasite of humans required a developmental phase in an insect to complete its life cycle occurred only 120 years ago. Sir Patrick Manson, working in China in 1877, showed that the human filarial parasite *Wuchereria bancrofti* required an obligatory period of development in the mosquito *Culex pipiens fatigans* (*Cx. pipiens quinquefasciatus*). Since that time, many important disease pathogens of humans have been shown to depend on insects to complete their transmission cycles.

The pathogens transmitted to humans by insects fall into five main categories of microorganisms: nematodes or roundworms, protozoa, bacteria, rickettsiae, and viruses. Some are true parasites of humans (e.g., *W. bancrofti*) but most are zoonotic, with other primary vertebrate hosts (reservoirs). Humans in this case become an incidental host, and although they may contribute to the transmission cycle on a temporary basis, they are not required for survival of the pathogen in nature.

DISEASE TRANSMISSION. An arthropod may transmit a disease agent from one person or animal to another in one of two basic ways.

Mechanical Transmission. This consists of a simple transfer of the organism on contaminated mouthparts or feet. No multiplication or developmental change of the pathogen on or in the insect takes place during this type of transmission. Examples include various enteroviruses, bacteria, and protozoa of humans that have a direct fecal-oral transmission cycle. Insects, e.g., houseflies, may become contaminated with these pathogens while feeding on feces and may transport them directly to the food of humans.

Biologic Transmission. The second and most important type of transmission by insects is biologic. As the name implies, the pathogen must undergo some type of development in the body of the insect vector in order to complete its life cycle. There are three types of biologic transmission.

Propagative Transmission. This type occurs when the organism ingested with the blood meal undergoes simple multiplication in the body of the insect. Examples are the arboviruses, which replicate extensively in the tissues of the insect.

Cyclopropagative Transmission. In this type of transmission, the pathogen undergoes a developmental cycle (changes from one stage to another) as well as multiplication in the body of the insect. The best example of this type is malaria, in which a single zygote may give rise to >200,000 sporozoites.

Cyclodevelopmental Transmission. In this third type of biologic transmission, the pathogen undergoes developmental changes from one stage to another but does not multiply. With the filariae, for example, a single microfilaria ingested by a mosquito may result in only one infective larva. In most instances, however, the number of infective larvae is significantly lower than the number of microfilariae ingested.

Extrinsic Incubation Period. In all types of biologic transmission, time is required for development of the pathogen to the infective stage that can be transmitted. With arboviruses, this means infection and replication in the salivary glands; with the malaria parasite, it means invasion of the salivary glands by the infectious sporozoites; and with filariae, it means development of the juvenile worms to the active stage III larvae. This period, called the *extrinsic incubation period*, generally lasts 7 to 14 days, depending on the pathogen, the vector, and various environmental factors, including temperature.

Transovarial Transmission. Some viral and rickettsial disease agents are transmitted from the female parent arthropod through the eggs to the offspring. If the pathogen actually infects the developing egg, this is termed *transovarial transmission*. With some arboviruses, however, only the ovarial sheath and oviduct are infected, and the egg is infected as it passes down the oviduct and is inseminated. This type is distinguished from transovarial transmission and is called *vertical transmission*. In either case, the newly hatched insect larval stages are infected with the pathogen, which is then transmitted to subsequent developmental stages of the arthropod (transstadial transmission). Finally, veneral transmission of certain viruses has been documented. Thus, male mosquitoes that become infected transovarially or vertically can transfer the infective virus to uninfected female mosquitoes in the seminal fluid during copulation. These latter types of transmission have obvious epidemiologic importance in the ultimate infection of humans or other animals and in the maintenance of the pathogen in nature.

Factors Influencing Transmission. The ability of insects to transmit a disease agent is dependent on many complex factors. Successful mechanical transmission depends on the degree of contact insects have with humans and on feeding behavior. For example, the domestic housefly has been incriminated as a mechanical vector of various intestinal pathogens, primarily because this insect breeds in large numbers, lives in intimate contact with humans, and has the bad habit of feeding on both feces and food. Tabanid flies are efficient mechanical vectors of both viruses and protozoa because of frequent interrupted blood feeding.

The ability to transmit a pathogen biologically varies greatly among species of insects and even among geographic strains within a species. Significant variation in susceptibility to become infected and subsequently to transmit an etiologic agent has been demonstrated in a number of insect vectors. Most work, however, has been done with mosquitoes, and variation in vector competence has been documented with all of the major diseases they transmit (i.e., malaria, filariasis, and arbovirus infections). Thus, within a single mosquito species, it is common to find geographic strains that are good vectors and other strains of that same species that are poor vectors. Because this general susceptibility to infection and growth of the pathogen in the tissues of the insect are genetically controlled, it may be expected to change as a result of selective pressure over time.

In addition to innate susceptibility to infection, the overall vectoral capacity of an insect is influenced by other biologic and behavioral characteristics of the insect population. The degree of contact the species has with humans is influenced by the host preference, the intrinsic blood-feeding and resting behavior of the insect, and the population density of both insect and humans. Longevity, resting behavior, flight behavior, and oviposition (breeding) behavior of the insect population are important intrinsic factors, which are influenced by extrinsic environmental factors, e.g., temperature, humidity, wind, and rainfall.

Finally, other extrinsic factors may influence whether an individual insect becomes infected with a pathogen. For example, it has been shown that mosquitoes ingesting blood containing both microfilariae and Rift Valley fever virus have a higher viral infection rate because disseminated virus infection is facilitated by microfilariae escaping from the midgut into the hemocoel. Other factors may also influence this "leaky gut" phenomenon and thus susceptibility to infection.

In temperate regions, insect transmission of disease is usually seasonal and can be correlated with temperature and day length. In the tropics, transmission generally occurs year round, but increased seasonal transmission is most frequently correlated with rainfall.

Systematics. Table 138–1 outlines the orders and lower taxa of the class Insecta that are known to transmit disease pathogens of humans. Mites and ticks are not included, as they are discussed elsewhere (Chapter 137). The order Diptera is by far the most important in terms of disease transmission, primarily because of the family Culicidae (mosquitoes).

Importance. Collectively, insects are responsible for hundreds of millions of cases of disease each year. In the past 20 years, the world has experienced a resurgence and expanding geographic distribution of vector-borne diseases, e.g., malaria, leishmaniasis, dengue hemorrhagic fever, yellow fever, Japanese encephalitis, and epidemic polyarthritis, and several

TABLE 138–1. Taxonomic Groups of the Class Insecta That Transmit Human Disease

Order	Family	Important Genera
Siphonaptera	Pulicidae	Pulex
		Xenopsylla
		Ctenocephalides
	Ceratophyllidae	Nosopsyllus
		Diamanus
	Leptopsyllidae	Leptopsylla
Anoplura	Pediculidae	Pediculus
Hemiptera	Cimicidae	Cimex
	Reduviidae	Triatoma
		Rhodnius
		Panstrongylus
Diptera	Ceratopogonidae	Culicoides
	Psychodidae	Phlebotomus
		Lutzomyia
		Sergentomyia
	Simuliidae	Similium
		Prosimulium
		Austrosimulium
	Culicidae	Aedes
		Anopheles
		Culex
		Mansonia
		Haemagogus
		Psorophora
		Sabethes
	Tabanidae	Tabanus
		Chrysops
	Glossinidae	Glossina
	Muscidae	Musca
		Fannia
		Muscina
	Chloropidae	Hippelates
		Siphunculina
	Calliphoridae	Calliphora
		Lucilia
		Phaenicia
		Phormia
		Chrysomyia
		Cochliomyia
	Sarcophagidae	Sarcophaga
Dictyoptera	Blattidae	Blatta
		Periplaneta
		Blattella

new diseases have emerged, e.g., Barmah Forest in Australia, a yet unnamed flavivirus that causes hemorrhagic disease in Saudi Arabia, and Lyme disease and ehrlichiosis in the United States. A major problem is that the most important vector-borne diseases occur in the tropics, usually in the areas where resources are most limited and surveillance is poor. The shrinking world, with highly increased human mobility due to air travel and commerce using containerized shipping, however, has made these diseases not just problems of the tropics; they present the world community with possibly its greatest health problem today. For example, an average of about 1000 reported cases of malaria are imported into the United States each year, and there are several fatalities, mainly because of late diagnosis. Many areas of the United States still have the anopheline mosquito vectors of this parasite, and recent sporadic local transmission has been documented in California, Arizona, New Jersey, Georgia, and Florida. Similarly, many cases of dengue fever are imported into the United States each year. The principal vector mosquito, *Aedes aegypti*, still occurs in most Gulf Coast states, and in 1985, another important vector mosquito, *Ae. albopic-*

tus, was found in Texas. This species subsequently spread throughout the eastern United States; it currently is found in 26 states. The first indigenous dengue transmission since 1945, secondary to imported disease, was documented in Texas in 1980 and again in 1986, 1995, and 1997. This underscores the need for physicians in nonendemic areas to be aware of these diseases and to be knowledgeable about where they occur and how to recognize and treat them.

The resurgence of some insect-borne viral diseases has become more acute in the 1990s. The incidence of dengue has increased dramatically in all major regions of the tropics, occurring not only as larger and more frequent epidemics but also in countries where the disease had not occurred before (Chapter 29.1). Moreover, the severe and fatal form of disease, dengue hemorrhagic fever, has moved out of Southeast Asia and is now occurring in many Pacific and American countries. Other viruses, e.g., yellow fever, Japanese encephalitis, Ross River, West Nile, Venezuelan equine encephalitis, Rift Valley fever, and o'nyong-nyong have expanded their geographic distribution and caused major epidemics. The reinfestation of the American tropics by *Ae. aegypti* has put that region at the highest risk for urban epidemics of yellow fever in >50 years.

■ DISEASE TRANSMISSION BY INSECT GROUPS

FLEAS (ORDER SIPHONAPTERA)
Biology. Fleas make up the order Siphonaptera. The adults are small, wingless, laterally flattened, obligate bloodsuckers that parasitize a wide variety of vertebrate hosts (Fig. 139–11). There are approximately 2375 species and subspecies of fleas, with representatives on all continents, including the Arctic and Antarctic; 94% of species parasitize mammals, and the remainder parasitize birds. Only a relatively few species are of importance in transmitting disease to humans (Table 138–2; Fig. 128–1).

The developmental cycle of fleas from egg to adult normally takes place in the nest of the host. Eggs are generally laid in the nest, where the normally free-living, legless, eyeless, and wormlike larvae feed on organic material, e.g., scales, dried blood, and feces deposited by the adults. After 2 to 3 weeks, the fully grown larvae spin a cocoon and pupate. The pupal stage may last 1 to 2 weeks, after which the adult emerges, often after the stimulus of movement or vibration caused when a host enters the nest. The entire period of development may last 3 to 4 weeks or longer, depending on temperature in the nest. The larvae require high humidity.

Most fleas are not strictly host specific and therefore attempt to feed on almost any animal. Because adults can go without feeding for considerable periods, they can search for new hosts after the nest has been vacated or the host has died.

Disease Transmission. Fleas are important natural vectors of two diseases of humans—plague and murine typhus. In addition, they were shown experimentally to transmit *Bartonella henselae*, the agent of cat-scratch disease, and have been implicated as but not proved to be vectors of various other diseases, e.g., tularemia, pseudotuberculosis, erysipeloid, hemorrhagic nephrosonephritis, boutonneuse fever, and Q fever. They are known intermediate hosts for at least two tapeworms (Table 138–2).

Plague. Caused by *Yersinia pestis*, plague is a typical zoonosis of rodents and small mammals that exists in much of the world in a flea-rodent-flea transmission cycle (Chapter 61). Large epidemics of plague, which in the past caused millions of deaths, no longer occur. However, smaller epidemics and

TABLE 138–2. Important Species of Fleas That Transmit Human Diseases

Flea Species	Principal Host	Geographic Distribution	Diseases
Xenopsylla cheopis	Rats	Tropicopolitan	Plague, murine typhus, rat tapeworm
X. brasiliensis	Rats	Africa, South America, India	Plague
X. astia	Rats	Asia	Plague
Nosopsyllus fasciatus	Rats, mice, swine, domestic animals	Europe, North America	Plague, murine typhus, rat tapeworm
Pulex irritans	Humans, domestic animals	Cosmopolitan	Plague
P. simulans	Humans	North and South America	Plague
Leptopsylla segnis	Rats, mice	Cosmopolitan	Plague, murine typhus
Ctenocephalides canis	Dogs, cats	Cosmopolitan	Dog tapeworm
C. felis felis	Dogs, cats	Cosmopolitan	Dog tapeworm
Diamanus montanus	Ground squirrels	Western United States, Mexico	Plague

sporadic human cases continue to occur each year in many parts of the world where plague exists in enzootic foci. Called *sylvatic* or *rural plague*, this type is maintained in nature by >200 species of rodents that are known hosts of plague bacilli and by many species of fleas that normally feed on these rodents. Humans become involved accidentally when they invade the plague focus, usually for hunting, trapping, or recreational purposes.

Epidemics still occasionally occur after long periods of no disease. For example, in Kenya, after an absence of plague for 10 years, 166 cases with 9 deaths were reported in 1978. In Peru, several thousand cases occurred in 1993 and 1994. An epidemic of plague occurred in Mahrastra, India, in 1994 after nearly 30 years of no reported cases. Factors responsible for periodic epizootics and/or epidemics are not well understood and are peculiar to each natural plague focus.

Urban plague usually occurs during the course of an epizootic when commensal rodents become involved. The infection is then maintained in the urban rat population by several species of fleas that parasitize these rodents (Table 138–2). Humans may become involved when urban rats begin to die of plague and infected fleas search for new hosts (Fig. 135–1). Urban plague epidemics have been rare in the past 50 years, but in 1994, a small, relatively focal outbreak in Surat, Gujarat State, India, caused an international health emergency because it was thought to be pneumonic plague and there was concern about transportation of this severe form of plague via infected persons on jet airplanes to urban areas all over the world.

Transmission of plague by fleas can occur in several ways, most importantly by the bite of an infected flea. Fleas become infected by ingesting plague bacilli with the blood meal taken from a rodent with bacteremia. The bacteria undergo multiplication in the stomach of the flea and frequently move forward to the proventriculus, resulting in partial or complete blockage. Fleas with a blocked proventriculus can take blood only with difficulty and frequently regurgitate in an attempt to get blood past the blocked area. In the process, plague bacilli are inoculated into the host. Because of the difficulty in getting blood past the proventricular obstruction, infected fleas become starved and biting frequency increases, making these fleas important in transmission. Factors that influence proventricular blockage include strain of pathogen, species of flea, temperature, and type of blood ingested.

Although it is a less important means of transmission, fleas have also been known to transmit plague bacilli in their feces. In this case, the organism is rubbed into the bite wound, other skin abrasions, or mucous membranes. Transmission has also been reported when infected fleas are crushed between the teeth. Finally, pneumonic plague is transmitted from person to person in respiratory droplets.

Murine Typhus. Murine or flea-borne typhus is a rodent zoonosis caused by *Rickettsia typhi (mooseri)* (Chapter 66.2). This is a disease primarily of rats and mice and has a worldwide distribution, mainly in the tropics. Clinically, it is similar to epidemic or louse-borne typhus but somewhat milder. The rash is the same.

The infection is maintained in nature by a rat-flea-rat cycle. The usual vertebrate reservoirs are *Rattus rattus* and *R. norvegicus*, and the principal insect vector is the tropical rat flea *Xenopsylla cheopis*, although other species of fleas can become infected (Table 138–2).

Humans become infected incidentally by a flea that has strayed from its host. Rickettsiae are ingested by fleas with a blood meal from an infected rat. The organisms multiply within the gut and are passed in the feces of fleas. The mechanism of transmission is by rubbing infected feces into skin abrasions or by transfer to mucous membranes. Transmission may also occur by inhalation of dust contaminated with infected flea feces.

Cestode Infections. In addition to serving as vectors, fleas also act as intermediate hosts for at least two tapeworms that may infect humans, *Dipylidium caninum* of dogs (Chapter 123.4) and *Hymenolepis diminuta* of rats (Chapter 123.3). Eggs of both parasites are passed in the feces of their respective vertebrate hosts and are ingested by larval fleas feeding on detritus in the nest. They hatch, and the cysticeroids develop in the body cavity of the immature flea. The adult flea is thus infected at the time of emergence from the pupa, and transmission occurs when the flea is ingested or crushed between the teeth of a dog, rat, or person.

Dog and cat fleas, *Ctenocephalides canis* and *C. felis*, are the most important intermediate hosts of *D. caninum*, whereas *X. cheopis* and *Nosopsyllus fasciatus* are important intermediate hosts for *H. diminuta* (Table 138–2).

SUCKING LICE (ORDER ANOPLURA)

Biology. Sucking lice are small, wingless, obligate ectoparasites of mammals belonging to the order Anoplura. The body is flattened, and the legs, in part, are adapted for clinging to hairs and feathers. Most species are very host specific, and the entire life cycle is spent on one host.

There are about 225 species of Anoplura, but only 3 are parasites of humans. These are the human body louse, *Pediculus humanus corporis* (Fig. 139–1); the head louse, *P. humanus capitis*; and the crab or pubic louse, *Phthirus pubis* (Fig. 139–2). All have a worldwide distribution.

The life cycle of all three species is incomplete, takes about 3 weeks, and is completed on the human host. Head and crab lice glue their eggs to hairs, whereas body lice lay eggs in the seams of clothing.

Disease Transmission. Only the body louse is of known importance in the transmission of human disease. This species lives in the clothing of humans, where it makes close contact with the skin. Heavy infestations of up to 10,000 lice can build up on an individual during cold months and times of poor hygiene. In general, all louse-borne diseases described in the following sections require the same epidemiologic conditions and are seen only when conditions are favorable for maintenance of large louse populations.

Epidemic (Louse-Borne) Typhus. Epidemic typhus is caused by *Rickettsia prowazekii* (Chapter 66.1). The disease has a wide distribution in Europe, Africa, Asia, and the Western Hemisphere. Large epidemics are generally associated with cooler temperatures during times of war, famine, and natural disasters, when people are crowded together in conditions of poor sanitation and hygiene.

Epidemic typhus has a human-louse-human cycle. A person is usually infectious during the febrile period, and lice become infected when taking a blood meal at that time. The rickettsiae enter the epithelial cells of the louse midgut and multiply to such an extent that the cells rupture in 3 to 5 days, releasing large numbers of rickettsiae into the lumen of the intestine, from which they are then passed in the feces of the louse. Humans become infected when infectious feces are rubbed into abrasions of the skin caused by scratching or into mucous membranes. Less commonly, infectious rickettsiae can be released from lice by crushing. Lice feces may dry in the clothing and can remain infectious for 60 to 90 days. As a result, the feces may become airborne, causing transmission by inhalation. Transmission of *R. prowazekii* does not occur by the bite of lice.

Epidemic transmission of louse-borne typhus is facilitated by the fact that lice are sensitive to changes in temperature. They immediately abandon hosts with high fevers and those who have died, seeking out other hosts and thus transferring the infection with them. Unlike many insect-borne diseases, *R. prowazekii* infection is also fatal to the lice, which eventually succumb to the damage caused by ruptured midgut epithelial cells.

Humans are apparently the principal reservoir of *R. prowazekii*. Asymptomatic carriers of the agent may remain infective to lice for many years and thus may provide sources of infection in areas where the rickettsiae have been absent. Another characteristic of louse-borne typhus is that it has a tendency to recrudesce, producing a disease known as Brill-Zinsser disease as long as 50 years after the initial infection. Evidence suggests that certain tree squirrels in Virginia may also be reservoir hosts of *R. prowezekii*.

Trench Fever. Trench fever is caused by *Rickettsia quintana*. It takes its name from the trenches of World War I, when it was first described and was a major problem. It was reported again in Eastern Europe during World War II. Trench fever has been reported from Europe, Africa, Mexico, and Central and South America but is an uncommon disease today (Chapter 68).

Lice become infected with *R. quintana* when taking a blood meal from an infected person. The rickettsiae do not enter the midgut epithelial cells but rather multiply in the lumen of the louse intestine. As a result, this infection is not fatal to the lice. Like epidemic typhus, however, transmission to humans is via infected louse feces, with the rickettsiae entering the body through abrasions in the skin or mucous membranes or by inhalation.

Epidemic (Louse-Borne) Relapsing Fever. Epidemic, or louse-borne, relapsing fever is caused by a spirochete, *Borrelia recurrentis* (Chapter 71). Various other species of *Borrelia* are associated with certain species of soft ticks that cause endemic, or tick-borne, relapsing fever. It is likely that *B. recurrentis* originated from one of the tick-borne strains of *Borrelia*, because some of these can also infect and be transmitted by lice.

Relapsing fever has been known clinically since the days of Hippocrates, who called it *ardent fever*. It has a worldwide distribution in its various forms, but *B. recurrentis*, once widespread, now appears to be limited primarily to East Africa.

Transmission of epidemic relapsing fever is strictly by a human-louse-human cycle. Lice become infected by taking a blood meal from an infected person. The spirochetes enter the hemocoele of the louse and multiply there instead of in the intestine. Transmission occurs only when an infected louse is crushed, releasing infective spirochetes, which may then enter the human host via skin abrasions or mucous membranes. In some areas, lice are frequently crushed with the teeth, resulting in transmission. The louse feces are not infective. Because *B. recurrentis* can be transmitted only by crushing infected lice, large louse populations are required before epidemic transmission can occur.

There has been considerable discussion in the popular press about insect transmission of HIV, including speculation about lice. Although no field or experimental work has implicated lice in transmission, lice have biologic and behavioral characteristics that would allow transmission either mechanically or biologically.

BUGS (ORDER HEMIPTERA). Members of the order Hemiptera are the true bugs and are recognized by the characteristic forewing, the basal half of which is membranous. The mouthparts are of the piercing-sucking type and are segmented. The proboscis is attached anteriorly and is kept folded back between the coxae of the first pair of legs. The life cycle is simple, with all instars requiring a meal of blood, hemolymph, or plant juices, depending on whether the species is hematophagous, predaceous on other insects, or phytophagous. Medically important bugs belong to two families in the order Hemiptera. These are the families Cimicidae (bedbugs) and Reduviidae (triatome bugs).

Family Cimicidae (Bedbugs)
Biology. Of the many species of bedbugs that are obligate ectoparasites primarily of birds, poultry, and bats, only two are parasites of humans. These are *Cimex lectularius*, the common bedbug, and *C. hemipterus*, the tropical bedbug (Fig. 138–1; Fig. 139–10). The former has a cosmopolitan distribution but is more common in temperate regions, whereas the latter has a wide distribution in the tropics.

Disease Transmission. Bedbugs meet all the criteria for human disease transmission: They are obligate bloodsucking parasites that have close and frequent contact with humans. They are most commonly found in beds in hotels and lounge chairs in public places, e.g., transportation terminals, where they have contact with many different hosts. Experimentally, they become infected with various pathogens, but to date, they have not been incriminated in transmission of any human disease. Work has shown that the swallow bug, *Oeciacus vicarius*, is a vector of Fort Morgan virus in swallows in the western United States. Mechanical transmission of hepatitis B virus by *C. lectularius* has been demonstrated experimentally. Considering the epidemiology of hepatitis B virus in the tropics, the stability of the virus outside the host, the high viremia levels associated with this infection in humans, and the biting habits of bedbugs, it is possible that bedbugs have a role as mechanical vectors of this virus. The bedbug has been considered as a possible vector of HIV. Experimental studies, however, have shown that HIV does not replicate in bedbug tissues and that mechanical transmission is unlikely. Moreover, HIV has not been detected in the feces of bedbugs, making it unlikely that transmission could occur by scratching fecal material into the bite wound.

Family Reduviidae (Triatomine Bugs)
Biology. The family Reduviidae consists of a large number of species that are primarily entomophagous and thus feed on other insects (assassin bugs). One predominantly Ameri-

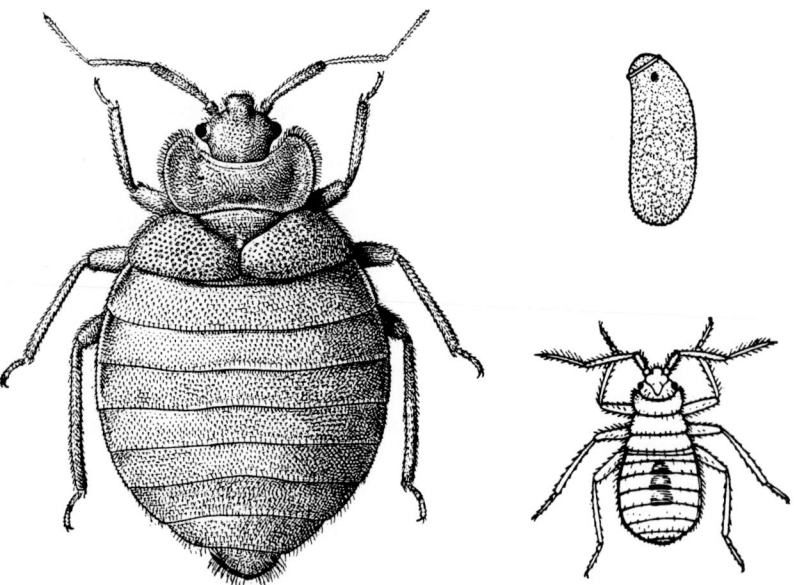

Figure **138-1.** The bedbug. *Cimex lectularius*—egg, nymph, and adult. (Courtesy of the Wellcome Foundation.)

can subfamily, Triatominae, feeds only on the blood of various vertebrate animals, including humans.

Triatomine bugs are relatively large (1 to 4 cm) and can be recognized by the elongate, cylindric, or cone-shaped head bearing a pair of long, four-segment antennae situated apically and bulging compound eyes situated laterally (Fig. 139–9). The proboscis, consisting of three-segment mouthparts, is carried flexed beneath the head, projecting posteriorly when at rest but projecting forward when feeding.

Most species of triatome bugs are sylvatic and live in close association with various wild animals such as armadillos, opossums, mice, rats, bats, and squirrels. Others live in close association with humans and their domestic animals. The bugs usually lay their eggs in or near the habitation of the host. The eggs hatch in 10 to 30 days, depending on the temperature and species. The life cycle is incomplete, with five nymphal instars, each requiring a blood meal before molting occurs. There is usually only one generation per year. Overwintering can occur in any stage, depending on the species. The adults can fly considerable distances in search of new hosts. The nymphs cannot fly.

Disease Transmission

CHAGAS DISEASE (AMERICAN TRYPANOSOMIASIS). The etiologic agent of Chagas disease is the protozoan *Trypanosoma cruzi*. This is a disease only of the American tropics and subtropics, with a wide distribution in South and Central America. It occurs sporadically in the southwestern United States (Chapter 94).

The bugs become infected with *T. cruzi* when they take a blood meal from a person or from a reservoir host with parasitemia. They may also become infected by cannibalism. The trypanosomes remain in the gut of the bugs and develop into infective metacyclic forms in 7 to 14 days. The infective trypanosomes are located in the hindgut and are passed in the feces. Transmission is usually associated with the bite of the bug, which often takes 10 to 20 minutes to engorge and frequently defecates during or shortly after the feeding process. Infection of the new host is usually accomplished by scratching the infective trypanosomes passed in the feces into the bite wound or into other skin abrasions or, most commonly, by transferring the agents on fingers to the highly receptive conjunctiva of the eye or to the mucosa of the mouth or nose.

Many species of triatomine bugs are susceptible to infection by *T. cruzi*, and more than half of these species from the Americas have been found naturally infected. However, relatively few species are associated with humans and their domestic animals, an essential condition for efficient transmission of this parasite. Those bugs known to be vectors of human infection are listed in Table 138–3.

Factors that influence the evolution of domesticity on the part of triatome bugs include physiologic and ecologic adaptability of the insects, availability of alternate hosts (domestic animals), climate, and location and type of construction of houses. The last is important, because the bugs are nocturnal and seek out cracks and crevices for hiding in during the day. The triatomes that are most highly domesticated are associated with poorly constructed houses that provide daytime resting places.

Trypanosoma rangeli infection: *Trypanosoma rangeli* is another parasite of humans and other mammals transmitted by triatome bugs. Because it is often found in the same areas as *T. cruzi* and has a similar morphology in both human and insect stages, it may cause some confusion. However, it is apparently nonpathogenic to humans (Chapter 94.1). *Rhodnius prolixus* is the most important vector of *T. rangeli*, but unlike the case with *T. cruzi*, development in the insect occurs in the hemolymph after a period in the gut. The infective trypomastigotes eventually invade the salivary glands, and transmission occurs through the bite of the triatome.

TABLE 138–3. Important Species of Triatome Vectors of American Trypanosomiasis

Species	Geographic Distribution
Panstrongylus megistus	Brazil
Rhodnius prolixus	Venezuela, Colombia, Central America
R. pallescens	Panama
Triatoma maculata	Venezuela, Colombia
T. infestans	Southern Brazil, Uruguay, Chile, Paraguay, Argentina, Bolivia
T. dimidiata	Central America, Mexico
T. barberi	Mexico

FLIES (ORDER DIPTERA)

Biology. The flies constitute the largest and single most important group of insects that cause or transmit human disease. They make up the order Diptera, which is characterized by having only one pair of wings instead of two like most other insects. The second pair of wings are called *halters*, small knoblike structures situated behind the functional wings and used for stability during flight. Most species have large compound eyes and three simple eyes, or ocelli, arranged in a triangular formation at the top of the head. Mouthparts are always of the sucking type, having undergone considerable evolution in the bloodsucking or hematophagous groups, with stylets used for piercing or lacerating the flesh of animals.

All Diptera undergo a complete metamorphosis with egg, larval, pupal, and adult stages. Eggs, depending on the species, are laid in various places, including all types of water, decaying vegetation, soil, feces, and both dead and live animal tissues. The term *myiasis* is given to the invasion of human and animal tissues by fly larvae (Chapter 128.2).

Systematics. The most commonly used classification divides the Diptera into three suborders (Table 138–4). The Nematocera are the most primitive and are most important medically. This suborder includes the midges, gnats, sandflies, black flies, and mosquitoes; all members are characterized by a simple filamentous type of antennae, represented by the Culicidae in Figure 138–2. Only the females of Nematocera are hematophagous; the males feed on nectars and other plant juices. The suborder Brachycera generally comprises large flies and includes the medically important horseflies and deer flies (family Tabanidae). This suborder is characterized by shorter three-segment antennae, the last segment of which is largest and may be annulated (Fig. 138–2). The last suborder, Cyclorrhapha, includes the higher Diptera. Members of this suborder are generally what most laypersons consider to be flies and include houseflies, stable flies, blowflies, and tsetse flies. They are characterized by having short three-segment antennae, the last segment of which bears a bristle called the *arista*, as represented by the Muscidae in Figure 138–2. The larvae of Cyclorrhapha are headless, usually having a pair of mouth hooks in the place of the head.

Suborder Nematocera
Family Ceratopogonidae (Biting Midges)

Biology. The biting midges are among the smallest hematophagous flies (Fig. 139–16). There are approximately 50 genera of Ceratopogonidae, of which only 4—*Culicoides, Forcipomyia, Leptoconops,* and *Austroconops*—feed on humans and other vertebrates and are therefore of medical importance.

TABLE 138–4. Taxonomic Subdivisions of Medically Important Diptera

Suborder	Family	Common Name
Nematocera	Ceratopogonidae	Biting midges, gnats
	Psychodidae	Sandflies
	Simuliidae	Black flies
	Culicidae	Mosquitoes
Brachycera	Tabanidae	Horseflies, deer flies
	Rhagionidae	Snipe flies
	Athericidae	Athericids
Cyclorrhapha	Glossinidae	Tsetse flies
	Muscidae	Houseflies, stable flies, face flies
	Calliphoridae	Blowflies
	Sarcophagidae	Blowflies
	Chloropidae	Eye gnats

ANTENNAE OF DIPTERA

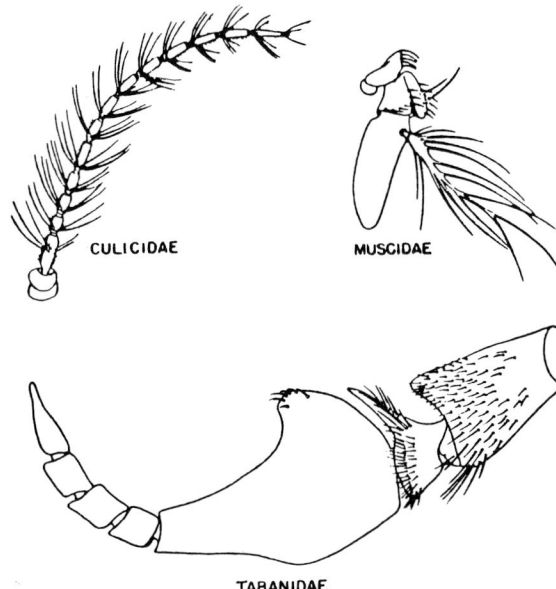

Figure 138–2. Types of antennae of the suborders of Diptera: Nematocera (Culicidae), Brachycera (Tabanidae), and Cyclorrhapha (Muscidae).

Culicoides is by far the most important genus and is the only one incriminated in disease transmission to humans.

Ceratopogonids have worldwide distribution, with >800 species described. Most species lay their eggs in batches in mud, wet soil, decaying leaves or other vegetation, manure, rotting banana tree stumps, or similar sites. The eggs usually hatch within a week or 10 days. The larvae, which may be aquatic or terrestrial, develop to the pupal stage in 2 to 3 weeks, feeding on a variety of decaying organic debris. There are four larval instars. The pupal stage usually lasts 3 to 4 days but may last as long as 10 days. In temperate regions, ceratopogonids may overwinter in the egg or larval stages, depending on the species.

The adults feed on plant juices and nectars, and females also require blood. They frequently occur in swarms, biting around the head and other unprotected parts of the body. The blood-feeding periodicity varies with the species. Many feed throughout the day, some feed in the early evening and night, and others feed primarily during early morning hours. Most species are exophilic and are not strong fliers, and adults remain within the vicinity of the breeding sites.

Disease Transmission. Ceratopogonidae are generally not important vectors of human disease. Although they are vectors of various animal filariae, protozoa, and arboviruses, few of these are pathogens of humans.

VIRUSES. Ceratopogonids are documented vectors of arboviruses of animals such as blue tongue. A total of 34 viruses have been isolated from *Culicoides* sp. Oropouche virus is a cause of febrile illness in Brazil and other South American countries, with periodic epidemics occurring primarily in the Amazon region and as far north as Panama (Chapter 29.9). This virus apparently exists in a sylvatic cycle with primates and sloths as the vertebrate hosts. The sylvatic vector is unknown. Epidemiologic evidence collected during epidemic investigations suggested that *Culicoides paraensis* was involved in urban transmission of this virus. Successful experimental transmission of Oropouche virus by this species has now been documented.

FILARIAL INFECTIONS. Flies of the genus *Culicoides* are the principal vectors of three filarial parasites of humans. *Mansonella ozzardi* occurs in Central and South America and some Caribbean islands (Chapter 109.1). The principal vector is *C. furens*. Filariae that are indistinguishable from *M. ozzardi* have also been described from *Simulium* (black flies) in Africa. *Mansonella perstans* is a common filarial parasite of humans in tropical Africa and certain countries of South America (Chapter 109.2). It is transmitted by *C. grahami* and *C. milnei* (*austeni*) in Africa and by other *Culicoides* species in the Americas. A third filarial parasite, *Mansonella streptocerca*, occurs primarily in West and Central Africa and is also transmitted by *C. grahami* and *C. milnei* (Chapter 109.3).

All three of the aforementioned filarial parasites are generally considered nonpathogenic to their human hosts. They are essentially nonperiodic, with the microfilariae present in the peripheral blood at all times of the day. Microfilariae ingested with the blood meal invade the thoracic muscles of the fly and undergo two molts to become active third-stage larvae in 10 to 12 days. These infective larvae eventually migrate to the head and are deposited on the skin of humans when the midge takes a subsequent blood meal.

Family Psychodidae (Sandflies)

Biology. The family Psychodidae contains one major subfamily, Phlebotominae, which is important in human disease transmission (Fig. 139–7). There are >600 species in the subfamily, but most of the important vectors of human pathogens belong to three genera. *Phlebotomus* is an Old World genus containing many important vectors of leishmaniasis and the phlebotomus fever group of viruses. *Sergentomyia* is also an Old World genus but is less important in the transmission of human disease. The genus *Lutzomyia* is found only in the Western Hemisphere.

Phlebotomine sandflies lay their eggs in small batches in protected places with high humidity and a high content of organic matter. Examples are cracks in walls, rodent burrows, tree buttresses, and under dead leaves on the forest floor. Depending on the temperature, the eggs hatch in 6 to 17 days or longer. The larvae are scavengers and feed on various organic matter. There are four instars, and larval development may last 3 to 6 weeks. The pupal stage may last another 8 to 10 days, and the entire life cycle requires from 5 to 12 weeks. In temperate regions, the flies overwinter in the larval stage.

Only females suck blood, which is taken from various vertebrate animals, including amphibians, reptiles, and mammals. The genera *Phlebotomus* and *Lutzomyia* most commonly feed on humans. Most species are nocturnal feeders, but some may feed during the day in dark rooms or in forests on dark days. Phlebotomine sandflies are weak fliers; they rarely fly more than a few meters from their breeding sites. Most fly in short hopping motions and can be repelled with the use of a good fan.

Disease Transmission. Phlebotomine sandflies are important vectors of *Leishmania*, the phlebotomous fever group of arboviruses, and bartonellosis.

LEISHMANIASIS. Leishmaniasis is a disease of humans caused by species of *Leishmania* that are natural parasites of various animals, both wild and domestic. The type of disease, parasite, geographic distribution, reservoir hosts, and principal phlebotomine sandfly vectors are presented in Table 95–1. Leishmaniasis is primarily a zoonosis, although in some areas of the world (e.g., India) there is no known animal reservoir host and the parasite is thought to exist in a human-sandfly-human cycle.

The principal mode of transmission of leishmaniasis is by the bite of infective sandflies. The amastigote stage of *Leishmania* is found in macrophages of the host and is ingested when the sandfly takes a blood meal. The amastigotes are released from the cells into the lumen of the sandfly gut, where they elongate and become promastigotes, which then multiply in the insect intestine by asexual reproduction. These infective promastigotes eventually move forward to the esophagus and mouth parts of the sandfly and are injected into a new host when a subsequent blood meal is taken. The injected promastigotes are then phagocytized by macrophages of the new human host. The salivary glands of sandflies are not involved in the transmission of leishmaniasis.

SANDFLY FEVER. Sandfly fever (phlebotomus or pappataci fever) is caused by arboviruses belonging to the genus *Phlebovirus*, family Bunyaviridae (Chapter 29.11). Natural hosts for these viruses probably include various rodents and wild animals, but seven viruses have been isolated from humans or have been implicated in causing disease in humans. These include SF-Naples and SF-Sicily, the original sandfly fever viruses that are transmitted by phlebotomine sandflies. Two other viruses, Chagres and Punta Toro, have been isolated from both humans and sandflies in Panama and are probably arboviruses. A fifth member of this virus group has been isolated in Brazil from persons with an illness compatible with sandfly fever, but the vector is not known.

SF-Naples and SF-Sicily viruses are the most widespread; isolation records suggest that they are endemic around the Mediterranean, the Middle East, central Asia, and the Indian subcontinent, in arid areas that have suitable breeding habitats for phlebotomine sandflies. The disease is generally mild in endemic areas. Epidemics usually occur only when a large population of susceptible individuals, such as an army, moves into the endemic area. Transmission generally occurs during the spring and summer months in the northern latitudes. *Phlebotomus papatasi* is the principal vector in most endemic areas, although the Naples virus has also been isolated from flies of the genus *Sergentomyia*. The sandflies become infected while taking a blood meal from a viremic animal or person, usually in the first 4 days of illness. The extrinsic incubation period is as short as 7 days but usually is 10 to 14 days, depending on the temperature.

The viruses have been isolated from male sandflies of the genera *Phlebotomus* and *Sergentomyia* that were collected in endemic areas. This, plus experimental evidence, suggests the viruses are transmitted transovarially from the female fly to her offspring, thus making the flies reservoir hosts. Epidemiologic evidence supports this mechanism as important in the maintenance of the viruses in nature.

The phlebotomine sandflies also are important vectors of other arboviruses in Central and South America. Six viruses of the Changuinola group (family Reoviridae, genus Orbivirus) have been isolated from sandflies, and one of these, Changuinola, has also been isolated from humans. Serologic evidence suggests that some of the other viruses of this group also infect humans, although associated illness is not known. A total of 42 viruses belonging to 7 antigenic groups have been isolated from phlebotomine sandflies.

BARTONELLOSIS. Bartonellosis (Chapter 60.1) is caused by the bacterium *Bartonella bacilliformis* and is a disease of humans in the mountainous areas of Peru, Ecuador, and Colombia. The disease has two forms—the highly fatal visceral form known as *Oroya fever* and the milder cutaneous form known as *verruga peruana*. There are no other known hosts of this bacterium, and because it can be isolated from asymptomatic individuals, humans are the likely reservoir host.

Bartonellosis is transmitted by sandflies of the genus *Lutzomyia*. *L. verrucarum* is the principal vector throughout its geographic range. Other species are also probably involved, but the mechanism of transmission has not been well studied.

The bacteria are associated with the red blood cells of the host and are ingested when the fly takes a blood meal. It is not known whether multiplication occurs in the fly or whether transmission occurs as a result of proboscis contamination.

Family Simuliidae (Black Flies)

Biology. The Simuliidae are small, stout-bodied, humped-back flies, and >1300 species have been described worldwide (Fig. 139–15). They are fierce biters and, in addition to disease transmission, are important as pests in many areas of the world, especially in temperate regions, where they occur in large swarms (Chapter 128.2).

The breeding habitat of all known species is flowing water, usually a river or stream. Fast-flowing white water is preferred by many species, whereas others prefer slow-moving water. In either case, female flies deposit masses of eggs just below the water line on objects protruding from the water. Female flies are frequently attracted to small sections of the stream for oviposition, resulting in a concentration of large numbers of larvae in a small area. The eggs hatch within a few days, and larvae attach to objects in the water by means of a posterior sucker. There are six to eight larval instars, which may last 7 to 14 days. Pupation takes 2 to 6 days, and adults emerge to the water surface in protective bubbles of gas.

Adults are strong fliers and may travel considerable distances from the breeding site in search of a blood meal. Only the female fly feeds on blood, and most species are zoophilic. Of the 12 or more genera described, only 3 are important in human disease transmission, mainly because of their human-biting habits. These are *Simulium*, *Prosimulium*, and *Austrosimulium*, the first being the most important.

Disease Transmission. The black flies are important vectors of only one major human disease, onchocerciasis, but are also important vectors of both protozoan and filarial infections of animals. In addition, they are important pest insects over much of their geographic range.

ONCHOCERCIASIS. Onchocerciasis, or river blindness, is caused by the filarial worm *Onchocerca volvulus* and is characterized by three cardinal features: subcutaneous nodules containing adult worms, pruritic dermatitis, and blindness. It occurs in tropical Africa and in South and Central America and affects an estimated 40 million people. In some savanna areas of West Africa, blindness due to onchocerciasis affects the majority of older adults in entire villages.

The adult worms live in the skin and subcutaneous tissue of humans. They produce microfilariae that migrate throughout the body, primarily in the skin. Black flies, being pool feeders, tear or cut the skin of the host to rupture the blood vessels. Microfilariae are ingested with the blood meal, penetrate the gut wall, and migrate to the thoracic muscles (Fig. 108–5). They enter the muscle cells and develop to third-stage infective larvae over 7 to 14 days. The infective larvae break out of the muscle cells, migrate to the head and proboscis of the fly, and escape onto the skin when a subsequent blood meal is taken. They enter the human host, generally through the bite wound, and develop to the adult stage.

The localization of the subcutaneous nodules (onchocercomas) containing adult worms varies with geographic region and with the species of black fly vector. In Africa, where members of the *Simulium damnosum* complex are the principal vectors (Fig. 108–3), nodules are localized in the lower parts of the body, primarily around the pelvis and, occasionally, on the lower legs. In Venezuela, the onchocercomas are also located on the lower part of the body. Both *S. metallicum*, the principal vector in Venezuela, and *S. damnosun* prefer to feed on the lower part of the body. In Central America, however, nodules are primarily on the upper part of the

body, and the principal vector, *S. ochraceum*, also feeds on the upper part of the body. This species breeds in streams at relatively high altitudes (1000 to 1500 m), and persons there (e.g., coffee plantation workers) generally are well covered, in contrast to people in Africa, who usually wear less clothing.

Table 138–5 lists the major black fly vector species and their distribution. The *S. damnosum* complex now consists of nine sibling species, the distribution of which closely coincides with the distribution of onchocerciasis in West and Central Africa. The *S. neavei* group has nine species, but only three—*S. neavei*, *S. woodi*, and *S. ethiopiense*—are important vectors. *S. neavei* and *S. woodi* have an interesting biology in that they have an obligatory phoretic relationship with river crabs, with the larvae and pupae completing development while attached to the crabs.

Family Culicidae (Mosquitoes).

Mosquitoes are by far the most important group of insects in terms of human disease transmission; more people die each year of mosquito-borne diseases than of any other single cause. There are >3000 described species in 34 genera, but only relatively few are important in disease transmission. The most important genera, *Aedes*, *Culex*, and *Anopheles*, contain vector species for viruses, protozoa, and filariae of humans. Diseases transmitted by mosquitoes occur worldwide and affect hundreds of millions of people each year.

Biology. Mosquitoes belong to the family Culicidae, suborder Nematocera. Taxonomically, the family is broken into three subfamilies: Toxorhynchitinae, large non–blood-feeding mosquitoes; Anophelinae, the anopheline mosquitoes that transmit malaria (Fig. 139–4); and Culicinae, by far the largest subfamily, with 30 genera (Fig. 139–6).

Most mosquitoes are small and slender (Fig. 138–3) and may vary in color from drab brown to black and white to metallic colors. They inhabit nearly every part of the globe, being limited only by the availability of breeding sites. All species are aquatic in the larval stage. Some breed in tundra or alpine pools, others in collections of water in desert areas, and still others in nearly all conceivable natural and artificial

TABLE 138–5. Principal Onchocerciasis Vectors and Their Geographic Distribution

Species	Geographic Distribution
***Simulium damnosum* Group**	
S. damnosum	Widespread in West, Central, East, and South Africa
S. sirbanum	Mali, Ivory Coast, Guinea, Burkina Faso, Ghana, Nigeria
S. sudanense	Mali, Ivory Coast, Guinea, Burkina Faso, Ghana, Nigeria
S. squamosum	Cameroon, Burkina Faso, Ivory Coast
S. soubrense	Benin, Guinea, Ivory Coast, Liberia
S. sanctipauli	Ivory Coast, Liberia
S. yahense	Guinea, Ivory Coast, Liberia
S. kilibanum	Burundi, The Congo, Tanzania, Uganda
S. dieguerense	Mali
***Simulium neavei* Group**	
S. neavei	Angola, The Congo, Uganda, Kenya
S. woodi	Malawi, Tanzania
S. ethiopiense	Ethiopia
S. ochraceum	Bolivia, Colombia, Ecuador, Guatemala, southern Mexico, Panama
S. metallicum	Widespread in Central, North, and South America
S. callidum	Colombia, Guatemala, Mexico
S. exiguum	Colombia, Ecuador, Venezuela
S. gulanense	Venezuela, Brazil

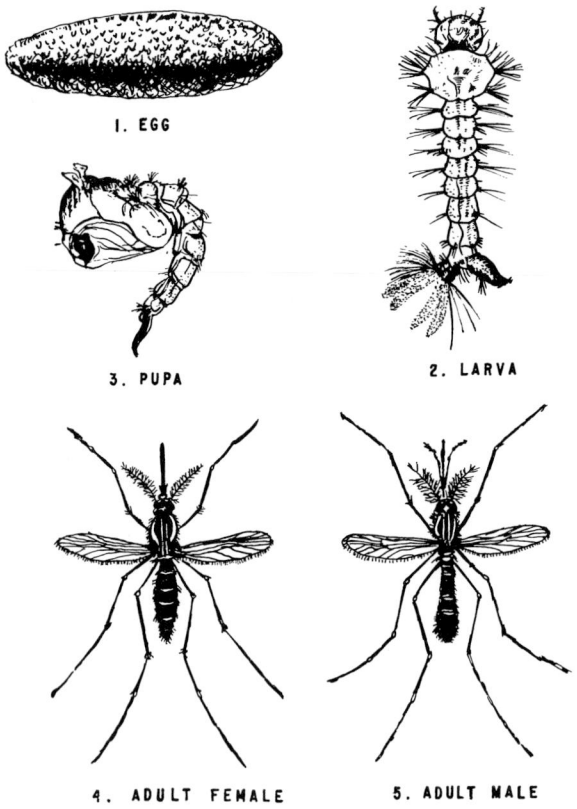

I. EGG

3. PUPA

2. LARVA

4. ADULT FEMALE

5. ADULT MALE

Figure 138–3. The yellow fever mosquito, *Aedes aegypti*.

containers holding water in between these two environmental extremes.

The majority of adult female mosquitoes are obligate bloodsuckers, requiring blood to develop their eggs. Both sexes feed on plant juices and nectars. Some species have evolved the capability of developing the first batch of eggs without a blood meal (autogenous development), an obviously advantageous survival mechanism. Animals that provide blood for mosquitoes include all major groups (e.g., fish, amphibians, reptiles, birds, and mammals). Many species of mosquitoes have evolved strict host requirements and feed only on a certain group of animals. Others have broader host ranges and feed on various animals, including humans. Those that feed exclusively on animals are called *zoophilic*, whereas those that prefer to feed on humans are called *anthropophilic*. The degree of anthropophilic behavior in zoophilic species is a major factor in human disease transmission because it allows for the transfer of animal diseases to humans (zoonoses).

After an adult female has taken a blood meal, eggs begin to develop, and within 3 to 7 days she seeks an oviposition site, which is generally quite specific to the species. Eggs, laid individually or in batches, may be deposited directly on the water, just above the water line, or in damp soil on a flood plain. Hatching usually occurs in 24 to 72 hours after contact with water, and first-stage larvae emerge. There are four larval stages, with the larvae feeding on various microorganisms in the water. Pupation occurs in 5 to 14 or more days, and the adults emerge 2 to 5 days later, depending on the species and environmental conditions. The newly emerged adults usually mate and begin to feed. If hosts are available, most female mosquitoes take their first blood meal within 1 to 4 days of emergence. Adult mosquitoes have survived in the laboratory for >4 months, but in nature, they

are generally short lived, with the majority not surviving the 10- to 14-day extrinsic incubation period required for transmission of most pathogens. Survival obviously depends on the species and environmental conditions.

In temperate regions, mosquitoes overwinter in the egg, larval, or adult stage, depending on the species. Depending on the location, there may be one generation per year (tundra) or a new generation every 10 to 14 days (tropics). In temperate regions, the cycle usually continues as soon as the ice melts; adult blood-feeding mosquitoes are usually present from about March to October. In the tropics, mosquitoes are present year round, but in some areas where the dry season is extended, mosquitoes may estivate as adults or in the egg stage.

Disease Transmission

VIRUSES. At least 262 viruses have been isolated from mosquitoes, mostly from culicines. Of these, 73 have also been isolated from humans, and serologic evidence shows that many more infect humans in nature. Most of these viruses are natural pathogens of other animals. Humans usually become involved in the transmission cycle accidentally and are a dead-end host for most of these viruses. Nevertheless, they can cause serious illnesses when people become infected.

A few viruses cause serious endemic and epidemic disease in humans, primarily because the mosquito vectors are closely associated with the domestic habitats. Table 138–6 lists the most important mosquito-borne viral diseases of humans, their distribution, and the principal vectors.

Alphaviruses: Chikungunya virus is one of the most widespread and one of the most important alphaviruses in terms of human health (Chapter 29.3). This virus, first described in Africa, probably exists there in a mosquito-primate-mosquito cycle involving forest mosquitoes. Humans are also susceptible and may carry the virus back to the village, where a human–*Ae. aegypti*–human transmission cycle may exist. The virus is endemic and widespread in the large urban areas of Asia, where it exists in this type of cycle. Transmission may periodically occur in epidemic form.

Another alphavirus, Ross River virus, which may eventually have a similar epidemiology, causes a disease known as *epidemic polyarthritis* in humans and has been limited to the Australia–New Guinea area (Chapter 29.6). This virus has been known clinically for > 50 years in Australia but was not isolated until 1963 and then only from mosquito pools. The mosquito vectors were *Culex annulirostris* and *Aedes vigilax*. Although many attempts were made, only a single isolate was made from human serum, leading to speculation that the polyarthritis was caused by virus-antibody complexes and that humans generally had low viremia. In 1979 and 1980, major epidemics of polyarthritis occurred on several South Pacific islands. During these epidemics, it was shown that humans did have viremia high enough to infect mosquitoes, and epidemiologic and experimental evidence suggested that *Stegomyia* mosquitoes, especially *Ae. polynesiensis*, *Ae. albopictus*, and *Ae. aegypti*, were efficient vectors of the virus. Furthermore, it has been demonstrated by Australian workers that *Ae. vigilax* can experimentally transmit Ross River virus transovarially. With these new developments and with increased air travel by people, epidemic polyarthritis may move west into Asia and east into the Caribbean and Central and South America.

Other alphaviruses have more complex cycles involving several mosquito species as vectors and both avian and mammalian reservoir hosts. Examples are the equine encephalitis viruses in North and South America (Table 138–6; see Fig. 30–7). The cycle of western equine encephalitis (Fig. 138–4) is an example. The virus is maintained with spring and

TABLE 138–6. Important Mosquito-Borne Viral Diseases of Humans and Known Vectors

Virus	Geographic Distribution	Vectors
Alphaviruses		
Chikungunya	Africa, Asia	*Aedes aegypti*, other *Aedes* species
Eastern equine encephalitis	North America, South America	*Culiseta melanura* *Aedes taeniorhynchus* *Aedes sollicitans*
O'nyong-nyong	Africa	*Anopheles funestus* *Anopheles gambiae* *Mansonia* spp
Ross River	Australasia, Pacific Islands	*Culex annulirostris* *Aedes vigilax* *Aedes polynesiensis* *Aedes aegypti*
Sindbis	Africa, Asia, Australasia, Europe	*Culex univittatus* *Culex tritaeniorhynchus*
Venezuelan equine encephalitis	North and South America	*Culex melanacom* species *Psorophora confinnis*
Western equine encephalitis	North and South America	*Culex tarsalis* *Aedes* species
Flaviviruses		
Japanese encephalitis	Asia, New Guinea	*Culex tritaeniorhynchus* group, *Culex annulirostris* *Culex annulus*
Murray Valley encephalitis	Australia, New Guinea	*Culex annulirostris* *Culex bitaeniorhynchus*
Rocio	South America	*Aedes scapularis*
St. Louis encephalitis	North and South America	*Culex pipiens* complex *Culex tarsalis* *Culex nigripalpus* *Culex restuans* *Culex salinarius*
West Nile	Africa, Asia, Europe	*Culex univittatus* *Culex pipiens* complex *Culex vishnui* subgroup
Dengue	Tropicopolitan	*Aedes aegypti* *Aedes albopictus* *Aedes polynesiensis* *Aedes hensilli* *Aedes scutellaris* complex
Yellow fever	Africa	*Aedes aegypti* *Aedes africanus* *Aedes simpsoni* *Aedes furcifer-taylori*
	Americas	*Aedes aegypti* *Haemagogus janthinomys* *Haemagogus spegazzinii* *Haemagogus leucocelaenus* *Sabethes chloropterus*
Zika	Africa, Asia	*Aedes aegypti* *Aedes africanus*
Bunyaviruses		
La Crosse	North America	*Aedes triseriatus*
Tahyna	Africa, Asia, Europe	*Aedes vexans*
Oropouche	South America	*Culex* species
Phleboviruses		
Rift Valley fever	Africa	*Culex pipiens* complex *Aedes* species

summer amplification in a *Culex tarsalis*–nestling and juvenile bird–*Cx. tarsalis* cycle in the western United States. For reasons that are not fully understood, epidemic Western equine encephalitis occurs, and humans and horses may occasionally become involved. However, both are dead-end hosts that

contribute nothing to the maintenance cycle of the virus. The overwintering mechanism is not known but possibly involves migrating birds, persistence of the virus in overwintering mosquitoes, or even transovarial transmission, which has recently been demonstrated.

Flaviviruses: Flaviviruses are considerably more important to human health than any other group of arboviruses. The most important include dengue, yellow fever, and Japanese encephalitis (JE) viruses. All have a wide distribution and are transmitted by species of mosquitoes that may have close human contact.

Dengue fever: Dengue fever is an acute infection characterized by sudden onset of fever and various nonspecific symptoms in its classic form (Chapter 29.1). These viruses also have the potential to cause severe and fatal disease in humans, and large epidemics of dengue hemorrhagic fever (DHF) are common in Asia. This form of disease primarily affects younger age groups and is one of the ten leading causes of hospitalization and death among children in Southeast Asia. Epidemic dengue, often associated with hemorrhagic disease, has also become a major health problem in the South and Central Pacific and the Caribbean Islands, South and Central America, Africa, and the Middle East.

There are four serotypes of dengue viruses, all closely related antigenically. The viruses have a tropicopolitan distribution that is closely linked to the distribution of the principal vector, *Ae. aegypti*. Today, more people (approximately 2.5 billion) are at risk for dengue virus infection than for any other arbovirus infection. Each year there are 50 to 100 million cases of dengue fever and >500,000 cases of DHF that occur on a global basis. The average case-fatality rate of DHF is about 5%.

The viruses probably originated in the jungles of the Malay Peninsula and/or in Africa. In Malaysia, they exist in a mosquito-monkey-mosquito cycle involving species of the *Ae. niveus* complex of mosquitoes and leaf monkeys. Evidence obtained by French workers suggests that a similar cycle exists in Africa. The importance of these jungle maintenance cycles to human health is not considered great, because all four dengue serotypes coexist in most of the large urban centers of the tropics in an *Ae. aegypti*–human–*Ae. aegypti* cycle. In rural and some urban areas of Asia and the Pacific, two other *Stegomyia* species, *Ae. albopictus* and *Ae. polynesiensis*, are important vectors. Vertical transmission of these viruses has been demonstrated in all three species of mosquito, with the domestic *Ae. aegypti* being least efficient. Mosquitoes become infected with dengue virus by feeding on a viremic human host and, depending on the species and strain of mosquito, the strain of virus, and environmental

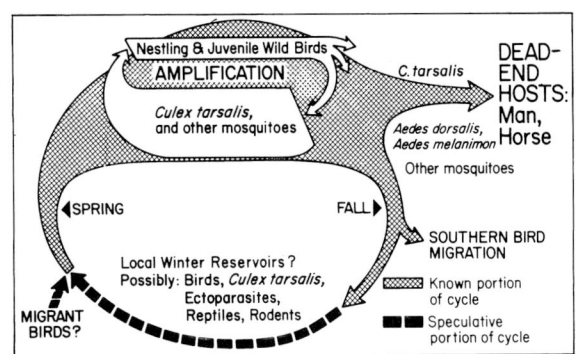

Figure 138–4. Maintenance cycle of western equine encephalitis virus in the western United States. (Courtesy of the Centers for Disease Control and Prevention.)

factors, can transmit the virus to a new host after an extrinsic incubation period of about 10 to 14 days.

Studies have shown that not all geographic strains of *Ae. aegypti* or *Ae. albopictus* are efficient vectors of dengue viruses. Some strains are refractory to oral infection with dengue viruses, a trait that is genetically controlled. Other work has shown variation among strains of dengue viruses in their epidemic potential. This variation among different strains of mosquito and dengue viruses could help explain why some areas or cities that appear to be permissive to dengue virus transmission do not have large epidemics of either dengue fever or DHF, whereas others do.

Yellow fever: Yellow fever is a flavivirus that is closely related to the dengue viruses ecologically, antigenically, and clinically. Antigenically, there is considerable cross reaction between dengue and yellow fever viruses, although there is not complete cross-protective immunity. Clinically, yellow fever is characterized by sudden onset of fever and various nonspecific symptoms similar to those of dengue fever. This may be followed by a more severe disease involving jaundice, hemorrhagic manifestations, and death (Chapter 31.1).

The virus is maintained in the jungles of Africa and South America in mosquito-monkey-mosquito cycles. In Africa, species of cercopithecoid monkeys are the vertebrate hosts, and transmission is generally by forest canopy mosquitoes, *Ae. africanus* and *Ae. furcifer-taylori*. Vertical and transstadial transmission of yellow fever virus occurs in both forest species and in *Ae. aegypti* (Fig. 139–5). This may be an even more important maintenance mechanism during long dry periods.

In Africa, humans can become infected with jungle yellow fever in two ways: Infected canopy-dwelling mosquitoes may transmit the virus to people when they are working in the jungle (Fig. 135–2). These workers may not get sick until they are back in the village or city where *Ae. aegypti* is present. Probably, a more common way yellow fever gets out of the jungle is by the monkeys themselves. They may frequent banana groves where another mosquito breeds in the banana leaf axils. These mosquitoes feed on the monkeys when they raid the banana plantations and can subsequently transmit the virus to humans when they visit the plantation to harvest bananas and work.

In South America, a similar cycle involves forest monkeys and canopy mosquitoes belonging to the genus *Haemagogus*. Forest workers may be infected as in Africa and carry the virus back to the village or city where *Ae. aegypti* is present. In both Africa and the Americas, major urban epidemics may be transmitted by *Ae. aegypti*.

Yellow fever virus is found only in Africa, where it probably originated, and in South America, where it was most likely introduced with the slave trade in the 1600s. The virus has never been documented in Asia and the Pacific, where *Ae. aegypti* is widespread and abundant. The reason for this lack of spread is not known but is probably the high prevalence of heterotypic flavivirus antibody from other closely related viruses, e.g., dengue, JE, and West Nile viruses. Although not cross protective, heterotypic flavivirus antibody may modulate yellow fever infection, resulting in milder illness and lower viremia titers. Other studies have suggested that the Asian strains of *Ae. aegypti* may be less competent vectors of yellow fever. Thus, even though the virus has probably been introduced to Asia in the past, the combination of cross-protective immunity from other flaviviruses and low vector susceptibility probably prevented subsequent transmission and spread.

Large urban epidemics of yellow fever have not occurred in Central and South America for many years as a result of combined *Ae. aegypti* control programs and yellow fever vaccination in many countries of the region. *Ae. aegypti* was eradicated in many countries, and yellow fever now occurs only in the jungle and in a few rural areas. In recent years, however, *Ae. aegypti* has reinvaded many urban areas of South and Central America, putting them at highest risk in >50 years for epidemic transmission. Africa still experiences large epidemics transmitted by *Ae. aegypti*: For the first time in >40 years, a major epidemic of urban yellow fever occurred in West Africa in 1987; the frequency of epidemic yellow fever has increased in West Africa in the past 10 years; and in 1992 to 1993, the first epidemic of yellow fever occurred in Kenya.

Japanese encephalitis (JE) virus: JE virus is another important flavivirus that is related antigenically to dengue and yellow fever viruses (Chapter 30.3). It is strictly an Asian virus, ranging from India in the west to Japan and Siberia in the east. It is primarily a rural disease, but in Asia, where there are dense human populations, large epidemics occur periodically. Thousands of cases have occurred in India, especially in West Bengal and Bihar State, and in Nepal. In 1990, a small outbreak occurred in Saipan, Western Pacific, and in 1995, an outbreak of JE was documented in the Torres Strait of Australia, expanding its geographic distribution. The illness in humans ranges from inapparent infection to severe encephalitis and death.

Transmission of JE virus is seasonal in the northern part of its range. Thus, it occurs only during the summer months in Japan, Korea, and China. In tropical areas, e.g., Indonesia, the virus is transmitted sporadically year round. The large epidemics of JE virus have occurred in the northern part of its geographic range. The exact maintenance cycle of JE virus is not known but most likely involves birds as the principal reservoir hosts and mosquitoes of the genus *Aedes* as the maintenance vector (Fig. 30–8). The virus overflows from this maintenance cycle to farms, where pigs may act as amplification hosts. The principal epidemic vectors are members of the *Culex tritaeniorhynchus* complex of mosquitoes, which breed in rice fields, barrow pits, and other standing water. Humans usually become involved as a result of contact with farm areas where there are pigs, and large epidemics of JE usually occur in areas with large pig populations.

Humans have been considered a dead-end host for JE because the virus has been infrequently isolated from human sera. Human viremia may occur, however, before onset of symptoms or early in the illness, when it would not be detected. Mosquitoes are most likely infected by feeding on viremic birds or pigs, although it has been documented experimentally that vertical transmission of JE virus can occur in *Cx. tritaeniorhynchus*. This could be an important maintenance mechanism for the virus, especially in northern temperate regions, where overwintering would be a problem.

Control of JE virus is difficult because it is a rural disease. In Japan, Korea, People's Republic of China, and Taiwan, however, epidemic JE has been reduced considerably by a combination of vaccination and water management practices.

St. Louis encephalitis virus: St. Louis encephalitis (SLE) virus is the most important arbovirus in North America and has caused major epidemics periodically since it was first described in 1933 (Chapter 30.5). This is strictly an American virus and has been documented in Central and South America as well as North America. As with JE, epidemics of SLE occur primarily in the temperate areas of its distribution.

SLE virus is maintained in nature in a bird–*Culex* mosquito–bird cycle (Fig. 134–1). The species of birds and mosquitoes may vary depending on the area. In the central and eastern United States, for example, various domestic and peridomestic birds, e.g., house sparrows, pigeons, blue jays, and robins, are the important maintenance and amplifying hosts. *Culex pipiens pipiens* and *Cx. pipiens quinquefasciatus*, which breed in storm drains, sewage treatment ponds, and other polluted water, are the principal mosquito vectors. Both vertebrate and mosquito hosts bring the virus into the human habitat, where transmission to humans may occur. Other *Culex* species, e.g., *Cx. restuans* and *Cx. salinarius* are efficient vectors of SLE virus and are probably important maintenance hosts in locations such as the Ohio-Mississippi River basin, where they are involved in enzootic transmission. In Florida, *Cx. nigripalpus* is the important epidemic vector. In the western United States, however, SLE is primarily a rural infection. The principal vector there is Cx. *tarsalis*, which breeds in clear or foul water, irrigation ponds, ditches, and other sources of ground water in areas fed by irrigation systems. Although mosquitoes of the *Cx. pipiens* complex are common in the western United States and may transmit SLE virus, they are not the principal vectors in that part of the country.

An important question that remains to be answered is how the virus survives the cold winter season, when mosquitoes do not feed. Studies have demonstrated repetitive foci in the central United States where SLE virus transmission occurs every year, even during interepidemic periods, suggesting that the virus is indigenous and not introduced. Other work has demonstrated that this virus is also transmitted vertically in *Culex* species and that it can survive the winter months in hibernating *Culex* mosquitoes. Thus, there may be more than one mechanism for the virus to overwinter and be available for spring amplification. Furthermore, biologic and biochemical studies suggest that there are epidemic strains of SLE virus that produce higher viremia in birds. Thus, a combination of factors is probably involved in maintenance of the virus in nature and its subsequent epidemic transmission (Fig. 134-1).

Limited experimental work suggests that HIV does not replicate in mosquito tissues, and the epidemiologic disease pattern is not compatible with biologic transmission of HIV by mosquitoes. Finally, the low viremia in humans infected with HIV makes it unlikely that mechanical transmission would occur.

PROTOZOA. Of the protozoan parasites of humans transmitted by insects, the malarial parasites are by far the most important. A combination of insecticide resistance in the mosquito vectors and drug resistance by the malarial parasites has resulted in a resurgence of malaria in most major endemic areas of the tropics (Fig. 92-1).

All malarial parasites of humans and lower primates have *Anopheles* mosquitoes as vectors. Table 138-7 lists the principal malaria vectors found in each of the major geographic areas of the world. In addition, many more species of anophelines are important vectors locally. Malaria has been controlled or eradicated from some of these areas, and therefore, transmission may no longer occur. The mosquito species listed, however, are documented vectors and could transmit malaria in the future if the parasite should be reintroduced.

The life cycle of all malarial parasites is similar and involves a human-*Anopheles*-human transmission cycle (Fig. 92-2). There is an exogenous sexual phase with multiplication in the mosquito and an endogenous asexual phase with multiplication in humans. Mosquitoes become infected when they ingest microgametocytes and macrogametocytes while taking a blood meal from a person with parasitemia.

After exflaggelation and fusion of the gametes, the zygote makes its way through the gut epithelium and encysts on the outside wall of the mosquito midgut. The oocyst forms, and in 10 to 14 days, >200,000 sporozoites may develop, break out of the oocyst, and migrate to all parts of the body, including the salivary glands. The parasites in the salivary

TABLE 138–7. Important Vectors of Malaria by Geographic Region

Geographic Region	Vector Species
North America	*Anopheles quadrimaculatus* complex
	An. freeborni
Central America	*An. albimanus*
	An. aquasalis
	An. bellator
	An. pseudopunctipennis
South America	*An. albimanus*
	An. darlingi
	An. nuneztovari
	An. pseudopunctipennis
	An. aquasalis
Northern Europe	*An. atroparvus*
	An. claviger
	An. labranchiae
	An. beklemishevi
Mediterranean and North Africa	*An. sacharovi*
	An. sergentii
	An. pharoensis
Africa (south of Sahara)	*An. gambiae* complex (six species)
	An. funestus
	An. moucheti
	An. nili
Indo-Persian region	*An. stephensi*
	An. culcifacies complex
	An. fluviatilis
	An. pulcherrimus
Indo-Chinese region	*An. dirus* complex
	An. minimus
	An. anthropophagus
	An. sinensis
Southeast Asia	*An. balabacensis*
	An. dirus complex
	An. minimus
	An. aconitus
	An. campestris
	An. sundaicus
	An. barbirostris
	An. flavirostris
Australasia	*An. farauti* complex
	An. koliensis
	An. punctulatus complex

glands can then be transmitted to a new person when the mosquito takes a subsequent blood meal.

The exogenous or sexual phase of the cycle in the mosquito is termed *sporogony*. The infecting sporozoites enter the blood, and some eventually invade the liver parenchyrna cells. There they multiply asexually, with each sporozoite giving rise to 10,000 to 20,000 progeny called *merozoites*. Liver merozoites are discharged and enter the blood system and penetrate erythrocytes. In the latter cells, they multiply asexually, producing more merozoites, the number being characteristic for each malarial parasite. This asexual or endogenous part of the cycle is termed *schizogony*. For reasons that are not fully understood, some tropozoites in the erythrocytes do not undergo schizogony but instead develop into a gametocyte; when these are ingested by a mosquito, the cycle begins again. The incubation period in malaria coincides with the prepatent period. Some *Plasmodium vivax* and *P. ovale* infections, however, may have a protracted incubation period of 9 months or more.

Many factors influence the transmission of malarial parasites. These include those associated with the mosquito population (e.g., susceptibility to infection, longevity, feeding and resting behavior, population density, breeding habits, and flight range), factors associated with the human population (e.g., susceptibility to infection, occupation, type of housing, population density, and migrations or movement of people), and factors associated with the environment (e.g., topography of the area, weather, and climate). The combination of these factors that exists in malarious areas determines the extent of interactions among parasite, humans, and vector, and this interaction in turn determines whether an area has stable or unstable malaria.

Malaria transmission often occurs indoors because of the feeding and resting behavior of the mosquitoes. This single factor made malaria controllable with residual insecticides and was responsible for the control successes of the 1960s. However, it also produced selection pressures that resulted in insecticide resistance in many species of *Anopheles* and in behavioral changes in some species. These changes in the mosquito populations, along with drug resistance, are the main factors responsible for the resurgence of malaria since the 1970s.

FILARIASIS. Three species of filaria of humans are transmitted by mosquitoes: *Wuchereria bancrofti*, *Brugia malayi*, and *Brugia timori*. In addition, many other mosquito-borne filariae parasitize other animals. These include some species in monkeys that can also infect humans, the common heartworm of dogs, and other species that infect various mammals, birds, reptiles, and amphibians.

Mosquito-borne human filariasis is widely distributed throughout the tropics and subtropics of the world. *W. bancrofti*, the most widely distributed, is basically a tropicopolitan species (Fig. 106–3). *B. malayi* is widespread in Asia from India and Sri Lanka in the west to Indonesia, the Philippines, and Japan in the east (Fig. 106–3). *B. timori* has a limited distribution and has been documented only in several eastern Indonesian islands from Timor to Sumba. Table 138–8 lists the three species of filarial parasites and the different strains of each, along with the geographic distribution and important mosquito vectors.

The basic life cycle is the same for all filarial parasites (Fig. 106–1). The embryonic microfilariae circulating in the peripheral blood (Fig. 106–1) are ingested by the mosquito when they take a blood meal. The microfilariae immediately exsheathe, penetrate the midgut wall, and migrate to the thorax of the mosquito, where they enter a muscle cell and begin to develop. The juvenile filariae molt twice during a development period of 10 to 14 days and emerge from the muscle cells as active third-stage or infective larvae. These larvae migrate throughout the body of the mosquito, including the proboscis or mouthparts. When the infective mosquito takes a subsequent blood meal, the larvae escape from the labium onto the skin and penetrate it.

The epidemiology of mosquito-borne filariasis varies with the strain and species of parasite and with the species of mosquito vector.

Periodic bancroftian filariasis: Filariasis caused by *W. bancrofti* in Asia is essentially an urban disease. The parasite is the nocturnally periodic form, which means that the microfilariae are found circulating in the peripheral blood only at night. This strain of *W. bancrofti* is transmitted in most urban areas by the night-biting common house mosquito, *Cx. pipiens quinquefasciatus*. This mosquito breeds in sewage-contaminated water in drains, tanks, and other ground water close to human habitations. It is a highly domesticated species and lives in intimate contact with humans. In tropical America, *W. bancrofti* is also transmitted by *Cx. pipiens quinquefasciatus*, but in Africa, the principal vectors are *An. gambiae* and *An. funestus*, which also transmit malaria. In rural rain forest communities of Asia, this parasite may be transmitted by forest mosquitoes of the genus *Aedes* or *Anopheles*.

Subperiodic bancroftian filariasis: Another strain of *W. bancrofti* found only in the South Pacific shows little or no microfilarial periodicity. This form, known as *subperiodic* or *aperiodic W. bancrofti*, has microfilariae circulating in the peripheral blood with little variation throughout the 24-hour day. Nearly coincident with subperiodic bancroftian filariasis

TABLE 138–8. Mosquito-Borne Filarial Parasites of Humans

Parasite	Distribution	Rural	Urban
Wuchereria bancrofti (periodic form)	Tropicopolitan (except Polynesia)	*Anopheles gambiae* *An. funestus* *An. flavirostris* *An. punctulatus* complex *An. barbirostris* *An. balabacensis* *Aedes niveus* *Ae. kochi* *Ae. poecilius* *Ae. togoi*	*Culex pipiens quinquefasciatus* *Cx. pipiens pallens*
W. bancrofti (subperiodic form)	Polynesia, New Caledonia	*Ae. polynesiensis* *Ae. tabu* *Ae. vigilax*	
Brugia malayi (periodic form)	Thailand Asia—India to Japan	*Ae. harinasutai* *Mansonia annulifera* *M. indiana* *M. uniformis* *Ae. togoi* *Ae. barbirostris* *An. anthropophagus* *An. sinensis* *An. donaldi* *Anopheles* species	
B. malayi (subperiodic form)	Swamp forests of Southeast Asia	*M. dives* *M. bonneae* *M. annulata* *M. uniformis*	
B. timori	Indonesia—Timor to Sumba	*An. barbirostris*	

is the distribution of *Ae. (Stegomyia) polynesiensis*, the principal vector throughout its range. Transmission by this species is associated with the peridomestic environment and coconut plantations on most islands. *Ae. polynesiensis*, which breeds in various natural and artifical containers (e.g., coconut shells, crab holes, and stored water containers) feeds by day on people working in these areas. On some islands, e.g., Tonga, Rotuma, and Niue, other *Stegomyia* species that are closely related to *Ae. polynesiensis* transmit filariasis, and in New Caledonia, *Ae. vigilax* is the principal vector.

Subperiodic brugian filariasis: B. malayi is the most common filaria of humans throughout most of rural Southeast Asia. It is most frequently associated with mosquitoes of the genus *Mansonia*, immature stages of which are associated with water plants of the genera *Pistia, Eichornia,* and *Salvinia*. Mansonia mosquitoes may feed during the day, but most blood feeding occurs in the evening and may take place indoors or outdoors. The subperiodic form of *B. malayi* is found primarily associated with swamp forests in Southeast Asia, where it occurs in macaques, leaf monkeys, and wild and domestic cats as well as in humans. Transmission thus occurs, via mosquito bite, from person to person, from humans to monkeys and cats, and from these animals to humans.

Periodic brugian filariasis: The periodic form of *B. malayi* is also transmitted by *Mansonia* species, but certain species of *Aedes* and *Anopheles* are the principal vectors in some areas. Therefore, the epidemiology varies considerably from area to area. In India and Sri Lanka, *M. uniformis* is the principal vector, and transmission is associated with coconut plantations; in areas of Indonesia, *An. barbirostris* is the vector, and transmission is associated with rural village areas and rice culture; and in Japan and Korea, *Ae. togoi* is the vector, and transmission is associated with coastal areas, where this mosquito breeds in rock pools. The periodic form of *B. malayi* is not known to have any vertebrate host other than humans. The extent to which animal reservoirs influence the epidemiology of brugian filariasis and the extent to which they complicate the problem of control remain to be determined.

The epidemiology of *B. timori* is similar to that of periodic *B. malayi* in certain areas of Indonesia because both parasites are transmitted by *An. barbirostris*. Reservoir hosts other than humans are not yet known.

Suborder Brachycera, Family Tabanidae (Deer Flies)

Biology. The Tabanidae are large, robust flies belonging to the suborder Brachycera (Fig. 139–14). They are divided taxonomically into four subfamilies, of which two, Chrysopsinae and Tabaninae, are of medical importance. More than 3000 species of tabanids are described worldwide. Only three genera (*Chrysops, Tabanus,* and *Haematopota*) contain species of medical importance, and only one of these, *Chrysops*, is important in the transmission of disease to humans.

As with the mosquitoes, only the females take blood meals from a wide variety of animals. The mouthparts are the cutting-lacerating type and thus produce pooled blood on which flies feed. The female flies deposit their eggs on the underside of leaves, rocks, and branches over the larval habitat, which may be a pond with clear or brackish water, or over muddy or semiaquatic sites. The eggs hatch in 7 to 14 days; the larvae drop to the underlying mud or water and usually burrow into the mud and begin to feed on organic matter, including other insect larvae. Tabanid larvae are commonly found along the edges of ponds, marshes, rice fields, and ditches and in rotting vegetation. Depending on the species, the temperature, and other environmental factors, larval development may last as long as 2 to 3 years. Most species, however, produce one generation or more per year. The mature larvae move to drier soil to pupate, usually an

inch or two below the surface. The pupal period may last 1 to 3 weeks, after which the emerging adults make their way to the surface.

Most species are diurnal and thus feed during the day. They are strong fliers and may be found a considerable distance from their breeding sites. Because of the type of mouthparts these flies have, their bite is painful, and they are frequently interrupted from feeding. This facilitates mechanical transmission, because the flies may bite several hosts in a short time before completing the blood meal.

Disease Transmission

BACTERIA. Two bacteria may be transmitted mechanically by species of tabanids. These are *Bacillus anthracis* and *Francisella tularensis*. The former has been documented only on rare occasions, but experimental and circumstantial evidence suggests that horseflies may be a mechanical vector of this bacillus. The other bacterium, which causes tularemia, exists in a natural cycle involving rabbits, mice, squirrels, beavers, and various other animals, including birds. The natural transmission cycle in the western United States involves ticks, but both field and experimental evidence implicates several species of *Chrysops* as mechanical vectors in outbreaks of tularemia (deer fly fever) in humans. Important species are *C. discalis, C. fulvaster,* and *C. aestuans*.

LOA LOA. Deer flies of the genus *Chrysops* are most important as biologic vectors of *Loa loa*, the African eye worm of humans (Chapter 107). This filaria occurs in the tropical rain forests of West and Central Africa and is transmitted from person to person by *C. dimidiata* and *C. silacea*. The adult worms live in the subcutaneous tissues and migrate to various parts of the body, including the eye. They produce microfilariae that have a dirunal periodicity in the peripheral blood. The microfilariae are ingested with the blood meal of the day-feeding flies, after which they penetrate the gut wall, migrate to the thoracic muscles, enter a muscle cell, and develop to third-stage infective larvae, much like the other filariae in mosquitoes. Transmission may occur in 10 to 14 days.

Another filaria that is morphologically identical to *L. loa* but that is found in monkeys and has a nocturnal microfilarial periodicity is transmitted by the night-biting tabanids *C. centurionis* and *C. langi*. Whether this is a new species or just a variant of *L. loa* and whether it can infect humans are not yet known.

Suborder Cyclorrhapha (Muscoid flies).
The muscoid flies represent the most specialized Diptera. They are readily distinguished from the other suborders by the adult antennae (Fig. 138–2), the presence of the frontal (ptilinial) suture, and larvae that have no distinct head capsule. The muscoid flies have a worldwide distribution and breed in feces, decaying vegetation, or dead animal tissues. Three families are important in the transmission of human disease.

Family Glossinidae (Tsetse Flies).
Tsetse flies are considered part of the family Muscidae by some investigators, but biologic as well as morphologic differences justify their elevation to family status. *Glossina* is the only genus in the family. They occur only in Africa but are widely distributed between 14 degrees North and 29 degrees South latitudes.

BIOLOGY. Tsetse flies are medium sized, robust, and strong fliers. They are readily identifiable by the saber-like proboscis that projects forward and the cleaver-shaped cell in the wing (Figs. 93–3 and 139–13). Both male and female flies suck blood and bite humans as well as various other animals. Although some species have preferred hosts, tsetse flies generally have broad host ranges and feed on several kinds of animals.

Unlike most other Diptera, tsetse flies do not have a free-living larval stage in their development. Instead, after a blood meal, the inseminated female fly produces a single egg, which is fertilized and hatches in the uterus. The eggshell is passed, and the young larva feeds on fluid from accessory glands. Regular blood meals must be taken every 2 to 5 days for the female to support development of the larva. After three molts during an 8- to 12-day development period, the mature third-stage larva is deposited by the female in loose, shaded soil. The larva immediately burrows into the soil, and the larval skin begins to harden and forms a reddish-brown puparium.

The pupation period generally lasts 3 to 5 weeks, depending on the temperature, but during cool periods, this time may be extended to 8 to 10 or more weeks. After pupation is complete, the adult emerges, crawls through the soil to the surface, and is ready to fly within 15 to 20 minutes.

Three groups of tsetse flies are differentiated on the basis of morphology and ecology. The *Glossina fusca* group is the largest but is the least important medically. These are primarily forest species that rarely feed on humans and therefore do not transmit disease. The *Glossina morsitans* group of species prefers the thornbush vegetation associated with the savanna and its edges in East and Central Africa. The *Glossina palpalis* group of species is found in wetter regions, primarily in the fringing woodland along rivers in West and Central Africa. The ecology of each of these groups has led to the commonly used terms *forest tsetses (G. fusca), savanna tsetses (G. morsitans),* and *riverine tsetses (G. palpalis)* when discussing African trypanosomiasis. The distribution of all of the aforementioned groups of tsetse flies expands and contracts during the rainy and dry seasons, respectively, as favorable and adverse conditions occur.

DISEASE TRANSMISSION. The only disease of humans transmitted by tsetse flies is African trypanosomiasis. This disease alone, however, has probably had a greater negative impact on the economic development of Central Africa than any other. African trypanosomiasis (African sleeping sickness) is caused by protozoan parasites belonging to the genus *Trypanosoma.* Two species affect humans, *T. brucei rhodesiense* and *T. brucei gambiense.* Another species, *T. brucei brucei,* does not infect humans but causes a disease called *nagana* in animals. All three species of *Trypanosoma* are morphologically identical but are biologically distinct. All have a similar developmental cycle in *Glossina.*

The tsetse fly ingests the trypanosomal form of the parasite with the blood meal (Figs. 93–2 and 93–7). In the midgut, the parasites multiply by binary fission. From the midgut, the parasites migrate forward again to the proboscis, enter the salivary duct, and finally reach the salivary glands, where the infective metacyclic forms develop. Alternatively, it has been shown that the parasites can also penetrate the gut wall and enter the salivary glands from the hemocoel. The extrinsic incubation period is about 20 days but may be as long as 30 days, depending on the species and environmental conditions. Transmission occurs when the tsetse fly takes a blood meal after metacyclic forms are present in the salivary glands.

The ecology and distribution of African sleeping sickness are closely tied to the tsetse fly (Fig. 93–4). Thus, the distribution of disease also expands and contracts along with that of the flies. Rhodesian sleeping sickness, caused by *T. brucei rhodesiense,* is primarily an East African disease and is transmitted by species of the *G. morsitans* group. These flies and the disease are associated with the savanna, where human populations are sparse. The principal animal reservoirs for the parasite are various game animals and domestic ungulates. Because *G. morsitans, G. swynnertoni,* and *G. pallidipes,* the principal vectors, prefer to feed on animals rather than on people, human disease is more sporadic and seldom occurs in epidemic form.

West African sleeping sickness, caused by *T. brucei gambiense,* is found in West and Central Africa. The disease is associated with river ecologies, where human population density is usually highest and where the principal vectors, *G. palpalis, G. tachinoides,* and *G. fuscipes,* occur. The disease is more chronic, and persons with parasitemia are seldom bedridden during the early stages of infection. Therefore, transmission may be more intense, and epidemics of this form are common. *T. brucei gambiense* has no known animal reservoirs, although some evidence shows that domestic pigs may have a role.

Family Muscidae (Houseflies). The family Muscidae contains the common housefly, *Musca domestica* (Figs. 138–5 and 139–8), and a number of other synanthropic species that live in intimate association with humans. Although the family contains several species that have evolved the bloodsucking habit, none of them have been incriminated in biologic transmission of human disease agents. The importance of houseflies lies in their indiscriminate feeding habits, which may

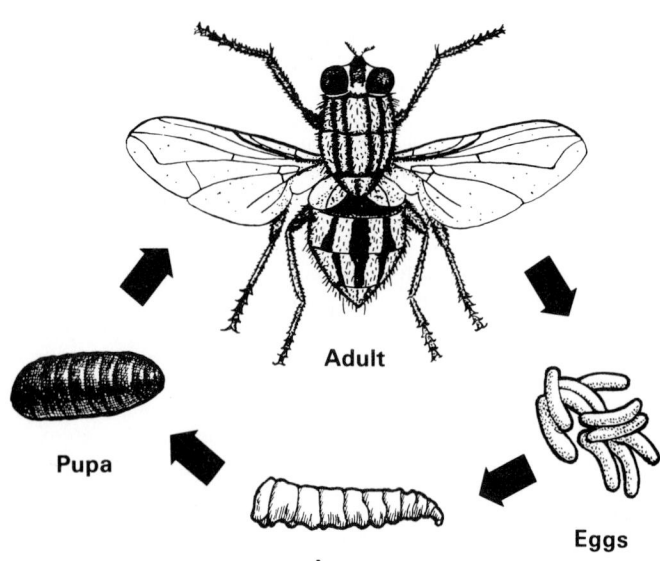

Adult

Pupa

Larva

Eggs

Figure 138–5. Life cycle of the housefly, *Musca domestica.*

TABLE 138–9. Human Pathogens Mechanically Transmitted by Houseflies and Their Relatives

Agent	Classification	Source
Virus	Poliomyelitis	Feces
	Coxsackievirus	Feces
	Hepatitis A	Feces
	Enteroviruses	Feces
Rickettsia	*Coxiella burnetii*	Milk
Bacterium	*Chlamydia trachomatis*	Conjunctiva
	Shigella species	Feces
	Salmonella species	Feces
	Salmonella typhi	Feces
	Escherichia coli	Feces
	Vibrio cholerae	Feces
	Helicobacter pylori	Feces
	Bacterial conjunctivitis	Conjunctiva
Spirochete	*Treponema pertenue*	Skin ulcers
Protozoon	*Entamoeba histolytica*	Feces
	Entamoeba coli	Feces
	Giardia lamblia	Feces
	Toxoplasma gondii (oocyst)	Feces
Cestode (eggs)	*Taenia solium*	Feces
	Dipylidium caninum	Feces
	Diphyllobothrium latum	Feces
Nematode (eggs)	*Ascaris lumbricoides*	Feces
	Trichuris trichiura	Feces
	Enterobius vermicularis	Feces

include feces of humans and animals and the food of humans. They are thus capable of mechanically transmitting many organisms, primarily enteric pathogens belonging to a number of taxonomic groups (Table 138–9).

Their success in the mechanical transmission of organisms is directly related to the behavior of the housefly and its relatives and the type of feeding that occurs. These flies are strong fliers and may be feeding or resting on uncovered food only moments after having visited feces. Transfer of the organisms can be by simple contamination of the mouthparts, feet, and body hairs or by ingestion and subsequent regurgitation or defecation on food. Although there is little doubt that houseflies have a role in the transmission of various human pathogens, their actual importance in the epidemiology of the diseases is hard to assess.

Family Chloropidae (Eye Gnats). These are small, robust flies that are attracted to various body secretions and sores of humans and animals. They are strong fliers and are persistent in their feeding habits, continuing to return after being brushed away. Breeding sites are usually in loose, sandy soil that has a high content of organic material.

Two genera are of medical importance. The genus *Hippelates* is American, ranging from Canada in the north to Argentina in the south. *Siphunculina* is similar in biology and habits but is an Asian genus, ranging from India through Southeast Asia.

The medical importance of both genera is mechanical transmission of conjunctivitis and yaws. Although these flies are not bloodsuckers, their habits of frequenting sores, wounds, the eye, and other secretions make them ideal for mechanical transmission. It is probable that *Hippelates* and *Siphunculina* species have important roles in the transmission of both bacterial and viral conjunctivitis, outbreaks of which usually occur during the fly season. Chloropid flies have also been implicated in the transmission of streptococcal and staphylococcal skin infections and yaws. The latter is a rural disease caused by the spirochete *Treponema pertenue* (Chapter 48.2). It is widespread in the tropics and results in large ulcerating sores. Both *Hippelates* and *Siphunculina* feed on sores of this kind and may ingest *T. pertenue*. *H. flavipes* may

regurgitate active spirochetes during subsequent feedings within 2 days of the original infection. Most of these diseases have a broader geographic distribution than the flies, and all can be transmitted directly by contact and by fomites.

COCKROACHES (ORDER DICTYOPTERA). Other insects, e.g., cockroaches (Fig. 139–12), are also capable of mechanical transmission of various organisms, but in general, the evidence for this is circumstantial. They are not as important as flies in this respect because of their less frequent contact with feces. Their presence in a building may cause allergies.

Bibliography

Busvine JR: Insects and Hygiene. The Biology and Control of Insect Pests of Medical Importance, 2nd ed. London, Methuen & Co, 1966.

Greenberg B: Flies and Disease, Vol II (Biology and Disease Transmission). Princeton, Princeton University Press, 1971.

Gubler DJ, Kuno G: Dengue and Dengue Hemorrhagic Fever. London, CAB International, 1997.

Harwood RF, James MT: Entomology in Human and Animal Health, 7th ed. New York, Macmillan, 1979.

Horsfall WR: Mosquitoes: Their Behavior and Relation to Disease. New York, Ronald Press, 1955.

Horsfall WR: Medical Entomology, Arthropods and Human Disease. New York, Ronald Press, 1962.

Hubbert WT, McCulloch WF, Schnurrenberger PR (eds): Diseases Transmitted from Animals to Man, 6th ed. Springfield, IL, Charles C Thomas, 1975.

Jamnback H: Simuliidae (Blackflies) and Their Control. WHO/VBC 6.653, Geneva, World Health Organization, 1976.

Knight KL, Stone A: A Catalog of the Mosquitoes of the World (Diptera: Culicidae). College Park, Thomas Say Foundation, Entomological Society of America, 1977.

Lewis DJ: The biology of Phlebotomidae in relation to leishmaniasis. Annu Rev Entomol 19:363, 1974.

Monath TP (ed): St. Louis Encephalitis. Washington, DC, American Public Health Association, 1980.

Monath TP (ed): Arboviruses: Epidemiology and Ecology. Vols I, II, III, IV, V. Boca Raton, FL, CRC Press, 1988.

Poland JD, Barnes AM: Plague. In Steele JH (ed): CRC Handbook Series in Zoonoses. Boca Raton, FL, CRC Press, 1979.

Pollitzer R: Plague. WHO Monograph Series, No. 22, Geneva, World Health Organization, 1954.

Service MM: A Guide to Medical Entomology. London, Macmillan, 1980.

Shelly AJ: Vector aspects of the epidemiology of onchocerciasis in Latin America. Annu Rev Entomol 33:337, 1988.

Smith KGV (ed): Insects and Other Arthropods of Medical Importance. London, British Museum of Natural History, 1973.

World Health Organization: Epidemiology of Onchocerciasis. Report of a WHO Expert Committee. WHO Tech Rep Ser 597, 1976.

139 *Control of Arthropods of Medical Importance**

Leon L. Robert

GENERAL PRINCIPLES. Some of the most common diseases in the world are vector borne. Most of them, transmitted by insects, ticks, and mites, are predominantly tropical and most common in underdeveloped countries with limited health services. In many cases, the disease has no simple cure or preventive vaccine. These diseases could often be controlled by simple changes in the habits and customs of the people or by community efforts to create conditions unfavorable for transmission. Personal protective measures, e.g., suitable clothing and footwear, screening for houses, arthropod repellents, and mosquito nets are available only to the minority. Adequate housing, water supply, and sanitation

---

*All the material in this chapter is in the public domain, with the exception of any borrowed figures or tables.

can only come from a buoyant economy, as can major environmental preventive measures. Thus, it is easy to conclude that the control method giving the greatest benefit to the greatest number of people in the shortest period of time is control of the vector.

Control methods may be aimed at vector eradication, reduction to low numbers, or disease eradication. Eradication is for vectors that are mechanical carriers of disease pathogens, e.g., flies and cockroaches. When the pathogen undergoes a cycle of development in the vector, control is directed toward reducing life expectancy to less than the time needed for completion of this intrinsic cycle and before the vector is capable of passing on the infection. For eradication, methods with a maximum effect on insect numbers, usually an integration of antilarval and antiadult measures, are necessary. This may combine source reduction methods with chemical control. Therefore, efficient housefly control may comprise the proper disposal of refuse, the use of insecticides to spray garbage collections, and the use of residual spot sprays or space sprays against adult flies. Transmission control generally involves application of residual insecticides onto the surfaces where the insect usually rests. On a few occasions when the vector rests predominantly indoors (e.g., *Anopheles darlingi*, the malaria vector in coastal Guyana, and *A. funestus* in tropical Africa), this has led to vector eradication. In most cases, however, the objective has been to interrupt transmission of the disease, eradicating the pathogen.

COLLECTING AND TRAPPING. Two simple, direct methods of vector control are collecting and trapping, which are seldom used separately because they only rarely contribute significantly to control by themselves. Thus, the search for and collection of the larger venomous arthropods (e.g., scorpions and spiders) in households may be helpful if the points of entry are dealt with at the same time. The removal of ticks causing paralysis is an obvious remedy once the symptoms are recognized. Using sticky flypapers to collect flies accidentally entering screened premises may be preferable to the use of insecticides. A combined attractant and trapping device may be useful, both indoors (e.g., for the control of cockroaches) and outdoors (e.g., to catch houseflies and tsetse flies). The potential of specific attractants has long been recognized, but few have been isolated for use against pests of medical importance. Bait-trapping of rodents has long been practiced as a supplement to flea control measures to combat plague outbreaks.

ENVIRONMENTAL CONTROL. Environmental control methods aimed at the breeding and assembly areas of pests can produce long-lasting effects and, in some cases, permanent solutions. These were the methods of choice before modern chemicals, which almost invariably need repeated applications. Good environmental sanitation is a prerequisite for the prevention of insects that breed in refuse and sewage, e.g., houseflies and mosquitoes, e.g., *Culex quinquefasciatus*. Proper storage, collection, and disposal of garbage and sewage are the only ways to avoid these pests. Removal or prevention of unnecessary water collections helps a great deal to control mosquito-borne and certain other vector-borne diseases. Such measures include drainage, canalization, filling in, water-level fluctuation, flushing, salinity change, pollution, and induced sunshine or shade. With a thorough knowledge of the life history and biology of the pest, it may be possible to produce habitat changes unfavorable to survival. Removal of vegetation may result in the disappearance of some species (e.g., tsetse flies), whereas its growth and the concomitant production of shade may be detrimental to others (e.g., some mosquito species). Therefore, one must be certain that what is unfavorable to the pest in question does not encourage another.

INSECTICIDES. Chemical methods of control, especially those involving the use of residual insecticides, form a convenient and rapid means of destroying vectors. Used indoors, they have a minimal effect on the environment and nontarget organisms. It is their widespread, often indiscriminate use outdoors in controlling agricultural pests that may cause environmental damage. This has produced some of the resistance in human disease vectors by the contamination of breeding and resting places.

Types of Insecticides. Insecticides are of three main types: those that act as stomach poisons (e.g., Paris green or copper acetoarsenite, sometimes used for the control of mosquito larvae); those that act as fumigants (e.g., ethyl formate, used for the delousing of clothing); and those that act through external contact with the arthropod exoskeleton (e.g., the nonresidual pyrethrum flowers and the true residuals, e.g., dichlorodiphenyltrichloroethane [DDT]). Some compounds can act in all three ways. Dichlorvos is an organophosphorus compound that is volatile and can therefore act as a fumigant. Applied in solution or emulsion in water, it can act as a stomach poison to mosquito larvae, and applied to solid surfaces, it can act through contact. The contact insecticides are particularly useful in vector control. Some contact insecticides act as physical toxicants that mechanically block a physiologic process, such as oils used to control mosquito larvae by blocking or clogging the respiratory openings or gills. Other physical toxicants are the inert abrasive dusts, e.g., boric acid, diatomaceous earth, silica gel, and aerosilica gel. These compounds kill insects by adsorbing waxes from the insect cuticle, causing continuous loss of water from the insect body. Death is caused by rapid dehydration.

The active ingredients of pyrethrum flowers, mainly pyrethrins, and now some synthetic relatives (e.g., bioresmethrin and bioallethrin), produce extremely rapid knockdown effects through contact but have little or no residual effect. They make safe space sprays for domestic use, with almost immediate alleviation of biting nuisances in closed spaces, and are often combined with residuals to flush out hiding pests. Dissolved in propellant liquefied gases, they form the basic ingredient of the modern aerosol dispenser (fly spray). They are also constituents of aerosols used outdoors for containment of epidemics of fly-borne diseases and mosquito-borne viral infections.

Four main groups of chemicals make up the residual insecticides: organochlorines, organophosphates, carbamates, and pyrethroids. The organochlorines DDT, hexachlorocyclohexane (HCH), and dieldrin transformed the control of vectors after World War II and were responsible for saving millions of people from malaria and other vector-borne diseases. Unfortunately, many vectors have become resistant to this group of compounds, and it is now necessary to use the less efficient and more expensive organophosphates (e.g., malathion), carbamates (e.g., propoxur), and pyrethroids (e.g., permethrin).

Table 139–1 presents a list of compounds that have been used against arthropods of medical importance, classified according to their general chemical grouping.

Application Methods. All the modern residual insecticides are effective in minute quantities. Dilution is usually necessary in a formulation suitable for a particular method of application. Formulations and application methods differ for different pests and situations.

Surface Spraying. Insecticide is most frequently applied to internal surfaces of human dwellings and other buildings, usually walls and roofs but sometimes floors as well. Three formulations are available: (1) solutions, which usually require special solvents, e.g., kerosene for their dilution; (2) emulsions; and (3) wettable powders, which require water

TABLE 139–1. Residual Insecticides

Organo-chlorines	Organo-phosphates	Carba-mates	Pyrethroids
aldrin	bromophos	bendiocarb	allethrin*
chlordane	chlorfenvinphos	carbaryl	bioallethrin*
chlordecone	chlorphoxim	dimetilan	bioresmethrin*
dicofol	chlorpyrifos	propoxur	cypermethrin
dieldrin	chlorpyrifos-		decamethrin
DDT	methyl		deltamethrin
endosulfan	diazinon		fenvalerate
endrin	dichlorvos		natural
heptachlor	dimethoate		pyrethrins*
HCH	dioxathion		permethrin
lindane	fenchlorphos		phenothrin*
(γ HCH)	fenitrothion		resmethrin*
methoxychlor	fenthion		tetramethrin*
mirex	jodfenphos		
toxaphene	malathion		
	naled		
	parathion		
	parathion-methyl		
	phoxim		
	pirimiphos-		
	methyl		
	temephos		
	tetrachlorvinphos		
	trichlorphon		

*Nonpersistent.

for dilution. Solutions and emulsions are normally used only where the surfaces should not be marked, but they are too readily absorbed (and lost from action) by some surfaces for general use. The most common formulation is the wettable powder, which, on dilution, produces a suspension of solid particles that remains on the surface of absorbent materials. Application is by a direct spray coarse enough to thoroughly wet the surface, delivered at a pressure low enough to give maximum adherence. The machine generally used for the application is the cylindrical, pneumatic, knapsack-type sprayer having a capacity of 9 to 14 L, operating at 40 psi (2.8 bar), and delivering 760 mL of spray per minute through a fan-jet nozzle with an 0.8-mm diameter. Held 45 cm from the surface to be sprayed, with a flat fan-spray with a spray angle of 80 degrees, this produces a swath 75 cm wide. Spraying is done in bands slightly less than this width to ensure uniformity, and those performing the spraying are trained to cover 19 m^2 in 1 minute (or 40 mL/m^2). Dilution of 75% DDT wettable powder at the rate of 67 g/L of water results in a deposit of 2 g/m^2, which gives a persistently high kill on most surfaces for about 6 months. γ HCH (lindane) diluted at a quarter of this rate may produce comparable results on absorbent surfaces but not on nonabsorbent ones. The organophosphates and carbamates are usually applied at 2 g/m^2, although some may be applied at 1 g/m^2. Their persistence on nonabsorbent surfaces is usually about 3 months but is considerably shorter on absorbent ones.

These details apply to the spraying of houses for malaria control. Such spraying of course kills other insects such as other mosquito species, sandflies, houseflies, bedbugs, triatomine bugs, cockroaches, fleas, and ticks. If these, rather than anopheline mosquitoes, are the main pests, spraying can be concentrated on those areas where insects congregate, such as beds (bedbugs), the bases of walls (cockroaches), and the floor (fleas).

Other Formulations and Applications. In addition to the formulations used to spray buildings with residual insecticides,

numerous other methods of dispersion of residual insecticides exist.

DUSTS. Historically, dusts have been the simplest formulations of pesticides to manufacture and the easiest to apply. These are mixtures of insecticides and finely ground, light, inert diluents such as china clay, talc, finely shredded paper, or even locally sieved road dust or wood ash. DDT dusts usually contain 5 to 10% of the insecticide; 10% DDT in talc is commonly used for the control of body lice. HCH dusts contain 0.5% of the gamma isomer, and malathion dust contains 1% of the insecticide. Dusts are commonly used in the control of agricultural pests and against cockroaches, fleas (especially in rodent burrows), fly maggots, and lice whose precise location is known. Dusts are also useful as mosquito larvicides on breeding waters containing emergent or floating vegetation, where control by oil films is not possible. Various methods of dust distribution are used, ranging from the simplest, by hand, to the use of aircraft. However, despite their ease in handling, formulation, and application, dusts are the least effective and, ultimately, the least economical of the pesticide formulations.

AEROSOLS OR FOGS. These are dispersions of solutions of insecticides in fine droplet form (usually <50 μm in diameter) that remain suspended in the atmosphere for a considerable time. They are produced in various ways from several kinds of machines:

1. *Atomizer,* in which a stream of air is made to impinge on a stream of insecticide solution, as in the ordinary Flit gun.
2. *Aerosol dispenser,* in which the insecticide is dissolved in or mixed with liquefied gases under pressure. When the pressure is released, the carrier liquid boils off, dispersing a cloud of insecticide solution droplets.
3. *Fogging machines,* in which larger machines generate aerosols containing droplets whose diameters are usually <10 μm but >1 μm. They are of two types: Thermal foggers use flash heating of an oil solvent to produce a visible vapor or smoke, and ambient foggers atomize a tiny jet of liquid in a Venturi tube through which passes an ultra–high-velocity air stream.
4. *Aircraft,* in which the insecticide may be gravity- or pump-fed into a boom beneath the aircraft wings bearing nozzles at intervals along its length. The spray is further broken up in the slipstream of the aircraft. Insecticide solution may also be distributed by introduction into the exhaust system of an aircraft, similar to the production of a thermal aerosol from a fogging machine.

Ultra–low-volume (ULV) application is a development in aerosol dispersion involving the distribution of low volumes of high insecticide concentration with a narrow range of droplet size. Insecticides are usually applied without further dilution, by special ground or aerial spray equipment that limits the volume from 0.6 L/hectare to a maximum of 4.7 L/hectare, as an extremely fine spray. The concentration depends on the activity level of the insecticide and the ease of dispersion of small volumes. Special ground machinery exists for this dispersion, or it can be applied from slow-flying aircraft. This technique has proved extremely useful where insect control is desired over vast areas.

Aerosols are primarily used where rapidity and good penetration are required and where residual effect is not of major importance. The persistent suspension of fine droplets is effective against flying insects; pyrethrins are often added to residual insecticides dispersed in this form to stimulate resting insects to fly. Aerosols have been effective in controlling insect pests of stored products (e.g., grain, tobacco, and hides), as well as in controlling insects resting in dense vegetation (e.g., mosquitoes, black flies, and tsetse flies). They have also proved efficient for the control of epidemics of fly-borne infections and plague where rapid applications both indoors and outdoors are considered more essential than the slower methods of applying residual deposits.

SMOKE GENERATORS. In smoke generators, the insecticide is mixed with a slow-burning chemical that, when ignited, produces a smoke bearing fine particles, droplets, or vapor of insecticide. Smokes have similar uses to liquid aerosols, without the elaborate production, but usually are not as effective. One reason is that a proportion of the insecticide is decomposed by the heat producing the smoke. The pyrethrum coil is a smoke generator designed to burn for an entire night and repel biting insects in bedrooms.

VAPORS. Naturally volatile compounds can be used in the vapor phase as slow-release insecticides. Plastic strips impregnated with dichlorvos, a volatile organophosphate insecticide, can be used in houses and in closed sewage systems to control houseflies, cockroaches, and mosquitoes. In addition, less volatile compounds may be deliberately vaporized by heating.

INSECTICIDAL WHITEWASHES, DISTEMPERS, RESINS, AND PAINTS. Mixing of insecticides with whitewashes and distempers has no advantage over spraying the insecticides onto such surfaces, because the insecticide is diluted and masked by the whitewash or distemper. In addition, lime causes slow decomposition of many insecticides. With oil-bound paints, the insecticide is lost in solution in the paint and thus is not available to affect insects. However, with a high concentration of insecticide (i.e., more than sufficient to saturate the paint oils), "blooming" crystals of insecticide occur on the surface and are highly toxic to alighting insects. This principle of blooming from supersaturated solution has been successful in surface coatings of urea-formaldehyde resins. Blooming from such surfaces continues for long periods and withstands the usual methods of cleaning (in fact, rubbing the surface encourages blooming). This method is favored for the "band treatment" of cockroach runs in hospital and restaurant kitchens.

SLOW-RELEASE FORMULATIONS. Mostly used as mosquito larvicides, these formulations take the form of combinations of insecticide in sand granules, clay pellets, briquettes, or capsules that disintegrate slowly in water, prolonging the insecticide's effect.

HIGH-SPREADING OILS. The control of mosquito larvae by a continuous film of ordinary oil required some 20 to 25 gallons/acre (>200 L/hectare) in the past. The addition of spreading agents (e.g., certain resins) increases the oil's spreading pressure and allows a reduction in the quantities to cover a given area. The addition of small amounts of residual insecticides greatly increases the toxicity of such thin films. The dispersion of such small quantities over large areas presents problems, however. Spraying from the air can be the answer only where large areas of water are involved and where economically feasible. For small collections of water such as rainwater pools, a small oiler is more satisfactory.

BAITS. A combination of insecticide with some substance that attracts the pests makes a useful method of control. Specific attractants derived from the pests themselves are ideal. At present, most baits are animal protein or sugar in one form or another. Bait-insecticide combinations are commonly used to control synanthropic flies and cockroaches. Spot application, such as placing bait in selected places accessible only to the target species, permits the use of very small quantities of toxic materials in a totally safe manner, with no environmental disruption.

Toxic Hazards. All insecticides are poisonous to humans to some extent. Persons most at risk are those handling the

undiluted formulations and the applicator and those who are continuously exposed to dusts or droplets, often within the confines of dwellings. Dermal penetration is of greater importance than inhalation or swallowing; hence, the need for protective clothing. In tropical climates, this must be simple, must cover most of the skin (e.g., lightweight overalls and a broad-brimmed hat), and must be able to be easily washed after each spraying occasion. The mixer of undiluted formulations should wear gloves and an apron and should stand upwind of the mixing container. Facilities for washing with soap and water should be on hand at all times.

An arbitrary classification of toxicities has been made by the World Health Organization (WHO), based on LD_{50} values (mg/kg body weight) when the insecticide is administered to rats orally or dermally and depending on whether it is a solid or liquid. The classification is by hazard, which is defined as "the acute risk to health" (Table 139–2).

Insecticide Resistance. One major effect of the widespread use of chemicals for pest control has been the selection of those arthropods genetically endowed with protective mechanisms against the chemicals used. The persistence of these arthropods and their offspring results in eventual replacement of a mixed population (one with some members susceptible to insecticides) by a resistant one. Among arthropods of medical importance, >150 species have shown resistance of one kind or another. In fact, the only major group of species not yet showing resistance is tsetse flies.

Various genetic, physiologic, and biochemical processes enable insects and related arthropods to overcome the intoxication characteristically produced by insecticide action. These mechanisms vary from enzymes that break the insecticide down into harmless metabolites, to reduced sensitivity of the target site of action of the insecticide (usually the central nervous system), to reduced penetration, or to an increased excretion rate of the insecticide. Some of these mechanisms are specific for particular groups of chemicals, and others protect against more than one group. The enzyme carboxylesterase metabolizes those organophosphates with a carboxylester band in the molecule (e.g., malathion) but not those without it (e.g., nearly all the other organophosphates). An insensitive acetylcholinesterase enzyme, on the other hand, imparts cross-resistance to a wide range of organophosphates and carbamates. Another group of enzymes, the mixed-function oxidases, are the principal enzymes involved in pyrethroid metabolism and may be involved in the metabolic breakdown of some organophosphates and carbamates.

Standard susceptibility tests designed to detect and monitor the spread of resistance for most of the major arthropod vectors of disease are distributed by the WHO. The pests are exposed to standard concentrations of the various insecticides known to normally kill the species (discriminating or diagnostic dosages), and their survival rate is monitored. New biochemical tests now being developed, however, will virtually eliminate all the ambiguities of the current, somewhat crude WHO susceptibility tests. They should eventually be able to identify actual resistance mechanisms in single insects and indicate directly what cross-resistance is likely to be shown and to what alternative compounds they will still be susceptible.

When resistance first appears as a mutation in the population, it is rare and in the heterozygous state. Only if heterozygotes survive the field dosage of insecticide and mate can a homozygote appear. Therefore, the degree of resistance imparted by the gene and its dominance characteristics are important in the process of resistance selection, because resistance is dependent on survival of the heterozygote. Leaving part of the environment unsprayed and using more than one (independently acting) insecticide either in mixture or in

TABLE 139–2. WHO Classification of Insecticide Toxicities

Extremely Hazardous	Highly Hazardous	Moderately Hazardous	Slightly Hazardous	Unlikely to Present an Acute Hazard in Normal Use
chlorfenvinphos	aldrin	bendiocarb	allethrin	bioresmethrin
parathion	dichlorvos	bioallethrin	bromophos	borax
parathion-methyl	dieldrin	carbaryl	dicofol	chlorphoxim
	dimetilan	chlordane	malathion	chlorpyrifos-methyl
	dioxathion	chlordimeform	pirimiphos-methyl	diflubenzuron
	endrin	chlorpyrifos	resmethrin	jodfenphos
	fenthion	cypermethrin	trichlorphon	methoprene
	Paris green	DDT		permethrin
		deltamethrin		phenothrin
		diazinon		temephos
		dimethoate		tetrachlorvinphos
		endosulfan		tetramethrin
		fenchlorphos		
		fenitrothion		
		fenvalerate		
		γ HCH		
		heptachlor		
		naled		
		phoxim		
		propoxur		
		pyrethrins		
		toxaphene		

	LD_{50} for the Rat (mg/kg Body Weight)*			
	Oral		**Dermal**	
Class	Solids†	Liquids†	Solids†	Liquids†
Ia Extremely hazardous	5 or less	20 or less	10 or less	40 or less
Ib Highly hazardous	5–50	20–200	10–100	40–400
II Moderately hazardous	50–500	200–2000	100–1000	400–4000
III Slightly hazardous	Over 500	Over 2000	Over 1000	Over 4000

*The LD_{50} value is a statistical estimate of the number of mg of toxicant per kg of body weight required to kill 50% of a large population of test animals.
†The terms *solids* and *liquids* refer to the physical state of the product or formulation being classified.

rotation encourage the survival of susceptible genes. The rationale for the use of mixtures of insecticides is that when resistance genes are rare, the likelihood of finding an individual insect with two genes affecting two differently acting insecticides is remote. The rationale for using insecticides in rotation is that resistance genes are less fit than their susceptible counterparts; thus, without insecticide selection, they tend to decline in the population. However, once selected for, genes controlling resistance seem to have very lengthy persistence in wild insect populations.

OTHER CHEMICALS. A number of alternatives to conventional residual insecticides are now commercially available, and many others are under investigation, mainly as mosquito larvicides.

Monolayers. These are substances that produce thin, continuous films over open water, denying mosquito aquatic stages access to the air. High-molecular-weight alcohols such as lauryl alcohol, lipids such as lecithin, and semisynthetic surfactants such as Monoxci are biodegradable and nontoxic. They are also harmless to those organisms that do not have to penetrate the water surface film to breathe air (i.e., gill-breathers).

Insect Growth Regulators. These compounds closely resemble or are identical to chemicals produced by insects and related arthropods. Thus, they are truly selective insecticides with extremely low toxicity to mammals.

Juvenile Hormones. Juvenile hormones and their synthetic counterparts, of which methoprene (Altosid) is the best-known example, act by affecting or preventing the molt from the last larval instar to pupa or that from pupa to adult. Because they affect only these late developmental stages, they have to be either applied repeatedly or delivered from some slow-release formulation. Methoprene is biodegradable and functional against mosquito larvae at 0.1 parts per million or less and has little effect on other organisms. Houseflies and *C. quinquefasciatus*, however, have already developed resistance to it.

Chitin Inhibitors. Diflubenzuron (Dimilin) is the most widely used substance that affects the fundamental processes of chitinization and melanization. Unlike juvenile hormones, these substances operate against all life stages, causing almost complete inhibition of adult emergence.

Precocenes. These substances antagonize the synthesis of natural juvenile hormones and thus interfere with metamorphosis from larva to pupa to adult. Precocenes cause premature metamorphosis, producing precocious sterile adults with incompletely developed reproductive systems. One precocene compound is currently undergoing commercial development for tick control.

Avermectins and Ivermectin. These compounds were isolated from fermentation products of *Streptomyces avermitilis* fungi. Avert, an avermectin cockroach bait, is commercially available. Ivermectin is a modified fungal product that is very effective at low doses as an acaricide against red spider mites, in bait for imported fire ant control, as a parasiticide for *Onchocerca volvulus* (Chapter 108), and as a general veterinary parasiticide.

ALTERNATIVES TO CHEMICALS. Chemicals require extensive tests for biologic activity and safety. Such evaluations involve direct toxicity tests on laboratory animals and extended tests for mutagenicity, teratogenicity, and carcinogenicity. Even after expensive testing, the end product may have only a short marketable life because of the development of resistance. The increase in the frequency, extent, and complexity of chemical resistance, the reluctance to pollute the environment with long-lasting chemicals, and the rising cost of developing new chemicals have led to alternatives to chemicals for vector control.

The three main alternatives to chemical control are environmental management measures (which have already been discussed), biologic control agents, and genetic control methods.

Biologic Control. This consists of the use of one plant or animal to control another, thus exploiting predator-prey and parasite-host relationships either by introducing new predators and parasites or by artificially increasing the proportions of existing ones.

Although many biologic control agents have been the subject of intensive scientific study, only two agents are currently being used in operational vector control programs. The bacterium *Bacillus thuringiensis* subspecies *israelensis (B.t.i.)* and the larvivorous fish *Gambusia affinis* are commercially available and are effective against mosquito larvae.

G. affinis is a small (4 to 6 cm long) top-feeding minnow that originated in the United States and has been used for many years to control mosquito larvae. It breeds rather rapidly; a single female may produce 200 to 300 offspring in 1 year, and its mass production and distribution present few difficulties. It is most efficient at a density of about 5000/ acre. However, where vegetation is dense, as favored by mosquito larvae, it may not gain access to its prey. Other limitations are that it will not thrive everywhere, is subject to diseases and predation itself, and may produce undesirable changes in the ecosystem by eating desirable organisms. However, where mosquito breeding places are suitable, *G. affinis* has produced useful control.

B.t.i. is a spore-forming bacterium that produces a crystal of toxic protein (δ-endotoxin). When spores and crystals are ingested by mosquito larvae, the mouth parts and gut are paralyzed and the gut epithelium destroyed. The crystal itself appears to be most important, but death due to bacterial septicemia can also occur. Because the crystals are insoluble in water, it is a particulate insecticide, usually formulated as a wettable powder or emulsion. Mass production in culture with isolation and extraction of endotoxin is now possible. Thus, *B.t.i.* is a biologic larvicide. Trials against both culicine and anopheline mosquito larvae, as well as those of the black fly (*Simulium* species), have produced favorable results.

Numerous other predators and pathogens (viruses, bacteria, protozoa, fungi, and nematode worms) are under investigation, with the following currently undergoing field evaluation: *Poecilia reticulata* and *Aplocheilus* species (fish); *Toxorhynchites* species (nonbiting mosquitoes whose larvae prey on other mosquito larvae); *Bacillus sphaericus* (another spore-forming bacterium); *Culicinomyces clavosporus, Langenidium giganteum,* and *Coelomomyces* species (fungi); *Nosema algerae, Amblyspora* species, and *Lambornella* species (protozoans); *Mesocyclops* and *Macrocyclops* species (copepods); and *Romanomermis culicivorax* and *R. iyengari* (nematode worms).

Genetic Control

Sterility. Genetic manipulation of arthropods to render them sterile, partially sterile, more susceptible to conventional methods of control, or harmless to humans has been the subject of laboratory and field research since the early 1950s. The impetus came from successful eradication of the screwworm fly *(Cochliomyia hominivorax)* by mass rearing of the insect and sterilization of male pupae by γ irradiation. These pupae were then introduced into the wild population just before adult emergence. The emerging sterile males mated with the wild females to produce dramatic reductions in fly numbers and eventual eradication in certain areas.

Sterility of arthropods can also be achieved by exposure to chemosterilants and, in some mosquito complexes, by crossing closely related species to produce sterile hybrid offspring. Several chemosterilants have been used in the field with moderate to good success for experimental housefly control around garbage and trash dumps. However, no chemosterilants are currently commercially available. In the *Culex pipiens* and *Aedes scutellaris* complexes, cytoplasmic incompatibility between certain populations of mosquitoes is evident, with the sperm of one dying in the cytoplasm of the other before fertilization. Such matings produce only sterile eggs; thus, the release of incompatible males into a wild population could lead to elimination of that population. Partial sterility can be achieved by the production of chromosome translocations from irradiation at lower doses than those causing complete sterility. When this occurs in only one of a pair of homologous chromosomes, the resulting individual produces a proportion of chromosomally imbalanced gametes, which, when mated with normal individuals, produce eggs of which only a portion hatch. If this inherited sterility is high enough, population depression follows. Another phenomenon, known only in the yellow fever mosquito, *Aedes aegypti,* and in *C. quinquefasciatus,* the tropical house mosquito, is sex ratio distortion in favor of the male sex. When strains producing more than nine males to every female are released, the numbers of females (the biting and disease-transmitting sex) and the reproductive potential of the population are reduced.

Population Replacement. For effective population suppression of highly reproductive pests (nearly all arthropods of medical importance, with the exception of tsetse flies), large releases of sterile or partially sterile insects over considerable time and areas are necessary. Therefore, more attention is being paid to genetic control techniques resulting in population replacement, in particular introduction of strains that are not carriers of disease or that are more amenable to control by other means. In its simplest form, population replacement can be achieved by prolonged release of fertile males carrying the gene or genes considered desirable to introduce into the population. The release of both sexes of a bidirectional, cytoplasmically incompatible strain or of those with a homozygous translocation (involving both chromosomes of a homologous pair) to produce nonviable matings could be used.

Desirable genes could be those affecting the continued existence of the pest population, such as temperature-sensitive lethal genes or insecticide-susceptibility genes, or those that can render the pest incapable of supporting and transmitting disease agents. Temperature-sensitive lethal genes have been isolated in both the housefly and *Culex tritaeniorhynchus,* the vector of Japanese encephalitis. They have not yet been used for field control purposes. Release of males carrying genes for susceptibility to insecticides has been advocated in areas of insecticide resistance so that inexpensive and efficient compounds such as DDT can continue to be used. Examples of strains of insects no longer capable of supporting development of the pathogen are to be found in the mosquito vectors of viruses, malarial parasites, and filarial worms. No one has yet tried replacing wild populations with the strains, although some long-term population cage trials have been carried out.

Requirements for Genetic Control Systems. The success of any genetic control system is dependent on a number of requirements. It must be possible to rear the pests in large numbers, and they must survive, disperse, and mate competitively with their wild counterparts. Fitness and competitiveness may be affected by the sterilization procedure or by the genetic manipulation to produce the particular control system. γ Irradiation and chemosterilants attempt to achieve a high degree of sterility without serious effect on fitness, a goal less easily obtained with radiation. The developmental stage of the insect at which sterilization is most conveniently performed is a consideration, as is the maturity of the gonads.

SEXING TECHNIQUES. With most pests of medical importance, the female sucks blood and transmits disease; therefore, for genetic control purposes, it is preferable to release only the male sex, because even a sterile female transmits disease. Thus, an efficient sexing technique is essential. With some pests, size differences between the sexes can be used as well as a sieving process. However, these seldom result in perfect separation of the sexes. In several mosquito species, much greater accuracy is obtained from actual genetic sexing techniques in which insecticide-resistant genes or temperature-sensitive lethal genes are translocated by irradiation onto the male sex chromosomes. Dieldrin resistance has been used in *Anopheles gambiae*, *A. arabiensis*, and *A. culicifacies*, and propoxur resistance has been used in *A. albimanus*. Partially resistant males carrying translocated chromosomes survive a small amount of the appropriate insecticide placed into the water where the eggs are laid. When these males mate with females, they transmit resistance at the heterozygous level to their sons, but their daughters remain susceptible. Thus, partially resistant males could be released into a sprayed area where resistance is present and survive to introduce susceptibility into the population.

ARTHROPOD ECOLOGY. For their efficient application, genetic control methods demand a detailed knowledge of pest ecology. A knowledge of flight range, longevity, population size, reproductive potential, and seasonal changes in these variables is essential for decisions on when and where to release genetically manipulated arthropods, how many to release, and over what area and period. It might be thought that the best time for release is when the target population is at its lowest level and least able to expand. However, the adverse conditions responsible for this low level may be even more adverse to the pest population being released, which, in the interests of mass production, has been reared under optimal conditions. The ideal might be to integrate the release with some other method of population reduction at the time of year when the release material is most likely to be effective. The other method of suppression could be conventional insecticide use, in which case it would be an advantage if the released arthropods were resistant to the particular insecticide.

CONTROL OF SPECIFIC ARTHROPODS OF MEDICAL IMPORTANCE. The following are descriptions of methods used for control of insects and other arthropods living on humans and those commonly found in people's houses and in outdoor situations.

Sucking Lice (Order Anoplura). Three different kinds of lice parasitize humans—body, head, and crab lice. The last two stay on the body continuously. The first, except when feeding, is found in the clothing. Infections pass from person to person through social and sexual contact.

Body Lice (Fig. 139–1). Regular laundering with hot water

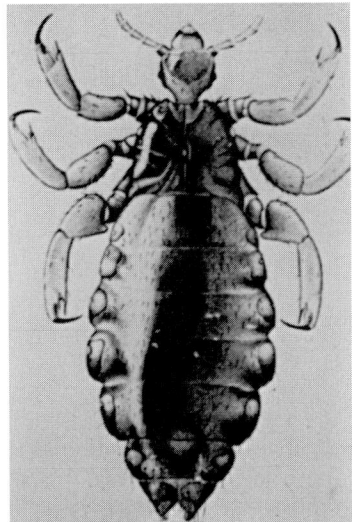

***Figure* 139–1.** Body louse.

and detergent and changing of clothing minimize the likelihood of body lice infestations, which are usually associated with poverty or with mass congregations and migrations of people such as during wars, famines, and other disasters. The old methods of clothing decontamination by heat or fumigants have been replaced by the use of dusts containing residual insecticides. These can be distributed by plunger-type dust guns with long nozzles for insertion beneath clothes without the need for undressing. During World War II, 10% DDT in talc was used in this way to combat typhus epidemics. Alternatively, sifter-top cans can be issued for individual use. A 1% lindane (γ HCH) powder may be used where DDT resistance is evident, although a second application of lindane within 7 to 10 days of the first may be necessary. Where resistance to both DDT and lindane has arisen, 1% malathion, 2% temephos, 1% propoxur, or 5% carbaryl dusts can be used. Resistance to malathion is now evident in Burundi, Ethiopia, and Egypt.

Head Lice. These are best controlled with insecticide lotions rubbed into the hair. Those containing malathion (0.5%) or carbaryl (0.5%) kill eggs as well as nymphs and adults. If 1% lindane shampoo (Kwell) is used, a weekly treatment for 3 weeks is recommended. Although resistance to the organochlorines is known in head lice, no resistance to organophosphates or carbamates has yet been recorded. Treatment with 0.2% synergized pyrethrins is also effective. Education emphasizing frequent bathing and hair washing can help avoid reinfestation.

Crab Lice (Fig. 139–2). These are controlled in the same way as head lice. Although usually confined to the pubic region, they can extend to other parts of the body, such as the axillae, chest hair, and even beards and eyelashes. Manual removal from eyelashes is preferable to insecticidal treatment. No resistance has yet been found in this species.

Scabies Mite (Order Astigmata, Family Sarcoptidae) (Fig. 139–3). A lotion containing 1% lindane applied to the entire body from the neck down is the most common method of treatment for scabies. The lotion should not be washed off for 24 hours, and if the hands are washed, the lotion should be reapplied. A second application 7 days later is desirable. Also used is 25% benzyl benzoate emulsion, which should be applied after a bath and left on the body for 24 hours. A repeat treatment on the third day is essential, and another on the fifth day is desirable.

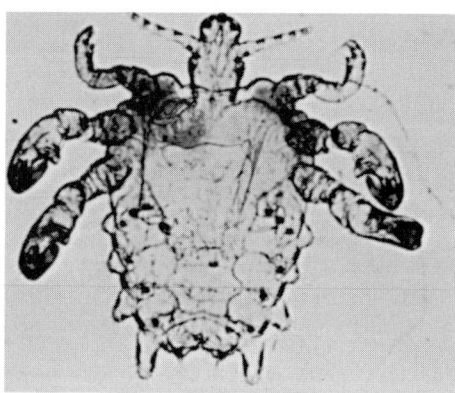

Figure 139–2. Crab louse.

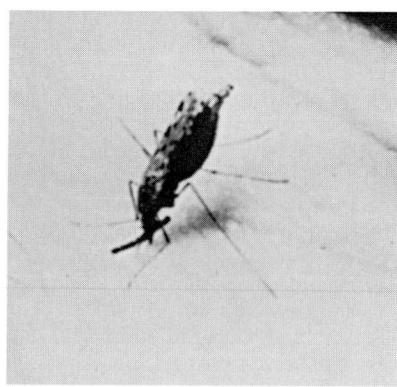

Figure 139–4. Anopheline mosquito.

Scabies is so highly contagious that it is essential to treat all members of a family or closely associated group; otherwise, reinfestation soon occurs.

Mosquitoes (Order Diptera, Family Culicidae). Most mosquitoes feed on blood, constituting a major biting nuisance; many transmit diseases as well. Individual control may alleviate the biting problem, but communitywide control is necessary to reduce disease transmission (Fig. 133–1). Personal protection using repellents (*N*, *N*-diethyl-3-methylbenzamide [deet], dimethyl phthalate, and 2-ethyl-1,3-hexanediol), clothing treatments (0.5% permethrin aerosol), bed nets (insecticide-impregnated bed nets are more effective), space sprays, and the screening of houses provide individual control. Other personal protective methods are the use of residual house sprays and perhaps attacking breeding places if these are few, small enough, and localized.

On a community basis, the use of residual insecticides, either in houses or in and around breeding sites, is the usual method of control, along with environmental measures directed against the breeding places. The following sections present methods adopted for the control of diseases carried by four groups of mosquitoes.

Anopheles Species (Fig. 139–4). Some 60 species of *Anopheles* are important malaria vectors.

ADULTS. The normal method of control is by spraying the walls and roofs or ceilings of the houses where they rest with a specific, uniform dose of a residual insecticide. Where the species are partly zoophilic, animal shelters should be sprayed as well. Other control measures must be adopted for some species that spend little or no time in houses. For

example, anophelines of the Kerteszia group (e.g., *A. bellator* and *A. cruzii* of South America), whose larvae breed in water held in the axils of the leaves of epiphytic bromeliad plants, bite predominantly outdoors. Removal or treatment of these plants is the method of attacking these vectors. *A. balabacensis* of the Far East spends little time indoors, although control of malaria transmitted by this species in Vietnam is claimed to have been achieved by spraying both the inside and outside (around the eaves) of houses with DDT.

A WHO Study Group recently concluded that DDT (2 g/m²) is still safe and effective for indoor residual spraying for control of malaria vectors. However, all the following conditions must be met: It is used only for indoor spraying; it is effective; the material is manufactured to WHO specifications; and the necessary precautions are taken in its use and disposal. DDT is irritating to most insects, however, and causes some to depart from a treated surface before they receive a lethal dose. Lindane (0.5 g/m²) is an alternative but is volatile and has a shorter persistence on nonabsorbent surfaces. For safety reasons, dieldrin is no longer recommended for house spraying. When organochlorine resistance is evident, malathion (2 g/m²) is the popular alternative, with fenitrothion (2 g/m²), pirimiphosmethyl (2 g/m²), and chlorphoxim being other possibilities among the organophosphates, propoxur and bendiocarb (1–2 g/m²) among the carbamates, and deltamethrin (0.05 g/m²) and permethrin (0.5 g/m²) among the synthetic residual pyrethroids. DDT can be expected to remain active for at least 6 months; the other compounds remain active for up to 3 months.

Smoke generators, cold aerosols, thermal fogs, and ULV sprays all have been used for exterior space treatments, especially during malaria epidemics produced by partially exophilic vectors and in large temporary gatherings of people such as religious pilgrimages. Malathion or some of the pyrethroids are usually favored as exterior space sprays.

LARVAE. Larvicides may be added where indoor residual insecticide spraying is insufficient to interrupt disease transmission. It is also used in urban or semiurban areas where indoor residual insecticide spraying is not practical or where breeding sites are relatively limited in number and size. If both adult and larval chemical control is being used against the same species, it is advisable to use differently acting insecticides for each control method to avoid the appearance of resistance. Organochlorine insecticides are not recommended as larvicides because of possible environmental toxicities attributable to their stability and persistence. The organophosphates temephos, malathion, fenthion, chlorpyrifos, jodfenphos, fenitrothion, and pirimphosmethyl and the pyrethroids permethrin and deltamethrin all have been recommended for use against anopheline larvae. They may be

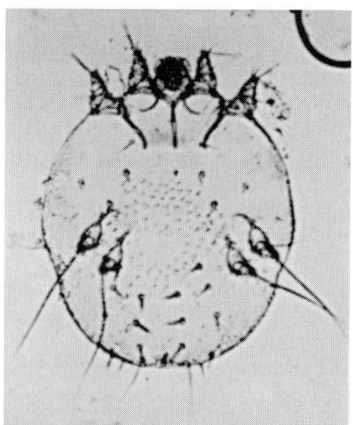

Figure 139–3. Scabies mite.

applied in solution with oils, as emulsions, wettable powders, or dusts, or in a special slow-release formulation. Various types of ground and aerial equipment are used for their distribution. The treatment cycle is usually every 10 to 14 days, but longer effect has been recorded. Temephos has proved to be particularly efficient and safe, but all larvicides present some hazard to fish and other aquatic life. The insect growth regulators methoprene and diflubenzuron have also been used as anopheline larvicides; they affect only arthropods.

RESISTANCE. At least 52 of the 60 important anopheline vectors of malaria are resistant to one insecticide or another in one or more parts of their distribution. Nearly 30 of them are resistant to three of the four chemical groupings to which the common insecticides belong (viz., organochlorines, organophosphates, carbamates, and pyrethroids). Eight species have acquired resistance to all types of these compounds. Of particular concern are multiple resistances in *A. albimanus* in most of the Central American countries, *A. sacharovi* in Turkey, *A. culicifacies* in the Indian subcontinent (now known to be a complex of at least three sibling species), *A. sinensis* in China, and *A. stephensi* in Iraq, Iran, Pakistan, and India. These complicated resistances have been attributed in some instances, particularly in *A. albimanus*, *A. sacharovi*, and *A. sinensis*, to the contamination of the mosquito breeding places by drift from the numerous different insecticides used for agricultural purposes (mainly against pests of cotton and rice).

OTHER CONTROL MEASURES. Environmental measures, e.g., water management aimed at the removal or alteration of existing breeding places, are alternatives to chemicals. Biologic control agents and genetic control methods have also been used. Of the biologic methods, the greatest emphasis has been on the use of larvivorous fish and the bacterial agent *B.t.i.* Various fish have been tried, of which *G. affinis* is the best known. Where breeding places are suitable for the fish and are the main or only sources of the mosquitoes, they have proved useful. Some 30 countries are using fish alone or as part of an integrated program of mosquito control. *B.t.i.* has proved efficient in both the laboratory and field against anophelines. Two trials of genetic control of anophelines have been done. The first involved the release of sterile hybrid males produced by crossing two sibling species of the *A. gambiae* complex against a third species of the same complex in an isolated village in Upper Volta in West Africa. It was unsuccessful because the sterile males failed to mate with the wild females. A larger trial with *A. albimanus* in Central America had some success. Sterilization was achieved by immersing pupae in the chemosterilant bisazir. At the peak of the trial, >1 million sterile males were released daily in an area of 150 km². Eradication was not achieved, however.

Aedes Species. *Ae. aegypti* (Figs. 138–3 and 139–5) is the most important vector and has been responsible for nearly all urban epidemics of yellow fever, dengue, and dengue hemorrhagic fever. *Ae. albopictus* is mainly involved with dengue transmission in Southeast Asia and the western Pacific. *Ae. simpsoni* is widespread in Africa and is a vector of yellow fever. *Ae. polynesiensis*, *Ae. pseudoscutellaris*, *Ae. vigilax*, *Ae. niveus*, and *Ae. togoi* all are vectors of filariasis (bancroftian and brugian) in the Far East. All breed in small collections of water, natural (e.g., leaf axils or crab holes) or artificial (e.g., tin cans or discarded tires). The adults are largely day feeders and have a limited flight range.

CHEMICAL CONTROL. These measures are directed more toward larval breeding places and their vicinity (perifocal spraying in the case of the domestic *Ae. aegypti*) or toward exterior space spraying rather than house spraying. Nonpotable water may be treated with malathion, fenitrothion, fen-

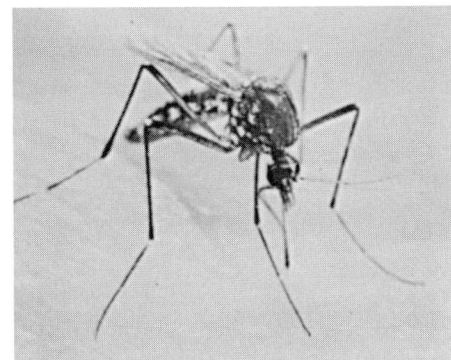

***Figure* 139–5.** *Aedes aegypti.*

thion, temephos, pirimiphos-methyl, or methoprene applied as solutions, emulsions, or granules. For potable water, only temephos in the form of 1% sand granules is used at a dose of 1 mg/L. Hand or power sprayers are used to apply the insecticides as a peripheral spray in and around nonpotable water containers and adjacent surfaces. The resulting insecticide residue is supposed to destroy present and subsequent larval infestations as well as adults that frequent the sites. A syringe or pipette can be used for treating indoor or outdoor flowerpots and ant traps. Exterior space treatments may be from the ground or from the air and are justifiable where epidemic conditions prevail. Malathion, naled, fenitrothion, and pirimiphos-methyl all have been used from thermal fog and ULV machines and are best applied up to a 400-m radius from houses.

Many of the common *Aedes* species show resistance to both organochlorines and organophosphates, and pyrethroid resistance occurs in *Ae. aegypti* in Thailand.

BIOLOGIC CONTROL. Most biologic control methods operate against the larval stages of mosquitoes. The problem in the case of *Aedes* species, which inhabit small collections of water, is delivering the agent to the breeding place. The larva of the large nonbiting *Toxorhynchites* mosquito occurring naturally in some *Aedes* habitats is an efficient predator.

GENETIC CONTROL. These methods, some highly sophisticated, have been tried in limited field trials against *Ae. aegypti* in India and Africa. They have included the release of males sterilized by irradiation and chemosterilants and the release of males carrying translocated chromosomes and meiotic-drive sex-ratio distortion systems.

The obvious solution to control of *Aedes* species that breed in small, usually synthetic containers is proper disposal of such containers. A piped water supply to houses eliminates the necessity for water storage in pots.

Other *Aedes* species (e.g., *Ae. nigromaculis*, *Ae. sollicitans*, and *Ae. taeniorhynchus* in the United States and *Ae. caspius*, *Ae. detritus*, and *Ae. cantans* in Europe) breed in extensive marshy sites, often coastal, brackish, and subject to periodic drying and flooding. Eggs laid in the dry season remain viable until the following rainy season. Insecticides or insect growth regulators must be delivered in a form (e.g., granules) that will remain active and release the compound when flooding occurs.

A new group of nontoxic synthetic materials called superabsorbent polymers have proved effective in field trials as controlled-release larvicides. One of these polymers, Culigel, when introduced into standing water at 5.5 kg/hectare, absorbs water and swells to form a hydrogel from which microbial, insect growth regulators, or other surface film can diffuse out. In granular, pellet, or briquette form, this material can be used in tires, potholes, and basins that are dry at

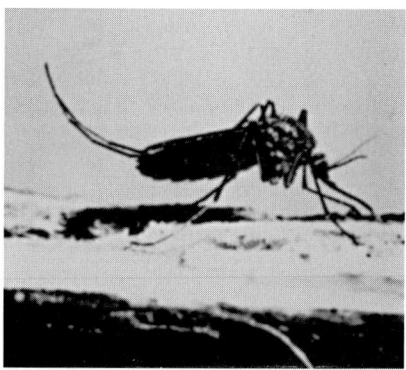

Figure 139–6. Culicine mosquito.

the time of application but flood later, thus activating the substance. After these areas dry out again, the hydrogel persists until reactivated by the next flooding.

Culex Species (Fig. 139–6). The common tropical house mosquito *C. quinquefasciatus,* which is found all over the world, is a vector of bancroftian filariasis in many urban areas. Its near relative of more temperate climates, *C. pipiens,* has been linked with the transmission of epidemic Rift Valley fever. Other vectors include *C. tritaeniorhynchus,* which transmits Japanese encephalitis in the Far East; *C. tarsalis,* which transmits St. Louis encephalitis in the United States; and *C. annulirostris,* which transmits Murray Valley encephalitis and Ross River fever in Australia.

INSECTICIDES. Methods for the control of *Culex* species are usually directed against the aquatic stages rather than the adult. Many species that habitually bite humans breed in well-defined waters, often heavily polluted and quite near habitations (e.g., cesspools and open drains). Control by prevention of access to or by removal or treatment of these breeding places is often relatively simple; the difficulty lies in locating them. In general, insecticidal emulsions, suspensions, and pellets are better larvicides than oil solutions, especially where organic matter in the water prevents the spread of oil. Higher doses than those used for the control of anopheline larvae are usually required, and allowance must be made for the effects of dilution in deep water, because culicines are not as confined to surface feeding as anophelines. Organophosphates, especially chlorpyrifos, are particularly effective in highly polluted water. In addition, tetramethrin among the pyrethroids, methoprene and diflubenzuron, Flit MLO, malariol, gas oil, and Paris green all have been used successfully against *C. quinquefasciatus* in polluted drains and pit latrines.

For those species that occupy extensive breeding areas (e.g., *C. tritaeniorhynchus,* typically a rice field breeder, and *C. tarsalis*), dusts, fogs, and ULV applications are used from ground-based equipment or from the air.

Organochlorine and organophosphate resistances are common in all the *Culex* species except *C. annulirostris. C. pipiens* and *C. quinquefasciatus* also show resistance to many organophosphates and carbamates, and resistance to methoprene and pyrethroids has been produced in the laboratory. Organophosphate resistance also occurs in *C. tritaeniorhynchus* and *C. tarsalis.*

ENVIRONMENTAL CONTROL. Environmental measures against *C. pipiens* and *C. quinquefasciatus* involve proper construction of sewage systems and prevention of access to them by gravid female mosquitoes. Pit latrines should have tight-fitting lids and screened vent pipes. Soakage pits and roadside drains should also be covered; a useful safeguard in

such closed systems is the hanging at intervals of plastic strips impregnated with the volatile organophosphate dichlorvos. Expanded polystyrene beads in sufficient quantity to cover the water surface completely have proved an extremely efficient way of preventing pit-latrine breeding, and a single application can last for years. Small collections of water near houses should always be discouraged.

BIOLOGIC CONTROL. Biologic control methods have included the use of predatory fish. *Poecilia reticulata* can survive high degrees of pollution. Pathogens tried on a small scale include *B. thuringiensis israelensis,* microsporidia, and the mermithid worm *Romanomermis culicivorax.*

GENETIC CONTROL. Many attempts have been made to control *C. quinquefasciatus* by genetic means. The phenomenon of cytoplasmic incompatibility is exhibited in this species and *C. pipiens* and consists of different strains of the Rickettsiaceae *Wolbachia pipientis* occurring in the cytoplasm of the different populations. Sperm die in the cytoplasm of the ovum of incompatible females. Control can be achieved by the release of incompatible males. The release of males sterilized by irradiation or chemosterilants has also been tried with some success, as has the release of males carrying translocated chromosomes. A combination of the latter with cytoplasmic incompatibility (an "integrated" strain) has shown great promise.

Mansonia Species. Several species of *Mansonia* are important vectors of filariasis, transmitting both *Wuchereria bancrofti* and *Brugia malayi. M. uniformis* is the most widely distributed species. The larvae and pupae of this genus attach themselves to the roots of aquatic plants (e.g., *Pistia, Eichornia, Scirpus,* and *Salvinia*) and breathe through the air system of the plant. Control is usually directed toward destruction of the plants with herbicides, which are generally applied from ground equipment, with the spray directed vertically onto the plants. In the case of *Pistia,* treatment should be done before seed formation. Two annual applications usually suffice.

The adults of some species (e.g., *M. uniformis* and *M. annulifera*) rest in houses and can be controlled by house spraying in the same way as endophilic anophelines. Organochlorine resistance is known in *M. indiana, M. annulifera,* and *M. uniformis* in Thailand.

Sandflies (Order Diptera, Family Psychodidae) (Fig. 139–7). These delicate moth flies, the vectors of leishmaniasis, bartonellosis, and viral sandfly fever, either may be outdoor feeders and resters or may frequent the indoors. The latter type are readily controlled when houses are sprayed with residual insecticides, although this is seldom done specifically for sandfly control. Where outside resting places are well known, such as termite hills in the case of *Phlebotomus*

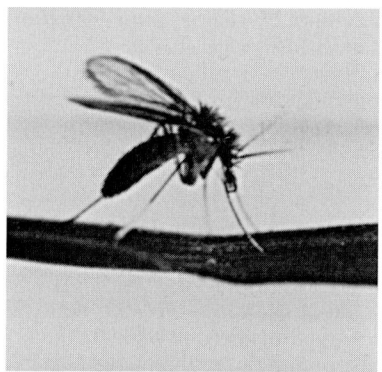

Figure 139–7. Sandfly.

martini, a vector of kala-azar in Kenya (Chapter 95), these may also be treated with residual insecticides. The larval habitat is often difficult to identify, and measures against it are seldom attempted. The use of mosquito repellents and sandfly nets (which have smaller holes than mosquito netting and are more uncomfortable in hot climates) provide personal protection. Larger mesh that has been treated with repellents or insecticide is more comfortable and works well.

Resistance to DDT, the first example of insecticide resistance in sandflies, has been established in *P. papatasi* in North Bihar. However, *P. argentipes* is the vector of kala-azar in this area.

Houseflies, Related Flies, and Stable Flies (Order Diptera, Family Muscidae). The synanthropic (associated with humans) flies include not only species in the family Muscidae but also some of those species in the families Calliphoridae and Sarcophagidae that breed on carrion and that cause myiasis. The Muscidae include the common housefly *(Musca domestica)* (Figs. 138–5 and 139–8), the greater housefly *(Muscina stabulans)*, the lesser housefly *(Fannia canicularis)*, the latrine fly *(Fannia scalaris)*, and the bloodsucking stable fly *(Stomoxys calcitrans)*. Because of their habits of visiting both excreta and food and their regurgitatory feeding methods, these flies may be mechanical vectors of viral, bacterial, protozoan, and helminthic diseases.

Breeding Sites. These flies prefer the excreta of humans or their domestic animals, decomposing animal or vegetable matter, and farm manure for egg laying and larval breeding. Control measures (e.g., construction of closed sewage disposal systems and correct disposal of animal excreta and refuse) are largely directed toward the prevention of access to this excreta or refuse so that it is no longer available for breeding. Good standards of hygiene and sanitation are basic to fly control and are becoming more important because these insects have developed resistance to a wide variety of chemicals. The common housefly has more resistant populations to more groups of insecticides than any other insect species. Populations present in both the Old World and the New World are resistant to organochlorines, organophosphates, carbamates, pyrethroids, and insect growth regulators. A particularly disturbing feature is cross-resistance between a certain type of DDT resistance and the new synthetic residual pyrethroids.

Indoor Control. Screening denies flies access to both food and potential breeding areas. A 10-mesh net from 32 SWG wire or plastic with an aperture of 2.17 mm is adequate. Particularly attractive items of foodstuffs, (e.g., milk and sugar) may need their own gauze protection. Occasional invaders of screened premises can be dealt with by insecticidal space sprays, sticky traps (fly papers), electrocution traps (usually an ultraviolet lamp behind an electrified grid), electric vaporizers (a small electrically heated surface to which

insecticide can be added), or residual fumigants (polyvinyl chloride strips impregnated with a volatile insecticide, usually dichlorvos). There may, however, be objection to the last two methods on the grounds of overconcentration of toxic insecticide in small enclosed domestic premises. Space sprays are usually composed of 0.035 to 0.1% pyrethrins in deodorized kerosene with a residual insecticide added. A simple contribution that householders can make to prevention of fly breeding is the addition every week or two of 60 g of *para*-dichlorobenzene to the garbage can.

Surface spraying of residual insecticides is directed against those areas where flies tend to congregate rather than against the entire insides of houses, as is usually done for the control of endophilic mosquitoes. Places sprayed to control adult flies include doors, windows, sills, and some of the outside surfaces of houses, kitchens, porches, latrines, animal shelters, and fences as well as around the grids of drains. Larval control is aimed at refuse dumps and accumulations of animal excrement and their vicinity. Spraying such dumps does not always kill breeding fly larvae but does kill flies attempting to lay their eggs and new adults as they emerge. It must be emphasized, however, that no insecticidal treatment can replace efficient methods of rubbish and excrement disposal.

At present, emphasis is on the use of organophosphates for fly control, with some restrictions on their use in milk rooms (dairy barns), restaurants, food-processing plants, and food stores. There are no restrictions on the use of bromophos, fenchlorphos, fenitrothion, jodfenphos, trichlorphon, pirimiphos-methyl, diazinon, or malathion. Dimethoate and naled (Dibrom) should not be used in milk rooms, although the latter is considered safe enough to spray in poultry houses without removing the birds. It is helpful to add attractants (e.g., sugar or molasses) to these insecticides.

Cords and strips impregnated with insecticide and hung high in infested buildings are an accepted form of control. Five millimeter cords dipped in 25% diazinon-xylene solution and installed at the rate of 1 m of cord/m² of floor area are effective for several months. Care is needed in the handling and preparation of these cords (gloves are essential). They should be marked to show what they are and to prevent their being used for other purposes.

Both organophosphates and carbamates have been incorporated in liquid (0.1 to 0.2% insecticide) and dry (1 to 2% insecticide) baits for spot treatments against flies. Dichlorvos, methomyl, and trichlorphon are the most widely used insecticides for this purpose, with the bait being some form of sugar or perhaps the housefly pheromone muscalure. Viscous paint-on baits are also used and are composed of an insecticide (2 to 6%), a binder, and sugar. These are applied by paintbrush as spot treatments to posts and walls.

Outdoor Control. Outdoor space treatments may be necessary where fly populations are excessive, especially during epidemics of enteric diseases. They are also useful in market areas where foods are on display and in large human assemblies. Power units are usually used to produce ULV mist sprays or thermal aerosols. The latter have the disadvantage of reducing visibility in traffic areas. The equipment is often mounted on vehicles that move at 8 to 16 km/hr and dispense the formulations at 24 to 48 L/km. Application rates of organophosphates vary from 200 to 700 g/hectare. The synthetic pyrethroids are also effective in ULV applications.

Triatomine Bugs (Order Hemiptera, Family Reduviidae) (Fig. 139–9). Variously known as cone-nose bugs, assassin bugs, barbeiros, kissing bugs, or vinchucas, several species are carriers of Chagas disease in Mexico and Central and South America. The main genera concerned in the transmission of the disease to humans are *Triatoma, Panstrongylus,*

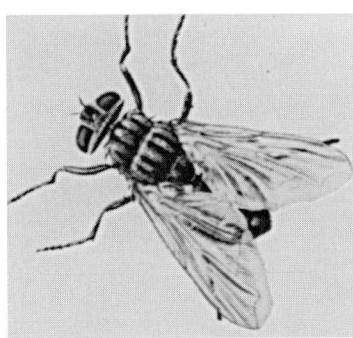

Figure 139–8. Housefly.

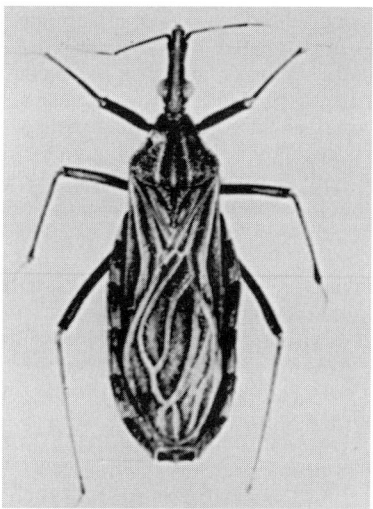

Figure 139–9. Triatomine bug.

and *Rhodnius.* Numerous animal species such as armadillos, opossums, domestic and wild rodents, birds, dogs, and squirrels act as reservoirs of the disease.

These bugs dwell in cracks and crevices in human habitations and in animal haunts and bird nests. House spraying with residual insecticides with special attention to cracks and crevices (pyrethroids may be added to flush them out) is the usual method of control. This is often combined with treatment of peridomestic sites of infestation (e.g., chicken houses, pigeon lofts, and piggeries). HCH and permethrin at doses used for malaria control, have been used rather than DDT. Dieldrin is no longer recommended for domestic use, and resistance to it and to HCH has been recorded in Venezuela. Organophosphates, carbamates, and residual pyrethroids all are possible alternatives. Plastering wall cracks and elimination of thatch roofs are encouraged. The scelionid parasitic wasp. *Telenomus fariai,* is an effective natural enemy.

Bedbugs (Order Hemiptera, Family Cimicidae) (Figs. 138–1 and 139–10). Strictly nocturnal, these bloodsucking insects spend their daylight hours in cracks and crevices in walls, floors, and roofs, behind pictures, and in bed springs, slats, mattresses, and furniture. Sprays of residual insecticides directed at these daytime resting places constitute the best method of control and will give good control for several weeks. The addition of 0.1 or 0.2% pyrethrins or synthetic pyrethroids (e.g., bioresmethrin) flushes the bugs from their hiding places, causing them to come into contact with the

residuals. Resistance to the original residual, a 5% DDT emulsion or solution, has forced a change to 0.5% lindane or, where resistance to both groups of organochlorines is evident, to 2% malathion, 1% pirimiphosmethyl, fenchlorphos, carbaryl, or propoxur, or 0.5% diazinon. Some *Cimex lectularius* have developed organophosphate resistance, but control is still satisfactory with the carbamates carbaryl and propoxur. Infants' beds and bedding should not be treated with residual insecticides. Care must be taken in applying these chemicals to adults' bedding.

When spray treatments are not desirable, infestations may be eliminated by fumigation with hydrogen cyanide (using 280 g of sodium or calcium cyanide per 28 m³ of space). While traveling, it is advisable to carry a small bottle of pyrethrum powder to be sprinkled over the bed under the sheets if bedbugs are suspected or found in the room. This treatment usually gives protection from bites for the night.

Fleas (Order Siphonaptera) (Fig. 139–11). Adult fleas are transient ectoparasites of animals, whereas the immature stages live in the nests, burrows, or other resting places of the animals. Control is directed more against the latter than the former, preferably with dusts containing residual insecticides. While killing the fleas, the dusts also contaminate the animal host; in sufficient concentration, they may kill the animal. In plague and murine typhus control, it is important to kill the fleas before the rats. Killing rats by rodenticides alone may cause disease-carrying fleas to move from rodents to humans. Dusts commonly used are 2% concentrations of diazinon, fenitrothion, and pirimiphos-methyl; 3% γ HCH; 5% carbaryl, malathion, and propoxur; and 10% DDT. They are directed against the resting places and runs of the animals. Resistance to the organochlorines is known in several species, including three species of *Xenopsylla.*

The fleas of domestic pets are a modern nuisance, especially in homes with central heating and fitted carpets. Regular vacuum cleaning helps to reduce infestations, but application of insecticides to the animal and to its kennel and bedding may be necessary. Care must be taken in applying insecticides to pets, however, especially cats, which lick their fur, and young animals. Pyrethrum dust (0.2% pyrethrins + 2% synergist) is safer than the synthetic residual insecticides for this purpose. Plastic collars impregnated with the volatile organophosphate dichlorvos or pyrethroids have proved useful for both cats and dogs.

Cockroaches (Order Orthoptera). Cockroaches are habitually associated with dirt, human excrement, and human food and have been suspected of transmitting diseases. An estimated 16 species are involved in different parts of the world. The three most common ones in temperate climates are the Oriental (*Blatta orientalis),* the German (*Blatella germanica)* (Fig. 139–12), and the American (*Periplaneta americana)* cockroaches. The tropical cockroaches include some large species in the genus *Blaberus.* Those of most concern to humans are

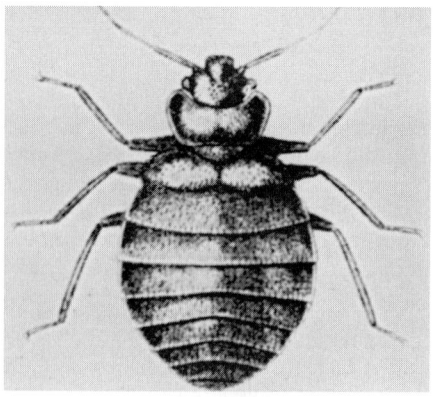

Figure 139–10. Bedbug.

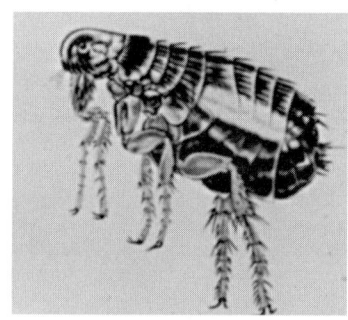

Figure 139–11. Flea.

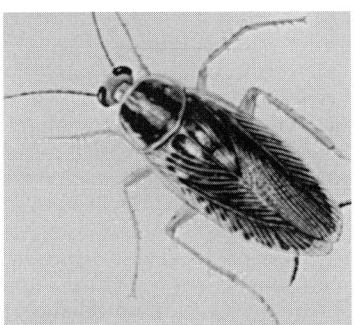

***Figure* 139–12.** German cockroach.

associated with sewage systems, food stores, and home and restaurant kitchens.

Control should be directed toward denying the insects access to food, sewage, and dirt, including strict cleanliness of food stores and kitchens and proper sealing of service ducts supplying these premises. Insecticides should be used with care to prevent food contamination. Chemical control is usually directed at the specific runs and resting places of the insects—that is, around baseboards and door frames; under fixed furniture, sinks, stoves, and refrigerators; in cupboards and drawers; around and beneath dustbins and drain grids; and in and around cracks and crevices. The formulations used may be liquid sprays, lacquers, or gels; dusts; or baits. Sprays and dusts are favored for good penetration into small spaces; sprays are less unsightly, whereas dusts require less elaborate machinery to apply. Lacquers or gels include insecticide dissolved in urea-formaldehyde resins or methylcellulose and are painted in bands on appropriate places (e.g., on baseboards and around door frames) where insects are likely to cross. Baits are usually combinations of insecticide, cereal, and some form of sugar. Jodfenphos (an organophosphate), hydromethylnon, and avermectin are the favored insecticides for baits, but boric acid seems to be equally popular. Organophosphates, carbamates, and the pyrethroid permethrin are also used for cockroach control. Organochlorine resistance is common in all three main species of cockroaches, with some species also resistant to organophosphates, carbamates, and the pyrethroids.

Alternatives to chemical control are under investigation. Pheromone attractants used in trapping devices seem particularly promising. Formulations of insect growth regulators (i.e., hydroprene or fenoxycarb) will reduce cockroach populations over long periods and are most appropriately used after heavy infestations have been reduced by other control methods. Genetic control methods involving chromosome translocations that produce partial sterility are being developed in *B. germanica*. Also, several species of parasitic wasps have been suggested as a biologic means for controlling cockroaches. The egg parasite *Comperia merceti* has given practical control of the brown-banded cockroach.

Tsetse Flies (Order Diptera, Family Glossinidae) (Fig. 139–13). Tsetse flies are confined to tropical Africa, where five species are responsible for the transmission of human sleeping sickness and ten for the transmission of trypanosomal diseases of animals. The adult fly is the only stage amenable to vector control measures; the transient larval stage buries itself in the soil to pupate. Fortunately, all species remain susceptible to insecticides, which, distributed from the air or the ground, have led to control and even complete eradication of tsetse flies from large areas. DDT, HCH, dieldrin, and endosulfan have been used, with the last two being preferred. The use of organophosphates, carbamates, and

pyrethroids is now being considered to alleviate the fear of environmental pollution from the widespread use of organochlorines.

Spraying. Two spraying techniques have been developed. One aims at producing residual deposits of insecticides on the known resting sites of adult flies. The vegetation bordering rivers and streams favored by the sleeping sickness vectors, *Glossina palpalis* and *G. tachinoides*, can be sprayed with a conventional knapsack sprayer. For control of the savanna-type species (e.g., the *G. morsitans* group responsible for animal trypanosomiasis), those parts of trees and bushes that the flies favor as resting places are selectively sprayed. Thus, in northern Nigeria, only certain branches of the doka tree at certain heights and angles are sprayed with residual insecticides. A more indiscriminate spraying technique uses aerial application as either an aerosol or a ULV spray. Repeated applications by this method are necessary because the pupal stage, which can last as long as 5 weeks, is not affected. In Botswana, for example, endosulfan has been applied from fixed-wing aircraft five times at 21-day intervals at a total cost for fly eradication of 70 to 75 dollars/km².

Trapping. The use of trapping devices impregnated with insecticide has had success in the control of riverine tsetse fly species in West Africa, where biconical traps impregnated with deltamethrin have reduced fly populations by >99%. Commonly, visual (the colors royal blue or black) and/or olfactory (bovine urine, carbon dioxide, acetone, 4-methyl phenol or octenol) attractants are used to improve the performance of traps treated with a lethal insecticide. Costs are low, and there are no harmful environmental effects.

Genetic Control. Genetic control by the release of mass-reared male flies sterilized by irradiation or by exposure to chemosterilants has been tried against both savanna and riverine tsetse fly species with some success, but difficulties in mass production of these male flies pose problems for large-scale application.

Environmental Control. Vegetation clearance can also lead to the disappearance of tsetse flies, especially when followed by human occupation and use of reclaimed land.

Horseflies and Deer Flies (Order Diptera, Family Tabanidae). Control of these biting flies, including the vectors of tularemia and loiasis (Fig. 139–14), is seldom attempted because of their extensive and often ill-defined breeding places, usually in marshy areas but sometimes in environments with relatively dry soil. Effective trapping devices treated with the

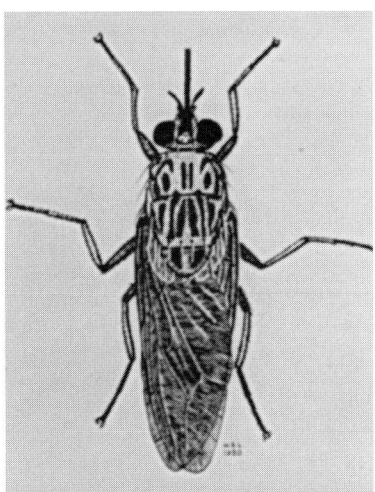

***Figure* 139–13.** Tsetse fly.

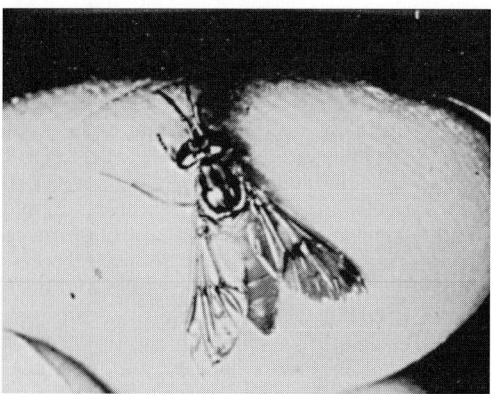

Figure 139–14. *Chrysops dimidiata* (tabanid).

attractant octenol can catch adults, but significant control with them is doubtful. Deet is fairly effective as a repellent.

Black Flies (Figs. 139–8; Fig. 139–15) **or Buffalo Gnats (Order Diptera, Family Simuliidae).** The immature stages of these flies characteristically breed in rapidly flowing water. The adults, which are outdoor daytime biters, are often numerous. They are a tremendous nuisance to humans and animals not only in the tropics, where they may be vectors of onchocerciasis, but also in colder parts of the world (e.g., northern Canada and Siberia).

Individual protection can have an important role when encountering black flies. A double layer of clothing, however light, is desirable, with the clothing secured at boot tops, neck, and wrists. Gloves and head veils should also be worn, if possible. Locating tents or camps on high, dry, and windy spots, away from underbrush, lessens attacks.

Control is usually directed against the aquatic stages, using insecticides delivered at the water head in quantities sufficient to give concentrations downstream of 0.01 to 5 parts per million for periods of 5 to 30 minutes. The actual quantities required depend on the depth and flow rate of the water. Delivery may be by drip feed, from fixed-wing aircraft flying across the water source, or from helicopters. DDT, which was used initially, has been largely replaced by the environmentally safe methoxychlor and temephos (Abate).

The onchocerciasis control program of the Volta River basin in West Africa, which was started in 1975, covers an area of 700,000 km². Of the 10 million inhabitants there, about 1 million were afflicted with onchocerciasis, with some 70,000 being either blind or nearly so. Resistance to temephos and to the substitute chlorphoxim has occured in some parts of

the area in some species of the *Simulium damnosum* complex but has so far been satisfactorily dealt with by a change to permethrin in the rainy season and to serotype H14 of *B. thuringiensis israelensis* in the dry season. This program, which is very expensive, must be continued for as many years as it takes for the adult worm *(O. volvulus)* to die out in the human population. Some success in control of the adult flies has been obtained with the use of aerosols and ULV sprays applied to vegetation bordering breeding areas.

Black flies are less easily repelled by deet than are mosquitoes, but considerable relief has been obtained by those wearing special jackets impregnated with the repellent.

Biting Midges or No-See-Ums (Order Diptera, Family Ceratopogonidae). The true biting midges, including the genera *Culicoides* (Fig. 139–16), *Leptoconops,* and *Styloconops,* are not known to be of great importance as disease vectors. However, they constitute severe biting nuisances because they occur in large numbers and are small enough to pass through the finest house screening and sandfly netting. Because these midges do not rest indoors for long periods, house spraying with residual insecticides does not contribute to their control, although painting screens with insecticides is useful. The treatment of nets with repellent or permethrin aerosol may also be helpful.

Breeding grounds, almost invariably extensive swampy areas, can be controlled by drainage or insecticide treatment. This is extremely expensive, as is repetitive use of thermal fogs or ULV applications in attempts to kill adult midges resting in vegetation.

Ticks (Order Metastigmata, Families Argasidae and Ixodidae). Ticks are vectors of many viral, rickettsial, and bacterial diseases. Most ticks parasitize a wide range of host animals. Each stage, the larva, nymph, and both sexes of adult, requires a blood meal. They often remain attached to the host animal for long periods and are usually difficult to remove because their mouth parts become fully embedded. Simple pulling often leaves these parts behind, causing irritation and secondary infection. They can be best removed carefully using tweezers.

Personal protection starts with tucking the pants legs into socks, making a continuous barricade that prevents ticks from reaching the skin. In addition, clothing should be

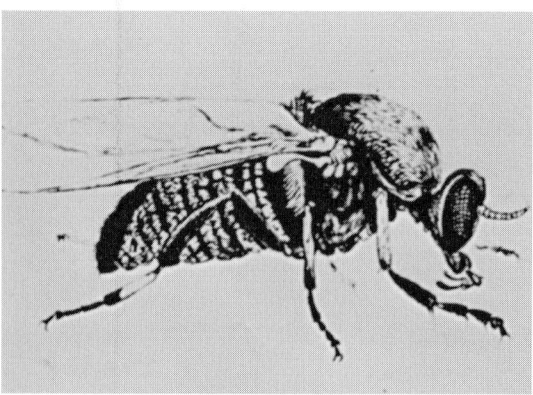

Figure 139–15. Black fly *(Simulium)*.

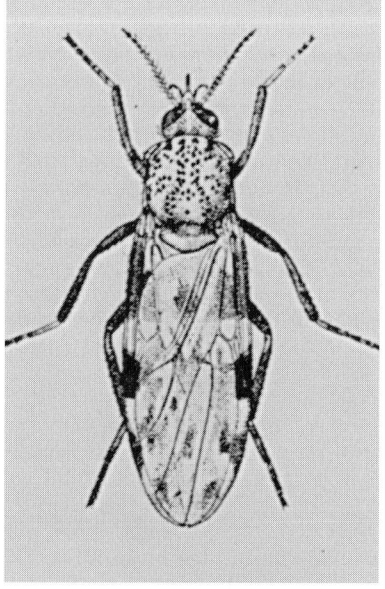

Figure 139–16. *Culicoides.*

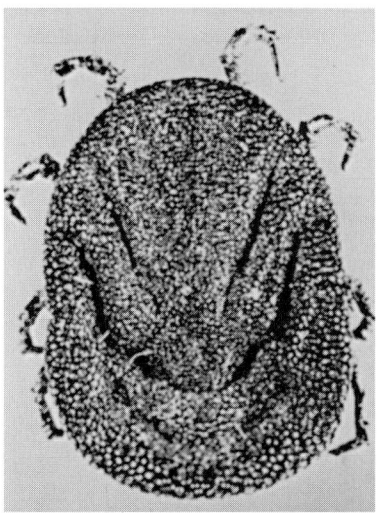

Figure 139–17. Soft tick (*Ornithodoros*).

treated with permethrin aerosol. Repellents such as dimethyl phthalate, dibutyl phthalate, and deet can prevent infestation and are strongly recommended for those exposed to infested vegetation. Performing a thorough visual check of one's body after leaving a tick-infested area is one of the most effective ways to prevent tick-borne diseases. Many ticks search the body for several hours before becoming attached and potentially transmitting disease agents. Therefore, a thorough examination of the entire body at the end of each day is recommended to decrease the chance of disease transmission.

Soft Ticks. The soft ticks (Argasidae) include the vectors (*Ornithodoros* species [Fig. 139–17]) of relapsing fever caused by *Borrelia (Treponema) duttonii*. These ticks live in the earthen floors of houses and manmade or natural shelters for animals. Control can be achieved by spraying or dusting infested areas with residual insecticides. γ HCH is a favored one, and the highest dose (3 g/m²) is claimed to last as long as 1 year. There is no evidence yet of resistance in this genus.

Hard Ticks. The hard ticks (Ixodidae) (Fig. 139–18) include vectors of Lyme disease, ehrlichiosis, Colorado tick fever, Rocky Mountain spotted fever, the tick-borne encephalitis of central Europe, Kyasanur Forest disease, certain hemorrhagic fevers, and tularemia. The genera *Ixodes, Dermacentor, Haemaphysalis, Hyalomma, Amblyomma, Rhipicephalus,* and *Boophilus*

are involved in their transmission. Primarily ectoparasites of domestic animals and pets, particularly dogs, these ticks can be controlled by treating the animals with insecticide washes, sprays, dips, or dusts or by treating the tick haunts (e.g., pasture vegetation or animal sleeping areas). Large-scale exterior treatments with ground and aerially produced fogs or ULV sprays are sometimes necessary. Tick invasion of houses may also necessitate spot applications to baseboards, floors, and wall cracks.

Organochlorines, organophosphates, carbamates, chlordimeform, and pyrethroids all have been used for tick control, with resistance to the first three of these groups now common in a number of genera and species. Some of the new synthetic pyrethroids, especially deltamethrin, permethrin, and cypermethrin, are proving to be efficient alternatives, although cross-resistance between DDT and pyrethroids has been established in *Boophilus microplus* in Australia.

Scrub Typhus Mites (Order Prostigmata, Family Trombiculidae). The medically important species belong to the genera *Leptotrombidium* and *Trombicula,* (e.g., *T. alfreddugesi, L. akamushi* and the *L. deliense* group of species). They are vectors of scrub typhus caused by *Rickettsia tsutsugamushi*, a disease restricted to Southeast and East Asia, northern Australia, and most of the islands located between these areas. Only the larval stage (Fig. 139–19) is parasitic, and normally it feeds only once in its life.

Control is directed against infested terrain, usually by spraying with a residual insecticide such as HCH, malathion, or propoxur. Dieldrin is extremely effective but is generally proscribed because of environmental toxicity. Personal protection against these and related mites is afforded by repellents, particularly dibutyl phthalate, diethyltoluamide, and benzyl benzoate, applied either to the skin or to the clothing of areas likely to be bitten, e.g., the legs.

Stinging and Biting Arthropods (Scorpions, Centipedes, Spiders, Bees, Wasps, and Caterpillars). Arthropod venoms applied to the body can produce bodily pain and illness in a number of ways: (1) by stinging (i.e., penetrating the skin with an organ located near the tip of the abdomen), (2) by biting (i.e., with the mouthparts), (3) by nettling with hollow poison hairs located on the dorsal surface of certain caterpillars, (4) by applying of caustic or corrosive fluids to the skin, and (5) by poisoning when accidentally swallowed (Chapter 128).

Spiders and other crawling arthropods (i.e., centipedes and scorpions) are best controlled by residual applications of 0.5% chlorpyrifos or diazinon, 1.0% propoxur, or 0.25% bendiocarb sprayed directly on floors and walls, inside latrines, and on other areas harboring pests. These treatments should remain effective for periods as long as a month or more. Bee swarms

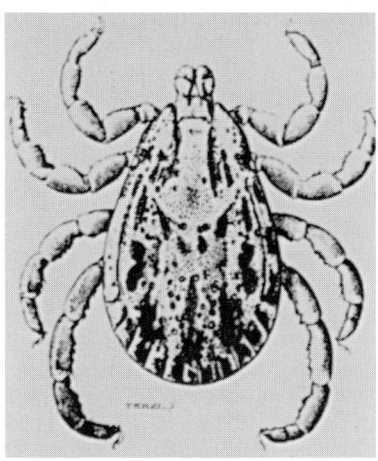

Figure 139–18. Hard tick.

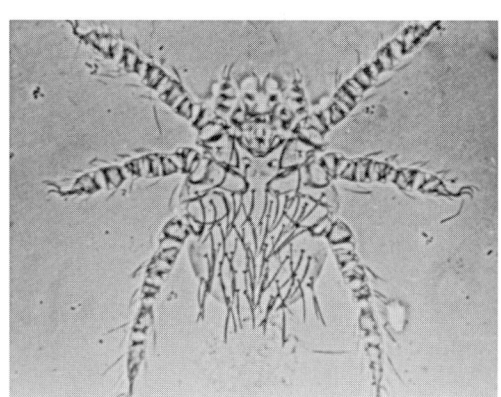

Figure 139–19. Scrub typhus mite larva.

are a common sight in certain parts of the tropics. Bees are not defensive when swarming and are easily eliminated with approved insecticides or by spraying with a 5% soapy water solution. A high volume of spray achieves the best effect.

Bibliography

Burges HD, Fontaine RE, Nalim S, et al: World Health Organization research on the biocontrol of vectors of disease: Present status and plans for the future. *In* Laird M (ed): Biocontrol of Medical and Veterinary Pests. New York, Praeger Publishers, 1981.

Burgess NRH, Cowan GO: A Colour Atlas of Medical Entomology. London, Chapman & Hall Medical, 1993.

Busvine JR: Insects and Hygiene, 3rd ed. London, Chapman & Hall, 1980.

Chemical Methods for the Control of Arthropod Vectors and Pests of Public Health Importance. Geneva, World Health Organization, 1984.

Clark GG (ed): Prevention of Tropical Diseases: Status of New and Emerging Vector Control Strategies. Am J Trop Med Hyg 50(Suppl):1, 1994.

Crampton JM, Warren A, Lycett GJ, et al: Genetic manipulation of insect vectors as a strategy for the control of vector-borne disease. Am Trop Med Parasitol 88:3, 1994.

Davidson G: Insecticides. Bulletin No. 1. London, The Ross Institute, London School of Hygiene and Tropical Medicine, 1988.

Eldridge BF, Service MW (eds): Vector control without chemicals: Has it a future? A symposium. J Am Mosq Control Assoc 11:247, 1995.

Environmental Management for Vector Control. Fifth report of the WHO Expert Committee on Vector Biology and Control. WHO Tech Rep Ser No. 649, 1980.

Equipment for Vector Control, 3rd ed. Geneva, World Health Organization, 1990.

Hayes LT, Laws ER: Handbook of Pesticide Toxicology, Vol 1. San Diego, Academic Press, 1991.

Kettle DS: Medical and Veterinary Entomology. New York, John Wiley & Sons, 1984.

Matthews GA: Pesticide Application Methods. London, Longman, 1979.

Metcalf RL, Metcalf RA: Destructive and Useful Insects: Their Habits and Control, 5th ed. New York, McGraw-Hill, 1993.

Olkowski W, Daar S, Olkowski H: Common-Sense Pest Control. Newtown, Taunton Press, 1991.

Safe Use of Pesticides. 14th Report of the WHO Expert Committee on Vector Biology and Control. WHO Tech Rep Ser No. 813, 1991.

Service MW: A Guide to Medical Entomology. London, Macmillan, 1980.

Specifications for Pesticides Used in Public Health, 5th ed. Geneva, World Health Organization, 1979.

The WHO Recommended Classification of Pesticides by Hazard and Guidelines to Classification 1988–1989. Division of Vector Biology and Control. WHO/VBC/88.953. Geneva, World Health Organization, 1988.

Vector Control: Guide to chemical methods for the control of vectors and pests. WHO Wkly Epidemiol Rec 60:218, 1985.

Vector Control for Malaria and other Mosquito-Borne Diseases. Report of a WHO Study Group. WHO Tech Rep Ser No. 857, 1995.

Vector Resistance to Pesticides. 15th report of the WHO Expert Committee on Vector Biology and Control. WHO Tech Rep Ser No. 818, 1992.

140 *General Principles*

Jay S. Keystone

Increasing numbers of North Americans and Europeans are embarking on travel to the developing world for business purposes or in the pursuit of sun, sand, surf, and sex. It has been estimated that >8 million Americans travel to the developing world each year, many of whom are exposed to infectious diseases that occur infrequently, if at all, in North America. For health care providers to advise on appropriate vaccinations and precautions for international travelers, it would be worthwhile for them to know the health risks that their patients are likely to encounter overseas (Chapter 149).

HEALTH RISKS FOR TRAVELERS. Steffen and colleagues in Switzerland have compiled the most comprehensive data on health problems encountered during travel to developing countries. A summary of the results of their 1984 study of more than 10,000 short-term travelers and a review of the medical literature up to 1987 are depicted in Figure 140–1. What is notable about the data in this figure is the absence of "exotic" tropical infections (e.g., filariasis, leishmaniasis, and schistosomiasis). The message here is that helminth in-

fections and other diseases of rural life are rarely acquired by short-term travelers to the developing world. On the other hand, temporary residents such as Peace Corps volunteers and missionaries are at greater risk of acquiring infections endemic in nationals of developing countries.

Traveler's Diarrhea. Traveler's diarrhea affects some 30% to 50% of visitors to developing countries. The highest risk appears to be in Latin America, Asia, the Middle East, and Africa (see Chapter 144). Although enterotoxigenic *Escherichia coli* (ETEC) is the most common cause of traveler's diarrhea globally, studies have shown that various other pathogens, including *Cyclospora* and *Cryptosporidium*, may also have small but important roles. In some areas of the world, depending on the season, *Campylobacter* sp. is a more important cause of traveler's diarrhea than is ETEC. As new causes of traveler's diarrhea are discovered, so are new remedies being made available for prevention and treatment. For instance, the quinolone group of antibiotics is effective in treatment courses as short as one dose and is more effective when combined with an antimotility agent such as loperamide. However, recent studies, particularly in Thailand, have demonstrated significant *Campylobacter* resistance to ciprofloxacin; in this setting, azithromycin was an effective alternative.

Typhoid Fever. The risk of typhoid fever for travelers varies from 0.035 per 1000 short-term (1 month) visitors to developing countries to as high as 12 per 100,000 in travelers to India and Pakistan. Although the efficacy of the new typhoid vaccines approximates that of the older killed vaccines, they are more convenient to administer and have fewer adverse effects. The live attenuated vaccine using the Ty21a mutant of *S. typhi* can be administered orally, whereas the purified Vi-capsular-polysaccharide of *S. typhi* can be given in one intramuscular dose (Chapters 75 and 142).

Hepatitis. The risk of hepatitis of all types has been shown by Steffen and associates to be 1 to 3 per 1000 visitors for a 2- to 3-week stay in a developing country. Another study from Sweden quotes a risk of 6 to 10 cases of hepatitis A per 1000 travelers during a mean stay of 2 weeks. With the declining incidence of hepatitis A in developed countries, it is estimated that < 20% of children born now will have natural antibodies to this infection by the time they are 50 years of age (Chapter 28). Of concern in this older population is the significant risk of death from hepatitis A (3% mortality over the age of 50). The risk of hepatitis A in travelers has been reduced with the introduction of three new safe and effective vaccines that provide prolonged protection (Chapter 142). A combined hepatitis A and B vaccine is now available in many countries.

Human Immunodeficiency Virus Infection and AIDS. The risk of AIDS for visitors to developing countries has not yet been ascertained, but it is certainly a concern for the traveling public. The most likely routes of infection are by blood transfusion after a motor vehicle accident, by injection with contaminated needles and syringes, and by unprotected sexual activity with infected nationals. At the end of 1995, 1.3 million cumulative AIDS cases had been reported from 193 countries (Chapter 22). By the year 2000, the World Health Organization estimates that 26 million persons will be infected with HIV, >90% of whom will be in developing countries (Chapter 149). The infection rate among some prostitute groups currently ranges from 27 to 88% in Africa and is

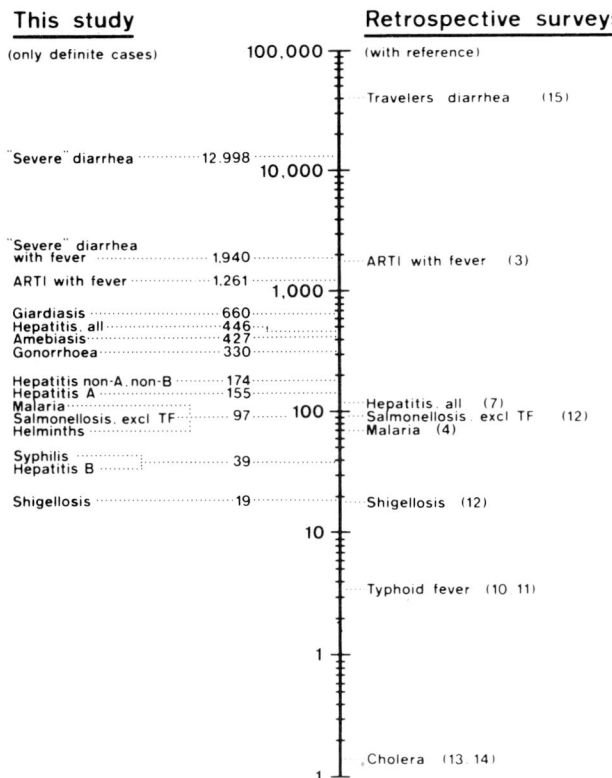

Figure 140–1. Incidence of infections per 100,000 travelers for a stay of 1 month in a developing country. ARTI = acute respiratory tract infection; TF = typhoid fever. (From Steffen R, et al: J Infect Dis 156:84–91, 1987.)

increasing steadily in parts of Asia, notably India and Thailand.

Malaria. The dramatic spread of drug-resistant *Plasmodium falciparum* malaria to almost all areas of the world where the infection is endemic has increased the risk of malaria for travelers. To compound the problem, chloroquine-resistant *Plasmodium vivax* has become an increasing problem in Indonesia, particularly Irian Jaya, and appears to be spreading in Central and South America. Also, for the first time, primaquine-resistant strains from Africa were documented in U.S. soldiers during political unrest in Somalia. Chloroquine-resistant *P. falciparum* malaria, primarily from Africa, continues to be the predominant species of malaria detected among returned U.S. civilians infected abroad (Chapters 92 and 149).

Although mefloquine appears to be the best current choice for malaria prevention, adverse drug effects and increasing *P. falciparum* resistance have thrown some doubt on the usefulness of this drug in the long term. However, recent chemoprophylaxis studies using primaquine, azithromycin, and the atovaquone/proguanil combination have brought renewed hope for the availability of effective and safe drugs to prevent malaria in travelers. Unfortunately, initial evaluations of candidate malaria vaccines have proved disappointing. Personal protection measures against mosquito bites will continue to have an important role in the prevention of malaria.

Motor Vehicle Accidents. Assessment of health risks for travelers to the developing world would be incomplete unless the causes of fatalities during overseas travel were considered. Hargarten and Barker have shown, in a 20-year analysis of Peace Corps volunteers, that 70% and 24% of fatalities were due to unintentional injury and illness, respectively. Motor vehicle accidents accounted for almost 50% of the injury deaths, whereas malaria, rabies, and pneumonia were the most frequent infectious causes of fatal illness. In a broader study looking at deaths of all American travelers during the years 1975 and 1984, the same researchers showed that cardiovascular disease accounted for almost 50% of deaths. Unintentional injury was responsible for 22% and infectious disease for only 1% of deaths. Motor vehicle accidents caused almost one third of the injury deaths. Although the risk of serious injury in a motor vehicle accident is relatively small for most travelers, it is likely to approximate that of serious infectious disease.

INTRODUCTION. The chapters in Part X supply readers with current guidelines for establishing a travel clinic (Chapter 141); for providing pretravel health advice (Chapter 142); and a problem-oriented approach to illness in short-term and long-term (Chapter 143) travelers and to diarrhea (Chapter 144), fever (Chapter 145), dermatitis (Chapter 146), and eosinophilia (Chapter 147) in returning travelers; and for dealing with diseases of immigrants (Chapter 148). The chapter on global epidemiology of infectious disease by those at WHO responsible for this function should assist practitioners in advising travelers of their risks of infectious disease and help in the diagnosis of illness in returning travelers and immigrants (Chapter 149). Because the geographic distribution of diseases in the developing world is constantly changing, as are the drugs and vaccines used to control them, it is wise to have up-to-date information when preparing international travelers for departure and when attending to those who return ill.

Bibliography

Bernard KW, Graitcher PL, Van der Vlugt T, et al: Epidemiological surveillance in Peace Corps volunteers: A model for monitoring health in temporary residents of developing countries. Int J Epidemiol 18:220, 1989.
Hargarten SW, Barker TD, Guptill K: Overseas fatalities of United States citizen travelers: An analysis of deaths related to international travel. Ann Emerg Med 20:622, 1991.
Ivanoff B, Levine MM, Lambert PH: Vaccination against typhoid: Present status. Bull WHO 72:957, 1994.
Quinn TC: Global burden of the HIV pandemic. Lancet 348:99, 1996.
Steffen R, Kane MA, Shapiro CN et al: Epidemiology and prevention of hepatitis A in travelers. JAMA 272:885, 1994.
Steffen R, Lobel HO: Epidemiologic basis for the practice of travel medicine. J Wilderness Med 5:56, 1994.
Steffen R, Rickenbach M, Wihelum U, et al: Health problems after travel to developing countries. J Infect Dis 156:84, 1987.
White NJ: Treatment of malaria. N Engl J Med 335:800, 1996.

141 Establishing a Traveler's Clinic

Eileen Hilton

INTRODUCTION. More people are traveling from developed to developing countries for business and pleasure. These individuals may come into contact with diseases that would be considered exotic in their own country. Many of these illnesses can be prevented with appropriate pretrip counseling and immunizations. It is becoming increasingly difficult for physicians to stay abreast of the rapidly changing health conditions in other countries. Clinics or centers that specialize in pretravel health advice and post-travel care are increasing in number. This chapter is designed to help practitioners set up and run a traveler's clinic.

HOW TO GET STARTED. First, physicians considering starting a traveler's clinic should assess the demographics of the area proposed for the clinic to determine whether the community can support such a specialized center. A professional consultant may be hired to undertake a feasibility study. This may be valuable but can be expensive. Alternatively, an informal feasibility study could be performed. In general, traveler's clinics are successful if located in areas of high population density, near corporations with international operations, and with access to major airports. Canvassing

TABLE 141–1. Resources for Start-up

Government	Phone Number
Centers for Disease Control (CDC)	(404) 639-3311
General Advice on Traveler's Health Issues	(404) 332-4559
Traveler's Fax Service	(800) 777-7751/
	(404)-332-4565
Malaria Hotline	(404) 332-4555
Malaria Prevention and Prophylaxis Division	(404) 639-1610
Parasitic Diseases Drug Service	(404) 639-3670
Rabies Branch	(404) 639-3095
Meningitis and Special Pathogens Branch	(404) 639-3534
Dengue Branch	(809) 781-3636
Health Information for International Travel Superintendent of Documents U.S. Government Printing Office Washington, DC 20402	(202) 783-3238
U.S. Department of State Overseas Citizens' Emergency Center Blue Sheet— Updates the health information for international travel, published biweekly	(202) 647-5226

TABLE 141–2. Information Sources

International Society of Travel Medicine
Journal of Travel Medicine
P.O. Box 15060
Atlanta, GA 30333-0060

Travel Advice for International Travellers
8 Old Lodge Place, St. Margarets Road
Twickenham, TW1 1RQ

The American Society of Tropical Medicine and Hygiene
60 Revere Dr., Suite 500
Northbrook, IL 60062
The American Journal of Tropical Medicine and Hygiene
Tropical Medicine and Hygiene News
Health Hints for the Tropics

International Association for Medical Assistance to Travellers (IAMAT)
417 Center Street
Lewiston, NY 14092
(716) 754-4883
or
1287 St. Clair Avenue West
Toronto, M6E 1B8

Divers Alert Network
(919) 648-8111

Hospital for Tropical Diseases Healthline–England
(0839) 337-733

Journal of Wilderness Medicine
Chapman and Hall Inc.
29 West 35th Street
New York, NY 10001-2291

Royal Society of Tropical Medicine and Hygiene
Manson House, 26 Portland Place
London W1N 4EY, United Kingdom
Transactions of the Royal Society of Tropical Medicine and Hygiene
Bulletin of Tropical Medicine and International Health

Newsletters
Morbidity and Mortality Weekly Report (MMWR)

The Diabetic Traveler
P.O. Box 8223 RW
Stamford, CT 06905

Travel Medicine Advisor
American Health Consultants
P.O. Box 740056
Atlanta, GA 30374
1-800-688-2421

Travelling Healthy Newsletter
108-48 70th Road
Forest Hills, NY 11375
(718) 268-7290

World Health Organization Publications
49 Sheridan Avenue
Albany, NY 12210
(518) 436-9686
or
1211 Geneva 27, Switzerland

of the area can be done by calling local travel agencies, corporations, and airlines. Because most travel centers do not operate with a high profit margin, the prospective clinicians must do their homework before embarking on what may turn out to be an expensive and revenue-losing project.

Practitioners should familiarize themselves with the literature available on travel medicine. Some of the resources that

travel clinics use include: *Health Information for International Travel*, put out annually by the Centers for Disease Control (CDC); *Travel Medicine Advisor*, published by American Health Consultants; *Traveling Healthy Newsletter; Morbidity and Mortality Weekly Review* from the CDC; and the World Health Organization (WHO) publications (Table 141–1). Specialized societies, journals, and newsletters may serve as resources (Table 141–2). Books on the subject include *Health Issues of International Travelers* from the *Infectious Diseases Clinics of North America; Health Hints for the Tropics; Travel and Tropical Medicine Manual; Traveler's Health;* and *Traveler's Medical Resource*. Many travel centers have opted to contract with computerized databases (Table 141–3).

SPACE, PERSONNEL, AND SUPPLIES. A great deal of office space is not required to start a traveler's clinic. Even for a busy travel center seeing 3000 to 4000 patients a year, one examination room and one interview room or even one examination room with a desk for interviewing may be adequate. It is essential that facilities for appropriate refrigeration and, in some cases, freezing of vaccines be available. If emergency generators are available, a special electrical outlet may be installed and connected to the generator, which is activated during power outages. Disruption of electrical power can be expensive, because many vaccines are heat sensitive. In addition, the refrigerator should be kept secured to prevent vaccine loss through robbery. For most travel clinics, it is not feasible to distribute prescription medications but rather to use a nearby pharmacy to do so. On the other hand, some clinics sell travel health products such as insect repellents, water purifiers, and bed nets.

STAFFING. Until the size of the client population has been determined, the most prudent approach is to start small.

TABLE 141–3. Computerized Databases

CATIS
The Travel and Inoculation Clinic
The Toronto Hospital
200 Elizabeth St.
Toronto, Ontario, Canada M5G2C4

EDISAN
CD Conseil
18 Rue Le Sueur
France 75016

Immunization Alert
93 Timber Drive
Storrs, CT 06268
(800) 584-1999

Medical Advisory Services for Travellers Abroad Ltd. (MASTA)
London School of Hygiene and Tropical Medicine
Keppel Street
London, WE1E 7 IIT England
(071) 631-4408

The Tropical Traveler
Hobbit Software
P.O. Box 308
Victoria Station
Montreal, Quebec, Canada, H3Z2V8

TRAVAX
1417 N. Wauwatosa Ave., Suite 201
Milwaukee, WI 53213-2646
(800) 755-2301

Travel Care
9559 Poole Street
La Jolla, CA 92037
(619) 455-1484

Hours should be chosen for patients' convenience; evening or weekend hours should be considered. Staffing should depend on the regulations of licensing bodies in your area. For instance, in some countries, states, or provinces, only a physician or a nurse may give injections. In others, anyone can give injections after appropriate instruction. The most frugal approach is to hire one person who will interview, counsel, and administer vaccinations. For writing prescriptions and provision of post-travel care, a physician, physician's assistant, or nurse practitioner must be present. When the travel clinic becomes more successful, an additional person can be hired as a designated interviewer while the other may specialize as the vaccinator. However, because of the repetitive nature of either activity, it might be ideal if the two jobs could be shared. Most travel centers start out with part-time employees, 1 to 2 days a week.

CLERICAL SUPPORT. In addition to the interviewer and vaccine administrator, clerical support is necessary for scheduling appointments and billing patients. Although it is possible that one employee can do all of these tasks, it is unlikely that the operation will be successful if scheduling is limited to a few days a week. If the clinic is associated with an established practice, clerical personnel working in the practice can be trained to determine vaccination requirements by telephone and then schedule the patients. Patients should be told to bring with them any past immunization records.

SUPPLIES. A list of vaccine suppliers is provided in Table 141–4. Many vaccines can be obtained from one wholesaler. Most offices keep a large supply of 22- and 25-gauge needles as well as 1- and 3-mL syringes. A travel clinic should maintain emergency equipment in the event of an allergic response to a vaccination. A well-stocked emergency box should include the following: Ambu bag, oral/nasopharyngeal airways, stethoscope, sphygmomanometer, diphenhydramine, epinephrine, and ammonia inhalants. Fruit juices should be available for patients who feel lightheaded before or after being immunized.

Additionally, the International Certificate of Vaccination as approved by the WHO can be obtained from the U.S. Government Printing Office in Washington, DC, at (202) 783–3238. An efficient approach is to set up an account. It is essential to have a supply of these cards, because certificates of vaccinations are required for entry into certain countries. In the United States, yellow fever vaccine cannot be administered unless a clinic is licensed as an official vaccination center. Special stamps that show your site license number are used in a patient's international certificate. In addition to the yellow fever stamp, the practitioner should have stamps

TABLE 141–4. Vaccine Sources

Pharmaceutical Companies

Wyeth-Ayerst Laboratories
  (800) 666-7248
Connaught Laboratories, Inc.
  (717) 839-7187
Berna Products
  (800) 533-5899
Merck & Company
  (800) 637-2579
SmithKline Beecham Pharmaceuticals
  (800) 366-8900

Wholesalers

AmeriSource Corporation
  (800) 562-2526
Neuman Distributors
  (800) 777-1780

prepared for the other vaccinations. This decreases the time that support staff must spend documenting the numerous vaccinations.

Other time-saving tips include preparation of preprinted prescription pads for frequently used agents (e.g., antimalarial drugs), antibiotics to treat diarrheal illness, and medication for preventing altitude sickness. It is wise for a travel center to offer its patients an information brochure detailing ways to avoid traveler's diarrhea and other common travel-associated ailments. This pamphlet may also include information on sun blocks, insect repellents, jet lag, and traveler's health insurance. Some centers give clients a list of English-speaking physicians in other countries. Patients should be told that these are unconfirmed suggestions and that the doctor's credentials have not been reviewed by anyone from your travel center. A list of overseas physicians is available from for-profit and nonprofit organizations (e.g., International Association of Medical Assistance to Travellers [IAMAT]).

SIDE EFFECT INFORMATION. It is useful to have a handout detailing the possible vaccine side effects and their remedies. For instance, intramuscular injection may result in a painful, swollen arm, which could be treated by applying ice to the area and taking nonsteroidal anti-inflammatory medications. One copy of this form can be given to the patient with instructions on who to call if a severe reaction occurs, and one copy kept in the chart as source documentation of counseling.

INTAKE INFORMATION. It is often very useful and efficient to have travelers provide important pretravel information by means of a questionnaire. This questionnaire, to be answered by travelers before interview, should include occupation, departure date, return date, countries to be visited, purpose of travel, whether they are traveling on their own or with an organized tour, going to rural areas or camping, prior international trips and any associated illnesses, and any medical problems that might cause difficulties. A detailed immunization history should be taken, with the most recent immunizations listed as well as type (oral or injectable).

Patients frequently lose or misunderstand their own handwritten instructions. It is advisable to prepare a preprinted sheet with instructions about their prescriptions. This may be organized by category of medication. For instance, with regard to malaria prophylaxis, instructions for administration of chloroquine, doxycycline, and mefloquine can be printed on one form. The practitioner can then circle the appropriate medication or check off a box adjacent to it.

ECONOMIC CONSIDERATIONS. Most traveler's centers are combined with other practices, either primary care, walk-in medical clinics, or the specialties of infectious disease and tropical medicine. The revenue generated from travel medicine is seldom sufficient to support a full-time operation. For a prospective American travel clinic, the penetration of managed care into the target area should also be considered. Managed care companies have contracts with individual hospitals or health care practitioners who supply coverage packages for their clients. An increasing number of these contracts include immunizations. The reimbursement allowance may barely meet the cost of the vaccines and the time spent by the practitioner and/or nurse for travel advice and vaccine administration.

In the past few years, the cost of vaccines has markedly increased; therefore, vaccine pricing should be recalculated frequently. The number of patients to be seen in the first year should be estimated. The cost of the vaccines, personnel, clinic space, printed material and publications, and computerized databases should be calculated. For a nonprofit organization, the vaccine should be priced such that overhead costs should equal the amount of estimated revenue for the first year. If applicable, a profit factor should then be added to the price of the vaccine. If you are in competition with other travel centers in the area, it is wise to assess their charges before start-up. Many travel centers charge a consultation fee in addition to vaccination fees. Prices for your vaccine and services should be re-evaluated at quarterly intervals.

MARKETING STRATEGIES. Advertising in local newspapers, on the radio, and on television is an excellent but expensive method to market your travel clinic. Lectures to health professionals, the community, and travel agent groups are inexpensive alternatives. Letters to travel agents have been successfully used by travel clinics and should include a listing of the services that your center offers. Rolodex cards or business cards can be sent to potential clients and to travel agents. A clinic newsletter with helpful hints for travelers can be published and mailed on a regular basis. Many periodicals have public service announcements that may be useful in developing a patient referral base. Local corporations should be contacted to offer your services to their employees making foreign travel. City, county, and state health offices are a good source of referrals, as are local physicians.

142 *Advice to Travelers*

Elaine C. Jong

International travel has become an increasingly common activity among diverse segments of the population. The spectrum of motivation for travel, ranging from tourism, education, sports, politics, and business to missionary and volunteer efforts, means that the population of travelers seeking health advice includes people of all ages, people in variable states of health, and people traveling under markedly different standards of accommodation.

The basic body of health advice applicable to all travelers covers three main areas: (1) vaccine-preventable diseases, (2) malaria, and (3) traveler's diarrhea. The health advice given in each of these areas must be personalized for each traveler, taking into account age, underlying health, and anticipated level of geographic risk. Other health concerns of travelers include chronic health conditions, insect precautions, high-altitude sickness, jet lag, motion sickness, pregnancy, birth control, safe sexual practices, blood transfusions, personal injury prevention, and environmental hazards. A comprehensive discussion of these other health concerns is beyond the scope of this chapter, but information on specific topics may be found in the bibliography at the end of this chapter.

VACCINE-PREVENTABLE DISEASES

Standard Routine Immunizations. The routine immunizations that all adults should be up to date on include tetanus, diphtheria, poliomyelitis, measles, mumps, and rubella.

Tetanus/Diphtheria. The tetanus/diphtheria (Td) vaccine that is used for immunization of patients 7 years of age and older needs to be boosted every 10 years to maintain immunity after the primary series is completed.

Poliomyelitis. Although primary immunization against poliomyelitis with oral poliomyelitis vaccine (OPV), a live attenuated viral vaccine, is recommended for healthy persons <18 years of age, enhanced potency inactivated poliovirus vaccine (eIPV) is recommended for unimmunized adults (18

years and older) (Chapter 27.1). If travel plans do not permit at least two doses of eIPV given 4 weeks apart to be received by a traveler departing for a poliomyelitis endemic area, a single dose of OPV or eIPV should be given. In either case, primary immunization with eIPV should be completed after the trip. If primary immunization with OPV or the old-type inactivated polio vaccine (IPV) was incomplete, the primary series can be completed with OPV or eIPV regardless of the interval since the last dose or the type of vaccine previously used. If a primary vaccine series with either OPV or IPV was completed >5 years before anticipated travel into an area with poliomyelitis, a single additional dose of OPV or eIPV should be used to boost immunity in travelers of all ages. Persons who should not receive OPV include patients with compromised immunity or those living in households with such patients. Pregnancy is a relative contraindication.

Measles/Mumps/Rubella. The primary immunization with measles/mumps/rubella (MMR) vaccine is customarily given as a single injection at 15 months of age or older. A booster dose of MMR or single-antigen measles vaccine is recommended at 5 to 12 years of age. However, if the MMR vaccine was given before 15 months of age, or if the patient received this vaccine (before 1967), or if the patient never received the vaccine and did not contract the natural viral infections, MMR vaccine is recommended for adults before travel in developing countries.

Other Immunizations. In subsets of the general population at risk because of underlying medical conditions, occupation, or age, the viral influenza vaccine, the pneumococcus vaccine, the *Haemophilus* b conjugate vaccine, and the hepatitis B vaccine should be given before travel.

Special Immunizations for Travelers. The vaccines traditionally given for travel may be divided into two groups: those regulated by the World Health Organization (WHO) and those that are recommended but not required for travel.

YELLOW FEVER. Yellow fever vaccine is the only vaccine currently regulated by the WHO that may be required. Yellow fever virus is transmitted by the bites of *Aedes aegypti* mosquitoes in equatorial Africa and South America (Chapter 31.1). The virus can cause a severe and often fatal hepatitis. Many countries in yellow fever endemic zones do not require travelers to be vaccinated if they are arriving from nonendemic areas. However, if there are no medical contraindications, a prudent traveler should be immunized before going to an endemic area, regardless of official requirements, because an outbreak of yellow fever could occur at any time without warning. In addition, valid proof of yellow fever vaccination is often required when travelers enter a tropical country after travel in other countries in the yellow fever endemic zones. A single injection of this attenuated live virus vaccine stimulates protective immunity lasting 10 years, beginning 10 days after the first dose.

Receipt of the vaccine from an Official Vaccination Center (designated by the public health department at the state, provincial, or national level) must be documented by an official stamp on the yellow fever certificate page contained in the International Certificates of Vaccination. Yellow fever vaccine is purified from chick embryo cultures, so people with a history of anaphylactic reaction to eggs or egg products may not be able to tolerate this vaccine. If the history is questionable, a test dose of the vaccine (according to manufacturer's directions) can be given. If the reaction to the test dose is positive or if the history is unequivocal for serious egg allergy, the standard vaccine dose should not be given, and WHO member countries will accept a signed letter on letterhead stationery from a physician stating that for medical reasons, yellow fever vaccination is contraindicated for that traveler. Unless there are time constraints, cholera and yellow fever vaccines should be administered at least 3 weeks apart. Live virus vaccines are generally contraindicated during pregnancy. However, if travel to a known yellow fever zone were unavoidable by a pregnant woman, the remote theoretical risk to the fetus from the vaccine might be outweighed by the expected protection derived by immunization against this life-threatening disease. The vaccine can be given to infants 6 months of age or older.

SMALLPOX AND CHOLERA. Smallpox and cholera vaccines are no longer regulated by the WHO. There has been no natural transmission of smallpox virus anywhere in the world in 20 years (Chapter 25.2). Although the current cholera pandemic still affects native populations of Asia, Africa, and Latin America, the old parenteral cholera vaccine in common use offers little protection to the usual traveler, whose risk of cholera is negligible (Chapter 41). A new oral live cholera vaccine is available in Europe and Canada, and its release in the United States is anticipated. The oral cholera vaccine contains attenuated strain *Vibrio cholerae* 01CVD 103-HgR. After a single dose, good protection is obtained for 6 months. Cholera vaccine may be considered for travelers with known risk factors that promote cholera infection in otherwise healthy people: achlorhydria, gastric resection, or any other condition decreasing gastric acidity. However, advice on selection of safe food and water while traveling and self-treatment with oral rehydration salts and antibiotics would probably be reasonable alternatives to the vaccine for prevention of cholera in travelers at risk.

TYPHOID FEVER. The older injectable typhoid fever vaccine is a purified bacterial vaccine, which causes inflammation and tenderness at the site of injection in many people (Chapter 75). This vaccine has largely been replaced by newer, better tolerated preparations. However, all three available typhoid vaccines have a demonstrated protective efficacy of approximately 70%.

The oral typhoid vaccine has fewer side effects than the old parenteral vaccine but may have compliance problems because it is self-administered by travelers. The vaccine is contraindicated in immunocompromised patients. This vaccine is made from attenuated *Salmonella typhi* Ty21a bacteria, and taking an enteric-coated capsule on days 1, 3, 5, and 7 gives protection commencing 2 weeks after the fourth dose and lasting for at least 5 years.

In recent years, a newer injectable preparation, the typhoid Vi capsular polysaccharide vaccine, has become available. After a single dose, protection lasting 2 to 3 years is elicited in vaccine recipients 2 years of age and older.

HEPATITIS A. Immunization with hepatitis A vaccine is recommended for most international travelers, because national reported rates of this infection do not adequately reflect pockets of high risk within a given country (Chapter 28). With increasing globalization of food supplies and international migration of workers in food-handling occupations, outbreaks of hepatitis A can occur even in countries with a high socioeconomic standard of living and reported low rates of hepatitis A incidence.

Only about one of three adults tests seropositive for hepatitis A antibody in studies of North American and Western European populations; thus, the majority of adult travelers in these populations are susceptible to hepatitis A infection. At least one half of reported cases of hepatitis A in American travelers occurred during standard tourist itineraries. This implies that the risk of hepatitis A exposure for the individual traveler cannot be predicted on the basis of quality of accommodations, rural versus urban itineraries, or food preferences.

The hepatitis A vaccines in predominant use around the world are made from inactivated hepatitis A virus derived from tissue cultures. The vaccines are safe and highly efficacious. After the first dose, given intramuscularly, protective immunity lasting 6 to 12 months is elicited in >95% of vaccinees. A second dose, given after 6 to 12 months, results in protective antibody levels lasting >10 years, according to mathematical models.

IMMUNE GLOBULIN. Immune globulin purified from pooled human serum and given as an intramuscular injection can provide protection against hepatitis A for a period of 3 to 5½ months, depending on the dose given (Chapter 28). This can be given at the same time as most travel vaccines at a separate injection site but should be given at least 3 to 4 weeks after a dose of MMR, OPV, eIPV, or *H. influenzae* b vaccine.

Owing to concern about the safety of blood products with regard to HIV transmission, many people express reluctance to receive immune globulin prophylaxis for travel. Concerned travelers need to be reassured about the safety of immune globulin: Unlike the fresh blood used for transfusion of cells or clotting factors, immune globulin is a highly purified blood product, and the purification process destroys any HIV theoretically present in the original serum pool. This is borne out by a long record of product safety in clinical practice.

MENINGOCOCCAL INFECTIONS. Meningococcal Polysaccharide Vaccine (quadrivalent groups A/C/Y/W-135) is a purified polysaccharide vaccine that is given as a single injectable dose to people 3 years of age and older (Chapter 52). The vaccine is recommended for those who plan to live or work in the Sahel region of Africa, in Brazil, and in other areas where epidemics of meningococcal meningitis recur. Since 1985, there have been reports of meningococcal meningitis among travelers trekking in Nepal, and the vaccine is highly recommended for such individuals. More recently, immunization has been recommended for travelers to Kenya and Tanzania.

HEPATITIS B VACCINE. Hepatitis B vaccine is available as a recombinant DNA yeast antigen product (Chapter 28) and is given as a primary series of three injections, the first 2 given 1 month apart, and the third given 6 months after the first dose. An alternative schedule for the Engerix recombinant hepatitis B vaccine is four doses at 0, 1, 2, and 12 months. Hepatitis B vaccination has had widespread use in the United States among health care workers and intimate contacts of known hepatitis B–infected persons. Travelers who plan to live or work among native populations in Africa and Asia or people who may be involved in high-risk activities in these countries (sexual contact, acupuncture, tattoos, ear-piercing, and so on), should be advised to be immunized. However, because activities that involve a high risk of hepatitis B acquisition are also a risk for HIV transmission, travelers should be advised to avoid these activities if possible, regardless of their hepatitis B vaccination status. A new, three-dose, combined hepatitis A and B vaccine is now available in Europe.

RABIES. Travelers to Mexico, Central and South America, Africa, and Asia need to be warned about rabid dogs and the need to avoid contact with stray animals (Chapter 30.1). Other animals e.g., bats, monkeys, foxes, wolves, and livestock in these countries may also be rabid. If an animal bite occurs, travelers need to know that this could be an emergency situation requiring postexposure treatment with rabies immune globulin (RIG) and rabies vaccine. They should ask for help from their nearest consulate or embassy. In some cases, emergency evacuation may be appropriate, as the most effective treatments may not be available.

Travelers planning extensive trips, prolonged residence, or work that involves animal contact in rabies endemic countries should receive the pre-exposure series of the human diploid cell vaccine (HDCV) for rabies, which consists of three injections given on days 0, 7, and 21 or 28. A small intradermal dose (0.1 mL) can be used if the series can be completed before chloroquine prophylaxis for malaria is instituted. If the time period is not adequate, a larger dose (1.0 mL) of HDCV given IM on the same schedule should be used. Receipt of the pre-exposure rabies vaccine series obviates the need for RIG after a high-risk bite and decreases the number of postexposure HDCV doses given (two over 1 week instead of five over 1 month).

JAPANESE ENCEPHALITIS VACCINE (JEV). This is a purified killed virus vaccine prepared from brain tissue of infected laboratory mice. The JEV (Biken) vaccine manufactured in Japan has been efficacious and safe in the first 15 years of its widespread use. Adverse reactions consisting of urticaria and/or angioedema occurring immediately or as long as 2 weeks after a JEV dose have been reported rarely. Persons with a history of urticaria may be at somewhat higher risk for this reaction.

Although many travelers go to areas in Asia where epidemics of Japanese encephalitis (JE) routinely cause morbidity and mortality among native populations (Korea, People's Republic of China, Philippines, Indonesia, Malaysia, Thailand, India, Sri Lanka, and Burma), most short-term travelers on the usual tourist routes are not at risk for infection through the bites of *Culex* mosquitoes (Chapter 30.3). However, students, educators, missionaries, agricultural advisors, and others traveling intensively or residing in rural areas where JE is a risk should obtain three doses of JEV given 1 week apart before travel.

PLAGUE AND TYPHUS. Immunization against plague is rarely recommended, except for travelers planning to camp in rural, mountainous, or upland areas in Africa, Asia, and the Americas where plague is reported and for persons whose occupation may lead them to direct or indirect exposure to wild animals (Chapter 61). Two injections are given at 4-week intervals, and the third dose is given 3 to 6 months after the second dose. Typhus is rarely seen in North American travelers (Chapter 66). The vaccine is no longer available in the United States.

BACILLE CALMETTE-GUÉRIN (BCG) IMMUNIZATION. Tuberculosis is very common in developing countries (Chapter 77). Persons who intend to live and work there are at increased risk of exposure. BCG, a live vaccine derived from a strain of *Mycobacterium bovis*, has been recommended by some for persons with a negative tuberculin skin test result who are planning an extended stay in a developing country. The efficacy of the currently available BCG vaccine is questionable, as exemplified by the negative results in a large-scale BCG trial in India. Side effects, ranging from draining abscesses at the site of immunization (common) to disseminated infection (rare), must be weighed against the individual's risk of active tuberculosis—a risk that varies directly with the intimacy of contact with the indigenous population. BCG vaccination usually results in a positive tuberculin skin test; the size of the reaction decreases over years. BCG vaccine is contraindicated in those who are immunocompromised.

Instead of providing immunization with BCG, most North American consultants recommend that long-stay travelers should have a tuberculin skin test before departure and, if results are negative, every 1 to 2 years during exposure.

MALARIA. The itinerary and the local climate at the time of the trip are primary malaria risk determinants (Chapter 92). Advice to travelers on malaria prevention falls into three categories: personal behavior, mosquito repellents, and chemoprophylaxis.

Personal Behavior and Mosquito Repellents. Travelers in malarious areas should try to stay indoors in screened rooms between dusk and dawn, when anopheline mosquitoes, which transmit malaria, are most likely to bite. When outdoors during these hours, clothing that covers the arms and legs and the use of insect repellent on exposed body areas decrease the risk of mosquito bites. Before going to sleep, the room should be inspected for mosquitoes on the walls and ceilings. Use of a spray insecticide or burning insect coils usually reduces the number of mosquitoes. Field studies suggest that sleeping under bed nets impregnated with permethrin (an insecticide) greatly reduces the likelihood of bites by mosquitoes as well as other insects and ectoparasites (Chapter 92).

Malaria Chemoprophylaxis. This has become an increasingly complex issue because of the emergence of chloroquine-resistant *Plasmodium falciparum* (CRPF) malaria (Chapter 92). In some areas, CRPF strains are also resistant to sulfadoxine-pyrimethamine (Fansidar) and mefloquine. In addition to a malarial chemoprophylaxis regimen appropriate for a given geographic area, successful prevention of malaria may depend on the use of personal protection measures against mosquito bites. No matter which chemoprophylactic regimen is used, breakthrough attacks of resistant malaria can occur. Travelers to remote areas may be required to self-diagnose malaria by clinical symptoms and to initiate treatment when medical services are not available.

Table 142–1 lists major geographic areas where malaria is endemic and suggests regimens that might be appropriate. Regimens 1 through 5 summarize the malaria chemoprophylaxis in current use (1999) throughout the world. Although not widely appreciated, recent studies in Africa and Indonesia have shown that primaquine, in an adult dose of 30 mg/day, is a well-tolerated and effective chemoprophylactic agent. Because the drug is a potent oxidant, glucose-6-phosphate dehydrogenase levels must be determined before use to avoid hemolytic anemia in those who are deficient in this enzyme.

Some antimalarial drugs may be unavailable or contraindicated for a given traveler. Alternatively, an acceptable strategy in some situations is to take standard chloroquine phosphate prophylaxis and to carry a treatment dose of drugs with efficacy against CRPF for emergency self-treatment of a suspected attack. Regimen 6 is the Centers for Disease Control (CDC) recommendation for emergency self-treatment should a traveler elect to take the weekly chloroquine regimen in a CRPF area. However, in view of increasing Fansidar resistance in Africa and South America and Fansidar's lack of efficacy in Southeast Asia and Oceania, this self-treatment option should be used with caution. The new drug combination of atovaquone and proguanil (Malarone), not yet available in North America, may prove to be an excellent self-treatment regimen when administered as 1 g of atovaquone plus 400 mg of proguanil daily for 3 days.

Several antimalarial drugs and drug combinations being used by international travelers from Western Europe, Australia, and Southeast Asia in areas of drug-resistant falciparum malaria are not available to North American travelers. In some cases, it may be appropriate for travelers to obtain and use these alternative drugs for malaria prevention in the areas of risk, even though the drugs are not licensed and approved for use in the United States or Canada. As with any medication, the relative benefits and risks of a given drug must be carefully reviewed by the physician with the patient. Mefloquine has become the drug of choice for the prevention of CRPF malaria in most endemic areas of the world (Chapter 92).

Although Table 142–1 lists recommended antimalarial regimens by country, the actual risk of malaria and of drug

TABLE 142–1. Malaria Chemoprophylaxis Regimens

Geographic Area	Suggested Regimen(s)*					
	1	2	3	4	5	6
Mexico	X					
Central America, Haiti	X					
South America		X	X		X	X
North Africa, Turkey, Middle East					X	X
Sub-Saharan Africa		X	X	X	X	X
Nepal					X	X
India					X	X
People's Republic of China	X	X			X	X
Thailand (rural and border), Laos, Cambodia, Vietnam, rural Philippines, Indonesia, Malaysia, Papua New Guinea		X	X		X	

*See text in this chapter and Chapter 92 for discussion; see Chapter 149 for more exact description of geographic locations of drug-resistant plasmodia.

1. Chloroquine phosphate (Aralen), 500 mg PO once a week, beginning 1 week before travel, continuing once a week on the same day during travel and for 4 weeks after travel in a malaria risk area.

2. Doxycycline (Vibramycin), 100 mg PO every day of the trip and daily for 4 weeks after travel, in a CRPF risk area.

3. Chloroquine phosphate (take as described in 1); *plus* dapsone, 100-mg tablet; *plus* pyrimethamine (Daraprim), 12.5-mg tablet: take both latter medications at the same time once a week, beginning 1 week before travel, continuing on the same day weekly during travel and for 4 weeks after travel. This combination of dapsone and pyrimethamine is sold as Maloprim in some countries.

4. Chloroquine phosphate (take as described in 1) *plus* daily proguanil (Paludrine), 100-mg tablet: 2 tablets (200 mg) of proguanil PO every day during the trip and for 4 weeks after in addition to weekly chloroquine phosphate.

5. Mefloquine (Lariam), 250-mg tablets: 1 tablet (250 mg) PO once a week beginning 1 week before travel and continuing up to and including 4 weeks after departure from a malarious area.

6. Chloroquine phosphate (take as described in 1) *plus* a treatment dose of sulfadoxine 500 mg–pyrimethamine 25 mg (Fansidar): Adults should take 3 Fansidar tablets as a single oral dose to treat an attack of suspected CRPF malaria.

resistance may be quite variable within each country. For example, there is no malaria risk in most urban centers of Southeast Asia or South America, and in rural areas travelers are at risk only if they remain overnight. However, in other regions e.g., sub-Saharan Africa and Haiti, malaria transmission occurs in both urban and rural areas. In some countries, China for example, CRPF is located in certain regions, whereas in other areas, only chloroquine-sensitive strains are transmitted.

Self-Treatment for Malaria. Because no current drug regimen guarantees protection against malaria, travelers, particularly those to remote areas, should be instructed about self-diagnosis of malaria. Any illness with high fever associated with headache, muscle aches, nausea, and abdominal discomfort occurring during or after travel in a malarious area must be considered to be malaria until proved otherwise. Although there are other important causes of fever in the tropics, urgency of therapy is often not as crucial as it is for malaria. Prompt self-treatment of malaria could be lifesaving if medical care is not readily accessible (Chapter 92). On the other hand, in case of fever on return home, travelers should be reminded to inform their health care providers that they have been exposed to malaria, that their antimalarial prophylaxis may not have provided complete protection and that

TABLE 142–2. Food and Water Precautions

Eat foods that are thoroughly cooked and served piping hot.
Avoid raw or undercooked fish, shellfish, and meat.
Avoid green salads and other salads served cold.
Avoid dairy products, e.g., milk, ice cream, cheese, and yogurt, which may be unpasteurized in some countries or improperly stored.
Drink bottled carbonated beverages, canned fruit juices, or beverages e.g., tea, coffee, or bouillon that have been prepared with boiled water. Beer and wine are usually safe.
Avoid ice cubes in cold beverages, including alcoholic beverages.
Use a water purification method when in doubt about tap water.
Use safe water for brushing teeth and for taking medications.

they wish to have thick and thin blood films examined for malaria.

CHEMOPROPHYLAXIS FOR OTHER SYSTEMIC PARASITES

African Trypanosomiasis. Chemoprophylaxis against trypanosomiasis has rarely been used in the past for workers living in endemic areas in rural West or Central Africa, where they may be exposed to Gambian trypanosomiasis (Chapter 93). A single intramuscular injection of 250 mg of pentamidine protects an adult for about 6 months. Pentamidine may not be available in parts of Africa where it is needed and is not available for preventive use in the United States. Chemoprophylaxis is not recommended for the usual safari visitor, who has very low exposure and is more likely to be exposed in East and South Africa to Rhodesian trypanosomiasis.

Filariasis. Most travelers to areas endemic for filariasis will not have sufficient exposure to acquire disease. For some persons planning an extended stay (e.g., Peace Corps volunteers), prophylactic diethylcarbamazine (DEC) may be recommended (Chapter 106). Untoward drug effects are rare in uninfected persons. The dose is 5 mg/kg taken once each month. For prophylaxis for human *Loa loa* infections in equatorial West and Central Africa, the DEC dose is 300 mg PO once a week. Ivermectin may replace DEC for these purposes in a few years.

TRAVELER'S DIARRHEA. Up to 50% of travelers to a tropical climate experience traveler's diarrhea. Although the illness is usually self-limited, lasting an average of 3 to 5 days, the frequent watery bowel movements and abdominal cramps associated with this condition can cause significant discomfort and interfere with travel plans. The majority of cases of traveler's diarrhea are thought to be caused by toxigenic strains of the bacteria *Escherichia coli* (Chapter 42). Other bacteria, viruses, and parasites cause traveler's diarrhea but are detected less frequently.

Preventive strategies for avoiding traveler's diarrhea include food and water precautions, daily doses of bismuth subsalicylate (BSS), or daily doses of a broad-spectrum antibiotic such as a quinolone (ciprofloxacin, norfloxacin, ofloxacin) or trimethoprim-sulfamethoxazole (TMP/SMX).

Food and Water Precautions. Although following the food and water precautions listed in Table 142–2 decreases the transmission of enteric pathogens and the occurrence of food poisoning in areas where unsanitary food preparation and storage may be a problem, no evidence shows that strict adherence to the precautions guarantees prevention of traveler's diarrhea.

Chemoprophylaxis. Prophylaxis against traveler's diarrhea by taking daily doses of BSS (Pepto-Bismol) or antibiotics has been shown to be effective. In one study, 2 tablets of BSS PO q.i.d. decreased the incidence of traveler's diarrhea by 60% in American students in Mexico. Trimethoprim-sulfamethoxazole double-strength tablets, or ciprofloxacin 500 mg, norfloxacin 400 mg, or ofloxacin 300-mg tablets taken once a day also are effective for traveler's diarrhea prophylaxis. Of great concern are the recent studies that have shown a dramatic increase in trimethoprim-sulfamethoxazole resistance by enteric organisms and marked resistance of *Campylobacter jejuni* to ciprofloxacin in Thailand. These drugs should be started prior to arrival in the tropics and continued for 2 days after departure.

However, the National Institutes of Health's National Travelers' Diarrhea Consensus Conference did not endorse prophylactic use of BSS or antibiotics against traveler's diarrhea for the usual traveler. The effectiveness of the various prophylactic routines was studied for relatively short periods of 3 weeks or less. The prophylactic routines may cause problems for some travelers owing to salicylate intolerance or adverse effects related to broad-spectrum antibiotics (drug allergy, skin rashes, yeast infections, antibiotic-associated diarrhea). Some of the drugs are not approved by the Food and Drug Administration for use in children or during pregnancy. However, some experts in travel medicine recommend antibiotic or BSS prophylaxis for individuals who are at particularly high risk for traveler's diarrhea or its sequelae. Such groups of individuals include persons with achlorhydria, diabetes, inflammatory bowel disease, or immunosuppressive disorders or those with a history of frequent gastrointestinal problems associated with travel.

Chemoprophylaxis of the common intestinal parasites causing diarrhea, e.g., amebiasis and giardiasis, is less useful than for bacterial diarrhea.

Patients need to be warned about buying antibiotics for prevention or treatment of diarrhea in foreign countries; in some countries, potentially dangerous drugs, e.g., chloramphenicol and iodochlorhydroxyquin, are available from pharmacies without a prescription.

Self-Treatment of Diarrhea with Antibiotics. The alternative to antibiotic prophylaxis is empirical self-treatment of diarrhea that develops during travel. If a traveler is stricken by a typical case of traveler's diarrhea, the use of an agent for symptomatic relief (BSS) or antiperistaltic drugs (e.g., loperamide, diphenoxylate, paregoric) and empirical self-treatment with an antibiotic (double-strength TMP/SMX, ciprofloxacin, ofloxacin, norfloxacin) for 3 to 5 days at appropriate therapeutic doses (usually twice daily) may contribute to a rapid recovery. Several studies have shown that a single dose of these drugs (usually double the daily dose for the 3- to 5-day regimen) is equally effective for self-treatment. The use of antiperistaltic drugs is contraindicated for those with diarrhea accompanied by a high fever and/or bloody or mucoid stools. These cases require the care of a physician, although travelers in remote areas may need to initiate antibiotic treatment if access to medical care is not possible.

The selection of the antibiotic for the treatment (or prevention) of diarrhea depends on the geographic location of the trip: drug-resistant strains of diarrhea-causing bacteria are present in areas where there has been widespread use of a given drug. For instance, TMP/SMX-resistant strains of bacteria are an increasing problem in Mexico and the Middle East. Tetracycline resistance is widespread among bacterial enteric pathogens in Central and South America and the Middle and Far East.

Oral Rehydration. No matter what drugs are used by travelers for self-treatment of traveler's diarrhea, prevention of dehydration by increasing the usual oral fluid intake to approximate the volume lost through watery bowel movements is of prime importance. Canned fruit juices, carbonated beverages, clear soups, and other drinks made with boiled or purified water can be used. If available, reconstituted powdered oral rehydration salts (formulated according to the WHO recipe) or the CDC oral fluids program provides replacement of fluid and electrolytes closely matching intestinal losses due to diarrhea. However, it is good to remember that rehydration with impure water is better than no rehydration at all!

HEALTH CARE ABROAD. Medical emergencies can occur at home and abroad. Prudent travelers should carry, in addition to the International Certificates of Vaccination, a summary of the health history, a list of current medications (including generic or chemical name and dosage), and pertinent data if an underlying medical condition is under treatment (e.g., allergies; cardiovascular problems, including hypertension, ischemic heart disease, artificial heart valves, and artificial pacemakers; pulmonary problems, including emphysema and asthma; diabetes mellitus; malignancies). Should the need for medical treatment arise while a person is traveling, such information would be invaluable to the treating physician. Travelers should also check with their health insurance provider to find out provisions for illness abroad. Even a traveler in perfect health could accidentally break a leg.

HEALTH CARE AFTER RETURN HOME. Travelers should be advised to consult a knowledgeable physician on return home if they have experienced any significant change in their health while abroad. The development of a high fever in the weeks to months after a trip in a malarious area, even if malaria chemoprophylaxis was taken, should raise the question of malaria, because no chemoprophylactic regimen can be considered to be 100% protective (Chapter 145). Changes in gastrointestinal function (Chapter 144) and skin lesions (Chapter 146) are other post-trip health problems that often require medical care.

SUMMARY. Although travelers to urban areas of developed countries may need only general advice for maintenance of health, travelers planning to visit rural areas, especially in tropical and developing countries, may need extensive preparation. Physicians who advise travelers must help them tread the thin line between caution and neurosis. The advice given and the emphasis with which it is presented should be weighed according to the personality of the patient and the anticipated health risks of the trip.

Bibliography

Barry M: Medical considerations for international travel with infants and older children. Infect Dis Clin North Am 6:389, 1992.

Bia FJ: Medical considerations for the pregnant traveler. Infect Dis Clin North Am 6:371, 1992.

Centers for Disease Control: Health Information for International Travel, 1995 (HHS Publication No. (CDC) 95–8280). Atlanta, GA, US Department of Health and Human Services, Public Health Service, 1995 (updated annually).

DuPont HI: Travelers' diarrhea: Which antimicrobial. Drugs 6:910, 1993.

DuPont HL, Ericsson CD, Johnson PC, et al: Prevention of travelers' diarrhea by the tablet formulation of bismuth subsalicylate. JAMA 257:1347, 1987.

Ericsson CD, DuPont HL: Traveler's diarrhea: Approaches to prevention and treatment. Clin Infect Dis 16:616, 1993.

Hoke CH, Nisalak A, Sangawhipa N, et al: Protection against Japanese encephalitis by inactivated vaccines. N Engl J Med 319:608, 1988.

Johnson PC, Ericsson CD, DuPont HL, et al: Comparison of loperamide with bismuth subsalicylate for treatment of acute travelers' diarrhea. JAMA 255:767, 1986.

Jong EC, McMullen R (eds): The Travel and Tropical Medicine Manual, 2nd ed. Philadelphia, WB Saunders, 1995.

Lackritz EM, Lobel HO, Howell BJ, et al: Imported *Plasmodium falciparum* malaria in American travelers to Africa—implications for prevention strategies. JAMA 265:383, 1991.

Levine MM, Black RE, Ferreccio C, et al: Large-scale field trial of Ty21A live oral typhoid vaccine in enteric-coated capsule formulation. Lancet 1:1049, 1987.

Nutman TB, Miller KD, Mulligan M, et al: Diethylcarbamazine prophylaxis for human loaiasis. N Engl J Med 319:752, 1988.

Steffen R, Rickenbach M, Wilhelm U, et al: Health problems after travel to developing countries. J Infect Dis 156:84, 1987.

Travelers' Diarrhea Consensus Conference. JAMA 253:2700, 1985.

Wilson ME, von Reyn CF, Fineberg HV: Infections in HIV-infected travelers: Risks and prevention. Ann Intern Med 114:582, 1991.

World Health Organization: Vaccination Certificate Requirements and Health Advice for International Travel, 1995. Geneva, World Health Organization, 1995 (updated annually).

143 *Screening of the Long-Term Traveler*

Douglas W. MacPherson and Phyllis E. Kozarsky

This chapter reviews the health screening procedures that may be used for the long-term (>3 months) or the particularly adventuresome traveler (backpacker, aid worker) returning from the developing world. Unfortunately, there are no uniformly accepted guidelines for screening of returning travelers and few data on the beneficial effects of screening. Some returning travelers are screened to reveal latent infections that may give rise to symptoms later on; some are screened to reduce the risk of contagion to contacts; others require screening to determine their fitness to return to work in the tropics. Practice guidelines for screening asymptomatic returned travelers need to reflect not only the patient's age and gender but also his or her risk profile. Studies of Peace Corps volunteers and missionaries have provided some information on the incidence of diseases in returnees from long-term posting in the developing world. A review of German expatriates who lived in developing countries for up to 10 years revealed that almost one third reported a severe illness while abroad. Most problems in this group, however, were due to underlying cardiovascular disease, and there were no deaths from tropical illnesses, although a significant number had malaria and hepatitis. In most groups studied, anxiety and depression were major causes of early repatriation.

■ THE BASIS FOR POST-TRAVEL SCREENING

Screening tests are applied to an asymptomatic traveler to detect later or occult disease or to notify the individual at risk of developing disease in the future. Screening may lead to a more extensive diagnostic evaluation or may be diagnostic on its own.

PARASITIC INFECTIONS. The most comprehensive review of screening tests for helminthic infections was carried out on 1600 asymptomatic returned travelers who attended a tropical medicine center in Montreal. The author's conclusions confirmed previous studies—that the eosinophil count was relatively insensitive as a screening device for helminthic

infections (sensitivity of 27%). On the other hand, three stool examinations, together with parasite serologies for strongyloidiasis, schistosomiasis, and filariasis, had a sensitivity of 89%. An earlier study in 1993, in which 1000 consecutive, asymptomatic returnees to the United Kingdom were screened for intestinal parasites, showed that 20% of travelers were found to be infected, most frequently with *Entamoeba histolytica/dispar* or *Giardia lamblia*.

VIRAL HEPATITIS AND STD. There are no data on the value of screening for viral hepatitis antibodies or sexually acquired infections (STDs), including the human immunodeficiency virus (HIV). While it is reasonable to screen for hepatitis exposure in those with abnormal liver function tests, it is probably unnecessary to perform these tests unless the history reveals risk factors. Using liver function tests as a marker for subclinical hepatitis is unreliable, since persons infected with hepatitis B or C can progress to chronic liver disease in the face of normal liver function tests (Chapter 28). Because of their risk for blood-borne infections it has been recommended that the following groups of returned travelers be screened by serology for HIV and viral hepatitis (depending on the immunization history): health care professionals; those who received inoculations, dental treatment, transfusions, tattoos, or body piercing; and those who participated in unprotected sex with casual contacts.

STDs are potential consequences of international travel. In studies of men and women attending genitourinary medicine clinics in the United Kingdom and STD clinics in Sweden, 20 to 27% of women and 42.5% of men reported casual sexual contact while traveling abroad. Results such as these have been seen in other studies reported from France and Australia. Therefore, in those at risk, syphilis serology should be added to the screening for viral hepatitis and HIV. Also, genital/pelvic examinations should be done in this group, looking especially for genital warts, asymptomatic ulcers, and chlamydial infections.

TUBERCULOSIS (TB). The rates of *Mycobacterium tuberculosis* infection in some parts of the world may exceed the risk in low-endemic areas by more than 100 times. The PPD conversion rate of U.S. soldiers serving in Vietnam was 3.3% after an average stay of just 7 months. Preliminary results of a prospective Canadian study in 47 travelers who had spent a mean of 3 months in hyperendemic transmission zones yielded 6 new infections, 2 of which represented active disease. Although there are no data on the routine use of post-travel screening chest x-rays, asymptomatic tropical pulmonary infections in returning travelers are so rare that they would not be cost effective.

■ LACK OF CONSENSUS

In an effort to obtain consensus on what practitioners of clinical tropical medicine and traveler's health are doing in the way of post-travel screening, a survey of two professional societies was conducted in 1996 by electronic mail. This study showed tremendous variability in screening practices, with >75% of these experts favoring only three screening tests: a CBC, schistosomiasis serology, and TB skin testing.

The value of post-travel screening has been questioned as "overmedicalizing" travel. It has been pointed out that general physicians should be able to use screening tests, e.g., schistosomiasis, syphilis, and HIV serologies, for those who may have been exposed to these infections. However, primary care physicians may have little knowledge of the geographic distribution of disease, the mode of acquisition of screenable diseases, and the appropriate tests for screening. In addition, the exposure history, which determines risk,

TABLE 143–1. Screening Tests for At Risk Returned, Asymptomatic Long-Term International Travelers*

	Condition	Test
Recommended	Tuberculosis	Tuberculin skin test (by Mantoux technique, PPD 5TU)
	Intestinal parasites	Stools for ova and parasites
Weakly recommended	Disorders of white cells, (including eosinophils and platelets), anemia	Complete blood counts (routine hematology)
	Psychological disorder	Various screening tools, e.g., Profile of Mood State
Recommended only if history of exposure	Sexually transmitted disease	Serology for HIV, hepatitis B, and syphilis *Chlamydia trachomatis* culture, antigen, or probe *Trichomonas vaginalis* examination, culture
	Strongyloides infection	Specific serology + / − stools for *Strongyloides* culture and O & P
	Schistosomiasis	Specific serology
	Filariasis	Specific serology
	Hepatitis B and C	Specific serology

*Individuals who have no clinical complaint and no abnormal physical findings but who potentially have had a significant exposure (due to duration of travel, specific activity, or concurrent health condition) in a geographic area endemic for the condition. A detailed travel history and knowledge of the risk factors for acquisition of the condition are prerequisites for screening.

requires specific knowledge, e.g., duration and style of travel and the effects of the individual's profile on disease risk.

Some argue that it is difficult to justify even basic screening tests, e.g., stool examinations for protozoa or helminths, when most organisms found will clear spontaneously or not cause chronic problems. The finding of *E. histolytica* or *G. lamblia* may not be clinically significant, since in 90% of asymptomatic cases the former has been shown to be the nonpathogen *E. dispar* and it does not require treatment.

■ RECOMMENDATIONS

All returning long-term travelers should have a clinical evaluation including a history and physical examination, but little additional testing need be done, except as indicated by risk. Even if the individual is asymptomatic, a detailed history should be obtained about itinerary, lifestyle, and exposures. During physical examination, special attention should be paid to the skin, lymph nodes, lungs, liver, and spleen. Laboratory tests that might be performed include those in Table 143–1. Examination of three stools for O & P collected on different days is recommended. A 5TU PPD should be placed on those with a history of a negative PPD prior to travel; if positive, a chest x-ray should be taken. Depending upon the history, it may be appropriate to perform serologic tests for parasite and HIV infections or other specialized blood tests or procedures (see Table 143–1). Since malaria and other illnesses may become symptomatic after the initial post-travel period, all returnees should be educated about nonspecific signs and symptoms that may develop later, especially fever during the first few months after return. The important message to convey is that they must inform health care professionals seen in the future about their travel history.

Although the focus of post-travel screening is to detect problems that may cause physical impairment, attention should also be paid to mental health. Many long-term travelers fail to make a successful transition to their country of posting or to their home country on return. Emotional problems may not be readily apparent, and the returnee may be hesitant to voice these concerns because of confidentiality issues or embarrassment. Health care professionals need to specifically inquire about exhaustion, anxiety, and depression as well as alcohol or drug use. Debriefing sessions, increased relaxation time, and a period for readjustment and re-adaptation should be encouraged.

■ CONCLUSIONS

There are no simple algorithms for post-travel assessment of the adventuresome or long-term traveler who is asymptomatic. The cost effectiveness of diagnosing an occult asymptomatic parasitic infection, e.g., schistosomiasis or filariasis, is not known. In addition, there is little information on the sensitivity, specificity, and cost effectiveness of our diagnostic tests. Post-travel screening should be viewed as one part of a comprehensive health maintenance plan for travelers that also should include education and assessment prior to departure and while abroad, as necessary.

Bibliography

Arvidson M, Hellberg D, Mardh, PA: Sexual risk behaviour and history of sexually transmitted diseases in relation to casual travel sex during different types of journeys. Acta Obstet Gynaecol Scand 75:4904, 1996.

Churchill DR, Chiodini PL, McAdam KP: Screening the returned traveller. Br Med Bull 49:465, 1993.

Fryatt RJ, Teng J, Harries L, et al: Intestinal helminthiasis in expatriates returning to Britain from the tropics: A controlled study. Trop Geogr Med 42:119, 1990.

Hawkes S, Hart GJ, Betsoe E, et al: Risk behaviour and STD acquisition in genitourinary clinic attenders who have travelled. Genitourin Med 71:351, 1995.

Libman LD, MacLean JD, Gyorkos TW: Screening for schistosomiasis, filariasis and strongyloides among expatriates returning from the tropics. Clin Infect Dis 17:353, 1993.

Parenti DM: Sexually transmitted diseases and travelers. Med Clin North Am 76:1499, 1992.

Struve J, Norrbohm O, Stenbeck J, et al: Risk factors for hepatitis A, B and C virus infection among Swedish expatriates. J Infect 31:205, 1995.

144 *Diarrhea in Travelers*

Bradley A. Connor

Acute Diarrhea

ETIOLOGY. Diarrhea is the most common travel-related ailment among the 20 million people who travel annually from industrialized to developing countries. Diarrhea in travelers is usually an acute illness resolving with or without specific therapy within 3 to 5 days. However, subacute or chronic diarrheal syndromes are not uncommon; in 8 to 15% of travelers, diarrhea persists for >1 week and in 2% continues >1 month. Rarely diarrhea may persist for years following the initial attack.

Approximately 85% of traveler's diarrhea is caused by bacterial enteropathogens. This explains the highly effective reduction in attack rates by prophylactic use of a wide range of antimicrobial agents as well as the highly efficacious therapeutic effects of antibacterial drugs. The bacterial organisms that predominate in different geographic regions vary, but numerous studies have shown the principal agents to be enterotoxigenic *Escherichia coli* (ETEC), *Shigella* and *Salmonella* species, *Campylobacter jejuni*, *Aeromonas* species, *Plesiomonas shigelloides*, and vibrios (usually *Vibrio parahaemolyticus* or other non-01 cholera vibrios) (Table 144–1). Seasonal variation is well documented; in North Africa and Mexico ETEC, *Salmonella*, and *Shigella* are the most frequent causes of traveler's diarrhea in the rainy summer season, whereas *Campylobacter jejuni* is more common in the drier winter season. Noncholera vibrios predominate in certain coastal areas of Asia. Other less frequent pathogens include enteroadherent, enteroinvasive, and verotoxin-producing *E. coli*; the parasites *Giardia lamblia*, *Cryptosporidium* sp., *Isospora* sp., *Cyclospora cayetanensis*, and *Entamoeba histolytica*; and viral agents, e.g., rotavirus and Norwalk virus. Helminths are rarely a cause of diarrhea in travelers.

EPIDEMIOLOGY. Several prospective studies have shown that for any 2-week visit an attack rate of 20 to 50% might be expected. The incidence depends on the country of origin and destination. When destination is considered, the risk of diarrhea is lowest (<10%) in Canada, the United States, northern Europe, Australia, and New Zealand; moderate (~20%) in southern Europe, Israel, South Africa, and the Caribbean; and highest (20 to 50%) for travel to Africa, Latin America, the Middle East, and most parts of Asia. Although gender does not affect the risk of travelers' diarrhea, age does; young adults and children are most prone to illness.

CLINICAL MANIFESTATIONS. The onset of traveler's diarrhea typically occurs between 5 and 15 days after arrival in a risk area. Illness is generally characterized by malaise, anorexia, nausea, abdominal cramps, and watery diarrhea consisting of 3 to 10 unformed stools daily. Illness is usually self-limited, lasting 2 to 5 days. Symptoms may also appear on return home, usually during the first 7 to 10 days. Although mortality is exceedingly rare during traveler's diarrhea, 1% are admitted to hospital, 20% are confined to bed for 1 to 2 days, and 40% are forced to change their travel itinerary.

DIAGNOSIS

Differential Diagnosis. Often the likely cause of traveler's diarrhea may be ascertained from a detailed clinical history and physical examination. Sudden onset of small-volume diarrhea, associated with tenesmus and lower abdominal cramps and accompanied by fever, suggests an invasive bacterial pathogen e.g., *Salmonella* (Chapter 76), *Shigella* (Chapter 40), *Campylobacter* (Chapter 43), or *Yersinia* (Chapter 44.1). Amebic dysentery classically has a gradual onset, progressively worsening symptoms, and low-grade fever (Chapter 86). Bloody diarrhea is noted in less than half of those who are infected with invasive pathogens. Noninvasive bacterial pathogens, e.g., ETEC, enteroadherent *E. coli* (EAEC) (Chapter 42), and vibrios (Chapter 41), tend to produce large-volume diarrhea, midabdominal cramps in the absence of fever, and tenesmus. The insidious onset of large-volume diarrhea, bloating, nausea, flatulence, and excessive fatigue is typical of parasitic causes of diarrhea, almost exclusively due to giardiasis, cyclosporiasis, isosporiasis, and cryptosporidiosis.

Another clue to the etiology of traveler's diarrhea is the time of onset of illness. Bacterial- and viral-induced diarrheas usually have short incubation periods and therefore may occur as early as 2 to 3 days following arrival in a risk area. Diarrhea from intestinal protozoa invariably begins at least 3 or 4 days after exposure. Amebic dysentery, on the other hand, may occur months after leaving an endemic area.

"Nontropical" causes of traveler's diarrhea must always be a consideration, particularly in those with persistent symptoms. A history of recent antibiotic use should prompt testing for *Clostridium difficile* cytotoxin. Where risk factors for AIDS are present, opportunistic infections, e.g., herpes and cytomegalovirus, require investigation.

A single stool culture will detect most bacterial pathogens. However, *Vibrio cholerae* will be missed unless a culture on alkaline media is requested. Intestinal parasites are intermittently excreted, and therefore several stool examinations for parasites (usually three) may be necessary to detect the causative pathogen. Since many diagnostic laboratories do not

TABLE 144–1. Geographic Distribution of Pathogens in Travelers' Diarrhea

Organism	Latin America (%)	Asia (%)	Africa (%)	Middle East (%)
Enterotoxigenic *Escherichia coli* (ETEC)	17–70	6–37	8–42	29–33
Enteroinvasive *E. coli* (EIEC)	2–7	2–3	0–2	1
Other *E. coli* (EAEC, EHEC, EPEC)	5–15	1	2–7	NA
Shigella spp.	2–30	0–17	0–9	8–26
Salmonella spp.	1–16	1–33	4–25	2
Campylobacter jejuni	1–5	9–39	1–28	1–2
Aeromonas spp.	1–5	1–57	0–9	1
Plesiomonas shigelloides	0–6	3–13	3–5	1
Vibrio cholerae non-01	0–2	1–7	0–4	2
Yersinia spp.	NA	0–3	NA	1
Rotavirus	0–6	1–8	0–36	NA
Entamoeba histolytica	NA	5–11	2–9	NA
Giardia lamblia	1–2	1–12	0–1	NA
Cryptosporidium	NA	1–5	2	NA
No pathogen identified	24–62	10–56	15–53	50–51

From Peltola H, Gorbach SL: Travelers' diarrhea: epidemiology and clinical aspects. *In* DuPont H, Steffen R (eds): Textbook of Travel Medicine and Health. Hamilton, Ontario, Canada, BC Decker, 1997, pp 78–86.
EAEC, enteroadherent *E. coli*; EHEC, enterohemorrhagic *E. coli*; EPEC, enteropathogenic *E. coli*; NA, not available.

TABLE 144-2. Antibiotic Treatment of Traveler's Diarrhea*

Drug	Dose	Frequency	Duration
Norfloxacin	400 mg	b.i.d.	3 days
Ciprofloxacin	500 mg	b.i.d.	3 days
Ofloxacin	300 mg	b.i.d.	3 days
TMP-SMZ†	160/800 mg	b.i.d.	3 days
Single Dose			
Norfloxacin	800 mg	once	
Ciprofloxacin	500 mg–1 g	once	
Ofloxacin	600 mg	once	
TMP-SMZ†	320/1600 mg	once	

*When combined with loperamide efficacy may be improved.
†Trimethoprim-sulfamethoxazole.

routinely perform modified acid-fast stains for *Cyclospora* (Chapter 89) and *Cryptosporidium* sp. (Chapter 88), it is important to ask specifically that this technique be applied during microscopic examinations of feces for parasites. Unfortunately, newer diagnostic techniques, e.g., gene probes and polymerase chain reaction (PCR) testing for DNA, and monoclonal antibody testing for pathogen antigens, largely remain research tools and are not available for the routine investigation of traveler's diarrhea. With the exception of amebic antibody detection, serology is not a useful diagnostic tool for traveler's diarrhea.

Diagnostic Tests. Invasive enteric pathogens can often be distinguished from noninvasive ones by stool examinations for occult or gross blood, or leukocytes. Leukocytes can be found most easily by methylene blue staining or lactoferrin antigen detection in fresh stool.

TREATMENT

Oral Rehydration and Dietary Recommendations. The mainstay of therapy for traveler's diarrhea is the maintenance of adequate fluid and electrolyte balance. A variety of oral rehydration solutions are available, especially for children, which contain a mixture of glucose or sugar with an electrolyte solution (Chapter 16). Although Gatorade, cola, apple juice, and orange juice are electrolyte-poor, the juices are high in potassium. Continued food intake is likely to be beneficial. Travelers with diarrhea should withhold solid foods during the acute phase of illness; when illness is improving, carbohydrates (e.g., breads, potatoes, rice, and bananas) and white meats (e.g., fish and chicken) may be taken. Fruits, vegetables, red meat, and milk products should be added only when symptoms have resolved.

Antibiotic Therapy. Effective antibiotic therapy often reduces the duration of traveler's diarrhea by more than 50%, and in some cases to a few hours. Quinolones, ciprofloxacin and norfloxacin, are the most effective antibiotics for the treatment of bacterial diarrheas (Table 144–2). Trimethoprim-sulfamethoxazole, which was widely used as the drug of choice for traveler's diarrhea, fell out of favor in the early 1990s because of the worldwide development of resistance to this drug by *Shigella* and ETEC. In addition, the recognition of *Campylobacter* spp. as an important cause of traveler's diarrhea favored the use of fluoroquinolones to which they are usually sensitive (Chapter 43). However, they may still be an effective agents for traveler's diarrhea acquired in Mexico. Because of widespread, high-grade resistance, doxycycline is no longer recommended. A single dose of antibiotic (often combined with loperamide) is an effective form of therapy for traveler's diarrhea; however, most practitioners continue to recommend a full 3-day course of therapy.

Quinolone resistance has recently been reported for *Campylobacter* isolates in Southeast Asia. Azithromycin, which exhibits excellent in vitro activity against multiple bacterial pathogens, has been used successfully to treat *Campylobacter* infections in northern Thailand; however, the drug was less effective against other pathogens and resistance to it has been noted as well. Also, nonabsorbable antibiotics such as bicozamycin and aztreonam have been effective in the treatment of traveler's diarrhea.

Nonantibiotic Therapy. Bismuth subsalicylate (BSS), 30 mL or two tablets every 30 to 60 minutes, as needed, to a maximum of eight doses per 24 hours, reduces the number of unformed stools by approximately 50%. This is most likely an effect of the antisecretory action of the salicylate moiety, although BSS also has antibacterial and anti-inflammatory properties.

By virtue of its antimotility action, loperamide reduces both the frequency of bowel movements and the duration of illness by up to 80%. Reports in the 1960s and 1970s recommended avoiding loperamide in patients with fever or dysentery; however, recent reports suggest this risk is overstated. As an adverse effect of reducing the number of bowel movements, antimotility agents may worsen abdominal cramping. Although the results of recent studies are conflicting about the increased efficacy of adding loperamide to antibiotic therapy, the combination provides rapid symptomatic relief while eradicating the offending organism. The risk of toxic megacolon from antimotility drugs may be eliminated with combination therapy.

Silicate clay (kaolin, attapulgite), hydrophilic agents (methylcellulose, psyllium, and polycarbophil), and probiotics (acidophilus, lactobacillus) have demonstrated little value in the treatment of acute traveler's diarrhea.

PREVENTION

Dietary Restrictions. Careful attention to food and beverage selection can reduce, but not totally eliminate, the likelihood of developing traveler's diarrhea. This is especially true for the long-term traveler or one who is traveling on a more adventurous itinerary where it may be almost impossible to avoid fecally contaminated food or beverage. General advice with respect to food and water centers around avoidance of salads and undercooked foods of any type, and the selection of foods that are fresh, well cooked, and served piping hot. Ice cubes made with tap water should be considered contaminated even when added to alcoholic beverages. However, dietary restrictions are of little value in preventing traveler's diarrhea; the primary problem is not the value of dietary restrictions in preventing infection, but rather the unwillingness of the traveler to adhere to them. This failure of motivation or "compliance" with dietary restrictions has stimulated much discussion about the use of nonantibiotic and antibiotic prophylaxis for traveler's diarrhea.

Antimicrobial Prophylaxis. Fluoroquinolones and BSS will reduce the incidence of traveler's diarrhea by 90 and 65%, respectively, during short-term travel in a developing country (Table 144–3). Minor side effects from their use in this situation are infrequent (1 to 3%) and severe reactions are rare (0 to 0.01%). To be effective, BSS must be taken four times each day; it can cause blackening of stools and the

TABLE 144-3. Prophylaxis for Traveler's Diarrhea

(One dose daily during exposure and for the following 2 days)	
Norfloxacin	400 mg
Ciprofloxacin	500 mg
Ofloxacin	300 mg
TMP-SMZ*	160/800 mg
Bismuth subsalicylate	Two tablets chewed q.i.d.

*Trimethoprim-sulfamethoxazole.

tongue and lead to tinnitus. Adverse reactions to antibiotics range from mild gastrointestinal upset to death from anaphylaxis. Because of the potential for side effects, increasing antibiotic resistance, and the ease of self-treatment of traveler's diarrhea, a National Institutes of Health consensus conference concluded that prophylactic antibiotic use is generally not recommended. Most travelers should be given loperamide and a self-treatment course of antibiotics to use at the onset of symptoms. Nevertheless, some experts continue to recommend prophylaxis in high-risk situations in which the traveler cannot afford even a short illness (e.g., military and diplomatic personnel and athletes) or is at risk of serious illness because of an underlying medical problem (e.g., AIDS, brittle diabetes mellitus, renal insufficiency, or inflammatory bowel disease).

Persistent Traveler's Diarrhea

ETIOLOGY AND INCIDENCE. There are limited data on the incidence, natural history of, and predisposing factors for chronic traveler's diarrhea. In a study of 4607 Peace Corps volunteers from the United States who were stationed in Central and West Africa, Haiti, and Nepal, 1.7% reported persistent diarrhea of >30 days. In a study of Swiss who traveled outside their country for ≤3 months, persistent diarrhea lasting >30 days was reported in 0.9% (73 of the 7886 persons). When persistent traveler's diarrhea is defined as a diarrheal illness lasting >14 days, 2 to 3% of those having acute traveler's diarrhea develop this complication. Although the etiology of persistent traveler's diarrhea is not well worked out, empirically postinfectious phenomena e.g., lactose intolerance and irritable bowel syndrome appear to be the most frequent causes (Chapter 4).

Infectious Causes. Intestinal pathogens are found in a small proportion of those with persisting traveler's diarrhea. Although most bacterial pathogens have been detected in those with prolonged gastrointestinal upset, it is unclear whether they are responsible for the symptoms or are present during the convalescent phase of illness. Enteroadherent, enteroaggregative, enteropathogenic, and enterohemorrhagic *E. coli* are pathogens found in children with persistent diarrhea in developing countries. On the other hand, enteric parasitic infections, notably giardiasis, cryptosporidiosis, cyclosporiasis, and amebiasis, are culprits that frequently produce prolonged gastrointestinal symptoms. *Entamoeba histolytica* is frequently blamed for causing chronic diarrhea; however, recent studies showing the existence of a microscopically indistinguishable nonpathogen, *Entamoeba dispar*, would suggest otherwise (Chapter 86).

Clostridium difficile should be ruled out in those who have received antimicrobial agents or, less frequently, antimalarial drugs. Persistent diarrhea in the returning traveler may be the result of human immunodeficiency virus (HIV) enteropathy. Enteric opportunistic infections in the immunocompromised host with organisms e.g., microsporidia, cytomegalovirus, or cryptosporidium may be the initial manifestation of HIV disease. In many cases of persistent diarrhea in the returning traveler, no microorganism is identified. Since the clinical pattern resembles an infectious disease, enteric pathogens not yet recognized may elude our best currently available diagnostic capabilities.

Parasites responsible for chronic diarrhea and malabsorption include *Giardia lamblia*, *Strongyloides stercoralis*, *Isospora belli*, *Ascaris lumbricoides*, *Capillaria philippinensis*, *Metagonimus yokogawai*, and *Cyclospora cayetanensis*.

Postinfective Malabsorption. One potential pitfall is the assumption that all chronic diarrhea from tropical countries is infectious. In a retrospective review of 129 inpatients at

the Hospital for Tropical Diseases in London from 1978 to 1984 who had bloody diarrhea acquired ≤2 weeks of return from the tropics, 25% had inflammatory bowel disease or colon cancer. If a workup for enteric pathogens and malabsorption is negative, especially in older persons, stool for occult blood and colonoscopic evaluation may be indicated.

An attack of acute infectious diarrhea may precipitate intestinal disaccharidase deficiency as a result of widespread damage to the intestinal mucosa; lactase deficiency is the most common followed by sucrase deficiency, which causes diarrhea when fruit or preserves are ingested. Symptoms of lactase deficiency include chronic diarrhea, abdominal pain, gaseous distention, and flatulence (Chapter 4). Postinfective malabsorption is frequently seen after acute enterovirus or rotavirus enteritis in infants and children (Chapter 27.2), whereas in adults the problem usually follows giardiasis (Chapter 87). Lactase deficiency may be temporary, resolving within a few weeks, or less commonly may become permanent. The latter may be the result of a preexisting genetic subclinical disaccharidase deficiency that becomes manifest after an infection.

In some parts of the world, notably the Caribbean and East Asia, tropical sprue is relatively common, but it is rare in travelers to these areas. It is more common in expatriates living abroad for at least 1 year, but may affect short-term travelers as well. Tropical sprue, caused by an overgrowth of bacteria in the small intestine, is associated with a chronic malabsorption syndrome characterized by anorexia, diarrhea, weight loss, and floating and foul-smelling stools (Chapter 4). Less commonly, underlying celiac sprue may be unmasked by an acute episode of traveler's diarrhea.

Diagnostic Testing. Diagnostic tests used to investigate chronic malabsorption include D-xylose absorption, Sudan stain of fecal fat in stool, 72-hour fecal fat, or ^{14}C-triolein breath test. In addition, serum albumin, carotene, and vitamin B_{12} levels may be reduced. A small bowel aspirate and biopsy are appropriate diagnostic interventions to characterize the cause of malabsorption. An aspirate may yield *Giardia*, *Strongyloides*, *Cyclospora*, or bacterial overgrowth. A biopsy of the small bowel may reveal the characteristic crypt hyperplasia and villous atrophy associated with malabsorption from any of the aforementioned causes (Fig. 4–3 and 89–3).

Variable and usually mild degrees of malabsorption occur in indigenous healthy persons living in the tropics in a condition commonly known as subclinical tropical malabsorption. A decreased absorption of D-xylose and glucose may be found associated with mild changes in small bowel architecture. The condition appears to be seasonal and invariably remits when the traveler returns to a temperate climate.

Inflammatory Bowel Disease. Unmasking of a previously asymptomatic gastrointestinal disorder may follow a bout of traveler's diarrhea. For example, inflammatory bowel disease, specifically ulcerative colitis, may be indistinguishable from amebic colitis or postdysenteric colitis. Before steroid therapy is considered for idiopathic ulcerative colitis it is imperative to rule out *Entamoeba histolytica* infection with stool examinations and serology (Chapter 86).

Irritable Bowel Syndrome. One of the most frequent disorders following acute traveler's diarrhea is an irritable bowel–like syndrome. Patients complain of crampy abdominal pain and intermittent diarrhea that occasionally alternates with constipation, bloating, and flatulence. The cause of this complication may be a postinfectious irritable bowel syndrome or an exaggeration of preexisting symptoms. It may represent a primary alteration in gut motility or be secondary to or exacerbated by the acute infection.

DIAGNOSIS AND MANAGEMENT
Clinical Evaluation. Chronic traveler's diarrhea is due to multiple syndromes with a variety of etiologies. An evalua-

tion of the patient with persistent traveler's diarrhea begins with a detailed medical and travel history. Particular attention should be paid to the onset and nature of symptoms and the response or lack of response to antibiotics and dietary items. The initial workup should include a bacterial culture and three stool specimens for ova and parasite examination. Stools might be tested for *Giardia* and *Cryptosporidium* antigens. Even if a bacterial culture is negative, empirical therapy with an antibiotic, e.g., a quinolone, might be appropriate since pathogenic *E. coli* cannot be diagnosed by most laboratories. If bacterial causes can be ruled out by culture or presumptive treatment, and symptoms persist, empirical therapy with metronidazole for giardiasis may be appropriate. If weight loss persists in the absence of an infectious etiology, a D-xylose or fecal fat test may be obtained to document malabsorption.

Empirical Therapy. When attempts to elucidate the cause of persistent traveler's diarrhea are unrewarding, some clinicians resort to empirical antimicrobial or antigiardial therapy, whereas others focus on dietary alteration as the initial therapy of choice. Many patients with a presumptive diagnosis of irritable bowel syndrome respond dramatically to psyllium hydrophilic mucilloid (Metamucil) or methylcellulose (Citrucel), given as 1 or 2 tablespoons/day. Natural bran works equally well but compliance may be an issue because patients do not consider it medication. Dietary manipulation in the form of a lactose-free diet is often very helpful in modulating some of the more distressing symptoms. Empirical treatment with digestive enzymes (e.g., pancreatic enzymes, lactase) may be of benefit in some individuals. A recent report suggests that cholestyramine may be useful when upper gastrointestinal dysmotility produces bile enteritis characterized by green-colored watery stools. Finally, some patients respond to antispasmodics, e.g., chlordiazepoxide/clidinium or chlordiazepoxide/amitriptyline, hyoscyamine, or scopolamine.

Bibliography

Addiss DG, Tauxe RV, Bernard KW: Chronic diarrheal illness in U.S. Peace Corps volunteers. Int J Epidemiol 19:217, 1990.

Anand AC, Reddy PS, Saiprasad GS, Kher SK: Does non-dysenteric intestinal amoebiasis exist? Lancet 349:89, 1997.

Bhan MK, Raj P, Levine MM, et al: Enteroaggregative *Escherichia coli* associated with persistent diarrhea in a cohort of rural children in India. J Infect Dis 159:1061, 1989.

Connor BA, Shlim DR, Scholes JV, et al: Pathologic changes in the small bowel in nine patients with diarrhea associated with a coccidia-like body. Ann Intern Med 119:377, 1993.

Cook GC: Aetiology and pathogenesis of postinfective tropical malabsorption (tropical sprue). Lancet 1:721, 1984.

DuPont HL, Capsuto EG: Persistent diarrhea in travelers. Clin Infect Dis 22:124, 1996.

DuPont HL, Ericsson CD: Prevention and treatment of traveler's diarrhea. N Engl J Med 328:1821, 1993.

Fung WP, Monteiro EH, Ang HB, et al: Ulcerative postdysenteric colitis. Am J Gastroenterol 57:341, 1972.

Giannella RA: Chronic diarrhea in travelers: diagnostic and therapeutic considerations. Rev Infect Dis 8:S223, 1986.

Harries AD, Myers B, Cook GC: Inflammatory bowel disease: a common cause of bloody diarrhoea in visitors to the tropics. Br Med J 291:1686, 1985.

Hoge CW, Shlim DR, Echeverria P, et al: Epidemiology of diarrhea among expatriate residents living in a highly endemic environment. JAMA 275:533, 1996.

Hoge CW, Shlim DR, Rajah R, et al: Epidemiology of diarrheal illness associated with coccidian-like organism among travellers and foreign residents in Nepal. Lancet 341:1175, 1993.

Klipstein FA: Tropical sprue in travelers and expatriates living abroad. Gastroenterology 80:590, 1981.

McKendrick MW, Read NW: Irritable bowel syndrome—post salmonella infection. J Infect 29:1, 1994.

Osterholm MT, MacDonald KL, White KE, et al: An outbreak of a newly recognized chronic diarrhea syndrome associated with raw milk consumption. JAMA 256:484, 1986.

Schumacher G, Kollberg B, Ljungh A: Inflammatory bowel disease presenting as travellers' diarrhoea. Lancet 341:241, 1993.

Steffen R, van der Linde F, Gyr K, Schar M: Epidemiology of diarrhea in travelers. JAMA 249:1176, 1983.

Taylor DN, Houston R, Shlim DR, et al: Etiology of diarrhea among travelers and foreign residents in Nepal. JAMA 260:1245, 1988.

Tomkins AM, James WPT, Walters JH, Cole ACE: Malabsorption in overland travellers to India. Br Med J 3:380, 1974.

Trier JS, Moxey PC, Schimmel EM, Robles E: Chronic intestinal coccidiosis in man: intestinal morphology and response to treatment. Gastroenterology 66:923, 1974.

145 *Fever in Travelers*

Alan J. Magill and G. Thomas Strickland

More tropical infectious diseases are being encountered in temperate climates because of the marked increase in movement of peoples (international travel, immigration, dislocations) and importation of food items within a global economy. Owing to the speed of air travel, travelers can return to their home countries within the incubation period of most infectious agents. For example, a febrile patient could have been on an East African camera safari 3 or 4 days previously. Therefore, the differential diagnosis must include falciparum malaria, African trypanosomiasis, Rift Valley fever, and other exotic infections. Travel to nontropical lesser developed countries (LDCs) still carries a high risk for food- and water-borne illness but usually has a lower risk for vector-borne illness than does travel in the tropics.

Individuals who have traveled in LDCs are possibly exposed to the usual causes of fever occurring in temperate climates (e.g., influenza, pneumococcal pneumonia, streptococcal pharyngitis); conditions endemic to the tropics or subtropics (e.g., malaria, visceral leishmaniasis, amebiasis, dengue, yellow fever); and other infections with a higher prevalence in LDCs (e.g., tuberculosis, viral hepatitis, salmonellosis).

It is not necessary to travel outside the country to be infected with exotic microbes. Cutaneous anthrax can be acquired by domestic textile workers from contaminated hides or yarn imported from Asia or South America; outbreaks of cyclospora enteritis have resulted from contaminated imported berries; and autochthonous vivax malaria has been documented in California, Georgia, Michigan, New Jersey, New York, and Texas within the last decade.

In general, the risk of acquiring a febrile illness during international travel depends on the area visited (Chapter 149), length of stay, season, and choice of accommodation, food and drink, and travel. Within each LDC, the risk of acquiring disease can vary greatly. Travelers venturing to smaller cities off the usual tourist routes and those who spend time in villages or rural areas for extended periods are at much greater risk of acquiring infectious diseases; this is because of greater exposure to the disease-transmitting insect vectors and to contaminated water and food as well as closer contact with local residents who might harbor infectious organisms. Therefore, it is not sufficient to ask, "Where have you been?" The physician must also ask, "Where did you go in the country?" and "How long did you stay?" and "What did you do?"

EVALUATION OF FEVER IN TRAVELERS. A history of recent travel in the tropics complicates and extends the differential diagnosis of fever.

Guiding Points in Management. Some infections (e.g., falciparum malaria, typhoid fever, meningococcemia) can be rapidly fatal if not quickly diagnosed and treated. Some infections (e.g., tuberculosis, viral hemorrhagic fevers) are highly contagious and require isolation of the patient to prevent secondary cases. Rickettsial infections and leptospirosis require early empirical therapy based on clinical suspicion before specific diagnostic test results are available in order to minimize morbidity and mortality.

Epidemiology. Clinical experience from two published series has shown that about 35% of patients with a significant febrile illness who recently traveled to malaria-endemic areas are proven to have malaria, 25% remain undiagnosed, and the remaining 40% have other infectious and noninfectious causes of their fever. Points useful in narrowing the differential diagnosis are the incubation period, vaccination and prophylaxis history, length of stay and living conditions, fever pattern, associated signs and symptoms, and geographic location of exposure.

Incubation Period. Knowledge concerning the time of exposure helps in making the correct diagnosis (Table 145–1). Some infectious diseases can be excluded if the time when the patient left the endemic area is known. In the case of malaria, this time usually ranges from as little as 10 to 15 days for falciparum malaria to 1 month or longer for *Plasmodium malariae* infection. However, this interval is frequently prolonged in patients who have received antimalarial suppressive therapy or who have partial immunity. Some strains of *P. vivax* can also have prolonged incubation periods (Chapter 92). Exposure does not have to be recent. The incubation period for many viral illnesses is measured in days; bacterial infections can be days to weeks; and parasitic infections can be days to months. The incubation periods for some illnesses, e.g., hepatitis A and E (20 to 45 days) and hepatitis B and C (45 to 90 days) have been well documented. Symptoms due to febrile arboviral infections usually occur within 1 week of the infecting bite, whereas the incubation period for the hemorrhagic fevers is usually longer.

Vaccination History. A history of vaccination for hepatitis A or B or yellow fever virtually excludes these diagnoses. Immunization with the currently available typhoid vaccines provides partial protection, usually quoted as between 50 and 70%. Childhood immunization for poliomyelitis, diphtheria, and tuberculosis may not provide protection in adults unless they received boosters or had natural exposure.

Prophylaxis History. Immune globulin provides partial protection for hepatitis A that decreases as the time following administration increases. Although faithful use of an effective antimalarial is likely to prevent malaria, failures of chemoprophylaxis occur with any regimen used (Chapter 92).

Length of Patient's Stay and Living Conditions. Exposures are heavily influenced by living conditions and length of stay. Tourists who stay for brief periods in first-class hotels in capital cities or tourist centers have different and less intense exposure than backpackers or volunteer workers who live on the economy with the local population and who often stay for longer periods in rural areas. These latter groups have a higher likelihood of acquiring diseases, e.g., tuberculosis, filariasis, visceral leishmaniasis, and schistosomiasis as well as malaria, diarrheal illness, and intestinal parasites.

Temperature Pattern. The maximum temperature and the type of temperature curve can assist in the differential diagnosis. Infections that characteristically have high fever spikes, frequently in the 105 to 106°F (40.5 to 41°C) range, are falciparum malaria, pneumococcal pneumonia, encephalitis, measles, and meningococcemia. The maximum fever in other infections, e.g., influenza, typhoid fever (Fig. 145–1A), tuberculosis (Fig. 145–1B), vivax malaria (Fig. 145–1C), African trypanosomiasis, pyelonephritis, brucellosis, relapsing fever, leptospirosis, dengue, the viral hemorrhagic fevers, is usually in the 103 to 104°F (39.5 to 40°C) range. Lower fever spikes (101 to 102° F [38.5 to 39°C]) are usually noted in most other viral infections, diphtheria, nontyphoidal salmonella infections, and familial Mediterranean fever.

The type of fever pattern is sometimes helpful in making the correct diagnosis (Fig. 145–1). A continuous fever (Fig. 145–1A) is one in which the temperature curve remains elevated without significant diurnal variation. Untreated typhoid fever and typhus often have this type of pattern. A remittent fever (Fig. 145–1B) has a curve with daily fluctuations of 2°C or more, with the low point in the day approaching but not reaching the normal level. This is the most common fever pattern and is characteristically found in pulmonary tuberculosis, bacterial septicemias, and African trypanosomiasis. An intermittent fever (Fig. 145–1C) is one in which the temperature drops to normal or below normal each day, with a wide variation between the peak and the nadir. This pattern is often seen in malaria, pyogenic abscesses, and miliary tuberculosis. A relapsing fever (Fig. 145–1D) is one in which febrile periods alternate with several days of normal temperature. This pattern is sometimes seen in quartan malaria, dengue fever, and relapsing fever caused by *Borrelia recurrentis*.

Associated Signs and Symptoms. Abrupt onset of pyrexia, high temperature (102°F [39.5°C] or greater), and chills are particularly suggestive of an infectious etiology. Other nonspecific but common symptoms are malaise, myalgia, arthralgia, headache, and photophobia. Signs and symptoms that may help in pinpointing the site of infection and agent(s) are nausea, vomiting, diarrhea, lymphadenopathy, splenomegaly, dysuria, urinary frequency, flank pain, sore throat, coryza, cough, pleuritic pain, and nuchal rigidity. Fever with diarrhea suggests an invasive bowel pathogen, e.g., *Shigella*, *Campylobacter*, invasive *Escherichia coli*, *Entamoeba histolytica*, or rotavirus infection. Frequent loose stools may occur with malaria, dengue, scrub typhus, leptospirosis, and enteric fever. However, constipation is frequently present in the last named. The viral hemorrhagic fevers can cause bloody diarrhea, as can the bowel pathogens. Chills occur occasionally in many infectious diseases; however, they are common in diseases characterized by rapid proliferation of the infecting

TABLE 145–1. Incubation Periods for More Common Infections Causing Fever in Travelers to Lesser Developed Countries

Short (<10 days)	
Campylobacter enterititis	Dengue fever (and other
Enteric fevers	arboviral infections)
Leptospirosis	Influenza
Salmonellosis	Rickettsial infections
Toxigenic *E. coli* infection	Shigellosis
Medium (10–21 days)	
Cytomegalovirus	Enteric fevers
Leptospirosis	Malaria (all)
Measles	Toxoplasmosis
Long (>21 days)	
Acute HIV infection	Acute schistosomiasis
African trypanosomiasis	Amebic liver abscess
Brucellosis	Cytomegalovirus
Filariasis	Infectious mononucleosis
P. falciparum (with use of	(acute EBV)
antimalarials)	*P. vivax*, *P. ovale*, and *P. malariae*
Secondary syphilis	infections
Visceral leishmaniasis	Viral hepatitis

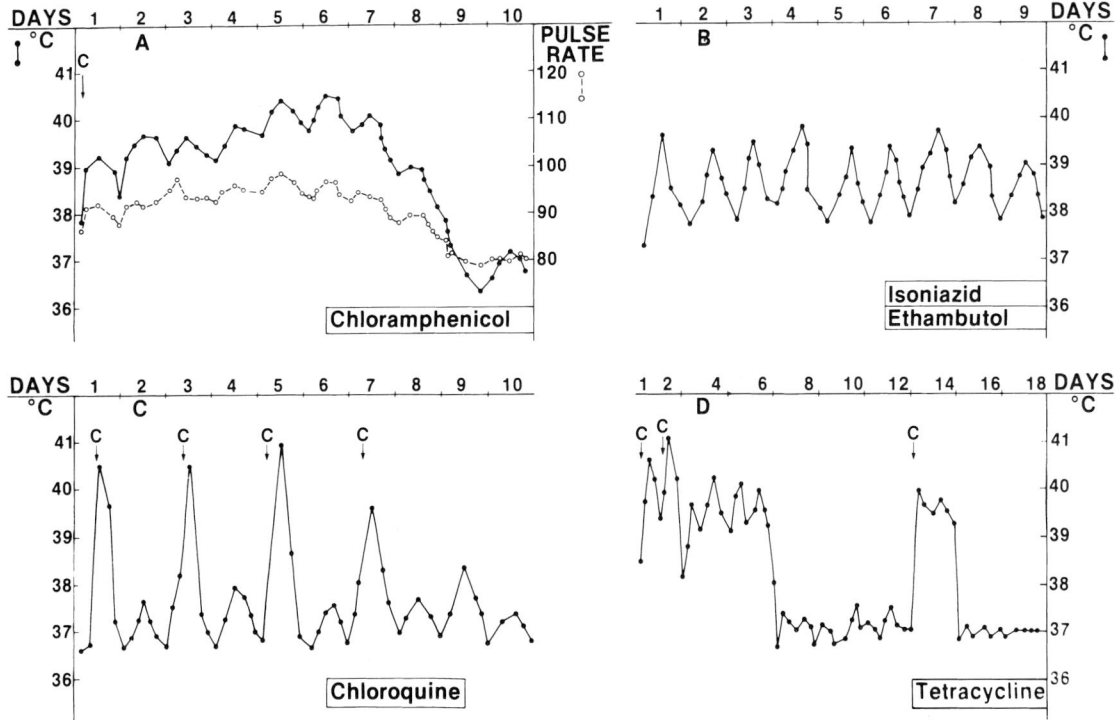

Figure 145–1. Four examples of fever patterns. *A, Continuous fever.* Temperature and pulse curve in a 26-year-old Indonesian male with typhoid fever who had a single chill (c) and clinical response to chloramphenicol therapy. *B, Remittent fever.* Temperature curve in a 27-year-old Indian woman with pulmonary tuberculosis who was treated with isoniazid and ethambutol. She was chilly every afternoon during the temperature elevation but did not have a rigor. *C, Intermittent fever.* Temperature curve of a 14-year-old Filipino female with established vivax malaria. She had shaking chills (c), each time associated with temperature elevations, and had an excellent response to chloroquine therapy. *D, Relapsing fever.* Temperature curve of a 22-year-old Ethiopian man with *Borrelia recurrentis* infection. He had chills (c) associated with temperature elevations and was treated with tetracycline.

agent (Table 145–2). Lymphadenopathy occurs so frequently that it is often not a useful diagnostic finding; however, malaria and the enteric pathogens seldom cause lymph node enlargement. Splenomegaly (Table 145–3), rash (Table 145–4), and jaundice (Table 145–5) can be useful findings in narrowing the differential diagnosis.

Geographic Location of Exposure. There are areas of the world where exposures to specific infectious agents are rather common (Table 145–6 and Chapter 149). Malaria, typhoid fever, and infectious hepatitis are widespread throughout the tropics and must be considered in every febrile patient. However, the geographic distribution of many other infectious diseases is quite localized. For example, Ebola fever, Marburg disease, Lassa fever, and African trypanosomiasis are limited to certain locations in Africa.

Work-Up of Fever. A patient with fever and a recent history of travel to tropical areas should have a thorough evaluation (Fig. 145–2). This should be done even though there is a reasonable likelihood that the cause of the fever is nontropical and self-limiting.

History. The usual historical questions as well as a travel-related history are important. A careful history should help rule out noninfectious causes of fever, including allergic reactions to drugs or serum, an exaggerated circadian temperature rhythm, and factitious fever. A travel history emphasizing the exposure history (Table 145–7) can help focus the diagnostic possibilities, and the associated signs and symptoms can lead to the correct diagnosis.

Physical Examination. Recording the vital signs; auscultation of the chest and heart; palpation of the liver, spleen, and lymph nodes; visual inspection of the skin for rash and the eyes for icterus, conjunctival injection, or suffusion; and a more extensive examination of any organ system associated with symptoms are the minimal requirements during the initial screening examination.

Laboratory Tests. Minimal laboratory tests to be performed include complete blood count and urinalysis. Other tests that should be performed, if historical, physical, or other

TABLE 145–2. Infectious Diseases Characteristically Associated with Chills

Malaria	Plague
Lobar pneumonia	Typhus fever
Influenza	Pyelonephritis
Typhoid fever	Bacterial abscess
Bacterial septicemia	Dengue
Cholangitis	Chikungunya

TABLE 145–3. Infections Causing Fever and Splenomegaly

Viruses	Bacteria	Parasites
Infectious mononucleosis	Enteric fever	Malaria
	Typhus	Visceral leishmaniasis
Cytomegalovirus (CMV)	Endocarditis	African trypanosomiasis
	Tuberculosis	Acute schistosomiasis
HIV infection	Brucellosis	Toxoplasmosis
	Leptospirosis	Acute American
	Relapsing fever	trypanosomiasis

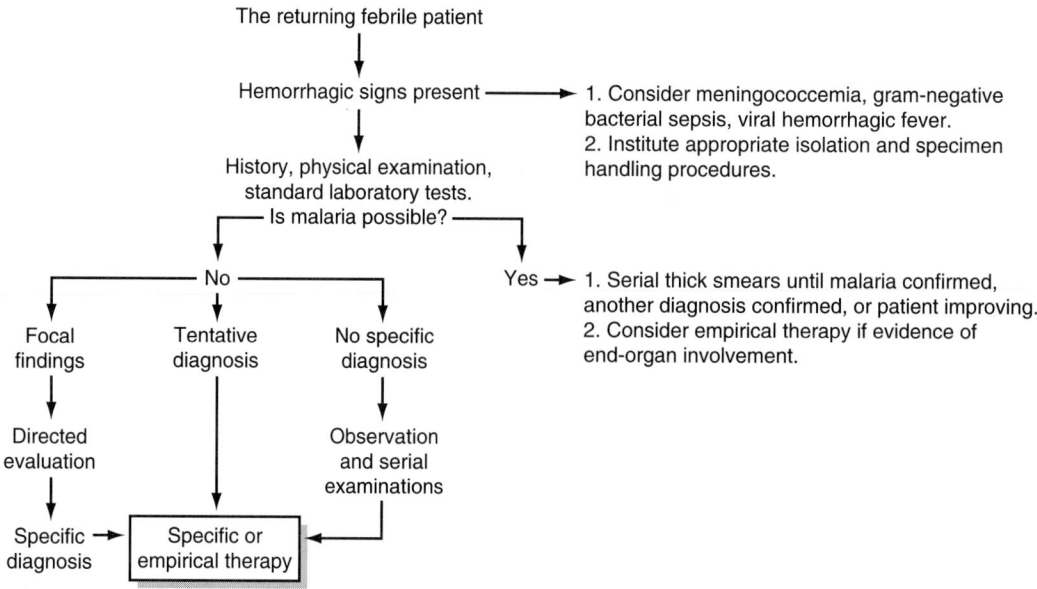

Figure 145–2. Algorithm for evaluation of a febrile patient who has been in the tropics.

laboratory findings suggest that they are indicated, include malaria blood film; chest radiograph; blood, stool, and urine cultures for bacteria; sputum smears and cultures for acid-fast bacilli; determinations of serum ALT and AST enzymes and alkaline phosphatase; and selected serologic tests.

If viral hemorrhagic fever is suspected, the communicable diseases branch of the local state health department should be informed, and all nonessential laboratory tests should be withheld until the situation has been thoroughly reviewed. In addition, the patient should be managed using strict barrier nursing techniques (i.e., gown, gloves, mask, separate room) until these highly contagious and serious infections have been ruled out.

Follow-Up. If the initial evaluation and findings are inconclusive and a serious illness is not believed to be present, the patient may be sent home and advised to chart his or her temperature and return in 2 or 3 days if the fever persists (sooner if feeling sicker). If there are positive or suspected positive findings, the patient should be hospitalized and treated. A young college student with an unremitting fever of 103°F, a pulse of 90, headache, chills, cough, constipation, and splenomegaly who had been working on a ranch in Mexico until 2 weeks before the onset of symptoms may have typhoid fever. This patient should be hospitalized, and blood, stool, and urine cultures should be performed. However, not everyone who has an established diagnosis will need to be hospitalized. For example, most patients with vivax malaria can be treated as outpatients.

Most patients sent home following the initial evaluation have a self-limiting viral infection and experience a spontaneous resolution of their illness. Serial observation and evaluation is required for those who remain febrile. If they have been keeping a temperature chart, this could be of diagnostic assistance. Laboratory tests, invasive procedures (biopsies), and imaging studies are performed as clinically indicated.

Empirical Chemotherapy. In rare cases, a diagnosis will not be made following a comprehensive evaluation, and a therapeutic trial may be indicated. Chemotherapy can be started for tuberculosis if this is suspected and specimens have been collected for cultures. Often, a patient may become afebrile and have considerable improvement in clinical symp-

TABLE 145–4. Infections Causing Fever and Rash

Infection	Cutaneous Manifestations
Measles	Maculopapular
Rubella	Maculopapular
Dengue	Diffuse erythematous or scarlatiniform; petechiae and ecchymoses in a few
Viral hemorrhagic fevers	Petechiae, ecchymoses
Infectious mononucleosis	Maculopapular
Monkey pox	Maculopapular, vesicular, pustular
HIV infection	Morbilliform
Spotted fevers	Diffuse macular or maculopapular; petechiae
Epidemic typhus	Diffuse macular or maculopapular
Scrub typhus	Eschar; diffuse macular or maculopapular
Secondary syphilis	Papular (copper penny)
Lyme disease	Maculopapular, erythematous
Typhoid fever	Rose-colored papules on trunk
Gonococcemia	Pustular, hemorrhagic, necrotic
Meningococcemia	Maculopapular, petechiae, ecchymoses
Plague	Macules, pustules, vesicles, petechiae
Bartonellosis	Erythematous papules
Scarlet fever	Maculopapular
Visceral leishmaniasis	Dark pigmentation, papule or ulcer
African trypanosomiasis	Chancre; erythematous

TABLE 145–5. Infections Causing Fever and Jaundice

Viruses	Bacteria	Parasites
Cytomegalovirus	Leptospirosis	Fascioliasis
Viral hepatitis	Relapsing fever	Malaria (severe
Yellow fever	Typhoid	P. falciparum)
	Paratyphoid	Toxoplasmosis
	Typhus	Trypanosomiasis

TABLE 145–6. Selected Diseases Causing Fever in the Tropics

Common with Wide Distribution
Malaria
Tuberculosis
Arboviral infections
  Dengue
Enteric fevers
  Typhoid fever
Less Common with Wide Distribution
Amebic liver abscess
Infectious hepatitis
Brucellosis
Poliomyelitis
Toxoplasmosis
Schistosomiasis
Filariasis
Less Common with Limited Distribution
Visceral leishmaniasis
Leptospirosis
Scrub typhus
Louse-, flea, and tick-borne typhus
Relapsing fever
African trypanosomiasis
Hemorrhagic fevers
  Ebola hemorrhagic fever
  Lassa fever
  Marburg disease
  Hantavirus infections
Plague
Melioidosis
Yellow fever
HIV infection
Noninfectious Conditions
Rheumatic fever
Sickle cell anemia
Familial Mediterranean fever
Rheumatoid arthritis
Systemic lupus erythematosus
Factitious conditions

toms within 2 weeks of institution of specific antituberculosis therapy. Patients with bacterial endocarditis, typhoid fever, and other bacterial septicemias who have previously received antibiotics may have repeatedly negative blood cultures. These individuals should be treated with the most appropriate antibiotic(s), with a therapeutic response suggesting that the presumptive diagnosis was correct. Rarely, patients with malaria (particularly individuals with *P. malariae* infections and those receiving incomplete treatment), visceral leishmaniasis, and amebiasis might need to be treated before the diagnosis is confirmed. Again, a response to therapy suggests, but does not prove, that the clinical impression was correct.

CAUSES OF FEVER IN TRAVELERS. It must be stressed that people who have visited or lived in the tropics can have all the usual causes of fever that occur in temperate climates, and the majority of febrile episodes will have nonexotic etiologies.

Common Infections. Many febrile episodes are not specifically diagnosed and are caused by cosmopolitan viruses and common pathogenic bacteria. Epstein-Barr virus (EBV, the cause of infectious mononucleosis in adolescents) and cytomegalovirus (CMV), influenza, and bacterial infections leading to abscesses, endocarditis, pneumonia, osteomyelitis, pyelonephritis, and infections of the biliary tract are as common in the tropics as in temperate climates. Systemic fungal infections, including histoplasmosis and cryptococcosis, can be causes of fever of unknown origin (FUO).

Noninfectious Causes of Infection. Malignancies (e.g., Hodgkin's disease, non-Hodgkin's lymphomas, leukemia, cancers of the colon, liver, pancreas, and kidney); atrial myxomas; collagen vascular diseases (e.g., systemic lupus erythematosus, rheumatoid arthritis, juvenile rheumatoid arthritis, idiopathic vasculitis, polymyalgia rheumatica); and granulomatous diseases (e.g., sarcoidosis, granulomatous hepatitis, inflammatory bowel disease, temporal arteritis) may all cause an unexplained fever. Drug fever and serum sickness may be more common in travelers because of greater use and exposure. Other nontropical causes of fever include pulmonary embolization, cirrhosis of the liver, alcoholic hepatitis, central nervous system tumors or vascular lesions, septic thrombophlebitis, cyclic neutropenia, and familial Mediterranean fever (FMF).

The collagen vascular diseases and granulomatous diseases are rare in residents of the tropics. However, cirrhosis of the liver and primary hepatoma are common. Other associated signs and symptoms should suggest these problems. Liver function tests and hepatic scanning and sonography should focus on the lesion; a liver biopsy is confirmatory.

Infectious Diseases Associated with Tropical Exposure. There is a group of diseases rarely transmitted in temperate climates and almost exclusively associated with exposure in the tropics.

Malaria. By all historical and current measures, malaria is responsible for much of the preventable morbidity and mortality in returning travelers. Tragic stories of previously healthy travelers dying of this infection are heard every year. Since 1990 about 1000 to 1200 cases per year of imported malaria have been reported to the United States Centers for Disease Control and Prevention (CDC). Between 1991 and 1993, *P. vivax* was the cause in 48% of cases and *P. falciparum* was the cause in 36% of cases. Between 1980 and 1992, there were 45 fatal malarial infections among U.S. civilians, 44 of which were caused by *P. falciparum*. Thirty-six of these fatal cases were acquired in sub-Saharan Africa. Most of these cases were associated with the failure to use chemoprophylaxis, use of suboptimal chemoprophylactic regimens, delays in seeking medical attention, and delays in clinical and laboratory diagnosis. Immigrants or expatriates visiting relatives in their home country, especially West Africa, are at higher risk.

TABLE 145–7. Exposures Suggesting Specific Infectious Agents

Ingestion of Unpasteurized Milk	Ticks or Mites
Brucellosis	Crimean hemorrhagic fever
Salmonellosis	Colorado tick fever
Tuberculosis	Kyasanur Forest disease
Fresh Water	Russian spring-summer
Leptospirosis	encephalitis
Schistosomiasis	Spotted fevers
Dracontiasis	Typhus
Animal Contact	Scrub typhus
Rabies	Q fever
Viral hemorrhagic fevers	Rickettsial pox
Q fever	Tularemia
Leptospirosis	Lyme disease
Tularemia	Relapsing fever
Plague	Babesiosis
Brucellosis	**Injections or Transfusions**
Babesiosis	Hepatitis B and C
	HIV infection
	Malaria
	Chagas' disease
	Toxoplasmosis

All febrile patients from endemic areas must be considered to have malaria until proved otherwise. The diagnosis must be confirmed or excluded by performing serial blood films. There are no pathognomonic clinical signs or symptoms for malaria (Chapter 92). A typical presentation in the nonimmune individual who has not taken any medication that could affect the malaria parasite consists of the abrupt onset of a paroxysm of rigors followed by fever and diaphoresis associated with profound malaise, fatigue, and severe headache. When accompanied by low white blood cell and platelet counts, the diagnosis of malaria is highly probable. However, many presentations are not typical and can mimic other illnesses, including gastroenteritis and respiratory infections.

Once malaria is considered in the differential diagnosis, it can be confirmed or excluded by performing serial Giemsa-stained blood films (Chapter 151). However, lack of experience with the optimal preparation, staining, and interpretation of malarial blood smears, especially thick blood films, in most laboratories of nonendemic countries continues to lead to errors and delays in diagnosis. Clinics and health care professionals who see returning travelers must either become proficient in the microscopic diagnosis of malaria themselves or identify a laboratory with qualified personnel before a crisis occurs.

A new generation of rapid, point-of-care, nonmicroscopic tests based on detection of specific malaria antigens in whole blood promises to improve the accuracy of diagnosis, especially in the hands of those inexperienced with microscopy. Two tests that detect *P. falciparum* infection are currently available commercially: Parasight Pf (Becton Dickinson Microbiology Systems, Sparks, MD, USA) and ICT Pf (AMRAD ICT, New South Wales, Australia). Sensitivity and specificity are over 90% when compared with microscopy.

When can malaria be excluded from the differential diagnosis of a febrile patient? The majority of symptomatic patients will have a positive blood film when first seen. In a case series from London, the first smear prepared on presentation was positive for 82 inpatients with malaria. In a second study of 482 cases of imported malaria, the diagnosis of malaria was confirmed in 98% on the first malaria smear. However, on occasion, the diagnosis can be delayed owing to very low parasitemias associated with an early clinical presentation in nonimmune patients or the use of antimalarial drugs that suppress blood stage infection. Patients who took chemoprophylaxis during travel may have less severe clinical disease. These individuals may present with a less acute illness of more insidious onset and atypical symptoms, e.g., intermittent low-grade fever, lumbosacral muscle pain, fatigue, malaise, and nonspecific gastrointestinal symptoms. Afebrile cases have also been rarely reported, and attenuated severity has been associated with prolonged prepatent periods when drugs taken for chemoprophylaxis had long half-lives. These patients may present weeks or months after returning from endemic areas.

Malaria in travelers frequently has the following characteristics: (1) Careful taking of prophylactic drugs does not always prevent malaria. (2) Vivax and ovale malaria may occur several weeks after exposure and be difficult to diagnose in individuals who have received suppressive prophylaxis but not causal prophylaxis with primaquine. (3) These individuals and others, who have partial immunity or have received incomplete prophylaxis, may develop clinical malaria long after returning from the tropics. Three fourths of patients with falciparum malaria have the onset of symptoms within 1 month of return from the tropics, whereas only 45% of those with vivax and the other forms of malaria have symptoms within the first month. With falciparum malaria, there is almost never onset of symptoms 6 months or more after

exposure, whereas one of four patients with vivax and ovale malaria has initial symptoms 6 months or more following return from the tropics. (4) Malaria often causes signs and symptoms in paroxysms; therefore, it should be suspected in patients with intermittent fever and symptoms. However, falciparum malaria is frequently not paroxysmal early in its course. It usually takes several days for infection to develop a rhythm. Therefore, continuous or minimal fluctuation in fever is also compatible with malaria.

Arboviral Infections. Viruses transmitted by arthropods are more common in the tropics or are limited to the tropics. Dengue is the most prevalent arboviral infection worldwide. Dengue is particularly prevalent in Brazil, Mexico, Puerto Rico, Colombia, Oceania, and Southeast Asia, where it is a hazard to tourists who are bitten by mosquitoes (Chapter 29.1). Serologic studies have shown that dengue and chikungunya are common causes of fever in nonimmune adults in Southeast Asia. Clinical features that suggest the diagnosis of dengue are chills, headache, malaise, anorexia, backache, myalgia, lymphadenopathy, and leukopenia. Generally, fever and other symptoms occur 5 to 8 days after exposure and then subside within 5 days. When it occurs, the classic "saddleback" relapsing fever curve (2 to 3 days of high fever followed by 1 to 3 or 4 days of no fever, relapsing to another few days of high fever), is a helpful diagnostic sign. Chikungunya infection is characterized by chills, arthralgias, malaise, myalgia, headache, arthritis, lymphadenopathy, and a macular rash. There are many other arboviruses that cause brief undiagnosed febrile illnesses in travelers who have recently returned from the tropics (Chapter 29.3).

Amebic Liver Abscess. A history of a recent visit to the tropics is not essential to make the diagnosis of amebic abscess of the liver. Cases have occurred in individuals who have not been in the tropics for 5 or more years and, in rare cases, in persons who have never left a temperate climate. Associated symptoms and signs that suggest amebic liver abscess are anorexia, weight loss, right upper quadrant abdominal pain, hepatomegaly, hepatic tenderness and leukocytosis. Hepatomegaly without splenomegaly is a helpful clue. The patient is often a male who drinks alcohol. Amebic serologic tests and a hepatic scan (Figs. 86–8 and 86–9) or sonography (Fig. 86–7) and a chest radiograph showing right-sided pleural effusion or elevation of the diaphragm (Fig. 86–10) help in making a presumptive diagnosis. Sometimes, hepatic aspiration is required to rule out a bacterial abscess.

Visceral Leishmaniasis. Visceral leishmaniasis is an uncommon cause of fever in a traveler to the tropics. However, sporadic cases, especially among more extensive travelers in the Mediterranean area, are seen (Chapter 95). The incubation period can be prolonged, up to several years. Commonly associated findings of weight loss, hepatosplenomegaly, anemia, leukopenia, and elevated IgG suggest the diagnosis later in the course, but early disease can be nonspecific and associated with marked fatigue and malaise with few physical findings. The diagnosis is best made by demonstration of the organisms in a Giemsa-stained smear or in culture from a bone marrow aspirate. To demonstrate the organism, splenic aspiration or liver biopsy is sometimes necessary.

Miscellaneous Viral Illnesses. The viral hemorrhagic fevers, although rare, are important because of their high mortality and infectivity (Chapter 31). Sporadic cases and small outbreaks of Korean hemorrhagic fever have been occurring in U.S. military troops during training exercises in Korea. The infection, also called hemorrhagic fever with renal syndrome (HFRS), is caused by a Hantavirus and is acquired during exposure to infectious rodent urine and feces (Chapter 31.6). Visitors to West, Central, and South Africa could be exposed to Ebola hemorrhagic fever, Lassa fever, Crimean-Congo hemorrhagic fever, or Marburg disease. Yellow fever can be prevented by vaccination (Chapter 31.1).

Rarely, in the United States and Europe, immigrants or travelers from developing countries have symptomatic rabies. Rabies should always be suspected in febrile patients with unexplained encephalitis who have been exposed to dogs where canine rabies still occurs (Chapter 30.1).

Rickettsial Infections. The rickettsial infections, transmitted by mites, fleas, ticks, and lice, are often divided into three groups: the spotted fever group (Rocky Mountain spotted fever, tick typhus, boutonneuse fever, and rickettsialpox (Chapter 67); the typhus group (epidemic typhus, murine typhus, and scrub typhus (Chapters 66 and 69); and the agents of Q fever and trench fever (Chapters 34 and 68). Characteristic findings are exposure to arthropod vectors, macular rash or eschar, high temperatures, malaise, chills, headache, myalgia, backache, lymphadenopathy, and a dramatic response to tetracycline therapy.

Serologic tests are the best method of establishing the diagnosis; however, in most settings they can provide only a retrospective diagnosis that is of little help to the clinician at the time of illness. Although mortality is low, empirical use of doxycycline in suspected cases can be lifesaving and is indicated whenever a rickettsial infection is suspected.

Diarrheal Illnesses. Fever in association with diarrhea is common in returning travelers. Although bacterial pathogens, e.g., *Shigella* (Chapter 40), *Salmonella* (Chapters 75 and 76), and *Campylobacter* (Chapter 43), are the most frequent etiologic agents, malaria and systemic viral infections must be considered, especially in children, who often develop diarrhea with febrile illnesses.

Sexually Transmitted Diseases. Sexually transmitted diseases have a very high prevalence in some areas of the tropics. An individual with lymphadenopathy and/or rash with fever and a homosexual or heterosexual exposure a few weeks to a few months previously could have primary human immunodeficiency virus (HIV) infection (Chapter 22) or secondary syphilis (Chapter 48.1). HIV and hepatitis B or C virus can also be parenterally transmitted by injections, transfusions of blood or blood products, and sharing of needles for intravenous drug injection. In these circumstances, an accurate and candid medical history is essential.

Miscellaneous Bacterial Infections. Brucellosis is a frequent cause of fever in endemic populations of Southwest Asia, particularly in Saudi Arabia and other Gulf States; however, it is uncommon in returning travelers. Brucellosis should be considered in someone with a history of eating or drinking unpasteurized dairy products and having fever and prominent musculoskeletal complaints (Chapter 64). The organisms are difficult to culture. Serologic tests demonstrating a rising antibody titer are helpful for establishing a diagnosis. Granulomas can be demonstrated in biopsy specimens.

Melioidosis has been associated with prolonged fever and generalized infection in individuals returning from Southeast Asia. The incubation period can be prolonged (Chapter 37). Plague is another cause of fever and severe illness. With the most common bubonic form, the patient has the characteristic fluctuant lymph nodes that can be aspirated. The organisms may be either visualized in stained smears of this aspirate or cultured (Chapter 61).

Miscellaneous Parasitic Infections. *Schistosoma mansoni* and *S. japonicum* can cause fever during the acute invasive stage (also known as Katayama fever). This is usually associated with diarrhea, blood in the stool, and marked peripheral eosinophilia. Parasitologic diagnosis may be difficult early in the course of infection because ova are either absent or present in very small numbers in the feces. Sensitive and specific serologic assays are available in the United States from the CDC (Chapter 152). This syndrome is more likely to occur in a nonimmune expatriate than in a national of the endemic country (Chapter 118). A number of cases in travelers returning from Africa have been reported; these are associated with freshwater exposure (i.e., swimming, wading, rafting) in ponds in the Dogon region of Mali, West Africa, and Lake Malawi. There is an increased incidence of pyelonephritis in patients with *S. haematobium* infections, and chronic salmonellosis has also been associated with schistosomiasis. No freshwater body of water in Africa is without the risk of schistosomiasis.

Filariasis has a wide distribution in the tropics. Febrile episodes lasting about a week and associated with lymphadenitis and lymphangitis occur frequently in subjects with bancroftian and Malayan filariasis (Chapter 106). The incubation period is at least 6 months, and clinical disease may not occur in those with brief exposures to infectious mosquito bites. Eosinophilia and perhaps some changes associated with lymphatic obstuction can be seen. The diagnosis is usually suggested by the presence of eosinophilia; it is established by demonstrating the microfilariae on a Giemsa-stained blood film. Serologic tests can help in confirmation (Chapter 152).

Rarely, African trypanosomiasis can be a serious cause of fever in returning travelers or emigrants from Africa. The bite of the vector, the tsetse fly, is usually memorable. There may be a chancre at the site of the bite (50%), transient skin rash, and lymphadenopathy. Hepatosplenomegaly, anemia, and elevated serum or cerebrospinal fluid IgM levels are characteristic in the later stages. The diagnosis is confirmed by demonstrating the trypanosome in the blood, in a lymph node aspirate, or in the spinal fluid (Chapter 94).

Infectious Diseases with Increased Prevalence in the Tropics. Some diseases are much more common in the tropics. Therefore, travel to these areas increases the chance of exposure to these infections.

Tuberculosis. Tourists to LDCs are rarely infected with *Mycobacterium tuberculosis*. However, tuberculosis is a common cause of fever in immigrants and should be suspected in individuals of all age groups who have prolonged fever, weight loss, and cough (Chapters 77 and 148). In Asian immigrants to the United States, tuberculosis is recognized in 40% within the first year of arrival and in almost half by the end of the second year. Half of these are under the age of 35 years. Chest radiographs are essential when tuberculosis is suspected. Positive tuberculin skin tests in children not previously given bacille Calmette-Guérin (BCG) immunization is strong evidence of infection. The diagnosis is confirmed by demonstrating acid-fast bacilli in sputum smears or by culturing the organism in sputum, urine, gastric washings, or other specimens. Sometimes, the patient must be treated in advance of bacteriologic confirmation of the diagnosis.

Enteric Fever. Enteric fever is most commonly associated with infection with *Salmonella typhi* (Chapter 75) or *S. paratyphi A* and *S. paratyphi B* (Chapter 76). Half of patients with enteric fever diagnosed in temperate climates have a history of recent travel to the tropics. Nineteen of 27 patients reported from a single hospital in Montreal had traveled in the tropics during the month prior to the onset of symptoms. Typhoid fever should be suspected in a febrile overseas traveler or immigrant who has many of the following symptoms and signs: headache, chills, cough, constipation or diarrhea, nausea, abdominal pain, unremittent fever (Fig. 145–1A), splenomegaly, elevated hepatic enzymes, and anemia. The diagnosis is confirmed by a positive blood, stool, or urine culture.

Infectious Hepatitis. Viral hepatitis is very common in LDCs, and nonimmune individuals traveling to these areas can be heavily exposed, particularly to hepatitis A and E, which are fecally-orally transmitted and often contaminate the water supply. Hepatitis B, C, and D are usually parenterally transmitted. They may contaminate blood products and are also sexually transmitted (Chapter 28). Vaccines for hepatitis A and B are available and provide excellent protection, although they are expensive. Often viral hepatitis will initially present with fever and other nonspecific symptoms before the patient becomes jaundiced. An elevated serum ALT suggests the correct diagnosis, which can be confirmed by serologic tests.

Toxoplasmosis. Toxoplasmosis can cause an acute febrile illness that is often associated with lymphadenopathy, myalgia, leukopenia, and anemia and that is difficult to differentiate from infectious mononucleosis or CMV infection (Chapter 97). It is more prevalent in LDCs, where food and water are more likely to be contaminated with cat feces containing the highly contagious oocyst, than in developed countries. A history of exposure to cats or the ingestion of rare or raw meat helps in establishing the diagnosis. The diagnosis is usually made with serologic tests.

Miscellaneous Infections. Poliomyelitis has been eradicated from the Americas since 1991. However, wild polio virus is still transmitted in parts of Africa and Asia, and individuals traveling to these areas may still be exposed to polio (Chapter 27.1). Very rarely, an adult immunized as a child may develop acute poliomyelitis following exposure in the tropics.

Leptospirosis is a cosmopolitan zoonosis, more common in LDCs than in North America or Europe (Chapter 72). Infected wild and domestic animals excrete the causative spirochete in urine. Humans become infected when leptospires enter through abraded skin, mucous membranes, or conjunctivae following contact with water or soil contaminated with infectious urine. Infected individuals often have a history of contact with dogs; swimming, rafting, or wading in fresh surface water; or farming and gardening in soil contaminated with leptospires. Symptoms, in addition to fever, suggesting leptospirosis include severe headache, myalgia, nausea, abdominal pain, conjunctival suffusion, an abnormal urine sediment, proteinuria, polymorphonuclear leukocytosis, and abnormal liver function tests. Serologic testing confirms the diagnosis. However, empirical therapy with a tetracycline derivative is sometimes indicated.

People who have eaten undercooked meat and who have fever, myalgia, and eosinophilia may have trichinosis (Chapter 111). There were two outbreaks of horsemeat-associated trichinosis in France in 1985.

Noninfectious Causes of Fever in the Tropics. Pyrexia is not always caused by infection. Fever caused by malignancies, collagen vascular diseases, and granulomatous diseases is infrequently diagnosed in the tropics. There are some noninfectious diseases associated with fever that have a higher prevalence in LDCs than in temperate climates but these are not unique risks for travelers.

Rheumatic Fever. Acute rheumatic fever is more prevalent in LDCs than in developed countries. The diagnosis should be suspected when carditis and migratory polyarthritis are also present. Subcutaneous nodules, erythema marginatum, chorea, and positive throat cultures for hemolytic streptococci are reported less frequently than in descriptions of the classic disease in temperate climates. Valvular heart disease is common, occurs at an early age, and is often rapidly progressive (Chapter 3).

Sickle Cell Anemia. Fever is a common complication of sickle cell anemia (Chapter 6). Homozygotes for SS hemoglobin have an increased incidence of infections and multiple pulmonary embolizations, accounting for their pyrexia. Sickled erythrocytes cause microthrombi and macrothrombi, leading to recurrent vaso-occlusive phenomena. Occasionally, the resulting pulmonary, bone, and other infarcts are secondarily infected. Repeated infarcts of the spleen impair splenic function. This, along with a defect in opsonin antibodies, interferes with the immune response to some bacteria.

Familial Mediterranean Fever (FMF)

ETIOLOGY AND EPIDEMIOLOGY. FMF is a syndrome manifested by self-limited episodes of fever along with abdominal, chest, and joint pains. Almost all individuals with FMF are of Mediterranean or Middle Eastern ethnic origin (Jewish, Armenian, Turkish, and Arab). It is inherited as a single autosomal recessive trait, with an incidence in homozygotes of 1:2000 in Israel. There is a 20% incidence of consanguinity and a 50% incidence of positive family history; 60% of the patients are male. Recurrent polyserositis is the principal pathophysiologic finding. FMF is clearly polymorphic, with several phenotypes, and the inheritance has some variables that are not fully discernible. In addition, cases of a similar disease have been described among non–Middle Eastern families. However, a physician working with travelers would most likely see fever caused by FMF in immigrants or visitors from the Middle East.

PATHOLOGY AND CLINICAL MANIFESTATIONS. Pathologic findings are nonspecific. Peritonitis, pleuritis, and arthritis are manifested by exudates containing a predominance of polymorphonuclear leukocytes. Biopsies demonstrate acute inflammatory changes. The age at onset of symptoms is usually between 5 and 15 years. The duration and frequency of attacks vary. The usual episode lasts 24 to 72 hours but sometimes is prolonged for 7 to 10 days, with the usual frequency being every 2 to 4 weeks. Spontaneous remissions lasting for years have been reported. During the acute attack, the temperature is usually between 100 and 102°F (38 and 39°C) and is often associated with symptoms and signs of peritonitis, pleuritis, arthritis, and, occasionally, erysipelas-like skin rashes on the dorsum of the foot and the anterior aspect of the lower leg or thigh. The peritonitis varies in severity. The pain sometimes involves the entire abdomen and is associated with nausea, vomiting, and abdominal distention, rigidity, rebound tenderness, and evidence of paralytic ileus. Many patients have undergone exploratory laparotomy before the diagnosis of FMF was suspected and confirmed. Other complications include amyloidosis, which is progressive and usually leads to death from renal failure. Narcotic addiction and emotional disturbances are frequent problems. Splenomegaly is the most common physical abnormality noted between episodes. Laboratory abnormalities during attacks include elevation of the erythrocyte sedimentation rate, white blood cell counts, and acute phase reactants (C-reactive protein and IgM).

DIAGNOSIS. The diagnosis is suspected in individuals of appropriate ethnic origin with the characteristic self-limited attacks, particularly if they have a positive family history. The rare patient who has only fever requires a complete workup for FUO in addition to prolonged observation. Febrile Egyptian patients with FMF were rapidly diagnosed by their characteristic history and physical findings and their response to colchicine; 35 of 299 patients admitted to an Abassia Fever Hospital-NAMRU-3 study for fever from 1971 to 1975 had FMF.

TREATMENT. Many therapeutic measures, including corticosteroids and a low-fat diet, have been used to prevent and treat the acute attacks of FMF. Colchicine can reduce the number of acute attacks and, in some patients, abort them. It is usually given in a dosage of 0.6 mg 3 times daily. If this dosage causes gastrointestinal symptoms, it is reduced to 0.6

mg 2 times daily. To abort attacks, the dosage used is 0.6 mg every hour for 4 hours starting at the first prodromal symptom. This is followed by the same dose every 2 hours twice, and then every 12 hours for 2 days. Colchicine probably interferes with the inflammatory response and thus reduces or prevents symptoms. It may also prevent the development of amyloidosis.

References

Centers for Disease Control: Hepatitis E among U.S. travelers, 1989–1992. MMWR 42:1, 1993.

Centers for Disease Control: Update: Management of patients with suspected viral hemorrhagic fever—United States. MMWR 44:475, 1995.

Centers for Disease Control: Outbreak of leptospirosis among white-water rafters—Costa Rica, 1996. MMWR 46:577, 1997.

Cunha BA: The clinical significance of fever patterns. Infect Dis Clin North Am 10:33, 1996.

Day J, Behrens R: Delay in onset of malaria with mefloquine prophylaxis. Br Med J 345:398, 1995.

Day J, Grant A, Doherty J, et al: Schistosomiasis in travelers returning from sub-Saharan Africa. Br Med J 313:268, 1996.

Doherty JF, Grant AD, Bryceson AD: Fever as the presenting complaint of travellers returning from the tropics. Q J Med 88:277, 1995.

Doherty JF, Moody AH, Wright SG: Katayama fever: An acute manifestation of schistosomiasis. Br Med J 313:1071, 1996.

Felton JM, Bryceson AD: Fever in the returning traveller. Br J Hosp Med 55:705, 1996.

Hall AJ: Hepatitis in travellers: Epidemiology and prevention. Br Med Bull 49:382, 1993.

Kumar A, Keystone J: Evaluating fever in travellers returning from tropical countries. Br Med J 312:953, 1996.

Kain KC, Harrington MA, Tennyson S, et al: Imported malaria: Prospective analysis of problems in diagnosis and management. Clin Infect Dis 27:142, 1998.

Lewis S, Davidson R, Ross E, Hall A: Severity of imported falciparum malaria: Effect of taking antimalarial prophylaxis. Br Med J 305:741, 1992.

Liu LX, Weller PF: Approach to the febrile traveler returning from Southeast Asia and Oceania. Curr Clin Top Infect Dis 12:138, 1992.

MacLean J, Lalonde R, Ward B: Fever from the tropics. Trav Med Adv 5:27.1, 1994.

Magill AJ: Fever in the returned traveler. Infect Dis Clin North Am 12:445, 1998.

Maguire JH: Epidemiologic considerations in the evaluation of undifferentiated fever in a traveler returning from Latin America or the Caribbean. Curr Clin Top Infect Dis 13:26, 1993.

Oster CN, Tramont EC: Fever in a recent visitor to the Middle East. Curr Clin Top Infect Dis 13:57, 1993.

Schwartz E, Mendelson E, Sidi Y: Dengue fever among travelers. Am J Med 101:516, 1996.

Smoak BL, McClain JB, Brundage JF, et al: An outbreak of spotted fever rickettsiosis in U.S. Army troops deployed to Botswana. Emerg Infect Dis 2:217, 1996.

Strickland GT: Fever in the returned traveler. Med Clin North Am 76:1375, 1992.

Svenson JE, Gyorkos TW, MacLean JD: Diagnosis of malaria in the febrile traveler. Am J Trop Med Hyg 53:518, 1995.

Svenson JE, MacLean JD, Gyorkos TW, Keystone J: Imported malaria. Clinical presentation and examination of symptomatic travelers. Arch Intern Med 155:861, 1995.

van Crevel R, Speelman P, Gravekamp C, Terpstra WJ: Leptospirosis in travelers. Clin Infect Dis 19:132, 1994.

Wyler DJ: Evaluation of cryptic fever in a traveler to Africa. Curr Clin Top Infect Dis 12:329, 1992.

146 *Skin Lesions in Travelers*

Kevin C. Kain and Jay S. Keystone

GENERAL PRINCIPLES. Skin lesions developing in association with travel pose a difficult diagnostic dilemma for physicians from temperate regions. This chapter provides a practical lesion-based approach to this diagnostic problem and, for each lesion, outlines the important causes and the steps in reaching a diagnosis.

As with other clinical problems in returning travelers, a detailed epidemiologic and exposure history of the traveler is essential in reaching a diagnosis. Identifying what individuals did while traveling is as important as elucidating which countries were visited and permits an assessment of what infectious diseases, vectors, and environmental hazards travelers were potentially exposed to. Most exotic dermatoses are acquired by low-budget adventurous travelers who visit rural areas or wander off the usual tourist routes.

The duration of stay also determines the possible exposure to agents causing tropical dermatoses. Short-term (<3 weeks) travelers do not acquire diseases e.g., leprosy, yaws, filariasis, Buruli ulcers, and cysticercosis. These disorders usually are seen only in immigrants and are unusual even in long-stay (>3 months) travelers or overseas workers. The arrival and departure dates in the tropics should be ascertained to establish an incubation period. The cause of lesions developing immediately after a short trip is different from the cause of those developing several weeks or months after a prolonged stay. The location (e.g., limbs vs. trunk; exposed vs. nonexposed skin), lesion type (e.g., papules, nodules, ulcers, linear), description and progression of lesions, and associated symptoms (e.g., fever, pruritus) are useful when formulating a diagnosis.

Dermatoses remain an important problem for travelers, accounting for approximately 10% of medical referrals to tropical disease units, and are reported to be the fifth most frequent travel-related problem. Recent reviews of returning travelers report the most common skin disorders to be cutaneous larva migrans (~25%), pyodermas (~18%), persistent or secondarily infected insect bites (~10%), myiasis (~9%), tungiasis (~6%), urticaria (~5%), fever and rash (~4%), and leishmaniasis (~3%). Exacerbations of pre-existing chronic dermatoses (e.g., eczema, psoriasis) are also common, often precipitated by hot, humid climates.

PAPULES

Arthropod Bites. The most frequent papular lesions seen in returning travelers are arthropod bites, frequently caused by mosquitoes, midges, sandflies, bedbugs, and fleas, all of which have a worldwide distribution. The appearance of individual bite reactions is usually nondiagnostic, but the configuration of numerous bites may provide a useful clue to the cause. Bites caused by fleas, bedbugs, and reduviid bugs are frequently grouped in clusters (often in threes) or have a linear distribution (Fig. 146–1). Finding flecks of blood

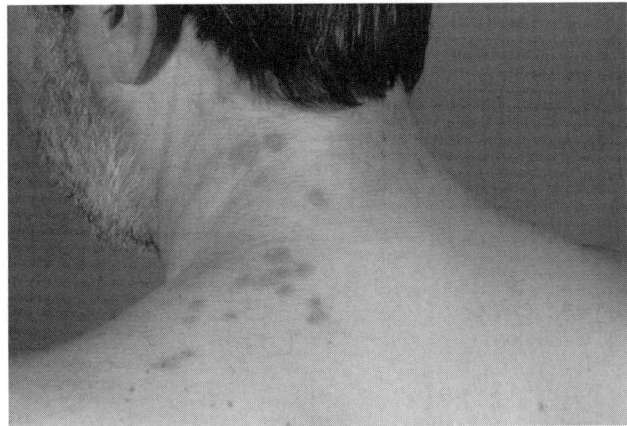

Figure 146–1. Linear and grouped papular lesions from bedbug bites.

on the bed linen suggests bedbug infestation. Most arthropod bites are pruritic, but the bites of the deer, tsetse, and black flies are also painful (Figs. 128–3 and 128–4). Bites from stinging arthropods such as scorpions, brown recluse spiders, and hymenoptera (bees, wasps, and fire ants) must also be considered in the differential diagnosis of painful bites (Fig. 128–12).

It is not uncommon for patients to complain of pruritic insect bites that come and go for weeks or months after return from the tropics. These prolonged reactions are most often associated with bedbug and flea bites. Papular urticaria is a more severe and persistent hypersensitivity reaction to insect bites occurring primarily in young children. The clinical findings are urticarial wheals, often with a central hemorrhagic punctum, papules, papulovesicles, and residual hyperpigmented spots. Most lesions are excoriated because pruritus is severe. Adults may develop this condition when they experience bites from arthropods to which they have not been previously exposed.

Scabies. Caused by the mite *Sarcoptes scabiei*, scabies is very frequent in the tropics. It is more commonly seen in backpacking, adventurous, or sexually active travelers. The cardinal features of scabies are (1) characteristic distribution of lesions, (2) nocturnal pruritus, and (3) mite burrows (Fig. 128–8). The mite burrow is typically a gray or skin-colored linear, raised ridge measuring a few millimeters to 1.5 cm and most frequently found on the finger webs (Fig. 128–9), wrists, genitalia, axillary folds, and nipples. Generalized pruritic urticarial papules due to parasite sensitization appear 6 to 8 weeks after the initial infestation. Scabies is diagnosed by unroofing a burrow with a needle or scalpel blade coated with oil and microscopically examining scrapings for mites and their ova. Crusted scabies is an extremely contagious variant found in HIV-infected or other compromised hosts; it is characterized by generalized crusted lesions containing thousands of mites. The combination of oral ivermectin and topical permethrin has been shown to be very effective in treating crusted scabies.

Miliaria Rubra. Prickly heat is a frequent disorder of travelers to tropical environments, particularly travelers who are unacclimatized. It is caused by maceration of sweat gland ducts, resulting in obstruction and leakage of sweat into the epidermis. It is characterized by tiny pruritic vesicles or papules on a red base (Fig. 17–2). The eruption spares hair follicles and is usually confined to covered areas of the body.

Other Etiologies. In long-stay travelers, particularly from West and Central Africa, onchocerciasis and streptocerciasis are two forms of filariasis that usually present with a pruritic papular rash, most often on the trunk or lower extremity. Because these patients are usually lightly infected, they have a mild pruritic rash (Fig. 108–9A); they do not have the advanced skin atrophy of onchocercal dermatitis that is reported in endemic populations (Fig. 108–5 and 108–9B–F). The diagnosis is made by identifying microfilaria that migrate out of skin snip biopsy specimens.

Because most travelers carry medications to be used prophylactically or therapeutically for tropical disorders (e.g., for self-treatment of traveler's diarrhea and malaria), it is important to inquire about drug use in any returning traveler who presents with a papular or urticarial rash.

PAPULOSQUAMOUS. The most commonly seen papulosquamous lesions in returning travelers are superficial fungal infections and exacerbations of pre-existing eczema and psoriasis.

Cutaneous Mycoses. The heat, humidity, and hygiene level in the tropics promote the development of new fungal infections or the progression of ones present before travel.

Dermatophyte infections of the skin (tinea corporis, pedis, and cruris) are characterized by erythema and scaling in an annular or diffuse pattern (Figs. 81–1 to 81–4). Lesions vary from asymptomatic to severe pruritus and burning. Nail and hair involvement is common. The diagnosis is made by potassium hydroxide examination and culture of scrapings from affected areas. Although exceedingly rare in returning travelers, nontuberculous mycobacterial infection, leishmaniasis, leprosy, yaws, and secondary syphilis may present as scaly erythematous lesions.

Candidiasis, usually found in intertriginous areas, presents with beefy red erythema and small pustules. Gram stain and culture of a skin swab taken from the lesion confirm the diagnosis, although a clinical diagnosis usually suffices.

Phytodermatitis. Contact with some plants may result in dermatitis characterized by erythema, desquamation, and bullae. These plant-induced dermatitides may result from a primary irritant produced by the plant, as in pineapple contact dermatitis. Allergic phytodermatitis results from contact with antigenic components contained in the essential oil or oleoresin of the sap or pollen. Contact with well-known toxicodendron plants (i.e., poison ivy, oak, and sumac) causes erythema, edema, papules, vesicles, and bullae with a characteristic linear streaking. Other plants of the same family that may cause similar reactions include the Japanese lacquer tree, India marking nut tree, and plant matter such as raw cashew shells, fruit from the female gingko tree, and skin of the mango fruit. Mango dermatitis ("mango mouth") is extremely common in the tropics and is seen mainly in and around the mouth after eating unpeeled fruit.

ULCERS

Pyodermatitis. The most frequent cutaneous ulcer experienced by travelers is ecthyma, a shallow, painful, purulent ulcer resulting from skin trauma or insect bites that have become secondarily infected with a pyogenic organism, most commonly *Staphylococcus aureus*, group A streptococci, or both. When such pyodermas are superimposed on pre-existing dermatoses, a superficial impetigo-like condition results. Impetigo is the most common of the pyodermas. This contagious superficial bacterial infection (usually initiated by β-hemolytic streptococci and secondarily invaded by *S. aureus*) usually occurs on the face as thin-walled vesicles that break down and form yellow crusts. A bullous type of impetigo in which an exfoliative toxin induces an intraepithelial cleavage resulting in blister formation occurs in the tropics. Overall, approximately 2% of pyodermas are associated with poststreptococcal glomerulonephritis. Erysipelas, cellulitis, furuncles, and carbuncles all are common in the tropics; recurrent furunculosis associated with nasal carriage of *S. aureus* is not infrequent in returning travelers in association with hot weather and poor hygiene (Chapter 8).

Chronic Ulcerations. All other types of tropical ulcers are rare. Although uncommon in travelers, cutaneous leishmaniasis is important to recognize (Figs. 95–10, 95–12, and 95–13). *Leishmania* ulcers are typically indolent and painless (unless secondarily infected), with a granulomatous or crusted base and heaped-up margins. Leishmaniasis may occasionally present in a linear lymphocutaneous fashion with ulcers, nodules, and regional adenopathy spreading proximally, resembling sporotrichosis (Chapter 82.2), cat-scratch disease, or *Mycobacterium marinum* infections (Fig. 79–3).

Diagnostic clues in the history or examination may point toward the cause of an ulcer; the granulomatous ulcer seen in *M. marinum* infection (swimming pool granuloma) is associated with exposure to fresh or salt water, particularly swimming pools or fish tanks. It grows as a reddish-purple, verrucous, hyperkeratotic growth on the extremities. Paracoccidioidomycosis infection caused by *Paracoccidioides brasiliensis* should be considered in travelers from South

America, especially Brazil (Chapter 83.4). This deep fungal infection is seen mainly in agricultural workers who initially inhale this saprophytic fungus; pulmonary infection is followed by dissemination to skin and mucosal surfaces. The first clinical lesions are usually painful buccal mucosal plaques that ulcerate; skin lesions and regional adenopathy involving the head and neck generally follow. The combination of pulmonary, mucosal, skin, and lymph node lesions is characteristic, as is the recognition of the typical "mariner's wheel" fungal elements in scrapings or discharge from the lesions.

Tick eschars are relatively common in people who have visited game parks or lived in the bush. Eschars, seen with boutonneuse fever or tick typhus infections (Fig. 67–2), scrub typhus (Fig. 69–1), and rickettsial pox, start as erythematous macules at the bite site and progress through papular, vesicular, and necrotic stages to form painless small (0.5 to 1 cm diameter), crusted black lesions surrounded by an erythematous halo, the so-called cigarette burn lesion. Regional adenopathy is common. Three to 7 days later, a cutaneous rash may develop. The skin eruption of louse, tick, and scrub typhus is usually macular or maculopapular, involving the trunk and abdomen (Fig. 66–2). The rickettsial pox rash is maculopapular or vesicular and resembles atypical varicella. It may be generalized and involve the mucous membranes.

Cutaneous amebiasis is a rare complication of *Entamoeba histolytica* infection resulting from an extension of intestinal or liver amebiasis to skin by contiguous spread or by metastasis. The skin breaks down to produce a very painful, rapidly extending perianal or genital ulcer with purulent drainage. Amebic trophozoites may be found in the lesion margins or discharge.

Anthrax is most likely to affect agricultural workers or those handling animal hides owing to inoculation of *Bacillus anthracis* spores into the skin. A single lesion is usually present on the face or upper extremity. It is a pruritic, erythematous macule that progresses to a vesicle that breaks down to a black eschar surrounded by extensive edema (Fig. 55–1).

The bite of the brown recluse spider (*Loxosceles* sp.), although often initially painless, may evolve into an edematous, irregular, violaceous lesion surrounded by a larger erythematous halo (Fig. 128–11). After 24 to 72 hours, a central blister may appear and become a black eschar, which sloughs in 2 to 5 weeks, leaving a deep ulcer. Systemic symptoms such as fever, chills, headache, and nausea may occur within 24 hours of envenomation.

Investigation of a cutaneous ulcer acquired in the tropics begins with a swab of the base for bacterial culture. Mycobacterial and fungal infections are diagnosed by histopathology, special stains (including acid-fast, silver, and periodic acid–Schiff stains), and culture for bacteria, mycobacteria, and fungus of a portion of the specimen taken from the lesion margin. If the patient has been in a rural area where leishmaniasis is endemic, amastigote parasites may be detected by Giemsa stain and culture (most sensitive) or histologic examination of ulcer material. Specimens taken by aspiration, slit skin smear, or biopsy from the edge of the ulcer are most likely to yield positive results (Fig. 95–12).

LINEAR LESIONS. Linear lesions can be divided into those that are serpiginous and those that are straight. Serpiginous lesions include cutaneous larva migrans due to dog and cat hookworms, *Strongyloides stercoralis*, and *Gnathostoma spinigerum*.

Creeping Eruptions. Cutaneous larva migrans is the most frequent serpiginous lesion seen in returning travelers, especially from the Caribbean. Lesions are produced by the entry and migration of the larval stage of the dog or cat hookworm. These hookworm larvae are usually acquired while walking barefoot or sitting on the beach. Marked pruritus and the migratory, serpiginous nature of the track, most commonly found on the foot and buttock, are helpful diagnostic clues (Fig. 115–1). In the early stages, only papular or vesicular lesions may be seen (see Fig. 146–2 in color section); these may be confused with dermatophytosis or eczema. A diagnosis can usually be made from the clinical history and the appearance of the lesion.

Strongyloides stercoralis larvae produce a faster-moving track, larva currens, traveling at a rate of 5 to 10 cm/hr compared with 2 to 3 cm/day for the cat and dog hookworm. This urticarial wheal surrounded by a flare is intensely itchy and often transient, lasting only a few hours. The lesions, seen on the buttocks, groin, and trunk, tend to occur in crops over a few days, with symptom-free periods lasting weeks in between. The parasite can maintain infection in the same host by autoinfection for many years.

Gnathostomiasis, a very rare infection of travelers, is caused by a nematode of felines and canines acquired when humans consume inadequately cooked fish, shellfish, or amphibians. The presentation in humans has both visceral and cutaneous manifestations. The migratory, serpiginous, cutaneous track of gnathostomiasis is much longer than that of the dog and cat hookworm (Fig. 113–5).

Chemical Dermatitis. The chemical dermatitis produced by contact with blister beetles and plants presents as straight linear lesions at the point of contact of the chemical with the skin. These lesions may result from direct skin contact with coelomic fluid or plant toxin (the earlier discussion of papulosquamous lesions) or from a phytotoxic reaction associated with the chemical on the skin. Blister beetle dermatitis is the result of a chemical burn by cantharidin released from the coelomic cavity of these insects crushed onto the skin (Fig. 128–2). Droplets of cantharidin produce the linear track. If the beetle is crushed in a skin fold such as the popliteal fossa, mirror-image lesions are seen on either side of the fold. Lesions generally stop itching by the fifth day and desquamate over the following week. Residual hyperpigmentation may remain for months.

Phytophotodermatitis. This results from exposure to a psoralen-containing compound, such as lime juice. It appears as painless, nonpruritic pigmented straight streaks or droplets that are particularly alarming because of their cosmetic effects (see Fig. 146–3 in color section). Photodermatitis results from intercalation of the psoralen with skin DNA in response to ultraviolet A. The initial sunburn in the area where the psoralen was in contact with skin is often mild and goes unnoticed. Patients first notice linear streaks of postinflam-

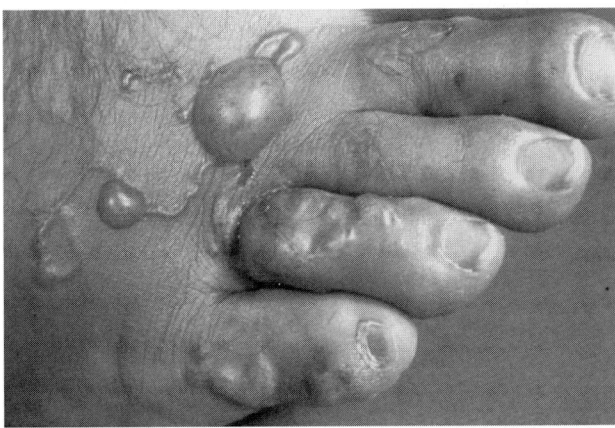

Figure 146–4. Cutaneous larva migrans on the foot of an individual who had recently visited the Caribbean.

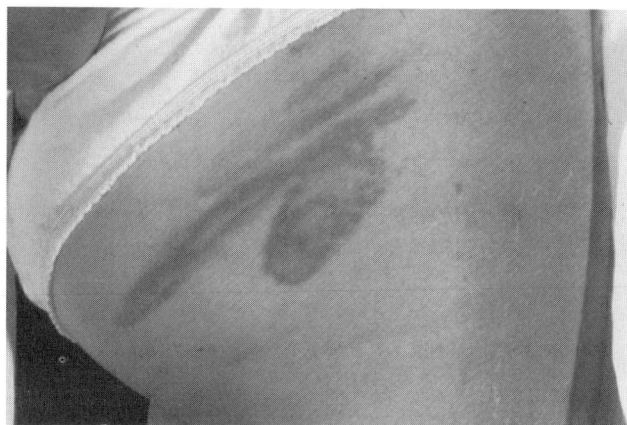

Figure 146–5. Lesions of phytophotodermatitis on a young woman following accidental lime juice exposure.

matory hyperpigmentation that resemble brown paint that has been dripped or streaked onto the skin with fingers.

Other skin lesions found in linear configurations include the lymphocutaneous ulcers of leishmaniasis, sporotrichosis, nocardiosis, cat-scratch disease (Fig. 60–2), and *M. marinum* and the papular insect bites of bedbugs, reduviid bugs, and fleas. The diagnosis of most linear lesions is usually determined by their clinical appearance.

DISORDERS OF PIGMENTATION. Skin pigmentation changes in travelers may result from an increase or decrease in skin pigment. Hyperpigmented lesions include pityriasis (tinea) versicolor, postinflammatory hyperpigmentation, pinta (rarely seen in travelers), the sequelae of phytophotodermatitis (lime juice, wild parsnips, cow parsnips, wild carrot, and bishop's weed), tinea nigra, and of course suntan.

Cutaneous Mycoses. Tinea nigra is a superficial fungal infection caused by the dematiaceous molds *Exophiala werneckii*, in South and Central America, and *Cladosporium mansonii* in Asia (Chapter 81.5). The lesions are typically asymptomatic, clearly defined hyperpigmented macules without scaling that involve the palms and rarely the soles. Tinea nigra must be distinguished from junctional nevus and melanoma.

Pityriasis (tinea) versicolor is the most common superficial mycotic infection in the tropics and the most frequent cause of either hypopigmented or hyperpigmented lesions in returning travelers. Tinea versicolor is caused by *Pityrosporum orbiculare* (also called *Malassezia furfur*), a normal skin commensal, which in humid environments may spread and become noticed by the traveler. Well-defined hypopigmented or hyperpigmented patches covered with a light scale are typically found on the upper trunk and neck (Fig. 81–8). The lesions are usually asymptomatic, and pruritus is absent. The diagnosis is most easily made by applying a piece of clear cellulose acetate tape to the lesions, peeling it off (with the surface scales attached), and then applying it, sticky side down, to a drop of methylene blue on a microscope slide. When viewed immediately under 4 × 10 magnification, the spaghetti-and-meatballs hyphae and spores are readily visualized. Lesions exhibit yellow florescence under Wood's lamp. Pityriasis (tinea) versicolor must be distinguished from vitiligo (milky whiteness without scaling) and indeterminant leprosy (hypoesthetic or anesthetic lesions without scaling).

Leprosy. This is usually seen in immigrants and only very rarely in long-stay travelers. Leprosy should be suspected when there is evidence of skin and nerve involvement. Skin lesions are usually hypopigmented patches (copper colored

in dark skin) that show a detectable loss of cutaneous sensation to pinprick or light touch (Figs. 78–4 and 78–5). The finding of thickened peripheral nerves supports the clinical diagnosis (Fig. 78–6). The presumptive diagnosis of leprosy is confirmed by biopsy and/or by finding acid-fast bacilli in slit skin smears.

SUBCUTANEOUS SWELLINGS AND NODULES. Subcutaneous swellings may be classified into three groups: fixed and painful, fixed and painless, and migratory swellings. Common causes of fixed, painful subcutaneous swellings in travelers include myiasis, tungiasis, and boils or furuncles.

Myiasis. Furuncular myiasis is secondary to skin invasion by larval maggots of various diptera species including *Cordylobia anthropophagia* (tumbu fly) in Africa and *Dermatobia hominis* (botfly) in South and Central America (Figs. 128–6 and 128–7). Tumbu fly eggs are deposited in shady soil or on clothing that is left on the ground or hanging out to dry. Botfly eggs are deposited on the underside of mosquitoes or other arthropods, which then transfer them to human skin during feeding. Myiasis lesions most closely resemble boils but with two important differences. The myiasis lesion has a central opening through which the maggot is able to breathe and protrude a portion of its body (Fig. 146–6), and patients with myiasis often feel movement within the larval burrow and experience intermittent sharp, lancinating pains. The diagnosis and management of myiasis are by extrusion of the larva. This may be accomplished by various strategies but least traumatically by suffocation of the maggot with an occlusive dressing of petroleum jelly or paraffin held in place by a cap (e.g., toothpaste cap) over the breathing opening for several hours. The larva attempts to exit the skin in search of air and subsequently may be extruded by firm lateral pressure on the lesion.

Tungiasis. "Jiggers" or "chigoes" is another cause of fixed, painful subcutaneous swellings in travelers to South and Central America, Africa, and India. The lesions are caused by invasion of the female sand flea, *Tunga penetrans*, into the skin between the toes, the nails, and the soles of the feet (Fig. 128–5). *T. penetrans* is widely distributed in sandy soil, particularly around pigsties and cow sheds. Skin invasion by the flea causes intense irritation and the formation of a small black dot. An inflammatory nodule 1 to 2 mm in diameter subsequently forms and breaks down, with discharge of eggs. Tungiasis is diagnosed and managed by surgical extraction of the flea. Complications include secondary bacterial infection with lymphangitis, gas gangrene, and tetanus.

Chancres. Other painful, fixed subcutaneous masses in-

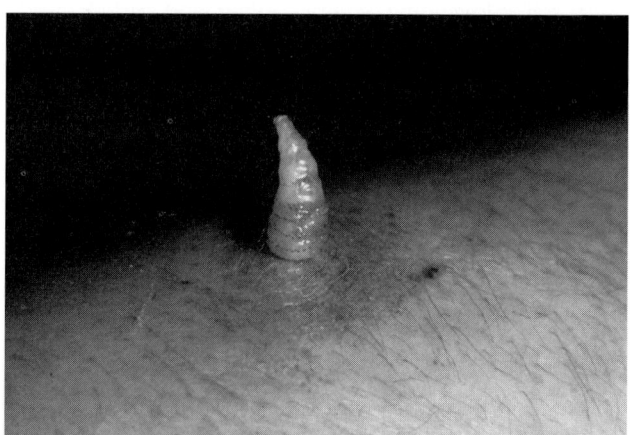

Figure 146–6. Furuncular myiasis caused by *Dermatobium hominus*, on the arm of a traveler recently returned from Central America.

clude the inoculation site of the South American and African forms of trypanosomiasis, the chagoma and trypanosoma chancre, respectively. The latter is rarely reported because patients usually assume it to be an infected insect bite. More characteristic of African trypanosomiasis is the irregular, evanescent erythematous macular rash. A subcutaneous inflammatory nodule may also be produced by ingesting the sparganum fish infected with the tapeworm larva of *Spirometra* species found in Southeast Asia (Chapter 123.5). It may develop into an abscess or produce conjunctivitis and periorbital edema when it is adjacent to the eye. The painless nodules of cysticercosis and onchocerciasis are very rare in returning travelers. Both lesions are relatively fixed in the subcutaneous tissues of the host.

Infection with the West African filarial worm *Loa loa* produces two characteristic clinical features: Calabar swellings, which are migratory, localized areas of angioedema on the extremities (Fig. 107–1), and eye worm, the subconjunctival migration of the adult worm (Fig. 107–2). Expatriates infected with *L. loa* may have frequent, severe, and pruritic Calabar swellings and more nonspecific pruritic rashes.

AQUATIC DERMATITIS. Aquatic dermatitides result from exposure to organisms in salt or fresh water. Common aquatic skin problems include sea bather's eruption and seaweed and cercarial dermatitis, which produce a generalized pruritic rash, and inadvertent contact with a venomous marine creature resulting in a painful localized lesion that may be accompanied by systemic symptoms.

Sea Bather's Eruption. Both sea bather's eruption and seaweed dermatitis are most easily recognized because the rash is generally localized to skin surfaces covered by the bathing suit. Sea bather's eruption has been associated with exposure to larval forms of sea anemones (*Edwardsiella lineata*) and jellyfish (*Linuche unguiculata*) of the phylum Cnidaria (formerly Coelenterata), members of which contain stinging nematocysts triggered by a physical or chemical stimulus. The eruption is characteristically a pruritic, erythematous papular rash that develops within minutes to hours of exposure to salt water. It may be aggravated by subsequent exposure to fresh water, which stimulates nematocyst discharge. The buttocks, genitals, and female breasts are the areas most often affected. The rash and pruritus typically last 3 to 7 days but may persist as long as 6 weeks in severe cases. Therapy is symptomatic, with topical antihistamines and corticosteroids.

Seaweed dermatitis results from persistent skin contact with blue-green algae living on seaweed in the Caribbean, Pacific, and Indian Oceans. The rash is usually seen in spring and summer and is burning and erythematous, developing within minutes to hours after exposure. In severe cases, bullous desquamation may occur in the genital, perineal, and perianal regions. Lesions may be prevented by washing with soap and water after exposure.

Cercarial Dermatitis. Swimmer's itch results from penetration of the skin by both human (anthropophilic) and nonhuman (zoophilic) schistosome cercariae. The rash from zoophilic schistosomiasis, usually due to avian schistosoma, is more common and severe than that associated with the anthropophilic forms (Fig. 118–14). Because cercarial dermatitis is the result of sensitization, symptom onset and severity increase with repeated exposures. The first attack may be a mild papular rash 8 to 13 days after exposure, whereas with re-exposure, a pruritic urticarial rash may begin within minutes to hours of exposure and pass within 48 to 96 hours through macular, papular, vesicular, and occasionally pustular stages, surrounded by a zone of erythema. The rash occurs on exposed surfaces of the body and may last for up to 2 weeks.

Venomous Coelenterates. Travelers are also at risk of developing other dermatologic conditions after contact with other hazardous marine animals. These conditions are generally puncture or bite wounds experienced in the aquatic environment or contact with Cnidaria sea creatures, including Portuguese man-of-war, jellyfish, fire coral, and sea anemones. This phylum, found worldwide in tropical and subtropical waters, is characterized by stinging nematocysts on appendages or tentacles. Each nematocyst contains a spirally coiled thread with a toxin-containing barbed end. After physical or chemical stimulation, the thread is uncoiled and forcibly ejected into the skin.

Jellyfish. Contact with jellyfish and the Portuguese man-of-war produces an immediate, proximally radiating stinging sensation, sometimes with burning numbness and paresthesia. Skin lesions follow the pattern of the tentacle contact (usually linear) and vary from urticarial to vesicular to ulcerative, depending on the species involved. In addition to skin lesions, envenomations may be associated with systemic symptoms including hypotension, muscle spasm, and respiratory paralysis, which may progress to death in as many as 20% of cases. Most notable for causing this problem is the box jellyfish, *Chironex fleckeri*, which can cause full-thickness skin necrosis, cardiopulmonary arrest, and death (Fig. 125–1). Healed lesions may appear as pigmented striae, which last for weeks or months; linear eruptions occasionally recur 1 to 4 weeks after envenomation.

Sea Anemones. These possess finger-like appendages containing nematocysts, which can sting a victim who accidentally brushes against them or handles them. An initial stinging or burning pain is immediately followed by painful pruritus. The most frequent initial lesion is a central pale area with a halo of erythema and petechial hemorrhage, which may progress with edema and diffuse ecchymosis. Severe envenomation may result in local hemorrhage, vesiculation, necrosis, and skin ulceration. Mild envenomations resolve within 48 hours, whereas severe envenomations may lead to eschar formation and pigmentation changes. Systemic symptoms may include fever, malaise, nausea, vomiting, and weakness.

Fire Coral. A fire coral sting produces burning followed by intense, painful pruritus. Urticaria develops within 30 minutes, reaching maximal size within an hour. The pain usually resolves within 1.5 hours and the urticaria within 48 hours. An area of hyperpigmentation may persist for 1 to 2 months. Delayed reactions to Cnidaria envenomation may occur in the area of the skin contact, and erythema nodosum–like reactions accompanied by systemic symptoms (fever, arthralgias, or arthritis) may recur frequently for 1 to 2 months.

Venomous Echinoderms. Sea urchins are echinoderms that have a flattened body covered with venomous spines and venom-secreting pincers located near to the mouth (pedicellariae) (Chapter 125.1). Sea urchin spines may produce numerous puncture wounds with associated erythema and edema. The initial wound may be followed by severe local muscle ache with accompanying systemic symptoms including muscle weakness, paralysis, hypotension, abdominal pain, and respiratory distress, particularly if a pedicellariae envenomation has also occurred. A diffuse delayed cutaneous reaction that may later develop is presumed to be secondary to residual toxins. Deep puncture wounds may result in focal bone erosion and, if a joint space is entered, bony destruction and synovitis. Spines may enter and exit, leaving only a brown discoloration (tattooing). If spine fragments are retained, however, they can initiate a granulomatous response that appears as flesh-colored intradermal or subcutaneous nodules 2 to 12 months after the initial injury.

Bibliography

Auerbach PS: Marine envenomations. N Engl J Med 325:486, 1991.
Auerbach PS (ed): Management of Wilderness and Environmental Emergencies, 3rd ed. St. Louis, CV Mosby, 1995, p 1417.
Brubaker ML, Binford CH, Trautman JR: Occurrences of leprosy in US veterans after service in endemic areas abroad. Public Health Rep 84:1057, 1969.
Canizares O, Harmon R (eds): Clinical Tropical Dermatology, 2nd ed. London, Oxford University Press, 1992.
Caumes E, Carriere J, Guermonprez G, et al.: Dermatoses associated with travel to tropical countries: A prospective study of the diagnosis and management of 269 patients presenting to a Tropical Disease Unit. Clin Infect Dis 20:542, 1995.
Elgart ML: Flies and myiasis. Dermatol Clin 8:237, 1990.
Freudenthal AR, Joseph PR: Seabather's eruption. N Engl J Med 329:542, 1993.
Lockwood DNJ, Keystone JS: Skin problems in returning travelers. Med Clin North Am 76:1393, 1992.
Meinking TL, Taplin D, Hermida JL, et al: The treatment of scabies with ivermectin. N Engl J Med 333:26, 1995.
Orkin M, Maibach HI (eds): Cutaneous Infestations and Insect Bites. New York, Marcel Dekker, 1985.
Wong DE, Meinking TL, Rosen LB, et al: Seabather's eruption. Clinical, histological, and immunological features. J Am Acad Dermatol 30:399, 1993.

147 Eosinophilia in Travelers and Immigrants

Surgheel H. Choudhri and Jay S. Keystone

Eosinophilia in returning travelers and newly arrived immigrants from developing countries is one of the more common problems encountered by clinicians who practice travel medicine. Although eosinophilia in itself is rarely harmful, it is often a clue to an underlying parasitic infection that may cause significant morbidity or even death. The challenge for the clinician is to determine, if possible, the cause of the eosinophilia, thereby ensuring that a potentially harmful illness does not go untreated. The approach to the diagnosis of eosinophilia in returning travelers and immigrants should be a stepwise process that hinges on the answers to several questions: (1) Is the absolute eosinophil count elevated? (2) Is the eosinophilia associated with the patient's travels or present symptoms? (3) If travel related, which parasitic infections are likely? (4) What are the most appropriate diagnostic steps? (5) What should be done if the cause of the eosinophilia cannot be determined?

IS THE ABSOLUTE EOSINOPHIL COUNT ELEVATED? The clinician must first determine whether there is a significant elevation of the eosinophil count. Eosinophils normally constitute 3 to 6% of the granulocytes in peripheral blood. Contrary to what is observed in many scientific papers, the absolute eosinophil count should be considered in determining the presence or absence of eosinophilia. Using the relative eosinophil count (percentage of eosinophils) alone is fraught with error. For example, an individual with 10% eosinophils does not have eosinophilia if the total white blood cell (WBC) count is below $4000 \times 10^9/L$. Normally, there are up to 350 eosinophils $\times 10^9/L$ in the peripheral blood. As a general rule, the absolute count should be greater than $450 \times 10^9/L$ to be considered a significant elevation.

With the introduction of electronic WBC counters, which have a high degree of accuracy, the absolute eosinophil count is most readily and cost effectively determined by multiplying the percentage of eosinophils detected in the differential count by the total WBC count. The degree of eosinophilia may be arbitrarily classified as being minimal (<1000 eosinophils $\times 10^9/L$), moderate (1000 to 3000 eosinophils $\times 10^9/L$), or high (>3000 eosinophils $\times 10^9/L$).

Eosinophil counts exhibit a diurnal variation, with the highest levels occurring at midnight and the lowest at midday. Levels are known to be affected by glucocorticoids, epinephrine, and estrogen. Studies have shown that individuals with parasite-induced eosinophilia may have counts that vary from day to day by as much as 100 to 200%.

IS THE EOSINOPHILIA RELATED TO THE PATIENT'S TRAVEL OR PRESENT SYMPTOMS? After eosinophilia has been confirmed, the next problem is to determine if the eosinophilia is related to the patient's travel or present complaints. It may be helpful to review pretravel differential WBC counts, if they are available, to ascertain whether the patient's eosinophilia was present prior to the trip abroad. Does the patient have any preexisting medical conditions (e.g., hay fever or asthma) that could account for the eosinophilia? It is crucial to keep an open mind and consider the possibility that the patient's signs and symptoms may be unrelated to the eosinophilia. This is likely to occur in a national from a developing country where a significant proportion of the population is infected with intestinal helminths. Thus, an immigrant may have a light helminth infection causing eosinophilia that is unrelated to his or her complaints.

Parasitic causes of eosinophilia are emphasized, as these are the most important considerations in a traveler or immigrant arriving from the tropics. However, there are many other conditions in which the eosinophil count may be elevated (Table 147–1). Eosinophilia associated with allergies (e.g., hay fever and asthma) is usually minimal. However, high eosinophilia counts may occur in those with drug allergy, patients with pulmonary infiltrates with eosinophilia (PIE) syndrome, and aspirin-sensitive asthmatics.

IF TRAVEL RELATED, WHICH PARASITIC INFECTIONS ARE LIKELY TO CAUSE EOSINOPHILIA? In a returning traveler or immigrant with eosinophilia, a parasitic cause is most

TABLE 147–1. Nonparasitic Causes of Eosinophilia

Allergy: asthma, seasonal rhinitis, atopic dermatitis, pulmonary aspergillosis, drug allergy, episodic angioedema with eosinophilia, organic dust hypersensitivity, eosinophilia-myalgia syndrome (L-tryptophan consumption)
Skin disorders: pemphigus, pemphigoid, herpes gestationis, dermatitis herpetiformis, eosinophilic cellulitis (Well's syndrome)
Pulmonary disorders: Löffler's syndrome, pulmonary infiltrates with eosinophilia
Gastrointestinal disorders: inflammatory bowel disease, eosinophilic gastroenteritis, chronic pancreatitis, eosinophilic cholangitis
Neoplastic disorders: lymphomas, carcinomas, acute lymphoblastic leukemia, immunoblastic lymphadenopathy, eosinophilic leukemia
Rheumatic disorders: Churg-Strauss vasculitis, rheumatoid arthritis, Wegener granulomatosis, polyarteritis nodosa, scleroderma, eosinophilia-myalgia syndrome
Immunodeficiency syndromes
Hereditary eosinophilia
Endocrine disorders: hypoadrenalism
Nonparasitic infections: coccidioidomycosis, HIV-1/HIV-2, tuberculosis, scabies, resolving scarlet fever
Miscellaneous: hypereosinophil syndrome, angiolymphoid hyperplasia with eosinophilia, Kimura disease, sarcoidosis, cholesterol embolization

HIV, human immunodeficiency virus.

likely. However, as a screening tool for parasites, the eosinophil count is a poor test. Its sensitivity in Southeast Asian refugees and North American expatriates was shown to be 67% and 38%, respectively, with a positive predictive value of 55% and 17%, respectively. The negative predictive value of eosinophilia in the review of refugees was only 73% and in the expatriate travelers, 95%. The following general guidelines should help to focus on the probable etiologies.

Protozoan Infections. Malaria, amebiasis or giardiasis, and most protozoan infections are not associated with eosinophilia. The three exceptions generally quoted in the literature are isosporosis, toxoplasmosis, and *Dientamoeba fragilis* infection. Unfortunately, those who have reported such findings have usually not ruled out other causes of eosinophilia.

Helminth Infections. On the other hand, helminth infections are the primary cause of parasite-related eosinophilia. It is important to remember that the degree of eosinophilia is a function of the extent of tissue invasion by the parasite. For example, tapeworms and adult roundworms, which do not invade the intestinal mucosa and remain in the bowel lumen, are associated with little or no eosinophilia. In contrast, migrating larval ascarids *(Toxocara canis)* or filaria may give rise to marked eosinophilia because these organisms have in their life cycle a significant degree of tissue invasion. However, clinicians should keep in mind that some infections, e.g., ascariasis and clonorchiasis, may produce high levels of eosinophilia transiently during their initial larval migration phase, with subsequent resolution when adult worms are fully developed. Figure 147–1 provides an outline of the magnitude of eosinophilia usually associated with various parasitic infections. This is meant only as a guideline to the degree of eosinophilia because the range is wide and exceptions occur. It is most important to know those infections that cause extremely high eosinophilia and those that are not usually associated with eosinophilia.

WHAT IS THE BEST APPROACH TO DETERMINE THE ETIOLOGY OF TRAVEL-ASSOCIATED EOSINOPHILIA?

History. The medical history should take into consideration both parasitic and nonparasitic causes of eosinophilia. Patients should be questioned in detail about their history of drug ingestion, atopy, and immune disorders (e.g., rheumatoid arthritis and inflammatory bowel disease). A particular

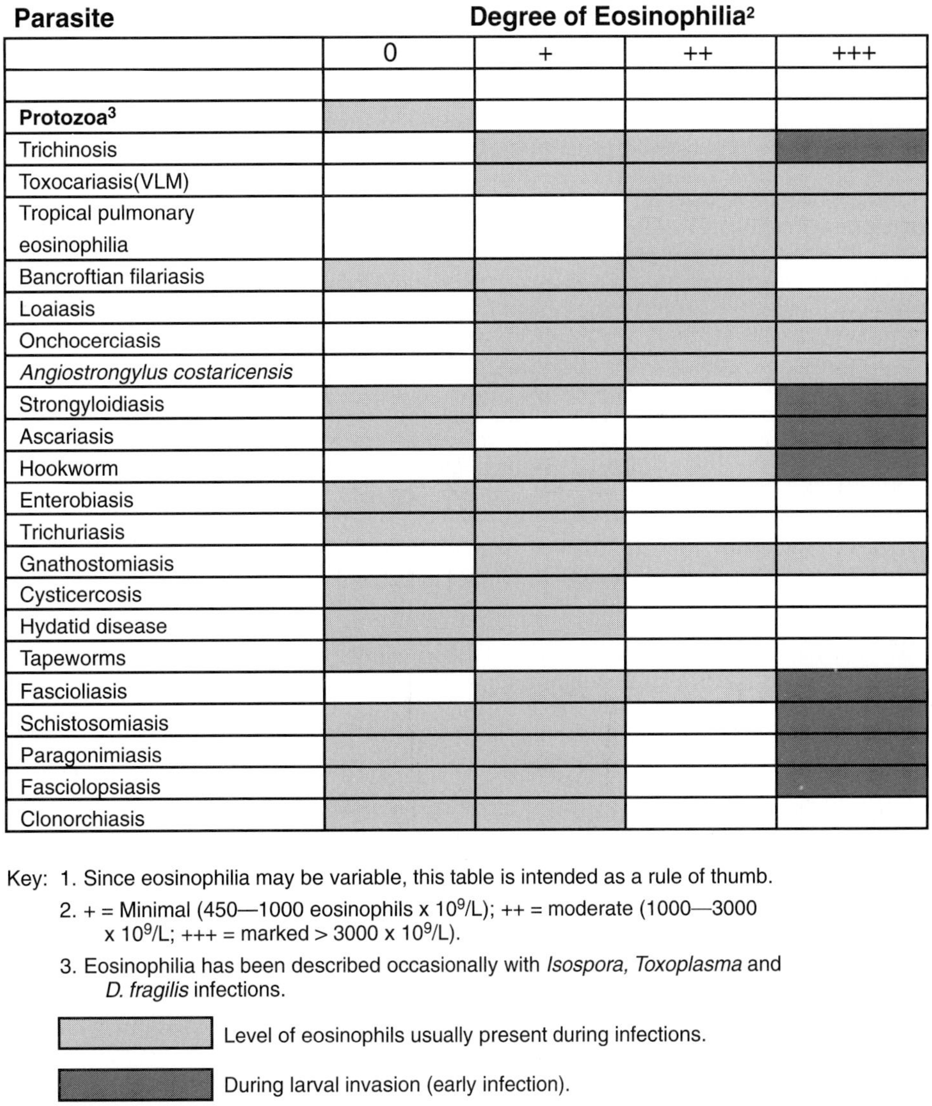

Parasite	Degree of Eosinophilia[2]			
	0	+	++	+++
Protozoa[3]	░			
Trichinosis		░	░	█
Toxocariasis(VLM)		░	░	░
Tropical pulmonary eosinophilia			░	░
Bancroftian filariasis	░	░	░	
Loaiasis		░	░	
Onchocerciasis		░	░	
Angiostrongylus costaricensis		░	░	
Strongyloidiasis	░	░	░	█
Ascariasis	░	░		█
Hookworm		░	░	█
Enterobiasis	░	░		
Trichuriasis	░	░		
Gnathostomiasis		░	░	
Cysticercosis	░	░	░	
Hydatid disease	░	░		
Tapeworms	░			
Fascioliasis			░	█
Schistosomiasis	░	░	░	█
Paragonimiasis		░	░	
Fasciolopsiasis	░			█
Clonorchiasis	░	░		

Figure 147–1. Eosinophilia associated with selected parasitic infections.[1]

Key: 1. Since eosinophilia may be variable, this table is intended as a rule of thumb.

2. + = Minimal (450—1000 eosinophils x 10^9/L); ++ = moderate (1000—3000 x 10^9/L; +++ = marked > 3000 x 10^9/L).

3. Eosinophilia has been described occasionally with *Isospora, Toxoplasma* and *D. fragilis* infections.

░ Level of eosinophils usually present during infections.

█ During larval invasion (early infection).

note of the countries visited, as well as the duration and extent of exposure to parasitic infections, should be made. Many parasitic infections (e.g., filariasis and schistosomiasis) have well-defined distributions, whereas others (e.g., hookworm, whipworm, and roundworm) have little geographic specificity. For the geographic history to have any relevance, a knowledge of the distribution of parasitic infections is required (Chapter 149).

In addition to places where the individual has traveled, the exposure history is often crucial. Individuals who travel to tropical areas but remain in resorts or urban areas and stay in first-class accommodations are not likely to acquire soil or arthropod-transmitted nematode infections. For example, if they have not walked in their bare feet in soil contaminated with human excrement, travelers are unlikely to acquire hookworm or *Strongyloides* infections. The possibility of schistosomiasis should be entertained only if there was exposure to fresh water in endemic areas. Parasitic infections, e.g., loiasis, onchocerciasis, hydatid disease, and schistosomiasis can usually be excluded in the absence of a history of travel to rural areas. Dietary history may be helpful in making or excluding a diagnosis of trichinosis, toxoplasmosis, or tapeworm infections.

The duration of stay in the tropics can help to establish or rule out some parasitic infections. For example, short-term travelers (<3 months) rarely acquire filariae (bancroftian filariasis, onchocerciasis), larval tapeworms (hydatid disease, cysticercosis), and most trematodes (paragonimiasis, clonorchiasis) with the exception of schistosomiasis. Prolonged stay or travel in the tropics should raise the index of suspicion for infections that are usually found in the indigenous population, having been acquired with extensive exposure.

Physical Examination. In asymptomatic individuals with eosinophilia, results of examination most often are normal. Some filariae *(Loa loa, Onchocerca volvulus, Mansonella streptocerca)* can cause subcutaneous swellings or dermatitis. Examination of the liver and spleen may be helpful in the diagnosis of schistosomiasis, hydatid disease, or toxocariasis.

Laboratory Investigations. Laboratory investigations should proceed in a stepwise manner. A recommended approach to the investigation of eosinophilia is summarized in Table 147–2 and detailed below.

Before initiating investigations, the incubation period of various helminth infections must be considered. Eosinophilia in travelers who have recently returned from the tropics might be due to the migrating larval stage of an intestinal nematode infection that could not be diagnosed for several months, until eggs are present in the stool. Similarly, eosinophilia might occur during the incubation period of a filarial infection that would not produce symptoms or microfilariae in skin or blood for at least 6 months after exposure. On the other hand, because *Strongyloides stercoralis* infection may last for the lifetime of the host, eosinophilia may be related to an infection that was acquired in the tropics many years before its discovery.

Initial investigations for patients with eosinophilia include the following:

1. A total WBC count, differential count, and hemoglobin and platelet count. The eosinophil count should be repeated if it is elevated initially to confirm whether the elevation is reproducible and persistent.
2. Examination of 3 stool specimens for ova and parasites. Because most parasite eggs and larvae are excreted intermittently, at least 3 specimens collected 48 hr apart should be examined by direct smear and a concentration technique (e.g., formalin-ether, zinc flotation) (Chapter 150). Negative stool examinations do not exclude a para-

TABLE 147–2. Approach to Investigation of Eosinophilia in a Returning Traveler

History	Allergy
	Drugs and vitamins (L-tryptophan)
	Geographic and exposure
Physical examination (areas of concentration)	Skin, subcutaneous tissues
	Liver/spleen
Investigations	*Baseline:*
Step 1	Complete blood count and differential white blood cell count
	Stool examination for ova and parasites (× 3)
	Urinalysis
	Examination of midday urine for ova and parasites (× 3) (Africa, Middle East)
Step 2	*Assuming appropriate geographic and exposure history:*
	Strongyloides culture and serology
	Duodenal aspirate/Entero-Test (strongyloidiasis, hookworm)
	Serology (*Schistosoma*, filariae, etc.)
	Day/night blood films (filariasis)
Step 3	*If history and physical examination suggest a specific diagnosis:*
	Skin snips (onchocerciasis)
	Mazzotti test (onchocerciasis)
	Liver biopsy (schistosomiasis, fascioliasis)
	Chest x-ray (hydatid, tropical pulmonary eosinophilia, paragonimiasis)
	Soft tissue x-ray (cysticercosis)
	Sputum examination for ova and parasites (paragonimiasis)
	Abdominal ultrasound (hydatid)
	Cystoscopy with or without biopsy (schistosomiasis)
	Rectal snips (schistosomiasis)

sitic cause of eosinophilia. Helminths invade a variety of tissues, including blood and subcutaneous tissue (e.g., filariasis), muscle (e.g., trichinosis), and liver (e.g., visceral larva migrans). As noted above, most helminth infections have a prepatent period of several weeks to months before eggs or larvae are detectable in body fluids or excreta.

3. Urinalysis and examination of three midday urine specimens for parasites and ova. The latter should be performed only on individuals with a history of freshwater exposure who have traveled to *Schistosoma haematobium* endemic areas (Middle East or Africa).

The following additional investigations for specific parasites might be included in the initial evaluation of a patient who has had potential exposure to these parasites in endemic areas (e.g., indigenous population, long-term residents, or adventurous travelers).

1. *Strongyloides* culture. This procedure concentrates the living strongyloides larvae and is best accomplished by the Baermann or blood agar techniques (Chapter 150).
2. *Strongyloides* serology (enzyme-linked immunosorbent assay [ELISA]). This has high sensitivity (88%) and specificity (80%) (Chapter 152).
3. *Schistosoma* serology (indirect fluorescent antibody test [IFA], indirect hemagglutination [IHA], ELISA, immunoblot). These tests have a high degree of sensitivity and specificity, particularly the immunoblot which can

differentiate schistosome species and human from non-human infections (Chapter 152).

4. Filaria serology (IHA, IFA, ELISA). This test is usually not specific because filaria antibodies are elevated in a variety of different helminth infections (Chapter 152). However, high titers may be more predictive of infection; specific antigens to detect filaria-specific IgG4 antibodies are being used in some research laboratories.

5. Day and night bloods for filaria. Concentrated midday blood counts should be examined for *Loa loa, Mansonella perstans,* or *Mansonella ozzardi* (Chapter 151). Blood should be taken at midnight for *Wuchereria bancrofti.* If a night blood specimen is difficult to obtain, a single 100-mg dose of diethylcarbamazine (DEC) may be administered and the blood examined for microfilariae 1 hr later. For bancroftian filariasis, this challenge test significantly increases the yield from daytime blood specimens.

A number of other diagnostic procedures that are parasite specific may be helpful if clinical findings suggest a particular diagnosis. These are dealt with in turn.

1. Duodenal aspirate, Entero-Test, and/or biopsy. Examination of the small bowel and its contents may be helpful in making a diagnosis of *S. stercoralis, Trichostrongylus,* hookworm, *Clonorchis sinensis,* or *Fasciola hepatica* infections (Chapter 151).

2. Rectal and bladder biopsy (snips). In the diagnosis of *Schistosoma mansoni* or *Schistosoma japonicum,* a rectal biopsy is one of the most sensitive diagnostic tests (Chapter 151). *S. hematobium* also can be diagnosed by this method, and ova can also be detected in bladder biopsies taken during cystoscopy (Fig. 118–23). The biopsy specimen should be crushed in a drop of saline between two glass slides and microscopically examined for eggs under low power.

3. Plain radiography. A chest x-ray film may be helpful during the larval migration phase of *Ascaris lumbricoides* or in the diagnosis of tropical pulmonary eosinophilia. In ascariasis, pulmonary infiltrates on the chest x-ray film associated with bronchospasm and eosinophilia constitute Löffler's syndrome, of which parasites are only one cause. *Echinococcus granulosus* may show up as one or more well-defined spherical masses (Fig. 124–7) or as a calcified liver cyst on chest x-ray (Fig. 124–9). On the other hand, *Echinococcus multilocularis* may presumptively be diagnosed by finding a pathognomonic "Swiss cheese" pattern of calcification in the liver, which may be detected on a flat plate of the abdomen. Typical coin lesions may be seen in dirofilariasis. Paragonimiasis can cause hilar masses and pulmonary infiltrates (Figs. 121–4 and 121–5). Occasionally, skull films (Fig. 124–3) or soft tissue x-rays of the arms and thighs (Fig. 124–1B) are helpful in the diagnosis of cysticercosis.

4. Sputum for ova and parasites. Sputum examination may be helpful by detecting ova of *Paragonimus westermani.* Rarely, one might find larval stages of *Toxocara canis* or *A. lumbricoides* or hooklets of *E. granulosus.* Larvae of *S. stercoralis* may be seen in sputum during hyperinfection (Chapter 151).

5. Skin snips. If onchocerciasis is suspected, a diagnosis may be made by finding microfilariae in the epidermis and upper dermis (Chapter 151).

6. Mazzotti test. This test may be helpful in making a presumptive diagnosis of onchocerciasis when microfilariae are too few to be found in skin snips (Chapter 108). An intense pruritic reaction occurs within 24 hr of the administration of a 50-mg dose of DEC and is considered to be diagnostic of infection. Skin snips should always precede a Mazzotti test because in heavy infections anaphylaxis may result from drug-induced killing of microfilariae. The test may be positive in other forms of filariasis, particularly in nonimmune hosts who are exposed to the parasite for the first time.

7. Muscle biopsy. Although a diagnosis of trichinosis can be confirmed by muscle biopsy, serodiagnosis has replaced this invasive test except early on in infections (Chapters 111, 151, and 152).

8. Other serologic tests. Blood tests for hydatid disease, cysticercosis, trichinosis, toxocariasis, and fascioliasis may be diagnostic. (Chapter 152).

WHAT SHOULD BE DONE IF THE CAUSE OF EOSINOPHILIA CANNOT BE DETERMINED? Even after extensive investigations, it is not unusual for the cause of eosinophilia in a returning traveler or immigrant to remain elusive. If the clinical findings do not warrant further investigations, a 3- to 6-mo waiting period might prove useful because the eosinophil count may return to normal during observation. If eosinophilia persists, stool, urine, and blood examinations for parasites should be repeated. Recent studies in refugees from Southeast Asia have documented hookworm and *Strongyloides* infections to be the most common causes of cryptic eosinophilia.

If the patient remains asymptomatic, two options exist. Some tropical disease specialists recommend a course of thiabendazole (or albendazole) for strongyloidiasis to prevent hyperinfection should the patient become immunocompromised at a later date (Chapter 105.2). If a treatment trial is not instituted, patients should be informed of the possibility that they might be harboring a parasite that has the potential to create health problems. They should be warned of the need to have their eosinophil count checked before receiving immunosuppressive therapy. If eosinophilia is present in such cases, an empirical course of treatment for strongyloidiasis should be given.

Morbidity is directly proportional to worm burden, and helminth infections are usually self-limited. Therefore, a lightly infected individual with eosinophilia caused by parasites is not likely to come to harm if the infection remains untreated, except in the case of strongyloidiasis and, rarely, schistosomiasis. Long-term clinical follow-up of these patients has shown that undiagnosed travel-related eosinophilia is not a significant health hazard for the returning traveler.

Challenging Problem. The problem of eosinophilia in a returning traveler is certainly challenging. After initial basic investigations, the approach requires knowledge of the geographic distribution of disease and the epidemiology and clinical presentations of helminth infections. Nontropical causes of eosinophilia are part of the differential diagnosis and influence decisions for more extensive investigations.

Bibliography

Harries AD, Myers B, Bhattacharrya D: Eosinophilia in Caucasians returning from the tropics. Trans R Soc Trop Med Hyg 80:327, 1986.

Libman MD, MacLean JD, Gyorkos T: Screening for schistosomiasis, filariasis and strongyloidiasis among expatriates returning from the tropics. Clin Infect Dis 17:353, 1993.

Mawhorter SD: Eosinophilia caused by parasites. Pediatr Ann 23:405, 1994.

Nutman TB, Ottesen EA, Ieng S, et al: Eosinophilia in South East Asian refugees: Evaluation at a referral centre. J Infect Dis 155:309, 1987.

Spry CJF: Eosinophilia. Practitioner 226:79, 1982.

Teo CG, Singh M, Ting WC, et al: Evaluation of the common conditions associated with eosinophilia. J Clin Pathol 38:305, 1985.

Weller PF: Eosinophilia in travelers. Med Clin North Am 76:1413, 1992.

Wilson ME: Eosinophilia. *In* A World Guide to Infections: Diseases, Distributions, Diagnosis. New York, Oxford University Press, 1991, pp 154–175.

Wolfe MS: Eosinophilia in the returning traveler. Infect Dis Clin North Am 6:489, 1992.

148 *Diseases of Immigrants*

Alison Holmes and James H. Maguire

In 1996, over 70% of the 9 million legal immigrants to the United States were Latin-Americans or Asians, and over two thirds of the 5 million undocumented aliens living in the United States were from Mexico and Central America. Overall, 20 million persons or 8% of the U.S. population were foreign-born according to the 1990 census.

EVALUATION OF RECENT ARRIVALS. The health problems of immigrants reflect their countries of origin and status as refugees, legal immigrants, or undocumented aliens. Health problems at the time of arrival are different from those several years later. An imported infectious disease may be the reason for a first encounter with the health care system, but often other problems are more pressing, e.g., a dental emergency, an ear infection, or the need for immediate vaccination or tuberculin skin testing before starting school or a new job. Such first visits provide the opportunity to begin a general evaluation and arrange for follow-up.

Required Health Assessment. Many immigrants will have received a medical examination overseas in order to obtain a visa for permanent residency. The purpose of the overseas examination is to identify not all physical and mental disorders, but primarily those that might prove harmful to the immigrant or the general population. By U.S. law (Immigration and Nationality Act), medical conditions that exclude persons from entry include (1) communicable diseases of public health significance, including infection with human immunodeficiency virus (HIV), active tuberculosis, infectious syphilis, chancroid, gonorrhea, granuloma inguinale, lymphogranuloma venereum, and leprosy; (2) failure to present documentation of having received vaccination against vaccine-preventable diseases, including mumps, measles, rubella, polio, tetanus, diphtheria, pertussis, *Haemophilus influenzae* type B, hepatitis B, and any other vaccinations recommended by the Advisory Committee for Immunization Practices; (3) physical or mental disorders or associated behavior harmful to the alien or others; or (4) drug abuse or addiction.

Less well defined reasons for exclusion include disorders that may prevent the immigrant from working, studying, or caring for himself or herself or may require extensive medical treatment or institutionalization in the future. The guidelines for the overseas medical examination, as formulated by the Centers for Disease Control and Prevention (CDC), include a medical history, physical examination, chest radiograph, and, for persons 15 years of age or older, screening tests for antibodies to HIV and syphilis. Younger children may have a tuberculin skin test instead of the chest radiograph, but radiographs are mandatory for Southeast Asian children ≥ 2 years of age. Smears of sputum are examined if there are radiographic signs suggestive of active tuberculosis. Persons with smear-positive tuberculosis become eligible for immigration only after treatment is begun and three smears are negative. Persons with active syphilis or other sexually transmitted diseases must be fully treated, and persons with leprosy must complete at least 6 months of treatment. Mandatory follow-up is required after arrival in the United States for persons with these and a wide range of other health conditions identified during the overseas examination.

Refugees undergo a similar evaluation overseas, often in a country of temporary asylum. In addition, there is a mandatory domestic health assessment on arrival in the state in which resettlement is to occur. The purpose is to follow up on conditions identified during the overseas examination and eliminate health-related barriers to successful resettlement. This assessment varies according to state and locality, but as a minimum usually includes a tuberculin skin test or repeat chest radiograph and screening tests for hepatitis B, parasitic infections, pregnancy, anemia, and visual, auditory, and dental problems. Many states require examinations for lead poisoning and chronic conditions such as diabetes or hypertension.

Additional Health Screening. For refugees and other immigrants who entered the country through legal channels, the results of the required overseas and domestic assessments should be reviewed, and supplementary screening should be performed as necessary. For instance, tuberculin skin testing may be required, since it is not part of the standard overseas medical evaluation.

Undocumented immigrants should receive a complete health evaluation similar to the mandatory overseas and domestic assessments described previously. Details of the evaluation vary according to country of origin, living conditions, exposures, medical conditions, and prior treatments. Immediate health problems should be addressed, and the status of chronic illnesses should be reviewed, including the adequacy of current supplies of medications. Information about smoking, alcohol consumption, and illicit drug use should be obtained. Assessment of immunization status should take into account the fact that many immigrants have not received complete series of vaccines or have no documentation of prior immunization. A history of having received bacille Calmette-Guérin (BCG) should be noted.

The physical examination should be thorough and include an evaluation of blood pressure, vision, hearing, and dentition; determination of height, weight, and nutritional status; and assessment of growth and development in the case of children. Attention should be paid to the skin for scabies and other common dermatologic diseases. Women often are in need of a Pap smear. Evidence of physical and psychologic trauma, including signs of depression, anxiety, or post-traumatic stress disorder, should be sought. Refugees, in particular, may have witnessed or experienced violent assault, fled from war zones, lost family members, or been imprisoned or detained in camps for many months.

Tuberculin skin testing is indicated for persons who do not have symptoms or signs of active tuberculosis. Persons with reactive tests or a history of tuberculosis should have a chest radiograph, and, when necessary, sputum smears and cultures. A complete blood count to exclude anemia and eosinophilia, tests for hepatitis B, and stool examination for ova and parasites are appropriate for persons from developing countries. Pre- and post-test counseling should be part of the evaluation for HIV infection. Screening for parasitic diseases other than intestinal parasites is indicated when there is a history of exposure, peripheral blood eosinophilia, or other compatible clinical picture. For instance, hematuria in a person who came from an area endemic for *Schistosoma haematobium* should prompt microscopic examination of the urine.

Provision of Health Care to Immigrants. The initial health needs of recently arrived immigrants include treatment of infections and other illnesses detected by screening and administration of vaccines and prophylactic medications. Infection control measures or contact tracing may be required if a contagious disease is detected. Prompt referrals to dentistry, ophthalmology, nutrition, obstetrics, gynecology, or psychiatry are provided as needed.

Assistance on accessing the local health care system and obtaining primary care services should be given. This may be easier for refugees, because the agency that arranged their asylum also arranges for the domestic health assessment and introduction to a clinic or physician. Immigrants frequently are unaware of services that are available to them or do not use available services because of concerns about being undocumented or uninsured. Social workers and outreach workers familiar with local regulations and health facilities can help immigrants obtain health care and financial assistance. Appropriate utilization of health services should be encouraged.

Health care facilities that best serve immigrant populations are family-oriented and provide pediatric and adult services, prenatal care, and maternal and child health care. Ideally, a bilingual and bicultural staff is available that can address specific health beliefs and cultural issues. There should be links with a multicultural psychiatric unit, support groups, and English classes. Educational efforts should address health maintenance and risk avoidance. Advice about immunizations and malaria prophylaxis should be provided for immigrants who return to their homeland for brief visits.

INFECTIOUS DISEASES OF IMMIGRANTS. Although an acutely ill immigrant may acquire an infection just prior to emigration or during a short visit to his or her native country, acute infections of immigrants more often originate in the adoptive country. After arrival, migrant farm workers and other indigent immigrants may experience overcrowding, poor sanitation, or other conditions that are conducive to the spread of infections. The source of infection often is another immigrant, as has been documented in outbreaks of imported malaria and measles. Imported foods or unsafe culinary practices have been responsible for outbreaks of brucellosis and trichinosis.

The majority of imported infections of immigrants are chronic and reflect prolonged exposure to poor living conditions in tropical climates. Some are latent and do not become evident unless reactivated by immunosuppressive therapy or an underlying illness, e.g., AIDS. Other infections are indolent and produce few symptoms until a threshold of organ damage or dysfunction is reached. An immigrant's risk of becoming ill diminishes as pathogens die off or persists indefinitely if the pathogen is long-lived or can replicate within the host.

In considering the geographic distribution and incubation period of infections, the clinician should be aware that some persons, particularly refugees, have spent long periods of time in countries other than their own. Genetic factors and immunity acquired through prior exposure determine an immigrant's susceptibility to infection and may modify the manifestations of disease. Cultural practices or beliefs may increase the risk of exposure to some infections and affect the interpretation of illness and willingness to seek and adhere to medical treatment.

Febrile Illnesses. The differential diagnosis of fever in an immigrant is lengthy, and first priority should be given to illnesses that can be rapidly fatal if not treated or that pose a threat to public health. For example, a delayed diagnosis of falciparum malaria, meningococcemia, or typhoid fever can be fatal, and unrecognized hepatitis, measles, or tuberculosis may lead to secondary cases.

Malaria. Immigrants account for a large proportion of imported cases of malaria each year (Chapter 92). Persons who return to their native countries for a short visit often are at high risk for infection because they fail to take prophylaxis or do not employ measures to prevent mosquito bites. Some immigrants are unaware that the malaria situation in their countries of origin deteriorated after they emigrated, whereas others erroneously believe that immunity acquired in the past will continue to protect them even years after their last exposure to the parasite.

In the United States during the first half of the 1990s, the highest rates of malaria occurred among immigrants from sub-Saharan Africa and Asia who had recently immigrated or returned from a short visit. Persons arriving from West Africa and Haiti mainly had *Plasmodium falciparum* infections, whereas persons from Somalia, the Indian subcontinent, Central America, and Mexico primarily had vivax malaria. Refugees from Southeast Asia were infected with either, and sometimes both, species. Most persons with *P. falciparum* infections developed symptoms within 1 month of arrival, whereas *Plasmodium vivax* infections usually became apparent between 1 month and 1 year of arrival.

Malaria in partially immune immigrants may have a longer incubation period and less intense symptoms than malaria in nonimmune travelers. Although subclinical infections have led to episodes of transfusion-induced, introduced, and congenital malaria, asymptomatic immigrants as a rule are not screened for malaria. Exceptions occur, e.g., in 1992, when screening of a group of Montagnard refugees being resettled in North Carolina showed that approximately one half were infected. Frequent episodes of malaria during their prolonged residence in remote camps along the Vietnam-Cambodia border probably led to substantial immunity, and many infected persons were asymptomatic. Their relocation had occurred rapidly and with minimal medical evaluation before arrival in the United States.

Bacterial Causes of Febrile Illnesses. Typhoid fever (Chapter 75) and enteric fever due to nontyphoidal *Salmonella* species (Chapter 76) are endemic throughout the developing world and are occasionally the source of fever in immigrants, either at the time of initial entry or following a visit to their country of origin. In the United States, most cases among immigrants originate in Mexico, elsewhere in Latin America, the Indian subcontinent, and the Caribbean. Typhoid has been common among immigrants from Ethiopia to Israel, and there have been cases among refugees from Bosnia-Herzegovina. In industrialized countries, symptomatic and asymptomatic immigrants have been the source of outbreaks of salmonellosis. Multidrug-resistant strains of *Salmonella typhi* may be imported from various areas, and strains that are resistant to ciprofloxacin, chloramphenicol, ampicillin, and trimethoprim-sulfamethoxazole have emerged from the Indian subcontinent.

Brucellosis, an unusual cause of fever in immigrants, can cause acute or insidious fevers anywhere from weeks to years after exposure (Chapter 64). The diagnosis is often elusive until appropriate serologic tests are requested, or the fastidious organism is isolated from blood, tissues, or other body fluids. Brucellosis remains a health problem in Latin American countries, the Mediterranean region, and Asia. Cases may be acquired in the immigrant's country of origin or result from ingestion of imported dairy products, e.g., unpasteurized goat's milk contaminated with *Brucella melitensis*.

Meningococcal infections are endemic in parts of sub-Saharan Africa and Nepal, and epidemics occur sporadically in other parts of the developing world (Chapter 74). Meningococcemia or meningococcal meningitis should be considered in recently arrived immigrants with febrile illnesses or central nervous system symptoms (Chapter 52).

Melioidosis, due to *Pseudomonas pseudomallei*, occurs in Southeast Asia and other regions between 20° North and South latitude (Chapter 37). Bacteremia, localized abscesses, or pulmonary disease may develop within several days of exposure to the organism in soil or water or may become manifest only after years of silent infection. Tropical pyomyositis, a purulent infection of striated muscle usually due to *Staphylococcus aureus*, has been reported in immigrants from

Latin America and other developing regions (Chapter 58). The extremely rare case of anthrax in industrialized countries is more likely to be the result of contact with imported animal products than of an imported human infection (Chapter 55). Partly because of the short incubation period and relatively short duration of illness, acute rickettsial infections and leptospirosis would also be unusual among immigrants. Recurrent louse-borne typhus or Brill-Zinsser disease may develop years after immigration (Chapter 66.1), and relapsing fever (Chapter 71) has been a consideration in refugee camps in Ethiopia.

HIV and Human T-Cell Lymphotropic Virus Type I (HTLV-I) Infections. Over 90% of the world's HIV-1 and HIV-2 infections occur in the developing world (Chapter 22). While an immigrant experiencing an acute retroviral infection may present with fever, most febrile illnesses in HIV-infected immigrants are due to opportunistic pathogens. In the United States, foreign-born AIDS patients have a higher incidence of tuberculosis, toxoplasmosis, and salmonellosis than U.S.-born AIDS patients. Latent paracoccidioidomycosis, histoplasmosis, Chagas' disease, visceral leishmaniasis, and *Penicillium marneffei* infection may reactivate in HIV-infected immigrants from endemic areas.

HTLV-I, the retrovirus associated with adult T-cell leukemia and lymphoma (ATL), tropical spastic paraparesis, and HTLV-I–associated myelopathy, is endemic in Japan, the Caribbean, parts of Central and South America, and Africa (Chapter 23). Fever with lymphadenopathy and skin lesions or opportunistic infections may be the initial presentation of ATL.

Other Viral Infections. An inadequately immunized immigrant has been the occasional source of imported vaccine-preventable diseases, e.g., measles (Chapter 25.1) and rubella. Secondary cases have occurred frequently among other unvaccinated immigrants. Of the many arboviruses and agents of viral hemorrhagic fevers that could be imported by arriving immigrants, only dengue appears to have caused introduced infections in the United States in recent years (Chapter 29.1). Nevertheless, the infectivity of lethal viruses such as Lassa and Ebola makes it critical that they be considered in the differential diagnosis of fever in an arriving immigrant (Chapter 31).

Parasitic Causes of Fever. Unlike expatriate visitors to areas endemic for schistosomiasis, infected immigrants from such areas are extremely unlikely to present with signs of acute schistosomiasis following arrival in an industrialized country. In contrast, lymphatic filariasis occurs after prolonged residence in an endemic area and is unlikely to be seen in short-term travelers. Filarial fevers, often with retrograde lymphangitis or lymphadenitis, may recur for years after the patient has left an endemic area (Chapter 106). Certain immigrant groups are susceptible to trichinosis even after arrival because of customs related to food preparation and pig-rearing practices (Chapter 111). In recent years in the United States, immigrant groups from Southeast Asia in particular have experienced outbreaks and sporadic cases of trichinosis.

Acute toxoplasmosis, an occasional cause of mononucleosis or asymptomatic lymphadenopathy, has resulted in congenital infections of infants born of immigrant mothers, usually from Southeast Asia (Chapter 97). Because the prevalence of chronic toxoplasmosis is high in tropical areas, reactivation toxoplasmosis is common among immigrants with AIDS. Imported cases of acute Chagas' disease and visceral leishmaniasis are exceptionally rare, and reactivated cases of chronic infections in persons with AIDS or another immunosuppressing condition are only slightly more common.

Pulmonary Diseases

Tuberculosis. Tuberculosis is undoubtedly the most important pulmonary infection of immigrants and refugees. In the United States, 30% of active cases of tuberculosis occur among the foreign-born population, up from 15% in 1977 (Chapter 77). Mexico, the Philippines, and Vietnam, the countries providing the greatest numbers of recent immigrants, account for the largest numbers of cases. It is unlikely that HIV co-infection has contributed dramatically to the rising rates of tuberculosis among immigrants, in part because of the legal restrictions that bar persons with HIV infection from entering the United States.

The majority of foreign-born persons who develop tuberculosis do so within the first 5 years after entry. Physicians caring for immigrants should consider even immigrants cleared during the legal immigration process to be at risk of active tuberculosis, since screening focuses on the identification of smear-positive persons. However, a high rate of negative sputum smears has been noted among actively infected Southeast Asian immigrants considered to have "nonprogressive" tuberculosis by radiograph. Any pulmonary parenchymal abnormality other than a calcified granuloma that is compatible with tuberculosis should be evaluated by sputum smears and cultures, even if the radiograph suggests inactive disease or remains unchanged over several months. Thoracentesis and pleural biopsy should be performed for the diagnosis of tuberculous pleural effusions, which can occur in the absence of parenchymal disease.

Drug resistance and poor compliance may complicate treatment of active tuberculosis in immigrants. Foreign-born patients have higher rates of multidrug-resistant tuberculosis than those born in the United States. Rates of isoniazid resistance are high in certain groups and have exceeded 20% in immigrants from Southeast Asia. A variety of social, economic, and cultural reasons underlie poor adherence to treatment regimens. Directly observed therapy should be administered whenever possible.

In the United States, the Public Health Service publishes recommendations for the evaluation and management of immigrants with a reactive tuberculin skin test. A reaction is always considered positive if there is induration ≥ 15 mm. Induration ≥ 10 mm is classified as positive if the immigrant arrived within 5 years from a country with high rates of tuberculosis or is at risk because of an underlying medical condition or risky living situation or exposures. Induration ≥ 5 mm is considered positive in HIV-infected persons, persons with recent close contact with a person with active tuberculosis, and persons who have fibrotic lesions on chest radiographs. In interpreting the tuberculin reaction a history of BCG vaccination should be disregarded. Vaccination does not prevent all cases of tuberculosis and may not result in a reactive skin test; moreover, a positive reaction may wane with time.

Isoniazid remains the agent of choice for preventive therapy. Failures may occur because of poor compliance or infection with isoniazid-resistant organisms. Rifampin appears to be effective prophylaxis for persons exposed to isoniazid-resistant strains. Combinations of agents, e.g., pyrazinamide and rifampin or ciprofloxacin, are under evaluation for prophylaxis against multidrug-resistant mycobacteria. Combinations of drugs may also permit shorter courses of prophylaxis.

Fungal Infections. Immigrants from areas endemic for histoplasmosis, coccidioidomycosis, or blastomycosis may present with illnesses that resemble tuberculosis, such as cavitary pneumonia, localized extrapulmonary disease, or disseminated infections (Chapter 83). Often the illness is the result of reactivation of latent infection in the setting of an underlying condition such as AIDS. *Histoplasma capsulatum* is widely distributed in the Caribbean, Latin America, and Southeast Asia. In Africa, a variant strain, *Histoplasma capsulatum* var. *duboisii* involves skin and bones rather than the lungs. Parts of Mexico and Central and South America are endemic for *Coccidioides immitis*. Paracoccidioidomycosis is endemic in southern Mexico and South and Central America, and there have been reports of infection with *Blastomyces dermatitidis* from Africa, Central America, and Mexico.

Other Respiratory Infections. The unusual case of melioidosis (Chapter 37) or paragonimiasis (Chapter 121) in immigrants from Southeast Asia and elsewhere may also produce a syndrome of chronic productive cough and cavitary pulmonary infiltrates suggestive of tuberculosis. Marked eosinophilia ($>3000/mm^3$) in an immigrant with recurrent cough and wheezing may be a clue to tropical pulmonary eosinophilia (Chapter 106.3). The illness occurs most commonly among persons from South and Southeast Asia, and less frequently elsewhere in the tropics. Unusual parasitic causes of peripheral blood eosinophilia and pulmonary infiltrates in an immigrant would include trichinosis, toxocariasis, and the migratory stage of *Ascaris* and hookworm infections. Pulmonary infiltrates in an immigrant receiving corticosteroids or other immunosuppressive medications should raise the question of hyperinfection due to strongyloidiasis, even if there is no peripheral blood eosinophilia (Chapter 105.2). Immigrants from the Middle East and other sheep-raising parts of the world may harbor hydatid cysts of the lung that can reach a large size without producing symptoms (Chapter 124.2).

Diphtheria, rhinoscleroma, leprosy, syphilis, mucocutaneous leishmaniasis, paracoccidioidomycosis, and histoplasmosis are among the infections of immigrants that can involve the nose or oropharynx. Immigrants with diphtheria have been responsible for outbreaks among unvaccinated persons (Chapter 33).

Gastrointestinal Diseases

Common Viral, Bacterial, and Protozoal Infections. Acute diarrheal disease due to viruses, *Escherichia coli*, *Salmonella* species, *Shigella*, and *Campylobacter* are infrequent imported problems of immigrants and, when seen, are more likely among children than adults. Sporadic cases of *Salmonella arizonae* infection among immigrants from Mexico have been caused by ingestion of capsules of dried rattlesnake meat (Chapter 76). The capsules were obtained in Mexico or illegally in the United States for treatment of AIDS, cancer, and other illnesses. Cholera is unlikely among immigrants but can be imported in shellfish (Chapter 41). Chronic diarrhea may accompany intestinal tuberculosis. *Helicobacter pylori* infections are extremely prevalent in the developing world, and should be considered in persons with symptoms of gastritis or peptic ulcer (Chapter 45).

Asymptomatic carriage of intestinal protozoa is more common than diarrheal illness due to these pathogens. Rates of carriage of *Cryptosporidium* (Chapter 88) and *Giardia* (Chapter 87) are higher among young children than adults. Because these agents can be spread from person to person, microscopic examination of the stool is indicated in cases of persistent diarrhea in immigrant families. Cryptosporidiosis, isosporiasis, and cyclosporiasis as causes of chronic diarrhea complicating HIV infection are more common among immigrants from the developing world than natives of industrialized countries.

Invasive amebiasis usually presents within several months of departure from endemic areas and occurs frequently in young men (Chapter 86). More cases of amebic dysentery or liver abscess in the United States originated in Mexico than in other countries, but other Latin American countries, South Africa, India, and Southeast Asia also have high rates of amebic disease. Asymptomatic carriers should receive treatment because of the risk of invasive disease, the potential for person-to-person transmission, and the current lack of readily available tests that distinguish *Entamoeba histolytica* from the nonpathogenic *Entamoeba dispar*. Other nonpathogenic intestinal protozoa are common in stool specimens of immigrants and do not require treatment. Rare cases of colitis due to the ciliate *Balantidium coli* have occurred among immigrants (Chapter 90.1). Dysphagia or prolonged constipation may raise the suspicion of chronic Chagas' disease among immigrants from Latin America south of the equator.

Intestinal Helminths. Infection with intestinal nematodes is extremely common among immigrants from developing countries, many of whom are infected with multiple species of parasites. The risk of complications due to *Ascaris*, *Trichuris*, and hookworm is as a rule greater in children than adults because of their greater worm burdens, and the probability of illness diminishes with time as worms die off. Light infections tend not to produce symptoms; however, even a single *Ascaris* organism can produce symptoms as it leaves the body through the anus or upper airways or obstructs the hepatobiliary tree or the appendix (Chapter 104).

Strongyloides stercoralis can persist for the lifetime of the host because of its autoinfectious cycle and should be considered in immigrants from the developing world, who may complain of chronic diarrhea, epigastric pain, or larva currens (Chapter 105.2). Persons at risk for the hyperinfection syndrome, such as those who receive corticosteroids or other immunosuppressant therapy or persons with HTLV-I infection, should be screened by stool examination and serology, even in the absence of peripheral blood eosinophilia or typical symptoms. Immigrants with beef, pork, or fish tapeworm infections usually have few symptoms besides passage of segments (Chapter 123). Identification of carriers of *Taenia solium* should be identified and treated because of the risk of giving household members cysticercosis (Chapter 124.1). Other common intestinal flatworms that occasionally cause diarrhea include *Hymenolepis nana*, schistosomes, and other flukes.

Viral Hepatitis and Other Hepatobiliary Diseases. Although acute hepatitis A is unusual in older immigrants from developing countries because of prior infection, vaccination should be considered for younger family members who have not been infected, especially if they plan to visit their country of origin (Chapter 28). The prevalence of hepatitis B surface antigenemia is high throughout the developing world and may exceed 20% in parts of Africa and Southeast Asia. To prevent acute infections, immigrants who do not have evidence of prior infection should be vaccinated. Persons with chronic hepatitis B antigenemia require close follow-up for chronic hepatitis, cirrhosis, and hepatoma. They should receive education about preventing spread of infection to others and avoiding infection with the delta virus.

Periportal fibrosis sometimes is detected by ultrasound in immigrants with schistosomiasis mansoni, japonica, or mekongi, but portal hypertension is unusual (Chapter 118). Other causes of liver disease to consider in immigrants include amebic abscesses, hydatid cysts, and cholangitis complicating ascariasis, clonorchiasis, or opisthorchiasis.

Neurologic and Ophthalmologic Infections. Acute infections of the central nervous system occurring around the time of arrival include bacterial meningitis, cerebral malaria, and viral encephalitides. Other acute infections such as trichinosis, congenital toxoplasmosis, or toxocariasis are more likely to result from dietary practices after immigration. Seizures, neurologic deficits, and hydrocephalus may develop after years to several decades of silent neurocysticercosis (Chapter

124.1). Major endemic areas include Mexico and other Latin American countries, Haiti, the Dominican Republic, Cape Verde, sub-Saharan Africa, India, China, the Philippines, Korea, and Southeast Asia. Reactivation of latent infection can cause tuberculous meningitis or tuberculoma, or, in the setting of AIDS or immunosuppression, toxoplasmosis, Chagas' disease, or strongyloidiasis. Gambian sleeping sickness may not become apparent in an African national up to 1 or 2 years after leaving the endemic area. Transverse myelitis and cerebral involvement are unusual complications of imported schistosomiasis or paragonimiasis. Arriving immigrants may show sequelae of poliomyelitis or already have a slowly progressing tropical spastic paraparesis due to HTLV-I infection. Tetanus has been acquired by unimmunized immigrants living in industrialized countries.

Onchocerciasis and cysticercosis are chronic infections that can affect the eye; loiasis is also chronic but presents acutely when an adult worm migrates across the conjunctiva. Relapses of toxoplasmic chorioretinitis, usually congenitally acquired, can be vision-threatening. Trachoma may leave permanent sequelae or cause relapses among immigrants from the Middle East, Africa, and Asia.

Cardiac Disease. Immigrants may present with one of the complications of rheumatic heart disease, which remains common in parts of the developing world (Chapter 3). Poor and crowded living conditions have been associated with sporadic cases and outbreaks of acute rheumatic fever among immigrant populations in New York and other large cities. An estimated 100,000 Latin Americans infected with *Trypanosoma cruzi* currently live in the United States. Most are asymptomatic, but up to 20 to 30% may develop congestive heart failure, arrhythmias, or heart block years to decades after entry (Chapter 94). Reactivation of chronic Chagas' disease may occur in persons with AIDS, persons who receive heart transplants for chronic Chagas' cardiomyopathy, and other immunosuppressed individuals. Asymptomatically infected immigrants have been the cause of transfusion-induced Chagas' disease. Pericardial diseases among immigrants include acute or restrictive tuberculous pericarditis, and, rarely, rupture of an amebic liver abscess into the pericardium. Aortic aneurysm, aortic insufficiency, and coronary ostia stenosis raise the possibility of cardiovascular syphilis.

Genitourinary Infections. Gonococci resistant to ciprofloxacin and other fluoroquinolones as well as to penicillin and tetracycline are becoming more common in parts of Asia and the Pacific Rim (Chapter 49). Ceftriaxone, cefixime, or spectinomycin should be used to treat immigrants who may have become infected in these areas. The diagnosis of syphilis, which is prevalent among some immigrant groups, may be complicated by serologic cross reactions due to infection with one of the nonvenereal treponematoses endemic in the developing world (Chapter 48). Chancroid, granuloma inguinale, and lymphogranuloma venereum are considerations in immigrants from endemic areas of the developing world. Amebiasis can be transmitted sexually and cause ulcerative lesions of the genitalia or anus.

Schistosoma haematobium may be the cause of hematuria, recurrent urinary tract infections, and other urinary symptoms in immigrants from Africa and the Middle East (Chapter 118). Granulomas around schistosome eggs occasionally cause lesions in the vagina, uterus, prostate, or external genitalia. Cystocele or chyluria should raise a suspicion of lymphatic filariasis in immigrants from endemic areas.

Diseases of Skin. In the United States, many cases of leprosy have been among immigrants from Mexico and Southeast Asia; others have originated in other endemic areas including Africa, India, and Central and South America (Chapter 78). Leprosy usually comes to medical attention within the first year of arrival, but some persons present only after a decade. Family members of patients with leprosy should be examined for characteristic lesions. Erythema nodosum occurs in association with leprosy, tuberculosis, and infections with dimorphic fungi.

Recurrent episodes of bacterial cellulitis and chronic lichenification are complications of the lymphedema of lymphatic filariasis. The differential diagnosis of ulcerative lesions of the skin among immigrants includes unusual conditions such as cutaneous diphtheria, anthrax, amebiasis cutis, cutaneous leishmaniasis, mycetoma, and mycobacterial infections, as well as the more common sexually transmitted diseases (Chapter 8). Subcutaneous nodules may represent cysticerci, onchocercomas, or migrating helminths, e.g., *Loa loa, Paragonimus, Fasciola, Gnathostoma,* or spargana. More superficial migratory lesions are characteristic of cutaneous larva migrans (Chapter 115) and larva currens. Pruritus and excoriations from scratching are typical of onchocerciasis, pinworm infection, and insect bites. Areas of depigmentation are seen with leprosy, yaws and other treponematoses, and onchocerciasis. Tinea versicolor and other dermatophyte infections are common among some immigrants (Chapter 81). Scabies is common among immigrant children, and lice are a problem of persons who have been in refugee camps or other substandard living conditions (Chapter 128.2). Myiasis and tungiasis would be expected only in recent arrivals.

NONINFECTIOUS DISEASES OF IMMIGRANTS. A variety of noninfectious disorders are prevalent among certain immigrant groups; many are genetic in origin or acquired because of exposures or customs. Common hemoglobinopathies include sickle cell anemia and hemoglobin C disease among Africans, hemoglobin E disease among Southeast Asians, and the thalassemias among persons from the Mediterranean, Africa, and Asia (Chapter 6). Enzyme deficiencies of red blood cells include most notably glucose-6-phosphate dehydrogenase deficiency among Africans, Mediterraneans, and Asians. Other causes of anemia include nutritional disorders, hookworm disease, and chronic infections.

Familial Mediterranean fever is a genetic disorder that may be seen among immigrants from the Middle East and Mediterranean and is characterized by recurrent episodes of fever, arthritis, and polyserositis. There have been cases of porphyria variegata among South African whites. Other groups may be predisposed to developing chronic medical diseases, such as hypertension among Africans, and ischemic heart disease or insulin-resistant diabetes among certain Asian immigrants.

Malignancies among immigrants may be related to chronic infections; examples include hepatoma, carcinoma of the cervix, squamous cell carcinoma of the bladder, cholangiocarcinoma, nasopharyngeal carcinoma, Burkitt lymphoma, Kaposi sarcoma, adult T-cell leukemia, and HIV-associated lymphomas (Chapter 12). Genetic predisposition and environmental exposures may lead to increased rates of other malignancies, e.g., skin cancers among albinos and other fair-skinned persons, or carcinoma of the stomach in persons residing in mountainous regions of East Africa and Colombia. Detection of cervical and breast carcinomas has been delayed among Hispanics and other immigrants because of a lack of routine gynecologic care.

Malnutrition and stunting of growth may be especially severe in immigrant children and refugees as a result of food deprivation and infections (Chapter 130). Malabsorption may result from intestinal protozoan infections or, rarely, tropical sprue; lactose intolerance is common among African and certain Asian immigrant groups (Chapter 4). Children may present with specific nutritional disorders such as xerophthalmia, endemic goiter, and deficiencies of vitamin D and other vitamins and minerals (Chapters 131 and 132).

Depression and stress are common among immigrants who are adapting to a new culture and language and have been separated from family and friends (Chapter 9). Post-traumatic stress disorder and other psychiatric problems are not uncommon among refugees, especially those who have experienced torture, rape, and other physical trauma. African women who have undergone circumcision require particular sensitivity when they receive gynecologic or obstetric care. There have been increased rates of suicides among several immigrant groups, e.g., young Asian women in Britain and Ethiopian immigrants to Israel.

CONCLUSION. The approach to health problems in immigrants includes an assessment of infectious and noninfectious diseases as well as a consideration of "functional" illness related to adjustment to a foreign culture and environment, loss of family and other social networks, and a previous history of physical and psychologic trauma. A knowledge of geographic medicine is crucial to the diagnosis of complex cases, particularly the global distribution of infectious diseases (Chapter 149). Malaria and tuberculosis are the two most important life-threatening infectious diseases of immigrants when a febrile illness begins within the first few months and years, respectively, after their arrival in an industrialized nation.

Bibliography

Evans CA Jr: Immigrants and health care: mounting problems. Ann Intern Med 122:309, 1995.

Iralu J, Maguire JH: Pulmonary infections in immigrants and refugees. Semin Respir Infect 6:235, 1991.

Kreiss JK, Castro KG: Special considerations for managing suspected human immunodeficiency virus infection and AIDS in patients from developing countries. J Infect Dis 162:955, 1990.

Liu LX, Weller PF: Approach to the febrile traveller returning from Southeast Asia and Oceania. Curr Clin Top Infect Dis 12:138, 1992.

Maguire JH: Epidemiologic considerations in the evaluation of undifferentiated fever in a traveler returning from Latin America or the Caribbean. Curr Clin Top Infect Dis 13:26, 1993.

Nelson KR, Bui H, Samet JH: Screening in special populations: a "case study" of recent Vietnamese immigrants. Am J Med 102:435, 1997.

Paxton LA, Slutsker L, Schultz LJ, et al: Imported malaria in Montagnard refugees settling in North Carolina: implications for prevention and control. Am J Trop Med Hygiene 54:54, 1996.

Sandler RH, Jones TC: Medical Care of Refugees. New York, Oxford University Press, 1987.

U.S. Department of Health and Human Services. Public Health Service: Screening for tuberculosis and tuberculosis infection in high-risk populations. MMWR 44 (RR-11):19, 1995.

Wilson ME: A World Guide to Infection: Diseases, Distribution, Diagnosis. New York, Oxford University Press, 1991.

Zuber PL, McKenna MT, Binkin NJ, et al: Long-term risk of tuberculosis among foreign-born persons in the United States. JAMA 278:304, 1997.

149 Global Epidemiology of Infectious Diseases

Guénaël R. Rodier, Michael J. Ryan, and David L. Heymann

■ GENERAL PRINCIPLES

The human population continues to expand and to interact with its environment in new and complex ways. Despite progress in economic development in many countries, poverty and its associated ill health remain a major burden worldwide. International travel and transport of goods globally has dramatically increased, bringing many places on earth "closer" to each other. Changes in the food chain, both industrial and international, and scientific successes in medicine, biology, and agriculture have led to unprecedented opportunities for biologic interaction. At the same time, over 1000 individual species of viruses, bacteria, fungi, and parasites known to infect humans, and many thousand more that live in close association with other species, are under new pressures associated with manmade transformations. All are susceptible to changes, including genomic mutations that will lead, in a few of them, to durable shifts and adaptation to new circumstances of living. As a result of these numerous and complex interactions, the epidemiology and geographic distribution of infectious diseases, once thought to be relatively stable, has become subject to rapid and significant changes.

The Changing Patterns of Infectious Disease Epidemiology

A characteristic of the epidemiology of infectious diseases is its potential for change. Examples of such changes include the spread of diseases to newly susceptible groups, such as the shift of measles from children to unvaccinated young adults following childhood immunization and changes in the geographic distribution of disease vectors (e.g., spread of *Aedes* spp., vector of dengue, in the Americas). An example associated with successful control programs is the disappearance or sharp decline of common infectious diseases from large regions (poliomyelitis in the Americas) or small areas (dracunculiasis-free villages in West Africa). A more dramatic illustration of epidemiologic change is the re-emergence of diseases in large epidemics, e.g., cholera in South America, and world-threatening outbreaks, e.g., pneumonic plague in India (Fig. 149–1). Resurgent epidemics can involve common agents (*Mycobacterium tuberculosis, Plasmodium falciparum*) as well as newly recognized infectious organisms. Ebola virus, Sin nombre virus, and prion-associated diseases are among these. Human immunodeficiency virus (HIV) is one of several newly recognized infectious agents that have been responsible for major pandemics.

Emerging and re-emerging diseases are not restricted to the developing world. Diseases, e.g., Lyme disease, AIDS, new variants of Creutzfeldt-Jakob disease, salmonellosis, and group A *Streptococcus* infections, also strike prosperous industrialized countries. Furthermore, the increasing number of diseases imported from endemic to nonendemic areas (cholera and yellow fever imported to Europe and North America) emphasizes the international consequences of epidemiologic changes.

Changes in the microbial world are also illustrated by the steady increases in infectious agents that have become resistant to antimicrobial drugs (e.g., multidrug-resistant strains of *Mycobacterium tuberculosis* and *Shigella dysenteriae*). These antibiotic-resistant organisms have often been associated with nosocomial infections, a problem increasingly recognized in the developed world and thought to be dramatically increasing in developing countries. Most of these changes have been of significant public health importance and have seriously hampered major control programs, including malaria and tuberculosis control.

THE DETERMINANTS OF CHANGE. The three major determinants of change in the epidemiology of infectious diseases are (1) changes in the susceptibility to infectious diseases; (2) increased opportunities for infection; and (3) the rapid adaptation of the microbial world. The conjunction of these factors on a worldwide scale has produced a situation charac-

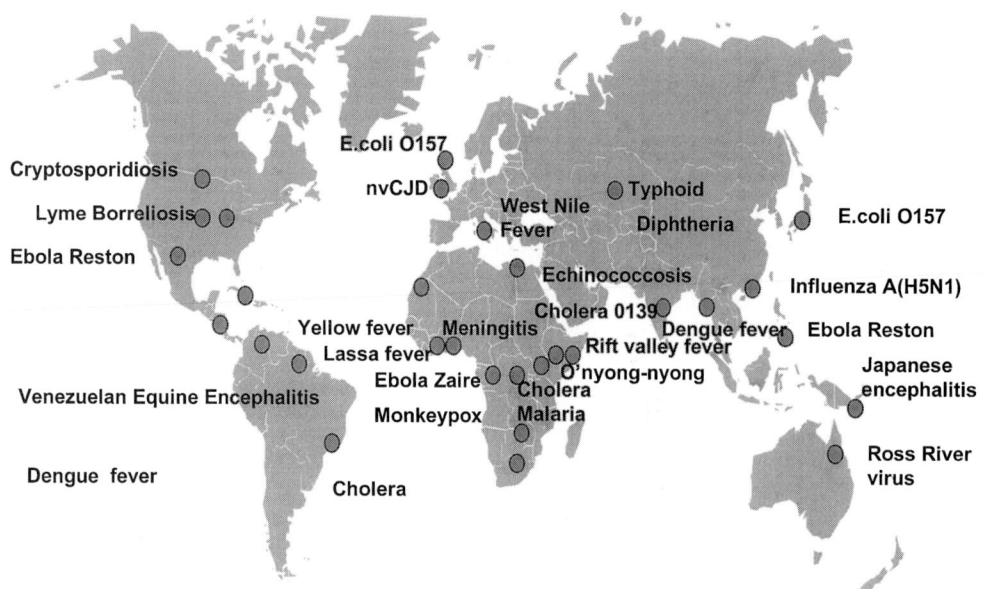

Figure 149–1. Examples of reported outbreaks worldwide, 1996–1997.

terized by a global increase in the threat of infectious diseases. Because susceptibility to infectious diseases and opportunities for infection rapidly increase with poverty, poverty remains the variable most frequently associated with the occurrence of infectious diseases.

CHANGES IN THE SUSCEPTIBILITY TO INFECTIOUS DISEASES. Changes in the susceptibility to infectious diseases have been influenced by various factors, including demographic changes, the worldwide spread of modern medicine through immunization policies, and better access to sophisticated health care. The important demographic changes of the last 30 years include spectacular population growth and changes in the ratio of old to young individuals with the shift to large populations of aged persons, who are more susceptible to infectious diseases as the immune system ages. Modern medicine has contributed to the emergence of large groups of immunocompromised individuals, particularly in developed countries, as the number of patients with chronic diseases (e.g., diabetes, cancer) and those who benefit from immunosuppressant drugs (e.g., steroids, cancer therapy) has increased. The AIDS pandemic has further increased the population of immunocompromised patients.

In contrast with the rise of large groups of nonimmune individuals, national, regional, and worldwide immunization campaigns have greatly increased the number of individuals immune to most vaccine-preventable diseases. In 1990, up to 80% of all children below 2 years of age had been vaccinated against diseases covered by the World Health Organization's (WHO) Expanded Program of Immunization (EPI). However, significant disparities in population immune status have been created, as immunization policy varies between and within countries. In addition, some population groups are no longer vaccinated. This is because either eradication programs have been successful—e.g., with smallpox worldwide and poliomyelitis in the Americas—or, at the other extreme, because they have collapsed or been ineffective, as with EPI in some African countries. The resurgence of epidemics of vaccine-preventable diseases is thus facilitated, as seen by the diphtheria epidemic in the newly independent states of Eastern Europe and meningococcal meningitis and yellow fever in sub-Saharan Africa.

INCREASED OPPORTUNITIES FOR INFECTION. Increased opportunities for infection have paralleled world population growth, which has dramatically increased the number of individuals at risk for infection. The marked shift from rural to urban living has resulted in newly experienced population density in some areas. Socioeconomic and cultural disruptions have been associated with lifestyle changes including diet, social behavior, and use of illicit drugs. Crowded urban environments provide optimal conditions for the transmission of person-to-person diseases (e.g., tuberculosis, HIV, and sexually transmitted diseases [STDs]). Poor hygiene education together with the collapse or absence of sewage and water systems has created ideal conditions for the occurrence of fecal-oral transmission of diseases, e.g., shigellosis, intestinal parasites, and cholera. The rapid development of important belts of poverty around large urban centers has occurred in both developing and developed countries. These give rise to new ecological niches particularly suitable for the re-emergence of infectious diseases associated with poor hygiene (louse-borne diseases). Further, diseases, e.g., malaria and Chagas' disease, once typically rural, have been imported with their vectors to poor urban areas. In many poor countries, the absence of efficient urban vector control programs has further supported the spread of diseases, e.g., dengue and plague, in the urban environment.

The frequent occurrence of disasters has resulted in the rapid deterioration of living conditions for millions of people. The consequences of natural disasters (e.g., floods and earthquakes) and manmade disasters (e.g., civil war, international embargoes and economic collapse) have often led to mass migration. As a consequence of the poor hygiene, low nutritional status, high population density, and inappropriate health infrastructure that often follow, diseases, e.g., cholera, shigellosis, measles, and tuberculosis have become closely associated with disaster.

The spread of diseases via human migration is not new. Examples are tuberculosis imported from Europe to the Americas, yellow fever and malaria spread from Africa to South and Central America, and the regional spread of African trypanosomiasis associated with European colonization of the Congo basin in the 1890s. However, the extraordinary development of rapid international travel and movement of goods has now made possible, in a matter of hours, the rapid and worldwide spread of diseases and their vectors. In this remarkable new environment, the food chain has rapidly taken on an international dimension of great complexity. Tracing the origin of all meal ingredients has become virtually impossible, constituting an enormous challenge for the control of food-borne diseases.

Not least, the rapid development of modern medicine, e.g., the worldwide distribution of blood and blood products for transfusion, the progress of sophisticated surgery, including organ transplants, and the development of intensive care units, has opened the microbial world, creating unprecedented opportunities for nosocomial transmission of infectious agents to new, atypical hosts.

ADAPTATION OF MICROORGANISMS. Adaptation of microorganisms is one factor contributing to the changing pattern of infectious disease. The steady emergence of bacterial strains resistant to antimicrobial drugs is another. Penicillin-resistant *Streptococcus pneumoniae*, vancomycin-resistant enterococcus, and methicillin-resistant *Staphylococcus aureus* are examples of a resistance problem that has become a serious public health concern. Some strains have become resistant to virtually all available drugs, e.g., multiresistant strains of *Shigella dysenteriae* type 1 and multidrug-resistant strains of *Mycobacterium tuberculosis*.

The emergence of drug-resistant organisms in humans has also been, in part, associated with antibiotic use in the veterinary industry. The interrelations between humans and animals must also be considered when addressing microbial threats. Vancomycin-resistant enterococci linked with the extensive use of paromomycin in poultry as a growth promoting agent highlights this connection. Although poorly understood, the adaptation of infectious agents to their new environment, including durable drug pressure, constitutes the greatest challenge for effective disease control. In addition, other changes in the environment have led to the emergence of new pathogenic strains (e.g., *Vibrio cholerae* serogroup 0139) and the introduction among human populations of infectious agents usually confined to a specific ecological niche (e.g., the Ebola virus).

The capacity of some infectious agents to display antigen variation (e.g., *Borrelia* spp.) is another example of microbial adaptation, in this case against the host immune response. This dynamism is exemplified by RNA viruses (e.g., influenza), which have an exceptionally high mutation rate. This allows the rapid emergence of new strains through genetic interaction with a new host, as well as the emergence and selection of mutants resistant to antiviral agents (e.g., HIV strains resistant to zidovudine).

Nosocomial infection is a leading emergent public health threat. The recent development of xenotransplants (i.e., transplant to humans of nonhuman primate organs) has raised the legitimate fear that unknown animal infectious agents may cross the species barrier and cause new human disease. Deforestation, climate changes, and pollution also constitute new environmental pressures to both human hosts and infectious agents.

In the face of this challenge of a dynamic microbial world, the remarkable development of molecular technologies and computer sciences has revolutionized our capacity to understand the invisible events that, until now, epidemiology could not properly investigate.

THE REVOLUTION OF MOLECULAR EPIDEMIOLOGY. The occurrence of diseases is but the visible part of a much larger collection of events that may, or may not, lead to symptoms. Laboratory investigation has thus become more and more important. In addition to symptoms and diseases classically used for surveillance (e.g., disease incidence and prevalence, mortality data, and description of outbreaks), the silent interplay between infectious organisms and their hosts has been increasingly documented. This has been done primarily

through specific serologic tests and isolation techniques, which allow, e.g., the detection of asymptomatic cases and healthy carriers.

For control purposes, it is crucial to understand whether different outbreaks are linked or independent, or if what appears to be a pandemic is in fact a juxtaposition of independent epidemics. The introduction of molecular epidemiology has provided a precise tool for strain characterization and epidemiologic tracking. More generally, it has allowed the exploration of relationships among genetic diversity and taxonomy, virulence, resistance to drugs, antigenic variation, and host and vector specificity. It has already provided unique insights into our understanding of the epidemiology of infectious diseases. For example, it has revealed the different regional epidemics underlying the cholera pandemic and the genetic relationship between *Plasmodium* species showing that *P. falciparum*, the agent of malignant malaria, is more closely related to *P. reichenowi*, a chimpanzee parasite. Where relevant, molecular epidemiologic information has been included in the presentation of the geographic distribution of infectious diseases.

Global Trends in Infectious Disease Epidemiology

Successful Control Programs

The last decade has seen some notable successes in the control of infectious diseases. These successes have been made possible through the integration of measures to prevent disease by vaccination, vector control, or treatment of patients with programs effectively reaching the populations at risk. In the area of vaccine-preventable diseases the achievement of high vaccine coverage has resulted in a dramatic fall in the incidence of poliomyelitis, measles, and neonatal tetanus. Successes in the control of dracunculiasis (guinea worm), onchocerciasis (river blindness), and American trypanosomiasis have largely come as a result of vector control, effective treatment of patients, and health education on the avoidance of infection.

AMERICAN TRYPANOSOMIASIS (Chapter 94). Chagas' disease remains endemic in 21 countries of Latin America with 16 to 18 million people infected and about 45,000 deaths each year. The rural-to-urban migration movements that occurred in Latin America in the 1970s and 1980s also transformed Chagas' disease into an urban infection. With vector control measures and improving housing, as well as the systematic screening of blood donors from endemic countries for *Trypanosoma cruzi*, the incidence of Chagas' disease has been greatly reduced. In 1991 Argentina, Bolivia, Chile, Paraguay, and Uruguay (which account for 60% of total cases on the continent) launched the Southern Cone Initiative aimed at eliminating the disease as a public health problem. Impressive progress has been made toward the elimination of *Triatoma infestans*, the main vector of *Trypanosoma cruzi*, and the elimination of Chagas' disease as a public health problem in the Americas by the year 2000 is now achievable in most countries. In Brazil, an international commission has been appointed to start the process of certification of the elimination of vectorial and transfusional transmission of Chagas' disease.

DRACUNCULIASIS (Chapter 110). Guinea worm disease is the only parasitic disease that may be eradicated from the world in the near future. Although widely distributed at the beginning of the 20th century, the disease is now found only in sub-Saharan Africa, the Arabian peninsula, and India. It is still endemic in 18 countries, of which 16 are in Africa. Approximately 122,000 cases were reported from fewer than 8000 endemic villages in 1995, as compared with 3.5 million in 1986 and 1 million in 1989. The population still at risk of infection is estimated at 120 million in Africa and 10 million in Asia.

LEPROSY (Chapter 78). In 1996, there were an estimated 2.4 million people with leprosy in 79 countries. Over half a million new cases are detected each year. The total number of new cases has dropped 67% from the estimate of 5.5 million in 1991 and by 85% since 1985, when there were an estimated 12 million cases. India, Myanmar, and Brazil represent 59% of the cases worldwide. Southeast Asia has half of the cases, with approximately 1.26 million cases reported in 1996. There are 220,000 people with leprosy in Africa and the Americas, 70,000 in the Western Pacific, 60,000 in the Eastern Mediterranean, and 6000 in Europe. Leprosy is targeted for *elimination as a public health problem* by the year 2000. This means a prevalence not exceeding one case per 10,000 population. Success in leprosy control has resulted from the availability of effective multidrug therapy and intensive case finding and treatment.

MEASLES (Chapter 25.1). Measles remains one of the major childhood killers, accounting for more deaths than any other vaccine-preventable disease. WHO estimates that in 1995 about 42 million cases of measles occurred worldwide causing more than a million deaths among children. The vast majority (98%) occur in developing countries. Globally, the disease accounts for over 10% of deaths in children under 5 years old. WHO set two targets in 1990: a reduction by 95% in the number of measles deaths, and a reduction of 90% in the number of measles cases by 1995. These targets have not yet been met but by the end of 1994 the number of deaths was down by 85% globally and the estimated number of cases by 78%. It is estimated that by the end of 1995 just over a third of all countries had achieved a 90% reduction in cases and over a half had cut the number of deaths by at least 95%. However, there are wide disparities between individual regions and countries. In the Americas every country reached the 1995 targets with transmission interrupted in Chile, Cuba, and the English-speaking Caribbean islands. Elimination of measles by the year 2000 is now a goal of the WHO Regional Office for the Americas (AMRO). By contrast, only two countries in WHO's Southeast Asia region and five in the Africa region have succeeded in reducing the number of cases by 90%.

NEONATAL TETANUS (Chapter 53). Neonatal tetanus has been eliminated from 97 countries around the world through the promotion of clean childbirth and cord care, routine tetanus immunization of pregnant women, and the use of a risk approach to target higher-incidence areas. Despite this success, in 1995 neonatal tetanus killed 450,000 newborns, primarily in developing countries.

ONCHOCERCIASIS (Chapter 108). Onchocerciasis remains the second leading infectious cause of blindness and the source of debilitating skin disease in 34 countries of Africa, the Arabian peninsula, and the Americas. Success at controlling onchocerciasis in West Africa has been achieved by the Onchocerciasis Control Program (OCP) through the strategy of vector control using larvicides to interrupt transmission. The development of safe, effective drug therapy has led to a new global strategy for controlling onchocerciasis based on yearly administration of ivermectin to affected populations. Prioritization of areas for treatment is based on the level of disease prevalence as determined by rapid epidemiologic mapping techniques. The Onchocerciasis Elimination Program for the Americas (OEPA) involves six countries: Brazil, Colombia, Ecuador, Guatemala, Mexico, and Venezuela.

POLIOMYELITIS (Chapter 27.1). Poliomyelitis has been virtually eradicated from the Americas; the last case of wild virus poliomyelitis was in 1991 in Peru. An increasing number of countries in the Old World are now reporting zero incidence of the disease. Global end of transmission of wild poliovirus by the year 2000 is now the goal of WHO. Worldwide, the number of cases is down by over 80% since the eradication effort began in 1988 (from 31,000 in 1988 to 4074 in 1996, although WHO estimates that one case in 10 is actually reported). The use of mass immunization campaigns to halt the circulation of wild poliovirus is increasing. By the end of 1997, 110 polio-endemic countries had conducted at least one national immunization day (NID). In China the number of reported cases dropped from 5000 in 1990 to zero in 1995 following two successful NIDs in 1993 and 1994, when 83 million children were immunized. Even more ambitious was MECACAR, a co-coordinated campaign of NIDs in 18 adjoining countries from the Middle East, Caucasus, and the Central Asian Republics, which targeted 56 million children. Most of the countries involved succeeded in immunizing over 95% of children under 5 years of age.

Re-emerging Public Health Threats

In contrast to some of the successes in the control of infectious diseases mentioned previously, there have been some serious failures of major control programs, e.g., the former worldwide eradication programs against malaria and tuberculosis. These diseases are re-emerging as public health threats.

AFRICAN TRYPANOSOMIASIS (Chapter 93). Sleeping sickness remains a persistent public health problem in areas corresponding to the distribution of the tsetse fly in West, Central, and East Africa. The existence of domestic and wild animal reservoirs for *Trypanosoma brucei rhodesiense* remains a major obstacle to achieving human disease control. With *Trypanosoma brucei gambiense*, humans are the major reservoir. Large numbers of cases go unreported in extensive war-torn and out-of-control areas in sub-Saharan Africa (e.g., Angola, Liberia, the Democratic Republic of the Congo, and Sudan). Almost all foci now reportedly active were considered eradicated in the 1960s. The resurgence started in the early 1980s with the decline of most surveillance and control activities. A regional coordination of control activities against human African trypanosomiasis has recently been set up in Central Africa.

CHOLERA (Chapter 41) **AND OTHER EPIDEMIC DIARRHEAL DISEASES.** Diarrheal diseases remain major public health problems, causing more than 3 million deaths in 1995, of which more than 80% were among children under 5 years of age. There has been a dramatic resurgence of cholera, with outbreaks occurring in Asia, Africa, the Americas, and Eastern Europe. Cholera cases were notified from 71 countries in 1996. Since 1991, over 1 million cases and 9000 deaths have occurred in Latin America. In 1992, the emergence in India of epidemic cholera produced by a non-01 cholera serogroup, *Vibrio cholerae* 0139 (Bengal), has raised fears that a new pandemic could be under way. However, the 0139 strain has not spread beyond South Asia and now seems less likely to become a global threat. *Shigella dysenteriae* type 1 (Sd1) is an unusually virulent enteric pathogen that causes endemic or epidemic dysentery with high death rates (Chapter 40). Over the last decade many African countries have experienced epidemics superimposed on endemic disease. Resistance to multiple antibiotics has become an increasingly serious problem.

Food-borne diseases have emerged as a more important cause of the global diarrheal disease burden than previously thought. Industrialized countries have been confronted with important increases in the incidence of food-borne disease caused by organisms such as *Salmonella* spp. (Chapter 76), *Campylobacter* spp. (see Chapter 43), and *Escherichia coli* spp.

(Chapter 42) (e.g., *E. coli* 0157 outbreak in Japan, 1996). These increases have been due to changes in the way food is produced, processed, and prepared. The intensification and centralization of food production and its international distribution have increased the risk of large food-borne outbreaks following food contamination.

DENGUE (Chapter 29.1). Dengue, dengue hemorrhagic fever (DHF), and dengue shock syndrome (DSS) constitute the most significant and rapidly increasingly arthropod-borne viral disease. The dengue pandemic began in Southeast Asia after World War II. Today prevalent in over 100 countries, dengue threatens 2.5 billion people. It is estimated that each year 500,000 people are hospitalized with DHF/DSS, 90% of whom are children under 15 years of age. Because *Aedes aegypti* eradication campaigns deteriorated during the 1970s and 1980s and air travel developed rapidly, dengue, including DHF/DSS, has emerged as a significant public health problem in the Pacific region, the Caribbean (e.g., Cuba, 1981), and Central and South America (e.g., Venezuela, 1989–1990). Dengue reached the African coast of the Indian Ocean (i.e., Kenya, Somalia, Djibouti) in the late 1980s following the spread of *A. aegypti* in all large coastal cities and is now spreading further along the Red Sea and the Arabian peninsula. In Southeast Asia, dengue continues to spread in new areas with significant epidemics (e.g., Delhi, India, 1996).

DIPHTHERIA (Chapter 33). Diphtheria was a leading cause of death in childhood until the introduction of a vaccine in the 1950s. Mass immunization has made it extremely rare in industrialized countries. In the early 1980s diphtheria incidence began to increase in the former Soviet Union because of disruption of immunization programs for children and adults. By the early 1990s the problem had become an epidemic in Russia and the Ukraine. In 1994 there were more than 39,000 cases of diphtheria with 1100 deaths in the Russian Federation. These recent epidemics are a warning that this disease can make a deadly comeback if immunization is not maintained.

JAPANESE ENCEPHALITIS (Chapter 30.3). Initially recognized in 1924 and eliminated by mass childhood vaccination in most developed Asian countries (i.e., Japan, Korea, Singapore, Taiwan), Japanese encephalitis (JE) has re-emerged as a major public health concern, causing an estimated 30,000 to 50,000 cases annually in the region. In the mid-1990s it has surpassed poliomyelitis as the leading cause of childhood infection of the central nervous system in Asia while spreading westward (e.g., India, Nepal, Sri Lanka) and southward. Well established in Bali and Papua New Guinea, JE has emerged in northern Australia (Torres Strait islands, 1995). The hypothesis of global climate warming has raised concern, as this will give JE mosquito vectors a much larger territory supporting further spread of the disease.

MALARIA (Chapter 92). Malaria, particularly malaria caused by *Plasmodium falciparum*, remains the world's most serious tropical parasitic disease. It is still a major health threat both to people living in endemic areas and to travelers to these areas. Although the geographic area affected by malaria has shrunk considerably over the past 50 years, the malaria eradication program has failed globally due to the complexity of malaria epidemiology, the collapse of vector control measures in most countries, and rapid environmental changes (e.g., uncontrolled urbanization, international travel). Malaria control has become more difficult. Gains obtained in the last 30 years are being eroded. In addition, the number of malaria cases imported to malaria-free areas, including transient local malaria transmission (airport malaria) has sharply increased, whereas the emergence of resistant strains has greatly limited options for both treatment and prophylaxis in many areas. Today more than 90 countries, inhabited by a total of some 2.4 billion people, are affected. Worldwide annual malaria prevalence is estimated to be in the order of 300 to 500 million clinical cases, with 1.5 to 2.7 million deaths per year. Sub-Saharan Africa accounts for 80% of all malaria cases. Two thirds of the remaining cases are concentrated in six countries: India, Brazil, Sri Lanka, Vietnam, Colombia, and the Solomon Islands, in decreasing order of prevalence.

MENINGOCOCCAL MENINGITIS (Chapters 52 and 74). Meningococcal meningitis occurs worldwide, causing sporadic disease or small clusters of cases with a seasonal increase in the winter period. Some countries have reported an increasing annual incidence over the last decade. Large epidemics continue to occur in sub-Saharan Africa with an increase in size and frequency and a tendency to spread southeastward, beyond the classic meningitis belt. One of the largest epidemics occurred in West Africa in 1996 causing more than 100,000 cases and 10,000 deaths. Control through mass immunization campaigns has not yet been successful.

PLAGUE (Chapter 61). Plague continues to be a threat to public health because of vast areas of persistent wild rodent infection. Wild rodent plague exists in the western half of the United States, in large areas of South America, in north-central, eastern, and southern Africa, in Madagascar, and in central and Southeast Asia. Human plague has occurred in several countries in Africa. Plague is endemic in China, Indonesia, Mongolia, Myanmar, India, and especially Vietnam. Although urban human plague has been controlled in most of the world, human plague still occurs sporadically in rural areas, usually in small clusters. However, in 1994 a limited but acute outbreak of pneumonic plague occurred in the city of Surat, Gujarat State, India, illustrating the permanent threat of urban plague where rodent populations are not controlled.

TUBERCULOSIS (Chapter 77). Industrialized countries had steady downward trends of tuberculosis mortality and morbidity since the end of the 19th century, and tuberculosis was further controlled with the availability of effective antibiotherapy after World War II. However, in the 1980s, reported cases plateaued or even increased as more cases were reported from the elderly and the poorest communities. In many less developed countries, tuberculosis still remains one of the most serious public health problems. In 1996, worldwide there were an estimated 7.2 million new cases and 2.9 million deaths caused by tuberculosis, 95% of which occurred in low-income countries. Tuberculosis notifications have trebled in parts of sub-Saharan Africa in the past decade, much of this increase being attributed to the HIV epidemic. Today, the conjunction of major population growth, rapid uncontrolled urbanization, inadequate tuberculosis control programs, AIDS-associated tuberculosis, and the emergence of multidrug resistance dramatically hampers many national tuberculosis control programs.

YELLOW FEVER (Chapter 31.1). Transmission, essentially sylvatic or in rural areas, is restricted to tropical regions of Africa and Latin America where 1000 to 1500 cases occur annually. However, it has been more and more frequently reported since the early 1990s, particularly in sub-Saharan Africa where yellow fever constitutes one of the most important re-emerging diseases with numerous outbreaks reported in a large array of countries (e.g., Benin, Cameroon, Gabon, Kenya, Liberia, Nigeria, Senegal, and Sierra Leone). More importantly, the threat of an urban epidemic of yellow fever has become a great concern as *Aedes aegypti* is now well established in most, if not all, large African cities. In South America, although less than 200 cases of yellow fever were reported per year from 1990 to 1993, the incidence increased to 515 in 1995, owing largely to an outbreak in Peru.

WORLD FIGURES IN INFECTIOUS DISEASES FOR THE YEAR 1995. These estimates are from the World Health Report, 1996.

THE TEN MOST PREVALENT INFECTIOUS DISEASES. In 1995, diarrheal diseases constituted the most frequent cause of infectious disease worldwide with an estimate of almost 4 billion episodes. Tuberculosis ranked second with an estimated 1.9 billion carriers of *Mycobacterium tuberculosis* and 8.9 million new cases. Intestinal parasite came third with about 1.4 billion persons infected at any time, followed by malaria with 500 million new cases, and viral hepatitis, including 350 million chronic carriers of hepatitis B virus and 100 million chronic carriers of hepatitis C virus. Acute respiratory infections were responsible for an estimated 395 million episodes and STDs counted for at least 330 million new illnesses. In addition, there were about 42 million cases of measles and 40 million cases of whooping cough, as well as about 350,000 cases of meningococcal meningitis.

THE TEN FIRST CAUSES OF DEATH BY INFECTIOUS DISEASES. Acute respiratory infections, with 4.4 million deaths, remained the leading cause of death in 1995, followed in decreasing order by diarrheal diseases and tuberculosis (3.1 million each), malaria (2.1 million), hepatitis B (1.1 million), AIDS and measles (>1 million each), neonatal tetanus (500,000), whooping cough (355,000), and roundworm and hookworm (165,000 together).

THE DISTRIBUTION OF TRANSMISSION ROUTES IN INFECTIOUS DISEASES. In 1995, the total number of deaths was estimated to be 51.9 million, of which 17.3 million (33%) were associated with infectious diseases. Among the latter, 11.2 million (65%) were infectious diseases transmitted person to person; 3.7 million (22%) were transmitted through food, water, or soil; 2.3 million (13%) were insect-borne; and 60,000 (0.3%) were animal-borne.

NEWLY IDENTIFIED INFECTIOUS AGENTS. Since the early 1970s, several hundreds of microbial agents have been identified. These discoveries were primarily due to the remarkable progress of the biotechnologies, particularly in virology and molecular biology. Tools, inconceivable a few decades ago (e.g., polymerase chain reaction technique), explain most of the exponential number of newly recognized organisms, some of which have been the cause of emerging human infectious diseases (Table 149–1).

DRUG-RESISTANT ORGANISMS. Antimicrobial resistance has become one of the most serious emergent problems in infectious disease control, as antimicrobial agents no longer kill many strains of bacteria. Recently developed antiviral drugs are also facing drug-resistant viral strains. In bacteria alone, over 100 resistant genes have been identified.

After the discovery of sulfonamides and penicillin earlier in the 20th century, the years between 1940 and 1970 saw the "golden age" of discovery of new antimicrobial agents. As a result, many infections that were once serious and potentially fatal could now be treated and cured. However, such past successes are now being challenged, as many microorganisms have become resistant to antimicrobial agents. This has complicated the choice of appropriate antibiotics, increased the cost of treatment, and prolonged illness.

Antimicrobial resistance was first detected to the sulfonamides in the 1940s, soon after their introduction. After each agent became widely used, a gene expressing resistance to it eventually emerged. That strain could then multiply even in the presence of the antimicrobial agent and spread to replace sensitive strains. It might also transfer its resistance gene to a second strain. Today, all families of antibiotics, including those that were at one time considered infallible, are becoming ineffective for some infections, such as penicillin for

streptococcal infections and the quinolones for shigellosis and gonorrhea.

Development of antimicrobial resistance is facilitated by indiscriminate use of antibiotics, by insufficient dosages prescribed by health workers, and by the medication-taking practices of patients. The prophylactic use of antimicrobials in animal husbandry may increase the pressure on the selection of resistant bacterial strains. Resistance rates are higher in the developing world. This is particularly problematic, as treatment choices are limited by drug availability and cost. Further, there is a lack of reliable laboratory susceptibility test results. At the same time, pharmaceutical companies are less willing to take the risk of developing new antimicrobials because of the high cost of research and development and the potential of rapidly developing resistance.

The challenge posed by antimicrobial resistance calls for a multifaceted response. This will include (1) reducing the need for antimicrobials by preventing infection and transmission of infectious diseases; (2) making better use of existing drugs by using appropriate drugs in proper doses and combinations; and (3) developing new drugs with novel mechanisms of action. There is a need for worldwide surveillance of antimicrobial resistance patterns of the etiologic agents causing major infectious diseases. Local and national patterns of antimicrobial resistance must be known to plan cost-effective treatment strategies and to curtail the evolution of resistance.

GEOGRAPHIC DISTRIBUTION OF INFECTIOUS DISEASES

The purpose of this chapter is to illustrate, from a public health perspective based on disease transmission patterns, the main epidemiologic features, changes, and trends observed in the various regions of the world. Information on disease occurrence is provided region by region and disease by disease. Diseases are assembled first, according to their main route of transmission and, second, by category of infectious agents. Finally, they are listed in alphabetical order with the name of the corresponding infectious agent(s).

The reader should be aware that this presentation by geographic regions and categories of infectious organisms may produce a static picture of what is, in fact, constantly changing. Hence, it is essential to stress that the dynamic relationship among host, infectious agent, and the environment may vary rapidly with time and place. This may occur particularly with changes in population patterns, migration, economic development, transformation of the environment (including natural or manmade disasters), and, eventually, as the microbial world adapts itself to these changes. Consequently, information and data on trends and the geographic distribution of diseases are subject to changes. The objective of this chapter is not to give a comprehensive list of infectious organisms distributed by geographic area but to highlight, for each region, the infectious diseases of public health importance and their current trends. These are illustrated by selected reference to significant and recent outbreaks or epidemics.

The geographic areas listed in this section are based primarily on similar climate characteristics as presented in the WHO *International Travel and Health* annual publication. Such geographic areas are less subject to change than regions based on similar population patterns or comparable economic features.

TABLE 149–1. Principal Newly Identified Infectious Organisms Associated With Diseases

Year	Newly Identified Organism	Disease (Year and Place of First-Recognized or Documented Case)
Diseases Primarily Transmitted by Food and Drinking Water		
1973	Rotavirus	Infantile diarrhea
1976	*Cryptosporidium parvum*	Acute enterocolitis
1977	*Campylobacter jejuni*	Enteric pathogens
1982	*Escherichia coli* 0157:H7	Hemorrhagic colitis with hemolytic-uremic syndrome
1983	*Helicobacter pylori*	Gastritis, peptic ulcer, and gastric cancer
1986	*Cyclospora cayatanensis*	Persistent diarrhea
1989	Hepatitis E virus	Enterically transmitted non-A, non-B hepatitis (India, 1979)
1992	*Vibrio cholerae* 0139	New strain of epidemic cholera (India, 1992)
Unclear Modes of Transmission, Thought to Be Primarily Transmitted by Drinking Water		
1985	*Enterocytozoon bieneusi*	Diarrhea
1991	*Encephalitozoon hellem*	Systemic disease with conjunctivitis in AIDS patients
1993	*Encephalitozoon cunicali*	Parasitic disseminated disease, seizures (Japan, 1959)
	Septata intestinalis	Persistent diarrhea in AIDS patients
Diseases Primarily Transmitted by Close Contact With Infectious Individuals		
1974	Parvovirus B19	Fifth disease
1980	HTLV-1	T-cell lymphoma leukemia
1982	HTLV-II	Hairy cell leukemia
1988	HHV-6	Roseola subitum
1995	HHV-8	Associated with Kaposi sarcoma in AIDS patients
1997	Influenza A/H5N1 virus	Severe acute respiratory infection
Sexually Transmitted Diseases		
1983	HIV-1	AIDS (1981)
1986	HIV-2	Less pathogenic than HIV-1 infection
Nosocomial and Related Infections		
1981	*Staphylococcus* toxin	Toxic shock syndrome
1988	Hepatitis C	Parenterally transmitted non-A, non-B hepatitis
1995	Hepatitis G viruses	Parenterally transmitted non-A, non-B hepatitis
Human Zoonoses and Vector-Borne Diseases, Including Viral Hemorrhagic Fevers		
Diseases Transmitted by Close Contact with Animals or Animal Products		
1977	Hantaan virus	Hemorrhagic fever with renal syndrome (1951)
1990	Reston strain of Ebola virus	Human infection documented but without symptoms (1990)
1991	Guanarito virus	Venezuelan hemorrhagic fever (1989)
1992	*Bartonella henselae*	Cat-scratch disease (1950s)
1993	Sin nombre virus	Hantavirus pulmonary syndrome (1993)
1994	Sabià virus	Brazilian hemorrhagic fever (1955)
Tick-Borne		
1982	*Borrelia burgdorferi*	Lyme disease (1975)
1989	*Ehrlichia chaffeensis*	Human monocytic ehrlichiosis
1991	New species of *Babesia*	Atypical babesiosis
1993	*Ehrlichia* spp. (HGE agent)	Human granulocytic ehrlichiosis
Unknown Animal Vector		
1977	Ebola virus	Ebola hemorrhagic fever (1976, Democratic Republic of Congo)
1994	Ivory Coast strain of Ebola virus	Ebola hemorrhagic fever
Soil-Borne or Airborne Diseases, and Diseases Associated With Recreational Water With No Evidence of Direct Person-to-Person Transmission		
1977	*Legionella pneumophila*	Legionnaires' disease (1947)

HHV, human herpesvirus; HIV, human immunodeficiency virus; HTLV, human T-cell lymphotropic virus.

■ **NORTH AMERICA** (Bermuda, Canada, Greenland, Saint Pierre and Miquelon, and the United States of America including Hawaii)

From north to south, North America includes Arctic islands, tundra, boreal forests interspersed with lakes and large rivers, central prairies, the Atlantic coastal plain, the Appalachians, the Rocky Mountains, and the subtropical cays of the southern United States and Hawaii. Although temperature and rainfall vary greatly in the region, the population is primarily concentrated in areas of temperate climate, and, to a lesser extent, in the tropical areas of the south and southeast United States. Thanks to the high economic development and high hygiene standard of the region, the incidence of communicable diseases is low and usually limited to susceptible groups. However, these groups tend to become more and more important as poverty spreads, and as a significant aging population, a highly sophisticated health system, and the spread of AIDS has led to a significant increase of immunocompromised patients. The region also reports numerous cases of diseases that are not locally endemic but imported by a large community of migrants, primarily from Latin America and Asia.

Diseases Primarily Transmitted by Food and Drinking Water

Although the region is of high hygiene standard, the food chain, essentially industrial and highly complex, allows the rapid international distribution of perishable food originating from other regions. This is in part to accommodate significant changes in eating habits, including a higher consumption of fresh foods and vegetables. Food-borne outbreaks are increasingly reported and constitute a model of emerging infections in the region.

VIRUSES. Hepatitis A: endemic; community outbreaks of hepatitis A are not uncommon and regional epidemics have been observed in 1961, 1971, and 1989. **Hepatitis E**: imported cases (e.g., travelers from endemic areas). **Norwalk and Norwalk-like viruses**: a common cause of diarrhea in children and adults; frequent outbreaks (e.g., associated with consumption of raw shellfish).

BACTERIA. **Cholera** (toxicogenic *Vibrio cholerae* serogroup 01): sporadic cases associated with seafood are episodically reported from the U.S. Gulf Coast where an El Tor biotype strain of *V. cholerae* 01 is endemic; also, increased frequency of imported cholera cases (e.g., coconut milk imported from Thailand; seafood salad from Peru), including cases of *V. cholerae* 0139. **Diarrhea caused by *Campylobacter jejuni***: endemic, reported outbreaks (e.g., outbreak in Canada caused by contamination of a municipal well). **Diarrhea caused by *Escherichia coli***: endemic with multiple outbreaks; enterohemorrhagic *E. coli* (EHEC) frequently involved in food-borne outbreaks since 1990, including *E. coli* 0157:H7 since 1982 (e.g., 1991 epidemic in the Inuit communities of the Canadian Northwest Territories and various outbreaks associated with hamburger meat; 1993 multistate outbreak, United States; Georgia and Tennessee outbreak, June 1995). **Listeriosis** (*Listeria monocytogenes*) has not been involved in major outbreaks since the 1981 epidemics in Nova Scotia, Canada, but remains a public health threat. **Salmonellosis**: increased frequency of notable outbreaks (e.g., *Salmonella poona* epidemic in summer 1991 in 23 states of the United States and Canada; 1994 nationwide outbreak of *Salmonella enteritidis* in the United States associated with the consumption of ice cream following the ability of *S. enteritidis* to contaminate chicken eggs; outbreak of *S. typhimurium* associated with raw ground beef, Wisconsin, 1994). **Shigellosis** (*Shigella* species): endemic, limited outbreaks. **Streptococcal diseases** (group A *Streptococcus*): increasing reports of explosive but limited outbreaks of streptococcal sore throat associated with milk and eggs. **Typhoid** (*Salmonella typhi*) and **paratyphoid** (three bioserotypes of *S. enteritidis*): low endemicity; most cases are imported but the number of reported outbreaks has recently increased, particularly in the United States (e.g., six outbreaks reported from 1980–1989 vs. seven in 1990).

PROTOZOA. **Amebiasis** (*Entamoeba histolytica*): low en-demicity but clusters of infections in households and institutions, particularly with low hygiene standards. **Cryptosporidiosis** (*Cryptosporidium parvum*): primarily in immuno-compromised patients but some significant outbreaks have been reported in the general community (e.g., March-April 1993, large-scale cryptosporidosis outbreak associated with contaminated municipal water, Milwaukee, Wisconsin, and September 1995, Blue Earth County, Minnesota). **Diarrhea caused by *Cyclospora*** (*Cyclospora cayentanensis*): common in immunocompromised individuals (AIDS patients); multiple outbreaks in 1996 and 1997 associated with raspberries imported from Guatemala. **Giardiasis** (*Giardia lamblia*): the most prevalent protozoal disease in the region. **Toxoplasmosis** (*Toxoplasma gondii*): low endemicity but an important disease in immunocompromised patients (e.g., brain lesions in AIDS patients) and notable outbreaks reported (e.g., Victoria, British Columbia, Canada, 1995, associated with contaminated water supply).

FUNGI. **Candidiasis** (*Candida albicans*): highly endemic; a major opportunistic infection in immunocompromised patients (e.g., oral thrush in AIDS patients).

HELMINTHS. **Anisakiasis** (larval nematodes of Anisakinae): rare, usually found in Hawaii. **Ascariasis** (*Ascaris lumbricoides*): endemic, commonly found in children and migrants recently arrived from developing countries. **Echinococcosis** (*Echinococcus multilocularis*): reported in Canada, Alaska, and north-central United States. **Enterobiasis** (*Enterobius vermicularis*): common in children and elderly, especially in institutions. **Fascioliasis** (*Fasciola hepatica*): rare cases; foci of *Fasciola gigantica* in Hawaii. **Taeniasis**: beef tapeworm (*Taenia saginata*) uncommon but pork tapeworm (*Taenia solium*) reported with increasing frequency in the United States, including rare cases of cysticercosis, particularly in immigrants from Latin America, Asia, and Africa; fish tapeworm (*Diphyllobothrium* spp.) cases in Alaska and western Canada. **Trichinellosis** (*Trichinella spiralis* spp.): reported particularly from Alaska and western Canada; and in migrants (e.g., outbreaks in Southeast Asian refugees). **Trichuriasis** (*Trichuris trichiura*): low endemicity, more common in the warm and moist areas of the south.

OTHER. Food poisoning outbreaks caused by **ciguatera** reported in southern California.

Diseases Primarily Transmitted by Close Contact With Infectious Individuals

Most diseases transmitted by close contact with infected individuals have dramatically decreased in the region, particularly since World War II. However, the sharp decrease in the prevalence of tuberculosis, the virtual eradication of poliomyelitis due to indigenous wild poliovirus (last American case in Peru, 1991), and the success of measles control in North America should not hide the resurgence of diseases such as tuberculosis in both poor communities and immunocompromised individuals. Outbreaks of vaccine-preventable diseases, e.g., pertussis, mumps, rubella, and serogroup C of meningococcal meningitis, have all been reported since 1990.

VIRUSES. Most diseases of this group are childhood and

vaccine-preventable diseases. They have sharply declined in incidence with the wide use of vaccines since the late 1960s, while a shift toward older children, adolescents, and young adults has been observed (e.g., chickenpox, measles, mumps, and rubella). **Chickenpox** and **herpes zoster**: highly endemic with seasonal outbreaks common in school and college populations; zoster more common in elderly and immunocompromised individuals (e.g., AIDS patients). **Influenza** (influenza virus types A, B, and C): widespread, sporadic, and seasonal epidemics. **Measles**: has become rare in the region but is still a public health threat with a shift in age groups. Significant outbreaks reported (e.g., Quebec City, 1989; Juneau, Alaska, 1996). **Mumps**: has sharply declined in the region but outbreaks still reported; shift in age groups.

Poliomyelitis: virtually eradicated; rare cases of vaccine-associated poliomyelitis. Importation to local community reported (e.g., from the Netherlands into a religious community that refuses immunization, Canada, 1992; detection in Canada of imported wild poliovirus from the Indian subcontinent, 1996). **Rotavirus**: endemic with sporadic or seasonal outbreaks (e.g., daycare settings); a major cause of severe gastroenteritis in infants and young children. **Rubella**: has declined but is still endemic with outbreaks reported in institutions, college and military populations, and in some non-vaccinated groups (e.g., outbreak in Amish community, Pennsylvania, United States).

BACTERIA. Acute bacterial conjunctivitis (*Haemophilus influenzae*): endemic, seasonal (i.e., summer and early autumn), usually confined to southern rural areas of the region. **Leprosy** (*Mycobacterium leprae*): few cases, primarily diagnosed in immigrants but limited endemic foci exist in California, Hawaii, Louisiana, Texas, and Puerto Rico. **Meningococcal meningitis**: community outbreaks of serogroup C of *Neisseria meningitidis* in children, adolescents, and young adults increasingly reported in the region. Group B *N. meningitidis* is also endemic and of increasing incidence (e.g., Oregon, 1994). Group A is less rarely involved. **Nontuberculous mycobacterial diseases**: infection with *Mycobacterium avium* complex organisms is the most common disease among AIDS patients in the region. **Pertussis** (*Bordetella pertussis*): endemic with some significant outbreaks of whooping cough (e.g., 1991 outbreak in Alberta, Canada). **Pneumonia caused by *Mycoplasma pneumoniae***: endemic with epidemics reported in all age groups. **Pneumonia caused by *Pneumocystis carinii***: constitutes a notable emerging opportunistic infection responsible for pulmonary infection that affected about 60% of AIDS patients in the region before the recent use of routine prophylactic drugs. **Pneumonia caused by *Streptococcus pneumoniae***: endemic, sporadic outbreaks; invasive penicillin-resistant *S. pneumoniae*, first identified in 1967, is now widespread in the region (e.g., 26% prevalence reported in Alaska).

Streptococcal diseases (group A *Streptococcus*): endemic with a limited re-emergence of the disease since the early 1990s despite the virtual elimination of acute rheumatic fever, streptococcal impetigo, scarlet fever, and erysipelas reported; rare outbreaks. **Tuberculosis** (*Mycobacterium tuberculosis*): in 1994, tuberculosis incidence was about 9.4/100,000 population in the United States resulting from both reactivation of latent foci and recent infections. Tuberculosis outbreaks, including, since 1990, outbreaks of multidrug-resistant strains of *M. tuberculosis*, are significantly reported from nursing homes, homeless shelters, hospitals, and prisons.

Sexually Transmitted Diseases

STDs, including HIV infection, remain an important public health concern, particularly in high-risk groups, e.g., those of low socioeconomic level.

VIRUSES. Hepatitis B: endemic; it is estimated that 5% of the adult population of the region has anti-HBc antibody; prevalence is much higher in high-risk groups (e.g., injecting drug users) and in the indigenous populations of Alaska and Canada. **Hepatitis C**: endemic; anti-HCV antibody in about 1% of the population, with a higher prevalence in high-risk groups (e.g., injecting drug users, transfused patients); accounts for about 20% of acute viral hepatitis; parenteral transmission of hepatitis C constitutes a notable concern. **HIV infection**: endemic. Rapidly spread in homosexual communities and intravenous drug users in the 1980s; slower but steady spread among heterosexual individuals; AIDS incidence in African Americans and Hispanics is six and three times higher, respectively, than among whites. HIV/AIDS control programs have been relatively successful in homosexual communities, with a lower incidence of HIV infection since the early 1990s. The cumulative number of AIDS cases officially reported in the United States and Canada was 561,429 and 14,836, respectively, as of June 30, 1997. **Human herpesvirus (herpes simplex virus, type 2)**: common with higher prevalence in high-risk groups. **Papillomavirus**: common and increasingly recognized.

BACTERIA. Gonococcal infection (*Neisseria gonorrhoeae*): endemic but in general decline since the early 1980s; the emergence of drug-resistant strains is of real concern; rare reports of gonococcal conjunctivitis in newborns. **Syphilis** (*Treponema pallidum*): endemic, including congenital syphilis, especially in high-risk groups (e.g., lower socioeconomic classes or urban areas); notable outbreaks in the 1980s (e.g., 1981–1987 syphilis outbreak in Alberta, Canada) followed by an increase until 1990 and a subsequent steady decline. In some areas, syphilis remains a major public health concern (e.g., 97% increase of reported primary and secondary syphilis cases in Baltimore, Maryland, 1993–1995). **Chlamydia: Chlamydial infections** (*Chlamydia trachomatis*): highly endemic with increased recognition of the disease since the 1970s.

FUNGI. Candidiasis (*Candida albicans*): extremely common, particularly in women.

Nosocomial Infections

The sophisticated health care system of the region has become increasingly confronted by nosocomial infections frequently associated with drug-resistant organisms.

VIRUSES. Viral nosocomial infections rarely reported but thought to occur (e.g., rotavirus in pediatric wards). Exceptional cases of rabies following corneal transplant.

BACTERIA. Numerous reports of nosocomial bacterial agents including *Acinetobacter baumanii*, *Clostridium difficile* (e.g., diarrheal diseases among elderly hospitalized patients). *Pseudomonas* species (e.g., outbreak of *Burkholderia cepacea* respiratory infection in mechanically ventilated patients. *Staphylococcus aureus* (frequently reported from neonatal nurseries) and **tuberculosis** (e.g., several outbreaks in health care workers) including drug-resistant strains of *Mycobacterium tuberculosis* (e.g., strain resistant to seven antibiotics reported in New York, 1991).

FUNGI. Nosocomial fungal infections frequently involve *Candida albicans* (e.g., following cardiac surgery), more rarely other species such as *C. parapsilosis* (e.g., hospital outbreak associated with contaminated parenteral nutrition production facility, Colorado, 1995).

Human Zoonoses and Vector-Borne Diseases, Including Viral Hemorrhagic Fevers

Although zoonoses and vector-borne diseases have been successfully controlled in the region, they remain a potential threat to public health, although they are usually distributed in well-defined foci.

Diseases Transmitted by Close Contact with Animals or Animal Products

VIRUSES. Hantavirus pulmonary syndrome (Sin Nombre virus): constitutes a notable emerging anthropozoonosis of the region since the April 1993 epidemic, Four Corners area, southwestern United States. **Rabies**: rare and mainly associated with bats, raccoons, or imported cases.

BACTERIA. Brucellosis: particularly due to *Brucella abortus*, is occasionally reported, including outbreaks (e.g., United States pork packing plant, 1992, North Carolina). **Cat-scratch disease** (*Bartonella henselae*): not uncommon. **Leptospirosis** (*Leptospira interrogans*): not uncommon. **Rickettsia: Q fever** (*Coxiella burnetii*): outbreaks of Q fever recently reported (e.g., eastern Maine).

Flea-Borne

BACTERIA. Plague (*Yersinia pestis*): wild rodent plague in western United States. Exceptional report of human cases (eight cases, including one death, reported in 1995).

Louse-Borne

BACTERIA. Trench fever (*Bartonella quintana*): since 1990, has emerged among louse-infected homeless people.

Mosquito-Borne

VIRUSES. Dengue fever: intermittently reported from southeastern Texas but notably spreading in adjacent Central America and the Caribbean; constitutes a real threat to the southern part of the region. **Mosquito-borne meningoencephalitis**: rare but endemic to the region, including eastern equine encephalomyelitis (reported from eastern and north-central United States and adjacent Canada), California encephalitis (coastal Canada, Alaska, western Ohio), La Crosse encephalitis (southern Canada and the United States from Minnesota and Texas east to New York and Georgia), Saint Louis encephalitis (usually limited to rural areas of northern United States and southern Canada, especially Ontario; small urban outbreaks reported), Venezuelan equine encephalomyelitis (southern Florida and southern Texas), snowshoe hare encephalitis, Jamestown Canyon encephalitis, and western equine encephalomyelitis (western and central United States and southern Canada).

PROTOZOA. Malaria (*Plasmodium falciparum, P. vivax*): malaria vectors are endemic in southern United States and malaria is sporadically reported, primarily from imported cases but also from exceptional local transmission (e.g., recurrent reports of "airport malaria"; New York City malaria outbreak).

Phlebotomine-Borne

VIRUSES. Vesicular stomatitis: reported from Indiana and New Jersey. Notable epizootics reported in the early 1980s (e.g., 1982–1985, Colorado, New Mexico, Georgia).

PROTOZOA. Cutaneous leishmaniasis: rare reports of *Leishmania mexicana* infection in southern Texas.

Tick-Borne

VIRUSES. Colorado tick fever: endemic in the Rocky Mountains and western Canada. **Powassan**: rare human cases reported from southern Canada and northern United States.

BACTERIA. Lyme disease (LD) (*Borrelia burgdorferi*): first recognized in 1978, continues to steadily spread in the region. Is endemic along the northern Atlantic coast, from Massachusetts to Maryland; also endemic in the upper Midwest (Wisconsin, Minnesota) and some endemic foci in the West (northern California, Oregon). In 1995, 11,603 cases were reported from 43 states, and the District of Columbia. **Tick-borne relapsing fever** (various strains): outbreaks reported, particularly from western United States to British Columbia, Canada. **Tularemia** (*Francisella tularensis*): endemic in the area from 30° to 71° North latitude.

RICKETTSIA. Rocky Mountain spotted fever: occasional reports; appears to be increasing in incidence since 1996 in the mid-Atlantic states. Infections with two species of ehrlichiae have emerged as a cause of "spotless-spotted fever" in the mid-South, the mid-Atlantic, and upper Midwest states in the 1990s.

Transmitted by Reduviidae *spp.*

PROTOZOA. Chagas' disease (*Trypanosoma cruzi*): exceptional human cases (e.g., Texas, California), some associated with blood transfusion; animal infection reported in southern United States.

Soil-Borne or Airborne Diseases and Diseases Associated With Recreational Water With No Evidence of Direct Animal-to-Human or Direct Person-to-Person Transmission

BACTERIA. Legionellosis (*Legionella* serogroups): since the 1957 outbreak in Minnesota, it has been identified throughout North America, outbreaks being more common in summer and autumn (e.g., Pontiac fever, Santa Clara County, California, 1988). **Tetanus** (*Clostridium tetani*): endemic but uncommon; few cases reported, mainly in people above 60 years of age and in rural areas.

FUNGI. Coccidioidomycosis (*Coccidioides immitis*): rare outbreaks reported (e.g., military unit, California, 1991). **American histoplasmosis** (*Histoplasma capsulatum*): outbreak in a paper factory (Michigan, 1993); hyperendemic in Ohio and Mississippi rivers.

HELMINTHS. Hookworm disease (*Necator americanus, Ancylostoma duodenale*): rare, found primarily in migrants from tropical areas, particularly Asian migrants. **Strongyloidiasis** (*Strongyloides stercoralis*): rare, usually associated with poor hygiene.

Diseases of Unknown Route of Transmission

Creutzfeldt-Jakob disease: very rare, steady incidence (e.g., about 19 cases per year, United States, 1991–1995).

■ MAINLAND MIDDLE AMERICA (Belize, Costa Rica, El Salvador, Guatemala, Honduras, Mexico, Nicaragua, and Panama)

This region includes countries with terrain ranging from coastal plains to rugged mountains and desert areas in the north to tropical rain forests in the southeast. Temperature and rainfall vary, increasing from north to south. Economic development lags behind that of North America with high population growth. The spectrum of infectious diseases reflects both the environmental conditions, the socioeconomic status, and the health infrastructure.

Disease Primarily Transmitted by Food and Drinking Water

Standards of hygiene vary widely between and within countries in the area where, overall, food- and drinking water–related diseases are common.

VIRUSES. Hepatitis A: highly endemic. **Hepatitis E:** reported in Mexico. **Enteroviruses:** common.

BACTERIA. Cholera (*Vibrio cholerae* 01) has had a resurgence with all countries reporting cholera to the WHO in 1993–1995, excepting Panama in 1995. **Diarrhea caused by** *Campylobacter* **spp.** frequent. **Enterotoxic and enteropathogenic** *E. coli:* common, mainly in children. **Listeriosis:** rare outbreaks (e.g., neonatal unit, Costa Rica, 1989). **Salmonellosis** (*Salmonella* spp.): endemic, frequent community outbreaks; high prevalence of *S. typhimurium* (Mexico, 1980–1989). **Shigella** (*Shigella* spp.): endemic, frequent outbreaks (e.g., Guatemala, 1991), including multiresistant strains (e.g., *Shigella sonnei* outbreak, pediatric daycare setting, Mexico). Many *Shigella dysenteriae* type 1 infections from mainland Middle America have been caused by drug-resistant enterobacteria. **Staphylococcal disease** (*Staphylococcus aureus*): one of the most frequent causes of food poisoning in the region. **Typhoid** (*Salmonella typhi, S. paratyphi*): endemic, drug-resistant strains; frequently reported (e.g., *S. typhi* infections, Mexico).

PROTOZOA. Amebiasis (*Entamoeba histolytica*): high endemicity (e.g., 3% of adult and 10% of pediatric diarrheas, with amebic hepatic abscess accounting for 1% of hospital admissions, Mexico). **Cryptosporidiosis:** common cause of diarrhea especially in the immunosuppressed. Outbreaks reported (e.g., pediatric hospital, Mexico, 1991). **Giardiasis:** highly endemic.

HELMINTHS. Ascariasis (*Ascaris lumbricoides*): common. **Fascioliasis** (*Fasciola hepatica*): rare. **Paragonimiasis** (*Paragonimus* spp.): rare cases reported in Costa Rica, Honduras, and Panama. **Taeniasis** (*Taenia solium, T. saginata*): common. Cysticercosis not uncommon. **Trichinosis:** endemic, outbreaks reported (e.g., Mexico; city of Delicias, 1992, associated with undercooked sausages).

OTHER. Paralytic shellfish poisoning: outbreaks common, usually associated with red tide (algae bloom).

Diseases Transmitted by Close Contact With Infectious Individuals

VIRUSES. Acute viral respiratory infections: an important cause of death in children under 5 years of age. **Acute hemorrhagic conjunctivitis:** occasional outbreaks. **Chickenpox and herpes zoster:** endemic. **Influenza (types A, B, and C):** endemic. **Measles:** transmission greatly reduced, vaccine coverages over 90% sustained over many years. Elimination of measles is possible in this area in the next few years. **Poliomyelitis:** No cases of wild poliovirus infection detected since 1990. **Rotavirus:** commonest cause of diarrhea in children under 5 years of age. **Rubella:** endemic. **Viral meningitis:** spring/summer epidemics affecting young children (e.g., ECHO 30 virus outbreak, Mexico, 1992).

BACTERIA. Diphtheria (*Corynebacterium diphtheriae*) incidence decreasing due to high immunization coverage. **Leprosy** (*Mycobacterium leprae*): incidence is declining but still prevalent. **Meningococcal meningitis** (*Neisseria meningitidis*): sporadic cases, occasional epidemics. **Pertussis** (*Bordetella pertussis*): endemic. **Pneumonia caused by** *Streptococcus pneumoniae:* common. **Streptococcal disease** (group A streptococcus): endemic. **Tuberculosis:** Countries in the area experience medium incidence of tuberculosis (e.g., Honduras 77 per 100,000 population). BCG coverage in infants is over 90%.

ECTOPARASITES. Pediculosis (*Pediculus humanus capitis*): very common. **Scabies** (*Sarcoptes scabiei*): very common.

Sexually Transmitted Diseases

STDs are common in the region, more prevalent in urban areas.

VIRUSES. Hepatitis B: endemic. **HIV infection:** endemic, continued spreading, not confined to high-risk groups. **Human herpesvirus (HSV-2):** endemic. **Papillomavirus:** endemic.

BACTERIA. Gonococcal disease (*Neisseria gonorrhoeae*): highly endemic. **Syphilis** (*Treponema pallidum*): very common. **Chlamydia: Chlamydial infections** (*Chlamydia trachomatis*): common.

FUNGI. Candidiasis (*Candida albicans*): very common.

ECTOPARASITES. Phthiriasis (*Phthirus pubis*): common.

Nosocomial Infections

As health services develop in the area, nosocomial infections are becoming more common although they are underreported.

VIRUSES. Hepatitis C: endemic; blood transfusion and other nosocomial transmission certainly underreported. **Respiratory syncytial virus (RSV):** outbreaks reported (e.g., neonatal intensive care unit, Mexico).

BACTERIA. *Klebsiella pneumoniae* and *Serratia marcescens* outbreaks, neonatal intensive care unit, Mexico. **Gram-negative bacteremia** outbreak, neonatal intensive care unit, Guatemala.

Human Zoonoses and Vector-Borne Diseases, Including Viral Hemorrhagic Fevers

Diseases Transmitted by Close Contact With Animals or Animal Products

VIRUSES. Lymphocytic choriomeningitis virus (arenavirus): rare reports. **Rabies:** endemic; stray dogs are the main reservoir; bats also contribute.

BACTERIA. Anthrax (*Bacillus anthracis*): endemic. **Brucellosis** (*Brucella abortus, B. melitensis, B. suis*): endemic, particularly in northern part of the region. **Cat-scratch disease** (*Bartonella henselae*): rare. **Leptospirosis:** endemic; outbreak reported (e.g., Nicaragua, 1995). **Rat-bite fever** (*Streptobacillus moniliformis*): rare. **Chlamydia: Psittacosis** (*Chlamydia psittaci*): endemic; rare reports. **Rickettsia: Q fever** (*Coxiella burnetii*): endemic.

Culicoides-Borne

VIRUSES. Oropouche disease: rare reports from Panama.

Fly-Borne

HELMINTHS. Onchocerciasis (*Onchocerca volvulus*): two small foci in the south of Mexico and four dispersed foci in Guatemala.

Louse-Borne

BACTERIA. Trench fever (*Bartonella quintana*): endemic foci in Mexico. **Rickettsia: Epidemic typhus** (*Rickettsia prowazekii*): foci in mountainous regions (e.g., Mexico area).

Mosquito-Borne

VIRUSES. Dengue. Marked increase in the incidence of dengue and dengue hemorrhagic fever (DHF) in the Americas. During 1993 Panama and Costa Rica, the last tropical Latin American countries that remained free of dengue, reported indigenous transmission of the disease. Cases have also been reported from Nicaragua (DHF epidemic, 1994), Mexico, Honduras, and throughout the region in 1995. This re-emergence has been due to the collapse of vector control programs, resulting in *Aedes aegypti* having a distribution similar to that before the eradication programs of the 1960s and 1970s. **Eastern equine encephalitis** (*Alphavirus*): scattered reports from Mexico, Guatemala, Honduras, and Panama. **Western equine encephalitis** (*Alphavirus*): epizootics in animals in Mexico (no human cases reported). **Yellow fever**: Panama is the only country in the area to be included in the yellow fever zone. No reports of cases to WHO since 1974. The spread of *Aedes aegypti* may herald a return of the disease to areas that have been free of the disease for decades. **Venezuelan equine encephalitis** (*Alphavirus*): endemic foci reported (e.g., El Salvador and Panama, 1989–1994). In 1993–1996, epizootics reported in Venezuela, Colombia, Mexico, and northern Peru after 20 years of absence.

PROTOZOA. **Malaria** (*Plasmodium vivax, P. falciparum*): holoendemic and increasing in all countries in areas below 1500 m of altitude. *P. vivax* accounts for the vast majority of cases.

HELMINTHS. **Lymphatic filariasis** (*Wuchereria bancrofti*): reported from Costa Rica.

Phlebotomine-Borne

PROTOZOA. **Cutaneous** and **mucocutaneous leishmaniasis** (*Leishmania mexicana* complex, *L. viannia braziliensis* complex): endemic foci, primarily in southern countries. **Visceral leishmaniasis** (*L. donovani chagasi*): endemic foci in El Salvador, Guatemala, Honduras, and Mexico.

VIRUSES. **Vesicular stomatitis**: epizootic, 1982–1985, Mexico.

Transmitted by Reduviidae spp.

PROTOZOA. **Chagas' disease** (*Trypanosoma cruzi*): rural foci in all eight countries but of decreasing incidence. Seropositivity in blood donors ranges from less than 1% in Costa Rica to between 6% and 8% in Honduras.

Tick-Borne

BACTERIA. **Tularaemia** (*Francisella tularensis*): reported (e.g., northern Mexico). **Tick-borne relapsing fever**: sporadic cases, occasional outbreaks. **Rickettsia: Rocky Mountain spotted fever** (*Rickettsia rickettsii*): reported (e.g., central Mexico, Panama, Costa Rica).

Soil-Borne or Airborne Diseases and Diseases Associated With Recreational Water With No Evidence of Direct Animal-to-Human or Direct Person-to-Person Transmission

BACTERIA. **Melioidosis** (*Pseudomonas pseudomallei*): rare reports (e.g., Panama, El Salvador, Puerto Rico, Mexico).

FUNGI. **Coccidioidomycosis** (*Coccidiodes immitis*): rare reports (e.g., desert areas of northern Mexico, other areas of mainland Middle America). **Blastomycosis** (*Blastomyces dermatitidis*): reported from Mexico.

HELMINTHS. **Hookworm**: common. **Strongyloidiasis** (*Strongyloides stercoralis*): common.

■ CARIBBEAN MIDDLE AMERICA (Antigua and Barbuda, Aruba, Bahamas, Barbados, British Virgin Islands, Cayman Islands, Cuba, Dominica, Dominican Republic, Grenada, Guadeloupe, Haiti, Jamaica, Martinique, Montserrat, Netherlands Antilles, Puerto Rico, Saint Kills and Nevis, Saint Lucia, Saint Vincent and the Grenadines, Trinidad and Tobago, Turks and Caicos Islands, and the [U.S.] Virgin Islands)

These island nations have terrain ranging from coastal plains to rugged mountains 1000 to 2500 m high. The climate is subtropical to tropical moderated by trade winds with little seasonal variation in temperature. However, there is seasonal variation in rainfall with heavy rainstorms and high winds occurring at certain times of the year. Economic development and infrastructure vary greatly.

Diseases Primarily Transmitted by Food and Drinking Water

Standards of hygiene vary widely between and within countries in the area. Food- and drinking–water related diseases are common and have a similar spectrum to those in mainland Middle America except for the following.

BACTERIA. **Cholera**: no cases have been reported in the Caribbean.

HELMINTHS. **Fascioliasis** (*Fasciola hepatica*): Cuba has the highest endemicity for the Americas (48% of all reported cases, 1969–1989).

Diseases Transmitted by Close Contact With Infectious Individuals

VIRUSES. **Acute viral respiratory infections**: common in children. **Acute hemorrhagic conjunctivitis**: outbreaks reported (Dominican Republic, 1993). **Chickenpox and herpes zoster**: endemic. **Influenza** (types A, B, and C): endemic. **Measles**: transmission greatly reduced owing to vaccine coverages over 90% sustained over many years. Elimination of measles is possible in this area in the next few years. **Poliomyelitis**: no wild poliovirus transmission. **Rotavirus**: commonest cause of diarrhea in children under age 5. **Rubella**: low incidence due to high vaccination coverage. **Viral meningitis**: spring/summer epidemics affecting young children.

BACTERIA. **Diphtheria** (*Corynebacterium diphtheriae*): incidence decreasing due to high immunization coverage. **Leprosy** (*Mycobacterium leprae*): important decline but autochthonous transmission remains in some areas (e.g., Cuba, Haiti). **Meningococcal meningitis** (*Neisseria meningitidis*): sporadic cases, occasional epidemics. Type C outbreaks frequent in Cuba. **Pertussis** (*Bordetella pertussis*): endemic. **Pneumonia caused by** *Streptococcus pneumoniae*: common. **Streptococcal disease** (group A streptococcus): endemic. **Tuberculosis**: countries in the area experience medium incidence. Bacille Calmette-Guérin (BCG) coverage in infants is over 90%.

ECTOPARASITES. **Pediculosis** (*Pediculus humanus capitis*): common. **Scabies** (*Sarcoptes scabiei*): common.

Sexually Transmitted Diseases

STDs are common and have a spectrum similar to mainland Middle America.

Nosocomial Infections

Poorly documented in the region with no reported outbreaks in 1990–1996 but estimated to be common.

Human Zoonoses and Vector-Borne Diseases, Including Viral Hemorrhagic Fevers

Diseases Transmitted by Close Contact With Animals or Animal Products

VIRUSES. **Lymphocytic choriomeningitis virus** (arenavirus): rare, probably underdiagnosed. **Rabies**: endemic. Dogs are the main reservoir although the small Indian mongoose (*Herpestes auropunctatus*) is important in Cuba, the Dominican Republic, Grenada, Haiti, and Puerto Rico. Bat-related rabies has been reported (e.g., Trinidad).

BACTERIA. **Brucellosis** (*Brucella abortus, B. melitensis, B. suis*): endemic. **Leptospirosis**: endemic, outbreaks reported (e.g., Cuba). **Chlamydia: Psittacosis** (*Chlamydia psittaci*): endemic. **Rickettsia: Q fever** (*Coxiella burnetii*): endemic.

Mosquito-Borne

VIRUSES. Dengue. Endemic since it reached the region in the 1970s and the first DHF/DSS outbreak outside Southeast Asia (Cuba, 1981); increased activity in the 1990s throughout the region with great epidemic potential. All four serotypes introduced with at least two being endemic in each country. Outbreaks still reported (e.g., Puerto Rico, 1991). **Eastern equine encephalitis** (*Alphavirus*): scattered endemic foci. **Venezuelan equine encephalitis** (*Alphavirus*): outbreaks reported (e.g., Trinidad). **Yellow fever**: intermittently reported in Trinidad.

PROTOZOA. Malaria (*Plasmodium falciparum, P. vivax*): endemic only in Haiti and parts of the Dominican Republic, *P. falciparum* almost exclusively.

HELMINTHS. Lymphatic filariasis (*Wuchereria bancrofti*): occurs in Haiti and the Dominican Republic.

Phlebotomine-Borne

PROTOZOA. Cutaneous leishmaniasis: diffuse form of the disease recently described in the Dominican Republic.

Tick-Borne

BACTERIA. Tularaemia (*Francisella tularensis*): rare reports from Haiti.

Soil-Borne or Airborne Diseases, and Diseases Associated With Recreational Water With No Evidence of Direct Animal-to-Human or Direct Person-to-Person Transmission

BACTERIA. Melioidosis (*Pseudomonas pseudomallei*): rare reports (e.g., Haiti, Puerto Rico, Aruba).
HELMINTHS. Hookworm: endemic. **Schistosomiasis** (*Schistosoma mansoni*): endemic in the Dominican Republic, Guadeloupe, Martinique, Puerto Rico, and St. Lucia; sporadic in other islands. **Strongyloidiasis** (*Strongyloides stercoralis*): endemic.

■ TROPICAL SOUTH AMERICA (Bolivia, Brazil, Colombia, Ecuador, French Guiana, Guyana, Paraguay, Peru, Suriname, and Venezuela)

This region includes countries with a wide variety of terrain and climate. It covers the narrow coastal strip on the Pacific Ocean, the high Andean range with numerous peaks 5000 to 7000 m high, and the tropical rain forests of the Amazon basin, bordered to the north and south by savanna zones and dry tropical forest or scrub. Economic development varies with rapid growth of large urban centers due to migration from rural areas. This had led to worsening problems of overcrowding and poverty. The spectrum of infectious disease reflects both the environmental and economic conditions and state of health and hygiene infrastructure.

Disease Primarily Transmitted by Food and Drinking Water

Food- and drinking water–related diseases are common. However, mortality from diarrheal disease has decreased in recent years. For example, in Venezuela the number of infant deaths from diarrheal disease fell from 2538 in 1990 to 1210 in 1992.

VIRUSES. Hepatitis A: endemic with high seroprevalence. **Enteroviruses**: common.

BACTERIA. Cholera: endemic in most countries since the 1991 epidemic, which started in Peru. In 1995 Bolivia, Brazil, Colombia, Ecuador, and Peru reported autochthonous cases. Limited outbreaks have been reported (e.g., Bolivia, early 1997). **Diarrhea caused by *Campylobacter***: a frequent cause of sporadic gastroenteritis. **Enterotoxic and enteropathogenic *Escherichia coli***: common cause of watery diarrhea mainly in children. **Salmonellosis**: common cause of sporadic food-borne gastroenteritis as well as outbreaks. In southeast Brazil *Salmonella typhimurium* was isolated in 13 of 25 outbreaks of food-borne illness studies between 1982 and 1991. An *S. agona* outbreak was reported from a pediatric hospital in Rio de Janeiro, Brazil, in 1994. **Shigellosis**: endemic. **Typhoid and enteric fevers**: common.

PROTOZOA. Amebiasis: common cause of adult and childhood diarrhea, particularly common in Colombia. **Cryptosporidiosis**: common cause of diarrhea especially in the immunosuppressed. **Giardiasis**: common.

HELMINTHS. Ascariasis: common. **Echinococcosis** (*Echinococcus granulosus*): particularly in Peru. **Fascioliasis**: occurs in sheep and cattle raising areas. Rare outbreaks (e.g., Aymar Indians, Bolivian altiplano, May 1991). **Taeniasis**: common. **Trichinosis**: endemic.

TREMATODES. Paragonimiasis: rare reports (e.g., Ecuador, Peru, Venezuela).

Diseases Transmitted by Close Contact With Infectious Individuals

VIRUSES. Acute viral respiratory infections: frequent and an important cause of death in children under 5 years of age. **Acute hemorrhagic conjunctivitis**: occasional outbreaks. **Chickenpox and herpes zoster**: endemic. **Influenza** (types A, B, and C): endemic. **Measles**: transmission has been greatly reduced due to vaccine coverages over 90% sustained over many years. Elimination of measles is possible in this area in the next few years. **Mumps**: endemic. **Poliomyelitis**: no wild poliovirus transmission. **Rotavirus**: commonest cause of diarrhea in children under age 5. **Rubella**: endemic. **Viral meningitis**: occasional outbreaks mainly affecting young children.

BACTERIA. Diphtheria (*Corynebacterium diphtheriae*): incidence decreasing due to high immunization coverage. **Leprosy** (*Mycobacterium leprae*): Brazil has the highest rates of leprosy (1992 prevalence rate of 143 per 100,000). Other countries with high prevalence include Suriname, Colombia, Venezuela, and Paraguay. Ecuador and Paraguay have already achieved prevalence rates of under 10 per 100,000. **Meningococcal meningitis** (*Neisseria meningitidis*): sporadic disease with occasional epidemics. Epidemics are common in Brazil and mainly caused by group C. **Pertussis** (*Bordetella pertussis*): endemic. Incidence falling due to improved vaccination coverage with diphtheria-pertussis-tetanus (DPT) vaccine. **Pneumonia caused by *Streptococcus pneumoniae***: common cause of community acquired pneumonia. **Streptococcal disease** (group A streptococcus): endemic. **Tuberculosis**: Reported rates vary widely. In 1994 rates varied from 28 per 100,000 in Belize to 130 per 100,000 and 208 per 100,000 in Bolivia and Peru, respectively. BCG coverage in infants is over 90%.

ECTOPARASITES. Pediculosis (*Pediculus humanus capitis*): common. **Scabies** (*Sarcoptes scabiei*): common.

Sexually Transmitted Diseases

Common in the region.

VIRUSES. Hepatitis B and **D**: endemic. Amazon basin highly endemic for hepatitis B and D. **Hepatitis C**: endemic.

HIV infection: increasing incidence. **Herpes simplex virus (HSV-2)**: endemic. **Papillomavirus infection**: common.

BACTERIA: Gonococcal infection *(Neisseria gonorrhoeae)*: endemic. **Syphilis** *(Treponema pallidum)*: endemic. **Chlamydia: Chlamydial infection** *(Chlamydia trachomatis)*: endemic.

FUNGI. Candidiasis *(Candida albicans)*: common.

ECTOPARASITES. Phthiriasis *(Phthirus pubis)*: common.

Nosocomial Infections

Poorly documented.

PROTOZOA. Chagas' disease *(Trypanosoma cruzi)*: estimated to be 10,000 to 20,000 cases of infection due to blood transfusion per year in Brazil (1992).

Human Zoonoses and Vector-Borne Diseases, Including Viral Hemorrhagic Fevers

Diseases Transmitted by Close Contact With Animals or Animal Products

VIRUSES. Guanarito (Venezuelan) hemorrhagic fever *(Arenavirus)*: first and only identified in Venezuela, 1989–1991 (outbreak followed by sporadic cases in Guanarito area). **Lymphocytic choriomeningitis virus** *(Arenavirus)*: rare reports. **Machupo (Bolivian) hemorrhagic fever** *(Arenavirus)*: sporadic epidemics in small villages of rural northern Bolivia (e.g., nine cases including seven deaths reported in 1994). **Rabies**: endemic, usually associated with dog bite. Unusual and significant outbreak reported from the Amazonian jungle, Peru, 1991, related to vampire bats.

BACTERIA. Anthrax *(Bacillus anthracis)*: endemic. **Brucellosis** *(Brucella abortus, B. melitensis, B. suis)*: endemic and common. **Cat-scratch disease** *(Bartonella henselae)*: rare. **Leptospirosis**: endemic. **Rat-bite fever** *(Streptobacillus moniliformis)*: rare. **Chlamydia: Psittacosis** *(Chlamydia psittaci)*: occurs in all countries. **Rickettsia: Q fever** *(Coxiella burnetii)*: occurs in all countries.

CESTODES. Echinococcosis: frequent in Peru.

Culicoides-Borne

Oropouche virus disease: endemic foci (e.g., rural areas of Brazil and Peru).

Flea-Borne

BACTERIA. Plague *(Yersinia pestis)*: wild foci in northeastern Brazil (Bahia State), Ecuador, the Andean region of Peru (Cajamarca, Lambayeque, La Libertad Departments since 1992), and Bolivia. Significant outbreak reported in Peru, 1992–1994 (1299 cases diagnosed).

Fly-Borne

HELMINTHS. Onchocerciasis *(Onchocerca volvulus)*: isolated foci in rural areas in Colombia, Ecuador, Venezuela, and northern Brazil. Elimination targeted for the year 2007.

Louse-Borne

BACTERIA. Relapsing fever *(Borrelia recurrentis)*: endemic foci in highland areas. **Trench fever** *(Bartonella quintana)*: endemic foci in Bolivia. **Rickettsia: Typhus** *(Rickettsia prowazekii)*: endemic foci in mountainous regions of Colombia, Peru, Ecuador, and Bolivia.

Mosquito-borne

VIRUSES. Dengue: endemic since *Aedes aegypti* reinvaded South America. In the 1980s, Bolivia, Brazil, Ecuador, Paraguay, and Peru, which had no recorded cases of dengue for several decades, faced explosive outbreaks. Incidence increased since the mid-1980s including outbreaks (e.g., Brazil, 1986–1987; Brazil and Venezuela, 1995). Venezuela suffered a serious outbreak in 1989–1990 with 5990 DHF cases and 70 deaths. **Eastern equine encephalitis** *(Alphavirus)*: reported from Brazil, Peru, Colombia, and Ecuador. **Western equine encephalitis** *(Alphavirus)*: epizootics in animals in Brazil (no recent human cases reported). **Yellow fever**: endemic foci in the Amazon region where jungle and urban cycles are now physically juxtaposed in many areas. Sharp increase of cases in 1995 due largely to an outbreak in Peru. Cases also reported from Bolivia, northern and western states of Brazil, Ecuador, and Colombia. **Venezuelan equine encephalitis** *(Alphavirus)*: Occasional epizootics and epidemics (1993–1996) after 20 years of absence. Endemic foci reported from Venezuela, northern Peru, Colombia, Brazil, Bolivia, Ecuador, and Paraguay.

PROTOZOA. Malaria *(Plasmodium vivax, P. falciparum)*: endemic in all 10 countries. In 1997, *P. vivax* accounted for three times as many cases as *P. falciparum*.

HELMINTHS. Filariasis *(Wuchereria bancrofti)*: endemic foci in Brazil, Guyana, and Suriname.

Phlebotomine-borne

BACTERIA. Bartonellosis (Oroya fever) *(Bartonella bacilliformis)*: reported from arid river valleys on the western slopes of the Andes, up to 3000 m.

PROTOZOA. Cutaneous and mucocutaneous leishmaniasis *(Leishmania braziliensis, L. mexicana, L. guyanensis, L. amazonensis, L. peruviana)*: occurs in all 10 countries with species-specific geographic distribution. There has been an increase of mucocutaneous leishmaniasis in Brazil and Paraguay. Outbreak of cutaneous leishmaniasis reported (e.g., Rio Doce Valley, Brazil, 1991). **Visceral leishmaniasis** *(L. chagasi)*: endemic rural foci, primarily in Brazil (e.g., northeast Brazil). Less frequent in Colombia and Venezuela, rare in Bolivia and Paraguay, and unknown in Peru.

Transmitted by Reduviidae spp.

PROTOZOA. Chagas' disease *(Trypanosoma cruzi)*: endemic throughout the region but with decreasing incidence. Primarily a rural problem.

Tick-Borne

BACTERIA. Tick-borne relapsing fever: sporadic disease in scattered foci. **Rickettsia: Rocky Mountain spotted fever** *(Rickettsia rickettsii)*: reported from Brazil and Colombia.

Soil-Borne or Airborne Diseases, and Diseases Associated With Recreational Water With No Evidence of Direct Animal-to-Human or Direct Person-to-Person Transmission

BACTERIA. Melioidosis *(Pseudomonas pseudomallei)*: rare. Has been reported from Brazil.

FUNGI. Coccidioidomycosis *(Coccidioides immitis)*: rare. Reports from the arid and semiarid areas of Venezuela, Paraguay, and Colombia. More frequent in the summer.

HELMINTHS. Hookworm: common. **Strongyloidiasis** *(Strongyloides stercoralis)*: common. **Schistosomiasis** *(Schistosoma mansoni)*: rare endemic foci (e.g., Brazil, Suriname, north-central Venezuela).

■ **TEMPERATE SOUTH AMERICA** (Argentina, Chile, Falkland Islands [Malvinas], and Uruguay)

This region covers the Mediterranean climatic area of the western coastal strip, the Andes, the steppes and deserts of

Patagonia in the south, and the prairies of the northeast. The climate varies from dry arid to Mediterranean, temperate, and subarctic. Economic development is generally ahead of the rest of South America.

Diseases Primarily Transmitted by Food and Drinking Water

Food- and drinking water–related diseases are common.
VIRUSES. Hepatitis A: endemic. **Enteroviruses**: common.
BACTERIA. Cholera: reported from Argentina, 1992–1995, with a peak in 1993 (2080 cases reported) and Chile, 1991–1994 (peak in 1992, 73 cases). **Diarrhea caused by *Campylobacter***: endemic. **Enterotoxic and enteropathogenic *Escherichia coli***: common in children. **Salmonellosis**: most common cause of sporadic food-borne gastroenteritis outbreaks. *Salmonella enteritidis* most commonly isolated serotype in Argentina with a significant increase since 1986. **Shigellosis**: endemic. **Typhoid and enteric fevers**: not common in Argentina, more frequently reported from Chile and Uruguay.
PROTOZOA. Amebiasis: common. **Cryptosporidiosis**: common. **Giardiasis**: common.
HELMINTHS. Ascariasis: common. **Echinococcosis** (*Echinococcus granulosus*): reported from all countries but Argentina. **Fascioliasis**: endemic foci in sheep- and cattle-raising areas. **Taeniasis**: common in Chile and Uruguay. **Trichinosis**: endemic; outbreaks reported (e.g., Purranque County, Chile, 1992, associated with infected pork).

Diseases Transmitted by Close Contact With Infectious Individuals

VIRUSES. Similar spectrum of disease as mainland Middle America and tropical South America. **Influenza** (influenza virus types A, B, and C): notable increase in incidence in summer 1996.
BACTERIA. Diphtheria (*Corynebacterium diphtheriae*): incidence low due to high immunization coverage. **Leprosy** (*Mycobacterium leprae*): countries in the area have achieved rates of leprosy of less than 10 per 100,000. **Meningococcal meningitis** (*Neisseria meningitidis*): sporadic disease with occasional epidemics (e.g., type B outbreak, Chile, 1993). **Pertussis** (*Bordetella pertussis*): falling incidence due to high vaccination coverage. **Pneumonia caused by *Streptococcus pneumoniae***: common. Incidence and mortality generally lower than the rest of South America. **Streptococcal disease** (group A *Streptococcus*): endemic. **Tuberculosis**: medium endemicity; reported incidence in 1993 was 21.9, 33.3, and 41.9 per 100,000 in Uruguay, Chile, and Argentina, respectively.
ECTOPARASITES. Pediculosis (*Pediculus humanus capitis*): endemic. **Scabies** (*Sarcoptes scabiei*): endemic.

Sexually Transmitted Diseases

Situation similar to that of tropical South America with increasing prevalence of **AIDS**. Up to December 1995, Argentina had reported the highest number of AIDS cases (2249) followed by Chile (886), and Uruguay (385).

Nosocomial Infections

Poorly documented. **Methicillin-resistant *Staphylococcus aureus*** reported from Chile.

Human Zoonoses and Vector-Borne Diseases, Including Viral Hemorrhagic Fevers

Diseases Transmitted by Close Contact With Animals or Animal Products

VIRUSES. Hantavirus: rare reports (e.g., pulmonary syndrome, Argentina, 1996). **Junin (Argentinian) hemorrhagic fever** (*Arenavirus*): endemic in pampas areas of Argentina primarily from March to October. **Lymphocytic choriomeningitis virus** (*Arenavirus*): rare reports. **Rabies**: endemic, main reservoir is dogs. Increasingly reported from Argentina but the trend is downward for human cases in all the other countries since the 1970s.
BACTERIA. Anthrax (*Bacillus anthracis*): endemic; an occupational hazard in Argentina, Chile, and Uruguay. **Brucellosis** (*Brucella abortus, B. melitensis, B. suis*): endemic and common. Urban outbreak reported from Buenos Aires, Argentina, associated with unpasteurized goat cheese. **Cat-scratch disease** (*Bartonella henselae*): rare. **Leptospirosis**: endemic. **Rat-bite fever** (*Streptobacillus moniliformis*): rare. **Chlamydia**: **Psittacosis** (*Chlamydia psittaci*): occurs in all countries. **Rickettsia**: **Q fever** (*Coxiella burnetii*): endemic in all countries.
CESTODES. Echinococcosis: low endemicity.

Louse-Borne

BACTERIA. Relapsing fever (*Borrelia recurrentis*): endemic foci in highland areas. **Rickettsia**: **Typhus** (*Rickettsia prowazekii*): endemic foci in mountainous regions (e.g., Argentina, Chile).

Mosquito-Borne

VIRUSES. Eastern equine encephalitis (*Alphavirus*): reported from Argentina. **Western equine encephalitis** (*Alphavirus*): no recent human cases reported; epizootics in Argentina.
PROTOZOA. Malaria (*Plasmodium vivax*): endemic seasonal foci in Argentina (below 1200 m, from May to October, particularly along the borders of Bolivia and Paraguay), almost exclusively caused by *P. vivax*.

Phlebotomine-Borne

PROTOZOA. Cutaneous leishmaniasis (*Leishmania braziliensis*): reported from northeastern Argentina.

Transmitted by Reduviidae *spp.*

PROTOZOA. Chagas' disease (*Trypanosoma cruzi*): endemic throughout the region but with decreasing incidence.

Tick-Borne

BACTERIA. Tick-borne relapsing fever: sporadic, scattered foci.

Soil-Borne or Airborne Diseases, and Diseases Associated With Recreational Water With No Evidence of Direct Animal-to-Human or Direct Person-to-Person Transmission

BACTERIA. Melioidosis (*Pseudomonas pseudomallei*): rare. Has been reported from Brazil.
FUNGI. Coccidioidomycosis (*Coccidioides immitis*): rare reports (e.g., northern Argentina). More frequent in the summer.
HELMINTHS. Hookworm (*Necator americanus, Ancylostoma duodenale*): common. **Strongyloidiasis** (*Strongyloides stercoralis*): common.

■ NORTHERN AFRICA (Algeria, Egypt, Libyan Arab Jamahiriya, Morocco, and Tunisia)

This region includes a Mediterranean, generally fertile, coastal area while the Sahara Desert composes most of the interior area with the exceptions of the oases and the Nile valley.

This region is also characterized by its recent and important population growth, leading to very high population density in some cities, and its low economic development. Consequently, hygiene is often insufficient and diseases transmitted by the fecal-oral route (i.e., mostly water-borne and food-borne diseases) are common. The region had, and still maintains, significant population movements with Europe (e.g., France and Belgium for workers from Morocco, Algeria, and Tunisia) and the Middle East (e.g., Saudi Arabia and Iraq for Egyptian workers). Tourism also contributes significantly to permanent population contacts (e.g., Europeans visiting Morocco, Tunisia, Egypt).

Diseases Primarily Transmitted by Food and Drinking Water

Enteritis agents, including intestinal worms, are highly endemic and outbreaks of food-borne diseases occur throughout the region.

VIRUSES. Hepatitis A: hyperendemic. **Hepatitis E**: reported from Egypt (very high prevalence) and Morocco. **Norwalk and Norwalk-like viruses**: rarely reported but thought to be common.

BACTERIA. Cholera (toxinogenic *Vibrio cholerae* serogroup 01): cases reported intermittently. **Botulism** (*Clostridium botulinum*): outbreaks sporadically reported (e.g., outbreak of type E botulism associated with traditional salted fish in Cairo, Egypt, 1991). **Diarrhea caused by *Campylobacter jejuni***: common. **Diarrhea caused by *Escherichia coli***: extremely frequent. **Listerosis** (*Listeria monocytogenes*): endemic but poorly documented. **Salmonellosis**: highly endemic with numerous outbreaks. **Shigellosis** (*Shigella* species): hyperendemic; frequent outbreaks. **Typhoid** (*Salmonella typhi*) and **paratyphoid** (three bioserotypes of *S. enteritidis*): common with an increase of *S. typhi* strains resistant to antibiotics, particularly to chloramphenicol (e.g., outbreak of typhoid resistant to chloramphenicol in Gharbeya Governorate, Egypt, 1990).

PROTOZOA. Amebiasis (*Entamoeba histolytica*): high endemicity. **Cryptosporidiosis** (*Cryptosporidium parvum*): endemic. **Giardiasis** (*Giardia lamblia*): extremely common. **Toxoplasmosis** (*Toxoplasma gondii*): endemic.

FUNGI. Candidiasis (*Candida albicans*): hyperendemic.

HELMINTHS. Ascariasis (*Ascaris lumbricoides*): very common. **Capillariasis** (*Capillaria philippinensis*): rare cases in Egypt. **Echinococcosis** (*Echinococcus granulosus*): endemic throughout the region. Rare report of *E. multilocularis* (e.g., Egypt). **Enterobiasis** (*Enterobius vermicularis*): very common. **Fascioliasis** (*Fasciola hepatica*): reported throughout the region, with an especially high prevalence in Egypt. **Paragonimiasis** (*Paragonimus* spp.): rare reports. **Taeniasis**: beef tapeworm (*Taenia saginata*) common throughout the region; the pork tapeworm (*T. solium*), including cysticercosis, is endemic essentially in Egypt. **Trichinellosis** (*Trichinella spiralis* spp.): common in Egypt. **Trichuriasis** (*Trichuris trichuria*): high endemicity.

OTHER. Pentastomid infection (*Linguatula serrata*): rare reports.

Diseases Primarily Transmitted by Close Contact With Infectious Individuals

Diseases with person-to-person transmission, particularly those associated with poor hygiene, are highly endemic throughout the region.

VIRUSES. Chickenpox and **herpes zoster**, **influenza** (influenza virus types A, B, and C), **measles**, and **mumps** are all highly endemic throughout the region. Frequent epidemics occur. **Poliomyelitis**: endemic but dramatic decline of incidence; no cases reported from Algeria, Libya, Morocco, and Tunisia since 1990, 1991, 1989, and 1992, respectively. **Rotavirus**: extremely common and a major cause of severe epidemic diarrhea in infants and children. **Rubella**: endemic.

BACTERIA. Diphtheria (*Corynebacterium diphtheriae*): cutaneous diphtheria is endemic. **Leprosy** (*Mycobacterium leprae*): rare foci, primarily in Egypt. Sharp prevalence decline since 1985. **Meningococcal meningitis** (*Neisseria meningitidis*): endemic; frequent in Egypt; all serogroups involved. **Nonvenereal syphilis**: endemic, particularly in poor and desert areas. **Pertussis** (*Bordetella pertussis*): endemic. **Staphylococcal diseases** (*Staphylococcus aureus*): hyperendemic, particularly in Egypt, with multidrug-resistant strains frequently reported. **Streptococcal diseases** (group A *Streptococcus*): common, with considerable rheumatic heart disease. **Tuberculosis** (*Mycobacterium tuberculosis*): endemic throughout the region with increasing reports of multidrug-resistant strains (e.g., Egypt). **Chlamydia. Trachoma** (*Chlamydia trachomatis*): endemic in the nomadic population of the Sahara.

Sexually Transmitted Diseases

The actual prevalence of STDs in the region is poorly documented.

VIRUSES. Hepatitis B and **delta agent** infections are common, with sporadic outbreaks reported (e.g., 1985–1987 hepatitis B outbreak, Egypt). **Hepatitis C**: endemic with particularly high prevalence in Egyptian rural areas. **HIV infection**: low endemicity but spreading in high-risk groups (e.g., intravenous drug users). **Herpes simplex virus (HSV-2)**: common. **Papillomavirus**: common.

BACTERIA. Chancroid (*Haemophilus ducreyi*): reported. **Gonococcal infection** (*Neisseria gonorrhoeae*): common; neonatorum gonococcal conjunctivitis reported. **Syphilis** (*Treponema pallidum*): endemic. **Chlamydia: Chlamydial infections** (*Chlamydia trachomatis*): thought to be highly endemic. **Lymphogranuloma venereum** reported.

FUNGI. Candidiasis (*Candida albicans*): hyperendemic.

Nosocomial Infections

Although rarely well documented or systematically reported, nosocomial infections are thought to be frequent and increasing in the region with some significant outbreaks documented.

VIRUSES. Poorly documented (e.g., rotavirus) with few exceptions (e.g., HIV infection associated with hemodialysis, Egypt, 1992).

BACTERIA. Thought to be frequent including various hospital-acquired tuberculosis infections, including multidrug-resistant strains of *Mycobacterium tuberculosis* and numerous other bacterial nosocomial infections, particularly with *Salmonella* spp. (e.g., nursery outbreak of *S. mbandaka*, Algeria, 1989; hospital-acquired pediatric epidemics caused by antibiotic-resistant *Salmonella* serovar Wien Tunis, 1982 and 1989).

Human Zoonoses and Vector-Borne Diseases, Including Viral Hemorrhagic Fevers

Zoonoses are frequent in the region, which maintains important populations of cattle, sheep, and goats usually in close contact with households.

Transmitted by Close Contact With Animals or Animal Products, Excluding Primarily Food-Borne Diseases

VIRUSES. Rabies: notably endemic, frequently urban, with large regional population of stray dogs.

BACTERIA. Anthrax (*Bacillus anthracis*): human infection reported. **Brucellosis** (*Brucella abortus, B. melitensis*): very common. **Leptospirosis** (*Leptospira interrogans*): endemic. **Rat-bite fever** (*Streptobacillus moniliformis*): rare. **Chlamydia: Psittacosis** (*Chlamydia psittaci*): reported. **Rickettsia: Q fever** (*Coxiella burnetii*): endemic.

Culicoides-Borne

HELMINTHS. Microfilarial infection (*Mansonella perstans*): rare reports (e.g., Algeria, Tunisia).

Flea-Borne

BACTERIA. Plague (*Yersinia pestis*): rare cases reported from the western Sahara.

Louse-Borne

BACTERIA. Epidemic typhus (*Rickettsia prowazekii*): occasionally reported from the desert regions (e.g., Sinai peninsula, Libya).

Mosquito-Borne

VIRUSES. Rift Valley fever: first significant epidemic in the region occurred in Egypt in 1977. Almost endemic in Upper Egypt since the 1993 outbreaks. **Sindbis, West Nile fever**, and **Zika**: endemic, particularly in the Nile valley. Recent outbreaks of West Nile fever reported (i.e., Algeria, Timimoun region, central Sahara, 1994; Morocco, 1996, primarily in horses).
PROTOZOA. Malaria: essentially *Plasmodium vivax*, some *P. malariae*, present in foci (e.g., El Faiyum and southern half of Nile in Egypt; Ihrir, Blida, and Annaba in Algeria; southwest Libya, western half; and northern Morocco. *P. falciparum* malaria is endemic in Egypt (e.g., El Faiyum, Upper Egypt) and is slowly spreading northward with reported outbreaks (e.g., Suez Canal, Upper Egypt); all large cities of the region are considered risk-free of malaria.
HELMINTHS. Lymphatic filariasis (*Wuchereria bancrofti*): rare but endemic in some foci (e.g., some urban areas of the Nile delta).

Phlebotomine-Borne

VIRUSES. Sandfly fevers (Naples and Sicilian types): endemic, usually seasonal.
PROTOZOA. Cutaneous leishmaniasis (*Leishmania tropica* complex, *L. major* complex): endemic, particularly along the coastal area. **Visceral leishmaniasis** (*L. infantum*): endemic in small rural foci along the Mediterranean, particularly in northern Tunisia and neighboring Algeria. Epidemics reported. Wild canidae and domestic dogs are the main reservoir.

Tick-Borne

VIRUSES. Crimean-Congo and **Thogoto**.
BACTERIA. Tick-borne relapsing fever (various *Borrelia* strains): reported.

Soil-Borne or Airborne Diseases, and Diseases Associated With Recreational Water With No Evidence of Direct Animal-to-Human or Direct Person-to-Person Transmission

BACTERIA. Legionellosis (*Legionella* serogroups): reported. **Tetanus** (*Clostridium tetani*): incidence has sharply declined in the region but remains endemic. Neonatal tetanus relatively common in some rural areas.
HELMINTHS. Hookworm disease (*Necator americanus, Ancylostoma duodenale*): endemic. **Cutaneous larva migrans** (*An-*

cylostoma braziliense, A. caninum): endemic. **Schistosomiasis** (*Schistosoma haematobium, S. mansoni*): highly endemic in Egypt, with an increasing prevalence of infection due to *S. mansoni*, initially limited to Nile but now also found in Upper Egypt. *S. haematobium* is endemic in Middle and Upper Egypt and in several oases in Egypt, Algeria, Tunisia, and Libya. **Strongyloidiasis** (*Strongyloides stercoralis*): endemic. **Toxocariasis** (*Toxocara canis, T. cati*): endemic.

■ SUB-SAHARAN AFRICA (Angola, Benin, Burkina Faso, Burundi, Cameroon, Cape Verde, Central African Republic, Chad, Comoros, Congo, Democratic Republic of Congo [Ex-Zaire], Djibouti, Equatorial Guinea, Eritrea, Ethiopia, Gabon, Gambia, Ghana, Guinea, Guinea-Bissau, Ivory Coast, Kenya, Liberia, Madagascar, Malawi, Mali, Mauritania, Mauritius, Mozambique, Niger, Nigeria, Réunion, Rwanda, Sao Tome and Principe, Senegal, Seychelles, Sierra Leone, Somalia, Sudan, Togo, Uganda, United Republic of Tanzania, Zambia, and Zimbabwe)

In this area, entirely within the tropics, temperature is high throughout the year but rainfall varies considerably, leading to a wide variety of vegetation. The north, with the Sahel and Sudan savannas, is essentially a hot and desert area with sparse rainfall. In the west and center, the tropical rain forest, although under severe deforestation, remains an important reservoir of wildlife as well as the moist orchard savanna north of the equator. East of the Rift Valley with its north-south chain of lakes are the wooded steppes of the Horn of Africa and the Indian Ocean coastal area. A notable exception to the relatively low elevation of the region are the highlands of Ethiopia and Kenya and the mountains and fertile hills of the Rift Valley (e.g., Rwanda, Burundi, Malawi).

The region is also characterized by its low economic development, the poor condition of its infrastructures, and, for the last 20 years, both a rapid population growth and a massive and uncontrolled urbanization. Significant areas of the region have been, or still are, sites of civil war or severe civil unrest leading to mass migration and large displaced populations. Most of the population of the region is concentrated along the Atlantic coastal area, particularly in Nigeria, and in the fertile regions of East and central Africa (e.g., Ethiopia, Kenya, Rwanda, Burundi, and Malawi).

Infectious diseases remain the leading cause of death in the region, particularly in infants and children below 5 years of age. Infectious disease–associated cancers (e.g., hepatocarcinoma, Kaposi sarcoma) and diseases such as tuberculosis represent a significant cause of mortality in adults. The disease surveillance systems in the region are poor and many cases and outbreaks of communicable diseases go unreported. The lack of proper reporting of disease occurrence precludes a definitive statement on their current prevalence. Many data and information originate from occasional reports, published research, or expert views (e.g., WHO estimates).

Diseases Primarily Transmitted by Food and Drinking Water

Enteric infections are hyperendemic in the region, often associated with malnutrition, especially in infants and young children. Of particular public health concern is the emergence of numerous antibiotic-resistant strains among enteric bacteria.

VIRUSES. Hepatitis A: natural immunity to hepatitis A is virtually universal. **Hepatitis E**: reported with particularly high prevalence and marked seasonal patterns in the Horn of Africa region (hepatitis E outbreak, Somalia, 1988; hepatitis E outbreak in military personnel, Ethiopia, 1988–1989). **Norwalk and Norwalk-like viruses**: endemic but poorly documented.

BACTERIA. Cholera (toxicogenic *Vibrio cholerae* serogroup 01): endemic and continues to spread throughout the region. All countries have reported cholera cases within the last 10 years but none has identified strains of *V. cholerae* 0139. Outbreaks and epidemics are numerous (e.g., Shaba, Democratic Republic of Congo [DRC], 1981; Mozambican refugee, Malawi, 1988; recurrent epidemic in Angola since 1987; Benin, 1991; Burundi and Zimbabwe, 1992–1993; Djibouti, 1993; Rwandan refugees, DRC, 1994; Nigeria, 1992; Senegal, 1995–1996; Chad, 1996). In 1996, there were about 80,000 cases in 26 African countries causing at least 5000 fatalities. **Botulism** *(Clostridium botulinum)*: outbreaks sporadically reported. *Clostridium perfringens* **food intoxication**: reported (type C, Uganda). **Diarrhea caused by *Aeromonas hydrophila***: rare reports (e.g., Ivory Coast) or *Edwardsiella tarda*: rare reports (Mali, Chad, DRC). **Diarrhea caused by *Campylobacter* spp.**: endemic. **Diarrhea caused by *Escherichia coli***: Enterotoxigenic *E. coli* (ETEC) is a common agent of enteritis, including outbreaks (e.g., Luanda, Angola, 1991–1993; enterohemorrhagic *E. coli* (EHEC) identified as causal agent of epidemic hemorrhagic colitis (e.g., Malawi, 1992). **Listeriosis** *(Listeria monocytogenes)*: endemic, poorly documented. **Salmonellosis**: hyperendemic with increased drug-resistant strains and frequent community outbreaks. **Shigellosis** *(Shigella* spp.): hyperendemic. Emergence of strains of *S. dysenteriae* type 1 resistant to virtually all locally available antibiotics responsible, since its first identification in 1979, for a continental epidemic (primarily East and central Africa) of severe dysentery with significant mortality (e.g., Mozambique, 1993; Burundi refugees in Rwanda, 1993–1994; similar outbreak among local residents of coastal Kenya, 1994). **Staphylococcal disease** *(Staphylococcus aureus)*: common cause of food poisoning outbreaks. **Streptococcal diseases** (group A *Streptococcus*): reports of food-borne sore throat outbreaks (e.g., Djibouti, 1993). **Typhoid** *(Salmonella typhi)* and **paratyphoid** (three bioserotypes of *S. enteritidis*): endemic.

PROTOZOA. Amebiasis *(Entamoeba histolytica)*: highly endemic. **Cryptosporidiosis** *(Cryptosporidium parvum)*: endemic, poorly documented. **Giardiasis** *(Giardia lamblia)*: hyperendemic. **Toxoplasmosis** *(Toxoplasma gondii)*: endemic.

FUNGI. Candidiasis *(Candida albicans)*: hyperendemic. **Unspecified fungi**: cause of outbreaks usually with seasonal patterns (e.g., cassava-associated outbreaks; seasonal ataxia caused by the consumption of larvae of *Anaphe venata*, southwestern Nigeria).

HELMINTHS. Angiostrongyliasis *(Angiostrongylus cantonensis)*: rare reports from Madagascar and Réunion. **Ascariasis** *(Ascaris lumbricoides)*: highly endemic throughout the region. **Dracunculiasis** *(Dracunculus medinensis)*: although rapidly disappearing from many West African traditional foci, remains important in some western foci, but more importantly in southern Sudan with outbreaks reported (e.g., Mazmum, central Sudan). **Enterobiasis** *(Enterobius vermicularis)*: hyperendemic in children. **Fascioliasis** *(Fasciola gigantica)*: endemic in some sheep-rearing areas. **Taeniasis**: beef tapeworm *(Taenia saginata)*, pork tapeworm *(Taenia solium)*: endemic, particularly in Ethiopia. Cysticercosis is common. **Trichinellosis** *(Trichinella spiralis* spp.): frequent. **Trichuriasis** *(Trichuris trichiura)*: endemic.

OTHER. Paragonimiasis *(Paragonimus africanus, P. uterobilateralis)*: reported from Cameroon, Gabon, Nigeria and recently in equatorial Guinea; very rare elsewhere (e.g., Liberia, Guinea).

Diseases Primarily Transmitted by Close Contact With Infectious Individuals

VIRUSES. Acute viral respiratory infections are frequent and are an important cause of death in children below 5 years of age. **Chickenpox** and **herpes zoster**: endemic. **Coxsackievirus**: occasional outbreaks of acute hemorrhagic conjunctivitis, usually seasonal (e.g., coxsackievirus A24, Ghana, 1987). **Influenza** (influenza virus types A, B, and C): endemic. **Measles**: a severe disease of infants and young children with significant mortality rate and recurrent outbreaks throughout the continent, particularly in large cities (e.g., N'Djamena, Chad, 1993). **Mumps**: endemic. **Poliomyelitis**: Although poliomyelitis prevalence has significantly decreased in the region, it remains endemic at a low level in most countries; outbreaks of poliomyelitis are reported from time to time (e.g., Gambia, 1986; DRC and Zambia, 1995). Most of the reported cases originate from Ethiopia, Kenya, and Nigeria with eastern African countries reporting only a few cases (in 1992, zero cases reported from Rwanda, Malawi, Tanzania, Zimbabwe). **Rotavirus**: hyperendemic. A major cause of severe diarrhea in young children. **Rubella**: endemic.

BACTERIA. Acute bacterial conjunctivitis *(Haemophilus influenzae)*: endemic. **Diphtheria** *(Corynebacterium diphtheriae)*: endemic throughout the region, involving primarily young children. **Leprosy** *(Mycobacterium leprae)*: Although still endemic throughout the region, there has been a sharp overall reduction in the number of registered cases during the last 10 years. In 1995, the detection rate of leprosy cases was still above 10 per 100,000 in Benin, Central African Republic, Chad, Ivory Coast, Gabon, Guinea, Madagascar, Mali, Mauritius, Mozambique, Niger, Sierra Leone, and DRC. **Meningococcal meningitis** *(Neisseria meningitidis)*: periodic epidemics in the meningitis belt area, which seem to occur more frequently, and in new areas (e.g., Burundi, Malawi, Kenya, Tanzania, Uganda, DRC, Zambia, 1996); the 1996 epidemics have been the most severe causing more than 150,000 cases, including more than 16,000 deaths; most affected countries were Nigeria and Burkina Faso but also Niger, Mali, and Chad. The epidemic resurged in early 1997. **Pertussis** *(Bordetella pertussis)*: endemic. **Pneumonia caused by *Streptococcus pneumoniae***: endemic. **Streptococcal diseases** (group A *Streptococcus*): endemic. **Tuberculosis** *(Mycobacterium tuberculosis)*: endemic throughout the region. Tuberculosis incidence has increased in most countries, partly associated with the AIDS epidemics, with the highest prevalence in the Horn of Africa (e.g., Somalia, Ethiopia). Lack of patient compliance has led to an increasing report of multidrug-resistant strains of *M. tuberculosis*. **Yaws** *(Treponema pallidum* subspecies *pertenue)*: has resurfaced in the north and parts of equatorial and western areas.

ECTOPARASITES. Pediculosis *(Pediculus humanus capitis)*: very common. **Scabies** *(Sarcoptes scabiei)*: very common.

Sexually Transmitted Diseases

The past 15 years have seen a significant increase in STDs in most cities, particularly among women and the poor.

VIRUSES. Hepatitis B: hyperendemic. High incidence of associated liver cancer. **Hepatitis C**: endemic. **HIV infection**: endemic with highest prevalence in urban centers and central-east Africa (e.g., Kenya, Rwanda, Uganda, DRC). Despite continuous spread in most African countries, recent evidence suggests, since 1990, a decline in HIV infection in countries that first suffered from the AIDS pandemic (e.g., Uganda). **Herpes simplex virus (HSV-2)**: endemic. **Papillomavirus**: endemic.

BACTERIA. Chancroid *(Haemophilus ducreyi)*: endemic. **Gonococcal infection** *(Neisseria gonorrhoeae)*: high endemicity.

Emergence of *N. gonorrhoeae* strains resistant to multiple antibiotics (e.g., Djibouti, DRC). Outbreaks of *N. gonorrhoeae* conjunctivitis also reported (e.g., North Omo district, Ethiopia, 1987–1988). **Syphilis** *(Treponema pallidum)*: common, including congenital syphilis. **Chlamydia: Chlamydia infections** *(Chlamydia trachomatis)*: urethral infection very common. **Lymphogranuloma venereum** frequent.

FUNGI. Candidiasis *(Candida albicans)*: hyperendemic.

ECTOPARASITES. Phthiriasis *(Phthirus pubis)*: very common.

Nosocomial Infections

Nosocomial infections are thought to be extremely common and largely underreported.

VIRUSES. Blood-borne pathogens including **HIV, HBV, HCV,** and since 1976, **Ebola** virus (e.g., Yambuku, DRC, 1976; Kikwit, DRC, 1995; Gabon and South Africa, 1996). Hospital person-to-person transmission of **Lassa fever** also reported.

BACTERIA. Tuberculosis and **enteric agents** thought to be common. Multidrug-resistant **enteropathogenic *E. coli* (EPEC)** (e.g., neonates, Nairobi, Kenya). Multidrug-resistant *Klebsiella pneumoniae* (e.g., Addis Ababa, Ethiopia, 1990; neonatal septicemia, Ibadan, Nigeria, 1991; intravenous cannula–associated septicemia, Kilifi district hospital, Kenya, 1992). *Pneumococcus* **meningitis** (hospital outbreak, DRC, 1996).

FUNGI. *Candida albicans*: common.

Human Zoonoses and Vector-Borne Diseases, Including Viral Hemorrhagic Fever

Diseases Transmitted by Close Contact With Animals or Animal Products

VIRUSES. Lassa fever: endemic in West Africa (e.g., Guinea, Liberia, Nigeria, Sierra Leone) with sporadic outbreaks (e.g., Sierra Leone, 1996); about 100,000 cases, including 5000 fatalities, are estimated to occur each year in the region. **Monkeypox**: rare human cases, sporadic in rain forest areas. Outbreak reported in DRC (oriental kasai) in summer 1996. **Rabies**: endemic throughout the region, stray dogs being the main animal reservoir.

BACTERIA. Anthrax *(Bacillus anthracis)*: endemic in animals particularly in the west and north, with rare human outbreaks (e.g., Pecixe Island, Guinea Bissau). **Brucellosis** *(Brucella abortus, B. melitensis)*: endemic, especially in the east. **Leptospirosis** *(Leptospira interrogans)*: endemic. **Q fever** *(Coxiella burnetii)*: endemic. **Rat-bite fever** *(Streptobacillus moniliformis)*: occasionally reported. **Chlamydia. Psittacosis** *(Chlamydia psittaci)*: rare reports. **Rickettsia: Murine typhus** *(Rickettsia mooseri)*: rare, foci along the west coast from Nigeria to Senegal.

CESTODES. Echinococcosis: widespread in animal-breeding areas (e.g., Turkana region, Kenya).

Flea-Borne

BACTERIA. Plague *(Yersinia pestis)*: wild foci in central and eastern parts of the region (e.g., Angola, Malawi, Kenya, Madagascar, Mozambique, Tanzania, Uganda, Zimbabwe, DRC), including urban areas where it has become a serious public health threat (e.g., Antananarivo, Madagascar, 1995). Outbreaks of bubonic plague recently reported (e.g., Tanzania, 1991; DRC, 1992; Mozambique, 1995; Zambia, 1996–1997).

Fly-Borne

Myiasis is common and flies play a role in the transmission of enteric agents (e.g., *Shigella*).

PROTOZOA. African trypanosomiasis: *Trypanosoma brucei gambiense*; endemic foci classically found from Senegal to eastern DRC and northern Uganda; *T. brucei rhodesiense* foci in Uganda, Kenya, Tanzania, Rwanda, Burundi, and Zambia. Today poorly documented despite its recurrence in many areas (e.g., *T. brucei gambiense* in Nigeria, Uganda, Ivory Coast). Epidemics occasionally reported (e.g., DRC, southeastern Uganda). Transmission rate high in southern Sudan, Uganda, Angola, and DRC.

HELMINTHS. Onchocerciasis *(Onchocera volvulus)*: endemic areas in West Africa along the Volta River basin, additional foci in Ethiopia, Angola, and Malawi. Sharp decrease in incidence (specific regional control program). **Loiasis** *(Loa loa)*: endemic in the Congo River basin (e.g., Gabon, Angola, DRC).

Louse-Borne

BACTERIA. Relapsing fever *(Borrelia recurrentis)*: reported from Ethiopian (e.g., Jimma, 1991) and Kenyan highlands and occasional outbreaks in refugee camps in the east (e.g., transit camp for prisoners of war, Ethiopia, 1991; Sudan, 1994). **Trench fever** *(Bartonella quintana)*: endemic foci in Ethiopia and Burundi. **Rickettsia: Epidemic typhus** *(Rickettsia prowazekii)*: persists in the mountainous areas of Ethiopia and much of northeastern and central Africa. Epidemic typhus also reported from Nigeria; additional cases recognized in Kenya, Gambia, Gabon, Angola, Zambia, Zimbabwe, Rwanda, and Burundi. In 1996–1997, a large outbreak occurred among refugees in Burundi in the provinces of Bujumbura, Gitega, Kayanza, Muramvya, and Ngozi.

Mosquito-Borne

VIRUSES. Dengue fever: dengue (primarily dengue 2 virus) reached East Africa in the early 1980s (e.g., Kenya, 1982) and has continued to spread, particularly along the Indian Ocean and the Red Sea (e.g., dengue 2 epidemic, Djibouti, 1991; dengue 1, Grand Comoro Island, 1993; Somalia, coastal Kenya, 1985) without outbreak of dengue hemorrhagic fever although it has become a serious threat. In West Africa, the presence of dengue 2 has been documented in mosquitoes (e.g., Senegal, 1990). **O'Nyong-nyong fever**: rare reports from East Africa (e.g., Uganda, Kenya, Tanzania, southern Sudan). **Rift Valley fever**: globally spreading in the region with outbreaks increasingly reported since the 1987 Mauritanian outbreak (Mauritania, Senegal, Madagascar). **Sindbis** and **West Nile**: common in East Africa. **Yellow fever**: rapidly re-emerging as a major public health concern since the early 1990s. In 1994, Nigeria reported 91% of all African cases. Outbreaks increasingly reported (e.g., Ethiopia, 1961–1962; Cameroon, 1990 and 1994; Kenya, 1992–1993, which was its first outbreak in 26 years; Ghana 1992–1994; Senegal, 1995 and 1996; Gabon, 1994, and Liberia, 1995, although both countries had not reported any cases since 1950; Sierra Leone, 1995; Benin, 1996).

PROTOZOA. Malaria *(Plasmodium falciparum, P. vivax, P. malariae)*: falciparum malaria is endemic through most of the region with different transmission patterns. It is responsible for an important mortality in infants and young children; its incidence is increasing in areas of normally low risk and malaria has recently spread to areas of usually low endemicity leading to severe epidemics (e.g., Balcad, Somalia, 1986–1988; Burundi highlands, 1990–1991; southern Madagascar outbreak, 1994) including many urban areas, particularly the suburbs of rapidly growing cities (e.g., Djibouti). There has been increased reports of malaria cases from the East Africa highlands (e.g., falciparum malaria epidemics in Kenya highlands, 1990; local transmission of falciparum malaria reported in Addis Ababa, Ethiopia; malaria epidemic in the central highlands of Madagascar, 1987). Resistance to chloroquine has been reported virtually from all countries since the initial reports from East Africa in the 1980s but is not yet a real public health problem in the west and south. *P. vivax*, the second malaria species in the region, is rare in West and central Africa but is endemic in East Africa. *P. ovale* and *P. malariae* are present but less often reported. No endemic falciparum malaria reported from the islands of Mauritius and Réunion.

Phlebotomine-Borne

PROTOZOA. Cutaneous leishmaniasis *(Leishmania major, L. aethiopica)*: uncommon in most of the region (e.g., West and central Africa, foci of *L. major*), more frequent in East Africa where there are foci of *L. aethiopica* (Ethiopia, Eritrea, Sudan, Kenya) with rare reports of outbreaks (e.g., Khartoum, Sudan, 1985–1986). **Visceral leishmaniasis** *(L. infantum* complex, *L. donovani)*: low endemicity but significant recrudescence in East Africa, particularly in eastern and southern Sudan where a large kala-azar epidemic has been recognized since 1991.

Tick-Borne

VIRUSES. Crimean-Congo hemorrhagic fever: central and East Africa. **Bhanja, Dhori, Dugbe Nairobi sheep disease, Quaranfil, Thogoto** (e.g., Kenya). **BACTERIA. Tick-borne relapsing fever** (various strains): uncommon but endemic throughout the region. **Tularemia** *(Francisella tularensis)*: rare reports from West Africa (e.g., Cameroon). **Rickettsia: African tick typhus** *(Rickettsia conorii)*: endemic in the east.

Unknown Animal Vectors

VIRUSES. Ebola hemorrhagic fever: first recognized during the 1976–1977 epidemics in southern Sudan and northern DRC and since rarely reported (Sudan, 1979) until recently (e.g., Ivory Coast, 1994–1995; DRC, 1995; Gabon, 1995–1996) including a major epidemic in the city of Kikwit, DRC, 1995. **Marburg virus** isolated from monkeys from Uganda, 1967; and human cases from Zimbabwe and Kenya.

Soil-Borne or Airborne Diseases, and Diseases Associated With Recreational Water With No Evidence of Direct Animal-to-Human or Direct Person-to-Person Transmission

BACTERIA. Melioidosis *(Pseudomonas pseudomallei)*: rare. Reported from Ivory Coast, Chad, Burkina Faso, Madagascar. **Tetanus** *(Clostridium tetani)*: Neonatal tetanus incidence has dramatically decreased in most regions but remains endemic throughout Africa. **Chlamydia: Trachoma** *(Chlamydia trachomatis)*: endemic in dry desert areas.
FUNGI. African histoplasmosis *(Histoplasma duboisii)*: rare, primarily found in the rain forest areas (Cameroon, Congo, DRC but also reported from the east (e.g., Uganda, Madagascar). **Blastomycosis** *(Blastomyces dermatitidis)*: sporadic cases (e.g., DRC, Tanzania). **Chromomycosis** (several species): rare but particularly high prevalence in Madagascar *(Fonsecaea pedrosoi* in forest areas and *Cladophialophora carrionii* in desert areas), which represents the most important focus of this fungal disease in the world. **Mycetoma** (several species): rare. Madura foot primarily reported from Ethiopia and Somalia. **Rhinoentomophthoromycosis**: rare reports (e.g., Nigeria, Cameroon).
HELMINTHS. Hookworm disease *(Necator americanus, Ancylostoma duodenale)*: highly endemic. **Schistosomiasis** *(Schistosoma haematobium, S. mansoni)*: endemic in foci throughout

the region. *S. mansoni* is globally spreading, particularly with the development of large irrigation projects (e.g., large epidemic of intestinal schistosomiasis, Senegal River Basin, 1988). Outbreaks also reported among nonimmune individuals (e.g., resettlers in Nigeria, 1988–1989; travelers returning from Mali, 1992). **Strongyloidiasis** *(Strongyloides stercoralis, S. fulleborni)*: endemic in the rain forest area and other foci in the east (e.g., Ethiopia, eastern Rwanda, Zambia, Zimbabwe). **Visceral larva migrans**: endemic.
ECTOPARASITES. Jiggers *(Tunga penetrans)*: endemic in West and East Africa.

■ SOUTHERN AFRICA (Botswana, Lesotho, Namibia, Saint Helena, South Africa, Swaziland)

The southern tip of Africa varies physically from the Namib and Kalahari deserts to fertile plateaus and plains and to the more temperate climate of the southern coast. The climate is temperate and the economic development more advanced than in other sub-Saharan African countries. The region enjoyed modern and reliable infrastructure, particularly in the South African Republic. The population includes significant minorities of European and Indian descent. The prevalence of infectious diseases is higher among the poorer black communities. The region is experiencing a significant increase in economic migrants from the north, especially South Africa since the end of its apartheid isolation.

With the exception of zoonoses and vector-borne diseases, the epidemiologic situation of infectious diseases in southern Africa is similar to the other sub-Saharan countries. Only information specific to the region or notably different is mentioned.

Diseases Primarily Transmitted by Food and Drinking Water

VIRUSES. Coxsackievirus: outbreaks reported (e.g., South Africa, 1984). **Hepatitis A** and **E**: limited outbreaks reported in South Africa.
BACTERIA. Cholera (toxinogenic *Vibrio cholerae* serogroup 01): cholera epidemic in South Africa, 1980–1987, and recent cholera outbreaks (e.g., Zululand, 1993). **Diarrhea caused by** *Escherichia coli*: water-borne hemorrhagic colitis epidemic caused by *E. coli* 0157 in Swaziland and South Africa, 1992. **Shigellosis** *(Shigella* spp.): epidemic. *Shigella dysenteriae* type 1, first isolated in 1994 in South Africa, has now spread and caused outbreaks in Natal. **Typhoid** *(Salmonella typhi)* and **paratyphoid** (three bioserotypes of *S. enteritidis)*: remain endemic in many parts of the region, including South Africa; multiresistant strains of *S. typhi* identified (e.g., typhoid outbreak, Natal, South Africa, 1991).
PROTOZOA. Amebiasis *(Entamoeba histolytica)*: lower endemicity but outbreaks recently reported in normally nonendemic areas (e.g., Cape Town area, South Africa).
HELMINTHS. Pork tapeworm *(Taenia solium)*: frequent, including cysticercosis, particularly in South Africa. **Dracunculiasis** *(Dracunculus medinensis)*: absent.

Diseases Primarily Transmitted by Close Contact With Infectious Individuals

VIRUSES. Measles: incidence has decreased in the region but outbreaks still reported (e.g., South Africa, 1992 epidemic). **Poliomyelitis**: since the Natal/Kwazulu 1987–1988 outbreak and the last confirmed case in Namibia, 1988, poliomyelitis has actually re-emerged in the region (e.g., outbreak in Namibia, 1993–1994).

BACTERIA. Diphtheria (*Corynebacterium diphtheriae*): rare, but epidemic reported (Lesotho, 1989). **Leprosy** (*Mycobacterium leprae*): rare endemic foci (e.g., South Africa). **Meningococcal meningitis** (*Neisseria meningitidis*): endemic, limited outbreaks. **Pertussis** (*Bordetella pertussis*): outbreaks reported (e.g., Cape Town, 1988–1989). **Pneumonia caused by Streptococcus pneumoniae**: endemic. **Streptococcal diseases** (group A *Streptococcus*): endemic. **Tuberculosis** (*Mycobacterium tuberculosis*): endemic, primarily among the poor and AIDS patients.

Sexually Transmitted Diseases

Situation similar to the other sub-Saharan countries, particularly among the poorer black communities.

Nosocomial Infections

Certainly underreported.
VIRUSES. Outbreak of hepatitis A among hemophiliacs (South Africa).
BACTERIA. Outbreak of septicemia caused by *Serratia odorifera* associated with contaminated intravenous parenteral nutrition (Johannesburg, South Africa, 1992).

Human Zoonoses and Vector-Borne Diseases, Including Viral Hemorrhagic Fevers

Diseases Transmitted by Close Contact With Animals or Animal Products

VIRUSES. Rabies: has recently become endemic in the entire region since it spread from Natal to Lesotho in 1982 and reached the Ciskei by 1990. Rabies-related viruses (i.e., Lagos bat, Mokola, Duvenhage) identified in Zimbabwe.
BACTERIA. Anthrax (*Bacillus anthracis*): rare. **Brucellosis** (*Brucella abortus, B. melitensis*): endemic. **Leptospirosis** (*Leptospira interrogans*): endemic. **Q fever** (*Coxiella burnetii*): endemic, particularly South Africa. **Chlamydia: Psittacosis** (*Chlamydia psittaci*): rare reports.

Flea-Borne

BACTERIA. Plague (*Yersinia pestis*): Wild foci (e.g., Namibia, South Africa); epidemics reported (Botswana, 1989–1990).

Fly-Borne

PROTOZOA. African trypanosomiasis (*Trypanosoma brucei rhodesiense*): endemic foci in northern Botswana and northeastern Namibia.

Louse-Borne

Rickettsia: Epidemic typhus (*Rickettsia prowazekii*): rare reports (e.g., South Africa).

Mosquito-Borne

VIRUSES. Dengue fever: imported cases. **Rift Valley fever:** endemic (e.g., eastern South Africa, eastern Namibia, northern Botswana). **West Nile fever:** endemic, rare outbreaks. **Yellow fever:** imported cases.
PROTOZOA. Malaria (*Plasmodium falciparum, P. vivax*): *P. falciparum* is the predominant species. Malaria transmission is generally seasonal and limited to endemic foci (e.g., lowlands of the Northern Providence, Eastern Transvaal, northeastern Kwazulu/Natal in South Africa; northern region and along the Kavango River in Namibia; northern Botswana; low veld areas of Swaziland). Epidemics occur (e.g., Natal, Zululand). Resistance to chloroquine reported.

Tick-Borne

VIRUSES. Crimean-Congo hemorrhagic fever: occasional outbreaks (e.g., Namibia, South Africa, 1996).

BACTERIA. Tick-borne relapsing fever (various strains): rare. **Rickettsia: African tick typhus** (*Rickettsia conorii*): endemic.

Unknown Animal Vectors

VIRUSES. Ebola and Marburg hemorrhagic fevers: exceptional imported cases (e.g., Marburg, South Africa, 1975; Ebola, South Africa, 1996).

Soil-Borne or Airborne Diseases, and Diseases Associated With Recreational Water With No Evidence of Direct Animal-to-Human or Direct Person-to-Person Transmission

BACTERIA. Legionellosis (*Legionella*): reported (e.g., South Africa). **Melioidosis** (*Pseudomonas pseudomallei*): rare. **Tetanus** (*Clostridium tetani*): endemic.
HELMINTHS. Hookworm disease (*Necator americanus, Ancylostoma duodenale*): endemic. **Schistosomiasis** (*Schistosoma haematobium, S. mansoni*): endemic foci in Botswana, Namibia, South Africa, and Swaziland. **Strongyloidiasis** (*Strongyloides stercoralis, S. fulleborni*): rare. **Visceral larva migrans**: endemic (e.g., South Africa).

■ NORTHERN EUROPE (Belarus, Belgium, Czech Republic, Denmark and Faroe Islands, Estonia, Finland, Germany, Iceland, Ireland, Latvia, Lithuania, Luxembourg, Netherlands, Norway, Poland, Republic of Moldova, Russian Federation, Slovakia, Sweden, Ukraine, and the United Kingdom (United Kingdom) Including the Channel Islands and the Isle of Man)

This large region includes the temperate maritime areas of the west, the mixed forests and plains of central Europe, the subarctic conditions of the far north, the steppes of the Russian Federation and the Ukraine, the tundras of Siberia, and finally the Pacific coast.

Economic development varies widely in the region with the western countries having highly developed economies and sophisticated health infrastructure. The collapse of communism in Eastern Europe and the former Soviet Union has led to economic hardship in many countries and significant deterioration in public health in some areas. Diseases related to the increasing intensification of food production are on the rise as are hospital-acquired infections. Diseases continue to be imported by returning travelers and immigrants.

Diseases Primarily Transmitted by Food and Drinking Water

Food- and drinking water–related diseases are common and reflect the pattern in North America.
VIRUSES. Hepatitis A: endemic, more common in eastern countries. Outbreaks reported from western countries (Germany, Belgium, United Kingdom, Ireland, the Netherlands). **Enteroviruses:** common. **Small round structured virus (SRSV):** increasingly recognized as a cause of sporadic disease and outbreaks.
BACTERIA. Cholera: imported cases in western and northern areas. Re-emergence in Ukraine (large outbreak, 1994), the southern part of the Russian Federation (e.g., Autonomous Republic of Dagestan, 1994), and the Republic of Moldova (e.g., 240 cases reported in 1995). *Campylobacter*: a frequent cause of sporadic gastroenteritis that is increasing as a public health problem (e.g., United Kingdom, 1992–1994). **Enterohemorrhagic** *Escherichia coli* **(EHEC) and verotoxin-**

producing *E. coli* (VTEC): increasingly important causes of diarrhea, especially in young children. Hemolytic-uremic syndrome reported in association with various serogroups, mainly *E. coli* 0157 (e.g., outbreaks in United Kingdom and Germany). Increase in VTEC incidence also noted, particularly in the United Kingdom. **Listeriosis**: reported from United Kingdom and Sweden. **Salmonellosis**: common cause of sporadic food-borne gastroenteritis as well as outbreaks. Huge increases in incidence (e.g., United Kingdom, Germany, Czech Republic) involving many *Salmonella* serotypes (e.g., *S. enteritidis, S. typhimurium*). Increase in *S. enteritidis* mainly due to *S. enteritidis* PT4; antibiotic-resistant strains of *S. typhimurium* DT104 have also emerged (e.g., United Kingdom) probably because of the use of antibiotics in farm animals. Large outbreaks increasingly reported (e.g., nationwide outbreak, Germany, 1993). **Shigella**: common. Pattern of infection in western countries has changed from an endemic situation to periodic outbreaks (e.g., Manchester, 1991–1992). **Streptococcus group A**: two food-borne outbreaks reported from Sweden in 1992; nationwide outbreaks (*S. pyogenes* group A, m1) in Norway, 1987–1988 and 1992. **Typhoid and paratyphoid fevers**: decreasing incidence in the area but still a problem in eastern countries. Small family outbreaks reported in immigrant families (e.g., United Kingdom, Norway). **Yersiniosis** (*Yersinia* spp.): commonly reported cause of gastroenteritis.

PROTOZOA. Cryptosporidium: increasingly recognized gastrointestinal infection in the general population especially in immunocompromised individuals (over 14,000 laboratory reports in England and Wales, 1992–1994). Water-borne outbreaks also reported (e.g., United Kingdom).

Diseases Transmitted by Close Contact With Infectious Individuals

Epidemiology in Western Europe is similar to that of North America.

VIRUSES. Acute viral conjunctivitis: reported in outbreaks throughout the area. Mainly due to adenoviruses and coxsackieviruses. **Parvovirus B19**: emerging infectious disease causing a febrile illness with rash and occasionally reported to cause arthralgia, aplastic anemia, or fetal loss. Outbreaks reported from the United Kingdom and Sweden. **Influenza**: winter epidemics are a major cause of morbidity especially among the elderly across the region. **Measles**: decreasing incidence due to high vaccine coverage. Outbreaks continue to occur even in adequately vaccinated populations due to the accumulation of susceptible individuals (e.g., Scotland, 1993). Viral transmission has been interrupted in England and Wales after mass vaccination of all children in 1994. **Rubella**: outbreaks reported in young adult males especially in universities and military units. Congenital rubella now rare. **Poliovirus**: rare infection due to high vaccination coverage; few notable outbreaks (Finland, 1984–1985; religious community, Netherlands, 1992–1993; Chechnya, 1995). **Respiratory syncytial virus (RSV)**: causes large winter epidemics (bronchiolitis) among young children each winter. Major cause of childhood morbidity.

BACTERIA. Diphtheria: incidence of toxigenic diphtheria is very low due to high vaccination coverage. A large outbreak occurred in the Russian Federation and the Ukraine and spread into neighboring countries due to falling vaccine coverage. Incidence of nontoxigenic disease appears to be increasing across the region. **Leprosy** (*Mycobacterium leprae*): imported disease only. **Meningococcal meningitis** (*Neisseria meningitidis*): sporadic disease with occasional epidemics. **Pertussis** (*Bordetella pertussis*): disease incidence has decreased gradually due to vaccination. However, vaccine cov-

erage varies widely and some countries have experienced increased incidence (Sweden). **Pneumonia caused by *Streptococcus pneumoniae***: rarely isolated but probably a common cause of community-acquired pneumonia. **Pneumonia caused by *Chlamydia pneumoniae***: reported as a cause of community-acquired pneumonia and in outbreaks from Finland. Outbreak also reported in 1995 from the United Kingdom. **Streptococcal disease** (group A *Streptococcus*): endemic. Invasive disease is rarely reported outside the health care setting. Outbreaks are occasionally reported from institutions such as schools. **Tuberculosis**: wide variation in incidence rates across the region. After decades of decline, resurgence in the late 1980s and early 1990s with occasional outbreaks (e.g., Kullorsuaq, Greenland, 1994) linked to increasing numbers of people in high-risk groups (e.g., homeless, HIV positives, immigrants, intravenous drug users). Although the situation is now improving in western countries, eastern countries and the Russian Federation are still facing significant problems with tuberculosis control, particularly in the Siberian region.

ECTOPARASITES. Pediculosis (*Pediculus humanus capitis*): common. **Scabies** (*Sarcoptes scabiei*): common.

Sexually Transmitted Diseases

Similar disease epidemiology to that of North America. Incidence of STDs has generally fallen probably in response to safer sexual practices in response to the HIV epidemic.

VIRUSES. Hepatitis B: endemic, highly prevalent among intravenous drug users. A number of outbreaks related to health care workers have been reported from the United Kingdom (12 between 1970 and 1990). **Hepatitis C**: endemic. Recent problems related to parenteral administration of contaminated immunoglobulin to prevent Rh sensitization after pregnancy have been reported from Germany and Ireland. **HIV infection**: endemic and increasing. **Herpes simplex virus (HSV-1 and HSV-2)**: endemic. **Papillomavirus**: endemic.

BACTERIA. Gonococcal infection (*Neisseria gonorrhoeae*): highly endemic. **Syphilis** (*Treponema pallidum*): falling incidence. **Chlamydia: Chlamydial infections** (*Chlamydia trachomatis*): common.

FUNGI. Candidiasis (*Candida albicans*): common.

Nosocomial Infections

Similar disease epidemiology to that of North America. The main concerns are the increase in methicillin-resistant *Staphylococcus aureus* in health care settings. In addition, the increasing sophistication of medical interventions has led to a number of outbreaks related to medical equipment and instrumentation. Those most at risk are the immunocompromised who represent a growing proportion of inpatients across the region.

BACTERIA. *Acinetobacter* infection: outbreak of multiresistant infection reported in 1995 from an intensive care unit (ICU) in the United Kingdom. *Clostridium difficile*: an increasingly common infection especially among hospitalized elderly patients in Europe. Mainly due to use of oral antibiotics. A large outbreak involving three hospitals in Manchester, England, occurred in 1991–1992. *Haemophilus influenzae*: outbreak of amoxicillin-resistant infection in a respiratory ward reported from the Netherlands in 1991. *Klebsiella oxytoca*: outbreak of septicemia related to invasive blood pressure monitoring equipment reported from Sweden in 1992. **Methicillin-resistant *Staphylococcus aureus* (MRSA)** is an increasingly important problem. Endemic in many hospitals across the area. Outbreaks reported from Austria, United Kingdom, Germany, Ireland, and the Netherlands. **Pneumococcus**: outbreak of penicillin-resistant infection in a respiratory ward in the Netherlands reported in 1994. *Pseudomonas* *aeruginosa*: two outbreaks have been reported from Denmark among immunocompromised patients related to contamination of fiberoptic equipment (reported 1994) and irrigation tubing (reported 1993); an outbreak reported from Northern Ireland in an ICU (1993). *Serratia marcescens*: outbreak ascribed to contaminated blood transfusion bags in Denmark reported in 1993; outbreak associated with a contaminated bronchoscope in an ICU in the Netherlands in 1993. **Invasive group A streptococcal** nosocomial infections: rising incidence in Scandinavian countries. Outbreak in a nursing home reported from the United Kingdom in 1995. **Multidrug-resistant tuberculosis**: an outbreak of hospital-acquired infection was reported from an HIV unit in London in 1995. **Vancomycin-resistant enterococci (VRE)**: increasingly recognized problem in the United Kingdom; 500 isolates from 44 hospitals in the United Kingdom between 1987 and 1994.

PROTOZOA. *Cryptosporidium*: nosocomial infections among immunocompromised patients have been reported (e.g., outbreak reported in AIDS patients from Denmark, 1990).

Human Zoonoses and Vector-Borne Diseases, Including Viral Hemorrhagic Fevers

Diseases Transmitted by Close Contact With Animals or Animal Products

VIRUSES. Hantavirus: Serologic evidence of infection throughout most of the region; hemorrhagic fever with renal syndrome reported from Europe west of the Urals. Cases reported from Belgium, Holland, Germany, and the Russian Federation. **Orf virus disease**: reported in man and reindeer in Finland. **Rabies**: animal rabies endemic (mainly foxes), except for the United Kingdom and Ireland. Human rabies cases reported from the Russian Federation (seven in 1994).

BACTERIA. Anthrax *(Bacillus anthracis)*: endemic in eastern countries. **Brucellosis** *(Brucella abortus, B. melitensis, B. suis)*: endemic. Mainly an occupational disease related to animal husbandry or slaughter. **Cat-scratch disease** *(Bartonella henselae)*: rare. **Leptospirosis**: endemic. **Chlamydia: Psittacosis** *(Chlamydia psittaci)*: endemic. **Rickettsia: Q fever** *(Coxiella burnetii)*: endemic. Outbreaks reported from the United Kingdom and Germany. **Murine typhus** *(Rickettsia typhi)*: rare.

Mosquito-Borne

VIRUSES. Snowshoe hare encephalitis *(Bunyavirus)*: rare reports (e.g., Russian Federation).

Tick-Borne

VIRUSES. Louping ill: rare. Occurs mainly in United Kingdom and Ireland. **Crimean-Congo hemorrhagic fever**: reported from Crimea in the Ukraine and the Astrakhan region of Russia (June to September). Most cases are animal husbandry workers or medical personnel. **Omsk hemorrhagic fever virus**: rare reports (e.g., forest steppe regions of western Siberia), seasonal. **Powassan virus encephalitis**: rare reports (e.g., Russian Federation). **Tick-borne encephalitis**: constitute the most important viral *(Flavivirus)* infection of the central nervous system in central Europe since its clinical description in 1934. Sporadic reports of two subtypes: the central European subtype mainly in forested areas of central Europe, and the Far Eastern subtype in the Asian part of the Russian Federation (Russian spring-summer encephalitis).

BACTERIA. Lyme disease *(Borrelia burgdorferi)*: endemic in forest areas (in Scandinavia, the British Isles, western and central Europe, the Balkans and Russia) having the tick vectors.

Soil-Borne or Airborne Diseases, and Diseases Associated With Recreational Water With No Evidence of Direct Animal-to-Human or Direct Person-to-Person Transmission

VIRUSES. Lymphocytic choriomeningitis virus *(Arenavirus)*: rarely reported but probably underdiagnosed.

BACTERIA. Legionnaires' disease: outbreaks reported from Germany, UK, Netherlands, Sweden, and the Russian Federation.

Diseases of Unknown Route of Transmission

Creutzfeldt-Jakob disease (prions): very rare in all countries but new variant identified since 1995 (18 in UK and one in France, as of June 1997) and suspected to be linked to bovine spongiform encephalopathy.

■ SOUTHERN EUROPE (Albania, Andorra, Austria, Bosnia and Herzegovina, Bulgaria, Croatia, France, Gibraltar, Greece, Hungary, Italy, Liechtenstein, Malta, Monaco, Portugal, including Azores and Madeira, Romania, San Marino, Slovenia, Spain and the Canary Islands, Switzerland, the former Yugoslav Republic of Macedonia, and Yugoslavia)

This is a temperate and relatively fertile area with broadleaf forests and a part of the southern Alps in the northwest, the Pyrenees and the plateaus of the Iberian Peninsula in the southwest, and, in the southeast, Italy and the mountains of the Balkans. Rainfall is evenly distributed throughout the year. The vegetation ranges from the forest and prairies of France and northern Italy to the scrub vegetation of the Mediterranean.

Although the population is widely scattered in the region, it is significantly concentrated in large urban areas (e.g., Paris, Lyon, Milan, Turin, Madrid, Barcelona, Athens) and along most of the coastal areas. Economic development and infrastructure is generally good throughout the region but varies from well-developed France and northern Italy to the poorly industrialized Albania; since 1989, the war has destroyed most of the health infrastructure in former Yugoslavia.

Diseases Primarily Transmitted by Food and Drinking Water

Globally increasing in the region, particularly in the newly independent states of southeastern Europe.

VIRUSES. Enterovirus: occasional outbreaks (e.g., ECHO 9 meningitis, 1993, Burgos, Spain; coxsackievirus B5 meningitis, Cyprus, 1996). **Hepatitis A**: endemic with an incidence of icteric hepatitis A in adults and an increased prevalence in the poorer eastern and southern countries (e.g., Albania, Bulgaria). Epidemics now rare but more extensive (e.g., France, 1992; hemophiliac patients, Italy, 1989–1992; Genoa, Italy, 1993). **Hepatitis E**: primarily imported cases. **Norwalk and Norwalk-like viruses**: endemic. Rare outbreaks (e.g., Spain, 1989). **Rotavirus**: endemic. Epidemics responsible for gastroenteritis in elderly community more frequently reported (e.g., France).

BACTERIA. Cholera (toxinogenic *Vibrio cholerae* serogroup 01): imported cases only. **Botulism** *(Clostridium botulinum)*: rare reports. **Diarrhea caused by** *Campylobacter jejuni*: endemic, outbreaks reported (e.g., Spain). **Diarrhea caused by** *Escherichia coli*: enterotoxigenic *E. coli* (ETEC): endemic, occasional outbreaks (e.g., military ship, former Yugoslavia). Significant outbreaks reported (e.g., associated with non-0157 verotoxin-producing *E. coli*, e.g., Italy, 1992; hemolytic-uremic syndrome in children associated with *E. coli* 0157, northern Italy). **Listeriosis** *(Listeria monocytogenes)*: endemic. Outbreaks not uncommon (e.g., nationwide, France, 1992; Grand Canary, Spain, 1991–1993; Valencia, Spain, 1989). **Salmonellosis**: endemic, limited outbreaks frequent throughout the region (e.g., *S. enteritidis*, Spain; Tenerife, flight passengers, 1991, Greece). **Shigellosis** *(Shigella* spp.): endemic; outbreaks not uncommon, particularly in the south (e.g., *S. sonnei*, Spain, 1991). **Staphylococcal disease** *(Staphylococcus aureus)*: rare reports of food-borne poisoning. **Streptococcal diseases** (group A *Streptococcus*): rare outbreaks of group A food-borne streptococcal pharyngitis (e.g., wedding banquet, Italy, 1986). **Typhoid** *(Salmonella typhi)* and **paratyphoid** (three bioserotypes of *S. enteritidis*): sporadic cases and limited outbreaks. Incidence has greatly fallen (e.g., Spain) but remains significant in the southeastern part of the region (e.g., *S. enterica* serotype paratyphi b associated with goat milk cheese, France, 1993; Bages county, Barcelona, Spain, 1994).

PROTOZOA. Amebiasis *(Entamoeba histolytica)*: few endemic foci in the southeastern part of the region. **Cryptosporidiosis** *(Cryptosporidium parvum)*: endemic. **Giardiasis** *(Giardia lamblia)*: endemic, particularly in the south. **Toxoplasmosis** *(Toxoplasma gondii)*: endemic. High prevalence in France where brain abscess caused by *T. gondii* is a common complication of AIDS.

FUNGI. Candidiasis *(Candida albicans)*: common in infants and immunocompromised individuals.

HELMINTHS. Ascariasis *(Ascaris lumbricoides)*: endemic, particularly in the south. **Echinococcosis** *(Echinococcus multilocularis)*: rare reports, primarily from east and southeast (e.g., eastern France, Austria, Balkans). **Enterobiasis** *(Enterobius vermicularis)*: very common. **Fascioliasis** *(Fasciola gigantica)*: rare reports, primarily from southern Europe. **Taeniasis**: beef tapeworm *(Taenia saginata)*, pork tapeworm *(Taenia solium)*: endemic primarily in southern countries; rare reports of cysticercosis. **Trichinellosis** *(Trichinella spiralis* spp.): endemic foci with small occasional outbreaks, usually associated with home-prepared pork products, including wild boar meat (e.g., Auvergne, France; Spain; former Yugoslavia; central Italy); notable outbreaks in France associated with imported horse meat. **Trichuriasis** *(Trichuris trichiura)*: rare.

Diseases Primarily Transmitted by Close Contact With Infectious Individuals

VIRUSES. Chickenpox and **herpes zoster**: endemic. **Coxsackievirus**: endemic. **Epstein-Barr virus infection**: endemic; mononucleosis common. Epidemic infantile papular acrodermatitis reported from Italy. **Influenza** (influenza virus types A, B, and C): endemic, seasonal, recurrent epidemics throughout the region, some particularly severe (e.g., Croatia, 1957; Italy and Romania, 1988–1989). **Measles**: Eliminated as a public health problem for northern countries (e.g., France) but outbreaks still a problem in the southeast and southwest (e.g., Bulgaria; Hungary, 1988–1989; Spain; Portugal). **Mumps**: endemic; limited epidemics common. **Pneumonia caused by respiratory syncytial virus (RSV)**: consecutive epidemics of RSV infection in infants (e.g., France). **Poliomyelitis**: Has sharply decreased since the 1960s and been virtually eliminated from the northwestern part of the region but has re-emerged as a serious public health concern since significant outbreaks in newly independent states (e.g., Bulgaria and Albania, 1996, which spread to Greece and the Federal Republic of Yugoslavia). **Rotavirus**: endemic. **Rubella**: incidence has sharply decreased in the north; outbreaks in the south (e.g., Rijeka, Croatia, 1989; Cadiz, Spain, 1991).

BACTERIA. Diphtheria *(Corynebacterium diphtheriae)*: im-

ported cases. Concern raised in the southern part of the region since the 1994 Ukraine epidemic. **Leprosy** *(Mycobacterium leprae)*: imported cases; rare endemic foci in the south (e.g., Greece, Portugal, Spain, Croatia). **Meningococcal meningitis** *(Neisseria meningitidis)*: occasional reports of community outbreaks (e.g., schools), primarily of groups C and B. **Pertussis** *(Bordetella pertussis)*: marked decline during the last 40 years; occasional outbreaks (e.g., Spain, 1989). **Pneumonia caused by *Mycoplasma pneumoniae***: endemic, rare outbreaks (e.g., family outbreak, Sevilla, Spain, 1993). **Pneumonia caused by *Streptococcus pneumoniae***: endemic; outbreaks reported (e.g., men's shelters, France, 1988–1989). **Tuberculosis** *(Mycobacterium tuberculosis)*: endemic; recent increase in incidence associated with the AIDS pandemic and a recrudescence of the disease among the poor and the elderly (e.g., France, Spain). Community-based outbreaks not uncommon (e.g., school outbreak, Spain; Italy, all in 1992–1993). **Chlamydia: Pneumonia caused by *Chlamydia pneumoniae***: possibly the third cause of epidemic bacterial pneumopathies in France; outbreak in former injection-drug users (e.g., Italy, 1991).

ECTOPARASITES. Pediculosis *(Pediculus humanus capitis)*: endemic, especially in low-socioeconomic groups. School outbreaks common. **Scabies** *(Sarcoptes scabiei)*: common in the south; occasional outbreaks (e.g., Spain).

Sexually Transmitted Diseases

STDs are endemic in the region, primarily among the poor and high-risk groups.

VIRUSES. Hepatitis B: endemic, especially in the south; outbreaks reported. **Hepatitis C**: endemic. **HIV infection**: endemic throughout the region, primarily among high-risk groups. High but recent stabilization of prevalence in France, Spain, and Italy. Epidemic more recent and still spreading in southeastern countries. **Herpes simplex virus (HSV-2)**: endemic. **Papillomavirus**: endemic.

BACTERIA. Gonococcal infection *(Neisseria gonorrhoeae)*: endemic; decreasing incidence in the most developed countries. **Syphilis** *(Treponema pallidum)*: endemic. **Chlamydia: Chlamydial infections** *(Chlamydia trachomatis)*: endemic.

FUNGI. Candidiasis *(Candida albicans)*: hyperendemic.

ECTOPARASITE. Phthiriasis *(Phthirus pubis)*: endemic.

Nosocomial Infections

Nosocomial infections have been increasingly reported in the most developed countries of the region and have attracted significant public health attention. They are certainly underreported in the less developed countries.

VIRUSES. Large nosocomial **HIV infections** reported (e.g., associated with blood transfusion received before 1991, between 3300 and 4400 infected recipients, France; HIV infection in children, 1989–1991, Romania). Outbreak of **rotavirus** gastroenteritis (e.g., neonatal ICU, Bulgaria, 1993).

BACTERIA. Numerous reports (e.g., hospital outbreak due to imipenem-resistant *Acinetobacter baumanii*, France, 1995; spinal cord injury unit, Spain, 1990–1992), *Clostridium difficile*–associated diarrhea among AIDS patients (e.g., France, 1992; Spain, 1992, where it represents the main cause of antibiotic-associated diarrhea). *Enterobacter cloacae*: resistant to third-generation cephalosporins and all aminoglycosides, except amikacin (e.g., neonatal unit, France, 1989; ventilated neonates, France, 1992). Antibiotic-resistant *Klebsiella pneumoniae* (e.g., neurologic unit, France, 1993–1994). **Legionnaires' disease** (e.g., hemodialysis unit, Spain, 1983). Multidrug-resistant *Mycobacterium bovis* (e.g., HIV-infected patients, France). *Pseudomonas aeruginosa* (e.g., burn unit and hematology unit, Paris, 1989; Italy, 1988; multiresistant strain, Spain, 1987–1988). **Salmonellosis** (e.g., 22 hospital outbreaks in England and Wales, 1992–1994). Extended-spectrum β-lactamase producing *Serratia marcescens* (e.g., ICU, Italy, 1991–1992). *Staphylococcus aureus* resistant to methicillin (e.g., France, Spain, since 1989). Drug-resistant *Staphylococcus epidermidis* (e.g., France, 1990). *Streptococcus* group G (e.g., hemodialysis associated, Nimes, France).

FUNGI. Candida albicans (e.g., neonatal ICU, Rennes, France, 1990s).

PROTOZOA. *Pneumocystis carinii* **pneumonia** (e.g., renal transplant unit, France, 1990s).

OTHER. Creutzfeldt-Jakob disease: transmission by prion-contaminated growth hormone (e.g., France, 1980s).

Human Zoonoses and Vector-Borne Diseases, Including Viral Hemorrhagic Fevers

Diseases Transmitted by Close Contact With Animals or Animal Products

VIRUSES. Hantavirus: endemic foci with occasional epidemics (e.g., northeastern France, 1992–1993; nationwide outbreak, Yugoslavia, 1989, primarily Bosnia and Herzegovina). **Rabies**: rare human cases. General decline of animal rabies in areas of fox immunization campaign (e.g., eastern France). Foxes are primary reservoir in the eastern part of region and difficult to control (e.g., reappearance of sylvatic rabies in Austria, 1966). Dogs are primary reservoir in the Iberian peninsula. Rabid bats occasionally reported.

BACTERIA. Anthrax (*Bacillus anthracis*): exceptional reports. **Brucellosis** (*Brucella abortus, B. melitensis*): endemic, particularly in the Mediterranean area; occasional accidental outbreaks (e.g., microbiology laboratory workers, Spain, 1993). **Leptospirosis** (*Leptospira interrogans*): endemic foci (e.g., eastern and central France), rare outbreaks (e.g., Italy, 1984). **Q fever** (*Coxiella burnetii*): endemic, particularly in the south; epidemics reported (e.g., Spain, 1990). **Rat-bite fever** (*Streptobacillus moniliformis*): uncommon. **Chlamydia: Psittacosis** (*Chlamydia psittaci*): rare reports (e.g., family outbreak, Spain, 1990).

Louse-Borne

BACTERIA. Trench fever (*Bartonella quintana*): exceptional reports.

Mosquito-Borne

VIRUSES. Dengue fever: imported cases only. **West Nile fever**: rare cases from endemic foci in the south (e.g., Camargue, France); recent outbreaks (e.g., Bucharest, Bulgaria, 1996).

PROTOZOA. Malaria (*Plasmodium falciparum, P. vivax*): steady increase in number of imported cases; occasional airport-associated cases. Declared eradicated from Spain in 1964.

Phlebotomine-Borne

VIRUSES. Sandfly fevers (Naples and Sicilian): endemic foci along the Mediterranean coast.

PROTOZOA. Cutaneous leishmaniasis (*Leishmania major*): sporadic cases in southern France (e.g., Cevennes, Languedoc) and along the Mediterranean (Calabria; coastal Adriatic, Italy). **Visceral leishmaniasis** (*L. infantum* complex): endemic foci along the Mediterranean coast. Reported from eastern Austria. Numerous AIDS-associated cases in Spain.

Tick-Borne

VIRUSES. Central European tick-borne encephalitis (refer to tick-borne viruses section for northern Europe): rare reports from endemic foci in rural areas of eastern countries (e.g., Austria).

BACTERIA. Lyme disease (*Borrelia burgdorferi*): Recently identified in the region (e.g., Spain, 1977; Italy, 1983); endemic foci, particularly in northeastern France, Austria, and northern Italy. **Tick-borne relapsing fever** (various strains): rare; occasional outbreaks in southern countries (e.g., Spain). **Tularemia** (*Francisella tularensis*): endemic foci in most rural areas (e.g., eastern and central France); occasional outbreaks (e.g., water-borne outbreak, Arezzo, Italy, 1992). **Rickettsia: Mediterranean spotted fever** (*Rickettsia conorii*): rare reports (e.g., family outbreak, Spain).

Soil-Borne or Airborne Diseases, and Diseases Associated With Recreational Water With No Evidence of Direct Animal-to-Human or Direct Person-to-Person Transmission

BACTERIA. Tetanus (*Clostridium tetani*): not uncommon, particularly in the elderly. **Legionnaires' disease**: occasional outbreaks (e.g., Valencia, Spain, 1983). **Unknown bacteria**: outbreak of pneumonia and meningitis associated with hot spring spa, caused by an unknown gram-negative bacterium, France, 1987.

FUNGI. Rhinosporidiosis: rare reports (e.g., outbreak, northern Serbia, 1992).

HELMINTHS. Hookworm disease (*Necator americanus, Ancylostoma duodenale*): low endemicity. **Strongyloidiasis** (*Strongyloides stercoralis*): rare autochthonous cases (e.g., northern France, northern Italy).

■ WESTERN SOUTH ASIA (Bahrain, Cyprus, Iraq, Israel, Jordan, Kuwait, Lebanon, Oman, Qata, Saudi Arabia, Syrian Arab Republic, Turkey, the United Arab Emirates, and Yemen)

The area ranges from the mountains (e.g., Turkey, northern Iraq) and steppes of the northwest to the large deserts and dry tropical scrub of the south. Most of the population lives in the coastal areas, along the fertile plains watered by few rivers (e.g., Tiger, Euphrates) and in few oases. In the eastern part of the Arabic peninsula, the highlands of Yemen and its high population density contrast with the Arabian desert.

The distribution of communicable diseases in the region varies significantly with the population density and the level of economic development (e.g., Israel, Kuwait, Saudi Arabia vs. Iraq, Yemen). Although generally satisfactory, the regional health infrastructure has been hampered by the former war in Lebanon and the Gulf War, including the still prevailing economic blockade of Iraq.

Diseases Primarily Transmitted by Food and Drinking Water

Prevalence of diseases transmitted by food and drinking water is higher in countries of higher population density and poorer infrastructure (e.g., Yemen, Iraq, Turkey).

VIRUSES. Hepatitis A: highly endemic throughout the region. **Hepatitis E**: reported. **Rotavirus**: endemic.

BACTERIA. Cholera (toxinogenic *Vibrio cholerae* serogroup 01): Sporadic cases in the region (e.g., Iraq, Yemen); many imported (e.g., Somali refugees in Yemen, 1993). **Botulism** (*Clostridium botulinum*): rare; occasional outbreaks (e.g., associated with imported fish, Israel, 1987). **Diarrhea caused by** *Campylobacter jejuni*: endemic. **Diarrhea caused by** *Escherichia coli*: enterotoxigenic *E. coli* (ETEC), and enterohemorrhagic *E. coli* (EHEC): endemic. **Listeriosis** (*Listeria monocytogenes*): endemic. **Salmonellosis**: endemic; frequent outbreaks (e.g., food handler–associated outbreak, Jordan University Hospital, 1989). **Shigellosis** (*Shigella* spp.): endemic, outbreaks frequent (water-borne *Shigella sonnei* outbreak in communal settlement, Israel, 1990). **Staphylococcal disease** (*Staphylococcus aureus*): occasional food poisoning. **Streptococcal diseases** (group A *Streptococcus*): endemic; occasional outbreaks (e.g., streptococcal throat infection, military unit, Israel, 1988). **Typhoid** (*Salmonella typhi*) and **paratyphoid** (three bioserotypes of *S. enteritidis*): high endemicity.

PROTOZOA. Amebiasis (*Entamoeba histolytica*): endemic. **Cryptosporidiosis** (*Cryptosporidium parvum*): endemic; occasional outbreaks (e.g., young children, agricultural community, Israel, 1990). **Diarrhea caused by** *Blastocystis hominis*: endemic; epidemic reported (children, northern Jordan, 1993). **Giardiasis** (*Giardia lamblia*): high endemicity. **Toxoplasmosis** (*Toxoplasma gondii*): endemic.

FUNGI. Candidiasis (*Candida albicans*): very common.

HELMINTHS. Ascariasis (*Ascaris lumbricoides*): endemic. **Dracunculiasis** (*Dracunculus medinensis*): small foci in Sanaa Governorate, Yemen). **Echinococcosis** (*Echinococcus multilocularis*): some endemic foci. **Enterobiasis** (*Enterobius vermicularis*): common. **Fascioliasis** (*Fasciola gigantica*): endemic foci (e.g., Iraq, Yemen, Turkey). **Taeniasis**: reported from many countries in the area, involving primarily beef tapeworm (*Taenia saginata*); pork tapeworm (*T. solium*) found primarily in Christian communities with rare reports of cysticercosis (e.g., Lebanon, Cyprus). **Trichinellosis** (*Trichinella spiralis* spp.): occasional outbreaks among Christian communities (e.g., southern Lebanon, 1982, attributed to raw pork); has become uncommon in Israel although some small outbreaks reported, usually associated with boar meat. **Trichuriasis** (*Trichuris trichiura*): endemic.

OTHER. Pentastomid infection (*Linguatula serrata*): rare reports of halzoun (e.g., Lebanon, Israel).

Diseases Primarily Transmitted by Close Contact With Infectious Individuals

VIRUSES. Chickenpox and **herpes zoster**: endemic. **Coxsackievirus**: endemic; occasional outbreaks (e.g., epidemic meningitis, Cyprus, 1996). **Human parvovirus B19**: caused aplastic crisis in patients with sickle cell disease, Dhahran, Saudi Arabia, 1991–1992. **Influenza** (influenza virus types A, B, and C): endemic. **Measles**: endemic, has declined in some areas (e.g., Kuwait), re-emerged in others with occasional outbreaks (Turkey, 1988 and 1993; Oman; epidemic cycles at interval of 2 to 4 years in Israel). **Mumps**: endemic. **Poliomyelitis**: important decline in the region. Almost eliminated in Israel (last case in 1988), Kuwait, Bahrain, United Arab Emirates. Low incidence in most other countries (e.g., rare reports from Lebanon, Jordan, Oman, Saudi Arabia, Cyprus, Iraq), except Turkey and Yemen. Notable outbreaks in Gizan, Saudi Arabia, 1989; Oman, 1988–1989 (poliovirus type 1, strain imported from South Asia) and 1991 (wild type 3 poliovirus, association with DTP vaccination); and Jordan, 1991–1992. **Rotavirus**: endemic. **Rubella**: endemic; occasional outbreak (e.g., Oman).

BACTERIA. Diphtheria (*Corynebacterium diphtheriae*): rare reports. **Leprosy** (*Mycobacterium leprae*): no autochthonous transmission in Israel but imported cases (e.g., Ethiopian refugees). Sharp decline in the region (e.g., Saudi Arabia, Kuwait, Lebanon) but endemic foci remain significant primarily in Yemen. **Meningococcal meningitis** (*Neisseria meningitidis*): occasional community outbreaks, some associated with imported cases (e.g., serogroup A, Mecca, Saudi Arabia, 1987, and serogroup A clone III-1, Mecca, Saudi Arabia, 1992). **Pertussis** (*Bordetella pertussis*): low endemicity, rare outbreaks (e.g., kibbutz, Israel, 1987). **Pneumonia caused by**

Streptococcus pneumoniae: endemic, including penicillin-resistant strains. **Streptococcal diseases** (group A *Streptococcus*): endemic. **Tuberculosis** (*Mycobacterium tuberculosis*): endemic, particularly in Lebanon, Yemen, Iraq, and Turkey. Epidemics reported (e.g., northern Lebanon, 1990). **Chlamydia: Trachoma** (*Chlamydia trachomatis*): endemic.

ECTOPARASITES. Pediculosis (*Pediculus humanus capitis*): endemic. **Scabies** (*Sarcoptes scabiei*): endemic.

Sexually Transmitted Diseases

With the exception of Israel, the situation is poorly documented but estimated to be similar to North Africa.

VIRUSES. Hepatitis B: endemic. Specific information on notable outbreaks includes penile condylomata caused by **human papillomavirus** (e.g., Israel, early 1990s). **Hepatitis B** virus mutant associated with an epidemic of fulminant hepatitis (Haifa, Israel, 1986).

BACTERIA. Gonococcal infection (*Neisseria gonorrhoeae*): outbreak of penicillin-resistant *N. gonorrhoeae* in southern Israel, 1987–1989.

Nosocomial Infections

Nosocomial infections are not well documented in the region although they seem to be of increasing importance. Reported nosocomial outbreaks are as follows.

VIRUSES. Chickenpox: British military personnel, field hospital, Kuwait, 1991; diarrhea caused by **rotavirus** serotype 1, pediatric ward, Israel.

BACTERIA. *Acinetobacter baumanii*, Lebanese medical center, 1984. Multiresistant *Klebsiella pneumoniae*, neonatal intensive care unit, Israel. Methicillin-resistant *Staphylococcus aureus*, neonatal ICU, Saudi Arabia (nasal carriage among staff member).

FUNGI. Outbreak of *Candida tropicalis* fungemia in a neonatal ICU, Haifa, Israel.

Human Zoonoses and Vector-Borne Diseases, Including Viral Hemorrhagic Fevers

Diseases Transmitted by Close Contact With Animals or Animal Products

VIRUSES. Rabies: no human rabies in Israel since 1960 and Saudi Arabia since 1982. Kuwait, Oman, and Cyprus are virtually rabies-free but human rabies remains important in Turkey, Yemen, and some rural areas of the West Bank of Jordan (e.g., Galilee). Dogs are the main animal reservoir.

BACTERIA. Anthrax (*Bacillus anthracis*): endemic. **Brucellosis** (*Brucella abortus, B. melitensis*): endemic. **Leptospirosis** (*Leptospira interrogans*): rare reports since the 1970s (e.g., Galilee, Israel). **Rickettsia: Murine typhus** (*Rickettsia mooseri*): endemic; best documented in Israel. **Q fever** (*Coxiella burnetii*): endemic.

Flea-Borne

BACTERIA. Plague (*Yersinia pestis*): exceptional; last outbreak in the region was along the Yemen and Saudi Arabia border, 1969.

Fly-Borne

HELMINTHS. Onchocerciasis (*Onchocerca volvulus*): endemic foci in Yemen and southwestern Saudi Arabia only (Wadi Ghayl, Kima, Nasyan, Zabid).

Louse-Borne

Rickettsia: Epidemic typhus (*Rickettsia prowazekii*): rare reports (e.g., Iraq).

Mosquito-Borne

VIRUSES. Dengue fever: has recently spread to the southwestern part of the region (e.g., Oman, Yemen, Saudi Arabia). Outbreaks reported (e.g., Jeddah, Saudi Arabia, 1994). **Sindbis** and **West Nile**: endemic in Cyprus, Israel, Lebanon, and Saudi Arabia.

PROTOZOA. Malaria (*Plasmodium falciparum, P. vivax*): low transmission and mainly seasonal in the region although the epidemiologic situation may vary significantly from one place to the other. *P. falciparum* primarily found in the southwest (e.g., Yemen, Oman, Saudi Arabia), and *P. vivax* in the northeast (e.g., Iraq, Syria, Turkey). Risk almost year-round in endemic areas of Saudi Arabia. Areas free or virtually free of malaria include the highlands of Yemen, Bahrain, Lebanon, Jordan, Qatar, Kuwait, Israel, Cyprus, the Dubai, and Jeddah and Medina areas. However, imported cases are common in the region.

Phlebotomine-Borne

PROTOZOA. Cutaneous leishmaniasis (*Leishmania major, L. aethiopica*): reported throughout the area. **Visceral leishmaniasis** (*L. infantum* complex, *L. donovani*): although rare in most of the area, it is relatively common in central Iraq, southwest Saudi Arabia, the northwest part of the Syrian Arab Republic, southeast of Anatolia in Turkey, and in the west of Yemen.

Tick-Borne

VIRUSES. Crimean-Congo hemorrhagic fever: rare reports; limited outbreaks; endemic in Iraq.

BACTERIA. Tick-borne relapsing fever (various strains): rare reports (e.g., Cyprus, Iraq, Jordan, Lebanon, Israel, Kuwait). **Tick-borne typhus**: rare. **Tularaemia** (*Francisella tularensis*): rare endemic foci (e.g., Turkey).

Soil-Borne or Airborne Diseases, and Diseases Associated With Recreational Water With No Evidence of Direct Animal-to-Human or Direct Person-to-Person Transmission

BACTERIA. Tetanus (*Clostridium tetani*): endemic, higher incidence in Yemen, Iraq, Turkey. **Legionellosis**: rare reports since 1985 (e.g., Israel).

HELMINTHS. Hookworm disease (*Necator americanus, Ancylostoma duodenale*): endemic. **Schistosomiasis** (*Schistosoma haematobium, S. mansoni*): endemic foci (e.g., Yemen, Iraq, Saudi Arabia, Syrian Arab Republic). **Strongyloidiasis** (*Strongyloides stercoralis*): endemic.

■ MIDDLE SOUTH ASIA (Afghanistan, Armenia, Azerbaidjan, Bangladesh, Bhutan, Georgia, India, Islamic Republic of Iran, Kazakhstan, Kyrgyzstan, Maldives, Nepal, Pakistan, Sri Lanka, Tajikistan, Turkmenistan, and Uzbekistan)

The region varies in topography from mountains in the north to steppes and desert in the west and tropical rain forests in the east and south. Countries usually have poor economic infrastructure, since there are either developing countries or economies in transition and since many of them have recently experienced limited or widespread armed conflicts.

Diseases Primarily Transmitted by Food and Drinking Water

These diseases are certainly underreported in the region. Sanitation and water supply vary but are generally of poor standard. Although some of the newly independent countries in the region have extensive infrastructure, inability to regularly maintain water purification and sewer systems has been increasingly reported, especially in areas afflicted by war, rebellions, or civil unrest (e.g., Afghanistan, Tajikistan, Sri Lanka).

VIRUSES. Hepatitis A: hyperendemic. **Hepatitis E**: endemic; large outbreaks reported or suspected since the 1960s (e.g., India, Pakistan): recent non-A, non-B hepatitis outbreak in rural areas of northern Rajasthan, India, 1994. **Norwalk and Norwalk-like viruses**: endemic.

BACTERIA. Cholera (toxinogenic *Vibrio cholerae* serogroup 01): endemic; outbreaks reported (e.g., Afghanistan, 1995). Since 1992, cholera caused by *V. cholerae* 0139 strain has emerged (India, Bangladesh) including new cases recently reported (Calcutta, India, 1996). **Diarrhea caused by *Campylobacter jejuni***: endemic but poorly documented. **Diarrhea caused by *Escherichia coli***: endemic. **Enterotoxic and enteropathogenic *E. coli***: endemic. **Listeriosis** (*Listeria monocytogenes*): endemic. **Salmonellosis**: highly endemic, with frequent epidemics (Tajikistan, 1996). **Shigellosis** (*Shigella* spp.): endemic. **Streptococcal** diseases (group A *Streptococcus*): endemic. **Typhoid** (*Salmonella typhi*) and **paratyphoid** (three bioserotypes of *S. enteritidis*): highly endemic; has recently become a serious public health problem with large epidemics reported (e.g., Calcutta, India, 1995; Tajikistan, 1996–1997; Turkmenistan, 1997).

PROTOZOA. Amebiasis (*Entamoeba histolytica*): high endemicity. **Giardiasis** (*Giardia lamblia*): common in all countries. **Toxoplasmosis** (*Toxoplasma gondii*): endemic.

FUNGI. Candidiasis (*Candida albicans*): hyperendemic.

HELMINTHS. Ascariasis (*Ascaris lumbricoides*): very common. **Dracunculiasis** (*Dracunculus medinensis*): rare; few remaining foci only in India currently being eliminated by the National Guinea Worm Eradication Program (six cases reported in 1996, from Rajasthan district). **Echinococcosis** (*Echinococcus multilocularis*): endemic in many countries in the area. **Enterobiasis** (*Enterobius vermicularis*): hyperendemic. **Fascioliasis** (*Fasciola hepatica*): endemic foci. **Fasciolopsiasis** (*Fasciolopsis buski*): endemic foci in the east (e.g., India). **Taeniasis**: beef tapeworm (*Taenia saginata*) and pork tapeworm (*T. solium*) are common. **Trichinellosis** (*Trichinella spiralis* spp.): common. **Trichuriasis** (*Trichuris trichiura*): common.

OTHER. Food poisoning outbreaks, including botulism.

Diseases Primarily Transmitted by Close Contact With Infectious Individuals

VIRUSES. Most viral diseases, including vaccine-preventable viral diseases, are endemic throughout the region. **Chickenpox** and **herpes zoster**: endemic. **Influenza** (influenza virus types A, B, and C): endemic. **Measles**: recently caused an epidemic in Sri Lanka among unvaccinated youth. **Mumps**: endemic. **Poliomyelitis**: overall decrease in incidence but remains of relatively high endemicity in all countries but Bhutan and the Maldives; recent outbreaks (e.g., Pakistan, 1990–1991). **Rotavirus**: highly endemic. **Rubella**: endemic.

BACTERIA. Acute bacterial conjunctivitis (*Haemophilus influenzae*): endemic. **Diphtheria**: endemic with frequent epidemics as childhood immunization programs have broken down (e.g., Azerbaidjan, Georgia, Kazakhstan, Kyrgyzstan, Tajikistan, Turkmenistan, and Uzbekistan). **Leprosy** (*Mycobacterium leprae*): remains significantly endemic in Bangladesh, India (50% of worldwide cases), and Nepal. **Meningococcal meningitis**: endemic. **Streptococcal diseases** (group A *Streptococcus*): high endemicity, including acute rheumatic fever, streptococcal impetigo, scarlet fever, and erysipelas. **Tuberculosis** (*Mycobacterium tuberculosis*): highly endemic in most countries. **Chlamydia: Trachoma** (*Chlamydia trachomatis*): common in Afghanistan and in parts of India, the Islamic Republic of Iran, Nepal, and Pakistan.

Sexually Transmitted Diseases

STDs are poorly documented in the region but are thought to have significantly increased in some newly independent countries, particularly in populations at higher risk.

VIRUSES. Hepatitis B: endemic. **Hepatitis C**: endemic. **HIV infection**: increasing throughout the region in populations at risk. **Human herpesvirus** and **papillomavirus**: endemic.

BACTERIA. Gonococcal infection (*Neisseria gonorrhoeae*): endemic. **Syphilis** (*Treponema pallidum*): endemic. **Chlamydia: Chlamydial infections** (*Chlamydia trachomatis*): endemic.

FUNGI. Candidiasis (*Candida albicans*): highly endemic.

Nosocomial Infections

Although poorly documented in the region, nosocomial infections are thought to be common or even very common in most countries of the region.

VIRUSES. Rotavirus (outbreaks in pediatric wards). **Hepatitis B** and **hepatitis C**.

BACTERIA. Nosocomial transmission certainly common; actual occurrence of hospital-acquired antibiotic-resistant bacterial infections is unknown.

FUNGI. Candidiasis (*Candida albicans*): documented following cardiac surgery; more rarely other species such as *C. parapsilosis*.

Human Zoonoses and Vector-Borne Diseases, Including Viral Hemorrhagic Fevers

Diseases Transmitted by Close Contact With Animals or Animal Products

VIRUSES. Rabies: endemic among nomadic and animal-raising populations throughout the region; main reservoir is the dog.

BACTERIA. Brucellosis: endemic. **Leptospirosis** (*Leptospira interrogans*): endemic foci. **Anthrax**: endemic; rare reports. **Rickettsia: Q fever** (*Coxiella burnetii*): endemic.

HELMINTHS. Echinococcosis (*Echinococcus granulosus*): endemic among nomadic and animal-raising populations throughout the region.

Flea-Borne

BACTERIA. Plague (*Yersinia pestis*): natural foci in wild rodent populations with increased activity reported (e.g., Kazakhstan and India). Isolated cases of bubonic plague not uncommon. Important outbreak of bubonic and pneumonic plague in Mararashtra State and the city of Surat, respectively, India, 1994.

Louse-Borne

Rickettsia. Typhus (*Rickettsia prowazekii*): endemic foci in Afghanistan and India.

Mosquito-Borne

VIRUSES. Dengue fever/DHF: current regional spread with the emergence of large urban epidemics (e.g., Delhi, India, 1996). Outbreaks frequently reported from Bangladesh, Pakistan, and Sri Lanka, with occasional reports of DHF (e.g., eastern India; Sri Lanka; Karachi, Pakistan, 1994; Delhi, India, 1996). **Japanese encephalitis**: endemic primarily in the east-

ern part of the region but spreading westward with reports of significant epidemics (e.g., Nepal, 1996). **Crimean-Congo hemorrhagic fever**: rare reports from the western part of the region.

PROTOZOA. Malaria (*Plasmodium falciparum, P. vivax*): endemic in all countries except Georgia, Kazakhstan, Kyrgyzstan, and Uzbekistan. Small foci in Azerbaidjan, Tajikistan, and Turkmenistan with a tendency to spread to usually malaria-free area, including urban areas. The resurgence of malaria in the area has been particularly important since 1995.

HELMINTHS. Lymphatic filariasis (*Wuchereria bancrofti*): common in Bangladesh, India, and the southwestern coastal belt of Sri Lanka.

Phlebotomine-Borne

VIRUS. Sandfly fever (*Phlebovirus*): increasing reports from the region.

PROTOZOA. Visceral leishmaniasis: endemic with markedly increased incidence (e.g., Bangladesh, India, Nepal, and northern Pakistan). **Cutaneous leishmaniasis**: endemic; epidemics more frequently reported (e.g., Afghanistan; Rajasthan, India; the Islamic Republic of Iran; and Pakistan). Small endemic foci in Azerbaidjan and Tajikistan.

Tick-Borne

VIRUSES. New tick-borne hemorrhagic fever reported in forest areas in Karnataka State, India, and in rural Rawalpindi district, Pakistan.

BACTERIA. Tick-borne relapsing fever (various strains): reported from Afghanistan, India, and the Islamic Republic of Iran. **Tularemia** (*Francisella tularensis*): rare endemic foci in the northern part of the region.

Soil-Borne or Airborne Diseases, and Diseases Associated With Recreational Water With No Evidence of Direct Animal-to-Human or Direct Person-to-Person Transmission

BACTERIA. Legionellosis (*Legionella* serogroups): poorly documented. **Melioidosis**: rare reports. **Tetanus** (*Clostridium tetani*): endemic, with neonatal tetanus remaining a serious problem in some areas. **Chlamydia. Trachoma**: endemic in dry and dusty areas of Afghanistan, India, Islamic Republic of Iran, Nepal, and Pakistan.

HELMINTHS. Strongyloidiasis (*Strongyloides stercoralis*): endemic foci. **Schistosomiasis** (*Schistosoma haematobium*): rare foci (e.g., Islamic Republic of Iran). **Toxocariasis** (*Toxocara canis*): endemic.

▪ EASTERN SOUTH ASIA (Brunei, Darussalam, Cambodia, Indonesia, Lao People's Democratic Republic, Malaysia, Myanmar, the Philippines, Singapore, Thailand, and Vietnam)

The region includes tropical rain and monsoon forests in the northwest and in the islands bordering the South China Sea, and savanna and dry tropical forests in the Indochina peninsula. Although the health infrastructure and economic development remain poor in most countries of the Indochina peninsula, they are of the highest standard in countries such as Brunei and Singapore.

Diseases Primarily Transmitted by Food and Drinking Water

Although water supplies and sanitation are, for the most part, well established and in good condition, diseases transmitted by food and drinking water remain particularly common in the rural Indochina peninsula and Myanmar.

VIRUSES. Hepatitis A and **hepatitis E**: endemic with documented outbreak of hepatitis E (e.g., military recruits, Myanmar and Indonesia, 1991; southwestern Vietnam, 1994). **Norwalk and Norwalk-like viruses**: endemic.

BACTERIA. Cholera (toxinogenic *Vibrio cholerae* serogroup 01): endemic in most countries. **Diarrhea caused by *Campylobacter jejuni***: endemic. **Diarrhea caused by *Escherichia coli***: endemic. **Enterotoxic and enteropathogenic *E. coli***: endemic. **Listeriosis** (*Listeria monocytogenes*): endemic. **Salmonellosis**: endemic; common outbreaks. **Shigellosis** (*Shigella* spp.): endemic; common outbreaks. **Streptococcal diseases** (group A *Streptococcus*): endemic. **Typhoid** (*Salmonella typhi*) and **paratyphoid** (three bioserotypes of *S. enteritidis*): reported from all countries in the area.

PROTOZOA. Amebiasis (*Entamoeba histolytica*): may occur in all countries in the area. **Giardiasis** (*Giardia lamblia*): endemic. **Toxoplasmosis** (*Toxoplasma gondii*): endemic.

FUNGI. Candidiasis (*Candida albicans*): highly endemic.

HELMINTHS. Anisakiasis (larval nematodes of Anisakinae): rare reports from coastal areas. **Angiostrongyliasis** (*Angiostrongylus cantonensis*): endemic foci (e.g., Indonesia, Malaysia, the Philippines, Thailand, Vietnam). **Ascariasis** (*Ascaris lumbricoides*): high endemicity. **Clonorchiasis** (*Clonorchis sinensis*): endemic in the Indochina peninsula. **Echinococcosis** (*Echinococcus granulosus*): endemic in the Indochina peninsula. **Enterobiasis** (*Enterobius vermicularis*): highly endemic. **Fascioliasis** (*Fasciola hepatica*): endemic in the Indochina peninsula. **Fasciolopsiasis** (*Fasciolopsis buski*): may be acquired in most countries in the area, particularly in pig-rearing areas. **Gnathostomiasis** (*Gnathostoma spinigerum*): rare endemic foci (e.g., Thailand). **Opisthorchiasis** (*Opisthorchis felineus*): endemic in the Indochina peninsula, the Philippines, and Thailand. **Paragonimiasis** (*Paragonimus westermani, P. skrjabini*, and other species): endemic in most countries. **Taeniasis**: beef tapeworm (*Taenia saginata*): endemic. **Trichinellosis** (*Trichinella spiralis* spp.): endemic. **Trichuriasis** (*Trichuris trichiura*): endemic.

Diseases Primarily Transmitted by Close Contact With Infectious Individuals

VIRUSES. Coxsackie (Coxsackie A 24): outbreaks of keratoconjunctivitis periodically reported (e.g., Malaysia, Singapore). **Chickenpox** and **herpes zoster**: endemic. **Influenza** (influenza virus types A, B, and C): endemic with frequent epidemics throughout the region. **Measles**: endemic. **Mumps**: endemic. **Poliomyelitis**: endemic in countries of the Indochina peninsula. Cases still reported from Cambodia, Indonesia, the Lao People's Democratic Republic, Myanmar, and Vietnam. Incidence low in Malaysia, the Philippines, and Thailand. **Rotavirus**: endemic. **Rubella**: endemic.

BACTERIA. Diphtheria: rare outbreaks (e.g., Saraburi province, Thailand, 1994). **Leprosy** (*Mycobacterium leprae*): endemic foci in Cambodia, Laos, and Vietnam. **Meningococcal meningitis**: endemic; outbreaks reported. **Pertussis** (*Bordetella pertussis*): endemic. **Streptococcal diseases** (group A *Streptococcus*): endemic, particularly in the Indochina peninsula, including acute rheumatic fever, streptococcal impetigo, scarlet fever, and erysipelas. **Tuberculosis** (*Mycobacterium tuberculosis*): endemic, particularly among the poor and urban areas.

Sexually Transmitted Diseases

Poorly documented in the Indonesia peninsula but thought to be common.

VIRUSES. Hepatitis B: highly endemic. Mainly sexually transmitted in the most developed countries of the region. **HIV infection**: increasingly prevalent in the region, despite some successful control interventions (e.g., Thailand). **Herpes simplex virus (HSV-2)**: endemic. **Papillomavirus**: endemic.

BACTERIA. Gonococcal infection (*Neisseria gonorrhoeae*): endemic. **Syphilis** (*Treponema pallidum*): endemic. **Chlamydia: Chlamydial infections** (*Chlamydia trachomatis*): common.

FUNGI. Candidiasis (*Candida albicans*): very common.

Nosocomial Infections

Certainly underreported in the region.

VIRUSES. Parenterally transmitted **hepatitis B, hepatitis C**, and, to a lesser extent, **HIV infection**, remain a constant threat throughout the region, particularly in less developed countries.

BACTERIA. Outbreaks of **methicillin-resistant *Staphylococcus aureus*** reported (e.g., hospital settings in Malaysia and Singapore). Nosocomial transmission of other drug-resistant bacteria, including multidrug-resistant *Mycobacterium tuberculosis*, thought to occur.

FUNGI. *Candida albicans* frequently reported.

Human Zoonoses and Vector-Borne Diseases, Including Viral Hemorrhagic Fevers

Diseases Transmitted by Close Contact With Animals or Animal Products

VIRUSES. Hantavirus: endemic foci (e.g., Thailand). **Rabies**: endemic in most countries of the region; stray dogs are the main reservoir.

BACTERIA. Brucellosis (*Brucella abortus, B. suis, B. melitensis*): sporadic. **Leptospirosis** (*Leptospira interrogans*): endemic foci. **Anthrax**: rare reports (e.g., Thailand, 1997). **Rickettsia: Q fever** (*Coxiella burnetii*): rare.

Flea-Borne

BACTERIA. Plague (*Yersinia pestis*): wild rodent endemic foci in Myanmar and Vietnam (e.g., Gialay-Kontum and Daklak provinces).

Louse-Borne

Rickettsia: typhus (*Rickettsia prowazekii*): sporadic reports.

Mite-Borne

Rickettsia: scrub typhus (*Rickettsia tsutsugamushi*): endemic in deforested areas of most countries (e.g., Indochina peninsula).

Mosquito-Borne

VIRUSES. Dengue fever/Dengue hemorrhagic fever: endemic (e.g., Indonesia, Myanmar, Thailand); seasonal outbreaks in both urban and rural areas have been associated with DHF (e.g., Malaysia, June 1996). **Japanese encephalitis**: endemic and of increasing incidence as it spreads to new areas (e.g., Indonesia, Papua New Guinea); seasonal epidemics in both urban and rural areas.

PROTOZOA. Malaria (*Plasmodium falciparum, P. vivax*): endemic in most rural areas throughout the region (e.g., Indochina peninsula, Thailand) and a significant cause of morbidity except for Brunei and Singapore, where cases are primarily imported.

HELMINTHS. Lymphatic filariasis (*Wuchereria bancrofti, Brugia malayi, B. timori*): endemic foci in many parts of the region, especially in rural areas where significant numbers of the adult population remain infected.

Soil-Borne or Airborne Diseases, and Diseases Associated With Recreational Water With No Evidence of Direct Animal-to-Human or Direct Person-to-Person Transmission

BACTERIA. Legionellosis (*Legionella* serogroups): sporadic reports. **Melioidosis** (*Pseudomonas pseudomallei*): rare reports throughout the region. **Tetanus** (*Clostridium tetani*): endemic throughout the region, including neonatal tetanus in poor areas. **Chlamydia: trachoma**: present in Indonesia, Myanmar, Thailand, and Vietnam.

FUNGI. Candidiasis: hyperendemic.

HELMINTHS. Cutaneous larva migrans (*Ancylostoma braziliense, A. caninum*): endemic. **Hookworm disease** (*Necator americanus, Ancylostoma duodenale, A. ceylanicum*) and **Strongyloidiasis** (*Strongyloides stercoralis*): endemic foci throughout the region.

Water-Snail-Borne

HELMINTHS. Schistosomiasis (*Schistosoma japonicum*): endemic foci (e.g., southern Philippines, central Sulawesi, Indonesia, and the Mekong delta).

■ **EAST ASIA** (China, including Taiwan, the Democratic People's Republic of Korea, Hong Kong, Japan, Macao, Mongolia, and the Republic of Korea)

The area includes the high mountains, deserts, and steppes of the west and the various forest zones of the east, including subtropical forests in the southeast. Temperature and rainfall vary greatly according to terrain. Japan has a temperate climate with alpine climate in mountainous areas. Some countries of the region have undergone rapid economic development with excellent health services (e.g., Japan, Hong Kong, the Republic of Korea, Taiwan, and parts of China), whereas health infrastructure remains poor or insufficient in others (e.g., Mongolia, the Democratic People's Republic of Korea, Macao, and rural China). Population density is particularly high in some areas (e.g., eastern China, Japan) with many cities having populations in excess of 1 million people. However, the population remains primarily rural (72%, 1995) in China. The region remains prone to natural disasters such as floods, earthquakes, and landslides.

Disease Primarily Transmitted by Food and Drinking Water

Food- and drinking water–related diseases are common and reflect either the extent of high population density or the high economic development. In the most developed countries of the area (e.g., Japan, Hong Kong) the pattern is similar to that of North America and Europe. In less developed areas, infections such as amebic and bacillary dysentery, typhoid, and hepatitis A are more common.

VIRUSES. Hepatitis A: endemic in all countries. Large outbreaks reported in China (e.g., Shanghai, China, 1988, affecting 290,000 people and related to the consumption of clams). **Hepatitis E**: endemic, seasonal epidemics (e.g., western China). **Small round structured virus (SRSV)**: outbreaks reported from Japan. **Astrovirus**: large outbreak reported in schools (Osaka, Japan, 1991).

BACTERIA. *Bacillus cereus*: common cause of food poisoning (often related to rice). **Cholera**: endemic in China and Korea. Re-emergence in Japan through imported cases, as well as in Hong Kong (e.g., Vietnamese refugees, 1991 and 1994). Notable cholera outbreak in Selenge Province, Mongo-

lia, 1996. *Campylobacter* spp.: common. *Escherichia coli* spp.: common. *E. coli* 0157:H7: an emerging public health issue in the region with several outbreaks reported from Japan (e.g., Sakai City, 1996). **Enterohemorrhagic *E. coli* (EHEC)**: endemic. **Enteropathogenic *E. coli* (EPEC)**: endemic; outbreaks reported (e.g., Chongqing, China, 1987). **Enterotoxigenic *E. coli* (ETEC)**: endemic; outbreaks reported (e.g., Akita, Japan, 1995). Japan also increasingly reports **verotoxin-producing *E. coli* (VTEC)**. **Salmonellosis**: common cause of sporadic food-borne gastroenteritis and outbreaks (e.g., water-borne outbreak, Takotoh, Japan, 1989). **Shigellosis**: common cause of outbreak (e.g., military barracks, Shanghai, 1990–1991). **Typhoid** and **paratyphoid fevers**: endemic. *Vibrio parahaemolyticus*: common cause of food poisoning (e.g., Japan).

PROTOZOA. Amebic dysentery: common in the poor areas.

HELMINTHS. Globally highly endemic in the region. **Clonorchiasis (oriental liver fluke)** and **paragonimiasis** (oriental lung fluke): reported from China, Japan, Macao, and Korea). **Fascioliasis** (giant intestinal fluke): reported in China. **Gnathostomiasis** (*Gnathostoma* spp.): four gnathostoma species associated with infections in humans; *G. hispidum, G. doloresi*, and *G. spinigerum* widely distributed. Outbreaks related to consumption of undercooked fish (e.g., China, Japan). **Fish tapeworm** (*Diphyllobothrium latum*): endemic (e.g., Japan, Korea, China). **Pork tapeworm** (*Taenia solium*): endemic foci (e.g., northern China, mountainous areas of Taiwan). **Trichinellosis** (*Trichinella spiralis* spp.): sporadic (three outbreaks in Japan reported since 1974).

Disease Transmitted by Close Contact With Infectious Individuals

The epidemiology of these diseases in the most developed countries of the region is similar to that of North America and Europe.

VIRUSES. Acute hemorrhagic conjunctivitis: common outbreaks; major causes are Coxsackie and enteroviruses (e.g., four sequential outbreaks in Taiwan, 1985–1989, related to Coxsackie virus A 24). **Acute viral meningitis**: endemic; outbreaks reported (e.g., echovirus 30, Shanghai, China, and Gifu, Japan, 1991; echovirus 11, Japan, 1994). **Measles**: decreasing incidence due to successful immunization programs but outbreaks still reported from China (e.g., Taiwan), Japan, and Korea. Major outbreak in Hong Kong, 1988. **Mumps**: endemic; outbreaks reported (e.g., Akita, 1993, and Keshima Island, Japan, 1994–1995). **Poliomyelitis**: dramatic decrease in incidence (of about 80% since 1988) linked to mass immunization campaigns (e.g., in 1995, China had zero virologically confirmed indigenous cases but one case of wild poliovirus imported from Myanmar; rare outbreaks reported in some areas (e.g., Mongolia); Japan is polio-free. **Rubella virus**: endemic.

BACTERIA. Diphtheria: falling incidence due to vaccination; outbreak reported from Hubei, China, in 1988–1989. **Leprosy** (*Mycobacterium leprae*): endemic foci. **Meningococcal meningitis** (*Neisseria meningitidis*): endemic; some significant outbreaks (e.g., Mongolia). **Pertussis** (*Bordetella pertussis*): endemic. **Acute bacterial pneumonia**: pneumococcus, *Chlamydia pneumoniae*, and *Mycoplasma pneumoniae* are common causes of community-acquired pneumonia. Large outbreak caused by *M. pneumoniae* in Hong Kong, 1988. **Streptococcal disease** (group A *Streptococcus*): endemic. **Tuberculosis**: medium to low endemicity; reported rates have globally and significantly decreased since the 1970s (e.g., Japan, China). *Yersinia pseudotuberculosis*: rare but large outbreak reported (e.g., Aomori, Japan, 1991). **Chlamydia: Trachoma** *(Chlamydia trachomatis)*: reported in China and Mongolia.

ECTOPARASITES. Pediculosis *(Pediculus humanus capitis)*: common. **Scabies** *(Sarcoptes scabiei)*: common.

Sexually Transmitted Diseases

Similar disease epidemiology to that of North America and Europe for the most developed countries of the region (e.g., Japan); poorly documented in other countries (e.g., China, Mongolia).

VIRUSES. Hepatitis B: highly endemic. **Hepatitis C**: endemic. **HIV infection**: low prevalence but steady increase since the early 1990s, particularly, but not exclusively, among high-risk groups; constitutes a new and major public health concern for the region. **Syphilis** *(Treponema pallidum)*: endemic. **Chlamydia:** *Chlamydia trachomatis*: common genital infection.

Nosocomial Infections

Similar patterns to that of North America and Europe for the most developed countries (e.g., Japan, Hong Kong, the Republic of Korea, Taiwan); poorly documented in others (e.g., China, Democratic People's Republic of Korea, Mongolia).

VIRUSES. Adenovirus: pharyngoconjunctival fever outbreaks in hospitalized children (e.g., Fukouoka, Japan, 1988). **Hepatitis B** and **hepatitis C**: thought to occur, particularly where health infrastructure is poor. **HIV**: a regional emerging threat of nosocomial infection.

BACTERIA. Methicillin-resistant *Staphylococcus aureus* **(MRSA)**: increasingly reported (e.g., Taiwan, Hong Kong, and Japan). *Clostridium difficile*: outbreak in neonatal ICU, Gifu, Japan, 1994. *Pseudomonas cepacia*: outbreak in hospitalized immunocompromised patients related to contaminated nebulizer equipment (Kagawa, Japan, 1991). *Pseudomonas picketti*: outbreak in hospitalized patients related to the contamination of NaCl solution, Taiwan, 1990. *Serratia marcescens* outbreak reported in mechanically ventilated patients, Taiwan, 1994.

PROTOZOA. *Pneumocystis carinii*: outbreak in hospitalized children, Hong Kong, 1994; opportunistic infection in AIDS patients.

FUNGI. *Candida tropicalis*: reported in peritoneal dialysis unit, Hong Kong, 1992.

Human Zoonoses and Vector-Borne Diseases, Including Viral Hemorrhagic Fevers

Diseases Transmitted by Close Contact With Animals or Animal Products

VIRUSES. Rabies: endemic in China, Mongolia, and Korea. Not reported from Japan, Hong Kong, and Taiwan.

BACTERIA. Anthrax *(Bacillus anthracis)*: sporadic reports in animals. **Brucellosis** *(Brucella abortus, B. melitensis, B. suis)*: endemic (e.g., rural China). **Leptospirosis** *(Leptospira interrogans)*: endemic foci (e.g., rural China); outbreaks reported (e.g., American military personnel, Okinawa, Japan, 1991). **Chlamydia: Psittacosis** *(Chlamydia psittaci)*: endemic. Familial outbreaks reported (e.g., Japan). **Rickettsia: Q fever** *(Coxiella burnetii)*: exceptional reports.

Flea-Borne

BACTERIA. Plague *(Yersinia pestis)*: endemic foci of wild rodents (e.g., Qinghai Province and Xizang autonomous region of China, Mongolia).

RICKETTSIA. Murine typhus *(Rickettsia typhi)*: rare foci (e.g., Korea).

Mite-Borne

Scrub typhus *(Rickettsia tsutsugamushi)*: endemic foci (e.g., southern China, some valleys of Japan, the Republic of Korea). Epidemics reported (e.g., military personnel, Matsu Peikang Island, China, 1990).

Mosquito-Borne

VIRUSES. Crimean-Congo hemorrhagic fever: reported in western China. **Dengue**: endemic. Epidemics common (e.g., southern China). **Japanese encephalitis**: endemic (e.g., Korea, China, Japan).

PROTOZOA. Malaria: endemic foci in China, predominantly *Plasmodium vivax* (e.g., Guangdong, Guizhou, Yunnan, Guangxi, Hainan, Sichuan, and Fujian). Foci of falciparum malaria in Hainan and Yunnan; sporadic cases in Guangxi; low endemicity in other areas (e.g., Anhui, Hubei, Hunnan, Jiansu, Jiangxi, Shandong, Shanghai, and Zhejiang).

HELMINTHS. Lymphatic filariasis *(Wuchereria bancrofti, Brugia malayi, B. timori)*: remaining foci in southern China.

Phlebotomine-Borne

PROTOZOA. Cutaneous leishmaniasis: recently reported from Xinjiang, Uygur autonomous region, China. **Visceral leishmaniasis** *(Leishmania infantum)*: foci remaining in northeastern China, but resurgence reported.

Tick-Borne

Rickettsia: North Asian tick fever *(Rickettsia siberica)*: reported from northern China and Mongolia.

Soil-Borne or Airborne Diseases, and Diseases Associated With Recreational Water With No Evidence of Direct Person-to-Person Transmission

VIRUSES. Hemorrhagic fever with renal syndrome (Hantaan virus): endemic foci (e.g., China with 40,000 to 100,000 cases reported annually; the Republic of Korea with about 1000 cases annually). Rare cases in Japan. Mongolia is the only nonendemic country of the region. **Lymphocytic choriomeningitis virus** (arenavirus): rare reports.

BACTERIA. Legionnaires' disease *(Legionella pneumophila)*: outbreaks reported (e.g., Japan, China).

HELMINTHS. Visceral larva migrans *(Ascaris suum)*: endemic; outbreaks reported (e.g., Kyushu, Japan, 1994–1995).

Water-Snail-Borne

HELMINTHS. Schistosomiasis *(Schistosoma japonicum)*: endemic foci in China (e.g., Yangtze River basin, Szechwan). Active foci no longer exist in Japan.

■ OCEANIA: MAINLAND (Australia, New Zealand, and the Antarctic)

In Australia, the large mainland has tropical monsoon forests in the north and east; dry tropical forests, savanna, and large deserts in the center; and Mediterranean scrub and subtropical forests in the south. New Zealand has a temperate climate but the North Island is characterized by subtropical forests and the South Island by steppe vegetation and hardwood forests.

Disease Primarily Transmitted by Food and Drinking Water

Food- and drinking water–related diseases reflect the pattern of North America and Europe.

VIRUSES. Hepatitis A: endemic; outbreak reported (e.g., child care center, Victoria State, Australia, 1995). **Enteroviruses**: common.

BACTERIA. Cholera: rare imported cases (e.g., five in Australia and two in New Zealand in 1995). **Diarrhea caused by** *Campylobacter*: a frequent cause of sporadic gastroenteritis (e.g., 10,117 reports from Australia in 1994). Water-borne outbreaks reported from New Zealand. **Enteropathogenic** *Escherichia coli* (**EPEC**) and **enterohemorrhagic** *E. coli* (**EHEC**): uncommon. However, hemolytic-uremic syndrome (HUS) has been reported associated with various serogroups. HUS in Australia seems more often associated with *E. coli* of the serotype 0111 than with the serotype 0157. **Listeriosis**: occurs in both Australia and New Zealand (e.g., 34 reported cases in Australia in 1994). **Salmonellosis**: common cause of sporadic food-borne gastroenteritis as well as outbreaks. Nineteen reported outbreaks of salmonellosis in Australia in 1994 (37% were *Salmonella typhimurium*, a 43% increase since 1993). **Shigella**: commonly reported in Australia. **Typhoid** and **paratyphoid fevers**: small numbers. **Yersiniosis** (*Yersinia* spp.): common cause of gastroenteritis.

Diseases Transmitted by Close Contact With Infectious Individuals

Similar epidemiology to that of North America and Europe.

BACTERIA. Leprosy (*Mycobacterium leprae*): both endemic and imported diseases in Australia (e.g., 67 cases notified in Queensland, Australia 1982–1994). **Meningococcal meningitis** (*Neisseria meningitidis*): sporadic; occasional epidemics (e.g., serogroups B and C, Australia, 1994). **Pertussis** (*Bordetella pertussis*): endemic. **Pneumonia caused by** *Streptococcus pneumoniae*: rare isolates but probably a significant cause of community-acquired pneumonia. **Streptococcal disease** (group A *Streptococcus*): endemic. **Tuberculosis**: Low incidence in both Australia and New Zealand (5.7 and 10.0 cases per 100,000 population, respectively, 1994).

ECTOPARASITES. Pediculosis (*Pediculus humanus capitis*): common. **Scabies** (*Sarcoptes scabiei*): common.

Sexually Transmitted Diseases

Epidemiology similar to that of North America and Europe.

VIRUSES. Hepatitis B: endemic. **Hepatitis C**: endemic (e.g., 37,077 reports in Australia, 1991–1995), primarily among intravenous drug users. **HIV infection**: endemic, particularly in high-risk groups. **Herpes simplex virus** (**HSV-1** and **HSV-2**): endemic. **Papillomavirus**: endemic.

BACTERIA. Gonococcal infection (*Neisseria gonorrhoeae*): highly endemic; drug resistance reported. **Syphilis** (*Treponema pallidum*): endemic in high-risk groups. **Chlamydia: Chlamydial genital infections** (*Chlamydia trachomatis*): common.

FUNGI. Candidiasis (*Candida albicans*): very common.

ECTOPARASITES. Phthiriasis (*Phthirus pubis*): common.

Nosocomial Infections

Patterns similar to that of North America and Europe. **Methicillin-resistant** *Staphylococcus aureus* (**MRSA**): increasingly reported; Australia-wide outbreak of bacteremia due to *Pseudomonas picketti* related to the contamination of sterile water for injection, 1990.

Human Zoonoses and Vector-Borne Diseases, Including Viral Hemorrhagic Fevers

Diseases Transmitted by Close Contact with Animals or Animal Products

VIRUSES. Rabies: Australia and New Zealand are rabies-free. Animal cases reported from the Antarctic.

BACTERIA. Anthrax (*Bacillus anthracis*): endemic; rare human cases. **Brucellosis** (*Brucella abortus, B. melitensis, B. suis*): rare reports (e.g., Queensland, Australia). **Cat-scratch disease** (*Bartonella henselae*): rare. **Leptospirosis**: endemic foci; outbreak reported (e.g., east Otago, New Zealand, 1992, caused by *Leptospira hardjo*). **Chlamydia: psittacosis** (*Chlamydia psittaci*): endemic. **Rickettsia: Q fever** (*Coxiella burnetii*): endemic (e.g., New South Wales and Queensland, Australia). Cases peak in May and June.

Flea-Borne

Murine typhus (*Rickettsia typhi*): reported from western Australia in 1994.

Mosquito-Borne

VIRUSES. Barmah forest virus: reports of human disease in Australia since 1988 when it was shown to cause pathogenic infection in humans. Cases reported from Queensland, Northern Territory, western Australia, and Victoria. **Dengue**: endemic with periodic epidemics (e.g., Northern Territory and Queensland, Australia, usually dengue 2 or 1). Recent outbreak in December 1996 ended in January 1997. **Japanese encephalitis**: remains virtually absent but its emergence in northern Australia in 1995 is of considerable public health importance. **Murray Valley encephalitis** (*Flavivirus*): foci in Australia. **Ross River virus**: endemic with occasional outbreaks; concentrated in the coastal areas of the north and east and in the southwest of western Australia.

PROTOZOA. Malaria: the region is malaria-free; all reported cases are imported (700 to 800 cases per year in Australia).

Tick-Borne

Rickettsia: Queensland tick typhus (*Rickettsia australis*): endemic foci in Australia (e.g., Queensland, New South Wales, Tasmania, and coastal areas of eastern Victoria).

Soil-Borne or Airborne Diseases, and Diseases Associated With Recreational Water With No Evidence of Direct Animal-to-Human or Direct Person-to-Person Transmission

VIRUSES. Equine morbillivirus: outbreak reported in 1994 in Australia; a previously undescribed virus, involving humans and horses. **Lymphocytic choriomeningitis virus** (*Arenavirus*): rare reports. **Orf**: important occupational disease in New Zealand.

BACTERIA. Melioidosis (*Pseudomonas pseudomallei*): rare; reports from the tropical north of the Northern Territory, Queensland, and western Australia (e.g., Northern Territory, 21 cases reported in 1994–1995, 28 cases in 1993–1994, and 33 cases in 1990–1991).

▪ OCEANIA: MELANESIA AND MICRONESIA-POLYNESIA (American Samoa, Cook Islands, Eastern Island, Fiji, French Polynesia, Guam, Kiribati, Marshall Islands, Micronesia (Federated States of), Nauru, New Caledonia, Niue, Palau, Papua New Guinea, Samoa, Solomon Islands, Tokelau, Tonga, Trust Territory of the Pacific Islands, Tuvalu, Vanuatu, and the Wallis and Futuna Islands)

The area covers an enormous expanse of ocean with the largest, mountainous, tropical, and monsoon rain-forest–covered islands of the west giving way to the smaller, originally volcanic peaks and coral islands of the east. The climate is tropical marine moderated by trade winds. In contrast to the size of the area, the population is scarce and scattered on numerous islands. Economic development is overall poor, ranging from very poor (e.g., Papua New Guinea) to relatively high (e.g., New Caledonia).

Diseases Primarily Transmitted by Food and Drinking Water

Food- and drinking water–related diseases are common and have a similar epidemiologic pattern as mainland Oceania. Biointoxication may occur from raw or cooked fish and shellfish. **Typhoid** is notably endemic in some areas (e.g., Papua New Guinea).

Diseases Transmitted by Close Contact With Infectious Individuals

Similar epidemiology to that of mainland Oceania.
VIRUSES. Measles: there tend to be two annual peaks in measles incidence each year in the area (March/April in the west and July/August in the east). The rate of measles is falling gradually in the area due to vaccination. Peaks in incidence are seen approximately every 4 years. The last measles outbreak in the region was reported in August 1993 in the Solomon Islands.
BACTERIA. Pneumonia is the most commonly notifiable disease. It is the most important cause of childhood morbidity and mortality. **Tuberculosis**: rates of tuberculosis vary widely in the area (e.g., in 1994, incidence ranged from 21 per 100,000 in the Cook Islands to 329 per 100,000 in Kiribati).

Sexually Transmitted Diseases

Similar disease epidemiology to that of mainland Oceania.

Nosocomial Infections

Poorly documented in the region. No reported outbreaks in 1990–1996.

Human Zoonoses and Vector-Borne Diseases, Including Viral Hemorrhagic Fevers

Diseases Transmitted by Close Contact With Animals or Animal Products

Little information available on zoonoses in the region.
BACTERIA. Brucellosis: Low endemicity or absent in most islands. **Leptospirosis** (*Leptospira icterohaemorrhagiae, L. hardjo*): endemic foci, important in some islands (e.g., New Caledonia).
VIRUSES. Rabies: rare reports. Papua New Guinea is considered rabies-free.

Mosquito-Borne

VIRUSES. Dengue: endemic; recurrent outbreaks, including hemorrhagic dengue (e.g., New Caledonia, 1971–1980, with the appearance of dengue 3 in 1985; French Polynesia, Cook Islands, 1997). **Japanese encephalitis**: rare but now emerging in the region (e.g., Papua New Guinea). **Murray Valley encephalitis** (*Flavivirus*): foci in Papua New Guinea. **Ross River virus**: reported from Papua New Guinea, Fiji, Tonga, the Cook Islands, and American Samoa.
PROTOZOA. Malaria (*Plasmodium falciparum*): holoendemic in Papua New Guinea, Solomon Islands, and Vanuatu; high resistance to chloroquine.

Soil-Borne or Airborne Diseases, and Diseases Associated With Recreational Water With No Evidence of Direct Animal-to-Human or Direct Person-to-Person Transmission

BACTERIA. Melioidosis (*Pseudomonas pseudomallei*): rare reports (e.g., Papua New Guinea, Guam).
HELMINTHS. Strongyloidiasis (*Strongyloides stercoralis*): endemic. *S. fulleborni* reported from Papua New Guinea.

■ INTERNATIONAL SURVEILLANCE OF COMMUNICABLE DISEASES

THE NEED FOR INTERNATIONAL SURVEILLANCE. Surveillance of communicable diseases is increasingly gaining international importance because of the potential of communicable diseases for rapid international spread either through travel of infected individuals (e.g., cholera, dengue, Ebola hemorrhagic fever) or through the importation of contaminated food products (e.g., cholera, hepatitis A), including livestock (e.g., anthrax, bovine spongiform encephalopathy) and accompanying small animals (e.g., rodents) and insects. These diseases have not only public health implications but also political and economic consequences (e.g., impact of epidemics on tourism industry, impact of restricted traffic on business and trade). As an example, the 1994 suspected plague outbreak in Surat cost India an estimated U.S. $1.7 billion, and the 1991 cholera outbreak in Peru caused an estimated U.S. $700 million loss from trade barriers and about $70 million loss in tourist revenue. In light of this, there have been increasing efforts to establish international surveillance of communicable diseases in order to provide early warnings of outbreaks and to better coordinate national responses.

CURRENT EFFORTS IN INTERNATIONAL SURVEILLANCE AND CONTROL. Countries usually coordinate disease surveillance activities in Ministries of Health or specialized national communicable disease control centers, e.g., the Centers for Disease Control and Prevention (CDC) in the United States, the Laboratory Center for Disease Control (LCDC) in Canada, the Public Health Laboratory Services (PHLS) in the United Kingdom, and the Reseau National de Sante Publique (RNSP) in France. The basis of these surveillance systems is the routine identification of specified communicable diseases by health care centers or laboratories. The centers use specific case definitions and reporting mechanisms coordinated at the national level. Reporting is either immediate or periodic, usually weekly or monthly. An example of a national surveillance system based on a network of physicians who report specific diseases or syndromes is SentiWeb, INSERM, France, for the rapid monitoring of influenza epidemics.

International initiatives for disease surveillance and control have existed for years under the auspices of the WHO. All were set up to support the specific needs of international control programs. Diseases targeted for eradication, elimination, or for lower transmission (e.g., poliomyelitis, dracunculiasis, measles, leprosy, HIV/AIDS) have been systematically monitored. A monitoring system for antimicrobial resistance (WHONET) has also been developed, based on approximately 200 hospital diagnostic laboratories. WHONET provides standard information on drug-resistant organisms. The WHO Influenza Network involves 110 laboratories in 80 countries and three WHO Collaborating Centers for Reference and Research on Influenza. Weekly reports from participating laboratories during the influenza season contribute each year to essential data regarding antigens to be included in the next influenza vaccine. The European Working Group for *Legionella* Infections (EWGLI) maintains an international system for the surveillance of legionnaires' disease. Examination of travel-associated cases across many countries allows for the identification of common risk factors (e.g., specific hotels). Another example of laboratory-based systems is SAL-MET, PHLS, in the United Kingdom, which uses a network of laboratories to report *Salmonella* isolates and has now taken an international dimension.

The International Health Regulations (IHR) are another international tool for disease surveillance and control. It is the only international public health legislation and it requires WHO member states to report severe infectious diseases with a potential for international spread. The agreed-upon code of practice for controlling the international spread of diseases currently covers cholera, plague, and yellow fever. However, since the adoption of the IHR in 1969, two problems have arisen: reporting from member countries is far from complete and major changes have occurred in disease epidemiology. Additional diseases have become of international concern, and there has been a massive increase in international trade and travel. The ongoing revision of the IHR will allow reporting of clinical syndromes of potential international importance such as hemorrhagic fever.

SOURCES FOR UPDATED EPIDEMIOLOGIC INFORMATION. In addition to various printed journals and bulletins such as the *WHO Weekly Epidemiological Record* or the *CDC Mortality Morbidity Weekly Report* (MMWR), or many national or regional epidemiologic bulletins, there is an ever-increasing number of sources of electronic information on infectious diseases. Specialized software provides searchable databases for information on infectious disease epidemiology, diagnosis, and treatment (e.g., software developed for travel medicine and library searchable databases). In addition, electronic communications have allowed the rapid development of user groups who share information on infectious diseases via e-mail distribution groups. Access to these groups is either open (e.g., ProMed) or restricted (e.g., WHO rumor/outbreak list). Finally many Internet sites have been established by international (e.g., WHO, United Nations Children's Fund [formerly UNICEF]), governmental (e.g., CDC in the United States), and nongovernmental agencies (e.g., universities) that provide relevant unrestricted information. Lists of such sites can be obtained by searching the Internet using freely available Internet search engines.

PART XI
Laboratory Diagnosis of Parasitic Diseases

General Principles

John H. Cross

In the majority of cases, parasitic diseases cannot be diagnosed on clinical grounds alone. Clinical signs and symptoms, together with the patient's travel history, may enable the clinician to use laboratory and other diagnostic aids more judiciously, but confirmation of a suspected diagnosis usually depends on the results of appropriate laboratory studies. The physician in practice in North America and Europe is increasingly confronted with exotic infections as a result of increased international travel and immigration from developing countries. The AIDS pandemic has brought with it an increased prevalence of many of the more common parasitic infections as well as some (e.g., microsporidiosis, pneumocystosis) that seldom cause symptomatic infections in immunocompetent persons.

Thus, competence of the laboratory becomes important. The techniques described (Chapters 150 and 151) should be available in the clinical parasitology laboratory, and many can be performed by the clinician in the field or in an emergency when technical assistance may not be at hand. A few of the techniques listed are not in general use in the clinical laboratory but have applicability in the field. At times it is not possible to make a diagnosis by isolation and identification of the parasite. Other techniques, such as x-ray studies, ultrasound, and magnetic resonance imaging, may be helpful in specific instances, such as in neurocysticercosis and hydatid disease (Chapter 21). Serologic tests, which in recent years have become increasingly sensitive and selective, are often used to make the diagnosis or follow the results of treatment (Chapter 152). Many serologic tests can be performed successfully in the clinical laboratory or the field, whereas others require referral to specialized laboratories.

150 Examination of Stool and Urine Specimens

John H. Cross

Many methods, some of general applicability, others serving only limited purposes, have been described for examination of stool specimens. For routine examination, it is best to employ standard techniques in order to become familiar with their advantages and limitations. Time may be lost by using methods for purposes for which they were not intended, and identification of a parasite becomes difficult or impossible unless the correct method of examination is employed.

PHYSICAL CHARACTERISTICS OF THE SPECIMEN. The consistency of an unpreserved stool specimen is important,

giving an indication of the organisms that it may contain. Trophozoites of the intestinal protozoa are usually found in liquid or soft stools but almost never in fully formed ones. Protozoan cysts are rarely seen in liquid stools, unless these are the result of administration of a cathartic, in which case both trophic and cystic forms may be present. Cysts will usually be found in fully formed specimens. Helminth eggs may be present in either liquid or formed stools, but as the liquid stool is usually very dilute, they may be difficult to detect in such specimens.

If the unpreserved specimen is available, its surface should be examined for macroscopic parasites. Pinworms may be seen on the surface, and tapeworm proglottids may be found there or in its interior. The stool should be broken up with applicator sticks to check for helminths. If bright red blood is seen on the surface of formed stools, it is most frequently a sign of bleeding hemorrhoids; bloody mucus in loose or liquid specimens is suggestive of amebic ulcerations in the large intestine, although it may be due to other conditions. Patches of mucus on the surface of a specimen, particularly if blood-tinged, should always be examined carefully for trophic amebas. Occult blood in a stool may be a result of intestinal bleeding caused by parasites, but it is more likely to be indicative of other gastrointestinal disorders.

The age of an unpreserved specimen is of great importance. Freshly passed specimens are essential for the detection of trophic amebas or flagellates. All liquid or soft stools are best examined *within one-half hour of the time of passage.* If this is impossible, part of the specimen should be preserved within this time for subsequent examination. The immediate examination of fully formed specimens is not as critical, but when they cannot be examined within 3 to 4 hours they should be preserved.

Examination of a freshly passed stool specimen is impractical in the field and often difficult to accomplish in an urban laboratory setting. Many laboratories now rely exclusively on specimens preserved immediately after passage in various fixative solutions. The specimens may then be submitted to the laboratory for examination at a convenient time. Kits containing these solutions are commercially available or may be prepared by the laboratory for distribution to patients. Some kits also allow for submission of an unpreserved portion of the specimen.

TECHNIQUES OF STOOL EXAMINATION. Unfortunately, no single technique of stool examination will yield satisfactory results, as none of the methods is equally applicable to the detection of trophic protozoa, cysts, and helminth eggs. For this reason, a combination of two or more is desirable.

Direct Wet Film. This method is most useful for the detection of trophic forms of amebas and flagellates but should be reserved for the examination of freshly passed liquid or soft stools or the mucoid portion of formed specimens. It allows the study of motility of the organisms, which is often characteristic and of value in making a precise identification. Protozoan cysts and helminth eggs may also be seen on wet film if they are present in large enough numbers; however, concentration methods are more efficient for their detection.

In the preparation of a wet film, a small portion of feces is mixed with a drop of normal saline on a clean slide; a coverslip is placed on the preparation and it is first examined unstained. In making the wet film, it is best to take small amounts of material from several parts of the stool specimen. The film should not be too thick. A convenient rule of thumb is to prepare the film just thin enough so that ordinary newsprint can easily be read through it. After the wet film has been thoroughly checked for trophic amebas and flagellates, under low power of the microscope and using a low intensity of illumination, an iodine stain may be prepared.

Iodine stains the cysts of amebas and other protozoa, revealing some details that cannot be seen in the unstained preparation. Trophozoites are rapidly killed and are sometimes unidentifiable after iodine staining; the stain should not be applied until after the specimen has been thoroughly examined in the unstained condition. Gram's iodine or Lugol's solution will give satisfactory results, but modified D'Antoni iodine solution is preferable.

A separate iodine stain may be prepared by the addition of a small drop of this reagent to a wet film of fecal material before it is covered, or the iodine may be added to the edge of the coverslip so that it gradually diffuses into the saline mount. It should be borne in mind that a concentrate of the stool may also be stained with iodine and will reveal, in larger numbers, any organisms that may be seen by direct examination of the iodine-stained specimen. Organisms present in such small numbers that they may not be seen at all on direct examination can at times be detected with ease after concentration of the specimen. The Merthiolate-iodine-formaldehyde (MIF) stain will fix and stain both trophozoites and cysts; iodine stains will shrink and distort trophic amebas or flagellates.

Concentration Techniques. Concentration methods attempt the separation of protozoan cysts and helminth eggs from the bulk of fecal matter through differences in specific gravity (Fig. 150–1). With the various sedimentation methods, eggs and cysts, which are heavier than the suspending liquid, become concentrated in the bottom of a tube. Flotation of eggs and cysts involves use of a heavy liquid, and the lighter parasites rise to its surface. The formalin-ether sedimentation technique of Ritchie is excellent for the concentration of both cysts and eggs and may be used with preserved specimens

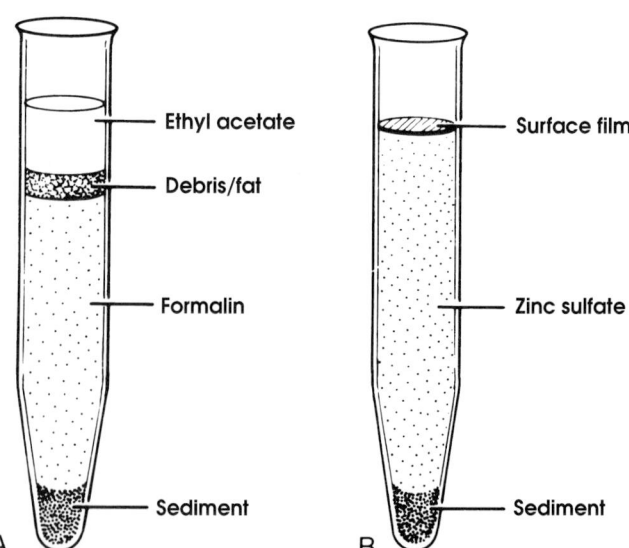

Figure 150–1. Fecal concentration procedures: various layers seen in tubes after centrifugation. *A,* Formalin-ether (or ethyl acetate). *B,* Zinc sulfate (the surface film should be within 2 to 3 mm of the tube rim). (Illustration by Nobuko Kitamura. From Garcia LS, Bruckner DA: Diagnostic Medical Parasitology, 3rd ed. New York, Elsevier, 1990.)

(Chapter 117). None of the sedimentation methods results in as good a separation of fecal debris from the eggs and cysts as can be achieved by a flotation method; the one recommended is a modification of the zinc sulfate centrifugal flotation method of Faust. The zinc sulfate flotation is also excellent for the recovery of protozoan cysts and most eggs, but it does not work well with trematode eggs or those of the broad fish tapeworm. Eggs of other types and protozoan cysts will be concentrated relatively free from fecal debris by this method. The laboratory worker should be familiar with both techniques.

After concentration, the diagnostic material is transferred to a microscope slide, and a drop of iodine is added to stain any protozoan cysts that may be present. Complete examination of every concentrate under low power of the microscope is required. A little practice will make it possible to recognize even the smaller protozoan cysts at this magnification, although for specific identification, magnification of a stained slide at high power may be necessary. Oil-immersion magnification serves no useful purpose, as the structural differentiation produced by iodine or MIF stains is not improved by higher magnification.

Stained Slides. Frequently it is impossible to make an exact identification of certain protozoa with a combination of the foregoing techniques. In such cases, the cytologic detail revealed by one of the permanent stains is essential. Such a stain will reveal significantly higher percentages of *Entamoeba histolytica* and other protozoan parasites than are detected when only direct examination and concentration methods are used. It is widely held that a report of *E. histolytica* infection should be made *only* when confirmed by a permanent stain.

When fresh stool specimens are used, a small quantity of feces is transferred to a clean slide with an applicator stick. The material is then streaked out in a thin uniform film. With a little practice, films of the correct thickness can be made regularly. Generally, formed stools are of the proper consistency for making films, but if the specimen is hard, it may be necessary to add a small amount of saline.

A liquid stool will sometimes fail to adhere to the slide; in such cases a thin layer of serum or of egg albumin, as used in mounting tissue sections, will increase adherence. When using fresh specimens, it is essential that the film be placed in fixative immediately after it is made; if it dries at any time, it will be useless.

When polyvinyl alcohol (PVA)–fixed material is used, slides are prepared as follows: The preserved specimen is again thoroughly mixed and may be strained through gauze to remove large particulate matter. After sedimentation, a portion of the fecal matter is removed with applicator sticks and placed on absorbent material, such as blotting paper, to remove the excess PVA. The material is then streaked onto slides, and the slides are allowed to dry for about 2 hours at room temperature or 1 hour at 37°C. They may then be stained or stored dry for subsequent staining.

Gomori trichrome stain, originally intended for histologic use, has been adapted for use in staining intestinal protozoa and is the method most frequently used at present. It is not generally recognized that helminth eggs can be identified in the trichrome-stained fecal film, but with a little experience it is possible to recognize most by this method. More precise cytologic detail may be obtained with the use of iron hematoxylin, which is preferable for staining sodium acetate–acetic acid–formalin (SAF)–preserved material. However, this stain requires considerable technical competence, whereas trichrome will give satisfactory results even in the hands of relatively inexperienced persons.

Artifacts. When examining stool specimens, it is possible to confuse some yeast, plant, or tissue cells or other commonly occurring objects with diagnostic forms of helminths or protozoa, especially with amebic cysts. A number of objects commonly found in the feces that may be mistaken for parasites are illustrated in Figure 150–2.

NUMBER OF SPECIMENS TO BE EXAMINED. The number of stools that should be examined will depend on the purpose for which the examination is made. If one is interested only in determining the presence or absence of intestinal or hepatic helminth parasites, one or two examinations may be sufficient if concentration methods are used, as these methods are very efficient in the detection of small numbers of eggs. On the other hand, Sawitz and Faust (1942) stated that a single stool examination, even if a combination of techniques is used, will uncover somewhat under 50% of *E. histolytica* infections, and that at least six examinations are necessary if over 90% accuracy is to be obtained. This is

shown graphically in Figure 150–3. These percentages apply to normally passed stools only. Many authorities recommend the routine use of purged stools if one is searching for *E. histolytica*, since purged specimens may increase the chances of finding parasites. Purged specimens must be examined or placed in a fixative solution immediately, or they are worthless. If one has the facilities to collect purged specimens and *examine them immediately after they have been passed*, this procedure should increase the percentage of positive results. A saline purge of Epsom salts or Fleet's Phospho-Soda is recommended. Parasites in the first bowel movement will probably be distorted; those in the second and subsequent movements will most likely be recognizable.

SUBSTANCES THAT INTERFERE WITH STOOL EXAMINATIONS. Castor oil or mineral oil should not be administered prior to the collection of stool specimens. Antibiotics that

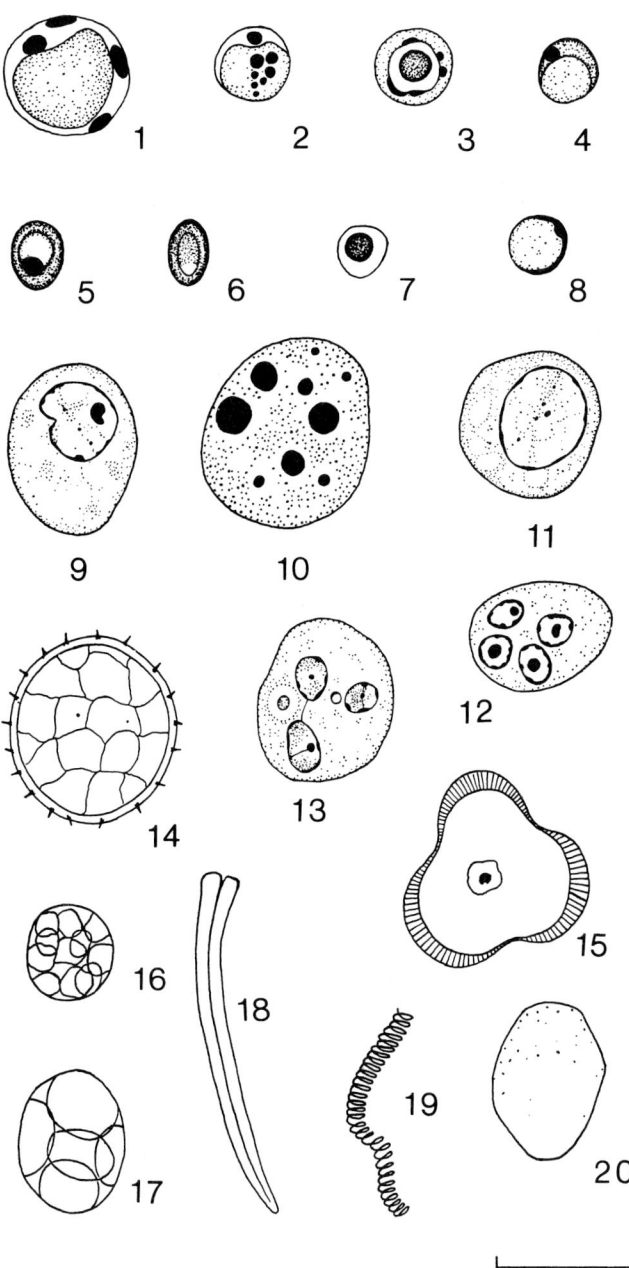

Figure 150–2. Various structures seen in stool preparations: *1, 2, 4, Blastocystis hominis; 3, 5, 6, 7, 8,* various yeasts; *9, 11,* squamous cells from rectal mucosa; *10,* deteriorated macrophage without nucleus; *12, 13,* polymorphonuclear leukocytes; *14, 15,* "pollen grains"; *16, 17,* aggregates of starch granules; *18,* plant hair; *19,* vegetable spiral; *20,* amorphous vegetable material, superficially resembling helminth egg or protozoan cyst. (From Markell EK, Voge M, John DT: Medical Parasitology, 7th ed. Philadelphia, WB Saunders, 1992.)

10μ

DETECTION OF E. HISTOLYTICA IN SERIAL STOOL EXAMINATIONS

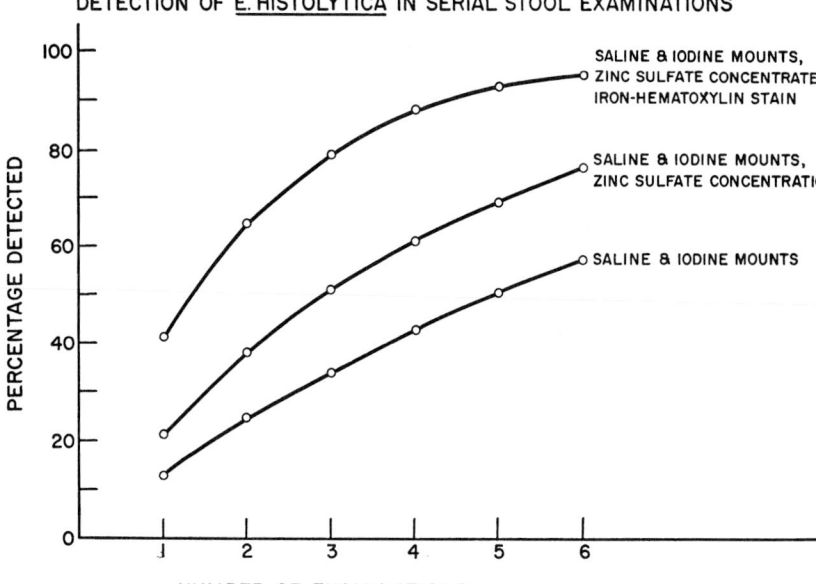

Figure 150–3. Probability of detecting *Entamoeba histolytica* by successive stool examinations, using various techniques. (Based on figures from Sawitz and Faust, 1942. From Markell EK, Voge M, John DT: Medical Parasitology, 7th ed. Philadelphia, WB Saunders, 1992.)

affect the intestinal flora, administered within the preceding month, will decrease the chances of finding intestinal protozoa, as will some antimalarials, e.g., chloroquine. Stools passed for about a week after the administration of barium cannot be examined for parasites, as the barium interferes with microscopy. Enemas of any type should be avoided. Compounds containing kaolin and bismuth, milk of magnesia, and antacids will also interfere with the examination for parasites, as will the presence of urine in the specimen.

PRESERVATION OF STOOL SPECIMENS. The trophic protozoa contained in a stool specimen begin to deteriorate almost as soon as the stool is passed. If the specimen cannot be examined promptly, a portion should be preserved for subsequent use. MIF solution will preserve the specimen for some months and also stain it for examination. A permanent preparation cannot be made from MIF-preserved material, and identification must be made on the basis of detail revealed by thimerosal (Merthiolate) and iodine.

If one desires to make permanent stains at a later date, PVA or SAF fixative solutions should be used. PVA-preserved material retains excellent staining properties for at least a month, after which time it slowly deteriorates. SAF fixative has the advantage of not containing mercuric chloride but is technically a little more difficult to use. If a helminth infection is suspected, a portion of the specimen should be preserved in formol-saline.

STAINS FOR DIRECT SMEARS
Modified D'Antoni Iodine Solution
Distilled water	100 mL
Potassium iodide	1 g
Powdered iodine crystals	1.5 g

The potassium iodide solution should be saturated with iodine, with some excess remaining in the bottle. Store in brown, glass-stoppered bottles in the dark. The solution is ready for use after 4 days, and sufficient quantity for daily use is decanted into a brown glass dropping bottle and discarded after 1 day. The stock solution remains good as long as an excess of iodine remains in the bottle.

Lugol's Solution
Distilled water	100 mL
Potassium iodide	10 g
Iodine crystals	5 g

Gram's Iodine
Lugol's solution	1 part
Distilled water	14 parts

MIF Stain-Preservative Solution
Stock MF Solution
Distilled water	250 mL
Tincture of Merthiolate	200 mL
Formaldehyde	25 mL
Glycerin	5 mL

This solution is stored in brown glass bottles. For use, it is combined with fresh Lugol's solution (not over 1 week old) in the following manner:

1. Measure 2.35 mL of stock MF solution into a small test tube, and stopper with a cork.
2. Measure 0.15 mL of Lugol's solution into a second tube, and close with a rubber stopper.

The two solutions are combined immediately before addition of the fecal specimen. The amount of fecal material to be added to this volume of preservative should be about 0.25 g. Break up the specimen in the MIF solution and mix thoroughly. The specimen may be examined immediately or stored in a well-stoppered tube; it will retain a good stain for some months. After storage, it will be found that most protozoa and helminth eggs occur in the upper layers of sedimented feces. A drop of mixed supernatant fluid and feces is withdrawn, placed on a slide, and covered with a coverslip.

PRESERVATIVE SOLUTIONS
PVA Fixative Solution.* This fixative, which consists of polyvinyl alcohol, glycerin, glacial acetic acid, and Schaudinn's solution, will keep indefinitely but must not be subjected to extremes of temperature. It is convenient to dispense the PVA fixative solution in screw-capped bottles, in approximately 5-mL quantities. To this volume of fixative, approximately 1 g of feces may be added. It must be well broken up and thoroughly mixed with the preservative solution. The solution preserves both trophozoites and cysts of protozoa;

---

*Obtainable from Medical Chemical Corporation, P.O. Box 445, Santa Monica, CA 90404; Marion Scientific, 30 Encore Ct., Newport Beach, CA 92663. However, many commercial stool-collection kits containing PVA fixative solution are now available.

most eggs are recognizable after PVA preservation. Protozoa remain stainable for at least 1 month. To prepare slides for staining, shake the preserved specimen well or mix contents with two applicator sticks. Pour some of the PVA mixture onto blotting paper and allow to stand for a few minutes. Apply stool material to slide in the manner described earlier, and dry for 2 hours at 37°C, or overnight at room temperature, before staining. The dry unstained slides may be mailed in this condition if necessary. This method is particularly useful because outpatients may be given vials containing PVA fixative and given instructions on how to fix their own stool specimens immediately after passage. If desirable, an entire series of specimens may be brought in at one time after all have been collected.

Schaudinn's Solution
Mercuric chloride, saturated aqueous . . . . 2 parts
Ethyl alcohol, 95% . . . . 1 part

Glacial acetic acid is added to Schaudinn's solution in the proportion of 1 part acetic acid to 19 parts of stock immediately before use.

SAF Fixative Solution
(Yang and Scholten, 1977). Like PVA, the sodium acetate–acetic acid–formalin (SAF) fixative-preservative may be used for the preservation of material, which can then be concentrated by the formalin-ethyl acetate technique or made into permanent stained smears. The fixative is more liquid than PVA, and the preserved specimen must be centrifuged after straining through gauze and the sediment used to prepare smears for staining; adherence to the glass slide may be improved if the slide is coated with albumin or possibly Silane solution (Surgipath Medical Industries). After drying, the slides may be placed in 70% alcohol.

SAF fixative solution is made up as follows:
Sodium acetate . . . . 1.5 g
Acetic acid, glacial . . . . 2.0 mL
Formaldehyde, 40% . . . . 4.0 mL
Distilled water . . . . 92.5 mL

CONCENTRATION METHODS. Concentration of stool specimens to demonstrate cysts and eggs present in small numbers should be a routine part of the parasitologic examination. Special techniques have been devised for the concentration of nematode larvae in the stool. These are rather simple to perform and should be used whenever the presence of these parasites is suspected if they cannot be demonstrated by more direct forms of examination.

Modified Zinc-Sulfate Flotation
Zinc sulfate, USP . . . . 330 g
Distilled water . . . . to make 1 L

This is only an approximation of the correct solution, which should have a specific gravity of 1.180. A reliable battery hydrometer must be used in adjusting to the correct specific gravity by the addition of zinc sulfate or water. Specific gravity is critical and must be checked frequently.

Procedure
1. Prepare a fecal suspension of approximately 1 mL of feces (more if dilute) in 10 to 15 times its volume of tap water.
2. Strain through two layers of wet gauze in a funnel, into a small test tube. Fill with water to about 1 cm from top of tube.
3. Centrifuge for 45 seconds at approximately $2000 \times g$. Break up any "plug" that may have formed at the top, and decant supernatant.
4. Add 2 to 3 mL of tap water, shake or tap tube to resuspend sediment, and fill tube with tap water to 1 cm from top. Centrifuge as before.

5. Decant supernatant, add 2 to 3 mL of zinc sulfate solution, resuspend, and fill tube with zinc sulfate solution to about 0.5 cm from top.
6. Centrifuge at $2000 \times g$ for 2 minutes. Do not "brake" the centrifuge or jar the tubes.
7. Without removing tubes from centrifuge, remove several loopfuls of material floating on surface (be careful not to go below surface film with wire loop), place on a slide with a drop of iodine solution, and cover with a coverslip.

Current's Modification of Sheather's Sugar Flotation for *Cryptosporidium*
Sheather's Sugar Solution
Sucrose . . . . 500 g
Tap water . . . . 320 mL
Phenol . . . . 6.5 g

Procedure
1. Boil sugar solution until clear. *Carefully* add phenol and stir. (Use fume hood.) Cool to room temperature.
2. Place 1 to 2 mL of fecal suspension in 12-mL conical centrifuge tube.
3. Add Sheather's sugar solution until tube is ¾ full.
4. Stir vigorously with applicator stick.
5. Fill tube to 1 to 2 cm from top.
6. Centrifuge at $300 \times g$ for 5 to 10 minutes.
7. Transfer surface material to microscope slide by means of wire loop.
8. Cover with a coverslip and observe with phase-contrast microscopy.

The rounded oocysts, 4 to 6 μm in diameter, contain crescentic sporozoites that are best seen by this method.

STAINED SMEARS. For many years the somewhat laborious iron hematoxylin stain, in various forms, was the only one available for permanent stains of stool specimens. It is seldom used nowadays. The trichrome stain has supplanted iron hematoxylin in most laboratories; the detail obtained is sufficient for diagnostic purposes, and the stain is easier to use.

Gomori's Trichrome Stain
Chromotrope 2R* . . . . 0.6 g
Light green SF* . . . . 0.3 g
Phosphotungstic acid . . . . 0.7 g
Acetic acid, glacial . . . . 1.0 mL
Allow to stand for 30 to 60 minutes, then
   add distilled water . . . . 100.0 mL

Slides may be prepared from fresh or PVA- or SAF-preserved material. If PVA-preserved material is used, start with step 3 of the procedure; with SAF-preserved stools, start with step 4.

Procedure
1. Fix in Schaudinn's solution with acetic acid added 30 minutes.
2. Wash in 70% alcohol for 15 minutes.
3. Wash in 70% alcohol to which sufficient iodine has been added to produce a port-wine color after 3 minutes.
4. Wash in 70% alcohol, two changes, each 1 minute.
5. Stain in Gomori's trichrome for 8 to 15 minutes.
6. Rinse in 90% alcohol with 1% acetic acid for 1 to 2 seconds.
7. Dip twice in 100% alcohol.
8. Dehydrate in a second change of 100% alcohol for 30 seconds.

---

*Manufactured by National Aniline Division, Allied Chemical and Dye Corp., New York, NY.

9. Place in xylene for 1 minute.
10. Mount in Permount or other mounting medium.

Although excellent for all other stool protozoa, neither of the foregoing methods will stain coccidia well. These organisms are acid-fast and stain well with a modified acid-fast stain (Garcia et al., 1983).

Cryptosporidium is a common pathogen. Formol-saline or formalin-preserved specimens may be used in preparing the stained smears, although the technique works well on slides prepared from a fresh stool specimen. If the formalin-preserved material is used, approximately 1 mL of the preserved material should be added to 10 mL of 10% formalin in a centrifuge tube. The mixture is centrifuged at 300 × *g* for 2 minutes, the supernatant decanted, and the sediment spread in uniform thin layers on glass microscope slides.

Modified Acid-Fast Stain for *Cryptosporidium Cyclospora*, and *Isospora*

Kinyoun's Carbol-Fuchsin

Basic fuchsin	4 g
Phenol (liquified)	8 g
Ethyl alcohol, 95%	20 mL
Distilled water	100 mL

Dissolve fuchsin in alcohol, add liquified phenol and mix well, then add water.

EXAMINATION OF URINE AND VAGINAL SECRETIONS.

Eggs of *Schistosoma haematobium* and on occasion, microfilariae of *Wuchereria* and *Onchocerca* may be found in the urine. *Trichomonas vaginalis* may be found in the urinary sediment of both males and females and in prostatic and vaginal secretions.

Schistosome eggs and microfilariae are best recovered by examination of centrifuged or membrane-filtered (Nucleopore) urine specimens. Ten milliliters of a fresh, midday urine specimen is preferred for *S. haematobium*; microfilariae of *Wuchereria* are found in the urine of patients exhibiting chyluria, whereas those of *Onchocerca* are usually seen immediately following treatment with diethylcarbamazine. The hatching test may demonstrate the presence of small numbers of schistosome eggs, if viable.

T. vaginalis may be recognized in a fresh specimen of urine or in vaginal or prostatic exudate by its jerky motility or (under high dry magnification) by the movement of its undulating membrane (see Fig. 91–1). It may also be seen in Pap smears.

SPECIAL DETECTION METHODS

Baermann Apparatus for Recovery of *Strongyloides* Larvae. *Strongyloides* larvae do not always concentrate well with either of the concentration techniques, although they may be detected by those methods. The Baermann technique yields a good concentration of the *living* larvae of *S. stercoralis*. It should be used when there is a high index of suspicion and routine stool examinations are negative, and for following the results of therapy.

1. A glass funnel with a diameter of 10 cm or greater is set up in a ring stand, with a short piece of rubber tubing attached to its stem and a pinchcock closing the tubing.
2. A wire circle, of slightly smaller diameter than the top of the funnel, is covered with two layers of gauze. The edges of the gauze are folded under the ring, which is fitted into the funnel.
3. The funnel is filled with lukewarm water to a level just covering the gauze, and a specimen of stool is placed on the gauze, partially in contact with the water.
4. Allow apparatus to stand at room temperature for 8 to 12 hours, then draw off a few drops of fluid through the tubing into a small glass dish.
5. Examine for larvae under low power of the microscope.

Agar Plate Culture for *Strongyloides* Larvae (Arakaki et al., 1990). Agar medium (beef extract, 0.5%; peptone, 1%; sodium chloride, 0.5%; agar, 1.5%) is poured in a thin layer into a 9-cm Petri dish, covered and hardened overnight. A few grams of feces are placed into the center of the agar and incubated for 48 hours at 28°C. Plates are always handled with disposable gloves. Tracks made in the agar by the larvae and free-living adult *Strongyloides* are examined under a dissecting microscope. The parasites are recovered by Pasteur pipette and placed onto a glass slide and identified under higher magnification.

Filter Paper Strip Procedure for Recovery of Hookworm *Strongyloides* or *Trichostrongylus* Larvae. This method takes too long for clinical usefulness but is well adapted for field or survey use, where quick results are not essential. The technique, originally described by Harada and Mori in 1955, requires minimal equipment.

A 20 × 13 mm filter paper strip, in the center of which is placed 0.5 to 1.0 g of feces, is inserted into a 15-mL centrifuge tube containing 3 to 4 mL of distilled water. The tube is placed upright or in a slightly slanted position, such that the filter paper is kept moist by capillary flow. Water may be added as needed to maintain the original fluid level. After 5 to 10 days a small amount of fluid is withdrawn from the bottom of the tube and examined for larvae. The preparation should be handled carefully, as the larvae may be in the infective stage.

Cellophane Tape Swab for *Enterobius* and *Taenia* Eggs. A number of commercial pinworm detection kits are now available, but the test is easily performed with cellophane.

Procedure

1. Fold together sticky surfaces of a piece of cellophane tape, 1 × 8 cm in length, for about 1 cm at each end.
2. Stretch tape, sticky side out, over butt end of a test tube, holding nonsticky ends firmly with thumb and forefinger.
3. Apply tape to anal area, rocking back and forth to cover as much of the mucosa and mucocutaneous area as possible.
4. Remove tape and apply to microscope slide, sticky side down. Press firmly into position.
5. Examine for eggs under low-power microscope. Pinworm eggs, which are generally deposited at night, will be found scattered around the perianal region. The tape should be used in the morning before the patient has washed or defecated.

Use of the clear type of cellophane tape is essential. Tape with a frosted appearance obscures the eggs. A number of commercial kits are available, e.g., the Swube Paddle (Falcon Plastics), a smooth plastic paddle coated on one side with an adhesive that collects and holds the specimen. The paddle can be examined directly under the microscope.

Schistosomal Hatching Test. If feces containing viable schistosome eggs is diluted with approximately 10 volumes of water, the eggs will hatch within a few hours, releasing miracidia. The miracidia are positively phototropic.

Procedure

1. A stool specimen is homogenized by shaking in normal saline and is then strained through two layers of gauze.
2. The material is allowed to sediment, the supernatant is decanted and the sediment resuspended in saline. This process is repeated at least twice.
3. The saline is decanted and replaced with distilled water, and the suspension is placed in a side-arm or Erlenmeyer flask. The side-arm flask is covered with black

paper, aluminum foil, or black paint, except for the side arm. If an Erlenmeyer flask is used, it is covered to 1 cm below the level of fluid in the neck of the flask. Additional water is added if necessary.

4. The flask is allowed to stand at room temperature for several hours in subdued light.
5. The side arm, or water in the neck of the flask, is then illuminated strongly from the side.
6. The illuminated area is examined with a magnifying glass to detect the presence of free-swimming miracidia.

Eggs of *Schistosoma haematobium* in the urine may also be hatched in this manner, but they are more easily concentrated by centrifugation or membrane filtration.

DUODENAL SAMPLING AND BIOPSY. Sampling and examination of duodenal contents is a reliable means of recovery of *Strongyloides* larvae and other small intestinal parasites, e.g., *Giardia, Isospora, Cryptosporidium,* and *Cyclospora.* Specimens may be obtained by intubation or by use of the enteric capsule or string test (Enterotest). A No. 00 gelatin capsule containing a 90-cm line (Fig. 150–4), composed of a 20-cm silicon rubber–covered thread and a 70-cm soft nylon yarn, is swallowed by the patient while the thread, which protrudes from a hole in the capsule, is held firmly. To the end of the nylon yarn is attached a 1-g weight, which eventually helps carry the string into the duodenum. The free end of the line is taped to the patient's neck or cheek and may be pulled up after 4 hours. The bile-stained mucus adhering to its distal end is examined under the microscope. The weight becomes disengaged in the intestine at the time the thread is withdrawn.

Biopsy of the small intestinal mucosa may reveal *Giardia, Cryptosporidium,* and microsporidia as well as *Strongyloides* larvae.

CULTURE METHODS. Many of the intestinal protozoa

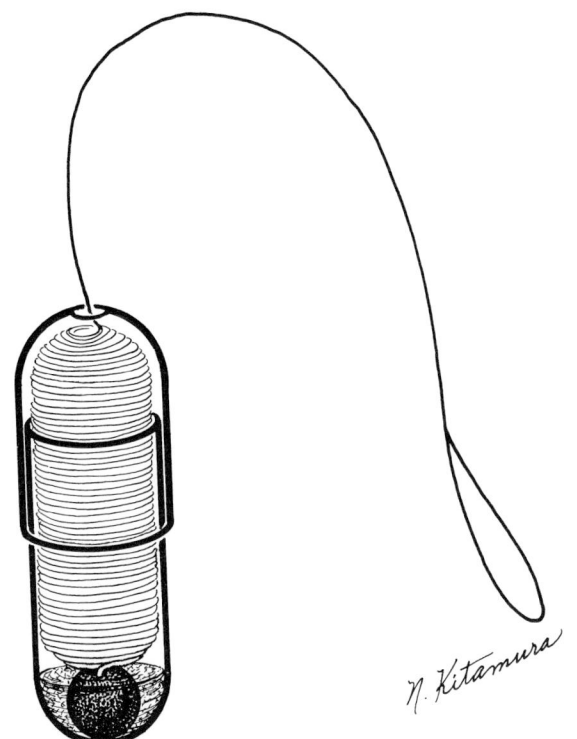

Figure 150–4. Enteric capsule for sampling duodenal content. (From Garcia LS, Bruckner DA: Diagnostic Medical Parasitology, 3rd ed. New York, Elsevier, 1997.)

have now been successfully cultured. Cultivation of the nonpathogenic amebas, the flagellates, and *Balantidium* falls into the category of research procedures, requiring too much material and time to be of diagnostic usefulness.

Entamoeba histolytica can be cultivated on a variety of media, some of which may be purchased in the dehydrated form and prepared with a minimum of effort. Various authorities advocate the use of *E. histolytica* cultures in the diagnostic laboratory as a screening procedure. Others suggest that the cultures be employed in every suspected case of amebiasis when the microscopic examination yields negative results. A third viewpoint is that expressed by certain workers who have determined the number of *E. histolytica* cysts that must be present per gram of feces to ensure a high percentage of successful cultures. Results of these studies indicate that the number of cysts necessary for viable cultures is sufficiently large to be detectable by ordinary microscopic methods, and thus cultures are superfluous.

The success with which *E. histolytica* is cultivated will depend largely on familiarity with the techniques involved. For this reason, sporadic use of culture techniques is not recommended; they should be undertaken only in laboratories where the number of specimens examined is sufficiently large to justify considerable time being spent on their maintenance and examination. Likewise, culture methods should never be used as a substitute for routine and thorough microscopic examination by the various methods outlined previously. Diamond's medium may be obtained freeze-dried for reconstitution as a liquid medium; Boeck and Drbohlav's Locke egg serum (LES) medium is solid with a liquid overlay and can be prepared in the laboratory.

Diamond's Medium for Axenic Culture of *Entamoeba*. Now obtainable as TYI-S-33 Medium, freeze-dried, from the American Type Culture Collection,* it is prepared as follows:

TYI-S-33 broth base with 10% bovine
    serum . . . . 1 bottle
Distilled water . . . . 55 mL

Dispense 13 mL of medium per tube into 16 × 125 mm screw-cap culture tubes. It may be stored at ambient temperature ($\pm 25°C$) for up to 90 days, but for longest shelf life it is recommended that it be stored at 2° to 8°C. Some strains of *E. histolytica* require 15% bovine serum, necessitating the addition of an extra 5% by volume of bovine calf serum, inactivated at 56°C for 30 minutes, prior to use.

Inoculate with a portion of stool the size of a small pea, adding to the medium before inoculation 100 units of penicillin and 100 µg of streptomycin/mL. Gentamicin 50 µg/mL may substitute for penicillin and streptomycin. Incubate at 37°C and examine after 2, 3, and 4 days of incubation by removing a small amount of sediment by pipette. The sediment is transferred to a slide, covered, and examined under low-power microscope. Primary isolation may yield few organisms, whereas subsequent transfers show a considerable increase in numbers. It should be unnecessary to use antibiotics for successive transfers after primary isolation.

Boeck and Drbohlav's Locke Egg Serum (LES) Medium for Amebas

Locke's Solution

NaCl	9.0 g
CaCl$_2$	0.2 g
KCl	0.4 g
NaHCO$_3$	0.2 g

*American Type Culture Collection, 10801 University Blvd., Manassas, VA 20110-2209.

Glucose . . . . 2.5 g
Distilled water . . . . 1 L

This solution should be autoclaved before storage

Procedure

1. Wash four eggs, brush with alcohol to sterilize, and break into a sterile flask containing glass beads.
2. Add 50 mL of Locke's solution; shake until homogeneous.
3. Dispense in test tubes a sufficient quantity to produce a 2½- to 3½-cm slant in bottom of tube.
4. Slant plugged tubes and place in inspissator at 70°C until slants are solidified. If an inspissator is not available, a substitute may be devised by leaving the door of the autoclave partly open.
5. When slants have become solidified, autoclave at 15 pounds pressure for 20 minutes. If any slants are badly broken, discard them.
6. Cover slants to a depth of about 1 cm with mixture of 8 parts of sterile Locke's solution to 1 part sterile inactivated human blood serum. Sterility of mixture of Locke's solution and serum should be ensured by filtration sterilization followed by incubation at 37°C for 24 hours or longer before use.

A loopful of sterile rice starch or powder is added to each tube before inoculation. Inoculate with a portion of stool the size of a small pea, break up well in medium, and incubate at 37°C. Examine as noted for Diamond's medium. Note that this is not an axenic medium and that antibiotics are not added.

METHODS FOR ESTIMATION OF WORM BURDEN. Estimates of daily egg output have been made for a number of hepatic and intestinal worms. If one can estimate the total number of eggs in a 24-hour stool specimen, it is possible to calculate the approximate number of adult worms present. This makes it possible to follow the results of therapy in a somewhat quantitative manner by periodic egg counts, affording a basis for comparison of the efficacy of various medications.

Estimates on numbers of eggs laid per female worm vary considerably and depend to some extent on the numbers of worms present. The Chinese liver fluke may lay 2400 or so eggs within 24 hours and an *Ascaris* female about 200,000 during the same period. Thus, from 1000 to 2000 eggs would be found per gram of feces in a 24-hour specimen from a patient infected with one pair of *Ascaris*. The egg-laying capacity of a single *Necator* female may vary from 12 to 44 eggs per gram of feces in a 24-hour period. *Ancylostoma* females lay about twice as many eggs as *Necator*. *Trichuris* females presumably lay about 14,000 eggs in 24 hours, but egg-laying capacity seems to vary inversely with total numbers of worms present.

Stoll Egg-Counting Technique

Procedure

1. Save entire 24-hour stool specimen, and determine weight in grams.
2. Weigh out accurately 4 g of feces.
3. Place feces in calibrated bottle (Stoll flask) or large test tube; add sufficient N/10 sodium hydroxide to bring volume to 60 mL.
4. Add a few glass beads and shake vigorously to make a uniform suspension. If specimen is hard, the mixture may be placed in a refrigerator overnight before shaking, to aid in its comminution.
5. With a Stoll pipette, remove immediately 0.15 mL of the suspension and drain onto a slide.
6. A coverslip is not needed but if preferred a 22 × 30

mm coverslip can be used. Eggs that escape from under the coverslip should be counted. Place slide on mechanical stage and count *all* the eggs on the slide.

7. Multiply egg count by 100 to obtain the number of eggs per gram of feces, and by weight of specimen to get total number of eggs per 24-hour specimen.

Kato Thick-Smear Technique. This technique has undergone a number of modifications since its introduction. Martin and Beaver (1968) suggest examination of a standard 50-mg sample of fresh feces, pressed between a microscope slide and a strip of wettable cellophane soaked in glycerin. After the fecal film has cleared, eggs in the entire film are counted (Fig. 118–22). The fecal sample may be weighed, but these investigators found that with some practice it was possible to estimate sample size with an acceptable degree of reliability. Samples taken from various portions of the specimen do not differ greatly in the number of eggs that they contain. Materials needed for this method are wettable, medium-thickness cellophane coverslips, 22 × 30 mm. They are soaked for at least 24 hours in a solution of 100 mL of pure glycerin, 100 mL of water, and 1 mL of 3% malachite green (the last is optional).

Feces are transferred to a clean slide and covered with a presoaked cellophane coverslip. The slide is inverted and pressed against an absorbent surface until the fecal mass covers an area 20 to 25 mm in diameter. The preparation is left for 1 hour at room temperature to allow clearing of the fecal material (but *not* of the eggs); it should then be examined promptly.

Peters and Kazura (1987) have found that for eggs of *Schistosoma mansoni* longer periods of clearing (24 hours) are needed. If left too long, eggs of hookworm and *Schistosoma japonicum* will gradually dissolve and disappear. To obtain 10-, 20-, or 50-mg samples they use metal templates containing holes calibrated to deliver those amounts of feces.

SPECIAL METHODS FOR INTESTINAL HELMINTHS

Platyhelminths. If gravid proglottids are found in a stool specimen or brought in for identification, *Diphyllobothrium* can usually be identified by the presence of a uterine rosette in the middle of each segment. If no rosette is seen, the segments are probably those of *Taenia*. To differentiate between the two species, segments should be rinsed in tap water and placed between two microscope slides that are separated at the edges by thin pieces of cardboard. The preparation may then be fastened by means of rubber bands at each end of the slides so that the segments become somewhat flattened. The uterine branches should be clearly visible under the low power of a dissecting microscope.

Species identification on the basis of uterine structure of gravid segments may be greatly facilitated by injection of segments with India ink. A little ink is drawn into a 1-mL tuberculin syringe, a No. 26 hypodermic needle is inserted into the distal end or into the genital pore of the proglottid or in the central uterine stem, and a small amount of ink is slowly injected. The branches of the uterus will become black and can be easily counted (Fig. 123–3). This procedure works best with fresh specimens but may at times be successful with formalin-fixed segments.

Nematodes. Generally, nematodes found in the feces can be readily recognized, but anisakids coughed up and brought to the laboratory or recovered by endoscopy must be identified by their internal structure (Fig. 116–4). This may be made visible by clearing in glycerin.

If the worms are still alive, they should be fixed by immersion in 70% alcohol heated to 75°C. Otherwise, transfer to a relatively large volume of 10% glycerin in 70% alcohol in a Petri dish. Cover the dish with an index card in a dust-free location, allowing the alcohol to evaporate over several days.

The specimen may then be mounted on a slide in glycerin and covered with a coverslip for microscopic examination.

Bibliography

Arakaki T, Iwanaga M, Kinjo F, et al: Efficacy of agar-plate culture in detection of *Strongyloides stercoralis* infection. J Parasitol 73:425, 1990.

Ash L, Orihel T: Parasites: A Guide to Laboratory Procedures and Identification. Chicago, ASCP Press, 1987.

Brooke MM, Goldman M: Polyvinyl alcohol–fixative as a preservative and adhesive for protozoa in dysenteric stools and other liquid material. J Lab Clin Med 34:1554, 1949.

Garcia LS, Bruckner DA: Diagnostic Medical Parasitology, 3rd ed. New York, Elsevier, 1996.

Garcia LS, Bruckner DA, Shimizu RY: Techniques for the recovery and identification of *Cryptosporidium* oocysts from stool specimens. J Clin Microbiol 18:185, 1983.

Harada Y, Mori O: A new method for culturing hookworm. Yonago Acta Med 1:177, 1955.

Hiatt RA, Markell EK, Ng E: How many stool examinations are necessary to detect pathogenic intestinal protozoa? Am J Trop Med Hyg 53:36, 1995.

Markell EK, Voge M, John DT: Medical Parasitology, 7th ed. Philadelphia, WB Saunders, 1992.

Martin LK, Beaver PC: Evaluation of Kato thick-smear technique for quantitative diagnosis of helminth infections. Am J Trop Med Hyg 17:382, 1968.

Peters PAS, Kazura JW: Update on diagnostic methods for schistosomiasis. Clin Trop Med Commun Dis 2:419, 1987.

Sawitz WG, Faust EC: The probability of detecting intestinal protozoa by successive stool examinations. Am J Trop Med 22:131, 1942.

Yang J, Scholten T: A fixative for intestinal parasites permitting the use of concentration and permanent staining procedures. Am J Clin Pathol 67:300, 1977.

151 Examination of Blood, Other Body Fluids, Tissues, and Sputum

John H. Cross

EXAMINATION OF FRESH BLOOD. Microscopic examination of fresh blood is not undertaken routinely but is useful for the detection of two types of parasites. Trypanosomes and microfilariae may easily be recognized by their characteristic motility in fresh blood. For specific identification of these organisms, however, a permanent stain is essential. When fresh blood is to be examined, it is important to make a sufficiently thin preparation so that the relatively small protozoan parasites are not masked by several layers of blood corpuscles. A small drop of blood is placed on a slide and covered with a coverglass to prevent clotting. If the preparation is too thick, it may be diluted with normal saline. For the detection of trypanosomes, the high-dry objective with reduced illumination is most suitable. During a search for microfilariae, the low power of the microscope should be employed. Whiplike motions of microfilariae and the rapid undulating and twisting movements of trypanosomes are usually seen before the precise shape of the organism is apparent. Organisms may quickly attract one's attention through their movements even when they are so few that a long search may be required to reveal them in fixed preparations.

STAINED PREPARATIONS. The preparation of good blood films will depend to a large extent on the cleanliness of the microscope slides and coverglasses employed. All glassware must be free of dust and oil. It is essential that both slides and coverglasses be washed in alcohol and dried with a clean towel before a blood film is prepared. Even slides taken from a newly opened box may be covered with an invisible oily film that prevents proper adherence, particularly of thick blood films.

Many methods have been described for the preparation and permanent staining of blood films. Correct initial handling of the blood is essential if good stains are to be obtained, regardless of the specific methods used. It is preferable to use peripheral blood, from fingertip or earlobe. The skin should be cleansed with alcohol before an incision is made, in order to remove all fatty substances, and the incision should be sufficiently deep so that blood flows freely. Blood that has been "milked" from the finger is mixed with tissue fluids, which dilute the parasites and make their detection more difficult. Films should be prepared as quickly as possible to prevent clotting. If venous blood must be employed, a small amount of heparin or other anticoagulant must be added, but preparations made from such blood will usually show some distortion.

The Thin Film. Thin blood films are used for the specific identification of malarial parasites (Chapter 92), trypanosomes (Chapters 93 and 94), and microfilariae (Chapters 106 to 109). A thin film should consist of *one* layer of evenly distributed blood cells. Since malaria parasites are intracellular, a piling-up of red blood cells makes specific identification of these parasites difficult, if not impossible. Specific identification of blood parasites rests on their morphologic characteristics. The chief advantage of a thin film is that it preserves the structure of the parasites and red cells with a minimum of distortion.

There are several ways in which to make a thin blood film. Although the procedure adopted will vary with individual preference, the following is recommended. Place a small drop of blood near one end of a microscope slide; raise the end of the slide farthest from the drop of blood by placing the end of the slide on your finger as your hand rests on a steady surface. Taking a second slide for a spreader, hold your hand so that the second slide makes an angle of approximately 30 degrees with the first. Draw back the supporting finger to move the slide back until the blood touches the spreader slide and begins to run out toward the edges. Before the blood has a chance to reach the edges of the spreader, move the finger that supports it forward in an even quick motion, so that the drop is drawn out into a thin film. Ideally, this should not reach the edges of the slide and should taper off into a "comet's tail" toward the end of the slide. After the film has been air-dried, it may be stained.

The stains commonly used are of two general types. One of these has the fixative incorporated in the staining solution so that fixation and staining of the dried film are accomplished simultaneously. An example is Wright's stain, in which methyl alcohol acts as a fixative. Wright's stain will give only fair results in staining malaria parasites and is *not* recommended for parasitologic use. More precise detail is seen in slides prepared with Giemsa's stain. Since this stain does not contain a fixative, thin films must be fixed in absolute methyl alcohol and air-dried before they are placed in the staining solution. It is important to dry slides in a vertical position after removal from either fixative or stain. As soon as the stained films are dry, they may be examined under oil immersion of the microscope. Immersion oil may be placed directly on the uncovered blood film and, when no longer needed, carefully removed with xylene and lens paper. Slides that one desires to keep for a permanent collection should always have the protection of a coverglass; a mounting medium, such as Permount (Fisher Scientific, 711 Forbes Ave., Pittsburgh, PA 15219-9919) or Acrytol (Surgipath Canada Inc., 1401 Church Ave., Winnipeg, Manitoba R2X 1G5, Canada) should be used.

Thick Blood Films. The thick film may also be used in identification of malaria parasites, trypanosomes, and microfilariae. As a thick layer of blood is used in this method, many more parasites will be present in each field. Increased distortion of the parasites is a disadvantage of this method, but experience enables one to recognize them readily.

To make a thick film, place three drops of blood, each of about the size that would be used to make a thin film, close together near one end of the slide. With one corner of another absolutely clean slide, stir the blood, mingling the three drops over an area 2 cm in diameter. Continue stirring for at least 30 seconds; this prevents the formation of fibrin strands, which otherwise tend to obscure the parasites. Allow the films to dry normally; do not heat, because this will fix the blood. After the films are thoroughly dry they must be laked to remove the hemoglobin. This can be done by immersion in buffer solution, prior to staining, or in Giemsa's stain itself. Thick films that cannot be stained immediately should be laked in buffer solution before storage, because removal of hemoglobin becomes increasingly difficult with time. When Giemsa's stain is used for thick films, the procedure is exactly the same as that employed with thin films, except that fixation in methyl alcohol is omitted. Staining times for thick and thin films are similar, but if separate preparations are made, different staining times may be required for optimal results. Thick and thin films may, however, be made on the same slide and stained simultaneously with Giemsa's stain. To accomplish this, the thin portion of the slide is fixed for 1 minute in methyl alcohol and then dried before staining.

Another method that may be used in the staining of thick films is that described by Field. It is very rapid and gives satisfactory, although not outstanding, results. Field's stain has been used extensively for survey purposes and when large numbers of slides must be prepared, but it is not recommended for routine use.

Blood Concentration Procedures. The thick film is itself a type of concentration technique and the only one applicable to the identification of parasites within the red cell. Buffy coat films serve to concentrate the white cells, in which *Leishmania* may be found, and are useful for detection of trypanosomes and microfilariae. A triple-centrifugation technique is also used to check for trypanosomes when they are too sparse to be found even in thick blood films. The presence of small numbers of microfilariae in the blood can be detected by means of a membrane filtration technique.

EXAMINATION OF CEREBROSPINAL FLUID. Trophozoites of *Naegleria* (Chapter 99) and trypanosomes (Chapter 93) may be found in the cerebrospinal fluid (CSF). *Trichinella* larvae may be found in the CSF of patients with severe infections; they also may be isolated from the blood (Chapter 111). CSF eosinophilia may be caused by parasites such as *Angiostrongylus* and *Gnathostoma*, which will not be found in the blood. Larvae, however, may be found in the CSF of children with *Angiostrongylus cantonensis* infection. Transverse myelitis caused by *Schistosoma mansoni* or *Schistosoma haematobium* may result in an eosinophilic CSF pleocytosis. Ova are rarely seen in the CSF.

The CSF must be examined promptly, as trypanosomes will survive for only about 20 minutes, and *Naegleria* may become rounded and nonmotile. The CSF may be centrifuged (7000 × *g* for 10 minutes), the supernatant removed, and the sediment examined under reduced illumination. Motility of *Naegleria* may be enhanced by use of a warm stage, and culture of the CSF or its sediment may be effective in isolation of this organism. A membrane filter will increase the chances of finding migrating larvae in blood or CSF in severe *Trichinella* infections.

TISSUE IMPRESSIONS. The detection of intracellular parasites such as *Leishmania* and *Toxoplasma* is greatly facilitated by examination of tissue impression smears stained with Giemsa's stain. Fresh lymph nodes, liver biopsy material, or bone marrow is lightly impressed on a clean microscope slide; the film is allowed to dry at room temperature and is stained in the manner of a thin blood film. Whole cells, with organisms showing little if any distortion, may be clearly distinguished in such preparations. When dealing with lymph nodes or other fairly solid tissue, it is best to prepare the smear from a freshly cut surface. The remaining tissue can then be fixed for conventional pathologic procedures or be used as desired.

BIOPSY AND ASPIRATION. Spleen, liver, and bone marrow biopsies are extensively used in the diagnosis of visceral leishmaniasis. Organisms may be demonstrated directly in the biopsy material, which also may be used for culture or animal inoculation to isolate the organism or for polymerase chain reaction (PCR) to detect the parasites' DNA. Sternal marrow aspiration is approximately as productive as the more hazardous splenic or hepatic biopsy. *Leishmania tropica* cannot be recovered from the surface of an oriental sore; if a hypodermic syringe is introduced through normal tissue at the side of the ulcer to the area below the ulcer bed, intracellular parasites may be demonstrated in the fluid that is withdrawn after instillation of a few drops of normal saline (Fig. 95–13). Aspiration of enlarged posterior cervical or other involved lymph nodes will at times reveal trypanosomes when the blood is apparently free of them. The lymph nodes are less often involved in Rhodesian sleeping sickness than in the Gambian form or in Chagas disease. Biopsy of enlarged nodes from patients having the latter disease may reveal intracellular (amastigote) forms of the parasite.

Aspiration of fluid from a hydatid cyst (a dangerous procedure unless done with ultrasonographic guidance) may reveal hydatid sand, but it must be remembered that certain hydatid cysts are sterile, so that the absence of scoleces or hooklets from the sediment, centrifuged or put through a membrane filter, is not evidence against the parasitic nature of the cyst. Aspiration of an amebic abscess will often demonstrate a thick reddish brown fluid, but amebas are seldom seen, as they occur chiefly in the tissue surrounding the abscess cavity (Fig. 86–15).

Eggs of *Schistosoma mansoni* and *Schistosoma japonicum* may be found in tissue taken from the rectal mucosa when they cannot be recovered from the stool; mucosa from the bladder wall, taken at cystoscopy, or a rectal snip biopsy may likewise reveal eggs of *S. haematobium* (Fig. 117–23). Larval *Trichinella spiralis* may be found in any voluntary muscle, but biopsies are usually taken from the gastrocnemius. Larvae may be most abundant in the diaphragm, and a search may be made for them in this muscle at autopsy (Fig. 111–1*B*). Microfilariae of *Onchocerca volvulus*, *Mansonella ozzardi*, and *Mansonella streptocerca* may be demonstrated in skin snips (Figs. 109–1*A* and 109–3).

EXAMINATION OF THE SPUTUM. Examination of the sputum is indicated when there is a question of pulmonary paragonimiasis, although the swallowed eggs are often found in the feces. *Entamoeba histolytica* may appear in the sputum of patients with pulmonary abscesses. *Pneumocystis carinii* may be found in the sputum but is more readily seen in bronchial aspirates or in impression smears of lung biopsy material (see Figs. 98–1 and 98–2). Migrating larvae of *Ascaris*, hookworm, and *Strongyloides* are rarely seen. *Entamoeba gingivalis* may multiply in bronchial mucus and *Trichomonas tenax* is usually an oral contaminant. *Cryptosporidium* has been found in both sputum and lung biopsy material. Ruptured hydatid cysts may be recognized by the presence of hooklets in the sputum.

Sputum specimens should be induced, if possible. Early-morning specimens, uncontaminated with saliva, also are acceptable. They should be examined by wet mount while fresh, or preserved in polyvinyl alcohol (PVA) fixative for protozoa and formol-saline for other organisms or eggs. If the specimen is very viscid, it should be diluted with an equal quantity of 3% NaOH, mixed thoroughly, and centrifuged before examination or preservation. Sodium hydroxide will, of course, destroy any amebas or flagellates that might be present.

Giemsa's Stain. Giemsa's stain is sold commercially as a concentrated stock solution. The product is quite variable, and each new lot should be thoroughly tested before being put into use. In general, if the coloration of the red and white cells seems satisfactory, it can be assumed that the stain will be adequate for the demonstration of malarial and other parasites.

Procedure (for Thin Films)
1. Fix blood films in absolute methyl alcohol for 1 minute.
2. Allow slides to dry.
3. Immerse slides in a solution of 1 part of Giemsa stock to 30 to 50 parts of buffered water (pH 7.2). Stain 30 minutes to 1 hour.
4. Dip slides briefly in buffered water, drain quickly and thoroughly, and air-dry.

The procedure to be used with thick films is the same, except that steps 1 and 2 are omitted. If the slide has a thick film at one end and a thin film at the other, fix only the thin portion, then stain both parts of the film simultaneously.

Method for Estimating Numbers of Malaria Parasites in Blood. Determine the patient's white blood cell count. On a thick blood smear, count the number of parasites seen per 100 white blood cells; the total number per cubic millimeter of blood can then be determined.

The Earle-Perez (1932) method of enumeration is more accurate. A known quantity of blood (5 µL) measured in a pipette is spread over an area of 3×15 mm as a thick smear and stained. The parasites are counted in a band of the smear. Every fifth band is counted and the number of parasites counted will be in 0.33 µL of blood.

Quantitative Buffy Coat. The QBC II developed by Becton Dickinson is a rapid diagnostic method for malaria and other blood parasites (microfilariae, trypanosomes). Blood is collected in an acridine orange–coated capillary tube with an internal float. Malaria parasites take up the acridine orange and become concentrated in the erythrocyte-granulocyte interface after centrifugation. Under fluorescent microscopy and ultraviolet (UV) light the stained parasite DNA fluoresces. It is all provided in a kit containing capillary tubes, centrifuge, UV adapter, and paraviewer.

Dipstick Test for Malaria. Becton Dickinson has developed a simple antigen detection test for *Plasmodium falciparum* (Parasight R-F). Histidine-rich protein (PF HRP-2) is released by the parasite and can be detected on a nitrocellulose and glass fiber dipstick pretreated with a mouse monoclonal antibody against HRP-2. The dipstick is placed in hemolyzed blood followed by a drop of reagent and visually read as instructed.

Rapid Methenamine Silver Stain for P*neumocystis carinii*. A number of stains, including periodic-acid–Schiff and Giemsa, have been used for the demonstration of *Pneumocystis* in sputum, brushings, and biopsy specimens. The best results are obtained by means of a methenamine silver impregnation technique. Fungi will be sharply delineated in black. *Pneumocystis carinii* will have a delicately stained wall, usually brownish or grayish, and rather transparent. Structures described as "parentheses" are often seen and stain black. Mu-

cin will be taupe to dark gray, the inner parts of mycelia and hyphae will be old rose, and the background will be pale green.

Membrane Filtration Method for Microfilariae (Dennis and Kean, 1971)

Procedure
1. Blood is collected in tubes containing 3.8% sodium citrate (20% by volume of blood specimen).
2. A Nuclepore* filter of 5-µm pore size is placed in a Swinney adapter; a 20- to 50-mL disposable plastic syringe is attached to the adapter.
3. Several milliliters of normal saline are added to the upright barrel.
4. About 2 to 4 mL of the blood specimen is added to the saline, and the mixture of blood and saline is forced through the filter.
5. Following several washes of small amounts of saline or distilled water, the filter may be removed from the adapter, placed on a microscope slide, and examined for living microfilariae; it can also be dried, fixed, and stained as for a thin blood film.

Gradient Centrifugation Technique for Concentration of Microfilariae

Procedure
1. Thirty milliliters of 50% Hypaque is mixed with 14 mL of distilled water; 1 part of this mixture is added to 2.4 parts of 9% Ficoll.
2. The Ficoll-Hypaque mixture, 4 mL, is placed in a 17×100 mm plastic centrifuge tube and overlaid with 4 mL of heparinized venous blood.
3. The tube is centrifuged at $400 \times g$ for 40 minutes.
4. Microfilariae will be found in the middle Ficoll-Hypaque layer, which separates the overlying plasma and white cell layers from the underlying red cells.

Buffy Coat Films for Leishmanias. This method is useful for the detection of *Leishmania donovani* if present in the circulation and will also reveal *Histoplasma capsulatum* and, rarely, *Toxoplasma gondii*. Microfilariae and trypanosomes also may be found in the buffy coat.

Procedure
1. Obtain 5 mL of blood and deliver into a tube containing oxalate crystals (prepared as for the Wintrobe hematocrit method).
2. Transfer blood with a capillary pipette into a Wintrobe tube. Cap to prevent evaporation, and centrifuge for 30 minutes at $2500 \times g$.
3. With a fine capillary pipette, withdraw the cells of the buffy coat, which lies between the packed red cells and the overlying plasma.
4. Spread out as thin film, dry, and stain with Wright's or Giemsa's stain.

Triple Centrifugation Method for Trypanosomes

Procedure
1. Deliver 9 mL of blood, obtained by venipuncture, into a centrifuge tube containing 1 mL of 6% citrate solution.
2. Centrifuge at $300 \times g$.
3. Remove supernatant fluid to another centrifuge tube; recentrifuge at $600 \times g$ for 10 minutes.
4. Remove supernatant fluid once more to a clean centrifuge tube; centrifuge at $1800 \times g$ for 10 minutes.
5. Examine sediment as a wet film, or make a thin film and stain with Giemsa's stain.

---

*This method is unsatisfactory for the isolation of *Mansonella perstans* microfilariae because of their small size. Other filters of similar pore size are not as satisfactory as the Nuclepore.

CULTURE METHODS. *Acanthamoeba* and *Naegleria* (Chapter 99), the leishmanias (Chapter 95), *Trypanosoma cruzi* (Chapter 94), and *Toxoplasma* (Chapter 97) can be cultured with relative ease. Cultivation of other blood and tissue parasites either has not been successful or (as in the case of the plasmodia) remains a research procedure.

Culbertson's Medium for *Acanthamoeba*. For the isolation of *Acanthamoeba* from tissues, Culbertson et al. (1965) recommend the following procedure.

Materials

1. Prepare a neomycin sulfate solution, 0.56% in sterile distilled water.
2. Prepare a sterile nystatin suspension in distilled water containing 1500 units per milliliter.
3. Prepare agar stock, 3 g of Bacto-Agar per 100 mL of 1.7% NaCl.
4. Prepare suspension of *Enterobacter aerogenes* in trypticase soy broth, giving 40% transmission on a Coleman Junior spectrophotometer against uninoculated broth. Since both live and killed bacteria are to be used in medium preparation, place at least 5 mL of the suspension in a sealed ampule and immerse in a water bath at 65°C for 30 minutes to kill the organisms. Keep refrigerated until use.

Procedure

1. To a mixture consisting of 5 mL of each antibiotic solution, 5 mL of killed bacterial suspension, and 85 mL of sterile distilled water, add 100 mL of melted and cooled 3% agar and combine all ingredients at 56°C in water bath.
2. Pour mixture into Petri plates, 8 mL per plate; allow excess moisture to evaporate by inverting bottom plate and resting it at a slight angle.
3. Place 0.05 mL of live *Enterobacter* suspension in center of plate and spread over an area 25 to 40 mm in diameter. Allow surface to dry at room temperature or at 4°C overnight.

Inoculation. Place drops of fluid or small pieces of tissue suspected of containing amebas near center of plate. Check for presence of amebas at edges of inoculum during the following 4 or 5 days.

Modified Nelson's Medium for *Naegleria*. The following procedure is for the isolation of *Naegleria* from the CSF.

Materials

1. Make up the following in Page's saline solution: 0.1% liver infusion (Oxoid, Wilson 1:20, or Panmede) and 0.1% glucose.

Page's Solution

MgSO₄•7HOH	0.4 mg
CaCL₂•2HOH	0.4 mg
Na₂HPO₄	14.2 mg
KH₂PO₄	13.6 mg
NaCl	12.0 mg
Distilled water	100.0 mL

$MgSO_4 \cdot 7HOH$ .... 0.4 mg
$CaCL_2 \cdot 2HOH$ .... 0.4 mg
Na_2HPO_4 .... 14.2 mg
KH_2PO_4 .... 13.6 mg
NaCl .... 12.0 mg
Distilled water .... 100.0 mL

2. Prepare non-nutrient agar: Page's saline with liver and glucose, 100 mL, and Difco agar 1.5 g. Dissolve agar in Page's saline with gentle heating. Aliquot 20-mL quantities into 20 × 150 mm screw-cap tubes. Autoclave at 15 psi for 15 minutes. Store in refrigerator.

Procedure

1. Prepare non-nutrient agar plates from above as needed, or store in refrigerator (up to 3 months) and warm to 37°C before use.
2. Add 2 or 3 drops of a suspension of *Escherichia coli* in Page's saline to the surface of the plate, and spread with a bacteriologic loop.

Inoculation. Inoculate a few drops of CSF sediment onto plate. Incubate at 35° to 37°C, and examine daily under low power. Cysts may appear within 4 to 5 days and trophozoites earlier.

OTHER CULTURE METHODS. *Acanthamoebaa, Naegleria,* and *Balamuthia* may be established in axenic cultures as well as in cell culture.

Novy–Mac Neal–Nicolle (NNN) Medium for *Leishmania* and *Trypanosoma cruzi*

Materials

Agar	14 g
NaCl	6 g
Distilled water	900 mL

Procedure

The water is brought to the boiling point and the salt and agar added and dissolved in it. It is then distributed in test tubes filled to about one-third capacity. The test tubes are plugged and sterilized in the autoclave in the usual manner. Tubes containing the agar base may be stored in the refrigerator and used as needed.

For use, the tubes are placed in hot water to melt the agar, after which they are cooled to 48° to 50°C. To each tube is added approximately one third as much sterile defibrinated rabbit's blood as the volume of agar. The blood and agar are thoroughly mixed by rapid rotation of the tube, and the tube is then placed in a slanting position, on ice, and cooled. After the tubes are cool, they are placed in an upright position and incubated for 24 hours at 37°C to determine sterility.

Blood may be obtained from the rabbit by cardiac puncture, sterile precautions being observed. The blood so obtained is placed in a sterile flask containing glass beads and defibrinated by shaking.

Peripheral blood, or material obtained by biopsy or marrow aspiration or from cutaneous ulcers by aspiration from below the ulcer bed, may be cultured on this medium, which gives excellent results. The tubes are kept at room temperature, as close to 22°C as possible. The organisms develop in the water of condensation, which collects at the bottom of the slanted agar. Cultures should be examined every other day for a month before being discarded as negative. If leishmanias are present in the inoculum in some numbers, culture forms will usually be found within 2 to 10 days, but if scarce, they may require much longer to develop in sufficient numbers to be detected. Leishmanias will not grow in the presence of bacterial contamination.

Tissue Culture of *Toxoplasma gondii*. A method for culture of *Toxoplasma* has been described by Shepp et al. (1985) and is applicable to blood, CSF, placental and other tissues.

Procedure

1. Collect 10 mL of blood in preservative-free heparin tubes; allow to sediment by gravity.
2. Remove the buffy coat with aseptic precautions; centrifuge at 800 × *g* for 10 minutes.
3. Wash buffy coat cells three times with Eagle's minimal essential medium.*
4. Inoculate washed buffy coat material onto complete human foreskin fibroblast monolayers, and observe weekly for cytopathologic effects.

Other tissues may be inoculated directly onto the tissue culture. If more than 1 mL of CSF is available, it may be centrifuged at 500 × *g* for 10 minutes and the sediment used for the inoculum.

ANIMAL INOCULATION. *Trypanosoma brucei gambiense* and *T. brucei rhodesiense* infections can be established in a number of laboratory animals. White rats, white mice, and guinea

---

*Grand Island Biological Co., Grand Island, NY.

pigs are most useful for diagnosis and the maintenance of laboratory strains. Young animals are most readily infected, and *T. brucei rhodesiense* is more virulent than *T. brucei gambiense*. Rats infected with *T. brucei gambiense* will survive for several months with a low-grade parasitemia; if infected with *T. brucei rhodesiense*, they die within a short time with an overwhelming parasitemia. *Trypanosoma rangeli* multiplies in common laboratory animals but does not cause apparent disease. Young white rats and white mice can be infected with *Trypanosoma cruzi*; the white mouse is best for diagnostic inoculation. When first isolated, this trypanosome is quite virulent, but after repeated animal passage it loses its virulence and may become noninfective. Intraperitoneal or subcutaneous inoculation should be used; amounts up to 2 mL of blood are injected, depending on the size of the animal used. It is important to check rats for the presence of their common parasite, *Trypanosoma lewisi*, before inoculation.

For isolation of leishmanias, the hamster is most satisfactory; other laboratory animals are infected only with difficulty. Following intraperitoneal or intratesticular inoculation, hamsters will develop a generalized infection with any form of *Leishmania*, and the organisms may be demonstrated in spleen impression smears or in testicular aspirates. This infection develops slowly, and culture methods are generally regarded as being superior for diagnostic use.

Toxoplasma gondii, a parasite that shows little host specificity, will infect all common laboratory animals. White rats and mice are generally used; rats develop a chronic infection and are good for maintenance of the strain, whereas intraperitoneal infection of mice results in tremendous proliferation of the organisms in the ascitic fluid and death of the mice within a few days. Mouse peritoneal fluid, rich in organisms, is used as a source of toxoplasmas for the dye test and other diagnostic procedures.

Xenodiagnosis may be considered a special case of animal inoculation; the term was originally applied to the diagnosis of Chagas disease by feeding uninfected reduviid bugs on a patient suspected of having the disease. Subsequent examination of the bugs will reveal developmental stages of the parasites if the test result is positive. Recently the term "xenodiagnosis" has been used for the diagnosis of trichinosis by feeding rats with muscle tissue from patients suspected of having the infection.

Bibliography

Ash LR, Orihel TC: Parasites: A Guide to Laboratory Procedures and Identification. Chicago, ASCP Press, 1987.

Culbertson CG, Ensminger PW, Overton WM: The isolation of additional strains of pathogenic *Hartmanella* sp. (*Acanthamoeba*). Proposed culture method for application to biological material. Am J Clin Pathol 43:383, 1965.

Dennis DT, Kean BH: Isolation of microfilariae: report of a new method. J Parasitol 57:1146, 1971.

Earle WC, Perez M: Enumeration of parasites in the blood of malaria patients. J Lab Clin Med 17:1124, 1932.

Gillespie SH, Hawkey PM: Medical Parasitology: A Practical Approach. Oxford, England, Oxford University Press, 1995.

Jones TC, Mott K, Pedrosa LC: A technique for isolating and concentrating microfilariae from peripheral blood by gradient centrifugation. Trans R Soc Trop Med Hyg 69:243, 1975.

Markell EK, Voge M, John DT: Medical Parasitology, 7th ed. Philadelphia, WB Saunders, 1992.

Shepp DH, Mackman RC, Conley FK, et al: *Toxoplasma gondii* reactivation identified by detection of parasitemia in tissue culture. Ann Intern Med 103:218, 1985.

Shiff CJ, Minjas J, Premji Z: The Parasight R-F Test: A simple rapid manual dipstick test to detect *Plasmodium falciparum* infection. Parasitol Today 10:494, 1994.

Spielman A, Perrone JB, Teklehaimanot A, et al. Malaria diagnosis by direct observation of centrifuged samples of blood. Am J Trop Med Hygiene 39:337, 1988.

Yu PKW, Uhl JR, Anhalt JP: Rapid methenamine silver stain. Arch Pathol Lab Med 113:111, 1989.

152 *Parasitic Immunodiagnosis**

Marianna Wilson and Peter M. Schantz

GENERAL PRINCIPLES. For parasitic diseases in which identification of parasites in host tissue or excreta is neither practicable nor always rewarding, detection of antibodies or antigens can be very useful as an indicator that an individual has been infected with a specific parasite. Immunodiagnostic methods should not be used as replacements for morphologic diagnosis for those infections in which parasites are easily detectable, e.g., *Ascaris*, hookworm, *Cryptosporidium*, *Giardia*, or malaria. If infection with a parasite is suspected and blood film, stool, or urine examinations are either not indicated or are negative, then the appropriate serology test for specific IgG antibodies should be requested. Tests for parasite-specific IgM, IgA, or IgE are generally not useful for diagnosis and should not be requested.

Detection of antibodies to parasitic diseases only indicates infection at some indeterminate time and not necessarily acute or current infection. A positive result in a person with no exposure to the parasite prior to recent travel in a disease-endemic area may be interpreted as indicating recent infection. However, detection of specific antibodies in a person native to an area where the parasite is endemic may reflect only a past infection unrelated to current clinical status. Levels of antibodies to parasites slowly decline after the patient is cured of the infection but generally last for 6 months to many years, depending on the infecting parasite, and thus are usually not reliable indicators of successful cure.

The past decade has seen changes in the availability of parasitic immunodiagnostic procedures (Table 152–1). Several private laboratories in the United States perform tests that were previously available only at the Centers for Disease Control and Prevention (CDC). Commercial kits for the detection of several parasitic diseases are now available. During the past 10 years antigen detection systems have been devel-

*All the material in this chapter is in the public domain, with the exception of any borrowed figures or tables.

TABLE 152–1. Antibody and Antigen Detection Tests Available in 1998 for Parasitic Diseases

Disease	Antibody Tests*	Antigen Tests
Amebiasis	EIA	EIA
Babesiosis	IFA	
Chagas disease	EIA, IFA	
Cryptosporidiosis		EIA, DFA, IFA
Cysticercosis	EIA, IB	
Echinococcosis	EIA, IB	
Fascioliasis	EIA	
Filariasis	EIA	
Giardiasis		EIA, DFA, IFA
Leishmaniasis	IFA	
Malaria	IFA	
Paragonimiasis	EIA, IB	
Schistosomiasis	EIA, IB	
Strongyloidiasis	EIA	
Toxocariasis	EIA	
Toxoplasmosis	EIA, IFA	
Trichinellosis	BF, EIA	
Trichomoniasis		DFA, EIA, DNA probe

*BF, bentonite flocculation; DFA, direct fluorescent antibody; EIA, enzyme immunoassay; IB, immunoblot; IFA, indirect fluorescent antibody.

oped, resulting in commercially available reagents for *Cryptosporidium parvum, Entamoeba histolytica, Giardia lamblia,* and *Trichomonas vaginalis.* Parasites for which immunodiagnostic tests are not available commercially but are possibly available by special request are listed in Table 152–2.

Although molecular biology techniques show promise for improving the diagnosis of acute parasitic infections, they are currently research tools and, with the exception of *Toxoplasma,* probably will not be commercially available for routine use in clinical diagnostic laboratories in the foreseeable future.

SPECIMEN REQUIREMENTS

Specimens for Antibody Detection. For all antibody detection tests for parasitic diseases, serum and plasma are acceptable specimens. For toxocariasis and toxoplasmosis, aqueous and vitreous eye fluids can be tested by some laboratories when accompanied by a serum specimen. For central nervous system infections e.g., cysticercosis or toxoplasmosis, cerebrospinal fluid (CSF) accompanied by a serum specimen may be tested. Not all laboratories are prepared to test eye fluids or CSF, so check with your laboratory for availability prior to shipment. All specimens may be shipped at room temperature to arrive at their destination within several days, but if the specimen volume is small (<1.0 mL), shipment with dry ice ensures that the specimen does not evaporate in transit. In general, acute and convalescent specimens are not required; valid results generally can be obtained by testing only one specimen because parasitic diseases are usually past the acute stage when initially considered.

Specimens for Antigen Detection. Fresh or formalin-fixed stool samples are acceptable for antigen detection testing with most kits, but ask your laboratory for the recommended procedure for the kit used by that facility.

AFRICAN TRYPANOSOMIASIS (Chapter 93). Immunodiagnostic tests for the detection of *Trypanosoma brucei rhodesiense* or *T. brucei gambiense* infections are not available in the United States. If African trypanosomiasis is suspected, call the Division of Parasitic Diseases at the CDC for information.

AMEBIASIS (Chapter 86). Detection of antibodies to *Entamoeba histolytica* is most useful in patients with extraintestinal disease, i.e., amebic liver abscess, when organisms are not generally found on stool examination. Antigen detection may be useful as an adjunct to microscopical diagnosis in detecting parasites and perhaps to distinguish between pathogenic and nonpathogenic infections.

The indirect hemagglutination (IHA) test has been the standard for routine serodiagnosis of amebiasis. The IHA test detects antibody specific for *E. histolytica* at titers of ≥1:256 in approximately 95% of patients with extraintestinal amebiasis, 70% of patients with active intestinal infection, and 10% of

TABLE 152–2. Parasites for Which Antibody- or Antigen-Detection Tests Have Been Reported But Are Not Commercially Available*

Organism
Ancyclostoma caninum
Angiostrongylus
Anisakis
Baylisascaris
Gnathostoma
Microsporidia
Opisthorchis
African *Trypanosoma*

*Contact the Centers for Disease Control and Prevention for information at (770) 488-7760.

asymptomatic persons who are passing cysts of *E. histolytica.* Positive titers may persist for years after successful treatment, so the presence of a titer does not necessarily indicate acute or current infection. Specificity is excellent: false positive reactions rarely occur at titers ≥1:256.

Enzyme immunoassays (EIA) are as sensitive and specific as the IHA test and have replaced the IHA in most laboratories. Although the immunodiffusion (ID) test is specific, it is slightly less sensitive than the IHA and EIA and requires a minimum of 24 hours to obtain a result, in contrast with 2 hours required for the IHA or EIA tests. Although detection of IgM antibodies specific for *E. histolytica* has been reported, sensitivity is only about 64% in patients with current invasive disease.

Recent studies indicated improved sensitivity and specificity of *E. histolytica* fecal antigen assays with the use of monoclonal antibodies, resulting in commercial availability of EIA kits. Perhaps the best use of tests for fecal antigen detection will be for differentiation of pathogenic *E. histolytica* from nonpathogenic *Entamoeba dispar* infections by detection of galactose-inhibitable adherence protein, which appears necessary for pathogenesis.

BABESIOSIS (Chapter 96). Diagnosis of *Babesia* infection should be made by observation of parasites in patients' blood films. However, antibody detection tests are useful for detecting infected individuals with very low levels of parasitemia, e.g., asymptomatic blood donors in transfusion-associated cases, for post-therapy diagnosis after parasitemia is no longer detectable, and for discrimination between *Plasmodium falciparum* and *Babesia* infection in patients whose blood film examinations are inconclusive and whose travel histories cannot exclude either parasite.

The indirect immunofluorescence test (IFA) is quite sensitive for *Babesia microti* infection. Patients' titers generally rise to ≥1:1024 during the first weeks of illness and decline gradually over 6 months to titers of 1:16 to 1:256, but may remain detectable at low levels for a year or more. Specificity is 100% in patients having other tick-borne diseases or persons not exposed to the parasite. Cross reactions may occur in serum specimens from patients with malaria infections, but generally titers are highest with the homologous antigen. The extent of cross reactivity between *Babesia* species is variable; a negative result with *B. microti* antigen for a patient exposed on the U.S. West Coast may be a false negative reaction. Natural transmission of *B. microti* occurs in the coastal areas of the northeastern United States, and rarely in Minnesota and Wisconsin. Recently, human infection on the West Coast with a *Babesia* species which is antigenically and genotypically distinct from *B. microti* was reported. Because the tick vector also transmits the causative agent of Lyme disease, dual infections of *B. microti* and *Borrelia burgdorferi* have been reported.

CHAGAS DISEASE (Chapter 94). Infections with *Trypanosoma cruzi* are common in Central and South America. Many immigrants from areas where Chagas disease is endemic reside in the United States and are potential sources for parasite transmission via infected blood. During the acute stage of illness, blood film examination generally reveals the presence of trypomastigotes. During the chronic stage of infection, parasites are rare or absent from the circulation; immunodiagnosis is the method of choice for determining whether the patient is infected.

The IFA and EIA tests are employed by many laboratories. Although IFA is very sensitive, cross reactivity occurs with sera from patients with leishmaniasis, which is endemic to the same geographic areas as *T. cruzi.* Sensitivity and specificity of EIA tests that use crude antigens are similar to those of the IFA test. Although differentiating between acute and chronic infection is very important in determining therapy, serology cannot be used for this purpose. A positive titer indicates only infection at some unknown time, and not acute infection. The immunoblot assay shows promise as a confirmatory test.

CRYPTOSPORIDIOSIS (Chapter 88). Tests for antibody detection in human *Cryptosporidium parvum* infection are not currently recommended due to lack of sensitivity and specificity. However, an immunoblot assay has shown specific antigen-antibody banding patterns in individuals suspected of infection, but this test is not available for general use.

Organism or antigen detection in stools is the current immunodiagnostic test of choice and provides equal or increased sensitivity over microscopy. A number of commercial kits are available for both direct fluorescent antibody (DFA) and EIA tests; all have sensitivities and specificities of 94% or greater. These tests do not take the place of routine stool examinations, but they may be very useful when trying to confirm *Cryptosporidium* infection in a symptomatic person excreting few oocysts in the stool. Antigen detection tests are less sensitive in formed specimens than in diarrheal specimens.

CYCLOSPORIDIASIS (Chapter 89). There are currently no immunodiagnostic tests available for cyclosporidiasis.

CYSTICERCOSIS (LARVAL *Taenia Solium*) (Chapter 124.1). The CDC enzyme-linked immunoelectrotransfer blot (CDC-EITB) with purified *Taenia solium* antigens has been acknowledged by the World Health Organization and the Pan American Health Organization as the immunodiagnostic test of choice for confirming a presumptive diagnosis of neurocysticercosis. It is 100% specific and has a sensitivity superior to that of any other test yet evaluated. Serum specimens from 97% of 108 parasitologic confirmed cases of cysticercosis had detectable antibodies. No serum samples from 376 patients with other microbial infections reacted with any of the *T. solium*–specific antigens. The most important factors identified as determining positive immunoblot reactions are the numbers and stage of development of cysticerci. Cumulative clinical experience has confirmed that in patients with more than two lesions, the test has more than 90% sensitivity. Seropositivity in biopsy-confirmed patients with a single, enhancing parenchymal cyst was <50%; in clinically defined patients with a single cyst but who were not biopsied sensitivity was 70%. Seropositivity in serum and CSF of patients with multiple but only calcified cysts was 82% and 77%, respectively. In all patients, regardless of their clinical presentation, the immunoblot assay is slightly more sensitive in serum than in CSF specimens: consequently, there is no need to obtain CSF solely for use in the immunoblot assay.

Assays employing crude antigens for the detection of antibody are not always reliable for the identification of this disease; all positive results and any negative results strongly suspected of cysticercosis should be confirmed by immunoblot. Currently available antibody detection tests for cysticercosis do not distinguish between active and inactive infections and thus are not useful in evaluating the outcomes and prognoses of medically treated patients.

ECHINOCOCCOSIS. Immunodiagnostic tests can be very helpful in the diagnosis of echinococcal disease, and should be used before invasive methods. However, the clinician must have some knowledge of the characteristics of the available tests and the patient and parasite factors associated with false positive results. False positive reactions may occur in persons with other helminthic infections, cancer, and chronic immune disorders. Negative test results do not rule out echinococcosis because some cyst carriers do not have detectable antibodies. Detectable immune responses have been associated with the location, integrity, and vitality of the larval cyst. Cysts in the liver are more likely to elicit antibody response than cysts in the lungs and, regardless of localization, antibody detection tests are least sensitive in patients with intact hyaline cysts. Fissuration or rupture of a cyst is followed by an abrupt stimulation of antibodies. Often a patient with senescent, calcified, or dead cysts is seronegative.

Cystic Hydatid Disease (*Echinococcus granulosus*) (Chapter 124.2). IHA, IFA, and EIA are sensitive tests for detecting antibodies in the serum of patients with cystic hydatid disease (CHD); sensitivity rates vary from 60 to 90%, depending on the characteristics of the cases. At present, the best available serologic diagnosis is obtained by using combinations of tests. EIA or IHA is used to screen all specimens; a positive reaction should be confirmed by immunoblot assay or one of the variety of gel diffusion assays that demonstrate the echinococcal "Arc 5." Although these confirmatory assays give false positive reactions with sera of 5 to 25% in persons with neurocysticercosis, the clinical and epidemiologic presentation of neurocysticercosis patients should be rarely confused with that of cystic echinococcosis.

Circulating antigens have been detected in the sera of only about half of patients with cystic echinococosis; however, these antigens may be detectable in the sera of patients with negative or borderline antibody titers. Therefore antigen assays, which are not yet available in the United States, might be useful as additional tests for those patients with no detectable *Echinococcus* antibodies.

Antibody responses have also been monitored as a way of evaluating the results of treatment, but with mixed results. Following successful radical surgery, antibody titers decline and sometimes disappear; titers rise again if secondary hydatid cysts develop. Tests for Arc 5 or IgE antibodies appear to reflect antibody decline during the first 24 months after surgery, whereas the IHA and other tests remain positive for at least 4 years. Chemotherapy has not been followed by consistent declines in antibody titers. Consequently, the usefulness of serology to moniter the course of disease is limited; imaging techniques provide a more accurate assessment of the patient's condition.

Alveolar Hydatid Disease (*Echinococcus multilocularis*) (Chapter 124.3). Most patients with alveolar hydatid disease (AHD) are positive in serologic tests using heterologous *E. granulosus* or homologous *E. multilocularis* antigens. With crude *Echinococcus* antigens, nonspecific reactions create the same difficulties as described previously for diagnosis of CHD; however, immunoaffinity-purified *E. multilocularis* antigens (Em2) used in EIA give positive serologic reactions in more than 95% of AHD cases. Comparing serologic reactivity to Em2 antigen with that to antigens containing components of both *E. multilocularis* and *E. granulosus* permits discrimination of patients with AHD from those with CHD. As in cystic echinococcosis, Em2 tests are more useful for postoperative follow-up than for monitoring the effectiveness of chemotherapy.

FASCIOLIASIS (Chapter 120.3). The acute manifestations of human fascioliasis may precede the appearance of eggs in the stool by several weeks; immunodiagnostic tests may be useful for early indication of *Fasciola* infection as well as for confirmation of chronic fascioliasis when egg production is low or sporadic and for ruling out "pseudofascioliasis" associated with ingestion of parasite eggs in sheep or calves' liver.

The current tests of choice for immunodiagnosis of human *Fasciola hepatica* infection are EIA with excretory-secretory (ES) antigens combined with confirmation of positive results by immunoblot. Specific antibodies to *Fasciola* may be detectable within 2 to 4 weeks after infection, which is 5 to 7 weeks before eggs appear in stool. Sensitivity for the Falcon assay screening test–enzyme-linked immunosorbent assay (FAST-ELISA) was reported to be 95%, whereas sensitivity for the immunoblot using 12-, 17-, and 63-kDa antigens appeared to be 100%. However, some cross reactivity occurs in the FAST-ELISA with serum specimens of patients with schistosomiasis. Antibody levels decrease to normal 6 to 12 months after chemotherapeutic cure and can be used to predict the success of therapy.

FILARIASIS

Lymphatic Filariasis (*Wuchereria bancrofti* and *Brugia* spp.) (Chapter 106). Parasitologic diagnosis of human filariasis is often difficult due to low parasite burden, parasite periodicity, and parasite sequestration. Sensitive and specific immunodiagnostic tests could be useful to indicate the presence of filaria and microfilaria. Antigen preparations employed in the past have been crude and fractionated extracts of filarial worms of other mammals, e.g., *Dirofilaria immitis,* the dog heartworm. Such antigens are usually reactive with serum samples of patients with filariasis but are completely lacking in specificity. ES or surface antigens of homologous *Wuchereria* or *Brugia* parasites are more specific than whole-worm somatic extracts, but supplies of such material are limited because of the lack of animal models and difficulties of in vitro cultivation.

Most residents of filarial endemic regions have been sensitized to filarial antigens through years of exposure to infected mosquitoes; filarial antigens may also cross react with those of other nematode parasites found in these areas. Thus, a positive immunodiagnostic test is necessary but not definitive for the diagnosis of brugian or bancroftian filariasis. Conversely, a negative test result in an American or European whose symptoms suggest lymphatic filariasis after travel in an area where filariasis is endemic strongly suggests no infection.

Antibody detection methods cannot distinguish past exposure from current infection nor is there any correlation of antibodies with worm burden. Detection of parasite material (antigen or other products) in blood or urine offers potential advantages for assessing the state of individual infections. Although circulating antigens can be detected in patients with bancroftian filariasis, positive results were initially confined almost exclusively to serum specimens from persons with microfilaremia detectable by blood film examination. However, many of the lymphatic filarial syndromes are not associated with microfilaremia and so would not be detected.

Onchocerciasis (Chapter 108). Diagnostic methods (detection of parasites in the skin or eye or the presence of suggestive clinical changes) are crude, laborious, and insensitive. Current immunodiagnostic tests generally lack specificity. IgG and IgE antibodies that react with onchocercal antigens are readily detected in sera of infected persons; however, they are not specific for the presence or extent of the infection, nor do they allow discrimination between onchocerciasis and other filarial infections. Tests based on IgE detection are more specific than those based on IgG. EIA restricted to detection of IgG4 antibodies and employing purified, surface-derived, low-molecular-weight onchocercal antigens is highly sensitive and specific, although tests still cross react with serum specimens of some patients with *W. bancrofti* infection. Antibodies directed against a 16-kDa *Onchocerca volvulus* antigen have been reported to be species-specific and to indicate active infection. Antigen detection methods are feasible, but these and antibody assays require refinement of the reagents to control specificity.

GIARDIASIS (Chapter 87). *Giardia lamblia* is one of the most common human intestinal protozoan pathogens in the United States and is an important cause of diarrhea in children and adults. Outbreaks of disease are common within daycare centers as a result of person-to-person contact and may also occur in communities as a result of drinking water contaminated by infected human or animal feces. Tests for antibody detection in human *Giardia* infection are not currently recommended due to lack of sensitivity and specificity.

Antigen detection in stools is the current immunodiagnostic test of choice and provides equal or increased sensitivity over microscopy. A number of commercial kits are available for both DFA and EIA assays; all have sensitivities and specificities of 94% or greater. Infected persons often excrete *Giardia* cysts intermittently, so multiple stools collected over at least several days must sometimes be examined to detect the parasite; use of antigen detection assays are very useful in confirming infections.

LEISHMANIASIS (Chapter 95). The IFA test is used for detection of antibodies to *Leishmania.* This procedure can differentiate leishmaniasis from other clinically similar conditions, but cannot determine the species of *Leishmania.* Cross reactions occur in patients with antibodies to *Trypanosoma cruzi* (Chagas disease), which is also endemic in some of the same Central and South American countries as leishmaniasis. If visceral leishmaniasis is suspected, antibody detection tests can be a very useful adjunct to clinical findings. Sensitivity is very good (>90%) for visceral leishmaniasis. Sensitivity of antibody tests for cutaneous leishmaniasis is poor: most patients do not develop a detectable circulating antibody response to the parasite. Although biochemical, immunologic, and molecular biology techniques have been used extensively in *Leishmania* research, molecular probes for the detection and identification of parasites are not yet available.

MALARIA (Chapter 92). The serodiagnosis of malaria is not recommended except for screening blood donors involved in cases of transfusion-induced malaria when the donor's parasitemia may be below the detectable level of blood film examination and for testing a patient with a febrile illness who is suspected of having malaria and from whom repeated blood smears are negative. IFA tests with organisms of the four human *Plasmodium* species for malarial antibody detection are very sensitive and specific, but the presence of antibodies indicates that infection occurred at some time in the past and does not necessarily indicate current infection.

PARAGONIMIASIS (Chapter 121). Pulmonary paragonimiasis is the most common presentation of patients infected with *Paragonimus* spp., although extrapulmonary (cerebral, abdominal) paragonimiasis may occur. Detection of eggs in sputum or feces of patients with paragonimiasis is often very difficult; therefore, serodiagnosis may be very helpful in confirming infections and for monitoring the results of chemotherapy. In the United States, detection of antibodies to *Paragonimus westermani* has helped physicians differentiate paragonimiasis from tuberculosis in Indochinese immigrants.

EIA tests have replaced the complement fixation (CF) test as the standard test for pargonimiasis. The CF test was highly sensitive for diagnosis and for assessing cure after therapy, but because of the technical difficulties of CF, EIA tests were developed as a replacement. The immunoblot (IB) assay performed with a crude antigen extract of *P. westermani* has been in use at CDC since 1988. Positive reactions, based on demonstration of an 8-kDa antigen-antibody band, were obtained with serum samples in 96% of patients with parasitologically confirmed *P. westermani* infection. Specificity was ≥99%; of 210 serum specimens from patients with other parasitic and nonparasitic infections, only one serum sample from a patient with *Schistosoma haematobium* reacted. Antibody levels detected by EIA and IB decline after chemotherapeutic cure but not as rapidly as those detected by the CF test. Most reports concern pulmonary paragonimiasis due to *P. westermani* although in some geographic areas other

Paragonimus species cause similar or distinct clinical manifestations in human infections. Cross reactivity between species occurs, but at varying levels for different species.

SCHISTOSOMIASIS (Chapter 118). Antibody detection can be useful to indicate schistosome infection in patients who have traveled in schistosomiasis endemic areas and in whom eggs cannot be demonstrated in fecal or urine specimens. Test sensitivity and specificity vary widely among the many tests reported for the serologic diagnosis of schistosomiasis and are dependent on both the type of antigen preparations used (crude, purified, adult worm, egg, cercarial) and the test procedure.

At CDC, a combination of tests with purified adult worm antigens are used for antibody detection. All serum specimens are initially tested by FAST-ELISA using *Schistosoma mansoni* adult microsomal antigen (MAMA). A positive reaction (greater than 8 units/μL serum) indicates infection with *Schistosoma* species. Sensitivity for *S. mansoni* infection is 99%, 95% for *Schistosoma haematobium* infection, and ≥50% for *Schistosoma japonicum* infection. Specificity of this assay for detecting schistosome infection is 99%. Because test sensitivity with the MAMA is reduced for species other than *S. mansoni*, immunoblots of the species appropriate to the patient's travel history are also tested to ensure detection of *S. haematobium* and *S. japonicum* infections. Immunoblots with adult worm microsomal antigens are species-specific and so a positive reaction indicates the infecting species. The presence of antibody is indicative only of schistosome infection at some time and cannot be correlated with clinical status, worm burden, egg production, or prognosis.

STRONGYLOIDIASIS (Chapter 105.2). Immunodiagnostic tests for human infections with *Strongyloides stercoralis* are indicated when the infection is suspected and the organism cannot be demonstrated by duodenal aspiration, string tests, or by repeated examinations of stool. Although IFA and IHA tests have been used, EIA is currently recommended because of its greater sensitivity (84 to 92%). Immunocompromised persons with disseminated strongyloidiasis usually have detectable IgG antibodies despite their immunodepression. Cross reactions in patients with filariasis and some other nematode infections may occur. Important test limitations are that 8 to 16% of *Strongyloides* carriers are seronegative and antibody test results cannot be used to differentiate between past and current infection. A positive test warrants continuing efforts to establish a parasitologic diagnosis followed by anthelmintic treatment. Serologic monitoring may be useful in the follow-up of immunocompetent treated patients: antibody titers decrease markedly within 6 months after successful chemotherapy.

TOXOCARIASIS (LARVA MIGRANS) (Chapter 112). Antibody detection tests are the only means of confirmation of a clinical diagnosis of visceral larva migrans (VLM), ocular larva migrans (OLM), and covert toxocariasis (CT), the most common clinical syndromes associated with *Toxocara* infections. The currently recommended serologic test for toxocariasis is an EIA with larval stage excretory-secretory (TES) antigens released in vitro by cultured infective larvae.

Evaluation of the true sensitivity and specificity of serologic tests for toxocariasis in human populations is not possible because of the lack of parasitologic methods to detect *Toxocara* parasites. These inherent problems result in underestimations of sensitivity and specificity. Evaluation of the *Toxocara* EIA in groups of patients with presumptive diagnoses of VLM or OLM indicated a sensitivity of 78 and 73%, respectively, at a titer of ≥1:32. When the cutoff titer for OLM cases was lowered to 1:8, sensitivity was increased to 90%. Further confirmation of the specificity of the serologic diagnosis of OLM can be obtained by testing aqueous or vitreous humor samples for antibodies. Specificity has been reported to be >90% at a titer of ≥1:32.

When interpreting the serologic findings, clinicians must be aware that a measurable titer does not necessarily indicate current clinical *Toxocara canis* infection. In the United States, 2.8% of 9000 randomly tested persons were positive, thus indicating the occurrence of asymptomatic toxocariasis; the percentage varied significantly according to age, race, and socioeconomic status.

TOXOPLASMOSIS (Chapter 97). *Toxoplasma* antibody detection tests are now performed by a large number of laboratories with commercially available kits. Comparisons of kits indicated that most perform comparably in detecting *Toxoplasma*-specific IgG antibodies but vary markedly in detecting *Toxoplasma*-specific IgM antibodies.

The IFA and EIA tests for IgG and IgM antibodies are the tests most commonly used today. Persons should be initially tested for the presence of *Toxoplasma*-specific IgG antibodies to determine their immune status (Fig. 152–1). A positive IgG titer indicates infection with the organism at some time. If more precise knowledge of the time of infection is necessary, then an IgG-positive person should have an IgM test performed by a procedure with minimal nonspecific reactions, such as IgM-capture EIA. Newborn infants suspected of congenital toxoplasmosis should be tested by both an IgM- and an IgA-capture EIA. Detection of *Toxoplasma*-specific IgA antibodies is more sensitive than IgM detection in congenitally infected babies. *Toxoplasma*-specific IgM antibodies may be detected by EIA for as long as 18 months after acute acquired infection, but high levels may indicate infection within the past 3 to 4 months.

A major problem with *Toxoplasma*-specific IgM testing is lack of specificity. Two situations occur frequently: (1) persons with positive IgM but negative IgG results and (2) persons with positive IgG and IgM results. In the first situation, a positive IgM result with a negative IgG result in the same specimen should be viewed with great suspicion; the patient's blood should be redrawn 2 weeks after the first test

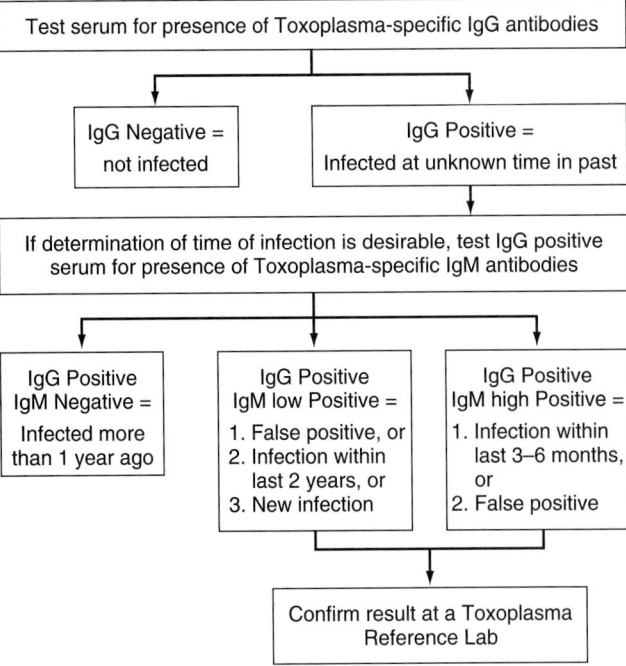

Figure 152–1. Algorithm for the serodiagnosis of toxoplasmosis in the United States.

and tested together with the first specimen. If the first specimen was drawn very early after infection, the patient should have highly positive IgG and IgM antibodies in the second sample. If the IgG is negative and the IgM is positive in both specimens, the IgM result should be considered to be a false positive and the patient should be considered to be not infected. In the second situation, a second specimen should be drawn and both specimens submitted together to a reference laboratory that uses a different IgM testing system for confirmation. All IgM positive results should be verified by a reference laboratory with experience in toxoplasmosis such as the CDC or the Toxoplasmosis Lab, Palo Alto Medical Research Foundation, Palo Alto, CA.

Toxoplasma-specific IgG antibody levels in AIDS patients with active central nervous system toxoplasmosis often are low to moderate, but occasionally no specific IgG antibodies can be detected. Tests for IgM antibodies are generally negative. Detection of circulating antigen in AIDS patients has been evaluated, but the procedure lacks sensitivity.

TRICHINELLOSIS (Chapter 111). Immunodiagnostic tests currently available in the United States include EIA and bentonite flocculation (BF). Positive reactions are detectable at some time during infection in serum samples of 80 to 100% of patients with clinically symptomatic trichinellosis. Antibody levels are often not detectable until 3 to 5 weeks after infection, well after the onset of acute-stage illness. Antibody development is also affected by the infecting dose of larvae: the higher the infecting dose, the faster the patient's antibody response will develop. Multiple serum specimens should be drawn several weeks apart to demonstrate seroconversion in patients whose initial specimen was negative. IgG, IgM, and IgE antibodies are detectable in many patients; however, tests based on IgG antibodies are most sensitive. Antibody levels peak in the second or third month after infection, and then decline slowly for several years.

EIA with ES antigen detects antibodies earlier than BF in 25% of serum specimens from patients with acute infection, but the EIA also remains positive for longer periods after infection than the BF, and is reactive in a larger proportion of persons with no clinical evidence of trichinellosis. The EIA test is used for routine screening; all EIA-positive specimens are then tested by BF for confirmation. A positive result in both tests indicates infection with *Trichinella* spp. within the past several years.

TRICHOMONIASIS (Chapter 91). Trichomoniasis, an infection caused by *Trichomonas vaginalis*, is a common sexually transmitted disease. Diagnosis is made by detection of trophozoites in vaginal secretions or urethral specimens by wet mount microscopic examination, DFA staining of specimens, or culture. Sensitivity of the assays was reported as 60% for wet mounts and 86% for DFA when compared with cultures. A kit which employs fluorescein isothiocyanate or enzyme-labeled monoclonal antibodies for use in a DFA or EIA procedure is available for detection of whole parasites in fluids. A latex agglutination test for antigen detection in vaginal swab specimens is available; the manufacturer's evaluation indicated good sensitivity and specificity. The Affirm VP Microbial Identification Test system was designed for use in clinics, physicians' offices, or clinical laboratories. The system uses synthetic oligonucleotide probes for the simultaneous detection of *T. vaginalis* and *Gardnerella vaginalis* from a single vaginal swab. Sensitivity for detection of *T. vaginalis* infection was 100% compared with wet mount examination but only 80% when compared with culture.

Bibliography

Berman JD: Human leishmaniasis: clinical, diagnostic, and chemotherapeutic developments in the last 10 years. Clin Infect Dis 24:684, 1997.

Boustani MR, Gelfand JA: Babesiosis. Clin Infect Dis 22:611, 1996.

Cetron MS, Chitsulo L, Sullivan JJ, et al: Schistosomiasis in Lake Malawi. Lancet 348:1274, 1996.

Garcia LS, Shimizu RY: Evaluation of nine immunoassay kits (enzyme immunoassay and direct fluorescence) for detection of *Giardia lamblia* and *Cryptosporidium parvum* in human fecal specimens. J Clin Microbiol 35:1526, 1997.

Genta RM: Predictive value of an enzyme-linked immunosorbent assay (ELISA) for the serodiagnosis of strongyloidiasis. Am J Clin Pathol 89:391, 1988.

Hillyer GV, Soler de Galanes M, Rodriguez-Perez J, et al: Use of the Falcon assay screening test–enzyme-linked immunosorbent assay (FAST-ELISA) and the enzyme-linked immunoelectrotransfer blot (EITB) to determine the prevalence of human fascioliasis in the Bolivian Altiplano. Am J Trop Med Hygiene 46:603, 1992.

Lightowlers MW, Gottstein B: Echinococcosis/hydatidosis: antigens, immunological and molecular diagnosis. *In* Thompson RCA, Lymbery AJ (eds): Echinococcus and Hydatid Disease. Wallingford, England, CAB International, 1995, pp 355–410.

Murrell KD, Brueschi F: Clinical trichinellosis. Prog Clin Parasitol 4:117, 1994.

Ottesen EA: Filarial infections. Infect Dis Clin North Am 7:619, 1993.

Ravdin JI: Amebiasis. Clin Infect Dis 20:1453, 1995.

Slemenda SB, Maddison SE, Jong EC, et al: Diagnosis of paragonimiasis by immunoblot. Am J Trop Med Hygiene 39:469, 1988.

Smith HV: Antibody reactivity in human toxocariasis. *In* Lewis JW, Maizels RM (eds): Toxocara and Toxocariasis: Clinical, Epidemiological, and Molecular Perspectives. London, Institute of Biology and British Society of Parasitology, 1993, pp 91–109.

Sulzer AJ, Wilson M: The indirect fluorescent antibody test for the detection of occult malaria in blood donors. Bull WHO 45:375, 1971.

Tsang VCW, Wilkins PP: Immunodiagnosis of schistosomiasis: screen with FAST-ELISA and confirm with immunoblot. Clin Lab Med 11:1029, 1991.

White ACJ: Neurocysticercosis: A major cause of neurological disease worldwide. Clin Infect Dis 24:101, 1997.

Wilson M, McAuley JB: Laboratory diagnosis of toxoplasmosis. Clin Lab Med 11:923, 1991.

Index

Note: Page numbers in *italics* indicate illustrations; those followed by t refer to tables.

A

Abacavir, in human immunodeficiency virus infection, 191t
Abdomen, actinomycosis of, 317
  distention of, causes of, 17, 17t
  imaging of, 168–169
  pain in, causes of, 17, 17t
  in sickle cell disease, 43
  surgery on, *112,* 112–113
  tuberculosis of, 503–504
Abortifacients, plant, 888t
Abortion, bovine, tick transmission in, 999
  in beta-thalassemia major, 47
Abrus precatorius, abortifacient effects of, 888t
  purgation from, 887t
  toxicity of, *884*
Abscess, brain, 76
  amebic, 76t
  Nocardia asteroides infection and, 318, *318*
  filarial, 747, *748*
  rupture of, 748, *749*
  hepatic, amebic. See *Amebiasis, hepatic abscess in.*
  multiple, in melioidosis, 315,
  surgery in, 111
Absidia species, 569
Acanthamoeba species, culture of, 1116
  infection by, 705
  tissue isolation of, 1116
Acanthaster planci, envenomation by, 891, 891t
Acanthocheilonema perstans, 770
Acanthophis species, 896t
  bites by, antivenom for, 905t
Acanthuridae, envenomation by, 894, 894t
Acari, 992
  classification of, 993–996, *993–996, 1000,* 1000–1001
Acariasis, *918,* 918–919, *919,* 920t
Acariformes, 993
Acarus siro, dermatitis from, 919, 920t
  in host dust allergies, 920t
Acclimatization, in heat-associated illness, 142
Acid-base balance, in malaria, *621,* 621–622
Acid-fast stain, of *Cryptosporidium cyclospora,* 1110
  of *Isospora,* 1110
Acidosis, metabolic, in malaria, *621,* 621–622, 628
Acinetobacter species, infection by, in northern Europe, 1092
Acinetobacter baumanii, infection by, in southern Europe, 1094
  in western south Asia, 1096
Acne, 72
Aconitum napellus, poisoning from, 886t
Acquired immunodeficiency syndrome (AIDS), 176–192. See also *Human immunodeficiency virus (HIV) infection.*
  American trypanosomiasis in, treatment of, 663
  antiretroviral therapy in, 188–189, 190t

Acquired immunodeficiency syndrome (AIDS) *(Continued)*
  bacterial infections in, prophylaxis against, 188, 188t, 189t
  blastomycosis in, 557
  care across continuum in, 187
  childhood, immunization in, 139
  coccidioidomycosis in, treatment of, 556
  cryptococcosis in, 561, 562
  treatment of, 563–564
  cryptosporidiosis in, 594, *595, 596*
  diarrhea in, 598
  prevention of, 600
  definition of, 176, 176t, 177t
  diarrhea in, 16
  disseminated histoplasmosis in, treatment of, 551
  drug therapy in, 187, 188t
  epidemiology of, 36, *178,* 178–181, 179t, *180*
  etiology of, 177–178
  gastrointestinal tract in, 17–18, 18t
  global surveillance of, 179
  helminthic infections in, 715
  hematologic complications of, 37
  history of, 176–177
  home care in, 188
  hospitalization in, 187, 187t
  in Africa, 179–180, 179t, *180*
  in eastern Europe, 179t, 180
  in Latin America, 179t, 180
  in south/southeastern Asia, 179t, 180
  in temperate South America, 1085
  in the Caribbean, 179t, 180
  in travelers, 1035–1036
  Kaposi sarcoma in, 100–101, *102,* 199
  management of, 37, 187–189, 187t–191t
  in resource-poor settings, 188
  microsporidiosis in, 710–711, *711*
  mycoses in, 566
  opportunistic infections in, prophylaxis against, 188, 188t, 189t
  oral candidosis in, 534
  treatment of, 535
  pneumocystosis in, prophylaxis against, 188, 188t, 189t
  pneumonia in, 5
  progression to, from human immunodeficiency virus infection, 182
  regional distribution of, 178, 179t
  Salmonella infection in, 488
  specialist care in, 188–189, 189t, 190t
  Strongyloides infection in, 715
  syndromic care in, 187–188, 187t, 188t
  toxoplasmosis in, 696, *696*
  prophylaxis against, 188, 188t, 189t
  transmission of, blood transfusion in, 36–37
  tuberculosis in, 504
  prophylaxis against, 188, 188t, 189t
  visceral leishmaniasis in, 674
  zinc deficiency in, 962
Acremonium species, 538, 538t
Acropora palmata, cuts by, 890t, 891
Actineida, 1000–1001, *1001*

Actinomadura madurae, 538, 538t
Actinomadura pelletieri, 538, 538t
Actinomyces israelii, filaments of, 316, *316*
  infection by, 316
Actinomycetes, in mycetoma, 538, 538t
Actinomycetoma, clinical manifestations of, 538–539, *539*
  macroscopic features of, 538t
  prognosis of, 540
  treatment of, 540
Actinomycosis, 316–317
  abdominal, 317
  central nervous system, 317
  cervicofacial, 316–317
  thoracic, 317, *317*
Adder, burrowing, 897
  puff, bites by, disseminated intravascular coagulation in, 59
Adenitis, tuberculous, 113, *114,* 499, *499*
Adenocarcinoma, breast, 102–103
  gastric, 98
  lung, 99
Adenopathy, cervical, in diphtheria, 303
  in pulmonary tuberculosis, 496, *497*
Adenovirus, 211t, 212t, 213
  diarrhea from, 224–225, *225*
  in atypical pneumonia, 4
  in east Asia, 1101
  vaccine for, 214
Adrenocortical response, in protein-energy malnutrition, 929
Adult respiratory distress syndrome, in malaria, 628
  miliary tuberculosis in, 501
Adult T-cell leukemia/lymphoma, 194–195
  acute, 195
  chronic, 195
  human T-lymphotropic virus type I and, 192
  lymphoma type, 195
  smoldering, 195
Aedes species, alphavirus transmission by, 1012
  as *Wuchereria bancrofti* vector, 745
  control of, 1027
  genetic control of, 1027–1028
  Rift Valley fever transmission by, 254
  Venezuelan equine encephalitis transmission by, 263
  yellow fever transmission by, 979–980, *981*
Aedes aegypti, 1027
  Chikungunya fever transmission by, 247
  control of, 1027–1028
  sex ratio distortion in, 1024
  dengue fever transmission by, 240, 241, 1013–1014
  yellow fever transmission by, 272, *1012,* 1014
Aedes africanus, yellow fever transmission by, 273, 1014
Aedes albopictus, dengue fever transmission by, 1014
Aedes furcifer-taylori, yellow fever transmission by, 1014

ISBN 0-7216-6223-4

90038

9 780721 662237